Oxford Textbook of
Medicine

VOLUME 3

Oxford Textbook of
Medicine

FIFTH EDITION
Volume 3: Sections 20–33

Edited by

David A. Warrell

Emeritus Professor of Tropical Medicine, Nuffield Department of Clinical Medicine; Honorary Fellow, St Cross College, University of Oxford, Oxford, UK

Timothy M. Cox

Professor of Medicine, University of Cambridge; Honorary Consultant Physician, Addenbrooke's Hospital, Cambridge, UK

John D. Firth

Consultant Physician and Nephrologist, Addenbrooke's Hospital, Cambridge, UK

Sub-editor Immunological Mechanisms and Disorders of the Skin
Graham S. Ogg
Reader in Cutaneous Immunology, MRC Senior Clinical Fellow; Consultant in Dermatology, Churchill Hospital, Oxford, UK

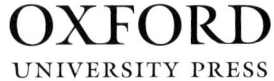

OXFORD
UNIVERSITY PRESS

Great Clarendon Street, Oxford OX2 6DP

Oxford University Press is a department of the University of Oxford.
It furthers the University's objective of excellence in research, scholarship,
and education by publishing worldwide in

Oxford New York

Auckland   Cape Town   Dar es Salaam   Hong Kong   Karachi
Kuala Lumpur   Madrid   Melbourne   Mexico City   Nairobi
New Delhi   Shanghai   Taipei   Toronto
With offices in
Argentina   Austria   Brazil   Chile   Czech Republic   France   Greece
Guatemala   Hungary   Italy   Japan   Poland   Portugal   Singapore
South Korea   Switzerland   Thailand   Turkey   Ukraine   Vietnam

Oxford is a registered trade mark of Oxford University Press
in the UK and in certain other countries

Published in the United States
by Oxford University Press Inc., New York

© Oxford University Press, 2010

First edition published 1983
Second edition published 1987
Third edition published 1996
Fourth edition published 2003
Fifth edition published 2010

British Library Cataloguing in Publication Data
Data available
Library of Congress Cataloging in Publication Data
Data available
Typeset by Cepha Imaging Pvt. Ltd., Bangalore
Printed in Italy by LegoPrint s.p.A.
9780199204854 (three volume set)
volume 1: 9780199592852
volume 2: 9780199592869
volume 3: 9780199592876
Available as a three volume set only
1 3 5 7 9 10 8 6 4 2

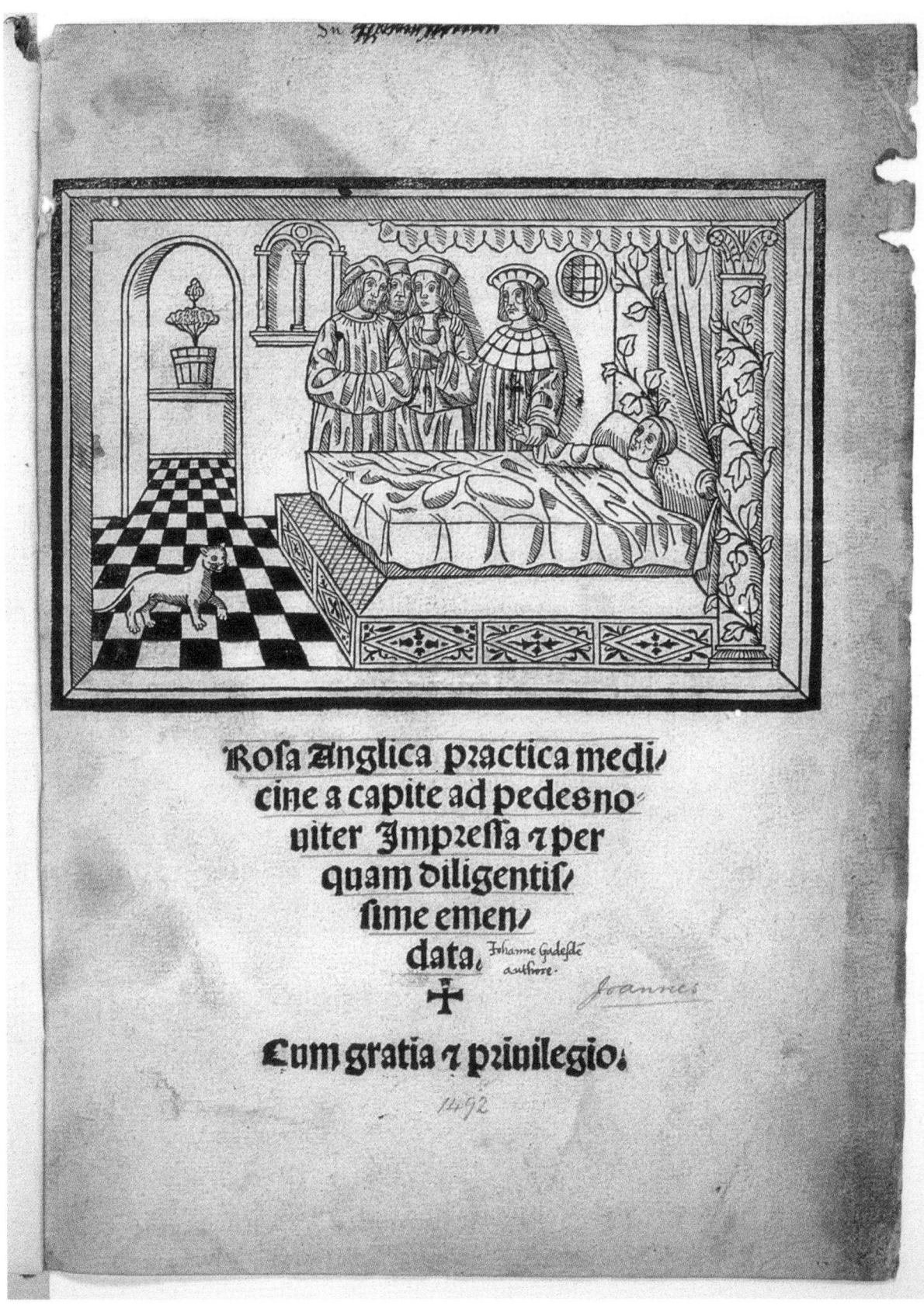

The title page of the 1492 edition of *Rosa Anglica* by John of Gaddesden (1280–1361), which was probably written in 1314. The author was a well known physician attached to Merton College, Oxford in the early part of the 14th century. His famous book was probably the first 'Oxford Textbook of Medicine'. The author was the model for the unsavoury Doctor of Physick in Chaucer's *Canterbury Tales*.

Foreword

by Professor Sir Aaron Klug OM FRS

Since it first appeared 25 years ago, the *Oxford Textbook of Medicine* has established itself as an authoritative source for doctors to consult in everyday practice, particularly when questions arise outside their experience. The coverage is comprehensive and covers diseases and problems that occur anywhere in the world. It is very respected and has become a standard reference in the United Kingdom for journalists and for legal disputes in the courts.

In a book with such wide coverage, it is important for the practising physician to be able to find the topic of current interest speedily. The book seems to me to be less discursive than, say, *Harrison's Principles of Internal Medicine*. Indeed, the layout of the book is such that one can efficiently look up something specific. This is facilitated by a good index, with the right degree of cross-referencing.

The book begins with the basic biological science underlying medicine, cell and molecular biology, and the genomic basis of medicine. Despite these big issues, the text does not lose sight of the clinical implications of the science being presented, in keeping with the underlying philosophy of the book that the material must be of practical value to the physician. Thus the advances in understanding the modification of proteins by kinases, which add phosphate groups to selected amino acids, has led to the development of chemical inhibitors of the kinases. An example of such a successful designer drug is imatinib for chronic myologenous leukaemia.

A totally new modality for the treatment has appeared in recent years, namely monoclonal antibodies with high selectivity against protein targets. Originally developed in mice, they could not be used in patients because of the anaphylactic response to a foreign protein, but over the years they have been 'humanized', i.e. their relatively small, specific antigen- or immunogen-recognition regions have been fused to a human framework, which make up most of the antibody. Examples include palivizumab, against respiratory syncytial virus, and bevacizumab, against colorectal cancer, now in widespread use. Even more striking is the development of fully human antibodies, synthesized out of the cloned repertoire of the human genes making up the constituent antibody domains. The antibody adalimumab, released a few years ago, not only relieves the pain of rheumatoid arthritis, but also stops the progress of the disease.

These new modalities are of course costly, as are many of the new anticancer drugs such as Herceptin: their introduction is changing the setting in which medicine is practised, particularly in the United Kingdom where the National Health Service (NHS) is free at the point of delivery, and in the United States of America where the Health Maintenance Organizations (HMOs) are insurance based. As recognized by David Weatherall in his foreword to the fourth edition of this textbook, none of the richer countries has got to grips with the problem of financing the increasing number and costs of new treatments. In the United Kingdom where the decision to allow the use of a licensed drug is made by the local Health Authority, there is no uniformity of practice, so leading to the term 'postcode availability' of a drug. There is also the question of individuals receiving treatment under the NHS but wishing to top up privately with other or new drugs not available under the NHS. Despite much controversy, this practice has recently been allowed by the NHS.

Another issue likely to arise out of the sequencing of the human genome is the prospect of personalized and preventive medicine. This is fast becoming a potential reality with the decreasing cost of rapid DNA sequencing to determine an individual genome. The supporting clinical data to interpret individual susceptibility to disease is likely to come from 'genome-wide association' studies. These represent a powerful approach to the identification of genetic variations involved in common human diseases. In 2007, there appeared in the journal *Nature* a genomic study of seven common diseases, including coronary artery disease, type 1 and type 2 diabetes, hypertension, and bipolar disorders. This large study involved 14 000 cases and 3000 shared controls. Similar studies have been carried out in several forms of cancer. The association of a particular locus in the genome with a disease is still very modest. The overall increase in risk conferred by the genetic factors identified is of the order of 1.2- to 1.5-fold, and so thus far does not provide a clinically useful prediction of disease. But the work must be recognized as an important first step towards dissecting the genomic basis of common diseases. By the time of the next edition of the *Oxford Textbook of Medicine*, we may well see the results of these powerful genomic tools becoming available or already in use.

Preface

"Naught for your comfort"

Trevor Huddleston

The fruits of medical research

Publication of this new edition of the *Oxford Textbook of Medicine* prompts consideration of the precepts and practices of medicine in a world that faces unprecedented challenges. There is much to celebrate, and—with many new contributors—we have sought throughout the book to reflect the revolutionary effects of discovery in the medical sciences on clinical practice. Spectacular advances have been made at the most fundamental level and these continue to inspire our belief that improved prevention, diagnosis and treatment of disease will eventually relieve suffering. The popular term, 'translational medicine', reflects the shared optimism of many research agencies.

The Fifth edition has been rigorously revised and updated. It differs most blatantly from previous editions in having the gift of colour throughout and the inclusion of 'Essentials' (mostly written and all edited by John Firth) that summarize the main points of each chapter. The introductory Sections 2 and 3 include eight new chapters on topics ranging from the future of clinical trials, the evaluation and provision of effective medicines, to health promotion. This expansion reflects the ever burgeoning successes, constraints and frustrations of modern medicine. New sciences like stem cell biology, and emerging pathogens such as SARS, H1N1 and drug-resistant bacteria and malaria parasites, are well represented in our pages, and we have introduced some highly topical themes, notably Darwinian Medicine and the context of Human Disasters

Darwinian Medicine

Evolutionary medicine has a firm place in this book (Randolph Nesse and Richard Dawkins—Evolution: medicine's most basic science—Chapter 2.1.2), consistent with the 200th anniversary of Charles Darwin's birth and the 150th anniversary of the publication of *On the Origin of Species* in 2009. Darwin's remarkable synthesis (subtended in part by Gregor Mendel's later discoveries in heredity) has salient implications for understanding disease, rendering outmoded the crude analogy of the diseased body as a 'broken machine'. Much illness results from conflict between a person and the external influences to which he or she is uniquely maladapted at a particular time. Given that genetic and environmental variations are biological characteristics, the evolutionary concept has profound implications for any full description and understanding of disease.

But while we have prodigious methods for determining genetic variation, our ability to measure environmental changes and interactions—or predict environmental disasters—is rudimentary.

Human disasters: political, sociological, and historical context

Human populations are dependent on the natural environment for food and water but exquisitely vulnerable to its storms, earthquakes and tsunamis. As demonstrated by one of our Nobel Laureate authors, Amartya Sen (Human disasters—Chapter 3.5), the effects of natural disasters are, irrespective of their origin, invariably magnified by dire socioeconomic circumstances resulting from human conquest. An agonising recent example was the seismic horror in Haiti, affecting a society dysfunctional and impoverished as an historical consequence of the European slave trade and more recent political interferences. Such disasters, including those attributable to wars, are also the province of medicine: in such catastrophes, doctors are needed to provide emergency treatment but, through proper involvement with governments, they are also critical for public health planning and the restoration of appropriate infrastructure and clinical services. In response to another human tragedy, the AIDS pandemic, and to mounting pressure on the industry, one of the world's largest pharmaceutical companies has recently agreed to cut the prices of its medicines in the poorest countries and to donate some of its profits to local hospitals and clinics. This initiative might be a bit late but is a significant first step taking other 'Big Pharmas' in a direction that improves access to treatments for stricken patients in poor countries.

The teaching and practice of medicine: a fine tradition betrayed

Irrespective of the political dimension of medicine, the care of patients and the prevention of disease depend on practising clinicians; the medicine of the future relies not only on scientific advances but on the education of doctors. Since the last edition, leaders of our profession in Britain have presided over, and in some cases acquiesced to the partial dismantling of arguably one of the finest systems of medical education. The implementation of a national process for the appointment of junior doctors has disaffected many trainees and their clinical mentors, who feel that they have become pawns in a bureaucratic political game. More important, if they understood the full implications, we believe that the British public and patients would be horrified. Within Europe, matters have been compounded by implementation of the European Working Time Directive, which threatens the professional apprenticeship and mentoring relationships between junior and senior doctors that best nurture young colleagues. The frequently heard mantra of the 'consultant-led service' is all very well, but the ideal will be short-lived if training is put in jeopardy.

We, the editors of this textbook, learnt how to practise as clinicians from such 'hands-on' apprenticeships and ask: how can young doctors accumulate adequate working knowledge and acquire essential skills if their clinical work is restricted to 48 hours each week? One might pose the question: would a patient prefer to be treated by a fully rested but inexperienced doctor whom they had never seen before, or a tired doctor with immense medical experience who knew them and their illness? We know whom we would prefer, as does Christopher Booth (On being a patient—Chapter 1.1). Short hours and other radical changes in the organization of clinical teams impair the continuity of medical care, an element of key importance for the patient but also critical for clinical education through time-honoured individual experience. Many countries are seeking to improve their systems of medical education, but for those who might consider adopting the current UK training timetables, we humbly offer advice—don't. It would be better to provide their medical students and young doctors with sufficient time and resources to acquaint themselves with the principles and practice of modern scientific medicine that are emphasized in this book.

Decline and fall of clinical trials evidence

How the profession responds to these old and new threats to the practice of medicine will influence the translation of new knowledge and scientific understanding into clinical benefit. Our contemporary environment is contaminated by countless man-made chemicals, including drugs and other medicinal products: many of the latter have untested effects on human health. One foundation of good practice is the evidence provided by clinical trials, but this is under threat from powerful self-interest groups. On one hand are those promoting alternative and so-called traditional treatments, which are ineffective and supported at best by what Robert Park has termed 'Voodoo Science', and who mount sustained attacks on anyone who might be brave enough to say so, including one of our authors, Edzard Ernst (Complementary and alternative medicine—Chapter 2.5). On the other hand are those who promote expensive health care, of which they take a financial cut: scaremongering occurs at every opportunity, and with the intensity that only billions of dollars can bring. Already most clinical trials are sponsored by pharmaceutical companies and instances where prompt release of all the results has been suppressed for commercial reasons continue to scandalize the profession.

Clinical trials require proper regulation, but burgeoning bureaucracy has become disproportionate; it is stifling the discipline and greatly discourages investigator-led clinical trials. Yet another vacuous meta-analysis, performed in the absence of sufficient data and therefore allowing of no conclusions, will be no substitute. We plead also for simplification of the legal and regulatory framework in which therapeutic trials and medical research can be conducted by individual doctors; for without the freedom ethically to test hypotheses prompted by the immediacy of clinical necessity, many imaginative advances will be thwarted.

Inalienable personal liberty versus the public good

The tension between the right to personal liberty and the desire for public good is ever more acute and is manifest in many ways. For the world as whole, population control (or lack thereof), is the most pressing issue. Even when we thought medicine might have solved a problem, the activities of the anti-vaccination lobby that resulted in the anti-MMR scandal reminded us that old battles sometimes need to be fought again. Many people in diverse populations are suffering because of this phenomenon and from the misguided public assessment of risk and disregard for specialist advice.

Bureaucratic targets

Well chosen targets are a good way of managing complex systems, but there is grave danger when those who set targets for clinical practice are intrinsically suspicious of doctors, take very selective advice, choose inappropriate limits, and compound the error by specifying crude and inappropriate mechanisms by which they should be achieved. What is being measured becomes of overwhelming importance, and the patient with the most pressing clinical need may not get the priority that he or she deserves. Many will suffer unless this state of affairs is remedied.

The future

Against a background of such uncertainty, we believe that sound clinical experience, combined with knowledge of the subject, based on authoritative books and peer-reviewed publications, remain the rocks upon which clinical management is based. The doctor whom doctors want to see, when they or their family are ill, is the one they recognize as having great knowledge, great experience, and good judgement, of patients and their disease. We have asked such doctors to write for this book, so that it will be of most value to those seeking a 'higher medicine'. Despite the many adverse factors detailed above, we are reassured that many bright young men and women training in medicine are motivated, hungry for knowledge, and prepared to challenge dogma in the struggle to provide the best care for their patients. We trust that this edition of the book hits the mark and will help those who use it to achieve this aim.

Our debts

This edition is a tribute to our long-suffering but ever-patient contributors who, faced by delays in publication, had to update their work or risk instant obsolescence.

We remember with gratitude seven authors who have died since publication of the 4th edition, but who contributed to the present edition, Richard S. Doll (Chapter 6.1), Ernest Beutler (Chapter 22.5.11), Philip A. Poole-Wilson (Chapter 16.1.2), Pauline de la Motte Hall (Chapter 15.22.7), Peter ('PK') Thomas (Chapter 24.16),

M. Monir Madkour (Chapter 7.6.21), and Richard Edwards (Chapter 24.24.4). Sir Richard S. Doll, who died in 2005, a giant of Oxford and World Medicine and a marvellous friend and inspiration to many, was a great supporter of this book. As a guest of the popular radio programme 'Desert Island Discs', he delighted us by choosing the *Oxford Textbook of Medicine* for his reading material.

Graham S. Ogg contributed his special skills and experience to the planning and editing of the sections on Immunological mechanisms and Disorders of the skin for which we are most grateful. We thank our wives, Mary, Sue, and Helen, and dedicated secretaries, Eunice Berry and Joan Grantham. In the publication team, we are particularly grateful to Helen Liepman, Anna Winstanley, Kate Wilson, Kathleen Lyle, and Aparna Shankar.

David A. Warrell
Timothy M. Cox
John D. Firth

Oxford and Cambridge
February 2010

Contents

SECTION 19
Rheumatological disorders

SECTION 22
Disorders of the blood

Contributors

P. Aaby Bandim Health Project, National Institute of Health, Guinea-Bissau
7.5.6: Measles

Steven G. Achinger Attending Nephrologist, Watson Clinic, Lakeland, Florida, USA
21.2.1: Disorders of water and sodium homeostasis

Dwomoa Adu Consultant Nephrologist, Department of Medicine, Korle Bu Hospital, Accra, Ghana
21.8.3: Minimal-change nephropathy and focal segmental glomerulosclerosis; 21.8.4: Membranous nephropathy; 21.10.3: The kidney in rheumatological disorders

Raymond M. Agius Professor of Occupational and Environmental Medicine and Honorary Consultant in Occupational Medicine, University of Manchester, Manchester, UK
9.4.1: Occupational and environmental health

Syed M. Ahmed Health Manager UK, Mediterranean & Shipping, Shell International, London, UK
9.5.10: Noise

Michael J. Aldape Assistant Research Scientist, Infectious Diseases Section, Veterans Affairs Medical Center, Boise, Idaho, USA
7.6.24: Botulism, gas gangrene, and clostridial gastrointestinal infections

Graeme J.M. Alexander Consultant Hepatologist, Cambridge University Hospitals, Cambridge, UK
15.22.5: Liver transplantation

Michael E.D. Allison Consultant Hepatologist, Cambridge University Hospitals, Cambridge, UK
15.22.5: Liver transplantation

Chris Andrews Mt Ommaney Family Clinic, Brisbane, Australia
9.5.7: Lightning and electrical injuries

Emmanouil Angelakis Faculté de Médecine et de Pharmacie, Université de la Méditerranée, Marseille Cedex, France
7.6.42: Bartonellas excluding B. bacilliformis

Gregory M. Anstead Associate Professor, Division of Infectious Diseases, Department of Medicine, University of Texas Health Science Center at San Antonio, and Medical Director, Immunosuppression and Infectious Diseases Clinics, South Texas Veterans Healthcare System, San Antonio, Texas, USA
7.7.3: Coccidioidomycosis

Clive B. Archer Consultant Dermatologist and Honorary Clinical Senior Lecturer, University Hospitals Bristol NHS Foundation Trust; The University of Bristol, UK
23.15: Skin and systemic diseases

Mark J. Arends University Reader and Honorary Consultant in Histopathology, Division of Histopathology, Department of Pathology, University of Cambridge, Addenbrooke's Hospital, Cambridge, UK
4.6: Apoptosis in health and disease

J. Arendt Professor Emeritus of Endocrinology, School of Biological Sciences, University of Surrey, Guildford, UK
13.13: The pineal gland and melatonin

Alison Armitage Consultant in Nephrology, The Richard Bright Renal Unit, Southmead Hospital, Bristol, UK
21.13: Urinary tract infection

James O. Armitage The Joe Shapiro Professor of Medicine, Section of Oncology/Hematology, University of Nebraska Medical Center, Nebraska Medical Center, Omaha, Nebraska, USA
22.4.3: Lymphoma

Frances M. Ashcroft Royal Society Research Professor, Department of Physiology, Anatomy and Genetics, University of Oxford, Oxford, UK
4.4: Ion channels and disease

Caroline Ashley Lead Specialist Pharmacist, Centre for Nephrology, Royal Free Hospital, London, UK
21.19: Drugs and the kidney

S.Q. Ashraf Academic Clinical Lecturer and Specialty Registrar, John Radcliffe Hospitals, Oxford UK
15.14: Colonic diverticular disease

Tar-Ching Aw Head of Department of Community Medicine, Faculty of Medicine & Health Sciences, United Arab Emirates University, Al-Ain, United Arab Emirates
9.5.10: Noise; 9.5.11: Vibration

Juan Carlos Ayus Director of Clinical Research, Renal Consultants of Houston, Texas, USA
21.2.1: Disorders of water and sodium homeostasis

Trevor Baglin Consultant in Haematology, Department of Haematology & Eastern Region Haemophilia Comprehensive Care Centre, Cambridge University Hospitals NHS Trust, Addenbrooke's Hospital, Cambridge, UK
22.6.2: Evaluation of the patient with a bleeding tendency

M. Bagshaw Director of Aviation Medicine, King's College, London, UK
9.5.5: Aerospace medicine

C. Baigent Clinical Trial Service Unit & Epidemiological Studies Unit (CTSU), University of Oxford, UK
2.3.3: Large-scale randomized evidence: trials and meta-analyses of trials

I. Banerjee Department of Paediatric Endocrinology, Royal Manchester Children's Hospital, UK
13.9.2: Puberty

Adrian P. Banning Consultant Cardiologist, John Radcliffe Hospital, Oxford, UK
16.3.2: Echocardiography; 16.14.1: Thoracic aortic dissection

George Banting Department of Biochemistry, University of Bristol, Bristol, UK
4.1: The cell

T.M. Barber Oxford Centre for Diabetes, Endocrinology and Metabolism, Churchill Hospital, Oxford, UK

13.12: Hormonal manifestations of nonendocrine disease

D.J.P. Barker Professor of Clinical Epidemiology, University of Southampton; Professor in Cardiovascular Medicine, Oregon Health & Science University

16.13.3: Influences acting in utero *and in early childhood*

Roger A. Barker University Reader in Clinical Neuroscience & Honorary Consultant, Cambridge Centre for Brain Repair and Department of Neurology, University Department of Clinical Neuroscience, Addenbrooke's Hospital, Cambridge, UK

24.3.1: Lumbar puncture; 24.7.3: Movement disorders other than Parkinson's disease

D. Barlow Consultant Physician, Department of Genitourinary Medicine, Guy's and St Thomas' Hospitals, London, UK

7.6.6: Neisseria gonorrhoeae

M.P. Barnes Professor of Neurological Rehabilitation, Hunters Moor Neurorehabilitation Ltd

24.13.2: Spinal cord injury and its management

Jonathan Barratt Senior Lecturer, University of Leicester; Honorary Consultant Nephrologist, University Hospitals of Leicester, UK

21.8.1: Immunoglobulin A nephropathy and Henoch–Schönlein purpura

John G. Bartlett Professor of Medicine, Johns Hopkins University School of Medicine, Baltimore, Maryland, USA

7.6.23: Clostridium difficile; 18.4.2: Pneumonia in the normal host; 18.4.3: Nosocomial pneumonia

Buddha Basnyat Oxford University Clinical Research Unit, Patan Hospital, Nepal

7.6.8: Typhoid and paratyphoid fevers; 9.5.4: Diseases of high terrestrial altitudes

M.F. Bassendine Professor of Hepatology, Institute of Cellular Medicine, Newcastle University, Newcastle upon Tyne, UK

15.21.3: Primary biliary cirrhosis

D.N. Bateman Professor in Clinical Toxicology, National Poisons Information, Edinburgh, UK

9.1: Poisoning by drugs and chemicals

David Bates Professor of Clinical Neurology, Newcastle University, UK

24.5.5: The unconscious patient; 24.9: Brainstem syndromes

Robert P. Baughman University of Cincinatti Medical Center, Cincinatti, Ohio, USA

18.12: Sarcoidosis

Peter J. Baxter Institute of Public Health, University of Cambridge, Cambridge, UK

9.5.12: Disasters: earthquakes, volcanic eruptions, hurricanes, and floods

Harald Becher Consultant Cardiologist and Honorary Senior Lecturer, Department of Cardiology, John Radcliffe Hospital, Oxford, UK

16.3.3: Cardiac investigation—nuclear and other imaging techniques

Diederik van de Beek Department of Neurology, Center of Infection and Immunity Amsterdam (CINIMA), University of Amsterdam, Amsterdam, The Netherlands

24.11.1: Bacterial infections

D. Gareth Beevers Professor of Medicine, University Department of Medicine, City Hospital, Birmingham, UK

16.17.5: Hypertensive urgencies and emergencies

John R. Benson Consultant Surgeon, Cambridge Breast Unit, Addenbrooke's Hospital, Cambridge, UK; Fellow and Director of Clinical Studies, Selwyn College, Cambridge, UK

6.2: The nature and development of cancer

Malcolm K. Benson Oxford Pleural Unit, Oxford Centre for Respiratory Medicine, John Radcliffe Hospital, Oxford, UK

18.19.4: Mediastinal cysts and tumours

Anthony R. Berendt Consultant Physician, Bone Infection Unit, Nuffield Orthopaedic Centre NHS Trust, Oxford, UK

19.7: Pyogenic arthritis; 20.3: Osteomyelitis

David de Berker Department of Dermatology, Bristol Royal Infirmary, Bristol, UK

23.13: Hair and nail disorders

Nancy Berliner Chief, Division of Hematology, Brigham and Women's Hospital, Professor of Medicine, Harvard Medical School, Baltimore, Maryland, USA

22.4.1: Leucocytes in health and disease; 22.4.2: Introduction to the lymphoproliferative disorders

Gordon R. Bernard Melinda Owen Bass Professor of Medicine, Division of Allergy, Pulmonary, and Critical Care Medicine; Associate Vice Chancellor for Research, Senior Associate Dean for Clinical Sciences, Vanderbilt University School of Medicine, Nashville, Tennessee, USA

7.1.2: Physiological changes, clinical features, and general management of infected patients

J.M. Best Emeritus Reader in Virology, King's College London, UK

7.5.13: Rubella

Delia B. Bethell Armed Forces Research Unit of Medical Sciences, Bangkok, Thailand (Clinical Trials Investigator); Oxford Radcliffe Hospital NHS Trust, Oxford, UK (Honorary Consultant Paediatrician)

7.6.1: Diphtheria

Ernest Beutler† Molecular and Experimental Medicine, The Scripps Research Institute, La Jolla, California, USA

22.5.11: Erythrocyte enzymopathies

Kaustuv Bhattacharya Staff Specialist, Metabolic Genetics Department, Western Sydney Genetics Program, The Children's Hospital at Westmead, Australia, NSW

12.3.1: Glycogen storage diseases

Rudolf Bilous Professor of Clinical Medicine, Newcastle University, Academic Centre, James Cook University Hospital, Middlesbrough, UK

21.10.1: Diabetes mellitus and the kidney

D. Bilton Consultant Physician, Royal Brompton Hospital and Honorary Senior Lecturer, Imperial College, London, UK

18.9: Bronchiectasis

A.E. Bishop Reader, Stem Cells & Regenerative Medicine, Department of Experimental Medicine & Toxicology, Imperial College Faculty of Medicine, Hammersmith Hospital, London, UK

15.9: Hormones and the gastrointestinal tract

Carol M. Black Professor of Rheumatology, Royal Free and University College Medical School, London, UK

19.11.3: Systemic sclerosis

S.R. Bloom Professor of Medicine, Imperial College, London, UK

13.10: Pancreatic endocrine disorders and multiple endocrine neoplasia; 15.9: Hormones and the gastrointestinal tract

Lotta von Boehmer Department of Oncology, University Hospital Zurich, Zurich, Switzerland

6.4: Cancer immunity and clinical oncology

Roland M. du Bois National Jewish Health, Denver, Colorado, USA

18.11.5: The lung in vasculitis

Christopher Booth Wellcome Centre for the History of Medicine, University College, London, UK

1.1: On being a patient

T.C. Boswell Consultant Medical Microbiologist, Nottingham University Hospitals, Nottingham, UK

7.6.38: Legionellosis and legionnaires' disease

Marina Botto Professor of Rheumatology, Rheumatology Section, Imperial College London, London, UK

5.1.2: The complement system

---

† It is with regret that we report the death of Professor Ernest Beutler during the preparation of this edition of the textbook.

S.J. Bourke Consultant Physician, Royal Victoria Infirmary, Newcastle upon Tyne, UK

18.14.5: Pulmonary Langerhans' cell histiocytosis;
18.14.6: Lymphangioleiomyomatosis; 18.14.12: Radiation pneumonitis;
18.14.13: Drug-induced lung disease

I.C.J.W. Bowler Consultant Microbiologist and Clinical Lead, Department of Medical Microbiology, Oxford Radcliffe Hospitals NHS Trust, Oxford, UK

7.2.3: Nosocomial infections

Paul Bowness Consultant Rheumatologist, Nuffield Orthopaedic Centre NHS Trust and Reader in Immunology, Nuffield Department of Medicine, Oxford University, UK

5.1.1: The innate immune system

S.M. Bradberry National Poisons Information Service and West Midlands Poisons Unit, City Hospital, Birmingham, UK

9.1: Poisoning by drugs and chemicals

Marcus Bradley Consultant in Radiology, Frenchay Hospital, Bristol, UK

24.3.3: Imaging in neurological diseases

Thomas Brandt Klinikum Groshadem, Neurologische Klinik, Munchen, Germany

24.6.2: Eye movements and balance

P. Brandtzaeg Department of Paediatrics, Oslo University Hospital, Oslo, Norway

7.6.5: Meningococcal infections

H.R. Branley Consultant in Respiratory Medicine, Whittington Hospital, London, UK

18.11.4: The lung in autoimmune rheumatic disorders

Philippe Brasseur Emeritus Professor of Parasitology, Faculty of Medicine of Rouen (France) and Research Unit (UMR 198), Institute of Research for Development, Dakar, Senegal

7.8.3: Babesiosis

J. Braun Rheumazentrum Ruhrgebiet, Herne, Germany; Ruhr University, Bochum, Germany

19.6: Ankylosing spondylitis, other spondyloarthritides, and related conditions

Sydney Brenner The Salk Institute, University of California, San Diego, California, USA

4.2.1: The human genome sequence

J.A. Bridgewater University College London Cancer Institute and UCLH/UCL Comprehensive Biomedical Centre, London, UK

15.16: Cancers of the gastrointestinal tract

F. Bridoux Department of Nephrology, Hopital Jean Bernard, Poitiers, France

21.10.4: Renal involvement in plasma cell dyscrasias, immunoglobulin-based amyloidoses, and fibrillary glomerulopathies, lymphomas, and leukaemias

Paul H. Brion Rheumatologist in Private Practice, Vista, California, USA

19.9: Osteoarthritis

Maries van den Broek Department of Oncology, University Hospital Zurich, Zurich, Switzerland

6.4: Cancer immunity and clinical oncology

Anthony F.T. Brown Professor of Emergency Medicine, Discipline of Anaesthesiology and Critical Care, School of Medicine, University of Queensland, Brisbane, Australia; Senior Staff Specialist, Department of Emergency Medicine, Royal Brisbane and Women's Hospital, Brisbane, Australia

17.2: Anaphylaxis

Arthur E. Brown Colonel, U.S. Army, Armed Forces Research Institute of Medical Sciences, Bangkok, Thailand

7.6.20: Anthrax

Kevin E. Brown Consultant Medical Virologist, Virus Reference Department, Centres for Infection, Health Protection Agency, London, UK

7.5.20: Parvovirus B19

Michael Brown Senior Lecturer, Department of Infectious & Tropical Diseases, London School of Hygiene & Tropical Medicine, London, UK

7.9.4: Strongyloidiasis, hookworm, and other gut strongyloid nematodes

Morris J. Brown Professor of Clinical Pharmacology, University of Cambridge, Addenbrookes Centre for Clinical Investigation (ACCI), Addenbrookes Hospital, Cambridge, UK

16.17.3: Secondary hypertension

Amy E. Bryant Research Scientist, Infectious Diseases Section, Veterans Affairs Medical Center, Boise, Idaho; Affiliate Assistant Professor, University of Washington School of Medicine, Seattle, Washington, USA

7.6.24: Botulism, gas gangrene, and clostridial gastrointestinal infections

A.D.M. Bryceson London School of Hygiene and Tropical Medicine, London, UK

7.8.12: Leishmaniasis

Camilla Buckley MRC Clinician Scientist and Honorary Consultant, Department of Clinical Neurology, University of Oxford, Oxford, UK

24.22: Autoimmune limbic encephalitis and Morvan's syndrome

Susan Burge Consultant Dermatologist, Oxford Radcliffe Hospitals NHS Trust, UK

23.7: Cutaneous vasculitis, connective tissue diseases, and urticaria

David J. Burn Professor in Movement Disorder & Neurology & Honorary Consultant, Institute for Ageing and Health, Newcastle University; Director, Clinical Ageing Research Unit, Campus for Ageing and Vitality, Newcastle upon Tyne, UK

24.7.3: Movement disorders other than Parkinson's disease

Alan Burnett Co-Director of the Center for Refugee and Disaster Response, Johns Hopkins, Department of Haematology, University of Wales College of Medicine, Cardiff, UK

22.3.4: Acute myeloid leukaemia

Gilbert Burnham Co-Director of the Center for Refugee and Disaster Response, Johns Hopkins, Department of International Health, Baltimore, Maryland, USA

7.9.1: Cutaneous filariasis

Aine Burns Consultant Nephrologist and Director of Postgraduate Medical Education, Centre for Nephrology, Royal Free NHS Trust and University College Medical School, London, UK

21.19: Drugs and the kidney

Jacky Burrin Department of Endocrinology, St Bartholomew's and the Royal London School of Medicine and Dentistry, London, UK

13.1: Principles of hormone action

N.P. Burrows Consultant Dermatologist and Associate Lecturer, Department of Dermatology, Addenbrooke's NHS Trust, Cambridge, UK

20.2: Inherited defects of connective tissue: Ehlers–Danlos syndrome, Marfan's syndrome, and pseudoxanthoma elasticum

Andrew Bush Consultant Physician, Royal Brompton and Harefield NHS Trust, London, UK

18.10: Cystic fibrosis

K. Bushby Professor of Neuromuscular Genetics, Institute of Human Genetics, International Centre for Life, Newcastle upon Tyne, UK

24.24.2: Muscular dystrophy

Valai Bussaratid Assistant Professor of Tropical Medicine, Department of Clinical Tropical Medicine, Mahidol University, Bangkok, Thailand

7.9.7: Gnathostomiasis

Anthony Busuttil Regius Professor of Forensic Medicine Emeritus, Forensic Medicine Section, University of Edinburgh, Edinburgh, UK

27.1: Forensic medicine and the practising doctor

Geoffrey A. Butcher The Malaria Centre, Department of Life Sciences, Imperial College London, London, UK

7.8.2: Malaria

Gary Butler Consultant in Paediatric and Adolescent Medicine and Endocrinology, University College London Hospital; Honorary Professor in Paediatric Endocrinology, UCL Institute of Child Health, Hospital for Children, London, UK

13.9.1: Normal growth and its disorders

W.F. Bynum Professor Emeritus of History of Medicine, Wellcome Trust Centre for the History of Medicine at University College London, UK

2.1.1: Science in medicine: when, how, and what

S.M. Cacciò Department of Infectious, Parasitic and Immunomediated Diseases, Istituto Superiore di Sanità, Viale Regina Elena, Rome, Italy

7.8.5: Cryptosporidium and cryptosporidiosis

P.M.A. Calverley Professor of Respiratory Medicine, School of Clinical Sciences, University of Liverpool, UK

18.15: Chronic respiratory failure

Louis R. Caplan Professor of Neurology, Harvard Medical School; Senior Neurologist, Beth Israel Deaconess Medical Center, Boston, Massachusetts, USA

2.3.2: Evidence-based medicine—does it apply to my particular patient?

Jonathan R. Carapetis Director, Menzies School of Health Research, Charles Darwin University, Darwin, Australia

16.9.1: Acute rheumatic fever

Simon Carette Professor of Medicine, University of Toronto; Deputy Physician-in-Chief, Education UHN/MSH; Head, Division of Rheumatology UHN/MSH, Toronto, Ontario, Canada

19.4: Back pain and regional disorders

M. Cariati Lecturer in Surgery, King's College London, UK

13.8.3: Breast cancer

R. Carter Consultant Surgeon, Lister Department of Surgery, Royal Infirmary, Glasgow, UK

15.24.1: Acute pancreatitis

Tim E. Cawston Professor of Rheumatology, Musculoskeletal Research Group, Institute of Cellular Medicine, The Medical School, Newcastle University, Newcastle upon Tyne, UK

19.1: Structure and function: joints and connective tissue

Bruce A. Chabner Clinical Director, Massachusetts General Hospital Cancer Center and Professor of Medicine, Harvard Medical School, Boston, Massachusetts, USA

6.6: Cancer chemotherapy and radiation therapy

Richard E. Chaisson Professor of Medicine, Epidemiology and International Health, Johns Hopkins University School of Medicine and Bloomberg School of Public Health, Baltimore, Maryland, USA

7.6.25: Tuberculosis

S.J. Challacombe Consultant in Oral Medicine, Guy's Hospital, London, UK

15.6: The mouth and salivary glands

Siddharthan Chandran MRC Centre for Regenerative Medicine, University of Edinburgh, UK

4.8: Stem cells and regenerative medicine; 24.10.2: Demyelinating disorders of the central nervous system

Badrinath Chandrasekaran Specialty Registrar in Cardiology, Wessex Cardiothoracic Unit, Southampton General Hospital, Southampton, UK

16.5.1: Clinical features and medical treatments

R.W. Chapman Consultant in Gastroenterology, Department of Gastroenterology, John Radcliffe Hospital, Oxford, UK

15.21.4: Primary sclerosing cholangitis

V. Krishna Chatterjee Professor of Endocrinology, Institute of Metabolic Science and Department of Medicine, University of Cambridge, Addenbrooke's Hospital, Cambridge, UK

13.1: Principles of hormone action

K. Ray Chaudhuri Co-director National Parkinson Foundation Centre of Excellence, Lead Neuroscience Research and Development Strategy, London South Representative, NIHR Nervous Systems Committee, Kings College/University Hospital Lewisham, Kings College and Institute of Psychiatry, London, UK

24.7.2: Parkinsonism and other extrapyramidal diseases

P.F. Chinnery Professor of Neurogenetics and Director of Newcastle, NIHR Biomedical Research Centre for Ageing and Age-related Disease, Institute for Ageing and Health, Newcastle University, Newcastle upon Tyne, UK

24.24.5: Mitochondrial encephalomyopathies

Lydia Chwastiak Assistant Professor, Department of Psychiatry, Yale University, Connecticut, USA

26.5.5: Anxiety and depression

Stefan O. Ciurea Assistant Professor, Department of Stem Cell Transplantation, Division of Cancer Medicine, The University of Texas MD Anderson Cancer Center, Houston, Texas, USA

22.3.8: The polycythaemias; 22.3.10: Thrombocytosis

P. Jane Clarke Consultant Breast Surgeon, Oxford Radcliffe Trust, Oxford, UK

13.8.4: Benign breast disease

P.E. Clayton Consultant in Paediatrics, Royal Manchester Children's Hospital, Manchester, UK

13.9.2: Puberty

S.M. Cobbe Consultant Cardiologist, Glasgow Royal Infirmary; former BHF Walton Professor of Medical Cardiology, University of Glasgow, Scotland

16.2.2: Syncope and palpitations; 16.4: Cardiac arrhythmias

Fredric L. Coe Professor of Medicine, Nephrology Section MC5100, University of Chicago, Chicago Illinois, USA

21.14: Disorders of renal calcium handling, urinary stones, and nephrocalcinosis

J. Cohen Dean of Medicine and Professor of Infectious Diseases, Brighton & Sussex Medical School, Brighton, UK

7.2.4: Infection in the immunocompromised host

R.D. Cohen Emeritus Professor of Medicine, University of London; Queen Mary University of London, Centre for Diabetes, Blizard Institute of Cell & Molecular Science, Bart's & The London School of Medicine & Dentistry, London, UK

12.11: Disturbances of acid–base homeostasis

J. Collier Consultant in General Medicine, John Radcliffe Hospital, Oxford, UK

7.5.22: Hepatitis C

R. Collins Clinical Trial Service Unit & Epidemiological Studies Unit (CTSU), University of Oxford, UK

2.3.3: Large-scale randomized evidence: trials and meta-analyses of trials

Alastair Compston Professor of Neurology, University of Cambridge, Cambridge, UK

24.1: Introduction and approach to the patient with neurological disease; 24.10.2: Demyelinating disorders of the central nervous system

Juliet Compston Professor of Bone Medicine, University of Cambridge School of Clinical Medicine, Cambridge, UK

20.4: Osteoporosis

C.P. Conlon Reader in Infectious Diseases and Tropical Medicine, University of Oxford; Consultant Physician, John Radcliffe Hospitals, Nuffield Department of Medicine, John Radcliffe Hospital, Oxford, UK

7.4: Travel and expedition medicine; 7.5.23: HIV/AIDS

Graham Cooper Consultant Cardiac Surgeon, Sheffield Teaching Hospitals NHS Foundation Trust, UK

16.13.7: Coronary artery bypass surgery

John E. Cooper The University of the West Indies, St Augustine, Trinidad & Tobago, West Indies; Department of Veterinary Medicine, University of Cambridge, Cambridge, UK

7.8.7: Sarcocystosis (sarcosporidiosis)

Susan J. Copley Consultant Radiologist and Reader in Thoracic Imaging, Imperial NHS Trust, London, UK

18.3.2: Thoracic imaging

Minerva Covarrubias Division of Allergy, Pulmonary and Critical Care Medicine, Vanderbilt University School of Medicine, Nashville, Tennessee, USA

14.8: Chest diseases in pregnancy

Philip J. Cowen Professor of Psychopharmacology, Warneford Hospital, Oxford, UK

26.6.1: Psychopharmacology in medical practice

Martin R. Cowie Professor of Cardiology, Imperial College London; Honorary Consultant Cardiologist, Royal Brompton Hospital, London, UK

16.5.1: Clinical features and medical treatments

Timothy M. Cox Professor of Medicine, University of Cambridge, Honorary Consultant Physician, Acting Head of Department, Addenbrooke's Hospital, Cambridge, UK

12.1: The inborn errors of metabolism: general aspects; 12.3.2: Inborn errors of fructose metabolism; 12.3.3: Disorders of galactose, pentose, and pyruvate metabolism; 12.5: The porphyrias; 12.7.1: Hereditary haemochromatosis; 12.8: Lysosomal diseases; 13.13: The pineal gland and melatonin; 15.10.5: Disaccharidase deficiency; 22.5.4: Iron metabolism and its disorders; 33.1: Acute medical presentations; 33.2: Practical procedures

S.E. Craig Research Fellow and Respiratory Medicine Specialty Registrar, Oxford Sleep Unit, Churchill Hospital, Oxford, UK

18.1.1: The upper respiratory tract; 18.5.1: Upper airways obstruction; 18.5.2: Sleep-related disorders of breathing

Robin A.F. Crawford Consultant Gynaecological Oncologist, Addenbrooke's Hospital, Cambridge, UK

14.17: Malignant disease in pregnancy

Adrian Crisp Consultant in Rheumatology and Metabolic Bone Diseases, Addenbrooke's Hospital, Cambridge, UK

20.5: Osteonecrosis, osteochondrosis, and osteochondritis dissecans

Nigel Crisp Independent Member of the House of Lords and London School of Hygiene and Tropical Medicine (formerly NHS Chief Executive and Permanent Secretary of Department of Health)

2.4.3: Priority setting in developed and developing countries

Derrick W. Crook Infectious Disease and Clinical Microbiology, Nuffield Department of Medicine, John Radcliffe Hospital, Oxford, UK

7.6.12: Haemophilus influenzae

Paul Cullinan Faculty of Medicine, Imperial College, London, UK

18.7: Asthma

Peter F. Currie Consultant Cardiologist & Clinical Lead for Cardiology, Perth Royal Infirmary & Ninewells Hospital, Perth, UK

16.9.3: Cardiac disease in HIV infection

Tim Dalgleish Senior Scientist, Medical Research Council, Cognition and Brain Sciences Unit, Cambridge, UK

26.5.1: Grief, stress, and post-traumatic stress disorder

Chi V. Dang Professor of Medicine, Cell Biology, Oncology & Pathology;Professor Vice Dean for Research, Johns Hopkins University School of Medicine, Baltimore, Maryland, USA

22.3.7: Myelodysplasia

Norman Daniels Mary B Saltonstall Professor and Professor of Ethics and Population Health in the Department of Global Health and Population at Harvard School of Public Health, Massachusetts, USA

2.4.2: Reasonableness and its definition in the provision of health care

Christopher J. Danpure Professor of Molecular Cell Biology, University College London, London, UK

12.10: Hereditary disorders of oxalate metabolism—the primary hyperoxalurias

A. Davenport Centre for Nephrology, University College London Medical School, London, UK

21.4: Clinical investigation of renal disease

Gail Davey Associate Professor, School of Public Health, Addis Ababa University, Ethiopia

9.5.8: Podoconiosis (nonfilarial elephantiasis)

Alun Davies Professor of Vascular Surgery, Imperial College School of Medicine, London, UK

16.14.2: Peripheral arterial disease

P.D.O. Davies Consultant Physician, Liverpool Heart and Chest Hospital and Aintree University Hospital, Liverpool, UK

7.6.26: Disease caused by environmental mycobacteria

R. Rhys Davies Consultant in Anaesthesia, Frenchay Hospital, Bristol, UK

24.3.1: Lumbar puncture

Robert J.O. Davies Professor of Respiratory Medicine, Oxford Centre for Respiratory Medicine, NIHR Oxford Biomedical Research Centre, University of Oxford and John Radcliffe Hospital, Oxford, UK

18.17: Pleural diseases; 18.19.3: Pleural tumours; 18.19.4: Mediastinal cysts and tumours

Simon Davies Professor of Nephrology and Dialysis Medicine, Institute of Science and Technology in Medicine, Keele University; Consultant Nephrologist, University Hospital of North Staffordshire, Stoke-on-Trent, UK

21.7.2: Peritoneal dialysis

Richard Dawkins Charles Simonyi Professor for the Understanding of Science, University of Oxford, Oxford, UK

2.1.2: Evolution: medicine's most basic science

Chris P. Day Institute of Cellular Medicine, Newcastle University, Newcastle upon Tyne, UK

15.22.1: Alcoholic liver disease; 15.22.2: Nonalcoholic steatohepatitis

Colin Dayan Head of Clinical Research and Reader in Medicine, Henry Wellcome Laboratories for Integrative Neuroscience and Endocrinology, University of Bristol, UK

13.11.1: Diabetes

Linda Dayan Senior Staff Specialist and Director of Sexual Health Services, Royal North Shore Hospital, Sydney; Clinical Lecturer, School of Public Health, University of Sydney, Sydney, Australia

7.6.36: Syphilis

Marc E. De Broe Professor of Medicine, Laboratory of Pathophysiology, University of Antwerp, Belgium

21.9.2: Chronic tubulointerstitial nephritis

Kevin M. De Cock Centers for Disease Control and Prevention, Nairobi, Kenya

7.5.24: HIV in the developing world

Menno D. De Jong Department of Medical Microbiology, Academic Medical Center, University of Amsterdam, Amsterdam, The Netherlands

24.11.2: Viral infections

Pauline de la Motte Hall[†] Late Professor, Division of Science, Murdoch University, Murdoch, Australia

15.22.7: Hepatic granulomas

P.B. Deegan Consultant in Metabolic Medicine, Department of Medicine, Addenbrooke's Hospital, Cambridge, UK

12.8: Lysosomal diseases

Barbara A. Degar Assistant Professor of Pediatrics, Dana-Farber Cancer Institute, Children's Hospital Boston, Harvard Medical School, Boston, Massachusetts, USA

22.4.2: Introduction to the lymphoproliferative disorders

D.M. Denison Emeritus Professor of Clinical Physiology, Royal Brompton Hospital and Imperial College London, London, UK

9.5.5: Aerospace medicine; 9.5.6: Diving medicine

Christopher P. Denton Professor of Experimental Rheumatology, Centre for Rheumatology, Division of Medicine, UCL Medical School, Royal Free Hospital, London, UK

19.11.3: Systemic sclerosis

Ulrich Desselberger Director of Research, Department of Medicine, Addenbrooke's Hospital, Cambridge, UK

7.5.8: Enterovirus infections; 7.5.9: Virus infections causing diarrhoea and vomiting

Michael Doherty Professor of Rheumatology, University of Nottingham, UK

19.3: Clinical investigation; 19.10: Crystal-related arthropathies

Richard S. Doll[††] Emeritus Professor of Medicine and Honorary Member, Cancer Studies Unit, Nuffield Department of Medicine, Radcliffe Infirmary, Oxford, UK

6.1: Epidemiology of cancer

[†] It is with regret that we report the death of Professor Pauline de la Motte Hall during the preparation of this edition of the textbook; [††] it is with regret that we report the death of Professor Richard S. Doll during the preparation of this edition of the textbook.

Clare Dollery Divisional Clinical Director, Consultant Cardiologist, The Heart Hospital, UCLH NHS Foundation Trust, London, UK
16.13.1: Biology and pathology of atherosclerosis

Michael Donaghy Department of Clinical Neurology, John Radcliffe Hospital, Oxford, UK
24.15: The motor neuron diseases

Basil Donovan Professor of Sexual Health, National Centre in HIV Epidemiology and Clinical Research, University of New South Wales; Senior Staff Specialist, Sydney Sexual Health Centre, Sydney Hospital, Sydney, Australia
7.6.36: Syphilis

Philip Dormitzer Senior Director, Senior Project Leader, Viral Vaccine Research, Novartis Vaccines and Diagnostics, Cambridge, Massachusetts, USA
7.5.9: Virus infections causing diarrhoea and vomiting

H.M.P. Dowson Consultant General and Laparoscopic Surgeon, Frimley Park Hospital, Surrey, UK
15.4.2: Gastrointestinal bleeding

Tilman B. Drüeke Division of Nephrology and Inserm U845, Necker Hospital, Paris, France
21.6: Chronic kidney disease

Patrick C.A. Dubois MRC Clinical Research Training Fellow, Specialty Registrar in Gastroenterology, Barts and The London School of Medicine and Dentistry, Queen Mary University of London, London, UK
15.10.3: Coeliac disease

Christopher Dudley Consultant Renal Physician. The Richard Bright Renal Unit, Southmead Hospital, North Bristol NHS Trust, Bristol, UK
16.14.3: Cholesterol embolism

D.W. Dunne Department of Pathology, University of Cambridge, Cambridge, UK
7.11.1: Schistosomiasis

Stephen R. Durham Professor of Allergy and Respiratory Medicine; Head, Section of Allergy and Clinical Immunology, National Heart and Lung Institute, Imperial College and Royal Brompton Hospital, London
18.6: Allergic rhinitis

P.N. Durrington Professor of Medicine, Cardiovascular Research Group Division of Clinical and Laboratory Sciences, University of Manchester Core Technology Facility, Manchester, UK
12.6: Lipid and lipoprotein disorders

J. Dwight Consultant Cardiologist, John Radcliffe Hospital, Oxford, UK
16.2.1: Chest pain, breathlessness, and fatigue

Patrick C. D'Haese Associate Professor, Laboratory of Pathophysiology, University of Antwerp, Belgium
21.9.2: Chronic tubulointerstitial nephritis

Ian Eardley Consultant Urologist, Leeds Teaching Hospital Trust, Leeds, UK
13.8.5: Sexual dysfunction

M. Eastwood Post-Retirement Honorary Fellow, Department of Medical Sciences, Western General Hospital, Edinburgh, UK
11.2: Vitamins and trace elements

Tim Eden Honorary Professor of Paediatric and Adolescent Oncology, University of Manchester, UK
22.3.3: Acute lymphoblastic leukaemia

Mark J. Edwards Sobell Department of Motor Neuroscience and Movement Disorders, Institute of Neurology, University College London; National Hospital for Neurology and Neurosurgery, London, UK
24.7.1: Subcortical structures: the cerebellum, basal ganglia, and thalamus

Richard Edwards[†] Late Emeritus Professor of Medicine, Liverpool University, UK
24.24.4: Metabolic and endocrine disorders

Rosalind A. Eeles Professor of Oncogenetics, The Institute of Cancer Research; Honorary Consultant in Cancer Genetics & Clinical Oncology, Royal Marsden NHS Foundation Trust, Sutton, UK
6.3: The genetics of inherited cancers

Perry Elliott The Heart Hospital, University College London, UK
16.7.2: The cardiomyopathies: hypertrophic, dilated, restrictive, and right ventricular; 16.7.3: Specific heart muscle disorders

Christopher J. Ellis Consultant Physician, Department of Infection and Tropical Medicine, Heartlands Hospital, Birmingham, UK
7.2.1: Clinical approach

Monique M. Elseviers Associate Professor, Department of Nursing Sciences, University of Antwerp, Belgium
21.9.2: Chronic tubulointerstitial nephritis

Caroline Elston Consultant Physician, Respiratory Medicine and Adult Cystic Fibrosis, King's College Hospital, London, UK
18.10: Cystic fibrosis

M.A. Epstein Nuffield Department of Clinical Medicine, John Radcliffe Hospital, Oxford, UK
7.5.3: Epstein–Barr virus

Wendy N. Erber Consultant Haematologist and Clinical Director of Haematology, Addenbrooke's Hospital, Cambridge, UK
22.3.2: The classification of leukaemia

E. Ernst Professor of Complementary Medicine, Peninsula Medical School, Universities of Exeter and Plymouth, Exeter, UK
2.5: Complementary and alternative medicine

David Eschenbach Professor and Chair, Department of Obstetrics and Gynecology, University of Washington, Seattle, Washington, USA
8.5: Pelvic inflammatory disease

Andrew P. Evan Chancellor's Professor, Department of Anatomy and Cell Biology, Indiana University School of Medicine, Indianapolis, Indiana, USA
21.14: Disorders of renal calcium handling, urinary stones, and nephrocalcinosis

Martin J. Evans School of Biosciences, Cardiff University, Cardiff, UK
4.7: Discovery of embryonic stem cells and the concept of regenerative medicine

Timothy Evans Professor of Intensive Care Medicine, Imperial College; Department of Anaesthesia and Intensive Care Medicine, Royal Brompton Hospital, UK
17.5: Acute respiratory failure

Pamela Ewan Consultant Allergist, Department of Medicine, Addenbrooke's Hospital, Cambridge, UK
5.3: Allergy

Christopher G. Fairburn Wellcome Principal Research Fellow and Professor of Psychiatry, Department of Psychiatry, University of Oxford, Oxford, UK
26.5.6: Eating disorders

Jeremy Farrar Oxford University Clinical Research Unit, Wellcome Trust Major Overseas Programme Vietnam; South East Asia Infectious Disease Clinical Research Network, Ho Chi Minh City, Vietnam
7.5.15: Dengue; 24.11.1: Bacterial infections; 24.11.2: Viral infections

Ken Farrington Consultant Nephrologist, Lister Hospital, Stevenage, UK
21.3: Clinical presentation of renal disease; 21.7.1: Haemodialysis

John Feehally Consultant Nephrologist, University Hospitals of Leicester; Honorary Professor of Renal Medicine, University of Leicester, UK
21.8.1: Immunoglobulin A nephropathy and Henoch–Schönlein purpura; 21.8.2: Thin membrane nephropathy

Eleanor Feldman Consultant Liaison Psychiatrist, John Radcliffe Hospital Oxford; Consultant in Eating Disorders, Warneford Hospital Oxford; Honorary Senior Clinical Lecturer in Psychiatry, University of Oxford, UK
26.2: Taking a psychiatric history from a medical patient; 26.3: Acute behavioural emergencies

Peter J. Fenner Associate Professor, School of Public Health, Tropical Medicine and Rehabilitation Sciences, James Cook University, Townsville, Australia
9.5.3: Drowning

[†] It is with regret that we report the death of Professor Richard Edwards during the preparation of this edition of the textbook.

Robert Ferrari Department of Medicine, University of Alberta, Edmonton, Alberta, Canada

19.2: Clinical presentation and diagnosis of rheumatic disease

C. ffrench-Constant Professor of Medical Neurology, MRC Centre for Regenerative Medicine, Centre for Multiple Sclerosis Research, The University of Edinburgh, Queen's Medical Research Institute, Edinburgh, UK

24.18: Developmental abnormalities of the central nervous system

Richard E. Fielding Locum Consultant Nephrologist, Brighton and Sussex University Hospital Trust, Brighton, UK

21.3: Clinical presentation of renal disease

R.G. Finch Professor of Infectious Diseases, Nottingham University Hospitals NHS Trust, Nottingham, UK

7.2.5: Antimicrobial chemotherapy

H.V. Firth Consultant Clinical Geneticist, Addenbrooke's Hospital, Cambridge, UK

24.18: Developmental abnormalities of the central nervous system

John D. Firth Consultant Physician and Nephrologist, Cambridge University Hospitals NHS Foundation Trust, Cambridge, UK

14.5: Renal disease in pregnancy; 14.12: Neurological disease in pregnancy; 16.15.3: Pulmonary oedema; 16.16.1: Deep venous thrombosis and pulmonary embolism; 16.19: Idiopathic oedema of women; 17.3: The clinical approach to the patient who is very ill; 21.2.2: Disorders of potassium homeostasis; 21.5: Acute kidney injury; 21.6: Chronic kidney disease; 21.10.9: Atherosclerotic renovascular disease; 33.1: Acute medical presentations; 33.2: Practical procedures

Rebecca Fitzgerald Honorary Consultant Gastroenterologist, Cambridge University Hospitals NHS Foundation Trust, Cambridge, UK

15.7: Diseases of the oesophagus

R. Andres Floto Wellcome Trust Senior Clinical Fellow, Cambridge Institute for Medical Research, University of Cambridge; Honorary Respiratory Consultant, Papworth & Addenbrooke's Hospitals, Cambridge, UK

4.5: Intracellular signalling

Edward D. Folland Chief of Clinical Cardiology, UMassMemorial Medical Center, Worcester, Massachusetts; Professor of Medicine, University of Massachusetts Medical School, Worcester, Massachusetts, USA

16.3.4: Cardiac catheterization and angiography; 16.13.6: Percutaneous interventional cardiac procedures

Keith A.A. Fox British Heart Foundation Professor of Cardiology, Centre for Cardiovascular Sciences, University of Edinburgh, Edinburgh, UK

16.13.5: Management of acute coronary syndrome

Ross S. Francis Transplantation Research Immunology Group, Nuffield Department of Surgery, University of Oxford, John Radcliffe Hospital, Oxford, UK

5.5: Principles of transplantation immunology

Stephen Franks Professor of Reproductive Endocrinology, Imperial College London, Hammersmith Hospital, London, UK

13.8.1: Ovarian disorders

Keith N. Frayn Professor of Human Metabolism, Oxford Centre for Diabetes, Endocrinology and Metabolism, University of Oxford, Oxford, UK

11.1: Nutrition: macronutrient metabolism

A.H. Freeman Consultant Radiologist, Addenbrooke's Hospital, Cambridge, UK.

15.3.3: Radiology of the gastrointestinal tract

Izzet Fresko Professor, Division of Rheumatology, Department of Medicine, Cerrahpasa Medical Faculty, University of Istanbul, Istanbul, Turkey

19.11.5: Behçet's syndrome

Peter S. Friedmann Emeritus Professor of Dermatology, University of Southampton, Southampton, UK

23.6: Dermatitis/eczema; 23.16: Cutaneous reactions to drugs

Peggy Frith Consultant Ophthalmic Physician, John Radcliffe Hospital, Oxford and University College Hospital London, UK

25.1: The eye in general medicine

David A. Gabbott Consultant Anaesthetist, Gloucestershire Hospitals NHS Foundation Trust UK; Chairman, Research subcommittee, Resuscitation Council (UK) Executive Committee Resuscitation Council (UK)

17.1: Cardiac arrest

Patrick G. Gallagher Professor of Pediatrics and Genetics, Yale University School of Medicine, New Haven, Connecticut, USA

22.5.10: Disorders of the red cell membrane

Hector H. Garcia Professor, Department of Microbiology, Universidad Peruana Cayetano Heredia, Lima, Peru; Head, Cysticercosis Unit, Instituto de Ciencias Neurológicas, Lima, Peru

7.10.1: Cystic hydatid disease (Echinococcus granulosus); 7.10.3: Cysticercosis

Lawrence B. Gardner Assistant Professor of Medicine and Pharmacology, Division of Hematology and the NYU Cancer Institute, New York University School of Medicine, New York, USA

22.3.7: Myelodysplasia

J.S. Hill Gaston Consultant in Rheumatology, Department of Rheumatology, University of Cambridge, Cambridge, UK

19.8: Reactive arthritis

Sarah Germain Senior Registrar in Obstetric Medicine, Guy's & St Thomas' Foundation Trust, London, UK

14.14: Autoimmune rheumatic disorders and vasculitis in pregnancy

G.J. Gibson Emeritus Professor of Respiratory Medicine, Newcastle University Newcastle upon Tyne, UK

18.3.1: Respiratory function tests

J. van Gijn Emeritus Professor of Neurology, University Medical Centre, Utrecht, The Netherlands

24.10.1: Stroke: cerebrovascular disease

I.P. Giles Centre for Rheumatology, Department of Medicine, University College London, London, UK

19.11.1: Introduction

Robert H. Gilman Professor, Department of International Health, Johns Hopkins Bloomberg School of Hygiene and Public Health, Baltimore, Maryland, USA

7.10.3: Cysticercosis

Ian Gilmore President, Royal College of Physicians, London, UK

15.24.3: Tumours of the pancreas

Alexander Gimson Consultant Physician and Hepatologist, Liver Transplantation Unit, Cambridge University Hospitals Foundation NHS Trust, Cambridge, UK

14.9: Liver and gastrointestinal diseases in pregnancy; 15.19: Structure and function of the liver, biliary tract, and pancreas; 15.26: Miscellaneous disorders of the bowel and liver

Paul P. Glasziou Department of Primary Health Care, University of Oxford, Oxford, UK

2.3.1: Bringing the best evidence to the point of care

Fergus V. Gleeson Oxford Pleural Unit, Oxford Centre for Respiratory Medicine, John Radcliffe Hospital, Oxford, UK

18.17: Pleural diseases

M.A. Glover Medical Director, Hyperbaric Medicine Unit, St Richard's Hospital, Chichester, UK

9.5.6: Diving medicine

Peter J. Goadsby Headache Group, Department of Neurology, University of California, San Francisco, California, USA

24.8: Headache

D. Goldblatt Professor of Vaccinology and Immunology, Consultant in Paediatric Immunology, Head, Immunobiology Unit, Director, Clinical Research and Development and, Director, NIHR Biomedical Research Centre, Great Ormond Street Hospital for Children NHS Trust and Institute of Child Health, University College London, UK

7.3: Immunization

Ann-Marie J. Golden Research Worker, Medical Research Council, Cognition and Brain Sciences Unit, Cambridge, UK

26.5.1: Grief, stress, and post-traumatic stress disorder

John M. Goldman Professor of Haematology (Emeritus), Imperial College, London, UK
22.3.6: Chronic myeloid leukaemia

Armando E. Gonzalez Dean, School of Veterinary Medicine, Universidad Nacional Mayor de San Marcos, Lima, Peru
7.10.1: Cystic hydatid disease (Echinococcus granulosus)

Timothy H.J. Goodship Professor of Renal Medicine, Newcastle University, UK
21.10.5: Haemolytic uraemic syndrome

Sherwood L. Gorbach Tufts University, Nutrition/infection Unit, Boston, Massachusetts, USA
15.18: Gastrointestinal infections

E.C. Gordon-Smith Emeritus Professor of Haematology, St George's, University of London, London, UK
22.3.11: Aplastic anaemia and other causes of bone marrow failure;
22.8.2: Haemopoietic stem cell transplantation

Eduardo Gotuzzo Instituto de Medicina Tropical Alexander von Humboldt Universidad Peruana Cayetano Heredia Av. Honorio Delgado, San Martín de Porres, Lima, Peru
7.5.25: HTLV-1, HTLV-2, and associated diseases

P. Goulder Wellcome Senior Clinical Fellow & Honorary Consultant Paediatrician, University of Oxford, Oxford, UK
7.5.23: HIV/AIDS

Jan Tore Gran Professor and Head, Department of Rheumatology, Oslo University Hospital, Rikshospitalet, Oslo, Norway
19.11.4; Polymyalgia rheumatica and temporal arteritis

J.M. Grange Visiting Professor, University College London, Centre for Infectious Diseases and International Health, London, UK
7.6.26: Disease caused by environmental mycobacteria

Alison D. Grant Department of Paediatrics, University of Auckland, Auckland, New Zealand
7.5.24: HIV in the developing world

Cameron Grant Department of Paediatrics, University of Auckland, Auckland, New Zealand
7.6.14: Bordetella infection

David Gray Reader in Medicine & Honorary Consultant Physician, Department of Cardiovascular Medicine, Nottingham University Hospitals NHS Trust, Nottingham, UK
16.3.1: Electrocardiography

R. Gray Clinical Trial Service Unit & Epidemiological Studies Unit (CTSU), University of Oxford, UK
2.3.3: Large-scale randomized evidence: trials and meta-analyses of trials

John R. Graybill Professor Emeritus, Division of Infectious Diseases, Department of Medicine, University of Texas Health Science Center at San Antonio, San Antonio, Texas, USA
7.7.3: Coccidioidomycosis

Manfred S. Green Professor and Head, School of Public Health, University of Haifa, Haifa, Israel
9.5.13: Bioterrorism

Roger Greenwood Consultant Nephrologist, Lister Hospital, Stevenage, UK
21.7.1: Haemodialysis

I.A. Greer Professor of Obstetric Medicine & Dean, Hull York Medical School, UK
14.7: Thrombosis in pregnancy

Christopher Griffiths Professor of Dermatology, Salford Royal NHS Foundation Trust, The University of Manchester, Manchester, UK
23.5: Papulosquamous disease

William J.H. Griffiths Consultant Hepatologist, Department of Hepatology, Addenbrooke's Hospital, Cambridge, UK
12.7.1: Hereditary haemochromatosis; 15.22.6: Liver tumours—primary and secondary

David I. Grove Formerly Director of Clinical Microbiology and Infectious Diseases, The Queen Elizabeth Hospital, Woodville and Clinical Professor, University of Adelaide, South Australia, Australia
7.9.5: Gut and tissue nematode infections acquired by ingestion;
7.10.4: Diphyllobothriasis and sparganosis; 7.11.2: Liver fluke infections;
7.11.4: Intestinal trematode infections

J.P. Grünfeld Université Paris Descartes, Department of Nephrology, Necker Hospital, Paris, France
21.12: Renal involvement in genetic disease

D.J. Gubler Director, Program on Emerging Infectious Disease, Duke-NUS Graduate Medical School, Singapore; Asian Pacific Institute of Tropical Medicine and Infectious Diseases, University of Hawaii, Honolulu
7.5.12: Alphaviruses; 7.5.14: Flaviviruses excluding dengue

Richard L. Guerrant Hunter Professor of International Medicine, Division of Infectious Diseases and International Health; Director, Center for Global Health, University of Virginia, Charlottesville, Virginia, USA
7.6.11: Cholera

John Guillebaud Emeritus Professor of Family Planning and Reproductive Health, University College, London, UK
8.6: Principles of contraception; 14.19: Benefits and risks of oral contraception

Mark Gurnell University Lecturer in Endocrinology, Institute of Metabolic Science and Department of Medicine, University of Cambridge, Addenbrooke's Hospital, Cambridge, UK
13.1: Principles of hormone action

Alejandro Gutierrez Instructor of Pediatrics, Harvard Medical School, Dana-Farber Cancer Institute and Children's Hospital Boston, Massachusetts, USA
22.3.1: Cell and molecular biology of human leukaemias

M.R. Haeney Consultant Immunologist, Salford Royal NHS Foundation Trust, Salford, UK
15.5: Immune disorders of the gastrointestinal tract

Davidson H. Hamer Associate Professor of International Health and Medicine, Boston University Schools of Public Health and Medicine; Director, Travel Clinic, Boston Medical Center, Adjunct Associate Professor of Nutrition, Tufts University Friedman School of Nutrition Science and Policy, Center for International Health and Development, Boston, Massachusetts, USA
15.18: Gastrointestinal infections

P.J. Hammond Consultant in Endocrinology, Harrogate District Hospital, Harrogate, UK
15.9: Hormones and the gastrointestinal tract

Y. Han Staff Physician, Transfusion Medicine, City of Hope Medical Center, Duarte, California, USA
22.8.1: Blood transfusion

M.G. Hanna Consultant Neurologist, National Hospital for Neurology and Institute of Neurology, London, UK
24.24.1: Structure and function of muscle

David M. Hansell Consultant Radiologist and Professor of Thoracic Imaging, Royal Brompton and Harefield NHS Trust, London, UK
18.3.2: Thoracic imaging

J.M. Harrington Emeritus Professor of Occupational Medicine, The University of Birmingham, Birmingham, UK
9.4.1: Occupational and environmental health

Nicholas K. Harrison Respiratory Unit, Morriston Hospital, Swansea, Wales, UK
18.11.3: Bronchiolitis obliterans and cryptogenic organizing pneumonia

Tina Hartert Associate Professor of Medicine, Vanderbilt University School of Medicine, Institute for Medicine and Public Health, Center for Health Services Research, Nashville, Tennessee, USA
14.8: Chest diseases in pregnancy

Adrian R.W. Hatfield Hepatobiliary Unit, The Middlesex Hospital, London, UK
15.3.2: Upper gastrointestinal endoscopy

Philip N. Hawkins Professor of Medicine, National Amyloidosis Centre and Centre for Acute Phase Proteins, UCL Medical School, London, UK

12.12.2: Hereditary periodic fever syndromes; 12.12.3: Amyloidosis

Keith Hawton Professor of Psychiatry, Centre for Suicide Research, Department of Psychiatry, University of Oxford, Oxford, UK

26.5.2: The patient who has attempted suicide

Roderick J. Hay Professor of Cutaneous Infection, Dermatology Department, King's College Hospital, London, UK

7.6.30: Nocardiosis; 7.7.1: Fungal infections; 23.10: Infections and the skin

Catherine E.G. Head Consultant Cardiologist, Guy's and St Thomas' NHS Foundation Trust, London, UK

14.6: Heart disease in pregnancy

Eugene Healy Professor of Dermatology, Dermatopharmacology, University of Southampton, Southampton General Hospital, UK

23.8: Disorders of pigmentation; 23.16: Cutaneous reactions to drugs

Nick Heather Emeritus Professor of Alcohol & Other Drug Studies, School of Psychology & Sport Sciences, Northumbria University, UK

26.7.2: Brief interventions against excessive alcohol consumption

David W. Hecht The John W. Clarke Professor and Chairman, Department of Medicine, Loyola University Medical Center, Maywood, Illinois, USA

7.6.10: Anaerobic bacteria

David A. van Heel Professor of Gastrointestinal Genetics, Honorary Consultant Gastroenterologist, Barts and The London School of Medicine and Dentistry, Queen Mary University of London, London, UK

15.10.3: Coeliac disease

Harry Hemingway Professor of Clinical Epidemiology, Department of Epidemiology and Public Health, University College London Medical School, London, UK

16.13.2: Coronary heart disease: epidemiology and prevention

Janet Hemingway Director, Liverpool School of Tropical Medicine, Liverpool, UK

7.8.2: Malaria

D.J. Hendrick Emeritus Professor, University of Newcastle upon Tyne, Consultant Physician Royal Victoria Infirmary, Newcastle upon Tyne, UK

18.14.1: Pulmonary haemorrhagic disorders; 18.14.2: Eosinophilic pneumonia; 18.14.3: Lymphocytic infiltrations of the lung; 18.14.4: Extrinsic allergic alveolitis; 18.14.5: Pulmonary Langerhans' cell histiocytosis; 18.14.6: Lymphangioleiomyomatosis; 18.14.7: Pulmonary alveolar proteinosis; 18.14.8: Pulmonary amyloidosis; 18.14.9: Lipoid (lipid) pneumonia; 18.14.10: Pulmonary alveolar microlithiasis; 18.14.11: Toxic gases and aerosols; 18.14.12: Radiation pneumonitis; 18.14.13: Drug-induced lung disease

Michael Henein Professor of Cardiology, Umea University, Sweden; Canterbury Christ Church University, UK

16.6: Heart valve disease; 16.8: Pericardial disease

Martin F. Heyworth Staff Physician and Adjunct Professor of Medicine, VA Medical Center and University of Pennsylvania, Philadelphia, Pennsylvania, USA

7.8.8: Giardiasis, balantidiasis, isosporiasis, and microsporidiosis

Tran Tinh Hien Vice Director, Centre for Tropical Diseases (Cho Quan Hospital), Ho Chi Minh City, Vietnam

7.6.1: Diphtheria

Katherine A. High Professor of Pediatrics, University of Pennsylvania School of Medicine, Children's Hospital of Philadelphia, Abramson Research Center, Philadelphia, Pennsylvania, USA

22.6.4: Genetic disorders of coagulation

Sharon Hillier Professor, Department of Obstetrics, Gynecology and Reproductive Sciences, University of Pittsburgh School of Medicine, Pittsburgh, Pennsylvania, USA

7.8.13: Trichomoniasis

David Hilton-Jones Clinical Director, Muscular Dystrophy Campaign, Muscle & Nerve Centre, Department of Clinical Neurology, John Radcliffe Hospital, Oxford, UK

24.23: Disorders of the neuromuscular junction; 24.24.3: Myotonia; 24.24.4: Metabolic and endocrine disorders

N. Hirani Consultant in Respiratory Medicine, Royal Infirmary, Edinburgh, UK

18.11.2: Idiopathic pulmonary fibrosis

Gideon M. Hirschfield Assistant Professor of Medicine, University of Toronto Liver Centre, Toronto Western Hospital, Toronto, Ontario, Canada

15.22.5: Liver transplantation

Moshe Hod Director, Division of Maternal Fetal Medicine, Helen Schneider Hospital for Women, Rabin Medical Center, Sackler Faculty of Medicine, Tel Aviv University, Petah-Tiqva, Israel

14.10: Diabetes in pregnancy

John R. Hodges Federation Fellow and Professor of Cognitive Neurology, Prince of Wales Medical Research Institute, Sydney, Australia

24.4.1: Disturbances of higher cerebral function; 24.4.2: Alzheimer's disease and other dementias

H.J.F. Hodgson Sheila Sherlock Chair of Medicine, University College London, London, UK

15.10.6: Whipple's disease; 15.21.1: Viral hepatitis—clinical aspects; 15.21.2: Autoimmune hepatitis

H. Hof Labor Limbach, Heidelberg, Germany

7.6.37: Listeriosis

A.V. Hoffbrand Consultant in Haematology. Department of Haematology, Royal Free Hospital, London, UK

22.5.6: Megaloblastic anaemia and miscellaneous deficiency anaemias

Ronald Hoffman Albert A. and Vera G. List, Professor of Medicine, Division of Hematology/Oncology, Director, Myeloproliferative Disorders Program, Tisch Cancer Institute, Departments of Medicine, Mount Sinai School of Medicine, New York, USA

22.3.8: The polycythaemias; 22.3.10: Thrombocytosis

Georg F. Hoffmann Chairman, University Children's Hospital, Department of General Pediatrics, Heidelberg, Germany

12.2: Protein-dependent inborn errors of metabolism

P. Holloway Consultant Chemical Pathologist and Honorary Senior Lecturer in Metabolic Medicine, Site Lead Clinician in Chemical Pathology and Immunology, St Mary's Hospital, Imperial College Healthcare NHS Trust, Medical School, London, UK

32.1: Biochemistry in medicine—reference intervals: the use of biochemical analysis for diagnosis and management

L. Holmberg Professor of Cancer Epidemiology, King's College London, UK

13.8.3: Breast cancer

Tony Hope Professor of Medical Ethics, University of Oxford; Fellow of St Cross College; and Honorary Consultant Psychiatrist

2.2: Medical ethics

Julian Hopkin Rector, Medicine & Health, School of Medicine, Swansea University, UK

18.2: The clinical presentation of respiratory disease

Bala Hota Division of Infectious Diseases, Department of Medicine, John H. Stroger Jr. Hospital of Cook County; Assistant Professor, Rush University Medical Center, Chicago, Illinois, USA

7.6.4: Staphylococci

Andrew R. Houghton Consultant Physician & Cardiologist, Grantham & District Hospital, Grantham, UK, and Visiting Fellow, University of Lincoln, Lincoln, UK

16.3.1: Electrocardiography

Laurence Huang Professor of Medicine, University of California San Francisco; Chief, AIDS Chest Clinic, HIV/AIDS Division, San Francisco General Hospital, San Francisco, California, USA

7.7.5: Pneumocystis jirovecii

H.C. Hughes Specialty Registrar (Infectious diseases/Microbiology), University Hospital of Wales, UK
7.5.29: Newly discovered viruses

I.A. Hughes Head of Department, Department of Paediatrics, Addenbrooke's Hospital, Cambridge, UK
13.7.2: Congenital adrenal hyperplasia; 13.9.3: Normal and abnormal sexual differentiation

R.A.C. Hughes Emeritus Professor of Neurology, King's College, London; Visiting Professor of Neurology, University College London; Cochrane Neuromuscular Disease Group, MRC Centre for Neuromuscular Disease
24.12: Disorders of cranial nerves; 24.16: Diseases of the peripheral nerves

P.J. Hutchinson Honorary Consultant Neurosurgeon and Senior Academy Fellow, Addenbrooke's Hospital, Cambridge, UK
24.5.6: Brain death and the vegetative state

Lawrence Impey Consultant in Obstetrics and Fetal Medicine, The John Radcliffe Hospital, Oxford, UK
14.15: Infections in pregnancy

C.W. Imrie Consultant Surgeon, Lister Department of Surgery, Royal Infirmary, Glasgow, UK
15.24.1: Acute pancreatitis

P.G. Isaacson Consultant in Histopathology, Department of Histopathology, Royal Free and University College Medical School, London, UK
15.10.4: Gastrointestinal lymphoma

David A. Isenberg Professor of Rheumatology, Centre for Rheumatology, Department of Medicine, University College London, London, UK
19.11.1: Introduction; 19.11.2: Systemic lupus erythematosus and related disorders

C. Ison Director, Sexually Transmitted Bacteria Reference Laboratory, Health Protection Agency Centre for Infections, London, UK
7.6.6: Neisseria gonorrhoeae

Alan A. Jackson Consultant in General Medicine, Southampton General Hospital, Southampton, UK
11.3: Severe malnutrition

Robin Jacoby Professor Emeritus of Old Age Psychiatry, University of Oxford; Department of Psychiatry, The Warneford Hospital, Oxford, UK
29.2: Mental disorders of old age

Dean Jamison Professor of Global Health, Department of Global Health, University of Washington, Seattle, Washington, USA
3.1: Global burden of disease: causes, levels, and intervention strategies

David Jayne Consultant in Nephrology and Vasculitis, Renal Unit, Department of Medicine, Addenbrooke's Hospital, Cambridge, UK
21.10.2: The kidney in systemic vasculitis

K.J.M. Jeffery Consultant Virologist, Oxford Radcliffe NHS Trust, John Radcliffe Hospital, Oxford, UK
7.5.22: Hepatitis C

Jørgen Skov Jensen Mycoplasma Laboratory, Copenhagen, Denmark
7.6.45: Mycoplasmas

D.P. Jewell Emeritus Professor of Gastroenterology, University of Oxford; Honorary Consultant Physician, John Radcliffe Hospital, Oxford, UK
15.12: Ulcerative colitis

Vivekanand Jha Additional Professor of Nephrology; Co-ordinator, Stem Cell Research Facility, Postgraduate Medical Institute, Chandigarh, India
21.11: Renal diseases in the tropics

Alexis J. Joannides Department of Clinical Neurosciences, University of Cambridge, UK
4.8: Stem cells and regenerative medicine

Anne M. Johnson Professor of Infectious Disease Epidemiology, Centre for Sexual Health and HIV Research, Research Department of Infection and Public Health, University College London, London, UK
8.2: Sexual behaviour

D. Joly Université Paris Descartes, Department of Nephrology, Necker Hospital, Paris, France
21.12: Renal involvement in genetic disease

E. Anthony Jones Former Chief of Hepatology, Academic Medical Center, Amsterdam, The Netherlands
15.22.4: Hepatocellular failure

Islam Junaid Consultant Urologist Barts and London NHS Trust Hospitals
21.17: Urinary tract obstruction

Summerpal S. Kahlon Melbourne Internal Medicine Associates, Melbourne, Florida, USA
7.5.16: Bunyaviridae

P.A. Kalra Consultant in Nephrology, Salford Royal NHS Foundation Trust, Salford, UK
21.10.9: Atherosclerotic renovascular disease

Kenneth C. Kalunian Professor of Medicine, Division of Rheumatology, Allergy and Immunology, University of California, San Diego School of Medicine, La Jolla, California, USA
19.9: Osteoarthritis

Eileen Kaner Institute of Health and Society, Newcastle University, UK
26.7.2: Brief interventions against excessive alcohol consumption

Niki Karavitaki Locum Consultant in Endocrinology, Department of Endocrinology, Oxford Centre for Diabetes, Endocrinology and Metabolism, Churchill Hospital, Oxford, UK
13.2: Disorders of the anterior pituitary gland; 13.3: Disorders of the posterior pituitary gland

Fiona E. Karet Professor of Nephrology, Honorary Consultant in Renal Medicine, University of Cambridge, UK
21.15: The renal tubular acidoses

Wayne J. Katon Professor and Vice-Chair, Department of Psychiatry & Behavioral Sciences, University of Washington, Washington, USA
26.5.5: Anxiety and depression

David Keeling Oxford Haemophilia & Thrombosis Centre, Churchill Hospital, Oxford, UK
16.16.2: Therapeutic anticoagulation

Jonathan Kell Department of Haematology, University Hospital of Wales and Cardiff University, Cardiff, UK
22.3.4: Acute myeloid leukaemia

David P. Kelsell Centre for Cutaneous Research, Blizard Institute of Cell and Molecular Science, Barts and the London School of Medicine and Dentistry, Queen Mary University of London, London, UK
23.3: Inherited skin disease

John G. Kelton McMaster University Medical Center, Hamilton, Ontario, Canada
22.6.3: Disorders of platelet number and function

Christopher Kennard Professor of Clinical Neurology, Head of Department, Department of Clinical Neurology, John Radcliffe Hospital, Oxford, UK
24.6.1: Visual pathways

R.S.C. Kerr Neurosurgery Consultant, John Radcliffe Hospital, Oxford, UK
24.11.3: Intracranial abscesses

M.G.W. Kettlewell Emeritus Consultant Colorectal Surgeon, John Radcliffe Hospital, Oxford, UK
15.14: Colonic diverticular disease

Maurice King Honorary Research Fellow, University of Leeds, Leeds, UK
3.4.2: A sinister pathogen corrupts two disciplines: the demographic entrapment of Middle Africa

Paul Klenerman Nuffield Department of Medicine, University of Oxford, Oxford, UK
5.1.3: Adaptive immunity; 7.5.22: Hepatitis C

Steve Knapper Department of Haematology, University Hospital of Wales and Cardiff University, Cardiff, UK
22.3.4: Acute myeloid leukaemia

Richard Knight Associate Professor of Parasitology (retired), Department of Microbiology, University of Nairobi, Kenya
7.8.1: Amoebic infections; 7.8.9: Blastocystis hominis infection; 7.9.2: Lymphatic filariasis; 7.9.3: Guinea worm disease (dracunculiasis); 7.9.6: Parastrongyliasis (angiostrongyliasis); 7.10.2: Cyclophyllidian gut tapeworms

Daniël Knockaert General Internal Medicine, University Hospital Gasthuisberg, Leuven, Belgium

7.2.2: Fever of unknown origin

Nine V.A.M. Knoers Professor in Clinical Genetics, Department of Human Genetics, Radboud University, Nijmegen Medical Centre, Nijmegen, The Netherlands

21.16: Disorders of tubular electrolyte handling

Alexander Knuth Department of Oncology, University Hospital Zurich, Zurich, Switzerland

6.4: Cancer immunity and clinical oncology

Yasushi Kobayashi Department of Immunobiology, Yale University School of Medicine, New Haven, Connecticut, USA

16.14.4: Takayasu's arteritis

G.C.K.W. Koh Honorary Specialist Registrar, Department of Medicine, University of Cambridge, Cambridge, UK

7.6.7.2: Pseudomonas aeruginosa

Stefan Kölker Consultant, Pediatric Metabolic Medicine, University Children's Hospital, Heidelberg, Department of General Pediatrics, Division of Inborn Metabolic Diseases, Heidelberg, Germany

12.2: Protein-dependent inborn errors of metabolism

Edwin H. Kolodny Bernard A. and Charlotte Marden Professor and Chairman, Department of Neurology, New York University School of Medicine, New York, USA

24.17: Inherited neurodegenerative diseases

Michael D. Kopelman Professor of Neuropsychiatry, Consultant Neuropsychiatrist, King's College London, St Thomas' Hospital, London, UK

26.4: Neuropsychiatric disorders

Christian Krarup Professor of Clinical Neurophysiology, Department of Clinical Neurophysiology, Rigshospitalet; Faculty of Health Science, University of Copenhagen, Copenhagen, Denmark

24.3.2: Electrophysiology of the central and peripheral nervous systems

D. Kumararatne Addenbrooke's Hospital, Cambridge, UK

5.2: Immunodeficiency

Robert A. Kyle Mayo Clinic, Rochester, Minnesota, USA

22.4.5: Myeloma and paraproteinaemias

Helen J. Lachmann Senior Lecturer, National Amyloidosis Centre and Centre for Acute Phase Proteins, University College London Medical School, London, UK

12.12.2: Hereditary periodic fever syndromes

R. Lainson Ex Director, The Wellcome Parasitology Unit, and research-worker, Department of Parasitology, Instituto Evandro Chagas, Rodovia, Bairro Levilândia, Ananindeua, Pará, Brazil

7.8.6: Cyclospora and cyclosporiasis

Peter C. Lanyon Consultant Rheumatologist, Nottingham University Hospitals Trust, UK

19.3: Clinical investigation

A.J. Larner Consultant Neurologist, Cognitive Function Clinic, Walton Centre for Neurology and Neurosurgery, Liverpool, UK

24.5.4: Syncope; 24.13.1: Diseases of the spinal cord

Malcolm Law Professor of Epidemiology and Preventive Medicine, Wolfson Institute of Preventive Medicine, St Bartholomews' and the Royal London School of Medicine and Dentistry, Queen Mary University of London, UK

3.3.2: Medical screening

T.P. Lawrence Neurosurgery Registrar, John Radcliffe Hospital, Oxford, UK

24.11.3: Intracranial abscesses

Stephen Lawrie Consultant in Psychiatry, Royal Edinburgh Hospital, Edinburgh, UK

26.5.7: Schizophrenia, bipolar disorder, obsessive–compulsive disorder, and personality disorder

N.F. Lawton Consultant Neurologist, Wessex Neurological Centre, Southampton General Hospital; Honorary Senior Lecturer, University of Southampton, UK

24.10.5: Idiopathic intracranial hypertension

Ramanan Laxminarayan Senior Fellow and Director, Center for Disease Dynamics, Economics, and Policy, Resources for the Future, Washington, DC, USA

3.1: Global burden of disease: causes, levels, and intervention strategies

Alison Layton Harrogate District Hospital, Harrogate, UK

23.11: Sebaceous and sweat gland disorders

John H. Lazarus Emeritus Professor of Clinical Endocrinology, Centre for Endocrine and Diabetes Sciences, School of Medicine, Cardiff University, Cardiff, UK

14.11: Endocrine disease in pregnancy

J.W. LeDuc Professor, Microbiology and Immunology, Robert E. Shope M.D. and John S. Dunn Distinguished Chair in Global Health, Deputy Director, Galveston National Laboratory, University of Texas Medical Branch, Galveston, USA

7.5.16: Bunyaviridae

Susannah Leaver Clinical Research Fellow/Specialty Registrar Respiratory and Intensive Care Medicine, Imperial College and Royal Brompton Hospital, London, UK

17.5: Acute respiratory failure

Philip Lee Lately Reader, Charles Dent Metabolic Unit, The National Hospital for Neurology and Neurosurgery, London, UK

12.3.1: Glycogen storage diseases

Y.C. Gary Lee Oxford Pleural Unit, Oxford Centre for Respiratory Medicine, John Radcliffe Hospital, Oxford, UK

18.17: Pleural diseases; 18.19.3: Pleural tumours

T. Lehner Professor of Basic & Applied Immunology, Kings College London at Guy's Hospital, London, UK

15.6: The mouth and salivary glands

Irene M. Leigh Vice Principal and Head of College, College of Medicine, Dentistry and Nursing, Ninewells Hospital and Medical School, Dundee, UK

23.3: Inherited skin disease

G.G. Lennox Consultant in Neurology, Addenbrooke's Hospital, Cambridge, UK

14.12: Neurological disease in pregnancy

Elena N. Levtchenko Pediatric Nephrologist, Radbound University Nijmegen Medical Centre, Nijmegen, The Netherlands

21.16: Disorders of tubular electrolyte handling

Jeremy Levy Imperial College Kidney and Transplant Institute, Imperial College Healthcare NHS Trust, London, UK

21.8.7: Antiglomerular basement membrane disease

Siong-Seng Liau Specialty Registrar in Hepatopancreatobiliary (HPB), Surgery, HPB Unit, Department of Surgery, Addenbrooke's Hospital Cambridge, UK

6.2: The nature and development of cancer

Peter Libby Chief, Cardiovascular Medicine, Brigham and Women's Hospital, Mallinckrodt Professor of Medicine, Harvard Medical School, Massachusetts, USA

16.13.1: Biology and pathology of atherosclerosis

Oliver Liesenfeld Professor of Medical Microbiology and Infection Institute for Microbiology and Hygiene, Charité Medical School Berlin, Berlin, Germany

7.8.4: Toxoplasmosis

Aldo A.M. Lima Professor of Medicine and Pharmacology, Faculty of Medicine, Federal University of Ceará, Fortaleza, CE, Brazil

7.6.11; Cholera

D.C. Linch Head of Department of Haematology, University College London, London, UK; Director of CRUK Cancer Centre at University College London, UK

22.2.2: Haemopoietic stem cell disorders

M.J. Lindop Consultant, John Farman Intensive Care Unit, Addenbrooke's Hospital, Cambridge, UK

17.8: Discontinuing treatment of the critically ill patient; 17.9: Brainstem death and organ donation

Gregory Y.H. Lip Consultant Cardiologist and Professor of Cardiovascular Medicine, Director, Haemostasis Thrombosis & Vascular Biology Unit, University of Birmingham Centre for Cardiovascular Sciences, City Hospital, Birmingham, UK

16.17.5: Hypertensive urgencies and emergencies

P. Little Professor of Primary Care Research, School of Medicine, University of Southampton, UK

18.4.1: Upper respiratory tract infections

William A. Littler Consultant Cardiologist, The Priory Hospital, Birmingham, UK

16.9.2: Infective endocarditis

A. Llanos-Cuentas School of Public Health & Administration and School of Medicine, Universidad Peruana Cayetano Heredia, Lima, Peru

7.6.43: Bartonella bacilliformis infection

Diana N.J. Lockwood Professor of Tropical Medicine, London School of Hygiene and Tropical Medicine, and Consultant Leprologist, Hospital for Tropical Diseases, London, UK

7.6.27: Leprosy (Hansen's disease); 7.8.12: Leishmaniasis

Jay Loeffler Herman and Joan Suit Professor, Harvard Medical School; Chair, Department of Radiation Oncology, Massachusetts General Hospital, Boston, Massachusetts, USA

6.6: Cancer chemotherapy and radiation therapy

Thomas Lom Senior Director, BBDO NY, New York, USA

3.3.3: The importance of mass communication in promoting positive health

David A. Lomas Department of Medicine, University of Cambridge; Cambridge Institute for Medical Research, Wellcome Trust, Cambridge, UK

12.13: α_1-Antitrypsin deficiency and the serpinopathies

Martin Lombard Liver and Pancreato-Biliary Unit, Royal Liverpool University Hospital, Liverpool, UK

15.24.3: Tumours of the pancreas

A. Thomas Look Professor of Pediatrics, Harvard Medical School; Vice Chair for Research, Department of Pediatric Oncology, Dana-Farber Cancer Institute, Boston, Massachusetts, USA

22.3.1: Cell and molecular biology of human leukaemias

Elyse E. Lower University of Cincinnati Medical Center, Ohio, USA

18.12: Sarcoidosis

Katharine Lowndes Specialty Registrar, Department of Haematology, Salisbury District Hospital, Wiltshire, UK

14.16: Blood disorders specific to pregnancy

James R. Lupski Baylor College of Medicine, Houston, Texas, USA

4.2.2: The genomic basis of medicine

Linda M. Luxon Professor of Audiovestibular Medicine, UCL Ear Institute and Consultant Neuro-otologist, National Hospital for Neurology and Neurosurgery, London, UK

24.6.3: Hearing

Lucio Luzzatto Chairman, Department of Human Genetics, Memorial Sloan-Kettering Cancer Center, New York, USA

22.3.12: Paroxysmal nocturnal haemoglobinuria;
22.5.12: Glucose-6-phosphate dehydrogenase (G6PD) deficiency

Graz A. Luzzi Consultant in Genitourinary Medicine and Honorary Senior Clinical Lecturer, University of Oxford, Wycombe Hospital, High Wycombe, UK

7.5.23: HIV/AIDS; 8.3: Sexual history and examination

David Mabey Professor of Communicable Diseases, Department of Infectious and Tropical Diseases, London School of Hygiene and Tropical Medicine, London, UK

7.6.44: Chlamydial infections; 8.1: Epidemiology of sexually transmitted infections

J.T. Macfarlane Lately Professor of Respiratory Medicine, University of Nottingham, and Consultant Respiratory Physician, Nottingham University Hospitals, Nottingham, UK

7.6.38: Legionellosis and legionnaires' disease

Kenneth T. MacLeod Reader in Cardiac Physiology, National Heart and Lung Institute (NHLI) Division, Faculty of Medicine, Imperial College London, London, UK

16.1.2: Cardiac myocytes and the cardiac action potential

William MacNee Professor of Respiratory and Environmental Medicine/Honorary Consultant ELEGI Colt Laboratories, MRC Centre for Inflammation Research, The Queen's Medical Research Institute, Edinburgh, UK

18.8: Chronic obstructive pulmonary disease

M. Monir Madkour‡ Consultant Physician, Military Hospital, Riyadh, Saudi Arabia

7.6.21: Brucellosis

C. Maguiña-Vargas Instituto de Medicina Tropical Alexander von Humboldt, Universidad Peruana Cayetano Heredia, Lima, Peru

7.6.43: Bartonella bacilliformis infection

Hadi Manji Consultant Neurologist and Honorary Senior Lecturer, National Hospital for Neurology and Neurosurgery, London, UK

24.11.4: Neurosyphilis and neuro-AIDS

J.I. Mann Professor of Human Nutrition and Medicine, University of Otago, Dunedin, New Zealand

11.4: Diseases of overnourished societies and the need for dietary change

J. Mansi Consultant Medical Oncologist, Guy's & St Thomas NHS Foundation Trust, London, UK

13.8.3: Breast cancer

David Mant Professor of General Practice, Department of Primary Health Care, University of Oxford, Oxford, UK

3.3.1: Preventive medicine

Vincent Marks Professor of Clinical Biochemistry Emeritus, Postgraduate Medical School, University of Surrey, Guildford, UK

13.11.2: Hypoglycaemia

Michael Marmot Professor of Epidemiology, Director of International Institute for Society and Health at University College London, Research Department of Epidemiology and Public Health, London, UK

16.13.2: Coronary heart disease: epidemiology and prevention

T.J. Marrie Dean, Faculty of Medicine, Dalhousie University, Clinical Research Centre, Halifax, Nova Scotia, Canada

7.6.41: Coxiella burnetii infections (Q fever)

C.D. Marsden* Late Professor of Neurology, National Hospital for Neurology and Neurosurgery, London, UK

24.19: Acquired metabolic disorders and the nervous system

Judith C.W. Marsh Professor of Clinical Haematology/Honorary Consultant Haematologist, Department of Haematology, St George's Hospital, St George's University of London, London, UK

22.3.11: Aplastic anaemia and other causes of bone marrow failure

Kevin Marsh Director, KEMRI Wellcome Research Programme, Kilifi, Kenya

7.8.2: Malaria

Steven B. Marston Professor of Cardiac Biochemistry, National Heart and Lung Institute (NHLI) Division, Faculty of Medicine, Imperial College London, London, UK

16.1.2: Cardiac myocytes and the cardiac action potential

N.M. Martin Consultant in Endocrinology, Hammersmith Hospital, London, UK

13.10: Pancreatic endocrine disorders and multiple endocrine neoplasia

Duncan J. Maskell Head of Department and Marks & Spencer Professor of Farm Animal Health, Food Science & Food Safety, Department of Veterinary Medicine, University of Cambridge, Cambridge, UK

7.1.1: Biology of pathogenic microorganisms

Jay W. Mason Professor of Medicine, Cardiology Division, University of Utah College of Medicine, Salt Lake City, Utah, USA

16.7.1: Myocarditis

---

† It is with regret that we report the death of Dr M. Monir Madkour during the preparation of this edition of the textbook.

*Deceased.

V.I. Mathan Vice-Dean and Campus Director, ICDDR.B, Dhaka, Bangladesh

15.10.8: Malabsorption syndromes in the tropics

Christopher J. Mathias Professor of Neurovascular Medicine and Consultant Physician, Imperial College at St Mary's and the National Hospital for Neurology and Neurosurgery, Institute of Neurology, University College London, UK

24.14: Diseases of the autonomic nervous system

Peter W. Mathieson Dean of the Faculty of Medicine & Dentistry, University of Bristol, Professor of Medicine and Honorary Consultant Nephrologist at North Bristol NHS Trust, UK

21.8.5: Proliferative glomerulonephritis; 21.8.6: Mesangiocapillary glomerulonephritis

Mary E. McCaul Professor, Department of Psychiatry & Behavioral Sciences, Johns Hopkins University School of Medicine, Baltimore, Maryland, USA

26.7.1: Alcohol and drug dependence

Brian W. McCrindle Professor of Pediatrics, University of Toronto, Staff Cardiologist, The Hospital for Sick Children, Toronto, Canada

19.11.8: Kawasaki's disease

A.D. McGavigan Associate Professor of Cardiovascular Medicine, Flinders University, South Australia, Australia

16.2.2: Syncope and palpitations; 16.4: Cardiac arrhythmias

John A. McGrath Professor of Molecular Dermatology, St John's Institute of Dermatology, King's College London (Guy's Campus), London, UK

23.1: Structure and function of skin

Jane McGregor Senior Lecturer and Honorary Consultant Dermatologist, Barts and the London NHS Trust, UK

23.9: Photosensitivity

Iain B. McInnes Professor of Experimental Medicine and Honorary Consultant Rheumatologist, Glasgow Biomedical Research Centre, University of Glasgow, Glasgow, UK

4.3: Cytokines

William J. McKenna The Heart Hospital, University College London, UK

16.7.2: The cardiomyopathies: hypertrophic, dilated, restrictive, and right ventricular; 16.7.3: Specific heart muscle disorders

A.J. McMichael Professor and NHMRC Australia Fellow, National Centre for Epidemiology and Population Health, ANU College of Medicine, Biology and Environment, Australian National University, Canberra, Australia

3.2: Human population size, environment, and health

Martin McNally Consultant Orthopaedic Surgeon, Nuffield Orthopaedic Centre NHS Trust, Oxford, UK

20.3: Osteomyelitis

K. McNeil Professor of Medicine, University of Queensland, CEO Metro North Health Service, Brisbane, Australia

18.16: Lung transplantation

Henry McQuay Nuffield Department of Anaesthetics, University of Oxford, Oxford, UK

30.1: Dealing with pain

Jill Meara Deputy Director/Public Health Consultant, Health Protection Agency Centre for Radiation, Chemical and Environmental Hazards, Chilton, UK

9.5.9: Radiation

David K. Menon Head, Division of Anaesthesia, University of Cambridge; Consultant, Neurosciences Critical Care Unit, BOC Professor, Royal College of Anaesthetists, Professorial Fellow, Queens' College, Cambridge, Senior Investigator, National Institute for Health Research

17.6: Management of raised intracranial pressure

Catherine H. Mercer Senior Lecturer in Sexual Health Research, Centre for Sexual Health and HIV Research, Research Department of Infection and Public Health, University College London, London, UK

8.2: Sexual behaviour

Vinod K. Metta Research and Clinical Registrar for Neurology and Movement Disorders, Kings College Hospital NHS Trust and University Hospital, London, UK

24.7.2: Parkinsonism and other extrapyramidal diseases

J. ter Meulen Executive Director Vaccine Basic Research, Merck Research Laboratories, West Point, Pennsylvania, USA

7.5.17: Arenaviruses; 7.5.18: Filoviruses

Wayne M. Meyers Visiting Scientist, Department of Environmental and Infectious Disease Sciences, Armed Forces Institute of Pathology, Washington DC, USA

7.6.28: Buruli ulcer: Mycobacterium ulcerans *infection*

Anna Rita Migliaccio Dirigente de Ricerca in Transfusion Medicine, Laboratory of Clinical Biochemistry, Istituto Superiore doi Sanità, Rome, Italy

22.5.1: Erythropoiesis and the normal red cell

M.A. Miles Professor of Medical Protozoology, Pathogen Molecular Biology Unit, Department of Infectious and Tropical Diseases, London School of Hygiene and Tropical Medicine, London, UK

7.8.11: Chagas disease

Robert F. Miller Professor, Reader in Clinical Infection, Centre for Sexual Health and HIV Research, University College London, London, UK

7.7.5: Pneumocystis jirovecii

Dawn S. Milliner Division of Nephrology, Departments of Pediatrics and Internal Medicine, Mayo Clinic, Rochester, Minnesota, USA

12.10: Hereditary disorders of oxalate metabolism—the primary hyperoxalurias

K.R. Mills Department of Clinical Neurophysiology, King's College Hospital, London, UK

24.3.4: Investigation of central motor pathways: magnetic brain stimulation

Philip Minor Division of Virology, National Institute for Biological Standards and Control, South Mimms, UK

7.5.8: Enterovirus infections

Pramod K. Mistry Department of Pediatrics, Yale School of Medicine, New Haven, Connecticut, USA

12.7.2: Inherited diseases of copper metabolism: Wilson's disease and Menkes' disease

Andrew R.J. Mitchell Consultant Cardiologist, Jersey General Hospital, Jersey, UK

16.3.2: Echocardiography; 16.14.1: Thoracic aortic dissection

Andrew J. Molyneux Consultant in Neuroradiology, The Manor Hospital, Oxford, UK

24.3.3: Imaging in neurological diseases

D.H. Molyneux Centre for Neglected Tropical Diseases, Liverpool School of Tropical Medicine, Pembroke Place, Liverpool, UK

7.9.2: Lymphatic filariasis

Kevin Moore Professor of Hepatology, Department of Medicine, University College London, London, UK

15.22.3: Cirrhosis and ascites

Marina S. Morgan Consultant Medical Microbiologist, Royal Devon & Exeter Foundation NHS Trust, UK

7.6.18: Pasteurella

Pedro L. Moro Immunization Safety Office, Centre for Disease Control and Prevention, Atlanta, Georgia, USA

7.10.1: Cystic hydatid disease (Echinococcus granulosus)

Nicholas W. Morrell British Heart Foundation Professor of Cardiopulmonary Medicine, University of Cambridge School of Clinical Medicine, Addenbrooke's and Papworth Hospitals, Cambridge, UK

16.15.1: Structure and function; 16.15.2: Pulmonary hypertension; 16.15.3: Pulmonary oedema

Emma Morris Senior Lecturer and Honorary Consultant, UCL Medical School, University College London, London, UK

22.8.2: Haemopoietic stem cell transplantation

N.J. McC. Mortensen Professor of Colorectal Surgery, University of Oxford and Consultant Colorectal Surgeon, John Radcliffe Hospitals, Oxford, UK

15.14: Colonic diverticular disease

Peter S. Mortimer Professor of Dermatological Medicine to the University of London, Consultant Skin Physician to St George's Hospital, London and the Royal Marsden Hospital, London, UK

16.18: Chronic peripheral oedema and lymphoedema; 23.12: Blood and lymphatic vessel disorders

Tariq I. Mughal Professor of Medicine and Hematology/Oncology, University of Texas Southwestern School of Medicine, Dallas, Texas, USA
22.3.6: Chronic myeloid leukaemia

David R. Murdoch Professor and Head of Pathology, University of Otago, Christchurch, New Zealand
9.5.4: Diseases of high terrestrial altitudes

Jean B. Nachega Associate Scientist, Department of International Health, Johns Hopkins University, Bloomberg School of Public Health, Baltimore, Maryland, USA; Extraordinary Professor, Department of Medicine, and Director, Centre for Infectious Diseases, Stellenbosch University, Tygerberg, Cape Town, South Africa
7.6.23: Tuberculosis

Robert B. Nadelman Division of Infectious Diseases, Department of Medicine, New York Medical College, Valhalla, New York, USA
7.6.32: Lyme borreliosis

N.V. Naoumov Immunology and Infectious Diseases, Novartis Pharma AG, Basel, Switzerland, and Honorary Professor of Hepatology, University College London, UK
7.5.21: Hepatitis viruses (excluding hepatitis C virus)

Ravinder Nath Maini Emeritus Professor of Rheumatology, The Kennedy Institute of Rheumatology Division, Imperial College London, UK
19.5: Rheumatoid arthritis

David Neal Professor of Surgical Oncology, Honorary Consultant Urological Surgeon, University of Cambridge; Department of Oncology, Addenbrooke's Hospital, Cambridge, UK
21.18: Malignant diseases of the urinary tract

Graham Neale Department of Surgery, Imperial College, London, UK
15.2: Symptomatology of gastrointestinal disease; 15.17: Vascular and collagen disorders

Catherine Nelson-Piercy Consultant Obstetric Physician, Guy's & St Thomas' Foundation Trust and Imperial College Healthcare Trust, UK
14.14: Autoimmune rheumatic disorders and vasculitis in pregnancy

Randolph M. Nesse Professor of Psychiatry and Psychology, Research Professor, Research Center for Group Dynamics, ISR, Director, Evolution and Human Adaptation Program, The University of Michigan, Ann Arbor, Michigan, USA
2.1.2: Evolution: medicine's most basic science

Peter J. Nestor University Lecturer in Cognitive Neurology, University of Cambridge, Department of Clinical Neurosciences, Cambridge, UK; Honorary Consultant Neurologist, Addenbrooke's Hospital, Cambridge, UK
24.4.1: Disturbances of higher cerebral function

J. Neuberger Honorary Consultant Physician, Liver Unit, Queen Elizabeth Hospital, Birmingham, UK; Honorary Professor of Medicine, University of Birmingham, UK; Associate Medical Director, Organ Donation and Transplantation, NHS Blood and Transplant, Bristol, UK
15.22.8: Drugs and liver damage; 15.22.9: The liver in systemic disease

A.J. Newman Taylor Consultant in Respiratory Medicine, Faculty of Medicine, Imperial College, London, UK
18.7: Asthma

A.G. Nicholson Consultant Histopathologist, Royal Brompton and Harefield NHS Trust; Professor of Respiratory Pathology, National Heart and Lung Institute, Imperial College School of Medicine, London, UK
18.11.2: Idiopathic pulmonary fibrosis

Perry Nisen Senior Vice President, Cancer Research, GlaxoSmithKline, Philadelphia, Pennsylvania, USA
2.3.4: The future of clinical trials

Jerry P. Nolan Consultant in Anaesthesia and Intensive Care Medicine, Royal United Hospital Bath, UK; Co-Chair International Liaison Committee on Resuscitation
17.1: Cardiac arrest

John Nowakowski Division of Infectious Diseases, Department of Medicine, New York Medical College, Valhalla, New York, USA
7.6.32: Lyme borreliosis

Paul Nyirjesy Professor of Obstetrics and Gynecology and of Medicine, Drexel University College of Medicine, Philadelphia, Pennsylvania, USA
8.4: Vaginal discharge

Kunle Odunsi Professor and Research Program Director, Roswell Park Cancer Institute, Buffalo, New York, USA
6.4: Cancer immunity and clinical oncology

Graham S. Ogg Reader in Cutaneous Immunology, MRC Senior Clinical Fellow; Consultant in Dermatology, Churchill Hospital, Oxford, UK
23.7: Cutaneous vasculitis, connective tissue diseases, and urticaria

Yngvild K. Olsen Assistant Professor, Department of Medicine, Johns Hopkins University School of Medicine, Baltimore, Maryland, USA
26.7.1: Alcohol and drug dependence

Petra C.F. Oyston Defence Science and Technology Laboratories in the Biomedical Sciences Department, Dstl Porton Down, Salisbury, UK; Chair at the University of Leicester in the Department of Infection, Immunity and Inflammation
7.6.19: Francisella tularensis infection

Nigel O'Farrell Consultant Physician, Ealing Hospital, London, UK
7.6.13: Haemophilus ducreyi and chancroid

Donncha O'Gradaigh Consultant Rheumatologist, Waterford Regional Hospital, Ireland
19.12: Miscellaneous conditions presenting to the rheumatologist; 20.5: Osteonecrosis, osteochondrosis, and osteochondritis dissecans

Kevin O'Shaughnessy Senior Lecturer/Consultant, Clinical Pharmacology Unit, Department of Medicine, Addenbrooke's Hospital, Cambridge, UK
10.1: Principles of clinical pharmacology and drug therapy

Edel O'Toole Centre for Cutaneous Research, Blizard Institute of Cell and Molecular Science, Barts and the London School of Medicine and Dentistry and Department of Dermatology, Barts and the London NHS Trust, London, UK
23.14: Tumours of the skin

Aparna Pal Centre for Diabetes, Oxford Endocrinology and Metabolism, Churchill Hospital, Oxford, UK
13.3: Disorders of the posterior pituitary gland

Jacqueline Palace Consultant in Neurology, The Horton Hospital, Banbury, UK
24.23: Disorders of the neuromuscular junction

Thalia Papayannopoulou Professor of Medicine (Hematology), University of Washington, Division of Hematology, Seattle, USA
22.5.1: Erythropoiesis and the normal red cell

Jayan Parameshwar Consultant Cardiologist, Transplant Unit, Papworth Hospital, Cambridge. UK
16.5.2: Cardiac transplantation and mechanical circulatory support

S. Parish Clinical Trial Service Unit, University of Oxford, Oxford, UK
2.3.3: Large-scale randomized evidence: trials and meta-analyses of trials

Gilbert Park Consultant in Anaesthesia and Intensive Care, Addenbrooke's Hospital, Cambridge, UK
17.7: Sedation and analgesia in the critically ill

P. Parker Head of Division of Cancer Studies, King's College London, UK
13.8.3: Breast cancer

David Parkes SGDP Research Centre, Institute of Psychiatry and Neurosciences Department, King's Healthcare, Denmark Hill, London, UK
24.5.2: Narcolepsy

Miles Parkes Consultant Gastroenterologist, Inflammatory Bowel Disease Genetics Research Unit, Addenbrooke's Hospital, Cambridge, UK
15.11: Crohn's disease

Philippe Parola Unité de Recherche en Maladies Infectieuses et Tropicales Emergentes, WHO Collaborative Centre for Rickettsioses and other Arthropod borne Bacteria, Faculté de Médecine, Université de la Mediterraníe, Marseilles, France

7.6.39: Rickettsioses

C.M. Parry Oxford University Clinical Research Unit, Hospital for Tropical Diseases, Ho Chi Minh City, Vietnam

7.6.8: Typhoid and paratyphoid fevers

J. Paul Regional Microbiologist, Health Protection Agency, South East Region, Regional Microbiologist's Office, Royal Sussex County Hospital, Brighton, UK

7.6.46: A check list of bacteria associated with infection in humans; 7.12: Nonvenomous arthropods

S.J. Peacock Professor of Clinical Microbiology, Department of Medicine, University of Cambridge Cambridge, UK

7.6.7.2: Pseudomonas aeruginosa; 7.6.15: Melioidosis and glanders

Roger Pedersen MRC Centre for Stem Cell Biology and Regenerative Medicine, University of Cambridge, UK

4.8: Stem cells and regenerative medicine

Malik Peiris Department of Microbiology, The University of Hong Kong, Queen Mary Hospital Pokfualm, Hong Kong SAR

7.5.1: Respiratory tract viruses

Hugh Pennington Emeritus Professor of Bacteriology, University of Aberdeen, UK

7.6.7.1: Enterobacteria and bacterial food poisoning

M.B. Pepys Head, Division of Medicine, Royal Free Campus, University College London; Director, UCL Centre for Amyloidosis & Acute Phase Proteins; UK NHS National Amyloidosis Centre, UK

12.12.1: The acute phase response and C-reactive protein; 12.12.3: Amyloidosis

S.P. Pereira Senior Lecturer in Gastroenterology, University College, London Medical School, London, UK

15.16: Cancers of the gastrointestinal tract

G.D. Perkin Emeritus Consultant Neurologist, Charing Cross Hospital, London, UK

24.5.1: Epilepsy in later childhood and adulthood

P.L. Perrotta Associate Professor of Pathology, Director of Clinical Laboratories, West Virginia School of Medicine, West Virginia, USA

22.8.1: Blood transfusion

David J. Perry Consultant Haematologist, Department of Haematology, Addenbrooke's Hospital, Cambridge, UK

14.16: Blood disorders specific to pregnancy

Hans Persson Senior Consultant Physician, Swedish Poisons Centre, Stockholm, Sweden

9.3.1: Poisonous plants and fungi

Michael C. Petch Consultant Cardiologist, Queen Elizabeth Hospital, Kings Lynn, UK

16.13.8: The impact of coronary heart disease on life and work

Eskild Petersen Department of Infectious Diseases, Aarhus University Hospital, Skejby, Aarhus, Denmark

7.8.4: Toxoplasmosis

L.R. Petersen Director, Division of Vector-borne Infectious Diseases, Centers for Disease Control and Prevention, Fort Collins, Colorado, USA

7.5.12: Alphaviruses; 7.5.14: Flaviviruses excluding dengue

R. Peto Clinical Trial Service Unit & Epidemiological Studies Unit (CTSU), University of Oxford, UK

2.3.3: Large-scale randomized evidence: trials and meta-analyses of trials; 6.1: Epidemiology of cancer

T.E.A. Peto Professor of Infectious Diseases, University of Oxford; Consultant Physician, Oxford Radcliffe Hospitals, Nuffield Department of Medicine, John Radcliffe Hospital, Oxford, UK

7.5.23: HIV/AIDS

A.O. Phillips Consultant in Nephrology, University Hospital of Wales, Cardiff, UK

21.1: Structure and functions of the kidney

Wendy Phillips Specialty Registrar in Neurology, Cambridge University Hospitals Foundation Trust, Cambridge, UK

24.3.1: Lumbar puncture

G. Pichert Consultant Clinical Geneticist, Guy's & St Thomas' NHS Foundation Trust, London, UK

13.8.3: Breast cancer

J.D. Pickard Professor of Neurosurgery, Academic Neurosurgery Unit, Department of Clinical Neurosciences, University of Cambridge, Addenbrooke's Hospital, Cambridge, UK

24.5.6: Brain death and the vegetative state

V.V. Pillay Chief, Poison Control Centre, Head, Analytical Toxicology, Amrita Institute of Medical Sciences, Cochin, Kerala, India

9.3.2: Common Indian poisonous plants

S. Pinder Professor of Breast Histopathology, King's College London, Consultant Histopathologist, Guy's & St Thomas NHS Foundation Trust, London, UK

13.8.3: Breast cancer

Michael R. Pinsky Professor of Critical Care Medicine, Pittsburgh, Pennsylvania, USA

17.4: Circulation and circulatory support in the critically ill

Mervi L.S. Pitkanen Consultant Neuropsychiatrist, Neuropsychiatry and Memory Disorders Clinic, Adamson Centre, London, UK

26.4: Neuropsychiatric disorders

R.J. Playford Professor of Medicine, Clinical Gastroenterologist, Vice Principal NHS Liaison and Deputy Warden, Barts and The London School of Medicine and Dentistry, UK

15.10.7: Effects of massive small bowel resection

J.M. Polak Emeritus Professor, Division of Investigative Science, Imperial Colllege London, London, UK

15.9: Hormones and the gastrointestinal tract

Eleanor S. Pollak Associate Professor, Hospital of the University of Pennsylvania, Children's Hospital of Philadelphia and the Philadelphia VA Medical Center, Abramson Research Center, Philadelphia, Pennsylvania, USA

22.6.4: Genetic disorders of coagulation

Andrew J. Pollard Professor of Paediatric Infection and Immunity, Department of Paediatrics, University of Oxford, Oxford, UK

9.5.4: Diseases of high terrestrial altitudes

Aaron Polliack Emeritus Professor of Hematology, and Head of Lymphoma, Leukemia Unit, Department of Hematology, Hadassah University Hospital and, Hebrew University Medical School Jerusalem, Israel; Senior Consultant, Emeritus Professor of Hematology, Department of Hematology and Bone Marrow Transplantation, Tel Aviv Sourasky Medical Center, Tel Aviv, Israel

22.3.5: Chronic lymphocytic leukaemia and other leukaemias of mature B and T cells

Philip A. Poole-Wilson‡ British Heart Foundation Simon Marks Professor of Cardiology, National Heart and Lung Institute (NHLI) Division, Faculty of Medicine, Imperial College London, London, UK

16.1.2: Cardiac myocytes and the cardiac action potential

Françoise Portaels Mycobacteriology Unit, Department of Microbiology, Institute of Tropical Medicine Nationalestraat, Antwerpen, Belgium

7.6.28: Buruli ulcer: Mycobacterium ulcerans infection

Jerry Posner Evelyn Frew American Cancer Society Clinical Research Professor—George C. Cotzias Chair of Neuro-oncology—Professor of Neurology and Neuroscience, Weil Medical School of Cornell University Department of Neuro-oncology, Memorial Sloan-Kettering Cancer Center, New York City, New York, USA

24.21: Paraneoplastic neurological syndromes

---

‡ It is with regret that we report the death of Professor Philip A. Poole-Wilson during the preparation of this edition of the textbook.

William G. Powderly Professor of Medicine and Therapeutics, Dean of Medicine, UCD School of Medicine and Medical Sciences, University College Dublin, Dublin, Ireland

7.7.2: Cryptococcosis

J. Powell-Tuck Emeritus Professor of Clinical Nutrition, Barts and the London School of Medicine and Dentistry, UK

11.2: Vitamins and trace elements

Janet Powell Department of Surgery & Cancer, Imperial College, London, UK

16.14.2: Peripheral arterial disease

Amy Powers Instructor, Harvard Medical School and Beth Israel Deaconess Medical Center, Boston, Massachusetts, USA

22.5.9: Haemolytic anaemia—congenital and acquired

J.W. Powles Department of Public Health and Primary Care, University of Cambridge, Cambridge, UK

3.2: Human population size, environment, and health

Michael B. Prentice Professor of Medical Microbiology, Department of Microbiology, University College Cork, Cork, Ireland

7.6.16: Plague: Yersinia pestis; 7.6.17: Other yersinia infections: yersiniosis

A. Purushotham Professor of Breast Cancer, King's College London, Consultant Breast Surgeon, Guy's & St Thomas NHS Foundation Trust, London, UK

13.8.3: Breast cancer

Charles Pusey Imperial College Kidney and Transplant Institute, Imperial College London, UK

21.8.7: Antiglomerular basement membrane disease

Anisur Rahman Professor of Rheumatology, University College London, UK

19.11.2: Systemic lupus erythematosus and related disorders

S. Vincent Rajkumar Professor of Medicine, Division of Hematology, Mayo Clinic, Rochester, Minnesota, USA

22.4.5: Myeloma and paraproteinaemias

M. Ramsay Consultant Epidemiologist, Immunisation, Hepatitis and Blood Safety Department, HPA Centre for Infections, London, UK

7.3: Immunization

A.C. Rankin Professor of Medical Cardiology, BHF Glasgow Cardiovascular Research Centre, University of Glasgow, UK

16.2.2: Syncope and palpitations; 16.4: Cardiac arrhythmias

Didier Raoult Faculté de Médecine et de Pharmacie, Université de la Méditerranée, Marseille Cedex, France

7.6.39: Rickettsioses; 7.6.42: Bartonellas excluding B. bacilliformis

Michael D. Rawlins National Institute for Health and Clinical Excellence, London, UK

2.4.1: The evaluation and provision of effective medicines

Paul J. Reading Consultant in Neurology, Department of Neurology, The James Cook University Hospital, Middlesbrough, UK

24.5.3: Sleep disorders

C.W.G. Redman Emeritus Professor of Obstetric Medicine, University of Oxford; Honorary Research Fellow, Lady Margaret Hall, Oxford Nuffield Department of Obstetrics and Gynaecology, John Radcliffe Hospital Oxford, UK

14.4: Hypertension in pregnancy

Jeremy Rees Consultant Neurologist, National Hospital for Neurology and Neurosurgery, London, UK

24.10.4: Intracranial tumours; 24.21: Paraneoplastic neurological syndromes

Shelley Renowden Consultant in Neuroradiology, Frenchay Hospital, Bristol, UK

24.3.3: Imaging in neurological diseases

Todd W. Rice Assistant Professor of Medicine, Division of Allergy, Pulmonary, and Critical Care Medicine, Vanderbilt University School of Medicine, Nashville, Tennessee, USA

7.1.2: Physiological changes, clinical features, and general management of infected patients

J. Richens Centre for Sexual Health and HIV Research, Research Department of Infection & Population Health, University College London, London, UK

7.6.9: Intracellular klebsiella infections (donovanosis and rhinoscleroma)

A.B. Rickinson Institute for Cancer Studies, University of Birmingham, Birmingham, UK

7.5.3: Epstein–Barr virus

B.K. Rima Deputy Head of the School of Medicine, Dentistry and Biomedical Sciences, Belfast, Ireland

7.5.5: Mumps: epidemic parotitis

Eberhard Ritz Department of Internal Medicine, Division of Nephrology, Heidelberg, Germany

21.6: Chronic kidney disease

Harold R. Roberts Sarah Graham Kenan Distinguished Professor of Medicine, Department of Medicine; Division of Hematology/Oncology, University of North Carolina, Chapel Hill NC and Attending Physician, University of North Carolina Hospitals, North Carolina, USA

22.6.1: The biology of haemostasis and thrombosis

T.A. Rockall Director MATTU, University of Surrey, Guildford, UK

15.4.2: Gastrointestinal bleeding

Kenneth Rockwood Professor of Geriatric Medicine, Dalhousie University, Halifax, Nova Scotia, Canada

29.1: Medicine in old age

Edward Roddy Specialty Registrar in Rheumatology, Nottingham City Hospital, Nottingham, UK

19.10: Crystal-related arthropathies

Simon D. Roger Director of Renal Medicine, Gosford Hospital, Gosford, NSW, Australia; Clinical Associate Professor, Department of Medicine & Health Sciences, Newcastle University, Newcastle, NSW, Australia

21.9.1: Acute interstitial nephritis

Jean-Marc Rolain Faculté de Médecine et de Pharmacie, Université de la Méditerranée, Marseille Cedex, France

7.6.42: Bartonellas excluding B. bacilliformis

P. Ronco Professor of Renal Medicine, University Pierre et Marie Curie, Tenon Hospital, and Inserm Unit UMR_S702

21.10.4: Renal involvement in plasma cell dyscrasias, immunoglobulin-based amyloidoses, and fibrillary glomerulopathies, lymphomas, and leukaemias

Antony Rosen Mary Betty Stevens Professor of Medicine, Professor of Pathology, Director, Division of Rheumatology, Johns Hopkins University School of Medicine, Baltimore, Maryland, USA

5.4: Autoimmunity

Mark J. Rosen Chief, Division of Pulmonary, Critical Care and Sleep Medicine, North Shore University Hospital and Long Island Jewish Medical Center, Professor of Medicine, Hofstra University School of Medicine, New York, USA

18.4.4: Pulmonary complications of HIV infection

Peter Rubin Professor of Therapeutics, Division of Therapeutics & Molecular Medicine, University of Nottingham, Nottingham, UK

14.18: Prescribing in pregnancy

Simon M. Rushbrook Consultant Hepatologist, Department of Hepatology Norfolk and Norwich University Hospitals NHS Foundation Trust, Norfolk, UK

15.19: Structure and function of the liver, biliary tract, and pancreas; 15.22.6: Liver tumours—primary and secondary

Anthony S. Russell Professor Emeritus, Rheumatic Disease Unit, University of Alberta, Edmonton, Alberta, Canada

19.2: Clinical presentation and diagnosis of rheumatic disease

Nikant Sabharwal Consultant Cardiologist, Department of Cardiology, John Radcliffe Hospital, Oxford, UK

16.3.3: Cardiac investigation—nuclear and other imaging techniques

I. Sadaf Farooqi Metabolic Research Laboratories, Institute of Metabolic Science, Addenbrooke's Hospital, University of Cambridge, Cambridge, UK

11.5: Obesity

Hesham Saleh Consultant Rhiniologist/Facial Plastic Surgeon, Charing Cross Hospital and Royal Brompton Hospital, Honorary Senior Lecturer, Imperial College, London, UK

18.6: Allergic rhinitis

Nilesh J. Samani British Heart Foundation Professor of Cardiology, Department of Cardiovascular Sciences, University of Leicester, Leicester, UK

16.17.4: Mendelian disorders causing hypertension

Swati Sathe Assistant Professor of Neurology, New York University School of Medicine, New York, USA

24.17: Inherited neurodegenerative diseases

Brian P. Saunders Wolfson Unit for Endoscopy, St Mark's Hospital for Colorectal Disorders, Harrow, London, UK

15.3.1: Colonoscopy and flexible sigmoidoscopy

S.J. Saunders Division of Hepatology, University of Cape Town Medical School, University of Cape Town, South Africa

15.22.7: Hepatic granulomas

E. Sawyer Consultant Clinical Oncologist, Guy's & St Thomas NHS Foundation Trust, London, UK

13.8.3: Breast cancer

K.P. Schaal Emeritus Professor of Medical Microbiology; Member of the Expert Committee of the Federal Ministry of Labour and Social Affairs Institute for Medical Microbiology, Immunology and Parasitology, University Hospital, Bonn, Germany

7.6.29: Actinomycoses

Michael L. Schilsky Associate Professor of Medicine, Medical Director, Adult Liver Transplant, Yale-New Haven Transplantation Center, Department of Internal Medicine, Yale School of Medicine, New Haven, Connecticut, USA

12.7.2: Inherited diseases of copper metabolism: Wilson's disease and Menkes' disease

Neil Scolding University of Bristol Institute of Clinical Neurosciences, Department of Neurology, Frenchay Hospital, Bristol, UK

24.19: Acquired metabolic disorders and the nervous system; 24.20: Neurological complications of systemic disease

Anthony Scott Wellcome Trust Senior Research Fellow in Clinical Science, KEMRI Wellcome Trust Research Programme, Kilifi, Kenya; Nuffield Department of Clinical Medicine, University of Oxford, Oxford, UK

7.6.3: Pneumococcal infections

A. Seaton Honorary Senior Consultant, Institute of Occupational Medicine, Edinburgh, UK and Emeritus Professor of Environmental and Occupational Medicine, University of Aberdeen, Aberdeen, UK

18.13: Pneumoconioses

Amartya Sen Lamont University Professor and Professor of Economics and Philosophy, Harvard University, Cambridge, Massachusetts, USA

3.5: Human disasters

G.R. Serjeant University of West Indies, Kingston, Jamaica

21.10.6: Sickle-cell disease and the kidney

Nicholas J. Severs Professor of Cell Biology, National Heart and Lung Institute (NHLI) Division, Faculty of Medicine, Imperial College London, London, UK

16.1.2: Cardiac myocytes and the cardiac action potential

Keerti V. Shah Department of Molecular Microbiology and Immunology, Johns Hopkins Bloomberg School of Public Health, Baltimore, Maryland, USA

7.5.19: Papillomaviruses and polyomaviruses

Pallav L. Shah Consultant Physician, Royal Brompton Hospital, London, UK, Chelsea & Westminster Hospital, London, UK

18.3.3: Bronchoscopy, thoracoscopy, and tissue biopsy

Michael Sharpe Professor of Psychological Medicine, Psychological Medicine Research, School of Molecular and Clinical Medicine, University of Edinburgh, UK

26.1: General introduction; 26.5.3: Medically unexplained symptoms in patients attending medical clinics; 26.5.4: Chronic fatigue syndrome (postviral fatigue syndrome, neurasthenia, and myalgic encephalomyelitis); 26.6.2: Psychological treatment in medical practice

Maire P. Shelly Consultant in Intensive Care, Wythenshawe Hospital, Manchester, UK

17.7: Sedation and analgesia in the critically ill

Jackie Sherrard Consultant in Genitourinary Medicine, Churchill Hospital, Oxford, UK

7.6.6: Neisseria gonorrhoeae; 8.3: Sexual history and examination

M.A. Shikanai-Yasuda Professor of Department of Infectious and Parasitic Diseases, Endemic Diseases Group/Infections in Immunosupressed Host Programme, Faculdade de Medicina, University of São Paulo, Brazil

7.7.4: Paracoccidioidomycosis

John M. Shneerson Director, Respiratory Support & Sleep Centre, Papworth Hospital, Cambridge, UK

18.18: Disorders of the thoracic cage and diaphragm

C.A. Sieff Division of Hematology, Karp 080006C, Children's Hospital Boston, Boston, Massachusetts, USA

22.2.1: Stem cells and haemopoiesis

J. Sieper Free University, Berlin, Germany

19.6: Ankylosing spondylitis, other spondyloarthritides, and related conditions

Udomsak Silachamroon Assistant Professor of Tropical Medicine, Department of Clinical Tropical Medicine, Faculty of Tropical Medicine, Mahidol University, Bangkok, Thailand

7.11.3: Lung flukes (paragonimiasis)

Leslie Silberstein Professor, Harvard Medical School, Children's Hospital Boston, Dana-Farber Cancer Institute, Brigham and Women's Hospital, and Harvard Stem Cell Institute, Boston, Massachusetts, USA

22.5.9: Haemolytic anaemia—congenital and acquired

Rod Sinclair Professor of Dermatology, University of Melbourne, Director of Dermatology, St. Vincent's Hospital, Director of Research and Training, Skin and Cancer Foundation, Fitzroy, Australia

23.17: Management of skin disease

Robert E. Sinden The Malaria Centre, Department of Life Sciences, Imperial College London, London, UK

7.8.2: Malaria

Joseph Sinning Harold Leever Regional Cancer Center, Waterbury, Connecticut, USA

22.4.1: Leucocytes in health and disease

Thira Sirisanthana Professor of Medicine, Chiang Mai University, Thailand

7.6.20: Anthrax; 7.7.6: Penicillium marneffei infection

J.G.P. Sissons Regius Professor of Physic, Director, Cambridge University Health Partners, School of Clinical Medicine, University of Cambridge, Cambridge, UK

7.5.2: Herpesviruses (excluding Epstein–Barr virus)

Geoffrey L. Smith Wellcome Principal Research Fellow, Section of Virology, Faculty of Medicine, Imperial College London, London, UK

7.5.4: Poxviruses

R. Smith Emeritus Professor of Rheumatology, Nuffield Orthopaedic Centre NHS Trust, Oxford, UK

20.1: Skeletal disorders—general approach and clinical conditions

Robert W. Snow Head, Malaria Public Health Group, KEMRI/Wellcome Trust Programme and Advisor, National Malaria Control Programme, Ministry of Health, Nairobi, Kenya

7.8.2: Malaria

E.L. Snyder Professor, Laboratory Medicine, Yale University School of Medicine, New Haven, Connecticut, USA

22.8.1: Blood transfusion

Jasmeet Soar Consultant in Anaesthesia and Intensive Care Medicine, Southmead Hospital Bristol, UK; Chair, Resuscitation Council (UK)

17.1: Cardiac arrest

Krishna Somers Consultant Physician in Cardiovascular Medicine, Royal Perth Hospital, Perth, Australia

16.9.4: Cardiovascular syphilis

M.W. Sonderup Division of Hepatology, University of Cape Town Medical School, University of Cape Town, South Africa

15.22.7: Hepatic granulomas

R.L. Souhami Emeritus Professor of Medicine, University College London, London, UK

6.5: Cancer: clinical features and management

C.W.N. Spearman Division of Hepatology, University of Cape Town Medical School, University of Cape Town, South Africa.
15.22.7: Hepatic granulomas

G.P. Spickett Consultant Clinical Immunologist, Regional Department of Immunology, Royal Victoria Hospital, Newcastle upon Tyne, UK
18.14.1: Pulmonary haemorrhagic disorders; 18.14.2: Eosinophilic pneumonia; 18.14.4: Lymphocytic infiltrations of the lung

S.G. Spiro Professor of Respiratory Medicine and Honorary Consultant Physician Royal Brompton Hospital, London, UK
18.19.1: Lung cancer; 18.19.2: Pulmonary metastases

Jerry L. Spivak Division of Hematology. The Johns Hopkins University School of Medicine, Baltimore, Maryland, USA
22.3.9: Idiopathic myelofibrosis

U. Srinivas-Shankar Consultant Physician, Department of Diabetes & Endocrinology, St Helens & Knowsley Teaching Hospitals NHS Trust, St Helens, UK
13.8.2: Disorders of male reproduction

Paweł Stankiewicz Assistant Professor, Department of Molecular and Human Genetics, Baylor College of Medicine
4.2.2: The genomic basis of medicine

Paul D. Stein Visiting Professor, Department of Internal Medicine, Michigan State University, College of Osteopathic Medicine, East Lansing, Missouri, USA
16.16.1: Deep venous thrombosis and pulmonary embolism

Dennis L. Stevens Chief, Infectious Diseases Section, Veterans Affairs Medical Center, Boise, Professor of Medicine, University of Washington School of Medicine, Seattle, Washington, USA
7.6.2: Streptococci and enterococci; 7.6.24: Botulism, gas gangrene, and clostridial gastrointestinal infections

Tom Stevens Consultant Psychiatrist, Lambeth Hospital, South London and Maudsley NHS Foundation Trust, London, UK
26.4: Neuropsychiatric disorders

J.C. Stevenson Department of Metabolic Medicine, Imperial College London, Royal Brompton Hospital, London, UK
14.20: Benefits and risks of hormone replacement therapy

P.M. Stewart Professor of Medicine and Director of Research and Knowledge Transfer, University of Birmingham, Birmingham, UK
13.7.1: Disorders of the adrenal cortex

Stephen F. Stewart Institute of Cellular Medicine, Newcastle University, Newcastle upon Tyne, UK
15.22.1: Alcoholic liver disease; 15.22.2: Nonalcoholic steatohepatitis

August Stich Department of Tropical Medicine, Medical Mission Institute, Würzburg, Germany
7.8.10: Human African trypanosomiasis

Heather Stoddart Principal Clinical Scientist, Department of Chemical Pathology and Immunology, St Mary's Hospital, Imperial College Healthcare NHS Trust, London, UK
32.1: Biochemistry in medicine—reference intervals: the use of biochemical analysis for diagnosis and management

John H. Stone Associate Professor of Medicine, Harvard Medical School, Director, Clinical Rheumatology, Massachusetts General Hospital, Massachusetts, USA
19.11.7: Polymyositis and dermatomyositis

J.R. Stradling Professor of Respiratory Medicine & Consultant Respiratory Physician, Oxford Centre for Respiratory Medicine, John Radcliffe Hospitals, Oxford, UK
18.1.1: The upper respiratory tract; 18.5.1: Upper airways obstruction; 18.5.2: Sleep-related disorders of breathing

Frank J. Strobl Director of Scientific Affairs, Therakos, Inc. RandCD, Exton, Pennsylvania, USA
22.5.9: Haemolytic anaemia—congenital and acquired

M.A. Stroud Senior Lecturer in Medicine, University of Southampton, UK
9.5.1: Heat; 9.5.2: Cold

Michael Strupp Department of Neurology, Ludwig-Maximilians University, Munich, Germany
24.6.2: Eye movements and balance

Peter H. Sugden Professor of Cellular Biochemistry, National Heart and Lung Institute (NHLI) Division, Faculty of Medicine, Imperial College London, London, UK
16.1.2: Cardiac myocytes and the cardiac action potential

J.A. Summerfield St Mary's Hospital, London, UK
15.23: Diseases of the gallbladder and biliary tree; 15.25: Congenital disorders of the liver, biliary tract, and pancreas

Joseph Sung Professor of Medicine, Head, Shaw College, Associate Dean (General Affairs), Chairman, Department of Medicine & Therapeutics, Director, Institute of Digestive Disease, Faculty of Medicine, The Chinese University of Hong Kong
15.8: Peptic ulcer disease

Pravan Suntharasamai Mahidol University, Bangkok, Thailand
7.9.7: Gnathostomiasis

P. Sweny Emeritus Consultant Nephrologist, Royal Free NHS Trust, London, UK
21.7.3: Renal transplantation

A.J. Swerdlow Professor of Epidemiology, Institute of Cancer Research, University of London, UK
6.1: Epidemiology of cancer

D. Swirsky Consultant Haematologist, St James's University Hospital, Leeds, UK
22.4.4: The spleen and its disorders

Penelope Talelli Sobell Department of Motor Neuroscience and Movement Disorders, Institute of Neurology, University College London; National Hospital for Neurology and Neurosurgery, London, UK
24.7.1: Subcortical structures: the cerebellum, basal ganglia, and thalamus

C.T. Tan Professor, Department of Medicine, University of Malaya, Kuala Lumpur, Malaysia
7.5.7: Nipah and Hendra virus encephalitides

David Taylor-Robinson Emeritus Professor of Genito-Microbiology and Medicine, Imperial College London, Division of Medicine, London, UK
7.6.44: Chlamydial infections; 7.6.45: Mycoplasmas

Henri A. Termeer Chairman and Chief Executive Officer, Genzyme Corporation, Cambridge, Massachusetts, USA
2.4.4: Sustaining innovation in an era of specialized medicine

R.V. Thakker May Professor of Medicine, Academic Endocrine Unit, Nuffield Department of Clinical Medicine, University of Oxford; Oxford Centre for Diabetes, Endocrinology and Metabolism, Churchill Hospital, Oxford, UK
13.6: Parathyroid disorders and diseases altering calcium metabolism

David G.T. Thomas Department of Neurological Surgery, Institute of Neurology, London, UK
24.10.3: Traumatic injuries to the head

P.K. Thomas‡ Emeritus Professor of Neurology, Royal Free Hospital School of Medicine and Institute of Neurology, London, UK
24.12: Disorders of cranial nerves; 24.16: Diseases of the peripheral nerves

D.G. Thompson Professor of Gastroenterology, Epithelial Sciences Research Group, School of Translational Medicine, University of Manchester, Clinical Sciences Building, Salford Royal Hospitals Salford, UK
15.1: Structure and function of the gut; 15.13: Irritable bowel syndrome and functional bowel disorders

R.P.H. Thompson Gastrointestinal Laboratory, The Rayne Institute, St Thomas's Hospital, London, UK
15.20: Jaundice

S.A. Thorne Consultant Cardiologist, University Hospital, Birmingham, UK
16.12: Congenital heart disease in the adult

---

‡ It is with regret that we report the death of Professor P.K. Thomas during the preparation of this edition of the textbook.

C.L. Thwaites Oxford University Clinical Research Unit, Ho Chi Minh City, Vietnam

7.6.22: Tetanus

Guy E. Thwaites Department of Microbiology, Imperial College, London, UK

24.11.1: Bacterial infections

Adam D. Timmis Professor of Clinical Cardiology, London Chest Hospital, London, UK

16.13.4: Management of stable angina

Charles Tomson Consultant Nephrologist, Richard Bright Renal Unit, Southmead Hospital, Bristol, UK

21.13: Urinary tract infection

P.A. Tookey Senior Lecturer, MRC Centre of Epidemiology for Child Health, UCL Institute of Child Health, London, UK

7.5.13: Rubella

Peter Topham Consultant Nephrologist, John Walls Renal Unit, University Hospitals of Leicester NHS Trust Leicester, UK

21.8.2: Thin membrane nephropathy

P.P. Toskes Professor of Medicine, University of Florida College of Medicine, Gainesville, Florida, USA

15.10.2: Small-bowel bacterial overgrowth; 15.24.2: Chronic pancreatitis

G. Touchard Professor, Department of Nephrology, Poitiers University Hospital, Poitiers, France

21.10.4: Renal involvement in plasma cell dyscrasias, immunoglobulin-based amyloidoses, and fibrillary glomerulopathies, lymphomas, and leukaemias

Thomas A. Traill Adult Cardiology Faculty, Johns Hopkins, Hospital, Baltimore, Maryland, USA

16.10: Tumours of the heart; 16.11: Cardiac involvement in genetic disease

A.S. Truswell Emeritus Professor of Human Nutrition,University of Sydney, Australia

11.4: Diseases of overnourished societies and the need for dietary change

Wai Y. Tse Consultant Nephrologist and Senior Lecturer, Renal Unit, Derriford Hospital, Plymouth, UK

21.10.3: The kidney in rheumatological disorders

D.M. Turnbull Professor of Neurology and Director Newcastle Centre for Brain Ageing and Vitality, Institute for Ageing and Health, Newcastle University, Newcastle upon Tyne, UK

24.24.5: Mitochondrial encephalomyopathies

A. Neil Turner Consultant in Nephrology, Royal Infirmary, Edinburgh, UK

21.10.7: Infection-associated nephropathies; 21.10.8: Malignancy-associated renal disease

J.A. Vale Director, National Poisons Information Service (Birmingham Unit) and West Midlands Poisons Unit; City Hospital, Birmingham, UK

9.1: Poisoning by drugs and chemicals

Patrick Vallance Senior Vice President Drug Discovery, GlaxoSmithKline, London, UK

2.3.4: The future of clinical trials; 16.1.1: Blood vessels and the endothelium

Steven Vanderschueren General Internal Medicine, University Hospital Gasthuisberg, Leuven, Belgium

7.2.2: Fever of unknown origin

Sirivan Vanijanonta Emeritus Professor of Tropical Medicine, Department of Clinical Tropical Medicine, Faculty of Tropical Medicine, Mahidol University, Bangkok, Thailand

7.11.3: Lung flukes (paragonimiasis)

Patrick J.W. Venables Professor of Viral Immunorheumatology, Kennedy Institute of Rheumatology. Imperial College, London, UK

19.11.6: Sjögren's syndrome

B.J. Vennervald DBL-Centre for Health Research and Development, Faculty of Life Sciences University of Copenhagen, Thorvaldsensvej, Denmark

7.11.1: Schistosomiasis

Vanessa Venning Consultant Dermatologist, Department of Dermatology, Churchill Hospital, Oxford, UK

23.2: Clinical approach to the diagnosis of skin disease

Anilrudh A. Venugopal Clinical Instructor, Division of Infectious Diseases, St. John Hospital and Medical Center, Detroit, Missouri, USA

7.6.10: Anaerobic bacteria

Kristien Verdonck Institute of Tropical Medicine Antwerp Nationalestraat, Antwerp, Belgium; Instituto de Medicina Tropical Alexander von Humboldt Universidad Peruana Cayetano Heredia Av. Honorio Delgado, San Martín de Porres Lima, Peru

7.5.25: HTLV-1, HTLV-2, and associated diseases

C.M. Verity Consultant Paediatric Neurologist, Child Development Centre, Addenbrooke's Hospital, Cambridge, UK

24.18: Developmental abnormalities of the central nervous system

Angela Vincent Consultant in Immunology, John Radcliffe Hospital, Oxford, UK

24.21: Paraneoplastic neurological syndromes; 24.22: Autoimmune limbic encephalitis and Morvan's syndrome

Raphael P. Viscidi Department of Pediatrics, Johns Hopkins University School of Medicine, Baltimore, Maryland, USA

7.5.19: Papillomaviruses and polyomaviruses

Peter D. Wagner Professor of Medicine & Bioengineering, Department of Medicine, University of California, San Diego, La Jolla, California, USA

18.1.2: Airways and alveoli

Nicholas Wald Professor of Environmental and Preventive Medicine, Wolfson Institute of Preventive Medicine, St Bartholomews' and the Royal London School of Medicine and Dentistry, Queen Mary University of London, UK

3.3.2: Medical screening

J.A. Walker-Smith Professor of Paediatric Gastroenterology, University Department of Paediatric Gastroenterology, Royal Free and University College Medical School, London, UK

15.15: Congenital abnormalities of the gastrointestinal tract

Mark J. Walport Director, The Wellcome Trust, London, UK

5.1.2: The complement system

Julian R.F. Walters Consultant Gastroenterologist and Reader, Imperial College, London UK

15.3.4: Investigation of gastrointestinal function; 15.10.1: Differential diagnosis and investigation of malabsorption

Gary S. Wand Professor, Department of Medicine Johns Hopkins University School of Medicine, Baltimore, Maryland, USA

26.7.1: Alcohol and drug dependence

T.E. Warkentin Professor, Department of Pathology and Molecular Medicine and Department of Medicine, Michael G. DeGroote School of Medicine, McMaster University, Hamilton, Ontario, Canada

22.6.5: Acquired coagulation disorders

David A. Warrell Emeritus Professor of Tropical Medicine, Nuffield Department of Clinical Medicine; Honorary Fellow, St Cross College, University of Oxford, Oxford, UK

7.4: Travel and expedition medicine; 7.5.10: Rhabdoviruses: rabies and rabies-related lyssaviruses; 7.5.11: Colorado tick fever and other arthropod-borne reoviruses; 7.5.27: Orf; 7.5.28: Molluscum contagiosum; 7.6.31: Rat-bite fevers; 7.6.33: Relapsing fevers; 7.6.35: Nonvenereal endemic treponematoses: yaws, endemic syphilis (bejel), and pinta; 7.8.2: Malaria; 7.13: Pentastomiasis (porocephalosis, linguatulosis/linguatuliasis); 9.2: Injuries, envenoming, poisoning, and allergic reactions caused by animals; 24.11.2: Viral infections; 24.24.6: Primary (tropical) pyomyositis; 33.1: Acute medical presentations; 33.2: Practical procedures

M. J. Warrell Oxford Vaccine Group, University of Oxford, Centre for Clinical Vaccinology & Tropical Medicine, Churchill Hospital, Oxford, UK

7.5.10: Rhabdoviruses: rabies and rabies-related lyssaviruses; 7.5.11: Colorado tick fever and other arthropod-borne reoviruses

Paul Warwicker Consultant in Nephrology, Lister Hospital, Stevenage, UK

21.10.5: Haemolytic uraemic syndrome

John A.H. Wass Professor of Endocrinology, University of Oxford Department of Endocrinology Oxford Centre for Diabetes, Endocrinology and Metabolism, Churchill Hospital, Oxford, UK

13.2: Disorders of the anterior pituitary gland; 13.3: Disorders of the posterior pituitary gland; 13.12: Hormonal manifestations of nonendocrine disease

Lawrence Waterman Director, Sypol Limited, Aylesbury; Head of Health and Safety, Olympic Delivery Authority, London
9.4.2: Occupational safety

Laurence Watkins Consultant in Neurosurgery, The National Hospital for Neurology and Neurosurgery, London, UK
24.10.3: Traumatic injuries to the head

Chris Watson Reader in Surgery and Honorary Consultant Surgeon, University of Cambridge Department of Surgery, Addenbrooke's Hospital, Cambridge, UK
15.4.1: The acute abdomen

George Watt Associate Professor of Medicine, University of Hawaii at Manoa, John A. Burns School of Medicine, Hawaii, USA
7.6.34: Leptospirosis; 7.6.40: Scrub typhus

Richard W.E. Watts Retired Professor & Honorary Consultant Physician, Imperial College School of Medicine, Hammersmith Hospital, London, UK
12.1: The inborn errors of metabolism: general aspects; 12.4: Disorders of purine and pyrimidine metabolism

D.J. Weatherall Regius Professor of Medicine Emeritus, University of Oxford; Weatherall Institute of Molecular Medicine, Oxford, UK
22.1: Introduction; 22.5.2: Anaemia: pathophysiology, classification, and clinical features; 22.5.3: Anaemia as a challenge to world health; 22.5.5: Normochromic, normocytic anaemia; 22.5.7: Disorders of the synthesis or function of haemoglobin; 22.7: The blood in systemic disease

D.K.H. Webb Consultant Paediatric Haematologist, Great Ormond Street Hospital for Children, London, UK
22.4.7: Histiocytoses

Lisa J. Webber Consultant in Reproductive Medicine, St Mary's Hospital, London, UK
13.8.1: Ovarian disorders

Kathryn E. Webert Assistant Professor, Haematology and Thromboembolism, McMaster University, Hamilton, Ontario, Canada
22.6.3: Disorders of platelet number and function

Bee Wee Consultant and Senior Clinical Lecturer in Palliative Medicine, Oxford Radcliffe Hospitals NHS Trust, and Fellow of Harris Manchester College, University of Oxford, UK
31.1: Palliative care

Anthony P. Weetman Professor of Medicine, Department of Human Metabolism, University of Sheffield, Sheffield, UK
13.4: The thyroid gland and disorders of thyroid function; 13.5: Thyroid cancer

Robert A. Weinstein The C. Anderson Hedberg Professor of Internal Medicine, Rush Medical College, Interim Chair, Department of Medicine, John H. Stroger Jr. Hospital of Cook County, Professor, Rush University Medical Center, Chicago, Illinois, USA
7.6.4: Staphylococci

R.A. Weiss Professor of Viral Oncology, Division of Infection and Immunity, University College London, London, UK
7.5.26: Viruses and cancer

Peter F. Weller Professor of Medicine, Harvard Medical School, Professor of Immunology and Infectious Diseases, Harvard School of Public Health, Chief, Infectious Disease and Allergy and Inflammation Divisions Beth Israel Deaconess Medical Center, Boston, Massachusetts, USA
22.4.6: Eosinophilia

A.U. Wells Interstitial Lung Disease Unit, Royal Brompton Hospital, London, UK
18.11.1: Diffuse parenchymal lung disease: an introduction; 18.11.2: Idiopathic pulmonary fibrosis; 18.11.3: Bronchiolitis obliterans and cryptogenic organizing pneumonia; 18.11.4: The lung in autoimmune rheumatic disorders; 18.11.5: The lung in vasculitis

Simon Wessely Professor, King's College, London, UK
26.6.2: Psychological treatment in medical practice

Gilbert C. White Executive Vice President for Research, Director, Blood Research Institute, Richard H. and Sara E. Aster Chair for Medical Research BloodCenter of Wisconsin; Associate Dean for Research, Professor of Medicine, Pharmacology, and Biochemistry Medical College of Wisconsin, USA
22.6.1: The biology of haemostasis and thrombosis

Joseph White Luxenberg Family Professor of Public Policy, Department of Political Science, Case Western Reserve University, Cleveland, Ohio, USA
3.4.1: The cost of health care in Western countries

H.C. Whittle Visiting Professor, London School of Hygiene and Tropical Medicine, MRC Laboratories, The Gambia, West Africa
7.5.6: Measles

Anthony S. Wierzbicki Department of Metabolic Medicine/Chemical Pathology Guy's & St Thomas Hospitals London, UK
12.9: Disorders of peroxisomal metabolism in adults

David E.L. Wilcken Emeritus Professor of Medicine, University of New South Wales, Prince of Wales Hospital, Sydney, Australia
16.1.3: Clinical physiology of the normal heart

Gordon Wilcock Professor of Clinical Geratology, University of Oxford, UK
29.1: Medicine in old age

James S. Wiley Professor of Haematology, Nepean Clinical School, University of Sydney, Penrith, Australia
22.5.8: Anaemias resulting from defective maturation of red cells

R.G. Will Professor of Clinical Neurology, Department of Clinical Neurosciences, University of Edinburgh, Edinburgh, UK
24.11.5: Human prion diseases

Bryan Williams Professor of Medicine, Department of Cardiovascular Sciences, University of Leicester School of Medicine, UK
16.17.1: Essential hypertension—definition, epidemiology, and pathophysiology; 16.17.2: Diagnosis, assessment, and treatment of essential hypertension

Christopher B. Williams Honorary Physician, Wolfson Unit for Endoscopy, St Mark's Hospital for Colorectal Disorders, London, UK
15.3.1: Colonoscopy and flexible sigmoidoscopy

David J. Williams Consultant Obstetric Physician, Institute for Women's Health, University College London Hospitals, London, UK
14.1: Physiological changes of normal pregnancy; 14.2: Nutrition in pregnancy; 14.3: Medical management of normal pregnancy

Gareth Williams Professor of Medicine, School of Clinical Science, University of Bristol, UK
13.11.1: Diabetes

J. David Williams Institute of Nephrology, University of Wales College of Medicine, Cardiff, UK
21.1: Structure and functions of the kidney

Bridget Wills Hospital for Tropical Diseases, Oxford University Clinical Research Unit, Wellcome Trust Major Overseas Programme, Vietnam, Ho Chi Minh City, Vietnam
7.5.15: Dengue; 24.11.2: Viral infections

R. Wilson Consultant Radiologist, Royal Marsden Hospital, London, UK
13.8.3: Breast cancer

Fenella Wojnarowska Professor Emeritus, University of Oxford, UK
14.13: The skin in pregnancy; 23.4: Vesiculobullous disease

Roger L. Wolman Consultant in Rheumatology and Sport and Exercise Medicine, Royal National Orthopaedic Hospital, Stanmore, UK
28.1: Sports and exercise medicine

Kathryn J. Wood Transplantation Research Immunology Group, Nuffield Department of Surgery, University of Oxford, John Radcliffe Hospital, Oxford, UK
5.5: Principles of transplantation immunology

Nicholas Wood Galton Professor of Genetics, Head of Department of Molecular Neuroscience, UCL Institute of Neurology, UK
24.7.4: Ataxic disorders

H.F. Woods Division of Molecular and Genetic Medicine, University of Sheffield School of Medicine, Sheffield, UK

12.11: Disturbances of acid–base homeostasis

Jeremy Woodward Consultant Gastroenterologist, Addenbrooke's Hospital, Cambridge, UK

11.6: Artificial nutrition support

Elaine M. Worcester Professor of Medicine, University of Chicago, Section of Nephrology, Chicago, Illinois, USA

21.14: Disorders of renal calcium handling, urinary stones, and nephrocalcinosis

B.P. Wordsworth Professor of Rheumatology, Nuffield Department of Orthopaedics, Rheumatology and Musculoskeletal Sciences, Nuffield Orthopaedic Centre, Oxford, UK

20.1: Skeletal disorders—general approach and clinical conditions

Gary P. Wormser Division of Infectious Diseases, Department of Medicine, New York Medical College, Valhalla, New York, USA

7.6.32: Lyme borreliosis

V.M. Wright Professor of Paediatric Gastroenterology, University Department of Paediatric Gastroenterology, Royal Free and University College Medical School, London, UK

15.15: Congenital abnormalities of the gastrointestinal tract

F.C.W. Wu Department of Endocrinology, Manchester Royal Infirmary, Manchester, UK

13.8.2: Disorders of male reproduction

Andrew H. Wyllie Head of Department, Department of Pathology, Cambridge, UK

4.6: Apoptosis in health and disease

Muhammad M. Yaqoob Professor of Nephrology, Barts and London NHS Trust Hospitals and School of Medicine and Dentistry, UK

21.17: Urinary tract obstruction

Hasan Yazici Professor and Chief, Department of Medicine and Division of Rheumatology, Cerrahpasa Medical Faculty, University of Istanbul, Istanbul, Turkey

19.11.5: Behçet's syndrome

Lam Minh Yen Hospital of Tropical Disease, Ho Chi Minh City, Vietnam

7.6.22: Tetanus

Jenny Yiend Research Scientist, Department of Psychiatry, University of Oxford, Oxford, UK

26.5.1: Grief, stress, and post-traumatic stress disorder

Yariv Yogev Director, Division of Maternal Fetal Medicine, Helen Schneider Hospital for Women, Rabin Medical Center, Sackler Faculty of Medicine, Tel - Aviv University, Petah-Tiqva, Israel

14.10: Diabetes in pregnancy

Sebahattin Yurdakul Professor, Division of Rheumatology, Department of Medicine, Cerrahpasa Medical Faculty, University of Istanbul, Istanbul, Turkey

19.11.5: Behçet's syndrome

A. Zeman Professor of Cognitive and Behavioural Neurology, Peninsula Medical School, Exeter, UK

24.2: Mind and brain: building bridges linking neurology, psychiatry, and psychology

Clive S. Zent Consultant Hematologist, Associate Professor of Medicine, Mayo Clinic, Rochester, Minnesota, USA

22.3.5: Chronic lymphocytic leukaemia and other leukaemias of mature B and T cells

SECTION 20

Disorders of
the skeleton

Skeletal disorders—general approach and clinical conditions

R. Smith and B.P. Wordsworth

Essentials

Bone is made up of (1) cells—osteoblasts, osteoclasts, and ostoe-cytes; and (2) extracellular mineralized matrix—roughly one-third organic (90% type I collagen) and two-thirds inorganic (mainly hydroxyapatite). Bone modelling occurs during growth and remodelling throughout life due to the constant processes of osteoclastic bone resorption and osteoblastic bone formation, which are closely linked and regulated within bone multicellular units. In the adult, the replacement of old bone with new occurs at an annual turnover rate of 25% in cancellous bone, and 2 to 3% in cortical bone.

Common presentations of bone disease include (1) deformity and short stature; (2) bone pain and fracture; (3) myopathy—in osteomalacia and rickets; (4) features of underlying disease—e.g. renal failure, myeloma. A full general medical history, carefully taken family history, and thorough physical examination—with particular emphasis on the musculoskeletal system—may be crucial in making the correct diagnosis. Many generalized disorders of the skeleton have entirely normal routine biochemical values, while in others changes are diagnostic. Radiographic imaging can be diagnostic in some cases, with MRI and CT imaging increasingly employed in addition to conventional ('plain') radiographs and bisphosphonate-labelled isotope scans. Bone biopsy is required for diagnosis in some circumstances.

An enormous variety of conditions can have skeletal manifestations: this chapter emphasizes those in which impact on the skeleton is a substantial feature.

Classic metabolic bone diseases

Osteomalacia and rickets—most frequently result from a lack of vitamin D or a disturbance of its metabolism, with the main histological feature of osteomalacia being defective mineralization of bone matrix. Causes are (1) nutritional—e.g. low dietary intake; (2) malabsorptive—e.g. coeliac disease; (3) renal—including renal tubular disorders, e.g. inherited hypophosphataemias, and chronic kidney disease; (4) miscellaneous—e.g. anticonvulsant drugs. Dominant symptoms are bone pain and tenderness, skeletal deformity, and proximal muscle weakness, often accompanied by the features of the underlying disorder and by those of hypocalcaemia. Biochemical changes depend on the cause, but in vitamin D deficiency or malabsorption there are low plasma calcium and phosphate, low urinary calcium excretion, and an increase in plasma alkaline phosphatase; a low plasma 25(OH)D level is a good indication of vitamin D deficiency. The radiological hallmark of active osteomalacia is the Looser's zone, a ribbon-like area of defective mineralization that is most often seen in the long bones, pelvis, ribs, and around the scapulae. Where there is doubt about the diagnosis, a bone biopsy examined before and after decalcification will demonstrate failure of mineralization and wide osteoid seams. Rickets and osteomalacia should respond rapidly to vitamin D (or one of its metabolites) in appropriate doses, and the response may be a useful way of confirming the diagnosis.

Paget's disease of bone—a common disorder (3–4% of people >40 years of age), characterized by excessive and disorganized resorption and formation of bone. Predominantly of genetic cause, with the most frequent mutation being in the gene coding for the ubiquitin-binding protein sequestosome. The condition is often asymptomatic, but symptoms of Paget's include pain, deformity, fracture, deafness and nerve compression; bone sarcoma arises in 1% or less of symptomatic patients. There is a marked increase in the level of plasma alkaline phosphatase, and the most characteristic radiological appearance is an increase in size of the affected bone. Many patients do not require any treatment. Bone pain should initially be treated with simple analgesics. If these are ineffective, or there are pagetic complications, treatment with a bisphosphonate is indicated, which can induce almost complete and permanent suppression of disease without significant side effects.

Parathyroid bone disease—hyperparathyroidism—see Chapters 13.6 and 21.6; hypoparathyroidism—see Chapter 13.6.

Osteoporosis—see Chapter 20.4.

Synthetic defects in the major components of the organic bone matrix and connective tissue

Osteogenesis imperfecta—involves those tissues that contain the main fibrillar collagen, type I. Manifest as a spectrum of disease, including (1) type II—the most severe; commonly arises from single base changes in COL1A1 or COL1A2 genes; nearly always lethal; to

(2) type III—causes severe and progressive disability; patients rarely walk and have very short stature; sclerae may be blue in infancy but may take on a normal colour in childhood; to (3) type I—the commonest and least serious form; appears to be caused by a null allele for collagen I, so that only 50% of collagen is produced, but this is of normal composition; fractures sometimes occur in the perinatal period but may be delayed until the menopause; other features can include hypermobility and dislocation of joints, dentinogenesis imperfecta, and cardiac valve disease (e.g. aortic incompetence); blueness of the sclerae is characteristic. In the first few years of life nonaccidental injury, 'battered baby syndrome', is the main differential diagnosis. Cyclic intravenous pamidronate may alleviate symptoms, increase bone density and reduce fracture rate in severe disease.

Skeletal dysplasias—a term used to cover a wide range of generalized disorders of the skeleton affecting both cartilage and bone. Can be classified into families on the basis of (1) clinical features—e.g. bodily proportions—achondroplasia is the prototype of the short-limbed, short-stature phenotype; spondyloepiphyseal dysplasias have prominent spinal involvement and short stature is partly due to shortness of the trunk; or (2) biochemical features/genetic analysis.

Inherited defects of connective tissue—see Chapter 20.2.

Skeletal disorders caused by enzyme defects

Homocystinuria—caused by cystathionine β-synthase deficiency; ocular, skeletal, central nervous, and vascular manifestations; skeletal features similar to Marfan's syndrome and include long, thin body habitus, pectus excavatum, scoliosis, and genu valgum. See Chapter 12.2.

Alkaptonuria—caused by decreased activity of homogentisate 1,2-dioxygenase; should be suspected when there is premature disc degeneration and/or early degenerative arthritis; characteristic features include abnormal dark pigmentation of the cartilage of the ear and nose, the sclerae, and of the urine. See Chapter 12.2.

Hypophosphatasia—caused by reduction in tissue nonspecific alkaline phosphatase; varies from a lethal perinatal disorder to an asymptomatic disease in adults, but adults may present with progressive stiffness, pain in the bones, and apparent 'stress' fractures.

Lysosomal storage diseases—a large group of conditions due to various inborn errors that affect the function of specific lysosomal enzymes normally responsible for the breakdown of a variety of complex molecules. Can cause a wide range of musculoskeletal problems, including some with devastating consequences, e.g. odontoid hypoplasia can lead to atlantoaxial instability, compression of the long spinal tracts, and paraplegia in Morquio's syndrome. See Chapter 12.8.

Intrinsic disorders of bone cells

Osteopetrosis ('marble bone disease')—a group of disorders with a range of severity that best known cause is of increased bone density. (1) Severe osteopetrosis—widespread increased density of the bones without modelling or remodelling, producing Erlenmeyer-flask deformity of the metaphyses; other features include leucoerythroblastic anaemia and hepatosplenomegaly, nerve compression, blindness, and deafness. (2) Mild osteopetrosis—affected individuals may be asymptomatic or affected by increased number of fractures affecting both the long bones and the small bones of the hands and feet. (3) Carbonic anhydrase II deficiency—features include mental retardation, growth failure, dental malocclusion, osteopetrosis, renal tubular acidosis, and cerebral calcification.

Fibrous dysplasia—a postzygotic activating mutation in GNAS1, the gene for the α subunit of the G-protein signalling system, leads to areas of immature fibrous tissue, either single or multiple, within the skeleton. Radiology reveals a smooth-walled translucent area within the bone, often with thinning of the cortex and sometimes with associated deformity. (1) Monostotic fibrous dysplasia—lesions may occur in any bone; the most frequent presenting symptom is bone pain; fracture may occur. (2) Polyostotic fibrous dysplasia—multiple bone lesions; frequently associated with pigmentation and sexual precocity, especially in females (McCune–Albright syndrome).

Ectopic ossification—this may be acquired at the site of injury, or in tumours and in a variety of other disorders. Inherited ectopic ossification is a major and disabling feature of two conditions: fibrodysplasia ossificans progressiva and progressive osseous heteroplasia.

Physiology of bone

The past decade has seen fundamental advances in our understanding of bone cell biology and in the noncollagen as well as the collagen components of the organic matrix of bone and the associated soft tissues. This is reflected in major discoveries in bone diseases such as osteoporosis, osteopetrosis, osteogenesis imperfecta, and Paget's disease. Outstanding discoveries in bone physiology include the identification and elucidation of the functions of the parathyroid-hormone-related protein (PRrP) and the bone morphogenetic proteins (BMP). The causes of many rare skeletal disorders have also now been discovered (Table 20.1.1). Examples are Marfan's syndrome (mutations in fibrillin), vitamin D dependent rickets type II (mutations in the 1,25-dihydroxycholecalciferol receptor), pseudohypoparathyroidism and fibrous dysplasia (abnormalities in the G-protein signalling system), osteogenesis

imperfecta (mutations in collagen type I), chondrodysplasias (some with similar mutations in collagen type II), the osteopetroses with mutations in the osteoclast acidification pathway, and fibrodysplasia ossificans progressiva (due to activating mutations in the BMP receptor, activin). The identification of the calcium-sensing receptor in the parathyroid and other tissues explains many rare disorders of mineral metabolism. Important new bone cell signalling systems continue to be identified, particularly that involving Wnt, an important controller of bone mass, and low density lipoprotein receptor-related protein 5 (LRP5). Further advances have been made in our understanding of the development of the osteoblast from stromal cell precursors and the ways in which the osteoblast controls osteoclast development and function (see below).

The mammalian skeleton serves two main functions, the demands of which sometimes conflict. The first is to provide a rigid structure; the second is to act as an accessible mineral store.

Table 20.1.1 Molecular basis of some metabolic disorders of bone and related tissues

Disorder	Affected gene protein
Familial high bone density	LRP5/lipoprotein receptor related protein 5
X-linked hypophosphataemia	PHEX
Autosomal dominant hypophosphataemic osteomalacia	FGF23/fibroblast growth factor 23
X-linked nephrolithiasis (Dent's disease)	CLCN5/chloride channel 5
Vitamin D dependent rickets type I	25OHD 1α-hydroxylase
Vitamin D dependent rickets type II	1,25(OH)$_2$D receptor
Oncogenic rickets (OM)	FGF23
Paget's disease	SQSTM1/sequestosome
Familial expansile osteolysis	RANK/TNFRSF11A
Expansile skeletal hyperphosphatasia	RANK/TNFRSF11A
Juvenile Paget's disease	OPG/TNFRSF11B
Multiple endocrine neoplasia type I	MEN1
Multiple endocrine neoplasia type II	RET
Familial hypocalciuric hypocalcaemia	CASR/calcium sensing receptor
Neonatal hyperparathyroidism	CASR
Pseudohypoparathyroidism	GNAS1
Jansen's metaphyseal dysplasia	PTH/PTHrP receptor
Blomstrand's chondrodysplasia	PTH/PTHrP receptor
Osteogenesis imperfecta	COL1A1, COL1A2
Osteoporosis pseudoglioma	LRP5
Marfan's syndrome	FBN1/fibrillin 1
Congenital contractural arachnodactyly	FBN2/fibrillin 2
Loeys–Dietz syndrome	TGFBR1/2
Ehlers–Danlos syndrome (EDS)	
EDS type I	COL5A1
EDS type IV	COL3A1
EDS type VI	PLOD1/lysyl hydroxylase
EDS type VIIA and B	COL1A1, COL1A2
Other	Tenascin XB
Homocystinuria	Cystathionine β-synthase
Hypophosphatasia	TNAP/alkaline phosphatase
Alkaptonuria	HGD/homogentisate 1,2-dioxygenase
Menkes' syndrome	ATP7A/copper transporting ATPase
Gaucher's disease	β glucosidase
Mucopolysaccharidoses	Multiple lysosomal enzymes
Achondroplasia	FGFR3/fibroblast growth factor receptor 3
Thanatophoric dysplasia	FGFR3
Hypochondroplasia	FGFR3
Spondyloepiphyseal dysplasia (SED)	COL2A1
Spondyloepiphyseal dysplasia tarda, (X-linked)	SEDLIN

Table 20.1.1 (*Cont'd*) Molecular basis of some metabolic disorders of bone and related tissues

Disorder	Affected gene protein
Stickler's syndrome	COL2A1, COL11A1
Kniest's dysplasia	COL2A1
Achondrogenesis	COL2A1
Multiple epiphyseal dysplasia	COL9A1, 2, 3, COMP, SLC26A2 (DTDST), MATN3 (matrilin 3)
Pseudoachondroplasia	COMP/cartilage oligomeric matrix protein
Metaphyseal chondrodysplasia (type Schmid)	COL10A1
Diastrophic dysplasia	SLC26A2 (DTDST)
Campomelic dysplasia	SOX 9
Apert's syndrome	FGFR2
Osteopetrosis (marble bone disease)	TC1RG1, CLCN7, CA2
Pycnodysostosis	CTSK/cathepsin K
Camurati–Engelmann disease	TGFB1
Sclerosteosis	SOST/sclerostin
Fibrous dysplasia	GNAS1 G$_s$ α-protein subunit
Familial hyperphosphataemic tumoral calcinosis	FGF23, GALNT3
Fibrodysplasia ossificans progressiva	ACVR1/activin receptor 1
Familial chondrocalcinosis	ANKH
Progressive osseous heteroplasia	GNAS1

Modified from Smith R, Wordsworth P (2006). *Clinical and biochemical disorders of the skeleton.* Oxford University Press, Oxford.

Both depend on the activities of specialized bone cells, which are controlled by genetic, mechanical, nutritional, and hormonal influences and by a host of short-acting messengers produced by cells, collectively known as cytokines.

Structure

Bone tissue consists of cells and an extracellular mineralized matrix (35% organic and 65% inorganic). Some 90% of the organic component is collagen type I. The remainder includes many noncollagen products of the osteoblast, such as osteocalcin, osteonectin, and proteoglycans. The mineral is present mainly as a complex mixture of calcium and phosphate in the form of hydroxyapatite.

Two anatomical types of bone may be defined: trabecular (cancellous) and cortical. The proportion of these differs from one bone to another; e.g. vertebral bodies are predominantly trabecular and the shafts of the long bones are cortical. Such variation is related both to the functions of the bones and to the development of disorders of them, such as osteoporosis. Trabecular bone contains more metabolically active surfaces in a given volume than cortical bone. Cellular activities take place on the surfaces of trabecular bone and through resorbing channels (cutting cones) in cortical bone. The fine structure of bone is dealt with in anatomical texts.

Bone is often assumed to be inert because of its structural rigidity and persistence after death, and to be composed entirely of mineral because it contains 99% of the calcium in the body. These assumptions are superficially reasonable but neither is correct.

Bone cells

Conventional histological sections of bone demonstrate three types of bone cell which are clearly different (Fig. 20.1.1): (1) osteoblasts, which may be plump and apparently active, or flat and apparently inactive—otherwise called bone-lining cells; (2) multinucleate osteoclasts, which most often occupy areas of resorption; and (3) osteocytes within lacunae in the mineralized bone, apparently in contact with other osteocytes and bone cells through their extensions in the canaliculi. All these cells are in close contact with the bone marrow, which contains their precursors and brings them into close relationship with the immune system.

Bone cells are at the centre of an information system of astonishing complexity and it is this complexity of bone that provides both the challenge and the fascination for those interested in its disorders. Histological techniques have been developed to study sequential cellular events in bone tissue and the techniques of cell biology are used to study the origin and functions of different types of cells and the communications between them. All bone cells communicate with each other to control bone modelling during growth and remodelling throughout life. The constant processes of osteoclastic bone resorption and osteoblastic bone formation that achieve this are closely linked and take place in bone multicellular units. The cellular cycle of such units begins with the activation of multinucleate osteoclasts from their macrophage-like mononuclear cell precursors; these produce resorption (Howship's) lacunae on the surface of trabecular bone or cutting cones in cortical bone. These are identical processes; in cancellous (trabecular) bone, the bone multicellular unit may be looked upon as a sagittal section of a cortical bone multicellular unit. Resorption is followed by a reversal phase, during which a cement line is deposited, and new bone matrix is formed by osteoblasts, which is subsequently mineralized. In the young adult, when the bone mass is constant and there may be several million resorbing sites in the skeleton at any one time, the amount of newly formed bone equals that resorbed.

In childhood, more bone is formed than is resorbed and in later years there is an imbalance between the two processes favouring resorption which eventually leads to osteoporosis.

Estimates of the time scale of the remodelling cycle are only approximate. In the adult, the replacement of old bone with new occurs at an annual turnover rate of 25% in cancellous bone and from 2% to 3% in cortical bone. In the bone multicellular unit, resorption takes from 1 to 2 weeks and new bone formation about 7 weeks. A complete cycle, including reversal and mineralization, takes several months. The turnover of bone at a given site is determined by the frequency with which bone multicellular units are activated and the rates of function of individual cells. Bone loss and gain depend on both factors and the mechanism of bone loss is different in different disorders. Although the existence of the bone multicellular unit system is widely accepted, it is far from understood: e.g. what factors lead to activation of the osteoclasts to initiate the resorbing cycle; how do cells talk to each other; and what links osteoblast and osteoclast activity?

It is clear that osteoblasts occupy a central position in bone physiology (Fig. 20.1.2a). They are derived from the mesenchymal–stromal cell system within the bone marrow. This system is multipotential and the stromal cells can give rise to osteoblasts, fibroblasts, chondrocytes, myocytes, and adipocytes. Under the influence of the differentiation factor identified as RUNX2 (runt-related transcription factor 2, also known as CBFA1), osterix (transcription factor Sp7) and LRP5, stromal cells develop into osteoblasts. Osteoblasts respond to humoral factors, both systemic and local (cytokines), and to mechanical stress. They synthesize the organic bone matrix (mainly collagen) and noncollagen proteins and they control bone mineralization. Importantly, they also appear to direct the activity of other cell types, particularly the osteoclasts. In this respect they may also activate the bone-resorbing cycle. One of the main factors that controls osteoclast differentiation has been identified as RANKL, the ligand for the receptor activator of

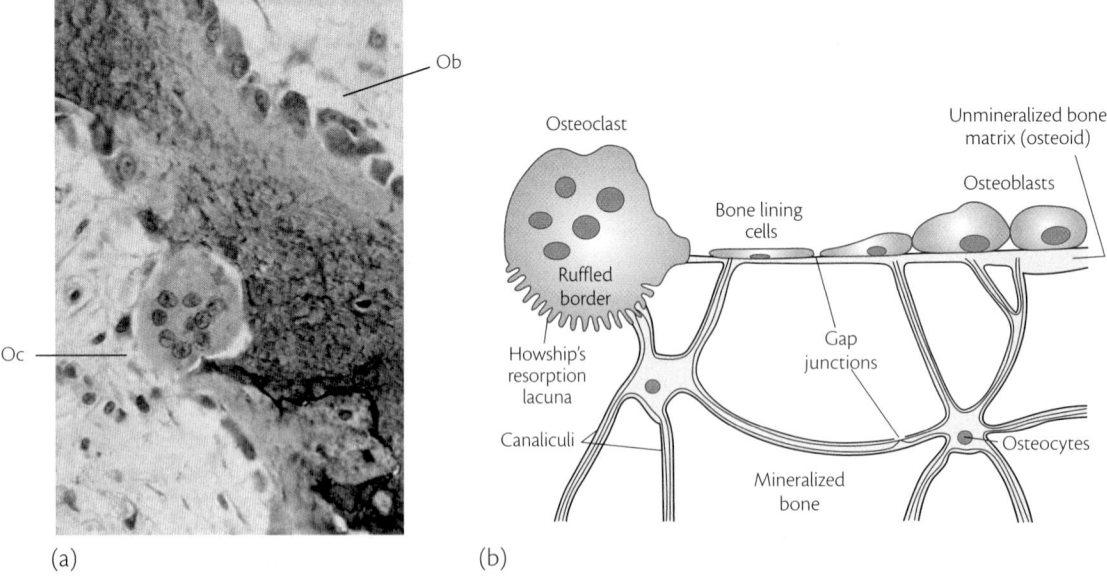

(a)   (b)

Fig. 20.1.1 Bone cells (a) The histological appearance: a multinucleated osteoclast (centre, arrow) is present on a Howship's resorption lacuna along one surface of a bone trabecula; a row of plump osteoblasts lie on the opposite surface (right, arrows) (haematoxylin and eosin, magnification ×400); and (b) a diagram to show the main connections of the osteocyte. Ob, osteoblast; Oc, osteoclast.
(From Smith and Wordsworth 2005, Clinical & Biochemical Disorders of the Skeleton. Oxford University Press with permission.)

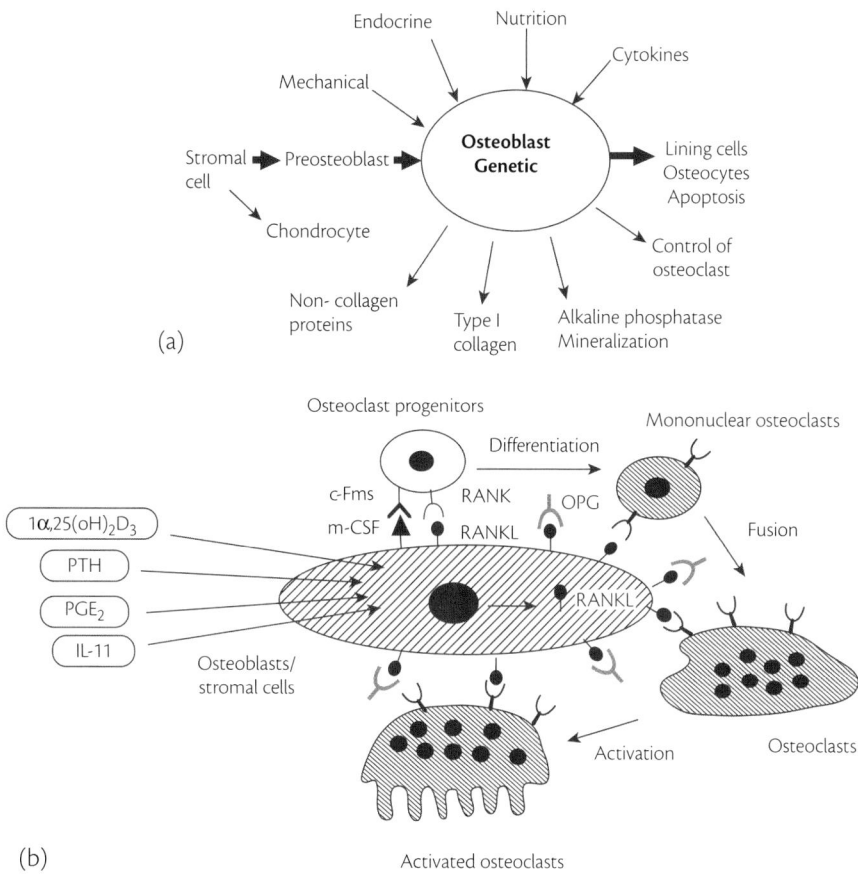

Fig. 20.1.2 The osteoblast (a) The central position of the osteoblast in bone physiology. Broad arrows show the origin of the osteoblasts from preosteoblasts, themselves derived from stromal cells, and of the lining cells and osteocytes. Endocrine influences include calciotropic hormones, oestrogen, and cortisol. Cytokines and hormones all act through specific receptors. The way in which mechanical forces and nutrition affect the osteoblast is not well defined. Most cytokines influence the activity of the osteoclast via the osteoblasts. Others bypass the osteoblasts and have a direct effect on osteoclasts. (b) The close interactions between the osteoblast and the origin and function of the osteoclast. Together, macrophage colony-stimulating factor (M-CSF) and RANKL act throughout osteoclast differentiation. Osteoprotegerin strongly inhibits all the effects of RANKL. Note that 1,25(OH)$_2$D, parathyroid hormone, PGE2 (prostaglandin E$_2$), and IL-11 (part of the IL-6 family) are shown to act via the osteoblasts, but there is evidence of direct cytokine effects on the osteoclasts.
(From Smith R, Wordsworth P (2006). *Clinical and biochemical disorders of the skeleton.* Oxford University Press, Oxford, with permission.)
(From Takahashi *et al.* 2002, Principles of Bone Biology, Academic Press, San Diego, with permission from Elsevier.)

NF-κB (RANK), found on the surface of osteoclast precursors. RANKL, also variously known as osteoclast differentiation factor (ODF), osteoprotegerin ligand (OPGL), tumour necrosis factor (TNF) related activation-induced cytokine (TRANCE), and TNF ligand superfamily member 11 (TNFSF11) is a soluble factor produced by osteoblasts, which plays an important role in controlling the formation and activation of osteoclasts through its effect on the osteoclast receptor RANK (Fig. 20.1.2b). It is possible that these many functions are divided between different osteoblasts. The bone-lining cells—resting osteoblasts—may not be as inactive as they appear since they may provide a cellular barrier separating the so-called bone fluid from the general extracellular compartment. The existence of a separate bone fluid has yet to be established.

Osteocytes, also derived from osteoblasts, occupy lacunae within the mineralized bone and communicate with each other through gap junctions via their processes within the canaliculi. They probably have an important function in the detection of mechanical forces and the resultant response of bone to them.

Osteoclasts have a different origin from osteoblasts since the former are multinucleated cells derived from the haemopoietic system. The osteoclasts resorb bone after attaching themselves to its

surface via integrins (vitronectin receptor) and forming a seal to isolate their area of activity (Fig. 20.1.3). Within this sealed zone they produce a very acid environment, with the aid of an osteoclast-specific proton pump linked to the enzyme carbonic anhydrase II, to enable digestion of whole bone by lysosomal enzymes, including cathepsin K. The absence of carbonic anhydrase II is linked to a rare form of osteopetrosis (see below). Other inherited defects of the acidification machinery lead to different forms of osteopetrosis. Osteoclasts have receptors to calcitonin that, when occupied, directly suppress their activity; the existence of any other hormone receptors is controversial. However, they are activated by prostaglandins. The osteoclastic resorptive effects of parathyroid hormone and of 1,25-dihydroxycholecalciferol are probably mediated through the osteoblast.

Bone formation

The factors that control bone formation are complex and not fully understood, but they must act largely through the osteoblast. The stromal precursors of osteoblasts are found in the periosteum and the endosteal surfaces close to the bone marrow. The local remodelling stimulus for new bone formation appears to come from

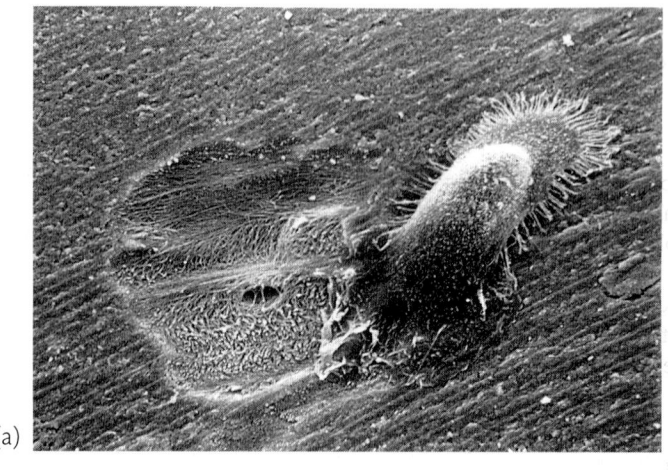

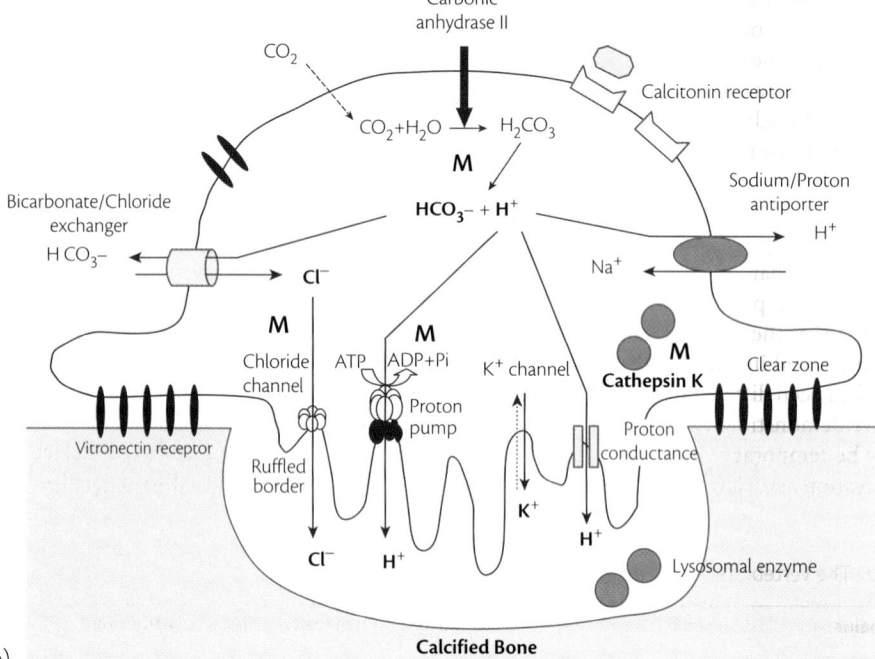

Fig. 20.1.3 The osteoclast (a) The appearance of damaged bone under the scanning electron microscope: the osteoclast has removed part of the mineralized surface and is presumed to be moving on to digest further bone; and (b) the cellular events and ion exchanges that occur within it. M, positions of gene mutations described in human osteopetrosis for carbonic anhydrase II (CA II), vacuolar ATP' (ATPase), chloride channels (Cl⁻), and cathepsin K (cysteine proteinase). (Adapted from Rouselle A-V, Heymann D (2002). Osteoclastic acidification pathways during bone resorption. *Bone*, **30**, 533–40, with permission).

some product or products of bone resorption, which could, for instance, be a group of polypeptide growth factors or BMPs liberated from resorbed bone. Such substances are included in the category of cytokines. A cytokine may be defined as a peptide produced by a cell which acts as an autocrine, paracrine or endocrine mediator. This definition includes a large number of substances with effects on the metabolism of bone and cartilage. Such effects have largely been demonstrated in experimental (and artificial) situations and their physiological role is unknown. Many cytokines have alternative names and multiple actions, featuring both synergism and antagonism. They include interleukins (IL-1 and IL-6), TNF, γ-interferon, platelet-derived growth factor, fibroblast growth factors (FGFs), insulin-like growth factors, transforming growth factor-β (TGFβ), and BMPs.

Since bone cells contain, synthesize, and respond to many cytokines, they are part of a complex network. As an example, TGFβ appears to comprise a family of multifunctional regulatory peptides and bone is probably their most abundant source. Not only do osteoblasts synthesize TGFβ, but they also have high-affinity receptors for it and are mitogenically stimulated by it. Strikingly, most of the BMPs belong to the TGFβ superfamily.

Bone resorption

Osteoclasts are controlled by systemic and local factors but there is no direct evidence that they are influenced by mechanical stress. Calcitonin directly inhibits the osteoclast, temporarily abolishes the active ruffled border, and suppresses the generation of new osteoclasts. Bone resorption is increased by parathyroid hormone and 1,25-dihydroxycholecalciferol. Since the osteoclast contains no receptors for either of these hormones it is proposed that their resorbing effect is mediated via the osteoblast. It is now realized that the balance between osteoprotegerin and RANKL is central to osteoblast–osteoclast interaction. The number and activity of the osteoclasts are also increased by a variety of cytokines produced by lymphocytes and monocytes (lymphokines and monokines, respectively) and by peptide growth factors such as epidermal growth factor. In myeloma, the malignant plasma cells release IL-1, IL-6, and TNF, all of which stimulate osteoclastic destruction of bone.

Bone mass (see also osteoporosis)

The development of the skeleton and its eventual size and density are influenced by important genetic factors modified by mechanical stress, nutrition, the systemic effects of endocrine hormones, and local factors produced by the bone cells themselves. These determine the balance between resorption and formation and their relative contribution varies with age.

Recent research emphasizes the importance of the genetic contribution to bone mass. Apart from the obvious differences in bone mass between races, the heritability of bone mass is demonstrated by the relative similarities between monozygotic twins compared to dizygotic twins. Clearly, mutations in the structural collagen type I genes will have a considerable effect on bone mass, as in osteogenesis imperfecta (see below). The contribution of vitamin D receptor gene polymorphisms and genetic changes in the promoter region of the collagen type I gene has been widely discussed (see osteoporosis). Since mutations in the gene for LRP5 can cause both low and high bone density, this protein—which is involved in Wnt signalling—is clearly important in the control of bone mass. Recent population studies suggest that LRP5 is also involved in the determination of bone mass in the normal population.

The main function of the skeleton is mechanical and bone is laid down along its lines of stress. Although the way in which this occurs is obscure, early in vitro experiments showed that osteoblasts may respond to mechanical stress by an increase in levels of cAMP and phosphoinositol, partly mediated by prostaglandins. It is also common sense that the size and density of the skeleton should be related to nutritional intake, particularly of calcium, protein, and energy. This has been difficult to prove, but twin studies in growing children have demonstrated a significantly greater density of bone (which may be temporary) in those taking calcium supplements, and the starvation associated with anorexia nervosa reduces bone mineral content. This may also be due to oestrogen deficiency and emphasizes the important effect of reproductive hormones on the skeleton. The sex hormones testosterone and oestrogen encourage new bone formation. Oestrogen-deficient men have osteoporosis, and the skeleton depends on a full complement of sex steroids for its integrity. Growth hormone is an important anabolic skeletal agent during the early years of life, partly through the local production of somatomedins (insulin-like growth factors). Several hormones that influence bone resorption may also have anabolic actions mediated by osteoblasts. One is parathyroid hormone, which under certain circumstances increases the proliferation of osteoblast precursors. This is relevant to the treatment of osteoporosis.

Collagen

Collagen is the principal extracellular protein in the body, more than half of which is contained within the skeleton, and is the main product of the osteoblast. There are many different molecular types, with different functions, each encoded by distinct genes (Table 20.1.2). Collagen in bone is type I. This heterotrimer is composed of two α-1(I) chains and one α-2(I) chain. The general structure of the α-1(I) chain is $(Gly–X–Y)_{338}$, where X and Y are often proline or hydroxyproline. The α-chains are synthesized as precursors within the osteoblasts and undergo a number of synthetic steps, including posttranslational hydroxylation of proline and lysine residues; certain hydroxylysine residues are further modified into aldehydes and are also glycosylated (Fig. 20.1.4).

After removal of their extensions, the triple-helical molecules form an exact structure with a quarter-stagger overlap that is subsequently crosslinked. The so-called 'hole zones' within this structure provide a template for early mineralization. Mutations in the collagen genes and defects in posttranslational modification cause inherited disorders of connective tissue, of which osteogenesis

Table 20.1.2 The vertebrate collagens

Type	α-chains	Most common molecular form	Tissue distribution
I	α-1(I), α-2(I)	$[\alpha$-1(I)$]_2\,\alpha$-2(I)	Most connective tissues, e.g. bone, tendon, skin, lung, cornea, sclera, vascular system
II	α-1(II)	$[\alpha$-1(II)$]3$	Cartilage, vitreous humour, embryonic cornea
III	α-1(III)	$[\alpha$-1(III)$]3$	Extensible connective tissues, e.g. lung, vascular system
IV	α-1(IV), α-2(IV), α-3(IV), α-4(IV), α-5(IV)	$[\alpha$-1(IV)$]_2\,\alpha$-2(IV)	Basement membranes
V	α-1(V), α-2(V), α-3(V)	$[\alpha$-1(V)$]_2\,\alpha$-2(V)	Tissues containing collagen type I, quantitatively minor component
VI	α-1(VI), α-2(VI), α-3(VI)	α-1(VI) α-2(VI) α-3(VI)	Most connective tissues, including cartilage
VII	α-1(VII)	$[\alpha$-1(VII)$]_3$	Basement-membrane-associated anchoring fibrils
VIII	α-1(VIII), α-2(VIII)	$[\alpha$-1(VIII)$]_2\,\alpha$-2(VII)?	Product of endothelial and various tumour cell lines
IX	α-1(IX), α-2(IX), α-3(IX)	α-1(IX) α-2(IX) α-3(IX)	Tissues containing collagen type II, quantitatively minor component
X	α-1(X)	$[\alpha$-1(X)$]_3$	Hypertrophic zone of cartilage
XI	α-1(XI), α-2(XI), α-3(XI)a	α-1(XI) α-2(XI) α-3(XI)	Tissues containing collagen type III, quantitatively minor component
XII	α-1(XII)	$[\alpha$-1(XII)$]_3$	Tissues containing collagen type I, quantitatively minor component
XIII	α-1(XIII)	$[\alpha$-1(XIII)$]_3$?	Quantitatively minor collagen, found, e.g. in skin, intestine
XiV	α-1(XIV)	$[\alpha$-1(XIV)$]_3$?	Tissues containing collagen type I, quantitatively minor component

[a] Closely related to α-1(II).

From Smith R (1998). Bone in health and disease. In: Maddison PJ, et al. (eds) Oxford textbook of rheumatology, 2nd edition, pp. 421–40. Oxford University Press, Oxford.

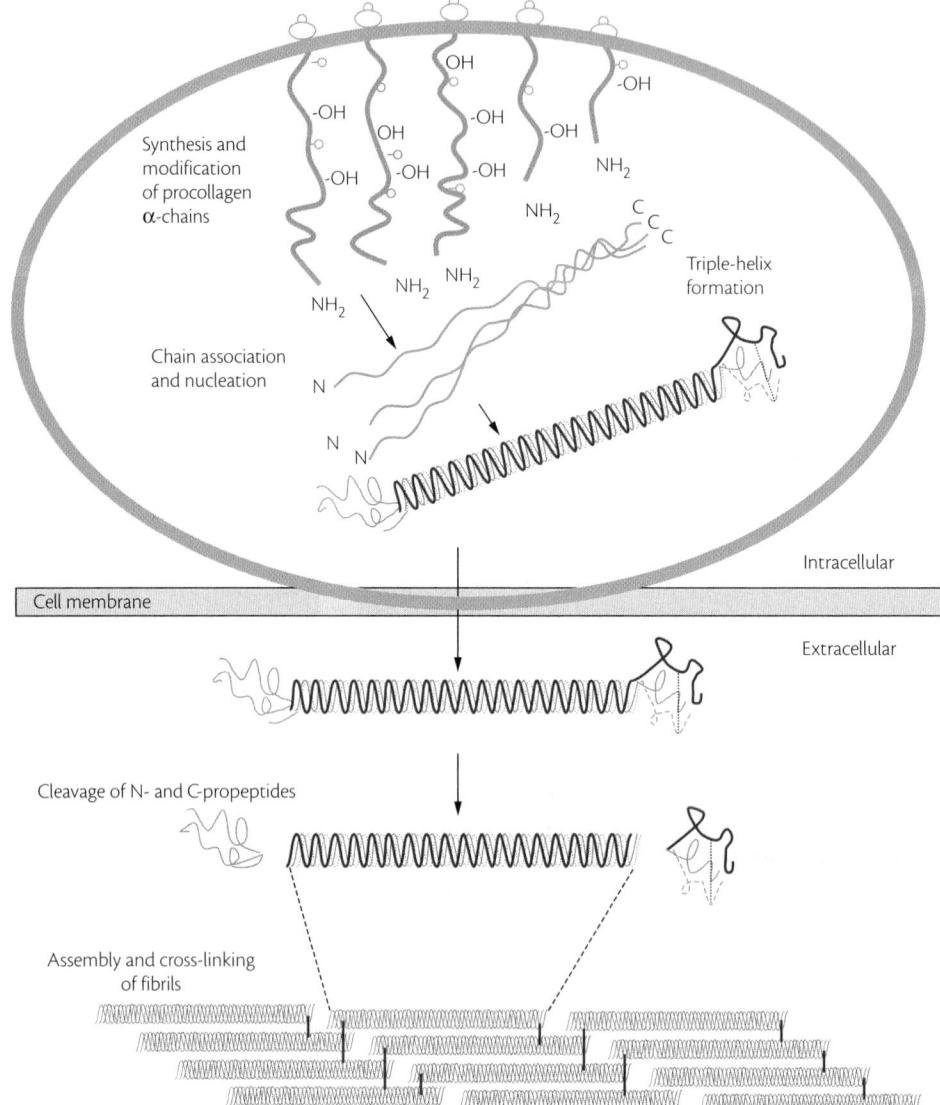

Fig. 20.1.4 Collagen: the synthetic pathways. The individual polypeptide chains are synthesized on the ribosomes of the rough endoplasmic reticulum. They undergo complex enzymic modifications before chain association and triple helix formation. The newly formed procollagen molecules are secreted into the extracellular space and proteinases remove the N- and C-propeptides. In the fibril, collagen molecules overlap (in a quarter-staggered array) and form specific covalent cross-links. (From Kielty and Grant, 2002. Connective Tissue and its Heritable Disorders, New York: Wiley Liss, pp. 159–221, with permission).

imperfecta (collagen type I) and the vascular form (type IV) of Ehlers–Danlos syndrome (collagen type III) are examples (Table 20.1.1). The fibrillar collagens are quantitatively the most important, but many other minor collagens exist, playing important roles in regulating fibre diameter and interactions with other matrix proteins. Renal excretion of hydroxyproline peptides is an indicator of bone collagen turnover. Excretion of pyridinium compounds is a measure of bone resorption (see below).

Noncollagen proteins

Many such proteins may be extracted from bone, although their abundance differs according to the starting material and the methods used. They include osteocalcin (bone Gla protein, see below), sialoproteins, various phosphoproteins, such as osteonectin and osteopontin, the bone morphogenetic proteins, and bone-specific proteoglycans.

The nature of noncollagen substances sequestered in bone matrix is complex and most are synthesized by the osteoblasts. Few, if any, are unique to bone, since they can be expressed transiently in other tissues. To date, no unambiguous function has been determined for any of these proteins. Osteonectin is the major noncollagen protein produced by human osteoblasts. It binds strongly to calcium ions, hydroxyapatite, and native collagen, but it is not limited to mineralizing tissue, being also found in human platelets. Although osteonectin mRNA is widely distributed in developing tissues, osteonectin is most abundant in bone. Two bone sialoproteins, BSP1 and BSP2, are now recognized. Their relative amounts vary with the species studied: e.g. BSP1 is a minor component of human bone but a major contributor to total sialoprotein in rat bone. The protein contains an RGD (Arg–Gly–Asp) cell-attachment motif and is therefore called osteopontin. The major human sialoprotein is BSP2.

There are two Gla-containing proteins in bone: osteocalcin (bone Gla protein; BGP) (osteocalcin) and matrix Gla protein. The term Gla refers to the γ-carboxylated glutamic acid residues, formed by the vitamin K-modulated, posttranslational carboxylation of peptide-bound glutamic acid. These proteins have some sequence homology but are products of different genes. Matrix Gla protein is also a cartilage protein and is found at an earlier developmental stage than osteocalcin. The function of osteocalcin is unknown. Osteocalcin biosynthesis is regulated by 1,25-dihydroxycholecalciferol (1,25(OH)$_2$D) (and no other hormone), which enhances its nuclear transcription and eventual secretion from bone cells. Plasma osteocalcin has been linked to the rate of bone formation or, less specifically, bone turnover.

Proteoglycans are proteins with one or more attached glycosaminoglycan chains. They vary widely in form and function. Those of bone, which include decorin and biglycan, have been studied less extensively than those of cartilage and differ in their small overall size and relatively larger amounts of protein. Such small proteoglycans are thought to interact with growing collagen fibrils in a precise manner and to regulate their growth, maturation, and interactions. Collagen type IX, one of a family of fibril associated collagens with interrupted triple helices (FACIT), is found on the surface of collagen type II fibrils in cartilage. It facilitates interactions between the collagen and proteoglycans in the cartilage matrix through the chondroitin sulphate glycosaminoglycan chain on the α-2(IX) chain.

It has been known for many years that demineralized bone matrix contains substances capable of inducing ectopic bone formation. Because they are present in such small amounts, their extraction and isolation have presented great difficulties, but these bone morphogenetic proteins have now been isolated and their corresponding genes cloned.

Bone mineral and mineralization

Mineralization occurs on bone matrix collagen. The way in which it occurs has been long debated, but there is now good evidence that, in most mineralized tissues, calcifying vesicles derived from chondrocytes or osteoblasts provide a focus for mineralization. These vesicles are easily demonstrable in cartilage, but their function in the organized matrix of bone is controversial. The precipitation of calcium within these vesicles may be controlled by the action of a pyrophosphatase that locally destroys pyrophosphate, itself an inhibitor of mineralization. Alkaline phosphatase is the most important pyrophosphatase and is readily demonstrable both

in osteoblasts and in mineralizing vesicles. Its deficiency in hypophosphatasia causes defective mineralization. It is possible, for the purpose of clarity, to consider two types of mineralization: (1) homogeneous nucleation from amorphous calcium phosphate to form crystalline hydroxyapatite, which occurs in the lumen of the matrix vesicles; and (2) heterogeneous nucleation, which is collagen-mediated and may partly rely on adsorbed noncollagen proteins as nucleators. After this first phase (mediated either by vesicles or collagen), there is a second phase of rapid spread of mineralization, initially in the hole zones and later the overlap regions of the collagen matrix.

Abnormal calcification or ossification may occur in many pathological states and also as a consequence of ageing. Thus abnormal calcification of articular cartilage (chondrocalcinosis) may occur with increasing age, in inflammatory states, as a result of trauma, or due to perturbations of inorganic pyrophosphate levels. Such lesions are not exclusively limited to the musculoskeletal system and may be manifest, for example, as ectopic mineralization in blood vessels.

Calcium and phosphorus balance (see also Section 12)

Much has been written about calcium balance and the main hormones that control it. Phosphate balance is less well understood (see Chapter 21.8). The circulating level of plasma calcium is determined by the amount of calcium that is absorbed by the intestine, the amount that is excreted by the kidney, and the exchange of mineral with the skeleton. The relative importance of these exchanges alters during growth and in different pathological states. Total plasma calcium concentration is closely maintained between 2.25 and 2.60 mmol/litre, of which nearly half is in the ionized form (47% ionized, 46% protein bound, and the remainder complexed). The skeleton contains approximately 1 kg (25 000 mmol) of calcium. The main fluxes of calcium in the young adult are shown in Fig. 20.1.5.

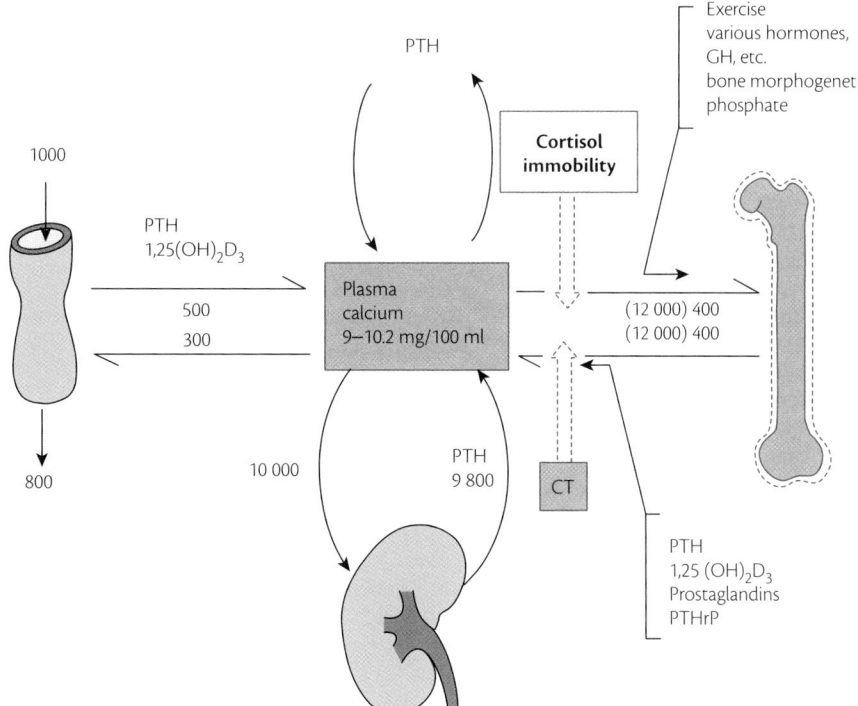

Fig. 20.1.5 Calcium homeostasis in the adult. The main daily changes in external calcium balance (figures refer to mg Ca/day). The interrupted line around the bone suggests a bone envelope across which rapid calcium exchange (12 000 mg/day) may occur. The complete interwoven effects of cytokines and molecules are not shown.
(From Smith, 1997, Oxford Textbook of Rheumatology 2nd edition, Oxford: Oxford University Press, pp. 421–440, with permission.)

Parathyroid hormone (see also Chapter 13.6)

Parathyroid hormone (PTH) is synthesized as a large precursor, in the way of proteins packaged for export, and its secretion is stimulated by a reduction in the plasma ionized-calcium concentration. Small changes in plasma calcium are detected by a G protein-coupled calcium sensing receptor (CASR) in the parathyroid gland. CASR can cause hypocalcaemic and hypercalcaemic syndromes (Table 20.1.1). Increase in PTH secretion leads to an increase in calcium absorption through the gut, an increase in calcium resorption through the kidney, and an increase in bone resorption. Intestinal calcium absorption is mediated by the active metabolite of vitamin D, $1,25(OH)_2D$, and the 1α-hydroxylation of 25-hydroxycholecalciferol (25OHD) in the kidney is stimulated by parathyroid hormone, so that the effect of parathyroid hormone on increasing intestinal calcium absorption is indirect. In contrast, the renal effect of parathyroid hormone on calcium resorption is direct. The cellular effects of parathyroid hormone on kidney and bone involve two cellular systems, namely cAMP and inositol triphosphate. PTH encourages osteoclastic bone resorption by its effects on the osteoblast (as previously described). Peripheral resistance to the effect of PTH due to inherited loss-of-function mutations in the G-protein signalling system occurs in pseudohypoparathyroidism (see below and Chapter 13.6).

Vitamin D

Vitamin D is synthesized either as vitamin D_3 (cholecalciferol) within the skin from its precursor 7-dehydrocholesterol under the influence of ultraviolet light (usually as sunlight) or taken in with food, either as vitamin D_3 or D_2 (ergocalciferol) (Fig. 20.1.6). It is transported to the liver by a binding protein where it undergoes 25-hydroxylation; 25-hydroxy-vitamin D (25OHD)

is then hydroxylated in the 1α-position by the renal 1α-hydroxylase. $1,25(OH)_2D$ is the active metabolite of vitamin D and has widespread effects, the full extent of which are only just being appreciated. These are mediated through a widely distributed vitamin D receptor that has DNA- and hormone-binding components. In addition to its classic effect on intestinal calcium transport, vitamin D is linked with the immune system and the growth and differentiation of a wide variety of cells. Measurement of the plasma 25OHD concentration has proved to be a useful indicator of vitamin D status and work on $1,25(OH)_2D$ and its receptors has illuminated the cause of the rarer forms of inherited rickets (see below). The kidney is the main source of $1,25(OH)_2D$ but it is now clear that this metabolite can also be synthesized by macrophages in a variety of granulomas, providing an explanation for the hypercalcaemia of sarcoidosis, disseminated tuberculosis, and, occasionally, lymphomas. There is also evidence that some cell types, including myocytes, can synthesize $1,25(OH)_2D$ locally without influencing the systemic concentrations of this metabolite.

Calcitonin

Calcitonin, a 32-amino-acid peptide, is just one product of the extensive calcitonin gene family. It is produced by alternative splicing of the primary gene transcript also responsible for the production of calcitonin gene-related peptide. The main effect of calcitonin is to reduce bone resorption by the direct and reversible suppression of osteoclasts and by inhibition of their production from precursors. The role of endogenous calcitonin is uncertain, although it is thought to protect the skeleton during physiological stresses such as growth and pregnancy. Recent work has shown that its receptor is widely distributed.

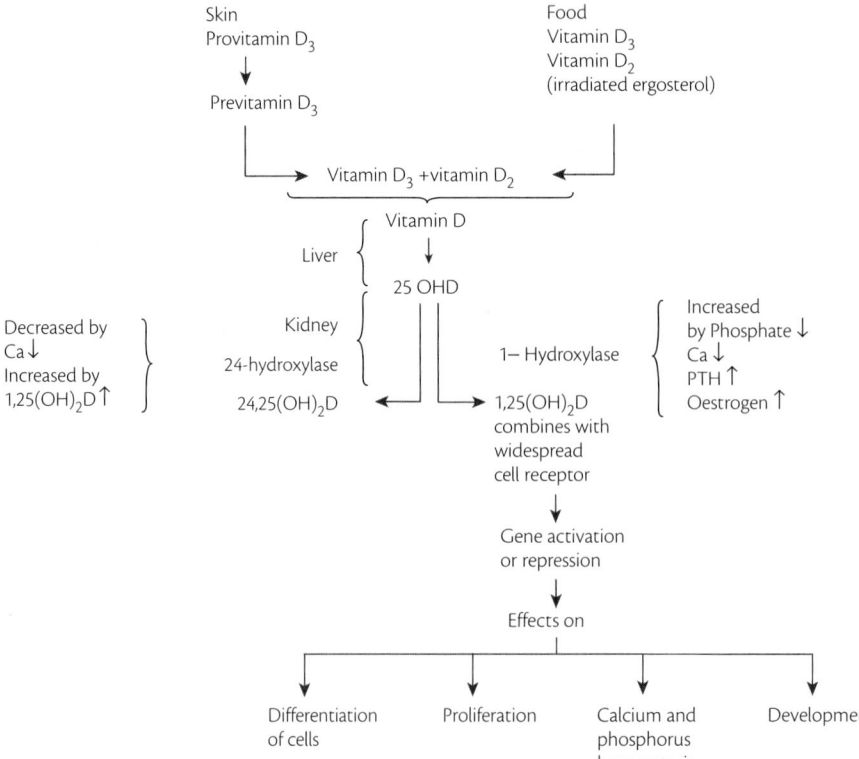

Fig. 20.1.6 The origin, synthetic pathways, and molecular and cellular effects of $1,25(OH)_2D$.
(From Smith, 1997, Oxford Textbook of Rheumatology 2nd edition, Oxford: Oxford University Press, with permission).

Parathyroid-hormone-related protein (PRrP)

This hormone was discovered through studies on patients with nonmetastatic hypercalcaemia of malignancy. PRrP has close sequence homology to PTH at the amino-terminal end of the molecule and has very similar effects. Its gene is located on the short arm of chromosome 12 and is thought to have arisen by a duplication of chromosome 11, which carries the human *PTH* gene. It has been detected in a number of tumours, particularly of the lung. There is also evidence that it may have a role in fetal physiology, controlling the calcium gradient across the placenta to maintain the relatively higher concentrations in the fetal circulation. PTH and PRrP have the same receptor. Activating mutations of this receptor can cause Jansen's metaphyseal chondrodysplasia (OMIM 156400) while inactivating mutations cause the Blomstrand's chondrodysplasia (OMIM 215045), indicating that PRrP is crucially involved in the early development of the skeleton.

Other hormones

Apart from the recognized calciotropic hormones, the skeleton is influenced by corticosteroids, sex hormones, thyroxine, and growth hormones. The main effect of excess corticosteroids (either therapeutic or in Cushing's syndrome) is to suppress osteoblastic new bone formation, although there is also an element of secondary hyperparathyroidism. Androgens and oestrogens promote and maintain skeletal mass. Osteoblasts have receptors for oestrogens, although they are not abundant. Thyroxine increases bone turnover and increases resorption in excess of formation; thyrotoxicosis thus leads to bone loss. Excess growth hormone leads to gigantism

Table 20.1.3 Biochemical measurements used to assess the rate of bone turnover

Measurement	Comment
Formation indicators	
Alkaline phosphatase (S)	Bone specific enzyme useful when total not greatly increased
Osteocalcin (S)	Variable methods and ranges
	Unstable on storage
Collagen propeptides (S)	PICP and PINP
Resorption indicators	
Hydroxyproline (U)	Useful if considerably increased
	Influenced by gelatin in diet
Pyridinium compounds (S, U)	Pyridinoline and deoxypyridinoline; HPLC tedious but still gold standard
Crosslinked telopeptides of collagen type I	
N-terminal (NTX-1) (S, U)	Osteomark: very variable
C-terminal (CTX-1) (S, U)	Crosslaps: very variable
C-terminal (CTX-MMP; ICTP) (S)	
Hydroxylysine glycosides (U)	Galactosyl hydroxylysine from skeletal collagens
Tartrate-resistant acid phosphatase (S)	
Bone sialoprotein (S)	

HPLC, high performance liquid chromatography; S, serum; U, urine.
From Smith R, Wordsworth P (2006). *Clinical and biochemical disorders of the skeleton.* Oxford University Press, Oxford, with permission.

and acromegaly (according to the age of onset) with enlargement of the bones. Absence of growth hormone will lead to proportional short stature; where there is general pituitary failure, the reduction in gonadotropins will also induce bone loss.

Biochemical measures of bone turnover

Knowledge of bone physiology allows one to interpret biochemical measures of bone turnover. These include plasma bone-derived alkaline phosphatase, osteocalcin, collagen-derived propeptides, and the urinary total hydroxyproline and crosslinked collagen-derived peptides (Table 20.1.3). Since formation and resorption are closely linked, such measurements are also related to each other and to overall bone turnover.

Total plasma alkaline phosphatase (largely derived from osteoblasts) provides a crude but readily accessible index of bone formation, being increased during periods of rapid growth and particularly when bone turnover is greatly increased, as in Paget's disease. Early measurements of serum osteocalcin gave widely variable results and depended on the origin, sensitivity, and stability of the antibodies used. Total urinary hydroxyproline excretion is influenced by dietary collagen (gelatin) and reflects both resorption and new collagen synthesis. The development of methods for the measurement of urinary collagen-derived pyridinium crosslinks gives a reliable indication of bone resorption rate, unrelated to new collagen formation and uninfluenced by diet. There are two forms of crosslinked peptide—pyridinoline and deoxypyridinoline, depending on whether they originate from oxidized hydroxylysine or lysine residues. Previous assays were dependent on high-pressure liquid chromatography of urinary peptides after hydrolysis with acid. Simple and more direct immunoassays have now been developed to measure collagen-derived fragments, both in the urine and plasma.

Correct interpretation of collagen-derived fragments depends on knowledge of collagen's metabolic pathway (Fig. 20.1.4). Soon after export from the cell, the amino- and carboxypropeptide extensions are cleaved from the helical central part of the collagen chain. Measurement of these fragments in the plasma indicates the collagen formation rate. Once the collagen chains are crosslinked, measurement of different crosslinked fragments in the urine and plasma indicate (mainly bone) collagen resorption (Table 20.1.3).

Diagnosis of bone disease

The diagnosis of bone disorders increasingly depends on specialized investigation, with the result that important clinical points tend to be forgotten.

History

Deformity, pain, and fracture are common features. To these may be added proximal myopathy (in osteomalacia and rickets) and the symptoms of any underlying systemic disease. The family history is always relevant.

Deformity and short stature

Deformity suggests an underlying skeletal disorder or previous skeletal disease, especially if there is also disturbance of growth. Short stature and disproportion are more frequent than excessive height. In children, knowledge of the normal growth patterns is essential: in the normal adult, height and span are approximately

Table 20.1.4 Some examples of short stature

Description	Disorder
Proportionate	
Genetic	Familial
Endocrine	Growth-hormone lack
	Hypothyroidism
Metabolic	Lysosomal storage diseases
	Renal glomerular failure
	Cystic fibrosis
Nutritional	Coeliac disease
	Starvation
Chronic disease	Cyanotic heart disease
Intrauterine	Low birth weight dwarfism
Chromosomal	Turner's syndrome
Social	Emotional deprivation
Disproportionate	
Short limbs	
Lethal	Type II osteogenesis imperfecta
	Thanatophoric dwarfism
	Achondrogenesis
Nonlethal	Achondroplasia
	Inherited hypophosphataemia
	Metaphyseal dysplasias
Short spine	Spondyloepiphyseal dysplasia

equal and the crown to pubis measurement is roughly equal to the pubis to heel length; and in children under the age of 10 years, the upper body segment is typically greater than the lower body segment. Short stature (defined as below the 0.4th centile) can be divided into proportionate and disproportionate forms, of which the most frequent is caused by short limbs. Proportionate short stature may occur in children who appear to be otherwise normal, whereas subjects with disproportionate short stature usually (but not always) appear abnormal from birth. Children below the 0.4th centile for height or who have sequential measurements of height that cross successive centile bands should be further investigated. About three-quarters of children exhibiting short stature either have familial short stature or constitutional delay of growth and puberty; others have chronic disease (10%), syndromic short stature (6%), chromosomal abnormalities (5%), skeletal dysplasias (1%), or growth hormone or other hormone deficiencies (1–2%). Some causes of short stature are given in Table 20.1.4. Skeletal dysplasias are dealt with further below.

Kyphosis, with loss of trunk height, as in osteoporosis and osteomalacia, is the commonest acquired deformity of adult life. It is often noticed because clothes no longer fit. During childhood, vertebral collapse will slow the growth rate. Other deformities are characteristic of the underlying disease: e.g. active childhood rickets produces knock knees, bowed legs, enlarged epiphyses, and bossing of the skull; Paget's disease produces asymmetric thick limb bones and an enlarged skull vault; and severe osteogenesis imperfecta produces very short limbs and deformity.

Bone pain and fracture

The cause of bone pain is not well understood. In osteomalacia it may be generalized and associated with tenderness on pressure. It may be due to excessive vascularity, with stretching of the periosteum; certainly it can be rapidly relieved by appropriate treatment, such as calcitonin for Paget's disease or parathyroidectomy for parathyroid bone disease. Fractures of different sorts occur: e.g. partial, multiple, and painful microfractures (fissure fractures) on the convexity of pagetic bone, the Looser's zones on medial borders of osteomalacic bones, and the multiple vertebral compression fractures of osteoporosis.

Myopathy

The cause of the proximal muscle weakness in osteomalacia and rickets remains unknown. The symptoms include a waddling gait and inability to rise from a chair, to lift objects off high shelves, or to climb stairs. Limbs may be described as stiff rather than weak. In contrast, myopathy does not occur in subjects with inherited hypophosphataemia.

Underlying disease

It is necessary to be alert for the symptoms of the underlying disease, such as renal failure, steatorrhoea, or myeloma, and to enquire particularly about previous abdominal operations, including hysterectomy and oophorectomy.

Physical signs

It is important to see the patient out of bed so that an abnormal gait or stature is not missed. The appearance may give vital clues: e.g. the large vault of Paget's disease; the coarse features, large nose, big lower jaw, and widely spaced teeth of acromegaly; and the round face, simplicity, and cataracts of pseudohypoparathyroidism. Endocrine disorders affecting the skeleton, such as hypogonadism and hypopituitarism, are readily recognizable. Special facial features should receive attention; these include the eyes for such signs as corneal calcification (hypercalcaemia), arcus juvenilis (osteogenesis imperfecta), and lens dislocation shown by the shimmering of the unsupported iris (iridodonesis; Marfan's syndrome). Other examples are corneal clouding (some mucopolysaccharidoses) and cystine crystals (cystinosis). Typically, the sclerae are blue in mild forms of osteogenesis imperfecta. In dentinogenesis imperfecta, often found with osteogenesis imperfecta, the teeth are abnormal in shape, tend to be opalescent, and vary in colour from yellow to grey. Enamel defects occur in hypoparathyroidism, teeth are lost early in hypophosphatasia, and dental abscesses are common in hypophosphataemic rickets.

Hands and feet need particular attention. The fingers may be abnormally long and thin (Marfan's syndrome) or excessively short and mobile (pseudoachondroplasia); alternatively, they may be short, wide, and stiff in some mucopolysaccharidoses or the hands may have short metacarpals (pseudohypoparathyroidism) or additional digits (Ellis–van Creveld syndrome, OMIM 225500). The monophalangic big toe (and, less often, short thumbs) is characteristic of fibrodysplasia ossificans progressiva. Abnormal body proportions are common: the spine is relatively short after vertebral collapse. Scoliosis often dates from adolescence and occasionally it may be a clue to an inherited connective tissue disorder. A thoracolumbar gibbus is a particular (though not exclusive) feature of the mucopolysaccharidoses. Spinal deformity produces secondary changes; thus, a young patient with severe osteoporosis will develop a prominent sternum with ribs that impinge on the iliac crest and a transverse crease across the front of the abdomen. Spontaneous tetany is a rare symptom, but there are two recognized bedside tests for latent tetany: of these, Chvostek's sign is more convenient, but that of Trousseau more reliable. The first involves tapping the branches of the facial nerves as they spread out from within the parotid gland; a positive sign is twitching of the appropriate facial muscle. In the second, the forearm is made ischaemic with a sphygmomanometer cuff for up to 3 min; if positive, carpal spasm will occur.

Investigations
Biochemistry

Plasma

Many generalized disorders of the skeleton, such as postmenopausal osteoporosis, osteogenesis imperfecta, and the chondrodysplasias, have normal routine biochemical values; in others, changes are diagnostic (Table 20.1.5). In normal persons, the fasting plasma calcium concentration remains virtually constant through life, the plasma phosphate, typically higher in children, declines in adolescence to adult levels while the plasma alkaline phosphatase increases temporarily during rapid adolescent growth. Since total plasma calcium includes a protein-bound fraction, it is usual to relate it to the plasma albumin level and, if necessary, correct it to a plasma albumin of 40 g per litre. Acceptable corrections include: corrected calcium (mg per 100 ml) = measured calcium—albumin (g per 100 ml) + 4; or for SI units: 0.02 mmol/litre for every 1 g/litre change of albumin from 40 g/litre. The fasting plasma calcium is normal in osteoporosis and also in Paget's disease unless the patient is immobilized. It is increased in primary hyperparathyroidism, various neoplasms (including humoral hypercalcaemia of malignancy), sarcoidosis, vitamin D overdosage, and, sometimes, a number of other states such as acromegaly and thyrotoxicosis (Table 20.1.5). It is often low in osteomalacia, but may be restored towards normal by secondary hyperparathyroidism, and it is low in parathyroid insufficiency. Normal values are to be expected in inherited untreated hypophosphataemia and in other forms of renal tubular rickets.

Since the main determinant of the fasting plasma phosphate concentration is its renal tubular resorption, hypophosphataemia occurs in primary hyperparathyroidism and in the humoral hypercalcaemia of malignancy, and it is also low in inherited hypophosphataemic

Table 20.1.5 The main symptoms, biochemical findings, and other features of disorders of the skeleton

Disorder	Most common symptoms	Plasma concentrations			Urine concentrations		Other biochemical features	Comments
		Ca	P	ALP[a]	Ca	THP[b]		
Osteoporosis	Fracture	N	N	N	N	N or H	Usually none but depends on cause	Hypercalciuria if immobilized
Osteomalacia (and rickets)	Bone pain; proximal muscle weakness; deformity	N or L	L	N or H	L	N or H	Depends on cause	Plasma P increased in renal glomerular failure
Paget's disease	Pain; deformity	N	N	H	N	H		Hypercalcaemia if immobilized; some have mutations in SQSTM1 gene
Idiopathic hyperphosphatasia: 'juvenile Paget's disease'	Large head; bowing of long bones; occurs in childhood	N	N	Very high	N	Very high		Similar to Paget's disease; very rare; osteoprotegerin deficiency; mutation in TNFRSF11B
Hyperparathyroidism (with bone disease)	Bone pain; hypercalcaemic symptoms	H	L	H	H	H	Aminoaciduria	AP and THP normal if clinical bone disease absent
Hypoparathyroidism	Tetany; ectopic calcification	L	H	N	N	N		May be acute or chronic
Pseudohypoparathyroidism`	Simple; short metacarpals; subcutaneous ossification	L	H	N	N	N		Some are biochemically normal (see text)
Neoplastic bone disease	Bone pain; fracture	N or H	N or L	N or H	N or H	N or H		Biochemistry depends on metastases and/or effects of PRrP
Osteogenesis imperfecta	Brittle bones; blue sclerae	N	N	N	N	N		Hypercalciuria may occur; most mutations in COL1A1, COL1A2

(Continued)

Table 20.1.5 (Cont'd) The main symptoms, biochemical findings, and other features of disorders of the skeleton

Disorder	Most common symptoms	Plasma concentrations			Urine concentrations		Other biochemical features	Comments
		Ca	P	ALP[a]	Ca	THP[b]		
Osteoporosis pseudoglioma syndrome	Loss of sight; fracture	N	N	N	N	N		Mutation in *LRP5*
Marfan's syndrome	Tall with scoliosis; dislocated lenses; aortic dissection	N	N	N	N	N or H		Dominant inheritance; clinically variable; mutations in *FBN1*
Homocystinuria	Intellectual disability; look like Marfan's syndrome	N	N	N	N	N	Homocystine in urine	Venous thrombosis may occur; variable deficiency of cystathionine synthase
Alkaptonuria	Back pain; early arthritis; dark urine	N	N	N	N	N	Homogentisic acid in the urine	Calcified intervertebral discs
Mucopolysaccharidosis	Short stature; thoracolumbar gibbus; intellectual disability (depends on type)	N	N	N	N	N	Characteristic mucopolysaccharide in urine	Varies with type (see text)
Hypophosphatasia	Lethal short-limbed dwarfism; bone disease like rickets	N	N	L	N	N	Phosphoethanolamine increased in urine	Sometimes hypercalcaemia in infancy; fractures in adult; multiple *ALPL* mutations
Chondrodysplasias	Short limbed; short stature; many types	N	N	N	N	N	Hypercalcemia in Jansen's metaphyseal dysplasia	Different biochemical families (see text and tables)
Osteopetrosis (marble bone disease)	Anaemia; deafness (extreme form); fractures; variable phenotype	N	N	N	L	N	Increase in acid phosphatase in some forms	Mild form fractures only; rarely carbonic anhydrase lack with systemic acidosis; mutations in chloride channel and H⁺ATPase genes
Fibrous dysplasia	Fracture; sexual precocity in girls; pigmentation	N	N	Slight increase	N	Slight increase	Biochemical changes in polyostotic form only	Mutations in *GNSA1*; occasional hypophosphataemic osteomalacia
Fibrogenesis imperfecta ossium	Fracture	N	N	Increased	N	Slight increase	Monoclonal proteinuria	Excessively rare; nonbirefringent osteoid
Fibrodysplasia ossificans progressiva	Pain and swelling in muscles; fixation of joints	N	N	Increased during acute episodes	N	N		Mutation in *ACVR1* monophalangic big toe; other patterning defects
Progressive osseous heteroplasia	Progressive soft tissue ossification/calcification, often asymmetrical	N	N	N	N	N		Rarely mutation in *GNSA1*

ALP, alkaline phosphatase; H, high; L, low; N, normal; PRrP, parathyroid-hormone-related protein; THP, total hydroxyproline.

[a] The changes in alkaline phosphatase refer to total alkaline phosphatase; bone specific measurements are useful where changes in total alkaline phosphatase are minor. The changes in osteocalcin are usually in the same direction but not always.

[b] THP = total hydroxyproline. The same changes occur in cross-linked collagen-derived peptides (CTX-1, NTX-1; see Table 20.1.3).

rickets. Both oral aluminium hydroxide and prolonged intravenous nutrition also lower plasma phosphate levels. Hyperphosphataemia occurs in hypoparathyroidism, in renal glomerular failure, and in the very rare, recessively inherited form of tumoral calcinosis (OMIM 211900).

Total plasma alkaline phosphatase and bone-derived alkaline phosphatase is normally increased in adolescence and in osteomalacia, particularly in the young, but it may be near normal in renal tubular osteomalacia. Increases occur in primary hyperparathyroidism, but only where there is demonstrable bone disease.

The highest values for plasma alkaline phosphatase are found in young patients with active Paget's disease and in idiopathic hyperphosphatasia, and the lowest in hypophosphatasia.

Other plasma measurements, which have application in particular circumstances and in research, include tartrate-resistant acid phosphatase (a product of the osteoclast and therefore an indication of bone resorption), osteocalcin (a product of the osteoblast and therefore sometimes useful as an indicator of bone formation), and the N- and C-propeptide extensions of collagen (again indicators of bone formation rate).

Urine

The amount of calcium excreted in the urine is related both to the plasma levels and to the percentage of the filtered load resorbed through the renal tubules, itself altered by parathyroid hormone. Hypocalcaemia therefore causes hypocalciuria, particularly in osteomalacia and rickets. Hypercalcaemia leads to hypercalciuria, especially when this is due to rapid bone loss as in neoplastic disease of the skeleton, leukaemia, myeloma, and immobilization. Since parathyroid hormone increases the renal tubular resorption of calcium, the normal relationship between plasma and urine calcium is disturbed in parathyroid disease; however, most hypercalcaemic hyperparathyroid patients excrete more calcium than normal. Urine phosphate excretion is increased in hyperparathyroidism but is also increased in certain genetic disorders associated with renal tubular dysfunction. These include various forms of inherited phosphaturia and oncogenic rickets (see below).

Total hydroxyproline in the urine (after acid hydrolysis of the peptides) is a good indicator of bone breakdown and collagen turnover, provided the patient is ingesting a low-gelatin diet. The physiological changes in hydroxyproline excretion are striking, with a particularly sharp peak in adolescence coinciding with the maximum height velocity. The highest values are seen in active Paget's disease, where the excretion may be up to 50-fold the normal value. Hydroxyproline excretion correlates well with plasma alkaline phosphatase and is therefore increased in some forms of osteomalacia and in hyperparathyroidism with bone disease. Since thyroxine increases collagen turnover, urinary hydroxyproline is also abnormally high in thyrotoxicosis and abnormally low in myxoedema (either primary or secondary).

Hydroxyproline excretion can be most usefully expressed as the amount in a 24-h urine sample in a patient on a gelatin-free diet or in a fasting urine sample in relation to creatinine. However, hydroxyproline peptide excretion is related both to newly formed and mature collagen and is not, therefore, a direct measure of bone resorption. The urinary excretion of pyridinium compounds (see above) from the lysyl- and hydroxylysyl-derived crosslinks of mature collagen is a direct measure of bone resorption, irrespective of dietary collagen. These cross-linked peptides may now be conveniently measured in the serum (Table 20.1.3). Finally, glucose in the urine of a patient with inherited rickets suggests multiple renal tubular defects and proteinuria is an important clue to myelomatosis.

Radiology

The diagnosis of bone disease often depends on the radiographic appearances, especially where there are no demonstrable biochemical changes. A particular example is in the differential diagnosis of perinatal lethal dwarfism. Conventional radiographs demonstrate structural changes such as fractures, deformity, areas of resorption, and alteration in size, but they are unreliable for the assessment of bone density. As radiographic techniques develop, increasing use is made of isotope bone scans, CT scans, and MRI scans. Bisphosphonate-labelled scanning agents are selectively taken up in areas of increased vascularity or turnover. They are very useful in demonstrating the skeletal extent of Paget's disease of bone, the presence of bony metastases, the pathological fractures of osteoporosis, and Looser zones in osteomalacia. An isotope scan is preferable to multiple radiographs to assess the distribution (but not the structure) of abnormal bone.

CT scanning can also be very useful in bone disease. Examples include the delineation of ectopic ossification, of spinal cord compression, and of bone tumours. MRI is very effective at defining soft tissue abnormalities but is also usually the investigation of choice in detecting bony pathology. Methods for measuring bone mass are considered under osteoporosis (see below).

Bone biopsy

Direct examination of bone is a valuable but underused investigation. Bone can be taken by a transiliac trephine (using a local anaesthetic) and sections should be examined with and without decalcification. Ideally the bone should be labelled with tetracycline to allow an estimate of formation rates. In the various metabolic bone diseases, the appearances are characteristic: the excess osteoid of osteomalacia; the disorganized mosaic pattern, excessive cellular activity, and fibrosis of Paget's disease; and osteitis fibrosa cystica of hyperparathyroid bone disease. In mild osteogenesis imperfecta, there is typically an increase in the number of osteocytes, and, in the more severe form, a considerable increase in the amount of woven bone. A normal biopsy will exclude these diseases except where the pathological changes are patchy. Where possible, histological examination should now include transmission and scanning electron microscopy and the report should include quantitative histomorphometry. More details are given in larger texts (see Further Reading).

Further investigations

Measurement of the external calcium and phosphorus balance is a classic way of investigating generalized bone disease and the effects of treatment upon it, but it is also tedious. The use of isotopes to measure calcium absorption, apparent bone formation, and resorption rates is less direct and also depends on a number of assumptions. This leaves a large number of measurements available for specific problems. Important examples (in the plasma) are intact PTH assays (to investigate hyper- and hypocalcaemia), PRrP (particularly for suspected hypercalcaemia of malignancy), and 25OHD and $1,25(OH)_2D$ (for the investigation of rickets and osteomalacia). In inherited disorders, analysis of DNA or biochemical studies of cultured skin fibroblasts can be diagnostic but require specialist facilities.

Concluding remarks on diagnosis

The diagnosis of a skeletal disorder is not difficult where there are clear biochemical disturbances (Table 20.1.5), although, as in osteomalacia, the causes may be many. An exact diagnosis may be impossible when the standard biochemical results are normal, and this is particularly so in some of the rare heritable disorders. Guidance based on the age of the patient and frequency of the disorder is given in Table 20.1.6.

Table 20.1.6 Diagnosis of disorders of the skeleton

Age	Main presenting symptom	Most likely diagnosis	Frequency	Exclude
Over 50 years	Pain in the back; loss of height; fracture	Osteoporosis, most common in women	Common	Myeloma (especially in men); secondary deposits; coexistent osteomalacia
	Deformity of long bones; pain in hips; pathological fracture; deafness	Paget's disease of bone; most common in men	Common	Osteomalacia; hyperparathyroid bone disease; skeletal metastases;
	Bone pain and tenderness; difficulty in walking; unable to climb stairs; pathological fracture	Osteomalacia	Uncommon, especially in the adult	Carcinoma; polymyalgia rheumatica
	Bone pain and deformity; thirst; nocturia; depression; vomiting; constipation	Osteitis fibrosa cystica; most common in women	Rare	Carcinoma with hypercalcaemia; myeloma
20–50 years	Loss of height; bone pain	Probably secondary deposits; or myeloma	Rare	Osteomalacia; accelerated osteoporosis
	Muscle weakness; loss of height; bone pain	Osteomalacia	Rare	Late muscular dystrophy; neoplastic neuromyopathy; Cushing's syndrome
0–20 years	Bowing of bones; deformity; weakness	'Nutritional' rickets	Most common Asian immigrants in northern cities	Other causes of rickets; hypophosphatasia
	Multiple fractures; bruising at different times	Non-accidental injury	Not uncommon	Osteogenesis imperfecta
	Bone pain; ill health	Leukaemia	Uncommon	Osteomyelitis; rickets
	Pain in back; difficulty in walking; pain in ankles; less rapid growth	Juvenile osteoporosis	Rare	Leukaemia; osteogenesis imperfecta
	Failure to grow (short stature)	Many causes (Table 20.1.4)	Common	Particularly hypothyroidism; Turner's syndrome; coeliac disease
	Excessive or disproportionate growth	Several causes, often familial	Less common than short stature	Particularly pituitary tumour; Marfan's syndrome; homocystinuria; hypogonadism and chromosomal abnormalities
	Fracture and deformity at birth (often lethal)	Severe osteogenesis imperfecta	Uncommon	Hypophosphatasia; achondrogenesis; thanatophoric dwarfism

Osteomalacia and rickets

Osteomalacia most frequently results from a lack of vitamin D or a disturbance of its metabolism; in the growing skeleton it is referred to as rickets and the terms are often used interchangeably (Table 20.1.7). Very rarely, severe calcium deficiency can lead to rickets. Inherited hypophosphataemia and several other renal tubular disorders may also cause rickets without clear evidence of abnormal vitamin D metabolism. The causal mutations in inherited hypophosphataemia have now been identified.

The main histological feature of osteomalacia is defective mineralization of bone matrix (Fig. 20.1.7). Our present understanding of osteomalacia relies on advances in knowledge of vitamin D metabolism (Fig. 20.1.8). For clinical purposes, two aspects of the physiology of vitamin D require emphasis. The first is the quantitative importance of vitamin D synthesis in the skin in comparison with that in the diet and the second concerns the relative role of different vitamin D metabolites. The measurement of circulating concentrations of 25OHD as an index of vitamin D status has identified those groups (Asian immigrants and older people) most at risk from vitamin D deficiency; importantly it has also shown the large amounts of vitamin D that can be synthesized in the human skin when exposed to ultraviolet light. The causes of osteomalacia can now be partly understood in terms of its metabolites and the major importance of $1,25(OH)_2D$ is established. The effects of giving vitamin D can probably not be ascribed solely to the actions of $1,25(OH)_2D$ alone and may include other biologically active derivatives such as 25OHD and, possibly, 24,25-dihydroxycholecalciferol $(24,25(OH)_2D)$.

Pathophysiology

The features of osteomalacia can be predicted largely from the known calciotropic effects of vitamin D. Examination of undecalcified bone shows wide osteoid seams with many birefringent lamellae of collagen (Fig. 20.1.7b) covering more of the bone surface than normal and absence of the 'calcification front'. The absence of this front is important since excessive osteoid may also be found in conditions other than osteomalacia, such as hypophosphatasia, Paget's disease of bone, and thyrotoxicosis, where the calcification front is normal; in these disorders, the increase tends to be in the amount of bone surface covered rather than in the thickness of osteoid. Excess osteoid also occurs when etidronate or aluminium accumulate in the skeleton. In rickets the main change is disorganization of the growth plate.

Since there is intestinal malabsorption of calcium in vitamin D deficiency, both the plasma and urine calcium levels are lower than normal; absorption of phosphorus is also defective, with resultant hypophosphataemia. As hypocalcaemia stimulates the secretion of parathyroid hormone, this will correct the low plasma calcium level and exaggerate hypophosphataemia. In osteomalacia, osteoblastic

Table 20.1.7 The main causes of osteomalacia and rickets

Cause	Effect
Lack of vitamin D	Defective synthesis in the skin
	Low dietary intake
	Increased requirement
Malabsorption	Gluten-sensitive enteropathy (coeliac disease)
	Gastric surgery
	Bowel resection
	Intestinal bypass surgery
	Biliary cirrhosis
	Pancreatic insufficiency
Renal disease	
Renal tubular disorders	X-linked inherited hypophosphataemia (Vitamin D resistant rickets)
	Others (see Table 20.1.9)
Renal glomerular failure	Renal osteodystrophy
	Bone disease with dialysis and transplantation
Others	Tumour rickets (oncogenic osteomalacia
	Vitamin D dependent rickets (types I and II)
	Phosphate deficiency rickets
	Anticonvulsant osteomalacia
	Calcium deficiency rickets

From Smith R, Wordsworth P (2006). *Clinical and biochemical disorders of the skeleton.* Oxford University Press, Oxford.

activity is increased and the plasma alkaline phosphatase is therefore also increased. There appears to be no difficulty in laying down bone matrix collagen, but it cannot be properly mineralized. One should recall that the effects of vitamin D are not confined to the skeleton, although they are clinically most obvious

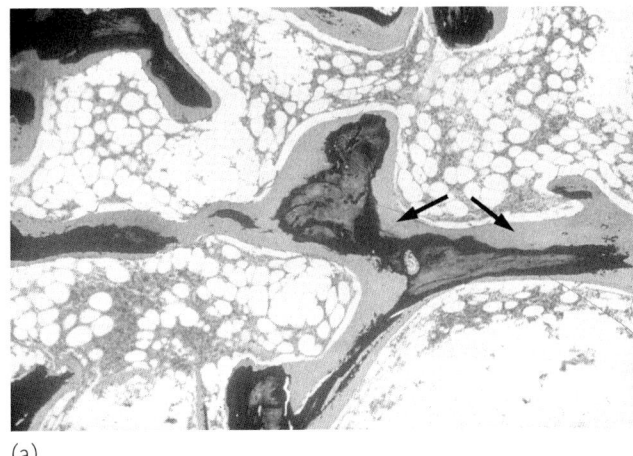

(a)

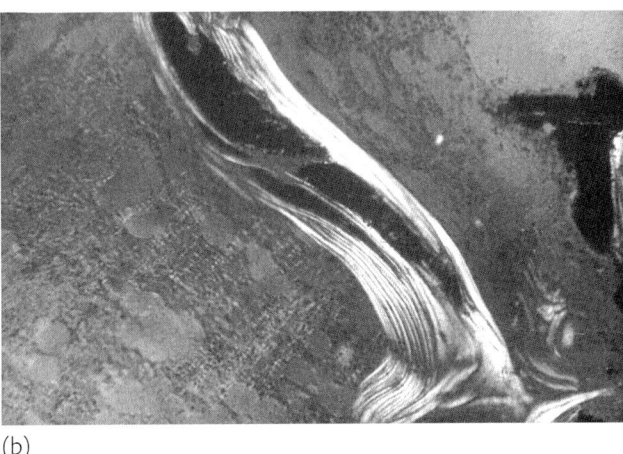

(b)

Fig. 20.1.7 (a) Bone from a patient with osteomalacia showing the appearance of excessive osteoid under polarized light; excessive unmineralized osteoid is arrowed. (b) There are regular lamellae of double refractile collagen fibres.

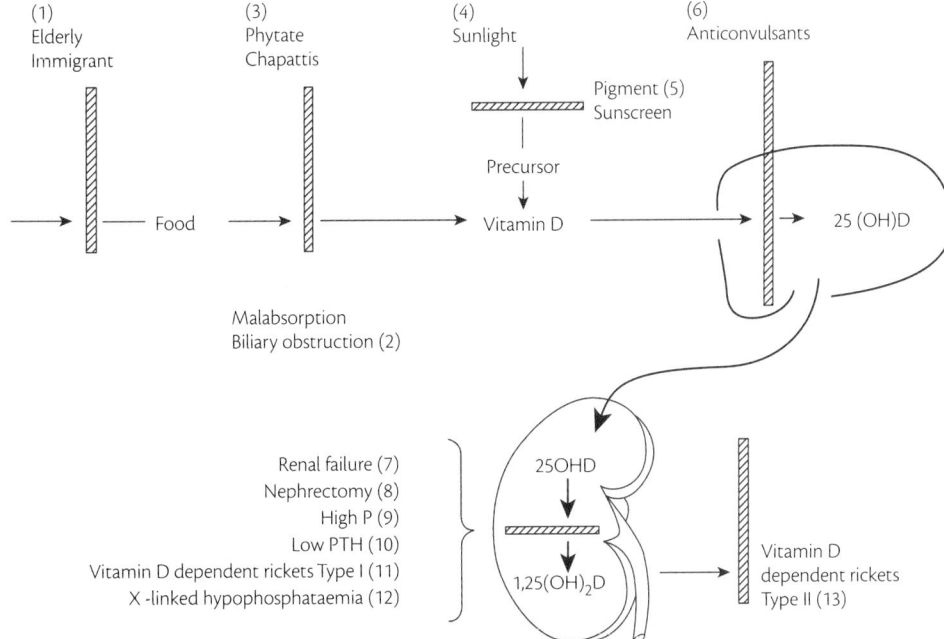

Fig. 20.1.8 The causes of rickets and osteomalacia in relation to vitamin D physiology. (1–5) Reasons for vitamin D deficiency; (6) anticonvulsants may reduce hepatic 25 hydroxylation of vitamin D; (7–11) some causes for reduced 1α-hydroxylation of 25OHD, which do not always cause rickets; (12) formation of 1,25(OH)$_2$D is inappropriately low in X-linked hypophosphataemia, due to mutations in *PHEX*; and (13) resistance to 1,25(OH)$_2$D in type II vitamin D dependent rickets.

in this tissue—thus vitamin D has important effects on cellular differentiation, on the immune system, and on striated muscle.

Causes

There are many causes of osteomalacia (and rickets), some of which are very rare. They may conveniently be divided into three main groups: nutritional, malabsorptive, and renal (Table 20.1.7). Most can be understood in terms of vitamin D metabolism (Fig. 20.1.8). In older people and immigrant populations, the food intake of vitamin D is often deficient and the requirements may be increased; the absorption of vitamin D is poor in coeliac disease, after partial gastrectomy, intestinal resection, or bypass, and in biliary disease. The intestinal absorption of calcium is reduced by phytate, as in chapattis, which may also increase vitamin D requirements (see below). Endogenous synthesis of vitamin D in the skin is reduced, especially in town and city communities in high northern latitudes; it is further reduced by skin pigmentation. The 25-hydroxylation of calciferol may be impaired in some chronic liver diseases and anticonvulsants may induce hepatic enzymes that degrade vitamin D. The 1α-hydroxylation of 25OHD is reduced or absent in renal failure, after nephrectomy, in hyperphosphataemia (which suppresses the activity of the enzyme 1α hydroxylase), parathyroid insufficiency, in type I vitamin D dependent rickets, and, probably, in some bone tumours. Many patients have more than one cause for their osteomalacia; older people often have poor vitamin D intake, limited exposure to sunlight, and progressive renal glomerular failure. Reduced exposure to sunlight is an indirect consequence of physical immobility and may contribute to osteomalacia in rheumatoid arthritis and other chronic diseases.

The effects of renal glomerular failure on the skeleton are complex (Chapter 21.6). Two main events occur: one is an increase in the plasma phosphate level, which leads to a fall in plasma calcium and secondary hyperparathyroidism with excessive bone resorption; the other is the reduced renal formation of $1,25(OH)_2D$, with defective intestinal absorption of calcium and defective bone mineralization. The combination of these events rapidly produces severe deformity, especially in the growing skeleton. In patients receiving dialysis, renal osteodystrophy may be complicated by aluminium intoxication.

Clinical features

The main symptoms of osteomalacia are bone pain and tenderness, skeletal deformity, and proximal muscle weakness, often accompanied by the features of the underlying disorder and of hypocalcaemia. In severe osteomalacia, all the bones are painful and tender, sometimes sufficiently so as to disturb sleep. The tenderness can be particularly marked in the lower ribs and may also be accentuated over Looser zones. Deformity is most often seen in rickets when the effects of vitamin D deficiency are superimposed on a growing skeleton; the linear growth rate is reduced, there is bowing of the long bones, enlargement of the costochondral junctions ('rickety rosary'), and bossing of the frontal and parietal bones. Later, osteomalacia may produce a triradiate pelvis, a gross kyphosis, and corresponding deformities of the chest. Indeed it has been suggested that osteomalacic pelvic deformity and the resulting abnormality of the birth canal may have been the most potent evolutionary stimulus to the development of a pale skin in some European populations in as little as 40 000 years, thereby allowing efficient vitamin D synthesis.

Proximal muscle weakness is an important symptom. Its cause is unknown, although myoblasts require $1,25(OH)_2D$ *in vitro* and the development of myofibrils in animals without the vitamin D receptor may be abnormal. It is more marked in some forms of osteomalacia than in others. Most commonly, there is a waddling gait and difficulty in getting up and down stairs, out of low chairs, and in and out of small cars. In older people, weakness may make

Table 20.1.8 Biochemical changes in rickets and osteomalacia

Main groups

Disorder	Plasma concentrations			Comments
	Ca	P	ALP	
Vitamin D deficient	↓	↓	↑	25OHD low; PTH increased
Malabsorption	↓	↓	↑	If severe may also have magnesium deficiency
Renal tubular				
Inherited hypophosphataemia	N	↓	↑	X-linked most frequent
Renal tubular acidosis	↓	↓	↑	Systemic acidosis
Fanconi's syndrome	↓	↓	↑	Generalized aminoaciduria; glycosuria
Renal glomerular osteodystrophy				
Renal glomerular	↓	↑	↑	Biochemistry of renal failure $(1,25(OH)_2D$ low)
Dialysis and transplantation	?	?	↑	Very variable. Aluminium excess important.
Oncogenic osteomalacia	N	↓	↑	$1,25(OH)_2D$ ↓, FGF23 ↑
Vitamin D dependent				
Type I	↓	↓	↑	$1,25(OH)_2D$ ↓
Type II	↓	↓	↑	$1,25(OH)_2D$ ↑
Phosphate deficiency	N	↓	↑	$1,25(OH)_2D$ ↑

Hypophosphataemic syndromes

Disorder	Plasma			Urine	Plasma $1,25(OH)_2D$
	Ca	P	ALP	Ca	
XLH	N	↓	↑ or N	↓	(↓)
HHRH	N	↓	↑ or N	↑	↑
ADHR	N	↓	↑ or N	↓	(↓)
Dent's disease	N	↓ or N	↑ or N	↑	(↓)
Oncogenic osteomalacia	N	↓	↑ or N	↓	↓

ADHR, autosomal dominant hypophosphataemic rickets; ALP, alkaline phosphatase; HHRH, hereditary hypophosphataemic rickets and hypercalciuria; N, normal; PTH, parathyroid hormone; XLH, X-linked hypophosphataemia.
Note that the serum 25OHD concentration is normal in all these disorders. (↓) indicates that the $1,25(OH)_2D$ concentration is decreased relative to serum phosphorus.

walking impossible thereby suggesting paraplegia. In younger subjects, even muscular dystrophy may be simulated.

Features of the underlying disorder include anaemia, tiredness and steatorrhoea (coeliac disease), and pigmentation, thirst, and nocturia in renal failure. Occasionally, hypocalcaemia may cause spontaneous tetany; the manifestations of carpopedal spasm, stridor, and fits are more dramatic in the child than the adult.

Examination of the patient with osteomalacia or rickets confirms the main symptoms. Measurement of the body proportions is useful. Thus patients with inherited hypophosphataemia and rickets have relatively short limbs, whereas those with late-onset osteomalacia may have a relatively short trunk due to vertebral collapse. It is important to look for clues as to the cause of the osteomalacia, such as the scars of previous gastric or intestinal surgery.

Investigations

Biochemistry

Since there are many causes of osteomalacia, the detailed biochemical changes differ from one to another (Table 20.1.8). In vitamin D deficiency or malabsorption, there are low plasma calcium and phosphate levels, a low urine calcium level, and an increased plasma alkaline phosphatase level. However, these may vary with the stage of the disease. Initially, hypocalcaemia may be the only abnormality. Later, with secondary hyperparathyroidism, the plasma calcium level returns towards normal, the plasma phosphate level falls, and the alkaline phosphatase level increases. In inherited X-linked hypophosphataemia (vitamin D-resistant rickets), plasma phosphate is low, but the plasma calcium is normal and the alkaline phosphatase may also be normal. Renal glomerular failure causes an increase in plasma phosphate, urea, and creatinine, and hypocalcaemia, and, in the rare renal tubular syndromes, there may be a marked systemic acidosis. In patients with osteomalacia, the urine should always be examined for the presence of glucose and protein. If these are present, it is important to check for the amino acid and low molecular weight proteinuria characteristic of renal tubular disorders. Some of these are associated with specific tubular defects,

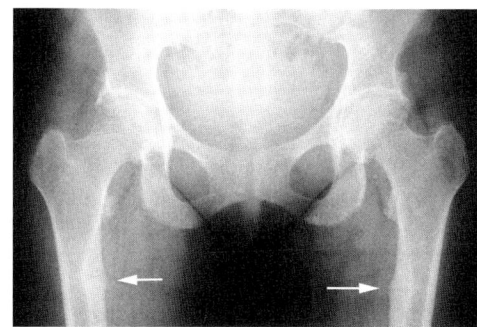

Fig. 20.1.10 Osteomalacia due to adult Fanconi's syndrome. Bilateral Looser zones (arrowed) on the medial border of the femora in a woman.

such in the chloride channel CLCN5 in Dent's disease (OMIM 300009) and related disorders (Chapters 21.15 and 21.16).

The measurement of vitamin D metabolites is now routine and a low plasma 25OHD level is a good indication of vitamin D deficiency. Estimation of plasma $1,25(OH)_2D$ is important to elucidate the very rare causes of rickets and particularly to distinguish between type I (low $1,25(OH)_2D$) and type II (high $1,25(OH)_2D$) vitamin D dependent rickets.

Radiology

The radiological appearances differ according to whether growth has ceased or not. In rickets, the main abnormalities are at the ends of the long bones, where the width of the growth plate is increased and the metaphysis is widened, cupped, and ragged (Fig. 20.1.9). Osteomalacia may show the deformities previously described, but the radiological hallmark of active osteomalacia is the Looser's zone (Fig. 20.1.10). This is a ribbon-like area of defective mineralization, which may be found in almost any bone but is seen particularly in the long bones, the pelvis, and the ribs, and also around the scapulae. Looser's zones may be bilateral and symmetrical; in bones such as the femur, they occur on the medial border of the shaft or neck and are usually single, which contrasts with the multiple fissure fractures on the lateral convexity of the bone in Paget's disease. In osteomalacia, the vertebral bodies are often uniformly biconcave, to produce an appearance likened to a fish spine. Additionally, in renal glomerular osteodystrophy, the endplates may become relatively more dense than the rest of the vertebral body, to produce the so-called 'rugger jersey' spine. In the adult with inherited hypophosphataemia, the bones may also become deformed, buttressed, and dense; in this disorder, calcification/ossification of the tendons and ligaments at their insertions (enthesopathy) and of the vertebral ligaments can produce an appearance similar to that of ankylosing spondylitis. Ossification of the ligamenta flava narrows the spinal canal and compresses the spinal cord and its roots. This is well shown on CT scans. In patients with osteomalacia and hypocalcaemia, the radiological features of secondary hyperparathyroidism appear with subperiosteal bone resorption that affects the phalanges, the pubic symphysis, and the outer ends of the clavicles. In rickets, periostitis of the distal ends of the long bones, such as the radius and ulna, often occur.

The most extreme effects of parathyroid overactivity are seen in the skeleton of the child with renal osteodystrophy, where the region of the growth plate and metaphyses may fracture (an appearance likened to a rotting stump). A bone scintigram may be very useful in cases of osteomalacia, demonstrating multiple

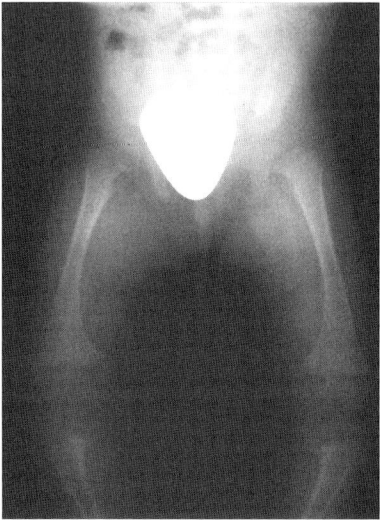

Fig. 20.1.9 The radiological appearance of rickets in a child with inherited hypophosphataemia. The growth plates are widened and the metaphyses are cupped and ragged.

pathological fractures often not seen on the plain films. The appearance is similar to that of bony metastases, for which it may be readily mistaken.

Bone biopsy

The diagnosis of osteomalacia is often clear without examining the bone. Where doubt exists, a transiliac biopsy examined before and after decalcification will demonstrate the failure of mineralization and the wide osteoid seams. It is important to take all surgical opportunities to examine bone histologically, particularly during operations on fractured femurs in older people.

Other investigations

Further investigation is not usually needed to diagnose osteomalacia, but may be necessary to identify its cause. Thus patients with vitamin D-deficient rickets and osteomalacia will have a low plasma 25OHD, but not all subjects with such low levels have osteomalacia. In the very rare condition of vitamin D dependent rickets (VDDR), measurement of circulating $1,25(OH)_2D$ will be necessary to distinguish the absence of 1α-hydroxylase (type I VDDR) from resistance to $1,25(OH)_2D$ (type II VDDR). Further, CT and MRI scanning may help to identify the presence of an FGF23-secreting mesenchymal tumour causing hypophosphataemic osteomalacia (oncogenic rickets, see below).

Diagnosis

Osteomalacia is not difficult to diagnose once it has been thought of. It should be distinguished from other forms of metabolic bone disease (Table 20.1.5), from other causes of proximal muscle weakness, and from other disorders causing bone pain. In patients with proximal muscle weakness, polymyalgia rheumatica, thyrotoxic myopathy, muscular dystrophy, neoplastic neuropathy, dermatomyositis, and polymyositis all need to be considered. Multiple myeloma and leukaemia should be excluded as causes of pain. Provided that the plasma calcium, phosphate, and alkaline phosphatase levels are always measured in patients with these symptoms, those with osteomalacia should be easily identified. Patients with psychological illness may have an abnormal gait and complain of pain and weakness in their limbs, but the biochemistry will be normal in such patients. In practice, symptoms of pain and stiffness often first lead the patient with osteomalacia to a rheumatologist.

Treatment

Rickets and osteomalacia should respond rapidly to vitamin D (or one of its metabolites) in appropriate doses and the response may be a useful way of confirming the diagnosis. Increased mobility with an increase in muscle strength may be the first clinical response, despite a temporary increase in bone pain. Biochemically, plasma phosphate and urine hydroxyproline levels are the first to increase. The alkaline phosphatase level may show a temporary rise and then fall slowly to normal levels. As the plasma calcium and 25OHD concentrations increase towards normal, the parathyroid hormone concentration falls.

The effective dose and the particular vitamin D preparation depends on the cause of the osteomalacia. That due to vitamin D deficiency will respond to microgram doses ($1\mu g = 40\,IU$), but it is often useful to give considerably more than this, such as calciferol 1.25 mg daily for 1 or 2 weeks only. Where there is doubt about compliance, vitamin D may be injected intramuscularly in one large dose (up to 15 mg, 600 000 units). Unfortunately this may not be efficiently absorbed from the injection site. Lack of a response to microgram doses suggest that the osteomalacia is not due to simple vitamin D deficiency but, for example, to malabsorption or renal failure. It is particularly in the last group that the 1α-hydroxylated metabolites of vitamin D are effective (see Chapter 21.6). Clearly, underlying disorders must be treated at the same time: e.g. patients with coeliac disease will need a gluten-free diet.

Particular forms of osteomalacia and rickets

Nutritional osteomalacia

In the United Kingdom and other northern European countries, so-called nutritional osteomalacia occurs particularly amongst older people and in Asian immigrants of all ages. In older people, the high incidence of osteomalacia is mainly due to their poor exposure to sunlight and a low intake of vitamin D; it may also be exacerbated by the effects of drugs such as anticonvulsants and by increasing renal glomerular failure. Since older people are often housebound, they may develop osteomalacia despite a sunny climate. Certainly, the prevalence of osteomalacia in the older population is significant. The frequency of osteomalacia in patients with fractures of the femoral neck is also higher than previously suspected. Osteomalacia should always be excluded in older people with bone disease, and particularly in those with femoral neck fractures. Where possible this should include histological examination of bone taken at operation or by biopsy. Vitamin D status should be assessed routinely. In the geriatric population, the mean concentration of 25OHD is much lower than in younger patients; the usual seasonal variation, with lowest values in the winter and early spring and highest values in late summer, may not occur in those who spend their time indoors.

Asian immigrants to more northerly latitudes develop osteomalacia and rickets more often than the indigenous population. There are probably several reasons for this. They tend to live in northern cities away from sunlight and, especially in women, do not expose their skin to the limited ultraviolet light. Where dermal synthesis of vitamin D is limited, dietary factors become more important and it is particularly those on a meat-free diet containing chapattis who develop osteomalacia. The role of chapattis and the phytates that they contain is not yet fully understood. Phytates bind to calcium so preventing its absorption and it can be shown, at least experimentally, that reduced calcium absorption increases the vitamin D requirement by increasing its parathyroid-mediated breakdown. It has been suggested that such a mechanism of reduced calcium absorption may also contribute to the osteomalacia of malabsorptive syndromes, such as that following partial gastrectomy.

Pigmentation of the skin can be shown experimentally, using a standardized dose of ultraviolet light, to reduce vitamin D synthesis, but in practice this is of little significance. Since north European immigrants of Afro-Caribbean descent have a lower incidence of rickets than Asians in the same environment, it is clear that factors other than skin colour are important.

As in older people, 25OHD levels can be very low, especially in Asian immigrants. They increase in the summer, when there may be spontaneous healing of rickets. Important work in Glasgow has shown that Asian rickets can be prevented by fortifying food such as chapatti flour with vitamin D, although the incidence of osteomalacia in Asian adults remains unaffected. Other local lifestyle changes will also influence the diet of children.

Osteomalacia and malabsorption

Coeliac disease (gluten-sensitive enteropathy) (Chapter 15.10.3) is a relatively common cause of osteomalacia, approaching 1% in the United Kingdom. Recent surveys demonstrate the high incidence of coeliac disease in the population. It should be suspected at any age and confirmed by the presence of circulating endomysial antibody and, if necessary, by a small intestinal biopsy showing an atrophic mucosa. Other causes of malabsorption vary in their frequency according to surgical practice. Thus, it is well established that osteomalacia follows classic partial gastrectomy, but the actual incidence is debated and its cause is probably multifactorial. Postgastrectomy subjects tend to take little vitamin D in their diet and there is defective calcium absorption. Available evidence suggests that clinical osteomalacia is rare after vagotomy and pyloroplasty. Osteomalacia can also follow the removal of long segments of small intestine for conditions such as Crohn's disease and complicates some intestinal bypass operations used for extreme obesity.

Osteomalacia and liver disease

Osteomalacia is uncommon in those with liver disease; in theory it may be due to a number of factors such as malabsorption of vitamin D and its defective 25-hydroxylation. Most research has concerned the osteomalacia of biliary cirrhosis, and osteomalacia in chronic liver disease appears to be a complication related to prolonged cholestasis.

Osteomalacia and renal disease

It is important to distinguish the osteomalacia and rickets of renal glomerular failure from that attributable to renal tubular disorders. Bone disease in renal glomerular failure (renal glomerular osteodystrophy) is dealt with elsewhere (see Chapter 21.6); this includes bone disease in the dialysis patient and the effects of aluminium. Renal glomerular osteodystrophy is a complex disease with excessive bone resorption, defective bone mineralization, and, in some cases, osteoporosis. Previously, it was treated with large doses of native vitamin D; more effective current therapy now includes the metabolites 1α-hydroxycholecalciferol or 1,25(OH)$_2$D.

Many renal tubular disorders lead to osteomalacia (Chapters 21.15 and 21.16; Tables 20.1.8 and 20.1.9). Of these, the most common is X-linked hypophosphataemia, so-called vitamin D-resistant rickets (OMIM 307800), which is normally inherited as an X-linked dominant trait; here, the main abnormality is hypophosphataemia due to a reduction in the maximum renal tubular resorption rate of phosphate. It exhibits substantial clinical heterogeneity; some patients in a family will have hypophosphataemia alone, whereas others will have hypophosphataemia with accompanying bone disease. It is now known that many cases of inherited hypophosphataemia are caused by mutations in the *PHEX* gene, the cognate protein of which has the features of an endopeptidase. Endopeptidases degrade or activate peptide hormones but it is not yet known for certain how *PHEX* mutations produce the defect in phosphate homeostasis. However, recent evidence suggests that the effects may be mediated through one of the fibroblast growth factors (FGF23), levels of which may be increased in X-linked hypophosphataemia. *PHEX* mutations alter the ability of this endopeptidase to cleave and inactivate the biologically active form of FGF23. In this regard, a rare human autosomal dominant form of hypophosphataemia caused by *FGF23* mutations is particularly interesting (OMIM 193100); these mutations abolish the PHEX catabolic cleavage site on FGF23, thereby increasing the biological activity of this potent hypophosphataemic mediator (as is also seen with the raised FGF23 levels in oncogenic osteomalacia; see below).

Since the 1,25(OH)$_2$D levels are normal where the plasma phosphate is low, it is also proposed that the sensitivity of the 1α-hydroxylase enzyme is reduced. Children with hypophosphataemic rickets or osteomalacia are unlike patients with other forms of rickets. They present with deformity but are otherwise well and without muscle weakness; however, growth is defective and their eventual height is usually less than 150 cm. Apart from hypophosphataemia, there may be no other abnormality in the biochemical values routinely available and the plasma alkaline phosphatase level can be normal for age. Radiographs show severe rickets and, later, the bones are often dense with buttressing and exostoses. The enthesopathy with ossification of the ligamenta flava can cause spinal nerve root compression and even paraplegia. Spinal stiffness may be profound, mimicking spondyloarthropathy. There may be profound ossification of the joint capsules restricting movement. Total hip replacement can be very effective in such cases. Ligamentous calcification may also contribute to deafness. Finally, abnormal teeth in this disorder cause periapical translucencies and may lead to abscesses.

The treatment of inherited hypophosphataemia is controversial. Early diagnosis is important to implement effective treatment promptly and to minimize growth retardation and deformity. For many years, its mainstay was large doses of vitamin D; this posed a continuous danger of vitamin D poisoning and did not correct the eventual short stature. There is an improvement in growth rate when oral phosphate is given in addition to vitamin D, but the condition does not appear to respond to phosphate alone. It has now been shown that combined 1,25(OH)$_2$D and oral phosphate (in up

Table 20.1.9 Renal tubular disorders, rickets, and osteomalacia

Description	Disorder
Vitamin D-resistant rickets	X-linked hypophosphataemia
Renal tubular acidosis (RTA)	
Inherited	Proximal (bicarbonate wastage)
	Distal (H$^+$ gradient defect)
Acquired	Ureterosigmoid anastomosis
Some multiple renal tubular defects (Fanconi's syndrome)	
Inherited	Cystinosis
	Oculocerebrorenal syndrome (Lowe's syndrome)
	Wilson's disease
	Galactosaemia
Acquired	Multiple myeloma
	Cadmium poisoning
	Ifosfamide toxicity
Other rare renal tubular defects	X-linked hypercalciuric nephrocalcinosis (Dent's disease)
	Hereditary hypophosphataemic rickets and hypercalciuria
	Autosomal dominant hypophosphataemic rickets

to five doses in 24 h) produces healing of epiphyseal and trabecular bone and this is now the recommended treatment. This combination not only produces bone healing but also increases eventual stature. However, it is still unusual for affected patients to have an eventual height of much more than 1.5 m (5 feet). Accounts of the effects of medical treatment on deformity and height differ; the necessity for corrective osteotomy on the lower limbs is less than previously, but discussion with an orthopaedic surgeon is important since the deformity may be complex.

It is also important that the parents should know the genetics of this condition. Because the defect in phosphate transport is inherited as a dominant on the X chromosome, an affected mother transmits the condition to 50% of her children regardless of their gender. All the daughters of an affected father will have the disease, but none of his sons. Affected sons may have more severe disease and some affected daughters may be asymptomatic. Diagnosis can be made from birth but this demands accurate knowledge of the normal plasma phosphate level at that age. Now that more is known about the exact gene location, prenatal diagnosis is possible. More than 100 mutations have been described in the *PHEX* gene but only about half of the patients with X-linked hypophosphataemia have a demonstrable mutation.

Hypophosphataemic animal models continue to help in understanding this disorder. The murine *gy* mutation, in which hypophosphataemia is associated with abnormal gyratory movement, has no clear human equivalent. Other renal tubular osteomalacic syndromes include hypophosphataemic osteomalacia presenting in adult life, which may be due to a tumour (see below), inherited and acquired forms of renal tubular acidosis and rickets associated with multiple renal tubular defects, and generalized aminoaciduria (Fanconi's syndrome). Renal tubular acidosis may be proximal or distal, with an inability to resorb bicarbonate or to acidify the urine. The osteomalacia may be cured by giving bicarbonate, alone or with vitamin D. A persistent acidosis with resultant osteomalacia may also result from ureterosigmoid anastomosis. The commonest cause of Fanconi's syndrome in childhood is nephropathic cystinosis, or cystine-storage disease, where there is a widespread deposition of cystine crystals throughout the tissues and in which thirst, polyuria, dehydration, photophobia, and loss of weight begin at about the age of 1 year. The rickets will heal with the correction of the acidosis and the administration of phosphate and 1α-hydroxycholecalciferol; renal transplantation corrects the renal failure and prolongs survival but does not prevent nonrenal complications. Amongst the rare renal tubular defects associated with rickets, mutations in the *CLCN5* chloride channel gene cause Dent's disease (X-linked recessive hypercalciuric nephrolithiasis). In this condition there is also low molecular weight proteinuria, which reflects a failure of endocytosis of these proteins in the brush border of the proximal renal tubule cells; this is normally mediated by the multiligand proteins megalin and cubilin, which are themselves physically associated with CLCN5 but are absent from the brush border in Dent's disease.

Other rare causes of renal tubular rickets and osteomalacia with generalized aminoaciduria are inherited, such as Wilson disease and the X-linked oculocerebral renal syndrome, or acquired, such as multiple myeloma, cadmium poisoning, and the toxic effects of ifosfamide used in the treatment of childhood malignant disease.

Anticonvulsant osteomalacia

In patients treated with anticonvulsants, the incidence of rickets and osteomalacia is higher than normal. This has been attributed to the induction by the anticonvulsants of hepatic enzymes that metabolize vitamin D to biologically inactive derivatives. However, epileptic patients in institutions are often vitamin D deficient because they are also deprived of sunlight; osteomalacia in such patients probably has several causes.

Tumour rickets

An unusual form of hypophosphataemic rickets or osteomalacia, oncogenic rickets or oncogenic osteomalacia, occurs in patients who have mesenchymal tumours, often of a particular histological type, namely sclerosing haemangiopericytomas or nonossifying fibromas. A tumour should be considered in any adult who develops hypophosphataemic osteomalacia, particularly with prominent myopathy. The disorder is improved by oral phosphate and cured by removal of the tumour. The way in which the tumour induces hypophosphataemia and subsequent osteomalacia is unclear but is likely to be multifactorial. Current evidence suggests that it interferes with the renal 1α-hydroxylation of 25OHD, since the circulating levels of 1,25(OH)$_2$D are abnormally low but rapidly return to normal when the tumour is removed. In this form of osteomalacia, an increase in the circulating level of FGF23 has been noted. Precisely how this promotes phosphaturia is incompletely understood but the mechanism appears to involve interactions with a membrane protein known as klotho and an isoform of the FGF receptor 1 expressed in the renal tubule. Oncogenic osteomalacia has also been described in cases of prostatic cancer and in small-cell carcinoma of the lung. Hypophosphataemic osteomalacia also occurs in adults with neurofibromatosis and polyostotic fibrous dysplasia.

Vitamin D dependent rickets (VDDR)

Patients with these very rare, recessively inherited forms of rickets show the features of severe rickets without vitamin D deficiency. There are at least two types of VDDR. In type I VDDR (OMIM 264700), the activity of the renal 1α-hydroxylase is reduced so that the concentration of 1,25(OH)$_2$D is abnormally low. However, it can be increased by large doses of the native vitamin, which shows that the enzyme block is not complete. In type II VDDR (OMIM 277440), there is an end organ resistance to 1,25(OH)$_2$D, which is present in high concentrations, due to mutations in the vitamin D receptor. In both forms, there is severe rickets and myopathy from infancy; in type II VDDR, lifelong total alopecia is a striking feature. Type I VDDR responds to very large doses of vitamin D or physiological doses of 1,25(OH)$_2$D. Type II VDDR may also respond to large doses of vitamin D or its metabolites or to prolonged intravenous calcium, but some recorded cases suggest that recovery occurs spontaneously with age.

Recent work on type II VDDR (otherwise known as hereditary 1,25(OH)$_2$D-resistant) shows that the 1,25(OH)$_2$D receptor defects, which are responsible for the end organ resistance in this disease, are due to a variety of point mutations, either in its steroid- or DNA-binding domains.

Phosphate-deficiency rickets

If patients ingest large amounts of phosphate-binding drugs, such as aluminium hydroxide, a form of hypophosphataemic osteomalacia may develop. This differs clinically from inherited hypophosphataemic osteomalacia by the presence of severe muscle weakness. Other biochemical features include increased calcium absorption with hypercalciuria, associated with an increase above normal in the concentration of 1,25(OH)$_2$D.

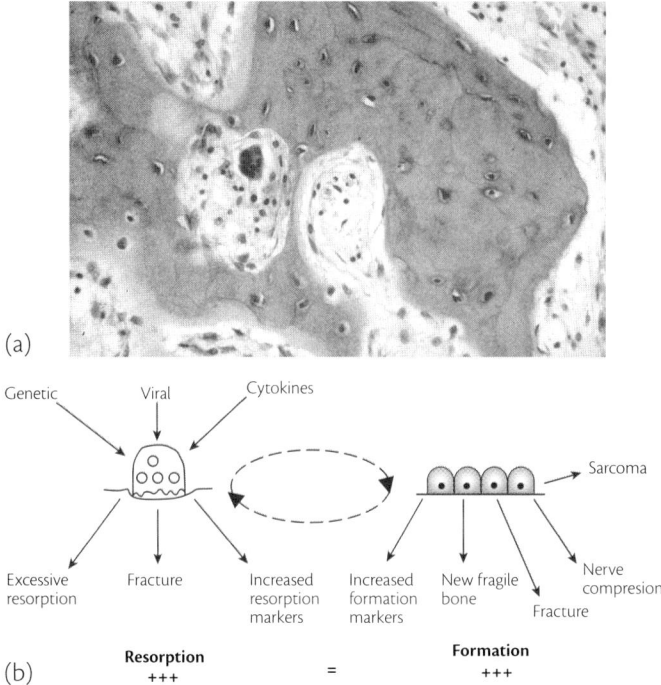

Fig. 20.1.11 Paget's disease of bone. (a) Histological appearance of bone in Paget's disease: cellular activity is increased with many large multinucleated osteoclasts and there is, in addition, fibrosis in the marrow and a mosaic pattern in the mineralized bone; and (b) diagram to show the causes and effects of Paget's disease of bone; the interrupted curves demonstrate the continued 'coupling' of resorption and formation even when cellular activity is very much increased.

Paget's disease of bone

Paget's disease of bone, osteitis deformans, was first described more than a century ago. It is the most common of the so-called metabolic bone diseases after osteoporosis. Its hallmark is excessive and disorganized resorption and formation of bone (Fig. 20.1.11). Its cause is multifactorial, but recent studies on pagetic osteoclasts and genetics studies have provided important insights. The new generation of bisphosphonate drugs now provide highly effective treatment. Rare related disorders include familial expansile osteolysis, expansile skeletal hyperphosphatasia, and idiopathic hyperphosphatasia (juvenile Paget's disease) (see below).

Pathophysiology

Historically there has been great interest in the observations that Paget's disease behaved in many respects like a multicentric neoplasm or a slow virus disease that begins in young adult life. Viruslike inclusion bodies have been seen in the osteoclasts of patients with Paget's disease. Some studies have suggested that various viruses, including measles, respiratory syncytial virus, or canine distemper virus might be involved, but confirmation has been elusive. In contrast, there is now overwhelming evidence of a genetic contribution to Paget's disease, with the most frequent mutation in the gene coding for the ubiquitin-binding protein, sequestosome1, a scaffold protein in the RANK/nuclear factor kappa B signalling pathway. Several related disorders are also caused by genes acting in this pathway. These include familial expansile osteolysis—the *RANK* (*TNFRSF11A*) gene; juvenile Paget's disease (OMIM 602080)—the osteoprotegerin gene (*TNFASF11B*); and inclusion body myopathy with early onset Paget's disease (OMIM

167320)—the clathrin gene (*VCP*). All result in overactivity of the osteoclast.

Histology shows multinucleate osteoclasts that appear to be resorbing bone and busy osteoblasts that appear to be replacing it; these activities are closely linked and both cell types are involved. There is also excess fibrosis in the marrow. The bone matrix is laid down in all directions and loses its birefringence and strength. Mineralization may be defective, probably because of the excessive rate at which the organic bone matrix is laid down. The cement lines and the mosaic appearances of the bone result from the tidemarks of resorption followed by formation. Osteosarcoma, which occurs in Paget's disease, is presumably the result of the excessive and prolonged activity of the bone cells. Pagetic bone is large, vascular, and deformed. Its physical characteristics depend on the stage of the disorder and it may be hard or soft. In any event, it fractures more readily than normal.

Incidence

Paget's disease occurs in about 3% or 4% of subjects over 40 years of age, is more common in men than in women, and its frequency increases with age. It is not unknown in younger people. In the United Kingdom, about 750 000 people may have Paget's disease, of whom fewer than 5% have symptoms. It appears to be a peculiarly Anglo-Saxon affliction, being very rare in Scandinavian countries and Japan. The high frequency of the P392L mutation in *SQSTM1* in familial and sporadic cases of Paget's disease represents strong evidence for a genetic founder effect. Within England, early radiological surveys in the 1970s showed that it occurred most often in Lancashire towns and in northern industrial regions (Table 20.1.10). It is also more frequent in recent British immigrants to Western Australia than in the indigenous population, but less frequent than in those relatives who remained in the United Kingdom. Such studies do not distinguish between the effect of environment and heredity. As many as 40% of individuals may have an affected relative but, clearly, for such a common disease this may often be due to chance. Recent data show a significant reduction in the prevalence of Paget's disease, which emphasizes the importance of (unknown) environmental factors.

Table 20.1.10 Radiological prevalence of Paget's disease in the United Kingdom

Town	Men (%)	Women (%)
Preston	8.6	6.3
Bolton	7.7	6.4
Blackburn	8.8	3.8
Bradford	7.9	3.6
Hull	7.6	3.1
Southampton	6.6	3.6
Bath	5.3	4.7
Stoke	4.7	4.2
York	5.8	2.5

These data are based on more than 500 patients in each town. The age-standardized incidence is always higher in men than in women. The high incidence in Lancashire towns is not explained. Modified from Barker DJP, *et al.* (1977). Paget's disease of bone in 14 British towns. *Br Med J*, **1**, 1181–3. Recent data suggest a decline in radiological prevalence (see Further reading).

Clinical features

Many subjects with Paget's disease have no symptoms.

Pain, deformity, fracture

In Paget's disease, the bone itself may be painful or pain may be due to arthritis of a nearby joint, to an associated fracture, or to the development of sarcoma. It has been suggested that there is a specific type of hip joint disorder associated with Paget's disease. Bone pain could be due to stretching of the periosteum, since this part of the bone (and the vessels within bone) contains nerves sensitive to pain. Clinically, the affected bones are enlarged, deformed, and warm. The enlargement is clearly seen in bones such as the tibia and the skull; in the former, the bone is typically bowed forwards; the latter shows a characteristic enlargement of the vault that is said to look like a soft beret or tam-o'-shanter, which appears to descend over the ears. Other long bones may become bent and a kyphosis may develop. Although any bone can be affected, including the maxilla and the phalanges, the most common sites for Paget's disease are the pelvis and the spine. Fracture may be the first symptom of undiagnosed Paget's disease.

Deafness and nerve compression

Deafness in Paget's disease is one of its most disabling symptoms and responds little to treatment. It has many causes, of which nerve compression is only one.

Most nerves can be compressed by enlarging pagetic bone. The spinal cord is particularly at risk, due to the combined effects of increased bone size, vertebral collapse, and excessive vascularity. Paraplegia or cauda equina lesions may occur. Alterations in the shape of the skull may produce multiple cranial nerve palsies and brainstem lesions, with dysphagia, dysarthria, and ataxia. Basilar invagination with obstruction of cerebrospinal fluid drainage can lead to internal hydrocephalus, raised intracranial pressure, and confusion.

Heart failure

In severe Paget's disease, cardiac output may be increased by the excessive vascularity of the affected bones, but there is no convincing evidence of large arteriovenous shunts within the skeleton. The heart failure that results may be of the high-output variety, but this is excessively rare. Since heart failure and Paget's disease of bone are common in older people, their occurrence together is almost always coincidental.

Associated disorders

Paget's disease is said to be associated with other disorders such as osteoarthritis, gout, vascular calcification, and articular chondrocalcinosis. Since all these occur more often in older people, the associations have little significance.

Investigations

Biochemistry

There is a marked increase in the level of plasma alkaline phosphatase, derived from the overactive osteoblasts, which is roughly related to the extent of clinical and radiological involvement with Paget's disease. In contrast, the acid phosphatase (derived partly from osteoclasts) level is only slightly increased. The rapid turnover of bone matrix collagen increases urinary hydroxyproline (and hydroxylysine) in proportion to the increase in alkaline phosphatase and also the urinary excretion of crosslinked collagen-derived peptides. Plasma calcium and phosphate levels are normal;

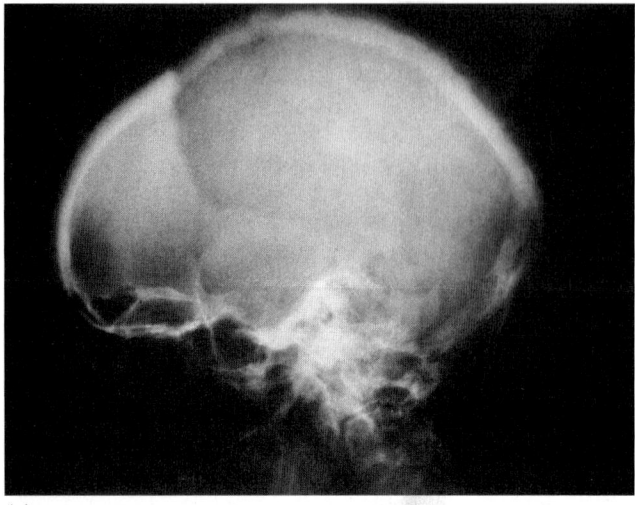

(a)

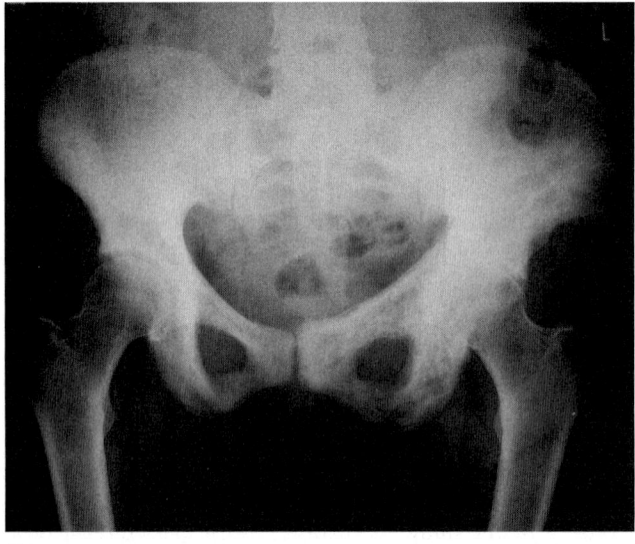

(b)

Fig. 20.1.12 Paget's disease of bone. (a) A resorbing front replacing normal bone in the skull vault, 'osteoporosis circumscripta'; and (b) Paget's disease of the pelvis demonstrating enlargement of the bones and disordered trabecular architecture in the left hemipelvis.

hypercalcaemia suggests coexistent hyperparathyroidism, malignant disease, or immobility.

Radiology

The radiological appearances of Paget's disease are legion. The most characteristic is an increase in size of the affected bone. Resorption predominates early in the disease and in the young patient. A resorbing front may be seen in a long bone or in the skull (Fig. 20.1.12a). Excessive resorption is inevitably followed by disordered bone formation and, at this stage, the bone becomes thick and deformed (Fig. 20.1.12b). In older subjects, the affected bone may be very osteoporotic and liable to fracture. Multiple partial fractures (microfractures, fissure fractures) are common on the deformed convex surface of long bones (see Fig. 20.1.13), particularly the femur and tibia.

The use of bone-scintigraphic agents (such as 99m-technetium-labelled disodium etidronate) has been particularly informative in

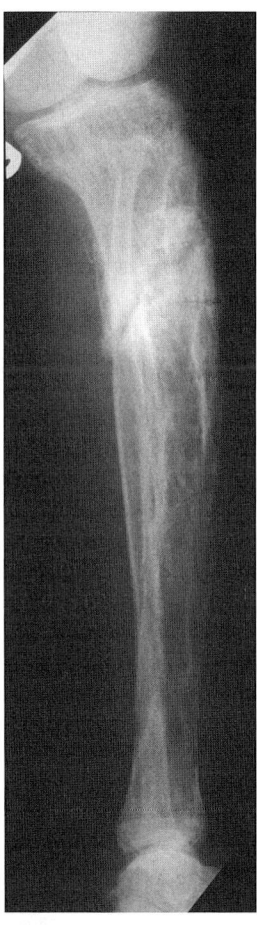

Fig. 20.1.13 Paget's disease of bone. Fissure fractures are seen in the proximal tibia, predominantly on the convex border of the area of grossly abnormal bone.

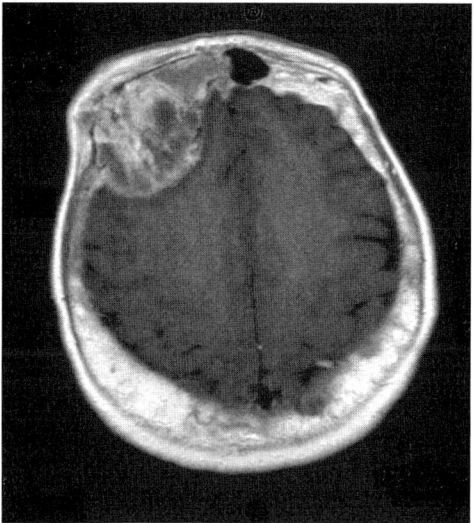

Fig. 20.1.14 Paget's disease of bone. Sarcomatous change in the skull is demonstrated on MRI scan. The presenting symptom was proptosis.

Paget's disease. Affected bones take up the isotope avidly, which demonstrates both the extent of the bone lesions and the effects of treatment. In one study, 180 patients with Paget's disease underwent whole-body scintigraphy and 826 lesions were identified—one-third of the patients had only one lesion and only 10 patients had no symptoms. The increase in plasma alkaline phosphatase and urinary total hydroxyproline was proportional to scintigraphic involvement and patients with skull involvement had the highest values. Apart from the number of sites involved, any distinction between monostotic and polyostotic disease appeared to be artificial.

Diagnosis

The diagnosis of Paget's disease is usually obvious. Bone biopsy is useful to exclude other generalized bone diseases, such as osteomalacia, as well as to confirm Paget's disease. Paget's disease may initially be confused with osteomalacia because of the high plasma alkaline phosphatase level; rarely, an elevated plasma calcium should suggest additional hyperparathyroidism or malignant disease. In prostatic carcinoma with osteoblastic bone secondaries, the dense bones are not enlarged (in contrast to Paget's disease) and the acid phosphatase level is considerably and disproportionately increased in relation to that of alkaline phosphatase. Of many other conditions with similar radiological appearance, fibrous dysplasia (see below), in which the alkaline phosphatase may also be slightly increased, may be difficult to distinguish; in the generalized

form of fibrous dysplasia (polyostotic), the asymmetric bone lesions, skin pigmentation, and sexual precocity (in women) are characteristic. Another very rare disorder usually mistaken for Paget's disease is fibrogenesis imperfecta ossium (see below), where the bone trabeculae are thickened without bony enlargement and there are multiple abnormal fractures.

Sarcoma

The incidence of sarcoma in Paget's disease has sometimes been overestimated in the past; it probably occurs in 1% or less of those with symptoms. Sarcoma should be considered in a patient known to have Paget's disease if pain has developed for the first time, or has worsened, or if deformity has altered. Radiologically, the appearance of the pagetic bone alters, with evidence of bone destruction (Fig. 20.1.14); the tumours occur most often in the medulla. A review of 85 bone sarcomas associated with Paget's disease confirmed the humerus as a high-risk site: rapidly worsening pain was the main symptom; lytic lesions were more common than sclerotic; periosteal reaction was uncommon; and radionuclide bisphosphonate scintigraphy usually showed areas of decreased uptake (contrasting with the underlying pagetic bone).

Treatment

Many patients with Paget's disease require no treatment, but it may be required for symptoms, to suppress the activity of the disease and to prevent its further progress. Indications include bone pain, nerve compression, and the suppression of vascularity before elective orthopaedic surgery. Since medical treatment is now so effective, these indications may be widened especially in young people.

Medical treatment

Patients with painful Paget's disease should first be treated with a simple analgesic. Where possible, it should be determined whether the pain is directly due to the bone disease or to associated arthritis. Specific treatment aimed at the pagetic bone should be considered for those who have pain due to bone disease despite analgesia or who have the complications of deformity, nerve compression, deafness, or, very rarely, heart failure. This treatment should also be considered in the young person with Paget's disease to prevent further progression. There is no evidence that the rapid course of pagetic sarcoma is altered by any treatment. Of the many agents previously tried in Paget's disease, such as aspirin, fluoride, corticosteroids, and mithramycin, only two are currently in use, the bisphosphonates and calcitonin.

The bisphosphonates are a series of compounds with a P–C–P structure resistant to the naturally occurring phosphonates and pyrophosphatases. They are effective both orally and parenterally and reduce excessive bone turnover in Paget's disease. Disodium etidronate, one of the early bisphosphonates, also interferes with mineralization if given in high doses (20 mg/kg body weight); subsequent derivatives such as dichloromethylene diphosphonate (clodronate) and 3-amino-hydroxypropylidene-L,L-bisphosphonate (pamidronate) do not appear to do this. According to their dose, the bisphosphonates may take up to 6 months to produce their effect on symptoms, histology, and biochemistry. Many new bisphosphonates have now been developed based on side-chain substitutions in the basic P–C–P structure. The aminobisphosphonates are particularly effective. These new bisphosphonates are many times more potent than etidronate. They include pamidronate, tiludronate, alendronate, risedronate, ibandronate, and zoledronate. Oral alendronate and intravenous pamidronate are equally effective. They may produce almost complete and permanent suppression of Paget's disease without significant side effects. A single intravenous dose of zoledronate (5 mg) suppresses the overactivity of Paget's disease for at least 2 years, judged biochemically. The long-term effects of such compounds on progression of the bone disease and its complications are unknown. The details of their dose regimes and expected responses are dealt with in larger reviews. One important possible side effect particularly of the powerful intravenous bisphosphonates, is osteonecrosis of the jaw.

Calcitonins are now rarely used for the treatment of Paget's disease. Salmon calcitonin is the most effective commercially available form. Various dose regimens can be used, for which 100 IU given three times a week is average. Injected calcitonin may produce nausea and vomiting; if side effects are troublesome, it is best given in the evening together with an antiemetic. Indications for the use of bisphosphonates and calcitonins are different. Calcitonin is particularly useful to treat bone pain and osteolytic Paget's disease and for preoperative treatment. Some evidence suggests that it may halt the progression of deafness. Spinal cord compression is also alleviated. Thus treatment of eight patients with paraparesis due to pagetic vertebrae with either calcitonin or bisphosphonate produced marked clinical improvement, at least comparable to the results of surgical decompression. Calcitonin can also be given by the nasal route (200 IU daily), which is more acceptable to the patient but less effective.

Surgical treatment

Fractures through pagetic bone require the usual surgical treatment, although union may be delayed. Where fracture occurs through a deformed bone, this deformity should be corrected. In addition, elective osteotomy with intramedullary nailing or Ilizarov correction may be considered for a severe long-bone deformity. Spinal cord compression not responding to medical treatment requires surgery. In patients with hip of spine pathology, diagnostic infiltration of structures such as the hip joints or lumbar nerve roots with local anaesthetic may be valuable. Rarely, hydrocephalus may require a ventriculojugular shunt. Whatever form of surgery is undertaken, it is important that the period of immobility is as short as possible, to avoid the development of hypercalciuria and hypercalcaemia.

Familial expansile osteolysis (OMIM 174810)

This rare condition is similar to Paget's disease. Bone pain from early life is associated with progressive focal expansion in the long bones with pathological fractures. The pelvis and skull are not affected. Hearing loss begins from childhood. Inheritance is autosomal dominant and the activating mutations have been identified in *TNFRSF11A*, the gene encoding RANK that plays a central role in osteoclast differentiation and activation.

Juvenile Paget's disease (OMIM 239000)

This rare condition, which simulates Paget's disease, has autosomal recessive inheritance and is due to homozygous deletion in the TNFRSF11B gene, which encodes osteoprotegerin, the decoy receptor for RANKL (the cognate ligand for RANK). The phenotype is variable but typically there is severe deformity from childhood associated with high bone turnover and a considerable increase in plasma alkaline phosphatase. Treatment with recombinant osteoprotegerin has been shown to be effective in small studies.

Parathyroids and bone disease

Knowledge of the biochemistry of parathyroid hormone has increased so rapidly that it now occupies a large and deserved part of any clinical description of parathyroid disorders (see Chapter 13.6). The close relationship between these endocrine glands and the skeleton has become less obvious with increasing recognition of the many other ways in which parathyroid disease presents. However, primary hyperparathyroidism was first identified because of its effects on bone and only later was it realized that it might more often present with renal stones, pancreatitis, and the signs and symptoms of hypercalcaemia, or that it might be a chance discovery as a result of multichannel biochemical analysis. The subject is discussed further in Chapter 13.6.

Molecular advances

With the discovery of the calcium-sensing receptor and extensive work on the cause of the multiple endocrine neoplasia syndromes, our understanding of the rarer causes of abnormal plasma calcium levels has considerably increased. Thus missense mutations of the *CASR* gene cause both familial benign hypocalciuric hypercalcaemia and neonatal hyperparathyroidism, whereas gain-of-function mutations in this receptor can cause familial hypoparathyroidism. Multiple endocrine neoplasia syndromes have traditionally been divided into two types: type I multiple endocrine neoplasia presents with hyperparathyroidism, pituitary adenomas, insulin- and gastrin-secreting tumours of the pancreas, and gastric hyperacidity (Zollinger–Ellison syndrome); type II, also known as Sipple's syndrome, presents with hyperparathyroidism, medullary carcinoma of the thyroid, and phaeochromocytoma. The molecular elucidation of these differences has identified subgroups. In type I multiple endocrine neoplasia, the principal genetic abnormality involves mutations in the *MEN1* gene together with loss of alleles

Table 20.1.11 The causes of hypercalcaemia according to their frequency

Cause	Disorder
Common	Primary hyperparathyroidism
	Malignant disease
Less common	
Drug induction	Vitamin D toxicity
	Lithium
	Thiazide diuretics
Endocrine	Thyrotoxicosis
	Addison's disease
Granulomatous disease	Sarcoidosis
Immobilization	
Rare	
Drug induction	Milk-alkali syndrome
Endocrine	Familial hypocalciuric hypercalcaemia
Granulomatous disease	Tuberculosis
Others	Lymphoma
	Vitamin A overdosage
	Hypophosphatasia
	Renal failure
	Total parenteral nutrition
	Aluminium intoxication
	Jansen's metaphyseal dysplasia
	Williams' syndrome

From Smith R, Wordsworth P (2006). *Clinical and biochemical disorders of the skeleton.* Oxford University Press, Oxford, with permission.

on chromosome 11; in type II multiple endocrine neoplasia (both A and B subgroups), there are mutations in the *RET* proto-oncogene on chromosome 10.

Hypercalcaemia

Of the known causes of hypercalcaemia in hospital inpatients, neoplasm is the most important (Table 20.1.11). It should always be considered and excluded clinically. The relative frequency of the causes of hypercalcaemia varies according to the population studied. In apparently healthy outpatients, primary hyperparathyroidism is the most frequent cause. In those patients with primary hyperparathyroidism, with hypercalcaemia, hypophosphataemia, hyperphosphatasia, and radiological evidence of osteitis fibrosa, and without clinical evidence of neoplasm, little further investigation is needed. Since only a few patients with hyperparathyroidism have clinical bone disease, further differentiation from other causes of hypercalcaemia is usually necessary. In practice, this means the exclusion of neoplasm, sarcoidosis, thyrotoxicosis, vitamin D overdosage, treatment with lithium or thiazide diuretics, or the 'milk alkali' syndrome. The subject is addressed further in Chapter 13.6.

Secondary (and tertiary) hyperparathyroidism

Where hypocalcaemia is prolonged, as in renal glomerular failure or gluten-sensitive enteropathy, the parathyroid glands increase both their size and activity in an attempt to restore the plasma calcium level to normal. This increases bone resorption and is a particular feature of renal glomerular osteodystrophy. Occasionally hypercalcaemia develops and persists in such patients, despite correction of the underlying disease. It has been proposed that one of the hyperplastic parathyroid glands becomes autonomous and, thus, the label 'tertiary hyperparathyroidism' has been given. Hypercalcaemia may also occur after renal transplantation (see Chapter 21.7.3).

Hypoparathyroidism (see also Chapter 13.6)

Parathyroid insufficiency may occur after surgical removal of the parathyroids, in idiopathic hypoparathyroidism, and in a familial form of hypoparathyroidism that is often associated with manifestations of autoimmune disease, including systemic candidiasis, malabsorption, thyroid and adrenal failure, and pernicious anaemia. In such patients, the levels of immunoreactive PTH are undetectably low but the cAMP response to exogenous PTH is maintained. This distinguishes parathyroid insufficiency from pseudohypoparathyroidism, in which the biochemical features of hypoparathyroidism are associated with characteristic skeletal abnormalities, including short fourth and fifth metacarpals (Albright's hereditary osteodystrophy). Pseudohypoparathyroidism is inherited as an autosomal dominant trait. In the most common form, the cAMP response to exogenous PTH is defective and the circulating level of immunoreactive PTH is high. Patients who have the skeletal manifestations of pseudohypoparathyroidism but with normal biochemistry may be found in families with pseudohypoparathyroidism; to them the term 'pseudopseudohypoparathyroidism' is applied. Investigation has shown that the end organ resistance to parathyroid hormone is due to loss of function mutations in *GNAS1*, which encodes the α-protein subunit of the G_s protein signalling system.

So far as the skeleton is concerned, the most striking changes are found in pseudohypoparathyroidism. Clinical features include intellectual disability, short stature, round face, short neck, and abnormal metacarpals (or metatarsals), of which the most common change is shortness of the third, fourth, and fifth. The bones may be excessively dense, and widespread ectopic calcification and ossification may also occur, in the basal ganglia and the subcutaneous tissues, respectively. Treatment of the hypocalcaemia is the same as for idiopathic hypoparathyroidism, with 1α-hydroxycholecalciferol.

Osteogenesis imperfecta: the brittle bone syndrome

This disorder, which has emerged from the status of an obscure osteopathy to a metabolic bone disease, provides remarkable lessons concerning the effects of mutations in the collagen genes. The correlation between genotype and phenotype is by no means exact and leaves interesting problems.

Osteogenesis imperfecta affects about 1 in 20 000 births; since the milder forms may never be diagnosed, this could be an underestimate. It is a leading cause of lethal short-limbed dwarfism and crippling skeletal dysplasia. There is no convincing evidence of different racial frequency. Many patients with osteogenesis imperfecta do not fit easily into the Sillence classification (Table 20.1.12) and in some cases hypermobility and features of the Ehlers–Danlos syndrome (see below) are dominant.

Table 20.1.12 Clinical classification of osteogenesis imperfecta

Type	Main clinical features	Inheritance	Main biochemical abnormality	Approximate relative frequency (% of all patients)
I	Mild bone fragility, blue sclerae, early-onset deafness, near normal height, normal teeth (IA); dentinogenesis imperfecta (IB)	AD	Non-functional allele for *COL1A1*	60
II	Severe bone disease; multiple fractures; perinatal lethal; dark sclerae; broad long bones (IIA)	AD	Most frequent single base mutations in *COL1A1, COL1A2*, replacing glycine	10
	Ribs show some modelling; small head with proptosis due to shallow orbits (IIB)	AR	Deficient cartilage associated protein (*CRTAP*) required for posttranslational hydroxylation of collagen	(~3% of type II)
	Ribs and long bones thin with many fractures (IIC)			
III	Progressive deforming disorder; scoliosis; very reduced height; sclerae often white	AD, rarely AR	Similar to type II; Very rare absence of α-2(I) chain, leading to α-1(I) trimers	20
IV	Moderate bone disease and deformity; sclerae often white	AD	Mutations often linked to α-2(I) chain	10[a]
Other	Osteogenesis imperfecta with hyperplastic callus (type V)	AD	No collagen mutation detected	Rare
	Osteogenesis imperfecta with excess osteoid (type VI)		No collagen mutation detected	Rare
	Rhizomelic osteogenesis imperfecta (type VII)	AR	Linked to chromosome 3; Deficient cartilage-associated protein (*CRTAP*) as in OI IIB (above)	Very rare
	Type VIII osteogenesis imperfecta	AR	Deficient prolyl-3-hydroxylase	Very rare

AD, autosomal dominant; AR, autosomal recessive.

[a] The frequency of type IV osteogenesis imperfecta is difficult to establish because of its heterogeneity.

Pathophysiology

Osteogenesis imperfecta involves those tissues that contain the main fibrillar collagen, type I. These include particularly bone and dentine, but also the sclerae, joints, tendons, heart valves, and skin. The pathology in bone varies with the type and severity of the disease and with age, previous fracture, and surgery. The skeletal effects of osteogenesis imperfecta are most severe in the lethal forms (type II) and at the region of the growth plate. There is faulty conversion of apparently normal mineralized cartilage to defective bone matrix. The collagen fibres are thin but show the normal striated pattern. The endoplasmic reticulum of the osteoblasts is dilated by retained mutant collagen. The bone structure is completely disorganized and structurally useless. In type III osteogenesis imperfecta, which is less severe, there are variable amounts of woven immature bone, with disorganized trabeculae and an apparent excess of osteocytes—as in other forms of the disorder. At the growth plate, there are multiple islands of cartilage in the epiphyses and metaphyses. Accounts of the bone pathology in type IV are sparse. Defective mineralization is described in a rare form of osteogenesis imperfecta (type VI).

In the so-called mild type I osteogenesis imperfecta, there is a reduction in the amount of bone (and hence in measured bone mineral density) and of defective bone formation at the cellular level, such that the osteoblasts each make approximately half as much bone collagen as normal. The result is an osteoporotic bone with an apparent excess of osteoblasts and osteocytes. This appearance of 'hyperosteocytosis' suggests (to some) an increase in bone turnover rate. The overall bone structure is otherwise normal, apart from occasional woven bone. In affected dentine, the odontoblasts produce short, branched dentinal tubules and fill in the dental pulp. In the ear, the auditory ossicles may be imperfect or fractured.

The reduction in collagen is repeated in nonskeletal tissues. Thus, the sclerae are thin (leading to their blueness since the pigmented coat of the choroid becomes visible), the tendons are gracile and weak, the thin heart valves may become incompetent, and the aortic root dilated.

Clinical features

Type I osteogenesis imperfecta is the most frequent and least serious form and it accounts for 60% of all patients with the disorder. Fractures sometimes occur in the perinatal period but equally may be delayed even until the early menopause. After the menopause, the overall fracture rate has been recorded at seven times more than in the normal population and the vertebral bone mineral content in adults with type I osteogenesis imperfecta is about 70% of normal.

Childhood fractures in type I osteogenesis imperfecta may be numerous but rarely lead to deformity unless treated inappropriately. Any type of fracture can occur but they become less frequent with age. Overall, fractures are more frequent in the lower limbs. Significant scoliosis is rare. The skull shows interesting changes; in addition to multiple Wormian bones (Fig. 20.1.15) (which can occur in other disorders, such as pycnodysostosis, cleidocranial dysostosis, Menkes' syndrome, Prader–Willi syndrome, progeria, and, rarely, in normal subjects), the vault may overhang the base, leading to basilar impression requiring surgical correction.

Clinical dentinogenesis imperfecta occurs in only some patients; the appearance varies widely and affects some teeth more than others; the teeth are discoloured and the enamel (which is normal) fractures easily from the dentine, leading to rapid erosion of both the first and second dentition. Blueness of the sclerae is a particularly

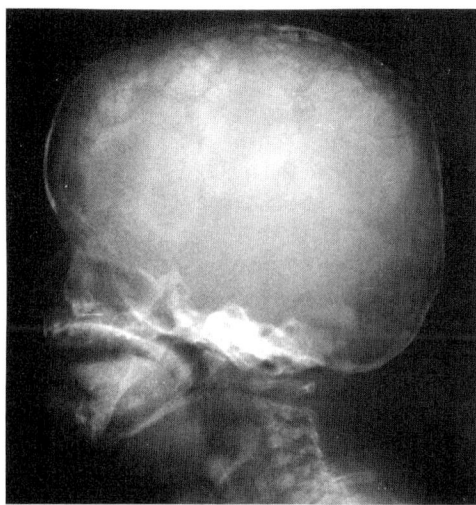

Fig. 20.1.15 Osteogenesis imperfecta. Innumerable centres of ossification are found in the vault of the skull (Wormian bones) in an infant with severe deforming (type III) osteogenesis imperfecta. Wormian bones are usually most obvious in the occipital region.

important physical sign of osteogenesis imperfecta. The cause of the frequently early (juvenile) arcus is unknown: limited investigation excludes hypercholesterolaemia. The cardiac manifestations of osteogenesis imperfecta are also important, not only because of their effects but because tissue fragility makes surgery dangerous. Aortic incompetence, aortic root widening, and mitral valve prolapse all occur. Patients with osteogenesis imperfecta often show hypermobility of joints, with resultant flat feet, hyperextensible large joints, and dislocation.

Type II osteogenesis imperfecta is nearly always lethal, but the severity does differ: some children may be born dismembered, whereas others may (rarely) survive the perinatal period to later merge into the type III form. Not all infants with multiple fractures at birth succumb immediately. It is possible to give a prognosis

from the extent of ossification of the skull, the shape of the long bones and ribs, and the number of fractures. In the most frequent form of lethal osteogenesis imperfecta (IIA), the infant is short with disproportionately short and deformed limbs, the skull is deformed and soft, and the sclerae are often deep grey blue. Whole-body radiographs, which distinguish osteogenesis imperfecta from other forms of lethal short-limbed dwarfism, show grossly defective mineralization of the skull, short broad limbs with multiple fractures, and broad ribs with innumerable fractures (Fig. 20.1.16). In type IIB, the ribs have some structure; in IIC, the long bones are narrow and beaded at the site of fractures and show some evidence of modelling. Perinatal death results from the mechanical uselessness of the skeleton, which leads to respiratory failure or intracranial haemorrhage.

Type III osteogenesis imperfecta causes most clinical difficulty, since the disability is severe and progressive. During the early years of life, progressive deformity affects the skull, the long bones, and the spine, chest, and pelvis; the deformity is associated with fractures but can probably occur without them. The radiological appearance of the bones changes rapidly with age. The face appears triangular, with a large vault, prominent eyes, and small jaw. The sclerae may be blue in infancy but take on a normal colour in childhood. Eventual disability and deformity is considerable. Such patients rarely walk, even after multiple operations, and have a very short stature (4–6 standard deviations below the mean). The changes in the long bones are often bizarre, with long, thin diaphyses and comparatively wide metaphyses. Cartilaginous islands often develop at the end of the long bones in the epiphyses and the metaphyses, spreading into the diaphysis, giving the appearance of 'popcorn' bone. Early death may occur from respiratory infections superimposed on the restrictive reduction in vital capacity associated with severe lordoscoliosis (Fig. 20.1.17). Progressive deformity requires specialized orthopaedic care.

Type IV osteogenesis imperfecta is clinically intermediate between type I and type III and is inherited as a dominant trait. The sclerae are of normal colour after infancy. Overall stature is reduced and disability is variable. The rare complication of hyperplastic callus occurs most often in this form (Fig. 20.1.18). This begins with a swollen, painful, and vascular swelling, most often

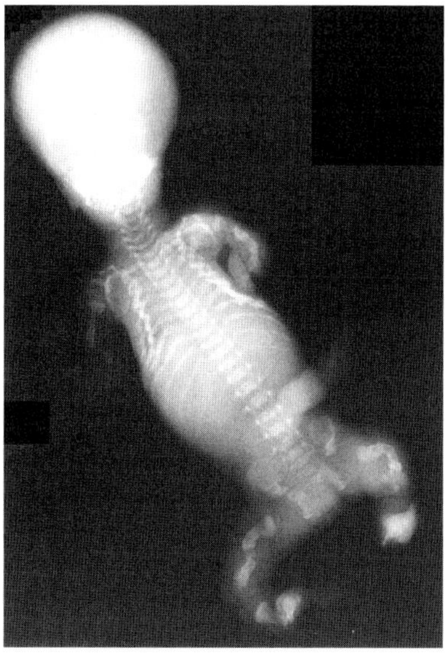

Fig. 20.1.16 Whole-body perinatal radiograph of lethal (type II) osteogenesis imperfecta. The vault of the skull is not calcified and the ribs and long bones show multiple fractures. There was no family history.

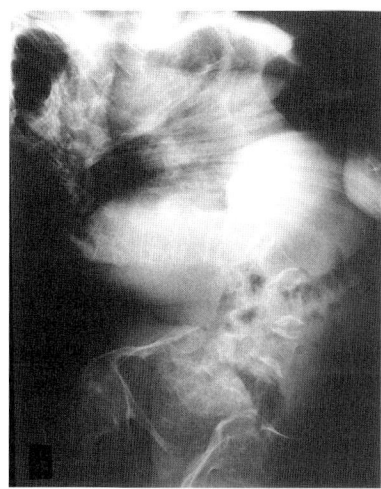

Fig. 20.1.17 Severe lordoscoliosis in type III osteogenesis imperfecta.

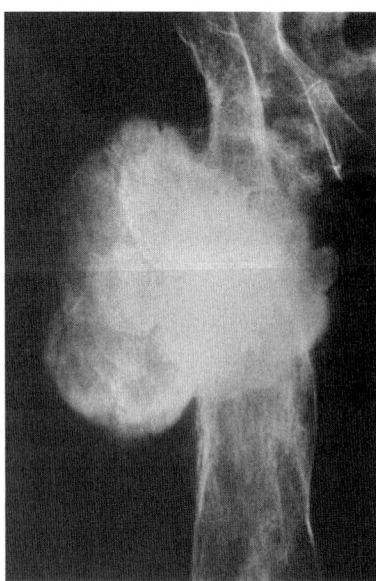

Fig. 20.1.18 The radiological appearance of hyperplastic callus in osteogenesis imperfecta (type V). The densely mineralized mass is recent. The apparently thickened femoral shaft is probably due to incorporation of previous episodes of excess callus formation.

over the long bones, an increase in plasma alkaline phosphatase, and, sometimes, a systemic illness. Recent investigations of osteogenesis imperfecta-affected families with hyperplastic callus have failed to find collagen mutations in affected children. Some classify this form as type V osteogenesis imperfecta (Table 20.1.12).

Other rare forms of brittle bone disease have been recently characterized. These include: type VI in which there is excess osteoid and indeterminate inheritance; type VII, a recessive rhizomelic form with coxa vara, minimally blue sclerae, congenital fractures, and major ambulatory problems in adulthood; and type VIII, a severe/lethal autosomal recessive variant with white sclerae, round face, and barrel chest. No distinguishing mutations have been found for type VI, but in type VII there are mutations in *CRTAP*, which encodes cartilage associated protein that is part of a complex that includes cyclophilin B and *P3H1*, which encodes prolyl-3-hydroxylase 1 that is required for the prolyl-3-hydroxylation of collagen. Mutations in this gene can also cause the recessive lethal type IIB, accounting for 3% of all lethal cases. Finally, type VIII is caused by mutations in *P3H1* that leads to abnormal posttranslational modification of collagen.

Diagnosis

In the perinatal period, the concern is with alternative causes of lethal, short-limbed dwarfism. These include severe hypophosphatasia (see below), achondrogenesis (see below), thanatophoric dwarfism, and the asphyxiating thoracic dystrophies. A perinatal whole-body radiograph is essential.

In the first few years of life, nonaccidental injury, 'battered baby syndrome', is the main differential diagnosis. This is suggested by multiple fractures at different sites and of different ages, especially if associated with clinical signs of neglect. Some fractures, such as metaphyseal 'corner' fractures and posterior rib fractures, are more often seen in nonaccidental injury, but any type of fracture can occur in osteogenesis imperfecta. The distinction between osteogenesis imperfecta and nonaccidental injury is legally important and can be difficult.

Idiopathic juvenile osteoporosis needs to be distinguished during late childhood and adolescence. This begins during growth, with fractures of the long bones, reduction in growth rate (due to vertebral collapse), and metaphyseal compression fractures. In adult life, mild osteogenesis imperfecta may go unrecognized.

In the recessively inherited osteoporosis pseudoglioma syndrome, there is severe osteoporosis leading to fracture and near blindness from infancy. This very rare disease used to be classified as a form of osteogenesis imperfecta. It is now known to result from mutations in the *LRP5* gene (Table 20.1.1).

Biochemistry

It is impossible to generalize about the clinical effect of a collagen gene mutation but some patterns are emerging. In type I osteogenesis imperfecta, there appears to be a null allele for collagen type I, so that only 50% of collagen is produced but this is of normal composition. Lethal osteogenesis imperfecta (type II) results most commonly from single base changes in *COL1A1* or *COL1A2*. Such changes convert a glycine codon to one for another amino acid with a side chain. The effect on the triple helix of incorporating such a mutant chain appears to be most marked when the substitution occurs near the C-terminal end of the chain (the helix winds up from this end), when the substituting amino acid is large, and when it occurs in the α-1 rather than the α-2 chain. Such mutations delay helix formation and render collagen mechanically unsound by causing overhydroxylation and overmodification of the lysine residues, which is detectable by the slowing and widening of the α-chains run on conventional polyacrylamide gels. Such abnormalities are common in type II osteogenesis imperfecta and less well defined in type III, which may rarely result from a failure to synthesize α-2 chains. Type IV osteogenesis imperfecta is more often due to changes in the α-2 chain. Such information can provide the basis for accurate prenatal diagnosis using fetal DNA derived from a chorionic villus biopsy. Mutations in *COL1A1* or *COL1A2* can be found in up to 90% of individuals with osteogenesis imperfecta in specialist centres using DNA sequencing methods and in about 80% using protein chemistry, thereby allowing more definitive diagnosis to be achieved in many cases.

Genetic advice

Parents who have already had an infant with osteogenesis imperfecta need accurate advice about further pregnancies. This can be difficult, because the facts are not clear. Where the mutant gene is dominant (type I and IV) and where one parent is affected, the likelihood of affected children is 50%. Difficulties arise where neither parent is clinically affected and with the lethal and progressive deforming varieties of the brittle bone syndrome. It is impossible to give a statistically accurate prediction of the likelihood of another affected child, particularly since the strict application of mendelian principles may be inappropriate because of the possibility of germline and somatic cell mosaicism. However, there are some guidelines. Where one offspring of clinically unaffected parents has a form of osteogenesis imperfecta that fits into type I or type IV, this is likely to be a new dominant mutation (50% of whose offspring will be affected) and the risk of a further affected sibling is little more than in the general population. It used to be considered that infants with the severe lethal form of osteogenesis imperfecta (type II) had inherited a mutant gene from both clinically normal parents and were, therefore, homozygous recessives, so that the risk of a further affected infant was 25%. The evidence is now that the great majority of cases (but not all) result from a new autosomal dominant (and lethal) mutation. It is now clear that some (~3%) lethal forms of the disease (type IIB) are recessively inherited due to *CRTAP* mutations (see above). These have some phenotypic differences from the more common type IIA (caused by collagen type I mutations), including relatively small head circumference, a degree of proptosis due to shallow orbits and relatively normal coloured sclerae. Such clinical features may help to raise the suspicion of an unusual phenotype and prompt a detailed genotypic analysis. To allow for the possibility of some recessives, the likelihood of phenotypically normal parents having a second baby with lethal osteogenesis imperfecta is often put empirically at approximately 7% (more than normal, but significantly less than 25%).

The precise recurrence risk in progressively deforming osteogenesis imperfecta is unknown and sometimes difficult to predict. A small minority of cases are recessively inherited and the overlap between types III, IV, VII, and VIII does generate some confusion. Most cases are felt to represent new dominant mutations in *COL1A1* or *COL1A2* (with a correspondingly low recurrence risk) but the possibility of recessive mutations in *CRTAP* or *P3H1* should be considered and, if confirmed, would correspond to a recurrence risk of 25%.

It is now also recognized that germline and somatic-cell mosaicism are important factors in the inheritance and expression of osteogenesis imperfecta and probably in many other disorders. In brief, germline mosaicism means that the spermatozoa or ova of an apparently normal person may contain a proportion of mutant genes for lethal or other forms of osteogenesis imperfecta. This accounts for those pedigrees where a phenotypically normal man has two or more babies with lethal osteogenesis imperfecta by separate partners. Somatic mosaicism, with variable proportions of mutant cells in different tissues, likewise provides one (but not the only) explanation for phenotypic variability and differing tissue expression. The many factors that control the regulated expression of the vertebrate collagen genes in different tissues are only partly understood.

Prenatal diagnosis

This may be done by analysis of fetal DNA from a chorionic villus biopsy in the first trimester and by ultrasound examination and appropriate radiographs from the second trimester. The appropriateness of such an investigation depends on the information previously available. In a dominantly inherited form of osteogenesis imperfecta, analysis of DNA from affected and unaffected family members can establish linkage to a particular collagen gene polymorphism. In such a situation, analysis of chorionic villus DNA is the most direct approach. Alternatively, the cells from such a biopsy may be cultured and the synthesized collagen examined for abnormalities. Where the collagen mutation is known in a previously affected family member, this method may directly confirm the presence of the mutation in the fetus. Except in well-organized laboratories, culture of cells and analysis of collagen will introduce unacceptable delays. Further, it is usually not possible to exclude an affected fetus merely on the grounds of apparently normal collagen since these techniques are only 80% sensitive even in the

best hands. The rapid direct detection of the mutation in DNA from the chorionic villus is an eventual aim and offers a sensitivity of about 90%.

Amniocentesis also provides amniocytes for DNA linkage analysis and mutation detection. Amniotic fluid cells tend to produce an α-1(I) homotrimer and are not, therefore, appropriate for collagen analysis.

Diagnosis by ultrasound examination is possible only in the more severe forms of osteogenesis imperfecta (types II and III). Since the severe forms of osteogenesis imperfecta are sporadic and therefore unsuspected, it is important to be able to detect them early and rapidly by routine scanning. Ultrasonographic features suggestive of osteogenesis imperfecta are shortness and deformity of the limbs, an abnormal skull shape with lack of mineralization, which makes the intracranial structures abnormally visible, and deformity of the ribs leading to a 'champagne cork' appearance on the anteroposterior projection.

Prognosis and management

For an infant born with manifest osteogenesis imperfecta, important questions are asked: how long will he or she survive; and what will be the likelihood of further offspring being affected? The immediate prognosis may already be answered by perinatal death, so that it remains to deal with the prognosis of survivors. Not all born with multiple fractures succumb immediately and radiographic appearances can give a good guide to outcome.

It is in those severely affected survivors that are classified as type III that management will be a lifelong and specialized problem. Such individuals are of normal intelligence and prolonged admission to hospital, either for repeated surgery or for investigation, should not necessarily take precedence over education. Intramedullary rodding and osteoclasis to correct deformity and improve mobility should be very selective since the bones are often so abnormal as to take no advantage from such procedures. An organized programme of rehabilitation is important. Analysis of life expectancy and cause of death in osteogenesis imperfecta shows that survival is normal in type I osteogenesis imperfecta and near-normal in type IV. It is those with type III who have the shortest lifespan and the most disability, of which basilar impression with neurological complications is a newly recognized problem. There is no convincing evidence that fluoride or calcitonin is beneficial, but the use of cyclic intravenous pamidronate is a considerable advance to alleviate symptoms, increase bone density, and reduce fracture rate particularly in severe osteogenesis imperfecta. The indications for the use of pamidronate in osteogenesis imperfecta and the reasons why it is effective in a disorder that is primarily due to osteoblast failure have yet to be agreed. Observational studies of oral bisphosphonates in milder forms of osteogenesis imperfecta also show beneficial effects on bone density. Attempts to transplant normal stromal cells from bone marrow into severely affected infants with osteogenesis imperfecta have also been reported.

Marfan's syndrome (see Chapter 20.2) (OMIM 154700)

Marfan's syndrome is most often regarded as an inherited disorder of connective tissue rather than as a metabolic bone disease. Where connective tissue disorders significantly affect the skeleton, this distinction is blurred. For many years, it was thought that the basic defect in Marfan's syndrome involved collagen but this was excluded by the demonstration of pathogenic mutations in *FBN1*, encoding fibrillin 1, one of the major components of the 10 nm microfibrils found in elastic tissues. However, any suggestion that Marfan's syndrome merely represents a simple structural failure of these tissues due to defective fibrillin has subsequently proved too simplistic. Recent research has implicated deranged TGFβ signalling with resultant abnormal elastic fibre genesis and, to bring the wheel full circle, excessive rather than reduced collagen in the affected tissues.

Pathophysiology

It is now recognized that Marfan's syndrome is most often caused by mutations in the epidermal growth factor-like regions of *FBN1*. Fibrillin is the major constituent of the microfibrillar system and of the suspensory ligament of the lens, and it is also associated with elastin-containing tissues such as the aorta. This explains the association between dislocation of the lens and dissection of the aorta. The aorta dilates at its proximal part at the sinuses of Valsalva and returns to normal diameter below the innominate artery, unless a dissection is present. The cusps of the aortic valve do not close efficiently. Dissection is most often above the aortic valves in the area of greatest dilatation. The dissection may progress forwards or backwards. Retrograde dissection may tear the attachment of the coronary arteries and rupture into the pericardial sac. Histopathology shows a reduction in elastic fibres, which are swollen and fragmented. The valve cusps are usually diaphanous and redundant. In the eye, the suspensory ligament of the lens is disorganized. Other aspects of the condition have always been more difficult to explain; the tall stature, dysmorphic facial features, reduced muscle mass, and abnormalities of the lung architecture mimicking emphysema are more suggestive of an abnormality of growth and development, not easily attributable to fibrillin at first glance.

Most of the *FBN1* mutations described in the Marfan's syndrome are consistent with qualitative or quantitative defects of fibrillin; many of the observed clinical abnormalities, such as aortic aneurysm and lens dislocation, can also be understood on this basis. However, it is increasingly apparent that the capacity of fibrillin to bind to TGFβ also plays a key role in several clinical features, such as the growth disturbance, vascular fragility, and other developmental abnormalities found in the Marfan's syndrome and related disorders. TGFβ commonly exists in an inactive form bound to latent TGFβ binding protein in the extracellular matrix of many tissues, which binds particularly to the epidermal growth factor-like domain of fibrillin, thereby targeting TGFβ to fibrillin-containing tissues and maintaining it in the inactive state. The loss of fibrillin microfibrils in Marfan's syndrome causes an increase in the amount of active TGFβ present in these tissues; this can lead to the generation of abnormal matrix in the elastic tissues of the aorta, abnormal septation of the developing lung alveoli, and abnormal muscle mass. In the *fbn1* knockout mouse model of Marfan's syndrome, these phenotypic effects can be reversed by using neutralizing antibodies to TGFβ. There is also substantial interest in the use of angiotensin II type 1 receptor blockers, such as losartan, since these have clinically relevant TGFβ antagonism. Encouraging results from animal studies have led to the establishment of trials of these agents in humans, the results of which are awaited with considerable interest.

Table 20.1.13 Major and minor organ involvement in Marfan's syndrome (Ghent criteria 1996)

Organ	Feature
Major involvement	
Eye	Lens dislocation
Cardiovascular	Aortic dilatation >2 standard deviations above mean (including sinus of Valsalva)
	Dissection of ascending aorta
Dura	Lumbo-sacral dural ectasia by MRI or CT
Skeleton (4/8 criteria)	Pectus carinatum
	Severe pectus excavatum
	Reduced upper body:lower body ratio (≤0.86) or excessive arm span:height ratio (≥1.05)
	Wrist and thumb signs
	Scoliosis >20° or spondylolisthesis
	Elbow contracture (≥15°)
	Pes planus with medial displacement of medial malleolus
	Protrusio acetabuli
Family history	Unequivocal clinical evidence of Marfan's syndrome in first-degree relative
Genetics	Linkage in family to *FBN1* or *FBN1* mutation known to be associated with Marfan's syndrome
Minor involvment	
Musculoskeletal	Moderate pectus excavatum
	Joint hypermobility (Beighton score ≥4/9)
	High arched palate and dental crowding
	Typical facial appearance
Ocular	Flat cornea (by optometry)
	Increased axial length of globe (by ultrasonography)
	Hypoplastic iris
Cardiovascular	Mitral valve prolapse ± regurgitation
	Dilated main pulmonary artery (<40 yrs)
	Calcification of mitral annulus (<40 yrs)
	Dilated/dissected descending thoracic/ abdominal aorta (<50 yrs)
Pulmonary	Spontaneous pneumothorax
	Apical blebs on chest radiograph
Skin	Striae not associated with weight change, physical stress, pregnancy (typically over shoulders and lumbar region)
	Recurrent or incisional hernias

Involvement of two major components plus at least one minor component equates with a diagnosis of Marfan's syndrome. See also Fig. 20.1.19.

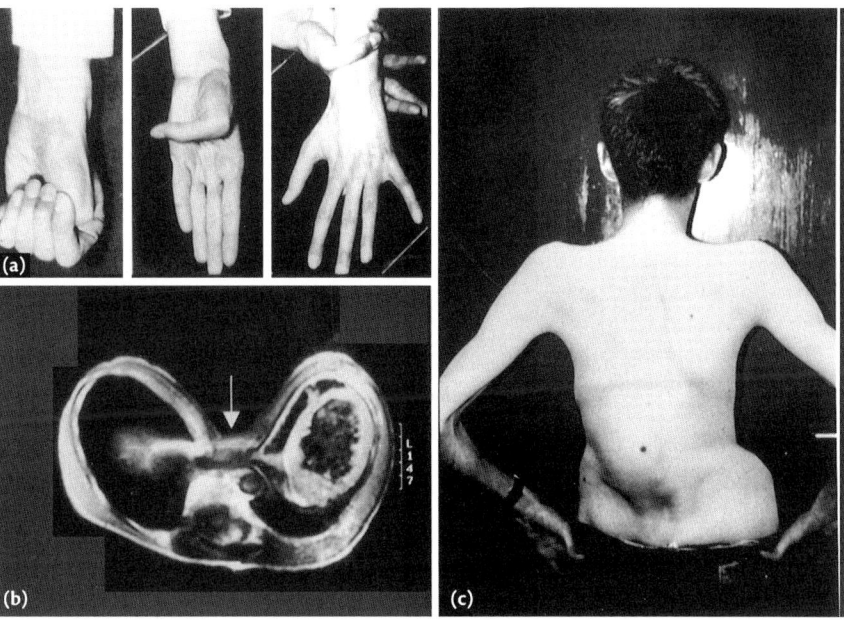

Fig. 20.1.19 Some of the characteristic major musculoskeletal criteria for Marfan's syndrome. (a) Positive wrist and thumb signs; (b) MRI showing severe pectus excavatum; and (c) severe localized thoracolumbar scoliosis.

Clinical features

Marfan's syndrome is dominantly inherited. Its main effects are on the skeleton, cardiovascular, and ocular systems (Table 20.1.13). There is considerable phenotypic variation. In the typical patient with Marfan's syndrome, overall height is increased (relative to unaffected siblings or a matched population) and the limbs are long relative to the trunk (so that the crown to pubis measurement is markedly less than pubis to heel). Long, thin fingers (arachnodactyly) are common. Together with hypermobility, this disproportion forms the basis of clinical signs of variable utility. However, not all patients with Marfan's syndrome are long and thin. The skeletal phenotype differs from one family to another and also differs within families. Asymmetric anterior chest deformity is associated with either depression or prominence of the sternum. Scoliosis is common, may be severe, and worsens during preadolescent growth as in the idiopathic form (Fig. 20.1.19). The hard palate is often narrow and high-arched (gothic), leading to dental crowding.

Dislocation of the lens is the main ocular feature of Marfan's syndrome (Fig. 20.1.20). Typically, this occurs upwards or sideways (somewhat in contrast to the downward dislocation often seen in homocystinuria) and it may be present at birth or occur later, but it rarely becomes apparent for the first time after 10 years of age. Dislocation causes the unsupported iris to wobble on movement (iridodonesis). Other important ocular features are myopia and retinal detachment. The axial length of the globe is increased and the cornea tends to be flattened (keratoconia).

The most severe complication of Marfan's syndrome is dilatation of the ascending aorta leading to aortic incompetence and dissection. Progressive widening of the aorta can be readily measured by serial echocardiography. Less serious manifestations of Marfan's syndrome include cutaneous striae, hernias, spontaneous pneumothorax, and dural ectasia. The mean life expectancy in those with Marfan's syndrome is significantly reduced, predominantly due to cardiovascular catastrophe. However, elective cardiac surgery has considerably improved the outlook for those at greatest risk. It is difficult to estimate the overall reduction in life expectancy given that milder variants of the condition are now recognized and that previous estimates suggesting a 50% reduction were based on patients with particularly severe and largely untreated disease.

Diagnosis

At present, even with the best biochemical and DNA techniques, there is no absolutely certain way of excluding or confirming Marfan's syndrome. In those with few clinical features and no family history, the diagnosis of Marfan's syndrome can still be difficult. Formal assessment of the musculoskeletal system should be undertaken to identify major criteria for the disease (often including full length radiographs of the spine to detect less severe forms of scoliosis and pelvic radiographs to identify acetabular protrusion). Slit lamp examination of the eye is essential to exclude minor degrees of lens subluxation (formal optometry is in practice rarely required); MRI of the lumbar spine and chest is often valuable to detect dural ectasia and to obtain accurate measurements of the aortic root; and two-dimensional echocardiography should be

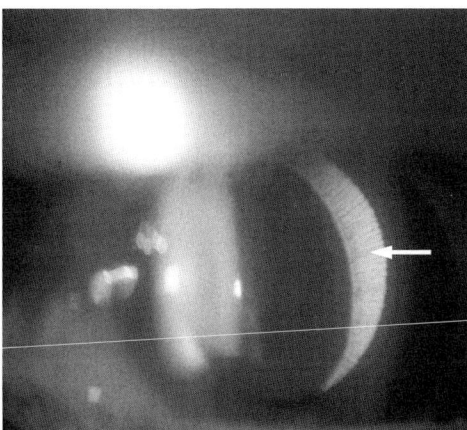

Fig. 20.1.20 Marfan's syndrome showing dislocation of the ocular lens (slit-lamp appearance). The redundant strands of the suspensory ligament are shown (arrows).

undertaken routinely in those suspected of having Marfan's syndrome and forms the basis of routine cardiology follow up (with increased frequency during pregnancy).

The requirements for the diagnosis of Marfan's syndrome have been revised (Ghent criteria 1996) (Table 20.1.13). Where the family history is not helpful, it is necessary to have major involvement of at least two different organ systems and at least minor involvement of a third. Where there is an unequivocally affected relative or an *FBN1* mutation known to cause Marfan's syndrome has been detected, major involvement of one organ system with minor involvement of a second is sufficient for the diagnosis. The criteria have now been further revised to place additional emphasis on cardiac and ocular manifestations in the Brussels criteria (Loeys *et al.* 2010). Homocystinuria (see below), which has a recessive mode of inheritance, should be excluded. Other important alternative diagnoses include congenital contractural arachnodactyly (Beal's syndrome), familial tall stature, isolated mitral valve prolapse, familial or isolated annuloaortic ectasia, and Stickler's syndrome (see under chondrodysplasias). The latter is a dominantly inherited connective tissue disorder that affects the eyes, ears, and skeleton with severe myopia in childhood, sensorineural hearing loss from adolescence, and degenerative arthritis from early adult life. The diagnosis can be made at birth if cleft palate and micrognathia are present. There is considerable phenotypic variation. In some families the disorder is linked to the collagen type II gene and in others to collagen type XI.

Contractures can occur in Marfan's syndrome but are of a late onset. In congenital contractural arachnodactyly, which is inherited as an autosomal dominant trait, contractures involving the hands, feet, and larger joints are present from birth and tend to improve. Abnormal ears are described and developmental abnormalities, such as duodenal atresia or structural cardiac defects, are more common than in Marfan's syndrome. This disorder results from mutations in another fibrillin gene, *FBN2*, on chromosome 5.

Of particular importance is a group of disorders related to Marfan's syndrome in which there may also sometimes be demonstrable *FBN1* mutations, but which do not necessarily carry the same adverse cardiac prognosis. These include the following in which there is major organ involvement of one system but not others: isolated ectopia lentis, isolated Marfan's-like body habitus, and familial thoracic aneurysm. In contrast, some individuals exhibit an array of minor signs often associated with Marfan's syndrome but do not have the MASS phenotype (major involvement of any system; typically including mitral valve prolapse, aorta in the upper end of the normal range, minor skeletal signs, and striae). It is important to recognize individuals that do not exhibit the MASS phenotype since they probably have an altogether milder condition that can usually be distinguished from Marfan's syndrome and does not carry the same adverse consequences for health or insurance.

Finally, it has recently been recognized that certain individuals, previously thought to have atypical forms of Marfan's syndrome, have a quite separate condition now known as Loeys–Dietz syndrome (OMIM 609192). This is characterized clinically by aortic aneurysms, generalized arterial tortuosity, hypertelorism, cleft palate, and bifid uvula; it is caused by mutations in the TGFβ receptor genes (*TGFBR1* or *TGFBR2*), which alter TGFβ signalling, with implications for extracellular matrix biology, including disarray of elastic fibres and excessive collagen.

Treatment

There is no specific treatment yet for the underlying defect, but many of the clinical manifestations require attention. Scoliosis may be progressive and severe, particularly in adolescence. Bracing is largely ineffective and operative stabilization may be necessary. Excessive height in girls may be prevented by giving oestrogen together with progestogen in the prepubertal years. Marked sternal deformity may need correction for cosmetic or cardiopulmonary reasons, but opinions on the value of surgery vary widely. The potential conflict between anterior chest wall surgery undertaken for largely cosmetic reasons and the subsequent need for cardiac surgery for aortic disease is one clear example. In the eyes, it is rarely necessary to remove dislocated lenses unless they prolapse into the anterior chamber, but myopia should be corrected. The main decisions concern the management of the cardiovascular problems: when and if to operate on the dilated ascending aorta or to replace incompetent valves, and whether aortic dilatation can be prevented by reducing the intermittent force on its walls due to left ventricular systole. As far as the second point is concerned, giving a β-blocker such as atenolol reduces the rate of aortic dilatation to some extent although the results in individual cases are highly variable. As regards surgery on the aorta, it is clear that progressive aortic widening (measured regularly by echocardiography), together with progressive aortic incompetence and left ventricular strain, provides strong indications for surgery of the proximal aorta. There is substantial debate about the timing and nature of the surgery that should be undertaken and whether the aortic valve can be preserved in those undergoing surgery to protect the aortic arch. However, it is evident that the risk of dissection or rupture increases dramatically when the maximum proximal aortic root diameter rises to 5.5 cm or more; in these circumstances, prophylactic surgery is usually justified. Mitral valve replacement may also be necessary and it is more commonly required in children then aortic surgery. There are some encouraging early results from the use of angiotensin inhibition from small studies. However, it remains to be demonstrated whether these agents have a major role to play in prophylaxis against cardiovascular complications of the disease (see above). Large trials care in progress.

Since both aortic and mitral valves are susceptible to endocarditis, prophylactic antimicrobials must be given at the time of dentistry in those with audible murmurs.

Genetic advice

Genetic advice is at present based on clinical observations and the knowledge that inheritance is of the autosomal dominant pattern. Numerous mutations in the fibrillin genes have now been described, allowing the application of DNA based techniques for prenatal diagnosis where it is required. However, 30% of cases arise from new dominant mutations and the possibility of parental mosaicism should be remembered. There is no clear relationship between genotype and phenotype although mutations occurring between exons 20 and 28 of *FBN1* tend to be associated with more severe disease. Where there is a suspicion of Loeys–Dietz syndrome or an overlapping phenotype, sequential analysis of *FBN1*, *TGFBR2*, and *TGFBR1* is justified.

Ehlers–Danlos syndrome (see Chapter 20.2)

Ehlers–Danlos syndrome (EDS) initially included only those conditions with the common clinical features of abnormal velvety

Table 20.1.14 Classification and main features of the different Ehlers–Danlos syndromes (note that only types VI and VII have significant effects on the skeleton)

Villefranche classification (1997)	Main features	Inheritance	Collagen or other gene affected	Biochemistry	Former classifications
Classic	Hyperextensible skin; hypermobile joints; wide atrophic scars	AD	V	Haploinsufficiency of collagen type V usually	Types I & II, gravis and mitis
Hypermobility	Marked hypermobility of joints	variable	Usually known Sometimes I	Not known	Type III, joint hypermobility
Vascular type	Rupture of middle-sized arteries, also bowel and uterus; premature aging in some	AD	III	Abnormal collagen type III synthesis, secretion or structure	Type IV, arterial (Sack Barabas)
Oculoscoliotic type	Scoliosis; fragile eyes with keratoconus	AR		Lysyl hydroxylase deficiency	Type VI, oculoscoliotic
Arthrochalasis	Congenital dislocation of the hips; short stature	AD	I	Exon 6 deletion; removes cleavage site for N-terminal peptide from collagen type I	Type VIIA and B
Dermatosparaxis	Severe fragility; osteoporosis	AR	I	Procollagen type I N-protease deficiency	Type VIIC
Occipital horn syndrome[a]	Soft skin; bladder diverticula; occipital horns	XLR	ATP7A	Defective Cu^{2+} transporting ATPase; secondary defect of Cu-dependent lysyl oxidase	Type IX, EDS with occipital horns
Fibronectin defect[a]	Similar to type II EDS	AR		Fibronectin defect	Type X
Tenascin X deficiency[a]	Similar to EDS II but without atrophic scars	AR	TNXB	Absence of tenascin-X	

AD, autosomal dominant; AR, autosomal recessive; EDS, Ehlers–Danlos syndrome; XLR, X-linked recessive.
[a] These types are not formally included in the 1997 classification.

hyperelastic skin that healed poorly, hyperextensible joints, and lax ligaments. However, the disorders included in this syndrome have now been increased and have brought with them additional specific features, amongst which is vascular rupture, especially in type IV (vascular) EDS, associated with various mutations in collagen type III (OMIM 130050). This variant carries the most adverse prognosis with premature death from rupture of hollow viscera including blood vessels commonly occurring before midlife. Pregnancy is particularly dangerous for these individuals. It is important to establish the precise type of EDS affecting the patient because the prognosis for many individuals with the condition is good; patients with the vascular form of the disease are uncommon and can be distinguished relatively easily from others on clinical grounds or, where necessary, by DNA analysis. In the currently expanded EDS classification, the skeleton is particularly affected in types VI and VII EDS (Table 20.1.14).

In type VI EDS (oculo–scoliotic type), the first disorder in which an inborn error of collagen metabolism was identified, the clinical features are due to lysyl hydroxylase deficiency (OMIM 225400). Since hydroxylation of peptide-bound lysine is an essential posttranslational step in collagen synthesis and a necessary precursor to crosslink formation, this defect weakens collagen structure. The main clinical features are severe scoliosis, microcornea, and ocular fragility.

In type VII EDS (arthrochalasia), there is excessive mobility, perinatal joint dislocations (especially of the hips), and short stature (OMIM 130060). There is persistence in the tissues of collagen type I molecules with a retained amino-terminal propeptide that leads to defective fibrillogenesis.

Classic EDS (types I and II) is associated with cigarette paper scars, pronounced joint hypermobility, redundant skin folds, and pronounced hyperelasticity of the skin (OMIM 130000). Most cases result from dominant mutations in the collagen type V genes, COL5A1 and COL5A2, although a small minority reflect mutations at collagen type I loci. Collagen type V is a quantitatively minor component of collagen fibrils in skin compared to collagen type I and it has a particular influence on regulating collagen fibre size. Up to one-quarter of patients with the classic and hypermobility forms of the disease have some evidence of dilatation of the proximal aorta although dissection or aortic valve dysfunction is uncommon, in contrast to Marfan's syndrome. Where there is evidence of dilatation, periodic monitoring by echocardiography is appropriate.

Type III EDS (benign joint hypermobility type-OMIM 130020) is without doubt the most commonly seen EDS variant but to what extent it truly reflects a disease state or is merely a normal variant is not always clear. Some patients with this condition report chronic joint pains, widespread musculoskeletal symptoms, and other somatic symptoms of the sort often described in fibromyalgia. However, whether these symptoms are truly caused by joint laxity is not entirely clear. Combinations of cognitive therapy and physical treatments particularly aimed at improving proprioception and aerobic fitness may be helpful.

One recently described variant of Ehlers–Danlos syndrome deserves mention. Recessively inherited deficiency of tenascin-X, an essential regulator of the deposition of collagen in the extracellular matrix, causes a syndrome of joint hypermobility and hyperelasticity of the skin but without the tendency to form atrophic scars

(OMIM 606408). It can be detected by the absence of tenascin-X from the serum. Given the proximity of the *TNXB* locus to *CYP21A2*, the steroid 21-hydroxylase locus in the major histocompatibility complex, it is unsurprising that 10% of the deletions underlying 21-hydroxylase deficiency are associated additionally with tenascin-X deficiency.

Homocystinuria (see also Chapter 12.2)

Homocystinuria (OMIM 236200) is phenotypically similar to Marfan's syndrome but with a different cause and additional important complications. It is due to a deficiency of cystathionine β-synthase, an enzyme whose gene is located on chromosome 21, and firmly bound pyridoxal phosphate (vitamin B_6) is a feature. Homocystinuria is inherited as an autosomal recessive condition. The amount of residual cystathionine synthase activity varies from 0% to 10% in patients and, in obligate heterozygotes, it is less than 50% of normal. It is generally rare (<1:350 000) but has a higher prevalence in Ireland (1:65 000) and can be screened at birth by measuring blood methionine levels.

Pathophysiology

Homocysteine lies at the crossroads of two metabolic pathways and is converted to cystathionine by the addition of serine. This reaction is controlled by cystathionine β-synthase. The alternative fate of homocysteine is methylation to methionine. Cystathionine β-synthase activity is controlled by pyridoxine, but not all patients with cystathionine-deficient homocystinuria are pyridoxine sensitive, although this sensitivity or dependency is constant in sibships. In homocystinuria, there is an increase in both homocysteine and homocystine, which accumulate proximal to the metabolic block. Cystathionine, normally present in the brain, is no longer detectable and cysteine (normally made from methionine) becomes an essential amino acid.

The pathological findings include fraying and disruption of the zonular fibres of the ocular lens, defective bone formation, and multiple central nervous system infarcts. It is not known how the biochemical changes lead to the clinical features. The increased thrombotic tendency is not fully explained by changes in platelet function, cellular endothelium, or soluble factors, although abnormalities have been described in all of them. The neurological abnormalities and intellectual disabilities have not been proven to be due to the biochemical consequences of cystathionine β-synthase deficiency or to repeated vascular thromboses. Homocyst(e)ine may increase the solubility of collagen and interfere with its synthesis; for some, this explains the dislocation of the lens due to failure of the ciliary zonule. Since it is now known that this structure is composed largely of fibrillin, a further explanation is required. There is current interest in the possibility that young adults with premature vascular disease may be heterozygotes for a mutant cystathionine synthase gene. Elevated plasma homocysteine levels are a risk factor for coronary heart disease.

Clinical features

The clinical features of cystathionine β-synthase deficiency develop some time after birth and involve four systems; ocular, skeletal, central nervous, and vascular. The main ocular manifestation is downward dislocation of the lens. Myopia, glaucoma, retinal degeneration, and detachment also occur, and cataracts, optic atrophy, and corneal abnormalities are described. Some skeletal features suggest Marfan's syndrome. They include a long, thin habitus, pectus excavatum, scoliosis, and genu valgum. There is often radiological osteoporosis and abnormal modelling of the long bones with epimetaphyseal widening. Many subjects with homocystinuria have learning difficulties (average IQ ~80) and may also have seizures and strokes. It is unknown how closely these follow the increased tendency to thrombosis or the biochemical changes, especially a lack of cystathionine. Thromboembolism may occur in any vessel and at any age and has been documented in as many as 25% of affected individuals after surgery.

Any patient who has the phenotypic features of Marfan's syndrome associated with thrombosis, intellectual disability, and affected siblings should have a cyanide–nitroprusside test performed on their urine, together with an amino acid analysis of the urine and plasma.

The outlook for patients whose biochemical abnormalities are corrected by large amounts of pyridoxine (i.e. those with pyridoxine-sensitive homocystinuria) is usually better than those who are pyridoxine resistant. The main cause of death is thromboembolism.

The management of patients with homocystinuria differs according to the time of diagnosis and whether or not the patient responds to pyridoxine. In pyridoxine-responsive patients diagnosed after the newborn period, giving pyridoxine in doses that vary from 250 to 1200 mg a day appears to prevent thromboembolism.

When homocystinuria is detected in the newborn infant (most are discovered by screening and are pyridoxine nonresponsive), a diet low in methionine appears to reduce the incidence of low intelligence. After the newborn period, in those who are unresponsive to pyridoxine, methionine restriction and the administration of betaine (as a methyl donor) are also possibly useful lines of approach.

Alkaptonuria (see also Chapter 12.2)

This condition (OMIM 203500) has a special place in the history of medicine as one of the first recognized inborn errors in which mendelian recessive inheritance was proposed, by Garrod more than 100 years ago. In this rare autosomal recessive disorder, decreased activity of homogentisate 1,2-dioxigenase (HGD) leads to accumulation of homogentisic acid in the urine and increased pigmentation (ochronosis) in cartilage and connective tissues. Alkaptonuria, the classic sign of darkening of the urine (which is not always present) is due to the presence of 2,5-dehydroxyphenylacetic acid derived from the oxidation and polymerization of homogentisic acid. Polymerization increases in alkaline urine and is slowed down by antioxidants such as vitamin C. The structure of the pigment that causes ochronosis is not known. It is granular or homogeneous and may occur within or outside the cell. It is said to be associated with a reduction in lysyl hydroxylase in the tissue concerned and an impairment of the crosslinks of collagen.

Alkaptonuria has a general prevalence of around 1:250 000 but is more frequent in Slovakia and the Dominican Republic than elsewhere. It is recessively inherited by mutations in the *HGD* gene on chromosome 3q2. Abnormal pigmentation is found in the cartilage of the ear (which may be calcified), the nasal cartilage, and the sclerae. The most important effects of this disease are on the skeleton and cardiovascular system; initially the spine (Fig. 20.1.21) and

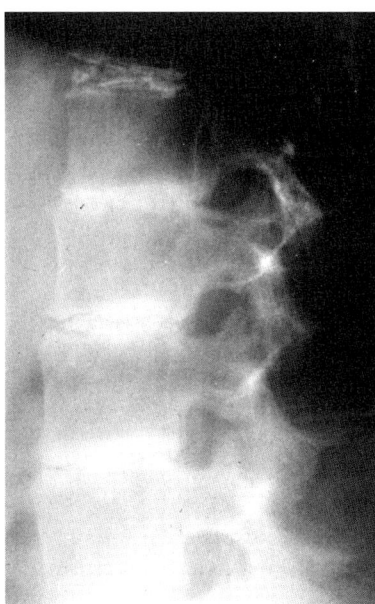

Fig. 20.1.21 The appearance of the spine in a man with alkaptonuria. There is universal calcification of the intervertebral discs.

subsequently the larger joints are affected. The intervertebral discs lose height and later calcify; they may also herniate acutely. The spine becomes rigid and short, and the lumbar lordosis is lost. In the large joints, such as the knees, shoulders, and hips, there are effusions and loose bodies. The symphysis pubis may be affected but not the sacroiliac joints. Calcification of the aorta may occur and cardiac valve surgery may be necessary. In addition around one-third of patients develop renal stones.

The diagnosis of alkaptonuria—often made late—should be suspected where there is a premature disc degeneration, even if there is no excessive darkening of the urine. Early degenerative arthritis suggests the disease, confirmed by finding deeply pigmented articular cartilage at the time of operation. In those patients with lifelong discoloured urine, the differential diagnosis is from other rare causes of urinary pigmentation. An increase in homogentisic acid in the urine and plasma confirms the diagnosis. The arthritis associated with alkaptonuria typically accelerates after the age of 30 and is more pronounced in women. It is characterized by excessive calcium pyrophosphate deposition that, in addition to causing chronic joint changes, may be punctuated by episodes of acute inflammation (pseudogout).

In theory, it should be possible to reduce the amount of homogentisic acid, and presumably the side effects, by cutting down protein intake to 30 or 40 g/day, thereby reducing tyrosine intake. High doses of vitamin C, which inhibits HGD activity, have also been advocated. But there is no convincing evidence that either of these measures has a significant effect. The herbicide nitisinone, licensed by the Food and Drug Administration for the treatment of tyrosinaemia, may reduce the excretion of homogentisic acid but its place in the treatment of alkaptonuria remains to be evaluated systematically.

Hypophosphatasia

This rare disorder has similarities with rickets and osteomalacia with considerable phenotypic variation. It is due to a reduction in the tissue nonspecific alkaline phosphatase (TNAP), which leads to

defective mineralization and a triad of biochemical disturbances: increased urinary phosphoethanolamine, plasma pyrophosphate, and plasma pyridoxal phosphate.

Studies on members of the Mennonite sect in Manitoba, in whom the incidence of hypophosphatasia is high, initially linked the defective gene to chromosome 1 and, subsequently, to the identification of numerous mutations in the *TNAP* gene. Although TNAP is widely distributed, its absence leads to lesions only in the bone and teeth.

Pathophysiology

The characteristic biochemical changes result directly from the alkaline phosphatase deficiency. Increased urinary pyrophosphate excretion is more reliable than urinary phosphoethanolamine as a marker for carriers of the hypophosphatasia gene. Occasionally there is hypercalcaemia and hypercalciuria in childhood and up to half of affected children and adults have increased plasma phosphate levels. Hyperphosphataemia is also described in some carriers of the hypophosphatasia gene. The recorded plasma alkaline phosphatase level must be compared with age-matched control values.

Histological examination of bone shows an excess of osteoid with abnormal tetracycline labelling without evidence of secondary hyperparathyroidism. Matrix vesicles do not contain alkaline phosphatase or hydroxyapatite crystals. The primary dental defect is in the cementum; additionally, the predentine is widened and the dentinal tubules are enlarged and few.

Clinical features

Hypophosphatasia occurs in all races. Since it is inherited as an autosomal recessive trait, it is more frequent where there is consanguinity. It has been estimated that hypophosphatasia occurs in 1 in 100 000 live births in Toronto. The four clinical types provide a continuous spectrum, from a lethal perinatal disorder to an asymptomatic syndrome in some adults.

The first is an important cause of lethal, short-limbed dwarfism (see above). Some newborn infants survive for a few days, but fever, failure to thrive, anaemia, seizures, and intracranial haemorrhages occur. Radiographs show grossly defective mineralization, especially in the skull, where only the base may be mineralized, and in diaphyses of the long bones which, rarely, may have bony spurs.

In the infantile form (within the first 6 months), hypotonia, failure to thrive, hypercalcaemia, and hypercalciuria occur. Clinical rickets is noticed and the fontanelle appears wide, but there is a functional synostosis. Craniostenosis can produce optic atrophy, exophthalmos, and raised intracranial pressure requiring surgery.

The most variable expression occurs in childhood. Early loss of deciduous teeth, due to defective cementum, may be the only feature (ondontohypophosphatasia). The pulp chambers are enlarged and the root canals are short (shell teeth). If bone disease is present, walking is delayed and deformities occur, e.g. bow legs, knock knees, short stature, and enlargement of the epiphyses at the wrist, knees, and ankles.

In adults, progressive stiffness, pain in the bones, and apparent 'stress' fractures can occur (Fig. 20.1.22). Approximately 50% of such patients have a childhood history of bone disease resembling rickets or premature loss of deciduous teeth or both. There may also be premature shedding of adult teeth, short stature, and abnormal skull shape. Recurrent poorly healing metatarsal fractures occur. Partial fractures of the long bones characteristically occur on the

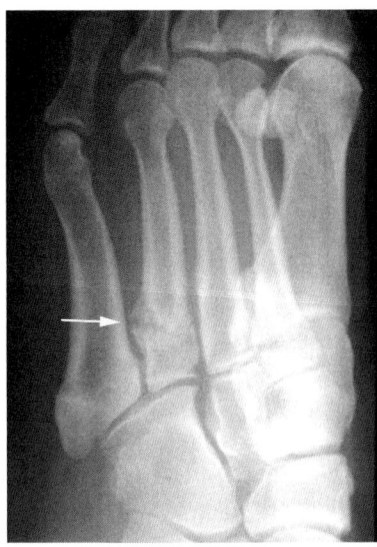

Fig. 20.1.22 Hypophosphatasia in the adult. A pathological ununited fracture in the bones of the foot (arrowed). The woman had lost her teeth in early childhood.

convex outer surface (in contrast to the concave inner position of the Looser's zones in osteomalacia), most often in the upper one-third of the femoral shaft, and are often bilateral; other sites include the ribs, tibias, and ulnas. They may be unaltered for years or they may increase in size and eventually fracture. Secondary hyperparathyroidism is not seen. Chondrocalcinosis is common and, in a proportion, is associated with clinical pyrophosphate gout (pseudogout).

Management

In the management of hypophosphatasia, premature synostosis leading to raised intracranial pressure requires surgical relief. Hypercalcaemia may be dealt with by reducing dietary calcium and by giving prednisolone. Intramedullary rods may prevent and treat fractures of the long bones. Dental abnormalities, which can occur in biochemically normal members of hypophosphatasia families, may require treatment.

Prenatal diagnosis of a severely affected child can be made by ultrasound examination, and mutations in *TNAP* may be detected. There is also reduced alkaline phosphatase activity in the amniotic fluid cells.

Lysosomal storage diseases (see also Chapter 12.8)

This large group of diseases is due to various inborn errors that affect the function of specific lysosomal enzymes normally responsible for the breakdown of a variety of complex molecules. As a result, these molecules, or their partially degraded derivatives, accumulate in the lysosomes and the tissues that contain them. The effect of this accumulation varies from one tissue to another according to the particular disorder and the skeleton is significantly involved in only a proportion of them. They include some mucopolysaccharidoses and Gaucher's disease.

Mucopolysaccharidoses

Failure of the normal lysosomal breakdown of complex carbohydrates leads to their accumulation in the tissues and produces many clinical abnormalities. The disorders may be divided into two main groups according to the chemistry of the accumulated substance, namely the mucopolysaccharidoses (MPS), and the mucolipidoses. Specific biochemical defects are described elsewhere in this book (see Section 11). Since some of these disorders have a prominent effect on the skeleton, some of them are briefly mentioned here: they are Hurler's syndrome (MPS type IH), Hunter's syndrome (MPS type II), and Morquio's syndrome (MPS type IV). With certain exceptions, the bone changes themselves do not permit precise diagnosis of the type of dysplasia or distinction from the mucolipidoses.

Hurler's syndrome (MPS type IH) (OMIM 607014)

This is the most severe type of mucopolysaccharidosis and causes death at an early age. The enzyme defect is recessively inherited and all patients have the same appearance, to which the term 'gargoylism' was previously applied. Affected infants appear to develop normally in the first few months of life, but then deteriorate mentally and physically. Death often occurs in late childhood, commonly due to pneumonia or to coronary artery disease associated with mucopolysaccharide deposits.

The physical features include proportionate short stature (Table 20.1.4), a typical facial appearance, a short neck with a lumbar gibbus and chest deformity, and a protuberant abdomen. The facial features are coarse, with flattening of the nasal bridge, with large open mouth and tongue, and, often, with hypertrophied gums over enlarged alveolar ridges. The eyes are prominent with corneal clouding. There is noisy breathing and variable deafness. The vault of the skull may show scaphocephaly or acrocephaly. Other striking features include the stiff, broad, trident hands and the large abdomen with hepatosplenomegaly. Radiographs show the abnormal shape of the skull, the slipper-shaped sella turcica, the beaking of the vertebrae with the thoracolumbar kyphosis, and the bullet-shaped phalanges.

Hunter's syndrome (MPS type II) (OMIM 309900)

This has similar but less severe features to Hurler's syndrome but is inherited as an X-linked recessive trait. Two forms of the disease are described: the more severe form, associated with intellectual disability and progressive physical disability, typically causes death by the age of 15; the less severe form is compatible with survival into adult life with slowly progressive cardiac valve disease. Both forms are associated with mutations in the enzyme iduronate-2-sulphatase.

Morquio's syndrome (MPS type IV) (OMIM 253010)

In this disorder, the orthopaedic manifestations are striking but intelligence is normal. In the first years of life, the child becomes progressively more deformed and dwarfed. Characteristically the neck is short, the sternum is protuberant, and there may be a flexed stance with knock knees. There is a striking loss of muscle tone in comparison to the stiffness of MPS type IH; hypermobility and a loose skin are features. Radiographs in infancy show a spine similar to that seen in those with Hurler's syndrome, but later flattening of the vertebrae with anterior beaking lead to relative shortening of the trunk. The small bones of the hands are different from those of MPS type IH and the metacarpals show diaphyseal constriction (Fig. 20.1.23). Importantly, the odontoid may be hypoplastic, leading to atlantoaxial instability, compression of the long spinal tracts, and paraplegia.

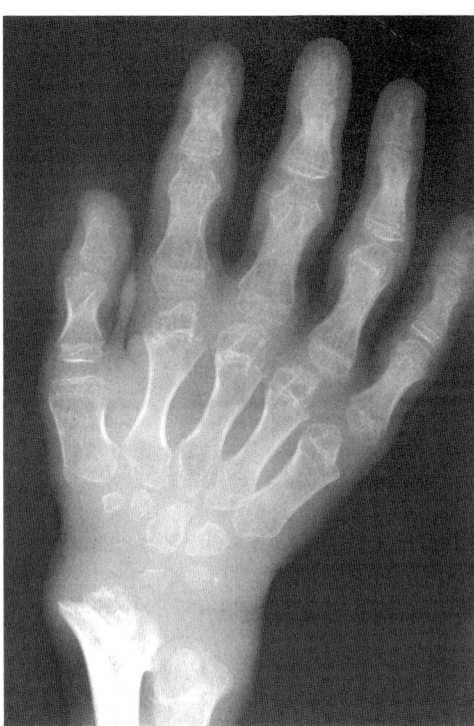

Fig. 20.1.23 The appearance of the hand in MPS type IV (Morquio's syndrome). The bases of the metacarpals are conical, the tubular bones are short, and the growth plates of the radius and ulna are inclined towards each other.

Gaucher's disease (see also Chapter 12.8)

This is a rare lysosomal storage disorder in which glucocerebroside-containing macrophages accumulate within the bone marrow, spleen, liver, and other organs. This accumulation is the result of deficiency of the enzyme β-glucocerebroside. Gaucher's disease is recessively inherited and overrepresented in Ashkenazi Jews, where the incidence of the adult form (type I) is about 1 in 2500 births. The skeletal manifestations are often severe and disabling. They vary from a characteristic but clinically insignificant failure of remodelling in the lower femora (Erlenmeyer-flask appearance) to a diffuse and localized bone loss and osteosclerotic and osteonecrotic lesions, which cause pain and pathological fracture and often require precocious joint replacement surgery. Enzyme replacement is an established but expensive form of treatment.

Skeletal dysplasias

The term 'skeletal dysplasia' has traditionally been used to cover a wide range of generalized disorders of the skeleton, often of unknown cause, affecting both cartilage and bone. One can now distinguish the chondrodysplasias, which are primarily due to mutations affecting cartilage, from conditions such as diaphyseal dysplasia and assorted dense bone diseases, where the causes are less well known. Since osteopetrosis is caused by well-defined deficiencies of osteoclast function, it is dealt with separately (see below).

The mutations in many of the skeletal dysplasias have been described (Table 20.1.1) and the skeletal dysplasias can now be classified into biochemical families according to their causes (Table 20.1.15). The supposition that many of them could be due to mutations in specific collagens has been partially confirmed with mutations found in

Table 20.1.15 Mutations in the skeletal dysplasias

Mutant gene	Disease family
Collagen mutations	
COL1A1 and COL1A2	Osteogenesis imperfecta and EDS type VII
COL2A1	Achondrogenesis type II
	SED
	Kniest's dysplasia
	Stickler's syndrome (with ocular manifestations: type I)
COL3A1	Vascular EDS (type IV)
COL5A1	Classic EDS (types I and II)
COL9A1, 2, 3	Multiple epiphyseal dysplasia (types 2 and 3)
COL10A1	Metaphyseal chondrodysplasia (type Schmid)
COL11A2	Stickler's syndrome (without ocular manifestations; type II)
Noncollagen mutations	
COMP	Pseudoachondroplasia
	Multiple epiphyseal dysplasia (type 1)
SLC26A2 (DTDST)	Diastrophic dysplasia
	Atelosteogenesis type II
	Achondrogenesis type IB
	Multiple epiphyseal dysplasia (type 4)
PTH–PRrP receptor	Jansen's metaphyseal chondrodysplasia
	Blomstrand's chondrodysplasia
SOX9	Campomelic dysplasia
Arylsulphatase E	Chondrodysplasia punctata
CDMP1	Acromesomelic chondrodysplasia
FGFR3	Achondroplasia
	Thanatophoric dysplasia
	Hypochondroplasia
	Crouzon's syndrome with acanthosis nigricans
FGFR2	Crouzon's syndrome
	Apert's syndrome
	Jackson–Weiss syndrome
	Pfeiffer's syndrome
FGFR1	Pfeiffer's syndrome
RUNX2 (CBFA1)	Cleidocranial dysostosis
Cathepsin K	Pyknodysostosis
Tumour suppressor genes (EXT1, EXT2)	Multiple hereditary exostoses
SEDLIN	Spondyloepiphyseal dysplasia tarda (X-linked)
RMRP	Metaphyseal chondrodysplasia McKusick's type (cartilage hair hypoplasia)
EVC (on chromosome 4)	Chondroectodermal dysplasia (Ellis–van Creveld syndrome)
WISP3	SED tarda with progressive arthropathy
Matrilin 3	Multiple epiphyseal dysplasia (type 5)

EDS, Ehlers–Danlos syndrome; PRrP, parathyroid-hormone-related protein; PTH, parathyroid hormone; SED, spondyloepiphyseal dysplasia congenita.

collagen types I, IX, X, and XI. Achondroplasia is a striking example of a skeletal dysplasia caused by a noncollagen mutation, i.e. a mutation in FGF receptor 3 (*FGFR3*). Mutations in *FGFR2* can cause craniosynostoses (e.g. Apert's and Pfeiffer's syndromes). Further details can be found in reviews (see Further Reading).

Clinical features

The physician confronted by a patient with a skeletal dysplasia is unlikely to make the correct diagnosis without additional help unless it is clearly one of the more distinctive forms, such as achondroplasia. Accurate classification of the dysplasias is important and has contributed to the rapid advances in clinical and biochemical understanding of these conditions. The most convenient simple classification is a clinical one. Most patients with skeletal dysplasias have restricted growth and most are short-limbed. The bodily proportions of people with skeletal dysplasias usually provide a clue about whether mainly the limbs or the spine, or both, are affected. In the short-limbed group, achondroplasia and achondroplasia-like dwarfs are the most typical. Other disorders, often with less conspicuous dwarfing, include various inherited epiphyseal dysplasias, diaphyseal dysplasias, and some, but not all, metaphyseal dysplasias. An alternative classification, not based on height, groups the dysplasias according to whether they are predominantly epiphyseal or metaphyseal, whether the spine is predominantly involved, and whether single limbs or segments are involved. Radiographs, taken as early in life as possible and, where possible, consecutively, are essential to determine whether the metaphyses of the long bones or the epiphyses are primarily affected.

For the purpose of this Section, osteopetrosis (marble bones disease) is dealt with separately as a disorder of bone-cell biology. Other sclerosing disorders of bone, in which biochemical abnormalities have been described (e.g. Camurati–Engelmann and van Buchem's diseases), receive brief mention.

Achondroplasia (OMIM 100800)

This is the prototype of short limbs and short stature. It is dominantly inherited and due to a highly specific recurrent mutation in the *FGFR3* gene encoding the FGF-receptor 3. Activation of this receptor exerts an inhibitory effect on the proliferating columns of chondrocytes in the growth plate. The characteristic glycine for arginine substitution at amino acid 380 in the transmembrane region of the receptor facilitates its dimerization and activation after engaging the FGF ligand, thereby causing overactivity and inhibition of chondrocyte proliferation in the growth plate and reduced longitudinal growth. There is strong evidence that the *FGFR3* mutation is exclusively paternally derived and that it reflects processes specific to spermatogenesis but not oogenesis. As the clinical definition of achondroplasia has not always been exact, its true incidence and natural history are not well defined. There is a failure of the epiphyseal growth of cartilage and bulbous masses of cartilage appear at the ends of the long bones. In contrast, periosteal and membrane bone formation and bone repair are normal. This selective effect on growth cartilage accounts for the skeletal deformity.

Achondroplasia can be diagnosed at birth or within the first year of life, when the disparity between the large skull and short limbs becomes obvious. There is a striking disproportion between the normal length trunk and the short arms and legs. Thus, the fingertips may only come down to the iliac crest. The shortness of the limbs particularly affects the proximal segment. The limbs themselves look very broad, with abnormally deep creases, and the hands are trident-like. In contrast to the short limbs is the enlarged bulging vault of the skull, the small face, and flat nasal bridge or 'scooped out' glabella. There is a marked lumbar lordosis and also, sometimes, some wedging of the upper lumbar vertebrae, which may later lead to a thoracolumbar kyphosis. Radiological features include metaphyseal irregularity and flaring in the long bones, irregular and late-appearing epiphyses, a narrow pelvis in its anteroposterior diameter, with short iliac wings and deep sacroiliac notches, and a spine that shows progressive narrowing of the interpedicular distance from above downwards, which is the reverse of normal. This may cause spinal stenosis. A highly characteristic radiographic observation in young children is the presence of a thoracolumbar gibbus clinically, associated with anterior wedging of the first lumbar vertebra radiographically. Any temptation to correct this surgically should be resisted since it usually corrects itself as the child starts walking by the age of 5 years.

Children with achondroplasia are of normal intelligence and the complications of this disease arise particularly from the skeletal disproportion. This may lead to early osteoarthritis, obstetric difficulties and the need for caesarean section, hydrocephalus, and paraplegia. Eventual height typically varies between about 120 and 150 cm. Recent reviews emphasize how often narrowing of the spinal canal produces symptoms of spinal stenosis; this may require surgical decompression, sometimes at multiple levels.

Homozygous achondroplasia (the occasional offspring of two affected parents) is severe and lethal. In the condition of hypochondroplasia, which is included in the same *FGFR3* molecular family, the skeletal disproportion and the spinal abnormalities are less severe than in achondroplasia and the skull is unaffected.

Achondroplasia-like dwarfism

For details of these and other causes of short-limbed dwarfism, the reader should consult more specialized texts. Those that most closely resemble achondroplasia at birth are thanatophoric dwarfism (also caused by *FGFR3* mutations), achondrogenesis (caused by *COL2A1* mutations), severe hypophosphatasia, and type II osteogenesis imperfecta. All can be distinguished radiologically from neonatal radiographs.

Spondyloepiphyseal dysplasias

This is a heterogeneous group of disorders in which there is prominent spinal involvement, with the short stature partly due to shortness of the trunk. The most severe type is spondyloepiphyseal dysplasia (SED) congenita; milder forms are often collectively referred to as SED tarda. There are various forms of inheritance. Some forms are due to mutations in collagen type II.

SED tarda (OMIM 313400) often has an X-linked recessive mode of inheritance so that only men are affected and women are carriers. Causal mutations in the *SEDL* gene have been identified. In affected men, the disproportionately short trunk becomes obvious at adolescence. Failure of ossification in the anterior part of the so-called ring epiphyses leads to central and posterior humps on the upper and lower parts of the flattened bodies. The condition needs to be distinguished from multiple epiphyseal dysplasia, which involves other major joints more than the spine.

SED congenita (OMIM 183900) can be diagnosed at birth because of the short stature associated with a short trunk. It is due to mutations in *COL2A1*. There may be a close resemblance to Morquio's disease (MPS type IV, see above). The severe form may be distinguished from the age of about 4 years. The appearance of the capital femoral epiphyses is delayed (in some patients it may never be seen except by arthrography). Marked lumbar lordosis, waddling gait, back pain, and progressive disproportion may occur. The odontoid is hypoplastic, kyphoscoliosis may develop, and the interpedicular distances of the vertebrae do not increase in the lumbar region. Paraplegia may occur as a result of all these changes. In this disorder there is often myopia and retinal detachment.

There is a form of SED, pseudoachondroplasia (OMIM 177170), which resembles achondroplasia because of the short limbs, but here the facial appearance is normal. The short stature only becomes obvious from about 2 years of age. Lumbar lordosis and scoliosis may develop. The tubular bones are short with irregular metaphyses and small, deformed epiphyses. Joint hypermobility is marked with additional striking hyperelasticity of the skin; early osteoarthritis, particularly of the hips, is common. Characteristic mutations in the COMP gene, interfering with calcium-binding domains in cartilage oligomeric matrix protein, disrupt its secondary structure.

Proportionate dwarfism

Although it is clinically important to classify short stature into proportionate and disproportionate, there are many conditions in which this distinction is difficult to make. Hypophosphataemic rickets, mucopolysaccharidoses, vitamin D dependent rickets, and osteogenesis imperfecta may come into both categories.

Bone dysplasias without conspicuous short stature

The height of patients with multiple epiphyseal dysplasia may be only slightly reduced. Although many epiphyses are affected, the spine is virtually normal. There are also variable forms of inheritance. A variety of clinical types are recognized caused variously by mutations in collagen type IX, COMP, matrilin 3, and SLC26A2 (encoding a sulphate transporter, deficiency of which causes undersulphation of proteoglycans).

In patients with multiple hereditary exostoses, often referred to as diaphyseal aclasis (OMIM 133700), stature is typically normal; there is a juxta-epiphyseal disorder of bone growth limited to bones developed in cartilage, which gives rise to cartilage-capped exostoses that point away from the joint. Inheritance is autosomal dominant caused by mutations in the genes EXT1 and EXT2, which are tumour suppressor genes involved in cartilage growth. Malignant change may lead to chondrosarcoma in 0.5% or 2% of cases but this is rare before the age of 10 or after the age of 50.

The metaphyseal disorders are rare; some, such as Jansen's metaphyseal dysplasia (associated with a mutation in the gene for the PTH/PRrP receptor) do cause severe dwarfing. In others with less severe growth disturbance, such as metaphyseal chondrodysplasia type Schmid (due to a mutation in the collagen type X gene, COL10A1), rickets is simulated and confusion with inherited hypophosphataemia is possible.

Cleidocranial dysplasia (OMIM 119600)

In this rare condition, the clavicles are hypoplastic or absent, the fontanelles remain open, there are supernumerary teeth, and there may be Wormian bones in the skull. Heterozygous mutations in RUNX2, encoding the osteoblast transcription factor CBFA1, are responsible (see above). In the mouse cbfa1 knockout, there is failure of the skeleton to mineralize, which is consistent with the key role of this transcription factor in triggering osteoblast activity.

Disorders of increased bone density

There are two main causes for the inherited dense bone diseases, namely excessive bone formation and reduced bone resorption. Apart from marble bone disease, most physicians' experiences of these conditions are limited by their extreme rarity.

Increased bone formation

Camurati–Engelmann disease (progressive diaphyseal dysplasia; OMIM131300) This rare autosomal dominant condition is inherited through mutations in the TGFβ1 gene but penetrance is variable. Mutations are clustered at the C-terminal end of the latency associated peptide domain of TGFβ1, probably affecting its activation (cf. Marfan's syndrome above). The condition affects the muscles as well as the skeleton, where the main feature is a variable but progressive endosteal and periosteal thickening of the diaphyses of the long bones (Fig. 20.1.24). In severely affected subjects, the spine, skull, and axial skeleton are all affected. In addition, there is a waddling broad-based gait, muscle wasting and weakness, loss of subcutaneous tissues, and pain in the legs during childhood, so that distinction from muscular dystrophy may be necessary. The appearance is characteristic; the head is large with a prominent forehead and proptosis, the muscle mass is reduced, and the bones are palpably thickened with fusiform swelling of the bones below the knees. Cranial nerve palsies, deafness, and blindness with raised intracranial pressure can occur. Puberty is delayed. Bone pain resistant to analgesia is often a presenting and troublesome feature. Anaemia, leukopenia, hepatosplenomegaly, and elevation of the erythrocyte sedimentation rate are described.

Radiographic appearances vary, from limited thickening of the diaphyses (often in the lower extremities) to widespread new bone formation that affects all bones including the skull, demonstrated by scintigraphy.

The increased bone turnover causes a moderate increase in plasma alkaline phosphatase and urinary hydroxyproline levels. There may be a markedly positive calcium balance, associated with hypocalcaemia and hypocalciuria. Hyperphosphataemia has been recorded.

Pathological examination confirms gross thickening of the bone with disorganization of internal structure and external shape. The peripheral subperiosteal new bone is woven. The muscles show nonspecific, type II fibre atrophy.

In the differential diagnosis, the proximal myopathy and abnormal gait simulate muscular dystrophy. The radiographic appearances are diagnostic, although idiopathic hyperphosphatasia may present some difficulties.

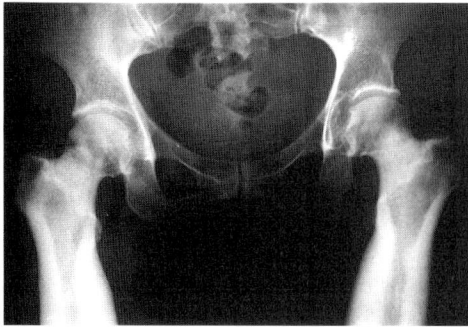

Fig. 20.1.24 Radiographic appearances of the long bones in Camurati–Englemann disease with pronounced thickening of the femoral diaphyses.

The course of this disorder is unpredictable and remission of symptoms may occur during adolescence or adult life, so it is difficult to assess treatment. Symptom onset is usually before the age of 30 and, often, before the age of 10. Bone pain may respond to corticosteroids in small, alternate-day doses and there is also evidence that the bone changes may be reduced. Etidronate (20 mg/kg daily) has produced hypocalcaemic tetany, but intermittent administration is reported to reduce pain. Limb pain may be relieved by surgical removal of a cortical window in the diaphysis.

Sclerosteosis (OMIM 269500) This condition is an autosomal recessive trait caused by mutations in the gene for sclerostin, a BMP antagonist. It has a particularly high prevalence in the Afrikaner population of South Africa. There is progressive overgrowth and sclerosis of the skeleton, including the skull and the mandible. There are similarities to van Buchem's disease (endosteal hyperostosis) but the skeletal problems are more severe, and there is often also syndactyly. Prophylactic craniotomy may be necessary to reduce the increased intracranial pressure.

van Buchem's disease (OMIM 239100) In this rare hyperostosis, endosteal thickening of the shafts of the long bones is associated with generalized hyperostosis, including the base of the skull, mandible, clavicle, and ribs. Bilateral facial nerve weakness, deafness, and optic atrophy may ensue. Deletions in the regulatory elements of the *SOST* gene have been described. A milder variant of endosteal hyperostosis (Worth type; OMIM 144750) is sometimes associated with activating mutations in the *LRP5* gene. This gene, which is associated with both the syndrome of familial high bone mass and osteoporosis pseudoglioma (see above), has also been linked to the determination of bone mass in the general population.

Decreased bone resorption

There are several genetic causes of reduced bone resorption that typically result in generalized increase in bone density but also increased fracture risk.

Osteopetrosis (marble bone disease)

Among those disorders with increased bone density, marble bone disease, or osteopetrosis (also known as Albers–Schönberg disease), is the best known. It is a heterogeneous disorder with a widespread increase in bone density. The classic bone-within-bone appearance (endobone) is not always apparent (Fig. 20.1.25). In most cases, the basic defect lies in the osteoclasts, which, for various

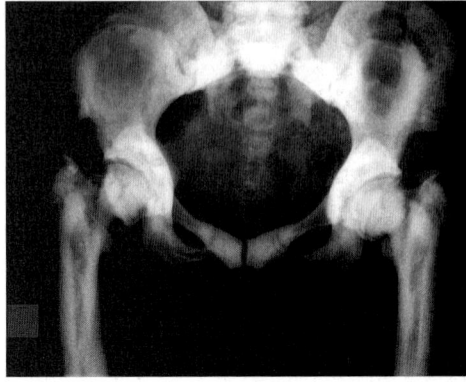

Fig. 20.1.25 Osteopetrosis. The classic bone-within-bone (endobone) appearance of the bones in a woman with type II dominantly inherited osteopetrosis (ADDO II).

reasons, are unable to resorb mineralized bone. Many animal models of osteopetrosis exist.

Until recently, two main forms were distinguished: recessively inherited severe osteopetrosis, causing death in childhood; and the dominantly inherited mild form, in which the diagnosis is often made on radiological grounds alone. This distinction is not absolute—two distinct dominantly inherited forms are recognized as well as intermediate forms. Deficiency of carbonic anhydrase II can also cause osteopetrosis associated with cerebral calcification, mild systemic acidosis, growth failure, and learning difficulties. Pycnodysostosis (see below) is another form of osteopetrosis also caused by a deficiency in the enzyme cathepsin K. The mutations that cause different types of osteopetrosis have now been identified (Table 20.1.16). They occur in the acidification pathways of the osteoclast. Mild dominantly inherited type II osteopetrosis results from mutations in the chloride channel gene *CLCN7* and severe recessive osteopetrosis from mutations in the gene *TCIRG1*, encoding a component of the vacuolar H+ATPase involved in acidification.

Severe osteopetrosis

In severe recessively inherited osteopetrosis (OMIM 259700), there is widespread increased density of the bones without modelling or remodelling. This produces the Erlenmeyer-flask deformity of the metaphyses. The increase in bone density is often intermittent, producing alternating bands of sclerosis. The failure of resorption leads to a reduction in bone marrow space with a leukoerythroblastic anaemia and hepatosplenomegaly. It can also produce nerve compression, blindness, and deafness. Other clinical features in this severe form can include hydrocephalus, delayed tooth eruption, and osteomyelitis. Fracture of the dense bones is common. The affected infant is short with an apparently large head with frontal bossing and with knock knees. The plasma calcium level appears to alter with the dietary intake and may be sufficiently low to contribute to rickets. The acid phosphatase concentration (derived from the defective osteoclasts) is increased. Secondary hyperparathyroidism leads to an increase in calcitriol levels. Apart from transplantation of bone marrow, as a source of normal osteoclasts, other forms of medical treatment deal only with complications; these include surgery for fractures, blood transfusions for anaemia, and antibiotics for frequent infections.

Mild osteopetrosis

The mild forms vary from subjects with an increased number of fractures affecting both the long bones and the small bones of the hands and feet to those in which the disorder is so mild that the diagnosis is made by radiology alone (accounting for apparently unaffected generations with the dominant form of the disease). There are more severe forms of dominantly inherited osteopetrosis with nerve compression, deafness and blindness, and anaemia at times of increased physiological requirement, such as pregnancy. Other established features include osteomyelitis and facial nerve palsy.

Recent studies of Danish families define two dominantly inherited forms (Table 20.1.16). In the first (OMIM 607634), mutations have been described in *LRP5*; it has uniformly dense bones with sclerosis of the cranial vault and the spine and no increase in the plasma acid phosphatase level. The second (OMIM 166600) is caused by mutations in *CLCN7*; it has variable bone density (giving rise to an endobone appearance, Fig. 20.1.25) and lack of

Table 20.1.16 Different types and clinical features of the osteopetroses

Type	Clinical features	Radiology	Plasma biochemistry	Chromosome locus	Gene
Mild dominantly inherited type I	Fractures; cranial nerve compression; variable anaemia; osteomyelitis of the jaw	Bones uniformly dense; sclerosis of the skull; enlarged thick cranial vault	Acid phosphatase normal	11	*LRP5* mutations in some
Mild dominantly inherited type II	As above	Variable bone density; endobones; sandwich vertebrae; lack of modelling	Acid phosphatase increased; calcium and PTH may be increased	16	*CLCN7* mutations most frequent
Severe infantile recessively inherited	Short stature; severe anaemia; cranial nerve palsies; fractures; deformity; hepatosplenomegaly	Uniform increased bone density; lack of modelling	Increased acid phosphatase; calcium may be low	11	TCIRG1
Carbonic anhydrase II deficiency, recessive	Cerebral calcification; growth retardation	As in other forms	Systemic acidosis	8	CA2
Pyknodysostosis; cathepsin K deficiency, recessive	Disproportionate short stature; blue sclerae; open anterior fontanelle; kyphoscoliosis	Uniform osteosclerosis; Wormian bones; acro-osteolysis	Normal	1	CTSK

modelling, with a significant increase in the plasma acid phosphatase level. Sometimes *CLCN5* mutations can also give rise to the severe infantile form of the disease.

Carbonic anhydrase II deficiency (OMIM 259730)

The association of carbonic anhydrase II deficiency with osteopetrosis, renal tubular acidosis, cerebral calcification, some degree of intellectual disability, growth failure, and dental malocclusion is of considerable interest because of the clues about the normal function of carbonic anhydrase II in bone resorption. Carbonic anhydrase II is part of the carbonic anhydrase gene family and is widely distributed. It is found in the kidney, brain, red cells, and elsewhere. Its gene is on chromosome 22. Deficiency of carbonic anhydrase II is autosomal recessively inherited and apparently normal parents of affected offspring have 50% of normal carbonic anhydrase II levels within their red cells. The bone disease is not distinguishable from other forms of osteopetrosis and fractures occur until adulthood. There is always growth retardation, and height may be more than four standard deviations below the mean. The bone age is also delayed. Radiographic appearances improve in adult life.

The renal tubular acidosis is mixed, both proximal and distal. Cerebral calcification affects the basal ganglia within the first decade. It increases during childhood to include the cortical grey matter and is similar to that occurring in idiopathic or pseudohypoparathyroidism. Bone histology shows unresorbed calcified cartilage and osteoclasts without a ruffled border.

The diagnosis of carbonic anhydrase II deficiency should be considered in any neonate with renal tubular acidosis. Genetic counselling is possible since adult heterozygotes have reduced levels of the enzyme in their red cells. However, the concentration of carbonic anhydrase II is normally very low at birth and cannot be used as a reliable neonatal test for the affected homozygote.

The treatment of carbonic anhydrase II deficiency is symptomatic. It is possible that correction of the renal tubular acidosis temporarily increases the rate of growth.

In the differential diagnosis of osteopetrosis, there are many disorders with an excessive amount of bone in various parts of the skeleton. These include other skeletal dysplasias, Caffey's disease (infantile cortical hyperostosis), which causes a temporary increase in bone density from birth and myelofibrosis, renal glomerular osteodystrophy, inherited hypophosphataemia, and fluorosis in adult life.

Pycnodysostosis (OMIM 265800)

Pycnodysostosis has an autosomal recessive mode of inheritance, with parental consanguinity in some 30% of subjects. It is caused by mutations that lead to deficiency of cathepsin K, an enzyme necessary for osteoclast function. Marked reduction in stature with short limbs is a particular clinical feature.

The vault of the skull is large, the face and chin small, the palate high-arched, and the teeth crowded, with retained deciduous teeth. The anterior fontanelle (and other cranial sutures) remain unfused. The painter Toulouse-Lautrec is regarded as a typical example of this disease. The fingers may appear to be clubbed because of associated acro-osteolysis. The chest is deformed with kyphoscoliosis and pectus excavatum. Recurrent fractures of long bones and, occasionally, rickets occur. Radiologically, there are similarities to osteopetrosis with generalized osteosclerosis and fractures. However, the osteosclerosis is uniform; there are no defects of modelling and no endobones. In addition to delayed closure of the cranial sutures, there are also Wormian bones; the bony fragility, Wormian bones, and blue sclerae simulate osteogenesis imperfecta.

Fibrous dysplasia

Fibrous dysplasia of bone is a condition in which areas of immature fibrous tissue, either single or multiple, are found within the skeleton (Fig. 20.1.26). The underlying genetic cause is a postzygotic activating mutation in *GNAS1*, the gene for the α-subunit of the G-protein signalling system. The extent to which this activating mutation affects the bone and other tissues depends on the degree of mosaicism, in other words the proportion and distribution of cells that carry the mutation. It is proposed that such a mutation in the germline would be lethal; certainly the condition is not inherited.

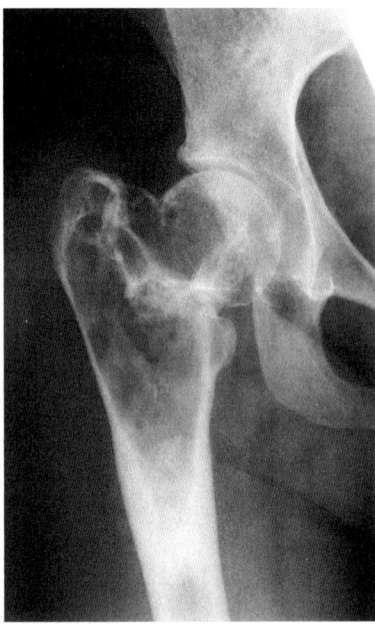

Fig. 20.1.26 Polyostotic fibrous dysplasia in a 23-year-old woman. A large cyst in the upper femur led to a spontaneous fracture that subsequently united with conservative treatment. Two ribs on the same side of the body show similar abnormalities. Puberty was precocious but pigmentation absent.

Monostotic fibrous dysplasia

This disorder is relatively common in orthopaedic practice. Although the lesions may occur in any bone and particularly in the facial bones and ribs, the most frequent presenting symptom at any age is a fracture, often of the upper end of the femur. The biochemistry is usually normal (although the alkaline phosphatase and other bone turnover markers may be elevated in active disease) and the diagnosis is usually made from the radiographic and pathological appearances. There is a smooth-walled translucent area within the bone, often with thinning of the cortex and, sometimes, with associated deformity. Pathologically, areas of disorganized fibrous tissue are found, associated with woven bone and wide osteoid seams. This represents mosaic tissue with some normal mesenchymal cells and some carrying the mutation. The differential diagnosis is from other causes of bone cysts, from Paget's disease, and from hyperparathyroidism with osteitis fibrosa cystica. In the monostotic form, treatment is largely orthopaedic. However, the large size of some of the defects in the shafts of the long bones may make conventional stabilization of fractures very difficult. Treatment with pamidronate or other bisphosphonates is reported to improve pain and reduce osteoclast overactivity.

Polyostotic fibrous dysplasia

Interest in this condition (OMIM 174800), in which the bone lesions are multiple, arises from its frequent association with pigmentation and sexual precocity, especially in women (McCune–Albright syndrome). The bone lesions and the brown pigmentation are typically associated in position (but not in extent) and may be restricted to one side of the body. Sexual precocity is present in about 50% of women with polyostotic disease and is then the presenting complaint. It may occur at a very early age, with menstruation, and with the appearance of secondary sexual characteristics from infancy. Where sexual precocity is not a feature, deformity

and fracture are often the first symptoms. Gross deformity of the upper femur and femoral neck produces the 'shepherd's crook' appearance. Asymmetry of the long bones and of the skull are also seen and, in about half of the cases, the base of the skull is thickened. The macular pigmentation tends to have smooth borders (in contrast to those of neurofibromatosis) and often does not cross the midline. In a recent long-term follow-up of 15 patients with two or more features of the McCune–Albright triad, the bone lesions tended to increase in size and number, but less rapidly after growth had ceased. Skin lesions were generally bilateral and did not correlate with the site of the bone lesions. There are a number of other features that, like the sexual precocity, are explained by the activating mutation. These include thyrotoxicosis, acromegaly, and Cushing's syndrome. The skeletal lesions may cause complications such as spinal cord compression and may be associated with hypophosphataemic osteomalacia. Sarcoma formation has been reported, but only after irradiation.

In the polyostotic disease, both the plasma alkaline phosphatase and the urinary hydroxyproline levels may be slightly increased and that of plasma phosphate slightly reduced. The pathology is similar to the monostotic form, but it is said that cartilage- and fluid-filled cysts are more common. Microscopically, there is an abundance of woven bone and an increase in osteoblasts and osteoclasts. The cortex and marrow may be virtually replaced by fibrous tissue, so that the bones are fragile. Healing is rapid with abundant callus formation. Radiologically, the bones are deformed, the cortex may be difficult to detect, and the medullary bone takes on a 'ground glass' or 'smoky' appearance.

In polyostotic fibrous dysplasia, the main differential diagnosis is from osseous neurofibromatosis; in the former condition, there is also pigmentation, bone deformity, and, sometimes, hypophosphataemic osteomalacia. The borders of the pigmentation are less smooth than in fibrous dysplasia. There are other cutaneous features of neurofibromatosis; the bone deformity in neurofibromatosis can be quite bizarre, with overgrowth or undergrowth of isolated bones; the characteristic spinal change is a very sharp upper thoracic kyphoscoliosis; and, finally, neurofibromatosis often shows clear evidence of dominant inheritance pattern.

The medical treatment of the McCune–Albright syndrome is complex. As for the monostotic form, polyostotic fibrous dysplasia may be improved by pamidronate.

Ectopic mineralization

Deposition of calcium in the soft tissues (ectopic calcification) and on ectopic bone matrix (ossification) has many causes (Table 20.1.17). These are nearly always pathological, but often the cause is unknown. In older people, calcification in the tissues such as the arteries is so common that it may be regarded as a feature of ageing, in the same way as age-related bone loss. There are some disorders in which calcification and/or ossification are associated with biochemical abnormalities.

Ectopic calcification without bone formation

Calcification can result from previous damage in soft tissues (dystrophic calcification) or from an increase in the circulating concentration of calcium or phosphate (metastatic calcification, e.g. in advanced renal osteodystrophy). Chondrocalcinosis is a particular example of ectopic mineralization.

Table 20.1.17 Causes of ectopic mineralization

Type	Cause	Disorder	Tissue distribution
Ectopic calcification			
Dystrophic (damaged tissue, biochemistry normal)	Unknown nucleators and inhibitors	Inflammation	In damaged tissues
		Haemorrhage	In damaged tissues
		Injury	In damaged tissues
		Age	Blood vessels, costal cartilages
		Systemic sclerosis	Particularly around phalanges
		Dermatomyositis	Sometimes in sheets associated with muscles
Metabolic (undamaged tissue, biochemistry abnormal)	High calcium	Hyperparathyroidism	Blood vessels, soft tissues
		Excessive vitamin D	Cornea, conjunctivae
		Excessive vitamin A	Tendons and ligaments
		Sarcoidosis	Nephrocalcinosis
	Low calcium	Hypoparathyroidism	Basal ganglia
		Pseudohypoparathyroidism	Subcutaneous (ossification)
	High phosphate	Renal glomerular failure	Blood vessels, soft tissues
		Inherited hyperphosphataemia	Periarticular soft tissues
	Low phosphate	Inherited hypophosphataemia	Tendons, ligaments (also ossification)
Chondrocalcinosis	Multiple (includes nucleators, deranged pyrophosphate transport, enzyme disorders)	Age	Joint cartilages
		Damaged cartilage	
		Hyperparathyroidism	
		Hypophosphatasia	
		Familial pyrophosphate arthropathy	
		Haemochromatosis	
		Wilson's disease	
		Hypomagnesaemia	
Ectopic ossification	**Acquired**		
	Local injury		
	Hip replacement		
	Traumatic paraplegia		
	Tumours		
	Others	Diffuse idiopathic skeletal hyperostosis (DISH)	
		Ossification of the posterior spinal ligament (OPLL)	
		Ankylosing spondylitis	
		Etretinate therapy	
		Some metabolic enthesopathies (eg X-linked hypophosphataemia, Dent's disease)	
	Inherited	Albright's hereditary osteodystrophy (AHO)	
		Fibrodysplasia (myositis) ossificans progressiva (FOP)	
		Progressive osseous heteroplasia (POH)	

Dystrophic calcification

This occurs in inherited and acquired disorders involving connective tissue, such as alkaptonuria (intervertebral discs), pseudoxanthoma elasticum (blood vessels), systemic sclerosis, and dermatomyositis (particularly in childhood), and also after infection, tumours, and trauma. In systemic sclerosis, subcutaneous calcification, often around the phalanges (calcinosis circumscripta), may be part of the CREST syndrome (calcinosis, Raynaud's phenomenon, oesophageal dysmotility, sclerodactyly, telangiectasia) (see also Chapter 19.11.3). The calcific deposits may sometimes ulcerate through the skin, discharging as toothpaste-like material. In dermatomyositis, sheets of subcutaneous calcification can be deposited some time after the initial inflammatory episode, characterized by a systemic illness and painful weak muscles; the calcification can be very extensive (calcinosis universalis) but can also disappear rapidly, sometimes in adolescence. Rarely this is associated with hypercalcaemia.

Metastatic calcification

The distribution of the calcification varies inexplicably with its cause (e.g. in hypoparathyroidism there is subcutaneous and basal ganglia calcification; and in hyperparathyroidism there is vascular calcification), suggesting that metastatic calcification is not only related to the Ca:P product. Calcification and ossification may also coexist.

Calcification and hypocalcaemia

This occurs in idiopathic and postsurgical hypoparathyroidism, as well as in pseudohypoparathyroidism. There may be extensive ectopic calcification, calcification within the basal ganglia (and outside it) and cataract formation. Pseudohypoparathyroidism is inherited as an autosomal dominant disorder with variable expression; additional clinical features include learning difficulties, round face, short stature, and short third and fourth metacarpals. An important feature is subcutaneous endochondral ossification. End organ resistance to parathyroid hormone may be due to mutations in the gene responsible for one component ($G_s\alpha$) of the G-protein signalling system (Table 20.1.1).

Calcification in hyperphosphataemia

Familial idiopathic hyperphosphataemia is a rare autosomal recessive disorder, with an increase in the maximal tubular resorption of phosphate and an inappropriate increase in the plasma $1,25(OH)_2D$ concentration. Masses of ectopic mineral, which form around the joints from childhood (tumoral calcinosis), may discharge through the skin. Treatment with large oral doses of aluminium hydroxide or other phosphate-binding agents can reduce the plasma phosphate level and the size of the deposits. A loss of function mutation in *FGF23* has been reported (cf. hypophosphataemic rickets, above) but mutations in *GALNT3* (involved in posttranslational protein glycosylation) also cause a recessive form of the condition.

Calcification in inherited hypophosphataemia

A particular feature of X-linked inherited hypophosphataemia is the widespread calcification and ossification of ligaments and tendons at their insertions into the periosteum (so-called Sharpey's fibres). This is termed an enthesopathy. Calcification and new bone formation in the ligamenta flava may produce spinal cord compression.

Idiopathic soft-tissue calcification

This includes calcific tendinitis and so-called calcinosis circumscripta.

Chondrocalcinosis

In chondrocalcinosis, crystals of calcium pyrophosphate dihydrate are deposited in the fibrocartilage of the knees, the triangular cartilage of the wrists, the symphysis pubis, and elsewhere. Calcium pyrophosphate dihydrate may also form as linear deposits in the hyaline cartilage parallel to the subchondral bone. It is most commonly an age-related phenomenon but may also reflect an underlying metabolic disturbance, such as haemochromatosis (OMIM 235200), hypophosphatasia, or hyperparathyroidism. Familial forms of chondrocalcinosis also exist; one florid polyarticular form presents with early-onset destructive arthritis (OMIM 118600) resulting from excessive accumulation of calcium pyrophosphate dihydrate in the extracellular tissues as a result of activating mutations in the *ANKH* gene, encoding a transmembrane transporter of inorganic pyrophosphate. Similar activating mutations have also now been described in sporadic cases of pyrophosphate arthritis.

Ectopic ossification

Acquired ectopic ossification may occur at the site of injury, such as after hip replacement, or at a distance from it (e.g. following paraplegia), or in tumours and in a variety of other disorders. Fibrodysplasia (myositis) ossificans progressiva (OMIM 135100) is a very rare autosomal dominant disorder caused by activating mutations in activin, a receptor for bone morphogenetic proteins (see below).

Acquired ectopic ossification

Posttraumatic ossification

Local ossification can occur after total hip replacement. The quoted incidence varies widely, depending on the method used to detect it. It is said to occur more often in men than in women and in certain individuals; e.g. where ossification follows hip replacement on one side, it is likely to occur if the contralateral hip is also replaced. The reason for this is unknown. The bone mainly forms in the hip abductors and ossification is classified according to its severity. Disodium etidronate may delay mineralization but only while it is being given, and nonsteroidal anti-inflammatory drugs are also useful. A small dose of radiotherapy may also delay ectopic ossification after total hip replacement.

Ossification after neurological injury

Extensive myositis ossificans can also occur from 1 to 4 months after injuries to the head or spinal cord in muscles distant from the injury such as the major muscles of the thigh. Affected muscles become swollen, red, and warm and, unless the cord lesion is complete, pain and tenderness also occur. At this time the differential diagnosis may include cellulitis, arthritis, and thrombophlebitis. Radiological calcification is initially absent (appearing at about 6 weeks or more after the injury), but an isotope bone scan will show increased uptake before that. Later there is progressive mineralization, with the eventual appearance of organized bone. Because the bone affects the major periarticular muscles, it leads to joint fixation, particularly of the hips. The plasma alkaline phosphatase level may be increased in the early stages.

Attempted surgical removal of ectopic bone is technically difficult and produces little increase in movement. The ectopic bone recurs, especially if it is removed too early. Oral disodium etidronate at full dose (20 mg/kg body weight per day) may delay the onset of mineralization but only while it is being given. Likewise, the prevention of further ectopic bone formation after its removal may be delayed by nonsteroidal anti-inflammatory drugs or radiotherapy, which should be commenced as soon as possible.

Myositis ossificans can also occur after other neurological diseases, such as poliomyelitis and meningitis, and also after prolonged coma. The reason why ectopic ossification occurs after head injury is unknown; interestingly, head injury is associated with an increased rate of fracture healing and excessive callus formation. In such patients, the serum contains increased mitogenic activity for osteoblast-like cells; the source of this activity is unknown, but there could be an increase in bone morphogenetic proteins.

Ossification can coexist with calcification and extensive ossification of the spinal ligaments in hypoparathyroidism can lead to progressive stiffness. The enthesopathy in inherited hypophosphataemia (vitamin D-resistant rickets) is a form of ectopic ossification. Ossification of the posterior longitudinal ligament and sternoclavicular hyperostosis is particularly described in Japan. Ligamentous ossification has been noted in patients treated with vitamin A analogues, such as etretinate, for dermatological disorders. Finally, ectopic bone may complicate varicose veins, chronic venous insufficiency, and surgical incisions.

Inherited ectopic ossification

The inherited causes of ectopic ossification (Table 20.1.17) are rare. In two disorders, fibrodysplasia ossificans progressiva and progressive osseous heteroplasia, ossification is a major and disabling feature.

Fibrodysplasia ossificans progressiva

Fibrodysplasia ossificans progressiva (OMIM 135100) is rare, with an incidence of between 1 and 2 per million, which increases with paternal age. Since patients rarely reproduce, most cases represent new mutations. However, the very few familial cases investigated worldwide have allowed genetic linkage analysis to identify activating mutations in the activin receptor gene, *ACVR1*, encoding a BMP type 1 receptor. This discovery is clearly consistent with the known abnormality of ossification in the condition but it is not clear why this should occur in discrete episodes. Diagnosis depends on the combination of progressive myositis, leading to ossification in the major skeletal muscles and characteristic bony skeletal abnormalities.

Pathophysiology Initially there is oedema and cellular infiltration throughout the muscle, with myofibrillar breakdown. Later endochondral ossification leads to mature bone, within which is haemopoietic marrow. Information on the earliest histological appearances is scanty because biopsies are often taken after the acute phase of myositis; for this reason there is still doubt about the primary lesion. Ectopic ossification occurs when mesenchymal or stromal cells take on the behaviour of osteoblasts. This form of cell differentiation could result from an increase in bone-inducing substances or (for unknown reasons) a change in stromal-cell expression. Although the timing of myositis differs widely from one affected patient to another, there is a specific order in which

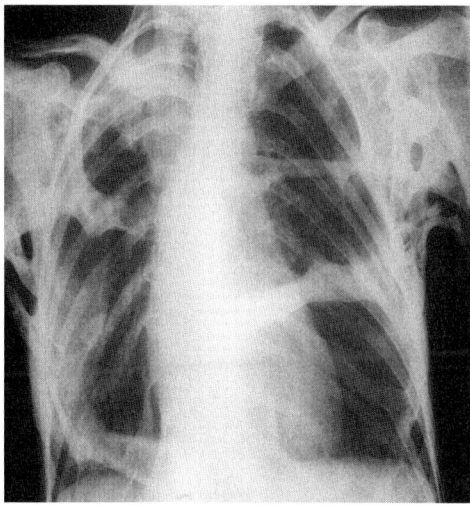

Fig. 20.1.27 Fibrodysplasia ossificans progressiva. Widespread ectopic ossification of the muscles around the thorax. The chest is completely fixed but the diaphragm is unaffected.

they are affected, from the upper paraspinal to the lower, and from the centre to the periphery.

Clinical features Episodes of myositis are the nonskeletal hallmark of this disease. Typically, the affected muscle becomes swollen and hard, sometimes following injury; after a week or two these features subside, but the apparent improvement is followed in a month or so by ossification within the muscle and progressive joint fixation. Myositis usually begins in the upper paraspinal muscles. By late childhood or adolescence, ossification will have occurred within the muscles around the shoulders, hips, and knees to fix these joints and to complete the disability (Fig. 20.1.27). The large, striated muscles are affected; ossification does not involve the small muscles of the hands and feet, the diaphragm, or the cardiac or smooth muscles. Ossification in the muscles around the jaw may fix it almost completely. Although the overall sequence of ossification is characteristic from large upper paraspinal to lower limb muscles, it varies considerably in its rate. For instance, neonates may have sufficient ossification to produce torticollis while, in contrast, late and slow ossification producing stiffness may delay the correct diagnosis until adolescence. Likewise, there may be long symptom-free periods.

The diagnostic skeletal abnormalities affect the big toes (Fig. 20.1.28), the cervical spine (Fig. 20.1.29), and, to a lesser extent, the thumbs. The big toes are always abnormal; in the infant, bony changes produce bilateral hallux valgus, and, in the adult, fusion produces a short fixed monophalangic big toe. In the cervical spine, the vertebral bodies are small and the laminae large. Both are variably fused; this fusion is independent of nearby ossification of the cervical muscles. The appearance of the cervical spine probably represents a failure of development of the zygapophyseal joints (cf. the monophalangeal great toe) rather than fusion resulting from new bone deposition. Finally, the femoral necks are short and wide and there are exostoses from the metaphyses.

Differential diagnosis Bilateral hallux valgus in the neonate should suggest the possibility of fibrodysplasia ossificans progressiva. In childhood, myositis may be mistaken for soft-tissue

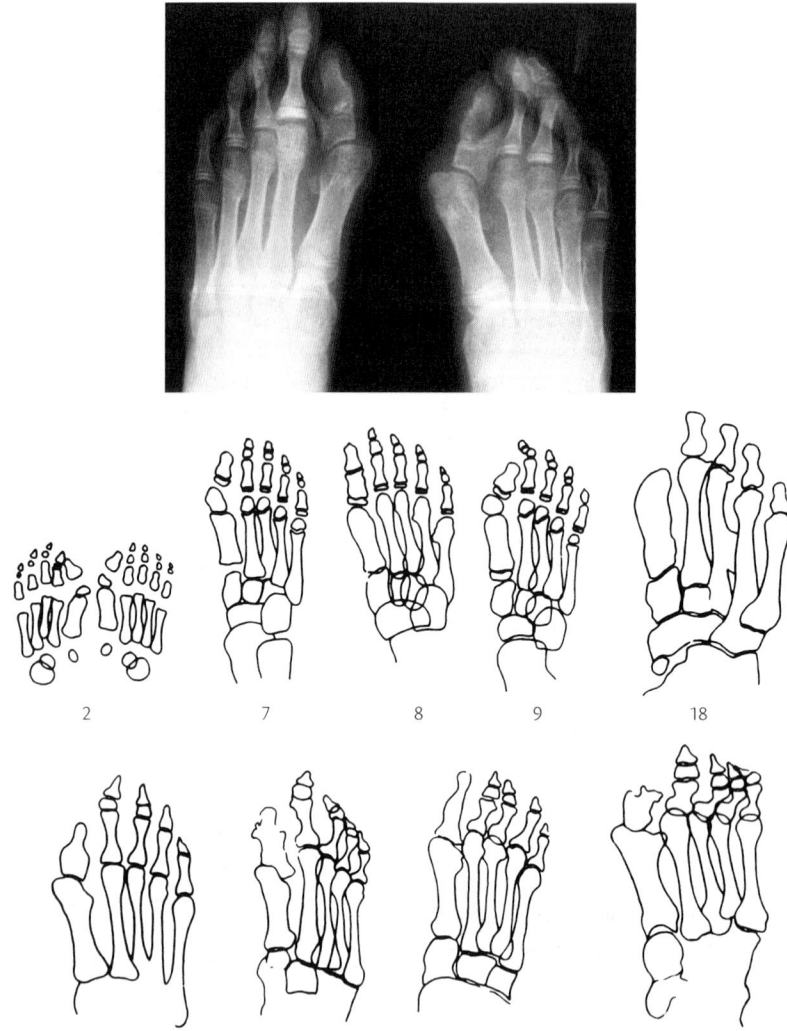

Fig. 20.1.28 Fibrodysplasia ossificans progressiva. (a) Abnormal first toes and (b) appearances in nine patients of different ages, traced from X-rays. The abnormal phalanges of the first toes, present at birth, later fuse into one unusual phalanx. Age in years are shown beneath each tracing.

sarcoma and a biopsy showing oedema and increased cellularity may support this or suggest an aggressive fibromatosis. Painful swelling of the masticatory muscles simulates mumps and progressive stiffness with a fixed abnormal neck suggests the Klippel–Feil syndrome or childhood rheumatoid arthritis.

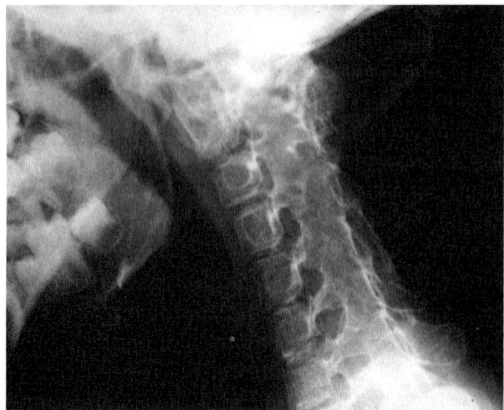

Fig. 20.1.29 Fibrodysplasia ossificans progressiva. Complete fusion of the posterior elements of the cervical spine. The vertebral bodies appear relatively small.

Management Once the diagnosis has been made, and this is often delayed, there are four main questions: can the myositis be prevented; if myositis does occur, can subsequent ossification be prevented; what will be the eventual disability; and should ectopic bone be removed?

Since the onset of myositis is quite unpredictable, it is almost impossible to assess the effect of any form of therapy. Corticosteroids have been used, sometimes associated with symptom-free periods. They are most appropriate in short high-dose regimes to reduce swelling in acute myositis. Myositis often follows injury, which should be avoided where possible. It seems likely, but difficult to prove, that myositis is normally followed by ossification. Although the bisphosphonate etidronate can suppress mineralization of bone, there is no evidence that it is effective in the long term in this condition; the newer bisphosphonates lacking this effect are not indicated. Surgical removal of ectopic bone is technically difficult and recurrence at the site of surgery may worsen the disability.

The eventual disability produced by fibrodysplasia ossificans progressiva is severe. The body moves as in one piece with the legs usually fixed in partial flexion. All major joints can become completely fixed. The help of a specialized rehabilitation centre is essential.

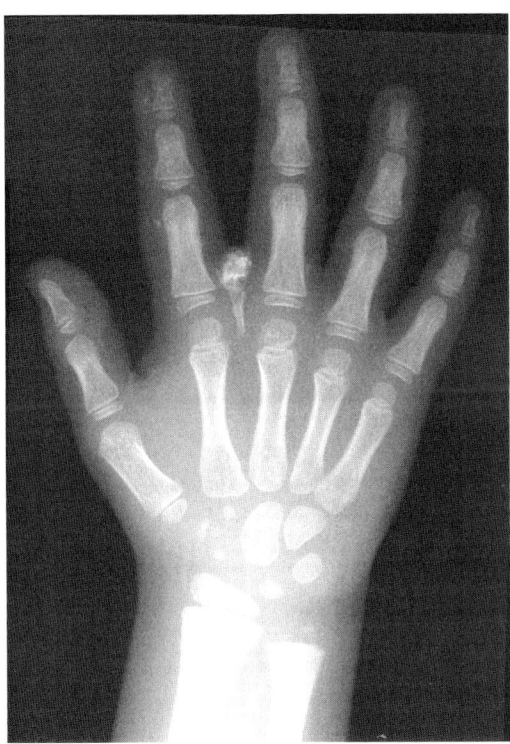

Fig. 20.1.30 Progressive osseous heteroplasia. Ossification in the second web space of the hand in a boy with a paternally inherited inactivating mutation of GNAS1.

Progressive osseous heteroplasia (OMIM 166350)

In this disorder, there is extensive and progressive heterotropic ossification affecting many tissues including subcutaneous fat, connective tissue, and muscles (Fig. 20.1.30). Typically ossification begins in the subcutaneous tissues of one limb in childhood; these may be preceded by maculopapular rashes at the site of future ossification. The ossification is progressive and surgery may be necessary.

Progressive osseous heteroplasia is inherited as an autosomal dominant disorder with very wide clinical expression. The mutation is in GNAS1, the gene coding for the $G_s\alpha$ protein. There is an overlap between progressive osseous heteroplasia and Albright hereditary osteodystrophy (AHO), which also has an inactivating mutation in GNAS1.

Miscellaneous bone disorders

The skeleton is affected in many systemic diseases (e.g. scurvy and the haemoglobinopathies), by the methods used to treat them (e.g. parenteral nutrition), and by excessive ingestion of minerals, vitamins, and metals (e.g. fluorosis, overdose of vitamins A and D, and metal poisoning). In some, the skeletal changes are clinically important; in others, they are a minor aspect of the general illness. This Section ends with a brief description of the obscure disorder fibrogenesis imperfecta ossium.

Scurvy

Vitamin C (ascorbic acid) is necessary for intracellular hydroxylation of peptide-bound proline. In its absence, formation of the collagen molecule is defective, structurally incompetent precursors accumulate within the cell and collagen-containing tissues are weak. The function of osteoblasts is impaired and spontaneous fractures occur in mutant mice with vitamin C deficiency. Scurvy is very rare, occurring most often in neglected infants who do not receive fruit juice or ascorbic acid for several months. Extensive subperiosteal haemorrhage leads to pain and immobility; the legs are held in a 'frog-like' position. In the adult, there is perifollicular haemorrhage, purpura, and bleeding gums. Radiographs in infancy show a widened zone of provisional calcification in the metaphyses, with a proximal disordered area representing the destroyed primary spongiosa and failure of new bone formation. The edges of the metaphyses may show small spurs and epiphyseolysis may occur. With healing the subperiosteal haematoma calcifies.

The clinical picture of scurvy may suggest nonaccidental injury, but scurvy is far less common. Similar radiographic appearances have been described in cases of copper deficiency.

The haemoglobinopathies

In the inherited disorders of haemoglobin (see Section 22), the skeleton is often abnormal. This may result from a hyperplastic bone marrow and overactivity of the osteoblasts, so that the skull, facial bones, and long bones are thickened. Additional features include collapse of the weight-bearing bones and disorganization of the joints following bone infarction. This is especially seen in sickle-cell disease, haemoglobin C disease, and haemoglobin SC compound heterozygotes. In β-thalassaemia, an increase in osteoid thickness has been described which resembles that of osteomalacia.

Parenteral nutrition

Prolonged parenteral nutrition can produce a form of bone disease with similarities to osteomalacia. The main symptom is periarticular bone pain, particularly in the ankles. Histology shows impaired mineralization of bone and biochemistry reveals an increase in plasma alkaline phosphatase, in urinary calcium, and, sometimes, in plasma calcium. The radiographic appearances suggest osteoporosis. Since patients on total parenteral nutrition are invariably ill to begin with and many have malabsorption, there are several probable causes for this disorder; aluminium intoxication may contribute.

Fluorosis

Deposition of excess fluoride in the skeleton can result from an excess in the diet (endemic fluorosis), from industrial exposure (during the manufacture of aluminium, steel, and glass and from exposure to the dust of fluoride-containing rock), and from the administration of sodium fluoride in treatment. The most severe effects are seen in endemic fluorosis, well described from the Punjab. In Asia, skeletal fluorosis may result from the consumption of inferior quality 'brick tea'. Similarly, excessive consumption of instant tea and obsessive use of fluoride-containing toothpaste can cause fluorosis.

There is considerable disability, with spinal rigidity, restricted movements of the joints, and flexion deformities of the hips and knees. There is a generalized increase in bone density (with loss of the normal corticomedullary junction) and the tendons, ligaments, and, sometimes, muscles may be mineralized. This can produce compression of the spinal cord and its roots, with progressive neurological disability. Mineralization of tendon insertions may be seen in other situations, such as inherited hypophosphataemia (see above), retinoid treatment, and fibrogenesis imperfecta ossium (see below).

Increased levels of fluoride can affect the enamel of developing teeth, producing chalky white patches, yellow-brown discoloration, and other defects.

The diagnosis of fluorosis depends on the radiographic changes and an increased urinary excretion of fluoride (which is an index of current exposure). When a bone biopsy is performed (most often to exclude other causes of increased bone density), histology shows an increase in new bone formation with an increase in the width of osteoid borders. There is also an increase in fibrous tissue and bone resorption. When the biopsy includes an area of tendinous insertion, this may be mineralized.

Sodium fluoride has been given widely to treat osteoporosis and it increases vertebral density. This does not increase vertebral bone strength and may cause an increase in appendicular bone fracture. The main effect of the fluoride ion is to stimulate new bone formation, while fluoroapatite may also reduce resorption. The new bone appears to be mainly woven in character and imperfectly mineralized. Although there is no doubt about the anabolic effects of fluoride on bone, current controversies about its clinical usefulness depend, in part, on the dose used.

Vitamin A

Retinoic acid and its derivatives have profound effects on osteoblast function. Vitamin A poisoning produces characteristic periostitis in the young skeleton and therapeutic retinoids (such as etretinate) causes widespread ligamentous calcification. Acute and chronic forms of vitamin A overdosage are described. In infants, it is uncommon under the age of 1 year. There is anorexia and failure to thrive; other features include pruritus, hepatosplenomegaly, jaundice, alopecia, dry skin, and fissures around the lips. Hard, tender masses appear in the limbs and radiographs show periosteal new bone formation, especially in the diaphyses of the tibias, which later blends into the cortex. A number of other radiological features include shortening of the shafts of the long bones, splaying of the metaphyses, enlargement, and premature fusion of the ossification centres and flexion deformities of the legs.

The prolonged use of retinoids for the treatment of skin disease, such as psoriasis and ichthyosis, leads particularly to calcification of the spinal ligaments, causing stiffness, and reduced mobility. There is a resemblance to Forestier's disease (diffuse idiopathic skeletal hyperostosis).

Vitamin D

Vitamin D poisoning can result from inappropriate therapeutic overdosage or accidental overconsumption. This leads to the features of hypercalcaemia (see Chapter 13.6) without detectable effects on the skeleton. The main opportunities for overdose exist when potent preparations of vitamin D are used inappropriately (e.g. to treat skin conditions and tuberculosis). Chronic vitamin D overdosage leads to soft-tissue calcification, especially in the arteries and kidneys. After several years, progressive stiffness in the spine, major joints, and feet lead to difficulty in walking. Radiographs show ligamentous calcification. Another cause of hypercalcaemia is an excess of $1,25(OH)_2D$ produced by granulomas, especially those of sarcoidosis following exposure of the skin to sunlight. The biochemical effects are the same as those of vitamin D poisoning. The $1,25(OH)_2D$ concentration increases with that of 25OHD and the hypercalcaemia of sarcoidosis often occurs during the spring in persons with outdoor jobs (such as farmers and window cleaners) or after foreign holidays in the sun. Treatment with corticosteroids and removal from sunlight rapidly reduces the hypercalcaemia and the elevated $1,25(OH)_2D$ levels.

Idiopathic hypercalcaemia can occur in infancy. Now named Williams' syndrome, it is associated with an unusual 'elfin face', intellectual disability, and congenital heart disease. Radiographs of the long bones show increased density of the metaphyses. The cause is not fully understood, but the concentration of 25OHD may be increased when the patients are hypercalcaemic. Deletion of the elastin locus on chromosome 7 has also been described and may explain the cardiac abnormalities.

Lead (see also Chapter 9.1)

Lead has unique effects on the skeleton, which may be combined with the other manifestations of lead intoxication. Lead deposition in the growing skeleton produces a radiologically dense line near the growth plate. When exposure to lead has been intermittent or the condition has been treated, this may be a single, relatively narrow line, which is superseded by apparently normal bone. If exposure to lead recurs, a further line will appear.

Lead poisoning due to industrial pollution is thought to be widespread, but the skeleton is affected only when lead exposure has been considerable. In children, one recognized source is lead-containing paint. Other sources include contaminated water from old lead pipes, eye blackener used by Asian women (which contains up to 88% lead sulphide), inhalation of lead fumes from burning old battery cases, and alcoholic drinks stored in vessels of lead glass or coated by lead enamel glaze. Environmentally-derived lead accumulates in chronic renal insufficiency.

Clinical features involve: the gastrointestinal tract (abdominal pain, colic with constipation, and a blue pigmentation of the gingival margin); the neuromuscular system, with weakness; and encephalopathy, with restlessness, irritability, and lethargy. Renal manifestations are described in Section 20.

Characteristic radiological features include widened skull sutures (due to raised intracranial pressure in infants), dense deposits in the gastrointestinal tract indicating heavy-metal ingestion, and dense lines in the metaphyses (lead lines). Such lines are an important clue to lead poisoning in infants and children up to about the age of 6 years. They occur most commonly around the knees, wrists, and ankles, and appear after about a month of chronic poisoning. The diagnosis of lead poisoning is confirmed by an increase in plasma and urinary lead levels. There are other causes of radiologically dense metaphyses. These include: other heavy metals (bismuth, mercury, or phosphorus); vitamin D intoxication and idiopathic hypercalcaemia of infancy; intermittent intravenous pamidronate (as in osteogenesis imperfecta); cretinism; and healing rickets. In practice, there is often difficulty in deciding on the significance of dense metaphyses due to excessive calcium in an otherwise well child, since this appearance can occur in the normal growing skeleton.

Aluminium (See also Chapter 9.1)

Aluminium in water is not significantly absorbed through the intestine, but this barrier was effectively removed in the early days of haemodialysis treatment for endstage renal failure. The resultant accumulation of aluminium in the skeleton in patients in some units where the aluminium content of tap water was high led to the occurrence and recognition of 'dialysis bone disease'. There was a close clinical association with dialysis dementia, also related to aluminium poisoning. The clinical features of this bone disease were proximal myopathy, multiple painful spontaneous fractures with radiographic evidence of osteopenia (osteoporosis), histological evidence of excess osteoid with aluminium deposition near the calcification front, and an absence of response to vitamin D metabolites.

In renal glomerular failure, aluminium may also accumulate in patients given oral aluminium hydroxide to reduce plasma phosphate (in order to lessen hypocalcaemia and subsequent secondary hyperparathyroidism). Aluminium bone disease can also occur in patients on prolonged parenteral nutrition.

The pathology of aluminium bone disease is not fully understood, but it seems likely that in some instances aluminium reduces osteoblast activity. Two different forms are described: in the first, there is excessive osteoid (with an appearance like that of osteomalacia); and in the second, there is little increase in osteoid with reduced osteoblastic activity. It is likely that the different histological features are related to the amount of aluminium in the bones.

Cadmium (See also Chapter 9.1)

Contamination of drinking water by cadmium and its accumulation in the body causes renal tubular damage with multiple biochemical defects. Cadmium intoxication is one of the acquired causes of Fanconi's syndrome, which leads to rickets or osteomalacia. Industrial exposure to cadmium fumes can produce hypophosphataemic osteomalacia.

Exceptionally, chronic lead poisoning can also produce osteomalacia by the same mechanism as cadmium and copper 'poisoning' causes Fanconi's syndrome and bone disease with Wilson's disease.

Fibrogenesis imperfecta ossium

This is a very rare, apparently acquired disorder, characterized by excessive bony fragility due to the replacement of normal bone with a fibre-deficient, poorly mineralized matrix. The cause is unknown. In recorded cases, the main clinical feature has been pathological fractures first presenting in adult life. In most patients, progressive disability has followed, with more fractures that fail to unite. Radiologically, the trabeculae throughout the skeleton appear to be thickened. There is also ectopic mineralization around large joints and tendon insertions. Biochemically, plasma calcium and phosphate levels are normal, but the alkaline phosphatase level is moderately raised. In the urine, monoclonal light chains may be present. The diagnosis is confirmed by the examination of undecalcified bone. This shows defective mineralization and wide osteoid seams, suggesting severe osteomalacia, but the osteoid is not birefringent under polarized light and the normal structure of bone collagen under electron microscopy is absent. The differential diagnosis is from those disorders that produce widespread coarse trabeculation throughout the skeleton and those that produce the histological changes of osteomalacia. In the first category, Paget's disease of bone, renal glomerular osteodystrophy, and fluorosis should be excluded, and in the second, axial osteomalacia has some similarities; in this very rare osteosclerotic disorder, both histology and radiographs suggest that the osteomalacia is limited to the spine, pelvis, and ribs.

Since the cause of fibrogenesis imperfecta ossium is unknown, treatment to date has been largely empirical. The occasional finding of an excess of plasma cells in the bone marrow or a monoclonal gammopathy, or light chain proteinuria, has led to apparently successful treatment with melphalan and prednisolone. Where surgery is indicated for fractures, particularly of the femoral neck, this is difficult because of the extreme fragility of the bones.

Although it seems likely that the defect may be related to an acquired disorder of bone collagen, no consistent abnormality has been detected.

Further reading

Introduction

Smith R, Wordsworth P (2006). *Clinical and biochemical disorders of the skeleton*. Oxford University Press, Oxford.

Physiology of bone

Bilezikian JP, Raisz LG, Rodan GA (2002). *Principles of bone biology*, 2nd edition. Academic Press, San Diego CA.

Brown EM (2007). Clinical lessons from the calcium-sensing receptor. *Nat Clin Pract Endocrinol Metab*, **3**, 122–33.

Harada S-I, Rodan G (2003). Control of osteoblast function and regulation of bone mass. *Nature*, **423**, 349–55.

Horton WA (2003). Skeletal development: Insights from targeting the mouse genome. *Lancet*, **362**, 560–9.

Johnson ML, et al. (2004). LRP5 and Wnt signaling: A union made for bone. *J Bone Miner Res*, **19**, 1749–957.

Royce PM, Steinmann B (2002). *Connective tissue and its heritable disorders*, 2nd edition. Wiley-Liss, New York.

Scriver CR, et al. (eds) (2001). *The metabolic and molecular bases of inherited disease*, 8th edition. McGraw Hill, New York.

The diagnosis of bone disease

Favus MJ (2003). *Primer on the metabolic bone diseases and disorders of mineral metabolism*, 5th edition. American Society for Bone and Mineral Research, Washington.

Meier C, Seibel MJ, Kraanzlin ME (2009). Use of bone turnover markers in the real world: are we there yet? *J Bone Miner Res*, **24**, 386–8.

Osteomalacia and rickets

Parfitt AM (1998). Osteomalacia and related disorders. In: Avioli LV, Krane SM (eds) *Metabolic bone disease*, 3rd edition, pp. 327–86. Academic Press, San Diego.

Shimada T, et al. (2004). FGF-23 is a potent regulator of vitamin D metabolism and phosphate homeostasis. *J Bone Miner Res*, **19**, 429–35.

Wharton B, Bishop N (2003). Rickets. *Lancet*, **362**, 1389–400.

Paget's disease of bone

Barker DJP, et al. (1977). Paget's disease of bone in 14 British towns. *Br Med J*, **1**, 1181–3.

Cavey JR, et al. (2005). Loss of ubiquitin-binding associated with Paget's disease of bone p62(SQSTM1) mutations. *J Bone Miner Res*, **20**, 619–24.

Cundy T, et al. (2005). Recombinant osteoprotegerin for juvenile Paget's disease. *N Engl J Med*, **353**, 918–23.

Deftos LJ (2005). Treatment of Paget's disease—taming the wild osteoclast. *N Engl J Med*, **353**, 872–75.

Hosking D, et al. (2007). Long-term control of bone turnover in Paget's disease with zoledronic acid and risedronate. *J Bone Miner Res*, **22**, 142–8.

Kanis JA (1998). *Pathophysiology and treatment of Paget's disease of bone*, 2nd edition. Martin Dunitz, London.

Lucas GJA, et al. (2004). SQSTM1 mutations in Paget's disease: evidence for a founder effect of an ancestral chromosome bearing the P392L mutation. *J Bone Miner Res*, **19**, 1033 [abstract].

Naot D, et al. (2007). Differential gene expression in cultivated osteoblasts and bone marrow stromal cells from patients with Paget's disease of bone. *J Bone Miner Res*, **22**, 298–309.

Reid IR, et al. (2005). Comparison of a single infusion of zoledronic acid with risedronate for Paget's disease. *N Engl J Med*, **353**, 918–23.

Roodman GD, Windle JJ (2005). Paget disease of bone. *J Clin Invest*, **115**, 200–8.

Woo SB, *et al.* (2006). Bisphosphonates and osteonecrosis of the jaws. *Ann Intern Med*, **144**, 753–61.

Parathyroids and bone disease

Bilezikian JP, Siverberg SJ (2004). Asympomatic primary hyperparathyroidism. *N Engl J Med*, **350**, 1746–51.

Thakker RV (2001). Genetic developments in hypoparathyroidism. *Lancet*, **357**, 974–6.

Osteogenesis imperfecta: the brittle bone syndrome

Barnes AM, Chang W, Morello R *et al.* (2006). Deficiency of cartilage-associated protein in recessive lethal osteogenesis imperfecta. *N Engl J Med*, **355**, 2757–64.

Rauch F, Glorieux FH (2004). Osteogenesis imperfecta. *Lancet*, **363**, 1377–85.

Marfan's syndrome

Gelb BD (2006). Marfan's syndrome and related disorders—more tightly connected than we thought. *New Eng J Med*, **358**, 841–4.

Ho NCY, *et al.* (2005). Marfan's syndrome. *Lancet*, **366**, 1978–81.

Judge DP, Dietz HC (2005). Marfan's syndrome. *Lancet*, **366**, 1965–81.

Mizuguchi T, *et al.* (2004). Heterozygous *TGFBR2* mutations in Marfan syndrome. *Nat Genet*, **36**, 855–60.

Ehlers–Danlos syndrome

Beighton P, *et al.* (1998). Ehlers Danlos syndrome: revised nosology, Villefranche 1997. *Am J Med Genet*, **77**, 31–7.

Byers PH (2001). An exception to the rule. *N Engl J Med*, **345**, 1203–5.

Pyeritz RE (2000). Ehlers-Danlos syndrome. *N Engl J Med*, **342**, 730–2.

Loeys B, *et al.* (2010). Revised Ghent nosology for Marfan's syndrome. *Am J Med Genet*, in press.

Homocystinuria

Raisz LG (2004). Homocysteine and osteoporotic fractures—culprit or bystander?. *N Engl J Med*, **350**, 2089–90.

Skovby F, Kraus JP (2002). The homocystinurias. In: Royce PM, Steinmann B (eds) *Connective tissue and its heritable disorders*, 2nd edition, pp. 627–50. Wiley-Liss, New York.

Alkaptonuria

La Du BN (2002). Alkaptonuria. In: Royce PM, Steinmann B (eds) *Connective tissue and its heritable disorders*, 2nd edition, pp. 809–25. Wiley-Liss, New York.

Nickkels AF, Piérard GE (2001). Medical mystery, the answer. *N Engl J Med*, **344**, 1642–3.

Phorphutkul C, *et al.* (2003). Natural history of alkaptonuria. *N Engl J Med*, **347**, 2111–21.

Hypophosphatasia

Whyte MP (2002). Heritable forms of rickets and osteomalacia. In: Royce PM, Steinmann B (eds) *Connective tissue and its heritable disorders*, 2nd edition, pp. 765–87. Wiley–Liss, New York.

Lysosomal storage diseases

Leroy JG (2002). Disorders of lysosomal enzymes: clinical phenotypes. In: Royce PM, Steinmann B (eds) *Connective tissue and its heritable disorders*, 2nd edition, pp. 849–99. Wiley–Liss, New York.

Staba SL, *et al.* (2004). Cord-blood transplants from unrelated donors in patients with Hurler's syndrome. *N Engl J Med*, **350**, 1960–9.

Skeletal dysplasias

Horton WA, Hecht JT (2002). Skeletal dysplasias, chondrodysplasias: general concepts and diagnostic and management considerations. In: Royce PM, Steinmann B (eds) *Connective tissue and its heritable disorders*, 2nd edition, pp. 901–8. Wiley–Liss, New York.

Spranger JW, *et al.* (2002). *Bone dysplasias. An atlas of genetic disorders of skeletal development*, 2nd edition. Oxford University Press, Oxford.

Unger S, *et al.* (2007). Chondrodysplasias. In: Rimoin D, Connor M (eds) *Principles and practice of medical genetics*, 5th edition, pp. 3709–53. Churchill Livingstone, Philadelphia.

Osteopetrosis (marble bone disease)

Boyce BF (2003). Bad bones, grey hair, one mutation. *Nat Med*, **9**, 395–6.

Boyle WJ, *et al.* (2003). Osteoclast differentiation and activation. *Nature*, **427**, 337–42.

Rouselle A-V, Heymann D (2002). Osteoclastic acidification pathways during bone resorption. *Bone*, **30**, 533–40.

Tolar J, Teitelbaum SL, Orchard PJ (2004). Osteopetrosis. *N Engl J Med*, **351**, 2839–49.

Fibrous dysplasia

Lania AG, Mantovani G, Spada A (2006). Mechanisms of disease: mutations of G proteins and G-protein-coupled receptors in endocrine diseases. *Nat Clin Pract Endocrinol Metab*, **2**, 681–93.

Levine MA (2002). Molecular and clinical characteristics of the McCune-Albright syndrome. In: Wass JAH, Shalet SM (eds) *Oxford textbook of endocrinology and diabetes*, pp. 923–30. Oxford University Press, Oxford.

Ectopic mineralization

Chefetz I, *et al.* (2005). A novel homozygous missense mutation in *FGF23* causes familial tumoral calcinosis associated with disseminated visceral calcification. *Hum Genet*, **118**, 261–6.

Connor JM, Evans DAP (1982). Fibrodysplasia (myositis) ossificans progressiva. The clinical features and natural history of 34 patients. *J Bone Joint Surg*, **64**, 76–83.

Juppner H (2002). The genetic basis of progressive osseous heteroplasia. *N Engl J Med*, **346**, 128–30.

Shore EM, *et al.* (2006). A recent mutation in the BMP type 1 receptor ACVR1 causes inherited and sporadic fibrodysplasia ossificans progressiva. *Nat Genet*, **38**, 525–7.

Williams C, *et al.* (2002). Autosomal dominant familial calcium pyrophosphate dihydrate deposition disease is caused by mutation in the transmembrane protein ANKH. *Am J Hum Genet*, **71**, 985–91.

Miscellaneous bone disorders

Carr AJ, *et al.* (1995). Fibrogenesis imperfecta ossium. *J Bone Joint Surg*, **77**, 820–9.

Kurland ES, *et al.* (2007). Recovery from skeletal fluorosis (an enigmatic, American case). *J Bone Miner Res*, **22**, 163–70.

Marsden PA (2003). Increased body lead burden—cause or consequence of chronic renal insufficiency. *N Engl J Med*, **348**, 345–7.

Mohan S, *et al.* (2005). Spontaneous fractures in the mouse mutation *sfx* are caused by deletion of the gulonolactone oxidase gene, causing vitamin C deficiency. *J Bone Miner Res*, **20**, 1597–610.

Whyte MP, *et al.* (2005). Skeletal fluorosis and instant tea. *Am J Med*, **118**, 78–82.

Inherited defects of connective tissue: Ehlers–Danlos syndrome, Marfan's syndrome, and pseudoxanthoma elasticum

N.P. Burrows

Essentials

The inherited disorders of connective tissue are all conditions in which structural defects in collagen or other extra cellular matrix proteins lead to its fragility, with the commonest sites of involvement being the skin, ligaments and vasculature.

Ehlers–Danlos syndrome (EDS)

EDS is a heterogeneous group of disorders resulting from abnormalities in collagen synthesis and processing, or of other extracellular matrix proteins. They can be classified on the basis of descriptive clinical phenotype and/or underlying molecular cause. Most cases are autosomal dominant, but 30 to 50% may be sporadic.

Clinical features—the cardinal manifestations are cutaneous hypextensibility, soft texture ('doughy consistency') and fragility, ligamentous laxity, and easy bruising. (1) Classical EDS (types I and II)—commonly caused by mutations in *COL5A1*; notable features include epicanthic folds and blue sclerae. (2) Hypermobile EDS (type III)/benign joint hypermobility syndrome—the commonest subtype of EDS; caused by haploinsufficiency of tenascin-X in some cases; manifest with joint hypermobility but minimal skin changes; persistent arthralgia may be difficult to treat. (3) Vascular EDS (type IV)—mutations in *COL3A1* lead to reduction of collagen III in blood vessels and bowel in this life threatening condition; about half of arterial ruptures involve medium/large thoracic or abdominal arteries, but any site can be affected; most bowel perforations affect the sigmoid colon; significant risk of uterine rupture in pregnancy. (4) Kyphoscoliotic EDS (type VI)—may be due to defective function of a post-translational modification enzyme, lysyl hydroxylase. (6) Arthrochalasis EDS (type VII)—due to deficient processing of collagen I; characterised by severe joint hypermobililty, congenital bilateral hip dislocations and recurrent subluxations.

Marfan's syndrome

Marfan's syndrome is caused by autosomal dominant mutations in the human fibrillin-1 (*FBN1*) gene, with *de novo* mutations occurring in about 25% of cases. Criteria for diagnosis include aortic root dilatation, aortic dissection, lens dislocation, dural ectasia, and the presence of skeletal features including pectus carinatum, pectus excavatum requiring surgery, reduced upper to lower segment ratio or arm span to height ratio >1.05, wrist and thumb signs, scoliosis or spondylolisthesis, reduced extensions at the elbows, pes planus, and protrusio acetabulae. The main causes of death in Marfan's syndrome are cardiovascular complications, in particular aortic rupture (see Chapters 16.11 and 16.14.1). It is possible that early treatment with angiotensin II receptor blockade will prevent this by slowing the progression of aortic root dilatation, and it may also help other noncardiovascular complications.

Pseudoxanthoma elasticum (PXE)

PXE is caused by molecular defects in the transporter gene (*ABCC6*) that lead to calcification of elastic fibres and manifestation with complications including (1) cutaneous—yellowish papules appear in flexures, leading to a 'plucked chicken' or 'gooseflesh' appearance; (2) ocular—fundoscopy reveals mottled *peau d'orange* pigmentation, progressing to breaks in Bruch's membrane when angioid streaks are seen; retinal haemorrhages, neovascularization and chorioretinitis can all lead to loss of central vision; and (3) cardiovascular—calcification of arterial elastic media and intima affects predominantly peripheral arteries; intermittent claudication is the commonest symptom.

Introduction

The inherited disorders of connective tissue, Ehlers–Danlos syndrome, pseudoxanthoma elasticum, and Marfan's syndrome, are a diverse group of conditions with variable manifestations from minor symptoms to life-threatening complications. All share structural defects in collagen or other extracellular matrix proteins leading to fragility of connective tissue. The commonest sites of involvement are the skin, ligaments, and vasculature, although any organ can be affected and share common clinical features.

Subtle inherited defects of connective tissue may exert their effects at different stages of life. Molecular interactions between structural proteins and the extracellular matrix are important early in embryogenesis, and inherited defects of protein constituents in connective tissues may thus disturb many tissues during development and organogenesis. In the ageing population, increased fragility of the skin, rupture of blood vessels, and laxity of ligaments, as well as defects of cartilage and bone, may occur. Such degenerative disorders include osteoporosis, osteoarthritis, and arterial aneurysms. In the light of recent advances in the understanding of the molecular structure and genetics of connective tissue components, it seems likely that many aspects of medicine hitherto ascribed to age-related degeneration will ultimately prove to have strong genetic components. A valid, molecular understanding of these processes may well emerge. It also appears likely that the discrete clinical conditions now recognized as Ehlers–Danlos syndrome, Marfan's syndrome, and pseudoxanthoma elasticum will prove to have diverse and genetically determined counterparts that are responsible for the so-called degenerative disorders in the population at large.

Ehlers–Danlos syndrome (EDS)

The first detailed description of EDS was provided by a Russian dermatologist, AN Tschernogubow, at the inaugural meeting of the Moscow Dermatological and Venereological Society in 1891. The eponymous title was proposed 30 years later following further delineation of features by Edvard Ehlers and, subsequently, Henri-Alexandre Danlos. The cardinal manifestations of the syndrome are cutaneous hyperextensibility; soft texture ('doughy consistency') and fragility; ligamentous laxity; and easy bruising (Fig. 20.2.1). These features vary in severity and may coexist with additional involvement of other organ systems due to abnormal collagen structures (Table 20.2.1). The most recent (Villefranche) classification (Table 20.2.2) delineates six subtypes but recognizes that other less well-defined types exist. The simplified classification provides major and minor features and is based primarily on the underlying molecular cause. The types are referred to in descriptive rather than numerical categories. It is estimated that EDS affects between 1:5000 and 1:560 000, the variable phenotype perhaps being reflected in these figures.

After the original description, it was realized that some patients with EDS were susceptible to spontaneous arterial rupture with its associated lethal consequences. Affected women experienced fetal prematurity, and examination of their skin showed a depletion of collagen and an increase in elastin fibres. This particular condition, which is associated with early fatality from vascular rupture, is correlated with defects in a collagen type III, as shown below. There are obstetric, rheumatological, orthopaedic, and abdominal complications of this vascular form of Ehlers–Danlos syndrome,

known as type IV, as well as an appreciable incidence of bladder-neck obstruction and ureteric reflux. Representative clinical features of EDS subtypes are illustrated in Figs. 20.2.1 and 20.2.2.

Clinical genetics

Collagen synthesis and assembly is complex. Collagen type III is an example of a homotrimer with three identical α chains whereas many of the other collagen molecules are composed of two or more α chains. Mutations in a single glycine located in the collagen helices disrupt up to 88% of the assembled homotrimers and 75% of collagen heterotrimers, depending on the particular stoichiometry. For these reasons, collagen defects of this type behave as autosomal dominant traits, while the enzymatic deficiencies of collagen formation segregate as autosomal recessive traits with little or no expression in heterozygotes.

Until recently, only three dermal fibrillar collagens, types I, III, and V, and their processing enzymes had been implicated in EDS. However, the latest EDS subtype to be defined, autosomal recessive hypermobile EDS, is caused by deficiency of the noncollagenous, extracellular matrix protein tenascin-X. Tenascin-X, encoded by the gene TNXB, plays a crucial role in the organization of extracellular matrices, and deficient states lead to reduced dermal collagen with abnormal elastic fibres. This illustrates the importance of collagen interactions with other extracellular matrix proteins. Haploinsufficiency of tenascin-X may account for up to about 5% or 10% of hypermobile EDS but this has only been found in women. Several other candidate proteins, such as decorin, lumican, and fibromodulin, have been implicated in EDS from studies in transgenic mice but, to date, no human example has been reported.

Autosomal dominant types

The majority of subtypes are autosomal dominant but it is estimated that from 30% to 50% of cases may be sporadic. Mutations in COLA1 and COLA2 genes encoding pro-α-1 and pro-α-2 chains of collagen type I, respectively, lead to a failure to remove the N-terminal procollagen extensions of collagen and the features of arthrochalasis EDS (type VII). Mutations in COL3A1 lead to reduction of collagen type III in blood vessels and bowel and a vascular EDS (type IV) phenotype. COL5A1 mutations cause abnormalities of the quantitatively minor collagen type V and lead to classical EDS (types I and II). Haploinsufficiency of tenascin-X due to heterozygous TNXB mutations manifests as hypermobile EDS in some women. It is not known why this does not appear to lead to the same phenotype in men.

Autosomal recessive types

Kyphoscoliosis EDS (type VI) is caused by recessively inherited mutations in PLOD leading to deficiency of lysyl hydroxylase and under hydroxylation of collagen molecules. This can be identified by electrophoresis of radiolabelled collagens from cultured fibroblasts. The rare autosomal recessive subtype VIIC, also known as dermatosparaxis, is caused by deficiency of the enzyme ADAMTS2, which leads to the inability to cleave off the N-terminal of procollagen types I, II, and III.

Deficiency of tenascin-X causes an autosomal recessive hypermobile type of EDS. Affected patients have marked bruising and hyperextensible skin but without scarring. Some may have been previously considered sporadic cases.

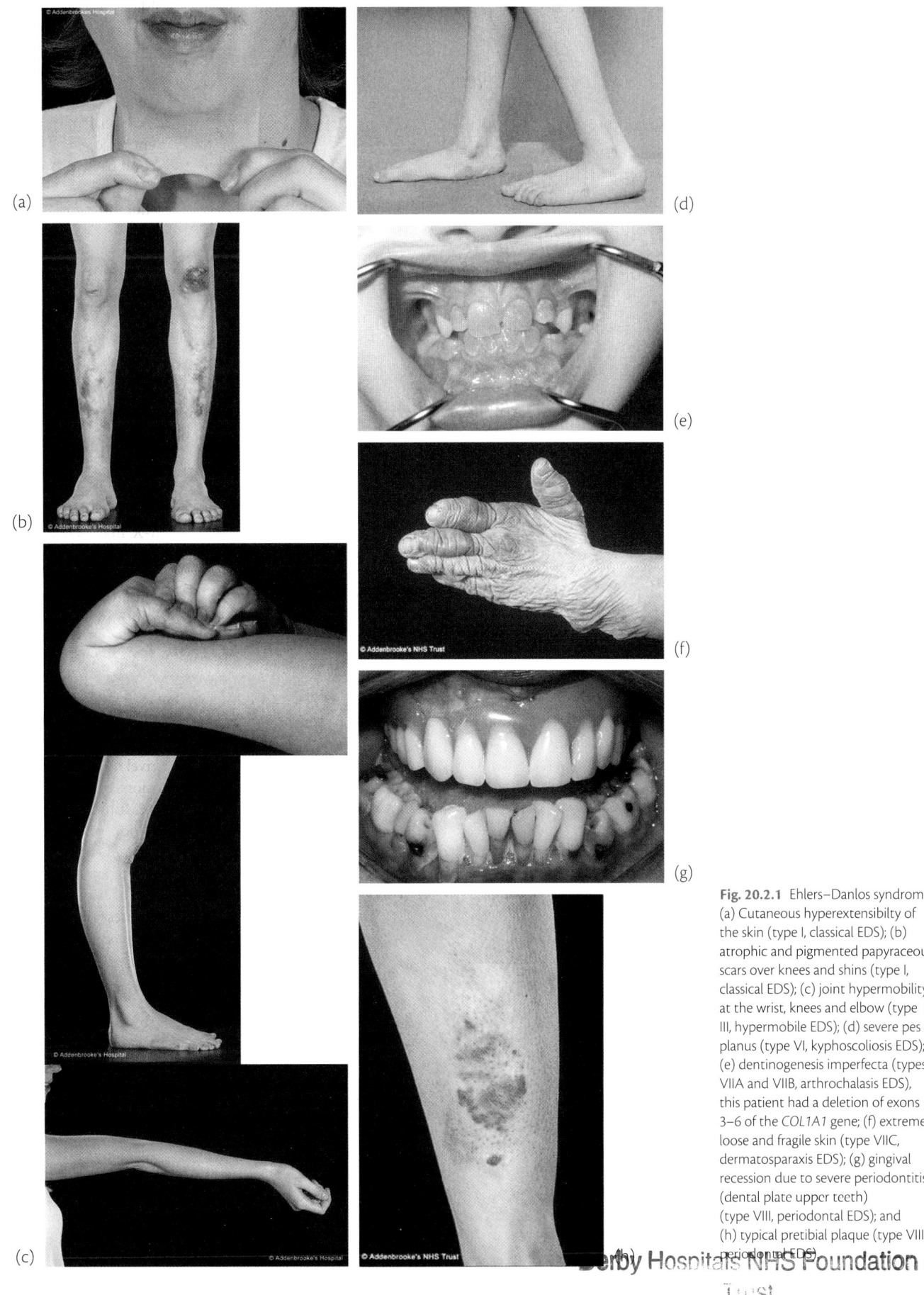

Fig. 20.2.1 Ehlers–Danlos syndrome.
(a) Cutaneous hyperextensibilty of
the skin (type I, classical EDS); (b)
atrophic and pigmented papyraceous
scars over knees and shins (type I,
classical EDS); (c) joint hypermobility
at the wrist, knees and elbow (type
III, hypermobile EDS); (d) severe pes
planus (type VI, kyphoscoliosis EDS);
(e) dentinogenesis imperfecta (types
VIIA and VIIB, arthrochalasis EDS),
this patient had a deletion of exons
3–6 of the *COL1A1* gene; (f) extremely
loose and fragile skin (type VIIC,
dermatosparaxis EDS); (g) gingival
recession due to severe periodontitis
(dental plate upper teeth)
(type VIII, periodontal EDS); and
(h) typical pretibial plaque (type VIII,
periodontal EDS).

Table 20.2.1 Clinicopathological correlations in Ehlers–Danlos syndrome

Tissue	Abnormality	Clinical effect
Skin	Increased elasticity, fragility/thinning, abnormal collagen ultrastructure	Atrophy with papyraceous scars, striae and keloid formation, nodules, spherules, tears/splits
Blood vessels	Fragility of veins and arteries	Premature varicose veins, aneurysms of small or medium arteries
Eyes	Visual/refractive errors	Corneal curvature, retinal detachment, scleral rupture
Joints	Hypermobility	Arthralgia, instability/dislocation
Skeleton and teeth	Osteoporosis	Distortion, soft tissue injury, dysplastic dentine, occasional fractures
Miscellaneous	Pleuroperitoneal Diverticulae Hernias	Pneumothorax Intestinal perforation Peritonitis, strangulation, rectal/pelvic prolapse

X-linked type

A single family with X-linked transmission has been described but its molecular basis remains uncertain.

Investigations

Skin biopsy for haematoxylin and eosin staining or immunohistochemistry will not detect abnormalities of collagen, although may demonstrate thinning of the dermis in vascular EDS (type IV). Ultrastructural analysis (transmission electron microscopy of dermal collagens) is necessary to delineate the variable patterns of collagen fibril pathology. Although not specific, 'cauliflower' fibrils are seen in classical EDS (types I and II) and represent abnormal fibrillogenesis due to defects in collagen type V, which regulates fibril formation (Figs. 20.2.3a, b). The result is abnormally large and loosely bound fibrils giving the end appearance of 'frayed rope'. Vascular EDS reveals more subtle changes with bimodal distribution of large and small fibrils (Fig. 20.2.3c). More specific features are seen in arthrochalasis (types VIIA and VIIB) with the presence of angulated fibrils and in dermatosparaxis (type VIIC) with hieroglyphic fibrils (Fig. 20.2.3d).

Further analysis of collagen synthesis and secretion can be performed on cultured, usually dermal, fibroblasts (Fig. 20.2.4). The collagen proteins are visualized by incorporating radiolabelled proline and separated on a polyacrylamide gel. Radioimmunoassay can also be used. Protein chemistry analysis is helpful particularly for those subtypes in which consistent molecular defects lead to abnormal synthesis or processing of collagens as occurs in vascular EDS (type IV), kyphoscoliosis EDS (type VI), and arthrochalasis EDS (type VII). It is less likely to detect aberrations in collagen for classical EDS despite the molecular evidence that up to 50% are due to collagen type V mutations. No consistent finding is present for hypermobile or the other types of EDS.

Classical Ehlers–Danlos syndrome (types I and II)

Following the discovery of identical mutations in both EDS types I and II, it is now realized that they are expressions of the same disease and are now referred to as classical EDS. This form is the most common after the hypermobile type. Classical EDS is associated with the cardinal features outlined in Table 20.2.2. The skin is hyperextensible but retains its normal elastic recoil. Skin fragility manifests once the child is mobile, at trauma-prone sites such as knees, elbows, forehead, and chin. The scars are 'fish-mouth' or gaping and their atrophic nature produces 'cigarette paper-like' scars. Fibrous nodules (molluscoid pseudotumours) may arise at sites of repetitive trauma. Calcification is seen on radiographs in some cases along the shins or forearms due to subcutaneous, firm, small, cyst-like nodules (spheroids). They probably represent subcutaneous fat lobules that have fibrosed due to the loss of blood supply and subsequent calcification. Other notable features of the condition include epicanthic folds and blue sclerae. Mitral valve prolapse is probably more common but does not usually result in dilatational rupture of the valve. Some degree of proximal aortic root dilatation is a common finding although the clinical significance is unclear and further longitudinal studies are required. Venous varicosities, premature bilateral hallux valgus, and distortion of the cornea leading to astigmatism, as well as premature osteoarthritis, are common. Bladder diverticulae are more common in men. Approximately half of the families with classical EDS show linkage to the collagen type V α-1 (*COL5A1*) or, less commonly, type V α-2 (*COL5A2*) genes; which are located, respectively, on human chromosomes 9q34 and 2q31. Mutation analysis usually reveals substitutions of glycine and exon-skipping events. In up to a third of instances, null alleles lead to the deficiency of collagen type V. Defects in the interactive properties of the N-terminal of collagen type V, which normally protrudes from the surface compound fibres comprising collagen types I, II, and V, impair normal interactions with other matrix components. Misdirection of the collagen fibrils leads to the generation of the so-called 'cauliflower' fibrils of classical EDS (Figs. 20.2.3a, b). The clinical consequences are fragile skin, ligaments, tendons, and corneas, as well as defective articular surfaces. Inter- and intrafamilial phenotype variability is observed but no genotype–phenotype correlation can be made.

Hypermobile Ehlers–Danlos syndrome (type III)/ benign joint hypermobility syndrome

This is the most common subtype of Ehlers–Danlos syndrome. The hallmark is joint hypermobility but with minimal skin changes and for this reason the diagnosis is frequently overlooked. It is clear that hypermobile EDS and benign joint hypermobility syndrome overlap phenotypically and are likely to be the same condition. Varying degrees of hypermobility are a common feature of many other disorders of connective tissues namely, osteogenesis imperfecta, Marfan's syndrome, and pseudoxanthoma elasticum. Persistent arthralgia without evidence of inflammatory joint disease is not uncommon and is difficult to treat. It is unknown whether hypermobile EDS patients have defective pain receptors. A subset of these also report the failure of local anaesthetic agents. Many patients complain of easy fatigue and other symptoms of orthostatic intolerance. It is likely that the underlying cause for this subtype is heterogeneous. Haploinsufficiency of tenascin-X has been identified in some autosomal dominant hypermobile patients but other, as yet uncharacterized, defects in extracellular matrix proteins and connective tissue-modifying enzymes may be responsible for the hypermobility of joints and other manifestations in this EDS type (Fig. 20.2.1c). Patients with Marfan's

Table 20.2.2 Diagnostic criteria of Ehlers–Danlos syndrome

Subtype	Synonym	Villefranche classification[a]	Molecular defect	Clinicopathological features
All subtypes (cardinal manifestations)				
				Soft, velvety, doughy, and hyperextensible skin; atrophic, papyraceous scars, especially over bony protuberances; easy bruising, especially on the legs; and hypermobile joints, dislocations, and pain
I	Gravis	Classical	COL5A1 and COL5A2 mutations result in abnormal fibrillogenesis	Severe cardinal manifestations
II	Mitis	Classical	COL5A1 and COL5A2 mutations result in abnormal fibrillogenesis	Milder cardinal features. Both show cauliflower-like collagen fibrils on TEM
III	Hypermobile	Hypermobility type	Haploinsufficiency of TNXB in some female patients may cause aberrant collagen deposition	Marked joint hypermobility, moderate skin extensibility. No scarring. Overlaps with benign joint hypermobility syndrome
IV	Acrogeric or ecchymotic	Vascular type	COL3A1 mutations result in reduced collagen type III	Thin skin with prominent venous patterns visible, pretibial haemosiderosis, variable hypermobility, colonic perforation, and acrogeric facies and extremities, with variable fibril diameters on TEM
VI	Ocular–scoliotic	Kyphoscoliosis type	Lysyl hydroxylase deficiency due to PLOD mutations leads to underhydroxylated collagen	Severe cardinal features, and severe motor delay
VIIA and VIIB	Arthrochalasis multiplex	Arthrochalasis type	Specific loss of exon 6 mutations in COL1A1 (VIIA) and COL1A2 (VIIB) results in inability to cleave N-terminal of procollagen 1	Severe cardinal features, short stature, early recurrent hip dislocation, dentinogenesis imperfecta, and angulated collagen fibres on TEM
VIIC	Dermatosparaxis	Dermatosparaxis type	ADAMTS2 deficiency results in inability to cleave N-terminal of procollagens	Very severe skin fragility, with redundant sagging skin, short stature, bruising, joint laxity, hernia, and blue sclera
Other types of EDS				
VIII	Periodontitis	Other form	Linked to chromosome 12p13	Variable cardinal features, aggressive periodontitis, and early tooth loss
V	X-linked	Other form	No molecular abnormality detected	Only one family described to date. Moderate cardinal features. Diagnosis based on X-linked inheritance
X	Fibronectin deficient	Other form	Abnormal platelet aggregation corrected by fibronectin	Phenotype resembles classical EDS type I but striae may occur in pregnancy
–	Progeroid	Other form	Galactosyl transferase I activity is reduced due to mutations in XGPT1 gene. Leads to defect in synthesis of glycosaminoglycans	Mild features of EDS with progeroid facies, short stature, osteopenia, and mental retardation
–	Autosomal recessive hypermobile	–	Deficiency of tenascin-X due to truncating mutations or deletions in TNXB is associated with abnormal deposition of collagen and abnormal elastic fibres	Discovered after Villefranche classification. Hypermobile joints, easy bruising, and hypermobile skin but without atrophic scars

TEM, transmission electron microscopy.

Beighton P, et al. Ehlers–Danlos syndrome: revised nosology, Villefranche, 1997. Am J Med Genet, 77, 31–7.

syndrome may show features of extensible skin and osteoporosis that overlap with hypermobile, kyphoscoliosis and arthrochalasis types of EDS.

Treatment of joint symptoms includes physiotherapy, rest, and graded exercise combined with conventional pain relief. Later, joint-stabilizing exercises or supports combined with proprioceptive enhancement, and cognitive therapy may be beneficial.

Vascular Ehlers–Danlos syndrome (type IV)

This autosomal dominant form of EDS is life threatening due to severe arterial and gastrointestinal fragility. Approximately half of arterial ruptures involve medium or large thoracic or abdominal arteries, although any site can be affected. The diagnosis should be considered in any young adult presenting with an unexplained cerebral vascular event. Most bowel perforations affect the sigmoid colon. A useful clue to the diagnosis is the history or presence of easy bruising typically accompanied by pretibial ecchymoses over the knees and shins as well as acrogeria (Fig. 20.2.2). Acrogeria refers to prematurely aged appearance of the extremities with thinning of the skin on the dorsum of the hands, feet, and shins. These features are combined with the so-called 'Madonna' facial appearance of large eyes, nasal thinning with lengthened philtrum, and small earlobes. Some patients may have a marfanoid appearance. Rarely there is acro-osteolysis, unexplained androgenic alopecia in women, congenital talipes, hip dislocations, and tendon contractures. Displacement of the metacarpophalangeal joints in the hands

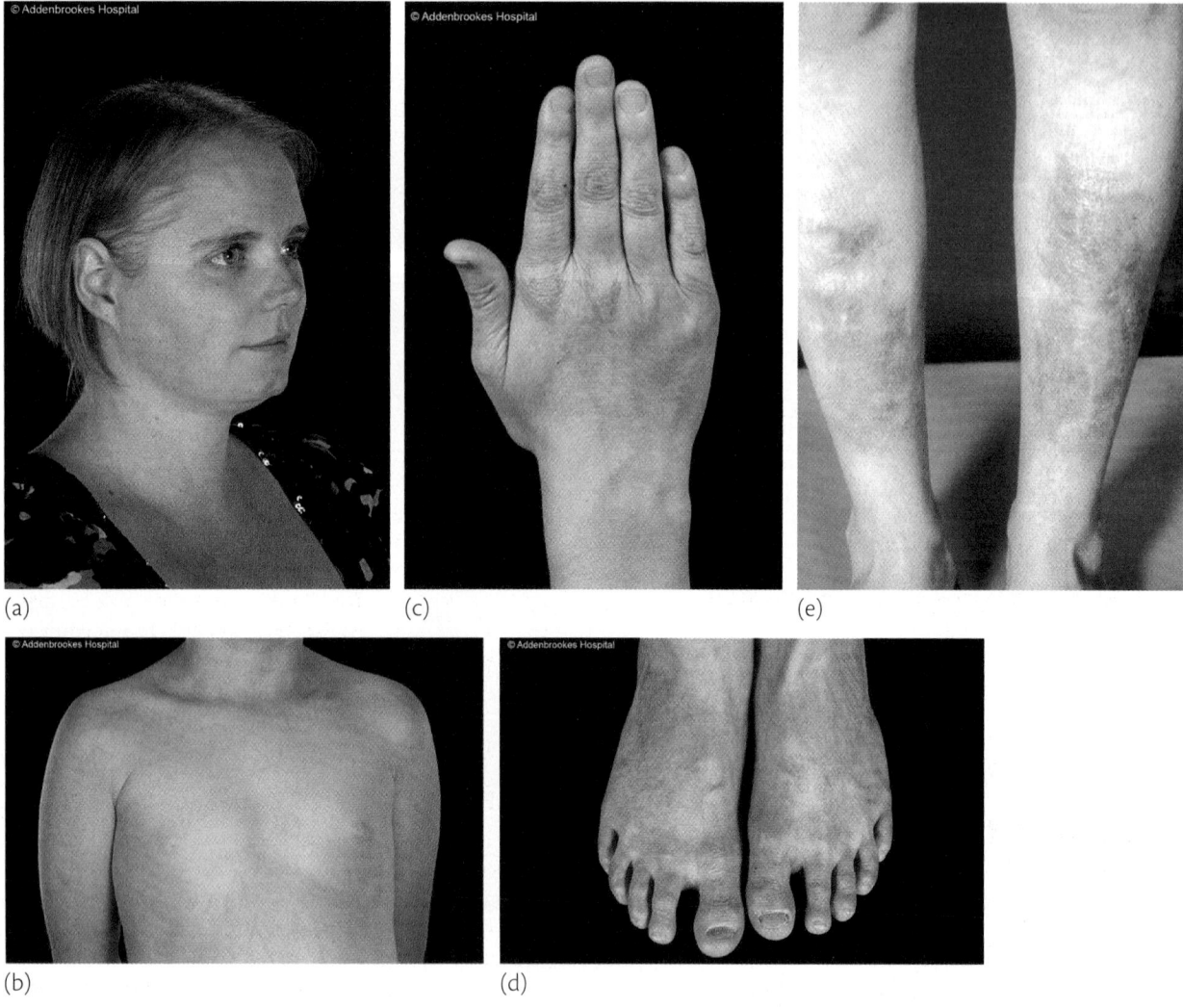

Fig. 20.2.2 Vascular EDS type IV. (a) Acrogeria, a specific clinical feature of vascular EDS, note the large eyes, thin, short nose (Madonna face), lobeless ears and scar over the chin. (b) obvious visible network of veins on upper chest due to cutaneous atrophy in 7-year-old boy; (c) premature atrophy and wrinkling on the dorsum of the hands (acrogeria) affecting the same child; (d) similar features present on the dorsum of feet; and (e) pretibial bruising and haemosiderosis.

may superficially resemble the changes of rheumatoid arthritis. Fragility of pleuroperitoneal membranes leading to pneumathoraces may complicate this and other types of EDS, including the classical and hypermobile types.

Angiographic studies may reveal a dilatated and tortuous arterial tree, including the carotid bifurcation, and major aortic or iliac disease. Conventional angiography should be avoided, if possible, because of the high risk of dissection.

Pepin and colleagues have reported the largest review of the medical and surgical complications in vascular EDS patients involving 220 index patients and 199 of their affected relatives with biochemically confirmed vascular EDS. The underlying *COL3A1* mutation was identified in 135 propositi. One-quarter of the index patients had had a first complication by the age of 20 and more than 80% had at least one complication by the age of 40. Most deaths resulted from arterial rupture, but bowel rupture, usually of the sigmoid colon, is frequent. It was noteworthy that in 81 pregnant women with vascular EDS, 12 died as a result of disease complications during pregnancy. Overall, the median lifespan of the whole group was reduced to 48 years.

In 2005, a new autosomal dominant disorder, Loeys–Dietz syndrome, was described. The major features of aortic aneurysms, arachnodactyly, and dural ectasia overlap clinically with Marfan's syndrome. Loeys–Dietz syndrome type I patients also have craniofacial involvement consisting of cleft palate, craniosynostosis or hypertelorism. Loeys–Dietz syndrome type II patients may have a bifid uvula (but no other craniofacial abnormalities) and features overlapping with the vascular EDS phenotype. In a cohort of 40 patients with a presentation suggestive of vascular EDS but normal collagen type III, Loeys and colleagues found mutations in the transforming growth factor-β receptor genes *TGFBR2* and *TGFBR1* in eight and four patients, respectively. The extent of vascular and skin involvement was similar to patients without *TGFBR* mutations although hypermobility was more pronounced in those with *TGFBR* mutations. The median overall survival of Loeys–Dietz patients is 37 years compared to 48 years for vascular EDS patients. However the survival during or immediately after vascular surgery is dramatically lower in Loeys–Dietz patients compared to vascular EDS patients (4.8% versus 45%, respectively). This illustrates one of the important reasons for genotyping such patients.

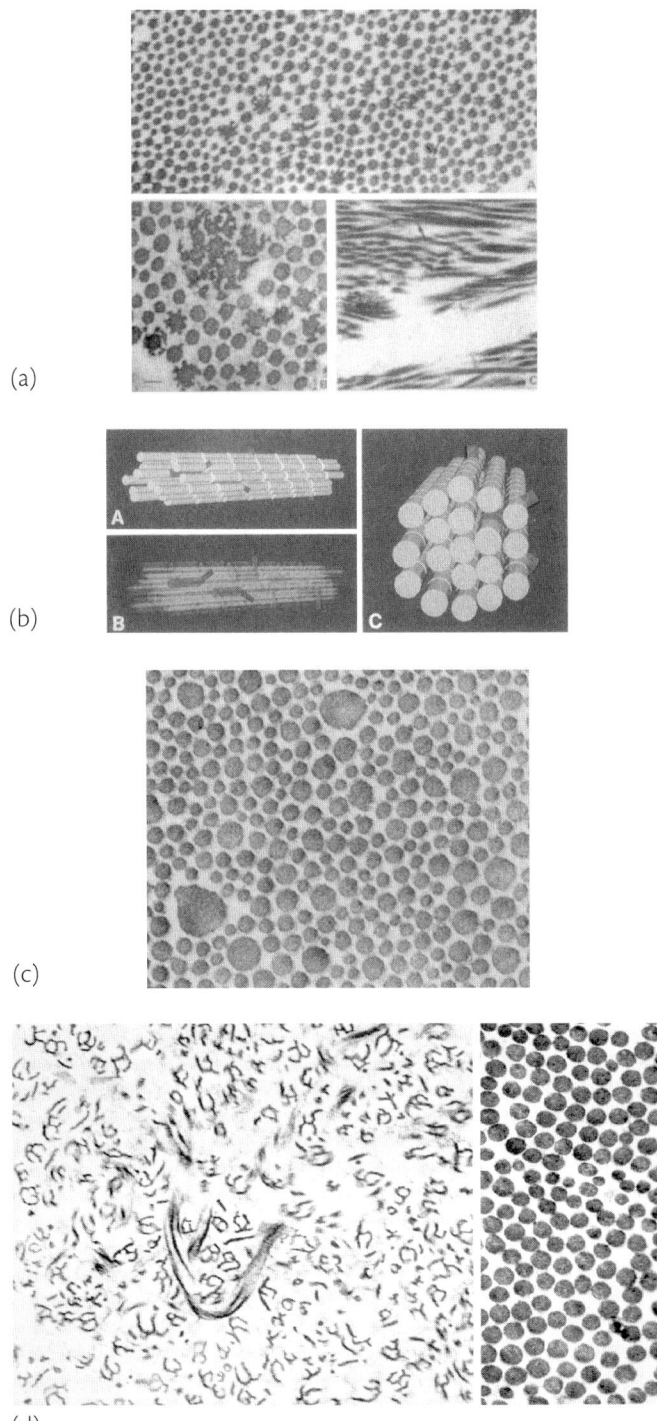

(a)

(b)

(c)

(d)

Fig. 20.2.3 Ultrastructural abnormalities of collagen in EDS. (a) Misassembled 'cauliflower' fibrils of skin and ligaments in classical EDS, resembling transversely sectioned cauliflower heads, the left panel showing transversely fused fibres, which appear to splay distally in longitudinal sections; (b) diagrammatic representation (A) of compound collagen types I and III fibres, composed of quarter-staggered individual triple helices, and dark collagen type V molecules (B), which regulate fibril diameter, and their protruding N-termini (C), which can interact with other matrix components; (c) dual distribution of large and small collagen fibres in vascular EDS; and (d) 'hieroglyphic' collagen fibres in EDS type VII, indicating very severe disruption of fibril packing in comparison with the healthy collagen shown on the right of the figure.
(a) Reproduced from J Med Genet, Nicholls AC *et al*, 33, 940–6, 1996 with permission from BMJ Publishing Group Ltd. (b) Reproduced from Birk DE, *et al*. (1990), J Cell Sci, 95, 649–57.

Molecular pathology

Histological examination of the skin reveals dermal thinning with depletion of dermal collagen and an overproliferation of elastic fibres. Examination of the skin by electron microscopy usually reveals marked variability in collagen fibril size (Fig. 20.2.3c).

Collagen type III is the dominant collagen in skin, blood vessels, tendons, ligaments, gastrointestinal tract, and pleuroperitoneal cavity linings, which thus explains the diverse multisystem phenotype of vascular EDS. Disturbed assembly, as well as haploinsufficiency of collagen type III, explains the wide-ranging severity of vascular EDS, although some affected patients have a mild clinical phenotype resembling hypermobile EDS. Numerous mutations in the collagen type III gene have been found; most are private, although several mutations are associated with hot spots in the complex collagen gene structure, which are located in exons 7, 16, and 24. The complications of vascular EDS cannot be predicted from the nature of the specific mutations in *COL3A1*. Measurement of serum N-terminal propeptide of procollagen type III may provide a useful marker of disease. Prenatal diagnosis is technically feasible but obtaining tissue is hazardous due to inherent tissue fragility. If vascular EDS is still suspected despite normal collagen type III or *COL3A1* analyses then subsequent screening of *TGFBR* genes should be undertaken.

Kyphoscoliosis EDS (type VI)

In addition to the manifestations of classical EDS, affected individuals with this autosomal recessive subtype have a propensity to kyphoscoliosis and serious ocular complications. There is reduced activity of the posttranslational modification enzyme, lysyl hydroxylase, in type A, whereas normal enzyme levels are present in type B. Lysyl hydroxylase catalyses the hydroxylation of lysine side chains, which are critical for cross-links between adjacent triple-helical collagen molecules. The cross-links confer stability and tensile strength to collagen fibrils. Homozygous or compound heterozygous mutations occur in the gene encoding lysyl hydroxylase (*PLOD*).

Arthrochalasis EDS (type VII)

This subtype is characterized by severe joint hypermobililty, congenital bilateral hip dislocations, and recurrent subluxations. Deficient processing of collagen type I results from heterozygous deletion of exon 6 of *COL1A1* (type VIIA) and *COL1A2* (type VIIB). This is the site of cleavage by the enzyme ADAMTS2 (a disintegrin and metalloproteinase with thrombospondin motifs), which excises the aminopropeptide of procollagen type I.

An extremely rare autosomal recessive form, dermatosparaxis (type VIIC) arises due to deficiency of ADAMTS2 but leads to a strikingly different phenotype of loose, sagging skin with extreme fragility (Fig. 20.2.1f), joint laxity, umbilical hernia, and blue sclera.

Other forms

Patients with periodontitis EDS (type VIII) show some overlap between the classical and vascular subtypes but with the addition of periodontitis and periodontal friability (Fig. 20.2.1g). Pretibial pigmented scars typically occur (Fig. 20.2.1h). Linkage has been identified to chromosome 12p13 in some families suggesting that this is a distinct phenotype.

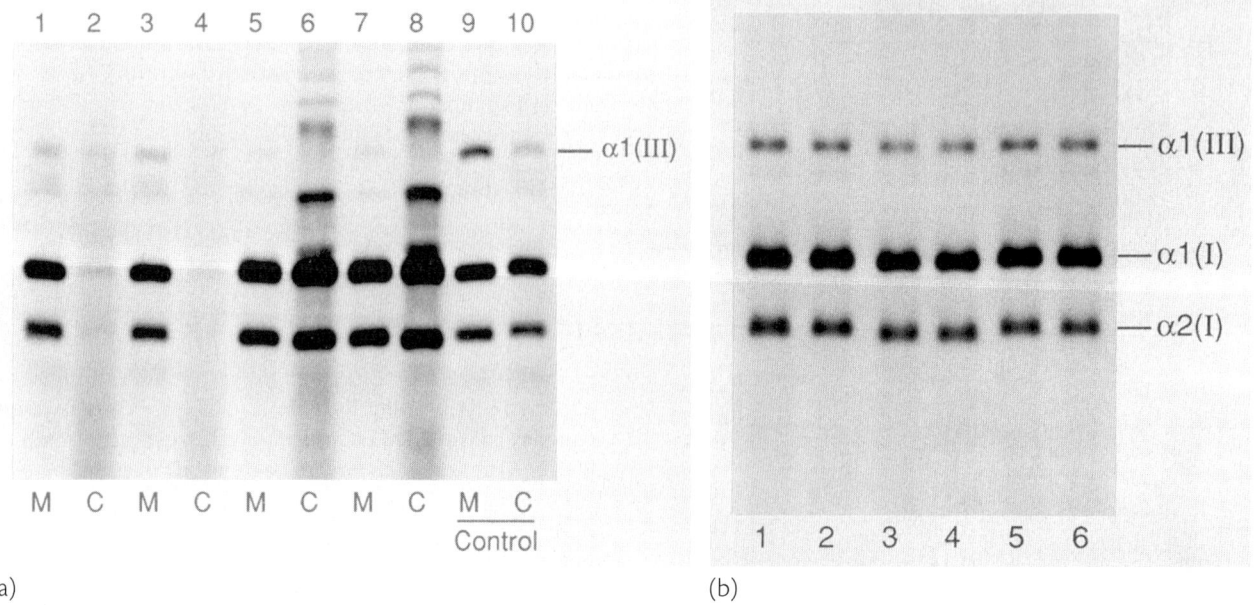

Fig. 20.2.4 Molecular analysis of collagen in EDS. (a) Typical collagen type III electrophoretic profile in fibroblasts after biosynthetic labelling in culture. There is virtually complete deficiency (tracks 5–8) or haploinsufficiency (tracks 1–4) compared with the normal pattern (9–10); and (b) electrophoresis of radiolabelled collagen proteins in fibroblasts obtained from a patient with severe pes planus due to kyphoscoliosis type EDS, showing accelerated migration (tracks 3–4) of underhydroxylated, compared with normal, collagen molecules (tracks 1–2; 5–6). C, collagen recovered from cells; M, collagen in culture medium.

Fibronectin deficient EDS (type X) has only been identified in one family with autosomal inheritance. The skin and joint changes are mild and the platelet defect can be corrected *in vitro* by adding fibronectin.

Progeroid EDS patients lack the full phenotype of progeria, but progeroid facies, short stature, osteopenia, and mental retardation may be present. Galactosyl transferase I activity is reduced due to mutations in *XGPT1* gene.

Marfan's syndrome

Marfan's syndrome affects both sexes with a prevalence of about 1 in 5000. It has a high penetrance with marked inter- and intrafamilial variability and is characterized by defects of connective tissue causing skeletal, cardiovascular, and ocular disease. Patients with Marfan's syndrome are disproportionately tall and thin with abnormally long extremities and, often, a cadaverous physique (Fig. 20.2.5). Abraham Lincoln was possibly affected. Marfan's syndrome overlaps with other inherited connective tissue disorders including hypermobile EDS/benign joint hypermobility syndrome, pseudoxanthoma elasticum, osteogenesis imperfecta, homocystinuria, and Loeys–Dietz syndrome. Marfan's syndrome is caused by autosomal dominant mutations in the human fibrillin 1 gene (*FBN1*) with *de novo* mutations occurring in about 25% of cases. Recent research has shown that abnormal fibrillin 1 exerts its detrimental effect by disrupting binding to transforming growth factor-β (TGFβ) resulting in increased expression of TGFβ. This appears to account for some of the more diverse features of Marfan's syndrome, which should now be considered part of a group of developmental disorders with defects in morphogenesis, homeostasis, and organ function.

Diagnostic criteria

Typically, there is joint hypermobility, hyperextensibility of the skin with striae, blue sclerae, and tall stature. The diagnostic criteria were revised in 1996. Without a positive family history, it is a requirement for diagnosis that major criteria in at least two different organ systems and involvement in a third are present. In families in which Marfan's syndrome is known to occur, only one major criterion is required. The major features necessary for the diagnosis include the following: aortic root dilatation, aortic dissection, lens dislocation, dural ectasia, and the presence of at least four major skeletal features (Table 20.2.3).

Marfan's syndrome shares features with other type I fibrillinopathies: mitral valve prolapse syndrome, aortic aneurysms, dominant ectopia lentis, Shprintzen–Goldberg syndrome (craniosynostosis and retarded neurodevelopment, with marfanoid features), Weill–Marchesani syndrome (short stature, brachycephaly, and other facial abnormalities) as well as Beals' syndrome (congenital contractural arachnodactyly) due to fibrillin 2 mutations.

Clinical features

Classical Marfan's syndrome arises from mutations in fibrillin 1. Typically, there are long fingers and toes (arachnodactyly), long slender limbs (dolichostenomelia), scoliosis, pectus excavatum, or pectus carinum (Fig. 20.2.6). Up to 80% have lens dislocation (ectopia lentis) (Fig. 20.2.7), usually bilateral and upwards due to rupture of the ciliary zonules, often in early childhood. Ectopia lentis is not unique to Marfan's syndrome: homocystinuria, Weill–Marchesani syndrome, and familial ectopia lentis need to be excluded. Mitral valve prolapse and aortic dilatation (Fig. 20.2.8) with dissection is the commonest cause of premature death. Rarely, dissection and rupture of the pulmonary artery occurs in Marfan's syndrome.

Since homocystinuria and Marfan's syndrome are distinct disorders—and because many patients with homocystinuria respond to specific therapies, e.g. pyridoxine supplements—clear distinction is necessary. Confusion between these two conditions

Table 20.2.3 Diagnostic criteria for Marfan's syndrome

System	Major criteria	Minor criteria	Diagnostic requirement
Skeletal	Pectus carinatum and pectus excavatum requiring surgery; reduced upper-to-lower segment ratio or arm-span-to-height ratio >1.05, wrist and thumb signs, scoliosis >20°, or spondylolisthesis; reduced extensions at the elbows (<170°); medial displacement of the medial malleolus causing pes planus; and protrusio acetabulae of any degree (ascertained on radiographs)	Pectus excavatum of moderate severity; joint hypermobility; highly arched palate with crowding of teeth; facial appearance (dolichocephaly, malar hypoplasia, enophthalmos, retrognathia, and down-slanting palpebral fissures)	At least two major criteria or one major and two minor criteria
Ocular	Ectopia lentis	Abnormally flat cornea (as measured by keratometry); increased axial length of globe (as measured by ultrasound); hypoplastic iris or hypoplastic ciliary muscle causing reduced miosis	At least two minor criteria
Cardiovascular	Dilatation of the ascending aorta, with or without aortic regurgitation, and involving at least the sinuses of Valsalva; and dissection of the ascending aorta	Mitral valve prolapse with or without mitral valve regurgitation; dilatation of the main pulmonary artery, in the absence of valvular or peripheral pulmonic stenosis or any other obvious cause, below the age of 40 years; calcification of the mitral annulus below the age of 40 years; and dilatation of dissection of the descending thoracic or abdominal aorta below the age of 50 years	One major or minor criterion
Pulmonary	None	Spontaneous pneumothorax; apical blebs (ascertained by chest radiography)	One minor criterion
Skin and integument	None	Stretch marks not associated with marked weight changes, pregnancy or repetitive stress; and recurrent or incisional hernias	One minor criterion
Dura	Lumbosacral dural ectasia by CT or MRI	None	One major criterion
Family/genetic history	Having a parent, child or sibling who meets these diagnostic criteria independently; presence of a mutation in *FBN1* known to cause Marfan's syndrome; presence of a haplotype around *FBN1*, inherited by descent, known to be associated with unequivocally diagnosed Marfan's syndrome in the family	None	One major criterion

Diagnosis in the absence of a positive family history requires major criteria in at least two different organ systems and involvement in a third. In families with an unequivocally affected first-degree relation, only one major criterion is required. Urine amino acid analysis (in absence of pyridoxine supplementation) must confirm the absence of homocystinuria (Godfrey 1993). De Paepe A, et al. (1996), Am J Med Genet, 62, 417–26.

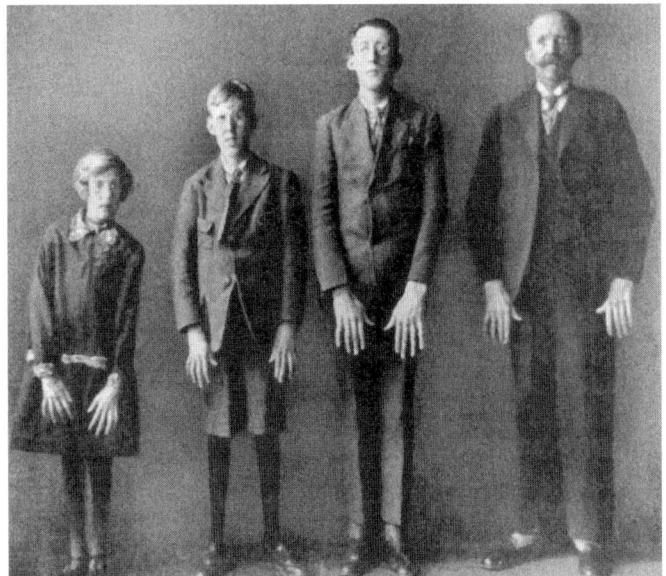

Fig. 20.2.5 Inheritance of Marfan's syndrome. Early illustration of a family with skeletal and ophthalmic features transmitted from the affected father to his daughter and two sons.

is particularly likely in tall young patients with ectopia lentis. Except in unequivocal cases, patients with suspected Marfan's syndrome should always undergo appropriate analysis (in patients not receiving vitamin B₆ supplements) for homocystinuria due to cystathionine β-synthase deficiency or other causes.

Genetics

Marfan's syndrome is typically inherited as an autosomal dominant trait (Fig. 20.2.5) and belongs to that group of genetic diseases in which a strong paternal-age effect occurs. The mean age of fathers of individuals who appear to harbour 'new' mutations is from 5 to 10 years greater than average. Approximately 25% of all patients with Marfan's syndrome are sporadic cases.

The role of fibrillin 1

Mutations in *FBN1* (chromosome 15) encoding fibrillin 1, an elastin-associated microfibril, are responsible for Marfan's syndrome (Fig. 20.2.9). A separate gene *FBN2* (chromosome 5) is responsible for Beals' syndrome (congenital contractural arachnodactyly that is not associated with defects in the ciliary zonules).

The fibrillins are elastin-associated microfibrils, which assemble autonomously to form beaded microfilaments with ordered

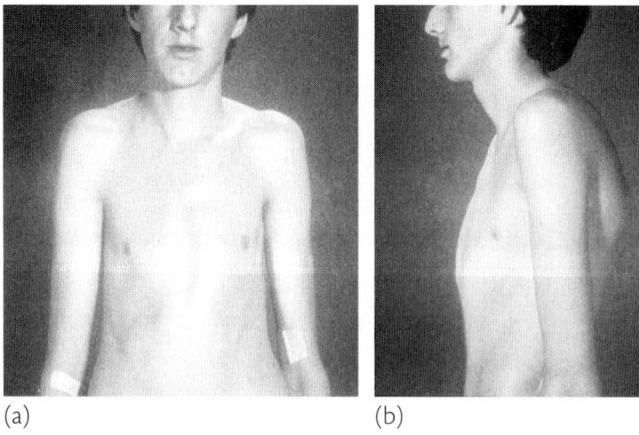

(a)   (b)

Fig. 20.2.6 Chest deformity in Marfan's syndrome. (a) Frontal and (b) lateral views showing pectus deformity and mild kyphosis. The abnormal sternum and ribs are laterally compressed.

quasicrystalline structures that can be studied by electron microscopy and other methods. The fibrillin 1 gene has a complex multiexon organization and encodes calcium-binding epidermal growth-factor-like and noncalcium binding epidermal growth-factor regions. The gene encodes 65 exons encoding several conserved cysteines, and in 1991 common mutations were identified as responsible for Marfan's syndrome. Of the mutations between exons 59 and 65, 40% are responsible for mild Marfan's syndrome without aortic dilatation. Patients with neonatal and atypically severe Marfan's syndrome have mutations clustered between exons 24 and 32. Despite this, mutations associated with classic Marfan's syndrome also occur in the same region and it is currently not possible to predict the phenotype for a given *FBN1* mutation.

Most mutations in fibrillin 1 are private, and the large and complex genetic structure greatly impedes the molecular analysis of the fibrillin gene in patients with suspected Marfan's syndrome.

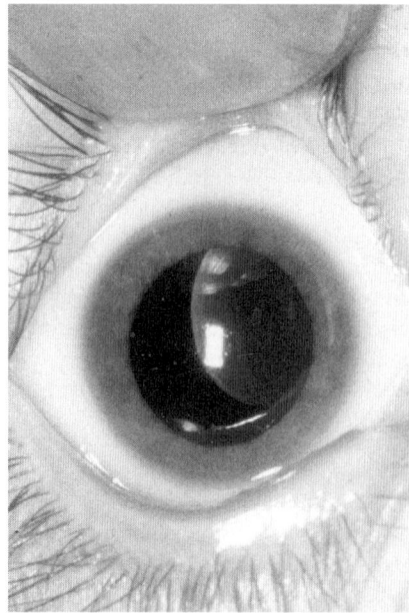

Fig. 20.2.7 Ectopia lentis in Marfan's syndrome. The lens is displaced upwards and medially. Typically, strong concave spectacle (aphakic) lenses are required to correct the extreme myopia.

The role of TGFβ

Until recently, the various structural defects observed in Marfan's syndrome were understood to occur by the dominant-negative effect of mutant fibrillin 1 on normal tissues. However, the lack of genotype–phenotype correlation and clinical features that would suggest abnormal morphogenesis, such as bone overgrowth, has been difficult to adequately explain. It is now clear that changes in growth factor signalling are critical in Marfan's syndrome. The fibrillins share similar modular domain structures with the latent TGFβ binding protein (LTBP) family of glycoproteins. These proteins have a structural role as well as the ability to bind to TGFβ, controlling its secretion and activity. Fibrillin binds to TGFβ and LTBPs and increased levels of active TGFβ are found in the presence of abnormal fibrillin (Fig. 20.2.10). Furthermore, mutations in the genes for the TGFβ receptors (*TGFBR1* and *TGFBR2*) have been identified in a number of disorders with phenotypic overlap with classical Marfan's syndrome. Examples are the newly described arterial tortuosity syndrome, with aortic aneurysm, bifid uvula, or cleft palate, and hypertelorism as well as craniofacial and skeletal abnormalities (Loeys–Dietz syndrome), which is caused by heterozygous mutations in *TGFBR1* and *TGFBR2*. Interestingly, some of these patients have cutaneous features indistinguishable from vascular EDS. *TGFBR2* mutations have also been identified in some nonsyndromic individuals with familial thoracic aortic aneurysms and dissections.

Treatment

The main causes of death in patients with Marfan's syndrome result from cardiovascular disease and complications elsewhere in the vascular system. Vigorous and regular surveillance is recommended with careful monitoring of aortic root width and of the function of aortic and mitral valves by transthoracic echocardiography and periodic electrocardiography.

Adrenergic β-blockers are widely used as prophylaxis in patients with Marfan's syndrome to reduce the mean arterial pressure and pulse rate. Whilst many studies have shown reduction in the development of aortic complications by β-blockers, in 2007 a meta-analysis of six studies, of which only one was randomized, found no improvement in the endpoints measured of aortic dissection, rupture, cardiovascular surgery, or death for patients taking β-blockers. The use of β-blocker therapy instituted during childhood may need to be reassessed.

The two most important determinants of risk of dissection of the aorta are the maximal dimension and family history of dissection. In adults, surgery is recommended when the aorta reaches 50 mm. For patients with evidence of progressive aortic disease, including dilatation of the ascending aorta and valve ring, a Dacron graft, with or without an artificial or reconstituted aortic valve (the Bentall procedure), may be considered. After excision of a terminally dilatated aorta, insertion of a Dacron graft to the aortic valvular ring requires reimplantation of the coronary arteries; in the best hands, the mortality rate of this procedure is less than 5%, with more than three-quarters of patients surviving 5 years. Gott and colleagues from Johns Hopkins Hospital, in the United States of America described the highly successful results of aortic root replacement in 271 patients with Marfan's syndrome over the period from 1976 to 2000. Most (>85%) patients underwent the Bentall procedure involving composite graft replacement of the aortic root. Mid-term results from valve-sparing, modified Dacron

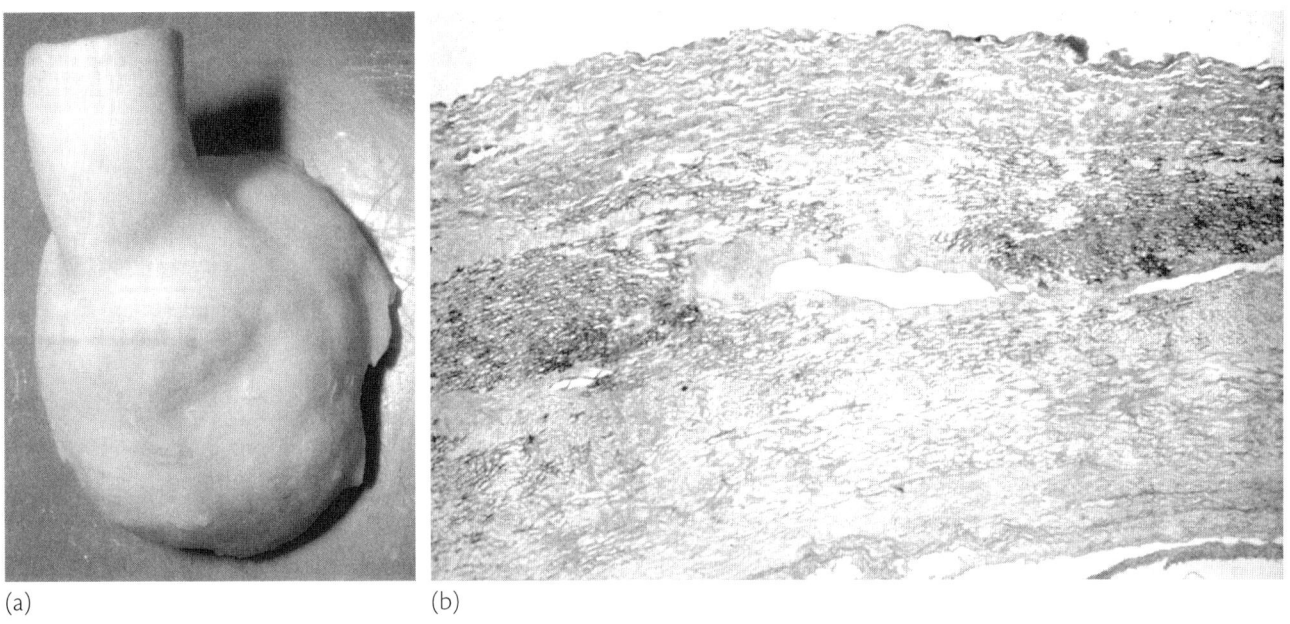

(a)   (b)

Fig. 20.2.8 Aortic disease in Marfan's syndrome. (a) Excised dilatated aortic root; and (b) histological section of the aorta showing elastic degeneration of the aortic media.

grafts, which allow annular stability and recreating sinuses that minimize leaflet stress, also look promising.

In managing the cardiovascular complications of young patients with Marfan's syndrome, there is a need to balance advice regarding restrictive lifestyle, drug therapy, the benefit of long-term monitoring, and the maturation and development of an often asymptomatic child.

Recent advances in our understanding of the molecular pathology of Marfan's syndrome have opened up the possibility of alternative treatment strategies. Different fibrillin deficient mice have been shown to lead to variable impairment of distal alveolar septation, myxomatous changes in the mitral valve and myopathy through increased TGFβ signalling. These pathological changes can be prevented by perinatal, systemic administration of TGFβ neutralizing antibody. This is clearly not practical in humans. Mice heterozygous for a common Marfan's syndrome mutation (cysteine substitution in the epidermal growth-factor-like domain of *FBN1*) develop progressive aortic root dilatation. Dietz and colleagues have elegantly shown, in mice, that postnatal administration of losartan, an angiotensin II type 1 receptor antagonist, which antagonizes TGFβ signalling, can reverse these aneurismal changes

as well as partially reversing the noncardiovascular complications. It is worth noting that muscle regeneration was also seen in a dystrophin deficient mouse treated with losartan. A retrospective study of 18 paediatric Marfan's syndrome patients (aged 1–16 years) treated with angiotensin II receptor blockers (17 patients received losartan and 1 received irbesartan) has shown that the blockers significantly slowed the rate of progression of aortic root dilatation. All patients had received β-blockers but the treatment was either ineffective or poorly tolerated. These important results require confirmation and a randomized control comparing losartan with atenolol is underway.

The discovery of excess TGFβ in the walls of aortic aneurysms in Loeys–Dietz syndrome and arterial tortuosity syndrome (due to *GLUT10* mutations) raises the broader possibility of anti-TGFβ therapy for more diverse vasculopathies.

Lens dislocation can be generally managed conservatively. Surgical removal is indicated if cataract, secondary glaucoma, or diminished visual acuity that cannot be corrected with spectacles occurs. This can be followed by artificial lens implantation.

Other complications of Marfan's syndrome, including unstable joints, dislocation of the patella, progressive kyphoscoliosis, and

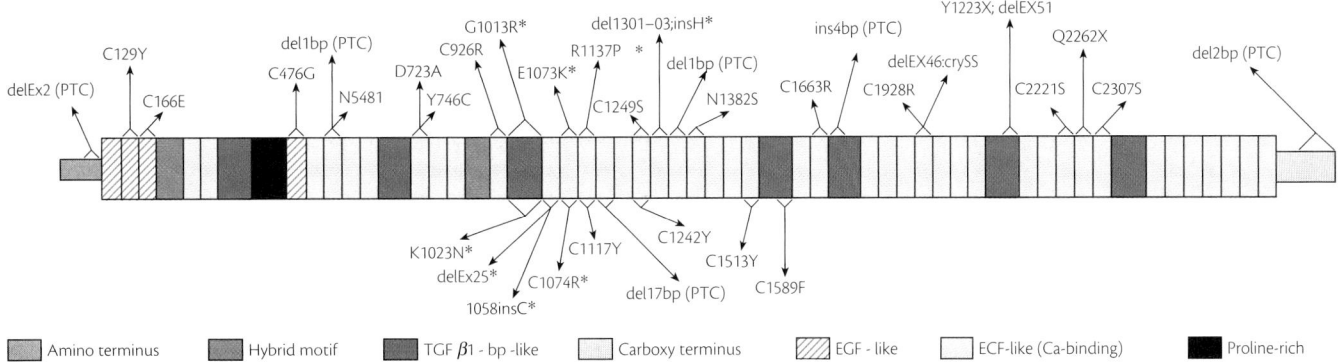

Fig. 20.2.9 Organization of the human fibrillin 1 gene. Mutations associated with Marfan's syndrome are depicted.

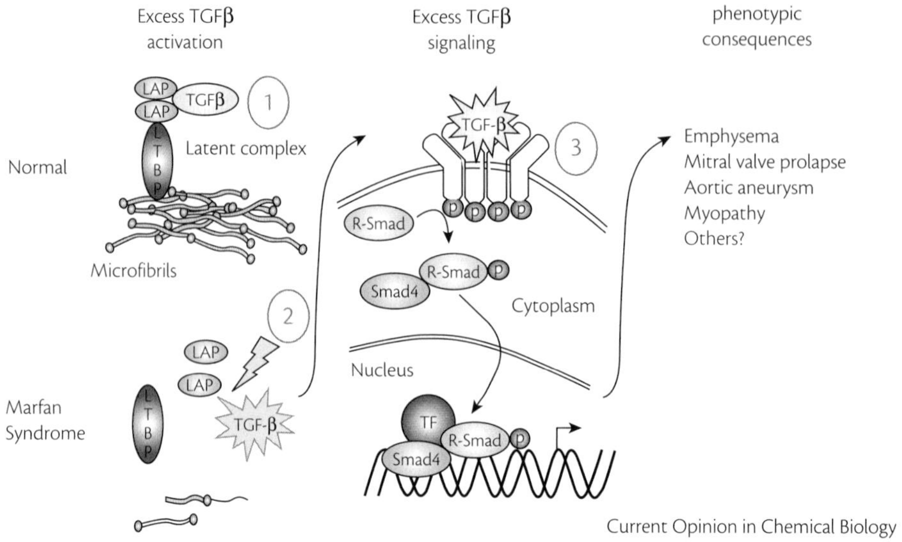

Fig. 20.2.10 The role of TGFβ in Marfan's syndrome. (1) Normal regulation of TGFβ; (2) microfibril (fibrillin 1) deficiency in Marfan's syndrome; and (3) excess TGFβ signalling, which gives rise to variable phenotypic consequences. From Ramirez F, Dietz HC. (2007). Marfan's syndrome: from molecular pathogenesis to clinical treatment. *Current Opinion in Genetics& Development*, **17**, 252–8.

recurrent pneumothoraces, with frequently complicating emphysema, require surgical intervention. Clearly, many patients with Marfan's syndrome will require support with the psychological aspect and in the light of their diminished life expectancy. Women with Marfan's syndrome require counselling, not only about the genetic risk to their offspring but also because of the intrinsic risks of carrying a pregnancy to term. In addition to cardiovascular complications, pregnancy is associated with a high rate of premature deliveries, premature rupture of membranes, and increased mortality in the offspring.

Prognosis

Patients with Marfan's syndrome have a reduced life expectancy, principally as a result of the cardiovascular complications. Indeed, about 80% of all deaths are due to aortic dilatation and its complications; the mean age of death in a series of 257 patients published in 1972 was 32 years. However, with the introduction of β-blocking agents and improvements in vascular and cardiac surgery, the prognosis has improved greatly and the early cohort studies were almost certainly subject to bias, since outcome was better in patients ascertained on the basis of family studies compared with those with sporadic disease.

Men with Marfan's syndrome have a lower survival rate than affected women—a conclusion based on several cohort studies. In a study of patients with Marfan's syndrome in Wales and Scotland between 1970 and 1990, the median survival for men was 53 years and for women, 72 years; the median age at death was 45±16.5 years. Patients with Marfan's syndrome are at risk if they participate in competitive athletics. Indeed, the presence of Marfan's syndrome is a common cause of fatal aortic dissection and rupture in young adults.

Pseudoxanthoma elasticum (Grönblad–Strandberg syndrome)

Pseudoxanthoma elasticum (PXE) has an estimated prevalence of from 1 in 25 000 to 1 in 100 000 with a predominance in women, although the latter may reflect presentation bias. It is an inherited disorder, caused by mutations in the ABC transporter gene (*ABCC6*) gene that affects the skin, eyes, and cardiovascular system. Clinical problems arise as a result of fragmentation and ultimately calcification of elastic fibres. Premature arterial stiffening and calcification leads most commonly to lower leg claudication, hypertension, and, rarely, cerebral haemorrhage. Gastrointestinal bleeding and retinal disease causing visual loss are among the most frequent complications of PXE.

Clinical genetics

The mode of transmission of PXE has been controversial over the last few years. At one time, five different genetic groups were postulated but clarification following mutation testing has confirmed only autosomal recessive inheritance (OMIM 264 800). Heterozygotes for an *ABCC6* mutation are probably relatively common (0.8% prevalence for R1141X mutation in a Dutch population) and instances in which the disease occurs in two generations can be attributed to pseudodominance due to matings between an affected (homozygote or double heterozygote) and randomly distributed heterozygotes. Carriers of a heterozygous mutation in *ABCC6* are usually asymptomatic but may have mild ocular and cutaneous findings.

Clinical features

The full syndrome consists of the distinctive skin lesions, retinal changes (particularly angioid streaks), and vascular involvement. The characteristic skin changes and angioid streaks have also been reported as isolated findings, but this is unusual. The diagnosis is often delayed by at least 20 years after the onset of skin lesions, which appear first, because many patients do not seek medical advice until ophthalmic complications occur.

Cutaneous

The average age of onset of the characteristic skin lesions is 13 years. Yellowish papules appear at flexural sites with predilection for neck and axillae antecubital fossae, inguinal folds as well as the umbilicus. The papules (1–3 mm) develop in a linear or reticular pattern and subsequently in confluent plaques resembling goose flesh or the skin of a plucked chicken (Fig. 20.2.11). Examination of the palate and mucous membranes may show similar changes. Endoscopy of the stomach may reveal nodular submucosal lesions comparable to those present in peripheral skin. Sometimes the skin changes are very subtle but in severe cases the skin may become inelastic, leading to increased folds and a hound-dog appearance to the face, neck, and groins, due to secondary cutis laxa. These changes may be aggravated by sun exposure and smoking. Less commonly reticulate pigmentation on the abdomen may occur and acneiform lesions have been reported.

Ophthalmic

Ophthalmoscopy is necessary to detect the typical ocular features. (Fig. 20.2.12). The first retinal change seen in most patients is a mottled *peau d'orange* pigmentation due to irregularity of elastic fibres in the pretinal Bruch's membrane. Progression leads to 'salmon spots', or drusen, reflecting hyaline degeneration, and when breaks occur in the Bruch's membrane, angioid streaks are seen. These retinal streaks vary in colour from dark red or maroon to black. Angioid streaks occur in at least 85% patients above the age of 50 years but only in about one-third of patients under 10 years.

Retinal haemorrhage, neovascularization, and chorioretinitis can all lead to loss of central vision and around half of patients will have some visual impairment. Myopia is more common in PXE patients.

Cardiovascular

Pseudoxanthoma elasticum is associated with disease of both large and small arteries, as shown in the retina. Calcification of arterial elastic media and intima affects predominantly peripheral arteries. Intermittent claudication is the most common cardiovascular symptom and reduced pulses of both arms and legs helps differentiate from ordinary atherosclerosis. Occasionally, ischaemic features develop in the hands that are associated with resorption of digital tufts. Symptoms of intermittent claudication of the lower limbs occur in 30% of patients by the age of 30 years.

Renovascular hypertension is not uncommon in patients with PXE and increases the risk of bleeding, which may also be associated with premature arterial calcification in peripheral arteries as well as coronary vessels.

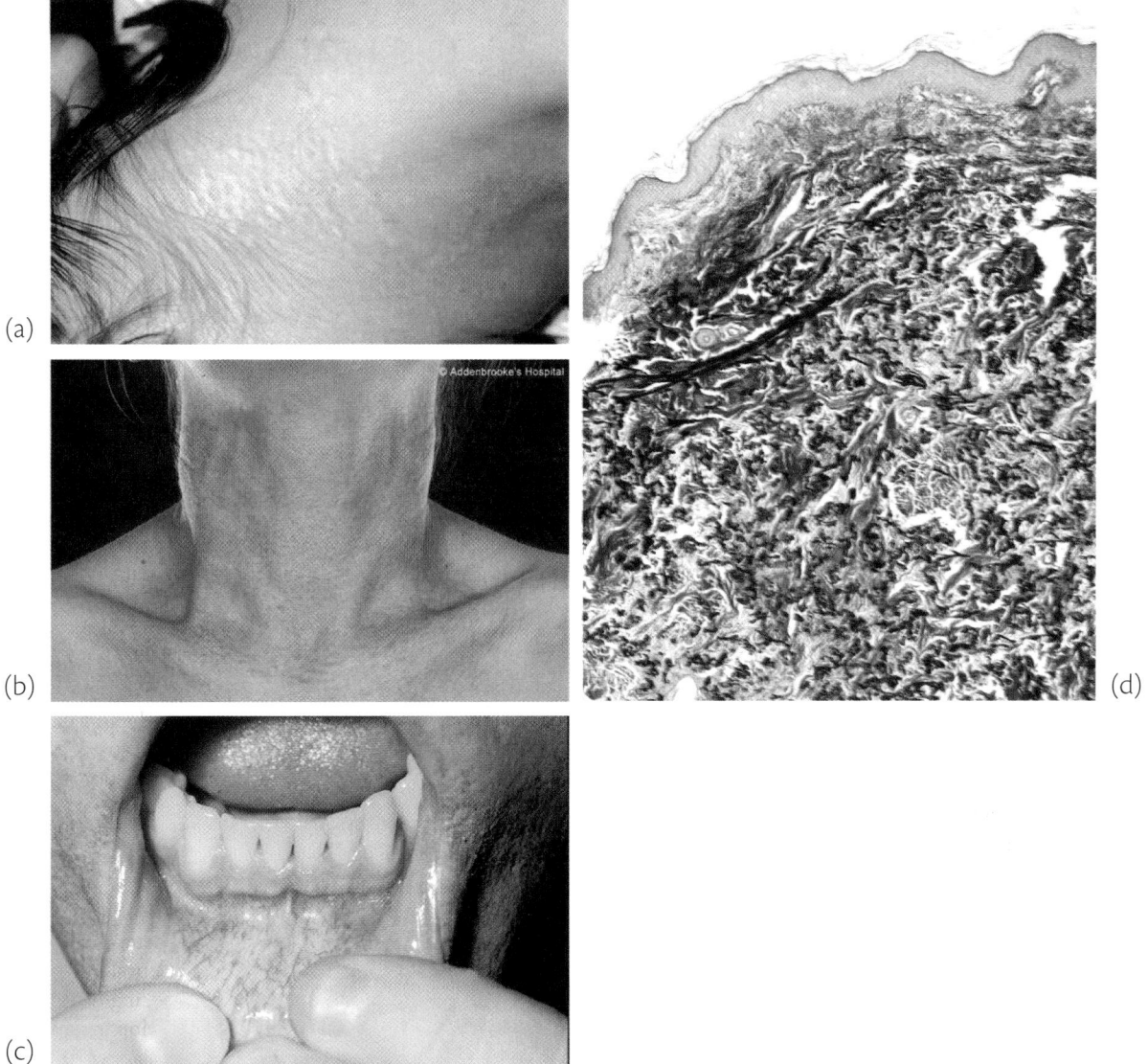

Fig. 20.2.11 Skin lesions in pseudoxanthoma elasticum (PXE). (a) Typical flexural skin lesions of PXE of the lateral neck; (b) more widespread changes on anterior neck with secondary cutis laxa; (c) mucosal infiltration of the lower lip in PXE; and (d) an elastic ponceau S stain of skin biopsy (magnification X10) showing mid-dermal elastic fibre fragmentation and degeneration.

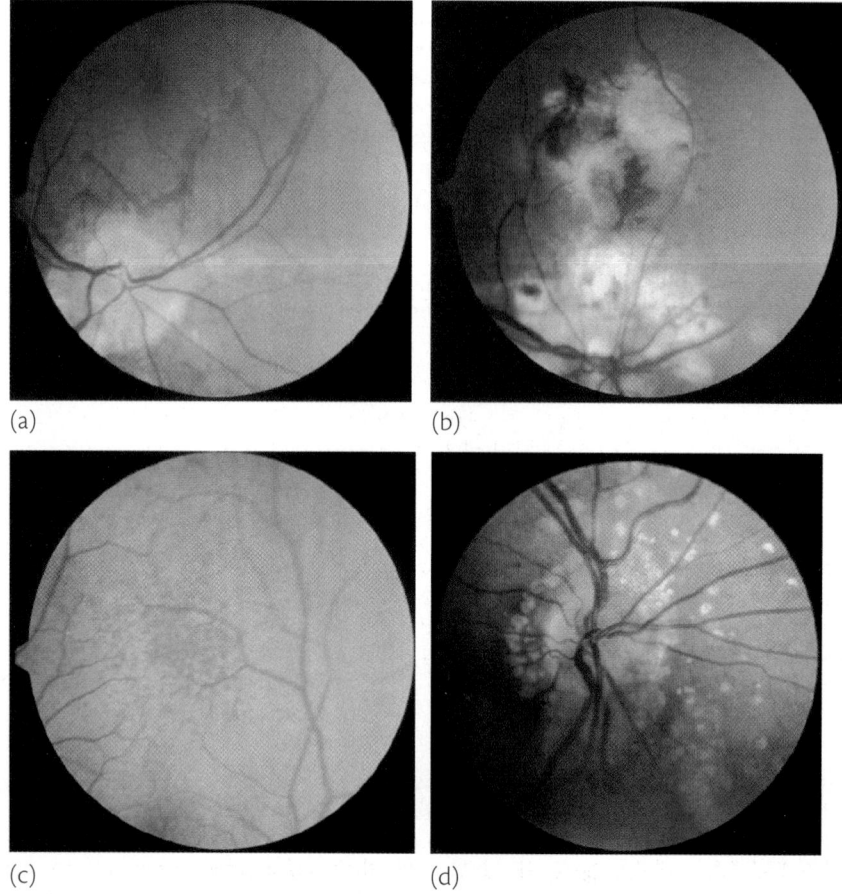

Fig. 20.2.12 Retinal changes in pseudoxanthoma elasticum (PXE). (a) Angioid streaks caused by fracture of the retroretinal Bruch's membrane—an early feature; (b) macular haemorrhage with consequential choroideretinitis; (c) specked *peau d'orange* mottling; and (d) salmon spotting (drusen).

Ischaemic heart disease has been reported in a child as young as 9 years. Other cardiac abnormalities identified in PXE include endocardial calcification, mitral valve prolapse and stenosis, restrictive cardiomyopathy, atrial septal aneurysm, and abnormal left ventricular diastolic function.

Additional features include episodic and often severe gastrointestinal haemorrhage usually from the stomach with, or without, a coincidental hiatal hernia or peptic ulcer. Bleeding may occur at other points including the renal, retinal, uterine, bladder, or subarachnoid spaces. Hyperechogenic dots representing calcified vessels can be detected by ultrasonography in the kidneys as well as the spleen and pancreas.

Diagnosis

Whilst a number of clinical criteria for the diagnosis of PXE have been defined, the most recent consensus by Lebwohl and colleagues, published in 1994, delineates three major and two minor features. However, this classification was proposed before the advent of molecular testing. If an individual has all three major criteria then the diagnosis is certain. However, as children rarely have eye complications, the most important criteria are the presence of the typical skin eruption with histological evidence of elastic degeneration and calcification. In a study of 18 patients with angioid streaks, a skin biopsy of normal-looking skin did

Table 20.2.4 Features of pseudoxanthoma elasticum (PXE) in different tissues.

Tissue	Feature
Skin	Classical flexural eruption[a]
	Elastic fragmentation and calcification and/or central elastic fibre calcification (by electron microscopy)[a]
	Increased cutaneous extensibility (heterozygotes)
	Occasional striae
Blood vessels	Decreased elasticity, hypertension
	Arteriosclerosis, claudication
	Medial calcification, venous varicosities
	Gastrointestinal haemorrhage
Eyes	Late-onset macular degeneration, macular central visual loss[a]
	Angioid streaks[a]
	Altered corneal geometry, myopia, blue sclerae
	Peau d'orange changes[b]
Miscellaneous	Positive family history of PXE[b]
	Mitral valve prolapse
	Pleural/parenchymal calcification

[a] Major diagnostic criteria.
[b] Minor diagnostic criteria.

not yield any additional diagnostic information. The major and minor criteria are set out in Table 20.2.4; any two major, or one major and two minor, criteria are sufficient to diagnose the disease.

Differential diagnosis

Angioid streaks occur without any systemic associations in about 50% of cases. However, they may be seen in Paget's disease, haemoglobinopathies, particularly sickle cell anaemia, acromegaly, and Ehlers–Danlos syndrome. They are rarely as florid as those occurring in pedigrees affected by PXE. Rarely, diabetic retinopathy may be associated with angioid streaks. Angioid streaks have also been reported in patients with neurofibromatosis and tuberous sclerosis. Cutaneous manifestations of PXE may resemble those of extreme solar injury to skin associated with ageing. Late onset PXE-like phenotypes have been observed in patients with β-thalassaemia and sickle cell disease, with no evidence of mutations in *ABCC6*. Characteristically, long-term penicillamine therapy leads to a syndrome that is a close phenocopy of pseudoxanthoma elasticum (pseudo-pseudoxanthoma elasticum). Elastosis serpiginosa perforans may also be present. Saltpeter, calcium salts, L-tryptophan, and chronic renal failure (periumbilical) can all induce pseudoxanthomatous skin changes.

Pathology

Pseudoxanthoma elasticum is diagnosed principally because of the occurrence of the constellation of clinical features, the family history, and a skin biopsy that reveals a characteristic fragmentation and disruption as well as calcification of the elastic fibres of the middle and deep zones of the dermis. The use of von Kossa's stain, which identifies carbonate and phosphate complexes of calcium, together with van Gieson's stain for elastic fibres is diagnostic; electron microscopy usually reveals electron-dense deposits throughout elastin fibres in the skin with a central core of minerals as well as altered collagen fibres.

Molecular genetics

The gene for PXE, *ABCC6*, was identified in 2000 and maps to chromosome 16p31.1 (Fig. 20.2.13). It encodes the multidrug

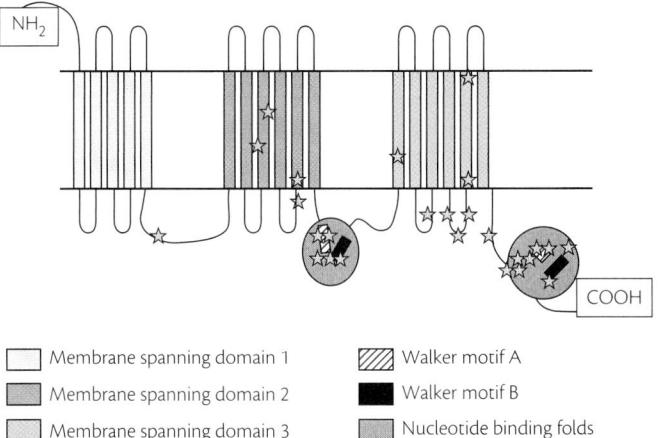

Fig. 20.2.13 Organization of the human *PXE* gene. *ABCC6* is a member of the ABC transmembrane ion transporter family. There are three membrane-spanning domains and two nucleotide-binding folds.

resistance-associated protein 6 (MRP6) and is an ATP-binding cassette transporter gene belonging to the same family as the cystic fibrosis transmembrane regulator gene, *CFTR*. *ABCC6* is expressed primarily in the liver and to a lesser degree in the proximal tubules of the kidneys and it is present, if at all, in very low levels in the skin. There are a number of lines of investigations to suggest that PXE is likely to be a primary metabolic disorder due to an imbalance of serum factors. The endogenous substrate for this transporter is unknown although it has been hypothesized that it may be related to vitamin K. Therefore the absence of the transporter activity could lead to reduced vitamin K, or one if its derivatives, both in the circulation and cells such as dermal fibroblasts. This in turn would result in the reduction of some vitamin K dependent reactions, most notably activation of the matrix gla protein (MGP) which is a major systemic inhibitor of mineralisation. Reduced MGP activity would then allow progressive calcification of tissues characteristic of PXE.

Affected individuals are either homozygous or compound heterozygous for loss of function mutations (most commonly missense mutations) clustering in exons 24 to 28 corresponding to the second nucleotide binding fold and the last intracellular domain. No genotype–phenotype correlation exists but recently polymorphisms in the SPP1 promoter region and the xylosyl transferase genes have been identified as possibly secondary genetic risk factors.

Treatment and management

With time, patients with PXE are prone to premature ageing in their skin and they experience cosmetic embarrassment as a result. Excess exposure to ultraviolet light should be avoided as far as possible and sunscreen lotions should be used when this is not possible. Patients with PXE may benefit from plastic surgery to remove redundant skin around the neck and groins, abdomen, and breasts. This is particularly applicable to women who become embarrassed by rapid cutaneous changes after pregnancy or the menopause. The skin is not fragile in PXE but keloid formation may complicate such cosmetic surgery and it is advisable that those who operate are apprised of this risk in PXE.

Although the skin and vascular lesions of PXE are associated with calcification, there is no evidence that calcium restriction influences the development of the disease. Nonetheless, some authorities recommend restricting calcium intake without evidence that this impedes the progression of the disorder. If a low calcium diet is adhered to, osteoporosis should be excluded, particularly in postmenopausal women. Because of their risk of severe systemic arterial disease, patients with PXE are advised to undergo regular monitoring of their vascular integrity and blood pressure. The rapid onset of severe systemic hypertension that is refractory to treatment may be due to unilateral renal artery stenosis—a well-described abnormality in PXE. Regular light exercise, maintaining normal body weight and avoidance of cigarette smoking are simple measures that also likely to be beneficial.

Contact sports, including boxing, and arduous exercise such as cross-country running should be avoided. Regular monitoring by a cardiologist and ophthalmologist may be beneficial, in that the occurrence of new vessel formation in relation to angioid streaks can be arrested by ocular laser therapy to prevent or diminish the risk of retinal haemorrhage. Similarly, regular blood pressure monitoring with the prompt use of β-blockers for hypertension where possible may delay the onset of peripheral vascular insufficiency and coronary heart disease.

Prompt treatment of systemic hyperlipidaemia, which may independently complicate the arteriopathy of PXE, is indicated to arrest arterial narrowing and prevent thrombosis. Antiplatelet drugs such as aspirin and nonsteroidal anti-inflammatory drugs are contraindicated because of the increased risk of visual loss due to retinal bleeding and of gastrointestinal haemorrhage. Coronary bypass surgery is as successful and no riskier than for the general population; there is little evidence to judge the outcome of vascular surgical procedures that may be indicated for stenoses of carotid or other major peripheral arteries.

Pregnancy

Whilst it has generally been recommended to limit pregnancies, apart from the increased risk of first trimester miscarriage and the cosmetic deterioration of the abdominal skin, pregnancy usually proceeds with only minimal difficulties. The theoretical risks of recurrent gastrointestinal haemorrhage and perineal tearing at delivery result only rarely in adverse outcomes in women with PXE. Maternal PXE does not appear to increase the risk of fetal abnormalities. However, monitoring of systemic arterial blood pressure with additional eye checks are recommended in pregnant patients with this disorder and during the peripartum period.

Prognosis

In some patients with PXE, premature death results from vascular disease, which may cause critical occlusion of the arterial supply to essential organs or fatal bleeding. Death from a recurrent massive gastrointestinal haemorrhage was recorded in a 13 year-old patient and severe bleeding due to PXE has been reported in younger children. McKusick has shown that many patients may live beyond 70 years and die of conditions unrelated to their connective tissue disorder; his study of 52 patients with PXE from the case records of the Johns Hopkins Hospital in the early 1970s showed that the median survival of this selected cohort was about 46 years.

Further reading

Beighton P (1993). The Ehlers–Danlos syndromes. In: Beighton P (ed) *McKusick's heritable disorders of connective tissue*, 5th edition, pp. 189–252. Mosby Year Book, St. Louis.

Beighton P, et al. (1998). International nosology of heritable disorders of connective tissue. *Am J Med Genet*, **29**, 581–94.

Beighton P, et al. (1999). Ehlers–Danlos syndrome: revised nosology, Villefrache, 1997. *Am J Med Genet*, **77**, 31–7.

Bergen AA, et al. (2000). Mutations in ABCC6 cause pseudoxanthoma elasticum. *Nat Genet*, **25**, 288–31.

Birk DE, et al. (1990). Collagen fibrillogenesis *in vitro*. Interaction of types I and V collagen regulates fibril diameter. *J Cell Sci*, **95**, 649–57.

Brooke BS, et al. (2008). Angiotensin II blockade and aortic-root dilation in Marfan's syndrome. *N Engl J Med*, **358**, 2787–95.

Brown SJ, et al. (2007). Pseudoxanthoma elasticum: biopsy of clinically normal skin in the investigation of patients with angioid streaks. *Br J Dermatol*, **157**, 748–51.

Buntinx IM, et al. (1991). Neonatal Marfan syndrome with congenital arachnodactyly flexion contractures and severe cardiac valve insufficiency. *J Med Genet*, **28**, 267–73.

Burrows NP, et al. (1996). The gene encoding collagen alpha 1 type V (COL5A1) to type II Ehlers–Danlos type I/II. *J Invest Dermatol*, **106**, 1273–6.

Byers PH, et al. (1979). Clinical and ultrastructural integrity of type IV Ehlers–Danlos syndrome. *Hum Genet*, **47**, 141–50.

De Paepe A, et al. (1996). Revised diagnostic criteria for the Marfan syndrome. *Am J Med Genet*, **62**, 417–26.

Dietz HC, et al. (1991). Marfan syndrome caused by a recurrent de novo missense mutation in the fibrillin gene. *Nature*, **352**, 337–9.

Elejalde BR, et al. (1984). Manifestations of pseudoxanthoma elasticum during pregnancy: a case report and review of the literature. *Am J Med Genet*, **18**, 755–62.

Gersony DR, et al. (2007). The effect of beta-blocker therapy on clinical outcome in patients with Marfan's syndrome: a meta-analysis. | *Int J Cardiol*, **114**, 303–8.

Godfrey M (1993). The Marfan syndrome. In: Beighton P (ed) *McKusick's heritable disorders of connective tissue*, 5th edition, pp. 51–135. Mosby Year Book, St Louis.

Gott VL (2002). Aortic root replacement in 271 Marfan patients: a 24-year experience. *Ann Thorac Surg*, **73**, 438–43.

Grahame R (2000). Heritable disorders of connective tissue. *Baillieres Clin Rheumatol*, **14**, 345–61.

Gray JR, et al. (1998). Life expectancy in British Marfan syndrome populations. *Clin Genet*, **54**, 124–8.

Habashi JP, et al. (2006). Losaratan, an AT1 antagonist, prevents aortic aneurysm in a mouse model of Marfan syndrome. *Science*, **312**, 117–21.

Jiang Q, et al. (2008). Pseudoxanthoma elasticum is a metabolic disease. *J Invest Dermatol*, **129**, 348–54.

Kielty CM, Shuttleworth AC. (1994). Abnormal fibril assembly by dermal fibroblasts from two patients with the Marfan syndrome. *J Cell Biol*, **124**, 997–1004.

Lebwohl M, et al. (1994). Classification of pseudoxanthoma elasticum: report of a consensus conference. *J Am Acad Dermatol*, **30**, 103–7.

Le Saux O, et al. (2000). Mutations in a gene encoding an ABC transporter cause pseudoxanthoma elasticum. *Nat Genet*, **25**, 223–7.

Le Saux O, et al. (2006). Serum factors from pseudoxanthoma elasticum patients alter elastic fiber formation in vitro. *J Invest Dermatol*, **126**, 1497–505.

Li Q, et al. (2009). Pseudoxanthoma elasticum clinical phenotypes, molecular genetics and putative mechanisms. *Exp Dermatol*, **18**, 1–11.

Loeys BL et al. (2005). A syndrome of altered cardiovascular, craniofacial, neurocognitive and skeletal development caused by mutations in *TGFBR1* and *TGFBR2*. *Nat Genet*, **37**, 275–81.

Loeys BL, et al. (2006). Aneurysm syndrome caused by mutations in the TGF-beta receptor. *N Engl J Med*, **355**, 788–98.

Malfait F, De Paepe A (2005). Molecular genetics in classic Ehlers-Danlos syndrome. *Am J Med Genet C Semin Med Genet*, **139C**, 17–23.

McGrath JA, et al. (2004). Anatomy and organization of human skin. In: Burns T, et al. (eds) *Textbook of dermatology*, 7th edition, pp. 3.1–3.84. Blackwell Science, Oxford.

Miksch S, et al. (2005). Molecular genetics of pseudoxanthoma elasticum: type and frequency of mutations in ABCC6. *Hum Mutat*, **26**, 235–48.

Neldner KH (1988). Pseudoxanthoma elasticum. *Clin Dermatol*, **6**, 1–159.

Neptune ER, et al. (2003). Dysregulation of TGF-beta activation contributes to pathogenesis in Marfan syndrome. *Nat Genet*, **33**, 407–11.

Nicholls AC, et al. (1996). An exon-skipping mutation of the type V collagen gene (COL 5A1) in Ehlers–Danlos syndrome. *J Med Genet*, **33**, 940–6.

Palz M, *et al.* (2000). Clustering of mutations associated with mild Marfan-like phenotypes in the 3-prime region of FBN1 suggests a potential genotype–phenotype correlation. *Am J Med Genet*, **91**, 212–21.

Pepin M, *et al.* (2000). Clinical and genetic features of Ehlers–Danlos syndrome type IV, the vascular type. *N Engl J Med*, **342**, 673–80. [This is the largest series of vascular EDS patients published and is extremely informative.]

Pope FM, Burrows NP (1997). Ehlers–Danlos syndrome has varied molecular mechanisms. *J Med Genet*, **34**, 400–10.

Pope FM, *et al.* (1975). Patients with Ehlers–Danlos syndrome type IV lack type III collagen. *Proc Natl Acad Sci U S A*, **72**, 1314–16.

Ramirez F, Dietz HC (2007). Marfan syndrome: from molecular pathogenesis to clinical treatment. *Curr Opin Genet Dev*, **17**, 252–8. [This is an excellent review article of the recent molecular advances and potential therapies.]

Shores J, *et al.* (1994). Progression of aortic dilatation and the benefit of long-term beta-adrenergic blockade in Marfan's syndrome. *N Engl J Med*, **330**, 1335–41.

Trip MD, *et al.* (2002). Frequent mutation in the ABCC6 gene (R1141X) is associated with a strong increase in the prevalence of coronary artery disease. *Circulation*, **106**, 773–5.

Viljoen DL (1993). Pseudoxanthoma elasticum. In: Beighton P (ed) *McKusick's heritable disorders of connective tissue*, 5th edition, pp. 335–65. Mosby Year Book, St Louis.

Viljoen DL, Beatty S, Beighton P. (1987). The obstetric and gynaecological implications of pseudoxanthoma elasticum. *Br J Obstet Gynaecol*, **94**, 884–8.

Zweers MC, *et al.* (2004). Joint hypermobility syndromes: The pathophysiologic role of tenascin-X gene defects. *Arthritis Rheum*, **50**, 2742–9.

20.3

Osteomyelitis

Anthony R. Berendt and Martin McNally

Essentials

Bacteria can obtain access to bone from a contiguous focus of infection (e.g. a diabetic foot ulcer) or by haematogenous spread. Osteomyelitis is most commonly caused by *Staphylococcus aureus*, β-haemolytic streptococci, and—in some situations—aerobic Gram-negative rods. An acute inflammatory response causes oedema within bone and soft tissue, and thrombosis in vessels that can result in bone infarction. Pus may form within cancellous bone and beneath the periosteum, stripping it from the bond and leading to extensive necrosis that sometimes involves an entire bone. The process may become chronic and relapsing.

Diagnosis—certain diagnosis of osteomyelitis requires the culture of bacteria from reliably obtained samples of bone, accompanied by histological evidence of inflammation, but this cannot be achieved in many cases and diagnosis is commonly made on the basis of clinical features and imaging. MRI is the standard and best method.

Acute osteomyelitis

Clinical features—the condition predominantly affects the metaphyses adjacent to large weight-bearing joints, presenting as rapid onset of pain and loss of function in the affected limb, usually accompanied by high fever and malaise.

Treatment—acute osteomyelitis is an orthopaedic and medical emergency. Antibiotics (probably for at least 4 weeks) should be initiated on clinical suspicion, with appropriate initial regimens in most cases being a cephalosporin, a β-lactam/β-lactamase combination, or the combination of an antistaphylococcal penicillin and gentamicin. Vancomycin or an alternative will be necessary if the patient has risk factors for infection with methicillin-resistant *S. aureus*. Surgery is indicated if abscesses are present, or if the patient is failing to respond to medical measures.

Chronic osteomyelitis

Clinical features—presentation is more variable than acute osteomyelitis, but is typically painful unless there is underlying neuropathy. Wound or sinus tract drainage is usually present when the condition complicates ulceration, instrumentation, or other surgery. Bone may be visible, palpable with a gloved finger, or located with a sterile metal probe in the base of an ulcer or sinus.

Treatment—chronic osteomyelitis usually requires both (1) surgery—to remove dead bone and soft tissue, drain abscesses, eliminate cavities, ensure skeletal stability, and restore soft-tissue cover; and (2) antibiotics—as above, but guided by culture results, for weeks to many months.

Prognosis—a positive and coordinated approach from a multidisciplinary team can produce good results (90% cure rate with acute osteomyelitis and 80 to 90% with chronic osteomyelitis), a fact that stands in contrast to the negative experiences or views of many patients, carers, and health care workers.

Introduction and historical perspective

Osteomyelitis is an ancient disease with a formidable reputation for persistence and relapse. The changes of chronic osteomyelitis are even apparent in some dinosaur fossils, most notably in the fibula of a *Tyrannosaurus rex* specimen displayed in Chicago. It has been diagnosed in human fossil remains from the late Neolithic and was described by many classical medical writers including Hippocrates. While the term indicates inflammation of the marrow (the suffix 'myelitis') due to infection, it will be used here to indicate any infection of bone, even if confined to the cortex (sometimes called 'osteitis').

Management of osteomyelitis should, whenever possible, be multidisciplinary and involve orthopaedic surgeons, specialists in infection, radiologists, pathologists, therapists with skills in physical rehabilitation, and—as appropriate—adult physicians or paediatricians.

Aetiology, pathogenesis, and pathophysiology

The pathogens causing osteomyelitis are dominated by *Staphylococcus aureus*, but there are many other known causes as shown in Fig. 20.3.1.

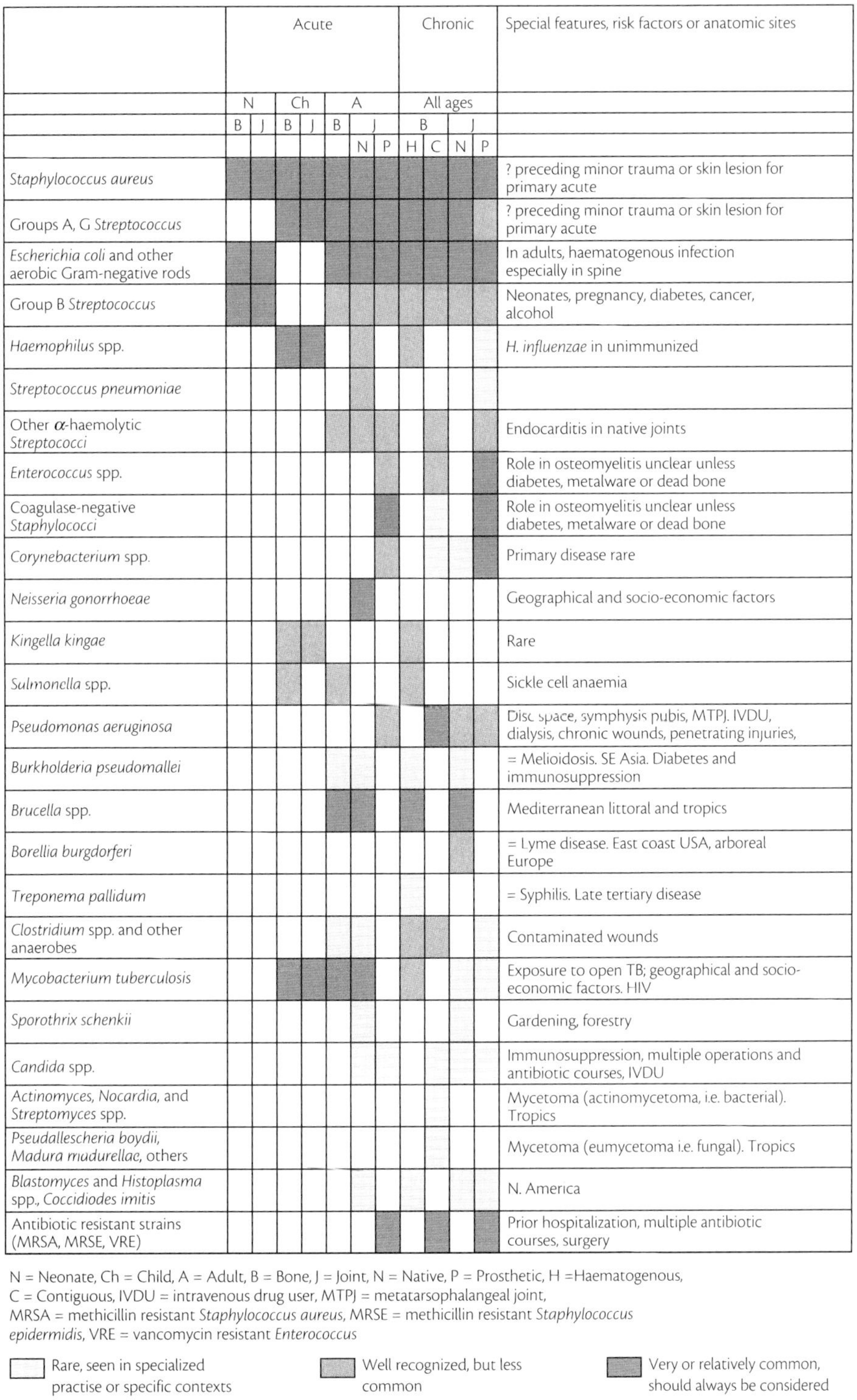

	Acute							Chronic				Special features, risk factors or anatomic sites
	N		Ch		A			All ages				
	B	J	B	J	B	J		B		J		
						N	P	H	C	N	P	
Staphylococcus aureus	▓	▓	▓	▓	▓	▓	▓	▓	▓	▓	▓	? preceding minor trauma or skin lesion for primary acute
Groups A, G Streptococcus			▓	▓	▓	▓	▓	▓	▓	▓	▓	? preceding minor trauma or skin lesion for primary acute
Escherichia coli and other aerobic Gram-negative rods	▓	▓			▓	▓	▓	▓	▓	▓	▓	In adults, haematogenous infection especially in spine
Group B Streptococcus	▓	▓			░			░		░		Neonates, pregnancy, diabetes, cancer, alcohol
Haemophilus spp.			░	░	░			░				H. influenzae in unimmunized
Streptococcus pneumoniae												
Other α-haemolytic Streptococci						░						Endocarditis in native joints
Enterococcus spp.						░				░		Role in osteomyelitis unclear unless diabetes, metalware or dead bone
Coagulase-negative Staphylococci							▓				░	Role in osteomyelitis unclear unless diabetes, metalware or dead bone
Corynebacterium spp.							░					Primary disease rare
Neisseria gonorrhoeae						▓						Geographical and socio-economic factors
Kingella kingae			░	░								Rare
Salmonella spp.			░		░							Sickle cell anaemia
Pseudomonas aeruginosa						░		░				Disc space, symphysis pubis, MTPJ, IVDU, dialysis, chronic wounds, penetrating injuries,
Burkholderia pseudomallei					░							= Melioidosis. SE Asia. Diabetes and immunosuppression
Brucella spp.					▓	▓		▓				Mediterranean littoral and tropics
Borellia burgdorferi										░		= Lyme disease. East coast USA, arboreal Europe
Treponema pallidum												= Syphilis. Late tertiary disease
Clostridium spp. and other anaerobes								░				Contaminated wounds
Mycobacterium tuberculosis			▓	▓	▓			▓				Exposure to open TB; geographical and socio-economic factors. HIV
Sporothrix schenkii						░						Gardening, forestry
Candida spp.							░				░	Immunosuppression, multiple operations and antibiotic courses, IVDU
Actinomyces, Nocardia, and Streptomyces spp.								░				Mycetoma (actinomycetoma, i.e. bacterial). Tropics
Pseudallescheria boydii, Madura madurellae, others								░				Mycetoma (eumycetoma i.e. fungal). Tropics
Blastomyces and Histoplasma spp., Coccidiodes imitis							░				░	N. America
Antibiotic resistant strains (MRSA, MRSE, VRE)							▓		▓		▓	Prior hospitalization, multiple antibiotic courses, surgery

N = Neonate, Ch = Child, A = Adult, B = Bone, J = Joint, N = Native, P = Prosthetic, H = Haematogenous,
C = Contiguous, IVDU = intravenous drug user, MTPJ = metatarsophalangeal joint,
MRSA = methicillin resistant Staphylococcus aureus, MRSE = methicillin resistant Staphylococcus epidermidis, VRE = vancomycin resistant Enterococcus

☐ Rare, seen in specialized practise or specific contexts   ▨ Well recognized, but less common   � Very or relatively common, should always be considered

Fig. 20.3.1 Microbiological causes and contexts in pyogenic arthritis and osteomyelitis.

The critical step in pathogenesis is the access of bacteria to the bone. This may occur from a contiguous focus such as chronic ulceration, surgery, trauma, or soft tissue infection. Alternatively, the route may be haematogenous, with bacteria reaching bone via the circulation. The exact mechanism by which this occurs is uncertain. It is believed that the tortuous capillary loops in the metaphyses of the long bones, a favoured site for haematogenous osteomyelitis, are particularly vulnerable to thrombosis, which provides a site for bacterial seeding. This is supported by a history of recent blunt trauma to the affected part in some 30% of haematogenous cases and by observations that in most animal models it is necessary to injure bone to infect it. Even minor bone and soft tissue trauma exposes components of blood clots, the extracellular matrix, and the bone matrix to the bloodstream. Many pathogens, notably S. aureus, can adhere to such host proteins through specific receptors and, hence, to tissues and cells, including endothelial cells and osteocytes.

An acute inflammatory response is elicited once bacteria gain access to bone and begin to multiply. This causes oedema within bone and soft tissue, and the procoagulant effect of inflammation may also cause thrombosis in vessels. The result can be bone infarction, possibly contributed to by bacterial toxins.

As infection progresses, it propagates within the bone marrow and through the cortical bone via the haversian canals. Pus may form within cancellous bone and beneath the periosteum (see Fig. 20.3.2 for a schematic diagram). It may break into the soft tissues and even extend to the surface as a sinus tract. Subperiosteal pus under pressure will strip off the overlying periosteum, tracking along the length of the bone and around its circumference. The vascular consequences of this are critical to the evolution of the disease, since the outer aspect of the cortical bone is vascularized by the periosteum, the inner by the endosteal circulation. If the endosteal blood supply is already compromised by the infection, periosteal stripping causes bone death. Thus, large pieces of bone, segments, or even whole long bones can die as the infection progresses.

Dead bone can potentially be revascularized and remodelled, but only if it remains in physical continuity with living bone. However, the action of bone-resorbing cells, recruited and activated by inflammation and some bacterial products, is frequently to separate dead from healthy bone. This produces a detached piece of dead bone called a sequestrum. Small sequestra can be extruded from sinuses or wounds and the episode of osteomyelitis may arrest spontaneously; larger sequestra result in continuing infection

and inflammation. Over time, more bone tends to be involved, sometimes resulting in new sinuses, with extension into soft tissues and contiguous joints. As bone is resorbed and killed, the resulting loss of strength may lead to pathological fracture.

Chronicity and relapse result both from this host response and from features of bacterial physiology. The body cannot mount effective inflammatory responses in dead tissue or chronic abscesses. Bacteria adhere to the inanimate surfaces of dead bone and, as in implant-related infections, form complex structures in which they are enmeshed in an antiphagocytic polysaccharide matrix, the whole being known as a biofilm. Their growth state alters within this, rendering them phenotypically resistant to almost all antibiotics. They may even be able to persist as metabolically crippled forms called small-colony variants: these can exist within cells and are also resistant to many antibiotics that would otherwise kill wild-type organisms.

If periosteum has been stripped and remains viable, it produces new bone called the involucrum. This may develop circumferentially, producing a shell of living bone around the dead segment, thus preserving mechanical strength. Defects in the involucrum, through which sinuses communicate with sequestra, are called cloacae.

Variations on this theme occur when flat bones or those of the spine are involved in haematogenous infection. In discitis and vertebral osteomyelitis, infection of the disc space is rapidly followed by involvement of the two adjacent vertebral bodies. The infection may arrest as disc material is replaced by granulation tissue, eventually leading to fusion of the two involved vertebral bodies. In flat bones such as the pelvis or the skull, infection can spread very rapidly in the cancellous bone between the two tables before exciting a periosteal reaction.

The inside-to-out nature of haematogenous osteomyelitis is in distinction to the outside-to-in nature of contiguous focus osteomyelitis. In this case, periosteum is destroyed as part of the same process that has destroyed the overlying soft tissues. Cortical bone is killed and infection can enter the medullary cavity, thereafter extending as for haematogenous disease. Sequestra may separate and be discharged, but the adverse biological factors that led to the initial soft tissue loss may impair subsequent healing and permit further bone infection to occur.

Epidemiology

Classical acute haematogenous osteomyelitis has its peak incidence in childhood. Men are more commonly affected than women. In children, a greater incidence in the southern hemisphere and among certain racial groups (e.g. aboriginal Australians) has been described, with rates varying from 10 to 100:100 000/year. Socioeconomic factors may contribute to this variation. Acute osteomyelitis is also seen as a complication of infections of fractures and trauma, commonly seen in victims of military conflict and road traffic accidents or after orthopaedic instrumentation. Most acute bone infections now arise through these routes.

Chronic osteomyelitis is such a diverse disease that an overall incidence and prevalence rate is not available, but incidence rises with age due to numerous causes including diabetes, peripheral vascular disease, infirmity, and ulceration. Chronic osteomyelitis also results whenever acute osteomyelitis is not treated successfully. The global diabetes pandemic is particularly noteworthy,

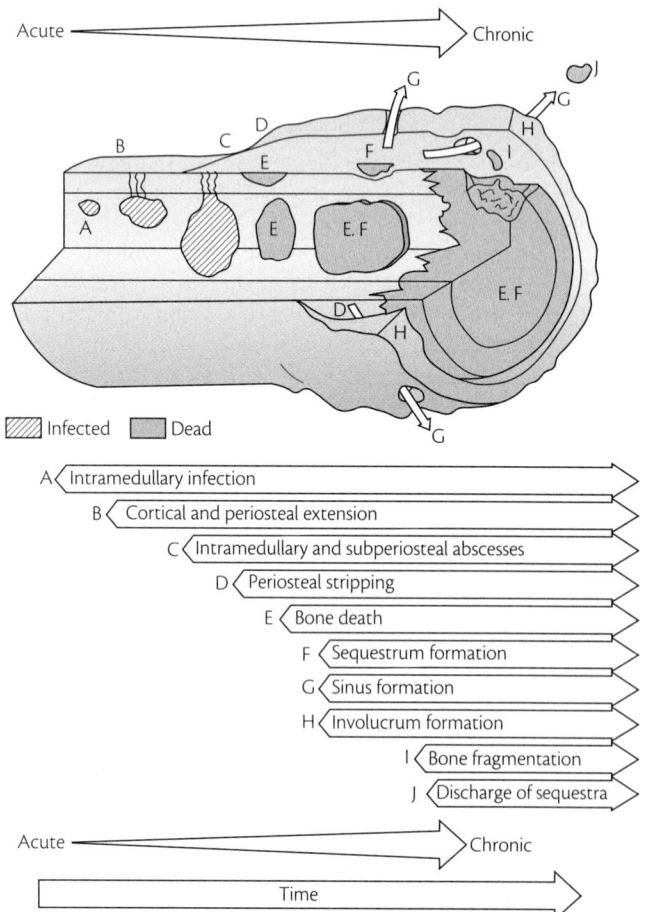

Fig. 20.3.2 Schematic diagram showing the evolution from acute to chronic osteomyelitis, with progressive necrosis, sequestration, and sinus formation.

with an estimated 252 million people affected in 2007, leading to a huge burden of chronic osteomyelitis of foot bones complicating diabetic neuropathic ulceration.

Prevention and control

There are no proven means of preventing haematogenous osteomyelitis, but prompt treatment can prevent chronicity. Contiguous osteomyelitis can be prevented by the appropriate management of open fractures and of infective foci or chronic wounds whenever these are close to a bone or joint. Pressure-area care for immobile patients and appropriate foot care for people with diabetes can prevent ulceration and subsequent osteomyelitis.

Clinical features

Acute osteomyelitis presents as rapid onset of pain and loss of function in the affected limb, usually accompanied by high fever and malaise. It predominantly affects the metaphyses adjacent to the large weight-bearing joints, but any bone can be involved. Prostration, sweating, rigors, and vomiting from bacteraemia, which accompany 50% of cases, may also be present. In neonates and infants, an acute septic arthritis (Chapter 19.7) can be an early complication or a presenting feature of an acute osteomyelitis because the joint capsule encloses not only the joint but also the metaphyseal growth plate; infection may therefore track out from the bone into the joint cavity. In older children, the joint capsule is much tougher and inserts at the growth plate. In both age groups, the cartilage of the growth plate forms a barrier to the direct passage of infection from the metaphysis to the epiphysis and the joint.

Chronic osteomyelitis presents more variably. Pain is the rule, unless there is underlying neuropathy, and there may be severe disability in the context of an ununited fracture or when the spine is involved. Wound or sinus tract drainage is usually present when osteomyelitis complicates ulceration, instrumentation, or other surgery. Bone may be visible, palpable with a gloved finger, or located with a sterile metal probe in the base of an ulcer or sinus. There may be evidence of soft tissue swelling or induration and bony tenderness on palpation or percussion. Some patients experience repeated flares of fever and acute illness due to inadequate drainage of deep pus or rapid extension into previously uninvolved soft tissue or bone. Minor ill health is common, manifesting as loss of weight or appetite, general malaise, or poor glycaemic control in people with diabetes. This is often only noticeable in retrospect when infection has been treated.

Patients with vertebral osteomyelitis may present with bacteraemia and acute back pain (raising the possibility of spinal epidural abscess and the need for urgent diagnosis and treatment), but more often they present with chronic back pain and nonspecific illness. Differential diagnoses of degenerative back pain, osteoporotic fracture, metastatic disease, and myeloma should be considered. The presence of severe back pain at rest, or of night pain, should prompt consideration of the diagnosis. Pain is often of a deep and unremitting character that patients can distinguish from previous back pains. Spinal tenderness is an unreliable sign. Deformity and the development of neurological signs are late features suggestive of loss of mechanical stability or the formation of paraspinal or epidural collections or masses.

Osteomyelitis in the diabetic foot presents with overlying chronic ulceration. The location of the infection is linked to the biomechanical changes produced by neuropathy that cause ulcers in high pressure areas related to metatarsal heads, phalanges, interphalangeal joints, or—more rarely—the calcaneum or plantar area.

Special forms of osteomyelitis include chronic multifocal osteomyelitis (this presents with pain but, despite radiological and histological features of osteomyelitis, is culture-negative), unifocal osteomyelitis with a similar behaviour, and Brodie's abscess (a well-defined chronic abscess in bone with a very indolent presentation).

Differential diagnosis

Primary or metastatic tumours or fractures may mimic acute or chronic infection. Charcot's neuro-osteoarthropathy can be difficult to distinguish from infection in patients with underlying neuropathy, a problem that is very common in diabetic foot osteomyelitis. A chronic periosteal reaction can arise from many causes, but commonly in the lower leg due to chronic venous insufficiency. Whilst a periosteal reaction in this situation is common, osteomyelitis is rare and is usually evident from other features such as massive soft tissue loss with obvious exposure of bone.

Clinical investigation

The white-cell count, erythrocyte sedimentation rate, and C-reactive protein, although generally elevated in acute infection and flares of chronic disease, are nonspecific and occasionally normal in chronic disease. It is helpful to see elevated inflammatory markers fall after treatment, but this may take several weeks. The alkaline phosphatase level is of no value, being neither sensitive nor specific for bone infection. Blood cultures are essential in acute infection, when they may be the only means of obtaining a microbiological diagnosis. Serological tests are useful for the diagnosis of syphilis, yaws, brucellosis, and occasionally bartonellosis.

Plain radiography of chronic osteomyelitis typically shows patchy osteopenia or frank bone destruction, loss of definition of the cortex, areas of sclerosis, or periosteal reaction with new bone formation. These changes take many weeks to develop fully. In acute infection, the earliest change visible on plain radiography is soft tissue swelling (minimum 2–3 days), which is followed by periosteal reaction (7 days) and (lastly) bone destruction (10 days). If radiographs are abnormal, the changes need to be distinguished from those of tumour, trauma, or degenerative bone disease. Repeat imaging at an interval (2–4 weeks) can sometimes help as osteomyelitis is usually an aggressive process with rapidly evolving radiology. For more rapid clarification of diagnosis, however, specialized imaging is needed.

Ultrasound can identify subperiosteal collections and soft tissue abscesses and can demonstrate sinuses. CT scanning may be able to identify cortical erosion that has been missed on plain films and can demonstrate sequestra within bone. Reformatted images make it possible to produce sagittal or coronal images (e.g. to view vertebral body endplates and the spinal canal in patients unable to undergo MRI scanning) and three-dimensional images for surgical planning. Soft tissue collections are easily identified. Other than a lack of sensitivity early in the disease, the principal pitfalls of CT scanning are the radiation dose, its lack of ability to determine the extent or activity of infection, and its sensitivity to image degradation from orthopaedic metalware.

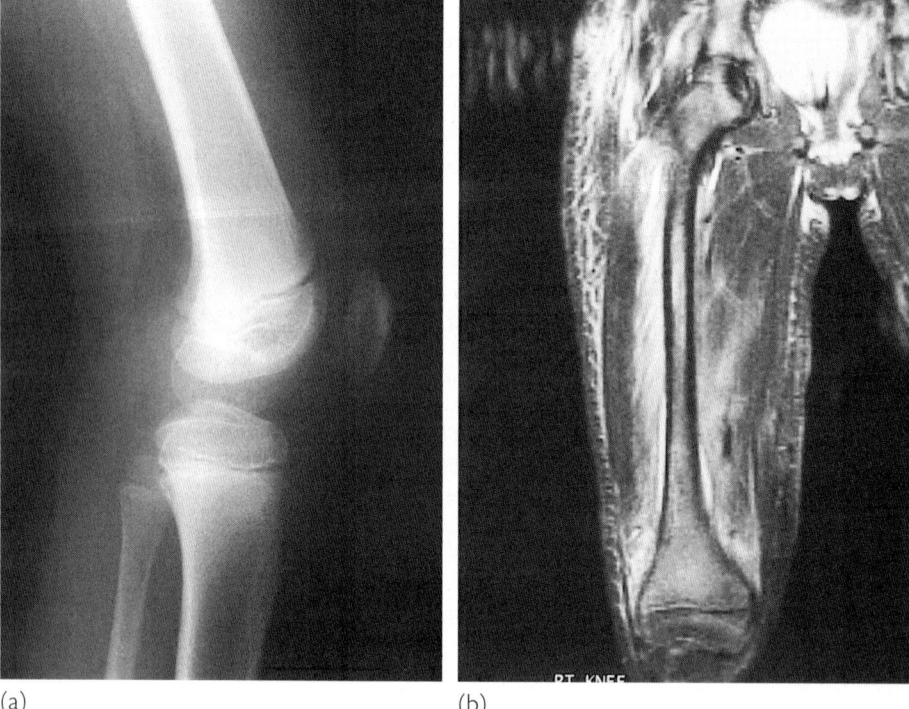

Fig. 20.3.3 Acute osteomyelitis of the femur in a child. (a) The plain radiograph, after 1 day of illness, is normal. *S. aureus* was isolated from blood cultures. (b) MRI scan (short T1 inversion recovery sequence) of the same patient on day 2. There is marked soft tissue and intraosseous oedema (high signal). Subperiosteal abscesses can clearly be seen as linear areas of high signal just outside the cortex, tracking proximally up the femur from the metaphysis.

(a)   (b)

Isotope scanning is widely used, but there is a lack of consensus on the utility of various tests. Conventional, three-phase, technetium bone scans are sensitive but nonspecific. Specificity may be increased by the addition of labelled leucocyte scanning. Other reagents include labelled immunoglobulins, antileucocyte monoclonal antibodies, and even radiolabelled antibiotics.

MRI is the standard and best method for diagnostic imaging of osteomyelitis (Figs. 20.3.3 and 20.3.4). It can detect intra- and extraosseous oedema, abscesses, dead bone, and sinus tracts. It can distinguish active from inactive infection. MRI has the advantages

that its costs are rapidly falling and its availability is increasing, but its use can be problematic, mainly because of its extreme sensitivity to physiological changes that may persist long after surgery or treatment and to metal artefacts from orthopaedic implants (and even to microscopic metallosis when implants have been removed).

The microbiological standard for the diagnosis of osteomyelitis is the growth of bacteria from samples of bone, taken with precautions to prevent contamination from superficial flora. Pus or soft tissue associated with infected bone may be acceptable, but sinus tract or wound swab cultures are not. The bacteria isolated from

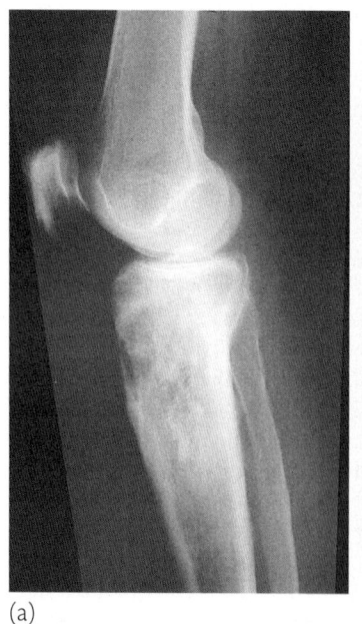
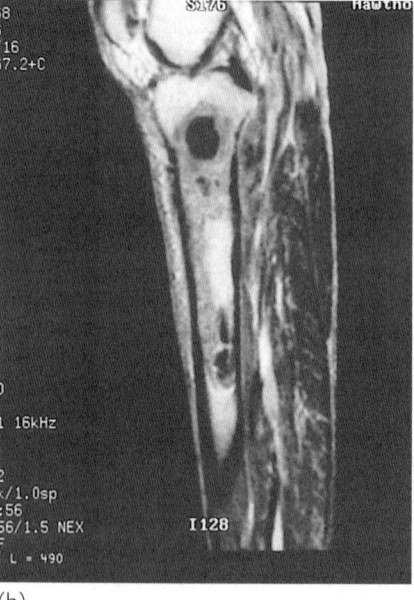

Fig. 20.3.4 (a) A plain radiograph showing chronic osteomyelitis of the proximal tibia in an adult, with patchy sclerosis and lysis, and (b) MRI of the same patient (short T1 inversion recovery sequence) showing oedema (low signal) in the area corresponding to plain film changes, but also an additional, distal, intramedullary satellite lesion.

(a)   (b)

wounds are poorly predictive of the deep flora because of asymptomatic colonization. Cultures of this kind should be reserved for detecting multiresistant organisms (such as methicillin-resistant *S. aureus* (MRSA)) for infection control purposes. Fluid for microscopy and culture can be aspirated from periosteal or subperiosteal abscesses. In infants, needle aspiration of bone itself is safe and well tolerated if performed by someone experienced in the technique. Bone biopsy can be performed surgically or percutaneously (by needle biopsy). In neuropathic ulcers, bone can be obtained by curettage following debridement of the overlying ulcer material. The laboratory must be made aware of the importance and nature of any specimen sent so that it can be appropriately processed and interpreted. As epidemiologically appropriate, cultures for mycobacteria, brucellae and fungi may need to be requested.

Bone histology is also an important diagnostic test: the presence of inflammatory cells, dead bone, and active bone remodelling are hallmarks of infection. They may provide the only confirmation of infection in cases where the culture results are unhelpful and may suggest specific pathogens if the changes are granulomatous rather than pyogenic.

Criteria for diagnosis

Formal criteria, as defined for endocarditis and many inflammatory disorders, have not been agreed by consensus. The criterion standard is considered to be the culture of bacteria from reliably obtained samples of bone, accompanied by histological evidence of inflammation. However, these criteria can be difficult to satisfy in many cases, so it is common to make a clinical diagnosis based on a range of clinical and imaging features.

Treatment

Acute osteomyelitis

Acute osteomyelitis is an orthopaedic and a medical emergency that may respond to antibiotics alone, with good outcomes if treated before the onset of bone death or abscess formation. Treatment should be initiated on the basis of the clinical diagnosis, with investigations used to confirm the diagnosis once treatment has begun. Following blood cultures, high-dose intravenous antibiotics effective against *S. aureus*, β-haemolytic streptococci, and—in some situations—aerobic Gram-negative rods, should be given. Appropriate regimens include a cephalosporin, a β-lactam/β-lactamase combination (amoxicillin/clavulanate or ampicillin/sulbactam), or the combination of an antistaphylococcal penicillin and gentamicin. Vancomycin or an alternative will be necessary if the patient has risk factors for infection with MRSA. Antibiotics can be modified based on culture results. For patient comfort, the limb should be splinted and elevated and analgesia should be given.

Surgery is indicated if abscesses are present or if the patient is failing to respond to medical measures. Abscesses must be drained and, although controversial, drilling of the bone allows free drainage of contained pus. In acute infection, the surgeon aims to minimize damage to living bone and soft tissues and thereby avoid further devascularization and consequent excessive bone death.

The necessary duration of antibiotic therapy is unclear, but treatment for less than 4 weeks is associated with higher rates of relapse. In children, oral therapy can be considered when all of the following criteria are met: (1) the patient is afebrile after the initial

48 h to 72 h of intravenous treatment; (2) there is no evidence of abscess formation, metastatic infection, or bacteraemia; (3) there is no suspicion from the history or imaging that, prior to treatment, infection has been prolonged or is associated with dead bone; (4) the organism is sensitive to reliably bioavailable oral antibiotics; and (5) compliance with therapy can be assured.

Less information is available for adults. The greatly lower rates of bone blood flow and turnover make the revascularization and absorption of necrotic bone and the delivery of antibiotics and white cells less certain. Adult acute osteomyelitis may be treated with intravenous therapy for periods of at least 4 weeks (outpatient parenteral antibiotic therapy (OPAT) programmes are useful for this), but certain drugs, notably clindamycin and ciprofloxacin, are highly bioavailable and have proved useful in the oral treatment of osteomyelitis. There are no randomized studies to inform decisions about the necessary duration of intravenous therapy or total duration of antibiotic treatment.

Chronic osteomyelitis

To achieve long-term arrest of infection, the management of chronic osteomyelitis usually requires multiple, coordinated inputs. The aims of treatment are to:

- remove dead bone and soft tissue
- drain abscesses
- eliminate cavities (which act as surgical 'dead spaces')
- ensure skeletal stability
- restore soft tissue cover (if necessary using plastic surgery)
- define pathogens from high-quality specimens and administer appropriate antibiotics
- correct adverse local and systemic host factors
- support the patient physically and psychologically
- reconstruct the skeleton if need be
- rehabilitate the patient

Surgery

Detailed consideration of surgical methods is beyond the scope of this book, but the importance of an expert surgical opinion in managing chronic osteomyelitis cannot be overstated, even if the conclusion of that input is that a surgical approach is not technically possible or in the patient's overall interests. Recent major surgical advances include the use of free-tissue transfer and bone transport techniques to close very large bony and soft tissue defects. These permit much more radical approaches to the resection of diseased and dead tissues. In this way, surgery can potentially convert chronic infected wounds with dead bone and soft tissue into contaminated wounds of living bone with healthy soft tissue cover. This allows a reduction in the duration of antibiotic therapy in some situations and offers a greater range of patients the possibility of long-term arrest of infection.

Antibiotics

These play an important role after surgery, although the 'added value' they confer is uncertain and may depend on the extent of

SECTION 20 DISORDERS OF THE SKELETON

surgical resection. Some conditions often respond well without surgery, including:

- discitis and vertebral osteomyelitis—surgery is reserved for abscess formation, progressive pain or deformity, instability, spinal cord compression, or persistent sepsis
- tuberculous osteomyelitis—surgery is reserved for mechanical complications, pain, or persistent infection
- osteomyelitis of small bones such as the phalanges
- patients with diabetic foot osteomyelitis—some authorities quote that chronic osteomyelitis can be arrested in about 70% or 80% of cases with only by limited podiatric debridement of bone

Antibiotics may also help when the patient refuses surgery, when there is no clearly definable surgical target, or when the risks and consequences of surgical resection would be worse than the disease itself.

The choice of antibiotics should be guided by the culture results. Intravenous therapy may need to be prolonged (for up to 6 weeks) where there is thought to be a risk of unreliable compliance, poor absorption, or lack of efficacy of oral therapy. As above, OPAT programmes are valuable for shortening the hospital stay for such patients. Periods of total antibiotic treatment vary from weeks to many months, but there is a growing trend to shorten the duration of treatment when an expert surgeon has achieved a radical surgical clearance, provided that local and systemic host factors are favourable. Antibiotics can also be delivered locally, by implanting antibiotic-loaded bone cement or collagen fleece at the time of surgery. The relative efficacies of intravenous, oral, or local antibiotics have received little attention and treatment protocols vary widely.

Adjunctive treatment

It is important to assess for, and if possible control, factors that may affect wound and bone healing. These include ischaemia due to peripheral vascular disease, anaemia, diabetes, hypoxia from respiratory or cardiac failure, peripheral oedema, poor nutrition, and smoking. Where neuropathy has contributed to ulceration, appropriate pressure relief is essential for healing and for secondary prevention. This must be continued indefinitely through the provision of specialist footwear, cushions, or beds. The patient must be taught about neuropathy and trained in methods to prevent further ulceration. Hyperbaric oxygen therapy has been widely employed with anecdotal success, but its effectiveness and its precise role are unclear, with definitive randomized trials still awaited. Given its expense, establishing a clear evidence base for hyperbaric oxygen should be a prerequisite for its commissioning and use.

Prognosis

More than 90% of cases of acute osteomyelitis that are amenable to medical treatment can be arrested. Chronic osteomyelitis can be arrested in about 80% or 90% of cases, usually when expert surgery has been combined with antibiotic treatment. Recurrence is most common within the first year, but may occur at any time, and recurrences have been described over 50 years after an initial infection has apparently been treated successfully. This poses major difficulties for the design of clinical trials, as extended follow-up is needed to make definitive statements about success or failure. Longstanding active chronic osteomyelitis may be associated with the eventual development of squamous metaplasia or carcinoma in a sinus and with the deposition of amyloid, but both these events are rarities, albeit important to consider.

Occupational, quality of life, and psychosocial aspects

Pain, chronic sepsis, and physical disability have a significant impact on quality of life. Psychological well being is further affected by issues common to all chronic diseases, together with anxiety and depression over risks of death, paralysis (e.g. in spinal infection), and limb loss, stigmatizing effects of chronic discharging wounds, and feelings of anger or failure where infection has resulted from an accident or surgery. The multidisciplinary team caring for the patient must have awareness and experience of dealing with these issues and access to appropriate rehabilitation resources to optimize long-term function and quality of life.

Likely developments in the near future

The rise in antimicrobial resistance is likely to make the antibiotic treatment of osteomyelitis more challenging and require the use of new agents, notably against MRSA. A major worldwide drive to decrease health care associated infections may bear fruit but be offset by increasing numbers of patients being injured through conflict or the effects of climate change. The aging populations of the industrialized world and the rising prevalence of diabetes are likely to result in further increases in the burden of diabetic foot and pressure sore osteomyelitis. For those able to afford them, there may be balancing advances in diagnosis using the polymerase chain reaction to detect microbial nucleic acid, microarrays to detect infection-specific host responses, and improved surgical reconstructive methods including the use of bone morphogenetic proteins to restore bone loss.

Further reading

Bachur R, Pagon Z (2007). Success of short-course parenteral antibiotic therapy for acute osteomyelitis of childhood. *Clin Pediatr (Phila)*, **46**, 30–5.

Berendt T, Byren I (2004). Bone and joint infection. *Clin Med*, **4**, 510–18.

Chihara S, Segreti J (2010). Osteomyelitis. *Dis Mon*, **56**, 5–31.

Cierny, III G, Mader JT (1984). Adult chronic osteomyelitis. *Orthopaedics*, 7, 1557–64.

Conterno LO, da Silva Filho CR (2009). Antibiotics for treating chronic osteomyelitis in adults. *Cochrane Database Syst Rev*, **8**, CD004439.

Gristina A, *et al.* (1985). Adherent bacterial colonisation in the pathogenesis of osteomyelitis. *Science*, **228**, 990–3.

Harik NS, Smeltzer MS (2010). Management of acute hematogenous osteomyelitis in children. *Expert Rev Anti Infect Ther*, **8**, 175–81.

Klenerman L (2007). A history of osteomyelitis from the Journal of Bone and Joint Surgery: 1948 TO 2006. *J Bone Joint Surg Br*, **89**, 667–70.

Le Saux N, *et al.* (2002). Shorter courses of parenteral antibiotic therapy do not appear to influence response rates for children with acute hematogenous osteomyelitis: a systematic review. *BMC Infect Dis*, **2**, 16.

Lew DP, Waldvogel FA (2004). Osteomyelitis. *Lancet*, **364**, 369–79.

McNally MA, *et al.* (1993). Two-stage management of chronic osteomyelitis of the long bones. The Belfast technique. *J Bone Joint Surg Br*, **75**, 375–80.

Miller AO, Henry M (2009). Update in diagnosis and treatment of diabetic foot infections. *Phys Med Rehabil Clin N Am*, **20**, 61–25.

Rega EA, Brochu CA (2001). Paleopathology of a mature *Tyrannosaurus rex*. *J Vert Paleontol*, **21**, 92A.

Stengel D, *et al.* (2001). Systematic review and meta-analysis of antibiotic therapy for bone and joint infections. *Lancet Infect Dis*, **1**, 175–88.

Swiontkowski MF, *et al.* (1999). A comparison of short and long course i.v. antibiotic therapy in the post-operative management of adult osteomyelitis. *J Bone Joint Surg*, **81B**, 1046–50.

Verdier I, *et al.* (2005). Contribution of a broad range polymerase chain reaction to the diagnosis of osteoarticular infections caused by Kingella kingae: description of twenty-four recent pediatric diagnoses. *Pediatr Infect Dis J*, **24**, 692–6.

Wininger DA, Fass RJ (1996). Antibiotic-impregnated cement and beads for orthopaedic infections. *Antimicrob Agents Chemother*, **40**, 2675–9.

Osteoporosis

Juliet Compston

Essentials

Osteoporosis is characterized by a reduction in bone mass and disruption of bone architecture, resulting in increased bone fragility and fracture risk, with fractures of the distal radius (Colles' fracture), spine and proximal femur being most characteristic. One in two women and one in five men over the age of 50 years will suffer an osteoporotic fracture during their remaining lifetime, with massive cost to health care services.

Pathogenesis—bone mass in later life depends both on (1) peak bone mass achieved in early adulthood—strongly influenced by genetic factors, also sex hormone status, nutrition and physical activity; and (2) rate of age-related bone loss—oestrogen deficiency is a major factor in menopausal bone loss in women.

Diagnosis—dual energy X-ray absorptiometry (DXA) is the best method for measuring bone mineral density (BMD) in the spine and hip, with osteoporosis defined as present when the BMD is 2.5 standard deviations or more below normal peak bone mass (T-score ≤ −2.5).

Risk assessment—an algorithm to estimate 10-year fracture probability (FRAX) uses (1) clinical risk factors—including age, glucocorticoid therapy, a previous history of fracture, a family history of hip fracture, current smoking, alcohol abuse, and certain diseases associated with osteoporosis, e.g. rheumatoid arthritis; with or without (2) BMD measurements. This enables intervention thresholds to be based on absolute risk rather than on BMD T-scores.

Treatment—appropriate levels of exercise should be recommended, and smoking and alcohol abuse discouraged. In postmenopausal women with osteoporosis, reductions of around 30 to 50% in vertebral fracture are seen after 3 years treatment with most drug interventions, with the current consensus being that this should be continued for a minimum of 5 years. (1) First-line treatments—for postmenopausal women these would generally be regarded as alendronate, risedronate, zoledronate (all bisphosphonates) and strontium ranelate, with a particularly strong evidence base for strontium ranelate in very elderly patients. (2) Second-line treatments—raloxifene (a selective oestrogen-receptor modulator) or ibandronate. (3) Other considerations—(a) intravenous zoledronate—the treatment of choice when oral medication cannot be given or will not be absorbed; (b) parathyroid hormone peptides—use limited to women with severe vertebral osteoporosis who are intolerant of or unresponsive to other treatments; (c) hormone replacement therapy—an appropriate option in younger postmenopausal women at high risk of fracture; (d) calcium and vitamin D—should be coprescribed with other treatments; (e) glucocorticoid-induced osteoporosis—primary prevention with a bisphosphonate is recommended for patients committed to any oral dose of prednisolone for > 3 months who are > 65 years or who have sustained a previous fragility fracture. Other patients taking oral glucocorticoids for > 3 months should have their BMD measured, and those with a T-score of—1.5 or lower should be considered for treatment.

Introduction

Osteoporosis is characterized by a reduction in bone mass and disruption of bone architecture, resulting in increased bone fragility and an increase in fracture risk. These fractures are widely recognized as a major health problem in the elderly population, resulting in an estimated annual cost to United Kingdom health services of £1.8 billion. One in two women and one in five men over the age of 50 years will have a fracture due to osteoporosis during their remaining lifetime. Demographic changes during the first half of the 21st century are predicted to lead to at least a doubling in the number of these fractures, largely as a result of increased longevity.

Epidemiology

Osteoporotic fractures are termed fragility fractures (defined as occurring after a fall from standing height or less). They may occur at a number of skeletal sites but fractures of the distal radius (Colles' fracture), spine, and proximal femur are most characteristic. The incidence of osteoporotic fractures increases markedly with age; in women, the median age for Colles' fracture is 65 years and for hip fracture, 80 years. The age at which incidence of vertebral fractures reaches a peak is less well defined but is thought in women to be between 65 and 80 years. In men, no age-related increase in forearm fractures is seen but incidence of hip fracture rises exponentially after the age of 75 years. The prevalence of vertebral fractures rises with age in men, although less steeply than in women.

Clinical features

Colles' fractures typically occur after a fall forwards on to the outstretched hand. They cause considerable inconvenience, usually requiring from 4 to 6 weeks in plaster and long-term adverse sequelae are seen in up to one-third of patients. These include pain, sympathetic algodystrophy, deformity, and functional impairment.

Vertebral fractures (Fig. 20.4.1) may occur spontaneously or as a result of normal activities such as lifting, bending, and coughing. A minority of vertebral fractures (possibly around one-third) present with acute and severe pain at the site of the fracture, often radiating around the thorax or abdomen. The natural history of this pain is variable; in general, there is a tendency for improvement with time but resolution is often incomplete. Multiple vertebral fractures result in spinal deformity (kyphosis), height loss, and corresponding alterations in body shape with protuberance of the abdomen and loss of normal body contours. These changes are commonly associated with loss of self-confidence and self-esteem, difficulty with daily activities, and increased social isolation. The clinical impact of vertebral fractures is thus substantial, although often underestimated.

Of all the osteoporotic fractures, hip fractures cause the greatest morbidity and mortality. They almost always follow a fall, either backwards or to the side, and require admission to hospital and surgical treatment. Because hip fractures characteristically affect frail elderly people, postoperative morbidity and mortality are high; at 6 months after fracture, mortality rates from 12 to 20% have been reported. Only a minority of older people who have had falls regain their former level of independence following a hip fracture and up to one-third require institutionalized care.

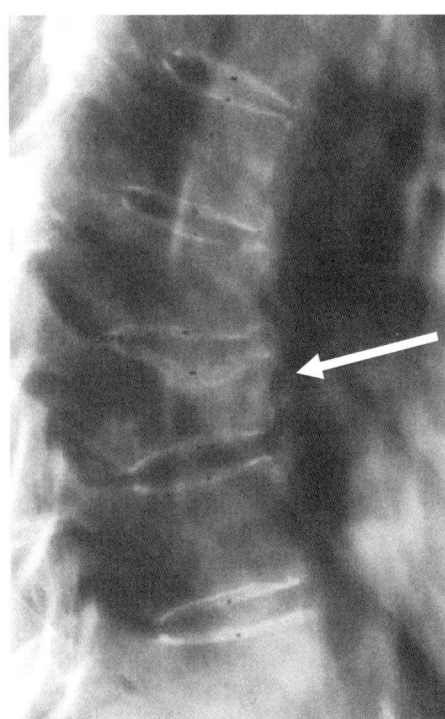

Fig. 20.4.1 Vertebral fracture (arrowed).

Pathogenesis

Lifetime changes in bone mass are shown in Fig. 20.4.2. Peak bone mass is attained in the third decade of life and age-related bone loss is believed to start in both men and women around the beginning of the fifth decade; thereafter bone loss continues throughout life. In women, there is an acceleration of the rate of bone loss around the time of the menopause, the duration of which is poorly characterized but may be from 5 to 10 years.

Bone mass in later life thus depends both on the peak bone mass achieved in early adulthood and on the rate of age-related bone loss. Genetic factors strongly influence peak bone mass, accounting for up to 70 or 80% of its variance. A number of genes are likely to be involved; these include the collagen type I α-1 gene (*COL1A1*), a polymorphism of which is associated both with low bone mineral density (BMD) and fracture risk. Sex hormone status, nutrition, and physical activity also influence peak bone mass.

In women, oestrogen deficiency is a major pathogenetic factor in menopausal bone loss. In older men, oestrogen status is also significantly related to BMD, whereas the relationship between age-related bone loss and declining testosterone levels is less prominent. In older people, vitamin D insufficiency and secondary hyperparathyroidism are common and contribute to age-related bone loss. Other potential pathogenetic factors include declining levels of physical activity and reduced serum concentrations of insulin-like growth factors.

Pathophysiology

The mechanical competence of the skeleton is maintained by the process of bone remodelling, in which a quantum of bone is removed by osteoclasts followed by the formation of new bone, in the cavity so created, by osteoblasts. Under normal circumstances, resorption always occurs before formation and the amounts of bone resorbed and formed within each bone-remodelling unit are similar.

In menopausal bone loss, there is an increase in the number of bone remodelling units on the bone surface (along with an increased remodelling rate), resulting in a higher number than normal of remodelling units undergoing resorption at any one time. In addition, within each of these units, less bone is formed than is resorbed, leading to a negative remodelling imbalance. It is believed that one of the early, and probably transient, effects

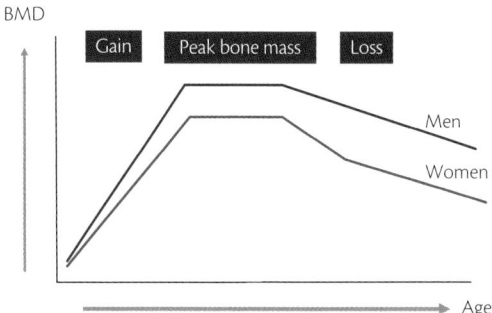

Fig. 20.4.2 Schematic representation of lifetime changes in bone mass in men and women.
(From Compston JE (1995). Review article: osteoporosis, corticosteroids and inflammatory bowel disease. *Aliment Pharmacol Ther*, **9**, 237–50.)

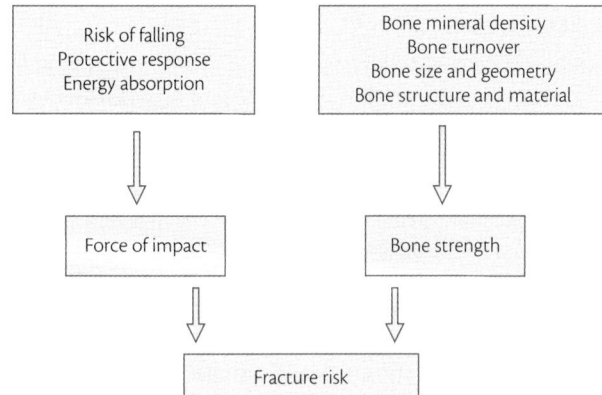

Fig. 20.4.3 Pathogenetic factors for osteoporotic fractures.

of oestrogen deficiency is to increase the activity of osteoclasts, at least in part by suppressing apoptosis. Increased osteoclastic activity causes an increase in the depth of erosion of bone by these cells, contributing to the trabecular penetration and disruption of bone architecture that characterizes postmenopausal osteoporosis.

Although bone mass and architecture are important determinants of bone strength and fracture risk, other aspects of bone composition and structure also contribute. These include composition of the bone matrix, mineral constituents, bone size, and bone geometry. In addition, increased bone turnover *per se* contributes to bone fragility independently of its effects on bone mass (Fig. 20.4.3).

The pathophysiology of other forms of osteoporosis remains to be fully defined. In glucocorticoid-induced osteoporosis, reduced bone formation and low bone turnover predominate in those being treated for the long term, but there is evidence that in the early stages of treatment there is an increase in bone turnover and osteoclast activity. The alterations in bone remodelling responsible for osteoporosis in men have not been established, but the lesser degree of structural disruption of cancellous bone during ageing suggests that reduced bone formation plays a greater role in age-related bone loss in men than women. Whether this applies to men with osteoporosis, however, is uncertain.

In recent years, a number of signalling pathways central to the regulation of bone remodelling have been defined. These include the receptor activator of NF-κB ligand/osteoprotegerin pathway, which plays a major role in the regulation of osteoclast development and activity and is being exploited in the development of a human monoclonal antibody to the receptor activator of NF-κB ligand for the treatment of osteoporosis and other diseases associated with excessive bone resorption. Another is the Wnt signalling pathway, which regulates bone formation. Inactivating mutations of sclerostin, which inhibits the pathway and activating mutations of LRP5, which is a coreceptor in the pathway, are associated with high bone mass and increased bone strength.

Diagnosis and risk assessment

Measurement of BMD

Bone mass can be assessed by a number of techniques, of which dual-energy X-ray absorptiometry (DXA) is the gold standard and provides measurements of BMD in the spine and hip. According to the World Health Organization (WHO) classification, osteoporosis is present when the BMD is 2.5 standard deviations or more below normal peak bone mass (i.e. a T-score of –2.5 or less). Established osteoporosis is defined as a T-score of –2.5 or less in association with a previous fragility fracture.

Other approaches to assessment of bone mass include broadband ultrasound attenuation and peripheral DXA. The T-scores generated by these methods differ according to the device used and so cannot be used to diagnose osteoporosis in the same way as central DXA. Nevertheless, low values obtained using these methods indicate increased fracture risk and are regarded as an indication for DXA measurements of the hip and spine.

Clinical risk factors

In clinical practice, BMD values are used to predict fracture risk in much the same way that blood pressure is used to predict stroke. Other clinical risk factors can also be used to improve prediction of fracture risk, since some of these act independently of BMD. These include age, glucocorticoid therapy, a previous history of fracture, a family history of hip fracture, current smoking practice, alcohol abuse, and certain diseases associated with osteoporosis, e.g. rheumatoid arthritis (Table 20.4.1). A World Health Organization-supported algorithm that uses these risk factors, with or without measurements of BMD, to estimate a 10-year fracture probability has been developed (FRAX; http://www.shef.ac.uk/FRAX) and enables intervention thresholds to be based on absolute risk rather than on T-scores of BMD.

Other risk factors that are associated with low BMD include untreated premature menopause, other causes of hypogonadism including treatment with aromatase inhibitors or gonadotropin-releasing hormone analogues, low body mass index, hyperthyroidism, and malabsorption. Recently, proton-pump inhibitors, thiazolidinediones, and selective serotonin receptor uptake inhibitors have been associated with increased fracture risk, although it is uncertain whether their effects are mediated solely through reduced BMD.

Risk factors for falling are major determinants of fracture risk, particularly for hip fractures in older people (Fig. 20.4.3). Their recognition is important since many are modifiable. They include poor visual acuity, neuromuscular weakness and incoordination,

Table 20.4.1 Risk factors for osteoporosis

Independent of bone mineral density	Dependent on bone mineral density
Age	Untreated hypogonadism
Previous fragility fracture	Malabsorption
Maternal history of hip fracture	Endocrine disease
Oral glucocorticoid therapy	Chronic renal disease
Smoking	Chronic liver disease
Alcohol intake ≥ 3 units/day	Chronic obstructive pulmonary disease
Rheumatoid arthritis	Immobility
Body mass index ≤ 19 kg/m²	Drugs, e.g. aromatase inhibitors, androgen deprivation therapy
Falls	

Table 20.4.2 Pharmacological interventions used in the prevention of osteoporotic fractures

Intervention	Dosing regimen	Route of administration
Alendronate	70 mg once weekly 5 or 10 mg once daily	Oral
Etidronate	400 mg daily for 2 weeks every 3 months	Oral
Ibandronate[a]	150 mg once monthly	Oral
Ibandronate[b]	3 mg once every 3 months	Intravenous injection
Risedronate	35 mg once weekly 5 mg once daily	Oral
Zoledronate	5 mg once yearly	Intravenous infusion
Raloxifene	60 mg once daily	Oral
Strontium ranelate	2 gm once daily	Oral
Teriparatide	20 μg once daily	Subcutaneous injection
Preotact	100 μg once daily	Subcutaneous injection

reduced mobility, cognitive impairment, and the use of sedatives, tranquillizers, and alcohol. There are also many environmental hazards that increase the risk of falling, such as uneven paving stones, poor lighting, and loose carpets and wires.

Radiology

Radiology plays an important role in the diagnosis of osteoporosis, particularly in the case of vertebral fractures. Since only approximately 20 or 30% of these fractures come to medical attention, lateral radiographs of the spine may be the only means of diagnosis. Even though vertebral fractures may be asymptomatic in some individuals, their diagnosis is important because of the high risk of future fractures, both in the spine and elsewhere, and the consequent need for treatment.

Table 20.4.3 Spectrum of antifracture efficacy of pharmacological interventions for osteoporosis

	Vertebral fracture	Nonvertebral fracture	Hip fracture
Alendronate	+	+	+
Etidronate	+	nae	nae
Hormone replacement therapy	+	+	+
Ibandronate	+	+*	nae
Preotact	+	nae	nae
Raloxifene	+	nae	nae
Risedronate	+	+	+
Strontium ranelate	+	+	+[a]
Teriparatide	+	+	nae
Zoledronate	+	+	+

nae, not adequately evaluated.
[a] Post hoc analysis in subset of patients.

Biochemical markers of bone turnover

Biochemical markers of bone resorption (such as urinary deoxypyridinoline, pyridinoline, and N-terminal and C-terminal crosslinked telopeptides of type I collagen) and formation (such as osteocalcin, bone-specific alkaline phosphatase, and C-terminal propeptide of type I procollagen) have been shown to be useful in the prediction of fracture risk, particularly when combined with measurements of BMD, and have potential use in the monitoring of response to treatment. However, their role in clinical practice has not been firmly established.

Differential diagnosis

Secondary causes of osteoporosis should be excluded where appropriate. A full blood count, liver function tests, serum calcium and phosphate levels, thyroid function tests, plasma immunoelectrophoresis, and Bence–Jones protein determination should be performed in the first instance, with further investigation if indicated. In men, in whom secondary causes are more common, determination of serum testosterone, gonadotropin, and prolactin concentrations and tests for 24-h urinary cortisol and/or dexamethasone suppression should also be performed.

Pharmacological interventions: general considerations

Interventions that are approved for the prevention and treatment of osteoporosis are shown in Table 20.4.2. Most of these are approved only for the treatment of postmenopausal osteoporosis, but alendronate, etidronate, risedronate, zoledronate and teriparatide also have licences for the prevention and/or treatment of glucocorticoid-induced osteoporosis, and alendronate, risedronate, zoledronate and teriparatide are approved for treatment of osteoporosis in men.

Calcitonin and calcitriol are also approved for osteoporosis in postmenopausal women but are little used and will not be considered further.

Positioning of treatments

Since there have been no head-to-head studies of these interventions in which fracture has been a primary end point, no direct comparisons can be made of the magnitude of fracture reduction between drugs. However, in the case of vertebral fracture, reductions from about 30 to 50% are seen in postmenopausal women with osteoporosis after 3 years of treatment with most interventions. The evidence base for antifracture efficacy at nonvertebral sites does, however, differ between interventions, as shown in Table 20.4.3. Thus only alendronate, risedronate, zoledronate, and strontium ranelate have been shown to reduce vertebral and nonvertebral fractures, including hip fractures. This distinction is important because, once a fracture occurs, the risk of a subsequent fracture at any site is increased independently of BMD and, hence, an intervention that covers all major fracture sites is preferable.

Because of their broader spectrum of antifracture efficacy, alendronate, risedronate, zoledronate, and strontium ranelate are generally regarded as front-line options in the prevention of fractures in postmenopausal women. Strontium ranelate has a particularly strong evidence base in women aged 80 years or more and is the treatment of choice in frail individuals who are unable to comply with the dosing instructions for bisphosphonates.

Since a reduction in hip fracture risk has not been shown for raloxifene or ibandronate, these drugs are generally considered as second-line options. Where intravenous therapy is required, e.g. in patients with malabsorption, intravenous zoledronate is now the treatment of choice because it has a strong evidence base and requires only once-yearly infusion. Finally, the use of parathyroid-hormone peptides is limited by their cost to women with severe vertebral osteoporosis who are intolerant to or appear to be unresponsive to other treatments.

Reduction in fracture risk has been shown to occur within 1 year of treatment for bisphosphonates and strontium ranelate. This is particularly important in the case of vertebral fractures because, after an incident vertebral fracture, there is a 20% risk of a further fracture occurring within the next 12 months, which emphasizes the importance of prompt treatment once a fracture has occurred.

Duration of therapy

The optimum duration of treatment is uncertain. There are potential concerns that long-term treatment with potent antiresorptives may increase bone microdamage and suppress its repair, possibly resulting in increased bone fragility. However, this concern has to be counterbalanced against the possibility that increased bone turnover and bone loss after withdrawal of therapy may result in increased fracture risk. The current consensus is that treatment should be continued for a minimum of 5 years; in those who remain at high risk (based on BMD and/or incident fractures during treatment), longer treatment periods may be indicated.

Compliance and persistence

Compliance and persistence with treatment for osteoporosis are poor; approximately 50% of patients do not follow their prescribed treatment regimen and/or discontinue treatment within 1 year. Patient education is important in this respect and nurse-led monitoring early in the course of treatment has been shown to improve compliance. Whether monitoring of BMD or biochemical markers of bone turnover provides additional benefits has not been established.

Current pharmacological therapeutic options for osteoporosis

Bisphosphonates

The bisphosphonates are synthetic analogues of the naturally occurring compound pyrophosphate and inhibit bone resorption.

Oral bisphosphonates are generally well tolerated. Upper gastrointestinal side effects may occur with nitrogen-containing bisphosphonates (alendronate, risedronate, and ibandronate), particularly if the dosing regimen is not adhered to. It is therefore important that patients take the drug according to the instructions, specifically in the morning with a full glass of water, 30 min before food, drink, or other medications, and remaining upright for about 30 to 60 min after the dose.

Ibandronate is available as an oral or intravenous formulation. The latter is given every 3 months as an injection lasting from 15 to 30 s. Zoledronate is given once yearly in a dose of 5 mg by intravenous infusion over a minimum of 15 min. An acute-phase reaction may occur with intravenous bisphosphonate administration, particularly with the first injection, resulting in flu-like symptoms for 1 or 2 days; the severity and frequency of this can be reduced by administration of paracetamol on the day of the infusion and the subsequent 1 or 2 days.

Strontium ranelate

Strontium ranelate is composed of two atoms of stable strontium with ranelic acid as a carrier. Although its mechanism of action remains to be fully defined, there is evidence that it increases bone strength by altering bone material properties . Treatment is associated with a substantial increase in BMD in the spine and hip, although part of this increase is artefactual and due to incorporation of strontium into bone.

Strontium ranelate is taken as a single daily dose and is generally well tolerated. There is a small increase in the frequency of diarrhoea, nausea, and headache.

Raloxifene

Raloxifene is a selective oestrogen receptor modulator that has oestrogenic (antiresorptive) effects in the skeleton without the unwanted effects of oestrogen in the breast and endometrium. It is taken orally as a single daily dose. Adverse effects include leg oedema, leg cramps, hot flushes, and a two- to threefold increase in the risk of venous thromboembolism. Its use is associated with a significant decrease in the risk of breast cancer.

Parathyroid-hormone peptides

Teriparatide (recombinant human 1-34 parathyroid-hormone peptide) and Preotact (recombinant human 1-84 parathyroid-hormone peptide) are administered by subcutaneous injection in daily doses of 20 μg and 100 μg, respectively. They have anabolic effects on bone, increasing bone formation and producing large increases in BMD in the spine. Side effects include nausea, headache, and dizziness; in addition, transient hypercalcaemia and hypercalciuria may occur.

Hormone replacement therapy

Because the risk–benefit balance of hormone replacement therapy is generally unfavourable in older postmenopausal women, it is regarded as a second-line treatment option. However, it is an appropriate option in younger postmenopausal women with a high risk of fracture, particularly those with vasomotor symptoms.

Calcium and vitamin D

Available evidence does not support a role for calcium and vitamin D alone in the prevention of osteoporotic fractures except in the institutionalized elderly population. However, calcium and vitamin D supplements should be coprescribed with other treatments for osteoporosis since the evidence base for their antifracture efficacy is derived from studies in which calcium and vitamin D were routinely administered.

Nonpharmacological interventions

Falls have an important role in the pathogenesis of fragility fractures, particularly in frail and older people. Multiple medical and environmental factors increase the risk of falling and many of these are modifiable. Multifaceted interventions have been shown to reduce the frequency of falling, although a reduction in fractures has not been shown.

A number of lifestyle measures improve bone health, including adequate dietary calcium intake and maintenance of a normal vitamin D status. Appropriate levels of exercise should be recommended and smoking and alcohol abuse discouraged. Physiotherapy and pain relief play important roles in the management of fractures.

Glucocorticoid-induced osteoporosis

Osteoporosis is a common complication of oral glucocorticoid therapy. Bone loss is most rapid during the first few months of therapy, during which there is also a rapid increase in fracture rate. Observational data indicate that increased fracture risk is seen at all doses of oral prednisolone, even those below 5 mg daily; however, higher doses are associated with more rapid bone loss and higher fracture risk.

The effects of inhaled glucocorticoids on bone are less certain but are potentially of great importance given their high level of use in the population. Cross-sectional data indicate that adverse effects on BMD may occur, particularly when high doses are administered on a long-term basis. In both adults and children, a small increase in relative risk of fracture has been demonstrated with inhaled glucocorticoid use, but because similar increases are seen in those using only bronchodilators, it is likely that the underlying illness rather than the glucocorticoids *per se* is responsible for the observed increase.

In the context of glucocorticoid induced osteoporosis, the term 'primary prevention' is used to denote initiation of bone protective therapy at the time that glucocorticoids are initiated, whereas 'secondary prevention' implies that bone protection is started later in the course of glucocorticoid therapy. This distinction is important because of the rapid onset of bone loss and increase in fracture risk after glucocorticoid initiation, providing a strong rationale for early intervention in high-risk individuals.

Although a number of interventions have been evaluated in the prevention and treatment of glucocorticoid-induced osteoporosis, the evidence base is much less robust than that which exists in postmenopausal women. Nevertheless, there is reasonable evidence that alendronate, risedronate, etidronate, zoledronate and teriparatide are effective and these are approved for this indication.

Guidelines for the management of glucocorticoid-induced osteoporosis have been produced by the Royal College of Physicians. Primary prevention with a bisphosphonate is recommended in men and women committed to any oral dose of prednisolone for 3 months or more who are over the age of 65 years or who have sustained a previous fragility fracture. Bone densitometry is not required in such individuals. In others taking oral glucocorticoids for 3 months or more, bone densitometry is recommended and those with a T-score of −1.5 or less should be considered for treatment. In addition, treatment should be advised for any individuals who sustain a fragility fracture during treatment.

Further reading

Avenell A, *et al.* (2005). Vitamin D and vitamin D analogues for preventing fractures associated with involutional and post-menopausal osteoporosis. *Cochrane Database Syst Rev*, CD000227.

Bischoff-Ferrari HA, *et al.* (2005). Fracture prevention with vitamin D supplementation: a meta-analysis of randomized controlled trials. *JAMA*, **293**, 2257–64.

Boonen S, *et al.* (2005). Effect of osteoporosis treatments on risk of non-vertebral fractures: review and meta-analysis of intention-to-treat studies. *Osteoporos Int*, **16**, 1291–8.

Compston JE, Seeman E. (2006). Compliance with osteoporosis therapy is the weakest link. *Lancet*, **368**, 973–4.

Cranney A, *et al.* (2006). Clinical Guidelines Committee of Osteoporosis Canada. Parathyroid hormone for the treatment of osteoporosis: a systematic review. *CMAJ*, **175**, 52–9.

Cummings SR, Melton III LJ. (2002). Epidemiology and outcomes of osteoporotic fractures. *Lancet*, **359**, 1761–7.

Guidelines Working Group for the Bone and Tooth Society, National Osteoporosis Society, Royal College of Physicians. (2002). *Glucocorticoid-induced osteoporosis: guidelines for prevention and treatment*. Royal College of Physicians, London.

Johnell O, Kanis JA. (2006). An estimate of the worldwide prevalence and disability associated with osteoporotic fractures. *Osteoporos Int*, **17**, 1726–33.

Kanis JA. (2002). Diagnosis of osteoporosis and assessment of fracture risk. *Lancet*, **359**, 1929–36.

Nguyen ND, Eisman JA, Nguyen TV. (2006). Anti-hip fracture efficacy of bisphosphonates: a Bayesian analysis of clinical trials. *J Bone Miner Res*, **21**, 340–9.

Lock CA, *et al.* (2006). Lifestyle interventions to prevent osteoporotic fractures: a systematic review. *Osteoporos Int*, **17**, 20–8.

O'Donnell S, *et al.* (2006). Strontium ranelate for preventing and treating postmenopausal osteoporosis. *Cochrane Database Syst Rev*, CD005326.

Pennisi P, Trombetti A, Rizzoli R. (2006). Glucocorticoid-induced osteoporosis and its treatment. *Clin Orthop Relat Res*, 443, 39–47.

Poole KE, Compston JE. (2006). Osteoporosis and its management. *Br Med J*, **333**, 1251–6.

Rosen CJ. (2005). Clinical practice. Postmenopausal osteoporosis. *N Engl J Med*, **353**, 595–603.

Seeman E, *et al.* (2006). Anti-vertebral fracture efficacy of raloxifene: a meta-analysis. *Osteoporos Int*, **17**, 313–16.

Siris ES, *et al.* (2004). Bone mineral density thresholds for pharmacological interventions to prevent fractures. *AMA Arch Intern Med*, **164**, 1108–12.

Stevenson M, *et al.* (2005). A systematic review and economic evaluation of alendronate, etidronate, risedronate, raloxifene and teriparatide for the prevention and treatment of postmenopausal osteoporosis. *Health Technol Assess*, **9**, 1–160.

20.5

Osteonecrosis, osteochondrosis, and osteochondritis dissecans

Donncha O'Gradaigh and Adrian Crisp

Essentials

Osteonecrosis—this can be caused by a range of conditions including trauma, drugs (e.g. corticosteroids), metabolic/endocrine (e.g. Cushing's disease, Gaucher's disease), sickle cell disease. It occurs particularly in patients with inherited procoagulant disorders (e.g. resistance to activated protein C). The epiphyses of the femoral head or condyles, or the head of the humerus, are particular affected. There are no specific features on history or examination, but the condition may present with pain and disability. MRI is required for diagnosis. Treatment may involve approaches designed to ameliorate vascular occlusion (vasodilators, low-molecular-weight heparin), promote bone repair (bisphosphonates), revascularize (e.g. surgical core decompression), or other surgical techniques (e.g. osteotomy, joint replacement).

Osteochondrosis and osteochondritis dissecans—osteochondrosis can occur at any epiphysis; osteochondritis dissecans is a distinct form of osteochondral injury through the articular cartilage in a diarthrodial joint, particularly the knee or elbow. Usual presentation is with progressive activity-related pain. Initial treatment includes modification of activities, analgesia, and a stretching regime to release traction on apophyseal sites; surgery is required for refractory cases.

Introduction

Osteonecrosis describes death of bone tissue, including the bone marrow, and is synonymous with avascular necrosis, although the former term is preferred. Osteochondritis dissecans and osteochondrosis are somewhat contentiously attributed to ischaemia of bone and cartilage.

Osteonecrosis

Pathophysiology

Systemic factors (Box 20.5.1) may result in osteonecrosis in several bones in the same individual. Common sites include the epiphyses at the femoral heads and the condyles, and the head of the humerus. The small bones of the foot or wrist are less commonly affected. Within weeks of ischaemic injury, a connective tissue matrix is formed at the interface between necrotic and viable bone, with increased vascularity in this area promoted by the inflammatory response. This matrix becomes calcified and the necrotic segment remains as an unresorbed sequestrum of bone. The overlying joint surface may collapse, with the development of degenerative joint changes.

Genetic factors

Osteonecrosis reflects an interaction between genetic predisposition and exposure to precipitating causes. A mutation in the *COL2A1* gene, which encodes collagen, is associated with increased risk, whereas expression of the multidrug resistance gene (for P-glycoprotein, which accelerates the excretion of drugs from cells) confers a reduced risk of steroid-associated osteonecrosis. A mutated alcohol dehydrogenase enzyme is associated with a reduced risk of alcohol-related osteonecrosis. Finally, osteonecrosis is increasingly attributed to several inherited procoagulant states (see below).

Vascular interruption

Ischaemia of bone may be due to an intraluminal occlusion or increased pressure within the inexpansile marrow compartment. Examples of the former include fat, amniotic fluid and cholesterol emboli, sickle-cell crisis, and caisson disease (also called dysbaric bone necrosis or 'the bends'). Caisson disease is due to occlusion by the formation of nitrogen bubbles during rapid returns to the surface after underwater diving with pressure-regulated breathing devices.

In a series of patients with osteonecrosis, 83% had one or more positive results for a range of procoagulant disorders. Of these, resistance to activated protein C (APC-R) and anticardiolipin antibodies were the most common, affecting 50% and 26.7% of the study group versus 7.5% and 1% of healthy controls, respectively.

Steroid-associated osteonecrosis is attributed to raised intramedullary pressure by the accumulation of lipid in marrow adipocytes. With treatment of less than 2 g of prednisolone equivalent, osteonecrosis is rare. Changes in bone imaging may be detected

Box 20.5.1 Conditions associated with avascular necrosis (incidences where available)

- Trauma—fractures, orthopaedic procedures
- Drugs—corticosteroids (2–5%), alcohol, cocaine, oral contraceptives (rare)
- Metabolic and endocrine disorders—Cushing's disease, Gaucher's disease (60%), pancreatitis, hyperlipidaemia (type IV), diabetes mellitus, pregnancy
- Systemic lupus erythematosus (occurring in 16% of those taking steroids)
- Transplantation
- Sickle-cell disease (5%; 40% with MRI)
- Dysbarism (caisson disease) (4%)
- Radiotherapy, thermal injury
- HIV, AIDS

within 3 months of commencing steroid treatment. No cases were detected in a large, prospective series after more than 12 months of steroid treatment. The accumulation of lipid also occurs in storage disorders (e.g. Gaucher's disease). Alcohol increases the risk of osteonecrosis 3-, 10-, and 15-fold in those consuming, per week, 40 units, from 41 to 100 units, and more than 100 units, respectively. The association between HIV/AIDS and osteonecrosis is attributed to the expression of anticardiolipin antibodies (50–80% of HIV/AIDS cases), the use of megesterol acetate for wasting syndrome, or highly active antiretroviral therapy agents (although case series suggest this is the least likely mechanism).

Epidemiology

There are 15 000 new cases of adult avascular necrosis annually in the United States of America. Males are more commonly affected (8:1), the majority under 50 years of age, with the exception of spontaneous osteonecrosis of the knee, which particularly affects women over the age of 50 years and has a prevalence of over 9% in imaging studies in women aged over 65 years.

Clinical and imaging features

There are no specific features on history or examination to indicate the diagnosis of osteonecrosis. Microfracture, damage to articular surfaces, and swelling of the bone marrow can each result in pain and disability. However, in early, potentially reversible stages, the diagnosis will only be made if suspicion prompts a request for the definitive test, MRI.

In a group of patients commencing high-dose steroid therapy, the first indication of osteonecrosis is the appearance of a lucent line (a linear high signal with a specialized, fat-suppression MRI technique (STIR images)). Later, bone scintigraphy shows increased uptake in a linear distribution surrounding a low-uptake area—this will occur somewhat later than the first MRI changes. A rim of sclerosis may be visible on conventional radiology with a radiolucent subchondral crescent where the necrotic bone lies. However, these changes can be subtle and, often, conventional radiography does not suggest the diagnosis of osteonecrosis until

some deformity has occurred, with collapse of the subchondral bone and degenerative arthrosis.

Treatment

Complex staging schemes are described for each bone that is commonly affected by osteonecrosis, based on the progressive imaging findings described above. Broadly, three groups can be recognized:

- early presentation with reversible causes (e.g. intraluminal occlusion)
- early presentation with repair or revascularization possible (i.e. before the collapse of the subchondral bone)
- late presentation with collapse or arthrosis, where joint salvage is the main aim of treatment

Small lesions that are detected with MRI typically do not progress and conservative measures are appropriate. Vasodilators (e.g. nifedipine and the prostacyclin analogue iloprost) have been used in sickle-cell crises to provide relief from bone pain. Daily treatment with low-molecular-weight heparin for 12 weeks resolves the majority of cases of osteonecrosis with a proven hypercoagulability state. Bisphosphonates have been successfully used to limit subchondral bone loss and the collapse of joint surfaces, e.g. progression to collapse of the femoral head occurred in only two out of 29 hips in those receiving 70 mg alendronate once per week compared with 19 out of 25 controls. Decompression chambers are the standard of care for dysbaric bone necrosis.

Various revascularization techniques are described. Detailed imaging is required to assess the risk of joint collapse and the feasibility of revascularization. Core decompression involves removing bone from the medullary cavity or drilling multiple smaller holes through the bone surface. The cavity may be then filled with a vascularized fibular graft or by nonvascularized cortical bone. More recently, stem-cell implantation in the marrow space has been reported with success in early femoral head lesions.

Osteotomy attempts to shift the weight from the necrotic segment. Subsequent joint replacement is technically more difficult. Limited joint replacement (hemiresurfacing) preserves the bone for later conventional arthroplasty and is the preferred option for collapsed joints in a younger patient.

Other issues and anticipated developments

Coincidental statin therapy reduces the incidence of osteonecrosis in patients starting long-term steroids, but there is no evidence that instituting statin therapy when steroid-induced osteonecrosis is first detected will alter the outcome. Better predictions of those at risk may allow an acceptable protocol to be developed. Bone morphogenetic proteins are used to stimulate bone repair in nonunion and other orthopaedic situations, with very limited experience in osteonecrosis to date.

Osteochondrosis and osteochondritis dissecans

Osteochondrosis can occur at any epiphysis and involves the articular surface, the epiphyseal plate, or apophysis (at a secondary ossification centre, site of ligament, or musculotendinous attachment). Osteochondritis dissecans is a distinct form of osteochondral injury through the articular cartilage in a diarthrodial joint.

Table 20.5.1 Classification of osteochondroses

Type	Site (eponym)	Comments
Articular	Metatarsal head (Freiberg's)	Especially second metatarsal head
		Uncommon
		Bilateral in 10%
	Hip (Legg–Calvé–Perthes)	4–10 years of age
		More complications over 8 years of age
		Bilateral in 10%
	Navicular (Köhler's)	3–7 years of age
		Male:female ratio 5:1
		Uncommon
		May be bilateral
	Talus (Mouchet's)	
	Lunate (Kienböck's)	Rare < 15 years of age
		Males especially
		Trauma
		May be associated with short ulna relative to radius
	Vertebra (Scheuermann's)	13–17 years of age
		Male:female ratio equal
		Usually lower thoracic more than upper lumbar
		Often several vertebrae affected (3–5)
Non-articular	Tibial tubercle (Osgood–Schlatter)	10–15 years of age
		More often in males than females
		Bilateral in 25%
	Lower pole of patella (Sinding–Larsen–Johansson)	10–14 years of age
		'Jumper's knee'
(i1) At tendon attachments (apophysitis)	Greater trochanter of hip (Mandl's disease)	
	Base of fifth metatarsal (Iselin's)	
(ii2) At ligament attachments	Ulnar collateral (Panner's)	'Little leaguer's elbow'
		4–16 years of age
		Especially occurs in males
(iii3) At impact sites	Femoral condyles (Ahlback's)	
	Calcaneus (Sever's)	9–15 years of age
	Sesamoids (Treve's)	
Physeal	Medial/proximal tibia (Blount's)	1–3 years of age, occasionally in adolescents
		Bowing of the tibia with sharp angulation and metaphyseal beaking
		Unilateral or asymmetrical

Pathophysiology

The definitive pathogenetic cause is unclear. Ischaemia of the underlying bone has long been proposed, although more sophisticated imaging has recently refuted older observations. In histological studies, features include chondrocyte hypertrophy, fibrous degeneration associated with collagen type I deposition, and chondrocyte dedifferentiation. Dissected fragments obtained at surgery often contain large numbers of viable cells.

Epidemiology

Growing children and adolescents are most commonly affected, with males being affected about twice as often as females (29 and 19 cases per 100 000, respectively). Osteochondritis dissecans occurs increasingly in young athletes due to earlier participation in competitive sports, particularly in the knee and the elbow. Osteochondroses are classified into articular, nonarticular, and physeal disorders (Table 20.5.1).

Clinical features and diagnosis

Detachment of the osteochondral fragment may precipitate effusion and mechanical symptoms of locking, catching, and giving way. The disorder usually presents with progressive activity-related pain. Local swelling may be evident if trauma has occurred. MRI shows cartilage disruption, subchondral bone cysts, and a linear high signal beneath the lesion. A defect in the hyaline cartilage represents displacement of an unstable lesion. Later, plain radiographs of the knee may detect changes (a tunnel view is essential).

Irregular ossification is a radiological differential diagnosis, typically very prevalent (66% of boys and 41% of girls in one series) in younger children (3–12 years of age). Scintigraphy is normal in such cases.

Treatment

Osteochondrotic lesions and most juvenile osteochondritis dissecans respond well to nonoperative care. Measures include modification of activities, analgesia, and a stretching regime to release traction on apophyseal sites. Failure to heal within 6 months requires further treatment. Compliance with conservative treatment may be poor, because symptoms typically recede long before bone healing has occurred.

Both adult and juvenile cases with unstable lesions require arthroscopic drilling into the affected areas (to promote healing), usually with autologous cortical bone grafting. Arthroscopic fixation of the fragment employs autologous osteochondral plugs or bioabsorbable polymer screws (which slowly degrade, allowing healing of the fixed fragment). Whether to excise or to reattach loose bodies remains controversial. A viable fragment requires at least 3 mm of subchondral bone. Removing large lesions from weight-bearing areas does not achieve a good outcome in most studies unless accompanied by curettage, drilling, or placement of osteochondral plugs (mosaicplasty).

Anticipated developments

Newer techniques, such as chondral resurfacing techniques, are expected to offer a better outlook for those who have not reached skeletal maturity. Hyaluronan-based scaffolds seeded with autologous chondrocytes are a viable treatment for damaged articular surfaces in the knee. The type of repaired tissue demonstrates histological characteristics similar to normal articular (hyaline) cartilage. Long-term investigations are needed to determine the durability of the repair produced with this technique.

Further reading

Lafforgue P (2006). Pathophysiology and natural history of avascular necrosis of bone. *Joint Bone Spine*, **73**, 500–7.

Mont MA, Jones LC, Hungerford DS (2006). Nontraumatic osteonecrosis of the femoral head: ten years later. *J Bone Joint Surg Am*, **88**, 1117–32.

Wall E, Von Stein D (2003). Juvenile osteochondritis dissecans. *Orthop Clin North Am*, **34**, 341–53.

SECTION 21

Disorders of the kidney and urinary tract

Structure and function of the kidney

J. David Williams and A.O. Phillips

Essentials

The kidney is responsible for control of water, electrolyte (particularly sodium and potassium), and acid–base balance and for excretion of metabolic wastes, and it has important functions as an endocrine organ, including key roles in renin, vitamin D, and erythropoietin production or metabolism.

The nephron—beginning at the glomerulus, the functional unit of the kidney is the nephron, through which glomerular filtrate passes to be finally excreted as urine. The nephron is divided into anatomically and functionally distinct sections that work together to maintain homeostasis.

Renal function—in simple terms, in an adult human under no particular physiological or pathophysiological stress, about 100 ml

of glomerular filtrate is generated from plasma each minute, 99 ml of which is reabsorbed, leaving a urinary volume of 1 ml/ min. Metabolic wastes within the plasma (e.g. urea and creatinine) are not reabsorbed (or only some fraction of them), hence they are concentrated in the urine, and some wastes are also secreted into the urine by the renal tubules. The bulk of sodium and water is reabsorbed in the proximal tubules, as are other small molecules that the body retains (e.g. glucose and amino acids), with fine-tuning of sodium and water excretion effected in the distal part of the nephron under the influences of aldosterone and ADH, respectively.

Introduction

The kidney is engaged in many tasks, including control of water, electrolyte (particularly sodium and potassium), and acid–base balance and excretion of metabolic wastes, and it has important functions as an endocrine organ, including key roles in renin, vitamin D, and erythropoietin production or metabolism. Most recently its role in the production of key growth factors during development has been highlighted.

The kidney is formed by the fusion of a number of lobes. In coronal section, the outer rim of the kidney (cortex) containing all the glomeruli and convoluted tubules can easily be distinguished from the pyramidal shaped medulla containing the loops of Henle and the collecting ducts that project into the renal pelvis as the papillae.

The nephron

The functional unit of the kidney is the nephron, which begins at the glomerulus (Fig. 21.1.1). The urinary space (the cavity between the glomerulus and its surrounding Bowman's capsule) leads into the proximal tubule, which itself can be subdivided into a convoluted segment and a straight segment. The straight segment of the proximal tubule descends into the medulla and changes abruptly into the descending limb of loop of Henle. This loop penetrates for

varying distances into the medulla before returning to the cortex. The longer loops pass all the way into the inner medulla, while the short loops only reach the outer medulla. Generally speaking, long loops belong to nephrons of glomeruli lying adjacent to the medullary region, while the shorter loops belong to the more superficial glomeruli. The descending limb of loop of Henle bends sharply back at its lowest point to form the ascending limb, which at another abrupt transition forms the medullary part of the thick ascending limb. This leads up into the cortex where it becomes convoluted and comes into close contact with the vascular pole of its own glomerulus, forming the juxtaglomerular apparatus. Further along the nephron, the thick ascending limb becomes the distal convoluted tubule and then the connecting tubule, which joins the cortical collecting duct. Each collecting duct receives connecting tubules from about a dozen nephrons and then opens onto the surface of a papilla.

The renal blood supply

Structure

The renal artery divides into the interlobar arteries and enters the renal substance at the columns of Bertin (the area between adjacent lobes). At the junction of the cortex and medulla, the arteries divide again and form the arcuate arteries (Fig. 21.1.1). Each arcuate artery

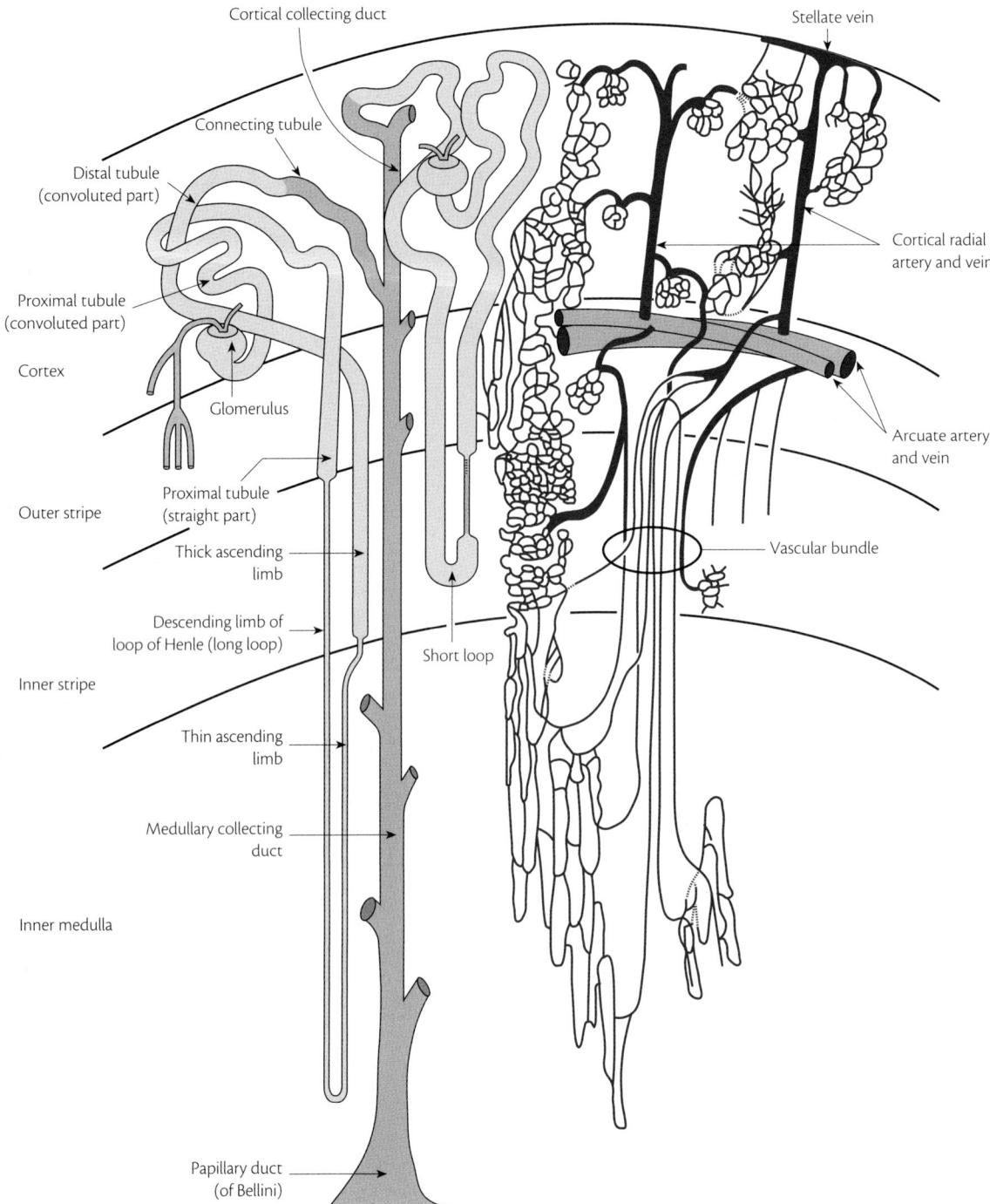

Fig. 21.1.1 The nephron and its blood supply.
Williams JD, *et al*. Clinical atlas of the kidney. Gower Publishing, London.

gives rise to cortical radial arteries that ascend through the cortex: there is no direct arterial supply to the medulla. The afferent glomerular arteries arise from the cortical radial arteries and directly supply the glomeruli. Efferent glomerular arteries drain the glomeruli and then supply the peritubular capillaries of the cortex and medulla, a unique arrangement meaning that the peritubular capillary supply is exclusively postglomerular. Efferent glomerular arteries can be divided into two types: those from the superficial and midcortical glomeruli supply the capillary plexus of the cortex and those from juxtamedullary glomeruli form the blood supply to the renal medulla. Within the outer stripe, they divide into the descending vasa recta, which penetrate the inner stripe in vascular bundles. The renal medulla is drained by the ascending vasa recta, which traverse the inner stripe within the vascular bundle and then join the cortical radial veins. The vascular bundles of the medulla represent the vascular component of the countercurrent exchange mechanism between the blood entering and leaving the medulla. Interestingly, the vascular bundles are organized such that the perfusion of the inner medulla is kept totally separate from the perfusion of the outer medulla. The cortical radial veins join the arcuate veins to eventually form the interlobular veins, which run alongside corresponding arteries.

Function

Renal blood flow is influenced by intrarenal and extrarenal factors. Autoregulation within the kidney maintains a relatively stable blood flow to the glomerulus over a range of arterial pressure. This phenomenon seems to be mediated by events intrinsic to the kidney since it has been demonstrated in both denervated and isolated kidney preparations.

The glomerulus

Structure

On entering the glomerulus (Fig. 21.1.2a), the afferent arteriole divides into primary capillary branches, each of which gives rise to an anastomosing capillary network that forms a glomerular lobule. These capillaries then coalesce into the efferent arteriole within the tuft. The structural organization of the capillaries is unlike that found in any other part of the body, with the capillary basement membrane (glomerular basement membrane) forming the barrier across which filtrate is generated. Embryologically, the glomerulus is the interface between the ureteric bud (or hollow nephrogenic vesicle) and the metanephrogenic cap, which develops into the capillary plexus. The result of this is a basement membrane formed by the fusion of the basement membrane of the capillaries and the basement membrane of the nephrogenic vesicle. This glomerular basement membrane forms the skeletal framework of the glomerular tuft.

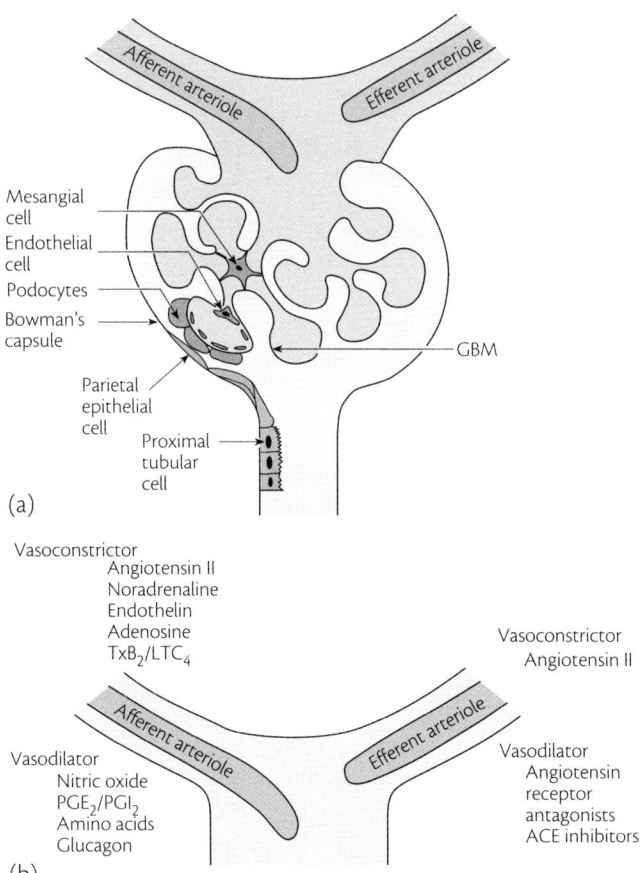

(a)

(b)

Fig. 21.1.2 The glomerulus: (a) structure; and (b) regulation of glomerular blood flow by vasoactive agents.

Although on electron microscopy the glomerular basement membrane appears as a three-layer structure with a central lamina densa and outer lamina rara interna and externa, this is probably an artefact. Freeze–fracture studies have suggested uniformity in the basement membrane from its outer to inner aspects. The major components of the membrane include a framework of type IV collagen linked by heparan sulphate proteoglycans and laminin, the basement membrane charge being provided by the heparan sulphate component (subtypes of which include perlican and agrican). Type IV collagen consists of a triple helix of fibres with a large noncollagenous globular domain at the C-terminal end (called NC1). This NC1 domain of the collagen molecule is the target for Goodpasture's disease, and mutations of the collagen chains are responsible for Alport's syndrome.

The endothelial cells, the basement membrane, and the podocytes form the filtration barrier. The endothelial cells are fenestrated (60 and 100 nm in diameter) and the lack of a diaphragm across the fenestrations exposes the basement membrane directly to the glomerular capillary contents. The luminal surface of the endothelial cells is negatively charged by polyanionic glycoproteins, but these are not present on the fenestrae. The capillary loops are incomplete (a tube of fenestrated endothelial cells surrounded only on its epithelial aspect by a basement membrane) and are held together on their inner aspect by the mesangial cells. Thus the basement membrane has an opening on its mesangial aspect so that the endothelial cells are in direct contact with the mesangium. At the vascular pole of the glomerulus the capillary basement membrane is reflected to form the parietal epithelium of Bowman's capsule.

The outer aspect of the filtration barrier is provided by the epithelial cells (podocytes), which interdigitate on the surface of the glomerular lobules. The foot processes of adjacent podocytes are separated by the filtration slits, which are bridged by the slit diaphragms and are the sites through which the glomerular filtrate passes. The pores have a central proteinaceous core with side arms linking to each adjacent cell, forming a structure with a zipper-like appearance and a width of about 40 nm. The luminal surface of the podocyte and the slit diaphragm are rich in negative charge, being covered in glycoproteins. The podocyte surface adjacent to the basement membrane expresses a number of adhesion proteins that ensure firm anchorage to the membrane.

The mesangium forms the pillar to which the glomerular basement membrane scaffold is attached. The interaction between the mesangial cells and the basement membrane provides the mechanism for the contractility of the glomerular tuft, and the means whereby the surface area of the tuft can be varied. The spaces between the mesangial cells are filled by the mesangial matrix that consists of a number of different collagens, as well as glycoproteins, fibronectin, and proteoglycans. This mesangial matrix provides a channel for the migration of a variety of molecules from the glomerular capillaries, with trafficking centrally towards the vascular pole of the glomerulus.

Function

The glomerular filtration barrier, consisting of the endothelial pores, the glomerular basement membrane, and slit diaphragms, will exclude molecules on the basis of size, shape, and charge. Size selectivity is imparted by the matrix of the glomerular basement membrane itself, as well as by the integrity of the podocytes. The matrix, formed by the type IV collagen molecules, consists of a series of interlinking pores, the narrowest of which determines the size of molecules that can pass through. Thus any pathological change to the structure of the matrix is likely to result in a greater permeability of the glomerular basement membrane. The resistance to the movement of water and small molecules is provided by the endothelial pores, the basement membrane, and the available surface area of the slit diaphragms, with the last of these probably being the effective barrier. The charge barrier, whose efficiency is disputed, is provided by the negative charge of the basement membrane and to a lesser extent by the surface of the endothelial and epithelial cells.

The effectiveness of the filtration barrier is dependent not only on the integrity of the basement membrane but also on the function of the epithelial cells. Most studies have demonstrated that changes in barrier function are closely correlated with significant alteration to the podocytes. These include changes in the surface area of the slit diaphragm (slit diaphragm frequency) as well as detachment of podocytes from the basement membrane. There is now a large body of evidence to suggest that heparan sulphate proteoglycans are involved in both the charge- and size-selective properties of the glomerular basement membrane and, furthermore, that alterations in glomerular basement membrane heparan sulphate proteoglycans may be important in the development of proteinuria.

Production of glomerular filtrate

The number of functioning glomeruli and the filtration rate at each single glomerulus determine the glomerular filtration rate (GFR). There are approximately a million glomeruli per human kidney, of which 90% are in the outer two-thirds of the cortex and fairly homogeneous in terms of structure and function. The remaining 10%, which are located in the juxtamedullary region, are larger, with a higher single-nephron GFR (SNGFR) compared with cortical glomeruli.

SNGFR is determined by a number of factors. First, the pressure of blood in the glomerular capillary and the hydrostatic pressure of the fluid in Bowman's space determine the pressure difference that drives the movement of fluid across the glomerular capillary wall, the transglomerular hydrostatic pressure difference or ΔP. Second, the gradient in colloid osmotic pressure, also known as the oncotic pressure ($\Delta \pi$), across the filtration barrier: this is equal to the colloid osmotic pressure within the glomerular capillary less the colloid osmotic pressure in Bowman's space (which, in effect, is zero). The difference between ΔP and $\Delta \pi$ is the net ultrafiltration pressure. Other determining factors are water permeability (K) and f (the area available for filtration, namely the surface area of the slit pores between podocytes), these two being combined as the glomerular filtration coefficient or ultrafiltration coefficient (Kf). Hence:

$$SNGFR = (\Delta P - \Delta \pi) \times Kf$$

SNGFR can be regulated by alterations in the ultrafiltration coefficient Kf, the net ultrafiltration pressure, or both. A change in the net ultrafiltration pressure may arise owing to a change in the hydraulic pressure ΔP, the capillary plasma oncotic pressure $\Delta \pi$, and/or the initial glomerular capillary plasma flow rate (which dictates changes in protein concentration with distance along a capillary network and hence affects colloid osmotic pressure).

Glomeruli contain receptors for a number of hormones that are capable of modifying the GFR (see Fig. 21.1.2b). These include vasoconstrictors such as adenosine, angiotensin II, and endothelin, as well as vasodilators such as dopamine, bradykinin, prostacyclin, and nitric oxide. Some of these vasoactive molecules are produced within the kidney, whereas others are delivered by the systemic circulation, and many studies have examined the effects of hormones on glomerular ultrafiltration. It is clear from the preceding discussion that, in addition to ΔP (i.e. change in hydraulic pressure), the GFR is dependent on the capillary plasma flow rate and the ultrafiltration coefficient (Kf), all of which may be altered by hormones. Vasoconstrictor substances such as angiotensin II and noradrenaline are capable of producing substantial reductions in renal plasma flow, generally with little change in GFR. Angiotensin II, for example, causes constriction of both afferent and efferent arterioles, with a resultant decrease in capillary plasma flow and a reduction in Kf, but little change in the SNGFR due to an increase in ΔP. Increased afferent arterial tone caused by endothelin or adenosine will decrease renal blood flow, decrease ΔP, and therefore decrease GFR. By contrast, dilatation of the afferent arteriole by nitric oxide or prostaglandins will also cause an increase in ΔP, but with an increase in renal blood flow and hence an increase in GFR.

In the normal adult human, water is filtered by the glomerulus at a rate of 80 to 200 ml/min. The GFR is critically related to all functions of the kidney and is closely regulated by mechanisms that maintain a constant high value for GFR. In practical clinical terms, the estimation of GFR is achieved by measuring the serum creatinine and employing an algorithm that allows for the age and sex of the patient (eGFR), or by estimating the renal clearance of a substance that is freely filtered at the glomerulus and not absorbed or secreted by the renal tubules. For a discussion of the methods of measuring GFR in clinical practice, see Chapter 21.4.

The proximal convoluted tubule

Structure

The main function of the proximal tubule is to reabsorb the bulk of filtered water and solutes, and its structure shows numerous adaptations for this purpose. Proximal tubular epithelial cells are tall and columnar with a well-developed brush border, resulting in a 40-fold increase in the apical surface area of the cells (Fig. 21.1.3). In addition, they possess extensive basolateral interdigitation, increasing the basolateral cell surface area. The apices of the cells are held together by junctional complexes: these are called 'tight junctions' (zona occludens), of the leaky variety, with a low electrical resistance that allows some transepithelial transport. The bases of the cells rest on the tubular basement membrane, which separates them from the peritubular capillaries. Another characteristic feature is the presence of large numbers of mitochondria, intimately associated with the basolateral cell membranes where the Na^+,K^+-ATPase is located, and whose function is to provide the energy source for fluid and electrolyte reabsorption.

Function

Sodium and water reabsorption

About seven-eighths of the volume of the glomerular filtrate is reabsorbed in the proximal tubule. Sodium enters the proximal tubular cells passively from the tubular fluid down an electrochemical gradient that is the driving force for fluid and electrolyte reabsorption. This gradient is produced by the action of the Na^+,K^+-ATPase

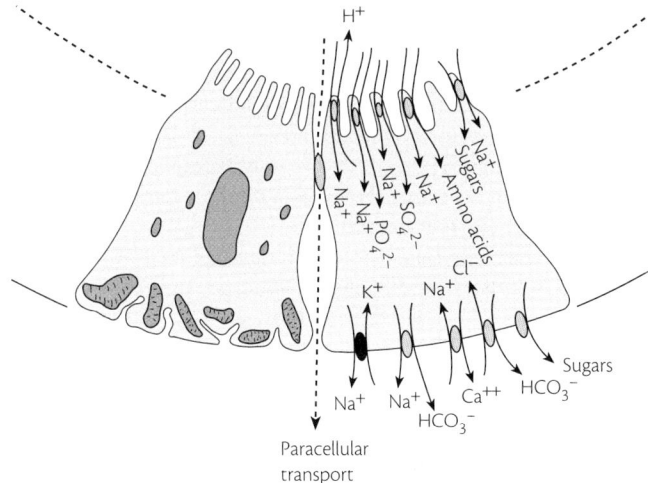

Fig. 21.1.3 Proximal tubular cell function. Principal transport processes of the proximal tubular cell.

on the basal surface, which transports sodium out of the cell in excess of the potassium transported into the cell, thereby generating a transmembrane potential of $-70\,\mathrm{mV}$. Chloride ions follow the same route by cotransport with Na^+, and the resulting increase in osmolality in the intercellular spaces results in the absorption of water by osmosis, such that the volume of the filtrate in the renal tubule is substantially reduced by the time it reaches the beginning of the loop of Henle, although its net osmolality does not change. In addition to this transcellular route for the transport of salt and water, there is also a paracellular route through the 'leaky' tight junctions.

Reabsorption of other substances

The proximal tubule is also responsible for the reabsorption of other substances such as glucose, phosphate, amino acids, and organic anions, including citrate and lactate. These enter the proximal tubular cells across the apical membrane by a series of cotransport systems, each of which binds one or more sodium ions and its specific substrate, and carries them across the cell membrane (Fig. 21.1.3). Thus, the rate of sodium entry into the cell is linked by cotransport systems to the reabsorption of these substances.

The energy for secondary active transport or cotransport of substances (glucose, phosphate, etc.) against their concentration gradient is therefore provided indirectly by Na^+,K^+-ATPase, which is responsible for the concentration gradient for sodium across the cell membrane. This is illustrated by the reabsorption of glucose, which involves brush-border, Na^+-coupled glucose transporters, termed SGLT, and basolateral facilitated glucose transporters (GLUT). In the human, the main site for glucose reabsorption is the early S1 segment of the proximal tubule, where 90% of the filtered glucose is reabsorbed, such that only a small fraction of the filtered load reaches the S2 and S3 segments. Glucose reabsorption in the S1 proximal tubular segment is mediated by a low-affinity, high-capacity, Na^+/glucose cotransporter, SLGT2, and reabsorption in the later segments is mediated by a high-affinity, low-capacity SGLT1. Similarly, the high rate of glucose efflux characteristic of the early proximal tubular segment is mediated by the low-affinity, facultative glucose transporter GLUT2 and high-affinity GLUT1, whereas only GLUT1 is produced in the late proximal tubule where a minor portion of the filtered glucose load is reabsorbed.

The kidneys are also involved in maintenance of the acid–base balance of the body by regulating the serum bicarbonate concentration to approximately 24 mmol/litre. The proximal tubule reabsorbs between 80 and 90% of the filtered bicarbonate, largely by the following mechanism. H^+ is secreted by the Na^+/H^+-exchanger on the luminal membrane. It then reacts with the filtered HCO_3^- to form H_2CO_3, which is converted to CO_2 and H_2O catalysed by carbonic anhydrase present on the luminal brush-border membrane. H_2O diffuses passively into the cell where it is split to yield the H^+ that is secreted and OH^-, and the hydroxyl ion then reacts with CO_2 (catalysed by carbonic anhydrase) to yield HCO_3^-, which exits the cell via a Na/HCO_3 synporter, thus restoring filtered HCO_3^- to the plasma.

Handling of protein

In addition to its role in fluid and electrolyte balance, almost all the protein that is filtered at the glomerulus is reabsorbed by the proximal tubule via a process of endocytosis. To date, four major routes of tubular handling of peptides have been identified: (1) reabsorption of filtered protein/peptides by endocytosis and intracellular lysosomal degradation, (2) luminal hydrolysis and reabsorption of free amino acids, (3) carrier-mediated reabsorption of small intact peptides, and (4) peritubular uptake of peptides. The most important of these is probably the endocytotic route.

In recent years, there has been considerable interest in the role of proteinuria in the progression of renal disease. Among the hypotheses currently under investigation are those that focus on the effect of excess protein trafficking on the generation of profibrotic factors by proximal tubular cells and the subsequent initiation of interstitial fibrosis. These theories suggest that cells of the proximal tubule play a role in maintaining the normal architecture of the renal interstitium. In support are numerous studies demonstrating that tubular cells are a rich source of many components of the extracellular matrix, which may modify matrix turnover by alterations in the synthesis of both matrix-degrading enzymes and their inhibitors, as well as through the production of cytokines. More recent studies have suggested that cells of the proximal tubule may migrate into the interstitium and transdifferentiate into the cortical fibroblasts during conditions of inflammation.

Interplay between the regulation of GFR and proximal tubular function

One aspect of the control of renal function is the correlation between the volume of filtrate produced by the glomerulus and the reabsorptive capacity of the renal tubule. The movement of sodium and water from the proximal tubular lumen into the capillary network depends on the hydrostatic pressure of the blood in the peritubular capillary complex, as well as the osmotic pressure of the blood within those capillaries. An increased hydrostatic pressure will reduce reabsorption, but an increased oncotic pressure will enhance reabsorption. Thus, increased systemic blood pressure will increase the pressure within the interstitium and result in the movement of sodium from the interstitial fluid into the lumen (pressure natriuresis).

The loop of Henle

The loop of Henle begins where the straight (S3) part of the proximal tubule changes abruptly in diameter to become the descending thin limb. Long loops pass into the inner medulla, before performing a hairpin bend and returning as the thin ascending limb, when an abrupt transition at the inner stripe of the outer medulla marks the beginning of the thick ascending limb, which is structurally distinct from its thin counterpart. In the case of the short loops, the transition to ascending thick limb takes place before the bend, so that the thick part of the tubule forms the loop.

Although there are only minor structural differences between the thin segments of descending and ascending limbs, there are major differences in their permeability properties. The thin descending limb, like the proximal tubule, is highly permeable to water as a result of the presence of aquaporin 1, whereas the thin ascending limb is impermeable to water. By contrast, the descending limb is impermeable to sodium, whereas significant sodium and urea reabsorption occurs in the thin ascending limb. This allows an osmotic gradient to be established in the medulla, which is the basis of the countercurrent multiplier mechanism (Fig. 21.1.4).

The juxtaglomerular apparatus

The juxtaglomerular apparatus comprises the macula densa, the extraglomerular mesangium, the terminal portion of the afferent

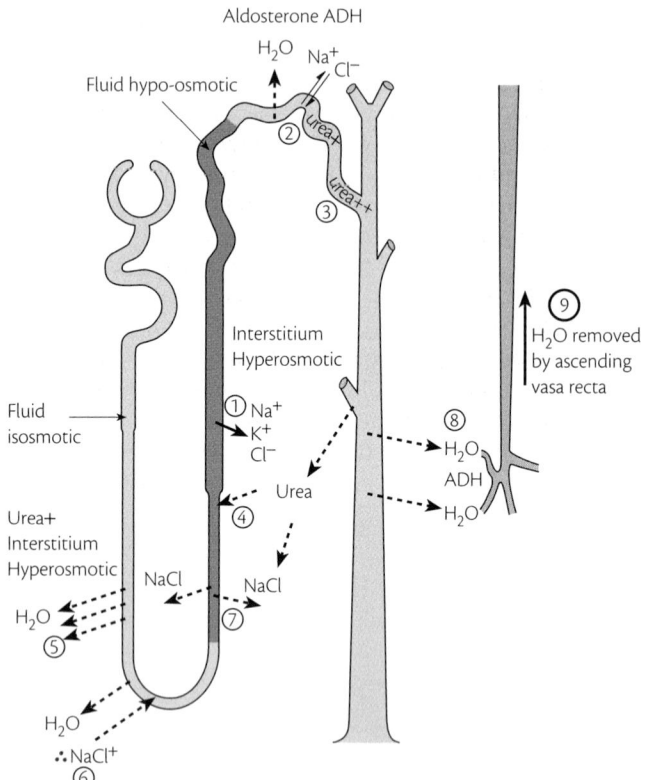

Fig. 21.1.4 Diagram to illustrate the mechanism of concentration of the urine. The darkened part of the nephron is impermeable to water. 1, Active transport of Na^+ and Cl^- into the insterstitium; 2, reabsorption of Na^+ and Cl^-; passive absorption of water under ADH control; 3, increased concentration of urea in tubule following reabsorption of water; 4, urea passes into the interstitium, thereby increasing osmolality; 5, the increased interstitial osmolality results in more water being extracted; 6, this leads to an increased salt concentration in the loop of Henle; 7, in the ascending limb, salt diffuses into the interstitium, further increasing its osmolality; 8, in the presence of ADH, the permeability of the distal nephron and collecting ducts is increased and water is reabsorbed; 9, water is removed from the interstitium by vasa recta.
Williams JD, *et al.* Clinical atlas of the kidney. Gower Publishing, London.

arteriole with its renin-producing granular cells, and the early portions of the efferent arteriole.

The thick ascending limb of the loop of Henle returns to its own glomerulus, where the cells that lie nearest to the glomerulus become taller to form the macula densa, the most obvious structural feature being that these cells are tightly packed and have large nuclei. The basal aspect of the macula densa is firmly attached to the extraglomerular mesangium.

The granular cells (also termed the juxtaglomerular cells) are assembled in clusters within the terminal portion of the afferent arteriole. These are modified smooth muscle cells containing cytoplasmic granules in which renin is stored. This enzyme is responsible for controlling the synthesis of angiotensin II by converting angiotensinogen to angiotensin I, which is in turn converted to angiotensin II by the action of the angiotensin-converting enzyme.

Granular cells appose the extraglomerular mesangial cells, adjacent smooth muscle cells, and endothelial cells, and are densely innervated by sympathetic nerve terminals. The secretion of renin by the granular cells is controlled by signals generated intrarenally (such as perfusion pressure and tubular fluid composition) and extrarenally, owing to changes in sympathetic output and by stimuli that decrease the extracellular fluid volume and blood pressure. Many factors may therefore be involved in the control of renin release, a particularly important one of these being an intrarenal baroreceptor mechanism that causes renin secretion to increase when the intrarenal arteriolar pressure at the granular cells is decreased. A major level of control also lies in the macula densa, where renin secretion is inversely proportional to the concentration of Cl^- or Na^+ in the tubular fluid. Decreased delivery of Na^+ and Cl^- to the macula densa is associated with increased renin secretion. Angiotensin II, by contrast, inhibits renin secretion by its direct action on the granular cells; it is also a major stimulant of aldosterone secretion, thereby stimulating sodium retention (see below), which closes the renin–angiotensin–aldosterone negative-feedback loop. In addition to these factors, increased activity of the sympathetic nervous system increases renin secretion, both by increased circulating catecholamines and by way of the renal sympathetic nerves.

It has been postulated that the intrarenal renin–angiotensin mechanism is the prime hormonal mediator of the tubuloglomerular feedback system, whereby a stimulus perceived at the macula densa, presumably related to luminal flow or ion concentration, influences filtration rate (Fig. 21.1.5). Evidence for this is inconclusive and it is almost certainly not the sole mediator of this feedback mechanism.

The distal tubule and collecting duct

The bulk of sodium and water reabsorption occurs in the proximal tubule, but fine regulation is necessary to maintain precise sodium and water balance. The distal tubule and the collecting duct are responsible for the necessary final adjustments that ultimately determine the rate of urinary water and sodium excretion, a mechanism substantially influenced by ADH (also known as vasopressin) and aldosterone, respectively.

Structure

The distal convoluted tubule begins just beyond the macula densa and ends at the cortical collecting duct. Its structure is similar to

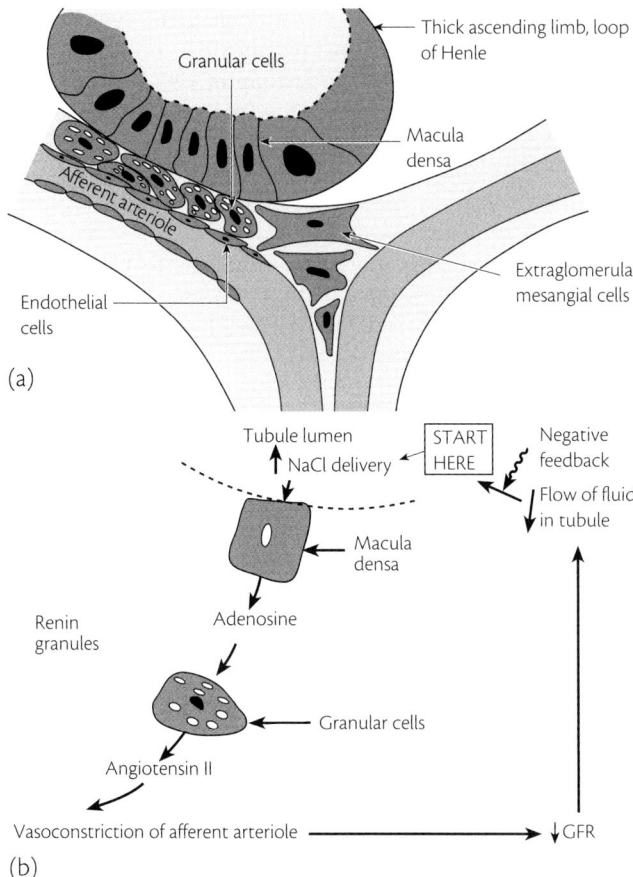

(a)

(b)

Fig. 21.1.5 Tubuloglomerular feedback: (a) anatomical basis; and (b) putative mechanism.

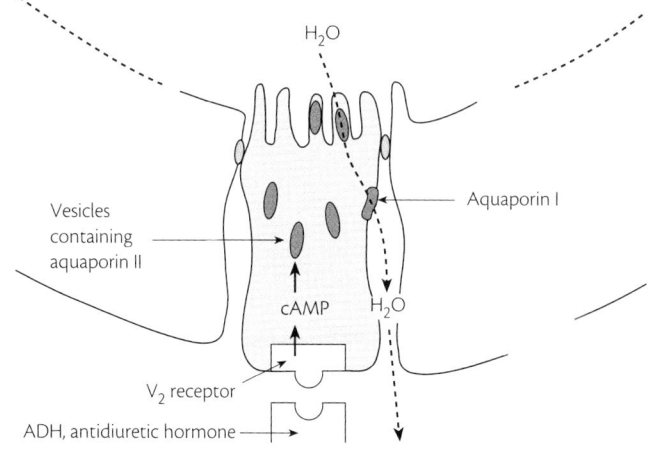

Fig. 21.1.6 Action of ADH.

that of the main part of the thick ascending limb of the loop of Henle. The collecting duct system includes the connecting tubule and the cortical and medullary collecting ducts. The connecting tubule and the collecting ducts, unlike the distal tubule, are lined by two cell types: principal cells, with small basal infoldings, some mitochondria, and small microvilli; and intercalated cells with darkly staining cytoplasm that contains mitochondria, smooth endoplasmic reticulum, and prominent Golgi apparatus. There are at least two types of intercalated cells, distinguished on the basis of immunocytochemical and functional characteristics: type A cells express H$^+$-ATPase at their luminal membrane and secrete H$^+$ ions, whereas type B cells express H$^+$-ATPase at their basolateral membrane and secrete HCO$_3^-$ ions.

Function

Cells of both the connecting tubule and the collecting duct are sensitive to ADH, but only those of the collecting duct are sensitive to mineralocorticoids. The renal concentrating and diluting processes are ultimately dependent on the ability of ADH to modulate the water permeability of collecting ducts. Regulation of ADH is dependent on osmoreceptors in the hypothalamus, which recognize changes in extracellular fluid osmolality, but release of ADH can be stimulated in the absence of changes in plasma osmolality, e.g. by intravascular volume depletion, pain, and nausea. Once released from the posterior pituitary, ADH exerts its biological action on water excretion by binding to receptors in the basolateral

membrane of the collecting duct (Fig. 21.1.6), resulting in increased adenylate cyclase activity, increased cAMP formation, and ultimately insertion of aquaporin 2 channels into the apical (luminal) cell membrane that make it more permeable to water.

The principal cells of the collecting duct are responsible for the modulation of sodium reabsorption. Entry of sodium into these cells occurs down a concentration gradient through specific sodium ion channels in the luminal membrane. This creates a negative potential difference in the lumen, which promotes either the secretion of potassium or the reabsorption of chloride via the paracellular route. These processes, which are the final regulators of sodium balance, are under the control of aldosterone, which increases the number of open sodium ion channels in the luminal membrane (Fig. 21.1.7). As previously discussed, angiotensin II is a major stimulant of aldosterone secretion. Hence activation of the renin–angiotensin system during periods of volume depletion leads to increased aldosterone production and sodium retention, whereas, when volume-replete, the system is suppressed and renin release and aldosterone secretion are reduced, resulting in natriuresis. Although the acute production of aldosterone is linked to the renin–angiotensin system, other mechanisms (including some

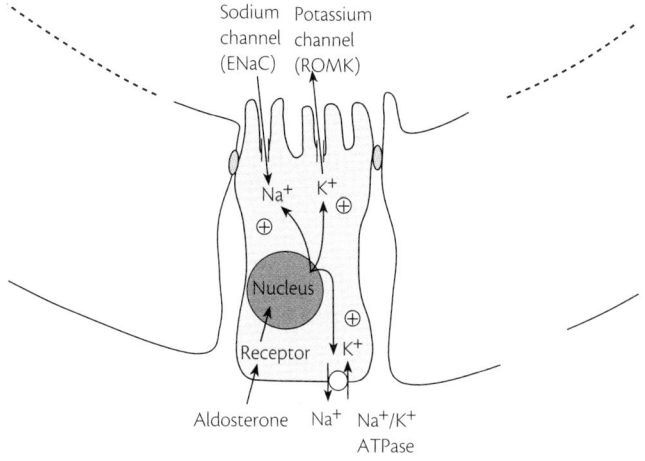

Fig. 21.1.7 The action of aldosterone on the collecting duct. Aldosterone stimulates an increase in the numbers and activity of apical ENaC and ROMK, and of basolateral Na$^+$,K$^+$-ATPase by direct and indirect effects.

relating to sodium or potassium balance) can also affect the ability of the adrenal glands to produce aldosterone.

The intercalated cells of the collecting duct are involved in maintenance of the acid–base balance. The method by which they excrete acid by generating ammonium ions is discussed in Chapter 12.11.

The interstitium

The renal interstitium is the space that is not occupied by the glomeruli and nephrons, and the vasculature of the kidney can be thought of as lying within it. The interstitium amounts to some 5 to 7% of the volume of the cortex, 3 to 4% of the outer stripe, 10% of the inner stripe, and up to 30% of the inner medulla. It is involved in virtually all functions of the healthy kidney, as well as in many pathological events. The transit of molecules from the tubules to the blood necessitates a crossing of the interstitial space, and vice versa, hence changes to the interstitium have a profound effect on the function of the tubules and indeed of the nephron itself.

The cells of the interstitium are not homogeneous but comprise different cell types that vary anatomically within the kidney and between health and disease. The main cellular component is the fibroblast, but there is evidence to suggest that there is a significant difference between the phenotype of the cortical fibroblast and that of the inner medullary fibroblast. Fibroblasts are important for the integrity of the interstitial matrix and are considered to be the source of matrix component production, as well as being responsible for their turnover. The renal fibroblasts also have endocrine functions: those of the cortex are the source of erythropoietin; the inner medullary fibroblasts produce significant amounts of prostaglandins, primarily prostaglandin E_2, and have a function in modifying electrolyte transport. Renal fibroblasts may have a pivotal role in renal interstitial fibrosis; it is now well established that the progression of renal disease is intimately linked to the degree of renal interstitial fibrosis, and it is likely that the key cell involved in this is the cortical fibroblast.

Dendritic cells are present in small numbers throughout the interstitium and express major histocompatibility complex (MHC) class II receptors. In addition, there are a few macrophages as well as some large lymphocytes. Dendritic cells, macrophages, and lymphocyte-like cells mostly have immunological and defence-like functions.

Further reading

Alpern RJ, Herbert SC (eds) (2007). *Seldin and Giebisch's the kidney*: *physiology and pathophysiology*, 4th edition. Academic Press, London.
Brenner B (ed) (2007). *Brenner and Rector's The kidney*, 8th edition. Saunders, Philadelphia.

Electrolyte disorders

Contents

21.2.1 Disorders of water and sodium homeostasis

Steven G. Achinger and Juan Carlos Ayus

Essentials

Regulation of water balance and sodium disorders

Water intake and the excretion of water are tightly regulated processes that are able to maintain a near-constant serum osmolality. Sodium disorders (dysnatraemias—hyponatraemia or hypernatraemia) are almost always due to an imbalance between water intake and water excretion.

Understanding the aetiology of sodium disorders depends on understanding the concept of electrolyte-free water clearance—this is a conceptual amount of water that represents the volume that would need to be subtracted (if electrolyte-free water clearance is positive) or added (if negative) to the measured urinary volume to make the electrolytes contained within the urine have the same tonicity as the plasma electrolytes. It is the concentration of the electrolytes in the urine, not the osmolality of the urine, which ultimately determines the net excretion of water.

Hyponatraemia

Hyponatraemia, defined as serum sodium concentration of less than 135 mmol/litre, is a common electrolyte disorder. It is almost invariably due to impaired water excretion, often in states where ADH release is: (1) a normal response to a physiological stimulus

such as pain, nausea, volume depletion, postoperative state, or congestive heart failure; or (2) a pathophysiological response as occurs with thiazide diuretics, other types of medications, or in the syndrome of inappropriate diuresis; with both often exacerbated in hospital by (3) inappropriate iatrogenic administration of water (or 5% dextrose).

Clinical features—these can range from the patient who is entirely asymptomatic at one end of the spectrum to hyponatraemic encephalopathy—most commonly manifesting with nausea, vomiting, and headache—at the other. Cerebral demyelination is a serious complication associated with hyponatraemia and its treatment, at its worst manifesting as pseudocoma with a 'locked in' state. Children and premenopausal women are at particular risk of poor outcomes, as are those who are hypoxic at presentation.

Management approach—the first priority is to exclude a hyperosmolar state and verify whether the patient is hypotonic, by (when possible) measuring the serum osmolality. The diagnostic approach is further based on the history, clinical assessment of the patient's volume status, and estimation of urinary electrolytes. Key issues are to recognize that: (1) hyponatraemic encephalopathy is a medical emergency that should be diagnosed and treated promptly with hypertonic saline to prevent death or devastating neurological complications; but also (2) that patients who are asymptomatic do not require treatment with hypertonic saline, whatever their level of serum sodium. Precipitating causes (e.g. thiazide diuretics) should be withdrawn when possible.

Practical management—algorithms, even if complex, cannot accurately predict a patient's response to treatment of hyponatraemia: close monitoring of serum sodium is essential. Patients with severe manifestations of hyponatraemic encephalopathy (active seizures or respiratory failure) should be given a bolus of 100 ml of 3% saline (over 10 min) to abruptly increase the serum sodium by about 2 to 4 mmol/litre, following which an infusion of 3% saline should be given at a rate of 1 ml/kg body weight per hour with the aim of raising the serum sodium to a mildly hyponatraemic level, but the total change in serum sodium should not exceed 15 to 20 mmol/litre over 48 h. For patients with less severe neurological manifestations, the bolus should be omitted.

Cerebral demyelination—this is a serious complication that has been associated with the correction of hyponatraemia, hence all patients receiving an infusion of 3% saline should have their serum sodium measured at least every 2 h until they are clinically stable and the serum sodium values are stable, with appropriate modification of treatment in response to the measurements. Failure to do so, and reliance on a calculated infusion rate, can lead to significant patient injury.

Prevention—hyponatraemia is usually iatrogenic and can be avoided or detected as follows: (1) hypotonic fluids should never be administered following surgery unless used to correct a free-water deficit—0.9% (normal) saline (NaCl) should be given postoperatively if parenteral fluids are indicated; (2) all hospitalized patients should be considered at risk for the development of hyponatraemia and should not be given hypotonic fluids unless a free-water deficit is present or if ongoing free-water losses are being replaced; (3) patients taking thiazide diuretics, especially older people, should be weighed before and after starting therapy and serum electrolytes monitored to detect water retention and the development of hyponatraemia.

Hypernatraemia

Hypernatraemia, defined as serum sodium concentration greater than 145 mmol/litre, is a common electrolyte disorder that occurs when water intake is inadequate to keep up with water losses. Since the thirst mechanism is such a powerful stimulus, the almost invariable context is illness and care that restrict the patient's access to water.

Clinical features—these are mainly related to central nervous system dysfunction caused by cerebral dehydration and cell shrinkage.

Management approach—the first step in evaluation is to take a detailed history focusing on fluid intake and losses. To assess urinary water losses, it is necessary to measure the urinary cationic electrolytes (sodium and potassium) and the urinary osmolality, remembering that the urinary osmolality alone cannot always determine the presence or absence of electrolyte-free water losses in the urine, the reason being that water can be excreted with nonelectrolyte osmoles or with electrolyte osmoles.

Practical management—needs to be guided by the following principles: (1) correction of underlying deficits in circulatory blood volume by infusion of 0.9% saline; (2) correction of chronic hypernatraemia at a pace that avoids therapy-induced cerebral oedema, which requires an understanding of both the initial water deficit and of ongoing water losses if the patient is polyuric; (3) administration of water by drinking or feeding tube is preferable to treatment with intravenous fluids if possible; (4) glucose-containing solutions should be avoided if possible; (5) as for the treatment of hyponatraemia, algorithms cannot accurately predict the response to treatment of hypernatraemia, hence regular monitoring of serum sodium with appropriate adjustment of treatment in response to the values obtained is mandatory.

Prevention—(1) patients with impaired access to water (e.g. infants, elderly, and hospitalized patients) should be considered at risk for the development of hypernatraemia, and their serum sodium should be monitored; (2) urinary electrolytes should be measured in conjunction with urinary osmolality in patients with polyuria to assess water losses in the urine and urinary concentrating ability.

Disorders of water metabolism

Hyponatraemia and hypernatraemia occur when there is a breakdown of the normal homeostatic mechanisms that keep water intake and excretion precisely balanced to prevent the development of disturbances in the serum sodium. There are numerous causes of impairment in this homeostatic function, such as renal failure, use of diuretics, and nonosmotic release of ADH due to nausea, pain, or other stimuli. Poor outcomes are still common among patients with hypernatraemia and hyponatraemia, in many cases due to failure to promptly recognize a life-threatening condition and initiate appropriate treatment. In this chapter the pathophysiology of sodium disturbances is addressed, with a focus on understanding clinical presentations of the diseases.

Regulation of water balance

Dysnatraemias (hyponatraemia or hypernatraemia) occur when there is an imbalance between water intake and water excretion. Extracellular fluid tonicity is reflected by the concentration of the serum sodium. Nearly all cell membranes are permeable to water, hence water will equilibrate between the intracellular space and the extracellular space to maintain the same osmolality in both compartments, and intracellular electrolyte concentrations will approximate the extracellular electrolyte concentrations. This means that the serum sodium concentration (Na_{se}) is proportional to the total body exchangeable sodium (Na_e) plus the total body exchangeable potassium (K_e):

$$(Na_e + K_e)/ \text{total body water} \propto Na_{se} \quad \text{(Equation 21.2.1.1)}$$

Water intake and the excretion of water are tightly regulated processes and therefore a near-constant serum osmolality is maintained (Fig. 21.2.1.1). Because of this tight regulation, disturbances in serum sodium are nearly always caused by perturbations in water balance, not of electrolytes.

Renal water handling

It is through the actions of ADH (also known as AVP) that the kidney regulates water excretion. The normal kidney has the ability to vary urinary concentration significantly, from as low as 50 mOsm/kg to as high as 1200 mOsm/kg when ADH activity is maximal, although when there is renal insufficiency (especially tubulointerstitial disease) this range is much more restricted. This means that the kidney can either excrete a large water load in very dilute urine or conserve water significantly. A mathematical illustration can make this clear. If a daily solute load is taken to be 800 mOsm (mainly electrolytes and urea, the latter due to protein catabolism), then this amount must be excreted in 24 h in order to maintain solute balance. Under conditions of maximal urinary concentration this could be excreted in approximately 667 ml of urine ($[800\,mOsm/1200\,mOsm] \times kg^{-1}$), which would be the expected response to a hypernatraemic state. Conversely, under conditions of maximal urinary dilution this osmolar load would be excreted in 16 litres of urine ($[800\,mOsm/50\,mOsm] \times kg^{-1}$), which would be an expected response to water intoxication or could occur in the setting of diabetes insipidus. Therefore, the body has the ability, under normal conditions, to achieve water balance across a very wide range of water intake. Disorders in water balance usually occur when there is a disruption in these processes that allow water intake and water excretion to be exquisitely matched.

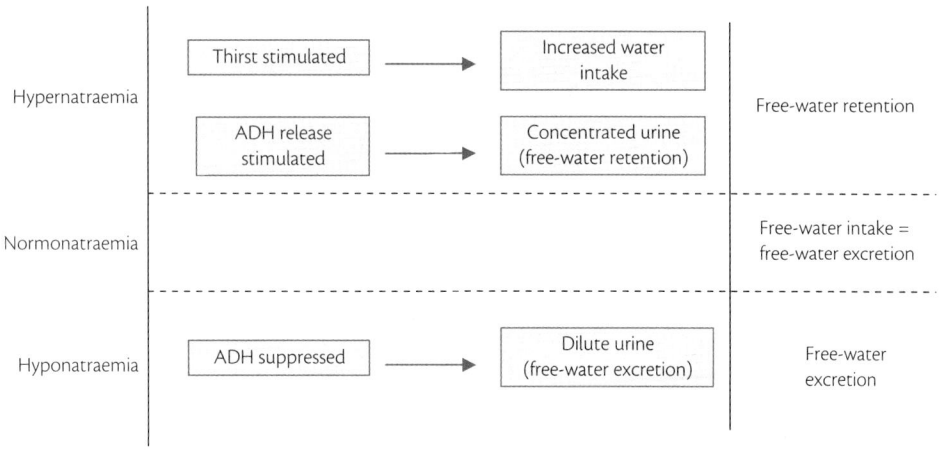

Fig. 21.2.1.1 Regulation of water intake and excretion to maintain normonatraemia.
Achinger, S.G., Ayus J.C. Fluid and Electrolytes. In *Civetta, Taylor, and Kirby's Critical Care*, 4th edition.

The concept of electrolyte-free water

The concept of electrolyte-free water is a good approach to understanding patients with disturbances in water balance. The electrolyte-free water clearance is a conceptual amount of a fluid that represents the volume that would need to be subtracted (if electrolyte-free water clearance is positive) or added (if negative) to the measured urinary volume to make the electrolytes contained within the urine have the same tonicity as the serum electrolytes (Fig. 21.2.1.2):

$$[1-([Na^+]_u+[K^+]_u)/([Na^+]_{se}+[K^+]_{se})]\times \text{volume of urine (ml)}$$

$$= \text{electrolyte-free water clearance} \quad \text{(Equation 21.2.1.2)}$$

where $[Na^+]_u$ is urinary sodium concentration, $[K^+]_u$ is urinary potassium concentration, $[Na^+]_{se}$ is serum sodium concentration, and $[K^+]_{se}$ is serum potassium concentration.

The electrolyte-free water represents the amount of water lost in excess of electrolytes and which would therefore—if not replaced—have an effect on serum osmolality. A few key points must be made about the electrolyte-free water. First, it is truly a conceptual volume because, as can be seen in Equation 21.2.1.2, it can take on a negative value, which occurs when the electrolyte concentration in the urine exceeds that in the serum: when the electrolyte-free water clearance is negative, there is net retention of electrolyte-free water. Second, the concept of electrolyte-free water clearance highlights the fact that it is the concentration of the electrolytes in the urine, not the osmolality of the urine, which ultimately determines the net excretion of water. In other words, the urine osmolality may be high but, if the urine contains mainly urea and very few electrolytes, there will still be a net loss of water. Electrolyte-free water clearance can therefore be calculated as shown in Equation 21.2.1.2 as a convenient clinical tool for assessing water need in a patient.

Clinical utility of electrolyte-free water clearance

A critical point to understand is that the urine electrolytes and not the urine osmolality determine the amount of free water excreted in the urine. Typically, if the relationship between the serum electrolytes and the urine electrolytes is understood, it is not necessary to calculate a value for the electrolyte-free water clearance. In the case where the concentration of electrolytes in the urine exceeds the concentration of electrolytes in the serum, then free water is not being excreted in the urine. Conversely, when the concentration of electrolytes in the urine is less than that in the serum, then free water is being excreted in the urine. Fig. 21.2.1.3 illustrates this relationship: much can be learned regarding water excretion by simply examining the concentration of the electrolytes in the urine.

Hyponatraemia

Hyponatraemia is defined as serum sodium lower than 135 mmol/litre, which is a common condition in hospital settings and is increasingly recognized in outpatients. Hyponatraemia can be asymptomatic, although careful neurological evaluation has detected subtle abnormalities in patients with chronic hyponatraemia and serum sodium as high as 132 mmol/litre. At the other end of the spectrum, presentation with hyponatraemic encephalopathy (central nervous system symptoms secondary to cerebral oedema) is a medical emergency that must be diagnosed promptly and treated quickly, or death or devastating neurological complications can result. It is critical to differentiate between these two extremes because the management is much different, depending on the symptoms. It is recognized that risk factors for hyponatraemic

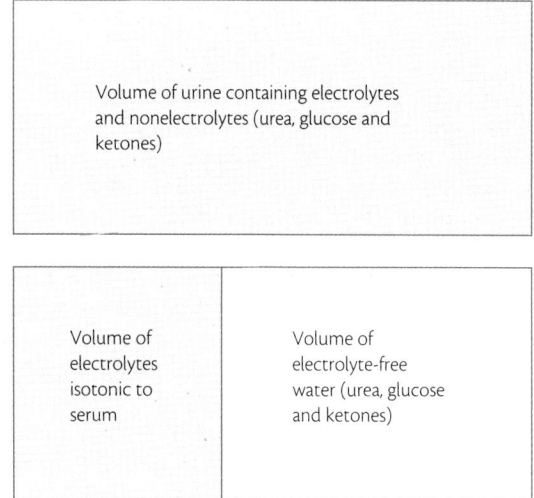

Fig. 21.2.1.2 Resolution of urinary volume into a proportion of electrolytes isotonic to serum, with the remainder as 'electrolyte-free water'.

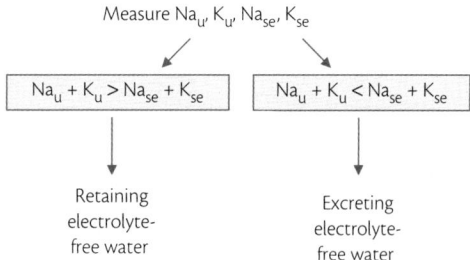

Fig. 21.2.1.3 Measurement of serum and urinary electrolytes can determine whether the patient is retaining or excreting electrolyte-free water. Na_u, urine sodium (spot); K_u, urine potassium (spot); Na_{se}, serum sodium; K_{se}, serum potassium.

encephalopathy play a critical role in the determining whether or not patients are likely to develop this condition as a consequence of hyponatraemia, these risk factors for poor outcome being young age, premenopausal women, and hypoxia. The pathogenic mechanisms that are responsible for these risk factors are discussed later in this chapter.

Pathogenesis

The main defence against the development of hyponatraemia is the ability of the kidney to dilute the urine and excrete free water. The typical adult (assuming normal renal function) can excrete approximately 15 litres of free water per day in the urine, hence excess ingestion of water as the sole cause of hyponatraemia is rare outside of the setting of mental illness. An underlying condition that impairs free-water excretion (Box 21.2.1.1) is typically necessary in conjunction with free-water intake for the development of hyponatraemia. States of impaired water excretion are often states where ADH release is a normal response to a physiological stimulus such as pain, nausea, volume depletion, postoperative state, or congestive heart failure. ADH release may also be pathophysiological such as occurs with thiazide diuretics or with other types of medications such as antiepileptic drugs, or in the syndrome of inappropriate diuresis.

Brain defences against cerebral oedema

Hyponatraemia leads to an osmotic gradient favouring water movement intracellularly, which—if allowed to act unopposed—could lead to cerebral oedema and severe neurological injury. The first-line defence against this is the blood–brain barrier, which impedes the entry of water. This starts with tight junctions between vascular endothelial cells of the brain capillaries and their interface with the foot processes of astrocytes, the latter being a highly specialized subtype of glial cell that performs many supporting functions in maintenance of the fluid environment and electrolyte milieu of the extracellular space of the brain.

The astrocytes are the main regulator of brain water content: they swell during hypotonic stress, whereas neurons do not, with this capacity largely due to the presence of a water channel specific to astrocytes, aquaporin 4. Mice with targeted deletion of aquaporin 4 are protected from cytotoxic cerebral oedema caused by water intoxication, brain ischaemia, or meningitis, but are particularly vulnerable to vasogenic cerebral oedema caused by e.g. cerebral abscess or tumour, or hydrocephalus. The response of the astrocyte is critical in determining the degree of cerebral oedema in response to hypo-osmolar stress, and modulation of aquaporin 4 production or function may prove useful in the management of a variety

---

Box 21.2.1.1 States where water excretion is impaired

Volume-depleted states
- Volume depletion
- Diuretics

States where volume is normal
- Syndrome of inappropriate diuresis
- Pain
- Postoperative state
- Nausea
- Hypothyroidism

Volume-expanded states
- Congestive heart failure
- Renal failure
- Cirrhosis

---

of cerebral disorders, including those associated with hyponatraemia, in the future.

However, progressive and increasing swelling of astrocytes in the face of hyponatraemia would not protect the brain against adverse consequences, and there are several other protective mechanisms. There is shunting of cerebrospinal fluid from within the brain: this is a rapid response, but its capacity to buffer significant volume change is limited. Ultimately, cell volume regulatory mechanisms in the cerebral astrocytes must be active to decrease the brain size. This is accomplished by reduction in cellular osmolyte content (mainly electrolytes) using an ATP-dependent mechanism that requires Na^+,K^+-ATPase to extrude ions (electrolytes) from within, with water obligatorily following to reduce brain volume. In animal models of acute hyponatraemia, brain water content is returned to near the baseline value 6 h after induction of acute hyponatraemia. As will be discussed later, several clinical factors have been shown to impair these glial cell adaptive responses, and these are the chief risk factors for poor patient outcome.

Clinical manifestations

The symptoms of hyponatraemia are attributable to osmotic swelling of the brain, with pressure on the brain parenchyma arising because of the rigid structures encasing the central nervous system. The manifestations can be varied and not necessarily related to the degree of decrease in serum sodium concentration, which is frequently less than 120 or 115 mmol/litre in congestive heart failure and in cirrhosis with very few—if any—overt symptoms. Conversely, life-threatening cerebral oedema can be the presentation of a patient with a serum sodium as high as 128 mmol/litre. Hyponatraemic encephalopathy is defined as symptomatic cerebral oedema secondary to hyponatraemia: the early signs are usually nonspecific—nausea, vomiting, headache—and can often go unrecognized, but brainstem herniation and death can occur if they are left untreated.

Hyponatraemic encephalopathy

Risk factors

Not all patients are equal in terms of risk of morbidity and mortality following the development of hyponatraemia. Children are at particular risk for poor outcome following the development of hyponatraemia due to their high ratio of brain size to skull size, the skull not reaching its full size until age 16 years, whereas the brain reaches its adult size at approximately age 6 years. This means that children cannot accommodate as much increase in brain size as adults: there is less capacity for brain expansion before pressure is exerted on the brain parenchyma. For this reason, the long-standing practice of administering hypotonic fluids to children is being challenged: normal (0.9%) saline is the most appropriate fluid to use to prevent the development of iatrogenic hyponatraemic encephalopathy in children.

Premenopausal women are another significant risk group in terms of neurological outcomes following hyponatraemia, being 25 times more likely to die following hyponatraemic encephalopathy than other groups of patients. This striking difference is not accounted for by differences in clinical presentation, and anatomical factors in terms of the brain size—cranial vault size ratio (as is seen with children)—cannot explain the disparity in outcomes. Differences in adaptive responses to hyponatraemia must exist. As described above, it is known that ATP-dependent mechanisms are important for the response to hypo-osmolar stress in the brain. Oestrogens have a similar steroidal structure to ouabain and other cardiac glycosides (such as digoxin), which are known to inhibit the Na^+,K^+-ATPase, and female sex hormones have been shown to inhibit the activity of this pump in diverse tissues such as mammalian heart, diaphragm, red blood cells, and liver. Sex steroids and gender also play a significant role in brain adaptation and in animal models of hyponatraemia. There is increased morbidity from hyponatraemia in female rats, and isolated synaptosomes from female hyponatraemic rats have increased uptake of sodium compared with male hyponatraemic rats, suggesting impairment in sodium extrusion. Regulatory volume decrease is also inhibited by the presence of oestrogen/progesterone in rat astrocytes treated in vitro. These studies support the notion that the presence of female sex hormones can impair the critical energy-dependent astrocyte cell volume regulatory processes, with this impairment leading to more severe cerebral oedema. Finally, female rats have more intense vasoconstriction than male rats in response to ADH, which may lead to tissue hypoxia, which is another possible factor in producing poor outcomes.

Role of hypoxia

Animal studies have demonstrated that survival is severely impaired and brain adaptation is significantly impaired following hyponatraemia and simultaneous brain hypoxia. Epidemiological studies have shown that patients with hypoxia at presentation of hyponatraemic encephalopathy have poor outcome compared with those who are not hypoxic, even after adjustment for comorbid conditions. Since impairment of astrocyte adaptive mechanisms can explain poor outcome in premenopausal females, it has been proposed that hypoxia may similarly have an effect on astrocyte volume regulation. Impairment of energy utilization in the brain—a common phenomenon following asphyxiation or cardiac arrest—can lead to diffuse cerebral oedema, termed 'cytotoxic' cerebral oedema, related to the impairment of cell-volume regulatory mechanisms. Hence, if hyponatraemia—which will by itself induce cerebral oedema—is compounded with impairment in volume regulatory mechanisms through hypoxia, then this is likely to lead to more severe cerebral oedema than if hypoxia were not present and a poor outcome.

Hypoxia develops in patients with hyponatraemic encephalopathy through two mechanisms: hypercapneic respiratory failure and neurogenic pulmonary oedema. Hypercapneic respiratory failure is secondary to central respiratory depression and is a first sign of impending brainstem herniation, with the hypoxaemia that then develops being due to the central respiratory depression further worsening astrocyte cell-volume regulatory mechanisms and leading to worsening of brain oedema. Neurogenic pulmonary oedema, caused by increased vascular permeability and increased catecholamine release that occurs secondary to elevated intracranial pressure, is a complication of cerebral oedema and can occur in the setting of hyponatraemic encephalopathy as well. This form of noncardiogenic pulmonary oedema is known as the Ayus-Arieff Syndrome, and is secondary to increased intracranial pressure due to cerebral oedema. Hypoxaemia is therefore both a risk factor and a pathogenic mechanism in severe cerebral oedema, as once hypoxaemia is established the underlying cerebral oedema will worsen because the hypoxia will initiate a vicious cycle that—unless broken—results in worsening of the underlying cerebral oedema (Fig. 21.2.1.4).

Diagnostic approach to hyponatraemic patients

With a patient with hyponatraemia, the first priority is to exclude a hyperosmolar state and verify that a hypotonic state exists by (when possible) measuring the serum osmolality. An osmotically active substance confined to the extracellular fluid—most typically glucose, mannitol, or glycine—leads to translocation of water from the intracellular space and to a decreased serum sodium concentration despite a net increase in serum osmolality. In assessing for a disturbance of sodium when hyperglycaemia is present, the serum sodium must be 'corrected' for the presence of hyperglycaemia by adding 1.4 mmol/litre for every 5 mmol/litre increase of the serum glucose above 5 mmol/litre (or 1.6 mmol/litre for every 100 mg/dl above 100 mg/dl).

The possibility of pseudohyponatraemia should also be kept in mind. Hyperproteinaemia and hyperlipidaemia can lead to spuriously low serum sodium measurements if samples are diluted prior to measurement of the serum sodium. By contrast, pseudohyponatraemia due to hyperproteinaemia and hyperlipidaemia alone is not a concern when a potentiometric method is used. Measured serum osmolality will be normal if pseudohyponatraemia is present.

The diagnostic approach is further based on the history, urinary electrolytes, and clinical assessment of the patient's volume status (Fig. 21.2.1.5), which will be further demonstrated in the case discussions to follow.

Treatment of hyponatraemic encephalopathy

Hyponatraemic encephalopathy is a life-threatening medical emergency that must be treated appropriately and in a timely manner to avoid death or severe neurological impairment. As described above, early symptoms are headache, nausea, and vomiting, with seizures commonly seen if cerebral oedema worsens. The final stages, if not corrected, are coma, respiratory arrest, and death.

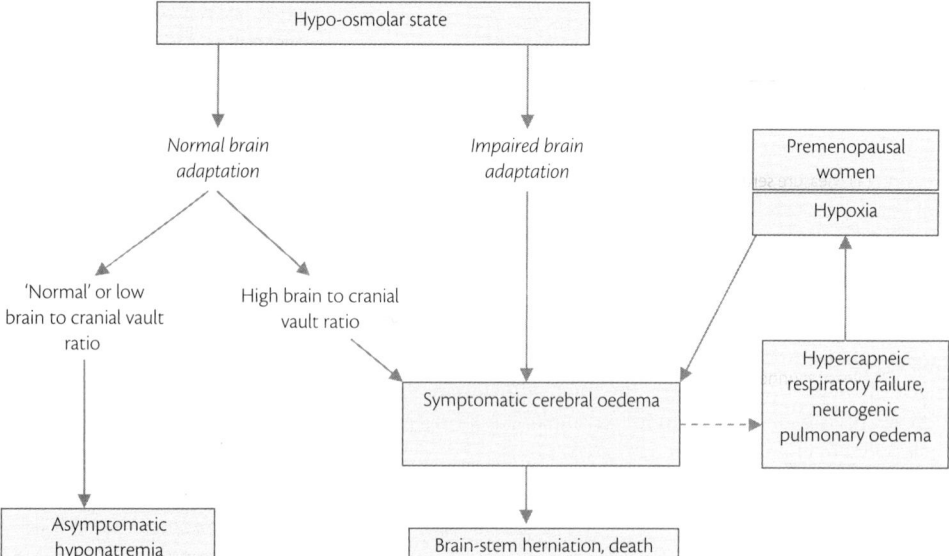

Fig. 21.2.1.4 The possible clinical outcomes of a hypo-osmolar state. Achinger, S.G., Ayus J.C. (2008). Fluid and Electrolytes. In *Civetta, Taylor, and Kirby's Critical Care*, 4th edition.

The aim of treatment of hyponatraemic encephalopathy is to: (1) remove patients with severe manifestations of cerebral oedema from immediate danger, (2) correct serum sodium to a mildly hyponatraemic level, and (3) maintain this level of serum sodium to allow for the brain to adapt to the change in serum osmolality (Fig. 21.2.1.6).

Prompt treatment is essential in all patients with hyponatraemic encephalopathy. Those with severe manifestations (active seizures or respiratory failure) can be treated with a bolus of 100 ml of 3% saline (given over 10 min) to abruptly change the serum osmolality, the goal of this action being to increase the serum sodium by approximately 2 to 4 mmol/litre. If seizures or respiratory failure are refractory to the first bolus, another bolus of 50 to 100 ml of hypertonic saline may be given. Following the bolus, an infusion of hypertonic saline should be given with the aim of raising the serum sodium to a mildly hyponatraemic level, but the total change in serum sodium should not exceed 15 to 20 mmol/litre over 48 h. For patients with hyponatraemic encephalopathy who do not exhibit ongoing seizures or respiratory arrest, an infusion of 3% saline without a bolus is appropriate initial management. The goal of treatment to clinically stabilize the patient and raise the serum sodium to a mildly hyponatraemic level, but again the total change in serum sodium should not exceed 15 to 20 mmol/litre over 48 h.

A few precautionary points must be understood to prevent therapy-induced brain injury: (1) the serum sodium should never be corrected to a normonatraemic or hypernatraemic level in a patient treated for hyponatraemic encephalopathy; (2) following correction, patients should be maintained at mildly hyponatraemic levels for a few days following hyponatraemic encephalopathy (this maintenance period will allow the patient to adjust to the new serum tonicity); and (3) if the patient has decreased cardiac output and pulmonary oedema may develop with vigorous saline volume expansion, then furosemide should be given in addition to hypertonic saline—this should prevent volume overload and pulmonary oedema, but such a patient requires very close monitoring.

Appropriate treatment of hyponatraemic encephalopathy with hypertonic saline is safe and effective, but improper therapy can have severe consequences. Some authors describe formulas of varying complexity to guide treatment of hyponatraemia: these should not be used at all when determining the amount of hypertonic saline to give because they are fundamentally flawed. Ongoing water losses are unpredictable, and formulas are not able to take these into account because they are based on a closed system assumption (i.e. no ongoing water losses). Significant overcorrection can occur if saline is prescribed according to formula when a patient undergoes a spontaneous water diuresis, which can easily occur when the stimulus for water retention is removed and the body begins to respond appropriately to hypotonicity by suppressing ADH release and excreting dilute urine. The first sign that this is occurring is a precipitous increase in urine output, hence hourly urine output should be followed closely. The key is to monitor the patient very carefully. In addition to measurement of urinary volume, all patients receiving an infusion of 3% saline for hyponatraemic encephalopathy should have frequent monitoring of serum sodium (at least every 2 h) until they are clinically stable and the serum sodium values are stable. Failure to do so and reliance on a calculated infusion rate can lead to significant patient injury. Furthermore, any patient with severe manifestations of hyponatraemic encephalopathy must be treated in an intensive care unit setting.

As a guide for initial therapy, in lieu of a calculated infusion rate, an assumption that can be useful is that an infusion of 3% saline of 1 ml/kg body weight will raise the serum sodium by approximately 1 mmol/litre. Thereafter, the rate of infusion should be titrated based on measured serum sodium values and clinical response of the patient. Fluid restriction as a sole treatment is not appropriate for a patient with hyponatraemic encephalopathy. Early recognition of hyponatraemic encephalopathy and institution of prompt treatment are the factors most associated with good neurological outcomes.

Risk factors for the development of cerebral demyelination

Cerebral demyelination is a serious complication that has been associated with the correction of hyponatraemia. The symptoms often become apparent days to weeks following correction of hyponatraemia, and can vary from being minimal or none to as severe as a pseudocoma with a 'locked-in stare'. A key point is that the hourly rate of correction of serum sodium by itself is not predictive of cerebral demyelination, whereas the absolute change in

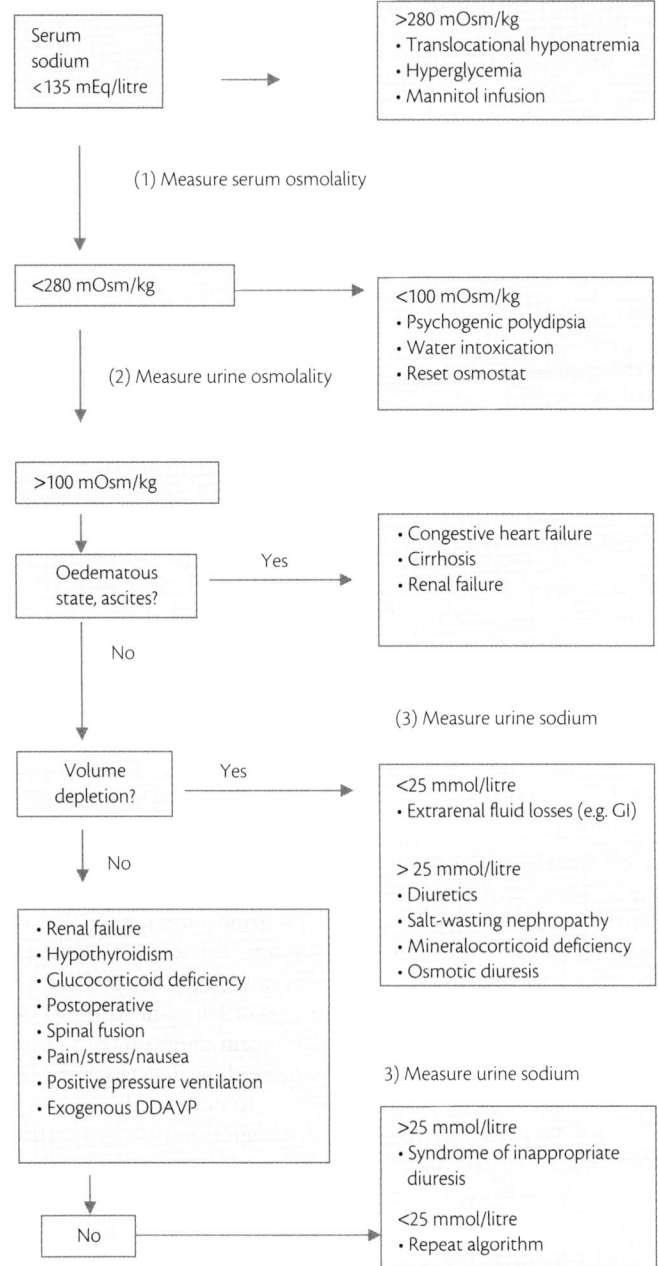

Fig. 21.2.1.5 Diagnostic approach to hyponatraemia. DDAVP, deamino-D-arginine vasopressin; GI, gastrointestinal. Adapted from MKSAP 2006.

serum sodium over 48 h is predictive. This is important because it is not appropriate to treat a patient with respiratory arrest due to hyponatraemic encephalopathy with a 'slow' infusion of hypertonic saline to increase the serum sodium by 0.5 to 1 mmol/litre per hour. This type of patient—with impending brainstem herniation—should be treated with a bolus of hypertonic saline to quickly reduce brain volume, after which the hourly rate of correction can be more modest as long as the total change in serum sodium does not exceed 15 to 20 mmol/litre over 48 h and the patient is not corrected to normonatraemic levels. Additionally, there are other clinical factors not related to degree of correction

such as liver disease and hypoxia that increase the risk of cerebral demyelination, and particular care must be exercised in treating these patients, for whom the safe degree of correction over 48 h is not known but might be less than 15 to 20 mmol/litre over 48 h.

Treatment of asymptomatic hyponatraemia

Regardless of the underlying aetiology and irrespective of the absolute level of the serum sodium, asymptomatic hyponatraemia does not require treatment with hypertonic saline. The underlying cause should be addressed and precipitating medications such as thiazide diuretics and anticonvulsants discontinued when necessary.

Fluid restriction may be helpful in some cases, but this is often not enough where electrolyte-free water excretion is minimal or negative, as is often the case in severe syndrome of inappropriate diuresis or cirrhosis. If hyponatraemia is refractory to fluid restriction, demeclocycline can be used to lower urine osmolality and increase free-water excretion. Vasopressin receptor (V_2) blockers are newly available agents that show promise and may become the mainstay of therapy in the future.

Case discussions

Case 1: postoperative hyponatraemia

A 29-year-old woman without significant medical history undergoes an elective laparoscopic cholecystectomy. During the procedure, 5% dextrose in quarter-strength normal saline (0.22% NaCl) is started and maintained at 125 ml/h. There was some bleeding during the procedure, but blood transfusion was not required. The patient is kept in the hospital for observation because of the bleeding. She does not tolerate oral intake, and the intravenous fluids are continued at the current rate. At 4 a.m. the following day the woman complains of headache and she is given paracetamol by the on-call physician. At 10.30 a.m. the attending doctor is notified that the serum sodium is 128 mmol/litre: no new orders are received. The woman is found to be lethargic by the nursing staff and an order is received to withhold pain medications. That afternoon the woman has a seizure and goes into respiratory failure. She is placed on mechanical ventilation and transferred to the intensive care unit. At the time of transfer, the serum sodium is 124 mmol/litre.

Discussion

The patient has several nonosmotic stimuli for ADH secretion (postoperative, volume depletion, pain, nausea) and the administration of a hypotonic fluid was not appropriate. Postoperative hyponatraemia can be prevented by the administration of 0.9% saline when parenteral fluids are indicated, with avoidance of the use of hypotonic fluids in a postsurgical patient. The induction of hyponatraemic encephalopathy is iatrogenic in this case and therapy needs to be instituted immediately, as described above and in Fig. 21.2.1.6, to try to prevent death or severe neurological impairment.

Case 2: exercise-associated hyponatraemia

A 24-year-old woman collapses 20 min after completing a marathon and is brought to the Emergency Department for evaluation. She has a decreased level of consciousness and is very short of breath. Cardiological examination is normal, but there are crackles in all lung fields. Neurological examination reveals a depressed

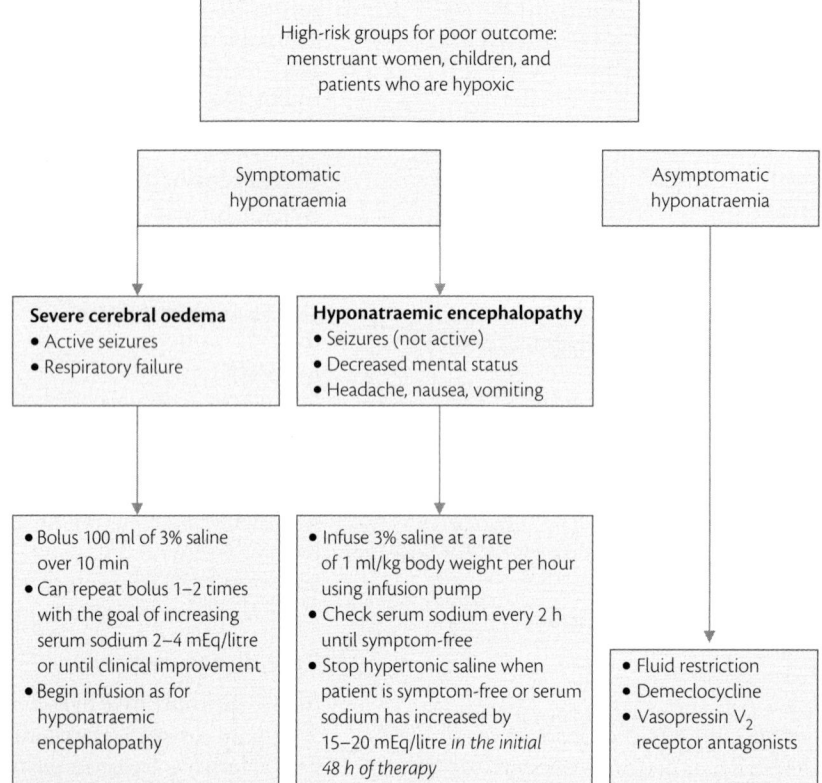

Fig. 21.2.1.6 Treatment of hyponatraemia.
Adapted with permission with permission from Achinger, S.G., Moritz, M.L., Ayus J.C. Dysnatremias: Why are patients still dying? South Medical J 2006; 99(4): 353–362.

mental status with no focal signs. The chest radiograph is consistent with pulmonary oedema. Serum electrolytes include sodium of 125 mmol/litre and potassium of 3.3 mmol/litre.

Discussion

Exercise-associated hyponatraemia has been reported in marathon runners, with those at risk for this problem consuming large amounts of water throughout the course of the race. It is thought that significant amounts of this water remain unabsorbed, sequestered in the gut because blood flow is directed away from the splanchnic circulation while exercising vigorously. At the end of the race the sequestered water is absorbed and hyponatraemia develops rapidly, with water excretion being inhibited by high levels of ADH release secondary to extreme physical exertion.

As with Case 1, treatment needs to be started immediately. This condition can be prevented by limiting fluid intake during endurance running: salt consumption or the use of hypotonic electrolyte sports drinks do not appear to be effective in prevention.

Case 3: DDAVP withdrawal

A 39-year-old man with a history of central diabetes insipidus following resection of a pituitary tumor is brought into the Emergency Department after a generalized seizure. He has previously been taking deamino-D-arginine vasopressin (DDAVP) 10 µg intranasally twice a day for his condition. In the Emergency Department he is found to be lethargic and unresponsive, with pulse 80 beats/min and blood pressure 135/80 mmHg, and his serum sodium is 119 mmol/litre and serum potassium 4.0 mmol/litre. It is not clear when the patient was last given a dose of DDAVP. Urine sodium is 125 mmol/litre and urine potassium 20 mmol/litre, with urine osmolality 585 mOsm/kg.

The man is given 2 litres of 0.9% saline in the Emergency Department. Six hours after presentation, the serum sodium is 127 mmol/litre and the man is admitted for management of hyponatraemia. The admitting physician continues to withhold the DDAVP and stops the intravenous fluids. The urine output increases significantly over the ensuing night, and the following morning the serum sodium is 158 mmol/litre, urine sodium 17 mmol/litre, urine potassium 10 mmol/litre, and urine osmolality 70 mOsm/kg.

Discussion

DDAVP by itself is not a cause of hyponatraemia. DDAVP will cause retention of free water and therefore dosing must be titrated in conjunction with the patient's fluid intake. The patient must be closely monitored and the serum electrolytes closely followed. If DDAVP is withheld following DDAVP-associated hyponatraemia, then a free-water diuresis will ensue and dangerous overcorrection of the serum sodium hypernatraemia may occur, as observed here. This is especially a concern in a patient such as this who has central diabetes insipidus and can rapidly excrete a large volume of dilute urine.

An appropriate approach to this patient with diabetes insipidus and hyponatraemic encephalopathy due to DDAVP-associated hyponatraemia would have been to continue DDAVP and restrict all enteral fluid intake. To correct the patient to the desired serum sodium level, 3% saline could have been used, and then discontinued. During this time, absolutely no hypotonic fluids would be given, and the patient would be monitored closely to restrict all enteral intake. A slow infusion of 0.9% saline could have been continued after the 3% saline was stopped if necessary to support volume status. This approach, coupled with frequent monitoring of the serum sodium, would have prevented overcorrection secondary to water diuresis as happened in this case.

Case 4: hyponatraemia due to syndrome of inappropriate diuresis

A 28-year-old man with HIV and a CD4 count of 75 is seen in follow-up 3 days after being discharged from the hospital where he had been diagnosed with pneumonia, suspected to be due to *Pneumocystis jirovecii*. His serum sodium had been decreased throughout the hospitalization, which was managed with fluid restriction. Current medications include a taper of prednisone and co-trimoxazole. He is significantly improved since hospital discharge, with physical examination revealing that he is afebrile, with pulse 84 beats/min, blood pressure 104/55 mmHg, and no abnormalities in the cardiac or respiratory systems—the lungs are clear and there is no peripheral oedema. Laboratory values from the morning of the clinic visit reveal the following:

- serum—sodium 113 mmol/litre, potassium 3.9 mmol/litre, creatinine 64 µmol/litre (0.7 mg/dl), glucose 6.2 mmol/litre (112 mg/dl), osmolality 248 mOsm/kg
- urine—sodium 105 mmol/litre, potassium 18 mmol/litre, osmolality 590 mOsm/kg

Discussion

This presentation is consistent with syndrome of inappropriate diuresis, which is defined as hypotonic hyponatraemia, with a urine osmolality above 100 mOsm/kg, in the absence of volume depletion, adrenal insufficiency, congestive heart failure, hypothyroidism, cirrhosis, and/or renal impairment. The laboratory values support syndrome of inappropriate diuresis as the serum osmolality is decreased, which rules out hyperosmolar hyponatraemia (also known as dilutional hyponatraemia) and pseudohyponatraemia, and the urine osmolality is high.

If this man were responding normally to the hypotonicity of the serum, the urine should be dilute. The fact that the urine is concentrated is abnormal, but it is important be sure that the patient does not have another cause of a water-retentive state that is a physiological response. These are most commonly congestive heart failure, cirrhosis, and volume depletion. In these conditions, the low effective circulating blood volume initiates both sodium and water-retentive mechanisms. Hence a similar set of laboratory values may be seen in these conditions, with the exception that the urine sodium should not be 105 mmol/litre. When the kidney is conserving sodium, the urinary sodium is typically below 20 mmol/litre, but many patients with cirrhosis and congestive heart failure receive diuretics and interpretation of the serum sodium must be done cautiously in this setting. The presence of severe congestive heart failure and cirrhosis is typically obvious based on history and physical examination. Volume depletion (not due to diuretic use) can be distinguished from syndrome of inappropriate diuresis based on the urine sodium, which should be less than 20 mmol/litre. Other conditions leading to ADH release should also be considered and ruled out before syndrome of inappropriate diuresis is diagnosed: these include postoperative stress, medications, trauma, pain, and nausea. Pulmonary disease, especially pneumonia, is a common cause of syndrome of inappropriate diuresis, as seen in this case: other causes are given in Table 21.2.1.1.

Despite the profound hyponatraemia, this man is clinically well and thus he does not require treatment with hypertonic saline.

Table 21.2.1.1 Causes of the syndrome of inappropriate antidiuresis

Neoplastic disease

Carcinoma (bronchus, pancreas, bladder, prostate, duodenum)

Thymoma

Mesothelioma

Lymphoma, leukaemia

Ewing's sarcoma

Carcinoid

Bronchial adenoma

Neurological disorders

Head injury, neurosurgery

Brain abscess

Brain tumour

Meningitis, encephalitis

Guillain Barré syndrome

Cerebral haemorrhage

Cavernous sinus thrombosis

Hydrocephalus

Cerebellar and cerebral atrophy

Shy-Drager syndrome

Peripheral neuropathy

Seizures

Subdural haematoma

Alcohol withdrawal

Chest disorders

Pneumonia

Tuberculosis

Emphyema

Cystic fibrosis

Pneumothorax

Aspergillosis

Drugs

Chlorpropamide

Opiates

Vincristine, cis-platinum

Vinblastine

Thiazides

Dopamine antagonists

Tricyclic antidepressants

MAOIs

SSRIs

'Ecstasy' (3,4-MDMA)

Anticonvulsants

Miscellaneous

Idiopathic

Psychosis

Porphyria

Abdominal surgery'

MAOIs = monoamine oxidase inhibitors; SSRIs = selective serotonin reuptake inhibitors; 3,4-MDMA, 3,4-methylenedioxymetamphetamnine.

The diagnosis of the syndrome of inappropriate diuresis is often made incorrectly: the syndrome is a diagnosis of exclusion and it is essential that the diagnostic approach described in Fig. 21.2.1.5 is rigorously applied to prevent wrong diagnosis and treatment.

Fluid restriction should be advised, with regular monitoring of the serum sodium, which should increase as syndrome of inappropriate diuresis resolves with recovery from pneumonia. If hyponatraemia is persistent and refractory to fluid restriction, then demeclocycline (or a V2 blocker) should be considered.

Case 5: hyponatraemic encephalopathy in an elderly woman presenting with a fall

A 77-year-old woman is brought to the Emergency Department after falling at home. Her past medical history is significant only with regard to osteoporosis, but the patient's daughter states that 2 weeks ago she was started by her primary care physician on a blood pressure medication and that she has been slightly confused over the last few days. Physical examination reveals that she is afebrile, with pulse 70 beats/min and blood pressure 120/60 mmHg. She is confused and not answering questions appropriately, but cardiac examination is normal, the lungs are clear, and she does not have any pedal oedema.

Laboratory investigation reveals the following:

- serum—sodium 110 mmol/litre, potassium 2.7 mmol/litre, creatinine 118 μmol/litre (1.3 mg/dl), urea 7.9 mmol/litre (22 mg/dl), glucose 6.2 mmol/litre (108 mg/dl), chloride 78 mmol/litre, bicarbonate 20 mmol/litre

Discussion

Hydrochlorothiazide can lead to significant hyponatraemia and is one of the more common causes of hyponatraemia in an outpatient setting. Thiazide diuretics (but not loop diuretics) act at the level of the distal convoluted tubule and impair urinary concentrating capacity. ADH secretion is stimulated by a state of relative volume depletion, and the result is increased urinary concentration and water retention. Loop diuretics, by contrast, act in the ascending limb of loop of Henle on the $Na^+/K^+/2Cl^-$ cotransporter and lead to impairment of both urinary concentrating and diluting capacity and are less likely to lead to hyponatraemia.

Depending on the degree of this woman's confusion, her immediate management could either be with fluid restriction or by infusion of hypertonic saline as described in Fig. 21.2.1.6. Her thiazide should be stopped, (almost) needless to say.

Depending on definition, about 10% of patients develop hyponatraemia when given a thiazide, and older people are particularly susceptible. A proposed measure to detect those who might be retaining water and thereby becoming hyponatraemic is to have the patient weigh themselves before and 48 h after starting the medication. If they fail to lose weight, or they actually gain weight, then the medication should be stopped and serum electrolytes checked; and all patients given thiazide diuretics should have their electrolytes measured after the onset of therapy or dose adjustments.

Hypernatraemia

Hypernatraemia, defined as serum sodium of greater than 145 mmol/litre, is a commonly encountered problem. It occurs when water intake is inadequate to keep up with water losses, and, since the thirst mechanism is such a powerful stimulus, restricted access to water is nearly always necessary for its development. This occurs in a variety of settings, usually in the very young or very old, or in patients whose illness inhibits their access to water.

Several other clinical factors typically seen in the hospital setting can contribute to hypernatraemia, including water losses due to solute diuresis (typically urea or glucose), loop diuretics, gastrointestinal fluid losses, and excessive hypertonic sodium bicarbonate administration. Most patients who develop hypernatraemia have some combination of factors that lead to both impaired access to water and ongoing free-water losses. Hypernatraemia is common in the hospital setting and is frequently iatrogenic during critical illness, typically involving the failure to recognize significant water losses in the urine and to provide the appropriate amount of replacement in either parenteral or enteral solutions.

Pathogenesis

When water intake falls below the level of ongoing water losses, the relative amount of exchangeable electrolytes in the body compared with water increases, and this leads to hypernatraemia. The thirst mechanism and the kidney's ability to concentrate the urine are the defences against this. However, in patients with normal mental status it is rare for hypernatraemia to develop, irrespective of the degree of ongoing water losses, if access to water is not limited because the thirst mechanism will lead to increased water intake to match ongoing losses. The common causes of hypernatraemia are shown in Box 21.2.1.2.

Hypernatraemia leads to osmolar forces that cause movement of water out of cells, which in particular subjects the brain to stress that can lead to significant damage. The brain attempts to counteract the osmolar stress during hypernatraemia through a series of adaptations, the principal among these being accumulation of osmotically active ions and *de novo* generation of osmotically active idiogenic osmoles. The earliest response involves accumulation of the osmotically active cations sodium and potassium. Idiogenic osmoles are a heterogeneous group of substances—including glycerophosphocholine, choline, myoinositol, and sorbitol—that are generated intracellularly to exert an osmotic effect and counteract osmotic forces favouring water removal from the cells. These responses are seen very quickly, and after 1 week of hypernatraemia no further changes in brain osmolality are observed. They serve to maintain brain volume during elevations in serum osmolality and prevent significant decrease in brain size due to osmotic water losses. During correction of chronic hypernatraemia it must noted that idiogenic osmoles are not rapidly dissipated, and correction of

---

Box 21.2.1.2 Common causes of hypernatraemia

Lack of water intake

- Decreased thirst, e.g. dementia, neurological impairment
- Bowel rest/nasogastric suction
- Dependent on others, e.g. mechanical ventilation, infants

Increased water losses

- Solute diuresis, e.g. hyperglycaemia, urea loading from tube feeds, or hyperalimentation
- Loop diuretics
- Gastrointestinal water losses
- Diabetes insipidus

chronic hypernatraemia over 24 h can lead to cerebral oedema. For this reason, chronic hypernatraemia should be treated cautiously to prevent the development of cerebral oedema.

Clinical manifestations

Clinical manifestations are mainly related to central nervous system dysfunction as cerebral dehydration and cell shrinkage occurs. Hypernatraemia, perhaps owing to the underlying conditions that lead to its development, is associated with an overall mortality between 40 and 70%. Groups at particular risk for complications and poor outcomes from hypernatraemia are older people and patients with endstage liver disease. In the latter case, the use of lactulose in the treatment of hepatic encephalopathy frequently leads to an osmotic diarrhoea and significant water losses in the stool: if this is not appreciated and free water is not given (many encephalopathic patients are obtunded and unable to drink), then hypernatraemia can develop quickly and lead to severe morbidity. It is therefore mandatory to monitor the serum electrolytes closely in this setting, particularly given that patients with liver disease are at increased risk for cerebral demyelination during changes in the serum sodium.

Diagnostic approach to hypernatraemic patients

The first step in evaluating a patient with hypernatraemia is to take a detailed history focusing on fluid intake and losses. Various potential sources of water loss need to be assessed. This is generally straightforward in the outpatient setting, where these are mainly in the urine, but in the patient in hospital many sources of water losses may need to be considered (Fig. 21.2.1.7): from the gastrointestinal tract (diarrhoea, nasogastric suction, bowel fistulae), from the urine, and from insensible losses (fever, sepsis, massive diaphoresis, burns). Whenever practical, these losses should be calculated or estimated. To assess urinary water losses it is necessary to measure the urinary cationic electrolytes (sodium and potassium) and the urinary osmolality, these pieces of information giving complementary but different information. However, a word of caution is necessary in the interpretation of urinary osmolality as errors are frequent in this area. The urinary osmolality alone cannot always determine the presence or absence of electrolyte-free water losses in the urine, the reason for this being that water can be excreted with nonelectrolyte osmoles or with electrolyte osmoles. Both of these contribute to the osmolality of the urine, but their excretion will have different effects on water balance. Recall the relationship that the serum sodium is proportional to

total body electrolytes relative to total body water (Equation 21.2.1.1). Therefore, when water is excreted with very few electrolytes, the loss of water is in excess of the loss of electrolytes and hypernatraemia can develop if this water is not adequately replaced. This situation of a high urine osmolality, but very few electrolytes in the urine, most typically occurs when there is a significant amount of urea or glucose (e.g. with poorly controlled diabetes) in the urine. By contrast, when water is excreted with a significant amount of electrolyte osmoles, this will tend not to affect the serum sodium, as long as the concentration of electrolytes in the urine and serum are similar, because loss of water is proportional to the loss of electrolytes and therefore the value of the serum sodium does not change.

When there is a high urea or glucose load, tremendous quantities of water can be lost in the urine despite maximal urinary concentration. This is what occurs during a solute diuresis and such a patient is typically polyuric. However, if there is a failure to concentrate the urine during a time of hypernatraemia when the patient does not have a solute diuresis, then this should raise suspicion of a urinary concentrating defect. The most common causes of such urinary concentrating defects are renal failure, loop diuretics, tubulointerstitial renal disease, and diabetes insipidus.

Treatment of hypernatraemia

Patients with hypernatraemia typically have significant intravascular volume depletion, hence the initial goal of treatment is to restore this, which is best accomplished with 0.9% saline or colloid. Focus then switches to correction of the serum sodium with free-water replacement (Box 21.2.1.3). The rate of fluid administration required by the patient will depend significantly on the degree of ongoing water losses, so that the appropriate amount of replacement water can be given for these in addition to that required for correction of the hypernatraemic state. If there are extrarenal fluid losses, these will need to be estimated because accurate monitoring is typically not possible, and it is necessary to assess any ongoing water losses in the urine to determine whether the kidneys are appropriately conserving water, or whether they are inappropriately continuing to excrete it. As described previously, electrolyte-free water losses in the urine can be calculated with the formula:

$$[1-([Na^+]_u + [K^+]_u)/([Na^+]_{se} + [K^+]_{se})] \times \text{urinay output rate (ml)}$$
$$= \text{rate of urinary water loss}$$

where $[Na^+]_u$ is urinary sodium concentration, $[K^+]_u$ is urinary potassium concentration, $[Na^+]_{se}$ is serum sodium concentration, and $[K^+]_{se}$ is serum potassium concentration.

Patients with hypernatraemia may be insulin resistant such that hyperglycaemia can result if dextrose-containing solutions are given. For this reason, glucose-containing solutions are potentially harmful and should be avoided if possible, but if they must be used (e.g. 5% dextrose in water), then plasma glucose should be monitored closely. When possible, the enteral route should be used before use of parenteral fluid administration.

As with the treatment of patients with symptomatic hyponatraemia, patients with neurological impairment due to hypernatraemia require serial measurement of electrolytes, every 2 h, until they are neurologically stable. In patients without evidence of

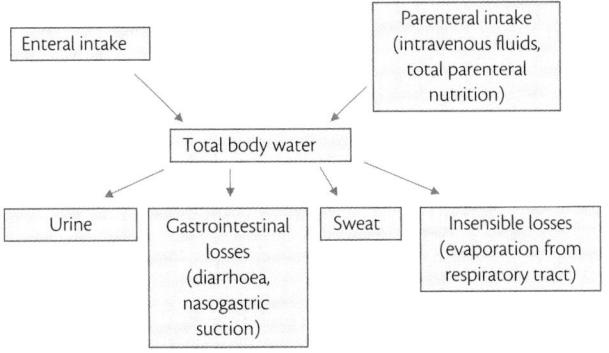

Fig. 21.2.1.7 Sources of water intake and loss.

Box 21.2.1.3 Treatment of hypernatraemia

1 Correct deficit of intravascular volume with colloid solution, 0.9% saline, or plasma—infuse rapidly until postural hypotension is abolished and the jugular venous pulse can be seen at the base of the neck.

2 Estimate water deficit—because of the many variables in clinical practice, there is no sense in trying to make a very precise estimate of the patient's water deficit, but in very approximate terms this is equal to [(serum sodium concentration −140)/140] × total body water. For total body water, 0.5 × body weight is a close enough working approximation. Hence an 80-kg man with serum sodium of 160 mmol/litre has a water deficit of [(160 − 140)/140] × 40 = 5.7 litres.

3 Replacement of ongoing water losses, estimated as described in the text, will be required in addition to that required to correct deficit.

4 Aim of treatment—to decrease serum sodium concentration by 0.5–1 mmol/litre per hour and by no more than 15 mmol/litre in the first 24 h. In severe hypernatraemia (>170 mmol/litre), serum sodium should not be corrected to below 150 mmol/litre in the first 48–72 h.

5 Give hypotonic fluid:

  a. Route and fluid—preferably water by mouth or nasogastric tube (or other feeding tube), but if parenteral treatment is required the usual replacement fluid is 0.45% saline (77 mmol/litre NaCl); a lower sodium concentration may be needed if there is a renal concentrating defect or sodium overload. Glucose-containing solutions should be avoided.

  b. Volume—using the incorrect assumption of a closed system (see discussion of treatment for hyponatraemia), and using the example described above in this box, to reduce the patient's serum sodium by 10 mmol/litre in the first 24 h would require administration of (10/140) × 40 = 2.85 litres of water in addition to fluids required to accommodate ongoing loses. This could be administered as water by drinking or by feeding tube, or by intravenous infusion of twice the volume of 0.45% saline (given 77 mmol/litre NaCl, half of the volume of a bag of 0.45% saline can be regarded as 'free water'). In practice, if the patient cannot drink freely, does not have a feeding tube, and it is not possible or desirable to place one, then it is reasonable to give 0.45% saline at 250 ml/h, adjusting the rate appropriately in response to repeated monitoring. If 5% dextrose is used (125 ml/h, all of which can be regarded as 'free water'), then it is essential to monitor blood glucose regularly.

6 Monitoring—serum electrolytes should be measured every 2 h until the patient is neurologically stable, and every 4 h while they remain on an intravenous infusion of hypotonic saline or 5% dextrose.

---

encephalopathy, the serum sodium should not be corrected more quickly than 0.5 to 1 mmol/litre per hour or 15 mmol/litre over 24 h, and, in severe cases (serum sodium above 170 mmol/litre), sodium should not be corrected to below 150 mmol/litre in the first 48 to 72 h.

Case discussions

The evaluation of a polyuric patient and differentiation of primary polydipsia, central diabetes insipidus, nephrogenic diabetes insipidus (Table 21.2.1.2), and hypernatraemia due to a solute diuresis can be complex and daunting to the general physician, but should be approached as described in the following case studies.

Case 6: primary polydipsia

A 27-year-old man with schizophrenia is being evaluated prior to admission to a psychiatric hospital. His only complaint is of frequent urination, approximately 15 times per day according to his family, and that he is always thirsty. He has had no recent seizures and his level of consciousness is normal. Routine physical examination is unremarkable. Laboratory values are as follows:

1 serum—sodium 131 mmol/litre, potassium 4.0 mmol/litre, chloride 96 mmol/litre, bicarbonate 24 mmol/litre, urea 5.7 mmol/litre (16 mg/dl), creatinine 118 μmol/litre (1.3 mg/dl), glucose 5.4 mmol/litre (98 mg/dl)

2 urine—sodium 10 mmol/litre, potassium 8 mmol/litre, osmolality 65 mOsm/kg

Discussion

This patient is very likely to be polyuric, given the history. Blood tests reveal mild hyponatraemia and near-normal renal function (CKD stage 3). Urinary parameters are consistent with a water diuresis. Calculation of the electrolyte-free water clearance shows that he is losing significant amounts of water in the urine (Equation 21.2.1.2): $([Na^+]_u + [K^+]_u)/([Na^+]_{se} + [K^+]_{se}) = (10 + 8)/(131 + 4) = 0.13$. This means that 87% of the patient's urine output is electrolyte-free water. The low urinary osmolality signifies that this is a water diuresis, rather than being driven by the presence of nonelectrolyte solute, e.g. glucose.

The question now becomes whether the water diuresis is an appropriate response to excessive water intake or whether it is is pathological, leading to excessive water losses that must then be replaced. In this case, the most likely answer is excessive water intake because of the hyponatraemia and decreased serum osmolality. If a urine concentrating defect were the primary cause of the polyuria, then the patient should not be hyponatraemic unless they had both a urinary concentrating defect and excessive water intake.

Case 7: primary polydipsia vs diabetes insipidus

A 39-year-old mother is concerned because her 12-year-old daughter has noted frequent urination and says that she is always thirsty. The patient is a well-adjusted adolescent with no past medical history and normal development up to this point. Her physical examination is normal. She also has had no recent seizures and her level of consciousness is normal. Serum electrolytes and the results of a 24-h urinary collection are as follows:

◆ serum—sodium 140 mmol/litre, potassium 4.5 mmol/litre, chloride 103 mmol/litre, bicarbonate 25 mmol/litre, urea

Table 21.2.1.2 Causes of polyuria-polydipsia syndromes

Cranial diabetes insipidus

Familial

Autosomal dominant inheritance

DIDMOAD* (autosomal recessive)

Acquired

Idiopathic

Inflammatory (lymphophocytic infiltration, sarcoidosis, histiocytosis X autoimmunity, Guillain Barré syndrome)

Trauma (neurosurgery, head injury)

Neoplasmsa (craniopharyngioma, germinoma, pinealoma, hypothalamic metastasis, large pituitary tumour)

Infection (meningitis, encephalitis)

Vascular (sickle cell anaemia, aneurysms of anterior communicating artery, Sheehan's syndrome)

Pregnancy (associated with vasopressinase)

Nephrogenic diabetes insipidus

Familial

X-linked inheritance

Autosomal recessive inheritance

Acquired

Idiopathic

Metabolic (hypercalcaemia, hypokalaemia)

Vascular (sickle cell disease)

Osmotic diuresis (glycosuria, post-obstructive uropathy)

Chronic renal disease (renal failure, amyloid, myeloma, sarcoidosis, pyelonephritis)

Drugs (lithium, demeclocycline, amphotercin, glibenclamide, methofluorane)

Primary polydipsia

Unknown aetiology

Psychogenic (compulsive water drinking)

Psychotic (schizophrenia, mania)

Idiopathic

Secondary

Granuloma (sarcoidosis)

Vasculitis

TB meningitis

Multiple sclerosis

Drugs (phenothiazines, tricyclic antidepressants)

*DIDMOAD=diabetes insipidus, diabetes mellitus, optic atrophy, deafness (Wolfram syndrome).

5.4 mmol/litre (15 mg/dl), creatinine 109 μmol/litre (1.2 mg/dl), glucose 5.7 mmol/litre (103 mg/dl)

• urine (24 h)—total volume 9 litres, sodium 15 mmol/litre, potassium 8 mmol/litre, osmolality 70 mOsm/kg

Discussion

The 24-h urinary collection volume clearly demonstrates that this girl is polyuric, and the urinary studies—similar to Case 6—are consistent with a water diuresis. However, the patient is normonatraemic and thus the serum electrolytes are not helpful in reaching a diagnosis: based on the information that we currently have, it is impossible to tell whether her polyuria is due to excessive water

intake or to a urinary concentrating defect, which is an important determination to make in this seemingly healthy adolescent. In order to distinguish between these two possibilities, a water deprivation test can be performed. This is usually done in a hospital setting because a patient with diabetes insipidus can rapidly develop hypernatraemia if water intake is restricted. The details of different protocols for water deprivation tests are beyond the scope of this chapter, but a typical test and its interpretation are shown in Box 21.2.1.4, the basic principle being that if a patient with diabetes insipidus is deprived of water and allowed to become mildly hypernatraemic, then such a patient will not have concentrated urine at that time. By contrast, a patient with primary polydipsia will begin to concentrate the urine if allowed to become mildly hypernatraemic.

Box 21.2.1.4 Procedure and interpretation of a water deprivation test

Procedure

1 The patient is encouraged to drink normally in the evening/night before the test.

2 In the morning, at the beginning of the test, the patient is weighed and baseline measurements made of urinary volume, and urinary and serum osmolality.

3 All fluid intake is withheld for 8 h, with the patient weighed and urine and blood samples taken and analysed every 1–2 h. The test is stopped if the patient loses more than 5% of their initial body weight, or if urinary osmolality above 750 mOsm/kg is achieved.

4 DDAVP (2 μg) is given by intramuscular injection, and the patient is allowed to drink (sensibly) and eat.

5 Urinary samples are collected for the next 16 h.

Interpretation

Urine osmolality (mOsm/kg)		Diagnosis
After dehydration	After DDAVP	
>750	>750	Normala
<300	>750	Cranial diabetes insipidus
<300	<300	Nephrogenic diabetes insipidus
300–750	<750	Partial cranial diabetes insipidus, partial nephrogenic diabetes insipidus, or primary polydipsiab,c

DDAVP, deamino-d-arginine vasopressin.
a Assuming that serum osmolality remains in the normal reference range of 285–295 mOsm/kg.
b The distinction of cranial or nephrogenic partial diabetes insipidus from each other and from primary polydipsia is difficult; measurement of plasma ADH may help in this circumstance.
c Assuming significant urinary output, if the patient does not lose weight over 8 h and serum osmolality does not rise, then they must be drinking. The period of 'water deprivation' can be extended, but this is unlikely to be helpful if the patient has not abstained from drinking from the beginning of the test. In this situation, a hypertonic saline infusion test may be helpful. The diagnosis is likely to be primary polydipsia, but it may be difficult, if not impossible, to exclude mixed pathology.

Case 8: nephrogenic diabetes insipidus

A 41-year-old man presents for a routine physical examination. His past medical history is significant only for bipolar disorder, for which he has taken lithium carbonate for the last 15 years. This information leads to further questioning, and he admits to frequent urination and excessive thirst, but denies any symptoms of hesitancy or dysuria. His physical examination is normal. Serum chemistry profile and urine studies are as follows:

- serum—sodium 147 mmol/litre, potassium 3.8 mmol/litre, chloride 110 mmol/litre, bicarbonate 26 mmol/litre, urea 5.4 mmol/litre (15 mg/dl), creatinine 73 μmol/litre (0.8 mg/dl), glucose 6.9 mmol/litre (124 mg/dl)

- urine—sodium 25 mmol/litre, potassium 22 mmol/litre, osmolality 160 mOsm/kg

Discussion

The laboratory data in this case are most consistent with diabetes insipidus. The history suggests polyuria, and, as nephrogenic diabetes insipidus is a complication of lithium therapy, it is appropriate to rule out this diagnosis in a patient such as this. In contrast with Case 7, we have a definite differentiation between primary polydipsia and diabetes insipidus because the serum sodium is mildly elevated and the urinary osmolality is simultaneously low, which confirms the diagnosis of diabetes insipidus. In a sense, by demonstrating the failure to concentrate the urine despite having hypernatraemia, we have the results of a water deprivation test. However, it is important to note that—based solely on the information given above—it is not known whether the patient has central or nephrogenic diabetes insipidus, although the latter would clearly be anticipated in a patient taking lithium. To make this distinction would require formalized testing to assess the response to exogenously administered DDAVP: if the patient fails to concentrate the urine following administration of DDAVP, then they have nephrogenic diabetes insipidus.

Case 9: central diabetes insipidus

A 28-year-old man is brought to the Emergency Department by ambulance following a car accident during which he sustained severe head trauma. His past medical history is significant only for asthma as a child and a previous appendicectomy. He is taken immediately to surgery for evacuation of an acute epidural haematoma. During the course of surgery, his urinary output increases from 35 ml/h to over 300 ml/h. Blood tests taken immediately on admission to hospital reveal serum sodium 141 mmol/litre; the findings on serum chemistry profile and urine studies taken just after surgery when he arrives on the intensive care unit are as follows:

- serum—sodium 148 mmol/litre, potassium 4.5 mmol/litre, chloride 112 mmol/litre, bicarbonate 26 mmol/litre, urea 6.8 mmol/litre (19 mg/dl), creatinine 127 μmol/litre (1.4 mg/dl), glucose 6.4 mmol/litre (115 mg/dl)

- urine—sodium 17 mmol/litre, potassium 13 mmol/litre, osmolality 120 mOsm/kg

Discussion

The history is highly suggestive of central diabetes insipidus due to head trauma as the cause of polyuria. The urinary studies, as in the three previous cases, show a water diuresis, and, as in Case 8, we have a definite diagnosis of diabetes insipidus because the patient is simultaneously hypernatraemic and undergoing a water diuresis. Again, based solely on the information above, it is not possible to say whether the patient has central or nephrogenic diabetes insipidus, but since the history is so suggestive of a central cause it is prudent to simply administer DDAVP and assess the response. If the patient fails to concentrate the urine following administration of DDAVP, then he has nephrogenic diabetes insipidus, whereas if the urine becomes concentrated—as would be anticipated in this case—then the diagnosis is central diabetes insipidus. When DDAVP is administered, water intake should be adjusted appropriately to avoid precipitation of significant hyponatraemia, and serum electrolytes should be monitored closely during dose titration.

Central diabetes insipidus should always be suspected when the urine is not concentrated in the setting of hypernatraemia. Severe hypernatraemia can develop rapidly in an individual who has restricted access to fluids, such as a patient in an intensive care unit, and hence early recognition is vital.

Case 10: solute diuresis from excess urea load

A 58-year-old man with long history of alcohol abuse and chronic liver disease is admitted with necrotizing pancreatitis. Among other manoeuvres, a urinary catheter is inserted, which demonstrates that his urinary output is 30 ml/h. Admission laboratory test results are as follows:

- serum—sodium 138 mmol/litre, potassium 3.9 mmol/litre, chloride 103 mmol/litre, bicarbonate 21 mmol/litre, urea 11.8 mmol/litre (33 mg/dl), creatinine 136 μmol/litre (1.5 mg/dl)

The patient is ordered to have no enteral intake overnight, and he receives 5 litres of 0.9% (normal) saline volume expansion. His abdominal pain worsens 24 h after admission and he is continued without enteral intake. Repeat laboratory tests show that his serum sodium has risen to 146 mmol/litre. Over the following 24 h his urinary output increases and infusion of 0.9% saline is continued at 100 ml/h. Total parenteral nutrition is initiated with a daily regimen that comprises a total volume of 1.5 litres, including 120 mmol of sodium and high amino acid content. Repeat laboratory tests are as follows:

- serum—sodium 151 mmol/litre, potassium 3.2 mmol/litre, chloride 117 mmol/litre, bicarbonate 26 mmol/litre, urea 22.5 mmol/litre (63 mg/dl), creatinine 100 μmol/litre (1.1 mg/dl), glucose 7.0 mmol/litre (126 mg/dl)

- urine—volume 150 ml/hour; sodium 50 mmol/litre, potassium 13 mmol/litre, osmolality 650 mOsm/kg

Discussion

What has occurred in this case is very typical of a solute diuresis leading to hypernatraemia in the critical care setting. The patient is significantly polyuric and has become progressively more and more hypernatraemic. It is important to recognize that, in contrast to previous cases discussed, the urinary osmolality is high, meaning that ADH activity is present and it must be concluded that the patient is losing 'free water' (which has to be the situation because the serum sodium is increasing in the absence of administration of any hypertonic sodium solution).

The loss of free water occurring at the same time that the urine is highly concentrated may appear paradoxical, but the answer is evident when the electrolyte-free water is calculated. The ratio of the (sodium + potassium) in the urine to the (sodium + potassium) in the serum is $63/159 = 0.39$, hence at his current urinary output he is losing water at a rate of (0.61×150) or $91.5\,ml/h$. Water replacement must be given at least equal to this rate to replace the ongoing urinary water losses. The low urinary sodium and potassium at a time when the urine osmolality is high signifies that there must be a nonelectrolyte osmole in the urine that is 'obligating' water loss. The patient is undergoing an osmotic diuresis secondary to a high urea load, this probably being secondary both to the hypercatabolic state of critical illness/stress (protein breakdown is increased, leading to significant urea generation) and to the high amino acid content of the total parenteral nutrition. This scenario is commonly seen in critical illness and is easily preventable if the responsible clinician appreciates the possibility of free-water loss in a patient who becomes polyuric.

Further reading

Abbott NJ, Ronnback L, Hansson E (2006). Astrocyte–endothelial interactions at the blood–brain barrier. *Nat Rev Neurosci*, **7**, 41–53.

Achinger SG, Moritz ML, Ayus JC (2006). Dysnatremias: why are patients still dying? *South Med J*, **99**, 1–12.

Agre P, *et al.* (1993). Aquaporin CHIP: the archetypal molecular water channel. *Am J Physiol*, **265**, F463–76.

Amiry-Moghaddam M, Ottersen OP (2003). The molecular basis of water transport in the brain. *Nat Rev Neurosci*, **4**, 991–1001.

Arieff AI, Ayus JC (1993). Endometrial ablation complicated by fatal hyponatremic encephalopathy. *JAMA*, **270**, 1230–2.

Arieff AI, Ayus JC (1993). Pathogenesis of hyponatremic encephalopathy. Current concepts. *Chest*, **103**, 607–10.

Arieff AI, Ayus JC, Fraser CL (1992). Hyponatraemia and death or permanent brain damage in healthy children. *BMJ*, **304**, 1218–22.

Ayus JC, Achinger SG, Arieff AI (2008). Brain cell volume regulation in hyponatremia: role of sex age, vasopressin, and hypoxia. *Am J Renal Physiol*, **295**, F619–F624.

Ayus JC, Arieff AI (1995). Pulmonary complications of hyponatremic encephalopathy. Noncardiogenic pulmonary edema and hypercapnic respiratory failure. *Chest*, **107**, 517–21.

Ayus JC, Arieff AI (1999). Chronic hyponatremic encephalopathy in postmenopausal women: association of therapies with morbidity and mortality. *JAMA*, **281**, 2299–304.

Ayus JC, Armstrong D, Arieff A (2006). Hyponatremia with hypoxia: effects on brain adaptation, perfusion and histology in rodents. *Kidney Int*, **69**, 1319–25.

Ayus JC, Krothapalli RK, Arieff AI (1987). Treatment of symptomatic hyponatremia and its relation to brain damage. A prospective study. *N Engl J Med*, **317**, 1190–5.

Ayus JC, Moritz ML (2010). Bone Disease as a New Complication of Hyponatremia: Moving Beyond Brain Injury. *Clin J Am Soc Nephrol*, F1–F2.

Ayus JC, Varon J, Arieff AI (2000). Hyponatremia, cerebral edema, and noncardiogenic pulmonary edema in marathon runners. *Ann Intern Med*, **132**, 711–14.

Ayus JC, Wheeler JM, Arieff AI (1992). Postoperative hyponatremic encephalopathy in menstruant women. *Ann Intern Med*, **117**, 891–7.

Dolman D, *et al.* (2005). Induction of aquaporin 1 but not aquaporin 4 messenger RNA in rat primary brain microvessel endothelial cells in culture. *J Neurochem*, **93**, 825–33.

Heilig CW, *et al.* (1989). Characterization of the major brain osmolytes that accumulate in salt-loaded rats. *Am J Physiol*, **257**, F1108–16.

Hew-Butler T, *et al.* (2005). Consensus statement of the 1st International Exercise-Associated Hyponatremia Consensus Development Conference, Cape Town, South Africa 2005. *Clin J Sport Med*, **15**, 208–13.

Lien YH, Shapiro JI, Chan L (1990). Effects of hypernatremia on organic brain osmoles. *J Clin Invest*, **85**, 1427–35.

Manley GT, *et al.* (2000). Aquaporin-4 deletion in mice reduces brain edema after acute water intoxication and ischemic stroke. *Nat Med*, **6**, 159–63.

Moritz ML, Ayus JC (1999). The changing pattern of hypernatremia in hospitalized children. *Pediatrics*, **104**, 435–9.

Moritz ML, Ayus JC (2003). Prevention of hospital-acquired hyponatremia: a case for using isotonic saline. *Pediatrics*, **111**, 227–30.

Moritz ML, Ayus JC (2003). The pathophysiology and treatment of hyponatraemic encephalopathy: an update. *Nephrol Dial Transplant*, **18**, 2486–91.

Moritz ML, Ayus JC (2004). Dysnatremias in the critical care setting. *Contrib Nephrol*, **144**, 132–57.

Moritz ML, Ayus JC (2005). Preventing neurological complications from dysnatremias in children. *Pediatr Nephrol*, **20**, 1687–700.

Nielsen S, *et al.* (1997). Specialized membrane domains for water transport in glial cells: high-resolution immolunogold cytochemistry of aquaporin-4 in rat brain. *J Neurosci*, **17**, 171–80.

Nzerue CM, *et al.* (2003). Predictors of outcome in hospitalized patients with severe hyponatremia. *J Natl Med Assoc*, **95**, 335–43.

Papadopoulos MC, Verkman AS. Aquaporin-4 and brain edema. *Pediatr Nephrol*, **22**, 778–84.

Schrier RW, *et al.* (2006). Tolvaptan, a selective oral vasopressin V2-receptor antagonist, for hyponatremia. *N Engl J Med*, **355**, 2099–112.

Simard M, Nedergaard M (2004). The neurobiology of glia in the context of water and ion homeostasis. *Neuroscience*, **129**, 877–96.

21.2.2 Disorders of potassium homeostasis

John D. Firth

Essentials

The normal range of potassium concentration in serum is 3.5 to 5.0 mmol/litre and within cells it is 150 to 160 mmol/litre, the ratio of intracellular to extracellular potassium concentration being a critical determinant of cellular resting membrane potential and thereby of the function of excitable tissues.

Hypokalaemia

Hypokalaemia is defined as serum potassium concentration lower than 3.5 mmol/litre, which is the most common electrolyte abnormality seen in clinical practice, found in about 20% of hospital inpatients.

Clinical features and investigation—mild hypokalaemia is asymptomatic, but a variety of nonspecific symptoms develop with more severe disturbance, and serious neuromuscular problems sometimes arise at serum potassium concentration lower than 2.5 mmol/litre.

Extensive testing of patients with mild hypokalaemia is almost certainly inappropriate and likely to be fruitless if pursued.

Emergency management—this is rarely required, but intravenous infusion of potassium (maximum 1 mmol/min by volumetric pump, with close monitoring) should be given in the rare circumstances of life-threatening cardiac arrhythmia or muscular paralysis.

Aetiology—there are a very large number of possible causes of hypokalaemia, but in most instances the diagnosis is immediately apparent, the most common causes being: (1) diuretics—particularly thiazides; (2) vomiting—where the renal response to metabolic alkalosis leads to hypokalaemia due to renal loss of potassium; and (3) diarrhoea—with direct loss of potassium in stool. Patients with unexplained severe hypokalaemia are a considerable challenge for both diagnosis and management, with the differential diagnosis usually comprising: (1) various abnormalities of tubular potassium transport; (2) concealed vomiting and/or usage of purgatives—which are strongly supported by the finding of a low plasma chloride concentration with the virtual absence of chloride from the urine; and (3) concealed ingestion of diuretics—which should be tested for if urinary chloride is greater than 20 mmol/litre.

Renal tubular causes of hypokalaemia—the most common genetic cause is Gitelman's syndrome, an autosomal recessive condition caused by mutations in the Na–Cl cotransporter (NCCT) in the distal convoluted tubule. It may be asymptomatic, but can cause nonspecific symptoms, and is associated with hypotension, alkalosis, hypomagnesaemia, hypocalciuria, and hypermagnesuria. Management is with potassium and magnesium supplements. Other causes of tubular wasting of potassium include: (1) Bartter's syndrome—four types are recognized, due to mutations in different tubular cotransporters, channels, or associated proteins (NKCC2, ROMK, CLCNKA, CLCNKB, and barttin); and (2) mineralocorticoid excess—real or apparent, each of various types.

Altered internal balance causing hypokalaemia—there are several rare conditions in which hypokalaemia is associated with episodes of extreme weakness/paralysis, including: (1) thyrotoxic periodic paralysis—mainly affects Asian men; attacks are treated with β-blocker (propranolol) and prevented by treatment of hyperthyroidism; and (2) familial hypokalaemic periodic paralysis—caused by mutations in one of three genes (*CACNL1A3*, *SCN4A*, and *KCNE3*); attacks are treated with intravenous potassium and prevented by carbonic anhydrase inhibitor (dichlorphenamide).

Hyperkalaemia

Hyperkalaemia, defined as serum potassium concentration of greater than 5.0 mmol/litre, is asymptomatic, and severe hyperkalaemia (>7 mmol/litre) is the most serious of all electrolyte disorders because it can cause cardiac arrest.

Clinical assessment—the electrocardiogram (ECG) is the best guide to the significance of hyperkalaemia in any particular individual—as the serum potassium rises the following changes are seen: (1) tenting of the T wave; (2) P-wave flattening, prolongation of the P–R interval, and widening of the QRS complex; and (3) a 'sine wave' pattern as a prelude to ventricular fibrillation and death.

Emergency management—patients with ECG manifestations more severe than tenting of the T waves should be given intravenous calcium gluconate (10 ml of 10%) followed by intravenous insulin and glucose, or nebulized salbutamol (see Chapter 21.5 for further discussion).

Aetiology—there are many causes of hyperkalaemia, but by far the most common are: (1) renal failure—acute kidney injury or chronic kidney disease; and/or (2) drugs—in particular potassium supplements, potassium-sparing diuretics, angiotensin converting enzyme (ACE) inhibitors, and angiotensin II receptor blockers.

Other causes of hyperkalaemia—these include: (1) hyporeninaemic hypoaldosteronism—patients with tubulointerstitial renal disease or diabetes often have a high serum potassium despite a glomerular filtration rate (GFR) that should be sufficient to maintain normokalaemia; the reason for this is not known, and diagnostic criteria are not well defined; treatment is with dietary potassium restriction and avoidance of drugs that can cause hyperkalaemia; (2) other drugs—nonsteroidal anti-inflammatory agents, heparin, calcineurin inhibitors, and trimethoprim–sulfamethoxazole; and (3) renal transport abnormalities—type IV renal tubular acidosis and pseudohypoaldosteronism types 1 and 2 (Gordon's syndrome).

Altered internal balance causing hyperkalaemia: (1) exhaustive exercise; (2) acidosis; (3) drugs—including digoxin and depolarizing muscle relaxants; and (4) hyperkalaemic periodic paralysis (very rare).

Potassium homeostasis

Potassium is the most abundant cation in the body. Total body potassium ranges between 37 and 52 mmol/kg body weight, and of this 98% is found within cells, where its concentration is 150 to 160 mmol/litre. By contrast, the normal range of potassium concentration in serum is 3.5 to 5.0 mmol/litre. The ratio of intracellular to extracellular potassium concentration is a critical determinant of cellular resting membrane potential and thereby of the function of excitable tissues, particularly the nerves and muscles. Potassium tends to leak out of cells through a variety of ion-selective potassium channels found in all cell membranes. The maintenance of the intracellular to extracellular gradient is largely dependent on the ubiquitous enzyme Na$^+$,K$^+$-ATPase, which pumps two potassium ions into the cell for every three sodium ions extruded.

The mechanisms of potassium homeostasis can be considered in terms of internal balance (the relationship between intracellular and extracellular potassium concentration) and external balance (which determines total body potassium).

Internal balance

A wide variety of factors modulate the distribution of potassium between the intracellular and extracellular fluid compartments. These factors either alter the function of the Na$^+$,K$^+$-ATPase or the rate of efflux of potassium from cells, which together dictate intracellular potassium concentration. In view of the importance of the ratio of internal to external potassium concentration for critical neuromuscular functions, some of these mechanisms serve as essential acute defence mechanisms to counteract life-threatening hyperkalaemia. Factors modulating internal potassium balance are shown in Box 21.2.2.1.

Box 21.2.2.1 Factors modulating internal potassium balance

Acid–base status

Acidosis (excepting renal tubular acidosis) tends to diminish potassium uptake by cells and to cause hyperkalaemia; alkalosis has the opposite effect. The relationship between pH and serum potassium is not simple, but in metabolic acidosis the serum potassium can rise by up to 0.7 mmol/litre for each 0.1 unit fall in blood pH, and alkalosis reduces serum potassium by up to 0.3 mmol/litre per 0.1 pH unit rise.

Pancreatic hormones

Insulin release is stimulated by hyperkalaemia and inhibited by hypokalaemia. It induces cellular uptake of potassium by activating the Na^+, K^+-ATPase directly. Glucagon can increase serum potassium concentration.

Catecholamines

β_2-Adrenergic agonists promote cellular potassium uptake by activating the Na^+, K^+-ATPase via a cAMP-dependent mechanism. α-Adrenergic agonists have the opposite effect.

Exercise

Exercise results in loss of potassium from muscle cells, which causes local vasodilatation and increases regional blood flow. Serum potassium can increase by as much as 50% after 10 to 15 min of vigorous exercise, falling precipitately in the recovery period.

Aldosterone

The most important actions of aldosterone are on external balance, but there is also evidence of effect on internal balance.

Osmolality

Hyperosmolality increases the serum potassium concentration.

Total body potassium

The distribution of potassium between intracellular and extracellular compartments is influenced by the total amount of potassium in the body. Changes in the extracellular compartment are always proportionately greater than those in the intracellular compartment. The mechanisms are not known.

External balance

Dietary potassium intake in people in Western societies typically varies between 50 and 150 mmol/day, but balance can be attained with intake of up to 500 mmol/day if homeostatic mechanisms are intact. In normal circumstances potassium excretion in the stool is not regulated, but amounts to only 5 to 15 mmol/day. When renal function is compromised, the absolute magnitude as well as the proportion of potassium in the faeces is increased, but variation in renal excretion of potassium is usually the only means by which the body achieves external potassium balance by ensuring that excretion equals intake.

With normal intake of potassium, 10 to 20% of the potassium filtered at the glomerulus is excreted, but fractional excretion of potassium can vary from 1% when intake is restricted to over 100% when intake is excessive. Micropuncture studies have shown that the amount of potassium reaching the distal convoluted tubule does not vary in these circumstances, indicating that

---

Box 21.2.2.2 Factors that modify potassium excretion by the distal nephron

Aldosterone

Aldosterone is the dominant hormone regulating potassium homeostasis. An increase in serum potassium directly stimulates aldosterone secretion by the adrenal glands. In the principal cells of the collecting ducts, aldosterone binds to its intracellular mineralocorticoid receptor, is translocated to the nucleus, and induces production of basolateral Na^+, K^+-ATPase and the apical sodium channel. The effect is to increase intracellular potassium concentration and the electrochemical potential favouring potassium secretion into the tubular fluid and hence its excretion from the body. Under normal conditions, changes in sodium intake lead to changes in plasma aldosterone (an increase leading to decreased secretion) such that potassium homeostasis is preserved despite alteration in sodium and fluid delivery to the distal nephron.

Intravascular volume

Reduction of intravascular volume leads to a 'contraction alkalosis', stimulated largely by aldosterone, and which is associated with hypokalaemia.

Dietary potassium intake

Chronic alterations in dietary potassium intake induce profound modifications in the renal capacity to excrete or conserve potassium. A low-potassium diet leads to an enhanced renal capacity to conserve potassium and a high-potassium diet enhances the ability to excrete a potassium load. The mechanisms involved in these adaptations are poorly understood, although aldosterone is involved.

Serum potassium concentration

The potassium concentration gradient across the basolateral membrane modulates potassium uptake by the cell and/or passive back-leakage, hence hyperkalaemia leads to enhanced potassium excretion.

Acid–base status

Systemic pH modulates potassium uptake across the basolateral membrane and conductance of the luminal membrane, with acidosis inhibiting excretion. Chronic metabolic alkalosis is almost invariably associated with potassium depletion.

Urine flow rate

Increased flow of tubular fluid lowers potassium concentration in that fluid and favours secretion across the luminal membrane.

Sodium

Reduced delivery of sodium (<30 mmol/litre) to the distal nephron impairs potassium secretion by the cortical collecting duct.

Other factors

ADH, poorly reabsorbable anions (such as sulphates), glucocorticoids, and α-adrenergic agonists stimulate potassium secretion.

---

modulation of renal potassium excretion is normally a property of the distal nephron. Factors that modify potassium excretion by the distal nephron are shown in Box 21.2.2.2. These factors are clearly interrelated: it is rare that one is modified in isolation and the overall effect on potassium excretion is almost invariably the aggregate result of several complementary or competing stimuli.

Hypokalaemia

A low serum potassium concentration (≤ 3.5 mmol/litre) is the most common electrolyte abnormality seen in clinical practice, found in up to 20% of patients in hospital. Most have mild hypokalaemia, with serum potassium in the range 3.0 to 3.5 mmol/litre, but 5% have a level lower than 3.0 mmol/litre, and 0.03% (more in some series) have very severe hypokalaemia with serum potassium concentration less than 2.5 mmol/litre.

Clinical features

Patients with mild hypokalaemia often have no symptoms attributable to their low serum potassium concentration. A variety of nonspecific symptoms develop with more severe hypokalaemia, including lassitude, generalized weakness, and constipation. At a serum potassium level of less than 2.5 mmol/litre, serious neuromuscular problems sometimes arise. Rhabdomyolysis (see Chapter 21.5) can occur, and increases in serum creatine kinase activity indicative of muscle injury are frequently detectable in those with a serum potassium concentration below 3.0 mmol/litre. Hypokalaemia can cause intestinal ileus, and is particularly likely to do so in the postoperative period when other factors also conspire to prevent normal gut motility. Paralysis of skeletal muscle has been reported, most dramatically in cases of hypokalaemic quadraparesis, which appears to be more common in India than elsewhere. Paraesthesias and tetany have rarely been described.

Hypokalaemia can cause polyuria and polydipsia, as well as a metabolic alkalosis. Severe prolonged potassium depletion is associated with chronic interstitial nephritis, the presence of renal cysts, and the development of chronic renal failure. It is not always clear, however, whether hypokalaemia is the cause or effect of this condition.

Hypokalaemia may be suspected from the clinical context (e.g. the patient taking diuretics or vomiting copiously), but there are no specific physical signs. Alterations induced in the ECG include flattening of the T wave, depression of the ST segment, and the development of prominent U waves, which can give the impression of a prolonged QT interval. These changes, typically observed with a serum potassium concentration lower than 3.0 mmol/litre, provide a diagnostic clue to the presence of hypokalaemia, but do not have any serious clinical implications in a patient with a normal heart. However, hypokalaemia can cause problems in those whose heart is abnormal. There is a correlation between hypokalaemia and the development of ventricular tachycardia or fibrillation during the acute phase of myocardial infarction; hypokalaemia can provoke life-threatening arrhythmias in those receiving digoxin; and there is controversy as to whether the mild hypokalaemia often produced by diuretic therapy constitutes a risk factor for sudden cardiac death.

Management

In emergencies

Emergency treatment of hypokalaemia is rarely required. In the rare circumstances of life-threatening cardiac arrhythmia or muscular paralysis, intravenous infusion of potassium (usually potassium chloride) should be given immediately. This must be administered into a central vein (internal jugular, subclavian, or femoral) since solutions containing the necessary high concentration of potassium cause pain and phlebitis if given peripherally, and can cause chemical burns if they extravasate. There is no good evidence on which to base a recommendation regarding dose and rate, but the maximum rate of infusion usually employed is 1 mmol/min, which should be controlled with a volumetric pump. The main danger of giving potassium with such rapidity is the development of hyperkalaemia, hence the patient and their ECG should be observed continuously and the serum potassium checked frequently, and infusion should be slowed as soon as the life-threatening problem has resolved (arrhythmia settled, muscular power improved). In one study, administration of 40 mmol of potassium over 1 h was found to increase serum potassium concentration by an average of 1.1 mmol/litre in hypokalaemic patients with both normal and impaired renal function.

In cases that are not emergencies

In most circumstances, the management of a patient with hypokalaemia requires a methodical approach to establishing the diagnosis, which is often readily apparent (but not always so), rectification (if possible) of the underlying cause, and administration of potassium at a less hurried rate than that described above. In most cases of hypokalaemia, the fall in the serum potassium concentration represents the tip of an iceberg, a reduction of 0.3 mmol/litre typically reflecting a 100 mmol deficit in body stores. This relationship is variable, but it is important to remember that patients with even modest hypokalaemia may have a very considerable deficit of total body potassium that needs to be replaced.

Potassium can be given orally or intravenously. Foods with high potassium content are listed later in this chapter, but it should be noted that the potassium which they contain is almost entirely coupled with phosphate. In the absence of adequate chloride intake they are therefore ineffective in replenishing body potassium in the many and common causes of hypokalaemia associated with chloride depletion, such as use of diuretics or vomiting (see below for further discussion). Potassium chloride can be given in either liquid or tablet form, typically 2 to 4 g (c.25–50 mmol) daily in divided doses. Both are well absorbed, but the liquid preparations are unpalatable to many patients and slow-release tablets have been associated with gastrointestinal ulceration, bleeding, and stricture, such that they must be taken with fluid while sitting or standing and not just before retiring to bed for the night. If intravenous administration of potassium is required, infusions containing a concentration of 20 mmol/litre can usually be tolerated through a good peripheral line. If a higher concentration than this is required, central venous access will be necessary. Care must always be taken to monitor serum levels closely.

Common causes

There are a very large number of possible causes of hypokalaemia (Box 21.2.2.3), but in most instances the diagnosis is immediately apparent. Whenever this is not so, it is wise to remember that common things are the most likely, and also important to recognize that concealment of the cause is not infrequent, with diuretic abuse or covert vomiting more likely than the many more exotic and rare causes of hypokalaemia.

Box 21.2.2.3 Causes of hypokalaemia

Altered internal balance (redistribution of potassium from extracellular to intracellular compartment)

- Alkalosis
- Insulin (high doses)
- β_2-Adrenergic stimulants
- Vitamin B_{12} therapy of deficiency anaemia
- Intoxications:
  - Theophylline
  - Toluene (paint/glue sniffing)
  - Barium
- Periodic paralysis:
  - Thyrotoxic periodic paralysis
  - Sporadic periodic paralysis
  - Familial hypokalaemic periodic paralysis
- ?Aldosterone.

Altered external balance (low total body potassium)

Renal losses (urinary potassium >20 mmol/day)

- Appropriate renal response to alkalosis:
  - Vomiting[a]
- Mineralocorticoid excess:
  - Primary hyperaldosteronism (Conn's syndrome)
  - Fludrocortisone
  - Congenital adrenal hyperplasia
  - 11β-Hydroxylase deficiency
  - 17α-Hydroxylase deficiency
  - Renin-secreting tumours

- Ectopic ACTH production
- Cushing's syndrome
- Glucocorticoid-responsive aldosteronism
- Renovascular hypertension
- Accelerated (malignant)-phase hypertension
- Vasculitis
- Apparent mineralocorticoid excess:
  - Liddle's syndrome
  - Syndrome of apparent mineralocorticoid excess (hereditary 11β-hydroxysteroid dehydrogenase deficiency)
  - Acquired 11β-hydroxysteroid dehydrogenase deficiency: liquorice, chewing tobacco, carbenoxolone
- Impaired renal tubular ion transport:
  - Diuretics[a]
  - Bartter's syndrome
  - Gitelman's syndrome
  - Renal tubular acidosis (distal)
  - High-dose penicillins
  - magnesium depletion

Extrarenal losses (urinary potassium <20 mmol/day)

- Gastrointestinal losses:
  - Biliary loss
  - Lower gastointestinal loss: diarrhoea,[a] laxative abuse, villous adenoma
  - Fistula
  - Ureterosigmoidostomy
- Skin losses

[a]The most common causes are diuretics, vomiting, and diarrhoea—these should be excluded before rare conditions are pursued.

Hypokalaemia is not a prominent feature of many of the disorders listed in Box 21.2.2.3: discussion in this chapter is limited to those conditions that are common, or where hypokalaemia is an important manifestation. A pragmatic approach is first to consider the most frequent causes of hypokalaemia—diuretic ingestion and gastrointestinal fluid loss—and then proceed to a systematic analysis if these are not evidently the cause of the problem.

Diuretics

The most common cause of hypokalaemia is diuretic therapy. All diuretics other than those acting directly on the collecting duct (amiloride, triamterene, spironolactone) block some form of chloride-associated sodium transport. As a result, they increase the delivery of sodium to the collecting duct, where its reabsorption creates a favourable electrochemical gradient for and obligates potassium secretion. Hypokalaemia frequently occurs together with metabolic alkalosis (serum bicarbonate concentration

28–36 mmol/litre). In general, the hypokalaemia is mild, with serum potassium in the range 3 to 3.5 mmol/litre, the average fall after initiation of the usual doses of loop diuretics (furosemide, bumetanide, torasemide) being about 0.3 mmol/litre, somewhat more with the usual doses of thiazides (bendroflumethiazide, chlorothiazide, chlortalidone) at about 0.6 mmol/litre. In one analysis of publications on hypokalaemia and diuretics it was found that the fall in serum potassium was little influenced by the reason for prescription (hypertension or heart failure), or by the dose or duration of treatment.

The question of whether or not patients receiving diuretics prone to induce hypokalaemia should be prescribed potassium supplements or potassium-retaining diuretics has been much debated. There is no strong evidence on which to base recommendations. It seems common sense to monitor for and intervene to prevent hypokalaemia in those considered at particular risk of hypokalaemic complications, including those with a history of cardiac arrhythmia, those on digoxin, and those with liver disease in whom electrolyte imbalance might precipitate encephalopathy. Most patients do not fall into any of these categories, and here the balance is between an attempt to prevent a hypothetical but unproven hazard and the requirement for medication that is unpalatable to many and in rare cases can have significant side effects. As in many other aspects of medicine, the behaviour of the physician will say as much about them as about the condition that they are dealing with. Those that like all test results to be in the 'normal range' will prescribe, but short of stopping diuretic therapy, correcting diuretic-induced hypokalaemia is not easy. In one study that monitored adverse drug reactions in 5047 consecutive inpatients, 2439 were taking potassium-losing diuretics, in whom serum potassium was less than 3.5 mmol/litre in 21%, and below 3.0 mmol/litre in 3.8%. When the group taking potassium-losing diuretics was broken down into those taking them without any attempt to prevent hypokalaemia, those taking them in conjunction with potassium supplements, and those taking them together with a potassium-sparing diuretic, then serum potassium below 3.5 mmol/litre was found in 24.9, 19.7, and 15.2%, respectively.

Loss of gastrointestinal fluid

In one study of severe hypokalaemia (serum potassium <2.5 mmol/litre), gastrointestinal fluid loss was the main cause in 22% of cases.

Vomiting

The concentration of potassium in gastric and upper intestinal secretions is between 3 and 12 mmol/litre. Reduced intake and direct loss of potassium in vomit are not, therefore, the cause of hypokalaemia, which is due to increased renal excretion of potassium. This arises as a result of the kidney's response to metabolic alkalosis, which is the dominant metabolic problem. Aside from modest quantities of potassium, gastric juices contain sodium ions (30–90 mmol/litre), protons (90 mmol/litre), and chloride (50–125 mmol/litre). Loss of gastric acid (HCl) pulls the buffer equation

$$H_2CO_3 + Na^+ + Cl^- \Leftrightarrow Na^+ + HCO_3^- + H^+ + Cl^-$$

to the right, hence the main effect is metabolic alkalosis. Depletion of extracellular fluid volume also occurs, activating the renin–angiotensin–aldosterone system. As the bicarbonate concentration in the blood rises, more is filtered at the glomerulus and some is excreted in the urine, partly in conjunction with potassium, whose distal excretion is stimulated by high levels of aldosterone. Considerations of acid–base balance have taken precedence over those of potassium homeostasis, and hypokalaemia results.

An important point to note is that the combination of direct chloride loss in vomit and contraction of extracellular fluid volume lead to a situation where the kidney avidly retains chloride and the urinary concentration of chloride falls to a very low level (<10 mmol/litre, sometimes as low as 1–2 mmol/litre, when the normal range is 30–120 mmol/litre). This is of critical clinical significance because reabsorption of filtered sodium and potassium ions by the renal tubule can only be achieved in combination with an anion, usually chloride, hence if urinary chloride concentration is already close to zero there is no way in which sodium and potassium can be reabsorbed efficiently, meaning that sodium and potassium that are administered can only be retained if provided

in conjunction with chloride, and not if given as other salts. The renal response of chloride retention also means that measurement of urinary chloride concentration can be helpful in making the diagnosis of surreptitious vomiting (see later).

Resuscitation of a patient with hypokalaemia due to vomiting requires the intravenous infusion of 0.9% sodium chloride, together with potassium supplementation as described above. In severe cases the total body deficit of fluid may be in excess of 5 litres, and of potassium of many hundreds of millimoles.

Diarrhoea

The concentration of potassium in stool is 80 to 90 mmol/litre, hence—given normal stool weight of 100 to 200 g/day—faecal loss of potassium is usually in the range 5 to 15 mmol/day. The potassium concentration in the stool decreases as stool volume increases, but volume can increase massively, such that substantial potassium loss and profound hypokalaemia can complicate any severe diarrhoeal illness.

Potassium loss in diarrhoeal states is usually associated with loss of bicarbonate, resulting in a coexisting metabolic acidosis, such that serum levels of potassium may not reflect the true body deficit. In this circumstance, the renal excretion of potassium is broadly appropriate, and potassium deficiency is not due to a renal leak. However, in some situations, potassium in stool is lost in conjunction with chloride, resulting in a metabolic alkalosis and a picture similar to that seen with vomiting (see above).

A villous adenoma of the colon or rectum can rarely result in profound hypokalaemia. The mechanism seems to involve secretion of cAMP and prostaglandin E_2 by the tumour, leading to disturbance of ion transport in the normal colonic mucosa. Treatment with nonsteroidal anti-inflammatory agents (NSAIDs) can significantly reduce stool volume and help to correct both volume depletion and hypokalaemia. Similar disturbances probably underlie the hypokalaemia of patients with the watery diarrhoea, hypokalaemia, achlorhydria (WDHA) syndrome, caused by excess vasoactive intestinal peptide (VIP) secreted by certain tumours. In addition to treatment directed at the tumour itself, somatostatin or somatostatin analogues are effective in controlling symptoms.

Diagnosing the cause of hypokalaemia in difficult cases

The diagnosis of the cause of hypokalaemia is usually straightforward and explained by diuretic therapy or gastrointestinal fluid loss, as described above. In other patients, the abnormality is mild, with the occasional serum potassium concentration measured at just below the lower limit of the normal range, such that extensive investigation is almost certainly inappropriate (and likely to be fruitless if pursued). However, some patients present with unexplained severe hypokalaemia, and these represent a considerable challenge for both diagnosis and management. The differential diagnosis in these cases usually lies between various abnormalities of tubular potassium transport, concealed vomiting and/or usage of purgatives, and concealed ingestion of diuretics.

It is important to ask directly for a history of vomiting or diarrhoea, and about present or past use of any medications, particularly diuretics or purgatives. It is also worthwhile to ask about consumption of liquorice or chewing tobacco (see below). Examination is likely to be unremarkable in cases of unexplained hypokalaemia, but pay particular attention to body weight, height, and body mass index, and to any other features that might support the diagnosis of an eating disorder such as anorexia nervosa or bulimia nervosa (see Chapter 26.5.6).

One study reported the findings of extensive investigation of 27 adult patients (17 women) who presented with chronic hypokalaemia (serum potassium concentration less than 3.4 mmol/litre) that was sustained for over 5 years and which had previously eluded diagnosis. The following diagnoses were established: diuretic abuse (in 5 patients), surreptitious vomiting (8), laxative abuse (1), renal tubular acidosis (1), and Gitelman's syndrome (12). Medical work-up that had sought to make the diagnoses by measurement of plasma renin activity, plasma aldosterone concentration, and urinary potassium concentration failed to discriminate between these conditions. Investigations that were diagnostically helpful are given in Table 21.2.2.1, the most useful being the plasma pH and chloride concentration, urinary chloride concentration and screen for diuretics, and (in one case) stool weight.

The finding of a low plasma chloride concentration with the virtual absence of chloride from the urine supports the diagnosis of surreptitious vomiting. Screening the urine for diuretics is appropriate if the urinary chloride concentration is above 20 mmol/litre, and if no diuretics are found in samples with a chloride concentration of above 50 mmol/litre then Gitelman's syndrome is likely. Vomiting, diuretics, and Gitelman's syndrome all cause alkalosis, whereas laxative abuse is associated with acidosis, as is renal tubular acidosis. The diagnosis of renal tubular acidosis can be established by demonstrating an inability to produce acid urine in the presence of systemic acidosis (see Chapter 21.15 for further discussion).

The management of cases of surreptitious vomiting, or diuretic or purgative abuse is difficult. Many patients will fulfil diagnostic criteria for anorexia nervosa or bulimia nervosa, and issues other than those simply and directly related to potassium homeostasis will clearly need to be considered. The physician may well need to seek expert psychiatric help. See Chapter 26.5.6 for further discussion.

Rare causes of hypokalaemia due to altered external potassium balance

Mineralocorticoid excess

Hypokalaemia can be caused by a large number of causes of mineralocorticoid excess, as shown in Box 21.2.2.3. Primary aldosteronism is discussed in Chapters 13.7.1 and 16.17.4, congenital adrenal hyperplasia in Chapter 13.7.2, and glucocorticoid-remediable aldosteronism in Chapter 16.17.3. Hypokalaemia is rarely a prominent feature of the other conditions of mineralocorticoid excess listed, which are discussed elsewhere in this book.

Apparent mineralocorticoid excess

Activating mutations in the β- or γ-subunits of the epithelial sodium channel in the collecting duct causes Liddle's syndrome (OMIM 177200). Disabling mutations in the type 2 11β-hydroxysteroid dehydrogenase gene cause a deficiency of the enzyme, allowing cortisol access to the mineralocorticoid receptor and the syndrome of apparent mineralocorticoid excess. Acquired inhibition of the action of 11β-hydroxysteroid dehydrogenase can be caused by liquorice, carbenoxolone, and chewing tobacco. Hypokalaemia with low plasma concentrations of renin and aldosterone are features of all of these conditions, which are discussed in Chapter 16.17.4.

Renal tubular abnormalities of potassium transport

Patients with 'classic' distal renal tubular acidosis are prone to hypokalaemia, as are most patients with proximal renal tubular acidosis: these conditions are discussed in Chapter 21.15.

Table 21.2.2.1 Diagnostic clues in 27 cases of hypokalaemia that were hard to diagnose

Investigation	Normal range	Diagnosis				
		Diuretic consumption	Vomiting	Laxative consumption	Renal tubular acidosis	Gitelman's syndrome
Number of cases		5	8	1	1	12
Plasma/serum						
Chloride	97–108 mmol/litre	Low normal or low	Low	Low	Normal	Low normal or low
Bicarbonate	22–28 mmol/litre	High normal or high	High	Low	Low	High normal or high
Magnesium	0.8–1.1 mmol/litre	NR	NR	NR	NR	Low
Urinary						
Sodium	40–130 mmol/litre	Normal	Normal	Low	Normal	High normal or high
Potassium	30–110 mmol/litre	Normal	Normal	Normal	Variable	Normal
Chloride	30–120 mmol/litre	Normal	Very low (<10 mmol/litre)	Low	Normal	High
Calcium	2.5–8.0 mmol per 24 h	NR	NR	NR	NR	Low
Magnesium	2.5–7.5 mmol/litre	NR	NR	NR	NR	High
Diuretic screen		Positive	Negative	Negative	Negative	Negative
Stool						
Weight	100–200 g/day	Normal	Normal	High	Normal	Normal

NR, not reported.
Gladziwa *et al.* (1995) Nephrology, Dialysis, Transplantation 10, 1607.

In 1962, Bartter described "hyperplasia of the juxtaglomerular complex with hyperaldosteronism and hypokalemic alkalosis: a new syndrome". Well over 100 papers were subsequently written to describe features of what was believed to be the same eponymously named condition. The picture became immensely confused, but since 1995 has been clarified by the recognition of distinct phenotypes within the group of patients previously thought to have 'Bartter's syndrome' and the application of powerful molecular genetic methods to their study. These revealed that most adults previously thought to have Bartter's syndrome in fact have Gitelman's syndrome.

Gitelman's syndrome

Gitelman's syndrome (OMIM 263800) is the most common genetic cause of hypokalaemia. If it presents clinically, it typically does so in early adulthood with hypotension, alkalosis, and salt wasting, along with hypomagnesaemia, hypocalciuria, and hypermagnesuria (see Table 21.2.2.1). The marked similarity between this picture and that induced by thiazide diuretics, which are potent inhibitors of the Na–Cl cotransporter (NCCT) in the distal convoluted tubule of the nephron, led to a candidate gene approach to the condition as soon as the thiazide-sensitive *NCCT* gene had been cloned. Mutations in the *NCCT* gene are responsible for Gitelman's syndrome (Fig. 21.2.2.1), which is an autosomal recessive condition.

Since there are no dramatic clinical symptoms or signs, suspicion of the diagnosis of Gitelman's syndrome often arises only when hypokalaemia is found (or in screening of family members of a known case). However, when surveyed directly, patients with Gitelman's syndrome are found to be significantly symptomatic, reporting salt craving, musculoskeletal symptoms (cramps, muscle weakness, and aches), constitutional symptoms (fatigue, generalized weakness, and dizziness), nocturia, and polydipsia, with up

to 45% of patients considering their symptoms to be a moderate problem or worse.

Management is with potassium and magnesium supplements. The latter are often poorly tolerated, but it is important to recognize that in the face of magnesium depletion the kidney cannot retain potassium. Diuretics that block sodium reabsorption in the collecting duct (spironolactone, triamterene, and amiloride) can reduce urinary potassium excretion and raise the serum potassium concentration, but they often need to be accompanied by salt loading to prevent volume depletion and hypotension. NSAIDs can sometimes be helpful, but their mechanism of action is uncertain. The long-term prognosis of patients with Gitelman's syndrome is not known.

Heterozygote carriers of Gitelman's mutations have increased urinary sodium excretion (due to a self-selected higher salt intake), modestly lowered blood pressure (in childhood if not in adulthood), a serum potassium concentration towards the lower limit of the normal range, and increased susceptibility to hypokalaemia induced by diuretics. They also have increased bone density.

See Chapter 21.16 for further discussion, in particular of genetic aspects and matters related to hypomagnesaemia.

Bartter's syndrome

Bartter's syndrome is now classified into four types: each is an autosomal recessive disorder caused by mutation of an ion transporter or ion channel that is present in cells of the thick ascending limb of the nephron (Fig. 21.2.2.1).

Type I (*NKCC2* mutations; OMIM 600839) This was originally described in six consanguineous families, with affected individuals born prematurely after pregnancies complicated by polyhydramnios and developing severe dehydration in the first few days of life. All had severe hypercalciuria in addition to hypokalaemic alkalosis, and most had nephrocalcinosis. In all cases, disease was associated with destructive mutations in the *NKCC2* gene encoding the Na–K–2Cl cotransporter (NKCC2), which is localized to chromosome 15. Other clinical manifestations can include short stature, intellectual disability, rickets, generalized weakness, and muscle cramps. Other reported abnormalities on investigation can include hyperreninism, hyperaldosteronism, increased renal prostaglandin production, erythrocytosis, a platelet aggregation defect, impaired vascular responses to angiotensin II, and hypertrophy or hyperplasia of the juxtaglomerular apparatus. Management is supportive: dehydration must be avoided and potassium supplementation is needed; nonsteroidal anti-inflammatory agents may be helpful (although they tend to be more useful in type II disease). There is a high mortality rate before diagnosis, with infants often dying owing to volume depletion caused by intercurrent illness, but the prognosis in cases where the diagnosis is made and where care is taken to avoid volume depletion is not known.

Type II (*ROMK* mutations; OMIM 241200) Abnormality of the NKCC2 gene product was excluded in five families where individuals also presented with severe neonatal dehydration, hypercalciuria, and nephrocalcinosis. The only clinical distinction from Bartter's syndrome type I was that patients often had a transient initial hyperkalaemia, with serum potassium falling rapidly into the hypokalaemic range as soon as they were rehydrated. An obvious explanation was mutation in another gene or genes whose product interacted with NKCC2 in some way, and this was

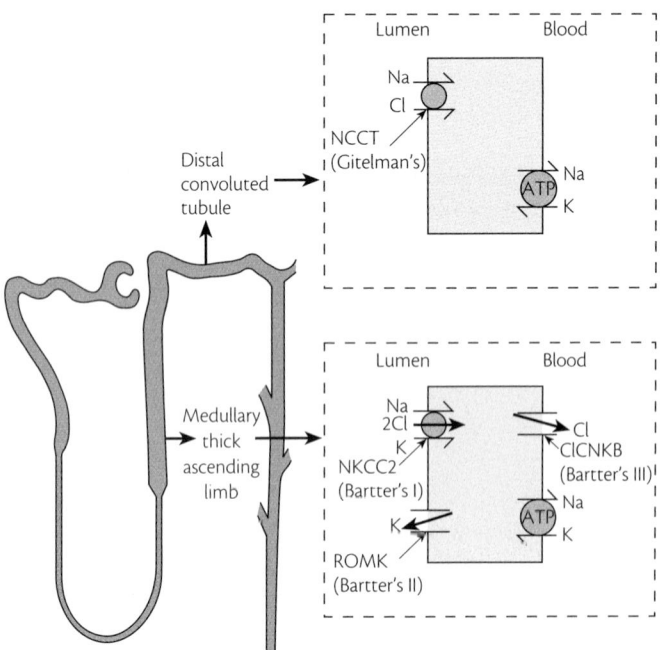

Fig. 21.2.2.1 Some genetic disorders of the renal tubule that cause hypokalaemia. Barttin (Bartter's syndrom type IV) colocalizes with the chloride channels. NCCT, Na–Cl cotransporter; NKCC2, Na–K–2Cl cotransporter; ROMK, ATP-regulated potassium channel; CLCNKB, kidney-specific chloride channel.

confirmed when functionally significant mutations of the *ROMK* gene—which encodes the apical ATP-sensitive potassium channel that recycles potassium back into the lumen and is critical for continued activity of the NKCC2 cotransporter—were identified in all affected individuals. Management and prognosis is as for Bartter's syndrome type I.

Type III (*CLCNKB* mutations; OMIM 607364) To determine whether mutation of other genes could account for the Bartter's phenotype, a large number of patients with inherited hypokalaemic alkalosis, normomagnesaemia, and normocalciuria or hypercalciuria were studied. Most (those in 44 of 66 families) did not have mutations in *NKCC2* or *ROMK*, with mutations in *CLCNKB*, which encodes a kidney-specific chloride channel, being the cause of the Bartter's syndrome in some. The clinical picture is more varied than that for types I or II Bartter's syndrome, ranging in severity from near-fatal volume depletion with hypokalaemic alkalosis and respiratory arrest, to mild disease presenting in a teenager with polyuria and weakness. None of the patients have nephrocalcinosis, distinguishing them phenotypically from those with *NKCC2* or *ROMK* mutations. Management is with potassium supplementation and care to avoid dehydration. Long-term prognosis is uncertain.

Type IV (OMIM 602522) This infantile variant of Bartter's syndrome is associated with sensorineural deafness and dysmorphism, and is due to mutations in the *BSND* gene (which encodes barttin, a protein that colocalizes with chloride channels in the kidney and inner ear) or simultaneous mutations in *CLCNKA* and *CLCNKB* genes.

Ureteric diversion into the colon

Surgical diversion of the ureters into the colon (ureterosigmoidostomy) was previously performed as a method of urinary drainage, most commonly in children for the treatment of bladder exstrophy and in adults following total cystectomy. The operation is now rarely (if ever) performed because of the metabolic consequences, which have driven improvement in surgical techniques for ileal conduits and alternative urinary diversions. However, the consequence of ureterosigmoidostomy is that urine remains in contact with the colonic mucosa for a long time, in which case its response is to reabsorb urinary ammonium and secrete bicarbonate, leading to hyperchloraemic acidosis, and also for there to be stimulation of colonic potassium secretion, resulting in hypokalaemia. Profound and life-threatening acidosis can occur with concurrent illness, and chronic renal failure can develop.

Rare causes of hypokalaemia due to abnormal internal potassium balance

Although there are many causes of hypokalaemia (see Box 21.2.2.3), there are relatively few causes of hypokalaemia associated with extreme weakness, the most common explanation for this rare presentation being hypokalaemic periodic paralysis. In Western countries most cases of hypokalaemic periodic paralysis are familial, termed familial periodic paralysis, whereas in Asian populations the most common cause is thyrotoxic periodic paralysis. In all forms of hypokalaemic periodic paralysis the hypokalaemia and paralysis result from an acute shift of potassium into cells, the mechanism for which is unknown, although there is speculation that it is due to a transient hyperadrenergic state.

One study reviewed the medical records of 97 patients who presented over a 10-year period to hospital in Taiwan with severe hypokalaemia (serum potassium less than 3.0 mmol/litre, mean 2.2 mmol/litre) and acute loss of muscle strength with inability to walk. The final diagnoses established are shown in Table 21.2.2.2.

Treatment of acute attacks of hypokalaemic periodic paralysis traditionally involves the administration of intravenous potassium. Some patients recover with as little as 20 mmol, but others require over 200 mmol. In all types of this condition, a paradoxical fall in serum potassium concentration can occur at the start of treatment, and rebound hyperkalaemia is also seen.

Thyrotoxic periodic paralysis

The diagnosis of thyrotoxic periodic paralysis is established if hyperthyroidism is present when hypokalaemic paralysis occurs. About 50% of patients give a history of thyrotoxic symptoms, but there is no family history of paralysis, although mutation in the *KCNE3* gene, which encodes a potassium channel subunit, has been reported in a sporadic case, and polymorphism of the *CACNA1S* gene, which encodes a calcium channel, has been associated. A variety of stimuli have been reported to provoke attacks, including large carbohydrate meals (perhaps via the mechanism of an exaggerated response to insulin), rest/sleep at night, hot weather, upper respiratory tract infection, and excessive physical activity. Physical findings during an attack include tachycardia (a useful

Table 21.2.2.2 Final diagnoses established in 97 patients initially diagnosed as having hypokalaemic periodic paralysis

Final diagnosis	Number	Mean age (years)	Male:female ratio
Patients with hypokalaemic periodic paralysis			
Thyrotoxic periodic paralysis	39	28	39:0
Sporadic periodic paralysis	29	26	23:6
Hypernatraemic hypokalaemic periodic paralysis[a]	3	18	3:0
Familial periodic paralysis	2	16	2:0
Patients who did not have hypokalaemic periodic paralysis			
Metabolic alkalosis			
Primary aldosteronism	6	39	2:4
Bartter's or Gitelman's syndromes	6	21	4:2
Diuretics	3	40	0:3
Hyperchloraemic acidosis			
Distal renal tubular acidosis	6	47	3:3
Toluene abuse	3	28	1:2

[a] Mean serum sodium concentration was 167 mmol/litre. Two patients had brain tumours and one patient had hypothalamic involvement with tuberculosis. It is possible that diabetes insipidus was the explanation for their presentation and there is insufficient evidence in the paper to justify the naming of a new syndrome.

Patients with hypokalaemic periodic paralysis do not have an acid–base disorder: arterial pH, Pco_2, and bicarbonate are all within the normal range. A key finding is that the urinary potassium concentration is low (mean 8 mmol/litre). There is also a low transtubular potassium concentration gradient (TTKG = (urine K/serum K)/(urine osmolality/serum osmolality)) of <3: the normal renal response to hypokalaemia of nonrenal origin being a TTKG <2, whereas a renal cause of hypokalaemia is usually associated with TTKG >5).

From Lin *et al.* (2001). *Quarterly Journal of Medicine* 94, 133–9.

diagnostic discriminator from sporadic periodic paralysis) and high blood pressure; signs of hyperthyroidism are absent in 20 to 40% of cases. In 39 patients reported from Taiwan, the mean serum T_3 concentration was 4.5 nmol/litre (range 2.3–8.4 nmol/litre, upper limit of normal being 3.0 nmol/litre), the mean serum T_4 concentration was 201 nmol/litre (range 154–299 nmol/litre, upper limit of normal being 154 nmol/litre), and the mean thyroid-stimulating hormone was less than 0.06 mU/litre (range less than 0.06 to 0.32 mU/litre; normal range 0.5–5.0 mU/litre). Hypophosphataemia and hypomagnesaemia are also found, the latter also being low in patients with Gitelman's syndrome.

Although treatment of thyrotoxic periodic paralysis conventionally involves administration of potassium, recent experience suggests that patients with this condition respond rapidly to the β-blocker propranolol (3 mg/kg body weight, given orally). This, rather than potassium, is now the preferred first-line treatment, with the expectation that serum potassium concentration will return to normal and paralysis will resolve within 2 h.

Effective treatment of hyperthyroidism prevents attacks, but about two-thirds of patients will have recurrent paralytic attacks, most commonly in the first 3 months after diagnosis, while their hyperthyroidism is brought under control.

Familial hypokalaemic periodic paralysis (OMIM 170400)

The diagnosis is established by finding a family history of attacks of flaccid weakness and hypokalaemia. These can sometimes be precipitated by administration of insulin or glucose and aborted by exercise, which induces an exaggerated rise in serum potassium concentration.

Familial hypokalaemic periodic paralysis can be caused by mutations in one of three genes: (1) *CACNL1A3*, which encodes a dihydropyridine receptor that functions as a voltage-gated calcium channel and is also critical for excitation–contraction coupling in a voltage-sensitive and calcium-independent manner; (2) *SCN4A*, which encodes for a sodium channel and is also the site of mutations causing hyperkalaemic periodic paralysis; or (3) *KCNE3*, which encodes a potassium channel. The conditions are autosomal dominant, with 100% penetrance in males, but much less in females.

Emergency treatment is with intravenous potassium: propranolol is ineffective. Dichlorphenamide (a carbonic anhydrase inhibitor) is effective at preventing attacks in most cases; acetazolamide (another carbonic anhydrase inhibitor) and pinacidil (a potassium channel opener) have also been used.

Sporadic periodic paralysis

The cause of sporadic periodic paralysis is not known: patients do not have a family history of hypokalaemic periodic paralysis and do not have hyperthyroidism. There are no obvious precipitating factors. Heart rate at presentation is lower than for those with thyrotoxic periodic paralysis (mean 76 compared with 105 beats/min). Treatment is as for familial hypokalaemic periodic paralysis.

Sudden unexplained death during sleep

Sudden unexplained death during sleep (SUDS), known in Thai as *lai-tai* and as the Filipino folk term *bangungut* (meaning 'to rise and moan during sleep'), is not uncommon in Asians and is a leading cause of death in young men in rural north-eastern Thailand. A recent survey in the Phillipines reported an annual incidence of 22 per 100 000 in the 20- to 39-year age group (mostly in men) and 43 per 100 000 overall. It has been recorded over the years as the cause of death of many hundreds of apparently healthy male Thai migrant workers in Singapore. Women are rarely, if ever, affected. Death occurs at rest and is nocturnal in most (84%) cases. In cases that are observed, witnesses often report that death is preceded by a few minutes of groaning, choking, coughing, and muscular spasticity or paralysis.

The cause of SUDS is not known. There is a family history of SUDS more often than would be expected by chance, and in some families there is inheritance of a Brugada syndrome ECG pattern (RSR′ and ST segment elevation in V1–3; see Chapter 16.4), but mutations in the cardiac sodium channel gene *SCN5A* that causes Brugada syndrome (OMIM 601144) have not been found in families of patients with SUDS. Other hypotheses include stress, other genetic factors, dietary deficiency (perhaps of thiamine), potassium deficiency, melioidosis, and sleep disorders. With regard to potassium, survivors of SUDS-like attacks and relatives of victims of SUDS have been reported to have significantly lower activity of erythrocyte Na^+,K^+-ATPase and lower serum potassium concentration than controls, but the reason for and significance of these findings is not certain.

Hyperkalaemia

Clinical features and treatment of hyperkalaemia

Hyperkalaemia is the most serious of all electrolyte disorders, despite being relatively infrequent, because it can cause cardiac arrest. Some patients report muscular symptoms such as weakness, stiffness, or simply a 'funny feeling', but the significance of these is rarely appreciated. A high serum potassium concentration leads to membrane depolarization in excitable tissues, making the initation of an action potential more likely, and to increased membrane potassium conductance, which impairs recovery after an action potential. The effect is to cause electrical instability with the risk of life-threatening arrhythmia. The likelihood of such an event increases as the serum potassium concentration rises, but some patients are more resistant to the cardiac effects of hyperkalaemia than others: for instance, those with endstage renal failure on long-term dialysis may be habitually hyperkalaemic (although this is not to be encouraged) and tolerate a serum potassium concentration that would kill a normal person if imposed acutely.

The best guide to the significance of hyperkalaemia in any particular individual is the impact that it is having on the ECG, and an ECG should be obtained immediately in any patient in whom the question of hyperkalaemia arises. The earliest change is tenting of the T wave, progressing as the serum potassium concentration rises to P-wave flattening, prolongation of the PR interval, widening of the QRS complex, and eventually a 'sine wave' pattern as a prelude to ventricular fibrillation and death. All involved in the care of acutely ill patients must be able to recognize this pattern of ECG changes and give effective emergency treatment for severe hyperkalaemia, as described in Chapter 21.5.

Causes of hyperkalaemia

There are many causes of a high serum potassium concentration (Box 21.2.2.4), but a survey of over 400 cases found that renal failure was present in 43% and potassium supplements or potassium-sparing diuretics had been taken by 37%. Life-threatening hyperkalaemia is almost exclusively seen in those with

---

Box 21.2.2.4 Causes of hyperkalaemia

Pseudohyperkalaemia (test-tube phenomena where measured potassium concentration does not reflect that in the patient's blood *in vivo*)

◆ Tight tourniquet with or without limb exercise

◆ Test-tube haemolysis

◆ Leukaemia with very high white cell count

◆ Thrombocytosis

Altered internal balance (redistribution of potassium from extracellular to intracellular compartment)

◆ Exercise

◆ Acidosis (inorganic)

◆ Massive tissue destruction:[a]
  · Crush injuries
  · Rhabdomyolysis
  · Burns
  · Tumour lysis

◆ Drugs/toxins:
  · Digoxin poisoning
  · Succinylcholine
  · Arginine
  · Fluoride intoxication
  · β-blockade

◆ Malignant hyperthermia

◆ Hyperkalaemic periodic paralysis

Altered external balance (high total body potassium)
Excessive ingestion[b]

◆ Consumption of high-potassium foods (Table 21.2.2.3)

◆ potassium supplements

◆ Low-salt diet (high in potassium)

◆ 'Salt substitutes' (contain potassium)

◆ Upper gastrointestinal haemorrhage ('blood meal')

Impaired excretion
General impairment of renal function

◆ Acute kidney injury

◆ Chronic kidney disease

Defects that specifically impair renal potassium excretion

◆ Mineralocorticoid deficiency:
  · Renin deficiency—hyporeninaemic hypoaldosteronism, which can be either idiopathic or drug induced (NSAIDs or calcineurin inhibitors such as tacrolimus and ciclosporin)
  · ACE inhibition—drug induced (lisinopril, ramipril, enalapril, etc.)
  · Angiotensin-II receptor blockade—drug induced (losartan, candesartan, etc.)
  · Defective aldosterone production—generalized adrenal failure (Addison's disease)

◆ Deficiency of aldosterone synthesis:
  · Drug induced (heparin)
  · Enzyme deficiencies
  · Idiopathic

Impaired tubular ion transport

◆ Drugs:
  · Potassium-sparing diuretics[c]
  · Trimethoprim
  · calcineurin inhibitors (ciclosporin, tacrolimus)

◆ Pseudohypoaldosteronism:
  · Type 1
  · Type 2 (Gordon's syndrome)

[a]Often associated with acute kidney injury.
[b]Note that it is very rare for hyperkalaemia to be caused by excessive ingestion if renal excretory mechanisms for potassium are working normally.
[c]These drugs should generally be avoided in patients with significant renal impairment.

---

renal failure, often in conjunction with another exacerbating cause. Common scenarios would be a patient with acute kidney injury who is hypercatabolic or who has extensive tissue destruction, as in rhabdomyolysis, or a patient with endstage renal failure who has missed a dialysis treatment, not adhered to a low-potassium diet (see Table 21.2.2.3), or suffered an upper gastrointestinal haemorrhage, thereby inadvertently consuming a high-potassium meal.

Hyperkalaemia is not a prominent feature of many of the conditions listed in Box 21.2.2.4: further discussion in this chapter is limited to disorders other than renal failure that are not discussed elsewhere in this textbook and in which hyperkalaemia is a common or important manifestation.

Pseudohyperkalaemia

Haemolysed samples show hyperkalaemia, which also occurs when there is considerable delay between venepuncture and separation of red cells and plasma or serum in the laboratory, allowing potassium to leak out of red cells after venesection. However, aside from these common and banal explanations, there are other reasons for pseudohyperkalaemia.

Potassium is released from white blood cells and platelets as blood coagulates, causing the serum potassium concentration to exceed, by a few tenths of a millimole per litre, that of plasma estimated in a parallel sample. This process is greatly exaggerated

Table 21.2.2.3 Potassium content of various foodstuffs

High-potassium foods (to be avoided in those with hyperkalaemia)	Suitable low-potassium alternatives
Dairy products	
Single cream	Reasonable daily allowance of milk
Condensed/evaporated milk	Various commercial coffee whiteners
Food drinks	
Meats	
Ready cooked meals in sauce	All kinds of meat
Fish	
Ready cooked fish pies, fish in sauce, etc.	All kinds of fish
Fruit	
All dried fruit	Apples
Apricots	Grapefruit
Avocado pears	Kiwi fruit
Bananas	Passion fruit
Cherries	Pears
Grapes	Satsumas
Melons	Tangerines
Oranges	Tinned fruit of all types—but after
Peaches	draining off the juice or syrup, which
Pineapples	contains a lot of potassium
Plums	
Raspberries	
Rhubarb	
Strawberries	
Vegetables	
Artichokes	Aubergines
Bamboo shoots	Beans—French, runner
Beans—baked, butter, haricot	Cabbage
Beetroot	Carrots
Cabbage—red	Cauliflower
Corn on the cob	Celery
Mushrooms	Courgettes
Peas—chick, split	Cucumber
Potatoes— jacket, chips, crisps, sweet	Lettuce
Spinach	Marrow
Tomato	Onions
Watercress	Peas
	Potato—boiled in plenty of water
	Radish
	Spring greens
	Sprouts
	Swedes
	Turnips
Cakes	
Any containing dried fruit or nuts	Dough
Chocolate	Fruit pies—if fruit not high potassium
Coffee	Jam tarts
Flapjacks	Meringue
Gingerbread	Scones—plain
Mince pies	Victoria sandwich—plain
Parkin	

Table 21.2.2.3 (*Cont'd*) Potassium content of various foodstuffs

High-potassium foods (to be avoided in those with hyperkalaemia)	Suitable low-potassium alternatives
Sweets and biscuits	
Any containing dried fruit or nuts	Chocolate
Barley sugar	Biscuits—plain
Fruit gums	Honey
Fudge	Humbugs
Liquorice	Jam
Marzipan	Marmalade
Toffee	Mints
Beverages	
Cocoa	Coca-Cola
Coffee—instant	Coffee—percolated
Drinking chocolate	Fruit squashes—unless with high juice
Fruit juices—if pure and containing any high-potassium fruit	content
Tea—instant	Lemonade and other fizzy drinks
	Soda water
	Tea—infusion
	Tonic water
Cereals	
Muesli and other cereals containing dried fruit or nuts	Bread
	Breakfast cereals—most types
	Pasta
	Rice
Other	
Salt substitutes	

This list is not exhaustive. If a patient with hyperkalaemia seems to be consuming an unusual diet, then obtain dietetic advice.

when gross leucocytosis or thrombocytosis is present, such that the serum potassium concentration can be over 2 mmol/litre higher than that in plasma. The plasma and not the serum potassium concentration should obviously be measured in this circumstance.

There is also the rare syndrome of familial pseudohyperkalaemia, first described in 16 members of 3 generations of a kindred from Edinburgh who had elevated serum potassium if the red cells were not separated promptly. Several other families have been described, in each of which there appears to be one of a variety of abnormalities in the temperature sensitivity of the ouabain-plus-bumetanide-resistant potassium flux, which reflects the passive leak. The blood film may show a few target cells, red cell survival is shortened, but there is no frank haemolysis. Other phenotypic abnormalities have been described in some families.

Abnormal external potassium balance

Mineralocorticoid deficiency

Hyporeninaemic hypoaldosteronism

It is not uncommon to find patients with chronic kidney disease who have hyperkalaemia despite a GFR that should be sufficient to maintain normokalaemia. Two-thirds of these will have the syndrome of hyporeninaemic hypoaldosteronism, which should be suspected in any patient with hyperkalaemia without other obvious explanation. Tubulointerstitial forms of renal disease predominate in this population and diabetes mellitus is common. Hyperkalaemia is usually asymptomatic, but presentation with cardiac arrhythmia and/or muscle weakness has been described.

Characteristics of the syndrome include low levels of plasma renin activity, which are unresponsive to sodium restriction or furosemide, low plasma and urinary aldosterone, hyperkalaemia, and hyperchloraemic metabolic acidosis. Fractional potassium excretion is low for the GFR, and the response to kaliuretic stimuli is blunted. Glucocorticoid metabolism is normal.

The cause of both hyporeninism and hypoaldosteronism is not known. Decreased renin secretion may be the result of pathological involvement of the juxtaglomerular apparatus, but this is not obvious histologically in cases where renal biopsies have been performed. Other hypotheses include defective prostacyclin production and disordered conversion of inactive (prorenin) to active renin, which is a well-documented observation in diabetes mellitus. Chronic expansion of extracellular fluid volume has also been blamed since plasma renin activity may be increased by prolonged sodium restriction or diuretic therapy. By contrast, acute salt restriction can worsen hyperkalaemia in these patients by diminishing the distal delivery of sodium without a concurrent rise in aldosterone secretion, and illnesses causing volume depletion can precipitate presentation with dangerous hyperkalaemia. Hypoaldosteronism is probably related to the low level of plasma renin activity, but the situation is more complicated than this since most patients secrete subnormal amounts of aldosterone in response to infusion of both angiotensin II and ACTH, suggesting a defect in the function of the adrenal gland.

Criteria for establishing the diagnosis of hyporeninaemic hypoaldosteronism are not well defined, and it is uncommon for patients to be intensively investigated in routine clinical practice since treatment is usually straightforward. However, establishing the diagnosis with certainty depends on demonstrating deficient responses of renin and aldosterone to sodium depletion. One study reported plasma renin and aldosterone concentrations in subjects in an upright posture after administration of 60 mg of intravenous furosemide: the renin concentration in those with hyporeninaemic hypoaldosteronism was 6 ± 2 ng/ml per minute (compared with 34 ± 6 ng/ml per minute in controls matched for degree of renal failure) and aldosterone concentration was 7 ± 2 ng/dl (compared with 28 ± 8 ng/dl in controls).

Therapy for hyporeninaemic hypoaldosteronism includes dietary potassium restriction and avoidance of drugs that can cause hyperkalaemia. Measures to increase urinary excretion of potassium, such as the use of thiazide or loop diuretics, can be useful. Cation exchange resins can be used to increase elimination of potassium from the gut, but compliance with long-term use of these medications is difficult to achieve. Although mineralocorticoid replacement (fludrocortisone, 0.2 mg/day) effectively treats the hyperkalaemia, sodium retention and worsening hypertension are often unacceptable side effects.

Effects of drugs on the renin–angiotensin–aldosterone system
NSAIDs Prostaglandin synthetase inhibitors produce hyporeninaemic hypoaldosteronism by interfering with prostacyclin-mediated renin secretion, with reduction in GFR and distal sodium delivery as potential contributory factors. These effects, as might be expected, become more important in the context of renal impairment: in one study approximately one-quarter of patients with chronic renal failure developed hyperkalaemia after treatment with indometacin.

ACE inhibitors and angiotensin-II receptor blockers These produce hyperkalaemia by impairing angiotensin II-mediated secretion of aldosterone. In one study, hyperkalaemia was found in 46 of 119 (39%) patients taking ACE inhibitors who were attending a renal clinic. The higher the serum creatinine concentration, the greater the chance of hyperkalaemia. Those with diabetes were also at particular risk. The treatment had to be stopped in 15 patients (13%). ACE inhibitors and spironolactone have been found to improve prognosis in heart failure, but care is needed when prescribing for those who might be prone to hyperkalaemia. One study reported life-threatening hyperkalaemia (mean serum potassium 7.7 mmol/litre) in 25 patients who had received this combination of medications.

Heparin Hyperkalaemia occurs in about 7% of patients given heparin, which is a potent inhibitor of aldosterone production. It can arise with doses as low as 10 000 units/day, but—as with most other hyperkalaemic stimuli—clinically important elevations in the serum potassium concentration are found only when more than one homeostatic mechanism for potassium is deranged. Patients with endstage renal failure who receive unfractionated heparin to provide anticoagulation during haemodialysis treatments have a higher predialysis serum potassium than those given low-molecular-weight heparin. The most important mechanism of aldosterone inhibition appears to involve reduction in both numbers and affinity of angiotensin II receptors in the zona glomerulosa, which is reduced in width by prolonged use of heparin. Direct inhibition of the enzyme 18-hydroxylase has also been postulated. Production of other corticosteroids is not affected.

Calcineurin inhibitors Hyperkalaemia is a well-documented complication of the immunosuppressive drugs ciclosporin and tacrolimus. Two mechanisms are possible, both of which may be exacerbated by reduction in GFR caused by nephrotoxicity: (1) drug-induced hyporeninaemic hypoaldosteronism, which is well documented with tacrolimus; and (2) in association with a distal tubular acidification defect that is caused (mechanism unknown) by both ciclosporin and tacrolimus.

Renal transport abnormalities
Tubulointerstitial renal disease
A few hyperkalaemic patients with chronic renal failure but a GFR that should be adequate for potassium homeostasis have normal levels of aldosterone and plasma renin activity and seem to have a primary defect in the ability of the distal nephron to excrete potassium. They also typically have tubulointerstitial types of renal diseases, the abnormality being documented in patients with obstructive uropathy, renal transplants, sickle cell disease, systemic lupus erythematosus, amyloidosis, and medullary sponge kidney—all of which can also be associated with hyporeninaemic hypoaldosteronism. In contrast to patients with hyporeninaemic hypoaldosteronism, their hyperkalaemia is unresponsive to mineralocorticoid replacement therapy.

Type IV renal tubular acidosis
Hyperkalaemia due to impaired renal excretion of potassium may be a feature of type IV or voltage-dependent renal tubular acidosis.

The lumen negative potential difference along the distal nephron normally facilitates the excretion of potassium and hydrogen ions, and hyperkalaemia and metabolic acidosis occur when this is reduced. This condition is discussed in Chapter 21.15.

Potassium-sparing diuretics

These are obviously likely to cause hyperkalaemia in patients with any predisposition to this condition, and they should only be used with great care in those with renal failure. The serum potassium concentration must be monitored closely in patients taking these agents who become acutely unwell.

Trimethoprim–sulfamethoxazole

A review of 80 patients treated with standard-dose trimethoprim (up to 320 mg/day) and sulfamethoxazole (up to 1600 mg/day) showed that this increased the serum potassium concentration by an average of 1.2 mmol/litre, whereas there was no change in a control group receiving other antibiotics. Some studies have shown a lesser effect than this, but even larger increases in serum potassium concentration have been reported in patients receiving high-dose trimethoprim–sulfamethoxazole to treat pneumocystis, and hyperkalaemia is also reported with use of pentamidine. Both trimethoprim and pentamidine block the apical sodium channel in the distal nephron in a manner similar to amiloride.

Pseudohypoaldosteronism type 1

There are autosomal recessive and autosomal dominant forms of this rare condition (see Chapter 16.17.4 for further discussion of the genetic abnormalities). The recessive form typically presents in infancy with vomiting and feeding difficulty. There are signs of volume depletion and laboratory findings of hyponatraemia, hyperkalaemia, and acidaemia. The plasma renin concentration is usually increased and plasma aldosterone concentration is markedly elevated. The sodium concentration in urine, sweat, saliva, and stool is high. Treatment is with salt supplements that must usually be continued into adulthood. By contrast, the autosomal dominant form has a milder phenotype, with symptoms that remit with age.

Pseudohypoaldosteronism type 2 (Gordon's syndrome)

This is a rare autosomal dominant condition (see Chapter 16.17.4 for further discussion of the genetic abnormalities) in which hypertension is accompanied by hyperkalaemia despite normal GFR. The condition is usually asymptomatic and detected fortuitously if serum potassium concentration is measured for any reason, or in the course of family studies, but it can rarely present in late childhood or adulthood with hyperkalaemic periodic paralysis. There is a hyperchloraemic acidosis, a low level of plasma renin activity, and normal or slightly low plasma aldosterone concentration. Giving exogenous aldosterone does not increase urinary potassium excretion or reduce hyperkalaemia. Because a kaliuresis can be provoked by infusion of sodium sulphate or sodium bicarbonate, but not sodium chloride, it has been suggested that enhanced reabsorption of chloride at a distal nephron site may underlie the abnormality in potassium secretion. Physiological abnormalities can be corrected with thiazide diuretics, which may provide effective treatment.

Abnormal internal potassium balance

Exercise

Exercise-related rises in the serum potassium concentration are a normal phenomenon and usually modest, but increases to 7 mmol/litre occur during acute, maximal, physical performance and levels as high as 10 mmol/litre have been reported with prolonged exhaustive exercise such as in marathons. Exercise-induced hyperkalaemia is accentuated by β-adrenergic blockade or α-adrenergic agonists, and in patients with chronic renal failure.

Acidosis

Acidosis diminishes potassium uptake by cells (see Box 21.2.2.1) and causes hyperkalaemia. The increase in the serum potassium concentration is greater with metabolic than respiratory acidosis, and occurs more markedly with hyperchloraemic than with organic acid-induced forms of metabolic acidosis. Stimulation of insulin release by organic acids appears to account for this divergent response, explaining the pathophysiology of disturbed potassium homeostasis in diabetic ketoacidosis. At presentation, when insulin is deficient, potassium is redistributed in a fashion comparable with mineral acid-induced metabolic acidosis and patients are hyperkalaemic. However, the preceding kaliuresis (caused by polyuria) has rendered the body enormously deficient in potassium, and the serum potassium concentration falls rapidly as soon as insulin is provided, allowing potassium to return to the cells. Indeed, dangerous hypokalaemia can develop if adequate potassium is not given during treatment.

Drugs

Several drugs can produce hyperkalaemia by altering the transcellular distribution of potassium. Digoxin and similar preparations diminish cellular potassium uptake by inhibiting the Na^+,K^+-ATPase pump, and substantial hyperkalaemia can accompany digoxin intoxication. Succinylcholine and other depolarizing muscle relaxants increase the potassium permeability of muscle: the serum potassium concentration typically increases by 0.5 to 1.0 mmol/litre, but hyperkalaemia can be more severe in patients with burns or neuromuscular diseases. Infusion of 30 g of the cationic amino acid arginine HCl increases serum potassium concentration by 0.5 to 1.0 mmol/litre and can produce life-threatening hyperkalaemia in individuals with deranged potassium metabolism. Fluoride intoxication appears to increase the serum potassium concentration by provoking leakage from the intracellular compartment, and associated hypocalcaemia enhances the cardiac risks of fluoride-induced hyperkalaemia.

Although $β_2$-adrenergic stimulants cause hypokalaemia and can be used to treat hyperkalaemia (see Chapter 21.5), the administration of β-blockers typically increases the serum potassium concentration only modestly (by 0.1 to 0.2 mmol/litre). However, the hyperkalaemic effect can be much more prominent when other potassium homeostatic mechanisms are deranged, e.g. in patients receiving intermittent haemodialysis, the predialysis serum potassium concentration is increased on average by 1.0 mmol/litre.

Hyperkalaemic periodic paralysis

Hyperkalaemic periodic paralysis is a rare autosomal dominant condition in which mutations in the sodium channel gene SCN4A are associated with episodes of flaccid generalized weakness (rather than paralysis) and elevation of the serum potassium concentration, typically into the range 6 to 8 mmol/litre. Mutations in the same gene can cause normokalaemic potassium-sensitive periodic paralysis, hypokalaemic periodic paralysis, and paramyotonia congenita. Attacks of weakness last from minutes to hours, occurring without any obvious precipitant, but sometimes following exercise or administration of potassium. Myotonia of the ocular muscles and tongue is sometimes observed both between and during attacks, the former demonstrable as slow opening of the lids after forced active closure of the eyes, or as myotonic lid lag lasting 15 to 20 s after elevation of the eyes. There can be generalized muscle wasting and progressive myopathy. In some families, cardiac arrhythmia, cardiac sudden death, short stature, microcephaly, and clinodactyly (typically a bent little finger) are reported. Treatment with β$_2$-agonists can be used to abort paralytic attacks, and dichlorphenamide is effective at preventing attacks in most cases (as with familial hypokalaemic periodic paralysis). Treatment with kaliuretic diuretics has also been used to prevent attacks, but without proof of efficacy.

Further reading

Brater DC (1998). Diuretic therapy. *New Engl J Med*, **339**, 387–95.

Cruz DN, et al. (2001). Gitelman's syndrome revisited: an evaluation of symptoms and health-related quality of life. *Kidney Int*, **59**, 710–17.

Cruz DN, et al. (2001). Mutations in the Na-Cl cotransporter reduce blood pressure in humans. *Hypertension*, **37**, 1458–64.

Ernst ME, Moser M (2009). Use of diuretics in patients with hypertension. *N Engl J Med*, **361**, 2153–64.

Gennari FJ (1998). Hypokalemia. *New Engl J Med*, **339**, 451–8.

Gervacio-Domingo G, et al. (2007). Sudden uenxplained death during sleep occurred commonly in the general population in the Philippines: a sub study of the National Nutrition and Health Survey. *J Clin Epidemiol*, **60**, 567–71.

Gladziwa U, et al. (1995). Chronic hypokalaemia of adults: Gitelman's syndrome is frequent but classical Bartter's syndrome is rare. *Nephrol Dial Transplant*, **10**, 1607–13.

Grier JF (1995). WDHA (watery diarrhea, hypokalemia, achlorhydria) syndrome: clinical features, diagnosis, and treatment. *Southern Med J*, **88**, 22–4.

Halevy J, et al. (1988). Life-threatening hypokalemia in hospitalized patients. *Miner Electrolyte Metab*, **14**, 163–6.

Hamill RJ, et al. (1991). Efficacy and safety of potassium infusion therapy in hypokalemic critically ill patients. *Crit Care Med*, **19**, 694–9.

Hsieh MJ, et al. (2008). Hypokalemic thyrotoxic periodic paralysis: clinical characteristics and predictors of recurrent paralytic attacks. *Eur J Neurol*, **15**, 559–64.

Kruse JA, et al. (1994). Concentrated potassium chloride infusions in critically ill patients with hypokalemia. *J Clin Pharmacol*, **34**, 1077–82.

Kung AW (2006). Clinical review: Thyrotoxic periodic paralysis: a diagnostic challenge. *J Clin Endocrinol Metab*, **91**, 2490–5.

Lin SH, Lin YF (2001). Propranolol rapidly reverses paralysis, hypokalemia, and hypophosphatemia in thyrotoxic periodic paralysis. *Am J Kidney Dis*, **37**, 620–3.

Lin SH, et al. (2001). Hypokalaemia and paralysis. *QJM*, **94**, 133–9.

Morgan DB, Davidson C (1980). Hypokalaemia and diuretics: an analysis of publications. *Br Med J*, **280**, 905–8.

Nadler JL, et al. (1986). Evidence of prostacyclin deficiency in the syndrome of hyporeninemic hypoaldosteronism. *New Engl J Med*, **314**, 1015–20.

Older J, et al. (1999). Secretory villous adenomas that cause depletion syndrome. *Arch Intern Med*, **159**, 879–80.

Oster JR, et al. (1995). Heparin-induced aldosterone suppression and hyperkalemia. *Am J Med*, **98**, 575–86.

Paice BJ, et al. (1986). Record linkage study of hypokalaemia in hospitalized patients. *Postgrad Med J*, **62**, 187–91.

Preston RA, et al. (1998). University of Miami Division of Clinical Pharmacology therapeutic rounds: drug-induced hyperkalemia. *Am J Ther*, **5**, 125–32.

Sansone V, et al. (2008). Treatment for periodic paralyses. *Cochrane Database Syst Rev*, **23**, CD005045.

Saperstein DS (2008). Muscle channelopathies. *Semin Neurol*, **28**, 260–9.

Scheinman SJ, et al. (1999). Genetic disorders of renal electrolyte transport. *New Engl J Med*, **340**, 1177–87.

Schepkens H, et al. (2001). Life-threatening hyperkalemia during combined therapy with angiotensin-converting enzyme inhibitors and spironolactone: an analysis of 25 cases. *Am J Med*, **110**, 438–41.

Seyberth HW (2008). An improved terminology and classification of Bartter-like syndromes. *Nat Clin Pract Nephrol*, **4**, 560–7.

Simon DB, Lifton RP (1998). Ion transporter mutations in Gitelman's and Bartter's syndromes. *Curr Opin Nephrol Hypertens*, **7**, 43–7.

Tosukhowong P, et al. (1996). Hypokalemia, high erythrocyte Na$^+$ and low erythrocyte Na$^+$,K$^+$-ATPase in relatives of patients dying from sudden unexplained death syndrome in north-east Thailand and in survivors from near-fatal attacks. *Am J Nephrol*, **16**, 369–74.

Widmer P, et al. (1995). Diuretic-related hypokalaemia: the role of diuretics, potassium supplements, glucocorticoids and β$_2$-adrenoceptor agonists. Results from the comprehensive hospital drug monitoring programme, Berne (CHDM). *Eur J Clin Pharmacol*, **49**, 31–6.

Wong ML, et al. (1992). Sudden unexplained death syndrome. A review and update. *Trop Geogr Med*, **44**, S1–19.

Clinical presentation of renal disease

Richard E. Fielding and Ken Farrington

Essentials

Renal disease may present in many ways, including: (1) the screening of asymptomatic individuals; (2) with symptoms and signs resulting from renal dysfunction; and (3) with symptoms and signs of an underlying disease, often systemic, which has resulted in renal dysfunction.

History and clinical signs—in many cases these are nonspecific or not apparent, and detection of renal disease relies on a combination of clinical suspicion and simple investigations, including urinalysis (by dipstick for proteinuria and haematuria, with quantification of proteinuria most conveniently performed by estimation of the albumin:creatinine ratio, ACR, or protein:creatinine ratio, PCR) and estimation of renal function (by measurement of serum creatinine, expressed as estimated glomerular filtration rate, eGFR).

Asymptomatic renal disease—this is common and most often detected as chronic depression of glomerular filtration rate (known as chronic kidney disease, CKD), proteinuria, or haematuria, either as isolated features or in combination.

Symptomatic renal disease—may present in many ways, including: (1) with features of severe chronic depression of glomerular filtration rate—'uraemia', manifesting with some or all of anorexia, nausea, vomiting, fatigue, weakness, pruritus, breathlessness, bleeding tendency, apathy and loss of mental concentration, and muscle twitching and cramps; (2) acute kidney injury—also known as acute renal failure; (3) with urinary symptoms—frequency, polyuria, nocturia, oliguria, anuria, and macroscopic haematuria; and (4) loin pain.

Specific renal syndromes—these include: (1) nephrotic syndrome—comprising oedema, proteinuria, and hypoalbuminaemia—caused by primary or secondary glomerular disease; and (2) rapidly progressive glomerulonephritis with acute renal failure.

Other conditions—renal disease may be associated with and present in the context of many underlying conditions, including: (1) diabetes mellitus; (2) renovascular disease; (3) myeloma and other malignancies; (4) infectious diseases, either as a nonspecific manifestation of the sepsis syndrome or as a specific complication of the particular infection, e.g. haemolytic uraemic syndrome, poststreptococcal glomerulonephritis, hantavirus infection, leptospirosis, HIV nephropathy; (5) systemic inflammatory diseases, e.g. systemic vasculitides, rheumatological disorders, sarcoidosis, amyloidosis; (6) drug-induced renal disease; and (7) pregnancy.

Introduction

Renal disease may present in a multitude of ways. In practice it is usually detected as a result of:

* screening of asymptomatic individuals

* symptoms and signs resulting from renal dysfunction

* symptoms and signs of an underlying disease, often systemic, which has resulted in renal dysfunction

Symptoms and signs of renal pathology are often absent or subtle, even in the presence of significant disease, hence the detection of renal problems requires careful evaluation of the history and clinical findings to assess the potential risk of underlying renal disease. This evaluation should focus on features of systemic and inflammatory disease as well as those relating directly to the renal tract, and similarly a drug and obstetric history may help elucidate the cause of renal disease. However, in many cases the history and clinical signs are nonspecific or not apparent, with detection of renal disease relying on a combination of clinical suspicion and simple investigations, including urinalysis and estimation of renal function.

Presentation of asymptomatic renal disease

Asymptomatic renal disease is common and may often remain stable and undetected. However, some patients with asymptomatic disease are at increased risk of developing renal failure with the passage of time or in the event of intercurrent illnesses. Active screening for subclinical disease is thus carried out in certain

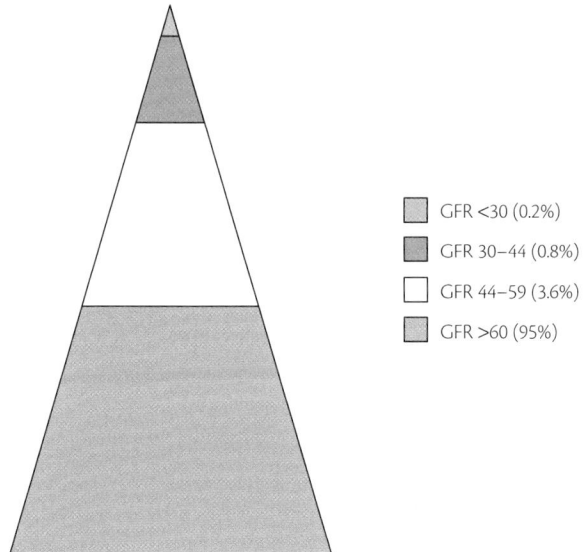

GFR <30 (0.2%)

GFR 30–44 (0.8%)

GFR 44–59 (3.6%)

GFR >60 (95%)

Fig. 21.3.1 Prevalence of chronic kidney disease in the general population. Patients with an eGFR 45–59 are classified as having CKD Stage 3A; eGFR 30–44 as having CKD Stage 3B; and those with eGFR below 30 as having CKD stages 4 (eGFR 15–30) and 5 (eGFR <15).

subpopulations with the result that patients may be identified with abnormal renal function or with abnormalities on urinalysis that may indicate significant renal pathology. Examples of such screening include:

◆ screening patients in primary care—general population screening via eGFR reporting (see below); monitoring of patients at 'high risk' of developing renal disease (e.g. hypertension, diabetes, multisystem disease); occupational and insurance medicals

◆ screening patients admitted to hospital with acute illnesses—as an incidental finding; as part of renal and electrolyte surveillance in patients at risk (e.g. in the presence of sepsis, hypovolaemia, and usage of nephrotoxic drugs)

◆ incidental finding on abdominal imaging—stones, cysts and tumours, reduced renal size

◆ screening of the family members of patients with inherited renal disease

Asymptomatic renal dysfunction and screening for chronic kidney disease

Traditionally, the basic means of assessing renal function has been estimation of the serum creatinine, and this can be used—with or without estimation of urinary creatinine excretion—to estimate the GFR, as described in Chapter 21.4. The Cockcoft–Gault equation, which estimates creatinine clearance from serum creatinine, weight, age, and sex, has largely given way as a screening tool to the Modification of Diet in Renal Disease (MDRD) formula, which in its simplest form generates an estimated glomerular filtration rate (eGFR) normalized to body surface area from serum creatinine, age, sex, and race. Using this method, population studies in the Western world have estimated that between 4 and 6% of the adult population have moderate to severe renal failure, with an eGFR of less than 60 ml/min per 1.73 m² body surface area (stage 3 to 5 chronic kidney disease (CKD), Fig. 21.3.1). Most of these are

Box 21.3.1   Summary of United Kingdom guidelines for serum creatinine measurement and estimation of GFR

Serum creatinine concentration should be measured at initial assessment and then at least annually in all adult patients with the following conditions:

◆ Previously diagnosed chronic kidney disease (CKD):
  · Persistent proteinuria
  · Unexplained haematuria
  · Identified renal pathology
◆ Conditions associated with a high risk of developing obstructive kidney disease:
  · Bladder voiding dysfunction (outflow obstruction, neurogenic bladder)
  · Urinary diversion surgery
  · Urinary stones
◆ Conditions associated with a high risk of silent development of parenchymal kidney disease:
  · Hypertension, diabetes, heart failure
  · Atherosclerotic vascular disease—coronary, cerebral, peripheral
◆ Conditions requiring long-term treatment with potentially nephrotoxic drugs:
  · ACE inhibitors, angiotensin receptor blockers, NSAIDs, lithium, mesalazine, ciclosporin, tacrolimus
◆ Multisystem diseases that may involve the kidney:
  · Systemic lupus erythematosus
  · Systemic vasculitides
  · Myeloma
  · Rheumatoid arthritis

elderly, and only very few of them (1–4%) progress to endstage renal failure when followed over a 5-year period, while over the same time many die owing to cardiovascular disease.

Population and 'risk group' screening for renal dysfunction
Population data suggest that most renal disease identified by screening is not progressive, but there are subpopulations in which progressive renal disease is more likely and in whom early intervention and optimal management may delay or prevent the need for dialysis. Hence in the United States of America and the United Kingdom guidelines have been drafted in which 'risk groups' are screened for renal dysfunction/CKD (Box 21.3.1). It is not yet known whether screening for renal dysfunction has any effect on outcome, but in the United Kingdom, data on the prevalence of CKD and associated information such as blood pressure measurement, its control, and the use of angiotensin converting enzyme (ACE) inhibitors in the CKD population, are now incorporated into the Primary Care Quality and Outcomes Framework, by which means funding is related to achievement of targets. As a consequence, there has been a substantial rise in the number of patients identified with asymptomatic renal dysfunction, and an increased

rate of referral to secondary care, especially of elderly patients. There is still considerable doubt about the validity and value of labelling many very elderly people as having moderate to severe renal failure, especially since in many patients an eGFR in this range seems to confer a very much higher risk of cardiovascular demise than of endstage renal failure.

Employment or insurance health screening

As well as targeted screening of 'at-risk' populations, asymptomatic renal disease may also be identified as a result of employment or insurance health screening. Common abnormalities identified are hypertension or abnormal urinalysis, such as proteinuria and microscopic haematuria. Patients identified in this way will often be referred for subsequent investigation.

Screening for renal dysfunction in secondary care

In the secondary care setting, patients in specialist clinics who are at risk of renal disease, such as patients with diabetes, are periodically screened for the development of hypertension, proteinuria, and renal dysfunction. Renal disease also often presents in acute medical and surgical patients. Up to 5% of acute patients have some acute deterioration in renal function during a hospital admission, mostly owing to hypotension, sepsis, or the use of nephrotoxic drugs (see Chapter 21.5). Monitoring renal function in such patients may help in the acute management of their illness and may also identify those with underlying chronic renal impairment who require long-term management.

Screening for drug-induced renal disease

Renal disease resulting from the use of nephrotoxic drugs is often asymptomatic, and CKD may develop as a result of long-term use of agents such as nonsteroidal anti-inflammatory drugs (NSAIDs), lithium, and calcineurin inhibitors. Often the only evidence for this is a progressive rise in serum creatinine and fall in eGFR, which may be progressive and—if not detected by routine screening—may present with advanced renal failure. Other drugs such as ACE inhibitors may cause an acute deterioration in renal function, screening for which is required, especially in high-risk groups.

Other incidental findings of renal disease

Subclinical renal disease may also present as an incidental finding on biochemical testing, e.g. abnormalities of potassium and acid–base homeostasis identified on a 'routine' sample may indicate a renal tubular acidosis and prompt further investigation for an underlying cause.

Renal disease identified incidentally with imaging

Advances in imaging technology combined with their widespread use have increased the number of incidental renal abnormalities identified. Many of these are anatomical abnormalities which are of little consequence, such as duplex ureters and isolated renal cysts, but significant pathology is sometimes found incidentally, such as polycystic kidneys, renal tumours, and asymmetrical kidneys.

Family screening for renal disease

Patients with a family history of inherited renal disease may also be identified with early, asymptomatic renal disease as a result of screening. The most common example is autosomal dominant polycystic kidney disease, which may be reliably identified by ultrasonography from the third decade onwards. The identification

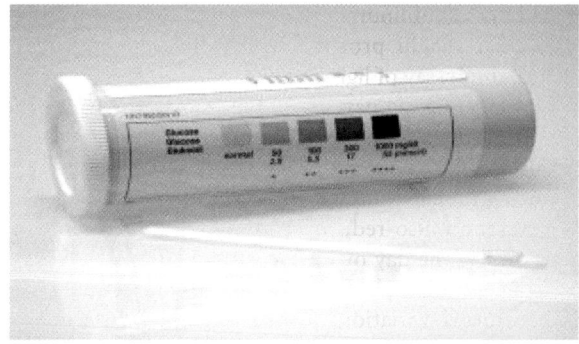

Fig. 21.3.2 Multireagent test strips used to screen patients for proteinuria and microscopic haematuria.

of disease genes for inherited renal diseases such as autosomal dominant polycystic kidney disease, tuberous sclerosis, von Hippel–Lindau disease, Alport's syndrome, and congenital nephrotic syndrome raises the possibility of future antenatal screening and earlydetection of these diseases long before they become clinically manifest.

Screening and management of asymptomatic proteinuria

The availability of reliable and cheap urine dipstick reagent strips has led to their widespread use to screen for and monitor renal disease in primary and secondary health care (Fig. 21.3.2). Within the general population, up to 5% of apparently healthy adults and 16% of those aged over 80 years have either a 'trace' or '+' of protein, but most of these do not have significant treatable disease, making routine population screening uneconomic and unnecessary. Guidelines aimed at identifying subclinical renal disease therefore suggest proteinuria screening only for patients at increased risk of renal disease. The 2005 United Kingdom guidelines are summarized in Box 21.3.2.

Detection of proteinuria

Most multireagent strips are sensitive to 100 to 200 mg/litre of protein, giving either a 'trace' or '+', although some designed to

---

Box 21.3.2 United Kingdom guidelines for proteinuria screening

Dipstick urinalysis for protein should be undertaken:

◆ As part of the initial assessment of patients with:
  · Newly discovered hypertension, haematuria, or reduced GFR
  · Unexplained oedema or suspected heart failure
  · Suspected multisystem disease, e.g. lupus, vasculitis, and myeloma
  · Diabetes mellitus

◆ As part of the annual monitoring of patients with:
  · Urologically unexplained haematuria or persistent proteinuria
  · Diabetes mellitus

◆ As part of routine monitoring for patients receiving nephrotoxic drugs, e.g. gold and penicillamine

screen for microalbuminuria are more sensitive. They do not detect low-molecular-weight proteins such as immunoglobulin light chains, and thus assay of light chains using urine immunoelectrophoresis is essential as part of the investigations for myeloma, primary amyloidosis, and light-chain glomerulopathy.

The kidney normally excretes less than 150 mg of protein in 24 h, mainly owing to failed tubular reabsorption of albumin. Urinary protein excretion also reduces overnight while recumbent, but increases during the day owing to posture and exercise. Urinary protein concentration also depends on urine flow rate. To overcome the diurnal variation, proteinuria has been traditionally evaluated from a 24-h urine collection, but these have been largely superseded by measuring the ratio of albumin or protein to creatinine in the urine (albumin:creatinine ratio, ACR; protein:creatinine ratio, PCR). This method has been validated against 24-h urinary collections and—as a rule of thumb—a urinary ACR of 70 mg/mmol or PCR of 100 mg/mmol equates approximately to a 24-h protein excretion of 1 g/24 h.

Management of asymptomatic proteinuria without haematuria

Proteinuria may be an early presentation of renal disease, but transient proteinuria is not associated with significant renal disease. A finding of proteinuria should lead the physician to take a history focusing on risk factors for renal disease (e.g. diabetes, drugs, multisystem disease, and family history), measure the blood pressure, and examine for oedema (Box 21.3.3).

In the absence of risk factors or signs of renal disease, transient proteinuria is not likely to indicate underlying renal disorder, hence an initial finding of proteinuria on dipstick testing should be repeated a week or so later, and any positive result confirmed and quantitated by estimation of ACR (or PCR). If postural or

---

Box 21.3.3 Approach to the patient with dipstick-positive proteinuria

Key features to establish

- Is there any evidence of diabetes or urinary infection?
- Are there any risk factors for or signs of renal disease?
- Is proteinuria transient or persistent?

Transient proteinuria

Causes include:

- Urinary tract infection
- Fever
- Exercise
- Orthostatic proteinuria

Persistent proteinuria

- Send urine for spot ACR (or PCR)
- Evaluate risk factors for renal disease:
  - Diabetes, hypertension, systemic inflammatory disease, myeloma, family history of renal disease
  - Are there any features of nephrotic syndrome (heavy proteinuria with oedema and low serum albumin)?

---

orthostatic proteinuria is suspected, an early-morning urine specimen should be sent for ACR (or PCR), in which case the diagnosis is substantiated by the finding of normal urinary protein excretion in this specimen.

Persistent proteinuria (ACR >70 mg/mmol, PCR >100 mg/mmol) on two or more occasions requires further investigation with:

- renal function (eGFR)
- serum albumin, for diagnosis of nephrotic syndrome
- serum paraprotein electrophoresis and urinary Bence Jones protein for myeloma
- immunological screen (antinuclear antibodies, complement, antineutrophil cytoplasmic antibodies (ANCA))
- renal ultrasonography
- consideration of renal biopsy if heavy proteinuria (ACR >150–200 mg/mmol, PCR >200–300 mg/mmol) or renal dysfunction

Management of asymptomatic proteinuria with microscopic haematuria

Proteinuria with haematuria on urinalysis indicates intrinsic renal disease. It may be the first sign of a severe glomerulonephritis and acute renal failure, hence this presentation must be considered seriously (see later). Patients with abnormal renal function, haematuria, and proteinuria require urgent referral to a nephrologist for investigation.

Apparently asymptomatic patients with normal renal function but persistent proteinuria and haematuria may describe subtle symptoms of multisystem disease on close questioning (e.g. myalgia, arthralgia, 'sinusitis', rash, or fever). These may be clues to an underlying disease, hence patients with such symptoms require screening for multisystem disease with urine microscopy for red cell casts, serum ANCA, antiglomerular basement membrane antibodies, antinuclear and anti-double-stranded DNA antibodies and complement levels, and referral to a nephrologist for further evaluation and consideration of renal biopsy.

Asymptomatic microscopic haematuria

Microscopic haematuria may potentially arise from anywhere in the urinary tract. As with renal dysfunction and proteinuria, isolated microscopic haematuria is common. Population studies indicate a prevalence between 0.2 and 16%, with a higher prevalence of 18% in men aged over 50 years. Studies of male army recruits screened and followed up for 12 years showed that 39% had microscopic haematuria on one occasion, and 16% had microscopic haematuria on two or more occasions. Although isolated microscopic haematuria may be associated with benign glomerular disease, in practice the main concern is the possibility of renal and urinary tract malignancy.

Urothelial and bladder carcinomas account for approximately 5% of microscopic haematuria. This risk increases with age, particularly in men over the age of 65 years. In contrast, underlying malignancy in those younger than 40 years is very rare, particularly in the absence of risk factors such as smoking and exposure to azo dyes.

Causes of microscopic haematuria

The causes of microscopic haematuria are summarized in Box 21.3.4. The true prevalence of intrinsic renal disease is unknown

Box 21.3.4 Causes of microscopic haematuria without proteinuria

Glomerular disease

- IgA nephropathy
- Thin basement membrane disease
- Hereditary nephritis (Alport's syndrome)
- Other glomerulonephritides (mesangiocapillary glomerulonephritis, vasculitis, lupus, etc.)

Nonglomerular renal disorders

- Nephrolithiasis
- Pyelonephritis
- Renal cell carcinoma
- Cystic kidney disease (polycystic and medullary sponge)
- Trauma
- Papillary necrosis
- Ureteric strictures
- Hydronephrosis
- Sickle cell disease
- Renal infarcts and arteriovenous malformations
- Renal tuberculosis

Lower urinary tract disorders

- Cystitis, prostatitis
- Bladder carcinoma
- Benign bladder and ureteral tumours and polyps
- Urethral strictures

Miscellaneous

- Exercise
- Overanticoagulation
- Factitious

because renal biopsies are not routinely performed in the absence of proteinuria or abnormal renal function. However, small biopsy studies of patients with no other cause for haematuria identified a glomerular cause in 16 to 30%. Within this group, IgA nephropathy and thin basement membrane disease are most common.

Management strategy for microscopic haematuria

The key to managing patients with asymptomatic microscopic haematuria is identifying risk factors for malignancy. In routine practice, patients older than 50 years, smokers, or those with an occupational history of dye exposure should be investigated for malignancy and referred to a urologist for cystoscopy.

Numerous different approaches to the management of patients with microscopic haematuria have been published, reflecting a lack of consensus and an insufficient evidence base. There are no indications for screening for microscopic haematuria as the positive predictive value for malignancy is as low as 5% in an elderly population, and early detection of disease has not been shown to improve prognosis.

Following the detection of microscopic haematuria without proteinuria on urine dipstick, menstruation, recent exercise, or sexual activity should be excluded, and the urine sent for microscopy and culture. Urinalysis should be repeated after 7 days: if this remains positive, further management depends on the patient's age:

- Patients over the age of 50 years or with risk factors for malignancy (e.g. smoking or occupational history of dye exposure) require measurement of renal function (eGFR), renal tract ultrasound (and/or intravenous urography or CT), and referral to urological services for cystoscopy (and subsequently to a nephrologist if renal function is impaired).

- Patients younger than 50 years with no risk factors for malignancy require measurement of renal function (eGFR). If this is abnormal, refer to a nephrologist for further investigation of possible intrinsic renal disease. If this is normal, monitor annually with urinalysis for blood and protein, blood pressure, and measurement of renal function, and refer if there is evidence of deteriorating renal function or development of persistent proteinuria.

Symptomatic renal disease

Many patients with renal disease remain asymptomatic, but others develop symptoms that may be nonspecific, e.g. due to the gradual onset of uraemia in patients with progressive CKD, renal-specific, e.g. loin pain or polyuria, or unrelated to the kidney and manifest as isolated 'nonrenal' symptoms or as a constellation of symptoms suggestive of a particular systemic condition. Key features to establish are the duration of symptoms, the presence of nonspecific symptoms possibly related to uraemia, the presence of specific renal symptoms, and the presence of symptoms possibly indicative of systemic disease.

Chronic kidney disease

The symptoms of CKD are attributed to the gradual onset of uraemia, anaemia, and salt and water retention. Patients often develop these slowly and may not report them until renal function is severely impaired, perhaps even an eGFR as low as lesss than 10 ml/min per 1.73 m^2 body surface area. The number of symptoms and their severity tend to increase as renal function declines, forming a spectrum from asymptomatic to overtly symptomatic uraemia. Symptoms and the level of eGFR may not correlate well: some patients with an eGFR of 15 to 20 ml/min per 1.73 m^2 may be symptomatic, whereas a few with an eGFR of less than 5 ml/min per 1.73 m^2 may be remarkably symptom free.

Most patients have some symptoms by the time that they require dialysis (CKD stage 5, eGFR <15 ml/min per 1.73 m^2) (Box 21.3.5). These include anorexia, nausea, and vomiting (in 76% of patients), fatigue and weakness (72%), pruritus (40%), breathlessness and orthopnoea (26%), bleeding tendency (14%), apathy and loss of mental concentration (12%), and muscle twitching and cramps (11%).

Factors contributing to the development of 'uraemia' and other symptoms include small-molecule nitrogenous substances, endproducts of protein metabolism, metabolic acidosis, salt and water retention, electrolyte disturbances (e.g. phosphate retention), malnutrition, and anaemia.

Some of these symptoms may be improved by treatment with agents such as erythropoietin, diuretics, and oral sodium bicarbonate,

---

Box 21.3.5 Features of uraemia and an eGFR less than 15 ml/min per 1.73 m² body surface area

- Anorexia and malnutrition
- Nausea and vomiting
- Tiredness
- Fluid overload with oedema, breathlessness, and orthopnoea
- Anaemia
- Pruritus
- Mental apathy and depression
- Muscle twitching, restless legs, and cramps
- Bleeding tendency—haematemesis, epistaxis
- Sexual dysfunction—loss of libido and impotence
- Cardiac—pericarditis

---

and dietary advice to improve malnutrition and phosphate control. Others respond to the initiation of dialysis. Some symptoms may persist in spite of all these measures.

It is unfortunately not uncommon for patients to present for the first time very late in the course of progressive CKD, with profound and symptomatic uraemia. This is the initial mode of presentation in 20 to 40% of patients entering dialysis programmes in the United Kingdom, who tend to be older, more dependent, and with greater comorbidities than those presenting earlier. Late presentation presents major problems: it is not possible to plan dialysis initiation, and patient choice of modality is limited, with haemodialysis being the default mode. Furthermore, it is often not possible to create definitive vascular access, hence patients often need to begin dialysis with temporary or semipermanent central venous lines. These and other features increase morbidity and mortality after late presentation.

It can be difficult and sometimes impossible to distinguish patients presenting late with advanced chronic renal failure ('crash-landers') from those with acute renal failure due to potentially reversible disease. Failure to become dialysis independent by 90 days after initiation is often taken as proof that the acute presentation was with endstage rather than acute renal failure. Patients who 'crash-land' are often extremely unwell and may be obtunded with uraemic encephalopathy. Fluid overload is common, with pulmonary and peripheral oedema. Metabolic acidosis is often present and if severe may cause Kussmaul's respiration as well as cerebral and cardiac depression. Patients may also show signs of muscle twitching, which may be a sign of hyperkalaemia or hypocalcaemia. A pericardial friction rub indicates uraemic pericarditis, which if unrecognized may lead to pericardial tamponade and occasionally to fatal pericardial haemorrhage.

See Chapter 21.6 for further discussion of chronic kidney disease.

Acute renal failure (acute kidney injury)

Acute kidney injury is discussed in detail in Chapter 21.5, but, in brief, causes can be classified as being prerenal (due to intrinsic renal disease) or postrenal (obstruction). In the general hospital setting, most cases (about 80%) are prerenal and occur as the result of reduced renal perfusion due to volume depletion, dehydration, cardiac failure,

and sepsis. Urinary tract obstruction accounts for 10% and acute glomerular disease and interstitial nephritis cause 5 to 10%.

Key features to establish sequentially when managing a patient with acute renal failure are as follows:

1 How ill are they? The condition of patients with similar biochemical abnormalities can range from the asymptomatic to the moribund: those with cardiorespiratory compromise need critical care support.

2 Does the patient need emergency haemodialysis or haemofiltration? The major indications are severe hyperkalaemia, pulmonary oedema, profound acidosis, and severe uraemia—the latter being defined more on clinical than biochemical grounds.

3 Is there a prerenal element that may respond to volume repletion or inotropic support? Clinical examination, perhaps supplemented by central venous pressure measurement, facilitates this decision.

4 Is the patient obstructed? Clinical features can be helpful, and a urinary tract ultrasound is usually diagnostic.

5 Is this acute or chronic renal failure? Sometimes this is difficult or impossible to determine on clinical grounds, but small kidneys on ultrasound signify chronic disease.

6 Is this intrinsic renal disease? Clinical features of systemic disease and relevant immunological tests (including ANCA and antiglomerular basement membrane antibody) must be pursued, and renal biopsy will usually be required to establish the diagnosis.

As with chronic kidney disease, many of the symptoms and signs attributed to loss of renal function are nonspecific and occur with advanced acute renal failure (GFR <15 ml/min per 1.73 m²). However, in contrast to CKD, the acute metabolic changes are often less well tolerated. The greatest danger is hyperkalaemia, which may develop quickly and is almost always asymptomatic until the onset of cardiac arrhythmias and cardiac arrest. Other potentially life-threatening features include pulmonary oedema, metabolic acidosis, and uraemic pericarditis.

The clinical context and history are of overriding importance in establishing the likely aetiology of acute renal failure. A patient developing acute renal failure postsurgery is likely to have prerenal and acute tubular injury due to a combination of hypovolaemia, sepsis, and analgesia with an NSAID. A patient presenting acutely after a prolonged period of unconsciousness following a drug overdose is likely to have rhabdomyolysis. A patient with a past history of lupus presenting with a recent fever, myalgia, and rash is likely to have rapidly progressive lupus nephritis. A patient with a history of lower urinary tract symptoms or of urinary stones is likely to have obstruction.

It is always important to consider the possibility of urinary tract obstruction as it may be readily reversible. Complete anuria is highly suggestive of total obstruction, although it may also occur in patients with rapidly progressive glomerulonephritis and those with acute obstruction of the renal arterial supply. However, urinary output is generally a poor guide to the presence of urinary tract obstruction, and a normal or even increased output does not exclude the diagnosis. All patients with unexplained acute renal failure should undergo ultrasound imaging of the kidneys and urinary tract. This permits the diagnosis or exclusion of obstruction in most cases, and also allows renal size to be assessed: small kidneys indicate chronic renal failure.

It is important to emphasize that, after stabilization, patients in whom the clinical features and initial investigations do not give sufficient clues to allow a diagnosis to be established will require a renal biopsy to avoid missing potentially reversible intrinsic renal disease. Details of important and common presentations of acute renal disease are discussed later in this chapter and in Chapter 21.5.

Urinary symptoms

Micturition

Most symptoms related to micturition relate to problems arising in the lower urinary tract. Bladder outflow obstruction is commonly associated with symptoms such as urgency, hesitancy, poor urinary stream, nocturia, dysuria, and dribbling. Recognition of these symptoms is important as outflow obstruction may result in complete obstruction with acute renal failure or chronic obstructive uropathy with CKD.

Patients may also describe discomfort or pain on micturition. This symptom of dysuria may also be associated with burning within the urethra or suprapubic pain during or after micturition. When associated with urinary frequency or fevers in young women, dysuria is likely to be caused by a urinary tract infection. However, dysuria occurring in isolation in men of any age suggests structural lesions within the prostate or bladder and warrants further investigation. Perineal or rectal pain associated with micturition suggests prostatic inflammation, such as prostatitis or malignancy.

Frequency

Patients may present with symptoms of increased frequency of micturition. In this situation, it is important to distinguish between frequent voiding of small volumes of urine and an overall increase in urinary volume with more frequent emptying of a full bladder. Charting urinary frequency and voided volumes over a number of days can allow these to be distinguished. The frequent passage of small volumes of urine suggests bladder irritation (from inflammation, stone, or tumour) or reduced volume from extrinsic compression or contraction (e.g. following radiotherapy). Increased frequency of emptying a full bladder is suggestive of polyuria, especially if the volume and frequency is unaffected during the night.

Polyuria

Polyuria (defined as a urinary output >3 litre/24 h) may result from solute diuresis, water diuresis, or a combination of both. Solute diuresis occurs in conditions such as hyperglycaemia and salt-losing states, e.g. overuse of diuretics and salt-losing nephropathies. Water diuresis may result from primary polydipsia, failure to synthesize or secrete ADH normally (congenital and acquired cranial diabetes insipidus), or failure of cortical and medullary collecting ducts to respond to ADH (congenital and acquired nephrogenic diabetes insipidus).

There are numerous causes of acquired nephrogenic diabetes insipidus, including chronic kidney disease (especially associated with ureteric obstruction, postobstructive states, and chronic interstitial nephritis), electrolyte abnormalities (hypercalcaemia and hyperkalaemia), nephrotoxic drugs (such as lithium and amphotericin), and many other miscellaneous conditions including sickle cell disease, Sjögren's syndrome, and sarcoidosis. Most patients with polyuria have associated thirst, polydipsia, and nocturia.

Polyuria needs confirmation by 24-h urinary collection as most patients are unclear as to their true daily urine output. Once it is established that the patient is polyuric, common causes such as hyperglycaemia and excessive diuretic use need to be excluded, after which investigations should focus on excluding primary polydipsia and distinguishing between cranial and nephrogenic diabetes insipidus, as discussed in Chapter 21.2.

Nocturia

Nocturia is defined as the need to get up once or more times for nocturnal voids. It may have a considerable negative impact on quality of life and in older people predisposes to falls. Three types of nocturia have been identified: low voided volume, nocturnal polyuria, and mixed origin. Nocturia due to low voided volumes occurs in patients with bladder outflow obstruction and those with hyperactive bladders from any cause. Nocturnal polyuria occurs when there is a reversal of the normal circadian pattern of voiding such that there is an increased nocturnal urine output. These types of nocturia are distinguishable by the use of voiding diaries. Elderly patients who void in excess of 33% of their total 24-h output between 11 p.m. and 7 a.m. are said to have nocturnal polyuria, the corresponding fraction in young adults being 20%. Factors predisposing to nocturnal polyuria include renal impairment, diabetes mellitus, congestive cardiac failure, sleep apnoea, and the mobilization of peripheral oedema due to any cause. In patients without predisposing causes, usually elderly, low nocturnal levels of ADH have been described.

Oliguria and anuria

Oliguria is arbitrarily defined as a urinary output of less than 400 ml/24 h or 0.5 ml/kg body weight per hour. Oliguria is the normal renal physiological response to reduced renal perfusion from any cause and is common in hospital inpatients, particularly those with acute illnesses associated with hypotension and reduced effective circulating volume. Monitoring of fluid balance and urinary output in such patients allows its early detection and treatment, which may help prevent progression to established acute renal failure. The recognition of oliguria should prompt an evaluation of the patient with attention to volume status, blood pressure and the detection/exclusion of sepsis, followed by appropriate management to optimize blood pressure and circulating volume.

Oliguria may also be a feature of intrinsic renal failure due to nephrotoxic drugs, acute glomerulonephritis, or interstitial nephritis, but it is a poor marker of intrinsic renal disease as urinary output often remains normal despite significantly impaired renal function.

The development of anuria, meaning the total absence of urine, is strongly suggestive of urinary tract obstruction, which may occur at any level in the urinary tract. A careful history, examination for an enlarged bladder and digital rectal examination for a prostatic or pelvic mass, should be followed by an urgent ultrasound of the kidneys and bladder. Very occasionally, anuria may be a manifestation of severe intrinsic renal disease, such as a rapidly progressive glomerulonephritis, cortical necrosis, or renal infarction.

Urine appearance and macroscopic haematuria

Macroscopic haematuria is the most common abnormality of the urine noted by patients. As little as 5 ml of blood in a litre of urine will lead to a visible change in urinary colour. Haematuria may arise from anywhere within the urinary tract, but bright red haematuria (with or without clots) is suggestive of lower urinary tract bleeding, whereas dark, smoky brown–black urine is more suggestive of renal pathology. Haematuria at the beginning of micturition, which then clears, suggests urethral pathology, whereas endstream haematuria is consistent with bladder pathology. Although the causes of haematuria are numerous (Box 21.3.6), infection, stones, and malignancy are the most common. Macroscopic haematuria warrants investigation in all patients.

Frank haematuria is uncommon in glomerular disease, with the notable exception of IgA nephropathy in which macroscopic haematuria classically occurs immediately following mucosal inflammation, typically an upper respiratory tract infection. In patients with polycystic disease, cysts may haemorrhage to cause loin pain and haematuria. This may be associated with infection of the cysts and usually resolves with conservative management, with antibiotics if there are signs of infection.

Red–brown–black urine is occasionally caused by haemo-globinuria due to haemolysis or myoglobinuria precipitated by rhabdomyolysis. Beetroot and food colouring may turn the urine pink, whereas drugs such as rifampicin may discolour the urine orange–red. Rarely, urine is found to darken following exposure to light, suggesting a diagnosis of porphyria or alkaptonuria.

Loin pain

The presence of pain in the renal angle (loin pain) is consistent with inflammation, obstruction, or stretching of the renal capsule by a mass lesion. Pain arising from acute obstruction is common and typically colicky in nature, with radiation into the groin and scrotum. The pain may be exacerbated by oral fluids, which increase urinary volume and pressure within the renal pelvis. Pyelonephritis typically causes renal angle pain on the affected side and is often associated with pyrexia and leucocytes in the urine. Similarly, a renal abscess extending into the renal capsule may present with loin pain or with isolated symptoms of diaphragmatic irritation or involvement of the psoas muscle, with pain on leg extension. Patients with polycystic kidneys may also develop loin pain as a result of infection or haemorrhage of single or multiple cysts.

Renal pain is an uncommon feature of glomerulonephritis and other intrinsic renal diseases: IgA nephropathy is very occasionally associated with renal pain, but active destructive glomerulonephritis and interstitial nephritis are invariably pain free.

Loin pain–haematuria syndrome

Rare patients may present with recurrent intermittent loin pain, haematuria (microscopic or macroscopic), and normal renal function, with no relevant structural abnormality of the renal tract. The cause of this condition, termed the loin pain–haematuria syndrome, is unknown: it is a diagnosis of exclusion which is most often seen in young women.

The pain—often described as 'deep', 'burning', or 'throbbing'—is usually felt in the loin, but can radiate in a typical renal pattern to the groin, genital area, and medial thigh. Some will describe a psychologically traumatic event before the onset of pain. The pain can sometimes be induced or exacerbated by exercise and affected by posture, e.g. sitting for a prolonged length of time can be uncomfortable, and in some cases there is associated nausea and vomiting. Some patients report continuous pain that never goes away, whereas others describe episodic pain that lasts more or less continuously for days or (more typically) weeks, interspersed with periods of remission. The pain is usually unilateral at presentation, but many patients eventually develop pain bilaterally. Many patients are taking large quantities of opioids and other analgaesics (e.g. amitriptyline, gabapentin) by the time they are referred to specialist services.

Urological investigation is unremarkable, or shows incidental abnormalities only. If renal biopsy is performed, the appearances may be normal, but thinning or thickening of the glomerular basement membrane has been reported in about 60% of cases in some series, and appearances of IgA nephropathy are sometime seem, but the relationship—if any—between these findings and symptomatology remains obscure.

Aside from loin pain, many patients will have other medically unexplained somatic symptoms, raising the possibility that this symptom is also a somatoform disorder. They may request nephrectomy and/or renal autotransplantation, which the wise physician will not accede to, preferring to help the patient by sympathetic discussion and referral to pain management services.

Box 21.3.6 Causes of macroscopic haematuria

- Infections:
  - Cystitis and pyelonephritis
  - Prostatitis
  - Urethritis
  - Schistosomiasis
- Urinary stones
- Tumours:
  - Renal cell
  - Transitional cell
  - Prostatic
  - Urethral
- Glomerular diseases:
  - IgA nephropathy
  - Alport's syndrome
  - Crescentic glomerulonephritis
- Interstitial and medullary renal diseases:
  - Polycystic kidneys
  - Interstitial nephritis
  - Papillary necrosis
  - Tuberculosis
- Miscellaneous causes:
  - Release of urinary obstruction
  - Trauma
  - Loin pain–haematuria syndrome
  - Arteriovenous malformations
  - Anticoagulation
  - Factitious

Specific renal syndromes

Nephrotic syndrome

Definition

Nephrotic syndrome is the triad of oedema, proteinuria, and hypoalbuminaemia (see Box 21.3.7 for an example). Proteinuria is usually greater than 3.5 g in 24 h, which equates approximately to an ACR of 250 mg/mmol or PCR of 350 mg/mmol. When patients have clinically apparent oedema, serum albumin is usually less than 25 g/litre (Fig. 21.3.3). However, in practice the definition is somewhat arbitrary, and the correlation between the degree of proteinuria, serum albumin, and presence of oedema is poor. Some patients (particularly older people) may develop oedema with

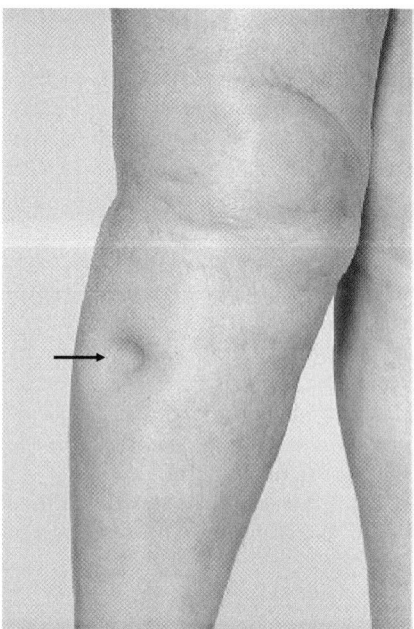

Fig. 21.3.3 Severe peripheral oedema of the lower legs with pitting below the right knee (arrow).

proteinuria less than 3.5 g, whereas others remain free of oedema despite having a serum albumin considerably less than 25 g/litre. Other patients may have heavy proteinuria but maintain a normal serum albumin and remain free of oedema.

Nephrotic syndrome indicates the presence of glomerular disease. Causes can usefully be divided into primary glomerular diseases and those arising secondary to systemic disease (Box 21.3.8), with the geographical context important in determining the most likely cause in any particular case. The most common cause of nephrotic syndrome in Western countries is diabetes mellitus, whereas in developing countries it is most commonly associated with infection. Nephrotic syndrome due to malaria and hepatitis are particularly common in sub-Saharan Africa, and poststreptococcal glomerulonephritis is also an important cause.

Clinical features

One of the earliest symptoms patients may report is that of frothy urine. This often occurs before the onset of oedema and may be a useful indicator of the onset of heavy proteinuria. As proteinuria develops and serum albumin falls, patients gradually develop oedema. This may be noticed first as periorbital swelling and 'puffiness' in the morning, or as ankle swelling in the evening due to the effects of gravity. Worsening leg oedema develops as salt and water retention increases, followed by abdominal distension from ascites. In men, scrotal oedema may be marked and very uncomfortable. Further fluid retention leads to pleural effusions, which are often bilateral but may be unilateral. Patients often feel lethargic, with a loss of appetite and nausea due to associated gut oedema.

Clinical examination of the patient's volume status may reveal a normal or low jugular venous pressure despite marked oedema. Although rare in untreated adult patients, it is important to identify intravascular volume depletion because the use of high-dose diuretic therapy in this setting may provoke circulatory collapse from hypovolaemia, or less dramatically may further reduce renal perfusion and exacerbate renal dysfunction. Conversely, a raised jugular venous pressure with a low blood pressure may suggest a

---

Box 21.3.7 Case illustration—proteinuria and oedema

A 54-year-old woman presents with worsening peripheral oedema. She had been diagnosed with type 2 diabetes 6 months earlier, but remained well until 4 weeks ago, when she suddenly noted frothy urine and mild peripheral oedema. Over the following weeks the oedema had worsened and she noted some abdominal distension. Her only regular medication is gliclazide.

Examination

- Pitting oedema to her lumbar spine, with bilateral small pleural effusions
- Jugular venous pressure not elevated and heart sounds normal
- Mild erythema over right ankle and lower leg

Investigations

- Urine dipstick test: protein 4+, no haematuria
- Urine albumin:creatinine ratio (ACR): 4520 mg/mmol
- 24-h urinary collection: 6.8 g proteinuria
- Serum albumin: 13 g/litre
- Serum creatinine: 82 μmol/litre
- Autoimmune and hepatitis serology: negative
- Renal ultrasonography and venous Doppler: normal
- Doppler ultra sonography of right leg: normal
- Renal biopsy: membranous nephropathy with subepithelial spikes on silver stain

Diagnosis

- Membranous nephropathy with nephrotic syndrome

Frothy urine, oedema, and hypoalbuminaemia indicate the onset of heavy proteinuria and nephrotic syndrome. The rapid onset of symptoms suggests a primary glomerular lesion rather than long-standing diabetic nephropathy. The presence of leg erythema may be due to infection or deep venous thrombosis, hence a Doppler ultrasound scan was requested. To make the diagnosis, a renal biopsy was performed, which showed membranous nephropathy. The patient was initially managed conservatively with diuretics and low-molecular-weight heparin as thromboembolic prophylaxis.

Box 21.3.8 Causes of nephrotic syndrome

◆ Primary glomerular diseases:
  · Minimal change
  · Focal segmental glomerulosclerosis (FSGS)
  · Membranous
  · Mesangiocapillary glomerulonephritis (MCGN)
◆ Secondary glomerular diseases:
  · Diabetes
  · Amyloid
◆ Drugs:
  · Gold, penicillamine, NSAIDs, captopril, heroin
◆ Systemic disease:
  · Lupus
◆ Infectious diseases:
  · Poststreptococcal glomerulonephritis
  · Hepatitis B and C
  · HIV
  · Malaria
  · Schistosomiasis
  · Filaria
◆ Malignancy:
  · Minimal change
  · Membranous
◆ Pre-eclampsia
◆ Hereditary:
  · Alport's syndrome
  · Nail–patella syndrome

Box 21.3.9 Case illustration—ANCA-associated vasculitis

An 80-year-old woman presents with a 2-week history of increasing malaise and lethargy. On close questioning she also reported arthralgia in the small joints of her hands, and numbness in her hands and feet in the last few months.

Examination

◆ Subtle purpuric rash on both legs
◆ Bibasal crepitations
◆ Reduced pinprick sensation in a glove and stocking distribution

Investigations

◆ Creatinine: 854 μmol/litre (56 μmol/litre 10 months before)
◆ Urea: 45 mmol/litre
◆ Hb: 8.3 g/dl
◆ Urine dipstick test: blood 3+, protein 2+
◆ Urine microscopy: red cell casts
◆ Serological testing: p-ANCA positive, with myeloperoxidase titre 78%
◆ Renal biopsy: focal necrotizing glomerulonephritis

Diagnosis

◆ Acute renal failure due to microscopic polyangiitis (an ANCA-associated vasculitis) with associated peripheral neuropathy

The history is nonspecific, except that the onset of symptoms is recent and suggestive of a systemic disorder. The presence of a purpuric rash makes the diagnosis of vasculitis a possibility. Dipstick testing of the urine and checking the renal function are critical in making the diagnosis of acute renal failure due to an inflammatory condition. Confirmation of a systemic vasculitis is made with a positive p-ANCA and renal biopsy.

---

significant pericardial effusion or underlying amyloid with cardiac involvement.

Patients may also present with complications associated with nephrotic syndrome. Thromboembolism may be difficult to detect clinically. Patients with marked peripheral oedema often have swollen legs of unequal size and associated erythema due to an increased susceptibility to cellulitis. These may mask the signs of deep venous thrombosis. Similarly, subtle symptoms of breathlessness, perhaps suggesting pulmonary embolism, or headache, perhaps suggesting cerebral venous sinus thrombosis, may be overlooked. In practice, a low threshold is required for investigation and treatment of suspected thromboembolism.

The combination of severe peripheral oedema and susceptibility to infection following skin breakdown often leads to cellulitis. Long-standing hypoalbuminaemia may lead to leuconychia. Severe hyperlipidaemia, which is a feature of nephrotic syndrome, may lead to cutaneous xanthomas.

Establishing a clinical diagnosis of nephrotic syndrome is often straightforward. The clinical history and examination may also provide clues to an underlying cause, which may be clear, such as in a patient with long-standing diabetes and progressive diabetic nephropathy. Alternatively, the immediate cause may only become apparent after a detailed history revealing long-standing use of drugs that may precipitate the condition (e.g. ACE inhibitors, NSAIDs, gold, or penicillamine). A history of chronic infections (such as hepatitis) may suggest an underlying membranous or mesangiocapillary glomerulonephritis, whereas a rash and arthralgia may lead to a diagnosis of an autoimmune condition such as systemic lupus erythematosus or cryoglobulinaemia. The presence of other long-standing inflammatory conditions, such as rheumatoid arthritis, raises the possibility of systemic amyloidosis. In older patients, an associated malignancy remains a possibility and should be sought in the history and examination, but does not warrant further investigation apart from a chest radiograph in the absence of clinical clues, e.g. disturbance of bowel habit would merit imaging of the colon. Very occasionally, a family history may reveal an inherited nephrotic syndrome such as familial focal segmental glomerulosclerosis.

Rapidly progressive glomerulonephritis with acute renal failure

Around 5% of cases of acute renal failure are caused by a rapidly progressive glomerulonephritis (RPGN). Recognizing this relatively

---

Box 21.3.10 Causes of a rapidly progressive glomerulonephritis

- Antineutrophil cytoplasmic antibody (ANCA)-associated vasculitis:
  - Wegener's granulomatosis
  - Microscopic polyangiitis
  - Churg–Strauss syndrome
- Other primary systemic vasculitides (ANCA-negative)
- Other systemic disorders:
  - Systemic lupus erythematosus
  - Cryoglobulinaemia
  - Henoch–Schönlein purpura
- Infection-related glomerulonephritis:
  - Postinfectious glomerulonephritis
  - Infective endocarditis
- Antiglomerular basement membrane disease (Goodpasture's syndrome)
- Crescentic phase of a primary glomerulonephritis:
  - IgA nephropathy
  - Mesangiocapillary glomerulonephritis

Table 21.3.1 Key features of specific systemic inflammatory diseases causing a rapidly progressive glomerulonephritis

Feature	Type	Disease
Skin rashes	Purpuric	Any vasculitis
	Lupoid	Lupus
Ear, nose and throat symptoms	Nasal crusting	Wegener's granulomatosis
	Deafness	Wegener's granulomatosis
	Oral ulceration	Any vasculitis or lupus
Eye symptoms	Scleritis and episcleritis	Any vasculitis, lupus, rarely Behçet's disease
Myalgia, arthralgia and arthritis		Any vasculitis, Henoch–Schönlein purpura, cryoglobulinaemia, lupus, rheumatoid arthritis, systemic sclerosis
Haemoptysis		Goodpasture's disease, any vasculitis, lupus
Neuropathy		Any vasculitis, lupus, cryoglobulinaemia

---

small group of patients is important because many of the causes respond well to treatment, provided the diagnosis is made early and treatment started promptly. The key to making a diagnosis is having a high index of clinical suspicion such that important features of the syndrome are identified (see Box 21.3.9 for an example).

The hallmarks of an RPGN are rapidly declining renal function, haematuria and proteinuria on urine dipstick testing, dysmorphic red cells or red cell casts on urine microscopy, and crescentic and focal necrotizing glomerulonephritis on renal biopsy.

Clinical presentation

An RPGN may present either *de novo* in a previously well patient or as a complication in a patient known to have a systemic disease (Box 21.3.10). Their clinical features may be diverse. Occasionally, patients may present with very few symptoms and signs, except for proteinuria and haematuria with a recent decline in renal function,

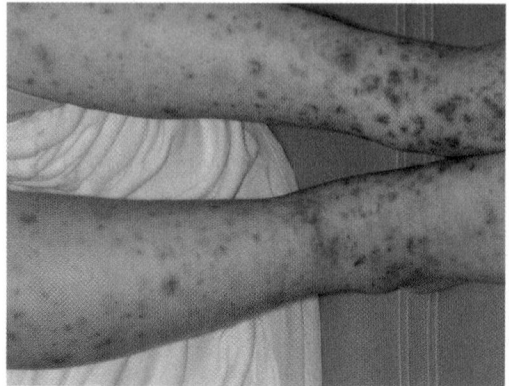

Fig. 21.3.4 Purpuric rash affecting the lower legs, consistent with a systemic vasculitis.

and at the other end of the spectrum patients may present with severe acute renal failure associated with features of uraemia. Importantly, patients may also present with clinical features of systemic inflammation that indicate an underlying cause for glomerulonephritis. These range from the subtle, such as arthralgia or myalgia, to the florid, such as a purpuric rash (Fig. 21.3.4), haemoptysis and peripheral neuropathy. Clinical features of specific inflammatory diseases associated with an RPGN are detailed in Table 21.3.1.

In practice, specific features to elicit in patients presenting with an acute decline in renal function include arthralgia and arthritis, myalgia and muscle tenderness, rashes, eye symptoms (pain and redness), ear, nose, and throat symptoms (epistaxis, nasal crusting, and new deafness), haemoptysis (important, as may be life-threatening if severe), and neuropathic symptoms and signs. Conversely, the clinician should have a high index of suspicion for an RPGN in patients presenting with any of the above features, and in this context suspicions are heightened by the presence of dysmorphic red cells and red cell casts on urinary microscopy (Fig. 21.3.5).

If an RPGN is suspected, then investigations should include ANCA, antiglomerular basement membrane (anti-GBM) antibodies, antinuclear and anti-double-stranded DNA antibodies, serum complement, antistreptolysin-O titre, and immunoglobulins and serum electrophoresis (including tests for cryoglobulins). It is almost certain that a patient with an RPGN will require a renal biopsy to confirm the diagnosis and to guide management, and thus all patients with suspected RPGN should be referred urgently to a nephrologist.

Presentation of renal disease associated with other underlying diseases

Renal disease is capable of presenting in many complex and diverse ways, and many renal problems arise as either direct or indirect complications of other disease. Examples include acute renal failure caused by sepsis, and progressive chronic kidney disease due to

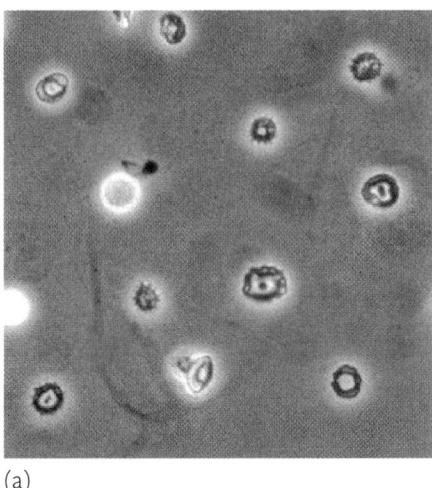
(a)

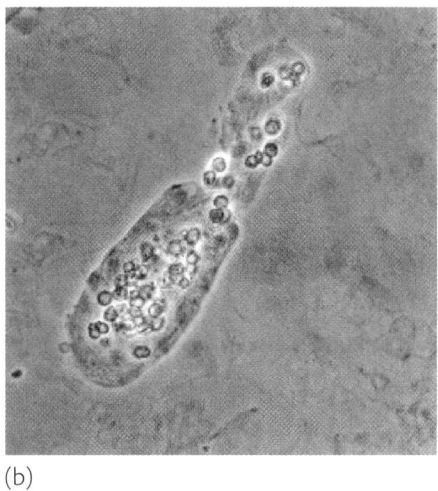
(b)

Fig. 21.3.5 Phase contrast micrographs showing dysmorphic erythrocytes (a) and a red cell cast (b) within the urine.

diabetes (Box 21.3.11). This section illustrates some common and important presentations of renal disease.

Diabetic nephropathy

In the Western world, diabetes is the most common cause of renal disease, accounting for 43% of endstage renal failure in the United States of America and 19% in the United Kingdom (Box 21.3.12). Diabetic nephropathy develops over the course of years and is preceded by a clinically silent phase of microalbuminuria, which is often detected as a result of diabetic screening programmes,

> **Box 21.3.11** Important and common presentations of renal disease
>
> ◆ Diabetic nephropathy with progressive chronic kidney disease
> ◆ Vascular disease:
>   • Renal atheroemboli
>   • Renal artery stenosis
> ◆ Underlying malignancy:
>   • Urinary tract obstruction
>   • Myeloma
>   • Hypercalcaemia
> ◆ Infection:
>   • Acute presentation with renal failure: (1) general syndromes—sepsis, rhabdomyolysis, haemolytic uraemic syndrome, postinfectious glomerulonephritis, tubulointerstitial nephritis; (2) specific syndromes—hantavirus, leptospirosis, malaria
>   • Chronic infections associated with renal disease: hepatitis B, hepatitis C, filaria, schistosomiasis, HIV
> ◆ Systemic inflammatory disease:
>   • Systemic vasculitides
>   • Systemic lupus erythematosus
>   • Sarcoidosis
> ◆ Drug-induced renal disease
> ◆ Pregnancy

enabling a targeted approach to management in which tight glycaemic control and blood pressure control with the use of agents to block the renin–angiotensin system aim to reduce the rate of progression of the nephropathy. As with other causes of progressive CKD, patients with diabetic nephropathy often only develop symptoms of kidney disease late in the course of their disease, but there is a tendency for those with this condition to become symptomatic, particularly in relation to anaemia and fluid retention, with lesser impairment of renal function than their nondiabetic counterparts. This leads to an earlier requirement for initiation of dialysis in patients with diabetic nephropathy.

Patients with diabetes are also subject to develop other microvascular and macrovascular complications, which may lead to superimposed renal atheroembolic disease and renal artery stenosis. These may present as an abrupt decline in renal function following the introduction of an ACE inhibitor or angiotensin receptor antagonist. Patients with diabetic nephropathy are also at increased risk of acute or chronic renal failure, with common causes for this including use of radiocontrast media for investigations such as coronary or peripheral angiography, surgery (especially cardiac surgery), and, in the context of diabetic emergencies, particularly diabetic ketoacidosis.

See Chapter 21.10.1 for further discussion of diabetic renal disease.

Renovascular disease

Many patients with diffuse atherosclerosis have evidence of renovascular disease, and a history of cerebrovascular, coronary, or peripheral vascular disease makes a diagnosis of renovascular disease likely. Up to 24% of patients presenting with peripheral vascular disease have stenoses in both renal arteries, and up to 50% have more than 50% stenosis in at least one renal artery. The absence of peripheral pulses and the presence of a femoral bruit make the diagnosis of renovascular disease extremely likely, although most of these patients remain asymptomatic from the renal point of view. Common presentations of renovascular disease are outlined in Box 21.3.13.

Myeloma and other malignancies

Myeloma can cause acute renal failure in several ways. Features suggestive of underlying myeloma in a patient presenting with unexplained renal failure are older age, bone pain (often nonspecific), hypercalcaemia (sometimes mild, and sometimes 'relative' considering the degree of renal impairment), anaemia (often inappropriately

Box 21.3.12 Case illustration—progressive chronic kidney disease due to diabetic nephropathy

A 66-year-old Asian man presents with nausea, anorexia, ankle swelling and breathlessness. He has a 25-year history of type 2 diabetes mellitus, a 14-year history of hypertension, and had coronary artery bypass grafts 3 years ago. Insulin, furosemide, and ramipril are his only regular medications.

Examination

- Cardiovascular—blood pressure 167/88 mmHg, jugular venous pressure +3 cm, cardiomegaly, bibasal crepitations, and peripheral oedema to sacrum
- Fundi—treated diabetic retinopathy
- Neurological—reduced pinprick sensation in stocking distribution to knees, with absent ankle reflexes, proprioception, and vibration sensation

Investigations

- Urine dipstick test: protein 4+, no haematuria
- Urine albumin:creatinine ratio (ACR): 1720 mg/mmol
- Serum creatinine: 568 µmol/litre (eGFR 9 ml/min per 1.73 m^2 body surface area)
- Serum bicarbonate: 15 mmol/litre
- Full blood count: Hb 9.8 g/dl
- Hb$_{A1C}$: 10.2%

Further history

Five years previously his blood pressure was 189/92 mmHg with creatinine of 154 µmol/litre and protein+ on urine dipstick. At the time of his coronary surgery, blood pressure was 165/86 mmHg with creatinine 210 µmol/litre. Over the last year he had felt well until the last 2 months, since when he had developed increasing lethargy, anorexia, and breathlessness on exertion, and noted increasing ankle swelling.

This man with long-standing diabetes presents with nonspecific symptoms and oedema. He also has evidence of end-organ damage, with cardiovascular disease, retinopathy, and neuropathy. Five years ago he had evidence of nephropathy with proteinuria and an eGFR of 43 ml/min (CKD stage 3). Since then his blood pressure and glycaemic control have been poor, which contributed to the progression of nephropathy to eGFR of 30 ml/min (CKD stage 3/4) 3 years ago, and now to CKD stage 5 with symptoms of uraemia.

Screening patients with diabetes for microalbuminuria and hypertension enables early diagnosis of complications and intensive management of glucose and blood pressure. As eGFR falls to 30 ml/min per 1.73 m^2 body surface area, patients should be referred to a nephrologist to plan for renal replacement therapy.

Box 21.3.13 Common presentations of renovascular disease

- As part of the investigation for acute, severe, or refractory hypertension
- An acute rise (>20%) in creatinine following introduction of an ACE inhibitor or angiotensin receptor antagonist
- Incidental finding of asymmetric kidney size on renal ultrasound
- As part of the investigation for progressive CKD.
- Symptomatically as acute ('flash') pulmonary oedema in the absence of cardiac failure or fluid overload
- Postoperative acute renal failure, especially following coronary artery bypass or aortic aneurysm surgery

Cast nephropathy accounts for 10% of all renal dysfunction in patients with myeloma and is characterized by the formation of tubular casts of excreted light chains and Tamm–Horsfall protein: these are thought to cause renal failure by obstructing the tubule and by direct tubular toxicity.

The key to the diagnosis is to maintain a high index of suspicion, particularly in elderly patients presenting with renal failure and hypercalcaemia. Serum electrophoresis and urinary Bence Jones proteins are the required investigations, followed—if either is positive—by bone marrow examination.

Other malignancies may present with renal involvement due to a number of mechanisms, including acute renal failure due to urinary tract obstruction by pelvic or retroperitoneal tumour. Other possible causes are outlined in Box 21.3.14.

See Chapters 21.10.4 (myeloma) and 21.10.8 (malignancy) for further discussion.

Renal presentation of infectious diseases

A wide range of systemic infections, resulting in either acute renal failure or chronic kidney disease, can affect the kidney. The presentation of infection-related kidney disease varies worldwide, and in the developing world—in contrast to the developed world—infectious diseases are the leading cause of acute and chronic kidney disease.

Acute renal failure may occur as part of a general systemic syndrome induced by infection, such as sepsis and septic shock,

Box 21.3.14 Renal presentations associated with malignancy

- Acute renal failure:
  - Urinary tract obstruction
  - Hypercalcaemia
  - Tumour lysis with urate nephropathy
  - Chemotherapy (e.g. cisplatin, ifosfamide)
  - Leukaemic infiltration
  - Microangiopathy
- Paraneoplastic glomerular disease:
  - Membranous
  - Amyloid
  - Mesangiocapillary glomerulonephritis

severe for the degree of renal impairment), abrupt decline in renal function after relatively minor prerenal 'insult', and unremarkable urine dipstick.

Up to 50% of patients presenting with myeloma have impaired renal function at the time of diagnosis. This may be reversible and due to hypercalcaemia, dehydration, hyperuricaemia, or infection.

haemolytic uraemic syndrome (HUS), rhabdomyolysis, postinfectious glomerulonephritis, and tubulointerstitial nephritis. Alternatively, an infectious agent may cause specific nephrotoxicity, e.g. hantavirus, leptospirosis, or malaria.

General systemic syndromes caused by infection

In Western countries, the most common infectious cause for renal disease is sepsis, which accounts for 10% of all hospital-acquired renal failure and, if severe, may lead to acute renal failure in the context of multiorgan failure.

Other general syndromes that may be induced by infection include HUS and rhabdomyolysis. For example, the verotoxin of *Escherichia coli* O157:H7 causes (D+) HUS, which is a thrombotic microangiopathy characterized by diarrhoea, acute renal failure, and thrombocytopenia. Patients with influenza, legionella, or streptococcal infection may present with fever, severe myalgia, and dark urine in the context of acute renal failure due to rhabdomyolysis.

Poststreptocccal glomerulonephritis is still one of the most common causes of acute renal failure in the developing world, although now seen rarely in the United Kingdom and developed countries. Typical presentation is 10 days to a few weeks following a streptococcal infection of the throat or skin with a 'nephritic' syndrome characterized by hypertension, oedema, haematuria and proteinuria, and acute renal failure.

Specific nephrotoxicity caused by infection

Hantavirus and leptospirosis

Hantaviruses are endemic in specific rodent reservoirs and are transmitted to man by inhalation of infectious aerosols or rodent excreta. In Europe, the main pattern of disease is haemorrhagic fever with renal syndrome (HFRS). The disease presents in four stages: (1) an abrupt febrile stage characterized by fever, loin or abdominal pain, nausea, vomiting, and periorbital oedema, lasting for 3 to 7 days; (2) a hypotensive phase associated with haemorrhages and ecchymoses, lasting hours to 2 days; (3) an oliguric phase for 3 to 14 days, with worsening acute renal failure due to a tubulointerstitial nephritis and haemorrhage; and (4) a polyuric phase as renal function returns to normal.

Leptospirosis may present with similar features to hantavirus. However, leptospirosis is endemic worldwide and is typically associated with jaundice and hepatomegaly. Acute renal failure occurs in 20 to 85% of patients owing to tubulointerstitial nephritis.

Malaria

Severe infection with *Plasmodium falciparum* occurs in nonimmune adults. Acute renal failure may occur either in the acute phase of the disease or in the recovery phase. Sequestration of parasitized erythrocytes in the renal vasculature and proinflammatory cytokine release cause tubular cell ischaemia and injury. Rarely, patients with falciparum malaria present with 'blackwater fever' due to massive intravascular haemolysis, which often occurs following quinine administration in association with glucose-6-phosphate dehydrogenase deficiency.

Infections and chronic kidney disease

In the developing world, CKD is commonly secondary to infectious disease, with the underlying infection often remaining subclinical until the presentation with renal manifestations. Examples of CKD secondary to infective agents include hepatitis B, hepatitis C, *Plasmodium malariae*, filaria, schistosomiasis, and HIV.

Hepatitis B is classically associated with nephrotic syndrome due to membranous nephropathy, but occasionally it may result in a mesangiocapillary glomerulonephritis. Hepatitis B virus infection is associated with the development of polyarteritis nodosa, although the reported frequency of this appears to be falling. Patients who develop such complications usually have chronic hepatitis, having contracted the virus in childhood.

Hepatitis C is increasingly recognized as a common cause for cryoglobulinaemia, but this remains asymptomatic in most patients, with only a few developing clinical evidence of vasculitis. The associated mesangiocapillary glomerulonephritis can present as nephrotic syndrome or chronic kidney disease.

Many infectious agents endemic in sub-Saharan Africa may also cause a mesangiocapillary glomerulonephritis presenting as nephrotic syndrome: most common is *P. malariae*, but filaria and schistosomiasis remain in the differential diagnosis.

HIV-associated nephropathy (HIVAN) is an increasingly recognized complication of HIV infection, and it now accounts for 1% of the dialysis population in the United States of America. Patients usually present with heavy proteinuria and nephrotic syndrome due a collapsing form of focal segmental glomerulosclerosis. HIVAN predominates in young African-American men and is rare in areas endemic for HIV.

See Chapters 21.5 (acute kidney injury), 21.10.7 (renal disease associated with infection) and 21.11 (renal disease in the tropics) for further discussion.

Systemic inflammatory diseases

Patients with systemic inflammatory disease are at risk of developing renal disease. Sometimes this may be the presenting feature of the condition, such as systemic vasculitis or systemic lupus, and on other occasions renal disease may develop as a complication later in the course of disease. Examples of systemic inflammatory diseases associated with renal involvement are detailed in Box 21.3.15. The presentation of an acute glomerulonephritis and progressive

---

Box 21.3.15 Systemic inflammatory diseases associated with renal involvement

◆ Typically associated with renal involvement:
  • Systemic vasculitides
  • Systemic lupus erythematosus
  • Sarcoidosis
  • Systemic sclerosis
  • Henoch–Schönlein purpura
  • Cryoglobulinaemia
◆ Unusually associated with renal involvement:
  • Relapsing polychondritis
  • Ankylosing spondylitis
  • Behçet's disease
  • Rheumatoid arthritis
◆ Renal complications of multisystem conditions:
  • Amyloidosis (of AA type)

renal failure due to systemic inflammatory diseases such as the vasculitides and systemic lupus erythematosus has been discussed earlier in the chapter, and further details can be found in Chapters 21.10.2 (vasculitides) and 21.10.3 (renal involvement in rheumatological disorders). Other inflammatory diseases may present in different ways.

Sarcoidosis

Renal disease is common in sarcoidosis and characterized histologically by granulomatous tubulointerstitial nephritis. The mean prevalence from biopsy studies is 35%, but this is likely to be an overestimate. Most renal disease is subclinical, but may be identified by the presence of proteinuria or tubular dysfunction with a renal tubular acidosis. However, sarcoidosis may present with acute renal failure, which may be caused by an acute tubulointerstitial nephritis associated with an eosinophilia and eosinophiluria, or be precipitated by hypercalcaemia, which may be more common in summer months owing to ultraviolet light exposure. The presence of extrarenal features of sarcoidosis (including bilateral hilar lymphadenopathy and erythema nodosum) helps to establish the diagnosis, but sometimes the diagnosis may only become apparent following a renal biopsy for unexplained renal impairment and measurement of serum ACE. See Chapter 18.12 for further discussion of sarcoidosis.

Systemic sclerosis

Systemic sclerosis may present with an acute crisis characterized by an abrupt rise in blood pressure (>160/90 mmHg) with hypertensive encephalopathy, acute renal failure, and a microangiopathic haemolytic anaemia. This may occur before the onset of the cutaneous features of the disease. Patients are typically tachycardic, with evidence of heart failure and a high systemic vascular resistance. This diagnosis should be suspected in any patient presenting with malignant-phase hypertension and acute renal failure. See Chapter 19.11.3 for further discussion of systemic sclerosis.

Systemic amyloidosis

Systemic amyloidosis is characterized by extracellular deposition of insoluble fibrillar proteins that lead to organ dysfunction. In AL amyloidosis this arises from light chains produced by a malignant plasma cell clone. AA amyloidosis occurs in the setting of longstanding inflammation, the amyloidogenic protein being an N-terminal fragment of serum amyloid A (SAA), an acute phase reactant. Patients may present with heavy proteinuria or nephrotic syndrome. Renal involvement can be demonstrated by serum amyloid P (SAP) scanning or by renal biopsy. See Chapter 12.12.3 for further discussion of the amyloidoses.

Box 21.3.16 Adverse effects of drugs on the kidney

Acute renal failure

- Acute tubular cell injury (acute tubular necrosis, ATN)
  - Aminoglycosides
  - Amphotericin
  - Cisplatin
  - Nsaids
  - Radiocontrast media
  - Paracetamol poisoning
  - Statins (by inducing rhabdomyolysis)
- Interstitial nephritis:
  - β-Lactam antibiotics (penicillins, cephalosporins)
  - NSAIDs
  - Furosemide
  - Allopurinol
  - Azathioprine
  - Sulphonamides
  - Aristolochic acid ('Chinese herb nephropathy')

Nephrotic syndrome

- Membranous:
  - High-dose captopril
  - Gold
  - Penicillamine
  - Phenytoin
- Minimal change:
  - NSAIDs
- Focal segmental glomerulosclerosis:
  - Pamidronate
  - Heroin

Tubular dysfunction

- Renal tubular acidosis:
  - Acetazolamide
  - Amphotericin
  - Lithium
- Nephrogenic diabetes insipidus:
  - Lithium
  - Demeclocycline

Others

- Renal papillary necrosis:
  - Aspirin with phenacetin
  - NSAIDs
- Crystalluria with tubular obstruction
  - Aciclovir
  - Indinavir
  - Methotrexate
  - Sulphonamides

Drug-induced renal disease

Numerous drugs have the potential for causing both acute renal failure and chronic kidney disease (Box 21.3.16). As well as prescribed and over-the-counter medication, renal disease may also arise from herbal and traditional Chinese medicines or illicit drugs. Mechanisms by which drugs cause renal disease include salt and water depletion, effects on renal perfusion, direct nephrotoxicity, and intrarenal obstruction.

Salt and water depletion

Acute renal failure may follow hypotension and reduced renal perfusion due to sodium and water depletion. This may be caused by excess diuretic use or diarrhoea and vomiting as a drug side effect.

Effect on renal perfusion and the regulation of intrarenal haemodynamics

Overdose of any hypotensive agent may compromise renal perfusion and interfere with renal function. Agents which block the renin–angiotensin system, the ACE inhibitors and angiotensin receptor blockers, require special consideration. These agents abrogate the effect of angiotensin II on efferent arteriole constriction, which is the normal adaptive response to any reduction in renal perfusion. A small and acceptable deterioration in renal function (up to a 20% increase in serum creatinine) often occurs following the introduction of an ACE inhibitor. A greater increase in serum creatinine may indicate underlying renal artery stenosis, for which further investigation may need to be carefully considered, and these agents are implicated in a significant proportion of cases of acute renal failure in patients with sepsis and dehydration. This is because renal perfusion is frequently compromised in these settings and the kidney is unable to autoregulate its blood flow in the presence of renin–angiotensin system blockade.

NSAIDs have numerous renal effects, including disturbances of autoregulation of intrinsic renal haemodynamics. These effects are mediated by inhibition of prostaglandin synthesis from arachidonic acid by nonspecific blocking of the enzyme cyclooxygenase. This may lead to vasoconstriction and reversible renal impairment in volume-contracted states. Long-term use of NSAIDs may cause chronic renal impairment, with selective COX-2 inhibitors seeming to confer no renal advantage.

Direct nephrotoxicity

The mechanisms of drug toxicity on the kidney include direct tubulotoxicity, drug-induced tubulointerstitial nephritis, tubular dysfunction, and glomerular disease. Common nephrotoxic drugs and mechanism are outlined in Box 21.3.16.

Tubulointerstitial nephritis is classically caused by penicillins and NSAIDs, but most drugs have the potential to cause the condition. Drug-induced tubulointerstitial nephritis usually occurs days to weeks after starting the drug. Symptoms may be nonspecific, with malaise, fatigue, and anorexia. A low-grade fever, fleeting rash, and arthralgia may also be reported. Investigations show a variable degree of renal dysfunction along with proteinuria and microscopic haematuria. Urine microscopy may show white and red cell casts, and there may be a blood eosinophilia. However, in practice the key is to suspect the diagnosis, stop the potentially offending drug (or drugs), and proceed with a renal biopsy if renal function does not improve.

Obstruction

Specific drugs, such as aciclovir and the protease inhibitor indinavir, may precipitate as crystals within the tubule, causing obstruction and sometimes renal failure. This is more likely to occur if the patient is dehydrated, hence adequate fluid input to achieve a high urinary volume is advised before these drugs are taken.

See Chapter 21.19 for further discussion of drugs and the kidney.

Pregnancy

Pregnancy provides a unique set of circumstances in which renal disease may present. Renal disease may be present before pregnancy and be detected as part of screening for proteinuria and hypertension during the first trimester. Alternatively, *de novo* renal disease may be precipitated by pregnancy and present with specific syndromes, such as nephrotic syndrome or acute renal failure due to pre-eclampsia. A summary of the presentation of renal disease in pregnancy is detailed in Box 21.3.17.

Box 21.3.17 Renal disease in pregnancy

Acute renal failure in pregnancy

- Hypovolaemia:
  - Hyperemesis
  - Haemorrhage
  - Sepsis
  - Abruption
- Infection:
  - Pyelonephritis
  - Septic abortion
  - Puerperal sepsis
- Obstruction:
  - Gravid uterus
- Endothelial dysfunction:
  - Pre-eclampsia
  - Acute fatty liver of pregnancy
  - Syndrome of haemolysis, elevated liver enzymes and low platelets (HELLP)
  - Haemolytic uraemic syndrome (HUS)

Exacerbation of pre-existing renal disease

- Any chronic kidney disease with deterioration of function, proteinuria, and pre-eclampsia
- Flare of systemic and renal disease (systemic lupus erythematosus and systemic sclerosis)

New-onset nephrotic syndrome

- Pre-eclampsia
- Systemic lupus erythematosus
- Minimal change disease

The clinical presentation of renal disease during pregnancy is often varied and nonspecific, but certain features may guide the diagnosis. Key points to note are as follows:

♦ Is there evidence of pre-existing renal disease?

♦ Were previous pregnancies complicated by hypertension or pre-eclampsia (PET)?

♦ What was the time of onset of renal disease during pregnancy? Onset in late pregnancy implies that the renal disease is likely to be pregnancy induced.

♦ Hypertension with proteinuria and oedema suggest PET or underlying renal disease (e.g. systemic lupus erythematosus).

♦ Hypotension and hypovolaemia suggest sepsis or haemorrhage.

See Chapter 14.5 for further discussion of renal disease in pregnancy.

Pre-eclampsia and HELLP

Pre-eclampsia classically presents with hypertension, oedema, and proteinuria. Other recognized features include elevation of serum urate, liver transaminases, and haematocrit, along with thrombocytopenia. However, patients may not be hypertensive or demonstrate other features, hence distinguishing pre-eclampsia from pre-existing renal disease may be difficult, and the condition may occasionally present with heavy proteinuria and nephrotic syndrome. The HELLP syndrome (haemolysis, elevated liver enzymes, and low platelets) is a severe variant of pre-eclampsia that is commonly associated with renal failure, severe haemolysis, and coagulopathy, and may progress to multiorgan failure. See Chapters 14.4 (hypertension in pregnancy) and 14.9 (liver and gastrointestinal disease in pregnancy) for further discussion.

Haemolytic uraemic syndrome and thrombotic thrombocytopenic purpura

Haemolytic uraemic syndrome and thrombotic thrombocytopenic purpura (HUS/TTP) are related disorders that are occasionally associated with pregnancy and can both cause acute renal failure. HUS usually occurs 2 days to 10 weeks postpartum and may cause severe renal failure. By contrast, TTP usually presents in the first or second trimester with predominant neurological features and only mild proteinuria and haematuria. See Chapters 21.10.5 (haemolytic uraemic syndrome), 22.6.3 (disorders of platelet number and function) and 22.6.5 (acquired coagulation disorders) for further discussion.

Further reading

Britton JP, et al. (1992). A community study of bladder cancer screening by the detection of occult urinary bleeding. *J Urol*, **148**, 788–90.
Burden RP, et al. (1979). The loin-pain/haematuria syndrome. *Lancet*, **1**, 897–900.
Cameron JS (1996). Nephrotic syndrome in the elderly. *Semin Nephrol*, **16**, 319–29.
Cohen RA, Brown RS (2003). Clinical practice. Microscopic hematuria. *N Engl J Med*, **348**, 2330–8.
de Lusignan S, et al. (2005). Identifying patients with chronic kidney disease from general practice computer records. *Fam Pract*, **22**, 234–41.
Denton CP, Black CM (2004). Scleroderma—clinical and pathological advances. *Best Pract Res Clin Rheumatol*, **18**, 271–90.
Dube GK, et al. (2006). Loin pain hematuria syndrome. *Kidney Int*, **70**, 2152–5.
Fairley KF, Birch DF (1982). Hematuria: a simple method for identifying glomerular bleeding. *Kidney Int*, **21**, 105–8.
Grossfeld GD, et al. (2001). Asymptomatic microscopic hematuria in adults: summary of the AUA best practice policy recommendations. *Am Fam Physician*, **63**, 1145–54.
Irish AB, Winearls CG, Littlewood T (1997). Presentation and survival of patients with severe renal failure and myeloma. *QJM*, **90**, 773–80.
Jayapaul MK, et al. (2006). The joint diabetic-renal clinic in clinical practice: 10 years of data from a District General Hospital. *QJM*, **99**, 153–60.
John R, et al. (2004). Unreferred chronic kidney disease: a longitudinal study. *Am J Kidney Dis*, **43**, 825–35.
Joint Specialty Committee on Renal Medicine of the Royal College of Physicians of London and the Renal Association. (2006). *Chronic kidney disease in adults: UK guidelines for identification, management and referral*. Royal College of Physicians of London, London.
Kamesh L, Harper L, Savage CO (2002). ANCA-positive vasculitis. *J Am Soc Nephrol*, **13**, 1953–60.
Levey AS, et al. (1999). A more accurate method to estimate glomerular filtration rate from serum creatinine: a new prediction equation. Modification of Diet in Renal Disease Study Group. *Ann Intern Med*, **130**, 461–70.
Liano F, Pascual J (1996). Epidemiology of acute renal failure: a prospective, multicenter, community-based study. Madrid Acute Renal Failure Study Group. *Kidney Int*, **50**, 811–18.
Little MA, Pusey CD (2004). Rapidly progressive glomerulonephritis: current and evolving treatment strategies. *J Nephrol*, **17**, S10–19.
National Kidney Federation. (2002). K/DOQI clinical practice guidelines for chronic kidney disease: evaluation, classification, and stratification. *Am J Kidney Dis*, **39**, S1–266.
Orth SR, Ritz E (1998). The nephrotic syndrome. *N Engl J Med*, **338**, 1202–11.
Perneger TV, Whelton PK, Klag MJ (1994). Risk of kidney failure associated with the use of acetaminophen, aspirin, and nonsteroidal antiinflammatory drugs. *N Engl J Med*, **331**, 1675–9.
Rossert J (2001). Drug-induced acute interstitial nephritis. *Kidney Int*, **60**, 804–17.
Ruggenenti P, et al. (1998). Cross sectional longitudinal study of spot morning urine protein:creatinine ratio, 24 hour urine protein excretion rate, glomerular filtration rate, and end stage renal failure in chronic renal disease in patients without diabetes. *BMJ*, **316**, 504–9.
Wingo CS, Clapp WL (2000). Proteinuria: potential causes and approach to evaluation. *Am J Med Sci*, **320**, 188–94.
Zager RA (1996). Rhabdomyolysis and myohemoglobinuric acute renal failure. *Kidney Int*, **49**, 314–26.

Clinical investigation of renal disease

A. Davenport

Essentials

An accurate history and careful examination will determine the sequence and spectrum of clinical investigations required to make a diagnosis or decide on prognosis or treatment.

Examination of the urine

Midstream urine (MSU) sample—this standard investigation requires consideration of: (1) macroscopic appearance—this may be suggestive of a diagnosis, e.g. frothy urine suggests heavy proteinuria; (2) stick testing—including for pH (<5.3 in an early-morning specimen makes a renal acidification defect unlikely), glycosuria, specific gravity (should be >1.024 in an early-morning or concentrated sample), nitrite (>90% of common urinary pathogens produce nitrite) and leucocyte esterase; and (3) microscopy—for cellular elements (in particular red cells, with the presence of dysmorphic red cells detected by experienced observers indicative of glomerular bleeding), casts (cellular casts indicate renal inflammation), and crystals.

Quantification of proteinuria—this is important because the risk for progression of underlying kidney disease to endstage renal failure is related to the amount of protein in the urine. Quantification by 24-h urinary collection is cumbersome and unreliable in many patients, and has been replaced by estimation of the urinary albumin:creatinine ratio (ACR; normal is <2.5 mg/mmol for men and less than 3.5 mg/mmol for women) or protein:creatinine ratio (PCR; normal is <13 mg/mmol) on a spot sample. An ACR of

100 mg/mmol approximately corresponds to proteinuria of 1.5 g/day, and 350 mg/mmol to nephrotic-range proteinuria.

Low-molecular-weight proteinuria—is caused by proximal tubular injury and can be detected with markers including α-glutathione-S-transferase, α_1-macroglobulin, and retinol-binding protein.

Estimation of glomerular filtration rate

Knowledge of the glomerular filtration rate (GFR) is of crucial importance in the management of patients, not only for detecting the presence of renal impairment, but also in the monitoring of all patients with or at risk of renal impairment, and in determining appropriate dosing of those drugs cleared by the kidney. Measurement of plasma creatinine remains the standard biochemical test used to assess renal function.

Estimating the glomerular filtration rate (eGFR)—from a measurement of plasma creatinine concentration, the standard method uses the simplified Modification of Diet in Renal Disease (sMDRD) formula, which requires knowledge of the patient's sex, age, and ethnicity (but not their weight). On the basis of the eGFR, stages of chronic kidney disease (CKD) are classified as follows:

Limitations of the eGFR—this has not been validated in people below 18 years of age, hospitalized patients, or those with acute kidney injury, pregnancy, oedematous states, muscle-wasting disorders, amputations, or malnourishment. Similarly, it has not

CKD stage[a]	eGFR (ml/min per 1.73 m² body surface area)
1	>90, with other evidence of renal disease
2	60–89, with other evidence of renal disease
3A	45–59
3B	30–44
4	15–29
5	<15, or receiving renal replacement therapy

[a] The suffix (p) can be used to denote the presence of proteinuria as defined by a spot urinary albumin:creatinine ratio (ACR) of ≥30 mg/mmol, which is approximately equivalent to a protein:creatinine ratio (PCR) of ≥50 mg/mmol (≥0.5 g/24 h).

been validated for extremes of age or body weight, or for ethnic groups other than whites of northern European origin and African-Americans.

Other methods of measuring GFR—isotopic methods can provide the most accurate determination of GFR, but are not often required in routine clinical practice. Estimation of creatinine clearance with a 24-h urinary collection remains a useful test, particularly when there is reason to doubt the validity of the eGFR.

Investigation of tubular function

Proximal tubule—analysis of excretion of the following substances can assist in the diagnosis of proximal tubular disorders: (1) glucose—the maximum reabsorption rate for glucose (T_mG) in the proximal tubule can be determined following infusion of 20% dextrose and is normally about 15 mmol/litre (T_mG/GFR); (2) phosphate—the theoretical maximum tubular threshold of phosphate (T_MP/GFR) can be estimated by formula from the plasma and urinary phosphate and creatinine concentrations, or can be measured directly following infusion of phosphate; and (3) amino acids—five types of renal aminoaciduria are distinguished: dibasic amino acids, neutral amino acids (monoaminomonocarboxylic acids), glycine and imino acids, dicarboxylic amino acids, and generalized amino aciduria (Fanconi's syndrome).

Distal tubule—a water-deprivation test can help to distinguish patients with primary or secondary nephrogenic or cranial diabetes insipidus from those with primary polydipsia, who may all present with polyuria.

Renal-induced electrolyte and acid–base imbalances— (1) estimation of urinary free-water clearance is useful in the analysis of patients with hyponatraemia (see Chapter 21.2.1); (2) estimation of transtubular potassium gradient (TTKG) is advocated by some as useful in analysis of disorders of potassium homeostasis (see Chapter 21.2.2); (3) tests of urinary acidification are discussed in Chapters 21.14 and 21.15.

Renal imaging

Ultrasonography—this noninvasive, safe, versatile and (relatively) inexpensive technique is the first-line method for imaging the kidney and urinary tract in many clinical circumstances.

Ultrafast multislice CT scanning—this allows resolution of 2 to 3 mm or less and has become the mainstay of renal imaging.

CT urography can be performed with a combination of unenhanced, nephrogenic-phase, and excretory-phase imaging: the unenhanced images are ideal for detecting urinary calculi; renal masses can be detected and characterized with the combination of unenhanced, nephrogenic- and excretory-phase imaging; the excretory phase provides imaging of the urothelium. CT angiography is the first-line investigation in the evaluation of acute renal trauma, assessment of tumour blood supply in cases of nephron-sparing surgery, and for the diagnosis of renal artery stenosis and/or aneurysms.

MRI—this is an alternative to CT scanning in patients who are allergic to conventional iodine-based radiocontrast media and has particular value in the staging of renal carcinoma and assessment of complex renal cysts. Magnetic resonance angiography (MRA) tends to overemphasize the significance of stenoses. Gadolinium contrast scanning should be carefully considered in patients with eGFR below 30 ml/min because of the risk of nephrogenic systemic fibrosis, which limits the utility of magnetic resonance techniques for many renal patients.

Renal nuclear medicine scanning—(1) dimercaptosuccinic acid (DMSA), used in estimation of differential renal function and detection of scarring (usually associated with reflux); (2) mercaptoacetyl-triglycine (MAG3), used in detection of functionally significant obstruction, estimation of differential renal function, screening for renal artery stenosis, and monitoring of renal transplants.

Invasive techniques—these can allow therapeutic intervention as well as diagnosis, including antegrade or retrograde ureteropyelography (insertion of stents to relieve urinary obstruction) and angiography (angioplasty or stenting of the renal artery).

Renal biopsy

A renal biopsy should be considered in any patient with disease affecting the kidney when the clinical information and other laboratory investigations have failed to establish a definitive diagnosis or prognosis, or when there is doubt as to the optimal therapy. However, renal biopsy has the potential to cause morbidity and (on rare occasions) mortality, hence its risk must be outweighed by the potential advantages of the result to the individual patient. Biopsies which would be 'of interest' but 'not in the patient's interest' should not be performed.

Introduction

The key to making any correct diagnosis depends on a careful history and thorough examination. In patients with kidney disease, the history and examination should attempt to differentiate acute from chronic kidney disease, single-organ system involvement from multisystem disease, and obstruction from intrinsic or prerenal disease. Kidney disease may be associated with preceding infections and the ingestion of drugs or herbal remedies. An accurate history and careful examination will determine the sequence and spectrum of clinical investigations required to make a diagnosis or decide on prognosis or treatment.

Examination of the urine

Urine collection

To minimize contamination, standard investigation is of a midstream urine (MSU) sample. Voiding from a full bladder containing at least 200 ml of urine should remove urethral organisms before the MSU is collected. Even so, in women, vaginal leucocytes and bacteria may contaminate the urine, and men should retract the foreskin to minimize contamination. Suprapubic aspiration is the technique of choice in babies and infants, and occasionally in adults who cannot cooperate to provide an MSU. The second urine of the morning is the best for microscopy as it is still acidic and concentrated, but without the overnight stay in the bladder that results in the degeneration of casts and cells. Cell lysis can occur in both hypotonic and alkaline urine. Only the first 10 ml of the stream should be collected in cases of suspected urethritis.

Macroscopic appearance

Fresh urine usually has a yellow colour due to the presence of urochromes, but occasionally it will have a milky appearance due to pus, spermatozoa, insoluble phosphates in alkaline urine (sometimes seen following heavy meals), or occasionally in cases of chyluria, or urate crystals in acid urine. Foamy or frothy urine is typical of heavy proteinuria. Certain agents and conditions can discolour urine.

Pink to red colouration

Haematuria may result in a range of colours from smoky pink through to port-wine red in cases of frank macroscopic haematuria. Other causes of a pink or red urine include eating sweets containing aniline dyes, beetroot or other foodstuffs containing anthocyanins; haemoglobin; myoglobin; some drugs such as phenindione and phenolphthalein; and (if the urine is left to stand) porphyrins in cases of acute intermittent porphyria.

Blue or green colouration

Blue or green colouration can be caused by pseudomonas urinary sepsis, methylene blue, biliverdin, triamterene, amitriptyline, chlorophyll-containing breath mints (Clorets), excessive use of mouthwash and deodorants, magnesium salicylate (Doan's pills), phenyl salicylate, guaiacol (in cough remedies), thymol (in volatile oils and horsemint), iodochlorhydroxyquin, tolonium, Evans blue, methocarbamol, Diagnex blue, indigo blue, resorcinol, azuresin, bromoform, and occasionally propofol. Phenol and lysol can result in a green or black discolouration.

Orange colouration

Orange colouration can be caused by anthraquinone-containing laxatives, rifampicin, and excess urobilinogen.

Yellow urine

Yellow urine may be found in patients prescribed mepacrine or phenacetin, those taking excessive amounts of riboflavin, and icteric patients with conjugated hyperbilirubinaemia.

Black or brown urine

Alkaptonuria results in black or brown urine, whereas myoglobin and melanin only lead to black urine on standing. Other causes of brown urine include bilirubin, l-dopa, niridazole, furazolidone, and phenazopyridine, and—after standing—haemoglobin and myoglobin. As mentioned above, phenol and lysol can result in a black or green discolouration.

Stick testing

The upper limit of normal for protein excretion in the urine is 128 mg/24 h. Although albumin is the largest single component, more than half of the protein content comprises low-molecular-weight proteins and protein fragments. Commercial sticks such as Albustix are very sensitive, detecting protein in urine starting at concentrations around 100 mg/litre. Since these sticks detect protein on a concentration basis using bromocresol green as an indicator dye, the results they give are affected by urine flow rate and urine dilution or concentration. The sticks are treated with a buffer to keep their pH constant: an elevated urinary protein concentration can erroneously be recorded if the buffer is washed off by leaving the stick in the urine for too long, and with very alkaline urine. Some antiseptics used to clean the skin, including cetrimide and chlorhexidine, may also react and cause a false-positive result. More recently, antibody-based dipsticks have been developed for detecting microalbuminuria.

pH

Normal urine is slightly acidic, but can vary between pH 4.5 and 8.0. If an early-morning urine specimen is under pH 5.3, then there is unlikely to be a significant defect in urinary acidification. Alkaline pH is often found in urine infected with urea-splitting bacteria. In some cases of urinary stone disease, particularly in cystinuria and urate nephropathy, crystal solubility is greater in alkaline urine, and patients should regularly check their urine pH. Haemoglobin and myoglobin are also more soluble in alkaline urine, hence maintaining a forced alkaline diuresis is important in the management of patients following tumour lysis and those with rhabdomyolysis or haemoglobinuria.

Glycosuria

The stick reaction is based on glucose oxidase, which releases hydrogen peroxide from glucose, so producing a graded colour change by oxidizing an indicator. This reaction is specific for glucose and does not detect other sugars. The reaction can be blocked by large doses of ascorbic acid. A positive stick test for glucose must be interpreted in light of the plasma glucose level as glycosuria may reflect a defect in renal tubular glucose absorption.

Specific gravity

Specific gravity is a measure of the number of particles dissolved in a litre, whereas osmolality is the number of particles per kilogram. Protein and glucose increase the specific gravity more than the osmolality as they are dense particles. In normal patients, the early-morning, or concentrated, urine sample should have a specific gravity of 1.024 or more.

Nitrite stick test

Nitrite sticks contain an aromatic amine that reacts with nitrites, which are produced by bacterial reduction of nitrate, to form a pink-coloured diazonium complex. More than 90% of the common urinary pathogens are nitrite-forming bacteria. However, pseudomonas, *Staphylococcus albus*, *Staphylococcus saprophyticus*, and *Enterococcus faecalis* may have minimal or no nitrite-producing capacity. Other false-negative results may be obtained in alkaline urine, in patients taking large doses of vitamin C, and with frequent voiding of dilute urine when the urinary nitrite concentration is too low.

Leucocyte esterase stick test

This stick test is based on the presence of a leucocyte esterase and is very specific for the presence of urinary leucocytes, both intact and lysed. This test may be more accurate than microscopy when the urine is alkaline or hypotonic. However, the test can be inhibited by high concentrations of glucose (20 g/litre or more), ketones, and antibiotics including cefalexin, cefalotin, nitrofurantoin, tetracycline, and tobramycin. The sensitivity of this test is also reduced when the specific gravity of the urine is high, for instance in the presence of a heavy proteinuria.

Urine microscopy

To obtain reproducible results, urine should be processed in a standard manner and examined under the microscope as soon as possible.

In our own institution, a few drops of acetic acid (10% v/v) are added to ensure a pH of 6.0 or less; then 10 ml of urine is centrifuged for 5 min at 1500 rev/min (750 g), following which 9.5 ml of supernatant is removed and the deposit resuspended. One drop (50 μl) is placed on a microscope slide and covered with a standard coverslip (24 × 32 mm). Although phase-contrast microscopy is an advantage in identifying red cells and casts, a standard microscope will suffice. A semiquantitative assessment of casts is made at low power (160×) and other elements at high power (400×), expressing the counts as numbers per field. Normal urine contains 1 or 2 leucocytes per high-power field (HPF), 1 erythrocyte per 2 or 3 HPF, 1 tubular cell per 10 HPF, and both hyaline casts (1 per low-power field, LPF) and granular casts (1 per LPF). Physical exercise can result in haematuria and cylindruria for several hours. Stains such as modified Sternheimer's stain (Sedi-stain) can be used to help differentiate renal tubular cells from leucocytes. To improve the detection of casts, urine can be filtered through a 5-μm Millipore filter, and the retained casts stained with Papanicolaou's stain.

Cellular elements

The morphology of the erythrocytes in the urine can give valuable information as to the source of bleeding. Those which have passed through the glomerulus and then along the renal tubule can become distorted or dysmorphic, whereas those originating from other sources within the urinary tract, such as the bladder, typically show much less evidence of damage so that they more closely resemble erythrocytes in the peripheral blood and are termed isomorphic. To establish a diagnosis of glomerular haematuria there should be a minimum of three different forms of dysmorphic erythrocytes present. One particular type of dysmorphic erythrocyte, the acanthocyte, is reported to have 52% specificity and 98% sensitivity for glomerular haematuria when the acanthocyte count is 5% or more. However, not all workers have found erythrocyte morphology to be useful in discriminating glomerular from nonglomerular bleeding, and the physician who only occasionally examines urine under the microscope is unlikely to obtain clear, reproducible, and useful discrimination between dysmorphic and isomorphic cells.

Some centres use automated haematological cell counters (Coulter counter) to assess red cell morphology in both urine and peripheral blood. The red cell size–distribution pattern for lower urinary tract haematuria is similar to that of the peripheral blood, with a relatively narrow size range and a high frequency distribution curve, whereas the typical pattern for dysmorphic haematuria is one of a broader range of red cell sizes, with a lower frequency distribution. To have any reliability, urine samples must be processed rapidly by those who do it regularly.

Microscopy may also reveal renal tubular epithelial cells. These cells are shed into the urine in acute tubular necrosis, in response to certain drugs (both nephrotoxic and ischaemic), and also in acute renal allograft rejection. In patients with nephrotic syndrome, these cells are seen as oval fat bodies, laden with lipid droplets. Squamous epithelial cells from the urethra and vagina and transitional cells from the ureter and bladder may also be present in normal urine. Urine cytology may reveal malignant transitional epithelial and/or metaplastic sqamous cells from the bladder.

During infection, the urine may contain large numbers of leucocytes and bacteria. When large numbers of leucocytes are present in the absence of bacteria (so-called sterile pyuria), then a variety of conditions should be considered: urinary stone disease, analgesic

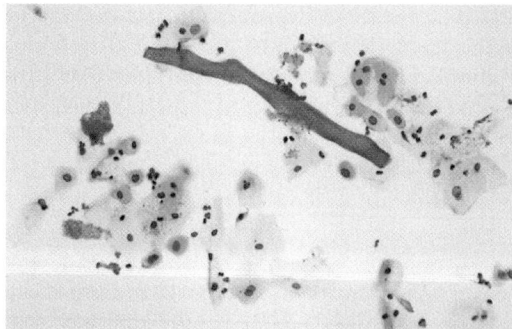

Fig. 21.4.1 Papanicolaou-stained urine showing a hyaline cast with both normal transitional and squamous cells and renal tubular cells.
(Courtesy of Dr Deery.)

nephropathy, interstitial nephropathy, proliferative glomerulonephritis (rarely), renal tuberculosis, schistosomiasis, and partially treated bacterial urinary tract infection. Phase-contrast microscopy can distinguish lymphocytes from neutrophils, but eosinophils can only be identified with specific stains (Hansel's stain). Urinary eosinophilia classically occurs in cases of acute interstitial nephritis, typically due to drugs, and also in cholesterol atheroembolic disease.

Urinary casts

Casts form from the transformation of Tamm–Horsfall glycoprotein, secreted by the distal tubular cells, into a gel matrix. They typically assume a tubular structure. Hyaline casts only contain Tamm–Horsfall glycoprotein and are found in a variable amount in the urine of normal subjects (Fig. 21.4.1). Fever, cardiac failure, strenuous exercise, and some drugs, such as furosemide and ethacrynic acid, increase hyaline cast excretion. During passage through the distal tubule and collecting duct, a variety of proteins, pigments, and cells can adhere to the Tamm–Horsfall protein, producing a wide variety of casts. Granular casts have deposits of either fine or coarse protein granules (Fig. 21.4.2). Although they may occur in normal subjects, or after exercise, they are typically found in cases of parenchymal renal disease. In patients with proteinuria, the protein deposited comes from the glomerulus, whereas in acute tubular necrosis, the protein comes from degenerate tubular cells. Broad waxy casts are much larger than normal casts and have clear-cut edges: they are formed in dilated hypertrophied tubules, as found in patients with chronic renal failure. Casts containing erythrocytes (red cell casts) indicate renal bleeding and are typically found when there is acute glomerular inflammation caused by glomerulonephritis or vasculitis (Fig. 21.4.3). White cell casts (containing leucocytes) can be found in proliferative glomerulonephritis, acute interstitial nephritis, and acute pyelonephritis.

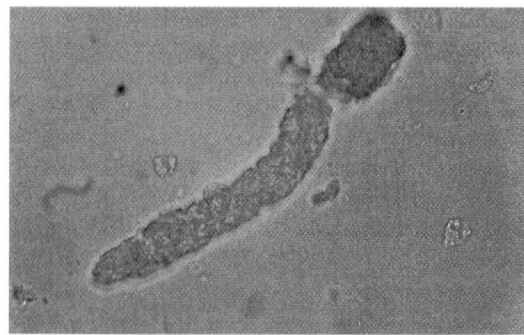

Fig. 21.4.2 Unstained urine specimen showing a granular cast.

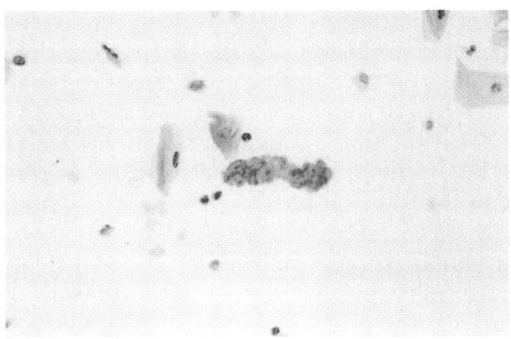

Fig. 21.4.3 Papanicolaou-stained urine deposit showing a red-cell cast.

Crystals

Urine may contain several types of crystals, depending on the pH. The presence of a few crystals of uric acid, calcium oxalate, or calcium phosphate is usually not clinically relevant, although thin hexagonal crystals of cystine are a marker of cystinuria. In a few cases, crystalluria may be associated with intratubular obstruction and acute kidney injury. Such cases would include acute uric acid nephropathy, ethylene glycol poisoning, and drugs including aciclovir, amoxicillin, indinavir, naftidrofuryl oxalate, sulfadiazine, and vitamin C.

Measurement of proteinuria

Quantification of proteinuria is important as the risk for progression of underlying kidney disease to endstage renal failure is related to the amount of protein in the urine. Traditionally, proteinuria has been measured using 24-h urine collections and expressed as grams per day. This has the advantage that it averages out protein excretion and is not therefore affected by its normal diurnal variation (less overnight and first thing in the morning) or urine concentration. Several different methods are used to measure the protein content of 24-h urine collections, ranging from the biuret method, which uses a copper-based method to precipitate proteins, to dye-binding methods using Coomassie Brilliant Blue as the indicator. These are more accurate than the turbidimetric methods, which use trichloroacetic or sulphosalicylic acid and measure turbidity with a densitometer. Radiocontrast media and some drugs (including penicillin, sulphonamides, and tolbutamide) may give false-positive results for proteinuria with the sulphosalicylic acid method. The biuret method measures total proteins, whereas the turbidimetric method provides different readings for albumin and globulins, as may do the dye-binding methods.

However, because of the inherent problems of accuracy and reliability with 24-h urine collections, the assessment of protein in spot urine samples has become the standard method of assessing proteinuria in routine clinical practice. Urinary albumin concentration is measured by a variety of methods based on an antibody technique for detecting serum albumin, including radioimmunoassay, nephelometry, immunoturbidity, and enzyme-linked immunosorbent assay (ELISA). Under resting conditions, urinary creatinine excretion is relatively constant throughout the day, hence to overcome the problems of timing of urinary collections, proteinuria in spot urine samples is expressed as an albumin:creatinine ratio (ACR, normal is less than 2.5 mg/mmol for men and less than 3.5 mg/mmol for women in a daytime urine or 24-h collection, and less than 1.5 mg/mmol for an overnight or early-morning sample). An ACR of 100 mg/mmol approximately corresponds to 1.5 g/day, and 350 mg/mmol to nephrotic-range proteinuria. However, albumin is not the only protein in urine and the relationship between albumin and total urinary protein is not linear, with a ratio of 50% albumin with a urinary protein of 300 mg/litre increasing to 70% at 1000 mg/litre.

As the measurement of protein in spot urine samples is cheaper than albumin, it has been suggested that, for patients with more than 1+ proteinuria on dipstick testing, the protein/creatinine ratio (PCR) should be used in routine clinical practice. The normal PCR is less than 13 mg/mmol, with a dipstick value of 1+ roughly equivalent to a PCR of 45 to 149 mg/mmol and ACR above 30 mg/mmol, a dipstick of 2+ to a PCR of 150 to 449 mg/mmol, and 3+ to 450 mg/mmol or more.

Aside from their use to replace 24-h urine collections, spot urine collections are particularly useful in the diagnosis of orthostatic proteinuria, in other words where the patient has a normal urinary protein excretion when recumbent, or overnight, but has marginally increased proteinuria in the ambulant or daytime sample.

The ACR should not be measured during acute illness, menstruation, or intercurrent illness as these will temporarily increase the degree of proteinuria.

Microalbuminuria

Various antibody based assays for albumin can detect an increased urinary albumin excretion in patients with normal levels of proteinuria. High-performance liquid chromatography (HPLC) detects more urinary albumin than the radioimmunoassay and other serum antibody-based tests. Normoalbuminuria is defined as an excretion rate of 20 µg/min or less. Proteinuria is usually detectable on dipstick testing at rates of over 200 µg/min, hence microalbuminuria is defined as an excretion rate between 20 and 200 µg/min. The albumin excretion rate (AER) is some 25% higher during the day than the night. The classification of abnormal urinary albumin excretion is shown in Table 21.4.1.

Table 21.4.1 Classification of abnormal urinary albumin excretion

	24-h urine albumin (mg/24 h)	Overnight albumin (µg/min)	Spot albumin (mg/litre)	Spot urine ACR (mg/mmol)	PCR (mg/mmol)
Normal	<15	<10	<10	M <1.25, F <1.75	<13
Microalbuminuria	30 to <300	20 to <200	20 to <200	M 2.5 -<25, F 3.5 to <35	16 to <160
Macroalbuminuria	>300	>200	>200	M >25, F >35	>160

ACR, albumin:creatinine ratio; F, female; M, male; PCR, protein:creatinine ratio.
The normal ACR ratio is lower in men than women owing to higher urinary creatinine excretion.

There is a good correlation between the morning AER and the ACR in the first urine sample of the morning. A further advantage of spot urines is that patients can provide a sample when they attend the clinic: provided these are taken at the same time and the patient's dietary intake is relatively constant, they are very useful in assessing patients over time. A further advantage of measuring the ACR instead of AER is that the former, but not the latter, eliminates the need for timing of urinary samples.

Microalbuminuria is not only an adverse factor for the progression of diabetic renal disease, but is also predictive of cardiovascular events in both the diabetic and nondiabetic population. In addition to those with diabetes, microalbuminuria may be found in patients with hypertension, cardiac failure, and following a pyrexial or viral illness. Similarly, microalbuminuria may be present in healthy subjects after exercise and during normal pregnancy.

Selectivity of proteinuria

Patients with glomerular disease typically have a nonselective proteinuria, with a similar clearance of both high- and low-molecular-weight plasma proteins. However, those with minimal change disease may have selective proteinuria, with clearance of predominantly low-molecular-weight proteins, the demonstration of which is useful in paediatric practice where patients are often treated with steroids without a renal biopsy.

Most laboratories compare the clearance of IgG as the large-molecular-weight protein (150 kDa) to that of albumin (or transferrin, 88 kDa) as the low-molecular-weight protein. Both plasma and spot urine samples are required. Protein concentrations are measured either by laser nephelometry or radial immunodiffusion. Nonselective proteinuria is taken as an $([IgG]_{urine}/[IgG]_{plasma}) \times ([transferrin]_{plasma}/[transferrin]_{urine})$ ratio of 0.2 or more, whereas selective proteinuria is taken as a ratio of 0.1 or less.

Spill-over proteinuria

Patients with myeloma, some types of amyloidosis, and those with reticuloendothelial disorders may have a spill-over proteinuria due to glomerular filtration of complete and incomplete κ and λ chains and immunoglobulin light chains. These low-molecular-weight proteins are not detected by simple urine stick testing, or by standard biochemical methods to determine urine protein concentration. Thus, when clinically appropriate, urine should specifically be sent for immunoelectrophoresis to exclude myeloma. However, light chains in particular may still not be detected, hence further investigation with specific antisera may be required if their presence is suspected.

Renal tubular proteinuria

Interstitial renal disease can result in proteinuria, usually of less than 2 g/day. Proximal tubular injury leads to increased low-molecular-weight proteinuria, characterized by an excess of intestinal alkaline phosphatase, N-acetylglucosaminidase, retinol-binding protein, tissue-specific alkaline phosphatase, α-glutathione-S-transferase (α-GST), α_1-macroglobulin, and β_2-microglobulin. By contrast, Tamm–Horsfall glycoprotein and α-GST are increased in distal tubular injury.

β_2-Microglobulin is freely filtered at the glomerulus and then reabsorbed in the proximal tubule, such that less than 1% of the filtered load is excreted in the urine of normal subjects (normal is <370 µg/24 h). Thus urinary β_2-microglobulin excretion has been used as a marker of proximal tubular damage. However, β_2-microglobulin is unstable in urine, and its excretion can be affected both by an increased production rate (found in cases of myeloproliferative disease, chronic inflammatory states, and acute liver disease) and by saturation of β_2-microglobulin tubular uptake due to an excess of dibasic amino acids.

More-reliable markers of tubular proteinuria are now available. These include α-GST, α_1-macroglobulin, and retinol-binding protein. Turbidimetric or enzyme assays are now available. Results are expressed as either excretion rates (e.g. normal α-GST is <12.5 ng/min or <11.5 µg/litre) or as a ratio to urinary creatinine (e.g. normal reference range for retinol-binding protein:creatinine is <0.019 mg/mmol). Typically in cases of renal tubular proteinuria the ratio of retinol-binding protein:creatinine is greater than that of albumin:creatinine.

These tests of renal tubular proteinuria are helpful in investigating patients with suspected Chinese herbal nephropathy, Asian subcontinent nephropathy, and Balkan nephropathy. Industrial workers exposed to heavy metals and organic chemicals, such as those used in the dry-cleaning industry, may develop interstitial renal disease characterized by increased urinary low-molecular-weight proteinuria.

Estimation of glomerular filtration rate

Biochemical tests

Knowledge of the GFR is of crucial importance in the management of patients, not only for detecting the presence of renal impairment but also in the monitoring of all patients with or at risk of renal impairment, and in determining appropriate dosing of those drugs cleared by the kidney. Measurement of plasma creatinine remains the standard biochemical test used to assess renal function. Unfortunately, the plasma creatinine concentration is not linearly related to the GFR, hence some 30% of patients with significantly impaired renal function still have a plasma creatinine value within the normal range (<120 µmol/litre).

Creatinine

Creatine, which is endogenously synthesized in the liver or exogenously supplied by meat in the diet, is transported to muscle and converted to creatinine by nonenzymatic dehydration. Muscle mass represents some 98% of the total body creatine pool. Thus gender, racial and age-related differences in body composition, physical training and exercise, muscle-wasting diseases, paralysis, and intercurrent illnesses will all affect the production rate of creatinine and therefore both the plasma creatinine concentration and urinary creatinine excretion (Table 21.4.2). Hence in young children there is a steady increase in the plasma creatinine level as their muscle mass increases. Dietary influences will affect plasma creatinine levels, with a reduction in strict vegans and increased values in those with a high meat intake (particularly stewed meat: cooking leads to the conversion of creatine to creatinine) or those taking creatine supplements. For any individual, the plasma creatinine level is relatively constant throughout the day, although there is a tendency for it to increase slightly in the afternoon.

Creatinine is not only freely filtered by the glomerulus but is also secreted into the renal tubule. Creatinine reabsorption may occur at low urinary flow rates, such as in congestive cardiac failure.

Table 21.4.2 Factors affecting creatinine generation

Factor	Effect on serum creatinine
Ageing	Decreased
Female sex	Decreased
Race or ethnic group (compared with white)	
Black	Increased
Hispanic	Decreased
Oriental	Decreased
Body habitus	
Muscular	Increased
Amputation	Decreased
Obesity	Decreased
Chronic illness	
Malnutrition, chronic inflammation, cancer, severe cardiovascular or respiratory disease, hospitalized patients	Decreased
Neuromuscular diseases	Decreased
Hypothyroidism	Increased
Diet	
Vegetarian diet	Decreased
Ingestion of cooked meat	Increased

The relative proportion of renal tubular creatinine secretion to that filtered increases as renal function declines. In addition, in oedematous states such as nephrotic syndrome, calculated creatinine clearance exceeds inulin clearance, suggesting increased tubular creatinine secretion. Several drugs are known to block the tubular secretion of creatinine and thus cause an increase in the serum creatinine level: these include the diuretics amiloride, spironolactone, and triamterene; also cimetidine, aspirin, probenecid, and trimethoprim.

The most accurate method of measuring plasma creatinine is by isotope dilution mass spectrometry (IDMS), followed by enzymatic methods, but these are costly compared with the standard Jaffé assay. Most laboratories therefore measure plasma creatinine using standard automated analysers that assess the chromogenic product of creatinine and alkaline picrate (Jaffé reaction). Table 21.4.3 lists

Table 21.4.3 Compounds that can affect the measurement of plasma or urinary creatinine concentration

Endogenous compounds	Exogenous compounds
Protein	Acetohexamide
Ketones	Cephalosporins
Ketoacids	5-Fluorocytosine
Glucose	Methanol metabolites
Fatty acids	Phenylacetylurea
Urate	
Urea	
Bilirubin	

some substances which in high concentration can act directly or indirectly as chromogens, or affect the background control blanks, and so result in a spurious increase in the plasma creatinine level. In clinical practice these may lead to an overestimation of creatinine in people with poorly controlled diabetes, and an underestimation in deeply jaundiced patients, such as those with primary biliary cirrhosis. Under these circumstances, a more accurate method is to determine the plasma creatinine level enzymatically.

Reciprocal creatinine or logarithm of creatinine values
As the plasma creatinine level roughly doubles for every 50% reduction in GFR, expressing (transforming) the results as the reciprocal or logarithm is useful in assessing serial plasma values, which changes the graph from an exponential to a straight-line plot. The advantage of using a straight-line plot of plasma creatinine is that it allows the rate of renal decline to be calculated, which can then be used to predict the onset of endstage renal failure and the requirement for dialysis treatment in many patients. The reciprocal creatinine plot assumes a constant rate of loss, whereas the logarithm a constant fractional loss of renal function.

Patients with diabetic nephropathy tend to have a faster rate of decline in renal function than those with glomerular disease, who tend to have a faster rate than those with tubulointerstitial renal disease. In addition, it is easier to assess the effect of treatment interventions on the progression of renal disease by analysing transformed data, and also to recognize when there has been a sudden and unexpected deterioration in function that requires urgent investigation.

Prediction of creatinine clearance from the plasma creatinine level and estimation of GFR (eGFR)
Despite the potential inaccuracies in the determination of plasma creatinine, variations in endogenous creatinine production rates, and the relative increase in renal tubular and intestinal creatinine secretion with deteriorating renal function, formulas based on the plasma creatinine level are used in clinical practice to estimate creatinine clearance. The first commonly used equation, validated in adults, was the formula of Cockcroft and Gault, later modified by Gault:

$$\text{Creatinine clearance}(\text{ml/min}) = \frac{(140-\text{age})\times \text{weight}(\text{kg})}{72\times \text{plasma creatinine concentration}(\text{mg/dl})}$$

or

$$\text{Creatinine clearance}(\text{ml/min}) = \frac{1.2\times(140-\text{age})\times \text{weight}(\text{kg})}{72\times \text{plasma creatinine concentration}(\mu\text{mol/litre})}$$

In the original formula there was a different equation for women, with a factor of 0.85 (instead of 1.2) to allow for the lower rate of creatinine production in women due to differences in their body composition. Similar equations were developed for children. Although these formulas may be helpful in clinical practice to provide an estimation of renal function (eGFR), they are not always accurate, particularly in people with diabetes and African-Americans (owing to differences in body composition).

Another equation was developed in 1999 following the Modification of Diet in Renal Disease (MDRD) trial, based on 1628 adult patients in the United States of America, and this was further revised in 2005 as the simplified MDRD equation (sMDRD):

$$eGFR \left(ml/min\ per\ 1.73m^2 \right)$$
$$= 175 \times \left[serum\ creatinine\ (mg/dl) \right]^{-1.154}$$
$$\times (age\ in\ years)^{-0.203} \times 0.742\ (if\ female)$$
$$\times 1.212\ (if\ black)$$

$$eGFR \left(ml/min\ per\ 1.73m^2 \right)$$
$$= 175 \times \left(\left[serum\ creatinine\ (\mu mol/litre)/1.004 \right] \times 0.011312 \right)^{-1.154}$$
$$\times (age\ in\ years)^{-0.203} \times 0.742\ (if\ female)$$
$$\times 1.212\ (if\ black)$$

The sMDRD equation has the advantage over the Cockcroft–Gault and many other formulas in that it does not require knowledge of the patient's weight, and their sex and age are routine demographics collected for sample identification. Use of the sMDRD equation has now been introduced into standard clinical practice in the United States of America, the United Kingdom, and Australia to define stages of chronic kidney disease, the intention being to encourage recognition of renal impairment at an early stage in the population at large, and therefore allow management of risk factors to reduce both renal progression and cardiovascular risk (Table 21.4.4).

The first problem in rolling out such a program of population screening was to standardize the measurement of plasma creatinine. For example, in the United Kingdom alone there were 31 different modifications of the standard Jaffé reaction used in routine clinical practice. Rather than each laboratory changing its method/analyser, each individual laboratory had to develop correction factors from the IDMS-traceable version of the MDRD equation. Thus in the United Kingdom the following equation is employed using an IDMS-based national external quality assessment service.

Table 21.4.4 The stages of chronic kidney disease (CKD)

CKD stage[a]	eGFR (ml/min per 1.73 m² body surface area)
1	>90, with other evidence of renal disease
2	60–89, with other evidence of renal disease
3A	45–59
3B	30–44
4	15–29
5	<15, or receiving renal replacement therapy

[a] The suffix (p) can be used to denote the presence of proteinuria as defined by a spot urinary albumin:creatinine ratio (ACR) of ≥30 mg/mmol, which is approximately equivalent to a protein:creatinine ratio (PCR) of ≥50 mg/mmol (≥0.5 g/24 h).
Patients with CKD stages 3A, 3B, 4, and 5 may or may not have any other evidence of renal disease.

$$eGFR\ (ml/min\ per\ 1.73m^2)$$
$$= 175 \times (([creatinine\ (\mu mol/l)\ -\ intercept]/slope) \times 0.011312)^{-1.154}$$
$$\times (age\ in\ years)^{-0.203} \times 0.742\ (if\ female)$$
$$\times 1.212\ (if\ black)$$

where intercept and slope are the individual laboratory correction factors for the IDMS method.

The eGFR has not been validated in people younger than 18 years, hospitalized patients, or those with acute kidney injury, pregnancy, oedematous states, muscle-wasting disorders, amputations, or malnourishment. Similarly, it has not been validated for extremes of age or body weight, or for ethnic groups other than whites of northern European origin and African-Americans.

In the United Kingdom, the value of the eGFR falls within 30% of the true GFR in 90% of patients. Typically, the eGFR underestimates true renal function in patients with hyperfiltration, with its accuracy improving as renal function deteriorates. In the United States of America, Australia, and Scotland, laboratories have been advised to report all eGFR values higher than 60 ml/min per 1.73 m² simply as '>60' because of increased inaccuracy at higher eGFR, whereas in the United Kingdom the advice to laboratories is to report values up to 90 ml/min per 1.73 m², and then '>90'.

Although the eGFR has inherent inaccuracies, it may prove useful in assessing stability or progression of renal function over time in the general population and allow a rational basis for referral to specialist renal physicians. It is most likely that, following the universal introduction of eGFR, further refinements to the predictive equation will be developed.

Creatinine clearance

In clinical practice, creatinine clearance is now being replaced by the eGFR, as the accuracy of the creatinine clearance method depends on patient compliance to provide an accurate 24-h urine collection. Even when patients are in a steady state, urinary creatinine excretion varies from day to day, and reliability can be increased by performing consecutive daily clearances.

Creatinine clearance is calculated as follows:

$$Creatinine\ clearance\ (ml/min)$$
$$= \frac{urine\ volume\ (ml/24\,h) \times urine\ creatinine\ concentration\ (\mu mol/litre)}{plasma\ creatinine\ concentration\ (\mu mol/litre)}$$
$$\times 24 \times 60$$

With regard to the use of the creatinine clearance measurement as an estimate of GFR, two errors tend to balance each other out. The chromogenic assay tends to overestimate the plasma, but not urinary, creatinine concentration, leading to an underestimation of GFR. By contrast, creatinine is not only excreted by glomerular filtration: some is secreted by the renal tubules, leading to an overestimation of the GFR. However, in patients with impaired renal function these contrasting effects are not balanced, and the relative increase in tubular creatinine secretion results in creatinine clearance exceeding GFR. This problem can be overcome by the administration of 400 mg of cimetidine to block renal tubular creatinine secretion, but this manoeuvre is rarely (if ever) performed in clinical practice solely for this purpose. By convention, creatinine clearance values are commonly corrected for body surface area to adjust for differences in muscle mass, assuming a fixed mathematical relationship between body surface area and the relative proportions of fat to muscle. However, body composition is not only age- and gender-dependent, but also varies from race to race, and other inaccuracies occur in oedematous states.

Cystatin C

Cystatin C is a low-molecular-weight basic protein (13.26 kDa) from the cystatin superfamily of cysteine proteinase inhibitors that is produced by all nucleated cells. It is freely filtered by the glomerulus and not reabsorbed, secreted or catabolised by the renal tubules during its passage into the urine. The generation of cystatin C appears to be less variable from person to person than creatinine, hence it has been advocated as a better marker for GFR than creatinine. Rapid and fully automated immunonephelometric assays are now available, but these are more costly than assays of creatinine.

As with creatinine, several formulae have been developed to estimate GFR from cystatin C measurements (in mg/litre) in adults:

- Larsson formula: $GFR = 77.329 \times \text{cystatin } C^{-1.2623}$
- Hoek formula: $GFR = -4.32 + 80.35 \times 1/\text{cystatin } C$
- Filler formula: $\log GFR = 1.962 + 1.123 \times \log (1/\text{cystatin } C)$

In most studies, the accuracy of cystatin C assessment of GFR is superior to that of creatinine-based eGFR (using the sMDRD formula) in those patients in the crucial CKD stage 3 and 4 groups, both in children and adults. However, evidence is accumulating that the serum concentration of cystatin C is influenced by corticosteroid use, sex, age, weight, height, smoking status, proteinuric states, chronic liver disease, malignancy, and the level of C-reactive protein, even after adjustment for creatinine clearance. Cystatin C has also been reported to be reduced in renal transplant recipients, with some drugs (including valsartan), in bone marrow transplant patients, following myeloablative chemotherapy, and in hypothyroid states, and to be increased in thyrotoxicosis.

Carbamylation

Urea accumulates with deteriorating renal function and in plasma can spontaneously dissociate to form a reactive cyanate species that can react with the terminal valine of haemoglobin α and β chains (and also similar valine molecules in other proteins). This reaction is termed 'carbamylation' and the product 'carbamylated haemoglobin' (or other protein). Whereas glycosylated haemoglobin has proved useful in clinical practice for assessing time-averaged diabetic control, carbamylated haemoglobin or carbamyl-lysine adducts have not been shown to be superior to simple serum creatinine measurements in determining stable renal function. However, they are useful in helping to differentiate acute from chronic renal failure, because of the time course of the carbamylation reaction, and also in the assessment of time-averaged urea levels in the dialysis patient with endstage renal failure. However, until the relevant assays are commercially available, their use will remain experimental.

Other methods

Isotopic methods

The GFR can be determined by the clearance of a compound which is freely filtered by the glomerulus and then passes through the nephron without tubular reabsorption or secretion. Traditionally,

inulin—a naturally occurring polyfructose—was given as a constant infusion to achieve a constant plasma concentration, and then clearance determined from timed urinary collections. This was a laborious technique. Furthermore, the biochemical estimation of inulin was initially tedious and difficult, with significant interassay variation, and accurate timed urine collections are unreliable in patients with urinary tract anomalies. To overcome these and other difficulties, compounds other than inulin are generally used to estimate GFR, and methods other than constant infusion.

Following a single bolus injection, depending on the compound used, the fall in plasma concentration follows either a single- or two-compartment model related to renal clearance. Chromium-labelled ethylenediaminetetraacetic acid ([51Cr]EDTA) is the most commonly used isotope. After the single injection, three timed plasma samples are taken to calculate the plasma decay rate and thereby the GFR. More recently it has been showed that only a single blood sample at 4 h is required for a GFR over 30 ml/min. At GFRs above 30 ml/min there is a very good correlation between inulin and [51Cr]EDTA clearance, but below 30 ml/min the accuracy of the isotope technique is reduced, there being some renal tubular reabsorption. Accuracy can be improved in this situation by taking a delayed (24-h) plasma sample.

Other isotopes that have been used to estimate GFR include [125I]iothalamate, which when given as a subcutaneous injection results in a constant plasma concentration equivalent to the infusion technique, and 99Tcm-diethylenetriaminepentaacetic acid (DTPA), which is less accurate because of its short half-life (6 h) and dissociation of DTPA from the radionuclide.

With all the isotopic methods, it is conventional for the GFR to be corrected for the size of the patient. This correction assumes a fixed relationship between the weight and height of an individual: hence serial estimations to detect a change in renal function are more likely to be accurate than single estimations.

Radiological methods

Iohexol is a nonionic, low-osmolality radiocontrast dye. It can be used to estimate GFR following a single bolus injection of between 2 and 5 ml. In patients with a clearance of over 30 ml/min, a single plasma sample taken 3 h after injection provides an accurate estimation, whereas additional later samples are required to improve the accuracy in those with severely impaired renal function.

Summary

Because of the difficulty in interpreting plasma creatinine concentrations below 150 μmol/litre as an assessment of renal function, the eGFR has been introduced in clinical practice in the United States of America, Australia, and the United Kingdom to detect patients with early stages of chronic kidney disease. It is an appropriate and adequate technique for most clinical purposes. When more precise estimation of GFR is required, an isotopic assessment is the most accurate method of determination, otherwise two 24-h urine collections with corresponding plasma samples should be used to calculate the GFR by creatinine clearance, although in some centres cystatin C has replaced creatinine for this purpose. To examine changes in renal function, where eGFR measurements are not available, plasma creatinine concentrations should be transformed to either the reciprocal or the logarithm to assess trends in serial results.

Estimation of renal blood flow

Renal blood flow can be estimated noninvasively using Doppler flow probes, provided there is a single renal artery and adequate imaging is possible. This is technically easier for a transplanted kidney than a native kidney. The recent development of contrast agents for ultrasonography may increase the reliability of these estimations. Alternatively, renal blood flow can be estimated from the measurement of the renal plasma flow and the haematocrit. However, the haematocrit of peripheral venous blood may not be the same as that entering the renal artery. More recently, the development of positron emission tomography (PET) coupled with CT has allowed assessment of renal blood flow using ^{15}O-labelled water, ^{82}Rb, and other tracers.

Renal plasma flow

Ideally, any compound used to assess renal plasma flow should have 100% uptake by the kidney, with any fraction not filtered by the glomerulus being extracted by the tubules and secreted. p-Aminohippurate is the most commonly used compound, but is only 85% extracted during a single passage through the kidney, and thus at best only provides an estimate of renal plasma flow. Continuous infusion of p-aminohippurate provides a more accurate estimation of renal plasma flow than single-injection techniques.

Renal blood flow varies in normal subjects with pain, stress, physical exercise, and normal pregnancy, and following a high-protein meal. In patients with impaired renal function, the decline in renal plasma flow generally corresponds to the decrease in GFR. However, in some conditions where there may be renal tubular hypoxia or toxicity, such as in patients with severe heart disease or those with ciclosporin nephrotoxicity, the reduction in estimated renal plasma flow is greater than that expected for the change in GFR, due to a reduction in the renal tubular uptake of p-aminohippurate. Similarly, p-aminohippurate uptake is reduced in small children. [^{125}I]o-Iodohippurate has also been used to estimate renal plasma flow, but this has a lower extraction than p-aminohippurate (75%), and is less reliable.

Investigation of tubular function

In a normal subject, some 180 litres of glomerular filtrate is produced each day and less than 3% of this is excreted, owing to reabsorption by the tubules. The proximal and distal tubules have different functions, and traditionally each is considered separately.

Proximal tubular function

Defects in proximal tubular function may be isolated or generalized, as in the Fanconi syndrome. Glucose, phosphate, amino acids, and organic ions are reabsorbed by the apical border of proximal renal tubular cells by sodium-dependent cotransporters, and are then transported across the basolateral membrane by different, sodium-independent, cotransporters.

Glucose

There is a maximum reabsorption rate for glucose (T_mG) in the proximal tubule of 15.1 ± 2.5 mmol/litre (T_mG/GFR), above which glycosuria will be present. To determine T_mG/GFR, a 20% dextrose infusion is administered at increasing rates to produce a slow rise in the plasma glucose up to a maximum of 30 mmol/litre, which is maintained for a minimum of 1 h. Plasma and urine samples are collected every 30 min. Renal function is determined by [^{51}Cr]EDTA-GFR. The glucose absorption rate is calculated as the difference between the filtered load in urine (urine volume × [glucose]$_{urine}$) and the filtered load in plasma (GFR × [glucose]$_{plasma}$). Patients with type A renal glycosuria typically have a reduced threshold of around 5 mmol/litre.

Phosphate

Phosphate is normally filtered at the glomerulus and reabsorbed in the proximal tubule, with only 10 to 20% of the filtered load being excreted. The normal tubular reabsorption of phosphate (TRP) is above 85% and can be calculated from:

$$\%TRP = \left(1 - [\text{phosphate clearance}/\text{eGFR}]\right) \times 100$$

If renal function is normal, then this can be simplified by collecting an early-morning specimen of urine, and:

$$\%TRP = \left(1 - \frac{[\text{phosphate}]_{urine} \times [\text{creatinine}]_{plasma}}{[\text{creatinine}]_{urine} \times [\text{phosphate}]_{plasma}}\right) \times 100$$

Alternatively, the theoretical maximum tubular threshold of phosphate (T_mP) can be estimated from:

$$T_mP/GFR = [\text{phosphate}]_{plasma} - \frac{[\text{phosphate}]_{urine} \times [\text{creatinine}]_{plasma}}{[\text{creatinine}]_{urine}}$$

or measured directly as for T_mG, following an infusion of phosphate (1.0 litre of 0.1 mol/litre sodium phosphate at pH 7.4) with a corresponding [^{51}Cr]EDTA-GFR.

Excessive urinary phosphate losses occur in proximal tubular disorders such as Fanconi's syndrome, primary and secondary hyperparathyroidism, and mitochondrial disorders, both primary and secondary, including those due to antiretroviral therapy. In the various forms of hypophosphataemic rickets, phosphaturia occurs with a characteristically reduced T_mP/GFR of less than 0.56 mmol/litre.

Amino acids

Apart from the reabsorption of histidine (90–95%), that of other amino acids is almost complete (97–99%). Although amidoaciduria can occur as a result of overflow when the plasma concentration exceeds the tubular transport maximum, this is very rarely the cause of aminoaciduria in adults. In general, five types of renal aminoaciduria are distinguished: dibasic amino acids, neutral amino acids (monoaminomonocarboxylic acids), glycine and imino acids, dicarboxylic amino acids, and generalized aminoaciduria in the case of Fanconi's syndrome. Generalized and specific aminoacidurias can be detected and quantified by thin-layer chromatography. In Fanconi's syndrome, amino acids from all four groups are present, whereas in glycinuria there is only excess glycine. Classic cases of cystinuria have increased urinary arginine, ornithine, lysine, and cystine; and patients with Hartnup's disease have an excess of neutral amino acids.

For more detailed discussion of other aspects of proximal tubular function and their diseases, see Chapter 21.16.

Distal tubular function

Patients with primary or secondary nephrogenic or cranial diabetes insipidus and those with primary polydipsia may present with polyuria. A water-deprivation test can help to differentiate between these conditions, and can be performed as follows. The patient should be admitted to a metabolic ward on the evening prior to the test, be weighed, and have samples taken for baseline plasma osmolality, chemistries, and AVP measurement. An osmolality above 295 mOsm/kg and a sodium concentration above 143 mmol/litre exclude a diagnosis of primary polydipsia. After midnight, no oral fluids are allowed until completion of the test. The early-morning urine osmolality is measured, and if it is above 800 mOsm/kg (normal response) the test is abandoned. Thereafter, the patient's weight, plasma and urine osmolality, and plasma AVP concentration should be recorded regularly. If weight loss exceeds 5%, then the test should be abandoned to prevent dangerous dehydration. Once urine osmolality reaches a plateau (an hourly increase of less than 30 mOsm/kg for 3 consecutive hours), then five units of aqueous vasopressin is administered subcutaneously and urine and plasma osmolality measured after a further 30 min, and then at hourly intervals.

Comparison of the last urine osmolality reading prior to the administration of vasopressin with the maximum osmolality following vasopressin is used to categorize patients. Those with nephrogenic diabetes insipidus will produce a urine osmolality under 300 mOsm/kg, with no response to exogenous vasopressin, and they will have high AVP levels. Those with severe cranial diabetes insipidus will have dilute urine, again less than 300 mOsm/kg, but they will respond to exogenous vasopressin by increasing urine osmolality by 50% or more, accompanied by low endogenous AVP levels. Both cranial and nephrogenic diabetes insipidus can occur as partial forms, which show some response to dehydration, but they can be discriminated by analysing the relative changes in endogenous AVP and the urinary and plasma osmolalities. Patients with primary polydipsia do not show pituitary suppression, and have little or no response to exogenous vasopressin.

Renally induced electrolyte imbalances

Sodium and water

There are many causes of hyponatraemia, as discussed in Chapter 21.2.1. Patients with cardiac failure, chronic liver disease, nephrotic syndrome, and prerenal acute renal failure will have a fractional excretion of sodium (FE_{Na}) of less than 1% (normal is 1–2%), where:

$$\%FE_{Na} = \frac{[sodium]_{urine} \times [creatinine]_{plasma}}{[sodium]_{plasma} \times [creatinine]_{urine}} \times 100$$

Those with the syndrome of inappropriate diuresis preferentially retain water and have a normal FE_{Na}, indeed the diagnosis cannot be made if FE_{Na} is low, but when interpreting measurements of FE_{Na} it must be remembered that this is increased by diuretic administration and in chronic renal failure.

Both those with reduced effective circulating plasma volume and those with the syndrome of inappropriate diuresis have impaired free-water excretion, which can be tested by giving the patient 20 ml/kg body weight of water to drink after voiding. More than 75% of the water load should be excreted within 3 h, and the urine osmolality should fall to under 100 mOsm/kg (specific gravity <1.003),

although this test can be affected by gastrointestinal disease, smoking, and emotional factors. The free-water clearance (Ch_2o) can be quantitated from:

$$C_{H_2O} = \text{urine volume in ml/min} - \frac{osmolality_{urine}}{osmolality_{plasma}}$$
$$\times \text{urine volume in ml/min}$$

A positive free-water clearance occurs when the urine is more dilute than plasma, and a negative free-water clearance when the urine is more concentrated. For further discussion of these issues, and the clinical approach to disorders of sodium and water homeostasis, see Chapter 21.2.1.

Potassium

To determine whether there is a renal tubular cause for potassium disturbances, the transtubular potassium gradient (TTKG) can be calculated. This attempts to estimate the potassium concentration in the cortical collecting duct as follows:

$$TTKG = \frac{[potassium]_{urine}}{[potassium]_{plasma}} \times \frac{osmolality_{plasma}}{osmolality_{urine}}$$

In a patient with hypokalaemia, a TTKG of less than 2 suggests a nonrenal cause, whereas a high TTKG (>10) is associated with mineralocorticoid excess, Liddle's syndrome, or drugs such as acetazolamide, fludrocortisone, and amphotericin. In a patient with hyperkalaemia, a TTKG above 10 implies a nonrenal cause and a low TTKG (<2) would be found in cases of potassium-sparing diuretics, hypoaldosteronism, and pseudohypoaldosteronism. However, while having some theoretical attraction, it is doubtful whether such analysis helps greatly in the diagnosis or management of patients with hypokalaemia or hyperkalaemia. For further discussion of these issues, and the clinical approach to disorders of potassium homeostasis, see Chapter 21.2.2.

For more detailed discussion of other aspects of distal tubular function and their diseases, including tests of urinary acidification, see Chapters 21.14 and 21.15.

Imaging of patients with renal disease

There are a number of techniques that can be used to image the kidney: a simple comparison of some of these is given in Table 21.4.5.

Plain radiography

Plain abdominal radiographs may demonstrate opaque urinary stones, nephrocalcinosis, and the renal outlines. Ultrafast, noncontrast CT scanning with three-dimensional reconstruction has generally replaced nephrotomograms for detecting low-opacity renal stones.

Chest radiography may be helpful in the diagnosis of pulmonary oedema, and also in demonstrating the cardiac silhouette and lung pathology sometimes associated with renal disease, such as pulmonary haemorrhage and cavitation. Multiple rib fractures may suggest multiple myeloma.

Intravenous urography

Intravenous urography (IVU) is no longer the standard investigation in nephrology, but still has an important place in the investigation

Table 21.4.5 Comparison of standard methods for radiological imaging of the kidney

Imaging method	Advantages		Disadvantages	
	General	Imaging	General	Imaging
Ultrasound	Noninvasive Safe Versatile Cost (cheap)	First-line imaging for excluding obstruction. Can be used to guide intervention	Operator/machine dependent. Dependent on patient having suitable body habitus	
Intravenous urography (IVU)	Cost (cheap)	Good for definition of upper tract anatomy	Contrast exposure	Good images not obtainable with eGFR <20 ml/min
Multislice 3-D CT	Widely available	High resolution, allowing best anatomical definition	Radiation dose	
CT KUB (kidneys, ureter, and bladder)	No contrast exposure	First-line imaging for urinary stones. Can detect nonrenal pathology	Limited study	Not good at detecting small blood clots
CT urography		First-line imaging for upper tract	Contrast exposure	Good images not obtainable with eGFR <15 ml/min. Limited for imaging of bladder pathology
CT angiography		First-line imaging of renal arteries.	Contrast exposure	
MRI without contrast	Noninvasive. Avoidance of radiation dose allows repeated studies	Good anatomical definition. Can visualize the whole of the urinary tract. Good for staging of renal carcinoma. Good for assessment of complex renal cysts	Patient needs to be able to hold their breath. Cost (expensive)	Not possible in all patients, e.g. prevented by cardiac pacemaker, cochlear implant, intracranial clips
MRI with contrast (gadolinium)— urography and angiography		Used to confirm normal vascular anatomy, e.g. in assessment of potential kidney donors	Careful consideration if eGFR <30 ml/min (nephrogenic systemic fibrosis)	Tends to overestimate the significance of stenoses. Likely to miss small accessory renal arteries
Renal angiography		The gold standard investigation for renal artery stenosis and brisk renal bleeding. Can be therapeutic as well as diagnostic, e.g. stent/angioplasty, embolisation by coiling/gel foam	Invasive. Contrast exposure. Requires considerable technical expertise	Risk of plaque rupture, vessel dissection, haemorrhage

Contrast nephrotoxicity with iodinated-based contrast agents is increased when eGFR <60 ml/min per 1.73 m^2.

of patients with suspected obstruction, particularly of the upper urinary tract. As with all radiographic procedures, potential fetal irradiation should be avoided. Bowel preparation is no longer standard, owing to the risks of dehydration in older people and of gaseous distension of the bowel obscuring the urinary tract. Even the newer nonionic lower-oncotic contrast media can cause nephrotoxicity in some patients, and care should be taken to ensure that those at risk (older people, and those with diabetes, myeloma, or pre-existing renal impairment) are adequately hydrated. Normal renal length is between three and four lumbar vertebrae, with a width approximately half that of the length.

The calyces and papillae are well demonstrated on the IVU, which may be diagnostic in cases of medullary sponge kidney, papillary necrosis, and sloughed papillae. Similarly, intraluminal radiolucent foreign bodies may be demonstrated surrounded by contrast, typified by radiolucent stones, blood clots, fungal ball, tumour, or sloughed papillae.

Abnormalities of the ureteric wall such as localized thickening are found in cases of transitional cell carcinoma, oedema, tuberculosis, and parasitic granuloma. The IVU may also demonstrate

external compression: this can be due to aberrant blood vessels in the upper tract, retroperitoneal fibrosis affecting the middle ureter, or prostatic pathology in the lower tract.

The IVU may provide valuable information about renal size and possible intrarenal masses. It retains a role for investigation of upper tract pathology to detect intraluminal tumours and blood clot, but has been replaced by other techniques, such as ultrasound and ultrafast CT scanning, to investigate renal colic.

Other conventional uroradiological techniques

Further information about the site and nature of any obstruction can be obtained by ureteropyelography. An antegrade study involves percutaneous puncture of the renal pelvis, with immediate relief of the obstruction by nephrostomy, and allows demonstration of the site of obstruction following an injection of contrast media (antegrade ureteropyelography) (Fig. 21.4.4). A retrograde study requires cystoscopy, allowing direct visualization of the distal ureter and the possibility of removing an obstructing stone, with injection of contrast media from below demonstrating the site of obstruction (retrograde ureteropyelography). Passage of a double

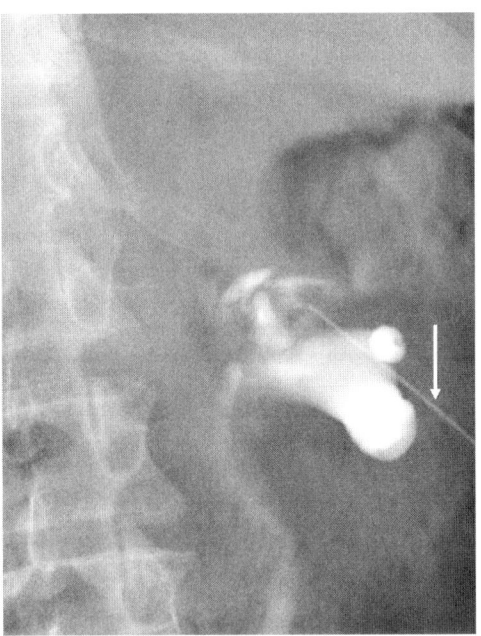
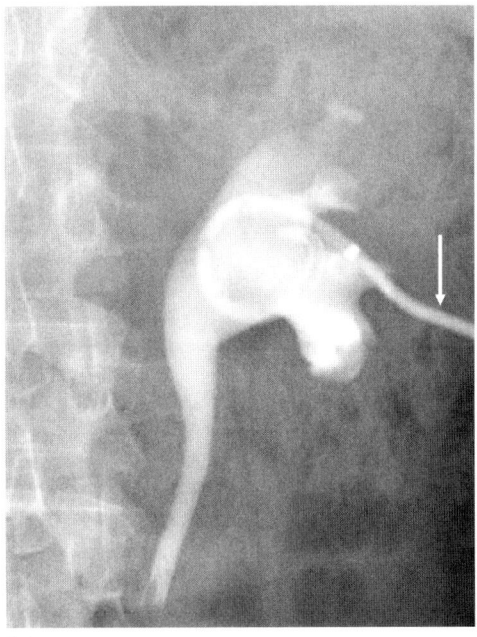

(a)   (b)

Fig. 21.4.4 Antegrade puncture of the collecting system of the left kidney: (a) the nephrostomy needle (arrowed) has punctured an upper pole calyx, confirmed by injection of contrast medium that can be seen outlining the dilated pelvicalyceal collecting system, with some flow into the upper ureter; and (b) the nephrostomy needle has been replaced by an antegrade nephrostomy tube (arrowed), with injection of contrast medium demonstrating a block to flow (due to retroperitoneal fibrosis in this case) in the mid ureter.

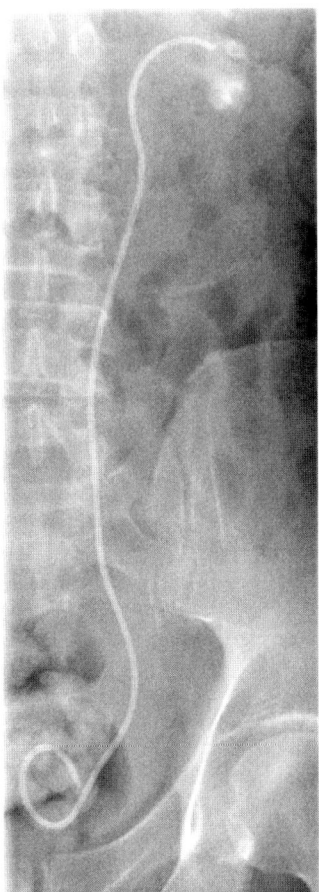

Fig. 21.4.5 Abdominal radiograph showing a double JJ stent placed in the left ureter. This was placed antegradely (from the kidney); some contrast medium from the preceding antegrade ureteropyelogram remains in the renal pelvis.

JJ stent from above (antegrade) or below (retrograde) can relieve obstruction by allowing internal drainage into the bladder (Fig. 21.4.5).

Antegrade techniques are usually more successful in relieving obstruction, particularly in those with pelvic malignancy or obstruction of a renal transplant. In cases when renal obstruction is considered, but investigation inconclusive, a pragmatic trial of antegrade stent insertion should be undertaken. Improvement of renal function confirms obstruction.

Retrograde urethrocystography is performed in women to detect lower urinary tract abnormalities, such as fistulas or urethral diverticulae. Sequential films taken during micturition may detect active reflux. In men, urethrocystography can be complicated by trauma and infection to the lower urinary tract, hence suprapubic bladder puncture is recommended.

Renal ultrasonography

The normal kidney and chronic kidney disease

The normal adult kidney is between 10 and 12 cm long, with a thin, bright capsule surrounded by highly reflective perinephric fat. The healthy cortex returns mid-level grey echoes, the pyramids are darker, and the renal sinus, containing fat and the major vascular pedicle, is bright with high reflectivity. Colour (flow) Doppler ultrasonography can be used to visualize the flow of urine from the native ureters into the bladder.

In most causes of chronic kidney disease, the kidneys become smaller, with reduced cortical thickness and increased cortical reflectivity when qualitatively compared with the liver. Diastolic blood flow is reduced on the Doppler scan. The renal ultrasound appearances are characteristic in some conditions, including focal segmental glomerular sclerosis secondary to HIV infection, in which the kidney is reported to be large and the cortex uniformly of a high reflectivity, greater than that of the renal sinus. Scars, either vascular or infective, may often be too small to be detected by ultrasound examination, especially in the neonate.

Renal masses

Ultrasonography is useful in the assessment of renal masses. Benign cysts have a smooth outline with well-demarcated borders and an echo-free centre, whereas renal tumours are usually irregular with heterogeneous echo reflectivity. Typical standard real-time two-dimensional B mode ultrasound may be able to detect renal masses and/or cysts as small as 2 to 3 mm in size, depending on the experience of the operator and the specification of the scanner, but this ability is reduced by several patient factors including high-density fat and muscle, and position, particularly when the kidneys are covered by the ribcage. Most tumours are vascular, with high flow during both systole and diastole on colour Doppler scanning, and adenocarcinomas in particular may be seen to extend into the renal vein. Renal transitional cell carcinomas are not readily detected unless large because ultrasound does not visualize individual calyces well. Angiolipomas may have a characteristic appearance due to their fat content which has high reflectivity, but confirmatory CT scanning is required.

In adult polycystic kidney disease, the kidneys are typically enlarged with multiple bilateral cysts. Middle-aged women (particularly but not exclusively) may also have hepatic cysts. It is important to remember that, if patients are scanned in their teenage years or before, then cysts may not have developed to a size detectable by ultrasound. Haemorrhage, infection, or malignant change all result in complex echoes within cysts, which cannot be differentiated by ultrasound scanning. Autosomal recessive polycystic kidney disease can be detected *in utero* with antenatal scanning.

There is an increased incidence of cystic change in the kidneys of patients with endstage renal failure, and occasionally these cysts may become malignant. It has been recommended that dialysis patients should be screened by ultrasound every 3 years, and then annually if cystic changes develop.

Urinary obstruction

In most centres, ultrasonography of the urinary tract is the first investigation performed when urinary obstruction is suspected. When urinary obstruction has been present for some time, the high reflectivity of the central renal sinus becomes replaced by echo-free urine, with distension of the calyces (Fig. 21.4.6). However, it is important to recognize that in acute obstruction, and in cases where the kidney and ureter are encased (usually the result of

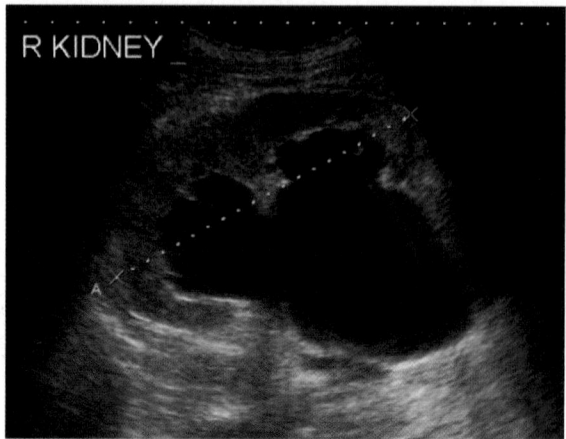

Fig. 21.4.6 Ultrasound scan of an obstructed kidney showing a massively dilated pelvicalyceal system.

tumour), the standard ultrasound examination may appear normal. In these circumstances, a colour Doppler scan may show reduced diastolic blood flow due to increased intrarenal pressure, and a difference in resistivity index (RI)—which equals (peak systolic velocity – end diastolic velocity)/peak systolic velocity)—of more than 0.1 between the two kidneys is thought to be a reliable parameter for diagnosing acute unilateral ureteric obstruction. Similarly, absence of the normal pulsatile jets of urine from the ureter into the bladder may be demonstrated on the side with acute obstruction.

Ultrasonography is not usually diagnostic of the cause of obstruction, but it may detect para-aortic nodes, a bladder mass, prostatic enlargement, or a ureterocele. Further investigation with transvaginal, transrectal, or transurethral ultrasound may confirm the cause of obstruction, with transrectal ultrasound being particularly useful in the detection of local invasion from prostatic carcinoma.

Urinary tract stones

Renal stones appear on ultrasonography as a bright echogenic focus with a distal acoustic shadow. Ultrasound can be used to follow up patients with renal calculus disease by assessing the number and size of stones. Nephrocalcinosis may result in an increase in medullary echoreflectivity due to calcium deposition, which usually affects the whole medulla, whereas calcification from papillary necrosis has an appearance more like that of a renal stone.

Renovascular disease

Colour Doppler can be used to investigate renal arterial and venous disease. Thrombosis of major vessels produces absent flow or changes to the intrarenal blood flow pattern. More recently, colour Doppler scanning has been used as a screening test for renovascular disease, as the higher the stenotic gradient in the renal artery, the slower and smoother the systolic upstream with identical diastolic velocity. This so-called 'parvus–tardus' flow results in a decrease in RI, which can be compared with the contralateral kidney, and an RI difference of more than 0.05 (based on three to six measurements) between the kidneys has been reported to be a reliable parameter to detect significant unilateral renal artery stenosis. Furthermore, one study suggested that assessment of the RI in patients with atherosclerotic renovascular disease had prognostic value: those patients with an RI above 0.8 did not improve following renal artery angioplasty.

Atherosclerotic renal artery stenosis occurs bilaterally in 20 to 30% of cases, and often affects the ostium, hence blood flow velocity at the ostium and along the renal artery should both be assessed. Thresholds ranging from 1.8 to 2.0 m/s (flow rate is accelerated in a narrowed stenotic artery) have been reported to have sensitivity and specificity of 70 to 90%, respectively, for renal artery stenosis, but the procedure is difficult and time-consuming, and even with an experienced operator it will be impossible to visualize the renal arteries adequately in some 20% of patients. Colour Doppler ultrasound is thus not a routine technique for screening for or investigating cases of renal artery stenosis, except in centres that have particular interest and expertise in the technique.

Renal transplantation

Ultrasound examination is an important investigation in the management of renal transplant recipients. Compared with the native kidney, the calyces and ureter are frequently visible in otherwise normal allografts, so experience is required in the interpretation of mild or even moderate calyceal dilatation. Early graft dysfunction mandates investigation to exclude a technical problem with either the renal artery or vein, or a urinary leak.

Colour Doppler scanning provides valuable information about the vascular supply of the graft (Fig. 21.4.7), and as with reno-vascular disease can be used to assess iliac artery and anastomotic stenoses. Estimation of the RI has been advocated to monitor early graft function, but acute tubular necrosis, acute rejection, acute renal vein thrombosis, and acute calcineurin toxicity all cause increased intrarenal pressure with reduced diastolic flow and increased RI. Similarly, by affecting the end-diastolic velocity, the RI can be reduced by tachycardia, and increased by bradycardia, compression of the transplant with the transducer, or Valsalva's manoeuvre through breath-holding. In addition, the RI is affected by vascular compliance, and older transplant recipients with stiffness of the prerenal vessels (aorta and iliac) will have an increased RI independently of graft function. Thus, the RI cannot be used solely to monitor graft function, but serial measurements can guide the timing of graft biopsy.

Fluid collections (commonly lymphoceles) appear as echo-free or echo-poor areas, and such perinephric collections can be drained under ultrasound guidance for diagnostic purposes or to relieve obstruction. As with the native kidney, percutaneous nephrostomy is the emergency treatment of choice for obstruction of a renal transplant. Colour Doppler scanning can detect the presence of arteriovenous fistulas, which are not uncommon following transplant biopsy.

Contrast agents for ultrasound

Colour Doppler ultrasonogrphy can detect bubbles present in injected contrast medium. Application of this technique can change the use of ultrasound from simple anatomical visualization of the kidneys to dynamic testing by assessment of the perfusion quotient. However, this remains an experimental investigation and not in routine clinical use, although it potentially has the capacity of allowing ultrasound to determine relative renal function, and improve investigation for obstruction, renovascular disease, and vascular rejection in renal transplants.

CT scanning

Ultrafast multislice CT scanning, with workstation reconstruction down to a resolution of 2 to 3 mm or less, has become the mainstay of renal imaging (Fig. 21.4.8). CT urography can be performed with a combination of unenhanced, nephrogenic-phase and excretory-phase imaging. The unenhanced images are ideal for detecting urinary calculi. Renal masses can be detected and characterized with the combination of unenhanced, nephrogenic- and excretory-phase imaging. The excretory phase provides imaging of the urothelium. As with the standard IVU, iodine-based contrast media may cause renal impairment, but only a single dose is required and contrast exposure is usually much less than that required for coronary angiography.

Unenhanced CT scanning

For patients with suspected renal colic due to stones, low-dose, unenhanced helical CT has become the gold standard investigation, particularly for patients with ureteric obstruction and kidney failure. CT allows both the cause and the level of the obstruction to be determined. Practically all stones (apart from indinavir) can be detected, hydronephrosis with perinephric stranding can usually be readily identified, and there may be hydroureter down to the level of the obstruction. In cases where a stone has passed, oedema may be noted at the vesicoureteric junction, with residual stranding around the ureter.

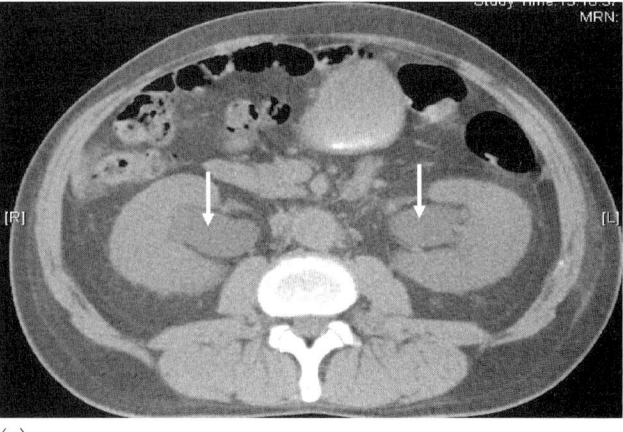

(a)

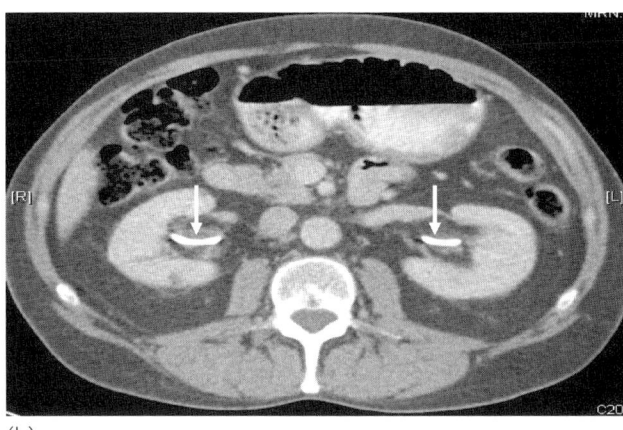

(b)

Fig. 21.4.8 CT imaging: (a) showing dilatation of both renal pelvices (arrowed) in a case of urinary obstruction; and (b) after relief of obstruction by placement of double JJ stents in both ureters (arrowed).

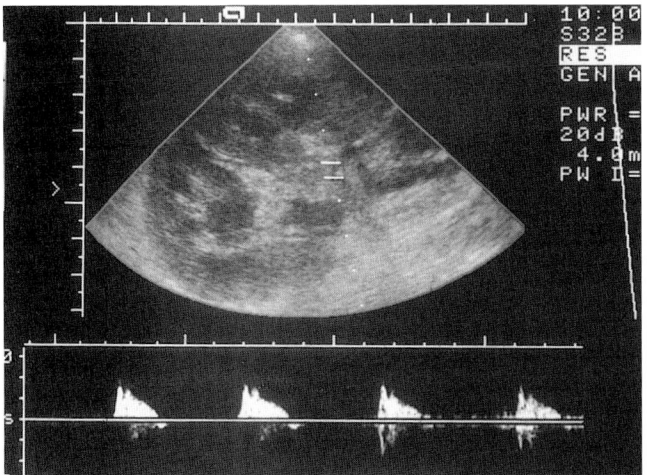

Fig. 21.4.7 Doppler ultrasound scan of a renal transplant showing normal systolic and diastolic waveform (resistivity index <0.65).

Other pathology may be identified in patients presenting with loin pain, such as renal enlargement with perinephric fat stranding, or oedema in cases of acute pyelonephritis, renal vein thrombosis, or acute arterial occlusion. Small blood clots can be difficult to identify. Other nonrenal pathology may be identified, including leaking abdominal aorta, diverticular disease, or appendicitis.

CT angiography

Contrast administration allows a CT angiogram phase to be acquired (Fig. 21.4.9). Compared with magnetic resonance angiography (MRA), CT angiography is more sensitive in detecting small accessory renal arteries and it does not overestimate the length and severity of stenoses, which appear greater during MRA owing to the combination of slower speed of data acquisition and blood flow. The main indications for CT angiography include the evaluation of acute renal trauma, tumour blood supply in cases of nephron-sparing surgery, the diagnosis of renal artery stenosis and/or aneurysms, defining the arterial supply in potential living renal donors, and prior to pyeloplasty for ureteropelvic junction obstruction, as endoluminal pyelomyotomy is not as successful as laparoscopic or open pyelomyotomy if there are posterior and/or anterior vessels. Some centres have used CO_2 as a contrast agent to reduce the risk of contrast nephropathy and volume loading, but the images are not as good as with conventional CT angiography and tend to overestimate strictures.

CT imaging of the renal parenchyma

Owing to the speed of data acquisition, there is a cortical phase followed by an exctretory phase, which allows imaging of both the cortex and then the medulla. Thus CT scanning is useful in the investigation of congenital and anatomical abnormalities of the renal tract (such as renal agenesis), nephrocalcinosis (before calcification can be detected on plain films), and papillary sloughing.

Apart from the investigation of cystic renal disease, CT scanning is used to investigate renal masses. Renal cell carcinomas vary in appearance: some show calcification both within and surrounding the tumour on nonenhanced scans, some are solid, and others are cystic or have necrotic centres. Most tumours are vascular and readily enhance with contrast, but those with heavy calcification may not. CT scanning is important in tumour staging and in determining the extent of perirenal spread, renal vein involvement,

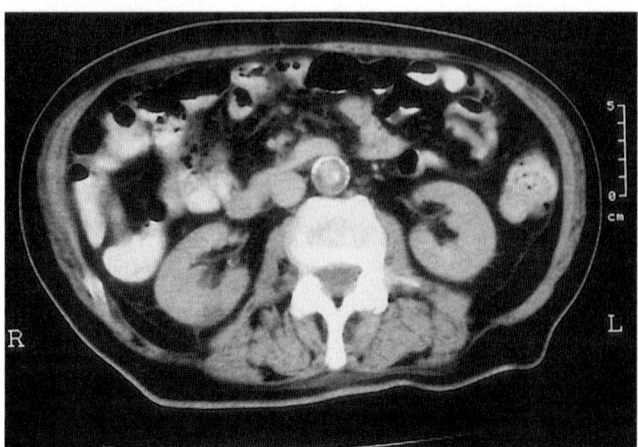

Fig. 21.4.9 Contrast-enhanced CT scan showing thrombosed aorta and renal arteries.

and enlargement of local lymph nodes. Occasionally, secondary deposits due to metastatic spread and secondary involvement in lymphomas and leukaemia can be found on contrast-enhanced renal scans. These are usually small, multiple intrarenal masses, often bilateral, typically homogeneous, and solid in lymphomas. Although ultrasound is used to screen and assess Wilms' tumours in children, CT scanning is important in excluding pulmonary metastases.

Angiolipomas can be recognized with ultrasound but should be confirmed on CT scanning as some renal cell carcinomas may contain small amounts of fat. In tuberous sclerosis, angiolipomas may be associated with renal cysts. Although angiolipomas are benign mesenchymal tumours, they can rarely rupture, especially those with intrarenal haematomas and aneurysms. Early detection by CT scanning allows prophylactic embolization of these vascular lesions.

Renal oncocytomas, another benign renal tumour, may have a central lucent area due to fibrosis on CT scanning. However, a proportion of oncocytomas may become malignant, hence any small renal lesion which is not a simple cyst or angiolipoma must be regarded as potentially malignant and surveillance with repeat CT scanning (or ultrasound) should be recommended.

Renal tract imaging in patients with acute pyelonephritis is usually requested to exclude the presence of obstruction, or when there has been an inadequate response to treatment. CT scanning defines the extent of disease better than ultrasound, detects abscesses, and can also exclude obstruction. Whereas focal acute bacterial pyelonephritis should respond to antibiotics, renal abscesses may require drainage. CT scanning may also detect gas bubbles within the renal parenchyma or perirenal space, which is characteristic of the emphysematous pyelonephritis that is typically found in people with diabetes Similarly, CT scanning may establish a diagnosis of xanthogranulomatous pyelonephritis, with an enlarged kidney containing areas of scarring, focal loss of renal parenchyma, and multiple low-density masses, often following recurrent infections in patients with staghorn calculi.

CT urography

Scanning during the excretory phase provides a CT urogram of high definition, which may detect filling defects within the collecting system, such as transitional cell carcinoma, blood clot, or stone, and also external compression due to vasculature. Review of three-dimensional formatted images allows surgical planning. The use of CT urography is currently limited to assessing local extravesicle extension or metastatic disease in the staging of bladder tumours. With further developments in computer software, it will be possible to perform virtual cystoscopy to detect intravesicle lesions of at least 5 mm or in size after distending the bladder with CO_2 or saline.

Functional CT

An estimate of GFR can be made using nonionic contrast media, which may be helpful when deciding on nephron-sparing surgery for renal tumours, and assessing patients with renovascular disease before and after interventional stenting.

MRI

CT scanning and ultrasound are good reliable techniques for detecting and evaluating renal masses. MRI is an alternative in patients who are allergic to conventional iodine-based radiocontrast media, but the current generation of MRI scanners does not have the resolution of the ultrafast three-dimensional CT scanners.

Gadolinium contrast used in MRI is taken up by the proximal tubule in a similar manner to aluminium. The dose of gadolinium-based contrast agent required is much less than those of standard iodinated contrast agents. Their biological half-life is increased in severe renal impairment, and they can result in spurious hypocalcaemia for up to 24 h after administration due to chelation with the commonly used automated assays for measuring serum calcium.

Although gadolinium-based contrast agents generally have a good safety profile, there are a few reports of acute kidney injury following their administration, in particular with high doses and intra-arterial administration, and they have also been found to cause nephrogenic systemic fibrosis/nephrogenic sclerosing dermopathy.

Nephrogenic systemic fibrosis

Nephrogenic systemic fibrosis is caused by exposure of patients with renal impairment to gadolinium-based contrast agents. The first cases were identified in 1997 and the condition first clearly described in 2000. Within weeks, months or (less commonly) years of exposure, patients develop a scleroderma-like disease, usually recognized with the development of areas of thickened and hardened skin that can progress rapidly to produce flexion contractures and joint immobility. The lungs, myocardium, and skeletal muscle can be involved. Gadolinium can be detected in skin biopsy specimens. Mortality is up to 30% in some series. There is no known effective treatment, and dialysis immediately after exposure does not prevent the condition.

It is difficult to determine the incidence of nephrogenic systemic fibrosis because mild cases undoubtedly go undetected. Release of free gadolinium ions (Gd^{3+}) appears to be crucial in pathogenesis, hence not all gadolinium-based contrast agents are equally culpable. Those with a cyclical structure are less likely to do so (and are therefore safer) than those with a linear ionic structure, which in turn are better than those with a linear nonionic structure. Most cases have been related to gadodiamide, with perhaps 2 to 4% of patients with significant renal impairment who received this agent developing the condition, although much higher rates (up to 25%) have been reported in some series.

Recognition of nephrogenic systemic fibrosis has led to the recommendation that cyclical gadolinium-based contrast agents should be cautiously used in patients with an eGFR of less than 30 ml/min (CKD stage 4 and CKD stage 5), and in patients with an eGFR of between 30 and 60 ml/min (CKD stage 3) the clinician should consider whether the necessary imaging information could better be obtained by another imaging technique.

Plain and conventional gadolinium-enhanced MRI

MRI is expensive, but does have some advantages over conventional CT. Tissues surrounded by fat, such as enlarged lymph nodes, or tumour extension into the renal vein, and angiomyolipomas are better demonstrated on MRI than CT. Thus MRI is useful in staging renal cell carcinoma, and by being able to distinguish blood from tissue can help to differentiate simple cysts complicated by haemorrhage from those that are malignant. The fact that MRI does not expose the patient to radiation also offers an obvious advantage over CT in those requiring repeated imaging.

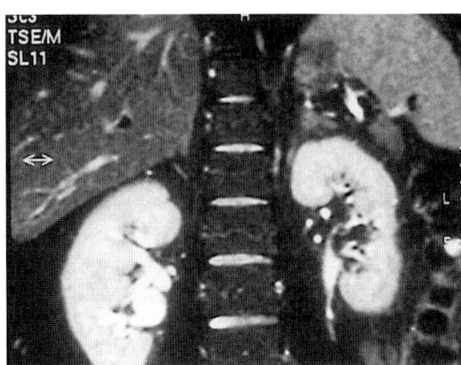

Fig. 21.4.10 Gadolinium-enhanced MRI showing left-sided pyelonephritic scarring, with a reduction in cortical thickness and scarring.

The whole of the urinary tract can be visualized, in a manner similar to an IVU, by using a heavily weighted T_2 fast spin–echo sequence. This rapid acquisition and relaxation enhancement scan can be used to assess potential live donors for renal transplantation, by demonstrating the renal vasculature, renal anatomy, and urinary drainage with one investigation. The quality of image provided by MRI can be very high (Figs. 21.4.10 and 21.4.11), and in general MRI can distinguish an acute process, such as pyelonephritis, from scarring from previous infections, but current MRI resolution is not as good as the new generation of ultrafast three-dimensional CT scanners.

In some cases, abnormal signal intensity on MRI is sufficiently characteristic to allow a specific radiological diagnosis. For example, low-signal MR images are seen in three main categories: haemolysis (e.g. paroxysmal nocturnal haemoglobinuria, cortical haemosiderin deposition from mechanical haemolysis, sickle cell disease, haemorrhagic fever with renal syndrome), vascular disease (renal arterial infarction, acute renal vein thrombosis, renal

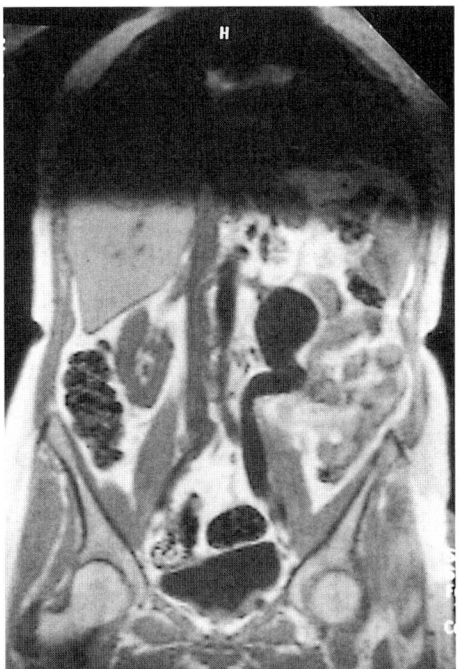

Fig. 21.4.11 Gadolinium-enhanced MRI showing a hydronephrotic left kidney and dilated upper two-thirds of the ureter following gynaecological surgery.

cortical necrosis, acute renal transplant rejection), and acute non-myoglobinuric renal failure.

As with the developments in CT, three-dimensional MRI scanners coupled with greater data acquisition are being developed to increase image resolution. New contrast agents such as gadolinium DTPA (see below) are being trialled with some success in a technique known as dynamic contrast magnetic resonance renography (MRR), which has the potential to provide complete anatomical and physiological kidney-specific evaluation. Similarly, blood oxygen level-dependent (BOLD) MRI has been developed to investigate oxygen uptake in the kidney in disease states and in response to drugs.

MRA

This technique overemphasizes any stenotic area or other vascular abnormality and may miss minor accessory renal arteries. MRA is useful in confirming normality, and is commonly employed in the preoperative assessment of living related kidney donors. A normal study of the renal arteries excludes renal artery stenosis and significant intrarenal vascular disease. Newer techniques are being developed to improve image acquisition and reduce respiratory artifacts to improve image resolution.

Magnetic resonance venography

As with MRA, magnetic resonance venography (MRV) using gadolinium contrast can be used to assess renal venous patency. Patients with nephrotic syndrome and those with renal adenocarcinoma may develop renal venous thrombosis, which can be difficult to positively diagnose with other imaging techniques.

Angiography and digital subtraction angiography

Although formal renal angiography remains the gold standard technique for assessing renovascular disease (Fig. 21.4.12), it has largely been replaced by ultrafast CT angiography and MRA in clinical practice. However, given that (as stated above) current MRA techniques overestimate stenosis, angiography is then often used to confirm the severity of a stenosis, allowing both the anatomy and direct pressure measurements to be assessed before proceeding to angioplasty/stenting.

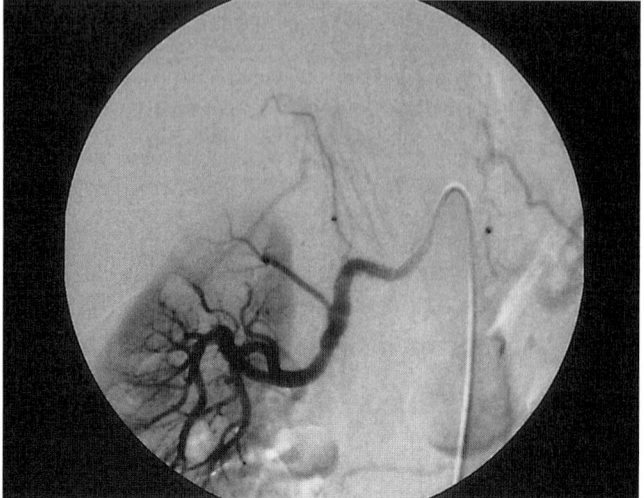

Fig. 21.4.12 Renal arteriogram showing fibromuscular hyperplasia of the renal artery.

Renal angiography is not without hazard: it involves an arterial puncture and the use of potentially nephrotoxic contrast agents, and carries the risk of dislodging aortic and renal artery plaques, which can result in intrarenal, intra-abdominal, and peripheral cholesterol embolization.

Aside from the investigation of suspected chronic renovascular disease, renal and coeliac arteriography can establish a diagnosis of classical macroscopic polyarteritis nodosa. Occasionally, renal angiography is helpful in assessing renal tumour vascularity, and in determining whether partial nephrectomy can be performed. In some cases of persistent nonglomerular haematuria, formal renal angiography reveals a vascular abnormality as the underlying cause.

Digital subtraction angiography (DSA) uses a venous injection of contrast and computer-derived images to view the major renal arteries and intrarenal vessels. High doses of contrast media may be required, but even so insufficient anatomical definition is obtained in between 5 and 20% of cases.

Interventional renal arteriography

Interventional renal arteriography should only be undertaken by experienced interventional radiologists with the support of vascular surgeons because it may be complicated by renal artery dissection or rupture. Embolization with gel foam or metal coils can be used to selectively control renal haemorrhage, which is particularly useful when this follows renal biopsy, and also in cases of arteriovenous malformation or tumour. Occasionally, a whole kidney is embolized. Some atheromatous renovascular stenotic lesions can be usefully treated by transluminal angioplasty and/or stenting.

Renal venography

Selective renal venous catheterization for blood sampling is still useful in patients with severe renovascular disease. The relative renal vein renin concentrations may aid the decision-making process in deciding whether to perform a surgical or medical nephrectomy in a patient with a small, poorly functioning kidney due to severe renal artery stenosis.

Nuclear medicine

The main uses of renal nuclear medicine scans are given in Box 21.4.1.

Static imaging—radiolabelled DMSA

Technetium-labelled dimercaptosuccinic acid (DMSA) binds to renal proximal tubular cells, and after an intravenous injection

---

Box 21.4.1 Main uses of renal nuclear medicine scans

- DMSA (dimercaptosuccinic acid):
  - Estimation of differential renal function
  - Imaging of scarring (reflux)
- MAG3 (mercaptoacetyltriglycine):
  - Detection of obstruction
  - Estimation of differential renal function
  - Screening for renal artery stenosis
  - Renal transplant monitoring

some 70% of the dose is taken up by viable tubules within 3 to 4 h. This can be detected by a gamma camera. DMSA scans provide information about the relative function of each kidney, and show areas of scarring due to renal stone disease, infection, and vascular disease. In children with urinary tract sepsis suspected of having reflux nephropathy, serial DMSA scans are used to assess progressive cortical scarring. During acute pyelonephritis, the DMSA scan may appear to show scars. These photopenic areas are due to inflammation and increased intrarenal pressure and can return to normal following resolution of infection. DMSA scans are also used to confirm the congenital absence of a kidney, to detect ectopic kidneys and other congenital malformations such as horseshoe kidney, duplex systems, and cross/fused ectopia, and to confirm absence of renal function.

More recently, the introduction of single-photon emission CT (SPECT) DMSA scans has improved resolution, although this starts to fade at GFR below 30 ml/min. These have shown that renal scars occur more frequently than previously thought, both in patients with acute pyelonephritis and also following lower urinary tract infection in renal transplant recipients.

Dynamic imaging—radiolabelled DTPA and MAG3

Technetium-labelled diethylenetriaminepentaacetic acid (DTPA) and mercaptoacetyltriglycine (MAG3) are both filtered by the glomerulus and then rapidly excreted by the kidney. MAG3 is now largely replacing DTPA as it has a better extraction efficiency and therefore offers improved image definition, particularly in patients with chronic kidney disease, with a lower absorbed radiation dose. The renograms produced have three phases: vascular, accumulation within the kidney, and excretion. Renal artery stenosis and acute tubular necrosis can reduce uptake, flattening the second and third phases of the renogram. Similarly, intrinsic renal disease flattens the second phase, and makes interpretation difficult when renal function is impaired.

Urinary obstruction

Radiolabelled DTPA and MAG3 scans are used to assess urological obstruction (Fig. 21.4.13), and can be useful in the management of patients with urinary calculi in assessing the functional significance of any obstruction, monitoring progress and the timing of intervention, uterocele, cases of differential obstruction such as a duplex kidney where obstruction is more likely to affect the upper pole, and possible obstruction following urinary diversion. Occasionally, patients with polycystic kidney disease present with severe pain due to the obstruction of a cyst, and DTPA/MAG3 scanning provides a dynamic test to confirm this. In cases of obstruction, the scan shows retention of tracer in the pelvicalyceal system, and the first change noted in the curve is a flattening of the third phase. When obstruction is established, the second phase is prolonged and the third phase continues to rise, and at worst all three phases are affected owing to ensuing poor renal function. In patients with dilated collecting systems, it is important to differentiate congenital megaureter from obstruction. Excretion may be slow owing to pooling in a dilated system, but obstruction is unlikely if there is a brisk washout following the administration of intravenous furosemide, although patients with impaired renal function may have a reduced response to furosemide, making interpretation of the renogram less reliable. Thus, in cases with impaired renal function, direct pressure measurement within the renal pelvis following percutaneous puncture may be required to exclude partial obstruction (Stamey test).

DTPA/MAG3 scans are also used to detect and monitor reflux in children, as reflux may be demonstrated during the 'emptying' phase of the renogram. If not, then an indirect micturating cystogram can be performed using the radioactivity which has passed into the child's bladder.

Hypertension

The main role of nuclear medicine in hypertension is the screening and diagnosis of renal artery stenosis (Fig. 21.4.14). Patients with renal artery stenosis may have a delay in uptake time (the time taken from injection to peak activity) and an increased intensity and duration of MAG3 accumulation (due to increased tubular salt and water reabsorption, not seen in the case depicted in

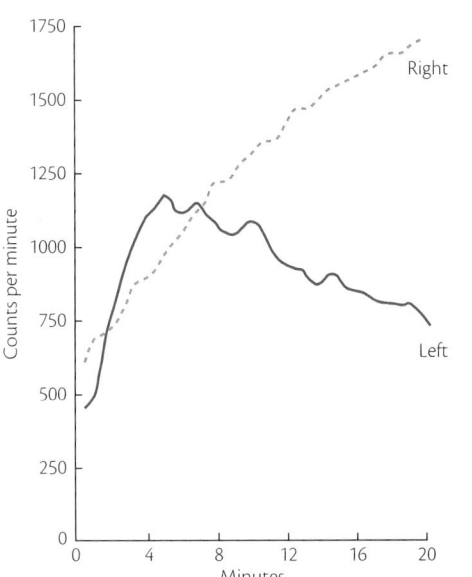

Fig. 21.4.13 DTPA renogram showing increasing uptake by the right kidney in a case of right-sided ureteric obstruction.

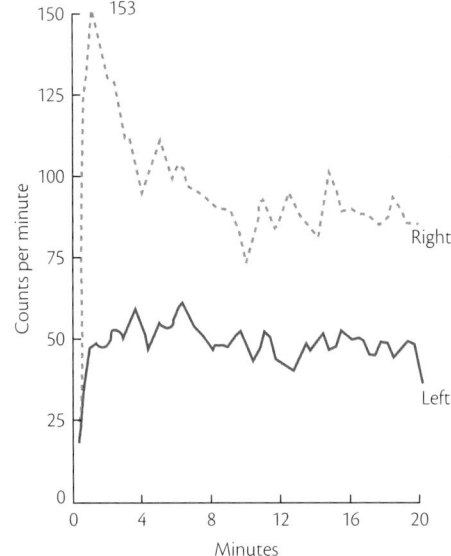

Fig. 21.4.14 MAG3 renogram demonstrating reduced uptake by the left kidney in a case of left-sided renal artery stenosis.

Fig. 21.4.14). If there is significant stenosis of a major branch artery, perfusion to one pole may be delayed.

Two scans are performed to improve the sensitivity and specificity of the MAG3 renogram in the detection of renal artery stenosis, one with and one without prior administration of captopril. The captopril–MAG3 renogram can also be used as a screening test to determine whether the use of angiotensin converting enzyme (ACE) inhibitors or angiotensin-II receptor blockers might be detrimental to renal function in patients with an increased risk of atheromatous renovascular disease, including those with severe cardiac failure or diabetes and elderly hypertensive patients, but it is rarely used for this purpose—the usual practice is to measure the serum creatinine before and 1 to 2 weeks after starting these drugs, and then stopping them (and considering imaging of the renal arteries) if this has risen by more than 20 to 30%.

As MAG3 can provide an assessment of divided renal function (although not as accurately as DMSA, particularly in infants), serial scanning may be helpful in monitoring patients over time to determine whether intervention with angioplasty or stenting is warranted, and similarly postintervention. Bilateral disease is more difficult to diagnose, but usually one kidney is more affected than the other.

Following kidney transplantation, serial MAG3 isotope scans can be used to monitor graft function. In cases of major arterial or venous thrombosis, and hyperacute rejection, the graft appears to have no perfusion. Acute tubular necrosis, rejection, and calcineurin toxicity may all have similar appearances. MAG3 scans may also reveal perirenal haematoma, lymphocele, and urinary leaks before they are clinically manifest. Later isotope scans may detect obstruction due to ureteric stenosis.

MAG3 can be used in anuric patients with acute renal failure to show vascular supply, such as those developing acute kidney injury after aortic surgery.

Other isotopes

Methyldiphosphonate (MDP) is filtered by the glomerulus, providing an immediate dynamic renogram. It is later taken up by inflamed muscles (found in patients with myositis and rhabdomyolysis) and the skeleton (detecting single or multiple bone metastases, and also metabolic bone disease in patients with endstage renal failure).

Combination techniques

Positron emission tomography (PET) scanning, using fluoride-labelled deoxyglucose, in combination with CT scanning was introduced to improve anatomical localization of tumours. Combining PET with standard CT improves lesion localization and characterization, and tumour staging. The role of PET/CT in primary staging of renal and prostate cancer has yet to be established, but it does have a role in detecting testicular tumours and in managing patients with advanced/metastatic renal and bladder cancer. However, PET/CT scanning also localizes areas of infection and inflammation and hence can be used to image and monitor response to treatment in a variety of circumstances, e.g. infected cysts in patients with adult polycystic kidney disease, large-vessel vasculitis in cases of Takayasu's arteritis, and retroperitoneal fibrosis.

Renal biopsy

Indications

A renal biopsy should be considered in any patient with disease affecting the kidney when the clinical information and other laboratory investigations have failed to establish a definitive diagnosis or prognosis, or when there is doubt as to the optimal therapy. However, renal biopsy has the potential to cause morbidity and (on rare occasions) mortality, hence its risk must be outweighed by the potential advantages of the result to the individual patient. Biopsies which would be 'of interest' but 'not in the patient's interest' should not be performed. Indications for renal biopsy must be considered on an individual basis, with the clinical presentations that warrant native renal biopsy given in Box 21.4.2.

Diabetic patients with proteinuria would not normally be biopsied unless they had other conditions suggesting there might be an alternative or additional diagnosis to diabetic nephropathy. Most paediatricians would treat small children presenting with nephrotic syndrome with steroids and only consider renal biopsy if they did not respond to treatment. Some conditions, in particular lupus nephritis and membranous glomerulonephritis, may change histological grading, so requiring repeat biopsy.

Renal biopsy is an important investigation in the management of patients with a renal transplant. Postoperative oliguria and/or deterioration in renal function requires urgent investigation to differentiate acute ischaemic tubular necrosis from calcineurin (ciclosporin or tacrolimus) or other drug toxicity, acute rejection (vascular and/or cellular), urinary obstruction and/or leakage, and even frank infarction. Serial biopsies may be required to monitor the response to antirejection therapy, and at a later stage to examine for recurrence of the original renal disease, or de novo glomerulonephritis in the graft.

Contraindications

Percutaneous renal biopsy should not be undertaken in patients with polycystic kidney disease. Similarly, patients with renal masses, such as tumours or cysts, should only be biopsied under direct vision, either by real-time ultrasonography or CT scanning, or by formal open surgical biopsy. Patients with a solitary (or solitary functioning) native kidney are normally considered only for open surgical biopsy, although the transjugular approach may be an option.

Haemorrhage is more likely to occur in patients with uncontrolled hypertension or hereditary or acquired coagulation disorders, and in those taking anticoagulants or antiplatelet agents. Blood pressure should be controlled and coagulation abnormalities treated before biopsy. Patients with renal amyloid also have an increased risk of haemorrhage, as may those with classic polyarteritis nodosa.

Patients with chronic renal failure and bilaterally small kidneys should not undergo biopsy. This would be technically difficult (the kidneys are small and hard) and the biopsy appearances of endstage renal failure are exceedingly unlikely to provide any information that might alter the clinical course or management. Percutaneous renal biopsy should not be performed in patients with untreated acute pyelonephritis due to the risk of developing a perinephric abscess.

Box 21.4.2 Indications for native kidney biopsy

♦ Asymptomatic proteinuria ≤1.5 g/day:
  · with controlled hypertension
  · with dysmorphic haematuria
  · with reduced GFR
  · with any combination of the above
♦ Asymptomatic proteinuria >1.5 g/day
♦ Nephrotic syndrome
♦ Microscopic or dysmorphic haematuria:
  · Hereditary condition
  · Insurance company requirement
  · Patient request
  · With proteinuria
  · With hypertension
  · With reduced GFR
♦ Acute kidney injury:
  · Exclude ischaemic ATN:
      with abnormal urinary sediment
      with proteinuria
      positive ANCA/ANA/anti-GBM
      severe hypertension
      no obvious cause
      prolonged history
  · Presumed ischaemic ATN:
      delayed recovery
♦ Chronic kidney disease (reasonable, equal-sized kidneys):
  · With proteinuria
  · With dysmorphic haematuria
♦ Known renal diagnosis (reasonable equal-sized kidneys):
  · Sudden unexplained reduction in GFR
  · Unexplained increase in proteinuria

ANA, antinuclear factor; ANCA, antineutrophil cytoplasmic antibody; ATN, acute tubular necrosis; GBM, glomerular basement membrane. Indications may be clear-cut (e.g. acute kidney injury of unknown cause with abnormal urinary sediment; adult with nephrotic syndrome) but they are not always so, and not all nephrologists would recommend biopsy in all of the circumstances listed (e.g. many would elect not to biopsy, but to arrange continued monitoring, for patients with asymptomatic proteinuria and stable renal function).

Technique

'Blind' biopsy of the native kidney, meaning biopsy without imaging for localization, should not be performed unless there are truly exceptional circumstances. It is possible to visualize the kidney and biopsy under fluoroscopic control after injection of radiocontrast medium as for an IVU, but the most commonly used method for directing biopsy is ultrasound guidance. This can either be used to record the depth of the lower pole from the skin and mark the surface position vertically above it on inspiration, or to provide real-time guidance. Occasionally, CT guidance is required.

Percutaneous renal biopsy should be carried out using sedation and local anaesthesia. Children may require general anaesthesia. For ultrasound-guided biopsy of the native kidney, the patient should be placed prone on top of pillows or folded sheets to compress the upper abdomen and lower ribs and fix (to some degree) the position of the kidneys. Under real-time ultrasound, the kidneys are visualized, the patient asked to take and hold a deep breath in inspiration, and the kidney which is thought to be technically the easiest to biopsy is targeted. To avoid major vessels, the aim should be for the lateral border of the lower pole. Either 14- or 18-gauge Tru-Cut-type needles are commonly used, with most centres now using an automated spring-loaded biopsy gun. Under direct vision, the needle tip is advanced to the renal capsule, and with the kidney fixed in inspiration, biopsy is performed. The advent of colour Doppler means that the operator can deliberately avoid the major intrarenal vessels.

Transjugular biopsy can be performed in patients who have an increased likelihood of bleeding complications. Technical developments have now allowed biopsy needles to be passed reliably from the renal vein into the renal cortex, such that in our own institution all such biopsies in the last 3 years have been diagnostic. Occasionally, open surgical biopsy is required, with the biopsy taken under direct vision and local bleeding controlled.

Renal transplants, usually placed in one or other iliac fossa, are biopsied in the supine position. Pillows can be placed under the side with the transplant to help move bowel and fat pad away from the transplant. Biopsies are taken from the lateral border of the upper pole, avoiding the major vessels and ureter.

The obvious risk of renal biopsy is haemorrhage. All patients should be placed on strict bed rest for at least 6 h after the procedure, and pulse and blood pressure should be checked frequently during this period. Hypotension, tachycardia, abdominal/back pain, and macroscopic haematuria are indications for urgent medical review.

Complications

Routine imaging after renal biopsy has shown that most patients develop a perirenal haematoma, which is usually asymptomatic. Arteriovenous fistulas may also develop acutely following biopsy, most of which disappear spontaneously with time, with only the occasional one requiring treatment by the interventional radiologist. Macroscopic haematuria occurs in fewer than 10% of patients, and bleeding sufficient to warrant blood transfusion in around 1%. Rarely, severe haemorrhage may necessitate treatment with the insertion of coils or gel foam embolization. Exceptionally, death may occur, usually due to failure to detect haemorrhage and provide appropriate resuscitation.

Complication rates are increased in patients with both acute and chronic renal failure. Uraemia prolongs the bleeding time, even when the conventional coagulation screening is normal (prothrombin time, activated partial thromboplastin time, and peripheral platelet count). The risk of uraemic haemorrhage can be at least partially reversed prior to biopsy by good dialysis to improve platelet function, correction of the haematocrit and any underlying coagulation defect, and by giving an infusion of deamino-d-arginine vasopressin (DDAVP) immediately prior to the procedure (0.3 µg/kg body weight, over 30 min), but vasopressin may cause cardiac ischaemia and should be avoided in patients with critical coronary artery disease.

Further reading

Urine microscopy

Birch DF, *et al.* (1994). *A color atlas of urine microscopy*, 1st edition. Chapman and Hall, London.

Fogazzi GB, *et al.* (1999). *The urinary sediment. An integrated view*, 2nd edition. Masson, Milan.

Renal function

Brenner BM, Rector FC. (2004). *Brenner & Rector's the kidney*, 7th edition. Saunders, Philadelphia.

Davison AM, *et al.* (2005). *Oxford textbook of nephrology*, 3rd edition. Oxford University Press, Oxford.

Schrier RW. (2003). *Renal and electrolyte disorders*, 6th edition. Lippincott Williams & Wilkins, Philadelphia.

Seldin DW, Giebisch G. (2000). *The kidney: physiology and pathology*, 3rd edition. Lippincott Williams & Wilkins, Philadelphia.

Valtin H, Schafer JA. (1995). *Renal function/mechanisms preserving fluid and solute balance in health*, 3rd edition. Little, Brown, Boston.

Creatinine/eGFR/cystatin C

Cockcroft DW, Gault MH (1976). Prediction of creatinine clearance from serum creatinine. *Nephron*, **16**, 31–41.

Grubb A, *et al.* (2005). Simple cystatin C based prediction equations for glomerular filtration rate compared with the modification of diet in renal disease prediction equation for adults and the Schwartz and the Counahan–Barrat prediction equations for children. *Clin Chem*, **51**, 1420–31.

Levey AS, *et al.* (2000). A simplified equation to predict glomerular filtration rate from serum creatinine. *J Am Soc Nephrol*, **11**, A0828.

Myers GL, *et al.* (2006). Recommendations for improving serum creatinine measurement: a report from the Laboratory Working Group of the National Kidney Disease Education Program. *Clin Chem*, **52**, 5–18.

National Kidney Foundation, K/DOQI (2002). *Clinical practice guidelines for chronic kidney disease: evaluation, classification, and stratification.* Part 5. Evaluation of laboratory measurements for clinical assessment of kidney disease. Guideline 4. Estimation of GFR. http://www.kidney.org/professionals/kdoqi/pdf/ckd_evaluation_classification_stratification.pdf

Randers E, *et al.* (1998). Serum cystatin C as a marker of the renal function. *Scand J Clin Lab Invest*, **58**, 585–92.

Stevens LA, *et al.* (2006). Assessing kidney function- measured and estimated glomerular filtration rate. *N Engl J Med*, **354**, 473–83.

Shlipak MG, Praught ML, Sarnak MJ (2006). Update on cystatin C: new insights into the importance of mild kidney dysfunction. *Curr Opin Nephrol Hyperns*, **15**, 270–5.

Renal imaging

Allan PL, Dubbins P, Pozniak MA. (1997). *Clinical Doppler ultrasound.* Churchill Livingstone, Edinburgh.

Ghantous VE, *et al.* (1999). Evaluating patients with renal failure for renal artery stenosis with gadolinium enhanced magnetic resonance angiography. *Am J Kidney Dis*, **33**, 36–42.

Helenon O, *et al.* (1997). Renovascular disease: Doppler ultrasound. *Semin Ultrasound*, **18**, 136–42.

Testa HJ, Prescott MC (1996). *Nephrourology, British Nuclear Medicine Society.* BPC Wheatons, Exeter.

Ultrasound scanning

Krumme B (2006). Renal Doppler sonography—update in clinical nephrology. *Nephron Clin Pract*, **103**, c24–28.

CT scanning

Read S, Allen C, Hare C (2006). Applications of computed tomography in renal imaging. *Nephron Clin Pract*, **103**, c 29–36.

MRI

Cowper SE (2008). Nephrogenic systemic fibrosis: an overview. *J Am Coll Radiol*, **5**, 23–8.

Laissy JP, *et al.* (2006). Magnetic resonance imaging in acute and chronic kidney diseases: present status. *Nephron Clin Pract*, **103**, c50–7.

Nuclear medicine

Hain SF (2006). Renal imaging. *J Roy Coll Phys*, **6**, 244–8.

21.5

Acute kidney injury

John D. Firth

Essentials

Definition—for practical clinical purposes, acute kidney injury is defined as a significant decline in renal excretory function occurring over hours or days. This is usually detected by a rise in the plasma concentration of creatinine. Oliguria—defined (arbitrarily) as a urinary volume of less than 400 ml/day—is usually present, but not always. More precise definitions, such as those of the Risk Injury Failure Loss and Endstage kidney disease (RIFLE) classification, or the modification of this definition as proposed by the Acute Kidney Injury Network (AKIN), are required for epidemiological or trial purposes.

Epidemiology—depending on precise definition, transient renal dysfunction complicates about 5% of medical and surgical admissions. Severe acute kidney injury (plasma creatinine >500 μmol/litre) affects 200 to 750 per million adult population per year in the United Kingdom.

Clinical approach

Diagnosis—all patients admitted to hospital with acute illness, but particularly older people and those with pre-existing chronic kidney disease, should be considered at risk of developing acute kidney injury. The most common precipitant is volume depletion—early detection of which requires careful monitoring of fluid input and output, lying and standing (or sitting) pulse and blood pressure, and daily weighing. Plasma creatinine and electrolytes should be measured on admission in all acutely ill patients, and repeated daily or on alternate days in those who remain so.

Assessment—after treatment of life-threatening complications, the initial assessment of a patient who appears to have acute kidney injury must answer three questions: (1) is the kidney injury really acute?—has plasma creatinine been measured previously?; (2) is urinary obstruction a possibility?—renal ultrasonography is required urgently when the diagnosis of acute kidney injury is not clear cut (but remember that 5% of cases of obstruction will have a misleading initial ultrasound report); and (3) is there a renal inflammatory cause?—stick testing of the urine is mandatory in any patient with acute kidney injury, with urinary microscopy for cellular casts if this reveals significant proteinuria or haematuria. Red-ell casts are found in acute glomerulonephritis, renal vasculitis, accelerated-phase hypertension, and (sometimes) in interstitial nephritis—their presence indicates the need for urgent specialist renal referral.

General aspects of management

The immediate management of a patient with renal impairment is directed towards three goals: (1) recognition and treatment of any life-threatening complications of acute kidney injury; (2) prompt diagnosis and treatment of hypovolaemia; and (3) specific treatment of the underlying condition—if this persists untreated then renal function will not improve.

Life-threatening complications—the greatest danger is hyperkalaemia, which can cause cardiac arrest without any preceding symptoms whatsoever. All doctors who work with acutely ill patients should be able to recognize the characteristic ECG appearances, which are a better indicator of cardiac toxicity in the individual patient than the plasma potassium level. As plasma potassium rises, the following changes occur progressively: (1) 'tenting' of the T wave; (2) reduction in size of P waves, increase in the PR interval, widening of the QRS complex; (3) disappearance of the P wave, further widening of the QRS complex; (4) irregular 'sinusoidal' ECG; and (5) asystole. Severe hyperkalaemic changes require immediate treatment with intravenous calcium (usually given as calcium gluconate, 10 ml of 10% solution, intravenously over 60 s), after which intravenous insulin/glucose or nebulized salbutamol can be used to reduce the plasma potassium for a few hours to allow time for renal excretion (in cases of renal failure that are rapidly treatable, e.g. bladder outflow obstruction) or initiation of renal replacement therapy.

Fluid management—a key part of the immediate assessment and management of any patient who is very ill, which will include many of those with acute kidney injury, is to make a correct assessment of their intravascular volume status and to resuscitate rapidly and effectively, as discussed in Chapter 17.3. Once this has been achieved, in the patient who remains oliguric, fluid intake should be limited to the volume of the previous day's urine output and gastrointestinal losses, plus 500 ml, but this allocation may need to be substantially increased in the presence of fever or in hot environments, when insensible losses may be much increased. To keep the patient in the optimal state of fluid balance, there is no substitute for careful, twice-daily clinical examination for signs of intravascular volume depletion or excess, supplemented by accurate daily weighing, to gauge the overall net fluid balance, and an intelligent flexible response to the findings.

Renal replacement therapy—mandatory indications for immediate instigation are: (1) refractory hyperkalaemia; (2) intractable fluid overload; (3) metabolic acidosis producing circulatory compromise; and (4) overt uraemia manifesting as encephalopathy, pericarditis, or uraemic bleeding. Modern practice is (whenever possible) to begin renal replacement therapy when the plasma creatinine reaches 500 to 700 μmol/litre, unless there is clear evidence that spontaneous recovery is occurring or there are other reasons to maintain a conservative approach.

Renal biopsy—should be considered when: (1) the history, examination, or laboratory tests suggest a systemic disorder that could cause acute kidney injury and could be diagnosed by renal biopsy; (2) the urinary sediment contains red cell casts; (3) the case history is atypical; and (4) renal failure is unusually prolonged (say beyond 6 weeks).

Specific causes of acute kidney injury

There are many possible causes of acute kidney injury, but in any given clinical context few of these are likely to require consideration. By far the most frequent are prerenal failure and acute tubular necrosis, which together account for 80 to 90% of cases of acute kidney injury seen by physicians.

Prerenal failure and acute tubular necrosis—these can best be regarded as a continuum of renal response to ischaemic injury, in much the same way that stable angina, non-ST-elevation myocardial infarction, and ST-elevation myocardial infarction are a continuum of cardiac response to ischaemia. Prerenal failure describes renal dysfunction that is entirely attributable to hypoperfusion, and where restoration of renal perfusion leads to rapid recovery. Acute tubular necrosis describes a clinical entity comprising acute kidney injury with three main characteristics: (1) it is seen in specific clinical contexts, frequently involving circulatory compromise and/or nephrotoxins; (2) urinary abnormalities usually suggest tubular dysfunction; and (3) recovery of renal function is expected within days or weeks, in most cases, if the patient survives the precipitating insult. There is no specific treatment for acute tubular necrosis, and it is a marker of severe illness with mortality around 15% in all cases, and 40 to 60% in series from intensive care units of patients receiving renal replacement therapy in the context of mechanical ventilation for respiratory failure.

Introduction

Definition

Review of the literature reveals literally dozens of definitions of acute renal failure, or—to label the condition by its preferred term—acute kidney injury. The two definitions most widely used are the Risk Injury Failure Loss and Endstage kidney disease (RIFLE) classification of the Acute Dialysis Quality Initiative (ADQI), and the more recent AKI staging system derived from this by the Acute Kidney Injury Network (AKIN) (Table 21.5.1). There is a great deal of overlap between these two classifications, and there has been much (often pretty sterile) debate over the precise details, but they have served the important purpose of emphasizing that acute changes in renal function that lead to small rises in plasma creatinine are associated with poorer patient outcome. Precise application of terminology is essential for high-quality epidemiological studies and clinical trial purposes, but determining whether or not a particular patient has AKI stage 1, 2, or 3 (or 'R', 'I', or 'F' of the RIFLE classification) is not clinically very important because it does not affect the approach to diagnosis, investigation, or management in any way.

For practical clinical purposes, acute kidney injury is defined as a significant decline in renal excretory function occurring over hours or days. This is usually detected clinically by a rise in the plasma concentration of creatinine. Oliguria—defined (arbitrarily) as a urinary volume of less than 400 ml/day—is usually present, but not always.

Epidemiology

Four population-based studies from the United Kingdom published between 2001 and 2005 reported that the incidence of severe acute kidney injury in adults (plasma creatinine above 500 μmol/litre) was between 202 and 736 per million population per year. The condition is much more common in older people, with a previous study showing the incidence rising from 17 per million in those under 50 years of age to 949 per million in those aged between 80 and 89 years. A study in 2000 from renal units and intensive care units in a defined geographical area of Scotland found that 131 patients per million population per year required renal replacement therapy for acute kidney injury, and more recent data from the same group revealed an incidence of milder forms of acute kidney injury (plasma creatinine above 150 μmol/litre in men and above 130 μmol/litre in women) to be 1811 patients per million population per year.

Acute kidney injury may arise as an isolated problem, but much more commonly occurs in the setting of circulatory disturbance associated with severe illness, trauma, or surgery. Depending on precise definition, transient renal dysfunction complicates about 5% of medical and surgical admissions.

Causes

There are many possible causes of acute kidney injury (Box 21.5.1), but in any given clinical context few of these are likely to require consideration. Table 21.5.2 shows the diagnoses made in 129 cases of acute renal impairment in 2216 consecutive medical and surgical admissions, and Table 21.5.3 shows the diagnoses established in 748 cases of acute kidney injury admitted to hospital in a prospective, multicentre, community-based study.

The frequency of particular causes of acute kidney injury will vary considerably depending on the population studied. An observational cohort study of 618 patients in 5 American intensive care

Table 21.5.1 Acute kidney injury defined by the RIFLE criteria and AKI stage

Criterion or stage	Urine output	Serum creatinine	GFR
RIFLE criteria			
Risk	<0.5 ml/kg body weight per hour for 6 h	1.5-fold increase	25% decrease
Injury	<0.5 ml/kg body weight per hour for 12 h	2-fold increase	50% decrease
Failure	<0.5 ml/kg body weight per hour for 24 h or anuria for 12 h	3-fold increase	75% decrease
Loss	Complete loss of kidney function (e.g. need for renal replacement therapy) for >4 weeks.		
Endstage renal disease	Complete loss of kidney function (e.g. need for renal replacement therapy) for >12 weeks.		
AKI stage			
1	<0.5 ml/kg body weight per hour for 6 h	Increase >0.3 mg/dl (26 µmol/litre) or 1.5- to 2-fold increase	
2	<0.5 ml/kg body weight per hour for 12 h	2- to 3-fold increase	
3	<0.3 ml/kg body weight per hour for 24 h or anuria for 12 h	Increase to >4 mg/dl (354 µmol/litre) with an acute increase of >0.5 mg/dl (44 µmol/litre) or >3-fold increase	

AKI, Acute Kidney Injury [Network]; RIFLE, Risk Injury Failure Loss and Endstage kidney disease.

The diagnostic criteria should be applied only after correction of intravascular volume depletion.

Urinary obstruction must be excluded as a cause of low urine output.

The most abnormal parameter—urine output, serum creatinine, or GFR—is used for classification.

It is not possible to calculate an increase in serum creatinine in the absence of a baseline value—the RIFLE authors suggested back-calculation of baseline serum creatinine assuming an eGFR of 75 ml/min per 1.73 m², but this will clearly not be correct in all cases; the AKI staging system is applied to changes observed within 48 h, which prevents strict application to cases of acute kidney injury before they have been monitored for >48 h.

Patients receiving renal replacement therapy are classified as having AKI stage 3.

Box 21.5.1 Some causes of acute kidney injury

◆ Prerenal uraemia

◆ 'Acute tubular necrosis':
   • Following haemodynamic compromise, commonly with sepsis or following exposure to nephrotoxins, including drugs, chemicals, rhabdomyolysis, or snake bite (see Table 21.5.5 and Box 21.5.3)

◆ Vascular causes:
   • Acute cortical necrosis
   • Large-vessel obstruction
   • Small-vessel obstruction: accelerated-phase hypertension and systemic sclerosis

◆ Glomerulonephritis and vasculitis

◆ Acute interstitial nephritis

◆ 'Haematological' causes:
   • Haemolytic uraemic syndrome/thrombotic thrombocytopenic purpura
   • myeloma

◆ Hepatorenal syndrome

◆ Urinary obstruction:
   • Intrarenal crystalluria
   • Postrenal—renal stones, papillary necrosis, retroperitoneal fibrosis, bladder/prostate/cervical lesions, massive lymphadenopathy (lymphoproliferative disorders, secondary carcinoma)

Clinical approach to patients with acute kidney injury

Diagnosis of the presence of acute kidney injury

A high index of clinical suspicion is required to diagnose acute kidney injury at an early stage of its development. This is because symptoms and signs attributable to the accumulation of fluid, electrolytes, acid, or uraemic wastes within the body are rarely apparent until the condition is far advanced. Furthermore, the symptoms and signs that may arise are not specific: unsuspected hyperkalaemia is the greatest danger, since this may produce no symptoms whatsoever before causing cardiac arrest.

All patients admitted to hospital with acute illness should be considered at risk of developing acute kidney injury. Those who have some pre-existing chronic impairment of renal function are particularly susceptible to acute exacerbations. This group includes all elderly patients, in whom a combination of low muscle mass and low dietary meat consumption may conspire to maintain an apparently 'normal' plasma creatinine level, despite a reduction in GFR to considerably less than 50% of that expected in a healthy young adult. Routine reporting of the eGFR following estimation of plasma creatinine has gone some way to alerting physicians to this issue, but it must be remembered that the calculated eGFR depends on the assumption that a patient is of normal weight for their age, and the reported figure will markedly overestimate kidney function if the patient is malnourished and frail.

units found that over 70% of cases were due to or associated with ischaemic and/or nephrotoxic (radiocontrast media, rhabdomyolysis) acute tubular necrosis, prerenal failure, cardiac failure, or liver disease, and that the patients had extensive comorbidities (chronic kidney disease 30%, coronary artery disease 37%, diabetes mellitus 29%, and chronic liver disease 21%). Reports based on data from biochemical laboratories (including cases both admitted to hospital and managed in primary care) find that urinary obstruction (mainly prostatic) typically accounts for 25% or more of cases of acute impairment of renal function. Obstetric causes account for around 1% of cases of acute kidney injury in developed countries, but in some parts of the world up to 30%, and for obvious reasons snake bite is a common cause of acute kidney injury in some places, but exceptionally rare in others (see Chapter 21.11 for further discussion of renal disease in the tropics).

Table 21.5.2 Causes of development of acute impairment of renal function in 2216 consecutive medical and surgical admissions

Cause	Number of patients
Acute tubular necrosis	
Hypovolaemia	22
Congestive cardiac failure	10
Sepsis	10
Nephrotoxins	25
Postsurgical	23
Other	12
Hepatorenal syndrome[a]	5
Obstruction	3
Vasculitis	2
Other/multifactorial/unknown	17
Total	129 (5.8% of admissions)

Acute impairment of renal function was diagnosed when the serum creatinine concentration rose by a predetermined amount (approximately one-third of the baseline) during the period of hospital admission.

During the period of study, 46 patients were excluded from analysis because they were either admitted specifically for treatment of acute renal failure or were recipients of long-term haemodialysis.

Dialysis was required in 10 cases.

[a] The frequency of hepatorenal syndrome was higher in this study than in routine clinical practice in most centres, presumably as a reflection of referral bias.

Modified from The American Journal of Medicine 74;2;6, Hospital-aquired renal insufficiency: A prospective study, Hou, Bushinsky, Wish, Cohen & Harrington © 1983, with permission from Elsevier.

For early recognition of acute kidney injury, the basic care of all acutely ill patients should include careful monitoring of fluid input and output, daily weighing, and lying and standing (or sitting) blood pressure, and regular estimation of plasma creatinine, urea, and electrolytes. It is important to emphasize that a single measurement of plasma creatinine does not give a rapid readout of kidney function and cannot in isolation be used to determine the severity of acute renal impairment: if a patient with plasma creatinine of 100 µmol/litre were to have both kidneys removed today, then the creatinine tomorrow would be only 150 to 200 µmol/litre.

Although it might seem to the inexperienced physician to be a simple matter to monitor fluid input and output, this is often not so in practice, excepting in patients who are restricted to parenteral fluids and who have a urethral catheter. Drinks may be spilt, extra drinks may be acquired from a variety of sources, urine may be spilt, and vomit and diarrhoea are often found in places where they are difficult to quantitate. These considerations mean that the most likely explanation for fluid balance charts being difficult to interpret is the erroneous recording of input or output. Daily weighing on accurate scales provides a much more reliable picture of net overall fluid balance. Patients who are acutely ill invariably lose flesh weight, commonly at a rate of up to a few hundred grams per day. If weight appears to fall at a rate faster than this, then negative fluid balance is likely, with the occurrence of greatly increased 'insensible' losses through the skin and lungs during fever being a common explanation. Aside from weight loss, the development of a postural drop in blood pressure (>20 mmHg fall in systolic blood pressure) or postural rise in pulse rate (>30 beats/min, or the development of

Table 21.5.3 Causes of acute kidney injury established in all cases (748) admitted to 13 tertiary-care hospitals in Madrid, Spain, over a 9-month period

Cause	Proportion of patients (%)
Acute tubular necrosis	45
Prerenal	21
Acute-on-chronic kidney disease	13
Urinary tract obstruction	10
Glomerulonephritis or vasculitis	4
Acute interstitial nephritis	2
Atheroemboli	1

Acute kidney injury was diagnosed when a sudden rise in serum creatinine to >177 µmol/litre was found in patients with previously normal renal function, or when there was a sudden rise of >50% in those known to have mild to moderate chronic renal failure.

Most cases of acute-on-chronic kidney disease were due to prerenal cause or acute tubular necrosis, and most cases of obstruction were due to prostatic disease in elderly men.

Dialysis was required in 36% of cases.

(Modified from Liano F, Pascual J. (1996). Epidemiology of acute renal failure: a prospective, multicenter, community-based study. Madrid Acute Renal Failure Study Group. *Kidney Int*, **50**, 811–18, with permission.)

severe postural dizziness) are reliable signs that a patient has developed significant intravascular volume depletion. If weight rises at any time, then this must be due to positive fluid balance, whatever the input/output charts may suggest. It may not be obvious from clinical examination where the fluid has gone: the possibilities of sequestration in the peritoneal cavity or in the tissue interstitium should be recognized.

Plasma creatinine and electrolytes should be measured on admission in all acutely ill patients, and repeated daily or on alternate days in those who remain so. These measurements will ensure that advanced acute kidney injury does not seem to have occurred 'suddenly' in patients already in hospital. However, many patients will be found to have significant renal impairment on admission, and many more will develop some degree of renal impairment while on the ward. In all cases, the physician must try to make a precise diagnosis of the cause.

Diagnosis of the cause of acute kidney injury

After treatment of life-threatening complications (see later), the initial assessment of a patient who appears to have acute kidney injury must answer three questions.

Question 1: Is the kidney injury really acute?

The only basis for excluding the possibility of pre-existing chronic renal impairment with absolute confidence is the knowledge of a previous normal measurement of renal function. In cases where there is uncertainty, a diligent search for previous notes and biochemical information may save the patient and the doctor the inconvenience (and occasionally hazard) of unnecessary investigation. The finding of two small kidneys on ultrasound examination indicates the presence of chronic kidney disease. Other clinical features are poor discriminators between acute and chronic renal impairment. A history of vague ill health of some months duration, of nocturia, of pruritus, or the findings of skin pigmentation or anaemia, would all suggest chronicity (see Chapters 21.3 and 21.6). However, anaemia is not invariable in chronic renal failure (e.g. in polycystic kidney disease the haemoglobin concentration may be normal), and anaemia can develop over a few days in acute kidney injury, as may hypocalcaemia and hyperphosphataemia. Radiological evidence of renal osteodystrophy is only found in patients with obviously long-standing renal failure and never aids the clinical distinction between acute and chronic renal failure.

Question 2: Is urinary obstruction a possibility?

One of the merits of the traditional division of the causes of acute kidney injury into prerenal, renal, and postrenal is that it encourages consideration of the possibility of urinary obstruction. It is extremely important that obstruction should not be missed, since most cases are readily treatable and delayed diagnosis may lead to permanent renal damage.

Obstruction is particularly likely to cause acute renal failure in those with a single functioning kidney, in those with a history of renal stones or of prostatism, and after pelvic or retroperitoneal surgery, but the possibility of obstruction should be seriously considered in all cases where another positive diagnosis cannot be made. The presence of anuria, or of alternating polyuria and oligoanuria, are helpful clues. However, it is not widely appreciated that a patient may pass normal or elevated volumes of urine despite significant obstruction, although this is extremely rare. The mechanism is poorly understood, but three factors present in obstruction tend to impair urinary concentrating ability, thereby leading to the preservation of urinary volume despite obstructive depression of the filtration rate. These factors are structural damage to the inner medulla and papilla, functional changes in the distal nephron resulting from increased intraluminal or interstitial pressure, and loss of medullary hypertonicity at low filtration rates.

Ultrasound examination of the kidneys and bladder is the usual first method of investigation for the presence of obstruction (Fig. 21.5.1). However, it is important to remember that the quality of the image obtained by renal ultrasonography is highly variable, depending on the patient, the equipment, and the operator. Furthermore, ultrasound detects calyceal dilatation, not obstruction, and the test may be 'negative' (because the calyces fail to dilate, or do so only minimally) in about 5% of cases of acute obstructive renal failure. If doubt as to the diagnosis persists in the clinician's mind, then the examination should be repeated, and

other investigations pursued if uncertainty still remains. If renal function is adequate (creatinine concentration less than about 250 µmol/litre) then diethylenetriaminepentaacetic acid (DTPA) or mercaptoacetyltriglycine (MAG3) renography with furosemide injection may be helpful, showing delayed excretion and clearance of radionuclide from the obstructed kidney(s). If renal function is severely impaired then imaging modalities that depend on renal excretion (including intravenous pyelography) are not useful, and percutaneous antegrade nephrostomy/pyelography or cystoscopy with retrograde ureteric catheterization and pyelography should be undertaken. (See Chapters 21.4 and 21.17 for further discussion.)

Obstruction, once diagnosed, must be relieved urgently by (as possible and appropriate) insertion of a urethral or suprapubic catheter, antegrade percutaneous nephrostomy, or cystoscopic insertion of ureteral stents, as a prelude to definitive treatment (where possible) of the underlying obstructive lesion. The most important causes of urinary obstruction are renal calculi, retroperitoneal fibrosis, and malignant diseases of the uterine cervix, prostate, bladder, and rectum (see Chapter 21.17).

Question 3: Is there a renal inflammatory cause?

Renal inflammatory conditions—including glomerulonephritis, interstitial nephritis, vasculitis, and other rarities—together account for fewer than 10% of cases of acute kidney injury. To make these diagnoses, which have critically important management implications, stick testing of the urine and microscopy of the urinary sediment is an essential part of the assessment of any patient with unexplained acute renal impairment. If stick testing indicates more than + of protein or more than a trace of blood, then a sample of urine should be examined under the microscope. This should be done by centrifuging 10 to 15 ml of urine at 1500 to 2500 rev/min (c.400–1120 g) for 5 min, carefully discarding all but 1 ml of the supernatant, and then resuspending the pellet. Examination should be made under high power, preferably after staining, which makes the cellular elements of casts more obvious. Urinary casts containing red blood cells (Fig. 21.5.2) are present in acute glomerulonephritis, renal vasculitis, accelerated-phase hypertension, and (sometimes) in interstitial nephritis, but not in other conditions. Their presence indicates the need for urgent specialist renal referral.

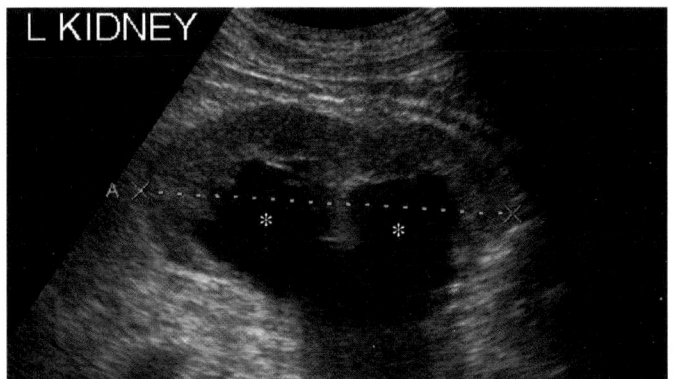

Fig. 21.5.1 Ultrasound image of an obstructed left kidney, showing pelvicalyceal dilatation (asterisks). The horizontal dotted line measures the length of the kidney (normal in this case), and the renal cortex is well preserved (not a thin rim), both of which suggest that there is a high likelihood that function will recover substantially when obstruction is relieved.

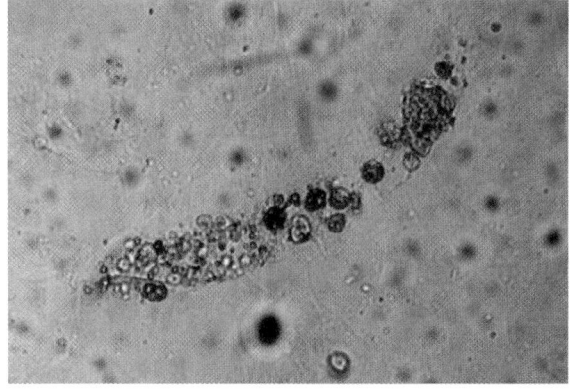

Fig. 21.5.2 A cellular urinary cast.

Clinical features of acute kidney injury

The early stages of acute kidney injury do not provide any obvious clinical features. Most patients who are unwell do not drink as much as usual and therefore pass less urine, and in any case as many as 50% of cases of acute kidney injury are not oliguric. The clinical picture is likely to be dominated by the primary condition, of which acute kidney injury is a complication, and by the effects of intravascular volume depletion, with dizziness caused by postural hypotension a common reason for patients being brought to medical attention.

In the later stages of acute kidney injury there are manifestations of uraemia with anorexia, nausea, vomiting (or occasionally diarrhoea), muscular cramps, and signs of encephalopathy—including a 'metabolic' flapping tremor (asterixis), progressing in extreme cases to depressed consciousness and grand mal convulsions. Skin bruising and gastrointestinal bleeding may occur. Uraemic haemorrhagic pericarditis is another potentially fatal complication, but this occurs much less frequently in acute kidney injury than in (neglected) chronic renal failure. For further discussion see Chapter 21.3.

Biochemical changes

The diagnosis of renal impairment, acute or chronic, is made when the plasma urea and creatinine concentrations rise. Other important biochemical changes include the development of hyperkalaemia, metabolic acidosis, hypocalcaemia, and hyperphosphataemia. Hyperkalaemia is due not only to reduced urinary excretion, but also to potassium release from cells—either as a consequence of cell death or as a result of metabolic acidosis. Particularly rapid rises are to be expected when there is extensive tissue damage or hypercatabolism, as in rhabdomyolysis, burns, and sepsis. Transfusion of stored blood is sometimes said to cause dangerous rises in plasma potassium concentration in oliguric patients. However, the transfused blood may not really be to blame, but the circumstances that demand transfusion. Loss of blood into the gastrointestinal tract or body tissues is followed by red cell lysis and the absorption of a considerable potassium load.

Protein catabolism produces sulphuric and phosphoric acids. These are normally buffered by bicarbonate and excreted by the kidney. In acute kidney injury these systems fail, leading to the development of acidosis. This is usually modest in degree (plasma pH 7.2–7.35), but can be more severe, manifesting as sighing Kussmaul's respiration and/or with circulatory compromise. Acidosis is sometimes the metabolic abnormality most obviously necessitating urgent institution of renal replacement therapy, but overzealous administration of bicarbonate should be avoided (see below).

Calcium malabsorption occurs early in acute kidney injury and is probably secondary to disordered vitamin D metabolism. Hypocalcaemia can develop with surprising rapidity. It is usually asymptomatic, but tetany and fits may be provoked by injudicious over-rapid correction of acidosis with resultant depression of ionized calcium. Profound hypocalcaemia and marked hyperphosphataemia, together with hyperuricaemia, is to be expected in rhabdomyolysis. Transient hypercalcaemia is frequently seen during the recovery phase from acute kidney injury, and this is particularly common after rhabdomyolysis, probably being caused by secondary hyperparathyroidism related to preceding hypocalcaemia.

The hypercalcaemic phase may be prolonged and accompanied by metastatic calcification in patients in whom there has been extensive muscle injury.

The plasma sodium concentration is usually normal in cases of acute kidney injury: any deficit of sodium is usually matched by that of water, thus leading to reduction of the extracellular fluid volume but with an unchanged plasma sodium concentration. However, on occasion the intake of water, either drunk in response to thirst or inflicted iatrogenically, may exceed the rate of excretion such that hyponatraemia results.

The retention of uric acid, sulphate, and magnesium occurs in renal failure, but these biochemical abnormalities are rarely clinically significant, with the exception of the grossly elevated levels of uric acid that can be seen in rhabdomyolysis and following tumour lysis.

General aspects of acute kidney injury

The immediate management of patients with renal impairment is directed towards three goals. The first is the recognition and treatment of any life-threatening complications of acute kidney injury. The second is prompt diagnosis and treatment of hypovolaemia. The third is specific treatment of the underlying condition: if this persists untreated then renal function will not improve.

Life-threatening complications

Hyperkalaemia

Hyperkalaemia, which is rarely a significant clinical problem in patients who do not have renal failure, is important in the context of acute kidney injury or chronic kidney disease because it can cause cardiac arrest. Patients may occasionally notice muscle weakness or paralysis, but the significance of these symptoms is rarely appreciated, and usually there are no symptoms whatsoever. All doctors who work with acutely ill patients should be able to recognize the characteristic ECG appearances, which are a better indicator of cardiac toxicity in the individual patient than the plasma potassium level. As plasma potassium rises, the following changes occur progressively:

1 'tenting' of the T wave

2 reduction in size of P waves, increase in the P–R interval, widening of the QRS complex

3 disappearance of the P wave, further widening of the QRS complex

4 irregular 'sinusoidal' ECG (Fig. 21.5.3)

5 asystole

Treatment of hyperkalaemia is described in Table 21.5.4.

Pulmonary oedema

The most serious complication of salt and water overload in acute kidney injury is the development of pulmonary oedema, which is usually iatrogenic, being caused by continued ill-advised intravenous infusion of fluids into patients who are anuric or oliguric. Severe cases are dramatic. The patient is terrified, restless, and confused. Examination reveals cyanosis, tachypnoea, tachycardia, widespread wheeze or crepitations in the chest, and a gallop rhythm (if the heart can be heard). Investigation demonstrates arterial

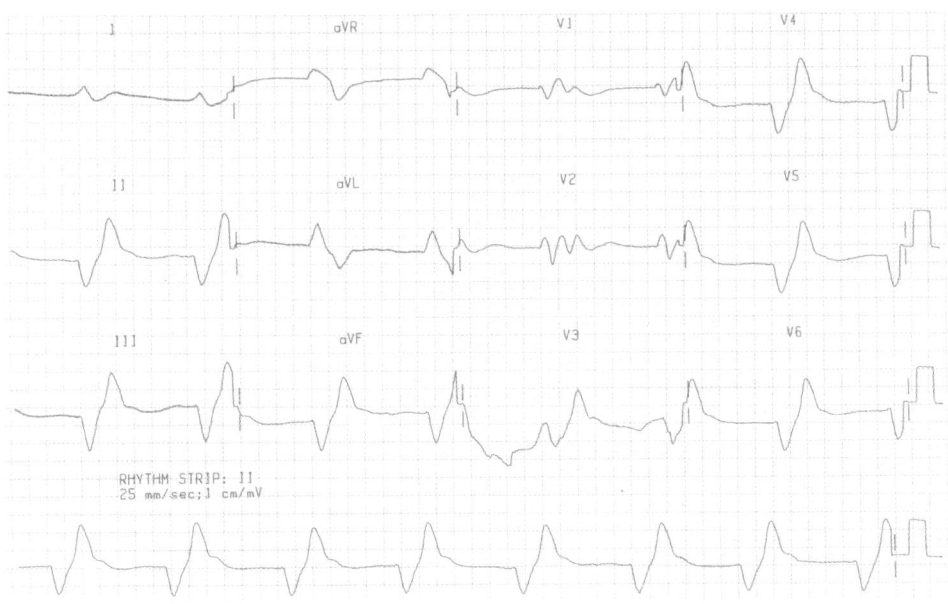

Fig. 21.5.3 An electrocardiogram showing severe hyperkalaemic changes in a patient with a plasma potassium level of 9.4 mmol/litre.

hypoxaemia and widespread interstitial shadowing on the chest radiograph. (See Chapters 16.15.3 and 17.3 for further discussion.)

The patient should be sat up and supported, and given oxygen by facemask in as high a concentration as possible using a reservoir bag. Furosemide may work as a venodilator but is unlikely to provoke a substantial diuresis in a patient with renal failure. Morphine can relieve symptoms rapidly and should be given (along with an antiemetic) in small (2.5–5 mg) doses, repeated if necessary and if tolerated, and with the opioid antagonist naloxone to hand in the event of respiratory depression. An intravenous infusion of a venodilator such as isosorbide dinitrate may be helpful.

The definitive treatment for pulmonary oedema caused by renal failure is the removal of fluid by haemodialysis or haemofiltration. Acute peritoneal dialysis is much less effective in this capacity and should only be considered in circumstances where haemodialysis and haemofiltration are not available. The immediate beneficial effects of venesection of 200 to 400 ml of blood from the patient *in extremis* should not be forgotten.

Table 21.5.4 Treatment of hyperkalaemia

	Treatment	Comment
1	Intravenous calcium (10 ml of 10% calcium gluconate, over 60 s, repeated until ECG improves)	Treatment to be given immediately if hyperkalaemia is associated with ECG changes more severe than tenting of the T wave. Acts instantly to 'stabilize' cardiac membranes (mechanism unknown). Does not alter plasma potassium concentration
2	Intravenous insulin and glucose (10–20 units of rapidly acting insulin plus 50 ml of 50% glucose, over 10 min)	Insulin stimulates Na^+,K^+-ATPase in muscle and liver, thus driving potassium into cells. Plasma potassium falls by 1–2 mmol/litre over 30–60 min
3	Nebulized salbutamol (10–20 mg)	β_2-agonists stimulate Na^+,K^+-ATPase in muscle and liver, thus driving potassium into cells. Plasma potassium falls by 1–2 mmol/litre over 30–60 min. Induces tremor and tachycardia, and sometimes nausea and vomiting
4	Intravenous sodium bicarbonate (50–100 ml of a 4.2% solution, over 10 min)	Traditionally thought to act by increasing blood pH, inducing exchange of intracellular protons for extracellular potassium. May not work in this manner since hypertonic saline has been shown to be effective. Only to be used if there is severe acidosis that merits treatment in its own right (see text for discussion). Glucose/insulin and salbutamol are equally effective and do not have the disadvantages of: (1) requiring a large sodium load, and (2) being severe chemical irritants ('burns' requiring surgical debridement and reconstruction can occur if concentrated bicarbonate gets into tissues from peripheral intravenous lines)
5	Cation exchange resins, e.g. sodium or calcium polystyrene sulphonate (15 g by mouth every 6 h or 15–30 g per rectum every 6 h)	Exchanges sodium or calcium for potassium in the gut lumen and thus induces loss of potassium from the body (unlike 1–3 above). Takes 4 h to produce an effect. Precautions against severe constipation are necessary
6	Haemodialysis/filtration	Except in those rare cases where renal function can be rapidly restored (e.g. relief of obstruction), it is likely that hyperkalaemia will recur and haemodialysis or high-volume haemofiltration will be required

Treatment with insulin/glucose and with β_2-agonists work in the same way, hence their effects in reducing plasma potassium are not additive and there is no benefit in giving both together. The side effects of β_2-agonist treatment mean that insulin/glucose is probably to be preferred if it can be administered easily.

Recognition and treatment of volume depletion

A key part of the immediate assessment and management of any patient who is very ill, which will include many of those with acute kidney injury, is to make a correct assessment of their intravascular volume status and to resuscitate rapidly and effectively. (See Chapter 17.3 for further details.)

Fluid and electrolyte requirements in established acute kidney injury

Fluid

Many patients with acute kidney injury are volume-depleted at the time of presentation. An urgent priority is to correct such depletion rapidly. Once this has been achieved—as judged by an improvement in peripheral perfusion, a fall in pulse rate, loss of postural drop in blood pressure, and a rise in jugular venous pressure—the perspective changes. In the absence of normal renal function the greatest care must be taken to regulate the intake of fluids and electrolytes to match losses in the urine, from the gastrointestinal tract, and from other 'insensible' sources. As a working rule, fluid intake is limited to the volume of the previous day's urine output and gastrointestinal losses, plus 500 ml, but this allocation may need to be substantially increased in the presence of fever or in hot environments, when insensible losses may be much increased. However, as discussed above, fluid-balance charts are frequently inaccurate and unthinking adherence to the 'output plus 500 ml' rule can lead to grief. To keep the patient in the optimal state of fluid balance, there is no substitute for careful, twice-daily clinical examination for signs of intravascular volume depletion or excess, supplemented by accurate daily weighing to gauge the overall net fluid balance, and an intelligent flexible response to the findings.

Sodium

In patients who are not being dialysed, the intake of sodium must also be matched to output. Requirements are usually very small in those who are oliguric, perhaps only 15 to 30 mmol/day, but if the patient is polyuric the requirements can be considerable, with a danger of volume depletion if these are not met. The urine of a patient with polyuric renal failure will usually contain sodium at a concentration of 50 to 70 mmol/litre, hence if urine output is 3 litres/day then over 200 mmol of sodium may be required. On occasion, the urine output in polyuric acute renal failure can be massive (even up to 1 litre/hour), and if the response is to administer an even greater quantity of fluid (output plus insensible losses), then it is possible to contrive a vicious cycle whereby an ever-increasing urinary output is rewarded by ever-increasing fluid infusion. To avoid this situation in a patient with polyuria, it is best to limit input to urinary output alone, thus allowing other fluid losses to establish a mild overall negative balance, only increasing fluid input if the patient develops significant postural hypotension, which should be checked for twice daily. For unknown reasons, an excess of sodium and water in patients with acute tubular necrosis leads to peripheral or pulmonary oedema, whereas in those with glomerulonephritis it tends to produce hypertension.

Potassium

Because hyperkalaemia is one of the most important problems in the management of patients with acute kidney injury, it is essential to check plasma potassium levels at least daily, and in those with hypercatabolism or gastrointestinal bleeding, or who require surgery, more frequent estimations are advisable. In oliguric cases, dietary consumption should be limited to the minimum compatible with an adequate intake of protein and amino acids (20–30 mmol/day).

Diuretics that work on the distal tubule (e.g. spironolactone, amiloride, and triamterene) promote potassium retention and should be stopped in all patients with acute kidney injury, and it is important when reviewing the drug chart to remember that these agents are frequent constituents of tablets containing a combination of diuretic/antihypertensive compounds. Angiotensin converting enzyme (ACE) inhibitors and angiotensin receptor blockers similarly increase plasma potassium and should generally be stopped, both because of their effect on potassium handling and because their haemodynamic effects are adverse in the context of most patients with acute kidney injury. Intravenous preparations of antimicrobial agents that contain large amounts of potassium should also be avoided whenever possible.

Excretion of potassium can sometimes be enhanced in those who are oliguric by the use of high doses of furosemide (0.5–1 g daily). Oral potassium-exchange resins (e.g. polystyrene sulphonate resins), prescribed concurrently with a laxative, can be useful in controlling plasma potassium for a few days or weeks, but they are not effective treatments for acute severe hyperkalaemia (see Table 21.5.4) and are usually found to be unpalatable for long-term use. By contrast, substantial losses of potassium can occur in polyuric acute kidney injury and need to be replaced. Measurement of the urinary potassium concentration can be helpful in estimating how much potassium is required.

Renal replacement therapy

Mandatory indications for immediate instigation of renal replacement therapy are:

- refractory hyperkalaemia
- intractable fluid overload
- metabolic acidosis producing circulatory compromise
- overt uraemia manifesting as encephalopathy, pericarditis, or uraemic bleeding

These indications will be present in some patients on their admission to hospital, but in many cases renal function will be seen to decline over a period of days or a few weeks when the patient is under observation in hospital. In this situation, there is no hard and fast rule as to when renal replacement therapy should be initiated. There is no level of nitrogenous waste at which the patient suddenly becomes susceptible to overt uraemic sequelae. Nevertheless, it is clearly not sensible to wait until an obvious uraemic complication (which might be fatal) arises. Many observational studies have reported better outcomes in patients who were started on renal replacement therapy earlier rather than later, but the fact that patients were not randomly allocated to treatment clearly confounds interpretation, and one randomized study in an intensive care context did not demonstrate any advantage of early treatment. Modern practice is (whenever possible) to begin renal replacement therapy when the blood urea reaches 25 to 35 mmol/litre and the plasma creatinine 500 to 700 μmol/litre, unless there is clear evidence that spontaneous recovery is occurring or other reasons to maintain a conservative approach. There are three basic options for renal replacement therapy: peritoneal dialysis, haemodialysis, and haemofiltration.

Peritoneal dialysis

Peritoneal dialysis is technically the simplest form of renal replacement therapy and is commonly used worldwide, although remarkably little has been published recently about its use in those with acute kidney injury. The principle is the same as that described for the long-term treatment of patients with chronic renal failure (see Chapter 21.7.2), the main differences being that: (1) catheters are used which can be inserted percutaneously using a metal stylet (although some use the same type of catheter as that used for continuous ambulatory treatment), and (2) smaller volume exchanges with shorter dwell times are the norm. The technique requires an intact peritoneum and is therefore precluded in the many patients whose renal failure is associated with abdominal surgery. Other problems include difficulties in maintaining dialysate flow, leakage, peritoneal infection, protein losses, and restricted ability to clear fluid and uraemic wastes. These limitations mean that, particularly in hypercatabolic patients, peritoneal dialysis is frequently unable to provide good dialysis of patients with acute kidney injury, and in the only randomized study it was shown to be inferior to haemofiltration in patients with infection-associated acute kidney injury. It is fair to say that peritoneal dialysis is virtually never the first choice modality for renal replacement therapy in an adult with acute kidney injury in those centres that have a range of techniques at their disposal.

Haemodialysis and haemofiltration

Haemodialysis is an intermittent technique, usually applied three times per week in the context of chronic renal failure (see Chapter 21.7.1), but often employed more frequently (up to every day) in the management of patients with acute kidney injury. By contrast, haemofiltration is a continuous technique, brief details of which are as follows: a mechanical pump (but sometimes the patient's own arterial pressure) drives blood through a haemofilter of high hydraulic conductivity. An ultrafiltrate of plasma is removed, usually at a rate of between 1 and 2 litre/h. This is replaced, minus the volume of other fluid inputs and the amount of 'negative balance' required, using (most commonly) a lactate/acetate-based substitution fluid. A large number of technical variations are possible—e.g. combination of filtration and dialysis elements (haemodiafiltration), and use of differing replacement fluids—but there is nothing to suggest that any one of these is better than another, excepting in those who are unable to metabolize lactate, when bicarbonate-based substitution fluid is essential.

Theoretical advantages of haemofiltration over haemodialysis in the management of patients with acute kidney injury include enhanced haemodynamic stability, increased ability to remove salt and water (allowing better prevention of volume overload and permitting improved nutrition), and greater clearance of inflammatory mediators (which may provide advantage in patients with sepsis). However, meta-analyses of trials that have compared intermittent with continuous treatments in the context of acute kidney injury have not shown important differences in outcomes, and usage depends on local custom and practice.

In the same way that there is no evidence on which to make firm recommendations as to when to start renal replacement therapy in those with acute kidney injury whose chemistry is gradually 'going off', there is also little information on which to base targets for the clearance of metabolic wastes that should be achieved by treatment. Most trials of daily haemodialysis vs thrice-weekly haemodialysis

have not shown advantage of daily treatment, provided that adequate dialysis dose (Kt/V >1.2) is delivered thrice weekly. With regard to continuous treatments, the standard of care is to provide an effluent (filtrate/dialysate) flow rate of 20–25 ml/kg body weight per hour, and exceeding this provides no clearly proven benefit.

Other issues in the management of patients with acute kidney injury

Indications for renal biopsy

Most cases of acute kidney injury are due to prerenal failure or to the clinical syndrome of acute tubular necrosis. They occur in an appropriate clinical setting and follow a typical time course, with recovery of renal function over a few weeks. In such instances, renal biopsy should not be performed since the information gained is exceedingly unlikely to influence management, and the risks of the procedure are therefore not warranted. There are, however, circumstances in which renal biopsy is essential to establish a correct diagnosis, with important implications for both management and prognosis. Biopsy should be considered when:

◆ the history, examination, or laboratory tests suggest a systemic disorder that could cause acute kidney injury and could be diagnosed by renal biopsy

◆ the urine sediment contains red cell casts

◆ the case history is atypical

◆ renal failure is unusually prolonged (say beyond 6 weeks), although in this context cortical necrosis (see below) is better diagnosed by CT scanning or angiography

Nutrition

Patients with acute kidney injury are invariably catabolic and derive a larger fraction of their energy expenditure from protein breakdown than normal. Insulin resistance, metabolic acidosis, the release of proteinases into the circulation, and changes in the metabolism of branched-chain amino acids have all been suggested as possible reasons. If nutrition is neglected, patients with acute kidney injury lose weight very rapidly, and those that lose most have the highest mortality, but it has not been proven in controlled trials that any form of nutritional support can generate a positive nitrogen balance, improve nutritional status, or alter mortality. Nevertheless, there is a consensus that early institution of nutritional support probably improves prognosis. Despite this, and almost certainly to the patient's detriment, action is frequently delayed or not taken at all, particularly if it is thought that the extra fluid load required will mandate the institution of dialysis or the need for additional dialysis sessions in an already busy unit.

There is very little good evidence on which to base recommendations. Enteral nutrition should be preferred to parenteral nutrition whenever possible, with typical recommended daily adult requirements for those with acute kidney injury being total energy 25 to 35 kcal/kg body weight (although some recommend less), including protein of 1 g/kg body weight. If patients with acute kidney injury are oliguric, the nutritional support should be given in a restricted fluid volume, with reduced amounts of sodium, potassium, and phosphate. For practical purposes, it is sensible to have enteral and parenteral fluids that satisfy these needs available routinely (a variety of commercial preparations are available): extra water and electrolytes can always be added when required. In the many patients who are too unwell to take adequate food by mouth, commonly those who need it most, tube feeding or parenteral nutrition should be started early. Protein restriction, aimed at moderating the rise of plasma urea, is not appropriate management for patients with acute kidney injury.

Bleeding

In uraemia the bleeding time is prolonged, and in acute kidney injury this summates with any abnormality of haemostasis that might be simultaneously induced by the precipitating condition. Better control of uraemia and the routine use of H_2-receptor antagonists have been associated with a greatly reduced risk of upper gastrointestinal bleeding, a previously frequent and grave occurrence. Impairment of haemostasis is not a cause of great clinical concern in most patients, but there are some who bleed—from anywhere and everywhere. Guidelines for the management of such cases are given in Box 21.5.2.

Sepsis

Overwhelming septicaemia is a common cause of acute kidney injury, and in such instances the diagnosis is often straightforward. However, in many more cases the role of sepsis is insidious and difficult to diagnose with certainty. There is often strong clinical feeling, but little in the way of hard proof, that sepsis underlies the slide towards worsening renal and multiorgan failure in patients who have been apparently successfully resuscitated from major trauma or surgery, and septicaemia is the most common cause of death in those with acute kidney injury. The index of clinical suspicion must therefore be very high: if a patient with acute kidney injury appears to be deteriorating in any way, the question must be asked 'is this sepsis?'. Unused intravenous lines and urinary catheters should be removed, and those that are necessary but in any way suspicious should be replaced. The patient should be examined regularly for signs of a septic focus. There should be a low threshold for repeated, thorough microbiological investigation. Proven infection should be treated promptly with appropriate antimicrobial agents (with the dose being modified as required). In many cases, however, it will be necessary to start treatment 'blind', having taken specimens for culture and having made an educated guess as to the likely pathogen, with the possibility of Gram-negative septicaemia high on the list.

Box 21.5.2 Practical strategies for the management of bleeding in acute kidney injury

1 Exclude the possibility of a heparin effect

2 Blood transfusion to obtain haematocrit >30% (very occasionally erythropoietin is of value)

3 Cryoprecipitate (10 bags) has its maximal effect between 1 and 2 h after administration. Its effect disappears at 24–36 h

4 Deamino-D-arginine vasopressin (DDAVP) (0.3 µg/kg intravenously) acts by increasing factor VIII coagulant activity. It has been shown in acute kidney injury to shorten prolonged bleeding time. Repeated doses have a lesser effect

5 Conjugated oestrogen: 0.6 mg/kg per day for 5 days. Shown to reduce bleeding time (for at least 14 days) in patients with chronic renal impairment and haemorrhagic tendency

---

In patients who appear 'obviously septic' or to be 'going off', but in whom no cause can be found, attention should be directed towards the abdomen, this being the most likely place for hidden mischief, either infective or ischaemic. Radiological investigations, in particular CT scanning, can be very useful in searching for abdominal sepsis or dead bowel, but are not infallible: surgical exploration may be required, both to diagnose and to treat, especially in patients whose renal failure follows previous abdominal surgical procedures.

Prescription of drugs

Many drugs are excreted by glomerular filtration or tubular secretion and must be given in reduced dosage or at longer intervals than normal in patients with renal failure (see Chapter 21.19). For patients with acute kidney injury, the following should not be given without very good reason: nonsteroidal anti-inflammatory drugs, ACE inhibitors, angiotensin-II receptor antagonists (all of which have adverse effects on renal perfusion and glomerular filtration), and aminoglycoside antibiotics (these are discussed later in this chapter). A note about two other drugs that may be given to patients with acute kidney injury is also appropriate here: both aciclovir and penicillins can cause encephalopathy if given in the doses used to treat severe infection in patients with normal renal function. The dose of aciclovir needs to be reduced from between 5 and 10 mg/kg every 8 h to between 2.5 and 5 mg/kg every 24 h in those receiving renal replacement therapy, and physicians should restrain themselves from prescribing the maximum recommended doses of penicillins. If in doubt, consult the manufacturer's data sheet before prescribing any drug to a patient with acute kidney injury.

Specific causes of acute kidney injury

A list of specific causes of acute kidney injury is given in Box 21.5.1: many of these are discussed in other chapters; those that are not are considered here.

Prerenal failure and acute tubular necrosis

Between 80 and 90% of the cases of acute kidney injury seen by physicians will fall into the categories of prerenal failure and acute tubular necrosis. The term 'prerenal failure' is used when renal dysfunction is entirely attributable to hypoperfusion, and where restoration of renal perfusion leads to rapid recovery. The term 'acute tubular necrosis' describes a clinical entity comprising acute kidney injury with three main characteristics:

1 It is seen in specific clinical contexts, frequently involving circulatory compromise and/or nephrotoxins.

2 Urinary abnormalities usually suggest tubular dysfunction.

3 Essentially complete recovery of renal function is expected within days or weeks in most cases if the patient survives the precipitating insult, with a period of polyuria commonly following oliguria.

The syndrome can be seen after virtually any episode of severe circulatory compromise, but not all causes of circulatory derangement are equally devastating to renal function. Primary impairment of cardiac performance, e.g. following myocardial infarction, may cause plasma creatinine to rise somewhat, but rarely causes renal failure of sufficient severity to require renal replacement therapy.

By contrast, an apparently similar haemodynamic upset caused by sepsis frequently does. Multiple insults are the rule rather than the exception. Circumstances associated with a particularly high risk of acute kidney injury include repair of a ruptured aortic aneurysm (20%, as opposed to 3% for elective repair), hepatobiliary surgery (10%), cardiac surgery (up to 20%, depending on case mix), pancreatitis (10%), and burns (2–38%, depending on the series).

Pathophysiology

The perfusion of the kidney seems to suffer more than that of any other organ when the circulation is compromised. In the face of modest underperfusion, the GFR is relatively preserved by a compensatory increase in the filtration fraction. This increase has repercussions on tubular function which, along with other factors, leads to the increased tubular reabsorption of sodium, water, and urea—a situation rapidly reversed by restoration of renal perfusion. However, following prolonged circulatory shock, renal function frequently deteriorates in a manner that is not immediately reversible, and it is not at all obvious why this should be so. Lack of a clear pathophysiological understanding has bedevilled attempts at the development of rational therapy. Under normal conditions the kidney enjoys high blood flow, exceeded on a volume/weight basis only by the carotid body, and oxygen tension in the renal venous effluent is high, suggesting that oxygen supply greatly exceeds demand. Such a situation might be expected to confer protection from the effects of circulatory compromise, but no such benefit is observed: indeed the kidney appears to be more susceptible to damage than other organs, with the typical histological features of acute tubular necrosis being effacement and loss of the brush border of the proximal tubule (particularly in the S3 segment), patchy loss of tubular cells, and casts in the distal tubule. Acute kidney injury similar to this can be produced in animal models by ischaemia, and the condition often arises clinically in the setting of profound haemodynamic disturbance, leading to the supposition that—despite apparently generous blood flow normally—renal ischaemia is the cause of renal failure in such circumstances.

At the 'whole organ' level, two main hypotheses, not necessarily mutually exclusive, have been proposed to explain the kidney's vulnerability to ischaemic damage. First, the specialized anatomical arrangement of the vasa rectae that is essential for the countercurrent mechanism involved in urinary concentration and dilution leads to arteriovenous shunting of oxygen and the presence of areas of profound hypoxia (Po_2 10–20 mmHg) within the normal kidney. These areas are operating on the verge of anoxia in the normal organ and hence might be susceptible to ischaemic damage in response to a modest compromise of whole-organ blood flow. Second, there is clinical and experimental evidence of intense constriction of renal vessels during shock, hence very severe reduction in renal blood flow (perhaps only transient) may be responsible for the initiation of ischaemic damage. The justification for many of the interventions proposed in the management of patients at risk of acute kidney injury, or with established acute kidney injury, is that they might preserve renal blood flow and/or reduce renal oxygen consumption, thus rendering the development of ischaemic injury less likely.

At a cellular level, a wide variety of pathophysiological mechanisms are involved. Endothelial cell injury arising directly from ischaemia or various inflammatory processes causes disruption of microvascular blood flow. Poor tissue oxygenation leads to epithelial cell injury via mechanisms including intracellular accumulation of calcium, generation of reactive oxygen species, activation of various proteases and phospholipases, and depletion of ATP. These lead to a range of consequences such as redistribution of tubular membrane proteins, sloughing of viable cells into the tubular lumen, and apoptosis. Recent work has drawn attention to the involvement of immunological factors (complement activation, intercellular adhesion molecules, inflammatory mediators) and receptors on tubular cells (peroxisome proliferator-activated receptor β, toll-like receptors, bradykinin receptors), some of which may in the future provide opportunity for therapeutic intervention.

Once damage to the kidney has been sustained, a variety of factors may be responsible for the persistence of excretory failure that is characteristic of the clinical syndrome of acute tubular necrosis. These include activation of tubuloglomerular feedback (increased delivery of sodium chloride to the macula densa leads to reduction in GFR), backleak of filtrate from damaged tubules, and tubular obstruction by casts. Even in experimental models it is very hard to determine what is happening at any time, and impossible to do so in clinical practice. However, many of the abnormalities have a structural as well as a functional basis, hence rapid reversal cannot be expected, there being good evidence that recovery from acute tubular necrosis depends on cellular regeneration.

Diagnosis

The diagnosis of prerenal failure/acute tubular necrosis is based on the clinical context, which often involves circulatory compromise, and the exclusion of obstruction or renal inflammatory conditions, usually by ultrasound examination of the kidneys and testing of the urine for blood and protein, respectively.

Prerenal failure and acute tubular necrosis can best be regarded as a continuum of renal response to ischaemic injury, in much the same way that stable angina, non-ST-elevation myocardial infarction, and ST-elevation myocardial infarction are a continuum of cardiac response to ischaemia. A simple analysis emphasizes that at the prerenal end of the spectrum the biochemical composition of the urine reflects the response of normal tubules to impaired renal perfusion. There is avid retention of sodium and water, leading to low urinary sodium and high urinary urea and creatinine concentrations, together with a high urinary osmolarity. By contrast, at the acute tubular necrosis end of the spectrum the tubules are damaged and unable to sustain large sodium or osmolar gradients, hence urinary sodium concentration is elevated and the urinary urea and creatinine concentrations and urinary osmolarity are relatively low. However, this simple analysis is flawed and biochemical analysis of the urine is rarely useful in clinical practice, as explained in Table 21.5.5. From a practical point of view, treatment is begun on exactly the same lines whether the expected diagnosis is of prerenal failure or of acute tubular necrosis. The response to resuscitation retrospectively defines the diagnosis—restoration of renal perfusion leads to rapid improvement in renal function in prerenal failure—and determines further management.

Over the past 20 years (and more), the measurement of urinary or plasma levels of a variety of proteins (e.g. urinary kidney injury molecule-1, plasma and urinary neutrophil gelatinase-associated lipocalin (NGAL), and many others) have been explored as possible early markers of acute tubular necrosis. None has yet been found useful in clinical practice.

Table 21.5.5 Urinary biochemical indices in prerenal failure and acute tubular necrosis

Index	'Typical' prerenal failure	'Typical' acute tubular necrosis
Urinary sodium (mmol/litre)	<20	>40
Urine osmolarity (mOsm/litre)	>500	<350
Urine:plasma urea	>8	<3
Urine:plasma creatinine	>40	<20
Fractional sodium excretion	<1%	>2%

There are several reasons why urinary biochemical indices are of very limited clinical use: (1) intermediate values are common; (2) 'typical' values do not reliably predict renal prognosis—it is recognized that cases that are otherwise indistinguishable from 'typical' acute tubular necrosis can have a low urinary sodium concentration; (3) diuretics and pre-existing tubular disease will impair the ability of tubules to retain sodium in prerenal failure; and (4) treatment is not dictated by urinary indices.

Two uncommon circumstances in which measurement of urinary sodium concentration may be helpful are: (1) hepatorenal syndrome, when urinary sodium concentration is low (<10 mmol/litre); and (2) acute renal artery occlusion (bilateral or of single functioning kidney) when urinary sodium concentration can equal that in plasma.

Circumstances predisposing to prerenal failure are almost invariably associated with raised plasma levels of ADH. This acts on the collecting duct to increase the tubular reabsorption of both water and urea, hence the plasma concentration of urea rises out of proportion to that of creatinine in prerenal failure. Plasma urea may also appear to be disproportionately raised in the presence of sepsis, steroids, tetracycline (catabolic effect), and gastrointestinal haemorrhage (protein meal).

Prevention

One of the main aims of the basic nursing and medical care provided to all acutely ill patients is to minimize the chances of the development of renal impairment. This can arise despite exemplary treatment, but poor care increases the likelihood. As described above, regular measurement of plasma creatinine will permit early recognition of declining renal function, but is not of itself therapeutic. The best way to prevent the development of prerenal failure or acute tubular necrosis is to maintain an optimal intravascular volume (as described above, with further information given in Chapter 17.3), and to avoid or reduce exposure to nephrotoxic agents.

One common clinical situation worthy of specific note is a patient about to undergo a major elective surgical procedure such as repair of an abdominal aortic aneurysm. The risk of acute kidney injury following such an operation is substantial if careful attention to fluid management is neglected, the aim being to avoid episodes of hypovolaemia before, during, and after the procedure. Preoperative treatment with intravenous fluids and/or inotropes to achieve predetermined goals for cardiac output and oxygen delivery may improve outcome, but the wherewithal to measure these is not available in many instances. In such circumstances, and even with the application of invasive measurements, it is generally regarded as good practice to maintain a diuresis, which can often be accomplished simply by infusion of crystalloid at moderate rate: this both demonstrates that the kidneys are receiving adequate perfusion, and may render them less susceptible to insult. Although the routine use of modest doses of diuretic agents

(e.g. furosemide 40–80 mg intravenously; mannitol 25 g intravenously) is advocated by some, they would appear to have no specific advantages over a simple crystalloid-induced diuresis in protecting the kidney, but very large doses of diuretic agents should not be given because they can provoke massive diuresis (urine output above 500 ml/h) and thereby lead to considerable difficulties in the control of electrolytes, especially potassium. A high-quality multicentre, randomized, double-blind, placebo-controlled trial of the use of dopamine in critically ill patients with evidence of early renal impairment did not show that this treatment was of any benefit.

In patients undergoing high-risk elective surgery, and certainly in patients about to undergo emergency surgery, drugs that might have adverse renal haemodynamic consequences (e.g. ACE inhibitors, angiotensin receptor blockers, nonsteroidal anti-inflammatory agents) should generally be temporarily discontinued, unless there are pressing reasons for not doing so.

For high-risk cases the insertion of a central venous pressure line preoperatively is a sensible precaution: the positioning of the patient for surgery and the presence of drapes may prevent proper intraoperative clinical assessment of cardiovascular status, and the risks of elective insertion of a central venous pressure line in the relative calm of the anaesthetic room are considerably less than those incurred if the attempt is made with the patient 'going off' on the operating table.

Clinical findings

There are no specific clinical features of prerenal failure or acute tubular necrosis. There may be symptoms of acute renal failure, as described previously, but these are also not specific and are rarely prominent, hence the clinical picture at presentation is likely to be dominated by signs of volume depletion and those of the precipitating condition.

If the patient does not die of acute kidney injury, either because the degree of uraemia is modest or renal replacement therapy is provided, then renal recovery occurs in the vast majority of those who survive the precipitating insult. This may begin at any time from a few days to a few months (median 10–14 days) after the onset of the condition, with a progressive increase in urinary volume typically preceding improvement in the plasma levels of creatinine and urea. Owing to a relatively persistent defect in renal tubular sodium reabsorption and concentrating ability, a period of polyuria may ensue, placing the patient at risk of sodium and water depletion.

Specific treatment

The importance of effective treatment of the underlying condition and of rapid correction of hypovolaemia are above clinical dispute, although neither has been subject to controlled trial as regards the outcome of prerenal failure or acute tubular necrosis. There is no good evidence that any other pharmacological agent is beneficial, and following the publication of a number of randomized controlled trials the use of agents such as loop diuretics (e.g. furosemide), dopamine, and mannitol is no longer recommended. In experimental models of acute tubular necrosis, the use of growth factors has been shown to speed renal recovery: this offers some hope for the future, but no benefit has yet been shown in clinical studies.

Prognosis

Having acute tubular necrosis is a marker of severe illness and poor prognosis. In one study of over 5 million Medicare beneficiaries,

Box 21.5.3 Some nephrotoxins that can cause acute kidney injury (excluding causes of interstitial nephritis)

Exogenous

- Antibiotics:
  - Aminoglycosides
  - Tetracyclines
  - Cephaloridine
  - Amphotericin B
  - Sulphonamides
  - Polymyxin/colistin
  - Bacitracin
  - Pentamidine
  - Vancomycin
- Radiocontrast media
- Anaesthetic agents:
  - Methoxyflurane[a]
  - Enflurane[a]
- Chemotherapeutic/immunosuppressive agents:
  - Ciclosporin
  - cis-Platinum
  - Methotrexate
- Organic solvents:
  - Glycols (e.g. ethylene glycol[a])
- Hydrocarbons (e.g. carbon tetrachloride, toluene)
- Poisons:
  - Venoms (snake bite, e.g. Russell's viper)
  - Stings
  - Insecticides/herbicides/rodenticides (including paraquat, copper sulphate, sodium chlorate)
  - Mushrooms (amanita)
  - Hemlock
  - Carp bile
  - Herbal medicines
- Drugs of abuse
- Heavy metals

Endogenous

- Pigments
  - Myoglobin
  - Haemoglobin
- Intrarenal crystal deposition:
  - Urate
  - Phosphate (tumour lysis syndrome)
- Tumour related:
  - Immunoglobulin light chains

In many instances, nephrotoxicity arises both from a direct toxic action on renal tissue and from indirect systemic effects.
[a]May be associated with intratubular precipitation of oxalate crystals.

the overall in-hospital death rate was 4.6% in cases without acute renal failure, 15.2% in cases where acute renal failure (mostly attributable to acute tubular necrosis) was the principal diagnosis, and 32.6% in cases where acute renal failure was a secondary diagnosis. Series from intensive care units of patients who require renal replacement therapy for acute tubular necrosis, commonly in the context of respiratory failure requiring mechanical ventilation, typically report mortality rates of 40 to 60%. Death should rarely be attributable to a primary sequel of renal failure, e.g. uraemia or hyperkalaemia, and the incidence of life-threatening gastrointestinal haemorrhage is much reduced: sepsis is the major killer. Patients die with but not directly of renal failure.

Assuming survival of the precipitating insult, complete recovery of renal function can be anticipated in almost all young (<65 years) patients with pre-existing normal renal function and acute tubular necrosis of short duration. This is not so for older patients, those with pre-existing chronic kidney disease, or those who have prolonged acute tubular necrosis (>4 week requirement for renal replacement therapy). In the largest reported series of patients with acute kidney injury, 11 to 12% of survivors of 'medical' or 'surgical' acute renal failure (presumed to have acute tubular necrosis) required long-term dialysis.

Nephrotoxins

Exogenous nephrotoxins

A wide variety of exogenous agents, including therapeutically prescribed drugs, can cause acute kidney injury (Box 21.5.3). Poisoning by drugs and chemicals are discussed in Chapter 9.1; envenoming and poisoning by animals or plants is discussed in Chapter 9.2; and those causes restricted (largely) to the tropics are discussed in Chapter 21.11. The following other causes are worthy of particular note.

Aminoglycosides

Gentamicin is nephrotoxic, as are tobramycin, amikacin, netilmicin and streptomycin to progressively lesser degrees. The risk of nephrotoxicity is increased by old age, pre-existing renal insufficiency, high dosage, prolonged treatment, combined treatment with other nephrotoxic drugs, renal ischaemia, and volume depletion. A 50% rise in plasma creatinine from baseline is seen in 10 to 20% of patients, even when monitoring optimally controls drug levels. Parenteral administration is not required for the development of toxicity: acute kidney injury can occur as a result of systemic absorption when aminoglycosides are used in irrigating or bowel-sterilizing solutions.

The typical clinical picture is of relatively mild nonoliguric renal failure coming on about 1 week after starting treatment. The urine typically shows low-level proteinuria, with hyaline or granular casts. Hypokalaemia, hypomagnesaemia, hypocalcaemia, and hypophosphataemia are sometimes seen, and also a Fanconi syndrome. Recovery typically occurs over about 3 weeks after the aminoglycoside is stopped, but this may be delayed or incomplete.

The nephrotoxicity of particular aminoglycosides is related to the strength of their positive charge. They are freely filtered by the glomeruli, with 90 to 95% passing into the urine, but 5 to 10% binding to negatively charged membrane phospholipids in parts S1 and S2 of the proximal tubule (and S3 in the presence of renal ischaemia), where they are delivered to megalin (the Heymann nephritis autoantigen, a member of the low-density lipoprotein (LDL) receptor family) in coated pits, endocytosed and trafficked to the endosome, where gentamicin—present within the proximal tubular cells at a concentration vastly exceeding the serum level—inhibits fusion *in vivo* and *in vitro*.

Aminoglycosides should only be used in the relatively uncommon circumstance that there is no suitable alternative antibiotic that is not nephrotoxic. The risk of nephrotoxicity can be reduced by choosing the least toxic aminoglycoside possible, ensuring that the patient is not volume depleted, correcting hypokalaemia and hypomagnesaemia, using a once-daily dosing regimen, adjusting the dose according to renal function, monitoring serum drug levels, limiting the duration of therapy to 7 to 10 days, and minimizing the use of other nephrotoxic drugs. Anionic polyaminoacids, e.g. polyaspartic acid, can interfere with the binding of cationic aminoglycosides to proximal tubular cell membranes and lysosomes and may be useful in preventing aminoglycoside nephrotoxicity, but this approach is not used clinically.

Radiographic contrast media

The incidence of acute kidney injury associated with the use of radiographic contrast media has been reported to vary between 0 and 50%. This extraordinary variability reflects differences in other risk factors in the populations under examination and in the definition of kidney injury used. Risk factors that are recognized include pre-existing chronic kidney disease, diabetic nephropathy with renal impairment, advanced cardiac failure, percutaneous coronary intervention, myeloma, and a high dose of contrast. Recent prospective studies, using nonionic contrast media and in which careful attention has been paid to the maintenance of adequate hydration, have shown a very low incidence of significant renal impairment—even in groups reported to be at high risk (diabetes, myeloma). When renal impairment does develop, it typically occurs 12 to 24 h after exposure, is nonoliguric and usually mild, and recovery begins within 3 to 5 days.

Concern about nephrotoxicity of radiocontrast media should very rarely, if ever, restrict the selection of imaging technique in a particular patient: if there is diagnostic uncertainty, then they require the imaging technique most likely to achieve a diagnosis; if there is no diagnostic uncertainty, then no imaging is needed.

Endogenous nephrotoxins

Myoglobin

Myoglobinuric acute kidney injury, the mechanism of which is incompletely understood (but probably involves a combination of volume depletion/renal ischaemia, tubular injury by free iron/haem,

---

Box 21.5.4 Some causes of rhabdomyolysis

- Direct muscle injury
- Ischaemic muscle injury:
  - Compression
  - Vascular occlusion
- Any cause of coma (e.g. opioid overdose, diabetes mellitus, cerebrovascular accident) or of prolonged restraint/immobility (e.g. following a fall in older people) can be associated with rhabdomyolysis owing to a pressure effect
- Excessive muscular activity:
  - Seizures
  - Sport, e.g. marathon running
- Inflammatory myositis:
  - Immunological, e.g. dermatomyositis, polymyositis
  - Infection, e.g. viral (influenza, coxsackie, HIV)
- Metabolic:
  - Hypokalaemia, hypophosphataemia
  - Myopathies, e.g. carnitine palmitoyltransferase (CPT) deficiency, myophosphorylase deficiency (McArdle's syndrome)
- Endocrine:
  - Diabetic ketoacidosis/nonketotic hyperglycaemia
  - Hypothyroidism
- Toxins/drugs:
  - Snake bite, carbon monoxide, alcohol, hemlock, paint/glue sniffing
  - clofibrate, aminocaproic acid, 3-hydroxy-3-methylglutaryl coenzyme A (HMG CoA) reductase inhibitors
- Others:
  - Sickle cell trait
  - Near drowning, hypothermia
  - Malignant hyperpyrexia
  - Neuroleptic malignant syndrome
  - Phaeochromocytoma 'storm'

---

and tubular obstruction by haem pigment casts), is typically associated with crush injury to muscle, most typically after patients have been trapped under rubble following earthquakes or explosions, but there are a large number of causes of nontraumatic rhabdomyolysis (Box 21.5.4).

A high index of suspicion is required to diagnose cases that are not obviously associated with muscle injury, since muscular pain, swelling, and tenderness may not be prominent features and can even be absent. The key to making the diagnosis is to detect myoglobin in the urine, or a very high level of enzymes released from muscle in the plasma. The former is recognized by the combination of dark-brown ('Coca-Cola') urine that tests positive for 'blood' on a reagent strip, but which does not contain red cells on microscopy, although pigmented 'muddy' granular casts are seen. The muscle enzyme usually measured in plasma is creatine kinase: the normal range of this is up to just below 200 U/litre; in rhabdomyolysis values above 10 000 U/litre are typical, a value of only 1000 to 2000 U/litre not being enough to establish the diagnosis of rhabdomyolytic acute kidney injury in the absence of other supporting evidence. Extremely high levels of plasma myoglobin, aldolase, and lactic dehydrogenase are also seen, all being released from damaged muscle.

Rhabdomyolysis can be associated with very high plasma levels of potassium, phosphate (above 2.5 mmol/litre), urate (above 750 μmol/litre), aspartate transaminase (in the many hundreds of U/litre, exceptionally in the thousands), and alanine transaminase (in the few hundreds of U/litre), and with an unusually low plasma calcium concentration (below 1.5 mmol/litre). Any of these findings should lead to serious consideration of rhabdomyolysis in any patient with unexplained acute kidney injury.

Aside from treatment (when possible) of the underlying cause, initial management involves correction of intravascular volume depletion, which may be massive owing to sequestration of fluid in damaged muscle, and provocation of a diuresis of around 200 ml/h while myoglobinuria persists, the intention being both to establish good renal perfusion and 'wash out' obstructing casts. This can be achieved by infusion of 0.9% saline or other balanced salt solution (e.g. Hartmann's), initially at a rate of 1 to 2 litre/h, titrated down at the first sign of fluid overload (pulmonary oedema) or—if and when the patient becomes massively polyuric—to maintain a urinary output of 200 to 300 ml/h. When this urinary output is achieved, many physicians would recommend additional infusion of bicarbonate and mannitol to sustain a forced alkaline-mannitol diuresis, with urinary pH above 6.5, the argument being that this might reduce the renal toxicity of myoglobin. The evidence that this is beneficial is not very substantial, and care must be taken to monitor for (with bicarbonate) hypokalaemia and hypocalcaemia, and (with mannitol) hypernatraemia and hyperosmolality. The plasma potassium concentration can rise by more than 1 mmol/litre per day, hence hyperkalaemia is the usual indication for renal replacement therapy.

Assuming that the patient survives the precipitating insult, hypercalcaemia develops in 20 to 30% of cases during the recovery phase. This is thought to be caused by mobilization of calcium from injured muscle, correction of hyperphosphataemia with improvement in GFR, and an increase in 1,25-dihydroxyvitamin D (mechanism uncertain).

Haemoglobin

Acute kidney injury can be seen in association with massive haemolysis in many circumstances, but these are relatively rare in the developed world, where ABO-mismatched blood transfusion is probably the most common cause. By contrast, intravascular haemolysis is a common feature of many cases in some countries, being found in over 20% of 325 patients receiving dialysis for acute kidney injury in Chandigarh (north India). This was most frequently seen in those with glucose-6-phosphate dehydrogenase deficiency, with copper sulphate poisoning and snake bite being the next most common causes. Malaria, arsine poisoning, burns, and as a complication of bladder irrigation with hypotonic solutions are other causes.

In each circumstance it is thought that the development of acute kidney injury is exacerbated by (if not solely caused by) the presence of large amounts of free haemoglobin within the circulation. As with rhabdomyolysis, the urine is coloured red to brown, with pigmented granular casts on microscopy, but the findings in the plasma are different: it is reddish in colour (whereas it is usually clear in rhabdomyolysis), creatine kinase is not elevated, haptoglobin levels are reduced, and the peripheral blood film is abnormal. The approach to renal management is as described above for rhabdomyolysis.

Urate and other endogenous nephrotoxins

The tumour lysis syndrome is associated with a rapid rise in plasma uric acid concentration (and almost certainly liberation of other nephrotoxins) as a complication of the treatment of lymphoma, leukaemia, myeloma, or other 'high-turnover' tumours. Hyperuricaemia and renal failure have been described on rare occasions after recurrent epileptic seizures. Prevention and management of tumour lysis syndrome are discussed in Chapter 21.10.4, as is acute kidney injury associated with myeloma.

Vascular causes

Acute cortical necrosis

Acute cortical necrosis is an uncommon cause of acute kidney injury, accounting for around 1% of cases in the developed world, but more (3.8%) in the experience of one large centre in the developing world (north India). However, these figures may be an underestimate, given that investigation is not pursued in many patients who fail to recover from what was presumed to be acute tubular necrosis, on the grounds that test results do not reliably predict prognosis or affect management, which is supportive.

Acute cortical necrosis presents in the same context as acute tubular necrosis, which is almost always the diagnosis made initially on clinical grounds. Suspicion should arise immediately if a patient without obstruction is anuric, as was found in 79% of 113 patients in the largest study reported, but cortical necrosis is often considered only when renal function fails to improve.

Most cases of acute cortical necrosis are the result of obstetric disasters, particularly postpartum haemorrhage, placental abruption, eclampsia, or septic abortion. Snake bite, haemolytic uraemic syndrome, acute gastroenteritis, pancreatitis, septicaemia (often with disseminated intravascular coagulation), trauma, and drug-induced intravascular haemolysis are risk factors in the nonobstetric population.

The pathological findings are of microvascular thrombosis, mainly affecting interlobular arteries, arterioles, and glomeruli, with complete infarction of affected areas of cortex. The medulla and a rim of juxtamedullary tissue are spared.

The best investigations to establish the diagnosis of acute cortical necrosis are renal angiography and contrast-enhanced CT scanning. The former reveals attenuation of interlobular arteries, an increase in the subcapsular vessels, and a negative outer cortical nephrogram; the latter shows enhancement of the renal medulla, but no enhancement of the renal cortex and no excretion of contrast. Biopsy necessarily samples only a very small piece of tissue and may mislead because of the patchy nature of renal damage. Radiopharmaceutical investigations that depend on renal excretion (e.g. dimercaptosuccinic acid (DMSA) scans) are unhelpful in patients with very poor renal function.

In the months or years after an episode of acute cortical necrosis, the kidneys tend to contract: cortical calcification, producing an eggshell or tramline appearance on the abdominal radiograph, is a characteristic sequel, but this is not useful in making the diagnosis acutely.

Return of renal function in cases of acute cortical necrosis occurs very slowly, if at all, and is attributable to the survival of islands of intact cortical tissue. About 50% of patients recover sufficiently to come off dialysis, but the GFR rarely exceeds 10 to 20 ml/min. Hypertension (including accelerated phase) may be a significant problem, and a subsequent decline in renal function with the necessity for a return to dialysis/transplantation is not uncommon.

Large-vessel obstruction

Arterial obstruction

Occlusion of the main renal arteries—or of the artery supplying a solitary functioning kidney—by trauma, dissection, thrombosis, or embolism may rarely be the reason for acute kidney injury. Loin pain sometimes occurs, and there is usually a low-grade fever, such that the clinical picture may mimic acute pyelonephritis, but symptoms can be notable by their absence. Proteinuria and haematuria may occur.

Diagnosis is important because thrombolysis and/or renovascular surgery can be surprisingly effective in restoring function, even when undertaken a considerable time after arterial occlusion (up to many weeks), in those with atherosclerotic renovascular disease in whom (prior to occlusion) a collateral blood supply to the renal parenchyma has developed. Suspicion should be aroused by complete, sudden anuria in the absence of urinary obstruction, especially if the clinical setting is appropriate, e.g. atrial fibrillation in an arteriopath. A useful pointer to the diagnosis is the finding of a urinary sodium concentration similar to that of plasma (see Table 21.5.5), but DTPA renography and renal angiography are the appropriate diagnostic tests if the diagnosis of renal artery occlusion is suspected. CT scanning may reveal wedge-shaped infarcts when occlusion is incomplete.

Venous obstruction

Renal vein thrombosis can cause acute kidney injury, most commonly in adults as a complication of nephrotic syndrome, but in infants and children as a result of abdominal sepsis or severe dehydration. Renal pain is common, as is increasing proteinuria and haematuria (which can be macroscopic), but there may be no symptoms. If there is clinical suspicion of the diagnosis, e.g. unexplained deterioration of renal function in a nephrotic patient, then appropriate investigation includes ultrasound/Doppler examination of the renal veins and inferior vena cava, CT/MRI scanning, or renal arteriography with late films taken specifically to look for filling of the renal veins. Treatment by anticoagulation is the usual practice.

Small-vessel obstruction

Accelerated-phase hypertension

'Accelerated-phase' hypertension (a term preferred to 'malignant' hypertension because the implication of malignancy is terrifying for patients) occurs when the blood pressure is elevated sufficiently to cause fibrinoid necrosis of blood vessels, leading to the development of haemorrhages and exudates in the ocular fundi. It may develop as a consequence of pre-existing renal disease, and is itself a potent cause of renal damage. Acute kidney injury is a common complication in those with previously normal renal function, and is associated with proteinuria, haematuria, and the presence of urinary red cell casts. The higher the creatinine at presentation, the poorer the prognosis for both patient survival and renal outcome: in one study only 9% of those with an initial plasma creatinine below 300 μmol/litre progressed to need renal replacement therapy, compared with two-thirds of those with a plasma creatinine above this level. The ability of the kidney to autoregulate perfusion is disturbed in accelerated-phase hypertension, hence the therapeutic lowering of arterial pressure may be associated with reduced renal perfusion and an abrupt decline in renal function. Accelerated-phase hypertension is one of the conditions in which renal function sometimes recovers after a lengthy period on dialysis. Renal failure was the cause of two-thirds of the deaths in patients with accelerated-phase hypertension in the days before dialysis was available. See Chapter 16.17.5 for further discussion.

Systemic sclerosis

This disease does not usually involve the kidney, but a syndrome resembling accelerated-phase hypertension and termed 'scleroderma renal crisis' is well recognized in patients with diffuse cutaneous systemic sclerosis. It usually occurs within the first 5 years of the disease, may be the presenting feature, and often appears during the winter months. Rapid worsening of skin manifestations may precede the crisis, but frequently there is no warning. The patient may develop headaches, visual disturbance, and convulsions. Arterial pressure is usually grossly elevated, but the renal syndrome can occur without a rise in arterial pressure. Haemorrhages and exudates are often seen in the ocular fundi. Renal failure, with proteinuria and haematuria, develops rapidly. A microangiopathic haemolytic anaemia may complicate the situation. Plasma levels of renin are grossly elevated. There have been a number of case reports of arrest or reversal of the syndrome after treatment with ACE inhibitors or nifedipine. These agents should be tried, but more in hope than expectation that they will prevent relentless progression to endstage renal failure. See Chapter 19.11.3 for further discussion.

Glomerulonephritic and vasculitic causes

A large number of glomerulonephritic and vasculitic diseases can cause acute kidney injury, sometimes in association with pulmonary haemorrhage. These are discussed in detail in the relevant subchapters of Chapter 21.8, and in Chapters 20.10.2 and 20.10.3. Together they form only 5 to 10% of cases of acute kidney injury, but making the correct diagnosis is of extreme importance because of the management implications. Regrettably, most nephrologists have seen cases where the diagnosis has been much delayed because renal impairment has incorrectly been attributed to acute tubular necrosis, and infiltrates on the chest radiograph to oedema or infection. This error, which can be catastrophic, should be avoided in patients in whom the cause of acute kidney injury is not obvious, by the procedure outlined in Box 21.5.5.

The possible presence of a rapidly progressive glomerulonephritis/vasculitis is a medical emergency. Anti-GBM disease responds well to immunosuppression with plasma exchange, steroids, and cyclophosphamide, but only if treatment is begun before dialysis is required. Immunosuppressive treatment should be given as early as possible in the course of acute kidney injury complicating microscopic polyangiitis/idiopathic rapidly progressive (crescentic)

Box 21.5.5 Diagnosis of glomerulonephritic and vasculitic causes of acute kidney injury

1 A history and examination specifically directed towards determining whether a glomerulonephritic or vasculitic illness might be present

2 Stick testing of the urine for blood and protein, followed (if positive) by microscopy to look for the presence of cellular casts

3 The following tests:

(a) Measurement of serum antiglomerular basement membrane (anti-GBM) antibodies—positive in Goodpasture's disease (see Chapter 21.8.7)

(b) Measurement of serum antineutrophil cytoplasmic antibodies (ANCA) (screening by indirect immunofluorescence test, specific tests for antiproteinase-3 and antimyeloperoxidase antibodies)—usually positive in microscopic polyangiitis and Wegener's granulomatosis (see Chapter 21.10.2)

(c) Estimation of serum complement levels (C3 may be depressed in postinfectious glomerulonephritis, mesangiocapillary glomerulonephritis, systemic lupus erythematosus) (see Chapters 21.8.5, 21.8.6 and 21.10.3)

(d) Measurement of serum antistreptolysin-O titre—elevated in poststreptococcal glomerulonephritis) (see Chapter 21.8.5)

(e) Serological tests for systemic lupus erythematosus (see Chapter 21.10.3)

(f) Estimation of serum immunoglobulins and testing for urinary light chains (see Chapter 21.10.4)

(g) Estimation of serum cryoglobulins (see Chapter 21.10.4)

4 Consideration of the possibility that pulmonary infiltrates in a patient with acute kidney injury might be due to haemorrhage; the chances of this are increased if there is a history of haemoptysis (associated with several forms of rapidly progressive glomerulonephritis), nasal discharge or bleeding (associated with Wegener's granulomatosis), or if anaemia is unusually profound and otherwise unexplained; lung function tests demonstrating an increase in carbon monoxide transfer factor can establish the diagnosis

5 An urgent renal biopsy in any patient with acute kidney injury and an active urinary sediment, unless the diagnosis is clear (e.g. a classical history of poststreptococcal nephritis, obvious infective endocarditis/shunt nephritis) or there is a strong contraindication, e.g. a single kidney or serious bleeding disorder

---

glomerulonephritis, Wegener's granulomatosis, and systemic lupus erythematosus. The urgency is such that it may well be appropriate to start these treatments while the results of blood tests and renal biopsy are awaited, and to stop them if the findings do not corroborate the initial clinical diagnosis. The management of these patients is complex and patients benefit from the judgement and expertise of specialists.

Acute interstitial nephritis

Acute interstitial nephritis is discussed in Chapter 21.9.1. Leptospirosis (Chapter 21.11) and hantaviral infection (Chapter 21.10.7) are both associated with acute kidney injury and acute interstitial nephritis: the account below is to aid the clinician in distinguishing between them.

Leptospirosis

The diagnosis of leptospirosis should be considered in any patient with unexplained acute kidney injury who has myalgias/muscle tenderness, conjunctival injection and/or haemorrhage and/or jaundice. Direct enquiry must be made as to whether any such patient has been exposed to rats. Blood tests commonly reveal a dramatic conjugated hyperbilirubinaemia (often above 250 µmol/litre) and thrombocytopenia (seen in 40% of cases), and there may also be elevation of plasma creatine kinase and a slight increase in plasma aspartate aminotransferase (AST). Anaemia may be severe owing to intravascular haemolysis. By contrast to most other causes of acute kidney injury, plasma potassium is often normal or low in cases of leptospirosis. Mild abnormalities of blood clotting tests can be seen, but disseminated intravascular coagulation is not a feature, which is an important point in distinction from bacterial septicaemia.

Hantavirus disease
In Europe
In Europe, the Puumala serotype of hantavirus produces an illness that can have many similarities to that produced by leptospirosis, although serological studies indicate that many patients must have a subclinical infection. In those that are symptomatic, high fever is typically followed within a couple of days by loin/abdominal pain and often by nausea and vomiting; photophobia and signs of meningeal irritation can also occur. Acute kidney injury follows when these symptoms have settled and is associated with conjunctival haemorrhage (20%), proteinuria (almost 100% of cases), microscopic haematuria (70%), thrombocytopenia (50%), and a transient mild rise in plasma liver enzymes. There may be a small increase in plasma bilirubin (maximum 40 µmol/litre). Mild abnormalities of blood clotting tests are seen, but disseminated intravascular coagulation is rare.

Renal biopsy, performed for the indication of unexplained acute renal impairment, shows interstitial nephritis. This has no pathognomonic features, leading in this clinical context to the differential diagnosis of leptospirosis and sometimes (depending on exposure) disease induced by nonsteroidal anti-inflammatory drugs (NSAIDs). Leptospirosis is much more likely if the plasma bilirubin is markedly elevated. NSAID-induced disease does not cause conjunctival haemorrhages or thrombocytopenia. The diagnosis of Puumala hantavirus infection is made on the basis of serological evidence. Prognosis is good: no deaths have been reported and renal function returns to normal.

In some areas of eastern and central Europe there is a more severe form of hantavirus infection, which is similar to that seen in Asia.

In Asia
The Hantaan and Seoul viruses cause hantavirus disease in Asia: the former causes more severe illness, but both are considerably

3902 SECTION 21 DISORDERS OF THE KIDNEY AND URINARY TRACT

more dangerous that the Puumala hantavirus seen in Europe. A total of five phases of disease are recognized:

- High fever and myalgias, followed by headache and severe abdominal/loin pain, often with an erythematous rash that may become petechial, also conjunctival haemorrhages

- Severe hypotension

- Gradual recovery of blood pressure, but associated with oliguria and renal failure with proteinuria and microscopic haematuria—one-third of patients in this stage have significant problems with bleeding: gastrointestinal, intracerebral or massive purpura (hence the terms epidemic or Korean haemorrhagic fever)

- Polyuria

- Convalescence

Differential diagnosis is from severe leptospirosis and other causes of haemorrhagic fever found in Asia, including dengue and murine typhus. The diagnosis is made serologically. Treatment is supportive. Mortality is between 3 and 7%; survivors recover completely.

'Haematological' causes

These are discussed in other chapters: haemolytic uraemic syndrome (Chapter 21.10.5); idiopathic postpartum renal failure (Chapter 14.5); and plasma cell dyscrasias, immunoglobulin-based amyloidoses, fibrillary nephropathies, lymphomas, and leukaemias (Chapter 21.10.4).

Hepatorenal syndrome

The hepatorenal syndrome consists of the association of severe and usually progressive liver disease with acute kidney injury. In one study of 229 patients with cirrhosis and ascites, it developed in 18% at 1 year and 39% at 5 years, and in another study it developed in 28 of 101 patients with acute alcoholic hepatitis.

The mechanism of renal failure in hepatorenal syndrome is uncertain, but it is associated with splanchnic vasodilatation and markedly reduced renal perfusion. These may be precipitated by acute insults such as gastrointestinal bleeding or infection. Presentation is typically with oliguria, an inactive urinary sediment, a very low urinary sodium concentration (<10 mmol/litre), and a rising plasma creatinine. Based on speed of onset, two forms are described: type 1 with rapid deterioration (creatinine clearance falling to less than 20 ml/min or plasma creatinine rising twofold to more than 221 µmol/litre (2.5 mg/dl) within 2 weeks); type 2 is less rapid.

Diagnostic criteria are unsatisfactory because they depend substantially on exclusion of other conditions, with particular difficulty in distinction from the effects of sepsis and acute tubular necrosis:

- Hepatic disease with advanced hepatic failure and portal hypertension

- Progressively rising plasma creatinine (>133 µmol/litre (1.5 mg/dl)) over days or weeks

- An inactive urinary sediment (no cellular casts, proteinuria <0.5 g/day)

- Exclusion of other cause of renal impairment (which requires a trial of volume expansion and discontinuation of nephrotoxins)

Hepatorenal syndrome is characterized by 'prerenal' urinary biochemistry, in particular a very low urinary sodium concentration (<10 mmol/litre) (Table 21.5.5), but this is not a diagnostic criterion. Histologically, the kidneys are normal, a fact emphasised by the fact that they work normally if transplanted (but by contrast, liver transplantation resulted in restoration of renal function in only 58% of patients in one study).

Distinguishing hepatorenal syndrome from prerenal disease and acute tubular necrosis is important, because the latter conditions are often reversible, whereas the prognosis of hepatorenal syndrome is extremely poor. In the presence of potentially reversible liver disease, or with the prospect of liver transplantation, intensive therapy and renal replacement therapy are justified. If these criteria are not met, then aggressive support may be inappropriate, although some success has been reported with the combination of midodrine (a selective α_1-adrenergic agonist) and octreotide (a somatostatin analogue), also with noradrenaline infusion. Transjugular intrahepatic portosystemic shunt (TIPS) procedures may provide short-term benefit.

The risk of hepatorenal syndrome can be reduced in patients with spontaneous bacterial peritonitis by administration of intravenous albumin in addition to antibiotics. Pentoxifylline may prevent the condition in patients with severe alcoholic hepatitis, and norfloxacin (400 mg once daily) may do so in some patients with cirrhosis and ascites.

Urinary obstruction

This is discussed in Chapter 21.17.

Further reading

Abassi ZA, et al. (1998). Acute renal failure complicating muscle crush injury. Semin Nephrol, 18, 558–65.

Ali T, et al. (2007). Incidence and outcomes in acute kidney injury: a comprehensive population-based study. J Am Soc Nephrol, 18, 1292–8.

Ash SR. (2001). Peritoneal dialysis in acute renal failure of adults: the safe, effective, and low-cost modality. Contrib Nephrol, 132, 210–21.

Bagshaw SM, et al. (2008). A comparison of the RIFLE and AKIN criteria for acute kidney injury in critically ill patients. Nephrol Dial Transplant, 23, 1569–74.

Bellomo R, et al. (2000). Low-dose dopamine in patients with early renal dysfunction: a placebo-controlled randomised trial. Australian and New Zealand Intensive Care Society (ANZICS) Clinical Trials Group. Lancet, 356, 2139–43.

Bhandari S, Turney JH (1996). Survivors of acute renal failure who do not recover renal function. QJM, 89, 415–21.

Brosius FC, Lau K (1986). Low fractional excretion of sodium in acute renal failure: role of timing of the test and ischemia. Am J Nephrol, 6, 450–7.

Brown CV, et al. (2004). Preventing renal failure in patients with rhabdomyolysis: do bicarbonate and mannitol make a difference? J Trauma, 56, 1191–6.

Chugh KS. (1989) Snake-bite-induced acute renal failure in India. Kidney Int, 35, 891–907.

Chugh KS, et al. (1977). Acute renal failure due to intravascular hemolysis in the North Indian patients. Am J Med Sci, 274, 139–46.

Chugh KS, et al. (1994). Acute renal cortical necrosis—a study of 113 patients. Ren Fail, 16, 37–47.

Cruz DN, Rizzi Z, Ronco C (2009). Clinical review: RIFLE and AKIN - time for reappraisal. Crit Care, 13, 211.

Davenport A, Stevens P (2008). Clinical practice guidelines. Module 5: Acute kidney injury. 4th Edition. UK Renal Association, Petersfield.

Denton MD, et al. (1996). 'Renal-dose' dopamine for the treatment of acute renal failure: scientific rationale, experimental studies and clinical trials. Kidney Int, 50, 4–14.

Feest TG, *et al.* (1993). Incidence of severe acute renal failure in adults: results of a community based study. *BMJ*, **306**, 481–3.

Firth JD. (1996). Acute irreversible renal failure. *QJM*, **89**, 397–9.

Gines P, *et al.* (2003). Hepatorenal syndrome. *Lancet*, **362**, 1819–27.

Hirschberg R, *et al.* (1999). Multicenter clinical trial of recombinant human insulin-like growth factor I in patients with acute renal failure. *Kidney Int*, **55**, 2423–32.

Ho KM, Sheridan DJ (2006). Meta-analysis of frusemide to prevent or treat acute renal failure. *BMJ*, **333**, 420.

Holt SG, Moore KP (2001). Pathogenesis and treatment of renal dysfunction in rhabdomyolysis. *Intensive Care Med*, **27**, 803–11.

Hou SH, *et al.* (1983). Hospital-acquired renal insufficiency: a prospective study. *Am J Med*, **74**, 243–8.

Jha V, *et al.* (1992). Spectrum of hospital-acquired acute renal failure in the developing countries—Chandigarh study. *QJM*, **83**, 497–505.

Liano F, Pascual J (1996). Epidemiology of acute renal failure: a prospective, multicenter, community-based study. Madrid Acute Renal Failure Study Group. *Kidney Int*, **50**, 811–18.

Liano F, *et al.* (1994). Use of urinary parameters in the diagnosis of total acute renal artery occlusion. *Nephron*, **66**, 170–5.

Lieberthal W, Nigam SK (1998). Acute renal failure. I. Relative importance of proximal vs. distal tubular injury. *Am J Physiol*, **275**, F623–31.

Lieberthal W, Nigam SK (2000). Acute renal failure. II. Experimental models of acute renal failure: imperfect but indispensable. *Am J Physiol*, **278**, F1–F12.

Liss P, *et al.* (2006). Renal failure in 57 925 patients undergoing coronary procedures using iso-osmolar or low-osmolar contrast media. *Kidney Int*, **70**, 1811–17.

Maillet PJ, *et al.* (1986). Nondilated obstructive acute renal failure: diagnostic procedures and therapeutic management. *Radiology*, **160**, 659–62.

Marik PE, *et al.* (2006). The course of type 1 hepato-renal syndrome post liver transplantation. *Nephrol Dial Transplant*, **21**, 478–82.

Mehta RL, *et al.* (2004). Spectrum of acute renal failure in the intensive care unit: the PICARD experience. *Kidney Int*, **66**, 1613–21.

Mehta RL, *et al.* (2007). Acute Kidney Injury Network: report of an initiative to improve outcome in acute kidney injury. *Crit Care*, **11**, R31.

Milligan SL, *et al.* (1978). Intra-abdominal infection and acute renal failure. *Arch Surg*, **113**, 467–72.

Molitoris BA. (1997). Cell biology of aminoglycoside nephrotoxicity: newer aspects. *Curr Opin Nephrol Hypertens*, **6**, 384–8.

Murphy SW, *et al.* (2000). Contrast nephropathy. *J Am Soc Nephrol*, **11**, 177–82.

Nigame S, Lieberthal W (2000). Acute renal failure. III. The role of growth factors in the process of renal regeneration and repair. *Am J Physiol*, **279**, F3–F11.

Parfrey PS, *et al.* (1989). Contrast material-induced renal failure in patients with diabetes mellitus, renal insufficiency, or both. A prospective controlled study. *New Engl J Med*, **320**, 143–9.

Pilmore HL, *et al.* (1995). Acute bilateral renal artery occlusion: successful revascularization with streptokinase. *Am J Nephrol*, **15**, 90–1.

Powell-Tuck J, *et al.* (2008). *British consensus guidelines on intravenous fluid therapy for adult surgical patients*. The Renal Association, Petersfield.

Ramsay AG, *et al.* (1983). Renal functional recovery 47 days after renal artery occlusion. *Am J Nephrol*, **3**, 325–8.

Rasmussen HH, Ibels LS (1982). Acute renal failure. Multivariate analysis of causes and risk factors. *Am J Med*, **73**, 211–18.

Remuzzi G. (1988). Bleeding in renal failure. *Lancet*, **1**, 1205–8.

Ronco C, *et al.* (2001). Acute dialysis quality initiative (ADQI). *Nephrol Dial Transplant*, **16**, 1555–8.

Salerno F, *et al.* (2007). Diagnosis, prevention and treatment of hepatorenal syndrome in cirrhosis. *Gut*, **56**, 1310–18.

Schiffer H, *et al.* (2002). Daily hemodialysis and the outcome of acute renal failure. *New Engl J Med*, **346**, 305–10.

Shilliday IR, *et al.* (1997). Loop diuretics in the management of acute renal failure: a prospective, double-blind, placebo-controlled, randomized study. *Nephrol Dial Transplant*, **12**, 2592–6.

Solez K, Morel-Maroger L, Sraer JD. (1979). The morphology of 'acute tubular necrosis' in man: analysis of 57 renal biopsies and a comparison with the glycerol model. *Medicine (Baltimore)*, **58**, 362–76.

Solez K, Racusen LC. (2001). Role of the renal biopsy in acute renal failure. *Contrib Nephrol*, **132**, 68–75.

Spital A, *et al.* (1988). Nondilated obstructive uropathy. *Urology*, **31**, 478–82.

Sponsel H, Conger JD. (1995). Is parenteral nutrition therapy of value in acute renal failure patients? *Am J Kidney Dis*, **25**, 96–102.

van Ypersele de Strihou C. (1998). Hantavirus infection. In: Davison AM, *et al.* (eds). *Oxford textbook of clinical nephrology*, pp. 1688–92. Oxford University Press, Oxford.

The RENAL Replacement Therapy Study Investigators. (2009). Intensity of continuous renal-replacement therapy in critically ill patients. *N Engl J Med*, **361**, 1627–38.

van Ypersele de Strihou C, Mery JP. (1989). Hantavirus-related acute interstitial nephritis in western Europe. Expansion of a world-wide zoonosis. *QJM*, **73**, 941–50.

Winearls CG, *et al.* (1984). Acute renal failure due to leptospirosis: clinical features and outcome in six cases. *QJM*, **53**, 487–95.

Xue JL, *et al.* (2006). Incidence and mortality of acute renal failure in Medicare beneficiaries, 1992–2001. *J Am Soc Nephrol*, **17**, 1135–42.

Chronic kidney disease

Eberhard Ritz, Tilman B. Drüeke, and John D. Firth

Essentials[1]

Definition—chronic kidney disease (CKD) is defined as kidney damage lasting for more than 3 months characterized by structural or functional abnormalities of the kidney, with or without decreased glomerular filtration rate (GFR).

Staging—CKD has been subdivided into five stages depending on the estimated GFR (eGFR), as described in Chapter 21.4, but in brief: CKD 1 is eGFR greater than 90 ml/min (per 1.73 m^2) with other evidence of renal disease; CKD stage 2 is eGFR 60 to 89 ml/min, with other evidence of renal disease; CKD stage 3 is eGFR 30 to 59 ml/min CKD stage 4 is eGFR 15 to 29 ml/min and CKD stage 5 is eGFR less than 15 ml/min. CKD 3 can be divided into 3A (eGFR 45–59) and 3B (eGFR 30–44), and the suffix 'p' can be added to any stage to denote proteinuria (ACR >30mg/mmol, PCR >50mg/mmol).

Epidemiology—mild CKD is common, with about 10% of the population of the United States of America having CKD 1, 2, or 3 (combined), but advanced CKD is relatively rare (about 0.2% are receiving renal replacement therapy). Patients with CKD 1, 2, or 3 are at relatively low risk of progressing to require renal replacement therapy, but are at high risk of death from cardiovascular disease.

Aetiology—the causes of chronic renal failure recorded in various national registries are diabetes mellitus (22–45%), glomerulonephritis (10–23%), hypertension (5–25%), chronic pyelonephritis (0.5 to 7%), adult polycystic kidney disease (2–7%), renal vascular disease (2–7%), other recognized conditions (13–15%), and unknown causes (4–26%). However, these data are flawed for many reasons: diagnoses are often allocated as 'best guesses' by clinicians, there is no universal agreement on the meaning of terms such as 'pyelonephritis', glomerulonephritis may be diagnosed without histological proof, and hypertension is often cited when it may be no more than a consequence of whatever caused the renal failure.

Pathophysiology

Compensatory mechanisms and their consequences—as kidney function gradually fails, these generally maintain acceptable health until the GFR is about 10 to 15 ml/min, and patients will not usually die of renal failure until the GFR is less than 5 ml/min. Despite a widened range of single-nephron GFR in damaged or diseased kidneys, glomerular and tubular function remains closely integrated in all individual nephrons (the 'intact nephron hypothesis'). However, the functional adaptations required to maintain overall homeostasis come at a price (the 'trade-off hypothesis'), with the 'hyperfiltration hypothesis' most clearly articulating how these adaptive changes lead, in the long run, to glomerulosclerosis and tubulointerstitial fibrosis and progressive decrease in GFR.

Pathophysiological changes—these include impairment in: (1) concentration and/or dilution of the urine; (2) excretion and/or conservation of sodium; (3) excretion of potassium, with hyperkalaemia often the immediate life-threatening consideration in the management of patients with renal failure; (4) excretion of acid; (5) calcium/phosphate/vitamin D/bone homeostasis; (6) erythropoietin production, leading to renal anaemia; (7) excretion of many substances and metabolites that act as 'uraemic toxins'; and (8) a wide range of endocrine functions.

The clinical presentation of CKD is discussed in Chapter 21.3 and investigation of patients with renal disease in Chapter 21.4.

Prevention of progression

Specific and general measures—in some patients, measures to conserve renal function may be specific to the cause of renal impairment, e.g. relief of obstruction, but it is probable that all patients will benefit from good blood pressure control and (when relevant) measures to reduce proteinuria, which is not only a marker but a promoter of progression of CKD.

Blood pressure and proteinuria—there is limited information on the target blood pressure to be achieved in patients with chronic kidney disease, but the consensus is that the lower the blood pressure, the better—as long as this can be achieved without unacceptable side effects. The European Society of Hypertension/European Society of Cardiology guidelines recommend a target of less than 130/80 mmHg, and even lower if there is significant proteinuria, which should be lowered as much as possible, preferably to less than 1g/24h (roughly equivalent to an albumin:creatinine ratio (ACR) of less than 60 mg/mmol or a protein:creatinine ratio (PCR)

[1] *Acknowledgement*: Dr C Winearls wrote on chronic renal failure in the fourth edition of this textbook: three figures and a small amount of his text are retained here.

of less than 100 mg/mmol). Combination therapy with several antihypertensive agents (including loop diuretics) is usually required, but there is good evidence that the regimen should contain an angiotensin-converting enzyme (ACE) inhibitor and/or angiotensin receptor blocker, which have antiproteinuric effects, if these can be tolerated (hyperkalaemia being the most common reason why they cannot be used in this context).

Medical management of the consequences of CKD

Diet—only patients with oliguric endstage renal failure need to restrict their fluid intake precisely. It is sensible to recommend modest dietary sodium restriction (100 mmol/day) in most cases. Patients with a tendency to hyperkalaemia should be offered advice regarding a low-potassium diet (with particular care taken if they are given medications that induce hyperkalaemia). Chronic acidosis will benefit from treatment with alkali. Malnutrition is common in advanced CKD, can be detected by serial monitoring of body weight and serum albumin concentration, and is best treated by initiating renal replacement therapy.

Chronic kidney disease mineral and bone disorders (MBD)—these including osteitis fibrosa, osteomalacia, adynamic bone disease, and osteopenia, the impact of which extends beyond the bones to cardiovascular structure and function, with increased mortality. Pathogenesis is complex but includes phosphate retention, deficiency of active forms of vitamin D, hypocalcaemia, and the development of hyperparathyroidism. Secondary hyperparathyroidism can be prevented by giving: (1) cholecalciferol 1000 U/day if serum 25-$(OH)D_3$ is low; (2) calcium carbonate 0.5 to 1.0 g with each meal if plasma calcium is decreased and/or plasma phosphate is increased; (3) calcium-free phosphate binder, e.g. sevelamer or lanthanum carbonate, if serum phosphate is increased and plasma calcium is normal or high; or (4) calcitriol 0.125 to 0.25 μg/day, or equivalent doses of alfacalcidol or other active vitamin D analogues, if serum intact parathyroid hormone (PTH) is consistently above target ranges and serum calcium/phosphate is normal (spontaneously or after intervention).

Advanced hyperparathyroidism can be treated by: (1) normalizing serum calcium and phosphate levels if serum intact PTH is constantly above target range; (2) reducing serum phosphate, if this is elevated, by using phosphate binders, dietary restriction, and increased dialysis; (3) reducing serum calcium if this is elevated by reducing/withdrawing calcium-containing phosphate binders and active vitamin D sterols, and by reducing dialysate calcium concentration; (4) if serum calcium and phosphate have been normalized and elevated intact PTH persists, by increasing dose or frequency of calcitriol or other active vitamin D sterols (e.g.

alfacalcidol, paricalcitol, doxercalciferol), or alternatively administering the calcimimetic cinacalcet, which renders the calcium receptor more sensitive to calcium; and (5) if serum intact PTH fails to decrease and/or hypercalcaemia/hyperphosphataemia develop or persist, then consider cinacalcet or surgical parathyroidectomy.

Anaemia—this is common in chronic kidney disease and is particularly marked in patients with diabetes. Partial correction of such anaemia by use of erythropoiesis-stimulating agents (ESAs) improves patients' physiological and clinical status, as well as quality of life. If a patient with chronic kidney disease has haemoglobin of less than 11 g/dl and symptoms that might be attributable to anaemia, then treatment to restore haemoglobin to the range 11 to 12 g/dl is warranted, but it has been convincingly shown in randomized studies that correction to a higher level ('normal or near normal') is associated with poorer outcomes and should be prevented. Treatment involves: (1) exclusion of other causes of anaemia; (2) optimization of iron status, which usually requires administration of intravenous iron; and (3) initiation and adjustment of dosage/frequency of administration of ESAs, with regular monitoring to achieve haemoglobin in the target range 11 to 12 g/dl.

Preparation for renal replacement therapy or conservative (palliative) management of terminal uraemia

Once endstage renal failure is inevitable, the patient must be prepared physically and psychologically for renal replacement therapy (see Chapters 21.7.1–21.7.3). In many cases it is possible to predict approximately when the endstage will be reached from consideration of the rate of renal deterioration, most easily demonstrated by plotting the reciprocal of the serum creatinine against time.

There are patients for whom dialysis is inappropriate, or who either choose not to start or to discontinue treatment. In frail patients, usually elderly and with multiple comorbidities, it is not likely that dialysis will greatly prolong life, although it can certainly lower the quality of it. The ethical and legal issues are complex and require that the patient makes the decision not to start or to discontinue treatment when fully informed and able to do so. They must be given a realistic account of what dialysis can achieve, what it cannot achieve, and at what cost—access, travel, restrictions, and complications. These conversations can be difficult and cannot be hurried, it being critically important that the patient (and their relatives/friends) does not get the entirely erroneous impression that dialysis means that 'the doctors care and I'll live for ever', whereas no dialysis means that 'the doctors don't care and I'll die soon'. Properly managed, death from uraemia is peaceful and free of suffering.

Definition

According to the Kidney Disease Outcomes Quality Initiative (K/DOQI) guidelines, chronic kidney disease (CKD) is defined as kidney damage lasting for more than 3 months characterized by structural or functional abnormalities of the kidney, with or without decreased glomerular filtration rate (GFR). CKD has been subdivided into five stages (Table 21.6.1).

◆ CKD stage 1—where there are pathological abnormalities or markers of kidney damage such as urinary abnormalities (albuminuria, proteinuria, abnormal urine sediment) or abnormal

imaging tests of the kidney, in the presence or absence of arterial hypertension, and GFR is above 90 ml/min per 1.73 m^2.

◆ CKD stage 2—defined by the presence of pathological abnormalities or markers of kidney damage, with or without high blood pressure, and GFR is in the range between 60 and 89 ml/min per 1.73 m^2. Note that CKD stage 2 is not defined just on the basis of GFR.

◆ CKD higher stages—defined by GFR below 60 ml/min per 1.73 m^2 for more than 3 months. Note that the serum concentration of creatinine can be elevated or, because of the limited sensitivity of serum creatinine, normal. Progressive decrease in

GFR may be associated with a variety of biochemical abnormalities and with abnormal imaging tests.

Table 21.6.1 summarizes the five stages of CKD suggested by the committee of the K/DOQI guidelines.

The issue of impaired renal function immediately raises the problem of which functional parameters are the most appropriate to define impairment. Currently the most frequently used index is the estimated GFR (eGFR), based on an update of the formula used in the Modification of Diet in Renal Disease (MDRD) study. This is based on standardized measurement of serum creatinine (a method which is easily disturbed by numerous confounders) and considers, in addition to serum creatinine, the age, gender, and ethnicity of the patient (see Chapter 21.4 for further discussion). The formula has acceptable accuracy only for eGFR below 60 ml/min per 1.73 m^2, and in the early stages of CKD it is inadequate as an estimate for follow-up examinations when particular precision is required, as documented in patients with diabetic nephropathy. A better indicator of decreased GFR is the serum concentration of the microprotein cystatin C, which is also a more accurate predictor of cardiovascular events than serum creatinine or eGFR, but the high cost of its measurement currently prevents its widespread use (see Chapter 21.4).

In addition to eGFR, information on urinary albumin/protein excretion is indispensable for the full assessment of renal dysfunction. At any given serum creatinine, the excretion in the urine of even small amounts of albumin (microalbuminuria) is indicative of a higher renal and cardiovascular risk. The renal risk is particularly elevated at protein excretion rates above 300 mg/day and increases progressively with increasing severity of proteinuria (for details, see below).

Prevalence and incidence of CKD

The enormous frequency of impaired renal function in the general population has been recognized only recently. Particularly at risk are prediabetic patients with metabolic syndrome, patients with diabetes mellitus, and individuals with many other conditions, e.g. advanced age, female sex, smokers, or patients receiving potentially nephrotoxic medications such as nonsteroidal anti-inflammatory drugs (NSAIDs).

Based on data of the National Health and Nutrition Examination Survey (NHANES) reported in 2003, it has become apparent that—in contrast to the relatively modest number of patients on renal replacement therapy (RRT) in the United States of America (300 000, i.e. less than 1% of the population of 175 million) —the estimated number of adults with CKD stages 1, 2, and 3 (combined) was 18.8 millions, i.e. 10–11% of the population. This observation is not only of academic interest, but also of major public health importance. The reason is shown in Table 21.6.2: in individuals with CKD stage 2 the risk of them living long enough to require RRT is 20 times lower than their risk of dying from cardiovascular causes. Even patients in the more advanced stage 4 of CKD are twice as likely to die from cardiovascular causes as they are to end up on RRT. From a public health perspective, there is therefore a great need to recognize CKD early to allow opportunity for therapeutic interventions, in particular to improve cardiovascular prognosis.

The prevalence and incidence of endstage renal disease is shown in Table 21.6.3, which gives the total number of patients on RRT worldwide at the end of 2004, i.e. 1.8 million, of whom 1.4 million were treated by haemodialysis or continuous ambulatory peritoneal dialysis (or other modalities of peritoneal dialysis) and 412 000 were alive with a functioning renal transplant. In Europe, an estimated total of 324 000 patients were on RRT and 149 000 were alive with a functioning renal graft. This gives a prevalence of 400 per million population for patients on dialysis (haemodialysis and peritoneal dialysis combined) and of 185 per million population for kidney transplant recipients.

Between 1990 and 1999 there was a dramatic increase in the adjusted incidence of RRT in Europe, rising from 73 per million population (range 58–101 per million population) in 1990–1991 to 117 per million population (range 92–145 per million population) in 1998–1999, i.e. by 4.8% per year (range 3.1–6.4%). The increase was greater in men than in women and did not flatten out at the end of the decade, except in the Netherlands. It is of note, however, that the incidence of end stage renal disease due to diabetic nephropathy (the commonest single cause of requiring RRT) has begun to flatten out in the general population of the United States of America. It has also done so in Pima Indians, in whom the cardiovascular risk is less than in whites, which excludes the possibility that failure to observe more diabetic patients reaching endstage renal disease was due to their more frequent death from cardiovascular causes before reaching endstage renal disease. A similar trend with regard to diabetic nephropathy as a cause of endstage renal failure has also been observed in Denmark, but there have been large differences in overall incidence and prevalence of RRT between European countries. Specifically, in the United Kingdom, the annual acceptance rate for RRT increased from 20 per million population in 1982 to 101 per million population in 2002, largely

Table 21.6.1 Classification of chronic kidney disease (CKD)

CKD stage[a]	eGFR (ml/min per 1.73 m^2 body surface area)
1	>90, with other evidence of renal disease
2	60–89, with other evidence of renal disease
3A	45–59
3B	30–44
4	15–29
5	<15, or receiving renal replacement therapy

Patients with CKD stages 3A, 3B, 4, and 5 may or may not have any other evidence of renal disease.

[a] The suffix (p) can be used to denote the presence of proteinuria as defined by a spot urinary albumin:creatinine ratio (ACR) of ≥30 mg/mmol, which is approximately equivalent to a protein:creatinine ratio (PCR) of ≥50 mg/mmol (≥0.5 g/24 h).

Table 21.6.2 Risk (percentage chance over 5 years) of death from CKD progression towards endstage renal disease (defined as need for renal replacement therapy, RRT) and risk of death from cardiovascular disease in 27 998 American patients with glomerular filtration rate (GFR) below 90 ml/min per 1.73 m^2 (for the period 1996–2001)

GFR (ml/min per 1.73 m^2)	Risk over 5 years (%)	
	RRT	Cardiovascular death
CKD stage 2 (60–89)	1.1	19.5
CKD stage 3 (30–59)	1.3	24.3
CKD stage 4 (15–29)	19.9	45.7

(From Keith DS, et al. (2004). Longitudinal follow-up and outcomes among a population with chronic kidney disease in a large managed care organization. *Arch Intern Med*, **164**, 659–63, with permission.)

Table 21.6.3 Global and regional overview of endstage renal disease (ESRD), dialysis, and transplant patient numbers, and prevalence values at year-end 2004 (numbers rounded)

Region	Patient numbers			Prevalence values (per million population)		
	ESRD	Dialysis (HD + PD)	Transplant	ESRD	Dialysis (HD + PD)	Transplant
Global	1 783 000	1 371 000	412 000	280	215	65
North America	492 000	337 000	154 000	1505	1030	470
Europe	473 000	324 000	149 000	585	400	185
(thereof EU)	(387 000)	(252 000)	(135 000)	(850)	(550)	(295)
Japan	261 000	248 000	13 000	2045	1945	100
Asia (excluding Japan)	237 000	196 000	41 000	70	60	10
Latin America	205 000	170 000	35 000	380	320	65
Africa	61 000	57 000	5000	70	65	5
Middle East	54 000	39 000	15 000	190	140	55

HD, haemodialysis; PD, peritoneal dialysis.
(From Grassmann A, et al. (2005). ESRD patients in 2004: global overview of patient numbers, treatment modalities and associated trends. Nephrol Dial Transplant, **20**, 2587–93, with permission.)

owing to higher acceptance rates of patients over 65 years of age and of those with comorbidities.

It has long been known that endstage renal disease is much more frequent in older people than in young people. Based on European Renal Association/European Dialysis and Transplant Association (ERA/EDTA) Registry data, Jager et al. found a four- to fivefold increase in the incidence and prevalence of RRT over the period 1985 to 1999, and in 1999 no fewer than 48% of new patients were above age 65 years, leading to their referring to RRT as an epidemic of ageing. In this context, it is also of interest that the long-term function of kidney grafts obtained from elderly donors, irrespective of whether they were live donors or cadaveric, is inferior to the function of kidney grafts from younger donors. As typical signs of senescence, telomere length is reduced, repair capacity is curtailed, and the kidneys of older people are generally hypoperfused as a consequence of vascular sclerosis.

It is of interest that the incidence of new patients requiring RRT does not parallel the prevalence of CKD stages 3 and 4. Despite similar prevalences of CKD stages 3 and 4, the incidence of CKD patients requiring RRT in Norway is significantly lower than in white patients in the United States of America. This is explained not by high mortality prior to endstage renal disease, but by more effective intervention with progression of CKD to stage 5, an observation that illustrates the great benefit of dedicated nephrological care for patients with advanced CKD.

Causes of CKD

The usual sources for descriptions of the causes of CKD are endstage renal failure databases. These are flawed for many reasons: diagnoses are often allocated as 'best guesses' by clinicians; there is no universal agreement on the meaning of terms such as 'pyelonephritis'; glomerulonephritis may be diagnosed without histological proof; hypertension is often cited when it may be no more than a consequence of whatever caused the renal failure. With these important caveats in mind, Table 21.6.4 lists the given causes of endstage renal failure in recent reports from the United Kingdom Renal Registry, the Australia and New Zealand Dialysis and Transplant Registry, and the US Renal Data Systems. Less common causes of chronic renal failure are given in Box 21.6.1. Note that

some causes of chronic renal failure that are uncommon from a global perspective, e.g. Balkan nephropathy and HIV nephropathy, may be very common in some populations.

As stated above, in most countries diabetic nephropathy has become the single most frequent cause of endstage renal disease. In contrast to previous years, the relative contribution of glomerulonephritis has substantially decreased, and the diagnosis of 'pyelonephritis', i.e. the concept that chronic bacterial colonization of the kidney and of the urinary tract causes chronic loss of renal function even in the absence of malformation or urological disease, has increasingly been abandoned on the basis of follow-up studies in cohorts of subjects with uncomplicated chronic urinary tract

Table 21.6.4 Percentage distribution of primary renal diagnosis in patients starting on renal replacement therapy

Diagnosis	UKRR[a]	ANZDATA[b]	USRDS[c]
Uncertain	26.2[d]	5	4
Diabetes[e]	22.2	32	44.8
Glomerulonephritis	10.4[f]	23[g]	8.5
Chronic pyelonephritis[h]	7.2	4	0.5
Renal vascular disease	6.8	Not specified	1.9[i]
Adult polycystic kidney disease	6.7	6	2.2
Hypertension[j]	5.4	15	25.2
Other[k]	15.3	15	13.3

ANZDATA, Australia and New Zealand Dialysis and Transplant Registry (2007 report); UKRR, United Kingdom Renal Registry (December 2007 report); USRDS, United States Renal Data Systems (2005 report).
[a] Data from 5343 patients beginning dialysis in United Kingdom renal units in 2006 for whom a primary renal diagnosis was reported.
[b] Data from all 2378 patients beginning dialysis in Australian renal units in 2006.
[c] Data from 484 998 incident patients from 1999 to 2003.
[d] Also includes "glomerulonephritis not proven by biopsy".
[e] It can be impossible to know whether diabetes is a cause of endstage renal failure or merely an association.
[f] 100% biopsy proven.
[g] 76% biopsy proven.
[h] Patients diagnosed as having "reflux nephropathy" are included under this heading.
[i] Classified as a subgroup of "hypertension".
[j] Reporting practices varied widely and variation in attribution of hypertension as a cause almost certainly does not reflect real differences in causation of endstage renal failure.
[k] Includes urinary obstruction.

Box 21.6.1 Less common causes of chronic renal failure

Metabolic
Cystinosis, cystinuria (stones), oxalosis, nephrocalcinosis, urate nephropathy.

Hereditary
Alport's syndrome, Fabry's disease, tuberous sclerosis, sickle cell disease, medullary cystic disease (and the metabolic conditions listed above).

Vasculitides and other multisystem disorders
Wegener's granulomatosis, microscopic polyangiitis, polyarteritis nodosa, Henoch–Schönlein purpura, systemic lupus erythematosus, scleroderma, sarcoidosis.

Malignancy
Renal cell cancer, von Hippel–Lindau disease, lymphoma.

Dysproteinaemias
Myeloma, primary (AL) and secondary (AA) amyloid, cryoglobulinaemia.

Structural/infection/interstitial
Cystic disease other than autosomal dominant polycystic kidney disease, congenital and acquired abnormalities of the lower urinary tract, tuberculosis and schistosomiasis, Balkan nephropathy, Chinese herb nephropathy, analgesic nephropathy, nephrotoxic metals, radiation nephropathy.

Other
Haemolytic uraemic syndrome, postpartum renal failure, acute cortical necrosis, accelerated ('malignant') hypertension, HIV nephropathy.

---

infection who failed to develop CKD in the absence of additional pathologies. It is of note, however, that in aboriginal populations the spectrum of renal disease is strikingly different, and this is also true for immigrant populations, including in the United Kingdom, who have an excess of diabetic nephropathy and a variety of renal diseases which are less frequently or rarely seen in white patients, e.g. renal tuberculosis, sickle cell anaemia nephropathy, and HIV nephropathy.

Detailed discussion of particular causes of CKD can be found in other chapters.

Pathophysiology of CKD

As kidney function gradually fails, compensatory mechanisms generally maintain acceptable health until the GFR is about 10 to 15 ml/min, and patients will not usually die of renal failure until the GFR is less than 5 ml/min. The remarkable capacity of renal function to adapt to maintain overall homeostasis in the face of such dramatic reduction in glomerular filtration is best understood on the basis of the 'intact nephron' hypothesis and the 'trade-off' hypothesis.

The intact nephron hypothesis, first articulated by Bricker, states that despite a widened range of single-nephron GFR in damaged or diseased kidneys, glomerular and tubular function remains closely integrated in all individual nephrons, both normal and damaged. As the GFR of the whole kidney falls, those nephrons that are still functioning produce an increased volume of filtrate (hyperfiltration), and their tubules respond appropriately for overall homeostasis by excreting fluid and solutes in amounts that maintain external balance, although the capacity for adaptation is variable. For sodium and potassium, compensation can occur down to GFR as low as 5 ml/min, but this cannot be achieved for phosphate and urate, plasma concentrations of which may be elevated when the GFR falls below 20 ml/min in some patients.

The trade-off hypothesis recognizes that the functional adaptations required to maintain overall homeostasis come at a price and that they contribute to changes characteristic of the syndrome of uraemia. The best example of such a trade-off is the generation of hyperparathyroidism. As GFR falls, leading (if there were no compensation) to a reduction in phosphate excretion and a rise in serum phosphate, the serum parathyroid hormone concentration rises and serves to maintain homeostasis by reducing tubular reabsorption of phosphate. However, a consequence is secondary (and sometimes tertiary) hyperparathyroidism, with adverse effects on blood vessels and bones.

Electrolyte, water, and acid–base homeostasis

An inability to concentrate the urine in the face of dehydration is sometimes the first symptom of chronic renal failure, manifesting as polyuria, nocturia and thirst. This is particularly likely in conditions that predominantly affect the renal medulla, e.g. obstructive uropathy, interstitial nephritides, medullary cystic disease. By contrast, urinary diluting capacity is preserved until renal failure is advanced, at which time urinary osmolality becomes fixed at around 300 mOsm/kg (roughly isotonic with plasma) and there is obligatory polyuria. It should be noted, however, that although urinary diluting capacity is maintained until late in chronic renal failure, large water loads are excreted more slowly than in normal subjects and excessive intake (by drinking or ill-advised iatrogenic infusion of dextrose-containing solutions) can lead to symptomatic hyponatraemia (see Chapter 21.2.1).

As renal function decreases, sodium balance and extracellular fluid volume are maintained until GFR is less than about 10 ml/min by an increase in the fractional excretion of sodium (the amount excreted in the urine as a fraction of that filtered at the glomerulus) from 1% (normal) to 30%. This capacity for adaptation is overwhelmed in advanced chronic renal failure, with sodium retention manifest as hypertension and/or oedema (peripheral and/or pulmonary). Such patients can also be at increased risk of sodium depletion as they are unable to restrict sodium excretion promptly in response to stimuli that would normally be expected to lead to such restriction, e.g. diarrhoea, vomiting. A few patients with modest impairment of GFR (e.g. CKD stage 3), usually with diseases affecting the medulla, may present with low blood pressure (often with a postural drop) due to sodium depletion caused by a urinary sodium leak: sodium supplements may be required.

Most patients maintain normal external potassium balance until their GFR is less than 5 ml/min, but their capacity to excrete potassium is limited and severe hyperkalaemia may follow a sudden reduction in GFR such as might be caused by intercurrent illness, excess dietary intake, or prescription of drugs that impair potassium excretion (ACE inhibitors, angiotensin receptor blockers, potassium-sparing diuretics). Some patients, particularly those with diabetes mellitus and/or interstitial nephritis, may develop hyperkalaemia due to hyporeninaemic hypoaldosteronism at levels of GFR that would not otherwise be expected to cause problems with potassium homeostasis. Hyperkalaemia is often the immediate life-threatening consideration in the management of patients with renal failure. See Chapters 21.2.2 and 21.5 for further discussion.

The kidney normally maintains acid–base homeostasis by reabsorbing filtered bicarbonate, acidifying urinary buffers, and excreting ammonia. Increasing acidosis tends to occur at a GFR of less than 10 ml/min, and is more likely to be an early feature in diseases that primarily affect the tubules and interstitium (aside from the renal tubular acidoses, where there are specific defects in acid–base homeostasis—see Chapter 21.15).

Abnormalities of calcium and phosphate homeostasis are discussed later in this chapter.

Endocrine dysfunction

In CKD, hormone concentrations may be elevated as a result of reduced degradation (e.g. insulin) or increased secretion in response to metabolic changes (e.g. parathyroid hormone), or reduced by impaired production (e.g. 1,25-dihydroxyvitamin D, erythropoietin, oestrogen, testosterone). Reductions in hormone-binding proteins, e.g. through protein losses in patients with nephrotic syndrome or on peritoneal dialysis, are common and may affect levels of free hormones circulating in the blood. Effects on vitamin D and erythropoietin are discussed later in this chapter.

Total thyroxine (T_4) and T_3 (tri-iodothyronine) may be low, with impaired peripheral deiodination of T_4 to T_3 and preferential diversion to inactive metabolites. However, patients are not clinically hypothyroid, and levels of thyroid-stimulating hormone (TSH) are generally normal and can be used in the usual way as a diagnostic test for hypothyroidism.

The kidney is the main site of growth hormone degradation and plasma levels of growth hormone are abnormally high in patients with renal failure because of this, and also because of alterations in hypothalamic–pituitary control. It is not clear whether or not this has any clinical impact in adults with renal failure, but in children with renal failure and growth restriction the impaired production of insulin-like growth factor 1 can be overcome by treatment with supraphysiological doses of recombinant growth hormone.

Decreased insulin clearances seems to be balanced by increased peripheral resistance to the effects of insulin, hence patients with renal failure are not prone to hypoglycaemia or diabetes, but there is a reduced requirement for exogenous insulin in people with diabetes as renal function declines.

Prolactin levels are high in renal failure and may contribute to gynaecomastia and sexual dysfunction in men and to infertility in women. Men with CKD may also have testosterone levels that are low to normal, with raised gonadotropins implying that testicular failure is the cause. The pituitary–ovarian access is disturbed in advanced renal failure, with many cycles anovulatory, causing oestrogen deficiency.

Middle molecules and the uraemic syndrome

Many of the clinical manifestations that are seen with progressive decline in renal function are attributable to derangements in fluid balance, electrolyte handling, and endocrine function as described above. However, these derangements do not provide adequate explanation for all clinical features, and it is assumed that those which are unexplained are due to retention of substances and metabolites that the failing kidney is unable to excrete. The nature of these 'uraemic toxins' is uncertain. Accumulation of urea itself has modest effects, and failure to excrete a variety of small water-soluble compounds, protein-bound compounds, and 'middle molecules' (meaning those whose molecular weight in the range 500–12 000 Da) is held responsible, although incriminating specific toxins has proved difficult. Among the small water-soluble compounds, those thought to have a role in the uraemic syndrome include various guanidine compounds, oxalate, phosphates and polyamines; and among the protein-bound compounds, p-cresol and p-cresylsulphate, homocysteine, various indoles, and furan-proprionic acid. The best-characterized example of a uraemic middle molecule is β_2-microglobulin, which is normally excreted by the kidneys, reaches a blood concentration 30 times higher than normal in dialysis patients, and accumulates as β_2-microglobulin amyloid in joints and bone. Many of the other middle molecules that have been incriminated have a proinflammatory effect, including a variety of advanced glycosylation endproducts that are probably attributable to increased concentrations of small carbonyl precursors in uraemia (and not to hyperglycaemia).

Progression of CKD

Brenner advanced the concept that the adaptive changes (described above) aimed at increasing the excretory capacity of the kidney are maladaptive in the long run, causing deterioration of renal function mainly as a result of glomerulosclerosis and tubulointerstitial fibrosis, the final result being endstage renal disease. The adaptive changes leading to single-nephron hyperfiltration, which sustains whole-kidney GFR in the short term, are mediated by a reduction of the resistance of the afferent preglomerular arterioles and an increase of the angiotensin-II-dependent resistance of the postglomerular efferent arterioles, which combine to raise intraglomerular capillary pressure (glomerular hypertension). Over time, however, GFR will decrease, driven by several pathogenic mechanisms, including proteinuria and oxidative stress.

This hypothesis led not only to the introduction of remarkably effective therapeutic and preventive approaches aimed at interfering with progression (see below), it also had repercussions concerning the relation between GFR and metabolic abnormalities in CKD. The Mild and Moderate Kidney Disease (MMKD) study found an increase in the plasma concentration of asymmetric dimethyl L-arginine (ADMA), even when whole-kidney GFR was still normal. The same was true for apolipoprotein abnormalities and sympathetic overactivity. A plausible explanation for these findings, despite normal whole-kidney GFR, is loss of nephrons with associated loss of metabolic capacity while whole-kidney GFR is still normal because of single-nephron hyperfiltration, hence having a normal GFR does not exclude functional renal abnormalities.

The rate of progression of CKD varies considerably depending on age, gender, type of underlying renal disease, genetics (family history of renal disease and cardiovascular disease), and many other factors. For a given primary kidney disease, the risk of progression is lower in premenopausal women than in men. Such gender difference is not found in children or postmenopausal women. This finding points to the role of sex hormones, which has also been documented in experimental studies. Testosterone aggravates renal disease, possibly by raising blood pressure and activating the renin–angiotensin system, whereas oestrogens ameliorate the evolution of renal disease.

Some types of renal disease tend to progress slowly and others rapidly: adult polycystic kidney disease, renal dysplasia, IgA-glomerulonephritis, and membranous glomerulonephritis usually progress slowly; rapid progression is anticipated in antiglomerular basement membrane glomerulonephritis and vasculitis; and intermediate rates of progression are typical in diabetic nephropathy.

Ethnicity also determines the renal risk for currently poorly understood reasons: in Australian aboriginals, Maoris, American Indians, and particularly individuals of African descent, the frequency of CKD and the rate of its progression are substantially higher than in white people. This has been particularly well documented in the immigrant population from south Asia living in the United Kingdom. A powerful predictor of the renal risk is a positive family history, not only of CKD but also of cardiovascular events in first-degree relatives, which is associated with a substantial increase in the risk of developing progressive kidney disease.

A relatively new insight is that a history of pre-eclampsia is associated with a dramatic increase in the risk of developing overt kidney disease later in life. Similarly, faulty prenatal programming *in utero* plays a role in the onset and progression of CKD. This is part and parcel of the Barker hypothesis, according to which interference with organogenesis in the prenatal period predisposes an individual at adult age to CKD, hypertension and the metabolic syndrome.

Although such non modifiable predictors are of some interest, more important clinically are modifiable predictors associated with a higher rate of progression (Box 21.6.2). It has been well documented that blood pressure has an adverse effect on progression of CKD, and this is true even for values below the former definition of hypertension (above 140/90 mmHg). This finding has greatly increased the ability to interfere with progression, and the same is true for measures to interfere with the activation of the renin–angiotensin system to reduce proteinuria.

Of major clinical importance is the fact that while renal function tends to deteriorate progressively in many (but not all) patients with CKD, almost exclusively this is true only in patients with albuminuria/proteinuria. The increased risk of cardiovascular events and cardiovascular death in patients with albuminuria/proteinuria has already been emphasized (Table 21.6.2).

Clinical presentation

The various presentations of renal disease are discussed in Chapter 21.3, but in brief the clinical presentation of CKD depends on the degree of renal dysfunction at the time that the condition is recognized.

Asymptomatic patients

At one extreme are patients with no symptoms whatsoever in whom an abnormal eGFR and/or proteinuria are detected on routine examination, such as an insurance medical. Such patients may be shocked when hearing for the first time that they have lost what might be a substantial amount of their kidney function. Counselling and persuading them to comply with follow-up and to

---

Box 21.6.2 Modifiable and nonmodifiable predictors of the rate of progression of CKD

Nonmodifiable predictors

- Age
- Gender
- History of pre-eclampsia
- Ethnicity
- Genetics (family history—renal and cardiovascular)
- Type of renal disease
- Prenatal programming (e.g. maternal hyperglycaemia, malnutrition, pre-eclampsia, low birthweight)

Modifiable predictors

- Elevated (systolic) blood pressure (particularly during the night)
- Activation of renin–angiotensin system
- Proteinuria
- Smoking
- Salt intake
- Obesity/metabolic syndrome
- Protein intake?

---

take medications occasionally proves difficult. Illnesses known to cause CKD, such as autosomal dominant polycystic kidney disease, other hereditary kidney diseases, or diabetic nephropathy, are generally easier to manage because these patients are more likely to understand the progressive nature of CKD and the benefit of treatment to prevent or slow progression.

Patients with associated disease

The presence of CKD may be diagnosed in many medical contexts in the absence of any symptoms pointing to the kidneys, e.g. outpatient clinics for hypertension, diabetes, cardiac disorders, or urological diseases.

Symptomatic presentation

In relatively few patients is the diagnosis of CKD made on the basis of symptoms or signs pointing to kidney disease, such as nocturia, foaming of the urine, facial or pedal oedema, or haematuria. Symptoms or signs pointing to advanced CKD include (among others) lethargy, personality change, changes in mentation, loss of appetite, nausea (often in the morning), and vomiting. These may or may not be accompanied by evidence of hypervolaemia, such as dyspnoea on exertion or at rest, swollen ankles/legs, elevated venous pressure, cardiomegaly, or basal crackles, and often only fluid removal can decide whether such manifestations are the result of fluid retention caused by renal failure, or by cardiac disease, and not infrequently they are the result of both. The final stage of uraemia is heralded by bleeding tendency, pericarditis, obtundation, and coma. See Chapter 21.3 for further discussion.

A relatively common clinical challenge to renal services is patients who present as an acute emergency requiring urgent RRT.

Box 21.6.3 Indications of chronic renal failure

History
More than 6 months' ill health, long-standing hypertension, proteinuria, nocturia for more than 6 months, sexual dysfunction, abnormalities previously detected during routine medicals and/or pregnancies, recurrent illness during childhood

Examination
Pallor, pigmentation, pruritus, brown nails, evidence of longstanding hypertension; the patient often appears 'well' for their very abnormal biochemistry

Investigations
Normochromic anaemia, small kidneys on ultrasound (except in diabetes, amyloid, myeloma, or adult polycystic kidney disease), renal osteodystrophy on radiography (this is rarely found but is conclusive evidence if present)

Box 21.6.4 Causes of acute deterioration in patients with chronic renal failure.

◆ Renal hypoperfusion:
  • Dehydration—diarrhoea, vomiting, excessive diuretics, inadequate fluid replacement (e.g. postsurgical)
  • Cardiac failure
  • Drugs—especially ACE inhibitors, angiotensin receptor blockers, NSAIDs
  • systemic infection
  • Renal vascular disease
  • Pericardial tamponade (rare)
◆ Obstruction and infection of the urinary tract:
  • Benign prostatic hypertrophy
  • Urinary stones
  • Cancer—particularly of prostate or bladder
  • Clot in the ureter
  • Papillary necrosis and sloughing—to be considered in patients with diabetes, sickle cell disease, and analgaesic nephropathy.
  • Polycystic cysts (rare)
◆ Metabolic and toxic:
  • Hypercalcaemia
  • Hyperuricaemia
  • Contrast media—especially in diabetes
  • Drugs—especially aminoglycosides
◆ Progression/relapse of underlying diseases:
  • Various nephritides and autoimmune/vasculitic conditions—look for an active urinary sediment with proteinuria, haematuria, and cellular casts, and also for serological evidence of disease activity
◆ Development of accelerated-phase hypertension
◆ Renal vein thrombosis—usually in severely nephrotic patients
◆ Pregnancy:
  • At the end of the pregnancy or after delivery, e.g. in patients with reflux nephropathy

ACE, angiotensin converting enzyme; NSAIDs, nonsteroidal antiinflammatory drugs.

This is not infrequently due to late referral, but it is not uncommon for there to be an acute deterioration of renal function in patients with pre-existing CKD as a result of intercurrent illness or medical interventions, e.g. cardiac decompensation from myocardial infarction or arrhythmia, hypovolaemia, exposure to radiocontrast media, or prescription of particular drugs. Regarding the latter, common culprits would be the new prescription of ACE inhibitors or angiotensin-II receptor blockers, particularly in patients with advanced CKD in the presence of hypovolaemia, heart failure, or other conditions activating the renin–angiotensin system. NSAIDs are also commonly incriminated, with other possibilities being nephrotoxic antibiotics (e.g aminoglycosides) and *cis*-platinum.

When a patient arrives in hospital as an 'acute uraemic emergency' it is important to determine whether the problem is acute kidney injury (acute renal failure, which may be entirely reversible), acute-on-chronic kidney failure (when recovery to previous baseline renal function may be possible), or the endstage of progressive chronic kidney failure (which by definition is not reversible). The only infallible method of determining whether a patient has CKD is to find documentation of previously reduced GFR indicated by past measurement of serum creatinine. When this is not available it is sometimes simply not possible to be sure of the situation at the time of presentation, although ultrasonography with documentation of small kidneys is often of great help in indicating chronicity.

Features that suggest the presence of chronic renal failure are shown in Box 21.6.3, and causes of acute deterioration of chronic renal failure are shown in Box 21.6.4.

Clinical assessment

Personal history

When taking the personal history, it is important to ask about nocturia (which may be the first, although nonspecific, sign of renal disease), foaming of the urine, past or present periorbital or pedal oedema, episodes of macroscopic haematuria, and whether or not urinary abnormalities (proteinuria, haematuria) have been detected previously, e.g. in medical examinations performed before military service or for occupational or insurance purposes. The information that the patient was told that they had 'a bit of protein/blood in the urine' many years ago (and almost certainly 'not to worry about it') clearly indicates long-standing renal pathology in the context of a patient presenting with renal impairment.

In women, information on proteinuria in pregnancy or preeclampsia is important. A history of pre-eclampsia greatly increases the risk of CKD later in life, and pregnancy often leads to the first manifestation or aggravation of pre-existing renal disease.

In elderly men, a history of prostatic disease or related lower urinary tract symptoms (problems with bladder emptying, dribbling, etc.) should raise the suspicion of obstructive nephropathy.

Also important when evaluating a patient with CKD are episodes of urinary tract infection before and after puberty, as well as a history of urolithiasis. A history of urinary stones may point to a urological cause of renal failure, and may also very occasionally be an indication of hyperparathyroidism.

In proteinuric patients with CKD of unknown origin, one should enquire for a history of chronic bacterial infection, e.g. bronchiectasis or osteomyelitis, and for a history of rheumatoid arthritis, all of which are potential causes of secondary amyloidosis. Particularly in older people with CKD of unknown origin, it is also important to ask regarding symptoms that might indicate multiple myeloma, which can cause renal impairment via a number of mechanisms (see Chapter 21.10.4).

The patient should be asked about the use of potentially nephrotoxic drugs, such as NSAIDs, analgesics (if taken regularly in high dose for prolonged periods, particularly compound preparations or those containing phenacetin, which has now been banned in many countries), nephrotoxic antibiotics (e.g. aminoglycosides), antineoplastic agents (*cis*-platinum), and herbal/alternative/homeopathic treatments (e.g. Chinese herbs; see Chapter 21.9.2). Covert drug intake, including laxatives and diuretics with or without surreptitious vomiting, may also cause chronic kidney disease. Since many drugs are excreted via the kidney, it is also important to ask patients with chronic kidney disease for a history of drug side effects.

Women with CKD may have menorrhagia or (in advanced CKD) amenorrhoea, and men with CKD not infrequently have erectile failure/impotence, but few will volunteer this information and it will only be discovered by the physician who asks directly.

Symptoms of advanced renal failure (uraemia)

With advancing renal failure to CKD stage 5, patients may develop anaemia and fluid retention manifested as breathlessness on exercise or even at rest, particularly at night-time, and they may notice swelling of their ankles and legs. The first symptoms pointing to the uraemic syndrome are anorexia with attendant loss of body weight and nausea and vomiting, frequently in the morning when brushing the teeth.

Further symptoms are superimposed if a patient enters the preterminal phase of uraemia, including severe dyspnoea as the combined result of metabolic acidosis and pulmonary congestion, pericarditic and pleuritic chest pains, bleeding tendency (bleeding mouth ulcers, gastrointestinal haemorrhage), numbness of the feet (polyneuropathy), and insomnia, headache, myoclonic jerks, and impairment of consciousness/coma.

Family history

It is important to ask for a family history of renal disease, the most common causes of familial nephropathy being autosomal dominant polycystic kidney disease and reflux nephropathy; see Chapter 21.13 for further discussion. If the patient has a history of hypertension, then concomitant proteinuria or diabetes should be sought, because very often these will be undiagnosed. Patients with type 2 diabetes who have a family history of diabetic nephropathy are at higher risk of nephropathy themselves.

A patient's risk of progressive kidney disease is greater if a first-degree relative has had any kind of CKD, even if this was not caused by the same kidney disease as that in the patient, suggesting that hereditary mechanisms are involved in the genesis of progression. Furthermore, the renal risk is higher if a first-degree relative has had essential hypertension or cardiovascular events.

Physical examination

Except in areas of world with very poor access to medical services, or in individuals who are severely neglected, the physician will rarely see the desperate case of terminal uraemia with coma, blindness from retinopathy, pericardial rub from uraemic pericarditis, massive gastrointestinal ulceration and bleeding, and urea frost covering the face. Patients with CKD stage 5 who are typically seen in Western countries may be pale (anaemic), have severe hypertension, and have fluid retention manifested as peripheral oedema and crackles/effusions in the lungs. As uraemia progresses, patients usually develop progressive hyperpigmentation of the skin, pruritus with excoriations and prurigo, xerosis, brown nails, and evidence of peripheral polyneuropathy.

Further signs are superimposed if a patient enters the preterminal phase of uraemia, including severe tachypnoea (before terminal cessation of breathing) with an acidotic sighing respiratory pattern and/or widespread crackles of pulmonary oedema, jerking movements (metabolic asterixis/flap/twitching), pericarditic and/or pleuritic rubs, impairment of consciousness/coma, red eyes, and evidence of bleeding (from mouth or rectum).

In routine outpatient practice, all patients presenting with CKD require a thorough general physical examination with particular attention to the features described in Table 21.6.5. Rarely there will be manifestations of systemic or genetic disorders associated with renal disease (see Chapters 21.10.1–21.10.9 and 21.12).

Investigation

Investigations required in the assessment of patients with CKD are shown in Table 21.6.6. See Chapter 21.4 for further discussion.

Management to prevent progression of CKD

In some patients, measures to conserve renal function may be specific to the cause of renal impairment, e.g. relief of obstruction, cessation of nephrotoxic drugs (e.g. lithium, ciclosporin, NSAIDs), relief of renal artery stenosis, and treatment of active autoimmune/vasculitic disorders. For further details, see the relevant specific chapters. However, the mechanisms of progression described briefly above are common to all forms of CKD, and insight into them has provided effective strategies aimed at slowing or—when started early—even halting progression of CKD. Since not all patients with primary kidney disease inevitably progress to end-stage renal disease, it is important to identify factors predisposing to an adverse renal outcome in individual patients—the main ones being high blood pressure (particularly at night-time), proteinuria, and reduced baseline eGFR—and to direct particular attention towards to such cases.

It is recommended that all patients with CKD stages 4 and 5 (also those with CKD stage 3 whose GFR is deteriorating rapidly—meaning by more than 5 ml/min per year—or who have significant proteinuria/haematuria), excepting those who are

Table 21.6.5 Features to look for on physical examination of patients with CKD

System	Feature	Comment
General	Pallor	Anaemia is a common feature of advanced CKD
	Pigmentation, scratch marks, brown nails	Indicate long-standing CKD
Cardiovascular/respiratory	Blood pressure	Hypertension is a common association (but uncommon cause) of CKD
	Elevated jugular venous pressure, enlarged heart, gallop rhythm, mitral regurgitant murmur, pulmonary crackles, peripheral oedema	Manifestations of fluid overload caused by CKD and/or cardiac failure associated with hypertension or 'uraemia'
	Aortic systolic murmur	Valvular calcification is more common in CKD
	Peripheral pulses, vascular bruits	Absence of pulses and/or presence of bruits increase the likelihood of renovascular disease as the cause of CKD
Abdominal	Palpable kidneys	Likely to indicate adult polycystic kidney disease in this context
	Palpable bladder, malignant-feeling prostate on digital examination	Consider urinary obstruction as cause of CKD
	Hernias	Require repair if peritoneal dialysis otherwise preferred as RRT
Neurological	Peripheral neuropathy	Indicates long-standing CKD
	Proximal myopathy	Indicates long-standing CKD
Rheumatological	Arthritis	Gout and pseudogout are associated with CKD
	Carpal tunnel syndrome	
Ocular fundi	Features of hypertension	

CKD, chronic kidney disease; RRT, renal replacement therapy.

terminally ill or for whom it would otherwise be inappropriate, are referred to and managed by or in conjunction with a nephrologist. This is important because appropriate timely intervention can reduce the rate of progression and also because the results of eventual dialysis and/or transplantation are better if the patient has been properly prepared (including blood pressure normalization, correction of anaemia, hepatitis B vaccination, creation of vascular access, and the search for a living kidney donor that might render pre-emptive transplantation possible).

Interventions to prevent progression of CKD should be initiated as early as possible, which justifies efforts to diagnose renal disease sooner rather than later. The best evidence comes from studies of patients with diabetes. Controlled trials in advanced diabetic nephropathy achieved reduction of progression by no more than about 30%. By contrast, in diabetic patients with early nephropathy, mostly at the stage of microalbuminuria, the DETAIL study had achieved by its fifth year a rate of loss of GFR that was virtually indistinguishable from that seen with advancing age. Even if progression is not completely halted, but only attenuated, the gain in years free of RRT is substantially greater if treatment is started early rather than late.

Blood pressure control

Although the adverse effects of high blood pressure on progression of renal disease had been recognized for many years, the first solid documentation of the importance of achieved blood pressure on progression was provided only in 1989, when a study of patients of the Kaiser Permanente cohort in the United States of America who had normal baseline urinary findings found that even within the range of normotensive values the risk of reaching endstage renal disease increased progressively with progressively higher blood pressure values at baseline (more so in patients with than without diabetes).

There is limited information on the target blood pressure and the role of different antihypertensive agents, but the consensus is that the lower the blood pressure, the better, as long as this can be achieved without unacceptable side effects. The guidelines of the European Society of Hypertension/European Society of Cardiology on treatment of hypertension state:

> Protection against progression of renal dysfunction has two major requirements: strict blood pressure control (<130/80 mmHg), and even lower if proteinuria is >1 g/day, and lowering of proteinuria to values as near to normal as possible. To achieve the blood pressure goal, combination therapy of several antihypertensive agents (including loop diuretics) is usually required. To reduce proteinuria, an angiotensin receptor blocker, and ACE inhibitor, or a combination of both are required.

It obviously needs to be considered whether such aggressive blood pressure lowering is safe. No excess of cardiovascular events or of mortality has been reported in nondiabetic patients and patients without coronary disease, although in older people limited tolerance and safety (orthostatic hypotension, falls) of intensive blood pressure lowering have to be taken into account. By contrast, higher mortality in patients with advanced diabetic nephropathy has been found with an achieved systolic blood pressure below 120 mmHg, and in nonrenal patients with coronary heart disease the rate of myocardial infarction has been reported to be increased if diastolic blood pressure is lowered to below 70 mm/Hg, hence some caution is indicated in populations at high cardiovascular risk, including those with CKD.

The most important predictor of progressive loss of renal function is the systolic blood pressure, not the mean or the diastolic blood pressure. Of particular concern in renal patients is the tendency for an attenuated decrease of blood pressure—or even a paradoxical increase—at night-time, recognition of which requires the use of ambulatory blood pressure measurements. Because of the complexity of blood pressure analysis and the limited accuracy of office blood pressure measurements, it is bad advice to stick only to fixed blood pressure targets—particularly since almost all studies have shown that the proportion of renal patients reaching target blood pressure values is disappointingly low, despite the use of multidrug regimens.

Table 21.6.6 Investigations required in the assessment of patients with CKD

Type of investigation/test	Comment
All patients	
Urine	
Dipstick	Screening for proteinuria, haematuria, glycosuria, nitrite, pyuria. Heavy proteinuria suggests glomerular disease
Microscopy	If abnormality on stick testing to detect bacteriuria, quantitate pyuria, look for cellular casts (indicative of renal inflammatory process)
Albumin:creatinine ratio (ACR)	To quantitate proteinuria
Culture	To detect urinary tract infection. For tuberculosis if clinically indicated (sterile pyuria)
Blood	
Creatinine	To quantitate level of renal function by eGFR
Electrolytes	Hyperkalaemia is the obvious concern
Urea	Elevated out of proportion to creatinine in dehydration and catabolism
Glucose	Exclusion of diabetes mellitus
Lipids	Assessment of cardiovascular risk
Full blood count	To detect anaemia
Liver and bone profile	Routine screen
Cardiac assessment	
ECG	Look for changes of ischaemia and/or left ventricular hypertrophy. Changes in morphology due to hyperkalaemia indicate the level of risk of cardiac arrhythmia and dictate treatment (see Chapter 21.5)
Chest radiograph	Assessment of heart size and evidence of fluid overload (pulmonary oedema, pleural effusion)
Renal imaging	
Ultrasonography of urinary tract	Expect to find two small and echogenic kidneys in CKD; exclude urinary obstruction; diagnose presence of renal cysts
In selected patients to diagnose particular causes of CKD	
Urine	
Bence Jones proteinuria	To detect myeloma when clinically appropriate
Blood	
Serum protein electrophoresis	To detect myeloma when clinically appropriate
Autoimmune/vasculitis screen—ANA, complement, ANCA, anti-GBM, cryoglobulins	To detect autoimmune (systemic lupus erythematosus) and vasculitic (Wegener's granulomatosis, microscopic polyangiitis) conditions, also Goodpasture's disease and cryoglobulinaemia, when clinically relevant
Renal imaging	
Plain abdominal film (KUB)	To look for urinary stones and/or renal calcification
CT scan	To determine cause of urinary obstruction
Renal angiography	If renal artery stenosis is likely
DMSA/MAG3 scan	To detect renal scarring
Renal biopsy	To be performed only in cases where there is diagnostic doubt and there is a reasonable likelihood that the result will affect the management of the particular patient. Should not be done otherwise
In patients with significantly impaired renal function (CKD stages 3B, 4, or 5) to look for complications of renal impairment and/or guide management	
Blood	
PTH	To diagnose hyperparathyroidism and monitor response to treatment
Bicarbonate	To detect acidosis and monitor response to treatment
Uric acid	In patients with gout associated with CKD
Haematinics—iron studies, vitamin B_{12}, folate	In patients with anaemia. Optimal response to erythropoietin (see later) requires plentiful iron stores (high normal/high ferritin)
Virology—screen for hepatitis C, hepatitis B, HIV	Relevant to RRT with dialysis or by transplantation
Virology—screen for CMV, HSV, HZV, EBV	Relevant to RRT by transplantation
Blood group	Relevant to RRT by transplantation

Table 21.6.6 (*cont'd*) Investigations required in the assessment of patients with CKD

Type of investigation/test	Comment
Cardiac assessment	
Echocardiogram	To assess left ventricular function. To exclude pericardial effusion when clinically appropriate
Tests for coronary heart disease—exercise tolerance test, radionuclide stress test, coronary angiography	If symptomatic. To assess risk of and fitness for renal transplantation
Imaging	
Radiographs of hands	To look for changes of renal osteodystrophy

ANA, antinuclear antibodies; ANCA, antineutrophil cytoplasmic antibodies; anti-GBM, antiglomerular basement membrane antibody; CKD, chronic kidney disease; CMV, cytomegalovirus; DMSA, dimercaptosuccinic acid; EBV, Epstein–Barr virus; ECG, electrocardiogram; HSV, herpes simplex virus; HZV, herpes zoster virus; KUB, kidneys, ureter, and bladder; MAG3, mercaptoacetyltriglycine; PTH, parathyroid hormone; RRT, renal replacement therapy.

Selection of antihypertensive agents

There is good evidence from experimental studies that activation of the renin–angiotensin system (RAS) and of the sympathetic nervous system play a major causal role in the genesis of progression. There has been some controversy over whether the effect of antihypertensive agents interfering with the activity of the RAS is exclusively explained by lowering of blood pressure. Considering controlled intervention trials where similar blood pressure lowering was achieved with antihypertensive agents that did and did not block the RAS, it is obvious that a definite but limited contribution to the slowing of progression is achieved by RAS blockade. An example of the finding of such a trial is shown in Fig. 21.6.1.

A head-to-head comparison, although somewhat underpowered, suggested that the effect of ACE inhibition and angiotensin receptor blockade is comparable in magnitude with respect to halting progression of renal disease. The blockade of the RAS is effective and safe, if properly supervised, but the risk of hyperkalaemia has to be taken into consideration, which is caused most frequently by excessive potassium intake and prescription of other drugs interfering with potassium excretion (β-blockers, potassium-sparing diuretics).

Patients with CKD are at high cardiovascular risk and, aside from renal benefit, ACE inhibition (if tolerated) has been shown in some trials to reduce cardiovascular mortality more effectively in those with impaired than in those with normal renal function.

Reduction of proteinuria

Proteinuria is not only a marker, but also an extremely important promoter of CKD progression, and it has therefore become an important additional treatment target. In patients with primary renal disease, the higher the baseline proteinuria, the greater the subsequent decline in GFR, and also the greater the risk of cardiovascular events.

Current guidelines recommend that proteinuria should be lowered as much as possible, preferably to less than 1 g/24 h (roughly equivalent to ACR <60 mg/mmol or PCR <100 mg/mmol). When this goal is not achieved, it is wise to check whether modifiable factors explain the limited efficacy of blood pressure lowering with RAS blockers, such as patient noncompliance, high sodium intake (which abrogates the antiproteinuric action of RAS blockade), high protein intake (which increases proteinuria), smoking, and poor glycaemic control in people with diabetes. If these factors have been excluded, there remain three strategies. First, one can attempt dose escalation of the ACE inhibitor or angiotensin receptor blocker above the dose licensed for blood pressure lowering. This strategy has been shown to be effective in slowing the progression of CKD, with angiotensin receptor blockers often preferred in this situation because of their better side effect profile. Second, postulating that ACE inhibitors and angiotensin receptor blockers might interfere with progression via different pathways, consider a combination of ACE inhibitor and angiotensin receptor blocker, but data in support of this strategy are somewhat less solid. Third, consider blockade of the mineralocorticoid receptor: aldosterone levels decrease immediately after the start of RAS blockade, but in many patients they subsequently rise again, a phenomenon known as 'aldosterone escape', which can be accompanied by failure to restrain proteinuria. Several studies have shown that, without further lowering of blood pressure, blockade of the mineralocorticoid receptor by low doses of spironolactone (25 mg/day) or

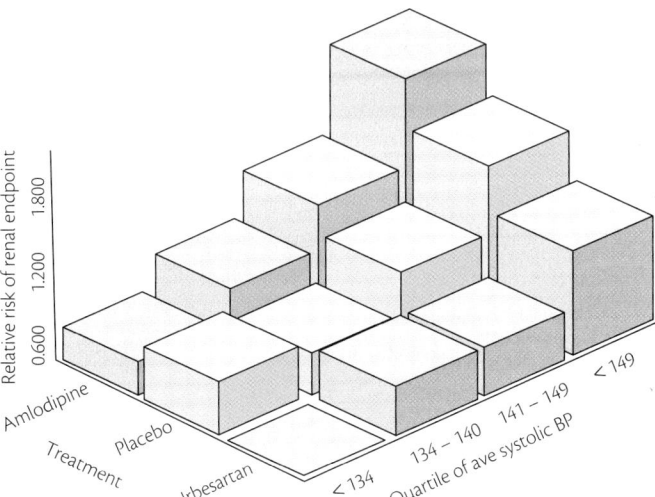

Fig. 21.6.1 The contribution of achieved blood pressure (BP) lowering and renin–angiotensin system (RAS) inhibition on the relative risk of reaching a renal endpoint (doubling of serum creatinine or endstage renal disease). At any given blood pressure level, patients on irbesartan (an angiotensin receptor blocker) had a lower renal risk than those on amlodipine (which does not block the RAS). (From Pohl MA, *et al.* (2005). Independent and additive impact of blood pressure control and angiotensin-II receptor blockade on renal outcomes in the irbesartan diabetic nephropathy trial: clinical implications and limitations. *J Am Soc Nephrol*, **16**, 3027–37, with permission.)

eplerenone can prevent such relapse. There is, however, a danger of precipitating hyperkalaemia, a risk that is justifiable only in patients who have received and accept appropriate dietary education and agree to close follow-up.

Other interventions

Dietary protein restriction

Reducing dietary protein intake may protect against progression of CKD by haemodynamically mediated reduction in intraglomerular pressure, by changes in cytokine profile, and/or by changes in matrix synthesis in the renal interstitium. It has been shown to be effective in attenuating progression of renal failure in several well-conducted animal studies. In clinical trials, numerous uncontrolled studies have also shown an apparently beneficial effect of low dietary protein intake on CKD progression, but the only major controlled prospective trial (the MDRD study) failed to document a significant effect. Although subsequent *post hoc* analyses were consistent with some benefit from dietary protein restriction, its magnitude does not compare with what can be achieved by lowering blood pressure and RAS blockade, and it is important to recognize that drastic lowering of protein intake carries the risk of malnutrition. In routine practice, most nephrologists do no more than to advise against high-protein diets, recommending limitation of protein (but not energy) intake only in CKD patients who have a gross excess of protein intake, e.g. more than 2 g/kg body weight per day, documented by urinary urea measurements. Those of a more interventionist persuasion may recommend a daily protein intake of 0.8 to 1 g/kg per day (and some even 0.7 g/kg per day), with careful monitoring to ensure that protein malnutrition does not develop and that there is adequate intake of calories.

Other dietary and lifestyle measures

As shown in Box 21.6.2, other modifiable progression promoters are smoking, high salt intake, obesity, and the metabolic syndrome. In diabetic patients, the risk of onset of microalbuminuria, and the progression from microalbuminuria to overt diabetic nephropathy, is higher in smokers, as is the rate of loss of GFR in smokers with advanced diabetic nephropathy. At least in diabetic patients, some evidence suggests that cessation of smoking slows the progression of CKD. Thus, in addition to the aim of reducing cardiovascular risk, this finding is another strong reason for patients with renal disease to stop smoking. Recent evidence even indicates that passive smoking increases albuminuria and is injurious to the kidney.

There is scant evidence in humans, in contrast to convincing evidence in animals, for an adverse effect of high salt intake on the progression of primary renal diseases. It is, however, important to recognize that high salt intake militates against control of hypertension and interferes with the antiproteinuric action of ACE inhibition, hence it seems sensible—in line with general recommendations accepted for the treatment of hypertension—to advise reduction in sodium intake from the usual (in developed countries) 150 to 200 mmol/day to 100 mmol/day (6 g of sodium chloride). In practice, this means the patient reducing the amount of processed food that they consume.

A further risk factor for the onset and promotion of CKD progression is visceral obesity and the metabolic syndrome. As shown in Fig. 21.6.2, the worse the metabolic syndrome, the greater the prevalence of CKD and of microalbuminuria in the general (American) population, and the degree of obesity at which renal

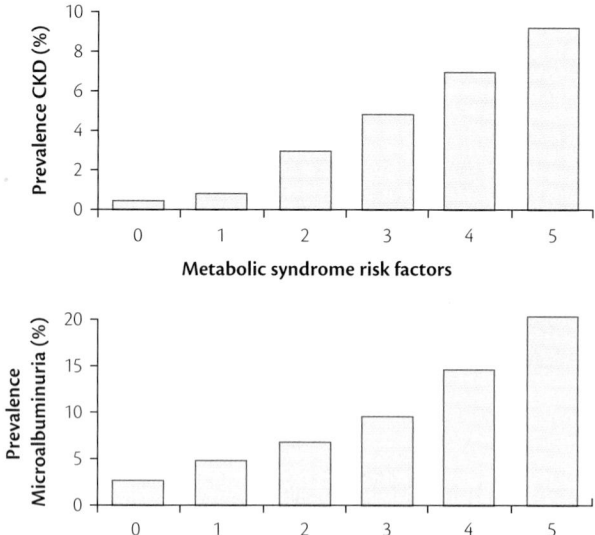

Fig. 21.6.2 The prevalence of CKD (GFR <60 ml/min per 1.73 m²) and of microalbuminuria (ACR 30–300 mg/g, approximately 3–30 mg/mmol) in relation to the number of metabolic risk factors that a patient has. The five metabolic risk factors considered were: (1) waist circumference >102 cm (men); (2) fasting glucose >110 mg/dl (>6.1 mmol/litre); (3) high-density lipoprotein cholesterol (HDL-C) <40 mg/dl (<1.03 mmol/litre); (4) triglycerides >140 mg/dl (>1.58 mmol/litre); and (5) blood pressure >130/80 mmHg.
Chen et al. Ann Int Med 2004; 140; 167–74 http://www.annals.org/content/vol140/issue3/

risk increases is surprisingly low (Fig. 21.6.3). Overweight patients with early CKD should therefore try to reduce their body weight, since this has proven to be effective in several studies. However, in more advanced stages of CKD—namely at an eGFR of approximately 30 to 50 ml/min—the situation is more complex, with higher body weight (even in the range of morbid obesity) lowering the risk of death for unknown reasons.

Other pharmacological interventions

Other interventions on top of ACE inhibition and/or angiotensin receptor blockade to attenuate CKD progression that are under evaluation include renin inhibitors, endothelin I blockers, glycosaminoglycans (increasing the electronegativity of the charge of the glomerular basement membrane), erythropoietin (effective in experimental studies), NSAIDs (potentially dangerous because of overshooting reduction of GFR), vitamin D analogues, and statins.

Medical management of the consequences of CKD

Water, electrolytes, acidosis, and nutrition

Only patients with oliguric endstage renal failure need to restrict their fluid intake precisely, when the usual recommendation (seldom complied with) is that the patient's daily intake should be a volume equal to their daily urinary output plus 500 ml for insensible losses. Most patients with CKD pass a normal volume of urine, but they need to avoid binge drinking because their ability to excrete free water is impaired, and also to be aware of the fact that they will need to drink more if they have other significant fluid losses, e.g. vomiting, diarrhoea, or excessive sweating, because their

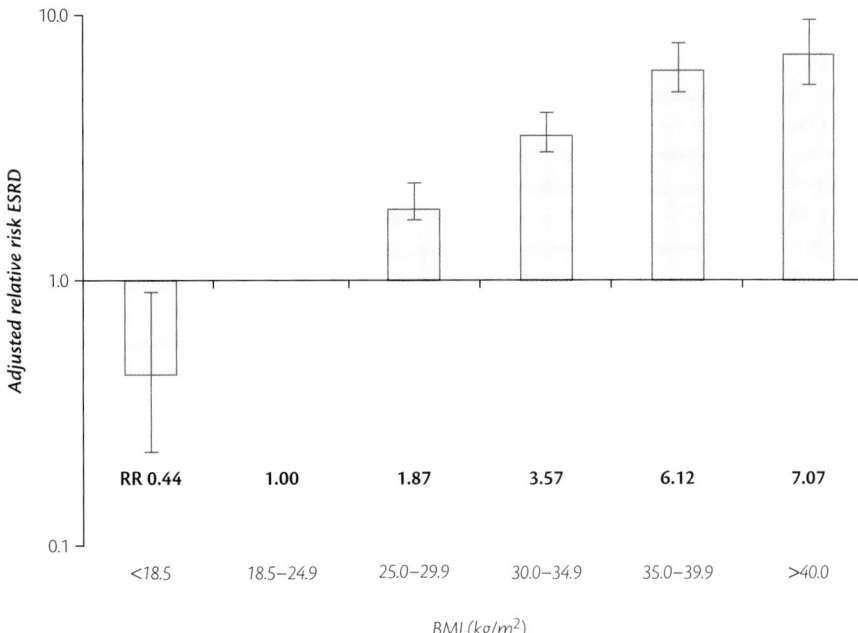

Fig. 21.6.3 Body mass index (BMI) is an independent predictor of endstage renal disease in the United States of America.
Hsu *et al.* Ann Int Med 2006; 144: 21–28
http://www.annals.org/cgi/content/full/144/1/21

kidneys will not be able to elaborate appropriately concentrated urine.

As stated above, it is sensible to recommend modest dietary sodium restriction (100 mmol/day) to patients with CKD. Reduction of sodium intake to around 60 mmol/day can be helpful in patients with fluid retention in the context of advanced CKD, but many patients find this unacceptable and the use of loop diuretics to encourage sodium excretion is more effective in most cases.

Hyperkalaemia is most commonly seen in the context of renal failure (acute or chronic) and can be life threatening. Emergency management is discussed in Chapter 21.5, but an important aim of medical management of patients with CKD is to avoid such excitement. Monitoring of the serum potassium must be routine whenever the creatinine is checked, and especially after introduction of drugs that are known to cause hyperkalaemia (including ACE inhibitors, angiotensin receptor blockers, and potassium-sparing diuretics). The patient should be offered dietary advice (see Chapter 21.2.2) if serum potassium is found to be in the range 5.5 to 6.5 mmol/litre, and the measurement should be repeated a few days later (unless they are known to have a stable potassium in this range). Dietary advice combined with stopping of all medications that might precipitate hyperkalaemia is appropriate if potassium is in the range 6.5 to 7 mmol/litre, again with repeated measurement a few days later. If the potassium is above 7 mmol/litre, the patient should be reviewed in hospital, with checking of the ECG for hyperkalaemic manifestations being an immediate priority, followed by consideration of possible precipitants, which include dietary indiscretion (fruit, chocolate, coffee) and gastrointestinal haemorrhage as well as more obvious intercurrent illness.

Chronic acidosis with serum bicarbonate in the range 12 to 20 mmol/litre is most common in patients with interstitial renal disease and will aggravate hyperkalaemia, inhibit protein anabolism, and accelerate calcium and phosphate loss from bone. Treatment with alkali to maintain the serum bicarbonate above 22 mmol/litre is recommended. Sodium bicarbonate (0.6–1.8 g three times a day) is the first-line treatment, with sodium citrate an alternative for those who cannot tolerate bicarbonate (usually because of abdominal bloating) as long as they are not taking aluminium-containing antacids (citrate enhances aluminium absorption).

Malnutrition is common in advanced chronic renal failure because of anorexia, impaired gut function, and acidosis. The most practical ways of detecting its insidious development is by serial monitoring of body weight and serum albumin concentration. Standard advice is that patients with CKD should have a diet containing about 30 to 35 kcal/kg body weight per day. Dietary supplements may be helpful in achieving this, but they are not a cure for the problem: a patient that is becoming malnourished needs to start RRT sooner rather than later.

Mineral and bone disorder

The mineral and bone disorder (MBD) associated with CKD is a major cause of disability in patients with endstage renal failure. It is mainly, but not exclusively, the consequence of abnormalities of the metabolism of calcium, phosphorus, parathyroid hormone (PTH), and vitamin D, and presumably also the novel phosphaturic hormones FGF23 and Klotho.

CKD-MBD is complex. Osteomalacia was first recognized as a major feature of bone disease in uraemic patients, and in the 1970s and 1980s aluminium-induced bone disease—secondary to high aluminium concentrations in the dialysate or ingestion of aluminium-containing phosphate binders—played an important role, but this iatrogenic complication has now virtually disappeared. Secondary hyperparathyroidism then became considered the major component of CKD-MBD, but with more efficient prevention and treatment of parathyroid overactivity, patients with advanced stages of CKD started to develop low bone turnover with increasing frequency, characterized by frequent episodes of hypercalcaemia, more or less permanent hyperphosphataemia, a high incidence of vascular calcification, and histologically by adynamic bone disease.

Clinicians have become increasingly aware of the potential impact of CKD-MBD on cardiovascular structure and function, as well as on parathyroid glands and bone. It is associated with an increased risk of arterial and valvular calcification, and increased cardiovascular and all-cause mortality, with the impact of severe renal secondary hyperparathyroidism on all-cause mortality best illustrated by the observation that actuarial survival is improved after parathyroidectomy. This adds a new dimension to the importance of CKD-MBD and its prevention or treatment in patients with impaired kidney function, and it is for this reason that we prefer the term CKD-MBD to renal osteodystrophy, which we restrict to usage in the context of the histological aspects of the various forms of renal bone disease.

Pathogenesis

Phosphate excess

In early stages of CKD, the plasma phosphate concentration remains normal or may be even low, which is achieved at the price of increased fractional clearance of phosphate. Hyperphosphataemia develops once the GFR has decreased to between 60 and 30 ml/min (CKD stage 3). Hyperphosphataemia aggravates secondary hyperparathyroidism by indirect mechanisms, such as inhibition of the synthesis of the active vitamin D metabolite 1,25-$(OH)_2$vitamin D_3 (1,25-$(OH)_2D_3$ or calcitriol) in tubular epithelial cells, and possibly also by inducing a tendency for hypocalcaemia. It has also been shown that phosphate directly stimulates PTH synthesis and secretion as well as parathyroid cell proliferation, independent of low serum 1,25-$(OH)_2D_3$ and hypocalcaemia. Increased PTH secretion reduces tubular phosphate reabsorption. In parallel, plasma FGF23 increases in CKD as a result of phosphate retention, and this in concert with Klotho also decreases renal phosphate reabsorption. The relative roles of PTH and FGF23 in the control of phosphate reabsorption are currently unclear.

1,25-$(OH)_2D_3$ deficiency

The hepatic vitamin D metabolite 25-(OH)vitamin D_3 (25-(OH)D_3) is transformed, mainly in renal tubular epithelial cells, to the most active vitamin D metabolite, 1,25-$(OH)_2D_3$, which acts as a circulating hormone (apart from paracrine actions of locally synthesized 1,25-$(OH)_2D_3$ in tissues such as activated macrophages, vascular cells, and others). Its synthesis is stimulated by PTH but inhibited by phosphate and FGF23, and even in early stages of CKD there is a tendency for 1,25-$(OH)_2D_3$ concentration to decrease, although it remains mostly within the normal range because such decrease is counteracted by increases in PTH. The average concentration of 1,25-$(OH)_2D_3$ falls progressively as CKD advances (Fig. 21.6.4).

One specific problem is that circulating vitamin D metabolites bound to vitamin D-binding protein may be lost in the urine of patients with heavy proteinuria, so that deficiency of vitamin D metabolites, such as 25-(OH)D_3 and 1,25-$(OH)_2D_3$, may ensue. The renal 1α-hydroxylase reaction is normally substrate independent, but with progression of CKD it becomes increasingly dependent on the availability of the substrate 25-(OH)D_3, with deficiency of this form of vitamin D further aggravating the impairment of synthesis of 1,25-$(OH)_2D_3$.

As also shown in Fig. 21.6.4, average serum levels of so-called intact PTH increase progressively as average serum 1,25-$(OH)_2D_3$ levels decrease with decreasing GFR in patients with various stages of CKD.

Hypocalcaemia

On average, plasma (total and ionized) calcium concentrations are maintained in the normal range until CKD stage 5. Nevertheless, for several reasons there is a permanent tendency towards hypocalcaemia, mainly because of reduced active intestinal calcium absorption as a result of insufficient active vitamin D generation and diminished release of calcium (skeletal resistance) in response to PTH and 1,25-$(OH)_2D_3$.

Skeletal resistance may well play an important role in the pathogenesis of secondary hyperparathyroidism, with another mechanism being impaired inhibition by extracellular Ca^{2+} of the parathyroid gland, which senses this cation via the calcium-sensing receptor (CaR), expression of which is decreased in CKD-MBD

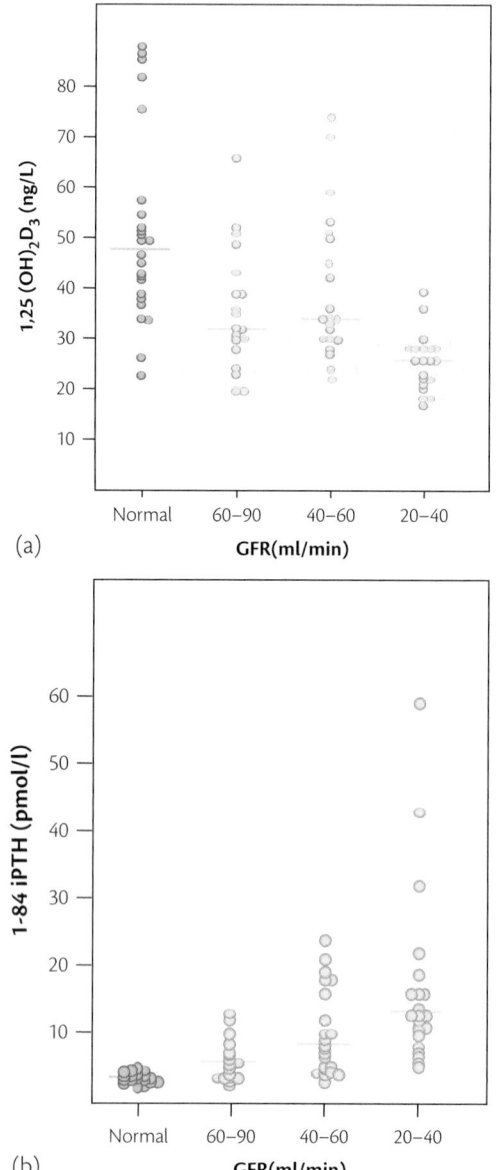

(a)

(b)

Fig. 21.6.4 1,25-$(OH)_2$vitamin D_3 (A) and intact plasma parathyroid hormone (B) values as a function of glomerular filtration rate (GFR) in patients with various stages of CKD.

Reproduced from Reichel *et al*, NDT 1991; 6: 162–9, with permission of Oxford Journals.

in parathyroid tissue. Some reports have showed abnormal Ca^{2+} sensing even in early stages of CKD. CaR down-regulation in the parathyroid can be reversed by low phosphate diet, calcimimetics, and other compounds.

Types of bone mineral disorder in CKD
The bone lesions discussed below, collectively known under the term renal osteodystrophy, are found in the skeleton of patients with CKD, in isolation or in combination (Box 21.6.5).

Osteitis fibrosa
This is characterized histologically by an increase in both osteoclastic bone resorption and osteoblastic bone apposition rates with (1) consecutive intense remodelling of bone trabeculae in the spongiosa, and (2) rarefaction and tunnelization of cortical and cancellous bone, with or without deposition of fibrous tissue (endosteal fibrosis) (Fig. 21.6.5). Typical radiological appearances are shown in Fig. 21.6.6.

Osteomalacia
Osteomalacia is characterized by a disparity between the rate of bone matrix synthesis and bone matrix mineralization, leading to widening of the seam of unmineralized bone matrix (osteoid), usually associated with signs of diminished numbers and activities of cells at the bone surface. Pure osteomalacia is rarely seen nowadays: 30 years ago it was mainly due to aluminium intoxication, and before that to overt vitamin D (cholecalciferol) deficiency.

Mixed lesions
In many patients with advanced stages of CKD, a combination of osteitis fibrosa and osteomalacia is present, which is commonly called mixed lesions or mixed renal osteodystrophy.

Adynamic bone disease
In patients with low or normal serum intact PTH concentrations, the number and activity of cells on the bone surface is strikingly reduced, as is bone turnover. This condition is most common in patients with CKD due to diabetes, those with poor nutritional

status, and those who have been overtreated with active vitamin D and/or calcium-containing phosphate binders. It predisposes to hypercalcaemia, hyperphosphataemia, and soft tissue calcification because the capacity of the skeleton to sequester calcium and phosphate is reduced. There is some evidence that adynamic bone may contribute to skeletal fractures in patients on dialysis, but it is not known whether there are more far-reaching clinical implications.

Osteopenia
The term osteopenia is preferred to osteoporosis because the pathophysiology of bone disease in CKD is strikingly different from that in idiopathic osteoporosis. Diminished bone mass (osteopenia), superimposed on uraemia-specific bony abnormalities, is very common in patients with advanced CKD. The most frequent causes are a history of treatment with steroids and (premature) menopause. It is not known whether the risk is aggravated by smoking and low calcium diets, or whether it can be prevented by substitution of oestrogens/gestagens or selective oestrogen receptor modulators.

Other bone-related pathologies
In patients with CKD, several bone pathologies unrelated to calcium metabolism may coexist with CKD-MBD (Box 21.6.5). Specifically, a dialysis-associated type of amyloidosis with preferential osteoarticular involvement, called β_2-microglobulin-related amyloidosis, must be considered in the differential diagnosis of bone pain and osteoarticular destruction.

Symptoms and signs
MBD in CKD is usually asymptomatic. Bone pain is not common, even in advanced osteitis fibrosa, although bones subjected to mechanical stress (spine, calcaneus, foot) may be painful. While fractures are uncommon, skeletal deformity, facial leontiasis, and avulsion of the patella may occur. By contrast, osteomalacia, particularly that secondary to aluminium intoxication, may be very painful, especially when Looser's zones (fatigue fractures) are present. Again, it is important to exclude alternative causes of bone pain, particularly myeloma and metastases (Box 21.6.6).

Severe extraosseous calcifications (Figs. 21.6.6–21.6.8), specifically periarticular, bursal, and visceral calcifications, are usually the consequence of severe hyperphosphataemia and high-normal serum calcium, with either high or low serum intact PTH concentrations. Tumoural tissue calcification is often triggered by trauma with haematoma formation and favoured by low bone turnover, which diminishes the capacity of the bone to sequester calcium and phosphate from the extracellular space.

Slowly progressing arterial and valvular calcifications may be associated with clinical evidence of cardiovascular disease, indeed cardiovascular mortality in dialysis patients is strongly predicted by the presence of coronary artery calcification detected by electron beam CT scanning.

Calciphylaxis, also called calcific uraemic arteriolopathy, is a rare medical emergency characterized by ischaemic eschars of the skin secondary to calcification of cutaneous arterial vessels. Predisposing factors, apart from secondary hyperparathyroidism, include diabetes, obesity, female gender, and (probably) treatment with warfarin. It can produce gangrene and may be fatal. It may respond to parathyroidectomy if serum PTH levels are elevated.

Box 21.6.5 Bone lesions in patients with CKD (renal osteodystrophy)

Bone lesions that may be found either in isolation or in combination

- Osteitis fibrosa
- Osteomalacia
- Mixed lesions
- Adynamic bone disease—overtreatment with calcium and/or vitamin D; rarely (today) from aluminium overload

Further pathologies that must be considered in atypical cases

- β_2-Microglobulin-related amyloidosis
- Sequelae of preceding corticosteroid therapy—fractures, osteonecrosis
- Osteopenia, particularly in postmenopausal patients
- Reflex sympathetic dystrophy
- Bony problems caused by primary disease leading to CKD—e.g. oxalosis

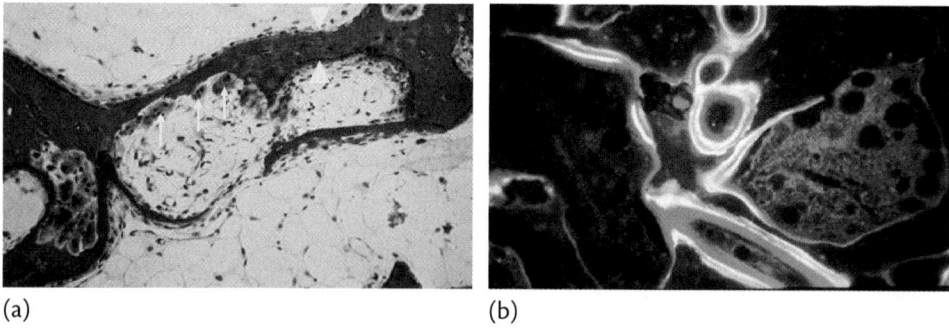

Fig. 21.6.5 Light microscopic images of osteitis fibrosa as the skeletal expression of severe secondary hyperparathyroidism in a patient with CKD stage 5 (Masson trichrome stain). Panel A—Increased osteoclastic bone resorption (arrows) and osteoblastic bone apposition with deposition of fibrous tissue (endosteal fibrosis). Widened osteoid seams (between large arrow heads). Panel B—Greatly enhanced mineralization activity, as evidenced by double fluorescent tetracycline bands (tetracycline stain).
Courtesy of ALM de Francisco MD.

Biochemical abnormalities

While patients with advanced stages of CKD left untreated usually have hypocalcaemia and hyperphosphataemia, patients with advanced secondary hyperparathyroidism are characterized by hypercalcaemia and hyperphosphataemia associated with an increase in serum total alkaline phosphatases and its bone-specific isoenzyme. The findings on serum biochemistry in patients with CKD-MBD are shown in Table 21.6.7, with the findings in the two main contrasting forms of MBD compared in Table 21.6.8. In patients with hypercalcaemia it is important to consider causes other than secondary hyperparathyroidism which necessitate specific treatment, as listed in Box 21.6.7.

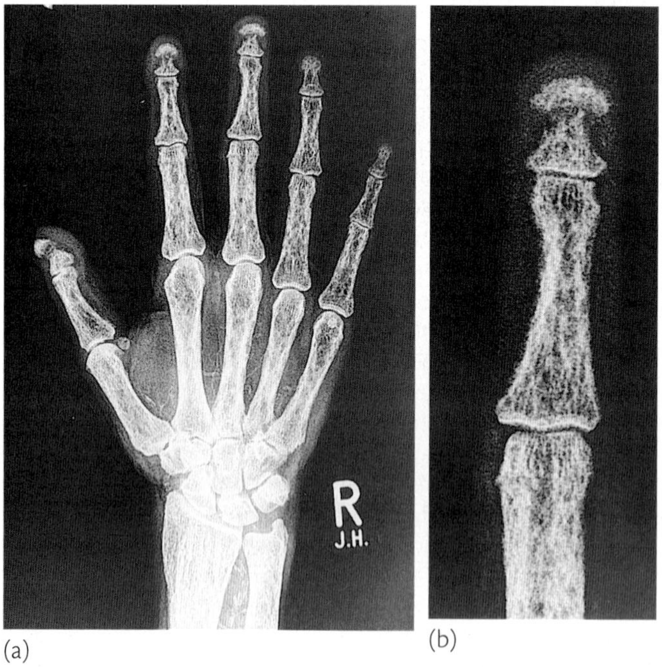

Prophylaxis and management of secondary hyperparathyroidism

Secondary hyperparathyroidism is the combined result of failing excretory function of the kidney (leading to phosphate retention) and failing endocrine function of the kidney (leading to calcitriol deficiency). Appropriate management requires prevention (whenever possible) and treatment of both abnormalities.

Approach to serum phosphate control

It is usually recommended that phosphate-lowering interventions should begin once plasma phosphate concentrations exceed the upper limit of the normal range, i.e. 1.45 mmol/litre. This is generally the case when GFR has decreased to about 30 ml/min and persists even when patients with CKD are on dialysis, which cannot (on a conventional thrice-weekly haemodialysis regimen, or by peritoneal dialysis) clear the amount consumed in a standard Western diet (50–100 mmol/day, of which 50–70% is absorbed).

The risk of soft tissue precipitation of calcium phosphate is particularly high if hyperphosphataemia is accompanied by hypercalcaemia and a high calcium × phosphate product (desirable target

Fig. 21.6.6 Radiographs of the hand. (A) Reduced mineral density as well as fluffy and mottled texture of the bones. Note (1) subperiosteal resorption zones at the radial side of the middle phalanges; (2) erosion cavities at the periosteal surface with overlying areas of calcification, so-called periosteal neostosis; (3) longitudinal striation of cortical bone (corresponding to enlarged Haversian channels); (4) thinning of cortical bone by endosteal bone resorption; (5) loss of the terminal lamella of the terminal phalanx; and (6) vascular calcification above the first digit and along the side of the radius. (B) A detail of the second digit, the terminal phalanx of which has collapsed such that the patient had 'pseudo-clubbing'.

Box 21.6.6 Differential diagnosis of bone pain in patients with advanced CKD or on dialysis

Mineral and bone disorders related to CKD

◆ Osteitis fibrosa—pain relatively rare

◆ Osteomalacia—secondary to vitamin D deficiency, or exceptionally aluminium accumulation

◆ β_2-Amyloidosis

Bone pathologies not directly caused by CKD

◆ Skeletal metastases, myeloma

◆ Osteomyelitis, mostly spondylodiscitis—may be related to infected vascular access

◆ Neuromelic pain after creation of arteriovenous fistula

◆ Bone infarction, osteonecrosis—related to corticosteroid treatment, sickle cell anaemia

◆ Osteopenia-associated infarctions and fractures

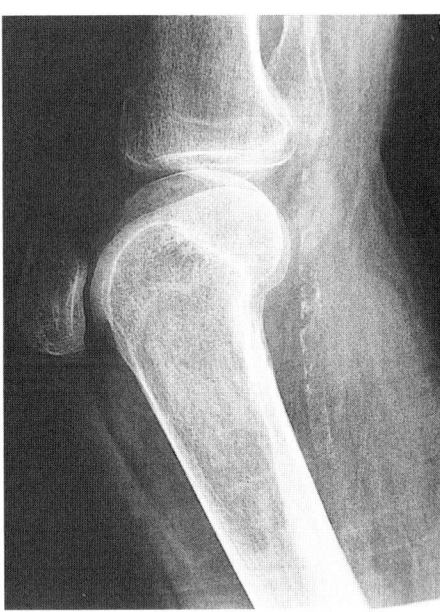

Fig. 21.6.7 Calcification of the popliteal artery in a patient with diabetes, CKD and severe secondary hyperparathyroidism.

below 5.6 mmol²/litre²). The K/DOQI guidelines propose an upper limit of serum phosphorus of 1.8 mmol/litre in dialysis patients.

Phosphate is present in virtually all foods, hence reduction of dietary intake is difficult without incurring the risk of malnutrition. Patients should be advised to avoid food items with very high phosphate content, e.g. some dairy products, and those to which phosphate is added, such as sausages and phosphate-rich soft drinks. A protein-restricted diet will reduce phosphate intake, but the merit or otherwise of protein restriction is debatable (see previous discussion). However, given that sufficient dietary restriction of phosphate is usually not feasible, patients with advanced CKD

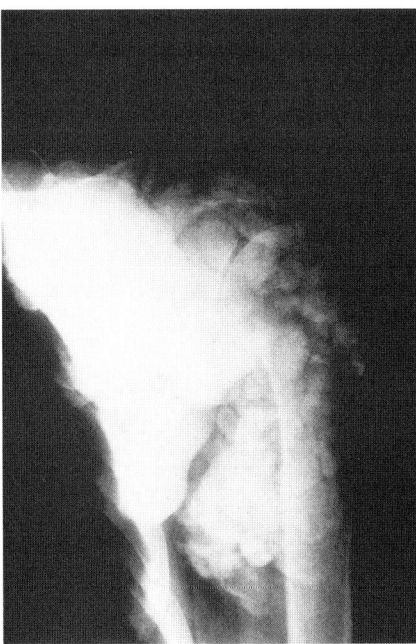

Fig. 21.6.8 Tumoral calcification around the left shoulder in a chronic haemodialysis patient with severe low-turnover bone disease.

remain in positive phosphate balance unless oral phosphate binders are administered.

All oral phosphate binders trap phosphate in the intestinal lumen by forming insoluble complexes with it, hence they must be taken together with meals, after which the phosphate concentration in the gut is highest. The agents most commonly used in the recent past as phosphate binders were calcium carbonate and calcium acetate, the prescription of aluminium-containing compounds having been abandoned by most nephrologists because of the risk of aluminium intoxication. However, calcium-containing phosphate binders cause positive calcium balance and perhaps promote vascular calcification. Recently, the calcium-free and aluminium-free phosphate binders sevelamer and lanthanum carbonate have been introduced into clinical practice. These allow similar control of plasma phosphate, while avoiding calcium and aluminium overload.

If hyperphosphataemia does not respond to medical intervention, then issues to consider include noncompliance, increased phosphate release from the skeleton (e.g. in severe osteitis fibrosa) and/or stimulation of intestinal phosphate absorption by excessive amounts of active vitamin D sterols, and (in patients on RRT) inadequate dialysis.

Approach to serum calcium control

The target range for serum total calcium (corrected for albumin) is 2.20 to 2.38 mmol/litre (8.8–9.5 mg/dl). If the corrected total serum calcium level exceeds 2.55 mmol/litre (10.2 mg/dl), then therapies that cause a rise in serum calcium should be adjusted and other potential causes of hypercalcaemia should be considered, in particular an inappropriately high dialysate calcium concentration and immobilization (see Box 21.6.7).

Reversal of deficiency of native vitamin D₃

Deficiency of the parent compound vitamin D_3 (cholecalciferol) is common among patients with CKD as a result of altered lifestyle, with insufficient sun exposure, hyperpigmentation of the skin, and loss of protein-bound vitamin D (metabolites) into proteinuric urine or peritoneal dialysis fluid. Vitamin D deficiency can be diagnosed, according to some authorities, when plasma 25-$(OH)D_3$ concentrations are below 40 nmol/litre (16 ng/ml), and vitamin D insufficiency when they are between 40 and 80 nmol/litre (16–32 ng/ml). The latter values are higher than recommended in the past, and are based on the recognition that still higher levels, although not providing further benefit in terms of calcium metabolism, may be necessary to achieve the recently recognized pleiotropic effects of vitamin D, e.g. on infection control, vascular biology, insulin sensitivity, and control of renin secretion.

In CKD, the synthesis of 1,25-$(OH)_2D_3$ depends on the concentration of the precursor substance 25-$(OH)D_3$. This explains why administration of at least 1000 IU vitamin D per day, possibly 2000 IU per day (which is 2–3 times the average daily intake with vitamin D fortified food), leads to an increase of serum calcitriol and a decrease of serum intact PTH in many patients with CKD. Serum 25-$(OH)D_3$ levels can usually be raised to a target of at least 75 nmol/litre (30 ng/ml) by supplementation with cholecalciferol or (less reliably) by sufficient sun exposure. Note, however, that treatment with pharmacological doses of native vitamin D is not appropriate in CKD: these are much less effective than its hydroxylated, more active metabolites (see below) and, if they do raise serum calcium and phosphate concentration, carry a substantial

Table 21.6.7 Serum biochemistry in the evaluation of CKD-MBD

Analyte	Comments	Normal range
Calcium	Low, normal, or elevated (elevated in severe HPT, vitamin D excess, therapy with calcium-containing phosphate binders, inappropriately high dialysate calcium, immobilization)	2.2–2.6 mmol/litre or 8.8–10.4 mg/dl
Phosphate	Elevated in advanced CKD (GFR <30 ml/min)	0.8–1.4 mmol/litre or 2.4–4.2 mg/dl
Intact PTH	Elevated in HPT; can be normal or even low (mostly in cases of aluminium intoxication, adynamic bone disease, overtreatment with calcitriol, after parathyroidectomy); beware of interassay variations of intact PTH measurements	1–7 pmol/litre or 10–65 pg/ml
25-(OH)D_3 (calcidiol)	Often low because of reduced sun exposure or low dietary intake; seasonal variation; if increased, check for exogenous source	50–200 nmol/litre or 20–80 ng/ml[a]
1,25-(OH)$_2D_3$ (calcitriol)	Usually low (if increased, check for calcitriol ingestion; rarely endogenous overproduction (granulomatous disease))	50–120 pmol/litre or 25–50 pg/ml[a]
Total alkaline phosphatases (AP)	Normal or increased; elevated in severe HPT (exclude concomitant liver disease by determination of γ-GT or bone-specific AP isoenzyme)	60–170 IU/litre
Osteocalcin	Diagnostic information analogous to AP; fragments accumulate in advanced CKD; probably no extra information in addition to intact PTH and bone isoenzyme of AP	c.3–8 µg/litre[b] (may depend on assay)
Magnesium	Normal or elevated (decreased renal excretion)	0.8–1.3 mmol/litre
Aluminium	Normal; elevated if aluminium-containing phosphate binders are taken or if dialysate is aluminium contaminated	<10 µg/litre

AP, alkaline phosphatase; CKD, chronic kidney disease; GFR, glomerular filtration rate; -GT, -glutamyl transferase; HPT, hyperparathyroidism; MBD, mineral and bone disorder; PTH, parathyroid hormone.
[a] Normal range varies depending on season (consult local laboratory guidance).
[b] In individual with normal renal function.

risk of inducing prolonged increases in serum calcium × phosphate product and soft tissue calcification.

Administration of active vitamin D sterols

If serum 25-(OH)D_3 levels are more than 75 nmol/litre (30 ng/ml) and intact PTH levels remain elevated, treatment with low doses of active vitamin D sterols (calcitriol, alfacalcidol, paricalcitol, or doxercalciferol) should be considered. In patients with CKD stage 5, whether on dialysis or not, complete return of intact PTH concentrations to normal is not desirable: in this condition, normal bone turnover requires that measured intact PTH concentrations be above the normal range. It is uncertain whether this reflects mainly PTH resistance of the skeleton, or problems with the second-generation intact PTH assay, which also measures inactive fragments of PTH. However, in reflection of these concerns, the K/DOQI guidelines advise variable target ranges for PTH dependent

on the stage of renal failure: 35 to 70 pg/ml (3.8–7.6 pmol/litre) in CKD stage 3; 70 to 110 pg/ml (7.6–11.8 pmol/litre) in CKD stage 4; and 150 to 300 pg/ml (16–32 pmol/litre) in CKD stage 5.

Box 21.6.8 provides an algorithm for the prophylaxis of secondary hyperparathyroidism. In experimental studies, continuous (daily) administration of calcitriol or alfacalcidol lowers intact PTH concentration and prevents parathyroid hyperplasia less effectively than intermittent (pulse) administration given at longer intervals, but there is no good evidence that this effect is of clinical importance.

Table 21.6.8 Typical serum biochemistry in the two main contrasting forms of renal bone disease

Analyte	Osteitis fibrosa	Adynamic bone disease
Calcium	Variable, high normal or elevated in advanced secondary hyperparathyroidism	Tendency to hypercalcaemia
Phosphate	Marked increase (dissolution of bone mineral)	No typical pattern, often elevated
Intact parathyroid hormone	Markedly elevated	Normal or low
Total alkaline phosphatases	Usually elevated	Tend to be low

Box 21.6.7 Differential diagnosis of hypercalcaemia in patients with advanced CKD or on dialysis

Related to CKD

◆ Severe hyperparathyroidism

◆ Intoxication with vitamin D sterols—cholecalciferol, ergocalciferol, calcidiol, calcitriol, or active vitamin D derivatives

◆ Excessive dose of calcium-containing phosphate binders

◆ Inappropriately high dialysate calcium concentration

Not directly caused by CKD

◆ Immobilization

◆ Cancer with bone metastases

◆ Myeloma

◆ Granulomatous disease—e.g. sarcoidosis, tuberculosis

◆ Other rare causes of hypercalcaemia—see Chapter 13.6

◆ Pseudohypercalcaemia—elevated total protein concentration

Box 21.6.8 Algorithm for prophylaxis of secondary hyperparathyroidism

Monitoring (serum biochemistry)

♦ calcium, albumin, phosphate, intact parathyroid hormone (PTH), 25-(OH)D₃, aluminium

Prophylactic measures

If serum 25-(OH)D₃ is low, i.e. below 75 nmol/litre (30 ng/ml)
→ give cholecalciferol 1000 U/day

If plasma calcium is decreased and/or plasma phosphate is increased
→ give calcium carbonate 0.5–1.0 g with each meal

If serum phosphate is increased and plasma calcium is normal or high
→ consider calcium-free phosphate binder, e.g. sevelamer or lanthanum carbonate

If serum intact PTH is consistently above target ranges (see text) and serum calcium/phosphate is normal (spontaneously or after intervention)
→ give calcitriol 0.125–0.25 µg/day or equivalent doses of alfacalcidol or other active vitamin D analogues.

Medical management of advanced hyperparathyroidism

The main side effects of treatment with active vitamin D sterols are hypercalcaemia and hyperphosphataemia. There has therefore been an intense search for new vitamin D analogues that suppress the parathyroid gland while causing less hypercalcaemia and hyperphosphataemia. Some of these—including paricalcitol (19-nor-1-α,25-(OH)₂D₂) and doxercalciferol—are available in some countries, but there is no firm evidence from clinical trials that they are clinically better than the parent compound, calcitriol, although observational studies in large dialysis patient cohorts suggest that treatment with active vitamin D compounds is associated with better outcome than no vitamin D treatment, and that treatment with novel active vitamin D derivatives may lead to better patient outcome than treatment with calcitriol.

Another method of affecting calcium balance in patients on dialysis is to manipulate the concentration of calcium in the dialysate. In the past, a dialysate calcium concentration of 1.75 mmol/litre (7 mg/100 ml) was recommended, such that net uptake of calcium occurred during the dialysis session to compensate for convective loss of calcium via ultrafiltration during, and negative intestinal calcium balance between, dialysis sessions. However, if calcium-containing phosphate binders or active vitamin D sterols are administered, then intestinal uptake of calcium is increased and patients may develop positive calcium balance, with or without hypercalcaemia. Lowering the dialysate calcium concentration to 1.5 mmol/litre (6 mg/100 ml) (and temporarily even to 1.25 mmol/litre (5 mg/100 ml)) counteracts this tendency, but it is essential to make absolutely sure that patients take their medication in this circumstance: if calcium carbonate and/or active vitamin D derivatives are omitted, then a negative calcium balance ensues with exacerbation of secondary hyperparathyroidism.

Another effective treatment for hyperparathyroidism is to use a calcimimetic, only one of which—cinacalcet—is in clinical use at present. This renders the CaR more sensitive to extracellular Ca²⁺ and has been shown to reduce both elevated serum intact PTH concentrations and the calcium × phosphorus product in dialysis patients with moderate or severe hyperparathyroidism. Its beneficial effect is maintained over prolonged time periods.

Tumour-like parathyroid growth and parathyroidectomy

Severe secondary hyperparathyroidism is a process that bears similarities to tumour growth. Nodular hyperplasia is usually found in patients whose estimated parathyroid mass exceeds 1 to 1.5 g, with the nodules exhibiting clonal growth, with microsatellite analysis showing loss of heterozygosity for many alleles, including putative tumour suppressor genes. The parathyroid tissue within these nodules is also characterized by reduced expression of vitamin D receptors (VDR) and CaR, which could explain—at least in part—the frequent lack of response to medical management. It appears that continuous stimulation of the parathyroid gland selectively favours cells with higher proliferative potential, so that the gland progressively escapes from growth-inhibitory control mechanisms. This is illustrated by the fact that regrowth, including locally invasive regrowth, occurs in many patients after subtotal parathyroidectomy or autotransplantation of parathyroid tissue.

Before the introduction of cinacalcet treatment, there was a tendency to consider parathyroidectomy in patients with marked elevation of serum intact PTH (>c.50 pmol/litre or 500 pg/ml) who failed to respond to medical treatment within 4 to 8 weeks, particularly in those with massive parathyroid enlargement on imaging procedures (estimated mass >1–1.5 g). Cinacalcet, when available, is now the treatment of first choice.

An absolute indication for parathyroidectomy is calciphylaxis (also called calcific uraemic arteriolopathy), namely ischaemic skin necrosis secondary to calcification of skin arteries, but only if associated with elevated serum intact PTH levels. Other indications are severe hypercalcaemia refractory to medical treatment, progressive and debilitating hyperparathyroid bone disease, and intractable pruritus or otherwise unexplained symptomatic myopathy associated with high intact PTH.

There has been a long-standing debate as to whether total parathyroidectomy or subtotal parathyroidectomy should be preferred, the latter with a remnant left *in situ* or autotransplanted into the subcutaneous abdominal fat or forearm musculature. There are no trial data to inform decision making. Leaving parathyroid tissue behind is associated with a relatively high risk of local recurrence, presumably because of the increased growth potential of parathyroid cells, although the risk can be reduced if only nonnodular parts of the gland are autotransplanted. Alcohol injection into the enlarged parathyroids under ultrasonographic guidance has been tried as an alternative to surgery, but this procedure has not found wide application except in Japan.

Box 21.6.9 summarizes the approach to the management of patients with advanced renal secondary hyperparathyroidism.

Anaemia

Pathogenesis

The physiological mechanisms controlling red-cell mass are shown in Fig. 21.6.9. The maintenance of a normal red-cell mass requires

---

Box 21.6.9 Treatment of advanced hyperparathyroidism

If serum intact parathyroid hormone (PTH) is constantly above target range (see text)
→ normalize serum calcium and phosphate levels.

If serum phosphate is elevated
→ give calcium carbonate, calcium acetate, or calcium-free phosphate binders with meals.
→ reduce excessive intake of dietary phosphate.
→ increase efficacy of dialysis (higher blood flow, longer dialysis sessions, more frequent dialysis sessions)

If serum calcium is elevated
→ reduce dialysate calcium to 1.5 mmol/litre (6 mg/dl) or—transiently—to 1.25 mmol/litre (5 mg/dl)
→ reduce or withdraw calcium-containing oral phosphate binders or active vitamin D sterols

If serum calcium and phosphate have been normalized and elevated intact PTH persists
→ increase dose of calcitriol (0.5–3 µg) or alternative active vitamin D sterols (e.g. alfacalcidol, paricalcitol, doxercalciferol)—these can be given one to three times per week, or daily, with dose and time interval depending on degree of elevation of serum intact PTH; alternatively, administer cinacalcet (initial dose 30 mg/day)
→ monitor serum calcium, phosphate, intact PTH, and total alkaline phosphatases

If serum intact PTH decreases below approximately 16.5 pmol/litre (150 pg/ml)
→ interrupt administration of calcitriol, measure intact PTH again, and decide whether low-dose long-term prophylaxis is necessary

If serum intact PTH fails to decrease and/or hypercalcaemia/hyperphosphataemia develop or persist
→ monitor parathyroid gland size (ultrasonography; MIBI scan before surgery to localize ectopic glands)
→ consider cinacalcet (initial dose 30 mg/day) or surgical parathyroidectomy

Note: active vitamin D sterols are contraindicated as long as plasma phosphate is elevated.

Note: active vitamin D sterols are contraindicated as long as serum calcium is elevated.

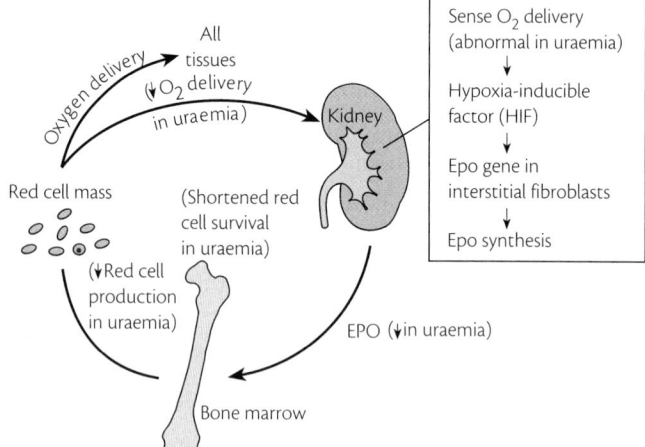

Fig. 21.6.9 The relationship between red-cell mass, oxygen delivery, erythropoietin synthesis, and red-cell production in the bone marrow. Erythropoietin production is reduced in uraemia because of defective sensing, reduced synthesis, or both.

women) is common in CKD, particularly in those with diabetes, but affects nearly 90% of all with CKD stages 4 and 5, many of whom will have haemoglobin below 10 g/dl. Renal anaemia, which is normochromic and normocytic, accounts for many of the symptoms that previously were attributed to uraemia, including lethargy, cold intolerance, and general fatigue. Population studies and registry data generally report higher mortality for dialysis patients with haematocrit 30 to 33% compared with those with haematocrit 33 to 36%, or for haemoglobin levels less than 11 g/dl or 11.5 g/dl than above.

Management

As a result of many trials of erythropoietin and other erythropoiesis-stimulating agents (ESAs), there is now general agreement that partial correction of anaemia in patients with CKD improves physiological and clinical status, as well as quality of life. This agreement has manifested itself in a plethora of clinical practice guidelines, including those produced by the National Kidney Foundation Dialysis Outcomes Quality Initiative (DOQI) in the

a rate of red-cell production by the bone marrow, with no substrate limitations and under the influence of an adequate amount of erythropoietin, which is sufficient to balance red-cell loss and destruction. All elements are disturbed in uraemia, and anaemia is one of the most obvious manifestations of the uraemic syndrome. Red-cell lifespan is shortened by accelerated destruction. Erythropoietin secretion is enhanced, but not to a sufficient level (Fig. 21.6.10).

Epidemiology and clinical significance

Anaemia (defined as a haemoglobin concentration <13 g/dl in adult men and postmenopausal women, and <12 g/dl in premenopausal

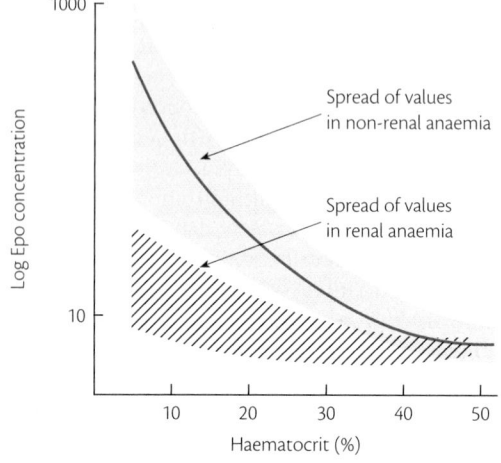

Fig. 21.6.10 In renal anaemia the erythropoietin concentration rises in response to anaemia, but to a much lower level than in comparably severe nonrenal anaemia.

United States of America, the European Renal Association/ European Dialysis and Transplant Association (ERA/EDTA), the Canadian Society of Nephrology, and the Japanese Society for Dialysis Therapy. There are minor differences between the particular guidelines, but they are all essentially very similar.

There is no particular haemoglobin concentration at which symptoms become manifest in all patients, hence the decision to start treatment in a particular patient is always a matter of judgement. As a rule of thumb, if a patient with CKD has haemoglobin below 11 g/dl and symptoms that might be attributable to anaemia, then treatment to restore haemoglobin to the range 11 to 12 g/dl is warranted if available, but it has been convincingly shown in randomized studies that correction to a higher level ('normal or near normal') is associated with poorer outcomes and should be prevented.

Before starting treatment with ESAs it is important to exclude other causes of anaemia: serum vitamin B_{12}, red-cell folate, and indices of iron status should be assessed in all patients, with other tests on the basis of clinical suspicion, e.g. an elderly patient presenting with renal impairment and marked anaemia may have myeloma. If a patient is significantly iron deficient, then standard clinical methods of history and examination followed by appropriate investigation may be required to determine the cause, but otherwise it is important to recognize that optimal response to ESAs requires plentiful iron, not simply a level that is not deficient. It is also important to ensure that blood pressure is reasonably controlled before ESAs are given. In the early days of erythropoietin treatment, rapid increases in haemoglobin concentration in combination with poorly controlled blood pressure precipitated hypertensive encephalopathy in some patients. The standard advice is thus that ESAs should not be started (or doses omitted) if blood pressure is above 160/100 mmHg.

Box 21.6.10 shows an algorithm whereby the patient's iron status is optimized before ESAs are administered. A range of ESAs are available: all are clinically effective, many can be administered intravenously or subcutaneously, patients may prefer one rather than another because of the particular method of delivery and frequency of administration (variable from once or twice a week to monthly), and those paying may wish to choose the cheapest. If the haemoglobin fails to respond, or falls after initially responding, then causes given in Table 21.6.9 need to be considered.

Complications of chronic renal failure

Chronic renal failure affects all parts of the body. Many of its complications have been discussed in this chapter, but a more complete—although not exhaustive—list is given in Table 21.6.10.

Preparation for renal replacement therapy

A point of seemingly minor but in fact crucial importance in any patient with advanced CKD who is likely to progress to endstage renal failure is to preserve superficial veins of the forearm for vascular access. Whenever possible, blood should only be drawn from the veins on the dorsal surface of the hand, or—if veins in the forearm or elbow must be punctured or cannulated—the nondominant arm must be kept free from assault for later formation of an arteriovenous dialysis fistula.

Once endstage renal failure is inevitable, the patient must be prepared physically and psychologically for RRT. In many patients

it is possible to predict approximately when the endstage will be reached from consideration of the rate of renal deterioration, most easily demonstrated by plotting the reciprocal of the serum creatinine against time (Fig. 21.6.11). This information is useful for the patient and those planning care, providing a guide for the timing of the creation of vascular access, placement of peritoneal dialysis catheters, or activating the patient on to a transplant waiting list. The temptation to delay starting dialysis for as long as possible should be avoided, as the quality of life and health of a well-dialysed patient is superior to that of a nondialysed, uraemic, malnourished one.

Box 21.6.10 Treatment of renal anaemia

Is anaemia due to CKD?
→ consider other causes.

Determine iron status
→ iron deficiency is defined by serum ferritin <100 μg/litre[a].
→ functional iron deficiency is defined by serum ferritin >100 μg/litre with hypochromic red cells[b] >6% or transferrin saturation <20%

Optimize iron status
→ aim to maintain serum ferritin >200 μg/litre with hypochromic red cells <6% (unless ferritin >800 μg/litre) or transferrin saturation >20% (unless ferritin >800 μg/litre).
→ it is likely that this will require intravenous iron (usually 600–1000 mg for adults)

Initiate erythropoiesis-stimulating agents (ESAs) and adjust dose and frequency
→ to maintain stable Hb in range 10.5–12.5 g/dl (to achieve the maximum number of patients within target range of 11–12 g/dl).
→ to keep the rate of increase of Hb between 1 and 2 g/dl per month

Maintain adequate iron levels
→ keep serum ferritin in the range 200–500 μg/litre with hypochromic red cells <6% (unless ferritin >800 μg/litre) or transferrin saturation >20% (unless ferritin >800 μg/litre).
→ it is likely that this will require regular but infrequent intravenous iron

Monitor
→ Hb every 2–4 weeks (induction phase, or after ESA dosage change) or every 1–3 months (maintenance phase).
→ iron status every 1–3 months (but not within a week of receiving intravenous iron)

Review
→ patient's clinical response
→ if there is any unexpected change in Hb level

[a]The 'normal' range for ferritin is usually quoted as 15–200 μg/litre
[b]Percentage of hypochromic red cells directly reflects the number of red cells with suboptimal haemoglobin content and may be determined by some automated analysers: <2.5% is normal and >10% indicates definite iron deficiency

Table 21.6.9 Causes of failure to respond to erythropoiesis-stimulating agents (ESAs)

Cause	Comment
Is the patient receiving the injections?	
Absolute or functional iron deficiency	Check serum ferritin and hypochromic red cells or transferrin saturation
Acute or chronic inflammatory states	These reduce the efficacy of ESAs
Other haematological conditions	Consider myeloma, other malignant diseases affecting the bone marrow, thalassaemia, vitamin B_{12} or folate deficiency
Chloramine in dialysis water	Can cause haemolysis presenting as apparent resistance to ESAs
Aluminium overload	Rare
Antierythropoietin antibodies	Rare, but a significant concern with one ESA preparation that led to its temporary withdrawal

The absolute indications for dialysis, other than in patients for whom such treatment would be inappropriate, are the development of complications that cannot be treated by conservative and pharmacological means. These are hyperkalaemia, fluid overload, severe hypertension, pericarditis, encephalopathy, and neuropathy. To wait for these is bad practice, but nephrologists generally do wait until the patient has some uraemic symptoms such as anorexia, lassitude and pruritus, if only because their relief reinforces the need to adjust to regular dialysis. Apart from the serum potassium concentration and the degree of acidosis, blood tests such as urea and creatinine do not provide a safe guide as to when to start. Nevertheless, it is advisable to start dialysis, even in the absence of symptoms, when GFR falls below about 10 ml/min. In small patients with little muscle bulk the urea concentration is often between 30 and 40 mmol/litre and the creatinine concentration between 650 and 800 μmol/litre; in larger subjects the blood urea concentration is typically 45 to 50 mmol/litre and that of creatinine above 1000 μmol/litre. Initiation of dialysis at lower blood levels of urea and creatinine is recommended in diabetic patients.

The choice of modality—haemodialysis, continuous ambulatory peritoneal dialysis, or renal transplantation—depends on many factors, not least their availability and the patient's preference (see Chapters 21.7.1–21.7.3 for further discussion). If transplantation is appropriate, there is no reason not to perform it before dialysis is required. If haemodialysis is chosen, vascular access should be created 4 to 6 months before it is needed. If continuous ambulatory peritoneal dialysis is to be used, the Tenckhoff catheter should be placed 2 to 3 weeks before dialysis needs to be started to allow it to seal.

Conservative management of terminal uraemia

There are patients for whom dialysis is inappropriate, or who choose either not to start treatment or to discontinue it. Because, intuitively, one would predict that instituting dialysis in a patient with renal failure and other comorbid conditions should result in some improvement by ameliorating at least one element of their clinical condition, many nephrologists find it very hard not to start. Some—often those who visit the floor of the dialysis unit relatively infrequently—argue that there is no harm done by starting because treatment can always be stopped, or the patient will die despite dialysis. However, haemodialysis is usually the only treatment modality possible in such circumstances, and the business of establishing access by (inevitably) insertion of central venous lines, the complications of such lines, the requirement for thrice-weekly transport to dialysis facilities for treatment that the frail body may

Table 21.6.10 Complications of chronic renal failure

Complication	Comment
Cardiovascular system	
Hypertension	Discussed in text
Left ventricular hypertrophy	Found in 75% of dialysis patients
Coronary atherosclerosis	Cardiovascular disease is responsible for about 50% of deaths of patients receiving RRT. High risk of acute myocardial infarction, but sudden arrhythmic death is the most common fatal cardiac event
Pericarditis	A feature of neglected uraemia, including inadequate dialysis; can lead to tamponade and death
Calcific valvular disease	Mitral valve calcification found in one-third of dialysis patients. Calcific aortic stenosis can progress very rapidly
Respiratory system	
Pulmonary oedema	Feature of fluid retention
Pleural effusion	Feature of fluid retention
Gastrointestinal system	
Anorexia, nausea and vomiting	
Poor oral hygiene	
Haemorrhage	Due to nonspecific gastric ulceration and/or angiodysplasia anywhere in the gastrointestinal tract; CKD renders normal bone marrow compensatory mechanisms less effective
Pancreatitis	Can be provoked by hypercalcaemia; long-term dialysis patients develop pancreatic fibrosis, but this does not seem to affect pancreatic function

Table 21.6.10 (*Cont'd*) Complications of chronic renal failure

Complication	Comment
Nervous system	
Encephalopathy	Typically presents with confusion, myoclonic muscular twitching, and impairment of consciousness; seizures are rare unless there is accelerated hypertension
Sensorimotor peripheral polyneuropathy	Presents as dysaesthesias, restless legs, eventually weakness with foot drop; dialysis leads to slow improvement, but patients are often left with motor disability
Autonomic neuropathy	Manifests as abnormal cardiovascular reflexes, particularly on dialysis
Carpal tunnel compression	Caused by β_2-microglobulin amyloid deposition; a feature in almost all patients who have been on dialysis for more than 10 years
Dialysis dementia	Presents as gradual deterioration in intellectual performance, progressing to dementia with abnormal movements. Due to aluminium intoxication. Should be of historical interest only
Musculoskeletal system	
Mineral and bone disorder	Discussed in text
Proximal myopathy	
Crystal arthropathy	Gout and pseudogout (pyrophosphate arthropathy) are common. Management of gout can be difficult: NSAIDs are best avoided if possible in patients with advanced CKD who are not on dialysis, although very short-term use is acceptable; diarrhoea caused by colchicine can lead to acute deterioration of CKD; a short course of oral prednisolone (20 mg/day) may be the best treatment for an acute attack; reduced dose of allopurinol required
Skin	
Pigmentation	
Pruritis	Can be a cause of significant distress. Associated with dry skin (xerosis), and worse when the skin is warm. Cause is uncertain—raised calcium × phosphate product, histamine sensitivity, and 'uraemia' have been blamed. Scratching can lead to infection and nodular prurigo. Treatments include starting/increasing dialysis, emollient lotions/creams, controlling plasma phosphate, keeping cool, antihistamines (e.g. chlorphenamine 4 mg at night), naltrexone, and ultraviolet phototherapy
Calciphylaxis	Discussed in text
Bullous eruptions	Pseudoporphyria, affecting sun-exposed areas. Thought to be due to accumulation of porphyrins in high-molecular-weight protein-bound complexes that are not removed by haemodialysis. Treatment is by avoidance of sun exposure, phlebotomy (for patients who are not anaemic and who have increased iron stores) and ESAs (which remove iron from stores by enhancing production of red blood cells)
Sexual function	
Men	Loss of libido and erectile impotence are common and of multifactorial cause. Sperm counts may be low leading to reduced fertility. Priapism is a rare complication of haemodialysis treatment
Women	Most women with severe CKD develop irregular periods or amenorrhoea and are infertile, with rare pregnancies almost always ending in miscarriage. For general discussion of pregnancy in women with kidney disease, see Chapter 14.5.
Psychological	
	Anxiety and depression are predictable and understandable consequences of loss of health, control, and pleasure. They tend to be most prominent in young patients. The best treatment is by sympathetic support of the dialysis multidisciplinary team. Psychotherapy/counselling can be helpful, but psychiatrists and/or medication have little to offer unless there is a specific mental illness
Metabolic	
Glucose intolerance	CKD causes resistance to insulin-mediated glucose uptake in skeletal muscle
Complex effects on lipids	Increased very-low-density lipoproteins (VLDL); increased high density lipoproteins (HDL)
Enhanced protein catabolism	Risk of malnutrition discussed in text
Haematological	
Anaemia	Discussed in text
Impaired platelet function	Platelet numbers are normal, but function impaired at the level of endothelial contact
Impaired T-cell immunity	Mechanism uncertain, but puts patients with advanced CKD at higher risk of reactivation of tuberculosis and herpes zoster, of failure to clear some viral infections (e.g. hepatitis B), and of failure to generate normal responses to immunization (e.g. hepatitis B vaccine)
Impaired neutrophil function	Mechanism uncertain, but may in part explain high incidence and severity of bacterial infections
Infective	
Blood-borne viruses	Dialysis is a risk factor for hepatitis C, hepatitis B and HIV
Methicillin-resistant *Staphylococcus aureus* (MRSA)	Dialysis patients are at high risk of acquiring MRSA because of their frequent contact with medical services, common requirement for invasive procedures/indwelling lines, and (perhaps) susceptibility to infection
Clostridium difficile infection	A problem on many renal units
Endocarditis	Bacteraemias in dialysis patients are often attributable to infection of vascular access sites, which, combined with high prevalence of calcific valvular disease, creates high risk of endocarditis, usually (70%) due to *S. aureus*

CKD, chronic kidney disease; ESA, erythropoiesis-stimulating agent; NSAID, nonsteroidal anti-inflammatory drug; RRT, renal replacement therapy.

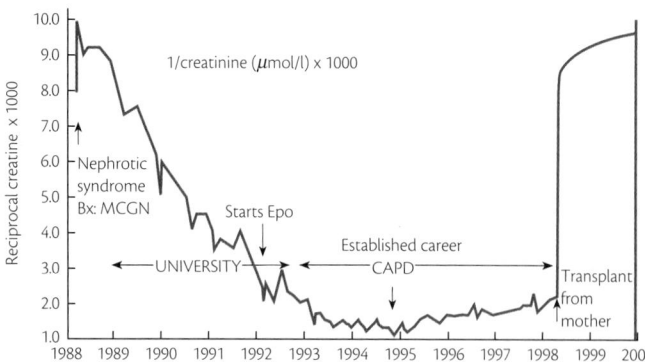

Fig. 21.6.11 A reciprocal creatinine plot showing the progressive decline in renal function in a patient with glomerulonephritis. The timing of the need to start dialysis could be predicted sufficiently well to allow planning of treatment.

find difficult if not impossible to tolerate, recovering only in time for the next dialysis session, can be truly miserable for the patient and all others concerned. Furthermore, in frail patients, usually elderly and with multiple comorbidities, it is not likely that dialysis will greatly prolong life, although it can certainly lower the quality of it. There have been no trials that have randomized such patients to treatment with RRT or to conservative (palliative) management, but one study reported the outcome of 63 patients who were recommended to receive palliative care after multidisciplinary assessment and counselling about treatment options. Ten of these patients opted for and received dialysis treatment, but their median survival after initiation of dialysis (8.3 months) was not significantly longer than survival beyond the putative date of dialysis initiation in the palliatively treated patients (6.3 months), and 65% of those treated with dialysis died in hospital, compared with 27% of those receiving palliative care.

Withdrawing dialysis or dying while on treatment is often traumatic for the patient, the patient's family and friends, and staff, but at least 10% of deaths in dialysis programmes follow withdrawal of treatment.

If one takes the view that dialysis is a treatment offered to allow a patient to continue living with a reasonable quality of life, as opposed to delaying death in the short term, then it will not be offered to patients with other immediately life-limiting conditions. One could argue that it should not be started when survival beyond 3 months outside hospital is unlikely. However, the ethical and legal issues are complex and require that the patient makes the decision not to start or to discontinue treatment when fully informed and able to do so. If possible, the physician should discuss with the patient the option of not starting before dialysis is actually needed. The patient needs to be given a realistic account of what dialysis can achieve, what it cannot achieve, and at what cost—access, travel, restrictions, and complications. These conversations can be difficult and cannot be hurried. They can often be helped by offering arrangements for the patient (and relative/friend) to visit the dialysis unit, and it is critically important that the patient (and their relatives/friends) does not get the entirely erroneous impression that dialysis means that 'the doctors care and I'll live for ever', whereas "no dialysis means that 'the doctors don't care and I'll die soon'.

Properly managed, death from uraemia is peaceful and free of suffering. It is important to ensure so far as is possible that the patient has peace of mind, that they are comfortable with their decision, and that their family members are understanding and supportive. They will be comforted to know that their doctor respects their decision. Several distressing symptoms may need to be controlled. Breathlessness from pulmonary oedema and acidosis is best controlled with a morphine infusion. Nausea and anorexia can be helped with regular chlorpromazine 25 mg four times daily, and ondansetron 8 mg twice daily can also be effective. Food and fluid should be offered in small, palatable helpings, with no pressure to eat or drink exerted on the patient. The mouth can become dry and crusted from mouth breathing and will smell foul from uraemic saliva, for which regular mouth washes and gum care will help. Pruritus is managed by keeping the skin cool, and soft with emollients. The patient may not be aware of myoclonic jerks, but these may distress the family: benzodiazepines, such as clonazepam, can be prescribed if needed.

Further reading

Brazy PC, Stead WW, Fitzwilliam JF (1989). Progression of renal insufficiency: role of blood pressure. *Kidney Int*, **35**, 670–4.

Chen J, *et al.* (2004). The metabolic syndrome and chronic kidney disease in U.S. adults. *Ann Intern Med*, **140**, 167–74.

Coresh J, *et al.* (2003). Prevalence of chronic kidney disease and decreased kidney function in the adult US population: Third National Health and Nutrition Examination Survey. *Am J Kidney Dis*, **41**, 1–12.

Grassmann A, *et al.* (2005). ESRD patients in 2004: global overview of patient numbers, treatment modalities and associated trends. *Nephrol Dial Transplant*, **20**, 2587–93.

Hallan S, *et al.* (2007). Association of kidney function and albuminuria with cardiovascular mortality in older vs younger individuals: The HUNT II Study. *Arch Intern Med*, **167**, 2490–6.

Hallan SI, *et al.* (2006). International comparison of the relationship of chronic kidney disease prevalence and ESRD risk. *J Am Soc Nephrol*, **17**, 2275–84.

Hsu CY, *et al.* (2005). Elevated blood pressure and risk of end-stage renal disease in subjects without baseline kidney disease. *Arch Intern Med*, **165**, 923–8.

Hsu CY, *et al.* (2006). Body mass index and risk for end-stage renal disease. *Ann Intern Med*, **144**, 21–8.

Jager KJ, *et al.* (2003). The epidemic of aging in renal replacement therapy: an update on elderly patients and their outcomes. *Clin Nephrol*, **60**, 352–60.

Keith DS, *et al.* (2004). Longitudinal follow-up and outcomes among a population with chronic kidney disease in a large managed care organization. *Arch Intern Med*, **164**, 659–63.

National Kidney Foundation. (2002). K/DOQI clinical practice guidelines for chronic kidney disease: evaluation, classification and stratification. *Am J Kidney Dis*, **39**, S1–S266.

Rossing P (2006). Diabetic nephropathy: worldwide epidemic and effects of current treatment on natural history. *Curr Diab Rep*, **6**, 479–83.

Smith C, *et al.* (2003). Choosing not to dialyse: evaluation of planned non-dialytic management in a cohort of patients with end-stage renal failure. *Nephron Clin Pract*, **95**, c40–6.

Progression of CKD and its prevention

Barnett AH, *et al.* (2004). Angiotensin-receptor blockade versus converting-enzyme inhibition in type 2 diabetes and nephropathy. *N Engl J Med*, **351**, 1952–61.

Brenner BM, Meyer TW, Hostetter TH (1982). Dietary protein intake and the progressive nature of kidney disease: the role of hemodynamically mediated glomerular injury in the pathogenesis of progressive glomerular sclerosis in aging, renal ablation, and intrinsic renal disease. *N Engl J Med*, **307**, 652–9.

Casas JP, *et al.* (2005). Effect of inhibitors of the renin–angiotensin system and other antihypertensive drugs on renal outcomes: systematic review and meta-analysis. *Lancet*, **366**, 2026–33.

Klahr S, *et al.* (1994). The effects of dietary protein restriction and blood-pressure control on the progression of chronic renal disease. Modification of Diet in Renal Disease Study Group. *N Engl J Med*, **330**, 877–84.

Lewis EJ, *et al.* (2001). Renoprotective effect of the angiotensin-receptor antagonist irbesartan in patients with nephropathy due to type 2 diabetes. *N Engl J Med*, **345**, 851–60.

Mancia G, Grassi G (2005). Joint National Committee VII and European Society of Hypertension/European Society of Cardiology guidelines for evaluating and treating hypertension: a two-way road? *J Am Soc Nephrol*, **16**, Suppl 1, S74–7.

Muntner P, *et al.* (2009). Hypertension awareness, treatment, and control in adults with CKD: results from the chronic renal insufficiency cohort (CRIC) study. *Am J Kidney Dis*, Dec 3.

Peterson JC, *et al.* (1995). Blood pressure control, proteinuria, and the progression of renal disease. The Modification of Diet in Renal Disease Study. *Ann Intern Med*, **123**, 754–62.

Pohl MA, *et al.* (2005). Independent and additive impact of blood pressure control and angiotensin-II receptor blockade on renal outcomes in the irbesartan diabetic nephropathy trial: clinical implications and limitations. *J Am Soc Nephrol*, **16**, 3027–37.

Remuzzi G, Chiurchiu C, Ruggenenti P (2004). Proteinuria predicting outcome in renal disease: Nondiabetic nephropathies (REIN). *Kidney Int Suppl*, S90–6.

Sarnak MJ, *et al.* (2005). The effect of a lower target blood pressure on the progression of kidney disease: long-term follow-up of the modification of diet in renal disease study. *Ann Intern Med*, **142**, 342–51.

Mineral and bone disorder

Arnold A, *et al.* (1995). Monoclonality of parathyroid tumors in chronic renal failure and in primary parathyroid hyperplasia. *J Clin Invest*, **95**, 2047–54.

Block GA, *et al.* (2004). Cinacalcet for secondary hyperparathyroidism in patients receiving hemodialysis. *N Engl J Med*, **350**, 1516–25.

Block GA, *et al.* (2007). Mortality effect of coronary calcification and phosphate binder choice in incident hemodialysis patients. *Kidney Int*, **71**, 438–41.

Eknoyan G, Levin A, Levin NW (2003). Bone metabolism and disease in chronic kidney disease. *Am J Kidney Dis*, **42**, 1–201.

Fine A, Zacharias J (2002). Calciphylaxis is usually non-ulcerating: Risk factors, outcome and therapy. *Kidney Int*, **61**, 2210–17.

Goodman WG, *et al.* (2004). Vascular calcification in chronic kidney disease. *Am J Kidney Dis*, **43**, 572–9.

Hollis BW (2005). Circulating 25-hydroxyvitamin D levels indicative of vitamin D sufficiency: implications for establishing a new effective dietary intake recommendation for vitamin D. *J Nutr*, **135**, 317–22.

Ketteler M, Gross ML, Ritz E (2005). Calcification and cardiovascular problems in renal failure. *Kidney Int*, **67**, S120–7.

London GM, *et al.* (2003). Arterial media calcification in end-stage renal disease: impact on all-cause and cardiovascular mortality. *Nephrol Dial Transplant*, **18**, 1731–40.

Massry SG, *et al.* (2003). K/DOQI clinical practice guidelines for bone metabolism and disease in chronic kidney disease. *Am J Kidney Dis*, **42**(4 Suppl 3), i–S201.

Moe S, *et al.* (2006). Definition, evaluation, and classification of renal osteodystrophy: A position statement from Kidney Disease: Improving Global Outcomes (KDIGO). *Kidney Int*, **69**, 1945–53.

National Institute for Health and Clinical Excellence (2007). *Cinacalcet for the treatment of secondary hyperparathyroidism in patients with end-stage renal disease on maintenance dialysis therapy.* NICE technology appraisal guidance 117, NICE, London.

Navaneethan SD, *et al.* (2009). Benefits and harms of phosphate binders in CKD: a systematic review of randomized controlled trials. *Am J Kidney Dis*, **54**, 619–37.

Razzaque MS. (2009). The FGF23-Klotho axis: endocrine regulation of phosphate homeostasis. *Nat Rev Endocrinol*, **5**, 611–9.

Ritz E (2005). The clinical management of hyperphosphatemia. *J Nephrol*, **18**, 221–8.

Ritz E, Gross ML, Dikow R (2005). Role of calcium-phosphorous disorders in the progression of renal failure. *Kidney Int*, 68, S66–70.

Schmitt CP, Odenwald T, Ritz E (2006). Calcium, calcium regulatory hormones, and calcimimetics: Impact on cardiovascular mortality. *J Am Soc Nephrol*, **17**, S78–80.

Teng M, *et al.* (2003). Survival of patients undergoing hemodialysis with paricalcitol or calcitriol therapy. *N Engl J Med*, **349**, 446–56.

Urena-Torres P, *et al.* (2007). Klotho: An antiaging protein involved in mineral and vitamin D metabolism. *Kidney Int*, **71**, 730–7.

Renal anaemia

Besarab A, *et al.* (2000). Optimization of epoetin therapy with intravenous iron therapy in hemodialysis patients. *J Am Soc Nephrol*, **11**, 530–8.

Drueke TB, *et al.*; CREATE investigators (2006). Normalization of hemoglobin level in patients with chronic kidney disease and anemia. *N Engl J Med*, **355**, 2071–84.

Hsu CY, Mcculloch CE, Curhan GC (2002). Iron status and hemoglobin level in chronic renal insufficiency. *J Am Soc Nephrol*, **13**, 2783–6.

Kaufman JS, *et al.* (2001). Diagnostic value of iron indices in hemodialysis patients receiving epoetin. *Kidney Int*, **60**, 300–8.

Kazmi WH, *et al.* (2001). Anemia: An early complication of chronic renal insufficiency. *Am J Kidney Dis*, **38**, 803–12.

Li S, Collins AJ (2004). Association of hematocrit value with cardiovascular morbidity and mortality in incident hemodialysis patients. *Kidney Int*, **65**, 626–33.

MacDougall IC, *et al.* (2009). A peptide-based erythropoietin-receptor agonist for pure red-cell aplasia. *N Engl J Med*, **361**, 1848–55.

National Collaborating Centre for Chronic Conditions (2006). *Anaemia management in chronic kidney disease: national clinical guideline for management in adults and children.* Royal College of Physicians, London.

Van Wyck D, *et al.* (2005). A randomized, controlled trial comparing IV iron sucrose to oral iron in anaemic patients with nondialysis-dependent CKD. *Kidney Int*, **68**, 2846–56.

Renal replacement therapy

Contents

21.7.1 **Haemodialysis**

Ken Farrington and Roger Greenwood

Essentials

Over the past four decades, maintenance haemodialysis has proved to be a highly successful treatment for patients with endstage renal disease. In the developed world, the haemodialysis population continues to increase and is becoming more elderly and dependent. However, despite considerable advances in haemodialysis technology and other significant improvements, such as those in renal anaemia management, the long-term clinical outcomes for patients remain much less good than those of other people with comparable characteristics but without renal failure.

Dialysis adequacy—working definitions are based on small-solute—typically urea—removal, which occurs mainly by diffusion. Current guidelines recommend targeting a normalized urea clearance (eKt/V) in excess of 1.2 per session for thrice-weekly treatment. Higher doses of dialysis delivered thrice weekly do not produce significant improvement in outcomes, but there is increasing interest in more frequent treatment as a means to adequately control uraemia and to improve survival, and there is also a need to incorporate more holistic approaches into the concept of adequacy.

Technical aspects of haemodialysis—high-flux membranes are needed to achieve significant removal of middle molecules, of which β_2-microglobulin is the prime example. Use of such membranes can slow the progression of dialysis-related amyloidosis, a complication of long-term haemodialysis related to β_2-microglobulin retention, but firm evidence of an effect on survival is lacking. The technique of haemodiafiltration adds a significant convective component to high-flux haemodialysis, providing improved β_2-microglobulin clearance, with observational studies suggesting a survival benefit.

Vascular access—the need to secure and maintain reliable vascular access is fundamental to achieving adequate dialysis and maintaining health. An arteriovenous fistula is the preferred option, with fewer complications and longer survival than other access options. The current overdependence on tunnelled lines contributes to morbidity and excess mortality, mainly from line-related sepsis, and represents a failure in access provision.

Complications of haemodialysis—the main acute complication of haemodialysis is intradialytic hypotension, resulting from an imbalance between the ultrafiltration rate and the rate of vascular refill. Underlying cardiovascular disease, antihypertensive drugs, autonomic dysfunction, shortened dialysis times, large interdialytic fluid gains, and inaccurate dry-weight assessment all predispose. Postdialysis headache is relatively common, as is prolonged bleeding from the fistula after needle removal. Dialyser reactions are less common. More serious bleeding problems with anticoagulation are rare. True heparin-induced thrombocytopenia (HIT-II) is very rare, but is potentially life threatening.

Comorbidities in patients on dialysis—the high mortality in the dialysis population is mainly due to accelerated cardiovascular disease. Traditional risk factors for atheroma such as hypertension and dyslipidaemia are common, but difficult to interpret: there seems to be a paradoxical relationship between blood pressure and mortality in patients on haemodialysis ('reverse epidemiology'), and there are questions about the appropriateness of current blood pressure targets in the absence of randomized interventional trials of the effect of blood pressure reduction in this population. Similarly, there are data to suggest that statins do not significantly affect overall cardiovascular morbidity and mortality in people with type 2 diabetes on haemodialysis. In addition, there are a myriad of less traditional risk factors operating in dialysis patients, including anaemia, disturbances of calcium and phosphate metabolism, hyperhomocysteinaemia, increased oxidative stress, and elevated inflammatory markers. It may be that the combined effect of all these risk factors outweighs the benefits of a single intervention, and more global approaches are required. It remains to be seen whether the improved control of the uraemic milieu possible with more frequent dialysis schedules will impact on survival.

Is haemodialysis in the best interest of the patient?—haemodialysis, although universally applicable, has its limitations. Dialysis initiation may not improve quality of life or survival for some very high-risk dependent patients, for whom supportive therapy, and not dialysis, may be the best treatment option.

Introduction

The availability of effective renal replacement therapy (RRT) has transformed the outlook for patients with endstage renal failure (ESRF) over the past 40 years, replacing certain and imminent death with the potential for long-term survival. The modalities of RRT comprise haemodialysis, peritoneal dialysis and renal transplantation. These therapies are appropriately regarded as complementary but, because of its very few contraindications, haemodialysis can be regarded as the default modality. Growing numbers of patients worldwide are now dependent on regular haemodialysis to sustain life, the escalating proportion of older and frailer patients being direct testimony to the flexibility of the treatment. Inevitably, this success needs qualification. (1) The functions of the kidney are many and diverse and dialysis provides only partial replacement for some, notably the excretion of nitrogenous waste products, and the control of water, electrolyte, and acid–base balance. Additional measures are required to manage problems such as anaemia and abnormal mineral metabolism (see Chapter 21.6). (2) Although there is agreement about the general aims of dialysis treatment—to maintain life and prevent or reduce morbidity from uraemia—there is no consensus on the best way to achieve these aims. There is still debate about what constitutes adequate dialysis and even about which parameters we should be trying to control. (3) Although dialysis undoubtedly prolongs life in patients with ESRF, mortality still far exceeds that in the general population. This is mainly due to cardiovascular disease, which is endemic and runs an accelerated course in dialysis patients, whatever the modality employed. This chapter outlines the scope of current practice in haemodialysis, stressing those aspects most relevant to clinical management.

Development of haemodialysis

The pioneers

The process of dialysis was discovered in the mid-19th century as a means of separating dissolved elements by diffusion through a semipermeable membrane (Graham, 1861). Subsequent evolution of the technique from the first use of an artificial kidney in experimental studies in dogs (by Abel and colleagues, 1913) to the first successful dialysis treatment of a patient with acute renal failure (by Kolff, 1943) followed technical advances in the development of the semipermeable membrane cellophane, which was originally introduced as sausage skin, and of anticoagulants—first hirudin, then heparin. The extension of the technique to the maintenance treatment of patients with ESRF followed the development in the 1960s of the

Scribner silastic shunt and the Brescia–Cimino arteriovenous fistula, which allowed safe and reliable long-term venous access.

Expanding services

Haemodialysis treatment was originally reserved for young and otherwise fit patients. Rigid selection criteria were applied, but ethical concerns, together with rising patient expectations, eventually led to more liberal policies. There were marked geographical differences, largely economically driven, in subsequent rates of expansion of dialysis programmes, in the modalities employed, and in the patterns of service provision. In the United States of America and most of Europe, haemodialysis was rapidly decentralized from the pioneering units into small but numerous hospital-based units and freestanding facilities in cities, towns, and rural areas (Fig. 21.7.1.1). By contrast, there was little decentralization in the United Kingdom from the 50 or so large metropolitan centres, and self-supervised home haemodialysis was the preferred means of expansion. Selection criteria remained tight.

The advent of continuous ambulatory peritoneal dialysis (CAPD) in the early 1980s was seized on as a means to liberalize access to treatment in the United Kingdom. CAPD became the dominant dialysis mode, engulfing the home haemodialysis programme and relegating centre-based haemodialysis to the status of rescue mode for those in whom CAPD was precluded or had failed. However, in the last 15 years the haemodialysis base in the United Kingdom has expanded, mainly through the building of satellite units, owing to the combined effects of an increasingly aged and frail dialysis population, many of whom are unable to cope with the requirements of CAPD or other peritoneal dialysis techniques, recognition that with loss of residual renal function peritoneal dialysis may not provide adequate treatment (see below), and also because of the flow of capital from commercial dialysis companies. This has led to a convergence towards the American/European pattern of provision (Fig. 21.7.1.2). Haemodialysis has become the dominant dialysis modality in the United Kingdom, with peritoneal dialysis falling to only 22% of prevalent patients.

Impact of adequacy

Although patients continued to dialyse thrice weekly, there was a general trend to reduce dialysis times in response to increasing

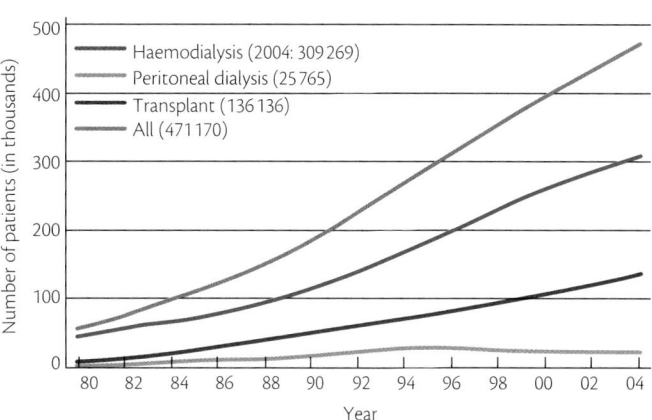

Fig. 21.7.1.1 Prevalent patient counts, by modality, for all patients receiving renal replacement therapy in the United States of America between 1980 and 2004. (Data from the United States Renal Data Systems (USRDS).)

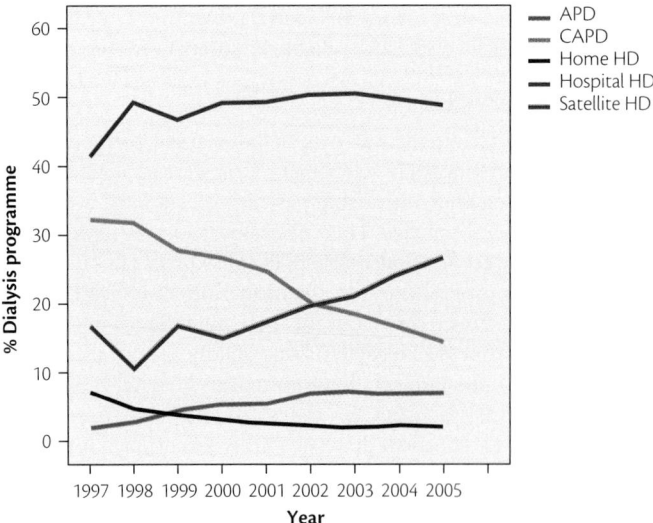

Fig. 21.7.1.2 Modality of renal replacement therapy in the United Kingdom between 1997 and 2005. APD, automated peritoneal dialysis; CAPD, continuous ambulatory peritoneal dialysis; HD, haemodialysis.

funding constraints and patient preference. 'Short dialysis' (<4 h/session) was held responsible for the excess mortality in American haemodialysis patients in the 1980s, which focused attention on the concept of dialysis adequacy. Most units now prescribe and monitor dialysis dose using the urea kinetic methods established at that time. The same concepts were also applied to CAPD, leading to recognition that CAPD adequacy is critically dependent on residual renal function, and that loss of residual renal function compromises adequacy, sometimes to the point of technique non-viability, especially in larger patients. This was a significant factor in the steady relative decline in the United Kingdom CAPD population during the 1990s (Fig. 21.7.1.2), a decrease that has been more than offset by increased centre-based haemodialysis provision. The automated peritoneal dialysis (APD) programme has also grown, but it remains small. In the last decade or so, dialysis practice in the United Kingdom has tended to converge to the American and European model.

Changing demographics

Demographic changes have placed increased demands on nephrological and other specialist resources. The median age of new patients commencing on dialysis in the United Kingdom has increased considerably over the last two decades and is now over 64 years, with around one-quarter over 75 years. Older people account for most of the increase in incidence and prevalence rates, which now exceed 100 and 600 patients per million population, respectively. The proportion of patients commencing dialysis with extrarenal comorbidities, particularly cardiovascular disease, has increased dramatically, and multiple pathologies are common. Around 20% of United Kingdom dialysis patients are diabetic, and in the United States of America this figure is around 50% (see Chapter 21.6). Many such patients have widespread micro- and macrovascular complications at the time of dialysis initiation.

Impact of transplantation

The haemodialysis population has continued to grow despite active transplant programmes. Two main factors account for this. First, the major growth in the dialysis population is among older people,

who tend to have a high comorbid load such that renal transplantation is contraindicated. Second, the donor pool is limited, despite initiatives to increase this, such as encouragement of living donation and use of asystolic donors (see Chapter 21.7.3).

Impact of conservative (nondialytic) management

There is increasing recognition that dialysis treatment may be of limited benefit to some elderly, dependent patients, many of whom have multiple comorbidities. In such patients, dialysis may not enhance quality of life or life expectancy and some may choose not to dialyse, opting instead for a conservative approach. Increased awareness of and provision of conservative management pathways and services may produce a small reduction in the rate of growth of the dialysis population. Where conservative management programmes have been established, up to 15% of patients reaching ESRF are supported by this modality.

Technical aspects of haemodialysis
Principles of dialysis

Dialysis is a physicochemical process allowing separation of the components of a complex solution by solute exchange across a semipermeable membrane. Such membranes act as molecular size-selective filters, the size threshold depending on the nature of the membrane. In haemodialysis, the membrane is interposed between the patient's bloodstream and a rinsing solution (dialysis fluid). Diffusive and convective mass transfer takes place across the membrane, allowing changes in the composition of body fluid compartments.

The rate of diffusive transport of a solute is dependent on its molecular weight, electrical charge, the blood–dialysis fluid concentration gradient, blood and dialysis flow rates, and membrane characteristics (membrane area and membrane mass transfer-area coefficient, K_oA). With current designs of dialysers, blood is perfused through a bundle of narrow capillaries with a total surface area between 1 and 1.5 m^2. Small molecules such as urea (60 Da) are cleared well, but larger molecules such as albumin (60 000 Da) cannot pass through the membrane. The clearance of middle molecules such as β_2-microglobulin (11 800 Da) can be improved somewhat by using high-flux membranes, which have pores of sufficient size to allow their passage, although fluid layering still presents a substantial barrier to slowly diffusing large molecules.

Convection involves the bulk movement of solvent and solute across the membrane. The driving force is transmembrane hydrostatic pressure, which can be adjusted by application of variable negative pressure to the dialysate side of the membrane. Solute transport (by solvent drag) is independent of diffusion. In general, convection contributes little to the clearance of rapidly diffusible small solutes such as urea, but can add significantly to the diffusive clearance of middle molecules by high-flux membranes. Convective movement of water from blood across the membrane is known as ultrafiltration, the rate of which depends on the hydrostatic pressure difference across the membrane and on its permeability to water (ultrafiltration coefficient, K_{uf}).

Membranes and dialysers

The original haemodialysis membranes were fashioned from regenerated cellulose, but technology has since proliferated and

Table 21.7.1.1 Haemodialysis membranes

Membrane class	Examples	Hydraulic permeability	β$_2$-Microglobulin clearance	Biocompatability
Regenerated cellulose	Cuprophane	Low-flux	–	Poor
Modified cellulose	Cellulose acetate Cellulose diacetate Cellulose triacetate	Low/high flux	–/+	Moderate
Synthetic	Polymethylmethcrylate Polyacrylonitrile Polysulphone Polyamide Polycarbonate	High/low flux	+/–	Good

there are now three major classes of membrane (Table 21.7.1.1). In dialysers, these semipermeable membranes are arranged to form separate adjacent paths for blood and dialysis fluid, which flow on opposite sides of the membrane in opposite directions to maximise diffusion gradients.

Dialysers are classified by design type (modern dialysers are usually of hollow-fibre design), membrane composition, surface area, and membrane permeability characteristics. Membrane permeability is defined in terms of dialyser clearance K_d for a range of solutes, and ultrafiltration coefficient K_{uf}, which is the water flux per unit of transmembrane pressure. A range of K_d values is normally quoted for a particular solute, these being derived from the dialyser's mass transfer-area coefficient K_oA for that solute at a variety of appropriate blood and dialysis fluid flow rates. In contrast to cuprophane, high-flux synthetic membranes are highly permeable (high K_{uf} and high K_d for middle molecules), remove β$_2$-microglobulin and other potentially toxic middle molecules, and tend to be more biocompatible, meaning that they cause less activation of inflammatory cells, the complement cascade, and contact pathways, and less cytokine production. However, in spite of numerous experimental demonstrations of such potentially beneficial effects, it is still unclear whether clinical use of biocompatible membranes translates into improved outcomes.

High-flux membranes permit high-volume ultrafiltration, which can be ulitised to combine convective clearance with the diffusive clearance offered by haemodialysis in the technique of haemodiafiltration (see later). As a consequence of the high flow rates employed and the countercurrent flow, there is an unavoidable movement of dialysis fluid into blood. This so called 'obligatory back-filtration' (Fig. 21.7.1.3) provides some useful convective clearance (internal haemodiafiltration), but also underscores the need to use ultrapure water in the preparation of dialysis fluid. Most would argue that this is highly desirable anyway. The observed absence of clinical sequelae from back-filtration may reflect the effectiveness of the membrane as a bacterial filter, but the absorptive capacity (for endotoxins) of the 'thick' matrix supporting the diffusing surface of the membrane may also be important.

Dialysis water and fluids

Patients on haemodialysis are intimately exposed to huge quantities of water. Normally people are exposed (by drinking and eating) to around 15 litres of water each week, from which they are protected by the gut. By contrast, haemodialysis patients are exposed to 300 to 600 litres/week and protected only by the dialysis membrane. The potential for poisoning by waterborne impurities is significant. Aluminium and chloramines are examples of proven toxins, which must be removed. Bacterial and endotoxin contamination can produce major acute problems, including intradialytic pyrexias and hypotension, and may also add to the inflammatory milieu, which is a feature of uraemia. Use of ultrapure water is important generally, but perhaps especially in high-flux modes in which dialysis fluid is infused, passively (back-filtration) or actively (online haemodiafiltration), directly into the patient's bloodstream. Mains water supplied to the renal unit is purified by a combination of techniques which include softening and deionization, carbon adsorption, reverse osmosis, ultraviolet irradiation, and ultrafiltration. Regular monitoring is required to ensure that chemical and microbiological standards are maintained. Currently, the latter accept low levels of endotoxin and bacterial growth on culture; ultrapure water is defined by the absence of both.

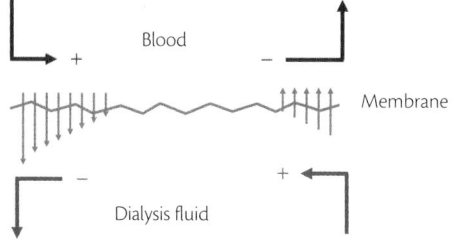

Fig. 21.7.1.3 'Obligatory back-filtration' across a high-flux dialysis membrane. At the 'arterial' end of the dialyser (left side) there is convective movement of ultrafiltrate from blood to dialysis fluid, but at the 'venous end' (right side) the situation is reversed and some dialysis fluid moves across the membrane and into the blood.

Table 21.7.1.2 Bicarbonate dialysis: concentrate composition achieved in the dialysate

Ion	Acid (mmol/litre)	Base (mmol/litre)
Na$^+$	99–110	27–40
K$^+$	0–3	0
Ca^{2+}	1.25–1.75	0
Mg^{2+}	0.75	0
Cl$^-$	99–110	0
Acetate	0	0
HCO$_3^-$	0	27–40
Glucose	0–5.5	0

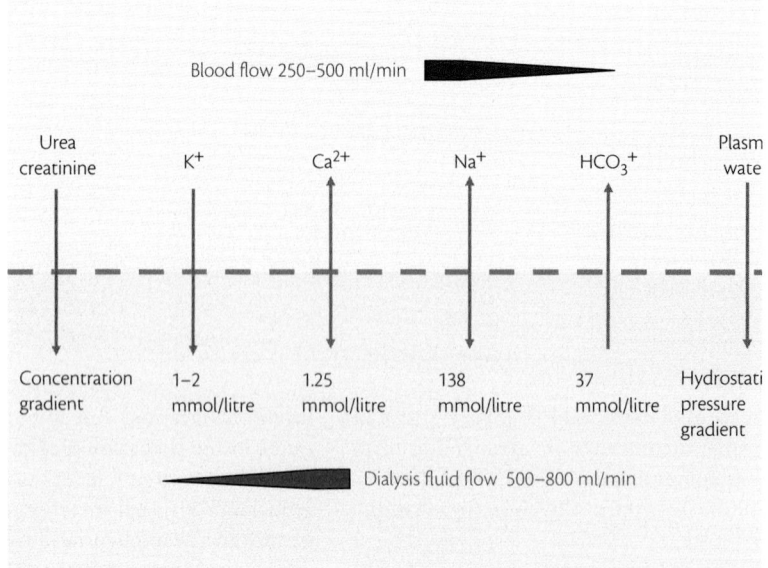

Fig. 21.7.1.4 Diffusive transport within a dialyser.

Acid and bicarbonate concentrates are mixed with treated water in a single-patient proportionating system within the dialysis machine to produce dialysis fluid of the desired composition (Table 21.7.1.2). Regulation of dialysis fluid composition is the main tool to maintain normal electrolyte and mineral concentrations and normal acid–base balance in body fluid compartments. The concentrations of substances in the dialysis fluid may be set to effect net diffusive loss (e.g. potassium), net diffusive gain (e.g. bicarbonate), or net zero balance (e.g. calcium). Sodium concentrations are generally set to achieve net zero diffusive balance with the required sodium removal being attained by ultrafiltration (Fig. 21.7.1.4). Although there is great potential for individualization, a programme-standard composition is typically adopted, which may be varied in particular circumstances.

The extracorporeal circuit

As illustrated in Fig. 21.7.1.5, blood is withdrawn from the patient via the 'A' needle inserted in the fistula (or the arterial limb of a dual-lumen dialysis catheter) by a peristaltic pump, circulated through the dialyser, and returned to the patient through the 'V' needle (or the venous limb of a dual-lumen dialysis catheter). The circuit is anticoagulated by heparin, which is infused downstream from the blood pump. The arterial pressure monitor (Pa) protects

the fistula or central vein by detecting excessive negative pressure. The venous pressure monitor (Pv) protects against blood loss from the circuit to the environment, although it is important to understand that leaks arising from dislodgement of the 'V' needle from the fistula may not be detected, since the major resistance to flow at this point in the circuit arises from the needle itself and not the fistula. Obstruction downstream of the needle or catheter does raise venous pressure. The bubble trap level detector protects against air embolus: a falling level activates a venous clamp and stops the blood pump.

The dialysis machine

The dialysis machine supplies dialysis fluid at the prescribed flow rate, temperature, and chemical composition in a fail-safe manner. It also monitors the extracorporeal circuit and in fail-safe mode activates the venous clamp and switches off the blood pump. Ultrafiltration is also controlled, volumes being preset by the operator (see below). In addition to housing the blood pump and heparin pump, most modern machines also incorporate additional devices allowing single-needle dialysis and haemodiafiltration (see below), and they may also include other technical advances such as blood temperature monitors, allowing control of thermal balance during dialysis (which may improve haemodynamic stability) and measurement of access recirculation, blood volume monitors, which detect changes in haematocrit during dialysis and are potentially useful in predicting episodes of hypotension, and devices for measuring ionic dialysance, which can allow online monitoring of adequacy parameters. The clinical usefulness of these recent technical developments remains to be fully established.

Control of ultrafiltration

Modern dialysis machines use volumetric methods that permit precise control of ultrafiltration. A balancing system placed in the dialysis fluid pathway in the machine balances dialysis fluid flow rates to and from the dialyser (Fig. 21.7.1.6). The ultrafiltration pump can be preset by the operator to remove fluid from the return limb from the dialyser, causing an equal volume to be drawn from the blood across the dialysis membrane into the dialysis fluid in order to maintain balance.

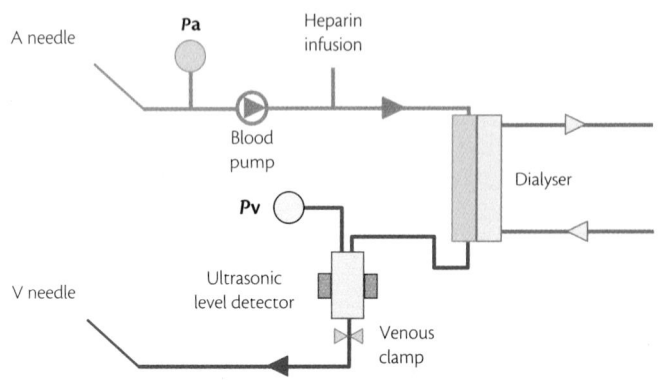

Fig. 21.7.1.5 A standard extracorporeal circuit. Pa, arterial pressure detector; Pv, venous pressure detector; A needle, arterial needle; V needle, venous needle.

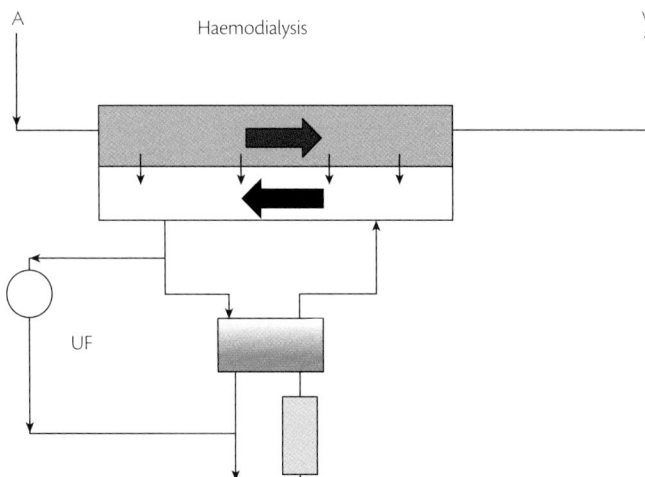

Fig. 21.7.1.6 The dialysis fluid pathway and the volumetric control of ultrafiltration. F1, filter; A, arterial line; V, venous line.

Anticoagulation

Unfractionated heparin (UFH) remains the standard anticoagulant. It is usually administered by initial intravenous bolus of 1000 to 2000 units and subsequent infusion at a similar hourly rate, stopping 30 min before the end of the session in patients with fistulas and grafts. Monitoring using whole-blood activated clotting times is possible, although many units reserve such measurements for problem situations. There is an increasing use of low-molecular-weight heparins (LMWH), which offer the advantage of single-bolus administration and appear to have a similar efficacy vs safety profile to UFH. However, measurement of anticoagulant effect is more difficult, requiring estimation of antifactor Xa inhibition, and—unlike with UFH—anticoagulation cannot be reversed with protamine. Heparin-free dialysis, employing regular saline flushes of the circuit, is the preferred strategy in patients at high risk of bleeding. In rare cases of heparin-induced thrombocytopenia (HIT), in which heparin-free dialysis is not possible, the direct thrombin inhibitor argatroban is probably the favoured option. LMWH should not be used in this situation.

Haemodialysis/filtration techniques

Conventional haemodialysis

Conventional haemodialysis uses low-flux membranes in standard circuits, producing diffusive but little convective solute removal. Smaller molecules such as urea are cleared efficiently, but middle-molecule clearance is poor. Previously, the definition would also have included the use of acetate as buffer, but bicarbonate dialysis is now the norm.

Haemofiltration

Haemofiltration is a purely convective treatment, the inefficiency of which for small-molecule clearance limits its applicability in the intermittent treatments required in chronic renal failure, but in continuous mode the technique has become established as a treatment of acute renal failure in the critical care setting. Highly permeable membranes are used, permitting high-volume ultrafiltration of 20 to 50 litres per session. Substitution fluid is delivered from commercially prepared bags, either on the arterial side of the filter (predilution) or into the venous bubble-trap (postdilution).

Middle-molecule clearance is excellent. There are a number of variants: continuous arteriovenous haemofiltration (CAVH), which required femoral artery cannulation, has given way to continuous venovenous haemofiltration (CVVH), which requires a pumped venous supply. Continuous venovenous haemodialysis (CVVHD) is a further variant. These continuous treatments are well tolerated haemodynamically and avoid the peaks and troughs in metabolic, electrolyte, acid–base, and volume control which are a feature of intermittent treatments. The inefficiency for small-molecule clearance may not be such a barrier for the use of haemofiltration in chronic renal failure if the current interest in more frequent (quotidian) dialysis continues (see below).

High-flux haemodialysis

Concerns about the biocompatibility of cuprophane, and its poor clearance of middle molecules, especially β_2-microglobulin, have fuelled the increasing use of high-flux membranes. High-flux haemodialysis uses highly permeable, usually biocompatible membranes, which provide good diffusive clearance of small solutes combined with much better diffusive removal of middle molecules than conventional dialysis. This is augmented by a convective contribution to middle-molecule clearance resulting from a degree of obligate back-filtration within the dialyser.

Haemodiafiltration

Haemodiafiltration is the addition of a prescribed convective component to the technique of high-flux haemodialysis. Adding a greater convective component (haemofiltration) to the diffusive and convective clearances offered by high-flux haemodialysis allows the benefits of both modalities to be maximized. In each high-flux session, 12 to 25 litres of ultrafiltrate is removed and replaced by substitution fluid. The cheap online production by the dialysis machine of ultrapure substitution fluid from dialysis fluid has allowed haemodiafiltration to become established as a viable routine therapy of ESRF (Fig. 21.7.1.7). Fluid is removed from the dialysis fluid pathway supplying the dialyser by a haemofiltration pump (HF), passed through an ultrafilter (F2), and infused in to

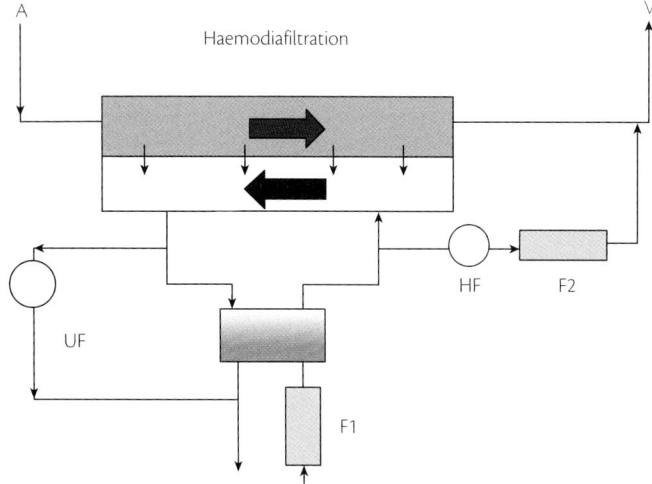

Fig. 21.7.1.7 The dialysis fluid pathway for online haemodiafiltration. Fluid is removed from the dialysis fluid pathway supplying the dialyser by a haemofiltration pump (HF), passed through an ultrafilter (F2), and infused into the 'V' venous line (postdilution) or the 'A' arterial line (predilution, not shown).

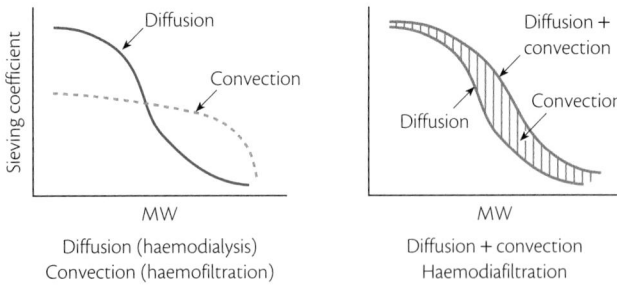

Fig. 21.7.1.8 Comparison of solute removal by diffusion and convection according to molecular weight. Convection has better middle-molecule clearance but much poorer clearance of small-molecular-weight solutes than diffusion. Haemodiafiltration combines the strengths of both techniques to broaden the spectrum of solute removal.

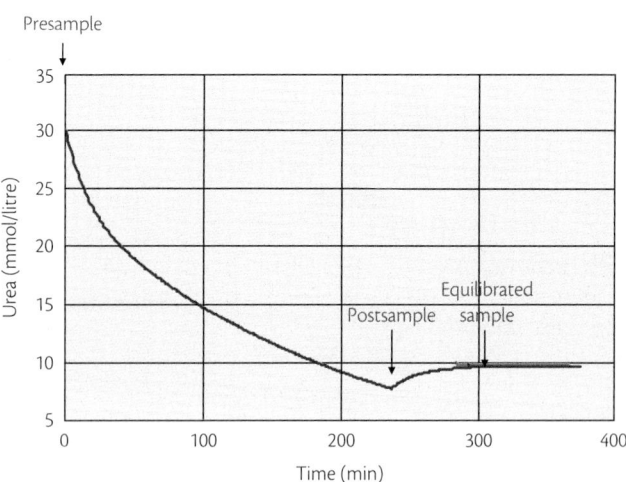

Fig. 21.7.1.9 Blood urea concentration during and after a haemodialysis session, showing an exponential decline during treatment with a postdialysis rebound due to two-pool effects.

the 'V' line (postdilution) or the 'A' line (predilution, not shown). To maintain balance in the fixed volume (volumetric) loop between the balance chamber and the dialyser, an equal volume of fluid is drawn from the blood across the dialysis membrane. The added convective component of haemodiafiltration produces a small improvement in small-solute clearance over that seen in high-flux dialysis, but a significant improvement in middle-molecule clearance (Fig. 21.7.1.8): serum β_2-microglobulin levels are reduced, and dialysis-related amyloidosis may be delayed; haemodynamic stability and survival may also be improved.

Adequacy of dialysis

The assessment of how much dialysis is required to maintain health is still controversial 40 years after its introduction for end-stage renal failure. We know that predialysis blood levels of urea and creatinine can be misleading as indicators of the adequacy of dialysis. Low levels are just as likely to indicate malnutrition and muscle wasting as good dialysis, and have been associated with increased mortality. Instead, dialysis dose is normally defined in relation to small-solute clearance, either by the urea reduction ratio (URR—the percentage reduction in blood urea during dialysis), or more commonly by urea kinetic modelling (UKM). UKM derives a normalized urea clearance, Kt/V, where K is the dialyser urea clearance, t is the duration of dialysis in minutes, and V is the urea distribution volume estimated as total body water from anthropomorphic data. This parameter, which derives from kinetic modelling of urea removal during dialysis (Fig. 21.7.1.9), can be used as a measure of dialysis dose or as a tool to prescribe the dialysis.

Urea reduction ratio

The URR is the simplest measure of dialysis adequacy and is given by:

$$URR = 100 \times (1 - C_{post}/C_0) \quad \text{(Equation 21.7.1.1)}$$

where C_0 is the initial blood urea concentration and C_{post} is the blood urea concentration in a blood sample taken immediately postdialysis. URR takes no account of urea generation, ultrafiltration, or residual renal function, but does correlate with outcome, testifying to its clinical utility. Most guidelines recommend a target URR of greater than 65%.

The urea kinetic modelling approach

Assuming urea is distributed in a single pool within the body and that the effects of urea generation and ultrafiltration during dialysis are small, the blood urea concentration (C_t) at any time (t) during the dialysis is given by:

$$C_t = C_0 e^{-Kt/V} \quad \text{(Equation 21.7.1.2)}$$

Hence, the delivered dose of dialysis, Kt/V, can be calculated from the expression

$$Kt/V = \ln(C_0/C_{post}) \quad \text{(Equation 21.7.1.3)}$$

The expression can be corrected for urea generation and ultrafiltration during dialysis according to a formula by Daugirdas:

$$Kt/V = \ln(R - 0.008T) + (4 - 3.5R)\Delta W/W \quad \text{(Equation 21.7.1.4)}$$

where $R = C_{post}/C_0$, T is the treatment time in hours, ΔW is the interdialytic weight gain, and W is the postdialysis weight.

The single-pool assumption (which is that all the urea in the body is in a pool that is equally accessible to removal by dialysis) is also an oversimplification. The rapid removal of urea (and other solutes) from the bloodstream during dialysis creates intercompartmental disequilibria: the intracellular concentration of urea exceeds the extracellular, and that in poorly perfused peripheral pools exceeds that in well-perfused body compartments. Urea exchange between these compartments continues after cessation of dialysis and causes a postdialysis rebound of blood urea concentration (Fig. 21.7.1.9). This rebound can be substantial in high-efficiency treatments and can cause overestimation of Kt/V delivery by as much as 20%, making the single-pool assumption untenable in these circumstances. There are a number of ways of dealing with this problem: the most straightforward is to incorporate a postdialysis sample which is delayed until rebound is complete (30–60 min)—the equilibrated postdialysis sample (though in practice patients find this inconvenient). Much more complex is to model the system as two pools, requiring the assumption of a number of physiological parameters and iterative solution by computer. There are a number of less complex approximations to equilibrated Kt/V (eKt/V), which are usually preferred and have been shown to produce equivalent results (Equations 21.7.1.5 and 21.7.1.6).

Box 21.7.1.1 Calculation of normalized protein catabolic rate (nPCR)

$$nPCR = 149.7 \times G/V + 0.17$$

where G is the urea generation rate given by

$$G/V = [C_{pre2}(V + w_g)/V - C_{post} + (V_u \times U_u)/V]/t_{id}$$

where C_{pre2} is predialysis blood urea concentration before succeeding dialysis, w_g is the interdialytic weight gain, V_u is the volume of interdialytic urinary collection, U_u is urinary urea concentration, and t_{id} is the duration of intradialytic urine collection (in minutes).

$$Kt/V = sp\ Kt/V - 0.6\ (K/V) + 0.03 \quad \text{Equation 21.7.1.5}$$

$$eKt/V = sp\ Kt/V\ (t/(t + 40)) \quad \text{Equation 21.7.1.6}$$

where sp Kt/V is the single pool Kt/V, and t is duration of dialysis session in minutes.

A further predialysis sample taken prior to the subsequent dialysis session allows an estimate of normalized protein catabolic rate (nPCR) to be calculated from the interdialytic rise in blood urea (see Box 21.7.1.1). This can provide valuable information about nutritional status.

Defining target *Kt/V*

In the early 1980s, the National Cooperative Dialysis Study (NCDS), a randomized controlled trial, established a *Kt/V* of 0.9 per session as the minimum threshold dose for thrice-weekly dialysis, provided the patients were adequately nourished as defined by an nPCR greater than 0.8 g/kg body weight per day. Lower doses were associated with increased short-term morbidity and mortality. It was also inferred from the study (perhaps inappropriately) that the duration of the dialysis session did not influence outcome provided small-solute clearance was adequate. Subsequently, a wealth of observational data suggested that higher delivered *Kt/V* levels produced improved outcomes. This debate culminated in the HEMO study, another randomized controlled trial, which found no additional benefit of high compared with standard doses (mean delivered two-pool *Kt/V* 1.53 vs 1.16), except perhaps in women. Neither was there a benefit of high-flux over conventional haemodialysis, certainly during the first few years of treatment. The HEMO study has probably defined the adequacy limits of thrice-weekly treatment and in doing so highlighted some of the limitations of the *Kt/V* concept. The target recommended by K/DOQI and the United Kingdom Renal Association is an equilibrated value (*eKt/V*) of at least 1.2 for thrice-weekly treatment (approximating to a single-pool *Kt/V* of 1.4).

Incremental dialysis

This approach recognizes that the target total urea *Kt/V* has dialysis (K_dt/V) and residual renal (K_Rt/V) components. As residual renal function declines during the first few years of dialysis, the dialysis component is gradually increased to ensure the target continues to be achieved. This allows a gentler initiation to dialysis and maximizes the use of scarce resources, but does require regular estimates of residual renal function, and also assumes an equivalence of renal and dialyser clearance, which holds for urea but not necessarily for other solutes, or other renal functions. It is relevant that the viability of CAPD as a renal replacement modality also depends on this assumption, and in practice the dosing of CAPD and peritoneal dialysis techniques are similarly incremental.

Adequacy, duration, and frequency

The relationship between small-solute clearance, session duration, and session frequency is complex. The concentrations in the blood of small solutes decline in an exponential fashion during a dialysis session (Fig. 21.7.1.9) Their rate of removal is thus maximal during the initial part of the session and increasing the duration of a dialysis session produces diminishing returns in terms of small-solute clearance, which is much greater if the same weekly duration (say 12 h) is configured as 6×2 h rather than 3×4 h. The standards discussed above for *Kt/V* are based on thrice-weekly dialysis. Comparing dialysis doses delivered by different frequency schedules and even different modalities is difficult and requires resort to other mathematical methods. The standard *Kt/V* (*sKt/V*) is such an approach, in which weekly doses delivered by any intermittent schedule can be compared after translation to an equivalent dose considered to have been delivered continuously over that week. Figure 21.7.1.10 shows the relationship between *Kt/V* per session, session frequency, and weekly *sKt/V*, illustrating the major benefits of increased frequency.

Other approaches to adequacy

Small-solute clearance is just one measure of the adequacy of dialysis. Adequate dialysis, by this criterion, can be delivered in short sessions using high blood flows and large dialysers to augment clearance, but it is difficult to control other parameters such as phosphate and blood pressure, which also affect morbidity and mortality. In addition, larger molecules such as β_2-microglobulin are certainly toxic in dialysed patients but do not figure in our currently accepted notions of adequacy. Broader concepts of adequacy are required which encompass these other factors impacting on the patient's global wellbeing.

Quotidian dialysis

Quotidian dialysis refers to schedules in which dialysis is carried out every day, or at least six times weekly. The HEMO trial effectively defined the limits of standard thrice-weekly dialysis. The prediction

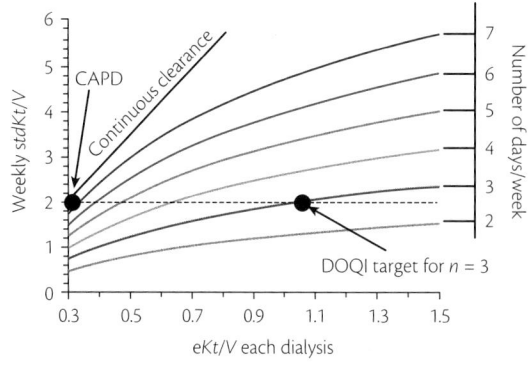

Fig. 21.7.1.10 Relationship between weekly standard *Kt/V*, sessional equilibrated *Kt/V*, and haemodialysis session frequency. CAPD, continuous ambulatory peritoneal dialysis.
Used with the permission of the Nature publishing Group.

is being borne out in practice that more frequent dialysis up to six times weekly, either overnight or short daily dialysis, not only enhances urea clearance to a degree which is not possible by extended thrice-weekly sessions but also provides excellent control of many other parameters. Patient wellbeing seems to improve markedly, and this and the freedom from dietary and fluid restriction more than compensates for the greater commitment required. How many patients will choose (and be allowed by health care systems that need to restrain costs) to enhance their long-term health prospects by quotidian dialysis remains to be seen.

Management of haemodialysis patients

Predialysis care and initiation of dialysis

The predialysis period, as discussed in Chapter 21.6, is an important time for planning and preparation. Ideally, patients will be referred to the renal services in good time to allow this. Embarking on a career of renal replacement therapy is a major life event. Patients and their families need to have the relevant information presented in an assessible way. They need the time to consider this and to discuss their options with members of the multidisciplinary team. The facts should be presented as clearly and as honestly as possible, and the patients allowed to choose whether or not they wish to receive dialysis treatment. In some cases, there are medical imperatives, which preclude some or occasionally all replacement options. For some patients, especially those who are frail and dependent, the modality choice offered should include conservative (nondialytic) management, it being particularly important to emphasize that conservative management is not 'no treatment' (Box 21.7.1.2). Patients opting for haemodialysis should be assessed early for fistula formation and the surgery planned 3 to 6 months before the putative initiation date. Vaccination against hepatitis B should also be carried out in this period: the earlier this occurs in the course of progressive renal failure, the greater the likelihood of a successful response. The prospects for pre-emptive (avoiding dialysis) transplantation should also be considered.

Unfortunately, there is still a very high incidence of late referral of patients with endstage renal disease to renal services, involving up to 30 to 40% of new patients in some areas, which precludes effective planning and increases morbidity and mortality.

Box 21.7.1.2 Goals of conservative (nondialytic) management

Improve/maintain quality of life

- Symptom control:
  - Maintain optimum fluid and electrolyte state
  - Prevent anaemia
  - Treat uraemic symptoms
- Provide appropriate end-of-life care
- Support patient and family throughout

Prolong life when appropriate

- Preserve residual renal function
- Treat underlying diseases

The timing of initiation of dialysis is subjective. The K/DOQI guidelines for dialysis initiation are now based on estimated GFR, with the recommendation that "the benefits, risks, and disadvantages of beginning kidney replacement therapy" should be evaluated when patients reach CKD stage 5 (estimated GFR less than 15 ml/min per 1.73 m^2). The decision needs to be individualized, taking into account factors such as age, general health, modality options, vascular access status, transport needs, and compliance, as well as symptoms, level of renal function, and the presence or absence of uraemic complications. Patients with comorbidities, such as diabetes and heart failure, tend to initiate dialysis therapy at higher levels of estimated GFR, probably because of the earlier development of symptoms.

Prescribing dialysis

Target Kt/V is normally 1.2 to 1.3. Patients with intercurrent illness require a higher target. The value of K is obtained from data sheets from the dialyser manufacturer, taking into account membrane area and blood and dialyser flow rates. The value of V is obtained empirically from age, sex, weight, and height, usually by the Watson formula. The dose of dialysis prescribed can be adjusted to achieve the target Kt/V by changing the surface area of the membrane, blood flow rate, dialysis fluid flow rate (these influence urea clearance by the dialyser), and dialysis duration. This logic allows adequate dialysis to be delivered in a shorter time using larger dialysers and high flow rates (high-efficiency dialysis). If the target Kt/V includes a component for residual renal function, then residual urea clearance should be measured monthly and dialysis time readjusted accordingly. Membrane type and flux should be specified. Use of high-flux synthetic membranes is increasingly standard, rather than restricted to patients showing evidence of amyloid deposition. Setting the dry weight (see below) allows the ultrafiltration requirement to be specified for each dialysis. The prescription should also refer to the heparin loading dose and maintenance infusion rate. Whether dialysis prescription is individualized in this manner or whether a unit approach is taken with standardization of modality, dialyser, and session duration, it is important to have a means of monitoring the effectiveness of delivery of the prescribed dose.

Monitoring dialysis delivery

Dialysis delivery should be monitored monthly. Prescription and monitoring protocols are now often computer based. Pre- and postdialysis blood sampling allows calculation of the URR, and single-pool Kt/V and eKt/V can be calculated using Equation 21.7.1.4, 21.7.1.5 and 21.7.1.6. Failure to reach adequacy targets needs investigation. There are many possible causes of underdelivery, including poor blood flows, inadequate vascular access, recirculation within the vascular access, clotting problems within the dialyser, multiple alarms and poor compliance, which both reduce actual dialysis duration. A low nPCR should provoke an evaluation of nutritional intake. It is vital to ensure correct sampling technique, particularly for the postdialysis sample, to avoid serious potentially misleading artefacts.

Dry weight

Regulation of salt and water balance is one of the key functions of the kidney. Renal failure results in salt and water retention, which along with activation of the renin–angiotensin–aldosterone system, contributes to hypertension, left ventricular hypertrophy, and dilatation, which are potent causes of morbidity and mortality. The removal of the excess fluid accumulated between dialysis sessions is a vital function of dialysis, so we need ways of estimating the degree of this excess. Dry weight is an important concept dating back to the early days of maintenance haemodialysis. It assumes that body weight at any time consists of two components: the dry weight or target weight, at which the patient's fluid compartments are normal in volume, and an excess weight consisting of surplus volume, which expands body fluid compartments and elevates blood pressure. The only way of defining dry weight is by trial and error. The protocol requires cessation of antihypertensive agents and weight reduction during successive dialyses during the first few weeks or months after initiation. The dry weight is the point at which the patient is oedema free and below which hypotension occurs on further fluid removal. The implicit assumption is that patients on dialysis have normal cardiovascular responses, which may have been reasonable in the highly selected dialysis population of 1970 but is much less tenable in the older, sicker patients on dialysis today. Applying such principles, most of the early patients on dialysis became normotensive without the need for antihypertensive agents. In most current patients, the target weight is likely to be the best achievable weight and hypertension is more likely. Shorter treatment times and less rigorous salt restriction have undoubtedly added to these difficulties. It is also vital to recognize that dry weight is not static: it changes over time, falling during periods of intercurrent illness and poor nutrition and increasing during recovery from such episodes, hence it requires regular clinical review. The potential adjunctive roles of methods such as natriuretic peptide measurement, ultrasonic inferior vena cava diameter estimation, blood volume monitoring, and bioimpedance spectroscopy in helping to define volume status in haemodialysis patients are still debated.

Hypertension

Many factors contribute to hypertension in patients on dialysis, including stimulation of the renin–angiotensin–aldosterone system and sympathetic overactivity, but the overriding factor is volume overload. In many units, 60% or more of patients receive antihypertensive agents. Insufficient emphasis on dietary sodium restriction and adequate ultrafiltration, coupled with a tendency for the early use of antihypertensive drugs, especially in patients with cardiac dysfunction, may render achievement of dry weight more difficult and further compromise blood pressure control. Hypertension is an important risk factor for cardiovascular disease mortality in the general population. However, unlike in the general population, many studies demonstrate a paradoxical relationship between blood pressure and mortality in haemodialysis populations—low to normal blood pressure being associated with poor outcome, and high pressure conferring a survival advantage ('reverse epidemiology'). This has been attributed to an increased incidence of cardiac failure in patients with low-normal blood pressure. Alternatively, the deleterious effects of hypertension may be being swamped by the numerous other toxic factors operating in endstage renal failure. There may also be a problem with the definition of hypertension in this setting. Fluid status varies throughout the dialysis cycle: predialysis patients are generally fluid overloaded, hence predialysis blood pressure is a reflection of the cardiovascular response to fluid overload; likewise, postdialysis blood pressure reflects the cardiovascular response to fluid removal. There are serious questions about the appropriateness of current United Kingdom Renal Association and K/DOQI blood pressure targets in the haemodialysis population (140/90 mmHg predialysis, 130/80 mmHg postdialysis) for which there is little or no evidence base. There are no randomized interventional trials of the effect of blood pressure reduction in this population and practice is essentially opinion based. We suggest targeting a 20-min postdialysis reading of 135/85 mmHg in patients younger than 65 years. Drug therapy is second-line treatment to be deployed after the achievement of optimal fluid status. No class of antihypertensive agent is contraindicated in dialysis patients, although the half-life of renally excreted drugs may be markedly prolonged and care is required with dosing schedules.

Vascular access

Securing and maintaining adequate, reliable, and robust vascular access is a major task, the importance of which cannot be overstated.

Temporary access

Beginning a career on maintenance haemodialysis with the need for temporary access should in most cases be regarded as a failure of adequate predialysis planning, although—as stated above—in a significant proportion of patients the initial presentation with end-stage renal failure is as a uraemic emergency. If acute access is required, temporary, noncuffed, dual-lumen catheters can be inserted into femoral, internal jugular, or subclavian veins. The femoral route is simplest, safest, and preferred in very sick patients, but the infection risk is high if femoral catheters are left *in situ* for more than a few days. Use of the subclavian route risks stenosis of the vein and compromises future ipsilateral fistula formation.

Permanent access

Options for permanent access include the subcutaneous arteriovenous fistula (AVF), arteriovenous polytetrafluoroethene (PTFE) grafts, and cuffed, tunnelled, internal jugular venous catheters. AVF are preferred: they have the lowest complication rate and the longest life span, and are created by end-to-side or side-to-side anastamosis, preferably of the radial artery and cephalic vein (Brescia–Cimino fistula) in the nondominant forearm. Use of other sites such as brachial artery and cephalic vein is common. After anastamosis, venous distension and arterialisation occur, and needling is usually possible by about 6 weeks. Primary nonfunction is unfortunately common, and attention to the preservation of these vessels in predialysis patients is important. Distal 'steal' resulting in critical underperfusion of the forearm and hand may occur with large brachiocephalic fistulae. Stenosis and thrombosis may occur, which, in addition to predisposing to premature fistula loss, may lead to access recirculation (see below). Access monitoring may help to avoid such problems, facilitating early diagnosis and pre-emptive radiological or surgical intervention. Fistula flow assessment by ultrasound dilution is probably the monitoring mode of choice.

The many patients that still present late for dialysis require primary central venous access by default, and tunnelled catheters are also required when other access options have been exhausted. They carry a high risk of infection, are prone to clotting, and provide much lower blood flow rates than the AVF. Despite this they are in common usage: a recent United Kingdom national survey carried found that only 31% of patients started their haemodialysis career with a native AVF and that around one-third of hospital admissions in haemodialysis patients are due to vascular access problems. Limiting the use of lines to the 15% or so of haemodialysis patients with no other option is an important quality target, which would make a significant impact on haemodialysis morbidity and mortality.

Recirculation

If there is a stenosis in a fistula severe enough to limit fistula blood flow to a level less than that demanded by the blood pump in the extracorporeal circulation, then blood returning from the dialyser to the fistula can be drawn directly from the 'V' needle to the 'A' needle and dialysed again. This is known as access recirculation, an effect that can also be produced by misplacement of fistula needles with the 'A' needle downstream to the 'V' needle. Also during dialysis, a proportion of the blood returning through the 'V' needle will pass directly to the 'A' needle after passage through the heart and lungs without traversing a capillary bed to be 'replenished' with solute. This is known as cardiopulmonary recirculation and is an inevitable consequence of having a fistula as the access. The higher the blood pump speed, the greater the degree of recirculation in all of these circumstances. Access recirculation is a major cause of underdelivery of prescribed dialysis dose, and unexplained reductions of monitored Kt/V or urea reduction ratios demand further investigation to exclude this. Recirculation can be detected and quantified by techniques such as ultrasound dilution, thermal dilution, and ionic dialysance. Significant recirculation (>10%), requires further investigation, which may include Doppler ultrasonography or fistulography. Fistuloplasty or surgical reconstruction may be required if stenotic lesions are identified.

Diet and nutrition

Malnutrition is common and is often due to underdialysis. The early signs are subtle and often masked by fluid overload, which can compound the problem. There are no simple, foolproof laboratory tests. Hypoalbuminaemia indicates the presence of inflammation as much as it reflects malnutrition. Monitoring of nPCR may be helpful, but cannot replace regular dietetic review. When malnutrition is identified, a range of oral nutritional supplements may be deployed, and there is a limited role for intradialytic parenteral nutrition.

Protein requirements in patients on haemodialysis are not well characterized but have been estimated at 1.2 g/kg ideal body weight per day, which is considerably more than the nonuraemic requirement. Intakes greatly in excess of this may cause problems unless dialysis dose is correspondingly increased. There is no role for protein restriction. The energy requirement of a moderately active patient on haemodialysis is about 35 kcal/kg body weight per day, which is similar to that of normal subjects. Attempts should be made to limit interdialytic fluid gains to 1 to 2 litres, which is difficult when residual renal function has been lost. The value of limiting sodium intake (40–80 mmol/day) to control thirst is often understated. Potassium restriction (to about 60 mmol/day) is usually required when residual renal function is minimal. The recommended intake of elemental calcium is 1 to 1.5 g/day, but achieving

this is seldom difficult given the extensive use of calcium salts as phosphate binders, although phosphate restriction to about 0.8 g/day of elemental phosphorus may reduce the requirement for these agents. There is no consensus on the need to supplement water-soluble vitamins (B and C), but the practice is widespread. Vitamin B_{12} supplements are recommended in high-flux treatments.

Hyperlipidaemia

Low-density-lipoprotein (LDL) cholesterol levels are normal or near-normal in haemodialysis patients, but the overall lipid profile is highly atherogenic and characterized by marked accumulation of apo B-containing triglyceride-rich particles. There are elevated very-low-density lipoprotein (VLDL) and intermediate-density lipoprotein (IDL) levels, decreased high-density lipoprotein (HDL) levels, and a shift of LDL particle size toward a small dense apo-B-rich LDL predominance. In the general population, primary and secondary prevention trials have shown significantly improved cardiovascular outcomes with statins, but the same may not be true in the haemodialysis population. In a recent large randomized controlled trial, atorvastatin did not significantly affect overall cardiovascular morbidity and mortality in people with type 2 diabetes on haemodialysis. This suggests that the continued action of other risk factors (traditional and nontraditional) may overwhelm any potential benefit from improved lipid profiles and that statin initiation in people with type 2 diabetes already on dialysis may come too late to affect cardiovascular outcome.

Infection control

Strict adherence to universal precautions is necessary to minimize the risk of cross-infection by blood-borne viruses. Transmission from contaminated external surfaces, rather than through the dialyser membrane, is the major cross-infection threat. Screening of patients about to start dialysis for evidence of prior infection with hepatitis B and C and HIV is routine, and should be repeated at least 3-monthly thereafter. Patients negative for hepatitis B surface antigen should be vaccinated: patients who are positive should be segregated and use a dedicated machine, as should those positive for hepatitis C or HIV.

Other aspects of care

Cardiovascular risk factors such as smoking should be addressed, and exercise encouraged, both during dialysis sessions and in general. Low-dose aspirin may be beneficial. Folate and vitamin B supplements may reduce elevated homocysteine levels. There is a high incidence of sexual dysfunction, especially in males: some may benefit from androgen replacement, sildenafil may be effective if not contraindicated, and skilled counselling may be helpful.

Complications of haemodialysis

Acute complications

Disequilibration

The severest forms of disequilibration occur shortly after dialysis initiation (dialysis disequilibrium syndrome). The main predisposing factors are late presentation with severe uraemia and aggressive dialysis initiation with lengthy dialyses and high solute clearance rates. Restlessness, headache, tremors, fits, and coma can result. Dialysis should not be initiated in this way. Cerebral oedema due to fluid shifts induced by intercompartmental differences in urea concentrations and paradoxical cerebrospinal fluid acidosis are among the suggested causes. Short initial treatments using dialysers of small surface area and low blood pump settings prevent the problem.

Postdialysis headache is a common symptom in patients undergoing regular haemodialysis and may be a minor manifestation of disequilibrium. Postdialysis fatigue is common in regular dialysis patients, lasting from a few minutes to many hours. It is reported that many of these symptoms are alleviated in quotidian dialysis.

Hypotension

Symptomatic hypotension occurs in up to 30% of dialysis sessions. Symptoms include nausea, vomiting, cramps, palpitations, dizziness, and syncope. The major cause is hypovolaemia, resulting from an imbalance between the rate of fluid removal from the circulation by ultrafiltration and the rate of vascular refilling from the interstitium. Underlying cardiovascular disease, the use of antihypertensive drugs, autonomic dysfunction, shortened dialysis times, excessive interdialytic fluid gains, and failure to reset dry weight after flesh weight gain all increase the likelihood. Accordingly, the mainstays of management are careful assessment and reassessment of target weight, limited use of antihypertensive agents, reduction of interdialytic weight gain by fluid and sodium restriction, and reduction of ultrafiltration rate. Newer dialysis machines have the capacity to monitor relative blood volume and to profile the sodium concentration of dialysis fluid throughout the dialysis session, techniques which may be useful in particular situations, but neither is yet used routinely. Convective therapies such as haemodiafiltration are associated with superior haemodynamic stability, possibly owing to blood cooling causing vasoconstriction. Episodes of hypotension may occasionally have more sinister causes such as primary myocardial events and heparin-induced bleeding. Cardiac arrhythmias are common, especially in patients with left ventricular hypertrophy and coronary artery disease, and are predisposed to by rapid intradialytic electrolyte fluxes, especially changes in serum potassium levels and in acid–base balance.

Dialyser reactions

Dialyser reactions are uncommon with the use of biocompatible membranes, and gamma- or steam-sterilised dialysers. Ethylene oxide, a device sterilant, has been implicated as a major cause of these reactions, along with other leachable materials. Type A reactions are anaphylactoid, rare, but life-threatening: symptoms usually begin in the first few minutes of dialysis but can be delayed for 20 min or more. Dialysis must be stopped, the lines clamped and discarded, and corticosteroids and antihistamines (adrenaline in very severe cases) administered. Type B reactions are less severe but more common: they occur 30 to 60 min after starting dialysis, which can be continued and the patient managed with supportive treatment. Reactions with reused dialysers are usually due to disinfectants, such as formaldehyde and peracetic acid, used in reprocessing. AN69 membranes may provoke anaphylactoid reactions, especially with concomitant angiotensin converting enzyme (ACE) inhibition, when bradykinin release by the negatively charged membrane and its reduced degradation due to ACE inhibition are responsible. A modified AN69 membrane is now available, coated with polyethyleneimine, which neutralises surface negative charge and decreases kinin generation.

Fevers

Febrile reactions occur occasionally. Use of disposable dialysers and the increasing use of ultrapure water have dramatically reduced their incidence, and they are now much more likely to be due to infection related to the use of tunnelled lines for access than to contaminated dialysis fluid.

Coagulation problems

Circuit clotting may be due to underanticoagulation, and prolonged bleeding from the fistula after needle removal may be due to overanticoagulation. More serious bleeding problems with anticoagulation are rare. Thrombocytopenia is common in patients on heparin and usually mild and transient (HIT-I). True heparin-induced thrombocytopenia (HIT-II) is a rare (1–4%) but potentially life-threatening syndrome caused by platelet-activating antibodies to complexes of platelet factor 4 (PF4) and heparin. Characteristic features are thrombocytopenia, a systemic reaction within 30 min of intravenous UFH administration, and a hypercoagulable state with a high risk of thromboembolic complications. Severe thrombocytopenia and/or thrombosis in a patient on UFH should raise strong suspicions. The presence of antiheparin/PF4 antibody is confirmatory in these circumstances, in which case UFH and LMWH should be avoided. The direct thrombin inhibitor argatroban is probably the anticoagulant of choice should heparin-free dialysis prove unsuccessful.

Other complications

Use of modern fail-safe dialysis machines and ultrapure water systems has fortunately rendered a number of previously well-described complications of haemodialysis exceedingly rare, including air embolism, severe hypercalcaemia due to dialysis against hard water, and acute haemolysis.

Chronic complications

Cardiovascular disease

Volume overload, hypertension, anaemia, hyperparathyroidism, excessive fistula flow rates, and uraemia itself all predispose to left ventricular hypertrophy, which is an independent risk factor for mortality. Correction of anaemia can favourably influence the natural history of left ventricular hypertrophy in patients on dialysis. Aortic pulse wave velocity predicts cardiovascular mortality, and is a major determinant of systolic hypertension. Haemodialysis patients also have a variety of other traditional risk factors, such as lipid abnormalities, and nontraditional risk factors, such as disturbances of calcium and phosphate metabolism, hyperhomocysteinaemia, increased oxidative stress, and elevated inflammatory markers.

Anaemia

Erythropoietin deficiency is the major cause of the anaemia of chronic kidney disease, but a number of additional causes of anaemia may arise from the haemodialysis process itself. Iron deficiency can result from the repeated loss of small amounts of blood in extracorporeal circuits. Intravenous iron saccharate is used in moderate doses (e.g. 100 mg on each of 10 successive dialyses) to correct iron deficiency, and as maintenance treatment (such as 50 mg weekly). Deficiencies of other haematinics can occur, particularly in high-flux treatments, when regular supplementation with vitamin B_{12} and folate is recommended. Mechanical and chloramine-induced haemolysis should not occur with modern techniques. There are other causes of erythropoietin resistance, the most potent being infection, in this context often arising from central venous lines. Some studies suggest that high-flux haemodialysis and haemodiafiltration may have beneficial effects on anaemia management, possibly related to removal of middle-molecule inhibitors of erythropoiesis. See Chapter 21.6 for more detailed discussion of the management of renal anaemia.

Bone disease

Haemodialysis patients have bone disease associated with chronic renal impairment, but may also develop skeletal complications of their treatment. Accumulation of β_2-microglobulin may cause dialysis-related amyloidosis which may be associated with significant bone problems, including bone cysts and spondyloarthropathy (see below). Control of serum phosphate levels is crucial in controlling secondary hyperparathyroidism and preventing metastatic calcification: this requires a three-pronged approach of dietary restriction, phosphate binders, and adequate dialysis, the importance of the latter being highlighted by the superb control gained, in the absence of phosphate restriction and binder usage, in patients on daily nocturnal dialysis. The setting of the dialysis fluid calcium concentration can significantly affect the spectrum of bone disease, high levels (1.75 mmol/litre) can suppress parathyroid hormone levels but risk adynamic bone disease and metastatic calcification; by contrast, levels of 1.25 mmol/litre or lower may be useful treatments of adynamic bone and relative hypoparathyroidism. Dialysis fluid magnesium concentrations may also impact on bone metabolism, but the clinical relevance of this is not established. The toxic effects of acid accumulation on the skeleton and other systems can be avoided by adequate dialysis and adjustment of the dialysis fluid bicarbonate concentration. The incidence of osteoporosis is increasing in the haemodialysis population, related to increasing age, low levels of physical activity, previous steroid therapy, and relative hypogonadism. The effects of heparin on bone are well established, but evidence for a specific role of heparin in the development of osteoporosis in this setting is sparse. Aluminium-related bone disease, along with other manifestations of aluminium accumulation, including progressive dementia and anaemia, occurred in 'epidemic' form due to aluminium contamination of dialysis water. Use of modern water purification methods has seen the disappearance of this problem and new cases should no longer be seen. See Chapter 21.6 for more detailed discussion of the management of renal mineral and bone disorders.

Amyloidosis

Dialysis-related amyloidosis is a serious complication of chronic dialysis. Its incidence increases with duration of haemodialysis and symptomatic involvement is almost universal after 15 years. Older patients are more susceptible. The syndrome manifests mainly as carpal tunnel syndrome and destructive arthropathy associated with bone cysts and a destructive spondyloarthropathy, but other organs can be involved. Deposits of amyloid, mainly composed of β_2-microglobulin fibrils, can be found at these and other sites. β_2-Microglobulin is an 11 800-Da protein that is part of the human class 1 major histocompatibility complex. It is 95% eliminated by glomerular filtration, hence levels are elevated in renal failure, and these are not cleared by low-flux membranes. Elevated plasma levels are the major predisposing factor to amyloid deposition, but other factors may also be important, including modification of β_2-microglobulin by advanced glycation endproducts and by oxidative and carbonyl stress, and it is also possible that β_2-microglobulin or modified β_2-microglobulin is directly toxic to tissues. Use of high-flux synthetic membranes, especially in haemodiafiltration mode, reduces plasma levels of β_2-microglobulin, although the levels remain about 10-fold higher than in those with normal renal function. High-flux dialysis and especially haemodiafiltration may prevent or delay the onset of symptomatic disease, and the use of ultrapure water may also be protective. Treatment options are limited for established disease, but renal transplantation may enable slow resorption of deposits.

Outcomes of haemodialysis

Dialysis undoubtedly prolongs the life of patients with endstage chronic renal failure, but survival remains markedly inferior to that of age-matched peers with normal renal function. Cardiovascular disease is the main cause of death, followed by infection. Comparison of outcome in the different eras of dialysis is fraught with problems, largely because of the dramatic differences in case mix of patients entering programmes. Age, comorbidity, and functional status are independent predictors of morbidity (rate of admission to hospital) and mortality. Late presentation for dialysis has a profound effect on survival; late planned initiation may also have an effect, perhaps mediated through malnutrition; and we have previously alluded to the effects of dialysis adequacy and nutrition on outcome. It is difficult to compare the outcome of patients treated with haemodialysis and peritoneal dialysis in any meaningful way. Data from single centres, multicentre studies, and analysis of registry data do not show consistent differences in survival between these modalities. There are a number of confounding factors. Patients initiated on CAPD are younger, have fewer coexisting nonrenal comorbidities, better functional status, and are less likely to have presented late. In addition, technique survival is poor in CAPD, and many patients require transfer to haemodialysis because of peritonitis, inadequate dialysis, or ultrafiltration failure. Quality-of-life assessments are similar in both groups, but both are inferior to those obtained in patients with successful transplants. It is probably safe to conclude that, in the early years of therapy at least, morbidity and mortality are similar on both modalities if risk-stratified groups are compared. There are few data to allow comparison of the outcome of conventional haemodialysis and more modern haemodialysis modes. The HEMO study demonstrated no overall survival benefit of high-flux over low-flux treatments, but there was a suggestion that patients whose dialysis vintage was greater than the mean 3.7 years fared better on high-flux treatment, and β_2-microglobulin correlated with survival. Observational data suggest improved survival with haemodiafiltation, although there are no controlled data. There is some evidence that high-flux modes and haemodiafiltration protect against the development of dialysis-associated amyloidosis. Daily dialysis is associated with improvements in morbidity, but again we await controlled data.

The future of haemodialysis

Haemodialysis is likely to remain centre based for the most patients. Technical advances will allow treatments to become more tailored to the specific requirements of the individual. Online dialysis quantification could guarantee the adequacy of each session. Online blood volume monitoring, possibly combined with bioimpedance spectroscopic monitoring of the extracellular fluid volume, coupled with algorithms to control ultrafiltration rate, dialysis fluid temperature, and sodium content on a minute-to-minute basis, could prevent intradialytic hypotension and allow patients to finish dialysis at their optimal achievable weight. Current concepts of the relationship between dialysis dose and sessional frequency, and the encouraging initial results with daily dialysis, suggest that the treatment may emerge as a self-supervised home modality, perhaps for a small proportion of younger, less dependent patients for whom transplantation or retransplantation is not an option. Vascular access is likely to remain the Achilles heel.

Further reading

Arieff AI (1994). Dialysis disequilibrium syndrome: current concepts on pathogenesis and prevention. *Kidney Int*, **45**, 629–35.

Bowry SK (2002). Dialysis membranes today. *Int J Artif Organs*, **25**, 447–60.

Canaud B, *et al.* (2006). Mortality risk for patients receiving hemodiafiltration versus hemodialysis: European results from the DOPPS. *Kidney Int*, **69**, 2087–93.

Chandna SM, *et al.* (1999). Is there a rationale for rationing chronic dialysis? A hospital based cohort study of factors affecting survival and morbidity. *BMJ*, **318**, 217–23.

Daugirdas JT (1993). Second generation logarithmic estimates of single-pool variable volume Kt/V: an analysis of error. *J Am Soc Nephrol*, **4**, 1205–13.

Daugirdas JT, Schneditz D (1995). Overestimation of hemodialysis dose depends on dialysis efficiency by regional blood flow but not by conventional two pool urea kinetic analysis. *ASAIO J*, **41**, M719–24.

Davenport A (2006). Intradialytic complications during hemodialysis. *Hemodial Int*, **10**, 162–7.

Dember LM, Jaber BL (2006). Dialysis-related amyloidosis: late finding or hidden epidemic? *Semin Dial*, **19**, 105–9.

Department of Health (2002). *Good practice guidelines for renal dialysis/transplantation units: prevention and control of blood-borne virus infection*. http://www.dh.gov.uk/PublicationsAndStatistics/Publications/PublicationsPolicyAndGuidance/PublicationsPolicyAndGuidanceArticle/fs/en?CONTENT_ID=4005752&chk=AVH6Zr

Eknoyan G, *et al.* (2002). Effect of dialysis dose and membrane flux in maintenance hemodialysis. *N Engl J Med*, **347**, 2010–19.

Feest TG, *et al.* (2005). Trends in adult renal replacement therapy in the UK: 1982–2002. *QJM*, **98**, 21–8.

Fluck R (2006). *Vascular access survey*. http://www.dh.gov.uk/assetRoot/04/13/05/09/04130509.pdf

Gotch FA (2001). Evolution of the single-pool urea kinetic model. *Semin Dial*, **14**, 252–6.

Gotch FA, Sargent JA (1985). A mechanistic analysis of the National Cooperative Dialysis Study (NCDS). *Kidney Int*, **28**, 526–34.

Guerin AP, *et al.* (2006). Cardiovascular disease in the dialysis population: prognostic significance of arterial disorders. *Curr Opin Nephrol Hypertens*, **15**, 105–10.

Hoenich NA, Ronco C (2007). Haemodialysis fluid: composition and clinical importance. *Blood Purif*, **25**, 62–8.

Jaeger JQ, Mehta RL (1999). Assessment of dry weight in hemodialysis: an overview. *J Am Soc Nephrol*, **10**, 392–403.

Mitra S, Chandna SM, Farrington K (1999). What is hypertension in chronic haemodialysis? The role of interdialytic blood pressure monitoring. *Nephrol Dial Transplant*, **14**, 2915–21.

National Kidney Foundation K/DOQI (2006). *Clinical practice guidelines for hemodialysis adequacy*. http://www.kidney.org/Professionals/kdoqi/guideline_upHD_PD_VA/index.htm

Owen WF Jr, *et al.* (1993). The urea reduction ratio and serum albumin concentration as predictors of mortality in patients undergoing hemodialysis. *N Engl J Med*, **329**, 1001–6.

Pickering TG (2006). Target blood pressure in patients with end-stage renal disease: evidence-based medicine or the emperor's new clothes? *J Clin Hypertens (Greenwich)*, **8**, 369–75.

Pierratos A, *et al.* (2006). Daily hemodialysis 2006. State of the art. *Minerva Urol Nefrol*, **58**, 99–115.

Smith C, *et al.* (2003). Choosing not to dialyse: evaluation of planned non-dialytic management in a cohort of patients with end-stage renal failure. *Nephron Clin Pract*, **95**, c40–6.

Sonawane S, Kasbekar N, Berns JS (2006). The safety of heparins in end-stage renal disease. *Semin Dial*, **19**, 305–10.

Tattersall JE, *et al.* (1996). The post-hemodialysis rebound: predicting and quantifying its effect on Kt/V. *Kidney Int*, **50**, 2094–102.

UK Renal Association (2006). *Clinical practice guidelines*. http://www.renal.org/Clinical/GuidelinesSection/Guidelines.aspx.

Wanner C, *et al.* (2005). Atorvastatin in patients with type 2 diabetes mellitus undergoing hemodialysis. *N Engl J Med*, **353**, 238–48.

21.7.2 Peritoneal dialysis

Simon Davies

Essentials

Peritoneal dialysis is achieved by repeated cycles of instillation and drainage of dialysis fluid within the peritoneal cavity, with the two main functions of dialysis—solute and fluid removal—occurring due to the contact between dialysis fluid and the capillary circulation of the parietal and visceral peritoneum across the peritoneal membrane. It can be used to provide renal replacement therapy in acute kidney injury or chronic kidney disease.

Practical aspects—choice of peritoneal dialysis as an effective modality for renal replacement in the short to medium term (i.e. several years) is, for most patients, a lifestyle issue. Typically, a patient on continuous ambulatory peritoneal dialysis (CAPD) will require three to five exchanges of 1.5 to 2.5 litres of dialysate per day. Automated peritoneal dialysis (APD) and use of the glucose-polymer dialysis solution icodextrin eables flexibility of prescription that can mitigate the effects of membrane function (high solute transport). Between-patient variability in membrane function influences patient survival.

Peritonitis—this remains the most common complication of peritoneal dialysis, presenting with cloudy dialysis effluent, with or without abdominal pain and/or fever, and confirmed (usually) by demonstrating a leucocyte count greater than 100 cells/µl in the peritoneal fluid. Empirical antibiotic treatment, either intraperitoneal or systemic, with cover for both Gram-positive and Gram-negative organisms, should be commenced immediately while awaiting specific cultures and sensitivities.

Encapsulating peritoneal sclerosis—this is a life-threatening complication of peritoneal dialysis, particularly if of long duration (15–20% incidence after 10 years) and if complicated by severe peritonitis, characterized by severe inflammatory thickening, especially of the mesenteric peritoneum, resulting in an encapsulation and progressive obstruction of the bowel. Extensive enterolysis is the only successful treatment in severe cases, but mortality is high.

Introduction

Peritoneal dialysis, along with haemodialysis and renal transplantation, is an effective form of renal replacement therapy. Worldwide it is used for both acute and chronic renal failure, although patterns of use vary considerably. In the treatment of chronic kidney disease (CKD), peritoneal dialysis should be considered as a short- to medium-term (several years) treatment option, to be used in the context of an integrated approach to renal replacement. For example, it is of value both before and after transplantation in a lifetime of treatment that might require more than one period on each of the renal replacement modalities. The only absolute contraindication is the lack of a peritoneal cavity.

Historical perspective

In the 1890s, Henry Starling, while conducting experiments from which he made his seminal observations on the forces that govern transcapillary fluid transport, provided evidence that the peritoneal membrane could be used to remove fluid and solutes—the fundamental requirements of renal replacement therapy. By the 1940s, peritoneal dialysis was established in the treatment of acute kidney injury, and a decade later intermittent treatments, typically twice weekly, were used to maintain patients with CKD. Critical to this was the development in 1968 of the Tenckhoff catheter, a soft silicone-based tube that could create permanent access to the peritoneal membrane. In 1978, Popovitch and Moncreif argued that peritoneal dialysis could be performed continuously in ambulant patients with permanent renal failure, coining the term 'continuous ambulatory peritoneal dialysis' (CAPD), following which peritoneal dialysis became established as a renal replacement modality that could be undertaken in the home environment. Modifications of this approach, using a device that delivers multiple exchanges of dialysis fluid overnight, so reducing the number of exchanges required during the daytime, is termed 'automated peritoneal dialysis' (APD). In addition to the reduced daytime burden of the treatment, the advantages of this approach are that it can facilitate delivery of care by a parent, partner, or assistant.

The use of peritoneal dialysis in renal replacement

Acute kidney injury

In a worldwide survey of 345 nephrology centres, peritoneal dialysis was used to treat acute kidney injury in 24%, as compared with 45% treating with continuous haemofiltration and 30% with intermittent haemodialysis. This distribution is not evenly spread across the world: there is much greater reliance on peritoneal dialysis in developing countries, the exception to this being in infants and small children in whom it remains the treatment of choice. Advantages of peritoneal dialysis in acute kidney injury include lack of reliance on a clean water supply, relatively stable haemodynamics, no need for vascular access, and the avoidance of anticoagulation and its complications.

Chronic kidney disease

The penetration of peritoneal dialysis as a treatment for CKD varies considerably throughout the world, ranging from about 5% in Japan to more than 80% in Mexico. The reasons for this are many, but, broadly speaking, in countries with predominantly private healthcare systems, especially when the nephrologists' reimbursement favours haemodialysis, penetration is low, whereas public health care provision is associated with greater use of peritoneal dialysis. Other factors include haemodialysis provision, the relative costs of labour vs consumables, and factors that favour the use of home therapies. Currently, the highest growth rates for peritoneal dialysis are seen in the developing world, especially Indo-Asia.

Predictors of survival

As for all types of renal replacement therapy, the most important factors associated with survival are age, inflammation, and comorbidity, the latter being weighted towards cardiovascular disease. The continued presence of residual renal function, a benefit that can be demonstrated with creatinine clearances as low as 1 to 2 ml/min, or just 250 ml/day of urinary volume, also improves survival. In addition, there is strong evidence that peritoneal membrane function has an effect. Membranes associated with less efficient fluid removal, due to high solute transport characteristics or low ultrafiltration capacity (see below), are associated with worse outcomes.

Comparison with haemodialysis

There is growing evidence that, when both haemodialysis and peritoneal dialysis are equally available, the choice between the therapies is largely determined by lifestyle issues (Table 21.7.2.1). The failure to date to perform a randomized controlled trial comparing modalities lies in the fact that most patients (96%) demonstrate a strong modality preference when the choice is made freely available. Modality comparisons have thus relied on observational studies from registry data, with adjustment for baseline factors. Generally, these analyses show equivalent 5-year survival. There appears to be a relative survival advantage for peritoneal dialysis during the first 2 years and for haemodialysis after 3 years, in keeping with an asymmetric pattern in modality switching. Technique failure is more likely to occur in peritoneal dialysis than haemodialysis, reflecting the effects of membrane damage associated with infection and long-term exposure to dialysis fluid as well as changes in a patient's circumstances, such that continuing with home treatment becomes untenable. The relative early survival benefits for peritoneal dialysis are best seen in the nondiabetic population. Taken overall, these survival differences are not sufficient

Table 21.7.2.1 Typical reasons for choosing peritoneal dialysis or haemodialysis as renal replacement modality

Reasons favouring peritoneal dialysis	Reasons favouring haemodialysis
No vascular access	No peritoneal access
Haemodialysis-induced hypotension	Multiple comorbidities
Preference for home treatment	Increasing age
Independence	Living alone
Distant from haemodialysis facility	Dependent
Family and work commitments	Close to haemodialysis facility
Dependent, when assisted APD performed by a carer or parent is available	Home haemodialysis option preferred and available

APD, automated peritoneal dialysis.

to override patient preferences associated with lifestyle choices, provided there is an understanding that modality switching may well be required. APD extends choice to the patient or their carer, so accommodating a variety of lifestyles; it is the preferred dialysis treatment for children.

Principles of therapy

Peritoneal dialysis is achieved by repeated cycles of instillation and drainage of dialysis fluid within the peritoneal cavity. The fluid is heat-sterilized, a process that requires an acidic pH; ideally a pH of 2 to 3 should be used, but this requires two or more dialysis bag compartments to enable reconstitution just prior to infusion. This approach enables a physiological pH solution with low concentrations of glucose degradation products as well as substitution of bicarbonate for lactate as the buffer. These more biocompatible solutions are not universally available, however, and most conventional peritoneal dialysis solutions have a pH of 5.2, with 35 to 40 mmol/litre of lactate as the buffer.

Typically, a patient on peritoneal dialysis will require three to five exchanges of 1.5 to 2.5 litres of dialysate per day. CAPD regimens usually comprise three 4- to 6-hour daytime exchanges and an overnight exchange; APD regimens may use up to six exchanges overnight and a long daytime dwell period. APD can be further augmented by adding an additional—typically evening—exchange, so increasing the dose of dialysis given. These volumes will be very different for children in whom they are adjusted according to body surface area.

The patient or their carer is trained in the sterile procedure of dialysis fluid exchange by a specialist peritoneal dialysis nurse, a process that generally takes a few days and can be achieved by a wide variety of individuals, despite physical and educational disabilities.

Peritoneal access

In order to drain peritoneal dialysis fluid in and out of the peritoneal cavity, a flexible permanent dialysis catheter is required, and this is also to be preferred when peritoneal dialysis is used for acute kidney injury. Correct insertion and subsequent catheter management is critical for the success of peritoneal dialysis. Insertion should be performed as a planned procedure by an experienced operator and may be achieved using either the Seldinger technique, open surgery, or with the use of a laparoscope. Catheters usually have two Dacron cuffs, one at each end of the subcutaneous tunnel: the deep cuff is placed at entry to the peritoneum, whereas the superficial cuff should be situated about 1.5 cm deep to the exit site, which should be positioned on the abdominal wall so that it is visible to the patient.

Peritoneal physiology

The two main functions of dialysis, solute and fluid removal, occur owing to the contact between dialysis fluid and the capillary circulation of the parietal and visceral peritoneum. In a typical adult, approximately 0.5 m^2 of the peritoneum is in contact with fluid, representing about one-third of the anatomical membrane.

Solute clearance

Removal of solute is predominantly by diffusion across the membrane and is thus governed by the concentration gradient, the number and density of capillaries in contact with dialysate (often termed effective peritoneal surface area), and the size of the solute in question. Equilibration time for urea is typically within 4 to 5 h, hence removal is limited by the drained dialysate volume rather than length of dwell. Equilibration is more time-limited for larger molecules such as creatinine and glucose, e.g. the average dialysate to plasma ratio of creatinine at 4 h is 0.65, with a range of 0.4 to 0.85 that is normally distributed. This measurement is termed the solute transport rate and is used to measure the diffusive component of membrane function in the 'peritoneal equilibration test'. The reasons for the large variability between patients in this measurement are mostly unknown.

Ultrafiltration

Fluid transport across the membrane is governed mainly by pressure gradients, including hydrostatic, osmotic, and oncotic, as well as some fluid reabsorption due to lymphatics. Instillation of fluid within the peritoneal cavity creates a positive pressure that is close to capillary pressure, resulting in little net fluid movement by this mechanism unless excessive intraperitoneal pressures are created. Conventional glucose-containing dialysis fluids create an osmotic pressure gradient proportional to glucose concentration (1.5–4.0%) that results in a peak net ultra-filtration volume between 2 and 4 h, depending on solute transport characteristics of the membrane (Fig. 21.7.2.1). It is by prescription of exchanges containing different glucose concentrations ('weak', 'medium' and 'strong' bags) that the patient's fluid status can be controlled to achieve the target weight specified by their physician. There are two pathways of water transport by this mechanism, intercellular and transcellular, each contributing about half the fluid removal, the latter being via aquaporins and thus water exclusive. Once the osmotic gradient has dissipated, fluid reabsorption occurs due to a combination of transcapillary oncotic (Starling) forces and lymphatics. Removal of ions such as sodium and calcium is predominantly by convection because the diffusion gradient is small (typical dialysate sodium concentration is 132 mmol/litre). Owing to the existence of the aquaporin pathway, there is uncoupling of water and sodium removal, termed sodium sieving, that is most pronounced in the early part of the dwell. As a consequence, peritoneal dialysis is always at risk of removing excess water compared with sodium, and treatment regimens that rely on too many short, hypertonic glucose exchanges are to be avoided. By the same token, lack of sodium sieving is an indicator of poor free-water transport and thus membrane failure.

Monitoring treatment quality

Solute clearance

Residual renal and peritoneal solute clearances are not equivalent in their impact on patient survival. To date, in CKD, no randomized study has been able to demonstrate an association between survival and peritoneal clearances, and there are no studies published in acute kidney injury. It is important, therefore, that both residual and peritoneal clearances are measured. Both urea (Kt/V_{urea}) and creatinine clearances can be used to monitor treatment, and there is general agreement in international guidelines—based on at least two large randomized trials—on minimum treatment targets. For Kt/V_{urea}, a combined residual and peritoneal clearance of 1.7 using the Watson formula to calculate V (total body

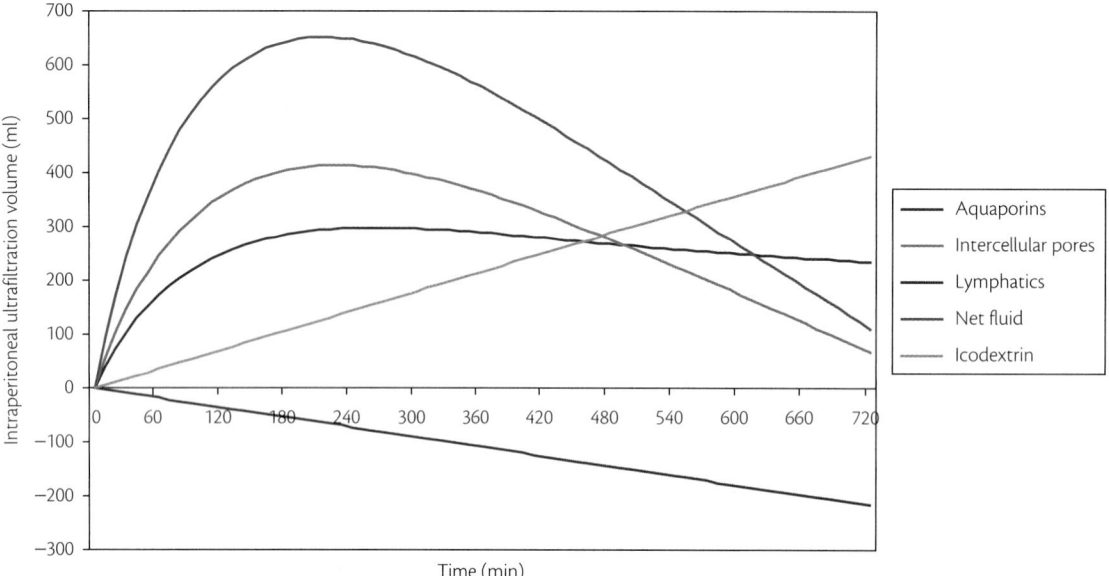

Fig. 21.7.2.1 Pathways of fluid transport across the peritoneal membrane. The net changes in intraperitoneal fluid volume and thus ultrafiltration achieved at each time point when using glucose (3.86%) as the osmotic agent are the result of fluid transport via at least three pathways: aquaporins (water exclusive), small intercellular pores, and lymphatic reabsorption. Fluid is reabsorbed once the intraperitoneal glucose has equilibrated with plasma. By contrast, when using the glucose polymer icodextrin, sustained ultrafiltration occurs for several hours.

water) should be achieved. Alternatively, a combined creatinine clearance of 50 litres/week per 1.73 m² can be used. In either case, however, dialysis dose should be increased in the presence of symptoms attributable to uraemia.

Ultrafiltration

Several observational studies have shown that a reduced peritoneal ultrafiltration and by implication sodium removal is associated with reduced survival, especially in anuric patients. Several reasons for this association have been proposed, but there is little doubt that a failure to remove adequate fluid owing to membrane characteristics that result in less good ultrafiltration or excessive fluid reabsorption are important. The simplest way to monitor membrane function is to perform a regular peritoneal equilibration test that measures solute transport rate and net ultrafiltration capacity in a standardised 4-h dwell. A membrane that results in less than 400 ml ultrafiltration using 3.86% or less than 100 ml using 2.27% glucose is unlikely to achieve adequate fluid removal. If this is associated with high solute transport (4-h dialysate:plasma creatinine ratio above 0.65), and thus early loss of the glucose gradient and more rapid fluid reabsorption, then a combination of APD delivering shorter exchanges overnight and icodextrin (a polydispersed glucose polymer derived from starch) in the long exchange will result in adequate fluid removal in most cases. Icodextrin achieves sustained ultrafiltration in the long dwell as it acts rather like a colloidal agent, thus counterbalancing Starling forces. It has been shown to improve fluid status, reduce peritoneal glucose exposure, and enhance diabetic control, and it represents a major advance in peritoneal dialysis therapy. Note, however, that icodextrin metabolites in blood can interfere with estimation of blood glucose by monitors that use glucose dehydrogenase, such that there is a risk of failing to diagnose hypoglycaemia.

Complications and their management

Peritonitis

Peritonitis is the most common and potentially serious complication of peritoneal dialysis, resulting in up to 50% of technique failures. With enhanced training, patients can be expected to have one episode of peritonitis for every 3 years of treatment. Presentation is with cloudy dialysis effluent, with or without abdominal pain and/or fever, and the diagnosis is confirmed (usually) when the leucocyte count is above 100/μl in the peritoneal fluid. Clinical assessment should include examination of the exit site and tunnel for infection, and the abdomen for signs of intraabdominal pathology. At least 20 ml of freshly drained dialysate should be sent for culture by appropriate methods, which are absolutely crucial. The technique recommended by the International Society for Peritoneal Dialysis (accessible at http://www.ispd.org) is for 50 ml of peritoneal effluent to be centrifuged at 3000 g for 15 min, followed by resuspension of the sediment in 3 to 5 ml of sterile saline and inoculation of material on both solid culture media and into a standard blood culture medium. With this method, fewer than 5% of cases should be culture negative.

Empirical antibiotic treatment, either intraperitoneal or systemic, with cover for both Gram-positive and Gram-negative organisms should be commenced immediately while awaiting specific cultures and sensitivities. The reader is again directed to the International Society for Peritoneal Dialysis website for detailed up-to-date guidelines on management, but most typically Gram-positive organisms will be covered by vancomycin or a cephalosporin, and Gram-negative infections by a third-generation cephalosporin, aminoglycoside or (if local sensitivities support such use) quinolone, with the regimen adjusted as and when results of culture and sensitivity of peritoneal fluid are available. A mixed bacterial growth, especially associated with anaerobes, should dictate early

Table 21.7.2.2 Classification and treatment of exit-site infections

Symptom	Points awarded		
	0	1	2
Swelling	Absent	At exit	Includes tunnel
Crust	Absent	<0.5 cm	>0.5 cm
Redness	Absent	<0.5 cm	>0.5 cm
Pain	Absent	Slight	Severe
Drainage	Absent	Serous	Purulent

An exit site with a score of 4 or greater, or a purulent discharge, should be treated with empirical antibiotics that cover coagulase-positive *Staphylococcus* and *Pseudomonas* until sensitivities are available.

surgical assessment, catheter removal, and laparotomy. Catheter removal is also likely if there is an associated tunnel infection or a failure to respond to antibiotics within a few days.

Exit-site infection

A simple scoring system has been devised to assess the exit site (Table 21.7.2.2).

Mechanical failure

Mechanical failure is common in the early stages of a patient's career on peritoneal dialysis, and can be due either to catheter displacement (outflow affected), wrapping of the catheter by the omentum (in- and outflow), or leakage. The latter can occur at the deep cuff or at any hernia site and may present as genital swelling. Diagnosis is either obvious or requires appropriate imaging, usually a CT scan with contrast introduced into the catheter.

Ultrafiltration failure

Changes can occur in membrane function with time on peritoneal dialysis that result in less good ultrafiltration. Drivers of this change appear to be early loss of residual renal function and use of more hypertonic glucose dialysis solutions. Most frequently, this is due to an increase in solute transport that can be addressed using APD and icodextrin (see above). In some patients, however, more serious membrane damage occurs which results in reduced osmotic conductance (efficiency) of the membrane for a given osmotic gradient. These patients require transfer to haemodialysis.

Encapsulating peritoneal sclerosis

Encapsulating peritoneal sclerosis is a relatively uncommon but life-threatening complication of peritoneal dialysis, characterized by severe inflammatory thickening, especially of the mesenteric peritoneum, resulting in an encapsulation and progressive obstruction of the bowel. Aetiological factors identified include prolonged time on treatment (incidence 15–20% after 10 years), severe and protracted peritonitis, acetate buffer in the early days of peritoneal dialysis, and contamination with particulate plastic. It may resolve slowly after stopping peritoneal dialysis, but often presents after modality transfer. Some advocate treatment with tamoxifen, although benefit is not proven. In severe cases—with life-threatening obstruction—extensive enterolysis is the only successful treatment, although mortality is high.

Further reading

Brimble KS, *et al.* (2006). Meta-analysis: peritoneal membrane transport, mortality, and technique failure in peritoneal dialysis. *J Am Soc Nephrol*, **17**, 2591–8.

Brown EA, *et al.* (2003). Survival of functionally anuric patients on automated peritoneal dialysis: the European APD Outcome Study. *J Am Soc Nephrol*, **14**, 2948–57.

Crabtree JH, Burchette RJ, Siddiqi NA (2005). Optimal peritoneal dialysis catheter type and exit site location: an anthropometric analysis. *ASAIO J*, **51**, 743–7.

Davies SJ (2004). Longitudinal relationship between solute transport and ultrafiltration capacity in peritoneal dialysis patients. *Kidney Int*, **66**, 2437–45.

Davies SJ (2004). Peritoneal dialysis solutions. In: Pereira BJ, Sayegh MH, Blake P (eds). *Chronic kidney disease, dialysis and transplantation – companion to Brenner and Rector's. The kidney.* 2nd edition. pp. 534–52. Elsevier Saunders, Philadelphia.

Gabriel DP, *et al.* (2006). Peritoneal dialysis in acute renal failure. *Ren Fail*, **28**, 451–6.

Jager KJ, *et al.* (2004). The effect of contraindications and patient preference on dialysis modality selection in ESRD patients in The Netherlands. *Am J Kidney Dis*, **43**, 891–9.

Piraino B, *et al.* (2005). Peritoneal dialysis-related infections recommendations: 2005 update. *Perit Dial Int*, **25**, 107–31.

Rippe B, *et al.* (2004). Fluid and electrolyte transport across the peritoneal membrane during CAPD according to the three-pore model. *Perit Dial Int*, **24**, 10–27.

Smit W, *et al.* (2004). Analysis of the prevalence and causes of ultrafiltration failure during long-term peritoneal dialysis: a cross-sectional study. *Perit Dial Int*, **24**, 562–70.

Vonesh EF, *et al.* (2004). The differential impact of risk factors on mortality in hemodialysis and peritoneal dialysis. *Kidney Int*, **66**, 2389–401.

21.7.3 Renal transplantation

P. Sweny

Essentials

Renal transplantation is the preferred option for the treatment of endstage chronic renal failure in patients for whom there are no major medical contraindications. In well-selected recipients, both life expectancy and quality of life are superior to treatment with long-term dialysis. However, as the dialysis population continues to grow, the gap between supply and demand for renal transplantation is widening. Attempts to bridge this gap have included (1) relaxation of the criteria for a suitable deceased donor (marginal donors); (2) reversion to the procurement of kidneys from non-heartbeating cadavers; and (3) encouragement of living donation—including techniques for desensitization of recipients, also paired exchanges, both to circumvent blood group incompatibilities or preformed antibodies that would otherwise bar transplantation.

Technical aspects

Surgery—the new kidney is placed in one or other iliac fossa, usually in an extraperitoneal position that allows ease of repeated biopsy to detect cause of graft dysfunction. Typically, the renal artery is anastomosed end to side to the common iliac artery or end to end to the internal iliac artery, the renal vein to the common iliac vein, and the transplant ureter is implanted into the bladder through a submucosal tunnel. The native kidneys are left *in situ* unless there are particular reasons for them to be removed in a separate pre-transplant operation.

Immunosuppression—excepting for transplants between HLA-identical twins, immunosuppression is required to prevent rejection, but there is no clear consensus on the best immunosuppressive regimen. Most centres use an induction antibody directed against CD25 (the IL-2 receptor), followed by what is now called standard triple therapy—comprising a calcineurin inhibitor (CNI) (ciclosporin or tacrolimus), combined with either mycophenolate mofetil or azathioprine, and steroids. Steroids are not infrequently tailed off rapidly in the early post-transplant period.

Transplant rejection

This can be classified into four main categories: (1) hyperacute—due to preformed cytotoxic antibodies, always leads to very rapid graft failure; (2) accelerated—a predominantly T-cell-mediated rejection crisis occurring within the first few days, cannot usually be treated satisfactorily; (3) acute cellular—due to a primary cell-mediated response, occurs in 10% to 20% of recipients, manifests histologically as tubulitis, first-line treatment (usually successful) with intravenous steroids; (4) humoral—antibody-mediated, manifest histologically as marked staining for the complement breakdown product C4d in peritubular capillaries, best treatment uncertain.

Complications of renal transplantation

Specific side effects of immunosuppressive agents—these are important causes of morbidity and (rarely) mortality, with steroids culpable for many of the complications of transplantation, and nephrotoxicity being the main drawback of CNIs. The desire to overcome these problems is one of the main drivers in the search for new immunosuppressants and immunosuppressive regimens.

Nonspecific side effects of immunosuppressive agents—all currently available immunosuppressive regimen are nonspecific in the sense that they suppress not only the immune response to the allograft, but also the immune response to infections and tumours.

Infective complications—transplant recipients are vulnerable to opportunistic infections including (1) viral infections—particularly cytomegalovirus (the main infectious complication in solid organ transplantation, with manifestation ranging from asymptomatic viraemia to life-threatening multiorgan failure), Epstein–Barr virus (EBV or HHV4), varicella zoster virus, herpes simplex, human polyomavirus (especially BK, which can lead to nephropathy and graft failure), human papillomavirus (HPV), and HIV; (2) bacterial infections—particularly mycobacterial, nocardia, nontyphoid salmonella, listeria; (3) fungal infections—including candidiasis and aspergillosis aspergillus and pneumocystis (a dreaded complication of transplantation before routine introduction of prophylaxis with co-trioazole or pentamidine); (4) parasitic infections—including *Strongyloides stercoralis*, scabies, and toxoplasmosis.

Malignant complications—post-transplant neoplasia is an important cause of morbidity and mortality. Particular conditions include (1) post-transplant lymphoproliferative disorder (PTLD)—driven by EBV, first-line treatment by stepwise reduction in immunosuppression; (2) Kaposi's sarcoma—caused by HHV8, first-line treatment by switch of immunosuppression to sirolimus; (3) HPV—responsible for skin, vulval, and anogenital warts, and some types are associated with carcinoma. After 20 years, most renal transplant recipients who are white will have cutaneous squamous cell carcinoma.

Other complications—these include hypertension, accelerated atherosclerosis, electrolyte, musculoskeletal, haematological, gastrointestinal, and cosmetic disorders.

Prognosis

The short-term outcome of renal transplantation has improved markedly over the last 30 years, with 1-year graft survival around 90%. However, the rate of chronic graft-loss remains at about 4% per year, with the descriptive term 'chronic allograft nephropathy' commonly (but unhelpfully, because it does not imply a mechanism or aid management) being applied to the failing graft. The commonest cause of insidious late graft failure is probably calcineurin toxicity, which by 10 years probably affects nearly all exposed grafts to some degree. Conversion from CNIs to either mycophenolate mofetil or sirolimus can prolong graft survival, and is being used increasingly in many centres.

Introduction

Renal transplantation is the preferred option for the treatment of endstage chronic renal failure in patients for whom there are no major medical contraindications. With improvements in immunosuppression and in the equally important general medical support of the immunocompromised patient, the age ranges and permissible comorbidities of recipients continue to be extended. In well-selected recipients, both life expectancy and quality of life are superior to long-term dialysis. The two impediments to the extension of transplantation are the shortage of donor organs and the side effects of the still crude immunosuppressive agents. Xenotransplantation may remove the first of these hurdles, but is likely to increase our dependence on potent immunosuppressive regimen. In humans, immunological tolerance to the graft with preservation of normal immunoresponsiveness to infections and tumours has not yet been achieved.

Supply, demand and kidney donation

In 2007 there were just over 6000 patients waiting for kidney transplantation in the United Kingdom, in comparison to an annual rate for renal transplantation which approaches 2000 per year. Approximately 1200 deceased donor kidneys are available for transplantation each year, with the remainder of kidneys coming from living donors. Living donation now accounts for about 30% of all renal transplants in the United Kingdom, but approximately 50% in the United States of America. The dialysis population continues to grow, with the gap between supply and demand for renal transplantation widening and the waiting list growing by about 3% per year. Attempts to bridge this gap have included a relaxation of the criteria for a suitable deceased donor (so called marginal donors), and the reversion to the procurement of kidneys from non-heart-beating cadavers.

In the United Kingdom, new legislation (the Human Tissue Act 2004) has helped facilitate living donation from both related and unrelated donors, and any significant increase in kidney transplantation seems most likely to come from increased living donation. It is now safe and effective to transplant across blood group incompatibility barriers by removal and suppression of recipient blood group antibodies using various combinations of antibody removal (plasma exchange or specific immunoabsorption) and suppression of antibody formation (most commonly with rituximab, an anti-CD20 monoclonal antibody) with or without intravenous immunoglobulin (IVIG). Transplantation can go ahead once antibody titres have been suppressed, but further cycles of treatment may be needed in the early post-transplant period.

The use of paired living donation is also increasing in many countries, including the United Kingdom. The principles are straightforward: A wishes to give a kidney to B, but is prevented from doing so because they are immunologically incompatible; C wishes to give a kidney to D, but again is prevented from doing so because of immunological incompatibility; however, A is not incompatible with D, and C is not incompatible with B, hence a paired exchange can be organized such that A gives to D and C to B, hence blood group incompatibilities or preformed antibodies that would otherwise bar transplantation are circumvented. Depending on local regulatory arrangements there can be several interlinked pairs.

A further possibility is altruistic donation, in which an individual offers a nondirected kidney for transplantation. It would theoretically be possible to use this to start a series of paired donations. Another proposal (not implemented) is that by donating a kidney to the national pool, a family member might secure the highest possible priority for the next suitable kidney for their relative.

Living donors

Every care must be taken to protect the interests of the donor. Informed consent is crucial. Potential donors must be aware that giving a kidney carries risks, albeit the mortality rate is only 0.01 to 0.03%, with most deaths attributable to acute pulmonary embolus. The other risks that are involved in a general anaesthetic and an abdominal operation must also be fully explained. Increasing use of laparoscopic kidney retrieval in live donors has done much to improve donor acceptability and speed postoperative recovery.

Needless to say, a donor should be in good general physical health and have normal kidney function and surgically acceptable renal anatomy. The assessments required are summarized in Box 21.7.3.1. Apart from exceptional circumstances, donors

---

Box 21.7.3.1 Assessment of the potential living donor

- Medical history
- Psychiatric and psychosocial history—including at-risk behaviour
- Physical examination
- Blood group (ABO)
- Tissue typing
- Lymphocyte crossmatch (recipient serum against donor lymphocytes)
- DNA testing to prove family relationship
- Urine:
  - Stick testing—blood, protein, glucose, leucocytes, nitrites
  - Culture and microscopy
  - Quantify protein excretion (albumin:creatinine ratio)
  - Creatinine clearance
- Blood:
  - Glucose—formal glucose tolerance test[a]
  - Electrolytes
  - Urea, creatinine, uric acid
  - Liver function tests
  - Full blood count
  - Glucose-6-phosphate dehydrogenase[a]
  - Haemoglobin, electrophoresis[a]
  - Sickle test[a]
  - Procoagulant screen[a]

- Infection screen:
  - HIV
  - HTLV 1 and 2
  - Cytomegalovirus (HHV5)
  - Epstein–Barr virus (HHV4)
  - Hepatitis B virus
  - Hepatitis C virus
  - Kaposi's sarcoma virus (HHV8)[a]
  - Syphilis
  - Toxoplasmosis
  - Schistosomiasis[a]
  - Malaria[a]
  - *Trypanosoma cruzi*[a]
  - *Strongyloides stercoralis*[a]
- Chest radiograph
- ECG
- Cardiac stress testing[a]
- Glomerular filtration rate estimation by isotopic method
- Renal imaging:
  - Ultrasound and DMSA scan
  - Donor renal arteriogram (MRA or CT)
- Informed consent, assessment by independent assessor (Human Tissue Act)

[a]Where clinically indicated, such as specific geographical or other risk.

outside the age limits of 18 to 70 years are not considered. It is usual to wait for a young female potential donor to complete her family.

Most studies have shown an increase in life expectancy of donors when compared with age-matched controls. A few donors will develop hypertension, but at a risk that is similar to that of the general population. A small number develop proteinuria, but this is usually less than 0.5 g/24 h and does not affect survival. Renal function usually returns to 75 to 80% of the predonation level.

The use of living kidney donors is driven not only by the shortage of cadaver organs for transplantation, but also by the fact that these kidneys do better than those from a deceased donor. This is partly due to better matching, with many related donors and recipients sharing one or two extended haplotypes, but an additional benefit—shared also by kidneys from living unrelated donors, which similarly out perform those transplanted from cadavers—is the physiological state of the organ when recovered under ideal and planned conditions, and without the necessity for prolonged cold storage.

Deceased donors

In this situation the prime responsibility is to the potential recipient. The kidney should be in as good a physiological state as possible, and there should be no obvious risk of transfer of infection or malignancy by the donor organ. The major contraindications to organ procurement are listed in Box 21.7.3.2. Marginal donors are increasingly being considered, particularly for older recipients and for those with a limited life expectancy. In some situations it may be appropriate to consider organs from hepatitis C (HCV)-positive or hepatitis B (HBV)-positive donors for positive recipients. Experience in parts of the world where safe long-term dialysis is not available have shown that an acceptable quality of life can be sustained with substandard kidneys, and—given the shortage of organs—marginal donors should not be discarded out of hand without discussion with the local transplant unit. Under some circumstances it may be appropriate to transplant two marginal donor kidneys ('en bloc') into the recipient in order to supply an adequate nephron mass. Prospective recipients of these marginal donors must be appropriately counselled.

Recipient assessment

Patients may be transplanted before the need for dialysis (pre-emptive transplantation) or from an established dialysis programme (haemodialysis or peritoneal dialysis). It is essential that all patients are fully assessed by both a transplant surgeon and transplant physician before being placed on the waiting list or offered a kidney, whether it be from a cadaver or a relative. Patients with chronic renal failure develop a multitude of complications that need assessment before surgery. Transplantation carries with it the risks of any major surgical procedure, together with the added risks of prolonged immunosuppression.

An additional consideration is that, given the shortage of organs for transplantation, it is important that the best use is made of all organs. Although everyone would agree with this in principle, making decisions in individual cases can be difficult. In some situations the general health and life expectancy of the potential recipient argue strongly against transplantation. Patients with congenitally abnormal lower urinary tracts can be difficult to transplant and ideally should be managed in centres with

---

Box 21.7.3.2 Contraindications to cadaver organ procurement

- Donor age:
  - <3 years (en bloc dual transplant possible)
  - >70 years[a]
- Cancer not confined to the central nervous system (CNS), but note:
  - Nonmelanoma skin tumours and carcinoma *in situ* of the uterine cervix are permissible
  - Cancer confined to CNS is acceptable, excepting medulloblastoma and glioblastoma
- Risk of transmissible infection:
  - At-risk behaviour
  - HCV
  - HBV
  - HIV
  - HTLV 1, 2
  - HHV8
  - Deep fungal infections
  - Parenchymal renal infection
  - Meningoencephalitic syndromes of unknown aetiology
  - Inadequately treated bacterial infection
  - Infection with resistant organisms (e.g. MRSA, VRE, ESBL)
- Diabetes mellitus[a]
- Acute renal failure[a]
- Hypertension[a]
- Chronic renal impairment
- Warm ischaemia >90 min
- Cold ischaemia >30 h[a]

ESBL, extended-spectrum β-lactamase producer; HTLV, human T-cell lymphocytotrophic virus; MRSA, methicillin-resistant *Staphylococcus aureus*; VRE, vancomycin-resistant enterococcus.
[a]Relative contraindication.

---

urological transplant expertise, some needing complex bladder augmentation or drainage procedures before transplantation.

Since the main cause of death post transplant is cardiovascular, it is important to screen at-risk patients for occult vascular disease (carotid, aortoiliac, peripheral, and cardiac). This is particularly true for patients with diabetes mellitus, for whom coronary angiography and appropriate intervention are particularly likely be required.

Recipient hepatitis (HCV or HBV) complicates transplantation. Without antiviral therapy, immunosuppression accelerates liver disease and death may occur within 5 to 10 years of transplantation, usually from sepsis or progressive liver disease, particularly in the case of HBV. The advent of effective antiviral therapy has greatly improved the outlook. Attempts should be made to clear hepatitis C prior to renal transplantation (the use of interferon after renal transplantation is contraindicated as it is likely to trigger acute allograft rejection.) There are now a number of effective oral agents for the treatment of HBV which can be used after renal transplantation particularly in combination. In the setting of advanced liver disease (cirrhosis and ascites) assessment for a combined liver and renal transplant may be appropriate.

Allocation of kidneys

Fully matched kidneys (zero A, zero B, and zero DR mismatch—denoted 0–0–0 mismatch) and DR identical kidneys do better than less well-matched organs, hence most countries have local or national kidney sharing schemes so that more recipients can receive the benefits of a well-matched organ. Use is increasingly being made of point scoring systems to allocate kidneys fairly, patients accruing points based on the degree of match as well as the length of time they have been waiting for a transplant.

Although there is no strict upper age limit for transplantation, it is relatively unusual to transplant patients over the age of 70 years because of increasing comorbidities. Whenever possible both age and size matching are important so that an adequate nephron mass is provided, but these are not features of most organ allocation algorithms.

Surgical technique

The new kidney is placed in one or other iliac fossa, usually in an extraperitoneal position that allows ease of repeated biopsy to detect cause of graft dysfunction. The renal artery is anastomosed end to side to the common iliac artery or end to end to the internal iliac artery. The renal vein is usually anastomosed to the common iliac vein. The transplant ureter only has a short distance to run before it can be implanted into the bladder, which is usually done through a submucosal tunnel to reduce the chances of reflux of urine from the bladder into the transplant. Some surgeons routinely place a vesicoureteric stent to reduce the risks of urine leakage and to promote healing. A drain is usually placed near the renal hilum. Lymphatics in the perihilar region are tied off. A urethral catheter and/or suprapubic bladder catheter is inserted and left *in situ* for about 5 days. The ureteric stent is removed at cystoscopy after a few weeks. Most units use prophylactic low-molecular-weight heparin (LMWH) routinely.

Note that in the standard renal transplant operation described above the native kidneys are left *in situ*. In some patients one or both may need to be removed (at a separate operation) before the patient can be listed for transplantation: mandatory indications for this include suspicion of renal tumour (usually in those with cystic disease), chronic renal infection, and massive organomegaly in patients with adult polycystic kidney disease, when there is literally no space in which to put a new kidney. Some would also advocate nephrectomy as a prelude to transplantation in those with gross ureteric reflux, persistent upper tract infection, renal stone disease, or analgesic nephropathy. Pretransplant nephrectomy is also recommended in patients with persistent gross nephrotic syndrome in order to correct the procoagulant state.

Retransplantation is increasingly being undertaken as the general medical care of patients with renal failure has improved.

Second transplants are now not uncommon, and even third and fourth transplants may be occasionally undertaken. Third and fourth transplants are more surgically demanding, as vessels available for anastomosis become limited. Aortic and venocaval anastomoses can be performed.

Ischaemia times

Warm ischaemia is defined as the time between circulatory arrest and renal artery cannulation for ice-cold perfusion, together with the time between the removal of the kidney from ice and release of the vascular clamps at implantation. With the beating heart donor, the first component is zero. The maximum permissible warm ischaemia time before irreversible damage occurs is 60–90 min.

Cold ischaemia time (preservation time) is defined as the time between ice-cold perfusion of the kidney and removal from the ice at the start of the implantation operation. Cold ischaemia times of up to 96 h have resulted in functioning grafts, but times in excess of 20 h are associated with a less favourable outcome. The permissible cold ischaemia time of 20 h allows for organ sharing and suitable operating times for the surgical teams.

Given the move back to the use of non-heart-beating donors, there is a trend for machine perfusion after procurement to attempt both to improve the graft and also to identify which kidneys are actually unsuitable for implantation.

Postoperative management

Excepting for transplants between HLA-identical twins, immunosuppression is required to allow transplantation. The first dose of this is often given pre- or intraoperatively. Details are discussed below.

Following implantation, the function of the new kidney is assiduously monitored. The use of dopamine and/or mannitol in the immediate postimplantation period has now virtually ceased as there is no evidence of benefit. Furosemide may be given to provoke a urine output for ease of management, but again there is no convincing evidence of benefit as far as improving glomerular filtration rate is concerned.

Hourly urinary volumes are closely monitored for the first few days. Fluid balance is usually maintained by a prescription that requires 100% replacement of urinary volumes and drain losses with crystalloid, and central venous pressure is monitored and maintained in the high normal range ($+10\,cmH_2O$) with blood or colloid.

Serum creatinine is measured daily. A failure to fall rapidly, or a 15% rise once it has fallen to a plateau, is evidence of graft dysfunction and requires prompt investigation. A kidney that fails to function initially, despite good perfusion on the table when the vascular clamps were removed, is usually suffering from acute tubular necrosis, which is expected to recover. A sudden cessation of urine flow usually means a surgical problem, e.g. clot obstruction, urinary leak, or vascular catastrophe. A slow tailing-off of the urinary volumes is more suggestive of rejection, hypovolaemia, or developing drug nephrotoxicity. Two of the major immunosuppressive agents, ciclosporin and tacrolimus, are nephrotoxic: doses have to be carefully adjusted to maintain the therapeutic range. Blood pressure should be returned to normal, obstruction excluded, and coagulation checked before any diagnostic biopsy is undertaken. Close and careful monitoring needs to continue for the first 6 months after transplantation as the risk of rejection is at its greatest during this period.

One of the 'holy grails' of transplant medicine is a method of determining the immunological relationship between the recipient and their transplanted organ, since this would allow tailoring of immunosuppression to immunological need. However, immunological monitoring of transplant recipients is still in its infancy: lymphocyte T- and B-cell subsets and activation markers can be of value, particularly when antilymphocyte preparations are being used; serial estimation of post-transplant anti-HLA antibodies can help predict patients at risk of humoral rejection. Much work continues to look for better ways of monitoring patients, such as testing for cytokine gene polymorphisms to predict those at highest risk of rejection, and examination of graft biopsies for alterations in gene expression and the expression of adhesion molecules, HLA, cytokines, and enzymes (e.g. granzyme, perforin) to better characterize the rejection process. Protocol biopsies may demonstrate subclinical rejection, and there is limited data that treatment of these may improve outcome. However, the optimum frequency and timing of protocol biopsies is yet to be determined, their benefits (if any) have to be weighed against their risks (certainly present), and they are not routine practice in most transplant centres. What is abundantly clear is that chronic damage and interstitial scarring with tubular atrophy is present within the first few months of transplantation, and that after 5 to 10 years evidence of nephrotoxic damage from the calcineurin inhibitors (CNI) is almost universal.

Complications of renal transplantation

Surgical

Table 21.7.3.1 summarizes the main surgical complications of transplantation, which include those of any general anaesthetic and laparotomy. Extra risk is added because patients on dialysis are immunosuppressed by uraemia *per se*, and transplant patients also require immunosuppressive drugs following surgery. Wound healing is significantly delayed in the early post-transplant period by steroids, and particularly by sirolimus, which for this reason is rarely used in transplantation practice until wounds have healed.

Some patients on dialysis will have a marked bleeding tendency related to defective platelet–endothelial cell interaction. The combination of uraemia, surgical stress, a bleeding tendency, and high-dose steroids produces an increased risk of bleeding peptic ulceration, which the routine use of H_2 or proton pump blockers has virtually abolished.

Many donor organs have small polar arteries that can be lost during or shortly after surgery, in which case the resulting segment of kidney will atrophy. Occasionally a polar infarct can lead to necrosis of a significant segment of renal cortex, causing a calyceal fistula and urinary leak. An area of ischaemia around a polar infarct may drive post-transplant hypertension. The ureteric artery derives from the main renal artery or its lower branch. If this is damaged at harvesting or surgery then an ischaemic necrosis of the ureter may develop, leading to an intrabdominal urinary leak all insidious scarring and late obstruction. Diagnosis is by renography (late films) or aspiration (urine has a creatinine concentration in mmol/litre, rather than μmol/litre as in serum or lymph).

Table 21.7.3.1 Complications of renal transplantation

Surgical	Medical
Wound infection (<1%)	Infections transmitted by graft
Wound haematoma	Opportunistic infections
Perirenal: (collections → infections)	Specific complications of immunosuppression
Lymph (1–5%)	Complex aetiologies:
Haematoma	Accelerated vascular disease
Urine	Hypertension
Vascular catastrophe: (arterial or venous)	Electrolyte disturbances
Haemorrhage	Cosmetic
Thrombosis (1% arterial/1–6% venous)	Thromboembolism
Segmental artery occlusions:	Erythrocytosis
Ischaemia → hypertension (2%)	Marrow suppression
Infarction → calyceal fistula	Liver dysfunction
Devitalization of ureter: (stripping)	Neoplasia
Sloughing	Metabolic bone disease
Ischaemic stricture	
Urinary leaks:	
Cystotomy	
Ureteric–bladder dehiscence	
Venous thromboembolism/PE (8%)	
Pancreatitis	
Urinary sepsis	

Perirenal collections of fluid (whether from inadequately tied-off perihilar lymphatics, haemorrhage, or a urinary leak) can become infected: these are best demonstrated by ultrasound, which can guide aspiration for estimation of creatinine and electrolytes, microscopy and culture, and drainage.

On review of a patient's predialysis and dialysis career it may be apparent that the patient has a procoagulant state (e.g. systemic lupus erythematosus, numerous thrombotic episodes involving vascular access, a past history of deep venous thombosis or pulmonary embolus). Such patients should have a full procoagulant work up before transplantation, and, if appropriate, be offered post-transplant anticoagulation. It is also of note that both the CNIs have a procoagulant effect.

Rejection

Rejection can be classified into four main categories (Table 21.7.3.2): these are not mutually exclusive and there is overlap in the pathological processes.

Hyperacute rejection

In the presence of preformed cytotoxic antibodies the new graft infarcts within minutes of insertion. This can occur if transplantation is attempted across ABO incompatibilities without appropriate antibody removal/immunosuppressive therapy. It is a rare event, as the lymphocyte crossmatch usually identifies pre-existing anti-HLA antibodies. Transplantation is not undertaken in the presence of a positive lymphocyte crossmatch, but hyperacute rejection can rarely occur in the presence of non-HLA cytotoxic antibodies. There is no treatment except nephrectomy.

Table 21.7.3.2 Classification of transplant rejection

	Hyperacute	Accelerated	Acute cellular	Humoral
Timing	Minutes	1–5 days	5 days–3 months	Variable
Mediators	Preformed antibodies Complement	Sensitized cells and antibodies	Primary cell-mediated response	Antibodies Complement
Histology	Infarction Platelets Fibrinogen Polymorphs	Tubulitis Endovasculitis (acute)	Tubulitis	Obliterative chronic endovasculitis Transplant glomerulopathy Splitting at tubular basement membrane
Treatment	Nephrectomy	Serotherapy salvage? Plasma exchange	High-dose intravenous steroids	Upgrade to tacrolimus and MMF Consider plasma exchange IVIg, rituximab

NB: Cellular and humoral rejection can coexist.

Accelerated rejection

A fierce, predominantly T-cell-mediated rejection crisis may occur within the first few days of transplantation. This is thought to be due to sensitization of the recipient by a previous pregnancy, blood transfusion, or a failed transplant. Patients present clinically with fever, an acutely swollen tender graft, and a rapidly rising serum creatinine. Salvage usually requires the combination of high-dose intravenous pulse methylprednisolone (10–15 mg/kg per day infused over 30 min on 3 successive days) and an antilymphocyte antibody such as antithymocyte (ATG) or antilymphocyte globulin (ALG), with the murine monoclonal antibody OKT3 used as an alternative. It is unusual to be able to reverse fully this type of severe rejection and long-term graft survival is compromised.

Acute cellular rejection

In most centres about 10 to 20% of patients will experience an acute cellular rejection, usually occurring between days 7 to 21, but up to 3 months after transplantation. Acute cellular rejection is often clinically silent, as the inflammatory component of the rejection is masked by immunosuppression. Fluid retention, increasing hypertension, and a sharp rise in creatinine are typical. Assessment of renal perfusion (Doppler ultrasonography or renography studies) may show a dramatic reduction in graft perfusion, but these tests are not sensitive or specific enough for a confident diagnosis of rejection. Most centres routinely take kidney biopsies for all episodes of graft dysfunction once infection, toxic levels of the CNIs and mechanical factors causing obstruction have been excluded. Obtaining a histological diagnosis is very important since several processes can mimic rejection, including drug nephrotoxicity, bacterial pyelonephritis, recurrence of original disease, BK virus-induced interstitial nephritis, and post-transplant lymphoproliferative disorder (PTLD). The hallmark of acute cellular rejection is tubulitis, in which the invading lymphocytes

have penetrated the tubular epithelial cell basement membrane and directly engage tubule epithelial cells. Late acute rejection episodes usually imply inadequate immunosuppression, sometimes due to poor compliance. Treatment is very effective and usually involves a bolus of intravenous steroid therapy as described above. Long-term graft survival is severely jeopardized if the rejection episode is not completely reversed. With some of the newer, very potent induction regimes, the incidence of acute rejection episodes can be reduced to less than 5 to 10%, but whether this will translate into a higher rate of infection and neoplasia awaits further follow-up.

Humoral rejection

Humoral rejection implies an antibody mediated attack on the graft. Histologically the biopsy reveals splitting and reduplication of tubular basement membrane, an hypercellular glomerulus with double basement membranes (so-called 'transplant glomerulopathy'), and a polymorph infiltration in the peritubular capillaries and glomeruli. Blood vessels show acute endothelial damage and may sometimes appear involved in a vasculitic process. Marked staining for C4d (a complement breakdown product) in the peritubular capillaries (involving >50%) is taken as evidence of an antibody-mediated attack on the graft. In some cases the patient may also have elevated levels of anti-HLA antibodies in the circulation, sometimes donor specific, which can now be detected by sensitive techniques. About 20% of patients develop circulating anti-HLA antibodies and these patients have a threefold increased rate of graft loss. Treatment may involve IVIG, increasing tacrolimus, adding in mycophenolate mofetil, and possibly plasma exchange. Some units have used rituximab, particularly if the rejection is acute.

'Chronic rejection'

The term 'chronic rejection' has been used for many years and is so poorly defined that it is of little value. Similarly, the term 'chronic allograft nephropathy' defines a light-microscopic appearance in the graft that has so many possible causes as to be of little practical help. Neither 'chronic rejection' nor 'chronic allograft nephropathy' represents a specific entity for which specific therapy can be prescribed. What is clearly of major importance is to define the pathological process in as much detail as possible so that appropriate therapy can be chosen.

Immunosuppressive regimens

There is no clear consensus on the best immunosuppressive regimen for renal transplantation, and for commercial reasons the large multicentre trials that the community of transplant physicians and surgeons would most like to see performed are unlikely ever to be funded. The choice of agents available is summarized in Table 21.7.3.3.

Most centres worldwide use what is now called standard triple therapy, comprising a CNI (ciclosporin or tacrolimus), combined with either mycophenolate mofetil or azathioprine, and steroids. Steroids are not infrequently tailed off rapidly in the early post-transplant period. Most units are using an induction antibody directed against CD25 (the interleukin 2 (IL-2) receptor).

Agents of established efficacy for induction therapy include polyclonal antibodies such as antithymocyte globulin (ATG) or antilymphocyte globulin (ALG), and the murine monoclonal antibody

Table 21.7.3.3 Choice of immunosuppressive agents in transplantation

Calcineurin inhibitors	Ciclosporin
	Tacrolimus
Purine antagonists	Azathioprine
	Mycophenolate mofetil
Antibodies	ALG
	ATG
	OKT3: muromonab
	Anti-CD20: rituximab
	Anti-CD52: alemtuzumab
	Anti-CD25 (IL2-receptor): basiliximab, daclizumab
Miscellaneous	Prednisolone
	Sirolimus

ALG, anti-lymphocyte globulin; ATG, anti-thymocyte globulin.

OKT3. Two anti-CD25 antibodies, daclizumab and basiliximab, which bind to the nonsignalling α-chain of the IL-2 receptor, have largely replaced these older agents. Both are heavily engineered antibodies, comprising a murine antigen-binding site and human immunoglobulin. Both are very effective and have been shown to reduce acute rejection episodes by about 30%.

A number of newer immunosuppressive regimen are in development to lessen our dependence on the nephrotoxic CNIs and steroids, which are responsible for much post-transplant morbidity. The potent monoclonal antibody alemtuzumab (anti-CD52) has been used as an induction agent followed by low-dose tacrolimus with or without mycophenolate mofetil and very early steroid withdrawal (or avoidance altogether). Preliminary results are very encouraging, with a low acute rejection rate and no apparent price to pay by way of increased infection or cancer. Rituximab (directed against the CD20 antigen) may have a role as an induction agent as well as in salvage from antibody-mediated rejection.

A variety of biological agents has been tried and is in development for blockade of the costimulatory pathways involved in the initiation of the immune response, the hope being that we can reduce our dependence on the nephrotoxic CNIs and use much less steroids to avoid later side effects and complications.

Many centres are now exploring the possibility of tailoring immunosuppression to the needs of the individual recipient, but as described above we are not good at assessing immunological risk. In practice this involves giving immunosuppressants that are perceived to be more powerful to those recipients perceived at greatest risk, e.g. using tacrolimus instead of ciclosporin, mycophenolate mofetil instead of azathioprine, or adding antibody induction. This would include patients who are highly sensitized, have rejected a previous transplant, or have suffered an acute rejection episode.

The best long-term immunosuppressive therapy is equally in doubt. This is partly due to the nephrotoxicity of two of the main agents employed for the prevention of rejection: both ciclosporin and tacrolimus can produce a nodular arterioleopathy resulting in ischaemic renal damage and graft loss. It is also clear that the morbidity and mortality from long-term steroid therapy is significant,

such that many centres are now attempting steroid-free immunosuppression or withdrawing steriods by day 5 to 10. Other centres are reducing or withdrawing steroids at 3 to 6 months despite the associated risk of rejection, which has been reported to be as high as 30% if background immunosuppression is inadequate. The risks of steroid withdrawal are less if induction therapy has been used and if patients are maintained on a CNI and an antiproliferative agent.

Unfortunately, it is not possible to predict who is going to reject on withdrawal of steroids, hence one of the main aims of those developing new immunosuppressive drugs and regimens is to devise agents or protocols that allow less dependence on steroids without increased rates of rejection or other unacceptable toxicities.

Specific side effects of particular immunosuppressive agents

Steroids

Steroids are responsible for many of the complications of transplantation (Box 21.7.3.3). In recent years the dose of steroids used has been safely reduced, thanks in part to the introduction of the CNIs, but attempts to produce totally steroid-free transplantation are only successful in about two-thirds to three-quarters of cases. One of the most significant side effects of steroids is that they mask

---

Box 21.7.3.3 Side effects of steroids

- Acne
- Hypertrichosis
- Redistribution of body fat
- Obesity
- Cushingoid facies
- Insulin resistance—diabetes mellitus
- Hypertension
- Hyperlipidaemia
- Proximal myopathy
- Osteoporosis—avascular necrosis of bone
- Tendon ruptures
- Poor wound healing
- Skin atrophy/fragility/easy bruising
- Scleromalacia
- Growth inhibition: premature fusion of the epiphyses
- Erythrocytosis
- Cataracts
- Benign intracranial hypertension
- Psychosis
- Peptic ulceration
- Colonic perforation
- Pancreatitis

the inflammatory response so that symptoms develop late, which is particularly important in cases of intra-abdominal catastrophy such as a perforated hollow viscus.

Calcineurin-blocking drugs

The main drawback of both ciclosporin and tacrolimus is nephrotoxicity (Table 21.7.3.4), which adds another level of complexity to the differential diagnosis and management of both acute and chronic graft dysfunction. Most consider tacrolimus to be more potent than ciclosporin, but perhaps more toxic (diabetes mellitus and neurotoxicity). It does, however, have real cosmetic advantages over ciclosporin, perhaps mediated by lower levels of transforming growth factor β (TGFβ). New-onset diabetes after transplantation (NODAT) occurs in about 10% of patients on ciclosporin but 15% of patients on tacrolimus.

Azathioprine and mycophenolate mofetil

Both agents block purine synthesis. The main side effects of azathioprine are hepatotoxicity and bone marrow suppression (Table 21.7.3.5). Mycophenolate mofetil is more potent and more specific than azathioprine, blocking purine synthesis in lymphocytes. Its most troublesome side effects are abdominal colic and diarrhoea: about 10% of patients are so badly affected that they are unable to

Table 21.7.3.4 Side effects of calcineurin inhibitors—relative risk

Side effect	Ciclosporin	Tacrolimus
Nephrotoxicity	++	++
Hypertension/sympathetic overactivity	++	+
Hyperuricaemia	++	++
Hyperkalaemia (type IV renal tubular acidosis)	+	+
Hypomagnesaemia (urine leak)	+	+
Haemolytic uraemic syndrome	+	+
Platelet hyperaggregability	+	?±
Insulin resistance → diabetes mellitus	+	+/++
Dislipidaemia	+	±
Hepatoxicity	+	+
Breast fibroadenosis	+	−
Coarsening of facial features	+	−
Gum hypertrophy	+	−
Hypertrichosis	+	−
Distal limb pain/periostitis	+	±
Cardiotoxicity	−	+
Neurotoxicity:	+	++
Fits	+	+
Ataxia	+	+
Posterior fossa leucoencephalopathy	+	+
Paraesthesiae		+
Tremor	+	i
Neoplasia	++	+
Infection	+	+

Table 21.7.3.5 Side effects of azathioprine and mycophenolate mofetil

Side effect	Azathioprine	Mycophenolate mofetil
Hepatotoxicity	++	+
Marrow suppression:	++	±
Platelets	±	±
Red cells	±	−
Granulocytes	++	±
Megaloblastic anaemia	+	−
Gut toxicity	±	++
Pancreatitis	+	−
Hypogammaglobulinaemia	±	+
Lung fibrosis	+	±
Alopecia	+	−
Infection	+	+/++
Cancer	+	±

tolerate the drug. A higher incidence of invasive cytomegalovirus (CMV) disease has been associated with mycophenolate.

Serotherapy

A range of antibodies to lymphocytes is available for clinical use (see Table 21.7.3.3). Side effects vary with the preparation used, but it is important to remember that the consequences of augmenting immunosuppression with serological agents may last many months, even though administration is usually limited to 10 to 14 days.

Polyclonal antilymphocyte preparations can cause a marked first-dose effect in which lymphocytes are activated and secrete cytokines. High fever, rigors, and muscle and back pains are common, and hypotension may occur. With successive doses this reaction subsides. The murine anti-CD3 antibody (OKT3) is particularly prone to produce a first-dose effect that can lead to a widespread capillary leak syndrome with noncardiogenic pulmonary oedema, hypotension, and shock. It should not be given to patients who are fluid overloaded. Aseptic meningitis and encephalitis are also seen occasionally. The toxicity profile of OKT3 has led to a dramatic reduction in its use.

By contrast, the humanized and chimeric anti-CD25 (anti-IL2 receptor) antibodies that have recently been introduced do not appear to have any short-term side effects. Although rituximab may cause a first-dose effect from cytokine release it appears remarkably safe: its place in transplantation is not yet clear, but it may have a role in the prevention and treatment of antibody mediated rejection. The recent introduction of alemtuzumab has enabled patients to be maintained on very low-dose tacrolimus, and in many cases also steroid free. Late rejections may be a problem, although with this sort of regimen early acute rejection rates are of the order of 5%, but long-term outcome data is not yet available.

General side effects of immunosuppression

It is important to remember that all currently available immunosuppressive regimen are nonspecific in the sense that they suppress not only the immune response to the allograft, but also the immune response to infections and tumours. All the agents used have significant side effects and toxicities, and to a very large extent the long-term complications of renal transplantation are those of the immunosuppressive agents used. Some side effects are more related to the total burden of immunosuppression rather than to any specific single agent, e.g. infections and cancer.

Opportunistic infections

The CNIs used for immunosuppression act to inhibit the T-helper cell (CD4) and prevent the elaboration of IL-2 and other cytokines. In some respects this is akin to the effects of HIV infection and it is therefore not surprising that the renal transplant recipient may develop the same range of opportunistic infections and tumours as is seen in patients with AIDS (see Chapter 7.5.23). Clinical features are often dramatic and rapidly evolving, hence prompt and precise microbiological diagnosis is essential. This requires early recourse to invasive techniques, e.g. biopsy, node aspiration, node excision, bronchoalveolar lavage, and even lung biopsy. Neurological symptoms and signs may herald CNS infection and require urgent CT or MRI and the examination of cerebrospinal fluid whenever possible. A brain biopsy may be the only route to a specific diagnosis. Any pyrexial episode in a transplant recipient should prompt a search for infection. Blood and urine cultures should be undertaken routinely.

Figure 21.7.3.1 summarizes the timetable of infections. In the first month, before immunosuppression is fully established, renal transplant recipients may develop the same sort of infection as seen after any general anaesthetic, abdominal operation, or urological procedure. From months 1 to 6, immunosuppression is maximal and the risk of opportunistic infections greatest. Thereafter, the risk of infection declines but remains greater than the general population, particularly in the patient with a poorly functioning graft.

Viral infections

Not all virus infections prove dangerous to the immunosuppressed renal transplant recipient. Those with particularly important clinical sequelae are summarized in Table 21.7.3.6. The most important group are the DNA viruses of the herpes group: infection with these is immunomodulating in its own right and further immunosuppresses the patient, hence they are not infrequently associated with superinfections, e.g. *Pneumocystis jiroveci*, listeria, and bacterial sepsis. Several of the viruses have proven oncogenic potential and are considered later. There has been a steady and dramatic fall in deaths from infection in the post-transplant period. This is due to many factors including better use of immunosuppressive agents, effective control of CMV, and major advances in the diagnosis and treatment of some infections.

Cytomegalovirus (CMV)

CMV is the main infectious complication in solid organ transplantation (Box 21.7.3.4), with a primary infection more likely to produce serious disease than either reinfection or reactivation. Viral load and the total burden of immunosuppression are the main determinants of disease. Use of potent serological agents, for either induction or rescue, is strongly associated with CMV disease, and as would be expected the total number of treated rejection episodes is an important risk factor. Diagnosis is usually by quantitative polymerase chain reaction (PCR) for viral DNA, or by an antigen assay (pp65) on peripheral blood leucocytes. Monitoring the serological response for diagnostic purposes is obsolete as it is far too insensitive, and routine cultures are too slow. A range of effective prophylactic regimen is available: oral valaciclovir or oral valganciclovir is effective. Another equally valid approach is careful monitoring combined with pre-emptive treatment of infection, where therapy can be given before clinical disease in vulnerable individuals, when 2 or 3 weeks of oral valganciclovir is usually effective. With this expectant approach only 40 to 50% of patients develop significant

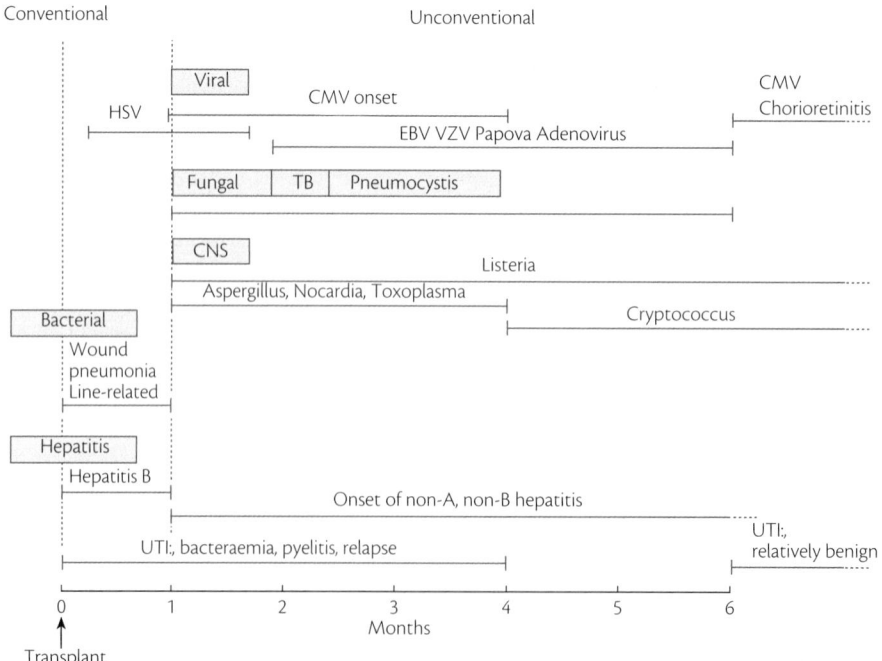

Fig. 21.7.3.1 Timetable of infections. Reproduced by permission from Rubin R.H. and Young L.S. (eds) 1994, Clinical approach to infection in the compromised host, 3rd edn. Plenum Medical Book Co., New York.

Table 21.7.3.6 Opportunistic infections in transplant recipients

Viruses	Human herpes viruses (HHV):
	Herpes simplex (HHV1, HHV2)
	Varicella zoster (HHV3)
	Epstein–Barr virus (HHV4)
	Cytomegalovirus (HHV5)
	Kaposi sarcoma virus (HHV8)
	Hepatitis viruses:
	Hepatitis B virus (HBV)
	Hepatitis C virus (HCV)
	Papovaviruses:
	Human papillomavirus (HPV)
	Polyomavirus (BK/JC)
	Human immunodeficiency virus (HIV)
Bacteria	Mycobacteria:
	Tuberculosis
	Atypicals
	Nocardia
	Listeria
	Nontyphoid salmonella
	Legionella
Fungi	Hospital acquired e.g.:
	Aspergillosis
	Community acquired e.g.:
	Candida
	Torulopsis
	Cryptococcus
	Mucormycosis
	Pneumocystis jiroveci
	Reactivation (geographically restricted) e.g.:
	Histoplasmosis
	Coccidioidomycosis
Parasites	Toxoplasmosis
	Cryptosporidium
	Geographically restricted:
	Strongyloides stercoralis
	Trypanosoma cruzi
	Malaria
	Leishmaniasis
	Schistosomiasis

viraemia and need pre-emptive therapy. Foscarnet is a more toxic (nephrotoxic) alternative that can be used in resistant CMV.

CMV may play a role in triggering or augmenting both acute and chronic rejection. If this is confirmed then more prolonged and universal prophylaxis may be indicated.

Epstein–Barr virus (EBV)

EBV-related syndromes (see Box 21.7.3.4) are an important cause of morbidity and mortality in renal transplant recipients, the most serious problem being so-called post-transplant lymphoproliferative disorder (PTLD), which is considered later.

Varicella zoster virus

Reactivation of latent varicella zoster virus (VZV) produces shingles, which is a common and unpleasant complication of transplantation. Immediate treatment with oral valaciclovir can limit spread and reduce postherpetic pain. Much more dangerous is a primary VZV infection in an immunocompromised individual: this can cause a fulminating disease with hepatitis, pneumonitis, and disseminated intravascular coagulation (DIC) occurring within a few days. Mortality is high. All patients who are to receive immunosuppression should have their VZV antibody status established. Those who are seronegative should be warned about exposure to chickenpox or shingles and should report any contact immediately. Vaccination is available, but being a live attenuated vaccine this can only be given pretransplant. If exposed, susceptible individuals should be given zoster immune globulin (ZIG) and monitored closely. High-dose intravenous aciclovir should be given at the first suggestion of disease.

Herpes simplex

Although the classic herpetic cold sore is common after transplantation, herpes simplex virus (HSV), particularly if a primary infection can produce a variety of serious clinical sequelae in the immunocompromised patient (see Box 21.7.3.4). Use of prophylactic valaciclovir or valganciclovir (primarily for CMV prophylaxis) dramatically reduces the risks of HSV infection. Treatment with valaciclovir is very effective.

Human polyomavirus (BK and JC)

Most adult recipients are already seropositive for these viruses, indicating childhood infection that is usually asymptomatic. Primary infection can occur from the allograft, and in most cases this is also asymptomatic. BK virus reactivation occurs in 20%, with urinary excretion of so-called decoy cells. Nephropathy occurs in 20% of patients excreting virus, with about one-half of the patients who develop BK nephropathy losing their graft despite reduction in immunosuppression, which is the main treatment strategy. The JC virus has been reported to cause a progressive multifocal leucoencephalopathy in renal transplant recipients, but this is very rare.

Human papillomaviruses (HPV)

HPV can cause an extensive range of viral warts in renal transplant recipients. Some types have been implicated in the pathogenesis of anogenital carcinomas and squamous cell carcinomas of the skin (see below). The management of viral warts in the immunocompromised patient is difficult when they are very extensive and consideration should be given to reducing immunosuppression. Localized lesions can be treated conventionally with topical agents such as glutaraldehyde or laser therapy, but widespread surgical excision is sometimes required. Local recurrence in scar tissue is common. A combination of oral isotretinoin (50 mg daily) and topical tretinoin cream (0.05%) can control the lesions in severe cases. Topical imiquimod can be useful, and cidofovir ointment is of value in anogenital disease.

HIV

Before the advent of highly active retroviral therapy (HAART), infection with HIV was considered an absolute contraindication to transplantation because the time to AIDS and death was very

---

Box 21.7.3.4 Clinical features of post-transplant viral infections

Cytomegalovirus (CMV)

- Asymptomatic
- CMV syndrome:
  - Fever
  - Wasting
  - Malaise
- Leucopenia
- Transaminitis
- Hepatitis
- Pseudolymphoma
- Retinitis
- Pneumonitis
- Colitis
- Gastroduodenitis
- Pancreatitis
- Myocarditis
- Superinfection, e.g. *Pneumocystis jeiruveci* pneumonia

Epstein–Barr virus (EBV)

- Asymptomatic
- Classic glandular fever
- Hairy leucoplakia
- Hepatitis
- Post-transplant lymphoproliferative disorder

Herpes simplex virus (HSV)

- Stomatitis
- Oesophagitis

- Anogenital ulcers
- Corneal ulcers
- Kaposi's varicelliform eruption
- Haemhorrhagic skin blisters
- Paronychia
- Pneumonitis
- Hepatitis
- Pancreatitis
- Meningoencephalitis

Varicella zoster virus (VZV)

- Reactivation:
  - Shingles
- Primary infection:
  - Pneumonitis
  - Hepatitis
  - Encephalitis
  - Pancreatitis
- Disseminated intravascular coagulation

Human papilloma virus (HPV)

- Cutaneous warts
- Condyloma acuminatum
- Bowen's disease
- Squamous cell carcinoma
- Anogenital carcinoma (e.g. cervical invasive neoplasia, vulvovaginal invasive neoplasia)

---

significantly shortened, particularly if HIV was acquired at or shortly after transplantation. However, intensive antiretroviral therapy for HIV infection has allowed safe transplantation, but, somewhat counterintuitively, HIV-positive patients have a higher incidence of rejection than might otherwise have been anticipated. It is important to remember that HIV infection, or behaviour considered to be at risk of contracting HIV or other viruses (lifestyle assessment), excludes such individuals from organ donation.

Bacterial infections

There are a limited number of bacterial infections that are significantly more common and more severe in the transplant population (see Table 21.7.3.6). However, there is little doubt that bacteraemias are more common in transplant recipients, usually as a result of urinary tract infections, and metastatic abscesses in joints, skin, muscles and the brain are also more frequent.

Mycobacterial infections

Reactivation of mycobacterial infection following transplantation is very common in the 'at risk' population, and most United Kingdom

units recommend prophylaxis with isoniazid (with pyridoxine to prevent neuropathy) in these groups, although some debate the need for this. Isioniazid should not be given to patients with underlying liver disease.

Experience in the Indian subcontinent suggests that pretransplant bacillus Calmette–Guérin (BCG) vaccination is not effective. Mycobacterial infections (both atypical and tuberculous) can present in many different guises, e.g. pneumonia, lymphadenopathy, intracranial space-occupying lesions, discharging sinus, pyrexia of unknown origin, and skin ulcers. Tissue biopsy, cultures, and smears employing special stains are essential. PCR, particularly of cerebrospinal fluid, is proving helpful. Gallium scanning may identify nodes that can be aspirated under CT guidance. Skin testing is unreliable in the immunocompromised patient.

Treatment is compromised by serious drug interactions between rifampicin and both the CNIs, prednisolone and sirolimus. Rifampicin is such a potent inducer of cytochrome P450 that subtherapeutic levels of the CNIs and steroids can develop within weeks. Graft loss from rejection will occur unless doses are increased: that of prednisolone is usually doubled, and the calcineurin blockers may have to be increased still further and given three times daily. Monitoring of drug levels is essential.

In many units a four-drug antituberculous regimen is recommended, comprising rifampicin, ethambutol, isoniazid, and pyrazinamide. This can be reduced when sensitivities become available. Treatment should be continued for at least a year, particularly in the case of atypical mycobacterial infections. Therapy may be further complicated by hepatotoxicity, for which the differential diagnosis is complex as many other factors can cause deranged liver function tests in renal transplant recipients (e.g. viral infections—HBV, HCV, CMV—and other drugs).

Nocardia

Nocardia typically produces either a pseudotuberculosis or a pseudostaphylococcal syndrome. CNS infections can occur. Dissemination is common, occurring in 25 to 30%. Diagnosis often requires a biopsy or aspiration, with cultures needing to be prolonged for at least 3 weeks. Prolonged treatment (at least 6 months) with co-trimoxazole is usually effective, following which long-term co-trimoxazole should continue indefinitely.

Nontyphoid salmonella

Nontyphoid salmonella infections are noteworthy because of their tendency to produce metastatic abscesses following bacteraemia. With control of the acute illness, the continued excretion of the organism may occur in stool or urine. Relapse is common, hence treatment needs to be prolonged. Suitable antimicrobials include ciprofloxacin, co-trimoxazole, and ampicillin.

Listeria

Listeria has a tendency to localize in the CNS following a bacteraemic phase. Neurological syndromes vary from meningitis and meningoencephalitis to space-occupying lesions, and listeria is the commonest cause of post-transplant meningitis. In the absence of evidence of raised intracranial pressure, all patients will require lumbar puncture and examination of cerebrospinal fluid. Delayed or inadequate treatment may result in permanent neurological deficit. Treatment usually includes high-dose ampicillin for at least 6 weeks, combined with gentamicin for the first week. The source of listeria is usually contaminated dairy products, chicken, or uncooked vegetables contaminated by manure.

Fungal infections

Oral candidiasis is a common post-transplant infection. Spread to the oropharynx and lungs may occur. All patients should receive prophylaxis (nystatin mouthwashes or amphotericin lozenges) for at least 6 weeks, but some practitioners would recommend longer courses, or even indefinite treatment in patients with diabetes. Intercurrent courses of antibiotics may need to be covered with oral prophylaxis against candida.

The spectrum of diseases produced by fungal infections is wide, ranging from mucocutaneous syndromes, severe pneumonias, and CNS syndromes, to skin or muscle abscesses. This variation in clinical presentation again highlights the need for aggressive invasive investigation. Outbreaks of aspergillus are usually related to hospital building projects and should prompt a search for the source. Deep-seated fungal infections carry a very high mortality. Dissemination is common. Specialist microbiological advice is usually required, but if the fungus is sensitive, then liposomal amphotericin is the drug of choice. The newer antifungals, e.g.

posaconazole, voriconazole, and caspofungin, have made a valuable contribution to the therapy of deep tissue or disseminated fungal infection in addition to amphotericin-B.

Pneumocystis jirovecii

Until the widespread introduction of prophylactic low-dose co-trimoxazole, *Pneumocystis jirovecii* pneumonia was a dreaded complication of solid organ transplantation. Oral co-trimoxazole or inhaled pentamidine (300 mg monthly) is effective prophylaxis. *Pneumocystis jirovecii* pneumonia is now most commonly seen in the setting of augmented immunosuppression (additional serotherapy) and in patients who already have developed CMV disease. Presentation is with fever, dry cough, and profound shortness of breath, occurring in the context of few added sounds in the chest and a remarkably clear chest radiograph. By the time the chest radiograph has altered, pulmonary fibrosis is occurring. Successful treatment demands on early diagnosis, such that the renal transplant recipient who complains of shortness of breath on exercise and who desaturates on exercise should be admitted and investigated as a medical emergency. Bronchoalveolar lavage is virtually mandatory under these circumstances.

Overall immunosuppression should be reduced in patients with *Pneumocystis jiroveci* pneumonia, but steroids may need to be increased to cover a stress response (e.g. prednisolone at 20–25 mg daily) and to limit pulmonary fibrosis. High-dose intravenous co-trimoxazole is given: 15 to 20 mg of trimethoprim and 75 to 100 mg of sulphamethoxazole per kg body weight per day, although these doses may need to be reduced in severe renal failure. Treatment should be continued for at least 2 weeks. It is essential to monitor respiratory effort carefully in the renal transplant recipient with an interstitial pneumonitis and intervene with continuous positive airways pressure or full ventilation if the patient tires or cannot protect his airways. Nutrition should be ensured, using total parenteral nutrition if necessary.

Parasitic infections

Some of the parasitic infections listed in Table 21.7.3.6 are geographically restricted and therefore only of specific relevance in those areas. Schistosomiasis, for example, can cause ureteric strictures and leaks following transplantation.

Strongyloides stercoralis

This is usually found in patients from the West Indies or East Asia: in the immunocompromised it can reactivate, complete its life cycle in the patient without need for an intermediate host, and produce a hyperinfestation syndrome. A pretransplant eosinophilia is sometimes present. Clinical presentation is with recurrent bouts of Gram-negative septicaemia as the worm penetrates the gut mucosa. Other clinical features include pruritus ani, haemorrhagic enteritis, larva currens, cough, wheeze, and a haemorrhaging bronchopneumonia. Meningitis may also occur. Diagnosis usually requires a duodenal aspirate. Treatment is with thiabendazole, which should be given pretransplant to patients at risk. Several courses of treatment may be needed to eradicate the infestation.

Scabies

This may occur in transplant recipients and can produce so-called 'Norwegian scabies' in which there may be many parasitic mites per burrow. In the immunocompromised patient, skin organisms are readily carried into the bloodstream, hence cellulitis and septicaemia are common.

Toxoplasma gondii

The transplant organ, particularly the heart, can transmit toxoplasmosis. The organism becomes widely disseminated, including into the CNS. Other clinical features may include low-grade fever, lymphadenopathy, pneumonia, myocarditis, retinopathy, and myositis, producing a picture that can mimic cytomegalovirus. Treatment is with pyrimethamine and sulphadiazine for at least 4 weeks. Prophylaxis with co-trimoxazole has greatly reduced the incidence of toxoplasmosis following solid organ transplantation.

Specific infective problems

Pulmonary disease

Recurrent chest infections are common. Many are viral and will be self-limiting, even in the immunosuppressed transplant recipient. An abrupt clinical onset with fever and a lobar pattern of lung infiltrates is likely to be due to a bacterial infection. A more insidious onset with scattered or diffuse pulmonary infiltrates is more likely to be due to an opportunistic infection. Blood and sputum should be cultured urgently. Sputum samples need careful microscopy, and cultures should be set up for mycobacteria, fungi, and legionella. PCR is available for *Mycobacterium tuberculosis*, *Pneumocystis jirovecii*, CMV, and most respiratory viruses. Antibiotics may be started pending culture results. A regimen that will cover most of the common organisms is penicillin V, clarithromycin (NB: drug interactions), and a third-generation cephalosporin.

Failure to respond promptly to therapy or a nonlobar pattern of infiltration is an indication for bronchoscopy and bronchoalveolar lavage, the diagnostic accuracy of which is about 80 to 90%. It is essential to examine the fluid thoroughly, which will involve viral and bacterial cultures, special stains, and PCR where available. In clinical practice it is often necessary to start therapy blindly in seriously ill patients. Sometimes this will involve the addition of high-dose co-trimoxazole and valganciclovir to conventional antibiotics. When the results of culture and sensitivity testing become available it may be possible to reduce the antimicrobial regimen or change to specific antituberculous or antifungal therapy.

The greatest mimic of a chest infection is pulmonary oedema: measurement of an elevated pulmonary capillary wedge pressure is diagnostic, and a therapeutic test of a potent diuretic sometimes produces a dramatic clearing of the chest radiograph. Other noninfectious causes of acute pulmonary syndromes that may occur in the renal transplant recipient are shown in Box 21.7.3.5.

Urinary tract infection

One-third of renal transplant recipients will develop urinary tract infection. In most this is related to postoperative bladder catheterization and usually resolves with removal of the catheter and a short course of antibiotics. There is an exponential relationship between the incidence of urinary tract infections and the duration of bladder catheterization. Some patients develop numerous recurrent infections, particularly in the first couple of years following transplantation. In some this can be related to a focus of infection in the native kidneys, when bilateral native nephroureterectomy may be indicated if sepsis is severe. A few patients will develop encrustation or even a stone in the bladder as a result of the surgical implantation of the ureter: a plain abdominal radiograph may reveal such calculi, which should be removed cystoscopically.

Box 21.7.3.5 Noninfective differential diagnoses of acute pulmonary syndromes in transplant recipients

- Pneumothorax
  - Central venous lines
- Pulmonary embolus
- Noncardiogenic pulmonary oedema:
  - Cytokine release syndrome
- Left ventricular failure:
  - Fluid overload
  - Tacrolimus cardiotoxicity
  - Unrecognized ischaemic heart disease
  - Acute arrhythmias—hypokalaemia, hypomagnesaemia
  - Uncontrolled hypertension
- Pulmonary fibrosis:
  - Mycophenolate mofetil (rare)
  - Azathioprine (rare)
  - Co-trimoxazole
- Interstitial pneumonitis:
  - Sirolimus
- Bronchospasm:
  - Allergic reactions—antilymphocyte serum
  - X-ray contrast media
- Pulmonary vasculitis:
  - Recurrence of original disease
- Pulmonary aspiration:
  - Diabetic coma
  - Fits
- Impaired ventilation:
  - Neuromuscular blockade
- Pulmonary infiltration:
  - Post-transplant lymphoproliferative disorder
  - Kaposi's sarcoma

More worrying is infection ascending into the transplant kidney itself during the intermediate period of post-transplantation immunosuppression when the patient is most immunocompromised. A severe bacterial pyelonephritis can develop in the transplant, presenting as would an acute rejection episode with a swollen kidney, low-grade fever, and deteriorating graft function. Such upper tract infections are frequently complicated by septicaemia, and it is always worth remembering that urinary sepsis is the commonest cause of post-transplant bacteraemia. It is essential that episodes of graft dysfunction due to upper tract infection are clearly diagnosed and aggressively treated with appropriate high-dose parental antibiotics. Misdiagnosis resulting in treatment with high-dose intravenous steroids for a presumed rejection episode can be catastrophic.

The advent of SPECT isotope scanning—single photon emission CT using dimercaptosuccinic acid (DMSA) labelled with technetium-99m—has enabled three-dimensional reconstructions of the grafted kidney to be produced. Progressive scarring can develop in some patients with recurrent infections and reflux to the graft, hence transplant recipients with recurrent urinary tract infections need full investigation and aggressive treatment. Every effort should be made to establish and maintain sterile urine. Long-term prophylactic low-dose antibiotics may be indicated.

Neurological syndromes

The main concerns are those of post-transplant lymphoproliferative disorder or an opportunistic infection producing progressive neurological deterioration due to an increasing space-occupying lesion. Examples of neurological syndromes seen in the renal transplant recipient and their common causes are given in Table 21.7.3.7. The range of infectious microorganisms that can cause CNS lesions is such that a diagnostic aspirate is usually essential. Tuberculosis is common in at-risk patients. Investigation should include CT with contrast or MRI, so that abscesses are not missed. In the absence of evidence of a raised intracranial pressure, cerebrospinal fluid should be examined. As with the processing of bronchoalveolar lavage fluid, close cooperation between clinician and the cytological and microbiological laboratories is essential.

Fits may occur in the early post-transplant period, when the cause is usually multifactorial, including hyponatraemia, hypertension, hypomagnesaemia, hypocalcaemia, and the toxic effects of CNIs. The rejection process itself can cause a rise in intracranial pressure, so-called rejection encephalopathy. Fits occurring after the first month should prompt a search for a serious intracranial space-occupying lesion.

Hepatological syndromes

Renal transplantation in the presence of liver dysfunction
The two main liver conditions encountered in patients on transplant waiting lists that give concern in the post-transplant period are HBV and HCV.

HBV usually causes persistent infection in patients with chronic renal failure. In many this may be subclinical, but in others a chronic hepatitis and cirrhosis can develop. Serology is of little help in assessing suitability for transplantation, which is contraindicated in the presence of cirrhosis and biopsy evidence of active hepatic inflammation since immunosuppression causes rapid viral replication and progressive liver disease. Death within 5 years of transplantation may occur in up to 50% of patients if wrongly transplanted, usually from extrahepatic sepsis. Long-term therapy with the newer antiviral agents before and after surgery has greatly improved the outlook and allows access to transplantation to those previously denied it.

Although HCV is now the most common cause of both pre- and post-transplant liver disease, the effects of immunosuppression on HCV seem much less dramatic than the effects on HBV. Occasional patients develop a fulminating hepatitis after transplantation, but overall HCV does not appear to have a major impact on the short- to medium-term outcome after renal transplantation. Nevertheless in the presence of detectable HCV RNA and active hepatitis every effort should be made to clear the virus before transplantation.

Table 21.7.3.7 Causes of neurological syndromes in transplant recipients

Syndrome	Causes
Psychosis	Steroids
Space-occupying lesions (focal)	Bacteria: Mycobacteria, Listeria, Nocardia; Fungi: Aspergillosis, Mucormycosis; Parasitic: Toxoplasmosis, Strongyloides; Other: PTLD
Meningitis: acute/subacute	Listeria
Meningitis: subacute/chronic	Mycobacteria, Cryptococcus, Coccidiodomycosis
Meningoencephalitis	Cryptococcus, OKT3
Encephalitis/multifocal	Herpes simplex and varicella zoster viruses, Toxoplasmosis
Progressive dementia	Primary measles, JC polyomavirus
Fits	Hypertension, Hyponatraemia, Calcineurin-inhibitors, Hypomagnesaemia, Acute rejection, Space-occupying lesions
Tremor/ataxia	Calcineurin-inhibitors
Peripheral neuropoathy	Diabetes mellitus, Pre-existing uraemic neuropathy
Myopathy	Steroids, Statins or fibrates

PTLD, post-transplant lymphoproliferative disorder.

Post-transplant liver dysfunction
Abnormal liver function tests following transplantation are common: both drugs and infectious agents may be responsible. Full investigation is required, including imaging of the liver, bile ducts, and gallbladder, as well as a liver biopsy. In some instances transient elevation of liver transaminases may herald CMV disease. In other situations raised liver enzymes can represent progressive HCV-or HBV- induced liver disease. It is important to remember that the donor organ can transmit most of the hepatotropic viruses. Treatment clearly depends on the cause. Where possible the offending drug (for instance azathioprine) should be withdrawn, and antiviral therapy may be appropriate in the case of viral hepatitis. Interferon therapy is contraindicated as it induces expression of

HLA antigens and may provoke acute rejection. In the case of HBV it is often possible to reduce the dosage of immunosuppressive agents significantly without precipitating a rejection episode.

Neoplasia

Post-transplant neoplasia is an important cause of morbidity and mortality. There is some debate as to whether some of the conditions often regarded as neoplastic can truly be classed as cancers, since several are clearly viral related and will regress with reduction of immunosuppression. Box 21.7.3.6 summarizes the tumours seen with increased frequency after transplantation. There is a marked geographical variation: for instance in Japan, renal, thyroid, and uterine cancers as well as lymphoma are common; in Saudi Arabia, Kaposi's sarcoma is the most common; in Australia squamous cell carcinoma of the skin is almost ubiquitous 20 years after transplantation (75%). It is also important to remember that the donor organ can transmit cancer.

Post-transplant lymphoproliferative disorder (PTLD)

PTLD is driven by EBV (HHV4) present in a latent form (episomal or circular DNA) in B lymphocytes. In nonimmunosuppressed individuals a normal T-cytotoxic lymphocyte response terminates infected proliferating B cells. In the presence of effective immunosuppression this does not happen and an unrestricted, increasingly monoclonal B-cell proliferation develops. The more potent the immunosuppressive regimen, the earlier PTLD occurs. In most centres, the incidence of this disorder is about 1–2%. The clinical features are summarized in Box 21.7.3.6. In common with many other infections following transplantation, a primary infection (i.e.

Box 21.7.3.6 Post-transplant neoplasia

- Post-transplant lymphoproliferative disorder (EBV driven)
  - Lymphadenopathy (33%)
  - Central nervous system (15–20%)
  - Graft infiltration
  - Gut (25%)
  - Skin masses (1%)
  - Scar infiltration (1%)
  - Pulmonary nodules/infiltrates
  - Widely disseminated (1–3%)
- Kaposi's sarcoma (HHV8 driven)
  - Local (60%)—skin-infiltrating nodules
  - Disseminated (40%)—lymphadenopathy, upper or lower gastrointestinal tract, lungs or pleura, bladder, oropharynx
- Anogenital carcinoma (HPV driven)
  - Cervical invasive neoplasia
  - Anal carcinoma
  - Vulvovaginal invasive neoplasia
- Squamous cell carcinoma of the skin (HPV driven)
- MALT lymphoma (*Helicobacter pylori* driven)

---

the recipient is naive or seronegative for EBV antibodies, while the donor is seropositive) leads more frequently to disease.

Diagnosis relies on tissue biopsy with expert processing of the tissue. PET scanning is the preferred imaging technique. Early diagnosis is important as the stepwise reduction of immunsuppression with careful monitoring of graft function can lead to regression of the tumour without graft rejection in over 50% of cases. It remains to be proven, but seems very likely, that carefully monitored stepwise reduction of immunosuppression may also be appropriate for other virally induced neoplasms in renal transplant recipients, for example Kaposi's sarcoma and squamous cell carcinoma. If PTLD does not regress with immunosuppression dose reduction, then rituximab may be given if the original tumour expresses CD20. Response occurs in over 50% of cases.

Conventional cytotoxic therapy should be introduced if PTLD progresses despite the withdrawal of immunosuppression, or the tumour is immediately life threatening. Chemotherapy (e.g. CHOP) is usually combined with rituximab, but this further suppresses the patient's immune system and death from overwhelming infection is all too common. Although exogenous EBV-specific cytotoxic T cells are effective, these are not widely available.

A few patients who have lost their grafts in the context of PTLD have been successfully retransplanted.

Kaposi's sarcoma

Kaposi's sarcoma is a vascular tumour composed of proliferating spindle cells (latently infected lymphatic endothelial cells) and thin-walled neovascular formations that is driven by the Kaposi's sarcoma virus (KSV), now redesignated HHV8. The incidence is less than 0.25% in Western countries, but in some areas, e.g. Saudi Arabia, the incidence is greatly increased. Aetiological factors are very similar to those of PTLD. Lesions may develop at almost any site on the skin, and visceral involvement is common. Prompt diagnosis and early reduction of immunosuppression may result in regression.

Sirolimus is an alternative immunosuppressant to the CNIs which blocks vascular endothelial growth factor (VEGF) and VEGF signalling, as well as arresting the cell cycle. These actions have an important anticancer effect and have been shown to result in the regression of cutaneous and visceral Kaposi's sarcoma in the transplant population. Not all respond, and recourse to chemotherapy (pegylated liposomal doxorubicin) may be required. As with PTLD, 'rejection' of the tumour may occur with rejection of the allograft. Retransplantation of a patient with proven Kaposi's sarcoma has usually resulted in recurrence. It is not yet known if sirolimus will allow safe retransplantation.

HPV-related carcinoma

HPV is responsible for skin, vulval, and anogenital warts, and some types are now clearly associated with carcinoma. Renal transplant recipients should therefore receive full dermatological and gynaecological examinations at regular intervals.

Aetiological factors for skin cancer include exposure to ultraviolet light (which may act by depletion of cutaneous Langerhans' cells as well as direct DNA damage), duration and intensity of immunosuppression, and the virus itself. The prevalence increases progressively with time, such that after 20 years most white renal transplant recipients will have cutaneous squamous cell carcinoma. Management should involve cautious dose-reduction of immunosuppressive agents. There is great interest in the role of combined oral and topical retinoids, which are associated with repopulation of the skin with Langerhans' cells and augmentation of natural killer cell activity, and may also act by blocking IL-6 pathways. Some cases of squamous cell carcinoma can metastasize, when reduction of immunosuppression dose, interferon-α therapy, and a willingness to abandon the graft should be considered before recourse to systemic cytotoxic chemotherapy. Sirolimus may also be of value after the development of squamous cell cancer. Pretransplant HPV vaccination is being explored.

Other post-transplant complications

Hypertension

The aetiology of post-transplant hypertension is complex (Table 21.7.3.8). Over 75% of renal transplant recipients will need drug therapy for hypertension in addition to lifestyle modification, and hypertension plays a crucial role in accelerating vascular disease and chronic allograft nephropathy (CAN). Most units aim for a systolic blood pressure of less than 145 mmHg and a diastolic pressure of less than 85 mmHg, but there is a lack of clear data regarding the ideal blood pressure. Tighter targets (125–130/70–75) are being recommended for patients with proteinuria.

Care should be taken with the choice of antihypertensive agents. On theoretical grounds, angiotensin converting enzyme (ACE) inhibitors or angiotensin I (AT-I) receptor antagonists appear a rational first choice in view of the multiple proinflammatory, profibrotic, and proproliferative actions of angiotensin II. There are overwhelming data showing reduction of proteinuria and a slowing of progression of renal disease in native kidneys treated with ACE inhibitors and by AT-I receptor-blocking drugs. However, the risks of using ACE inhibitors in patients with renal artery stenosis should not be forgotten, with transplant renal artery stenosis being most likely to develop between 3 and 12 months after transplantation, sometimes (but not always) associated with a bruit over the kidney. Serum creatinine must be carefully monitored, any substantial rise after ACE inhibition leading to withdrawal of the drug and consideration of angiography of the transplant renal artery.

It is preferable to avoid drugs that exacerbate dyslipidaemia, such as β-blockers and thaizides. Poor blood pressure control with short-acting dihydropyridine calcium-channel blockers may increase proteinuria and cardiovascular mortality. In refractory cases, or those where treatment is problematic, estimation of renin levels in the veins draining the native and transplant kidneys may help in the decision to proceed to a native kidney nephrectomy.

Accelerated atherosclerosis

In common with patients on dialysis, the major cause of death following renal transplantation is cardiovascular disease. Indeed, death with a functioning graft is now the major cause of late graft failure. Much of the cardiovascular disease that shortens life expectancy in renal transplant recipients will have developed and be established pretransplantation. Table 21.7.3.8 summarizes the pre- and post-transplant aetiological factors. Prevention and treatment of established vascular disease is essential. About one-third of renal transplant recipients will have hypercholesterolaemia and many will also be hypertensive. Lifestyle modification is important. All renal transplant recipients should be strongly advised not to smoke.

Table 21.7.3.8 Aetiological factors for accelerated atherosclerosis in transplant recipients

Factor	Cause
Hypertension	Insulin resistance (sympathetic overactivity)
	Drugs:
	CNIs
	Steroids
	Native kidneys
	Transplant kidneys (ischaemia, rejection)
Hyperlipidaemia	Dialysis and chronic renal failure
	Proteinuria
	Insulin resistance
	CNIs
	Steroids
	β-Blockers
	Thiazides
Proteinuria	Glomerular disease in native/transplant kidneys
Endothelial cell activation	Oxidized low-density lipoproteins
	Calcineurin-inhibitors
	Hypertension
	Smoking
Oxidized lipids	CNIs
	Proteinuria
Hyperhomocysteinaemia	Renal failure *per se*
	B$_{12}$ and folate deficiency
Platelet hyperaggregability	Nephrotic syndrome
	Calcineurin-inhibitors
Hyperfibrinogenaemia	Nephrotic syndrome
	Acute-phase response
Insulin resistance	Steroids, obesity
	Calcineurin-inhibitors
	Chronic renal failure per se
Diabetes mellitus	Primary renal disease
	Acquired post-transplant (e.g. steroids and CNIs)
Lifestyle	Smoking
	Excessive alcohol
	Diet
	Obesity
Inflammation	Original nephritis
	Haemodialysis *per se*
	Infection and rejection

CNI, calcineurin inhibitor.

Following transplantation, some 10% of transplant recipients become quite grossly obese. It is important to remember that the cardiovascular risk factors multiply rather than summate, hence the long-term management of renal transplant recipients has to address all cardiovascular risk factors. Treatment recommendations are by extrapolation from studies in the general population as there is little in the transplant literature to guide the physician.

Electrolyte disorders

Hypophosphataemia

In the presence of inadequately controlled secondary hyperparathyroidism a well-functioning transplant will waste phosphate, and in a few cases phosphaturia persists despite resolution of the secondary hyperparathyroidism. In some patients there is steroid-related malabsorption of phosphate. In the first few months after renal transplantation, phosphate wasting can be severe and oral supplements will be required. Untreated chronic hypophosphataemia can lead to bone fractures (hypophosphataemic rickets).

Hyperkalaemia

The CNIs cause hyperkalaemia, particularly when levels are toxic. This is thought to be due to type IV renal tubular acidosis in which distal tubular potassium secretion is reduced in response to a fall in renin secretion due to reduced renal prostaglandins. The addition of ACE inhibitors, AT-I receptor-blocking drugs, NSAIDs, or potassium-conserving diuretics can produce a brisk rise in serum potassium in renal transplant recipients. Dietary advice and loop diuretics are usually sufficient, but a few patients may require fludrocortisone (100–200 µg daily.)

Hypomagnesaemia

Renal tubular magnesium wasting is a component of the nephrotoxicity of the CNIs and can be exacerbated by diuretics and diarrhoea. Hypomagnesaemia may predispose to fits and cardiac arrhythmias in susceptible individuals. Levels should be monitored and oral supplements of magnesium glycerophosphate given if required.

Hypercalcaemia

Hypercalcaemia can develop after grafting if renal osteodystrophy has been poorly controlled and severe secondary hyperparathyroidism is present at the time of transplantation. The transplant kidney produces adequate amounts of 1,25-dihydroxycholecalciferol, which in the presence of high levels of parathyroid hormone will result in hypercalcaemia. Widespread metastatic deposition of calcium can occur if hypercalcaemia is severe.

Simple controlling measures include adequate fluids, sodium supplements, and the use of loop diuretics rather than thiazides. Occasional patients will require regular infusions of pamidronate (15–30 mg), which can be combined with intermittent doses of oral alphacalcidol (or other active vitamin D sterol) to suppress parathyroid hyperplasia. Cinacalcet is an alternative, but hyperparathyroidism tends to recur quickly once treatment has stopped. Parathyroidectomy is occasionally required. It may take 12 to 24 months for secondary hyperparathyroidism to resolve following renal transplantation, but it does not always do so.

Bicarbonate wasting

The transplant kidney may waste bicarbonate as well as phosphate. This may be due to persistent hyperparathyroidism, but can also reflect acute tubule damage from rejection. A chronic metabolic acidosis will contribute to post-transplant osteoporosis and should be treated with bicarbonate supplements.

Hyponatraemia

Hyponatraemia may develop, particularly in the early postoperative period. It is usually due to inappropriate intravenous fluids (excess 5% dextrose or dextrose saline) in the context of deteriorating graft function, and may be an important contributing factor to fits after transplantation.

Musculoskeletal

Tendon rupture

Steroids impair collagen synthesis. Tendons and tendon insertions are weakened and avulsions may occur, most commonly in the fingers or Achilles tendon.

Myopathy

An important complication of steroid therapy is proximal myopathy, which can be incapacitating in some patients. Physiotherapy plus vitamin D supplements and a rapid reduction of steroids (alternate-day prescription or even cessation) can produce improvement. Hypophosphataemia should be corrected. Acute rhabdomyolysis may develop if fibrates or statins are used with the CNIs. Care should be taken with colchicine and CNIs.

Avascular necrosis of bone

Avascular necrosis of bone, particularly of the weight-bearing ends of the long bones, causes an extremely painful joint. MRI is diagnostic. When the hips are involved, walking can become impossible and total hip replacement is the only treatment. Prevention may be possible by the careful control of secondary hyperparathyroidism before transplantation, and the early use of bisphosphonates to minimize post-transplant osteoporosis may be beneficial. The condition is now much less common (0.5%) with the reduction in the use of steroids.

Osteoporosis

Osteoporosis is a common and progressive complication of long-term steroid therapy, such that regular bone-density assessment should be part of long-term renal transplant follow-up. Fracture rates of 3 to 4% per year are common. The problem is particularly severe in postmenopausal women, in whom hormone replacement therapy is of benefit. Prophylaxis with intravenous pamidronate has been advocated in the first few months after transplantation, as this is the time when the greatest loss of bone mass occurs.

Renal osteodystrophy

Over half of patients with a functioning graft have persistent hyperparathyroidism. In the presence of a poorly functioning graft, control of parathyroid hormone (PTH) and the calcium × phosphate product (ideally to be kept at <5) is as important as it is in the pre-transplant patient with chronic renal failure (see Chapter 21.6). PTH levels should be kept at one to two times the upper limit of normal by the careful use of alphacalcidol (or other active vitamin D sterols) and calcium supplements. Serum phosphate should be kept at 1 to 1.5 mmol/litre using calcium carbonate as an oral phosphate binder, taking care to avoid hypercalcaemia. Uncontrolled post transplant hypercalcaemia has the potential to significantly damage graft function, should be avoided if possible, and treated promptly if it occurs.

Gout

The CNIs impair urate secretion in the proximal tubule, and urate retention is exacerbated by the concomitant use of diuretics, particularly in patients with poorly functioning grafts. Uric acid levels may rise dramatically and be associated with attacks of clinical gout as well as tophi. Management is complicated, both for acute attacks and for prophylaxis. For acute episodes the physician must choose between three treatments, all of which are problematic. NSAIDs are the usual first-line treatment for acute episodes in general medical practice, but in those with renal impairment—including many transplant recipients—they are best avoided, although COX-2 inhibitors may prove safer. Colchicine can be used for acute attacks, but the transplant recipient tolerates diarrhoea and the attendant hypovolaemia poorly. There is a risk of rhabdomyolysis with a combination of colchicine and CNI's. Oral prednisolone (20 mg daily) can be effective, but will clearly exacerbate steroid side effects, which are already a problem in many patients.

As regards prophylaxis, allopurinol is (relatively) contraindicated if the patient is receiving azathioprine (the dose of azathioprine should be reduced to about 25% of normal, with very careful monitoring for leucopenia). Most uricosuric agents work poorly in the presence of renal impairment. In some patients it may be helpful to stop azathioprine altogether and use mycophenolate mofetil in its place so that allopurinol can be used more safely.

Haematological

Venous thromboembolism is not uncommon following renal transplantation, with deep venous thrombosis/pulmonary embolus occurring in about 8% of patients. The local effects of surgery on the pelvic veins together with immediate postoperative bed rest contribute to the risk. The CNIs have an activating and procoagulant effect on endothelial cells and platelets. Nephrotic patients have a profound disturbance of many coagulation factors and represent an extremely high-risk group for perioperative venous thromboembolism. Prophylactic subcutaneous LMWH (e.g. enoxaparin at 20 mg daily) is standard practice, with higher doses (e.g. enoxaparin at 40 mg daily) in those at highest risk. LMWH is relatively contra-indicated in severe renal failure, but used in many units with the precaution of monitoring anti-Xa levels to guard against excessive dosing.

A direct endothelial effect of the CNIs can result in a *de novo* post-transplant haemolytic uraemic syndrome (HUS), and it seems likely that both ciclosporin and tacrolimus may increase the risk of recurrent HUS in patients with this as their primary disease. Unfortunately sirolimus has also been reported as a precipitant of HUS. Recurrence of HUS can occur aggressively post-transplant (e.g. factor H mutations) and the patient's original disease may have been misdiagnosed as severe hypertension rather than a thrombotic microangiopathy.

Bone marrow suppression may occur as a result of intercurrent viral infection and a variety of drugs. In the context of severe CMV infection it is safe to continue with valganciclovir or valaciclovir, but the bone marrow should be stimulated with granulocyte colony-stimulating factor. Profound bone marrow suppression may occur when allopurinol is used with azathioprine if the dose of the latter is not appropriately reduced (see above). Parvo B19 infection may occur post-transplant and cause severe anaemia.

An acute haemolytic anaemia can develop at any time following transplantation. Sometimes this is triggered by an intercurrent infection, but in many cases may be due to antibodies to minor blood antigens. Treatment consists of intravenous immunoglobulin and an increase in steroids.

Patients with a poorly functioning graft will become anaemic, just like their predialysis counterparts. Haematinics should be prescribed if patients are deficient, using intravenous iron if iron stores cannot be restored by oral supplements. Erythropoietin may be required.

About 20% of renal transplant recipients develop erythrocytosis. The mechanism is probably multifactorial. The transplant kidney may produce an excess of erythropoietin, occasionally stimulated by renal artery stenosis in the donor kidney. The use of diuretics may produce blood volume contraction. Reduction in erythrocytosis following administration of ACE inhibitors or AT-I receptor-blocking drugs suggests that angiotensin II may contribute to pathogenesis. In most cases the condition is self-limiting, but there is a risk of cerebrovascular occlusion if the haematocrit is grossly elevated and most practitioners recommend regular venesection (or ACE inhibitors) to keep the haemoglobin below 15 or 16 g/dl. A high haematocrit will also exacerbate hypertension.

Gastrointestinal

About 20% of patients have gastrointestinal complications, severe in 10%. Mouth ulcers are common and can be painful. Up to 25% of patients on sirolimus develop oral ulceration. Abdominal colic and diarrhoea complicate mycophenolate therapy and can be severe enough to interrupt therapy in 10% of cases. CMV (e.g. colitis), Kaposi's sarcoma and PTLD (intestinal obstruction) can present with gastrointestinal symptoms and signs. Diarrhoea in a transplant patient is often caused by an infectious agent and requires appropriate investigations.

Cosmetic

It is important not to underestimate the psychological importance of the cosmetic disfigurement that can be produced by some of the treatment regimens used in transplantation. They are an important contributing factor to noncompliance, particularly in adolescents, and can even lead to agoraphobia and suicide. With the currently available choices of immunosuppressive agents it should be possible to minimize cosmetic complications when these cause great distress, e.g. steroid withdrawal, substitution of tacrolimus for ciclosporin, and use of mycophenolate mofetil to reduce reliance on steroids and CNIs. The better cosmetic profile of tacrolimus is thought to be due to lower TGFβ production.

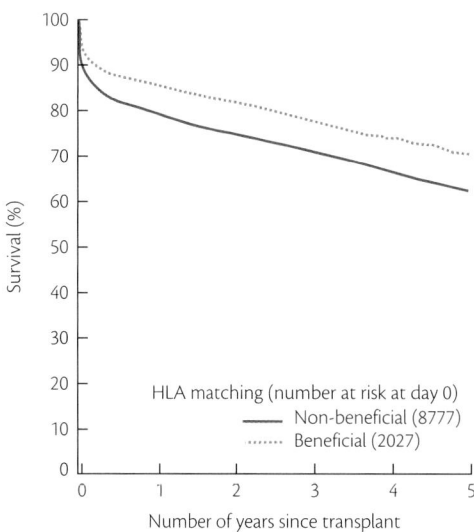

Fig. 21.7.3.2 Graft survival: first cadaver graft
Courtesy of UK transplant.

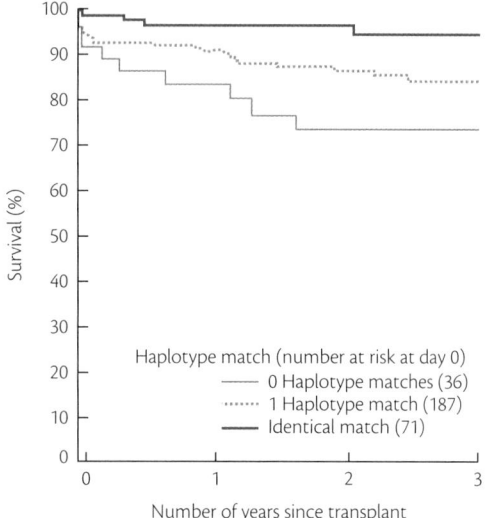

Fig. 21.7.3.3 Graft survival: living related grafts.
Courtesy of UK transplant.

Outcome of renal transplantation

Graft and patient survival

Figures 21.7.3.2 and 21.7.3.3 summarize the graft survival rates for first cadaver and living related transplants. The highest rate of graft loss is within the first few months. Graft losses due to technical factors should be less than 5%. The commonest cause of early graft loss continues to be acute rejection, but it is a matter of concern that the attrition of grafts following the first year has altered little, even with the introduction of newer, more potent immunosuppressive agents. Currently some 4% of grafts fail annually for a variety of causes loosely grouped together as chronic allograft nephropathy (see discussion below). As stated previously, death with a functioning graft is now the most common cause of late graft failure.

Factors affecting graft survival are summarized in Table 21.7.3.9. Even with potent immunosuppressive regimes, HLA matching remains extremely important, forming the rationale for local and national organ sharing schemes to ensure that the best possible matches can be obtained. Figure 21.7.3.2 indicates that beneficially matched cadaver kidneys (1–0–0 or 0–1–0 mismatch) fare significantly better than nonbeneficially matched, and well-matched living related transplants do best of all (Fig. 21.7.3.3).

Early studies indicated that an acute rejection episode had a major impact on long-term graft survival, reducing it by almost one-half, but if an acute rejection episode is completely reversed the effect on long-term graft survival is markedly reduced. Long-term graft survival can be clearly related to the creatinine level at 1 year, which has led to great emphasis on efforts to reduce the rate of early acute rejection episodes. One crucial observation that predicts those at increased risk is the presence of widely reactive anti-HLA antibodies to potential donors. Newer techniques allow the detection of individual specificities of anti-HLA antibodies at very low titres both before and after transplantation. The development of donor specific anti HLA antibodies post-transplant predicts a poor outcome.

Patients who have already rejected a kidney within 6 months of transplantation also do poorly on subsequent transplantation

Table 21.7.3.9 Factors affecting graft outcome

Adverse factors	Medical factors
Recipient factors	Organ matching policy
Obesity	Choice of immunosuppression
Poor compliance	Surgical and medical expertise
Recurrence of original disease	Nephrotoxicity of CNIs
Hypertension	Adequacy of control of hypertension
De novo glomerulonephritis	Control of CMV
Diabetes mellitus/insulin resistance	Repeated acute rejection episodes
High immune responsiveness (highly sensitized)	Poorly reversed acute rejections
Race: black individuals	Late acute rejections
Infections: CMV	Inadequate long-term immunosuppression
High creatinine at 1 year	
Proteinuria/hyperlipidaemia	
Smoking	
Donor factors	
Extremes of age (reduced nephron mass)	
Delayed graft function	
Size mismatch	
Long ischaemia times	
Poor donor organ quality	
Source: cadaver less good than living donor	
Agonal cytokine storm	

CMV, cytomegalovirus; CHI, calcineurin inhibitor.

unless immunosuppression is augmented. Increasingly potent induction regimens and combinations of drugs have been introduced, but in the absence of accurate predictors of the risk of rejection this has the effect that a significant number of patients will be grossly over-immunosuppressed, while others remain under-immunosuppressed. Poor long-term graft survival is also related to hypertension, proteinuria, hyperlipidaemia, and a high body mass index (Table 21.7.3.9).

In the early post-transplant period the main causes of death are related to cardiovascular complications of surgery, but with good patient selection the rate should be very low (1 in 300 perioperatively), despite the fact that increasingly older patients are being offered transplantation, as are those with significant comorbidities, e.g. diabetes mellitus in particular. In the first year the main cause of death is infection. Later on, death from neoplasia and accelerated vascular disease are more common (Fig. 21.7.3.4).

Chronic allograft nephropathy

First-year transplant losses from rejection have been dramatically reduced from about 40% in the 1970s to 5%. Similarly, early rejection rates can be reduced from around 50% to (using some immunosuppressive regimens) less than 10%. However, as stated above, the rate of chronic graft loss remains at about 4% per year. Some of these graft losses will be due to death with a functioning graft, but many patients present with an insidiously rising creatinine, increasing proteinuria, and worsening hypertension. The causes of this late graft dysfunction are multifactorial and involve many different

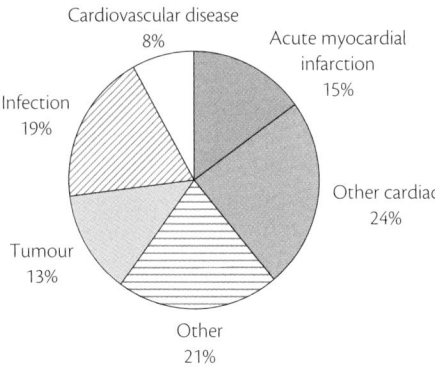

Fig. 21.7.3.4 Causes of death in renal transplant recipients.

conditions and several overlapping pathogenic pathways. Histologically, many of these kidneys will show tubular atrophy, interstitial scarring, and an obliterative vasculopathy of the intrarenal arteries and arterioles. Even with a transplant biopsy it is frequently not possible to define the pathological process.

Despite this uncertainty, every effort should be made to produce an accurate diagnosis. Obstruction due to ureteric ischaemia must be excluded by renography or ultrasound. A review of past urine cultures and a technetium-99 m labelled DMSA SPECT scan may reveal pyelonephritic scarring. Late graft dysfunction due to renal artery stenosis can be demonstrated by angiography.

It is possible that the single transplant kidney may simply have insufficient numbers of nephrons to cope with the work demanded of it, particularly if many nephrons have been lost early from acute rejection, manifest as a raised serum creatinine at 1 year. This situation may also arise if there is a very large size mismatch, with a very large recipient being given a kidney from a smaller donor, leading to the self-perpetuating inherently progressive cycle of hyperperfusion and hyperfiltration of the surviving nephrons (Brenner's hypothesis). Treatment is empirical but must involve control of blood pressure, preferably using an ACE inhibitor or an AT-I receptor blocker to reduce intraglomerular blood pressure.

Some features strongly suggest that late damage may be due to anti-graft antibodies, e.g. detection of donor-specific antibodies in the blood, deposition of C4d in the peritubular capillaries, transplant glomerulopathy, and reduplication of the tubular basement membrane.

The commonest cause of insidious late graft failure is probably CNI toxicity, which by 10 years probably affects nearly all exposed grafts to some degree. The newer agent mycophenolate mofetil may have a particular role to play in that it has been shown to reduce proliferation of smooth muscle cells, which may ameliorate the obliterative vasculopathy typical of the condition, and permit reduced reliance on long-term calcineurin-blocking agents. Conversion from the CNIs to either mycophenolate mofetil or sirolimus can prolong graft survival in patients with chronic allograft nephropathy, particularly if associated with CNI toxicity, and is being used increasingly in many centres.

Some pathogenic aspects of insidious graft loss are akin to atherosclerotic changes, and interventions designed to limit vascular damage may prolong the life of poorly functioning kidneys. The early use of ACE inhibitors (especially if there is proteinuria), aspirin, fish oils, and control of cholesterol may help.

Recurrence of original disease and *de novo* glomerulonephritis

Most of the primary glomerular diseases can recur in the transplant, but few are associated with graft loss. Overall, histologically demonstrable recurrence occurs in about 60% of patients, but less than 10% will lose their graft as a result. Accurate recurrence rates are difficult to determine, being roughly 2.5% at 2 years, 10% at 5 years, and perhaps as high as 20% by 8 years. Treatment of recurrent glomerulonephritis is not particularly effective but has usually involved intensive plasma exchange or an increase in immunosuppression. Rituximab may have a role to play.

Oxalosis will recur rapidly in the kidney unless a liver transplant is also done to correct the underlying enzyme defect. Transplantation in the presence of circulating antibody to glomerular basement membrane will result in the immediate recurrence of Goodpasture's disease. The dense deposit variety of mesangiocapillary glomerulonephritis, which is usually associated with hypocomplementaemia, predictably recurs and may destroy the graft. In paediatric practice, the nephrotic syndrome associated with focal segmental glomerulosclerosis may recur in the immediate post-transplant period and can be associated with massive proteinuria, hypovolaemia, and thromboembolism. The risk of recurrence should be taken into account when assessing patients for the possibility of a living related transplant.

Membranous glomerulonephritis can develop *de novo* (<2%) in patients in whom the original disease was demonstrably different. Attempts should be made to define the underlying defect (often genetic) in the thrombotic microangiopathies so that the risk of recurrence (often very high) can be assessed and live donor transplantation possibly avoided and in some circumstances a combined liver/kidney transplant undertaken to correct the underlying genetic defect.

Other aspects of medical management of transplant recipients

Drug interactions

Care has to be taken when prescribing drugs for renal transplant recipients. Renal function must be considered, as well as the potential for drug interactions between immunosuppressive agents and other pharmaceuticals. Table 21.7.3.10 summarizes the more common interactions. ACE inhibtors, AT-I receptor antagonists, and NSAIDs can compromise the perfusion of a single transplanted kidney, particularly if there is a degree of renal artery stenosis. Great care must be taken with potent enzyme inducers such as rifampicin as subtherapeutic levels of steroids and the CNIs can occur.

Diet

The help of a renal-trained dietitian is essential. Patients may eat voraciously after release from the restrictions of dialysis and, with the euphoric effects of steroids, some gain in excess of 20 kg in the first year. About 5% become grossly obese, which is associated insulin resistance, hyperlipidaemia, sympathetic overactivity, and hypertension. Overweight patients significantly increase their risk of developing new-onset diabetes mellitus after transplantation (NODAT), which reduces both graft and patient survival.

Hypercholesterolaemia is present post-transplant in about 30% of patients and is related to drugs, proteinuria, and diet. Patients should

Table 21.7.3.10 Common drug interactions in transplantation

Drugs	Interaction
Cytochrome P450 induction, e.g. Rifampicin Barbiturates Carbamazepam Phenytoin	Subtherapeutic levels of: CNIs Steroids Oral contraceptives Sirolimus
Cytochrome P450 inhibition, e.g. Macrolides, e.g. erythromycin Imidizoles, e.g. fluconazole Calcium channel blockers	Toxic levels of CNIs and sirolimus
Statins (or fibrates) plus CNIs	Rhabdomyolysis
Colchicine plus CNIs	Rhabdomyolysis
Allopurinol plus azathioprine	Toxic accumulation of 6-mercaptopurine Marrow suppression
ACE inhibitors (or AT-I receptor antagonists) CNIs NSAIDs Potassium-conserving diuretics	Risk of hyperkalaemia with combinations
Diuretics and CNIs	Hyperuricaemia, gout, tophi
Nephrotoxins	
NSAIDs	Nephrotoxins summate—risk of acute renal failure
CNIs	
Aminoglycosides	
Co-trimoxazole	

ACE, angiotensin converting enzyme; AT-I, angiotensin-I; CNI, calcineurin inhibitor, NSAID, nonsteroidal anti-inflammatory drug.

avoid a high intake of saturated fats. Sodium intake—easily gauged from monitoring the 24-h urinary sodium excretion—is often excessive, a desirable intake being less than 100 mmol per day. A high urinary sodium causes urinary calcium wasting and may contribute to post-transplant osteoporosis as well as making hypertension more difficult to control. All patients should spend time with the dietitian and be encouraged to adopt a healthy eating pattern. In addition to dietary advice, transplant recipients need education about the risks of contaminated food, e.g. with listeria, campylobacter, and cryptosporidium.

Additional therapy

The medical complications of renal transplantation are so numerous that many recipients will require many different drugs. The regimen may become intolerable and noncompliance can be a major problem. In the early post-transplant period it is necessary to give prophylaxis with co-trimoxazole, an H_2-antagonist or a proton pump inhibitor, and possibly a bisphosphonate, as well as an appropriate anti-CMV regime. Patients who are at risk of tuberculosis require isoniazid for the duration of immunosuppression. Hypertension needs aggressive control. In the early post-transplant period there is also the possibility of wasting of magnesium, phosphate, and bicarbonate, each requiring supplements. Uric acid

levels may be high and clinical gout may develop, requiring allopurinol. Long-term management needs to include regular vaccinations (influenza and pneumococcus). To reduce the risks of accelerated vascular disease, aspirins and statins may also be indicated.

In patients with poorly functioning transplants, medical management must include the same measures as would be undertaken in a low-clearance clinic for patients expected to start dialysis. Under these circumstances, treatment may include erythropoietin therapy, iron and vitamin supplementation, active vitamin D sterols, and oral phosphate-binders, as discussed in Chapter 21.6.

Follow-up

With an uncomplicated transplant operation, patients may only be in hospital for about 7 days. After discharge, patients will need to be seen two or three times a week for the first month, once or twice a week for the second month, and then weekly for the third month. At each visit blood pressure and graft function is checked. Many units undertake twice weekly CMV surveillance for at least the first 3 months after transplantation. After 3 months, outpatient visits are gradually reduced with patients eventually being reviewed only every 3 to 4 months. Particular attention has to be paid to cardiovascular risk factors, infections, and neoplasia. Ideally, all patients should have an annual dermatological examination, and women should have an annual cervical smear and colposcopy if indicated. Bone density should be monitored regularly. Even in an apparently stable transplant, some units perform a renogram every 1 to 2 years to detect deteriorating renal perfusion or obstruction from an ischaemic ureteric stenosis. Patients at risk of tuberculosis will require a regular chest radiograph. Vaccinations should be kept up to date. Many centres offer an anniversary clinic when these medical complications can be more fully assessed. Accelerated atherosclerosis will lead to early coronary and peripheral vascular disease. Increasingly, renal transplant recipients are being put forward for coronary revascularization procedures.

Pregnancy

A successful renal transplant restores fertility, and pregnancy with normal vaginal delivery (unless there are obstetric indications for caesarean section) is possible. Most recommend that pregnancy is not embarked upon in the first year or if the serum creatinine is above 150 μmol/litre or proteinuria greater than 2 g/day. Many successful pregnancies have been undertaken with renal function worse than this, but the risks are greater. Overall, 20% of patients show a deterioration in graft function and up to 10% in some series lose their grafts.

There is little evidence that immunosuppression with prednisolone, azathioprine and a CNI has a significant adverse effect on the fetus. To maintain therapeutic levels of the CNI, dosages may have to be considerably increased. CNIs may be associated with intrauterine growth retardation ('small for dates' babies) and prednisolone may produce neonatal adrenal suppression. Experience of pregnancy with mycophenolate mofetil and sirolimus is limited, but these drugs do not seem to be safe in pregnancy and patients should be advised not to become pregnant while taking them.

There is an increased risk of hypertension and pre-eclampsia in renal transplant recipients. Care has to be taken with the choice of antihypertensive agent. ACE inhibitors and AT-1 receptor blockers are contraindicated. Labetolol and methyldopa have withstood the test of time.

During delivery, intravenous fluid should be given and great care taken to avoid episodes of hypovolaemia and hypotension. It is usual to give an extra dose of steroid during the delivery, e.g. 100 mg of intravenous hydrocortisone, and to increase oral prednisolone for a few days afterwards. Regular midstream urine specimens should be sent in the postpartum period.

Further reading

General

Forsythe JLR (2006). *Transplantation:A companion to specialist practice*, 3rd edition. W B Saunders, Philadelphia.

Morris PJ , Knechtle SJ (2008). Kidney transplantation: principles and practice 6th Edition, Saunders.

Ponticelli C (2007). Medical complications of kidney transplantation Informa Health Care.

Rubin RH, Young LS (eds) (1994). *Clinical approach to infection in the compromised host*, 3rd edition. Plenum, New York.

Suthanthiran M, Strom TB (1994). Renal transplantation. *N Engl J Med*, **331**, 365–76.

Infections

Green M, Avery RK, Preiksaitis J (eds) (2004). Guidelines for the prevention and management of infectious complications of solid organ transplantation. *Am J Transplant*, **4** Suppl 6, 1–166.

Hirsch HH, *et al.* (2005). Polyomavirus associated nephropathy in renal transplantation: interdisciplinary analysis and recommendations. *Transplantation*, **79**, 1277–86.

Pescovitz MD (2006). Benefits of cytomegalovirus prophylaxis in solid organ transplantation. *Transplantation*, **82**, Suppl 2, S4–8.

Snydman DR (2006). The case for cytomegalovirus prophylaxis in solid organ transplantation. *Rev Med Virol*, **16**, 289–95.

Sweny P, Rubin R, Tolkoff-Rubin N (eds) (2003). *The infectious complications of renal disease*. Oxford Medical Publications, Oxford.

Malignancy

Andrés A (2005). Cancer incidence after immunosuppression treatment following kidney transplantation. *Crit Rev Oncol Hematol*, **56**, 71–85.

Antman K (2000). Kaposi's sarcoma. *N Engl J Med*, **342**, 1027–38.

Buell JF, Gross TG, Wood LE (2005). Malignancy after transplantation. *Transplantation*, **80**, S254–64.

Dreno B (2003). Skin cancers after transplantation. *Nephrol Dial Transplant*, **18**, 1052–8.

Little RF, Yarchoan R (2003). Treatment of gammaherpes-related neoplastic disorders in the immunosuppressed host. *Semin Haematol*, **40**, 163–71.

Morath C, *et al.* (2004). Malignancy in renal transplantation. *J Am Soc Nephrol*, **15**, 1582–8.

Opelz G, *et al.* (2006). Dissociation between risk of graft loss and risk of non-Hodgkin lymphoma with induction agents in renal transplant recipients. *Transplantation*, **81**, 1227–33.

Taylor AL, Marcus R, Bradley JA (2005). Post-transplant lymphoproliferative disorder (PTLD) after solid organ transplantation. *Crit Rev Oncol Hematol*, **56**, 155–67.

Yarchoan R (2006). Key role for a viral lytic gene in Kaposi's sarcoma. *N Engl J Med*, **355**, 1383–85.

Particular complications

Afzali B, *et al.* (2006). Anaemia after renal transplantation. *Am J Kidney Dis*, **48**, 519–36.

Aroldi A, *et al.* (2005). Natural history of hepatitis B and C in renal allograft recipients. *Transplantation*, **79**, 1332–6.

Cunningham J (2005). Post transplant bone disease. *Transplantation*, **79**, 629–34.

Kaisiske BL, *et al.* (1996). Cardiovascular disease after renal transplantation. *J Am Soc Nephrol*, **7**, 158–65.

Kasiske B, *et al.* (2004). Clinical practice guidelines for managing dyslipidaemias in kidney transplant patients. *Am J Transplant*, **4** Suppl, 1–53.

Kujovick JL (2004). Thrombophilia and thrombotic problems in renal transplant patients. *Transplantation*, **79**, 959–64.

Markell M (2004). New-onset diabetes mellitus in transplant patients: pathogenesis, complications and management. *Am J Kidney Dis*, **43**, 953–65.

Meier-Kriesch H-V, *et al.* (2004). Kidney transplantation halts cardiovascular disease progression in patients with end-stage renal disease. *Am J Transplant*, **4**, 1662–8.

Palmer SC, Strippoli GFM, McGregor DO (2005). Interventions for preventing bone disease in kidney transplant recipients:, A systematic review of randomized controlled trials. *Am J Kidney Dis*, **45**, 638–49.

Pontielli C, Passerini P (2005). Gastrointestinal complications in renal transplantation. *Transplant Int*, **18**, 643–50.

Wheeler DC, Steiger J (2000). Evolution and etiology of cardiovascular diseases in renal transplant recipients. *Transplantation*, **70**, 41–5.

Immunosuppression

Cianco G, Miller J, Gonwa T (2005). Review of major clinical trials with mycophenolate mofetil in renal transplantation. *Transplantation*, **80** Suppl 2, S191–200.

Cianco G, Warque ME, Miller J (2006). Efficacy of alemtuzumab in organ transplantation: current clinical status. *Biodrugs*, **20**, 85–92.

Danovitch GM (2000). Immunosuppressant-induced metabolic toxicities. *Transplant Rev*, **14**, 65–81.

Haller M & Oberbauer R. (2009).Calcineurin inhibitor minimization, withdrawal and avoidance protocols after kidney transplantation. *Transpl. Int.*, **22**(1), 69–77.

Kumar NSA, Heifets M, Moritz MJ (2006). Safety and efficacy of steroid withdrawal two days after kidney transplantation: analysis of results at three years. *Transplantation*, **81**, 832–9.

Kuypers DRJ, Vanrenterghem YFC (2004). Monoclonal antibodies in renal transplantation: old and new. *Nephrol Dial Transplant*, **19**, 297–300.

Matas A.J (2009).Minimization of steroids in kidney transplantation *Transpl. Int.*, **22**(1), 38–48.

Miller LW (2002). Cardiovascular toxicities of immunosuppressive agents. *Am J Transplant*, **2**, 807–18.

Samaniego M, Becker B, Djamali A (2006). Drug insight: maintenance immunosuppression in kidney transplant recipients. *Nature Clin Pract Nephrol*, **2**, 688–99.

Chronic allograft nephropathy

Cai J, Terasaki PI (2005). Humoral theory of transplantation: mechanism, prevention and treatment. *Human Immunol*, **66**, 334–42.

Dudley C, *et al.* (2005). Mycophenolate mofetil substitution for ciclosporine A in renal transplant, recipients with chronic progressive allograft dysfunction: The 'Creeping Creatinine' study. *Transplantation*, **79**, 466–75.

Joosten SA, *et al.* (2005). Chronic renal allograft rejection: pathological considerations. *Kidney Int*, **68**, 1–13.

Nankivelli BK, Chapman JR (2006). Chronic allograft nephropathy: current concepts and future directives. *Transplantation*, **81**, 643–54.

Nankivelli BK, *et al.* (2003). The natural history of chronic allograft nephropathy. *N Engl J Med*, **349**, 2326–33.

Outcomes and other topics

Choy BY, Chan TM, Lai KN (2006). Recurrent glomerulonephritis after transplantation. *Am J Transplant*, **6**, 2535–42.

Hariharan S, *et al.* (2002). Post transplant renal function in the first year predicts long-term kidney transplant survival. *Kidney Int*, **62**, 311–18.

Opelz G, Dohler B (2005). Improved long-term outcomes after renal transplantation associated with blood pressure control. *Am J Transplant*, **5**, 2725–31.

Stratta P, *et al.* (2003). Pregnancy in kidney transplantation: satisfactory outcomes and harsh realities. *J Nephrol*, **16**, 792–806.

Wolfe RA, Ashby VB, Milford EL (1999). Comparison of mortality in all patients on dialysis, patients on dialysis awaiting transplantation, and recipients of a first cadaveric transplant. *N Engl J Med*, **341**, 1725–30.

Glomerular diseases

Contents

21.8.1 Immunoglobulin A nephropathy and Henoch–Schönlein purpura

Jonathan Barratt and John Feehally

Essentials

Immunoglobulin A nephropathy (IgAN) is the commonest pattern of glomerulonephritis identified in areas of the world where renal biopsy is widely practised. It is defined pathologically by IgA deposition in the glomerular mesangium accompanied by a mesangial proliferative glomerulonephritis which may vary greatly in severity. Aetiology is uncertain, but abnormalities of IgA1 hinge-region O-glycosylation are consistently found.

Clinical features—IgAN can present with: (1) macroscopic haematuria, typically in children and young adults, developing within a day or two of upper respiratory tract infection ('synpharyngitic'); (2) asymptomatic microscopic haematuria/proteinuria; (3) nephrotic syndrome (less than 5% of cases); (4) acute kidney injury (uncommon); and (5) chronic renal failure with up to 25% of patients reaching endstage renal failure within 20 years of diagnosis. Henoch–Schönlein purpura (HSP) is a small vessel systemic vasculitis characterized by small blood vessel deposition of IgA that predominantly affects the skin, joints, gut, and kidney, with nephritis that may be histologically indistinguishable from IgA nephropathy.

Management—there is no treatment known to modify mesangial deposition of IgA. Treatment options are mostly directed at controlling blood pressure and limiting proteinuria through blockade of the renin–angiotensin–aldosterone axis. In the rare patient presenting with acute kidney injury in whom biopsy shows crescentic IgA nephropathy, a regimen such as those used for renal vasculitis and other forms of crescentic glomerulonephritis should be considered, e.g. oral prednisolone in combination with cyclophosphamide.

Introduction

Immunoglobulin A nephropathy (IgAN) was first described by Berger in 1968 and at one time was known as Berger's disease. It is defined by IgA deposition in the glomerular mesangium accompanied by a mesangial proliferative glomerulonephritis which may vary greatly in severity. Although recurrent macroscopic haematuria is the hallmark of the disease, the old term 'benign recurrent haematuria' is a discredited misnomer since it is now clear that IgAN is associated with a significant risk of progression to endstage renal failure. Henoch–Schönlein purpura (HSP) is a somewhat misleading historical term: the purpuric rash is in fact a cutaneous vasculitis, and the renal lesion (HSP nephritis) is a mesangial proliferative glomerulonephritis usually indistinguishable from IgAN.

Aetiology

In most cases the aetiology of IgAN remains unclear. The provocation of macroscopic haematuria by mucosal infection in IgAN and the presumption that the mesangial IgA represented deposited immune complexes led to the view that IgAN was a complication of infection. Cytomegalovirus and *Haemophilus parainfluenzae* have been most studied, but neither these nor any other viral or bacterial antigens have been consistently associated with development of the disease or identified in IgA immune complexes or mesangial deposits. Alternatively, it has been suggested that IgAN results from hypersensitivity to food antigens, in view of its association with gluten-sensitive enteropathy. There is some evidence that withdrawal of gluten from the diet of these specific patients may improve the renal disease, but there is little evidence for widespread hypersensitivity to food antigens in IgAN.

Genetics

Despite many studies of potential immunogenetic associations, the genetic basis for susceptibility to IgAN has not yet been identified. IgAN is familial in less than 10% of cases, but the true frequency of familial IgAN remains uncertain because there are no reliable serological markers for the disease. In one study, 23% of 'unaffected' relatives had urinary abnormalities; a significant minority also had high serum IgA and high levels of IgA-containing immune complexes. Genome-wide linkage analysis in 30 multiplex kindreds has demonstrated linkage to 6q22-23, but there are no obvious candidate genes within the linked interval, and no linkage was found in the same kindreds for several other candidate genes all implicated in the pathogenesis of IgAN. Further definition of the genes involved within the IGAN1 locus is still awaited.

Pathogenesis

Mechanism of mesangial IgA deposition

Mesangial proliferative glomerulonephritis such as is seen in IgAN and HSP nephritis may be the consequence of immune complex deposition, either due to trapping of circulating IgA immune complexes or the formation of complexes *in situ* by reaction of IgA with antigen which has already been deposited. No exogenous antigen has been consistently identified in the mesangial deposits in IgAN, which may indicate that the IgA complexes are a common response to different antigens, or that the initiating antigen has disappeared by the time of the renal biopsy. Alternatively, the IgA may be deposited by some mechanism independent of classic antigen–antibody interactions, such as a physicochemical abnormality of the IgA.

The frequent recurrence of both IgAN and HSP nephritis after renal transplantation strongly suggests that the abnormality resides in the host IgA immune system. The mesangial IgA deposits are polymeric IgA1 (pIgA1). Most pIgA is synthesized in the mucosa and the clinical association of macroscopic haematuria with mucosal infection originally led to the assumption that an exaggerated mucosal IgA response resulted in mesangial IgA deposition. But IgA production is in fact down-regulated in the mucosal immune system and up-regulated in the bone marrow, and exaggerated IgA1 responses to immunization in these patients are marrow rather than mucosally derived.

There is increasing evidence of abnormal glycosylation of both serum and mesangial IgA1 in patients with IgAN and HSP nephritis. The glycosylation abnormality may favour the development of immune complexes or may directly provoke mesangial deposition, but these putative mechanisms have not yet been further defined.

Progression of IgA nephropathy

IgA deposition may occur in many patients with mild disease with little mesangial injury. What decides the prognosis in any individual is the extent to which the IgA deposition is followed by mesangial proliferation, inflammation, and scarring. There is nothing to suggest that these subsequent mechanisms of damage and scarring are unique to IgAN, rather they are generic to many forms of glomerulonephritis.

Relationship of IgAN and HSP

There is much indirect evidence to suggest a close relationship between IgAN and HSP. Monozygotic twins have been described, one who developed IgAN and the other HSP at the same time. HSP developing on a background of proven IgAN has been described in both adults and children. Many abnormalities of the IgA immune system, including abnormal IgA1 glycosylation, have been described in both IgAN and HSP. IgAN is increasingly thought of as 'HSP without the rash'. Why some individuals get a renal-limited disease (IgAN) and others a systemic disease (HSP) is not known.

Pathology

Immune deposits

IgAN and HSP nephritis are defined by the presence of mesangial IgA detected by immunofluorescence or immunoperoxidase (Fig. 21.8.1.1). Complement C3 frequently accompanies IgA in the same mesangial distribution; IgG and IgM are less common. Electron microscopy identifies mesangial electron-dense deposits corresponding to the mesangial IgA (Fig. 21.8.1.2).

Light microscopy

Mesangial proliferative glomerulonephritis is the characteristic appearance, although when haematuria is the only clinical finding abnormalities on light microscopy may be minimal despite florid IgA deposition. Mesangial hypercellularity and matrix expansion are usually global (Fig. 21.8.1.3a) but may be focal and segmental (Fig. 21.8.1.3b,c). The hypercellularity is followed by increasing mesangial matrix deposition and eventual sclerosis (Fig. 21.8.1.3b). In acute kidney injury there may be severe glomerular inflammation with crescent formation. In advanced cases there is

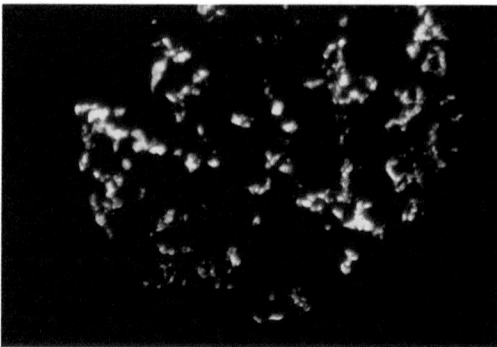

Fig. 21.8.1.1 Immunofluorescence of a glomerulus in IgAN. Bright fluorescent staining is seen within the mesangium with labelled antibodies to IgA. In some cases similar staining is also seen along capillary walls. A similar distribution of staining for C3 is commonly present. Antihuman IgA, magnification ×375.

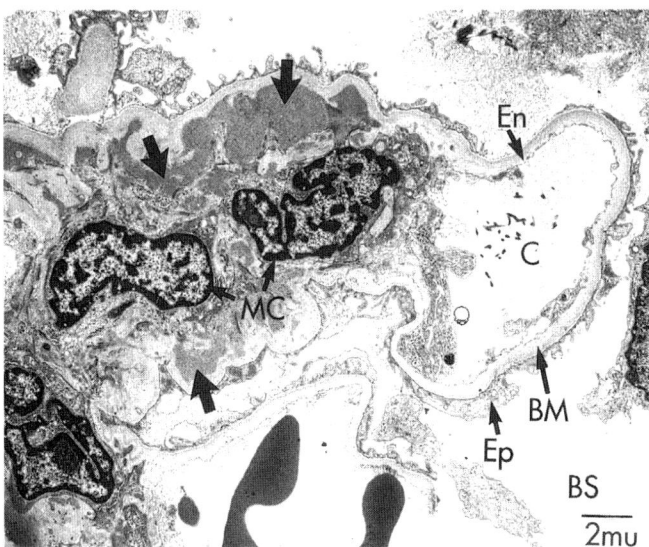

Fig. 21.8.1.2 Electron micrograph of glomerular capillary loop in IgA nephropathy. Numerous electron-dense deposits representing deposits of IgA (large arrows) are seen within the expanded mesangium. BM, basement membrane; BS, Bowman's space; C, capillary lumen; En, fenestrated endothelium; Ep, visceral epithelium; MC, mesangial cell nucleus. Magnification ×5200.

glomerulosclerosis and corresponding tubular atrophy and interstitial fibrosis; these are entirely nonspecific changes of 'endstage kidney'.

Epidemiology

IgAN is the commonest glomerulonephritis in countries where renal biopsy is widely used. It is typically found in 30% of biopsies with primary glomerular disease, but the apparent prevalence varies markedly around the world. It is commoner in the Pacific rim and Mediterranean countries, and less so in North America and northern Europe. At least part of this apparent difference is explained by the varying use of urine testing in health screening and varying attitudes to the value of renal biopsy in individuals with isolated haematuria or other minor clinical evidence of renal disease. For example, in Japan there is routine urine testing of schoolchildren and employed adults, the threshold for renal biopsy is low, and the reported prevalence of IgAN is high. There are also important racial differences in susceptibility. IgAN is uncommon in Afro-Caribbean people and also less common in Polynesian people than white people in Australasia, a particularly striking finding given the exaggerated susceptibility of Polynesian people to most forms of renal disease.

Clinical features

IgAN

IgAN can occur at any age, but the peak age of onset is in the second and third decades of life (Fig. 21.8.1.4). In western Europe IgAN is three times more common in males than females, but this gender difference disappears in the Pacific Rim.

Macroscopic haematuria

The characteristic clinical picture of recurrent macroscopic haematuria occurs in about 40 to 50% of cases. A child or young adult develops episodes of painless macroscopic haematuria occurring within a day or so of the onset of an upper respiratory tract

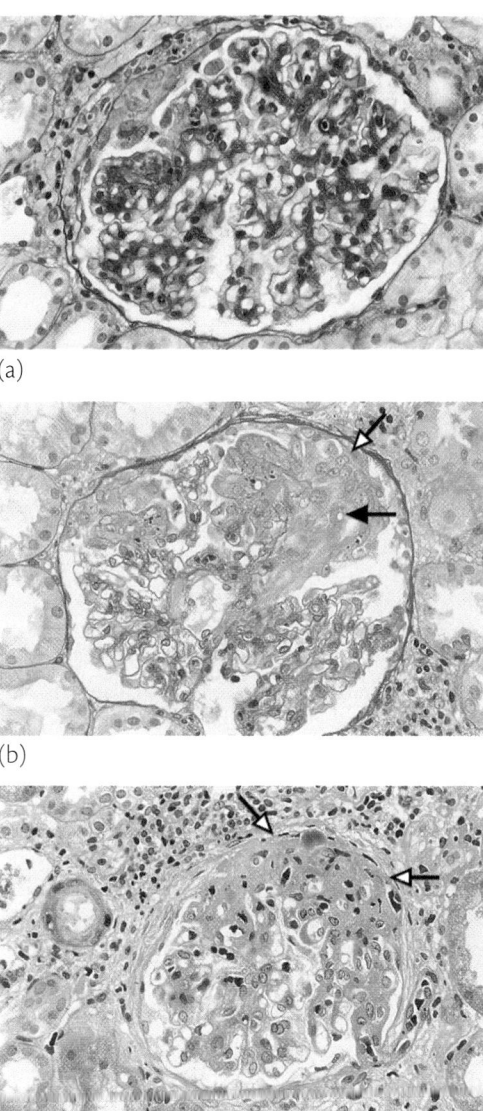

Fig. 21.8.1.3 Light microscopic appearances of IgA nephropathy. (a) Glomerulus showing global increase in mesangial matrix and cellularity. Alcian blue/PAS stain, magnification ×375. (b) Glomerulus showing segmental increase in mesangial matrix and hypercellularity with fibrinoid necrosis (solid arrow) and synechia formation (open arrow) between the segmental lesion and parietal epithelium of Bowman's capsule. Alcian blue/PAS stain, magnification ×375. (c) Glomerulus showing segmental increase in mesangial matrix and segmental sclerosis with synechia formation (open arrows) overlying Bowman's capsule. Masson's trichrome stain, magnification ×375.

infection, or occasionally infections of other mucosal or IgA-secreting surfaces such as gastrointestinal tract, bladder, or breast. The urine may be frankly bloody, but more often is brown (like Coca-Cola or tea without milk), there are no clots passed, and it is usually painless although there may be dull loin ache. The episodes settle spontaneously after 1 to 5 days and may be recurrent, but rarely for more than a year or two. Serum IgA is moderately elevated in 30% of cases, but serum complement C3 and C4 are normal. Between episodes there will be persistent microscopic haematuria. This presentation does not occur beyond the age of 40 years (Fig. 21.8.1.4).

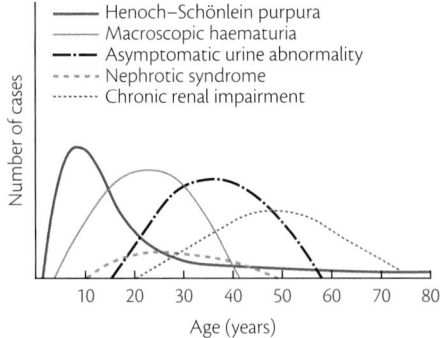

Fig. 21.8.1.4 Clinical presentations of IgA nephropathy and HSP in relation to age at diagnosis. HSP is most common in childhood but may occur at any age. Macroscopic haematuria is very rare over the age of 40 years. The importance of asymptomatic urine abnormality as the presentation of IgAN will depend on attitudes to routine urine testing and renal biopsy. It is uncertain whether those presenting with chronic renal impairment have a disease distinct from that of those presenting younger with macroscopic haematuria.

Asymptomatic haematuria/proteinuria

Thirty to 40% of cases of IgAN are identified by urine testing, when microscopic haematuria may be combined with proteinuria (usually <2 g/24 h). Since this is glomerular haematuria, dysmorphic red cells may be seen on phase contrast microscopy, but red cell casts are frequently absent in mild disease.

Nephrotic syndrome

Nephrotic syndrome is the presentation in only 5% of IgAN. Very occasionally in children or young adults this appears to be the consequence of coincidental minimal-change nephrotic disease; the proteinuria resolves completely with corticosteroid therapy, but haematuria and IgA deposits persist. More commonly nephrotic syndrome may develop in IgAN with overt mesangial proliferative glomerulonephritis, or may be a consequence of glomerular scarring in advanced IgAN.

Acute kidney injury

Acute kidney injury occurs for two reasons in IgAN. Episodes of macroscopic haematuria may produce acute tubular occlusion by red cells in the face of minor glomerular injury. Alternatively, there can be acute severe necrotizing glomerulonephritis with crescent formation, 'crescentic IgA nephropathy', which may be the presenting feature or occur on a background of known milder disease.

Chronic renal failure

IgAN may also present with hypertension and established renal impairment, often in older patients (Fig. 21.8.1.4). Too little is yet known about the pathogenesis of IgAN to understand whether this is a distinct disease entity or the same disease presenting much later because there was never an episode of macroscopic haematuria or a urine test to bring it to medical attention earlier.

Clinical associations with IgAN

The commonest secondary cause of IgAN is chronic liver disease, typically alcoholic liver disease, in which it is probable that IgA deposition is a consequence of impaired IgA clearance from the circulation via the liver. Most hepatic IgAN is asymptomatic, and progression to endstage renal failure is unusual. The other best established associations are with coeliac disease and dermatitis herpetiformis; with rheumatoid arthritis, ankylosing spondylitis, and Reiter's disease; and with HIV infection. Many other conditions have been reported occasionally with IgAN, but since IgAN is so common it is difficult to know if these are more than chance associations.

HSP nephritis

HSP can occur at any age but is commonest in the first decade of life (Fig. 21.8.1.4). There is a slight male preponderance. A palpable purpuric rash caused by cutaneous vasculitis is the presenting feature. It has a characteristic extensor surface distribution with sparing of the trunk and face (Fig. 21.8.1.5). Crops of rash, often provoked by intercurrent infection, may continue for some time, but rarely beyond a year from first presentation. Polyarthralgia is common. Abdominal pain, due to gut vasculitis, is usually mild and transient, but severe pain and bloody diarrhoea may develop due to intussusception.

Apart from intussusception, the major sequelae of HSP come from renal involvement. Much of the renal disease in HSP is transient, with asymptomatic haematuria or proteinuria disappearing in a few weeks. Of those with persistent evidence of renal disease, asymptomatic haematuria/proteinuria is the commonest clinical state, but 20% will have nephrotic syndrome. Serum IgA is raised in 50%, but complement C3 and C4 are normal. Acute kidney injury due to crescentic HSP nephritis usually occurs early and is commoner than crescentic IgAN.

Differential diagnosis

Macroscopic haematuria

Nonglomerular causes of haematuria, including renal stones and neoplasia, must always be considered and excluded where appropriate by urological investigation. While episodic macroscopic haematuria coinciding with upper respiratory tract infection in children and young adults is the hallmark of IgAN, it is not pathognomonic. Similar episodes can occur with other glomerular diseases, most commonly hereditary nephropathies such as Alport's syndrome and thin membrane nephropathy. The distinction of IgAN from postinfectious (usually poststreptococcal) glomerulonephritis is also important. In poststreptococcal glomerulonephritis there is a 10- to 14-day latency from the onset of infection and the development of symptomatic renal disease, contrasting with the immediacy of haematuria in IgAN, for which the term 'synpharyngitic haematuria' has been coined. The haematuria is usually less heavy in

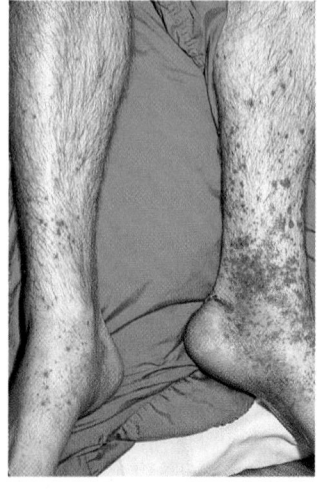

Fig. 21.8.1.5 Characteristic purpuric rash affecting the lower limbs in HSP.

poststreptococcal glomerulonephritis so that the urine is typically smoky rather than frankly bloody; hypertension, oedema, and other features of the acute nephritic syndrome are usually present. Serological evidence of recent streptococcal infection (such as antibodies to endostreptosin) and low C3 are not found in IgAN.

Nephrotic syndrome

The differential diagnosis when IgAN presents with nephrotic syndrome includes the usual range of glomerular disease known to cause nephrotic syndrome given the age of the patient.

Chronic renal failure

Advanced IgAN presenting with hypertension, proteinuria, and renal impairment is clinically indistinguishable from many other causes of chronic progressive renal disease. Renal biopsy can establish the diagnosis since mesangial IgA can often still be identified even when light microscopy shows 'endstage kidney', but should only be performed if there is a reasonable expectation that the result might benefit the particular patient.

HSP

In children HSP is the commonest form of vasculitis, and a clinical diagnosis is often made from the characteristic rash and abdominal pain. In adults the differential diagnosis is wider, including many other forms of small vessel vasculitis which must be distinguished on the basis of clinical, serological, and histopathological findings.

Clinical investigation

No accumulation of clinical and laboratory evidence has sufficient specificity and sensitivity to avoid the need for diagnostic biopsy in IgAN or HSP. IgA deposits are seen in blood vessels in affected skin, but this is not a universal feature. Raised serum IgA1 levels are found in 30 to 50% of all patients, but are less common in children and do not correlate with disease activity or severity. A high proportion of λ light chain, rather than the normal predominance of the κ isotype, is also a distinctive feature of serum IgA in IgAN, although the significance of this is unknown. Complement components C3 and C4, and CH_{50} in the serum, are usually normal, but there is some evidence of systemic complement activation with more specific testing. Circulating autoantibodies, including antiendothelial antibodies, have been described in IgAN, but none appear to be disease specific. Circulating IgA-rheumatoid factors and IgA-containing circulating immune complexes have been reported by many different assay methods but are not diagnostically useful, nor can they be reliably correlated with disease activity.

Secondary causes of IgAN must be identified. A thorough history and physical examination, along with laboratory checks for liver function and hepatitis B status are sufficient to exclude the common secondary associations with IgAN.

Criteria for diagnosis

IgAN

By definition, the diagnosis of IgAN requires a renal biopsy; no serological or other laboratory indices provide diagnostic information reliable enough to avoid the need for biopsy.

HSP

While the distribution of the vasculitic rash may be highly suggestive in HSP, ultimate confirmation requires identification of tissue

Table 21.8.1.1 Current recommendations for the treatment of IgAN

Clinical feature	Recommendation		
Microscopic haematuria	No treatment		
Macroscopic haematuria	No treatment—no indication for prophylactic antibiotics or tonsillectomy		
Acute kidney injury	Biopsy	Tubular occlusion	Supportive treatment only
		Crescentic IgAN	Prednisolone 0.5 mg/kg per day, reducing to 5–10 mg daily by 3 months Cyclophosphamide 2–3 mg/kg per day for 3 months, followed by azathioprine 2–3 mg/kg per day
Proteinuria <1 g/24 h	No treatment		
Nephrotic syndrome with minimal change on biopsy	Prednisolone 0.5 mg/kg per day for 8–12 weeks		
All other proteinuria >1 g/24 h	ACE inhibitor and ARB		
Hypertension	Target BP 125/75 mmHg if proteinuria >1 g/24 h, otherwise target BP 130/80 mmHg, using regimen including ACE inhibitor and ARB		

ACE, angiotensin-converting enzyme; ARB, angiotensin receptor blocker; BP, blood pressure.

IgA deposition which can be found in the vessels of affected skin as well as the kidney.

Treatment

IgAN

Treatment proposals for IgAN are summarized in Table 21.8.1.1. Only in very few patients with IgAN is there any evidence that drug therapy alters the natural history of the disease. Despite being so common among renal diseases, there is still a dearth of well-conducted prospective randomized controlled trials in IgAN on which to base therapeutic decisions.

Specific treatment for IgAN would either restrict the formation of relevant pathogenic IgA molecules or prevent their deposition in the mesangium. However, so little is understood about the pathogenesis of the disease that the prospect for such treatment is still remote.

Haematuria

There is no specific treatment for the great majority of patients with IgAN who have isolated haematuria with or without low-grade proteinuria (<1 g/24 h). Microscopic haematuria should merely be observed. Recurrent macroscopic haematuria settles without treatment; there is no role for prophylactic antibiotics as most precipitating infections are viral. Tonsillectomy will reduce the number of episodes of macroscopic haematuria, but there is no evidence that it reduces the risk of progressive renal failure.

Proteinuria

Those with proteinuria above 1 g/24 h as well as haematuria have a worse prognosis. Immunosuppressive therapies have been tried, although the frequent recurrence of IgAN in transplanted kidneys when patients are receiving immunosuppressive therapy argues against their value. Short-term randomized controlled trials of corticosteroids have shown no benefit. A controlled trial of 6 months of treatment with corticosteroids (prednisolone 0.5 mg/kg per day) showed a significant reduction in proteinuria and reduced risk of developing renal impairment at 10 years follow-up. This requires further confirmation, and corticosteroid treatment is not presently recommended except in the rare circumstance where the biopsy suggests coincidental minimal-change nephrotic syndrome which may be fully steroid responsive.

Other immune modulating drugs have been tried in IgAN, including cyclophosphamide, mycophenolate mofetil, azathioprine, ciclosporin, and pooled human intravenous immunoglobulin, but there are few properly controlled studies and for none is there consistent evidence of benefit or an acceptable risk–benefit ratio in most patients who have indolent slowly progressive disease.

Acute kidney injury

Renal biopsy is mandatory when acute kidney injury develops in IgAN. If this shows mild glomerular disease but tubular occlusion with erythrocytes and accompanying acute tubular necrosis, supportive treatment only is required while recovery is awaited. If there is crescentic IgAN, a regimen such as those used for renal vasculitis and other forms of crescentic glomerulonephritis should be considered unless the histological appearances are thought to be advanced and irreversible, e.g. oral prednisolone 0.5 mg/kg per day (reducing to a maintenance dose of 5–10 mg daily by 3 months) in combination with oral cyclophosphamide 2 to 3 mg/kg per day (replaced by azathioprine 2–3 mg/kg per day after 3 months). Plasma exchange has also been used. There are no randomized controlled trials of these treatments in crescentic IgAN. Although initial response to treatment is excellent, the medium-term outlook is much less good; 50% will be on long-term dialysis after 12 months.

Progressive renal impairment

Slowly progressive renal impairment due to IgAN requires a management approach common to any form of chronic renal failure. Rigorous control of blood pressure is the one established method of delaying progressive renal failure. Angiotensin-converting enzyme (ACE) inhibitors, often in combination with angiotensin II receptor blockers, are widely used as first-line therapy for their special role in lessening proteinuria for the same degree of blood pressure control. Fish oil therapy (which provides a supplement of $\omega - 3$ fatty acids) has effects likely to impact favourably on mechanisms of progressive renal damage and has been used in randomized controlled trials in IgAN, but there is no reason to expect its effects are specific for IgAN rather than other progressive diseases. One randomized controlled trial has shown a substantial reduction in the risk of progression to endstage renal failure, but other studies have not shown comparable benefit and at present the use of fish oil is not recommended until confirmatory studies are available.

HSP nephritis

There is very little information to guide treatment of HSP nephritis. There are no published randomized controlled trials and most therapeutic studies in IgAN exclude those with HSP, hence it is unclear whether their conclusions can be extrapolated to HSP.

Transient early nephritis requires no specific treatment. There is no evidence that corticosteroids or other immunosuppressive regimens alter the natural history of nephrotic syndrome or slowly progressive glomerular damage in HSP. Crescentic HSP nephritis is more common than crescentic IgAN. Regimens used for renal vasculitis have also been applied to crescentic HSP nephritis with apparent benefit, although there are no controlled trials.

Prognosis

Thirty per cent of children will have a spontaneous clinical remission with complete disappearance of haematuria within 10 years of diagnosis. But IgAN, despite the apparently benign presentation in many cases, is an important cause of endstage renal failure, with up to 25% of patients reaching this within 20 years of diagnosis. Where a lower risk of endstage renal failure is reported the series will contain larger numbers of patients with mild disease, such as those with isolated microscopic haematuria.

Perhaps unexpectedly a history of episodic macroscopic haematuria is a favourable prognostic feature. The prognosis for patients who present with microscopic haematuria and minimal proteinuria (<1 g/24 h) is very good, but not perfect; even in this group up to 5% of patients will develop worsening proteinuria and hypertension during follow-up and are at eventual risk of endstage renal failure. Consequently the long-term follow-up of any patient with biopsy-proven IgAN is mandatory. The risk of progressive renal failure can be predicted by clinical and pathological features at diagnosis (Table 21.8.1.2), but these predictive features are not specific to IgAN as they would identify the risk of progression in any glomerular disease.

Table 21.8.1.2 Prognostic markers at presentation in IgAN

Poor prognosis[a]	Good prognosis	No influence on prognosis
Clinical		
Increasing age	Recurrent macroscopic haematuria	Gender
Duration of preceding symptoms		Ethnicity
Severity of proteinuria		Serum IgA level
Hypertension		
Renal impairment		
Increased body mass index		
Serum uric acid		
Histopathological		
Glomerular sclerosis	Minimal light microscopic abnormalities	Intensity of IgA deposits
Tubular atrophy		Codeposition of IgG, IgM, and C3
Interstitial fibrosis		
Vascular wall thickening		
Capillary loop IgA deposits (some reports only)		

[a] Note that none of the clinical or histological adverse features are specific to IgAN, except capillary loop IgA deposits.

Both IgAN and HSP nephritis recur after renal transplantation. Mesangial IgA deposits appear within a few months in 60% of patients with IgAN. Initially this is benign, accompanied by little mesangial injury, but in the long-term recurrent disease will contribute to progressive graft loss in a number of patients. However, overall transplant success and graft longevity do not differ in IgAN or HSP from other primary renal diseases. The changes in immunosuppressive regimens used to prevent rejection over the last two decades have not altered the recurrence rate or its prognosis.

Further reading

Clinical

Barratt J, Feehally J (2005). IgA nephropathy. *J Am Soc Nephrol*, **16**, 2088–97.

D'Amico G (2004). Natural history of idiopathic IgA nephropathy and factors predictive of disease outcome. *Semin Nephrol*, **24**, 179–96.

Davin JC, Ten Berge IJ, Weening JJ (2001). What is the difference between IgA nephropathy and Henoch–Schönlein purpura nephritis? *Kidney Int*, **59**, 823–34.

Floege J (2004). Recurrent IgA nephropathy after renal transplantation. *Semin Nephrol*, **24**, 287–91.

Pouria S, Feehally J (1999). Glomerular IgA deposition in liver disease. *Nephrol Dial Transplant*, **14**, 2279–82.

Pathogenesis and genetics

Barratt J, Feehally J, Smith AC (2004). Pathogenesis of IgA nephropathy. *Semin Nephrol*, **24**, 197–217.

Coppo R, Amore A (2004). Aberrant glycosylation in IgA nephropathy (IgAN). *Kidney Int*, **65**, 1544–7.

Gharavi AG, et al. (2000). IgA nephropathy, the most common cause of glomerulonephritis, is linked to 6q22-23. *Nat Genet*, **26**, 354–7.

Hsu SI, et al. (2000). Evidence for genetic factors in the development and progression of IgA nephropathy. *Kidney Int*, **57**, 1818–35.

Treatment

Appel GB, Waldman M (2006). The IgA nephropathy treatment dilemma. *Kidney Int*, **69**, 1939–44.

Barratt J, Feehally J (2006). Treatment of IgA nephropathy. *Kidney Int*, **69**, 1934–8.

Donadio JV Jr, et al. (1999). The long-term outcome of patients with IgA nephropathy treated with fish oil in a controlled trial. Mayo Nephrology Collaborative Group. *J Am Soc Nephrol*, **10**, 1772–7.

Floege J (2006). Is mycophenolate mofetil an effective treatment for persistent proteinuria in patients with IgA nephropathy? *Nat Clin Pract Nephrol*, **2**, 16–17.

Nakao N, et al. (2003). Combination treatment of angiotensin-II receptor blocker and angiotensin-converting-enzyme inhibitor in non-diabetic renal disease (COOPERATE): a randomised controlled trial. *Lancet*, **361**, 117–24.

Pozzi C, et al. (2004). Corticosteroid effectiveness in IgA nephropathy: long-term results of a randomized, controlled trial. *J Am Soc Nephrol*, **15**, 157–63.

Samuels JA, et al. (2004). Immunosuppressive treatments for immunoglobulin A nephropathy: a meta-analysis of randomized controlled trials. *Nephrology*, **9**, 177–85.

Tumlin JA, Hennigar RA (2004). Clinical presentation, natural history, and treatment of crescentic proliferative IgA nephropathy. *Semin Nephrol*, **24**, 256–68.

21.8.2 Thin membrane nephropathy

Peter Topham and John Feehally

Essentials

Thin membrane nephropathy is a common autosomal-dominant glomerular disorder that results in persistent microscopic haematuria and is pathologically characterized by the presence of diffuse and uniform thinning of the glomerular basement membrane. Recent genetic studies have identified mutations in the *COL4A3* and *COL4A4* genes in 40% of affected families. There is no specific treatment. Prognosis is excellent for most people, but a few cases with progressive renal impairment have been described.

Introduction and definition

Thin membrane nephropathy (TMN) is an autosomal-dominant condition diagnosed by examination of a renal biopsy by electron microscopy, which shows glomerular basement membranes (GBM) that are thin but otherwise morphologically normal. The term 'benign familial haematuria' was previously used in an era before the GBM abnormality had been identified.

Aetiology, genetics, and pathogenesis

The similarity between the basement membrane changes seen in early Alport's syndrome and those seen in TMN suggested the presence of a similar underlying genetic defect. It has been demonstrated that 40% of families with TMN have haematuria that segregates with the *COL4A3/COL4A4* locus, and identical mutations have been described in both TMN and autosomal recessive Alport's syndrome such that patients with TMN with these mutations can be considered as carriers of autosomal recessive Alport's syndrome. Approximately 20 different *COL4A3* and *COL4A4* mutations have been identified in families with TMN, most being single nucleotide substitutions that are different in each family. In some families linkage with the *COL4A3* and *COL4A4* genes has not been found; some of these cases may be explained by *de novo* mutations or incomplete penetrance, but it is probable that the remainder are due to the presence of further TMN loci.

Pathology

The pathological findings in TMN are limited to diffuse thinning of the GBM which is otherwise morphologically normal (Fig. 21.8.2.1). This contrasts with Alport's syndrome in which the GBM is thickened and lamellated and the normal lamina densa of the GBM is disrupted. The normal range for GBM thickness must be determined in each laboratory because of the influence of techniques used for fixing the biopsy, but normal GBM thickness is typically 350 to 450 nm, and a reduction to less than 250 nm involving over 50% of the GBM is diagnostic of TMN.

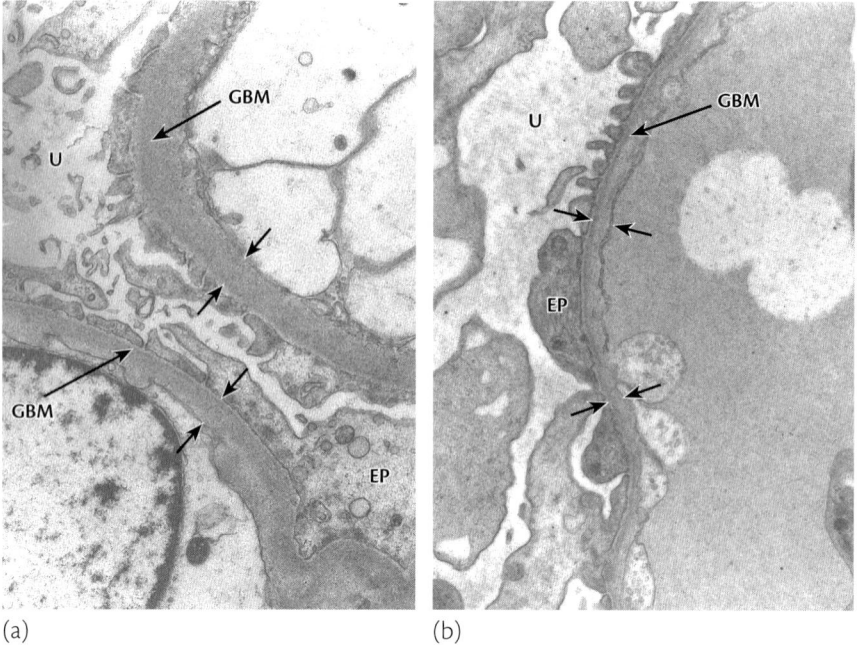

(a)   (b)

Fig. 21.8.2.1 Thin membrane nephropathy. Electron micrographs contrasting (a) GBM of normal thickness (350–450 nm) with (b) uniform membrane thinning (150–200 nm) in thin membrane nephropathy. Space between the heads of the short arrows defines GBM width. Ep, visceral epithelial cells; GBM, glomerular basement membrane; U, urinary space. Magnification ×20 000.

Clinical features

TMN is common and thought to be the diagnosis in 20 to 25% of patients presenting to a nephrologist with isolated microscopic haematuria. Autopsy and kidney transplant donor studies suggest it may be present in 5 to 9% of the population. It is an autosomal-dominant condition but may also be sporadic. Persistent microscopic haematuria is usually lifelong, and episodic macroscopic haematuria may also occur in up to one-fifth of patients. Flank pain occurs in up to 30% of patients and a small number of cases with loin-pain haematuria syndrome have been described. Hypertension may be more common than in the general population, although this is not confirmed in all studies. Proteinuria is uncommon and patients with nephrotic range proteinuria usually have a second, additional renal diagnosis. Progressive renal impairment is rare but has been described in several families. Deafness and other extrarenal manifestations seen in Alport's syndrome are absent. There is no specific treatment.

Differential diagnosis

TMN can only be distinguished from IgAN by renal biopsy. The coexistence of TMN and IgAN is well recorded and it is a matter of debate whether this merely represents the coincidence of two common glomerular diseases or is more than a chance occurrence.

TMN must be distinguished from Alport's syndrome (hereditary nephritis with deafness), of which the commonest form is X-linked. If there is a clear autosomal-dominant pattern of haematuria without renal insufficiency or extrarenal problems, then a clinical diagnosis of TMN may be established with reasonable confidence, but a renal biopsy in at least one family member is still preferable. Once the diagnosis is established in a kindred, biopsy is not required unless there are unexpected clinical changes. Differentiation from

the less common autosomal forms of Alport's syndrome is less straightforward. Subclinical deafness must be excluded by audiography if necessary, and the renal biopsy also requires careful assessment. In TMN there is uniform thinning, whereas early in the course of Alport's syndrome marked variability in GBM width is typical, even if the typical structural disruption of the GBM has not yet developed. Staining of GBM for the α-chains of type IV collagen is highly informative since in Alport's syndrome α3, α4, and α5 are absent, whereas normal α-chain distribution is preserved in TMN. Genetic testing for COL4A3 or COL4A4 mutations to diagnose TMN is clinically not practical because of the huge size of these genes, their frequent polymorphisms, and the likelihood of the existence of further gene loci.

Prognosis

The prognosis is excellent in the great majority of families with TMN, but there is a small but real risk of developing chronic renal failure, identified by the onset of proteinuria and hypertension. Long-term follow-up of those with TMN is therefore mandatory; urinalysis and measurement of blood pressure and renal function are recommended every 1 to 2 years.

Further reading

Dische FE, et al. (1990). Incidence of thin membrane nephropathy: morphometric investigation of a population sample. *J Clin Pathol*, **43**, 457–60.

Tiebosch AT, et al. (1989). Thin-basement-membrane nephropathy in adults with persistent hematuria. *New Engl J Med*, **320**, 14–18.

Nieuwhof CM, et al. (1997). Thin GBM nephropathy. Premature glomerular obsolescence is associated with hypertension and late onset renal failure. *Kidney Int*, **51**, 1596–601.

Tryggvason K, Patrakka J (2006). Thin basement membrane nephropathy. *J Am Soc Nephrol*, **17**, 813–22.

21.8.3 Minimal-change nephropathy and focal segmental glomerulosclerosis

Dwomoa Adu

Essentials

Minimal-change nephrotic syndrome

Minimal-change nephrotic syndrome (MCNS) is an immune-mediated condition, usually of unknown cause, but which can sometimes be associated with Hodgkin's disease or the use of nonsteroidal anti-inflammatory drugs. On light microscopy the glomeruli appear normal or small, and on electron microscopy there is effacement of epithelial-cell foot processes over the outer surface of the glomerular basement membrane. MCNS is the cause of about 80% of cases of nephrotic syndrome in children and 20% in adults.

Management and prognosis—treatment in adults is with prednisolone at an initial dose of 60 mg/day (then tapering), with 75% responding by 6 months. Up to 60% of patients who go into a remission have a relapse, and about 40% have frequent relapses, and in these patients treatment with cyclophosphamide induces a sustained remission in 60% over a 5-year period. Ciclosporin is also of benefit in frequent relapsers, but most patients relapse when this is discontinued. Just over 5% of patients remain nephrotic in the long term. Progression to renal failure is not expected and would call the diagnosis of MCNS into question.

Focal segmental glomerulosclerosis

Focal segmental glomerulosclerosis (FSGS) is not a specific disease entity but a histological lesion, often of unknown aetiology, which is characterized by segmental areas of glomerular sclerosis. It may be: (1) primary—which is by definition of unknown cause, but in about 30% of cases is associated with a circulating protein factor that causes an increase in glomerular permeability; or (2) secondary—the end product of a variety of pathological processes including glomerular hyperfiltration, healed glomerulonephritis, viral infection (HIV), and genetic mutation. Based on the site of the lesions and other histological features the primary condition can be divided into five variants: (1) perihilar; (2) glomerular tip; (3) collapsing variant; (4) cellular variant; and (5) 'not otherwise specified', when the other variants have been excluded. Most patients with FSGS present with nephrotic syndrome (FSGS is the diagnosis in 20% of adults with nephrotic syndrome), some with persistent proteinuria, and a few have haematuria as well as proteinuria.

Management and prognosis—patients with primary FSGS and nephrotic syndrome should be treated with prednisolone for 6 months (initially 60 mg/day, then tapering), and those who are resistant should receive ciclosporin for 26 to 52 weeks. Those who achieve a complete remission have a 5-year survival off dialysis of over 90%, as compared with about 50% of those who do not achieve remission. Patients with the glomerular tip lesion respond best; those with classic FSGS ('not otherwise specified') have an intermediate

response; and those with collapsing FSGS have the worst prognosis. The nephrotic syndrome recurs—often within days—after renal transplantation in 20 to 40% of patients with primary FSGS, leading to graft failure in approximately 50% of cases.

General considerations in the nephrotic syndrome

Classification of glomerulonephritis

The most helpful classification of glomerulonephritis is one based on histology. Careful clinical and pathological studies have established the histological patterns of glomerulonephritis in patients with a nephrotic syndrome inhabiting temperate regions of the world (Table 21.8.3.1). The aetiology and patterns of glomerulonephritis in tropical countries differ considerably and are considered elsewhere (see Chapter 21.11); discussion in this chapter refers to disease seen in temperate regions. Idiopathic glomerulonephritis accounts for 90% of all childhood cases of the nephrotic syndrome and for approximately 80% in adult patients. Although these histological changes are usually of unknown aetiology, they may also be secondary to well-defined aetiological factors.

General clinical approach

Children

In the original studies of the International Study of Kidney Diseases in Children (ISKDC), the diagnosis of minimal-change nephrotic syndrome (MCNS) was based on renal biopsies. From these and other studies it was established that for a child aged between 1 and 16 years with a nephrotic syndrome and highly selective proteinuria, and who did not have microscopic haematuria, hypertension, or renal impairment, the likely diagnosis was minimal-change nephropathy. When treated with steroids, such children had a greater than 90% chance of going into remission within 4 weeks. Based on these observations, children of this age with the features summarized above are no longer have a renal biopsy, but instead are treated with a trial of steroids. This leads to the term 'steroid-responsive nephrotic syndrome' of childhood and most, but not all, of such children will have MCNS. In neonates and in children under 1 year of age there is a high probability of the congenital nephrotic syndrome or diffuse mesangial sclerosis, and therefore renal biopsy should be considered as neither of these lesions respond to steroids.

Adults

Only 20% of adults with a nephrotic syndrome have MCNS and for that reason a renal biopsy is necessary to establish the type of glomerulonephritis. This provides useful information on the likelihood of response to treatment and also the prognosis. In skilled hands the dangers of renal biopsy are small and outweighed by those of steroid treatment given for disorders that will not respond.

General aspects of the management

Although steroids and immunosuppressants have been widely used in the treatment of the nephrotic syndrome, general measures remain an important part of the treatment of these disorders. Initial treatment of oedema is with salt restriction and, if there is hyponatraemia, with fluid restriction. Adults are commonly treated with loop diuretics such as furosemide, but this must be used with

Table 21.8.3.1 Histology of the nephrotic syndrome

Histology	Number of children[a] (%)	Number of adults[b] (%)
Minimal-change nephrotic syndrome	76	17
Mesangiocapillary glomerulonephritis	8	3
Focal segmental glomerulosclerosis	7	17
Proliferative (including diffuse mesangial proliferation)	2	0
Membranous	2	30
Other	5	9
Systemic lupus erythematosus	–	8
Amyloid	–	7
Diabetes	–	9

[a] From International Study of Kidney Disease in Children (1978). Prediction of histopathology from clinical and laboratory characteristics at time of diagnosis. *Kidney Int*, **13**, 159–65. [Excludes secondary causes of nephrotic syndrome, e.g. systemic lupus erythematosus, Henoch–Schönlein purpura; about 10%.]

[b] From Howie AJ, Pankhurst T, Sarioglu S, *et al.* Evolution of nephrotic-associated focal segmental glomerulosclerosis and relation to the glomerular tip lesion. Kidney Int 2005;67(3):987–1001.

care, particularly in children, because of the risk of volume depletion and consequent renal impairment.

Thromboembolic disease

The nephrotic syndrome may be complicated by venous and less commonly by arterial thromboembolism. Many coagulation abnormalities have been described, including raised serum levels of factors V, VII, and X, as well as fibrinogen and von Willebrand factor, and low serum levels of antithrombin III.

In adults the incidence of venous thrombosis has variously been reported in between 10 and 40% of patients, and less commonly in children (2–4%). Venous thrombosis may be complicated by pulmonary emboli. Renal vein thrombosis is now recognized as a complication of the nephrotic syndrome and not its cause, but is particularly common in membranous nephropathy, with a reported prevalence of about 30%, and it is also seen frequently in membranoproliferative glomerulonephritis, but less so in MCNS and focal segmental glomerulosclerosis (FSGS). Thrombosis may also occur in the arterial circulation, with the most common site being the femoral artery, often after this has been punctured.

The high incidence of thromboembolic disease raises the question of whether prophylactic anticoagulation is justified. A decision analysis justified prophylactic anticoagulation in patients with a nephrotic syndrome due to membranous nephropathy, but in the absence of data from randomized controlled trials of anticoagulation in the nephrotic syndrome it is difficult to make any firm recommendations. One could justify prophylactic anticoagulation in patients with an idiopathic nephrotic syndrome that is likely to be resistant to therapy, especially when the serum albumin is less than 20 g/litre. Obviously patients with identified thromboembolic disease should be given anticoagulants, with treatment continuing until the nephrotic syndrome is in remission.

Hypercholesterolaemia

Hypercholesterolaemia is a defining feature of the nephrotic syndrome and is due to increased levels of very low density cholesterol and low-density cholesterol. The mechanisms of this are unclear. One study showed that, as compared with matched controls (for smoking and hypertension), patients with a nephrotic syndrome had a relative risk for myocardial infarction of 5.5 and for death from coronary artery disease of 2.8. Statins (pravastatin or simvastatin) reduce low-density cholesterol and total cholesterol levels by 22 to 33% in patients with a nephrotic syndrome, but there are no studies showing that they confer survival benefit. Effects on triglyceride levels are less marked. Short-term studies report that statins are safe in patients with a nephrotic syndrome, but it is important to note that many statins are metabolized by the cytochrome P450 isoenzyme CYP3A4, and drugs that inhibit this enzyme such as ciclosporin increase drug levels and toxicity. This complication is less likely with pravastatin or fluvastatin.

Angiotensin blockade

Angiotensin converting enzyme (ACE) inhibitors and angiotensin-II receptor antagonists reduce proteinuria in patients with a nephrotic syndrome by up to 40%. There is evidence of an additive effect in proteinuria reduction with combined ACE inhibition and angiotensin-II blockade, but careful monitoring of serum potassium and renal function is required to make this approach safe.

Minimal-change nephropathy

Aetiology and pathogenesis

The responsiveness of the nephrotic syndrome of MCNS to steroids, cyclophosphamide, chlorambucil, and ciclosporin A is strong evidence that this disorder is immune mediated. The pathogenetic mechanisms remain obscure, but recent studies suggest a role for T lymphocytes, as originally suggested by Shaloub. Patients with MCNS show a T-lymphocyte repertoire that is biased towards a TH2 phenotype, with raised serum levels of IgE, interleukin (IL)-13 and IL-4. Subtractive cloning of T lymphocytes in remission and relapse show an increase in transcripts associated with T-cell receptor-mediated signalling. Numerous studies have examined major histocompatibility complex (MHC) associations with MCNS, but these are inconclusive, as are studies of polymorphisms in cytokine genes.

There is a well-recognized association between Hodgkin's lymphoma and MCNS. Nonsteroidal anti-inflammatory drugs can cause an interstitial nephritis, which in some cases is accompanied by a nephrotic syndrome with renal histology showing the changes of MCNS.

Pathology

The histological features are similar in both children and adults. On light microscopy the glomeruli appear normal or small (Fig. 21.8.3.1), and on electron microscopy there is effacement of epithelial-cell foot processes over the outer surface of the glomerular basement membrane. Some authors accept a minor degree of mesangial IgM deposition and mesangial proliferation as being consistent with this disorder.

Clinical features in children

Although this is textbook of adult medicine, an account of MCNS in children is appropriate because some will continue to be affected in adolescence and adulthood. MCNS is found in approximately 76% of children with an idiopathic nephrotic syndrome. Most affected

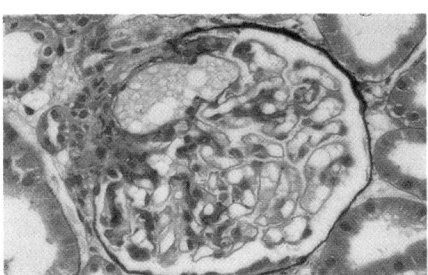

Fig. 21.8.3.1 Minimal-change nephropathy. The glomerulus looks normal on light microscopy. Periodic acid–methenamine silver staining, magnification × 64. By courtesy of Professor A. J. Howie.

children are under 6 years of age (80%), with a peak age of onset of 2 to 4 years. The condition is responsible for 59% of cases of nephrotic syndrome in those aged between 6 and 15 years. It is more common in boys than in girls, with a male to female childhood ratio of 2:1. Most cases are responsive to steroids, hence children with a nephrotic syndrome in temperate countries no longer require a renal biopsy and are defined on the basis of their responsiveness to steroids. In children (as in adults) a major problem is relapsing nephrotic syndrome, and recommended second-line treatments for this are (first) cyclophosphamide and (second) ciclosporin. The long-term prognosis for renal function is good in children.

Clinical presentation

The clinical presentation is with a nephrotic syndrome that is characterized by severe hypoalbuminaemia, with a serum albumin level of less than 10 g/litre in approximately 38% of cases. Microscopic haematuria is infrequent (22%), as is hypertension (9%). Renal impairment is infrequent at diagnosis, being found in approximately 10% of cases, and presentation in acute renal failure is rare. These children are prone to infections, in particular cellulitis and pneumococcal peritonitis.

Diagnosis

The role (or not) of renal biopsy has already been discussed. The current approach is to treat all children in temperate countries with a nephrotic syndrome with steroids, and then to define their illness as either steroid responsive or not steroid responsive. In most countries in the tropics, MCNS is uncommon in children and a renal biopsy is needed to establish the diagnosis.

Treatment

Steroids

Meta-analysis showed that treatment with prednisolone for 3 months or more during the first episode of a nephrotic syndrome in children significantly reduced the risk of relapse at 12 to 24 months, as compared with treatment for 2 months (relative risk (RR) 0.70; 95% CI 0.58–0.84). Treatment for 6 months as compared to 3 months reduced the number of subsequent frequent relapsers (RR 0.55; 95% CI 0.38–0.80). It is therefore recommended that children receive at least 6 weeks of treatment with daily oral prednisolone 60 mg/m^2, followed by 6 weeks of alternate day prednisolone 40 mg/m^2.

Frequent relapsers

In children presenting with a first episode of nephrotic syndrome, about 90% go into remission (meaning that proteinuria disappears)

with steroid treatment, but about 30 to 50% will have frequent relapses. An 8-week course of cyclophosphamide (2–3 mg/kg per day) or chlorambucil (0.2 mg/kg per day) significantly reduces the risk of further relapse as compared with prednisolone alone (RR 0.44; 95% CI 0.26–0.73 and RR 0.13; 95% CI 0.03–0.57, respectively). Approximately 50% of treated children are in remission at 2 years and 40% at 5 years. Cyclophosphamide has been carefully evaluated and is the drug of choice. Ciclosporin (6 mg/kg per day) is as effective as cyclophosphamide or chlorambucil, but the effect is maintained only during treatment. Levamisole has also been used and is more effective in reducing relapses than prednisolone alone (RR 0.60; 95% CI 0.45–0.79), but again the effect is restricted to the period of treatment. Levamisole can cause a reversible neutropenia.

Toxicity of cyclophosphamide and chlorambucil

The risk of gonadal toxicity is greater in boys than in girls. Gonadal toxicity occurs with chlorambucil at a cumulative dose of 8 to 10 mg/kg. The borderline dose for permanent gonadal toxicity with cyclophosphamide is a cumulative dose of 200 mg/kg. Bone marrow toxicity with both drugs means that the leucocyte count should be regularly measured during treatment. These drugs also increase the long-term risk of developing cancer. Other toxic side effects of cyclophosphamide include haemorrhagic cystitis and alopecia. At the doses and duration of treatment outlined above it is relatively safe.

Steroid-resistant nephrotic syndrome in children

The 10% or so of children who have steroid-resistant nephrotic syndrome will be found, if biopsied, to have MCNS, mesangioproliferative glomerulonephritis, or FSGS. In these patients ciclosporin is more effective in inducing complete remission than placebo or no treatment (RR for persisting nephrotic syndrome 0.64; 95% CI 0.47–0.88). There is no difference between oral cyclophosphamide and prednisolone compared with prednisolone alone (RR 1.01; 95% CI 0.74–1.36), or intravenous cyclophosphamide compared with oral cyclophosphamide (RR 0.09; 95% CI 0.01 1.39). Azathioprine and prednisolone are no better than prednisolone alone (RR 1.01; 95% CI 0.77–1.32). The ACE inhibitor fosinopril reduces proteinuria by 0.95 g/24 h (95% CI −1.21 to −0.69).

Long-term outcome

The risk of a future relapse is low for those children in whom the nephrotic syndrome goes into remission within 8 weeks of steroid therapy and who do not relapse for 6 months. Early relapse within 6 months is reported to be associated with a risk of relapses for up to 3 years, and approximately 5.5% of affected children continue to relapse into adult life, all of whom have presented with a nephrotic syndrome before the age of 6 years. Children with persistent proteinuria at 8 weeks have a 21% risk of developing endstage renal failure, and this increased to 35% if they still have proteinuria at 6 months. The long-term mortality rate in children ranges from 2.6 to 7.2%.

MCNS as part of a spectrum of glomerular disease

In temperate countries, most children with a nephrotic syndrome have MCNS, FSGS, or a mesangial proliferative glomerulonephritis (Table 21.8.3.1). Repeat renal biopsies performed if the character of illness changes, e.g. if patients become frequent relapsers, steroid dependent, or steroid resistant, sometimes show progression from MCNS or mesangial proliferative glomerulonephritis to FSGS.

One study showed that patients with presumed MCNS whose renal biopsies showed large glomeruli were more likely to develop FSGS. In general, those patients with MCNS who develop FSGS but remain steroid responsive have a good prognosis for renal function, while those who are steroid resistant develop progressive renal failure. The prognosis for renal function is therefore determined by the responsiveness to steroids and not by the histological lesion.

Clinical features in adults

About 20% of adults with a nephrotic syndrome have MCNS. The mean age of onset is 40 years, but the condition can occur at any age. The histology is identical to that found in children, with the exception of a higher incidence of globally sclerosed glomeruli that are a feature of ageing.

Clinical presentation

As in children, the clinical presentation is with a nephrotic syndrome, although this is not generally as severe. Profound hypoalbuminaemia (serum albumin level under 10 g/litre) is rare in adults. The disease is slightly more common in men than in women, with a male to female ratio of 1.3:1. More adults than children are hypertensive (30%), have microscopic haematuria (28%), and have renal impairment at diagnosis (60%). These abnormalities are more severe in patients aged over 60 years, who are also at particular risk of developing acute renal failure.

Diagnosis

A renal biopsy is essential to make the diagnosis in adults with a nephrotic syndrome.

Treatment

Treatment is with prednisolone at an initial dose of 60 mg/day, response to which takes longer than in children and is also less complete (75% at 6 months). Up to 60% of patients who go into a remission have a relapse, and about 40% have frequent relapses. In frequent relapsers treatment with cyclophosphamide induces a sustained remission in 60% over a 5-year period. Ciclosporin is also of benefit in frequent relapsers, but most patients relapse when this is discontinued. Patients who are steroid responsive or multiple relapsers are more likely to respond with complete or partial remissions (70–80%) than those who are resistant to steroids (40–50%).

Ciclosporin should be considered in those patients who develop steroid toxicity because they have multiple relapses or who are steroid dependent. However, relapses appear to recur with the same frequency after ciclosporin A has been discontinued as before, and for that reason it is still advisable to use cyclophosphamide as the first-choice treatment in patients with a multiple relapsing or steroid-dependent minimal-change nephropathy in the hope of inducing a sustained remission. Ciclosporin A appears to be effective at blood levels of between 100 and 200 ng/ml, and at these levels significant short-term nephrotoxicity and hypertension are uncommon. In this author's view, ciclosporin A can best be viewed as a steroid-sparing agent in patients with minimal-change nephropathy.

Mycophenolate mofetil and tacrolimus have also been reported in uncontrolled trials to be effective in inducing and maintaining remission in patients with steroid-resistant or relapsing minimal change disease, and in FSGS.

Long-term outcome

Approximately 6% of adult patients are still nephrotic after a mean follow-up of 7.5 years. The survival in patients over 60 years of age has been reported to be 50% at 10 years, and in those aged 15 to 59 years it was 90%.

Focal segmental glomerulosclerosis

FSGS was first described by Rich in 1957 at autopsy in children who died from a nephrotic syndrome. Fewer terms have generated more disagreement among pathologists and nephrologists as it is not a disease entity but a histological lesion that is often of unknown aetiology.

Types of FSGS

Secondary FSGS

Segmental scarring of glomeruli is the end product of a variety of pathological processes. These include, e.g. sickle cell anaemia, reduced renal mass, HIV infection, inherited mutations of podocyte-related genes, and immune complex nephritis (Table 21.8.3.2). Some of these causes lead to well-defined glomerular lesions, e.g. collapsing glomerulopathy in HIV-associated nephropathy, and prominent hilar segmental lesions in reduced renal mass.

Mutations in genes encoding slit diaphragm proteins are found in up to 20 to 30% of children with steroid-resistant nephrotic syndrome, but not in children with steroid-sensitive nephrotic syndrome, and they are uncommon in adults. Patients with a genetic cause for their nephrotic syndrome show no response to steroids or immunosuppressants, and these should not be used.

Patients with a secondary form of FSGS may have nephrotic or non-nephrotic range proteinuria. FSGS has also been found late on during the clinical course of patients with a nephrotic syndrome who had an initial renal biopsy showing MCNS.

Pathogenesis

Focal segmental sclerosis can develop from different pathogenic mechanisms in different experimental models, including toxic injury (puromycin nephropathy), immunological injury (anti-GBM nephritis), lupus-associated nephritis in NZB/NZW F1 mice, and hyperfiltration injury (five-sixths nephrectomy). Some of these models have clinical counterparts, and the diversity of pathogenic

Table 21.8.3.2 Aetiology of FSGS

Cause	Comment
Idiopathic	
Genetic	Mutations in α-actinin 4, podocin, nephrin, ion-receptor protein transient receptor potential cation channel 6 (*TRPC6*)
Healed glomerulonephritis	IgA nephropathy, vasculitis
Viral infection	HIV, parvovirus B19
Drugs	Heroin, pamidronate, lithium
Glomerular hyperfiltration (with or without reduced renal mass)	Reduced renal mass, reflux nephropathy, renal agenesis, sickle cell anaemia
Parasitic infection	*Schistosoma mansoni*

mechanisms may explain the variability in the clinical presentation and response to treatment.

Primary (idiopathic) FSGS

FSGS may be apparently idiopathic and found early on during the clinical course of patients with proteinuria or nephrotic syndrome. About 7% of children and 20% of adults with a nephrotic syndrome have FSGS. Even when FSGS is found early on in the course of a nephrotic syndrome there is no evidence to suggest that it represents a homogenous disease.

Pathogenesis

In about 30% of patients with primary FSGS there is a circulating factor that causes an increase in glomerular permeability *in vitro*, with the rapid development of heavy proteinuria following renal transplantation in 30 to 40% of patients with primary FSGS, strongly supporting the clinical importance of something in the circulation. The factor appears to be a protein with a molecular weight of between 30 and 50 kDa, and it is not an immunoglobulin. A 70% ammonium sulphate precipitate of serum from patients with recurrent FSGS following renal transplantation is reported to decrease tyrosine phosphorylation of the cytoskeleton-associated proteins focal adhesion kinase and paxillin, which may impair cell–cell interactions in the podocytes slit-pore junction leading to proteinuria.

Pathology

The histological lesions of FSGS comprise segmental areas of glomerular sclerosis with hyalinization of glomerular capillaries, the segmental areas usually being adherent to Bowman's capsule. In childhood FSGS, these lesions predominantly affect juxtamedullary glomeruli. One suggested classification is the Columbia FSGS classification, shown in Table 21.8.3.3; there is still a lack of agreement over the details, but it provides a useful framework for the management of patients. Several variants are described, based on the site of the segmental sclerosing lesion (perihilar variant and glomerular tip lesion), the presence of glomerular collapse (collapsing variant), and endocapillary cellularity with visceral epithelial cell hyperplasia (cellular variant), leaving 'FSGS (not otherwise specified)' when these have been excluded. This latter lesion is equivalent to classic nephrotic-associated FSGS, when the areas of segmental sclerosis are typically randomly distributed within the glomerular tuft, with a predilection for the hilar regions (Figs. 21.8.3.2, 21.8.3.3). Focal areas of tubular atrophy and interstitial nephritis are prominent. On immunofluorescence microscopy, deposits of IgM and complement C3 may be seen in the

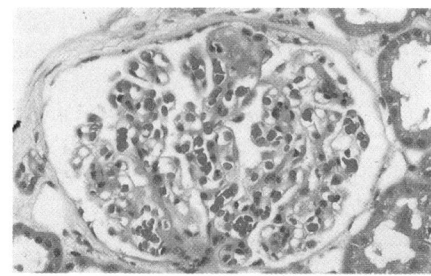

Fig. 21.8.3.2 Classic segmental sclerosing glomerulonephritis at an early stage. The glomerulus shows an erratic increase in mesangium with a segmental area of foamy cells and sclerosis opposite the vascular pole, next to the tubular origin. Haematoxylin and eosin staining, magnification ×50.
By courtesy of Professor A. J. Howie.

sclerotic areas. Electron microscopy shows diffuse foot-process effacement in apparently unaffected glomeruli.

Collapsing glomerulopathy

This is a type of focal segmental sclerosing glomerulonephritis, characterized by segmental or global collapse of glomerular capillaries with basement-membrane wrinkling and crowding of glomerular epithelial cells. These appearances represent a distinct subset of patients with FSGS, and were initially described in patients with HIV-associated nephropathy in the context of a severe nephrotic syndrome and rapid progression to endstage renal failure. Subsequent reports show that the condition may also be idiopathic. Presentation is with a nephrotic syndrome and renal impairment (70% of cases). Treatment with steroids or cytotoxic drugs has been ineffective in inducing remission or preventing the development of endstage renal failure. There is rapid deterioration of renal function and over 70% of patients are in endstage renal failure after a follow-up of 5 years.

Clinical presentation

Children

Approximately 7% of children presenting with an idiopathic nephrotic syndrome have FSGS. Boys and girls are equally affected and the peak age at onset is between 6 and 8 years. Most patients with FSGS (75%) present with a nephrotic syndrome, 20% have persistent proteinuria, and 5% haematuria as well as proteinuria. Clinically, these patients differ from children with MCNS in that two-thirds have microscopic haematuria, one-half have impaired renal function at diagnosis, and one-third are hypertensive. The proteinuria is usually poorly selective.

Table 21.8.3.3 Idiopathic FSGS, classification and treatment

Variant, based on site of segmental sclerosing lesion	Treatment
FSGS, not otherwise specified	Steroids if nephrotic
Perihilar variant	ACE inhibitors
Cellular variant	Steroids if nephrotic
Glomerular tip lesion	Steroids if nephrotic
Collapsing variant	ACE inhibitors

ACE, angiotensin converting enzyme.

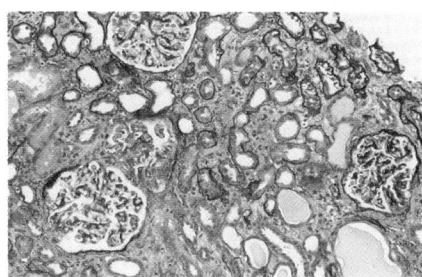

Fig. 21.8.3.3 Classic segmental sclerosing glomerulonephritis at a late stage. Four glomeruli show an erratic increase in mesangium and segmental lesions at various sites. Periodic acid–methenamine silver staining, magnification ×64.
By courtesy of Professor A. J. Howie.

Adults

The clinical presentation in adults does not differ in any significant respects from that in children. The mean age at onset is between 20 and 30 years, but FSGS has been found in patients aged over 70.

Treatment of primary ('classic') FSGS

The prognosis in patients with primary FSGS and proteinuria in the non-nephrotic range is good, and 80% of such patients survive for 10 years without developing endstage renal failure. These patients do not need treatment with either prednisolone or immunosuppressants and should be treated with general measures only.

The main problem is the treatment of patients with FSGS and a nephrotic syndrome. The different histopathological varieties of idiopathic FSGS vary in their clinical presentation, response to treatment, and progression to renal failure (Table 21.8.3.3). Patients with the glomerular tip lesion (probably an early form of classic FSGS) have a good response to prednisolone and only infrequently progress to endstage renal failure. Patients with classic FSGS ('not otherwise specified') have an intermediate response to prednisolone and are more likely to progress to renal failure. Patients with collapsing FSGS have the worst prognosis.

Steroids

There have been no randomized controlled trials of steroid therapy in FSGS. Cohort studies report that 40 to 60% of patients treated with a 6-month course of prednisolone go into complete or partial remission. Complete as well as partial remissions are associated with a significant reduction in the risk of developing endstage renal failure as compared with no remission. Adult patients who achieve a complete remission have a 5-year survival off dialysis of 94% as compared with 53% of those who do not achieve remission; children who achieve a complete remission have a 100% renal survival as compared with 92% with a partial remission and 47% with no remission. However, relapses are common and are found in 40 to 56% of patients.

All patients with primary FSGS and a nephrotic syndrome should be treated with prednisolone for 6 months. Children are treated with prednisolone at an initial dose of 60 mg/m^2 per day, and adults with a dose of 60 mg/day with tapering of the steroid dose.

Ciclosporin

Patients whose nephrotic syndrome is resistant to 6 months of treatment with prednisolone should receive ciclosporin for 26 to 52 weeks. A meta-analysis of three studies in patients with FSGS who were resistant to an 8-week course of prednisolone indicates that ciclosporin was more effective than prednisolone or placebo in inducing remission (RR for persisting nephrotic syndrome 0.34; 95% CI 0.18–0.69) and in preventing endstage renal failure (RR 0.45; 95% CI 0.21–0.97).

Other immunosuppressants

The evidence supporting the addition to prednisolone of cyclophosphamide or chlorambucil in the treatment of FSGS is not convincing.

ACE inhibition/angiotensin receptor blockade

In one retrospective study of childhood FSGS, angiotensin blockade (hazard rate (HR) 4.96; 95% CI 1.69–9.29) and calcineurin inhibitors (HR 2.54; 95% CI 1.20–5.35) were associated with remission of the nephrotic syndrome by univariate analysis, but by multivariate analysis only angiotensin blockade was significant (HR 3.35; 95% CI 1.42–9.75).

Prognosis

There is no difference in prognosis between adults and children. Adverse prognostic factors include tubulointerstitial fibrosis, renal impairment, and a failure of remission with treatment.

Recurrence after renal transplantation

The nephrotic syndrome recurs in 20 to 40% of patients with primary FSGS, often within days of renal transplantation, and this leads to graft failure in approximately 50% of cases. After recurrence in a first transplant the rate of recurrence in a subsequent transplant approaches 75%. Plasma exchange and protein immunoadsorption have resulted in a reduction of proteinuria or a remission of the nephrotic syndrome in some patients.

Further reading

General

Crew RJ, Radhakrishnan J, Appel G (2004). Complications of the nephrotic syndrome and their treatment. *Clin Nephrol*, **62**, 245–59.

Llach F (1985). Hypercoagulability, renal vein thrombosis, and other thrombotic complications of nephrotic syndrome. *Kidney Int*, **28**, 429–39.

Sarasin FP, Schifferli JA (1994). Prophylactic oral anticoagulation in nephrotic patients with idiopathic membranous nephropathy. *Kidney Int*, **45**, 578–85.

Minimal-change nephropathy

Bargman J (1999). Management of minimal lesion glomerulonephritis: evidence-based recommendations. *Kidney Int*, **55** Suppl 70, 3–16.

Day CJ, et al. (2002). Mycophenolate mofetil in the treatment of resistant idiopathic nephrotic syndrome. *Nephrol Dial Transplant*, **17**, 2011–13.

Durkan A, et al. (2005). Non-corticosteroid treatment for nephrotic syndrome in children. *Cochrane Database Syst Rev*, **2**, CD002290.

Ghiggeri GM, et al. (2004). Cyclosporine in patients with steroid-resistant nephrotic syndrome: an open-label, nonrandomized, retrospective study. *Clin Ther*, **26**, 1411–18.

Hodson EM, Habashy D, Craig JC (2006). Interventions for idiopathic steroid-resistant nephrotic syndrome in children. *Cochrane Database Syst Rev*, **2**, CD003594.

Hodson EM, et al. (2005). Corticosteroid therapy for nephrotic syndrome in children. *Cochrane Database Syst Rev*, **1**, CD001533.

International Study of Kidney Disease in Children (1978). Prediction of histopathology from clinical and laboratory characteristics at time of diagnosis. *Kidney Int*, **13**, 159–65.

Korbet SM, Schwartz MM, Lewis FJ (1988). Minimal-change glomerulopathy of adulthood. *Am J Nephrol*, **8**, 291–7.

Mak SK, Short CD, Mallick NP (1996). Long-term outcome of adult-onset minimal-change nephropathy. *Nephrol Dial Transplant*, **11**, 2192–201.

Mathieson PW (2003). Immune dysregulation in minimal change nephropathy. *Nephrol Dial Transplant*, **18** Suppl 6, vi26–9.

Nolasco F, et al. (1986). Adult-onset minimal change nephrotic syndrome: a long term follow-up. *Kidney Int*, **29**, 1215–23.

Ponticelli C, et al. (1993). Cyclosporin versus cyclophosphamide for patients with steroid-dependent and frequently relapsing idiopathic nephrotic syndrome: a multicentre randomized controlled trial. *Nephrol Dial Transplant*, **8**, 1326–32.

Tarshish P, et al. (1997). Prognostic significance of the early course of minimal changes nephrotic syndrome: report of the International Study of Kidney Disease in Children. *J Am Soc Nephrol*, **8**, 769–76.

Ueda N, Kuno K, Ito S (1990). Eight and 12 week courses of cyclophosphamide in nephrotic syndrome. *Arch Dis Childhood*, **85**, 1147–50.

Focal segmental glomerulosclerosis

Aucella F, *et al*. (2005). Molecular analysis of NPHS2 and ACTN4 genes in a series of 33 Italian patients affected by adult-onset nonfamilial focal segmental glomerulosclerosis. *Nephron Clin Pract*, **99**, c31–6.

Burgess E (1999). Management of focal glomerulosclerosis: evidence based recommendations. *Kidney Int*, **55** Suppl 70, 26–32.

D'Agati V (1994). The many masks of focal segmental glomerulosclerosis. *Kidney Int*, **46**, 1223–41.

D'Agati VD, *et al*. (2004). Pathologic classification of focal segmental glomerulosclerosis: a working proposal. *Am J Kidney Dis*, **43**, 368–82.

Detweiler R, *et al*. (1994). Collapsing glomerulopathy: a clinically and pathologically distinct variant of segmental glomerulosclerosis. *Kidney Int*, **45**, 1734–46.

Howie A, *et al*. (1993). Different clinicopathological types of segmental sclerosing glomerular lesions in adults. *Nephrol Dial Transplant*, **8**, 590–9.

Howie AJ, *et al*. (2005). Evolution of nephrotic-associated focal segmental glomerulosclerosis and relation to the glomerular tip lesion. *Kidney Int*, **67**, 987–1001.

Korbet S, Schwartz M, Lewis E (1994). Primary focal segmental glomerulosclerosis: clinical course and response to therapy. *Am J Kidney Dis*, **23**, 773–83.

Niaudet P, for The French Society of Pediatric Nephrology (1992). Comparison of cyclosporine and chlorambucil in the treatment of idiopathic nephrotic syndrome: a multicenter randomized controlled trial. *Pediatr Nephrol*, **6**, 1–3.

Rich A (1957). A hitherto undescribed vulnerability of the juxta-medullary glomeruli in lipoid nephrosis. *Bull Johns Hopkins Hosp*, **100**, 173–86.

Ruf RG, *et al*. (2004). Patients with mutations in NPHS2 (podocin) do not respond to standard steroid treatment of nephrotic syndrome. *J Am Soc Nephrol*, **15**, 722–32.

Savin V, *et al*. (1996). Circulating factor associated with increased glomerular permeability to albumin in recurrent focal segmental glomerulosclerosis. *N Engl J Med*, **334**, 878–83.

Stirling CM, *et al*. (2005). Treatment and outcome of adult patients with primary focal segmental glomerulosclerosis in five UK renal units. *QJM*, **98**, 443–9.

Troyanov S, *et al*. (2005). Focal and segmental glomerulosclerosis: definition and relevance of a partial remission. *J Am Soc Nephrol*, **16**, 1061–8.

21.8.4 Membranous nephropathy

Dwomoa Adu

Essentials

Membranous nephropathy, which accounts for 20 to 30% of cases of the nephrotic syndrome in adults, is defined histologically by the presence of subepithelial immune deposits on the outer surface of the glomerular basement membrane. The immune mechanisms that lead to this are uncertain, and most cases are of unknown cause (idiopathic), but the condition can be associated with autoimmune diseases (systemic lupus erythematosus), malignancy (in 10% of cases, most commonly lung and prostate cancer), drugs, and infections.

Management and prognosis—untreated membranous nephropathy evolves either to remission or to the development of chronic renal failure. Treatment is contentious, but: (1) steroids alone are of no benefit in inducing remission or preventing endstage renal failure; (2) cyclophosphamide or chlorambucil together with prednisolone lead to more complete and partial remissions than prednisolone alone, but have no beneficial effect in preventing endstage renal failure; (3) ciclosporin probably has similar effects to cyclophosphamide/chlorambucil with prednisolone.

Introduction

Membranous nephropathy accounts for between 20 and 30% of cases of the nephrotic syndrome in adults and about 2 to 5% of those in childhood. Histologically it is defined by the presence of subepithelial immune deposits on the outer surface of the glomerular basement membrane. No cause for this histological lesion is found in most patients living in temperate countries, and it is therefore termed idiopathic membranous nephropathy. A recent study however showed that 70% of these patients had autoantibodies to an M-type phospholipase A2 receptor found on podocytes. The aetiology of membranous nephropathy (where identifiable), genetic basis, frequency as a cause of the nephrotic syndrome, and clinical evolution with or without treatment differ substantially between studies from different countries. The treatment of idiopathic membranous nephropathy is unsatisfactory partly because there is a high rate of spontaneous remission and because the long term outcome of untreated membranous nephropathy is relatively good in terms of developing end stage renal failure.

Aetiology

In about 20 to 25% of adults and 35% of children with membranous nephropathy there is an identifiable associated condition (Box 21.8.4.1). The frequency of this varies in different parts of the world. Gold and penicillamine are no longer widely used and are now an infrequent cause; about 3% of all patients with membranous nephropathy have systemic lupus erythematosus; in northern Europe about 1% of patients with membranous nephropathy have positive hepatitis B serology, but this association is much more common in South-East Asia and in Africa, particularly in children.

Membranous nephropathy and malignancy

The association between membranous nephropathy and malignancy is well recognized. Approximately 10% of patients with membranous nephropathy have a malignancy, most commonly lung and prostate cancer (together accounting for 54% of cases). This is apparent at diagnosis in one-half of the patients and in the remainder within a year of diagnosis. The risk of cancer is higher in those aged over 65 years (25%) and lower in those aged less than 54 years (2%), such risks being significantly higher than an age-matched population with a standardized risk ratio of 9.8 (95% CI 5.5–16.2) for men and 12.3 (95% CI 4.5–26.9) in women. Remission of the cancer is associated with remission of the nephrotic syndrome, but the outlook for cancer-associated membranous nephropathy is poor, with an eightfold increase in mortality when compared with patients with idiopathic membranous nephropathy. Screening for malignancy should be considered in patients with membranous nephropathy who are aged over 65 years.

Box 21.8.4.1 Conditions associated with membranous nephropathy

Autoimmune diseases

◆ Systemic lupus erythematosus

◆ Rheumatoid arthritis

Drugs

◆ Gold

◆ Penicillamine

◆ Captopril

Malignancy

◆ Carcinoma (bronchus, colon, stomach, prostate, breast)

Infections

◆ Hepatitis B

◆ Syphilis

◆ Filariasis

◆ Leprosy

Miscellaneous

◆ Autoimmune thyroid disease

◆ Diabetes mellitus

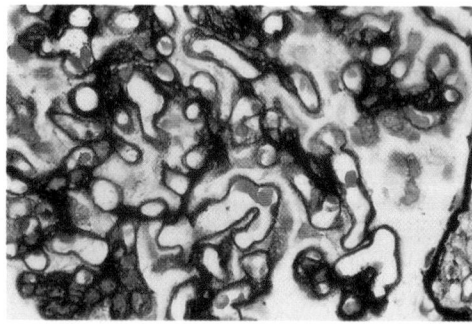

Fig. 21.8.4.1 Membranous nephropathy. There are regular short spikes on the outside of glomerular capillary loops. Periodic acid–methenamine silver staining, magnification ×80.

Pathogenesis

It has long been known that in rats, the administration of antibodies against renal tubular epithelial antigen leads to a membranous nephropathy that histologically resembles the human condition. The antibody responsible for this Heymann's nephritis in rats binds to an antigen called (megalin), which is found on renal tubular brush border and on glomerular epithelial cells. In glomeruli this leads to the development of subepithelial deposits through the *in situ* formation of immune complexes. However megalin is not found on human podocytes.

The observation that maternal-to-fetal transmission of antibodies to neutral endopeptidase (NEP), which binds to NEP on fetal podocytes, can lead to a membranous nephropathy provides an insight to the pathogenesis of this disease.

A recent study showed that 70% of patients with an apparently idiopathic membranous nephropathy had autoantibodies to the M-type phospholipase A_2 receptor (anti-PLA2R) which is found in podocytes. These antibodies were not present in secondary forms of membranous nephropathy due to lupus and hepatitis B. The anti-PLA$_2$R antibodies were predominantly IgG4 which is the isotype found in immune deposits in idiopathic membranous nephropathy. If confirmed these observations may allow monitoring of treatment and also explain the effect of immunosuppressants and B-lymphocyte depletion in membranous nephropathy.

Pathology

Idiopathic membranous nephropathy is characterized histologically by diffuse thickening of the glomerular basement on light microscopy, usually with argyrophilic subepithelial spikes (Fig. 21.8.4.1). On immunofluorescence or immunoperoxidase microscopy this thickening is shown to be due to the presence of immune deposits, usually consisting of IgG and complement C3, on the subepithelial surface of the glomerular basement membrane (Fig. 21.8.4.2). The size and extent of incorporation of immune deposits into the glomerular basement membrane on electron microscopy forms the basis of histological classification:

Stage 1: subepithelial deposits without spikes

Stage 2: large subendothelial deposits separated by spikes of basement membrane

Stage 3: deposits incorporated into a thickened basement membrane with many spikes

Stage 4: a very thick irregular basement membrane with no spikes and resorbed deposits

The presence of mesangial proliferation, mesangial immune deposits, and IgA and C1q on immunofluorescent microscopy raises the possibility that membranous nephropathy is secondary to systemic lupus erythematosus. Histology in malignancy-associated membranous nephropathy is characterized by a glomerular inflammatory infiltrate, which is uncommon in idiopathic membranous nephropathy.

Clinical presentation

In children, boys are affected 3 times as often as girls. In adults, most studies report a preponderance of men, with a male to female ratio of between 2:1 and 3:1. Most patients are aged between 30 and 50 years, although the condition has been described in patients aged up to 80 years. The clinical presentation is with the nephrotic syndrome in about 75% of cases, with the remainder having

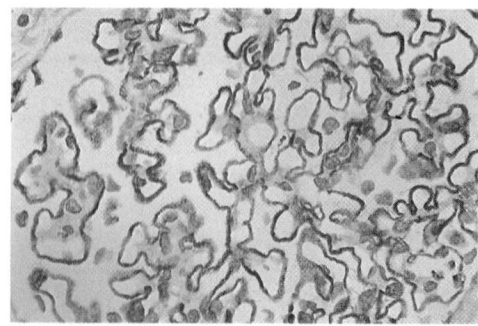

Fig. 21.8.4.2 Membranous nephropathy. Immunoperoxidase staining shows uniform granular deposits of IgG on the epithelial side of glomerular basement membranes. Magnification ×80.
By courtesy of Professor A. J. Howie.

proteinuria only. Microscopic haematuria is found in 50% of adults and 90% of children. Macroscopic haematuria is found in about 10 to 20% of children but is rare in adults. About 25 to 40% of adults and 6% of children are hypertensive at diagnosis, and between 10 and 30% of patients have a raised serum creatinine level.

Renal vein thrombosis

Patients with membranous nephropathy appear to be at particular risk of developing renal vein thrombosis, although this is not as high as originally suggested. Such patients are mostly asymptomatic, but they may present with pulmonary emboli. Detection is by Doppler ultrasonography of the renal veins, CT, or MRI. In practice a renal vein thrombosis should be looked for if there is a sudden deterioration of renal function in a patient with membranous nephropathy.

It is now known that renal vein thrombosis is a consequence of the hypercoagulable state of the nephrotic syndrome and not a cause of membranous nephropathy. Patients with a malignancy-associated membranous nephropathy are more likely to develop a thrombotic event (25% of patients).

Membranous nephropathy with a crescentic glomerulonephritis

About 5% of patients with a membranous nephropathy develop a crescentic glomerulonephritis with rapid deterioration of renal function. Most of these patients have antibodies to glomerular basement antigen or to neutrophil cytoplasmic antigens. Treatment has been with prednisolone and cyclophosphamide as for other patients with a crescentic glomerulonephritis.

Clinical evolution of untreated membranous nephropathy

In the long-term, untreated membranous nephropathy evolves either to remission or to the development of chronic renal failure. The rate at which either outcome occurs varies in different studies. After a mean follow-up of 4.5 to 6 years, between 9.5 and 22% of patients are in endstage renal failure, 9.5 to 19% have significantly impaired renal function, and 23 to 50% are in remission. The actuarial survival rate shows that about 75% of patients are alive at 10 years and 60% have functioning kidneys. Examination of the control untreated patients in recent treatment trials shows that, of 205 patients followed for between 2 and 5 years, 15% were in complete remission and 9% in endstage renal failure. Any study of treatment in membranous nephropathy must therefore address the difficulty of treating large numbers of patients who have little risk of developing endstage renal failure with toxic drugs.

Treatment options

The twin aims of treating membranous nephropathy are to induce remission of the nephrotic syndrome and to prevent the development of endstage renal failure. Despite several careful studies using steroids and immunosuppressants, there is still no agreement that these aims can be achieved.

Steroids

In the 1979 collaborative study, conducted in the United States of America, treatment with prednisolone reduced the rate at which renal function deteriorated. Two subsequent studies, the United Kingdom Medical Research Council (MRC) study and a Canadian study, showed no benefits in renal function or proteinuria. On balance these data indicate that short-term steroids are of no benefit in the treatment of membranous nephropathy.

Steroids and alkylating agents (chlorambucil or cyclophosphamide)

In an Italian multicentre study in which patients were randomized to symptomatic treatment only, or treatment with the following alternating regimen. Month 1: intravenous methylprednisolone, 1 g on each of 3 consecutive days, followed by oral methylprednisolone (0.4 mg/kg per day) or prednisolone (0.5 mg/kg per day) for 27 days; month 2: oral chlorambucil (0.2 mg/kg per day) alone for 1 month, the dose being lowered if the leucocyte count fell below 5×10^9/litre. Alternating monthly cycles of methylprednisolone and chlorambucil were given for a total of 6 months. After a mean follow-up of 31 to 37 months, significantly more treated than untreated patients were in remission (either total or partial): 23/32 (72%) versus 9/30 (30%). Furthermore, 8 of 30 controls showed a 50% rise in serum creatinine in contrast to none of the treated patients. The side-effects of treatment were minor and consisted of epigastric pain and leucopenia.

To answer the question of whether the beneficial effect of this regimen was due solely to the steroid component, a further study compared the effect of methylprednisolone alone with methylprednisolone and chlorambucil. Patients treated with the combination were more likely to have an early remission of the nephrotic syndrome, but this benefit was lost after 4 years. There was no difference in the rate of decline of renal function between the two therapies. A subsequent study compared cyclophosphamide and prednisolone with chlorambucil and prednisolone, the outcome being comparable and the former treatment had less toxicity.

Ciclosporin

Randomized controlled studies suggest that ciclosporin increases the likelihood of remission of the nephrotic syndrome, but not the risk of developing endstage renal failure.

Meta-analysis of treatment trials

There have been several meta-analyses on the treatment of idiopathic membranous nephropathy. These show that steroids alone are of no benefit in inducing remission or preventing endstage renal failure. Treatment with cyclophosphamide or chlorambucil together with prednisolone leads to more complete remissions (RR 2.37; 95% CI 1.32–4.25) and more partial remissions (RR 1.22; 95% CI 0.63–2.35) than prednisolone alone, but no beneficial effect is seen on endstage renal failure (RR 0.56; 95% CI 0.18–1.68). In this meta-analysis ciclosporin as compared with prednisolone or no treatment did not appear to be associated with any important clinical benefit. Our own analysis indicates that ciclosporin as compared with prednisolone or placebo increases the likelihood of remission, but does not reduce the risk of developing endstage renal failure.

Rituximab treatment of membranous nephropathy

Rituximab is a monoclonal antibody directed at the B lymphocyte antigen CD20 that leads to B lymphocyte depletion. Initially developed for the treatment of B lymphocyte lymphomas it has been widely used as an immunosuppressive agent in rheumatoid arthritis and also lupus nephritis. Several studies have examined the effect of rituximab in membranous nephropathy. A systematic review concluded that rituximab treatment of membranous nephropathy lead to a complete remission of 15 to 20% and partial remission of 35 to 40% with few side effects. The role of rituximab in the treatment of membranous nephropathy with a nephrotic syndrome remains to be established by randomized controlled trials.

Treatment: a pragmatic approach

The patient who remains nephrotic

Given that 40 to 60% of patients with membranous nephropathy and nephrotic syndrome go into spontaneous remission, our current strategy is to wait for 12 to 18 months and then only treat those patients who are still nephrotic with ciclosporin, or with prednisolone and cyclophosphamide. An ongoing MRC randomized controlled trial is testing the efficacy of this approach.

The patient with deteriorating renal function

Drug-induced interstitial nephritis, renal vein thrombosis, and crescentic glomerulonephritis should be excluded. In patients with deteriorating renal function due to the progression of membranous nephropathy, several uncontrolled studies have suggested that treatment with intravenous methylprednisolone, or with oral prednisolone and chlorambucil or cyclophosphamide, may reverse the rate of decline in renal function. These studies are difficult to interpret as renal function may stabilize or improve without treatment in some cases, but if the patient's renal function seems to be deteriorating inexorably it is hard to stand by and simply observe. Frank discussion of the uncertainties with the patient is required and most will decide that they wish to pursue a course of treatment, which the physician may need to advise stopping if the burden of side effects seems likely to outweigh any benefit.

Prognosis

Identifying those patients who at the onset of membranous nephropathy are likely to have a poor outcome for renal function would be helpful in deciding who to treat. Most studies show that adverse risk factors for the development of renal failure include male sex, a nephrotic syndrome, persistent heavy proteinuria, tubulointerstitial fibrosis, renal impairment at diagnosis, and deterioration of renal function in the first 2.5 years after diagnosis. In particular, patients with proteinuria of over 6 g/day for longer than 9 months were found to have a 55% likelihood of progressing to renal failure. Children appear to do better than adults; in one study, 42% of children went into complete remission and only 10% developed endstage renal failure after a mean follow-up of 4 years.

Further reading

Beck, L. H, et al. (2009). M-type phospholipase A2 receptor as target antigen in idiopathic membranous nephropathy. N Engl J Med, 361, 11–21.

Bomback, A. S, et al. (2009). Rituximab therapy for membranous nephropathy: a systematic review. Clin J Am Soc Nephrol, 4, 734–44.

Cattran D (2005). Management of membranous nephropathy: when and what for treatment. J Am Soc Nephrol, 16, 1188–94.

Honkanen E, Tornroth T, Gronhagen-Riska C (1992). Natural history, clinical course and morphological evolution of membranous nephropathy. Nephrol Dial Transplant, 7 Suppl 1, 35–41.

Imperiale T, Goldfarb S, Berns J (1995). Are cytotoxic agents beneficial in idiopathic membranous nephropathy? A meta-analysis of the controlled trials. J Am Soc Nephrol, 5, 1553–8.

Laluck BJ Jr, Cattran DC (1999). Prognosis after a complete remission in adult patients with idiopathic membranous nephropathy. Am J Kidney Dis, 33, 1026–32.

Lefaucheur C, et al. (2006). Membranous nephropathy and cancer: epidemiologic evidence and determinants of high-risk cancer association. Kidney Int, 70, 1510–17.

Muirhead N (1999). Management of idiopathic membranous nephropathy: evidence-based recommendations. Kidney Int, 55 Suppl 70, S47–55.

Pei Y, Cattran D, Greenwood C (1992). Predicting chronic renal insufficiency in idiopathic membranous nephropathy. Kidney Int, 42, 960–6.

Ruggenenti, P, et al. (2003). Rituximab in idiopathic membranous nephropathy: a one-year prospective study. J Am Soc Nephrol, 14, 1851–7.

Schiepatti A, et al. (1993). Prognosis of untreated patients with idiopathic membranous nephropathy. N Engl J Med, 329, 85–9.

Schieppati A, et al. (2004). Immunosuppressive treatment for idiopathic membranous nephropathy in adults with nephrotic syndrome. Cochrane Database Syst Rev, 4, CD004293.

Troyanov S, et al. (2004). Idiopathic membranous nephropathy: definition and relevance of a partial remission. Kidney Int, 66, 1199–205.

21.8.5 Proliferative glomerulonephritis

Peter W. Mathieson

Essentials

Proliferative glomerulonephritis—which occurs in many conditions—describes the finding of increased cellularity of the glomerulus, which may be due to proliferation of intrinsic glomerular cells, infiltration of leucocytes, or both. Patients will typically have haematuria, and this may be associated with proteinuria and/or impairment of excretory renal function and/or hypertension. Different subtypes of proliferative glomerulonephritis are recognized:

1 Proliferation of mesangial cells—most commonly seen in immunoglobulin A (IgA) nephropathy (see Chapter 21.8.1), but rare variants without IgA deposition may feature IgM or complement 3 (C3) deposition or no immune reactants. The behaviour of these variants is uncertain, but responsiveness to corticosteroid treatment is often seen.

2 Endocapillary proliferation—glomerular hypercellularity is confined within the glomerular capillary tuft; best described in the form of poststreptococcal glomerulonephritis, but can be provoked by other infections; treatment is directed at eradicating underlying infection; most cases recover, but haematuria and proteinuria can persist, and some cases (particularly nonstreptococcal) develop chronic renal failure.

3 Diffuse proliferative glomerulonephritis—some 'idiopathic' cases have no preceding history of infection, no evidence of other disease, and no atypical histological features; prognosis and treatment are uncertain.

4 Extracapillary proliferation—produces crescentic glomerulonephritis (discussed in Chapters 21.8.1, 21.8.4, and 21.8.7).

Introduction

The term proliferative glomerulonephritis covers a variety of conditions (Box 21.8.5.1) where there is increased cellularity of the glomerulus, either due to the proliferation of resident glomerular cells, or infiltration of leucocytes, or both. The proliferative changes may be focal (that is to say, they only affect some glomeruli) and/or segmental (in other words, only affecting parts of each glomerulus). Many of these entities are considered in other chapters, and only those not covered elsewhere (see Box 21.8.5.1) will be described here.

Mesangial proliferative glomerulonephritis

Patients will typically have haematuria and this may be associated with proteinuria and/or impairment of excretory renal function and/or hypertension. Most patients whose renal biopsies show only mesangial proliferation will have IgA nephropathy (see Chapter 21.8.1), but a few will have no IgA deposits and their classification is not straightforward; possibilities include IgM nephropathy, 'idiopathic' mesangial proliferative glomerulonephritis, and the recently described C3 glomerulonephritis.

IgM nephropathy

There is continuing controversy about this diagnostic entity. In patients with nephrotic syndrome, if the only abnormalities on the renal biopsy are in the mesangial region, with proliferation of mesangial cells and deposition of IgM, many authorities would

---

> **Box 21.8.5.1** Proliferative glomerulonephritis
>
> **1 Proliferation of mesangial cells**
> - IgA nephropathy ± Henoch–Schönlein disease
> - IgM nephropathy[a]
> - Systemic lupus erythematosus
> - Idiopathic[a]
>
> **2 Endocapillary proliferation**
> - Postinfectious glomerulonephritis[a]
> - Infective endocarditis
> - Other infections, including leprosy
>
> **3 Extracapillary proliferation (crescent formation)**
> - Small vessel vasculitides (Wegener's/microscopic polyangiitis)
> - Antiglomerular basement membrane disease
> - Henoch–Schönlein disease
> - Systemic lupus erythematosus
> - HIV nephropathy (proliferation of podocytes)
> - Idiopathic (rare)
>
> **4 Diffuse proliferative glomerulonephritis (may include elements of 1–3)**
> - Systemic lupus erythematosus
> - Idiopathic[a]
>
> [a]Conditions discussed in this chapter.

---

assign a diagnosis of minimal-change nephropathy (see Chapter 21.8.3) and advocate treatment with corticosteroids. Some would consider that these morphological features are markers for a poorer prognosis and a reduced likelihood of a response to corticosteroids, but others would consider the patient to have a completely different disease entity and give a diagnosis of IgM nephropathy.

Some of this confusion may be explained by methodological factors: assessment of the degree of mesangial hypercellularity is subjective, and reagents to detect IgM are notoriously unreliable since they may give high background staining. Mesangial IgM has been found in up to 60% of 'normal' kidneys donated for transplantation, and the diagnostic significance of IgM is also cast into doubt by its presence in over 75% of controls as well as in patients with various other forms of glomerulonephritis.

The best support for the existence of IgM nephropathy, as an entity distinct from minimal-change nephropathy, comes from the occurrence of a familial form; from the identification of this pattern of glomerular injury in patients who, after lengthy follow-up, have an appreciable risk of developing impaired excretory kidney function; and from a recent case report in which there was recurrence of IgM nephropathy after renal transplantation.

Idiopathic mesangial proliferative glomerulonephritis

This term may be applied if there is isolated mesangial proliferation without deposition of IgA or IgM. Again there is overlap with minimal-change nephropathy; if the patient presents with nephrotic syndrome, most nephrologists would not allow the presence of mesangial proliferation to deflect them from treating the patient with corticosteroids, although there is evidence that the presence of this histological finding is associated with a poorer response rate. If, however, the patient has haematuria and/or hypertension and/or impaired kidney function, none of which are typical features of minimal-change nephropathy, it is difficult to resist the need for another separate diagnostic category. Unfortunately there are no informative studies to guide treatment or give information on prognosis.

Glomerulonephritis with C3 deposition

A recent report describes a form of proliferative glomerulonephritis in which the only immune reactant detected in the glomerulus is deposition of C3, the third component of complement. This lesion was associated in some cases with mutations in complement regulatory genes factor H and/or factor I, and so may have aetiological similarities with other forms of glomerulonephritis seen in association with such genetic variants, i.e. haemolytic uraemic syndrome (see Chapter 21.10.5) and mesangiocapillary glomerulonephritis (see Chapter 21.8.6).

Endocapillary proliferative glomerulonephritis

Patients will often have impaired excretory function, haematuria, proteinuria, and hypertension, sometimes presenting acutely as a 'nephritic syndrome'. On renal biopsy, the glomerular hypercellularity is confined within the glomerular capillary tuft, which is probably due to the combination of a proliferation of intrinsic (endothelial and mesangial) cells together with an infiltration of inflammatory cells. This can occur in systemic lupus erythematosus (see Chapter 21.10.3) and as a complication of a variety of infections (see Chapter 21.10.7). Only postinfectious glomerulonephritis will be considered here, with the main focus on poststreptococcal glomerulonephritis.

Poststreptococcal glomerulonephritis

Most infection-related glomerulonephritis occurs concurrently with the infection. By contrast, postinfectious glomerulonephritis (of which poststreptococcal glomerulonephritis is the most frequent and best characterized) occurs, as the name implies, after the infection. In poststreptococcal glomerulonephritis the delay between the inciting infection and the onset of the renal complication may be long enough for the infection to have been forgotten, and this may contribute to diagnostic confusion. The typical case follows infection with streptococci of Lancefield group A (β-haemolytic streptococci, *Streptococcus pyogenes*), either causing pharyngitis or skin infection such as cellulitis or impetigo. Children are most commonly affected. Around 2 weeks later, sometimes longer after skin infections, the patient develops nephritis which may be sufficiently acute and severe to cause a nephritic syndrome with oliguria, hypertension, and oedema. If a renal biopsy is performed, it will show diffuse proliferative glomerulonephritis, with infiltration by neutrophil polymorphs often particularly prominent (Fig. 21.8.5.1). Immunohistology shows deposition of IgG, IgM, and complement in the mesangial and subepithelial areas, and electron microscopy shows large subepithelial deposits ('humps').

Serological tests

There are typical serological features which give clues to the pathogenesis and these include antibodies to streptococcal antigens and evidence of activation of the complement cascade. The antibodies are IgG; reactivity with numerous streptococcal antigens has been reported including streptolysin O, deoxyribonuclease B, hyaluronidase, and streptokinase. Antistreptolysin O is the most useful diagnostic test after pharyngitis; anti-Dnase B is best after skin infections.

Hypocomplementaemia (low C3 in most cases, also low C4 in some) reflects activation of both the alternative and the classic pathways (the complement system is discussed in more detail in Chapter 21.8.6). In poststreptococcal glomerulonephritis the alternative complement pathway may be activated by bacterial antigens and/or by IgG autoantibodies called nephritic factors, which resemble those seen in mesangiocapillary glomerulonephritis; the classic pathway may be activated by circulating immune complexes.

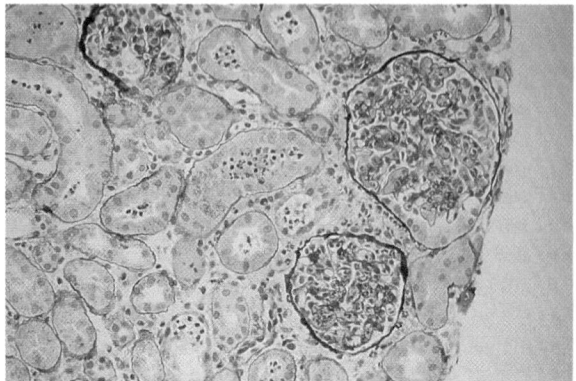

Fig. 21.8.5.1 Poststreptococcal glomerulonephritis.

Pathogenesis

It is believed that the pathogenesis of poststreptococcal glomerulonephritis can be explained as follows: streptococcal antigens are deposited in glomeruli by virtue of some aspect of their charge, size, or other physicochemical characteristics, during the early phase of the infection. After the 10 to 14 days necessary for the host to mount an immune response to the bacterial infection, circulating antibody appears and binds to the 'planted' antigens in the glomeruli. Complement is activated, leucocytes are attracted (by complement-activation products C3a and C5a among other chemoattractants), and an inflammatory reaction is provoked, injuring the glomeruli.

The precise nature of the streptococcal antigens that act in this nephritogenic manner remains controversial; only certain serological types of streptococci (referred to as M types and serotyped according to cell-wall protein antigens) are capable of inciting glomerulonephritis, but the M proteins themselves are not believed to be nephritogenic. In addition to the planted antigen mechanism, streptococci may lead to glomerulonephritis by their other complex effects on the immune response. These include the direct activation of T cells by a superantigen effect, whereby M proteins can bind to particular Vβ regions of the T-cell receptor and activate families of T cells sharing receptors of this 'family'. Antigenic crossreactivity ('molecular mimicry') similar to that thought to be responsible for rheumatic fever may also occur, so that antistreptococcal antibodies crossreact with, and therefore bind to, renal autoantigens such as laminin and collagen.

Management

Poststreptococcal glomerulonephritis is less common in the developed than in the developing world, possibly influenced by socioeconomic factors. Its general importance lies in the fact that early recognition allows appropriate treatment, with the prognosis often being very good, and also that the immunopathological mechanisms outlined above may be instructive in understanding other forms of glomerulonephritis where the inciting stimulus is not so evident.

Treatment of patients with poststreptococcal glomerulonephritis should be directed at eradicating the infection (a 10-day course of penicillin or erythromycin is advised even if the original infection appears to have resolved) and providing symptomatic relief of the consequences of the acute nephritis including aggressive treatment of hypertension, salt and water restriction with or without diuretics for oedema, and dialysis if necessary (which is uncommon). Recovery is the rule, although haematuria and proteinuria may persist, and some authors believe that in the long-term there is a risk of chronic renal failure.

Nonstreptococcal postinfectious proliferative glomerulonephritis

It is apparent that similar clinical and histopathological features occur without evidence of prior streptococcal infections in modern series of patients with infection-related glomerulonephritis. In one series from France describing 76 adult patients from suburban boroughs of Paris, including a high proportion of alcoholics and intravenous drug abusers, staphylococci and Gram-negative organisms were more commonly isolated than streptococci, and a poor renal prognosis was reported.

The importance of knowledge of local variations in prevalent infections or other environmental factors is further emphasized by the recent description of a novel form of eosinophilic

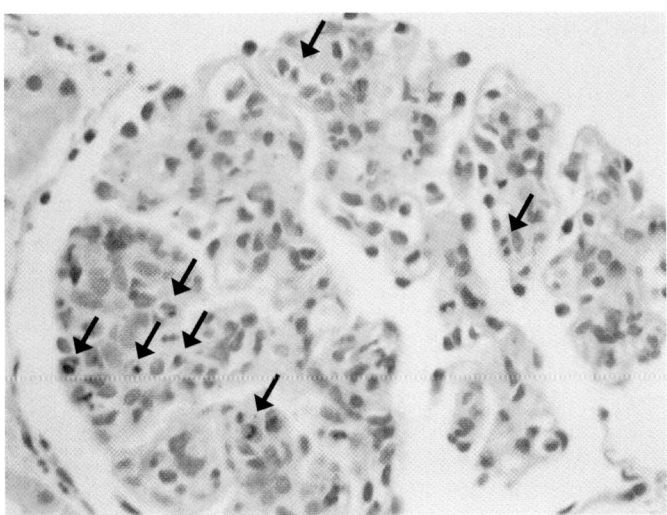

Fig. 21.8.5.2 Eosinophilic proliferative glomerulonephritis. Numerous eosinophils (some arrowed) expand the glomerulus.

glomerulonephritis in a large series of children from rural Uganda (Fig. 21.8.5.2). The cause of this is not known, but it does not seem to be attributable to streptococcal infection, or to HIV or malaria which are also locally prevalent. Symptomatic treatment allows most children to recover.

The basic principles of management of infection-related glomerulonephritis apply to these series including eradication of the infection if possible, supportive care during the acute phase, and moves towards prevention whenever possible by detailed investigation of underlying causes.

Idiopathic diffuse proliferative glomerulonephritis

A few cases will have no preceding history of infection, no evidence of lupus, and/or atypical features on the renal biopsy. These may be assigned the unsatisfactory 'idiopathic' sobriquet, with the implication that the prognosis and the appropriate treatment are uncertain.

Further reading

Ji-Yun Y, *et al.* (1984). No evidence for a specific role of IgM in mesangial proliferation of idiopathic nephrotic syndrome. *Kidney Int*, **25**, 100–6.

Myllymäki J, *et al.* (2003). IgM nephropathy: clinical picture and long-term prognosis. *Am J Kidney Dis*, **41**, 343–50.

Oliveira DBG (1997). Poststreptococcal glomerulonephritis: getting to know an old enemy. *Clin Exp Immunol*, **107**, 8–10.

Salmon AH, *et al.* (2004). Recurrence of IgM nephropathy in a renal allograft. *Nephrol Dial Transplant*, **19**, 2650–2.

Scolari F, *et al.* (1990). Familial IgM nephropathy: a morphologic and immunogenetic study of three pedigrees. *Am J Nephrol*, **10**, 261–8.

Servais A, *et al.* (2007). Primary glomerulonephritis with isolated C3 deposits: a new entity which shares common genetic risk factors with hemolytic uremic syndrome. *J Med Genet*, **44**, 193–9.

Walker A, *et al.* (2007). Eosinophilic glomerulonephritis in children in south western Uganda. *Kidney Int*, **71**, 569–73.

Watanabe-Ohnishi R, *et al.* (1994). Characterization of unique human TCR V beta specificities for a family of streptococcal superantigens represented by rheumatogenic serotypes of M protein. *J Immunol*, **152**, 2066–73.

21.8.6 Mesangiocapillary glomerulonephritis

Peter W. Mathieson

Essentials

Mesangiocapillary glomerulonephritis (MCGN)—which is synonymous with membranoproliferative glomerulonephritis—is diagnosed when renal biopsy reveals glomeruli with a characteristic lobular appearance. Immunohistology and electron microscopy allow further subdivision into three patterns, types I, II (also called dense deposit disease), and III. Clinical presentation is with proteinuria (sometimes nephrotic syndrome) and/or haematuria; hypertension and/or impairment of excretory kidney function may be associated.

Aetiology and pathogenesis—MCGN can be a primary idiopathic form of glomerulonephritis, but also (especially type I) occurs as a secondary complication, especially of infections, e.g. hepatitis C virus, or of systemic diseases, e.g. systemic lupus erythematosus. All forms are characterized by activation of the complement system, with the pattern of activation differing in the three types. There is good evidence that complement activation is of pathogenetic importance, at least in type II MCGN, which is closely associated with the presence of an IgG autoantibody called nephritic factor that activates the alternative pathway of complement. Such activation may also directly injure fat cells (leading to association with partial lipodystrophy), and possibly be responsible for drusen in the eye, which is associated with age-related macular degeneration.

Management and prognosis—the prognosis may be good if an underlying cause can be identified and eradicated, but there is no proven form of therapy for the 'primary' forms of the disease, although all patients should have their blood pressure aggressively managed. Overall, renal survival in MCGN is about 50% at 10 years from diagnosis. There is a high rate of recurrence of the disease in renal transplants.

Introduction

Mesangiocapillary glomerulonephritis (MCGN) is synonymous with membranoproliferative glomerulonephritis, the terms describing a morphological pattern of glomerular injury in which there is diffuse thickening of the glomerular basement membrane associated with increased cellularity, giving a characteristic lobular appearance to the glomeruli (Fig. 21.8.6.1). Renal biopsy is required for diagnosis.

As with other forms of glomerulonephritis, such as membranous nephropathy (see Chapter 21.8.4), the appearances on light microscopy are indistinguishable whether the lesion occurs as a primary idiopathic renal disease or secondary to an extrarenal/systemic disorder. Extra information is obtained with the use of immunohistology and electron microscopy, which allow further subdivision into three patterns. In type I MCGN there is typically IgG, IgM, and complement C3 in mesangial areas as well as along the glomerular capillary loops in a subendothelial or intramembranous location,

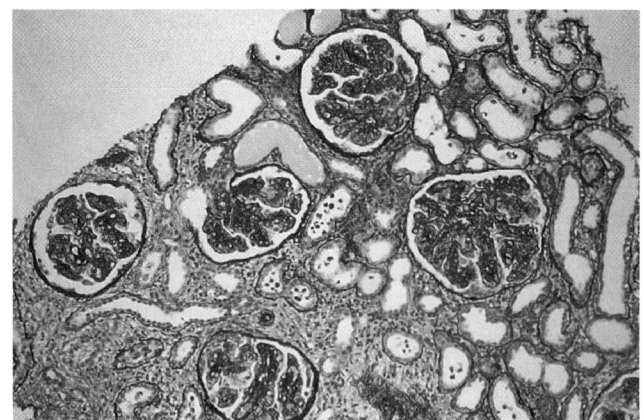

Fig. 21.8.6.1 MCGN. Note characteristic lobular appearance of expanded glomerulus.

and electron microscopy shows discrete electron-dense deposits in these regions. In type II MCGN there is typically no immunoglobulin deposited, but C3 is detected in a linear distribution along the capillary loops and often also in tubular and vascular basement membranes. Electron microscopy shows typical thick linear electron-dense material along these basement membranes, giving rise to the other term for type II MCGN, which is '(linear) dense deposit disease' (Fig. 21.8.6.2). Type III MCGN is similar to type I, excepting that there are subepithelial as well as subendothelial deposits and there may be disruption of the glomerular basement membrane with accumulation of new basement membrane material in layers. Most secondary forms of MCGN are of the type I pattern.

Pathogenesis

MCGN is typically associated with activation of the complement system and there is evidence, at least for some types of MCGN, that complement dysregulation may directly cause the renal lesion. The pattern of activation differs in the three subtypes of MCGN.

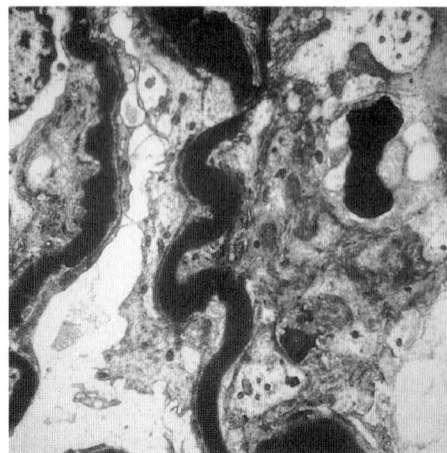

Fig. 21.8.6.2 Electron micrograph of type II MCGN, 'dense deposit disease'. Note linear electron-dense material along the glomerular basement membrane.

The complement system

Complement activation can occur via two main pathways, the classical and the alternative pathways (Fig. 21.8.6.3). A more recently described third pathway, the lectin or mannan-binding pathway, yields similar results to classical pathway activation and is of unknown relevance to nephritis. In general, classical pathway activation leads to depletion of plasma C3 and C4, whereas alternative pathway activation leads to a low C3 with normal C4. This is an oversimplification, since both C3 and C4 are acute-phase reactants whose synthesis is up-regulated in inflammation, hence there may be considerable complement activation without depletion of circulating levels due to compensation by increased production. Further complexity is introduced by the fact that genetic deficiencies of C4 are common. There are four C4 genes encoded within the major histocompatibility complex on chromosome 6, and it is estimated that only 60% of the population has all four normal C4 genes, with one or more null alleles commonly present, which result in no C4 protein production and therefore a reduction of circulating C4 concentration. Thus a single low C4 level must be interpreted with caution unless a previous 'normal' result is available for that individual; serial measurements are helpful since they give an indication of the level of C4 consumption.

The classical pathway is activated predominantly by immune complexes, which are immunoglobulin molecules linked to antigen. The alternative pathway is more concerned with host defence, being activated by bacteria or other foreign surfaces, and existing in a state of constant low-level activity, so-called tickover. This state of constant activity demands tight regulation to avoid excessive complement activation, and this is achieved by regulatory proteins factor H and factor I.

The classical and alternative pathways converge at the point at which C3 is cleaved. The enzyme formed by classical pathway activation is called the classical pathway C3 convertase, and denoted C4b2a. The enzyme formed by alternative pathway activation is the alternative pathway C3 convertase, denoted C3bBb. Each of these enzymes leads to the cleavage of C3, releasing C3a and leading to the formation of a C5 convertase enzyme which cleaves C5, thereby releasing C5a and leading to the formation of C5b–9, the membrane-attack complex (MAC).

Complement activation in MCGN

In MCGN, the pattern of complement activation (and therefore possibly the pathogenesis) is different in each of the three forms. In type I, the complement activation predominantly affects the classical pathway (causing low levels of both plasma C3 and C4); in type II it is the alternative pathway which is predominantly affected (low C3 with normal C4); and in type III there is activation of the terminal pathway leading to depletion of C5, sometimes associated with mild depletion of C3 and/or C4.

Secondary MCGN may occur in systemic lupus erythematosus, cryoglobulinaemia with or without hepatitis C, other viral infections such as hantavirus, bacterial infections such as infective endocarditis or other chronic bacteraemic states (e.g. 'shunt nephritis', originally described with infected ventriculoatrial shunts), or in association with neoplasms. In each of these situations there is activation of the classical pathway, which is presumed to be due to circulating immune complexes, and this is associated with a type I MCGN pattern.

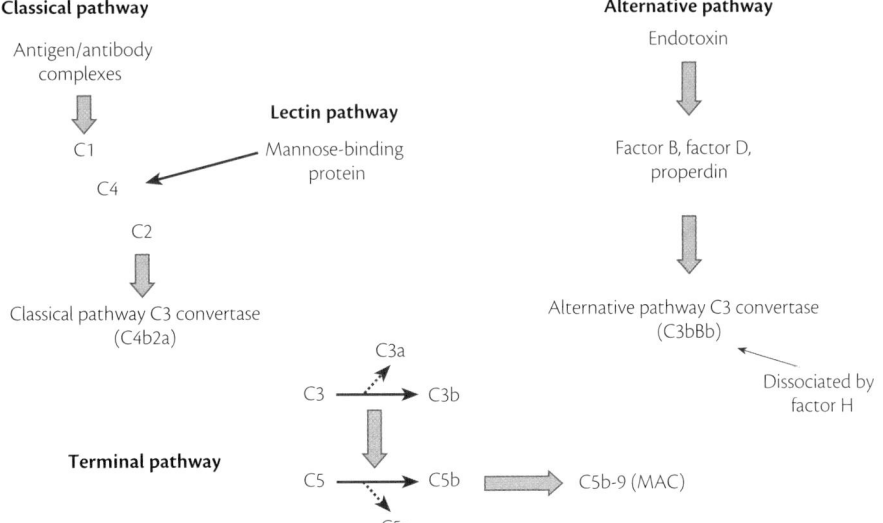

Classical pathway

Antigen/antibody
complexes

C1

C4

C2

Classical pathway C3 convertase
(C4b2a)

Lectin pathway

Mannose-binding
protein

Alternative pathway

Endotoxin

Factor B, factor D,
properdin

Alternative pathway C3 convertase
(C3bBb)

Dissociated by
factor H

C3a

C3 → C3b

Terminal pathway

C5 → C5b → C5b-9 (MAC)

C5a

Fig. 21.8.6.3 The complement
system.

In idiopathic type I MCGN, a variety of complement-activating factors have been described. There may be circulating immune complexes, some patients have antibodies to Clq which probably directly activate the classical pathway, and some have other autoantibodies which interfere with the normal regulation of the classical pathway.

In type II MCGN, the alternative pathway activation is due to the presence of an IgG autoantibody (known as C3 nephritic factor, C3NeF, or more simply as nephritic factor, NeF) which binds to a neoantigen formed when the alternative pathway C3 convertase enzyme C3bBb is assembled. The antibody stabilizes this enzyme and protects it from degradation by factor H. Thus the half-life of the enzyme is prolonged, and the normal regulatory mechanism is subverted. This type of nephritic factor has also been described in patients with type I and type III MCGN, but its presence is virtually invariable in type II MCGN.

In type III MCGN, the presence of a circulating factor which activates complement slowly in a properdin-dependent manner has been postulated, but the reasons for the preferential depletion of terminal pathway components and whether there is a direct relationship of this activation to the renal injury in type III MCGN remain unanswered questions.

The best evidence for a causative role of complement activation in MCGN comes in type II disease. As mentioned above, most patients with type II MCGN have the IgG autoantibody known as NeF, which allows unregulated alternative pathway activation. Two other situations in which there is similar overactivity of the alternative pathway, and an associated renal lesion with the appearances of type II MCGN, have been characterized. First, genetic deficiency of the regulatory protein known as factor H, which normally serves to degrade the alternative pathway C3 convertase, has been reported in a variety of inbred pigs and also in rare human cases. Second, there is a case report of an individual whose serum contained a monoclonal λ light chain which interacted with factor H *in vitro* and prevented its action, allowing unregulated alternative pathway activation. Therefore, in these three situations (the presence of NeF, genetic deficiency of factor H, or functional blocking of factor H), there is dysregulated alternative pathway activation, but due to completely different mechanisms. In each case, the renal lesion is

type II MCGN, strongly suggesting that it is the complement activation *per se* which leads to the renal injury. Importantly, in the factor H-deficient pigs, replacement of factor H leads to prevention of the excessive alternative pathway activation and an improvement in the MCGN. Mice whose factor H gene has been 'knocked out' spontaneously develop MCGN and are more susceptible to other forms of immune-mediated glomerular injury. These observations on the importance of factor H and of complement regulation in general have clear implications for the therapy of human MCGN (discussed further below).

Association with partial lipodystrophy

The NeF autoantibody and the resultant unregulated alternative pathway activation have another striking clinical association with partial lipodystrophy in which there is permanent loss of adipose tissue from the face and neck, and sometimes also from the upper trunk (Fig. 21.8.6.4). Such patients may also have type II MCGN and—as with the renal lesion—there is evidence to suggest that the complement activation directly causes the tissue injury; NeF-containing IgG can cause complement-mediated lysis of adipocytes *in vitro*. Furthermore, adipocytes are probably susceptible to this injury because they produce complement components, and these observations have contributed to a growing appreciation that the complement system plays a previously unsuspected role in the normal physiological regulation of adipose tissue.

Other associations

It has long been appreciated that MCGN, especially type II, may be associated with abnormalities in the eye, especially with prominent presence of drusen (deposits within Bruch's membrane). Recent observations provide a unifying explanation for this, and again involve regulation of the alternative pathway of complement. Age-related macular degeneration (ARMD) is the commonest cause of blindness in adults in the developed world. Recently it has been reported that variations in the gene encoding factor H, the regulator of the alternative complement pathway mentioned above, predispose to ARMD. Drusen are the hallmark lesions of ARMD, and histologically these lesions show evidence of local complement activation. It is therefore likely that drusen result from dysregulated

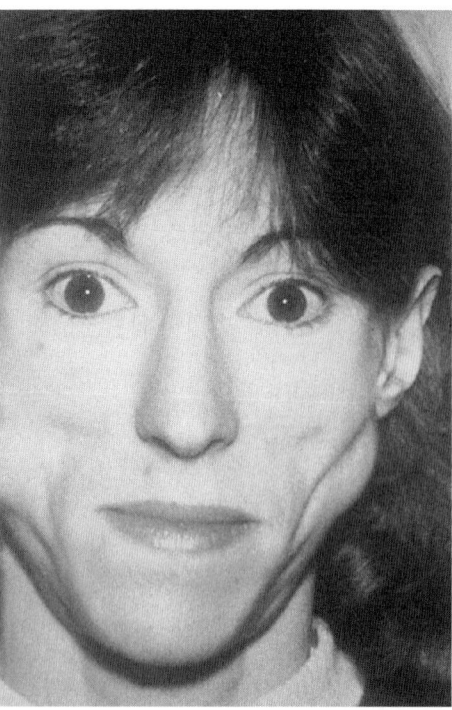

Fig. 21.8.6.4 Facial appearance in partial lipodystrophy. This patient has had silicone pads inserted into her cheeks, accounting for the bulges in the regions where adipose tissue has been completely lost.

complement activation in the subretinal pigment epithelial layer in exactly the same way as glomerular injury occurs when the alternative pathway escapes its normal tight regulation.

Mutations in complement regulatory genes, especially factor H but also factor I and factor B, predispose to another form of renal injury, haemolytic uraemic syndrome (HUS, see Chapter 21.10.5). There are many morphological similarities between the glomerular lesions of HUS and those of (especially early) MCGN, and it seems likely that there is pathogenetic overlap between these renal lesions, presumably explained by the shared importance of complement activation in their genesis.

Epidemiology

MCGN occurs in older children and in adults; it is rare under the age of 5 years. There is no obvious gender difference. Urinary screening programmes allow detection of asymptomatic renal disease. In large series from Japan and Korea of schoolchildren screened in this way, MCGN accounts for a small proportion of cases. In the developed world, the estimated annual incidence of nephrotic syndrome in children is between 2 and 7 cases per 100 000. MCGN typically accounts for 5 to 7% of these. It is generally believed that MCGN is becoming less common (possibly because of improved control of infectious diseases). One recent study estimated that the proportion of cases of nephrotic syndrome in adults explained by MCGN had halved in a 20-year period.

Clinical features

MCGN typically presents with proteinuria, which may be sufficiently severe to cause nephrotic syndrome, and/or haematuria, which—especially in children—may be macroscopic. Hypertension

and/or impairment of excretory kidney function may be associated. Acute presentation as a nephritic syndrome is recognized in children.

As mentioned above, type II MCGN may be associated with partial lipodystrophy, and the loss of adipose tissue can precede the onset of nephritis by many years. Drusen-like deposits and mottled pigmentation in the fundi may rarely be the presenting feature, and retinal neovascularization may occasionally threaten sight and require laser therapy.

Treatment

The forms of therapy that have been applied to MCGN are similar to those used in other forms of nephritis. Antiplatelet drugs, anticoagulants, corticosteroids, and alkylating agents have been used, alone or in various combinations. The studies tend to be small, with varying proportions of children and adults, and of the three subtypes of MCGN. There is a dearth of randomized controlled trials and reviews of the subject have usually concluded that there is no treatment of proven efficacy. Nevertheless, there are hints from some of the studies that certain drugs may have useful effects. In particular, high doses of prednisone, usually given on alternate days (especially in children) are favoured by some authors, especially the Cincinnati group which has published most extensively on this subject. However, high corticosteroid dosages are required for prolonged periods and the magnitude of benefit obtained may be too small to justify the risks of such treatment. Possibly by refining the dosage schedule and by applying the treatment only to high-risk groups, such as those with severe nephrotic syndrome, the risk:benefit ratio may be more favourable.

Since complement activation is so prominent in MCGN, therapy aimed at the complement system may be rational, and promising anticomplement agents are now becoming available, such as a soluble form of the regulatory complement receptor CR1 and drugs which neutralize the proinflammatory effects of C5, the initiator of the terminal complement pathway. So far there are no data on the use of these agents in MCGN. At present, the best strategy is to try to identify any underlying cause of complement activation and remove it if possible. As in other forms of glomerulonephritis, associated hypertension should be aggressively treated. Patients with proteinuria of any cause have their renal prognosis improved if they are treated with angiotensin-converting enzyme inhibitors. They are at increased cardiovascular risk, and attention should also be paid to other modifiable risk factors, especially cigarette smoking and hyperlipidaemia.

Prognosis

Overall, the renal survival in MCGN at 10 years from diagnosis is approximately 50%. Children tend to have a more acute presentation and a slower decline in renal function, although with lengthy follow-up the overall renal survival is similar to that in adults. The prognosis differs between the three subtypes of MCGN, with type II carrying the greatest risk of the development of endstage renal disease. In one study the median time to endstage renal disease in types I, II, and III was, respectively, 15.3 years, 8.7 years, and 15.9 years. Since presentation with the nephrotic syndrome carries a substantially increased risk of endstage renal disease compared to other milder clinical syndromes, the adverse prognosis of type II MCGN may simply reflect the greater likelihood of nephrotic presentation with this histological type. As in many other forms of glomerular disease, the presence of tubular atrophy and interstitial fibrosis indicate a worse prognosis, as do hypertension and/or impairment of excretory renal function at the time of presentation.

Recurrent MCGN in renal transplants

MCGN is one of the types of nephritis that tends to recur in kidney transplants: type I recurs in around 25 to 30% of grafts and type II recurs even more frequently, possibly in 85 to 90% of cases. However, recurrent MCGN only causes graft failure in a few cases, presumably because the antirejection immunosuppressive therapy modulates the damage done by the nephritis.

Further reading

Alexander JJ, Quigg RJ (2006). The simple design of complement factor H: looks can be deceiving. *Mol Immunol*, **44**, 123–32.

Cansick JC, et al. (2004). Prognosis, treatment and outcome of childhood mesangiocapillary (membranoproliferative) glomerulonephritis. *Nephrol Dial Transplant*, **19**, 2769–77.

Donadio JV, Offord KP (1989). Reassessment of treatment results in membranoproliferative glomerulonephritis, with emphasis on life-table analysis. *Am J Kidney Dis*, **14**, 445–51.

Haas M, et al. (1997). Changing etiologies of unexplained adult nephrotic syndrome: a comparison of renal biopsy findings from 1976–1979 and 1995–1997. *Am J Kidney Dis*, **30**, 621–31.

Levin A (1999). Management of membranoproliferative glomerulonephritis: evidence-based recommendations. *Kidney Int Suppl*, **70**, S41–6.

Mathieson PW (1998). Is complement a target for therapy in renal disease? *Kidney Int*, **54**, 1429–36.

Mathieson PW (1999). Mesangiocapillary glomerulonephritis. In: CD Pusey (ed) *Treatment of glomerulonephritis*, pp. 81–92. Kluwer Academic, Dordrecht.

Mathieson PW, Peters DK (1997). Lipodystrophy in MCGN type II: the clue to links between the adipocyte and the complement system. *Nephrol Dial Transplant*, **12**, 1804–6.

McEnery PT (1990). Membranoproliferative glomerulonephritis: the Cincinnati experience—cumulative renal survival from 1957 to 1989. *J Pediatr*, **116**, S109–14.

Varade WS, Forristal J, West CD (1990). Patterns of complement activation in idiopathic membranoproliferative glomerulonephritis, types I, II, III. *Am J Kidney Dis*, **16**, 196–206.

Zipfel PF, et al. (2006). Complement and diseases: defective alternative pathway control results in kidney and eye diseases. *Mol Immunol*, **43**, 97–106.

21.8.7 Antiglomerular basement membrane disease

Jeremy Levy and Charles Pusey

Essentials

Antiglomerular basement membrane disease (anti-GBM disease, also known as Goodpasture's disease) is a rare autoimmune disease caused by pathogenic autoantibodies directed against the noncollagenous,

C-terminal domain of the α-3 chain of type IV collagen (α3(IV) NC1). Immunohistology is characteristic, with linear deposition of IgG (sometimes with IgA or IgM) and complement C3 along the GBMs.

Clinical features—anti-GBM disease classically presents with pulmonary haemorrhage (in two-thirds of patients) and rapidly progressive glomerulonephritis (RPGN, with haematuria and proteinuria, urinary red cell casts, and typically severe acute renal failure). Haemoptysis can be triggered by cigarettes, inhaled toxins, fluid overload, and intercurrent infection. The condition must be distinguished from other cause of RPGN, especially antineutrophil cytoplasmic antibody (ANCA)-associated vasculitis, in particular because there is only a small window of opportunity in which to rescue renal function in patients with Goodpasture's disease. Key investigations are (for diagnosis) serological testing for anti-GBM antibodies and ANCA, and renal biopsy, and (for detection of pulmonary haemorrhage) chest radiology and estimation of carbon monoxide transfer factor (K_{CO}).

Management and prognosis—untreated anti-GBM disease is usually fatal, and renal function never recovers. Immunosuppressive treatment (plasma exchange, cyclophosphamide, oral steroids) is given immediately on diagnosis to patients with serum creatinine levels lower than 600 μmol/litre at presentation and/or with active pulmonary haemorrhage. In contrast, patients with serum creatinine levels more than 600 μmol/litre at presentation rarely recover renal function, hence immunosuppressive treatment in such cases would be restricted in most centres to those with pulmonary haemorrhage or in whom the renal biopsy suggested additional mechanisms of renal damage such as acute tubular necrosis. In recent series, 1-year patient survival is 66 to 92%, 1-year renal survival is 15 to 59%, with renal recovery in patients with initial creatinine levels greater than 600 μmol/litre of 0 to 21%. Patients do not need long-term immunosuppression, and the disease rarely recurs. Transplantation is safe if performed after autoantibodies have been suppressed or naturally disappeared.

Introduction

Antiglomerular basement membrane disease is an autoimmune disease in which patients develop pathogenic autoantibodies against the glomerular basement membrane (GBM). They typically present with renal failure and pulmonary haemorrhage, but isolated renal disease and more rarely isolated lung disease are well recognized. The triad of anti-GBM antibodies, rapidly progressive glomerulonephritis (RPGN), and pulmonary haemorrhage is referred to as Goodpasture's disease in the United Kingdom, while the term Goodpasture's syndrome describes patients with RPGN and pulmonary haemorrhage of various aetiologies.

Historical perspectives

The term 'Goodpasture's syndrome' was first used in 1958 by Stanton and Tange in their report of nine patients with pulmonary–renal syndrome, in which they referred to a patient with fulminant pulmonary haemorrhage and proliferative glomerulonephritis described by Goodpasture during the influenza pandemic of 1919. In retrospect, this original patient may have had systemic vasculitis, not anti-GBM disease. In recent years much has been learnt about the immune response in Goodpasture's disease, but despite huge advances in our understanding of the aetiopathogenesis, therapy has changed little in the last 25 years.

Aetiology and pathogenesis

The Goodpasture antigen

All patients with Goodpasture's disease have circulating antibodies that bind a GBM antigen, the α3 chain of type IV collagen (α3(IV)). Type IV collagen is found in all basement membranes, but the α-3, α-4, and α-5 chains are restricted in their distribution primarily to the GBM and alveolar basement membranes. The epitope for autoantibodies in Goodpasture's disease is carried at the N-terminus of the 230-amino acid, noncollagenous, C-terminal domain of the α-3 chain (α3(IV)NC1), which is normally hidden within the collagen network. The α3(IV)NC1 is also found in the basement membranes of the choroid plexus, the cochlea, Bruch's membrane in the eye, retinal capillaries, and the thymus. It is now clear that a very limited number of amino acids within this domain confirm antigen specificity on the structure, and that both B-cell and T-cell immune responses are driven by this protein.

Anti-GBM antibodies and the T-cell-mediated immune response

Transfer of antibodies from patients into squirrel monkeys initially confirmed the pathogenicity of the autoantibodies. Clinical studies report a correlation between antibody levels at presentation and disease activity, and the disease recurs immediately in renal transplants when the recipient still has circulating antibodies. All patients have antibodies against α3(IV)NC1, either circulating or bound to the GBM. A small number of patients develop antibodies against other GBM components, particularly the α-1 (15% of patients) or α-4 (4% of patients) chains of type IV collagen. In some cases it can be impossible to detect circulating antibodies using conventional assays, but antibody is found bound either to glomerular or alveolar basement membranes in all. However, anti-GBM antibodies are unlikely to be the only cause of glomerular injury, and a cell-mediated immune response is also important in inducing renal damage. In animal models it is possible to induce disease by immunizing with the Goodpasture antigen in the complete absence of B lymphocytes or immunoglobulin, although the damage induced in these cases by T lymphocytes and macrophages is less severe.

Alveolar haemorrhage generally requires a second insult, either local to the lungs (e.g. cigarette smoking or pulmonary oedema), or systemic with activation of cytokines and inflammatory mediators (e.g. sepsis).

Genetic predisposition

Goodpasture's disease has been reported in four sibling pairs and two sets of identical twins, but discordant twin pairs are also documented. More striking is the association with the HLA serotype HLA DR2, which is carried by more than 85% of patients with Goodpasture's disease, compared with 30% of controls. Molecular analysis of HLA alleles has confirmed the association with HLA DR15 (DRB1*1501 and -1502), and a weaker association with HLA DR4 (DRB1*04). A negative association with HLA DR7 (DRB1*07) has been demonstrated. These associations have been confirmed in several studies of different white populations. Thus, specific characteristics of the HLA molecules on antigen-presenting cells determine susceptibility to Goodpasture's disease.

Environmental factors

No specific pathogens or toxins have been identified that can initiate Goodpasture's disease, but many case reports have documented exposure to hydrocarbons before the development of clinical manifestations, and cigarette smoking undoubtedly precipitates pulmonary haemorrhage. It seems more likely that organic solvents trigger overt pulmonary damage (and possibly renal injury) in the presence of circulating autoantibodies than that hydrocarbons are involved in the initiation of autoimmunity. Several clusters of cases have been reported, but no clear associations with influenza virus or other infectious agents have been proven. In animal models it has been demonstrated that molecular mimicry between bacterial antigens and the Goodpasture antigen might be responsible for initiating disease. Thus, a single peptide derived from a *Clostridium botulinum* protein which shares crucial amino acids with the T-cell epitope in Goodpasture's disease can induce both glomerular injury and even pulmonary haemorrhage in rats, but, as stated above, evidence for specific infective causes in humans is lacking.

Disease associations

Anti-GBM disease is only rarely associated with other autoimmune disorders, apart from systemic vasculitides. Increasing numbers of patients (up to 30%) have been shown to have circulating antineutrophil cytoplasmic antibodies (ANCA), generally p-ANCA, in addition to anti-GBM antibodies. Conversely, only few patients with ANCA-associated vasculitis also have anti-GBM antibodies (2.5–8%). This is an important distinction since the 'double positive' patients tend to behave more like those with 'pure' Goodpasture's disease than systemic vasculitis.

Anti-GBM disease has been reported after lithotripsy and urinary tract obstruction, and in some patients with membranous nephropathy. In all these cases it is possible that disruption of the GBM in susceptible individuals can lead to a breakdown in tolerance to the α-3 chain of type IV collagen, with the development of autoantibodies and clinical disease. Patients with HIV infection are also described with anti-GBM antibodies, but almost never with Goodpasture's disease, these antibodies being nonpathogenic and usually of low titre. HIV is, however, associated with a variety of renal diseases, including membranous nephropathy, IgA disease, collapsing glomerulopathy, and immune complex disease.

Pathology

Immunohistology is characteristic (Fig. 21.8.7.1), with linear deposition of IgG (sometimes with IgA or IgM) and complement C3 along the GBMs. Rare patients have been reported with IgM or IgA alone. Less intense linear staining with IgG can occasionally be seen in diabetes, systemic lupus erythematosus, myeloma, and transplanted kidneys. The most characteristic morphological finding is severe crescentic glomerulonephritis, with almost all the glomeruli exhibiting cellular crescents, usually at the same stage of evolution. Segmental necrosis and cellular proliferation may occur. Blood vessels are usually normal, but rarely vasculitis has been reported,

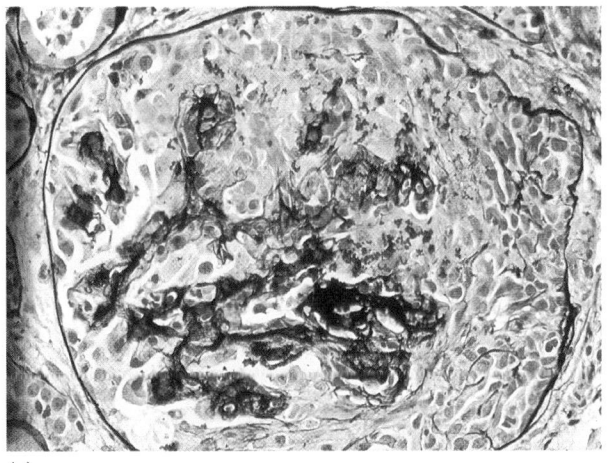

(a)

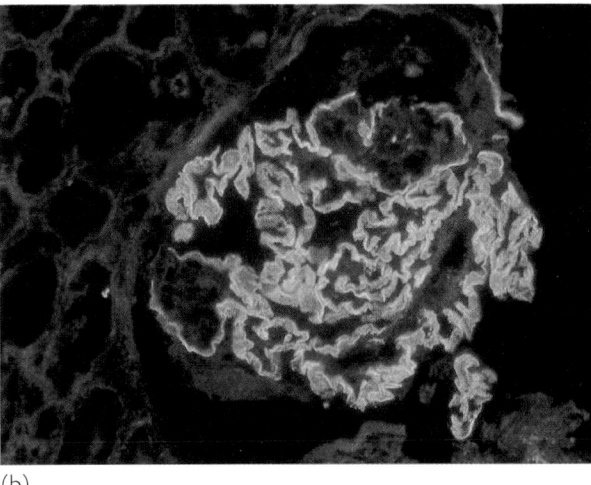

(b)

Fig. 21.8.7.1 Renal biopsy from a patient with Goodpasture's disease. (a) Light microscopy showing a single glomerulus with cellular crescent and focal necrosis. Silver stain. (b) Immunofluorescence of a single glomerulus with linear deposition of IgG along the GBM.
Figure by courtesy of Professor HT Cook.

Clinical features

Most patients present with RPGN or lung haemorrhage, or both. Some patients have isolated lung haemorrhage and never develop renal failure (although most of these have haematuria and proteinuria), and a few have mild isolated nephritis. General malaise, fatigue, weight loss, and anaemia are the commonest systemic features, while other signs and symptoms are much rarer than in patients with systemic vasculitis.

Pulmonary features

Pulmonary haemorrhage occurs in two-thirds of patients, more commonly in young men. It usually precedes presentation with acute renal failure, and is strongly associated with cigarette smoking. Patients often complain of breathlessness and cough. Haemoptysis can be triggered by cigarettes, inhaled toxins, fluid overload, and intercurrent infection, either local (pneumonia) or systemic (sepsis), but there is a poor relationship between overt haemoptysis and the degree of alveolar haemorrhage. Clinical signs are often indistinguishable from those of pulmonary oedema or infection. The most sensitive indicator is an elevated Kco (diffusing capacity for carbon monoxide), which identifies the presence of haemoglobin in alveolar spaces by increased binding of inhaled carbon monoxide. Radiographic features are not specific, but alveolar shadowing in the central lung fields is typically seen (Fig. 21.8.7.2).

Renal features

Patients can present with isolated haematuria, chronic renal failure, or mild renal insufficiency, but classically present with severe acute renal failure due to rapidly progressive glomerulonephritis. The clinical features of the nephritis are indistinguishable from any other cause of RPGN, with cellular casts in the urine, haematuria, and mild-to-moderate proteinuria (nephrotic range proteinuria is uncommon but reported). Hypertension and oliguria are late features. A few patients have relatively normal renal function at presentation, but always have abnormal urine findings and evidence of antibody deposition on renal biopsy.

even in the absence of detectable ANCA. There is often a prominent interstitial cellular infiltrate.

Histological specimens are rarely obtained from lungs, since transbronchial biopsy does not usually penetrate beyond the bronchial mucosa. Open-lung biopsy can reveal alveoli full of red blood cells, macrophages, and fibrin, interspersed between relatively normal alveoli. Immunofluorescence inconsistently reveals linear deposition of antibody.

Epidemiology

Limited epidemiological studies suggest that Goodpasture's disease has an incidence of 0.5 to 1 new case per million of the population per year. It is found in 1 to 2% of renal biopsies. In comparison, systemic vasculitides have an incidence of 15 to 30 new cases per million of the population per year. The disease is less common in Afro-Caribbean populations, but increasingly reported in Asian people. There is a bimodal age distribution, with peak incidence in the third and sixth decades, and a slight excess of men.

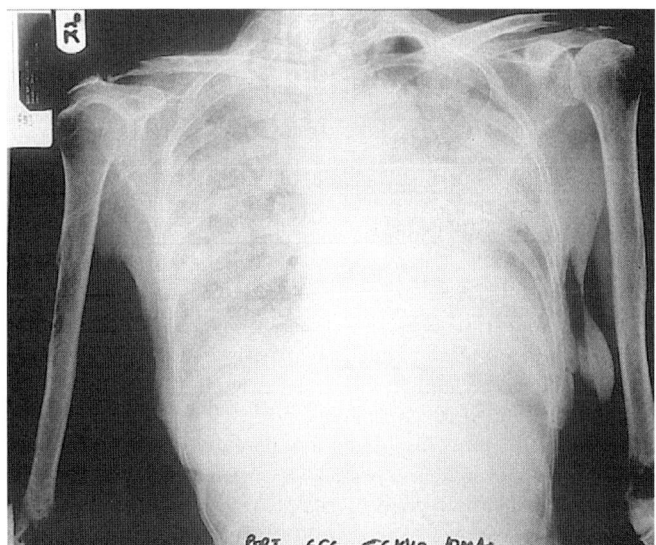

Fig. 21.8.7.2 Chest radiograph from a patient with Goodpasture's disease showing florid pulmonary haemorrhage.

Box 21.8.7.1 Pulmonary–renal syndromes

Renal and pulmonary failure without alveolar haemorrhage
More common

◆ Kidney disease (acute or chronic) of any cause with pulmonary oedema (fluid overload)

◆ Severe pneumonia and renal failure, especially legionella

◆ Cardiac failure with pulmonary oedema and secondary renal failure

◆ Infective endocarditis

Less common

◆ Pulmonary embolism and renal failure (often in nephrotic syndrome)

◆ Paraquat poisoning

◆ Organic solvents

◆ Hantavirus infection

Goodpasture's syndrome (alveolar haemorrhage and nephritis)
More common

◆ Microscopic polyangiitis

◆ Wegener's granulomatosis

◆ Anti-GBM disease (Goodpasture's disease)

◆ Systemic lupus erythematosus

Less common

◆ Churg–Strauss syndrome

◆ Henoch–Schönlein purpura

◆ Haemolytic uraemic syndrome

◆ Behçet's disease

◆ Essential mixed cryoglobulinaemia

◆ Rheumatoid vasculitis

◆ Penicillamine therapy

Differential diagnosis

It is crucial to distinguish anti-GBM disease from other causes of RPGN, and especially ANCA-associated vasculitis. There is only a small window of opportunity in which to rescue renal function in patients with anti-GBM disease, in contrast to systemic vasculitis in which renal failure can be reversed at a later stage. All patients with suspected RPGN, acute renal failure of unknown cause, or lung haemorrhage and urinary abnormalities, should have both anti-GBM antibody and ANCA assays performed urgently. Other differential diagnoses to consider include systemic lupus erythematosus, cryoglobulinaemia, haemolytic uraemia syndrome, and other causes of pulmonary–renal syndrome (see Box 21.8.7.1).

Clinical investigation

Serological testing for anti-GBM antibodies and ANCA is crucial for confirming the diagnosis, and a renal biopsy is almost always

warranted. Some healthy individuals exposed to inhaled oils, hydrocarbons, or solvents may have borderline raised anti-GBM antibody levels, and anti-GBM antibody has also been detected in HIV-negative patients with pneumocystis pneumonia. Other investigations are detailed in Table 21.8.7.1. Alveolar haemorrhage is an important cause of mortality and must be identified early. All patients should have baseline KCO and chest radiology, repeated as necessary.

Treatment

Untreated anti-GBM disease is usually fatal, and renal function never recovers. In most centres immunosuppressive treatment is given immediately on diagnosis to those with a serum creatinine concentration below 600 μmol/litre at presentation and/or with active pulmonary haemorrhage. Those with a serum creatinine concentration above 600 μmol/litre and without active pulmonary haemorrhage need more careful consideration before being treated since they have a small chance of recovery of renal function (see below).

Treatment with plasma exchange, cyclophosphamide, and corticosteroids, together with dialysis when required, can allow up to 90% of patients to survive, but only around 40% of survivors

Table 21.8.7.1 Investigation of patients with anti-GBM disease

Investigation	Comments
Urinalysis	Dipstick shows proteinuria and haematuria
	Microscopy shows numerous erythrocytes and red cell casts
Full blood count	Haemoglobin often reduced
	Monitor white blood cell count during immunosuppression
Urea and electrolytes	Severe acute renal failure common
C-reactive protein	Moderately elevated (less than in vasculitis)
Immunoglobulins	Normal or mildly raised
Anti-GBM antibodies	Always positive, usually IgG, but may be only mildly raised, even in typical disease
ANCA	Negative in true anti-GBM disease. If 'double-positive', may have a poor outcome from renal failure
ANA, dsDNA, complement, cryoglobulins, ASOT	Negative or normal
Chest radiography	Usually bilateral airspace shadowing. Difficult to distinguish infection and fluid overload from pulmonary haemorrhage
KCO	Raised in alveolar haemorrhage. Normal or reduced in pulmonary oedema or infection
Renal biopsy	Crescentic glomerulonephritis and linear IgG deposition along the GBM
Transbronchial biopsy	Not usually diagnostic (difficult to obtain alveoli; open biopsy more useful). Helpful in diagnosis of infection

ANA, antinuclear antibody; ANCA, antineutrophil cytoplasmic antibody; ASOT, antistreptolysin-O titre; dsDNA, double-stranded DNA; GBM, glomerular basement membrane; KCO, diffusing capacity for carbon monoxide.

will recover renal function. Daily plasma exchange removes circulating antibodies, while cyclophosphamide prevents further antibody synthesis. There has only been one controlled trial of plasma exchange, which utilized a low intensity of exchanges in a small number of patients and showed a nonsignificant trend towards an improved outcome. However, the dramatic improvement in overall mortality and renal function coincident with the introduction of a treatment regimen of the type described above has led to its widespread use. The regimen we use is shown in Box 21.8.7.2. An alternative to plasma exchange is protein-A immunoadsorption, which has not shown any benefit over plasma exchange in the most severely affected patients. Ciclosporin has been used in occasional patients unresponsive to other therapies, but is of doubtful benefit. Long-term treatment is unnecessary, and patients can stop taking cyclophosphamide after 2 to 3 months, and withdraw prednisolone over approximately 6 months.

Prognosis

The outcome of patients with Goodpasture's disease in published series is shown in Table 21.8.7.2. Most will now survive the acute illness, but pulmonary haemorrhage and infection remain important causes of death. In those with a serum creatinine concentration below 600 µmol/litre at presentation, the creatinine should begin to fall within 1 to 2 weeks of treatment, and most will recover renal function. However, patients with a creatinine concentration above 600 µmol/litre, or with oligoanuria, less commonly recover renal function. For this reason most centres would not give immunosuppressive agents to this group with the sole intention of trying to restore renal function, although they would for concurrent active pulmonary haemorrhage or if the renal biopsy suggests that tubular necrosis may be contributing to the severity of the renal failure (see above). Crescent scores over 50% and delay in diagnosis are also markers of a poor renal prognosis.

The prognosis in anti-GBM disease is in marked contrast to that of patients with a diagnosis of ANCA-associated RPGN. Renal recovery is to be expected in the latter group with immunosuppression, and around 70% of patients presenting with a creatinine concentration above 600 µmol/litre will recover renal function.

Relapses of pulmonary haemorrhage and worsening of renal function can occur early during the course of treatment in the presence of circulating autoantibodies, and can be triggered by smoking, infection, or fluid overload. True late recurrence is very unusual. Transplantation is safe once autoantibodies are no longer detectable, and is best delayed until between 6 and 12 months after the disappearance of anti-GBM antibody.

Anti-GBM disease in Alport's syndrome

Patients with X-linked Alport's syndrome have a mutation in the α5 chain of type IV collagen, but also have undetectable Goodpasture antigen in their kidneys despite a normal α3(IV) gene. Transplantation of a normal kidney into such recipients may allow the development of anti-GBM antibodies as a result of the exposure of the immune system to neoantigens to which tolerance has not developed. These antibodies are usually anti-α5(IV)NC1, but can also be anti-α3(IV)NC1 (classic Goodpasture autoantibodies).

Box 21.8.7.2 Treatment of anti-GBM disease

Initial treatment
Plasma exchange
- Daily, 4-litre exchange for 5% human albumin solution
- Use 300–600 ml fresh-frozen plasma within 3 days of any invasive procedure (e.g. biopsy) or in patients with pulmonary haemorrhage
- Continue for 14 days, or until antibody levels fully suppressed
- Withhold if platelet count $<70 \times 10^9$/ml, or haemoglobin <9 g/dl
- Watch for coagulopathy, hypocalcaemia, and hypokalaemia

Cyclophosphamide
- Daily oral dosing at 3 mg/kg per day (round down to nearest 50 mg; reduce to 2 mg/kg per day in patients over 55 years; maximum 200 mg)
- Stop if white cell count $<4 \times 10^9$/ml, and restart at lower dose when counts $>4 \times 10^9$/ml

Prednisolone
- Daily oral dosing at 1 mg/kg per day (maximum 60 mg)
- Reduce dose weekly to 20 mg by week 6, and then more slowly
- No evidence for benefit of intravenous methylprednisolone and may increase infection risk (possibly use if plasma exchange not available)

Prophylactic treatments
- Oral nystatin and amphotericin (or fluconazole) for oropharyngeal fungal infection
- Ranitidine or proton-pump inhibitor for steroid-promoted gastric ulceration
- Low-dose co-trimoxazole for *Pneumocystis jiroveci* pneumonia prevention
- Consider valganciclovir as cytomegalovirus prophylaxis
- Consider calcium/vitamin D for prevention of osteoporosis (but relatively short course of steroids)

Maintenance treatment
Prednisolone
- Reduce dose slowly from 20 mg at 6 weeks, to stop completely by 6 months

Cyclophosphamide
- Stop after 2–3 months
- No further cytotoxic agents necessary

Most patients do not develop overt nephritis, simply depositing antibody along the GBM without recruiting a glomerular inflammatory response, but a few develop severe glomerulonephritis. In the absence of lung antigen, pulmonary haemorrhage never occurs.

Table 21.8.7.2 Outcome of patients with Goodpasture's disease. Data from all published series

Series	Number of patients	1-year patient survival (%)	1-year renal survival (%)	Renal recovery[a] (% treated patients)	Notes
Benoit et al. (1964)	52	4	4	NA	No treatment. Patients with Goodpasture's syndrome of all causes
Wilson and Dixon (1973)	53	75	23	NA	Immunosuppression only
Beirne et al. (1977)	26	46	15	NA	Seven patients not treated. Remainder immunosuppression only
Teague et al. (1978)	29	62	31	NA	Excluded patients without lung haemorrhage
Briggs et al. (1979)	18	83	11	0	Seven patients not treated. Remainder immunosuppressed
Peters et al. (1982)	41	76	39	4	Hammersmith hospital single centre. All plasma exchanged
Simpson et al. (1982)	20	90	59	0	Excluded patients without pulmonary haemorrhage
Johnson et al. (1985)	17	94	45	0	Randomized prospective study of plasma exchange
Walker et al. (1985)	22	59	45	18	Australian single centre. All plasma exchanged
Savage et al. (1986)	59	75	8.5	NA	Data from multiple British centres
	49	84	35	11	Hammersmith hospital single centre
Williams et al. (1988)	10	90	20	NA	Single British unit. Patients presenting over 13 months
Bouget et al. (1990)	14	79	29	0	French single centre
Herody et al. (1993)	29	93	41	0	French single centre. Most plasma exchanged
Merkel et al. (1994)	35	89	40	3	Survival at time of analysis. All plasma exchanged
Daly et al. (1996)	40	–	20	0	All plasma exchanged
Levy et al. (2001)	71	77	53	21	Extended Hammersmith series. All plasma exchanged. Only 8% of patients requiring dialysis recovered renal function
Segelmark et al (2003)	79	66	59	0	Swedish series
Li et al. (2004)	10	70	15	0	Hong Kong Chinese patients. 80% plasma exchanged
Cui et al. (2005)	69	92	22	2	Chinese series. Only 45% plasma exchanged

NA, not available.

[a] Renal recovery if initial creatinine >600 µmol/litre.

Further reading

Cui Z, et al. (2004). Characteristics and prognosis of Chinese patients with anti-glomerular basement membrane disease. *Nephron Clin Pract*, **99**, 49–55.

Fisher EG, Lager DJ (2006). Anti-glomerular basement membrane glomerulonephritis. *Am J Clin Pathol*, **125**, 445–50.

Herody M, et al. (1993). Anti-GBM disease: predictive value of clinical, histological and serological data. *Clin Nephrol*, **40**, 249–55.

Hudson BG (2004). The molecular basis of Goodpasture and Alport syndromes: beacons for the discovery of the collagen IV family. *J Am Soc Nephrol*, **15**, 2514–27.

Hudson BG, et al. (2003). Alport's syndrome, Goodpasture's syndrome and type IV collagen. *N Eng J Med*, **348**, 2543–56.

Johnson JP, et al. (1985). Therapy of anti-glomerular basement membrane antibody disease: analysis of prognostic significance of clinical, pathological and treatment factors. *Medicine*, **64**, 219–27.

Lerner RA, Glassock RJ, Dixon FJ (1967). The role of anti-glomerular basement membrane antibodies in the pathogenesis of human glomerulonephritis. *J Exp Med*, **126**, 989–1004.

Levy JB, Pusey CD (2007). Plasmapheresis. In: Johnson R, Floege J, Feehally J (eds) *Comprehensive clinical nephrology*, 3rd edition, pp. 83.1–8. Mosby, London.

Levy JB, et al. (2001). Long-term outcome of anti-GBM antibody diseases treated with plasma exchange and immunosuppression. *Ann Int Med*, **134**, 1033–42.

Levy JB, et al. (2004). Clinical features and outcome of patients with both ANCA and anti-GBM antibodies. *Kidney Int*, **66**, 1535–40.

Lockwood CM, *et al.* (1976). Immunosuppression and plasma exchange in the treatment of Goodpasture's syndrome. *Lancet*, **i**, 711–15.

Merkel F, *et al.* (1994). Course and prognosis of anti-basement membrane antibody mediated disease, a report of 35 cases. *Nephrol Dial Transplant*, **9**, 372–6.

Saus J, *et al.* (1988). Identification of the Goodpasture antigen as the α3(IV) chain of collagen IV. *J Biol Chem*, **263**, 13374–80.

Savage COS, *et al.* (1986). Anti-GBM antibody mediated disease in the British Isles 1980–1984. *BMJ*, **292**, 301–4.

Stanton MC, Tange JD (1958). Goodpasture's syndrome, pulmonary haemorrhage associated with glomerulonephritis. *Australas Ann Med*, **7**, 132–44.

Tubulointerstitial diseases

Contents

21.9.1 Acute interstitial nephritis

Simon D. Roger

Essentials

Acute interstitial nephritis (AIN) is an inflammation of the tubules and interstitium within the kidney, associated with relatively sudden onset and fast decline in renal function. It is usually secondary to drugs (proton pump inhibitors being most commonly incriminated), with other causes being infections (classically streptococcal, but this is now less common) and immune disorders (systemic lupus erythematosus, sarcoidosis, and tubulointerstitial nephritis with uveitis).

Clinical features—the diagnosis of AIN should be considered in any patient with unexplained acute renal failure. Drug-induced AIN may present with a classic allergic response, including arthralgias, fever, rash, loin pain, and eosinophilia/eosinophiluria, but these are not invariable and their absence does not exclude the diagnosis. The urine typically shows low-grade proteinuria (<1 g/day). The only way of confirming or excluding the diagnosis is by renal biopsy.

Management and prognosis—treatment is by removing the offending agent, treating the concurrent infectious cause, or managing the immune aetiology, with or without steroids (typically prednisolone 1 mg/kg per day, tapered to zero over 6–8 weeks). Most patients with drug-induced AIN recover renal function, but some are left with chronic renal impairment, and a few even progress to endstage chronic kidney disease.

Introduction

Acute interstitial nephritis (AIN) is characterized by an interstitial infiltrate of inflammatory cells with relative sparing of the glomeruli and vessels, and presents as acute impairment of renal function. The term 'tubulointerstitial' nephritis is also applied, reflecting the damage that occurs to the tubular cells in addition to the interstitial changes.

Historical perspective

In 1898 Councilman described the first account of acute tubulointerstitial nephritis involving patients with scarlet fever or diphtheria, whose kidneys were sterile but had inflammatory infiltrates. Since then drug-induced AIN has surpassed infection as a more common cause of the condition in adults, especially with the widespread use of antibiotics.

Aetiology

The aetiology of AIN is usually divided into groups on the basis of the precipitating cause (Box 21.9.1.1).

Drugs

Drugs are now responsible for most cases of AIN. The proton pump inhibitors were first recognized as causing AIN in 1992 and are now the most common cause of drug-induced AIN. They induce AIN on rechallenge, with AIN being a class effect rather than due to specific drugs within the group. Other commonly implicated drugs are penicillins, cephalosporins, sulpha-based agents, nonsteroidal anti-inflammatory drugs (NSAIDs), and furosemide (frusemide). Some of the newer pharmaceutical agents that have appeared on the formulary over the past 20 years are possible culprits, including pamidronate, amlodipine, Chinese herbal agents, and perhaps also cocaine.

Infections

Many pathogenic organisms (bacterial, viral, protozoal, and fungal) have been implicated as causing AIN, and in children infection remains the most common cause of this condition. Several warrant specific mention:

◆ Streptococcal infection—previously a very common cause of AIN, but has now waned with the advent of and widespread use of antibiotics.

Box 21.9.1.1   Main causes of acute interstitial nephritis

Drugs

- Proton pump inhibitors
  - Esomeprazole
  - Lansoprazole
  - Omeprazole
  - Pantoprazole
  - Rabeprazole
- Antibiotics
  - Cephalosporin
  - Ciprofloxacin
  - Co-trimoxazole and other sulphonamides
  - Erythromycin
  - Methicillin
  - Other penicillin derivatives
  - Rifampicin
  - Vancomycin
- Nonsteroidal anti-inflammatory drugs
- Diuretics
  - Furosemide (frusemide)
  - Thiazides
  - Triamterene
- Others
  - Aciclovir
  - Allopurinol
  - Captopril
  - Clofibrate
  - Diphenylhydantoin
  - Fenofibrate
  - H_2-receptor blockers
  - Indinavir
  - Interferon-α
  - Paracetamol
  - Phenindione
  - Phenobarbital
  - Phenothiazine
  - Salicylate derivatives
  - Streptokinase
  - Valproate
  - Warfarin

Infectious diseases

- Bacterial
  - Brucellosis
  - Legionella
  - Leptospirosis
  - Mycoplasma
  - Rickettsia
  - Streptococci, including pneumococci
  - Syphilis
  - Tuberculosis
  - Typhoid fever
- Viral
  - BK virus
  - Coxsackievirus
  - Cytomegalovirus
  - Echovirus
  - Epstein–Barr virus
  - Hantavirus
  - HIV
  - Measles
  - Parvovirus B19
- Parasitic
  - Leishmania
  - Toxoplasma

Systemic diseases

- Sarcoidosis
- Sjögren's syndrome
- Systemic lupus erythematosus

Idiopathic

- Associated with unilateral or bilateral uveitis (TINU syndrome)
- Isolated

Adapted from Droz D, Chauveau D (2003). Acute interstitial nephritis. In: Warrell DA, *et al*, (eds). Oxford Textbook of Medicine, 4th edition. Oxford University Press, UK. P359.

- Legionella—although a relatively rare cause of AIN, the organism can be detected in renal tissue by immunofluorescence and electron microscopy; coexistent rhabdomyolysis may be present.

- HIV—AIN is present in up to 40% of autopsy series, typically with mononuclear cell infiltrate of predominantly CD8+ positive lymphocytes.

- Epstein–Barr virus—renal involvement is not uncommon; CD8+ T lymphocytes may predominate.

- Cytomegalovirus—a common cause in immunosuppressed patients (HIV-positive or organ transplant recipients) and may cause irreversible renal failure.

- Polyomavirus Bk—the renal transplant population are specifically at risk of BK virus inducing an AIN. This polyomavirus is present in the urothelium of 60 to 80% of people, with immunosuppression allowing it to become a significant pathogen in the renal transplant. Management generally involves reduction in immunosuppression, and ciprofloxacin is often given on the basis of small series where it has been thought to be helpful, but the outlook for graft function is not good.

- Toxoplasmosis—AIN is uncommon but can occur as part of systemic infection.

- Leishmaniasis—disseminated leishmaniasis (kala-azar) can present with acute renal failure from AIN, which tends to resolve.

- Mycobacteria—these have been recognized as inducing AIN and, along with toxoplasmosis and leishmaniasis, are a commoner cause of AIN than drug-induced cases in developing countries.

In septicaemia, bacteria such as *Escherichia coli* and staphylococci and fungal elements such as *Candida albicans* can directly invade the renal parenchyma and lead to the development of microabscesses, which are found on diagnostic renal biopsy.

Immune-mediated diseases

In systemic lupus erythematosus a tubulointerstitial infiltrate usually coexists with significant glomerulonephritis, but it has been found in isolation. Cellular infiltrates include mononuclear cells, but also sometimes neutrophils. In Sjögren's syndrome an AIN may be associated with renal tubular acidosis, and IgG and complement C3 may be detected on the tubular basement membrane on immunofluorescent staining.

In sarcoidosis there can be cellular infiltrate with typical granulomas in the renal interstitium, which—often in association with hypercalcaemia—can lead to dialysis-dependent renal failure.

A more specific entity was described by Dobrin in 1975 as the 'tubulointerstitial nephritis with uveitis' (TINU) syndrome, which is presumed to be an autoimmune condition. It most commonly affects pubertal girls, the ocular problems may precede or follow the renal dysfunction, and it responds to oral steroids but is prone to relapse.

Antitubular basement membrane antibodies have been reported in some cases of the rare idiopathic form of AIN.

A variety of primary glomerulonephritides may cause secondary tubulointerstitial inflammation and nephritis, e.g. in the context of antiglomerular basement membrane antibodies and coexistent antitubular basement membrane antibodies (occurring in 50%), or membranous glomerulonephritis.

Pathogenesis

There are two possible mechanisms by which AIN develops, antigen-driven immunogenicity and humoral immunogenicity. In antigen-driven immunogenicity AIN is classically associated with an infiltrate of T lymphocytes (both helper-inducer and suppressor-cytotoxic), T-cell-mediated hypersensitivity, and cytotoxic T-cell injury. Granuloma formation occurs via this pathway. The presence of transforming growth factor-β_1 (TGFβ_1) acts as a proinflammatory molecule and is the most important profibrotic factor. In humoral immunogenicity, although T cells are implicated in the pathogenesis, there is also evidence from experimental animal models to implicate the humoral immune system, in particular tubular basement membrane antibodies and complement, a process which is active in the TINU syndrome where there is an increase in IgG that has been reported as being reactive against a 125-kDa human kidney protein.

The exact pathogenesis of drug-induced AIN is not known. It is an idiosyncratic reaction, not dose related, whereby it is thought that the drug or its metabolites act either as haptens (mimicking renal antigens) or deposit as circulating immune complexes, leading to stimulation of a T-cell hypersensitivity reaction. Evidence for this hypothesis comes in part from the extrarenal manifestations of hypersensitivity (rash, arthralgias, and eosinophilia).

Whatever the mechanisms of initiation, it is thought that these induce interstitial fibroblasts to express a variety of growth factors and cytokines, such as TGFβ and platelet-derived growth factor (PDGF), which lead to inflammatory cascades and subsequent fibrotic change. This results in tubular destruction and glomeruli without tubules that subsequently sclerose, changes which can progress to the classic features of chronic interstitial nephritis.

Pathology

On light microscopy the renal biopsy typically shows an infiltrate within the interstitium of T lymphocytes (especially CD4+ and CD8+ cells), monocytes, macrophages (expressing CD14+ and CD68+ in addition to cell activation markers), and possibly polyclonal plasma cells and eosinophils (Fig. 21.9.1.1). The infiltrate may vary in intensity, and there may be extensive interstitial oedema. If granulomas have formed, then the differential diagnosis includes a drug reaction, sarcoidosis, tuberculosis, or acute bacterial infection. The tubules themselves may show necrosis or signs of regeneration.

In primary AIN, when the sample is examined by light microscopy or immunofluorescent techniques, the glomeruli and vessels are either unremarkable or show only minor change. Immunofluorescence of the tubules and interstitium may stain positive for antitubular basement membrane antibodies, IgG and IgM, in addition to fibrinogen. Linear IgG and C3 deposition is rarely found, although it has been associated with antibiotic-induced disease (β-lactams and ciprofloxacin). Electron microscopy reveals altered continuity of the tubular basement membrane.

Fibrosis within the interstitium has been detected within 2 weeks as a component of the reparative process.

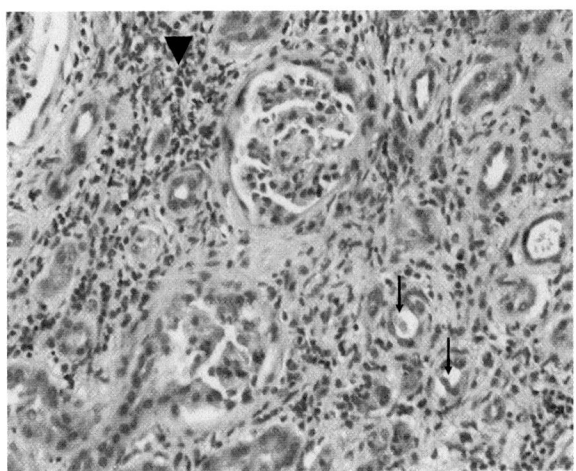

Fig. 21.9.1.1 Renal biopsy demonstrating AIN with cellular infiltrate (large arrow head) and sloughing of tubular epithelial cells (arrows). Haematoxylin and eosin stain.

Epidemiology

The incidence of AIN is difficult to gauge. It is not a common entity and is found in approximately 1 to 3% of unselected renal biopsy series, but series of renal biopsies performed for investigation of acute renal failure demonstrate AIN as the cause in 6 to 15% of cases. The prevalence is greater in biopsies where the cause of acute renal failure is unknown, or when the urinary sediment is inactive, i.e. there is no heavy proteinuria, no significant haematuria, and no dysmorphic red blood cells. In this setting the prevalence of AIN is reported as high as 27%.

Clinical features

The clinician should always consider AIN in any patient with unexplained acute renal failure, with or without specific tubular dysfunction. It is also important to consider AIN in a patient with chronic kidney disease whose renal function suddenly deteriorates at a rapid rate. A thorough drug history is essential, including over-the-counter medications, herbal compounds, and other nonprescription agents, and the dates/duration of exposure. Given that drug-induced AIN is an idiosyncratic reaction, it must be presumed that all are at risk.

Drug-induced AIN may present with a classic allergic response, as typically provoked by methicillin-including arthralgias (45% of cases), fever (30%), rash (20%), loin pain (20%), and eosinophilia/eosinophiluria. These systemic features may present early, 2 to 3 weeks after drug exposure, or up to a mean of 3 months afterwards following drugs such as the proton pump inhibitors, or up to years later with drugs such as the NSAIDS (although it can be difficult if not impossible to attribute causation after lengthy delay). In patients who are inadvertently rechallenged with an offending drug, the onset of AIN is rapid.

The following three classes of agents are the most common causes of iatrogenic AIN.

Proton pump inhibitors

Proton pump inhibitors are one of the most widely prescribed classes of drugs in the western world. All five drugs in the class have

been reported as causing AIN. The triad of fever, rash, and eosinophilia associated with classic methicillin-induced AIN is not prominent and even absent in proton pump inhibitor-induced AIN. The presenting complaints are nonspecific and include tiredness, nausea, and weight loss. The most common abnormalities on investigation, apart from raised serum creatinine, are proteinuria, pyuria, and eosinophiluria.

Due to the widespread availability of these drugs, both over the counter in some countries and on prescription, there is a high risk of inadvertent rechallenge unless patients are clearly counselled. This iatrogenic complication may be devastating, hence education of all prescribing doctors (including general practitioners, gastroenterologists, and surgeons) in addition to pharmacists is warranted.

Nonsteroidal anti-inflammatory drugs

This class of drugs rarely causes extrarenal manifestation, but concurrent nephrotic syndrome with heavy proteinuria and oedema is common, being present in up to 70% of cases. Macroscopic haematuria is rare. In Europe, fenoprofen accounts for up to 50% of cases. Precise history-taking is imperative. These medications are readily available over the counter, are usually taken on an 'as needed' basis, and many patients may not regard them as 'drugs' unless specifically asked about them by the clinician.

β-Lactam antibiotics

These agents cause the 'classic' allergic drug-induced AIN, which occurs within a few days or up to 2 months after starting treatment. Fever, skin rash, arthralgias, eosinophilia, and renal impairment are evident.

Differential diagnosis

The differential diagnosis of AIN includes other causes of acute renal failure, as discussed in Chapter 21.5. It may be impossible on clinical grounds to differentiate acute tubular necrosis from AIN, or to distinguish AIN from one of the acute glomerulonephritides or vasculitides; in these cases renal biopsy is the only test that will conclusively confirm or dismiss the diagnosis.

When assessing kidney biopsy specimens, any infiltrate of mononuclear cells needs to be differentiated from a monoclonal infiltrate that might be found be in renal lymphoma or leukaemia.

Clinical investigation

The urine typically has a low-grade proteinuria of less than 1 g/day, or albumin/creatinine ratio (ACR) less than 60 mg/mmol, or protein/creatinine ratio (PCR) less than 100 mg/mmol on a spot urine sample. There may be biochemical urinary changes reflecting tubular dysfunction, such as glycosuria, aminoaciduria, and uricosuria.

Serum urea and creatinine are likely to be elevated as a result of impairment of glomerular filtration rate. Other biochemical changes attributable to tubular dysfunction may include hypo- or hyperkalaemia, or alterations in serum bicarbonate. Either type I (distal) or type II (proximal) renal tubular acidosis patterns may predominate (see Chapter 21.15).

The full blood count may reveal a high eosinophil count, and microscopic examination of the urine stained with Wright's or Hansel's stains, which are pH dependent, may demonstrate eosinophils. Other causes of eosinophiluria include prostatitis, bladder carcinoma, eosinophilic cystitis, and cholesterol emboli. Eosinophils in the urine have been reported to have 40% sensitivity and 72% specificity for AIN, with a positive predictive value of 30%, but it may be argued that the series studied are too small for the development of accurate predictive parameters.

There may be nonspecific increases in inflammatory markers, including erythrocyte sedimentation rate, C-reactive protein, and serum globulin concentrations.

Gallium scans have been assessed as another diagnostic tool in helping to differentiate AIN from acute tubular necrosis, being positive in the former but negative in the latter, but they cannot provide a definitive diagnosis.

As stated previously, renal biopsy is the gold standard for making the diagnosis of AIN. The clinician is often faced with a patient who presents with an elevated serum creatinine and a reduced estimated glomerular filtration rate, an inactive urinary sediment, and a long list of possible culprit medications which may cause AIN. This means that a strong argument can be made for performing a renal biopsy in all cases of suspected AIN, with the exception being where the clinician is reasonably confident of the diagnosis and judges that biopsy in the particular patient would constitute a greater risk than that of stopping any likely offending drug and waiting, with or without giving steroids.

Treatment

The diagnosis of drug-induced AIN is vital, as prompt identification and discontinuation of the causative agent facilitates recovery of renal function.

There is no consensus as to whether simply removing the offending drug would be as effective as combining that with steroids. However, a recent retrospective study has suggested the use of corticosteroids in all patients with drug-induced AIN. If steroids are prescribed, then a standard regimen would be oral prednisone at 1 mg/kg per day, tapered to zero over a 6- to 8-week period. In cases that do not appear to respond to steroids, other immunosuppressants such as cyclophosphamide, ciclosporin, and mycophenolate mofetil have been used, but evidence of their efficacy is weak. Plasma exchange has been utilized in patients testing positive for tubular basement membrane antibodies.

Supportive treatment may be required if the degree of uraemia warrants, including renal replacement therapy with dialysis.

Prognosis

Significant recovery of renal function, with return of serum creatinine to baseline or near baseline, can be anticipated in most cases of AIN, but some patients retain a degree of renal impairment, and some even progress to endstage chronic kidney disease. The renal prognosis, as with other conditions such as glomerulonephritis, depends on the severity and degree of interstitial fibrosis demonstrated by biopsy. Other parameters that predict a less good outcome are high initial creatinine, renal impairment that has been present for more than 3 weeks, and granulomata or more pronounced interstitial cellular infiltrates on renal biopsy. The phenotype of inflammatory cells or the degree of tubulitis has not been shown to be helpful.

The pattern of recovery often follows two stages: a rapid improvement over 6 to 8 weeks and then a slower phase of improvement that may occur over the following 12 months.

Further reading

Bagnis CI (2004). Herbs and the kidney. *Kidney Int*, **44**, 1–11.

Clarkson MR, *et al.* (2004). Acute interstitial nephritis: clinical features and response to corticosteroid therapy. *Nephrol Dial Transplant*, **19**, 2778–83.

Councilman WT (1893). Acute interstitial nephritis. *J Exp Med*, **3**, 393–420.

Dobrin RS, Vernier RL, Fish AL (1975). Acute eosinophilic interstitial nephritis and renal failure with bone marrow lymph node granulomas and anterior uveitis: a new syndrome. *Am J Med*, **59**, 325–33.

Geevasinga N, *et al.* (2006). Proton pump inhibitors and acute interstitial nephritis. *Clin Gastroenterol Hepatol*, **4**, 597–604.

Gonzalez E, *et al.* (2008). Early steroid treatment improves the recovery of renal function in patients with drug-induced acute interstitial nephritis. *Kidney Int*, **73**, 940–6.

Kleinknecht D (1995). Interstitial nephritis, the nephrotic syndrome, and chronic renal failure secondary to non-steroidal anti-inflammatory drugs. *Semin Nephrol*, **15**, 228–35.

Linton AL, *et al.* (1985). Gallium 67 scintigraphy in the diagnosis of acute renal disease. *Clin Nephrol*, **24**, 84–7.

Randhawa P, Brennan DC (2006). BK virus infection in transplant recipients: an overview and update. *Am J Transplant*, **6**, 2000–5.

Rossert J (2001). Drug-induced acute interstitial nephritis. *Kidney Int*, **60**, 804–17.

Ruffenach SJ, Siskind MS, Lien YH (1992). Acute interstitial nephritis due to omeprazole. *Am J Med*, **93**, 472–3.

Ruffing KA, *et al.* (1994). Eosinophils in urine revisited. *Clin Nephrol*, **41**, 163–6.

21.9.2 **Chronic tubulointerstitial nephritis**

Marc E. De Broe, Patrick C. D'Haese, and Monique M. Elseviers

Essentials

Chronic tubulointerstitial nephritis is usually asymptomatic, presenting with slowly progressive renal impairment. Urinalysis may be normal or show low-grade proteinuria (<1.5 g/day) and/or pyuria. Diagnosis depends on renal biopsy, which reveals variable cellular infiltration of the interstitium, tubular atrophy, and fibrosis. There are many causes including sarcoidosis, drugs (prescribed and non-prescribed), irradiation, toxins, and metabolic disorders.

Sarcoidosis—hypercalciuria and hypercalcaemia are the commonest manifestations that affect the kidney, but sarcoidosis rarely causes a granulomatous interstitial disease that usually responds rapidly to steroid treatment.

Analgesic nephropathy—characterized by renal papillary necrosis and chronic interstitial nephritis. It is caused by the prolonged and excessive consumption of combinations of analgesics, mostly (but not always) including phenacetin. In the 1970s and 1980s this was the cause of endstage renal failure in up to 20% of patients on dialysis in some countries (including Australia and Belgium), but it is now a relatively rare condition following withdrawal of phenacetin (in most countries). It is associated with a high incidence of urothelial malignancy.

Nonsteroidal anti-inflammatory drugs—the most frequent cause of permanent renal insufficiency after acute interstitial nephritis, risk factors for irreversible failure being pre-existing renal damage, long-standing intake of the causative drug, slow oligosymptomatic disease development, and histological signs of chronicity.

5-Aminosalicylic acid—used in the treatment of chronic inflammatory bowel disease and causes clinical nephrotoxicity in approximately 1 in 4000 patients/year. Inflammation can persist in the renal interstitium for months or years after stopping the drug, and renal impairment can continue to worsen even after the drug is stopped.

Chinese herb nephropathy—first recognized in women presenting with renal failure, often near endstage, following exposure to a slimming regimen containing Chinese herbs. Renal biopsy reveals extensive interstitial fibrosis with atrophy and loss of the tubules, but with little cellular infiltration. It is caused in most cases (but perhaps not all) by aristolochic acid, and is associated with a high incidence of urothelial malignancy.

Lithium—most common renal side effect is to cause nephrogenic diabetes insipidus. Long-term treatment does not affect glomerular filtration rate in most patients, but 20% develop chronic renal insufficiency. It is likely that the serum concentration of lithium is important, and that renal damage is more probable if the serum concentration is consistently high, or if there are repeated episodes of lithium toxicity.

Endemic Balkan nephropathy—a chronic, familial, noninflammatory tubulointerstitial disease of the kidneys that is associated with a high frequency of urothelial atypia, occasionally culminating in tumours of the renal pelvis and urethra. Prevalence is very high in farmers living along the valley of the Danube and its tributaries. It has clear clinical and pathological similarities with Chinese herb nephropathy, and is likely to be caused in genetically predisposed people by exposure to aristolochic acid.

Radiation nephropathy—preventive shielding of the kidneys in patients receiving radiation therapy generally prevents radiation nephropathy, but total-body irradiation preceding bone marrow transplantation leads 20% to develop chronic renal failure in the long term.

Nephropathies induced by toxins. (1) Lead—a diagnosis of lead nephropathy should be considered in any patient with progressive renal failure, mild to moderate proteinuria, significant hypertension, a history of gout, and an appropriate history of exposure. (2) Cadmium—exposure to high levels of cadmium are clearly toxic to the kidneys, but in the environmentally exposed population its renal effects appear to be mild and not associated with progressive renal impairment.

Nephropathies induced by metabolic disorders. (1) Chronic hypokalaemia—can induce interstitial fibrosis, tubular atrophy, and cyst formation that is most prominent in the renal medulla. (2) Chronic urate nephropathy—persistent hyperuricaemia can lead to the deposition of microtophi of amorphous urate crystals in the interstitium, with a surrounding giant cell reaction ('gouty nephropathy'). However, clinical evidence linking chronic renal failure to gout is weak; renal dysfunction can be documented only when the serum urate concentration is more than 10 mg/dl (600 μmol/litre) in women and more than 13 mg/dl (780 μmol/litre) in men for prolonged periods.

Sarcoidosis

Sarcoidosis is a multisystem disorder of unknown aetiology characterized by the accumulation in many tissues of T lymphocytes, mononuclear phagocytes, and noncaseating granulomas. The pathogenesis and clinical features of the condition are discussed in Chapter 18.12.

Clinically important renal involvement is an occasional problem—hypercalciuria and hypercalcaemia are usually responsible, although granulomatous interstitial disease, glomerular disease, obstructive uropathy, and (rarely) endstage renal disease may also occur. The true incidence of renal involvement in sarcoidosis remains unknown, but several small series of renal biopsies suggest that some degree of renal involvement occurs in approximately 35% of patients with sarcoidosis.

Clinical features

Hypercalciuria, hypercalcaemia, nephrolithiasis, granulomatous interstitial nephritis, glomerular disease, and urinary tract disorders can all be observed in patients with sarcoidosis. Macrophages in sarcoid granulomas contain a 1α-hydroxylase enzyme, but not a 24-hydroxylase enzyme, capable of converting vitamin D to its active form. The resultant increase in the absorption of calcium from the gut, which occurs in up to 50% of those with sarcoidosis, leads to hypercalciuria and, in 2.5 to 20% of cases, to hypercalcaemia. Most patients remain asymptomatic, but nephrolithiasis, nephrocalcinosis, renal insufficiency, and polyuria are potential complications. Nephrolithiasis occurs in approximately 1 to 14% of patients with sarcoidosis and may be the presenting feature. Nephrocalcinosis, observed in over one-half of those with renal insufficiency, is the most common cause of chronic renal failure in sarcoidosis. The increase in urine output associated with hypercalcaemia and hypercalciuria is due to reduced responsiveness to antidiuretic hormone (ADH).

An interstitial nephritis with granuloma formation is common in sarcoidosis, but the development of clinical disease manifested by renal insufficiency is unusual. A survey of all renal biopsies over a 6-year period at three general hospitals found clinically significant sarcoid granulomatous interstitial nephritis in only four cases. Most affected patients have clear evidence of diffuse active sarcoidosis, although some present with an isolated elevation in the plasma creatinine concentration and no or only minimal renal manifestations. Renal biopsy reveals normal glomeruli, interstitial infiltration mostly with mononuclear cells, noncaseating granulomas in the interstitium, tubular injury, and—with more chronic disease—interstitial fibrosis.

Granulomatosis interstitial nephritis is also seen in other diseases, including allergic interstitial nephritis (mainly drug-induced, caused by nonsteroidal anti-inflammatory drugs (NSAIDs) and 5-aminosalicylic acid), Wegener's granulomatosis, berylliosis, and tuberculosis. The urinary manifestations of granulomatous interstitial nephritis are relatively nonspecific, with urinalysis typical of other chronic tubulointerstitial diseases, being normal or showing only sterile pyuria or mild proteinuria.

Glomerular involvement is rare in sarcoidosis. A variety of different lesions have been described in isolated cases, including membranous nephropathy, a proliferative or crescentic glomerulonephritis, and focal glomerulosclerosis. The presence of heavy proteinuria or red cell casts tends to differentiate these glomerulopathies from interstitial nephritis.

Occasionally, retroperitoneal lymph node involvement, retroperitoneal fibrosis, or renal stones may produce ureteric obstruction.

Diagnosis and treatment

Sarcoid nephropathy should be considered in any patient with unexplained renal failure and hypercalcaemia, nephrocalcinosis, renal tubular defect, or increased serum immunoglobulins. Patients with sarcoid nephropathy will often have signs and symptoms of pulmonary, ocular, and/or dermal involvement, but the presence of granulomas on renal biopsy, while not specific to sarcoidosis, should strongly suggest this diagnosis in an appropriate setting. In patients with known sarcoidosis, sarcoid nephropathy should be considered in the presence of renal failure, hypercalcaemia, nephrolithiasis, nephrocalcinosis, or renal tubular defects.

Granulomatous interstitial nephritis can be treated effectively with glucocorticoids, typically prednisolone 1 to 1.5 mg/kg per day initially, tapered off following resolution of symptoms or signs of disease activity. Patients often respond quickly with an improvement in renal function, but this depends greatly on the extent and severity of inflammation and fibrosis before treatment was initiated. There are no controlled trials regarding the dose or length of the treatment.

The hypercalcaemic/hypercalciuric syndrome also responds quickly to corticosteroids. In general the dose needed to treat this complication is significantly lower than that required to treat granulomatous interstitial nephritis, and can be as low as 35 mg prednisolone daily. Chloroquine, by decreasing the level of 1,25-dihydroxycholecalciferol, is also an effective therapy for the hypercalcaemic/hypercalciuric syndrome. Ketoconazole, an inhibitor of steroidogenesis, has been used in a single patient who could not tolerate corticosteroids and was effective in decreasing the level of active vitamin D as well as serum and urinary calcium.

Although uncommon in patients with sarcoidosis, endstage renal failure requiring renal replacement therapy is usually due to

hypercalcaemic nephropathy rather than granulomatous nephritis. Graft loss after renal transplantation due to disease recurrence has not been reported.

Drug-induced nephropathies

Three well-described forms of drug-induced chronic interstitial nephritis—analgesic nephropathy, 5-aminosalicylic acid nephropathy, and Chinese herb nephropathy—are compared and contrasted in Table 21.9.2.1, along with a fourth condition, endemic Balkan nephropathy.

Analgesic nephropathy

Analgesic nephropathy is a specific form of renal disease characterized by renal papillary necrosis and chronic interstitial nephritis caused by the prolonged and excessive consumption of analgesics. It is invariably caused by compound analgesic mixtures containing aspirin or other antipyretic agent in combination with phenacetin, paracetamol, or salicylamide and caffeine or codeine in popular over-the-counter proprietary medicines.

In the recent past, analgesic nephropathy was one of the commoner causes of chronic renal failure, particularly in Australia and parts of Europe. Estimates made before phenacetin was removed from over-the-counter analgesics and before the enactment of legislation making combined analgesic preparations only available by prescription (in Sweden, Canada, and Australia) suggested that analgesic nephropathy was responsible for 1 to 3% of cases of endstage renal disease in the United States of America as a whole, up to 10% in areas of North Carolina, and 13 to 20% in Australia and some countries in Europe (such as Belgium and Switzerland). During the 1990s, there was a clear decrease in the prevalence and incidence of the condition among patients undergoing dialysis in several European countries and Australia. Most authors have associated this decrease with the removal of phenacetin from analgesic mixtures, but it is impossible to draw definitive conclusions from the epidemiological observations since other factors, such as

Table 21.9.2.1 Differential diagnosis of some forms of chronic interstitial nephritis

	Analgesic nephropathy	5-Aminosalicylic acid nephritis	Chinese herb nephropathy	Endemic Balkan nephropathy
Course	>10–15 years	>6 months	6 months–2 years	>20 years
Kidney imaging	Shrunken, irregular contours, papillary calcifications	Slightly shrunken, smooth, no calcifications	Shrunken, irregular contours, no calcifications	Shrunken, smooth surface, no calcifications
Histology				
◆ Cellular infiltration	++	+++	+	+
◆ Fibrosis	++	++	++	++
◆ Atrophy	++	+	++	+++
Capillary sclerosis	+	?–	?/+	+
Apoptosis	?	?	?	+
Urothelial malignancies	+[a]	–	+	+
Familial occurrence	–	–	–	+
Aetiology	Analgesics + addictive substances	5-Aminosalicylic acid + additional factors	Aristolochic acid + vasoactive substances	?Aristolochic acid + genetic predisposition

[a] As long as phenacetin was part of the analgesic mixture.

eligibility criteria for dialysis treatment and the availability of remaining analgesic mixtures, may also have had an influence.

Pathogenesis and pathology

The aetiology of analgesic nephropathy remains controversial, and the question of which kinds of analgesic are nephrotoxic is still a matter of debate. Experimental studies, mainly using rats fed with large amounts of drugs, sometimes aggravating the renal effects by dehydration or by introducing sepsis, have produced results that have been difficult to interpret, but it could be concluded that renal papillary necrosis was most frequently observed after the administration of aspirin in combination with phenacetin or paracetamol.

In humans, the long-standing excessive use of analgesics observed in patients with analgesic nephropathy is preferentially that of analgesic mixtures rather than single agents, abusers taking these products for their mood-altering effects rather than for the relief of physical complaints, hence all these mixtures contain caffeine and/or codeine, substances that can create psychological dependence. In most of the early reports of analgesic nephropathy, nearly all patients had taken large amounts of analgesic mixtures containing phenacetin.

In a variety of case-control studies, patients with renal failure ranging from newly diagnosed chronic kidney disease (CKD, stages 1–3) to endstage renal disease, and the specific diagnosis of renal papillary necrosis, have been compared with a variety of controls. The definition of 'minimal analgesic abuse' has varied considerably, from a frequency of twice a week to daily, and from a period of 1 month to 1 year. However, overall the findings show that analgesic abuse is associated with an exceptionally high relative risk of 17.2 with regard to papillary necrosis, a risk of between 2.2 and 2.9 with regard to chronic kidney disease or endstage renal failure in four studies, and with nonconclusive results in other studies.

Most of these case-control studies also reported on the nephrotoxicity of different kinds of analgesics. Except for single analgesics, however, the products taken were part of analgesic mixtures, the composition of many of which changed considerably over the time period that they were available. Only Pommer *et al.* were able to calculate reliable risk ratios for the different analgesics in the combinations as they were marketed, and controlled for the use of other analgesics and for their 'historical' compositions. They found an overall relative risk of 2.4 (95% CI 1.8–3.4), with increased risks ranging from 2.6 to 4.8 for the different combinations (with or without phenacetin) marketed in Germany, and no increased risk for single ingredient analgesics. By contrast, the prospective controlled longitudinal epidemiological study of Dubach *et al.* demonstrated a high increased risk associated with the regular consumption of analgesic mixtures mostly containing phenacetin.

The Basle autopsy prevalence of analgesic nephropathy decreased continuously from approximately 3% in 1980 to 0.2% in 2000. Similarly, capillary sclerosis of the urinary tract, the initiating event in the pathophysiology of papillary necrosis and analgesic nephropathy and the histological hallmark of the effect of toxic metabolites of phenacetin in analgesic abusers, decreased from 4% of autopsy cases between 1978 and 1980 to a single case in a study observed at the end of 2000.

However, the withdrawal of phenacetin from analgesic mixtures in western Europe, Australia, and the United States of America gives rise to the question of the nephrotoxic potency of different kinds of products. Clinical observations in countries where analgesics without phenacetin have been on the market for more than 20 years (e.g. Australia, Belgium, Germany) have shown that identical renal pathology is observed in patients abusing analgesic mixtures that have never contained phenacetin. We observed a cohort of 226 patients with analgesic nephropathy diagnosed according to objective renal imaging criteria. Abuse of analgesic mixtures was documented in all except seven patients, and in 46 patients nephrotoxicity was found in the absence of any previous phenacetin consumption. These patients abused the combinations of aspirin and paracetamol; aspirin and pyrazolones; paracetamol and pyrazolones; and two pyrazolones.

The mechanisms responsible for renal injury are incompletely understood. Phenacetin is metabolized to acetaminophen and to reactive intermediates that can injure cells, in part by lipid peroxidation. These metabolites tend to accumulate in the medulla along the medullary osmotic gradient created by the countercurrent system. As a result, the highest concentrations are seen at the papillary tip, the site of the initial vascular lesions. The potentiating effect of aspirin with both phenacetin and acetaminophen may be related to two factors. First, acetaminophen undergoes oxidative metabolism by prostaglandin H synthase to reactive quinone imine that is conjugated to glutathione. If acetaminophen is present alone, there is sufficient glutathione generated in the papillae to detoxify the reactive intermediate. However, if acetaminophen is ingested with aspirin, the aspirin is converted to salicylate, which becomes highly concentrated and depletes glutathione in both the cortex and papillae of the kidney. With the cellular glutathione depleted, the reactive metabolite of acetaminophen then produces lipid peroxides and arylation of tissue proteins, ultimately resulting in necrosis of the papillae (Fig. 21.9.2.1). Second, aspirin (and other NSAIDs) suppress prostaglandin production by inhibiting cyclooxygenase enzymes. Renal blood flow, particularly within the renal medulla that normally exists on the verge of hypoxia, is highly dependent on the systemic and local production of vasodilatory prostaglandins. The final injury is therefore due to both the haemodynamic and cytotoxic effects of these drugs, resulting in papillary necrosis and interstitial fibrosis.

The renal damage induced by analgesics is most prominent in the medulla. The earliest changes consist of prominent thickening of the vasa recta capillaries (capillary sclerosis) and patchy areas of tubular necrosis; similar vascular lesions can be found in the renal pelvis and ureter, suggesting that the primary effect is damage to the vascular endothelial cells. Later changes include areas of papillary necrosis and secondary cortical injury, with focal and segmental glomerulosclerosis and interstitial infiltration and fibrosis.

Clinical features

The renal manifestations of analgesic nephropathy are usually nonspecific; renal function is normal or there is slowly progressive chronic renal failure, and urinalysis may be normal or may reveal sterile pyuria and mild proteinuria (less than 1.5 g/day). Hypertension and anaemia are commonly seen with moderate to advanced disease; more prominent proteinuria that can exceed 3.5 g/day can also occur at this time, a probable reflection of secondary haemodynamically mediated glomerular injury. Most patients have no symptoms referable to the urinary tract, although flank pain or macroscopic/microscopic haematuria from a sloughed or obstructing papilla may occur, or as a result of a transitional cell carcinoma. Urinary tract infection is also somewhat more common in women with this disorder.

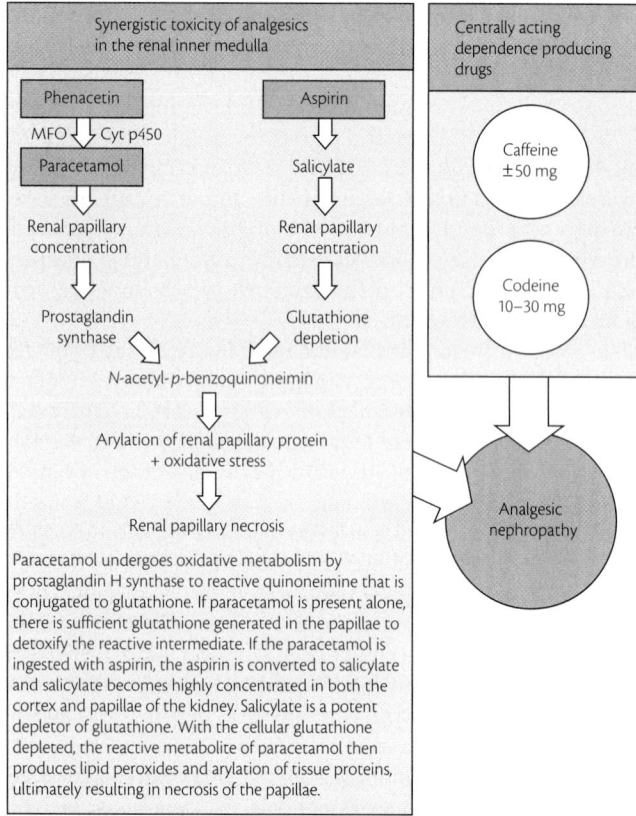

Fig. 21.9.2.1 Synergistic toxicity of analgesics in the renal inner medulla and centrally acting dependence-producing drugs leading to analgesic nephropathy. Reproduced with permission from Kincaid-Smith P, Nanra RS (1993). In: Schrier RW, Gottschalk CW, eds. Diseases of the kidney, pp 1099–129. Little, Brown and Company, Boston, MA, and Duggin G (1996). American Journal of Kidney Diseases 28/1 (Suppl. 1), S39–S47.

The tumours generally become apparent after 15 to 25 years of analgesic abuse, usually but not always in patients with clinically evident analgesic nephropathy. Most patients are still taking the drug at the time of diagnosis, but clinically evident disease can first become apparent several years after cessation of analgesic intake and even after renal transplantation. It is presumed that the induction of malignancy results from the intrarenal accumulation of N-hydroxylated phenacetin metabolites that have potent alkylating action. The highest concentration of these metabolites will be in the renal medulla, ureters, and bladder (as described above), possibly explaining the predisposition to carcinogenesis at these sites. The pathogenetic importance of phenacetin metabolites is suggested indirectly from the observation that the prolonged ingestion of other analgesics that can cause papillary necrosis, but do not form the same metabolites, such as acetaminophen and the NSAIDs, is not associated with tumour formation. The main presenting symptom of urinary tract malignancy in patients with analgesic nephropathy is microscopic or gross haematuria, hence continued monitoring is essential, and new haematuria should be evaluated by urinary cytology and, if indicated, cystoscopy with retrograde pyelography. The incidence of urothelial carcinoma after renal transplantation in patients with analgesic nephropathy is comparable to the general incidence (up to 10%) of urothelial carcinomas in patients with endstage renal failure due to analgesic nephropathy. Removal of the native kidneys before renal transplantation has been suggested, but the efficacy of this regimen has not been proven.

Diagnosis and treatment

The lack of reliable criteria for diagnosis and yet the apparent high prevalence of analgesic nephropathy during the 1980s in Belgium (17.9% in 1984) led us to perform a series of prospective multicentre controlled studies to define and validate the diagnostic criteria for this disease. We provided strong evidence that specific anatomical changes, best seen by noncontrast CT scan, have much greater sensitivity and specificity than other clinical signs and symptoms in the diagnosis of endstage renal disease due to analgesic nephropathy. These changes are: (1) decrease in renal volume, (2) bumpy renal contours, and (3) papillary calcifications. In a more recent study, these observations were validated in a representative sample of patients with analgesic abuse with endstage renal disease and extended to patients with moderate renal failure. In patients with endstage renal failure, decreased renal volume had the greatest sensitivity at 95%, while papillary calcification had the highest specificity, and contour or papillary necrosis had a sensitivity and specificity of 90%. In patients with moderate renal failure, papillary calcification was most sensitive at 92% and specific at 100%. The combination of papillary necrosis with either a bumpy renal contour or small kidneys did not improve sensitivity or specificity. In clinical practice, however, it is important to remember that the predictive value of this test, like any other diagnostic test, is very much dependent on the prevalence of the disease in the population under study. This test should therefore be utilized in patients with a reasonable risk for analgesic nephropathy and not as a general screening test.

As indicated above, patients with normal or only mildly/moderately impaired renal function should be strongly encouraged to stop taking analgesics in the hope that further deterioration in renal function can be avoided. Those with severe or endstage renal

Despite the nonspecific nature of the renal presentation, there are frequently other findings that point towards the presence of analgesic nephropathy. Most patients are between the ages of 30 and 70 years, and careful questioning often reveals a history of chronic headaches or low back pain that leads to the analgesic use. Also common are other somatic complaints (such as malaise and weakness), and ulcer-like symptoms or a history of peptic ulcer disease due in part to chronic aspirin ingestion.

The decline in renal function can be expected to progress if analgesics are continued, whereas renal function stabilizes or mildly improves in most patients if analgesic consumption is discontinued. However, if the renal disease is already advanced, then progression may occur in the absence of drug intake, presumably due to secondary haemodynamic and metabolic changes associated with nephron loss. The late course of analgesic nephropathy may also be complicated by two additional problems, malignancy and atherosclerotic disease. Urinary tract malignancy will develop in as many as 8 to 10% of patients with analgesic nephropathy, but in well under 1% of phenacetin-containing analgesic users without kidney disease. For example, in women under the age of 50, analgesic abuse is the most common cause of bladder cancer, an otherwise unusual disorder in young women. The potential magnitude of this problem has also been illustrated by histological examination of nephrectomy specimens obtained before renal transplantation, when the incidence of urothelial atypia approaches 50%.

failure are unlikely to recover renal function, although there may be other valid medical reasons for recommending that they stop ingesting large quantities of analgesics. The medical management of chronic renal failure is along conventional lines, as is provision of renal replacement therapy.

NSAIDs

NSAIDs are popular for treating a wide range of clinical conditions and are available both over the counter and on prescription. Despite their usefulness, there is substantial evidence from experimental and clinical studies that they have a variety of effects on the kidney. The most common renal disorder associated with NSAIDs is acute, largely reversible, insufficiency due to the inhibition of renal vasodilatory prostaglandins in the clinical setting of a stimulated renin–angiotensin system. Older age, hypertension, concomitant use of diuretics or aspirin, pre-existing renal failure, diabetes, and plasma-volume contraction are known risk factors for renal failure after the ingestion of NSAIDs. Rarely, NSAIDs may cause acute interstitial nephritis with proteinuria.

In contrast to the well-characterized acute effects of NSAIDs on the kidney, the chronic effects are less well documented. However, a recent report demonstrated that NSAIDs are the most frequent cause of permanent renal insufficiency after acute interstitial nephritis. Risk factors for irreversible failure are pre-existing renal damage, long-standing intake of the causative drug, slow oligosymptomatic disease development, and histological signs of chronicity with those of acute interstitial nephritis. Although renal papillary necrosis and chronic renal failure can occur after the prolonged use of NSAIDs, the actual risk of these serious complications is unknown. Furthermore, the frequency of renal papillary necrosis in the context of NSAID intake as a primary or contributing cause of endstage renal disease remains unknown.

5-Aminosalicylic acid

Over the past few years an association between the use of 5-aminosalicylic acid (5-ASA) in patients with chronic inflammatory bowel disease and the development of a particular type of chronic tubulointerstitial nephritis has been suggested.

For many years, sulfasalazine, an azo-compound derived from sulphapyridine and 5-ASA, the latter being the pharmacologically active moiety, was the only valuable noncorticosteroid drug in the treatment of inflammatory bowel disease. Since the therapeutically inactive sulphapyridine moiety was largely responsible for the mainly haematological side effects of sulfasalazine, this stimulated the development of several new 5-ASA formulations (mesalazine, olsalazine, balsalazide) for topical and oral use. These new 5-ASA products replaced sulfasalazine as the first-line therapy for mildly to moderately active inflammatory bowel disease. However, a literature search revealed 17 published cases of renal impairment associated with 5-ASA therapy in patients with inflammatory bowel disease, and in several it was shown that this did not recover completely on stopping the drug, even after a follow-up period of several years. In a retrospective study, nephrologists reported 40 patients with inflammatory bowel disease showing renal impairment, including 15 cases with interstitial nephritis and previous use of 5-ASA. Stimulated by these findings we started a European prospective registration study aiming to register all patients with inflammatory bowel disease and renal impairment and to control for a possible association with 5-ASA therapy. A cohort of 1449 patients with inflammatory bowel

disease seen during 1 year in the outpatient clinics of 28 European gastroenterology departments was investigated. Preliminary results showed 30 patients (2%) with decreased renal function, and a possible association with 5-ASA therapy was found in one-half of them. A recent study estimated the incidence of clinical nephrotoxicity in patients taking 5-ASA as 1 in 4000 patients/year.

However, determining the cause of renal disease in those with inflammatory bowel disease is not straightforward. The most frequent renal complications are oxalate stones and their consequences, such as pyelonephritis, hydronephrosis, and (in the long term) amyloidosis. Chronic inflammatory bowel disease is also associated with glomerulonephritis and minimal-change glomerulonephritis, membranous, membranoproliferative, and focal glomerulosclerosis, and proliferative crescentic glomerulonephritis have all been reported. As for many drugs, reversible acute interstitial nephritis has been described with the use of 5-ASA compounds. In view of this complexity, the association of 5-ASA and chronic interstitial nephritis in patients with inflammatory bowel disease can be difficult to interpret, since renal involvement may be an extraintestinal manifestation of the underlying disease. However, the particular form of chronic tubulointerstitial nephritis in patients with inflammatory bowel disease treated with 5-ASA is characterized by an important cellular infiltration of the interstitium with macrophages, T cells, and also B cells (Fig. 21.9.2.2).

Pathogenesis and pathology

That 5-ASA causes renal disease is supported by the number of case reports in the literature of patients with inflammatory bowel disease using 5-ASA as their only medication, the improvement (at least partially) of impaired renal function on stopping the drug, and a worsening after resuming 5-ASA use. Furthermore, the molecular structure of 5-ASA is very close to that of salicylic acid, phenacetin, and aminophenol, drugs with well-documented nephrotoxic potential (Fig. 21.9.2.1). Calder et al. found that necrosis of the proximal convoluted tubules and papillary necrosis developed in rats after a single intravenous injection of 5-ASA at doses of 1.4, 2.8, and 5.7 mmol/kg body weight (high pharmacological doses). The mechanism of renal damage, possibly caused by 5-ASA itself, may be analogous to that of salicylates by inducing hypoxia of renal tissues, either by uncoupling oxidative phosphorylation in renal mitochondria by inhibiting the synthesis of renal prostaglandins, or by rendering the kidney susceptible to oxidative damage by a reducing renal glutathione concentration after inhibition of the pentose phosphate shunt.

Clinical features

A typical case is shown in Fig. 21.9.2.2. An intriguing aspect of this type of toxic nephropathy is the documented persistence of the renal interstitium inflammation even several months/years after first taking the drug. The disease is more prevalent in men, with a male to female ratio of 15:2. The age of patients in reported cases ranges from 14 to 45 years. By contrast with analgesic nephropathy, where renal lesions are only observed after several years of analgesic abuse, interstitial nephritis associated with 5-ASA was observed during the first year of treatment in 7 out of 17 reported cases; most of these patients had started 5-ASA therapy with documented normal renal function. In several patients, particularly those in which there was a delayed diagnosis of renal damage, recovery of renal function did not occur, and some needed renal replacement therapy.

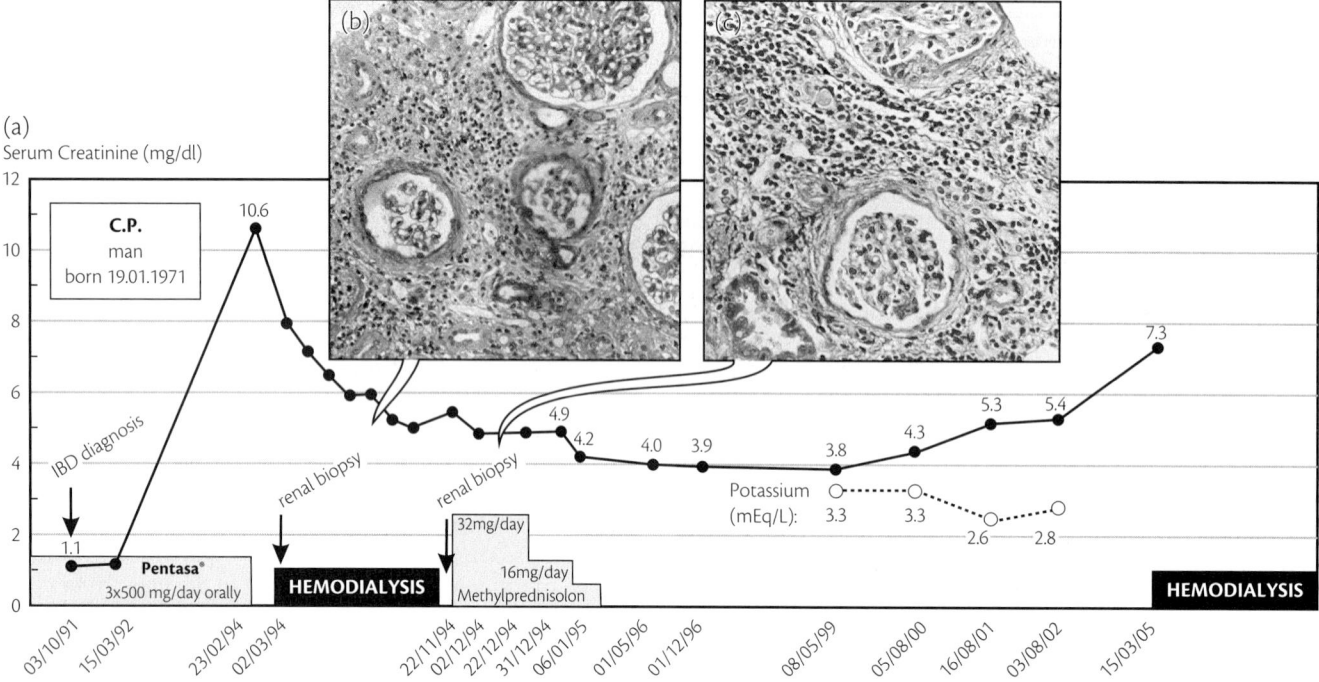

Fig. 21.9.2.2 Nephrotoxicity in a patient treated with 5-aminosalicylic acid for inflammatory bowel disease. (a) Evolution of renal failure. (b) First renal biopsy showing widening and massive cellular infiltration of the interstitium, tubular atrophy, and relative spacing of glomeruli. The cellular infiltration was identified using appropriate monoclonal antibodies and consisted not only of T cells and macrophages but also of B cells. (c) A second renal biopsy performed after the drug had been stopped for 8 months, when there was a modest improvement in renal function, again showed a significant cellular infiltration of the interstitium, tubular atrophy, and fibrosis. Thirteen years after the diagnosis of chronic interstitial nephritis was made in this young man, who had documented normal renal function at the start of treatment, haemodialysis had to be started. He is now on the waiting list for renal transplantation.

Diagnosis and treatment

Since this type of chronic tubulointerstitial nephritis produces few if any symptoms, and if diagnosed at a late stage progresses to irreversible chronic endstage renal disease, serum creatinine levels should be measured in any patient with inflammatory bowel disease treated with 5-ASA at the start of the treatment, every 3 months for the remainder of the first year, and annually thereafter. The use of concurrent immunosuppressive therapy, as is the case in severe forms of chronic inflammatory bowel disease, may necessitate extension to the period of intensive renal function monitoring. If serum creatinine increases, a renal biopsy is the only way to demonstrate the cause.

Chinese herb nephropathy/aristolochic acid nephropathy

In 1992, physicians in Belgium noted an increasing number of women presenting with renal failure, often near endstage, following their exposure to a slimming regimen containing Chinese herbs. An initial survey of seven nephrology centres in Brussels identified 14 women under the age of 50 who had presented over a 3-year period with advanced renal failure due to biopsy-proven chronic tubulointerstitial nephritis, nine of whom had been exposed to the same slimming regimen. As of early 2000, a total of more than 120 cases had been identified. The epidemiology is unknown, as is the risk for the development of severe renal damage, but the recent publication of case reports from several countries in Europe and Asia would seem to indicate that the incidence of herbal medicine-induced nephrotoxicity is more common than previously thought.

Pathogenesis and pathology

The aetiology of Chinese herb nephropathy is not fully understood. A plant nephrotoxin, aristolochic acid, was proposed as a possible aetiological agent, but this compound was not part of the herbal preparations used by all the patients. Furthermore, aristolochic acid (0.15 mg/tablet) has been used as an immunomodulatory drug for 20 years in Germany by thousands of patients, sometimes in doses comparable to the Chinese herb slimming regimen; despite this exposure, there is no report relating chronic tubulointerstitial nephritis to aristolochic acid.

In addition to aristolochic acid, patients with Chinese herb nephropathy also received the appetite suppressants fenfluramine and diethylpropion, which have vasoconstrictive properties, and acetazolamide, which alkalinizes the urine, thereby potentially enhancing the nephrotoxic effect of aristolochic acid, although a recent experimental study did not support this hypothesis.

Another uncertain factor is why only some patients exposed to the same herbal preparations develop renal disease. Women appear to be at greater risk than men, and other factors that might be important include toxin dose, batch-to-batch variability in toxin content, individual differences in toxin metabolism, and a genetically determined predisposition towards nephrotoxicity and/or carcinogenesis.

The main histological lesion, which is located principally in the cortex, is extensive interstitial fibrosis with atrophy and loss of the tubules (Fig. 21.9.2.3). Cellular infiltration of the interstitium is scarce. Thickening of the walls of the interlobular and afferent arterioles results from endothelial cell swelling. The glomeruli are relatively spared and immune deposits are not observed.

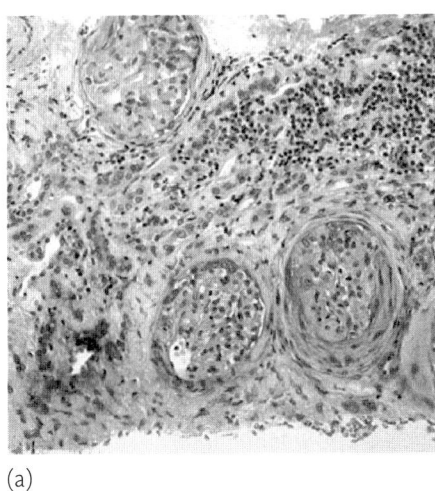
(a)

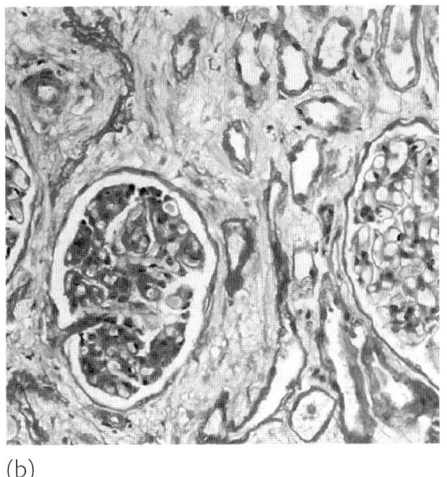
(b)

Fig. 21.9.2.3 Renal biopsy from a patient with Chinese herb nephropathy showing tubular atrophy, widening of the interstitium, cellular infiltration, and fibrosis, with glomeruli surrounded by a fibrotic ring. Masson staining (a), haematoxylin and eosin staining (b).

These findings suggest that the primary lesions may be centred in the vessel walls, thereby leading to ischaemia and interstitial fibrosis.

At one centre in Belgium, 19 native kidneys and ureters were removed in a series of 10 patients during and/or after renal transplantation. Multifocal, high-grade, flat, transitional cell carcinoma (carcinoma *in situ*) was observed in four (40%), while all had multifocal moderate atypia. Tissue samples revealed aristolochic acid-related DNA adducts, indicating a possible mechanism underlying the development of malignancy. In another study of 39 patients with Chinese herb nephropathy and endstage renal disease who underwent prophylactic removal of the native kidneys and ureters, urothelial carcinoma was discovered in 18 and mild to moderate urothelial dysplasia in 19. All atypical cells were found to overexpress a p53 protein, suggesting the presence of a mutation in the gene.

Clinical features

Patients present with renal insufficiency and other features indicating a tubulointerstitial disease. Blood pressure is either normal or only mildly elevated, and the urinary sediment reveals only a few red and white cells. The urine contains protein (less than 1.5 g/day), consisting of both albumin and low molecular weight proteins that are normally reabsorbed by the proximal tubules, hence tubular dysfunction—also marked by glycosuria—contributes to the proteinuria. The plasma creatinine concentration at presentation has ranged from 1.4 to 12.7 mg/dl (123–1122 µmol/litre). Follow-up studies have revealed relatively stable renal function in most patients with an initial plasma creatinine concentration below 2 mg/dl (176 µmol/litre) once the intake of the drug has been stopped. However, progressive renal failure resulting in eventual dialysis or transplantation may ensue in patients with more severe disease, even if further exposure to Chinese herbs is prevented.

A similar clinical and pathological process has been reported in a group of patients from Taiwan who had ingested a selection of uncontrolled traditional Chinese herbs that differed from those of the slimming regimen. Despite discontinuation of these remedies, progressive renal failure was common.

Diagnosis and treatment

There are no specific criteria for the diagnosis of this type of renal disease. The condition should be suspected in any patient with unexplained relatively rapidly progressive renal disease who is using/abusing herbal remedies. The presence of tubular proteinuria may be a clue to the diagnosis, particularly in the early stages. The histological appearances are not specific, but renal biopsy is necessary to exclude other conditions in this clinical context.

There is no proven effective therapy for this disorder, which typically presents with marked interstitial fibrosis without prominent inflammation, although an uncontrolled study suggested that corticosteroids may slow the rate of loss of renal function. The high incidence of cellular atypia of the genitourinary tract suggests that, as a minimum, these patients should undergo regular surveillance for abnormal urinary cytology. Whether more aggressive management strategies, such as bilateral native nephroureterectomies (particularly in those undergoing renal transplantation), are required is unclear. Findings from a recent report support the more aggressive option. Renal transplantation is an effective modality for those who progress to endstage renal disease; one report noted no recurrence in five patients.

Lithium

Lithium is used extensively in the treatment of patients with manic-depressive psychosis. Different forms of renal effects/injury have been described, most frequently nephrogenic diabetes insipidus, but also renal tubular acidosis, chronic interstitial nephritis, nephrotic syndrome, and focal segmental glomerular sclerosis/global glomerular sclerosis. Hyperparathyroidism is also observed in patients treated with lithium.

Pathogenesis and pathology

Lithium is eliminated from the body almost entirely by the kidney, being filtered at the glomerulus and reabsorbed in the proximal tubule, resulting in a clearance of one-third of the normal creatinine clearance. It moves in and out of cells only slowly and accumulates in the kidney, particularly in the collecting tubule, entering these cells through sodium channels in the luminal membrane. Hence, its principal toxicity relates to distal tubular function, where inhibition of adenylate cyclase and generation of cyclic AMP result in down-regulation of aquaporin-2, the collecting tubule water channel, and a decrease in ADH receptor density, leading to resistance to ADH. Further effects compound this. A low intracellular level of cyclic AMP leads to the increased cellular levels of glycogen observed in kidney biopsy specimens from patients taking lithium, as does the fact that lithium also directly inhibits enzymes involved in glycogen breakdown. The ensuing increased glycogen storage may interfere with distal tubular function and be responsible for the observation that polyuria and polydipsia in lithium-treated patients is due to nephrogenic diabetes insipidus.

The tubular defect in the distal nephron can also impair the ability to maximally acidify the urine. A lithium-induced decrease in the activity of the H^+-ATPase pump in the collecting tubule may be responsible for this defect.

Lithium treatment has been aetiologically related to parathyroid hypertrophy and hyperfunction, the latter seeming to be due to an upward resetting of the level at which the plasma calcium concentration depresses parathyroid hormone release. Persistent hypercalcaemia (in 5–10% of the patients) may exacerbate both the concentrating defect and the interstitial nephritis seen in lithium-treated patients.

Renal biopsies from patients taking lithium show a specific histological lesion in the distal tubule and collecting duct. On light microscopy there is swelling and vacuolization in cells associated with a considerable accumulation of periodic acid–Schiff-positive glycogen. This is present in all renal biopsies from patients taking lithium, appears within days after the administration of lithium, and disappears when lithium ingestion is ceased.

Hestbech *et al.* were the first to suggest that progressive chronic interstitial lesions occurred in the kidneys of patients receiving lithium. However, a controlled study showed no difference between biopsies from patients taking lithium and those from a group of patients who had affective disorders but were not doing so. Specifically, there was no difference in the incidence of glomerular sclerosis, interstitial fibrosis, tubular atrophy, cast formation, or interstitial volume, but there was a significant increase in the number of microcysts in the lithium-treated patients. One reason why it has been difficult to determine the nature of lithium-induced chronic renal damage has been the lack, until recently, of an animal model in which lesions similar to those noted in human biopsies could be demonstrated. However, a recent study on lithium nephrotoxicity carried out in the rabbit showed clear-cut evidence of progressive histological and functional impairment, with the development of significant interstitial fibrosis, tubular atrophy, glomerular sclerosis, and cystic tubular lesions. A recent publication by Markowitz *et al.* revealed chronic tubulointerstitial nephropathy in 100% of 24 patients who had received lithium for several years, associated with cortical and medullary tubular cysts or dilatation. There was also a surprisingly high prevalence of focal segmental glomerulosclerosis and global glomerulosclerosis, sometimes of equivalent severity to the chronic tubulointerstitial disease. Despite discontinuing lithium treatment, seven of nine patients with initial serum creatinine values above 2.5 mg/dl (225 μmol/litre) progressed to endstage renal disease.

A recent French follow-up study of lithium-treated patients demonstrated that the duration of lithium therapy and the cumulative dose of lithium were the major determinants of nephrotoxicity and estimated a prevalence of lithium-related endstage renal failure in 2 of 1000 dialysis patients. Twelve out of 74 patients in this study reached endstage renal failure at a mean age of 65 years, with an average latency between onset of lithium therapy and endstage renal failure of 20 years. Lepkifker *et al.* retrospectively studied 114 subjects with major depressive or schizoaffective disorders who had been taken lithium for 4 to 30 years from 1968 to 2000. Long-term lithium therapy did not influence glomerular function in most patients, but 20% of those receiving long-term lithium exhibited 'creeping creatinine' and developed chronic renal insufficiency.

Clinical features

Apart from acute lithium intoxication, chronic poisoning can occur in patients whose lithium dosage has been increased or in those with a decreased effective circulating volume, decreased sodium intake, diabetes mellitus, gastroenteritis, and renal failure, thereby resulting in an increase in serum lithium levels. Symptoms associated with poisoning include lethargy, drowsiness, coarse hand tremor, muscle weakness, nausea, vomiting, weight loss, polyuria, and polydipsia. Severe toxicity is associated with increased deep tendon reflexes, seizures, syncope, renal insufficiency, and coma. The commonest manifestation is altered mental status.

Chronic lithium poisoning is frequently associated with electrocardiographic changes, including ST-segment depression and inverted T waves in the lateral precordial leads. Lithium is concentrated within the thyroid and inhibits the synthesis and release of thyroxine, which can lead to hypothyroidism, and it may also cause thyrotoxicosis. Symptoms of hypercalcaemia may also be present, exacerbating the urinary concentrating defect already present in these patients.

In patients with glomerular lesions such as minimal-change or focal glomerular sclerosis, proteinuria generally begins within 1.5 to 10 months after the onset of therapy, completely or partially resolving in most patients within 4 weeks after lithium is discontinued. Reinstitution of lithium has led to recurrent nephrosis in some cases.

The hyperparathyroidism observed in patients receiving lithium treatment is characterized by elevated parathyroid hormone levels, hypercalcaemia, hypocalciuria, and normal serum phosphate levels, in contrast to primary hyperparathyroidism in which hypophosphataemia and hypercalciuria are seen.

Diagnosis and treatment

The severity of chronic lithium intoxication correlates directly with the serum lithium concentration and may be categorized as mild (1.5–2.0 mM/litre), moderate (2.0–2.5 mM/litre), or severe (>2.5 mM/litre).

Polyuria and polydipsia due to nephrogenic diabetes insipidus and other acute manifestations of the effect of lithium on the kidney usually disappear rapidly if lithium is withdrawn. The decision about management, however, usually revolves around the relative benefit of the lithium in controlling and preventing the manifestation of manic-depressive psychosis, and the disadvantage to the patient of the major side-effect of lithium, i.e. polyuria. In most cases the lithium is so clearly beneficial that the polyuria is accepted as a side-effect and treatment continued. It is likely that the serum concentration of lithium is important, and that renal damage is more probable if the serum concentration is consistently high, or if repeated episodes of lithium toxicity occur. The serum lithium concentration should therefore be monitored carefully (at least every 3 months) and maintained at the lowest level that will provide adequate control of psychiatric symptoms.

Much more difficult to handle is the situation where a patient on long-term lithium therapy is found to have impaired renal function for which there is no obvious alternative cause. As stated above, renal failure may progress even if lithium therapy is withdrawn, and in some patients the discontinuation of lithium can lead to a devastating deterioration in their psychiatric condition. The decision as to whether or not to discontinue lithium should therefore be made after frank and open discussion, admitting all uncertainties, with the patient, psychiatric colleagues, and (if appropriate) relatives/carers.

Endemic Balkan nephropathy

Endemic Balkan nephropathy (EBN) is a chronic, familial, noninflammatory tubulointerstitial disease of the kidneys which is associated with a high frequency of urothelial atypia, occasionally culminating in tumours of the renal pelvis and urethra.

As the name suggests, EBN is most commonly seen in southeastern Europe, including the areas traditionally considered to comprise the Balkans, i.e. Serbia, Bosnia and Herzegovina, Croatia, Romania, and Bulgaria. It is most likely to occur among those living in the valley of the Danube river and its tributaries, a region in which the plains and low hills generally have a high humidity and rainfall (Fig. 21.9.2.4). There is a very high prevalence in endemic areas, with rates ranging between approximately 0.5 and 4.4%, increasing to as high as 20% if the disorder is suspected and carefully screened for among an at-risk population. Two recent papers have demonstrated that the prevalence of EBN has remained stable over the last 40 to 50 years in two of the sites where the condition was first recognized. A striking observation is that nearly all affected patients are farmers.

Pathogenesis

The aetiology of EBN is unknown. Many environmental and genetic factors have been evaluated as potential underlying causes, with much emphasis recently on the possibility that aristolochic acid is responsible.

Environmental factors

Given that the condition is endemic to a specific geographic area, toxins and/or environmental exposures that are unique to the Balkans have been investigated. Much recent work has focused on the possibility is that aristolochic acid, a mutagenic and nephrotoxic alkaloid found in the plant *Aristolochia clematis*, may underlie

both Chinese herb nephropathy (see above) and EBN (see Table 21.9.2.1). There are striking pathological and clinical similarities between the progressive interstitial fibrosis observed in young women who have been on a slimming regimen containing Chinese herbs (as well as other agents) and EBN. The detection of aristolochic acid-specific DNA adducts in a number of patients with endstage renal disease and upper urinary tract malignancy coming from areas endemic for EBN also supports the hypothesis that chronic exposure to aristolochic acid is a risk factor for EBN and its associated cancers.

Two other environmental causes have to be considered. First, the mycotoxin hypothesis, which considers that EBN is produced by ochratoxin A. Second, the Pliocene lignite hypothesis, which proposes that the disease is caused by long-term exposure to polycyclic aromatic hydrocarbons and other toxic organic compounds leaching from low-rank coals into drinking-water in wells in the vicinity of settlements where EBN is endemic, although this hypothesis was not supported by a study of large numbers of water samples from endemic and nonendemic villages in Bulgaria.

Genetic factors

Support for a genetic aetiology includes observations that the disease clearly affects particular families, and that some ethnic populations who have lived in endemic areas for generations do not develop EBN. The mode of inheritance has not yet been established and possible causative gene(s) have not been identified, but a locus in the region between 3q25 and 3q26 has been incriminated. By contrast, some observations are inconsistent with a genetic basis for EBN. First, EBN is observed in individuals who have immigrated into the Balkan area from regions without the disorder, and in previously unaffected families who have lived for at least 15 years in endemic areas. Second, EBN does not develop in members from previously affected families who have left endemic areas early in life or who spent less than 15 years in these areas.

A unifying hypothesis may be that the disease most likely occurs in genetically predisposed individuals who are chronically exposed to a causative agent, probably aristolochic acid.

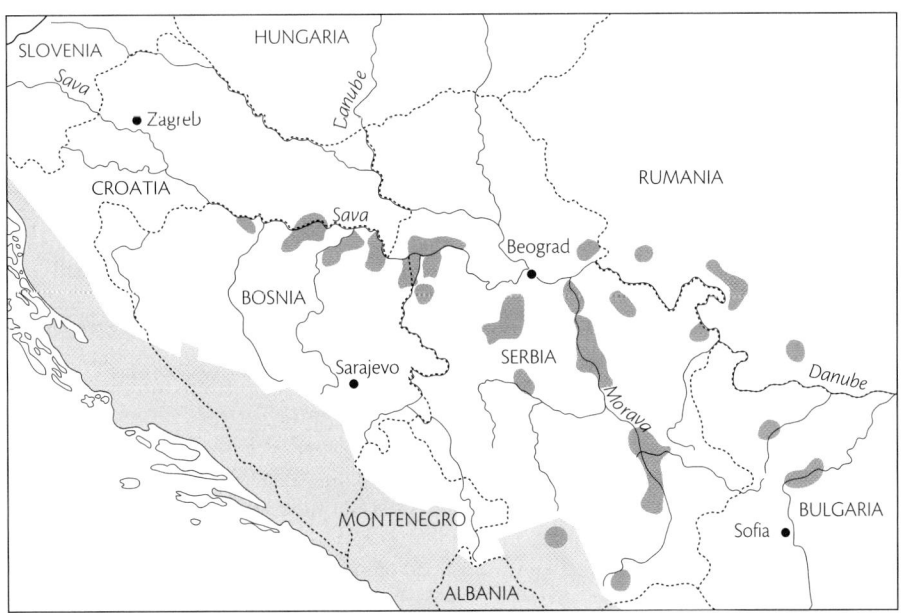

Fig. 21.9.2.4 Foci of endemic Balkan nephropathy.

Pathology

In the early stages of disease, renal histology reveals focal cortical tubular atrophy, interstitial oedema, and peritubuloglomerular sclerosis with limited mononuclear cell infiltration. Narrowing and endothelial swelling of interstitial capillaries (e.g. capillary sclerosis) is also described. In advanced cases, marked tubular atrophy and interstitial fibrosis develop along with focal segmental glomerular changes and global sclerosis. There is an extremely high incidence of cellular atypia and urothelial carcinoma of the genitourinary tract.

Clinical features

EBN is a slowly progressive tubulointerstitial disease that may culminate in endstage renal disease. Clinical manifestations first appear between 30 and 50 years of age, with findings before the age of 20 being extremely rare. One of the first signs is tubular dysfunction, which is characterized by an increased excretion of low molecular weight proteins (such as β2-microglobulin). Early tubular injury can also lead to renal glycosuria, aminoaciduria, and diminished ability to handle an acid load. Over a period of more than 20 years there is a progressive decrease in concentrating ability (resulting in polyuria) and in the glomerular filtration rate (resulting in endstage renal disease). Patients are usually without oedema and normotensive, with hypertension only developing with endstage disease. A normochromic normocytic anaemia occurs with early disease, which becomes increasingly pronounced as the disorder progresses. Urinary tract infection is rarely observed. Kidneys are of normal size early in the course of the disease, but a symmetrical reduction of kidney size with a smooth outline and normal pelvicalyceal system is subsequently observed in patients with late-stage disease. Intrarenal calcifications are not seen.

EBN is also associated with the development of transitional cell carcinoma of the renal pelvis or ureter, with studies noting a wide range in incidence (from 2 to nearly 50%). These tumours are generally superficial and slow-growing.

Diagnosis and treatment

The diagnosis of EBN is based on the presence of some combination of the following findings:

- Symmetrically shrunken kidneys with absence of intrarenal calcifications
- Farmers living in the villages where EBN occurs
- Familial history positive for EBN
- Mild tubular proteinuria, hyposthenuria
- Normochromic/hypochromic anaemia occurring in patients with only slightly impaired renal function

As with many other chronic tubulointerstitial diseases of unclear origin, there is no specific prevention or treatment. Therapy is therefore supportive, with renal replacement therapy being initiated in patients with endstage renal disease.

The high incidence of cellular atypia in the genitourinary tract suggests that regular surveillance should be performed for abnormal urinary cytologies. Whether bilateral native nephroureterectomies are required, particularly in those undergoing renal transplantation, is unclear.

Radiation nephropathy

Radiation nephropathy is a renal disorder caused by ionizing radiation. The kidney may be injured by radiation administered to tumours within the kidney or nearby tissues (testis, ovary, retroperitoneum). Clinicians were aware of the potential adverse effects of X-rays on renal function from the beginning of the 20th century, and between 1940 and 1960 a significant number of cases were reported. In 1953 Luxton established the clinical features of the condition and defined the tolerance of the kidney to irradiation, leading to preventive shielding of the kidneys in patients receiving radiation therapy and to a marked decline in the frequency of radiation nephropathy. In recent years, however, total-body irradiation preceding bone marrow transplantation has resulted in an increasing incidence of radiation nephropathy, with late chronic renal failure developing in 20% of patients who receive this treatment.

Pathogenesis and pathology

The radiation doses traditionally associated with radiation nephropathy were above 2000 rad (20 Gy) (less in children). By contrast, in patients receiving total-body irradiation preceding bone marrow transplantation, renal impairment was observed after doses of 1000 to 1400 rad (10–14 Gy). Fractionation, time, and effects of cytotoxic chemotherapy can probably explain the differences. In laboratory rodents, fractionation of the total dose into multiple separated doses decreases the risk, probably due to repair of sublethal radiation damage during the time between the fractionated doses. Total-body irradiation before bone marrow transplantation is usually administered over a short period, which does not allow sufficient time for the repair of radiation injury to the kidney. Moreover, the additional cytotoxic chemotherapy given to these patients potentiates the effects of ionizing radiation.

The precise pathogenesis of radiation nephropathy remains to be determined. The initial target of ionizing radiation within the kidney appears to be the endothelial cell. Radiation kills cells by damaging DNA, so that cell death after radiation is delayed until the cell divides. After the initial glomerular endothelial injury, vascular occlusion subsequently develops, leading to tubular atrophy. Because inflammatory cells are not seen in the renal parenchyma, the previously used terminology of 'radiation nephritis' is a misnomer.

The pathological features of radiation nephropathy comprise a continuous spectrum of changes that vary in relation to the dose of irradiation administered and the time elapsed after exposure. Large doses are followed by complete atrophy, thickening of basement membranes, and interstitial fibrosis.

Clinical features

Radiation nephropathy can take several forms. Acute radiation nephropathy occurs between 6 and 12 months after radiation therapy and presents with hypertension, anaemia, and oedema. The severity of hypertension ranges from mild to malignant, and more than one-half of the patients progress to chronic renal failure. Radiation nephropathy after total-body irradiation before bone marrow transplantation most closely corresponds to this acute form of radiation nephropathy.

A more insidious chronic form of radiation nephropathy develops over a period of several years and presents primarily with diminished glomerular filtration rate, hypertension, and (occasionally) proteinuria. Another subset of patients may develop hypertension within a few years of irradiation, evolving in some to malignant hypertension with accelerated loss of renal function. Isolated persistent or intermittent proteinuria may also occur, frequently developing more than a decade after radiation exposure.

Diagnosis and treatment

Radiographic studies may help in the diagnosis of acute radiation nephropathy. CT scans with contrast demonstrate sharply demarcated, dense, persistent nephrograms corresponding to the irradiated areas.

The treatment of radiation nephropathy is supportive. Aggressive treatment of hypertension may slow the progression of renal disease, and the use of angiotensin-converting enzyme (ACE) inhibitors may have its classic renoprotective effect independent of antihypertensive action. Hypertension due to unilateral disease may respond to nephrectomy.

Since radiation nephropathy is an irreversible process, preventive measures should be taken during the administration of radiation. This includes selective shielding of the kidneys and the use of fractionated doses. Patients exposed to additional nephrotoxins remain at an increased risk of toxic effects.

Toxins

Lead

Lead toxicity affects many organs, resulting in encephalopathy, anaemia, peripheral neuropathy, gout, and renal failure. It was the epidemic of lead nephropathy in Queensland (Australia) that provided the strongest link between lead and chronic tubulointerstitial nephritis. Henderson noted an excess mortality due to chronic interstitial nephritis in Queensland but not in other parts of Australia, and correlated the incidence of granular contracted kidneys at autopsy with the lead content of the skull in people from Queensland and Sydney, showing that this correlated closely with the incidence of renal failure. Exposure was due to the lead-based paints used between 1890 and 1930, but recently the source of lead is industrial exposure. This type of exposure is often insidious and occurs over a very long period. Two studies have shown an inverse relationship between low-level lead exposure and renal function in the general population. Recent studies have failed to show any effect on renal function 17 to 50 years after an episode of acute childhood plumbism, the difference with Henderson's findings reflecting the greater lead burden in his study compared to the recent ones. Although low-level lead exposure in the general population is associated with mild but significant depression of renal function, its role in the development of endstage renal disease is unclear.

Pathogenesis and pathology

The pathogenesis of renal disease seen in the context of lead exposure may be related to proximal tubule reabsorption of filtered lead, with subsequent accumulation in proximal tubule cells. Aminoaciduria, glycosuria, and phosphaturia representing the Fanconi syndrome are observed after lead exposure, and thought to be related to an effect of lead on mitochondrial respiration and phosphorylation. Since lead is also capable of reducing 1,25-dihydroxyvitamin D synthesis, prolonged hyperphosphaturia and hypophosphataemia caused by lead poisoning in children could result in bone demineralization and rickets. Chronic lead poisoning can affect glomerular function. After an initial period of hyperfiltration the glomerular filtration rate is reduced and nephrosclerosis and chronic renal failure may ensue. Protracted lead exposure also interferes with the distal tubular secretion of urate, leading to hyperuricaemia and gout.

Renal biopsies in patients with subclinical lead nephropathy and a mild to moderate decrease in glomerular filtration rate primarily show focal tubular atrophy and interstitial fibrosis with minimal cellular infiltration. Electron microscopy shows mitochondrial swelling, loss of cristae, loss of basal infoldings, and a lysosomal-like structure containing dense bodies in the proximal tubules. In Australian patients who died as a result of severe lead exposure, their kidneys were fibrotic and shrunken, the interstitium showed variable degrees of fibrosis with tubular dilatation, and the vessels had thickened muscular walls with subintimal hyaline deposition in afferent arterioles, but these findings in patients with endstage renal failure were nonspecific.

Clinical features

Renal failure becomes apparent years after exposure and is associated with gout in most, if not all, cases. Hypertension is also a very common feature of lead nephropathy, and an association between hypertension without renal failure and low-level lead exposure has gained increasing recognition in recent years. Although hyperuricaemia is common in renal failure, gout is less so and its presence should raise the possibility of lead nephropathy.

However, whether chronic lead nephropathy exists as a clinical entity has been questioned. Many studies of occupational lead poisoning have not taken into account the co-exposure to other toxins such as cadmium. Additionally, the relationship between early markers of renal tubular dysfunction, such as the urinary excretion of low molecular weight proteins or N-acetyl β-D-glucosaminidase, to the subsequent development of renal failure remains to be determined.

Diagnosis and treatment

The diagnosis of lead nephropathy should be considered in any patient with progressive renal failure, mild to moderate proteinuria, significant hypertension, history of gout, and an appropriate history of exposure.

As the blood lead level only reflects recent lead exposure, and is usually normal in patients with chronic renal failure due to their previously sustained low-level lead exposure, the diagnosis has to be based on measurement of the body lead burden. The test of choice is the ethylenediaminetetraacetic acid (EDTA) mobilization test. This involves the administration of 2 g of EDTA intramuscularly in two divided doses 8 to 12 h apart, and collection of three consecutive 24-h urine samples. A cumulative excretion of more than 600 μg is suggestive for a high body lead burden. Renal failure in itself does not increase body lead load but it does delay the excretion of lead.

There is very little experience of the therapeutic use of EDTA in patients with chronic renal failure. Wedeen et al. treated eight industrially exposed patients with EDTA injections three times weekly for 6 to 15 months, all having mild renal failure with glomerular filtration rates of around 50 ml/min before treatment; four patients improved with a 20% increase in their glomerular filtration rate.

Cadmium

Cadmium is a cumulative environmental pollutant and accumulates in the human body after inhalation or gastrointestinal absorption. Due to its various applications and increased industrial production, it has been released into the environment in much larger amounts from the 1950s onwards, particularly in Belgium and Japan, which are among the most important cadmium-producing countries worldwide. However, the atmospheric emissions of cadmium from zinc smelters have been reduced since the 1970s. At the present, normal cadmium values are set at 0.1 to 0.8 μg/litre (nonsmokers) in blood, and 0.02 to 0.7 μg/g creatinine in urine.

Cadmium is a highly toxic metal and it has long been recognized that high-level exposure after inhalation or ingestion can give rise to nephrotoxicity, and that this effect is usually considered to be the earliest and most important feature from the point of view of health. When exposed to high levels of cadmium in the workplace (cadmium in renal cortex >100–400 μg/kg wet weight), workers have developed tubular proteinuria, renal glycosuria, aminoaciduria, hypercalciuria, phosphaturia, and polyuria, and in a few severe cases (long-standing high exposure and urinary excretion >20 μg/g creatinine and β_2-microglobulin >1500 μg/g creatinine) renal damage may progress to an irreversible reduction in glomerular filtration. Signs of distal tubular damage such as a cadmium-induced inhibition of ADH-stimulated ion transport have also been reported.

The extent to which chronic low-level environmental exposure to cadmium affects renal function is much less clear. The Cadmibel study, in which a random sample of 1699 subjects was recruited from four areas of Belgium with varying degrees of cadmium pollution, showed that (after standardization for several confounding factors) five markers of renal dysfunction (retinol binding protein, N-acetyl-β-glucosaminidase, β_2-microglobulin, amino acids, and calcium) were significantly associated with urinary cadmium excretion. There was a 10% probability of these variables being abnormal when urinary cadmium levels exceeded 2 to 4 μg/24 h. However, in a 5-year follow-up of a subcohort from the Cadmibel study, the so-called Pheecad study, in which 593 individuals with the highest urinary cadmium excretion were re-examined on average 5 years later, it was demonstrated that the subclinical tubular effects previously documented were not associated with deterioration in glomerular filtration rate. Hence, in the environmentally cadmium-exposed population, the renal effects due to cadmium appear to be weak, stable, and even reversible. These findings in environmentally exposed subjects may reasonably be extrapolated to the current, moderately exposed, occupational population, where, in various epidemiological studies, increased cadmium levels/exposure have repeatedly been associated with disturbed levels of markers of early renal dysfunction, but without evidence for accelerated progression towards chronic renal failure.

Metabolic disorders

Chronic hypokalaemia

Several renal abnormalities, most of which are reversible with potassium repletion, can be induced by hypokalaemia. Vasopressin-resistant impairment of the ability to concentrate the urine, increased renal ammonia production, enhanced bicarbonate reabsorption, altered sodium reabsorption, and hyperkalaemic nephropathy have all been described.

Persistent hypokalaemia can induce a variety of changes in renal function, impairing tubular transport and possibly inducing chronic tubulointerstitial disease and cyst formation. Hypokalaemic nephropathy in humans produces characteristic vacuolar lesions in the epithelial cells of the proximal tubule and (occasionally) the distal tubule, abnormalities which probably require about 1 month to develop. More severe changes occur if prolonged hypokalaemia is maintained, including interstitial fibrosis, tubular atrophy, and cyst formation that is most prominent in the renal medulla. The pathogenesis of these changes is not well understood.

Renal growth accelerates when rats are placed on a potassium-deficient diet, and within 8 days there is a 25% increase in kidney mass. The changes are most prominent in the outer medulla, especially the inner stripe, where hyperplastic enlarged collecting duct cells form cellular outgrowths that project into the lumen causing partial obstruction. If the potassium-deficient state persists, then cellular infiltrates appear in the renal interstitial compartment and tubulointerstitial fibrosis develops. It has been proposed that some of these pathological changes may be initiated by the high levels of ammonia generated in potassium-deficiency states and may be mediated through the activation of the alternate complement pathway. In support of this hypothesis is the finding that bicarbonate supplementation sufficient to suppress renal ammoniagenesis attenuates the renal enlargement and tubulointerstitial disease: against it are reports that increased renal ammoniagenesis induced by acid loading causes renal enlargement without cellular proliferation or interstitial disease. A recent paper provides results consistent with a sustained role for insulin-like growth factor-1 (IGF-1) in promoting the marked tubular epithelial cell hypertrophy and hyperplasia that occurs in the inner stripe of the outer medulla of the kidney with chronic potassium depletion. The same study also showed that potassium depletion causes a selective increase in the renal expression of transforming growth factor-β (TGF-β) in the hypertrophied nonhyperplastic thick ascending limb, but, unlike IGF-1, it is absent from the hyperplastic collecting duct cells. This might be responsible for preventing the conversion of the mitogenic stimulus of IGF-1 into a hypertrophic one. It is possible that TGF-β causes the prominent interstitial infiltrate that develops in chronic hypokalaemia, since this growth factor is a well-known chemoattractant for macrophages.

A recent study has shown that angiotensin receptor blockade ameliorates tubulointerstitial injury induced by chronic potassium deficiency, and the same authors also showed that endothelin-1 can mediate hypokalaemic renal injury in two different ways, by directly stimulating endothelin-A receptors and by locally promoting endogenous endothelin-1 production via endothelin-B receptors, hence endothelin-A and -B receptor blockade may be renoprotective in hypokalaemic nephropathy.

Hyperoxaluria

Hyperoxaluria may be primary or acquired. The primary form is a rare inherited disorder due to an enzymatic abnormality in the metabolism of glyoxylic acid. The acquired forms of hyperoxaluria are more common and result either from the ingestion of oxalate precursors, such as ethylene glycol and ascorbic acid, and exposure to methoxyflurane anaesthesia, or from increased absorption from the intestinal tract in those with inflammatory bowel disease or who have undergone small-bowel resection.

Microcrystallization of calcium oxalate first occurs in the proximal tubules, where oxalate secretion occurs. However, the lesions that develop are more severe in the renal medulla, where the increasing concentration of the tubular fluid and its acidification promote the precipitation of calcium oxalate. If the overload is insidious and chronic, then inflammatory cell infiltration, oedema, interstitial fibrosis, tubular atrophy, and dilatation result in a chronic tubulointerstitial nephritis with progressive renal failure.

Hypercalcaemia

Prolonged elevation of urinary and serum calcium levels may result in the deposition of calcium in the kidney, which also occurs in some clinical conditions not associated with hypercalcaemia. Calcium is most concentrated in the medulla, where degeneration and tubular necrosis begins due to intracellular overload, with damage to mitochondria and other critical organelles. Reactive inflammatory changes occur in the adjacent interstitium, and necrotic cells may cause intratubular obstruction and tubular atrophy. The final results of these changes are focal areas of tubular atrophy, interstitial fibrosis, and a mononuclear cell infiltrate. See Chapter 21.14 for further discussion.

Hyperuricaemia/hyperuricosuria

There are three different types of renal disease induced by abnormal uric acid metabolism: acute uric acid nephropathy, chronic urate nephropathy, and uric acid stone disease, the last being discussed in Chapter 21.14.

The kidneys are mainly responsible for the excretion of uric acid and are a primary target organ affected in disorders of urate metabolism. Renal lesions result from the crystallization of uric acid either in the urinary outflow tract or in the renal parenchyma. The determinants of uric acid solubility are its concentration and the pH of the medium in which it is dissolved, hence the supersaturation of fluid within the renal tubules as excreted uric acid becomes concentrated in the medulla, and the acidification of the urine in the distal tubule, are both conducive to the precipitation of uric acid. The major sites of urate deposition are the renal medulla, the collecting tubules, and the urinary tract. The pK_a of uric acid is 5.7, and at the acid pH of the fluid in the distal tubule the bulk of filtered urate will be present in its nonionized form as uric acid, whereas at the more alkaline pH of the blood and interstitium it is in its ionized form as urate salts.

Acute uric acid nephropathy

Acute uric acid nephropathy is an uncommon condition caused by the precipitation of birefringent uric acid crystals in the collecting tubules, with consequent tubular obstruction, dilatation, and inflammation. This can occur in disorders associated with an increased production of uric acid, e.g. myeloproliferative or lymphoproliferative disorders, tumour lysis syndrome, chronic haemolytic anaemia, psoriasis, or the Lesch–Nyhan syndrome, or when there is increased renal clearance of uric acid, e.g. inherited or acquired defects of tubular urate transport or uricosuric drugs.

In those prone to acute uric acid nephropathy, management centres on prophylaxis with a plentiful fluid intake, with or without alkalinization of the urine, and pretreatment with allopurinol or recombinant urate oxidase enzyme (rasburicase). Presentation of acute uric acid nephropathy is with acute renal failure, with urine microscopy revealing plentiful birefringent crystals.

Chronic urate nephropathy

The principal renal lesion in chronic hyperuricaemia is the deposition of microtophi of amorphous urate crystals in the interstitium, with a surrounding giant cell reaction. This results in a secondary chronic inflammatory response similar to that seen with microtophus formation elsewhere in the body, potentially leading to interstitial fibrosis and chronic renal failure.

Recent evidence has incriminated uric acid as an independent risk factor for cardiovascular death and major clinical events. Hyperuricaemia induces endothelial dysfunction, and uric acid regulates critical proinflammatory pathways in vascular smooth muscle cells, possibly having a role in the vascular changes associated with hypertension and vascular disease. It also accelerates renal progression in the remnant kidney model via a mechanism linked to high systemic blood pressure and cyclooxygenase-2 (COX-2)-mediated thromboxane-induced vascular disease. These studies provide direct evidence that uric acid may be a true mediator of renal disease and progression, but clinical evidence linking chronic renal failure to gout is weak, and the long-standing notion that chronic renal disease is common in patients with hyperuricaemia has been questioned in the light of prolonged follow-up studies of renal function in people with this condition. Renal dysfunction could be documented only when the serum urate concentration was more than 10 mg/dl (600 μmol/litre) in women and more than 13 mg/dl (780 μmol/litre) in men for prolonged periods. Furthermore, the deterioration of renal function in those with hyperuricaemia of a lower magnitude has been attributed to the higher than expected occurrence of hypertension, diabetes mellitus, abnormal lipid metabolism, and nephrosclerosis. Nonetheless, it seems reasonable to prescribe allopurinol (in a dose appropriate to the level of renal function) to those very rare patients with biopsy evidence of 'gouty nephropathy', and possibly to patients with chronic renal failure who have a grossly elevated serum urate.

There is an association between severe lead intoxication, chronic renal failure, and gout (saturnine gout) (see above). It has also been suggested that there might be an association between renal disease and hyperuricaemia in those with a past history of exposure to lead and consequent subclinical lead toxicity (saturnine nephropathy). Evidence for this association is not clear-cut, nor is the mechanism whereby lead exposure might aggravate hyperuricaemia and renal failure.

Further reading

Sarcoidosis

Kettritz R, *et al.* (2006). The protean face of sarcoidosis revisited. *Nephrol Dial Transplant*, **21**, 2690–4.
Korzets Z, *et al.* (1985). Acute renal failure due to sarcoid granulomatous infiltration of the renal parenchyma. *Am J Kidney Dis*, **6**, 250–3.

Analgesic nephropathy

Blohme I, Johansson S (1981). Renal pelvic neoplasms and atypical urothelium in patients with end-stage analgesic nephropathy. *Kidney Int*, **20**, 671–5.
De Broe ME, Elseviers MM (2009). Over-the-counter analgesic use. *J Am Soc Nephrol*, **20**(10), 2098–103.
Duggin GG (1996). Combination analgesic-induced kidney disease: the Australian experience. *Am J Kidney Dis*, **28** Suppl 1, S39–47.

Fored CM, *et al.* (2001). Acetaminophen, aspirin, and chronic renal failure. *N Engl J Med*, **345**, 1801–8.

Henrich WL, *et al.* (2006). Non-contrast-enhanced computerized tomography and analgesic-related kidney disease: report of the national analgesic nephropathy study. *J Am Soc Nephrol*, **17**, 1472–80.

Ibanez L, *et al.* (2005). Case-control study of regular analgesic and nonsteroidal anti-inflammatory use and end-stage renal disease. *Kidney Int*, **67**, 2393–8.

Mihatsch MJ, Khanlari B, Brunner FP (2006). Obituary to analgesic nephropathy: an autopsy study. *Nephrol Dial Transplant*, **21**, 3139–45.

Mihatsch MJ, *et al.* (1983). Capillary sclerosis of the urinary tract and analgesic nephropathy. *Clin Nephrol*, **20**, 285–301.

Perneger TV, Whelton PK, Klag MJ (1994). Risk of kidney failure associated with the use of acetaminophen, aspirin, and nonsteroidal antiinflammatory drugs. *N Engl J Med*, **331**, 1675–9.

van der Woude FJ, *et al.* (2007). Analgesics use and ESRD in younger age: A case-control study. *BMC Nephrol*, **8**, 15.

5-Aminosalicylic acid

Calder IC, *et al.* (1972). Nephrotoxic lesions from 5-aminosalicylic acid. *BMJ*, **1**, 152–4.

Gisbert JP, González-Lama Y, Maté J (2007). 5-Aminosalicylates and renal function in inflammatory bowel disease: a systematic review. *Inflamm Bowel Dis*, **13**(5), 629–38.

Muller AF, *et al.* (2005). Experience of 5-aminosalicylate nephrotoxicity in the United Kingdom. *Aliment Pharmacol Ther*, **21**, 1217–24.

World MJ, *et al.* (1996). Mesalazine-associated interstitial nephritis. *Nephrol Dial Transplant*, **11**, 614–21.

Chinese herb nephropathy

Cosyns JP, *et al.* (1994). Chinese herbs nephropathy: a clue to Balkan endemic nephropathy? *Kidney Int*, **45**, 1680–8.

Cosyns JP, *et al.* (1999). Urothelial lesions in Chinese-herb nephropathy. *Am J Kidney Dis*, **33**, 1011–17.

Diamond JR, Pallone TL (1994). Acute interstitial nephritis following use of tung shueh pills. *Am J Kidney Dis*, **24**, 219–21.

Vanherweghem JL, *et al.* (1993). Rapidly progressive interstitial fibrosis in young women: association with slimming regimen including Chinese herbs. *Lancet*, **341**, 387–91.

Yang CS, *et al.* (2000). Rapidly progressive fibrosing interstitial nephritis associated with Chinese herbal drugs. *Am J Kidney Dis*, **35**, 313–18.

Lithium

Boton R, Gaviria M, Battle CD (1987). Prevalence, pathogenesis, and treatment of renal dysfunction associated with chronic lithium therapy. *Am J Kidney Dis*, **10**, 329–45.

Grünfeld JP, Rossier BC (2009). Lithium nephrotoxicity revisited. *Nat Rev Nephrol*, **5**(5), 270–6.

Lepkifker E, *et al.* (2004). Renal insufficiency in long-term lithium treatment. *J Clin Psychiatry*, **65**, 850–6.

Markowitz GS, *et al.* (2000). Lithium nephrotoxicity: a progressive combined glomerular and tubulointerstitial nephropathy. *J Am Soc Nephrol*, **11**, 1439–48.

Presne C, *et al.* (2003). Lithium-induced nephropathy: rate of progression and prognostic factors. *Kidney Int*, **64**, 585–92.

Wolf ME, *et al.* (1997). Lithium therapy, hypercalcemia, and hyperparathyroidism. *Am J Ther*, **4**, 323–5.

Endemic Balkan nephropathy

Arlt VM, *et al.* (2007). Aristolochic acid mutagenesis: molecular clues to the aetiology of Balkan endemic nephropathy-associated urothelial cancer. *Carcinogenesis*, **28**, 2253–61.

Batuman V (2006). Fifty years of Balkan endemic nephropathy: daunting questions, elusive answers. *Kidney Int*, **69**, 644–6.

Dimitrov P, *et al.* (2006). Clinical markers in adult offspring of families with and without Balkan endemic nephropathy. *Kidney Int*, **69**, 723–9.

Grollman AP, *et al.* (2007). Aristolochic acid and the etiology of endemic (Balkan) nephropathy. *Proc Natl Acad Sci USA*, **104**(29), 12129–34.

Stefanovic V, *et al.* (2006). Etiology of Balkan endemic nephropathy and associated urothelial cancer. *Am J Nephrol*, **26**, 1–11.

Voice TC, *et al.* (2006). Evaluation of the hypothesis that Balkan endemic nephropathy is caused by drinking water exposure to contaminants leaching from Pliocene coal deposits. *J Expo Sci Environ Epidemiol*, **16**, 515–24.

Radiation nephropathy

Cohen EP (2000). Radiation nephropathy after bone marrow transplantation. *Kidney Int*, **58**, 903–18.

Luxton RW (1961). Radiation nephritis: a long-term study of fifty-four patients. *Lancet*, **2**, 1221.

Toxins

Buchet JP, *et al.* (1990). Renal effects of cadmium body burden of the general population. *Lancet*, **336**, 699–702.

Farkas WR, Stanawitz T, Schneider M (1978). Saturnine gout: lead-induced formation of guanine crystals. *Science*, **199**, 786–7.

Hotz P, *et al.* (1999). Renal effects of low-level environmental cadmium exposure: 5-year follow-up of a subcohort from the Cadmibel study. *Lancet*, **354**, 1508–13.

Staessen JA, *et al.* (1992). Impairment of renal function with increasing blood lead concentrations in the general population. *N Engl J Med*, **327**, 151–6.

Staessen JP, *et al.* on behalf of the Working Groups (1996). Public health implications of environmental exposure to cadmium and lead: an overview of epidemiological studies in Belgium. *J Cardiovasc Risk*, **3**, 26–41.

Metabolic disorders

Benabe JE, Martinez-Maldonado M (1978). Hypercalcemic nephropathy. *Arch Intern Med*, **138**, 777–9.

Cremer W, Bock KD (1976). Symptoms and course of chronic hypokalemic nephropathy in man. *Clin Nephrol*, **7**, 112–19.

Duffy WB, Senekjian HO, Knight TF (1981). Management of asymptomatic hyperuricemia. *JAMA*, **246**, 2215–16.

Hestbech J, *et al.* (1977). Chronic renal lesions following long-term treatment with lithium. *Kidney Int*, **12**, 205–13.

Johnson RJ, *et al.* (1999). Reappraisal of the pathogenesis and consequences of hyperuricemia in hypertension, cardiovascular disease, and renal disease. *Am J Kidney Dis*, **33**, 225–34.

Kang DH, *et al.* (2002). A role for uric acid in the progression of renal disease. *J Am Soc Nephrol*, **13**, 2888–97.

Suga S, *et al.* (2002). Angiotensin II type 1 receptor blockade ameliorates tubulointerstitial injury induced by chronic potassium deficiency. *Kidney Int*, **61**, 951–8.

Torres VE, *et al.* (1990). Association of hypokalemia, aldosteronism, and renal cysts. *N Engl J Med*, **322**, 345–51.

The kidney in systemic disease

Contents

21.10.1 Diabetes mellitus and the kidney

Rudolf Bilous

Essentials

Diabetic nephropathy is the commonest cause of endstage renal disease in the developed world, causing about 50% of incident cases requiring renal replacement therapy in the United States of America and 20% in the United Kingdom. Most of these have type 2 diabetes, and in some countries the proportion of patients with endstage renal disease who have type 1 diabetes is falling.

Aetiology and pathology—causation is related to glycaemic control (e.g. glycation of proteins, sorbitol overproduction, alteration in growth factors), hypertension, genetic factors, and dietary and other environmental factors. Pathological hallmarks are thickening of the glomerular basement membrane and mesangial expansion, with or without nodule formation, secondary to an accumulation of extracellular matrix.

Staging and natural history—is classically described in terms of urinary albumin excretion rate (UAER): (1) normoalbuminuria—UAER less than 20 µg/min, albumin/creatinine ratio (ACR) less than 2.5 mg/mmol (men), less than 3.5 mg/mmol (women); (2) microalbuminuria (also called incipient nephropathy)—UAER 20 to 200 µg/min, ACR 2.5 to 30 mg/mmol (men), 3.5 to 30 mg/mmol (women); and (3) clinical proteinuria (sometimes called clinical nephropathy or overt nephropathy)—UAER greater than 200 µg/min, ACR greater than 30 mg/mmol. This staging does not map well onto that of chronic kidney disease based on estimated glomerular filtration rate (eGFR) (see Chapters 21.4 and 21.6).

Clinical features—most patients (>60%) will have a normal UAER throughout their diabetic life, but 1 to 2% of the remainder develop persistent microalbuminuria each year. Once UAER exceeds 200 µg/min, there tends to be a relentless increase in proteinuria, occasionally into the nephrotic range, and GFR declines progressively at a rate that largely depends on blood pressure control.

Prevention—in both type 1 and type 2 diabetes, tight glycaemic control can prevent microalbuminuria. In type 2 diabetes, intensive blood pressure control using angiotensin converting enzyme (ACE) inhibitors can prevent microalbuminuria. In both type 1 and type 2 diabetes, intensive blood pressure control using ACE inhibitors or angiotensin II receptor blockers (ARBs) slows progression from microalbuminuria to clinical proteinuria and slows the rate of decline in GFR (more so in type 1 than type 2).

Management—aims for: (1) good control of glycaemia (typical recommendations are for HbA1c level <7.5% in type 1 and 6.5–7.5% in type 2); (2) good control of hypertension (<130/80 mmHg, with even lower targets recommended in those with heavy proteinuria) using an ACE inhibitor and/or an ARB; and (3) other interventions, including some or all of serum lipid lowering, low-dose aspirin, smoking cessation and reduction of dietary protein and salt.

Prognosis—mortality is higher for people with diabetes and increased albuminuria compared to those with normoalbuminuria. In type 2 diabetes, the annual mortality is almost 5% for patients with clinical proteinuria, and almost 20% for those with a serum creatinine greater than 175 μmol/litre or in endstage renal disease. Survival on dialysis remains much worse for patients with diabetes compared to those without; around 25% are alive after 5 years. Cardiovascular disease is the commonest cause of death, and multifactorial cardiovascular risk-factor intervention has been shown to reduce mortality and morbidity in type 2 diabetes, and is mandatory for all patients with diabetic nephropathy.

Introduction

Diabetic nephropathy is the commonest single cause of endstage renal disease requiring renal replacement therapy in the United Kingdom and the United States of America, and the second most common cause in mainland Europe and Japan. Around 40% of patients with type 1 and 20% of those with type 2 diabetes develop nephropathy and consequently are at high risk of endstage renal disease. The incidence of diabetes worldwide is increasing, with an estimated prevalence of 380 million by 2025, hence the future personal and health economic burdens of diabetic endstage renal disease pose serious problems for health care providers.

Historical perspective

Proteinuria had been described in patients with diabetes in the 19th century, but its significance was only appreciated after the description of nodular glomerulosclerosis in the kidneys of diabetic patients by Kimmelstiel and Wilson in 1936. The specificity of these lesions for diabetes and the description of a more generalized accumulation of extracellular matrix material in the mesangium and glomerular basement membrane confirmed the pathological basis for proteinuria.

Lundbaek developed the concept of microangiopathy, linking the pathological features of retinal and glomerular lesions, and Root in 1953 coined the term triopathy to include retinopathy, nephropathy, and neuropathy. Microangiopathy is almost completely specific to diabetes and its presence has been used to define the blood glucose levels that diagnose diabetes. In the 1960s, the mean time from onset of proteinuria to endstage renal disease was 7 years; it is currently over 14 years. However, diabetic patients with nephropathy continue to have a greatly increased mortality from cardiovascular disease. The multifactorial aetiopathogenesis of nephropathy offers opportunities for treatment but also poses major problems for prevention.

Aetiology

Hyperglycaemia

Observational studies have shown that sustained poor glycaemic control is associated with a greater risk for the development of nephropathy in both type 1 and type 2 diabetes. There are several potential mechanisms by which hyperglycaemia may cause nephropathy. These are common to all the microvascular complications of diabetes and are listed in Box 21.10.1.1 (see also 'Glycaemic control').

Blood pressure

Systemic blood pressure is higher in patients with type 1 diabetes who subsequently develop microalbuminuria. One study has also found a stronger family history of hypertension in type 1 patients with diabetic nephropathy compared to those without.

In type 2 diabetes, a prediabetic mean arterial pressure higher than 97 mmHg (130/70 mmHg) strongly predicts the development of proteinuria in Japanese people and Pima Indians. Cohorts of normotensive (<140/90 mmHg) type 2 patients with microalbuminuria from Israel, Japan, and India showed little change in blood pressure over 7, 4, and 5 years, respectively, despite an increase in their urinary albumin excretion rate (UAER) over this time. The situation in Europid type 2 diabetes may be different. In the United Kingdom Prospective Diabetes Study (UKPDS), hypertension (defined as >160/90 mmHg or >150/85 mmHg on treatment) was present in over 30% of newly diagnosed patients. Only one-third of these had increased UAER.

The observed changes in blood pressure may therefore initiate the nephropathic process in type 2 diabetes but occur as a result of it in type 1, although this distinction is not absolute. What is certain is that progression of nephropathy is much faster in patients with higher systemic blood pressure, which is presumably transmitted to the intraglomerular capillary bed.

Haemodynamic factors

Glomerular filtration rate (GFR) is increased in newly diagnosed type 1 and type 2 diabetic patients. This phenomenon has been

---

Box 21.10.1.1 Aetiopathological factors for nephropathy

- Glycaemia related:
  - Glycation of proteins—formation of advanced glycation end products
  - Polyol pathway—sorbitol overproduction
  - Protein kinase C β activation
  - Altered glomerular haemodynamics
  - Increased production of growth factors/cytokines such as TGFβ, CTGF, NF-κβ, VEGF, PDGF, IGF-1, angiotensin II, and prostanoids
- Systemic hypertension
- Genetic factors
- Mechanical/structural factors
- Fetal programming
- Dietary factors, such as high protein intake and salt
- Smoking, other environmental factors

CTGF, connective tissue growth factor; IGF-1, insulin-like growth factor-1; PDGF, platelet-derived growth factor; TGFβ, transforming growth factor β; VEGF, vascular endothelial growth factor.

termed hyperfiltration and is thought to be due to a relative vasodilatation of the afferent glomerular arteriole, which leads to an increase in intraglomerular capillary pressure (Fig. 21.10.1.1) and thereby glomerulosclerosis. Hyperfiltration and raised intraglomerular capillary pressure are thought to be caused by activation of the local renin–angiotensin system, leading to an excess production of angiotensin II and thereby relative vasoconstriction of the efferent glomerular arteriole.

The evidence in humans is conflicting and not helped by differing definitions of an abnormally high GFR and the difficulty of obtaining an estimate of intraglomerular capillary pressure. It appears that the rate of decline of GFR in hyperfiltering type 1 patients with a normal UAER is greater than that seen in age-matched and duration-matched controls. More recent data suggest that there is a link between hyperfiltration and later development of microalbuminuria in adolescents, and a positive relationship between GFR and glomerular basement membrane thickening in younger adults. Pima Indians show an increase in GFR at or shortly after the development of type 2 diabetes, but their baseline values are not linked to the subsequent development of nephropathy.

Growth factors

In experimental animals an initial increase in kidney size observed in diabetes is preceded by an increase in renal production of insulin-like growth factor-1, and there are reports of increased circulating and urinary levels in people with diabetes. Other growth factors listed in Box 21.10.1.1 have been linked to matrix accumulation and development of proteinuria in experimental diabetes.

Increased whole kidney volume is also a feature of newly diagnosed type 1 diabetes in humans, but there is no conclusive link to subsequent development of nephropathy. Several of the growth factors listed in Box 21.10.1.1 have been found to have an increased production or gene expression in biopsies from patients

with diabetes compared to those from nondiabetic patients. It is unclear whether these changes are causative.

Mechanical and structural factors

Along with whole kidney volume, glomerular size is also increased at diagnosis of type 1 diabetes and is a feature of established clinical proteinuria in both type 1 and type 2 disease. These changes may be secondary to haemodynamic alterations in early disease or represent an adaptive response to loss of filtration surface in established diabetic nephropathy. A link between glomerular size and subsequent progression to sclerosis has been described in patients with minimal-change nephropathy, but the connection in diabetes is not proven.

Reductions of heparan sulphate proteoglycan in the extracellular matrix of diabetic patients and the glomerular basement membrane of those with microalbuminuria and clinical proteinuria have been reported. This finding has formed the basis of the so-called Steno hypothesis, which proposes that these alterations underpin the pathophysiology of nephropathy.

In vitro studies of mechanical stretch on cultured human mesangial cells and podocytes has demonstrated increased production of cytokines and growth factors associated with extracellular matrix accumulation. These studies provide a plausible mechanism whereby changes in intraglomerular capillary pressure may lead to glomerulosclerosis.

The discovery of glomerular epithelial cells (podocytes) in the urine of patients with proteinuria has led to extensive research into their possible role in progressive nephropathies, including diabetes. Reduced numbers of podocytes have been found in human diabetic glomeruli from patients with diabetic nephropathy, but it remains unclear whether these changes precede or result from developing glomerulopathy. There is a significant negative relationship between the numbers of podocytes per glomerulus and increasing proteinuria in patients with established diabetic nephropathy.

Fetal programming

The low birth weight–thrifty phenotype hypothesis proposes intrauterine malnutrition as a possible cause of adult hypertension and diabetes, perhaps mediated by reduced numbers of renal glomeruli or islets of Langerhans, respectively. Studies have failed to confirm lower glomerular numbers in white diabetic patients with nephropathy compared to those without, and no consistent relationship between birth weight and adult glomerular number has been demonstrated.

Other factors

Smoking rates are higher in diabetic patients with nephropathy, although a plausible mechanism of effect has yet to be defined. A link between raised blood lipids and the causation and progression of renal disease is still hotly debated. Both cross-sectional and prospective studies have shown an association between plasma total cholesterol and triglyceride levels and UAER and change in GFR, but the effects of therapy are inconsistent.

In experimental diabetes, dietary protein restriction can prevent glomerulosclerosis. Cross-sectional studies of patients with type 1 diabetes found that UAER increased in patients with a protein intake of more than 20% of their total food energy, while in type 2 diabetic and normal subjects, a 0.1-g/kg body weight per

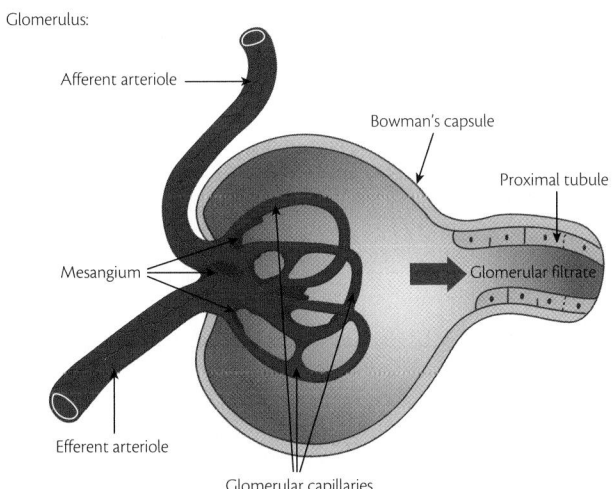

Fig. 21.10.1.1 Schematic of a glomerulus. In diabetes there is relative afferent arteriolar dilatation and angiotensin II induced efferent arteriolar constriction. This leads to increased glomerular capillary flow and pressure resulting in elevated GFR (hyperfiltration) and increased albumin filtration. Blockade of the renin-angiotensin system dilates the efferent arteriole and reduces GFR and capillary pressure.

day increase in protein intake was associated with a greater risk of developing microalbuminuria.

Abnormalities of endothelial function assessed by increases in plasma von Willebrand factor and homocysteine levels have been described in diabetic patients with normoalbuminuria who go on to develop microalbuminuria, and also in those with a persistently increased UAER at baseline. The EURODIAB investigators suggest that endothelial dysfunction provides a unifying hypothesis for the causation of microvascular and macrovascular disease in diabetes.

Genetics

There is a greater than 80% concordance for nephropathy and a more than 73% concordance for normoalbuminuria in diabetic siblings of probands with type 1 diabetes. In Pima Indians, the prevalence of diabetic nephropathy is 14% in the offspring of parents neither of whom have nephropathy, compared to 46% of offspring when both parents have the condition. These observations have led to many studies looking for a possible genetic cause of nephropathy, most of which have used the candidate gene approach with largely disappointing results. The most intensively studied genetic abnormality has been the insertion/deletion polymorphism in the angiotensin-converting enzyme (ACE) gene, but the results are inconsistent. A genome-wide scan has identified a possible locus on chromosomes 7 and 20 in the Pima Indians, and other loci have been described in different populations. Although some workers have suggested that the family observations are consistent with a major gene effect, none has yet been confirmed. It is very likely that genetics play a role, but this is almost certainly a polygenic rather than a monogenic effect.

Pathology and pathogenesis

Patients with newly diagnosed type 1 diabetes have large kidneys, and studies in experimental animals suggest that this enlargement is due to tubular hypertrophy and hyperplasia, together with an expansion of the tubulointerstitium. Proximal tubular cells appear loaded with glycogen (the Armanni–Ebstein lesion). These changes are probably a response to the increased filtration of glucose at the glomerulus and can be reversed in animals by glycaemic correction. Glomerular and tubular structure is otherwise normal at diagnosis in human type 1 diabetes.

The pathological hallmarks of diabetic nephropathy are thickening of the glomerular basement membrane and mesangial expansion, with or without nodule formation, secondary to an accumulation of extracellular matrix (mostly type IV collagen) (Fig. 21.10.1.2). This accumulation results from a combination of increased production and decreased breakdown of matrix proteins. Glomerular basement membrane thickening can be detected in nearly all patients with diabetes of more than 10 years' duration, irrespective of UAER. Those with clinical proteinuria almost invariably have glomerular basement membrane widths 2 to 3 times the upper limit of normal (350 nm). Mesangial volumes remain in the normal range in patients who have a normal UAER. Nodule formation, although virtually pathognomonic, is not invariable. A combination of mesangial expansion encroaching on the available filtration surface area and afferent arteriolar hyalinosis leading to glomerular ischaemia leads to eventual total glomerulosclerosis

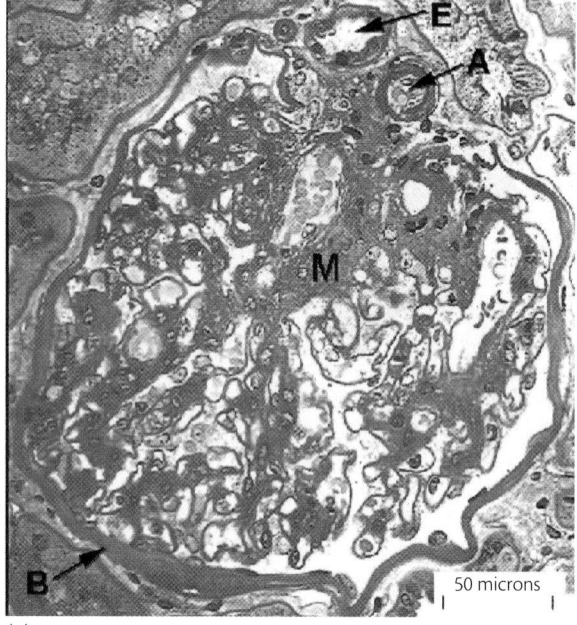

(a)

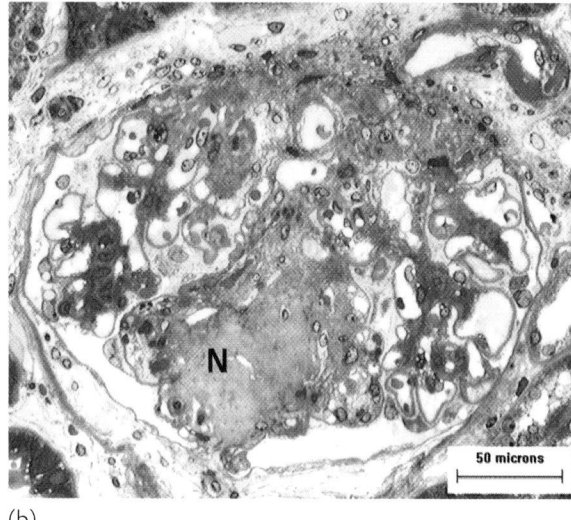

(b)

Fig. 21.10.1.2 Glomerulus from patient with type 1 diabetes and clinical proteinuria (haematoxylin and eosin stain). Note afferent (A) and efferent (E) arteriolar hyalinosis, thickened and split Bowman's capsule (B), and mesangial expansion (M) (b) Glomerulus from patient with type 1 diabetes and clinical proteinuria (toluidine blue stain) showing typical nodule (N). Note central accumulation of matrix material with surrounding nuclei.

and permanent loss of filtration capacity, ultimately resulting in endstage renal disease.

Patients with type 2 diabetes have been less well studied, but the pathological appearances of subjects with established diabetic nephropathy are very similar to those with type 1. However, pathological changes in patients with microalbuminuria are more heterogeneous, and a significant prevalence of nondiabetic pathology (c.10%) has been reported.

Latterly, changes to the podocyte including foot process effacement, podocyte loss, and subsequent adhesion of the glomerular basement membrane to Bowman's capsule have been linked to increasing UAER and are the subject of intensive research.

Tubulointerstitial expansion with fibrosis and tubular atrophy are also well described in patients with clinical proteinuria.

Epidemiology

Reported incidence and prevalence rates of nephropathy are heavily dependent on the diagnostic criteria (see below) and the population under study. Classically, nephropathy has been classified based on UAER into normoalbuminuria, microalbuminuria, and clinical proteinuria (Table 21.10.1.1). Selecting only population-based cohorts with good patient ascertainment gives prevalence rates for microalbuminuria of between 5 and 21% for type 1 and 11 to 42% for type 2 diabetes. Reported annual incidence rates are around 2% for type 1 patients (Table 21.10.1.2). For clinical proteinuria, the prevalence is 6.4% in type 1 patients in the United Kingdom, with a range from 5 to 33% worldwide for type 2. A cumulative incidence of approximately 20% after 20 years' duration was found in type 1 diabetic cohorts of the Steno Hospital in Denmark and Joslin Clinic in the United States of America, and similar figures have been reported for patients with type 2 diabetes in the United States (25%) and Germany (27%).

More recent data from patients prospectively studied from diagnosis of type 1 diabetes in Scandinavia have revealed lower cumulative incidences of 15% after 20 years (Denmark) and 11% after 30 years (Sweden). There have also been reductions in the numbers of patients with type 1 diabetes entering renal replacement therapy programmes in the United States of America (incident rate in 1995–1999 was 7.1% vs 3.9% in 2000–2004); and the cumulative incidence of endstage renal disease secondary to type 1 diabetes in Finland is only 7.8% after 30 years.

The situation for type 2 diabetes is less clear as far as microalbuminuria and clinical proteinuria are concerned, although the transition rates are similar to type 1 at 1 to 2% per year. A population-based study in the United States of America has suggested that fewer patients with type 2 diabetes presented with clinical proteinuria at diagnosis in the 1990s compared to 30 years previously. Recent analysis of the UKPDS cohort has suggested a cumulative incidence of a urinary albumin concentration between 50 and 299 mg/litre (microalbuminuria) of 42% at 20 years and of clinical proteinuria of 20% after 20 years. Endstage renal disease rates for type 2 diabetes continue to increase in Europe but have reached a plateau in the United States of America at around 50% incidence and 35% prevalence. Incidence rates are now declining in the Pima Indians but are continuing to increase in the United Kingdom and Europe.

There is a dramatic difference in the risk of microalbuminuria, clinical proteinuria, and endstage renal disease in ethnic subgroups. In the United States of America there is a fourfold increased prevalence of African American and native American patients on renal replacement therapy compared to white patients. The increase is threefold for those of Hispanic origin. A similar increased risk has been reported for South Asian populations in the United Kingdom.

Many countries have registers of patients entering renal replacement therapy and in 2003 Malaysia had the highest incident rate of patients with diabetes entering renal replacement therapy at over 50%. Close behind was New Zealand at 40%, but there were much lower numbers in Australia, almost certainly due to the differing ethnic mix. Pacific islanders and Maori people are much more prone to renal disease and diabetes than those of European extraction. The reasons for the excess risk of endstage renal disease in these groups is unclear but may be genetic, related to increased rates of hypertension, or the result of fetal programming. There are intriguing data suggesting that the number and size of glomeruli is different in Australian aborigines compared to white Europid patients.

Prevention
Glycaemic control

The association of glycaemia and development of nephropathy has led to numerous studies exploring the potential of glycaemic control in the prevention of increases in UAER. The two largest studies were the Diabetes Control and Complications Trial (DCCT) in type 1 and the UKPDS in type 2 (Table 21.10.1.3). Both compared the intensive management of hyperglycaemia using multiple injections of insulin in type 1 and early use of insulin in type 2 against more conventional control. Those in the intensively treated groups also had more frequent contact with health care professionals. The DCCT cohort was invited to continue surveillance for a further 8 years as part of the Epidemiology of Diabetes Interventions and Complications (EDIC) study.

Both DCCT and UKPDS demonstrated a significant reduction in numbers developing microalbuminuria, although there was still a substantial incidence of 15 and 19.2%, respectively, in the intensively treated cohorts (Table 21.10.1.3). Interestingly, the benefit

Table 21.10.1.1 Levels of proteinuria, albuminuria, and albumin/creatinine ratio (ACR) that define normal, microalbuminuria, and clinical proteinuria. Borderline results should be repeated on early morning samples or confirmed by a timed collection

| | 24h urine | | Timed overnight | 'Spot' sample[a,b] | | |
	Total protein (g/day)	Albumin (mg/day)	Albumin (μg/min)	Albumin concentration (mg/litre)	ACR (mg/mmol)	ACR (mg/g)
Normal	<0.15	<30	<20	<20	<2.5 male <3.5 female	<20 male <40 female
Microalbuminuria		30–300	20–200	50–300	2.5–30 male 3.5–30 female	20–300 male 40–300 female[c]
Clinical proteinuria	>0.5	>300	>200	>300	>30	>300

[a] False-positive results with diurnal variation, exercise, urine infection, other renal disease, haematuria, heart failure.
[b] False-negative results with dilution, diuresis.
[c] American Diabetes Association uses a definition of 30–300 mg/g for both males and females.

Table 21.10.1.2 Natural history of nephropathy in type 1 diabetes[a]

	Normal	↔	Microalbuminuria	→	Clinical proteinuria
UAER	<20 μg/min	1–2% p.a progress to microalbuminuria	20–200 μg/min (increasing by 20% p.a) (up to 25% type 1 revert to normal)	1–4% p.a progress to clinical nephropathy	>200 μg/min
GFR	Stable: declines at 1 ml/min per year from over 40 years of age		Age-related changes until UAER approaches 200 μg/min or if blood pressure increases		Declines at 10 ml/min per year (hypertensive), 4 ml/min per year (normotensive)
Blood pressure	Stable: significantly higher in those progressing to microalbuminuria		Initially stable, but higher than normal controls. Tends to increase with increasing UAER		Most patients hypertensive (>140/90 mmHg). Increases with declining GFR
Pathology	Large kidneys Tubular hypertrophy/hyperplasia Glomerular enlargement—normal ultrastructure, but glomerular basement membrane thickening 20 nm p.a.		Kidneys can remain large Glomerular basement membrane thickening 54 nm p.a. Mesangial expansion 4% p.a.		Kidneys tend to shrink Glomerular basement membrane 2–3 times normal thickness, but stable Nodule formation Global glomerulosclerosis Mesangial expansion c.7% p.a.

GFR, glomerular filtration rate; p.a., per annum; UAER, urinary albumin excretion rate.
[a] Fewer data in type 2 patients, many of whom are hypertensive at diagnosis.

of intensive treatment continued in the EDIC follow-up, despite a deterioration in HbA1c to levels close to those seen in the conventional group at 8.2%. Thus a prolonged period of good glycaemic control appears to confer benefit in terms of prevention of complications in the kidney (and the retina) for many years. Moreover, the intensive cohort who were normotensive at the beginning of the EDIC study showed a 32% reduction in the risk of developing hypertension (blood pressure >140/90 mmHg) compared to the conventional group.

There is continuing controversy as to whether intensive glycaemic control alone can prevent the progression of microalbuminuria to clinical proteinuria. Careful analysis of the DCCT cohort failed to show an impact. It is likely that other factors such as blood pressure control are of more importance for progression once UAER exceeds 30 to 40 mg a day. There are no conclusive data on the impact of improved glycaemic control on the development of endstage renal disease, decline in GFR, or death in patients with type 1 diabetes. The UKPDS showed a positive benefit of intensive therapy on the rate of doubling of serum creatinine at 12 years (0.91% vs 3.52%, $P<0.003$) in patients with type 2 diabetes, but the numbers were very small. Pancreas transplantation in type 1 patients has demonstrated that long-term (10 years) complete glycaemic normalization can reverse established pathological changes in native (nontransplanted) glomeruli. Thus glomerulopathy may take as long to reverse as it does to develop, and studies to date may have been of too short a duration and glycaemic correction inadequate.

Blood pressure control

There have been many studies of antihypertensive therapy in diabetic nephropathy. For clarity these will be dealt with under three headings: primary prevention (of microalbuminuria), secondary prevention (of clinical proteinuria), and tertiary prevention (of endstage renal disease and death).

Table 21.10.1.3 Comparison of intensive vs conventional therapy in the prevention of microalbuminuria in type 1 (DCCT + EDIC) and newly diagnosed type 2 (UKPDS) patients

Study	Number	Ethnicity	Duration of study (years)	Achieved HbA$_{1c}$		Microalbuminuria		
				Intensive (%)	Conventional (%)	Intensive (%)	Conventional (%)	RRR (%)
DCCT		European (96%)	9	7.2 (normal <6.05)	9.1	(UAER >40 mg/day)		
No retinopathy	726					15	27	44
Retinopathy	715					27	42	35
EDIC	1112		8	8.0	8.2	6.8	15.8	57
UKPDS	3867	European 81% Indian Asian 10% Afro-Caribbean 8%	9	7.0 (normal 6.2)	7.9	19.2 (UAC >50 mg/litre)	25.4	24

DCCT, Diabetes Control and Complications Trial; EDIC, Epidemiology of Diabetes Interventions and Complications Study; RRR, relative risk reduction; UAC, urinary albumin concentration, annual; UAER, urinary albumin excretion rate, annual 4-h collections (biannual for EDIC); UKPDS, United Kingdom Prospective Diabetes Study.

Primary prevention

The EURODIAB Controlled Trial of Lisinopril in Insulin-dependent Diabetes (EUCLID) studied normotensive type 1 diabetic patients with a UAER between 5 and 20 µg/min and demonstrated a significant reduction in albuminuria after 2 years, but no significant impact on the numbers developing microalbuminuria. This finding has been confirmed recently by the Diabetic retinopathy Candesartan Trials (DIRECT) study. The Bergamo Nephrologic Diabetes Complications Trial (BENEDICT) studied 1204 hypertensive type 2 patients with normoalbuminuria and demonstrated a significant reduction in the numbers developing microalbuminuria after 3 years on trandolapril (6%), compared to verapamil (11.9%), or placebo (10%). In the UKPDS, the number of hypertensive patients developing a urinary albumin concentration of more than 50 mg/litre at 6 years was 2.3% in the tight (blood pressure 144/82 mmHg) and 12.5% in the less tight (blood pressure 154/87 mmHg) groups ($P < 0.009$).

Secondary prevention

Most studies have shown a short- to medium-term benefit of antihypertensive therapy on UAER in the microalbuminuric range, with drugs blocking the renin–angiotensin system seeming to be more effective.

In mainly European patients with type 1 diabetes, a meta-analysis has shown an adjusted risk reduction of more than 60% for the development of clinical proteinuria comparing ACE inhibitors with placebo. More recently the angiotensin-II receptor blocker (ARB) irbesartan has demonstrated a similar magnitude of effect in microalbuminuric type 2 diabetic patients. Thus, blockade of the renin–angiotensin system by any means appears to confer benefit in terms of a reduction in the numbers of patients developing clinical proteinuria. Accurate data on GFR are not given in many of these studies, but in type 1 patients long-term ACE inhibitor therapy appears to stabilize renal function after an initial reduction. Interpretation of all these studies is complicated by the fact that the actively treated patients have nearly always had significantly lower blood pressures than the placebo groups. While statistical correction for these differences has been applied, it is uncertain whether mathematical correction can completely allow for the biological consequences of blood pressure reduction.

Tertiary prevention

Studies in the early 1980s established that lowering blood pressure in hypertensive type 1 patients with clinical proteinuria resulted in a more than 50% reduction in UAER and a significant slowing of the rate of decline of GFR from 10 to 3 ml/min per year. The Collaborative Study Group Trial in type 1 diabetic patients with a blood pressure below 140/90 mmHg and clinical proteinuria showed that the addition of captopril 100 mg a day resulted in a significant reduction in the numbers of patients doubling baseline serum creatinine compared to placebo (35% vs 78%; $P < 0.001$). This significance was confined to those with an entry serum creatinine concentration of more than 133 µmol/litre (1.5 mg/dl). There was a similar reduction in the numbers reaching a combined endpoint of death or the need for renal replacement therapy in the captopril-treated patients.

In patients with type 2 diabetes the results are complicated due to an increased cardiovascular comorbidity. Two large studies using ARBs in patients with clinical proteinuria have shown a reduction

of 25 to 33% in the rate of doubling of serum creatinine after 2 to 3 years treatment. This is considerably less than that seen in the captopril trial in type 1 patients, possibly because the type 2 patients had more advanced diabetic nephropathy at entry.

Taken together, the studies in type 1 and 2 patients support the use of drugs which block the renin–angiotensin system as first-line therapy in both microalbuminuric and clinically proteinuric patients and are recommended in all national and international guidelines.

Nonrenal outcomes

Although there are many large studies of the effects of antihypertensive therapy on cardiovascular mortality and morbidity in patient groups that have included sizeable cohorts of diabetic patients, their nephropathic status has rarely been specified. Most have shown that low blood pressure is associated with the reduction in overall mortality and stroke incidence, although the effect on myocardial infarction is inconsistent. Diabetic patients on the whole showed a greater benefit from active treatment.

Clinical features

Clinical progression is usually defined in terms of changes in UAER, GFR, and blood pressure. Much of our current understanding is based on cross-sectional data, although more long-term prospective studies of individual patients are being reported. Albuminuria is clearly a continuous variable and its separation into stages is artificial, but the distinction between microalbuminuria and clinical proteinuria has proved to be useful.

UAER

UAER may increase at diagnosis of type 1 diabetes and during acute hyperglycaemia, but usually returns to normal with glycaemic correction. Thereafter most patients (>60%) will have a normal UAER throughout their diabetic life, but the remainder develop persistent microalbuminuria at incident rates of between 1 and 2% per annum, usually preceded by intermittently positive tests. Interestingly, an inception cohort of Danish type 1 patients followed from diagnosis showed that UAER was significantly higher (but well within the normal range) in those subsequently going on to develop microalbuminuria after 15 to 20 years, compared to those who did not (11 vs 8 µg/min; $P = 0.002$). The rate of increase of UAER in patients with microalbuminuria is historically around 20% per annum, but this is lower in those commencing antihypertensive therapy or intensified insulin regimens (Table 21.10.1.2).

It is unusual to develop microalbuminuria within the first 5 years of diabetes onset, but it can develop at any time thereafter, even after 40 years. Most patients with type 1 diabetes and microalbuminuria will progress to clinical proteinuria unless treated; those with longer durations of diabetes before microalbuminuria tend to progress more slowly. More recent prospective studies have shown that up to 25% of type 1 microalbuminuric patients may spontaneously regress to normoalbuminuria. Around 12.5% may oscillate between normoalbuminuria and microalbuminuria for many years. The significance of these movements is unclear and is possibly the result of blood pressure-lowering therapies and short-term changes in glycaemic control.

Once UAER exceeds 300 mg/day there tends to be a relentless increase, occasionally into the nephrotic range. The rate of change varies between patients and is very dependent on systemic blood pressure. Historically the incidence of clinical proteinuria peaked after 15 to 17 years duration of diabetes, but more recent studies are showing a delay to 25 years or more.

Because the onset of type 2 diabetes is more difficult to define, the precise incidence of microalbuminuria is harder to estimate, although the UKPDS suggests that rates are similar to type 1 (Table 21.10.1.2). Up to 7% of newly diagnosed type 2 patients in the United Kingdom will have a urinary albumin concentration above 50 mg/litre (microalbuminuria), and 1% will be above 300 mg/litre (clinical proteinuria). Some studies have reported a reduction in UAER with initial glycaemic correction, but many patients have a sustained increased suggesting established nephropathology at diagnosis.

GFR

As previously mentioned, GFR at diagnosis of type 1 and type 2 diabetes is increased in 40 to 45% of patients. It returns to normal in most following glycaemic correction, although a significant minority maintain persistently high values (hyperfiltration). In humans the GFR declines by 1 ml/min per year after the age of 40, and it does so also in normotensive diabetic patients who have normal UAER. As the UAER approaches and exceeds the clinical proteinuria threshold, there tends to be a steady decline. This is particularly so in hypertensive patients, in whom the rate of loss of GFR varies considerably. In historical series in those with poorly controlled hypertension the average decline was 10 ml/min per year, leading to endstage renal disease 7 to 10 years after the onset of clinical proteinuria. More recently, the rate of decline is closer to 4 ml/min per year in patients with well-controlled systemic blood pressure, effectively delaying endstage renal disease by more than 10 years. It is now recommended that all people with diabetes have an estimate of GFR (eGFR) performed annually using the Modification of Diet in Renal Disease (MDRD) equation. Patients with type 2 diabetes and a normal UAER may still demonstrate a declining GFR with time.

Blood pressure

In patients with type 1 diabetes, blood pressure is virtually always normal at diagnosis. This is not the case in type 2 diabetes, where over one-third will have blood pressure higher than 160/95 mmHg and many more are hypertensive by recent criteria. Type 1 patients who go on to develop microalbuminuria have significantly higher blood pressures than those who remain with a normal UAER, although the averages remain below 140/90 mm Hg in both groups. Patients with newly developed microalbuminuria show a steady increase in blood pressure such that over 45% exceed 140/90 mmHg within 4 years. Most type 1 and type 2 patients with clinical proteinuria are hypertensive and on therapy.

Clinical concomitants of nephropathy

Many patients with diabetic nephropathy will also have retinopathy and neuropathy, which will tend to progress. Both of these complications can be reversed or at least ameliorated by improved glycaemic control. There is an increased incidence of cardiovascular, cerebrovascular, and peripheral vascular disease; intensive management of modifiable cardiovascular risk factors is essential (see below). Amputation rates in patients with diabetic nephropathy are high; careful foot surveillance and preventative podiatry are essential.

Differential diagnosis

It is important to remember that not all renal or urinary tract disease in diabetic patients is due to diabetic nephropathy. Urinary tract infection is more common in diabetic women compared to age-matched nondiabetic controls. Infection is often asymptomatic and culture should always be performed in any patient with an isolated positive urinalysis for protein, blood, leucocytes, or nitrite. A positive result is much more likely if two or more of these tests are positive.

Papillary necrosis has been described in women with long-standing type 1 diabetes and is a recognized complication of hyperosmolar coma in patients with both types of diabetes. Atheromatous renovascular disease is also common in diabetes, but the prevalence of functionally significant renal artery stenosis is uncertain.

Whereas the vast majority of type 1 patients with microalbuminuria have histologically proven diabetic glomerulopathy, the situation is less certain in type 2 diabetes. Up to 10% of such patients have evidence of nondiabetic pathologies, many have nonspecific ischaemic changes, and only a minority have classic diabetic lesions. The presence of diabetic retinopathy is partly helpful as those with it are almost certain to have diabetic lesions and those without it much less so. Even so, there are few cases of specifically treatable glomerulopathy in those with nondiabetic disease, hence management is unlikely to be significantly different, although those with nonclassic lesions tend to have slower rates of decline of GFR.

Clinical investigation

Type 2 diabetes is becoming more common and as a result the chance of concomitant nondiabetic renal or urological disease is increased. The need to exclude urinary tract infection has already been mentioned. Current United Kingdom guidelines suggest investigation and possible referral of all diabetic patients with persistent microscopic or macroscopic haematuria. An atypical presentation of proteinuria, or an unusually rapid clinical course such as rapidly deteriorating GFR, or the presence of features of other systemic diseases should prompt referral and investigation (Box 21.10.1.2). Current United Kingdom guidelines suggest expert review of all with an eGFR of loss than 60 ml/min per 1.73m².

Box 21.10.1.2 Clinical features suggestive of nondiabetic renal disease

- Increased UAER/clinical proteinuria/nephrotic syndrome in absence of retinopathy
- Low GFR with normal UAER
- Rapidly declining GFR
- Rapidly increasing proteinuria
- Refractory hypertension—consider renal artery stenosis
- Presence of active urinary sediment (red cells, cellular casts)
- Signs or symptoms of other systemic disease
- A greater than 30% reduction in GFR within 2–3 months of initiation of renin–angiotensin system blocking agents—consider renal artery stenosis

Criteria for diagnosis

Diabetic nephropathy is a clinical diagnosis based on the finding of proteinuria in a patient with diabetes and in whom there is no evidence of urinary infection. Conventionally, the level of proteinuria for a diagnosis of clinical proteinuria is 0.5 g/day, which is roughly equivalent to a UAER of 300 mg/day (Table 21.10.1.1). Patients with a UAER between 30 and 300 mg/day are defined as having microalbuminuria. Current United Kingdom guidelines suggest confirming the diagnosis with one or two repeat tests over the subsequent 1 to 6 months (Fig. 21.10.1.3).

Although timed urine collections remain the gold standard for diagnosis, they are cumbersome to use in routine clinical practice and most definitions depend on a spot urine sample and thus a test of albumin concentration. Levels above 50 mg/litre or above 300 mg/litre define microalbuminuria and clinical proteinuria, respectively. Sensitivity and specificity can be improved by using an early morning, first-voided specimen and correcting the urinary albumin level for creatinine concentration (an albumin/creatinine ratio, ACR). Defining levels are shown in Table 21.10.1.1.

It is unfortunate that the recent diagnostic and classification system for chronic kidney disease based on eGFR and now widely adopted does not map neatly to the more classic staging of diabetic nephropathy based on UAER (Table 21.10.1.4). eGFR estimated from the MDRD equation has not been validated in large diabetic cohorts, nor is it very accurate at values above 90 ml/min. As many newly diagnosed type 1 and type 2 patients have an elevated GFR, significant reductions may therefore pass undetected. Small retrospective cohorts using the MDRD equation have reported an underestimate of true GFR in diabetes and large prospective studies are urgently required.

Treatment

Glycaemic control and blood pressure

The roles of glycaemic control and blood pressure management have been discussed earlier in this chapter. Current target HbA1c levels from the National Institute of Health and Clinical Excellence (NICE) guidelines in the United Kingdom are less than 7.5% for type 1 and 6.5 to 7.5% for type 2 patients. Blood pressure targets are below 130/80 mmHg for type 1 and below 135/75 mmHg for type 2 patients with microalbuminuria. Because of the pivotal role that angiotensin II is thought to play in diabetic nephropathy development, all guidelines suggest using renin–angiotensin system blocking agents as first-line treatment. However, the UKPDS has shown that most type 2 patients will require two or more agents in order to achieve target. The British Hypertension Society guidelines suggest the addition of a diuretic as the next step, followed by a choice of calcium channel blocker, α-blocker, and then other agents. β-blockers are no longer recommended in diabetic patients, except for with postmyocardial infarction. The blood pressure target for patients with heavy proteinuria (>1 g/day) is 125/75 mmHg.

There has been increasing interest in using combined ACE inhibitor/ARB combinations, together with aldosterone antagonists such as spironolactone or eplerenone. The rationale is that each of these agents alone is not enough to completely block angiotensin II production. Studies to date have demonstrated a modest benefit on blood pressure and UAER, but have been too short to address endstage renal disease or rate of decline of GFR. It is also important to recognize that there is a real risk of significant hyperkalaemia on these regimens, and patients need to be monitored carefully and told to stop therapy during illnesses that may lead to dehydration such as diarrhoea and vomiting.

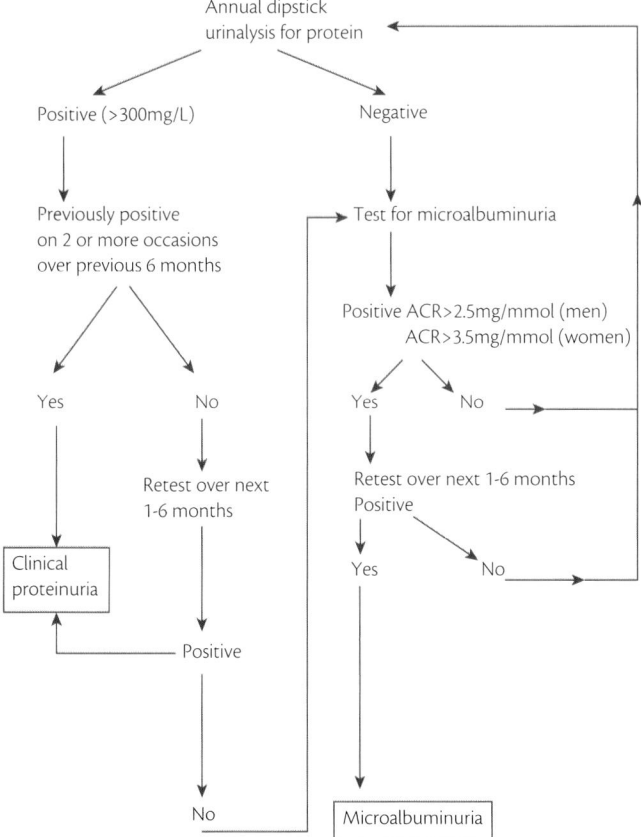

Fig. 21.10.1.3 Flowchart for diagnosis of microalbuminuria and clinical proteinuria.
NB: Assumes sterile urine throughout. Exclude infection when proteinuria first detected and at any time thereafter if a history of UTI.

Table 21.10.1.4 Cross-tabulation of different classification of diabetic kidney disease using classical staging by UAER and the CKD staging system

	eGFR ml/min/1.73m²		
	>60 (stage 1 and 2)	30–60 (stage 3)	<30 (stages 4 and 5)
Normoalbuminuria (<30 mg/day)	Possible DKD (at risk)	Possible DKD (could be DM + CKD)	Possible DKD (could be DM + CKD)
Microalbuminuria (30–299 mg/day)	Possible DKD (probable if DR)	Probable DKD (definite if DR)	Probable DKD (definite if DR)
Clinical proteinuria (>300 mg/day)	DKD	DKD	DKD

CKD, chronic kidney disease; DKD, diabetic kidney disease; DM, diabetes mellitus; DR, diabetic retinopathy, eGFR, estimated glomerular filtration rate; UAER, urinary albumin excretion rate.
NB: Staging by UAER may be confounded by proteinuria-lowering therapies such as renin–angiotensin system blockers. Wherever possible, classification by UAER should be based on pretreatment levels. A reduced GFR in the presence of normoalbuminuria is well described in both type 1 and type 2 diabetes; renal biopsy often shows DKD in such patients.

Achieving blood pressure targets is difficult, particularly in patients with type 2 diabetes and systolic hypertension. However, the UKPDS suggested significant benefit in terms of stroke and heart disease risk for any reduction in glycaemia and blood pressure, hence it is important to attain the lowest achievable and tolerated levels for both.

Other aspects

Low protein diets have been shown by meta-analysis to slow the rate of decline of GFR in diabetic patients, and a more recent study from Denmark has also shown benefit on mortality. Current dietary recommendations are for an intake of between 0.7 and 0.9 g protein/kg body weight per day.

Aspirin in a dose of 325 mg/day reduced myocardial infarction (RR 0.72; 99% CI 0.55–0.95) in 3711 type 1 and 2 patients with retinopathy. Although nephropathy status was not determined in this study, the use of low-dose aspirin is advised for all patients with an increased UAER (unless contraindicated) because of their high risk for cardiovascular disease. Lipid-lowering therapy should also be commenced.

Observational studies suggest that patients with better glycaemic control have a better overall survival on haemodialysis. Active foot surveillance and eye screening for these patients also confers benefit in terms of limb and sight preservation.

A multiple risk factor approach

Because the outlook for patients with diabetic nephropathy is poor, many national guidelines now suggest a multiple risk factor approach to management. However, many patients with advanced diabetic nephropathy referred to renal units in Europe and the United States of America have inadequate blood pressure control, low use of therapies of proven benefit, e.g. β-blockers, ACE inhibitors, lipid-lowering therapy, and low-dose aspirin, and poor assessment of comorbidities such as retinopathy and foot care.

The Steno 2 study in microalbuminuric type 2 diabetic patients involved a multifactorial intervention for 7 to 8 years that addressed glycaemia, blood pressure (using renin–angiotensin system blocking agents in all), serum lipid lowering, low-dose aspirin, smoking cessation, reduction of dietary fat and salt, exercise, and antioxidant vitamins. Compared to routine care this significantly reduced the development of clinical proteinuria and the composite cardiovascular outcome of fatal and nonfatal myocardial infarction and stroke, myocardial revascularization (surgical or percutaneous), and peripheral vascular surgery or amputation. There is, therefore, a real challenge for our patients as well as their carers to implement multiple therapies in a way that will facilitate compliance and deliver long-term benefit.

Prognosis

Microalbuminuric type 1 and type 2 patients have a two- to fourfold increased mortality, mainly from cardiovascular disease. The reported relative mortality for European 40-year-old type 1 patients with clinical proteinuria in Denmark was between 80 and 100 times that of the nondiabetic population, while the World Health Organization study revealed a three- to fourfold excess for clinically proteinuric patients with type 2 diabetes. Most of these deaths are due to stroke or myocardial infarction. In Finland, type 1 patients with nephropathy have a 10-fold relative risk for both stroke and myocardial infraction compared to nondiabetic controls. The UKPDS cohort demonstrated an annual mortality of 4.6% for those with clinical proteinuria, and almost 20% for those with a serum creatinine above 175 µmol/litre or in endstage renal disease (Fig. 21.10.1.4), cardiovascular disease being the main cause of death. Pima Indians also show an increase in mortality with increasing ACR. The causes of death are somewhat different to white Europid patients; vascular disease is much less prevalent in native Americans, although more frequent in those with diabetic nephropathy. A reduced eGFR of less than 60 ml/min per 1.73m² confers a more than 3.3-fold increased hazard ratio for cardiovascular mortality irrespective of albuminuria status.

Survival on dialysis remains much worse for patients with diabetes compared to those without; around 25% are alive after 5 years in both European and American registries. While 5-year survival has improved in recent years for those with nondiabetic renal disease, diabetic patients have shown only a modest improvement from 25 to 27%, and in the United States of America the death rate for never transplanted 20- to 44-year-old diabetic patients with endstage renal disease is nearly twice as great as that for nondiabetic controls. Overall survival for diabetic patients is best in those who have an early successful kidney transplant.

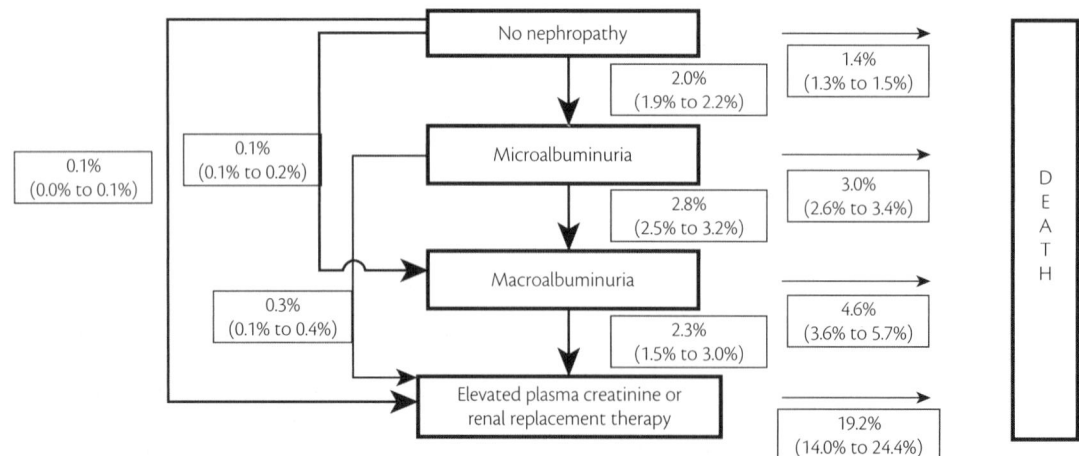

Fig. 21.10.1.4 Annual transition rates and 95% CI through stages of nephropathy in 5097 newly diagnosed type 2 diabetic patients in the UKPDS. (Reproduced with permission).

Areas of uncertainty or controversy

Should we screen for diabetic nephropathy?

Because of the strong associations between an increase in UAER and cardiovascular disease, a case for screening for diabetic nephropathy can be made with some confidence, although the evidence base for beneficial intervention at lower levels of albuminuria is not secure. Current recommendations from national diabetes associations advise at least annual screening, based on the diagnostic flowchart shown in Fig. 21.10.1.3. Extrapolating the known effects of ACE inhibitors on a reduction of UAER to a possible prevention of clinical proteinuria and thus endstage renal disease has led several authors to propose a potential cost benefit from the early use of these agents. However, only long-term prospective studies of primary prevention can conclusively answer this question, and no such trials are currently being undertaken.

Can glycaemic control reverse established nephropathy?

The DCCT was inconclusive, but data from pancreas transplant series suggest that glomerulopathology can be reversed in native kidneys after 10 years of normoglycaemia.

Why does intensive glycaemic control fail to completely prevent development of microalbuminuria?

Glycaemia is one of many factors leading to nephropathy. Moreover, even in the DCCT complete glycaemic normalization was not achieved. It is possible that newer insulins and delivery systems with continuous glucose monitoring may make sustained normoglycaemia more easily achievable.

Do drugs that block the renin–angiotensin system prevent or only delay the development of nephropathy? Can they reverse established nephropathy?

The data are not conclusive, partly because of the relatively short duration of many trials, but most studies show a benefit in terms of reduction of UAER. A meta-analysis published in 2005 raised concerns about the effectiveness of these drugs, but was itself flawed by the overwhelming influence of the Antihypertensive and Lipid-lowering Treatment to Prevent Heart Attack Trial (ALLHAT), which was not designed to study renal outcomes as a primary endpoint.

For those with established clinical proteinuria and chronic kidney disease stages 3 and beyond there is no doubt that renin–angiotensin system blocking drugs delay endstage renal disease. For microalbuminuria there are no studies of sufficient power to confirm benefit on hard clinical endpoints such as mortality or endstage renal disease. Primary prevention of microalbuminuria itself has only been shown in hypertensive type 2 patients.

Likely developments in the near future

Hyperglycaemia is thought to lead to nephropathy through several pathways, as outlined in Box 21.10.1.1. There are developments in most of these fields, with the following being studied in trials: pyridoxamine and other inhibitors of glycation; ruboxistaurin, a protein kinase Cβ inhibitor; avosentan and other endothelin inhibitors; and aliskirena direct rennin inhibitor.

Further reading

Adler AI, et al. (2003). Development and progression of nephropathy in type 2 diabetes: the United Kingdom Prospective Study (UKPDS 64). Kidney Int, 63, 225–32.

American Diabetes Association. (2009). Executive summary: standards of medical care in diabetes – 2009. Diabetes Care, 32 suppl 1, S6–S12.

Bilous R. (2008). Microvascular disease: what does the UKPDS tell us about diabetic nephropathy? Diabetic Med, 25 suppl 2, 25–29.

Bilous R, et al.(2009). Effect of candesartan on microalbuminuria and albumin excretion rate in diabetes: 3 randomised trials. Ann Intern Med, 151, 11–20.

British Cardiac Society, British Hypertension Society, Diabetes UK, HEART UK, Primary Care Cardiovascular Society, Stroke Association (2005). JBS 2: Joint British Societies' guidelines on prevention of cardiovascular disease in clinical practice. Heart, 91, Suppl 5, V1–52.

Cooper ME, Jandeleit Dahn K, Thomas MC (2005). Targets to retard the progression of diabetic nephropathy. Kidney Int, 68, 1439–45.

DCCT/EDIC Research Group. (2003). Sustained effect of intensive treatment of type 1 diabetes mellitus on development and progression of diabetic nephropathy. JAMA, 290, 2159–2167.

Diabetes Control and Complications Trial Research Group (1993). The effect of intensive treatment of diabetes on the development and progression of long term complications in insulin dependent diabetes mellitus. N Engl J Med, 329, 977–86.

Finne P, et al. (2005). Incidence of end stage renal disease in patients with type 1 diabetes. JAMA, 294, 1782–7.

Forbes JM, Coughlan MT, Cooper ME.(2008). Oxidative stress as a major culprit in kidney disease in diabetes. Diabetes, 57, 1446–54.

Fried LF, Orchard TJ, Kasiske BL, for the Lipids and Renal Disease Progression Meta-analysis Study Group (2001). Effect on lipid reduction on the progression of renal disease: a meta-analysis. Kidney Int, 59, 260–9.

Gaede P, et al.(2008). Effect of multifactorial interventions on mortality in type 2 diabetes. N Engl J Med, 358, 580–91

Gaston RS, et al. (2004). Transplantation in the diabetic patient with advanced chronic kidney disease: a task force report. Am J Kidney Dis, 44, 529–42.

Hansen HP, et al. (2002). Effect of dietary protein restriction on prognosis in patients with diabetic nephropathy. Kidney Int, 62, 220–8.

Hovind P, et al. (2004). Predictors for the development of microalbuminuria and macroalbuminuria in patients with type 1 diabetes mellitus: inception cohort study. BMJ, 328, 1105–8.

International Diabetes Federation (2006). Diabetes atlas, 3rd edition. www.eatlas.idf.org

Joint Specialty Committee on Renal Medicine of the Royal College of Physicians and the Renal Association and the Royal College of General Practitioners (2006). Chronic kidney disease in adults: UK guidelines for identification management and referral. Royal College of Physicians, London.

Marshall SM, Flyvbjerg A (2006). Prevention and early detection of vascular complications of diabetes. BMJ, 333, 475–80.

Molitch ME, et al., American Diabetes Association (2004). Nephropathy in diabetes. Diabetes Care, 27 Suppl 1, S79–83. [Updated at www.diabetes.org]

National Kidney Foundation (2007). KDOQI Clinical practice guidelines and clinical practice recommendations for diabetes and chronic kidney disease. Am J Kidney Dis, 49 Suppl 2, S2–180.

National Collaborating Centre for Chronic Conditions. (2004). Type 1 diabetes in adults: National Clinical Guideline for Diagnosis and Management in Primary and Secondary Care. London: Royal College of Physicians. Accessed by www.nice.org.uk/nicemedia/pdf/cg015_fullguideline_adults_development_section.pdf

National Collaborating Centre for Chronic Conditions.(2008). Type 2 diabetes: National Clinical Guideline for Management in Primary and Secondary Care (update). London: Royal College of Physicians. Accessed by www.nice.org.uk/nicemedia/pdf/cg66fullguideline0509.pdf

Olsen S, Mogensen CE (1996). How often is NIDDM complicated with non-diabetic renal disease? An analysis of renal biopsies and the literature. *Diabetologia*, **39**, 1638–45.

Pavkov ME, *et al.* (2006). Increasing incidence of proteinuria and declining incidence of end stage renal disease in diabetic Pima Indians. *Kidney Int*, **70**, 1840–6.

Rich SS (2006). Genetics of diabetes and its complications. *J Am Soc Nephrol*, **17**, 353–60.

Robertson LM, Waugh N, Robertson A.(2006). Protein restriction for diabetic renal disease. *Cochrane database of systematic reviews* 2006; issue 2. Art. No. CD002181DOI:10.1002/14651858.CD002181/pub2

Rossing P (2006). Prediction, progression and prevention of diabetic nephropathy. *Diabetologia*, **49**, 11–19.

Rossing K, *et al.* (2004). Progression of nephropathy in type 2 diabetic patients. *Kidney Int*, **66**, 1596–605.

Singh R, *et al.* (2001). Advanced glycation end products: a review. *Diabetologia*, **44**, 129–46.

Stehouwer CDA (2004). Endothelial dysfunction in diabetic nephropathy: state of the art and potential significance for non-diabetic kidney disease. *Nephrol Dial Transplant*, **19**, 778–81.

Strippoli GFM, *et al.* (2004). Effects of angiotensin converting enzyme inhibitors and angiotensin II receptor antagonists on mortality and renal outcomes in diabetic nephropathy: systematic review. *BMJ*, **329**, 828–40.

The Renal Association.(2008).UK Renal Registry 11th Annual Report 2008. www.renalreg.com/report/2008.htm

UK Prospective Diabetes Study Group (1998). Intensive blood glucose control with sulphonylureas or insulin compared with conventional treatment and risk of complications in patients with type 2 diabetes (UKPDS 33). *Lancet*, **352**, 837–53.

UK Prospective Diabetes Study Group (1998). Tight blood pressure control and risk of macrovascular and microvascular complications in type 2 diabetes (UKPDS 38). *BMJ*, **317**, 703–13.

U.S. Renal Data System.(2008). USRDS 2008 Annual Data Report: Atlas of Chronic Kidney Disease and End-stage Renal Disease in the United States, National Institutes of Health, National Institutes of Diabetes and Digestive and Kidney Diseases, Bethesda. www.USRDS.org/adr/htm

White SA, Shaw JA, Sutherland DER.(2009). Pancreas transplantation. *Lancet*, **373**, 1808–1817.

Wolf G (2003). Growth factors and the development of diabetic nephropathy. *Curr Diab Rep*, **3**, 485–90.

Wolf G, Chen S, Ziyadeh FN (2005). From the periphery of the glomerular capillary wall towards the centre of disease: podocyte injury comes of age in diabetic nephropathy. *Diabetes*, **54**, 1626–34.

21.10.2 **The kidney in systemic vasculitis**

David Jayne

Essentials

Systemic vasculitis can occur as a primary autoimmune disorder, or as a secondary manifestation of another disease process (e.g. related to infection, malignancy, chronic inflammatory disorder, or drugs). Primary systemic vasculitis is classified according to the predominant size of blood vessel involved and the presence of circulating antineutrophil cytoplasmic autoantibodies (ANCA). Incidence and

prevalence rates are between 15 and 20 per million and 200 to 400 per million population, respectively.

Small-vessel vasculitides—Wegener's granulomatosis (see Chapter 18.11.5), microscopic polyangiitis, and renal-limited vasculitis affect small vessels and are grouped together as the ANCA-associated vasculitides (AAV). Henoch–Schönlein purpura (see Chapter 21.8.1) and cryoglobulinaemia (see Chapter 21.10.4) also affect small vessels, but are ANCA negative.

Medium and larger vessel vasculitides—Churg–Strauss angiitis (30–50% are ANCA positive, see Chapter 18.11.5) and polyarteritis nodosa (ANCA negative) affect medium-sized vessels, as does Kawasaki's disease (see Chapter 19.11.8). Giant cell arteritis (see Chapter 19.11.4) and Takayasu's arteritis (see Chapter 16.14.4) affect larger vessels.

Aetiology and pathogenesis—the cause of primary systemic vasculitis is (by definition) unknown. The pathogenetic role of ANCA remains controversial because this pathology can occur without circulating ANCA, immune deposits are rarely present, and ANCA often persist without disease activity.

Pathology—the typical renal lesion of small vessel vasculitis is a glomerular capillaritis leading to segmental necrotizing glomerulonephritis with epithelioid crescent formation. Glomerular immune deposits are scanty or absent in AAV ('pauci-immune').

Clinical presentation—the diagnosis of vasculitis is often delayed for many months because initial symptoms such as fever, night sweats, polymyalgia, and weight loss are nonspecific. Patients with vasculitis present with: (1) persistent symptoms of constitutional disturbance; (2) nonrenal vasculitic manifestations, the nature of which may indicate a specific diagnosis, e.g. upper respiratory tract symptoms or signs (Wegener's granulomatosis), 'maturity-onset' asthma (Churg–Strauss angiitis), or mononeuritis multiplex (polyarteritis nodosa); or (3) uraemia. AAV is the most common cause of rapidly progressive glomerulonephritis—crescentic glomerulonephritis with renal failure—and should be considered in any unexplained case of acute renal impairment, especially when associated with microscopic haematuria and proteinuria and the kidneys are of normal size on ultrasound examination. Patients with renal-limited vasculitis present with more advanced renal failure than those with extrarenal disease because they are asymptomatic until uraemia develops.

Diagnosis—this depends on the triad of clinical features, serology, and histology, and the exclusion of secondary causes. ANCA positivity, confirmed by a positive proteinase 3 ANCA (PR3-ANCA) or myeloperoxidase ANCA (MPO-ANCA), has a predictive value of over 95% for the diagnosis of AAV with renal involvement in a patient with suspected nephritis. The diagnosis of polyarteritis nodosa is usually made by demonstration of aneurysms of medium-sized muscular arteries on angiography, or when biopsy of affected tissue reveals fibrinoid necrosis of involved vessels, accompanied by a marked inflammatory response. Other investigations determine the extent and severity of systemic disease.

Management—combination therapy with cyclophosphamide and high-dose oral prednisolone leads to control of active disease in 90% of patients, but is complicated by toxicity, in particular, cytopenias and severe infection. Azathioprine or methotrexate in combination with low-dose prednisolone are used to maintain remission after 3 to 6 months in order to avoid the malignancy and other late toxicities associated with cyclophosphamide, and they may also be considered for the induction of remission in mild presentations without renal impairment. High-dose intravenous methylprednisolone is widely used for initial therapy for renal vasculitis, and plasma exchange improves the chances of renal recovery in patients with severe renal impairment. Careful follow-up of patients in experienced centres with regular monitoring of blood counts, biochemical indices, inflammatory markers (erythrocyte sedimentation rate and C-reactive protein), and ANCA permits the prevention and early detection of drug-related toxicity and infection, and the early diagnosis and treatment of disease relapse.

Disease relapse—this is seen in 50% of patients by 5 years and is more common in Wegener's granulomatosis, in the presence of persisting ANCA positivity, and after withdrawal of immunosuppressive drugs. Agents used for relapsing or refractory disease include mycophenolate mofetil and leflunomide, high-dose intravenous immunoglobulin, and B-cell depletion with rituximab.

Prognosis—patient survival in AAV with renal involvement is 83% and 73% at 1 and 5 years, respectively, with a high serum creatinine at diagnosis, older age, and extensive extrarenal vasculitis indicating a poorer prognosis. Fifty per cent of those presenting with a serum creatinine greater than 500 µmol/litre will be alive and off dialysis at 1 year of follow-up.

Introduction

Systemic vasculitis occurs either as a primary autoimmune disorder, or as a secondary manifestation of another disease process (Table 21.10.2.1, Box 21.10.2.1). Primary systemic vasculitis is classified according to the predominant size of vessel involved and the presence of circulating antineutrophil cytoplasm autoantibodies (ANCA) (Table 21.10.2.2). Wegener's granulomatosis, microscopic polyangiitis, and renal-limited vasculitis are grouped together as the ANCA-associated vasculitides (AAV), and together represent 50% of presentations of systemic vasculitis. This grouping is justified by the similarity of many clinical and histological features, by a similar treatment response, by the putative role of ANCA in pathogenesis, and the frequent practical difficulty in discriminating between

Box 21.10.2.1 Secondary causes of vasculitis

Infection
- Endocarditis
- Chronic pulmonary infection (bronchiectasis, cystic fibrosis)
- Chronic viral infection (hepatitis B, hepatitis C, and HIV)
- Tuberculosis
- Other infections

Malignancy
- Lymphoma
- Renal cell carcinoma
- Other malignancies

Chronic inflammatory disorders
- Rheumatoid arthritis
- Systemic lupus erythematosus
- Sjögren's syndrome

Drugs
- Propylthiouracil
- Penicillamine
- Hydralazine
- Minocycline
- Cocaine

Wegener's granulomatosis (discussed in greater detail in Chapter 18.11.5) and microscopic polyangiitis in an individual patient.

Seventy per cent of patients with AAV have kidney involvement and are at risk of developing endstage renal disease. Kidney involvement is also frequent in the ANCA-negative small vessel vasculitides, Henoch–Schönlein purpura and cryoglobulinaemia, but is less common in medium and large vessel vasculitis.

The typical renal lesion of vasculitis is a glomerular capillaritis leading to segmental necrotizing glomerulonephritis with epithelioid crescent formation (Fig. 21.10.2.1). In AAV, glomerular immune deposits are scanty or absent ('pauci-immune'), whereas in Henoch–Schönlein purpura and cryoglobulinaemia, immune complex deposition is present. Isolated pauci-immune glomerulonephritis with crescents has been previously called idiopathic crescentic glomerulonephritis, but most cases occur in association with ANCA and have been redefined as renal-limited vasculitis and represent a 'forme fruste' of microscopic polyangiitis.

As a systemic disease, renal vasculitis occurs in conjunction with involvement of other organs, and features such as arthritis, purpura, or episcleritis in AAV, and especially ear, nose, and throat involvement in Wegener's granulomatosis, may precede renal disease and provide important clues for diagnosis. Fifty per cent of patients with AAV have pulmonary involvement and the simultaneous presentation of diffuse lung haemorrhage and renal vasculitis is the most common cause of the 'pulmonary–renal syndrome'.

Systemic vasculitis can be controlled by immunosuppressive and corticosteroid treatment and is a preventable cause of endstage renal

Table 21.10.2.1 Classification of primary systemic vasculitis according to the predominant size of blood vessel involvement and the presence or absence of ANCA

Predominant size of vessel involved	Usually ANCA positive (pauci-immune histology)	Usually ANCA negative
Small	Wegener's granulomatosis	Henoch–Schönlein purpura
	Microscopic polyangiitis	Cryoglobulinaemia
	Renal-limited vasculitis	
Medium	Churg–Strauss angiitis (30–50% ANCA positive)	Polyarteritis nodosa
		Kawasaki's disease
Large		Giant cell arteritis
		Takayasu's arteritis

Table 21.10.2.2 Disease definitions of primary systemic vasculitis syndromes that involve the kidney, according to the Chapel Hill Consensus Statement 1993

Disease	Definition
ANCA-associated vasculitis	
Wegener's granulomatosis	Granulomatous inflammation involving the respiratory tract, and necrotizing vasculitis affecting small to medium-sized vessels, e.g. capillaries, venules, arterioles, and arteries. Necrotizing glomerulonephritis is common
Microscopic polyangiitis	Necrotizing vasculitis with few or no immune deposits affecting small vessels, i.e. capillaries, venules, or arterioles. Necrotizing arteritis involving small and medium-sized arteries may be present. Necrotizing glomerulonephritis is very common. Pulmonary capillaritis often occurs
Churg–Strauss angiitis	Eosinophil-rich and granulomatous inflammation involving the respiratory tract and necrotizing vasculitis affecting small to medium-sized vessels, and associated with asthma and blood eosinophilia
Renal-limited vasculitis	Isolated pauci-immune necrotizing and crescentic glomerulonephritis, typically known as idiopathic rapidly progressive glomerulonephritis, has many features to suggest that it represents a renal-limited form of microscopic polyangiitis or Wegener's granulomatosis, including the presence of ANCA
Other primary systemic vasculitis syndromes	
Henoch–Schönlein purpura	Vasculitis with IgA-dominant immune deposits affecting small vessels, i.e. capillaries, venules, or arterioles. Typically involves skin, gut, and glomeruli, and is associated with arthralgias or arthritis
Cryoglobulinaemic vasculitis	Vasculitis with cryoglobulin immune deposits affecting small vessels, i.e. capillaries, venules, or arterioles, and associated with cryoglobulins in serum. Skin and glomeruli are often involved
Polyarteritis nodosa	Necrotizing inflammation of medium-sized or small arteries, without glomerulonephritis or vasculitis in arterioles, capillaries, or venules
Giant cell arteritis	Granulomatous arteritis of the aorta and its major branches, with a predilection for the extracranial branches of the carotid artery. Often involves the temporal artery. Usually occurs in patients older than 50 years and is often associated with polymyalgia rheumatica. Renal involvement is rare
Takayasu's arteritis	Granulomatous inflammation of the aorta and its major branches. Usually occurs in patients younger than 50 years
Kawasaki's disease	Arthritis involving large, medium-sized, and small arteries and associated with mucocutaneous lymph node syndrome. Coronary arteries are often involved. Aorta and veins may be involved. Usually occurs in children.

disease. Most clinical research has focused on AAV, with management of other primary systemic vasculitides often extrapolated from results in AAV. However, the age of many patients at diagnosis, late presentations with advanced renal failure, and the toxicity of current drugs contribute to poor outcomes, with endstage renal disease or death occurring in 17% of AAV patients at 1 year.

It has become increasingly clear that the incidence of renal vasculitis rises with age, and this disease is undoubtedly a commoner primary cause of renal failure in older people than previously thought. Because untreated renal vasculitis progresses to endstage renal disease, and steroid and immunosuppressive therapy can improve the outcome, early diagnosis and institution of therapy are particularly important. However, clinical decision making can often be very difficult as the toxicity of such treatments is increased in elderly patients, contributing both to morbidity and mortality. There is therefore a clear advantage in early diagnosis, when less intense treatment is effective, and on careful monitoring of therapy to minimize adverse recent risk. It is important that physicians continue to search for and evaluate safer alternative drugs.

Historical perspective

The subgroups within primary systemic vasculitis were initially described as discrete clinicopathological syndromes: Henoch–Schönlein purpura in 1837, polyarteritis nodosa in 1866, Takayasu's arteritis in 1910, microscopic polyangiitis in 1923, Wegener's granulomatosis in 1936, and Churg–Strauss angiitis in 1951. The American College of Rheumatology published diagnostic and classification criteria for vasculitis in 1990, but these ignored ANCA and microscopic polyangiitis and included a now discarded term, hypersensitivity vasculitis. International consensus on the definitions and terminology of vasculitis was subsequently achieved in Chapel Hill in 1992, and these definitions remain valid. Although there are no agreed diagnostic criteria for vasculitis in clinical practice, criteria have been determined by international clinical trial groups which have stood the test of time. An association of ANCA with Wegener's granulomatosis was first reported in 1985, and with microscopic polyangiitis in the following year. The target autoantigens for ANCA in systemic vasculitis, proteinase 3 (PR3-ANCA) and myeloperoxidase (MPO-ANCA), were identified in 1989. The availability of ANCA testing has been a major step in the diagnosis and monitoring of vasculitis and has provided insights into pathogenesis and classification.

Before 1960 systemic vasculitis with renal involvement was usually fatal. High-dose corticosteroids were partially effective in the short term, but it was the introduction of immunosuppressive therapy, and particularly cyclophosphamide, during the next decade which enabled sustained control of vasculitis to be achieved. An increasing awareness of the late toxicity of cyclophosphamide with infertility and bladder and haematological malignancies in the 1980s encouraged the development of strategies to minimize cyclophosphamide exposure. Several additional agents have been introduced with the aim of improving control of fulminant or refractory disease, or reducing steroid or immunosuppressive exposure, and these include plasma exchange, intravenous immunoglobulin, tumour necrosis factor-α (TNFα) blockade, and lymphocyte depletion. However, improving the sustained efficacy of therapy and reducing its toxicity remains a major challenge.

Aetiology, genetics, pathogenesis, and pathology

The cause of primary systemic vasculitis is unknown. Genetic associations have been reported with polymorphisms of cytotoxic

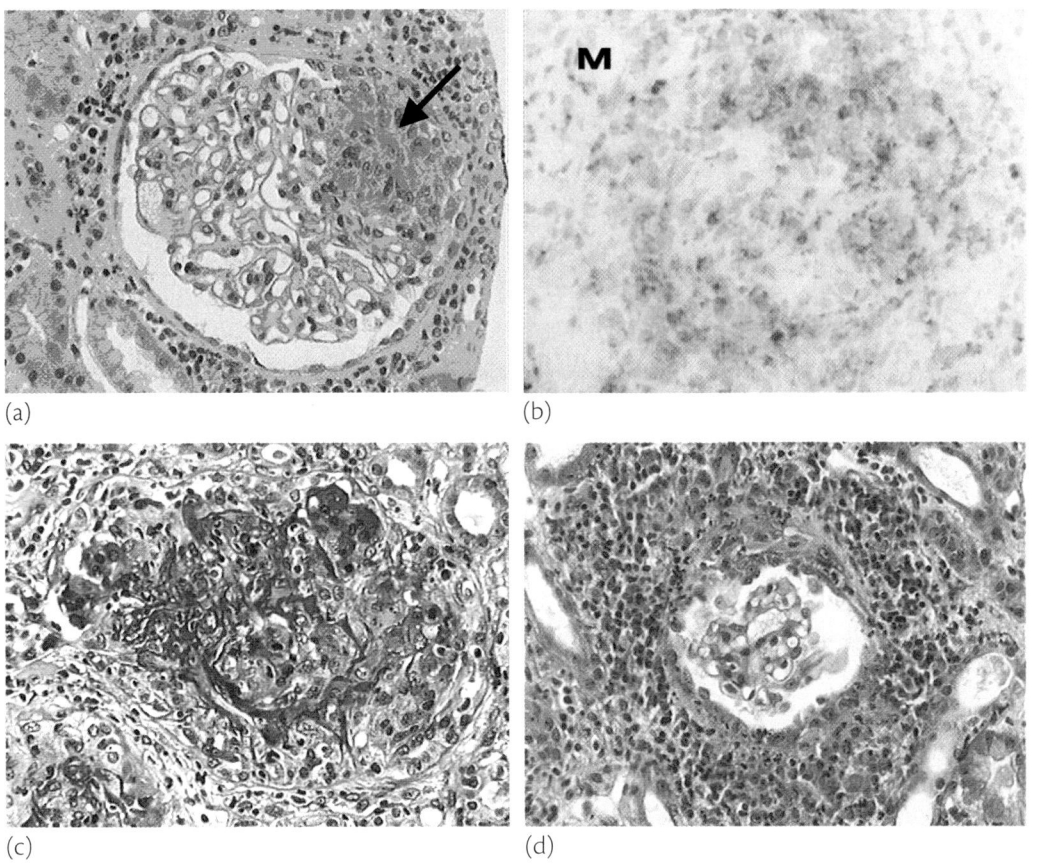

(a)

(b)

(c)

(d)

Fig. 21.10.2.1 Glomerular histology of ANCA-associated vasculitis. (a) A glomerulus showing focal necrosis with an early crescentic reaction (arrow). (b) Glomerular macrophage infiltration (brown) illustrated by CD68 staining. (c) Severe glomerular involvement with widespread necrosis, a circumferential crescent, and collapse of the glomerular tuft. (d) Massive periglomerular leucocyte infiltration occurring around an affected glomerulus.

T-lymphocyte associated antigen 4 (CTLA4), tyrosine-protein phosphatase nonreceptor type 2, the third complement component, and the FcγRIII immunoglobulin receptor. There has been no consistent associations with HLA genes. α1-antitrypsin-deficient phenotypes develop more aggressive PR3-ANCA-associated vasculitis.

Occupational exposure to silica and other industrial dusts increases the risk of MPO-ANCA vasculitis. An increased incidence of MPO-ANCA vasculitis was reported in Kuwait in 1991 after the first Gulf war, and also after the Kobe earthquake in 1995. Whether other occupational exposures are aetiologically related, such as to heavy metals or insecticides, is unclear.

AAV predominantly affects small blood vessels, capillaries, arterioles, and venules, but may also affect muscular arteries and rarely larger arteries. Capillaritis in the glomerular tuft results in capillary thrombosis and infarction. This appears on biopsy as segmental fibrinoid necrosis and a secondary crescentic reaction within Bowman's capsule, containing monocytes and epithelial cells (Fig. 21.10.2.1a,b), which progresses to involve the whole tuft and destroy the glomerulus (Fig. 21.10.2.1c). In addition there is periglomerular and tubulointerstitial inflammation, which may contain giant cells (Fig. 21.10.2.1d). Extraglomerular arteritis is seen in 15% of cases and frank granulomata occur rarely in Wegener's granulomatosis. There is considerable variety in the severity and proportion of fibrotic lesions between glomeruli. Obsolescent glomeruli and fibrotic crescents reflect previous vasculitic events and are associated with tubulointerstitial scarring. Capillaritis in pulmonary alveoli causes capillary rupture and haemorrhage into the alveolar space.

The pathogenetic role of ANCA remains controversial because this pathology can occur without circulating ANCA, immune deposits are rarely present, and ANCA often persist without disease activity. Experimental studies have demonstrated unequivocally that ANCA induce neutrophil activation, superoxide and cytokine release, and can cause neutrophil-mediated endothelial cytotoxicity. ANCA require neutrophil priming with tumour necrosis factor, which leads to translocation of proteinase 3 or myeloperoxidase from primary granules in the cytoplasm to the cell membrane. In addition to binding to cell surface autoantigen, ligation of the Fc component of the ANCA antibody to neutrophil Fc receptors is necessary for intracellular signalling and cell activation. Both spontaneous and induced animal models have demonstrated the ability of ANCA to cause a pauci-immune renal vasculitis in susceptible animal strains.

The ANCA autoantigen proteinase 3 is abundantly expressed in granulomatous lesions in close proximity to mature dendritic cells capable of antigen presentation. The inflammatory infiltrate at such foci is neutrophil rich, and interventions which deplete neutrophils, including experimental chemokine blockade or the drugs cyclophosphamide and deoxyspergualin, are effective therapies. T cells in granulomatous lesions are over-represented by a CD4+, CD28− subset which release γ-interferon and TNFα and have cytotoxic potential. A pathogenetic role for cytotoxic T cells has been shown in larger vessel arteritis, and similar mechanisms are also likely to be important in smaller vessel disease. Circulating markers of T-cell activation are elevated, including the soluble interleukin 2 receptor.

The efficacy of B-cell depleting therapies has focused attention on B cells, which are present in granulomata and at sites of vasculitic injury. They have specificity for ANCA autoantigens and demonstrate features of affinity maturation. Autoantibodies to endothelial antigens are found in over 50% of patients with vasculitis, but their targets have not been defined and their contribution to pathogenesis is unclear.

The involvement of the respiratory tract in Wegener's granulomatosis has led to interest in the interaction between respiratory tract infection and a dysregulated immune response. Colonization with *Staphylococcus aureus* is associated with a higher relapse rate in Wegener's granulomatosis, and bacterial strains expressing toxic shock staphylococcal toxin are particularly implicated. Damage to the respiratory tract resulting from vasculitic inflammation impairs its ability to eradicate microbial infection and a cycle of vasculitis and recurrent infection develops. Cytokine-induced up-regulation of endothelial adhesion molecules promotes leucocyte adhesion and injury, providing an additional mechanism by which inflammation secondary to infection can stimulate vasculitis.

The cause of polyarteritis nodosa is not known in most cases, but hepatitis B infection (particularly when due to intravenous drug abuse, and with presentation usually within 3–6 months of infection) and hairy cell leukaemia are recognized associations.

Epidemiology

The incidence of primary systemic vasculitis is 40/million population per year, with AAV comprising 15–20/million population per year. An apparent increased incidence of AAV has been explained by improved detection, especially in older people, and no increase in incidence has been seen where long-term epidemiological studies have been performed. Prevalence rates of ANCA vasculitis range from 90–400/million. Both Wegener's granulomatosis and microscopic polyangiitis are very rare in children and have an increasing incidence with age, the rising curve for Wegener's granulomatosis flattening off at age 60, but that for microscopic polyangiitis continuing to rise in the oldest age groups (Fig. 21.10.2.2).

Renal involvement is very common in microscopic polyangiitis, with over 90% of patients affected. In Wegener's granulomatosis the likelihood of renal involvement increases with age, with the proportion of kidney biopsies displaying a crescentic nephritis rising from 5% in those under 60 years of age to over 11% in those

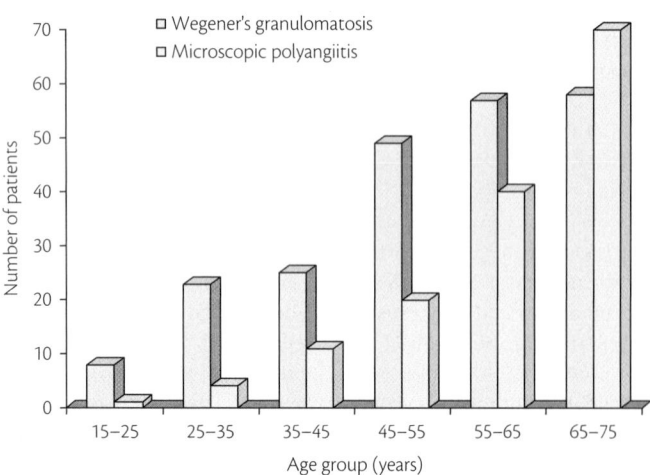

Fig. 21.10.2.2 Frequency of Wegener's granulomatosis and microscopic polyangiitis according to the patients' age at diagnosis.
Data from three clinical trials performed by the European Vasculitis Study Group.

over 60 years of age. Renal function at diagnosis is worse in older patients, indicating that not only is renal involvement more frequent, but it is also more aggressive.

The age association implies an aetiological contribution of an ageing immune system and the possible involvement of environmental factors. Silica exposure increases the incidence of microscopic polyangiitis, and an association with farming—especially with animals—has also been demonstrated. The relative frequencies of Wegener's granulomatosis and microscopic polyangiitis are influenced by latitude, with Wegener's granulomatosis being more frequent in colder climates in both the northern and southern hemispheres. In addition, there are ethnic differences, with Wegener's granulomatosis being less common in eastern Asian and black populations. The lack of a major immunogenetic contribution and the late age of onset differentiates ANCA-associated autoimmunity from other autoantibody-associated autoimmune diseases.

The epidemiology of polyarteritis nodosa is not well described, but the condition is rare, with incidence probably in the range 5 to 10/million population per year. It typically affects middle-aged men (male to female ratio 2:1).

Clinical features

Patients with primary systemic vasculitis vary in the pattern and severity of organ involvement, in their response to therapy, and in their subsequent disease course and prognosis. Clinical evaluation confirms the extent and severity of organ involvement, which permits the patient to be placed in a subgroup to guide therapy (Table 21.10.2.3). Appropriate treatment aims to obtain and sustain disease remission, but relapses are common and refractory disease or chronic, persisting low disease activity states are therapeutic challenges (Table 21.10.2.4).

Presentation

AAV

Following a prodromal phase of several months with constitutional symptoms such as fever, night sweats, polymyalgia, and weight loss, vasculitis patients present either with a nonrenal vasculitic manifestation, or symptoms of constitutional disturbance, or evidence of uraemia. Nonrenal manifestations result in referral to the appropriate specialty, when a high index of suspicion for vasculitis is required for the presence of renal involvement to be detected. Because renal vasculitis is asymptomatic until uraemia develops, the absence of specific symptoms of renal disease often results in diagnostic delay. In consequence, patients with renal-limited vasculitis present with more advanced renal failure than those with extrarenal disease.

The average delay from onset of symptoms to diagnosis is 6 months. During this phase urinary abnormalities will be present and should therefore be sought in all patients with unexplained illness, or where there is a suspicion of vasculitis. Glomerular haematuria and proteinuria is always present in renal vasculitis, but may be confused with prostatic disease or urinary tract infection. The presence of red cell casts on urine microscopy reflects severe glomerular injury and is usually associated with crescentic glomerulonephritis. Atypical presentations including 'failure to thrive' and unexpected asymptomatic renal impairment are more common in elderly patients. Certain clinical features should raise suspicion of a vasculitic illness (Box 21.10.2.2).

Table 21.10.2.3 Subgrouping of patients with AAV at diagnosis according to disease severity and treatment response. Randomized controlled trials performed by the European Vasculitis Study Group and average age at entry of each subgroup

Subgroup	Organ involvement	Constitutional symptoms	ANCA status	Serum creatinine (μmol/litre)	Average age at onset (years)
Localized	One site, typically the upper respiratory tract in Wegener's granulomatosis	No	±	<120	
Early systemic	Any, except renal or imminent vital organ failure	Yes	+	<120	51
Generalized (or renal)	Imminent vital organ failure or renal vasculitis	Yes	+	<500	56
Severe	Vital organ failure, typically renal	Yes	+	>500	66
Refractory	Progressive disease despite conventional therapy	Yes	⊥	Any	

Table 21.10.2.4 Definitions of disease state in primary systemic vasculitis according to a European League against Rheumatism (EULAR)/European Vasculitis Study Group (EUVAS) consensus statement

Activity state	Definition
Remission	Absence of disease activity attributable to active disease, qualified by the need for ongoing stable maintenance immunosuppressive therapy. The term 'active disease' is not restricted to vasculitis only, but also includes other inflammatory features such as granulomatous inflammation in Wegener's granulomatosis or tissue eosinophilia in the Churg–Strauss syndrome
Response	A 50% reduction of disease activity score and absence of new manifestations
Relapse	Reoccurrence or new onset of disease attributable to active vasculitis
Major relapse	Reoccurrence or new onset of potentially organ- or life-threatening disease
Minor relapse	Reoccurrence or new onset of disease which is neither potentially organ-threatening nor life-threatening
Refractory disease	Unchanged or increased disease activity in acute AAV after 4 weeks of treatment with standard therapy with cyclophosphamide and corticosteroids Or Lack of response, defined as ≤50% reduction in the disease activity score after 6 weeks of treatment Or Chronic, persistent disease—defined as the presence of at least one major or three minor items on the disease activity score list after ≥12 weeks of treatment
Low activity disease state	Persistence of minor symptoms (e.g. arthralgia, myalgia) that respond to a modest increase in the corticosteroid dose and do not warrant an escalation of therapy beyond a modest dose increase of the current medication

Renal vasculitis is more common in elderly patients, with AAV, being present in 95%. Pulmonary involvement, typically with radiological infiltrates, both in Wegener's granulomatosis and microscopic polyangiitis, reflects alveolar capillaritis. Pulmonary fibrosis may precede or be detected at the same time as AAV and it is uncertain whether it represents a vasculitic complication or separate but concurrent disease process. See Chapter 18.11.5 for further discussion of Wegener's granulomatosis.

Renal vasculitis most commonly presents with the syndrome of rapidly progressive glomerulonephritis, i.e. deteriorating renal function and crescentic glomerulonephritis on kidney biopsy. It accounts for 50 to 80% of cases of this syndrome and is differentiated from other causes by circulating immune reactants and renal immunofluorescence studies (Table 21.10.2.5).

AAV with anti-GBM disease

Approximately 5% of AAV patients present with simultaneous renal vasculitis and antiglomerular basement membrane (GBM) disease. They are older, have more severe renal disease, and are more likely to have pulmonary involvement than other AAV patients. The serology demonstrates ANCA positivity, usually MPO-ANCA, and anti-GBM antibodies. Renal histology reveals an aggressive crescentic glomerulonephritis, typically involving all glomeruli with linear IgG deposition on immunofluorescence. When presenting in renal failure, such patients are more likely to recover renal function than in pure anti-GBM disease. However, after the initial presentation, unlike in anti-GBM disease, they can follow a relapsing course with persisting ANCA positivity. See Chapter 21.8.7 for further discussion of anti-GBM disease.

Henoch–Schönlein purpura

Henoch–Schönlein purpura, although most frequent in children, occurs in adults, when it often pursues a relapsing course. By definition, extrarenal features of vasculitis including purpura, arthritis, and gastrointestinal involvement are present, but differentiation from other vasculitic syndromes requires the demonstration of IgA deposition on skin or renal biopsy. The renal presentation in Henoch–Schönlein purpura overlaps with that of IgA nephropathy but is more likely to pursue a rapidly progressive course and to have extracapillary glomerular necrosis with crescents on biopsy. See Chapter 21.8.1 for further discussion of Henoch–Schönlein purpura.

Box 21.10.2.2 Clinical features that should raise suspicion of vasculitis when persistent and unexplained

Constitutional disturbance

- Polymyalgia, polyarthralgia, flitting polyarthritis
- Fatigue, weight loss, fevers, night sweats

Ear, nose, and throat

- Nasal obstruction and epistaxis
- Recurrent sinusitis
- Deafness

Eye

- Episcleritis/scleritis
- Corneal ulcer
- Retinal vein thrombosis

Lung

- Haemoptysis
- 'Maturity onset' asthma
- 'Antibiotic-resistant pneumonia'

Heart

- Pericarditis

Skin

- Purpura
- Nonhealing ulcer

Kidney

- Haematuria and proteinuria
- Impaired renal function

Nervous system

- Headache
- Peripheral neuropathy (sensory or motor)

Table 21.10.2.5 Classification of rapidly progressive glomerulonephritis according to renal immunofluorescence and circulating immune reactants

Type	Renal immunofluorescence	Compatible serology	Diagnosis
I	Linear IgG	Anti-GBM antibodies	Anti-GBM disease
II	Granular IgG/IgA/IgM	ANA/anti-dsDNA/ low C3/4	Systemic lupus erythematosus
	Granular IgG/IgA/IgM	Low C3/4	Postinfectious glomerulonephritis
	Granular IgG/IgA/IgM	Low C3/4	Mesangiocapillary glomerulonephritis
	Granular IgG/IgA/IgM	Low C3/4, cryoglobulins	Cryoglobulinaemia
	Granular IgA	None	Henoch–Schönlein purpura
III	Pauci-immune (absent or scanty deposits)	ANCA	Vasculitis

ANA, antinuclear antibodies; ANCA, antineutrophil cytoplasmic autoantibodies; dsDNA, double-stranded DNA; GBM, glomerular basement membrane.

hypertension, and regional infarction—presenting with loin pain and haematuria—is rarely seen. Virtually any organ can be involved, with presentations ranging from myocardial ischaemia to orchitis.

The association of polyarteritis nodosa with microscopic vessel involvement, such as necrotizing glomerulonephritis, has been called 'polyangiitis overlap syndrome', but is now classified as microscopic polyangiitis.

Takayasu's arteritis

A few patients with Takayasu's arteritis have disease below the diaphragm (class IV), which may involve the renal arteries causing renal artery stenosis, hypertension, reduced renal size, and renal impairment (Fig. 21.10.2.3). See Chapter 16.14.4 for further discussion of Takayasu's arteritis.

Investigation

Diagnosis depends on the triad of clinical features, serology and histology, and the exclusion of secondary causes. ANCA positivity (Fig. 21.10.2.4) confirmed by a positive PR3-ANCA or MPO-ANCA has a predictive value above 95% for the diagnosis of AAV with renal involvement in a patient with suspected nephritis. However, 5 to 10% of patients with a pauci-immune necrotizing crescentic glomerulonephritis are ANCA negative, and ANCA will be negative in other immune-complex-mediated vasculitis syndromes, such as Henoch–Schönlein purpura, or in larger vessel vasculitis. ANCA positivity by indirect immunofluorescence (i.e. C-ANCA or P-ANCA) with negative PR3-ANCA and MPO-ANCA is still compatible with a diagnosis of AAV, but other chronic inflammatory processes that can produce a C-ANCA or P-ANCA need to be considered.

Renal histology enables a more secure diagnosis to be made, although there is sometimes debate as to the diagnostic necessity of renal biopsy when the PR3-ANCA or MPO-ANCA are positive and the clinical presentation is typical. However, biopsy also

Churg–Strauss angiitis

The kidney is involved in 15% of cases of Churg–Strauss angiitis. ANCA are usually present and the renal histology and disease course are similar to that seen in AAV. See Chapter 18.11.5 for further discussion of Churg–Strauss angiitis.

Polyarteritis nodosa

Patients usually present with constitutional features of weight loss, fever, and night sweats, with specific symptoms depending on the vessels involved. Myalgia and muscle tenderness due to muscle involvement is common, as is abdominal pain due to intestinal ischaemia. Involvement of the skin can produce livedo reticularis, bullous/vesicular eruptions, and ulcers, and aneurisms can sometimes form palpable nodules when they occur in subcutaneous tissues. Infarction of peripheral nerves presents with mononeuritis multiplex. Ischaemia in the kidney frequently manifests with

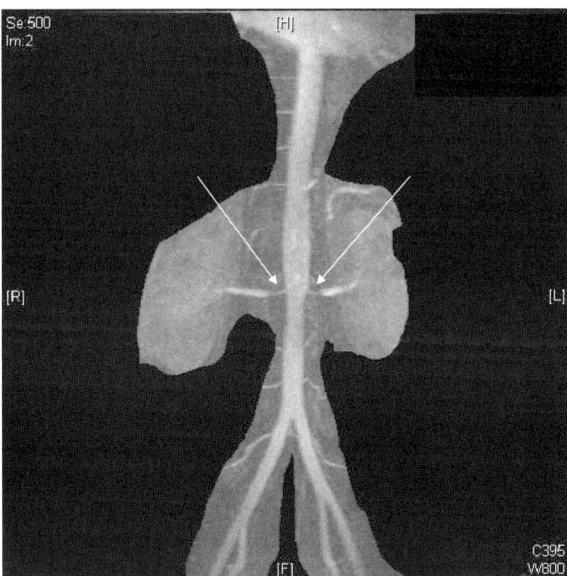

Fig. 21.10.2.3 Magnetic resonance angiogram demonstrating bilateral renal artery stenosis (arrows) in a patient with Takayasu's arteritis.

permits diagnosis of concurrent conditions, such as anti-GBM disease or IgA nephropathy, and carries prognostic significance. Biopsy is strongly recommended when PR3-ANCA or MPO-ANCA are negative.

The typical renal biopsy features in AAV are a pauci-immune necrotizing glomerulonephritis with crescent formation (Fig. 21.10.2.1). Microscopic polyangiitis is associated with more severe biopsy changes, with greater evidence of chronicity and scarring. In Wegener's granulomatosis acute tubular changes are more frequent, scarring is less apparent, and the prognosis is better. However, in an individual case, the predictive value of biopsy is not sufficiently robust to dictate therapy, and the presence of severe scarring does not exclude the possibility of a good renal outcome.

There are no agreed diagnostic criteria for primary systemic vasculitis syndromes, but consensus definitions are described in Table 21.10.2.2. Diagnosis of AAV relies on clinical presentation

supported by the results of ANCA testing and tissue biopsy. Diagnosis of other forms of primary systemic vasculitis relies on the clinical pattern supported by radiological or histological assessment.

The diagnosis of polyarteritis nodosa is usually made by demonstration of aneurisms of medium-sized muscular arteries on angiography, with studies of the hepatic circulation said to have the best diagnostic yield. Biopsy of affected tissue reveals fibrinoid necrosis of involved vessels, accompanied by a marked inflammatory response. Destruction of the internal elastic lamina and aneurisms may be seen (Fig. 21.10.2.5). Acute phase reactants are raised, but serological tests for autoimmune and vasculitic diseases are negative.

For incomplete presentations a period of observation and assessment of treatment response will increase or reduce confidence in the diagnosis. Overlaps between vasculitic syndromes occur, e.g. an ANCA-positive necrotizing glomerulonephritis in the context of giant cell arteritis.

Differential diagnosis

Secondary causes of vasculitis and diseases mimicking vasculitis need to be excluded before a diagnosis of primary systemic vasculitis can be made (Box 21.10.2.1). Chronic inflammatory disorders such as bacterial endocarditis or rheumatoid arthritis can mimic vasculitis, e.g. with constitutional symptoms and renal impairment, or induce a systemic vasculitis syndrome such as an AAV. Chronic bacterial infection may be obvious, as in cystic fibrosis or bronchiectasis, but occult endocarditis or abdominal sepsis should be considered. Tuberculosis and other nonvasculitic causes of pulmonary cavities can mimic Wegener's granulomatosis. When suspected, bronchoscopy and bronchoalveolar lavage are indicated. Lung biopsy is now rarely performed to confirm a vasculitic diagnosis but may be required if the serology is unhelpful and there is little extrapulmonary disease. Hepatitis C is the most common cause of cryoglobulinaemic vasculitis but has also been linked to other forms of vasculitis.

For those presenting with deteriorating renal function, other causes of rapidly progressive glomerulonephritis, myeloma kidney, atheroembolic renal disease, and other causes of acute renal failure

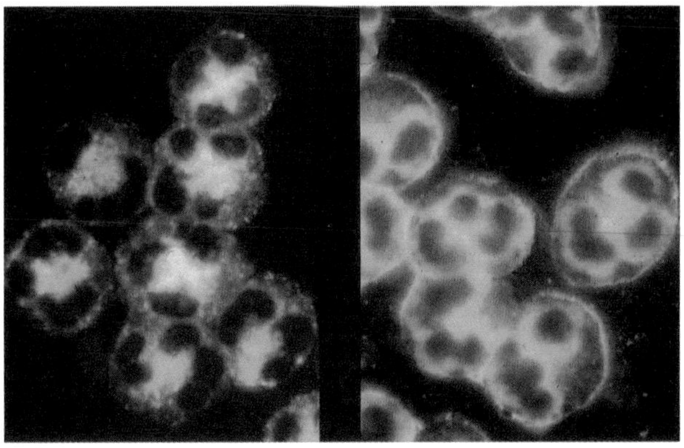

(a)   (b)

Fig. 21.10.2.4 Indirect immunofluorescence assay for ANCA. (a) Typical staining pattern of cytoplasmic ANCA that is usually due to antibodies to proteinase 3. (b) Typical staining pattern of perinuclear ANCA that is usually due to antibodies to myeloperoxidase.

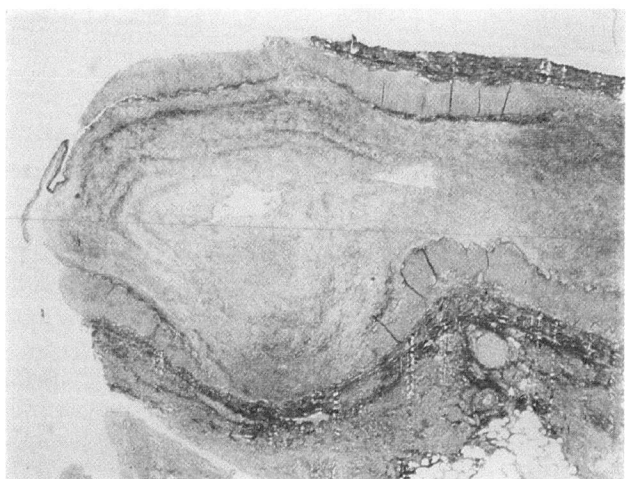

Fig. 21.10.2.5 A renal artery from a patient with polyarteritis nodosa. The elastic lamina has been destroyed and the artery has become aneurysmal.

need to be considered (Box 21.10.2.2). Radiological assessment of renal size is typically normal in vasculitis; reduced renal size points to more chronic causes of renal disease, such as hypertension or diabetes. The presence of microscopic haematuria and proteinuria is nonspecific, occurring in other forms of renal and lower urinary tract inflammation and infection. Nephrotic range proteinuria may be found during the recovery phase of AAV and in vasculitis associated with immune complexes, such as cryoglobulinaemia or Henoch–Schönlein purpura, but other causes of the nephrotic syndrome are more likely if this is the initial presentation.

Subgrouping by severity

Attempts have been made to subgroup patients with vasculitis according to the extent and severity of disease and several systems have been developed. The simplest is the concept of 'limited' Wegener's granulomatosis, when disease is restricted to the respiratory tract, in contrast to 'generalized' disease when extrarespiratory disease, especially renal, is present. The 'five-factor score' identified five factors predictive of a poor prognosis: proteinuria, impaired renal function, cardiac or gastrointestinal vasculitis, and central nervous system vasculitis.

The European Vasculitis Study Group (EUVAS) has subclassified ANCA vasculitis at presentation into three groups: 'early systemic', 'generalized', and 'severe', according to the presence and severity of renal disease (Table 21.10.2.3). In three concurrent studies the average age of each group rose with the severity of the vasculitis.

Treatment

Without therapy, renal vasculitis in the AAV will usually progress to endstage renal disease. Progression of renal disease in rarer vasculitides, such as in Henoch–Schönlein purpura, has been less well studied and the role of therapy less established. Current regimens aim to suppress manifestations of disease activity and achieve a 'remission' in order to avoid further vital organ damage, rescue renal function, and reduce constitutional disturbance. The induction phase of 3 to 6 months aims to control active features of vasculitis; therapy is then continued during the maintenance or remission phase of 2 to 4 years to consolidate disease control and prevent relapse. Treatment is then slowly withdrawn, but indefinite follow-up is required for the early detection of late relapse, and the management of irreversible damage caused by the disease and its treatment.

Induction therapy

The combination of cyclophosphamide and high-dose corticosteroids, introduced in the 1970s, remains the 'standard of care' for renal vasculitis. Cyclophosphamide is equally effective as a daily oral or pulsed intravenous preparation. The pulsed protocols expose the patient to a lower cumulative cyclophosphamide dose and permit bladder protection through rehydration and the use of mesna, and leucopenia—an important risk factor for severe infection—is more common with daily oral treatment. Cyclophosphamide is continued for 3 to 6 months, by which time vasculitis will have been controlled in 90% of patients. Improvement in renal vasculitis is mainly judged by improvement or stability of renal function, and control of extrarenal vasculitis and suppression of initially elevated C-reactive protein (CRP). Microscopic haematuria persists for many months after the onset of therapy, and

proteinuria typically increases during the recovery period, occasionally to levels sufficient to cause the nephrotic syndrome. ANCA levels are not used to guide the duration or intensity of induction therapy.

The elimination of cyclophosphamide and its active metabolites are influenced by age and renal function, hence doses must be reduced accordingly. Close monitoring of the full blood count is required for the early detection of cytopenias and appropriate dose adjustment. Prednisolone is commenced at high dose, 1 mg/kg per day, and reduced in steps to 5 to 10 mg/day by 6 months. Prophylaxis against *Pneumocystis jirovecii* pneumonia with low-dose sulfamethoxazole/trimethoprim is recommended, as is prophylaxis against fungal infections, peptic ulceration, and steroid-induced bone disease.

Additional treatment with intravenous methylprednisolone (between one and three doses of 500–1000 mg each) is widely used for renal vasculitis, and may be commenced on suspicion of the diagnosis before ANCA testing or renal histology is available. There is no strong evidence that this is beneficial.

Plasma exchange improves the chances of renal recovery in those presenting in renal failure with creatinine over 500 µmol, but it is uncertain whether it also has a role in renal vasculitis with deteriorating renal function below this level. It is also used in patients with severe nonrenal presentations, such as diffuse alveolar haemorrhage. The increasing evidence for the pathogenicity of ANCA in renal vasculitis provides a rationale for its use, but removal of coagulation factors, cytokines, or other substances may also be important. Plasma filtration or centrifugation appear equally effective, with a total of between 5 and 10 daily or alternate day exchanges most typically used. The procedure requires central vascular access, and may be complicated by haemorrhage and thrombocytopenia.

To avoid the toxicity of cyclophosphamide, weekly methotrexate has been shown to be as effective as cyclophosphamide for remission induction in 'early systemic' disease, including those with haematuria and proteinuria but without renal impairment. However, subsequent relapse rates, including renal relapses, are high after methotrexate induction.

Treatment intolerance and severe infection are the most common causes of treatment failure in the induction phase. Progressive disease is treated first with intravenous methylprednisolone and/or plasma exchange. If this fails, or there is treatment intolerance, or active disease persists beyond 6 months, then agents used for refractory vasculitis are employed (see below).

Maintenance therapy

Disease relapse occurs in 75% of those with Wegener's granulomatosis and 50% of those with microscopic polyangiitis by 5 years. The goals of maintenance therapy are to prevent disease relapse, with less risk of drug toxicity than during the induction phase. Cyclophosphamide is withdrawn and substituted by azathioprine or methotrexate, which are equally effective for remission maintenance. Azathioprine allergy or intolerance occurs in 5 to 10%, and testing for thiopurine *S*-methyltransferase activity identifies rare patients at risk of severe myelosuppression. Methotrexate is excreted by the kidneys and should be avoided in the presence of moderate or severe renal impairment. Although rare, concerns over methotrexate pneumonitis complicate its use in the presence of pulmonary vasculitis. Leflunomide and mycophenolate mofetil are alternative remission maintenance agents.

Prednisolone is either continued in conjunction with an immunosuppressive, or is withdrawn during the maintenance phase. Steroid withdrawal is probably associated with an increase in risk of relapse, but this has to be balanced against the toxicity of long-term administration.

Treatment withdrawal is the strongest predictor of relapse, with other predictors being a diagnosis of Wegener's granulomatosis, persisting ANCA positivity, a previous history of relapse, or nasal colonization with *Staphylococcus aureus* in patients with Wegener's granulomatosis. ANCA levels are not closely related to disease activity, but the persistence of ANCA at 6 months after induction therapy, or a rising ANCA level, indicate relapse is more likely. This is particularly useful when treatment is withdrawn, relapse being almost inevitable if ANCA remains positive; very prolonged low-dose immunosuppression should be considered in these cases.

Relapse of vasculitis is classified as minor or major depending on the threat to vital organ function, with the severity and consequences of relapse being dependent on how quickly the problem is detected. Relapse is usually associated with ANCA positivity and rises in erythrocyte sedimentation rate (ESR) and CRP. Infection may trigger relapse and can be difficult to distinguish from relapse. In Wegener's granulomatosis the two processes often occur together in the respiratory tract, hence if relapse is being considered, thorough microbiological assessment including studies for tuberculosis, fungi, and viral infections is required, and aggressive treatment of infection is necessary for vasculitis therapy to be effective. Minor relapses are treated by an increase in prednisolone and return of immunosuppression to full dosage if it has been reduced. Multiple minor relapses require a trial of an alternative immunosuppressive. Major relapse is treated by an increase in prednisolone and reintroduction of cyclophosphamide.

Adverse events of therapy

The main early risk of combined cyclophosphamide and prednisolone treatment is sepsis, often associated with leucopenia, which increases the septic risk more than fourfold. Cyclophosphamide dosing should aim to minimize the risk of neutropenia. Older age and uraemia greatly increase the risk of sepsis, in part due to the increased myelosuppressive effects of cyclophosphamide; impaired neutrophil function may also contribute to susceptibility to infection.

Steroid-related side-effects are very frequent and include fluid retention, weight gain, hypertension, diabetes, and steroid-induced bone disease. The treatment of elderly patients with severe renal disease is a particular challenge due to their high risk of infection and treatment intolerance.

Refractory vasculitis

Refractory vasculitis is rare during the induction phase, but more common later in the disease course when it is manifested by multiple relapses or a chronic state of persistent disease activity. The reintroduction of conventional agents including intravenous methylprednisolone, plasma exchange, and cyclophosphamide can control most acute cases of refractory disease. However, their use may be complicated by intolerance, intercurrent infection, or concern over a high cumulative exposure to cyclophosphamide. High-dose intravenous immunoglobulin reduces levels of vasculitic activity in persisting or relapsing vasculitis, reduces ANCA production, and is

a useful short-term additional agent permitting reduction in immunosuppressive or steroid dosing. This is desirable in the face of active infection, in patients at high risk of infection, such as on the intensive care unit, and in pregnancy. Blockade of TNFα with infliximab or etanercept has led to remission when used as an additional agent, but prolonged use appears ineffective and may increase the risk of infection.

B-cell depletion with rituximab, a chimeric anti-CD20 monoclonal antibody, has shown surprising efficacy in early studies in refractory vasculitis, and it appears to be safe. Immunosuppressives are withdrawn after rituximab, with retreatment at the time of ANCA rise or relapse usually being effective. Thus B-cell depletion carries the hope of improving control in vasculitis while reducing the risks associated with immune suppression. The therapeutic effect of rituximab may be delayed by 2 to 3 months, during which time increases in prednisolone or cyclophosphamide may be required. With rituximab protocols reflecting those used in non-Hodgkin's lymphoma or in rheumatoid arthritis, the average remission duration has been at least 1 year. T-cell depletion with antithymocyte globulin or alemtuzumab has also led to remissions in refractory disease, but carries a high risk of infective mortality in those over 60 years of age or in those with uraemia.

The variation in individual responses to immunosuppressive drugs suggests that if one is ineffective in maintaining remission, an alternative should be tested until satisfactory disease control is achieved. An alternative approach is to obtain remission in a refractory or relapsing patient with cyclophosphamide and then reintroduce the previous immunosuppressive. The biological agents discussed above should be considered when these strategies fail.

Endstage renal disease and transplantation

In renal-limited vasculitis, treatment with immunosuppression and prednisolone can be withdrawn once endstage renal disease is established. However, in Wegener's granulomatosis and microscopic polyangiitis continued therapy is required to control extrarenal vasculitic disease. Relapse rates of AAV are lower in patients with endstage renal disease, but relapse—especially of the respiratory tract—may still occur. Patients with vasculitis and endstage renal disease have a higher incidence of infection, which complicates therapy.

The success of renal transplantation in AAV is similar to that for other nondiabetic causes of endstage renal disease. Transplantation reduces the risk of vasculitic relapse and can proceed in the face of a persistently positive ANCA. Previous cyclophosphamide and corticosteroid exposure places patients with a history of vasculitis at increased risk of opportunistic infection after transplantation.

Management of other vasculitic syndromes involving the kidney

Henoch–Schönlein purpura

Although nephritis is not prevented by prednisolone, this is commonly used to treat active renal disease causing progressive deterioration in renal function, often in combination with an immunosuppressive (typically cyclophosphamide). Plasma exchange has the rationale of removing IgA and IgA-containing immune complexes and may be considered when deterioration in renal function is refractory, but there is no strong evidence that it is effective.

Polyarteritis nodosa

About 50% of cases of polyarteritis nodosa respond to corticosteroids alone, with cyclophosphamide most commonly added if the patient fails to respond, or from the beginning in those with more severe disease (e.g. mesenteric ischaemia, mononeuritis multiplex, and renal impairment).

Cryoglobulinaemic vasculitis

When associated with hepatitis C, therapy is directed at controlling viral replication. Prednisolone may be required for initial therapy of inflammatory manifestations such as nephritis. Hepatitis C-negative 'essential' cryoglobulinaemia is treated with glucocorticoids, with or without an immunosuppressive, and plasma exchange. Rituximab has led to remissions in refractory hepatitis C-associated and essential cryoglobulinaemia. See Chapter 21.10.4 for further discussion.

Takayasu's arteritis

Prednisolone and an immunosuppressive are used to arrest progression of vascular disease, but renal artery involvement requires specific therapy if there is evidence of functional decline in the affected kidney. The stenoses are less amenable to angioplasty and stenting than in atheromatous renovascular disease, but this option may still be effective. Renal autotransplantation appears to be a useful alternative. See Chapter 16.14.4 for further discussion.

Prognosis

Creatinine at presentation remains the strongest predictor of both patient and renal survival in renal vasculitis. Those presenting in renal failure have a particularly poor outcome, and earlier diagnosis is likely to improve outcome more than improved therapies. Mortality of AAV at 1 and 5 years is 10 and 40%, respectively; for those under 60 years of age it is 5% at 1 year, rising to 23% for those over 60, and 44% for those over 70 (Fig. 21.10.2.6). In part this is due to more advanced renal disease with more chronicity on renal biopsy in elderly patients, but intolerance of therapy and infections are significant contributors. If treatment of renal vasculitis is unsuccessful and the patient progresses to endstage renal failure, mortality is particularly high (over 50% after 1 year). Dual positive presentations of anti-GBM disease and vasculitis are associated with particularly aggressive pulmonary and renal disease and poor outcomes.

Specific predictors of endstage renal disease include a lack of response to therapy, a high level of proteinuria during the recovery phase, and on biopsy the proportion of fibrotic crescents, the presence of extraglomerular arteritis or arteriosclerosis, and the severity of tubulointerstitial scarring. In contrast, the finding on biopsy of a high proportion of normal glomeruli, the presence of glomeruli with active crescents, and demonstration of acute tubular necrosis are predictors of a good renal outcome. The overall disease activity at diagnosis, as measured by the Birmingham Vasculitis Activity Score, is predictive of the burden of irreversible damage the patient acquires and their mortality risk.

There is a gradual improvement in renal function over the first year in those presenting with renal impairment who respond to therapy. Glomerular filtration rate (GFR) may then remain stable for many years, even if recovery is to a GFR below 30 ml/min. In this setting, vasculitis relapse with renal involvement carries a

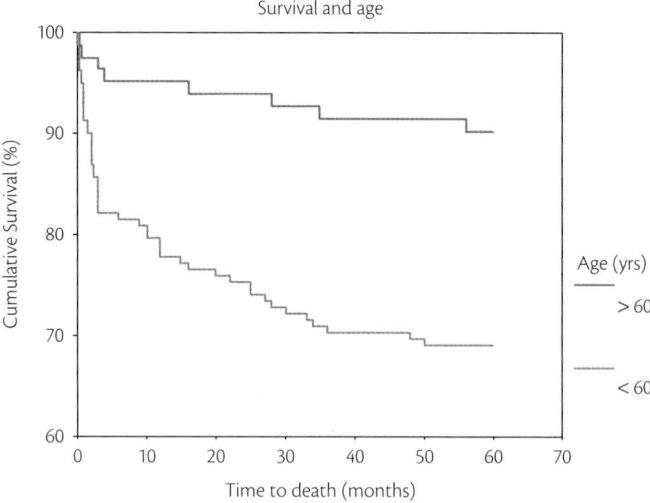

Fig. 21.10.2.6 Patient survival according age above or below 60 years for patients presenting with renal vasculitis in London between 1995 and 2000.

high risk of endstage renal disease. However, a few patients develop progressive glomerulosclerosis and lose renal function without reactivation of vasculitis; in these patients blockade of the renin–angiotensin system may improve renal outcome but requires further study.

Cardiovascular events are common during periods of active vasculitis and may be caused by the increased prothrombotic tendency. There is also an increased cardiovascular risk during follow-up, which may relate to more widespread vascular injury at the time of active vasculitis or the consequences of chronic renal failure and long-term medication. Malignancy rates at 5 years are 10 to 15%, which is an increase on those expected. A wide distribution of malignancies is seen, with bladder malignancies over-represented due to cyclophosphamide exposure, although the extent to which pulsed intravenous cyclophosphamide regimens increase the risk of bladder malignancy is not known.

Over 50% of relapses are mild, with no consequences on vital organ function. However, a protracted relapsing–remitting course, often seen in patients with ear, nose, and throat or pulmonary disease, does lead to progressive damage and a high cumulative drug burden. The risk of relapse declines with time, but follow-up should remain lifelong because late relapse can still occur with potentially devastating consequences.

The 5-year survival of untreated polyarteritis nodosa is in the range 10 to 15%, improving to around 80% with treatment, with renal failure and gastrointestinal and central nervous system involvement associated with a worse prognosis.

Quality of life and health economic aspects

The quality of life of patients with AAV is severely depressed when their disease is active, and physical activity remains reduced during follow-up when features of active vasculitis are no longer present. Respiratory function is often chronically impaired, and there are negative consequences on social and economic activity. Health utilization and treatment cost-effectiveness studies have not been performed. The development of national strategies for the unique demands of patients with vasculitis has begun in two European

Union countries. As a multisystem disease the care of patients can be disjointed, and access to appropriate expertise unavailable. The lack of pharmaceutical company interest in developing drugs for vasculitis is reflected in the slow and uncontrolled introduction of newer drugs into therapy.

Areas of uncertainty or controversy

The diagnosis of vasculitis is often delayed due to a poor understanding of many physicians as to when the possibility of a vasculitic illness should be considered, and a lack of diagnostic criteria both for vasculitis in general and for the specific vasculitic subgroups. The current classification systems are uncertain whether to regard Churg–Strauss angiitis as an AAV or as a separate entity, this heterogeneous subgroup often having overlapping features with AAV. There is also controversy as to how to classify patients with overlapping features of vasculitis syndromes, e.g. those with both muscular middle-sized arterial involvement and microscopic vasculitis. According to the Chapel Hill statement they should be regarded as microscopic polyangiitis, although features of polyarteritis nodosa are present.

Renal biopsy is recommended for all patients with potential renal vasculitis, but in the presence of ANCA positivity (both C-ANCA or P-ANCA and PR3-ANCA or MPO-ANCA) over 95% of biopsies will show renal vasculitis, hence it has been argued (as discussed previously) that biopsy is unnecessary for these patients. The prognostic value of renal biopsy for endstage renal disease may be helpful, but is not sufficiently well determined to influence treatment in a particular individual. Microscopic haematuria persists for many months after the commencement of therapy for renal vasculitis despite normalization of the inflammatory markers CRP and ESR. It is unclear how well haematuria correlates with histological activity and what the criteria for repeat biopsy should be.

Although ANCA testing is widely used for the diagnosis of vasculitis there is often confusion concerning the value of a negative result, this depending very heavily on the clinical context, and in the interpretation of marginally positive results. In part this is influenced by variable assay performance and differing referral practices. The role of ANCA in monitoring is more controversial, with the best evidence suggesting that ANCA positivity during the remission phase indicates a higher risk of subsequent relapse.

The first consensus treatment guidelines were published in 2007 and highlight areas where evidence is lacking and no clear direction can be given. The optimal route of administration of cyclophosphamide, daily oral or pulsed intravenous, is unclear. Local experience and health service issues will influence the choice. The duration of cyclophosphamide induction therapy has reduced to less than 6 months, but it is not known whether much shorter courses followed by an alternative immunosuppressive will be as effective. Similarly, corticosteroid dosing has not been formally tested, although there is a trend for doses to be reduced more rapidly. The duration of maintenance immunosuppression and corticosteroid therapy varies widely, between 6 months and over 4 years. The value and toxicity of prolonged therapy needs to be assessed. The short-term benefit of plasma exchange on renal recovery has been demonstrated, but it is not known whether this expensive intervention influences long-term mortality or likelihood of endstage renal disease; there is also controversy over its

role in other severe vasculitis presentations, such as in rapidly progressive glomerulonephritis without advanced renal failure and in lung haemorrhage with respiratory failure. Clinical trials with TNFα blockade have led to contradictory conclusions; this remains a potentially important induction agent that may permit steroid sparing, more rapid disease control, and less drug toxicity.

Most clinical trials focus on AAV and there is less evidence supporting treatment in the less common vasculitis subgroups. Henoch–Schönlein purpura in adults is a particular problem, with uncertainty as to the use of immunosuppressives, plasma exchange, and intravenous immunoglobulin.

Likely developments in the near future

It is hoped that patient identification will occur earlier in the disease course as vasculitis classification and triggers for suspicion of vasculitis become better understood and more widely known. There should be better determination of the long-term outcome of vasculitis from patient cohorts currently under study and patient registries. These will define the cardiovascular and malignancy risk of vasculitis, improve the value of prognostic markers at diagnosis and after induction therapy, and indicate the consequences of current medications.

New genetic associations and interactions of susceptibility genes will emerge from studies in large patient cohorts. The combination of genetic and gene expression studies will define the immune and inflammatory pathways involved in vasculitis and suggest further therapeutic targets. A better understanding of the influence of genetic polymorphisms on the pharmacodynamics of immunosuppressive drugs and improved biomarkers predicting future disease course will facilitate which drugs to use and how long to use them for.

Of the newer drugs under evaluation, B-cell depletion is emerging as both safe and effective for obtaining sustained disease remission and may replace current regimens with long-term immunosuppression and corticosteroids. However, there are currently no promising agents to accelerate remission induction in more severely affected patients and thereby reduce the high levels of drug toxicity seen in the first 12 weeks.

Finally, and more in hope than immediate expectation, improved organization of health care systems could facilitate earlier diagnosis and the delivery and monitoring of newer drugs, and increased pharmaceutical company involvement would accelerate the evaluation of newer drugs and lead to regulatory authorities issuing licenses and approving their use in vasculitis.

Further reading

Birck R, et al. (2003). 15-Deoxyspergualin in patients with refractory ANCA-associated systemic vasculitis: a six-month open-label trial to evaluate safety and efficacy. *J Am Soc Nephrol*, **14**, 440–7.

Boomsma MM, et al. (2000). Prediction of relapses in Wegener's granulomatosis by measurement of antineutrophil cytoplasmic antibody levels: a prospective study. *Arthritis Rheum*, **43**, 2025–33.

Booth AD, et al. (2003). Outcome of ANCA-associated renal vasculitis: a 5-year retrospective study. *Am J Kidney Dis*, **41**, 776–84.

Coppo R, Amore A, Gianoglio B (1999). Clinical features of Henoch-Schönlein purpura. Italian Group of Renal Immunopathology. *Ann Med Interne (Paris)*, **150**, 143–50.

de Groot K, Adu D, Savage CO (2001). The value of pulse cyclophosphamide in ANCA-associated vasculitis: meta-analysis and critical review. *Nephrol Dial Transplant*, **16**, 2018–27.

de Groot K, *et al.* (2005). Randomized trial of cyclophosphamide versus methotrexate for induction of remission in early systemic anti-neutrophil cytoplasmic antibody-associated vasculitis. *Arthritis Rheum*, **52**, 2461–9.

de Lind van Wijngaarden RA, *et al.* (2006). Clinical and histologic determinants of renal outcome in ANCA-associated vasculitis: a prospective analysis of 100 patients with severe renal involvement. *J Am Soc Nephrol*, **17**, 2264–74.

Fauci AS, Wolff SM, Johnson JS (1971). Effect of cyclophosphamide upon the immune response in Wegener's granulomatosis. *N Engl J Med*, **285**, 1493–6.

Ferrario F, Rastaldi MP (2005). Histopathological atlas of renal diseases: ANCA-associated vasculitis (first part). *J Nephrol*, **18**, 113–16.

Guillevin L, *et al.* (1991). Longterm followup after treatment of polyarteritis nodosa and Churg-Strauss angiitis with comparison of steroids, plasma exchange and cyclophosphamide to steroids and plasma exchange. A prospective randomized trial of 71 patients. The Cooperative Study Group for Polyarteritis Nodosa. *J Rheumatol*, **18**, 567–74.

Hamano Y, *et al.* (2006). Genetic dissection of vasculitis, myeloperoxidase-specific antineutrophil cytoplasmic autoantibody production, and related traits in spontaneous crescentic glomerulonephritis-forming/ Kinjoh mice. *J Immunol*, **176**, 3662–73.

Hauer HA, *et al.* (2002). Renal histology in ANCA-associated vasculitis: differences between diagnostic and serologic subgroups. *Kidney Int*, **61**, 80–9.

Hellmich B, *et al.* (2007). EULAR recommendations for conducting clinical studies and/or clinical trials in systemic vasculitis: focus on anti-neutrophil cytoplasm antibody-associated vasculitis. *Ann Rheum Dis*, **66**, 605–17.

Hewins P, Savage CO (2003). ANCA and neutrophil biology. *Kidney Blood Press Res*, **26**, 221–5.

Hoffman GS, *et al.* (1992). Wegener granulomatosis: an analysis of 158 patients. *Ann Intern Med*, **116**, 488–98.

Hogan SL, *et al.* (2007). Association of silica exposure with anti-neutrophil cytoplasmic autoantibody small-vessel vasculitis: a population-based, case-control study. *Clin J Am Soc Nephrol*, **2**, 290–9.

Jayne DR, Rasmussen N (1997). Treatment of antineutrophil cytoplasm autoantibody-associated systemic vasculitis: initiatives of the European Community Systemic Vasculitis Clinical Trials Study Group. *Mayo Clin Proc*, **72**, 737–47.

Jayne D, *et al.* (2003). A randomized trial of maintenance therapy for vasculitis associated with antineutrophil cytoplasmic autoantibodies. *N Engl J Med*, **349**, 36–44.

Jayne DR, *et al.* (2007). Randomized trial of plasma exchange or high-dosage methylprednisolone as adjunctive therapy for severe renal vasculitis. *J Am Soc Nephrol*, **18**, 2180–8.

Jennette JC, *et al.* (1994). Nomenclature of systemic vasculitides. Proposal of an international consensus conference. *Arthritis Rheum*, **37**, 187–92.

Keogh KA, *et al.* (2006). Rituximab for refractory Wegener's granulomatosis: report of a prospective, open-label pilot trial. *Am J Respir Crit Care Med*, **173**, 180–7.

Lane SE, Watts R, Scott DG (2005). Epidemiology of systemic vasculitis. *Curr Rheumatol Rep*, **7**, 270–5.

Lapraik C, *et al.* (2007). BSR and BHPR guidelines for the management of adults with ANCA associated vasculitis. *Rheumatology*, **46**, 1615–16.

Levy JB, *et al.* (2004). Clinical features and outcome of patients with both ANCA and anti-GBM antibodies. *Kidney Int*, **66**, 1535–40.

Metzler C, *et al.* (2007). Elevated relapse rate under oral methotrexate versus leflunomide for maintenance of remission in Wegener's granulomatosis. *Rheumatology (Oxford)*, **46**, 1087–91.

Sanders JS, *et al.* (2006). Prediction of relapses in PR3-ANCA-associated vasculitis by assessing responses of ANCA titres to treatment. *Rheumatology (Oxford)*, **45**, 724–9.

Savige J, *et al.* (1999). International consensus statement on testing and reporting of antineutrophil cytoplasmic antibodies (ANCA). *Am J Clin Pathol*, **111**, 507–13.

Schmitt WH, van der Woude FJ (2003). Organ transplantation in the vasculitides. *Curr Opin Rheumatol*, **15**, 22–8.

Sinico RA, *et al.* (2006). Renal involvement in Churg-Strauss syndrome. *Am J Kidney Dis*, **47**, 770–9.

Specks U (2001). Diffuse alveolar hemorrhage syndromes. *Curr Opin Rheumatol*, **13**, 12–17.

Stegeman CA, *et al.* (1994). Association of chronic nasal carriage of *Staphylococcus aureus* and higher relapse rates in Wegener granulomatosis. *Ann Intern Med*, **120**, 12–17.

van der Woude FJ, *et al.* (1985). Autoantibodies against neutrophils and monocytes: tool for diagnosis and marker of disease activity in Wegener's granulomatosis. *Lancet*, **1**, 425–9.

Walton EW (1958). Giant-cell granuloma of the respiratory tract (Wegener's granulomatosis). *BMJ*, **2**, 265–70.

Wegener F (1936). Uber generaliste, septische efaberkrankungen. *Verh Dtsch Ges Pathol*, **29**, 202–10.

Wegener's Etanercept Study Group (WGET). (2005). Etanercept plus standard therapy for Wegener's granulomatosis. *N Engl J Med*, **352**, 351–61.

Weyand CM, Goronzy JJ (2003). Giant-cell arteritis and polymyalgia rheumatica. *Ann Intern Med*, **139**, 505–15.

Xiao H, *et al.* (2002). Antineutrophil cytoplasmic autoantibodies specific for myeloperoxidase cause glomerulonephritis and vasculitis in mice. *J Clin Invest*, **110**, 955–63.

21.10.3 **The kidney in rheumatological disorders**

Wai Y. Tse and Dwomoa Adu

Essentials

Systemic lupus erythematosus (SLE)

Epidemiology and clinical features of renal disease—10 to 20% of patients with SLE have evidence of renal involvement at presentation, with this subsequently developing in about 40 to 50% of cases, typically during the first 5 years after diagnosis. Presentation is with proteinuria (causing nephrotic syndrome in c.50% of cases), microscopic haematuria, hypertension or rapidly deteriorating renal function.

Diagnosis and classification of renal lupus—the diagnosis of SLE is made on the basis of clinical features in combination with appropriate serological tests for autoantibodies (see Chapter 19.11.2), but precise renal diagnosis depends upon renal biopsy, which can reveal a wide range of appearances that are of prognostic significance. Six classes of lupus nephritis are described: (I) minimal mesangial; (II) mesangial proliferative; (III) focal; (IV) diffuse; (V) membranous; (VI) advanced sclerosing.

Class I and II lupus nephritis—typically present with proteinuria and microscopic haematuria, commonly with normal renal function and a low rate of progressive renal failure; often treated with prednisolone.

Class V lupus nephritis—presents with proteinuria, with nephrotic syndrome in 50%; intermediate prognosis; treated with prednisolone with or without other immunosuppressants (mycophenolate mofetil, ciclosporin, azathioprine).

Class III and IV lupus nephritis—present with active urinary sediment (proteinuria, haematuria, red cell casts) and high risk of progressive renal failure; remission induced by treatment with pulsed intravenous cyclophosphamide or oral mycophenolate mofetil and maintained with azathioprine or mycophenolate mofetil; toxicity of current drug regimens along with tendency of disease to relapse responsible for continuing search for better treatments; 90 to 95% 10-year patient survival, but 5 to 15% with endstage renal failure.

Systemic sclerosis

Scleroderma renal crisis develops in 8 to 19% of patients with systemic sclerosis and characterized by the abrupt onset of severe hypertension, usually with retinopathy, together with the rapid deterioration of renal function and heart failure. Renal impairment is usually accompanied by a microangiopathic haemolytic anaemia, with thrombocytopenia and fragmented red blood cells. On renal biopsy smaller arcuate and interlobular arteries are predominantly involved, showing intimal hyperplasia with concentric mucoid intimal degeneration, and there is fibrinoid necrosis of afferent arterioles and glomeruli, also glomerular thrombosis. Hypertension should be treated with an angiotensin converting enzyme inhibitor, use of which has improved survival from less than 10% to 70% at 5 years.

Rheumatoid arthritis

Rheumatoid arthritis can affect the kidneys in many ways, most commonly by causing amyloid A amyloidosis. This presents with proteinuria, often severe enough to cause nephrotic syndrome, with 50% progressing to end stage renal failure after 5 years (90% at 10 years). Renal vasculitis, mesangiocapillary glomerulonephritis, and mesangial IgA proliferative glomerulonephritis are also described.

Patients with rheumatoid arthritis are at high risk of drug nephrotoxicity, including (1) nonsteroidal anti-inflammatory drugs—can cause reversible haemodynamically mediated renal impairment, acute tubular necrosis, and acute interstitial nephritis with or without a nephrotic syndrome; and (2) gold and penicillamine (now rarely used)—can cause proteinuria, sometimes with nephrotic syndrome.

Primary Sjögren's syndrome

Renal involvement is most commonly mild and often subclinical, with asymptomatic proteinuria and haematuria. Some patients present with distal renal tubular acidosis, impairment of urinary concentration, hypokalaemia, or (rarely) with Fanconi's syndrome, in which cases renal biopsy reveals tubulointerstitial nephritis with interstitial lymphocytic infiltrates.

Lupus nephritis

Systemic lupus erythematosus (SLE) is a multisystem autoimmune disease that is characterized by the presence of antinuclear antibodies (ANA) (see Chapter 19.11.2). The overall survival of patients with SLE and nephritis has improved considerably in recent years, from less than 50% survival at 5 years in the 1960s to over 80% survival at 20 years in the 1990s. This improved survival is due to a combination of factors, including the wider use of corticosteroids and immunosuppressants, and the availability of more effective antihypertensive drugs, antibiotics, renal dialysis, and transplantation. Early deaths from extrarenal lupus and infection are now uncommon, but instead renal failure and cardiovascular disease have emerged as important determinants of morbidity and mortality.

Pathogenesis

The pathogenesis of SLE in general, and lupus nephritis in particular, is complex and multifactorial. Immunological dysregulation leads to the production of autoantibodies to nuclear (in particular double-stranded DNA) and other cellular antigens. Genetic factors seem to play a role in the pathogenesis, with HLA-DR2, HLA-DR3, C4A null alleles, and FcγIIa alleles all associated with the development of lupus. Several clinical observations further support the genetic basis of SLE, including the increased incidence of lupus in families of individuals with the disease, racial differences in the incidence and severity of lupus, and data showing a high concordance among identical twins for the disease. For further discussion see Chapter 19.11.2.

The renal lesions of lupus nephritis show glomerular and less often tubular deposits of immunoglobulins and complement in a granular pattern indicating immune aggregation. It now seems likely that this is due to *in situ* assembly of antigen–antibody complexes rather than the deposition of immune complexes from the circulation.

Clinical presentation

Renal disease may rarely be the presenting feature of SLE. At presentation 10 to 20% of patients with the condition have evidence of renal involvement, with this developing in about 40 to 50% of patients, typically during the first 5 years after diagnosis. While renal disease is a major complication of SLE, it is always important to recognize that lupus is a systemic disease and that nephritis typically occurs in patients with extrarenal symptoms such as a rash, arthralgia, Raynaud's phenomenon, and pleuropericarditis. Other major organ systems may be involved, including the central nervous system, heart, and lungs.

Proteinuria is a common finding, and in 50 to 60% of patients is heavy enough to lead to a nephrotic syndrome. Microscopic haematuria accompanies the proteinuria in about 80% of patients. Hypertension is found at presentation in 20 to 50% of patients. Approximately 20 to 30% present with rapidly deteriorating renal function that may occasionally be severe enough to lead to acute renal failure, and in such patients a diffuse crescentic nephritis, often with intracapillary glomerular thrombi, is frequently seen.

Diagnosis

Immunology

Patients with lupus almost invariably express antibodies to components of the cell nucleus (ANA), with a fluorescent antinuclear test being positive in greater than 95% of cases. A positive fluorescent ANA test is useful because of its sensitivity, although it lacks specificity and a positive fluorescent ANA test can be found in other connective tissue diseases. More specific but less sensitive findings include anti-double-stranded DNA (anti-dsDNA) and anti-Sm autoantibodies (for discussion of immunological tests for SLE see Chapters 19.3 and 19.11.2).

In general, anti-dsDNA antibody levels reflect disease activity, particularly if accompanied by falling complement levels. Reduced serum complement concentrations are useful both in diagnosis and in assessing disease activity. Many patients with SLE have activation of the classical pathway of complement cascade with consumption of C1q, C4, and C3. Patients with lupus nephritis have antibodies to phospholipids in approximately 30% of cases, resulting in prolongation of the partial thromboplastin time.

Pathology

A renal biopsy is justified when there is evidence of glomerular disease with a urinary sediment indicative of active nephritis—proteinuria (>200 mg/24 h or protein/creatinine ratio >100 mg/mmol), haematuria (>10 dysmorphic red blood cells per high power field), and/or casts of red and white blood cells—and/or renal insufficiency. Histology allows an assessment of disease activity and provides a basis for therapeutic options, as well as providing prognostic information.

A distinctive feature of lupus nephritis on light microscopy is the variability of the glomerular changes seen in a single biopsy, and sometimes within the same glomerulus. This makes classification of renal histology difficult, but that most widely used is the modified World Health Organization (WHO) classification, revised in 2003 by the International Society of Nephrology and the Renal Pathology Society (ISN-RPS) (Table 21.10.3.1). This revised classification preserves the simplicity of the original WHO classification, incorporates selective refinements concerning activity and chronicity, and introduces qualitative differences between class III and IV lesions. Segmental glomerular thrombosis, necrosis, and extracapillary proliferation (crescents) are frequently found in association with the proliferative type lesions (WHO/ISN-RPS classes III and IV). On immunofluorescent microscopy, there is often florid deposition of immunoglobulins IgG, IgA, and IgM, as well as complement proteins C3, C4, and C1q.

Patients with minimal changes or mesangial glomerulonephritis (WHO/ISN-RPS class I and II lesions) (Fig. 21.10.3.1) usually have an inherently low rate of progressive renal failure. Patients with membranous nephropathy (WHO/ISN-RPS class V) have an intermediate prognosis for renal function. In contrast, patients with focal or diffuse proliferative glomerulonephritis (WHO/ISN-RPS classes III and IV) (Fig. 21.10.3.2) have a high risk of progressive renal failure.

Table 21.10.3.1 The 1995 World Health Organization classification of lupus nephritis and abbreviated International Society of Nephrology and Renal Pathology Society (ISN-RPS) classification of lupus nephritis (2003)

Class	WHO	ISN-RPS
I	Normal glomeruli, with or without immune deposits	Minimal mesangial lupus nephritis, with immune deposits
II	Pure mesangial changes	Mesangial proliferative lupus nephritis (allowed rare small capillary wall deposits)
III	Focal segmental glomerulonephritis	Focal lupus nephritis, meaning <50% of all glomeruli involved[a]
IV	Diffuse glomerulonephritis	Diffuse lupus nephritis, meaning ≥50% of all glomeruli involved (IV-S if >50% of glomeruli have segmental lesions; IV-G when >50% of glomeruli have global lesions)[a]
V	Diffuse membranous	Membranous lupus nephritis—may be associated with class II, III, or IV
VI	Advanced sclerosing glomerulonephritis	Advanced sclerosing lupus nephritis, meaning 90% of glomeruli are globally sclerosed

[a] ISN-RPS class III and IV may be accompanied by active (a) or chronic (c) lesions.

General aspects of treatment

As with other proteinuric renal diseases, we recommend angiotensin-converting enzyme (ACE) inhibitors or angiotensin II receptor blockers in patients with lupus nephritis. Hyperlipidaemia should be treated with statins in view of the increased risk of vascular disease in patients with lupus. We use bone protection in the form of calcium and vitamin D supplements in patients on long-term steroids, but bisphosphonates are contraindicated in women of childbearing age and we avoid these drugs in our female patients with lupus. A key feature of the care of patients with lupus nephritis is close monitoring of the white cell count and renal function,

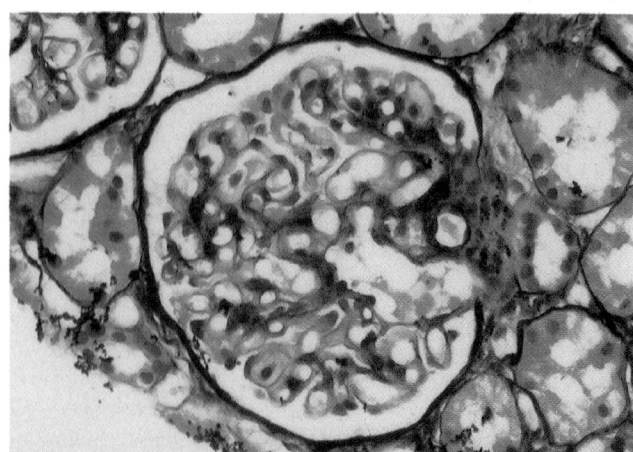

Fig. 21.10.3.1 Lupus nephritis. The glomerulus has mild mesangial increase (WHO class II). Periodic acid–methenamine silver staining, magnification ×50. (Courtesy of Professor A J Howie.)

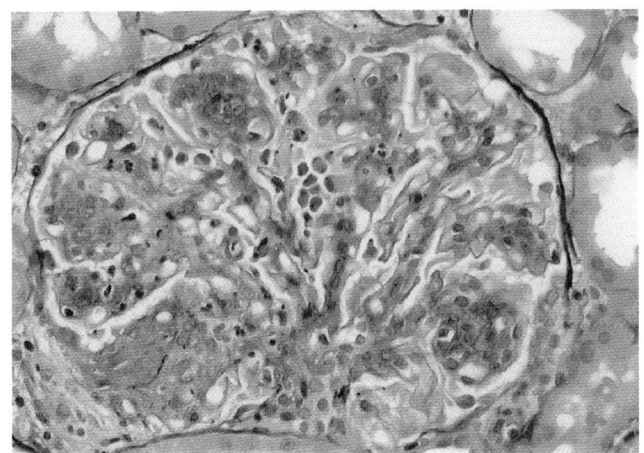

Fig. 21.10.3.2 Lupus nephritis. The glomerulus has marked mesangial increase with wire loops, a few doubled basement membranes, and segmental lesions (WHO class IV). Periodic acid–methenamine silver staining, magnification ×40. By courtesy of Professor A J Howie.

and detailed surveillance and management of infection, extrarenal lupus, and hypertension.

Immunosuppressive treatments for particular classes of lupus nephritis

There are several considerations in the approach to the treatment of patients with lupus nephritis: the histological severity of the renal lesion; the severity of the clinical presentation; and the choice of therapy for inducing remission of acute disease and for maintaining remission and treating relapses. The heterogeneity of the clinical course of lupus nephritis and the relatively few randomized controlled trials means that decision making is difficult, and there are still substantial disagreements regarding the optimum treatment. Steroids and or immunosuppressants are used, and the major toxicities of these drugs need to be offset against any benefit.

Mesangial proliferative glomerulonephritis (WHO class II)

Most such patients present with proteinuria and microscopic haematuria, often with little in the way of renal impairment. There are no controlled trials to guide treatment. We treat such patients with corticosteroids in the hope that this will prevent progression to a more severe glomerulonephritis, but this is not certain.

Membranous nephropathy (WHO class V)

In patients with lupus nephritis the frequency of membranous nephropathy is approximately 12% when the definition of the renal histology is confined to pure membranous nephropathy, with or without mild mesangial hypercellularity, expansion, and scattered deposits (WHO classes Va and Vb; ISN-RPS class V). With the new ISN-RPS classification, biopsies with focal segmental proliferative or diffuse proliferative glomerulonephritis in addition to membranous changes are now classified as class V plus class III, or class V plus class IV. This causes some difficulties in interpreting earlier studies where these appearances were classified as Vc and Vd.

The clinical presentation of lupus membranous nephropathy is with proteinuria, and in about 50% of cases a nephrotic syndrome. Patients with pure membranous nephropathy have a low rate of progressive renal failure. There are no controlled trials of treatment and thus there is no consensus. In some studies these patients have been treated with prednisolone, with a smaller proportion

also receiving pulses of methylprednisolone and oral cyclophosphamide or azathioprine. With these approaches to treatment the 10-year survival free of death and renal failure in WHO classes Va and Vb is 72 to 92%. Most nephrologists treat patients with pure lupus membranous nephropathy—with or without minor mesangial proliferation—with prednisolone, and consider adding in azathioprine, ciclosporin, or mycophenolate mofetil as a corticosteroid-sparing agent.

Focal and diffuse lupus proliferative glomerulonephritis (WHO classes III and IV; ISN-RPS classes III and IV)

Pulse cyclophosphamide—National Institutes of Health (NIH) regimen

A series of clinical trials from the NIH provided evidence of the effectiveness of intermittent intravenous cyclophosphamide together with oral prednisolone in preserving renal function in patients with severe lupus nephritis. This regimen is preferable to continuous oral cyclophosphamide as it leads to less bladder toxicity, although the frequency of gonadal toxicity is unaffected. It is not yet known whether pulse cyclophosphamide is less carcinogenic than continuous oral therapy, although this is unlikely. From the NIH data, monthly pulse cyclophosphamide ($0.5–0.75\,g/m^2$), adjusted for the glomerular filtration rate and leucocyte count at 10 to 14 days, is given monthly for the first 6 months and then quarterly for 18 to 24 months. The longer course of cyclophosphamide is associated with fewer relapses than a shorter 6-month course, but at the expense of greater gonadal toxicity. To reduce the bladder toxicity of intravenous cyclophosphamide patients should be hydrated either with oral or intravenous fluid and mesna given concomitantly.

Prednisolone is given in conjunction with the cyclophosphamide at an initial dose of 0.5 to 1 mg/kg per day for 6 to 8 weeks, with gradual tapering, preferably to an alternate day regimen to minimize toxicity.

Pulse cyclophosphamide—Euro-Lupus regimen

A recent study showed that a 12-week course of intravenous cyclophosphamide, 500 mg every 2 weeks, given with oral prednisolone and followed by azathioprine, was as effective as an abbreviated NIH regimen (6 monthly pulses of cyclophosphamide of $0.5\,g/m^2$ with oral steroids, followed by two quarterly pulses) in terms of remission induction and avoidance of endstage renal failure after a median follow up of 72 months. The Euro-Lupus regimen is now accepted as a reasonable alternative to the prolonged 2 years NIH high dose cyclophosphamide for the treatment of proliferative lupus nephritis.

Azathioprine

Azathioprine is a safe drug, and many have argued that it was safer than and probably as effective as cyclophosphamide in the management of lupus nephritis. A recent randomized controlled trial compared methylprednisolone, prednisolone, and azathioprine with prednisolone and intravenous cyclophosphamide in patients with mostly proliferative lupus nephritis. After a mean follow-up of 5.7 years, azathioprine was less effective than cyclophosphamide in reducing the risk of nonsustained doubling of serum creatinine and in reducing relapses.

Mycophenolate mofetil

The clinical benefit of mycophenolate mofetil was first confirmed in several small, uncontrolled studies, and then by larger randomized controlled trials. One study reported that mycophenolate mofetil and prednisolone was as effective as prednisolone and oral cyclophosphamide followed by azathioprine in patients with lupus nephritis. There was no significant difference in the rates of doubling of serum creatinine, endstage renal failure, and relapses. However, the risk of amenorrhoea was significantly lower with mycophenolate mofetil than with cyclophosphamide/azathioprine. A further study randomized 140 patients with lupus nephritis to treatment with 3 g/day mycophenolate mofetil and prednisolone or to intravenous cyclophosphamide 0.5 to 1.0 g/m^2 and oral prednisolone in a 24-week study. Complete remission (defined as a return to within 10% of normal values of serum creatinine, proteinuria, and urinary sediment) was achieved in 16 of 71 patients treated with mycophenolate mofetil (22.5%) and in 4 of 69 patients treated with cyclophosphamide (5.8%) ($P = 0.005$). On follow-up there was no difference in the rates of renal relapse, endstage renal failure, or of deaths. Both of these studies excluded patients with severe renal failure.

Another study, the Aspreva Lupus Management Study (ALMS), included 370 patients with either class III, IV or V nephritis, who were randomized to either mycophenolate 3g/day or intravenous cyclophosphamide 0.5-1g/month for 6 months. The trial was powered for superiority of mycophenolate over intravenous cyclophosphamide. The results showed no difference in renal response between groups, serious adverse events, or infections. The lack of a difference in adverse event rates with mycophenolate may be attributed to the higher target mycophenolate dose of 3g/day. Also there were more patients with severe renal impairment (<30ml/min/1.73m^2) in the mycophenolate group (20 patients) compared with the cyclophosphamide group (12 patients). Whilst superiority of mycophenolate was not shown, a subset analysis revealed a difference in response when ethnicity was factored in. Mycophenolate was significantly superior to intravenous cyclophosphamide in non-Caucasians, non-Asian (i.e. blacks and mixed race) patients, with a 60.4% response rate in the mycophenolate group compared with 38.5% in the intravenous cyclophosphamide group.

One can conclude from these studies that mycophenolate mofetil is probably as effective as and less toxic than cyclophosphamide in patients with new onset mild to moderate lupus nephritis. Further adequately powered randomized controlled studies are underway to confirm the role of mycophenolate mofetil in the management of lupus nephritis.

Remission maintenance—sequential regimen

A recent study assessed the role of mycophenolate mofetil or azathioprine or quarterly intravenous cyclophosphamide as maintenance therapy in patients with lupus nephritis (mainly classes III and IV), all of whom had received induction with intravenous cyclophosphamide given once a month for 6 months. Patient survival was higher in patients treated with azathioprine than in those on intravenous cyclophosphamide ($P = 0.02$). Although there were no significant differences in progression to renal failure, the event-free survival rates for the composite endpoints of death and chronic renal failure were higher in the mycophenolate mofetil and azathioprine groups than the cyclophosphamide group ($P = 0.05$ and $P = 0.009$, respectively). The cumulative probability of remaining relapse free was higher in the mycophenolate mofetil compared to the cyclophosphamide group after a median treatment duration of 29 and 25 months, respectively ($P = 0.02$). Hospitalization, amenorrhoea, and infections were lower in the mycophenolate mofetil or azathioprine groups, compared to cyclophosphamide.

Table 21.10.3.2 Treatment of lupus nephritis

Renal histology	Remission induction	Remission maintenance
Mesangial proliferative lupus nephritis (ISN-RPS class II)	Prednisolone[a]	Not known
Focal and diffuse lupus nephritis (ISN-RPS class III or IV)	NIH: intravenous cyclophosphamide every month for 6 months Or Euro-Lupus: intravenous cyclophosphamide every 2 weeks for six doses Or Mycophenolate mofetil 3 g/day for 6 months	Azathioprine or mycophenolate mofetil
Membranous nephropathy (ISN-RPS class V)	Prednisolone With or without Mycophenolate mofetil *or* ciclosporin *or* azathioprine[a]	Not known

[a] Not evidence based.

Treatment of proliferative lupus nephritis—conclusions

On the basis of the randomized controlled data, we feel that the choices for the initial treatment for severe lupus nephritis are three-fold, all of which require a reducing dose of prednisolone. First, the NIH protocol of monthly pulses of cyclophosphamide for 6 months followed by azathioprine or mycophenolate mofetil; second, the Euro-Lupus regimen of six 2-weekly pulses of cyclophosphamide, followed by azathioprine; and third, prednisolone and mycophenolate mofetil (Table 21.10.3.2).

Meta-analysis of treatment of lupus nephritis

In a recent meta-analysis of randomized controlled studies, cyclophosphamide and prednisolone reduced the risk of doubling of the serum creatinine (RR 0.59; 95% CI 0.4–0.88) when compared with prednisolone alone, while azathioprine did not (RR 0.98; 95% CI 0.36–2.68). Neither drug reduced the risk of developing endstage renal failure, although our unpublished meta-analysis shows that cyclophosphamide does so. However, azathioprine reduced the risk of death (RR 0.60; 95% CI 0.36–0.99), while cyclophosphamide did not (RR 0.95; 95% CI 0.53–1.82).

Lupus affects predominantly women of childbearing age, hence the documented gonadotoxicity of cyclophosphamide (RR 2.18; 95% CI 1.10–4.34) makes it an inherently unattractive agent for therapy and one that could only be justified by its effectiveness in reducing the risk of reducing renal failure.

Toxicities of 'standard' immunosuppressive treatments

Cyclophosphamide

Intravenous cyclophosphamide often causes nausea and vomiting, which can usually be controlled by giving serotonin antagonists such as ondansetron together with dexamethasone.

The most common toxic effect is depression of normal haematopoiesis, which is dose dependent and reversible on discontinuing therapy. A further major side-effect is an increased risk of infections, worsened by the concomitant use of corticosteroids. In particular, an increased incidence of herpes zoster is seen with cyclophosphamide.

Cyclophosphamide is metabolized to phosphoramide mustard and acrolein that are excreted by the kidneys. Acrolein can lead to a haemorrhagic cystitis, which is particularly common with oral cyclophosphamide. The use of intravenous cyclophosphamide with vigorous hydration and concomitant administration of sodium 2-mercaptoethane sulphonate (mesna) has essentially eliminated bladder complications. Prolonged oral cyclophosphamide is associated with an increased risk of malignancy and it is likely that intravenous cyclophosphamide also carries this risk.

Cyclophosphamide causes dose- and age-related gonadal toxicity, with oligospermia in men and premature ovarian failure in women. Few data on gonadal toxicity in men with lupus are available. In one study of six men treated with oral cyclophosphamide at a daily dose of 50 to 100 mg, germinal aplasia occurred after a cumulative dose of 9 to 18 g. All studies show that the risk of ovarian toxicity rises substantially with age and is correlated with the duration of treatment and the cumulative dose of cyclophosphamide. In patients aged less than 25 years, ovarian failure did not occur after 6 months of monthly intravenous cyclophosphamide, while a further 24 months of quarterly cyclophosphamide increased the risk to 17%. Comparable figures for women aged over 31 years were 25% and 100%, respectively. In contrast, one out of 20 patients (5%) treated with azathioprine developed ovarian failure.

Since lupus nephritis chiefly afflicts women of reproductive age, one must balance the risk of premature ovarian failure, which may be permanent, with the benefits of treatment. There is limited evidence that the administration of gonadotropin-releasing hormone agonist analogues (GnRHa), e.g. depot leuprolide acetate injected monthly to women during cyclophosphamide pulse treatment, can preserve fertility and protect ovarian function. In one study premature ovarian failure occurred in one of 20 women with SLE treated with leuprolide acetate as compared with six of 20 matched historical controls ($P<0.05$). A possible risk with this treatment is the development of a disease flare from hormonal stimulation. These observations need to be confirmed by randomized controlled trials. Cyclophosphamide, unlike azathioprine, is a potent teratogen and must not be used in pregnancy.

Azathioprine

Some patients are intolerant of azathioprine and develop nausea, vomiting, and diarrhoea. It also causes marrow suppression, which can be severe in individuals who have a deficiency of thiopurine S-methyltransferase. Other toxicities include an increased risk of infection and the development of malignancies with prolonged usage.

Mycophenolate mofetil

Mycophenolate mofetil is teratogenic in animal studies and is therefore contraindicated during pregnancy. In general, mycophenolate mofetil is well tolerated, and most of the adverse events responded to a reduction in dose. Gastrointestinal intolerance, particularly nausea and mild to moderate diarrhoea, occurred in up to 10 to 40% of patients. There is an increased risk of infections, which can be associated with leucopenia and lymphopenia.

Other therapeutic options

Plasma exchange

Several studies have examined the role of plasmapheresis in the treatment of patients with lupus nephritis. It was well tolerated, with few adverse effects, but the impact on renal function was disappointing, with controlled trials in patients with all types of proliferative or membranous glomerulonephritis showing no benefit over treatment with prednisolone and immunosuppressants alone.

Because removal of autoantibodies leads to a compensatory enhanced production of autoantibodies by pathogenic B-cell clones, the concept of synchronizing plasmapheresis with subsequent pulse cyclophosphamide to target proliferating B-cell clones was introduced. Initial studies showed good remission rates in patients with lupus nephritis, but the toxicity was high and hence this approach is not recommended. We currently use plasmapheresis only in patients with a severe diffuse proliferative glomerulonephritis and pulmonary haemorrhage whose disease has not responded to prednisolone and cyclophosphamide.

Intravenous immunoglobulin

Uncontrolled studies have shown a temporary benefit from the infusion of high doses of intravenous immunoglobulin in patients with SLE. However, there are limited data on the use of this treatment for lupus nephritis and it cannot be recommended.

Ciclosporin

Several studies have examined the effectiveness of ciclosporin in the treatment of lupus nephritis. None of these were controlled and it is difficult to discern whether it was of any benefit, and the nephrotoxicity of ciclosporin is a significant concern. There is some attraction in using ciclosporin for patients with a membranous nephropathy because of its efficacy in idiopathic membranous nephropathy.

Methotrexate

Methotrexate may be useful as a steroid-sparing agent in lupus with arthritis and serositis, and may have potential benefits in mild nephritis. However, methotrexate is excreted by the kidneys and cannot be used safely in patients with renal impairment.

Inhibition of costimulation

CD40 binding to CD40 ligand is one of the most important costimulatory signals on B cells, inducing activation and proliferation. The first open-label study of an agent that inhibited this interaction focused on 30 patients with lupus nephritis and showed improvement in serology, but it was halted because of unexpected thromboembolic events. A second double-blind placebo controlled trial of 85 patients with mild to moderate SLE failed to show clinical efficacy over placebo.

Other costimulatory targets in SLE include cytotoxic T-lymphocyte associated antigen 4 (CTLA4) receptors and their T-cell ligands, B7–1 and B7–2. The T-cell antigen CTLA-4 linked to murine IgGg2a (CTLA-4Ig) has been shown to block autoantibody production and prolong lifespan in NZB/NZW F_1 mice. However, the immunosuppressive properties of these classes of drugs have not been thoroughly tested in humans, and further information is required before any recommendations can be made regarding their efficacy in lupus nephritis.

B-lymphocyte depletion

Rituximab is a chimeric monoclonal antibody against the CD20 antigen that is found on pre-B lymphocytes and on mature B lymphocytes, but not on plasma cells. Rituximab leads to depletion of B lymphocytes and was originally developed to treat B-cell lymphomas. Several open label and case studies suggest that B-cell depletion with rituximab can be effective in treating SLE and lupus nephritis that is refractory to other agents. However, some patients developed elevated human antichimeric antibodies, and a recent report of two cases of JC polyoma virus induced progressive multifocal leucoencephalopathy in patients with SLE treated with rituximab suggests that caution should be used with this agent. Recently the uses of a humanized anti-CD20 antibody and a humanized anti-CD22 antibody have been explored in the treatment of SLE. Careful randomized controlled studies are required to establish the role of these B-lymphocyte-depleting agents in the management of lupus nephritis.

Oral tolerance therapy

Oral tolerance therapy may have a role in the treatment of SLE, if the offending antigens can be identified. A phase III trial of 317 randomized patients was recently completed using the B-cell tolerogen LJP394. Preliminary results indicate a sustained reduction in anti-dsDNA antibodies and improvement in health-related quality of life; additional studies are ongoing.

Immune ablation and stem cell transplantation

The role of autologous stem cell transplant using high-dose cyclophosphamide for SLE has not yet been determined and the treatment cannot be recommended. Procedure-related mortality varies between 5 and 12%.

Other modalities

Other potential treatments for lupus nephritis include neutralizing antibodies to anti-C5 complement, anti-B cell activation factor (BAFF), a chemokine receptor CCR1 antagonist, and human recombinant DNase. These are still in the preliminary stages of development.

Antiphospholipid antibody nephropathy in SLE

Antiphospholipid antibodies are associated with a syndrome (antiphospholipid syndrome) that includes arterial and venous thromboses and repeated miscarriages. These antibodies have reactivity against cardiolipin and the lupus anticoagulant. The antiphospholipid syndrome may be primary or associated with SLE, with antiphospholipid antibodies being found in 15 to 30% of patients with SLE. The renal manifestations include a thrombotic microangiopathy of glomerular capillaries and preglomerular arterioles, and also chronic vascular lesions that are superimposed on those of lupus nephritis and associated with impaired renal function, hypertension, and interstitial fibrosis. It is important to identify antiphospholipid antibody nephropathy as a cause of renal impairment in patients with lupus nephritis. Management is with good blood pressure control and, if there is evidence of extrarenal thrombosis, with anticoagulants.

Prognostic factors in lupus nephritis

The overall survival of patients with SLE and a proliferative glomerulonephritis has improved considerably in recent years. Nevertheless, 5 to 10% of patients will have died after 10 years of treatment, and a further 5 to 15% will have developed endstage renal failure. For reasons that are not clear, prognosis is much poorer in African Americans and Hispanic people than in American or European white peoples, and this needs to be acknowledged when considering the results of randomized controlled studies.

Patients with proliferative glomerulonephritis (WHO/ISN-RPS classes III and IV) tend to have a worse outcome for renal function than those with milder lesions, although with treatment this difference is now small. The combination of severe active and chronic histological changes on a renal biopsy adversely affects outcome. Even in the face of active lupus nephritis, patients without chronic histological changes have a lower risk of developing renal failure. Depending on how it is defined, a significant proportion of patients (30–50% or more) with lupus nephritis do not achieve complete remission despite treatment with cyclophosphamide, and in most studies failure to achieve a remission of the renal disease is associated with a significantly increased risk of developing endstage renal failure and of dying. In one study, 58% of patients did not achieve remission and of these 9% died or developed endstage renal failure. Further renal relapses were also more common in patients who failed to achieve remission. In most studies relapses develop in 20 to 40% of patients who achieve a complete remission of their renal disease over a mean follow-up of about 10 years, and these are associated with an increased risk of developing endstage renal failure.

Several clinical variables are also associated with a greater probability of renal progression in lupus nephritis, including low haematocrit, raised serum creatinine level at diagnosis, hypertension, heavy proteinuria, and poor socioeconomic status.

Long-term outcome

Renal failure can be treated by dialysis and transplantation and the main causes of death in lupus nephritis are treatment-related sepsis, which occurs early, and myocardial ischaemia, which occurs late. Both haemodialysis and continuous ambulatory peritoneal dialysis are well tolerated, and there is a tendency for the activity of lupus disease to diminish after the start of dialysis. We discontinue immunosuppressants in patients on dialysis if there is no overt disease activity, only persisting with a small dose of prednisolone. Overall survival on dialysis is good, being 75% at 10 years. After transplantation, graft survival and function in patients with lupus are comparable to those obtained in patients with other diseases, and recurrence of lupus nephritis is rare.

Renal disease in systemic sclerosis

Systemic sclerosis is a systemic disorder characterized by skin thickening due to the deposition of collagen in the dermis, autoimmunity, and extensive vascular damage involving multiple organs (see Chapter 19.11.3). Adverse prognostic features are renal, cardiac, and pulmonary involvement. A major complication is the development of scleroderma renal crisis, which is characterized by the abrupt onset of severe hypertension, usually with retinopathy, together with the rapid deterioration of renal function and heart failure. Scleroderma renal crisis develops in 8 to 19% of patients with diffuse systemic sclerosis, the most important risk factor being the rapid progression of diffuse skin disease. It usually occurs early, within 3 years of the onset of illness, and develops more commonly in the autumn and winter.

Pathogenesis

The pathogenetic mechanisms leading to renal damage in systemic sclerosis are not known. While plasma renin activity is almost always raised in scleroderma renal crisis, there is no evidence that this occurs before the development of this complication and plasma renin activity does not predict the problem. Patients with systemic sclerosis may show cold-induced reduction in renal perfusion and increased plasma renin activity, but this does not correlate with the presence of renal histological vascular abnormalities. There is evidence of endothelial activation in patients who develop renal damage, with raised serum levels of circulating endothelially derived adhesion molecules including s-ELAM, s-VCAM, and s-ICAM, but these are likely to reflect the presence of endothelial injury rather than being of pathophysiological significance. Transforming growth factor-β (TGFβ), connective tissue growth factor, and platelet-derived growth factor induce proliferation of fibroblasts, resulting in collagen accumulation and end-organ damage. Antitopoisomerase I (Scl-70) antibody is strongly associated with pulmonary fibrosis and anti-RNA polymerase III with severe skin involvement and renal crisis.

Antecedent hypertension does not increase the risk of development of scleroderma renal crisis, which is as common in men as in women, although systemic sclerosis is more common in the latter, with a female to male ratio between 3:1 and 4:1. In one retrospective case-controlled study the risk of scleroderma renal crisis was increased by prior treatment with steroids (more than 15 mg prednisolone/day), with an odds ratio of 4.37 (95% CI 2.03–9.42), and reduced by treatment with penicillamine (odds ratio 0.41; 95% CI 0.24–0.69). One report suggests that ciclosporin may predispose to the development of scleroderma renal crisis.

Pathology

The smaller arcuate and interlobular arteries are predominantly involved in scleroderma renal crisis, showing intimal hyperplasia with concentric mucoid intimal degeneration, but the internal and external elastic laminae remain intact. The adventitia of interlobular arteries shows an abnormal degree of fibrosis. There is fibrinoid necrosis of afferent arterioles and glomeruli, and also glomerular thrombosis. Ischaemia of the glomerular tuft leads to wrinkling and thickening of the glomerular basement membrane and glomerular sclerosis (Fig. 21.10.3.3). These lesions resemble those seen in accelerated hypertension or the haemolytic uraemic syndrome, although the vessels involved tend to be larger and adventitial fibrosis is not seen in accelerated hypertension.

Clinical presentation

Hypertensive scleroderma renal crisis

The clinical presentation is typically with symptoms of malignant hypertension, with headaches, blurred vision, fits, and heart failure. Renal function is impaired and deteriorates rapidly. The hypertension is almost always severe, with a diastolic blood pressure in excess of 100 mmHg in 90% of patients. In approximately 85% of patients there is hypertensive retinopathy, with exudates and haemorrhages and, sometimes, papilloedema.

Normotensive scleroderma renal crisis

Scleroderma renal crisis can also develop in individuals with a normal blood pressure. They are more likely to have a microangiopathic haemolytic anaemia (90% vs 38%), thrombocytopenia (83% vs 21%), and pulmonary haemorrhage than patients with hypertensive scleroderma renal crisis.

Diagnosis

The clinical presentation described above in a patient with the typical diffuse skin thickening of systemic sclerosis is diagnostic. Renal impairment is usually accompanied by a microangiopathic

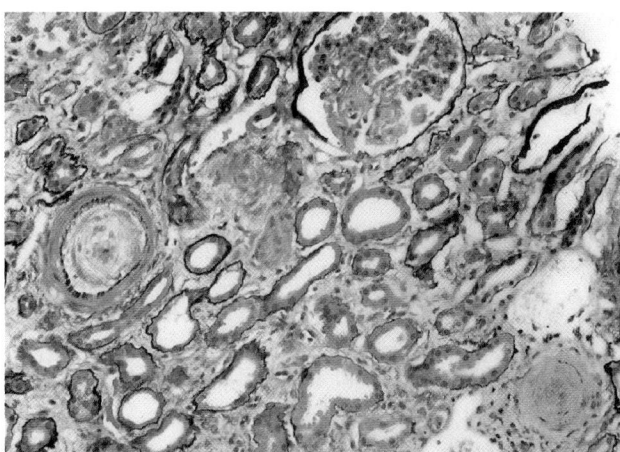

Fig. 21.10.3.3 Scleroderma kidney. A small artery has concentric mucoid intimal thickening, an arteriole has thrombosis and fibrinoid necrosis, and tubules and a glomerulus have ischaemic damage. Periodic acid–methenamine silver staining, magnification ×25.
By courtesy of Professor A J Howie.

haemolytic anaemia, with thrombocytopenia and fragmented red blood cells (schistocytes or burr cells). Once the blood pressure has been well controlled for at least 7 days then, if there is doubt, the diagnosis can be established by renal histology.

Treatment

Scleroderma renal crisis is a medical emergency. The hypertension should be treated with an ACE inhibitor, which can also help with the treatment of the heart failure. The aim should be for a slow and gradual reduction in blood pressure as an abrupt fall can lead to cerebral ischaemia or infarction, as it can in accelerated hypertension. Calcium channel blockers may be required in addition to ACE inhibitors. Deterioration of renal function in these patients is often rapid and they can precipitately develop pulmonary oedema, hence they should be treated in a hospital with facilities for renal replacement therapy.

Prognosis

Before the early 1970s scleroderma renal crisis was almost always a fatal illness, with most patients dying within a year. Survival improved slightly with the use of dialysis and better hypotensive agents, but it is only since the introduction of ACE inhibitors that prognosis has improved. Several large prospective observational studies show that survival has increased from less than 10% to greater than 70% at 5 years, and about 50% of patients who initially require dialysis are able to discontinue this while taking ACE inhibitors. However, other recent studies have reported 50% mortality, and hence scleroderma renal crisis is an important complication of the condition. ACE inhibitors should be started as soon as renal crisis is diagnosed, and continuing therapy with ACE inhibitors reduces the risk of development of chronic renal damage. Improved survival from renal crisis has made pulmonary fibrosis the most common cause of death in scleroderma.

Renal disease in rheumatoid arthritis

The main causes of renal disease in rheumatoid arthritis are secondary (amyloid A) amyloidosis and nephrotoxicity from drugs used in treatment (see Box 21.10.3.1 and Chapter 19.5). Nonsteroidal

---

Box 21.10.3.1 Renal disease in rheumatoid arthritis

Consequences of rheumatoid arthritis

- Amyloid A amyloidosis
- Vasculitic glomerulonephritis
- Mesangiocapillary glomerulonephritis
- Mesangial IgA proliferative glomerulonephritis

Drug nephrotoxicity
Nonsteroidal anti-inflammatory drugs

- Reversible haemodynamically mediated renal impairment
- Acute tubular necrosis
- Acute interstitial nephritis with or without a nephrotic syndrome

Gold and penicillamine

- Proteinuria
- Nephrotic syndrome
- Membranous nephropathy
- Rare reports of a crescentic glomerulonephritis

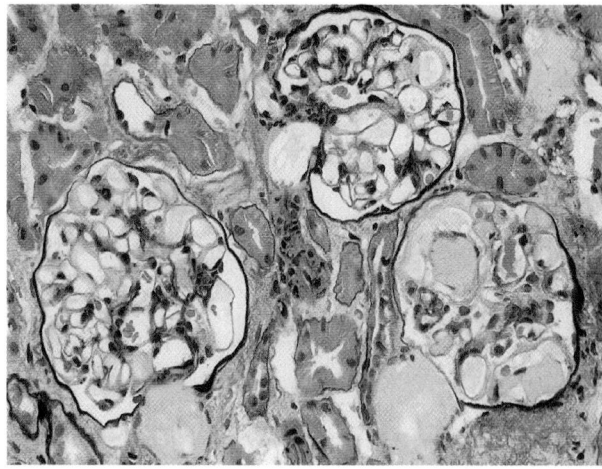

Fig. 21.10.3.4 Amyloidosis in rheumatoid arthritis. Arterioles and glomeruli contain acellular masses of amyloid. Periodic acid–methenamine silver staining, magnification ×40.
By courtesy of Professor A J Howie.

---

anti-inflammatory drugs (NSAIDs) are widely used for pain relief and are associated with the development of a variety of renal syndromes, ranging from a reversible reduction in glomerular filtration rate to acute renal failure, either due to an acute tubular necrosis or an acute interstitial nephritis, and the latter may be complicated by nephrotic range proteinuria. Renal vasculitis and glomerulonephritis are also described.

The pattern of renal disease in rheumatoid arthritis is changing. Gold and penicillamine are now infrequently used, hence nephrotoxicity from these causes is rare nowadays. The incidence of amyloid A amyloidosis and also of rheumatoid vasculitis has declined, probably as a result of early and more aggressive treatment of the disease.

Secondary amyloidosis

Secondary amyloidosis results from deposition of fibrils containing amyloid A protein that is antigenically related to the acute phase reactant serum amyloid A (see Chapter 12.12.3). Rheumatoid arthritis is the commonest disease producing secondary amyloidosis in developed countries. Prevalence rates of 8 to 17% are found at autopsy, while data from biopsy series show a lower prevalence of around 5 to 10%. There is some evidence for a decline in prevalence of amyloid in recent years, and since 2003 the incidence appears to have dropped dramatically. The reason for this is likely to be much more aggressive therapy of rheumatoid disease, with fewer patients being left with a persistently elevated acute phase response. Cases of crescentic glomerulonephritis superimposed on renal amyloidosis in patients with rheumatoid arthritis have been described.

Clinical features and diagnosis

The presentation of renal amyloid is with proteinuria that is often severe enough to cause a nephrotic syndrome. Renal vein thrombosis is particularly common. Diagnosis is established by renal biopsy (Fig. 21.10.3.4), where histological Congo red staining, which is birefringent in polarized light, is characteristic of amyloid. This staining is abolished by potassium permanganate in reactive amyloidosis but not in primary amyloidosis. Monoclonal and polyclonal antibodies that specifically bind amyloid A are now available and are of use for histological diagnosis. The diagnosis of amyloid has also been aided by the availability of scans using radiolabelled serum amyloid P (SAP) protein, utilizing the strong calcium-dependent affinity of SAP for amyloid fibrils of any protein type.

Treatment and prognosis

There is no specific therapy for amyloid A amyloidosis, the general principle being suppression of the underlying chronic inflammation. Uncontrolled evidence suggests that aggressive treatment of rheumatoid arthritis may be effective in delaying the deterioration of renal function in patients with renal amyloid, and aggressive treatment with prednisolone and cyclophosphamide or methotrexate can induce remission of the nephrotic syndrome due to amyloid in patients with this condition. More recently, treatment with antitumour necrosis factor-α (anti-TNFα) antibodies was reported to lead to remission of renal disease due to amyloidosis.

Renal amyloid leads to progressive renal failure; 50% of patients develop endstage renal failure after 5 years, rising to 90% at 10 years. Treatment of endstage renal failure from amyloid is by dialysis and renal transplantation.

Gold and penicillamine nephropathy

Clinical features and diagnosis

The most frequent presenting feature is proteinuria, which occurs in approximately 10% of patients receiving gold and up to 30% of those taking penicillamine. This progresses to the nephrotic syndrome in 30 and 16%, respectively. Haematuria is uncommon, although it is seen more frequently with penicillamine, and still requires the exclusion of other causes when occurring in the context of therapy with these drugs. Renal function is usually normal. Gold and penicillamine are no longer widely used to treat patients with rheumatoid arthritis and nephrotoxicity from these agents is correspondingly uncommon.

About 55 to 80% of patients who present with penicillamine- or gold-induced proteinuria will have a membranous glomerulonephritis. Minimal-change nephropathy is the next most frequently encountered histological lesion. Other less common renal lesions include mesangiocapillary glomerulonephritis and tubulointerstitial inflammation. Penicillamine may lead to the development of a rapidly progressive glomerulonephritis with crescents and pulmonary haemorrhage, resembling Goodpasture's syndrome but without antiglomerular basement membrane antibodies.

Treatment and prognosis

In general, gold and penicillamine should be discontinued when significant proteinuria develops (more than 0.5 g/24 h). After cessation of the drug, proteinuria peaks at around a month then gradually disappears, and most patients will have clear urine by 1 year and almost all will achieve this by 2 years. Renal function does not deteriorate in uncomplicated cases.

Nephrotoxicity of other drugs

Ciclosporin

The renal toxicity of ciclosporin in general and in rheumatoid arthritis is well documented, hence in these patients ciclosporin should be started at a dose of 2.5 mg/kg per day and not increased beyond 5 mg/kg per day. Ciclosporin is contraindicated in patients with renal dysfunction, and it should be used with caution in patients older than 65 years of age, also in those patients taking other drugs that may independently affect renal function. A reduction of ciclosporin dose is advised if creatinine rises by more than 30% from baseline values, and it should be discontinued if this is persistent. The most common histological changes in the kidney during treatment with ciclosporin are focal interstitial fibrosis, tubular atrophy, and arteriolar hyalinosis.

Nonsteroidal anti-inflammatory drugs

Nonsteroidal anti-inflammatory drugs are potentially nephrotoxic and in patients with rheumatoid arthritis may lead to a reversible reduction in glomerular filtration rate, acute tubular necrosis, an acute interstitial nephritis often with heavy proteinuria, renal papillary necrosis, and chronic tubulointerstitial nephritis.

Anti-TNFα antibodies and glomerulonephritis

Treatment with anti-TNFα antibodies can lead to autoimmunity with the development of ANA, anti-dsDNA antibodies, and anticardiolipin antibodies. Recently five patients with rheumatoid arthritis treated with anti-TNFα antibodies were reported to have developed lupus nephritis (n = 2), a pauci-immune necrotizing glomerulonephritis (n = 2), and a membranous nephropathy with renal vasculitis (n = 1). Patients treated with these agents should have their urine, renal function, and autoantibody levels carefully monitored.

Glomerulonephritis

The most commonly described glomerulonephritis in rheumatoid arthritis that is not related to drug use is a mesangiocapillary glomerulonephritis, which in many cases is accompanied by IgA deposits (IgA nephropathy). The other major type of glomerulonephritis reported in rheumatoid arthritis is membranous nephropathy.

Renal vasculitis

The clinical spectrum of rheumatoid arthritis includes a systemic necrotizing vasculitis with involvement of blood vessels ranging in size from capillaries to small and medium-sized arteries. With more aggressive treatment of rheumatoid arthritis, vasculitis from this cause is now uncommon. The clinical presentation includes nail fold infarcts, a leucocytoclastic vasculitis, a peripheral neuropathy, pericarditis, gastrointestinal infarcts, and renal vasculitis.

Renal abnormalities are found in about 25% of patients with rheumatoid vasculitis, usually microscopic haematuria, proteinuria, and renal impairment. Renal histology shows a large vessel renal arteritis and a segmental necrotizing glomerulonephritis with crescent formation (vasculitic glomerulonephritis) (Fig. 21.10.3.5). Treatment is with prednisolone and cyclophosphamide, usually leading to improvement of renal function.

Renal disease in juvenile chronic arthritis

Renal involvement in juvenile chronic arthritis is infrequent, but its presence is associated with a poor outcome. Proteinuria is found in 3 to 12% of patients and microscopic haematuria in 3 to 8%. The renal lesions reported are usually complications of the underlying rheumatic disease, such as amyloidosis, or those arising as side-effects of the drugs used (see above). Cases of necrotizing crescentic glomerulonephritis, focal segmental glomerulosclerosis, and mesangial glomerulonephritis have all been described in children with the condition.

Renal amyloid is found in 1.2 to 6.7% of patients with juvenile chronic arthritis, and affects patients with chronic and active disease, with a predilection for systemic onset disease. It typically presents with nephrotic range proteinuria. Aggressive treatment with chlorambucil has been shown to improve survival in patients with juvenile chronic arthritis and amyloid A amyloidosis.

Renal disease in primary Sjögren's syndrome

Sjögren's syndrome is characterized by a lymphocytic infiltration of exocrine glands leading to a dry mouth (xerostomia) and dry eyes (keratoconjunctivitis sicca) (see Chapter 19.11.6). It may be primary or secondary to a variety of autoimmune disorders, including rheumatoid arthritis, SLE, systemic sclerosis, and mixed connective tissue disorder.

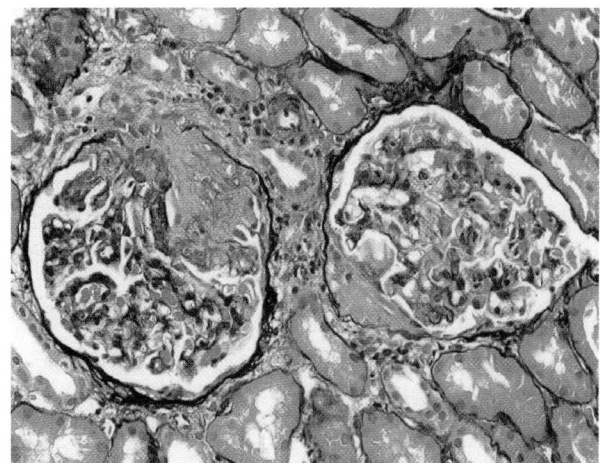

Fig. 21.10.3.5 Vasculitic glomerulonephritis in rheumatoid arthritis. Two glomeruli have sharply defined segmental lesions where there has been disruption of the tuft and partial obliteration of Bowman's space. Periodic acid–methenamine silver staining, magnification ×32.
By courtesy of Professor A J Howie.

Renal involvement in Sjögren's syndrome is most commonly mild and often subclinical, with asymptomatic proteinuria and haematuria, but clinically significant renal disease has been reported in about 10 to 25% of cases. Some patients present with distal renal tubular acidosis, impairment of urinary concentration, hypokalaemia, or rarely with the Fanconi syndrome. Clinical manifestations of these renal tubular disorders include the development of renal calculi, polyuria, and rarely hypokalaemic periodic paralysis. Renal biopsy in these patients shows tubulointerstitial nephritis with interstitial lymphocytic infiltrates.

Glomerulonephritis is rare in primary Sjögren's syndrome, and is most commonly mesangiocapillary glomerulonephritis or membranous glomerulopathy. Their pathogenesis is most probably attributed to immune complex deposition, with IgMκ rheumatoid factor, polyclonal IgG, and IgA. Patients can rarely have both an interstitial nephritis and a glomerulonephritis.

Overall, interstitial nephritis occurs early in the disease and glomerulonephritis as a late manifestation. Immunosuppressants have been used with beneficial effects in some patients with glomerulonephritis, while others progress to endstage renal failure.

Renal disease in mixed connective tissue disease

Some patients with a connective tissue disorder do not fit easily into the accepted definitions of a single disease. In patients with mixed connective tissue disease there is the sequential or concurrent development of the clinical features of SLE, systemic sclerosis, polymyositis, and less commonly of rheumatoid arthritis (see Chapter 19.11.2). While initial reports stressed the paucity of renal involvement in mixed connective tissue disorder, subsequent studies noted a higher prevalence of immune complex nephritis (10–50%). Renal presentation is asymptomatic proteinuria or haematuria and less commonly with a nephrotic syndrome, and patients with renal disease appear to have more systemic manifestations than those without.

Membranous nephropathy and a mesangiocapillary glomerulonephritis are the most common histological changes, found in 34 and 30% of cases, respectively. A focal or diffuse proliferative glomerulonephritis is found in 17%, a mixed lesion with membranous nephropathy in 5%, and in 7% renal histology is normal. Immunofluorescence microscopy of glomeruli in patients with mixed connective tissue disease has shown immunoglobulin and complement deposits; dense deposits are found on electron microscopy.

Treatment of renal disease in mixed connective tissue disease is with steroids, initially in high doses, subsequently tapering to a low maintenance dose over weeks. Treatment of patients with a nephrotic syndrome with high-dose steroids leads to a significant reduction of proteinuria in 62% of cases. Whether those with renal disease resistant to steroids would benefit from the addition of immunosuppressant drugs is not known. Approximately 14% of patients with mixed connective tissue disease and renal disease develop chronic renal failure.

Further reading

Adu D, et al. (eds) (2001). *Rheumatology and the kidney*. Oxford University Press, Oxford.

Appel G, et al. Mycophenolate mofetil versus cyclophosphamide for induction treatment of lupus nephritis. *J Am Soc Nephrol*, **20**, 1103–1112.

Lupus nephritis

Balow JE, et al. (1996). Management of lupus nephritis. *Kidney Int*, **53**, S88–92.
Cameron J (1999). Lupus nephritis. *J Am Soc Nephrol*, **10**, 1–17.
Chan TM, et al. (2005). Long-term study of mycophenolate mofetil as continuous induction and maintenance treatment for diffuse proliferative lupus nephritis. *J Am Soc Nephrol*, **16**, 1076–84.
Contreras G, et al. (2004). Sequential therapies for proliferative lupus nephritis. *N Engl J Med*, **350**, 971–80.
Contreras G, et al. (2005). Outcomes in African Americans and Hispanics with lupus nephritis. *Kidney Int*, **69**, 1846–51.
Daugas E, et al. (2002). Antiphospholipid syndrome nephropathy in systemic lupus erythematosus. *J Am Soc Nephrol*, **13**, 42–52.
Flanc RS, et al. (2004). Treatment for lupus nephritis. *Cochrane Database Syst Rev*, **1**, CD002922.
Ginzler EM, et al. (2005). Mycophenolate mofetil or intravenous cyclophosphamide for lupus nephritis. *N Engl J Med*, **353**, 2219–28.
Grootscholten C, et al. (2006). Azathioprine/methylprednisolone versus cyclophosphamide in proliferative lupus nephritis. A randomized controlled trial. *Kidney Int*, **70**, 732–42.
Houssiau FA, et al. (2004). Early response to immunosuppressive therapy predicts good renal outcome in lupus nephritis: lessons from long-term follow up of patients in the Euro-Lupus Nephritis Trial. *Arthritis Rheum*, **50**, 3934–40.
Howie AJ, et al. (2003). Powerful morphometric indicator of prognosis in lupus nephritis. *QJM*, **96**, 411–20.
Illei GG, et al. (2002). Renal flares are common in patients with severe proliferative lupus nephritis treated with pulse immunosuppressive therapy: long-term follow up of a cohort of 145 patients participating in randomized controlled studies. *Arthritis Rheum*, **46**, 995–1002.
Korbet SM, et al. (2000). Factors predictive of outcome in severe lupus nephritis. Lupus Nephritis Collaborative Study Group. *Am J Kidney Dis*, **35**, 904–14.
Lewis EJ, et al. (1992). A controlled trial of plasmapheresis therapy in severe lupus nephritis. *N Engl J Med*, **326**, 1373–9.
Mok CC, et al. (2004). Predictors and outcome of renal flares after successful cyclophosphamide treatment for diffuse proliferative lupus glomerulonephritis. *Arthritis Rheum*, **50**, 2559–68.
Pasquali S, et al. (1993). Lupus membranous nephropathy: long-term outcome. *Clin Nephrol*, **39**, 175–82.
Weening JJ, et al. (2004). The classification of glomerulonephritis in systemic lupus erythematosus revisited. *J Am Soc Nephrol*, **15**, 241–50.

Systemic sclerosis

DeMarco PJ, et al. (2002). Predictors and outcomes of scleroderma renal crisis: the high-dose versus low-dose D-penicillamine in early diffuse systemic sclerosis trial. *Arthritis Rheum*, **46**, 2983–9.
Helfrich D, et al. (1989). Normotensive renal failure in systemic sclerosis. *Arthritis Rheum*, **32**, 1128–34.
Steen V, Medsger TJ (1998). Case-control study of corticosteroids and other drugs that either precipitate or protect from the development of scleroderma renal crisis. *Arthritis Rheum*, **41**,1613–19.
Steen VD, Medsger TA Jr (2000). Long-term outcomes of scleroderma renal crisis. *Ann Intern Med*, **133**, 600–3.
Steen V, et al. (1984). Factors predicting development of renal involvement in progressive systemic sclerosis. *Am J Med*, **76**, 779–86.
Steen V, et al. (1990). Outcome of renal crisis in systemic sclerosis: relation to availability of angiotensin converting enzyme (ACE) inhibitors. *Ann Intern Med*, **113**, 352–7.

Rheumatoid arthritis

Adu D, et al. (1993). Glomerulonephritis in rheumatoid arthritis. *Br J Rheumatol*, **32**, 1008–11.

Boers M (1990). Renal disorders in rheumatoid arthritis. *Semin Arthritis Rheum*, **20**, 57–68.

Esteve V, *et al.* (2006). Renal involvement in amyloidosis. Clinical outcomes, evolution and survival. *Nefrologia*, **26**, 212–17.

Hall CL, *et al.* (1987). The natural course of gold nephropathy: long term study of 21 patients. *BMJ*, **295**, 745–84.

Hall CL, *et al.* (1988). Natural course of penicillamine nephropathy: a long term study of 33 patients. *BMJ*, **296**, 1085–6.

Harper L, *et al.* (1997). Focal segmental necrotizing glomerulonephritis in rheumatoid arthritis. *QJM*, **90**, 125–32.

Honkanen E, *et al.* (1987). Membranous glomerulonephritis in rheumatoid arthritis not related to gold or D-penicillamine therapy: a report of four cases and review of the literature. *Clin Nephrol*, **27**, 87–93.

Kuroda T, *et al.* (2006). Long-term mortality outcome in patients with reactive amyloidosis associated with rheumatoid arthritis. *Clin Rheumatol*, **25**, 498–505.

Kuznetsky KA, *et al.* (1986). Necrotizing glomerulonephritis in rheumatoid arthritis. *Clin Nephrol*, **26**, 257–64.

Stokes MB, *et al.* (2005). Development of glomerulonephritis during anti-TNF-alpha therapy for rheumatoid arthritis. *Nephrol Dial Transplant*, **20**, 1400–6.

Uda H, *et al.* (2006). Two distinct clinical courses of renal involvement in rheumatoid patients with AA amyloidosis. *J Rheumatol*, **33**, 1482–7.

Sjögren's syndrome

Moutsopoulos H, *et al.* (1978). Immune complex glomerulonephritis in sicca syndrome. *Am J Med*, **64**, 955–60.

Moutsopoulos H, *et al.* (1991). Nephrocalcinosis in Sjögren's syndrome. *J Intern Med*, **230**, 187–91.

Shearn M, Tu WH (1965). Nephrogenic diabetes insipidus and other disorders of renal tubular function in Sjögren's syndrome. *Am J Med*, **39**, 312–18.

Talal N, Zisman E, Schur P (1968). Renal tubular acidosis, glomerulonephritis and immune complex glomerulonephritis in Sjögren's syndrome. *Arthritis Rheum*, **11**, 774.

Mixed connective tissue disease

Kitridou RC, *et al.* (1986). Renal involvement in mixed connective tissue disease: a longitudinal clinicopathologic study, *Semin Arthritis Rheum*, **16**, 135–45.

21.10.4 Renal involvement in plasma cell dyscrasias, immunoglobulin-based amyloidoses, and fibrillary glomerulopathies, lymphomas, and leukaemias

P. Ronco, F. Bridoux, and G. Touchard

Essentials

Plasma cell dyscrasias are characterized by uncontrolled proliferation of a single clone of B cells which is responsible for the secretion of a monoclonal immunoglobulin (Ig) or Ig subunit that can become deposited in tissues. They can cause a wide range of renal diseases.

Light-chain amyloidosis—renal presentation is usually with proteinuria, often progressing to nephrotic syndrome. Progressive decline in renal function usually occurs, leading finally to endstage renal failure. Diagnosis is made by the detection of monoclonal gammopathy in serum and/or urine (90% of cases) in combination with biopsy evidence of amyloid- forming light chain deposits. Chemotherapy with oral mephalan plus dexamethasone should be considered as first line treatment.

Myeloma—renal failure is found at presentation in 20% of patients, occurs in 50% at some time, and is most commonly caused by cast nephropathy, diagnosis of which relies on the detection of a urinary monoclonal light chain, with renal biopsy typically showing 'fractured' casts. Chemotherapy, e.g. high-dose dexamethasone, combined with various drugs including bortezomib, and /or alkylating agents, and/or thalidomide.

Light-chain, light- and heavy-chain, and heavy-chain deposition disease—collectively known as monoclonal Ig deposition diseases, present with proteinuria and renal failure. Diagnosis is by renal biopsy which reveals nodular glomerulosclerosis, monotypic light- and/or heavy-chain deposits along glomerular and tubular basement membranes (by immunofluorescence), and nonfibrillar granular electron-dense deposits (by electron microscopy). Patients with myeloma (45% of cases) are treated with conventional chemotherapy or high-dose therapy followed by autologous stem cell transplantation in selected cases.

Fibrillary glomerulonephritis and immunotactoid glomerulopathy—usual presentation is with the nephrotic syndrome, microscopic haematuria, and hypertension. Diagnosis is by renal biopsy when electron microscopy reveals (respectively) fibrils (solid, diameter 12–22 nm, randomly arranged) or microtubules (hollow, diameter 10–60 nm, sometimes in parallel arrays). Cases associated with chronic lymphocytic leukaemia or lymphoma may respond to chemotherapy.

Cryoglobulinaemia—type II ('essential mixed'), which involves a monoclonal IgM with rheumatoid factor activity and a polyclonal IgG, may present with proteinuria, haematuria, hypertension, and gradually declining renal function, or with an acute nephritic picture. It should be suspected in the presence of an IgM rheumatoid factor and low complement C4, and confirmed by the finding of a cryoglobulin. It is often associated with hepatitis C. Renal biopsy typically reveals membranoproliferative glomerulonephritis with massive subendothelial deposits. The best treatment is uncertain, but it may involve antiviral agents and/or immunosuppression.

Tumour lysis syndrome—a life-threatening metabolic emergency that occurs in patients with haemopathies with high cell turnover, e.g. Burkitt's lymphoma and acute leukaemia, mostly at the onset of chemotherapy and/or radiation therapy. Prevention is by vigorous hydration with 0.9% saline before treatment with the addition of allopurinol (in low-risk cases) or the recombinant modified urate oxidase rasburicase (in high-risk cases). Treatment is by saline diuresis (if possible), rasburicase, and haemodialysis (if required).

Introduction

Plasma cell dyscrasias are characterized by uncontrolled proliferation of a single clone of B cells, usually with plasma cell differentiation, which is responsible for the secretion of a monoclonal immunoglobulin (Ig) or Ig subunit that can become deposited in tissues. The range of renal diseases in which it is recognized that there is deposition or precipitation of Ig-related material has expanded dramatically in recent years.

These conditions can be classified into two categories on the basis of their ultrastructural appearances (Table 21.10.4.1). Those with organized deposits include diseases with crystal formation, mainly myeloma cast nephropathy; diseases with fibril formation, mainly light-chain amyloidosis; and diseases with microtubule formation, including cryoglobulinaemia kidney and immunotactoid/microtubular glomerulonephritis (also called GOMMID for glomerulonephritis with organized microtubular monoclonal Ig deposits). A second category of diseases is characterized by the presence of nonorganized granular electron-dense deposits made of light and/or heavy chains along the basement membranes of many tissues, most importantly the kidney. First described by Randall and associates, these are referred to as monoclonal Ig deposition diseases (MIDD). More recently, glomerular diseases with amorphous monoclonal Ig deposits distinct from Randall-type MIDD have been described. It is now well established that the spectrum of plasma cell dyscrasia-related renal complications is due to intrinsic properties of the monoclonal component.

Except for myeloma cast nephropathy, diagnosis relies on careful analysis of a biopsy specimen taken from the kidney, which should systematically include immunohistochemical studies with specific antibodies and also electron microscopy in all ambiguous cases. Since most of these patients will develop renal failure, it is essential to identify the underlying plasma cell dyscrasia because appropriate treatment may halt the extension of visceral deposits, and even induce their regression. Except in patients with myeloma cast nephropathy, who usually present with a high-mass myeloma, 'malignancy' more often results from life-threatening visceral deposits than from the Ig-secreting clone itself.

Renal involvement in Ig light-chain amyloidosis

Definition and epidemiology

Amyloidosis is a general term for a family of diseases defined by morphological criteria and characterized by deposition in extracellular spaces of a proteinaceous material that stains with Congo red and is metachromatic. Amyloid deposits are composed of a felt-like array of 10-nm-wide rigid linear aggregated fibrils of indefinite length with a β-pleated sheet configuration. They occur in a variety of conditions including Alzheimer's disease and other neurodegenerative disorders, tumoural and inflammatory diseases, and plasma cell dyscrasias. The various types of amyloidosis differ essentially by the nature of the precursor protein that yields the main component of fibrils, and are classified accordingly (see Chapter 12.12.3 for further discussion).

Light-chain amyloidosis has become the most frequent form of amyloidosis with renal involvement. Amyloid deposits are found in approximately 10% of myeloma patients, their prevalence reaching 20% in those with pure light-chain myeloma (Fig. 21.10.4.1).

Clinical presentation

The main clinical features of light-chain amyloidosis at presentation are fatigue (62%) and weight loss (52%), followed by purpura (15%), pain (5%), and gross bleeding (3%). Hepatomegaly is found in 24% of patients, and macroglossia in 9%. A palpable spleen and lymphadenopathy can also be found.

Proteinuria is the usual symptom of renal amyloidosis, detected in 55% of patients at presentation and often progressing to a severe nephrotic syndrome, which can be complicated by renal vein thrombosis. Haematuria is uncommon, and when present should prompt examination for a bleeding lesion of the urinary tract. Progressive decline in renal function usually occurs, leading finally to endstage renal failure. In those rare patients in whom renal tubulointerstitial deposits predominate, renal failure may progress without a nephrotic stage, and in some of these patients renal tubular dysfunction may be the presenting problem, including Fanconi's syndrome, renal tubular acidosis, or even nephrogenic diabetes insipidus. Hypertension is uncommon but may develop concomitantly with renal failure. The kidneys may be of normal size or large, even when renal function is impaired.

Systemic light-chain amyloidosis can infiltrate almost any organ (except the brain) and thus be responsible for a wide variety of clinical manifestations. It frequently involves the tongue, gastrointestinal tract, peripheral nervous system, carpal tunnel, heart, and skin. Purpuric macules in the periorbital region are very typical of light-chain amyloidosis.

Diagnosis

Light-chain amyloidosis should be suspected when the clinical manifestations described above are associated with a monoclonal component in the serum or urine. Light-chain amyloidosis is always the result of the proliferation of a plasma cell clone; 56% of patients have an increased number of plasma cells in the bone marrow, and 15% have true myeloma. Monoclonal light chains are detected by immunoelectrophoresis of urine in around 73% of cases, with the λ isotype being twice as frequent as the κ isotype. An over-representation of the Vλ6 subgroup has been found in AL amyloidosis with renal involvement. With the use of more sensitive

Table 21.10.4.1 Pathological classification of diseases with tissue deposition or precipitation of monoclonal Ig-related material

Organized			Nonorganized (granular)	
Crystals	Fibrillar	Microtubular	MIDD (Randall-type)	Other
Myeloma cast nephropathy	Light-chain amyloidosis	Cryoglobulinaemia kidney	LCDD	Non-Randall-type proliferative GN
Fanconi's syndrome	Nonamyloid fibrillary GN	Immunotactoid GN/GOMMID	LHCDD	Waldenström's macroglobulinaemia
Other			HCDD	

GN, glomerulonephritis; GOMMID, glomerulonephritis with organized microtubular monoclonal Ig deposits; LCDD, LHCDD, HCDD, light-chain, light- and heavy-chain, heavy-chain deposition disease; MIDD, monoclonal immunoglobulin deposition disease.

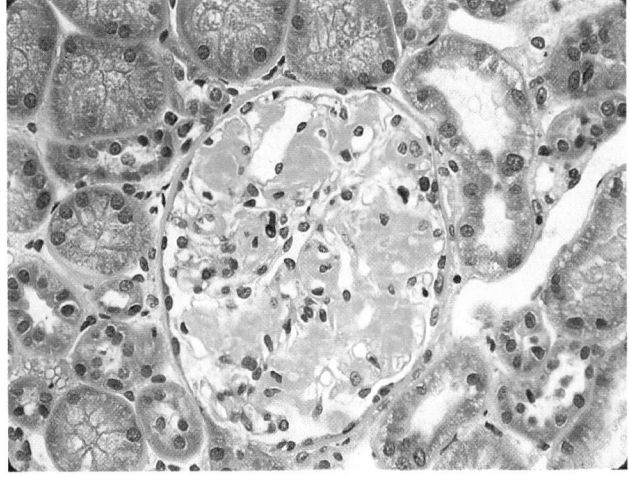

(a)

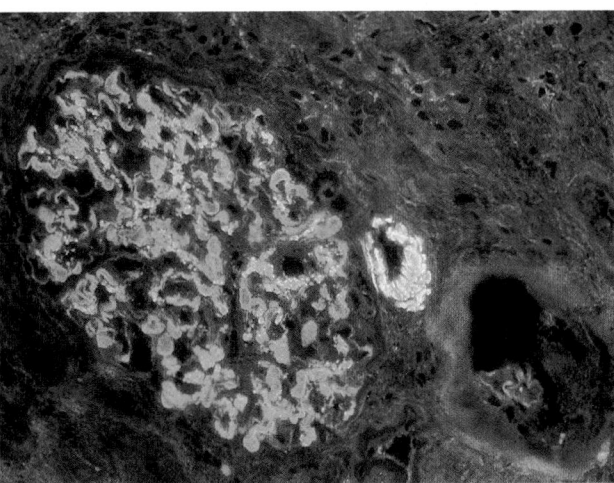

(b)

(c)

Fig. 21.10.4.1 Light-chain amyloidosis. (a) Amyloid deposits in a renal glomerulus. Masson's trichrome stain, magnification ×312. (b) Apple-green/yellow dichroism under polarized light. Congo red stain, magnification ×312. (c) Immunofluorescence with anti-λ antibody. Note glomerular and arteriolar deposits. Magnification ×312.
(From Béatrice Mougenot's personal collection.)

techniques such as immunofixation, a monoclonal Ig is found in the serum and/or the urine in nearly 90% of patients, but still not in all of them. The recent development of a sensitive nephelometric immunoassay for circulating free Ig light chains has been an important advance in the management of AL amyloidosis, allowing detection of abnormal serum free light chain levels in 98% of patients and reliable monitoring of response to chemotherapy.

However, it is important to recognize that detection of monoclonal gammopathy is insufficient for the diagnosis of AL amyloidosis, which should be established in all cases by taking a biopsy specimen from a superficial organ, including skin, salivary glands, and gum, or by aspiration biopsy of abdominal fat. These biopsies should be performed before biopsies of rectal mucosa (which should include vessels of the submucosa where amyloid deposits usually start) and/or of kidney, because of the risk of bleeding complications due to factor X deficiency or amyloid infiltration of vascular walls. After Congo red staining, amyloid deposits appear faintly red and show characteristic apple-green birefringence under polarized light. Congo red staining may be falsely negative if tissue sections are less than 5 μm in thickness. Metachromasia is also observed with crystal violet, which stains the deposits red. In the kidney, the earliest lesions are located in the mesangium, along the glomerular basement membrane, and in the blood vessels. Because there are specific diagnostic and therapeutic strategies depending on the type of protein deposited within tissues, immunofluorescence with specific antisera including anti-κ and anti-λ light chains should be performed routinely. When pathological confirmation of AL type cannot be obtained, genetic studies should be performed to exclude systemic hereditary amyloidosis caused by mutations in the genes encoding transthyretin, fibrinogen A α-chain, lysozyme or apolipoprotein A-I or A-II, all of which are frequently associated with renal involvement.

Treatment

Light-chain amyloidosis is a wasting disease with a mean survival of only 6 to 15 months in untreated patients. Cardiac involvement is a main prognostic factor, accounting for 30% of deaths. The aim of treatment is to suppress production of amyloidogenic free light chain with acceptable toxicity. Due to the lack of comparative clinical trials, treatment of AL amyloidosis is debated. Low-dose chemotherapy (oral melphalan and prednisone) was extensively used in the 1990s with modest increase in median survival (up to 18 months). Improved results have been obtained with intermediate-dose regimens, such as vincristine, doxorubicin, and dexamethasone (VAD), or, more recently, oral melphalan plus dexamethasone. These regimens, which induce rapid and higher rates of haematological response, have been shown to increase median survival to 40 to 50 months, with limited treatment-related mortality. Intensive therapy, i.e. high-dose intravenous melphalan followed by autologous stem cell transplantation, has been extensively used in recent years, resulting in complete clonal response in up to 40% of cases and median survival of 4.6 years. However, such intensive therapy is associated with high morbidity and treatment-related mortality, ranging from 12% in experienced centres to more than 40% in multicentre series. It is therefore limited to selected patients, usually on the basis of the following criteria: aged under 70 years, one or two organs involved, glomerular filtration rate above 50 ml/min, and absence of advanced amyloid cardiopathy. In a randomized controlled trial that enrolled 100 patients with systemic AL amyloidosis, oral melphalan plus dexamethasone resulted in improved overall survival compared to high-dose chemotherapy followed by autologous stem cell transplantation, suggesting that intensive therapy should be offered only to those refractory to conventional chemotherapy.

Results of chemotherapy in amyloidosis are difficult to document because there is no easy way to measure the amount of amyloid present. Resolution of the nephrotic syndrome does not necessarily reflect the disappearance of amyloid deposits, and the progressive deposition of amyloid can occur despite improved clinical and laboratory findings. Scintigraphy after the injection of ^{123}I-labelled serum amyloid P (SAP) may be helpful for monitoring the extent of systemic amyloidosis, but it is available only in a limited number of centres (see Chapter 12.12.3). The effects of chemotherapy are better evaluated by serial nephelometric measurements of serum free light chains. When remission of the underlying plasma cell disorder is achieved with chemotherapy, which is reflected by at least a 50% reduction in serum free light chain levels, survival is significantly increased. Serum levels of N-terminal pro-brain natriuretic peptide, a sensitive marker of myocardial dysfunction in AL amyloidosis, should be also monitored.

Among patients with the nephrotic syndrome, a normal serum creatinine and no echocardiographic evidence of cardiac amyloidosis are associated with a higher response rate (39%) to chemotherapy, as defined by a 50% reduction in proteinuria without an increase in serum creatinine. Amyloid nephropathy requires supportive therapy of the nephrotic syndrome and of renal failure. Depending on the burden of their extrarenal disease, patients in endstage renal disease are candidates for regular dialysis and/or kidney transplantation. Their prognosis is compromised by the risks of extension of extrarenal deposition, especially to the heart, and by recurrence of amyloidosis in the graft if suppression of the plasma cell disorder has not been obtained with appropriate treatment.

Renal involvement in myeloma

Definition and epidemiology

Renal failure is one of the main complications of myeloma, found at presentation in 20% of patients and occurring in 50% during the course of the disease. It is mostly due to cast nephropathy, although other forms of renal disease may occur, including light-chain amyloidosis (10% of myeloma patients), light-chain deposition disease (5%), Fanconi's syndrome, infiltration of renal interstitium by plasma cells, calcium precipitation, and renal infection. Myeloma cast nephropathy is due both to alterations in tubule cells induced by massive reabsorption of light chains in proximal tubule cells, and to cast formation involving light chains and Tamm–Horsfall protein in the distal tubule. The risk of developing renal failure is twice as high in patients with pure light-chain myeloma, and 5 to 6 times greater in patients with light-chain proteinuria of more than 2.0 g/day compared with those with proteinuria of less than 0.05 g/day.

Clinical presentation

Myeloma cast nephropathy usually presents as acute or subacute renal failure, often revealing myeloma with a high tumour burden

(found in 70–80% of myeloma patients with renal failure). Common triggering factors include hypercalcaemia, dehydration, infection, use of toxic compounds including radiocontrast media, nonsteroidal anti-inflammatory drugs, diuretics and angiotensin-converting enzyme inhibitors or angiotensin II receptor antagonists, all of which reduce renal perfusion, especially in those who are dehydrated.

Renal failure induced by cast nephropathy is remarkably silent. The clinical and urinary syndrome is characterized by nonspecific signs including weakness, weight loss, bone pain, and signs of infection, all due to myeloma, and by urinary excretion of a monoclonal light chain. It must be emphasized that urinary dipsticks do not detect the light chain, which is measured by quantitative tests of proteinuria. Light chain accounts for more than 70% of total proteinuria by urine electrophoresis.

Tubular dysfunction is rarely a presenting symptom. Fanconi's syndrome due to proximal tubule impairment may result from toxicity of intratubular inclusions of κ light chains, usually organized into crystals. This can lead to osteomalacia and in rare cases may precede the diagnosis of myeloma by several years.

Diagnosis

Diagnosis of myeloma cast nephropathy relies on the detection of a urinary monoclonal light chain in patients with subacute or acute renal failure of apparently unknown origin. In those patients with pure light-chain myeloma, diagnosis can be suspected before urinalysis on the basis of dramatic hypogammaglobulinaemia detected by serum electrophoresis.

A renal biopsy should not be performed routinely in patients with a presumed diagnosis of myeloma cast nephropathy. It can, however, be useful for several reasons: first, to analyse tubulointerstitial lesions and allow diagnosis and treatment of other potential causes of renal impairment in those with multiple possible precipitating factors (infection, drugs, etc.); second, to establish the diagnosis of Fanconi's syndrome; and third, to identify glomerular lesions in patients with albuminuria over 1 g/day and no evidence of amyloid deposits in 'peripheral' biopsies. Myeloma casts have unique characteristics, including a 'fractured' appearance due to crystal formation, polychromatism when stained with Masson's trichrome, and the presence of multinucleated giant cells. They are consistently associated with dramatic epithelial tubular lesions and interstitial inflammatory infiltrates.

Treatment

The first aim of treatment is to prevent or retard renal impairment in all patients with myeloma, most particularly those with light-chain myeloma, by prevention of dehydration, maintenance of a high urinary output and urine alkalinization, avoidance of nephrotoxic drugs, and control of hypercalcaemia (if present), which requires correction of salt and water deficit, steroids, and/or bisphosphonates, which are potent inhibitors of osteoclast activity but must be used with caution as they can be associated with acute renal failure.

Renal failure of recent onset should be promptly and vigorously managed. Intravascular depletion must be rapidly corrected by intravenous infusion of 0.9% saline, after which a high urinary output should be maintained whenever possible by continued saline and/or forced alkaline diuresis (which may help to prevent intratubular light-chain precipitation). Plasma exchange has been advocated to remove light chains more rapidly, but its value is unproven. In patients with oliguria, dialysis should be provided early. Recently, it has been shown that an extended haemodialysis protocol, using a new generation dialyser with very high permeability to proteins, was highly efficient in removing circulating free LC. In preliminary studies, this approach combined with chemotherapy, resulted in dialysis withdrawal in more than 60% of patients with myeloma cast nephropathy and severe renal failure.

Most patients with overt myeloma cast nephropathy should be promptly given chemotherapy to reduce the production of monoclonal light chains, which is justified because partial or complete recovery of renal function occurs in approximately one-half of patients. Only patients with refractory haematological disease should be given purely symptomatic treatment. However, median survival in those with progressive renal failure (about 2 years) remains shorter than that of patients without renal failure (3 to 4 years).

The optimum use of chemotherapy in patients with multiple myeloma and renal failure is uncertain. Conventional chemotherapies can induce remissions, but they have not markedly lengthened median survival. The low-dose oral melphalan–prednisone regimen has slow antitumour action, requires reduction of melphalan doses in patients with altered renal function, and melphalan interferes with any attempt at subsequent stem cell mobilization, hence this approach is reserved for older patients not eligible for more aggressive treatments. An intravenous regimen, such as VAD, induces earlier remission and is safer in those with renal failure because the drugs are metabolized in the liver, but the use of VAD has declined due to the neurotoxicity of vincristine. High-dose oral dexamethasone, which induces rapid decrease in serum free monoclonal light chains and has potent anti-inflammatory effects, can be introduced immediately after diagnosis and has the advantage of avoiding the use of a central line. It may be used alone or in combination with thalidomide, or with the proteasome inhibitor bortezomib, which appears to be well tolerated even in patients with severe renal failure. However, safety and efficiency of these protocols remain to be evaluated in controlled trials. Monitoring of serum free light chains should be performed to optimize therapy. In younger patients (those aged less than 60) with myeloma cast nephropathy and renal failure, high-dose chemotherapy with autologous stem cell transplantation should be considered because substantially longer survival can be achieved.

In patients with irreversible renal failure and in those whose renal function deteriorates later, regular dialysis may be indicated if allowed by the patient's general clinical condition. Recombinant human erythropoietin may be helpful to correct anaemia, although very high doses (and therefore great expense) are likely to be needed, and regular blood transfusion is often preferred.

Light-chain, light- and heavy-chain, and heavy-chain deposition disease

Definition and epidemiology

It has been known since the late 1950s that nonamyloidotic forms of glomerular disease resembling the lesion of diabetic glomerulosclerosis could occur in multiple myeloma. Randall and associates recognized the presence of monoclonal light chains in these lesions in 1976, defining light-chain deposition disease. Monoclonal heavy chains can also be found in association with light chains (defining light- and heavy-chain deposition disease), or occasionally in the absence of light chains (heavy-chain deposition disease). In clinical and pathological terms, light-chain deposition disease, light- and heavy-chain deposition disease, and heavy-chain deposition disease are similar and hence are also collectively referred to as (Randall-type) monoclonal Ig deposition disease (MIDD). They differ from amyloidosis by the lack of affinity for Congo red and fibrillar organization. MIDD occurs in a wide range of ages (31–79 years) with a slight male preponderance. Myeloma accounts for 45% of cases, but as in amyloidosis a monoclonal plasma cell proliferation can be found in virtually all patients by immunofluorescence examination of the bone marrow with specific anti-heavy and anti-light chain antisera.

Clinical presentation

Light-chain deposition disease is a systemic disease with deposition of Ig light chains along basement membranes in most tissues. However, deposition in tissues other than the kidney is often (but not always) totally asymptomatic and renal involvement dominates clinical presentation, mainly in the form of proteinuria and renal failure. In 23 to 67% of patients with light-chain deposition disease, albuminuria is associated with the nephrotic syndrome. In 25%, the urinary albumin output is less than 1 g/day, and these patients mainly exhibit a tubulointerstitial syndrome. Haematuria is more frequent (44%) than one would expect for a nephropathy in which cell proliferation is usually modest. Renal failure is remarkable for its high prevalence (89%), early appearance, and severity, irrespective of urinary albumin output. Hypertension occurs in approximately one-half of patients.

Diagnosis

Diagnosis of MIDD relies on the association of the clinical features described above with the finding of a monoclonal Ig component in the serum and/or the urine. Since this component cannot be detected even by immunofixation in 15 to 30% of patients, the diagnosis of MIDD is mostly made by renal biopsy. In virtually all patients with this condition tubular lesions are characterized by the deposition of periodic acid–Schiff-positive ribbon-like material along the basement membrane. This is usually associated with a marked interstitial fibrosis and nodular glomerulosclerosis (found in two-thirds of patients with light-chain deposition disease and in all patients with heavy-chain deposition disease reported so far). Nodules are composed of membrane-like material with nuclei at the periphery (Fig. 21.10.4.2). A key step in the diagnosis of the various forms of Randall-type MIDD is immunofluorescence examination of the biopsy specimen, revealing evidence of monotypic light- and/or heavy-chain deposits along glomerular and tubular basement membranes in all cases. By contrast with light-chain amyloidosis, the κ isotype is 2 to 3 times more frequent than the λ isotype, with a predominance of the Vκ4 subgroup. In those patients with heavy-chain deposition disease, a deletion of the first constant domain of the heavy chain can invariably be demonstrated by immunofluorescence analysis of the kidney specimen with specific antisera. Finally, nonfibrillar granular electron-dense deposits are visible by electron microscopy along tubular basement membranes and in glomerular lesions.

Treatment

The natural history of MIDD is more uncertain than that of light-chain amyloidosis because extrarenal deposits can be totally

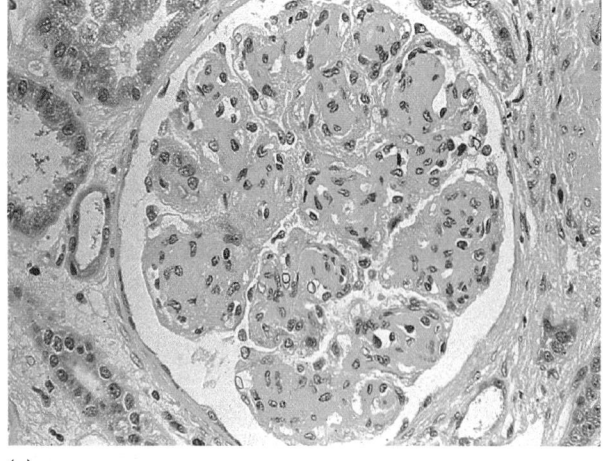

(a)

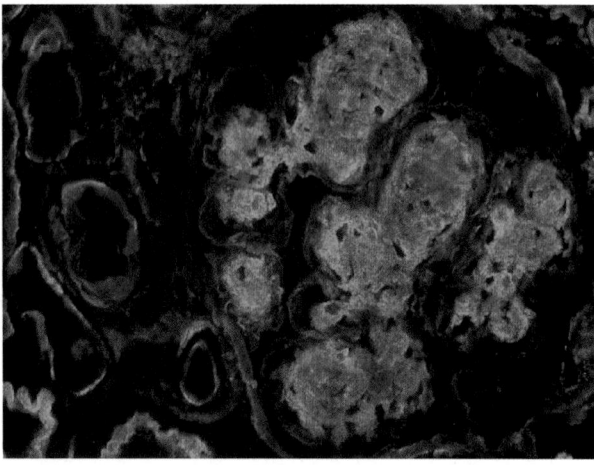

(b)

Fig. 21.10.4.2 Monoclonal Ig deposition disease. (a) Typical nodular glomerulosclerosis. Note the membrane-like material in the centre of the nodules and nuclei at the periphery. Some glomerular capillaries show double contours. Note also thickening of the basement membrane of atrophic tubules. Masson's trichrome stain, magnification ×312. (b) Bright staining of tubular basement membranes and mesangial nodules and, to a lesser extent, of glomerular basement membrane with anti-κ antibody in a case of κ light-chain deposition disease. Immunofluorescence, magnification ×312.

asymptomatic or cause severe organ damage, including severe heart failure, pulmonary disease, and occasionally hepatic insufficiency or portal hypertension. The 5-year actuarial rates for patient survival and survival free of endstage renal failure (with chemotherapy) are 70% and 39%, respectively.

Patients with MIDD and myeloma should be treated with conventional chemotherapy if they are over 60 years of age, but intensive chemotherapy with autologous stem cell transplantation should be discussed in younger patients (see above). The correct treatment for those without myeloma is uncertain, the rarity of the disease meaning that there are no controlled trials. Deposited light chains have disappeared in isolated instances after intensive therapy. A pragmatic approach is to use alkylating agents plus prednisone or dexamethasone in those with moderate but rapidly progressive renal insufficiency in an endeavour to prevent progression to endstage renal failure, but not to treat those with severe renal failure unless there are significant extrarenal complications.

Serial monitoring of serum free light chain concentrations using nephelometric immunoassay is mandatory to assess haematological response to therapy. Recurrence of the disease has usually been observed in the few patients who have received renal transplants.

Non-Randall-type MIDD

Few cases of proliferative glomerulonephritis with monoclonal Ig deposits that do not display the characteristic features of Randall-type MIDD have been described. Almost all patients present initially with renal failure, proteinuria, and microscopic haematuria, with nephrotic syndrome and hypertension in more than 50% of patients. Non-Randall-type MIDD is a renal-limited disease. Whereas a serum and/or urine monoclonal component is detected in 60% of patients, only 10% have evidence of associated lymphoproliferative or plasma cell disorder. Activation of the classical or alternative complement pathway is present in 25% of cases. Endocapillary proliferative glomerulonephritis or membranoproliferative glomerulonephritis are the most common patterns of glomerular lesions. Electron-dense granular deposits of nondeleted IgG, IgA, or light chain are located in mesangial and paramesangial areas, and in subendothelial and/or subepithelial areas of glomerular basement membranes. These deposits do not usually show significant organization at the ultrastructural level. At variance with Randall-type MIDD, deposits are not found around tubular basement membranes or in vascular walls around myocytes.

Nonamyloid fibrillary and immunotactoid/microtubular glomerulopathies

Definition and epidemiology

Fibrillary glomerulonephritis and immunotactoid glomerulopathy are characterized (respectively) by fibrillar and microtubular deposits in the mesangium and the glomerular capillary loops. These deposits do not have a β-pleated sheet organization and are readily distinguishable from amyloid by the larger thickness of fibrils and the lack of Congo red staining. Whether they are totally distinct entities has been the subject of considerable debate. However, it is now established that the distinction between the two diseases is of great clinical and pathophysiological interest in the context of plasma cell dyscrasias, because monotypic deposits are detected in 50 to 80% of immunotactoid/microtubular glomerulopathies (sometimes referred to as GOMMID), while they are found in fewer than 20% of fibrillary glomerulopathies.

The prevalence of glomerulopathy with nonamyloid deposition of fibrillary or tubular material in a nontransplant adult biopsy population is around 1%, but this is almost certainly an underestimate because insufficient attention is given to atypical reactions with histochemical stains for amyloid and also most specimens are not examined by electron microscopy. The age range extends from 10 to 80 years with a peak incidence between 40 and 60 years.

Clinical presentation

The usual presentation is with the nephrotic syndrome, microscopic haematuria, and hypertension. Extrarenal manifestations, including skin and peripheral nerve involvement, have been described, almost exclusively in immunotactoid/microtubular glomerulopathy, which—at variance with fibrillary glomerulopathy—often occurs in the setting of chronic lymphocytic leukaemia or lymphoma.

Diagnosis

Diagnosis relies entirely on analysis of the renal biopsy specimen by immunofluorescence microscopy with anti light chain and anti IgG subclass antibodies, and by electron microscopy. In immunotactoid/microtubular glomerulopathy this reveals either atypical membranous glomerulonephritis (often associated with segmental mesangial proliferation) or lobular membranoproliferative glomerulonephritis. Immunofluorescence shows coarse granular deposits of IgG and C3 along capillary basement membranes and in mesangial areas. Monotypic deposits composed of either IgG1, IgG2, or IgG3 (usually with a κ light chain) are common. Using sensitive techniques such as immunoblotting, a circulating monoclonal Ig is detected in approximately 60% of patients. Electron microscopy shows immunotactoid/microtubular glomerulopathy to be remarkable for the presence of organized deposits of thick-walled microtubules with a central hollow core, 10 to 60 nm in diameter (usually greater than 30 nm), at times arranged in parallel arrays (Fig. 21.10.4.3). When immunotactoid/microtubular glomerulopathy occurs in the setting of chronic lymphocytic leukaemia or related B-cell lymphoma, inclusions showing the same microtubular organization and containing the same IgG subclass and light-chain type as the renal deposits are often detected in the cytoplasm of leukaemic lymphocytes in the blood.

Mesangial proliferation and membranoproliferative glomerulonephritis are the commonest lesions observed in nonamyloid fibrillary glomerulonephritis. Immunofluorescence studies mainly show polyclonal IgG deposits of the γ4 isotype. Electron microscopy shows the fibrils, devoid of a central lumen, to be randomly arranged with a diameter varying between 12 and 22 nm. In almost all cases there is no evidence of associated lymphoproliferative disorder or monoclonal gammopathy.

Infection with hepatitis C virus has sometimes been reported in patients with nonamyloid fibrillary glomerulonephritis and immunotactoid glomerulopathy.

Treatment

In patients with GOMMID, especially in those with chronic lymphocytic leukaemia, corticosteroids and/or chemotherapy are associated with partial or complete remission of the nephrotic syndrome, parallel with improvement of the haematological condition. More variable results are obtained with these treatments in patients with crescentic fibrillary glomerulonephritis. Recurrence of these diseases has been reported in patients receiving a renal allograft.

Renal involvement in cryoglobulinaemia

Definition and epidemiology

Cryoglobulinaemia is a pathological condition in which the blood contains Igs that precipitate on cooling (4°C) and resolubilize on warming (37°C). According to Brouet's classification, there are three types of cryoglobulinaemia defined by their composition. Renal involvement is observed mainly in patients with mixed type II cryoglobulinaemia involving a monoclonal IgM (most often including a κ light chain) with rheumatoid factor activity and a polyclonal IgG. Type II cryoglobulinaemia can be associated with overt lymphoproliferative disorders of the B-cell lineage, although in many cases no underlying haematological disorder is found such that this type of cryoglobulinaemia has long been referred to as essential mixed cryoglobulinaemia. Glomerular disease may also occur in type I cryoglobulinaemia, composed of a single monoclonal Ig

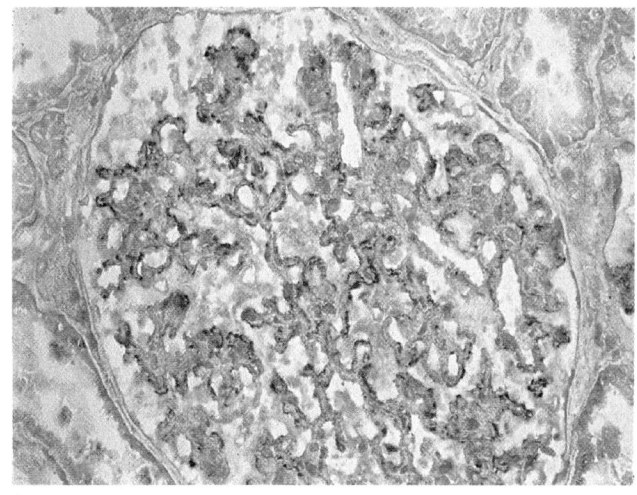
(a)

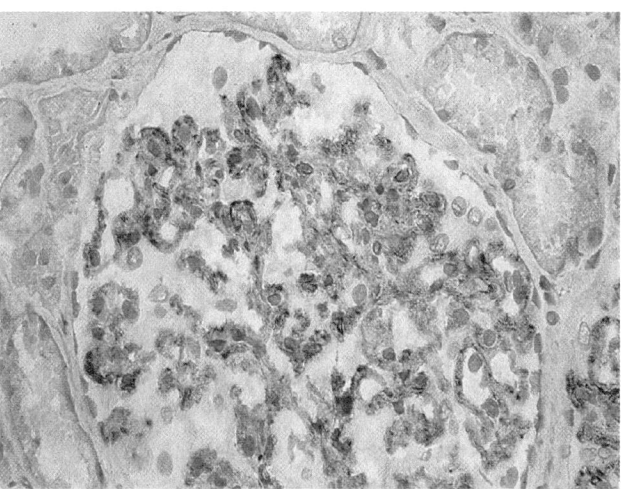
(b)

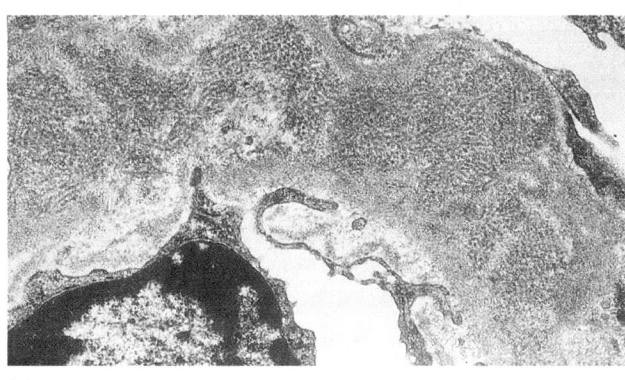
(c)

Fig. 21.10.4.3 Immunotactoid/microtubular glomerulopathy in a patient with chronic lymphocytic leukaemia. Atypical membranous glomerulonephritis showing exclusive staining of the deposits with anti-γ (a) and anti-κ (b) antibodies. Immunohistochemistry, alkaline phosphatase, magnification × 312. (c) Electron micrograph of glomerular basement membrane, showing the microtubular structure of the subepithelial deposits. Uranyl acetate and lead citrate, magnification × 12 000. (From Béatrice Mougenot's personal collection.)

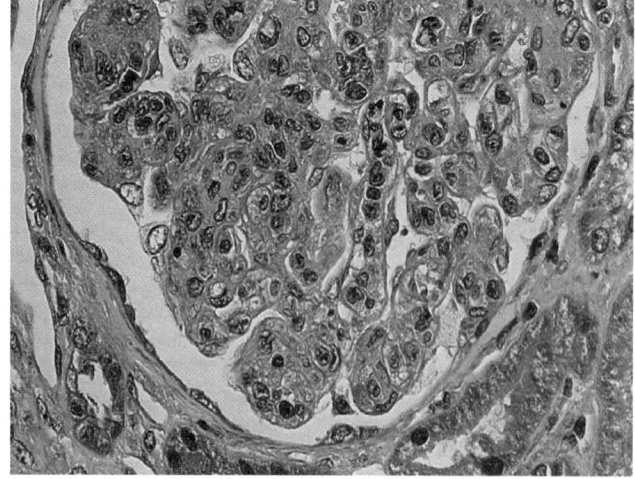

(a)

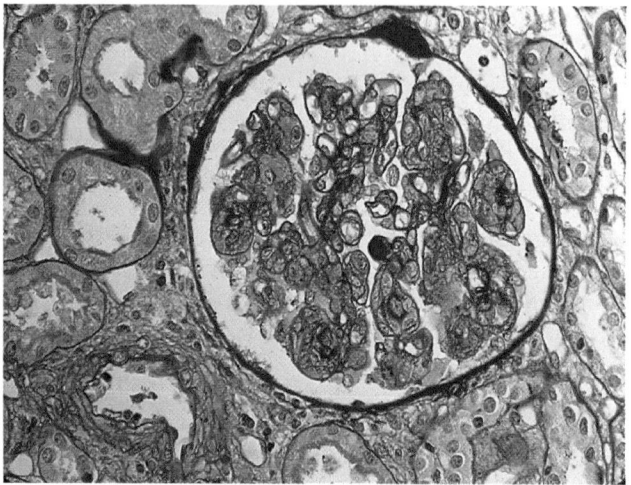

(b)

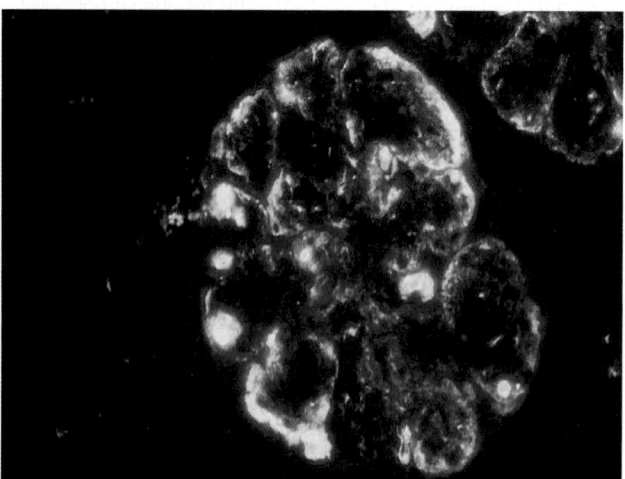

(c)

Fig. 21.10.4.4 Cryoglobulinaemic glomerulonephritis. (a) The glomerulus shows a marked endocapillary hypercellularity with massive infiltration of mononuclear leucocytes. Masson's trichrome stain, magnification × 500. (b) Frequent doublecontour aspect and intraluminal thrombi. Periodic acid–Schiff stain, magnification × 312. (c) Thrombi and segments of glomerular basement membrane are brightly stained with anti-IgM antibody. Immunofluorescence, magnification × 312. (From Béatrice Mougenot's personal collection.)

(mostly IgM or IgG), usually in the context of underlying lymphoproliferative or plasma cell disorder (see later).

Viral infections may trigger the formation of cryoglobulin. Whereas hepatitis B and Epstein–Barr virus infections have been implicated in the past, the role of hepatitis C virus infection is now recognized to be an important factor in the pathogenesis of type II cryoglobulinaemia. Antibodies to hepatitis C virus and hepatitis C virus RNA are found in the sera of most patients with type II cryoglobulinaemia, probably explaining the uneven geographical distribution of mixed cryoglobulinaemias, which predominate in southern Europe where hepatitis C infection is more prevalent.

The condition is commonest in adults in the fifth and the sixth decades of life, with a slight female predominance.

Clinical presentation

Renal disease most often occurs in patients with a long history of cryoglobulinaemia-related vasculitic symptoms, including palpable purpura (70%), arthralgias (50%), fatigue, Raynaud's phenomenon, peripheral neuropathy (22%), and hepatic involvement.

The renal disease may present as an acute nephritic syndrome (in 20 to 30% of patients) with gross haematuria, heavy proteinuria, hypertension, and renal failure of sudden onset, sometimes with oliguria (5% of patients). The pathological finding in these patients is membranoproliferative glomerulonephritis with the presence of numerous intraluminal thrombi and/or necrotic vasculitic lesions. Remission may occur spontaneously or during therapy, with relapses following in up to 20% of cases.

Most patients with mixed cryoglobulinaemia (55%) have an indolent and protracted renal course, presenting with proteinuria, haematuria, and hypertension. The usual renal lesion in this context is membranoproliferative glomerulonephritis, with some of the peculiarities described above.

Nephrotic syndrome affects another 20% of patients. Arterial hypertension is observed in more than 80% of patients at the time of onset of renal disease. Endstage renal disease develops in fewer than 10% of patients. It should be stressed that the overall risk of non-Hodgkin B-cell lymphomas is 35 times higher in patients with hepatitis C virus-related cryoglobulinaemia compared to the general population.

Diagnosis

Mixed type II cryoglobulinaemia should be suspected in patients with the clinical picture described above, an IgM rheumatoid factor, and a very low serum C4 fraction and total haemolytic activity of complement. In this context a careful search for the presence of cryoglobulin must be made, requiring that a blood sample from a fasting patient should be placed in warm water and taken promptly to the laboratory, which needs to be forewarned that such a sample will arrive.

Cryoglobulinaemia-related membranoproliferative glomerulonephritis usually shows several distinctive histological features, including massive subendothelial deposits filling the capillary lumen and forming so-called thrombi, and dramatic infiltration by leucocytes, mainly monocytes (Fig. 21.10.4.4). The thrombi are brightly stained with anti-μ and anti-κ antibodies and present a microtubular crystalline structure similar to that of the cryoprecipitate. These glomerular changes may be associated with acute vasculitis of the small and medium-sized arteries (33%) and lymphocytic infiltrates in the interstitium. Crescentic extracapillary proliferation is rare and always limited.

Treatment

The best treatment of mixed cryoglobulinaemia is not firmly established because the course of the disease is unpredictable and acute exacerbations may remit spontaneously. In patients with moderate renal and extrarenal manifestations, immunosuppressive agents are not indicated. In those with hepatitis C virus infection, combined pegylated interferon and ribavirin for at least 1 year appears to be the treatment of choice, the dose of the latter being adapted according to renal function to prevent haemolytic anaemia, which may require supplementary recombinant erythropoietin therapy. In more severe cases, particularly those with signs of systemic vasculitis, high-dose steroids, plasma exchange, and cyclophosphamide or monoclonal anti-CD20 antibody (rituximab) are indicated. Rituximab, which is usually well tolerated, appears to be as efficient as cyclophosphamide. Because ribavirin and pegylated interferon are not recommended in patients with advanced renal failure, standard interferon should be used for controlling virus replication enhanced by steroids and/or immunosuppressive agents. Hypertension needs to be carefully controlled because cardiovascular complications are the major causes of death.

Renal involvement in Waldenström's macroglobulinaemia

A glomerulonephritis with intracapillary thrombi of monoclonal IgM is rare, but is almost specific for Waldenström's macroglobulinaemia. It is characterized by periodic acid-Schiff-positive, noncongophilic endomembranous deposits in a variable number of capillary loops, which are sometimes so large as to occlude the capillary lumen either partially or completely, thus forming thrombi. There may also be a B-cell interstitial infiltrate. Renal presentation is with proteinuria or renal impairment. Some patients have a cryoglobulin, in others the amount of circulating IgM seems to be higher than that in patients with Waldenström's macroglobulinaemia without obvious renal involvement, or with amyloidosis, leading to the suggestion that hyperviscosity is important in the pathogenesis of the renal lesion. The haematological condition is treated on its own merits (see Chapter 22.4.5). In those with acute renal failure there is anecdotal experience that plasma exchange can be effective in restoring renal function at least temporarily, allowing time for other treatments to be applied.

Renal involvement in lymphomas and leukaemias

Renal complications of lymphomas and leukaemias are summarized in Box 21.10.4.1. All patients with unexplained renal failure should undergo ultrasound examination of the kidney, which should be arranged as a matter of urgency, to identify either enlarged kidneys due to tumour infiltration or hydronephrosis. The presence of heavy albuminuria in this setting is suggestive of paraneoplastic glomerulopathy.

Hodgkin's disease and non-Hodgkin's lymphoma

Glomerulonephritis is a rare complication of lymphoma, most often described in patients with Hodgkin's disease, of whom 0.4% have minimal-change disease and 0.1% have AA amyloidosis. This low incidence of amyloidosis in patients with Hodgkin's disease is

---

Box 21.10.4.1 Renal complications of lymphomas and leukaemias

- Mechanical complications
  - Infiltration of renal parenchyma
  - Obstructive uropathy (retroperitoneal fibrosis)
  - Compression of renal artery or vein
- Electrolyte disturbances and disseminated intravascular coagulation
- Glomerulopathies (including amyloidosis)
- Treatment-induced complications
  - Tumour lysis syndrome
  - Lithiasis and urate nephropathy
  - Radiation nephropathy
  - Drug-induced toxic nephropathy
  - Thrombotic microangiopathy and mesangiolysis

---

most likely attributable to modern treatment protocols that induce rapid remission. Hodgkin's lymphoma-related minimal-change disease shows features of a paraneoplastic glomerulopathy. The nephrotic syndrome usually appears early, revealing the haemopathy in about one-half of the cases; it rapidly disappears after effective treatment of the underlying condition; and it usually relapses simultaneously with the haemopathy. Cases of crescentic glomerulonephritis with rapidly progressive renal failure due to antiglomerular basement antibodies have also been reported.

Glomerulonephritis may also occur in patients with non-Hodgkin's lymphoma, including both T- and B-cell proliferations. In these conditions, unlike in Hodgkin's lymphoma, minimal-change disease is uncommon, and membranoproliferative glomerulonephritis and necrotizing crescentic glomerulonephritis with or without vasculitis are the most frequent lesions. Some cases are associated with type I cryoglobulinaemia or GOMMID. In other cases the association between non-Hodgkin's lymphoma and renal disease may be coincidental. Presenting renal symptoms are nephrotic syndrome and/or renal impairment. Full remission of these symptoms can be achieved in some patients by aggressive therapy of the lymphoma.

Chronic lymphocytic leukaemia and low-grade B-cell lymphoma

These haemopathies, particularly chronic lymphocytic leukaemia, have been reported in association with glomerular disease in about 50 cases. Most commonly the nephropathy, usually manifesting as nephrotic syndrome with impaired renal function, and the leukaemia are detected simultaneously. The most frequent glomerular disease is membranoproliferative glomerulonephritis with or without cryoglobulinaemia (mostly type I). In type I cryoglobulinaemic glomerulonephritis, glomerular monoclonal Ig deposits often display an ultrastructural organization into microtubules, and less frequently into crystals. In the absence of cryoglobulinaemia, a molecular link can be established between the haemopathy and the glomerulopathy when monotypic Ig deposits are found in the glomerulus, which can occur even in the absence of detectable circulating M component. As discussed previously, some of these patients present with typical immunotactoid/microtubular glomerulopathy or MIDD. Improvement of the nephropathy after treatment for the leukaemia is well described.

Acute leukaemias

Disseminated intravascular coagulation has been associated with acute progranulocytic leukaemia. Other renal complications are commonly due to treatment, most particularly the tumour lysis syndrome (see below).

POEMS syndrome

POEMS syndrome is a rare condition defined by the presence of peripheral neuropathy, organomegaly, endocrinopathy (excluding diabetes mellitus or hypothyroidism), monoclonal plasma cell disorder (IgA, IgG, or IgM, almost always associated with a λ light chain), and skin changes. The association of POEMS syndrome with osteosclerotic myeloma or Castleman's disease is common. Although the pathophysiology of the disease is unknown, POEMS syndrome is characterized by increased production of proinflammatory cytokines (interleukin-1 and 6, tumour necrosis factor-α) and vascular endothelial growth factor. Renal disease may occur, which usually manifests as proteinuria, haematuria, and renal failure that may progress to endstage renal failure. Kidney biopsy reveals lesions resembling thrombotic microangiopathy, with glomerular enlargement, cellular proliferation, and mesangiolysis with marked swelling of endothelial and mesangial cells, associated with endarteritis-like lesions in the small renal arteries. The monoclonal component is usually not deposited in kidney.

Tumour lysis syndrome

Tumour lysis syndrome is a life-threatening metabolic emergency. It occurs in patients with haemopathies involving a high cell turnover, such as Burkitt's lymphoma or acute leukaemia, mostly at the onset of chemotherapy and/or on radiation therapy. The ensuing massive cytolysis generates high levels of uric acid, phosphate, potassium, and xanthine (especially in patients treated with allopurinol), with a concomitant decrease in serum calcium concentration. Oliguric or anuric acute renal failure may occur, especially in those who are dehydrated or have pre-existing impairment of kidney function. This acute renal failure is mostly the consequence of acute precipitation of urate crystals in the tubular lumen, but in those with a moderate increase in uric acid concentration the role of severe hyperphosphataemia causing precipitation of calcium/phosphate complexes in renal interstitium and the tubular system has been assumed.

Prevention is better than cure, and intensive monitoring is mandatory to prevent the development and the consequences of this syndrome. Patients at risk of the tumour lysis syndrome should be vigorously hydrated with 0.9% saline (assuming normal or near normal baseline renal function, and with care taken to avoid inducing pulmonary oedema) before receiving chemotherapy or radiotherapy. Urinary alkalinization should be used with caution because it may induce phosphate precipitation. Reduction of urate production with allopurinol, which increases the risk of formation of xanthine nephropathy/stones due to accumulation of xanthine, should be reserved for patients at low risk for developing tumour lysis syndrome. In high-risk patients (high tumour burden, aggressive chemotherapy, hypovolaemia) with hyperuricaemia, recombinant modified urate oxidase (rasburicase) should be preferred, which rapidly reduces the uric acid pool, prevents accumulation of xanthine and hypoxanthine, and does not require alkalinization for effect. Rasburicase is also indicated in the treatment of established tumour lysis syndrome, associated with vigorous hydration with 0.9% saline to encourage urinary output in patients passing urine, with close clinical monitoring to prevent iatrogenic fluid overload. Patients with severe acute renal failure should be treated with haemodialysis, which allows recovery of renal function following the reduction of serum phosphate and serum uric acid concentrations.

Further reading

Touchard G (2003). Ultrastructural pattern and classification of renal monoclonal immunoglobulin deposits. In: Touchard G, *et al.* (eds) *Monoclonal gammopathies and the kidney*, pp. 95–117. Kluwer, Dordrecht.

Renal involvement in Ig light-chain amyloidosis

Comenzo RL, Gertz MA (2002). Autologous stem cell transplantation for primary systemic amyloidosis. *Blood*, **99**, 4276–82.
Guidelines Working group of UK Myeloma Forum; British Committee for Standards in Haematology; British Society for Haematology (2004). Guidelines on the diagnosis and management of AL amyloidosis. *Br J Haematol*, **125**, 681–700.
Jaccard A, *et al.* (2007). High-dose melphalan versus melphalan plus dexamethasone for AL amyloidosis. *N Engl J Med*, **357**, 1083–93.
Kyle RA, Gertz MA (1995). Primary systemic amyloidosis: clinical and laboratory features in 474 cases. *Semin Hematol*, **32**, 45–59.
Ronco PM, Aucouturier P, Moulin B (2010). Renal amyloidosis and glomerular diseases with monoclonal immunoglobulin deposition. In: Feehally J et Johnson R (eds) *Comprehensive Clinical Nephrology*, in press. Mosby, London.
Skinner M, *et al.* (2004). High-dose melphalan and autologous stem-cell transplantation in patients with AL amyloidosis: an 8-year study. *Ann Intern Med*, **140**, 85–93.

Renal involvement in myeloma

Chanan-Khan AA, *et al.* (2007). Activity and safety of bortezomib in multiple myeloma patients with advanced renal failure: a multicenter retrospective study. *Blood*, **109**, 2604–6.
Hutchison CA, *et al.* (2007). Efficient removal of immunoglobulin free light chains by hemodialysis for multiple myeloma: in vitro and in vivo studies. *J Am Soc Nephrol*, **18**, 886–95.
Korbet SM, Schwartz MM (2006). Multiple myeloma. *J Am Soc Nephrol*, **17**, 2533–45.
Ronco PM, Aucouturier P, Mougenot B (2005). Kidney involvement in plasma cell dyscrasias. In: Davison, Cameron, Grünfeld, Kerr et Ritz, Winearls (eds) *Oxford textbook of Clinical Nephrology*, 3rd edition, vol 2, pp. 709–32. Oxford University Press, Oxford.

Light-chain, light and heavy-chain, heavy-chain deposition disease

Heilman RL, *et al.* (1992). Long-term follow-up and response to chemotherapy in patients with light-chain deposition disease. *Am J Kidney Dis*, **20**, 34–41.
Lin J, *et al.* (2001). Renal monoclonal immunoglobulin deposition disease: the disease spectrum. *J Am Soc Nephrol*, **12**, 1482–92.
Moulin B, *et al.* (1999). Nodular glomerulosclerosis with deposition of monoclonal immunoglobulin heavy chains lacking C_H1. *J Am Soc Nephrol*, **10**, 519–28.

Pozzi C, et al. (2003). Light chain deposition disease with renal involvement: clinical characteristics and prognostic factors. *Am J Kidney Dis*, **42**, 1154–63.

Ronco PM, Aucouturier P, Moulin B (1999). Renal amyloidosis and plasma cell dyscrasia-related glomerulopathies. In: Feehally J, Johnson R (eds) *Comprehensive nephrology*, section 5, chapter 31, pp. 1–14. Mosby, London.

Royer B, et al. (2004). High dose chemotherapy in light chain or light and heavy chain deposition disease. *Kidney Int*, **65**, 642–48.

Non-Randall-type MIDD

Nasr SH, et al. (2004). Proliferative glomerulonephritis with monoclonal IgG deposits: a distinct entity mimicking immune-complex glomerulonephritis. *Kidney Int*, **65**, 85–96.

Touchard G (2003). Ultrastructural pattern and classification of renal monoclonal immunoglobulin deposits. In: Touchard G, et al. (eds) *Monoclonal gammopathies and the kidney*, pp. 95–117. Kluwer, Dordrecht.

Nonamyloid fibrillary and immunotactoid glomerulopathies

Brady HR (1998). Fibrillary glomerulopathy. *Kidney Int*, **53**, 1421–29.

Bridoux F, et al. (2002). Fibrillary glomerulonephritis and immunotactoid (microtubular) glomerulopathy are associated with distinct immunologic features. *Kidney Int*, **62**, 1764–75.

Fogo A, Qureshi N, Horn RG (1993). Morphologic and clinical features of fibrillary glomerulonephritis versus immunotactoid glomerulopathy. *Am J Kidney Dis*, **22**, 367–77.

Rosenstock JL, et al. (2003). Fibrillary and immunotactoid glomerulonephritis: distinct entities with different clinical and pathologic features. *Kidney Int*, **63**, 1450–61.

Touchard G, et al. (1994). Glomerulonephritis with organized microtubular monoclonal immunoglobulin deposits. *Adv Nephrol Necker Hosp*, **23**, 149–75.

Renal involvement in cryoglobulinaemia

Brouet JC, et al. (1974). Biologic and clinical significance of cryoglobulins. A report of 86 cases. *Am J Med*, **57**, 775–88.

D'Amico G (1998). Renal involvement in hepatitis C infection: cryoglobulinemic glomerulonephritis. *Kidney Int*, **54**, 650–71.

Matignon M, et al. (2009). Clinical and morphologic spectrum of renal involvement in patients with mixed cryoglobulinemia without evidence of hepatitis C virus infection. *Medicine (Baltimore)*, **88**, 341–48.

Saadoun D, et al. (2006). Antiviral therapy for hepatitis C virus-associated mixed cryoglobulinemia vasculitis. *Arthritis Rheum*, **54**, 3696–706.

Sansonno D, et al. (2003). Monoclonal antibody treatment of mixed cryoglobulinemia resistant to interferon alfa with an anti-CD20. *Blood*, **101**, 3818–26.

Renal involvement in Waldenström's macroglobulinaemia

Audard V, et al. (2008). Renal lesions associated with IgM-secreting monoclonal proliferations: revisiting the disease spectrum. *Clin J Am Soc Nephrol*, **3**, 1339–49.

Harada Y, et al. (2000). Nephrotic syndrome caused by protein thrombi in glomerulocapillary lumen in Waldenström's macroglobulinaemia. *Br J Haematol*, **110**, 880–83.

Veltman GA, et al. (1997). Renal disease in Waldenström's macroglobulinaemia. *Nephrol Dial Transplant*, **12**, 1256–59.

Renal involvement in lymphomas and leukaemias

Moulin B, et al. (1992). Glomerulonephritis in chronic lymphocytic leukemia and related B-cell lymphomas. *Kidney Int*, **42**, 127–35.

Ronco PM (1999). Paraneoplastic glomerulopathies: new insights into an old entity. *Kidney Int*, **56**, 355–77.

Renal involvement in POEMS syndrome

Nakamoto Y, et al. (1999). A spectrum of clinicopathological features of nephropathy associated with POEMS syndrome. *Nephrol Dial Transplant*, **14**, 2370–8.

Tumour lysis syndrome

Cairo MS, Bishop M (2004). Tumour lysis syndrome: new therapeutic strategies and classification. *Br J Haematol*, **127**, 3–11.

Haas M, et al. (1999). The spectrum of acute renal failure in tumour lysis syndrome. *Nephrol Dial Transplant*, **14**, 776–9.

Rampello E, et al. (2006). The management of tumor lysis syndrome. *Nat Clin Pract Oncol*, **3**, 438–47.

21.10.5 Haemolytic uraemic syndrome

Paul Warwicker and Timothy H.J. Goodship

Essentials

The haemolytic uraemic syndrome (HUS) is characterized by the triad of: (1) microangiopathic haemolytic anaemia, (2) thrombocytopenia, and (3) acute renal failure. Endothelial cell activation leads to a change in phenotype from an anticoagulant to a procoagulant state.

Diarrhoeal associated (D+) HUS—this accounts for over 90% of cases and is the commonest cause of acute renal failure in children. The usual pathogen is enterohaemorrhagic *Escherichia coli*, notably *E. coli* O157:H7, and the commonest vehicle for transmission is ground (minced) beef. Release of a microbial toxin (verocytotoxin) inhibits ribosomal function and causes severe illness (mortality of 3–5%, renal replacement therapy is required in 50%). Treatment is supportive as no specific treatment has yet been proved to be beneficial, although plasma exchange is often used.

Nondiarrhoeal (D–) HUS—this can be familial (with 60% of cases having mutations in various complement components), or related to drugs (ciclosporin, tacrolimus, various cytotoxic drugs, etc.), pregnancy (also known as postpartum renal failure), infections (e.g. HIV), systemic disorders (e.g. systemic lupus erythematosus), malignancies, or transplantation (e.g. renal), or is of unknown cause (idiopathic). Treatment is supportive, with plasma exchange also used in most cases. There is a 50% risk of recurrence after renal transplantation.

Introduction

The haemolytic uraemic syndrome (HUS) is characterized by the triad of microangiopathic haemolytic anaemia (Coombs' test negative), thrombocytopenia, and acute renal failure. Thrombotic thrombocytopenic purpura (TTP) is characterized by the same criteria but with the addition of neurological manifestations and fever. HUS can be divided into diarrhoeal-associated (D+) and nondiarrhoeal-associated (D−) disease (Box 21.10.5.1), the latter also being known as atypical (aHUS) or non-Shiga toxin HUS.

Pathogenesis of HUS

All the conditions listed in Box 21.10.5.1 are characterized by endothelial cell activation, which consists of five core changes: loss of vascular integrity, expression of leucocyte adhesion molecules, cytokine production, up-regulation of HLA molecules, and a change in phenotype from an anticoagulant to a procoagulant state. It is the latter that predisposes to the development of a thrombotic microangiopathy.

The factors that in the context of HUS result in endothelial cell activation include antiendothelial antibodies, immune complexes, lipopolysaccharide, toxins, complement, and drugs. The anticoagulant state of the endothelium is maintained by lack of constitutive expression of tissue factor, endothelial expression of heparin, tissue-plasminogen activator, and thrombomodulin, and local secretion of vasoactive substances preventing platelet aggregation, including nitric oxide, prostacyclin, and adenosine. After endothelial activation many of these changes are reversed, in particular both tissue factor and tissue-plasminogen activator inhibitor (tPAI) are expressed. In addition von Willebrand's factor (vWF) is synthesized and secreted in increased amounts, promoting platelet aggregation by binding to the $\alpha_{iiib}\beta_3$ integrins on the platelet surface and also to the endothelial matrix. Down-regulation of this process is achieved by endothelial secretion of a metalloproteinase (ADAMTS13) that cleaves vWF, rendering it inactive. There have been many descriptions previously of phenomena associated with HUS, such as complement activation and the secretion of ultralarge vWF, selectins, and tPAI-I, and a causal relationship has been proposed. In retrospect, many of these observations merely reflect

---

Box 21.10.5.1 A classification of HUS

D+ HUS

◆ *Escherichia coli* O157:H7

◆ Other infective causes

D− HUS

◆ Idiopathic

◆ Familial

◆ Transplantation

◆ Drug related

◆ Pregnancy related

◆ Malignancy related

◆ HIV related

◆ Other infective causes

◆ Immunological disorders

◆ 'HUS-like' syndromes:

　• Scleroderma renal crisis

　• Accelerated hypertension

　• Severe acute vascular rejection of renal allograft

---

a state of endothelial activation. However, if the mechanisms that are responsible for down-regulating the sequelae of endothelial activation are impaired, then it is possible that a procoagulant state will be maintained. This has been shown for both HUS (overactivity of the alternative complement pathway) and TTP (antibodies against and deficiency of ADAMTS13).

Histopathology

In D+ HUS it is predominantly the glomerular endothelium that is affected (hence termed thrombotic glomerulopathy), while in D− HUS it is the endothelium of the preglomerular vessels (hence termed arterial thrombotic microangiopathy). In addition, in some forms of D− HUS there is severe intimal proliferation and luminal stenosis affecting arterioles and interlobular arteries, and the subendothelial spaces are widened and may contain fibrin deposits.

Diagnosis and laboratory features

The diagnosis of HUS is based on demonstrating the aforementioned triad of microangiopathic haemolytic anaemia, thrombocytopenia, and acute renal failure. It should be considered and excluded in all cases of acute renal failure whose cause is not obvious, especially those associated with diarrhoea and/or severe hypertension.

The anaemia of HUS may be severe, with features of haemolysis, including raised lactate dehydrogenase which can be used as a marker of disease, a reticulocytosis, increased unconjugated bilirubin, and decreased haptoglobin. Coombs' test is negative. Careful examination of a blood film may reveal fragmented and deformed cells. Thrombocytopenia ranges from severe to mild; 50% of patients will have platelet counts greater than 100×10^9/litre. There may be an associated leucocytosis, the extent of which is correlated with disease severity in D+ HUS. Fibrinogen degradation products may be raised, but clotting tests are characteristically normal; if they are deranged, then septicaemia and disseminated intravascular coagulation should be considered. Urinalysis usually shows microscopic haematuria and proteinuria. Urine output may be reduced, although nonoliguric renal failure is also seen.

Hyponatraemia may complicate D+ HUS and may be associated with seizures. Hyperkalaemia is occasionally severe. Complement levels should be measured as C3 is often low in both D+ HUS, where it is associated with a poor prognosis, and D− HUS, where it is associated with recurring or familial types of disease. In appropriate risk groups HIV infection should also be considered.

Diarrhoeal (D+) HUS

Incidence

This is the commonest form of HUS, accounting for over 90% of cases in industrialized countries. It is the commonest cause of acute renal failure in children and is associated with a diarrhoeal prodrome, hence D+ HUS. The bloody diarrhoea is caused by bacterial infection, predominantly with strains of enterohaemorrhagic *Escherichia coli*, notably *E. coli* O157:H7. This strain has only recently become a significant health hazard, with the first descriptions of haemorrhagic colitis and HUS associated with it in 1983. Since then there has been a rapid increase in the number of cases reported. The usual vehicle for transmission is ground (minced) beef, but a wide variety of other agents can be responsible. One of the largest and most serious outbreaks was the Central Scotland outbreak of 1996, where 496 individuals were infected, 27 developed HUS, and 18 died. Other diarrhoeal pathogens, particularly *Shigella dysenteriae* type 1, can also cause D+ HUS.

Clinical features

E. coli is very virulent, with as few as 50 organisms causing disease. The bacteria adhere to the large bowel and release a toxin, known as verocytotoxin or Shiga toxin, into the blood stream. This toxin belongs to the ribosomal inhibitory protein group of proteins, which are among the most potent toxins known. They include ricin, which gained notoriety in 1978 when an iridium pellet containing trace amounts was injected with the aid of an umbrella into the calf of the Bulgarian dissident journalist, Georgi Markov, on Waterloo bridge in London. He subsequently died from multiorgan failure. These toxins consist of five β-subunits and a single α-subunit. The β-subunit binds to Gb3, a glycolipid found in the membranes of eukaryotic cells. After endocytosis, the α-subunit blocks protein synthesis at the ribosome.

The delay between exposure and illness is on average 3 days, typically starting with abdominal cramps and diarrhoea, which becomes bloody over the following 2 days. Most patients then recover, although late sequelae such as colonic strictures and chronic pancreatitis are seen, but between 3 and 20% go on to develop HUS of varying severity. Approximately 50% of D+ HUS patients require renal replacement therapy, 5% are left with chronic renal failure, and 3 to 5% die of the acute illness. Between 15 and 40% of those that recover show evidence of persistent renal damage with proteinuria and/or hypertension. Acute neurological complications such as cerebrovascular accident, seizures, and coma develop in approximately 25% of D+ HUS patients.

Diagnosis

E. coli O157:H7 infection is diagnosed by stool culture and subsequent detection of the O157:H7 antigen. It is also possible to detect antibodies to the O157 lipopolysaccharide in convalescent sera, although this is of limited use in acute illness and is not widely available.

Treatment

Identification of infection and early diagnosis of HUS is important. However, it is not clear whether antibiotics in the early stages are of benefit, and it is possible that they may increase the risk of developing HUS, as may antimotility agents. Treatment of D+ HUS is predominantly supportive, including careful fluid and electrolyte balance, control of hypertension, nutritional support, and renal replacement therapy if necessary. Vigilance should be maintained for complications such as ischaemic colitis, myocardial dysfunction, and pancreatitis. There is little evidence for the benefit of either plasma exchange or plasma infusion, but plasma exchange continues to be used, particularly in complicated and prolonged cases. No specific treatment has yet been found to be beneficial.

Prevention and good public health policies are likely to be of utmost importance in the future. The outbreak in Scotland led to the commissioning of the Pennington report, with recommendations for disease prevention ranging from the 'farm to the table'.

Nondiarrhoeal (D−) HUS
Types of D− HUS
Idiopathic

Idiopathic, also known as sporadic, HUS accounts for about 5 to 10% of cases. It is typically insidious, although it may present following an upper respiratory tract infection. All ages are affected, and there is no seasonal incidence. Severe hypertension is frequent and mortality is higher than in D+ HUS. Renal involvement is usually pronounced, with significant proteinuria and uraemia. The disease may recur in both native kidneys and allografts.

Familial HUS can present as an apparently sporadic case until the true diagnosis is revealed when other family members become affected. A search for a genetic predisposition for idiopathic HUS has focused on dysfunction of components of the complement pathway, case reports and series often revealing hypocomplementaemia for C3 indicating overactivity of the alternative complement pathway (see familial HUS).

Familial

HUS may be inherited in both autosomal recessive and autosomal dominant forms. In phenotype, familial HUS most closely resembles idiopathic HUS with severe hypertension a prominent feature, being found in approximately 80% of autosomal dominant and 40% of autosomal recessive cases. There is usually no diarrhoeal prodrome, prognosis is poor, mortality is high (often over 50%), and recurrence is common. Management includes aggressive control of blood pressure, particularly with angiotensin-converting enzyme (ACE) inhibitors, careful fluid balance, and plasma exchange (although it is often unsuccessful in reversing the disease).

Although familial HUS is rare, it has afforded an opportunity to elucidate underlying mechanisms predisposing to D− HUS. Genetic linkage of the familial form of the disease to chromosome 1q32 established that D− HUS is a disease of complement dysregulation. In 60% of patients mutations have been found in various complement components, including factor H (a soluble regulator), membrane cofactor protein (a transmembrane regulator), factor I (a serine protease that cleaves C3Bb), C3, and factor B. In addition, antifactor H antibodies have been described in some patients with D− HUS.

Transplantation

Both *de novo* and recurrent HUS are seen following renal transplantation. HUS is a well-established side-effect of both ciclosporin and tacrolimus, and other risk factors include acute rejection, cytomegalovirus (CMV) infection, and simultaneous kidney/pancreas transplantation. Treatment includes discontinuation of the drug, substitution of other immunosuppressive agents, and plasma exchange.

HUS is also seen in other forms of transplantation, particularly bone marrow, where 6 to 26% of patients show evidence of a microangiopathy. The aetiology is unclear, but may be related to endothelial damage secondary to total body irradiation, intensive conditioning chemotherapy, ciclosporin, CMV infection, or graft-versus-host disease. Management is supportive, including renal replacement therapy, aggressive treatment of hypertension with ACE inhibitors, and withdrawal of ciclosporin. Plasma exchange with fresh frozen plasma replacement may be of benefit, but in the more fulminant forms treatment is usually unsuccessful and prognosis is poor.

Drug related

Other drugs besides ciclosporin and tacrolimus are associated with HUS. In particular, several cytotoxic drugs used in chemotherapy can be complicated by the syndrome (so-called C-HUS or cancer chemotherapy HUS), including mitomycin C, 5-fluorouracil, and cisplatin, either alone or in combination with daunorubicin, vinblastine, and bleomycin. The disease may be associated with severe hypertension, pulmonary oedema (often after transfusion of blood products), neurological features, and a high mortality (60–75% in some series). With mitomycin C the disease is dose related, and it is rarely seen in patients receiving less than $30\,mg/m^2$, but more frequently at doses above $60\,mg/m^2$, with an incidence of 2 to 15% and presentation usually weeks or months after the last treatment, often when the patient is in clinical remission. Few treatments have proven effective, although staphylococcal protein A column perfusion to remove circulating immune complexes seems to be more effective than plasma exchange and may be of benefit in less severe forms of the disease.

Other drugs implicated in HUS include crack cocaine, ticlopidine, and quinine. Use of the oral contraceptive is also said to be associated with HUS, although with such a commonly prescribed formulation it is difficult to be certain whether the association is coincidental. However, it is wise to advise against its use in survivors of D− HUS and in families with inherited HUS.

Pregnancy related

HUS is seen in pregnancy with an incidence of approximately 1 in 25 000. Presentation is usually peripartum, or within several weeks postpartum (also known as postpartum renal failure). Changes in pregnancy that may predispose to HUS include increased concentrations of procoagulant factors, decreased fibrinolytic activity, and reduced expression of endothelial thrombomodulin. In women presenting in the third trimester, differentiation from severe forms of pre-eclampsia such as the HELLP syndrome (haemolysis, elevated liver enzymes, and low platelets) may be difficult. Pre-eclamptic syndromes tend to be associated with less severe forms of haemolytic anaemia, the presence of hepatocellular necrosis, and rapid improvement following delivery. Features of pregnancy-related HUS include severe hypertension, neurological symptoms, fever, and renal failure requiring renal replacement therapy. Although plasma exchange increases survival rates, maternal mortality remains between 5 and 20%, and preterm delivery and intrauterine fetal death (approximately 30%) are frequent complications. Long-term follow-up is important because of the later development of renal failure and hypertension. About 50% of patients will have a recurrence, not only during a further pregnancy but at other times as well, which suggests a genetic predisposition.

Malignancy related

HUS is associated with malignancy, particularly adenocarcinoma. Patients with a gastric primary and metastatic disease are at particular risk.

HIV related

There are several forms of nephropathy associated with HIV infection, including a thrombotic microangiopathy with features resembling both idiopathic HUS and TTP. Before the advent of highly active antiretroviral therapy (HAART) the incidence of HUS in HIV-infected patients was approximately 1%, usually presenting in later stages of the disease and occasionally being the first presentation. The incidence is now less, but the diagnosis should be considered in the differential diagnosis of HUS and TTP in high-risk groups and patients originating from a high prevalence area. The p24 antigen in endothelial cells may reflect either a direct cytopathic effect of the virus or functional impairment of the endothelium. Concurrent CMV infection has also been associated with HUS. Neurological involvement is common and severe hypertension is a prominent feature. Treatment with plasma exchange can lead to renal recovery, but overall prognosis is poor and few patients survive a year from diagnosis. ACE inhibitors are used in other forms of HIV-associated nephropathy and would seem a logical choice to treat the hypertension.

Other infective causes

Occasionally nondiarrhoeal bacterial infections are associated with HUS. Pneumococcus and some *Clostridia* spp. can produce neuraminidase which strips sialic acid from cell membranes, exposing the cryptic Thomsen–Friedenreich antigen on erythrocytes, platelets, and glomerular cells. An IgM antibody, present in most plasma, causes agglutination, endothelial injury, and HUS. Plasma exchange is therefore contraindicated and treatment consists of washed red cells and antibiotics. Difficulty in red cell typing and a blood film demonstrating both agglutination and red cell fragments may give a clue to diagnosis. Capnocytophaga sepsis from dog bites has also been associated with cases of HUS.

Systemic disorders

HUS has been reported in association with systemic lupus erythematosus, primary antiphospholipid syndrome, and cobalamin C disease. This last disease is characterized by methylmalonic aciduria and homocystinuria, and is the most common inborn error of cobalamin metabolism.

'HUS-like' syndromes

The renal crisis of systemic sclerosis can be clinically and histologically indistinguishable from idiopathic D− HUS, and a diagnosis of systemic sclerosis is often made retrospectively from serological markers or with the development of other features of the disease. Likewise, the thrombotic microangiopathy of accelerated hypertension may be difficult to distinguish from HUS. The most important aspect of treatment in these syndromes is good control of blood pressure, and ACE inhibitors or angiotensin II receptor antagonists should be prescribed early, balanced with the requirement to reduce blood pressure gradually. In the renal crisis of systemic sclerosis there may be late recovery of renal function, even when the patient has been established on dialysis for some weeks.

Treatment of D− HUS

There have been few randomized controlled trials in D− HUS, and in particular the use of plasma exchange remains controversial.

Supportive

This consists of careful fluid balance, blood transfusion, and renal replacement therapy. In oliguric patients care should be taken to prevent fluid overload, and central venous monitoring may be required. Platelet transfusions should be avoided, unless there is evidence of bleeding. Patients with deteriorating renal function should always be referred for specialist renal care.

Plasma treatment

Previous studies of the efficacy of plasma treatment in HUS are difficult to interpret because of the inclusion of patients with TTP who respond well to plasma exchange. Nevertheless, plasma exchange is recommended for most forms of D− HUS.

Corticosteroids

The use of corticosteroids is also controversial. There is evidence for efficacy in TTP, but in small retrospective studies of D− HUS there appears to be no significant effect on survival or the need for renal replacement therapy.

Hypertension

ACE inhibitors are the treatment of choice, with clear parallels existing with their use in the renal crisis of systemic sclerosis. Bilateral nephrectomy has been advocated for severe D− HUS with widespread manifestations not responding to plasma exchange. In a series of four patients, three of whom had ACE inhibitor resistant hypertension, bilateral nephrectomy led to complete haematological and clinical remission within 2 weeks.

Renal transplantation

Renal transplantation in patients with renal failure secondary to D+ HUS is safe, with little risk of recurrence of the disease. In contrast, patients with D− HUS have an approximately 50% risk of recurrence, usually within the first 2 months, and often within the first 2 weeks. Once recurrent HUS is established, most grafts are lost despite treatment with plasma exchange, which is reflected by the poor 2-year overall graft survival rate of 35%. Graft nephrectomy should not be delayed in this situation.

In those patients known to have a mutation in either the gene encoding factor H or factor I, the risk of losing the transplant to recurrent disease within 2 years of transplantation is approximately 80%. In these patients a combined liver/kidney transplant is a logical alternative as both factor H and factor I are synthesized predominantly by the kidney. Acute vascular rejection may be difficult to differentiate from recurrent HUS, both clinically and histologically.

Further reading

Artz MA, et al. (2003). Renal transplantation in patients with hemolytic uremic syndrome: high rate of recurrence and increased incidence of acute rejections. *Transplantation*, **76**, 821–6.

Becker S, et al. (2004). HIV-associated thrombotic microangiopathy in the era of highly active antiretroviral therapy: an observational study. *Clin Infect Dis*, **39** Suppl 5, S267–75.

Bresin E, et al. (2006). Outcome of renal transplantation in patients with non-Shiga toxin-associated hemolytic uremic syndrome: prognostic significance of genetic background. *Clin J Am Soc Nephrol*, **1**, 88–99.

Dashe JS, Ramin SM, Cunningham FG (1998). The long term consequences of thrombotic microangiopathy (thrombotic thrombocytopenic purpura and hemolytic uremic syndrome) in pregnancy. *Obstet Gynecol*, **91**, 662–8.

Dlott JS, et al. (2004). Drug-induced thrombotic thrombocytopenic purpura/hemolytic uremic syndrome: a concise review. *Ther Apher Dial*, **8**, 102–11.

Ducloux D, et al. (1998). Recurrence of hemolytic-uremic syndrome in renal transplant recipients: a meta-analysis. *Transplantation*, **65**, 1405–7.

George JN (2003). The association of pregnancy with thrombotic thrombocytopenic purpura-hemolytic uremic syndrome. *Curr Opin Hematol*, **10**, 339–44.

Kavanagh D, Goodship T (2007). Update on evaluating complement in hemolytic uremic syndrome. *Curr Opin Nephrol Hypertens*, **16**, 565–71.

Moake JL (2002). Thrombotic microangiopathies. *N Engl J Med*, **347**, 589–600.

Saland JM, et al. (2006). Favorable long-term outcome after liver-kidney transplant for recurrent hemolytic uremic syndrome associated with a factor H mutation. *Am J Transplant*, **6**, 1948–52.

Sutor GC, Schmidt RE, Albrecht H (1999). Thrombotic microangiopathies and HIV infection: report of two typical cases, features of HUS and TTP, and review of the literature. *Infection*, **27**, 12–15.

21.10.6 Sickle-cell disease and the kidney

G.R. Serjeant

Essentials

The vasa rectae system of the renal medulla is uniquely conducive to sickling, which leads to vascular damage and tubular dysfunction, including an inability to concentrate the urine. Renal presentations include nocturnal enuresis, haematuria (thought to be due to ischaemic lesions of the papillae, including papillary necrosis), and gradually progressive chronic renal failure, which is an important cause of morbidity and death in patients with homozygous sickle-cell disease over the age of 40 years.

Introduction

Homozygous sickle-cell (SS) disease results in anaemia, a hyperdynamic circulation, less deformable red blood cells, and probably widespread endothelial damage and dysfunction. These processes affect structure and function in the kidney: medullary and glomerular involvement occurs at different ages and with different implications for outcome. Other genotypes of sickle-cell disease such as sickle-cell haemoglobin C (SC) disease, sickle-cell β°-thalassaemia, and sickle-cell β⁺-thalassaemia manifest similar but less frequent and less severe changes, and even the sickle-cell trait is associated with some abnormalities of renal function.

Medullary involvement

Vascular damage

The vasa rectae system of the renal medulla with its low oxygen tension, high pH, and hypertonicity is uniquely conducive to sickling, causing disruption of the blood vessels and secondary damage to the renal tubules. Microradioangiographic studies have shown almost complete obliteration of the fine vessel system of the vasa rectae, the remaining vessels being distorted into spirals, dilatations, and appearing to end blindly. These changes have been observed in SS disease in childhood and occur to a lesser extent in the sickle-cell trait, in which haemoglobin S levels are only 20 to 45% of total haemoglobin.

Tubular dysfunction

The functional effect of these vascular changes is an inability to concentrate the urine normally, which becomes worse with age but can be improved by transfusion in children under 2 years of age. Proximal tubular functional abnormalities include an increased secretion of urate and creatinine, and an increased reabsorption of phosphate and of β_2-microglobulin. Distal tubular functional abnormalities include an inability to excrete an acid load, defective maximal potassium excretion, and occasionally evidence of hyporeninaemic aldosteronism. Clinically, these changes are reflected in hyposthenuria, with larger urinary volumes contributing to enuresis and possibly a tendency to dehydration.

Glomerular involvement

Large hypercellular glomeruli are characteristic of SS disease from the age of 2 years, with the size continuing to increase with age, even over the age of 40 years. The large glomeruli in childhood are associated with supranormal glomerular filtration rates, effective renal blood flows, and effective renal plasma flows. All these indices fall with age, and are below normal in many patients aged 30 to 40 years, with particularly rapid decline occurring in some patients who proceed to chronic renal failure. This functional deterioration is assumed to reflect progressive glomerular loss, the mechanism of which is unclear, but there may be contributions from immune complexes derived from renal tubular antigens and mechanical damage to the nephron from hyperfiltration. The notion that glomerular capillary hypertension might be involved gained support from the observation that angiotensin-converting enzyme inhibitors significantly reduce proteinuria in some proteinuric patients with SS disease.

Clinical syndromes

Nocturnal enuresis

Enuresis is common in SS disease, and in the Jamaican Sickle Cell Cohort study occurred at least two nights a week in 52% of boys and 38% of girls with SS disease aged 8 years, compared with values of 22% and 17%, respectively, in control children without SS disease. Enuretic children with SS disease have slightly higher urinary volumes and lower mean maximal functional bladder capacity than those without enuresis, and the ratio of overnight urine volume to bladder capacity was significantly greater in enuretic subjects. Enuresis alarms may be the most appropriate therapy but require testing in controlled studies.

Haematuria

Haematuria occurs in both SS disease and sickle-cell trait and is believed to result from ischaemic lesions of the renal papilla, varying from minute ulcerations to renal papillary necrosis. Treatment is conservative, although prolonged haematuria may require blood transfusion or (rarely) limited surgery. ε-Aminocaproic acid, which inhibits urokinase, has been effective in some cases, but promotes clots that may obstruct the ureters.

Urinary tract infections

The frequency of urinary tract infections is increased in subjects with the sickle-cell trait during pregnancy, and may be increased in SS disease, although no reliable data are available. *Escherichia coli*, klebsiella, and enterobacter are most commonly responsible.

Acute glomerular disease

Poststreptococcal glomerulonephritis in SS disease may occur at later ages than typical for the normal population. An association of proteinuria with leg ulceration raised the possibility that leg ulcers acted as a portal of entry for β-haemolytic streptococci, but further analysis did not support this hypothesis.

Nephrotic syndrome

It is unclear whether patients with SS disease are more prone to nephrotic syndrome, but the histological picture of membranoproliferative glomerulonephritis accounts for over one-half of adult cases. Nephrotic syndrome has been reported following parvovirus B19 infection, and B19-specific DNA has been demonstrated within renal biopsy tissue 1 year after the onset of nephrotic syndrome. If nephrotic syndrome is due to acute glomerulonephritis the prognosis is good, but it is not if the cause is otherwise, with a 50% mortality within 16 months in one study.

Chronic renal failure

Chronic renal failure is an important contributor to illness and death among adults with SS disease, especially those over 40 years of age. It is usually insidious in onset, manifested initially by a falling haemoglobin level attributable to lowered erythropoietin levels, hence renal function of older patients should be monitored regularly. In this regard it is important to recognize that serum creatinine levels tend to be lower than normal in steady-state SS disease, hence values within the accepted normal range should not be interpreted as indicating normal renal function, indeed in SS disease it is likely that levels of 60 to 70 μmol/litre reflect significant renal damage.

Since the early symptoms of chronic renal failure in those with SS disease are principally due to a low haemoglobin level, patients may be maintained in tolerable health for years by regular transfusion. The response to subcutaneous erythropoietin is unpredictable, large doses being required to induce a response, but some patients show dramatic increases in haemoglobin that may precipitate painful crises. Endstage renal failure may require long-term renal replacement therapy or renal transplantation, but there are conflicting data on outcome. Successful transplantation can be followed by striking increases in haemoglobin level, sufficient to precipitate painful crises, and recurrent sickle nephropathy may affect the transplanted kidney.

Further reading

Bakir AA, et al. (1987). Prognosis of the nephrotic syndrome in sickle nephropathy. A retrospective study. *Am J Nephrol*, **7**, 110–15.

Barber WH, et al. (1987). Renal transplantation in sickle-cell anemia and sickle disease. *Clin Transplant*, **1**, 169–75.

Bhathena DB, Sondheimer JH (1991). The glomerulopathy of homozygous sickle hemoglobin (SS) disease: morphology and pathogenesis. *J Am Soc Nephrol*, **1**, 1241–52.

Falk RJ, et al. (1992). Prevalence and pathologic features of sickle cell nephropathy and response to inhibition of angiotensin-converting enzyme. *N Engl J Med*, **326**, 910–15.

Morgan AG, Serjeant GR (1981). Renal function in patients over 40 with homozygous sickle cell disease. *BMJ*, **282**, 1181–3.

Readett DRJ, Morris J, Serjeant GR (1990). Determinants of nocturnal enuresis in homozygous sickle cell disease. *Arch Dis Child*, **65**, 615–18.

Statius van Eps LW, *et al.* (1970). Nature of concentrating defect in sickle-cell nephropathy. Microradioangiographic studies. *Lancet*, i, 450–2.

Thompson J, *et al.* (2007). Albuminuria and renal function in homozygous sickle cell disease: observations from a cohort study. *Arch Intern Med*, **167**, 701–8.

Wierenga KJJ, *et al.* (1995). Glomerulonephritis after human parvovirus infection in homozygous sickle cell disease. *Lancet*, **346**, 475–6.

21.10.7 Infection-associated nephropathies

A. Neil Turner

Essentials

Infection may be a primary cause of renal disease (e.g. postinfectious glomerulonephritis) or affect the kidneys on a background of debilitating illnesses and previous medical interventions. Renal disease may arise as a consequence of immune responses to a pathogen, direct invasion by the microorganism, or the effects of infection on the systemic or local circulations.

Glomerulonephritis—associated with chronic and acute bacterial infections. Shunt nephritis follows colonization of a ventriculoatrial shunt, most commonly with *Staphylococcus epidermidis*, which leads to constitutional symptoms, an acute inflammatory response, and (most characteristically) a type 1 mesangiocapillary glomerulonephritis; treatment requires removal of the shunt. Infective endocarditis and other deep-seated bacterial infections may produce a renal picture similar to shunt nephritis; they can mimic vasculitic syndromes and outcome is dependent on the response of the infection to treatment. Acute postinfectious glomerulonephritis—see Chapter 21.8.5.

Interstitial nephritis—bacteria that can cause this include leptospira (Weil's disease), *Rickettsia rickettsii* (Rocky Mountain spotted fever), legionella, and mycobacteria. Viral infections include hantaviruses (haemorrhagic fever with renal syndrome and nephropathia epidemica) and, almost exclusively following renal transplantation, cytomegalovirus and polyomavirus hominis type 1 (BK) virus.

HIV-associated renal disorders—these include HIV nephropathy, a focal segmental glomerulosclerosis of the 'collapsing' form, occurring almost exclusively in black patients; it is the third most frequent cause of endstage renal failure in black adults of working age in the United States of America.

Hepatitis B virus—chronic infection is strongly associated with membranous nephropathy; affected individuals are HBeAg and HBsAg positive, usually with coexistent hepatitis; seroconversion from HBeAg positive to HBeAb positive (naturally or induced by treatment) is associated with remission of the renal lesion.

Hepatitis C virus—chronic infection is the commonest cause of mixed essential (type II) cryoglobulinaemia in most populations; it is associated with mesangiocapillary glomerulonephritis, and reduction of viral replication has been associated with disease remission.

Introduction

Almost all renal lesions, particularly glomerular lesions, may be associated with infections. The pathways leading to these are sometimes understood, but often obscure. In the West, infection-associated nephritis was once predominantly recognized during acute infections occurring in apparently healthy individuals, and this is still the pattern in many countries. However, improvements in living conditions and health care have reduced the numbers of healthy people succumbing to complications of infection in developed countries. By contrast, infections occurring on a background of debilitating illnesses and previous medical interventions have become more common.

In this chapter glomerular diseases and interstitial diseases associated with infection are considered in turn. Particular attention is given to those glomerulopathies associated with bacterial endocarditis and other chronic bacterial infections, and three viral infections of worldwide importance, HIV, hepatitis B, and hepatitis C.

Pathogenesis

Infection-associated glomerular disease is usually attributed to trapping of circulating antigen–antibody complexes, or to immune responses to pathogen-derived antigens that become 'planted' in the glomerulus. The evidence for deposition of circulating immune complexes is strong for cryoglobulinaemia, and highly plausible for infections occurring within the vascular system such as bacterial endocarditis. In most other infections the evidence is less clear, and in general this is probably not a common mechanism of glomerular disease. A direct cytopathic effect on glomerular cells seems likely for some pathogens such as HIV and parvovirus, both of which have been associated with 'collapsing' focal segmental glomerulosclerosis.

Interstitial renal disease is often blamed on direct invasion by the microorganism, and for some, particularly viruses, there is evidence that this is true. The pathogen may cause injury directly, or indirectly by causing cells to express foreign antigens which generate an immune response. More speculatively, an immune response generated to an organism may cross-react with a remote self-antigen, triggering autoimmunity through molecular mimicry, but there are no unequivocal examples of this.

Infection may also involve the kidney by interfering with the circulation either generally (septic shock) or locally (e.g. by causing thrombotic microangiopathy, as for *Escherichia coli* O157 or *Capnocytophaga canimorsus* (previously DF-2)). On occasions toxins may be released that harm the kidney directly (e.g. haemoglobin in malaria). Medically administered toxins include antimicrobial agents that impair renal function by crystallization (e.g. aciclovir, indinavir) or by predictable toxicity (e.g. aminoglycosides, amphotericin), or by idiosyncratic reactions such as acute interstitial nephritis (e.g. penicillins).

Glomerulonephritis associated with chronic and acute bacterial infections

Classic acute postinfectious glomerulonephritis is considered in Chapter 21.8.5. This account considers subacute or chronic diseases, although other causes of a 'classic' picture are mentioned. Shunt nephritis was first recognized in the 1960s, and it remains the archetype of an immune complex nephritis. The glomerulonephritis occurring in association with infective endocarditis is very similar. Both are caused by subacute infection within the bloodstream, with constant shedding of antigen and formation of antigen–antibody complexes. Other bacterial infections may cause similar pictures.

Shunt nephritis

In shunt nephritis a ventriculoatrial shunt implanted for hydrocephalus becomes colonized by bacteria, usually of low pathogenicity. More common modern equivalents of this clinical syndrome are infected long-term central venous catheters and other intravascular devices. The syndrome does not occur with ventriculoperitoneal shunts, which are therefore now the preferred neurosurgical option. Although *Staphylococcus epidermidis* has been most commonly implicated, *Propionibacterium acnes* or other organisms are sometimes involved. Typically the diagnosis is only appreciated after weeks to months of symptoms of mild to moderate pyrexia and malaise associated with haematuria and proteinuria and progressive renal impairment. Fevers have often been attributed to urinary infection in patients with neurogenic bladders. There may be moderate splenomegaly. Investigations show complement consumption and an acute phase response with normochromic normocytic anaemia, and variable renal impairment. The renal lesion is characteristically a type 1 mesangiocapillary glomerulonephritis with deposition of multiple immunoglobulins and complement components beneath the endothelium, the classic appearance of a circulating immune complex nephritis. Sometimes the picture is more severe, showing a diffuse proliferative lesion, occasionally with crescents. In other cases the histological appearances are less pronounced with focal proliferative changes.

Antibiotic treatment alone is almost never adequate to cure these infections, which require removal of the shunt (or other device), followed by its replacement after an interval if it is still required. Delayed diagnosis and delayed removal may lead to more severe and irreversible renal damage, and sometimes to endstage renal failure, but substantial recovery often follows successful treatment.

Infective endocarditis

A similar syndrome occurs in infective endocarditis, as part of which minor degrees of glomerular disease are probably extremely common. Most symptoms and signs in these circumstances are common to shunt nephritis. Typical streptococcal infections are well represented in case reports, but there have been multiple reports involving 'slow' infections such as Q fever (*Coxiella burnetii*), and more unusual causes including chlamydia and fungi. Infection of prosthetic or native heart valves may be implicated. Right-sided endocarditis occurring in intravenous drug abusers may be particularly likely to present as nephritis, because the diagnosis is often delayed. Depletion of serum complement is again diagnostically useful, but, as for shunt nephritis, most other serological and haematological changes are nonspecific. Partial treatment with antibiotics makes diagnosis and management more difficult, as positive blood cultures are usually a key part of proving the diagnosis and prescribing appropriate therapy.

The pathological lesion is typically similar to that of shunt nephritis, but forms of endocarditis that are acute, rather than subacute (e.g. that associated with *Staphylococcus aureus*), are more likely to cause glomerulonephritis in a diffuse proliferative

pattern, sometimes with crescent formation. Focal changes that are indistinguishable from antineutrophil cytoplasmic antibody (ANCA)-associated vasculitis have been increasingly reported in recent literature, indeed in some cases ANCA have been detected. However immune deposits are usually present in glomeruli, in contrast to the primary small vessel vasculitides. Cutaneous vasculitis may be seen in association with bacterial infection, and this seems particularly likely in endocarditis (Fig. 21.10.7.1).

In most cases the outcome is dependent on the response of the endocarditis to treatment, but renal involvement is a poor prognostic factor for survival, which may be simply because it reflects long-lasting infection. Recovery from dialysis dependence may occur.

Patients with endocarditis are also prone to two other renal lesions: interstitial nephritis related to antibiotics and, in those with disease on the left side of the heart or with right–left shunts, renal emboli, although glomerulonephritis is probably a more common cause of urinary abnormalities.

Deep-seated bacterial infections

Amyloidosis is a well-recognized consequence of very chronic bacterial (including mycobacterial) and other infections, and is described in Chapters 12.12.3 and 21.10.4. As in reactive amyloidosis of other aetiologies, progression of the renal lesion may be prevented or even partially reversed by treatment of the cause.

Deep-seated infections, particularly abscesses, may also be associated with acute renal pathology. Although the mechanisms involved are presumably similar to those of shunt nephritis and nephritis associated with endocarditis, blood cultures have often been negative in reported cases. *Staphylococcus aureus* is the most frequently implicated organism. A specific type of renal disease in association with methicillin-resistant organisms (MRSA) has been postulated, but without strong support. A wide variety of renal lesions have been described, usually inflammatory/proliferative and with immunoglobulin deposition. Unsuspected abscesses or other deep-seated infections are occasionally found only after the renal biopsy appearances trigger a search. Such hidden abscesses are more likely in obese people, older people, and in those on corticosteroids or who are immunosuppressed by other means or by disease.

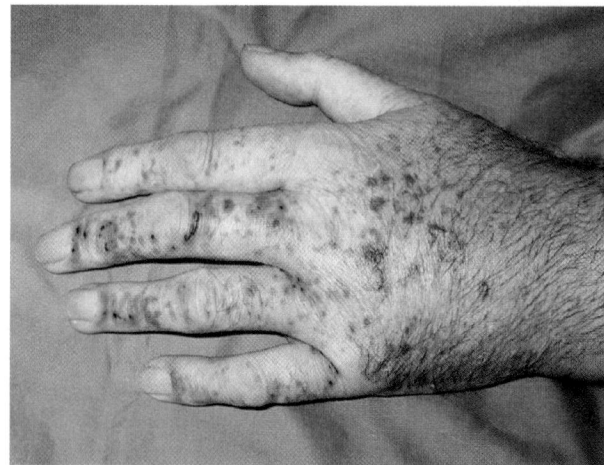

Fig. 21.10.7.1 Cutaneous vasculitis in a patient with *Staphylococcus aureus* endocarditis.

Acute glomerulonephritis and other infections

Acute glomerulonephritis resembling poststreptococcal nephritis has been reported in association with a large number of other organisms, including current (as opposed to recent) infection with staphylococci, streptococci, and other bacteria, and with acute viral infections that are usually self-limiting. These include Epstein–Barr virus, cytomegalovirus, varicella, measles, mumps, parvovirus, and coxsackieviruses. Some may cause a clinical syndrome that is very similar to poststreptococcal nephritis, while others typically cause a less florid 'nephritic' or mixed 'nephritic/nephrotic' picture.

Diagnostic difficulties in bacterial infection-related glomerulonephritis

Infection-related nephritis may present in a very similar manner to nephritis associated with other systemic diseases, notably microscopic polyangiitis and other small vessel vasculitides. As both types of disease process may be associated with fever, a systemic illness, and an acute phase response, it is important to consider the possibility of infection in all patients thought to have systemic vasculitis. Blood cultures should be routine. ANCA assays are extremely useful, but it is important to note that ANCA positivity has been recorded in many infections, both by fluorescence and by solid phase assays: ANCA are not diagnostic of small vessel vasculitides. Renal biopsy is often the most discriminating investigation. Infection-associated glomerulonephritis is usually associated with plentiful immunoglobulin deposition, although the pattern is variable, whereas small vessel vasculitis is characteristically pauci-immune. Nonglomerular causes of renal impairment (interstitial nephritis, acute tubular necrosis) are also distinguished by renal biopsy.

Interstitial nephritis associated with infections

Bacterial infections

Acute bacterial pyelonephritis is usually a florid and painful disorder associated with symptoms of urinary tract infection, as described in Chapter 21.13. Substantial renal impairment is usual only if a single functioning kidney is affected. Occasionally, however, the diagnosis is masked by immunosuppression (e.g. in a transplanted kidney), age, or other factors, and the diagnosis is made by the renal biopsy appearances of neutrophils in the interstitium and in tubules, which are rarely found in any other renal lesions.

Acute interstitial nephritis is a key feature of Weil's disease, a severe form of leptospirosis (see Chapter 7.6.34). Jaundice and renal failure follow a febrile illness caused by infection with *Leptospira interrogans*. The renal lesion comprises interstitial oedema with predominantly mononuclear infiltrates and foci of tubular necrosis. Renal failure is usually oliguric but may be polyuric. Dialysis may be required for days to weeks, and renal recovery may sometimes be incomplete.

Other bacterial infections that may cause a similar pathological picture include Rocky Mountain spotted fever (*Rickettsia rickettsii*), in which there may be an interstitial nephritis with foci of haemorrhage, and acute *Yersinia pseudotuberculosis* infection, in which an acute lymphocytic interstitial nephritis has been described in

several patients. Legionnaires' disease (*Legionella pneumophila*) has been reported to be associated with renal impairment, also with an interstitial nephritis, but in some instances may show a picture of acute tubular necrosis. The same is probably true of other severe pneumonias.

Mycobacteria can cause a chronic granulomatous interstitial nephritis; this is discussed below.

Viral infections

Hantaviruses

Hantaviruses are carried by small rodents, and have been associated with a range of human syndromes that involve the kidneys with varying severity. 'Haemorrhagic fever with renal syndrome' (HFRS) is characterized by oliguric renal failure, associated histologically with lymphocytic interstitial nephritis that may be haemorrhagic in severe cases, reflecting the systemic bleeding diathesis. Some patients have been reported to have persistent renal impairment after recovery.

HFRS was originally associated with Hantaan strains of hantavirus in Korea, while milder disease, with less frequent and usually less severe renal impairment and without haemorrhagic diathesis, was associated with the Seoul strain. Milder disease (nephropathia epidemica) recognized in northern Europe and subsequently more widely was associated with the Puumula strain. However, it has become apparent that there are many more subtypes of hantavirus, and the association of a serotype with a particular clinical picture is not rigid. Severe disease with shock, variable haemorrhage, and sometimes pulmonary impairment has been encountered in the Balkans and Greece. Disease with predominantly pulmonary manifestations and shock has been recognized, particularly in North America, although these geographical variations in clinical picture are no more rigid than the strain variations.

Ribavirin is active against hantaviruses *in vitro*, and therapy with ribavirin was found to be effective in HFRS caused by the classic Hantaan strain in China, but there are likely to be strain differences as no benefit could be demonstrated in trials in the pulmonary syndrome in North America.

Cytomegalovirus, polyomaviruses, and other viruses

Cytomegalovirus (CMV) may lie dormant in renal tubular cells, and during new or reactivated infection causes characteristic inclusion bodies. This rarely has significant impact on renal function outside the setting of renal transplantation, where CMV infection commonly occurs concurrently with acute rejection. Although there is evidence that CMV infection may precipitate rejection, it is also clear that the risk of CMV infection is greatly increased by most types of antirejection therapy. CMV may also rarely cause a florid glomerular lesion characterized by gross endothelial cell damage and swelling, resembling pre-eclampsia. This has again been recognized almost exclusively in renal transplants, where some believe that the appearances are due to, or complicated by, vascular rejection.

Human polyomaviruses (BK and JC) were previously believed to be benign passenger viruses which replicated without causing damage during immunosuppression. However, BK virus has been increasingly recognized as a cause of impaired renal transplant function, usually many months after transplantation. The histological changes of tubulitis closely resemble acute cellular rejection, but further immunosuppression favours further infective damage. Observation of typical inclusion bodies and immunohistochemical studies prove the true cause of the tubulitis, and renal function may improve after reduction of immunosuppressive agents. For reasons that are not clear, polyomavirus renal disease seems to be very rare in patients immunosuppressed for reasons other than renal transplantation.

A wide range of other viruses and microorganisms have been less regularly associated with interstitial lesions. HIV (considered below) may cause an interstitial nephritis. Another condition that is likely to be infective in origin, Kawasaki's disease, is associated with interstitial nephritis, although glomerular lesions have also been described occasionally.

HIV and renal disease

Renal impairment is commonly encountered at some stage of HIV infection. The largest single cause of serious renal disease in this group is the distinct entity of HIV nephropathy. However, this generalization is misleading as this specific diagnosis is largely restricted to black patients, and there are many other causes of renal disease in patients with HIV infection.

Focal segmental glomerulosclerosis associated with HIV infection (HIV nephropathy)

HIV nephropathy is characterized by heavy proteinuria and renal impairment. It has become the third most frequent cause of end-stage renal failure in black adults of working age in the United States of America. Although it has often been described as an initial manifestation of HIV infection, in these circumstances the infection is advanced, with high viral loads and low CD4 counts. Histologically the appearances are of focal segmental glomerulosclerosis (FSGS) of the 'collapsing' form, with injury and hypertrophy of glomerular epithelial cells accompanied by variable interstitial inflammation with oedema and microtubular dilatation. Without therapy the condition progresses to endstage renal failure rapidly, over weeks to months. Perhaps because it is associated with low CD4 counts, the medium-term prognosis in the past was poor despite renal replacement therapy. There is conflicting evidence as to whether HIV enters podocytes and is directly cytopathic to them.

Non-FSGS nephropathies in HIV infection

FSGS accounts for a minority of HIV-associated renal disease in most populations. An HIV immune complex glomerulonephritis (HIVICK) has been described, but so have other specific types of glomerular disease. A very wide range of diagnoses has been described encompassing almost all types of glomerular lesion, interstitial nephritis, cryoglobulinaemia, and thrombotic microangiopathy. IgA nephropathy has been frequently recorded. Some of these lesions may be directly caused by HIV infection while others are related to concurrent infections with other microorganisms, others may be related to therapy, while others again may be due to immune dysfunction. Aciclovir and indinavir have replaced sulphonamides as common causes of crystal nephropathy, tenofovir is known to be nephrotoxic, and adjusting the doses of these and other drugs in the setting of renal impairment is problematic. Idiosyncratic reactions to drugs may be more frequent in patients with HIV infection, but they also receive many drugs with predictable

nephrotoxicity. The occurrence of autoimmune phenomena in HIV infection may also be accompanied by an increase in immune-mediated primary glomerular diseases.

Highly active antiretroviral (HAART) and other therapies

HAART when instituted early may arrest the progression of FSGS as well as lowering the mortality of patients with endstage renal failure. Severity of chronic damage on biopsy is a better prediction of prognosis than serum creatinine. Its effect on non-FSGS nephropathies is uncertain. Short to medium term improvement may often be seen but it is rarely possible to discern how much this is a specific effect of antivirals. Patients with any diseases associated with proteinuria should be treated with angiotensin-converting enzyme (ACE) inhibitors. Treatment with corticosteroids should probably be considered in patients with HIV-FSGS who progress despite effective HAART and intensive renoprotective therapy with ACE inhibitors and blood pressure control.

The effectiveness of HAART makes it possible to consider patients with HIV infection for immunosuppressive therapies that would be indicated for their renal disease in the absence of HIV infection, and even for renal transplantation. Several national guidelines now accept that transplantation may be beneficial for patients whose prognosis is of many years.

Nephropathy associated with hepatitis B virus

Chronic infection with hepatitis B virus (HBV) is strongly associated with membranous nephropathy, and it is an important secondary cause of the lesion. A less clear relationship holds with membranoproliferative nephropathy, while for hepatitis C virus the converse is true.

Chronic HBV infection is much more common in some regions and racial groups, and the distribution of HBV-related nephropathy closely follows this distribution. The clinical picture may be complicated by the concurrence of HBV infection by infection with HCV, HIV, or with other organisms, or by the coincidence of significant renal and hepatic disease. HBV membranous nephropathy has a close relationship with virus multiplication, so affected individuals are HBeAg and HBsAg positive, and hepatitis usually coexists, although it may be minor and subclinical. Membranous nephropathy is a more common complication of HBV infection in children, but it is also more benign in this group. The lesion may be static, or in some cases (particularly in adults) associated with progressive deterioration to endstage renal failure.

Histopathology is typical of membranous nephropathy, and HBV antigens may be detectable in glomerular deposits. Animal models suggest that antibodies to podocyte surface molecules are a more likely way of producing the membranous lesion than trapping of preformed antigen–antibody complexes. It is possible that viral genes are expressed in renal cells, but this has not been proven.

Seroconversion from HBeAg positive to HBeAb positive is associated with remission of the renal lesion, whether the conversion occurs naturally or is induced by treatment. Spontaneous remission of the renal lesion is more likely in children. Antiviral treatment is the appropriate therapy when required, as immunosuppression may increase viral burden.

Recently acquired (within months) HBV infection has been associated with classic polyarteritis nodosa (PAN) in some populations, such as in France and North America, but even in these areas HBV-PAN is uncommon and apparently decreasing. Furthermore, the association of the two diseases is rare in some countries with low (e.g. the United Kingdom) and with high (e.g. Thailand) rates of HBV carriage, suggesting the involvement of a cofactor. Clinically, the disease is typical of PAN, affecting medium and somewhat smaller vessels but not capillaries, and therefore not usually associated with focal necrotizing or crescentic nephritis. ANCA are not usually detected. Treatment is difficult to balance as immunosuppression (usually with corticosteroids alone) is often indicated but favours viral replication and exacerbation of liver disease, while remission is associated with seroconversion from HBeAg positivity to HBeAb positivity.

Nephropathy associated with hepatitis C virus

Chronic hepatitis C virus (HCV) infection is the commonest cause of mixed essential (type II) cryoglobulinaemia in most populations. The clinical picture includes cutaneous vasculitis, glomerular pathology (mesangiocapillary glomerulonephritis, MCGN), and other manifestations. The cryoglobulins contain quantities of HCV antigens and bound antibody, in addition to monoclonal IgM rheumatoid factors. HCV may also be associated with MCGN in the absence of detectable cryoglobulins. A relationship with membranous nephropathy is also possible, but not proven.

As for HBV, reduction of viral replication has been associated with disease remission, but this is harder to achieve for HCV than for HBV with current therapies. Immunosuppression with corticosteroids and sometimes other agents may be required to control disease manifestations caused by vasculitis.

Renal sequelae of other chronic infections

Amyloidosis

Amyloidosis may be a consequence of all sorts of chronic infection, but of the 'tropical' infections is most frequently associated with schistosomiasis, filariasis, or leishmaniasis.

Mycobacteria

Mycobacterial infections cause a chronic granulomatous interstitial nephritis that is characteristically associated with inflammatory and fibrotic abnormalities in the ureters and lower urinary tract. Symptoms often relate to lower tract involvement, but the disease may be asymptomatic, and in the earliest stages involvement is presumed to be restricted to the kidneys, with subsequent spread to the lower tract. Sterile pyuria is the rule, and impaired renal function is common at presentation. Imaging by intravenous urography or other techniques will show blunting of calyces, progressing to changes typical of pyelonephritis or papillary necrosis, along with lower tract abnormalities such as ureteric strictures and scarring and contraction of the bladder. Amyloidosis is a well-recognized secondary complication of mycobacterial infections. Idiosyncratic reactions to antituberculous drugs are another common cause of late renal dysfunction.

Syphilis

Congenital syphilis may cause severe nephrotic syndrome with the histological pattern of membranous nephropathy. This is also the usual pattern when secondary syphilis rarely causes nephrotic syndrome. Both respond to antispirochaetal treatment.

Malaria

Plasmodium falciparum infections are an extremely important cause of acute renal failure worldwide. It occurs in 1 to 5% of infected patients native to a malarial area, but a higher proportion of nonimmune visitors, and is associated with high mortality (15–45%).

Recent series from Africa have cast doubt on the existence of a specific chronic malarial nephropathy that was described in earlier literature. Biopsy studies have shown a high incidence of infection-related glomerulonephritis and of FSGS, but have found little evidence of a distinct malarial disease.

Schistosomiasis

Schistosomiasis is best recognized for causing disease of the lower urinary tract, but chronic infections associated with hepatosplenomegaly may be associated with glomerular disease after many years. In *Schistosoma haematobium* infection this is often due to secondary infections with *Salmonella* spp. rather than directly associated with schistosomal infection. In *Schistosoma mansoni* infection the relationship is probably usually directly causal, producing a mesangiocapillary or mesangioproliferative picture.

Filariasis

Longstanding filariasis may also be associated with glomerular lesions. An acute syndrome with tubulointerstitial nephritis has also been described in association with the presence of microfilariae in renal capillaries.

Further reading

Alric L, et al. (2004). Influence of antiviral therapy in hepatitis C virus-associated cryoglobulinemic MPGN. *Am J Kidney Dis*, **43**, 617–23.

Bonarek H, et al. (1999). Reversal of c-ANCA positive mesangiocapillary glomerulonephritis after removal of an infected cysto-atrial shunt. *Nephrol Dial Transplant*, **14**, 1771–3.

Conlon PJ, et al. (1998). Predictors of prognosis and risk of acute renal failure in bacterial endocarditis. *Clin Nephrol*, **49**, 96–101.

Daghestani L, Pomeroy C (1999). Renal manifestations of hepatitis C infection. *Am J Med*, **106**, 347–54.

Daugas E, Rougier JP, Hill G (2005). HAART-related nephropathies in HIV-infected patients. *Kidney Int*, **67**, 393–403.

Doe JY, et al. (2006). Nephrotic syndrome in African children: lack of evidence for 'tropical nephrotic syndrome'? *Nephrol Dial Transplant*, **21**, 672–6.

Guillevin L, et al. (2005). Hepatitis B virus-associated polyarteritis nodosa: clinical characteristics, outcome, and impact of treatment in 115 patients. *Medicine (Baltimore)*, **84**, 313.

Haffner D, et al. (1997). The clinical spectrum of shunt nephritis. *Nephrol Dial Transplant*, **12**, 1143–8.

Huggins JW, et al. (1991). Prospective, double-blind, concurrent, placebo-controlled clinical trial of intravenous ribavirin therapy for hemorrhagic fever with renal syndrome. *J Infect Dis*, **164**, 1119–27.

Johnson RJ, Couser WG (1990). Hepatitis B infection and renal disease: clinical, immunopathogenetic and therapeutic considerations. *Kidney Int*, **37**, 663–76.

Jones JM, Davison AM (1986). Persistent infection as a cause of renal disease in patients submitted to renal biopsy: a report from the

Glomerulonephritis Registry of the United Kingdom MRC. *QJM*, **58**, 123–32.

Lai AS, Lai KN (2006). Viral nephropathy. *Nat Clin Pract Nephrol*, **2**, 254–62.

Majumdar A, *et al.* (2000). Renal pathological findings in infective endocarditis. *Nephrol Dial Transplant*, **15**, 1782–7.

McGuire BM, *et al.* (2006). Glomerulonephritis in patients with hepatitis C cirrhosis undergoing liver transplantation. *Ann Intern Med*, **144**, 735–41.

Montseny JJ, *et al.* (1995). The current spectrum of infectious glomerulonephritis: experience with 76 patients and review of the literature. *Medicine (Baltimore)*, **74**, 63–73.

Moudgil A, *et al.* (2001). Association of parvovirus B19 infection with idiopathic collapsing glomerulopathy. *Kidney Int*, **59**, 2126–33.

Naqvi R, *et al.* (2003). Outcome in severe acute renal failure associated with malaria. *Nephrol Dial Transplant*, **18**, 1820–3.

Neugarten J, Baldwin DS (1984). Glomerulonephritis in bacterial endocarditis. *Am J Med*, **77**, 297–304.

Nickeleit V, Mihatsch MJ (2006). Polyomavirus nephropathy in native kidneys and renal allografts: an update on an escalating threat. *Transpl Int*, **19**, 960–73.

Peters CJ, Simpson GL, Levy H (1999). Spectrum of hantavirus infection: hemorrhagic fever with renal syndrome and hantavirus pulmonary syndrome. *Ann Rev Med*, **50**, 531–45.

Post FA, et al .(2008). Predictors of outcome in HIV-associated nephropathy. *Clin Infect Dis*, **15**, 1282–9.

Szczech LA, *et al.* (2004). The clinical epidemiology and course of the spectrum of renal diseases associated with HIV infection. *Kidney Int*, **66**, 1145–52.

21.10.8 Malignancy-associated renal disease

A. Neil Turner

Essentials

Malignancies can affect the kidneys by direct invasion, metabolic and remote effects of tumour products, deposition of tumour products, triggering of immune reactions, and effects of treatment.

Particular malignancy-associated renal diseases discussed in this chapter include the following:

1 Thrombotic microangiopathy—particularly reported for malignancies of the stomach, pancreas, and prostate, and also with certain chemotherapeutic agents (e.g. bleomycin and mitomycin).

2 Minimal-change nephrotic syndrome—rarely caused by lymphoma, usually Hodgkin's disease.

3 Membranous nephropathy—associated with malignancy, usually of solid organs, in 5 to 11% of cases. Malignant disease is typically advanced and obvious when nephrotic syndrome or heavy proteinuria is recognized. Very few treatable and otherwise subclinical tumours are uncovered by investigation in routine clinical practice.

4 Focal necrotizing and crescentic nephritis—may rarely be associated with malignancy and are usually antineutrophil cytoplasmic antibody (ANCA) negative.

Introduction

Malignant disease may affect the kidney and urinary tract by five broad mechanisms (see Table 21.10.8.1).

Direct involvement of the urinary tract

Solitary kidney tumours in adults are usually caused by renal cell carcinoma (hypernephroma). Bilateral tumours may occur, but multicentric tumours should lead to suspicion of an inherited disorder, either von Hippel–Lindau syndrome (see Chapter 21.12; cystic and solid lesions, some malignant) or tuberous sclerosis (see Chapter 21.12; benign lesions), both having autosomal dominant inheritance. Lymphoma and leukaemia may occasionally invade the renal substance on a sufficient scale to cause renal impairment, but it is rare for other tumours to do so.

A rare and aggressive renal medullary tumour has been described in young patients with sickle-cell trait or disease. These are easily confused with tumours of the collecting system and carry a poor prognosis.

The collecting system and lower urinary tract may be affected by transitional cell tumours or by malignancies that may invade the tract bilaterally or below the bladder. Transitional cell tumours affecting the bladder are common, and sometimes cause renal manifestations if extensive. Lesions in the ureters and collecting system are less common. They occur multifocally in association with analgesic nephropathy, Chinese herb nephropathy, and Balkan nephropathy (see Chapter 21.9.2).

Metabolic effects of malignancies on the kidney

Hypercalcaemia is a feature of many malignancies, both with and without metastasis. Its renal effects are discussed in Chapter 21.14. Hypokalaemia may be a consequence of acute leukaemias or rectal tumours, and may occasionally be severe enough to cause renal dysfunction (see Chapter 21.2.2).

Severe hyperuricaemia (>900 µmol/litre) is characteristically associated with massive cell death occurring following chemotherapy of haematological or solid tumours (tumour lysis syndrome), when it is usually accompanied by hyperphosphataemia, often by hypocalcaemia, and high serum lactate dehydrogenase levels may also be diagnostically useful. Similar gross hyperuricaemia may also be seen following radiotherapy of radiosensitive tumours, or may occur without therapy in malignancies with a very high rate of cell turnover, particularly acute lymphocytic or acute myeloid leukaemia, or poorly differentiated solid tumours. Uric acid levels this high can lead to precipitation within renal tubules and acute renal failure. Prevention and treatment of tumour lysis syndrome is discussed in Chapter 21.10.4.

Remote effects of malignant tumours on the kidney

Thrombotic microangiopathy

Thrombotic microangiopathy occurring in association with malignant disease (also known as malignancy-associated TTP, see Chapters 22.6.3 and 22.6.5) is often attributed to chemotherapy. It is

Table 21.10.8.1 How malignant disease affects the kidney and urinary tract

Mode of involvement	Examples
Direct	Tumours of the renal substance
	Lymphoma, leukaemia deposits
	Remote metastases from solid tumours
	Tumours of the urinary tract, prostate gland, etc.
	Local invasion (cervix, colon)
Metabolic and remote effects	Hypercalcaemia
	Hypokalaemia
	Hyperuricaemia
	Thrombotic microangiopathy (tumour-associated thrombotic thrombocytopenic purpura)
Deposition of tumour products	Myeloma kidney (precipitation in tubules)
	Immunoglobulin deposition diseases
Immune reaction	Minimal-change disease (particularly with lymphomas)
	Membranous nephropathy (particularly with solid tumours)
	Rapidly progressive glomerulonephritis and small vessel vasculitis
Effect of treatment	Tumour lysis syndrome
	Direct toxicity of drugs
	Idiosyncratic (e.g. immune) response

particularly associated with certain agents (e.g. bleomycin, mitomycin), although isolated reports implicate others. However, in some instances the classic presentation with thrombocytopenia, microangiopathic haemolytic anaemia, and renal failure occurs in association with primary tumours. This has been particularly reported for malignancies of the stomach, pancreas, and prostate. The syndrome is occasionally the presenting sign of malignancy but often occurs in a patient known to have a tumour.

In the absence of specific evidence, tumour-related thrombotic microangiopathy is usually treated in the same way as thrombotic microangiopathy of other types, by plasma exchange for fresh frozen plasma. If the tumour itself is responsive to treatment, microangiopathy generally subsides in a similar manner. Renal function may be recoverable if the process is halted rapidly, an outcome that is most likely in prostatic carcinoma.

Tumour products

The protean effects of monoclonal overproduction of immunoglobulins, or their component parts, are considered elsewhere (Chapter 21.10.4). The tubulotoxic effects of freely filtered immunoglobulin light chains may be amplified by hypercalcaemia in myeloma, or by concurrent administration of other nephrotoxins, notably intravenous radiological contrast media or possibly loop diuretics. Amyloidosis is another possible consequence of monoclonal proliferation of B cells, devastating enough on its own but it may be associated with myeloma or progress to overt myeloma. A variety of other renal consequences may occur in B-cell disorders

with overproduction of immunoglobulin fragments, notably the light chain (and rarer heavy chain) deposition disorders.

Immune reactions

Malignant diseases are common, hence on occasions cancer will be associated with nephropathies by chance. There are many case reports in the literature, but some associations have been reported consistently and are beyond doubt. The best-supported linkages between malignancies and intrinsic renal diseases are for minimal-change disease and membranous nephropathy, glomerular conditions that are believed to be immunologically mediated, although the evidence is often circumstantial. There is also substantial evidence for an association of malignancy with various types of vasculitis, which, as with glomerulonephritis, is usually believed to be immunologically mediated, both because of the typical contexts in which it occurs and because of its usual response to immunosuppressive agents. By contrast, there is little evidence for association of malignancies with primary interstitial renal diseases.

Some malignancies are particularly likely to be associated with renal disease. Chronic lymphocytic leukaemia and similar low-grade B-cell tumours are associated with a variety of types of glomerulopathy. Thymomas have frequently been associated with glomerular lesions, usually causing nephrotic syndrome with a variety of histological patterns.

Minimal-change nephrotic syndrome

Lymphomas, usually Hodgkin's disease, are rarely associated with minimal-change nephropathy. The renal lesion is typical in pathological characteristics, and usually also in response to corticosteroid treatment. In exceptional cases this is the presenting sign of the lymphoma, and it may also herald relapse. More so than with other renal lesions that are putatively associated with malignancy, there is often a close temporal relationship between the occurrence of nephrotic syndrome and the presentation of the tumour. However, there is no way of proving the association in an individual patient, or of suspecting an underlying lymphoma in patients who present with nephrotic syndrome without systemic symptoms. As the association is very rare in comparison to the number of young patients with minimal-change disease, screening other than by clinical examination and simple investigations is not justified.

Less commonly, minimal-change disease has been associated with solid tumours, and particularly with malignant and benign thymomas.

Membranous nephropathy

Membranous nephropathy has often been associated with malignancies, but membranous nephropathy is not rare and occurs in older patients who are at relatively high risk of malignancy simply on account of their age. Series have shown rates of malignancy from 5 to 11%, although the risk is greater in older patients. However, variation in reporting practice makes published figures difficult to interpret, e.g. if tumours that are recognized long after the renal diagnosis are included. Most reported tumours are of solid organs, including almost all types, but haematological malignancies are also implicated. Very often the disease is advanced and obvious when nephrotic syndrome or heavy proteinuria is recognized. In some cases the nephrotic syndrome or proteinuria lessens after effective treatment of the malignancy. The use of alkylating agents or corticosteroids as treatment for the membranous nephropathy is not recommended in this setting, unless this would be appropriate for treatment of the malignancy itself.

There is controversy about the value of screening for malignancy in patients presenting with membranous nephropathy when malignancy is not apparent from initial investigations. Aside from routine haematological and biochemical investigations, chest radiography, and renal ultrasonography that are needed in all cases of nephrotic syndrome, in older patients it is appropriate to perform careful breast and rectal examination, faecal occult blood screening, and possibly mammography and sigmoidoscopy or colonoscopy. However, in routine clinical practice the number of treatable and otherwise subclinical tumours uncovered in this way is low.

Systemic vasculitis

Focal necrotizing and crescentic nephritis, with or without evidence of small vessel vasculitis affecting other organs, may occur in association with malignancy. Some cases may be chance associations of malignancy with typical small vessel vasculitis that is not uncommon in older people, but there are sufficient reports of unusual associations to strongly suggest that there is sometimes a causal relationship. As well as true vasculitis, cancer-related thrombotic microangiopathy and thrombotic events complicating disseminated intravascular coagulation in association with cancer may resemble systemic vasculitis and lead to diagnostic confusion.

The most common type of vasculitis to be associated with malignancy is small vessel cutaneous vasculitis. In other cases, bowel and other organs including the kidney have been involved by a small-to-medium vessel systemic vasculitis, which is usually antineutrophil cytoplasmic antibody (ANCA) negative. However, more typical ANCA-associated vasculitis has also been associated with malignancy, and there may be a particular relationship between Wegener's granulomatosis and renal cell carcinoma. Usually the kidney is not involved in cancer-associated systemic vasculitis, but when it is the appearances are indistinguishable from those of small vessel vasculitis of other aetiologies. Immune deposits in glomeruli are not usual (pauci-immune).

Atrial myomas have been associated with lesions of larger and smaller vessels, and it appears that embolization is not always the explanation for this.

Effects of treatment for malignancy

These include the tumour lysis syndrome (discussed above and in Chapter 21.10.4), as well as idiosyncratic or predictable reactions to therapeutic agents. On occasions minimal-change disease or other proteinuria-causing lesions have been associated with treatment with interferons.

Further reading

Bacchetta J, et al. (2008). Paraneoplastic glomerular diseases and malignancies. *Crit Rev Oncol Haematol*, **70**, 39–58.

Biava CG, et al. (1984). Crescentic glomerulonephritis associated with nonrenal malignancies. *Am J Nephrol*, **4**, 208–14.

Burstein DM, Korbet SM, Schwartz MM (1993). Membranous glomerulonephritis and malignancy. *Am J Kidney Dis*, **22**, 5–10.

Cosyns JP, et al. (1999). Urothelial lesions in Chinese-herb nephropathy. *Am J Kidney Dis*, **33**, 1011–17.

Dabbs DJ, et al. (1986). Glomerular lesions in lymphomas and leukemias. *Am J Med*, **80**, 63–70.

Dimashkieh H, Choe J, Mutema G (2003). Renal medullary carcinoma: a report of 2 cases and review of the literature. *Arch Pathol Lab Med*, **127**, e135–8.

Gordon LI, et al. (1999). Thrombotic microangiopathy manifesting as thrombotic thrombocytopenic purpura/hemolytic uremic syndrome in the cancer patient. *Semin Thromb Hemost*, **25**, 217–21.

Kurzrock R, Cohen PR, Markowitz A (1994). Clinical manifestations of vasculitis in patients with solid tumors. A case report and review of the literature. *Arch Intern Med*, **154**, 334–40.

Lesesne JB, et al. (1989). Cancer-associated hemolytic-uremic syndrome: analysis of 85 cases from a national registry. *J Clin Oncol*, **7**, 781–9.

Ronco PM (1999). Paraneoplastic glomerulopathies: new insights into an old entity. *Kidney Int*, **56**, 355–77.

Tatsis E, et al. (1999). Wegener's granulomatosis associated with renal cell carcinoma. *Arthritis Rheum*, **42**, 751–6.

Valli G, et al. (1998). Glomerulonephritis associated with myasthenia gravis. *Am J Kidney Dis*, **31**, 350–5.

21.10.9 Atherosclerotic renovascular disease

P.A. Kalra and John D. Firth

Essentials

Atherosclerotic renovascular disease (ARVD), a general term that describes atheromatous narrowing of one or both renal arteries, affects about 0.5% of people over the age of 67 years in the United States of America. Patients with this condition are at high cardiovascular risk because of the presence of concomitant non-renal arterial disease, with mortality between 8 and 9% per year. Many patients have chronic kidney disease, but after the diagnosis of ARVD this only deteriorates in the minority, suggesting that prior hypertensive and/or ischaemic renal parenchymal injury is the usual cause of renal dysfunction.

Management—patients should be encouraged/helped to stop smoking and offered antiplatelet agents, cholesterol-lowering medication, blood pressure control (especially renin angiotensin blockade – which might appear surprising), and (in those with diabetes) optimization of glycaemic control. On the basis of randomized controlled trial data, they should not be offered revascularization by angioplasty/stenting for the purpose of improving blood pressure control or stabilizing/improving renal function, with reasonable exceptions to this being patients with otherwise unexplained rapid decline in renal function, recurrent episodes of flash pulmonary oedema, and (perhaps) those with severe hypertension not adequately controlled by drug treatment.

Introduction

Atheromatous disease is common, indeed almost universal in elderly individuals in western countries, and many patients have atherosclerotic narrowings of their renal arteries, renal artery stenosis (RAS). When present, RAS may be responsible for important clinical complications, such as hypertension or progressive decline in renal function, but more often it is an incidental finding and not pathophysiologically important. The physician is faced with a considerable challenge in steering the correct course between: (a) neglect of useful investigation and intervention in a few cases, and (b) meddlesome investigation and ineffective intervention in many, with risk of harm and little likelihood of benefit.

The issue of investigation and treatment of RAS in the context of the patient presenting with hypertension is discussed in Chapter 16.17.3. This brief chapter focuses more on patients with impairment of renal excretory function (chronic kidney disease) with reduced (and falling) estimated glomerular filtration rate (eGFR) in association with atherosclerotic renovascular disease (ARVD).

The underlying aetiology, genetics, pathogenesis, and histopathology of the major macrovascular RAS lesions in ARVD are broadly as for atherosclerotic disease in general (Chapter 16.13.1). However, histopathology of the kidney in patients with chronic kidney disease (CKD) associated with ARVD can involve a spectrum of changes including hypertensive and ischaemic injury, as well as atheroembolic disease. The latter is a recognized cause of acute kidney injury occurring after renal revascularization.

Epidemiology

It is difficult to state the true incidence and prevalence of ARVD because of variability in both definition and in the enthusiasm with which the diagnosis is pursued. There is no uniform agreement about the precise degree of RAS which constitutes a haemodynamically significant lesion. However, in the context of the patient with gradually failing renal function, in which the causal mechanism might be 'ischaemic renovascular disease' (ischaemic nephropathy), many consider that the presence of significant high-grade RAS (>75% narrowing of both renal arteries, or of the artery to a single functioning kidney) is necessary to make the diagnosis. A study of claims data from the United States Medicare population over 67 years of age gave an incidence of 3.7/1000 patient years. The overall prevalence in such patients is around 0.5%. In various studies RAS has been demonstrated in 5 to 22% of patients with endstage renal disease aged over 50 years, but the presence of ARVD here does not always imply causality of the renal dysfunction.

Patients with ARVD usually have evidence of other macrovascular disease such as coronary (67%), peripheral arterial (56%), and cerebrovascular (37%) atherosclerotic disease. Incidental RAS is found unilaterally in about 5% and bilaterally in about 1% of patients undergoing coronary angiography. One prospective study of 100 patients presenting with symptomatic peripheral arterial disease found unsuspected bilateral renovascular disease in 24%.

Some atherosclerotic RAS lesions become worse with time, but this is not inevitable, especially since the advent of statin therapy. Serial imaging studies report progression in 30 to 60% over 5 years, and those developing more severe stenoses tend to have more significant deterioration in renal function than those that do not, but these were performed in the pre-statin era. Progression to complete renal artery occlusion is uncommon (3% risk over 3 years in one study).

Clinical features

The diagnosis of ARVD should be suspected in any patient with other manifestations of atherosclerosis who presents with stable CKD or progressive impairment of renal function, especially in the presence of hypertension that is particularly severe or difficult to control. Other clinical pointers are the presence of abdominal or iliofemoral bruits, significant deterioration in renal function after initiation of treatment with an angiotensin-converting enzyme inhibitor or an angiotensin receptor blocker, and asymmetry of renal size on imaging (>1.5 cm difference in length of the two kidneys). Flash (acute) pulmonary oedema is a well-described and 'classic' manifestation of ARVD, but pulmonary oedema in a patient with ARVD is more usually attributable to concurrent ischaemic cardiac disease. ARVD is now increasingly recognized in association with congestive cardiac failure.

Clinical investigation

ARVD can only be confirmed by some form of imaging and the main techniques used include duplex Doppler ultrasonography (very operator dependent), magnetic resonance (MR) angiography (which requires administration of gadolinium and is contraindicated in patients with eGFR <30 ml/min, see Chapter 21.4), CT angiography (which requires administration of contrast media), and digital subtraction angiography (which requires arterial puncture/instrumentation and administration of contrast media). The investigative approach will be determined by local availability and expertise, but MR angiography is the technique of choice in many centres for patients with an eGFR of more than 30 ml/min. Note that, with the exception of high-quality arterial Doppler studies, none of the above tests assess functional significance of the RAS lesion, which remains a major deficiency in the investigation and management of patients with ARVD.

The urine may contain some protein (albumin/creatinine ratio uncommonly >50 mg/mmol), but is bland, without red cells or casts.

Management

All patients with ARVD should receive interventions appropriate for any patient with known atherosclerotic disease, including encouragement of and assistance with smoking cessation, aspirin (or other antiplatelet agents), statin therapy, blood pressure control, and (in patients with diabetes) optimization of glycaemic control. In view of the intrarenal parenchymal injury that is frequently associated with large vessel RAS, and which is the main cause of CKD in patients with ARVD, as well as the associated heart disease, the agents of choice for hypertension treatment are angiotensin-converting enzyme inhibitors and angiotensin receptor blockers. However, a minority of patients with critical bilateral RAS, or severe RAS affecting a solitary functioning kidney, are at risk of acute kidney injury with such therapy.

Aside from these general measures, the key management question concerns whether renal revascularization with renal artery angioplasty/stenting is warranted. While there is no doubt that such interventional procedures can produce 'anatomical cure' of RAS (Fig. 21.10.9.1), they can also cause major debilitating complications ranging from groin haematoma and acute kidney injury (10% each) to cholesterol embolization, arterial dissection, and renal infarction; these last serious complications occur in 5 to 10% of patients undergoing revascularization. Hence, a vital consideration is whether or not anatomical improvement translates into clinically useful outcome for patients. Results from small randomized controlled trials show no clear evidence of benefit. The best data

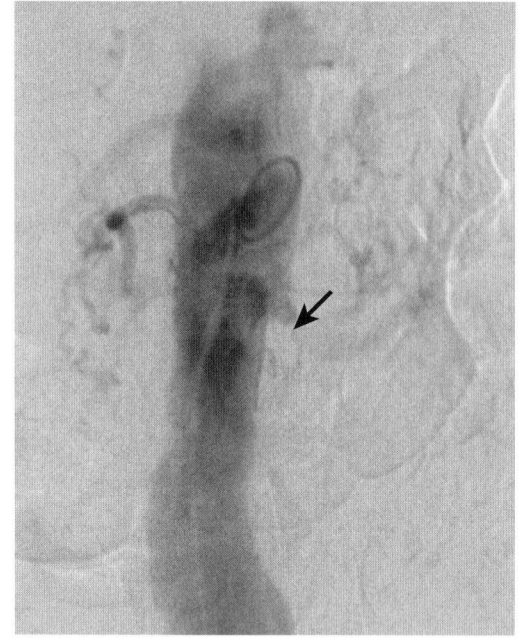

(a)

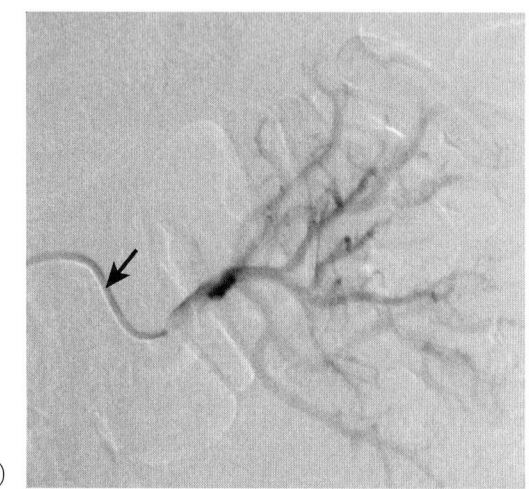

(b)

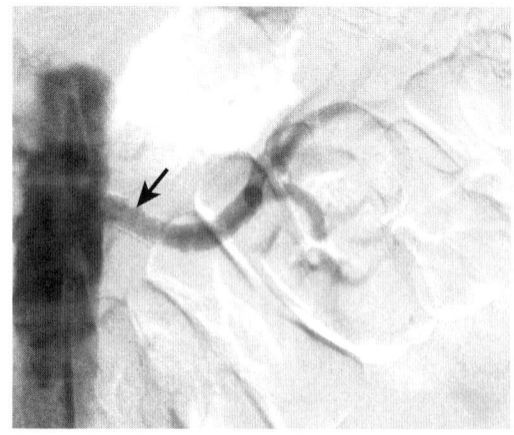

(c)

Fig. 21.10.9.1 An intra-arterial digital subtraction angiography series showing left renal angioplasty and stent placement. (a) Flush aortogram showing severe (>95%) left renal artery stenosis (arrow); the more distal circulation beyond the stenosis is just visible. (b) The angioplasty catheter (arrow) has traversed the renal artery stenosis. (c) A stent has been deployed (arrow).
(Courtesy of Professor J Moss, Gartnavel Hospital, Glasgow.)

come from the Angioplasty and Stenting for Renal Artery Lesions (ASTRAL) trial. Between November 2000 and October 2007 this recruited 806 patients (57 centres) with ARVD and significant RAS for whom the responsible clinicians were substantially uncertain as to whether to recommend that revascularization was definitely indicated. Patients were randomized in equal numbers between percutaneous revascularization (angioplasty and/or stenting) plus medical therapy or medical therapy alone. At baseline the average age for all patients was 70 years, eGFR 40 ml/min, creatinine 179 µmol/litre, blood pressure approximately 150/76 mmHg; 72% were current or previous smokers, 30% were diabetic, and 50% had pre-existing ischaemic heart disease; 60% of patients had a RAS of more than 70% and the average degree of RAS was 76%. At latest follow-up (mean duration 34 months) there was no difference in renal function (creatinine rose by 18 µmol/litre in the first year in both groups), blood pressure, renal events, and cardiovascular events between the two arms of the trial, and mortality was approximately 8% per year in both groups. Data from longer follow-up are awaited, as are the findings of another large study that is led by United States investigators, the Cardiovascular Outcomes with Renal Atherosclerotic Lesions [CORAL] study.

Our recommendation is that there is no benefit of screening asymptomatic patients with CKD and/or hypertension for ARVD, and that most patients found to have ARVD should generally not be referred for revascularization for the purpose of improving blood pressure control or stabilizing/improving renal function. Reasonable exceptions to this include those patients with severe RAS and with otherwise unexplained rapid decline in renal function, those with recurrent episodes of flash pulmonary oedema (not explained by cardiac disease), and perhaps those with severe hypertension not adequately controlled by multiple drug treatment (or in whom reduction in arterial pressure leads to significant decline in eGFR). Another subgroup who could justifiably be treated with revascularization are those who require angiotensin-converting enzyme inhibitors and angiotensin receptor blockers because of concomitant heart disease and/or renal parenchymal injury, but show intolerance of these drugs as manifest by acute kidney injury. It is not proven that revascularization is helpful to patients with RAS with these last clinical scenarios, but this is not the same as saying that there is evidence of no benefit.

Prognosis

Patients with ARVD are at high cardiovascular risk, with 34% mortality at 4 years in the ASTRAL study, but most (around 80%) have stable renal function over that time period. Indeed, in the United States Medicare population the risk of mortality during follow-up was almost 6 times that of requiring renal replacement therapy.

Likely future developments

It remains a concern that, while most patients with ARVD do not benefit from revascularization, there is undoubtedly a subgroup—yet to be categorically defined—who would, and that an excessively nihilistic approach will prevent such patients from being identified. It is possible that the combination of functional and structural imaging techniques, e.g. those which enable comparison of single kidney GFR with parenchymal volume of the kidneys, may allow recognition of kidneys supplied by functionally significant RAS which retain 'hibernating parenchyma' (i.e. kidney volume unusually large for a given single-kidney GFR, implying that the renal tissue is not already irretrievably damaged). Such kidneys might respond beneficially to revascularization, but this can only be determined if appropriate clinical trials are performed.

Further reading

Caps MT, *et al.* (1998). Prospective study of atherosclerotic disease progression in the renal artery. *Circulation*, **98**, 2866–72.

Cheung CM, *et al.* (2005). Dilemmas in the management of renal artery stenosis. *Br Med Bulletin*, **73**, 35–55.

Cheung CM, *et al.* (2006). MR-derived renal morphology and renal function in patients with atherosclerotic renovascular disease. *Kidney Int*, **69**, 715–22.

Kalra PA, *et al.* (2005). Atherosclerotic renovascular disease in United States patients aged 67 years or older: risk factors, revascularization, and prognosis. *Kidney Int*, **68**, 293–301.

The ASTRAL investigators. (2009). Revascularisation versus medical therapy for renal-artery stenosis. *N Engl J Med*, **361**, 1953–62.

Renal diseases in the tropics

Vivekanand Jha

Essentials

Kidney diseases encountered in tropical areas are a mix of conditions with worldwide distribution and those that are secondary to factors unique to the tropics, e.g. climatic conditions, infectious agents, nephrotoxic plants, envenomations, and chemical toxins. Important presentations are with nephrotic syndrome, acute renal failure, and progressive renal insufficiency. Cultural factors, illiteracy, superstitions, living conditions, level of access to health care, and nutritional status also affect the nature and course of disease. Knowledge of such conditions and issues is important for medical professionals in all parts of the globe, as ease of travel means that individuals and practices are exported with increasing frequency.

Glomerular diseases—important infection-related glomerulopathies include quartan malarial nephropathy in African children; schistosomal nephropathy in North Africa and South America; postinfectious glomerulonephritides in South America, Africa, and Asia; and filarial nephropathy in South-East Asia and Africa. An immunological basis secondary to prolonged exposure to microbial antigens is thought to be responsible. Once established, the course of disease is rarely modified by treatment of underlying infection, but the incidence of these conditions has shown a decline in some areas alongside the control of infection.

Acute kidney injury—diarrhoeal diseases, obstetric complications, intravascular haemolysis due to inherited red-cell enzyme deficiency, copper sulphate poisoning, ingestion of toxic plants, snake bites, insect stings, and infections specific to the particular region are the main causes of community-acquired acute renal failure in the tropics. Renal failure is often part of multiorgan failure, which significantly increases the risk of death. Falciparum malaria and leptospirosis are the most important infectious aetiologies.

Toxins—use of traditional medicines that include indigenous herbs and chemicals dispensed by faith healers are the most important toxic causes of acute renal failure in sub-Saharan Africa. Bites by venomous snakes belonging to viper and sea snake families, and stings by bees, hornets, and wasps, cause renal failure through a combination of direct nephrotoxicity, intravascular haemolysis, and rhabdomyolysis. Prompt antivenom administration and supportive treatment is the key to recovery from snake envenomation. Renal failure is irreversible in the few patients with obstetric complications and snake-bite who develop acute renal cortical necrosis.

Uncommon presentations of tropical kidney diseases include renal infarction (with acute renal failure in case of bilateral involvement) due to mucormycosis, chyluria due to filariasis, amyloidosis due to tuberculosis and leprosy, obstructive nephropathy due to lower urinary tract schistosomiasis, and progressive interstitial nephritis secondary to chronic ingestion of some tropical herbs.

Introduction

Kidney diseases in the tropical areas are a mix of globally encountered conditions and those specific to the tropics. The latter can be related to exposure to environmental factors unique to the tropics, e.g. climatic conditions, infectious agents, nephrotoxic plants, envenomations, and chemical toxins, or secondary to genetic predisposition in specific ethnic groups. A high prevalence of nephrolithiasis in some tropical areas, secondary to dehydration caused by a combination of exposure to high ambient temperatures and a high prevalence of diarrhoeal diseases is an example. Genetic factors that predispose to kidney disease in the tropics include glucose-6-phosphate dehydrogenase (G6PD) deficiency giving rise to intravascular haemolysis and pigment-induced acute renal failure; progressive kidney disease in haemoglobinopathies such as sickle cell anaemia and thalassaemias; and hypokalaemia, hypercalcaemia, hypocitraturia, and renal tubular acidosis due to inherited defects in tubular transport.

Cultural factors, illiteracy, superstitions, poor living conditions, and nutritional status also affect the nature and course of kidney disease. Lack of access to health care in underdeveloped regions of the tropics results in delayed diagnosis, and extreme presentations that have been eliminated in the developed world are still encountered. For example, it is not uncommon for children with distal renal tubular acidosis to present with marked skeletal deformities and severe growth retardation; and acute renal cortical necrosis following septic abortion and placental abruption continues to be seen regularly. Malnutrition exaggerates the impact of kidney disease; a lower degree of protein loss leads to more severe peripheral oedema and serous effusions. Delayed and suboptimal treatment increases morbidity and mortality.

Reliable statistics on renal diseases in the tropical countries are not available. Published data is mostly based on individual experiences and may not be accurate reflection of disease in entire regions.

Easy transcontinental movement of people, organisms, and materials has increased the need of awareness of tropical renal diseases among nephrologists other regions of the world. People who have migrated from the tropics continue to engage in habits that predispose to kidney disease even in their new location. Also, slowly progressive diseases due to past infections or exposure to toxins in the tropics may manifest much later.

This chapter highlights the important differences between different syndromes of kidney disease in the tropics and the rest of the world, and discuss certain specific renal diseases unique to the tropical regions.

Presentations of renal disease in the tropics

Glomerular diseases

The overall prevalence of glomerulonephritis is reported to be higher in tropical countries than in temperate regions. Hospital-based surveys from South Africa, Zimbabwe, Senegal, Uganda, Nigeria, Yemen, and Papua New Guinea show that nephrotic syndrome accounts for 0.2 to 4% of all hospital admissions. Primary glomerular diseases account for the majority, but secondary causes are responsible in 40 to 55% of patients in Zimbabwe and Jamaica.

Significant differences are noted in the epidemiology, aetiology, and natural history of glomerulonephritis between populations living in countries with tropical and temperate climates (Figs. 21.11.1 and 21.11.2). In particular, there is a high prevalence of infection-related glomerulonephritis in tropical regions; the pattern being

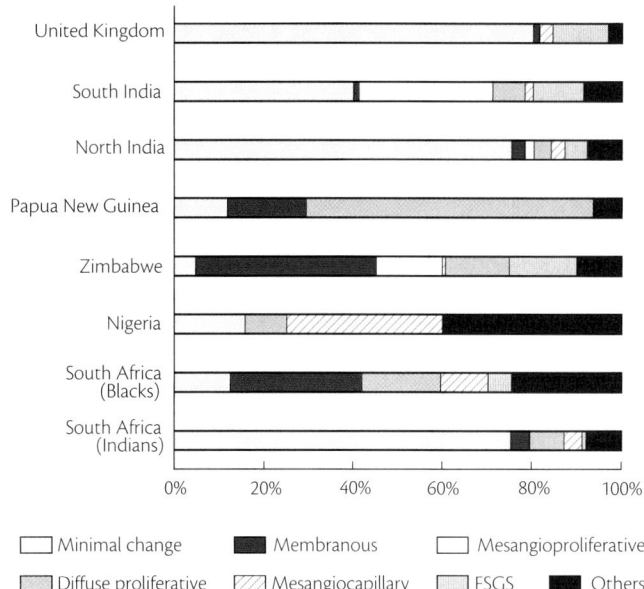

Fig. 21.11.2 Prevalence of different types of glomerular lesion in children with nephrotic syndrome in different parts of the world.

dependent upon the nature of the prevalent endemic infection in that region.

Minimal-change disease is as frequent in Asia and North Africa as in the developed world, but is seen less commonly in the rest of Africa. In a study from South Africa, minimal-change disease was responsible for nephrotic syndrome in 75% of children of Indian ancestry, whereas only 13.5% of black children showed this lesion. A high frequency of proliferative glomerulopathies and steroid resistance is described in pediatric patients from the Democratic Republic of Congo (formerly Zaire), Zimbabwe, Malawi, Nigeria, Kenya, and Uganda. Membranous nephropathy is seen with a high frequency in countries with a high hepatitis B carrier rate.

IgA nephropathy accounts for between 30 and 50% of all cases of primary glomerulonephritis in tropical East Asian countries, but is reported much less frequently from the Indian subcontinent, South America, and Africa. One explanation for this difference may be the lack of facilities for immunofluorescence studies.

Postinfectious glomerulonephritis, due to both streptococcal and nonstreptococcal organisms, continues to be encountered. In a study from Venezuela, the prevalence of poststreptococcal glomerulonephritis in Goajiro Indian community was twice that seen in other parts of the state.

Acute renal failure

Community-acquired acute renal failure is the commonest nephrological emergency encountered in the tropics. Referral patterns to dialysis units suggest a higher prevalence of community-acquired acute renal failure in the tropics than in Western countries with a temperate climate. In a large referral hospital in North India, 1.5% of all hospital admissions were referred to the nephrology service for management of moderate to severe acute renal failure. Medical causes predominate, with diarrhoeal diseases, intravascular haemolysis due to G6PD deficiency, ingestion of toxic plants, snake bites, insect stings, and infections specific to the region being responsible for most cases, although obstetric causes remain common in some parts of the world (Figs. 21.11.3 and 21.11.4).

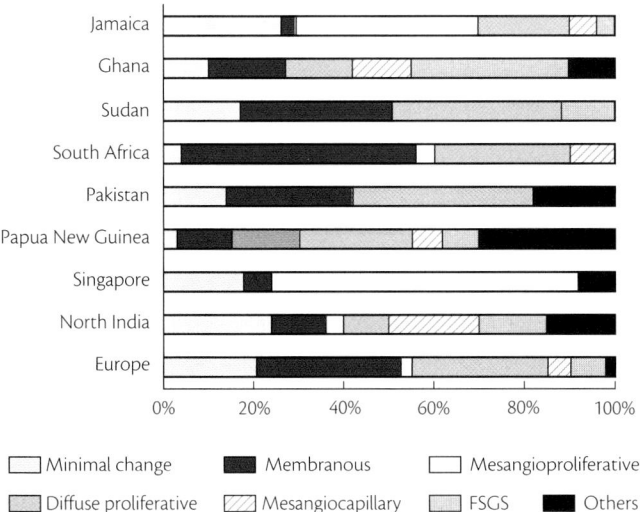

Fig. 21.11.1 Prevalence of different types of glomerular lesion in adults with nephrotic syndrome in different parts of the world.

Patients presenting with and receiving treatment for acute renal failure in tropical countries are relatively young; in one study the average age of patients dialysed for acute renal failure in India was 34.3 years. Frequently, acute renal failure is a part of multiorgan failure that includes liver failure, respiratory failure, neurological dysfunction, disseminated intravascular coagulation (DIC), and metabolic acidosis.

Because of lack of sufficient haemodialysis or haemofiltration facilities, established acute renal failure is treated by intermittent peritoneal dialysis using a rigid catheter in many units in underdeveloped tropical countries.

Chronic kidney disease

Several differences are described in the pattern of chronic kidney disease in topical populations compared to those in temperate zones (Fig. 21.11.5). Tropical patients with endstage renal disease are significantly younger, and infection-related glomerular diseases are reported to be the most frequent cause in many areas. The relative contribution of diabetic nephropathy is increasing in some parts of tropics as a result of increasing Westernization.

Many patients with endstage renal disease come to medical attention for the first time with advanced renal failure and few, if any, prior symptoms. Investigations reveal minimal proteinuria, bland urinary sediment, and smooth contracted kidneys. It has been postulated that these cases represent a form of chronic interstitial nephritis as a result of exposure to unknown nephrotoxins present in agricultural pesticides, or due to consumption of nephrotoxic plants, Chinese herb (aristolochic acid) nephropathy being a specific example of the latter (as discussed in Chapter 21.9.2).

Kidney diseases specific to the tropics

In addition to well-recognized nephropathies with worldwide distribution, several renal lesions have been described solely in residents of tropical countries. These can be broadly grouped under infectious and toxic categories. Causal relationships are initially suggested by epidemiological studies and then established by demonstrating the resolution of renal lesions following treatment of the infection or withdrawal of environmental insult. More

recently, improved diagnostic techniques and well-designed experimental studies have provided more concrete evidence of a cause-and-effect relationship. Confirmation has been obtained by the demonstration of either the organism or microbial antigens in the lesions, and elution of specific antibodies in the case of infections and toxic compounds in the case of plant and animal toxins. Animal models have been developed that provide insight into the genesis of the lesions.

Kidney diseases caused by infections in the tropics

The tropical ecobiology supports the growth of a variety of exotic microbes that are not encountered in temperate countries. Many of these have been associated with kidney disease (Table 21.11.1).

Malarial renal diseases

Malaria, caused by members of the protozoan *Plasmodium* genus, is endemic in the Indian subcontinent, Middle East, East Asia, sub-Saharan Africa, and Central America where the hot and humid tropical climate is conducive to multiplication of the disease vector, the anopheles mosquito. Of the four species that are pathogenic in humans—*P. vivax*, *P. ovale*, *P. malariae*, and *P. falciparum*—only the latter two are associated with clinically significant renal disease. Glomerulonephritis is observed with *P. malariae* (quartan malarial nephropathy), and less commonly with *P. falciparum* infection. Acute renal failure is the chief complication of falciparum malaria.

Malarial glomerulopathy

Quartan malarial nephropathy has been described amongst nephrotic children in western Nigeria, Uganda, Kenya, Côte d'Ivoire, Sumatra, New Guinea, and Yemen. Nephrotic syndrome is encountered with increased frequency in hospitals during periods of intense malaria transmission, with plasmodium positivity noted in 39–75% cases. The prevalence has shown a consistent decline with the eradication of malaria in many areas. Autopsy studies reveal glomerular lesions in about 18% of cases with *P. falciparum* malaria, but urinary abnormalities including nonselective proteinuria, microhaematuria and casts are noted in 20 to 50%.

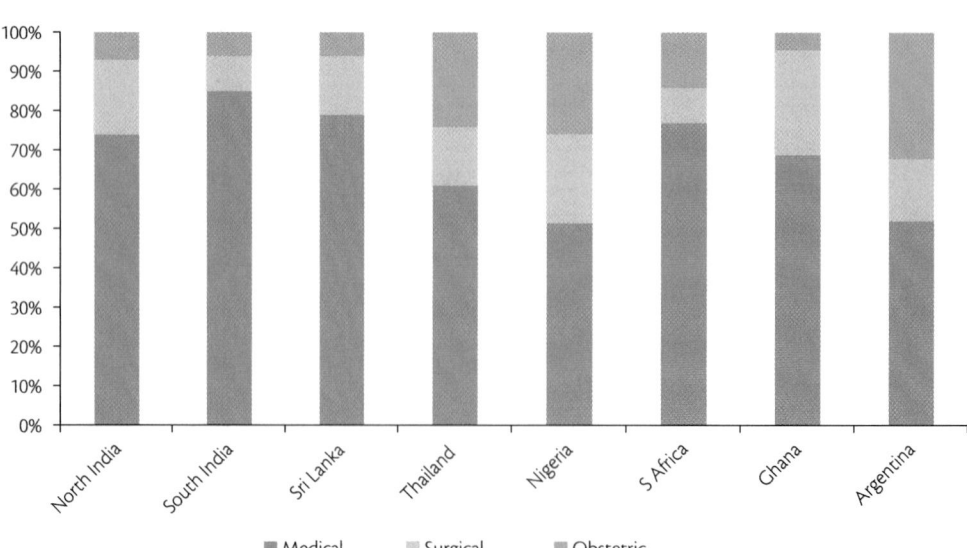

Fig. 21.11.3 Causes of acute renal failure in different tropical countries. Modified from Chugh, Satprija and Jha, Oxford Textbook of Clinical Nephrology, Oxford University Press, Oxford 2005.

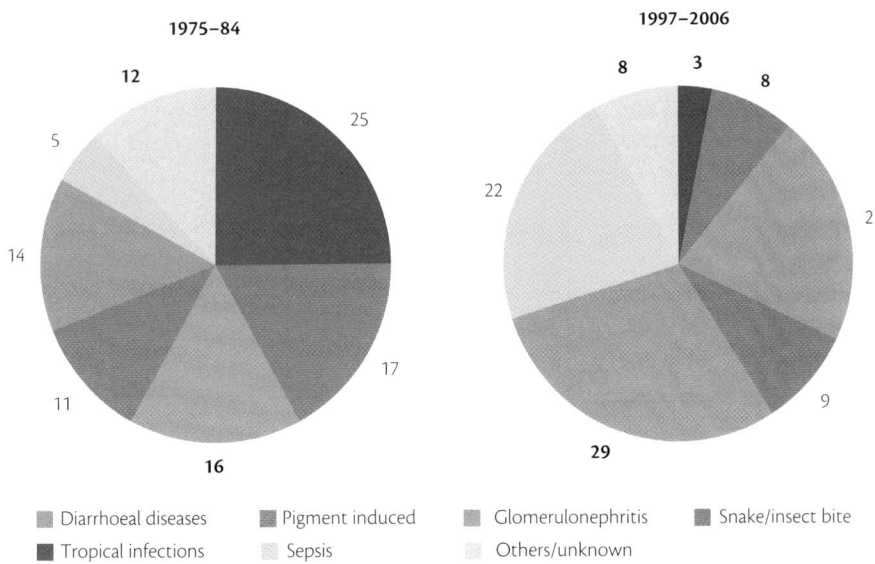

Fig. 21.11.4 Change in the causes of medical acute renal failure seen at the Postgraduate Institute of Medical Education and Research (Chandigarh, India) over two time periods, 1975–84 and 1997–2006.

Clinical features

Rare during the first 2 years of life, the peak incidence of quartan malarial nephropathy is noted between 5 and 8 years of age; sporadic cases are reported in adult life. The nephrotic syndrome develops several weeks after the onset of quartan fever. Proteinuria is nonselective, and microscopic haematuria is noted in about one-third of cases. Hypertension develops along with decline in renal function. Anaemia is universal, and hepatosplenomegaly is present in over 75% of cases. Hypoalbuminaemia is profound, with values commonly less than 1 g/dl. The serum cholesterol level tends to be normal or low, reflecting low dietary intake. Serum creatinine is usually normal at presentation. Serum complement (C3) is within the normal range.

Pathology

The predominant light-microscopic abnormality in quartan malarial nephropathy is segmental glomerular capillary wall thickening due to the subendothelial deposition of periodic acid–Schiff and silver stain-positive fibrils arranged in a plexiform manner. Laying down of new basement membrane material on the subepithelial side gives rise to the classic 'double contouring'. Focal in the early stages, the lesion becomes diffuse as the disease progresses. Eventually the capillary lumina are obliterated and global mesangial sclerosis supervenes. Proliferative lesions including fibroepithelial crescents have been described in adults. A mild endocapillary glomerulonephritis has been described in falciparum malaria.

Immunofluorescence shows deposits of IgG, IgM, and C3. Three patterns have been described: the commonest is a coarse, granular IgG3 deposition along the capillary walls; a few show diffuse, homogeneously distributed IgG2 deposits; and a mixed pattern is observed in the remaining cases. *P. malariae* antigen is detected in the deposits in about one-third of patients. Electron microscopy reveals subendothelial and intramembranous deposits.

Pathogenesis

Demonstration of malarial antigen in the deposits and binding of specific antibody to circulating malarial antigens suggest an immunological basis for the condition. The rhesus monkey (*Macaca mulatta*) develops an immune complex glomerulonephritis when infected with *P. inui*. Subendothelial location of the deposits indicates formation of immune complexes in the circulation rather than *in situ*. It has been suggested that environmental factors such

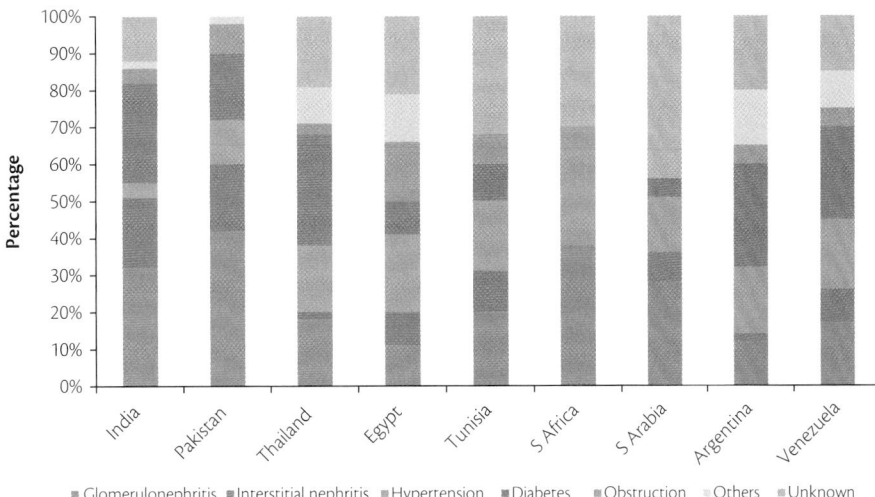

Fig. 21.11.5 Causes of endstage kidney disease in different countries. (Data from Barsoum R (2002). Overview: End-stage renal disease in the developing world. *Artif Organs*, **26**, 737; and Jha V, unpublished.)

Table 21.11.1 Tropical infections associated with glomerular lesions

Protozoal	Plasmodium malariae
	Plasmodium falciparum
	Schistosoma mansoni
	Wuchereria bancrofti
	Loa loa
	Onchocerca volvulus
Bacterial	Mycobacterium leprae
	Mycobacterium tuberculosis
	Salmonella typhi
	Shigella dystenteriae
	Brucella abortus
	Burkholderia pseudomallei
	Vibrio vulnificus
Viral	Dengue haemorrhagic fever
	Hantavirus infection
	Rift valley fever
	Yellow fever
	HIV
	Hepatitis B and C
Spirochete	Leptospira icterohaemorrhagica

as malnutrition or coinfection with Epstein–Barr virus (EBV) may be permissive, also that the liver may act as a source of continuous antigen supply by harbouring the parasite. Transient glomerular lesions akin to those in falciparum malaria can be induced in BALB/c mice and Sprague–Dawley rats infected with *P. berghei* and in *P. falciparum*-infected squirrel monkeys. CD4 cell subpopulations of the Th2 class may be playing a significant role, as renal cytokine expression strongly correlates with the severity of proteinuria in *P. berghei* infected mice.

Management

Treatment of quartan malarial nephropathy is highly unsatisfactory. Once established, the disease follows an inexorably progressive course, culminating in renal failure within 2 to 4 years. Antimalarial drugs such as chloroquine and pyrimethamine have been ineffective in controlled trials. Prednisolone is ineffective in inducing remissions and may lead to infections and worsening of hypertension. Remission of nephrotic syndrome has been reported occasionally with cyclophosphamide, but there is no improvement in survival. By contrast, glomerulonephritis associated with falciparum malaria resolves within a few weeks of eradication of infection.

Malarial acute renal failure

Less than 1% of all cases with *P. falciparum* infection develop acute renal failure, but the prevalence increases to 60% in those with severe infection. Nonimmune visitors to an endemic area are more likely to develop severe infection than local residents. Malarial acute renal failure has been reported from the Indian subcontinent, Thailand, Malaysia, and Africa.

Clinical features

The initial symptoms are nonspecific and consist of malaise, headache, fatigue, muscle aches, fever, and chills; classic malarial paroxysms with spiking fever and rigors are rare. Nausea, vomiting, and hypotension are more frequent in nonimmune individuals. Neurological involvement, noncardiogenic pulmonary oedema, shock, and disseminated intravascular coagulation indicate severe infection. Acute renal failure is usually seen by the end of first week and is nonoliguric in 50–75% of cases. Haemolytic anaemia and cholestatic jaundice are frequent accompaniments. The so-called 'blackwater fever' has seen a resurgence amongst nonimmune European expatriates, probably due to reintroduction of quinine and mefloquine into the treatment regimen. Renal failure lasts from a few days to several weeks, with an average of 2 weeks. Investigations show severe azotaemia, hyponatraemia, hyperkalaemia, and lactic acidosis. Diagnosis requires the demonstration of asexual forms of the parasite in peripheral blood smears stained with Giemsa stain or acridine orange.

Pathology

Acute tubular necrosis, characterized by cloudy swelling and degeneration of tubular cells and casts loaded with malarial pigment, is the most prominent finding. Tubular cells contain haemosiderin granules. Varying degrees of interstitial oedema and mononuclear cell infiltrate are also seen.

Pathogenesis

Renal failure is attributed to haemodynamic alterations produced by unique properties of the parasite, which produces haemorheological changes leading to renal ischaemia. *P. falciparum* merozoites consume and degrade erythrocyte proteins and alter the red-cell membrane, making the erythrocytes more spherical and less deformable. Cup-shaped, electron-dense structures that overlie accretions of histidine-rich *P. falciparum* erythrocyte membrane protein and extrude an adhesive protein of high molecular weight are expressed on the erythrocyte membrane and mediate attachment to CD36, PECAM-1/CD31, thrombomodulin, selectins, ICAM-1, and VCAM-1 present on endothelial cells, causing a phenomenon called 'cytoadherence'. Infected erythrocytes also adhere to uninfected red cells, platelets, monocytes, and lymphocytes. Finally, *P. falciparum* activates the alternate complement pathway and intrinsic coagulation cascade. Increased endothelin-1 levels, increased plasma viscosity secondary to an increase in plasma fibrinogen, and rhabdomyolysis also contribute to the acute renal failure. Studies from Thailand indicate that prior infestation with helminths is protective against malarial acute renal failure.

Management

Severe falciparum malaria requires intensive supportive care in combination with specific antimalarial treatment (see Chapter 7.8.2). Patients are at particular risk of pulmonary oedema due to capillary leak, hence fluid should be administered cautiously. Some studies have found dopamine and furosemide to be beneficial in maintaining renal blood flow and urine volume in patients with mild renal failure. Any form of dialysis, including peritoneal dialysis and continuous renal replacement therapy, can be used for managing these patients.

The mortality of malarial acute renal failure is 10 to 40%. Late referral, high parasitaemia, multiorgan involvement, and infection in previously unimmunized subjects portend a poor prognosis.

Renal disease in schistosoma infections

Schistosomiasis is a chronic infection caused by trematodes (blood flukes) and affects over 300 million people in Asia, Africa, and South America. Of the seven species pathogenic to humans, the most prevalent are *Schistosoma haematobium* (Africa and the Middle East), *S. mansoni* (South America and Africa) and *S. japonicum* (China and the Far East). *S. haematobium* primarily involves the lower urinary tract, whereas *S. mansoni* involves the gastrointestinal tract and portal system, leading to hepatic fibrosis and portal hypertension.

Schistosomal nephropathy

Glomerulonephritis has been described in association with hepatosplenic schistosomiasis produced by *S. mansoni*. Reports from autopsy series in Brazil during the 1960s were followed by clinical observations from endemic areas of Africa, Saudi Arabia, and Yemen. Proteinuria has been reported in 1 to 22% of patients infected with *S. mansoni* and 2 to 5% with *S. haematobium* infection. Subclinical glomerular lesions were found in about 40% of patients with hepatosplenic schistosomiasis.

Clinical features

Though described at all ages, glomerulonephritis is most frequent in young adults with overt hepatosplenic disease. Males are affected twice as frequently as females. Peripheral oedema and ascites are the hallmarks; hypertension is seen in 50% of cases, appearing late in the disease. Proteinuria is poorly selective and haematuria is uncommon in the absence of lower urinary tract involvement. Complement levels are usually low. Nonspecific antibody production is demonstrated by false-positive rheumatoid factor or the VDRL (Venereal Disease Research Laboratory) tests. It is important to exclude other causes of nephrotic syndrome before attributing the lesions to schistosomiasis. Diagnosis is confirmed by demonstrating viable eggs in the stool or egg-containing granulomas in rectal or liver biopsies.

Pathology

Five patterns of glomerular pathology have been described (Table 21.11.2). The class I lesion is the earliest and most frequent, and the principal lesion in renal allografts with recurrent schistosomal nephropathy. Class II lesions are more frequent in patients with concomitant salmonella infection. The frequency of class III lesions varies from 20% in asymptomatic patients to over 80% in those with overt renal disease. Electron microscopy shows subendothelial and epimembranous deposits in classes IIIA and IIIB, respectively. The class IV lesion, seen in 15 to 40% of cases, cannot be distinguished from idiopathic focal segmental glomerulosclerosis on the basis of light microscopy, but immunofluorescence reveals IgA deposition. Class III and IV lesions are seen in patients with fibrotic livers and associated with severe hypocomplementemia. Class V prevalence varies from 15 to 40%, with a higher frequency in African patients. This form is not usually affected by hepatic fibrosis. Schistosomal antigen is detected in a minority of cases.

Pathogenesis

Schistosomal glomerulopathy is caused by the immunological reaction to specific parasitic antigens. Out of over 100 immunological constituents extracted from various stages of the worm life cycle, the pathogenic antigens have been identified as arising from the gut of the adult worm. Schistosoma antigens have been demonstrated in the glomeruli of Kenyan baboons infected with *S. mansoni*, and circulating immune complexes have been documented in experimental animals and humans with hepatosplenic disease. Circulating complexes localize in mesangial and subendothelial locations, whereas the extramembranous deposits form *in situ*.

Portocaval shunting prevents normal hepatic processing of worm antigen and delivers it directly into the systemic circulation. Despite heavy infestation, glomerular disease is seen neither in humans with *S. haematobium* infection, nor in baboons with *S. mansoni* infection, who do not have portal fibrosis. IgM antibodies are seen in most patients with hepatosplenic schistosomiasis alone, but circulating mononuclear IgA-bearing cells and IgA antibodies predominate in those with glomerular involvement. An isotype switch from IgM- to IgA-producing B cells is believed to be responsible for this alteration.

A role for disordered autoimmunity is suggested by demonstration of antinuclear antibodies against the public anti-DNA idiotype 16/6 ID in the sera and glomerular deposits of humans and experimental animals.

The immune reaction may be modified by concomitant infection with salmonella, hepatitis viruses, staphylococci, and mycobacteria. Epidemiological studies have shown clearance of urinary abnormalities following therapy for salmonella alone, suggesting a permissive role of this infection in some cases.

Management

Treatment of schistosomal glomerulopathy is disappointing. Antischistosomal drugs like oxamniquine, hycanthone, or praziquantel are unsuccessful in altering the clinical course, which is one of inexorable progression to renal failure. Steroids or cytotoxic agents are ineffective: isolated reports of response to these agents have not been evaluated in controlled trials. Salmonella infection should be looked for and treated in all patients.

Schistosomiasis involving the lower urinary tract

The adult *S. hematobium* worm resides and lays eggs in the perivesical venous plexus, where they get trapped in the lower urinary tract mucosa and incite granuloma formation. Clinical manifestations appear when they coalesce into larger ganulomata or polyps that ulcerate and bleed. With passage of time, fibrosis and calcification set in. The presenting feature in the initial stages is painful haematuria, and characteristic ova with terminal spikes may be seen on urinary examination. Later stages are characterized by symptoms related to reduced bladder volume, obstruction to urine flow at the level of bladder outlet or ureterovesical junction, vesicoureteric reflux or urinary tract infection. Plain radiology may reveal linear or irregular calcification in the bladder wall, ureter, or seminal vesicles (Fig. 21.11.6). Cystoscopy confirms bladder cicatrization.

Vesical cancer is a complication of chronic schistosomal cystitis, and develops approximately three decades after the initial infection in about 5% of all infected individuals. In Egypt, schistosomal eggs are demonstrated in over 85% of resected specimens of bladder cancer.

Long-standing obstruction leads to progressive loss of kidney function; 7 to 20% of the endstage renal disease population in Egypt is secondary to lower tract schistosomiasis.

Table 21.11.2 Clinicopathological classification of schistosomal glomerulopathy

Class	I	II	III A	IIIB	IV	V
Light microscopic pattern	Mesangioproliferative	Exudative	Mesangio- capillary type I	Mesangiocapillary type II	Focal and segmental glomerulosclerosis	Amyloidosis
	(a) 'Minimal lesion'					
	(b) Focal proliferative					
	(c) Diffuse proliferative					
Immunofluorescence	Mesangial IgM and C3. Schistosomal gut antigens	Endocapillary C3 Schistosomal antigens	Mesangial IgG, IgA and C3, schistosomal gut antigen	Mesangial and subepithelial IgG and C3, schistosomal gut antigen (early), IgA(late)	Mesangial IgG, IgM, and IgA	Mesangial IgG
Asymptomaticproteinuria	+++	−	+	+	+	+
Nephrotic syndrome	+	+++	++	+++	+++	+++
Hypertension	±	−	++	+	+++	±
Progression to end stage renal disease	±	±	++	++	+++	+++
Response to treatment	±	+++	−	−	−	−

(modified from Barsoum R, *Kidney Int* 1993).

Renal disease in filarial infection

Filarial worms are nematodes that dwell in the subcutaneous tissues and lymphatics. These are transmitted to humans through arthropod bites. Clinical manifestations depend upon the location of microfilariae and adult worms in the tissues. Of the eight filarial species that infect humans, *Loa loa*, *Onchocerca volvulus*, *Wuchereria bacrofti*, and *Brugia malayi* are associated with glomerular disease.

Loiasis is prevalent in West and Central Africa and manifests with localized allergic inflammation and calabar swellings. Onchocerciasis (river blindness) is characterized by subcutaneous nodules, a pruritic skin rash, sclerosing lymphadenitis, and ocular lesions. Bancroftian and brugia infections cause febrile episodes associated with acute lymphangitis and lymphadenitis, leading to lymphoedema manifesting as hydrocele and elephantiasis. This form of filariasis is endemic in Africa and South-East Asia.

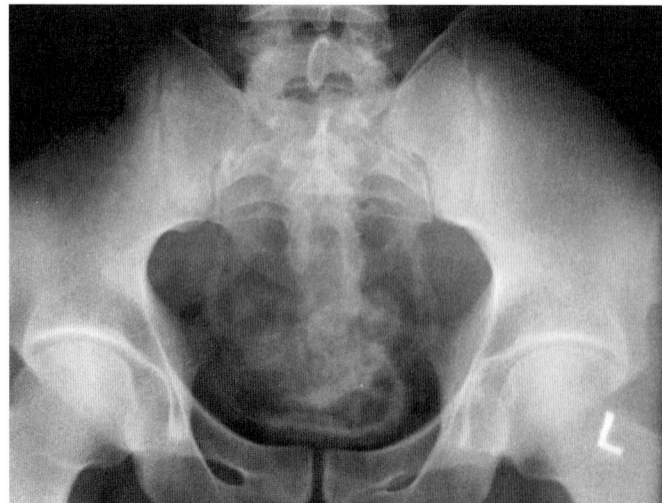

Fig. 21.11.6 Plain radiograph of a patient with *S. haematobium* infection showing calcification of bladder wall (courtesy Prof R Barsoum).

Filarial nephropathy

Clinical features

Urinary abnormalities have been described in 11 to 25% of cases of loiasis and onchocerciasis, with a nephrotic syndrome in 3 to 5%, this being more common in those with polyarthritis and chorioretinitis. Compared to controls, patients infected with *B. malayi* show a higher incidence of proteinuria. In a survey in an endemic area, proteinuria was detected in over 50% of patients with filariasis, with 25% showing a glomerular pattern of protein loss. The frequencies of proteinuria, microhaematuria, and hypertension are significantly higher in patients with chronic sclerosing filariasis than in those with an acute febrile illness or microfilaraemia. False-positive rheumatoid factor and anti-DNA and antiphospholipid antibodies have been described.

Pathology

Light microscopy reveals a gamut of lesions, including mesangial proliferative, mesangiocapillary, and chronic sclerosing glomerulonephritis, minimal-change disease, and the collapsing variant of focal segmental glomerulosclerosis. A diffuse basement membrane thickening with mild increase in the number of endocapillary cells is the commonest finding. Mononuclear interstitial infiltration and microinfarcts around blood vessels have been demonstrated in patients with loiasis. Microfilariae may be found in the glomerular capillary lumina, tubules, and interstitium. Electron microscopy shows widely spaced subepithelial, subendothelial, and intramembranous deposits and spikes. *O. volvulus* and *B. malayi* antigens have been demonstrated, along with IgM, IgG, and C3.

Pathogenesis

Filarial glomerulonephritis appears to be immune complex-mediated. The levels of circulating immune complexes correlate with the adult worm burden. Dogs infected with *Dirofilaria immitis* develop glomerular lesions similar to human filariasis. *In situ* immune complexes formation was suggested by a study that showed the development of glomerular lesions in kidneys after selective catheterization and infusion of *D. immitis* into one renal artery. The contralateral kidney either remained uninvolved or showed minor lesions.

Diethylcarbamazine treatment, by killing the parasite, may lead to antigen release into the circulation, thus exacerbating the immune process. A temporal relationship between the administration of this agent and the development of proteinuria has been noted.

Management

A good response to antifilarial therapy with diethylcarbamazine is observed in patients with nonnephrotic proteinuria and/or haematuria. The response is inconsistent in those with nephrotic syndrome, and deterioration of renal function may continue despite clearance of microfilariae with treatment.

Chyluria

Characterized by passage of milky white urine due to leakage of lymph, with or without haematuria, chyluria is encountered with increased frequency in individuals living in areas where *W bancrofti* infection is endemic. Rupture of dilated retroperitoneal lacteals into the urinary system secondary to fibrosis of the draining lymph glands is responsible. Prolonged chyluria may result in the loss of protein, fat, and lymphocytes in the urine and lead to protein malnutrition, vitamin deficiencies, and heightened risk of infections. Patients complain of backache, probably caused by distended vessels. Formation of chylous clots may result in acute urinary retention. About 80% of cases respond to treatment with diethylcarbamazine and dietary modification. Sclerotherapy using local instillation of povidone iodine, hypertonic dextrose or silver nitrate—or less commonly surgery—is required for resistant cases.

Renal disease in mycobacterial infections

Leprosy

Leprosy is a chronic granulomatous disorder caused by the acid-fast bacillus *Mycobacterium leprae*. Nephritis was an important cause of death until the 1950s, but is now rare. The main glomerular lesions encountered in leprosy are glomerulonephritis and secondary amyloidosis, but a few patients show other renal lesions, mainly tubulointerstitial nephritis.

Glomerulonephritis

The incidence of glomerulonephritis in leprosy is less than 2% on clinical evaluation, but increases to more than 50% if histology is examined. Glomerulonephritis is seen in both lepromatous and nonlepromatous forms, and is more common during episodes of erythema nodosum leprosum. Most patients present with asymptomatic urinary abnormalities, but nephrotic syndrome, acute nephritic syndrome, and rapidly progressive renal failure have all been described. Reduced creatinine clearance and impaired urinary acidification and concentration are noted in patients with erythema nodosum leprosum. Hypocomplementaemia is common, and circulating cryoglobulins may be present.

The most frequent histological findings are mesangial proliferative and diffuse proliferative glomerulonephritis. Acid-fast bacilli are seen rarely. Electron microscopy reveals electron-dense deposits in the mesangial and subendothelial regions, focal foot-process widening, glomerular capillary basement membrane reduplication with mesangial interposition, and endothelial cytoplasmic vacuolation. Immunofluorescence reveals granular IgG and C3 deposits in the mesangium and along capillary walls.

Circulating immune complexes can be detected in about one-third of those with lepromatous disease and over 75% of patients with active erythema nodosum leprosum. The antigen is thought to be derived from *M. leprae*, but there is also speculation about the role of a nonmycobacterial antigen derived from coinfecting microorganisms or dapsone:antidapsone antibodies. Alternate-pathway complement activation by cryoprecipitates can exacerbate the glomerular injury.

Steroids or antileprosy drugs have no effect on the course of glomerular disease. Prednisolone may hasten the recovery of renal function in patients with renal failure during episodes of erythema nodosum leprosum.

Amyloidosis

Amyloid was documented in 55% of cases in older autopsy and biopsy studies from the United States of America, 31% from Brazil, and less than 10% from Mexico, Africa, and India. The amyloid is of AA type and is far more frequent in lepromatous leprosy than nonlepromatous leprosy. Erythema nodosum leprosum further increases the risk as each episode is associated with a marked and persistent elevation of serum amyloid A protein. Patients with tuberculoid leprosy who have long-standing and infected trophic ulcers can also develop this complication.

Tuberculosis

Granuloma formation, interstitial nephritis, and caseous destruction are the main features of renal involvement in tuberculosis. An association with glomerulonephritis was postulated in the preantibiotic era, but only stray reports have described immune complex glomerulonephritis and dense-deposit disease in tuberculosis in recent times. A well-known complication, however, is amyloidosis, which is still seen in a significant proportion of patients in poor countries where the disease remains untreated for long periods. Once established, the course of amyloidosis is unaffected by treatment of the underlying tuberculosis.

Renal disease caused by leptospirosis

Leptospirosis, the most widespread zoonosis in the world, is prevalent throughout the tropics. The pathogenic *Leptospira interrogans* complex has 30 serogroups and 240 serotypes. The animal hosts (rats, mice, gerbils, hedgehogs, foxes, dogs, cattle, sheep, pigs, and rabbits) carry high number of organisms in their kidneys and shed leptospira in their urine for years. These can survive outside a host for several weeks at neutral or alkaline pH in a moist environment with low salinity. Human infection occurs upon exposure of abraded skin and exposed mucosae to the urine or tissue of an infected animal, or to contaminated water, soil, or vegetation. Leptospirosis is an occupational hazard in coal miners, in sewage, abattoir, and farm workers, and in the aquaculture industry.

Leptospiral acute renal failure
Clinical features

Leptospirosis occurs in both sexes and in all age groups. The peak incidence is seen between 11 and 40 years, with a male preponderance. The incidence increases during or soon after the rainy season, especially following floods.

Presentation varies from subclinical infection and self-limited anicteric febrile illness to severe and potentially fatal disease. Symptoms appear 7 to 13 days after exposure and are typically biphasic in character. The first (leptospiraemic) phase is characterized by high fever, chills, headache, severe muscle aches and tenderness, and dry cough; and terminates with defervescence after 4 to 10 days. The second or immune phase follows 1 to 3 days later. The recurrence of fever and constitutional symptoms is accompanied with renal and hepatic involvement and haemorrhagic manifestations. The combination of renal failure and cholestatic jaundice constitutes Weil's syndrome.

Acute renal failure occurs in 20 to 85% of cases and is oliguric in 40 to 60%. Volume and inotrope-unresponsive hypotension may be noted in 20 to 25%. Diuresis ensues by the end of the second week, and may last longer than that associated with other causes of acute renal failure. The renal failure is typically mild and nonoliguric in anicteric patients.

Diagnosis

Diagnosis is based on either culture or serology. The organisms can be grown on Fletcher's or Stuart's semisolid media from blood during the first phase and later from urine. Anti-leptospira antibodies are detectable in the second phase. A single titre of greater than 1:400 or a fourfold increase is taken as significant. The macroscopic agglutination test or the slide test can be used to screen patients, but is not specific. The benchmark is the complex microscopic agglutination test that requires maintenance of live leptospira cultures. Other tests include an IgM-specific dot-ELISA (enzyme-linked immunosorbent assay), complement fixation, serum and salivary ELISA, rapid IgM dipstick ELISA, and gold immunoblot tests.

Urinalysis during the leptospiraemic phase reveals mild proteinuria, and hyaline and granular casts. Conjugated hyperbilirubinemia and azotaemia are prominent in the second phase. Hypokalaemia secondary to increased tubular potassium excretion is observed in 45%, and thrombocytopaenia may be encountered in 40%.

Pathology

Grossly, the kidneys are swollen and bile stained. The main light-microscopic lesions are interstitial oedema and infiltration with mononuclear cells and eosinophils. Degeneration and necrosis of tubular epithelial cells and disruption of the basement membrane, and intraluminal bile casts and haemoglobin casts may be present. Mild and transient mesangial proliferative glomerulonephritis with C3 and IgM deposition is occasionally noted. The organisms may be demonstrated in renal parenchyma with a silver impregnation staining.

Pathogenesis

Renal involvement is thought to result from direct invasion of the renal tissue by the organism and liberation of bacterial enzymes, metabolites, and endotoxins. Addition of leptospira endotoxin to human macrophages induces induction of tumour necrosis factor $\alpha(TNF\alpha)$ release. The glycoprotein component of the endotoxin inhibits the renal Na$^+$,K$^+$-ATPase and apical Na$^+$–K$^+$–Cl$^-$ cotransporter, leading to potassium wasting. Leptospiral outer membrane proteins have been localized to proximal tubules and interstitium of infected animals. Pathogenic leptospires promote the binding of transcription factor NF-κB to DNA, leading to enhanced message for inducible nitric oxide synthase, monocyte chemoattractant protein-1 and TNFα.

The systemic haemodynamic changes of leptospirosis are similar to those seen in sepsis syndromes, and are accompanied by reduced renal blood flow.

Management

Leptospirosis is a self-limiting disease, and mild cases recover spontaneously. The emphasis is on symptomatic measures, together with correction of hypotension and fluid and electrolyte imbalance. Crystalline penicillin (1.5 million units intravenously every 6 h for 7 days) or doxycycline (100 mg orally twice daily for 7 days) shorten the duration of fever and hasten amelioration of leptospiruria. Administration of dopamine and furosemide increased urine flow and reduced the serum creatinine level within 24 h in a small series of patients with mild acute renal failure. Adverse prognostic factors include advanced age, pulmonary complications, hyperbilirubinaemia, diarrhoea, hyperkalaemia, and presence of other infections.

Other infective causes of renal disease

Mucormycosis

Mucormycosis is a rare opportunistic infection caused by zygomycete fungi of the order Mucorales and genera *Rhizopus*, *Absidia*, and *Rhizomucor*. Organ involvement occurs by vascular invasion leading to thrombosis of large and small arteries and infarction and necrosis of the affected organ. The main clinical forms are rhinocerebral, pulmonary, and gastrointestinal, but primary renal mucormycosis involving major renal vessels has been described from India. Patients present with high fever, lumbar pain, and pyuria, and bilateral involvement is characterized by oliguric acute renal failure. Ultrasonography and CT reveal enlarged kidneys with perirenal collections and/or intrarenal abscesses (Fig. 21.11.7). Characteristic broad, aseptate hyphae can be demonstrated in the material obtained by needle aspiration or at surgery. The only definitive treatment is extensive debridement of affected tissue, which may include bilateral nephrectomy, and systemic antifungal therapy with amphotericin B. Bilateral renal mucormycosis carries an extremely poor prognosis.

HIV infection

Even though most infected individuals live in the tropical countries of Africa and South Asia, little data is available on the pattern of kidney disease in this population. In one study from South Africa, 6% of over 600 HIV-infected individuals showed proteinuria. In a retrospective review of 99 biopsies in black HIV-infected Africans, lesions directly attributable to HIV, i.e. classic HIV-associated nephropathy (HIVAN) and HIV-immune complex kidney, were seen in 27% and 21% cases, respectively (see Chapter 21.10.7). The rest showed a variety of other renal lesions. Minimal-change disease was not seen in this population.

Kidney diseases caused by toxins

Animal toxins

Snake venoms

Most of the 450 venomous snake species are found in the tropical and subtropical regions. The World Health Organization estimates the global annual mortality from snake bite to be around 40 000, of which 23% occur in West Africa, 20% in South America, and 10% in India. Renal lesions have been reported following bites by snakes belonging to classes Viperidae (Russell's viper, saw-scaled viper, puff adder, pit viper, and rattlesnakes), Colubridae (boomslang, *Bothrops jararaca*, gwardar, dugite, and *Cryptophis nigrescens*), and Hydrophidae (sea snakes). Acute renal failure is the most frequent and clinically important effect of envenomation on the kidneys, with most cases seen following viper and sea snake bites. In India, about 13 to 32% of those bitten by *Echis carinatus* (Russell's viper) develop acute renal failure. The reported incidence from other countries varies between 1 and 27%.

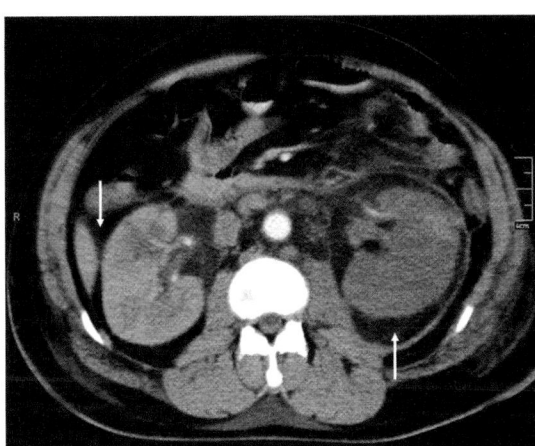

Fig. 21.11.7 Contrast-enhanced CT of the abdomen showing almost complete nonenhancement of the left and minimal patchy contrast enhancement of the right renal parenchyma (suggesting infarction), along with bilateral perinephric stranding (arrows) in a patient with acute renal failure due to bilateral mucormycosis.

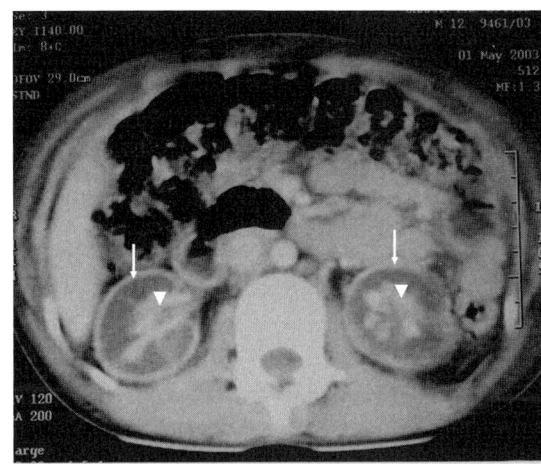

Fig. 21.11.8 Contrast-enhanced CT of the abdomen showing acute cortical necrosis. The nonenhancing zone of necrosed cortex is limited by the enhancing subcortical rim on the outside (arrows) and the medulla on the inside (arrowheads).

Clinical features

The initial symptoms are pain and swelling of the bitten part, followed by blister formation and ecchymosis. Bleeding—manifesting as ooze from fang marks, haematemesis, malaena, or haematuria—is seen in 65% of cases and indicates systemic poisoning. Sea snake bites cause myonecrosis, which manifests as muscle pains and weakness.

Renal failure sets in within a few hours to as late as 4 days after the bite, and is usually oliguric. A history of passage of 'Coca-Cola' coloured urine, indicating intravascular haemolysis, is obtained in about one-half of cases. Life-threatening hyperkalaemia may develop in patients with haemolysis or myonecrosis. With effective management, oliguria resolves in 5 to 21 days; persistence indicates the likelihood of renal cortical necrosis (Fig. 21.11.8). Nonoliguric renal failure is seen in less than 10% of cases.

Pathology

Grossly, the kidney may be swollen and exhibit petechial haemorrhages. Light microscopy shows acute tubular necrosis in 70 to 80% of cases. The tubular lumina contain desquamated cells and hyaline or pigment casts. Interstitial oedema, inflammatory cell infiltration and scattered haemorrhages may be seen. Electron microscopy reveals dense intracytoplasmic bodies in the proximal tubules representing degenerated organelles. Other lesions that have been described include acute interstitial nephritis, thrombotic microangiopathy, necrotizing arteritis of interlobular arteries, and crescentic glomerulonephritis (Fig. 21.11.9). Acute cortical necrosis is seen in about 20 to 25% of cases.

Pathogenesis

Renal damage is a cumulative effect of direct nephrotoxicity of venom, hypovolaemia, haemolysis, myoglobinuria, and DIC. Injection of snake venom leads to increased excretion of tubular enzymes in rats. Studies in the isolated perfused rat kidney showed a dose-dependent decrease in inulin clearance following administration of Russell's viper venom. Destruction of the glomerular filter, lysis of vessel walls, mesangiolysis followed by endo-and extracapillary proliferation, and tubular injury have been shown in experimental models. A vasculotoxic factor has been isolated from the venoms of *E. carinatus, Vipera palastinae, Agkistrodon halys,*

B. jararaca, and Habu snakes. Similarities have been noted between the structure of the potent vasoconstrictor endothelin-1 and the venom of the Israeli burrowing asp.

Hypotension and circulatory collapse can result from blood loss, release of kinins or depression of the medullary vasomotor centre or myocardium. Kininogenases are present in crotalid venom. *V. palastinae* venom produces depression of the medullary vasomotor centre, whereas *Bitis arietans* venom causes myocardial depression, arteriolar dilatation, and increased vascular permeability.

Phospholipase A and a basic protein called 'direct lytic factor' present in Russell's viper and *E. carinatus* venoms can lead to intravascular haemolysis or disseminated intravascular coagulation. Microangiopathic haemolytic anaemia can develop following *A. rhodostoma,* Russell's viper, Echis carinatus, puff adder, and gwardar bites. Viper venom activates the coagulation cascade at several levels, leading to rapid thrombin formation.

Management

The mainstay of management is prompt antivenom administration to cases with evidence of systemic envenomation or local

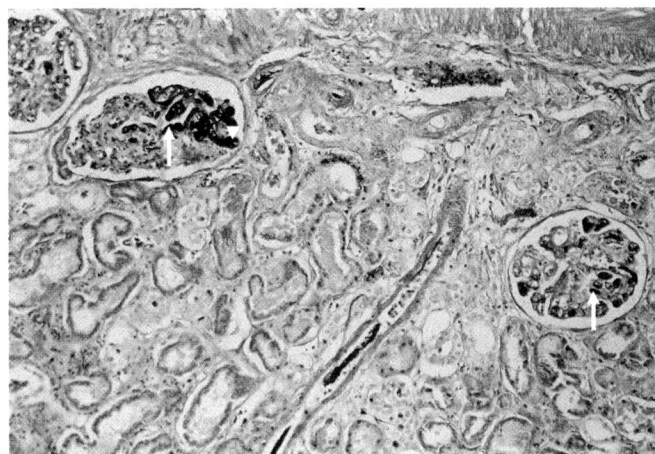

Fig. 21.11.9 Photomicrograph showing fibrin thrombi in the glomerular capillaries (arrows) and arterioles (arrowhead) in a patient with acute renal failure following snake bite. Also seen is diffuse shedding of tubular epithelial cells.

inflammation involving more than 50% of the limb circumference. Administration must be continued until the effects of systemic envenoming disappear. A simple way to monitor efficacy is by estimating whole-blood clotting time three to four times every day, with testing continuing for at least 3 days as coagulation defects can recur due to delayed absorption of the venom. Significant batch-to-batch variability is noted in antivenom activity: in one study 60 to 270 ml (average 120 ml) was required to reverse the clotting defect. Concomitant measures include replacement of lost blood, maintenance of electrolyte balance, administration of tetanus immunoglobulin, and adequate treatment of pyogenic infection. Maintenance of a high urinary output, as well as alkalinizing the urine, may attenuate renal damage in those with haemolysis. The mortality rate is up to 30%.

Bee, wasp, and hornet stings

Honey bees, yellow jackets, hornets, and paper wasps are stinging insects belonging to the order Hymenoptera and are found in most tropical countries. Systemic symptoms develop when an individual receives a large dose of the venom after being attacked by a swarm of insects. Manifestations include vomiting, diarrhoea, hypotension, and loss of consciousness. Acute renal failure is secondary to haemolysis, rhabdomyolysis, or both. Haemolysis results from the action of a basic protein fraction, melittin, and phospholipase A. Rhabdomyolysis has been attributed to polypeptides, histamine, serotonin, and acetylcholine. Experimental studies have suggested a direct nephrotoxic role of venom components. Renal biopsy invariably reveals acute tubular necrosis.

Carp and sheep bile

Acute hepatic and renal failure have been reported following consumption of the raw gallbladder or bile of freshwater and grass carps (*Ctenophryngodon idellus, Cyprinus carpio, Hypophythalmichthys molitrix, Mylopharyngodon pisceus,* and *Aristichthys nobilis*) in Taiwan, South China, Hong Kong, Japan, India and South Korea, and sheep bile in the Middle East. Initial symptoms include abdominal pain, nausea, vomiting, and watery diarrhoea. Hepatocellular jaundice and acute renal failure occur 48 h after ingestion. Haematuria is noted in 75% of cases. The duration of renal failure ranges from 2 to 3 weeks. Manifestations vary depending upon the varieties of carp and amount of bile ingested. Histology reveals acute tubular necrosis and interstitial oedema.

Other animal toxins

Acute renal failure has been reported following stings by the scorpion, jellyfish, and giant centipede. Scorpion stings results in DIC and internal bleeding, and these give rise to intravascular haemolysis.

Plant toxins

Many tropical communities consume products derived from locally grown plants, either as food or as medicines. Many of these contain nephrotoxic substances. Exposure may also be accidental, when a toxic plant is mistaken for an edible one. The insult can be identified quickly when the presentation is acute, but the cause–effect relationship may be harder to establish in the case of slowly progressive lesions.

Traditional medicines constitute a special class of nephrotoxins among poor populations in tropical Africa and Asia.

In South African hospitals, more than 75% of all deaths from acute poisoning and 25 to 60% of all acute renal failure from medical causes are due to traditional medicines. These agents are obtained from traditional healers ('witch-doctors'), people with considerable authority who also act as spiritual leaders and exorcists. Administration is either by the oral route or as enemas, the latter consisting of mixtures of herbs, barks, roots, leaves, and bulbs, administered through a truncated cow's horn or hollow reed. Increasing urbanization and industrialization have introduced the use of potent chemicals, e.g. paint thinners, turpentine, chloroxylenol, ginger, pepper, soap, vinegar, copper sulphate, and potassium permanganate. According to some estimates, members of the Zulu tribe receive up to three herbal enemas per week and Swazi infants 50 enemas per year. About 63% of patients admitted in Baragwanath Hospital (Soweto, Johannesburg, Republic of South Africa) admitted to being frequent enema users. Acute renal failure has been reported following the use of such enemas: detailed studies are not available, but histology usually shows acute tubular necrosis.

Callilepis laureola (impila) poisoning

Callilepis laureola, a herb with a tuberous rootstock, grows in South Africa, Zambia, the Democratic Republic of the Congo, Zimbabwe, and neighbouring countries. An extract of the tubers is taken orally, or as an enema or douche. According to one estimate this is used by over 50% of the population in Natal (South Africa), and poisoning is a common cause of acute renal failure in the black South African population. Symptoms appear within 24 h in 40% and within 4 days in 70% of patients. Children and older people show earlier and more severe abnormalities. Abdominal pain and vomiting are followed by hypoglycaemia, convulsions, and jaundice. Renal failure precedes hepatic dysfunction and is oliguric. Histology shows acute tubular necrosis with interstitial oedema and—occasionally—dense interstitial infiltration. Atractyloside, an alkaloid in the tuber of the plant, inhibits ATP synthesis and is believed to have nephrotoxic and hypoglycaemic effects. Gastrointestinal fluid loss contributes to the renal dysfunction. Treatment is supportive and includes correction of hypoglycaemia and volume and electrolyte replacement. The mortality rate is over 50%.

Djenkol bean poisoning

Djenkol beans (*Pithecolobium lobatum* and *Pithecolobium jiringa*, family Mimosaceae) are considered a delicacy in Indonesia, Malaysia, southern Thailand, and Myanmar (Burma), and are consumed raw, fried, roasted, or at the sprouting stage. Acute renal failure can occur when raw beans are consumed in large amounts with low fluid intake. Nephrotoxicity has been reported most commonly in the rainy season from Malaysia and Indonesia (Java and Sumatra). Symptoms appear soon after ingestion or as late as 36 h after consumption, and include dysuria, lumbar pain, hypertension, haematuria, and oligoanuria. The breath and urine emit a characteristic sulphuric odour. Urinalysis shows needle-like crystals of djenkolic acid. Individual susceptibility to the toxic effects is variable and is possibly related to the hydration status or interindividual variability in activity of metabolizing enzymes. Djenkolic acid is a sulphur-rich cysteine thioacetal of formaldehyde, which forms needle-like crystals in the concentrated acidic urine of the distal tubules. Chronic ingestion can lead to development of djenkolic acid stones. High fluid intake and urinary alkalinization

Table 21.11.3 Plant nephrotoxins in the tropics

Plant	Reported from	Active molecule	Renal manifestations	Other manifestations
Averrhoa carambola (Star fruit)	Hong Kong, Taiwan	Oxalate	Intratubular precipitation of oxalate crystals	Vomiting
Catha edulis (khat leaf)	East Africa, Arab peninsula	S-cathione, Ephedrine	ATN	Hepatotoxicity
Cleistanthus collinus (Oduvan)	India	Cleistanthin A and B, collinusin, diphylline	AKI	Hypotension, hypokalemia, arrhythmia
Colchicum autumnale (meadow saffron)	Turkey	Colchicine	ATN	Hemorrhagic gastroenteritis, muscle paralysis, respiratory failure
Crotalaria laburnifolia (Bird flower)	Zimbabwe, Sri Lanka	Pyrrolizidine alkaloids	ATN, HRS	Hepatic veno-occlusive disease, pulmonary injury, thrombocytopenia
Cupressus funebris Endl (Mourning Cypress)	Taiwan	Flavonoid	ATN, AIN	AHF, haemolytic anaemia, thrombocytopenia
Dioscorea quartiniana (yam)	Africa, Asia	Dioscorine, dioscin	ATN	Convulsions
Euphorbia metabelensis (spurge)	Zimbabwe	Irritant chemicals in plant latex	ATN	Thrombocytopenia
Glycyrrhiza glabrata (Liquorice)	Several countries	Glycyrrhizic acid	ATN	Rhabdomyolysis, hypokalemia, hypertension, cardiac arrhythmia
Larrea tridentate (chaparral)	Chile, South Africa	Nordihydroguaiaretic acid, s-quinone	Renal cysts, Renal cell carcinoma	Hepatic failure
Propolis	Brazil, Taiwan	Unknown	AIN	Contact dermatitis
Rhizoma rhei	Hong Kong	Anthraquinones (Emodin, Aloe-Emodin)	AIN	None
Securidacea longepedunculata (violet tree, wild wisteria)	Congo, Zambia, Zimbabwe	Methylsalicylate, securinine, saponins	ATN	Vomiting, diarrhoea
Sutherlandia frufesces (cancer brush), *Dodonaea angustifolia*	South Africa	Unknown	AIN	Pulmonary embolism
Takeout roumia	Morocco, Sudan	Paraphenylenediamine	ATN	Rhabdomyolysis
Taxus celebia (Chinese yew)	Asia	Flavonoid	ATN, AIN	Hepatitis, haemolysis, DIC
Thevetia peruviana (yellow oleander)	India, Sri Lanka	Cardiac glycosides	ATN, mesangiolysis	Liver failure, cardiac arrhythmias
Tripterygium wilfordii Hook F (Thunder god vine)	Taiwan	Triptolide	ATN	Diarrhoea, shock
Uncara tomentosa (Cat's claw)	Peru	Alkaloids, flavonols	AIN	Diarrhoea, hypotension, bruising, bleeding gums

ATN: acute tubular necrosis; AIN: acute interstitial nephritis; AKI: acute kidney injury; HRS: hepatorenal syndrome, AHF: acute hepatic failure; GI: gastrointestinal; DIC: disseminated intravascular coagulation.
(Modified from Burdmann E, Jha V and Sitprija V. *Comprehensive Clinical Nephrology*, 4th ed, Elsevier)

helps in dissolving the crystals. Most victims recover within a few days.

Mushroom poisoning

Less than 1% of all mushrooms are toxic. Acute renal failure has been observed following the ingestion of mushrooms of the genera *Amanita*, *Galerina*, *Cortinarius* and *Inocybe*. *Amanita phalloides* (deathcap) and *Amanita virosa* (destroying angel) are found commonly in the tropics. They grow commonly in lawns, pastures, and forests, on stumps and living trees, and in such locations as basements, plasterboard walls, and flower pots, and may be picked and ingested by inexperienced collectors and children in the mistaken belief that they are edible. Initial symptoms are related to the gastrointestinal tract and may result in dehydration and hypotension. The toxic compounds (phallotoxin, amatoxin) inhibit RNA polymerase. Hepatic and renal failure develops after a couple of days. Renal histology shows acute tubular necrosis. Management is supportive; charcoal haemoperfusion is effective in clearing α-amanitin from circulation and may improve outcome. Overall mortality is over 50%, and exceeds 70% in children.

Long-term ingestion of cortinarious mushrooms has been implicated in chronic renal failure.

Details of other toxic plants that have been associated with development of kidney diseases are described in Table 21.11.3.

Chemical nephrotoxins

Increasing industrialization has facilitated the access of the poor and ignorant populations of tropical countries to large number of chemicals. Poisonings have been reported after accidental ingestion or following attempted suicide or homicide. Acute renal failure is a manifestation of toxicity of many of these agents, such as copper sulphate, ethylene glycol, paraphenyl diamine (hair dye), paraquat, ethylene dibromide, and hexavalent chromium compounds.

Copper sulphate poisoning

Commonly used in the leather industry, copper sulphate is cheap and freely available in tropical countries. It has often been used as a mode of suicide by poor people in the Indian subcontinent. Poisoning also has been reported from Nigeria and among people of Nigerian origin living in other countries following ingestion of 'holy water' laced with copper sulphate given by spiritual leaders for cathartic purposes.

Copper sulphate is corrosive; initial symptoms consist of a metallic taste, increased salivation, burning retrosternal pain, nausea, vomiting, diarrhoea, haematemesis, and malaena. The presence of copper sulphate in the vomitus can be confirmed by observing a change in colour to deep blue on addition of ammonium hydroxide. Jaundice, hypotension, convulsions, and coma indicate severe poisoning. Acute pancreatitis, myoglobinuria, and methaemoglobinaemia have also been reported. Oliguric acute renal failure develops in 20 to 25% of cases and is frequently associated with passage of 'Coca-Cola' coloured urine, indicating intravascular haemolysis. Copper interferes with the activity of red blood cell enzymes such as ATPase, G6PD, glutathione reductase, and catalase, and sensitizes them to the effects of oxidants. Genetic G6PD deficiency increases the risk of haemolysis. Renal histology shows acute tubular necrosis with abundant pigmented haemoglobin casts indicating haemoglobinuria. Acute cortical necrosis can occur rarely. Survivors may develop corrosive oesophageal strictures.

Management entails gastric lavage with 1% potassium ferrocyanide solution. Egg white or milk can also be administered as an antidote. No attempt should be made to induce emesis. Correction of volume deficit and management of metabolic complication are required in those with features of systemic toxicity. The fatal dose of copper sulphate is 30 to 100 g, but deaths have been reported even with a dose as small as 1 g.

Ethylene glycol nephrotoxicity

Ethylene glycol is used as an organic solvent, antifreeze, preservative, and glycerine substitute. It is metabolized in the liver to glyoxylic acid and oxalate, which combines with calcium and gets deposited in the acid milieu of renal tubules as calcium oxalate crystals, leading to acute renal failure.

Epidemics of ethylene glycol poisoning in children as a result of substitution of nontoxic propylene glycol with toxic di- and polyethylene glycols as a vehicle in paediatric syrup preparations have been reported from tropical countries including India, Bangladesh, Nigeria, South Africa, and Haiti. The mortality is high due to underlying diseases and delayed diagnosis: 236 deaths were recorded amongst 339 children with acute renal failure in Bangladesh during one such epidemic.

Further reading

Abdul-Fattah MM, *et al.* (1995). Schistosomal glomerulopathy: a putative role for commonly associated Salmonella infection. *J Egypt Soc Parasitol*, **25**, 165–73.

Agnihotri N, *et al.* (1995). Role of reactive oxygen species in renal damage in experimental leprosy. *Lepr Rev*, **66**, 201–9.

Barsoum RS (2000). Malarial acute renal failure. *J Am Soc Nephrol*, **11**, 2147–54.

Barsoum R (2004). The changing face of schistosomal glomerulopathy. *Kidney Int*, **66**, 2472–84.

Barsoum R, *et al.* (1996). Immunoglobulin-A and the pathogenesis of schistosomal glomerulopathy. *Kidney Int*, **50**, 920–8.

Chijioke A (2001). Current concepts on pathogenesis of renal tuberculosis. *West Afr J Med*, **20**, 107–10.

Chugh KS (1989). Snake-bite-induced acute renal failure in India. *Kidney Int*, **35**, 891–907.

Chugh KS, *et al.* (1994). Acute renal cortical necrosis—a study of 113 patients. *Ren Fail*, **16**, 37–47.

Daher Ede F, *et al.* (2003). Acute renal failure after massive honeybee stings. *Rev Inst Med Trop São Paulo*, **45**, 45–50.

De Siati L, *et al.* (1999). Immunoglobulin A nephropathy complicating pulmonary tuberculosis. *Ann Diagn Pathol*, **3**, 300–3.

Eiam-Ong S, Sitprija V (1998). Falciparum malaria and the kidney: a model of inflammation. *Am J Kidney Dis*, **32**, 361–75.

Freire BF, *et al.* (1998). Anti-neutrophil cytoplasmic antibodies (ANCA) in the clinical forms of leprosy. *Int J Lepr Other Mycobact Dis*, **66**, 475–82.

Gerntholtz TE, Goetsch SJ, Katz I (2006). HIV-related nephropathy: a South African perspective. *Kidney Int*, **69**, 1885–91.

Jayakumar M, *et al.* (2006). Epidemiologic trend changes in acute renal failure—a tertiary center experience from South India. *Ren Fail*, **28**, 405–10.

Jha V, *et al.* (1992). Spectrum of hospital-acquired acute renal failure in the developing countries—Chandigarh study. *Q J Med*, **83**, 497–505.

Jha V, Chugh KS (2008). Acute kidney injury in Asia. *Semin Nephrol* **28**, 330–47.

Jha V, Rathi M (2008). Acute kidney injury due to natural medicines. *Semin Nephrol*, **28**, 416–28.

Langhammer J, Birk HW, Zahner H (1997). Renal disease in lymphatic filariasis: evidence for tubular and glomerular disorders at various stages of the infection. *Trop Med Int Health*, **2**, 875–84.

Nakayama EE, *et al.* (2001). Renal lesions in leprosy: a retrospective study of 199 autopsies. *Am J Kidney Dis*, **38**, 26–30.

Okoro BA, Okafor HU, Nnoli LU (2000). Childhood nephrotic syndrome in Enugu, Nigeria. *West Afr J Med*, **19**, 137–41.

Pakasa NM, Nseka NM, Nyimi LM (1997). Secondary collapsing glomerulopathy associated with *Loa loa* filariasis. *Am J Kidney Dis*, **30**, 836–9.

Pandey AP, Ansari MS (2006). Recurrent chyluria. *Indian J Urol*, **22**, 56–58.

Pinho FM, Zanetta DM, Burdmann EA (2005). Acute renal failure after *Crotalus durissus* snakebite: a prospective survey on 100 patients. *Kidney Int*, **67**, 659–67.

Prakash J, *et al.* (2006). Acute renal failure in pregnancy in a developing country: twenty years of experience. *Ren Fail*, **28**, 309–13.

Sakhuja V, *et al.* (1994). Chronic renal failure in India. *Nephrol Dial Transplant*, **9**, 871–872.

Sitprija V (1988). Nephropathy in falciparum malaria. *Kidney Int*, **34**, 867–77.

Ujah IA, *et al.* (2005). Factors contributing to maternal mortality in north-central Nigeria: a seventeen-year review. *Afr J Reprod Health*, **9**, 27–40.

Renal involvement in genetic disease

D. Joly and J.P. Grünfeld

Essentials

There are many inherited disorders in which the kidney is affected: this chapter is concerned with the commonest inherited diseases leading to renal failure.

Autosomal dominant polycystic kidney disease—accounts for about 7% of cases of endstage renal failure in Western countries. Inheritance is autosomal dominant, with mutations in polycystin 1 responsible for 85% of cases and mutations in polycystin 2 accounting for most of the remainder, these being transmembrane proteins that are able to interact, function together as a nonselective cation channel, and also induce several distinct transduction pathways. May present with renal pain, haematuria, urinary tract infection, or hypertension, or be discovered incidentally on physical examination or abdominal imaging, or by family screening, or after routine measurement of renal function. Commonly progresses to endstage renal failure at between 40 and 60 years of age. Extrarenal manifestations include intracranial aneurysms, liver cysts, and mitral valve prolapse.

Alport's syndrome—X-linked dominant inheritance in 85% of kindreds, with molecular defect involving the gene encoding for the α-5 chain of the type IV collagen molecule. Males typically present with macroscopic haematuria in childhood, followed by permanent microscopic haematuria, and later by proteinuria and renal failure. Extrarenal manifestations include perceptive deafness of variable severity, ocular abnormalities (bilateral anterior lenticonus

is pathognomonic), and (uncommonly) macrothrombocytopenia. Carrier women often have slight or intermittent urinary abnormalities, but may develop mild impairment of renal function late in life, and a few develop endstage renal disease. In the autosomal recessive form of Alport's syndrome, renal disease progresses to endstage before 20 to 30 years of age at a similar rate in both affected men and women.

Nephronophthisis—the most common genetic cause of endstage renal disease in children and young adults, this is a group of autosomal recessive tubulointerstitial nephropathies with multiple small medullary cysts that appear late in the course of the disease. Eighty per cent of cases are caused by homozygous deletions of the NPH1 gene, which codes for nephrocystin. Present with polyuria, polydipsia, and growth retardation in early childhood, progressing to endstage renal disease at a mean age of 14 years.

von Hippel–Lindau disease—due to mutation in the tumour suppressor gene VHL; renal cysts and bilateral multifocal renal cell carcinomas are found in 70% of cases. Carcinomas are often asymptomatic, should be screened for regularly, and occur at a mean age of 45 years.

Tuberous sclerosis—due to mutation of genes encoding for hamartin (TSC1) or tuberin (TSC2); characterized by renal angiomyolipomas, which are benign, often multiple and bilateral.

Introduction

The spectrum of inherited renal disorders (and of inherited diseases with kidney involvement) is summarized in Box 21.12.1. Attention will be focused in this section on the commonest inherited kidney diseases leading to renal failure.

Cystic kidney diseases

An overview of cystic kidney diseases is shown in Box 21.12.2.

Autosomal dominant polycystic kidney disease (ADPKD)

ADPKD is by far the most frequent inherited kidney disorder, accounting for approximately 7% of cases of endstage renal failure

in Western countries. It is one of the most frequent human inherited monogenic diseases (c.1 in 1000 individuals).

Diagnosis

The diagnosis of ADPKD is based on the two following features:

- Evidence for autosomal dominant inheritance
- Demonstration of multiple renal cysts in both kidneys, which are often enlarged, by ultrasonography (Fig. 21.12.1)

The latter criterion deserves further comment. Renal cysts are initiated in the fetal kidney and develop progressively in life over the course of years. They may be too small to be detected by ultrasonography in childhood, and kidney enlargement also progresses with age. Thus, the sensitivity of ultrasonography for detecting ADPKD is poor before 20 years of age (but the specificity is high

---

Box 21.12.1 Main groups of inherited kidney diseases

- Cystic kidney diseases (see Box 21.12.2)
- Alport's syndrome and variants
- Inherited metabolic diseases with renal involvement
  - With glomerular involvement (such as diabetes mellitus, genetic amyloidosis, Fabry's disease)
  - With nonglomerular involvement (such as cystinosis, primary hyperoxaluria)
- Other inherited diseases
  - With glomerular involvement (such as congenital nephrotic syndrome, nail–patella syndrome)
  - With nonglomerular involvement (such as nephronophthisis)
- Primary immune glomerulonephritis, occasionally familial (such as IgA nephropathy)
- Inherited tubular disorders
- Various renal diseases with 'genetic influence' (such as reflux nephropathy, haemolytic–uraemic syndrome)

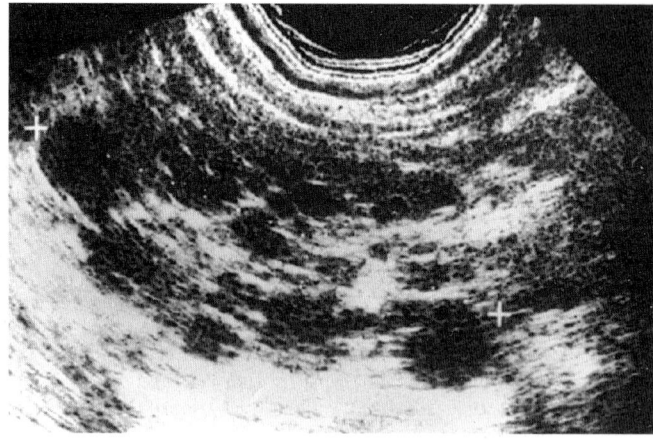

Fig. 21.12.1 Typical ultrasonographic findings in a patient with autosomal dominant polycystic kidney disease. The kidney is enlarged and contains multiple cysts of different sizes; the contralateral kidney had similar changes. The concentration of serum creatinine was 120 μmol/litre at the time of ultrasonography.
By courtesy of Dr O. Helenon.

since solitary renal cysts are very rare at this age, and bilateral cysts even more so). In families with the *PKD1* gene mutation, false-negative ultrasonographic diagnosis is very unlikely at ages above 30 years, and rare at ages 20 to 29 years. Routine screening of asymptomatic members of affected families should not be done before 20 years of age. By contrast, renal cysts, even bilateral, are relatively common in patients aged 50 years or more, hence strict criteria (multiple cysts in both enlarged kidneys and clear-cut inheritance) are required for diagnosing ADPKD in older patients.

Symptoms

Renal manifestations

In some patients, ADPKD is asymptomatic and discovered during family investigation, or by chance on abdominal ultrasonography. In most cases, however, there are symptoms and patients complain of one or more of the following at some time during their life: renal pain due to cyst development, or stone or blood clot migration; bleeding within a cyst, leading to flank pain, with the hyperdense cyst fluid then being visualized by CT; bleeding into the urinary tract, with gross haematuria occurring in approximately 30% of cases; fever due to upper urinary tract infection, which is more frequent in women, or to cyst fluid infection. Renal stones,

---

Box 21.12.2 Genetic cystic kidney diseases

- Autosomal dominant polycystic kidney disease
- Autosomal recessive polycystic kidney disease
- HNF-1β mutations (renal cysts and diabetes syndrome)
- Juvenile nephronophthisis–medullary cystic disease complex
- Associated with multiple malformation syndrome, such as phacomatoses (autosomal dominant): tuberous sclerosis, von Hippel–Lindau disease; or other rare syndromes

---

predominantly uric acid (for unknown reasons), develop in about 20% of the patients.

Hypertension is a common and early finding in ADPKD, occurring in about 30 to 50% of patients with normal renal function. Subsequently, with the development of renal failure, up to 80% of patients become hypertensive. Why hypertension develops is not known: it has been ascribed to compression and ischaemia of the normal renal parenchyma by cysts.

Renal failure is also a common finding in ADPKD. When it occurs, it usually progresses to endstage at between 40 and 60 years of age. However, in 30% of cases it reaches endstage later, and in 5% earlier, including very rare instances when it develops in the first years of life. Recent epidemiological studies have indicated that ADPKD may have a much more indolent course in a substantial number of cases: 25 to 50% of affected subjects are not in endstage renal failure by 70 years of age, and some patients may reach 80 or 90 years without the need for renal replacement therapy. This information is crucial for genetic counselling.

Genetic and nongenetic factors determine renal prognosis: the renal disease may progress more slowly in families with *PKD2* disease (mean age at endstage renal disease 55 years in *PKD1* disease, compared with 70 years in *PKD2* disease), it progresses more slowly in women than in men, and control of hypertension may reduce the rate of progression.

Extrarenal manifestations

Liver cysts develop in 70% of patients, usually later in life than renal cysts. They are more frequent and more diffuse in women than in men. They are usually asymptomatic but may be clinically palpable, and are typically detected by ultrasonography. Liver function tests are usually normal. Liver cyst infection may occur, particularly in patients on dialysis or in transplant recipients. Massive liver involvement can cause severe discomfort in some cases, mostly in women.

Cardiovascular abnormalities include intracranial aneurysms and mitral valve prolapse. Subarachnoid haemorrhage or intracerebral bleeding due to rupture of intracranial aneurysm are among the most severe complications of ADPKD and occur in approximately

1 to 2% of patients. Rapid diagnosis and urgent neurosurgical opinion are required. Diagnosis should be suspected early, before complete rupture, in patients with ADPKD with recent and severe headache, or with any transient focal neurological deficit.

In cross-sectional studies performed using noninvasive screening methods such as high-resolution CT or magnetic resonance angiography (MRA), intracranial aneurysms have been found in 7 to 8% of asymptomatic middle-aged patients with ADPKD. The prevalence is higher in those with a family history of intracranial aneurysm. The risk of rupture is largely dependent on aneurysm size. Routine screening by noninvasive methods is not indicated for all asymptomatic patients with ADPKD, but it seems reasonable in certain subgroups, in particular those with a family history of intracranial aneurysm or subarachnoid haemorrhage, those who have already bled from an aneurysm (since recurrent aneurysm is possible), and possibly those who are to undergo major elective surgery. In high-risk groups, screening should be repeated every 5 to 10 years since the cerebral vascular disease is progressive.

Mitral valve prolapse is discovered in 20% of patients with ADPKD by echocardiography, whereas it is found in only 2 to 3% of the general population. Other cardiac valve abnormalities and occasionally artery dissection or aneurysm may also be detected.

Other extrarenal abnormalities observed in ADPKD include pes excavatum, colonic diverticula, and abdominal hernias.

Pathogenesis

The mechanisms underlying cyst formation and progression are poorly understood: cysts develop only in a small percentage of nephrons and only focally, whereas all nephron cells carry the mutated gene. This has been explained by a two-hit phenomenon which postulates that renal tubular (or liver biliary) cells which are at the origin of cysts bear first the germinal *PKD* gene mutation, and then acquire a somatic *PKD* gene mutation involving the other allele, this event occurring at random in a limited number of cells. This explanation does not exclude other mechanisms. The link between the genetic event(s) and cystic fluid accumulation is not known.

The disease has an autosomal dominant mode of inheritance, so that the risk of any child of an affected parent carrying the abnormal gene is one in two, new mutations being very rare. Mutations affecting polycystin 1 (from the *PKD1* gene on the short arm of chromosome 16) are responsible for 85% of cases, with mutations affecting polycystin 2 (from the *PKD2* gene on the long arm of chromosome 4) accounting for most of the remainder. Polycystin 1 and polycystin 2 are transmembrane proteins that are able to interact, function together as a nonselective cation channel, and also induce several distinct transduction pathways. The 'polycystin complex' may have three different subcellular localizations and associated putative functions: at lateral membranes of the cells (with a role in cell–cell interaction); at the basal pole of the cell (with a role in cell–extracellular matrix interaction); and at the apical primary cilia of the cells (with a role in mechano-transduction of the urinary flux).

Treatment

High fluid intake and regular follow-up of blood pressure and renal function are indicated in all patients with ADPKD. The control of hypertension is an essential part of management, achieved with standard antihypertensive agents. Haematuria should be managed conservatively if at all possible, although bleeding may sometimes be prolonged over several days and even weeks.

The relief of pain or abdominal discomfort can be difficult. In addition to symptomatic treatment, surgical renal cyst decompression should be restricted to very selected cases. Surgery is rarely needed in the management of renal stones. Liver cyst aspirations by needle under CT guidance, fenestration, or resection may be needed when massive involvement gives rise to pain; and in very rare cases such patients have come to liver transplantation.

Kidney infection requires administration of antimicrobials appropriate for upper urinary tract infection (see Chapter 21.13). In some cases control of infection is not obtained, most probably because agents penetrate some infected cyst fluids poorly and do not achieve adequate concentration. Lipophilic drugs such as trimethoprim–sulphamethoxazole and ciprofloxacin have the best penetration into cyst fluid. Liver cyst infection also requires antimicrobials and drainage if infection is not controlled. Ciprofloxacin penetrates well into liver cyst fluid.

Standard medical management of chronic renal failure is indicated, as are renal replacement therapy and kidney transplantation when the patient reaches endstage, the results being similar to those obtained in other renal diseases.

Genetic counselling

The pattern of inheritance of ADPKD means that the offspring of an affected subject each have a 50% risk of having the disease. The disease has a highly variable clinical course, even within a given family. Prenatal diagnosis by gene linkage studies using material derived from chorionic villus sampling has been performed and can be considered if required and if adequate family information is available, but the demand for such prenatal diagnosis has been very low in Western countries. This is explained by the late onset and the variable clinical course of the disease, often relatively benign, which cannot yet be predicted by DNA analysis.

Ultrasonography may occasionally show renal cysts in the fetus, but late in pregnancy. Obviously, due to the slow and late development of macrocysts, negative ultrasonography in the fetus (as well as in a child) does not rule out the disease.

Autosomal recessive polycystic kidney disease (ARPKD)

ARPKD is a rare inherited disease (*c*. 1 in 40 000 individuals), the first manifestations of which appear early in childhood. Mutations at a single locus, polycystic kidney and hepatic disease 1 (*PKHD1*, located on chromosome 6), are responsible for all typical forms of ARPKD. The *PKDH1* gene product, fibrocystin, is a transmembrane protein localized to the cell primary cilia.

Three clinical features characterize this disease:

♦ Its recessive nature: both heterozygous parents are unaffected, with normal renal ultrasonography; parental consanguinity is found in some families

♦ Renal cysts derive from the collecting ducts, accounting for the striations in the dilated collecting system seen on intravenous pyelography

♦ The renal disease is invariably associated with congenital hepatic fibrosis: this may be responsible for portal hypertension due to presinusoidal block, or for bacterial angiocholitis due to intrahepatic bile duct dilatation

In children, ARPKD should be differentiated from ADPKD, which can be detected in childhood, even in neonates. Family history and renal ultrasonography in parents are decisive for correct diagnosis. In very rare families with *PKD1* disease, renal involvement may be revealed in neonates and may progress to endstage within the first year of life.

The diagnosis of ARPKD may be made before birth by antenatal ultrasonography, showing renal enlargement and increased echogenicity (as well as oligohydramnios). However, prenatal diagnosis may be uncertain and, since cystic changes occur in well-developed collecting ducts, these are detected only in the second half of pregnancy. When there is huge renal enlargement, pulmonary hypoplasia and respiratory distress may lead to death within hours after birth. With prolonged survival, liver and renal involvement becomes prominent. Gastrointestinal bleeding due to portal hypertension may be life threatening and necessitate surgical portocaval shunt. Systemic hypertension is a frequent finding in the first year of life but, surprisingly, it may regress in subsequent years. Urinary tract infection is common. The rate of progression of renal failure is variable: of those who survive the neonatal period, about 50% reach endstage in childhood, whilst this occurs in adulthood in the remainder.

Renal cysts and diabetes syndrome (RCAD)

Heterozygous mutations in the gene encoding hepatocyte nuclear factor (HNF)-1β, a DNA transcription factor, were initially described as one of the main molecular causes of maturity-onset diabetes of the young (MODY). It now appears that renal anomalies are the key feature of HNF-1β mutation phenotype and often precede the onset of diabetes. Renal cysts and progressive renal failure are frequent; glomerulocystic kidney disease and renal hypoplasia have been reported. Abnormal liver function tests, hyperuricaemia, pancreatic hypoplasia, and urogenital malformations have also been related to HNF-1β mutations.

Other cystic kidney diseases

Renal cysts may be found in von Hippel–Lindau disease and in tuberous sclerosis (see below). Renal medullary cysts are also found in juvenile nephronophthisis, but not early in the course (see below). By contrast, such cysts—well localized in adults by ultrasonography or CT—are seen early in autosomal dominant renal medullary cystic disease. This very rare condition progresses to endstage renal failure. Three different genetic loci have so far been localized.

Inherited diseases with glomerular involvement

Alport's syndrome

First described in 1927 by Dr Arthur Cecil Alport, this syndrome is characterized by the association of progressive haematuric hereditary nephritis and bilateral sensorineural hearing loss. Its prevalence is approximately 1 in 5000 individuals. In 85% of kindreds the mode of transmission is compatible with X-linked dominant inheritance. In the remaining families, autosomal dominant or recessive inheritance should be considered.

Symptoms

Renal manifestations

The first clinical manifestation is typically gross haematuria, occurring sometimes in the first year of life, recurring during childhood, and followed by permanent microscopic haematuria. Proteinuria appears later. A nephrotic syndrome, usually moderate, develops in 30 to 40% of patients. In other cases, moderate proteinuria and microscopic haematuria are the presenting symptoms in adulthood. The disease is progressive, leading to renal failure in all affected males, but the rate of progression is heterogeneous from one family to another, although usually homogeneous within a given family. In some endstage is reached at or before 30 years of age, sometimes in childhood; in others renal failure progresses to endstage between the ages of 30 and 60 years.

Carrier females of X-linked Alport's syndrome often have slight or intermittent urinary abnormalities. They may develop mild impairment of renal function late in life, but do not usually have progressive renal disease as occurs in males, although this does happen in a few cases. In the autosomal recessive form of Alport's syndrome, renal disease progresses to endstage before 20 to 30 years of age at a similar rate in both affected men and women.

Extrarenal manifestations

The hearing defect may lead to severe perceptive deafness, but it is often moderate or slight, only detected by audiometric testing. The hearing loss labels a given family, but is not found in all patients with renal disease. Familial haematuric progressive nephritis without hearing defect is documented in some kindreds, which forms one end of the spectrum of Alport's syndrome.

Eye abnormalities are detected in 30 to 40% of cases. These include bilateral anterior lenticonus detected by slit-lamp examination—a pathognomonic abnormality—and perimacular or macular retinal flecks that are seen by fundoscopic examination and do not alter visual acuity. Recurrent corneal erosions occur in some patients.

In some families, macrothrombocytopenia is associated with nephritis and hearing defect. In other rare kindreds the latter features are found in association with diffuse leiomyomatosis, mainly oesophageal, and congenital cataracts.

Pathogenesis

The primary defect in Alport's syndrome involves the glomerular basement membrane. By electron microscopy, this membrane can be abnormally thickened with splitting of the lamina densa, thinned with focal thickening, or diffusely thin in younger children. In some patients, antigenicity of the glomerular basement membrane is abnormal: antiglomerular basement membrane antibodies do not bind linearly along the Alport glomerular basement membrane, whereas they show linear fixation along the glomerular basement membranes of normal and diseased kidneys which contain the corresponding Goodpasture antigen (Goodpasture's syndrome is an autoimmune disorder characterized by the development of antiglomerular basement membrane antibodies directed against this antigen; see Chapter 21.8.7).

In X-linked Alport's syndrome the molecular defect involves the gene encoding for the α-5 chain of the type IV collagen molecule, which is a major component of basement membranes. Six α chains of type IV collagen have been identified so far, with each molecule of type IV collagen being made up of three of these chains, differently associated in various basement membranes. In Alport's syndrome, mutations have been identified in the gene encoding for the α-5 chain that maps to the long arm of the X chromosome. The Goodpasture antigen is located in the α-3 chain, the gene of which has been mapped on chromosome 2. Absence or severe alteration of the α-5 chain possibly prevents normal integration of the α-3 chain into the glomerular basement membrane, leading to the defect in antigenicity.

In the autosomal recessive form of Alport's syndrome, the genes encoding for α-3 or α-4 chains are mutated. Affected subjects are homozygotes in consanguineous families, or compound heterozygotes in other cases. In families with leiomyomatosis, α-5 and α-6 genes, located contiguously on the X chromosome, are both involved in a large deletion.

Skin biopsy has become valuable for diagnosis of Alport's syndrome. Epidermal basement membrane normally contains α-5 but not α-3/α-4 chains, hence negative α-5 staining by immunofluoresence is highly specific for X-linked Alport's syndrome, but is found in only 75% of cases because α-5 chains that are only slightly mutated can be detected. α-5 Staining is normal in the autosomal recessive forms of Alport's syndrome.

In the disease with macrothrombocytopenia, mutations involve the *MYH9* gene, encoding the nonmuscle myosin heavy chain IIA.

Genetic counselling and treatment

Genetic counselling first requires the correct identification of the mode of inheritance. If X-linked dominant inheritance is documented, affected men will not transmit the disease to their sons, whereas all their daughters will carry the mutant gene; affected women will transmit the mutant gene to 50% of either sons or daughters. DNA analysis may be helpful for genetic counselling in these families.

Treatment of hypertension and supportive management of renal failure are indicated in patients with progressive disease. The results of kidney transplantation are similar to those obtained in other renal diseases, but in rare cases antiglomerular basement membrane crescentic glomerulonephritis develops in the graft. It is assumed that this complication is related to alloimmunization to the 'missing antigen' introduced by the transplant.

Benign familial haematuria

This disease is characterized by isolated microhaematuria, without proteinuria or progression to renal failure, in both men and women. Renal biopsy usually shows a thin glomerular basement membrane and immunofluorescence studies are negative. The mode of transmission is compatible with autosomal dominant inheritance. In some families, subjects with microhaematuria are heterozygotes carrying mutations involving the α-3 or α-4 chain gene.

Congenital nephrotic syndrome of the Finnish type

This disease specifically affects the kidney and is characterized by massive proteinuria, which occurs already *in utero* and then persists in infancy. Intense therapy is needed to afford the children a chance of survival: nutritional support to compensate for protein loss; prevention of infection and thrombosis; bilateral nephrectomy; continuous peritoneal dialysis, and finally kidney transplantation.

It is an autosomal recessive disease caused by mutation of the nephrin gene whose product probably has a zipper-like structure, is localized at the slit diaphragm between podocyte foot processes (which are both absent in affected subjects), and plays a key role in the normal glomerular filtration barrier.

Nail–patella syndrome

This syndrome, also known as hereditary osteo-onycho dysplasia, is a rare autosomal dominant disorder, defined by the association of nail hypoplasia or dysplasia, bone abnormalities (including iliac horns), and renal disease. The latter is found in 50 to 60% of cases, progressing to endstage in approximately 15%. The hallmark of renal involvement is the detection by electron microscopy of fibrillar collagen bundles within the glomerular basement membrane. Open-angle glaucoma is a feature in rare families.

The mutated gene, *LMX1B* (located on 9q), belongs to a family of transcription factors that are involved in pattern formation during development. *LMX1B* is more specifically involved in the dorsoventral patterning of the limbs, and mice with a deletion in their *lmx1*-homologue exhibit skeletal defects similar to those observed in nail–patella syndrome and abnormal dorsoventral patterning of the extremities of the limbs.

Metabolic diseases with glomerular involvement

Anderson–Fabry disease

This disease, X-linked (prevalence *c.*1 in 40 000 individuals) and due to α-galactosidase A deficiency, results in glycosphingolipid deposition, mainly in the cardiovascular and renal system. The first manifestations in hemizygotes are painful acroparaesthesias, appearing in childhood and often prevented by administration of carbamazepine or phenytoin. Angiokeratomas, anhydrosis, and corneal deposits develop subsequently. Ischaemic cerebrovascular complications, cardiac valve abnormalities, myocardial deposition of glycolipids, and coronary events are the most severe manifestations, along with renal involvement.

In the kidney, glycolipid deposition involves glomerular epithelial cells, tubular cells, and endothelial and smooth muscle cells of intrarenal arteries. The latter changes are responsible for progressive renal ischaemia. Renal disease is revealed by proteinuria at around 20 years, and then progresses to endstage between 40 and 60 years of age, necessitating regular dialysis and/or kidney transplantation. Glycolipid deposition does not recur in the renal graft that contains normal α-galactosidase activity.

Most heterozygote females (80%) have corneal deposits. Symptoms are usually absent or moderate because of random X-chromosomal inactivation, but they may be severe in some cases, with cardiac changes and/or symptomatic renal disease.

Diagnosis is based on symptoms, familial history, measurement of α galactosidase activity in leucocytes, demonstration of typical inclusions on a tissue biopsy, and genetic analysis. Enzyme replacement therapy is available. All males with Fabry's disease and all females with substantial disease manifestations should receive this treatment as early as possible. See Chapter 12.8 for further discussion.

Lecithin-cholesterol acyl transferase (LCAT) deficiency

This is a very rare autosomal recessive disorder. LCAT is a key enzyme in the metabolism of cholesterol, responsible for its esterification. In affected subjects the proportion of cholesteryl ester to total cholesterol is very low. Lipid accumulation occurs in the eyes (causing corneal deposits), erythrocyte membranes (leading to low-grade haemolytic anaemia), arterial walls (contributing to premature atherosclerosis), and kidneys, predominating in glomerular mesangial cells and progressing to endstage renal disease.

LCAT is expressed primarily in the liver, hence liver transplantation would theoretically be the treatment of choice, but this has not so far been performed in this disease. Patients have received kidney transplants: lipid deposition recurs slowly in the graft. See Chapter 12.6 for further discussion.

Type I glycogen storage disease

Also named von Gierke's disease (see Chapter 12.3.1), this disease is due to glucose-6-phosphatase deficiency. Affected infants develop hypoglycaemia, growth retardation, and hepatomegaly. Fanconi's syndrome may occur as a consequence of glycogen deposition in the proximal tubule. Progressive renal involvement is not predominantly caused by glycogen accumulation, but related to the development of focal segmental glomerulosclerosis, the mechanism of which is unclear, usually after 20 years of age. This complication has only been recognized recently since children with severe hypoglycaemia have now survived to adulthood thanks to the progress achieved by paediatricians, dietitians, and families in providing adequate feeding and nutrition.

Familial primary glomerulonephritis

Familial focal segmental glomerulosclerosis with either autosomal dominant or autosomal recessive inheritance has recently been well characterized. Mutation of the *NPHS2* gene, which encodes podocin, causes recessive steroid-resistant nephrotic syndrome in some families, which can be of early or late onset. Podocin mutations are also detected in rare cases of sporadic steroid-resistant nephrotic syndrome. Mutations in *ACTN4*, which encodes α-actinin-4, cause autosomal dominant focal segmental glomerulosclerosis. Podocin and α-actinin 4 are both synthesized and exclusively secreted by the podocytes, and interact and regulate plasticity and slit diaphragm permselectivity with other podocyte proteins.

In most types of primary glomerulonephritis, familial cases have been anecdotally reported. The most frequent form, albeit rare, is probably familial IgA nephropathy, either primary (Berger's disease) or associated with Henoch–Schönlein purpura.

Inherited tubulointerstitial disorders

Juvenile nephronophthisis

Nephronophthisis is a group of autosomal recessive tubulointerstitial nephropathies with multiple small medullary cysts that appear late in the course of the disease. It is the most common genetic cause of endstage renal disease in children and young adults. Many patients have no obvious family history. Eighty per cent of cases are caused by homozygous deletions of the *NPH1* gene, which codes for nephrocystin. At least three other genes (*NPH2, 3,* and *4*) account for the remainder of the cases, and the respective encoded proteins (inversin, nephrocystin 3, nephrocystin 4) may interact in common signalling pathways downstream of primary cilia.

Polyuria, polydipsia, growth retardation, and urinary sodium leak are usually present before 4 years of age. Proteinuria is a late finding. Renal failure appears before 12 years of age in most cases and uniformly progresses to endstage renal disease before 20, with a mean age of 14 years. On ultrasound examination the kidneys have a normal or slightly reduced size with smooth outline, increased echogenicity, and loss of corticomedullary differentiation. Multiple small or large cysts at the corticomedullary junction are usually seen in advanced renal failure. Histology reveals atrophic tubules alternating with groups of dilated or collapsed tubules, and homogeneous or multilayered thickening of basement membranes is highly suggestive of nephronophthisis.

In about 10 to 15% of cases renal involvement is associated with retinal changes comprising tapetoretinal degeneration with or without retinitis pigmentosa, leading to blindness early or later in life (this association is referred to as the Senior–Loken syndrome, in most cases of which no deletion of the *NPH1* gene has been detected). Mental retardation, cerebellar ataxia, various bone anomalies, and hepatic fibrosis have been described in some families.

Detection of *NPH1* homozygous deletions allows diagnosis for the propositus and siblings without the need for renal biopsy, also prenatal diagnosis.

Uromodulin mutations

Hereditary mutations of *UMOD*, which codes for uromodulin (or Tamm–Horsfall protein), the most abundant protein in normal urine, lead to an autosomal dominant renal disease characterized by juvenile onset of gout; hyperuricaemia disproportionate to the age, sex, or degree of renal dysfunction, which is due to low renal fractional excretion of urate; corticomedullary cysts; and renal failure often recognized between 20 and 40 years of age. Renal biopsy shows nonspecific tubulointerstitial changes. This entity was previously called 'familial juvenile hyperuricaemic nephropathy' or 'medullary cystic kidney disease type 2'. Allopurinol is indicated to prevent gout, and perhaps to slow the progression of renal disease.

Genetic disorders with nephrolithiasis

Pertinent clinical data on these disorders are summarized in Table 21.12.1. Additional information can be found in Chapters 21.14, 21.15, and 21.16.

Other genetic diseases with kidney involvement

Phakomatoses

Two diseases of this group have significant renal involvement: von Hippel–Lindau disease and tuberous sclerosis.

In von Hippel–Lindau disease, renal cysts and bilateral multifocal renal cell carcinomas are found in 70% of the patients. Carcinomas are often asymptomatic, should be screened for regularly (Fig. 21.12.2), and occur at a mean age of 45 years. Nephron-sparing surgery (tumorectomy) or radiofrequency ablation is advocated when technically feasible.

The most typical renal lesion encountered in tuberous sclerosis is angiomyolipoma, which is a benign tumour, often multiple and bilateral. By ultrasonography this tumour is hyperechogenic, and by CT it is characterized by its fat content (Fig. 21.12.3). Bleeding is the main complication of renal angiomyolipoma, although multiple angiomyolipomas may rarely severely reduce renal mass and lead to renal failure. The development of segmental glomerulosclerosis may accelerate the progression to endstage. Renal cysts may also be found in *TSC2* forms (see below), and the incidence of renal cell carcinoma is slightly higher than in the general population.

Table 21.12.1 The main inherited disorders associated with nephrolithiasis

Disease	Mode of transmission	Type of stone	Chronic renal failure	Specific treatment
Cystinuria	AR	Cystine	No	Urine alkalinisation D-penicillamine or other chelators
Idiopathic hypercalciuria	Unknown	Calcium	No	Diet (normal sodium and protein intake) Thiazide
Primary hyperoxaluria type I	AR	Monohydrated calcium	Yes (nephrocalcinosis)	Vitamin B_6
		Oxalate		Liver transplantation
Dent's disease	XR	Calcium	Yes (nephrocalcinosis)	
Distal tubular acidosis	AR/AD	Calcium	No	Potassium citrate or bicarbonate
HPRT deficiency (Lesch–Nyhan syndrome)	XR	Uric acid	Yes	Urine alkalinisation Allopurinol
APRT deficiency	AR	2,8-dihydroxyadenine	Yes (rarely)	Allopurinol
Xanthinuria	AR	Xanthine	No	

AD, autosomal dominant; APRT, adenine phosphoribosyl transferase; AR, autosomal recessive; HPRT, hypoxanthine-guanine phosphoribosyl transferase; XR, X-linked.

The genes mutated in von Hippel–Lindau disease and tuberous sclerosis are tumour-suppressor genes. Two mutations ('two-hit' phenomenon) are required to trigger tumour formation: the first one is germinal, inherited, and the second one is somatic. The *VHL* gene has been cloned and located on 3p. Two somatic mutations of the same gene are involved in sporadic renal cell carcinoma. Two genes are identified in tuberous sclerosis: *TSC1* on chromosome 9q, encoding for hamartin, and *TSC2* on chromosome 16p, encoding for tuberin.

Cystinosis

Cystinosis (which is completely different from cystinuria that is due to defective reabsorption of cystine in the proximal tubule, see Chapter 21.14) results from defective carrier-mediated transport of cystine through the lysosomal membrane. The disease is transmitted as an autosomal recessive trait with an incidence of about 1 in 200 000 live-born babies and is due to mutations in the gene encoding cystinosine. The diagnosis is based on the findings of cystine crystals in tissues, such as the eyes, and on the elevated cystine content in leucocytes.

The clinical manifestations are due to progressive intralysosomal accumulation of cystine. In the infantile form, the first symptoms are related to the clinical consequences of Fanconi's syndrome (salt and water depletion, hypokalaemia, acidosis, rickets) appearing before 6 months of age. Renal failure develops later, reaching endstage generally before 12 years. Cystine accumulates in other

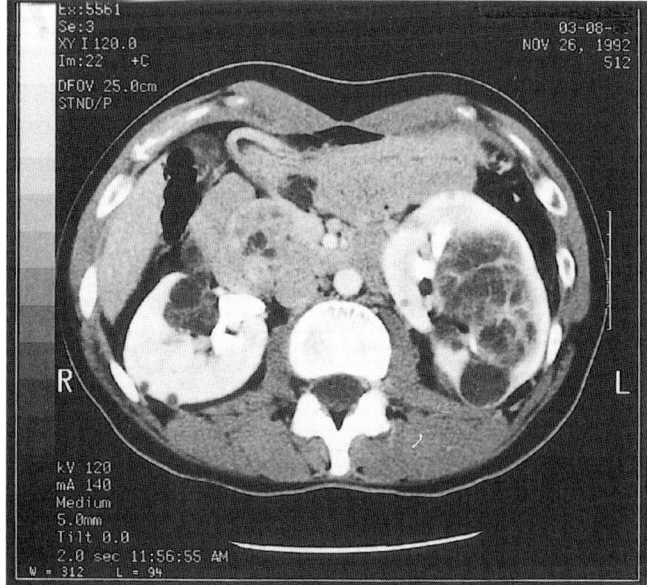

Fig. 21.12.2 CT of the kidneys in a patient with von Hippel–Lindau disease. In the right kidney, a solid tumour is found as well as cystic changes. In the left kidney, a voluminous multilocular tumour is detected with thick walls, corresponding to renal clear cell carcinoma, associated with other cystic lesions.

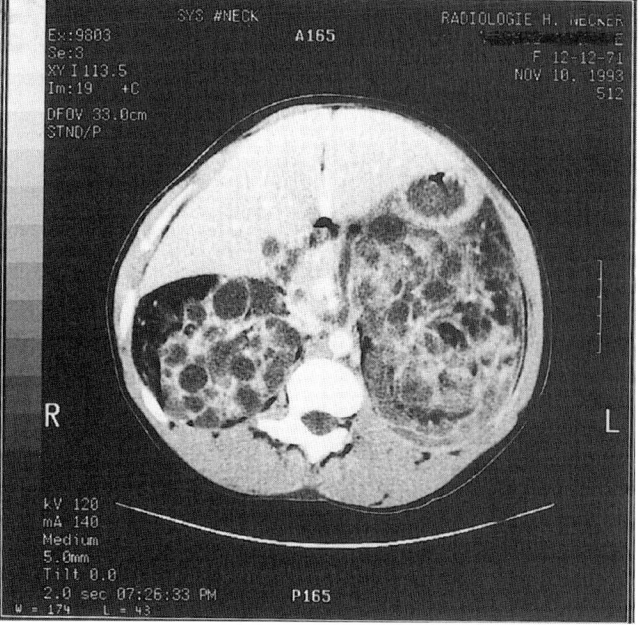

Fig. 21.12.3 Multiple bilateral renal angiomyolipomas in a patient with tuberous sclerosis (CT scan). Note the voluminous angiomyolipoma (with high content of fat that is black) at the periphery of the right kidney.

tissues, both before and after kidney transplantation: eyes (photophobia due to corneal deposits, then retinal depigmentation and visual impairment), thyroid gland (hypothyroidism), liver and spleen (portal hypertension), pancreas (diabetes mellitus), muscles, testis, and central nervous system (encephalopathy) (see Chapter 12.2).

In addition to symptomatic management, cysteamine has proved to be effective in cystinosis. It accumulates within lysosomes, promotes cystine outflow, and thus reduces tissue cystine content. Administration of this drug should be started as soon as the diagnosis is made. It may slow the rate of progression of renal failure and prevent most extrarenal complications. However, despite recent progress, tolerance of the drug is not good because of its offensive taste and odour, so compliance may be poor. Topical cysteamine prevents corneal crystal deposition.

Juvenile cystinosis is very rare, but can present in late childhood or early adult life with renal involvement.

Malformation syndromes with kidney involvement

The most frequent of these rare syndromes is Bardet–Biedl syndrome. This is a heterogeneous autosomal recessive condition for which six different genetic loci have been identified. Clinical features comprise obesity, hypogonadism (in males), polydactyly or dystrophic extremities, retinal dystrophy (leading to blindness), and renal abnormalities. The last have only been recognized recently as a cardinal feature in the syndrome. Renal imaging often shows the following abnormalities: calyceal clubbing and pronounced diverticula, and lobulated renal outlines of the fetal type. These changes are probably dysplastic in nature, and are characteristic when associated. Renal cortical and medullary cysts have also been found by ultrasonography, but the latter may be difficult to differentiate from calyceal diverticula. Approximately 25% of patients develop chronic renal failure, progressing to endstage, which is probably the major cause of death. The most important treatment is the provision of specialized education with low-vision aids. Symptomatic management of diabetes mellitus (found in 30%), hypertension, and renal failure is required.

Renal hypoplasia or unilateral renal agenesis is found in other malformation syndromes, such as the following.

- Kallmann's syndrome—with hypogonadism and hyposmia or anosmia; caused by mutation of the fibroblast growth factor-1 gene (or others).

- Branchio-oto-renal syndrome—where laterocervical fistulas or cysts and otic abnormalities, involving the outer, middle, or inner ear are found, and the *EYA1* gene, on the long arm of chromosome 8, is mutated. This gene is the homologue of a gene present in drosophila, the mutation of which leads to eye absence.

- Renal–coloboma syndrome—with optic nerve coloboma and sometimes hearing defect, and where the *PAX2* gene, located on 10q, is mutated.

- Alagille's syndrome—characterized by paucity of intrahepatic bile ducts leading to cholestasis, vertebral abnormalities (butterfly vertebra), and heart defects; caused by mutations of *JAG1* or *NOTCH2* genes.

All these genes implicated in malformation syndromes are involved normally in the control of kidney development.

Further reading

Cystic kidney diseases

Pirson Y, Chauveau D (1996). Intracranial aneurysms in ADPKD. In: Watson ML, Torres VE (eds) *Polycystic kidney disease*, pp. 530–47. Oxford University Press, Oxford.

Pirson Y, Chauveau D, Grünfeld JP (1998). Autosomal-dominant polycystic kidney disease. In: Davison AM, *et al.* (eds) *Oxford textbook of clinical nephrology*, pp. 2393–415. Oxford University Press, Oxford.

Wilson PD, (2004). Polycystic kidney disease. *N Engl J Med*, **350**, 151–64.

Alport's syndrome

Flinter FA, *et al.* (1988). Genetics of classic Alport's syndrome. *Lancet*, ii, 1005–7.

Grünfeld JP, Knebelmann B (1998). Alport's syndrome. In: Davison AM, *et al.* (eds) *Oxford textbook of clinical nephrology*, pp. 2427–37. Oxford University Press, Oxford.

Kashtan CE (2004).Familial hematuria due to type IV collagen mutations: Alport syndrome and thin basement membrane nephropathy. *Curr Opin Pediatr*, **16**, 177–81.

Inherited diseases with glomerular involvement

Eng CM, *et al.* (2006). Fabry disease. *Genet Med*, **8**, 539–48.

Lonser RR (2003). von Hippel-Lindau disease. *Lancet*, **351**, 2059–67.

Morgan SH, Grünfeld JP (1998). *Inherited disorders of the kidney*. Oxford University Press, Oxford.

Yates JRW (2006). Tuberous sclerosis. *Eur J Hum Genet*, **14**, 1065–73.

Inherited tubulointestinal disorders

Cameron JS *et al.* (1998). Inherited disorders of purine metabolism and transport. In: Davison AM, *et al.* (eds) *Oxford textbook of clinical nephrology*, pp. 2469–84. Oxford University Press, Oxford.

Hildebrandt F, Jungers P, Grünfeld JP (2001). Medullary cystic and medullary sponge renal disorders. In: Schrier RW (ed.) *Diseases of the kidney*, pp. 521–46. Little Brown, Boston.

Genetic diseases with kidney involvement

Parfrey PS (1998). Bardet–Biedl syndrome. In: Morgan SH, Grünfeld JP (eds) *Inherited disorders of the kidney*, pp. 321–39. Oxford University Press, Oxford.

Urinary tract infection

Charles Tomson and Alison Armitage

Essentials

Urinary tract infection (UTI) is a common condition, accounting for 1 to 3% of all primary care consultations in the United Kingdom. It affects patients of both sexes and all ages. The commonest organism causing uncomplicated community-acquired bacterial UTI is *Escherichia coli*.

Aetiology and pathogenesis

The occurrence and course of a UTI is influenced by the integrity of the host defence and by bacterial virulence factors. Disruption of the highly specialized transitional cell epithelium which lines the urinary tract, incomplete bladder emptying, anatomical abnormalities, and the presence of a foreign body, such as a urinary catheter, can all contribute to disruption of the host defence and increase the likelihood of infection. Sexual intercourse, use of condoms, and use of spermicides all increase the risk, and genetic factors influence the susceptibility of some people, e.g. girls with the P1 blood group are at increased risk of acute pyelonephritis. Bacterial characteristics that determine their ability to cause infection include specific mechanisms to adhere to the uroepithelium ('pili' or 'fimbrias' in the case of certain *E. coli*), or adaptations allowing them to colonize foreign surfaces, such as a urinary catheter (proteus), and subsequently cause infection.

Clinical features and diagnosis

Presentation—UTI can present in a number of ways, but most commonly with some combination of dysuria, urgency, frequency, polyuria, suprapubic tenderness, and haematuria. Asymptomatic infection is common, especially in older people, but it is not justified to send a urine sample from an asymptomatic patient for culture, with the notable exceptions of pregnant women and prior to invasive urological surgery when treatment is mandatory.

Diagnosis—acute uncomplicated UTI can often be diagnosed on symptoms alone and submission of a sample for microbiological testing is unnecessary (exceptions to this rule include pregnancy and those patients with abnormal host defences). Current United Kingdom and European guidelines on the level of bacterial counts required to diagnose 'significant' infection are variable and should not be used as the sole determinant of whether antibiotic treatment should be initiated.

Differential diagnoses ('culture negative syndromes')—these include (1) chlamydial infection, which must be identified and treated to avoid long-term complications such as infertility; also (2) urethral syndrome and (3) painful bladder syndrome (interstitial cystitis), which significantly affect a patient's quality of life and for which treatment is often unsuccessful.

Investigation—beyond microbiological testing, further investigation of women with uncomplicated UTI is seldom justified. In men, and those women with features indicating complicated infection, investigation for an underlying cause should be considered: diabetes must be excluded, and anatomical or functional abnormality of the urinary tract sought, as appropriate, by imaging, cystoscopy, and urinary flow studies.

Management

Antibiotics—trimethoprim remains the first choice for community-acquired UTI in most areas. Complicated UTI (see below) is caused by a wider spectrum of organisms, and recommendations for treatment differ. Guidelines on specific antibiotic treatment and duration of treatment are available, but with increasing antibiotic resistance (including of *E. coli* to Trimethoprim), local microbiological advice should be taken into account when choosing antibiotic treatment.

Prevention of recurrent uncomplicated UTI—many clinicians advise patients with such recurrence to take measures to improve perineal hygiene, to empty the bladder after sexual intercourse, to maintain a high fluid intake, and (if vesicoureteric reflux is suspected) to practise double voiding, but the evidence that these measures are effective is weak. Long-term antibiotic prophylaxis reduces the rate of recurrent UTI, but at the risk of adverse effects. Nightly, thrice weekly, and postcoital prophylaxis have all been shown to be of benefit, but there is no evidence to support the use of rotating antibiotic prophylaxis regimen. Cranberry products and methenamine hippurate are effective in some patients. Oestrogens are not recommended for the routine prevention of recurrent infection in postmenopausal women, but may be of benefit in those with marked atrophic vaginitis. Vaccines against uropathogenic bacteria can prevent recurrent UTI, but these are not widely used in routine clinical practice in the United Kingdom.

Complicated urinary tract infections

Complicated UTIs are those occurring in a patient with abnormal host defence. It is uncommon for any man with an anatomically normal urinary tract to suffer a UTI. An important differential diagnosis in men is prostatitis—an umbrella term used to describe a disparate group of conditions, the treatment of which is often unsatisfactory.

Urethral catheterization—UTI occurs after 2% of in/out urethral catheterizations and after 10 to 30% of 5-day indwelling catheterization, and is nearly inevitable in patients with long-term indwelling catheters. This is an important cause of hospital-acquired infection, significantly increasing the risk of Gram-negative septicaemia and mortality. However, management of patients unable to empty their bladder fully for reasons such as prostatic outflow obstruction or neurogenic bladder dysfunction because of spinal cord injury is often difficult without medium- or long-term urinary catheterization. Use of prophylactic antibiotics to cover short-term catheter insertion may be justified, but this is not the case in patients with long-term catheters, although regular bladder washouts and methenamine may be of some benefit. Treatment of asymptomatic bacteriuria in patients with anatomically abnormal urinary tracts or with indwelling urinary catheters is unjustified and likely only to lead to the emergence of antibiotic-resistant urinary infection. Clean, intermittent self-catheterization should be considered as an alternative where possible.

Urinary tract stones—these are an important cause of recurrent and relapsing UTIs that are difficult or impossible to treat with antibiotic therapy alone, repeated courses of which often encourage the development of resistant organisms. Removal of stones is often difficult and requires repeated interventions. Identification of the stone type and prevention of formation of further stones is an important part of any treatment plan (see Chapter 21.14).

Anatomically abnormal kidneys—inherited renal abnormalities such as polycystic kidneys are often complicated by UTI, which can be difficult to treat if the infection involves a cyst that may be difficult to identify and can be sheltered from antibiotic penetration. Renal transplant recipients are at an increased risk of UTI due to a variety of factors, including the anatomy of the transplant kidney, postoperative catheterization, and immunosuppressive medication. Unusual viral organisms such as polyoma (BK) virus may cause infection in this group of patients.

Vesicoureteric reflux—the normal bladder prevents reflux of urine into the ureters during micturition. Congenital abnormalities of the vesicoureteric junction can allow this to occur, as can acquired abnormalities such as bladder outflow obstruction, which disrupts normal host defence against ascending infection and thus makes children (particularly girls) more prone to ascending UTI. Cortical defects ('scars') in the upper and lower poles of the kidneys are frequently found in such children. These may be caused by ascending infection causing acute pyelonephritis, but similar appearances can occur in the absence of UTI and are likely due to renal dysplasia, inherited along with abnormal insertion of the ureters into the bladder. Progressive kidney failure may occur in such patients, but it is not clear whether this is due to the late effects of renal dysplasia and congenital reduction in renal mass, or to the effects of scarring caused by ascending infection. Clinical trials comparing long-term prophylactic antibiotics for the first 5 years of life vs surgical ureteric reimplantation have shown similar incidence of symptomatic UTI in both treatment groups; whether either treatment reduces the risk of progressive kidney failure remains uncertain.

Pregnancy—there is a significantly increased risk of acute pyelonephritis in pregnant women with untreated bacteriuria, many of whom will be asymptomatic. Late pyelonephritis is associated with an increased incidence of preterm delivery and low birth weight, hence the need in pregnancy to screen for and treat UTI promptly with antibiotics.

Ascending UTI is rarely complicated by unusual conditions such as acute papillary necrosis or perinephric abscess. These can lead to destruction of renal parenchymal tissue and long-standing renal impairment, usually in the context of abnormal host defence such as diabetes or urinary tract obstruction. Malakoplakia is an extremely rare complication of bacterial UTI, characterized by destructive tumour-like granulomatous infiltrates in the urinary bladder, kidneys, and (occasionally) other organs. Other causes of UTI may need to be considered depending on the patient's ethnic background and medical and travel history, e.g. fungal infections, tuberculosis, and schistosomiasis.

Introduction

Infection of the urinary tract is important for different reasons in different age groups. In infants and children, ascending infection is thought to be a preventable cause of renal parenchymal scarring and eventual renal failure, although it is controversial how frequently this occurs. In adult women, recurrent lower urinary tract infection ('cystitis') is a common cause of time off work. In all age groups, persistent or relapsing infection is an important indicator of abnormal host defences, usually due to abnormal anatomy or function of the urinary tract, and may result in irreversible renal damage unless the underlying cause is dealt with. Urinary tract infections (UTI) are the cause of over 50% of Gram-negative septicaemic episodes. In older people, nonspecific symptoms including toxic confusional states are often due to occult UTI.

'Urinary tract infection' refers to bacterial or fungal infection of the kidneys, renal pelvis, ureters, or bladder (viral infections may involve the urinary tract, as in Hantaan virus infection or BK virus nephropathy, but viruria more commonly reflects systemic viral infection). Infections primarily involving the urethra are nearly always sexually acquired and are dealt with elsewhere (see Section 8). 'Pyelonephritis' refers to infection primarily involving the kidneys and collecting systems. 'Cystitis' refers to infections localized to the urinary bladder. 'Recurrent' UTI are due to repeated reinfection, whether by similar organisms on each occasion or by different species; 'relapsing' and 'persistent' infections are due to the continued presence of the same organism, suppressed or not suppressed during antibiotic therapy. 'Uncomplicated' UTI occurs in an anatomically and functionally normal urinary tract; 'complicated' infection refers to all infections occurring in patients either with impaired host defence (e.g. diabetes), or with abnormal urinary tract function (e.g. pregnancy), or abnormal urinary tract anatomy (e.g. urinary tract obstruction).

Epidemiology

Symptomatic bacterial UTI is one of the commonest bacterial infections. Around 1% of boys and 3% of girls will develop a UTI during childhood, and 50% of women will be treated for at least one UTI during their lifetime, with recurrent infections in a significant minority. UTI is rare in men until after the age of 60, when the rising prevalence of impaired bladder emptying leads to an increased incidence of infection. Asymptomatic bacteriuria is found in about 10% of elderly men and in 20% of elderly women. UTI is one of the commonest bacterial infections managed in primary care, and is the cause of 1 to 3% of all primary care consultations in the United Kingdom. UTI is responsible for over 25% of all community-acquired bacteraemias, more than any other source of infection. The Nosocomial Infection National Surveillance System reported that in England (1997–2002), 8.5% of hospital-acquired bacteraemias were due to catheter-associated UTI and 5.2% due to non-catheter-associated UTI.

Aetiology

The commonest causative organisms in uncomplicated bacterial UTI are Gram-negative gut organisms, particularly *Escherichia coli* (Box 21.13.1). This reflects the fact that most infections reach the urinary tract via the urethra from the perineum. However, as discussed below, only some subtypes of *E. coli* and only some of the other species of gut organisms have the necessary virulence characteristics to enable infection of the normal urinary tract. *E. coli* is the third most common organism causing hospital-acquired bacteraemia. Complicated UTIs are caused by a broader spectrum of bacteria, including Gram-positive in addition to Gram-negative organisms and those with multiple resistance to antibiotics.

Pathophysiology

The occurrence and course of UTI are influenced by the integrity of the host defence and bacterial virulence factors.

Host defence

Most UTIs are acquired by ascent of the infecting organism up the urethra; only a very small minority result from haematogenous spread or—even less commonly—from vesicoenteric fistulas. The renal pelvis, ureters, bladder, and urethra possess a highly specialized

---

Box 21.13.1 Organisms commonly causing uncomplicated UTI

- *Escherichia coli*
- *Klebsiella pneumoniae*
- Proteus
- Pseudomonas
- Enterococcus
- *Staphylococcus saprophyticus* (in sexually active females)

---

transitional cell epithelium, which normally maintains complete impermeability to all components of urine, including toxins and water. This is maintained by tight junctions between the surface layers of epithelial cells, with a very high transepithelial electrical resistance. In the bladder, this impermeability has to be maintained despite repeated large changes in surface area as the bladder fills and empties. This is maintained by unfolding and refolding of the large, highly folded 'umbrella' cells that form the uppermost layer of the epithelium, together with insertion and endocytosis of vesicles, ready-lined with uroplakin, a hexagonal transmembrane protein found only on the surface of umbrella cells. In experimental models, infection is associated with a marked reduction in transepithelial resistance and loss of tight junctions, allowing components of urine to stimulate pain fibres and inflammatory cytokine release.

Ascending infection takes place in a series of steps, at each of which defective host defence increases the chance of successful establishment of infection (Fig. 21.13.1).

Frequency and completeness of bladder emptying

For an ascending infection to become established in the bladder, the number of organisms needs to reach a critical mass. The chance of this happening is reduced by increased urine flow rate, causing dilution of organisms within the bladder, and by frequent voiding, which also flushes the urethra and helps to prevent ascent of organisms into the bladder. This is termed 'hydrokinetic' defence. Habitual infrequent voiding is thought to be a risk factor for recurrent UTI for this reason. Patients with recurrent UTIs are routinely advised to increase fluid intake and frequency of voiding, and some

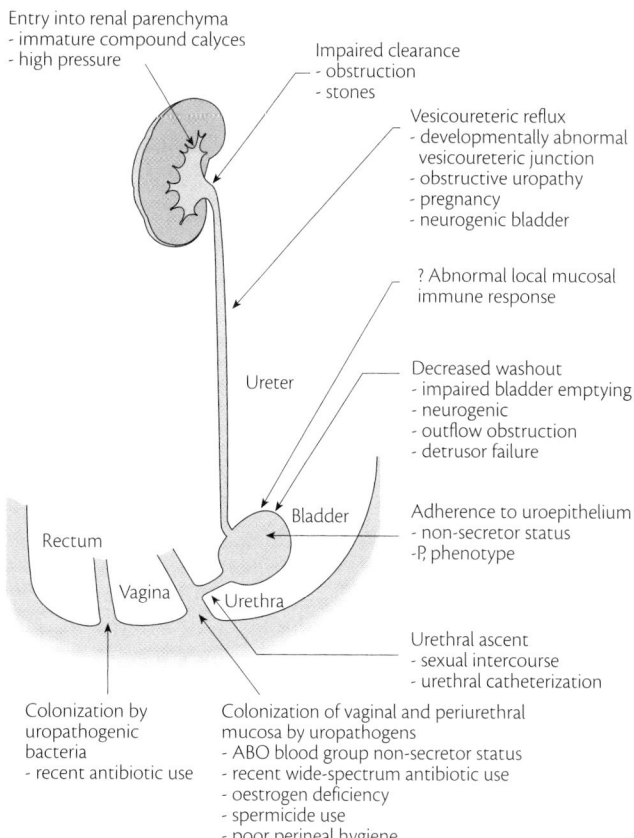

Fig. 21.13.1 Mechanisms allowing ascent of infection up the urinary tract.

women report that a high fluid intake alone is enough to clear symptomatic infection. Incomplete voiding, which may be present in both sexes and is not necessarily due to outflow obstruction (Box 21.13.2), is an important cause of increased susceptibility to urine infection.

Vesicoureteric reflux

During normal micturition urine is expelled into the urethra, while retrograde flow ('reflux') of urine into the ureters is prevented because muscular contraction of the bladder wall results in closure of the vesicoureteric junctions. Reflux of urine into the ureters can occur if this mechanism is defective, sometimes as far as the renal pelvis, followed by return to the bladder once bladder contraction has finished. The most common cause of reflux is abnormal insertion of the ureters into the bladder, which occurs as a relatively frequent developmental anomaly. The other major cause is abnormally high intravesical pressure, e.g. in high-pressure chronic retention of urine due to bladder outflow obstruction, or in neurogenic bladder in patients with partial spinal cord lesions. Whatever the cause, reflux of urine results in failure to expel all bladder urine during micturition and therefore significantly impairs host defence against infection, as well as being associated with a greatly increased risk of infection ascending to the kidneys and causing acute pyelonephritis. Vesicoureteric reflux is frequently found in children with UTI. The question of whether ascending infection is a cause of renal damage in children with reflux is discussed later in this chapter.

Foreign bodies, stones, and privileged sites

The presence of a foreign body, such as a urinary catheter or ureteric stent, or a stone within the urinary tract, creates a protected site where uropathogenic organisms can adhere and multiply, relatively protected from both hydrokinetic and mucosal defence mechanisms. In this situation it is often impossible to eradicate urine infection unless the foreign body or stone is removed, and prolonged use of antibiotics often results in the acquisition of resistance by the infecting organism. Urinary infection is nearly inevitable after a few weeks of bladder catheterization. Other 'privileged' sites include renal cysts (as in polycystic kidney disease, discussed below) and bladder diverticulae.

Sexual behaviour

Many women first experience acute cystitis shortly after becoming sexually active. Most women have transient bacteriuria after sexual

---

Box 21.13.2 Some causes of incomplete bladder emptying

- Bladder outflow obstruction
  - Benign prostatic hypertrophy
  - Prostate cancer
  - Strictures—bladder neck, urethral
  - Uterine prolapse
- Detrusor underactivity
- Abnormal bladder innervation
  - Spinal cord injury
  - Autonomic neuropathy, e.g. diabetes

---

intercourse, which develops into symptomatic cystitis only in a minority. In case–control studies of young women, the risk of UTI was associated with vaginal intercourse, and increased further by condom use. These findings are explained by the mechanical effect of intercourse encouraging ascent of organisms up the urethra, an effect that may be exacerbated by condom use, particularly without lubricants. The risk of UTI is also increased by a change in sexual partner, which may reflect male to female transmission of uropathogens. Use of spermicides as an adjunct to barrier contraceptive methods is also associated with an increased rate of periurethral colonization with *E. coli* and other uropathogens and with an increased risk of symptomatic UTI, probably because the active component in spermicides (nonoxynol-9) is bactericidal against lactobacilli. The protective effect of micturition soon after intercourse, based on the supposition that washout of recently introduced bacteria will prevent establishment of infection, remains unproven.

Vaginal and periurethral flora

Vaginal secretions are normally colonized by lactobacilli that appear to protect against colonization by uropathogenic bacteria such as *E. coli*. The mechanism of this protection is uncertain, but may in part be related to the maintenance of an acidic pH, which suppresses growth of some uropathogenic bacteria. Suppression of this normal vaginal colonization by antibiotic treatment or by spermicide use increases the risk of colonization of the periurethral mucosa by uropathogenic bacteria and subsequent ascending UTI. In addition, atrophic vaginitis caused by oestrogen deficiency is associated with the absence of lactobacillus colonization, which may be part of the reason for the increased risk of UTI in postmenopausal women.

Genetic factors

In laboratory studies, adherence of *E. coli* to both vaginal and buccal cells is greater in cells taken from women with recurrent UTI than in cells from healthy controls, and women with recurrent UTI more frequently have gut colonization by uropathogenic strains of *E. coli*, suggesting that they experience more frequent UTIs because they are more susceptible to colonization of the periurethral area by uropathogenic bacteria. It appears that this difference in susceptibility to colonization and infection, especially in patients in whom there is no other defect of host defence (such as vesicoureteric reflux), is due to genetically determined differences in the extracellular antigens to which bacteria adhere, in particular in the expression of blood group antigens.

The density of glycosphingolipids is higher in patients with the P1 blood group than those with the P2 blood group, and the P1 blood group is a risk factor for acute pyelonephritis among girls without vesicoureteric reflux. Expression of the large oligosaccharide A, B, H blood-group antigens on the cell surface partially or completely obscures the smaller glycosphingolipids, preventing them from being bound by type P pili, which is why women with the secretor phenotype, in which these antigens are both expressed on the cell surface and secreted, are less prone to most *E. coli* infections than nonsecretors. Nonsecretors also have an increased inflammatory response (fever and acute phase response) to urinary infection compared with secretors, and nonsecretors are over-represented among patients with urographic evidence of reflux nephropathy. However, some *E. coli* strains only bind to cells from subjects who are secretor-positive blood group A.

Local immunity

Another aspect of host defence is the local production of antimicrobial peptides, secreted by uroepithelial cells into the urine, and the secretion of immunoglobulin A into the urine. However, there is little convincing evidence that impaired local IgA secretion is responsible for increased susceptibility to UTI. Patients with defects in systemic immunity, whether cellular or humoral, do not appear to be at greatly increased risk of UTI; the risk of UTI with AIDS is only increased in homosexual men practising anal intercourse.

Bacterial virulence factors

The ability of a bacterium to colonize the gut and periurethral mucosa, and subsequently to adhere to the uroepithelium, is a major determinant of its ability to cause clinical infection, particularly if other host defences are intact. This ability to adhere is governed by specific interaction between bacterial adhesins, located on the tips of thin filaments ('pili' or 'fimbrias'), with genetically determined glycoproteins on the cell surface of the host cell. Type 1 fimbrias bind to mannose-containing glycoproteins that are present on the surface of uroepithelial cells, but also to Tamm–Horsfall protein, which is present in urine and can competitively inhibit binding of bacteria to cell surface glycoproteins. Type P pili bind the α-galactosyl-1,4-β-galactose disaccharide sequence present in some glycoproteins and glycosphingolipids, including the human P blood-group antigen system, and also on the cell surface of uroepithelial cells as well as red cells.

Some uropathogens are particularly adapted to colonizing foreign surfaces, particularly those coated by biofilm or mucin; for example, proteus are able to transform into a swarming phenotype with massive flagellas, organize into rafts, and move very rapidly against the flow of urine—they are therefore important causes of infection in patients with indwelling urinary catheters and those with ileal conduits. *Staphylococcus saprophyticus*, an important cause of UTI in sexually active young women, is probably better able to cause UTI than *S. aureus* or *S. epidermidis* because of its possession of a lactosamine adhesion, permitting adherence to uroepithelial cells.

Following adherence, fimbrias appear to retract, drawing the organism closer to the surface of the uroepithelial cell. Adherence is followed by apoptosis, exfoliation, and excretion of infected superficial cells and replacement by less differentiated cells, a process that may also contribute to host defence.

Bacterial adherence results in the local production of interleukin 8 (IL-8), which results in neutrophil migration through the uroepithelium into the bladder. Inflammatory cytokine release may also be promoted by soluble bacterial stimuli, such as lipopolysaccharide.

A few species of bacteria, collectively known as 'uropathogenic' bacteria, together account for most UTIs (Table 21.13.1); the presence of nonuropathogenic species suggests an abnormality of host defence. Within uropathogenic species there are strains that are capable of causing infection and other strains that are far less likely to do so: uropathogenicity is determined by expression of cell surface molecules determining adhesion to receptors on uroepithelial cells, toxin production, factors conferring resistance to the membrane attack complex, and virulence factors.

Table 21.13.1 Usefulness of inspection and dipstick testing in the diagnosis of UTI

Test	Utility	False positive	False negative
Cloudy appearance	Suggestive	Phosphate crystals	Common
Haematuria	Unreliable	Renal disease, stones, tumours	Common
Proteinuria	Unreliable	Renal disease	Common
Leucocyte esterase	Highly suggestive	Some antibiotics	Boric acid
Nitrite	Highly suggestive	Few	Gram +ve infection

Clinical features of UTI

Cystitis

The commonest presentation of UTI is with 'cystitis', a symptom complex associated with lower UTI in which many of the symptoms are directly attributable to increased bladder irritability caused by local infection. Typical symptoms—not all of which are specific for lower UTI—are listed in Box 21.13.3. Dysuria may be due to urethritis or vaginitis, but these are usually not associated with urinary frequency, and may be associated with vaginal discharge or itching and with specific findings on vaginal examination. There is considerable overlap between the symptoms of UTI (urgency, frequency, and urge incontinence) and idiopathic overactive bladder, but dysuria and haematuria are uncommon in this condition.

Genuine inflammation of the bladder wall may or may not be present, and it is important to remember that there may be noninfective causes of increased bladder irritability, such as chemical- or drug-induced cystitis and radiation cystitis, and pinworm/threadworm infection. Most patients with cystitis (bacterial infection confined to the bladder) do not have fever, nor is there evidence of an acute phase response.

Box 21.13.3 Common symptoms of lower UTI

- Severe dysuria, often described as 'scorching' or 'like peeing barbed wire', worse towards the end of or immediately after micturition
- Increased urinary frequency
- Urgency—the sensation of a strong desire to pass urine
- Strangury—the feeling of needing to pass urine despite just having done so
- Offensive-smelling urine, often described as 'strong' or 'fishy'
- Macroscopic haematuria
- Urge incontinence—leakage of urine associated with the desire to pass urine
- Constant lower abdominal aching, not just in the genital area but also in the back, flanks, and lower abdomen
- Nonspecific malaise, aching all over, nausea, tiredness, irritability, and cold sweats

Asymptomatic bacteriuria

By definition, this is an incidental finding in patients whose urine is cultured despite the absence of urinary tract symptoms. It is seldom justified to send a urine sample from an asymptomatic patient for culture, so this diagnosis should only rarely be made in clinical practice. Two important exceptions are during pregnancy and prior to invasive urological surgery (see below). Elderly patients with asymptomatic bacteriuria are also at increased risk of death, but this is probably because bacteriuria is a marker of poorer general health, and antibacterial treatment has not been shown to improve survival in this situation.

Acute pyelonephritis

The term 'acute pyelonephritis' denotes infection within the renal pelvis, with or without active infection within the renal parenchyma. The diagnosis is usually made on the basis of the presence of flank pain (usually unilateral), fever, rigors, raised C-reactive protein (or erythrocyte sedimentation rate (ESR) or plasma viscosity), neutrophilia, and evidence of urine infection on culture of a midstream urine sample. However, rigorous tests to localize the site of infection (discussed below) show that the correlation between the presence or absence of bacteriuria in the upper urinary tract and the presence or absence of flank pain, systemic symptoms, and an acute phase response is dismally poor; many patients with infection confined to the bladder have flank pain and fever, whereas over 60% of elderly women with asymptomatic bacteriuria have upper tract infection. The symptoms and signs of so-called 'acute pyelonephritis' are therefore in reality those of a marked host response to UTI, irrespective of whether organisms are multiplying in the renal pelvis or in the bladder.

Diagnosis

Inspection and dipstick testing

In a 'classic' case of established UTI the urine is cloudy, has an offensive smell, and is positive for blood, protein, leucocyte esterase, and nitrite on dipstick urinalysis. In this situation it is reasonable to make a diagnosis of UTI without further delay, and to institute empirical treatment. Whether a midstream urine sample should also be sent to the laboratory for confirmation and identification of the causative organism depends on the clinical situation, as discussed below. However, in many situations the diagnosis is not so obvious, and the diagnostic accuracy of inspection and dipstick testing less good.

Cloudy urine may be caused by bacteria and pyuria, but may also be caused by amorphous phosphate crystals that form in normal urine as it cools. Low concentrations of bacteria and white cells will not cause sufficient turbidity to be detected on visual inspection. An offensive, fishy smell is highly suggestive of UTI, but relatively infrequent.

Macroscopic haematuria can certainly occur as a result of severe cystitis, but is frequently absent in genuine UTI and is more often due to glomerular bleeding or urothelial bleeding as a result of tumours or stones. Dipstick detection of haematuria is neither sensitive nor specific for the detection of UTI. Proteinuria can occur in UTI as a result of the release of proteins from white cells, but is neither specific nor sensitive.

Leucocyte esterase is an enzyme released by white cells and a reliable test for pyuria, which is in most situations a major diagnostic

criterion for UTI, as discussed in the next section. A positive test indicates 10 white cells/ml. Note, however, that transport of urine samples in containers containing boric acid can result in false-negative leucocyte esterase tests, as the boric acid inhibits the enzyme.

Nitrite is produced by most uropathogens, which reduce urinary nitrate to nitrite, but not by Gram-positive organisms. A positive test for nitrite is highly suggestive of UTI. False-negative tests can be seen in patients with low dietary nitrate and in those taking high-dose ascorbic acid. The diagnosis of acute uncomplicated UTI is highly likely with a history of two urinary symptoms, and the likelihood is increased further with specific combinations of symptoms (e.g. dysuria and frequency without vaginal discharge), or a positive nitrite test.

A combination of visual inspection and dipstick testing is a reasonable screening test for patients in whom uncomplicated UTI is suspected on clinical grounds: in this situation, crystal-clear urine and negative dipsticks for nitrite and leucocyte esterase make the diagnosis of UTI very unlikely (Table 21.13.1). The worst that is likely to happen if the diagnosis is missed is that the patient will re-present with more obvious abnormalities due to progression of the UTI to a more severe stage. However, in situations in which it would be important not to miss the opportunity to start treatment early, e.g. in patients with known abnormalities of host defence, pregnancy, or previous acute pyelonephritis, or in suspected atypical infections, formal microscopy and culture of the urine is required. An algorithm for diagnosis of suspected uncomplicated UTI in adult women is shown in Fig. 21.13.2.

Microscopy and culture of urine

The diagnosis of bacterial infection in the urinary tract might appear straightforward, relying on culture of freshly voided urine. However, urine samples are very easily contaminated during voiding by bacteria from the perineal skin (or, to a lesser extent, the foreskin in males), resulting in false-positive results. The only certain way to circumvent this problem is to take urine directly from the bladder, either by suprapubic needle aspiration of urine from the bladder, which is invasive and seldom performed in clinical practice, or by urethral catheterization, which carries a 1 to 2% risk of introducing infection into the bladder. In men, contamination of the voided urine sample can largely be avoided by retraction of the foreskin prior to voiding. In women, the reliability of urine culture can be improved by instructing women to part the labia with one hand and ensuring collection of a midstream sample, without either the initial portion or the 'afterdrip', but is not improved further by perineal washing or antiseptic use. These precautions only reduce the risk of contamination, rather than abolishing it altogether.

Microscopy of urine samples allows quantification of pyuria—the presence of white blood cells in the urine. However, the methodologies used to report pyuria vary enormously: microscopy of urine that has been centrifuged and resuspended, with reporting of the number of cells per high-power field, gives results which bear little relation to leucocyte excretion rate or to counting cells from unspun urine in a counting chamber, when significant pyuria is usually defined as a urinary white cell count of 10 leucocytes/µl or more.

Bacterial UTI is by far the commonest cause of pyuria, and symptomatic patients with pyuria whose urine cultures are reported as showing no significant pathogens should be suspected either of having 'low-count' bacteriuria due to early infection, or infection

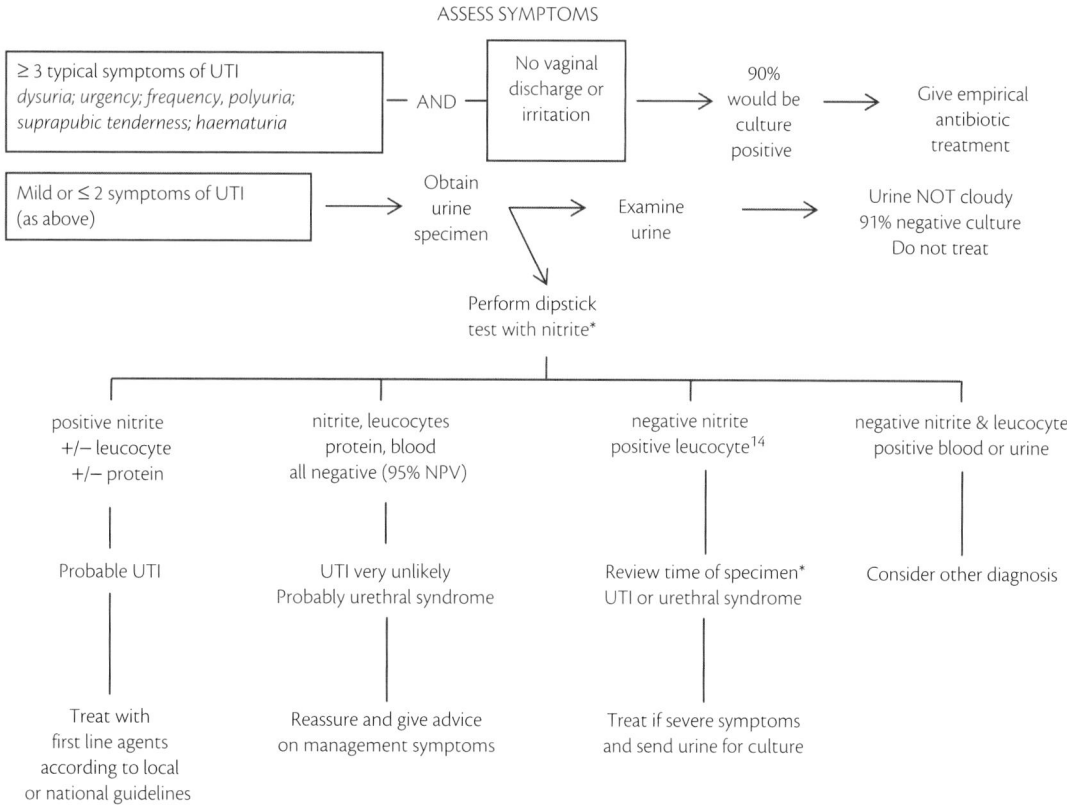

ASSESS SYMPTOMS

≥ 3 typical symptoms of UTI
*dysuria; urgency; frequency, polyuria;
suprapubic tenderness; haematuria* — AND — No vaginal discharge or irritation → 90% would be culture positive → Give empirical antibiotic treatment

Mild or ≤ 2 symptoms of UTI (as above) → Obtain urine specimen → Examine urine → Urine NOT cloudy 91% negative culture Do not treat

Perform dipstick test with nitrite*

positive nitrite +/− leucocyte +/− protein | nitrite, leucocytes protein, blood all negative (95% NPV) | negative nitrite positive leucocyte[14] | negative nitrite & leucocyte positive blood or urine

Probable UTI | UTI very unlikely Probably urethral syndrome | Review time of specimen* UTI or urethral syndrome | Consider other diagnosis

Treat with first line agents according to local or national guidelines | Reassure and give advice on management symptoms | Treat if severe symptoms and send urine for culture

*Nitrite is produced by the action of bacterial nitrate reductase in urine. As contact time between bacteria and urine is needed, morning specimens are most reliable. When reading test wait for the time recommended by manufacturer. NPV, negative predictive value.

Fig. 21.13.2 Algorithm for diagnosis of suspected acute uncomplicated UTI in adult women.
(Reproduced with permission from http://www.hpa.org.uk/infections/topics_az/primary_care_guidance/uti_guide.pdf)

Box 21.13.4 Causes of 'sterile pyuria'

◆ Partially treated bacterial UTI

◆ Bacterial UTI with a 'fastidious' organism

◆ Chlamydial urethritis

◆ 'False-negative' urine cultures due to contamination of midstream urine sample with antiseptic

◆ Contamination by vaginal leucocytes

◆ Chronic interstitial nephritis:
  · Analgesic nephropathy
  · Sarcoidosis (urinary white cells may be lymphocytes, not neutrophils)

◆ Urinary tract stones

◆ Acute interstitial nephritis, e.g. allergic interstitial nephritis (urinary white cells may be eosinophils)

◆ Papillary necrosis:
  · Diabetes
  · Sickle-cell disease

◆ Renal tract tuberculosis

◆ Fever

---

with a slow-growing organism, chlamydial infection, or one of the causes of sterile pyuria (Box 21.13.4). However, vaginal leucorrhoea can also result in 'false-positive' pyuria.

Microscopy also gives information on whether the urine sample is contaminated by cells from the periurethral area. Squamous cells are five to seven times larger than red cells and are easily recognized on microscopy: their presence in a midstream urine sample has conventionally been taken to indicate contamination, but they may originate from the urethra or from the epithelium of the vulva and vagina, as well as from areas of squamous metaplasia in the bladder, which is a common finding; and squamous cells are frequently seen in urine obtained by bladder catheterization, showing that their presence is not an absolute indicator of contamination.

Once a urine sample is obtained, the conditions under which it is cultured determine whether any organisms present grow. Standard laboratory culture conditions are designed to encourage the growth of recognized urinary pathogens (if present), but may not be optimal for the growth of atypical organisms or of those not usually recognized as urinary pathogens. Because small numbers of organisms are frequently cultured from urine as a result of contamination, growth of an organism is conventionally reported as a 'significant growth' if it meets several criteria. These are summarized in Box 21.13.5.

Genuine mixed growth of two or more bacteria may occur in complicated UTI (Box 21.13.6), as may the growth of an organism not usually associated with the urinary tract. The spectrum of

---

Box 21.13.5 Criteria for the diagnosis of UTI

◆ There is a pure growth, i.e. of a single organism

◆ The organism grown is a 'recognized' urinary pathogen

◆ Quantitative urine culture results in $>10^5$ cfu/ml

◆ There is significant pyuria on urine microscopy, and few if any squamous cells

---

organisms recognized as capable of causing genuine UTI is widening. *S. saprophyticus* was only fairly recently recognized as a cause of UTI in sexually active women, and it is possible that other true urinary pathogens are yet to be identified, perhaps accounting for some cases of the so-called urethral syndrome (see below). 'Low-count' bacteriuria may reflect genuine bladder infection, particularly in early UTIs, and may occur in patients who have increased their fluid intake and are 'diluting' their bacterial counts by generating a high urinary output; also in patients infected with slow-growing organisms such as *S. saprophyticus*.

The criterion of 10^5 cfu/ml was originally validated in asymptomatic women, but subsequent studies showed that nearly 50% of women presenting with frequency and dysuria had genuine bladder infection but with counts between 10^2 and 10^5 cfu/ml on culture of a midstream urine sample. If symptomatic women with counts of between 10^2 and 10^4 cfu/ml are left untreated, most will have persistent symptoms and counts of more than 10^5 cfu/ml 2 days later. Current European guidelines cite a lower cut-off (10^3 cfu/ml) specifically for *E. coli* and *S. saprophyticus*. In men, bacterial counts of 10^3 cfu/ml or more are very likely to reflect significant infection, as the potential for significant contamination is lower.

The presence of pyuria further increases the likelihood that low counts are significant, although pyuria is not always present in proven bladder infection, particularly if the sample is taken early after the onset. The traditional method of expressing urinary white cell counts as cells per high-power field is very poorly reproducible as the volume in a high-power field is extremely variable. If a counting chamber or equivalent is used, then a criterion of 10 white cells/mm^3 separates patients with genuine bacteriuria from those without.

Localization to upper or lower urinary tract

Tests to discover whether infection is confined to the bladder or whether it has spread to involve one or both kidneys are very

---

Box 21.13.6 Conditions in which genuine mixed-growth UTI may occur

◆ Ileal conduits

◆ Neurogenic bladder

◆ Vesicocolic fistula

◆ Urinary tract stones

◆ Renal abscesses

◆ Long-term indwelling urinary catheters or stents

---

seldom necessary, but may be required if, for example, surgical removal of a kidney because of recurrent infection is contemplated. The 'gold standard' for diagnosis of upper UTI is culture of urine obtained from each ureter by direct catheterization during cystoscopy, but such an invasive procedure can only be justified in exceptional circumstances, and even then may be difficult to interpret due to contamination of ureteric samples by bladder urine during passage of the catheters.

An alternative to ureteric catheterization is the Fairley test, which involves a bladder washout using neomycin and fibrinolytic enzymes. Urine is cultured following completion, to confirm eradication of bladder bacteria, and then at 10, 20, and 30 min after completion of the washout. Bacteriuria returns slowly, if at all, in patients with infection confined to the bladder, but because the washout procedure has no effect on bacteria in the upper urinary tracts, rapid reappearance of bacteriuria indicates upper UTI. Using this test it has been shown that both upper and lower UTI are frequently asymptomatic and that flank pain and fever are extremely unreliable indicators of the presence of upper UTI.

Detection (by immunofluorescence staining) of immunoglobulin-coated bacteria is suggestive of tissue invasion, but is not reliable compared with ureteric catheterization or Fairley tests. This may be partly because tissue invasion can also occur in severe lower UTI, such as that complicating urethral catheterization. Raised concentrations of urinary β_2-microglobulin occur in the presence of tubular damage due to ascending infection, but may also be found patients with chronic kidney disease. Renal excretory function usually remains unchanged during acute pyelonephritis unless obstruction is present, but acute renal failure is occasionally seen, often associated with coincident use of nonsteroidal anti-inflammatory drugs (NSAIDs) and diuretics. Abnormal appearances on contrast CT scanning and/or dimercaptosuccinyl acid (DMSA) scanning have been reported, including generalized renal swelling, focal areas of decreased parenchymal enhancement, and perirenal abscess formation, with the development of cortical scars and calyceal diverticulae if imaging is repeated on follow-up. In general, the more severe the infection is clinically (assessed by acute phase response, duration of fever, etc.), the more marked the radiological abnormality. However, significant loss of renal excretory function following acute pyelonephritis in patients without diabetes, obstruction or pre-existing reflux nephropathy/dysplasia, is remarkably uncommon even on long-term follow-up, and the significance of such scars is therefore uncertain.

Differential diagnosis of UTI

Occasionally patients may present with symptoms and signs highly suggestive of UTI, with or without pyuria, but with negative urine cultures. These patients may have 'false-negative' urine cultures, e.g. a low growth of a genuine pathogen; infection with a 'fastidious' organism, the presence of which is not detected by routine laboratory cultures; or they may have a noninfectious cause. It is dangerous to label symptoms in such patients as psychogenic; prolonged symptoms combined with numerous unsuccessful trials of antibacterials, or with different explanations from different doctors, may result in psychological stress, which in turn may amplify symptoms, and there is little evidence that psychological disease is the primary problem, even in a subgroup.

Urethral syndrome and chlamydial urethritis

The term 'urethral syndrome' was used in the past as a synonym for the typical symptoms of cystitis, namely frequency, urgency, and dysuria. More recently it has been applied to the subgroup of women with typical symptoms but in whom a recognized urinary pathogen cannot be cultured from the urine. A significant proportion of these patients, particularly those with pyuria, have chlamydial urethritis.

Chlamydial infection can be confirmed by culture of a urethral swab or by detection of chlamydia antigens on an endocervical or urethral swab or first-pass urine specimen by nucleic acid amplification techniques. It can be treated with tetracyclines, but as the infection may be sexually transmitted it is also important to treat the patient's sexual partner(s), who may be asymptomatic. Patients with confirmed chlamydial infection should also be tested for gonorrhoea.

Other patients with urethral syndrome have 'low-count' infection with a true bacterial urinary pathogen. Vaginal infection or atrophy should be excluded, as these can cause similar symptoms.

The pathogenesis and optimal management of the remaining patients with frequency and dysuria, but with no identifiable bacterial infection, remains controversial. There is controversy over the role of 'fastidious bacteria' that are difficult to grow in the laboratory, particularly lactobacilli. Empirical antibiotic treatment is equally successful in eradicating symptoms in women presenting to primary care whether or not urinary pathogens are found on urine culture, suggesting that the syndrome is frequently due to bacterial infection that is not detected by routine laboratory urine culture. However, a few women with persistent symptoms do not respond to antibiotics, and in these women repeated courses of antibiotics are likely to lead to the emergence of antibiotic-resistant organisms, which may later cause true infection that is difficult to treat. Psychological distress is common in patients with persistent lower urinary tract symptoms, but the prevalence of emotional or psychiatric disorders is no higher in women presenting to general practitioners with dysuria and frequency whose urine cultures are negative than in those with proven cystitis. Urologists often offer such women urethral dilatation on the assumption that the symptoms are due to urethral spasm or stricture, but there is minimal evidence beyond clinical anecdote that this procedure is of any benefit; one randomized controlled trial showed no difference in outcome between urethral dilatation and cystoscopy alone.

Women with recurrent episodes of frequency and dysuria, with or without pyuria, whose urine cultures remain sterile should be carefully evaluated for the presence of vaginitis (either infective or atrophic). It is justified in this situation to obtain urine direct from the bladder during an episode, preferably by suprapubic aspiration or alternatively by urethral catheterization, and ensure that this is cultured in conditions permitting the identification of fastidious or low-growing organisms. In urine obtained direct from the bladder, any growth of organisms is clinically significant. Any infection so detected should be treated, preferably with a prolonged course of an appropriate antibiotic to ensure complete eradication. If no infection can be detected, cystoscopy is required to exclude noninfective causes of cystitis.

Painful bladder syndrome/interstitial cystitis

Painful bladder syndrome/interstitial cystitis is a chronic bladder syndrome of unknown aetiology. It is characterized by bladder pain (which classically worsens on bladder filling and diminishes with bladder emptying), urgency, frequency, and nocturia, despite—by definition—sterile urine. Urine microscopy shows pyuria. Cystoscopy shows variable inflammation, sometimes with ulceration (Hunner's ulcers, first described in 1914). Bladder biopsies show a chronic inflammatory infiltrate; mast cell infiltration is common, but is also seen in infective cystitis. The condition may progress to cause contracture of the bladder.

Many of these features would be explained by an acquired defect in the barrier function of the uroepithelium, but the cause of such a defect remains unclear. It remains possible that infection by a fastidious organism is responsible for initiating the disease in some patients. Numerous therapies have been tried, including various oral drugs (amitriptyline, antibiotics, ciclosporin); instillation of intravesical agents including heparin, glycosoaminoglycans and bacille Calmette–Guérin (BCG); and most commonly hydrodistension. In severe cases, where all other therapeutic options have failed, bladder augmentation or cystectomy with urinary diversion may be necessary.

Drug-induced cystitis

This presents similarly, although often more acutely and with macroscopic haematuria. It may be caused by acrolein, a metabolite of cyclophosphamide and ifosfamide, and also by NSAIDs, particularly tiaprofenic acid, and by danazol.

Radiation-induced cystitis

Radiation-induced cystitis is seen in patients who have been treated for bladder or gynaecological malignancy.

Clinical investigation—distinction between uncomplicated and complicated UTI

The clinical approach to investigation and treatment of patients with UTI—including whether to send a urine sample for culture, how long to treat for, and whether to send a repeat sample to confirm eradication of infection—depends on making a distinction between 'uncomplicated' and 'complicated' UTI. Although this is sometimes straightforward—for instance, UTIs in pregnant women and in catheterized patients are, by definition, 'complicated'—sometimes the decision on whether to investigate for an underlying cause of 'complicated' UTI depends solely on the presenting features.

Most women with uncomplicated cystitis do not require investigation other than urine culture, and may even be treated empirically, the choice of antibiotic being based on locally prevalent sensitivity patterns of the most common uropathogens, rather than waiting for the results of culture and sensitivity. The yield in such women of investigation with cystoscopy and/or intravenous urography is low. Because minor abnormalities such as duplex collecting systems are common in the general population, these will often be found in women presenting with cystitis, but detection of such abnormalities does not lead to any change in treatment. Investigation of women should therefore be reserved for those with atypical features (Box 21.13.7).

In men, UTI is nearly always associated with an underlying abnormality of host defence, and all men with proven UTI should therefore be offered investigation.

Table 21.13.2 shows the important abnormalities that need to be excluded if investigation is thought to be necessary. Whether adults

Box 21.13.7 Indications for further investigation in females with UTI

- Genuine mixed growth
- Failure of standard antibiotic treatment to eradicate infection
- Relapsing infection (repeated detection of the same organism, as identified by antibiotic sensitivity pattern, or more detailed typing)
- Confirmed infection with organisms not usually recognized as uropathogens
- Infection with proteus
- Marked acute phase response (or symptoms of 'acute pyelonephritis'), suggesting tissue invasion
- Persistent haematuria after treatment of infection
- Asymptomatic bacteriuria, for no known cause

should be investigated for vesicoureteric reflux is open to doubt, as there is no good evidence that antireflux surgery (e.g. ureteric reimplantation, injection of Teflon around the ureteric orifice) is of benefit in preventing either ascending infection or renal damage.

Treatment

Uncomplicated asymptomatic bacteriuria

The only situations in which treatment of asymptomatic bacteriuria is mandatory are during pregnancy and prior to invasive urological surgery; these situations are discussed below.

Uncomplicated 'cystitis'

The two main aims of antibiotic treatment in UTI are to achieve rapid resolution of symptoms, and to prevent recurrent episodes of infection in the individual patient to minimize the emergence of antibiotic resistance of organisms. Rational treatment of UTI requires the physician to balance the costs and dangers of treatment (including cost of the drug, risk of unwanted side-effects, and the induction of resistance) with benefit.

Is treatment necessary at all? Many women with recurrent uncomplicated cystitis report that they can clear their own infections by increased fluid intake and frequent voiding. Many buy alkalinizing agents (e.g. potassium citrate) to ameliorate the symptoms, which

Table 21.13.2 Clinical investigation of UTI

Abnormality to be excluded	Investigation
Diabetes	Blood test
Urinary tract stones	Ultrasonography, plain radiography (KUB), intravenous urography, CT urography[a]
Anatomical abnormalities of the upper tract (e.g. papillary necrosis, reflux nephropathy)	
Urinary tract obstruction	
Bladder diverticulae	Cystoscopy
Impaired bladder emptying	Urinary flow studies

KUB, kidneys–ureters–bladder.
[a] Choice of imaging dependent on local facilities.

work by reducing bladder irritability. Placebo-controlled studies have confirmed that infection may clear spontaneously, although this may take several weeks or even months, and a small percentage of women remain infected until given antibiotics. There is therefore no justification in insisting on antibiotic treatment in those who wish to try to do without.

Choice of antibiotic
It is usually impracticable to await the results of culture and sensitivity testing, if these tests are justified at all. The choice of antibiotic is therefore usually empirical, based on the likelihood that the drug will clear the infection (efficacy), cost, side-effect profile, and the risk of selection of resistant organisms, both in the patient being treated and in the community.

The efficacy of antibiotics is not fully predictable from *in vitro* sensitivity testing, which is probably part of the reason why trimethoprim (with or without sulphamethoxazole) remains the first-line choice in many areas, despite an upward trend in resistance rates. This is at least in part because many antibiotics are concentrated in the urine to levels far greater than those found in tissues, and at these concentrations may remain active against organisms that are reported to be resistant to the concentrations found in tissues, which are usually used to define resistance *in vitro*. However, increasing resistance *in vitro* to trimethoprim is sure to lead sooner or later to increased clinical failure rates, as has already been observed for β-lactam antibiotics. Some of the clinical properties of the most commonly used antibiotics are reviewed in Table 21.13.3, with the target and mechanisms of actions of different antibiotic agents shown in Fig. 21.13.3. The most recent recommendations of the United Kingdom Health Protection Agency for treatment of UTI in primary care are summarized in Table 21.13.4.

Duration of treatment
A single high dose of an antibiotic will cure many women; it is simple, cheap, and may reduce the risk of side-effects and bacterial resistance. Single-dose treatment is thought to be popular amongst patients, although those paying for prescription medications may feel 'short-changed' by paying a full prescription fee for a single tablet. Treatment for 3 to 14 days is more likely to result in absence of persistent bacteriuria at 2 weeks than single-dose treatment, but there is no difference in long-term bacteriuria. The rate of adverse reactions also increases with duration of therapy, particularly for trimethoprim–sulphonamide combinations, which should therefore be given for no more than 3 days. Cure rates of UTIs caused by *S. saprophyticus* and in elderly women are low with 3-day regimens, and these infections should be treated with 7-day courses.

Alternatives to antibiotic therapy
Cranberry juice and tablets, methenamine hippurate, and treatment of atrophic vaginitis with topical oestrogens have all been used in the prevention of UTI (see below), but there is no proven role for any of these interventions in the treatment of an established UTI.

Uncomplicated 'acute pyelonephritis'
Choice of antibiotic
The antibiotic chosen in this situation needs good tissue penetration as well as high urinary excretion, and must be fully active against the infecting organism at typical serum concentrations. It is therefore much more important to identify the infecting organism

Table 21.13.3 Clinical properties of antibiotics commonly used for UTIs

Antibiotic	Advantages	Disadvantages
Trimethoprim	Cheap Well tolerated High concentrations in vaginal and periurethral fluid.	Increasing rates of *in vitro* resistance
Trimethoprim-sulphamethoxazole	As for trimethoprim Possible reduced risk of emergence of resistant strains.	Increasing rates of resistance Adverse reactions (e.g. rash) to sulphonamide component
β-lactams (e.g. amoxicillin, cephalosporins)	Cheap Well tolerated	High rates of resistance Less effective than trimethoprim in 3-day or single-day regimens Allergic reactions High risk of *Clostridium difficile* colitis
β-lactams with β-lactamase inhibitor (e.g. co-amoxiclav)	As for β-lactams Low rates of resistance	Cost Risk of selection of resistant strains Allergic reactions High risk of *Clostridium difficile* colitis
Nitrofurantoin	Cheap Does not induce resistance in bowel organisms	Nausea and vomiting (less with macrocrystalline preparations) Hepatic, neurological, haematological, and pulmonary toxicity (mostly seen with prolonged treatment)
Quinolones, e.g. ciprofloxacin	Well tolerated Broad antibacterial spectrum including many uropathogens	Cost High risk of *Clostridium difficile* colitis Achilles tendon damage

and its antibiotic sensitivity pattern by sending urine (or blood from patients in hospital) for culture. However, empirical treatment must be started while awaiting culture and sensitivity results, as acute pyelonephritis can evolve rapidly into a life-threatening illness.

Oral therapy with a quinolone antibiotic (ciprofloxacin, ofloxacin, norfloxacin) is probably the best choice, although trimethoprim or trimethoprim–sulphamethoxazole are alternatives if local rates of resistance among uropathogens remain low. Treatment with β-lactam antibiotics, even if the infecting organism is fully sensitive *in vitro*, is associated with a high rate of recurrence compared with treatment by other agents. Patients with septicaemia should receive a quinolone (for which oral administration is as effective as intravenous) or a combination of an aminoglycoside with ampicillin plus β-lactamase inhibitor, or an extended-spectrum cephalosporin with or without an aminoglycoside. Once-daily administration of aminoglycosides is as effective as thrice-daily and reduces the risk of toxicity.

Duration of therapy

It is widely recommended that acute pyelonephritis is treated with a significantly longer course of antibiotics than acute cystitis (Table 21.13.11). Since, as discussed above, the clinical distinction between acute pyelonephritis and cystitis relies on the presence of fever, flank pain, and an acute phase response, and since all of these may be present in acute cystitis with no involvement of the upper urinary tract and entirely absent in acute pyelonephritis, what these recommendations really mean is that those patients demonstrating a more marked host response should be treated more aggressively and for longer. It is therefore reasonable to suggest that in a patient with systemic symptoms (including flank pain) and fever; or leucocytosis, or a raised C-reactive protein, plasma viscosity, or ESR; antibiotic treatment should be continued until these abnormalities have disappeared. A 14-day course is as effective as a 6-week course in uncomplicated acute pyelonephritis, and a 7-day course may be sufficient for patients with mild illness.

Prevention of recurrent uncomplicated UTI

Lifestyle and personal hygiene

It is common practice to advise women with UTI to change their lifestyle, e.g. by voiding after intercourse, double micturition, wiping themselves from front to back after micturition, and increasing fluid intake. A systematic review concluded that the evidence for lifestyle advice was not based on good evidence, and stated "routine advice about adopting or discontinuing any particular lifestyle factors should not be offered to patients with bacterial UTI". However, absence of evidence of benefit is not the same as evidence of absence of benefit, and for individuals with recurrent and/or complicated UTI, individualized advice along these lines is reasonable.

Long-term prophylactic antibiotics

Some women with recurrent cystitis choose to have antibiotic treatment for each infection as it arises, particularly if they are allowed to self-administer treatment as soon as symptoms start. Others may opt for prophylactic treatment. Long-term low-dose antibiotic treatment is effective in reducing the rate of infection in such women, although not to zero, and with a significant risk of

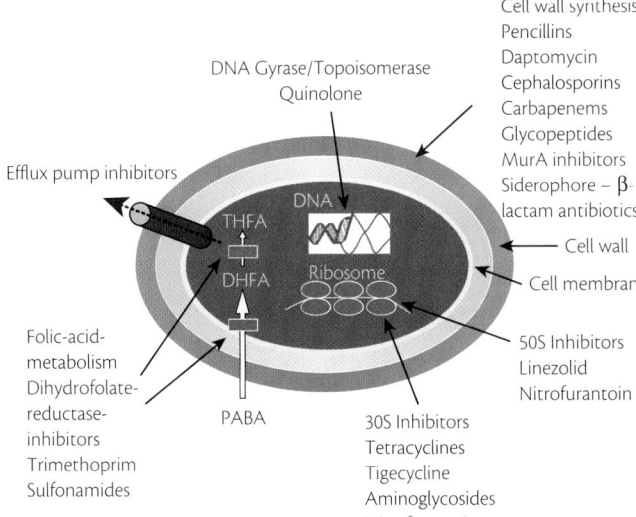

Fig. 21.13.3 Targets and mechanisms of actions of different antibiotic agents used in the treatment of UTI. DHFA, dihydrofolic acid; PABA, *p*-aminobenzoic acid; THFA, tetrahydrofolic acid.
EUROPEAN UROLOGY, V49(2): 235–244 © 2006 European Association of Urology.

Table 21.13.4 Health Protection Agency recommendations for the treatment of UTI in the community

Uncomplicated UTI, i.e. no fever or flank pain	Use urine dipstick to exclude UTI –ve nitrite and leucocyte 95% negative predictive value There is less relapse with trimethoprim than cephalosporins or pivmecillinam. Community multiresistant *E. coli* with extended-spectrum β-lactamase enzymes (ESBLs) are increasing so perform culture in all treatment failures. ESBLs are multiresistant but remain sensitive to nitrofurantoin	Trimethoprim OR nitrofurantoin	200 mg BD 50–100 mg QDS	3 days
		Second line—depends on susceptibility of organism isolated, e.g. nitrofurantoin, amoxicillin, cefalexin, co-amoxiclav, quinolone, pivmecillinam		
UTI in pregnancy and men	Send MSU for culture. Short-term use of trimethoprim or nitrofurantoin in pregnancy is unlikely to cause problems to the fetus	Nitrofurantoin OR trimethoprim Second line: Cefalexin OR amoxicillin	50–100 mg QDS 200 mg BD 500 mg BD 250 mg TDS	7 days 7 days 7 days 7 days
Children	Send MSU for culture and susceptibility Waiting 24 h for results is not detrimental to outcome	Trimethoprim OR nitrofurantoin OR cefalexin If susceptible, amoxicillin	See BNF for dosage	7 days
Acute pyelonephritis	Send MSU for culture. A recent randomized controlled trial showed 7 days ciprofloxacin was as good as 14 days co-trimoxazole If no response within 24 h—admit to hospital	Ciprofloxacin OR co-amoxiclav If susceptible, trimethoprim	500 mg BD 500/125 mg TDS 200 mg BD	7 days 14 days 14 days
Recurrent UTI women ≥3/yr	Post coital prophylaxis is as effective as prophylaxis taken nightly. Prophylactic doses	Nitrofurantoin OR trimethoprim	50 mg 100 mg	Stat postcoital OR OD at night

BD, twice daily; MSU, midstream urine; OD, once daily; QSD, four times daily; TDS, three times daily.
Note: Amoxicillin resistance is common, therefore only use if culture confirms susceptibility. In elderly people (>65 years), do not treat asymptomatic bacteriuria; it occurs in 25% of women and 10% of men and is not associated with increased morbidity.
In the presence of a catheter, antibiotics will not eradicate bacteriuria; only treat if systemically unwell or pyelonephritis is likely.

adverse effects (e.g. gastrointestinal symptoms, rash, vaginal irritation). Prophylactic treatment should be considered in women with at least two symptomatic infections per year and probably works by preventing colonization of periurethral tissues by uropathogens.

Trimethoprim (100 mg at night) is widely used for prophylaxis because it achieves very high concentrations in vaginal fluid and may therefore remain active against organisms that are resistant to the concentrations used in *in vitro* sensitivity testing. Nitrofurantoin (100 mg at night) has also been widely used, and may be more effective, but can cause rare but serious adverse effects (pulmonary and hepatic toxicity) with long-term therapy, making regular monitoring of liver enzymes and lung function tests necessary. Because both are well absorbed they do not reach high concentrations in the colon, hence emergence of resistant strains in colonic flora is uncommon, whereas this problem does arise with long-term use of β-lactam antibiotics. Long-term use of quinolones is expensive and associated with a significant risk of selection of resistant strains. A number of dosage regimens have been used, including nightly treatment, thrice-weekly treatment, and postcoital treatment, with no convincing evidence of the superiority of one regimen over another. There is no evidence to support the use of 'rotating' antibiotic prophylaxis.

Other treatments

Cranberry juice or tablets

Cranberry juice contains proanthocyanidin, which inhibits adherence of P-fimbriated *E. coli*. Cranberry products are not regulated and the concentration of the active ingredient varies considerably. On meta-analysis, cranberry juice or tablets significantly reduce the number of symptomatic UTIs in women over a 12-month period, but with a significant drop-out rate. No direct comparison of cranberry products and antibiotic prophylaxis in preventing UTI has been reported, but the number needed to treat to prevent one infection is higher for cranberry products than for nightly antibiotic prophylaxis, or postcoital antibiotic prophylaxis. Patients on coumarin anticoagulation should avoid cranberry products.

While cranberry juice and tablets may be effective in the prevention of UTI, there have been no trials assessing their use in treatment of UTI.

Methenamine hippurate

Methenamine is hydrolysed in acid urine to produce formaldehyde, a powerful antiseptic. Use of this drug is not associated with the emergence of antibiotic resistance. There is limited evidence that long-term methenamine treatment can reduce the rate of recurrent UTIs in women without upper tract abnormalities.

Treatment of atrophic vaginitis

There is significant heterogeneity in the results of trials examining the effects of topical oestrogens on prevention of recurrent UTI. This may be due to differences in inclusion criteria. Oestrogens are not recommended for the routine prevention of recurrent UTI in postmenopausal women, but they may be of benefit in individuals with marked atrophic vaginitis.

Probiotics

Attempts to prevent recurrent urinary infection by re-establishing colonization by lactobacilli have so far not yielded convincing results.

Vaccines

There are currently two vaccines available and recommended for patients with recurrent UTI. Uro-vaxom is an orally administered bacterial extract consisting of immunostimulating components derived from 18 uropathogenic *E. coli* strains. Studies have shown it to be effective in the prevention of UTI as compared to placebo, but no comparison to antibiotic prophylaxis has been made.

Strovac is a whole-cell bacterial extract which is administered intramuscularly. It is derived from a number of uropathogenic strains, including *E. coli*, *E. faecalis*, and *Proteus mirabilis*. There is some evidence to suggest it reduces the risk of reinfection compared to placebo, although further studies are needed.

Complicated UTI

As discussed previously, 'complicated' UTIs are those occurring in a patient with abnormal host defence, and as a result are often more severe.

UTI in men

In the first year of life, UTI is commoner amongst boys than girls; circumcision reduces the risk. UTI in men is uncommon, as the length of the urethra and the fact that the penile mucosa is seldom colonized with faecal organisms including uropathogens confer major protection against ascending infection. The occurrence of UTI in a man therefore suggests an abnormality of host defence, which may predispose to more severe infection and should be investigated unless the cause is immediately obvious (e.g. the presence of a urinary catheter). Risk factors that may be identified by investigation are listed in Box 21.13.8.

Prostatitis

Prostatitis is a common cause of visits in primary care and of urological referrals. It can cause considerable morbidity, and patients may remain symptomatic for years. The National Institutes of Health (NIH) consensus classification of prostatitis syndromes is summarized in Box 21.13.9.

Acute bacterial prostatitis

Acute bacterial prostatitis causes fever, rigors, backache, and dysuria, and may result in acute urinary retention. Symptoms and signs of epididymitis may also be present. Rectal examination reveals an enlarged, tender prostate. Bacteriuria and pyuria are related to the prostate and bladder. Untreated, acute prostatitis may culminate in prostatic abscess formation. The causative organism (commonly *E. coli*) can be identified on urine culture. An antibiotic which has good tissue penetration (e.g. trimethoprim, a tetracycline, or a quinolone) should be used and continued for 4 weeks, as it is thought that this reduces the risk of chronic prostatitis.

Chronic bacterial prostatitis

This is an uncommon syndrome caused by the persistence of a uropathogen (usually Gram-negative organisms or enterococcus) within the prostate, with repeated episodes of acute infection caused by the same organism on each occasion, and few if any symptoms between episodes. Obtaining bacteriological proof that the infecting

---

Box 21.13.8 Possible causes of UTI in men

◆ Bacterial prostatitis and prostatic calcification

◆ Lack of circumcision

◆ Impaired bladder emptying (particularly if this has resulted in bladder catheterization or instrumentation)

◆ Anal intercourse

◆ Urinary tract stones

◆ Reflux nephropathy

---

organism is 'hiding' in the prostate gland between acute episodes is difficult. The 'textbook' method described by Stamey and Mears involves culture of four specimens obtained during voiding of the bladder: the first 10 ml voided and a midstream sample are collected; the patient then interrupts the flow of urine, bends forward, and digital prostatic massage is performed, resulting (sometimes) in the collection of a few drops of 'expressed prostatic secretions'; finally, voiding is completed and a fourth sample collected. Prostatitis is diagnosed when bacterial counts are highest in the expressed prostatic secretions and the final voided urine sample; urethritis, by contrast, results in high counts in the first sample. Because of its complexity and the unpleasantness of performing digital prostatic massage *per rectum* during interrupted micturition, this test is very rarely performed in practice, and many patients are simply treated with a prolonged course of a quinolone antibiotic. α-Blockers have been shown to reduce recurrence rate, possibly by reducing reflux of urine into prostatic ducts during micturition.

Acute and chronic bacterial prostatitis are the best understood but least common of the prostatitis syndromes. More than 90% of symptomatic patients have chronic prostatitis/chronic pelvic pain syndrome.

Chronic prostatitis/chronic pelvic pain syndrome

Chronic urological pain is the primary component of this disorder. Patients may also complain of dysuria, strangury, urinary frequency, and pain during sexual intercourse, but have no evidence of bacterial infection on cultures of prostatic secretions, semen, or postmassage urine specimens. Certain conditions must be excluded, including active urethritis, urological cancer, significant urethral stricture, or neurological disease affecting the bladder.

Patients with this symptom complex may be further subclassified as having inflammatory or noninflammatory pelvic pain

---

Box 21.13.9 National Institutes of Health classification of prostatitis syndromes

◆ Acute bacterial prostatitis

◆ Chronic bacterial prostatitis

◆ Chronic prostatitis/chronic pelvic pain syndrome

  A Inflammatory

  B Noninflammatory

◆ Asymptomatic inflammatory prostatitis

Adapted from National Institutes of Health classification of prostatitis syndromes, with permission

syndrome according to the presence or absence of leucocytes in semen. Occasionally, patients are found to have evidence of prostatic inflammation on biopsy, or to have leucocytes in prostatic fluid in the absence of symptoms, in which case they are regarded as having asymptomatic inflammatory prostatitis.

Treatment

There is no gold standard for diagnosis, nor a clear understanding of the pathophysiology, no correlation between symptoms and prostatic histology, and no satisfactory treatment for this ill-understood group of conditions. As in the urethral syndrome in women, some cases may be caused by persistent infection by fastidious bacteria, such as chlamydia or mycoplasma; a prolonged trial of a tetracycline is therefore often used. Other treatments include regular prostatic massage, NSAIDs, α-blockers, and 5-α reductase inhibitors. α-Blockers have been shown to be of some benefit in all types of symptomatic chronic prostatitis in one randomized study.

Urethral catheterization

UTI occurs after 2% of in/out urethral catheterizations, after 10 to 30% of 5-day indwelling catheterization, and is nearly inevitable in patients with long-term indwelling catheters. It is an important cause of hospital-acquired infection, increasing the risk of Gram-negative septicaemia fivefold and carrying a threefold increase in mortality after adjustment for age, severity and type of underlying illness, duration of catheterization, and renal function. Organisms enter the bladder either by migration between the catheter and the urethral mucosa or by ascent up the column of urine in the lumen after entry into the drainage system following contamination at disconnection or drainage points. Although most infections are probably caused by ascent of the patient's own faecal flora, investigation of clusters of infections by highly antibiotic-resistant organisms showed that inadequate hand-washing by hospital staff may also cause some infections.

A sample obtained directly from the catheter (not from the drainage bag) represents bladder urine, when any bacterial growth should be considered as evidence of UTI; low-count infection (e.g. <10^2 cfu/ml) usually progresses within days to higher counts. Mixed growths are common in patients with long-term catheterization and may be associated with mixed-growth bacteraemia.

Risk factors for the acquisition of infection include increasing duration of catheterization, increasing age, female sex, renal impairment, diabetes mellitus, and the nature of the underlying illness. Use of prophylactic antibiotics is associated with a delay in the onset of infection and may be justified in high-risk patients requiring catheterization for at least 24h and up to 14 days, whereas in those with long-term catheters, use of prophylactic antibiotic simply increases the risk of emergence of antibiotic-resistant pathogens without any benefit. Use of silver alloy-coated catheters, or use of antibiotic-impregnated catheters, also reduces the risk of infection and may be justified in high-risk patients; no direct comparisons of these two interventions have been performed; both are more expensive than standard catheters, and the balance of cost and benefit remains uncertain. Progress is being made in the development of new catheter materials that may provide further resistance against colonization by microorganisms.

Urethral catheters should not be inserted unless absolutely necessary (is knowledge of hourly urinary output really going to change your management?). Early removal of urethral catheters reduces the risk of symptomatic UTI. Suprapubic catheters are associated with lower risks of UTI and a lower rate of recatheterisation in postsurgical patients, but their use may be associated with a higher risk of complications. If a urethral catheter is used, catheter care should follow appropriate guidelines (e.g. as provided by the National Institute for Health and Clinical Excellence in the United Kingdom).

Clean intermittent self-catheterization should be considered as an alternative to long-term urethral catheterization. Whether prophylactic antibiotics further reduce the risk of UTI amongst patients undertaking intermittent self-catheterization remains uncertain.

Condom drainage should be used as an alternative to urethral catheterization in men unless there is obstructive nephropathy; this form of bladder drainage reduces the risk of UTI fivefold and is better tolerated.

Treatment of asymptomatic bacteriuria in patients with anatomically abnormal urinary tracts or with indwelling urinary catheters is unjustified and is likely only to lead to the emergence of antibiotic-resistance urinary infection.

Abnormal bladder emptying

Incomplete bladder emptying, removing the 'washout' part of host defence, greatly increases the risk of UTI, as in patients with prostatic bladder outflow obstruction and those with neurogenic bladder due to spinal cord injury. Long-term catheterization only increases these risks. Where possible, the cause of incomplete bladder emptying should be treated. However, patients shown on urodynamic study to have underactive detrusor activity will not benefit from prostatectomy or α-blockade and may require long-term intermittent self-catheterization.

Bladder dysfunction in patients with neurogenic bladder, e.g. due to spina bifida or spinal cord injury, depends on the level of injury. Patients with lesions above T11 have hyperreflexic bladder activity, often with sphincter dyssynergia (failure of the sphincter to relax during detrusor contraction), resulting in a high-pressure system, often with high-pressure reflux, combined with impaired emptying. In combination with UTI, this frequently results in progressive renal damage. Those with lesions below L1 have decreased detrusor activity with large amounts of residual urine, which also increases the risk of UTI. Diabetic neuropathy may also cause decreased detrusor activity. The aim of treatment in both situations is to achieve a low-pressure bladder with low residual volumes. This may involve teaching patients to utilize reflexes to induce bladder contraction and sphincter relaxation, condom drainage for incontinence, anticholinergics to reduce detrusor overactivity, sphincterotomy, augmentation cystoplasty, and intermittent self-catheterization. Urethral catheterization should be avoided wherever possible.

There is no evidence that regular use of antiseptics to wash the perineum and urethral meatus are of benefit. Bladder washouts with saline or boiled (and then cooled to body temperature) water may be of benefit in eliminating mucus in patients with augmentation cystoplasties. Antiseptic bladder washouts are of minimal value in prevention, probably because uropathogens become embedded in a biofilm adherent to the bladder wall. Methenamine, a drug that releases formaldehyde into acidic urine, may be of some benefit in preventing infection.

Treatment of UTI in patients with abnormal bladder emptying should be reserved for those with evidence of invasive infection. The diagnosis is obvious in those with cloudy urine combined with fever, rigors, and flank pain, but it is important to remember that symptoms and signs—particularly flank pain, dysuria, urgency, and frequency—may be absent in those with neurological dysfunction.

Urological surgery

Patients with asymptomatic bacteriuria who undergo invasive urological procedures that are associated with mucosal bleeding are at high risk of postprocedure bacteraemia and clinical sepsis syndromes, and there is evidence that preoperative antibiotic treatment of asymptomatic bacteriuria (ideally, the night before the procedure, continued until completion or removal of an indwelling catheter, whichever is the later) reduces these risks.

Urinary diversion

Ileal or colonic conduits have been used for many years in patients requiring cystectomy for malignancy, and occasionally (although increasingly less frequently) for nonmalignant conditions such as neurogenic bladder. Such conduits are frequently complicated by urine infection as the bowel mucosa and the mucus it produces readily permits adherence of uropathogens. Upper urinary tract dilatation is common, irrespective of whether the ureteric anastomoses are designed to be nonrefluxing or not, and there is a high incidence of recurrent 'acute pyelonephritis' with flank pain, fever, and rigors. Diagnosis of UTI in patients with a conduit requires insertion of a catheter to the far end of the conduit and collection of urine via the catheter, rather than culture of urine collected from the conduit bag. Preventive measures include ensuring that the ileal segment is as short as possible at the time of surgery and ensuring a high fluid intake. The belief that cranberry juice reduces the incidence of UTI by reducing bacterial adherence is as yet unproven, although it seems likely that treatments designed to interfere with bacterial adherence or with mucin production are more likely than antibiotic treatment to help prevent symptomatic infection in these patients.

Renal tract stones

Renal tract stones are an important cause of persistent or relapsing UTI, as they provide a 'hiding place' in which organisms are protected from antibiotics. Management of such patients is complicated, as it may be impossible to eradicate infection without aggressive stone management (which may involve extracorporeal shock-wave lithotripsy, percutaneous and ureteroscopic stone removal). Attempts at stone removal may be complicated by septicaemia unless combined with antibiotic treatment, yet prolonged antibiotic therapy may encourage the emergence of resistance in the infecting organism.

Infection stones are caused by chronic infection with urease-producing organisms, usually *P. mirabilis*, and account for around 5% of urinary tract stones. These stones are made of struvite ($MgNH_4PO_4.6H_2O$), which forms as a result of the action of the alkaline pH caused by the production of ammonium and hydroxyl ions from the breakdown of urea by urease. Pure struvite stones may result from *de novo* UTI by a urease-producing organism, and are commoner in women and (probably) in patients with pre-existing anatomical abnormalities of the upper urinary tract such

as reflux nephropathy, pelviureteric junction obstruction, or urinary diversion. They may also form as a secondary complication of metabolic stones. Struvite stones often expand to fill the entire renal pelvis, forming 'staghorn' calculi, but such calculi should not be assumed to be due to infection (rather than a metabolic cause) without demonstration of chronic infection by a urease-producing organism and/or biochemical analysis showing that the stone is made of struvite. The usual presentation is with symptomatic 'acute pyelonephritis' and alkaline urine; renal colic is unusual due to the large size of the stones. Treatment is with a combination of antibiotics and stone removal, which is imperative to prevent stone recurrence. Urease inhibitors (acetohydroxamic acid, propionhydroxamic acid) may reduce stone recurrence but are too toxic for clinical use. See Chapter 21.14 for further discussion.

Encrusted cystitis and pyelitis occur as a result of chronic infection by urease-producing organisms, including corynebacterium, in immunosuppressed patients, causing deposition of struvite in the bladder wall.

Autosomal dominant polycystic kidney disease

Cystitis is common in women with polycystic kidney disease, and in 20% it is the presenting clinical finding, but there is no evidence that host defence in the lower urinary tract is abnormal. However, the risk of upper UTI is increased, and its diagnosis and treatment complicated. Acute parenchymal infection presents as acute pyelonephritis with flank pain, fever, and infected bladder urine, and usually responds to conventional therapy. Infection of cysts is more difficult to diagnose: the urine may be sterile and there may be no pyuria if the infected cyst does not communicate with the urinary space. Presentation is with fever and a discrete area of tenderness in the affected kidney. Blood cultures are the most reliable way of making a bacteriological diagnosis. Imaging studies, looking for cysts with increased fluid density, septations, and thick walls, are seldom conclusive, as similar appearances may occur normally or after previous cyst haemorrhage. The spectrum of causative organisms suggests that ascending infection rather than haematogenous spread is the usual route of infection. Hydrophilic antibiotics, including aminoglycosides and β-lactam antibiotics, penetrate poorly into those cysts which maintain large ionic gradients, whereas quinolones, trimethoprim–sulphamethoxazole, doxycycline, and clindamycin achieve better penetration. Prolonged courses of antibiotics are usually needed to eradicate infection, with surgical resection a last resort.

Renal transplantation

UTI is the commonest bacterial infection after renal transplantation. Risk factors include urethral catheterization in the early postoperative period, the use of ureteric stents, pre-existing abnormalities of bladder emptying (such as diabetic autonomic neuropathy, previous bladder outflow obstruction, small contracted bladders in anuric patients on dialysis), anatomical abnormalities in the upper urinary tract (such as reflux nephropathy), contamination of the transplanted organ during retrieval and storage, abnormal drainage of urine from the transplanted kidney, vesicoureteric reflux into the transplant, areas of renal infarction, and immunosuppression. The commonest causative bacteria are those found in the general population with UTI, but many organisms not usually considered as urinary tract pathogens may also cause significant infection in these patients. Many infections are asymptomatic. Prophylactic antibiotics may reduce the early post-operative risk and many centres use co-trimoxazole as it also reduces the risk of pneumocystis pneumonia. Antibiotic treatment must be chosen with care because of the risk of interactions with immunosuppressive treatment and of nephrotoxicity.

Infection with BK virus (a polyoma virus) may cause cystitis, ureteric stenosis, and interstitial nephritis (easily mistaken for acute rejection) in renal transplant recipients. The diagnosis may be suggested by recognition of infected transitional uroepithelial cells on urine cytology ('decoy' cells), quantitative PCR of blood and urine for BK virus, and confirmed by histological recognition of inclusion bodies on renal biopsy. Treatment is by reduction of immunosuppression, but this is often complicated by further rejection.

Pregnancy

Asymptomatic bacteriuria early in pregnancy is associated with the development of acute pyelonephritis in up to 30% of patients (20–30 times the risk in women without bacteriuria) if left untreated. It is commoner in women of lower socioeconomic status and is associated with an increased incidence of preterm delivery and low birth weight, particularly if the pregnancy is complicated by acute pyelonephritis towards term. The increased risk of pyelonephritis is attributed to ureteric dilatation caused primarily by progesterone-induced smooth muscle relaxation.

Antibiotic treatment of asymptomatic infection reduces the risk of acute pyelonephritis and of preterm delivery and low birth weight. Similar benefit is seen from a short course of treatment and from continued antibiotic prophylaxis. The optimum duration of antibiotic treatment for UTI in pregnancy is uncertain; the recent Health Protection Agency guidelines (Table 21.13.4) recommend a 7-day course. Whatever duration of treatment is used, follow-up urine cultures at each antenatal visit should be performed to ensure that bacteriological cure has been achieved. (See Chapter 14.5 for further discussion.)

Reflux nephropathy

Vesicoureteric reflux (retrograde flow of urine up into the ureters and, in severe cases, as far as the renal pelvis) is often found in children with recurrent UTI. At the time of first diagnosis of UTI or subsequently, a few such children are found to have a characteristic pattern of renal parenchymal scarring at the upper and lower poles, with underlying clubbing and distortion of calyces. This pattern of scarring has become known by a variety of terms, including 'reflux nephropathy' and 'chronic pyelonephritis'. Patients with reflux nephropathy have an increased risk of recurrent UTI, may develop infection or stones, and some develop hypertension, proteinuria, and progressive renal impairment with an inexorable progression to endstage renal failure. Under the age of 1 year, when only relatively severe cases come to clinical attention, slightly more boys than girls are affected; in older children the disease is diagnosed up to five times more frequently in girls, possibly because the disease is often discovered during investigation of UTI, which is commoner in females. Reflux nephropathy is commonly familial, best modelled by an autosomal dominant pattern of inheritance with variable penetrance. Linkage has been demonstrated to an area of chromosome 1 in some large pedigrees.

The diagnosis of reflux nephropathy is conventionally made in adults by intravenous urography, which permits the detection both of focal parenchymal scarring and the underlying calyceal abnormality

(Fig. 21.13.4). Ultrasound scanning can show focal scarring but does not allow visualization of the calyces. DMSA isotope scanning is the most sensitive test for the detection of parenchymal scars, and is widely used in children, as there are few alternative causes of focal scarring in this age group. Lateral displacement of the ureteric orifices can be demonstrated by Doppler ultrasound in most patients with reflux nephropathy. Demonstration of vesicoureteric reflux by direct or isotopic micturating cystography is commonly used to confirm the diagnosis in children, but is rarely justified in adults, as the absence of reflux could be due to spontaneous resolution of reflux with age (it often resolves in childhood), and its presence seldom justifies a change in clinical management. The histological appearances of 'chronic pyelonephritis' are well described and may occasionally be seen in patients with no scarring on urography or even DMSA scanning, probably because the scars are too small in these patients to be detected radiologically.

The conventional view is that reflux nephropathy is 'postinfectious focal renal scarring' and caused by the ascent of infected urine into the renal pelvis and then into the collecting ducts and renal parenchyma via compound papillas (papillas in which more than one collecting duct opens into the pelvis) that are found at the upper and lower poles, but not in the middle calyces—explaining the polar distribution of scars. Sequential radiological imaging studies in children with UTIs appear to support this theory, with the emergence of new scars up until the age of around 5 years, after which it is thought that maturation of the papillas prevents entry of infected urine into the renal parenchyma. Experimental infection in pigs causes a pattern of scarring very similar to that seen in human reflux nephropathy.

An alternative hypothesis is that at least some children with the radiological diagnosis of reflux nephropathy have congenital renal dysplasia, caused by abnormal nephrogenesis *in utero*, and associated with abnormal embryogenesis of the ureterovesical junction leading to vesicoureteric reflux. Vesicoureteric reflux is often found in the rare genetic syndromes that include renal dysplasia, and in nonsyndromic renal dysplasia or aplasia, vesicoureteric reflux in the contralateral ureter is commonly seen. This theory would explain the presence of classic reflux nephropathy

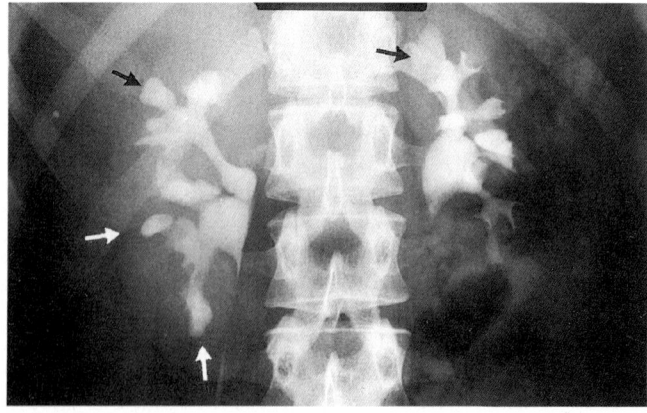

Fig. 21.13.4 Reflux nephropathy on intravenous urography, more marked on the right side than the left. Several focal scars (arrowed) involving the full thickness of the renal parenchyma and associated with calyceal clubbing are most obvious in the polar regions.
Bailey RR (1993). Vesicoureteric reflux and reflux nephropathy. In: Schrier RW, Gottschalk CW, eds. Diseases of the kidney, 5th edn, pp 689–727. Little, Brown, Boston.

in neonates and in children with no documented history of UTI. Even the emergence of new scars during the first 5 years of life could be due to differential growth around areas of renal dysplasia. The rarity with which acute pyelonephritis in adults results in renal impairment, even in the presence of radiological evidence of scar formation, is perhaps further evidence that progressive loss of renal function is more likely to be due to 'remnant nephropathy' in dysplastic kidneys rather than the result of postinfectious scarring alone.

These two hypotheses have different implications for the prevention of reflux nephropathy. Proponents of the 'postinfectious focal renal scarring' theory believe that diagnosis in infancy and treatment to prevent the ascent of infected urine into the renal pelvis until at least the age of 5 years should prevent the emergence of renal scarring and the later sequelae of hypertension, proteinuria, and progressive renal failure; by contrast, such treatment will not prevent these sequelae if reflux nephropathy is a disease of embryogenesis. Of course, the two theories are not mutually exclusive: in an individual patient reflux nephropathy may be due to the interaction of dysplasia and ascending infection during infancy. Antireflux surgery (ureteric reimplantation) and long-term prophylactic antibiotic treatment have been compared in several large randomized trials. Surgery is more effective at preventing episodes of acute pyelonephritis than medical treatment, but no other major differences in outcome were observed, and potential complications of antireflux surgery include ureteric obstruction, itself a potent cause of renal parenchymal damage. No trials have included an 'untreated' control group, so the benefits either of long-term antibiotic treatment or of antireflux surgery remain uncertain.

Eradication of asymptomatic infection in children with or without proven vesicoureteric reflux is widely practised in the hope that this will prevent ascending infection and renal damage. However, prophylactic treatment for 2 years of covert bacteriuria in schoolgirls without renal scarring has no effect on glomerular filtration rate at age 18, but is associated with lower fractional reabsorption of glucose and with a smaller increment in glomerular filtration rate and greater degrees of glycosuria during subsequent pregnancy. Screening for asymptomatic bacteriuria with the aim of preventing these minor abnormalities is not currently thought justified.

Whatever the cause of reflux nephropathy, there is little doubt that women with it are more prone to recurrent acute pyelonephritis than those with anatomically normal upper urinary tracts, particularly during pregnancy.

Invasive/destructive renal parenchymal infection

As discussed above, ascending infection may cause the clinical syndrome of 'acute pyelonephritis' but seldom causes significant renal parenchymal damage. However, this is not the case if there is further impairment of host defence against infection, particularly by diabetes or urinary tract obstruction.

Acute papillary necrosis

This is an unusual complication of acute pyelonephritis, but more likely to occur in older people and especially those with diabetes. It should be suspected, as should urinary stones, in the patient with symptoms and signs of acute pyelonephritis who also has pain suggesting renal colic. This situation requires immediate imaging, usually with ultrasonography, to exclude urinary obstruction, and

if obstruction is present then it must be relieved urgently, most often by antegrade nephrostomy.

The use of NSAIDs is associated with an increased incidence of chronic renal papillary necrosis, perhaps because they compromise the renal medullary circulation. It therefore seems reasonable to say that these agents should be discontinued, at least temporarily, in the presence of acute pyelonephritis.

Renal carbuncle

Renal carbuncle is the formation of renal cortical abscesses, often only in one kidney, caused by blood-borne infection, usually associated with untreated *S. aureus* septicaemia. It is most commonly seen in intravenous drug abusers and patients with diabetes. There is usually a significant time delay between the initial infection and presentation with renal carbuncle, typically 6 to 8 weeks. Presenting symptoms include fever, malaise, and abdominal or flank pain, and are often nonspecific. Because the infection is limited to the renal cortex and does not communicate with the collecting system, the urine is sterile and acellular. Blood cultures are usually negative. Radiological studies show a semisolid, thick-walled mass, percutaneous aspiration of which yields pus.

Pyonephrosis

Pyonephrosis is bacterial infection within a completely obstructed collecting system, for instance due to an obstructing ureteric stone. Patients usually present with fever, rigors, and flank pain, and have a marked neutrophilia and acute phase response. Radiological differentiation from hydronephrosis relies on the presence of echogenic material and/or septae in the pelvicalyceal system, and confirmation is by percutaneous aspiration; as with other localized UTIs, the voided bladder urine may be sterile. Untreated pyonephrosis rapidly results in complete destruction of the renal parenchyma, followed by death from complications of sepsis if nephrectomy is not performed; correction of obstruction and aggressive intravenous antibiotic therapy may prevent this if instituted soon enough.

Perinephric abscess

Perinephric abscess may complicate renal carbuncle or, more commonly, acute pyelonephritis—particularly if complicated by an anatomical or functional abnormality of the urinary tract. Typical presenting symptoms are those of acute pyelonephritis, with flank pain, fever, and rigors. If the abscess does not communicate with the collecting system, e.g. in abscesses caused by haematogenous spread or complicating obstruction or renal cysts, there may be no lower urinary tract symptoms, no pyuria, and the urine may be sterile. Response to antibiotic treatment is much less rapid than in patients with uncomplicated acute pyelonephritis. Diagnosis is by ultrasonography, urography, or CT, followed by percutaneous (or occasionally surgical) aspiration, drainage, and culture of the aspirate. Prolonged antibiotic treatment of the organism identified is needed, stopping only when there is evidence that the infection has resolved, based on resolution of fever and of the acute phase response, and repeated radiological studies. This may take as long as 8 weeks.

Xanthogranulomatous pyelonephritis

Xanthogranulomatous pyelonephritis is an atypical form of chronic infection of the renal parenchyma in which bacterial infection, usually in the presence of obstruction or staghorn calculi, results in formation of granulomas with the accumulation of lipid-rich foamy macrophages. The process may be multifocal and can be complicated by extension into the perinephric fat, causing perinephric abscess. Patients are typically febrile and ill, with a history of progressive weight loss, anaemia, and malaise, without lower urinary tract symptoms, and have a mass in the flank on examination. Radiologically, the multifocal mass crossing tissue planes may be indistinguishable from a renal cell carcinoma, which may also cause systemic symptoms such as fever, anaemia, and weight loss. Although both require surgical excision, radical surgery can be avoided if the diagnosis is made preoperatively.

Emphysematous pyelonephritis

Emphysematous pyelonephritis is a rare and life-threatening form of acute pyelonephritis in which there is tissue necrosis together with formation of hydrogen and CO_2, which accumulate in pockets in the renal parenchyma, perinephric space, and collecting systems—'gangrene of the kidney' (Fig. 21.13.5). The typical patient is an obese, elderly woman with type 2 diabetes; urinary tract obstruction is another important risk factor. Presentation is with fever, vomiting, and abdominal pain. The patient is often extremely ill with hypotension, neutrophilia, and renal impairment. The commonest causative organism is *E. coli*; clostridial infection has not been reported. Even with aggressive medical treatment the mortality is high, and although occasional successes with antibiotics combined with percutaneous drainage have been reported, the standard treatment is nephrectomy.

Malakoplakia

Malakoplakia (Greek: 'soft plaque') is a rare disease characterized by destructive tumour-like granulomatous infiltrates in the urinary bladder, kidneys, and occasionally other organs. Bladder involvement usually presents with haematuria, frequency, and dysuria; renal involvement presents with fever, flank pain, and renal enlargement, and may frequently be bilateral. The diagnosis may be suspected at cystoscopy or on renal imaging, but is confirmed histologically by detection of large eosinophilic granular macrophages containing characteristic intracellular lamellated 5- to 10-μm inclusion bodies. It is caused by bacterial UTI, commonly

E. coli, together with an ill-understood acquired defect of microtubule assembly within phagocytic cells, resulting in the accumulation within the cytoplasm of bacterial remnants that subsequently calcify. Treatment with bethanechol (to stimulate intracellular cGMP and thus microtubule assembly) and ascorbic acid (to stimulate the intracellular hexose monophosphate shunt, which is involved in phagocytosis) have been recommended on theoretical grounds, but seldom arrest the disease. The best chance of avoiding nephrectomy comes from the use of long-term quinolone antibiotics such as ciprofloxacin, which penetrate macrophages well.

Unusual infections

Tuberculosis

Genitourinary tuberculosis is an uncommon late manifestation of tuberculosis, and is often clinically silent, with few if any systemic symptoms. Most cases of renal tuberculosis probably result from haematogenous spread, although unilateral disease is common. Seeding of infection from above leads to ulceration and distortion of the collecting system, pelvis, and ureter, followed by stricture formation and calcification. Obstruction and parenchymal infection may eventually lead to 'autonephrectomy' (Fig. 21.13.6). The disease is usually detected either during investigation of asymptomatic sterile pyuria or during investigation of irritative lower urinary tract symptoms or haematuria due to bladder involvement. Reactivation of disease may result from acquired deficiency of 1,25-dihydroxyvitamin D. Occasionally, renal tuberculosis may present with a cold abscess in the flank. Chronic renal failure due to bilateral diffuse interstitial renal tuberculosis may occur, and may account for some of the excess of chronic renal failure in Asian immigrants in the United Kingdom.

Diagnosis of renal tuberculosis is by culture of early morning urine samples. Treatment is with rifampicin, isoniazid, pyrazinamide, and ethambutol for 2 months, followed by rifampicin and isoniazid for a further 4 months. It should be supervised by a physician experienced in the chemotherapy of tuberculosis, and with adjustment of the dose of ethambutol in the presence of renal impairment. Corticosteroids may help to prevent or reverse ureteric

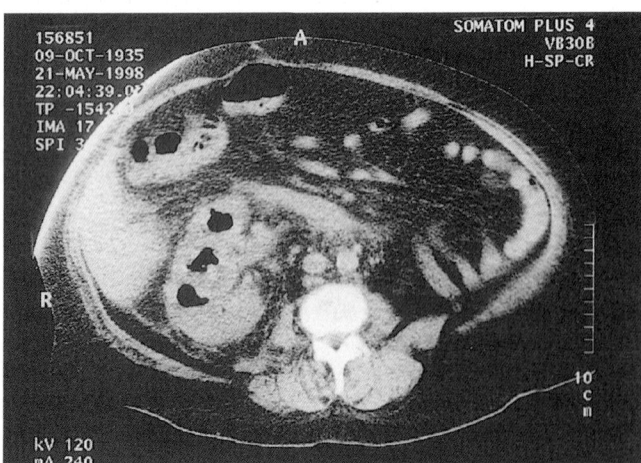

Fig. 21.13.5 Gas-forming infection, seen as the three black holes in the single remaining (right) kidney of a patient with diabetes. The left kidney had been removed 2 years earlier for a similar gas-forming infection. This infection was successfully treated by intravenous antibiotics and percutaneous drainage.

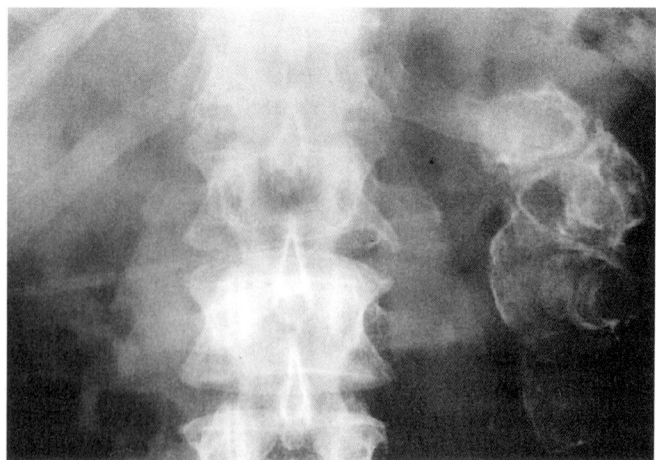

Fig. 21.13.6 Calcified 'autonephrectomy' as a result of long-standing tuberculous infection.
Reproduced by permission of Professor P. W. Mathieson.

obstruction, which may otherwise require stent insertion or surgery to prevent renal destruction. Nephrectomy is seldom necessary.

Schistosomiasis

Schistosoma haematobium infection in the venules of the urinary bladder may cause irritative symptoms and terminal haematuria, starting 2 to 3 months after the initial infection. Eosinophilia may be present. The diagnosis is made by detection of ova in a midday terminal urine specimen or by cystoscopy and biopsy. Treatment is with systemic anthelmintic drugs, currently praziquantel. See Chapter 21.11 for further discussion.

Fungal infections

Fungal UTIs typically occur in patients whose host defence is compromised by indwelling urethral catheters or ureteric stents, previous wide-spectrum antibiotic therapy, immunosuppressive drugs, or diabetes. Most infections are caused by candida. Many patients with funguria have asymptomatic colonization, but some develop life-threatening ascending disease. Severity of infection does not correlate with pyuria. It is important to differentiate funguria from contamination of voided urine by candida in patients with vaginal candidiasis. Many infections clear spontaneously on removal of the urethral catheter, although this can take many months.

Treatment options for patients thought to be at high risk of invasive infection (e.g. patients with diabetes with indwelling catheters, renal transplant recipients) include removal of the catheter or nephrostomy tube wherever possible; continuous bladder irrigation or antegrade perfusion via a nephrostomy tube with amphotericin B at 50 mg/litre if the tube cannot safely be removed; and oral fluconazole. For patients whose tube cannot safely be removed, a combination of amphotericin B irrigation and fluconazole is reasonable, but evidence comparing the options is very limited. Patients with clinical features of acute pyelonephritis require parenteral antifungal treatment, adjusted to *in vitro* sensitivities.

Fungaemia is often complicated by renal parenchymal infection, possibly because the hypertonic and hypoxic conditions in the renal medulla favour transformation of candida from the yeast to the mycelial phase. Infection starts with multiple cortical abscesses and progresses to invasion of the renal pelvis and ureter, with eventual obstruction by fungus balls.

Likely future developments

Current methods for prevention and treatment of uncomplicated and complicated UTI are unsatisfactory, with persisting high morbidity and mortality from complicated infection and increasing rates of antibiotic-resistant organisms. Development of new antibiotics is likely only to remain half a step ahead. We hope to see major advances in the prevention of UTI, perhaps with the development of substances designed to inhibit bacterial adherence to the uroepithelium, new compounds for vaccination, and the development of new catheter materials and of alternatives to urethral catheterization.

Further reading

Abrutyn E, *et al.* (1993). Does asymptomatic bacteriuria predict mortality and does antimicrobial treatment reduce mortality in elderly ambulatory women? *Ann Intern Med*, **120**, 827–33 [Erratum: Ann Intern Med (1994), **121**, 901].

Bailey RR (1993). Vesicoureteric reflux and reflux nephropathy. In: Schrier RW, Gottschalk CW (eds) *Diseases of the kidney*, 5th edition, pp. 689–727. Little, Brown, Boston.

Car J (2006). Urinary tract infections in women: diagnosis and management in primary care. *BMJ*, **332**, 94–7.

Cardenas DD, Hooton TM (1995). Urinary tract infections in persons with spinal cord injury. *Arch Phys Med Rehab*, **76**, 272–80.

Cattel WR (ed.) (1996). *Infections of the kidney and urinary tract*. Oxford University Press, Oxford.

Franz M, Horl WH (1999). Common errors in diagnosis and management of urinary tract infections. I: pathophysiology and diagnostic techniques. *Nephrol Dialysis Transplant*, **14**, 2746–53.

Franz M, Horl WH (1999). Common errors in diagnosis and management of urinary tract infections. II: clinical management. *Nephrol Dialysis Transplant*, **14**, 2754–62.

Gordon I (1995). Vesico-ureteric reflux, urinary-tract infection, and renal damage in children. *Lancet*, **346**, 489–90.

Hooton TM, *et al.* (1996). A prospective study of risk factors for symptomatic UTI in young women. *N Engl J Med*, **335**, 468–74.

Hunt GM, Oakeshott P, Whitaker RH (1996). Intermittent catheterisation: simple, safe, and effective but underused. *BMJ*, **312**, 103–7.

Krieger JN, *et al* (1999) NIH consensus definition and classification of prostatitis. *JAMA*, **282**, 236–7.

Kunin CM, White LV, Hua TH (1993). A reassessment of the importance of 'low-count' bacteriuria in young women with acute urinary symptoms. *Ann Intern Med*, **119**, 454–60.

McNulty CA, *et al.* (2006). Clinical relevance of laboratory—reported antibiotic resistance in acute uncomplicated urinary tract infections in primary care. *J Antimicrob Chemother*, **58**, 1000–8.

National Institute for Clinical Excellence (2003). *Prevention of healthcare-associated infection in primary and community care*. http://www.nice.org.uk/guidance/CG2

Nosocomial Infection National Surveillance Survey (NINSS) and Public Health Laboratory Service (PHLS). *Surveillance of hospital-acquired bacteraemia in English hospitals 1997–2002*.http://www.hpa.org.uk/webc/HPAwebFile/HPAweb_C/1194947379958

Platt R *et al.* (1982). Mortality associated with nosocomial urinary-tract infection. *New England Journal of Medicine*, **307**, 637–42.

Raz R, Stamm WE (1993). A controlled trial of intravaginal estriol in postmenopausal women with recurrent urinary tract infections. *N Engl J Med*, **329**, 753–6.

Saint S, Lipsky BA (1999). Preventing catheter-related bacteriuria: Should we? Can we? How? *Arch Intern Med*, **159**, 800–8.

Schaeffer AJ (1994). Urinary tract infections in men—state of the art. *Infection*, **22**, S121.

Smaill F, Vasquez JC (2007). Antibiotics for asymptomatic bacteriuria in pregnancy (Cochrane Review). *Cochrane Database Syst Rev*, **1**, CD000490.

Scottish Intercollegiate Guidelines Network (2006). *SIGN 88: Management of suspected bacterial urinary tract infections in adults*. http://www.sign.ac.uk/pdf/sign88.pdf

Stamm WE, Hooton TM (1993). Management of urinary tract infections in adults. *N Engl J Med*, **329**, 1328–34.

Stamm WE, *et al.* (1982). Diagnosis of coliform infection in acutely dysuric women. *N Engl J Med*, **307**, 463–8.

Stapleton A (1999). Prevention of recurrent urinary-tract infections in women. *Lancet*, **353**, 7–8.

Svanborg C (1993). Resistance to urinary tract infections. *N Engl J Med*, **329**, 802–3.

Wagenlehner FM, Naber KG, (2006). Treatment of bacterial urinary tract infections: presence and future. *Eur Urol*, **49**, 235–44.

Warren JW, *et al.* (1999). Guidelines for antimicrobial treatment of uncomplicated acute bacterial cystitis and acute pyelonephritis in women. *Clin Infect Dis*, **29**, 745–58.

Wong-Beringer A, Jacobs RA, Guglielmo BJ (1992). Treatment of funguria. *JAMA*, **267**, 2780–5.

Additional resources

The Cochrane database (http://www.cochrane.org) has numerous relevant reviews.

The NHS clinical knowledge summaries website (http://www.cks.nhs.uk) contains guidance on the management of lower UTI in men and women, on acute pyelonephritis, and on UTI in children. Patient information leaflets are also available.

Disorders of renal calcium handling, urinary stones, and nephrocalcinosis

Elaine M. Worcester, Andrew P. Evan, and Fredric L. Coe

Essentials

Renal stones are common, with a prevalence of about 5% in the United States of America. Acute stone passage almost always produces the severe pain of renal colic, but stones are often asymptomatic and discovered incidentally on imaging.

Investigation and general management

The initial evaluation of patients with renal colic optimally includes noncontrast CT, which can accurately visualize the size and location of stones in the urinary tract. Initial management of stones less than 5 mm in diameter in patients without anatomical abnormalities of the urinary tract is to provide adequate analgesia, followed by watchful waiting to allow time for stone passage. The presence of urinary tract infection, inability to take oral fluids, or obstruction of a single functioning kidney requires hospitalization and active management. Once the acute episode of stone passage or removal is over, thought should be given to diagnosis of the underlying causes of stones, and steps taken towards prevention. Stone analysis is the cornerstone of diagnosis.

Particular types of urinary stone and nephrocalcinosis

Most stones (66–76%) are formed of calcium oxalate: other types include calcium phosphate (12–17%), uric acid (7–11%), struvite (magnesium ammonium phosphate, 2–3%), and cystine (1–2%). They form because urine becomes supersaturated with respect to the stone mineral, and treatment to lower supersaturation can prevent recurrence.

Calcium oxalate stones—systemic diseases such as primary hyperparathyroidism, renal tubular acidosis, and hyperoxaluria should be ruled out, but most cases are idiopathic, when onset is often in early adulthood, with recurrence in 40% at 5 years. Stones typically form on suburothelial calcium phosphate deposits, called Randall's plaques, most commonly in the context of idiopathic hypercalciuria, which is a polygenic familial trait. Diets high in salt, protein, and sucrose may increase urinary calcium further. Treatments shown in randomized trials to decrease recurrence include increased fluid intake, a diet that is low in sodium and protein but with normal calcium intake, thiazide diuretics, and potassium citrate.

Calcium phosphate stones—form when hypercalciuria is combined with alkaline urinary pH, which is idiopathic in many cases. Treatment to lower urinary calcium excretion (thiazides, reduced protein and sodium intakes) can reduce the risk of recurrence.

Uric acid stones—most often the result of persistently low urinary pH, which decreases uric acid solubility. Poorly visualized on standard plain radiographs. Treatment with alkali can improve uric acid solubility and decrease stone recurrence.

Struvite stones—found in patients colonized with bacteria that possess the enzyme urease (e.g. proteus), which results in extremely alkaline urine with high levels of ammonia, leading to formation of stones made of magnesium ammonium phosphate. Individuals with chronic urinary tract instrumentation or neurogenic bladder are at particular risk. Effective treatment requires antibiotics and removal of all stone material.

Cystine stones—result from rare autosomal recessive abnormalities of cystine transport in the kidney, leading to high urinary cystine concentrations. Poorly visualized on standard plain radiographs. High fluid intake and alkali can increase cystine solubility, but may require treatment with drugs that chelate cysteine and form soluble hetero-dimers, such as D-penicillamine or tiopronin.

Nephrocalcinosis—this is defined as precipitation of calcium salts in renal tubules or interstitium. All calcium stones are accompanied by a small amount of such precipitation, but larger amounts are typically seen in diseases including distal renal tubular acidosis, primary hyperoxaluria, and a range of other monogenic conditions. Deposition of large amounts of mineral in medullary (and occasionally cortical) tissue may lead to renal failure.

Abnormalities of renal calcium handling

The plasma calcium concentration is tightly regulated by homeostatic mechanisms which control calcium fluxes between extracellular fluid and the gut, kidney, and bone. These fluxes are under the control of calcitropic hormones including parathyroid hormone (PTH), calcitriol, and calcitonin. The goal is maintenance of normal extracellular ionized calcium concentration and support of bone growth and remodelling. Renal tubule calcium reabsorption is up-regulated by PTH and down-regulated by the calcium sensing receptor found along the nephron; calcitriol affects calcium handling indirectly via its ability to regulate synthesis of PTH as well as the molecules involved in both intestinal calcium absorption and tubule calcium transport. Calcium reabsorption is linked to sodium at most sites in the nephron, the exception being the distal tubule, which is responsive to PTH. Abnormalities in PTH, calcitriol, sodium transport, or the calcium sensing receptor may lead to abnormal urine calcium excretion.

Urinary calcium excretion is the difference between net calcium absorption from food and net bone calcium balance; when urinary calcium exceeds net calcium absorption persistently, calcium must be leaving bone. Normal urinary calcium excretion is defined by the mean excretion ±2 standard deviations in a normal healthy population on an average calcium intake. This is usually less than 3.5 mmol/g creatinine (140 mg/g creatinine) daily, a definition that is also applicable to children, but wide normal ranges are quoted dependent on dietary intake. However, urinary calcium excretion in the normal range may be associated with long-term loss of calcium from bone while plasma calcium remains normal, because clinicians cannot measure gut calcium absorption in practice.

Abnormalities of renal calcium handling have not been identified as primary disorders, but as part of disorders presenting as hypercalcemia, nephrolithiasis or nephrocalcinosis, or chronic loss of bone mineral. Idiopathic (familial) hypercalciuria is the commonest disorder seen in patients with calcium stones (discussed below).

Urinary stones

Historical perspective

Descriptions of urinary stones and their treatment were recorded in the earliest medical writings, doubtless because of their acuity and severity. Mesopotamian texts (>1000 BC) advise: "If a man is sick with stone (treat with) black saltpetre, shell of ostrich egg, pine turpentine…" Ancient Indian, Chinese, and Persian texts also describe treatments for urinary stone disease. Urinary tract stones occur worldwide, although stone formation in more developed countries is almost entirely nephrolithiasis, while in less developed areas bladder stones also occur, often in children.

Epidemiology

Calcium-containing stones are composed mainly of calcium oxalate, as the monohydrate (whewhellite) or dihydrate (weddellite) salt, admixed with a small amount of calcium phosphate (hydroxyapatite), which may form the initiating nidus (Table 21.14.1). Less frequently, stones may be composed largely or entirely of calcium phosphate, as apatite or brushite (calcium monohydrogen phosphate), uric acid, cystine, or struvite (magnesium ammonium phosphate). For reasons that are unknown the incidence of phosphate stones has been increasing over the past three decades, but these

Table 21.14.1 Types of kidney stone and their frequencies

Stone type	University of Chicago[a] (2011 patients)			Hôpital Necker[b] (10 438 stones)		
	Males (1402)	Females (675)	Both	Males (7244)	Females (3194)	Both
Calcium oxalate	82%	66%	76%	72%	52%	66%
Calcium phosphate	8%	19%	12%	10%	31%	17%
Uric acid	8%	6%	7%	12%	7%	11%
Cystine	1%	4%	2%	1%	2%	1%
Struvite	1%	5%	2%	2%	5%	3%

[a] Major stone component for each patient with at least one analysis.
[b] Major stone component in each analysed stone (from: Daudon M, et al. (1995), Sex- and age-related composition of 10,617 calculi analyzed by infrared spectroscopy. Urol Res, **23**, 319–26.)
Very rarely, stones may be due to xanthine (in xanthinuria due to deficiency of xanthine oxidase); 2,8-dihydroxyadenine (in adenine phosphoribosyl transferase deficiency); silica (e.g. from excessive ingestion of the antacid magnesium trisilicate); or drugs (e.g. sulphonamides, triamterene, indinavir).

are associated with increased numbers of lithotripsy procedures and with alterations in renal pathology. Very rarely, stones may be due to xanthine (in xanthinuria due to deficiency of xanthine oxidase); 2,8-dihydroxyadenine (in adenine phosphoribosyl transferase deficiency); silica (e.g. from excessive ingestion of the antacid magnesium trisilicate); or drugs (e.g. sulphonamides, triamterene, indinavir).

Stones occur more often in men than in women (see Table 21.14.1) and stone type frequency varies somewhat between the sexes. In the United States of America, the prevalence of stones in both sexes has been rising over the past 30 years, and by the age of 74 almost 12% of white men and 6% of white women will report forming a stone; rates in Asians and African-Americans are lower. The peak age of onset is the third decade, whereas the highest incidence of stones is seen in the fifth and sixth decades.

Stone recurrence is common, particularly when stones are associated with systemic diseases. Idiopathic calcium stones have a recurrence rate of 40 to 50% at 5 years, and 50 to 60% by 10 years, but it is difficult to predict in which patients they will recur.

Clinical features

Presentation and initial management

Acute stone passage almost always produces severe pain, known as renal colic, triggered by movement of a stone from the renal pelvis into the ureter, which leads to ureteral spasm and possibly obstruction. Pain often starts in the flank area, and progresses downward and anteriorly into the genital region as the stone moves down the ureter. The pain is not alleviated by change of position, and may be accompanied by nausea and vomiting; haematuria is always present, but may be microscopic. If the stone is lodged at the ureterovesical junction, it may cause a sensation of frequency and urgency. Stones less than 5 mm in diameter will usually pass spontaneously, although it may require several weeks of conservative management, while 50% of stones larger than 5 mm require urologic intervention for removal.

The initial evaluation of patients with renal colic optimally includes noncontrast CT, which can accurately visualize the size and location of stones in the urinary tract. A kidney–ureter–bladder

(KUB) plain radiograph will often be able to visualize calcium-containing stones in the kidney or ureter, but uric acid stones may be radiolucent, and cystine stones often visualize poorly as well.

Initial management of stones less than 5 mm in diameter in patients without anatomical abnormalities of the urinary tract is to provide adequate analgesia, followed by watchful waiting to allow time for stone passage. Presence of any signs of urinary tract infection, inability to take oral fluids, or obstruction of a single functioning kidney requires hospitalization and active management. Some studies suggest that use of an α_1-adrenoreceptor antagonist such as tamsulosin may hasten the time to stone passage.

Sometimes large stones in the renal pelvis may be asymptomatic. Stones with a branched configuration filling two or more calyces are called staghorn calculi. Struvite stones often present in this fashion, as may cystine stones, and—occasionally—calcium phosphate and uric acid stones.

Urological management

Urological management of stones that cannot pass will depend on the size, location, and type of stone. Extracorporeal shock-wave lithotripsy, which uses sound waves to fragment stones into small pieces that can be easily passed, is effective for most stones less than 2 cm in size, although cystine stones and phosphate stones may be resistant to fragmentation. Larger stones, particularly those composed of cystine or struvite, can be removed via percutaneous access through a small flank incision, allowing direct visualization for stone disruption and removal. Ureteroscopy with laser lithotripsy is becoming increasingly useful for stones in the ureter and renal pelvis, and may be used with laser lithotripsy as well. The urologic societies in the United States of America (http://www.auanet.org) and Europe (http://www.uroweb.org) have developed evidence-based recommendations to guide the choice of modality. See Chapter 21.17 for further discussion.

Changes in renal function and blood pressure

Renal stone formers may have decreased renal function (Fig. 21.14.1); this is particularly true for those with systemic diseases such as primary hyperoxaluria, cystinuria, and renal tubular acidosis.

Stone formers, especially females, have an increased tendency to high blood pressure. Approximately 1 to 2% of cases of endstage renal failure are attributed to stone disease in both Europe and the United States of America.

General aetiology of urinary stones

Formation of stones is a consequence of the need to excrete poorly soluble minerals or metabolites such as calcium, oxalate, and uric acid in modest volumes of urine. For example, daily excretion of calcium and oxalate in the usual volume of urine often leads to concentrations that are above the known thermodynamic solubility product, when the urine is said to be supersaturated with respect to this salt. In the case of uric acid and calcium phosphate, the urine pH as well as the total excretion will determine solubility; the solubility of uric acid increases as urine pH rises above 6, while that of calcium phosphate falls. Supersaturation is generally expressed as the ratio of the concentration of the salt in the urine to its known solubility, which is most often calculated by computer algorithms that can account for the complexity of urinary solutions. A ratio greater than 1 indicates that crystals of the salt are able to form, while a ratio below 1 means that an added crystal would dissolve. The type of stone formed by a patient correlates with the type of supersaturation present in the urine. Evaluation of stone formers is aimed at discovering the cause of the supersaturation that is driving stone formation, and preventive treatment is designed to lower supersaturation, by lowering the urine concentrations of stone-forming salts, or increasing inhibitors or solubility, when possible.

Supersaturated conditions may persist without immediate crystal formation because of the presence of inhibitors of crystal formation in urine. Almost a dozen known inhibitors of calcium crystal nucleation, growth, and aggregation are found in urine, most of them macromolecules. Stone formers generally have higher levels of supersaturation with respect to stone-forming materials such as calcium oxalate, and decreased levels of crystal inhibition, compared to non-stone-formers. If conditions permit crystals to be retained in the kidney, stones can form and grow in the renal pelvis.

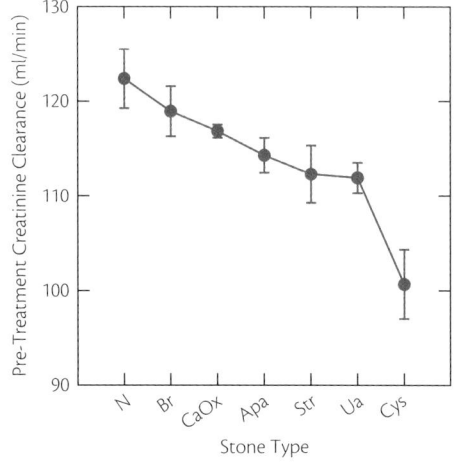
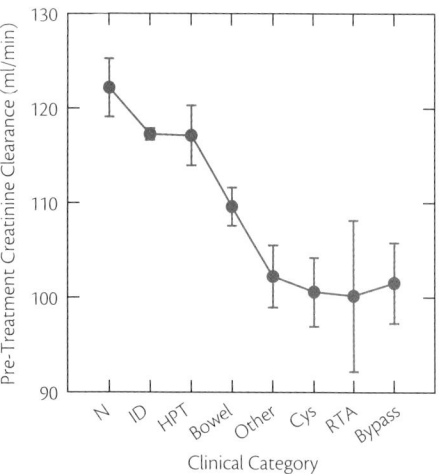

Fig. 21.14.1 Pretreatment creatinine clearances by stone type or clinical category, adjusted for age, weight, and gender, shown as means ± SEM; overall, 1856 stone formers, 153 normal subjects. N, normal; Br, brushite; CaOx, calcium oxalate; Apa, apatite; Str, struvite; Ua, uric acid; Cys, cystine; ID, idiopathic; HPT, hyperparathyroid; Bowel, bowel disease with or without surgery; Other, rare diseases such as sarcoid, drug stones; RTA, renal tubular acidosis; Bypass, obesity bypass.
(From Worcester EM, et al. (2006). Renal function in patients with nephrolithiasis. *J Urol*, **176**, 600–3, 2006, by permission of the American Urological Association.)

General evaluation of urinary stone formers

Once the acute episode of stone passage or removal is over, thought should be given to diagnosis of the underlying causes of stones, and steps taken toward prevention. Stone analysis is the cornerstone of diagnosis; urinalysis may reveal crystals, but is often unhelpful. Patients with noncalcium stones need preventive therapy, because uric acid, cystine, and struvite stones are prone to recur and can lead to kidney damage. For a first calcium stone, systemic diseases such as primary hyperparathyroidism, renal tubular acidosis, and hyperoxaluria should be ruled out, especially when stones present in childhood or adolescence.

A scheme for evaluation of first-time and recurrent stone formers is shown in Box 21.14.1. The most frequent abnormalities contributing to urine supersaturation and stone formation are listed in Box 21.14.2. Commercial laboratories provide testing specifically for stone formers, and include calculated supersaturations. An alternative for calcium stones is to calculate the urine calcium oxalate activity product index (an approximation of supersaturation) using the formula of Tiselius:

$$(1.9 \times calcium^{0.84} \times oxalate)/(citrate^{0.22} \times magnesium^{0.12} \times volume^{1.03})$$

where units are mmol/24 h, except for volume (litres/day). The equation makes clear that lowering supersaturation can be accomplished by decreasing concentrations of calcium and oxalate, and increasing citrate and volume (and magnesium to a lesser extent).

Calcium stones and nephrocalcinosis

Genetics and environment

Several rare monogenic disorders are associated with hypercalciuria or hyperoxaluria and formation of calcium stones (Table 21.14.2). Although a familial association is present in many cases of idiopathic calcium stone formation, the genes involved are not yet known.

Environment and diet also promote supersaturation and stone formation. High salt and sugar intakes can increase urinary calcium excretion. Likewise, very high protein intakes will increase calcium excretion, in part because of the acid production that occurs as the sulphated amino acids are metabolized. On the other hand, higher dietary calcium intake (1000–1200 mg/day) has been found to be protective, in both epidemiological and treatment trials, compared to low-calcium diets. Fluid intake is protective, and has been shown to lower stone recurrence in a trial of single stone formers (Table 21.14.5). Patients should be advised to increase water intake, and use a variety of other fluids in moderation, to keep urinary volume over 2 litres/day. Sodium intake should be about 100 mmol/day, and high protein intake avoided.

Pathology, pathogenesis and specific treatments

Idiopathic calcium oxalate stones form on the surface of the renal papillae, attached to suburothelial deposits of calcium phosphate and protein known as Randall's plaque (Fig. 21.14.2a). These deposits are found in the medullary interstitium (Fig. 21.14.2b), but crystals are not found in the lumen of renal tubules, and tubular cells are intact. The number of calcium oxalate stones formed varies directly with the amount of papillary surface covered by plaque, and amount of plaque varies directly with urinary calcium concentration and inversely with urinary volume.

Box 21.14.1 Evaluation of stone formers

First stone

- Rule out systemic diseases and stone types associated with frequent recurrence and damage to kidney (cystine, struvite, uric acid)
- Determine stone type:
  - Stone analysis by X-ray crystallography or infrared spectroscopy
  - Urinalysis (may identify crystal type, or infection with urea-splitting organism)
  - Qualitative screen for cystine (× 1) if stone type unknown
- Determine whether first stone or recurrent:
  - History of prior episodes
  - X-ray—other stones seen, or nephrocalcinosis noted
- Rule out systemic disease:
  - Normal serum calcium—primary hyperparathyroidism, other hypercalcaemic diseases unlikely
  - Normal serum bicarbonate—renal tubular acidosis unlikely
  - Normal urine oxalate—primary or secondary causes of hyperoxaluria unlikely
- No known anatomical renal abnormalities (single kidney, pelviureteric junction obstruction)
- No history of bowel disease or resection
- No urinary tract infection with organisms possessing urease
- If first episode of calcium oxalate stone—conservative treatment (fluids and dietary modification)

Recurrent calcium stone *or* stone type is uric acid, cystine, or struvite

Further workup needed to determine proper preventive therapy

- Calcium stone—24-h urine measurement of creatinine, calcium, oxalate, sodium, urea, uric acid, citrate, volume, pH (sulfate, ammonia, potassium, and supersaturation helpful)
- Uric acid stone—24-h urine measurement of creatinine, pH, uric acid, volume
- Cystine stone—24-hour urine measurement of creatinine, pH, volume, cystine, calcium, sodium, urea.
- Struvite stone—urine culture for identification of organism and antibiotic sensitivity. Surgical treatment needed. Some struvite stone formers have risk factors for other stone types, which may have become secondarily infected.

In contrast, calcium phosphate stones (both brushite and apatite) are associated with dense crystal deposits of calcium phosphate as apatite in the lumens of the ducts of Bellini (Fig. 21.14.2c). These crystal plugs may cause massive tubular dilation, and injury to lining cells is seen (Fig. 21.14.2d), as well as interstitial fibrosis. A similar but more extensive picture is seen in patients with distal renal tubular acidosis associated with phosphate stones. Thus, phosphate stones appear to be associated with more renal paren-

<table>
</table>

Box 21.14.2 Causes of stone formation

Calcium stones

- Hypercalciuria and hypercalcaemia
  - Primary hyperparathyroidism
  - Granulomatous diseases
  - Vitamin D excess
  - Malignancy (rare as cause of stone)
  - Hyperthyroidism
- Hypercalciuria with normocalcaemia (also see Table 21.14.2)
  - Distal renal tubular acidosis
  - Granulomatous diseases
  - Cushing's disease
  - Idiopathic hypercalciuria
- Hyperoxaluria
  - Primary hyperoxaluria—PH1, PH2
  - Enteric hyperoxaluria
  - Dietary hyperoxaluria
  - Low-calcium diet
- Hypocitraturia
  - Secondary to hypokalaemia
  - Secondary to metabolic acidosis
  - Idiopathic
- Hyperuricosuria
- Low urinary volume

Uric acid stones

- Low urine pH
  - Gouty diathesis
  - Idiopathic (insulin resistance)
  - Bowel disease (especially colon resection)
- Low urinary volume
- Hyperuricosuria

Cystine stones

- Elevated cystine excretion

Struvite stones

- Urinary tract infection with urea-splitting organism

---

chymal damage than do oxalate stones, and—as mentioned previously—are also associated with the need for more frequent procedures for stone removal.

Patients with nephrolithiasis and cystinuria or distal renal tubular acidosis also have plugging of Bellini ducts and inner medullary collecting ducts with apatite crystals, in addition to cystine crystals in cystinuric patients. More surprisingly, patients who form calcium oxalate stones due to enteric hyperoxaluria after jejuno-

ileal bypass have also been found to have apatite crystal plugs in inner medullary collecting ducts. Overall, all stone formers with papillary biopsies studied so far have had crystal deposition in renal medullary tubules, except idiopathic calcium oxalate stone formers, who have only interstitial crystal deposits.

Idiopathic hypercalciuria

The commonest disorder associated with calcium stones, idiopathic hypercalciuria, leads to elevated urinary calcium without associated systemic leads to and is found in approximately one-half of calcium stone formers of both sexes. The condition is familial, seemingly polygenic, and involves abnormalities of the gut, kidney, and bone. The conventional upper limits of normal calcium excretion are 6 mmol/day in women, and 7.5 mmol/day in men, near the 95th percentile for excretion in non-stone-formers. However, calcium excretion is a graded risk factor for stone formation, and even patients with excretions at the 75th percentile (4.25 mmol/day for women and 6.25 mmol/day for men) often benefit from treatment to decrease calcium excretion.

Patients with idiopathic hypercalciuria often have elevated serum 1,25-dihydroxy vitamin D levels and a resulting increase in intestinal calcium absorption. However, they also manifest a decreased ability of their kidneys to reabsorb filtered calcium, and if placed on low-calcium diet, may excrete calcium in excess of the amount absorbed; i.e. they are prone to go into negative calcium balance, losing calcium from bone. It is therefore not surprising that multiple studies have shown decreased bone density in patients with idiopathic hypercalciuria, and an increased fracture risk, primarily vertebral. High dietary salt, sucrose, or protein loads worsen urinary calcium excretion.

Treatment with a diet restricted in animal protein and salt, but with normal calcium intake (25 mmol/day), was found to be successful in reducing stone recurrence in males with idiopathic hypercalciuria (Table 21.14.3). Thiazide diuretics lower urinary calcium excretion and have decreased stone recurrence in three prospective randomized double blind trials; the mechanism appears to be, at least in part, an increase in calcium absorption in the proximal tubule, induced by volume contraction. In balance studies, thiazides resulted in a positive calcium balance.

Primary hyperparathyroidism

About 5% of calcium stone formers have increased PTH production, usually from an adenoma, which leads to high serum and urinary calcium levels. Increased serum calcium levels, often in the range of 2.5–3 mmol/litre, associated with elevated or unsuppressed PTH and very high urinary calcium excretion are the hallmark of this disorder. Removal of the overactive gland is curative of the hormonal disorder and greatly reduces stone recurrence.

Hyperoxaluria
Dietary hyperoxaluria

Mild dietary hyperoxaluria is not uncommon and may often be found in individuals on a low-calcium diet, or a diet unusually rich in oxalate-containing foods such as rhubarb, spinach, okra, beetroot, nuts, and chocolate, and it seems reasonable to advise patients with recurrent stones to avoid consuming excessive quantities of these. High protein intake may also provoke increased oxalate excretion.

Enteric hyperoxaluria

This occurs with all forms of small-bowel and pancreato-biliary disease that result in fat malabsorption, particularly ileal bypass or

Table 21.14.2 Monogenic disorders of nephrocalcinosis and stone formation

Disease	Inheritance	Gene/gene product	Function	Stones	NC	Phenotype
Dent's disease	X-linked	CLCN5/ClC-5	Endosomal Cl channel	+	+	Hypercalciuria, LMW proteinuria, CRF
Bartter's syndrome type I	AR	SLC12A1/NKCC2	Na-K-2Cl co-transporter		+	Hypercalciuria, hypokalaemic alkalosis
Bartter's syndrome type II	AR	KCNJ1/ROMK	K channel		+	Hypercalciuria, hypokalaemic alkalosis
Bartter's syndrome type III	AR	CLCNKB/ClC-Kb	Basolateral Cl channel	+	+	Hypercalciuria, hypokalaemic alkalosis
Bartter's syndrome type V	AD	CASR/CaSR (severe gain of function)	Calcium sensing receptor	+	+	Hypercalciuria, hypokalaemic alkalosis, CRF, hypocalcemia
Hypocalcemic hypercalciuria	AD	CASR/CaSR (gain of function)	Calcium sensing receptor		+	Hypercalciuria, CRF, hypocalcemia
Familial hypomagnesaemia with hypercalciuria	AR	PCLN1/Paracellin 1	Tight junction protein	+	+	Hypercalciuria, hypermagnesuria, CRF, hypomagnesemia
Hereditary hypophosphatemic rickets with hypercalciuria	AR	SLC34A3/NaPi-IIc	Sodium-phosphate co-transporter	Rare	Rare	Hypercalciuria, hypophosphataemia, rickets
Distal RTA	AD	SLC4A1/AE1	Cl-bicarbonate exchanger	+	+	Hypercalciuria, hypokalaemia, osteomalacia,
Distal RTA with hearing loss	AR	ATP6V1B1/B1 subunit of vacuolar H-ATPase	Proton secretion	+	+	Hypercalciuria, hypokalaemia, rickets
Distal RTA	AR	ATP6V0A4/A4 subunit of vacuolar H-ATPase	Proton secretion	+	+	Hypercalciuria, hypokalaemia, rickets
Cystinuria type A	AR	SLC3A1/rBAT	Heavy chain of dibasic aa transporter	+		Cystinuria, CRF
Cystinuria type B	Incomplete AR	SLC7A9/b⁰,⁺AT	Light chain of dibasic aa transporter	+		Cystinuria, CRF
Primary hyperoxaluria type I	AR	AGXT/alanine glyoxylate aminotransferase	Converts glyoxalate to glycine	+	+	Hyperoxaluria, CRF
Primary hyperoxaluria type II	AR	GRHPR/Glyoxylate reductase	Converts glyoxylate to glycolate	+		Hyperoxaluria, CRF

aa, amino acid; AR, autosomal recessive; CRF, chronic renal failure; LMW, low molecular weight; NC, nephrocalcinosis; RTA, renal tubular acidosis.

resection, provided that colon is present and receiving small-bowel effluent. Stool losses of fluid and citrate cause increased supersaturation with respect to both calcium oxalate and uric acid, leading to stone formation. Hyperoxaluria occurred in patients with jejuno-ileal bypass, a form of weight loss surgery no longer performed, and caused recurrent stones as well as renal insufficiency in some patients. Modern bariatric surgery also leads to an increase in urinary oxalate excretion, for uncertain reasons, and there are early reports of increased stone formation in such patients. Treatment measures include diets reduced in fat and oxalate, increased calcium intake with meals to bind oxalate and prevent absorption, and sometimes use of oxalate-binding agents such as cholestyramine. Potassium alkali may also be needed.

Primary hyperoxaluria

Primary hyperoxaluria types 1 and 2 arise from genetic disorders of oxalate synthesis (see Table 21.14.2). Urinary oxalate is 100–300 mg/day, and nephrocalcinosis and renal failure are common. Symptoms often begin in childhood. High doses of pyridoxine may lower urinary oxalate in some patients with type 1 primary hyperoxaluria, and neutral orthophosphate has also been used successfully in some patients. In type 1, liver transplantation is the definitive treatment; type 2 is milder, and renal failure is uncommon. There is an international registry for patients with primary hyperoxaluria

to improve diagnosis and treatment of these rare disorders (www.rarekidneystones.org).

Hypocitraturia

Diagnosed when urinary citrate is below 350 mg/day (males) or 500 mg/day (females), this common abnormality reduces both urinary calcium binding into soluble complexes and deprives urine of an established inhibitor of calcium crystal formation. Treatment with potassium citrate proved effective in two high-quality trials (Table 21.14.3). Urine pH should be monitored because values above 6.5 could promote calcium phosphate stones. Most cases of hypocitraturia are of unknown cause, but it may be seen in patients with distal renal tubular acidosis. Sometimes it arises from potassium depletion, which can occur with bowel disease and diarrhoea, or as a consequence of thiazide-induced renal potassium wasting. In either case, repletion with potassium alkali is a good therapeutic option.

Hyperuricosuria

An elevated urine uric acid excretion (>750 mg/day in women or 800 mg/day in men) may be seen in patients with calcium stones, often caused by a diet high in protein. Hyperuricosuria decreases the solubility of calcium oxalate, and promotes stones. Allopurinol was successful in decreasing stone recurrence in such patients

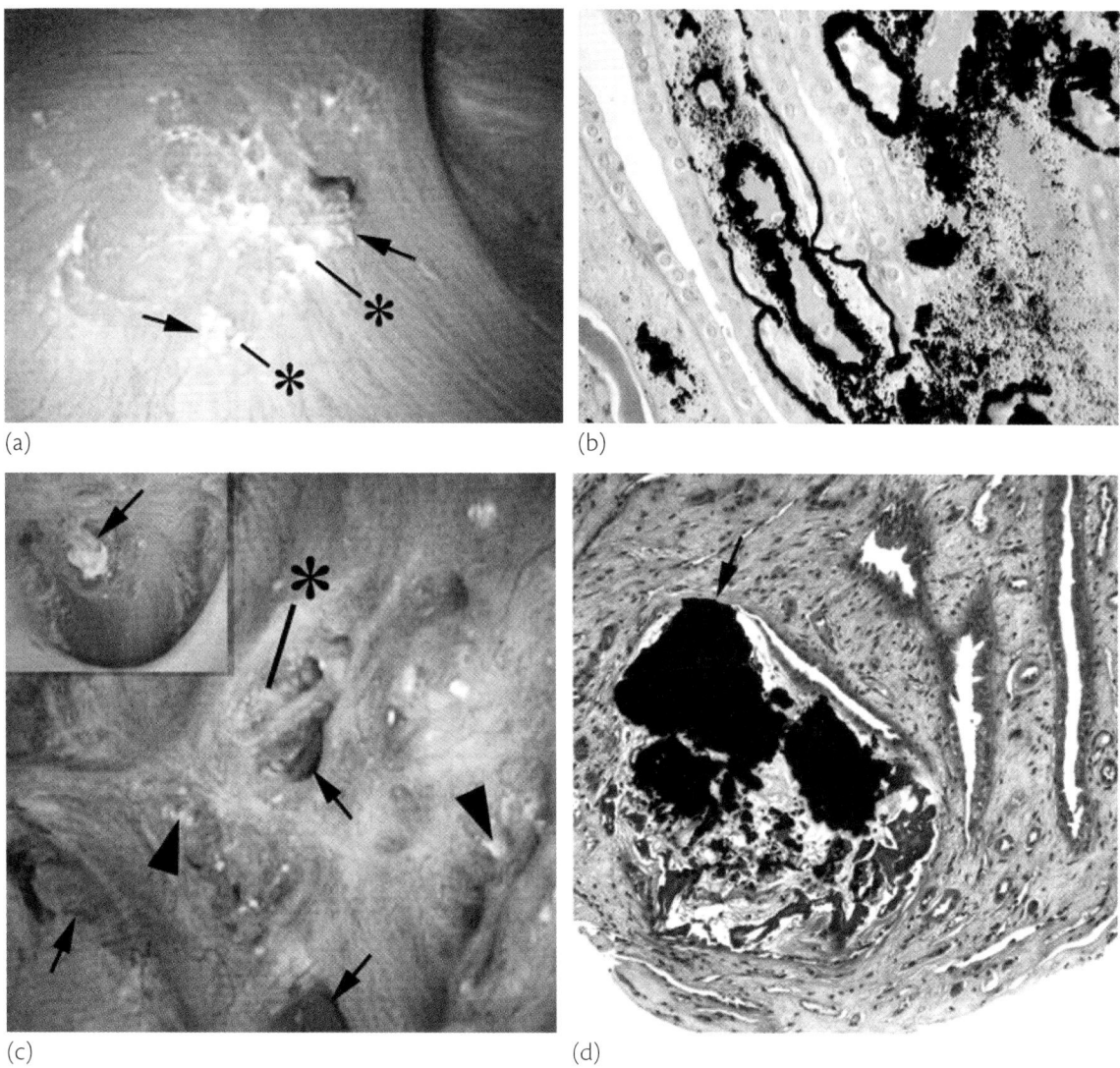

Fig. 21.14.2 Endoscopic and histological images from calcium stone formers. (a) Papilla from a calcium oxalate stone former, recorded at the time of stone removal. Scattered white Randall's plaque (asterisks) is accompanied by some small stones at the arrows. (b) On biopsy, tubular cells are normal under light microscopy; plaque, seen as dark deposits with Yasue stain, ranges from a fine dust to thick deposits, always interstitial. (c) The papillum of a brushite stone former no longer has recognizable normal landmarks, with depressions (arrows) near the papillary tip. At the asterisk a mass of crystals grows out of a dilated duct of Bellini. Arrowheads point to routine plaque. The inset shows an enlarged duct of Bellini with crystal material protruding from the duct, which may form an attachment site for stone. (d) On biopsy, a massively dilated Bellini duct is filled with apatite crystal deposit; all around it the interstitium is scarred. Tubular lining cells are injured or absent.

(Images c and d from Evan AP, et al. (2005). Crystal-associated nephropathy in patients with brushite nephrolithiasis. *Kidney Int*, **67**, 576–91, with permission).

(see Table 21.14.3), and a decrease in protein intake would be helpful as well.

Calcium phosphate stones

Calcium phosphate stones form when supersaturation for calcium phosphate (brushite) in the urine is elevated. The major determinant of this type of supersaturation is alkaline urine pH (>6.3), coupled with hypercalciuria. These stones are associated with a more destructive renal pathology, and often require more procedures for removal. The cause of the elevated urine pH in these patients is often unclear; few have true distal renal tubular acidosis. The use of alkaline citrate as a treatment for stones should be followed by careful follow-up to assure that supersaturation with respect to calcium phosphate is not rising, as formation of calcium phosphate stones may worsen.

Nephrocalcinosis

Nephrocalcinosis is defined as precipitation of calcium salts in renal tubules or interstitium. As noted above, all calcium stones are accompanied by at least some tissue precipitation of calcium phosphate, but the amount is not large, and not yet detectable by current radiological methods. Larger amounts of precipitation may be seen in certain disease states (see Table 21.14.2), and particularly in diseases such as distal renal tubular acidosis and primary hyperoxaluria, where deposition of large amounts of mineral in medullary (and occasionally cortical) tissue may lead to renal failure. Current radiological techniques cannot adequately distinguish between calcification in the renal pelvis and in renal tissue, which often coexist.

Table 21.14.3 Randomized trials of preventive treatment for calcium stones

Treatment	Dose	Controlled trial	Recurrence (%)	
			Treated	Control
Calcium stones—hypercalciuria (± mild hyperoxaluria, hypocitraturia)				
Fluid (single calcium oxalate stone formers)	Told to increase fluid intake to keep urine volume > 2l/day	5 years, high fluid intake vs usual intake n = 199	12	27
Diet (recurrent calcium oxalate stone formers)	Calcium 1200 mg/day Sodium 50 mmol/day, Protein 52 gm/day	5 years, study diet vs. 400 mg calcium diet, n = 120	20	38
Chlorthalidone	25 mg/day	3 years, drug vs placebo; n = 73	14	46
Hydrochlorothiazide	25 mg bid	3 years, drug vs placebo; n = 50	17	40
Indapamide	2.5 mg/day	3 years, drug vs placebo; n = 75	15	43
Calcium stones—hypocitraturia (and urine pH not alkaline)				
Potassium citrate	30–60 meq/day	3 years, drug vs placebo, n = 57	28	80
Potassium magnesium citrate	60 meq/day	3 years, drug vs placebo, n = 64	13	64
Sodium potassium citrate	Variable dose to keep urine pH 7–7.2	3 years, drug vs no drug, n = 50	69	73
Calcium stones—hyperuricosuria				
Allopurinol	100 mg tid	3 years, drug vs placebo, n = 60	31	58

bid, twice daily; tid, three times daily.

Uric acid stones

Aetiology and pathogenesis

Uric acid stones occur when urine pH is abnormally low. The solubility of undissociated uric acid is only 0.54 mmol/litre (90 mg/litre), and at pH below 5.35 (the pK_a) over half the uric acid present is in the undissociated form. Normal daily excretion of uric acid is 3 to 4.8 mmol/day (500–800 mg/day), depending on protein intake, so it is easy to see that acid urine will be supersaturated with respect to uric acid in most cases. Low urinary volume and high uric acid excretion will exacerbate the tendency to uric acid precipitation.

Patients with diarrhoea, especially with ileostomy, excrete concentrated, acid urine because of loss of water and bicarbonate in stool; uric acid stones are a common complication of this condition. Low urinary pH and uric acid stones also occur in patients with insulin resistance, as in diabetes or the metabolic syndrome, because insulin resistance is associated with decreased ability to synthesize ammonia, leading to lower urinary pH because of lack of this proton buffer. Increasing body weight is also associated with low urinary pH, perhaps because of insulin resistance. Diabetic stone formers have a 35 to 45% prevalence of uric acid stones, which is much higher than the 5 to 10% prevalence seen in the general population of stone formers. Patients with gout are frequently obese or diabetic; however, some forms of gout are associated with acid urine pH without the established need for insulin resistance. Certain forms of renal disease result in reduced ammonia production and low pH; chronic lead nephropathy is a well-known example (saturnine gout). Although low pH is common in most forms of progressive renal failure, uric acid stones are not.

Diagnosis and treatment

Uric acid stones are poorly visualized on standard plain radiographs, although they are easily seen on CT. On intravenous pyelograms they may be seen as filling defects. Alkali treatment to raise urinary pH above 6.2 will solubilize uric acid and can prevent stones. Use of potassium alkali is preferred, as sodium alkali (sodium citrate or sodium bicarbonate) will raise urinary calcium, and possibly blood pressure. Urine pH needs monitoring because excessive elevation may cause calcium phosphate stones, and serum potassium also needs to be monitored to avoid hyperkalaemia, especially in diabetics. Giving doses of 10 to 20 mmol of alkali 2 to 3 times a day is usually sufficient to keep urinary pH at 6 to 6.5. Dietary intake of purine should be limited if uric acid excretion is elevated, and increased fluids are a standard part of stone management.

Cystine stones

Aetiology and pathogenesis

Cystine stones form in patients with inherited defects of dibasic amino acid transport in the proximal tubule, which lead to increased excretion of cystine, ornithine, lysine and arginine in the urine. The only clinical outcome of this defect is cystine stones, because of the poor solubility of this amino acid, thus the defect has been termed cystinuria. Cystine stones are found in only 1 to 2% of stone formers, but they are often recurrent, and may become very large, leading to the need for many stone removal procedures. Cystine stones are poorly fragmented by extracorporeal shockwave lithotripsy, so alternative means of stone removal may be needed. Renal function is often reduced, perhaps as the result of the effects of stones and surgery. Stones are not well visualized using plain abdominal radiographs, although they are seen well with CT.

Cystinuria is an autosomal recessive disorder, which may be caused by defects in either of two genes, *SLC3A1* or *SLC7A9*. The proteins encoded by these genes form a heterodimer, which is responsible for cystine transport in the apical membrane of the proximal tubule, and in the small intestine. Defects in these two genes appear to explain most cases of cystinuria, and they are clinically indistinguishable with respect to age of stone onset, frequency of recurrence, or cystine excretion. Papillary biopsies show crystal deposits that contain cystine and also calcium phosphate in collecting ducts. The degree of interstitial fibrosis and tubular cell injury is quite marked, and accords with reduction of renal function that is more severe than in almost any other stone disease.

Cystine stones may begin in childhood, or even in infancy. In a large cohort study the median age of first stone was 12 years; males appear to be more severely affected than females for reasons that are unclear. Cystinuria should always be looked for when stones present in childhood or adolescence. Preventive therapy should be started as soon as stones are diagnosed, and continued lifelong because of high recurrence rates and severe kidney injury.

Diagnosis and treatment

Cystinuria may be diagnosed by stone analysis showing cystine, and the finding of characteristic hexagonal crystals in urine is pathognomonic. In addition, all stone formers should have at least one urine sample screened for cystine using the cyanide–nitroprusside qualitative test, which is positive when urine cystine concentration is above 75 mg/litre. Normal cystine excretion is only 30 mg/day (0.13 mmol/day); in comparison, patients with cystine stones usually excrete over 400 mg/day (1.7 mmol/day). Heterozygotes for cystinuria may excrete 250 mg (1 mmol) per day, but seldom form stones. Cystine excretion may be transiently elevated in infancy, and diagnosis in this age group is more difficult.

Lowering supersaturation of the urine with respect to cystine is the goal of treatment. Cystine solubility is pH dependent, and is higher at alkaline pH, but not very accurately predicted from nomograms. At a pH of 7 to 7.5, solubility can vary from 175 to 360 mg/litre (0.7–1.47 mmol/litre). A reasonable goal is to keep urinary cystine concentration below 243 mg/L (1 mmol/litre) and urine pH about 7.

Management begins with measurement of daily cystine excretion and urinary pH. High fluid intake is a cornerstone of treatment, and the amount needed to achieve a concentration of <1 mmol/litre can be calculated and prescribed, with fluid intake distributed throughout the day, and in the evening as well. Some patients will require potassium alkali, as potassium citrate or bicarbonate, in divided doses, to improve solubility. Potassium salts are preferred, as sodium intake can raise cystine excretion. Low sodium (100 mmol/day) and protein (0.8–1 g/kg per day) intake can reduce cystine excretion modestly.

If stones recur despite adequate hydration and increase of pH, a cysteine-binding drug should be added to fluids and alkali to decrease the concentration of cystine further. Cystine is formed by the linkage of two cysteine molecules by a disulphide bond. Cysteine binding drugs have sulphydryl groups that form mixed disulphides with cysteine, which are more soluble than the homodimer, cystine. D-Penicillamine (1–2 g/day, in 3 or 4 divided doses) is one such drug, the penicillamine–cysteine disulphide being 50 times more soluble than cystine. A second agent, α-mercaptopropionylglycine (tiopronin, 400–1200 mg/day in divided doses), is also effective. Both drugs have side effects, including fever, rash, dysgeusia, arthralgias, leucopenia, and proteinuria, but tiopronin is better tolerated, with a lesser incidence and severity of adverse reactions. Captopril has also been used with some success. Recurrent stones should be analysed, as patients may form stones containing calcium phosphate due to the alkaline urine pH, which require different treatment.

Struvite stones

Struvite (magnesium ammonium phosphate) stones may present with vague flank pain and gradual deterioration of renal function, rather than colic. They form when the kidney is infected with organisms that possess the enzyme urease, such as proteus, providentia, klebsiella, pseudomonas and enterobacter species. Urease hydrolyses urea to ammonia and CO_2, with the ammonia raising the pH of the urine and leading to production of bicarbonate and carbonate in the urine. Calcium carbonate coprecipitates with struvite, forming large, branched stones within the kidney. Bacteria adhere to the stone, where they are poorly reached by antibiotics, making urine sterilization impossible when stones are present, hence adequate treatment requires removal of all stone material in addition to appropriate antibiotics. Struvite stones are more common in settings with chronic urological instrumentation, or in patients with neurogenic bladders. In cases where removal of all stone material is not possible, acetohydroxamic acid, a urease inhibitor, has been used prevent stone recurrence and growth, but its use is limited by serious side effects, including headache, gastrointestinal upset, and thrombophlebitis.

Further reading

Abate N, et al. (2004). The metabolic syndrome and uric acid nephrolithiasis: novel features of renal manifestation of insulin resistance. *Kidney Int*, **65**, 386–92.

Asplin JR, et al. (1999). Reduced crystallization inhibition by urine from men with nephrolithiasis. *Kidney Int*, **56**, 1505–16.

Auge BK, Preminger GM (2002). Surgical management of urolithiasis. *Endocrinol Metabol Clin North Am*, **31**, 1065–82.

Barcelo P, et al. (1993). Randomized double-blind study of potassium citrate in idiopathic hypocitraturic calcium nephrolithiasis. *J Urol*, **150**, 1761–4.

Borghi L, et al. (1993). Randomized prospective study of a nonthiazide diuretic, indapamide, in preventing calcium stone recurrences. *J Cardiovasc Pharmacol*, **22** Suppl 6, S78–86.

Borghi L, et al. (1996). Urinary volume, water and recurrences of idiopathic calcium nephrolithiasis: a 5-year randomized prospective study. *J Urol*, **155**, 839–43.

Borghi L, et al. (2002). Comparison of two diets for the prevention of recurrent stones in idiopathic hypercalciuria. *N Engl J Med*, **346**, 77–84.

Coe FL, Evan A, Worcester E (2005). Kidney stone disease. *J Clin. Invest*, **115**, 2598–608.

Coe FL, Favus MJ, Asplin JR (2004). Nephrolithiasis. In: Brenner BM, Rector FC Jr (eds) *The kidney*, pp. 1819–66. Elsevier, Philadelphia.

Curhan GC, et al. (2001). Twenty-four-hour urine chemistries and the risk of kidney stones among women and men. *Kidney Int*, **59**, 2290–8.

Ettinger B, et al. (1986). Randomized trial of allopurinol in the prevention of calcium oxalate calculi. *N Engl J Med*, **315**, 1386–89.

Ettinger B, et al. (1988). Chlorthalidone reduces calcium oxalate calculous recurrence but magnesium hydroxide does not. *J Urol*, **139**, 679–84.

Ettinger B, et al. (1997). Potassium-magnesium citrate is an effective prophylaxis against recurrent calcium oxalate nephrolithiasis. *J Urol*, **158**, 2069–73.

Evan AP, et al. (2003). Randalls plaque of patients with nephrolithiasis begins in basement membranes of thin loops of Henle. *J Clin Invest*, **111**, 607–16.

Evan AP, et al. (2005). Crystal-associated nephropathy in patients with brushite nephrolithiasis. *Kidney Int*, **67**, 576–91.

Gambaro G, *et al.* (2004). Genetics of hypercalciuria and calcium nephrolithiasis: from the rare monogenic to the common polygenic forms. *Am J Kidney Dis*, **44**, 963–86.

Hofbauer J, *et al.* (1994). Alkali citrate prophylaxis in idiopathic recurrent calcium oxalate urolithiasis—a prospective randominzed study. *Br J Urol*, **73**, 362–5.

Laerum E, Larsen S (1984). Thiazide prophylaxis of urolithiasis: A double-blind study in general practice. *Acta Med Scand*, **215**, 383–9.

Lieske JC, *et al.* (2005). International registry for primary hyperoxaluria. *Am J Nephrol*, **25**, 290–6.

Maalouf NM, *et al.* (2004). Association of urinary pH with body weight in nephrolithiasis. *Kidney Int*, **65**, 1422–5.

Moe OW (2006). Kidney stones: pathophysiology and medical management. *Lancet*, **367**, 333–44.

Pak CY, *et al.* (1986). Management of cystine nephrolithiasis with alpha-mercaptopropionylglycine. *J Urol*, **136**, 1003–8.

Parks JH, *et al.* (2004). Clinical implications of abundant calcium phosphate in routinely analyzed kidney stones. *Kidney Int*, **66**, 777–85.

Ryall RL (2004). Macromolecules and urolithiasis: parallels and paradoxes. *Nephron Physiol*, **98**, 37–42.

Stamatelou KK, *et al.* (2003). Time trends in reported prevalence of kidney stones in the United States: 1976–1994. *Kidney Int*, **63**, 1817–23.

Taylor EN, Stampfer MJ, Curhan GC (2004). Dietary factors and the risk of incident kidney stones in men: new insights after 14 years of follow-up. *J Am Soc Nephrol*, **15**, 3225–32.

Worcester EM (2002). Stones from bowel disease. *Endocrinol Metab Clin North Am*, **31**, 979–99.

Worcester EM, *et al.* (2006). Reduced renal function and benefits of treatment in cystinuria vs other forms of nephrolithiasis. *Br J Urol Int*, **97**, 1285–90.

The renal tubular acidoses

Fiona E. Karet

Essentials

Renal tubular acidosis (RTA) arises when the kidneys either fail to excrete sufficient acid, or are unable to conserve bicarbonate, both circumstances leading to metabolic acidosis of varying severity with altered serum potassium. Proximal and distal types of RTA can be differentiated according to which nephron segment is malfunctioning. The condition may be secondary (e.g. associated with drugs, autoimmune disease, or diabetes mellitus) or inherited, and there may be renal tract calcification and—in chronic cases—metabolic bone disease.

Proximal RTA

Aetiology and diagnosis – the condition may be (1) secondary to generalized proximal tubular dysfunction (part of the renal Fanconi syndrome), or rarely (2) due to inherited mutation of a single transporter (NBC1) located at the basolateral surface of the proximal tubular epithelium. The combination of normal anion gap acidosis with other features of proximal tubular dysfunction such as renal phosphate wasting (and hypophosphataemia), renal glycosuria, hypouricaemia (due to uricosuria), aminoaciduria, microalbuminuria, and other low-molecular-weight proteinuria suggests the diagnosis.

Management—this requires large quantities of oral alkali (as bicarbonate or citrate), with (in most cases) potassium supplements to prevent severe hypokalaemia. Associated phosphate and vitamin D deficiencies may also require treatment. Precipitating drugs should be stopped if possible.

Distal RTA

Aetiology—two main classes are differentiated by whether (1) the acid-handling cells (α-intercalated cells) in the collecting ducts are themselves functioning inadequately, in which case there is associated hypokalaemia (this is 'classic' distal RTA); or (2) the main abnormality is of the salt-handling principal cells in the same nephron segment, in which case hyperkalaemia occurs and the acidosis is a secondary phenomenon. This is hyperkalaemic distal RTA, which is most often secondary to hyporeninaemic hypoaldosteronism (e.g. in diabetes mellitus or critical illness) but may also be reversibly precipitated by drugs such as trimethoprim or ciclosporin.

Diagnosis—the combination of normal anion gap acidosis with a urine pH higher than 5.5 suggests classic distal RTA, especially if renal tract calcification is present or there is coexistent autoimmune disease. Diagnosis may require an oral urine acidification test if the metabolic abnormalities are partially masked by compensatory mechanisms, when inability to achieve a urine pH less than 5.5 clinches the diagnosis of classic distal RTA. By contrast, urine-acidification capacity is normal in hyperkalaemic distal RTA.

Management—(1) Classic distal RTA—1 to 3 mg/kg per day of oral alkali (additional supplements should not be required); (2) Hyperkalaemic distal RTA—treatment is with sodium bicarbonate, but fludrocortisone and/or potassium-lowering measures may also be necessary. Precipitating drugs should be stopped.

Introduction

The kidney plays a key role in the regulation of acid–base balance and the term 'renal tubular acidosis' (RTA) refers to systemic acidosis arising from a tubular ion transport abnormality. On a mixed omnivorous diet, humans produce a net acid load of about 1 mmol/kg per day, which must be excreted. Through activity at two main sites in the nephron, the proximal convoluted tubule and the collecting duct, the kidney is able to vary bicarbonate reclamation and net acid excretion such that urine pH can range from about 4.5 to over 8, enabling systemic pH to be closely maintained at 7.4 ± 0.04. Failure of these tubular functions can cause very severe acidosis with pH below 7.

The traditional classification of the RTAs is an historical one, based on the order in which the defects were described, but in thinking about the different mechanisms involved it is least confusing to use a 'geographical' division to classify them, first considering the nephron segment affected:

- Proximal (former type 2)

- Distal, subdivided into 'classic' (type 1) and 'hyperkalaemic' (type 4)

- Mixed, which usually refers to carbonic anhydrase deficiency (type 3)

Note that RTA excludes the acidosis of chronic kidney disease, also that within each class of RTA there is then a division into primary (inherited) and secondary types. Primary RTA is directly due to inadequate function of a proton or bicarbonate transporter, and molecular genetic studies have identified a variety of these (as discussed below). In general, disorders associated with RTA that are inherited dominantly are clinically milder and give rise to over-activity or gain of abnormal function of a channel or transporter, whereas those that are recessively inherited are clinically more severe and due to loss-of-function genetic defects. Although all the recessive diseases described in this chapter are rare, they are encountered more commonly in areas of the world where parental consanguinity is prevalent, and the investigation of kindreds where affected children are the offspring of such union of unaffected parents has allowed us to investigate the genetic causes of such disorders, and to understand better the molecular pathophysiology involved.

In adult clinical practice, secondary causes of RTA are much commoner than primary, in particular hyperkalaemic dRTA in association with diabetes mellitus, and classic dRTA in autoimmune disease. Secondary RTA also describes metabolic acidosis arising from other renal ion transporter dysfunctions: the kidney does not carry out any of its myriad homeostatic functions in a vacuum, and interactions with these other systems form an important part of the overall picture. This is perhaps most marked in the context of salt homeostasis, where the endocrine system—particularly the mineralocorticoid axis—is closely involved, and defects in these pathways can cause hyperkalaemic RTA.

Physiology of renal acid–base homeostasis

To understand the pathophysiology of the different types of RTA, it is helpful to consider normal renal acid–base balance, again in a geographic way. Broadly, this consists of the combination of bicarbonate reabsorption (proximal tubule), proton secretion and bicarbonate generation (collecting duct), and ammonium generation and secretion (proximal tubule and medulla).

Proximal tubule

Since the total load of sodium and bicarbonate reaching the glomeruli is freely filtered, the proximal tubule has a considerable reabsorption task to perform, reclaiming 90% (3–4 mol) of bicarbonate daily from the tubular fluid, with Na^+, H^+ and HCO_3^- transport linked, as shown in Fig. 21.15.1. Citrate is also reabsorbed by the proximal tubule, which yields additional bicarbonate. Proximal tubular cells are also capable of generating 'extra' bicarbonate through the deamination of glutamine to glutamate, then forming α-ketoglutarate and eventually glucose (Fig. 21.15.1). This produces bicarbonate and ammonium - the former is reabsorbed and the latter secreted into the tubular lumen. This process is up-regulated in states of chronic acidosis of non-renal origin.

Collecting duct

Two cell types with distinctly different functions are present in the collecting duct (Fig. 21.15.2). These are principal cells (PC, responsible for salt handling) and intercalated cells (IC, acid–base). Within the IC population, many studies—mostly in rodents—have described at least two subtypes, α- and β-ICs. α-ICs are responsible for coupled apical secretion of protons into the urine and reclamation of bicarbonate across the basolateral surface (Fig. 21.15.2). On the apical surface, the multisubunit proton pump (H^+-ATPase) transfers H^+ into the urine. It is of the same type as the H^+-ATPases found ubiquitously in intracellular organelles such as lysosomes, which require a low pH for efficient function. H^+-ATPases are composed of at least 13 different subunits, organized into a membrane-anchored V_0 ('stalk') domain (subunits a–e), through which

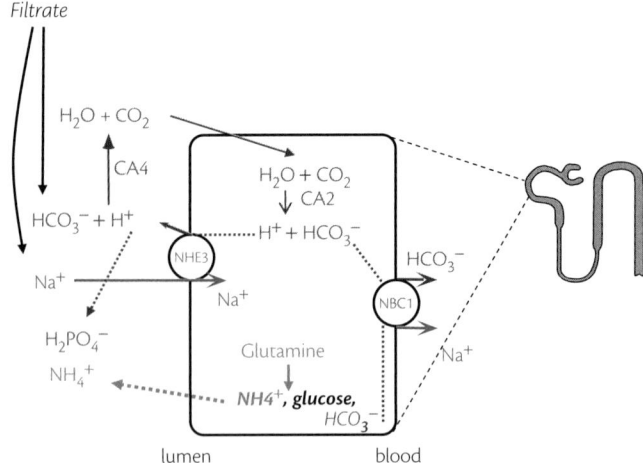

Fig. 21.15.1 Schema of proximal tubular acid–base movement. H^+/HCO_3^- movement pathways are shown in red, Na^+/Cl^- in blue, and ammonium in green. Na^+ is absorbed in direct exchange for H^+ by the sodium-proton exchanger NHE3. In the lumen, the H^+ and HCO_3^- rapidly form H_2O and CO_2 under the catalytic influence of membrane-bound carbonic anhydrase (CA 4). Having diffused into the cell, CO_2 undergoes a reverse reaction (via intracellular CA2) to re-form bicarbonate, which is then available for Na^+/HCO_3^- reabsorption into the interstitial fluid (and from there into the blood) via the sodium-bicarbonate transporter NBC1. Any excess luminal H^+ is buffered by filtered phosphate (HPO_4^{2-}). Proximal tubular cells also generate 'extra' HCO_3^- and ammonium through the deamination of glutamine as shown, the former being reabsorbed and the latter secreted into the tubular lumen. Dopamine and acetazolamide affect NHE3 and CA2 respectively.

protons are moved, and a V_1 'head' that hydrolyses ATP (subunits A–H). Apical and intracellular proton pumps can be differentiated by their subunit composition: the α-IC's apical renal pumps contain B1 rather than B2 subunits, and a4 instead of a1, whereas—being ubiquitously produced—B2 and a1 may be regarded as 'housekeeping' forms.

In α-ICs, apical H^+-ATPase function is coupled to basolateral bicarbonate exit (in exchange for chloride) via the anion exchanger AE1 (Fig. 21.1.5.2), which is structurally similar to the isoform present in the erythrocyte membrane, except that it is a little shorter at the N-terminal end. Chloride/bicarbonate exchange is 1:1.

β-ICs essentially reverse the processes of α-ICs, so they secrete bicarbonate into the urine. It remains unclear whether α- and β-ICs are molecular mirror images of each other or are separate cell types. Two other potential Cl^-/HCO_3^- exchangers, pendrin and AE4, which may reside apically in β-IC, have been reported in animals. Defects in pendrin cause Pendred's syndrome of deafness and goitre, but alkalosis is not a feature in either Pendred's patients or pendrin knockout mice. In any event, the acid load provided by an omnivorous human diet dictates that the great majority of ICs will be α-ICs.

There is a second, less structurally complex, P-type ATPase present apically in α-ICs, which exchanges protons for K^+. In humans, however, the overall contribution of H^+/K^+-ATPase to α-IC function is not clear.

Clinical presentation

RTA can range from being asymptomatic and undetectable without specialised biochemical tests, to presenting with a severe syndrome of failure to thrive in infancy. A list of causes of RTA is given

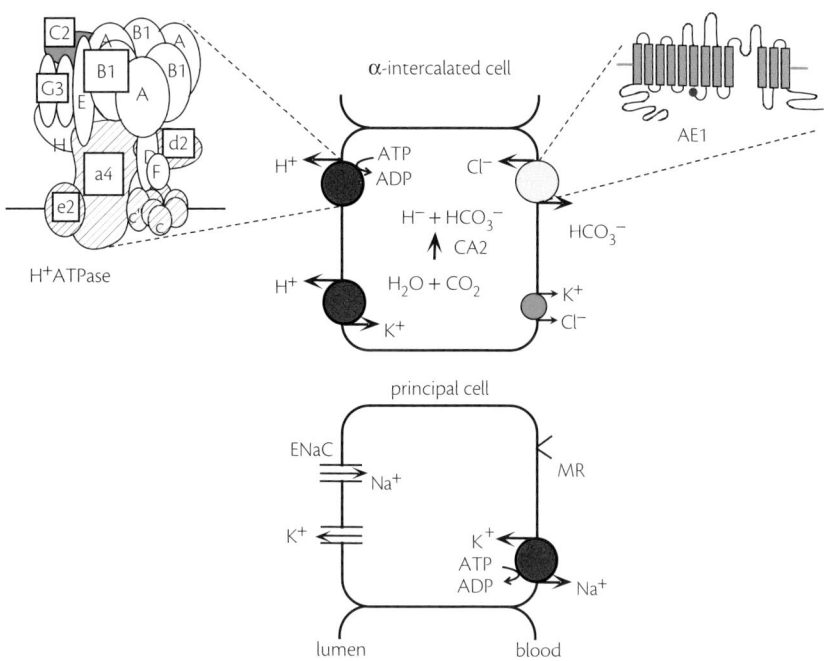

Fig. 21.15.2 Collecting duct acid–base regulation. Intercalated cells are responsible for coupled apical secretion of protons into the urine and reclamation of bicarbonate across the basolateral surface. On the apical surface, the multisubunit proton pump (H^+ATPase) transfers H^+ into the urine. The various subunits of this pump are shown on the left of the figure: mutations in B1 and a4 cause recessive dRTA. Basolateral bicarbonate exit (in exchange for chloride) occurs via the anion exchanger AE1. A cartoon of this exchanger is shown on the right of the figure, with R589—a mutational hotspot for dominant dRTA—marked with a red dot. There is a second, less structurally complex, P-type ATPase present on the apical surface and exit routes for K and Cl that are not yet well characterized in humans. The adjacent principal cells (responsible for salt handling) are depicted: electrogenic sodium reabsorption via the epithelial sodium channel ENaC takes place in exchange for K^+ secretion; this is under the control of aldosterone, acting via the basolateral mineralocorticoid receptor (MR).

in Table 21.15.1. The following patients should all be suspected of having RTA:

- Recurrent calcium-containing stone formers, especially if there is a family history
- Individuals with osteomalacia (rickets in children) without other clear explanation
- Patients with autoimmune disease, especially Sjögren's syndrome (see Chapter 19.11.6) and an unexplained low potassium and/or bicarbonate
- Infants with osteopetrosis
- Any with an unexplained metabolic acidosis

Biochemically, overt RTA is characterized by the presence of a normal anion gap (hyperchloraemic) metabolic acidosis in the setting of either reduced renal net acid secretion (distal RTAs) or bicarbonate wasting (proximal RTA), but otherwise normal or near normal renal excretory function. In distal RTA, similar molecular defects can cause mild or severe acidosis, the reason for which are not well understood. The clinical features of the various types of acidopathy are summarized in Table 21.15.2.

Proximal RTA

Clinical and biochemical features

The hallmark of proximal RTA is bicarbonate wasting into the urine. The consequent metabolic acidosis is often less severe than in other types of RTA, because as bicarbonate falls a larger proportion of it can be reabsorbed more distally, such that an equilibrium is reached at a venous bicarbonate level of around 15 mmol/litre.

The bicarbonate loss from the proximal tubule is usually accompanied by other features of proximal tubular dysfunction (i.e. the renal Fanconi syndrome), such as renal phosphate wasting (and hypophosphataemia), renal glycosuria, hypouricaemia (due to uricosuria), aminoaciduria, microalbuminuria, and other low-molecular-weight proteinuria (e.g. retinol binding protein or β_2-microglobulin, both of which can be measured in a spot urine sample). These patients also have rickets or osteomalacia (depending on age) because diminished proximal tubular protein reabsorption precludes sufficient vitamin D being reabsorbed, with conversion of $25OH-D_3$ to 1α-calcidol also being hampered.

The associated hypokalaemia may be severe, and this is attributed to up-regulated distal secretion of potassium, which may be exacerbated still further by the administration of alkali.

Cell biology and genetics

In adults, proximal RTA is usually discovered as a secondary manifestation of substances that interfere with tubular function such as myeloma proteins or drugs (e.g. cytotoxics or sodium valproate).

It may be a feature of renal transplant rejection, but in this context, general interstitial inflammation may also compromise distal nephron function.

Proximal RTA may be part of a renal Fanconi syndrome, (Table 21.15.1), either sporadic or inherited. The inherited syndromes - e.g. Lowe's (phosphatidylinositol 4,5- bisphosphate-5-phosphatase deficiency) and cystinosis - are often severe, are usually recognized

Table 21.15.1 Causes of RTA

		Proximal RTA	Classic distal RTA	Hyperkalaemic distal RTA
Acquired	Intrinsic renal disease	Hypokalaemic nephropathy Renal transplant rejection	Medullary sponge kidney Nephrocalcinosis	Diabetic nephropathy Interstitial nephritis
	Haematological disease	Myeloma	Myeloma	
	Drugs	Gentamicin Cisplatin Ifosfamide Sodium valproate Zidovudine	Amphotericin Lithium Ifosfamide	Trimethoprim Ciclosporin K-sparing diuretics ACE inhibitors/ARBs Heparin
	Heavy metals/toxins	Lead Cadmium Mercury Toluene (glue-sniffing)	Vanadate	
	Hormonal	Primary hyperparathyroidism	Pregnancy	
	Nutritional/other	Kwashiorkor (protein-energy malnutrition)	Autoimmunity (esp. Sjögren's syndrome)	
Inherited	Inherited renal disease	Autosomal dominant Fanconi syndrome Autosomal recessive proximal RTA X-linked (Dent disease, but acidosis usually mild and may be absent)	Autosomal dominant dRTA Autosomal recessive dRTA	Pseudohypoaldosteronism type 1 Gordon syndrome Hypomagnesaemia/hypercalciuria syndrome
	Inherited syndromes	Cystinosis Tyrosinaemia type 1 Galactosaemia Oculocerebrorenal syndrome (Lowe's syndrome) Wilson's disease Hereditary fructose intolerance	Sickle cell anaemia	

Table 21.15.2 Clinical and biochemical features of acidopathies

	Proximal RTA	Distal RTA—dominant/sporadic	Distal RTA—recessive	Mixed RTA	Hyperkalaemic RTA
Usual age of presentation	Childhood (primary) Adult (acquired)	Older/child/adult	Infancy/early childhood	Infancy/early childhood	Adult
Symptoms/signs	Variable including intellectual disability Rarely glaucoma/cataracts	Sometimes none Nephrolithiasis Nephrocalcinosis Sometimes rickets/osteomalacia	Vomiting/dehydration Poor growth Early nephrocalcinosis Rickets Sensorineural deafness	Fractures Poor growth Intellectual disability Blindness Osteopetrosis/fractures Conductive deafness Dental malocclusion	Related to underlying disorder e.g. diabetes complications
Biochemistry	Mild/moderate acidosis Normal/low K^+ (if Na^+ given)	Mild or compensated acidosis Low/normal K^+	Severe acidosis Low K^+	Severe acidosis Low K^+	Mild/moderate acidosis High K^+
Min urine pH	< 5.5	> 5.5	>5.5	>5.5	<5.5
Treatment	Much bicarbonate $\pm K^+$	Citrate/bicarbonate	Citrate/bicarbonate	Citrate/bicarbonate, bone marrow transplant	Sodium bicarbonate Fludrocortisone K^+-lowering drugs
Genes (primary disorders)	Loss of function *SLC4A4* Secondary: Fanconi syndromes	Mistargeting of *SLC4A1*	Loss of function *ATP6V1B1* or *ATP6V0A4*	Loss of function *CA2*	Loss of function *MR* or *CLDN16* Gain of function *WNK1* or *WNK4*

in infancy, and generally shorten life. Primary (autosomal recessive) proximal RTA is exceptionally rare, but serves to illustrate the importance of the basolateral sodium-bicarbonate transporter NBC1 (Fig. 21.15.1). It is due to mutations in *SLC4A4*, which encodes NBC1. The features here are isolated bicarbonate wasting with aberrant calcification within the eyes (known as band keratopathy), cataracts and intellectual disability. The corneal endothelium normally transports sodium and bicarbonate from corneal stroma to aqueous humour, hence this same sodium bicarbonate cotransporter is thought to play a role in preservation of corneal clarity.

In contrast, Dent disease is a rare X-linked condition that is an umbrella term for a group of allelic disorders including X-linked recessive nephrolithiasis, hypophosphataemic rickets, and low molecular-weight proteinuria syndrome. Boys or men presenting with features of proximal tubular dysfunction and stones or nephrocalcinosis may have Dent's. They usually have high levels of low-molecular weight proteinuria and phosphate wasting, but other proximal tubular features may be absent. Indeed acidosis is at worst usually mild. The defective gene is *CLCN5*, which encodes an intracellular chloride channel present both proximally and distally that participates in the acidification of subapical vesicular structures and not directly in cell surface proton movement, hence any observed acidosis is not fully accounted for.

Distal RTA with hypokalaemia (classic distal RTA)

Clinical and biochemical features

Classic distal RTA arises when the collecting ducts fail to excrete excess acid into the urine. It is therefore characterized biochemically by failure of the kidney to produce appropriately acid urine in the presence of systemic metabolic acidosis or following acid loading (e.g. with ammonium chloride). The spectrum of clinical severity is very wide, ranging from compensated mild acidosis, absence of symptoms, and the incidental finding of renal tract calcification or stones, to major effects in infancy with severe acidosis, impaired growth, and early nephrocalcinosis, eventually causing renal insufficiency. The combination of low systemic pH, a normal anion gap (see below) and a urinary pH above 5.5 is suspicious of distal RTA, particularly if K$^+$ is reduced. If the urine pH is as high as 8, infection with urea-splitting organisms must be excluded.

Mild cases of distal RTA may require formal acidification testing for confirmation, e.g. in the context of recurrent stone formation. Chronic dRTA is almost always accompanied by nephrocalcinosis and/or nephrolithiasis associated with hypercalciuria. Why some patients get stones while others calcify the parenchyma remains a mystery. Urinary citrate is low in dRTA because citrate reabsorption is up-regulated in the proximal tubule to provide new bicarbonate. Abnormal calcium deposition is attributable in large part to this hypocitraturia and to urine alkalinity, but the exact mechanisms are unclear.

Other biochemical findings in dRTA include hypokalaemia, which may be marked, and as with proximal RTA is attributed to increased compensatory distal K$^+$ secretion, but here it arises because protons are failing to be moved into the urine. Metabolic bone disease (osteomalacia or rickets) occurs in untreated cases; calcium and phosphate levels are usually normal.

Most commonly, dRTA is acquired in the context of immunological diseases and drugs (see Table 21.15.1) and should be reversible when disease remits or drugs are withdrawn. However, both autosomal dominant and autosomal recessive inheritance patterns

have been reported in hypokalaemic distal RTA (OMIM 179800, 267300, 602722). In general, though not invariably, patients with dominant distal RTA display a milder phenotype than do those with recessively inherited disease. In addition, among patients with recessive but not dominant disease, many have progressive and irreversible bilateral sensorineural hearing loss. Vestibular aqueductal widening is reported in association with recessive dRTA, but this abnormality is not pathognomonic, also being seen in branchio–oto–renal syndrome and Pendred's syndrome, and in isolation. Rarely, classic distal RTA arises in pregnancy and resolves with delivery of the fetus.

Cell biology and genetics

At the time of early descriptions, dRTA was thought to be due to 'back-leak' of normally secreted protons across a leaky tubular epithelium. It later became evident that, apart from in the case of amphotericin (where intercellular permeability is compromised and back-leakage does indeed occur), acid secretion itself is abnormal, due to failure of hydrogen ion secretion in the cortical collecting duct. It is now clear that defective function in at least three components of the α-IC's polarized membrane transporters can cause dRTA (Fig. 21.15.2). Mutations in genes encoding two different subunits of the apical proton pump that are tissue-specific forms (the B1 and a4 subunits) cause loss of pump function and recessive disease, usually but not always with progressive sensorineural hearing loss. This form of dRTA rarely presents for the first time beyond childhood. If treatment has been complied with, these patients reach adulthood and the renal clinic.

B1 and a4 are both expressed within the cochlea and endolymphatic sac. This is of interest because endolymph, the fluid that fills these compartments, has a unique ionic composition with a very high [K$^+$] of some 150 mmol/litre. Given that endolymph pH is less than 7.4 (rather than the predicted alkalinity), this implies a requirement for proton pumping into this fluid. Although it remains speculative in the absence of a suitable animal model, the idea is that defective H$^+$-ATPase function leads to raised endolymph pH and eventual irremediable functional loss of hair cells, which would explain why alkali therapy is of no help to the deafness of recessive dRTA.

At the basolateral cell surface, proper AE1 localization is essential for normal function, and heterozygous mutations that disrupt trafficking and/or targeting lead to dominant dRTA. It is notable that expression of various mutant AE1s in xenopus oocytes does not generally result in significant loss of function, suggesting that distal RTA is not due to haploinsufficiency. Indeed, mutations in the longer version of the same gene cause the dominant red-cell morphological diseases hereditary spherocytosis and ovalocytosis. Some of these would lead to severe disruption or absence of the encoded protein, but are not usually associated with dRTA. Recessive dRTA due to AE1 mutations is very rare and confined to Thailand. Much more prevalent in East Asia is an acquired form of distal RTA that is related to the high levels of vanadium found in soil, which inhibits the H$^+$/K$^+$-ATPase at the apical surface of α-ICs.

Distal RTA with hyperkalaemia

Clinical and biochemical features

When distal RTA is accompanied by hyperkalaemia, it is usually secondary to drugs or to hyporeninaemic hypoaldosteronism, which is itself most often found in the context of diabetes mellitus. (Table 21.15.1). The acidosis here is secondary to the kidney's failure to conserve sodium and secrete potassium (i.e. a failure of principal cell function). Drugs most commonly associated with hyperkalaemic RTA include trimethoprim, ciclosporin and angiotensin converting enzyme (ACE) inhibitors. Trimethoprim acts as an antagonist of the epithelial sodium channel, whilst ciclosporin inhibits the basolateral Na^+,K^+-ATPase, and ACE inhibitors directly interfere with the renin–angiotensin–aldosterone axis.

Cell biology and genetics

Inadequate sodium reabsorption in the collecting duct diminishes lumen negativity such that potassium and proton secretion are both inhibited. Hyperkalaemia inhibits the generation of ammonium, which contributes to the acidosis.

Rarely, this type of distal RTA is part of an inherited disorder, e.g. Gordon's syndrome or hypomagnesaemia/hypercalciuria syndrome. In Gordon's syndrome (also known as pseudohypoaldosteronism type 2) there is hypertension, hyperkalaemia, and metabolic acidosis with normal urine acidification capacity. Two responsible genes have been identified; these encode members of the 'with-no-lysine' (WNK) family that are regulators of a number of ion transporters. The result is an up-regulation of distal convoluted tubule reabsorption of Na^+ and Cl^-, the other biochemical changes being secondary to this. The defect in hypomagnesaemia/hypercalciuria syndrome is in an intercellular protein, paracellin, that acts as a magnesium and calcium channel in the loop of Henle. Again, electrochemical imbalance in the downstream nephron leads to metabolic acidosis.

Mixed RTA

The entity of transient mixed proximal/distal RTA arising just after birth enjoyed some popularity a few decades ago, but it is now thought not to represent a distinct disease process, but rather a developmental hiatus in that distal nephron function continues to mature after birth. However, RTA with the characteristics of both proximal and distal tubular dysfunction usually accompanies one form of autosomal recessive osteopetrosis (Guibaud–Vainsel syndrome or marble brain disease, OMIM 259730), when both defective urinary acidification and bicarbonate wasting may be present, although each has been reported individually. This condition is characterized by thickened bones that fracture, short stature, intellectual disability, dental malocclusion, visual impairment from optic nerve compression, and (sometimes) calcification of the basal ganglia. Loss of carbonic anhydrase 2 is the biochemical defect, and loss-of-function mutations in *CA2* have been described. The commonest of these involves loss of the splice donor site in intron 2, nicknamed the Arabic mutation. CA2 is expressed in both proximal and distal nephron segments, explaining the mixed acidosis, and in osteoclasts, whose loss of function results in the bone thickening.

Diagnosis of RTA

When considering the diagnosis of RTA in a particular case, it is helpful to proceed by asking the following questions or performing the following tests.

1 Is there acidosis? RTA should be suspected if the serum bicarbonate low without evidence of gastrointestinal losses. Measure arterial blood gases to confirm the type of acidosis.

2 Is the anion gap normal? Calculate $(Na^+ + K^+) - (Cl^- + HCO_3^-)$ in plasma, as long as the patient is not severely dehydrated. In RTA the anion gap is normal (12–16 mmol/litre, corrected for albumin).

3 What is the plasma potassium? If this is low, suspect classic dRTA or proximal RTA. If raised, measure plasma renin and aldosterone.

4 What is the urine pH? This must be measured in a freshly voided urine sample using a pH meter. If there is to be any delay in measurement, overlay urine with mineral oil to exclude air.

5 What is the urinary ammonium (NH_4)? Measurement of this may sometimes be necessary to differentiate types of RTA when urinary pH is high. Most labs are not able to measure this directly, when it must be calculated from the urine osmolal gap: $U_{NH4} = 0.5$(measured – calculated U_{osm}), with calculated $U_{osm} = 2U_{Na} + 2U_K + U_{glucose} + U_{urea}$ (but note that this calculation only applies if the serum creatinine is normal and the liver works). A normal value is about 100 mmol/litre.

6 Urine acidification testing. In some patients with hypokalaemic distal RTA the biochemical abnormalities are masked by compensatory mechanisms that are not well understood. The plasma bicarbonate may therefore be within the normal range, but the urinary pH will still be high, hence formal urine acidification testing may occasionally be necessary to reveal the dRTA (traditionally referred to as 'incomplete' dRTA). The 'gold standard' test of urine acidification relies on the ability of the kidneys rapidly to excrete an orally ingested acid load and thereby reduce urine pH to less than 5.5. Ammonium chloride (0.1 g/kg) is the traditional load, but it is highly unpalatable and may cause vomiting and other gastrointestinal discomfort such that the test is rarely used. As an alternative, the combination of fludrocortisone and furosemide should cause the collecting duct to receive more sodium such that it up-regulates acid extrusion sufficient to generate urine pH <5.5. However, patients may fail this test and need to go on to ammonium chloride testing, so we currently recommend it only as a screening tool to rule out dRTA.

7 Measure urinary citrate. This is low in distal RTA (requires 24-h collection into a vessel containing HCl).

8 Look for additional evidence of proximal tubular dysfunction. If proximal RTA is suspected: measure urinary phosphate and urate (high); dipstick test for glucose (with concomitant plasma glucose measurement); measure plasma urate; measure urinary low-molecular-weight protein excretion and quantify albumin excretion (albumin: creatinine ratio).

Box 21.15.1 Interpretation of investigations

◆ Acidosis + normal anion gap + alkaline urine + low urine citrate and NH_4 = classic distal RTA

◆ Acidosis + normal anion gap + high urine NH_4 = proximal RTA. Urine pH may be high or low depending on bicarbonate level; other tests of proximal function are usually abnormal

◆ Acidosis + normal anion gap + hyperkalaemia + low aldosterone and/or relevant drug history = hyperkalaemic distal RTA

Urine P_{CO_2} is often quoted as being low in distal RTA, but meaningful measurement requires intravenous bicarbonate loading and the test is very rarely used.

See Box 21.15.1 for interpretation of the results of these investigations.

Management

Provision of alkali is the mainstay of treatment in all forms of RTA, whether to replace losses or to buffer retained acid. Either bicarbonate or citrate can be used. Proximal RTA is more difficult to treat than distal because of the amount of bicarbonaturia, and very large quantities of alkali supplementation may be required. This often has the effect of further reducing the serum potassium, hence potassium supplements are frequently necessary, as may be supplementation of vitamin D and phosphate, which are often deficient in proximal tubular dysfunctional states.

Simple alkali replacement on its own is sufficient to reverse most of the biochemical abnormalities and associated bone disease in classic distal RTA, permitting resumption of normal growth and reversal of metabolic bone disease. Doses of 1–3 mEq/kg per day are usually sufficient. Potassium salts are preferable to sodium as the latter can exacerbate both hypokalaemia and hypercalciuria. However, while alkali administration prevents further renal tract calcium deposition, the deafness associated with some forms of distal RTA is not reversible, because (as described previously) orally administered alkali does not access the inner ear compartment. Compliance with treatment is important because uncontrolled stone formation (with associated obstruction), infection and/or nephrocalcinosis will eventually lead to renal impairment and sometimes endstage kidney disease.

Management of hyperkalaemic dRTA includes withdrawal of precipitating drugs and provision of sodium bicarbonate. Fludrocortisone and/or potassium-lowering measures such as oral resins may be necessary. Lowering potassium will have a beneficial effect on renal ammoniagenesis.

There is no specific treatment of CA2 deficiency other than alkali supplementation, although the osteopetrosis can be cured by bone marrow transplantation.

Further reading

Borthwick KJ, Karet FE (2002). Inherited disorders of the H⁺-ATPase. *Curr Opin Nephrol Hypertens*, **11**, 563–8.

Laing CM, Unwin RJ (2006). Renal tubular acidosis. *J Nephrol*, **19** Suppl 9, S46–52.

Quigley R (2006). Proximal renal tubular acidosis. *J Nephrol* **19**, Suppl 9, S41–5.

Wagner CA *et al.* (2006). Renal acid–base transport: old and new players. *Nephron Physiol*, **103**, 1–6. Doloreros alis eu feugiat. Ectet wisi.

Disorders of tubular electrolyte handling

Nine V.A.M. Knoers and Elena N. Levtchenko

Essentials

Glycosuria

Physiology—glucose reabsorption in the proximal tubule is carried out by two different pairs of apical Na^+-dependent (SGLT1 and 2) and basolateral Na^+-independent (GLUT1 and 2) glucose transporters.

Clinical disorders—abnormalities in renal glucose transport can be seen in association with other defects of proximal tubular transport (Fanconi syndrome, see below). Familial renal glycosuria is an autosomal recessive condition caused by mutations in the SGLT2-encoding gene, SLC5A2.

Phosphate-handling disorders

Physiology—the plasma concentration of inorganic phosphate depends on the balance between intestinal absorption, renal excretion, and the internal contribution from bone. Absorption in the small intestine is mainly mediated by the brush border membrane sodium-dependent transporter, isoform NaPi-IIb. In the kidney about 80% of filtered phosphate is reabsorbed in the proximal tubule. In the proximal tubules, phosphate reabsorption is mediated by two members of the SLC34 family, NaPi-IIa and NaPiIIc, which are specifically expressed in the brush border membrane of proximal tubular cells. Renal phosphate excretion is regulated by numerous hormones and other factors, with key regulators being parathyroid hormone (PTH) and fibroblast growth factor 23 (FGF23), both of which cause phosphaturia.

Clinical disorders—changes of serum phosphate levels can be caused by numerous inherited and acquired conditions (frequently during severe infections). Disorders associated with increased urinary phosphate excretion and low serum phosphate levels produce symptoms that mainly affect the bones: rickets in children and osteomalacia in adults.

X-linked hypophosphataemic rickets (XLH)—this is the most frequent (prevalence 1:20 000) and best-characterized inherited disorder of renal phosphate metabolism. It is caused by inactivating mutations of the cell-surface endopeptidase PHEX, is inherited as an X-linked dominant disorder, and presents with growth retardation, femoral and/or tibial bowing, rickets/osteomalacia, low serum phosphate, and inappropriately normal 1,25-dihydroxycholecalciferol (calcitriol; $1,25(OH)_2$ D) for the degree of hypophosphataemia. Treatment is with administration of phosphate and calcitriol.

Magnesium-handling disorders

Physiology—normal plasma magnesium concentration is achieved by variation of urinary magnesium excretion in response to altered uptake by the intestine. The main site of magnesium absorption is the small bowel, via paracellular simple diffusion at high intraluminal concentrations, and via active transcellular uptake through the magnesium channel TRPM6 (transient receptor potential channel melastatin 6) at low concentrations. Regulation and fine-tuning of serum magnesium concentration occurs primarily in the kidney: most filtered magnesium is passively reabsorbed in the thick ascending limb of Henle's loop through the paracellular pathway via claudin proteins; active and modulated reabsorption takes place in the distal convoluted tubule via the epithelial magnesium channel, TRPM6.

Clinical disorders—hypomagnesaemia is common in hospitalized patients, and often an acquired disorder resulting from deficient oral intake or accelerated urinary or intestinal loss. Genetic disorders of magnesium handling include Gitelman's syndrome, which is an autosomal recessive condition caused by loss-of-function mutations in the SLC12A3 gene that encodes the renal thiazide-sensitive sodium-chloride cotransporter NCCT. Most patients suffer from carpopedal spasms; paraesthaesias are frequent; some experience severe fatigue; a few develop chondrocalcinosis. Most patients remain untreated, but there is an argument for lifelong supplementation of magnesium; hypokalaemia can be treated by drugs that antagonize the activity of aldosterone (e.g. spironolactone) or block the epithelial sodium channel (ENaC) in the distal nephron (e.g. amiloride).

Aminoaciduria and renal Fanconi syndrome

Physiology—most amino acids (except for tryptophan, which is protein bound) are freely filtered by the glomerulus, after which 95% to 99.9% are reabsorbed in the proximal tubules by apical Na^+-dependent cotransporters (for neutral amino acids, aromatic neutral amino acids, and anionic amino acids) and Na⁺-independent cotransporters (H⁺-cotransporter for glycine and proline; heterodimeric exchanger bo,+AT-rBat for cystine, and cationic amino acids). Aminoaciduria is defined as urinary excretion of more than 5% of the filtered load of an amino acid.

Specific aminoacidurias—these include (1) cystinuria, which manifests with urinary stones (see Chapter 21.14); (2) Hartnup's disease, associated with defective renal and intestinal absorption of neutral amino acids (see Chapter 12.2); (3) Lysinuric protein intolerance, caused by defective dibasic amino acid transport and progressing to renal failure in some patients (see Chapter 12.2).

Renal Fanconi syndrome—this is characterized by generalized defect of both Na⁺-coupled and megalin-dependent proximal tubular transport. Symptoms manifest at various ages dependent on the underlying condition and comprise generalized aminoaciduria; glycosuria; renal sodium, potassium, urate and phosphate wasting; proximal tubular acidosis; and low-molecular-weight proteinuria and albuminuria. It can be caused by inherited (e.g. cystinosis) or acquired (e.g. Sjögren's syndrome, drugs) conditions.

Glycosuria

Physiology of renal glucose handling

The glomeruli filter about 180 g of glucose from the plasma each day, which is almost completely reabsorbed by the renal tubules under normal circumstances, with less than 0.05% excreted in the urine: 90% is reabsorbed in the proximal convoluted tubule, and the remainder in the proximal straight tubule, the loop of Henle, and—to some extent—in the collecting duct.

Transepithelial glucose reabsorption in the proximal tubule is carried out by two different pairs of apical Na⁺-dependent and basolateral Na⁺-independent glucose transporters. A low-affinity/high capacity Na⁺-glucose cotransporter, SGLT2, and a basolateral Na⁺-independent, low-affinity transporter, GLUT2, are responsible for the bulk of glucose reabsorption in the early, convoluted part of the proximal tubule. A high-affinity/low-capacity Na⁺-glucose cotransporter, SGLT1, coupled with the basolateral Na⁺-independent, high-affinity GLUT1 reabsorbs the remaining filtered glucose in the late pars recta of the proximal tubule. SGTL2 is almost exclusively expressed in the kidney proximal tubule, whereas SGLT1 is also strongly expressed in the small intestine.

Renal glycosuria

Familial renal glycosuria is an inherited renal tubular disorder, characterized by persistent glycosuria in the presence of normal fasting blood glucose levels and a normal glucose tolerance test. It is caused by mutations in *SLC5A2*, the gene encoding sodium/glucose cotransporter SGLT2. The disorder is inherited in an autosomal recessive pattern, although mild glycosuria in some heterozygous carriers has led some investigators to postulate codominant inheritance with variable penetrance. Individuals with familial renal glycosuria are generally asymptomatic, except for occasional cases in which polyuria has been described.

Renal glycosuria, although rather mild, is also found in patients with intestinal glucose–galactose malabsorption. This autosomal recessive disease is characterized by a neonatal onset of severe watery diarrhoea that results in death unless glucose and galactose are removed from the diet. It is caused by mutations in *SLC5A1*, the gene encoding sodium/glucose cotransporter SGLT1.

Abnormalities in renal glucose transport can also be seen in association with other defects of proximal tubular transport. Collectively these are designated as Fanconi syndrome, in which renal glycosuria is part of a general disorder of proximal tubular function, with aminoaciduria, phosphaturia, and renal tubular acidosis.

The Fanconi–Bickel syndrome, a very rare autosomal recessive condition characterized by hepatorenal glycogen accumulation, Fanconi syndrome, and impaired utilization of glucose and galactose, is caused by mutations in *SLC2A2*, the gene encoding GLUT2. Impaired function of the GLUT2 protein, which normally facilitates glucose efflux at the basolateral membrane of tubular cells, leads to an accumulation of free glucose and glycogen within the proximal tubular cell. By a mechanism not yet fully understood, this leads to Fanconi syndrome with disproportionately severe glycosuria.

Phosphate-handling disorders

Physiological control of plasma phosphate

The plasma concentration of inorganic phosphate (hereafter simply termed 'phosphate') depends on the balance between intestinal absorption, renal excretion, and the internal contribution from bone: it remains within the range 0.8 to 1.5 mmol/litre despite wide variation in intake. Active absorption of phosphate in the small intestine is mainly mediated by the brush border membrane sodium-dependent transporter, isoform NaPi-IIb (a member of the SLC34 family of solute carriers), and is regulated by active vitamin D metabolites. In plasma about one-half of the total phosphate is in an ionized form, and the rest either makes complexes with small solutes (c.40%) or is bound to protein (c.10–15%). In the kidney, free phosphate and that bound to small solutes is freely filtered by the glomerulus, about 80% is reabsorbed in the proximal tubule, about 10% by the distal tubule (especially in case of low-phosphate diet), and about 10% is finally excreted in the urine.

In the proximal tubules phosphate reabsorption is mediated by two members of the SLC34 family, NaPi-IIa and NaPiIIc, which are specifically expressed in the brush border membrane of proximal tubular cells. NaPi-IIa, preferentially transporting divalent phosphate with a Na⁺:phosphate stoichiometry of 3:1, is the main protein responsible for phosphate reabsorption in the adult kidney. NaPi-IIc is also expressed on the brush border membrane of proximal tubular cells, has a Na⁺:phosphate stoichiometry of 2:1, and seems to play a more important role in renal phosphate reabsorption during infancy and childhood.

The mechanism of the exit of phosphate across the basolateral membrane of both intestinal and proximal tubular epithelial cells is not yet known. The NaPi-III cotransporter on the basolateral membrane presumably mediates the uptake of phosphate rather than its exit.

Renal phosphate excretion is regulated by numerous hormones and other factors (Table 21.16.1), with parathyroid hormone (PTH) being the key regulator. Binding of PTH to apical and basolateral PTH receptors activates protein lipase C/protein kinase C and protein kinase A cascades, respectively. Both pathways lead to the endocytotic removal of NaPi from the apical membrane, thus reducing phosphate reabsorption.

In conditions where the body requires enhanced phosphate reabsorption, e.g. low-phosphate diet, more NaPi cotransporters

Table 21.16.1 Factors modulating renal phosphate excretion

Factors increasing renal phosphate excretion	Factors decreasing renal phosphate excretion
PTH	1,25(OH)$_2$ vitamin D
FGF23	High calcium intake
High dietary phosphate intake	Phosphate deprivation
High plasma phosphate	Insulin
Extracellular volume expansion	Alkalosis
Acidosis	Thyroid hormone
Glucocorticoids	Growth hormone
Calcitonin	
ANP	
Dopamine	
PTHrP	
Diuretics	
Acute renal denervation	

ANP, atrial natriuretic peptide; FGF23, fibroblast growth factor 23; PTHrP, parathyroid hormone related peptide.

are expressed at the apical membrane by mechanisms stabilizing the transporters and increasing the rate of their insertion into the brush border membrane. Vitamin 1,25(OH)$_2$ D up-regulates the cotransporters. High dietary phosphate intake decreases phosphate reabsorption without changes in PTH levels.

A novel hormone, fibroblast growth factor 23 (FGF23), has been recognized as an important player in several disorders of phosphate metabolism. This is predominantly expressed in the osteocytes and principally acts as a phosphaturic factor and a suppressor of 1α-hydroxylase activity in the kidney, inhibiting the synthesis of 1,25(OH)$_2$ vitamin D. FGF23 interacts with a family of FGF receptors, the activation of which requires the cofactor Klotho, determining tissue-specific actions of FGF23. Although Klotho is mainly expressed in the distal renal tubule, low levels of expression in the proximal tubule are suggested. Circulating FGF23 levels are regulated by an X-linked phosphate-regulating endopeptidase homologue (PHEX), dentin matrix protein 1 (DMP1), and matrix extracellular phosphoglycoprotein (MEPE), all synthesized in osteocytes, and also by phosphate and 1,25(OH)$_2$ D.

Changes of serum phosphate levels can be caused by numerous inherited and acquired conditions (frequently during severe infections). In this chapter the few clinically relevant disorders of renal phosphate handling are highlighted, most of which are linked to alterations in FGF23 levels (Table 21.16.2).

Disorders associated with increased urinary phosphate excretion

These disorders are characterized by low serum phosphate levels and inappropriate phosphaturia (Table 21.16.2). The tubular reabsorption of phosphate (TRP = 1 −C_{pi}/C_{cr}, where C_{pi} is the urinary clearance of phosphate and C_{cr} is the creatinine clearance, with normal TRP >80%) and tubular maximum transport for phosphate (T_m P$_i$/100 ml GFR = P_{pi} − (U_{pi} × P_{cr})/U_{cr}, where P_{pi} is plasma phosphate concentration and U_{pi} is urinary phosphate

concentration, with normal T_m P$_i$/GFR = 0.8–1.4) are decreased. Different age-dependent reference values should be applied for children.

Clinical symptoms vary in severity and mainly concern the bones: rickets in children and osteomalacia in adults.

Inherited disorders

X-linked hypophosphataemic rickets (XLH)
XLH is the most frequent (prevalence 1:20 000) and best characterized inherited disorder of renal phosphate metabolism, also known as vitamin D-resistant rickets, for which two murine models (*Hyp* and *Gy* mice) are available. It is caused by inactivating mutations of the cell surface endopeptidase PHEX, and is inherited in an X-linked dominant pattern. The disease manifests with growth retardation, femoral and/or tibial bowing, evidence of rickets and osteomalacia, low serum phosphate levels, and inappropriately normal 1,25(OH)$_2$ D for the degree of hypophosphataemia. Consistent with X-linked dominant inheritance, males are usually more severely affected than females and there is variable penetrance. Inactivation of PHEX leads to increased expression of FGF23, causing phosphaturia and the inhibition of 1,25(OH)$_2$ D synthesis. Treatment is with administration of phosphate and 1,25(OH)$_2$ D (calcitriol), which must be monitored closely because of the risk of nephrocalcinosis that might impair renal function.

Autosomal dominant hypophosphataemic rickets (ADHR)
ADHR is characterized by incomplete penetrance, delayed onset (adolescent or adult age), and occasional spontaneous resolution of phosphate wasting. The disease may also manifest in children, resembling XLH. ADHR is caused by mutations in the RXXR furin-like cleavage domain of the FGF23, which impairs proteolytic degradation of FGF23.

Autosomal recessive hypophosphataemic rickets (ARHR)
ARHR is caused by inactivating mutations of the dentin matrix acidic phosphoprotein DMP1, resulting in increased transcription of FGF23 in osteocytes.

Analogous to XLH, patients with ADHR and ARHR have elevated circulating FGF23 levels and inappropriately normal 1,25(OH)$_2$ D due to the inhibition by FGF23.

The therapy of ADHR and ARHR is similar to XLH and consists of the combination of oral phosphate and vitamin D.

Autosomal recessive rickets with hypercalciuria (HHRH)
Unlike other forms of hypophosphataemia, HHRH associates with elevated levels of 1,25(OH)$_2$ D, which leads to increased intestinal reabsorption of calcium and hypercalciuria. Because the phenotype of HHRH is similar to that of NaPi-IIa deficient mice, heterozygous mutations in NaPi-IIa cotransporter were initially suggested as the cause of this disorder, but later were not confirmed. Homozygous mutations in *SLC34A3*, the gene encoding the NaPi-IIc cotransporter, have been demonstrated in patients with HHRH, indicating a more critical role of this transporter in renal phosphate handling. Treatment is with phosphate supplementation.

Sporadic/acquired disorders

Oncogenic hypophosphataemic osteomalacia (OHO)
OHO, also known as tumor-induced osteomalacia, is a rare form of renal phosphate wasting associated with tumors of mesenchymal origin and likely to result from FGF23 production by the tumor.

Table 21.16.2 Inherited disorders of renal phosphate handling (note—this list of conditions is not exhaustive)

Disorder	OMIM	Gene/inheritance	Protein	Key clinical/biochemical features
Disorders associated with increased urinary phosphate excretion and low serum phosphate				
X-linked hypophosphataemic rickets (XLH)	307800	*PHEX*/XL-D	Cell surface endopeptidase Phex	Growth retardation. Rickets, bowing of extremities, osteomalacia. Normal 1,25(OH)$_2$ vitamin D
Autosomal dominant hypophosphataemic rickets (ADHR)	193100	*FGF23*/AD	Fibroblast growth factor 23	See those of XLH Delayed onset Incomplete penetrance
Autosomal recessive hypophosphataemic rickets (ARHR)	241520	*DMP1*/AR	Dentin matrix acidic phosphoprotein	See those of XLH. Severe presentation Dental defects Osteosclerosis
Autosomal recessive hypophosphataemic rickets with hypercalciuria (HHRH)	241530	*SLC34A3*/AR	NaPi-lic cotransporter	Growth retardation Rickets Hypercalciuria Elevated levels of 1,25(OH)$_2$ D
Disorders associated with decreased urinary phosphate excretion and elevated serum phosphate				
Hyperphosphataemic familial tumoral calcinosis (HFTC)	211900	*FGF23* Inactivating mutations/AR	Fibroblast growth factor 23	Elevated/normal serum phosphate levels Soft tissues calcifications Normal/elevated 1,25(OH)$_2$ D
		GLANT3/AR	Glycosyltransferase GalNAc. Decreased FGF23 stability,	
Pseudohypoparathyroidism Ia (PHP)	103580	*GNAS1*/AD (usually)	Guanine nucleotide binding protein, alpha-stimulating activity polypeptide 1, GNAS1 Gs, α subunit	Hypocalcaemia and elevated serum PTH Short stature, obesity, round facies, subcutaneous calcification, short metacarpals (particularly 5th and 4th), intellectual disability Normal serum calcium and PTH Other features as for PHP: both conditions may occur in same family

AD, autosomal dominant; AR, autosomal recessive; XL-D, X linked dominant.

Some other genes, including *MEPE*, have been implicated in the condition: this has been demonstrated to inhibit PHEX and can indirectly increase FGF23 levels and cause phosphaturia. Surgical removal of the tumor leads to normalization of FGF23 levels and disappearance of phosphate wasting.

McCune–Albright syndrome
McCune–Albright syndrome is caused by a somatic mosaicism for activating mutations in the *GNAS1* gene and is characterized by variable clinical symptoms including polyostotic fibrous dysplasia, pigmentary patches of the skin, and endocrine organ involvement including hyperthyroidism, Cushing's syndrome, pituitary gigantism, and precocious puberty. Approximately half of the patients have hypophosphataemia due to increased circulating levels of FGF23, presumably synthesized by the fibrodysplastic tissue.

Disorders associated with decreased urinary phosphate excretion
Inherited disorders
Hyperphosphataemic familial tumoral calcinosis (HFTC)
HFTC is a rare autosomal recessive disorder that is the clinical converse of ADHR. It is characterized by the progressive deposition of basic calcium phosphate crystals in periarticular spaces and soft tissues. Treatment is with dietary phosphate restriction and phosphate binders, with surgical excision of calcific masses when appropriate.

Pseudohypoparathyroidism (PHP)
PHP includes a heterogeneous group of disorders characterized by resistance to the action of PTH: see Chapter 13.6 for further discussion. Treatment is with phosphate binders and active vitamin D metabolites (e.g. alphacalcidol, calcitriol) as required.

Hypoparathyroidism
See Chapter 13.6.

Sporadic/acquired disorders
Severe depression of glomerular filtration rate of any cause is associated with depression of urinary phosphate excretion and hyperphosphataemia. Hypoparathyroidism can be acquired as part of a pluriglandular autoimmune condition (see Chapter 13.6): it is also the consequence of total parathyroidectomy, most commonly performed as treatment for tertiary hyperparathyroidism that is not responsive to medical treatment (see Chapter 21.0).

Magnesium handling disorders
Physiological control of plasma magnesium
Magnesium is the second most abundant intracellular cation and plays an essential role in a wide variety of biological activities. Normal plasma magnesium concentration (0.75–1.4 mmol/litre) is achieved by modulation of urinary magnesium excretion in response to altered uptake by the intestine. The main site of absorption is the

small bowel, where approximately one-third of dietary magnesium is absorbed: some additional absorption takes place in the large bowel. Absorption in the small bowel occurs via paracellular simple diffusion at high intraluminal concentrations and, at low concentrations, via active transcellular uptake through the magnesium channel TRPM6 (transient receptor potential channel melastatin 6), which is expressed along the brush border membrane of the small intestine. The TRPM6 protein belongs to a large family of transient receptor potential (TRP) cation channels which play an important role in a wide variety of physiological processes, ranging from thermal, tactile, taste, osmolar, and fluid flow sensing, to transepithelial calcium and magnesium transport. Detailed electrophysiological analyses and expression studies have demonstrated that TRPM6 is a magnesium-permeable channel that is specifically localized to the apical membrane of magnesium-reabsorbing tubular segments in the kidney (distal convoluted tubule) and the brush border membrane of the magnesium-absorptive cells in the small intestine.

Regulation and fine-tuning of serum magnesium concentration occurs primarily in the kidney. Approximately 2500 mg of magnesium is filtered per day, 96% of which is reabsorbed along the nephron. Only a small portion (5–15%) is reabsorbed in the proximal tubule. In the thick ascending limb of Henle's loop 50 to 72% of filtered magnesium is passively reabsorbed through the paracellular pathway via claudin proteins that create charge-selective channels in the tight junctions between the epithelial cells. Active reabsorption of magnesium takes place in the distal convoluted tubule and accounts for 10% of the total filtered load: this is the last site of magnesium reabsorption, hence the final urinary secretion of magnesium is determined here. The epithelial magnesium channel, TRPM6, is essential for the apical influx of magnesium (Fig. 21.16.1), but the mechanisms of cytosolic magnesium diffusion and basolateral transport of magnesium are not yet clear.

Disorders causing abnormal plasma magnesium

Hypomagnesaemia is a common finding in hospitalized patients, and often an acquired disorder resulting from deficient oral intake or accelerated urinary or intestinal loss. Renal magnesium wasting is commonly caused by drug therapy (i.e. diuretics, aminoglycosides, immunosuppressive agents), alcohol, and osmotic diuresis (i.e. diabetes mellitus). It has recently been described that hypomagnesaemia is also a frequent, and sometimes severe, side effect of cetuximab, a monoclonal antibody against the epidermal growth factor receptor (EGFR), used in the treatment of colorectal cancer.

Hypermagnesaemia is a rare and generally iatrogenic condition. Those at risk are elderly people and patients with bowel disorders or renal insufficiency. Hypermagnesaemia may also be found in familial hypocalciuric hypercalcaemia and neonatal severe hypoparathyroidism, resulting from inactivating mutations in the gene encoding the calcium/magnesium-sensing receptor.

Table 21.16.3 summarizes the presently known genetic disorders of magnesium handling, the most important of which are discussed below.

Gitelman's syndrome

Gitelman's syndrome is an autosomal recessive disorder characterized by hypomagnesaemia accompanied by hypocalciuria, hypokalaemia and metabolic alkalosis. Patients usually present after the age of 6 years, and in many cases the diagnosis is only made in adulthood. Most patients suffer from carpopedal spasms, especially

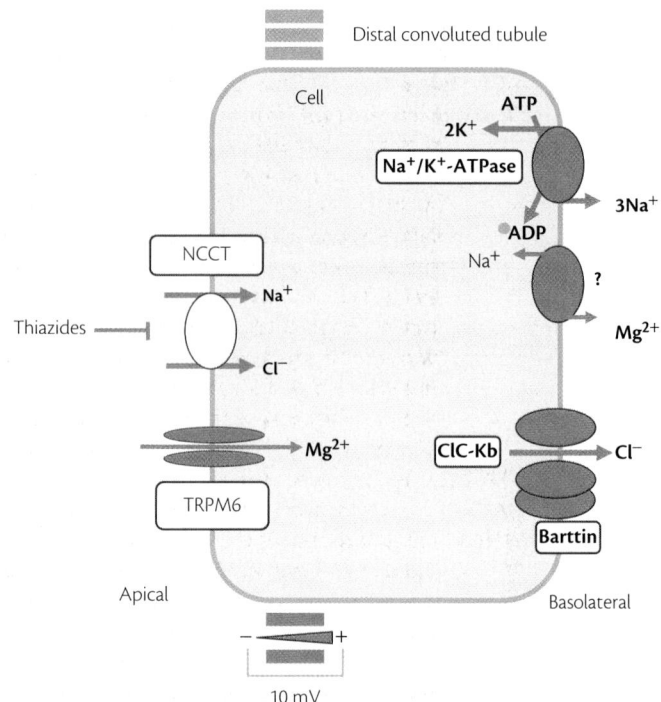

Fig. 21.16.1 Schematic model of transport mechanisms in the distal convoluted tubule. Sodium chloride (NaCl) enters the cell via the apical thiazide-sensitive Na$^+$-Cl$^-$ cotransporter (NCCT) and leaves the cell through the basolateral Na$^+$,K$^+$-ATPase, and the Cl$^-$ channel (ClC-Kb) respectively. Barttin is a subunit of ClC-Kb. Cl$^-$ also leaves the cell through the basolateral K$^+$,Cl$^-$ cotransporter (not shown). Indicated also are the apical magnesium channel TRPM6 and a putative Na/Mg exchanger in the basolateral membrane.
Knoers NVAM (2006), Gitelman syndrome. Advances in chronic kidney disease 13, 148–54.

during periods of fever or when extra magnesium is lost due to vomiting or diarrhoea. Paraesthesias, especially in the face, are frequent. Some patients experience severe fatigue that interferes with daily activities, whereas others never complain of tiredness. In contrast to Bartter's syndrome, a genetically distinct and clinically more severe tubular transport disorder (Table 21.16.3) which shares the hypokalaemic metabolic alkalosis of Gitelman's syndrome, growth retardation and polyuria are usually absent. Blood pressure is lower than in the general population, indicating that even the modest salt wasting of this disease reduces blood pressure.

The electrocardiogram reveals that the QT interval is slightly to moderately prolonged in about 50% of cases, but this is rarely associated with clinically relevant cardiac arrhythmias. A few patients with Gitelman's syndrome develop chondrocalcinosis, which is assumed to result from chronic hypomagnesaemia. Progression to renal insufficiency is extremely rare.

The serum magnesium concentration is low (<0.65 mmol/litre) in all patients. The best biochemical parameter to differentiate Gitelman's syndrome from Bartter's syndrome is a low urinary calcium excretion (molar ratio of urinary calcium to urinary creatinine <0.1). Prostaglandin excretion is normal in Gitelman's syndrome; plasma renin activity and plasma aldosterone concentration are elevated. Renal functional studies demonstrate normal or slightly decreased urinary concentrating capacity, but clearly reduced distal fractional chloride reabsorption during hypotonic saline infusion.

Table 21.16.3 Inherited disorders of magnesium transport

Disorder	OMIM	Gene/inheritance	Protein	Key clinical/biochemical symptoms
Bartter's syndrome type I	601678	*SLC12A1*/AR	Na-K-2Cl cotransporter NKCC2	Polyhydramnios/prematurity Polyuria/polydipsia Salt craving Failure to thrive Hypokalaemia Hypercalciuria/nephrocalcinosis
Bartter's syndrome type II	241200	*KCNJ1*/AR	Renal potassium channel ROMK	as in type I hyperkalaemia in neonatal period
Bartter's syndrome type III	607364	*CLCNKB*/AR	Renal chloride channel ClC-Kb	'Classic' Bartter syndrome; overlaps with type I/II or Gitelman's syndrome Normal serum magnesium or hypomagnesaemia. Hypokalaemia.hypercalciuria/(hypocalciuria)
Bartter's syndrome type IV	602522	*BSND*/AR	ClCKb/ClCka subunit Barttin	Polyhydramnios/prematurity Polyuria/polydipsia Salt craving Sensorineural deafness Hypokalaemia Hypercalciuria
Autosomal dominant hypocalcaemia	146200	*CaSR* (activating mutations)/AD	Calcium/magnesium sensing receptor CaSR	Tetany/seizures Nephrocalcinosis Polyuria Hypomagnesaemia in 50% Hypocalcaemia/hypercalciuria
Familial hypocalciuric hypercalcaemia	145980	*CaSR* (inactivating mutations; heterozygous/AD	Calcium/magnesium sensing receptor CaSR	Nephrolithiasis Pancreatitis
Severe neonatal hyperparathyreoidism	239200	Homozygous/AR		Failure to thrive Hypotonia Skeletal deformations Respiratory distress Hypermagnesaemia is some cases Hypercalcaemia/hypocalciuria
Gitelman's syndrome	263800	*SLC12A3*/AR	Na-Cl cotransporter NCCT	Muscle weakness/tetany/fatigue/ Chondrocalcinosis Hypokalaemia Hypomagnesaemia Hypocalciuria
Familial hypomagnesaemia with hypercalciuria and nephrocalcinosis	248250	*CLDN16*/AR *CLDN19*/AR	Claudin-16 Claudin-19	Polyuria Renal stones/nephrocalcinosis Ocular abnormalities Severe hypomagnesaemia Hypercalciuria
Autosomal dominant renal hypomagnesaemia with hypocalciuria/isolated renal Mg loss	154020	*FXYD2*/AD	γ-subunit Na$^+$,K$^+$ ATPase	Seizures Chondrocalcinosis Hypomagnesaemia Hypocalciuria
Familial hypomagnesaemia with secondary hypocalcaemia	602014	*TRPM6*/AR	Epithelial magnesium channel TRPM6	Tetany/seizures Hypomagnesaemia Hypocalcaemia

AD, autosomal dominant; AR, autosomal recessive.

Most cases of Gitelman's syndrome are caused by loss-of-function mutations in the *SLC12A3* gene, which encodes the renal thiazide-sensitive sodium-chloride cotransporter NCCT that is specifically expressed in the first part of the distal convoluted tubule, DCT1 (see Fig. 21.16.1). More than 100 different putative loss-of-function mutations in the *SLC12A3* gene have been identified in patients, including missense, nonsense, frame-shift, and splice-site mutations that are scattered throughout the protein. In general, there is extreme inter- and intrafamiliar phenotype variability, the latter emphasizing the lack of a correlation between the severity of symptoms in Gitelman's syndrome and the type of mutation in the *SLC12A3* gene.

A few patients with the Gitelman phenotype, including hypomagnesaemia and hypocalciuria, have been shown to have mutations in the *CLCNKB* gene encoding the renal chloride channel ClC-kb, located in the distal tubules (Fig. 21.16.1). The clinical phenotype in these patients can be highly variable, from an antenatal onset of Bartter's syndrome at one end of the spectrum, to a phenotype closely resembling Gitelman's syndrome at the other (see Table 21.16.1).

Both loss-of-function mutations in NCCT and mutations in CLC-kb lead to disruption of NaCl reabsorption in the distal convoluted tubule (Fig. 21.16.1). This leads to more sodium being delivered to the collecting duct and mild volume contraction, which activates the renin–angiotensin system. Elevated aldosterone levels give rise to increased electrogenic sodium reabsorption in the cortical collecting duct via the epithelial sodium channel (ENaC), defending salt homeostasis at the expense of increased secretion of potassium and hydrogen ions, thus resulting in hypokalaemia and metabolic alkalosis.

It has been shown that passive calcium reabsorption in the proximal tubule and reduced abundance of the epithelial magnesium channel TRPM6 explain thiazide-induced hypocalciuria and hypomagnesaemia, respectively. Since thiazides are known to inhibit NCCT, and in view of the phenotypic resemblance between Gitelman's syndrome and chronic thiazide treatment, it is very likely that similar mechanisms are involved in the pathogenesis of hypocalciuria and hypomagnesaemia seen in Gitelman's.

Most patients with Gitelman's syndrome remain untreated, but in view of the assumption that chondrocalcinosis is due to magnesium deficiency, there is a clear argument for lifelong supplementation of magnesium. The bioavailability of magnesium preparations is different: magnesium oxide and magnesium sulphate have significantly lower bioavailability than magnesium chloride, magnesium lactate and magnesium aspartate, but normalization of serum magnesium is difficult to achieve since high doses of these agents cause diarrhoea. Hypokalaemia can be treated by drugs that antagonize the activity of aldosterone (e.g. spironolactone) or block the sodium channel ENaC in the distal nephron (e.g. amiloride).

See Chapter 21.2.2 for further discussion, in particular differential diagnosis from other causes of hypokalaemia and clinical features.

Autosomal dominant renal hypomagnesaemia with hypocalciuria

Autosomal dominant renal magnesium wasting is a disorder characterized by hypomagnesaemia due to renal magnesium loss, associated with hypocalciuria. Patients may suffer from generalized convulsions, but may also be asymptomatic, except for the development of chondrocalcinosis at adult age. The genetic defect in a large Dutch family with this disorder appears to be a heterozygous missense mutation (G14R) in the *FXYD2* gene, encoding the γ subunit of the Na^+,K^+-ATPase that is expressed on the basolateral membrane of epithelial cells of the distal convoluted tubule. This γ subunit has an important role in modulating the activity of the Na^+,K^+-ATPase that maintains the membrane potential and the sodium gradient, and expression studies reveal that the mutation abolishes its interaction with the αβ subunits of the Na^+,K^+-ATPase, resulting in a failure of γ to traffic to the cell surface and to modulate pump kinetics.

The exact molecular mechanism of hypomagnesaemia and the associated hypocalciuria in patients with *FXYD2* mutations is not known. It has been speculated that abrogation of γ-mediated modulation of the Na^+,K^+-ATPase kinetics changes the electrochemical gradients of sodium and potassium, with a secondary reduction in magnesium reabsorption through the apical TRPM6 channel.

Familial hypomagnesaemia with hypercalciuria and nephrocalcinosis

Familial hypomagnesaemia with hypercalciuria and nephrocalcinosis (FHHNC) is an autosomal recessive renal disorder characterized by excessive renal magnesium wasting which results in persistent hypomagnesaemia, and by calcium wasting leading to early nephrocalcinosis. Also characteristic is multisystem involvement, with the most distinctive features being ocular abnormalities such as myopia, nystagmus, and chorioretinitis.

In most cases, FHHNC is caused by loss-of-function mutations in the *CLDN16* gene, encoding claudin-16 (formerly paracellin-1), an important tight junction protein located in the paracellular pathway of the thick ascending limb. In Germany and eastern European countries a founder mutation (Leu151Phe) that is present in approximately 50% of mutant alleles has been identified, a finding which greatly facilitates molecular diagnosis in patients originating from these countries. Some specific mutations in the PDZ domain of claudin 16 have been shown to result in isolated hypercalciuria and nephrocalcinosis. In a subset of families with FHHNC and severe ocular involvement (OMIM 248190), the disease is caused by mutations in *CLDN19*, which encodes another important tight junction protein, claudin-19.

The hypomagnesaemia is unresponsive to magnesium supplementation. Renal function declines progressively in approximately 30% of patients, many of whom reach endstage renal disease by teenage or young adult age. Thus, overall the prognosis of FHHNC is poor, and a definite cure can only be achieved by renal transplantation.

Familial hypomagnesaemia with secondary hypocalcaemia

Familial hypomagnesaemia with secondary hypocalcaemia (HSH) is an autosomal recessive disorder that manifests in the newborn period and is characterized by very low serum magnesium. It is caused by mutations in the *TRPM6* gene that lead to substantial truncations in the TRPM6 protein, which result in loss-of-function of TRPM6. In view of the fact that TRPM6 is expressed both in colon as well as in kidney, this leads to a combined defect of intestinal and renal (re)absorption. Hypocalcaemia is another characteristic feature and is a secondary consequence of parathyroid failure and parathyroid hormone resistance as a result of chronic, severe hypomagnesaemia. Affected patients show neurological symptoms of hypomagnesaemic hypocalcaemia, including seizures and muscle spasms. Untreated, the disease may be fatal or may lead to severe neurological damage. Treatment with high-dose magnesium supplementation can be effective in correcting the hypomagnesaemia and secondary hypocalcaemia.

Aminoaciduria and renal Fanconi syndrome
Physiology of proximal tubular amino acid handling

Reabsorption of amino acids is a major function of the kidney proximal tubule. The total concentration of amino acids in plasma is approximately 2.5 mmol/litre, these L-amino acids largely being absorbed from the gastrointestinal tract, although they may be products of protein catabolism or of the *de novo* synthesis of nonessential amino acids. Because amino acids (except for tryptophan) are mainly not bound to plasma proteins, they are freely filtered by the glomerulus, after which most (95–99.9%) of the filtered amino acid load (*c.*50 g daily) is reabsorbed in the proximal tubules, mainly by the apical Na^+-dependent cotransporters (for neutral amino acids, aromatic neutral amino acids, and anionic amino acids). Na^+-independent cotransporters mediate the uptake of the other amino acids (H^+-cotransporter for glycine and proline; heterodimeric exchanger bo,+AT-rBat for cystine and cationic amino acids). At the basolateral membrane most amino acids exit the cells via facilitated diffusion. In the late proximal tubule and more distal nephron segments basolateral membrane uptake of amino acids becomes important for the metabolism and nutrition of the cells. The function of most apical amino acid transporters is regulated by an integral membrane protein Tmem27, also known as collectrin. However, because of substantial complexity due to overlapping substrate selectivity, the absence of selective inhibitors, and the fact that several transporters function as more or less obligatory and symmetrical exchangers of amino acids, the genetic basis and physiology of amino acid transport is still incompletely understood.

Aminoaciduria is defined as urinary excretion of more than 5% of the filtered load of an amino acid. The most clinically relevant disorders in which the genetic defects have been identified (cystinuria, Hartnup's disorder, and lysinuric protein intolerance) are described in this chapter; other rare and frequently asymptomatic aminoacidurias are listed in Table 21.16.4.

Specific aminoacidurias

Cystinuria

Cystinuria is an inherited form of nephrolithiasis that can be transmitted as either an autosomal recessive or an autosomal dominant trait. The disease is characterized by impaired transport of cystine and dibasic amino acids lysine, ornithine, and arginine in the proximal tubular cells and in the epithelial cells of the intestine. Cystinuria occurs in approximately 1:7000 births and manifests with renal stones at various ages, including infancy (mainly before the age of 30 years). The diagnosis is made by the chemical analysis of the stone and by the quantitative measurement of urinary cystine output (usually >1000 μmol/g creatinine).

Two cystinuria genes have been identified: *SLC7A9* (solute carrier family 7 member 9), which encodes the luminal transport channel bo,+AT, and *SLC3A1* (solute carrier family 3 member 1), which encodes the rBAT transporter subunit. Patients with classical recessive cystinuria have two *SLC3A1* mutations, whereas patients with the dominant form of cystinuria have one *SLC7A9* mutation. Based on the genetic defect, recessive cystinuria can be classified into type A, caused by mutations in *SLC3A1* in both alleles, and type B, caused by mutations in *SLC7A9* in both alleles. Type A heterozygotes have normal urinary cystine concentration, whilst most type B heterozygotes have increased urinary cystine and a few even develop renal stones, although some (*c.*14%) have normal urinary cystine concentrations. Individuals with digenic inheritance (type AB) are very rare and generally behave as type B heterozygotes.

Hypotonia–cystinuria syndrome is characterized by generalized hypotonia at birth, failure to thrive, facial dysmorphism, growth

hormone deficiency, and nephrolithiasis followed by hyperphagia and rapid weight gain in later childhood. This syndrome is attributed to homozygous deletions disrupting the *PREPL* and SLC3A1 genes.

See Chapter 21.14 for discussion of treatment of patients with cystinuria.

Hartnup's disease

Hartnup's disease is characterized by a pellagra-like light sensitive rash, cerebellar ataxia, emotional instability, rarely intellectual disability, and defective renal and intestinal absorption of neutral amino acids alanine, asparagine, glutamate, histidine, isoleucine, leucine, methionine, phenylalanine, serine, threonine, tryptophan, tyrosine, and valine. The incidence of Hartnup's disease is 1:26 000 births. Most patients are asymptomatic and are mainly identified by neonatal screening programmes. The clinical symptoms are related to nicotinamide deficiency due to defective tryptophan reabsorption (nicotinamide being a metabolite of tryptophan) and can be triggered by inadequate dietary intake or increased metabolic requirements. The disease is inherited as an autosomal recessive trait and is caused by mutations in the *SCL6A19* gene, encoding the system b(o) neutral amino acid transporter 1. Symptomatic individuals are treated with nicotinamide (50–300 mg/day), usually leading to the disappearance of dermatitis and neurological symptoms. See Chapter 12.2 for further discussion.

Lysinuric protein intolerance

Lysinuric protein intolerance (LPI) is a rare autosomal recessively inherited disorder caused by defective dibasic amino acid transport. The incidence in Finland is 1:60 000 births; it is very rare elsewhere. Mutations in the *SLC7A7* gene, encoding renal and intestinal basolateral dibasic amino acid transporter y+LAT-1 have been identified in several families. Acute symptoms include nausea and vomiting after protein ingestion. Chronic symptoms include enlarged liver and spleen, growth retardation, muscle weakness, osteoporosis, pulmonary alveolar proteinosis, various immunological abnormalities, and renal failure in some patients. The explanation of these symptoms is incompletely understood. The disturbed intestinal absorption of arginine, ornithine, and lysine causes low plasma levels of these amino acids, leading to decreased activity of the urea cycle resulting in hyperammonaemia. Urinary excretion of lysine and all cationic amino acids is increased. Patients are treated with moderate protein restriction and citrulline (3–8 g/day), which can be converted to ornithine and arginine in the liver and replenishing the urea cycle. See Chapter 12.2 for further discussion.

Renal Fanconi syndrome

Apical proximal tubular reabsorption can be broadly divided into (1) Na^+-gradient dependent transport, which plays a central role in the reabsorption of amino acids, glucose, phosphate, and bicarbonate, and (2) receptor-mediated endocytosis, responsible for proximal tubular uptake of low-molecular-weight proteins, albumin, polypeptide hormones, and vitamin-binding proteins. Renal Fanconi syndrome (also called deToni–Debré–Fanconi syndrome) is characterized by generalized defect of both Na^+-coupled and megalin-dependent proximal tubular transport. Symptoms manifest at various ages dependent on the underlying condition and comprise generalized aminoaciduria; glycosuria; renal sodium, potassium, urate and phosphate wasting; proximal tubular acidosis; low-molecular-weight proteinuria and albuminuria. All these features are not necessarily present in all patients and

Table 21.16.4 Renal aminoacidurias

Disorder	OMIM	Gene/Inheritance	Protein	Key clinical/biochemical features
Cationic aminoacidurias				
Cystinuria/	220100	*SLC3A1*/AR	Solute carrier family 3 member 1(rBAT)	Renal stones
		SLC7A9/ADIP/AR	Solute carrier family 7 member 9 bo,+AT	
Isolated cystinuria	238200	*SLC7A9*/AD	Heterozygous carriers of *SLC7A9* mutations	
Hypotonia–cystinuria syndrome/	606407	*PREPL*/AR *SLC3A1*	Prolyl oligipeptidase rBAT	Hypotonia Failure to thrive Facial dysmorphism Growth hormone deficiency Renal stones
Hyperdibasic aminoaciduria type 1 (lysine, arginine, ornithine)	222690	?/AR	?	Intellectual disability or normal Hyperammonaemia Failure to thrive
Lysinuric protein intolerance (LPI) (hyperdibasic aminoaciduria type II)	222700	*SLC7A7*/AR	Dibasic amino acid transporter y+LAT-1	Failure to thrive Hyperammonaemia Acidosis Coma Osteoporosis
Neutral aminoacidurias				
Hartnup's disease	234500	*SCL6A19*/AR	System b(0) neutral amino acid transporter 1	Rash Cerebellar ataxia Psychiatric disorder
Histidinuria	235830	?/AR	?	Intellectual disability, convulsions or benign
Iminoaciduria/glycinuria				
Iminoglycinuria	242600	?/AR	?	Benign
Isolated glycinuria		?/AR	?	Benign
Dicarboxylic aminoaciduria	222730	EAAC1/AR	Glutamate transporter	Ophthalmoplegia Deafness Peripheral polyneuropathy Intellectual disability, or no symptoms

AD, autosomal dominant; AR autosomal recessive.

vary in individuals with specific defects (see Table 21.16.5). Treatment focuses on the replacement of electrolytes, phosphate and bicarbonate losses, and on specific treatment of the underlying disease.

Cystinosis

Cystinosis is the most frequent inherited cause of renal Fanconi syndrome, occurring in 1:200 000 births. The disease is caused by recessive mutations in the *CTNS* gene encoding the lysosomal cystine transport protein cystinosin, and is characterized by lysosomal cystine accumulation throughout the body. Most patients manifest with Fanconi syndrome during the first year of life and develop endstage renal disease around the age of 10 years. Extrarenal organs—including thyroid, pancreas, muscles, brain, and gonads—can be affected, usually after the first decade. Less than 5% of patients have milder degrees of proximal tubular dysfunction, and some only complain of photophobia caused by corneal cystine crystals. The diagnosis is made by the demonstration of elevated cystine content in blood polymorphonuclear cells. Corneal cystine

crystals are also pathognomonic, but generally do not appear during the first year of life. Specific treatment consists of the administration of the aminothiol cysteamine (1.3 g/m² daily in four doses, including one at night), which depletes intralysosomal cystine accumulation, slows the progression of renal disease, and postpones extrarenal complications. It has to be administered as early as possible and continued also after renal transplantation to protect extrarenal organs. Cysteamine eye drops (0.5%) are used topically to dissolve corneal cystine crystals. See Chapter 12.2 for further discussion.

Further reading

Glycosuria

Brown GK (2000). Glucose transporters: structure, function and consequences of deficiency. *J Inher Metabol Dis*, **23**, 237–46.

Wright EM (2001). Renal Na⁺-glucose transporters. *Am J Physiol Renal Physiol*, **280**, F10–18.

Table 21.16.5 Causes of renal Fanconi syndrome

(a) Inherited causes

Disorder	OMIM	Gene/inheritance	Protein	Key clinical/biochemical features
Cystinosis Infantile Juvenile	219800 219900	CTNS/AR	Cystinosin	Failure to thrive Rickets Metabolic acidosis, Renal failure
Dent's disease	300009	CLCN5/XL-R OCRL1/XL-R	Chloride channel 5 Phosphatidylinositol-4,5-biphosphate-5-phosphatase	LMW proteinuria Hypercalciuria Nephrocalcinosis, nephrolithiasis, renal failure
Lowe's syndrome*	309000	OCRL1/XL-R	Phosphatidylinositol-4,5-biphosphate 5-phosphatase	Short stature Intellectual disability Congenital cataract Seizures Elevated transaminases
Hereditary fructose intolerance	229600	ALDOB/AR	Aldolase B	Fructose intolerance Growth retardation
Galactosaemia	230400	GALT/AR	Gal-1-P uridylyl transferase	Hepatomegaly, liver disease Cataract Intellectual disability
Tyrosinaemia type 1	276700	FAHD2A/AR	Fumaryl-acetoacetate hydrolase	Hepatomegaly, cirrhosis Nephrocalcinosis, glomerulosclerosis Rickets Growth retardation
Wilson's disease	277900	ATP7B/AR	Copper-transporting ATPase, β subunit	Kayser–Fleischer rings(cornea) Hepatitis, cirrhosis CNS abnormalities
Fanconi–Bickel syndrome	227810	SLC2A2/AR	GLUT2	Hepatorenal glycogen accumulation, hepatomegaly Rachitis, osteomalacia Intellectual disability Growth retardation
Glycogen storage disease type 1	232400	G6PC/AR	glucose-6-phosphatase	glycogen deposition liver, kidney hypoglycemia
Mitochondrial disorders	diverse	diverse	diverse	diverse

AD, autosomal dominant; ADIP, autosomal dominant incomplete penetrance; AR autosomal recessive; CNS, central nervous system; LMW, low molecular weight; XL-R, X linked recessive.
* glucosuria might be absent

(b) Acquired causes

Intrinsic renal disease	Acute tubular necrosis
	Myeloma
	Sjögren's syndrome
	Renal transplant rejection
Drugs	Cisplatin
	Ifosfomide
	Gentamicin
	Valproic acid
	6-Mercaptopurine
Other exogenous toxins	Glue sniffing
	Heavy metals (mercury, lead, cadmium, uranium)
	Maleic acid (in experimental animals)
Nutritional	Kwashiorkor

Disorders of plasma phosphate

Agarwal R, Knochel JP (2000). Hypophosphemia and hyperphosphatemia. In: Brenner BM (ed.) *The kidney*, pp. 1071–125. W B Saunders, Philadelphia.

Forster IC, *et al.* (2006). Proximal tubular handling of phosphate: a molecular perspective. *Kidney Int*, **70**, 1548–59.

Liu S, Quarles LD (2007). How fibroblast growth factor 23 works. *J Am Soc Nephrol*, **18**, 1637–47.

Disorders of plasma magnesium

Knoers NVAM (2006). Gitelman syndrome. *Adv Chron Kidney Dis*, **13**, 148–54.

Konrad M, Weber S (2003). Recent advances in molecular genetics of hereditary magnesium-losing disorders. *J Am Soc Nephrol*, **14**, 249–60.

Nijenhuis T, *et al.* (2005). Enhanced passive Ca^{2+} reabsorption and reduced Mg^{2+} channel abundance explains thiazide-induced hypocalciuria and hypomagnesemia. *J Clin Invest*, **115**, 1651–8.

Thebault S, Hoenderop JG, Bindels RJ (2006). Epithelial Ca^{2+} and Mg^{2+} channels in kidney disease. *Adv Chron Kidney Dis*, **13**, 110–17.

Aminoaciduria and renal Fanconi syndrome

Bonnardeaux A, Bichet D (2000). Inherited disorders of the renal tubule. In: Brenner BM (ed.) *The kidney*, 6th edn, pp. 1656–98. W B Saunders, Philadelphia.

Gahl WA (2002). Cystinosis. *N Engl J Med*, **347**, 111–21.

Levtchenko EN, *et al.* (2006). Strict cysteamine dose regimen is required to prevent nocturnal cystine accumulation in cystinosis. *Pediatr Nephrol*, **21**, 110–13.

Palacin M, *et al.* (2005). The genetics of heteromeric amino acid transporters. *Physiology*, **20**, 121–4.

Website

NCBI. Online mendelian inheritance in man (OMIM) http://www.ncbi.nlm.gov/omim/

Urinary tract obstruction

Muhammad M. Yaqoob and Islam Junaid

Essentials

Obstructive nephropathy can manifest as either a sudden or an insidious decline in renal function, which can be can halted or even reversed by relief of obstruction. Obstruction can be due to anatomical or functional abnormalities of the urethra, bladder, ureter, or renal pelvis, which may be congenital or acquired, and it can also occur as a consequence of diseases extrinsic to the urinary tract. Although dilatation of the outflow system proximal to the site of obstruction is a characteristic finding, widening of the ureter and/or pelvicalyceal system does not necessarily indicate the presence of obstruction, and flow may be obstructed without such dilatation.

Calculi and pelviureteric junctional obstruction are common causes of unilateral obstruction, while prostatic enlargement, stone disease, and bladder and pelvic tumours account for about 75% of cases of bilateral obstruction in developed countries.

Acute upper urinary tract obstruction

Clinical features—typically gives rise to pain in the flank, which may radiate to the groin. Ultrasonography is useful for determining the presence or absence of obstruction, but not good for determining its cause, with unenhanced spiral CT the investigation of choice (or intravenous urography if CT is not available).

Management—this depends on the cause, and whether or not there is accompanying infection. Drainage must be established as a matter of urgency if the patient has clinical features of local or systemic sepsis, usually by percutaneous antegrade nephrostomy. Urinary stones less than 5 mm in maximum diameter will usually pass spontaneously: extracorporeal shock-wave lithotripsy and/or endoscopic manoeuvres are used when colic is persistent.

Acute lower urinary tract obstruction

Clinical features and management—symptoms of bladder outflow obstruction with hesitancy, poor urinary stream, and terminal dribbling often precede acute urinary retention. Suprapubic pain along with a palpable bladder is sufficient evidence for immediate catheterization, although ultrasonography will confirm or refute the presence of bladder distension if there is doubt about the diagnosis.

Chronic upper urinary tract obstruction

Clinical features and management—obstruction must be excluded in all patients with unexplained renal failure. Ultrasonography is the usual screening test, but this cannot distinguish between an obstructed distended system and a baggy, low-pressure dilated system. Furosemide renography can be helpful when there is doubt, but the 'gold standard' to determine whether or not there is functionally significant obstruction remains a trial of drainage (usually by antegrade nephrostomy). Specific management will depend upon the cause of obstruction.

Retroperitoneal fibrosis

Epidemiology and aetiology—this is a rare condition characterized by the presence of fibro-inflammatory tissue which typically surrounds the abdominal aorta and iliac arteries and extends into the retroperitoneum to entrap the ureters, causing unilateral or bilateral obstruction. Two-thirds of cases are idiopathic; the remainder are attributable to drugs, malignant diseases, or other causes.

Clinical features—early symptoms are constitutional upset, often accompanied by dull back, flank, and abdominal pain; later disease is characterized by symptoms related to the entrapment of retroperitoneal structures, most commonly ureteric obstruction.

Diagnosis—CT reveals findings typical of urinary tract obstruction together with a periaortic mass. CT-guided needle biopsy may be sufficient to diagnose lymphoma or carcinoma with confidence, but laparotomy is typically required to obtain a sufficiently large sample to exclude these conditions, the microscopic appearance of idiopathic retroperitoneal fibrosis being characterized by fibrotic tissue infiltrated with a mixture of mononuclear cells.

Management—the objective is to relieve ureteric obstruction (when present), suppress the acute phase reaction, halt the progression of fibrosis, and prevent relapse. Urgent relief of obstruction is generally recommended if there is significant renal dysfunction: this may be achieved by antegrade nephrostomy, retrograde insertion of ureteric stents, or open surgical ureterolysis, but these are not required if renal function is stable and normal. Standard medical treatment is to give corticosteroid therapy, typically beginning with prednisolone 1 mg/kg per day (maximum 60 mg/day) for 4 to

6 weeks and then gradually reducing at a rate determined by monitoring of the patient's symptoms, inflammatory markers (erythrocyte sedimentation rate (ESR), C-reactive protein (CRP), etc.) and repeated imaging. Recurrence of disease occurs in 10% to 30% of cases, usually within the first year but sometimes many years later, hence long-term surveillance is required.

Introduction

Obstructive nephropathy can manifest as either a sudden or an insidious decline in renal function, which can be can halted or even reversed by relief of obstruction, hence obstructive uropathy is a potentially curable cause of renal failure. Obstruction can be due to anatomical or functional abnormalities of the urethra, bladder, ureter, or renal pelvis, which may be congenital or acquired, and it can also occur as a consequence of diseases extrinsic to the urinary tract. Although dilatation of the outflow system proximal to the site of obstruction is a characteristic finding, widening of the ureter and/or pelvicalyceal system does not necessarily indicate the presence of obstruction, and flow may be obstructed without such dilatation. Causes of dilatation in the absence of obstruction include (1) anatomical variants—extra renal pelvis, megaureter (possible secondary to vesicoureteral reflux); (2) pregnancy—hormonal changes cause dilated ureters and renal pelvis; and (3) post obstruction—a 'baggy' system may remain long after relief of chronic obstruction.

Obstruction may be of the upper (at or above the ureter) or lower (at or distal to the bladder) tract, partial or complete, unilateral or bilateral. It is important to realise that all causes of lower-tract obstruction may lead to upper-tract obstruction, but the reverse is not the case. Complete obstruction is the commonest cause of anuria and is usually easy to diagnose because of straightforward findings on renal imaging, but diagnosis of partial obstruction is frequently difficult because of variable urinary output and imaging findings. Bilateral obstruction, obstruction of a single kidney, or lower-tract obstruction are a greater danger to the patient than unilateral obstruction, and obstruction associated with infection is a greater threat to kidney function and to life than obstruction in the absence of infection. Obstruction of the urinary tract should be considered in every uraemic patient, whether acute or chronic.

Incidence

The incidence, prevalence, and cost of obstructive uropathy are difficult to estimate because obstruction can occur in a wide variety of settings. It is common during childhood, when it is mainly due to congenital anomalies of the urinary tact; the incidence then declines until age 60 to 65 years, after which it rises, most particularly in men because of prostatic disease. Urinary tract obstruction is found in 3.8% of routine autopsies and up to 25% of autopsies carried out on uraemic patients. Up to 166 per 100 000 hospitalization episodes are coded as being due to obstructive nephropathy.

Urinary tract obstruction is a common cause of endstage renal disease in children. Obstruction in early gestation can cause renal dysplasia; late in gestation or after birth it can cause irreversible loss of renal function. Obstructive nephropathy accounts for about 3 to 4% of cases of endstage renal disease in adults, but the incidence and causes of obstructive uropathy vary with the gender and age of the patient. Calculi and pelviureteric junctional obstruction are common causes of unilateral obstruction, while prostatic enlargement, stone disease, and bladder and pelvic tumours account for about 75% of cases of bilateral obstruction in developed countries. Males outnumber females with endstage renal disease due to obstructive nephropathy, and whites are more susceptible than African Americans, Asians, and Native Americans. Wide geographic variations occur in the relative incidence of some causes of obstruction, e.g. schistosomiasis.

Causes

Obstruction may be caused by lesions within the lumen or the wall of the urinary tract or by pressure from outside (Table 21.17.1).

Calculi, particularly calcium oxalate stones, are the most common cause of urinary tract obstruction in the young adult male, in whom they are two to three times more common than in females. Common sites for impaction of stones are in the calyx, at the pelviureteric junction, at the pelvic brim, and at the vesicoureteric junction. Stones smaller than 0.5 cm in diameter usually pass spontaneously.

Table 21.17.1 Causes of urinary obstruction

Level of obstruction	Obstruction within the lumen	Obstruction within the wall	Extrinsic compression
Kidney	Stones Sloughed papillae	Cysts Tumours Anatomical abnormalities, e.g PUJ obstruction	Lower polar renal vessels crossing at PUJ
Ureter	Stones	Tumours. Stricture, e.g. malignant, post surgery or post-radiotherapy, tuberculous, schistosomiasis. Anatomical abnormalities, e.g. VUJ obstruction	Tumours Retroperitoneal fibrosis[a] Retrocaval right ureter (congenital) Pancreatitis (rare) Inflammatory bowel disease (rare)
Bladder/ bladder neck	Stones. Clot retention	Tumours Functional obstruction, e.g. diabetes, neurological damage to bladder, drugs	Pelvic tumours
Urethra	Stones. Blood clots (after catheterization or surgery)	Stricture, e.g. postinfective, postsurgical. Congenital urethral valves Tumours	Prostate enlargement

PUJ, pelvi-ureteric junction; VUJ, vesico-ureteric junction.
[a] Discussed in detail later in the chapter.

A calcified sloughed papilla in the urinary tract may mimic an opaque calculus, although the characteristic triangular shape of the opacity and the presence of a relevant underlying condition, e.g. diabetes, sickle cell disease, or analgesic abuse, should alert the clinician to the correct diagnosis.

Functional obstruction resulting from failure of normal peristalsis through a segment of the urinary tract usually results from an absence of smooth muscle fibres. In many cases no gross histological abnormalities are present. Classically, obstruction in childhood is seen at the pelviureteric junction (PUJ), which is usually bilateral when diagnosed before 1 year of age. The condition may be diagnosed *in utero*, but peak incidence is at age 5 years, and 20% of reported cases occur in adults over the age of 30 years. A functional defect of the vesicoureteric junction (congenital megaureter) is the second most common cause of obstruction in childhood, but is uncommon in adults. Males are more often affected than females, especially in childhood. The disease is sometimes claimed to be analogous to Hirschsprung's disease of the colon, but typical findings of a reduction in the number of muscle fibres and an increase in collagen fibres, together with preservation of the nerve ganglia, makes the analogy with Hirschsprung's disease invalid. Some studies have shown segmental up-regulation of transforming growth factor β (TGFβ) in the longitudinal muscle layer, suggesting segmental developmental delay of the terminal ureter.

Diseases of the retroperitoneal space commonly cause obstruction, particularly tumour invasion from cervix, prostate, bladder, colon, ovary, and uterus. In retroperitoneal fibrosis (see below) it is unclear whether obstruction results from extrinsic compression or failure of peristalsis resulting from encasement of the ureter within a fibrous exoskeleton. That the latter may be the case is suggested by the fact that contrast medium injected into the lower ureter typically passes freely up to the pelvicalyceal system despite the presence of clinical, radiological, and isotopic imaging evidence of functional urinary tract obstruction.

Functional obstruction may also occur at the bladder neck and at the level of the distal sphincter because of lack of coordination between bladder contraction and sphincter relaxation (detrusor sphincter dysenergia), resulting in either the bladder wall becoming noncompliant or detrusor hypertrophy. Common causes of functional outflow obstruction (neuropathic or neurogenic bladder) include diabetes mellitus, multiple sclerosis and spinal cord injuries, and meningomyelocele in childhood. Cerebrovascular disease and advanced Parkinson's disease are often associated with functional bladder outflow obstruction in older people. In some patients, particularly women, there appears to be a psychological component, but in some women an overactive external urethral sphincter is the cause of outflow obstruction (Fowler's syndrome). Certain drugs, including those with antimuscarinic activity (e.g. tricyclic antidepressants) and calcium channel blockers, have pharmacological effects on the bladder that may precipitate urinary retention.

Other causes of lower urinary tract obstruction include urethral strictures (following repeated instrumentation or surgery, or gonococcal infection), urethral tumours, and ureterocele. In children, urethral valves may be responsible for such obstruction. But in men by far the commonest causes of lower tract obstruction are benign prostatic enlargement and prostatic cancer. In women, pelvic malignancy is a common cause, with less common causes including uterine fibroids and complete procidentia.

Clinical approach to the patient with urinary obstruction

To the clinician, the first and most important question is whether urinary tract obstruction is of recent onset (acute obstruction) or long-standing (chronic obstruction). The pathophysiological changes, clinical features, approach to investigation and management, differ in important respects in these two circumstances, which will be discussed separately.

Acute upper urinary tract obstruction

Pathophysiology

Urine reaches the bladder as a result of three inter-related mechanisms: glomerular filtration pressure, ureteric and pelvic peristalsis, and gravity. Coordinated smooth-muscle contraction in the ureters directs urine toward the bladder, with maximum intraluminal pressures of 25 mmHg.

Acute ureteric obstruction causes delayed urinary transit, and over time leads to increased intratract pressures and declining blood flow to the kidneys, resulting in renal impairment. Histologically, tubular dilatation initially affects mainly the collecting duct and distal tubular segments; Bowman's space may be dilated at the later stages.

Clinical features

Acute upper-tract obstruction typically gives rise to pain in the flank, which may radiate to the iliac fossa, inguinal region, testis, or labium. The pain may be dull or sharp, intermittent or persistent, though waxing and waning in intensity. It may be provoked by a high fluid intake, alcohol, or diuretics, all measures that increase urinary volume and distend the collecting system. This is particularly noticeable when obstruction occurs at the pelviureteric junction. Loin tenderness may be detected and (rarely) an enlarged kidney may be palpable (in thin patients). Upper urinary tract infection with malaise, fever, and symptoms and signs of septicaemia may dominate the clinical picture.

Complete anuria is strongly suggestive of complete bilateral obstruction or complete obstruction of a single kidney. The differential diagnosis includes bilateral total renal cortical necrosis, acute anuric glomerulonephritis, and bilateral renal arterial occlusion. Intermittent anuria indicates the presence of intermittent complete obstruction.

Investigation

General investigation of the patient with suspected acute urinary obstruction will clearly include tests to determine renal function, e.g. serum creatinine, but specific investigation must allow the site and cause of obstruction to be identified rapidly, accurately, safely, and as economically as possible. A range of imaging tests may be employed.

Intravenous urography

In the developing world, emergency intravenous urography (IVU) is usually the preferred method of investigating the patient with suspected acute upper tract obstruction. It will confirm the diagnosis and will usually demonstrate the site, cause, and degree of obstruction, providing invaluable guidance for management. Ultrasonography, although demonstrating dilatation, cannot visualize the ureters adequately.

The initial sequence of intravenous urograms must include a full-length KUB (kidneys–ureter–bladder) film, which must be examined carefully for opaque calculi along the line of the ureter—calculi overlying bones are easily missed. Some obstructing calculi are very small and only faintly calcified or nonopaque. Ureteric calculi within the bony pelvis are often impossible to distinguish from calcified phleboliths on the plain film.

Contrast medium enters the pelvicalyceal system and ureter slowly in the presence of obstruction, hence delayed films are required, and opacification of the pelvicalyceal system and ureter may never be seen in severe acute obstruction. Furthermore, in acute ureteric obstruction the pelvicalyceal system and ureter may be only slightly dilated. Acute obstruction is characterized by increased excretion of contrast medium by the liver, leading to gallbladder opacification on delayed films.

Diagnosis is simple when typical obstructive changes are present, with a ureter dilated down to a calcified opacity. By contrast, diagnosis is more difficult if there is an obstructed nephrogram or dilatation of the pelvicalyceal system/ureter but no radiodense calculus is seen. If the history is of recent-onset pain, then the likely possibilities are recent passage of an opaque stone, uric acid stone, acute pelviureteric junction obstruction, blood clot, or sloughed papilla. Urography shows uric acid stones as lucent filling defects, and similar filling defects may be seen with transitional cell tumours or blood clots. Since most ureteric stones pass spontaneously, investigation of a possible transitional cell tumour or blood clot should be delayed, with CT imaging often very helpful if a persistent lucency is present.

Acute idiopathic pelviureteric junction obstruction should be suspected if there is a large soft tissue density inferomedial to the kidney on the plain film, produced by the distended pelvis. This usually fills on delayed films of the urogram, with no filling of the ureter.

Clot colic is always associated with macroscopic haematuria. When clot colic is suspected the urogram should be repeated after 2 weeks, by which time the clot should have lysed and any underlying lucent filling defect can be seen. Such patients require further investigation to define the cause of bleeding.

Sloughed papillae occur as a consequence of papillary necrosis. Abnormal calyces are typically seen in both kidneys, but papillary necrosis may occasionally be unilateral, usually as a result of a previous episode of infection associated with unilateral obstruction, especially in diabetics. Calcified papillae may occasionally mimic stones.

CT scanning (CT-KUB)

Unenhanced spiral CT is a fast, well-tolerated technique and the first-line investigation of choice in patients with urinary obstruction. It is more effective than intravenous urography in identifying ureteric calculi and is equally effective in detecting urinary obstruction (Fig. 21.17.1).

Ultrasonography

Ultrasonography is used as the first-line screening test to look for urinary obstruction in patients presenting with unexplained renal failure. It is a good investigation in such circumstances, with high sensitivity and specificity, but it must be remembered that about 5% of patients who subsequently prove to have urinary obstruction will have a false-negative initial ultrasound report. Furthermore, in patients with acute obstruction of the upper tract it is less informative than urography. It can demonstrate dilatation of the intrarenal collecting system and the upper third of the ureter, but dilatation of the middle and lower thirds of the ureter is not easily visible, and the dilated ureter cannot always be traced to the level of obstruction, although colour and pulsed Doppler can sometimes detect the presence or absence of ureteral jets to diagnose ureteric obstruction.

Ultrasonography may be preferred in the investigation of patients with acute obstruction if they are pregnant, have a history of contrast allergy, or are considered to be at particularly high risk of contrast nephrotoxicity, e.g. patients with diabetes or myeloma with moderate to severe renal impairment.

Antegrade and retrograde pyelography and ureterography

If the site of obstruction is not demonstrated by other techniques, then antegrade or retrograde examination may be helpful, both of which can be initiated as a method of diagnosis but then extended to provide a therapeutic role by providing drainage.

Magnetic resonance urography

Magnetic resonance (MR) urography using half-Fourier acquisition single-shot turbo spin-echo (HASTE) imaging can accurately and rapidly show the level and degree of ureteric obstruction. It can also be used to differentiate between acute and chronic obstruction on the basis of its ability to show perirenal fluid. Although IVU and CT are likely to remain the standard procedure for imaging the upper tract, MR urography enhanced by gadolinium and furosemide may be helpful if there is dilated system with no excretory function, in pregnant women, in children, and in those with contrast medium allergy, although the risks of nephrogenic systemic fibrosis need to be considered (see Chapter 21.4).

Radionuclide imaging

In cases where there is doubt as to whether or not there is obstruction, e.g. when structural imaging shows 'possible dilatation', then technetium mercaptoacetyltriglycine (MAG-3) radioisotope scanning can be used to differentiate obstructed from unobstructed kidneys.

Management

Stones

Most patients presenting with renal and ureteric colic have a stone in the lower third of the ureter. They can be managed conservatively if the stone is 5 mm or less in its maximum diameter. It is unusual for acute episodes of colic to persist for more than 72 h. Patients with ureteric colic are usually admitted to hospital, but this is often unnecessary since the only medical requirement is the provision of regular analgesia in the form of morphine, pethidine or nonsteroidal anti-inflammatory agents (NSAIDs) administered parenterally, orally, or *per rectum*.

With the advent of lithotripsy there is a tendency for earlier intervention. However, since most stones causing ureteric colic will pass spontaneously, the extent to which lithotripsy will hasten the process is difficult to establish. Stones almost anywhere in the ureter can be imaged and treated using a lithotripter that incorporates the additional facility of radiological imaging. Stone-free rates after *in situ* extracorporeal shock-wave lithotripsy (ESWL) have been reported to range from 81 to 96%. A larger number of shock waves at a higher voltage and an increased number of repeat sessions are required when a stone is within the ureter rather than in the kidney. Controversy remains as to whether upper ureteric

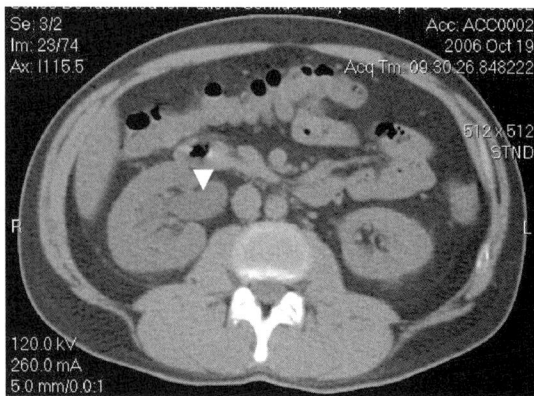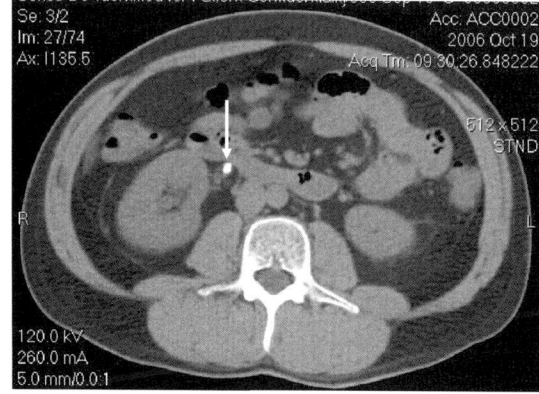

Fig. 21.17.1 Two images from a CT-KUB series showing a calculus in the PUJ/upper ureter (arrow) producing obstruction and hydronephrosis (arrowhead).

stones should be manipulated back into the kidney before ESWL, and the value of a JJ stent inserted alongside an impacted ureteric stone in both aiding fragmentation and enhancing the passage of stone fragments is unclear. Endoscopic manoeuvres, which are usually performed under general anaesthesia, are reserved for those patients with persistent colic.

Other causes

The two other relatively common causes of acute upper-tract obstruction are sloughed papillae and blood clots. The principles of management are similar to those for ureteric stones, but patients with papillary necrosis more commonly require intervention, usually with percutaneous antegrade nephrostomy, because of accompanying infection. Colic due to blood clot caused by renal parenchymal tumours and transitional cell tumours of the collecting system may require ablative open surgery. Bleeding arteriovenous fistulae, most often seen as a complication of renal biopsy, can be embolized with a high success rate. The most difficult cause of recurrent bleeding to manage is that associated with papillary necrosis in sickle cell trait or disease. Antifibrinolytic agents may be of value, but administration of such treatment during active bleeding may produce hard, rubbery clots, which fill the collecting system and require surgical removal.

Drainage of an obstructed system

If there is evidence of infection above an obstruction, i.e. the patient has clinical features of local or systemic sepsis, then drainage must be established as a matter of urgency. In most specialist centres insertion of a percutaneous antegrade nephrostomy tube under local anaesthetic and ultrasound/radiological guidance is the preferred option. Such a system may be used to provide drainage for weeks or even months if necessary. An alternative is retrograde insertion of a JJ ureteric stent, requiring general anaesthesia and radiological image intensifier screening in the operating theatre. Occasionally a retrograde catheter cannot be passed beyond the obstruction, in which case the diagnostic role of retrograde ureterography cannot be extended to a therapeutic one.

Acute lower urinary tract obstruction

Pathophysiology

Overstretching of smooth muscle fibres results in reduced mechanical efficiency, culminating in acute urinary retention. Factors such as sudden diuresis after alcohol ingestion or diuretic therapy for heart

failure, urinary tract infection, and drugs with antimuscarinic and calcium channel blocking activity may precipitate acute retention.

Clinical features

Symptoms of bladder outflow obstruction with hesitancy, poor urinary stream, and terminal dribbling often precede acute urinary retention. Acute retention is accompanied by severe suprapubic pain, but this may be absent if acute retention is superimposed on chronic retention or if there is an underlying neuropathy. Epidural anaesthesia may precipitate painless acute retention of urine: the pain from bladder overdistension is sympathetically mediated and will be abolished by a high epidural reaching to T10; obstetricians need to be particularly alert to this problem.

Chronic obstruction may result in muscle wall hypertrophy, sacculation and diverticulum formation: these in turn predispose to chronic lower urinary tract infection and occasionally to bladder stones. Epididymo-orchitis may also occur.

Investigation

Most patients presenting with acute urinary retention require no investigation before treatment. Suprapubic pain coexisting with a palpable bladder is sufficient evidence for immediate catheterization. Ultrasonography will confirm or refute the presence of a distended bladder if there is doubt about the diagnosis.

Flexible cystoscopy under local anaesthesia or a retrograde urethrogram may be performed if an attempt at urethral catheterization proves unsuccessful. This is done as an elective procedure after bladder drainage has been secured by suprapubic catheterization.

Management

The bladder may be catheterised *per urethram* or suprapubically. In women catheterization *per urethram* typically presents no difficulty, although a hypospadiac external urethral meatus may be difficult to locate on the anterior vaginal wall. Urethral catheterization may prove difficult in some men. Only an experienced operator should pass a urethral catheter on an introducer; the help of a urologist should be sought if there is difficulty.

Chronic upper urinary tract obstruction

Pathophysiology

Chronic ureteric obstruction causes dilatation of ducts of Bellini at first, followed by that of papillary structures and compression of renal cortical tissue with thinning of the renal parenchyma. Shrinkage of the renal parenchyma with reduction in size of the kidney (obstructive atrophy) is believed to result from the effects of compression of the renal parenchyma and from prolonged renal ischaemia. Slowly progressive partial obstruction tends to result in gross dilatation of the collecting system and gross atrophy of renal parenchyma.

Histologically, chronic obstructive uropathy is characterized by primary tubulointerstitial pathology and subsequent involvement of glomerular structures. Interstitial fibrosis a common consequence of long-standing obstruction (Fig. 21.17.2) and presumed to develop due to an imbalance between extracellular matrix synthesis/deposition and degradation. Work with experimental models of unilateral ureteral obstruction has demonstrated the involvement of tubular cell hypertrophy, proliferation, apoptosis, and atrophy; proliferation and activation of interstitial fibroblasts; accumulation of (myo)fibroblasts due to epithelial mesenchymal transdifferentiation; inflammatory cellular infiltration; increased extracellular matrix; deposition; and tubular atrophy. Studies in genetically modified animals have provided important information about the role of specific intracellular signalling pathways. In addition to confirming the pivotal role for angiotensin II and TGFβ in obstructive nephropathy, they have also led to the discovery of unexpected and often contradictory roles (both pro- and antifibrotic) for angiotensin II, matrix metalloproteinase 9 (an extracellular matrix degrading enzyme), activators or inhibitors of tissue plasminogen, the adhesion molecule osteopontin, and bone morphogenic protein 7. Further studies in these animals, in combination with pharmacological agents, may identify novel antifibrotic strategies in obstructive nephropathy and other progressive renal diseases.

Obstruction causes decline in GFR due to both a decrease in single-nephron GFR and in the number of filtering nephrons. It also leads to impaired ability to concentrate the urine due to acquired nephrogenic diabetes insipidus which is resistant to administration of antidiuretic hormone (ADH), and to partial distal renal tubular acidosis, often with associated hyperkalaemia. These specific consequences of obstructive uropathy are accompanied by general features of chronic kidney disease determined by the severity of renal failure, such as anaemia, renal osteodystrophy, and both hypertension or hypotension (secondary to salt wasting).

Clinical features

Patients may present with flank or abdominal pain, renal failure, or both; the symptoms and signs of urinary tract infection and septicaemia may be superimposed. Rarely, presentation is with hypertension or polycythaemia and their complications. Some patients are asymptomatic, obstruction being found during investigation of conditions such as haematuria, urinary infection, or hypertension.

Polyuria often occurs in chronic partial obstruction owing to impairment of renal tubular concentrating capacity. Intermittent anuria and polyuria indicate intermittent complete and partial obstruction.

Investigation

Obstruction must be excluded without undue delay in all patients with unexplained renal failure. In patients with known renal disease, rapid deterioration in renal function unexplained by the primary renal problem also demands investigation. Relapsing urinary tract infections should also raise the possibility of an associated obstructing lesion. The diagnosis of partial obstruction should not be discounted simply because urine volume is normal or increased.

The choice of imaging depends on the mode of presentation. As described previously, that initial investigation of a patient with unexplained impairment of renal function should include ultrasonography, together with plain abdominal radiographs. However, since ultrasound cannot distinguish between an obstructed distended system and a baggy, low-pressure dilated system, an abnormality on ultrasound should prompt further definitive investigation (Fig. 21.17.3). In very long-standing obstruction, generalized thinning of the renal parenchyma (obstructive atrophy) is seen: this is typically diffuse and symmetrical, with associated generalized calyceal dilatation.

The main value of CT in the investigation of chronic upper-tract obstruction is in defining the cause. A dilated collecting system appears as a multiloculate fluid collection of water density in the renal sinus. It is possible to distinguish the intrarenal collecting system from the extrarenal portion of the pelvis, which is important since obstruction can only be diagnosed on CT when there is dilatation of the intrarenal collecting system; a prominent extrarenal pelvis may be a normal variant. The whole dilated ureter is well shown on CT.

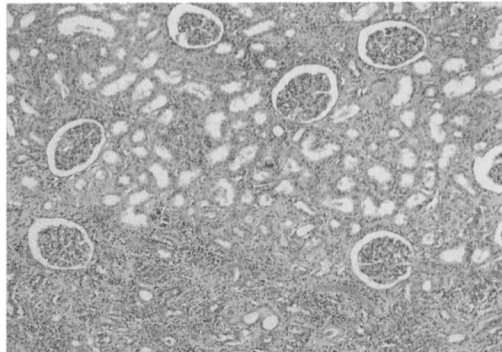

Fig. 21.17.2 Histological appearances in long-standing obstruction. Note dilated tubules, interstitial fibrosis and vessel wall thickening, but with preservation of glomeruli.

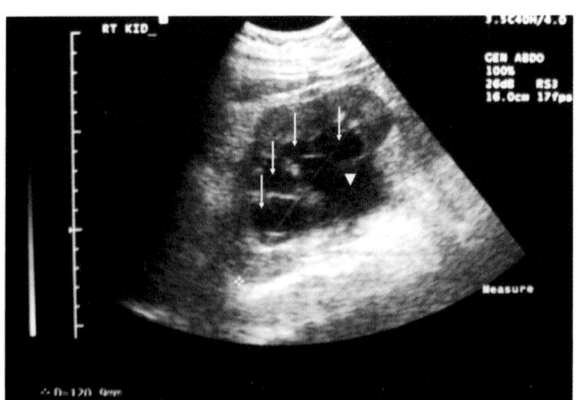

Fig. 21.17.3 Ultrasound scan of obstructed right kidney, showing dilated calyces (arrows) and pelvis (arrowhead) of the kidney.

Radionuclide scintigraphy is not appropriate as the first investigation in suspected obstruction, but—as described above in the context of acute obstruction—is useful in determining whether dilatation shown by other methods is obstructive. Dynamic renal scintigrams performed during diuresis, typically induced by furosemide, may be of value to ascertain whether prolongation of parenchymal transit time is due to retention of tracer within a large, baggy, low-pressure, unobstructed collecting system, or to genuine obstruction.

Antegrade (nephrostogram) and retrograde (ureterogram) studies are often necessary to define the exact site of obstruction and to arrive at a definitive diagnosis.

Differential diagnosis of nonobstructive collecting system dilatation

Vesicoureteric reflux may be associated with dilatation of the ureters, and the pelvicalyceal system may also be dilated in severe reflux. On urography the presence of reflux is suggested by variation in the degree of dilatation at different times during the examination, by dilatation which is greatest from the vesicoureteric junction upwards, and by a postmicturition film that shows a large bladder residual representing urine that has refluxed into the ureters during voiding and drained back into the bladder thereafter.

The decision of whether an operation is indicated for idiopathic pelviureteric junctional obstruction may be facilitated by furosemide urography or furosemide scintigraphy. In some patients the urographic findings are unremarkable during asymptomatic periods, while emergency intravenous urography during an episode of pain may define the condition.

Diagnosing significant incomplete chronic upper urinary tract obstruction

Incomplete obstruction is clinically important if it causes deterioration in kidney function that can be corrected by intervention. In patients with partial obstruction of a single functioning kidney or those with bilateral partial obstruction, a progressive rise in serum creatinine may suggest that obstruction is functionally significant, but there may clearly be other causes of a rising creatinine, and observing significant decline in renal function before taking action is clearly not ideal. Other proposed methods of detecting significant incomplete obstruction are shown in Table 21.17.2.

Management

The goals of treatment are to relieve symptoms, improve or conserve renal function, and avoid complications such as septicaemia.

Urinary stones are the commonest cause of chronic upper urinary tract obstruction. Management consists of stone removal by lithotripsy, endoscopic, or open surgical procedures, with or without ureteric stenting, details of which can be found in specialized urological texts. Attention must also be given to medical treatments to prevent stone recurrence (see Chapter 21.14).

Obstruction of the PUJ is the second most common cause of chronic obstruction in adults. The Anderson–Hynes pyeloplasty gives very satisfactory results and provides the standard against which other open and endoscopic techniques (such as endopyelotomy) must be assessed.

Renal prognosis

Long-term renal outcome after the relief of chronic obstructive uropathy has not been reported extensively. In one study of

Table 21.17.2 Techniques for detecting significant incomplete urinary obstruction

Technique	Comment
Furosemide urography	Urographic observation of distension of the renal pelvis induced by intravenous furosemide
Furosemide renography	Observation of the effect of intravenous furosemide on the isotope renogram
Retention function analysis	Comparison of activity/time curves after injection of ^{99}Tc- DTPA in whole kidney versus renal pelvis
Antegrade pressure flow measurement	Introduction of a needle into the renal pelvis with direct measurement of the pressure developing after infusion of fluid at a known flow rate
Antegrade nephrostomy	Placement of a drainage catheter directly into the renal pelvis, with observation of the effect on renal excretory function (serum creatinine)

Note: a trial of drainage by antegrade nephrostomy (or other method) is the 'gold standard': if renal function does not improve after such drainage, then obstruction is not the cause of renal impairment. The sensitivity and specificity of the other techniques in predicting the response to antegrade nephrostomy are not known.

67 patients with benign obstructive uropathy, 30 developed end-stage renal disease during a median follow-up of 58 months, and in 22 of the remaining 37 there was progressive decline in GFR of (median) 3 ml/min per year (range 0.9–9 ml/min per year). Chronic obstructive uropathy with advanced renal insufficiency (plasma creatinine >250 μmol/litre) is an important cause of endstage renal disease, especially in patients with significant proteinuria (>1 g/day). It remains to be seen whether angiotensin converting enzyme (ACE) inhibitors, AT1 receptor blockers, and endothelin receptor blockers will improve renal survival in obstructive uropathy.

Chronic lower urinary tract obstruction

In adults, chronic outflow obstruction to the bladder is most commonly due to benign prostatic hypertrophy, although prostatic malignancy and urethral strictures can also be responsible. Functional obstruction can also occur at the bladder neck and distal sphincter due to a failure of coordination of bladder contraction and sphincter relaxation, in which case the bladder may be highly compliant (low pressure, with no dilatation of the upper tracts) or poorly compliant (high pressure, with transmission of high pressure to the upper tracts, often leading to severe renal impairment).

There are no clinical features that differentiate high-pressure and low-pressure chronic retention: both are painless, and the bladder may be palpably distended in both.

Investigation typically includes ultrasonography of the upper and lower urinary tract, a plain abdominal radiograph, measurement of urinary flow rate, urine culture, and measurement of serum creatinine and electrolytes. Measurement of prostate-specific antigen (PSA) is appropriate if there is clinical evidence of prostatic malignancy (see Chapter 21.18). Full urodynamic studies may be needed in some cases.

The management of chronic bladder outflow obstruction is the remit of the urologist: details can be found in specialized urological texts.

Retroperitoneal fibrosis

Retroperitoneal fibrosis is a rare condition, first described in the French literature, with the classic description by Ormond in 1948. It is characterized by the presence of fibro-inflammatory tissue which typically surrounds the abdominal aorta and iliac arteries and extends into the retroperitoneum to entrap the ureters, causing unilateral or bilateral obstruction, usually at the junction between the middle and lower thirds of the ureter. The condition is progressive: the fibrous tissue is initially fairly cellular, but later it becomes relatively acellular.

Contrast medium injected into the lower ureter may pass freely up to the pelvicalyceal system despite the presence of clinical, radiological, and isotopic evidence of functional urinary tract obstruction, hence it is thought that obstruction is probably caused by loss of ureteric peristalsis.

Retroperitoneal fibrosis is idiopathic in two-thirds of cases, with the remainder attributable to drugs, malignant diseases (8–10% of cases), infections, and surgery (Table 21.17.3).

Epidemiology

The only epidemiological data about the incidence and prevalence of idiopathic retroperitoneal fibrosis are from a Finnish study which reported an incidence of 0.1 per 100 000 person-years and a prevalence of 1.38 per 100 000. Males outnumber females with a ratio of 2.5:1; the mean age at presentation is 50 to 60 years, but there are reports of children and older adults being affected; there is no clear ethnic predisposition. Familial clustering is rare, with anecdotal cases in twins and siblings reported.

Aetiology

The aetiology of idiopathic retroperitoneal fibrosis is unknown. It is significantly associated with HLA DRB1*03, an allele linked to various autoimmune diseases. Environmental factors such as smoking and occupational exposure to asbestos might play a part.

Pathogenesis

It is generally thought that idiopathic retroperitoneal fibrosis is an autoallergic condition. A popular hypothesis argues that periaortitis

Table 21.17.3 Causes of retroperitoneal fibrosis

Cause	Type of cause	Example
Idiopathic		
Secondary	Drugs	Methysergide, lysergic acid, bromocriptine, pergolide, ergotamine, methyldopa, hydralazine, β-blockers
	Malignant diseases	Carcinomas of the colon, prostate, breast, stomach, carcinoid, Hodgkin's and non-Hodgkin's lymphomas, sarcomas
	Infections	Tuberculosis, syphilis, histoplasmosis, actinomycosis, fungal infections.
	Surgical	Lymph node resection, colectomy, hysterectomy, aortic aneurysm repair.
	Other	Radiotherapy, retroperitoneal haemorrhage, histiocytoses, Erdheim–Chester disease, amyloidosis, sclerosing peritonitis (following peritoneal dialysis).

is driven by macrophages from atherosclerotic plaques presenting antigens such as oxidized low-density lipoprotein (LDL) and ceroid (a lipoprotein polymer resulting from LDL oxidation within plaque macrophages) to immunocompetent cells, which are recruited and activated in medial and adventitial aortic layers. Evidence in favour of this is that B cells producing antibodies to ceroid are found in close apposition to extracellular ceroid, with the inflammatory reaction then extending into the periaortic retroperitoneum. However, this is not the explanation in all cases: retroperitoneal fibrosis has been described in the absence of atherosclerosis, particularly in children. Moreover, some observations suggest that idiopathic retroperitoneal fibrosis is a manifestation of a systemic autoimmune disease rather than an exaggerated local reaction to atherosclerosis. An alternative 'autoimmune' hypothesis is that the condition is initiated as a vasculitis of the vasa vasorum in the aortic wall, which is often seen in chronic periaortitis. This inflammatory process can cause weakening of aortic wall with medial thinning, can promote atherosclerosis, and can also extend into the surrounding retroperitoneum, with a fibro-inflammatory reaction typical of chronic periaortitis. An autoimmune reaction to plaque antigens could be an epiphenomenon of this immune-mediated process.

Another potential pathogenetic mechanism may be activating antibodies against fibroblasts, which are detectable in about one-third of patients with idiopathic retroperitoneal fibrosis. Support for this hypothesis comes from the observation that patients with this condition have IgG4-bearing plasma cells, a common finding in sclerosing pancreatitis, which is sometimes associated with idiopathic retroperitoneal fibrosis.

Infiltrating B cells in idiopathic retroperitoneal fibrosis may show clonal or oligoclonal immunoglobulin heavy chain rearrangement, raising the possibility of the condition being a primary B-cell disorder.

Secondary retroperitoneal fibrosis

Secondary retroperitoneal fibrosis can be caused by many factors and clinical conditions with varying pathogenic mechanisms (see Table 21.17.3). The most common cause is certain drugs, particularly derivatives of ergot alkaloids, e.g. methysergide, which affect the retroperitoneum and also the pericardium, pleura, and lungs. Their effect probably mediated by serotonin.

Malignant retroperitoneal fibrosis results from a florid desmoplastic response to retroperitoneal metastases, or local release of mediators such as serotonin by carcinoids, or release of profibrogenic growth factors by other cancers.

Infective retroperitoneal fibrosis is probably due to local spread of an infectious focus such as tuberculosis from paraspinal abscesses. Other rare causes of secondary retroperitoneal fibrosis include abdominal surgery, radiotherapy, and proliferative disorders such as Erdheim–Chester disease. The latter is a rare form of non-Langerhans' cell histiocytosis that is characterized by osteosclerosis, exopthalmos, and diabetes insipidus. Retroperitoneal involvement is found in about 20 to 30% of cases, which can mimic retroperitoneal fibrosis but is characterized by xanthogranulomatous infiltration with foamy histiocytes nested in areas of fibrosis.

Clinical features

The clinical manifestations of retroperitoneal fibrosis vary with the stage of presentation. Early symptoms typically consist of mild fever, weight loss, weakness, nausea, vomiting, and malaise. There is often an associated dull back, flank and abdominal pain, with no specific radiation pattern, which generally does not respond to NSAIDs. Later disease is characterized by symptoms related to the entrapment of retroperitoneal structures, i.e. ureters (back and/or flank and/or abdominal pain, haematuria, polyuria/oliguria/anuria), renal arteries (renovascular hypertension), superior and inferior mesenteric vessels (bowel ischaemia), inferior vena cava (leg oedema and deep vein thrombosis), gonadal vessels (hydrocoele), and lymphatics, aorta, and common iliac arteries (lymphoedema, claudication, and rarely gangrene). The most frequent of these complications is ureteric obstruction, which can lead to acute or chronic renal failure.

In up to 15% of patients with retroperitoneal fibrosis the fibrotic process can also involve structures outside the retroperitoneum, supporting the hypothesis that this is a systemic disease. Mediastinal fibrosis, Riedel's fibrosing thyroiditis, sclerosing cholangitis, fibrotic orbital pseudotumor, fibrotic arthropathy, and pleural/pericardial/lung fibrosis have been reported.

Abnormalities demonstrated by laboratory tests include some degree of renal insufficiency in up to 75% of patients. Mild normochromic normocytic anemia and elevated inflammatory markers (ESR, CRP) are frequent, supporting the hypothesis that the disease process is inflammatory. Leucocytosis, thrombocytosis, hypergammaglobulinemia, and positive autoimmune/vasculitic serology (ANA, rheumatoid factor, P-ANCA, C-ANCA) are less common. Significant proteinuria and/or macroscopic haematuria are infrequent.

Diagnosis

Retroperitoneal fibrosis is more common than generally appreciated, particularly if subclinical forms of the condition are considered. Diagnostic delay is the rule: 6 to 12 months (or even longer) elapsed from the onset of symptoms to diagnosis in one series, perhaps explaining why bilateral rather than unilateral upper-tract obstruction was present in most patients.

Ultrasonography, isotopic methods, and IVU will reveal findings typical of urinary tract obstruction. The IVU may show medial deviation of the ureters (Fig. 21.17.4), but this may be present in normal subjects and is an unreliable guide to diagnosis. CT scanning will show the periaortic mass (Fig. 21.17.5). MRI produces findings comparable to those of CT.

Fluorodeoxyglucose-positron emission tomography (FDG-PET) is not useful for the diagnosis of retroperitoneal fibrosis because of low specificity. However, it allows whole-body imaging and can detect occult malignant or infectious foci, particularly in secondary retroperitoneal fibrosis. Furthermore, it can be used reliably to assess the metabolic activity of the retroperitoneal mass and thus be used to monitor the residual inflammatory component following medical therapy.

A histological diagnosis of retroperitoneal fibrosis should be obtained if at all possible. CT-guided needle biopsy of a mass may be sufficient to diagnose lymphoma or carcinoma with confidence (Fig. 21.17.6), but laparotomy is typically required to obtain a sufficiently large sample to exclude these conditions.

The microscopic appearance of idiopathic retroperitoneal fibrosis is characterized by fibrotic tissue infiltrated with a mixture of mononuclear cells, but the relative contribution of these two elements varies with disease stage. Initially, the tissue is often

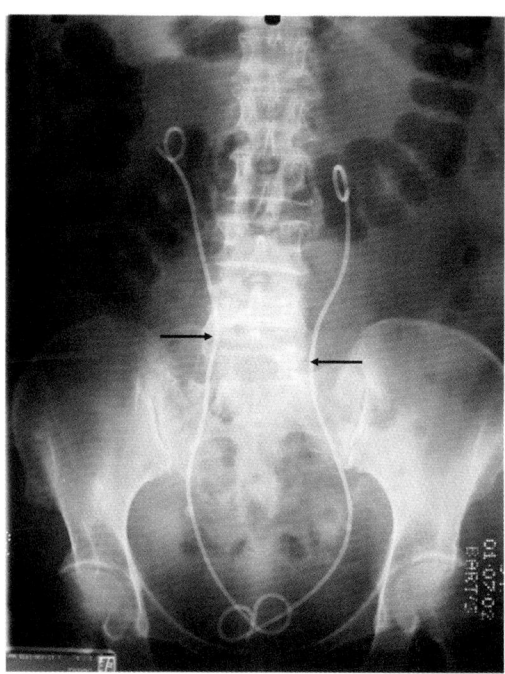

Fig. 21.17.4 JJ stents in the ureters of a patient with retroperitoneal fibrosis. Note the position of these stents, indicating medial deviation of the ureters (arrows).

oedematous and highly vascular, with an active chronic inflammatory component comprising large numbers of mononuclear cells (mainly CD20 +ve B cells, macrophages, plasma cells and eosinophils, with few CD4 +ve cells and an absence of neutrophils) within fibroblast and collagen bundles. In the late stages there is pronounced sclerosis and scattered calcifications (Fig. 21.17.7). Aside from lymphoma (Fig. 21.17.8), the differential diagnosis of retroperitoneal fibrosis includes the much rarer conditions of retroperitoneal fibromatosis (a condition associated with Gardner's syndrome characterized by homogenous proliferation of fibroblasts arranged in interlacing bundles) and inflammatory myofibroblastic tumour (which affects children and has distinct histological characteristics, mainly of myofibroblast proliferation).

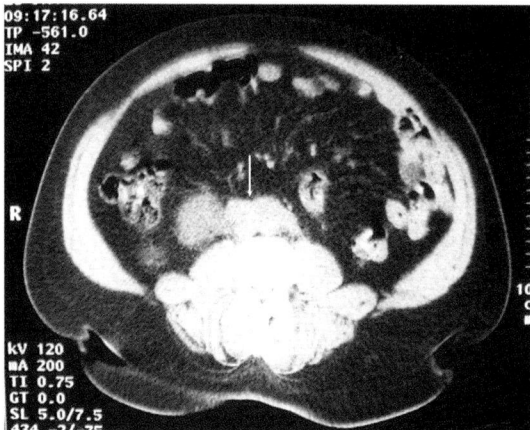

Fig. 21.17.5 CT scan of a patient with retroperitoneal fibrosis, showing periaortic fibrosis (arrow).

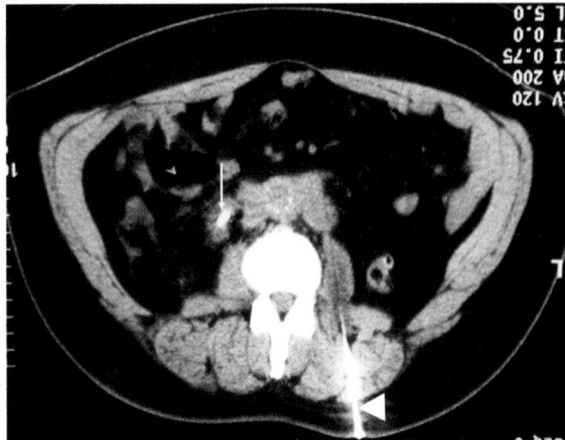

Fig. 21.17.6 CT guided needle biopsy of retroperitoneal fibrosis showing the needle (arrowhead) and its track. Note the arrow pointing at the stent in the right ureter.

Management

Management is empirical and controversial since controlled trials of treatment are lacking. The objective of any therapy includes relieving ureteric obstruction (when present), suppressing the acute phase reaction, halting the progression of fibrosis, and preventing relapse.

Urgent relief of obstruction is generally recommended if there is significant renal dysfunction, which may be achieved by antegrade nephrostomy, retrograde insertion of ureteric stents (see Fig. 21.17.4), or open surgical ureterolysis. This is not required if there is hydronephrosis but renal function is normal and stable: such cases will be managed medically, with close monitoring of serum creatinine and repeated ultrasound imaging to determine whether hydronephrosis is getting better or worse.

Treatment of secondary forms of retroperitoneal fibrosis requires dealing with the underlying cause. This may be straightforward, e.g. stopping of the culprit drug (usually in combination with corticosteroids, see below), but in some cases—e.g. untreatable cancer, trauma, major surgery, and radiotherapy—palliative surgical approaches are the only option, with relief of obstructive complications by the placement of ureteric stents and/or nephrostomies.

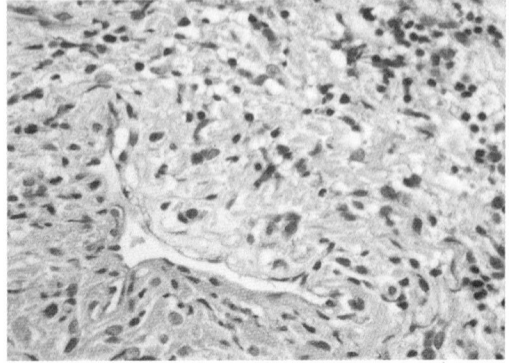

Fig. 21.17.7 Histological appearance of fibrocellular tissue consistent with retroperitoneal fibrosis.

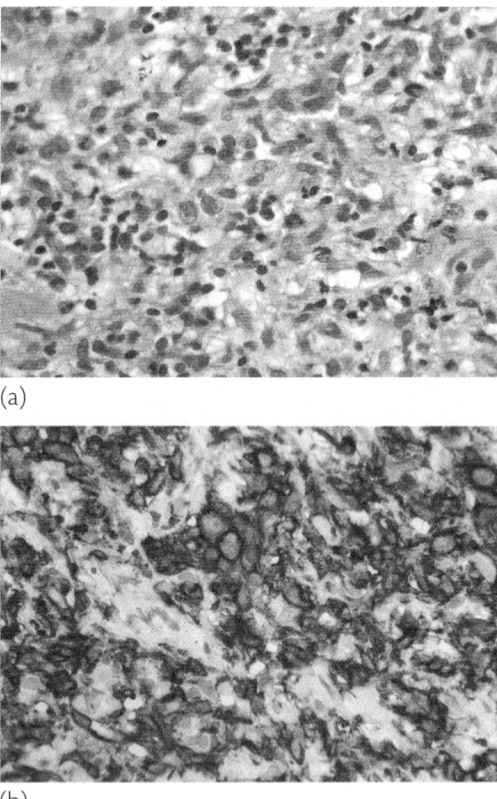

Fig. 21.17.8 Histological appearance of lymphoma presenting as retroperitoneal mass (a). Immunostaining reveals that the infiltrating cells are positive for CD 20, a cell surface marker for B lymphocytes (b).

Relief of obstruction

There have been no studies comparing antegrade nephrostomy, retrograde ureteric stenting, and open surgical ureterolysis in the management of patients with retroperitoneal fibrosis. The approach adopted is likely to depend upon availability of local expertise. However, open surgical ureterolysis, which requires mobilization of the ureters followed by their manipulation to try to prevent recurrent fibrotic encasement (by wrapping them in omental fat, transposing them laterally, or transplanting them intraperitoneally), is a difficult procedure with significant risks and complications (most obviously ureteric leakage). This should not be attempted by a surgeon who performs the procedure 'occasionally', and is perhaps best reserved for cases where (1) other methods of relieving obstruction have been unsuccessful or are particularly contraindicated, (2) there is significant unresolved concern that there is underlying malignancy and definitive diagnosis by surgical biopsy is required, or (3) medical treatment fails to achieve regression of the retroperitoneal fibrotic mass, which would leave the patient requiring long-term stents, although these are an option if the risks of surgery would be prohibitive (thermoexpandible metallic stents, Fig. 21.17.9).

Medical treatment

Standard practice is to give corticosteroid therapy, typically beginning with prednisolone 1 mg/kg per day (maximum 60 mg/day) for 4 to 6 weeks. Response of the inflammatory process is judged on the basis of changes in the patient's symptoms, inflammatory markers (ESR, CRP) and imaging (CT). If matters are improving

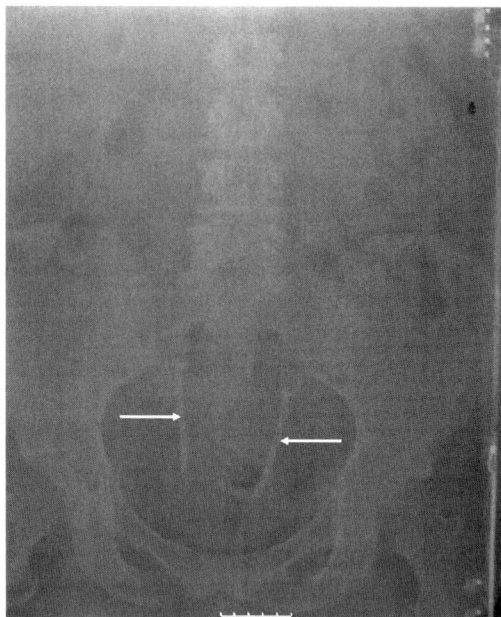

Fig. 21.17.9 'Memokath' metallic stents (arrows) placed in both lower ureters in a patient with retroperitoneal fibrosis.

the dose of prednisolone is then tapered to 10 mg/day over a few months, after which it is gradually withdrawn over the following year or so, with continued monitoring of symptoms and inflammatory markers (and imaging if appropriate). The diagnosis should be reviewed if matters do not improve after 4 to 6 weeks of oral prednisolone, but it remains possible that the patient does have idiopathic retroperitoneal fibrosis, but of a 'fibrotic' rather than an 'inflammatory' type.

If retroperitoneal fibrosis is refractory to corticosteroid treatment alone, it is common practice to add another immunosuppressive agent, e.g. azathioprine, cyclophosphamide, methotrexate, ciclosporin, mycophenolate. There are anecdotal reports of success.

The antioestrogen drug tamoxifen may result in the regression of benign fibrotic desmoid tumours, which has led to its use in patients with retroperitoneal fibrosis. Improvement was reported in 15 of 19 cases in one series, but there is no way of knowing whether this compares favourably with what would have been achieved with corticosteroids, and there is no data on long-term outcome.

Prognosis

Pain and constitutional symptoms usually resolve within a few days of starting corticosteroid treatment. Serum inflammatory markers fall rapidly and obstruction is typically relieved, with shrinking of the retroperitoneal mass, within a few weeks. Mortality is very low (in nonmalignant cases), but recurrence of disease is reported in 10 to 30% of cases in most series. This usually occurs within the first year but has been reported over 10 years later, hence long-term surveillance is required with annual measurement of blood pressure, serum creatinine, and inflammatory markers, and with a low threshold for repeat imaging.

Further reading

Obstruction

Jung P, *et al.* (2000). Magnetic resonance urography enhanced by gadolinium and diuretic: a comparison with conventional urography in diagnosing the cause of ureteric obstruction. *Br J Urol Int A*, **86**, 960–5.

Klahr S (2003). Obstructive nephropathy: pathophysiology and management. In: Schrier RW (ed) *Renal and electrolyte disorders*, 6th edition, pp. 498–538. Lippincott-Raven, Philadelphia.

McClelland P, *et al.* (1994). Obstructive uropathy and progression of renal failure. *Nephrol Dialysis Transplant*, **8**, 952A.

Sfakianakis GN, *et al.* (2000). MAG-3-F0 scintigraphy in decision making for emergency intervention in renal colic after helical CT positive for a urolith. *J Nuclear Med*, **41**, 1813–22.

Webb JA (2000). Ultrasonography and Doppler studies in the diagnosis of renal obstruction. *Br J Urol*, **86** Suppl 1, 25–32.

Yaqoob M, Junaid I (2004). The patient with urinary tract obstruction. In: Davison AM *et al.* (eds) *Oxford textbook of clinical nephrology*, 3rd edition, pp. 2449–470. Oxford University Press, Oxford.

Retroperitoneal fibrosis

Baker LRI, *et al.* (1988). Idiopathic retroperitoneal fibrosis. A retrospective analysis of 60 cases. *Br J Urol*, **60**, 497–503.

Bascands JP, Schanstra JP (2005). Obstructive nephropathy: insights from genetically engineered animals. *Kidney Int*, **68**, 925–37.

Bourouma R, *et al.* (1997). Treatment of idiopathic retroperitoneal fibrosis with tamoxifen. *Nephrol Dialysis Transplant*, **12**, 2407–10.

Moroni G, Dore R, Collini P (2005). Idiopathic retroperitoneal fibrosis. *J Nephrol*, **18**, 794–808.

Ormond JK (1948). Bilateral ureteral obstruction due to envelopment and compression by an inflammatory process. *J Urol*, **59**, 1072–9.

Ozener C, *et al.* (1997). Potential beneficial effect of tamoxifen in retroperitoneal fibrosis. *Nephrol Dialysis Transplant*, **12**, 2166–8.

Uibu T, *et al.* (2004). Asbestos exposure as a risk factor for retroperitoneal fibrosis. *Lancet*, **363**, 1422–26.

Vaglio A, Salvarani C, Buzio C (2006). Retroperitoneal fibrosis. *Lancet*, **367**, 241–51.

Vaglio A, *et al.* (2005). ^{18}F-fluorodeoxyglucose positron emission tomography in the diagnosis and follow-up of idiopathic retroperitoneal fibrosis. *Arthritis Rheum*, **53**, 122–25.

van Bommel EF, *et al.* (2006). Brief communication: tamoxifen therapy for nonmalignant retroperitoneal fibrosis. *Ann Intern Med*, **144**, 101–6.

Veyssier-Belot C, *et al.* (1996). Erdheim–Chester disease. Clinical and radiologic characteristics of 59 cases. *Medicine (Baltimore)*, **75**, 157–169.

21.18

Malignant diseases of the urinary tract

David Neal

Essentials

Urological cancers are an important cause of morbidity and mortality. Their treatment frequently involves a combination of surgery, radiotherapy, and chemotherapy, with patients needing both local therapy to treat the primary tumour and systemic therapy to decrease the risk of metastatic relapse.

Bladder cancer

Bladder cancer usually arises from the transitional epithelium and typically presents with haematuria, lower urinary tract symptoms, pelvic pain, or (metastatic disease) systemic symptoms. Most cases are sporadic and related to cigarette smoking. They are graded histologically as: 1 (low risk of future progression), 2, or 3 (high risk of progression/metastases), and staged according to the tumour–nodes–metastases (TNM) classification, with the most important issues being whether the tumour is muscle invasive (T2 or above) or localized to urothelium only (Ta), and whether there is metastatic disease.

Management—(1) Low-risk noninvasive cancers (TaG1 and TaG2) are treated by endoscopic resection. (2) High-risk non-invasive cancers (TaG3, T1G3, carcinoma *in situ*) are treated by endoscopic resection plus intravesical immunotherapy with BCG (bacille Calmette–Guerin). (3) Muscle-invasive cancers with no evidence of metastatic disease are treated with radical surgery (cystoprostatectomy or cystectomy/hysterectomy/oophorectomy, with both requiring urinary diversion) or radiotherapy. Systemic chemotherapy is an option as either neo-adjuvant or adjuvant treatment for muscle invasive disease.

Kidney cancer

Kidney cancer most commonly (75–85% of cases) arises from the epithelium of the proximal tubule (clear cell renal carcinoma). Most cases are sporadic, but the condition is common in the von Hippel–Lindau syndrome, and almost all sporadic tumours show mutations in the *VHL* tumour suppressor gene. Histologically they are graded into Fuhrman grades 1 (best prognosis) to 4 (worst), and staged according to the TNM classification. Typical presentation is with haematuria, but many cases are discovered incidentally on abdominal imaging.

Management—(1) Surgery (laparoscopic or open) is the primary treatment for localized renal cell carcinoma, which is not responsive to conventional chemotherapy and not radiosensitive. (2) Metastatic renal cell carcinoma has a poor outcome (median survival 8 months): treatments include biological response modifiers to stimulate the immune system (e.g. interleukin and interferon) and small molecules targeting pathways involved in tumour-cell proliferation and angiogenesis (e.g. sorafenib), but response is limited. (3) Small asymptomatic renal masses that are detected incidentally in older patients often grow very slowly and may not alter life expectancy.

Prostate cancer

Prostate cancer is the commonest malignancy in men in the United Kingdom and the United States of America. Diagnosis and treatment is not straightforward because some prostate cancers are indolent and very unlikely to progress, whereas others are highly aggressive.

Diagnosis, grading, and staging—early prostate cancer is asymptomatic: diagnosis is made by combining a digital rectal examination (DRE) with serum prostate-specific antigen (PSA) measurement linked to transrectal ultrasound scanning and biopsy. Symptomatic presentation of more advanced disease is typically with lower urinary tract symptoms, or with evidence of metastatic disease. Histologically graded by the Gleason score (well differentiated, 6 or less; moderately differentiated, 7; poorly differentiated, 8–10), and staged according to the TNM classification.

Management—(1) Disease localized to the prostate may be treated with curative intent, either with surgery or radiotherapy, or by 'active monitoring' (regular PSA testing and DRE, with treatment if there is evidence of progression). (2) Locally advanced disease can be managed using a combination of radiotherapy and neo-adjuvant hormone therapy. (3) Metastatic prostate cancer is incurable but dramatically responsive to androgen blockade, which is most commonly achieved with luteinizing hormone-releasing hormone (LHRH) agonists, although eventually the cancer develops into a hormone-independent state.

Testicular cancer

Typically presents with a painless testicular swelling that may grow rapidly. Ninety per cent are of germ-cell origin—either seminomatous or nonseminomatous. Staged according to the TNMs classification, where 's' designates the serum tumour marker (α-fetoprotein, β-human chorionic gonadotropin (β-hCG), and lactate dehydrogenase (LDH)) level.

Management—all solid testicular masses are usually treated with radical inguinal orchidectomy, after which treatment depends on histological type: (1) seminomas—Stage 1 may be offered para-aortic radiotherapy, or single-dose chemotherapy, or surveillance with chemotherapy given at the time of clinical relapse; Stage 2 is treated with radiotherapy or chemotherapy; (2) nonseminomatous germ cell cancer—Stage 1 may be offered surveillance with chemotherapy on relapse, prophylactic chemotherapy, or primary retroperitoneal lymph node dissection; metastatic disease is treated with chemotherapy.

Urothelial cancer

Bladder cancer is the eighth commonest cause of death from malignant disease in England and Wales and the fourth most common cancer in men (data from CRUK 2006). It usually arises from the transitional epithelium that lines the urinary tract from the tips of the renal papillae to the distal urethra, hence transitional cell carcinoma (sometimes known as urothelial cell cancer) may arise in the kidney, ureter, bladder, or urethra. The bladder is the commonest site of origin, where it usually presents with haematuria, lower urinary tract symptoms, pelvic pain, or—when there is metastatic disease—with systemic symptoms.

Other primary epithelial cancers of the bladder include squamous cell carcinoma, which arises in response to chronic inflammation/irritation of the bladder following exposure to schistosomiasis, radiotherapy, chronic infection, or long-term catheterization. Adenocarcinoma can arise from urachal remnants in the dome of the bladder, but more commonly is a consequence of locally invasive or metastatic disease where the bladder is invaded by direct extension from a sigmoid adenocarcinoma.

Risk factors

The risk factors for urothelial cell cancers are well established (Table 21.18.1) and include male sex, increasing age, and smoking. Occupational exposure to aromatic amines, dyes, and anilines increases the risk. The metabolism of aromatic amines involves acetylation through a polymorphic enzyme (*N*-acetyltransferase 2), with slow acetylator status appearing to be a risk factor. Chronic inflammation associated with schistosomiasis infection predisposes to squamous cell carcinoma and treatment with cyclophosphamide predisposes to bladder cancer. Radiotherapy to the pelvis for the treatment of gynaecological malignancy increases the risk of distal ureteric transitional cell carcinoma fourfold.

The vast majority of bladder cancer is sporadic and related to cigarette smoking, but one rare genetic syndrome (Lynch's syndrome—hereditary nonpolyposis colon cancer, OMIM 120435) caused by mutations in DNA mismatch repair genes increases the risk of right-sided colon cancer and transitional cell carcinoma of the upper urinary tract.

Table 21.18.1 Risk factors for transitional carcinoma

Risk factors for transitional cell carcinoma of the bladder	Additional risk factors for upper-tract transitional cell carcinoma
Smoking	Analgesic nephropathy
Increasing age	Papillary necrosis
Male gender	Chinese herb nephropathy
Chemical/occupational exposure	Balkan nephropathy
Cyclophosphamide treatment	
Chronic inflammation	
Schistosomiasis infection	
External beam radiation	
Genetic risk factors (rare)	

Some Chinese medicines containing aristocholic acid are a cause of Chinese herb nephropathy, and this agent is likely to be the cause of Balkan nephropathy, both of which are strongly associated with upper urinary tract urothelial cell carcinoma (see Chapter 21.9.2).

Genetic changes

Oncogenes and tumour suppressor genes are involved in the pathogenesis of bladder cancer, and there are mutually exclusive genetic alterations that lead to the development of either papillary noninvasive transitional cell carcinoma (stage pTa) or high-grade invasive carcinomas. The most common sporadic genetic mutations in low-grade transitional cell carcinoma are loss of heterozygosity of chromosome 9 and alterations in fibroblast growth factor (FGF) 3. By contrast, high-grade invasive cancers most frequently show loss of tumour suppressor genes which affect the cell cycle such as *TP53*, *RB*, and *E2F3*. Loss of chromosome 8p and alterations in methylation of cytosine residues of particular genes in DNA are also associated with tumour progression in this high-grade invasive group. In the future such alterations may lead to new biomarkers of bladder cancer.

Staging and grading

Histological grade is usually ascribed as grade (G) 1, 2 or 3, with grade 1 tumours being at low risk of future progression and—regardless of tumour stage—grade 3 disease being at high risk for progression and development of metastatic disease.

Clinical bladder cancer staging follows the TNM classification (Table 21.18.2; Fig. 21.18.1). The most important issues are whether the local tumour is muscle invasive (T2 or above) or localized to the urothelium only (Ta), or invading lamina propria (pT1)and whether there is any evidence of metastatic disease to pelvic lymph nodes, bone or lung. Traditionally, bladder cancers were described as either superficial (located in the urothelium or lamina propria—pTa or pT1) or muscle invasive. This division arose on the basis that superficial disease may be resected completely endoscopically via the urethra using electrocautery, but unfortunately this distinction does not truly reflect the risk to patients from a T1G3 bladder cancer or carcinoma *in situ*, up to one-third of whom will die of bladder cancer.

Low-risk noninvasive bladder cancer—TaG1, TaG2

These tumours comprise most of all new bladder cancers (60%), usually present with painless macroscopic haematuria, and are easily

Table 21.18.2 TNM classification of transitional cell carcinoma of the bladder

Bladder cancer stage	Stage descriptor
Primary tumour (T stage)	
Ta	Noninvasive papillary tumour
Tis/Cis	Carcinoma *in situ*
T1	Tumour invades lamina propria
T2a	Superficial muscularis propria invaded
T2b	Deep muscularis propria invaded
T3a	Microscopic perivesical fat invasion
T3b	Macroscopic perivesical fat invasion
T4	Tumour invades prostate, uterus, vagina T4a, pelvic side wall; T4b, abdominal wall
Nodal status	
N0	No lymph node metastases
N1	Single nodal metastasis, <2 cm in size
N2	Node 2–5 cm or multiple nodes
N3	Nodes >5 cm
Metastases	
M0	No distant metastases
M1	Distant metastases

diagnosed using flexible cystoscopy under local anaesthetic. Treatment is by endoscopic resection under either spinal or general anaesthesia: a cystoscope is inserted into the bladder through the urethra and electrocautery is used to remove the lesion.

The tumours are usually papillary and are often found on a stalk are fronded, but may be multifocal and will recur locally in the bladder in about 75% of patients in the long term. The risk of progression to muscle-invasive disease with TaG1 disease is extremely low. The risk of recurrent superficial disease can be reduced by the

instillation of chemotherapeutic agents (mitomycin C) into the bladder immediately following endoscopic resection. These chemotherapeutic drugs have a high molecular weight, which means that they are usually not absorbed through the bladder mucosa or associated with neutropenia or other systemic side effects.

Patients with noninvasive bladder cancer require long-term endoscopic surveillance of the bladder until they have been free of recurrence disease for 5 years.

High-risk superficial bladder cancer—TaG3, T1G3, carcinoma *in situ*

Poorly differentiated high-grade bladder tumours have a different genetic profile from low-risk tumours, more akin to muscle-invasive tumours. It is uncommon for a low-risk cancer (pTa, G1, or G2) to progress to a high-risk one, but progression of pT1 or pTa G3 disease to muscle invasion occurs commonly. Isolated TaG3 disease progresses to muscle-invasive disease in up to 40% of patients after 5 years in the absence of aggressive local therapy following endoscopic resection. Adjuvant treatment in the form of intravesical immunotherapy with BCG (bacille Calmette–Guérin) is offered to such patients. This is instilled in to the bladder once per week for 6 weeks, its mechanism of action being via stimulation of T cells that coordinate an immune response to destroy residual disease and reduce the risk of future recurrence. A diagnosis of T1G3 disease should prompt an early second endoscopic resection as some patients will have muscle-invasive disease. If no evidence of muscle invasion is found on repeat resection, a 6-week course of BCG with maintenance dosing every 3 months is advised.

Carcinoma *in situ* is an aggressive intraepithelial neoplasia with a high risk of progression to solid muscle-invasive tumours. It is also treated with intravesical BCG, to which up to 65% of people will respond. Recurrent disease should be treated by cystectomy, if the patient is fit.

Muscle invasive bladder cancer

One in four new bladder tumours are found to be muscle invasive on resection, and up to 50% of these have overt or covert metastases at presentation. Patients with muscle-invasive bladder tumour require staging with a bimanual rectal or vaginal examination at the time of resection to designate a clinical T stage. Staging is completed with a CT scan of the abdomen, pelvis, and chest (Fig. 21.18.2). Routine biochemistry should be checked and if the alkaline phosphatase is elevated a bone scan should be performed.

A patient with muscle-invasive bladder cancer and no evidence of metastatic disease requires aggressive local treatment. Treatment options for the local tumour include either surgery or radiotherapy. There are no recent randomized trials comparing the two treatments, but it is generally accepted that surgery provides better local control at the expense of higher risk. Some patients (e.g. those with small pT2 lesions away from the trigone of the bladder) will respond well to resection and radiation, or chemoradiation. Radical surgery involves cystoprostatectomy in men and cystectomy, hysterectomy, and oophorectomy in women (anterior exenteration). An extended pelvic lymph node dissection is also performed: this provides prognostic information and is therapeutic for patients with low-volume micrometastatic disease. Urinary diversion is then established by means of an ileal conduit (incontinent cutaneous diversion), or bladder substitution (folding 55 cm of small bowel into a sphere and anastomosing it to the

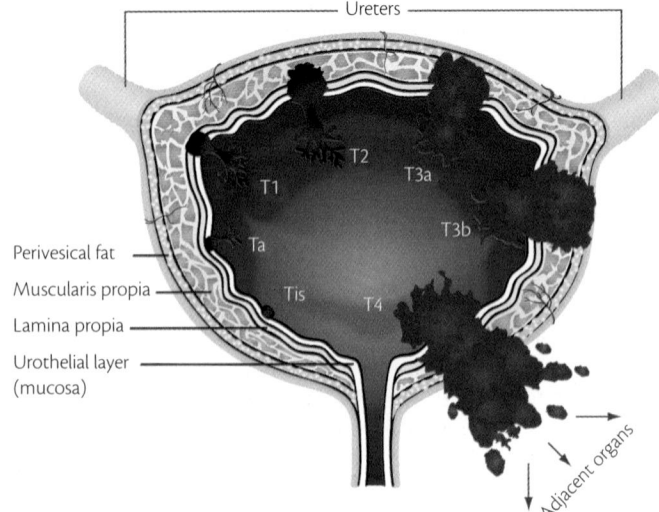

Fig. 21.18.1 Staging of bladder cancer.

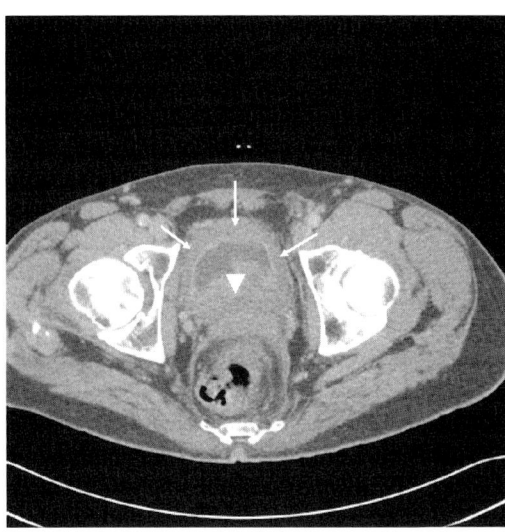

Fig. 21.18.2 CT scan of the pelvis showing a transitional cell carcinoma of the bladder (arrowhead) demonstrating muscle invasion (arrows).

urethra—continent urethral diversion), or a continent cutaneous reservoir (less common, as it frequently requires reoperation).

Alternative local therapy can be provided by means of radiotherapy to the bladder. The major benefit of this approach is that it allows bladder preservation, thereby avoiding the many long-term side effects of urinary diversion. However, it does place the patient at risk of developing a second muscle-invasive bladder cancer. Overall up to 50% of patients have persistent or subsequent recurrent disease in the bladder, and up to 30% will require a subsequent cystectomy.

Bladder cancer is moderately chemosensitive, hence systemic chemotherapy is an option as either neo-adjuvant or adjuvant treatment for patients with muscle-invasive bladder cancer. Neo-adjuvant treatment in the form of MVAC (methotrexate, vinblastine, adriamycin, and cisplatin) provides a 5 to 7.5% overall survival benefit for patients who subsequently undergo radical cystectomy or radiation treatment. Chemotherapy is also used in patients with node-positive disease or lymphovascular space invasion at the time of cystectomy, although many are too debilitated following surgery to receive chemotherapy.

Metastatic transitional cell carcinoma

Patients with regional metastatic disease to lymph nodes in the pelvis can be given chemotherapy if they are fit enough. This may result in complete radiological resolution, after which cystectomy can be performed. If residual active cancer is identified in the pelvic lymph nodes or there is invasion of the lymphovascular space, then the patient has a very poor prognosis.

Patients with nonregional metastatic disease to bones, liver, lungs, or abdominal lymph nodes have a very low 5-year survival. Chemotherapy can be offered if the patient has good performance status. Palliative radiotherapy to the bladder helps in local control and reduces haematuria, or ureteric obstruction which can lead to renal failure.

Transitional cell carcinoma of the kidney or ureter

Patients with high-grade bladder cancer are at risk of developing upper-tract transitional cell carcinoma (*c.*5%), but there are several other specific risk factors for its development, including phenacetin abuse, papillary necrosis, Balkan nephropathy, and Chinese herb nephropathy, as well as hereditary nonpolyposis colon cancer (HNPCC). Accurate staging, grading, and surveillance of the upper tracts is difficult and recurrence rates are high, hence these patients are generally best treated with nephroureterectomy if the contralateral kidney is normal. Annual cystoscopy is recommended thereafter because over 50% of patients with new upper-tract transitional cell carcinoma will go on to develop transitional cell carcinoma of the bladder.

Kidney cancer

In the United Kingdom renal cell cancer was the 10th commonest tumour in men and 15th commonest in women in 2004, with a 5:3 male:female incidence. The incidence is increasing in the United Kingdom and across the Western world, largely as a result of the routine use of abdominal imaging to evaluate abdominal pain. Most tumours detected in such a way are small and asymptomatic with an excellent prognosis. In the United Kingdom, however, there has also been an increasing mortality from kidney cancer that appears to be due to an increasing number of patients presenting with advanced and metastatic disease, which is a major concern when most other common cancers now have decreasing mortality rates.

Primary kidney cancer arises from the renal parenchyma in 90% of cases. There are different histological subtypes, each of which is important as they have different prognoses and different genetic causes. Kidney cancer that arises from the epithelium of the proximal tubule is known as conventional or clear cell renal carcinoma (75–85%). Other histological subtypes include papillary (15%), chromophobe (5%), collecting duct (<1%), and unclassified tumours. Some 5 to 10% of cancers in the kidney arise from the epithelium of the collecting system and are therefore classified as transitional cell carcinoma of the upper tract. Secondary tumours of the kidney occur in association with lymphoma, breast, and lung cancer. Primary renal cell carcinoma tends to metastasize to lung, lymph nodes, and bone (lytic lesions), and less commonly to liver, brain, and soft tissue.

Risk factors

The risk factors for sporadic renal cell carcinoma include increasing age, male sex, and cigarette smoking. Smoking conveys a relative risk of twofold for developing conventional renal cell carcinoma and is the most consistent of studied risk factors. Patients on dialysis may develop acquired cystic disease of the kidneys, which increases the risk of renal cell carcinoma between 5 and 30 times. Patients with a previous history of sporadic renal cell carcinoma treated with radical nephrectomy have a 1% risk per decade of developing a metachronous tumour. Other risk factors studied include obesity, which may be an important risk factor for women, and possibly hypertension. There is conflicting evidence as to whether hypertension increases the risk of renal cell carcinoma.

Patients with inherited cancer syndromes associated with renal cell carcinoma develop multifocal tumours at a younger age than those with sporadic renal cell carcinoma. Von Hippel–Lindau syndrome (OMIM 193300) has several different subtypes, with differing likelihood of developing renal cell carcinoma. Family members tend to develop renal tumours at the same age as the index case, hence screening is performed at the appropriate ages in younger probands.

Cumulative exposure to radiation is an important consideration in the long-term follow-up of such patients: wherever possible MRI and ultrasonography are used for screening.

Genetic changes

There are both sporadic and genetic (familial) forms of renal cell carcinoma. Genetic renal cell carcinoma is associated with Von Hippel–Lindau syndrome. Hereditary papillary renal cell carcinoma comes in two forms: type I associated with mutations in the receptor for hepatocyte growth factor, c-MET; and type II associated with mutations in the fumarate hydratase gene. Birtt–Hogge–Dube syndrome (OMIM 135150) is associated with chromophobe carcinoma, and there are other rare inherited syndromes. Knowledge of kidney cancer genetics has been derived mainly from studying these several rare inherited syndromes.

The genetic alterations in von Hippel–Lindau syndrome are found in a tumour suppressor gene located on chromosome 3 at locus 3p25–26. Individuals with von Hippel–Lindau syndrome inherit the abnormality of this tumour suppressor gene as a germline mutation, with tumours developing in an individual with subsequent knock-out of the single normal gene either by mutation, deletion, or methylation, hence this tumour follows Knudson's two-hit hypothesis (see Chapter 6.2). In sporadic renal cell carcinoma nearly 100% of tumours also show loss of 3p 25–26, with the mutations in chromosome 3 in sporadic RCC forming a wider spectrum than those seen in von Hippel–Lindau syndrome. A protein known as hypoxia inducible factor 1 α (HIF-1α) is part of the normal cellular mechanism for adaptation to hypoxia, allowing cells to grow and survive under hypoxic conditions (such as those seen with rapid growth of solid tumours) by inducing the expression of angiogenic growth factors such as VEGF. The von Hippel–Lindau tumour suppressor gene product normally targets HIF1-α for destruction in the proteosome by means of ubiquitinylation. In its absence the end result is that high levels of VEGF drive tumorigenesis, and drive the marked angiogenesis that is such a feature of renal cell carcinoma. Small-molecule inhibitors of VEGF have now been developed for clinical use.

There are also well-established genetic abnormalities for papillary renal cell carcinoma, including mutation in the c-*met* oncogene, gains in chromosomes 7 and 17, loss of chromosome Y, and mutations in fumarate hydratase. The genetic locus involved in the hereditary form of chromophobe renal cell carcinoma has recently been identified, which should allow further research in to the abnormalities found in sporadic chromophobe renal cell carcinoma.

Diagnosis, staging, and grading

Renal cell carcinoma is staged by the TNM classification. If a solid mass is detected in the kidney on ultrasonography, a contrast-enhanced CT scan of the abdomen and chest is performed to evaluate the mass, and to assess for metastatic disease. Solid masses in the parenchyma typically enhance with intravenous contrast, and more than 90% of such masses are malignant. Percutaneous biopsy is not accurate enough to reliably distinguish benign from malignant masses and is therefore not performed unless there is a strong suspicion that lymphoma may be responsible, or there is a suspicion that the renal lesion is metastatic, or where surgery may lead to renal failure because there is significant renal impairment.

Simple cystic masses with no internal echoes or septation occur in the renal parenchyma of 50% of 50-year-olds and are benign. Complex cysts (meaning those with septation, calcification, or solid elements) on ultrasonography require CT scanning to detect enhancing elements and are likely to be well-differentiated cystic renal cell carcinomas.

Clinical staging with CT allows identification of metastatic disease to lymph nodes, adrenal glands, liver, and chest. Renal cell carcinoma also frequently metastasizes to bone, where lytic lesions are typically found. A bone scan is performed if the patient has bone pain or an elevated alkaline phosphatase. Another important feature of renal cell carcinoma is the propensity for the tumour to invade the renal vein and subsequently the inferior vena cava (Fig. 21.18.3), even extending as far as the right atrium. Staging with multislice CT or MRI is important to determine the distal extent of the tumour thrombus as this affects the surgical approach required.

The Fuhrman grading system for renal cell cancer is a histological grading system based on the architecture and size of the nucleus assessed at low power. This is graded 1–4, with 4 designating a worse prognosis, and carries independent prognostic information.

Paraneoplastic phenomena

Paraneoplastic syndromes are common in renal cell carcinoma and include hypercalcaemia, polycythaemia from erythropoietin production, and weight loss/anaemia. Stauffer's syndrome comprises abnormal liver function tests and coagulation defects that normalize after nephrectomy. If suspected paraneoplastic syndromes do not disappear following nephrectomy, then it is likely that there is undiagnosed metastatic disease.

Treatment

Renal cell cancer is not responsive to conventional chemotherapy and is not radiosensitive. Surgery is therefore the primary treatment for localized renal cell carcinoma. Radical nephrectomy involves removal of the kidney within Gerota's fascia (renal fascia), with en bloc removal of the ipsilateral adrenal gland and hilar lymph nodes. Partial nephrectomy is increasingly used to excise small solid masses in patients with a solitary kidney, impaired renal function, or bilateral tumours, and also as primary treatment in

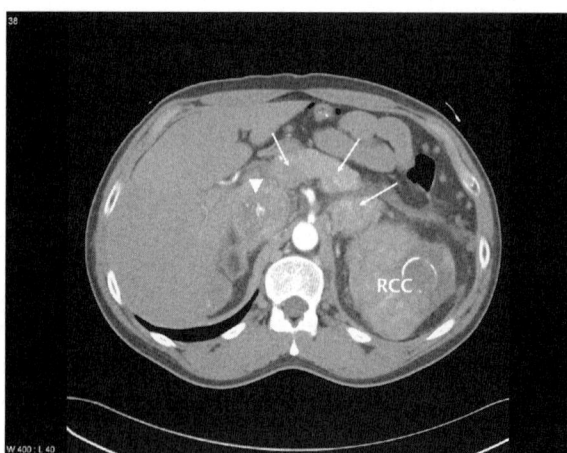

Fig. 21.18.3 Left renal cell cancer (RCC) spreading through the renal vein (arrows) into the inferior vena cava (arrowhead).

people with normal renal function. The surgical approach to the kidney may be with open or laparoscopic surgery.

Laparoscopic surgery

Laparoscopic nephrectomy was first performed in 1991, and this is now the gold standard for surgical treatment of T1 tumours. The oncological outcomes are equivalent to open surgery, and postoperative recovery is much faster, with shorter hospital stay, lower analgesic requirement, and earlier return to paid employment. The role for laparoscopic radical nephrectomy is expanding, with experienced surgeons now treating selected T2 tumours. Partial nephrectomy may also be performed laparoscopically by a skilled team, but this is a difficult procedure that is performed well only by a small number of surgeons throughout the world.

Open surgery

The approach to the kidney may either be through the abdomen (anterior), through the flank, or by a combined approach through the chest and abdomen (thoracoabdominal). Most T2 or more advanced localized cancers are treated with an anterior approach. Tumours that involve the renal vein and inferior vena cava (Fig. 21.18.3) may be treated surgically with good outcomes if the tumour thrombus has not invaded the wall of the cava (it usually projects as a floating tongue of thrombus inside the vessel). Such surgery involves mobilization of the liver and may require cardiac bypass if the tumour thrombus reaches the right atrium. Open partial nephrectomy is now the treatment of choice for small primary renal cell carcinomas.

Metastatic disease

Metastatic renal cell carcinoma has a poor outcome with very short median survival, although there are rare reports (0.8% of cases) of regression of metastatic disease following nephrectomy. Management varies according to the volume of metastatic disease, the sites of metastases, and patient's performance status. Those with metastases to the brain, liver, and bone tend to have a poor prognosis, whereas those with nonbulky lymph node disease and pulmonary metastases have a better outlook.

Patients with good performance status (meaning that they are systemically well) and low-volume metastatic disease have survival benefit if they undergo a nephrectomy. Given that renal cell cancer is not responsive to conventional chemotherapy, other treatment is with biological response modifiers that are used to stimulate the immune system, the response to which also appears to be better if a patient has had a nephrectomy. Interleukin has a better complete response rate than interferon, but is very toxic with significant side effects, hence the latter is the most commonly used biological agent. Interferon can be administered on an outpatient basis, three times a week via a subcutaneous injection, but the partial response is only 10 to 15%, with a complete response rate of 2%. The most exciting developments for the treatment of renal cell carcinoma are small-molecule therapies targeted at pathways involved in tumour-cell proliferation and angiogenesis. One such promising agent can be taken orally (sorafenib) and prevents angiogenesis via inhibition of Raf-kinase and VEGF receptors, pathways which are up-regulated in renal cancers because of loss of the von Hippel–Lindau gene (as described previously). Sorafenib and other similar drugs are not cytotoxic but are cytostatic: they have the potential to prevent progression of metastatic disease, thus potentially turning this into a chronic illness as opposed to a rapidly fatal condition.

Palliative treatment for metastatic renal cell carcinoma includes radiotherapy to painful bony metastases, prophylactic orthopaedic surgery where severe cortical bone loss has occurred in weight-bearing long bones, whole-brain irradiation for brain metastases, and blood transfusion. There is little role for palliative chemotherapy.

Prognosis

As for many malignancies, long-term prognosis in renal cell carcinoma is strongly dependent on the initial clinical stage. Table 21.18.3 shows 5-year survival according to the original Robson classification. The presence of metastatic disease portends a very poor prognosis, with a median survival of only 8 months. The AJCC 1997 classification of primary renal tumour size designated a cut-off point of 7 cm to differentiate between T1 and T2 tumours: T1 tumours have now been separated into T1a (<4 cm) and T1b (4–7 cm), reflecting the excellent prognosis of small renal masses that are detected incidentally.

The outcome of small asymptomatic renal masses that are detected incidentally ('incidentalomas') is not yet clear, but it appears that in many cases they grow very slowly and may not threaten an individual's life expectancy. Historically renal masses less than 3 cm in size were classified as renal adenomas, although histologically some of these were likely to have been papillary tumours. Elderly patients or others who would be high risk for surgery can be offered monitoring with 3-monthly ultrasonography when a small (<4 cm) mass is diagnosed: if the size (volume) of the tumour is unchanged over 12 months, then most such lesions appear to remain stable over time. However, this approach is not yet validated and should not be recommended for young patients with small solid renal masses, because once renal cell cancer has metastasized there is little chance of cure.

Prostate cancer

Prostate cancer is an important health problem: it is the commonest malignancy in men in the United Kingdom and the United States of America and is second only to lung cancer as a cause of death from malignancy. In England and Wales it results in over 10 000 deaths annually. In the United States the recognized incidence of prostate cancer rose sharply after the introduction of prostate-specific antigen (PSA) testing in the early 1990s, but despite this the mortality from the condition has remained relatively static over the same time period, recently demonstrating a small decrease which has been ascribed to treatment for early-stage disease. However, in the United Kingdom, where PSA testing is not routine, there has also been a small decrease in mortality from prostate cancer, making it unlikely that changes in death rates are solely due to aggressive treatment of early cancers.

Table 21.18.3 Survival from renal cell carcinoma according to Robson stage

Robson kidney cancer stage	5-year survival (%)
Stage I	60–95
Stage II	47–80
Stage III	35–50
Stage IV	<5 (median survival 8 months)

The diagnosis and treatment of prostate cancer is more complex than it immediately appears. Difficulties arise because some prostate cancers are rather indolent, have long latent periods, and are highly unlikely to progress and cause metastatic disease in a given individual; by contrast, other prostate cancers are highly aggressive, and some have an intermediate risk. The challenge is to diagnose prostate cancer while it is localized and to treat those people who have clinically significant disease that is likely to threaten longevity. This is difficult because there are no biomarkers that predict accurately whether a man is likely to die from prostate cancer. The natural history of untreated prostate cancer is also poorly defined: autopsy studies reveal microscopic foci of prostate cancer in up to 60% of 60-year-olds, yet only 3% of these men will eventually die of the disease.

Risk factors

Increasing age is a strong risk factor, but genetic risk factors are also important. Some men with first degree relatives affected by prostate cancer have a two- to threefold higher risk, the risk being higher if the first-degree relative is a brother as opposed to a father. Ethnicity also influences the risk of prostate cancer, with African-Americans having the highest risk and Asian men the lowest risk. Dietary factors may play a role: lycopene (found in tomatoes), selenium, and vitamin E are potentially protective; a Western-style high-fat diet is associated with a high risk for prostate cancer in the developed world, and probably plays a role in the increasing risk of such cancer in Japanese men who migrate to the United States of America. As for many cancers, it is likely that there is an interaction between environmental factors and an inherited genetic predisposition leading to prostate cancer.

Genetic changes

Around 5 to 10% of all prostate cancer is thought to be related to a highly penetrant genetic predisposition, and genetic factors may be responsible for as many as 40% of those prostate cancers appearing at an early age (diagnosed prior to age 50 years). Several different putative prostate cancer genes are under evaluation, including *HPC1* (chromosome 1), *HPC2* (chromosome 17), *MSR1* (macrophage scavenging receptor 1—chromosome 8), and *RNASEl*. Men from families harbouring a *BRAC2* mutation have a fivefold increase in risk of prostate cancer. Recent genome wide scans have found more than 30 predisposition alleles known as single nucleotide polymorphisms [SNPs]. Many prostate cancers demonstrate a translocation between the androgen-regulated *TMPRS2* gene and the ETS transcription factor, putting the latter under the control of an androgen-regulated promoter.

The androgen receptor plays an important role in cell signalling, progression, and metastases in prostate cancer, and androgen blockade (antitestosterone agents) can produce clinical regression of local and metastatic disease. Mutations in the androgen receptor leading to overexpression or altered ligand binding are associated with the development of later hormone independence.

Diagnosis, staging, and grading

The prostate is divided into different zones (peripheral, central, transitional, periurethral, and fibromuscular) based on different embryological origins, with most prostate cancers (75%) arising in the peripheral zone. Early prostate cancer does not give rise to any symptoms, whereas locally advanced disease may cause lower urinary tract symptoms or haematuria, and metastatic disease may present with bone pain from sclerotic metastases. As early prostate cancer is asymptomatic, diagnosis is currently achieved by combining a digital rectal examination (DRE) with a PSA measurement linked to transrectal ultrasound scanning and biopsy of the prostate (TRUSP).

PSA is a serum protease that is secreted by prostatic epithelium. It is not a specific marker for cancer as there are many nonmalignant processes that also elevate PSA, such as benign prostatic hyperplasia (BPH), urinary tract infection, urinary tract instrumentation, ejaculation, and traumatic catheterization. Age-adjusted norms for PSA are available to improve the sensitivity and specificity of the measurement in clinical practice, an alternative approach being to set a predetermined cut-off above which further evaluation is recommended. PSA kinetics may be more valuable in making treatment decisions than a single value: a rapidly rising PSA with a short doubling time (even if starting at a very low number) indicates that a man is likely to have high-risk prostate cancer.

If a man has an elevated PSA or an abnormal DRE and there is no evidence of urinary or prostatic infection which might explain the elevation, then it is recommended that the patient undergoes a transrectal ultrasound-guided needle biopsy of the prostate under local anaesthesia, taking about 10 separate biopsies which will detect 80 to 85% of clinically significant prostate cancers.

Histological analysis is carried out by Gleason grading. The architecture is graded into five categories (1–5) for the most prominent pattern, the second most prominent pattern is assigned a secondary Gleason score, and the two scores are added together to give a Gleason sum (e.g. 3 + 4 = 7). Well-differentiated disease has a Gleason sum of 6 or less, moderately differentiated disease is 7, and poorly differentiated disease 8 to 10. It is unusual to diagnose a Gleason sum of less than 6 on needle biopsy; very well differentiated prostate cancers (Gleason <5) may be diagnosed following a transurethral resection of prostate and are usually indolent. The Gleason score is predictive of outcome: large observational studies show that men with poorly differentiated disease have a 60 to 80% chance of dying from prostate cancer within 15 years of diagnosis. The biggest problem is predicting outcome in the individual with Gleason 6 or 7 disease.

Prostate cancer is staged using the AJCC system (Table 21.18.4). When prostate cancer metastasizes it frequently goes to the pelvis, to non-regional lymph nodes, other bones (sclerotic metastases), and also local pelvic structures. It rarely invades the rectum, with Denonvillier's fascia providing a natural barrier. Digital rectal examination provides clinical T stage, but MRI scanning of the pelvis is now the preferred way of local staging. A bone scan is performed to evaluate for metastatic disease.

Screening

Screening for prostate cancer is a controversial issue. There are several large trials currently evaluating whether prostate cancer screening should be recommended. In the United Kingdom screening is not recommended as it does not fulfil World Health Organization or United Kingdom national screening guidelines. There is no doubt that prostate cancer is an important health problem, but with PSA screening most cancers currently detected are low volume, well differentiated, often indolent, and do not threaten an individual's life expectancy.

Table 21.18.4 TNM classification of prostate cancer

Prostate cancer stage	TNM Descriptor
Primary tumour (T stage)	
T1a	<5% of TURP chips, Gleason score <7
T1b	>5% of chips or high grade prostate cancer
T1c	Biopsy detected in benign feeling gland
T2a	Nodule <50% one lobe of prostate
T2b	Nodule >50% of one lobe
T2c	Nodules both lobes
T3	Disease extends outside prostate
T4	Invades other local organs/structures
Nodal status	
N0	No metastatic disease to lymph nodes
N1	Single node <2 cm
N2	Single node 2–5 cm or multiple nodes
N3	Node >5 cm
Metastases	
M0	No metastases
M1a	Nonregional lymph node metastases
M1b	Bone metastases
M1c	Other sites

Several large observational studies have aided our understanding of the risk of prostate cancer death following diagnosis. Screening with a PSA and DRE is imperfect as there are many nonmalignant reasons for PSA elevation, thus subjecting many men to a potentially morbid prostate biopsy (with complications including sepsis, haemorrhage, pain, and urinary symptoms). Assigning age-derived normal PSA values with a cut-off point does not detect all clinically relevant prostate cancer, as shown in the prostate cancer prevention trial where a significant number of Gleason 3 + 4 cancers were found with a PSA between 0 and 2.5 ng/ml (normal).

Although there are well-established treatment options for screen-detected prostate cancer, there are no robust randomized trials demonstrating efficacy of treatment or revealing which option provides the best outcome. One important clinical trial randomized patients in a pre-PSA era to watchful waiting or radical prostatectomy, showing an improvement in overall and prostate cancer specific survival for patients treated with radical prostatectomy. The ProtecT (United Kingdom) and PIVOT (United States of America) trials should provide useful further information, but it must be remembered that treatments for prostate cancer are not without significant morbidity, including impotence and incontinence (discussed below). One recent large randomized trial of screening, the European Randomized Study of Screening for prostate cancer (ERSPC) has shown a 20% reduction in prostate cancer deaths. However this was at the price of considerable overdiagnosis and over treatment with 50 men required to be treated to save one life.

Treatment

Treatment options for prostate cancer are dependent on many factors, including patient age, life expectancy, stage, Gleason grade, PSA kinetics, and tumour volume. For practical purposes patients are classified into having localized disease, locally advanced disease, or metastatic disease. One very important factor in the choice of treatment for a man with low- or intermediate-risk localized prostate cancer is the patient's view of the risks and benefits of treatment.

Localized disease

Disease localized to the prostate may be treated with curative intent, with either surgery or radiotherapy. Patients are eligible for radical treatment if they have a life expectancy greater than 10 years, reflecting the fact that because prostate cancer is generally slow growing, the benefit from treatment of early-stage prostate cancer is not gained unless the patient lives at least another decade. More conservative approaches such as 'active monitoring' are very reasonable options for patients with low volume localized disease and favourable Gleason grade. This form of management involves regular PSA testing and rectal examination and aims to treat prostate cancer once there is evidence of progression (increasing PSA or increases in local stage on rectal examination), but before there is metastatic disease.

Radical surgery

Radical prostatectomy involves removal of the prostate gland and seminal vesicles, plus or minus a pelvic lymph node dissection, followed by anastomosis of the bladder to the urethra. This can be performed by open or laparoscopic surgery, and the latter can be performed using a robotic three-dimensional system with superior instruments and vision over standard laparoscopy (Figs. 21.18.4 and 21.18.5).

After surgery there should be no detectable PSA in the serum, with PSA recurrence (rising PSA after surgery) indicating either local recurrence or metastatic disease. The long-term outcomes for screen-detected prostate cancer are good, with 80 to 90% 5-year biochemical-free survival (undetectable PSA). Local recurrent disease may follow where there are positive margins on the radical prostatectomy specimens, the chances of which can be reduced by low-dose radiotherapy in men at high risk of this complication.

The neurovascular bundles which produce penile erection and a sense of orgasm run very close to the prostate and are at risk during the operation. Their preservation depends on the skill of the surgeon, and whether the stage and grade of the tumour argue for a more radical excision of periprostatic tissue. The seminal vesicles are removed with the prostate, hence ejaculation is invariably absent. The risks of urinary incontinence also depend on the skill of the surgeon. The best outcomes from surgery are achieved in centres where surgeons perform a large number of operations.

Radical radiotherapy

Radical radiotherapy may be delivered using either external beam treatment or internally via brachytherapy (radioactive seeds implanted into the prostate). The cancer cure rates for surgery and radiotherapy are similar, with patient choice being the most important factor in deciding which treatment option is preferred. Overall there is slightly less urinary morbidity from radiotherapy, but at the expense of a small risk of bowel dysfunction (bloody diarrhoea). There also appears to be an increase in the risk of secondary cancers following pelvic radiotherapy, including rectal carcinoma.

Locally advanced disease

Locally advanced disease is described as cT3 or cT4 using the TNM classification. The definition of T3 disease is that it has either invaded the seminal vesicles or has spread beyond the prostate capsule as suggested by MRI or DRE. T4 disease invades the bladder

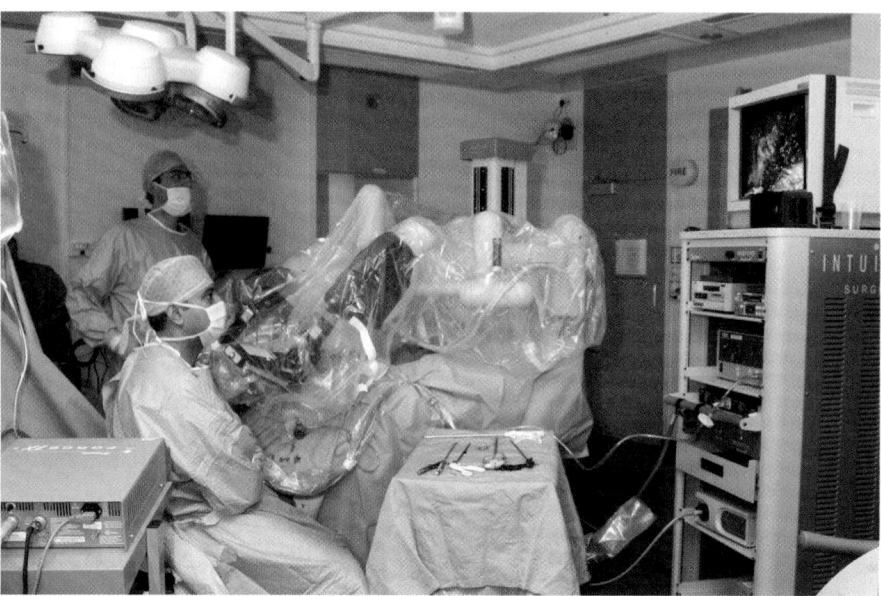

Fig. 21.18.4 Patient in theatre undergoing robotic prostatectomy.

base, urethral sphincter, or pelvic side wall. This is therefore a relatively heterogeneous group of patients, including some with early T3 disease and others with significant locally advanced disease. Some T3 patients can be managed using a combination of radiotherapy and neo-adjuvant hormone therapy. Patients with T4 disease are treated similarly, but also offered palliative radiotherapy as there is a high likelihood of both local recurrence and undetected micrometastatic disease. In the future multimodality treatment with chemoradiation and hormonal treatments, or combinations with radical surgery are likely to be tested in trials.

Metastatic prostate cancer

Metastatic prostate cancer is incurable but is dramatically hormone responsive. Androgens (testosterone, dihydrotestosterone, and

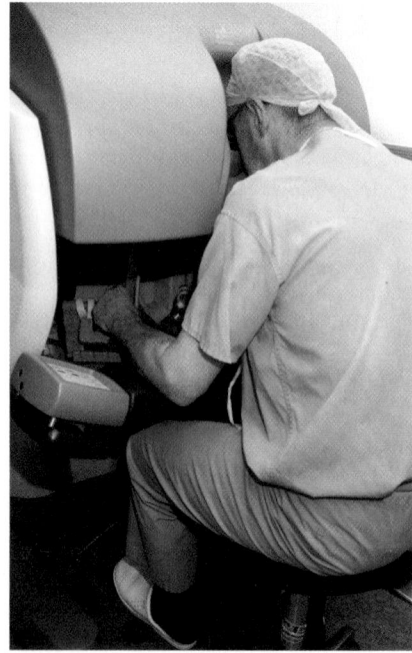

Fig. 21.18.5 The Author sitting at robotic console during radical prostatectomy.

dihydroepiandrostenedione—DHEA) drive prostate cancer growth via the androgen receptor. Androgen blockade at any point along the hypothalamic–pituitary axis results in tumour control, with temporary regression of local and metastatic disease in most men. Various forms of androgen blockade are available, including luteinizing hormone releasing hormone (LHRH) agonists, which work by providing a constant level of LHRH that prevents the physiological release of LH that is triggered by pulsatile gonadotropin releasing hormone (GnRH). Other options include orchidectomy or the use of antiandrogens. The most reliable forms of androgen blockade are LHRH agonists and orchidectomy. Patients are sometimes opposed to the latter for body image and psychological reasons, making LHRH agonists the most widely used form of castration.

Advanced prostate cancer treated by androgen ablation eventually develops into a hormone-independent state through selection of androgen-insensitive clones, or via further dedifferentiation of prostate cancer. Once a state of hormone independence is reached the median survival is less than 18 to 24 months. Second-line hormonal manipulations may result in PSA decline: these include the addition of an antiandrogen, or the use of oestrogens or ketoconazole, the latter being quite toxic. There is no proven survival benefit for such measures, but a decline in PSA may correlate with delayed progression. Chemotherapy with taxanes can result in modest improvements in overall survival in men with hormone-unresponsive disease and is now being trialled as an adjuvant treatment for high-risk early-stage prostate cancer.

Haematuria, lower urinary tract symptoms, and distal ureteric obstruction are common manifestations in patients with hormone-independent prostate cancer. Haematuria may be treated with palliative radiotherapy to the prostate bed, and symptoms suggestive of bladder outflow obstruction can be treated with a channel transurethral prostatic resection if the patient's performance status allows. Distal ureteric obstruction results in obstructive renal failure and may be treated with ureteric stenting in selected cases, but such intervention should not be pursued in a patient who is obviously terminally ill.

Bone metastases may cause pain, pathological fractures, or spinal cord compression. Radiotherapy in single fractions is useful in alleviating painful bone disease. Zoledronic acid, a potent bisphosphonate, can be used to reduce skeletal-related events.

Testicular cancer

Testicular cancer accounts for 1% of male malignancies and is unusual in that it occurs predominantly in young men, being the most common tumour in 15- to 44-year-olds in the United Kingdom. The peak incidence of 15 cases per 100 000 is in the fourth decade. Testicular cancer is also unusual for a solid tumour in that more than 90% of cases are curable using a combination of surgery, chemotherapy, and radiotherapy.

Testicular cancer is becoming commoner in the Western world, predominantly in white men, and there is geographical variation in incidence amongst white populations, with a higher incidence in northern European men.

Risk factors

Cryptorchidism (undescended testis) is a risk factor for the development of testicular cancer, with the risk in the undescended gonad increasing with the severity of maldescent. The risk is at least 10-fold increased for a testis descended to or below the inguinal canal, and even greater for testes with arrested descent in the abdomen. Such patients also have an increased risk (c.5%) of developing a tumour in the normally descended contralateral gonad, particularly if the testis is small and atrophic. Patients with inherited syndromes, including Kleinfelter's and Down's syndrome, are also at increased risk of testicular cancer. Between 1 and 3% of patients report a positive family history of testicular cancer.

The pathogenesis of testicular cancer is thought to involve a noninvasive precursor stage, termed intratubular germ cell neoplasia (IGCN) or carcinoma *in situ*. Although the natural history of this condition is not completely defined, it would appear that most men with it eventually progress to invasive testicular cancer.

Presentation and diagnosis

Patients present with a testicular swelling that is usually painless and may grow rapidly. Symptoms and signs including back pain, weight loss, lymphadenopathy, headache, shortness of breath, and haemoptysis all suggest metastatic disease. Clinical examination of scrotal swellings is crucial, with key questions being: (1) is it arising in the scrotum? (a hernia comes down from above); (2) is it confined to the body of the testis (a testis cancer is within the testis); and (3) does it transilluminate (i.e. is it cystic or solid). A solid swelling in the body of the testis is a testicular tumour until proved otherwise.

When a testicular mass is detected on clinical examination, a scrotal ultrasound examination is performed to determine if the mass is solid or cystic—cystic scrotal masses are benign and include epididymal cysts and hydroceles. Solid testicular masses are usually malignant, but may be difficult to differentiate from focal infection, infarction, and epidermoid tumours. Preoperative blood is taken for serum tumour markers—α-fetoprotein, β-hCG, and LDH.

About 5% of germ-cell tumours present at an extragonadal site, usually in either the retroperitoneum or mediastinum. Some such patients will have carcinoma *in situ* of the testis, or a burnt-out primary testicular tumour manifested as a focal testicular scar on ultrasonography.

Histological subtypes of testicular cancer

Over 90% of testicular cancer is of germ-cell origin: a few tumours are derived from stromal and supporting cells, either Leidig or Sertoli cell tumours. Testicular tumours in men over the age of 50 are commonly either lymphoma or metastatic, although a subtype of germ-cell cancers known as spermatocytic seminoma occur in older men. Germ-cell tumours are classified as shown in Table 21.18.5. For clinical purposes testicular cancer is divided into seminomatous or nonseminomatous germ cell tumours (NSGCT), the treatment of these two categories being different. Mixed tumours are classified as nonseminomatous tumours. Serum tumour markers for testicular cancer are very useful in diagnosis and in follow-up after orchidectomy.

Staging

Testicular cancer is initially staged with a CT scan of the abdomen, pelvis, and chest. Clinical stage is determined using the TNM classification. The degree of tumour marker elevation carries independent prognostic information and is incorporated into the TNM classification—'TNMs', where 's' designates the serum tumour marker level.

Testicular lymphatic drainage is based on the embryological origin of the testis from the mesonephric ridge in the retroperitoneum, hence the most common sites for metastatic disease are the retroperitoneal para-aortic lymph nodes and the chest (Fig. 21.18.6).

Treatment

A solid testicular mass is usually treated with radical inguinal orchidectomy through an inguinal incision, with excision of the testis, cord and all of their coverings (spermatic fascia). Testicular cancer is the model *par excellence* of a curable solid malignancy. Treatment strategies are tailored to the clinical stage and involve combinations of surgery, chemotherapy, and radiotherapy. The excellent overall cancer cure rates for the young men presenting with this disease mean that the long-term effects of chemotherapy and radiotherapy are potential significant issues (such as the development of secondary malignancy). Much effort is therefore placed

Table 21.18.5 Classification of testicular germ cell tumours

Histological subtypes of primary testicular cancer	Percentage of cases
Seminomatous germ-cell tumours	55.4
Classical	
Anaplastic	
Spermatocyctic	
Nonseminomatous germ-cell tumours	
Embryonal	13.5
Teratocarcinoma	11.5
Choriocarcinoma	1.8
Yolk sac	1.2
Mature teratoma	3.7
Mixed germ-cell tumour (e.g. embryonal and seminoma)	12.9

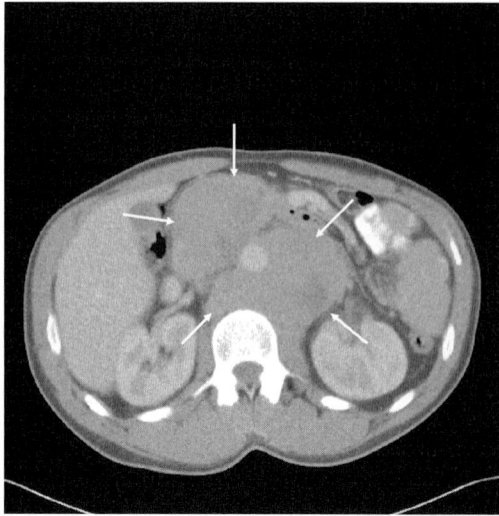

Fig. 21.18.6 CT scan showing a very large metastatic para-aortic lymph node mass (arrows) from a testicular seminoma.

Table 21.18.6 Prognostic groupings of germ-cell cancers according to the International Germ Cell Cancer Collaborative Group (IGCCCG)

Seminoma germ-cell tumour prognosis (IGCCCG classification)	Nonseminomatous germ-cell tumour
Good prognosis	
Any primary, no non-pulmonary visceral metastases, any tumour markers: 86% 5- year survival	Testicular or retroperitoneal primary, no nonpulmonary visceral metastases, slightly elevated tumour markers: 92% 5-year survival
Intermediate prognosis	
Any primary or tumour markers, nonpulmonary visceral metastases present (brain, liver, bone): 72% 5-year survival	Identical to good prognosis but intermediate elevation of tumour markers: 80% 5-year survival
Poor prognosis	
No seminoma patients are classified as poor prognosis	Primary mediastinal tumour, or nonpulmonary visceral metastases, or high serum tumour marker concentration: 48% 5-year survival

on minimizing side effects of treatment while maintaining excellent cure rates.

Seminoma

Stage I seminoma has a cure rate approaching 100%. About 12% of men with clinical stage I disease have occult disease in the retroperitoneal nodes and may be offered para-aortic radiotherapy, or single-dose chemotherapy, or surveillance with chemotherapy given at the time of clinical relapse. Patients at higher risk of relapse include those with tumours greater than 4 cm in size or those with invasion of the rete testis, and it is these patients who may chose to have adjuvant therapy.

Stage II seminoma has metastasized to the retroperitoneal lymph nodes and may either be low or high volume. Low-volume disease may be treated with radiotherapy or chemotherapy, whereas high-volume disease is best treated with three cycles of chemotherapy (bleomycin, etopiside, and cisplatin (BEP))

In the presence of advanced metastatic disease (stages III and IV), patients with seminoma are classified as having intermediate prognosis and have survival rates approaching 80% with the use of chemotherapy (Table 21.18.6). Following treatment patients may be left with a residual mass in the retroperitoneum, the treatment of which is discussed later.

Stage I nonseminomatous germ cell tumour (NSGCT)

About 25 to 30% of men who apparently have stage I NSGCT will relapse during follow-up, usually in the retroperitoneum. The risk is greatest when the patient has embryonal carcinoma, a large primary tumour (>6 cm), or lymphovascular space invasion. Despite this, long-term survival rates approach 98 to 99%. Treatment strategies following orchidectomy for stage I disease include (1) surveillance with chemotherapy on relapse; (2) prophylactic chemotherapy given as two cycles (as opposed to three cycles on clinical relapse); and (3) primary retroperitoneal lymph node dissection. The decision on which treatment strategy to employ is based on patient choice, the presence or absence of the above-mentioned risk factors, and whether the patient will reliably attend follow-up. The overall survival rates are equal using all options.

Metastatic NSGCT

Good-prognosis metastatic NSGCT is treated with three cycles of BEP chemotherapy and poor-prognosis disease with four cycles. Potential complications from bleomycin include pneumonitis that is occasional fatal, but omitting bleomycin from the regimen significantly lowers long-term cure and cannot be recommended.

Management of a residual retroperitoneal mass

Following treatment for metastatic disease with chemotherapy, a residual mass is often left in the retroperitoneum. This may be caused by fibrosis, residual cancer, or mature differentiated teratoma, which does not respond to chemotherapy. In the setting of NSGCT a retroperitoneal lymph dissection may be offered if the mass is greater than about 1 cm in size. A residual mass following the treatment of a seminoma is often diffuse and densely adherent to the aorta and vena cava, making surgical dissection difficult, even in experienced hands, but this is still indicated if the mass is discrete, globular, and more than 3 cm in size.

Penile cancer

Squamous-cell cancer of the penis is a rare primary malignancy in the United Kingdom and the United States of America, but more common in Asian and South American populations. Risk factors include lack of neonatal circumcision, phimosis, infection with human papillomavirus (in particular HPV 16), smoking, and penile conditions including balanitis xerotica obliterans.

Diagnosis and staging

Penile cancer presents either as *in situ* carcinoma or as invasive malignancy. The former presents as a red velvety lesion and the latter as a firm mass or as ulceration. Penile squamous-cell cancer most commonly arises from the glans penis or prepuce, but may also originate on the penile shaft. Delayed presentation is common because of embarrassment or neglect.

Histological diagnosis is achieved by way of a penile incision biopsy that also provides a T stage and grade. Squamous-cell cancer of the penis metastasizes in orderly fashion, without skip lesions, first to the superficial and then to the deep inguinal lymph nodes. The lymphatic drainage of the penis is bilateral and therefore laterality of the primary lesion is not relevant to the likely site of lymph node metastasis. Metastases also occur to bone and lungs.

Staging of penile cancer follows a TNM classification. A histological grade is also assigned. The combination of stage and grade helps to predict the risk of occult groin node metastases.

Treatment

This depends on the site, the clinical stage, and the grade of the lesion. In general the primary lesion should be treated by an adequate but relatively conservative approach, whereas the lymph nodes may require aggressive treatment if the cancer is high risk. Squamous-cell cancer *in situ* or superficial well-differentiated disease may be treated by local excision or laser therapy. Lesions exclusively located on the prepuce may be treated with a circumcision. A large bulky (T3) lesion may require total penectomy, which involves a perineal urethrostomy.

Patients refusing surgical management of the primary lesion may be treated with radiotherapy with local control rates of 60% at 5 years.

Lymphadenectomy

Penile cancer is a good example of where aggressive treatment of micrometastatic disease to local lymph nodes can result in good long-term cure rates. The difficulty lies in determining those men who have micrometastatic disease, with reluctance to perform a bilateral ilioinguinal lymph node dissection in everyone with penile cancer relating to the high morbidity of the procedure, including lymphoedema, flap necrosis, infection, and lymphocele formation. Novel staging strategies are being evaluated, including the use of lymphotrophic-nanoparticle MRI scanning.

Patients with palpable lymphatic groin nodes should undergo a lymph node dissection if fine-needle aspiration confirms the presence of cancer, the differential diagnosis for such palpable nodes being infection related to the primary tumour. If there is strong suspicion that infection is the cause of lymphadenopathy, then a 6-week course of antibiotics is given, with node dissection carried out if the nodes remain palpable afterwards.

Radiotherapy is a frequently employed treatment for both the primary lesion and the groin nodes in populations with a high incidence of penile cancer, but would appear to provide inferior cancer control at 5 years compared to surgery.

Further reading
Bladder
Jung I, Messing E (2000). Molecular mechanisms and pathways in bladder cancer development and progression. *Cancer Control*, **7**, 325–34.
Khadra MH, et al. (2000). A prospective analysis of 1,930 patients with hematuria to evaluate current diagnostic practice. *J Urol*, **163**, 524–7.
Stein JP, et al. (2001). Radical cystectomy in the treatment of invasive bladder cancer: long-term results in 1,054 patients. *J Clin Oncol*, **19**, 666–75.

Kidney
Maher ER, et al. (1990). Clinical features and natural history of von Hippel–Lindau disease. *Q J Med*, **77**, 1151–63.
Ono Y, et al. (2005). Laparoscopic radical nephrectomy for renal cell carcinoma: the standard of care already? *Curr Opin Urol*, **15**, 75–8.
Tsui KH, et al. (2000). Prognostic indicators for renal cell carcinoma: a multivariate analysis of 643 patients using the revised 1997 TNM staging criteria. *J Urol*, **163**, 1090–5.
Vogelzang NJ, Stadler WM (1998). Kidney cancer. *Lancet*, **352**, 1691–6.
Volpe A, et al. (2004). The natural history of incidentally detected small renal masses. *Cancer*, **100**, 738–45.

Prostate
Basch EM, et al. (2007). American Society of Clinical Oncology endorsement of the Cancer Care Ontario Practice Guideline on nonhormonal therapy for men with metastatic hormone-refractory (castration-resistant) prostate cancer. *J Clin Oncol*, **25**, 5313–18.
Bill-Axelson A, et al. (2005). Radical prostatectomy versus watchful waiting in early prostate cancer. *N Engl J Med*, **352**, 1977–84.
Cooperberg MR, Moul JW, Carroll PR (2005). The changing face of prostate cancer. *J Clin Oncol*, **23**, 8146–51.
Miller DC, et al. (2003). Prostate carcinoma presentation, diagnosis, and staging: an update from the National Cancer Data Base. *Cancer*, **98**, 1169–78.
NICE (2008) *Prostate cancer: diagnosis and treatment. Clinical guideline 58.*http://www.nice.org.uk/Guidance/CG58/Guidance/pdf/English

Testis
De Wit R, et al. (1997). Importance of bleomycin in combination chemotherapy for good-prognosis testicular nonseminoma: a randomised study of the European Organisation for Research and Treatment of Cancer Genitourinary Tract Cancer Cooperative Group. *J Clin Oncol*, **15**, 1837–43.
Huyghe E, Matsuda T, Thonneau P (2003). Increasing incidence of testicular cancer worldwide: a review. *J Urol*, **170**, 5–11.
Kondagunta GV, Sheinfeld J, Motzer RJ (2003). Recommendations of follow-up after treatment of germ cell tumors. *Semin Oncol*, **30**, 382–9.

Drugs and the kidney

Aine Burns and Caroline Ashley

Essentials

The kidney plays a critical role in the elimination of many drugs from the body, hence consideration should be given to a patient's renal function whenever any drug is prescribed. Much kidney disease is unrecognized, but the widespread reporting of estimated glomerular filtration rates (eGFR) has brought greater awareness of the prevalence of chronic kidney disease (CKD) and thereby encouraged medical practitioners to take account of reduced renal function when prescribing. CKD is very often one of many coexisting comorbid conditions, especially in elderly patients, when particularly careful thought must be given to appropriate drug dosing and the possibility of drug interactions.

A reduced GFR is the primary reason for reduced excretion of drugs in renal failure, but drug absorption, distribution, protein binding, metabolism, and pharmacodynamics may all be affected. Key general points are:

1 Both filtration and secretion of drugs appear to fall in parallel and in proportion to the GFR.

2 The clinical significance of a reduction in GFR and increased drug half-life depends on the relative importance of renal excretion and metabolism as a mode of elimination, and the therapeutic ratio of the drug.

3 If nonrenal clearance accounts for elimination of more than 50% of a drug, then no adjustment needs be made to dose or frequency of administration. Dosages of drugs which are mainly excreted in active form by the kidney (i.e. as unchanged drug or active metabolites) may need to be modified to avoid accumulation.

4 Potentially toxic drugs should only be used in patients with renal failure if there is a specific indication for their use and if therapy can be monitored appropriately. If dose adjustment is required, then dose, dose interval, or both can be adjusted to achieve the desired therapeutic profile.

Drug metabolism in normal and impaired kidney function

Drug metabolism in normal kidney function

It is necessary to understand how the normal kidney handles drugs to understand the consequences of renal impairment on the way the body handles drugs. Molecular size, protein binding, lipid-solubility, and charge are all important factors determining elimination of drugs by the kidney.

Non-protein-bound compounds up to a molecular size of 60 kDa are filtered through the glomerulus, with smaller molecules filtered more freely than bigger ones. Highly protein-bound substances may be filtered only if their protein binding is saturated, e.g. in salicylate poisoning.

Once filtered into the renal tubule, reabsorption of a drug may occur if it is nonpolar or lipid soluble, allowing it to diffuse readily across tubular cell membranes and back into the plasma, provided the concentration gradient permits. Polar or water-soluble drugs remain in the glomerular filtrate and are excreted in the urine. Many nonpolar drugs are metabolized in the liver to produce more water-soluble compounds which can then be eliminated effectively in the urine.

Some drugs can be actively secreted into the tubular fluid (e.g. cimetidine) or absorbed from it (e.g. gentamicin) independent of their water solubility and size. The tubular fluid/urinary pH can also enhance or retard drug elimination from the normal kidney: acidic compounds become less ionized and more soluble in alkaline urine, as do basic compounds in acidic urine. The amount of ionized drug at any particular pH is determined by its pK, which is the pH at which 50% of the drug is ionized.

Four other concepts are important in drug excretion by the kidney:

- volume of distribution (V_d)
- half-life ($t_{1/2}$)
- elimination rate constant (k_e)
- steady state concentration (C_{ss}) of a drug.

The relationship between these variables is discussed below. Finally, drugs present in tubular fluid may affect the elimination of other compounds, e.g. aspirin reduces methotrexate removal.

Drug handling with impaired kidney function

In considering the likelihood that excretion of an individual drug may be affected by kidney failure, a physician needs to consider the following:

◆ Size—molecules small than 60 kDa are filtered by glomerulus

◆ Protein binding—only unbound drug can be filtered, hence the more protein bound a drug is, the less that drug is available for filtration; proteins can become saturated, leaving unbound drug to be filtered depending on its size

◆ Polarity or water/lipid solubility—polar/water soluble drugs are usually not reabsorbed once filtered

◆ Charge—acidic drugs are excreted more efficiently in alkaline urine and basic compounds in acidic urine

◆ Volume of distribution (V_d)—a measure that relates the total amount of drug in the body to the concentration in the blood. It is the theoretical volume that would be required to contain all of the drug in the body if the drug were present at the concentration measured in the blood

◆ Half-life($t_{1/2}$)—the time taken for the plasma concentration of a drug to fall by half, after absorption and distribution is complete

◆ Elimination rate (k_e)—the proportion of the total amount of drug removed per unit time

◆ Proportion of the drug excreted by the kidney

◆ Extent of liver metabolism and renal excretion of metabolites

◆ Active secretion or reabsorption of drug by the kidney

However, in considering drug metabolism in chronic kidney disease (CKD), the most important and relevant point is that both filtration and secretion of drugs fall in parallel and in proportion to the GFR, hence accurate measurement of GFR is essential for appropriate dose or interval adjustments to be made. Issues relating to the estimation of GFR are discussed in Chapter 21.4, but for practical clinical purposes the value almost always employed is the eGFR as calculated by the modified MDRD (modification of diet in renal disease) equation, which is now routinely reported by many laboratories.

Drug kinetics and the effects of renal impairment

For most drugs, their rate of removal is proportional to their concentration (first-order kinetics), with the elimination rate constant (k_e) being the proportion of the total amount of drug removed per unit time. Most drugs thus display a simple exponential decline in concentration: the higher the drug concentration the more gets eliminated. The half-life is inversely proportional to the k_e (the more slowly the drug is eliminated the longer the half-life), which can be expressed as a mathematical formula: $t_{1/2} = 0.693/k_e$.

The volume of distribution of a drug is more complicated as a particular drug may be confined solely to the plasma, in which case the V_d would approximate to plasma volume, or V_d may be an apparent volume, defined as the volume in which the amount of drug administered would have distributed to produce the measured plasma concentration. This can be affected by binding of the drug to proteins and tissues, as well as lean body mass and changes in intra- and extravascular fluid volumes.

The serum concentration of a drug, at any time, is a product of the dose and frequency of administration, the volume of distribution, and the rate of elimination. The anticipated concentration or steady state concentration (C_{ss}) of a drug can be calculated using these parameters. The concentration is proportional to the dose and $t_{1/2}$, and inversely proportional to the V_d and dosage interval. C_{ss} can be reduced by either lowering the dose or increasing the dose interval.

Renal disease can also affect drug action by another mechanism. The activity of most drugs is usually related to the plasma concentration of unbound drug. When plasma albumin is decreased, or binding of drugs altered by renal disease (e.g. urea and some drugs compete for albumin binding sites in uraemia), the fraction of unbound drug may differ from that in individuals with normal renal function.

In CKD the following simple rules apply when tailoring drug doses:

◆ If nonrenal clearance accounts for elimination of more than 50% of a drug, then no adjustments need be made

◆ If dose amendment is required, then dose, dose interval, or both can be adjusted to achieve the desired C_{ss}. Here it is necessary to consider the desired therapeutic effect, e.g. where antibiotics are concerned and particular peak concentrations are required for optimal bactericidal or bacteriostatic effects, then small frequent doses may not be appropriate and the normal dose given less frequently may be required

Elimination of drugs by haemodialysis/filtration and peritoneal dialysis

The same principles of drug elimination apply to dialysis and filtration membranes as to native kidneys. Drug removal follows first-order kinetics, with the amount of drug removed determined by plasma concentration, the sieving coefficient or permeability of the membrane, the molecular mass of the drug, and the extent to which it is bound to plasma proteins. Haemodialysis generally removes drugs with a molecular mass less than 500 Da (although 'high flux' membranes can remove much larger molecules), whereas haemofilters remove molecules smaller than inulin (average molecular mass 5200 Da). Most drugs which are not protein bound are removed by haemodialysis, including most antibiotics, but drugs such as vancomycin (1800 Da), amphotericin (960 Da) and erythromycin (734 Da) behave differently in haemodialysis and haemofiltration. Just as in the native kidney, water-soluble drugs are more readily filtered than fat-soluble ones.

The plasma concentration of a drug is determined by its volume of distribution and tissue binding characteristics. Digoxin, phenytoin, and antidepressants, for example, have large volumes of distribution with only very low plasma concentrations and are therefore hardly influenced by dialysis or filtration.

Drugs are eliminated much less efficiently by the peritoneal membrane than by synthetic dialysis or filtration membranes. This poor permeability is used to advantage in treating peritonitis in patients on peritoneal dialysis, where antibiotics are injected into the peritoneal fluid. However, it should be remembered that the inflamed peritoneal membrane leads to the variable elimination of drugs, and also means that solutes within peritoneal dialysis fluid that are not usually absorbed systemically are now able to cross the peritoneum into the body, e.g. antibiotics and glucose, which can complicate diabetic control.

Practicalities of prescribing for patients with renal impairment

The following sections consider groups of drugs as grouped by the British National Formulary (BNF) classification according to systems. Only key information is included, and for more detailed guidance other reference sources should be consulted. A particularly good website for detailed information is http://www.emc.medicines.org.uk. This electronic Medicines Compendium (eMC) provides electronic Summaries of Product Characteristics (SPCs) and Patient Information leaflets (PILs) and is continuously updated with new and revised SPC and PIL information which, after approval by the licensing authorities, is submitted directly by pharmaceutical companies.

Gastrointestinal system

Patients with renal failure are not exempt from disorders of the gastrointestinal tract, indeed gastrointestinal sources of occult blood loss are common in renal patients and the investigation and treatment of these are particularly pertinent to the management of renal anaemia.

Dyspepsia and gastro-oesophageal reflux disease

Reflux is a particularly common problem in patients on peritoneal dialysis.

Antacids

These usually contain aluminium and magnesium compounds that are not excreted in renal failure and need to be avoided, unless carefully supervised, in moderate and severe renal impairment. Absorption of aluminium is increased by citrates, which are contained in many effervescent preparations. Both aluminium and magnesium preparations are occasionally used as phosphate binders in renal impairment but may accumulate in oligoanuric patients and should be used with care, monitoring serum magnesium and aluminium levels if necessary.

Compound alginates

These form a 'raft' intended to float on top of the stomach contents and prevent reflux. Many contain substantial amounts of sodium, which may contribute to fluid overload in patients with renal failure.

Antispasmodics and other drugs altering gut motility

These include antimuscarinics and smooth muscle relaxants, which are not contraindicated in renal failure but should be used cautiously in those with hypertension.

Ulcer-healing drugs and eradication of *Helicobacter pylori*

Nearly all duodenal ulcers and most gastric ulcers not associated with nonsteroidal anti-inflammatory drugs (NSAIDs) are caused by *Helicobacter pylori*. Regimens for eradication of *H. pylori* in patients with impaired renal function are, in general, no different from those employed in patients with normal renal function: 1 week

of triple therapy combining a proton pump inhibitor, amoxicillin, and either clarithromycin or metronidazole eradicates the infection in over 90% of cases. However, other regimens involving the use of tripotassium dicitratobismuthate, and tetracyclines should be avoided or used with caution in renal failure.

H₂-receptor antagonists

These should be used carefully in patients with renal impairment, and discontinued if signs of confusion develop. Ranitidine bismuth citrate should be avoided if the eGFR is less than 25 ml/min. Note also that cimetidine interferes with cytochrome P450, although the other H₂-receptor blockers do not. Cimetidine can also be used to inhibit active urinary creatinine secretion and thus improve the accuracy of 24-h urine collection measurements for creatinine clearance.

Proton pump inhibitors

Interstitial nephritis has been associated with usage of proton pump inhibitors, but is very rare. Proton pump inhibitors are widely used in nephrological practice and in general no dose restrictions apply, even in severe renal impairment.

Chelates and complexes

The two drugs in this category, tripotassium dicitratobismuthate and sucralfate (a complex of aluminium hydroxide and sulphated sucrose), should be used with extreme caution in moderately impaired renal function and avoided in severe renal failure, the former because of its potassium and the latter because of its aluminium content.

Prostaglandin analogues

Misoprostol is a synthetic prostaglandin analogue whose use is mainly limited to elderly and frail patients from whom NSAIDs cannot be withdrawn. It should be used with extra caution in this population, including those with reduced renal function, as they may be vulnerable to the effects of hypotension because of underlying cerebrovascular or cardiovascular disease. NSAIDs are contraindicated for most renal patients because of their detrimental effects on residual renal function and because their use is more frequently associated with gastrointestinal blood loss. Combining these adverse effects with the frequency of coexisting cerebrovascular or cardiovascular disease means that NSAIDs have hardly any role in nephrological practice.

Acute diarrhoea

Patients with underlying renal impairment are very susceptible to acute deterioration of renal function consequent to the fluid and electrolyte depletion that may occur during bouts of acute diarrhoea, hence prevention and reversal of volume depletion is a priority. Oral rehydration preparations can be used, but if acute tubular necrosis has occurred and the urine output fails to respond once intravascular volume status is optimized, then it is important to reassess the patient's clinical condition regularly to avoid fluid overload, particularly in those with underlying renal impairment or who are susceptible to congestive heart failure.

Adsorbents and bulk-forming drugs

These compounds, which contain agents such as ispaghula, methylcellulose and sterculia, are not recommended for acute diarrhoeas but can be useful in controlling the diarrhoea associated with diverticular disease. Diverticular disease is almost universally present in patients who have inherited adult polycystic kidney disease, and as the proportion of elderly patients being cared for by nephrologists grows it is useful to note that these agents may be safely prescribed for those with renal impairment.

Antimotility drugs

Codeine phosphate and loperamide used for uncomplicated chronic diarrhoea are safe and very commonly used in mild renal impairment. However, in severe renal failure all opioid agents must be used with caution and in reduced dosage to avoid increased and prolonged effects, such as severe constipation leading to hyperkalaemia, and respiratory depression.

Chronic bowel disorders

Maintenance of a liberal fluid intake as well as dietary manipulation is frequently recommended for patients suffering from chronic bowel disorders when malignancy has been ruled out. The former is contraindicated and the latter complicated in most patients with significant chronic kidney disease, making constipation one of the most trying symptoms for renal patients and their nephrologists.

The prevalence of Crohn's disease and ulcerative colitis is no different in patients with and without chronic renal failure. Effective management requires drug therapy, attention to nutrition and—in some circumstances—surgery. Aminosalicylates and corticosteroids form the mainstays of drug therapy. Short courses of ciclosporin, azathioprine, methotrexate, and (more recently) infliximab are also used for the acute management and maintenance of patients with moderate to severe disease. Aminosalicylates should be used sparingly in moderate renal impairment and avoided wherever possible in severe impairment, since the metabolites are renally excreted and highly nephrotoxic. When used in moderate renal failure a high fluid intake must be ensured to avoid crystalluria. Renal dysfunction secondary to interstitial nephritis and nephritic syndrome is very rare and usually reversible. Because of the risk of renal toxicity, patients on mesalazine should have renal function checked every 3 months for the first year then 6 monthly thereafter.

Laxatives

Constipation is a common complaint, particularly amongst patients receiving peritoneal dialysis, when it can impair fluid inflow and drainage such that good management of the problem is very important.

Bulk-forming laxatives

These relieve constipation by increasing faecal mass and stimulating peristalsis. Unprocessed wheat and oat bran are most commonly used, but methylcellulose, ispaghula, and sterculia are useful in coeliac patients and those who are otherwise intolerant of bran. Fybogel and mebeverine should be used with caution in severe renal failure. Care must also be exercised with fluid balance: use of bulk-forming laxatives requires a high water intake to avoid bowel obstruction, and if absorbed this could lead to pulmonary oedema in an oligo/anuric patient.

Stimulant laxatives

Stimulant laxatives including bisacodyl and senna can both be used safely in renal patients, although the latter colours urine red.

Osmotic laxatives

Osmotic laxatives increase the amount of water in the large bowel, either by drawing fluid from the body into the bowel, or by retaining the fluid they were administered with. These agents can cause profound dehydration and could thus exacerbate underlying renal

impairment. Lactulose, a semisynthetic disaccharide, is widely prescribed by nephrologists, but care must be taken to avoid dehydration. Magnesium and sodium salts as well as phosphate enemas are useful when rapid bowel evacuation is required, but these are not recommended in severe renal failure because of the risk of magnesium and sodium overload.

Bowel cleansing solutions

Phosphate-based bowel cleansing preparations (e.g. Fleet) should be avoided in severe renal impairment because their phosphate content can cause uncontrollable hyperphosphataemia. However, macrogol-based solutions (e.g. Klean-Prep) and those containing sodium picosulphate (Picolax) may be used, since their hyperosmolar effect pulls fluid into the bowel, rather than allowing absorption of fluid and electrolytes into the body.

Drugs affecting intestinal secretions

Drugs affecting biliary composition and flow

There are no contraindications to the use of ursodeoxycholic acid in renal impairment.

Bile acid sequestrants

The only caution to the use of cholestyramine is that, being a non-absorbed anion-exchange resin, it can interfere with absorption of a number of drugs.

Pancreatin

No contraindications, but hyperuricaemia and hyperuricosuria can be exacerbated with very high dosage.

Cardiovascular system

Positive inotropic drugs

Cardiac glycosides increase the force of myocardial contraction and reduce conductivity within the atrioventricular node.

Cardiac glycosides

Two agents are available in this category, digoxin and digitoxin. Digoxin has a long half-life and is renally excreted, hence dosage needs to be reduced—even in mild renal failure—and levels monitored to avoid toxicity. Hypokalaemia and hypomagnesaemia can both exacerbate toxic side effects. Digitoxin is mainly eliminated by liver metabolism but also has a prolonged half-life in severe renal impairment, when a lower dose should be used.

Phosphodiesterase inhibitors

Enoximone and milrinone are both used in treating congestive heart failure. Consideration of reduction of dose is advised in patients with known renal impairment, and in those with normal renal function monitoring of renal function is advised.

Diuretics

Diuretics are used both to reduce oedema in chronic heart and renal failure and to reduce blood pressure by promoting a negative sodium balance. Elderly patients are more susceptible to their side effects and should receive lower initial doses. Hypokalaemia is a risk with both thiazide and loop diuretics, but thiazides are more likely to cause this effect because of their longer duration of action.

Thiazides and related diuretics

These moderately potent diuretics work by inhibiting sodium reabsorption at the beginning of the distal convoluted tubule (Fig. 21.19.1). They act within 1–2 h of administration and their effects

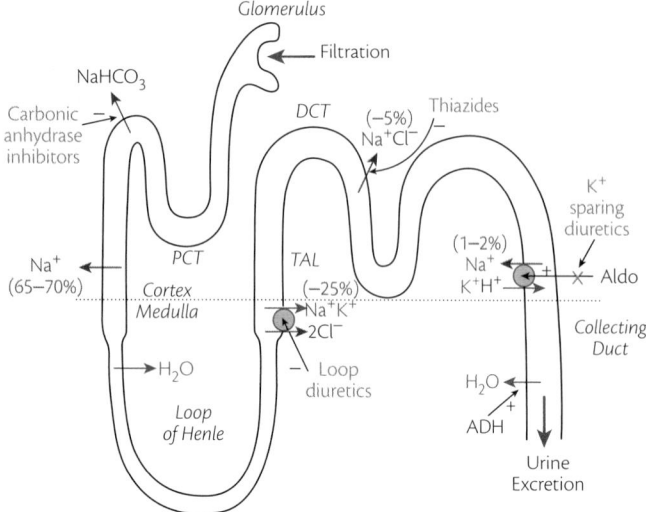

Fig. 21.19.1 Sites of action of diuretics on the renal tubule. ADH, antidiuretic hormone; Aldo, aldosterone; DCT, distal convoluted tubule; PCT, proximal convoluted tubule; TAL, (medullary) thick ascending limb.

last for 12 to 24 h. Low doses of thiazides produce a near maximal effect, and increasing the dose merely serves to increase the likelihood of side effects such as hypokalaemia, hyponatraemia, hyperglycaemia, hyperuricaemia, and gout. Bendroflumethiazide (bendrofluazide) is the most commonly used drug of this class, over which others in the class offer little advantage. The value of thiazides in patients with renal impairment is limited, as for the most part they are ineffective below a creatinine clearance of 30 ml/min (stage 4 CKD). Metolazone, however, is particularly effective—even in advanced renal failure—when combined with a loop diuretic and can be used (usually by specialists) when a profound diuresis is needed, but prescribers should be aware that excessive rapid diuresis can occur. Chlorthalidone has been linked to allergic acute interstitial nephritis.

Loop diuretics

These inhibit reabsorption of sodium from the thick ascending limb of the loop of Henle (Fig. 21.19.1) and are powerful diuretics. When administered intravenously for pulmonary oedema they produce relief faster than diuresis occurs, probably as a result of venodilator action. The two most commonly used agents are furosemide (frusemide) and bumetanide: both act within 1 h of oral administration and their effects last up to 6 h; following intravenous injection they have a peak effect in 30 min. Patients with severe renal impairment usually require very high doses (frequently 250–1000 mg/day for furosemide or equivalent of bumetanide, where 40 mg furosemide = 1 mg of bumetanide) to produce their effect. At these high doses there is a risk of deafness (usually the result of rapid parenteral administration in patients with background renal impairment), and bumetanide can cause myalgia.

In the past there was enthusiasm for giving high doses of loop diuretics by intravenous infusion to patients with acute renal failure presumed due to acute tubular necrosis. A number of randomized trials have failed to show clinically useful benefit, although it remains possible that a subset of patients (yet to be defined) could respond. Few nephrologists now recommend this treatment (see Chapter 21.5), but if it is to be given to patients with oliguric acute renal failure, it is very important that bladder outflow obstruction

is excluded and intravascular volume optimized before diuretic is administered. A standard regimen would be to give furosemide 250 mg over 1 h, perhaps continuing until a maximum of 1 g over 4 h is reached.

Potassium-sparing diuretics and aldosterone antagonists

These are weak diuretics if given alone, but can be used with thiazides or loop diuretics as an alternative to potassium supplementation. Care must be taken if they are coadministered with angiotensin converting enzyme (ACE) inhibitors or angiotensin II receptor blockers (ARBs) because hyperkalaemia may result, and they are relatively contraindicated in moderate to severe renal impairment for the same reason, although if used judiciously with regular monitoring of serum potassium they may have an additional beneficial role in treating patients with both heart and renal failure. Triamterene may cause blue fluorescence of urine and has been found in kidney stones.

Potassium-sparing diuretics with other diuretics

In renal failure fixed combinations of drugs should generally be avoided because they do not allow tailoring of the doses of the individual drugs to the patient's requirements.

Osmotic diuretics

Mannitol is used for the treatment and prevention of cerebral oedema. In the past some nephrologists advocated administration of mannitol in acute dialysis protocols with the aim of preventing precipitate falls in plasma osmotic pressure that might in part be responsible for dialysis disequilibrium. This is not required if an appropriate schedule is prescribed for the patient just starting on dialysis (short hours, small dialysis membrane, cooling of the dialysate temperature, higher dialysate potassium concentration).

Carbonic anhydrase inhibitors

The carbonic anhydrase inhibitor acetazolamide is a weak diuretic and is used for mountain sickness, but should be avoided even in mild renal impairment because of the risk of metabolic acidosis.

Diuretics with potassium

Most patients on diuretics do not need potassium supplementation, and the amount of potassium available in combined preparations may not be enough for the few who do, hence the use of these drugs is to be discouraged. There is no place for these drugs in the management of renal patients.

Antiarrhythmic drugs

Management of all cardiac arrhythmias requires precise diagnosis of the type of arrhythmia. There are very few extra precautions that need to be taken when treating arrhythmias in renal patients. In general, both cardiac arrhythmias and the proarrhythmogenic actions of many drugs are potentiated by hypokalaemia, and this should be kept in mind when choosing the dialysate potassium concentration for patients receiving haemodialysis, particularly when interdialytic or immediate postdialysis arrhythmia occurs. The various drugs available are listed in Table 21.19.1 according to the Vaughan Williams classification, together with any adjustments necessary in renal failure.

Antihypertensive agents

β-Blockers

The most water-soluble β-blockers (atenolol, celiprolol, nadolol, and sotalol) are less likely to enter the brain and may therefore have

Table 21.19.1 Antiarrhythmic drugs in renal failure

Class of antiarrhythmic	Examples	Comments
Ia	Quinidine Procainamide	Quinidine is mainly eliminated via cytochrome P450, although 20% is excreted via the urine; use with caution in severe renal impairment—overdosage causes cinchonism. Procainamide and its active metabolite both renally excreted; use with caution at decreased dose or increased dosing interval
Ib	Lidocaine Mexilitine	Use with caution in severe renal impairment Almost exclusively liver metabolized, hence no dose adjustment necessary in renal impairment
Ic	Flecainide Propafenone Disopyramide	If GFR <30 ml/min, flecainide should be used at half usual dose elimination of propafenone and its major metabolite is not affected by renal impairment 75% of dose excreted unchanged in the urine; increase the dosing interval in renal impairment; avoid long-acting preparations.
II	Esmolol Propranolol Metoprolol	Generally no need to reduce dose in renal impairment; titrate dose to required clinical response
III	Amiodarone Bretylium	No dose adjustment in renal impairment Renally excreted; use at reduced dose in moderate and severe renal impairmen
IV	Verapamil Diltiazem	Extensively metabolized in the liver, but 70% of the metabolites are excreted in the urine; use at normal doses in renal impairment, but monitor patient carefully. Extensively metabolized in the liver; use at normal dose and monitor response
V	Digoxin	Digoxin is renally excreted; risk of accumulation in renal impairment; reduce dose

fewer sleep-related side effects, but they are excreted by the kidneys and therefore dose reductions may be necessary in renal failure. The general rule with the prescribing of all β-blockers in patients with renal impairment is to start with a low dose and titrate upwards according to response. Those agents that are renally cleared may require lower than usual doses to achieve the desired effect. In severe renal impairment β-blockers may reduce renal blood flow and adversely effect renal function.

Vasodilator antihypertensive drugs

These can have a role in severe hypertension unresponsive to standard oral medication. Sodium nitroprusside is used at normal doses, although prolonged use should be avoided in CKD stages 4 and 5. Minoxidil at normal doses is useful in severe hypertension, together with a diuretic (to counteract fluid retention) and β-blocker (to counteract reflex tachycardia). Bosentan and sildenafil are both

indicated for pulmonary arterial hypertension, may be given at normal doses, although with sildenafil the dosing interval should initially be extended from 8 to 12 hours in CKD stages 4 and 5. Iloprost is used for pulmonary hypertension and (sometimes) for blood pressure control in scleroderma renal crisis: since it is very short-acting, the dose is as in normal renal function and titrated according to response. Drug-induced systemic lupus erythematosus (SLE) is a rare complication of hydralazine therapy, with occasional proteinuria and haematuria reported.

Centrally acting antihypertensive drugs

Methyldopa, clonidine, and moxonidine—start with small doses and increase slowly in CKD stages 4 and 5 because there may be increased sensitivity to hypotensive and sedative effects.

α-Adrenoceptor blocking drugs

Doxazocin, prazosin, terazosin and indoramin are all commonly used agents. Regardless of whether they are cleared renally or hepatically, the general rule is to dose as for normal renal function, starting with the lowest possible dose and titrating upwards according to clinical response.

Drugs affecting the renin–angiotensin system

The kidney eliminates all ACE inhibitors and ARBs, hence it is usually necessary to reduce initial doses in CKD and in elderly patients, in whom the GFR has declined often appropriately with age, but also sometimes in association with generalized atheroma. ACE inhibitors and ARBs can reduce or abolish GFR and cause severe and progressive renal failure in patients with severe bilateral renal artery stenosis or severe stenosis of the artery of a single kidney. Renal function and electrolytes should therefore be checked before starting these drugs, and 1 to 2 weeks after initiating them or increasing dosage. A rise of up to 20% in serum creatinine can be anticipated and tolerated (in anticipation of probable long-term benefit), but a rise greater than this should lead to the drug being stopped. With these provisos, the general rule for prescribing ACE inhibitors and ARBs in patients with renal impairment is to start at the lowest dose and titrate upwards according to response. Concomitant treatment with NSAIDs increases the risk of renal damage and potassium sparing diuretics increase the risk of hyperkalaemia. Anaphylactoid reactions can occur with ACE inhibitors and their use should be avoided during dialysis with high-flux polyacrylonitrile membranes and during LDL apheresis with dextran sulphate to minimize the risk.

Management of hypertension in patients with renal failure

The threshold for initiating antihypertensive treatment in patients with mild renal impairment or persistent proteinuria is a systolic blood pressure greater than 140 mmHg or a diastolic pressure greater than 90 mmHg. An optimal target blood pressure in patients with CKD is systolic blood pressure less than 130 mmHg and diastolic blood pressure greater than 80 mmHg (identical to that for diabetics). The choice of antihypertensive drug depends on the relevant indications or contraindications for the individual patient. However, most nephrologists would recommend ACE inhibitors or ARBs as the first-line agents for patients with established CKD, particularly if significant proteinuria is present, the two notable exceptions being where renovascular disease is present, and during pregnancy.

Most patients with CKD require a combination of antihypertensive drugs. In routine (nonrenal) practice a standard strategy for initiating and combining such drugs is articulated in the 'ABCD rule' (see Chapter 16.17.2), but there is little secure evidence related to patients with renal failure. The author's personal therapeutic hierarchy is as follows: begin with an ACE inhibitor or ARB or both for full angiotensin system blockade (assuming this is not prevented by hyperkalaemia), followed by an α-blocker, followed by a loop diuretic. I rarely use calcium channel blockers (except for patients of Afro-Caribbean origin) because of their tendency to cause peripheral oedema, which can confuse clinical judgement with regard to salt and water balance, and I usually avoid β-blockers because of side effects. Minoxidil, together with β-blockade and loop diuretic, can be used to control resistant hypertension. All patients should be counselled with regard to the importance of a low sodium diet, it being particularly important to point out the hidden sodium content of preprepared meals.

Antianginal drugs—nitrates, calcium channel blockers, and other agents

Nitrates, calcium channel blockers, and potassium channel activators have a vasodilating effect and are used in the treatment of angina and heart failure as well as hypertension. The nitrates (glyceryl trinitrate, isosorbide dinitrate/mononitrate) are generally used at normal dose in patients with renal dysfunction. Calcium channel blockers (e.g. amlodopine, diltiazem, nifedipine, felodipine, lacidipine) should be initiated at the lowest normal dose and titrated upwards according to clinical response.

Nicorandil (a potassium channel activator with nitrate component) and ivabradine (which slows the heart by its action on the sinus node) should be initiated at normal dose in patients in all stages of CKD, and increased as necessary.

Peripheral vasodilators, e.g. naftidrofuryl, pentoxifylline, cilostazol, and moxisylyte, are sometimes used for the symptomatic relief of claudication. They have no proven benefit, but doses should be reduced by 30 to 50% in CKD stages 4 and 5.

Sympathomimetics

Inotropic sympathomimetics

These act on β-receptors in cardiac muscle and increase contractility with little effect on heart rate. Dobutamine, dopamine and dopexamine are all very short-acting agents given by continuous infusion, and no adjustment is necessary for CKD.

Vasoconstrictor symphathomimetics

These raise blood pressure by acting on α-adrenergic receptors to constrict peripheral vessels. They are used in critically ill patients to raise blood pressure but may compromise perfusion of vital organs. Metaraminol, noradrenaline (norepinephrine), and phenylephrine require no dose adjustment in patients with CKD. Ephedrine hydrochloride should be avoided in CKD stage 4 and 5 as there is an increased risk of neurological toxicity.

Cardiopulmonary resuscitation

This should be conducted as for any adult regardless of renal function, but in a patient with renal failure the possibility of reversible electrolyte disturbance—particularly hyperkalaemia—should be considered early, as should the possibility of cardiac tamponade in the uraemic patients. Cardiac arrest in dialysis patients is most often secondary to volume depletion, although pulmonary emboli—including air embolus from central access lines—should

not be forgotten. The incidence of myocardial infarction is increased on dialysis days in haemodialysis patients.

Anticoagulants and protamine

Standard (unfractionated) heparin initiates anticoagulation rapidly but has very short duration of action. It is used as the routine anticoagulant in the maintenance of extracorporeal circuits for haemodialysis. The effects of heparin can be rapidly terminated by stopping the infusion, but most units have a policy of avoiding nonemergency surgical interventions for at least 4 h following dialysis sessions.

Heparin

In severe renal failure the risk of bleeding is increased. Inhibition of aldosterone secretion by heparin (including low-molecular-wight heparin) may result in hyperkalaemia in patients with CKD, also in those with diabetes. Heparin-associated antibodies with clinically important thrombocytopenia, also known as heparin-induced thrombocytopenia (HIT), should be considered in patients receiving heparin for more than 6 to 10 days who develop thrombosis or thrombocytopenia. It is more likely to occur in acute renal failure, with accompanying sepsis or underlying malignancy, and when higher doses of heparin are used. It is immune mediated and necessitates immediate discontinuation of the heparin. Alternative anticoagulants can be used if necessary, e.g. lepirudin or danaparoid, but both of these agents have greatly prolonged half-lives in end-stage renal failure and so there is a need for a much reduced dose and careful monitoring.

Low-molecular-weight heparins (LMWH)

These (e.g. dalteparin, enoxaparin, tinzaparin) are now generally the treatment of choice for medical and surgical thromboembolic prophylaxis, and in the treatment of deep vein thrombosis, pulmonary embolus, and acute coronary syndrome, as well as being used in some units as anticoagulation of the extracorporeal circuit for haemodialysis. However, all LMWH are renally cleared, so there is a serious risk of accumulation with associated bleeding in patients with CKD stages 4 and 5. This risk must be balanced against the difficulties of managing unfractionated heparin regimens, which are frequently associated with periods of under- or over-anticoagulation. Some nephrologists advise avoidance of LMWH in patients with CKD stage 5, and some even in CKD stage 4, whereas others allow usage with monitoring of antifactor Xa activity (typically from day 3 of a treatment regimen and day 5 of a prophylactic regimen).

Hirudins

Both bivalirudin and lepirudin have greatly increased half-lives in patients with severe renal impairment and so should be used with extreme caution in this patient group. The dose should be significantly reduced, and the dosing interval greatly increased, with close monitoring of the activated partial thromboplastin time (APTT).

Oral anticoagulants

As always, the decision to anticoagulate a patient depends on a balance of benefits and risks. Those prescribing warfarin for patients with severe renal impairment, especially those on dialysis, must recognize that the risk of significant haemorrhage is higher than in other patient groups, i.e. 10%/year for warfarinized patients on dialysis, as opposed to 2% for the normal population.

Antiplatelet drugs

Although the BNF advises that aspirin should be avoided in severe renal impairment, citing fluid retention, further reduction in GFR and increased risk of bleeding, in practice the drug is commonly used without problem. Clopidogrel, dipyridamole, eptifibatide, and tirofiban can be used in normal doses. However, care should be exercised when combining these agents in patients with renal failure, who by virtue of their uraemia already have poor platelet function and may have increased risk of bleeding.

Myocardial infarction and fibrinolysis
Initial and long-term management should proceed following the same principles as for patients without renal failure.

Antifibrinolytic drugs and haemostasis
Tranexamic acid may be used in patients with moderate to severe renal impairment, albeit at a reduced dose. Extra care should be exercised in dialysis-dependent patients because of the risk of clotting the vascular access. Desmopressin is sometimes used to reduce the risk of bleeding following renal biopsy in uraemic patients.

Lipid-regulating drugs
Premature cardiovascular mortality is well recognized in patients with CKD and on dialysis. There is debate as to whether the pathogenesis is identical to that of other groups, and it is likely that vascular calcification will prove to be an important factor. Trials are under way to demonstrate whether lipid lowering is beneficial to patients with CKD, but there is now wide experience of HMG-coenzyme A reductase inhibitors in patients with renal impairment. All statins may be initiated at normal doses, although it is recognized that they may cause myopathy, particularly in severe renal impairment or if used in conjunction with ciclosporin (which raises plasma statin levels) or gemfibrozil. All patients with known renal impairment should commence on low doses of these agents, be warned of the risk of muscle problems, and advised to stop the lipid-lowering agent should they develop muscle pains. The fibrates (gemfibrozil and benzafibrate) can be used at reduced dose in CKD stages 3 and 4, but are not recommended in stage 5.

Ezetimibe is a relatively new agent which is used to lower cholesterol in addition to dietary measures, either with or without a statin: it may be used safely in renal impairment. Nicotinic acid and $\omega - 3$ fatty acid compounds are safe in CKD.

Respiratory system

Bronchodilators
The selective β_2-agonists such as salbutamol and terbutaline are the safest and most effective treatment for asthma. These can be administered at normal doses to renal patients by inhalation, oral, or parenteral routes. Other adrenoceptor agonists such as ephedrine, and antimuscarinic bronchodilators such as ipratropium, are also safe in usual dosage. Theophylline and aminophylline, though difficult to use in hepatic failure, can be used in the normal manner in patients with CKD.

Corticosteroids
Steroid metabolism is not altered in renal impairment, hence steroids can be used in the usual manner.

Cromoglicate and leukotriene receptor antagonists
These drugs block the effect of cysteinyl-leukotrienes in the airways, and although they have very rarely been associated with the development of Churg–Strauss syndrome, no other caution need be noted in patients with renal impairment or on renal replacement therapy.

Antihistamine and allergic emergencies
Antihistamines are commonly used for the symptomatic relief of pruritus in patients with advance renal impairment. They differ in their duration of action, incidence of drowsiness (which may be potentiated in severe renal impairment), and antimuscarinic effects (which may aggravate bladder outflow obstruction). The most commonly used agents in renal failure are chlorphenamine maleate and hydroxyzine hydrochloride, which are generally used in normal dosage, with the proviso that the patient may experience excessive drowsiness. Allergic emergencies should be treated in a standard fashion regardless of renal function.

Cough preparations
Opiate-containing cough suppressants, e.g. codeine linctus, should be used with caution in renal impairment (as with all opiates—see 'Analgesics'). Simple linctus is harmless and inexpensive and suitable for all renal patients.

Systemic nasal decongestants
These should be used with caution when hypertension may occur, as in most renal patients. Pseudoephedrine should be avoided in severe renal impairment because of enhanced neurological toxicity and increased vasoconstriction leading to hypertension.

Central nervous system

Hypnotics and anxiolytics
These should be reserved for short courses because of the risk of physical and psychological dependence, as well as tolerance. In renal impairment the usual precautions need to be acknowledged, and the clinician should always start with small doses because of the risk of increased cerebral sensitivity. Chloral hydrate should be avoided in severe renal impairment because it is rapidly metabolized into trichloroethanol and trichloroacetic acid, both of which are renally excreted, and higher doses can depress respiration and blood pressure.

Amongst the benzodiazepines, oral clonazepam is used widely to counter the troublesome restless leg syndrome and myoclonic jerking associated with advanced renal impairment and renal replacement therapy. Pramipexole is now considered to be the most effective agent, followed by gabapentin. Barbiturate doses should be reduced in severe renal failure.

Drugs used in psychoses and related disorders
As with hypnotic and anxiolytic drugs, it is advised that initial doses be small because of reported increased cerebral sensitivity, with special caution being taken with amisulpride and sulpiride. Treatment at prolonged intervals can be given to patients on dialysis. Starting doses of olanzapine, quetiapine, and risperidone should all be reduced, with smaller than usual incremental increases as required. In the case of risperidone, a 25-mg depot preparation can be used every 2 weeks if the patient has tolerated a 1 to 2 mg oral dose. Clozapine should be avoided in severe kidney disease. Benzodiazepines, carbamazepine, and sodium valproate can be used in patients with renal impairment, although caution needs to be exercised with carbamazepine and valproic acid, with careful monitoring of drug levels needed in those with moderate and severe renal impairment.

Lithium and depression in renal disease
A recent review of symptoms in renal disease quotes prevalence rates of depression in patients with endstage renal disease of

between 26 and 49%. Lithium is a widely used and very effective treatment for bipolar affective disorders, but long-term treatment with lithium has been associated with several different forms of renal injury. Nephrogenic diabetes insipidus is the most common, but renal tubular acidosis, the nephrotic syndrome, and chronic interstitial nephritis have also been described, and lithium is a rare cause of hypercalcaemia. These side effects of lithium treatment need to be balanced against the risks associated with depression, and for many patients the judgement will come down in favour of continued lithium treatment, with close monitoring to ensure that levels remain in the therapeutic range and episodes of toxicity are avoided.

Concern has also been raised about possible adverse interactions between lithium and ACE inhibitors, leading to renal insufficiency that may be associated with lithium accumulation. Although it is unclear if this interaction is real, the serum creatinine concentration and lithium levels must be monitored particularly closely if a patient on lithium is begun on an ACE inhibitor.

Tricyclic agents, monoamine-oxidase inhibitors (MAOIs), and selective serotonin reuptake inhibitors (SSRIs) may all be used in patients with renal impairment, starting at the lowest dose and titrating upwards slowly. Venlafaxine, flupentixol (flupenthixol), reboxetine, and mirtazapine should all be used with caution, particularly venlafaxine, with agitation, aggression, hallucinations, abnormal dreams, and syncope all reported in patients with CKD stage 5 on this drug.

Drugs used in the treatment of obesity

Orlistat, which acts on the gastrointestinal tract to reduce the absorption of dietary fat, is safe in renal impairment but reduces the absorption of fat-soluble drugs, e.g. ciclosporin. Sibutramine should be used with caution in all patients with renal impairment, since it is contraindicated in uncontrolled hypertension, congestive cardiac failure, and coronary heart disease.

Drugs used in nausea and vertigo

Cinnarizine, cyclizine, prochlorperazine, and promethazine can all be used in normal dose in renal failure. Domperidone and metoclopramide can also be given in normal doses to patients with severe renal impairment, although theoretically there is an increased risk of extrapyramidal side effects. Serotonin (5HT$_3$) antagonists such as dolasetron, granisetron, ondansetron, palonosetron, and tropisetron need no adjustment. Similarly, the neurokinin receptor antagonists aprepitant and betahistine need no adjustment. However, the cannabinoid nabilone has been associated with hypertension, and hyoscine hydrobromide needs to be used with caution because of the increased risk of central nervous system depression.

Analgesics

NSAIDs are the most notorious analgesics in renal medicine, inducing vasoconstriction of afferent arterioles and with the potential to cause deterioration in renal function with salt and water retention even in the early stages of CKD. Topical NSAIDs have also been shown to reduce renal function. Sepsis, intravascular volume depletion, NSAID usage, and prescription of other nephrotoxic drugs are frequent partners in crime in patients in hospital who develop acute or acute-on-chronic renal failure. Renal impairment caused by acute NSAID usage is usually reversible, but long-term NSAID usage can cause permanent chronic renal impairment.

Phenacatin is no longer manufactured because of its association with renal papillary necrosis, and its carcinogenic properties (see Chapter 21.9.2).

Table 21.19.2 summarizes the hierarchy of analgesic use suitable for patients with renal impairment.

Antiepileptics

Phenytoin, carbamazepine, and valproic acid are given in the usual dosage, although it is standard practice with the latter two drugs to commence treatment with low doses and assess tolerability in each individual. Protein binding of phenytoin is reduced in CKD, leading to higher free circulating drug levels, but this is usually counteracted by increased excretion of free drug and thus dosages rarely need to be adjusted downwards. Care must be exercised when using lamotrigine as its metabolites may accumulate in renal impairment, while the dosage intervals of levetiracetam used both for adjunctive treatment of partial and myoclonic seizures should be extended in CKD stages 4 and 5.

Gabapentin and pregabalin are used to treat the neuropathic pain associated with advanced uraemia and dialysis associated neuropathy. Gabapentin is almost exclusively excreted renally and

Table 21.19.2 Analgesics in renal impairment

Class of Analgesic	Examples	Comments
Topical	Capsaicin cream	
Simple analgesics	Aspirin Paracetamol	Avoid high doses of aspirin
Compound analgesics	Co-codaprin Co-codamol Co-dydramol Co-proxamol	Very effective, although the side effects of the opiate components may be enhanced in patients with severe renal impairment
NSAIDs	Ibuprofen Naproxen Indomethacin Diclofenac	Use with great caution in patients with CKD stage 3, and avoid use in CKD stages 4 and 5, although may be used if the patient is dialysis-dependent (provided sufficient gastroprotective measures taken)
Weak opioid analgesics	Codeine Dihydrocodeine Tramadol	Usually well tolerated, but beware enhanced CNS effects of opiates, and constipation may exacerbate hyperkalaemia
Potent opioid analgesics	Morphine Diamorphine Oxycodone Alfentanyl Fentanyl Pethidine	Must be used at reduced dose and increased dosing interval. Morphine and diamorphine have active metabolites that are excreted via the kidney, hence very prolonged duration of action. Oxycodone and alfentanyl are much better tolerated. Pethidine may be used for 1–2 doses, but then accumulation of the active metabolite norpethidine is proconvulsant.

CNS, central nervous system; NSAID, nonsteroidal anti-inflammatory drug.

hence it should be commenced at one-third of the normal dose in CKD stage 5, and increased very gradually thereafter.

Endocrine system

Insulin requirements fall with declining renal function as a result of reduced catabolism of insulin by the kidney. Patients on peritoneal dialysis using sugar-based solutions may need introduction of insulin or dose adjustment. Insulin can be injected into peritoneal dialysis fluid, but this is rarely recommended because patients administering their insulin therapy in this way were found to have increased incidence of peritonitis (related to poor technique of injection). Oral hypoglycaemic agents are safe, although doses may need to be reduced for the reasons outlined above.

Obstetrics, gynaecology, and urinary tract disorders

A full discussion of contraception and other gynaecological disorders is beyond the scope of this chapter, but the widespread use of erythropoietin and better-quality dialysis has meant that many women on dialysis are now fertile and nephrologists are more often faced with managing pregnancies in their dialysis population. In the author's experience the Mirena coil has particular merit for female patients with menorrhagia, as well as for its contraceptive value, although expert advice should be sought for individual patients (and see Chapter 8.6).

Malignant disease and immunosuppression

Treatment of malignant disorders with chemotherapy is increasingly successful. There are many reliable websites (e.g. emc.medicines.org.uk) which can calculate the dose adjustments needed for each agent depending on renal function.

Renal transplant patients are more susceptible to virally mediated tumours of skin, cervix, and lymphoid tissues and should have regular surveillance.

Nutrition

Ensuring adequate and appropriate nutrition is a very important and often neglected aspect of the care of renal patients. A full discussion of this topic is beyond the scope of this chapter, but a few important points are worth making here. The first relates to salt intake, which should be reduced/minimized in most cases of renal impairment because of its detrimental effect on blood pressure control and the efficacy of antihypertensive therapy. Secondly, in the past the emphasis on dietary restrictions—particularly of phosphate and potassium, but in many instances protein as well—led to significant malnutrition amongst patients entering renal dialysis programmes. Today, however, most renal dietitians tend to concentrate on encouraging patients to eat within certain parameters determined by their individual circumstances, and in general a low–normal protein intake (0.75 g/kg body weight) is recommended in patients with CKD. Early nutritional intervention in patients with acute renal failure is important, with a number of low-sodium and low-phosphate liquid foods available for nasogastric administration.

Skin

Oral tacrolimus and ciclosporin are used in the management of psoriasis: both are nephrotoxic, and care must be taken to keep dosage to a minimum and to monitor drug levels to avoid this complication. Concern has been expressed about topical agents containing tacrolimus, but—although some absorption occurs—blood concentrations are 30-fold less than those seen with oral use, and further reduction in absorption can be expected as the skin improves with treatment.

Immunological products and vaccines

The United Kingdom government recommends that all renal patients receive annual influeza vaccine, as well as regular pneumococcus and *Haemophilus influenzae* B vaccinations. Likewise, hepatitis B vaccination is recommended for all nonimmune patients in whom dialysis is planned. The vaccination should occur as early as possible, before endstage renal failure is reached, to maximize the chances of seroconversion.

Renal transplant and other immunosuppressed patients should not receive live vaccines.

Treating common problems in patients with renal impairment

Hyperuricaemia and gout

Oxypurinol, the principal metabolite of allopurinol, is retained in renal impairment and causes some of the side effects of the drug (rash, gastrointestinal upset, and most importantly bone marrow suppression), hence the dose should be reduced to 100 mg/day when patients have stage 4 or 5 CKD. Hyperuricaemia is rarely a problem once dialysis has commenced because uric acid is a small and water-soluble molecule and therefore readily dialysed out. Allopurinol interferes with the metabolism of 6-mercaptopurine, which is an active metabolite of azathioprine, causing it to accumulate if the two drugs are combined with the potential for profound marrow toxicity. Use of allopurinol in conjunction with azathioprine should be avoided if possible, but if they are used together the dose of azathioprine should be reduced to 20 to 25% of normal and the white blood cell count monitored closely.

Probenecid inhibits secretion of acids in the proximal tubule and prevents reabsorption of urate from the tubular lumen. It prolongs the effects of penicillins, cephalosporins, naproxen, indomethacin, methotrexate, and sulphonylurea, causing accumulation and the potential for toxicity. It also inhibits tubular secretion and therefore activity of bumetanide and furosemide. It is used to prevent the toxicity associated with cidofovir usage. It becomes increasingly ineffective as renal function declines, hence is of little use in managing gout associated with CKD stage 5, and the same is true of sulfinpyrazone.

Colchicine is a very useful drug in managing acute gout in patients with renal impairment for whom NSAIDs are contraindicated. To minimize its unpleasant side effects it may be given every 4- to 6 h in CKD stages 4 and 5, rather than the usual 2-hourly.

Phosphate control

There is increasing awareness of the importance of phosphate control in CKD; it is likely that poor control contributes to vascular calcification and the increased cardiovascular mortality observed in this patient group. Phosphate is poorly removed during dialysis. Curtailing dietary phosphate intake helps but is not the ideal solution. Over the last four decades various oral phosphate-binding preparations have moved in and out of favour. None is particularly palatable, hence compliance is a major issue and hyperphosphataemia remains prevalent amongst dialysis patients. See Chapter 21.6 for further discussion.

The patient with advanced renal impairment

Table 21.19.3 details a typical prescription for a patient with advanced renal impairment.

Anaesthesia and the kidney

Surgery causes the release of catecholamines, renin, angiotensin, and AVP, leading to redistribution of renal blood flow and a decrease in GFR. Additionally, general anaesthesia often results in some degree of hypotension and depression of cardiac output, which further reduces renal perfusion and potentially jeopardizes renal function. A careful anaesthetic plan is imperative in the patient with renal insufficiency or failure because acute renal failure in the perioperative period is associated with high morbidity and mortality. Factors including advanced age, diabetes, underlying renal insufficiency, and heart failure place a patient at high risk for developing acute renal failure, and it is imperative to maintain euvolaemia, normotension, and cardiac output, and to avoid nephrotoxic agents, in an endeavour to optimize renal blood flow and renal perfusion as the best prevention of renal dysfunction.

Intravenous and inhalational anaesthetics can be used freely in patients with renal impairment, as can muscle relaxants, anticholinesterases, and local anaesthetics. The half-life of opioid analgesia, hypnotics, and anxiolytics is greatly prolonged in renal failure, which—along with increased cerebral sensitivity—needs to be taken into account when renal patients undergo surgery.

Renal transplantation

An in-depth review of this topic is beyond the scope of this chapter, but for reference a typical drug regimen for a patient immediately after transplantation is given in Table 21.19.4.

An important point to note is that having a renal transplant does not automatically restore 'normal' renal function to a recipient; they are still likely to have a degree of impairment of renal function, hence when prescribing for renal transplant patients the following points should be remembered:

◆ Avoid nephrotoxic agents wherever possible, and if they must be used, prescribe for the shortest time possible.

◆ Where drugs are renally excreted, all doses should be adjusted according to the level of renal function of the patient, especially if the drug has a narrow therapeutic index.

◆ If possible, measure plasma levels of drugs to avoid toxicity.

◆ Beware of drug–drug interactions with the immunosuppressive agents used to prevent graft rejection.

Table 21.19.3 A typical prescription of a patient with advanced renal impairment

Drug	Example	Comments
Antihypertensive agents	ACE inhibitor, ARB, α-blocker, β-blocker, calcium channel blocker, etc.	Treating hypertension in a patient with advanced renal disease often requires a combination of agents.
Vitamin D	1-Alfacalcidol, calcitriol, paricalcitol	To correct hypercalcaemia and reduce PTH
Phosphate binder	Calcium carbonate, calcium acetate, aluminium hydroxide, magnesium carbonate, sevelamer hydrochloride, lanthanum carbonate	Most units start therapy with Ca-containing phosphate binders and then progress to other agents as the PTH and Ca × P product rises.
Erythropoietin	Epoietin, darbepoietin	May be given IV or SC. Both agents are effective at treating renal anaemia
Iron	Oral: ferrous sulphateIV: iron dextran or iron saccharate	Renal patients are poor absorbers of oral iron supplements, hence IV iron supplementation is the preferred route
Diuretic	Furosemide, bumetanide	Useful especially if dialysis-dependent patient is still passing urine
H$_2$-blocker/proton pump inhibitor	Ranitidine/lansoprazole/omeprazole	Uraemic patients are at increased risk of developing gastric lesions
Vitamin supplements	Ketovite, Renovite, Orovite	Often prescribed as the renal diet is deficient in vitamin-containing foods, e.g. fruit and vegetables
Sodium bicarbonate		To correct metabolic acidosis. Probably not required if patient is adequately dialysed

ACE, angiotensin converting enzyme; ARB angiotensin receptor blocker; IV, intravenous; PTH, parathyroid hormone; SC, subcutaneous.

Table 21.19.4 A typical drug regimen for a patient who has recently received a renal transplant

Drug	Example	Comments
Immunosuppression Calcineurin inhibitor Antiproliferative agent Corticosteroid	Ciclosporin or tacrolimus Mycophenolate mofetil or azathioprine Prednisolone	See NICE guidance 2004 Blood levels must be closely monitored. Side effects include nephrotoxicity, hypertension. Some immunosuppression regimens are steroid sparing
Prophylaxis Antifungal Pneumocystis	Nystatin or amphotericin mouthwash lozenges Fluconazole Cotrimoxazole	Usually given for the first 4–14 weeks post-transplant Usually given for the first 6 months post-transplant
Others	Aspirin (low dose) Antihypertensives Epoietin Vitamin D analogue.	May be continued for a while post-transplant until the graft is producing adequate quantities of endogenous erythropoietin. May be continued for a while post-transplant until the graft is producing adequate quantities of endogenous active vitamin D

Table 21.19.5 Antimicrobials in renal impairment

Drug	Usual adult dose	GFR			CAVH/CVVH	Comments
		20–50 ml/min	10–20 ml/min	<10 ml/min		
Aciclovir IV	5–10 mg/kg every 8 h	5–10 mg/kg every 12 h	5–10 mg/kg every 24 h	2.5–5 mg/kg every 24 h	5–10 mg/kg every 24 h	
Amikacin	15 mg/kg every 24 h	8–12 mg/kg every 24 h	3–4 mg/kg every 24 h	2 mg/kg every 24–48 h	3–4 mg/kg every 24 h	Monitor serum trough levels. Trough level <5 mg/litre
Amoxicillin	500 mg–1 g every 8 h (max 6 g daily)	No change	No change	250–500 mg every 8 h	No change	
Amphotericin (liposomal)	1–3 mg/kg daily	No change	No change	No change	No change	
Azithromycin	500 mg daily	No change	No change	No change	No change	
Benzylpenicillin	600 mg–14.4 g per day in divided doses	No change	Max of 2.4 g every 6 h	Max of 1.8 g every 6 h	Max of 2.4 g every 6 h	Increased incidence of seizures in renal impairment
Caspofungin	70 mg stat, then 50 mg every 24 h	No change	No change	No change	No change	
Cefixime	200–400 mg daily	No change	150–300 mg every 24 h	100–200 mg every 24 h	150–300 mg every 24 h	
Cefotaxime	1–2 g every 8 h (max 12 g daily)	No change	No change	0.5–1 g every 8–12 h	1 g every 12 h	Reduce dose further if concurrent hepatic and renal failure
Cefradine	0.5–1 g every 6 h (max 8 g daily)	No change	No change	250 mg every 6 h	No change	
Ceftazidime	1–2 g every 8–12 h	1 g every 12 h	1 g every 24 h	0.5–1 g every 24 h	0.5 g -1 g every 8–12 h	
Ceftriaxone	1 g daily (severe infections 2–4 g daily)	No change	No change	No change	No change	Severe renal impairment max 2 g daily
Chloramphenicol	50 mg/kg per day in 4 divided doses	No change	No change	No change	No change	
Ciprofloxacin IV	200–400 mg every 12 h	No change	100–200 mg every 12 h	100–200 mg every 12 h	200–400 mg every 12 h	Excellent oral bioavailability
Clarithromycin	500 mg every 12 h	No change	250–500 mg every 12 h	250 mg every 12 h	250–500 mg every 12 h	
Clindamycin	0.6–4.8 g daily in 2–4 divided doses	No change	No change	No change	No change	Stop if patient develops diarrhoea
Co-amoxiclav IV	1.2 g every 8 h	No change	1.2 g every 12 h	1.2 g stat, then 600 mg every 12 h	1.2 g every 12 h	
Co-trimoxazole	120 mg/kg/day in 2–4 divided doses	No change	60 mg/kg every 12 h for 3 days, then 30 mg/kg every 12 h	30 mg/kg every 12 h (only give if haemodialysis available)	60 mg/kg every 12 h for 3 days, then 30 mg/kg every 12 h	Doses quoted are treatment doses for PCP
Doxycycline	200 mg stat, then 100–200 mg daily	No change	No change	No change	No change	
Ertapenem	1 g daily	1 g every 24 h[a]	1 g every 24 h[a]	0.5–1 g every 24 h[a]	1 g every 24 h[a]	
Erythromycin	25–50 mg/kg/day in 4 divided doses (max 4 g per day)	No change	No change	50–75% of normal dose; max 1.5 g daily	No change	Increased risk of ototoxicity in renal impairment
Ethambutol	15 mg/kg/day	No change	No change	7.5 mg/kg/day	No change	Perform baseline visual acuity test
Flucloxacillin	0.5–2 g every 6 h	No change	No change	Max of 4 g per day	No change	
Fluconazole	50–400 mg every 24 h	No change	No change	50% of normal dose	No change	

Table 21.19.5 (*Cont'd*) Antimicrobials in renal impairment

Drug	Usual adult dose	GFR			CAVH/CVVH	Comments
Flucytosine	200 mg/kg/day in 4 divided doses (doses of 100–150 mg/kg/day may be used)	50 mg/kg every 12 h	50 mg/kg every 24 h	50 mg/kg then dose according to levels. 0.5–1 g daily is usually adequate	50 mg/kg every 24 h (monitor levels)	Monitor blood levels 24 h after starting therapy. Pre-dose level 25–50 mcg/ml. Do not exceed 80 mcg/ml.
Foscarnet	60 mg/kg every 8 h–induction dose	28 mg/kg every 8 h	Seek specialist advice			
Fusidic Acid	>50 kg 500 mg every 8 h <50 kg 6–7 mg/kg every 8 h	No change	No change	No change	No change	
Ganciclovir	5 mg/kg every 12 h	If CrCl is 25–50 ml/min use 2.5 mg/kg every 12 h	If CrCl is 10–25 ml/min use 2.5 mg/kg every 24 h	1.25 mg/kg every 24 h	2.5–5 mg/kg every 24 h	
Gentamicin	7 mg/kg/day[b] sMonitor serum levels 6–14 h post dose Adjust dosing interval using the Hartford nomogram			2 mg/kg every 24 h[a] Check trough level at 24 h Aim for trough <2		
Isoniazid	>50 kg: 300 mg every 24 h <50 kg: 150 mg every 24 h	No change	No change	No change	No change	Give pyridoxine 25 mg daily to prevent peripheral neuropathy
Itraconazole	200 mg every 24 h	No change	No change	No change	No change	
Linezolid	600 mg every 12 h	No change	No change	No change	No change	
Meropenem	1 g every 8 h Meningitis: 2 g every 8 h	1 g every 12 h Meningitis: 2 g every 12 h	1 g every 12 h Meningitis: 2 g every 12 h	1 g every 24 h Meningitis: 2 g every 24 h	1 g every 12 h Meningitis: 2 g every 12 h	
Metronidazole	500 mg every 8 h	No change	No change	500 mg every 12 h	No change	
Moxifloxacin	400 mg every 24 h	No change	No change	No change	No change	
Nitrofurantoin	50–100 mg every 6 h	Contraindicated	Contraindicated	Contraindicated	Contraindicated	Avoid if GFR <60 ml/min. Ineffective and increased risk of neuropathy.
Ofloxacin	200–400 mg every 24 h, increased to every 12 h in severe infections	Normal loading dose, then 200 mg every 24 h	Normal loading dose, then 100–200 mg every 24 h	Normal loading dose, then 100 mg every 24 h	Normal loading dose, then 100 mg every 24 h	
Penicillin V	500 mg every 6 h	No change	No change	No change	No change	
Streptomycin	15 mg/kg every 24 h (max 1 g daily)	15 mg/kg every 24 h (max 1 g daily)	15 mg/kg every 24–72 h (max 1 g daily)	15 mg/kg every 72–96 h (max 1 g daily)	15 mg/kg every 24–72 h (max 1 g daily)	Monitor serum levels. Peak levels ≤20–25 µg/ml
Synercid	7.5 mg/kg every 8 h	5–7.5 mg/kg every 8–12 h	5–7.5 mg/kg every 8–12 h	5 mg/kg every 8–12 h	5–7.5 mg/kg every 8–12 h	
Tazocin	4.5 g every 8 h	No change	4.5 g every 12 h	4.5 g every 12 h	4.5 g every 12 h	
Teicoplanin	400 mg every 12 h for 3 doses, then 400 mg daily	Reduce dose from Day 4 to 400 mg every 48 h	Reduce dose from Day 4 to 400 mg every 72 h	Reduce dose from Day 4 to 400 mg every 72 h	Reduce dose from Day 4 to 400 mg every 48 h	
Trimethoprim	200 mg every 12 h	No change	No change	No change	No change	
Vancomycin	1 g every 12 h Monitor trough levels before 3rd or 4th dose.	1 g every 24 h Monitor trough levels before 3rd dose	1 g every 24–48 h Monitor trough levels before 2nd dose	Patients NOT on dialysis: 1 g stat Monitor trough level at 24 h and only give another dose when level <15 mg/litre	500 mg–1.0 g stat during last hour of dialysis. Monitor trough levels pre-dialysis and only give another dose when level <10 mg/litre	Monitor serum trough levels. Trough level 5–15 mg/litre (dependent on infection type)

[a] Unlicensed indication.
[b] Use ideal body weight to calculate doses.

Sepsis and antibiotic use in renal impairment

An in-depth discussion of this topic is beyond the scope of this chapter, but most of the important issues are summarized in Table 21.19.5.

Further reading

Bennett WM, *et al.* (1999). *Drug prescribing in renal failure: dosing guidelines for adults*, 4th edition, revised. American College of Physicians, Washington DC.

Bohler J, Donauer J, Keller F (1999). Pharmacokinetic principles during continuous renal replacement therapy: drugs and dosage. *Kidney Int*, **72**, S24–8.

Bonate PL, Reith K, Weir S (1998). Drug interactions at a renal level. *Clin Pharmacokinet*, **34**, 375–404.

Inui KI, Masuda S, Saito H (2000). Cellular and molecular aspects of drug transport in the kidney. *Kidney Int*, **58**, 944–58.

Masereeuw R, Russel FG (2001). Mechanisms and clinical implications of renal drug excretion. *Drug Metab Rev*, **33**, 299–351.

Website

electronic Medicines Compendium (eMC) http://www.emc.medicines.org. uk/ [Contains information about UK licensed medicines, providing updated Summaries of Product Characteristics (SPCs) and Patient Information leaflets (PILs).]

SECTION 22

Disorders of the blood

Introduction

D.J. Weatherall

Essentials

Almost all diseases can produce changes in the blood, and primary haematological disorders can affect any organ system. The general clinical approach to the patient with a haematological disorder involves the following:

History

This should place particular emphasis, depending on the presenting problem, on (1) symptoms of anaemia; (2) overt blood loss—gastrointestinal or menstrual; (3) dietary history and evidence of malabsorption; (4) weight loss, night sweats, bone pain, and pruritus—which may indicate a lymphoproliferative or myeloproliferative disorder; (5) drug ingestion—many drugs produce haematological side effects; (6) bruising/bleeding—has the patient bled significantly in the past following dental extractions or minor surgical procedures?; (7) family history—may give useful clues to the cause of bleeding or anaemia, as may the ethnic origin of the patient's ancestors.

Physical examination

Aspects of particular importance include (1) skin—for bruising, purpura, infiltration or ulceration; (2) mouth—for glossitis, ulceration, infection, bleeding, and tonsils; (3) lymph nodes—for enlargement; (4) abdomen—for hepatomegaly and splenomegaly; (5) eyes—for anaemia, haemorrhages, jaundice, and retinal haemorrhages (commonly seen in patients who have had a sudden fall in haemoglobin level); (6) musculoskeletal—recurrent bleeding into joints may produce a chronic deforming arthritis in patients with coagulation defects.

Laboratory investigation

The diagnosis and management of blood disease requires an examination of the blood and—if appropriate—the bone marrow, with the best chance of useful information being obtained if there is very close liaison between the laboratory and the ward or clinic.

Key investigations include (1) full blood count—which gives a wealth of information including packed cell volume, haemoglobin level, red cell indices, total and differential leucocyte count, platelet count, and (with appropriate analysers) reticulocyte count; (2) stained blood film—the most important investigation in haematology, allowing each of the cell types to be studied separately; (3) examination of the marrow—to assess the overall cellularity and for the presence of abnormal cells.

The study of blood is one of the most fascinating branches of clinical medicine. Almost all diseases produce changes in the blood at some time during their course. Furthermore, primary disorders of the blood and blood-forming tissues can give rise to clinical manifestations, which may involve any of the organ systems. Primary disorders of the blood and blood-forming organs account for only a small percentage of a haematologist's practice. Most patients who are referred with haematological abnormalities have diseases in other systems. Anaemia is a good example. Most anaemias are due to blood loss, infection, renal failure, malignant disease, or malnutrition or parasitic infestation. Anaemia may be the first indication of a chronic urinary tract infection, hypothyroidism, pituitary failure, bacterial endocarditis, polymyalgia rheumatica, or rarities such as atrial myxoma.

This section emphasizes primary diseases of the blood and blood-forming organs, but many of these conditions are relatively uncommon.

An approach to patients with haematological disorders

The diagnosis of blood diseases follows the same process as that for any other condition; expertise in the laboratory will never make up for an inadequate history and clinical examination. It should be remembered that many patients who are referred to hospital for a specialist opinion on their blood are worried about the possibility of leukaemia, although they will rarely say so. It is important to reassure them as soon as possible if this is not the diagnosis.

Where leukaemia is suspected, no time should be lost in determining an accurate diagnosis and a well worked out plan of management. The position can then be discussed frankly with the patient and their family; knowledge of what they face and precisely what form of treatment is to be instituted often engenders a great sense of relief after weeks or months of fearing the worst.

Clinical history

In taking a history from a patient who is suspected of having a haematological disorder, certain factors are of particular importance. The symptoms of anaemia are described in detail later in this section. However, a slowly developing anaemia may be completely asymptomatic, even when the haemoglobin concentration is extremely low. Individuals who are otherwise healthy should be able to compensate for a relatively mild anaemia; a young individual with a haemoglobin level of 10.5 g/dl who complains of tiredness and an inability to cope with life is more likely to have these symptoms because of chronic anxiety rather than the anaemia. Other general symptoms are of great importance, particularly weight loss, night sweats, bone pain, and pruritus. Moderate nocturnal sweating is common in anxiety states; drenching sweats requiring several changes of nightclothes and sheets are a more ominous symptom, often associated with infection or lymphoproliferative disease. Pruritus occurs in conjunction with many disorders of the blood. When associated with lymphoma it is nonspecific, but when pruritus accompanies the myeloproliferative disorders it is often precipitated by warmth such as getting into bed or a hot bath. A detailed drug history is essential; many drugs produce haematological side effects.

Although a complete systematic history must be taken, gastrointestinal and haemostatic functions are particularly relevant to diseases of the blood. A detailed dietetic history is essential when investigating anaemia, and it is important to ask specifically about symptoms such as a sore tongue, bleeding gums, dysphagia, dyspepsia, disturbance of bowel habit suggestive of malabsorption, and rectal bleeding. Patients are often referred to haematological departments for investigation of easy bruising. Many people, particularly women, bruise easily, and the key question is whether the bruising is unusual for them. Is it spontaneous or related to only mild trauma? It is also extremely helpful to enquire into certain key episodes in a patient's life that may provide a clue as to whether there is an inborn bleeding tendency. These include circumcision, dental extraction (was a return to the dentist for stitching or packing ever required?), menstruation, surgical procedures, and so on.

Assessment of menstrual blood loss is an important part of the history in women with iron deficiency, as well as for assessing haemostatic function. It is not enough to ask a woman whether she considers that her periods are normal. If she only uses internal tampons, she probably does not have menorrhagia. However, the use of one or more packets of the more absorbent brands of external pads, or the need to get up at night to change pads or to stay at home during the menstrual period, suggests a heavy loss.

Family histories are particularly important for the diagnosis of blood diseases. It is not only essential to ask for a family history of anaemia or bleeding disorders, but the ethnic origin of the patient's ancestors may also give valuable clues to the cause of anaemia. The long-forgotten Italian great-grandparent may have been the source of the thalassaemia gene that is responsible for a refractory hypochromic anaemia or the red-cell enzyme deficiency that leads to a haemolytic drug reaction. A detailed personal history is also essential. Cigarette or cigar smoking is probably the most common cause of mild polycythaemia. Alcohol can produce remarkably diverse haematological changes. A detailed occupational history may reveal exposure to industrial solvents or other agents responsible for bone marrow depression; unusual hobbies may also result in contact with toxic agents.

Physical examination

The examination of a patient with a haematological disorder follows the same pattern as any physical examination, but there are certain aspects of particular importance. On general inspection it is essential to examine the skin carefully for evidence of bruising, purpura, infiltration, or ulceration. The distribution and pattern of bruising or petechiae may be diagnostic, particularly in disorders such as Henoch–Schönlein purpura, senile purpura, scurvy, purpura due to venous obstruction, and the painful bruising syndrome. Thrombocytopenic purpura is often seen most easily over pressure areas; a few lesions in these regions are easily overlooked. Cutaneous lymphoma may mimic a variety of skin diseases. Chronic leg ulceration is a common finding in sickle cell anaemia; it occurs occasionally with other genetic haemolytic anaemias. The perianal region and perineum should be carefully inspected. There may be perianal infiltration, particularly in the monocytic leukaemias, and it is very important to recognize perianal infection early in neutropenic patients. Digital examination of the rectum should be avoided in neutropenia for fear of disseminating an infection.

Potential sites of infection in compromised patients must be examined daily. They include the skin, intravenous infusion sites, the mouth and throat, and the perineum. The mucous membranes, nail beds, and palmar creases should be examined carefully for pallor, always remembering that the clinical assessment of anaemia is very inaccurate. Pigmentation of the face is sometimes a feature of folic acid deficiency. Mild jaundice may be a useful indicator of haemolysis, while a greyish pigmentation of the skin is common in patients with iron overload, both primary and secondary to repeated transfusion. There is an association between vitiligo and pernicious anaemia. In patients with polycythaemia there may be suffusion of the conjunctivae, a high colour, and prominence of the vessels over the face, neck, and upper part of the chest. The nails should be examined for unusual fragility; flattened, spoon-shaped nails (koilonychia), which are supposed to be diagnostic of chronic iron deficiency, are now rarely seen.

An assessment of the size of the lymph nodes and an inspection of other lymphatic tissue are an important part of the examination of patients with haematological disorders. It is most important to develop a systematic approach to lymph node examination. Each group of nodes in the head and neck, axillae and groins, together with the epitrochlear nodes, must be examined in detail. In the head and neck it is useful to start with the occipital nodes, then move to the preauricular and postauricular nodes, and, finally, to examine systematically the anterior and posterior triangles and supraclavicular regions. In patients with enlarged occipital or posterior cervical nodes, the scalp should be inspected for signs of infestation and secondary infection due to scratching. A simple way of describing enlarged lymph nodes should be used, without the use of too many adjectives. Nodes should be labelled as hard, firm, or soft, and tender or nontender. Ambiguous terms such as 'rubbery' should be avoided. Soft, tender nodes usually indicate infection. Large, firm nodes are characteristic of lymphoma. Hard nodes occur in secondary carcinoma, although calcified nodes, matted together and attached to skin, are still encountered in patients with tuberculous adenitis. The approximate size of the nodes should be recorded, together with whether they are mobile, attached deep or superficially, and discrete or matted together. It is also very important to examine the tonsils and adenoids, particularly in a patient suspected of having a lymphoproliferative disease.

A detailed examination of the mouth should include the state of the tongue, mucous membranes, gums, teeth, and fauces. Glossitis, as evidenced by a smooth, depapillated tongue, occurs in iron-deficiency and megaloblastic anaemia. Small, black bullas (blood blisters) on the tongue or mucous membranes, which burst and leave superficial ulcers, are characteristic of thrombocytopenic purpura. Gingival hypertrophy is sometimes found in patients with acute leukaemia, particularly the monocytic type, and in some individuals with megaloblastic anaemia due to phenytoin therapy. Ulcers of the mouth and fauces occur in all forms of acute leukaemia. Oral infection, often associated with ulceration, is very common in neutropenic patients. Candidosis may be seen on the fauces, tongue, or mucous membranes. Candidal infection of the throat, associated with dysphagia, should raise the suspicion of oesophageal candidosis (-iasis). The teeth may be badly formed, and the bite may be abnormal in patients with severe forms of thalassaemia. Dental abscesses are common in patients with neutropenia; suspect teeth should be gently percussed for evidence of apical infection. Telangiectases may be found on the lips and oral mucous membranes of patients with hereditary telangiectasia.

On abdominal examination, the most important questions are the size of the liver, whether there is splenomegaly, and if there are any palpable para-aortic lymph nodes. It is not possible to learn how to examine the spleen from a textbook, but a few hints may be helpful. Large spleens can often be seen to move up and down on respiration if the abdomen is well illuminated and the observer stands at the end of the bed. Very large spleens tend to move downwards and medially towards the right iliac fossa and can be missed if the examiner does not start palpating from this region, moving upwards and medially towards the left subcostal region. A sure way to miss a moderately enlarged spleen is to go digging in with the fingers without eliciting the patient's help. With the left hand hooked round the region above the left costal margin, and the right hand resting lightly on the abdomen, the examining practitioner should ask the patient to gently breathe in and out through the mouth. The secret of success is to persuade the patient to breathe just deeply enough to move the spleen down without contracting the abdominal muscles. The examiner should wait for the spleen tip to meet their fingers rather than to try to find it by deep palpation. Once defined, the position of the lower border of the spleen should be recorded in centimetres, vertically below the costal margin. Manoeuvres designed to facilitate the palpation of a slightly enlarged spleen, such as turning the patient on their right side, while useful for impressing clinical examiners, are rarely of much help in practice. Be gentle! The author has seen enlarged spleens ruptured by overenthusiastic medical students. If there is pain over the spleen or referred to the left shoulder, do not forget to listen for a rub. Finally, remember that spleens come in all sizes and shapes, and often lie more laterally than expected. Do not be disappointed not to feel the much publicized notch; it happens once or twice in a clinical lifetime. The differential diagnosis of palpable masses in the region of the spleen is considered later in this section.

The eyes are a mine of information in patients with haematological disorders. Periorbital oedema is sometimes seen in infectious mononucleosis. The conjunctivae may show mild icterus not obvious in the skin, and there may be haemorrhages in bleeding disorders. Pingueculae of the conjunctivae are seen in Gaucher's disease. Retinal haemorrhages are common in patients who have had a sudden fall in haemoglobin level. They are less frequent in severely thrombocytopenic patients with normal haemoglobin levels; the combination of anaemia and thrombocytopenia is particularly likely to lead to severe retinal bleeding. Papilloedema occurs commonly in patients with leukaemia involving the central nervous system. Proliferative abnormalities of the retinal vessels are often seen in patients with sickling disorders, particularly haemoglobin SC disease. The hyperviscosity syndrome associated with macroglobulinaemia and some forms of myeloma is characterized by fullness of the retinal veins, which are sometimes broken up into segments like a string of sausages. These changes are often associated with widespread retinal haemorrhages. Optic atrophy may occur in patients with severe vitamin B_{12} deficiency. Unilateral exophthalmos occurs occasionally in patients with myeloma deposits or lymphoma involving the orbit.

Examination of the musculoskeletal system may be particularly rewarding in patients suspected of having genetic blood disorders. In patients with coagulation defects such as haemophilia or Christmas disease, recurrent bleeding into joints may produce a chronic deforming arthritis. Muscle haematomas are also common and are easily missed. For example, bleeding into the psoas sheath may produce a discrete swelling above the inguinal ligament, which may later be associated with nerve compression leading to weakness of the quadriceps and anaesthesia over the anterior aspect of the thigh. If muscle pain is the presenting symptom, it is very important to palpate the muscle groups carefully for the cystic swellings that may occur in haemophiliacs after bleeding into muscles. The joints have other important associations with blood disorders. A mild refractory anaemia is a very common accompaniment of rheumatoid arthritis. Painful arthritis of the large joints may be the presenting symptom of primary haemochromatosis. Gout is a common complication of all the myeloproliferative diseases; the ears should be examined carefully for tophi, in addition to a full assessment of the joints. The value of bone tenderness in the diagnosis of acute leukaemia has been overemphasized. When present it is best elicited by carefully palpating the sternum or tibias, or by rib compression. Be gentle, because sometimes the tenderness is quite exquisite. Bone tenderness or local swelling are also found in patients with myeloma or sickle cell anaemia. In children with thalassaemia or other hereditary haemolytic anaemias, there may be reduced growth, bossing of the skull, and facial deformities. A wide variety of skeletal changes may occur with congenital hypoplastic anaemia.

The use of the laboratory

The diagnosis and management of blood disease requires an examination of the blood and, if appropriate, the bone marrow. Clinicians will obtain the maximum information from their colleagues in the laboratory if they ask the right questions. Scribbling down 'full blood count' on a laboratory request form is useless. It is essential to ask for an examination of the blood film in any patient who is suspected of having a haematological disorder. More can be learned from the help of an experienced morphologist than from any other investigation in clinical haematology. Some haematological investigations are underused; others are requested far too often. For example, the often forgotten reticulocyte count is an invaluable guide to the response of the bone marrow to anaemia and for the recognition of bleeding or mild haemolysis. On the other hand, bone marrow examination is an unpleasant investigation and should only be requested with very clear indications. For example, clinicians should stop and think why they are ordering a bone marrow examination in an elderly patient with a peripheral blood lymphocyte count of 80×10^9/litre. This can only be chronic lymphatic leukaemia; the bone marrow will be infiltrated with lymphocytes. Why put the patient through this traumatic investigation? The result is predictable and will not help in their management.

It cannot be emphasized too strongly that the most useful information is obtained by very close liaison between the laboratory and the ward. Clinicians should visit the haematology laboratory regularly, review films and haematological data with their laboratory colleagues, and be very precise in setting out the reasons for the investigations they order. Much valuable information is lost because of the lack of good liaison between the bedside and laboratory.

Examination of the blood

Constituents of normal blood

Blood consists of several different types of cells suspended in plasma. The classification and morphological analysis of blood cells was made possible by the studies of Ehrlich, who, in 1877, described the use of aniline dyes for staining dried blood films. This approach has been refined over the years. The fine structure of the blood cells has been analysed in greater detail with the electron microscope and, more recently, with the scanning electron microscope (Fig. 22.1.1).

The formed elements of the blood, or blood cells, consist of the red cells, white cells, and platelets. The red cells are biconcave discs approximately 7 to 8 μm in diameter (Fig. 22.1.1). They consist of a membrane that contains a concentrated solution of haemoglobin and a variety of other proteins, salts, and vitamins. Normally they

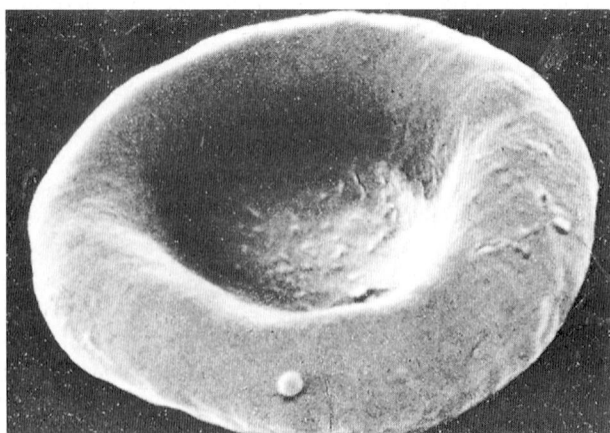

Fig. 22.1.1 A human erythrocyte as viewed through the scanning electron microscope.
(By kind permission of Dr S M Lewis.)

are of a uniform shape and size, and contain similar amounts of haemoglobin. On supravital staining, approximately 1% of the red cells show a reticular appearance. These are newly released cells and because of their staining characteristics are called reticulocytes.

The white cells are classified according to their morphological appearances into granulocytes (polymorphonuclear leucocytes (PMNs)), monocytes, and lymphocytes. The granulocytes and monocytes are phagocytic cells, while the lymphocytes are involved in a variety of immune mechanisms. The granulocytes can be further classified according to their maturity. In the newly produced forms, band cells or juvenile polymorphonuclear leucocytes, the nucleus is horseshoe-shaped but single. In a normal blood film the majority of the granulocytes have matured beyond this stage, and their nuclei consist of two or more lobes separated by thin, filamentous chromatin strands. These cells are about 12 to 15 μm in diameter. The granulocyte series is further classified according to the staining characteristics of the granules into neutrophils, eosinophils, and basophils. The monocytes are of similar size to the granulocytes but have oval nuclei with a slate-coloured cytoplasm, which may contain some fine granules.

There are two morphologically distinct forms of lymphocyte: a large cell with a diameter of 8 to 16 μm and a smaller one measuring 7 to 9 μm. Both forms are round and have a light blue cytoplasm. In the large lymphocytes the nucleus fills about half of the cell, whereas in the small lymphocytes it almost completely fills the cell.

The platelets are disc-shaped cells measuring approximately 2 to 3 μm in diameter. In normal blood they are relatively homogeneous in structure; their fine structure cannot be distinguished by conventional light microscopy.

More detailed descriptions of the structure and function of these different blood cells and their precursors appear later in this section.

The normal blood count

A full blood count is carried out on an anticoagulated blood sample. A stained blood film is prepared for examination of the morphology of the different cells. Using either chemical and physical methods, or the more accurate electronic cell counters, the relative volume of packed red cells and white cells, the haemoglobin level, and the red-cell, white-cell, and platelet counts can be determined. From a series of calculations relating the volume of packed cells, haemoglobin level, and red-cell count, it is possible to derive a series of absolute indices that provide useful information about the size and degree of haemoglobinization of the red cells. Finally, the relative numbers of reticulocytes and the erythrocyte sedimentation rate (ESR) can be determined.

The stained blood film

An examination of the stained blood film is the most important investigation in haematology. Each of the cell types is studied separately.

The red cells are examined to assess their degree of haemoglobinization and their shape; if both are normal, they are described as normochromic and normocytic. Disorders of the red cell are frequently associated with changes in their morphology or staining properties. These include variation in size or anisocytosis; an increase in size or macrocytosis; a reduction in size or microcytosis; variability in shape or poikilocytosis; pale staining or hypochromia, which suggests underhaemoglobinization; and variation in the degree of staining from cell to cell, which is called anisochromia. In addition to these changes there may be more specific alterations in the morphology of the red cells. Some of these, together with the different clinical disorders with which they are associated, are summarized in Table 22.1.1 and illustrated in Fig. 22.1.2.

The white cells may be abnormal in number or morphology. An increased white-cell count is called a leucocytosis. If this involves the polymorphonuclear series, it is called a polymorphonuclear leucocytosis or granulocytosis. An elevated eosinophil, basophil, monocyte, or lymphocyte count is called an eosinophilia, basophilia, monocytosis, or lymphocytosis, respectively. A reduced white count is called a neutropenia or lymphopenia, depending on the cell type involved. An absence of granulocytes in the blood is called agranulocytosis. Much can be learned by morphological examination of the white cells. A blood film is said to show a 'shift to the left' if there are relatively more 'young' polymorphonuclear leucocytes present than normal. This is reflected by an increased proportion of band forms and, in more extreme cases, by a variable number of myelocytes or metamyelocytes. In acute bacterial infections, vacuoles may appear in the cytoplasm of polymorphonuclear leucocytes. In addition, the granules may become morphologically abnormal; heavy granulation of this type is called toxic granulation. This change is sometimes associated with the presence of

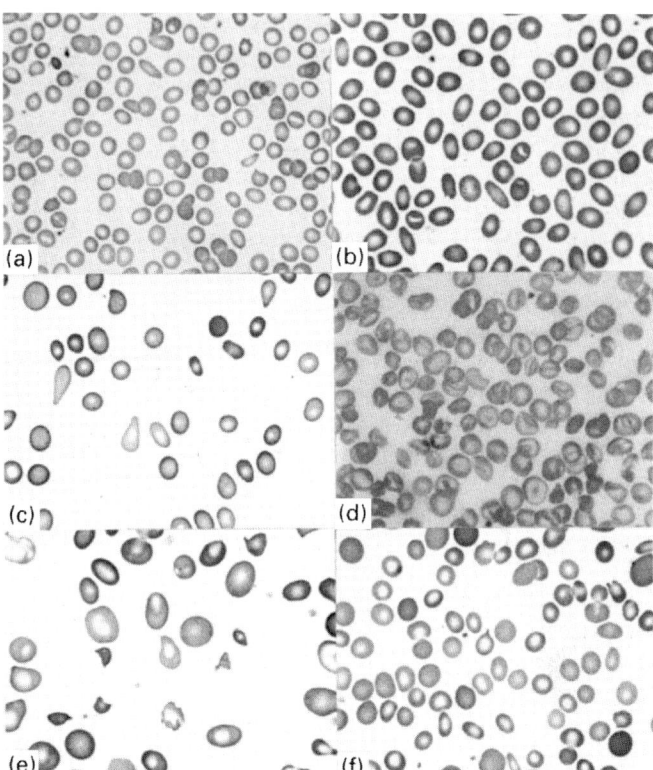

Fig. 22.1.2 Morphological changes of the red cells (magnification ×600–800): (a) hypochromia and microcytosis; (b) elliptocytosis; (c) poikilocytosis (myelosclerosis); (d) target cells and intracellular crystals (haemoglobin C disease); (e) macrocytosis and anisocytosis (pernicious anaemia); (f) dimorphic picture: normochromic and hypochromic (sideroblastic anaemia).

Table 22.1.1 Significance of morphological and staining variations of the red cells

Change	Clinical significance
Hypochromia	Defective haemoglobinization; usually iron deficiency or defective haemoglobin synthesis
Microcytosis	As above
Macrocytosis	Dyserythropoiesis or premature release; may indicate megaloblastic erythropoiesis or haemolysis
Anisochromia	Variability of haemoglobinization or presence of young red-cell populations, e.g. in haemolysis
Spherocytosis	Usually indicates damage to membrane; may result from a genetic disorder of the membrane or an acquired defect often due to antibody or other damage to the cell
Target cells	Large 'floppy' cells that occur with deficient haemoglobinization or in liver disease; also occur in hyposplenism
Elliptocytes	May result from a genetic defect in the red-cell membrane but also occur in a variety of acquired conditions including iron deficiency
Poikilocytes: include burr cells, helmet cells, schistocytes, fragmented forms etc.	Usually indicates trauma to red cells in microcirculation or severe oxidant damage
Sickle cells	Occur in sickling disorders
Acanthocytes	Occur in genetic disorders of lipid metabolism
Inclusions: iron granules(siderocytes), Howell–Jolly bodies and Cabot's rings (nuclear remnants), basophilic stippling, and Heinz bodies	Iron granules and nuclear remnants are often seen after splenectomy. Basophilic stippling indicates accelerated erythropoiesis or defective haemoglobin synthesis. It also occurs in some hereditary haemolytic anaemias. Heinz bodies are precipitated haemoglobin or globin subunits

small (1–2 μm) oval bodies called Döhle bodies. A variety of genetic changes of nuclear configuration or of the granules of the polymorphonuclear leucocytes has been described; these are discussed later in this section.

The packed cell volume, haemoglobin level, and red-cell indices

A great deal can be learned about the character of an anaemia from a few simple haematological tests. The volume of packed red cells (PCV or haematocrit) can be estimated either by centrifugation of a blood sample, or by a conductivity method in which it is derived from measurement of the red-cell volume and the number of red cells using an electronic counting system. The haemoglobin concentration is usually determined spectrophotometrically by comparing a test sample with a stable standard, usually of the cyanmethaemoglobin derivative. Red-cell counting has become part of a standard blood count because of the accuracy of electronic cell counters.

Normal values for the PCV, haemoglobin level, and red-cell count are shown in Table 22.1.2. It is important to become familiar with the variability of these figures between the sexes and at different stages of development (Table 22.1.3). Furthermore, it should be emphasized that the accuracy of these measurements relies very much on the method used for their determination. An electronic cell counter gives extremely reproducible results for all three measurements, whereas a red-cell count made with a counting chamber is of little value. The red-cell indices can be estimated by combining

Table 22.1.2 Haematological values for normal adults

Red-cell count	
Men	$5.0 \pm 0.5 \times 10^{12}$/litre
Women	$4.3 \pm 0.5 \times 10^{12}$/litre

Haemoglobin	
Men	150 ± 20 g/litre
Women	140 ± 20 g/litre

Packed cell volume (PCV; haematocrit value)	
Men	0.45 ± 0.05 (litre/litre)
Women	0.41 ± 0.04 (litre/litre)

Mean cell volume (MCV)	
Men and women	92 ± 10 fl

Mean cell haemoglobin (MCH)	
Men and women	29.5 ± 2.5 pg

Mean cell haemoglobin concentration (MCHC)	
Men and women	330 ± 15 g/litre

Red-cell diameter (mean values)	
Dry films	$6.7–7.7\,\mu$m
Red-cell density	1092–1100 g/litre
Reticulocyte count	0.5–2.0% ($25–85 \times 10^9$/litre)

Blood volume	

Red-cell volume	
Men	30 ± 5 ml/kg
Women	25 ± 5 ml/kg
Plasma volume	45 ± 5 ml/kg
Total blood volume	70 ± 10 ml/kg
Red-cell lifespan	120 ± 30 days
Leucocyte count	$7.0 \pm 3.0 \times 10^9$/litre

Differential leucocyte count	
Neutrophils	$2.0–7.0 \times 10^9$/litre (40–80%)
Lymphocytes	$1.0–3.0 \times 10^9$/litre (20–40%)
Monocytes	$0.2–1.0 \times 10^9$/litre (2–10%)
Eosinophils	$0.04–0.4 \times 10^9$/litre (1–6%)
Basophils	$0.02–0.1 \times 10^9$/litre (<1–2%)
Platelet count	$130–400 \times 10^9$/litre

Bleeding time	
Ivy's method	2–7 min
Template method	2.5–9.5 min
Prothrombin time	12–16 s
Partial thromboplastin time (PTT)	30–46 s
Thrombin time	15–19 s
Plasma fibrinogen	2.0–4.0 g/litre
Fibrinogen titre	≥128

Plasminogen	
Function	0.75–1.35 u/ml
Antigen	0.76–1.36 u/ml

Table 22.1.2 *(Cont'd)* Haematological values for normal adults

Euglobulin lysis time	90–240 min

Antithrombin III	
Function	0.86–13.2 u/ml
Antigen	0.79–1.11 u/ml
β-Thromboglobulin	<50 ng/ml
Platelet factor 4	<10 ng/ml
Protein C	<10 ng/ml
Function	0.70–1.40 u/ml
Antigen	0.61–1.32 u/ml

Protein S	
Total	0.78–1.37 u/ml
Free	0.68–1.52 u/ml
Heparin cofactor II	55–145%

Autohaemolysis (37° C)	
48 h, without added glucose	0.2–2.0
48 h, with added glucose	0–0.9%
Cold agglutinin titre (4° C)	<64
Serum iron	$13–32\,\mu$mol/litre (0.7–1.8 mg/litre)
Total iron-binding capacity	$45–70\,\mu$mol/litre (2.5–4.0 mg/litre)
Transferrin	1.2–2.0 g/litre

Ferritin	
Men	$20–300\,\mu$g/litre, median $100\,\mu$g/litre
Women	$15–150\,\mu$g/litre, median $30\,\mu$g/litre
Serum vitamin B$_{12}$	160–760 ng/litre
Serum folate	$3–20\,\mu$g/litre
Red-cell folate	$160–640\,\mu$g/litre
Plasma haemoglobin	10–40 mg/litre
Serum haptoglobin	0.6–2.7 mg/litre
HbA$_2$	2.2–3.5%
HbF	<1.0%
Methaemoglobin	<2.0%

Sedimentation rate (1 h at $20 \pm 3°$ C)	

(upper limits)	
Men	
17–50 years	10 mm
50–60 years	12 mm
61–70 years	14 mm
>70 years	30 mm

Sedimentation rate (1 h at $20 \pm 3°$ C)	

(upper limits)	
Women	
17–50 years	19 mm
50–60 years	19 mm

Table 22.1.2 *(Cont'd)* Haematological values for normal adults

61–70 years	20 mm
>70 years	35 mm
Plasma viscosity	1.50–1.72 mPa/s
25° C	1.16–1.33 mPa/s
37° C	<80
Heterophile (anti-sheep red cell agglutinin titre) after absorption with guinea-pig kidney	<10

Values are expressed as means ± SD (95% range), unless indicated otherwise.
(After Dacie JV, Lewis SM (2006). *Practical haematology*, 10th edition. Churchill Livingstone, Edinburgh.)

information obtained from these measurements. The mean cell haemoglobin (MCH), which is derived from the haemoglobin value and the red-cell count and is expressed in picograms (pg), gives a reliable indication of the amount of haemoglobin per cell. The mean cell haemoglobin concentration (MCHC) represents the concentration of haemoglobin in g/dl (g/100 ml) of erythrocytes. The mean cell volume (MCV), calculated in femtolitres (fl), gives an indication of the size of the erythrocytes. Hence it is elevated in patients with macrocytic disorders and reduced in the presence of microcytic red cells. The normal values at different stages of development are summarized in Table 22.1.3.

It should be emphasized that the red-cell indices give an indication of the average size and degree of haemoglobinization of the red cells. They are only of value if combined with an examination of a blood film to provide information about the relative uniformity of any changes in size or haemoglobin concentration. Although many modern electronic cell counters provide data on the red-cell distribution width (RDW) these data do not provide enough information to reduce the critical importance of a blood-film examination.

Reticulocyte count

Reticulocytes are newly released red cells that contain residual RNA that can be identified either by supravital staining or by automated methods that utilize fluorescent RNA-binding dyes. There is a reasonably good correlation between these two methods of assessing the reticulocyte count. More recently, automated analysers also provide data about reticulocyte indices and RNA content.

The total and differential leucocyte count

The leucocyte count can be determined either by using a counting chamber or electronically. The differential count is obtained from analysing the different types of white cells in a total of 200 to 300 cells, or more if the total white-cell count is unusually low. It should be remembered that the total white-cell count shows remarkable variability even in the same individual at different times. There are variations during the menstrual cycle and a marked diurnal rhythm with minimum counts in the morning with subjects at rest. Activity may increase the white-cell count slightly, as may emotional stress and eating. Furthermore, the differential white-cell count varies considerably during normal human development. There is a preponderance of lymphocytes during the first few years of life and of polymorphonuclear leucocytes during later development and in adult life. These normal variations are shown in Table 22.1.3.

The platelet count

This is most accurately determined with an electronic cell counter, although a rough approximation can be obtained by using a counting chamber. There is marked variation in the normal platelet count and the range in health is approximately 150×10^9 to 400×10^9/litre. A slight drop in the count occurs before menstruation, but on the whole it varies less within an individual than the white-cell count.

Table 22.1.3 Haematological values for normal infants and children

	At birth (full term)	Day 3	1 month	2–6 months	2–6 years	6–12 years
Red-cell count ($\times 10^{12}$/litre)	6.0± 1.0	5.3± 1.3	4.2± 1.2	3.8± 0.8	4.6± 0.7	4.6± 0.6
Haemoglobin (g/litre)	165± 30	185± 40	140± 30	115± 20	125± 15	135± 20
Packed cell volume/haematocrit	0.54± 0.10	0.56± 0.11	0.43± 0.12	0.35± 0.07	0.37± 0.03	0.40± 0.05
Mean cell volume (MCV) (fl)	110± 10	108± 13	104± 19	91± 17	81± 6	86± 8
Mean cell haemoglobin (MCH) (pg)	34± 3	34± 3	34± 6	30± 5	27± 3	29± 4
Mean cell haemoglobin concentration (MCHC) (g/litre)	330± 30	330± 40	330± 40	330± 30	340± 30	340± 30
Reticulocytes (%)	2–5	1–4.5	0.3–1	0.4–1	0.2–2	0.2–2
Leucocyte count ($\times 10^9$/litre)	18± 8	15± 8	12± 7	12± 6	10± 5	9± 4
Neutrophils ($\times 10^9$/litre)	5–13	3–5	3–9	1.5–9	1.5–8	2–8
Lymphocytes ($\times 10^9$/litre)	3–10	2–8	3–16	4–10	6–9	1–5
Monocytes ($\times 10^9$/litre)	0.7–1.5	0.5–1	0.3–1	0.1–1	0.1–1	0.1–1
Eosinophils ($\times 10^9$/litre)	0.2–1	0.1–2.5	0.2–1	0.2–1	0.2–1	0.1–1

Values are expressed as means ± 2 SD, or 95% range.
(After Dacie JV, Lewis SM (2006). *Practical haematology*, 10th edition. Churchill Livingstone, Edinburgh.)

4198 SECTION 22 DISORDERS OF THE BLOOD

Blood volume, red-cell mass, and plasma volume

Because the haemoglobin level or PCV may vary due to expansion or contraction of the plasma volume, it is occasionally necessary to measure the red-cell mass and plasma volume directly. This is usually done by radioisotope dilution. The red-cell volume (RCV) is measured by labelling the red cells with chromium-51 and the plasma volume (PV) by the use of isotope-labelled albumin. These measurements are fraught with difficulties because of the variation of vascularity and PCV between different organs, and because fat is a relatively avascular tissue. There is still considerable controversy about how best to express the results. A variety of correction factors has been derived, which attempt to relate the measured RCV or PV to an ideal body weight. In practice it is usual to simply calculate the RCV or PV in ml/kg. The wide range of normal values is summarized in Table 22.1.2.

The erythrocyte sedimentation rate (ESR)

The ESR is a measure of the suspension stability of red cells in blood. It is usually expressed in millimetres (mm) and is obtained by measuring the distance from the surface meniscus to the upper limit of the red-cell layer in a column of blood after 60 min. The ESR depends on the difference in specific gravity between the red cells and plasma but is influenced by many other factors, particularly the rate at which the red cells clump or form rouleaux. The increased sedimentation rate of clusters of cells reflects reduced fluid friction resulting from a decreased surface to volume ratio. Rouleaux formation is related to the concentration of fibrinogen and, to a lesser extent, of α_2- and γ-globulins in the plasma. Unfortunately, the ESR is also subject to many technical difficulties including the dimensions of the tube, the nature of the anticoagulant used, and any degree of tilt of the tube from the horizontal.

The ESR is still widely used as a nonspecific index of organic disease. It is elevated in many acute or chronic infections, neoplastic diseases, collagen diseases, renal insufficiency, and any disorder associated with a significant change in the plasma proteins. Anaemia may cause an increased rate of sedimentation. Although many attempts have been made to develop correction factors to allow for this variable, none is satisfactory. Like all haematological measurements, the ESR changes in certain physiological states, particularly in pregnancy and with increasing age. In men and women over the age of 60, a slightly elevated ESR is often found without an obvious cause, although it may indicate the presence of a monoclonal gammopathy (Table 22.1.2).

Other haematological investigations

The simple tests that have been outlined in this section form the general screening investigations for all haematological disorders. In later sections we will describe the more specialized investigations that are often required to diagnose specific disorders of the red cells, white cells, and platelets, or of haemostasis and coagulation. Normal values for some of these investigations are given in Table 22.1.2.

Examination of the marrow

Bone marrow can be examined by needle aspiration, closed needle biopsy, or open surgical biopsy. In adults the sites most easily available are the sternum and the anterior or posterior iliac crests, although the marrow at the iliac crests tends to become rather fatty in older people. In children under 1 year of age, the anterior surface of the tibia is the site of choice, but in older children the iliac crest or the lumbar vertebral spines are suitable. After aspiration of the marrow, films are made and stained with a Romanowsky stain. Needle or surgical biopsy samples are fixed and sectioned by standard methods.

The marrow films are initially examined under low power to assess the overall cellularity and for the presence of abnormal cells. It is sometimes useful to obtain a differential count and from this to determine the myeloid to erythroid (M/E) ratio. This is approximately 3:1 in health, although, if there is increased erythroid activity, it may fall to unity or less. It should be remembered that differential counts may be quite inaccurate because the precursors may be distributed homogeneously. This is a particular problem in disorders in which there are abnormal cells in the marrow. Having determined the overall cellularity, the morphology of the individual cells is examined. The degree of maturation of the red cells, white cells, and megakaryocyte series is assessed and the marrow examined carefully for the presence of any abnormal cells.

A biopsy specimen is particularly useful for looking at overall cellularity and relating the amount of haemopoiesis to the amount of fatty tissue. It is of particular value if an aspiration yields a 'dry tap' when it may show replacement by fibrous or tumour tissue, which may not aspirate readily. Using appropriate stains, it is possible to estimate the amount of iron and reticulin in the marrow.

Assessment of bone marrow activity and distribution

Some indication of marrow function is obtained from its morphological appearances and from the M/E ratio. It is also possible to measure the rates of production and turnover of the red-cell series using radioactive iron. It is sometimes necessary to attempt to estimate the distribution of the haemopoietic marrow, and this is usually done by using isotopes to produce scintigrams that show the distribution of erythropoietic or reticuloendothelial marrow throughout the body. Erythropoietic marrow can be visualized using the short-lived, positron-emitting isotope iron-52 with a scintillation camera. In health this shows erythropoietic marrow in the ribs, spine, pelvis, scapula, and clavicle, with a variable amount in the skull. The reticuloendothelial portion of the marrow can be labelled with a radiocolloid with an appropriate particle size; the most effective and commonly used is technetium-99m–sulphur colloid.

Further reading

Lichtman MA, *et al.* (eds) (2010). *Williams' hematology*, 8th edition. McGraw-Hill, New York.

Dacie JV, Lewis SM (2006). *Practical haematology*, 10th edition. Churchill Livingstone, Edinburgh.

Hoffman R, *et al.* (2005). *Hematology: basic principles and practice*, 4th edition. Churchill Livingstone, New York.

Orkin, S.H. *et al.* (eds) (2009). *Nathan and Oski's Hematology of Infancy and Childhood*, 7th edition, W.B. Saunders, Philadelphia.

Haemopoietic stem cells

Contents

22.2.1 Stem cells and haemopoiesis

C.A. Sieff

Essentials

Haemopoiesis is the process of the amplification and terminal differentiation of immature precursors of the formed elements of the blood. A complex but ordered process proceeds via stem cells, progenitor cells, and precursor cells to produce mature cells of many lineages—erythrocytes, platelets, basophils, polymorphonuclear leucocytes, monocyte/macrophages, eosinophils, and a variety of types of lymphocyte.

Mechanisms of haemopoiesis

Key elements—(1) Pluripotent stem cells—present at extremely low frequency in marrow (1 in 10^4–10^5 cells); capable of both self-renewal and multilineage differentiation under the influence of certain non-lineage-specific growth factors such as Flt-3 ligand, stem cell factor (SCF), interleukin 6, and thrombopoietin. (2) Committed progenitor progeny—present at frequency in marrow of 1 in 10^3 cells; the level in the process at which amplification of blood-cell production occurs; limited proliferative potential that depends upon the presence of specific growth factors. (3) An appropriate microenvironment for haemopoietic differentiation, which in normal adults is confined to the bone marrow.

Particular cell lineages—(1) Erythropoiesis—release of erythropoietin from specialized peritubular cells in the kidney by anaemia or hypoxia stimulates the division and differentiation of erythroid progenitors and erythroblasts. (2) Myelopoiesis—under the influence of unique colony-stimulating factors (CSF), granulocyte and monocyte progenitors differentiate into mature granulocytes and monocytes, the latter leaving the circulation and differentiating further to become fixed tissue macrophages. (3) Megakaryocytopoiesis—thrombopoietin induces lineage-restricted megakaryocyte progenitor proliferation and differentiation of megakaryoblasts to the megakaryocytes that in turn produce platelets.

Marrow anatomy—the melange of cells within the marrow exist in delicate fronds thrust into the venous sinuses. Cells are packed in close proximity within the fronds, held together by extensions of fibroblast cytoplasm and fibronectin. Such delicate anatomy is subject to many abnormalities that can disturb the orderly progress of cell–cell interactions that govern the system, with the multiple symptoms of bone marrow failure resulting from such disturbances.

Clinical use of haemopoietic growth factors

Several recombinant haemopoietic growth factors are in clinical use, including (1) erythropoietin—to treat the anaemia of advanced chronic kidney disease (and sometimes other anaemias); (2) G-CSF—to shorten the period of neutropenia following myelosuppressive anticancer chemotherapy, and for reduction of infection in some patients with nonmyeloid malignancies; (3) GM-CSF—to accelerate haemopoietic reconstitution after bone marrow transplantation (also G-CSF).

Introduction

Normal haemopoiesis in the adult depends on the production of blood cells from their recognizable precursors in the bone marrow, their survival in the vasculature, and their demise in the reticuloendothelial system, predominantly in the spleen, liver, lung, and the marrow itself. Though the concentration of cells in the blood varies widely, the values observed in normal individuals are remarkably consistent, particularly considering the vast differences in the lifespans of these cells. For example, the mean lifespan of granulocytes in the peripheral blood may be measured in hours. In contrast, platelets survive for 7 to 10 days. Though platelets are removed from the blood in part by random forces, most of their lifespan is dictated by metabolic changes within them that lead to predetermined death. Normally, red cells are lost by a process of metabolic decay that begins after the erythrocyte has attained an age of approximately 100 days. Lymphocytes have very dramatic differences in lifespan. Some are removed from the circulation in 2 or 3 weeks by a process that is not understood. Others, particularly certain T lymphocytes, appear to survive for the entire lifespan of the individual, carrying within them the programmes embossed upon them by the thymus.

The steady-state concentrations of blood cells vary from one another by three orders of magnitude or more, but the marrow production rates that maintain them are very similar. Approximately 5×10^4 red cells, 2×10^4 platelets, and 2×10^4 granulocytes are produced per microlitre of blood per day to maintain a normal blood count. Lymphocyte production must be considerably lower because the bulk of lymphocytes in the peripheral blood are long-lived T lymphocytes.

The relatively constant production rates of blood cells are regulated by a highly complex marrow tissue, characterized morphologically by recognizable, differentiating precursor cells. These are partially renewed by a variable population of invisible progenitor cells, some of which have the characteristics of stem cells. Precursor cells and their progenitors are packed together into fronds surrounded by endothelial cells that separate marrow cells from the venous sinuses. The completed blood cells find apertures through the endothelial cells and migrate between them to fall into the sinuses, the currents of which carry them into the peripheral blood.

In this chapter, critical aspects of the physiology of haemopoiesis in the marrow are described. To understand this process, we must first review its ontogeny and comparative development.

Phylogeny and ontogeny

In the developing human haemopoiesis moves through several overlapping anatomical and functional stages, beginning in the yolk sac, entering the hepatic phase at 6 weeks gestation, and the marrow phase at 20 weeks. Transfer to the bone marrow phase is generally complete at birth. These anatomical shifts are associated with marked alterations in functional properties, particularly with respect to the pattern of globin synthesis in the red cell. These changes are referred to as the 'fetal switch'. This transition is not a single event involving only the γ-chains of fetal haemoglobin; rather, it is polygenic, involving a series of changes regulated in a programmed fashion. The mechanism of this coordinated series of changes is mediated at the level of the progenitors of haemopoietic cells and involves interaction of an upstream locus control region with the promoters of the embryonic, fetal, and adult genes. Both gene competition and autonomous silencing appear to be involved.

Marrow anatomy

The relative red (active) marrow space of a child is much greater than that of an adult, presumably because the high requirements for red cell production during neonatal life demand the resources of the entire production potential of the marrow. During postnatal life the demands for red cell production ebb. Much of the marrow space is progressively filled with fat (Fig. 22.2.1.1). In certain diseases that are usually associated with anaemia, such as myeloid

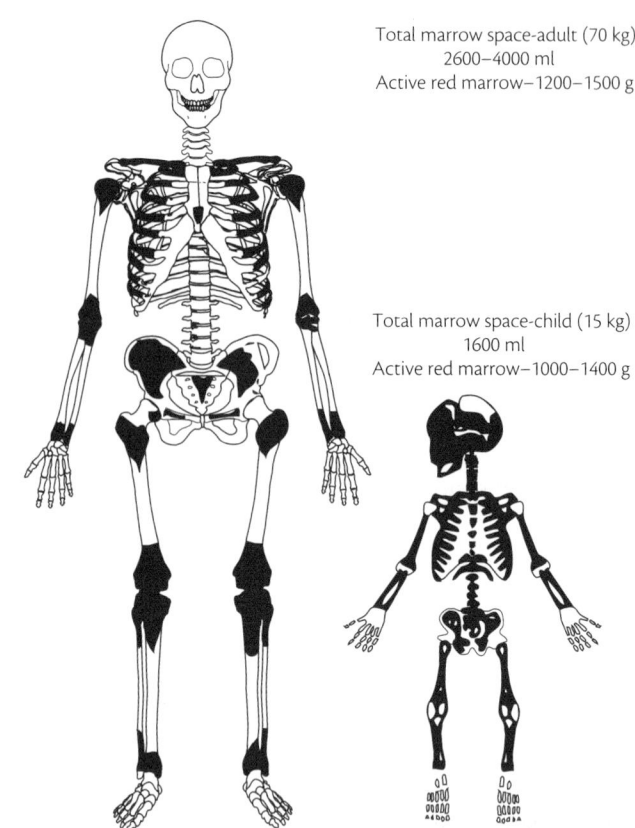

Total marrow space-adult (70 kg)
2600–4000 ml
Active red marrow–1200–1500 g

Total marrow space-child (15 kg)
1600 ml
Active red marrow–1000–1400 g

Fig. 22.2.1.1 A comparison of active red marrow–bearing areas in a child and adult. Note the almost identical amount of active red marrow in the child and adult despite a fivefold discrepancy in body weight.
(From MacFarlane RG, Robb-Smith AHT (eds) (1961). *Functions of the blood*, p. 357. Blackwell Scientific, Oxford, with permission.)

metaplasia, haemopoiesis may return to its former sites in the liver, spleen, and lymph nodes and may also be found in the adrenals, cartilage, adipose tissue, thoracic paravertebral gutters, and even the kidneys.

The microenvironment of the marrow cavity is a vast network of endothelial cell-lined vascular channels or sinusoids bounded by the endosteal (inner) surfaces of bone that separate clumps of haemopoietic cells, including fat cells, that reside in the intersinusoidal spaces. These two compartments are separated by reticular cells (derived from fibroblasts) that form the adventitial surfaces of the sinuses and extend cytoplasmic processes to create a lattice on which blood cells are found. The lattice is demonstrated by reticulin stains of marrow sections (Fig. 22.2.1.2). The conformation of the meshwork of cytoplasmic extensions and the placement of haemopoietic cells in the network of sinuses are best illustrated by scanning electron microscopy. Haemopoietic stem cells (HSCs) are found in two distinct niches: an endosteal niche where HSCs lie in close proximity to a subset of spindle-shaped, N-cadherin$^+$ osteoblasts; and a vascular niche lined by sinusoidal endothelial cells. The endosteal niche is thought to be important for the regulation of HSC self-renewal, while the vascular niche is important for proliferation, differentiation, and mobilization. The fibroblast–endothelial cell network provides two major functions: (1) an adhesive framework onto which the developing cells are bound by fibronectin and other integrins and (2) the production of haemopoietic growth factors by these cells. Cell–cell adhesion may

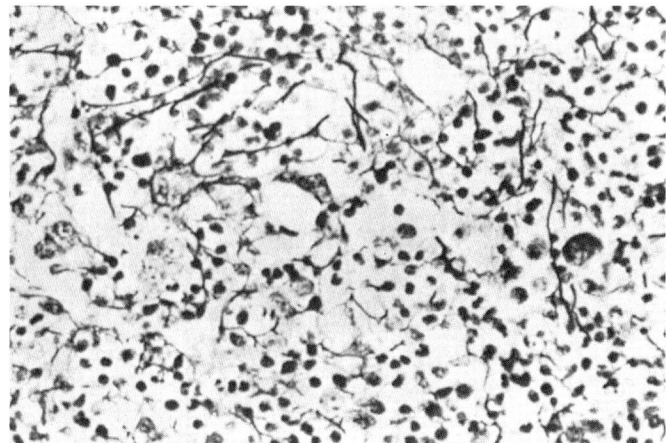

Fig. 22.2.1.2 Bone marrow biopsy sample of a patient with mild myelofibrosis. A slight increase in the number of reticulin fibres in a delicate discontinuous fibre network is present. Gomori stain, ×350.
(From Lennert K et al., 1975, Clinical Haematology **4**, 335, with permission.)

be mediated by binding of the haemopoietic VLA-4 integrin to stromal fibronectin or vascular cell adhesion molecule 1 (VCAM-1).

The central and radial arteries ramify in the cortical capillaries, which in turn join the marrow sinusoids and drain into the central sinus. Cells that egress from the marrow sinusoids then join the venous circulation through concomitant veins. The inner, or luminal, surface of the vascular sinusoids is lined with endothelial cells, the cytoplasmic extensions of which overlap, or interdigitate, with one another. The escape of developing haemopoietic cells into the sinus for transport to the circulation occurs through gaps that develop in this endothelial lining and even through endothelial-cell cytoplasmic pores.

The haemopoietic growth factors comprise a family of small glycoproteins that not only affect immature cells but also influence the survival and function of mature cells. They do so by binding to specific cell surface receptors. The genes for many of the growth factors and their receptors have been isolated. The cellular origin and the major sites of action of important members of the haemopoietic growth factor family are shown in Fig. 22.2.1.3. Three of the receptors—c-kit, the receptor for Steel factor (also called stem cell factor (SCF)); Flt-3, the receptor for Flt-3 ligand; and c-fms, the monocyte colony-stimulating factor (M-CSF) receptor—are members of the transmembrane tyrosine kinase family. In contrast, the receptors for the other haemopoietic growth factors such as interleukin 3 (IL-3), granulocyte–macrophage colony stimulating factor (GM-CSF), granulocyte colony-stimulating factor (G-CSF), IL-5, IL-6, erythropoietin (EPO), and thrombopoietin (TPO) are members of the haemopoietic growth factor receptor family. They share several structural features; lacking cytoplasmic tyrosine kinase domains, they activate cells by conformational change of preformed dimers or by multimer formation after binding their cognate ligands. This promotes the recruitment and activation of cytoplasmic tyrosine kinases such as members of the Janus kinase (JAK) family. The JAK proteins in turn activate members of the signal transducer and activator of transcription (STAT) family and phosphorylate tyrosines of the cytoplasmic domains of the receptor itself. This stimulates recruitment of other signalling or adaptor proteins that activate pathways, such as those involving Ras/MAP kinase and phosphatidylinositol-3 (PI-3) kinase.

The location of the different haemopoietic cells is not random. Clumps of megakaryocytes are found adjacent to marrow sinuses. They shed platelets, the fragments of their cytoplasm, directly into the lumen. This reduces the requirement for movement of bulky mature megakaryocytes, a mobility characteristic of the myeloid- and erythroid-differentiated precursors as they approach the point at which they egress from the marrow.

The formed elements of blood in vertebrates, including humans, continuously undergo replacement to maintain a constant number of red cells, white cells, and platelets. The number of cells of each type is maintained in a very narrow range in normal adults— approximately 5000 granulocytes, 5×10^6 red blood cells, and 150 000 to 300 000 platelets per microlitre of whole blood. The following section reviews the nature of the signals that affect the proliferation of the stem and progenitor cells, and the normal regulatory mechanisms that maintain balanced production of new blood cells.

Function of stem cells and progenitors

The progenitors of recognizable precursor cells are mononuclear 'blast' cells with large nuclei, prominent nucleoli, and basophilic cytoplasm devoid of granules. These primitive progenitors are present at extremely low frequencies, approximately 1 in 10^4 to 10^5 marrow cells for the stem cell population and 1 in 10^3 for their committed progenitor progeny. A single pluripotent stem cell is capable of giving rise, in a stochastic fashion, to increasingly committed progenitor cells according to the schema outlined in Fig. 22.2.1.3. These committed progenitors are destined to form differentiated recognizable precursors of the specific types of blood cells.

Pluripotent stem cells are defined as cells capable of both self-renewal and multilineage differentiation under the influence of certain non-lineage-specific growth factors such as Flt-3 ligand, SCF, IL-6, and TPO. Other factors such as Wnt, Jagged, bone morphogenetic protein (BMP), and angiopoietin-like growth factors are also important for HSC expansion. Their differentiation programme is random and leads to a broad array of more mature lineage-committed progenitors that are themselves responsive to broadly active factors such as IL-3, GM-CSF, IL-11, and subsequently to the more lineage-restricted growth factors, including EPO, TPO, G-CSF, IL-5, and M-CSF. Some of the lineage-restricted growth factors, particularly EPO, are produced in response to the circulating levels of differentiated blood cells.

Lineage-committed progenitors are characterized by limited proliferative potential that depends upon the presence of specific growth factors that interact with their cognate receptors on progenitor surfaces. Progenitors are not capable of indefinite self-renewal. In fact, they 'die by differentiation' to mature precursors of the blood cells. The maintenance of their numbers ultimately depends upon the presence of lineage-specific growth factors and on random influx into their pool from the pluripotent stem cell pool. Therefore, amplification of blood cell production occurs at the level of the committed progenitor pool, while maintenance of the progenitors depends upon the capacity of members of the pluripotent stem cell pool to differentiate into the committed progenitor pool.

Haemopoietic differentiation requires an appropriate microenvironment. In normal adults, this is confined to the bone marrow, whereas in the mouse it includes both the spleen and bone marrow.

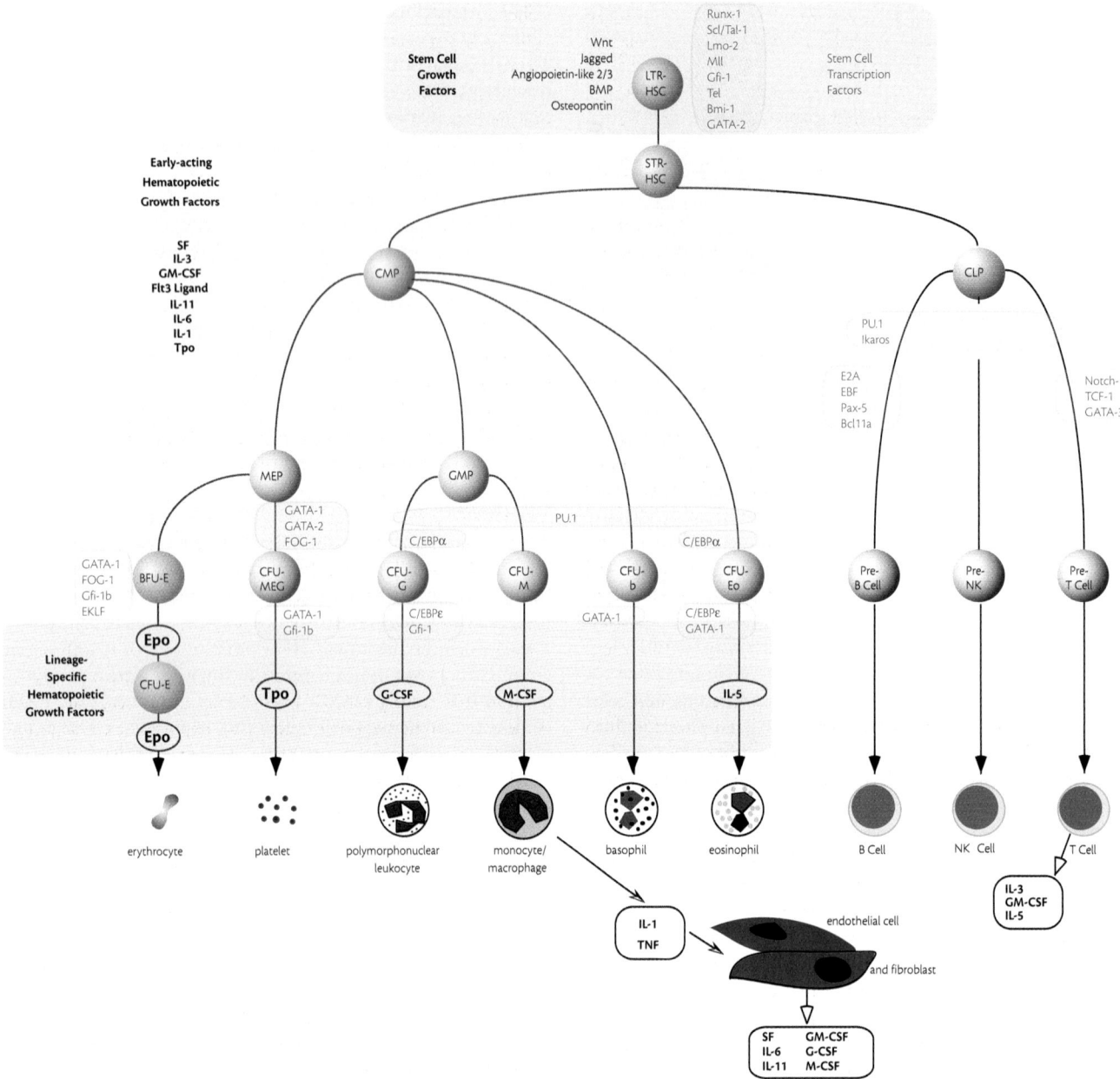

Fig. 22.2.1.3 Major cytokine sources and actions and transcription factor requirements for haemopoietic cells. Cells of the bone marrow microenvironment such as macrophages, endothelial cells, and reticular fibroblastoid cells produce M-CSF, GM-CSF, G-CSF, IL-6, and probably SCF after induction with endotoxin (macrophage) or IL-1/TNF (endothelial cells and fibroblasts). T cells produce IL-3, GM-CSF, and IL-5 in response to antigenic and IL-1 stimulation. These cytokines have overlapping actions during hematopoietic differentiation, as indicated, and for all lineages optimal development requires a combination of early- and late-acting factors. Transcription factors important for survival or self-renewal of stem cells are shown in red at the top, and stages of haemopoiesis blocked after the depletion of indicated transcription factors are shown for multipotent and committed progenitors. Abbreviations are spelled out in the text.

The existence of certain strains of mice that exhibit a deficiency in the haemopoietic microenvironment suggests that the interactions between haemopoietic cells and the bone marrow microenvironment involve very specific molecular mechanisms. Insight into the nature of one of these interactions has come from isolation of the genes that determine the *White Spotting (W)* and *Steel (Sl)* mutations in mice. Animals affected by mutations at both of these loci have a severe macrocytic anaemia associated with defects in skin pigmentation and fertility. The mutations, however, map to different chromosome loci (*W* to chromosome 5, *Sl* to chromosome 10). The *W* mutation is in stem cells whereas the *Sl* defect

is in the bone marrow microenvironment. The *W* gene is allelic with the c-*kit* proto-oncogene, a member of the tyrosine kinase cell surface receptor family; in contrast, the *Sl* mutation results in defective production of the ligand for this receptor (Steel factor, also known as SCF). Interestingly, SCF is produced in both a secreted and membrane-bound form by fibroblasts and other cells. The latter form may thus provide one molecular explanation for interactions between the stem cells and their microenvironment.

Progenitors can exist outside the marrow. Early haemopoietic cells, including the pluripotent stem cells and certain committed progenitor cells, have been demonstrated in the circulation of normal individuals and experimental animals. The capacity of haemopoietic stem cells to negotiate the circulation is especially significant in relation to stem cell transplantation. While this procedure is still often carried out by infusion of bone marrow from the donor into the circulation of the recipient, mobilized blood stem and progenitors cells are now frequently being used.

Both T and B lymphocytes and natural killer cells are derived from a common lymphoid progenitor (CLP), while a common myeloid progenitor (CMP) cell matures to form the committed progenitors of red blood cells, phagocytes, and megakaryocytes (Fig. 22.2.1.3).

The pluripotent stem cell

The concept that sustained haemopoiesis comes from pluripotent stem cells derives from the observation that mice can be protected from the lethal effects of whole-body irradiation by exteriorization and shielding of the spleen. This protective effect was shown to be cell-mediated as the injection of spleen cells could initiate recovery and re-establish haemopoiesis in irradiated animals. Till and McCulloch demonstrated that colonies of haemopoietic cells could be observed in the spleen in bone marrow–transplanted, irradiated recipient mice within 10 days after the transplant. These spleen colony-forming units (CFU-S) produce colonies that contain precursors of erythrocytes, granulocytes, macrophages, and megakaryocytes. Subsequent experiments using karyotypically marked donor cells confirmed the clonal origin of the differentiated cells. Experiments in which foreign genes have been inserted into spleen colony-forming cells have further substantiated this finding. Each colony contains a variable number of stem cells that could again form spleen colonies of differentiated progeny in a second irradiated recipient, indicating the self-renewal property of stem cells. The demonstration of a stem cell that can differentiate to form progenitor cells for erythropoiesis, granulopoiesis, and megakaryopoiesis is completely consistent with subsequent observations in diseases such as chronic myeloid leukaemia and polycythaemia vera in which a clonal origin of abnormal erythroid, granulocytic, and megakaryocytic precursor cells can be demonstrated (see Chapter 22.3.5). In addition, these studies of chronic myeloid leukaemia have demonstrated a pluripotent stem cell that gives rise to B cells as well as to the aforementioned blood cells.

Stem cells and lineage-committed progenitors form a continuum of cells with a decreasing capacity for self-renewal, increasing likelihood for differentiation, and increasing proliferative activity. The cells progress in a unidirectional fashion in this continuum. The most immature stem cell has the capacity for long-term haemopoietic reconstitution after bone marrow transplantation (LTR-HSC; Fig. 22.2.1.3). In the mouse, as few as 30 cells of a highly purified marrow population that lacks lineage-specific antigens but expresses Ly-6 (Sca-1) and low levels of Thy-1 (that is, lin− Sca-1+ Thy-1lo) can reconstitute haemopoiesis in 50% of lethally irradiated mice. This fraction appears to comprise virtually 100% CFU-S, but single-cell transfer experiments have shown that it is still heterogeneous. Indeed, cell elutriation studies have shown that most of the CFU-S population is contained within a more mature cell fraction that confers short-term radioprotective capacity (STR-HSC; Fig. 22.2.1.3).

Differences in physical properties and expression of the antigens CD34 and CD33/CD38 have been used to enrich for human stem cells. Most colony-forming cells express all three cell-surface molecules. Cells that give rise to colony-forming cells in long-term bone marrow cultures (i.e. long-term culture-initiating cells; LTC-IC) can be separated by their expression of CD34, lack of expression of CD33, CD38, and other lineage-specific markers, and intermediate forward light-scattering properties. The importance of CD34+ marrow cells is emphasized by in vivo simian studies. Like human bone marrow, the CD34 antigen is expressed by a minority of baboon cells. Infusion of these purified cells can reconstitute lymphohaemopoiesis in lethally irradiated baboons. The cloning of the murine CD34 cDNA has cast some doubt on expression of CD34 by LTR-HSCs. A monoclonal antibody raised to a murine CD34–GST fusion protein was used to separate marrow cells into CD34lo/−, CD34lo, and CD34+ fractions. Interestingly, long-term multilineage reconstitution was observed after transplantation of the CD34lo/− cells, whereas the CD34+ fraction gave early but unsustained multilineage reconstitution. These data are supported by experiments demonstrating that a tiny subset of murine bone marrow cells that exclude the Hoechst 33342 dye at blue and red wavelengths (called the side population) contains all the LTR-HSC activity, but is CD34−. Recent human studies have also raised the possibility that LTR-HSC do not express CD34. When primitive human lin− cells are separated into CD34+ and CD34− fractions, the capacity to reconstitute haemopoiesis in immunodeficient mice (called SCID repopulating cells or SRCs) is found in both cell fractions. A resolution to this controversy may come from the demonstration that resting murine haemopoietic stem cells are CD34−, while activated haemopoietic stem cells express the CD34 antigen.

Studies with purified populations of stem cells have shown that combinations of specific haemopoietic growth factors such as SCF, Flt-3 ligand, IL-6, and surprisingly, TPO can act at the stem cell level to induce cell cycling and proliferation. IL-3, produced by T cells and natural killer cells, and GM-CSF, a product of both stromal cells and T cells, appear to be factors essential for the survival in vitro of a class of stem cells that forms blast colonies in methylcellulose culture. These 'blast' colonies contain multilineage and unilineage progenitors. They are probably at the myeloid stem-cell stage of differentiation (Fig. 22.2.1.3). When isolated from bone marrow, these stem cells are mostly in a noncycling, quiescent state. The addition of IL-3, GM-CSF, or SCF or other stromally produced haemopoietic growth factors such as IL-6, IL-11, or G-CSF shortens the G_0 phase in these cultures, thus hastening the onset of blast colony formation.

The factors that control the fate of stem cells to undergo either self-renewal or commitment to differentiate down a lineage pathway are poorly understood. However, nuclear transcription factors have been shown to play a role in haemopoietic cell proliferation and lineage commitment (Fig. 22.2.1.3). The tal-1/SCL, Rbtn2/LMO2, and GATA family of transcription factors are important in this regard. In particular, tal-1/SCL, a basic helix–loop–helix (bHLH) transcription factor, is expressed in biphenotypic (lymphoid/myeloid) and T-cell leukaemias, and in both early haemopoietic progenitors and more mature erythroid, mast, megakaryocyte, and endothelial cells. Targeted disruption of the tal-1/SCL gene in murine embryonic stem cells leads to death in utero from absence of blood formation; a lack of in vitro myeloid colony formation suggests a role for this factor very early during haemopoiesis.

Another transcription factor implicated in T-cell acute lymphoblastic leukaemia (ALL) is the LIM domain nuclear protein rhombotin

2 (rbtn2/LMO2). Mice that lack this factor die *in utero* and have the same bloodless phenotype as the tal-1/SCL$^{-/-}$ animals. GATA-2 is expressed in the regions of the *Xenopus* and zebrafish embryos that are fated to become haemopoietic, and is highly expressed in progenitor cells. Overexpression of GATA-2 in chicken erythroid progenitors leads to proliferation at the expense of differentiation. Targeted disruption of the *GATA-2* gene by homologous recombination in embryonic stem cells leads to reduced primitive haemopoiesis in the yolk sac and embryonic death by day 10 to 11. Definitive haemopoiesis in liver and bone marrow is profoundly reduced with loss of virtually all lineages. *In vitro* differentiation data show a marked deficiency of SCF-responsive definitive erythroid and mast cell colonies and reduced macrophage colonies, suggesting that GATA-2 serves as a regulator of genes that control haemopoietic growth factor responsiveness or proliferation of stem and/or early progenitor cells. These data contrast with the later time of embryonic death from anaemia (day 15) in mice with targeted disruption of the c-*myb* or retinoblastoma (*Rb*) genes, or with severe forms of *W* and *Sl* mutations. Similarly, loss of function of the *RUNX1 (AML1)* gene, which encodes the α subunit of the heterodimeric core-binding factor, results in fetal death by day 12.5 due to failure of production of all definitive haemopoietic lineages. Core-binding factor recognition sequences are present in the IL-3, GM-CSF, M-CSFR, and T-cell antigen receptor promoters. The human *RUNX1* gene is frequently rearranged in acute myeloid leukaemia (AML) and childhood ALL, and is expressed in myeloid and lymphoid cells.

The survival of a particular stem cell in the marrow requires a 'niche'; thus isogeneic marrow infusions are not successful unless the recipient is irradiated or treated with sufficient doses of cytotoxic drugs to create an adequate number of niches. Therefore, reports of failure of engraftment in aplastic anaemia using identical twin donors but no radiation or other conditioning regimen do not necessarily implicate an immunological basis for the disease. Equally likely is persistence of nonfunctional pluripotent progenitors in the aplastic marrow niches. These abnormal cells must be destroyed to allow implantation of transfused normal progenitors.

The stem cell model of haemopoiesis has parallels in other organ systems. That rapidly self-renewing epithelial tissues like skin and intestine have stem cells that continually replenish the cells lost by differentiation is well described. It is likely that most epithelial tissues, e.g. liver and pancreas, also contain stem cells that are brought to bear after organ damage. The demonstration of the existence of neural stem cells in the adult brain has raised the possibility that many organ systems might retain a population of self-renewing stem cells. Muscle satellite cells also appear to fulfil this role.

Mesenchymal stem cells, derived from an adherent bone marrow cell population, express neither CD34 nor CD45, markers of haemopoietic cells. Mesenchymal stem cells are capable of marked expansion in culture, and can then be induced to differentiate into osteoblasts and osteocytes, chondrocytes, adipocytes, and myotubules.

Erythropoiesis

The rate of erythropoiesis is driven by anaemia or hypoxia. Both stimulate a class of peritubular kidney cell, through stabilization of a transcription factor called HIF-1α, to transcribe the *EPO* gene and release the hormone into the blood (Fig. 22.2.1.4). Under normoxic conditions a prolyl hydroxylase PHD2 hydroxylates HIF-1α, which leads to binding to the von Hippel–Lindau protein and ubiquitin-mediated destruction, while a second hydroxylation reaction inhibits binding to a transcriptional coactivator p300; under hypoxic conditions both hydroxylases are inhibited, leading to an increase in HIF-1α and recruitment of the p300 coactivator. The hormone binds to the EPO receptor in erythroblasts and erythroid progenitors to stimulate their division and differentiation. The least mature committed erythroid progenitor is known as an erythroid burst-forming unit (BFU-E), because when it differentiates *in vitro* it forms large colonies of erythroblasts and reticulocytes that may contain as many as 50 000 cells. The colonies, derived from single cells, have a burst-like appearance because they may be composed of multiple subcolonies. Thus one BFU-E may first divide in culture to form subcolony-forming cells, which then differentiate into colonies of erythroblasts and reticulocytes. BFU-E progressively mature during their sojourn in the marrow. In doing so they lose their capacity to divide and migrate *in vitro*, but gain in sensitivity to EPO until they reach the stage at which they are known as erythroid colony-forming units (CFU-E).

The regulated proliferation and maturation of erythroid progenitors depends on interaction with a number of growth factors. EPO is essential for the terminal maturation of erythroid cells. Its major effect appears to be at the level of the CFU-E during adult erythropoiesis. Recombinant preparations are as effective as the natural hormone. These very mature progenitors and proerythroblasts do not require 'burst-promoting activity' in the form of IL-3, GM-CSF, or SCF. Their dependence on EPO is emphasized by the observation that they will not survive *in vitro* in its absence.

SCF has also been shown to have marked synergistic effects on BFU-E cultured in the presence of EPO. Alone, it has no colony-forming ability. The majority of CFU-E are in cycle; their survival in the presence of EPO is probably tightly linked to their proliferation and differentiation to proerythroblasts and mature erythrocytes. EPO also acts on a subset of presumptive mature BFU-E that require it for survival and terminal differentiation. A second subset of BFU-E, presumably less mature, survive deprivation of EPO if 'burst-promoting activity' is present, either as SCF, IL-3, or GM-CSF.

Factors distinct from the classic colony-stimulating factors may positively regulate erythropoiesis, either directly or indirectly. Limiting dilution studies of highly purified CFU-E in serum-free culture show that insulin and insulin-like growth factor 1 (IGF-1) act directly on these cells. Dexamethasone also enhances erythropoiesis and may be particularly important during stress. The presence of EPO is also essential. CFU-E and mature BFU-E are highly responsive to the mitogenic effect of EPO as well as to its differentiating role. Therefore, in haemorrhagic or haemolytic anaemias with elevated levels of EPO, the numbers of CFU-E and mature BFU-E may rise remarkably in the marrow. Immature BFU-E are less responsive to the mitogenic effect of EPO, and therefore, the frequency of this subset of BFU-E changes little in anaemia.

Negative regulation of erythropoiesis

Subsets of lymphocytes with an immunological suppressor phenotype isolated from normal subjects can inhibit erythroid activity *in vitro*, but their role in the regulation of erythropoiesis *in vivo* is uncertain. Some patients with anaemia or granulocytopenia have an associated expansion of certain T-lymphocyte populations.

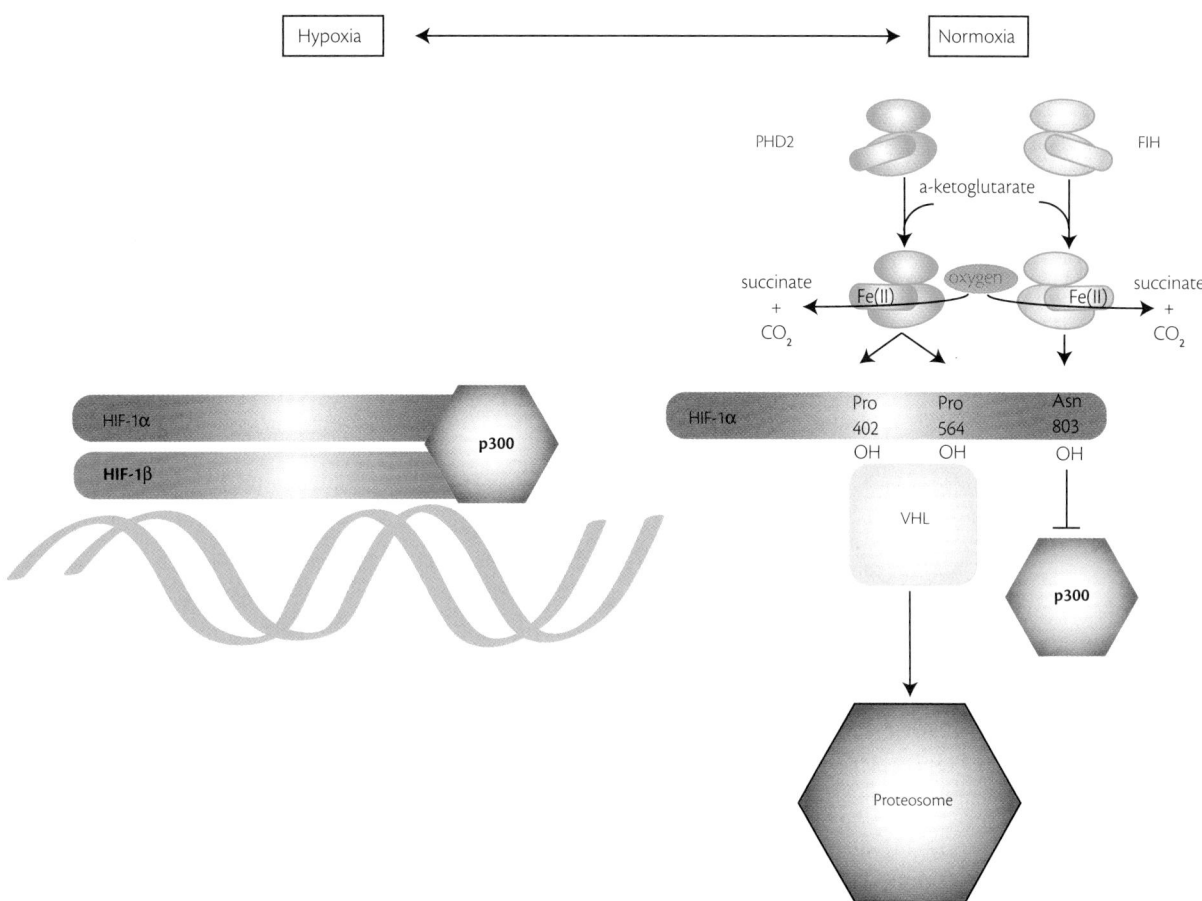

Fig. 22.2.1.4 Hypoxia-inducible regulation of EPO production. Under normoxic conditions, HIF-1α undergoes prolyl hydroxylation at proline 402 and proline 564 that leads to binding of HIF-1α to the von Hippel–Lindau (VHL) protein and subsequent ubiquitin-mediated destruction. This dioxygenase enzymatic reaction is catalysed by a prolyl hydroxylase termed prolyl hydroxylase domain 2 (PHD2). A second hydroxylation at asparagine 803 prevents binding of HIF-1α to its transcriptional coactivator p300, and is catalysed by a HIF asparaginyl hydroxylase called factor-inhibiting HIF (FIH). Both these reactions are dependent on oxygen, Fe(II), and a-ketoglutarate, which is oxidized to succinate with the release of CO_2. Under hypoxic conditions both hydroxylases are inhibited, leading to an increase in HIF-1α and recruitment of the p300 coactivator, which together with the ubiquitously expressed HIF-1β, activates transcription.

In the rare disorder 'T lymphocytosis with cytopenia', *in vitro* suppression of erythropoiesis (or granulocytopoiesis) has been correlated with the expansion of a T-lymphocyte population that may be the counterpart of the haemopoietic suppressor cells isolated from normal peripheral blood. The cell expanded in many of these cases and originally described as a 'Tγ' cell has been renamed a large granular lymphocyte (LGL), and these cells can be of either T cell (CD3+, T-cell receptor (TCR) αβ or γδ) or NK cell (CD3–, TCR–) origin.

Exactly how suppressor T cells interact with haemopoietic progenitors, and what surface antigens are 'seen' by the suppressors is not known. There is evidence to support the concept that suppression of erythroid colony expression *in vitro* can be regulated by T cells and may be genetically restricted. Certain phenotypes of T cells 'recognize' distinct classes of histocompatibility antigens on immunological cell surfaces. Thus, the observation that haemopoietic progenitors have a unique distribution of class II major histocompatibility complex (MHC) antigens on their cell surface suggests a role for these antigens in the cell–cell interactions that regulate haemopoietic differentiation.

Tumour necrosis factor (TNF) also suppresses erythropoiesis *in vitro*. The injection of peritoneal macrophages into animals infected with Friend murine leukaemia virus results in rapid but transient resolution of the massive erythroid hyperplasia associated with this disease. This may be due to elaboration by macrophages of IL-1α, which does not suppress erythropoiesis itself, but acts by the induction of tumour necrosis factor. This effect is reversed by EPO.

Proerythroblasts represent the ultimate stage of differentiation of committed erythroid progenitors. In contrast to the progenitors, which comprise less than 0.1% of the marrow cell population, proerythroblasts are present at 3 to 5%, and their daughters, the recognizable erythroid precursors, comprise 30% of the population.

Estimates of reticulocyte production and erythroblast content of marrows, together with measurements of the rate at which the proerythroblast compartment is renewed from the progenitor pool, suggest that approximately 10% of the daily reticulocyte production is derived from the terminal differentiation of proerythroblasts newly developed from the progenitor department. During anaemic stress, the rate at which progenitors differentiate to proerythroblasts may increase tenfold or more. This increase in the rate of proerythroblast formation from progenitors is associated with an increase in the production of fetal haemoglobin in a large fraction of the erythroid cells derived from them. The basis of this reactivation of fetal haemoglobin synthesis is not understood. The extent to which fetal haemoglobin may be increased in such settings could be genetically controlled. It is an important phenomenon because those with the capacity to develop large increases in fetal haemoglobin who are also homozygous for major β-chain haemoglobinopathies may have a remarkably mild course. Fetal haemoglobin elevation occurs in many forms of accelerated erythropoiesis and is a marker of such a condition.

Myelopoiesis

The development of a clonal assay for granulocyte and macrophage progenitors preceded the development of erythroid progenitor assays by nearly a decade, yet a clear understanding of the regulation of myeloid differentiation remains elusive. Fig. 22.2.1.3 describes the development and regulation of granulocyte, monocyte, and macrophage production from the pluripotent stem cell. The colony-forming unit–granulocyte-macrophage (CFU-GM) is derived from the pluripotent progenitor. It gives rise to separate granulocyte and monocyte progenitors (CFU-G and CFU-M), which, under the influence of unique colony-stimulating factors such as SCF, IL-3, GM-CSF, G-CSF, and M-CSF, differentiate to mature granulocytes and/or monocytes, respectively. Both IL-3 and GM-CSF affect a similar broad spectrum of human myeloid progenitor cells. This includes colonies that contain granulocytes, erythrocytes, monocytes, and megakaryocytes (CFU-GEMM), eosinophils (CFU-Eo), CFU-GM, CFU-G, and CFU-M.

Colony-stimulating factors also induce a variety of functional changes in mature cells. GM-CSF inhibits polymorphonuclear neutrophil migration, induces antibody-dependent cellular cytotoxicity (ADCC) for human target cells, and increases neutrophil phagocytic activity. Some of these changes may be related to GM-CSF–induced increase in the cell surface expression of a family of antigens that function as cell adhesion molecules. The increase in antigen expression is rapid and is associated with increased aggregation of neutrophils. Granulocyte–granulocyte adhesion can be inhibited by an antigen-specific monoclonal antibody. GM-CSF also acts as a potent stimulus of eosinophil ADCC, superoxide production, and phagocytosis. G-CSF acts as a potent stimulus of neutrophil superoxide production, ADCC, and phagocytosis, while M-CSF activates mature macrophages and enhances macrophage cytotoxicity.

Monocytes leave the circulation and differentiate further to become fixed tissue macrophages. These tissue macrophages include alveolar macrophages and hepatic Kupffer cells, dermal Langerhans cells, osteoclasts, peritoneal macrophages, pleural macrophages, and possibly brain microglial cells, though the origin of these is still uncertain. The wide variety of cells with diverse functions that must be supplied from the granulocyte–macrophage progenitor requires that this system be highly regulated at many levels of differentiation.

The granulocyte compartment itself is more complex than either the erythroid or megakaryocyte compartments. The circulating half-life of the newly rapidly deployed granulocyte is only 6.5 h. To meet sudden demands, an additional noncirculating granulocyte pool exists in the spleen, marginated around blood vessels, and in a readily releasable bone marrow pool. The rate at which new myeloblasts or monoblasts are produced by progenitors *in vivo* is not known, but exhaustion of progenitors in infection, particularly in the neonatal period, is associated with a fatal outcome due to a failure of granulocyte production.

Suppression of phagocyte production

An elaborate system exists for suppression of granulocyte and macrophage production. It involves T lymphocytes and their products, particularly interferon-γ, monocytes, and perhaps acidic isoferritins. In some circumstances, clones of T cells that suppress granulocyte production *in vitro* and *in vivo* have caused profound granulocytopenia. Clearly, a twin regulatory system exists that contributes to the fine control of phagocyte production by close control between progenitors and adventitial cells that secrete inducer and suppressor molecules. It is well established that T lymphocytes capable of the suppression of phagocyte colony formation may be present in human marrow and induce neutropenia.

Megakaryocytopoiesis

The cloning of TPO has greatly clarified our understanding of the regulation of megakaryocytopoiesis. Before the discovery of TPO, several factors including IL-3, IL-6, IL-11, SCF, and even EPO were shown to stimulate megakaryocytopoiesis and thrombopoiesis *in vitro* and *in vivo*. Hence, all of the above-mentioned haemopoietic growth factors, except EPO, can contribute collectively to 'megakaryocyte colony-stimulating activity' (Meg-CSA). Meg-CSA is therefore a 'soup' of growth factors that transduce three of the four classes of receptors that drive haemopoietic differentiation; these comprise the β common, tyrosine kinase, and gp130 families. All of these receptors, when engaged, drive early progenitor proliferation and partial differentiation to more mature progenitors. The final steps of lineage-committed mature progenitor development into recognizable marrow precursors require a lineage-specific growth factor: G-CSF for the granulocyte, M-CSF for the macrophage, IL-5 for the eosinophil, and EPO for the erythrocyte.

The discovery of TPO provides the final step of understanding of megakaryocytopoiesis because this factor, and probably none other, actually induces lineage-restricted megakaryocyte progenitor proliferation, differentiation of those committed progenitors to megakaryoblasts, and finally, differentiation of megakaryoblasts to the megakaryocytes that in turn produce platelets. Circulating TPO levels are high in hypoplastic thrombocytopenias, just as EPO levels are elevated in the erythroid hypoplasias. Administration of high doses of EPO is usually of little benefit in the latter conditions. Thrombopoietin may be just as unsuccessful in certain megakaryocyte hypoplasias because those conditions are often associated with severe depletion of lineage-specific or multipotent progenitors.

Thrombopoietin

Identification of the proto-oncogene *c-mpl* revealed an orphan haemopoietic growth factor receptor that proved to be crucial for megakaryocytopoiesis. In 1993, Methia and coworkers performed a critically important experiment, when they demonstrated that exposure of CD34+ progenitor cells in culture to oligonucleotides that were antisense to *c-mpl* inhibited the ability of these cells to form megakaryocyte, but not other haemopoietic colonies. In 1994 several laboratories cloned the all-important ligand for this receptor, the growth factor TPO, and important physiological studies of TPO were launched. The cloning and expression of the gene for TPO has provided new insight into the regulation of levels of platelets. Gene disruption studies of *c-mpl*, the receptor for TPO, in mice have shown that in the absence of the function of this pathway, mice have only 15% of the normal levels of circulating platelets. Thus, while redundancy among the growth factors, perhaps including SCF, IL-3, IL-6, and IL-11, can partially compensate for dysfunctional c-*mpl* signalling, Tpo, like Epo in the erythrocyte lineage, appears to be the major regulator of circulating platelet levels.

The *TPO* gene is localized on the long arm of chromosome 3. It contains five exons, the boundaries of which line up precisely with those of the *EPO* gene. The gene is widely expressed in liver, kidney, smooth muscle, endothelial cells, and fibroblasts. Thus TPO is produced at the site of stoma supporting haemopoiesis. Though its activity is increased in the blood during episodes of thrombocytopenia, it does not necessarily function as a hormone because it is produced directly at the site of thrombopoiesis. In this sense, it differs from EPO, which is not produced at all in marrow stroma. It is likely that the level of production of TPO is quite constant in all tissues. The blood levels may increase in thrombocytopenic states merely because circulating platelets and tissue megakaryocytes sop up the growth factor and carry it out of the circulation. This theory has received support from observations in mice with disruption of the murine transcription factor gene called *NF-E2*; although these animals are thrombocytopenic, they have an increase in megakaryocyte mass and no increase in serum TPO levels.

The TPO molecule is considerably longer than the other haemopoietic growth factor polypeptides. Its 5′ half bears 23% sequence homology to EPO, while the 3′ half bears no structural homology to any cytokine and may be removed by a proteolytic mechanism. Indeed, removal of this half does not ablate physiological function. The resemblance of the 5′ domain of the molecule to EPO may explain the synergy of TPO and EPO in megakaryocyte colony formation and platelet production. It is well recognized that splenectomized individuals with persistent anaemia usually have significant thrombocytosis, and many individuals with red cell aplasia and high EPO levels also have thrombocytosis and megakaryocytosis.

Circulating platelets

The differential diagnosis of thrombocytopenia rests first on evaluation of platelet morphology. In conditions in which megakaryocytopoiesis is accelerated, circulating platelet volume (and usually diameter) is increased. The reasons for this shift in volume are disputed. Some claim that young platelets are larger than old platelets, while others suggest that large megakaryocytes give rise to large platelets. Neither explanation satisfies all experimental and clinical conditions, but in general, thrombocytopenia secondary to increased destruction of platelets is associated with platelets of large volume. Thrombocytopenia related to decreased production of platelets is associated with platelets of normal size.

There are major exceptions to this rule. Patients with hyposplenism tend to have large platelets in their blood, whether thrombopoiesis is increased or not, and patients with primary abnormalities of platelet function, such as Wiskott–Aldrich syndrome or Bernard–Soulier syndrome, have small and large platelets, respectively, that bear no relationship to platelet production. TPO increases platelet production by increasing both the number and size of individual megakaryocytes. Though TPO is probably solely responsible for the later stages of recognizable megakaryocyte differentiation and proliferation of megakaryocyte progenitors, its function depends, at least in part, on the additional stimulation of earlier megakaryocyte progenitors with other growth factors, including IL-3, IL-11, and SCF.

Megakaryocyte progenitors in disease

A number of attempts have been made to relate diseases associated with elevated or depressed platelet counts to the number or the growth characteristics of megakaryocyte progenitors. Megakaryocyte progenitors in essential thrombocythaemia are similar in their growth characteristics to the expanded numbers of erythroid progenitors in polycythaemia vera. The latter develop into erythroid colonies without additions of EPO to the culture medium. The trace of EPO in the serum is sufficient to drive the sensitive receptor system in these progenitors. In a similar fashion, the numerous megakaryocyte colony-forming units in essential thrombocythaemia develop into megakaryocyte colonies in the absence of stimulation by aplastic anaemia serum. They are 'thrombopoietin independent' and many produce endogenous TPO.

Clinical studies with haemopoietic growth factors

Several recombinant haemopoietic growth factors are currently in use and under evaluation in a variety of clinical settings. Initial studies focused on EPO in the anaemia of chronic renal failure, and GM-CSF and G-CSF in both transient and long-standing bone marrow–failure syndromes. These three factors are now commercially available for clinical use.

Anaemia is a major complication of endstage renal failure, and is due primarily to a reduction in EPO production. Several phase I, II, and III studies have documented that recombinant human EPO can induce a dose-dependent increase in effective erythropoiesis. The extension of this treatment to patients who do not yet require dialysis has met with similar success. EPO may also be useful in the anaemia of chronic disease and in the anaemia that complicates azidothymidine treatment of patients with AIDS. EPO treatment has been associated with an increased risk of thromboembolic complications in adults, particularly when target haemoglobin (Hb) concentrations were in the normal range, with a possible adverse effect on breast cancer progression. Two randomized studies in which the targeted Hb level was either in the normal (>13.5 g/dl) or subnormal (10.5–11.5 g/dl) range showed an increased risk of adverse cardiovascular effects for the normal Hb groups. A 2006 update of a Cochrane review of 57 trials including more than 9000 patients showed strong evidence that epoetin and darbepoetin increased the risk of thromboembolic complications compared with controls. As a result of these and other studies, the United States Food and Drug Administration have recommended the lowest dose possible to increase the Hb to a level that avoids transfusion, not to exceed 12 g/dl or a rise of more than 1 g in any 2 weeks. A marked increase in pure red cell aplasia (PRCA) occurred from 1998 to 2004 due to the development of antierythropoietin (anti-EPO) antibodies, with reports of approximately 250 suspected or proven cases. The complication, characterized by reticulocytopenia, absence of erythroid precursors and severe anaemia, has occurred mostly in adults (a few children are included) with renal disease treated with epoetin alfa (Eprex) outside the United States of America, but cases have been reported in the United States as well. Differences in EPO glycosylation status, drug formulation, processing, storage and route of administration appear to affect the immunogenicity of EPO. Changes in drug formulation and drug monitoring programmes have led to an 80%

reduction in the incidence of PRCA, and EPO should not be withheld for this reason.

G-CSF has proven to be useful for shortening the period of neutropenia following myelosuppressive anticancer chemotherapy, and has been approved in the United States of America and Europe for reduction of infection in patients with nonmyeloid malignancies. GM-CSF and G-CSF can accelerate haemopoietic reconstitution after bone marrow transplantation, and GM-CSF has been approved for use in the United States in autologous transplantation. In the context of bone marrow failure, GM-CSF is a useful palliative treatment as it can increase the neutrophil count, particularly in mild acquired aplastic anaemia. The most severely affected patients respond poorly. GM-CSF can also increase neutrophils, eosinophils, and monocytes in AIDS. Most patients with Kostmann's syndrome, a rare inherited severe failure of neutrophil production, respond dramatically to G-CSF treatment. Patients with other defects of neutrophil production such as cyclic neutropenia and chronic idiopathic neutropenia have also responded to this factor.

Recombinant human TPO or its polyethylene glycol (PEG)–derivatized 163-residue N-terminus (PEG-MGDF) stimulates megakaryocyte proliferation and endoreduplication *in vitro* and is a potent inducer of megakaryocytopoiesis and platelet production *in vivo* in mice and nonhuman primates. Because of TPO's potent *in vitro* activity and its role as the factor essential for terminal megakaryocytic differentiation, analogous to EPO for the erythroid lineage, clinical studies designed to assess its affect on platelet production have been reported. Both recombinant human TPO and PEG-MGDF are safe and show no organ toxicity, and in normal volunteers a single bolus of 3 µg/kg per day PEG-MGDF doubles the blood platelet concentration by day 12 with a return to baseline by day 28. A stimulatory effect on platelet production was observed when TPO or PEG-MGDF was administered after chemotherapy to more than 100 cancer patients, with a decrease in the time for platelet counts to return to normal and elevated platelet nadirs. Further studies showed that TPO and PEG-MGDF are effective in malignancies treated with nonmyeloablative chemotherapy but were less effective in myeloablative regimes followed by stem cell transplantation used to treat leukaemia. Furthermore, PEG-MGDF has caused the development of antibodies to TPO that resulted in severe thrombocytopenia, and these cytokines have been withdrawn from clinical use. Small molecules, peptides, and a peptide-Fc antibody (AMG 531, a 'peptibody') that have no sequence homology with TPO but activate the receptor are under investigation.

Further reading

Bohlius J, *et al.* (2006). Erythropoietin or darbepoetin for patients with cancer. *Cochrane Database Syst Rev*, **3**, CD003407.

Cantor AB, Orkin SH (2002). Transcriptional regulation of erythropoiesis: an affair involving multiple partners. *Oncogene*, **21**, 3368–76.

Drueke TB, *et al.* (2006). Normalization of hemoglobin level in patients with chronic kidney disease and anemia. *N Engl J Med*, **355**, 2071–84.

Kaushansky K (2006). Lineage-specific hematopoietic growth factors. *N Engl J Med*, **354**, 2034–45.

Kirito K, Kaushansky K (2006). Transcriptional regulation of megakaryopoiesis: thrombopoietin signaling and nuclear factors. *Curr Opin Hematol*, **13**, 151–6.

Kondo M, *et al.* (2003). Biology of hematopoietic stem cells and progenitors: implications for clinical application. *Annu Rev Immunol*, **21**, 759–806.

Metcalf D, Moore MAS (1971). *Haematopoietic cells*. North-Holland Publishing Company, Amsterdam.

Metcalf D (2008). Hematopoietic cytokines. *Blood*, **111**, 485–91.

Osawa M, *et al.* (1996). Long-term lymphohematopoietic reconstitution by a single CD34– low/negative hematopoietic stem cell. *Science*, **273**, 242–5. [Original paper showing that murine long-term reconstituting stem cells do not express CD34.]

Pronk CJH, *et al.* (2007). Elucidation of the phenotypic, functional, and molecular topography of a myeloerythroid progenitor cell hierarchy. *Cell Stem Cell*, **1**, 428–42.

Shizuru JA, *et al.* (2005). Hematopoietic stem and progenitor cells: clinical and preclinical regeneration of the hematolymphoid system. *Annu Rev Med*, **56**, 509–38.

Sieff CA, Zon LI (2009). Anatomy and physiology of hematopoiesis. In: Orkin SH, Nathan DG, Ginsburg D, Look AT, Fisher DE, Lux SE (eds) *Hematology of infancy and childhood*. Saunders Elsevier, Philadelphia. [Comprehensive chapter that discusses haemopoiesis in more detail.]

Singh AK, *et al.* (2006). Correction of anemia with epoetin alfa in chronic kidney disease. *N Engl J Med*, **355**, 2085–98.

Stamatoyannopoulos G (2005). Control of globin gene expression during development and erythroid differentiation. *Exp Hematol*, **33**, 259–71.

Szilvassy SJ (2006). Haemopoietic stem and progenitor cell-targeted therapies for thrombocytopenia. *Expert Opin Biol Ther*, **6**, 983–92.

Yin T, Li L (2006). The stem cell niches in bone. *J Clin Invest*, **116**, 1195–201.

22.2.2 Haemopoietic stem cell disorders

D.C. Linch

Essentials

The term stem-cell disorder is usually understood to imply that a disease process has begun in a primitive cell with the potential to develop into cells of different lineages. Difficulties with such a definition include (1) malignant change in a very primitive cell does not necessarily lead to the production of mature cells of multiple lineages; (2) although an immature phenotype of a malignant cell may indicate transformation of a very early cell, it is possible that transformation could arise in a later cell with subsequent dedifferentiation.

Possible stem cell disorders—quantitative and qualitative abnormalities of haemopoietic stem cells could result in one or more of the following: (1) depletion of the stem cell population leading to failure of production of adequate mature progeny; (2) failure of proliferation of a normal number of stem cells also leading to a similar deficiency of end-cells; (3) production of normal numbers of defective end-cells; (4) malignant transformation of stem cells.

A pragmatic approach—the involvement of multiple lineages in a disease process is a ready indicator of a stem cell disorder. Such disorders include (1) myeloproliferative disorders—polycythaemia rubra vera, chronic myeloid leukaemia, myelofibrosis, and various intermediate/transitional forms are characterized by the predominant cell type produced by the malignant clone, but they all involve a primitive stem cell; (2) acute myeloid leukaemia—in adults, red cells and platelets are commonly involved in addition to myeloid cells; (3) aplastic anaemia—by definition refers to involvement of multiple myeloid lineages; (4) paroxysmal nocturnal haemoglobinuria—due to a somatic mutation in the haemopoietic stem cell in the X-linked phosphatidylinositol glycan-A (PIG-A).

Introduction

The haemopoietic stem cell is a poorly defined entity with an undifferentiated phenotype, which resides within the haemopoietic tissue. It has the ability to self-renew and the capacity to generate large numbers of mature progeny of multiple haemopoietic lineages (see Chapter 22.2.1), and recent studies indicate that stem cells may have far greater plasticity than previously appreciated. Within the adult marrow, stem cells have been found that can give rise not only to blood cells, but also to other mesodermally derived tissues such as endothelium and muscle, and to hepatic and neuronal cells traditionally thought to be derived from the endoderm and ectoderm, respectively. In some instances, the extensive repertoire may be due to the presence of nonhaemopoietic mesenchymal stem cells within the bone marrow, but there is also evidence that stem cells with haemopoietic potential can give rise to other tissue types, at least under experimental, nonphysiological conditions. In addition, stem cells within the brain have been shown to be capable of generating cells that are embryologically derived from all three germ layers, and this includes the generation of haemopoietic cells.

The implication of these findings is that either very undifferentiated multipotent stem cells persist in many adult tissues, or—under appropriate conditions—some stem cells can undergo dedifferentiation and reprogramming, although controversy remains as to the frequency and completeness of this process. The most dramatic evidence for the possibility of dedifferentiation came from the cloning of Dolly, the sheep, generated by the transfer of a mature cell nucleus into an enucleated egg. Clearly, the environment within the egg cytoplasm can re-program the genetic material within the nucleus, and it is conceivable that similar processes could be induced by an appropriate extracellular milieu. It is not yet clear whether these new insights into the potential of the stem cell will alter the way in which we consider the haemopoietic stem cell disorders, but some of the fundamental assumptions of recent decades may be challenged.

In practice, the definition of a stem cell disorder is often extremely difficult. Self-renewal, one of the hallmarks of a stem cell, may not alone be an adequate defining property of a stem cell in the context of malignant disorders, as any malignant clone, arising in any tissue, at any stage of differentiation, must have undergone immortalization and be capable of self-renewal. The term 'stem cell disorder' is usually used, therefore, to imply that the target cell for the disease process has occurred in a primitive cell with the potential to develop into cells of different lineages. Such a cell could be a relatively 'late' or 'lineage-restricted' stem cell capable, for example, of giving rise to phagocytes and erythrocytes, or it could be a very primitive stem cell capable of giving rise to all myeloid and lymphoid lineages. There are, however, a number of difficulties

with such a definition. First, malignant change in a very primitive cell does not necessarily lead to the production of mature cells of multiple lineages. It is a feature of the acute leukaemias that there is a block in differentiation; in some cases of acute myeloid leukaemia (AML), no mature progeny are produced by the malignant clone. In other cases of AML, neutrophils alone are produced. However, it cannot be assumed that the target cell of the original oncogenic event was not a cell with the potential to form all the myeloid elements, including the red-cell series. Second, whereas an immature phenotype of a malignant cell was always considered to be indicative of the transformation of a very early cell, we must now consider the possibility that transformation could arise in a later cell with subsequent dedifferentiation.

The concept of a haemopoietic stem cell disorder is, therefore, imprecise. Finally, it should be noted that tumour stem cells are now thought to be present in most forms of malignancy.

Detection of multilineage involvement

Pragmatically, the involvement of multiple lineages in a disease process is a ready indicator of a stem cell disorder. In the bone marrow hypoplastic states, stem cell involvement is obvious because of the pancytopenia that occurs. In the myeloproliferative disorders, examination of the blood count and blood film also reveals the involvement of multiple lineages; neutrophil leucocytosis may coexist with eosinophilia, basophilia, and thrombocytosis. A number of more sophisticated techniques have also been used to demonstrate that a particular cell lineage is involved in a clonal process (Table 22.2.2.1).

Analysis of nonrandom cytogenetic abnormalities represents one of the most long-standing techniques for examining cell-lineage involvement in the haematological malignancies. This approach was used in the investigation of AML to show that the large majority of T cells in the peripheral blood were not part of the malignant clone. The combination of this technique with immunophenotyping for lineage-specific markers provides a powerful addition to this approach. Conventional cytogenetic studies suffer the disadvantage that only cells in metaphase can be analysed, but techniques such as fluorescence in situ hybridization (FISH) (with or without immunophenotyping) allow cells in interphase to be examined.

Somatic mutations, from major chromosomal alterations to point mutations, can also be detected using nonmicroscopic methods employing recombinant DNA technology. Polymerase chain reaction (PCR) methods are particularly sensitive and make it possible to study small samples of cells, but it is difficult to make the techniques fully quantitative. Errors in interpretation can readily arise from minor contaminating cells in supposedly purified cell populations. Analysis of somatic mutations is subject to a further potential problem if the mutation is a secondary event in the disease process. Under these circumstances the mutation observed could have arisen in a subclone and not be present in all the malignant cells. In AML, mutations in N-*ras* or *FLT3* may be present in all or just a few of the leukaemic cells; sometimes a mutation detected at presentation cannot be found in relapse, indicative of the process of clonal evolution and the fact that the N-*ras* or *FLT3* mutation is not always an early event in the leukaemogenic process.

The use of polymorphic X-linked markers has been a very useful tool for examining clonality in informative females, and is not subject to the problems of clonal evolution. The original studies

Table 22.2.2.1 Assessment of clonality in haematological disorders

1. *Chromosome analysis by microscopy*
   Conventional cytogenetic analysis
   Dual cytogenetic analysis with surface immunophenotyping
   Fluorescent *in situ* hybridization (FISH) for specific chromosome translocations, and changes in chromosome number, e.g. trisomy 8
   Dual FISH and immunophenotyping

2. *Detection of somatic mutations by non-microscopic means*

Detection of chromosome loss	) RFLP analysis
Detection of translocations	) and
Detection of point mutations	) PCR
DNA fingerprinting	) methodology

3. *Lymphocyte gene rearrangements**
   Expression of surface light chains on B cells
   Rearrangement of immunoglobulin heavy- and light-chain genes
   Rearrangement of T-cell receptor genes (β, γ, δ)

4. *X- chromosome inactivation*
   Protein expression, e.g. isoforms of G6PD
   DNA expression:
     PGK
     HPRT
     M27B
     HUMARA
     MOA
     Fragile X (FMR1)
   mRNA expression:
     HUMARA
     G6PD
     IDS
     P55

*Detection of lymphocyte gene rearrangements is not usually applicable to the stem-celldisorders, but a small proportion of cases of acute myeloid leukaemia do havere arrangements of the immunoglobulin heavy chains or T-cell receptor genes.
RFLP, restriction fragment length polymorphism; PCR, polymerase chain reaction; G6PD, glucose-6-phosphate dehydrogenase; PGK, phosphoglycerate kinase; HPRT, hypoxanthine phosphoribosyl transferase; HUMARA, human androgen receptor; MOA, monoamineoxidase-A.

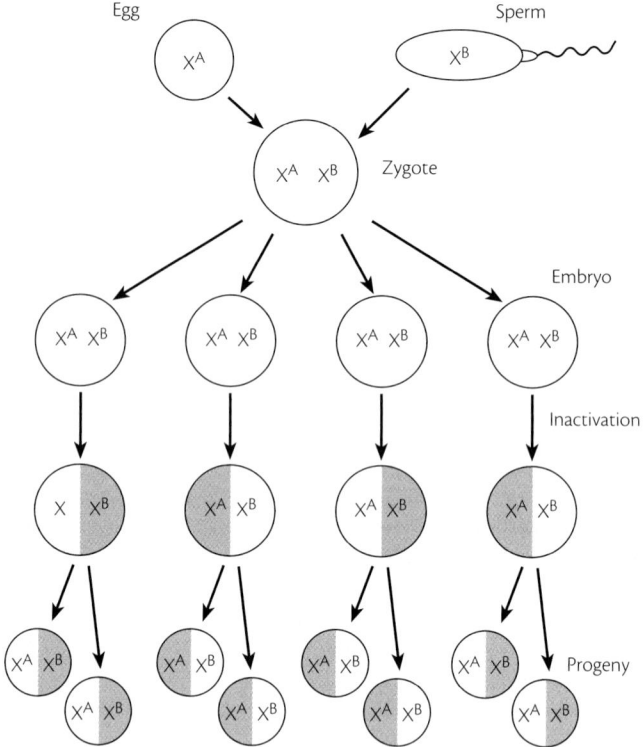

Fig. 22.2.2.1 X-chromosome inactivation.

were based on the presence of polymorphisms in the glucose-6-phosphate dehydrogenase (G6PD) enzyme. In populations of African descent, a common normal variant exists which is designated as A type. Although this variant only differs by one amino acid, it can be readily separated from the more frequent normal B type on starch-gel electrophoresis. Because the gene which codes for G6PD is on the X chromosome, individual cells of a heterozygous female (AB) express only one enzyme type, with approximately half the cells expressing type A and half type B (in other words, the individual is a mosaic). This restricted pattern of gene expression arises because of the process of random X inactivation, known as lyonization, which occurs in early embryonic life and is passed on to the progeny of those cells in a stable manner (Fig. 22.2.2.1). Malignant disorders nearly always arise in a single cell, and thus all the malignant cells in a particular patient will have the same X chromosome inactivated. In an informative G6PD female all the tumour cells will express either type A or type B enzyme. Analysis of the G6PD levels in blood cells of different lineages will help to determine whether they are involved in a haematological

malignancy. This technique is limited by the low frequency of informative polymorphisms in populations other than those of African descent.

Clonality can also be investigated using X-linked DNA polymorphisms which do not result in different protein products. This is based on the fact that the active and inactive genes are differentially methylated at specific cytosine residues. DNA samples are first digested with an appropriate restriction endonuclease to distinguish maternal and paternal copies of the gene, and subsequently with a restriction endonuclease sensitive to cytosine methylation in its recognition sequence to distinguish active from inactive copies of the gene. Useful genes to study include the hypoxanthine phosphoribosyl transferase (*HPRT*) gene and the phosphoglycerate kinase (*PGK*) gene (Fig. 22.2.2.2). The X-linked, multiple tandem repeat recognized by the probe M27B is highly informative (*c.*80% of females are heterozygous), but as this is not a gene it is not really correct to talk about active and inactive copies. None the less, it acts as a useful marker of the inactivated X-chromosome, and results with this probe are concordant with those obtained with HPRT or PGK. PCR-based assays have also been developed to

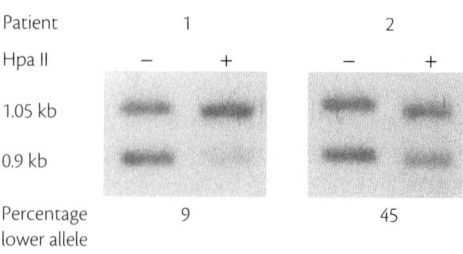

Fig. 22.2.2.2 Clonal analysis of PCK heterozygotes.

examine the methylation status of a number of genes, including the monoamine oxidase A gene (*MOA*), the human androgen-receptor gene (*HUMARA*), and the fragile X gene. These assays require far fewer cells than are required for techniques based on Southern blotting and hence are now more frequently used. The *HUMARA* gene is the most informative, with heterozygosity rates in white populations of about 90%. More recently a number of reverse transcriptase polymerase chain reaction (RT-PCR) assays have been introduced that enable direct analysis of the relative expression of the two alleles at the transcript level, which may circumvent the problem of complex DNA methylation patterns. Informative genes must contain polymorphisms in the coding sequence, although these do not necessarily have to lead to changes in the amino acid sequence. It is also essential that the gene to be analysed is expressed by the cell type being investigated.

The *HUMARA* gene is again the most informative gene as the polymorphic variable number tandem repeat (VNTR) is contained within the coding sequence. The two alleles can be readily distinguished on electrophoresis of the RT-PCR product, but unfortunately this gene is not expressed in all haemopoietic tissues. The transcripts most commonly studied in haematological samples include G6PD, iduronate-2-sulfatase (IDS), and the palmitoylated membrane protein p55 (p55). Together these three RNA transcripts are informative in about 70% of females. Once the mRNA has been reverse-transcribed into cDNA, the different alleles, which differ only by single base changes, are then detected by allele-specific PCR or allele-specific restriction analysis. Even with these genes, expression is not constant between different haemopoietic cell types. In one study, IDS expression was shown to be sixfold higher in T cells than in neutrophils. High sample purity is thus essential when using this methodology.

Clonality studies based on X-chromosome inactivation patterns have three main drawbacks. First, it must be appreciated that lyonization occurs early in embryogenesis when there are few stem cells destined to give rise to the different tissues. As a consequence of this and the random nature of X inactivation, considerable constitutive skewing away from the expected 50:50 expression of maternal and paternal alleles occurs in some individuals. An ill-defined inherited component may also contribute to this random process. In approximately one-quarter of females more than 75% of the expressed genes derive from the same allele, and in 3% of normal individuals more than 90%. It is therefore essential that X-chromosome inactivation patterns are interpreted with reference to normal tissue. This has frequently been omitted, and many of the reports in the literature are thus suspect. Furthermore, in the case of the haematological malignancies, it is not always easy to obtain appropriate control samples. Nonhaemopoietic tissues can be misleading controls, as X-inactivation patterns can vary between tissues. T cells are probably a good control in most myeloid malignancies, as they derive from the same stem cell pool as the myeloid cells, and it is unlikely that the majority of T lymphocytes will be involved in the malignant clone. Second, it has been clearly demonstrated that skewing of the myeloid lineages is acquired in a significant proportion of elderly women, so clonal analysis of haemopoietic lineages must be limited to females under 65 years of age. Third, it must be remembered that the study of X-inactivation patterns is an insensitive technique which will not necessarily detect a clonal population in a polyclonal background. If the constitutive X-chromosome inactivation pattern in an

individual is 50:50, then a clone representing 40% of the whole can be reliably detected. If the constitutive pattern, however, is 70:30 then it is possible to detect a 30% clone if it arises in a cell with the minor allele, but if it arises from a cell with the major allele, then reliable detection requires the mutant clone to represent 60% of the whole population.

Myeloproliferative disorders

The term 'myeloproliferative disorders' was invented by Dameshek and others in the 1950s in an attempt to explain the variability of the haematological findings in polycythaemia rubra vera, chronic myeloid leukaemia (CML), and myelofibrosis, and the existence of intermediate and transitional forms. The myeloproliferative disorders are characterized by the predominant cell type produced by the malignant clone, but they all involve a primitive stem cell (Fig. 22.2.2.3). AML frequently arises at the stem cell level, and diseases such as CML and polycythaemia rubra vera not infrequently terminate in 'blastic transformation'. By convention, however, the term 'myeloproliferative disorders' is usually reserved for the chronic malignancies where mature myeloid cells predominate.

Lineage involvement was first studied in chronic myeloid leukaemia because of the presence of the characteristic Philadelphia (Ph1) chromosome (t(9;22)(q34;q11)). Not only were all cells of the phagocytic- and red-cell series found to be involved, but some Epstein–Barr virus (EBV)–transformed B lymphocytes were also shown to contain the Ph1 chromosome, thus indicating that the target cell for malignant transformation was a primitive stem cell with both myeloid and lymphoid potential. This is confirmed by the fact that about one-third of blastic transformations are due to the accumulation of primitive B cells.

A similarly primitive stem cell is thought to be the cell of origin of polycythaemia rubra vera. A V617F mutation in JAK2 is characteristic of this disease, and can be found in nearly all of the cells of the different myeloid lineages, but not in mature lymphoid cells. The situation in essential thrombocythaemia (ET) is more complex. Clonality studies have revealed that a significant proportion of cases of ET are polyclonal and not malignant disorders, despite fulfilling the usual diagnostic criteria. Overall, JAK2 mutations are present in about 50% of cases, but these mutants may be in small clones on a polyclonal thrombocytosis background. The cause of

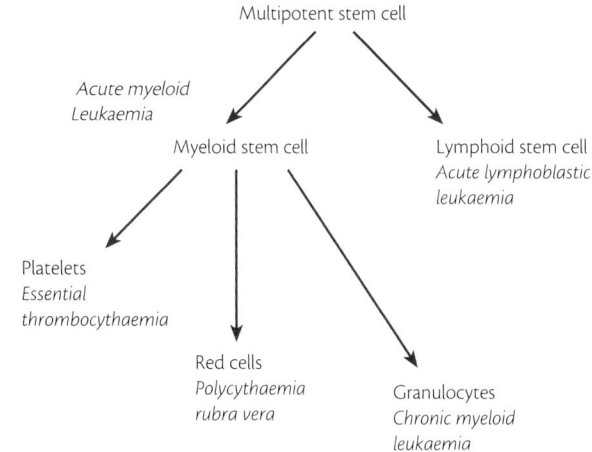

Fig. 22.2.2.3 The myeloproliferative disorders.

the dysregulated blood cell production in such cases is unknown. An important observation made by several groups is that people with the polyclonal forms of ET have a lower incidence of thrombosis.

Dameshek had considered that idiopathic myelofibrosis was part of the myeloproliferative disease spectrum, and indeed this is the case. The fibroblasts are not part of the malignant clone, however, but are a reaction to an underlying myeloid malignancy. The myeloid cells have been shown to be clonal, and in about 50% of cases there is a mutant V617F JAK2 and in a smaller proportion a mutant thrombopoietin receptor (MPL). Some studies suggest additional involvement of lymphoid cells. Fibrosis is particularly common when cells of the megakaryocytic series predominate, and may be due to the excessive local production of platelet growth factors such as platelet-derived growth factor (PDGF) and transforming growth factor-β (TGF-β).

Acute leukaemias

In children with AML, the red cells and platelets do not appear to be part of the malignant clone, whereas such trilineage involvement is frequent in adults. There is no convincing evidence of lymphoid involvement. Regardless of which cell lineages are part of the malignant clone, it is generally believed that the 'leukaemic hit' occurred in a cell more primitive than the majority of the blast cell population. In many cases of AML, the leukaemic cells will engraft in immunodeficient mice and the leukaemia-initiating cell can have a more undifferentiated phenotype than the majority of the blast cells. Few of these cells are cycling, reflecting the cell cycle status of normal stem cells. This has obvious clinical relevance as the noncycling stem cells may be less amenable to attack by cytotoxic agents, and their persistence then gives rise to relapse. If the 'leukaemic hit' occurs in such a primitive cell, the self-renewal programme is already operative, an essential requirement for leukaemogenesis. It is possible, however, that some cases of AML arise in a later cell and the 'leukamogenic hit' must then cause a reversion to self-renewal. If this occurs without generalized phenotypic dedifferentiation, then such cells might be susceptible to treatment with monoclonal antibodies recognizing antigens that are not expressed on the more primitive normal stem cells.

Myelodysplasia, which frequently precedes AML, often involves all myeloid lineages, as is evident from examination of the blood and bone marrow films. There is considerable controversy within the literature, but the majority of studies do not demonstrate involvement of the lymphoid series.

Acute lymphoid leukaemia (ALL) is usually restricted to the B-cell or T-cell lineage. An exception occurs in cases of Ph1-positive ALL, where the myeloid lineages are often involved. This entity is akin to CML presenting in lymphoid blast crisis.

Aplastic anaemia

Aplastic anaemia by definition refers to involvement of multiple myeloid lineages (pancytopenia). In severe cases, the lymphocyte count is also reduced, suggesting that the defect is at the level of stem cells with the potential to give rise to both myeloid and lymphoid elements. Although T-cell numbers tend to be relatively well preserved, it must be appreciated that many T cells are long-lived cells, and their numbers would not be expected to fall rapidly if their production from stem cells ceased. Furthermore, the basis

of immunological memory, and a characteristic difference between myeloid and lymphoid cells, is that the mature progeny of the lymphoid stem cells can undergo amplification-division and self-renewal.

In those patients who respond (at least partially) to immuno-suppression, with long-term follow-up there is a very high incidence of the development of clonal disorders such as paroxysmal nocturnal haemoglobinuria (PNH), myelodysplasia, and AML. In some patients at presentation, the few remaining granulocytes are clonal, although it is not clear how a clonal disorder can give rise to a hypoplastic bone marrow.

Paroxysmal nocturnal haemoglobinuria

PNH is a clonal disorder, due to a somatic mutation in the haemopoietic stem cell in the X-linked phosphatidylinositol glycan-A (PIG-A) responsible for the assembly of glycosyl phosphatidylinositol (GPI)–linked proteins on the cell surface of that cell and its progeny. This results in complement hypersensitivity and low-level expression of a number of antigens which are useful for defining lineage involvement. These include CD59 for red cells, platelets, and T cells; CD67 for granulocytes; CD14 for monocytes; and CD24 for B cells. Flow cytometric studies have revealed variable lineage involvement: red cells, granulocytes, and monocytes and natural killer cells are involved in most cases; B cells are involved in a proportion of cases, and there is one report of a subpopulation of T cells involved in the PNH clone. It is possible that the variable lineage involvement represents differences in the target cell for the initiating mutation. The immunophenotypic studies have also confirmed that there is variable persistence of normal haemopoiesis, and some patients have more than one PNH clone with different levels of expression of GPI-linked molecules. Major unresolved issues in PNH are how the PNH clone, which is not usually considered to be a malignancy, acquires a growth advantage over the normal haemopoietic tissue, and why some clones remain as stable subpopulations that do not continue to expand.

Further reading

Abrahamson G, *et al.* (1991). Clonality of cell populations in refractory anaemia using combined approach of gene loss and X-linked restriction fragment length polymorphism-methylation analyses. *Br J Haematol*, **79**, 550–5.

Adamson JW, *et al.* (1976). Polycythaemia vera: stem cell and probable clonal origin of the disease. *N Engl J Med*, **295**, 913–16.

Beutler E, Collins Z, Irwin LE (1967). Value of genetic variants of glucose-6-phosphate dehydrogenase in tracing the origin of malignant tumours. *N Engl J Med*, **276**, 389–91.

Bjornson CR, *et al.* (1999). Turning brain into blood: a haemopoietic fate adopted by adult neural stem cells *in vivo*. *Science*, **283**, 534–7.

Bonnet D, Dick JE (1997). Human acute myeloid leukaemia is organized as a hierarchy that originates from a primitive hematopoietic cell. *Nat Med*, **3**, 730–7.

Dameshek W (1951). Some speculations on the myeloproliferative syndromes. *Blood*, **6**, 392–5.

Fialkow PJ (1972). Use of genetic markers to study cellular origin of development of tumours in human females. *Adv Cancer Res*, **15**, 191–226.

Gale RE, Wheadon H, Linch DC (1991). X-chromosome inactivation patterns using HPRT and PGK polymorphisms in haematologically normal and post-chemotherapy females. *Br J Haematol*, **79**, 193–7.

Gale RE, *et al.* (1994). Tissue specificity of X-chromosome inactivation patterns. *Blood*, **83**, 2899–905.

Gale RE, *et al.* (2007). Long term serial analysis of X-chromosome inactivation patterns and JAKV617F mutant levels in patients with essential thrombocythaemia show that minor mutant clones can remain stable for many years. *Blood*, **109**, 1241–3.

Harrison C, *et al.* (1999). A large proportion of patients with a diagnosis of essential thrombocythaemia do not have a clonal disorder and may be at lower risk of thrombotic complications. *Blood*, **93**, 417–25.

Hillmen P, Richards SJ (2000). Implications of recent insights into the pathophysiology of paroxysmal nocturnal haemoglobinuria. *Br J Haematol*, **108**, 470–9.

Huntly BJ, *et al.* (2004). MOZ-TIF2 but not BCR-ABL confers properties of leukaemic stem cells to committed murine haematopoietic progenitors. *Cancer Cell*, **6**, 587–96.

Jamieson CH, *et al.* (2006). The JAK2 V617F mutation occurs in haematopoietic stem cells in polycythaemia vera and predisposes to erythroid differentiation. *Proc Natl Acad Sci U S A*, **103**, 6224–9.

Lyon MF (1961). Gene action in the X-chromosome of the mouse (*Mus musculus* L). *Nature*, **190**, 372–3.

Nissen C, *et al.* (1986). Acquired aplastic anaemia: a PNH-like disease? *Br J Haematol*, **64**, 355–62.

Pikman Y, *et al.* (2006). MPL W515L is a novel somatic activating mutation in myelofibrosis with myeloid metaplasia. *PloS Med*, **3**, e270.

Rowley JD (1973). A new consistent chromosomal abnormality in chronic myeloid leukaemia identified by quinacrine fluorescence and Giemsa staining. *Nature*, **243**, 290–3.

Turhan AG, *et al.* (1988). Molecular analysis of clonality and *bcr* rearrangements in Philadelphia chromosome positive acute lymphoblastic leukaemia. *Blood*, **71**, 1495–500.

van Kamp H, *et al.* (1991). Clonal haematopoiesis in patients with acquired aplastic anaemia. *Blood*, **78**, 3209–14.

Vogelstein B, *et al.* (1987). Clonal analysis using recombinant DNA probes from the X-chromosome. *Cancer Res*, **47**, 4806–13.

Weissman I (2000). Translating stem and progenitor cell biology to the clinic: barriers and opportunities. *Science*, **287**, 1442.

22.3

The leukaemias and other bone marrow disorders

Contents

22.3.1 Cell and molecular biology of human leukaemias

Alejandro Gutierrez and A. Thomas Look

Essentials

The human leukaemias arise when haematopoietic stem and progenitor cells acquire genetic alterations that lead to malignant transformation, following which affected cells can exhibit differentiation arrest in any lineage and at any stage of maturation.

Genetic alterations leading to leukaemia—a recurring theme is that the genes most frequently altered are those with evolutionarily conserved roles in the embryological development of various cell lineages and organ systems, including (but not limited to) genes that control normal haematopoiesis. The molecular genetic alterations that drive leukaemogenesis can generally be characterized into lesions affecting transcription factors and those that aberrantly activate signal transduction pathways, which often occur via activating mutations in tyrosine kinases.

The effects of leukaemogenic genetic alterations—some of these affect cell proliferation or survival, whereas others exert their primary effects on cell differentiation. The critical lesion almost always involves a 'master' transcriptional regulatory gene or tyrosine kinase signalling molecule that stands near the top of a hierarchy of gene control, such that leukaemia is efficiently instigated by a limited number of alterations rather than by multiple changes affecting tens of responder genes in the biochemical cascade.

Cell and molecular biology of particular leukaemias—(1) Acute lymphoblastic leukaemia and acute promyelocytic leukaemia—in most cases the initial lesion appears to affect progenitors at the same stage of differentiation as the predominant phenotype in the malignant clone. (2) Acute myeloid leukaemia and chronic myeloid

Acknowledgements: The authors would like to thank John Gilbert for editorial review and critical comments. Supported in part by NIH grant CA068484-12.

leukaemia—most cases appear to arise in a primitive haemopoietic stem cell rather than a committed myeloid progenitor, with subsequent blockade of differentiation at a later developmental stage that determines the morphological subtypes of myeloid leukaemia apparent at diagnosis; this may also be the situation in some cases of acute lymphoblastic leukaemia, at least those expressing the BCR-ABL1 fusion oncogene. (3) Chronic lymphocytic leukaemia—it is currently believed that defective apoptosis *in vivo* is the primary pathogenic abnormality.

Introduction

Attempts to understand the pathobiology of the human leukaemias have focused on clinical presentation, cell morphology, histochemistry, cell immunophenotype, cytogenetics, and, in recent years, molecular genetics. Clinical and cell-biological findings are useful in diagnosis and risk assessment; however, most insights into the mechanisms underlying leukaemic transformation have relied on analysis of genes involved in recurrent cytogenetic and molecular genetic abnormalities. The emerging picture of leucocyte transformation indicates that most cases of leukaemia involve chromosomal translocations that result in aberrantly expressed transcription factors or activated tyrosine kinases, which drive malignant conversion and maintain the leukaemic phenotype. Transcriptional control genes are frequently activated by chromosomal translocations, which lead either to the production of structurally abnormal transcription factors generated by the fusion of disparate gene fragments, or to the aberrant expression of structurally intact genes that have been placed in the vicinity of transcriptional control elements (promoters and enhancers) that are normally highly active in the cell that subsequently becomes transformed: for example, the T-cell receptor (*TCR*) or immunoglobulin (*IG*) gene regulatory elements in lymphoid leukaemias. Oncogenic transcription factors appear to act by either up-regulating critical target genes that co-ordinate normal cell proliferation or survival (gain of function), or by interfering with normal regulatory cascades controlling programmed cell death and differentiation (loss of function). Similarly, signal transduction pathways, which are typically activated through point mutations in receptor tyrosine kinases or other genes mediating growth factor receptor signalling, act through signal transduction cascades that ultimately dysregulate the transcriptional control of gene expression. This chapter provides an introduction to the cell and molecular biology of leukaemia, focusing on characteristic examples of molecular genetic alterations that drive malignant transformation in the human leukaemias. Whenever possible, we have attempted to link advances in the molecular biology of a particular leukaemia to unique implications for treatment and prognosis.

Acute lymphoblastic leukaemia

Approximately 5000 people in the United States, two-thirds of them children, develop acute lymphoblastic leukaemia (ALL) each year. More than 80% of children who are older than 12 months of age at ALL diagnosis achieve long-term event-free survival with modern risk-adapted therapy, attesting to the remarkable treatment advances that have been made over the past three decades. Unfortunately, fewer than 50% of adults become long-term survivors.

The marked differences in outcome across age groups may be explained in part by differences in the age-specific incidence of genetic features that have prognostic implications. For example, the *TEL-AML1* translocation, which is associated with an excellent prognosis, is detectable in 25% of children with ALL but is rare in infants and adults, while the *BCR-ABL1* chimaeric oncogene, which is associated with poor responses to conventional chemotherapy, is much more common in adults. Despite differences in the incidence of several molecular genetic abnormalities across age groups, most of these abnormalities occur in both children and adults, and data is accumulating that similar molecular defects share similar pathophysiology across age groups.

In most instances, the pathobiology of transformed B-lymphoid cells mirrors the altered expression of genes that contribute to the normal functioning of developing lymphocytes, or occasionally mature B cells, although it may involve the aberrant expression of normally quiescent genes. Approximately 80% of patients with ALL have lymphoblasts whose phenotypes correspond to those of B-cell precursors. Only 2 to 3% of these patients have mature B-cell leukaemia, which is thought to represent a disseminated form of Burkitt lymphoma.

B-lineage ALL

BCR-ABL1

The first constitutively activated tyrosine kinase described in ALL results from fusion of 5′ sequences of the *BCR* proto-oncogene to 3′ sequences of the *ABL* (also known as *ABL1*) kinase due to action of the t(9;22) translocation, leading to creation of the so-called Philadelphia (Ph) chromosome. Most investigators believe that the t(9;22) translocation occurs in haemopoietic stem cells possessing both lymphoid and myeloid differentiative potential. Differences in the incidence of *BCR-ABL1*+ leukaemias between children and adults are striking. Found in only 5% of newly diagnosed paediatric ALL cases, this translocation is present in at least 25% of adult cases. *ABL* encodes a nuclear protein with tyrosine kinase activity, the normal function of which remains incompletely understood. However, it may stimulate p53-dependent growth arrest, suggesting a role as a cell cycle checkpoint after damage to the cellular genome.

The *BCR-ABL1* translocation occurs both in ALL and in chronic myelogenous leukaemia (CML). In CML, the *BCR* breakpoints on chromosome 22 occur almost exclusively in the M-bcr (major breakpoint cluster region). In ALL, the *BCR* breakpoints tend to cluster in the m-bcr (minor breakpoint cluster region), although they also occur in the M-bcr. Breaks in the m-bcr region lead to fusion genes encoding a 190-kDa protein (p190), while those in M-bcr generate a 210-kDa protein (p210). Both the p190 and p210 forms of BCR-ABL1 are localized in the cytoplasm, have increased tyrosine kinase activity, and can transform haematopoietic cells in experimental systems. The precise mechanism by which BCR-ABL1 transforms human haemopoietic cells is incompletely understood, but this fusion kinase has been shown to activate several SRC family kinases and activate the RAS, PI3K, and JAK/STAT signal transduction pathways.

The expression of a *BCR-ABL1* fusion gene is one of the few situations in which bone marrow transplantation for patients with ALL in first remission is clearly beneficial. Additionally, several kinase inhibitors have been identified that target the ABL tyrosine kinase and are highly active in BCR-ABL1+ CML. Although imatinib, the first of these targeted kinase inhibitors, shows activity against BCR-ABL1+ ALL, success rates with this as a single agent in ALL have been disappointing, as resistance frequently emerges via mechanisms discussed in the CML section below. However, the addition of imatinib to standard chemotherapy has led to remarkable improvements in short-term event-free survival in pediatric BCR-ABL1+ ALL, raising the possibility that this combination may supplant the need for bone marrow transplantation in first remission.

TEL-AML1

The *TEL-AML1* (also termed *ETV6-RUNX1* or *ETV6-CBFA2*) translocation is present in 25% of cases of childhood ALL; however, it is not detectable by standard cytogenetic analyses and thus was discovered only relatively recently. The *TEL-AML1* translocation often arises prenatally and is probably the initiating lesion in ALL, although it is insufficient to cause leukaemia, because the incidence of detectable *TEL-AML1* translocations in normal newborns is approximately 100-fold greater than the incidence of ALL. This chimaeric oncogene is generated by a t(12;21) translocation, which leads to the fusion of the HLH domain of *TEL* to almost all of *AML1*. Both of these genes are transcription factors required for normal haematopoiesis, and both are involved in other leukaemia-related translocations. However, the precise oncogenic mechanisms mediating transformation by *TEL-AML1* remain incompletely understood.

The identification of the *TEL-AML1* translocation, which occurs almost exclusively in children, is associated with a particularly favourable prognosis, with event-free survival rates of approximately 90%. These cases appear to be particularly responsive to antimetabolite chemotherapy, perhaps as a result of decreased expression of the *MDR-1* multidrug resistance gene and of genes involved in purine biosynthesis. The presence of the *TEL-AML1* fusion identifies a large group of children that are excellent candidates for less intensive therapy.

E2A fusion genes

The *E2A* gene, which encodes a bHLH transcription factor on chromosome 19, is targeted by two recurrent translocations in patients with ALL—the t(1;19), found in 3 to 5% of all cases, and the t(17;19) found in approximately 0.5% of children. The former generates one of the best-characterized fusion oncogenes in ALL, in which the transcriptional transactivation domains of *E2A* are linked to the DNA-binding homeodomain of *PBX1*. *PBX1* is an orphan *HOX* gene that shares homology with the *exd* gene of *Drosophila*, which regulates segment identity through direct interaction of its product with specific HOM proteins of the *Bithorax* and *Antennapedia* complexes.

E2A-PBX1, which binds to DNA in a site-specific manner, is clearly oncogenic in fibroblast transformation assays, and appears to induce programmed cell death (apoptosis) in lymphoid cells. Like its exd homologue, PBX1 is directed to its consensus DNA-binding site by a subset of interacting HOX proteins, whether or not it is fused to E2A. Surprisingly, these site-specific recognition sequences of PBX1 are not required for the transforming activity of E2A-PBX1. How, then, would the chimaeric oncoprotein induce leukaemia, if not by disruption of gene expression normally regulated by HOX proteins? The answer appears to lie in a short peptide sequence that regulates the HOX-specific protein–protein interaction, and which is essential for leukaemogenic activity. The presence of the *E2A-PBX1* translocation was originally associated with

a poor prognosis; however, this translocation is no longer associated with inferior outcomes in the setting of modern risk-adapted therapy for childhood ALL.

The t(17;19) translocation generates the *E2A-HLF* fusion gene, consisting of the N-terminal transactivation regions of *E2A* and the C-terminal DNA-binding and dimerization domains of *HLF*, a member of the bZIP transcription factor gene family. E2A-HLF appears to mediate leukaemic transformation largely through the transcriptional activation of *SLUG*, which inhibits p53-mediated apoptosis. The *E2A-HLF* translocation, which occurs in less than 1% of cases of ALL, is typically seen in adolescents, associated with hypercalcaemia and disseminated intravascular coagulation at the time of diagnosis, and appears to have an unfavourable prognosis, perhaps as a result of *SLUG*-induced resistance to chemotherapy.

MLL fusion genes

Translocations involving the *MLL* (mixed lineage leukaemia) gene, located on chromosome band 11q23, are found in 80% of cases of infant leukaemia, whether ALL or acute myeloid leukaemia (AML), and in 5 to 10% of primary ALL and AML cases in older children and adults. Furthermore, *MLL* translocations occur in 85% of secondary AML cases that develop in patients treated with topoisomerase II inhibitors. The MLL protein is expressed in all haematopoietic stem and progenitor cells and is required for normal haematopoiesis. It contains multiple domains, including three N-terminal A–T hook DNA-binding motifs, a region with homology to DNA-methyltransferase, a transcriptional activation domain, and a C-terminal SET domain. The stability and localization of the MLL protein depend on proteolytic processing by Taspase1, a specialized protease that cleaves the MLL protein into N- and C-terminal fragments that remain associated through intramolecular protein–protein interactions. MLL binds DNA in a non-sequence-specific manner as part of large multiprotein complexes, and appears to act largely as a transcriptional activator.

More than 30 discrete chromosomal sites participate in 11q23 translocations, most commonly 4q21, 9p22, and 19p13, resulting in fusion of the *AF4*, *AF9*, and *ENL* genes to *MLL*. The leukaemogenic role of *MLL* fusions has been definitively demonstrated through the generation of mouse models, with mice expressing *MLL-AF9*, *MLL-ENL*, *MLL-ELL*, or *MLL-CBP* in their haematopoietic precursor cells developing leukaemias. As with *PBX1*, the dysregulation of *HOX* genes appears to play a prominent role in the pathogenesis of *MLL*-rearranged leukaemia. MLL is known to bind to and activate several *HOX* gene promoters, and leukaemias with *MLL* rearrangements characteristically show overexpression of specific *HOX* genes, including *HOXA9*, *HOXA10*, *HOXC6*, and the *HOX* gene regulator *MEIS1*. In particular, *HOXA9* has been shown to play critical functions in the transformation of haematopoietic precursors by *MLL* fusion oncogenes in murine models of leukaemia.

The *MLL-AF4*, *MLL-AF9*, and other *MLL* fusion genes predict a dismal outcome in patients with early B-lineage ALL treated with conventional therapy. Additionally, allogeneic bone marrow transplantation to intensify therapy for infants with *MLL*-rearranged ALL in first remission is not clearly beneficial, and limited evidence suggests that this may actually worsen outcomes when compared with chemotherapy alone. One notable exception to the worse risk implications of MLL translocations is the t(11;19)(q23;p13.3) translocation leading to the *MLL-ENL* fusion in the case of T-ALL. Although this translocation is associated with poor prognosis in

B-precursor ALL, the largest case series published to date shows a surprisingly good outcome in T-ALL patients treated with chemotherapy alone whose leukaemic cells harbour this translocation.

MYC

Chromosomal translocations in B-lineage cells can also mobilize proto-oncogenes to sites adjacent to normally active enhancer or promoter elements of *IG* genes, without structurally altering the oncogene involved. The prototype for this mechanism in B-lineage ALL is the t(8;14), which arises in mature B cells and places the *MYC* proto-oncogene on chromosome 8 under the control of *IG* heavy-chain gene regulatory sequences on chromosome 14. Similar repositioning of *MYC* adjacent to the light-chain regulatory sequences results from the t(2;8) or the t(8;22), which is seen in a much smaller percentages of cases. Through one of these translocations, *MYC* expression becomes highly up-regulated, leading to abnormally increased amounts of the MYC protein, a transcription factor that forms a DNA-binding complex with another cellular protein (MAX), and eventually leads to disruption of gene expression involved in the control of cell proliferation.

Although the coding region of *MYC* is not structurally altered by these translocations, point mutations commonly arise in these cases at codons 58 or 62 of the MYC protein. These point mutations disrupt phosphorylation sites involved in regulating the activity and stability of the MYC protein and not only lead to the accumulation of activated and stabilized MYC protein, but also impair the ability of MYC to activate an important tumour suppressor mechanism mediated by the *BIM* gene.

Children and adults with *MYC*-translocated mature B-cell ALL have extremely poor outcomes when treated with conventional regimens designed for the treatment of ALL. However, these patients have excellent responses to the relatively brief but intensive regimens designed for the treatment of Burkitt lymphoma, and most experts now consider mature B-cell ALL to be a disseminated form of Burkitt lymphoma. Thus, B-cell ALL was the first example of a subtype of ALL requiring tailored therapy with a vastly different drug regimen for effective disease control.

T-lineage ALL

First recognized as a distinct clinical entity in the early 1970s, T-ALL accounts for 10 to 15% of acute lymphoblastic leukaemias in children and 20 to 25% of cases in adults. The disease can arise in thymocytes at any stage of maturation, defined on the basis of reactivity with monoclonal antibodies (CD4/CD8 double-negative immature thymocytes, cytoplasmic CD3+, CD7+, CD2+, and CD5+; CD4/CD8 double-positive common thymocytes, cytoplasmic CD3+, CD1+, CD2+, CD5+, CD7+, CD10+, CD4+, and CD8+; and CD4/CD8 single-positive late thymocytes, cytoplasmic CD3+, CD2+, CD5+, CD7+, CD4+, or CD8+).

Dysregulated expression of oncogenic transcription factors

In contrast to the fusion oncogenes that drive the development of B-cell precursor ALL, oncogene activation in T-ALL typically reflects the overexpression of genes encoding structurally intact T-cell proto-oncogenes. Approximately 25% of cases of T-ALL have cytogenetically identifiable chromosomal translocations that typically mobilize intact proto-oncogenic transcription factors into the vicinity of transcriptionally active sites of the β or α/δ loci of the T-cell receptor genes (TCRβ or TCRα/δ). Among the genes that are aberrantly expressed in thymocytes and cause leukaemic transformation through this mechanism are those representing the

bHLH family of transcription factors (*TAL1/SCL1, TAL2/SCL2, LYL1,* and *BHLHB1*), the bHLH/ZIP family (*MYC*), other nuclear regulatory proteins (LMO1 and LMO2), homeobox proteins (HOX11), and a truncated and constitutively activated form of NOTCH1. The relationship of these genes to the pathogenesis of T-ALL has been established by their recurrent involvement in translocations that affect thymocytes or their precursors. Surprisingly, many of the T-cell oncogenes identified to date are not usually expressed in T cells; hence, their ability to induce leukaemia most likely reflects the misexpression of master transcriptional control genes with the disruption of normal T-cell developmental pathways. This is illustrated by *HOX11*, which is not normally expressed in lymphoid cells, but has been shown to be essential for normal development of the spleen.

Despite intensive cytogenetic research, chromosomal translocations have been identified in only about 25% of T-ALL cases. However, gene expression profiling has identified overexpression of many of the oncogenes found in recurrent T-ALL chromosomal translocations in most cases of ALL, even when such translocations are not present, suggesting that translocation-independent mechanisms are at work that disrupt these key transcriptional control networks in thymocyte development, leading to overt T-ALL.

NOTCH1 mutations

The *NOTCH1* gene was initially identified as a partner gene in a t(7;9) translocation in very rare cases of T-ALL, in which a truncated *NOTCH1* is placed under control of the T-cell receptor β locus. Despite the rarity of this translocation, a search for activating mutations in *NOTCH1* identified these in greater than 50% of cases of T-ALL. *NOTCH1* encodes a cell surface receptor that, upon ligand binding, undergoes proteolytic processing that culminates in the proteolytic release of an intracellular portion of the receptor known as intracellular NOTCH1 (ICN), which then moves to the nucleus where it is active as a transcription factor. The *NOTCH1* mutations found in T-ALL either lead to the ligand-independent proteolytic release of the ICN, or mutate the PEST domain of the ICN, thus leading to accumulation of nuclear ICN protein as a result of impaired proteolytic degradation.

The identification of *NOTCH1* mutations in T-ALL has generated considerable excitement for the application of γ-secretase inhibitors to the treatment of patients with T-ALL. γ-Secretase is required for the proteolytic activation of NOTCH receptors, and inhibitors of this enzyme, which have previously been developed due to the role of γ-secretase in Alzheimer's disease, effectively inhibit NOTCH receptor activation in experimental systems. Such γ-secretase inhibitors (GSIs) are currently undergoing clinical trials in patients with T-ALL. Although GSIs are effective against several human T-ALL cell lines harbouring activating *NOTCH1* mutations, some of these cell lines are resistant. Recent data demonstrate that the effect of GSIs in cultured T-ALL cell lines requires the *PTEN* tumour suppressor, and *PTEN* loss mediates resistance to these inhibitors in cultured T-ALL cells. Interestingly, pharmacological suppression of the AKT pathway, which is normally inhibited by PTEN, was effective against *PTEN*-null, *NOTCH1*-mutated T-ALL. Moreover, recent data has demonstrated that GSI therapy reverses glucocorticoid resistance in T-ALL cells, while glucocorticoids simultaneously prevent GSI-induced gastrointestinal toxicity in the mouse. Taken together, these data suggest that therapy with a NOTCH1 inhibitor, an AKT pathway inhibitor, and a glucocorticoid may prove to be a particularly effective combination in T-ALL.

Ongoing studies to clarify the molecular pathogenesis of T-ALL should greatly enhance the value of molecular genetics in predicting the clinical responses of patients with T-ALL and, ultimately, could provide additional effective targets for novel drug therapies.

Lesions activating tyrosine kinases, RAS, and PI3K signalling pathways in ALL

Oncogenic lesions leading to the aberrant activation of signal transduction pathways that normally mediate growth factor signalling are common events in both B-precursor and T-ALL. As previously described, the *BCR-ABL1* fusion oncogene, found in t(9;22)-translocated B-precursor ALL and chronic myeloid leukaemia, acts as a constitutively activated tyrosine kinase to activate a number of growth factor signalling pathways. Although *BCR-ABL1* fusions are rare in T-ALL, *NUP214-ABL1* fusions have recently been described in 6% of patients with T-ALL. These fusions arise via a mechanism in which a portion of chromosome band 9q34, which contains both *NUP214* and *ABL1*, is circularized in a manner leading to the fusion of these 2 genes, with the same breakpoint in *ABL1* as is seen in the *BCR-ABL1* translocation. Similar to the BCR-ABL1 fusion oncoprotein, the NUP214-ABL1 fusion has constitutive ABL1 tyrosine kinase activity that can be inhibited by the BCR-ABL1 kinase inhibitor imatinib.

FLT3 encodes a receptor tyrosine kinase that plays important roles in early haematopoietic precursors. Although activating mutations in this gene are rare in adult ALL, *FLT3* is commonly mutated or overexpressed in most cases of ALL that involve MLL gene rearrangements or hyperdiploidy, which are typically seen in childhood ALL. *FLT3* mutations also occur in AML and are discussed in more detail in that section below.

The RAS guanine nucleotide-binding proteins, which were originally identified due to their homology with viral oncogenes, are activated by haematopoietic cytokine receptors in response to ligand binding in normal haematopoietic precursors. Activating mutations of *NRAS* are found in approximately 10% of cases of ALL, while *KRAS* mutations occur in 5 to 10%. These mutations typically consist of single amino acid substitutions at codons 12, 13, or 61 of RAS, and lead to constitutive receptor-independent activation of downstream signal transduction pathways, including the MAPK and PI3K pathways. Activation of the PI3K pathway in T-ALL can also occur via loss of the *PTEN* tumour suppressor, an abnormality which is found in approximately 15% of cases of T-ALL.

Acute myeloid leukaemia

The estimated number of new cases of acute myeloid leukaemia (AML) occurring annually in the United States is vastly higher in adults than in children (20 000 vs 1000). Overall, prognosis remains poor in both age groups, although several cytogenetic and molecular genetic abnormalities have been found to have prognostic relevance and allow risk stratification into favourable, intermediate, and unfavourable subgroups. Additionally, evidence now suggests that bone marrow transplantation can improve outcomes for patients with higher-risk disease who have histocompatible donors and are young and healthy enough to tolerate this procedure. AML has traditionally been classified according to the developmental stage at which differentiation arrest occurs in the bulk of the myeloblast population, and differentiation stages in AML are best described in the context of the French-American-British (FAB)

classification system. However, evidence now suggests that the transformed cell in AML is a haematopoietic stem or primitive progenitor cell that retains the ability to differentiate into the more mature myeloid cells that form the bulk of the tumour. Many cases of AML can now be classified based on the presence of characteristic chromosomal translocations, several of which have prognostic and therapeutic implications.

Recurrent genetic abnormalities in AML frequently target several transcription factors involved in the regulation of haematopoietic stem and progenitor cell differentiation, including the core-binding factor (CBF) transcription complex, RARα, MLL, and transcriptional coactivators such as CBP and MOZ. These genetic aberrations typically lead to the activation of self-renewal pathways, including the WNT-CTNNB1, NOTCH, and BMI1 pathways, and these are believed to function at the level of the leukaemic stem cells that maintain the myeloid leukaemic cell population.

PML-RARα fusion

Promyelocytic leukaemia, defined as the clonal expansion of transformed myeloid cells blocked at the promyelocyte stage of development, is characterized by the presence of the t(15;17) translocation that generates the *PML-RARα* fusion gene. RARα (retinoic acid receptor alpha) is a member of the nuclear hormone–receptor superfamily, functioning as a ligand-dependent, zinc-finger transcription factor with a critical role in normal myeloid cell differentiation. The PML transcription factor is a tumour suppressor that regulates several apoptotic pathways via interactions with p53 and other proteins. The fusion PML-RARα protein contains nearly all the key functional domains of each molecule, including the protein–protein interaction motifs of PML and the DNA-binding, dimerization, ligand-binding, and transcriptional activation domains of RARα. The PML-RARα oncoprotein induces leukaemia by inhibiting, in a dominant fashion, the normal biological activities of both RARα and PML. The net effect is a blockade of differentiation with immortality and sustained proliferation among promyelocytes, the hallmark of acute promyelocytic leukaemia (M3 AML). Treatment of *PML-RARα*+ AML with pharmacological dosages of the RARα ligand *all-trans*-retinoic acid (ATRA) results in the release of corepressor complexes from the PML-RARα fusion protein, reversing the protein's inhibitory activity and enabling the leukaemic promyelocytes to proceed to terminal differentiation. The unique specificity of ATRA for the underlying molecular lesion in M3 AML has allowed marked improvements in outcomes for patients with promyelocytic leukaemia.

AML1-ETO

The *AML1-ETO* fusion gene (also known as *RUNX1-CBFA2T1*) results from the t(8;21) translocation, which is found in 10% of AML cases overall, particularly those of the FAB M2 subtype. This fusion oncogene consists of the N-terminal portion of AML1, involving the entire RUNT homology domain that mediates binding to the promoters of several haematopoietic genes, and the C-terminal portion of ETO, which mediates interactions with the nuclear corepressor complex. Thus, the AML1-ETO fusion exerts its leukaemic activity by recruiting nuclear corepressor complexes to the promoters of genes that are normally activated by the AML1-CBFβ complex, whose function is essential for the development of all haematopoietic lineages.

Patients whose myeloid blasts carry the *AML1-ETO* translocation have been shown to have a relatively favourable prognosis, and respond more readily to chemotherapy regimens involving high-dose cytarabine than most other patients with AML. Since AML-ETO is a dominant-negative chimaeric transcription factor that relies on corepressor complexes, novel treatments that disrupt the formation, stability, or activity of such complexes, such as histone deacetylase inhibitors, might reverse the leukaemic phenotype, as seen with the use of ATRA in patients with acute promyelocytic leukaemia carrying the *PML–RARα* oncogene.

CBFβ–MYH11

The *CBFβ-MYH11* fusion product, due to inv(16) or t(16;16), is seen in approximately 5% of newly diagnosed cases of AML. Once thought to be pathognomonic for cases with dysplastic eosinophilic precursors among myeloblasts and monoblasts (M4Eo subtype), this finding has since been made in acute myeloblastic leukaemia (M1 and M2 subtypes). These genetic rearrangements fuse most of CBFβ to a variable amount of the C-terminal α-helical rod domain of MYH11, a smooth-muscle, myosin heavy-chain protein that possesses both actin-binding and ATPase activity. Like AML1-ETO, the CBFβ-MYH11 fusion protein aberrantly associates with nuclear corepressor complexes and results in the recruitment of these corepressor complexes to the promoters of genes normally activated by the AML1-CBFβ complex. As with *AML1-ETO*, the expression of the *CBFβ-MYH11* fusion confers an increased probability of achieving a sustained remission with high-dose cytarabine-containing chemotherapy regimens.

MLL fusion genes

Translocations involving the mixed lineage leukaemia (*MLL*) gene are found in both AML and ALL, and the pathobiology of *MLL* fusion genes was reviewed in the ALL section earlier in this chapter. Interestingly, recent work has shown that, in a mouse model of MLL-rearranged acute myeloid leukaemia, the introduction of the oncogenic *MLL-AF9* fusion gene into committed granulocyte–macrophage progenitor cells leads these progenitors to re-activate a subset of genes that are highly expressed in normal haematopoietic stem cells, while their overall gene expression profile remains very similar to that of normal granulocyte–macrophage progenitors, suggesting that the primary transformed leukaemic stem cell in this disorder in humans may also be a committed progenitor rather than a pluripotent haematopoietic stem cell.

NPM mutations

Mutations in the nucleophosmin gene *(NPM)* were recently identified in approximately one-third of all primary cases of AML, and occur selectively in AML cases with a normal karyotype. The *NPM* gene encodes a protein that demonstrates nuclear-cytoplasmic shuttling and has a wide range of biologic activities. *NPM* mutations in AML occur in exon 12 and result in a frameshift involving the C terminus of the protein. Although several different frameshift mutations are found, these uniformly lead to disruption of at least one of the tryptophan residues at positions 288 and 290, which disrupts the protein's nuclear localization signal. Additionally, these frameshift mutations also introduce an aberrant nuclear export signal, resulting in abnormal subcellular localization with very high cytoplasmic and low nuclear levels of nucleophosmin.

NPM acts as a chaperone for proteins, nucleic acids, and histones. It is required for the assembly of mature ribosomal complexes, and it is thought to regulate protein synthesis and cell growth through its effects on the ribosome pool. NPM also maintains genomic stability through the regulation of DNA repair and centrosome duplication during mitosis, and it interacts with the key cell cycle regulators CDK2-cyclin E. Finally, NPM interacts with p53 and ARF to regulate the ARF-MDM2-p53 pathway. Although alterations in any of these functions could represent the mechanism driving selection for *NPM* mutations during leukaemogenesis, the precise mechanism(s) mediating the oncogenic effect of these *NPM* mutations is a matter of intense ongoing investigation.

Mutations activating tyrosine kinase and RAS signalling pathways in AML

Activating mutations leading to constitutive activation of growth factor receptor signalling pathways are common events in AML, as in ALL. The RAS guanine nucleotide–binding proteins, which were originally identified due to their homology with viral oncogenes, are activated in response to haematopoietic cytokine receptors in response to ligand binding in normal haematopoietic precursors. Point mutations in codons 12, 13, or 61 of *KRAS* and *NRAS* are found in the leukaemic cells of 25% and 15%, respectively, of patients with AML. These point mutations are oncogenic due to their constitutive, growth factor–independent activation of downstream signal transduction pathways, including the PI3K, MAPK, and RALGDS pathways. The data on the prognostic relevance of *RAS* mutations in AML remain inconclusive.

Mutations in the *KIT* tyrosine kinase, which is the receptor for the stem cell factor (SCF) ligand, are found preferentially in AML cases harbouring t(8;21), inv(16), or t(16;16), occurring in approximately 25% of these cases. These mutations typically involve the extracellular domain of the receptor or the catalytic domain, and result in spontaneous ligand-independent receptor activation. Mutations in the extracellular domain lead to activation of the MAPK and PI3K signalling pathways, while catalytic domain mutations have been shown to constitutively activate PI3K and STAT3 signalling. *KIT* mutations are associated with increased relapse rates in patients with the otherwise prognostically favourable t(8;21), inv(16), or t(16;16). However, imatinib and several newer tyrosine kinase inhibitors, originally designed to target the BCR-ABL1 fusion kinase, have also been found to be effective inhibitors of *KIT* signalling, and these small molecules may prove to have a role in the therapy of *KIT*-mutant AML.

The *FLT3* gene encodes a receptor tyrosine kinase that is highly expressed in haematopoietic precursors, where it plays important functional roles. Activating mutations in *FLT3* are typically either internal tandem duplications (ITD) in the juxtamembrane domain, or point mutations or insertions in the second tyrosine kinase domain. These mutations lead to ligand-independent autophosphorylation and activation of downstream signal transduction pathways. ITD mutations are found in 25% of cases of AML, while mutations in the kinase domain are found in 10% of these patients. Several studies now demonstrate that *FLT3* ITD mutations are associated with poor outcomes in AML, particularly in the setting of high *FLT3* allelic ratio. Experimental evidence suggests that the pharmacological inhibition of FLT3 has important antileukaemic effects, and several small molecule inhibitors of FLT3 are currently under clinical development.

Chronic myeloid leukaemia

Most patients with chronic myeloid leukaemia (CML), both children and adults, harbour the classic t(9;22) translocation in myeloid cells, giving rise to the Philadelphia chromosome and the *BCR-ABL1* fusion oncogene. The pathobiology of the BCR-ABL1 fusion oncoprotein, which also occurs in ALL, was discussed in that section of this chapter. In most untreated patients with CML, the resulting disease is biphasic, with an initial (chronic) phase that lasts 3 years on average, and a terminal (blast) phase that is highly refractory to therapy and is generally fatal within a median of 2 to 4 months. Allogeneic bone marrow transplantation is the only known curative treatment for CML. However, therapy for patients with CML who lack histocompatible donors or are otherwise not candidates for bone marrow transplantation was revolutionized with the introduction of imatinib, which has altered the natural history of this disease. Imatinib is a small molecule that inhibits BCR-ABL1 tyrosine kinase activity by targeting its ATP-binding site. Although experimental and clinical data suggest that BCR-ABL1 inhibitors are unlikely to be curative as single agents, long-term imatinib therapy can control chronic-phase CML for many years. Imatinib resistance can develop in chronic-phase CML, and it tends to develop particularly rapidly in late-stage CML and in BCR-ABL1+ ALL, typically through point mutations in the kinase domain that impair imatinib binding without disrupting kinase activity. Several newer 'second-generation' BCR-ABL1 inhibitors have now been developed, many of which also inhibit other kinases including the SRC family kinases, which are known mediators of BCR-ABL1 oncogenic signalling. Some of these newer inhibitors have been shown to target most imatinib-resistant BCR-ABL1 mutants, and indeed are active against CML after imatinib failure, although resistance to these second-generation inhibitors can also arise. Several novel small molecules targeting BCR-ABL1 via ATP-binding-site-independent mechanisms, or targeting a broader range of kinases, are currently undergoing clinical development in an effort to overcome drug-resistant BCR-ABL1 mutations.

Chronic lymphocytic leukaemia

Chronic lymphocytic leukaemia (CLL) is the most common leukaemia in Europe and North America, with an estimated incidence of 15 000 cases per year in the United States. Although rare before 50 years of age, the incidence of CLL rises relatively rapidly thereafter. The diagnosis of CLL rests on the identification of an absolute peripheral blood lymphocytosis ($>5 \times 10^9$ cells/litre) and an appropriate immunophenotype, and patients can also develop lymphomatous involvement of lymph nodes or other tissues. Interestingly, 3.5% of healthy individuals older than 40 years have a small but identifiable clonal population of lymphocytes with an immunophenotype consistent with CLL, although the clinical significance of this finding remains unclear. Despite the frequency of CLL, relatively little is known about its molecular pathogenesis, in large part due to difficulties in culturing these cells in the laboratory and bringing them into mitosis for karyotyping, and the lack of a suitable animal model for indolent CLL. The accumulation of mature B cells that have escaped apoptosis and undergone cell cycle arrest in G_0/G_1 is the hallmark of CLL, and these cells overexpress several of the antiapoptotic *BCL2* family members, including *BCL2* itself, *BCL-XL*, and *MCL1*. It is currently believed that defective apoptosis *in vivo* is the primary pathogenic abnormality in CLL,

and inhibitors of these antiapoptotic proteins, which effectively induce apoptosis in these cells, are currently under clinical development for the treatment of this disease.

Clinical summary

Several molecular genetic changes in leukaemic cells at diagnosis are sensitive markers of response to therapy, and therefore can be used as guides to treatment. Table 22.3.1.1 summarizes the clinical utility of recognized oncogenic transcription factors in the human leukaemias.

Table 22.3.1.1 Clinical applications of common oncogenic transcription factors in the human leukaemias

Altered gene	Leukaemia subtype*	Risk of treatment failure†	Recommended treatment‡
ALL			
TEL–AML1 (*ETV6–EBFA2*)	Pro-B cell	Low	Well-tolerated chemotherapy (antimetabolites primarily)
E2A–PBX1	Pre-B cell	Intermediate	Intensive chemotherapy (genotoxic drugs and antimetabolites)
MYC	B cell	High	Intensive chemotherapy (rotation of genotoxic drugs)
MLL–AF4	CD10– pro-B cell	Very high	Intensive chemotherapy or allogeneic stem-cell transplantation
BCR–ABL1	Pro-B cell (predominantly)	Very high	Allogeneic stem-cell transplantation
AML			
AML1–ETO	Acute myeloblastic leukaemia with maturation (M2 morphology)	Intermediate	Intensive chemotherapy (including high-dose cytarabine)
CBFβ–MYHII	Acute myelomonocytic leukaemia with eosinophils (M4Eo morphology)	Intermediate	Intensive chemotherapy (including high-dose cytarabine)
PML–RARα	Acute promyelocytic leukaemia (M3 morphology)	Intermediate	Intensive chemotherapy (including all-*trans*-retinoic acid and an anthracycline)

ALL, acute lymphoblastic leukaemia; AML, acute myeloid leukaemia.

* Subclassifications of AML are those of the French–American–British (FAB) cooperative group.

† As determined in standard programmes of chemotherapy (without haemopoietic stem-cell rescue). Treatment failure refers to either remission induction or remission maintenance, or both. The average rates of long-term, leukaemia-free survival in children and adolescents with ALL or AML range from 65–70 per cent and from 30–40 per cent, respectively.

‡ The choice of therapy is based on detection of the indicated fusion gene at diagnosis by cytogenetic analysis, Southern blotting, or RNA-polymerase chain reaction assays for chimeric mRNAs.

Thus far, only a few specific lesions, the *PML-RARα* fusion gene in acute promyelocytic leukaemia, the *BCR-ABL1* kinase in CML and ALL, the *NUP214-ABL1* kinase in T-ALL, and the *KIT* and *FLT3* mutations in AML have been productive targets for molecular-oriented therapy, but this number will likely increase as we continue to unravel the genetic mechanisms that transform normal blood cells and maintain leukaemic phenotypes.

Further reading

Armstrong SA, Look AT (2005). Molecular genetics of acute lymphoblastic leukemia. *J Clin Oncol*, **23**, 6306–15.

Bonnet D, Dick JE (1997). Human acute myeloid leukemia is organized as a hierarchy that originates from a primitive hematopoietic cell. *Nat Med*, **3**, 730–7.

Clark SS, *et al.* (1987). Unique forms of the abl tyrosine kinase distinguish Ph1-positive CML from Ph1-positive ALL. *Science*, **235**, 85–8.

de The H, *et al.* (1990). The t(15;17) translocation of acute promyelocytic leukaemia fuses the retinoic acid receptor alpha gene to a novel transcribed locus. *Nature*, **347**, 558–61.

Del Gaizo Moore V, *et al.* (2007). Chronic lymphocytic leukemia requires BCL2 to sequester prodeath BIM, explaining sensitivity to BCL2 antagonist ABT-737. *J Clin Invest*, **117**, 112–21.

Dighiero G, Hamblin TJ (2008). Chronic lymphocytic leukaemia. *Lancet*, **371**, 1017–29.

Falini B, *et al.* (2005). Cytoplasmic nucleophosmin in acute myelogenous leukemia with a normal karyotype. *N Engl J Med*, **352**, 254–66.

Ferrando AA, *et al.* (2002). Gene expression signatures define novel oncogenic pathways in T cell acute lymphoblastic leukemia. *Cancer Cell*, **1**, 75–87.

Frohling S, *et al.* (2005). Genetics of myeloid malignancies: pathogenetic and clinical implications. *J Clin Oncol*, **23**, 6285–95.

Golub TR, *et al.* (1995). Fusion of the TEL gene on 12p13 to the AML1 gene on 21q22 in acute lymphoblastic leukemia. *Proc Natl Acad Sci U S A*, **92**, 4917–21.

Gutierrez A, Look AT (2007). NOTCH and PI3K-AKT pathways intertwined. *Cancer Cell*, **12**, 411–13.

Hemann MT, *et al.* (2005). Evasion of the p53 tumour surveillance network by tumour-derived MYC mutants. *Nature*, **436**, 807–11.

Inaba T, *et al.* (1996). Reversal of apoptosis by the leukaemia-associated E2A-HLF chimaeric transcription factor. *Nature*, **382**, 541–4.

Krivtsov AV, Armstrong SA (2007). MLL translocations, histone modifications and leukaemia stem-cell development. *Nat Rev Cancer*, **7**, 823–33.

Krivtsov AV, *et al.* (2006). Transformation from committed progenitor to leukaemia stem cell initiated by MLL-AF9. *Nature*, **442**, 818–22.

Look AT (1997). Oncogenic transcription factors in the human acute leukemias. *Science*, **278**, 1059–64.

Okuda T, *et al.* (1996). AML1, the target of multiple chromosomal translocations in human leukemia, is essential for normal fetal liver hematopoiesis. *Cell*, **84**, 321–30.

Palomero T, *et al.* (2007). Mutational loss of PTEN induces resistance to NOTCH1 inhibition in T-cell leukemia. *Nat Med*, **13**, 1203–10.

Pui CH, *et al.* (2008). Acute lymphoblastic leukaemia. *Lancet*, **371**, 1030–43.

Rabbitts TH (1994). Chromosomal translocations in human cancer. *Nature*, **372**, 143–9.

Shtivelman E, *et al.* (1985). Fused transcript of abl and bcr genes in chronic myelogenous leukemia. *Nature*, **315**, 550–4.

Thirman MJ, *et al.* (1993). Rearrangement of the MLL gene in acute lymphoblastic and acute myeloid leukemias with 11q23 chromosomal translocations. *N Engl J Med*, **329**, 909–14.

Warrell RP Jr, *et al.* (1991). Differentiation therapy of acute promyelocytic leukemia with tretinoin (all-trans-retinoic acid). *N Engl J Med*, **324**, 1385–93.

Weisberg E, *et al.* (2007). Second generation inhibitors of BCR-ABL for the treatment of imatinib-resistant chronic myeloid leukaemia. *Nat Rev Cancer*, **7**, 345–56.

Weng AP, *et al.* (2004). Activating mutations of NOTCH1 in human T cell acute lymphoblastic leukemia. *Science*, **306**, 269–71.

22.3.2 The classification of leukaemia

Wendy N. Erber

Essentials

Leukaemia is a malignant neoplasm of haematopoietic cells originating in the marrow and spreading to the blood and other tissues, such as the lymph nodes, spleen, and liver. The characteristic feature of the neoplastic cells is that they retain the ability to proliferate but fail to differentiate normally into functional haematopoietic cells. This results in replacement of the normal bone marrow by the leukaemic cells.

General approach to classification of leukaemia

Leukaemias are subdivided into acute or chronic and lymphoid or myeloid on the basis of the cell lineage and stage of differentiation of the malignant cell. This is of fundamental importance because each subtype differs in clinical behaviour, prognosis, and response to treatment.

Clinical approach—morphological assessment of the blood film and (usually) bone marrow aspirate is essential. The cellular morphology may be diagnostic and is used to determine which ancillary tests are required for classification. Establishing the cell lineage and stage of differentiation is achieved by phenotyping the neoplastic cell using a panel of antibodies to cellular antigens associated with specific cell types (lymphoid or myeloid lineage; B-, T- or NK-cells) and degree of maturation. Determining the genotype of the malignant cell, e.g. by examination for chromosomal translocations and other genetic abnormalities, is the defining property for some acute leukaemias and can be prognostically significant.

WHO classification of acute and chronic leukaemias

The following classes of leukaemia are recognized: (1) precursor B- and T-cell neoplasms—lymphoblastic leukaemias/lymphomas; (2) acute myeloid leukaemias—including subtypes with recurrent genetic abnormalities, with myelodysplasia-related changes, therapy-related and 'not otherwise specified'; (3) acute leukaemias of ambiguous lineage; (4) mature B-cell neoplasms—including chronic lymphocytic leukaemia; (5) mature T-cell and NK-cell neoplasms—including T-cell prolymphocytic leukaemia; (6) myeloproliferative neoplasms—including chronic myelogenous leukaemia; (7) myelodysplastic/myeloproliferative neoplasms.

This classification of leukaemia cannot be regarded as fixed and definitive—it will certainly need to be revised as new discoveries are made and new disease subtypes defined.

Introduction

Over the past 40 years there have been several leukaemia classifications. For a classification to be useful it must be reproducible, clinically relevant, and able to be used worldwide. The French–American–British (FAB) classification of acute leukaemias, introduced in the mid-1970s, was widely applied because of its ease of use and clinical applicability. FAB was based on morphology of the neoplastic cells in the blood and bone marrow together with cytochemical reactivity. The classification was revised to include cell phenotype for some entities, and a classification for chronic lymphoid leukaemias was introduced. In the 1990s it was realized that clearer definitions of leukaemic subtypes could be achieved by combining genetic data with morphology and cell phenotype. The World Health Organization (WHO) classification of haematopoietic neoplasms, which incorporates all this information, has now replaced the FAB classification.

WHO classification

The *World Health Organization Classification of Tumours of Haematopoietic and Lymphoid Tissues* was published in 2001 and revised in 2008 (Box 22.3.2.1). This is a comprehensive consensus classification of all haematological malignancies, including the leukaemias. It stratifies neoplasms by cell lineage and defines clinicopathological entities by integrating clinical features, morphology, cell phenotype, and genotype. For many entities, especially those of lymphoid origin, the cell of origin and stage of differentiation are postulated. The lymphoid classification identifies B-cell, T-cell, and natural killer (NK) cell types, and stratifies the neoplasms into precursor and mature neoplasms. For myeloid neoplasms, the cell of origin is most commonly the pluripotent stem cell. The myeloid disorders are divided into acute myeloid leukaemia, myeloproliferative neoplasms (MPN), myelodysplastic syndromes (MDS), and MDS/MPN overlap syndromes.

To diagnose and classify acute and chronic leukaemias, morphological assessment of the blood film and, usually, bone marrow aspirate are essential. The cellular morphology may be diagnostic and is used to determine which ancillary tests are required to classify the leukaemia. Establishing the cell lineage and stage of differentiation by phenotyping the neoplastic cell is implicit in the classification. Phenotyping is performed using a panel of antibodies to cellular antigens associated with specific cell types (lymphoid

---

Box 22.3.2.1 The classification of acute and chronic leukaemias (extract from WHO Classification of Tumours of Haematopoietic and Lymphoid Tissues)

Precursor lymphoid neoplasms

- B lymphoblastic leukaemia/lymphoma
- T lymphoblastic leukaemia/lymphoma

Acute myeloid leukaemias

Acute myeloid leukaemia with recurrent genetic abnormalities

- AML with t(8;21)(q22;q22); *RUNX1-RUNX1T1*
- AML with inv(16)(p13.1q22) or t(16;16)(p13.1q22); *CBFB-MYH11*
- Acute promyelocytic leukaemia with t(15;17)(q22;q12); *PML-RARA*
- AML with t(9;11) (p22;q23); *MLLT3-MLL*
- AML with t(6;9)(p23;q34); *DEK-NUP214*
- AML with inv(3)(q21q26.2) or t(3;3)(q21;q26.2); *RPN1-EVI1*
- AML (megakaryoblastic) with t(1;22)(p13;q13); *RBM15-MKL1*
- *AML with mutated NPM1*
- *AML with mutated CEBPA*

Acute myeloid leukaemia with myelodysplasia-related changes

Therapy-related myeloid neoplasms

Acute myeloid leukaemia, not otherwise specified

- Acute myeloid leukaemia with minimal differentiation
- Acute myeloid leukaemia without maturation
- Acute myeloid leukaemia with maturation
- Acute myelomonocytic leukaemia
- Acute monoblastic and monocytic leukaemia
- Acute erythroid leukemia

- Acute megakaryoblastic leukaemia
- Acute basophilic leukaemia
- Acute panmyelosis with myelofibrosis

Myeloid sarcoma

Myeloid proliferations related to Down syndrome

Acute leukaemias of ambiguous lineage

Mature B-cell neoplasms

- Chronic lymphocytic leukaemia/small lymphocytic lymphoma
- B-cell prolymphocytic leukaemia
- Hairy cell leukemia
- Burkitt lymphoma

Mature T-cell and NK-cell neoplasms

- T-cell prolymphocytic leukaemia
- T-cell large granular lymphocytic leukaemia
- Aggressive NK cell leukaemia
- Adult T-cell leukaemia/lymphoma

Myeloproliferative neoplasms

- Chronic myelogenous leukaemia, *BCR-ABL1* positive
- Chronic neutrophilic leukaemia
- Chronic eosinophilic leukaemia, NOS

Myelodysplastic/myeloproliferative neoplasms

- Chronic myelomonocytic leukaemia
- Juvenile myelomonocytic leukaemia
- Atypical chronic myeloid leukaemia, *BCR-ABL1* negative
- Mast cell leukaemia

or myeloid lineage; B-, T-, or NK-cells) and stage of differentiation (Table 22.3.2.1). Chromosomal translocations and dysregulation of specific genes are important in the pathogenesis of leukaemia. Over 50% of leukaemias have genetic abnormalities, and many of these are associated with specific oncogenes in particular types of leukaemia. The genotype is the defining property for some acute leukaemias and can be prognostically significant. In this chapter the major acute and chronic leukaemia entities defined by the WHO will be described.

Acute leukaemias

Acute leukaemias occur as a result of malignant transformation of a progenitor or stem cell, leading to the unregulated proliferation of immature (blast) cells, without differentiation, in the bone marrow. Blood involvement is common, and there may be organ infiltration, particularly of the spleen, liver, and lymph nodes. The diagnosis requires blast cells to constitute 20% or more of all of the nucleated cells in the blood or bone marrow. Generally the marrow is hypercellular and diffusely replaced by leukaemic cells.

Table 22.3.2.1 Monoclonal antibodies used for the classification of acute and chronic leukaemias

Disorder/cell type	Monoclonal antibodies
B-cell malignancies **Pan B-cell antigens**	**CD19, CD20, CD22, CD79a, CD79b, IgM, κ, λ**
B-lymphoblastic leukaemia	CD10, CD34, CD45, TdT; myeloid antigens CD13, CD33
Chronic lymphocytic leukaemia	CD5, CD23, CD38, ZAP70
B-cell prolymphocytic leukaemia	CD5, CD23
Hairy cell leukaemia	CD11c, CD25, CD103, CD123
Burkitt lymphoma	CD10, BCL6
T-cell malignancies **Pan T-cell antigens**	**CD2, CD3, CD4, CD5, CD7, CD8**
T-lymphoblastic leukaemia	CD1a, TdT; myeloid antigens CD13, CD33
T-cell prolymphocytic leukaemia	CD26
T-cell large granular lymphocytic leukaemia	CD16, CD56, CD57, CD158a,b,e
Natural killer–cell leukaemia **NK-cell antigens**	**CD2, CD7, CD8, CD16, CD56, CD57, CD158a,b,e**
Acute myeloid leukaemia **Pan-myeloid antigens**	**CD13, CD33, CD34, CD117, HLA-DR, MPO**
AML with monocytoid differentiation	CD11b, CD14, CD64, CD68, lysozyme
Acute promyelocytic leukaemia	PML protein, CD2, CD9, CD68
Erythroleukaemia	CD235, haemoglobin A
Acute megakaryoblastic leukaemia	CD41, CD42, CD61

Red indicates those antibodies that are lineage-associated.

Acute leukaemia can be lymphoid or myeloid, based on blast cell lineage (Figs. 22.3.2.1 and 22.3.2.2).

Precursor lymphoid neoplasms

Precursor lymphoid neoplasms are clonal proliferations of immature lymphoid precursors or lymphoblasts of B- or T-cell lineage. Lymphoblasts have a high nuclear to cytoplasmic ratio, fine chromatin, inconspicuous nucleoli, and usually lack cytoplasmic granules. They have an immature lymphoid cell phenotype including the presence of the intranuclear DNA polymerase terminal deoxynucleotidyl transferase (TdT).

B-lymphoblastic leukaemia

B-lymphoblastic leukaemia, previously known as B-cell acute lymphoblastic leukaemia (B-ALL), is a leukaemia of lymphoblasts committed to the B-cell lineage. This is most commonly a disease of children (75% of patients are under 6 years of age). The blood and bone marrow are involved in all cases, and there may be involvement of lymph nodes, liver, spleen, and extranodal sites. When patients present with primarily organ involvement, it is termed B-lymphoblastic lymphoma. The lymphoblasts are uniform in their appearance but can vary in size. They express B-cell–associated antigens such as CD19, cytoplasmic CD22 and CD79a, are TdT-positive, and commonly express the CD34 stem cell–associated antigen. There can be variation in the degree of differentiation of the blast cells, and this can be ascertained by the pattern of expression of the CD10 antigen. Early or 'pro-B-ALL', the least differentiated, is CD10-negative (10% of childhood and 30% of adult B-ALL cases); 'common-ALL' is CD10-positive (75% of childhood B-ALL); and 'pre-B-ALL', the most differentiated, is CD10-positive and expresses cytoplasmic μ immunoglobulin (Ig) heavy chains. The blast cells do not express surface heavy or light chains of Ig.

Cytogenetic abnormalities are important in defining prognosis. Hyperdiploidy (51–65 chromosomes) is common in children and has a good prognosis. Translocation t(12;21)(q21;q22), present in 15 to 30% of paediatric cases, but rarely in infants and adults, also has a good prognosis. This translocation generates a chimaeric *TEL-AML1* fusion gene and is associated with aberrant myeloid antigen expression (e.g. CD13 or CD33). Other genetic abnormalities have a poorer prognosis. The t(1;19)(q23;p13) translocation, involving the *PBX1* and *E2A* genes, accounts for 25% of B-ALL cases, the majority being of the pre-B-ALL type. These frequently have organomegaly and central nervous system involvement. The poorest prognosis B-ALL cases are associated with t(9;22) and *MLL* 11q23 gene rearrangements. The t(9;22)(q34;q11), resulting in the Philadelphia (Ph) chromosome and the *BCR-ABL1* fusion gene, is more common in adult (20% of cases) than paediatric B-ALL where it is uncommon (2-5%) and the fusion gene generates a p190 chimaeric protein. In adults the fusion results in a p210 chimaeric protein, the same as seen in chronic myelogenous leukaemia (CML). Translocations involving the mixed lineage leukaemia (*MLL*) gene on chromosome band 11q23 have a particularly poor prognosis. These are commonly CD10 and TdT-negative (pro-B-ALL), and gene expression profiling has demonstrated that these are derived from an early haemopoietic progenitor cell. The most common translocation involving the *MLL* gene is t(4;11)(q21;q23) which generates a hybrid *MLL-AF4* gene. This is common in infants (70% of cases) with over half of all cases under 4 years of age. The t(4;11) is associated with organomegaly and high blast cell

Acute Leukaemias

Chronic Leukaemias

LYMPHOBLASTS

MATURE
LYMPHOCYTES

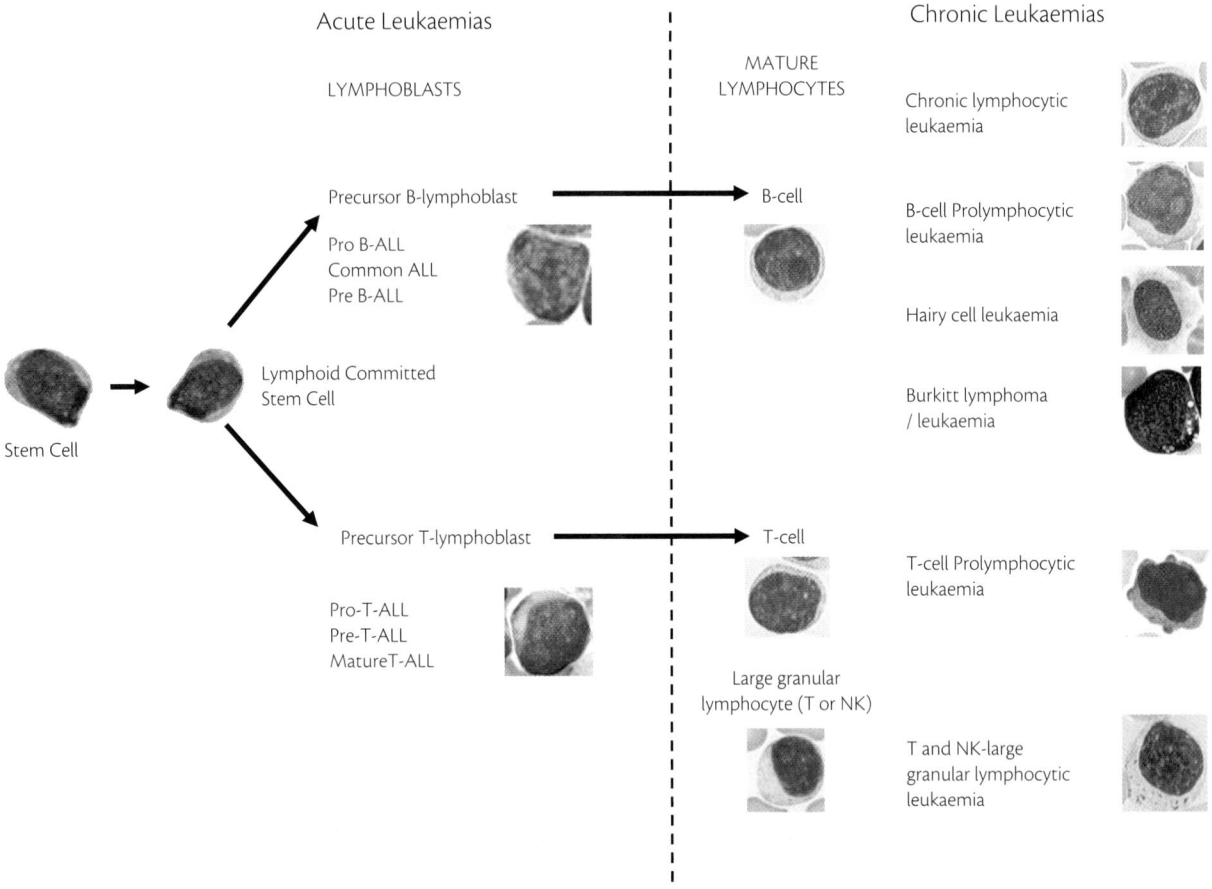

Fig. 22.3.2.1 A simplified schematic representation of lymphoid cell differentiation from the stem cell to mature lymphoid cells, showing the derivation of precursor lymphoid neoplasms (acute leukaemias) and mature lymphoid neoplasms (chronic leukaemias) of both B- and T-cell lineage.

counts at presentation. These patients go into complete remission but have an early and rapid relapse. The WHO classifies B lymphoblastic leukaemia based on these genetic features due to their distinct prognostic associations.

T-lymphoblastic leukaemia

T-lymphoblastic leukaemia or T-cell acute lymphoblastic leukaemia (T-ALL) is a leukaemia of lymphoblasts committed to the T-cell lineage. They comprise 15% of paediatric and 25% of adult ALL cases. T-ALL is more common in males than females, and is more common in adolescents than young children. It commonly presents with a high leucocyte count and organomegaly, particularly thymic enlargement, and can have less marrow involvement than B-ALL. When only nodal or extranodal sites are involved, it is termed T-lymphoblastic lymphoma. The blast cell morphology is similar to that of B-ALL. T-lymphoblasts have variable expression of T-cell–associated antigens, are TdT-positive, and rarely express CD34 antigen. T-ALL can be stratified into different stages of thymic differentiation by the pattern of T-cell antigens expressed. The most immature, or 'pro-T-ALL' (immature thymocyte), only express surface membrane CD7 and cytoplasmic CD3 antigens. Intermediate (common thymocyte), 'pre-T-ALL', express CD1a, CD2, CD5, CD7 and both CD4 and CD8 antigens. 'Mature T-ALL' (cortical thymocyte) express CD3 on the cell surface, are CD1a-negative and express either the CD4 or CD8 antigen. It remains controversial as to whether there are prognostic differences between

these subtypes. Approximately one-third of T-ALL cases have chromosomal translocations involving the *TCRα/δ* loci at 14q11 and the *TCRβ/γ* loci at 7q34. Examples include t(1;14)(p32;q11) involving the *TAL1* gene, t(10;14)(q24;q11) with the *HOX11* gene, and t(11;14)(p13;q11) involving the *RBTN2* gene. In 25% of T-ALL cases, the *TAL1* locus (1p32) is dysregulated by submicroscopic deletion.

Acute myeloid leukaemias

Acute myeloid leukaemia (AML) is a clonal expansion of myeloid blast cells (myeloblasts) in the bone marrow. Myeloblasts vary in size from slightly larger than a lymphoblast to the size of a monocyte (12-15 μm). They have variable amounts of basophilic or light grey cytoplasm which may contain azurophilic granules or Auer rods, the latter being myeloid-specific. The nuclei vary from round to ovoid, indented or convoluted, and the nuclear chromatin is fine with one or more nucleoli. The blast cell morphology is typical in some AML subtypes, such as acute promyelocytic leukaemia. Myeloperoxidase (MPO), Sudan Black B, and esterase (nonspecific and α-naphthyl acetate) cytochemical stains are variably positive. The most useful phenotypic markers are antibodies to myeloid lineage–associated antigens such as CD13, CD33, CD68, CD117, and MPO. CD34 is expressed in over 50% of cases. The AML categories in the WHO classification incorporate genetic data that define biological entities and predict clinical behaviour and outcome.

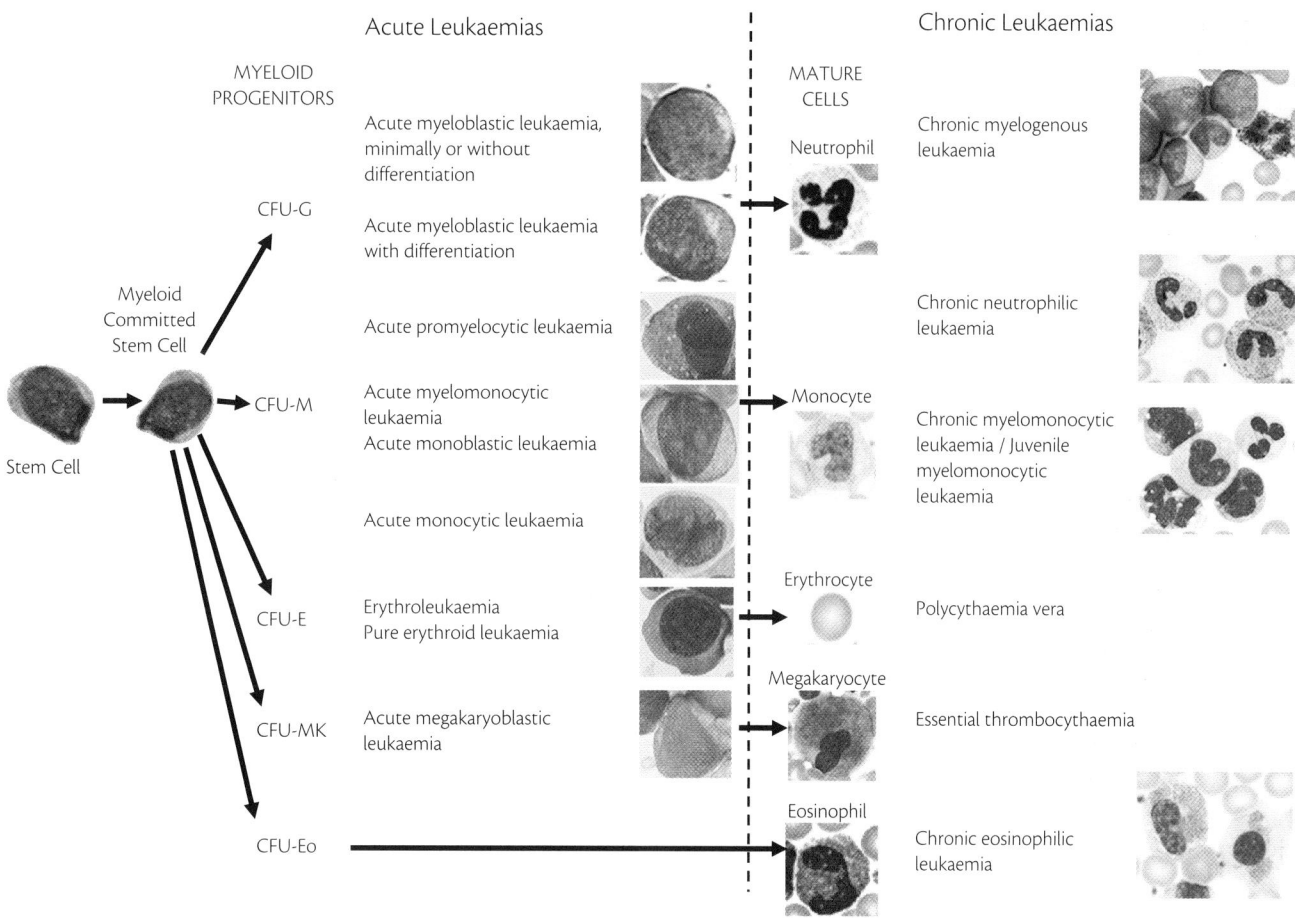

Fig. 22.3.2.2 A simplified schematic representation of myeloid cell differentiation from the stem cell to mature myeloid cells, showing the derivation of acute and chronic myeloid leukaemias.

Acute myeloid leukaemia with recurrent genetic abnormalities

This group includes AML with the recurrent genetic abnormalities t(8;21), t(15;17), inv(16) or t(16;16), t(9;11), t(6;9), inv(3) or t(3;3), t(1;22) and mutations of *NPM1* and *CEBPA*. Cases with t(8;21), t(15;17) or inv(16) represent 20 to 25% of all AML, and have a significantly better prognosis than those with normal karyotypes or other genetic abnormalities.

AML with t(8;21)(q22;q22);*AML1-ETO* occurs in 5 to 10% of AML cases, most commonly younger patients, has a high complete remission rate and long-term disease-free survival. In some cases, predominantly those in children, it presents as a myeloid sarcoma and may have little or no bone marrow involvement. The blast cells show evidence of myeloid maturation, with significant azurophilic granulation and frequent Auer rods, and there are maturing myeloid cells present in the marrow. The blast cells express myeloid-associated antigens (CD13, CD33, MPO) and are usually CD34-positive. The B-lymphoid lineage antigen CD19 (70% of cases) and CD56 are commonly expressed. The translocation involves the *AML1* (or *RUNX1*) and *ETO* genes.

AML with inv(16)(p13.1q22) or t(16;16)(p13;q22);*CBFB-MYH11* represents approximately 10% of AML cases, particularly in young adults, and has a high complete remission rate and favourable prognosis. The blast cells have both granulocytic and monocytic (myelomonocytic) differentiation. Auer rods may be present. There is a variable eosinophilia, and the eosinophils have abnormal large granules. In addition to myeloid antigens, the blast cells frequently express monocyte-associated antigens (CD11b, CD11c, CD14, CD64, and lysozyme). Both inv(16)(p13.1q22) and t(16;16) (p13;q22) result in the fusion of the *CBF*β gene (16q22) with the *MYH11* gene (16p13).

Translocation t(15;17)(q22;q12), occurs in acute promyelocytic leukaemia (APML), and accounts for 5 to 8% of AML cases, predominantly in middle-aged adults. The leukaemic cells have characteristic morphology being large with reniform or bilobed nuclei, heavily granulated cytoplasm, and may contain bundles of Auer rods ('faggot cells'). Less granulated cases occur and are called microgranular or hypogranular APML. The immunophenotype is characteristic with strong homogeneous CD33 expression, heterogeneous CD13, CD117, and MPO, and frequent expression of CD2 antigen. CD34 and HLA-DR are negative. The PML protein shows a nuclear microgranular pattern by immunofluorescent microscopy. The t(15;17) generates a *PML-RARA* fusion gene. APML is sensitive to all-*trans* retinoic acid, a differentiation-inducing agent, and has a favourable prognosis. Patients with less common variant translocations such as t(11;17)(q23;q12), which also involve *RARA*, usually lack the typical APML morphology and do not respond to all-*trans* retinoic acid.

AML with t(9;11); *MLL T3-MLL* have an intermediate prognosis. These occur in approximately 5% of AML cases and are most common in children, with a particularly high frequency in infants (aged under 1 year) and in therapy-related AML. They generally have monocytic and myelomonocytic morphology. The phenotype is nonspecific, expressing myeloid-associated antigens (CD13 and CD33) and monocyte-associated antigens (CD11b, CD14, CD64, and lysozyme); CD34 is negative. Variant MLL translocations also occur e.g. t(11;19); *MLL-ELL*.

In addition to chromosomal translocations, specific gene mutations also occur as recurrent genetic abnormalities in AML. Mutations in the *NPM1* gene occur in approximately one-third of AML and are associated with monocytoid morphology, CD34-negative and better prognosis. They occur most commonly in middle-aged females. *CEBPA* mutations occur in 6-15% of AML and have no gender or morphologic association. Mutations in *FLT3* are not associated with a specific AML type but have prognostic association.

Acute myeloid leukaemia with myelodysplasia-related changes

AML with myelodysplasia-related changes predominantly occur in elderly patients, presents with pancytopenia, and has a poor prognosis. It may evolve from a myelodysplastic syndrome or arise apparently *de novo*. In addition to blast cells, there is dysplasia in more than 50% of cells of two or more bone marrow lineages (i.e. erythroid, granulocyte, and megakaryocyte). The blast cells are generally CD34-positive myeloblasts (CD13, CD33 positive). The commonest chromosomal abnormalities are –5/del(5q–) and myeloid neoplasms –7/del(7q).

Therapy-related myeloid neoplasms

Therapy related AML occurs following exposure to cytotoxic chemotherapy and/or radiotherapy. These are thought to be the consequence of mutations secondary to cytotoxic therapy.

AML secondary to alkylating drugs or radiotherapy occur 5 to 6 years following exposure and may be preceded by myelodysplasia. Morphologically, these cases have over 20% myeloblasts and dysplasia of all myeloid cell lines. Abnormalities of chromosomes 5 and 7 are common.

AML following treatment with drugs targeting topoisomerase II (e.g. etoposide, teniposide, and anthracyclines) has a short latency (median 33 months) without a preceding myelodysplastic phase. Most cases have a monocytoid or myelomonocytic morphology and phenotype. They have balanced translocations and often involve the *MLL* gene.

Acute myeloid leukaemia not otherwise specified

This category in the WHO classification encompasses those cases that do not fulfil the criteria of the above-mentioned AML groups. They are largely classified according to FAB definitions, with some additions (Table 22.3.2.1; Fig. 22.3.2.2).

Acute myeloid leukaemia with minimal differentiation

These have no morphological or cytochemical evidence of myeloid differentiation. Their myeloid lineage can only be ascertained by the expression of one or more myeloid-associated antigens e.g. CD13, CD33. This entity, formerly known as FAB M0, comprises approximately 5% of AML cases, mostly adult.

Acute myeloid leukaemia without maturation

The blast cells are poorly differentiated (FAB M1) but do have some morphological (e.g. azurophilic granules and Auer rods) and cytochemical (MPO and Sudan Black B positivity) evidence of myeloid differentiation. They express myeloid-associated antigens but not monocyte antigens.

Acute myeloid leukaemia with maturation

The blast cells commonly have cytoplasmic granules and Auer rods, and there is morphological evidence of maturation to mature neutrophils (FAB M2). Many cases have t(8;21) and are therefore included in the group defined by the cytogenetic abnormality. Other cases may have a bone marrow basophilia together with abnormalities in chromosome 12p or t(6;9)(p23;q34) resulting in a chimaeric *DEK-CAN* fusion gene, one of the recurrent genetic abnormalities in AML.

Acute myelomonocytic leukaemia

This subtype (FAB M4) comprises 15 to 25% of AML cases and has blasts with both myeloblast and monoblast morphology. Neutrophils and their precursors, and monocytes and their precursors, each comprise at least 20% of marrow cells. Nonspecific genetic abnormalities are present in the majority of cases. Cases with inv(16) occur and are included in the group with recurrent genetic abnormalities.

Acute monoblastic and monocytic leukaemia

These are defined by over 80% of the blast cells having monocytoid features. In acute monoblastic leukaemia (FAB M5a) these are monoblasts, whereas in acute monocytic leukaemia (FAB M5b) they are more mature promonocytes. The blast cells may show haemophagocytosis. There is variable expression of monocyte-associated antigens; specifically CD64 is commonly expressed but CD14 only by more the mature monocytic cases. Chromosomal translocations involving chromosome band 11q23 are common.

Acute erythroid leukaemia

There are 2 rare AML subtypes with a predominant erythroid population (FAB M6). In erythroleukaemia (erythroid/myeloid) greater than 50% of cells in the marrow are erythroid progenitors, and, more than 20% of nonerythroid cells are myeloblasts. Pure erythroid leukaemia is a neoplastic proliferation of committed primitive erythroid cells (>80% of marrow cells) that express CD235 (glycophorin A) and haemoglobin A and in which there is no myeloblastic population.

Acute megakaryoblastic leukaemia

In this uncommon form of AML (FAB M7), the blast cell morphology is not diagnostic. The megakaryocyte lineage is identified by expression of one or more platelet glycoproteins (CD41, CD42, and CD61). In the marrow the blasts are commonly accompanied by dysplastic megakaryocytes.

Other acute myeloid leukaemias

Other rare forms of AML in the WHO classification are acute basophilic leukaemia, acute panmyelosis with myelofibrosis, and myeloid sarcoma, a myeloid tumour developing in an extramedullary site. Acute leukaemias of ambiguous lineage are leukaemias where the morphology, cytochemistry, and phenotype either lack sufficient evidence to ascribe lineage (acute undifferentiated leukaemia), or the blast cells are of mixed lineage (biphenotypic or bilineal).

Chronic leukaemias

Chronic leukaemias are the proliferation of mature-appearing malignant cells with morphology resembling normal blood cells. As in the acute leukaemias, these can be lymphoid or myeloid (Box 22.3.2.1; Figs. 22.3.2.1 and 22.3.2.2).

Mature B-cell neoplasms

Mature B-cell neoplasms include leukaemias (chronic B-cell leukaemias) and B-cell non-Hodgkin lymphomas. The chronic B-cell leukaemias are clonal proliferations of mature, surface immunoglobulin-positive B cells that involve the blood and bone marrow and are generally indolent. Four main types of chronic B-cell leukaemia, each with a relatively distinctive morphology and immunological profile will be described. Several types of B-cell non-Hodgkin lymphoma can present with, or evolve into, a leukaemic phase (i.e. circulating lymphoma cells >5×10^9/litre).

Chronic lymphocytic leukaemia

Chronic lymphocytic leukaemia (CLL) is the commonest leukaemia in the Western world and occurs in adults. It is characterized by monomorphic, small, round lymphocytes with clumped chromatin and minimal cytoplasm, together with a small number of prolymphocytes. The cells express B-cell antigens (CD19, weak CD20, and CD22), CD5, CD23, and weak IgM. Expression of ZAP70 and CD38, and genetic abnormalities (e.g. p53 and 11q deletions) assist in determining prognosis.

B-cell prolymphocytic leukaemia

B-cell prolymphocytic leukaemia (B-PLL) is rare in comparison with CLL. It presents in elderly patients, predominantly men, with marked splenomegaly and minimal lymphadenopathy, and has a poor prognosis. The neoplastic cell is larger than in CLL and is round with a centrally placed nucleus, single prominent nucleolus, and basophilic cytoplasm. The cells strongly express surface IgM and B-cell antigens; CD5 is present in one-third and CD23 is negative.

Hairy cell leukaemia

Hairy cell leukaemia (HCL) is a rare leukaemia that occurs primarily in middle-aged men, is indolent and potentially curable. It is typically associated with pancytopenia, splenomegaly, and fibrotic marrow. The leukaemic cells are of intermediate size due to abundant irregular grey cytoplasm with 'hairy' projections. The nuclei are eccentrically located and have a reniform shape. They have a characteristic phenotype with strong B-cell antigens, and express CD11c, CD103, CD123 and CD25 antigens. They have cytochemical tartrate-resistant acid phosphatase positivity.

Burkitt lymphoma

Burkitt lymphoma (BL), formerly classified as an acute leukaemia in the FAB classification, is a mature B-cell neoplasm derived from a germinal centre B-cell. It is highly aggressive, but potentially curable, and commonly has blood and bone marrow involvement. The cells are round, of intermediate size, and have intensely basophilic vacuolated cytoplasm and prominent nucleoli. They express B-cell associated antigens (CD19, CD20, strong Ig heavy and light chains), CD10, and BCL6. A characteristic feature of BL is that over 90% of cells are in cell cycle. They are TdT- and CD34-negative. BL is characterized by t(8;14)(q24;q32) resulting in a *MYC-IgH* fusion gene. Alternative translocations, t(2;8)(p12;q224) and t(8;22)(q24;q11), involve the *MYC* and κ and λ light chain genes, respectively. Gene expression profile analysis has shown BL to have a distinct molecular signature.

Mature T-cell and natural killer cell neoplasms

Mature T-cell neoplasms, derived from mature post-thymic T-cells, and NK-cell neoplasms are both rare and are grouped together in the WHO classification, as they are phenotypically similar. Those with a predominant leukaemic phase are termed chronic leukaemias. Sézary syndrome, a cutaneous T-cell lymphoma, and adult T-cell leukaemia/lymphoma are two T-cell non-Hodgkin's lymphomas that commonly develop a leukaemic phase.

T-cell prolymphocytic leukaemia

T-cell prolymphocytic leukaemia (T-PLL) is an aggressive leukaemia of mature post-thymic T-cells characterized by hepatosplenomegaly and high leucocyte counts. The disease has a progressive course, but indolent forms are also reported. The neoplastic cells are small with irregular outline, convoluted or indented nuclei with a nucleolus, and basophilic cytoplasm with protrusions. T-PLL cells express T-cell antigens (CD2, CD3, CD5, strong CD7) and are generally CD4-positive. In 30% of cases both CD4 and CD8 antigens are expressed, and rarely, they express CD8 and lack CD4. Up to 90% of T-PLL have inversions of chromosome 14 with breakpoints at 14q11, the *TCRα/β* locus, and 14q32, the *TCL1* and *TCL1b* loci.

Large granular lymphocytic leukaemias

Large granular lymphocytic leukaemias (LGL) of T- or NK-cell type are defined by a persistent (>6 months) unexplained lymphocytosis of large granular lymphocytes. T-LGL are associated with autoantibodies (25% of cases), have an indolent course, and morbidity is generally due to neutropenia. The cells resemble normal large granular lymphocytes, have a mature T-cell phenotype and have rearranged T-cell receptor genes. 80% of cases are CD8-positive and CD4-negative. They have variable expression of NK-cell–associated antigens, especially CD16 and CD57, and restricted expression of only one of the CD158 isoforms a, b, or e. Chronic NK-cell LGL has a similar morphology to T-cell LGL, expresses NK-associated antigens (CD16, CD56, CD57), but does not express T-cell–associated antigens or have rearranged T-cell receptor genes.

Aggressive NK-cell leukaemia

This is a rare, aggressive leukaemia, more common in Asia than the West, and the Epstein–Barr virus is thought to be pathogenic in many cases. The neoplastic cells are large and pleiomorphic with irregular hyperchromatic nuclei and basophilic granulated cytoplasm. They have variable expression of NK-cell antigens.

Chronic leukaemias of myeloid origin

Chronic leukaemias of myeloid origin fall into one of two WHO categories. The first, the myeloproliferative neoplasms (MPN), includes chronic myelogenous leukaemia (CML), chronic neutrophilic leukaemia (CNL), chronic eosinophilic leukaemia (CEL) and mast cell leukaemia. These are clonal haematopoietic stem cell disorders with essentially normal morphology of the endstage cell. The type of chronic leukaemia is defined by the lineage of the predominant proliferating cell. The second, the myelodysplastic/myeloproliferative neoplasms, consists of chronic myelomonocytic leukaemia (CMML), juvenile myelomonocytic leukaemia (JMML), and atypical chronic myeloid leukaemia (aCML). These all have dysplastic morphology as well as proliferative features.

Chronic myelogenous leukaemia, BCR-ABL1 positive

CML is a clonal myeloproliferative neoplasm defined by the presence of the hybrid *BCR-ABL1* fusion gene which results from the reciprocal t(9;22)(q34;q11) translocation. Splenomegaly is characteristic. The blood has a leucocytosis with granulocytic cells at all stages of differentiation present. Myelocytes and mature neutrophils predominate, basophilia is characteristic, and eosinophilia common. Blast cells are present but make up fewer than 5% of cells in the chronic phase of the disease. The bone marrow is markedly hypercellular with granulocytic hyperplasia (myeloid to erythroid ratio >10:1) with normal differentiation. Megakaryocytes are increased and are characteristically small ('dwarf') with bilobed nuclei. The diagnosis is confirmed by the presence of the Ph chromosome and BCR-ABL1. Accelerated phase of CML is defined by one or more of the following: progressive leucocytosis, increasing spleen size, an increase in blast cells (10–19%), basophilia, persistent thrombocytopenia or unresponsive thrombocytosis, and cytogenetic evidence of clonal evolution. Blast phase resembles acute leukaemia with over 20% of blast cells in the marrow and can be of myeloblastic or lymphoblastic type.

Chronic eosinophilic leukaemia

CEL is a rare myeloproliferative neoplasm characterized by a blood eosinophilia with atypia. The eosinophils are hypogranular with abnormal cytoplasmic distribution of the granules. An internal deletion of chromosome band 4q12, which results in a FIP1L1-PDGFRA fusion gene, defines CEL, and these patients generally respond to tyrosine kinase inhibitors. CEL cases with the FIP1L1-PDGFRA mutation are included in the WHO entity Myeloid and Lymphoid Neoplasms with Eosinophilia and abnormalities of PDGFRA, PDGFRB or FGFR1 due to the clinical and therapeutic relevance of these recently described genetic mutations associated with eosinophilia.

Chronic neutrophilic leukaemia

CNL is a rare, slowly progressive myeloproliferative disorder with a marked neutrophil leucocytosis without immature forms. Some cases have the t(9;22), but, in contrast to CML, the BCR-ABL1 rearrangement results in a p230, rather than a p210, protein product.

Mast cell leukaemia

This is a rare disorder where neoplastic mast cells account for 10% or more of peripheral blood leucocytes and over 20% of nucleated cells in the marrow.

Chronic myelomonocytic leukaemia and juvenile myelomonocytic leukaemia

CMML is characterized by a blood monocytosis ($>1 \times 10^9$/litre) with dysplastic features, granulocytic hyperplasia in the marrow, and less than 5% blast cells. It occurs in older adults, generally over 70 years. Although there are no characteristic chromosomal abnormalities, some patients have t(5;12) generating the PDGFRB-TEL fusion gene. Survival is variable and largely determined by the blast cell count. JMML occurs in children under 4 years of age, and the morphology is similar to CMML. Monosomy 7 occurs in 15% of cases, and 10% of affected children have neurofibromatosis. The prognosis of JMML is generally poor if untreated, and bone marrow transplantation is the only therapy that improves survival.

Atypical chronic myeloid leukaemia, BCR-ABL1 negative

Atypical CML defines those patients with high leucocyte counts who are Ph chromosome and BCR-ABL1 negative. The morphological features are more heterogeneous than CML, there is granulocytic dysplasia and a mild monocytosis, and, notably, there is no basophilia.

Conclusion

This chapter highlights that there are many subtypes of leukaemia which can be identified based on cell morphology and biological characteristics. It is important to distinguish between these entities because of therapeutic and prognostic differences. The WHO Classification has highlighted the significance of both cell phenotype and genetics in the definition of these diseases.

With the pace of progress of medical science, the WHO Classification will require periodical review and updating. New discoveries will continue to be made, and new disease subtypes will be defined, requiring inclusion in the classification. The WHO classification can, therefore, not be regarded as the definitive classification of leukaemia.

Further reading

Bain BJ, Fletch SJ (2007). Chronic eosinophilic leukemias and the myeloproliferative variant of the hypereosinophilic syndrome. *Immunol Allergy Clin North Am*, **27**, 377–88.

Bennett JM, et al. (1976). Proposals for the classification of the acute leukaemias. *Br J Haematol*, **33**, 451–8.

Bennett JM, et al. (1985). Criteria for the diagnosis of acute leukemia of megakaryocyte lineage (M7). *Ann Intern Med*, **103**, 460–2.

Bennett JM, et al. (1991). Proposal for the recognition of minimally differentiated acute myeloid leukaemia (AML-M0). *Br J Haematol*, **78**, 325–9.

Bullinger L, et al. (2007). Gene-expression profiling identifies distinct subclasses of core binding factor acute myeloid leukemia. *Blood*, **110**, 1291–1300.

Farahat N, et al. (1994). Demonstration of cytoplasmic and nuclear antigens in acute leukaemia using flow cytometry. *J Clin Pathol*, **47**, 843–9.

Falini B, et al. (2005). Cytoplasmic nucleophosmin in acute myelogenous leukemia with a normal karyotype. *N Engl J Med*, **352**, 254–66.

Hummel M, et al. (2006). A biologic definition of Burkitt's lymphoma from transcriptional and genomic profiling. *N Engl J Med*, **354**, 2419–30.

Jaffe ES, et al. (2001). World Health Organization classification of tumours: pathology and genetics of tumours of haematopoietic and lymphoid tissues. IARC Press, Dijon.

Löwenberg B, Downing JR, Burnett A (1999). Acute myeloid leukaemia. *N Engl J Med*, **341**, 1051–62.

Macdonald D, Cross NC (2007). Chronic myeloproliferative disorders: the role of tyrosine kinases in pathogenesis, diagnosis and therapy. *Pathobiology*, 74, 81–8.

Melo JV (1996). The diversity of BCR–ABL fusion proteins and their relationship to leukemia phenotype. *Blood*, **88**, 2375–84.

Oshimi K (2007). Progress in understanding and managing natural killer-cell malignancies. *Br J Haematol*, **139**, 532–44.

Preudhomme C, et al. (2005). Favorable prognostic significance of CEBPA mutations in patients with de novo acute myeloid leukemia: a study from the Acute Leukemia French Association (ALFA). *Clin Cancer Res*, **11**, 1416–24.

Rowley JD (2000). Molecular genetics in acute leukemia. *Leukemia*, **14**, 513–17.

Swerdlow SH, et al. (2008). WHO Classification of Tumours of Haematopoietic and Lymphoid Tissues. IARC Press, Lyon.

22.3.3 Acute lymphoblastic leukaemia

Tim Eden

Essentials

Genetic changes in key progenitor cells in acute lymphoblastic leukaemia (ALL) are typically either point mutations or (more frequently) translocation of proto-oncogenes to active promoter sites, with such genetic rearrangements leading to aberrant protein production. In most childhood disease the first genetic events arise *in utero*, with one or more further events usually being required to convert a preleukaemic clone or clones into overt ALL.

Clinical features and diagnosis

Clinical features—typical presentation is with manifestations including pallor, petechiae/bruising, fever with or without lymphadenopathy, and abdominal and/or limb pain (arising from organ or bone infiltration). Life-threatening risks include Gram-negative or -positive septicaemia and fungaemia, bleeding (especially into the brain), and tumour lysis.

Diagnosis—the key investigations are examination of peripheral blood and bone marrow for blast cell infiltration. Immunophenotyping, cytogenetics, and gene expression arrays are important in defining subsets with variable prognostic and drug resistance profiles.

Treatment and prognosis

Treatment—aside from supportive care, the key requirements are (1) induction and consolidation of remission—usually with steroids (dexamethasone), vincristine, and L-asparaginase, sometimes with the addition of an anthracycline in high risk patients; (2) or treatment directed to the central nervous system—repeated administration of intrathecal methotrexate. Only very high risk patients including some older adults now require cranial irradiation; (3) delayed intensification and maintenance of remission—long-term survival is improved by giving pulses of second-line drugs (e.g. cytarabine, cyclophosphamide), along with more steroids, vincristine and L-asparaginase; and sometimes (4) intensive therapy followed by allogeneic bone marrow transplantation—considered for patients whose disease is refractory or relapse quickly.

Prognosis—the single most important factor is the highest white cell count recorded at presentation before introduction of any intervention—those in whom it is >50 × 10^9/litre fare worse than those with lower counts. Most children with ALL can be cured, but 20 to 25% relapse, many unpredictably. Improvement in survival has been less marked in adults, but appears to be getting better with use of more sustained, continuous therapy rather than the previously adopted 'pulsed' regimen of cytotoxic treatment. Identification of minimal residual disease by new molecular technology and stratification of therapy consequently has enabled reduction of intensivity of therapy for low risk and escalation for high risk patients.

Introduction

After Sidney Farber and his team (1947/8) showed that the folic acid antagonist aminopterin could induce temporary remission in acute lymphoblastic leukaemia of childhood, the search for other active agents started. The therapeutic value of adrenal corticoid steroids (1949, especially prednisolone), thiopurines (1953), methotrexate (1956, replacing aminopterin) and vincristine (1962) heralded in the era of potential cure.

The concept of total therapy was pioneered by Pinkel *et al.* at St Jude Children's Research Hospital in Memphis (United States of America) and encompassed remission induction, consolidation of remission, central nervous system disease control, and maintenance or continuing therapy. Emphasis was on sustained, almost continuous therapy rigorously applied without significant gaps in therapy. The result has been an improvement in survival from little expectation of cure in the 1960s to over 80% survival for children in resource-rich countries in the 21st century. For teenagers and adults the success has been more limited but recent strict adherence to 'paediatric' protocols has improved their survival also by 15 to 20%. Previous approaches in adults involved more intermittent pulsed therapy which may have allowed malignant cell recovery as well as recovery from myelosuppression.

No 'curative' new agents have been identified since the early 1970s although a few 'possible' drugs are currently under investigation, some of which may offer the possibility of targeted therapy and toxicity reduction within protocols which are inevitably intensive and aggressive. Most emphasis has been on better delivery of standard drugs. Rapidity of blood and bone marrow clearance of leukaemic cells, more recently supplemented by molecular identification of minimal residual disease (not visible by conventional microscopy) has facilitated stratification of patients into standard, high, and very high risk groupings. Nevertheless, numerically most relapses still occur in standard-risk patients. Trying to understand why is the focus of much current research. Most adults with acute lymphoblastic anaemia (ALL) fit into the high or very high risk groupings. Current 'curative' therapy is also only available to about 20% of the children worldwide who acquire ALL. Most children and adults affected by acute leukaemia in the world do not even receive any supportive or palliative care.

Reduction in induction and remission deaths has contributed to the improved survival, and involves vigilance, early, and intensive support for febrile patients with antimicrobial prophylaxis, e.g. use of cotrimoxazole for prevention of pneumocystis infection.

Presentation and diagnosis

Historically, ALL has been diagnosed by clinical suspicion followed by peripheral blood and bone marrow examination for blast cell infiltration.

Growth and proliferation of lymphoid precursors arrested at an immature stage of differentiation suppress production of normal bone marrow cells. This causes thrombocytopenia and bleeding/petechiae, myelosuppression and immunosuppression increasing risk of infection, fever and anaemia. The classic presentation is with a constellation of signs and symptoms including pallor, petechiae/bruising, fever with or without lymphadenopathy (including mediastinal swelling in T cell ALL) and abdominal and/or limb pain. The latter arise from organ or bone infiltration with leukaemia. About 3 to 5% of patients present with overt central nervous system infiltration. Hepatosplenomegaly is variable but more frequently seen in childhood ALL (especially in T-ALL and mature B-ALL disease). Organ infiltration of the liver and kidneys can complicate diagnosis and induction of remission. Especially if the white cell count is high, tumour lysis syndrome (hyperkalaemia, hyperuricaemia, uraemia, hyperphosphataemia and hypocalcaemia) can occur before the start of treatment or concurrent with it. Presentation with joint swelling and pain can cause confusion with rheumatoid arthritis. Isolated lytic and/or sclerotic bone lesions are not unusually seen in childhood and may lead to vertebral body collapse.

At presentation and during the induction phase of treatment, there are several life-threatening risks: Gram-negative or -positive septicaemia and fungaemia; bleeding (especially into the brain) and tumour lysis. Childhood early death rates have fallen from 9 to 10% in the 1980s to about 1% currently.

Diagnosis should be prompt and appropriate measures put in place to hydrate and support the patient whilst blast cell typing is taking place.

The French–American–British (FAB) staging classification into three subtypes—L1 (small monomorphic cells), L2 (large heterogeneous cells), and L3 (Burkitt-like cells with deeply basophilic cytoplasm and vacuoles)—is useful in separating out mature B-cell leukaemia, which requires quite different treatment, but is no longer used for stratification of other subtypes. Immunophenotyping, (increasingly using flow cytometry), cytogenetics, and gene expression arrays have become more important in defining subsets with variable prognostic and resistance profiles. In childhood about 75% of cases are of precursor B cell type (CD10, CD 19, HLA DR, and Tdt positivity); in adults about 50%. Coexpression of one or more myeloid markers (e.g. CD 13, CD 33, CDw 65) is not of prognostic significance and does not denote a true mixed lineage leukaemia. About 10 to 15% of all ALL cases express cytoplasmic immunoglobulin and are designated pre-B-ALL. T-cell phenotype (CD 7, CD 2 and/or CD 1 positivity) accounts for 11 to 12% of childhood cases and roughly double that in adults. Mature B-cell leukaemia requires a completely different lymphoma-type therapeutic approach from that used in precursor B, pre-B-, and T-ALL, all of which respond to sustained continuous therapy.

The greatest advance in subtype definition and prognostication has come from the definition of the genetic subtypes which vary in frequency between children and adults. These represent aberrant expression of proto-oncogenes, fusion genes resulting from chromosomal translocations (usually encoding for transcription factors or kinases) and chromosomal replication (e.g. high hyperdiploidy with >50 chromosomes). In childhood B-ALL, high hyperploidy is seen in about 25% of cases; t(12;21) (*TEL-AML1* fusion gene) in 22%; both with favourable outcome on current therapy; and 3% with t(9;22) (*BCR-ABL1*); 8% with MLL rearrangements (especially t(4;11), t(11;19), or t(9;11) and 1% with hypodiploidy (<45 chromosomes); all with more adverse outcome. In adults the percentages are 7%, 2%, 25%, 10%, and 2%. The higher incidence of adverse prognostic groups goes some way to explain the poorer outcome in adult ALL. In T-ALL not only is the overall incidence higher in adults, but, in most, T-cell receptor genes are rearranged and there is an increased expression of certain *HOX* genes (50% *NOTCH1*). Given the relatively poor survival with standard treatment, especially in adults, the involvement of these genes is exciting interest as targets for novel therapeutic approaches. In the last few years a new subgroup with intrachromosomal amplification of chromosome 21 (iAMP21) which represents about 2% of ALL cases in childhood has been identified with an adverse prognosis, at least on standard therapy, but treatment intensification appears to have reduced relapse rates. How frequently this is seen in adults is as yet unknown.

Prognostic factors

The single most important prognostic factor is the highest white cell count recorded at presentation before introduction of any intervention. Those with a white blood cell count greater than 50×10^9/litre fare worse than those with lower counts. Patients under 1 year and over 10 years of age fare worse. As already mentioned, part of the reason for older patients having a worse prognosis is the increasing frequency of adverse molecular rearrangements with associated resistance patterns, but reports also suggest poorer tolerance of therapy, decreased adherence to therapy especially following greater experienced toxicity, and less effective treatment regimens, traditionally used in adults partially because of worries about such toxicity. The impact of genetic factors has been alluded to for leukaemias involving *BCR-ABL1*, *MLL* gene rearrangements, and hypodiploidy, and all three present a special therapeutic challenge. For all these subtypes treatment has improved and individual prognostic factors have altered in their significance.

Management

The key elements of successful management of ALL are good supportive care— induction of remission and consolidation of remission; treatment directed to the central nervous system; delayed intensification; and maintenance of remission with a total duration of therapy of 2 to 3 years for most patients. Treatment of any presenting infection, alkalinization of urine especially for high-risk patients, with the use of allopurinol or urate oxidase (to reduce the risks of hyperphosphataemia and hyperuricaemia respectively), are essential before treatment is started. Once diagnosis is established, transfusion of red cells and platelets for any mucosal haemorrhages or overt bleeding are important supportive measures. An initial platelet count less than 50×10^9/litre requires transfusion before the diagnostic lumbar puncture is carried out. The presence of blast cells in cerebrospinal fluid requires more aggressive intrathecal therapy with methotrexate and is one of the few current indications for cranial radiotherapy, especially in adult ALL.

The three most useful induction agents are steroids, vincristine, and L-asparaginase. Recent evidence suggests that dexamethasone is more effective than prednisolone (the traditional steroid used) especially because of its greater penetrance into brain tissue. Older patients appear to have greater steroid toxicity (especially avascular necrosis of weight-bearing joints, e.g. hips and knees) and either capping of dosage or intermittent high-dose courses are recommended for them. Traditionally steroids have been given for 4 weeks orally along with five to six doses of intravenous vincristine. L-Asparaginase is a crucial element of treatment but carries with it risks of overt anaphylaxis, silent neutralizing antibody production, coagulation disorders, and pancreatitis. The most effective formulation providing some protection against antibody production in induction is the peglyated form of *Escherichia coli* asparaginase, with a half life of 5.7 days. This means that fewer injections are required (two in induction rather than six to nine with native asparaginase) and more effective depletion achieved of the essential amino acid asparagine which appears essential for efficacy. The exact mechanism of action of L-asparaginase is still in doubt. A percentage of patients (20–25%), mostly with high-risk ALL, have blasts secreting proteases which cleave asparaginase, producing both greater risk of inactivation and anaphylaxis. Dexamethasone and asparaginase have some synergy. For high or very high risk patients the addition of an anthracycline, doxorubicin or daunorubicin, is recommended. In childhood ALL remission rates of 93 to 96% are now achieved, but rates are slightly lower in adults. The speed of early response is used for stratification of patients. Traditionally this is measured by peripheral blood and marrow clearance, but in the modern era minimal residual disease monitoring, by molecular or flow cytometric measures, has been added. Those with slow early responses require greater intensification of therapy, and very slow responders or refractory patients appear to benefit from subsequent bone marrow transplantation. However in childhood the proportion of patients who require such therapy is ever decreasing. In those with *BCR-ABL1*, hypodiploid, and *MLL* gene rearrangement ALL it is a more likely requirement for cure. For those under 1 year of age with *MLL* gene rearrangements (most commonly t 4:11) a combination of ALL and AML-type therapy appears to be yielding better results.

Intrathecal methotrexate given two or three times during induction at 2-weekly intervals (weekly if overt blasts are present) followed by ongoing intrathecal therapy during the first year of treatment has replaced traditional cranial irradiation (18–24 Gy) in childhood because of the latter's neurotoxicity and effects on growth. More effective delivery of steroids and asparaginase contributes to better control of disease in the central nervous system (failure rate now <2% in children and 5% in adults). There is more toxicity with triple intrathecal therapy (methotrexate, hydrocortisone, and cytosine arabinoside) without obvious benefit.

Post-remission consolidation and use of intensification pulses of sustained treatment principally with second-line drugs such as cytarabine and cyclophosphamide along with more steroids, vincristine, and L-asparaginase has improved long-term survival to 75 to 80% in children. For the reasons outlined before, results are still less favourable in teenagers and adults than in childhood. The reduction in use of pulsed therapy and adoption of 'childhood'-type protocols has been shown to increase survival in younger adults and is now being tested in those up to 50 years. Control of lymphoblastic leukaemia appears to be improved with sustained, almost continuous immunosuppression, without marked myelosuppression. Prolonged neutropenia enhances the risk of sepsis and death while at the same time affording leukaemic blasts time to recover. The number of intensification modules required is currently being tested in randomized clinical trials.

In childhood ALL any attempt to shorten the length of continuing therapy (maintenance) to less than 2 years has decreased survival. Its effectiveness using oral methotrexate weekly and daily thiopurine, (usually 6-mercaptopurine), probably reflects influences on immune function and/or on bone marrow stroma cells rather than any ability to kill blast cells directly.

Truly refractory patients and those relapsing early on treatment or within 6 months of stopping therapy are considered for intensive therapy followed by allogeneic bone marrow transplantation (BMT). No clear benefit from autologous BMT has been demonstrated in patients with ALL. Effective cytoreductive therapy, prevention of anti-graft-vs-host and infection control have improved disease and event-free survival after marrow transplantation, but still the risks outweigh the benefits in most childhood and young adult ALL patients, unless they have true refractory disease. A combination of relapses after BMT and death from infection/or graft-vs-host disease still result in 25 to 30% mortality; with matched related and unrelated donor BMT having similar outcomes in the modern era.

Continuing challenges

The remarkable success of what has essentially been empirical treatment has characterized much fruitful development, but we are left with the challenges of the unpredictable relapses among patients with 'low risk' features (numerically the largest group) and of very high risk ALL. Some of the 'unpredictable' relapses have been identified as being due to novel genetic rearrangements such as those occurring in the iAMP21 ALL group. For such patients intensive therapy and particularly the use of higher dose methotrexate and/or more effective asparaginase appears to have improved survival. Delivering each agent most effectively has improved disease control to its current high point, at least in childhood ALL. Can understanding of the genetic alterations leading to ALL also provide clues to novel ways of treatment?

Leukaemogenesis and novel therapies

It is now recognized that in most childhood ALL (and possibly AML) the first genetic events in key progenitor cells arise *in utero* but that one or more further events are usually required to convert a preleukaemic clone or clones into overt ALL. Response to infection may play a part in promoting development of ALL. Whether this sequence leads to ALL in older age is not yet known, but all events may occur postnatally. Those initial genetic changes alter cellular functioning, e.g. by facilitating unlimited capacity for self-renewal; altering the controls on proliferation; blocking partially or completely differentiation; and/or providing resistance to apoptosis. The BCR-ABL1 fusion protein seen in Philadelphia-positive ALL is a kinase that affects the signalling pathways which do indeed control cell proliferation, survival, and self-renewal. Identification of the kinase not only facilitates diagnosis of this form of ALL but an inhibitor of BCR-ABL1 tyrosine kinase has been produced (imatinib mesylate) which can inhibit blast growth and contribute to apoptosis. Alternative BCR-ABL1 kinase inhibitors are in trial. Good response rates (70%) in BCR-ABL1-positive ALL and in chronic myeloid leukaemia are observed with imatinib, but with time resistance can develop. Hence the search for alternative ways to inhibit the fusion product. Current trials are testing long-term efficacy of inhibition given in addition to standard ALL therapy.

Most of the genetic changes identified in ALL involve oncogenes rather than tumour suppressor malfunction. Such genetic rearrangement, due either to point mutations or, more frequently, translocation of proto-oncogenes to active promoter sites, leads to aberrant protein production.

The *TEL-AML1* fusion gene seen in 20 to 25% of childhood ALL cases but only in a small minority of adult ALL combines the *TEL* gene involved in the homing of progenitors to the marrow and *AML1*, which is a DNA-binding component of the heterodimeric transcription factor core binding factor (CBFα plus CBFβ), with its crucial role in haematopoiesis.

The HOX genes, so frequently involved in T-ALL, appear to function downstream of the transcriptional cascade initiated by CBF. This pathway is also targeted by MLL fusion proteins, seen especially in infancy and in pre-B-ALL carrying the 1;19 chromosomal translocation (*E2A-PBX1* rearrangement). The TEL-AML1 fusion protein inhibits the transcription normally activated when AML1 binds to a DNA region known as the core enhanced sequence. It recruits histone deacetylases which lead to closure of the chromatin structure and alter self-renewal and differentiation. Exploration of the use of small-molecule inhibitors of histone deacetylases has occurred usually in combination with cytotoxics. Similarly, investigation of other molecules along the HOX regulatory pathway as potential drug targets may yield a more targeted approach to therapy especially in T-ALL. Such work has focused on γ-secretase inhibition causing interference with NOTCH signalling. Another drug on trial in T-cell malignancies is nelarabine, a deoxyguanosine analogue.

As described earlier, the initiating genetic events in leukaemogenesis may require secondary changes to induce overt leukaemia. Primary changes which impair differentiation, e.g. *TEL-AML1*, require further mutations altering proliferation and survival of cells. For example, the commonest secondary change in *TEL-AML1* cells is deletion of the other *TEL* gene.

Another example is the overexpression of FLT3, a receptor tyrosine kinase (role in development stem cells) seen both in ALL with MLL rearrangements and in high hyperdiploidy. Inhibitors of the kinase are now being tested in clinical trials (e.g. PKC412, MLN518, CEP701).

Very frequently in ALL the complex pathways involving the tumour suppressor retinoblastoma protein (RB), p130, p107, and Tp53 are altered by deletion or epigenetic silencing of P16$^{ink 4a}$ or P15$^{ink 4b}$ (especially in childhood T-ALL). As in many cancers, components of the Tp53 pathway are frequently mutated. Similarly, some lymphoid malignancies overexpress *BCL2* with consequent blocking of apoptosis. All of these pathways are being investigated as potential drug targets, especially using small molecule inhibitors.

Sensitivity/resistance to chemotherapy

It has long been recognized that some subtypes of ALL have differential sensitivity/resistance to certain classes of cytotoxic drug. For example, hyperdiploid ALL appears to be very sensitive to antimetabolites (methotrexate especially). Such leukaemic cells accumulate high intracellular levels of methotrexate and its active polyglutamates following therapy. Most patients with high hyperdiploidy have three or more copies of chromosome 21 including the folate transporter gene for cellular influx of methotrexate. Effective therapy for such patients should include significant doses of systemic methotrexate. Only the blasts cells take up the methotrexate selectively. Conversely, T-ALL blasts appear to accumulate fewer active polyglutamates than B-lineage cells.

TEL-AML1 leukaemic blasts appear to be selectively sensitive to L-asparaginase; conversely, *BCR-ABL1* and iAMP21 cells are frequently not. In these latter two it has been recently identified that they more commonly over express proteases especially asparaginyl endopeptidase which can cleave *E. coli* L-asparaginase, and inactivate the drug.

It has been reported that t(4;11)-ALL in infants and adults is preferentially sensitive to high-dose cytarbine. This may relate to increased secretion of hENT1, another cell membrane transporter. Genetic polymorphism of key metabolizing genes have been implicated in causation and response to therapy/resistance, e.g. NAD(P)H quinine oxidoreductase for causation and thiopurine methyl transferase for response.

Gene expression arrays have facilitated identification of unique leukaemia-associated markers which are then available as response identifiers; the arrays have also enabled identification of differentially expressed genes in drug-sensitive and drug-resistant ALL. Patterns of resistance to one or more of the key induction drugs (steroids, vincristine, daunorubicin and L-asparaginase) have been identified and strongly correlated with survival. This methodology has uncovered new potential therapeutic targets, e.g. in steroid-resistant ALL, overexpression of the anti-apoptotic *MCL1* gene with subsequent attempts made to inhibit it using rapamycin. In addition, under-expression of several transcription genes was identified. The potential to modulate glycolytic pathways and increase steroid responsiveness has also emerged from such array studies. This research has emphasized the complexity of resistance mechanisms which formerly concentrated on studies of the multidrug-resistance gene product and its inhibition by calcium channel blocking agents.

Other potential targets

Methylation

An imbalance of DNA methylation, involving widespread hypomethylation, regional hypermethylation, and increased cellular capacity for methylation, is characteristic of human neoplasia. Beginning in preneoplastic cells, methylation becomes extensive in subsequent stages of tumour progression. This aberrant methylation, particularly of cytosine, may mark abnormalities of chromatin reorganization and mediate progressive loss of gene expression associated with tumour development.

Abnormal methylation sites have been detected in lymphoid malignancies but to date we have little evidence of affective use of agents aimed at interfering with such events in ALL. The drug decitabine is being tested for potential efficacy.

Marrow microenvironment

Increasingly there is scientific interest in what supports survival of leukaemic cells within the marrow and in extramedullary sites and what facilitates migration of cells.

The growth of leukaemic cells requires the aggressive infiltration of capillaries into nests of tumour in excess of that seen in normal bone marrow. Relative selectivity of this neovascularization results in selective tumour regression on administration of antiangiogenic agents that block the effects of vascular endothelial cell growth factor (VEGF). Other drugs act to block oncoprotein function by inhibiting signal transduction, e.g. Ras farnesyltransferase inhibitors. Such factors might inhibit the neovascularization and supply of blood to new tumour growth if given at the time of maximal leukaemia-cell reduction. To date, the application of such agents in ALL has been limited. The stromal cells which support such nests of cells are of increasing research interest. It has been speculated that the effectiveness of 'maintenance' therapy may depend on its impact on the stromal cell component rather than directly on the leukaemia blasts.

Moncolonal antibodies

Cell-surface-directed approaches are now in large clinical trials with some encouraging responses. Constructs aimed directly at receptors including monoclonal antibodies specific for the cell-surface receptors CD20, CD33, CD52, and CD22 linked with antibiotics or endotoxins are being tested. Monoclonal antibodies have achieved utility in the treatment of lymphoma particularly with the use of rituximab, an anti-CD20 chimeric murine–human monoclonal antibody.

Further reading

Appelbaum FR, *et al.* (2007). End points to establish the efficacy of new agents in the treatment of acute leukaemia. *Blood*, **109**, 1810–16.

Boissel N, *et al.* (2003). Should adolescents with acute lymphoblastic leukaemia be treated as old children or young adults? Comparison of the French FRALLE-93 and LALA-94 trials. *J Clin Oncol*, **21**, 774–80.

Cheok MH, Evans WE (2006). Acute lymphoblastic leukaemia; a model of the pharmacogenomics of cancer therapy. *Nat Rev Cancer*, **6**, 117–29.

Chessells JM, *et al.* (2004). The impact of age on outcome in lymphoblastic leukaemia; MRC UKALLX and XA compared: a report from the MRC. Paediatric and Adult Working Parties. *Leukaemia*, **12**, 463–73.

Eden TOB (2002). Translation of cure for acute lymphoblastic leukaemia to all children. *Br J Haematol*, **118**, 945–51.

Farber S, *et al.* (1948). Temporary remission in acute leukaemia in children prolonged by folic acid antagonist. *N Engl J Med*, **238**, 787–93.

Holleman A, *et al.* (2004). Gene-expression patterns in drug-resistant acute lymphoblastic leukaemia cells and response to treatment. *N Engl J Med*, **351**, 533–42.

Laone E, *et al.* (2007). Dexamethasone-induced apoptosis in acute lymphoblastic leukaemia involves differential regulation of BcL-2 family members. *Haematologica*, **92**, 1460–9.

Lamb J, Crawford ED, Peck D (2006). The connectivity map: using gene-expression signatures to connect small molecules, genes, and disease. *Science*, **313**, 1929–35.

Lennard L, *et al.* (1990). Genetic variation in response to 6-mercaptopurine for childhood acute lymphoblastic leukaemia. *Lancet*, **336**, 225–9.

Moorman AV, *et al.* (2007). Prognosis of children with acute lymphoblastic leukaemia (ALL) and intrachromosomal amplification of chromosome 21 (iAMP21). *Blood*, **109**, 2337–30.

Nachman MD, *et al.* (1993). Young adults 16–21 years of age at diagnosis entered on Children's Cancer Group acute lymphoblastic leukaemia and acute myeloblastic leukaemia protocols. *Cancer*, **71**, 3377–85.

Piller GJ (2001). Leukaemia—a brief historical review from ancient times to 1950. *Br J Haematol*, **12**, 282–92.

Pui C-H, Relling MV, Downing JR (2004). Acute lymphoblastic leukaemia—mechanism of disease. *N Engl J Med*, **350**, 1535–48.

Staal FJT, Langerak AW (2008). Signalling pathways involved in the development of T cell acute lymphoblastic leukaemia. *Haematologica*, **93**, 493–7.

Wei G, *et al.* (2006). Gene expression-based chemical genomics identifies rapamycin as a modulator of MCL1 and glucocortoid resistance. *Cancer Cell*, **10**, 331–42.

Wiemels JL, *et al.* (1999). Prenatal origin of acute lymphoblastic leukaemia in children. *Lancet*, **354**, 1499–1503.

Wiemels JL, *et al.* (1999). Lack of function NAD(P)H quinine oxidoreductase alleles are selectively associated with paediatric leukaemias that have MLL fusions. *Cancer Res*, **59**, 4095–9.

Yeoh E-J, *et al.* (2002). Classification, subtype discovery and prediction of outcome in pediatric acute lymphoblastic leukaemia by gene expression profiling. *Cancer Cell*, **1**, 133–43.

22.3.4 Acute myeloid leukaemia

Jonathan Kell, Steve Knapper, and Alan Burnett

Essentials

It is believed that acute myeloblastic leukaemia arises in a haematopoietic stem cell as a result of mutations which promote growth or inhibit apoptosis arising in association with mutations that inhibit differentiation. In most cases there is no obvious cause, but exposure to chemical and ionizing radiation may be relevant, including previous chemotherapy for solid tumours.

Clinical features and diagnosis

Clinical features—typical manifestations are those of marrow failure, most commonly symptoms and signs of anaemia and of bleeding (petechiae, purpura, from mucous membranes). Acute promyelocytic leukaemia is a medical emergency characterized by bleeding and disseminated intravascular coagulation.

Diagnosis—the key investigations are examination of peripheral blood and bone marrow for blast cell infiltration, with classification and prognosis of disease depending on morphology, immunophenotyping, karyotyping, and definition of particular molecular mutations.

Treatment and prognosis

General approach—aside from providing appropriate supportive care, the first clinical decision to be made in an individual patient is whether to undertake conventional intensive chemotherapy aiming for disease eradication, or to adopt a more palliative approach. Intensive chemotherapy is the norm up to age 60 years, but the biology of the disease tends to be less favourable above this age (e.g. more adverse cytogenetic abnormalities and expression of multidrug resistance genes), and patients develop comorbidities and become less generally fit.

Initial chemotherapy—(1) Intensive chemotherapy—this typically involves the combination of daunorubicin and cytosine arabinoside (cytarabine, ara-C), which achieves complete remission in 40 to 80% of cases, followed by consolidation chemotherapy comprising a second course of induction treatment and then courses of ara-C with or without additional agents (e.g. amsacrine, etoposide, mitoxantone). (2) Less-intensive chemotherapy—most often comprises hydroxycarbamide (hydroxyurea) or low doses of ara-C. (3) Acute promyelocytic leukaemia—this is exquisitely sensitive to all-*trans*-retinoic acid, which is given concurrently with chemotherapy.

Relapsed disease—more than 50% of patients will ultimately relapse and their overall outcome is generally very poor. The only curative option is allogeneic bone marrow transplantation if a second complete remission can be achieved with reinduction chemotherapy

Prospects for the future

Increasing knowledge of the underlying biology may allow treatment with small molecules that inhibit the effects of the more common molecular mutations. However, unlike chronic myeloid leukaemia (which is characterized by a single molecular abnormality), a single inhibitor is not going to offer corrective therapy.

Epidemiology and causation

The median age at presentation is 68 years. Acute myeloid leukaemia (AML) occurs at all ages, ranging in frequency from 3 per million up to 12 to 15 per million patients in their 70s and 80s (Fig. 22.3.4.1). This age range has implications for treatment. In most cases there is no obvious cause; however, it is known that chemical and ionizing radiation exposure can be leukaemogenic. Several diseases of older patients evolve from the related disorder myelodysplastic syndrome, and indeed the boundary between the diseases is sometimes hard to define. The current international consensus defines AML as over 20% blast cells in the bone marrow. At this level, marrow function is usually compromised requiring intervention. An increasing risk of chemotherapy in general is that it may be leukaemogenic, and the development of AML represents a late complication of treatment of solid tumours, which is becoming more often seen as chemotherapy becomes more successful.

At the molecular level it is believed that AML is an example of multi-hit pathogenesis, with mutations which promote growth or inhibit apoptosis, arising in association with mutations that inhibit differentiation. Molecular abnormalities that have such effects are being increasingly recognized.

Diagnosis

The heterogeneity of morphology which reflects the ability of the leukaemic blast to achieve some degree of differentiation gave rise to a commonly accepted morphological classification known as the French–American–British (FAB) classification. With the increasing availability of high-quality monoclonal antibodies, immunophenotypic confirmation gave some objectivity to the diagnostic process. Over 30 years ago it was being recognized that various chromosome abnormalities were present in the blast cells. These were nonrandom and comprised balanced translocations, deletions, and trisomies. In about 40% of cases only a normal karyotype could be found. Some of these abnormalities corresponded to the morphological subtype. It took a number of years for the clinical community to feel that this was useful knowledge. However, it is now recognized that the karyotype is the strongest predictor of response to therapy, and is now an essential part of the diagnostic process.

Currently a similar awakening is underway with the recognition that molecular abnormalities are often found. The most common are mutations of the *FMS* receptor FLT3, NPM1, CEBPα, RAS, and c-KIT. These represent in some cases additional strong independent prognostic factors, but may become the target of a new generation of molecular-based therapies.

Box 22.3.4.1 Prognostic factors

- Age
- Cytogenetics
- Presenting white cell count
- Secondary disease
- Performance score
- FLT3/NPM1 mutation status
- Expression of resistance phenotype
- Marrow response to first chemotherapy course

Prognostic factors

The following are among the main characteristics that independently predict how a patient will respond to treatment. Most apply to the prospect of initial treatment achieving complete disease remission, and to overall survival. Performance score is only useful for predicting response to induction treatment. It should be mentioned here that these factors have been defined in the setting of large clinical trials, into which poor performance patients may not be entered.

These factors are shown in Box 22.3.4.1. Cytogenetics has been most widely adopted, and can guide treatment decisions such as who should be subjected to allogeneic transplant. Grouping the more favourable abnormalities (t(8;21), inv(16), and t(15;17)) and the poorer group abnormalities (of chromosomes 5 or 7, 3q–, complex) leaves about 60% of patients as at standard risk. As can be seen in Fig. 22.3.4.2, this subdivision has a major impact on survival. One of the reasons that older patients respond less well to the same chemotherapy is that older patients tend to have a high proportion of adverse features, in contrast to younger patients.

Treatment of AML

General considerations

Because of the variation of disease and patient biology, treatment and the assessment of treatment is complex. Treatment outcomes have improved over the years in children and adults under 60 years (Fig. 22.3.4.3), but there is little sign of such progress in older patients. Chemotherapy has continued with similar chemotherapeutic agents over the years, and it is easy to attribute the better outcomes

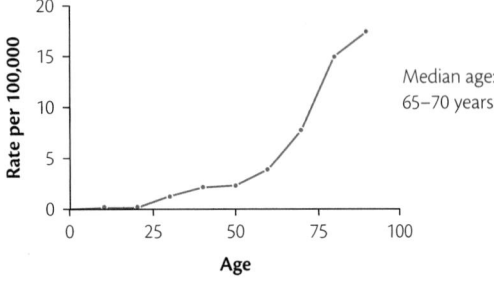

Fig. 22.3.4.1 Age-specific incidence of acute myeloid leukaemia (AML). (From Wingo PA, *et al.* (1995). Cancer statistics, 1995. *CA Cancer J Clin*, **45**, 8.)

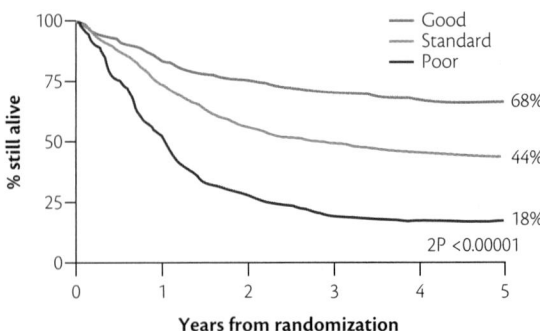

Fig. 22.3.4.2 Survival from complete remission (CR) by Medical Research Council (MRC) risk group.

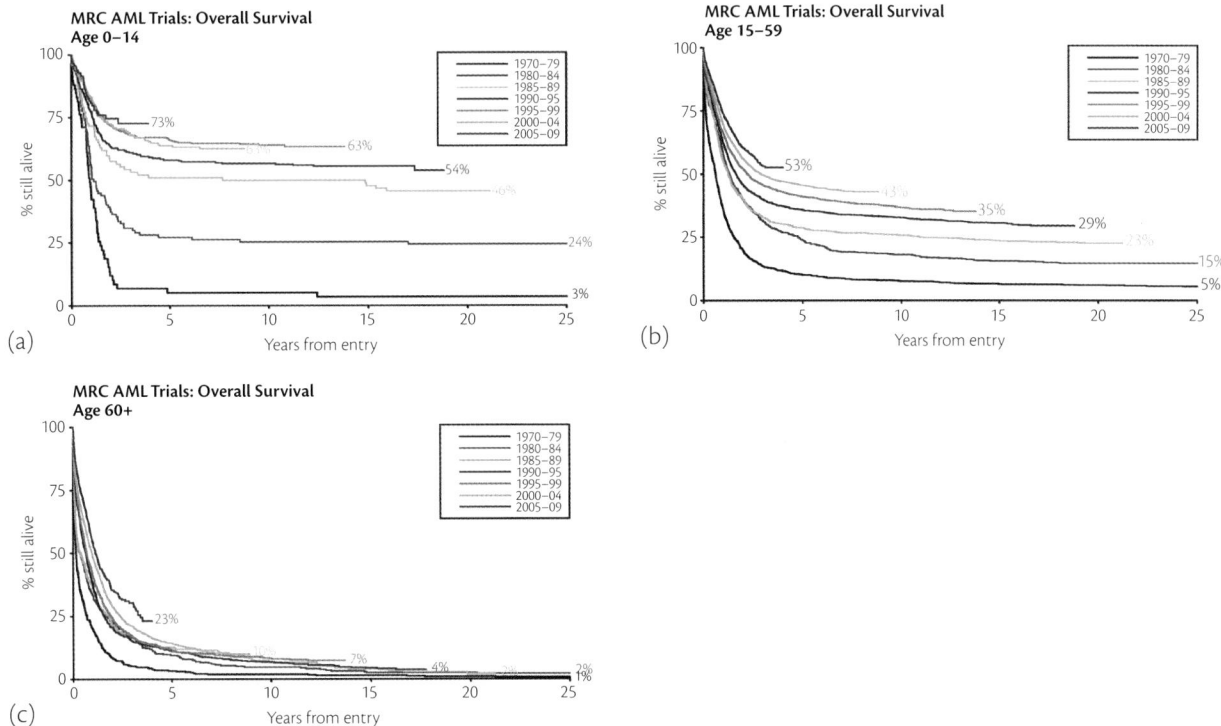

Fig. 22.3.4.3 Medical Research Council (MRC) trial results by patient ages. (a) 0 to 14 years (n = 1096); (b) younger adults, 15 to 59 years (n = 7704); (c) older patients, 60+ years (n = 3541).

to improved supportive care, which in turn has allowed treatment to be given in a more intensive way.

Definition of remission

The standard definition of 'remission' is that the bone marrow should show evidence of trilineage activity with less than 5% blasts, and peripheral blood counts should have returned to at least 100×10^9/litre for platelets and 1.0×10^9/litre for neutrophils. Molecular and other markers of disease still indicate the presence of the leukaemic clone, and it is well established that failure to deliver further courses of treatment to consolidate the response will result in rapid regrowth of disease.

The first clinical decision to be made in an individual patient is whether to undertake conventional intensive chemotherapy aiming for disease eradication, or to adopt a more palliative approach. The aim of intensive chemotherapy is to kill off the leukaemic population, which then enables normal haemopoiesis to re-establish itself.

Chemotherapeutic regimens

The combination of the anthracycline daunorubicin and the antimetabolite cytosine arabinoside (cytarabine, ara-C) has been the mainstay of treatment of AML for nearly 40 years with the intention of inducing complete remission (CR) and curing the disease. Such a combination is extremely myelosuppressive and is associated with a significant risk of infection and severe systemic toxicity. Among younger patients there is a risk of death during induction therapy of almost 10%, usually due to infection or bleeding. Such toxicity may limit the applicability of such a regimen to the treatment of older adults who constitute the majority of patients with AML. Patients who achieve CR will continue with further courses of chemotherapy, at approximately monthly intervals, to consolidate the remission and reduce the risk of relapse.

In the United Kingdom, initial induction therapy for younger people (<60 years of age) comprises 3 days of daunorubicin at doses of 45 to 50 mg/m² (usually given on days 1, 3, and 5) with 10 days of ara-C 200 mg/m² daily. In the United States of America this is usually shortened to a 7-day continuous infusion of ara-C, the so-called 3+7 approach. There are other apparent differences between the United States and the United Kingdom. Comparison of large national trials has not shown convincing evidence that the addition of a third drug, usually etoposide or thioguanine, improves the outcome of induction treatment in younger adults since the additional leukaemia cell kill is potentially offset by increased toxicity. Equally, attempts to improve outcomes with alternative anthracyclines (idarubicin or mitoxantrone) have shown no advantage. The United Kingdom Medical Research Council (MRC) AML12 trial compared mitoxantrone with daunorubicin, in combination with either etoposide or thioguanine, and found no overall difference in long-term outcome. In general, daunorubicin remains the anthracycline of choice.

Cytarabine remains one of the most active drugs in the treatment of AML. Several groups have increased the dose up to 3 g/m² in induction with mixed results. At these high doses there is significant skin, renal, and central nervous system toxicity. However, certain subsets of AML, particularly the core binding factor leukaemia associated with t(8;21) and inv(16), are particularly sensitive to ara-C and may benefit from this approach. Newer analogues of cytarabine such as clofarabine are now entering randomized trials.

Outcomes of treatment

Between 40 and 80% of patients will achieve CR with this approach. Factors influencing the chance of CR include age at diagnosis, cytogenetic abnormalities, and expression of multidrug resistance genes (p-glycoprotein). For example, 75 to 80% of patients under

60 will achieve a CR, compared with 45 to 55% of older patients given the same treatment schedule.

Indications for further chemotherapy

At least 70% of those attaining CR will do so after a single course of chemotherapy. The usefulness of adding a third drug to this conventional induction is disputed. However, in recent years, it has become feasible to conjugate chemotherapeutics with antibodies as a means of targeting the antileukaemic potential without increasing toxicity. The archetypal agent in AML is gemtuzumab ozogamicin, which is a CD33-targeted immunoconjugate of the anthracycline-like drug, calicheamicin. CD33 is a transmembrane protein expressed on the cells of 95% of patients with AML. On binding antibody, it is rapidly internalized, and free calicheamicin is released causing genotoxic damage. Early studies with the combination of gemtuzumab ozogamicin with conventional chemotherapy are reporting an improved level of disease control—i.e. reduced relapse risk in younger patients.

Consolidation of chemotherapy

Patients who achieve CR will require further consolidation chemotherapy. A second course of the initial induction treatment is followed by two or three further courses of alternative drugs. High doses of ara-C (1.5 g/m^2) are common in the United States of America, whereas the combination of ara-C with amsacrine, etoposide, or mitoxantrone is favoured in the United Kingdom. There is no clear difference in outcome rates with the two approaches, which have been compared directly in the United Kingdom MRC AML15 trial. It also remains unclear as to whether a total of four or five courses of treatment is ideal.

Treatment of older patients

Age is a major factor determining CR rates and long-term outcome. Older age is associated with the onset of significant comorbidities such as hypertension, lung disease, and renal impairment, which limit chemotherapy delivery. Similarly, the biology of leukaemia appears to change as people age, with a higher incidence of adverse genetic changes and multidrug resistance in older patients. Consequently, older people tend to do less well than younger patients with AML.

The age of 60 years is frequently taken as an arbitrary threshold for the use of the term 'older'. Up to this age there is little doubt that intensive chemotherapy should be the norm; however, with increasing age, patients develop comorbidities and become less generally fit. This makes intensive treatment more risky. In addition the biology of the disease is less favourable, with a higher proportion of patients with secondary AML, more with leukaemia that has associated resistance proteins within the leukaemic population, and a higher proportion with an adverse risk karyotype. A number of epidemiological studies indicate that as many as 40% of older patients are not treated with intensive chemotherapy and receive supportive care only with hydroxycarbamide (hydroxyurea). Older or less fit patients may do better with a more palliative approach to their disease. There has been much recent interest in the development of treatments for this patient group. A major national trial in the United Kingdom attempted to analyse which patients would benefit from these two approaches, but was unable to recruit adequate numbers of patients to the randomization. Nonetheless,

the same trial was able to demonstrate that low doses of ara-C given subcutaneously (20 mg twice daily for 10 days) repeated at 4- to 6-week intervals is superior to the orally active ribonucleotide reductase inhibitor hydroxyurea. Indeed, one in six patients will gain CR with this approach, although these remissions tend to be less durable than those seen in younger patients treated with conventional doses of chemotherapy. However, overall the outlook for older patients with AML remains very poor.

Treatment of relapsed AML

Despite 60 to 80% of patients with AML attaining CR with induction chemotherapy, more than 50% of these will ultimately relapse with their disease. Induction with intensive chemotherapy remains an option for these patients, but the overall outcome is generally very poor. Remission rates with reinduction are less than in first presentation, and remissions are generally of shorter duration. The only curative option is to proceed to an allogeneic bone marrow transplantation when in CR2. No randomized trial has shown a superiority of one reinduction regimen over another, but the combination of fludarabine (a purine analogue) with ara-C and idarubicin with granulocyte-colony stimulating factor (G-CSF) support is one favoured regimen.

Targeted therapy

In recent years the molecular-genetic heterogeneity of AML has become better understood. This is now introducing the era of targeted therapy, the prime example of which is the modern management of the APL subtype. Recently several genetic mutations have been described which influence prognosis and relapse risk. Fms-like tyrosine kinase 3 (FLT-3) is a type 3 tyrosine kinase receptor expressed in bone marrow, brain, and gonadal tissue. An activating tandem duplication resulting in the insertion of a variable number of in-frame base pairs has been described leading to a constitutively active protein resulting in increased cell survival pathways. This mutant, or an activating point mutation (D835Y), is present in approximately one-third of patients with AML and is associated with an adverse prognosis from an increased relapse risk. CEP-701 is an orally active inhibitor of FLT-3 and may decrease the relapse risk in early-phase clinical trials. Other potentially useful agents include tipifarnib (an inhibitor of farnesyl transferase which is required for RAS activation) and arsenic trioxide (which is active in APL, including relapsed disease, in combination with low doses of ara-C).

Maintenance chemotherapy and DNA methylation

In many human cancers, including leukaemia, genomic DNA is frequently hypermethylated. This methylation, occurring on CpG tandem repeats, results in gene silencing. The cytotoxic purine analogue 2-deoxyazacytidine is incorporated into DNA, but the nitrogen atom in the 5-position of the purine ring cannot be methylated. At low doses, this agent and its RNA dependent counterpart, azacytidine, result in demethylation of DNA allowing increased gene expression.

Traditionally, maintenance therapy has not been shown to be of benefit in AML, unlike in acute lymphoblastic leukaemia (ALL), where prolonged maintenance chemotherapy substantially reduces the risk of relapse, and, more recently, in APL as discussed above. However, the potential of these hypomethylating agents to induce epigenetic changes is now being explored as a maintenance treatment for older patients in remission after receiving intensive induction chemotherapy.

Bone marrow transplantation

Having entered remission, the main challenge is to prevent relapse. There is no doubt that the most effective approach is to administer myeloablative chemoradiotherapy followed by infusion of haematopoietic stem cells. These have been obtained from an HLA-matched sibling donor as bone marrow cells. This approach reduces the risk of disease relapse from 40 to 50%, to 10 to 15%. This powerful antileukaemic effect is partly due to the myeloablation and partly due to the associated 'graft versus leukaemia' mediated by donor T lymphocytes in the graft. Unfortunately, it has not been possible to fully realize the antileukaemic potential of allogeneic transplantation because to the associated risks of graft-versus-host disease and immunosuppression which usually involve a life-threatening risk of 30%. The risks increase with age and in the United Kingdom experience, there is no overall survival benefit seen in patients older than 35 years. The development of large donor banks has made the finding of a matched unrelated donor a practical possibility, and the results of this approach are now equivalent to those using a matched sibling. Allografting involving reduced intensity conditioning has become well developed. Here the mechanism is primarily immunological. It was initially thought that this approach would be more suitable for chronic lymphoproliferative diseases, but data now emerging suggest that this is also a feasible approach in AML in older patients up to the age of 70 years. There are, however, no controlled studies to provide information about how much better, if at all, this is than chemotherapy.

As discussed above, once patients enter remission, they are at differing risks of relapse, based on their cytogenetic group. It is unlikely that patients with favourable cytogenetics will benefit, because the additional reduction in relapse risk is more than outweighed by the treatment risks. For patients at intermediate risk, there are mixed opinions, but no convincing evidence of overall survival benefit in United Kingdom prospective trials. Most would accept that patients with bad risk disease should undergo a transplant as soon as the risk is known. Such patients will have a higher risk of relapse after the transplant, but they have a very poor outcome with chemotherapy alone.

For patients who relapse from chemotherapy and enter a second remission, the prospects for cure are poor and are largely dictated by the length of CR1. It is axiomatic that second remissions will be shorter that first remissions. Transplantation is the only treatment that can change this and is indicated for all patients who relapse, where it offers a 30 to 40% chance of salvage.

Supportive care in AML

The steady but significant improvements seen in disease survival rates over the last 30 to 40 years have been facilitated by the development of better supportive care strategies which have allowed the safer intensification of chemotherapy regimens.

Following diagnosis of AML, early mortality can result either directly from presenting complications of the disease, from the direct consequences of treatment initiation, or from problems arising during the 3 to 4 weeks of profound pancytopenia that inevitably follow remission induction chemotherapy. Effective supportive care during this period requires close coordination between specialists from a number of disciplines including haemato-oncologists, microbiologists, radiologists, intensivists, specialist nurses, pharmacists, and dieticians working in facilities dedicated to the care of this type of patient. Clear written standards should be adhered to, including local policies for infection prophylaxis and treatment, national guideline documents, and, where appropriate, clinical trial protocols.

Supportive care at the initiation of therapy

The presenting clinical features of AML vary according to both the depth of bone marrow failure and the rate of turnover of the leukaemic clone. Prompt chemotherapeutic intervention is required in cases with high rates of blast proliferation but, paradoxically, rapid cell kill may lead to life-threatening metabolic disturbances.

Hyperleucocytosis

Although a feature of only a minority of cases, a high presenting white cell count (WCC) is a well-established poor prognostic factor in AML. Patients with hyperleucocytosis (WCC > 100×10^9/litre) are at a threefold greater risk of early mortality (15%) than those with lower counts. Hyperleucocytosis predisposes to hyperviscosity and leucostasis. 'Sludging' in the microvasculature, particularly of the lungs and brain, clinically manifests most frequently as hypoxia and central nervous system dysfunction and carries significant risks of both thrombotic and haemorrhagic sequelae. The effects of hyperviscosity may be partially offset at presentation by the presence of concurrent anaemia: red cell transfusion should thus be delayed, unless absolutely unavoidable, until the WCC has been reduced. Oral hydroxycarbamide (hydroxyurea) may be of practical value in reducing the WCC prior to the commencement of formal induction chemotherapy. Leucapheresis is generally safe and, although evidence is lacking, may be considered in patients presenting with symptomatic hyperleucocytosis. However, leucapheresis may fatally exacerbate the presenting coagulopathy of APL and should be avoided in this setting.

Tumour lysis syndrome and metabolic complications

Acute tumour lysis syndrome (ATLS) describes a collection of metabolic abnormalities including hyperuricaemia, hyperphosphataemia, hypocalcaemia, and hyperkalaemia that result from the release of nuclear and cytoplasmic degradation products from malignant cells and may precipitate acute renal failure. It is vital that treating physicians are aware of the risks of ATLS, particularly when instituting cytoreductive therapy in AML patients with hyperleucocytosis or bulky extramedullary disease. Emergency haemodialysis may be required in the event of acute renal failure, rising potassium levels, or recalcitrant hyperphosphataemia.

Standard measures to prevent ATLS prior to the commencement of chemotherapy include use of the xanthine oxidase inhibitor allopurinol (300 mg daily) coupled with vigorous intravenous hydration and with meticulous monitoring of fluid balance and electrolyte levels as induction therapy commences. Alkalinization of the urine using intravenous bicarbonate has been used historically to reduce tubular uric acid crystal deposition, but it remains controversial as it carries the potential for both reducing tubular xanthine solubility and exacerbating calcium pyrophosphate deposition in organs including the heart. The recombinant urate oxidase enzyme rasburicase is able to rapidly reverse hyperuricaemia by promoting the breakdown of uric acid into allantoin. It is now the treatment of choice in patients with hyperleucocytosis at presentation, renal failure, or early evidence of evolving ATLS. Rasburicase also avoids any need for urinary alkalinization.

Hypokalaemia is also frequently encountered in AML patients, both at presentation (due to high serum lysozyme levels particularly in monocytic subtypes M4 and M5) or later as a consequence of prolonged diarrhoea or the renal tubular effects of amphotericin. Vigorous intravenous electrolyte supplementation is frequently required.

Other supportive measures prior to starting cytotoxic therapy

Secure central venous access is usually established through insertion of a tunnelled Hickman line or temporary central line, allowing safe administration of vesicant drugs, blood products, and intravenous antibiotics, as well as facilitating frequent blood-sampling procedures. Young men should be counselled regarding potential loss of fertility and, whenever possible, offered the opportunity to store sperm. Loss of fertility due to chemotherapy is less common in women: *in vitro* preservation of unfertilized ova is not yet undertaken routinely. There is a high risk of severe emesis with intensive chemotherapy, and strenuous efforts should be made to prevent this distressing complication. Serotonin antagonists (ondansetron or granisetron) are a standard first choice, although combination therapy is often necessary.

Supportive care during chemotherapy-induced pancytopenia

Clearance of leukaemic blasts by induction chemotherapy is achieved at the expense of 3 to 4 weeks of severe pancytopenia, and similar cytopenic episodes will follow subsequent courses of consolidation therapy. During these periods, patients remain at high risk: prompt access to blood product support and robust procedures to prevent and manage neutropenic infections are vital.

Blood product support

By the time of initial disease presentation, the ability of most patients to produce red cells and platelets is severely impaired. Due to the often rapid onset of anaemia, there may be little time for haemodynamic compensation making many patients symptomatic due to acute impairment of oxygen-carrying capacity. In the absence of hyperleucocytosis, red cells should be transfused promptly.

Following intensive chemotherapy, patients will inevitably be dependent on regular transfusional support until bone marrow recovery. Although there is no firm evidence to support a particular red cell transfusion threshold, many units operate a policy of transfusing as required to maintain haemoglobin levels in excess of 8 g/dl. All patients in whom allogeneic stem cell transplantation is a possibility should be transfused cytomegalovirus (CMV)–negative cellular products until their CMV status is known, while those treated with cytotoxic regimes containing purine analogues (fludarabine or clofarabine) should receive irradiated blood products to minimize the risk of transfusion-associated graft-versus-host disease.

In general, one adult therapeutic dose of platelets should be transfused whenever the platelet count falls to below 10×10^9/litre. Platelet survival may be further compromised by sepsis or the use of concurrent intravenous antibiotics, and in these situations or in the presence of additional haemostatic abnormalities a higher transfusion threshold of 20×10^9/litre is usually observed. Antifibrinolytic agents such as tranexamic acid may be useful for local mucosal bleeding but are contraindicated in the presence of haematuria due to the potential for ureteric clot formation.

Infection

The risk of infection in AML is influenced by both the degree and duration of neutropenia and increases markedly during episodes of chemotherapy-induced bone marrow aplasia. Changes to the bacterial flora as a consequence of broad-spectrum antibiotic use, and poor nutritional status following prolonged periods of hospitalization also contribute significantly. The vast majority of AML patients will become febrile at some point, although only a minority of these episodes will be accompanied by symptoms or signs of localizing infection. Sepsis should be suspected in the presence of any sudden nonspecific clinical deterioration; inflammatory responses may be muted in the neutropenic setting and may be associated with hypothermia, declining mental status, myalgia, or increasing lethargy. Potential portals of bacterial entry include indwelling lines and chemotherapy-induced breaches in the integrity of the bowel mucosa.

Neutropenic patients should be advised to pay particular attention to personal hygiene and dental care. Careful hand-washing and decontamination before patient contact is mandatory for health care workers. The role of prophylactic antibiotic therapy remains contentious. Prophylactic quinolone (ciprofloxacin or ofloxacin) use is widespread, and while there is a lack of evidence for any reduction in mortality or incidence of febrile episodes, there may be a reduction in the incidence and morbidity of Gram-negative infections.

Patients should be made aware of their susceptibility to infection and provided with emergency contact details to allow rapid clinical assessment. In the presence of neutropenic sepsis, the prompt institution of broad-spectrum antibacterial therapy is potentially life-saving. Patterns of infection and pathogen isolation will vary between hospitals, and clear written guidelines for the emergency management of patients with febrile neutropenia should be decided in discussion with local microbiologists. Examples of empirical antibiotic regimes include monotherapy with a third-generation cephalosporin or carbopenem, or combination therapy with a broad-spectrum antipseudomonal penicillin and aminoglycoside. Vancomycin or teicoplanin may be added to broaden Gram-positive coverage if there are particular clinical concerns regarding indwelling line infection. Mandatory investigations include central and peripheral blood cultures, cultures of urine and stool, and a chest radiograph. Further modifications to the initial antibiotic regime should be based on culture results and regular clinical examination, although surveys demonstrate that the rate of proven bacteraemia during episodes of febrile neutropenia has remained between 20 and 25% for many years. Persistent infection or blood culture isolation of Gram-negative organisms or candida should prompt indwelling central line removal.

The risk of invasive fungal infection is high in AML patients receiving intensive chemotherapy, and its incidence increases with the severity and duration of neutropenia, often occurring in the aftermath of bacterial sepsis. Established fungal infections carry a high mortality. The diagnosis of invasive fungal infection should be confirmed wherever possible, and there is an increasing move away from the empirical use of antifungal agents as treatment of fever of unknown origin. High resolution CT scanning of the chest in patients with persistent pyrexia refractory to antibiotic therapy, and screening of patients using the sandwich enzyme-linked immunosorbent assay (ELISA) for *Aspergillus galactomannan* aid the early detection of invasive pulmonary aspergillosis, allowing the targeted implementation of antifungal therapy with agents including liposomal amphotericin B and caspofungin. Azole antifungal agents are widely prescribed prophylactically during neutropenia in AML. Itraconazole is the drug of choice in this setting and has activity against a broader spectrum of fungal organisms than fluconazole which is inactive against moulds including aspergillus species.

A modest reduction in duration (but not depth) of neutropenia may be achieved with the use of recombinant growth factors (G-CSF or granulocyte-macrophage colony stimulating factor) following induction and consolidation chemotherapy. Large controlled trials show variable effects on the incidence of severe infection and no clear overall survival benefit. Routine growth factor use is not recommended, although there may be cost–benefit advantages in terms of reduction in both antibiotic usage and the duration of hospital admissions.

Acute promyelocytic leukaemia

Acute promyelocytic leukaemia (APL) is a medical emergency characterized by bleeding and disseminated intravascular coagulation (DIC). It usually presents with pancytopenia rather than a raised white cell count. The diagnosis is made on morphology with a typical hypercellular marrow with characteristic heavily granulated promyelocytes, and confirmed on immunophenotyping which shows a characteristic perinuclear speckled pattern on staining for PML and cytogenetic or molecular studies for the PML-RARa rearrangement of the t(15;17) translocation.

Treatment of APL

This disease is exquisitely sensitive to treatment with all-*trans*-retinoic acid (ATRA), a vitamin A analogue normally present in blood. The translocation renders cells resistant to physiological concentrations of ATRA, but sensitive to pharmacological doses. ATRA is given concurrently with chemotherapy, inducing higher rates of CRs and an excellent long-term prognosis with 5-year disease-free survival of around 80%. However, treatment is associated with an increased risk of bleeding in these patients, and intense support of the coagulation system is required with blood products. Very few patients with APL who attain CR subsequently relapse, and this risk is further reduced by maintenance chemotherapy for up to 2 years following the intensive induction and consolidation chemotherapy. Further, due to the specific nature of the molecular lesion in APL, monitoring of minimal residual disease by polymerase chain reaction (PCR) allows very sensitive detection of any impending relapse. Restarting chemotherapy at the time of molecular detection of disease recurrence improves overall outcome.

Supportive care issues specific to treatment initiation in APL

Although abnormalities of coagulation may contribute to a bleeding tendency at presentation in any subtype of AML, APL and more especially its hypogranular variant (M3v) are particularly associated with a high risk of early haemorrhagic death due to a combination of DIC and increased fibrinolysis. Eighty per cent of APL patients have clinically significant coagulopathy: this condition constitutes a genuine haematological emergency that requires rapid diagnosis and prompt initiation of therapy. There is now considerable evidence that the early introduction of 'differentiation therapy' with ATRA alongside anthracycline-based chemotherapy improves the coagulopathy associated with APL. The platelet count and coagulation profile should be checked at least twice daily during the early stages of treatment. By employing an aggressive transfusion policy, the platelet count should be maintained above 50×10^9/litre, and coagulation times kept within the normal range using fresh frozen plasma replacement. Cryoprecipitate or fibrinogen concentrates should be used to maintain a fibrinogen level close to 2 g/litre. The use of heparin is no longer recommended.

Complications of treatment in APL

Retinoic acid syndrome (RAS; also known as differentiation syndrome) is a potentially life-threatening complication of the use of ATRA or arsenic trioxide (ATO) therapy in APL. It is caused by cytokine release from differentiating APL cells and characterized by a rising WCC with accompanying features of fluid retention and capillary leak including pulmonary infiltrates, pleural and pericardial effusions, peripheral oedema, hypoxia, and progressive respiratory failure. Standard treatment on first suspicion of RAS is dexamethasone 10 mg intravenously twice daily, with interruption of ATRA therapy and provision of respiratory support until all symptoms and signs have resolved.

Further reading

Appelbaum FR, *et al.* (2006). Age and acute myeloid leukemia. *Blood*, **107**, 3481–5.

Burnett AK, Mohite U (2006). Treatment of older patients with acute myeloid leukemia—new agents. *Semin Hematol*, **43**, 96–106.

Estey EH (2001). Growth factors in acute myeloid leukaemia. In: Burnett AK (ed.) *Clinical Haematology*, pp. 175–87. Baillière Tindall, London.

Estey E, Dohner H (2006). Acute myeloid leukaemia. *Lancet*, **368**, 1894–1907.

Gale RE, *et al.* (2008). Med Res Council Adult Leukaemia Wo. The impact of FLT3 internal tandem duplication mutant level, number, size, and interaction with NPM1 mutations in a large cohort of young adult patients with acute myeloid leukemia. *Blood*, **111**, 2776–84.

Grimwade D, *et al.* (1998). The importance of diagnostic cytogenetics on outcome in AML: Analysis of 1,612 patients entered into the MRC AML:10 Trial. *Blood*, **92**, 2322–3.

Kantarjian H, *et al.* (2006). Results of intensive chemotherapy in 998 patients age 65 years or older with acute myeloid leukemia or high-risk myelodysplastic syndrome. *Cancer*, **106**, 1090–8.

Lowenberg B, Downing JR, Burnett A (1999). Acute myeloid leukemia. *N Engl J Med*, **341** (14), 1051–62.

Milligan DW, *et al.* (2006). Guidelines on the management of acute myeloid leukaemia in adults. *Br J Haematol*, **135**, 450–74.

Sanz MA, *et al.* (2009). Management of acute promyelocytic leukemia: recommendations from an expert panel on behalf of the European LeukemiaNet. *Blood*, **113**, 1875–91.

Wheatley K, *et al.* (2009). Prognostic factor analysis of the survival of elderly patients with AML in the MRC AML11 and LRF AML14 trials (p). *DOI:10.1111/j.1365-2141.2009.07663.x* (Abstract). *Br J Haematol*, **145**, 598–605.

22.3.5 Chronic lymphocytic leukaemia and other leukaemias of mature B and T cells

Clive S. Zent and Aaron Polliack

Essentials

Chronic lymphocytic leukaemia/small lymphocytic lymphoma (CLL) is the most prevalent lymphoid neoplasm in Europe and North America, but its cause remains unknown. The 'cell of origin' is a mature B lymphocyte that has rearranged its immunoglobulin gene, expresses surface immunoglobulin, and is characterized by defective apoptosis.

Clinical features

Most patients have no clinical features of disease and diagnosis is made incidentally on discovery of lymphocytosis. A few have rapidly progressive disease and develop symptoms from (1) tissue accumulation of lymphocytes—e.g. disfiguring lymphadenopathy, splenomegaly causing abdominal discomfort; or (2) effects of marrow failure cytopenias—e.g. anaemia, thrombocytopenia. Patients also have an increased risk of developing autoimmune cytopenias and of second malignancies.

Diagnosis and clinical staging

Diagnosis is usually made by analysis of the immunophenotype of malignant cells from the blood or (in rare patients without a detectable monoclonal B cell population in the blood) lymphocytes from the bone marrow, lymph nodes or spleen. Current diagnostic criteria have an arbitrary requirement for (1) B-lymphocyte count $>5 \times 10^9$/litre, or (2) clinically detectable adenopathy—at least 1 cm in diameter, or (3) organomegaly, or (4) over 30% bone marrow involvement by CLL cells. Staging is based on clinical examination and blood count evaluation.

Treatment and prognosis

Treatment—there is no standard curative therapy, and patients should not be treated until they have progressive and symptomatic disease or develop anaemia or thrombocytopenia due to bone marrow failure. If a decision is made to treat, then the best initial treatment is not certain: single-agent therapy with oral chlorambucil was until recently regarded as the standard of care, but (excepting in frail patients) current practice has moved towards regimen such as those employing purine-analogues, cyclophosphamide, and rituximab, although the only potential curative treatment is allogeneic stem cell transplantation.

Prognosis—this is highly variable and depends on the clinical stage of disease, biological characteristics of the malignant cells, and the general health of the patient. Those with advanced stage disease have a median survival of 4 to 6 years.

Introduction

The mature lymphocytic leukaemias were historically defined by light microscopic cell morphology and included a wide range of diseases derived from different classes of lymphocytes. In recent years there have been major improvements and advances in the understanding of lymphocyte biology resulting in the development of better diagnostic methodologies which are now routinely used in more accurate diagnosis, clinical management decisions, and subsequent follow-up. Individual diseases can now be defined and diagnosed at both a cellular and molecular level. Most patients with mature lymphocytic leukaemias in Europe and North America have chronic lymphocytic leukaemia/small lymphocytic lymphoma (CLL). The other less frequently encountered entities, which also need to be considered in the differential diagnosis of CLL, include the leukaemic phase of B-, T-, and natural killer (NK)-cell lymphomas, prolymphocytic leukaemias, and the nonclassified chronic lymphoproliferative disorders. This chapter concentrates on CLL, with only limited reference to the rarer malignancies of mature lymphocytes.

CLL, the most prevalent lymphoid neoplasm in Europe and North America, is a distinct B-cell malignancy. The disease has a protean clinical presentation, marked variation in the rate of disease progression, and an increasing number of new treatment options which have become available over the past 2 decades. The challenge to the medical practitioner is still to make an accurate diagnosis, recognize the significance of newer prognostic factors and the indications for treatment, and to be aware of and know how to manage the many potential complications of the disease. Although CLL is incurable with standard therapy and will eventually cause major morbidity and mortality in most patients who have the disease, good medical care can improve the quality of life and increase longevity for many patients with the disease.

Historical perspective

The leukaemias of mature lymphocytes were first recognized in the latter half of the 19th century. The subsequent recognition of the pivotal role of lymphocytes in the immune system led to the discovery and recognition of the different T, B, and NK subsets. This information has now been combined with a better understanding of lymphocyte biology to develop newer classifications of lymphoid malignancies—those of the Revised European-American Classification of Lymphoid Neoplasms (REAL) and the World Health Organization (WHO)—based on the presumptive normal counterpart of the malignant cells. CLL and the other leukaemias of mature lymphocytes with similar light microscopic cellular morphology are now recognized to be different diseases.

The clinical presentation of CLL has changed dramatically in the past few decades. The widespread use of automated cell counters providing rapid and accurate blood lymphocyte counts has greatly increased the incidental finding of lymphocytosis. In these patients, lymphocytes can be characterized on the flow cytometers in clinical pathology laboratories. This often results in a diagnosis of CLL. Among populations with access to these technologies, most CLL patients are thus now diagnosed early with asymptomatic disease. Presentation with symptomatic disease is indeed becoming less common.

CLL and small lymphocytic lymphoma (SLL) were previously considered to be different diseases. However, the recognition that CLL/SLL cells have the same immunophenotype with considerable overlap in presentation and progression, has led to inclusion of both of them in the CLL category in the REAL and WHO classifications. Clinical presentation of the disease with predominance of adenopathy vs high circulating numbers of leukaemic cells is likely to reflect differences in CLL cell trafficking and does not appear to have any major biological or clinical importance.

In the last 3 decades there has been a marked improvement in the treatment options available for patients with progressive CLL. Single-agent alkylator therapy has been supplemented with purine analogues and more recently lymphocyte-targeting monoclonal antibodies. Combinations of these therapies (chemoimmunotherapy (CIT)) have resulted in better and more durable responses to therapy, which are associated with longer disease-free periods and a subsequent improvement of the quality of life for these patients.

Aetiology, genetics, pathogenesis, and pathology

The aetiology of CLL remains essentially unknown. CLL is a familial disease in about 10% of patients who have a first-degree relative with CLL or another B-cell lymphoproliferative disorder (LPD). Additional evidence for a genetic predisposition for CLL is the marked ethnic variation in the incidence of the disease, which remains relatively unchanged after large population migrations. The highest rates of CLL are in patients of European descent, with a substantially lower risk in people of South-East Asian ancestry. The specific genetic defects in susceptible patients have not yet been clearly defined,

The role of environmental factors in the aetiology of CLL is poorly understood. Epidemiological studies raise concerns about the increased risk in patients with exposure to industrial and agricultural chemicals. Although CLL was previously not considered to be induced by radiation, more recent studies suggest that radiation exposure could increase the risk. The most compelling evidence for a possible environmental agent in the aetiology of CLL comes from recent studies of the variable region allele use in the immunoglobulin molecule expressed by CLL cells. These show a restricted gene usage and limited stereotypes which suggest a possible aetiological role for as-yet-undefined environmental or endogenous antigens. The ongoing study of the aetiology of CLL could be informative in eventually directing preventative measures.

The current model of B-cell lymphoid malignancies assumes that distinct diseases evolve from malignant transformation of lymphocytes at a specific stage of maturation. However, the 'cell of origin' of CLL is not yet fully defined. The culprit cell is a mature B lymphocyte that has rearranged its immunoglobulin gene and does express surface immunoglobulin. However, somatic hypermutation, the result of antigen-driven mutations in the germinal centre of the lymph node, occurs in only about 50% of cases of CLL, while the remaining cases are unmutated. Because somatic hypermutation is considered the basic hallmark of the passage of B lymphocytes through the germinal centre after antigen exposure, this discrepancy does limit the currently ability to determine the cell of origin of CLL. The difficulty relating to the classification of the cell of origin of CLL is exacerbated by the expression of CD5 by CLL cells. CD5 is expressed by most T lymphocytes but only a small subset of normal B cells which produce low-affinity autoreactive antibodies and generally do not undergo maturation in the germinal centre. The relationship between CLL and the normal CD5$^+$ B-cell population is still unclear.

CLL cells are characterized by defective apoptosis which is a major mechanism in this disease. However, the fundamental defect in apoptosis is as yet undefined. CLL cells have disrupted *BCL2* gene family expression with higher levels of antiapoptotic genes and lower levels of proapoptotic genes. The mechanism of increased *BCL2* expression is unknown, and translocations involving the *BCL2* gene are rare. CLL cells are characterized by several recurrent genetic defects which usually occur in subclones of the neoplastic cell population and are considered to be the result of clonal evolution. Of these, deletions of chromosome band 17p13 (loss of p53) and 11q22 (loss of ATM), could indeed impair the activity of an important cell control mechanism. The most common recurrent chromosomal defect is the deletion of 13q14 which results in the loss of the microRNA genes *miR15* and *miR16*, which could play a role in pathogenesis or progression of the disease. Recent studies of CLL cell kinetics using labelling with heavy water have shown that CLL cell turnover is higher than previously measured by less sensitive markers of cell proliferation. These studies showed that daily turnover of cells is in the range of 0.1 to 1%, which suggests a dynamic clone and relatively short CLL cell survival in some patients.

CLL cells are identified by immunophenotyping of membrane proteins. The lymphocytes are examined for expression of CD19 (pan-B-cell marker), light chain restriction (predominant expression of either the κ or λ immunoglobulin light chains), and coexpression of CD5, CD23, dim CD20, and dim expression of surface immunoglobulin/CD79b. These CLL cells usually accumulate in the bone marrow, lymph nodes, and spleen, and traffic between these sites in the blood and lymphatics. CLL cells are often found in viscera, serosal fluids, and cerebrospinal fluid even in early-stage CLL and can infiltrate any site of inflammation.

Pathological effects of CLL cells can be direct and indirect. The most common direct effects of accumulation of CLL cells are lymphadenopathy, splenomegaly, hepatomegaly, and bone marrow failure. Lymphadenopathy is an earlier event in disease progression followed by splenomegaly and hepatomegaly, and bone marrow involvement resulting in cytopenia is usually a late event. In contrast, the indirect effects of CLL are less predictable, and their mechanism is not well understood. Patients with CLL have an early-onset defect in humoural immunity characterized by decreased antibody levels and increased rates of infection with encapsulated organisms. T-cell function is usually well preserved in early-stage disease despite a skewed T-cell repertoire. Patients also have an increased risk (~5%) of developing autoimmune cytopenias during the course of their disease. These can present as autoimmune haemolytic anaemia (AIHA), immune thrombocytopenia (ITP), pure red blood cell aplasia (PRCA), or rarely autoimmune granulocytopenia. In addition, CLL is also associated with an increased risk of developing second malignancies. The most common second haematological malignancy is diffuse large cell lymphoma (Richter's transformation) which is often, but not always, clonally related to the CLL. The most common nonhaematological malignancies are squamous and basal cell carcinomas, which can be aggressive. Lung cancer risk is markedly increased in smokers with CLL, while the risk of most other common cancers is also increased. The reason for the increased risk of second malignancies is unknown, but contributing factors could include a genetic predisposition, immunosuppression, and shared environmental risk factors.

Epidemiology

CLL is the most prevalent lymphoid malignancy in Europe and North America, with a lower prevalence in Africa and lowest prevalence in the Far East. In most patients with access to modern medical care, CLL is an incidental diagnosis made during investigation of lymphocytosis. These patients usually have early-stage asymptomatic disease.

CLL is very rare in patients under the age of 30, and the median age at diagnosis is about 70 years. There is a 1.5 to 2:1 male to female predominance. Most patients with CLL will die of the disease or its complications. CLL is likely to decrease the overall survival of all patients who have the disease, even older patients with early-stage disease.

The improvement in diagnostic methods has resulted in an increased recognition of small monoclonal B-cell populations, often with a CLL immunophenotype, in patients with normal lymphocyte counts and no other evidence of CLL. This monoclonal B-cell lymphocytosis (MBL) increases in prevalence with age and can be detected in over 3% of Europeans over the age of 65 years. The natural history of MBL is not yet defined, but retrospective data suggest that only a minority of people will progress to CLL or other clinically relevant lymphoid malignancies.

Prevention

There are no known preventive measures to decrease the risk of CLL.

Clinical features

CLL has a highly variable clinical presentation and course. Most patients now have an incidental diagnosis on investigation of lymphocytosis with no clinical features of disease. These patients should have as complete an evaluation of the prognostic biological characteristics of their disease as possible. Although no treatment is indicated outside of clinical trials, this information is still very important for the planning of subsequent care and to allow the patients to adjust to their new diagnosis.

The clinical manifestations of CLL can be a direct consequence of the disease burden or the indirect effects of the CLL cells. The rate of progression of CLL is highly variable. A minority of patients have rapidly progressive disease and require treatment for symptoms or cytopenia within a few years of treatment. In contrast, about 20 to 30% of patients never need treatment for their CLL. Progressive adenopathy can cause disfigurement and abdominal distention and discomfort. Obstructions of the ureters or other viscera are rare but serious complications when encountered. Progressive splenomegaly can cause abdominal discomfort in the left upper quadrant, abdominal distention, and early satiety. Splenic infarcts can cause severe abdominal pain. Anaemia is usually the first manifestation of bone marrow failure caused by progressive infiltration

by CLL cells. This is often followed by the development of thrombocytopenia. However, the differential diagnosis of both anaemia and thrombocytopenia in patients with cytopenia includes AIHA, ITP, PRCA, and other unrelated causes. The lymphocyte count can increase to very high levels in patients with CLL, but complications of even extreme lymphocytosis are extremely rare. In patients with progressive disease, increased tumour burden can be associated with severe fatigue, drenching night sweats, fevers, and nondeliberate weight loss. These clinical features need to be carefully investigated to ensure that they are caused by CLL rather than other medical conditions.

Disruption of immune function by CLL causes both immunosuppression and an increase in autoimmune cytopenia. Because of the early suppression of humoral immunity, patients are at high risk of infections by encapsulated bacteria which can cause severe infections. Further deterioration of immune function including T-cell-mediated immunity will increase the risk of viral reactivation and opportunistic infections as the disease progresses or is treated with therapies that decrease immune function. Autoimmune complications of CLL usually cause cytopenia. The most common problems are AIHA and PRCA resulting in symptomatic anaemia and ITP which can cause bleeding. These abnormalities need to be carefully differentiated from cytopenia caused by bone marrow failure, which has a poorer prognosis and often requires different therapy.

Second malignancies are markedly increased in patients with CLL. CLL is associated with a significant increase in second lymphoid malignancies. The most common of these is diffuse large cell lymphoma which can cause dramatic weight loss, drenching night sweats, fevers, and rapid increases in the size of lymph nodes. Patients with CLL also have an increased risk of developing other second lymphomas including Hodgkin's lymphoma. CLL is also associated with a significant increase in the risk of nonhaematological malignancies. One of the most common is skin cancer, which can be locally aggressive and metastasize. There is also a substantial additional increase in the risk of lung cancer in smokers with CLL.

Differential diagnosis

The differential diagnosis of CLL depends on the presentation. Most patients present with sustained lymphocytosis. The differential diagnosis then includes benign aetiologies associated with lymphocytosis, which is some times atypical, and other lymphoid malignacies in leukaemic phase (Fig. 22.3.5.1). Benign lymphocytosis is usually caused by chronic infections (e.g. hepatitis C). The other lymphoid malignancies that most often present with lymphocytosis with mature small lymphocytes are the leukaemic phase of mantle cell, marginal zone, follicular, and lymphoplasmacytic lymphoma, hairy cell leukaemia, prolymphocytic leukaemia, and the unclassified chronic B-cell lymphoproliferative disorders. In patients presenting with lymphadenopathy and splenomegaly, the differential diagnosis includes a wide range of benign and malignant causes, and when malignant blood lymphocytes are not available for analysis, a bone marrow or lymph node biopsy, or even splenectomy could be required to establish the diagnosis.

Clinical investigation

CLL is most easily diagnosed by analysis of the immunophenotype of malignant cells from the blood. In rare patients without a detectable

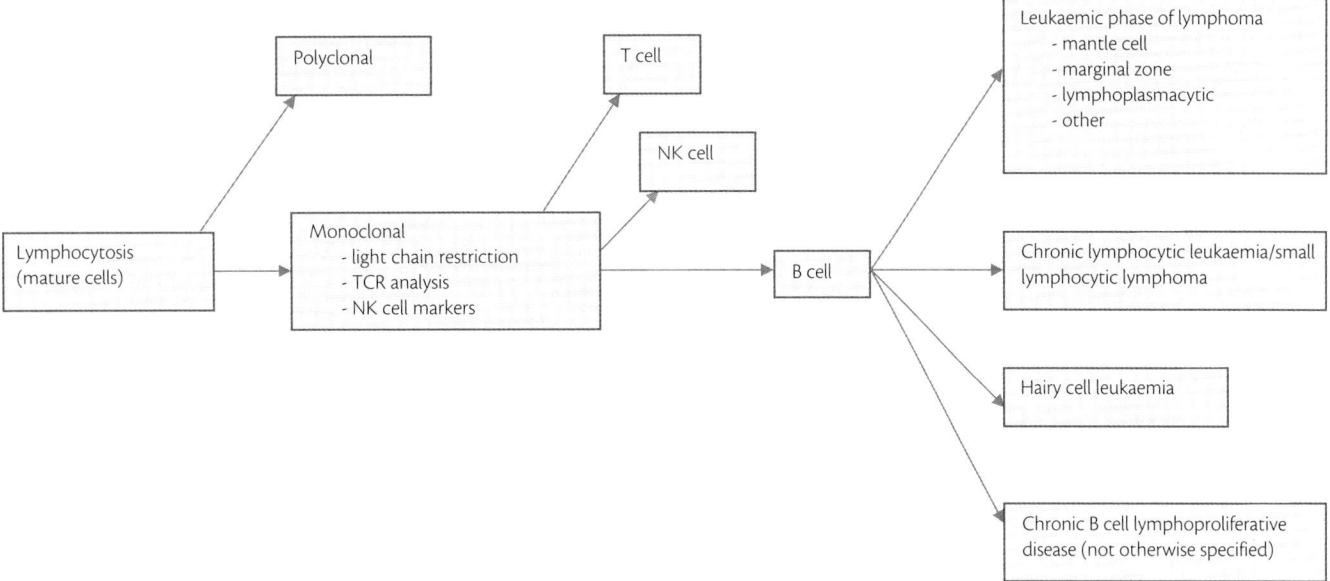

Fig. 22.3.5.1 Evaluation of chronic lymphocytosis. TCR, T-cell receptor.

monoclonal B-cell population in the blood, lymphocytes from the bone marrow, lymph nodes, or spleen can be examined. Staging is based on a clinical examination and blood count evaluation and does not require imaging studies or a bone marrow study (Box 22.3.5.1). Bone marrow studies are required to investigate the cause of cytopenias and are done prior to initiation of therapy by many physicians to ensure that patients do not have other causes of cytopenia and to determine tumour burden. Imaging studies are not required routinely in all patients, and their use can be limited to investigating specific concerns. However, an increasing number of treating physicians do CT scans before starting specific therapy as a baseline study to facilitate evaluation of the therapeutic outcome. These studies could be useful in planning subsequent management especially in younger patients with CLL. Testing for prognostic factors is important and is detailed in the section on staging CLL.

Criteria for diagnosis

The CLL cell typically coexpresses the B-cell surface antigen CD19 with CD5 and CD23 and has low levels of expression of surface immunoglobulin (and CD79b) and CD20. These characteristics are used for diagnosis by flow cytometric or immunohistochemical techniques. Interphase fluorescent in situ hybridization (FISH) examination of CLL cells with an IGH probe is very useful for excluding mantle cell lymphoma with its characteristic t(11;14). The current criteria for diagnosis of CLL have an arbitrary requirement for a B-cell lymphocytosis $>5\times10^9$/litre, clinically detectable adenopathy (at least 1 cm in diameter), organomegaly, or $>30\%$ bone marrow involvement by CLL cells.

Staging CLL

The clinical staging systems for CLL are based on readily available clinical data. The widely used Rai and Binet classifications use clinical examination and the complete blood count to determine tumour burden (Box 22.3.5.1). These simple methods are very effective at identifying patients with advanced-stage disease who have a poorer prognosis (median survival of about 4–6 years). However, clinical

staging using the Rai or Binet classifications does not provide any information on the risk of disease progression in the majority of patients who are diagnosed with early-intermediate-stage CLL.

Improvements in the diagnosis and management of CLL in the past few decades have increased the utility of determining prognosis at diagnosis in earlier-stage disease. This information can be very useful to health care providers and patients in planning medical care. There has been impressive progress in defining molecular determinants of

---

Box 22.3.5.1   Clinical staging of CLL

Rai classification

0   lymphocytosis

I   lymphocytosis and lymphadenopathy

II   lymphocytosis and palpable liver or spleen enlargement

III   lymphocytosis and anaemia (Hgb <110 g/litre)

IV   lymphocytosis and thrombocytopenia (platelets $<100\times10^9$/litre)

Modified Rai classification

Low risk   stage 0

Intermediate risk stages I–II

High risk   stages III–IV

Binet classification

A lymphocytosis and lymphadenopathy in <3 areas[a]

B lymphocytosis and lymphadenopathy ≥3 areas[a]

C anaemia (<100 g/litre) and/or thrombocytopenia ($<100\times10^9$/litre)

[a] Areas are cervical, axillary, and inguinal nodes (unilateral or bilateral), liver, and spleen (n = 5).

Table 22.3.5.1 Molecular prognostic factors and risk of disease progression in early-stage CLL

	Low risk	Intermediate risk	High risk
FISH	13q14- as sole abnormality	Nil, 12+	17p13-, 11q22-
IgVH mutation	Mutated (≥2%) except for VH3-21	Unmutated VH3-21 mutated	
ZAP-70 (≥20%)	Negative	Positive	
CD38 (≥30%)	Negative	Positive	

FISH, fluorescent *in situ* hybridization.

risk in CLL patients. These are direct measurements of critical biological parameters in the malignant CLL B cells rather than indirect measures of tumour progression. The best-studied novel parameters are immunoglobulin mutation sequence analysis (mutation status of IgV_H), specific chromosomal defects detected by using interphase FISH, expression of the intracellular protein ZAP-70, and membrane protein CD38 (Table 22.3.5.1). IgV_H mutation (≥2% difference from germline sequence) is associated with a significantly better survival in multiple retrospective analyses. FISH analysis is currently the most useful available clinical method of chromosome analysis in CLL and usually includes probes for detection of deletions at chromosome bands 13q14, 11q22, 17p13, and 6q21, trisomy 12 (12+), and abnormalities involving 14q32 (IgH locus). Deletion of 17q13 (17p13-) resulting in loss of p53 is associated with a shorter time to initial treatment, poor response to treatment, and very poor survival. Deletion of 11q22 (11q22-), resulting in loss of the *ATM* gene, is more common in younger patients and associated with more aggressive disease, bulky adenopathy, and a poorer prognosis. Patients with 12+ or no detected abnormality have an intermediate prognosis and patients with only deletion of 13q14 (13q14-) have the most favourable prognosis of all. ZAP-70 is an intracellular signalling molecule expressed at a high level by T lymphocytes but only in a small minority of normal B cells. ZAP-70 expression (≥20% positive cells) was originally predicted to be a surrogate marker for unmutated IgV_H. Although this predictive capability of ZAP-70 measurement was subsequently found to be limited, ZAP-70 expression is an independent marker of poor prognosis in CLL. Unfortunately, the assay for ZAP-70 expression is technically demanding and poorly reproducible, which limits its clinical application. CD38 is a cell membrane protein of uncertain function expressed by mature B cells and plasma cells. Expression of CD38 by ≥30% of CLL cells is an independent predictor of poor prognosis, but the expression of CD38 can change during the course of CLL, and there is still no consensus on the clinical application of this measurement. Additional biological markers of prognosis in early-stage CLL include serum β_2-microglobulin, soluble CD23, thymidine kinase, and the percentage of smudge cells on the peripheral smear (low numbers predict for poorer prognosis). The challenge is to combine a selection of these factors and other markers of prognosis into a practical prognostic formulation that will be easy to use and accessible to most patients with CLL.

Treatment

Currently, there is no standard curative therapy for CLL. Patients should not be treated until they have progressive and symptomatic disease or develop anaemia or thrombocytopenia due to bone marrow failure. In this regard, early treatment of all patients has not been shown to be of benefit and could even be detrimental to some patients.

Initial treatment

Patients are treated for progressive disease as defined by the National Cancer Center Working Group criteria of 1996 which were recently revised by the International Workshop for CLL (IWCLL). These recommend that patients should be treated only if they are symptomatic from progressive disease (severe fatigue, drenching night sweats, fever, >10% weight loss, discomfort from lymphadenopathy or splenomegaly), or if they develop anaemia (hemoglobin <11 g/dl) or thrombocytopenia (platelets $<100 \times 10^9$/ litre).

The best initial treatment for CLL is not yet defined and is likely to differ depending on the biology of the disease, patient comorbidities, and functional status of the patient. Single-agent therapy with oral chlorambucil was until recently regarded as the standard of care and still could have a role for initial treatment of frail patients or those with multiple comorbidities. The purine analogues (fludarabine, pentostatin, and cladribine) in use since the late 1980s, have achieved higher response rates than chlorambucil, but improvements in overall survival have been difficult to prove largely because of crossover of relapsing patients to other effective therapies. The German, British, and American trials have shown that results with a combination of fludarabine and cyclophosphamide are better than fludarabine alone. Therapy of CLL has been further improved by the introduction of the therapeutic monoclonal antibodies alemtuzumab (anti-CD52) and rituximab (anti-CD20). However, rituximab has limited efficacy as a single agent, and neither antibody is effective against bulky adenopathy or splenomegaly. Response rates for first-line therapy of CLL are currently highest with the use of chemoimmunotherapy using a combination of purine analogues, cyclophosphamide, and rituximab. The regimen with one of the highest response rates is fludarabine, cyclophosphamide, and rituximab (FCR), but its use is limited by myelotoxicity and infection, and the pentostatin, cyclophosphamide, and rituximab (PCR) regimen seems to be better tolerated. These regimens usually have a high response rate (*c.*90%) with a complete response rate ranging from 40 to 60%. The median duration of response is about 3 to 4 years. The initial reports of the large German CLL Group prospective randomized trial comparing initial treatment of progressive CLL with FCR vs FC show significantly better survival for those patients treated with FCR. Patients with the 17p13-, who generally have aggressive disease, are very often not responsive to purine analogue–based therapies but do usually respond to regimens employing alemtuzumab.

Relapsed/refractory disease

Patients with progressive disease usually do not need treatment until they once again fulfil the criteria for treatment. There is no standard therapy for this group of patients, and in those who have had an initial duration of response to their first-line treatment of at least 1 year, retreatment with the same regimen is reasonable and recommended by most physicians. In patients with initial treatment failure or earlier progression, treatment options depend on comorbidity and the biological characteristics of the CLL. Treatment options then include alemtuzumab-containing regimens or high-dose corticosteroids. There are an increasing number of drugs showing therapeutic value in these patients, including lenalidomide, flavopiridol, and the newer monoclonal antibodies such as ofatumumab. In patients with extensive comorbidity, treatment could be limited to palliative measures.

High-dose chemotherapy with autologous stem cell support has limited value in CLL. In contrast, allogeneic transplant can induce a therapeutic graft-vs-leukaemia effect and can potentially be curative in CLL. Myeloablative allogeneic transplantation is however associated with very high treatment-related mortality (c.30–40%) largely due to infection, and is thus of limited value. However, reduced intensity conditioning allogeneic transplantation appears to have a lower initial morbidity and mortality and could be an acceptable and reasonable alternative for some patients with aggressive CLL. Use of reduced intensity conditioning regimens requires a pretransplant regimen that can effectively decrease tumour bulk so that the transplanted immune system has sufficient time to develop a therapeutic graft-vs-leukaemia effect. Graft-vs-host disease is often delayed but can be severe and together with donor availability and cost are the major limitations to use of this treatment.

Management of complications of CLL

Autoimmune cytopenia is responsible for about 20% of anaemia and thrombocytopenia in patients with CLL. In CLL patients without a large CLL tumour burden, treatment should be directed at the autoimmune cytopenia. Initial management of severe anaemia or thrombocytopenia is usually corticosteroids but may also require the use of intravenous immunoglobulin (IVIG). Patients with ITP can benefit from splenectomy, but patients with AIHA are less likely to benefit from this measure. Many patients with AIHA and ITP will benefit from the use of rituximab. However, because about half of the cases of PRBCA involve a cellular immunity–mediated mechanism, rituximab is less likely to be effective treatment for this entity. Management of more advanced stage CLL complicated by autoimmune cytopenia requires regimens that can treat both the autoimmune disorder and the CLL. Purine analogue monotherapy can cause autoimmune complications and should be avoided. Effective regimens combine alkylating agents, corticosteroids, and rituximab. The use of purine analogue–containing regimens including rituximab and alkylating agents is controversial.

Infection is the most common direct cause of death in CLL. Even in early-stage CLL, patients have increased susceptibility to infections with encapsulated bacteria which can progress rapidly and prove fatal. CLL patients are also at increased risk of sinusitis and other respiratory tract infections. Patients should be educated about this risk and advised to seek early medical evaluation for all febrile illnesses. With disease progression and treatment, patients develop more severe defects in cellular immunity and become more susceptible to viral and opportunistic infections. Once again, patients need to be educated about the need for early antimicrobial treatment. Prophylactic treatment of patients with monthly IVIG does decrease the risk of bacterial infection but has not been shown to improve overall survival and is expensive and tedious. Use of prophylactic antiviral therapy in patients with recurrent herpes zoster and herpes simplex infections can be beneficial. Vaccination for influenza and pneumococcus are less effective than in immunocompetent subjects but are still useful and indicated.

Second malignancies

Patients with CLL require careful observation for second malignancies. This includes education about the symptoms of transformation including drenching night sweats, fever, and involuntary weight loss. Diffuse large B-cell lymphoma (Richter's transformation) or Hodgkin's lymphoma requires immediate treatment, but responses are usually poorer than those achieved by patients with primary lymphoma. CLL patients also need to be educated about skin care including avoidance of sun damage. They need careful observation for the development of skin cancers which should be treated aggressively when detected. An important measure to decrease the risk of other secondary cancers is the cessation of smoking. Careful routine checks for malignancy should be advised and can be beneficial.

Quality of life

A diagnosis of incurable CLL is stressful. This emotional burden is exacerbated by the absence of effective early intervention and the 'watch and wait' period of care. Management of this problem can be difficult. Measures of value in alleviating this problem include education, a simple and frank discussion of the disease and its complications, and acceptance of the validity of the patient's concerns.

Prognosis

The prognosis of patients with CLL is highly variable and depends on the clinical stage of disease, biological characteristics of the malignant cells, and the general health of the patient. Patients with advanced-stage disease have a poor prognosis with a median survival of 4 to 6 years. In contrast, patients with early-stage disease have a wide variation of median survival. This ranges from decades in the lowest risk cohort (mutated IgV_H, 13q14- as the sole abnormality on FISH analysis, negative for ZAP-70 and CD38) to a few years for patients with 17p13-.

Areas of uncertainty or controversy

Biology

The cause of CLL and the role of genetic susceptibility to the disease are topics of active research. One of the most interesting aspects is the role of the B-cell receptor and its antigen specificity in the aetiology and progression of CLL

Prognostic markers

The ability to use molecular markers to predict prognosis at diagnosis could be very helpful in the management of patients with CLL. However, the best practical way to combine these tests in clinical practice is still being evaluated.

Treatment

The standard of care is still to treat patients with CLL only when they have progressive disease causing clinical problems. However the ability to predict which patients are at high risk of disease progression could change this paradigm. Selection of a subgroup of patients with lower tumour burden for earlier treatment could in principle be more effective. In addition, the best use of currently available drugs is still undecided. Some of the most effective drugs such as the purine analogues and alemtuzumab are highly immunosuppressive, and the timing and optimal combination of therapy for treatment of each stage of CLL has not yet been defined.

Likely developments over the next 5 to 10 years

Biology

Current research will no doubt result in an improved understanding of the aetiology of the disease including the genetic defects contributing to CLL aetiology. Definition of the immune defects in patients with CLL could result in a much better understanding of the early defect in humoural immunity and help to explain why some patients develop autoimmune cytopenia.

Treatment

Risk-stratified approaches should provide optimal therapies for patients while potentially curative therapies could be developed from attempts to generate the graft-vs-leukaemia effect without transplantation.

Further reading

Auer RL, *et al.* (2007). Emerging therapy for chronic lymphocytic leukaemia. *Br J Haematol*, **139**, 635–44.

Binet JL, *et al.* (1981). A new prognostic classification of chronic lymphocytic leukemia derived from a multivariate survival analysis. *Cancer*, **48**, 198–205.

Brenner H, *et al.* (2008). Trends in long-term survival of patients with chronic lymphocytic leukemia from the 1980s to the early 21st century. *Blood*, **111**, 4916–21.

Byrd JC, *et al.* (2005). Addition of rituximab to fludarabine may prolong progression-free survival and overall survival in patients with previously untreated chronic lymphocytic leukemia: an updated retrospective comparative analysis of CALGB 9712 and CALGB 9011. *Blood*, **105**, 49–53.

Byrd JC, *et al.* (2007). Flavopiridol administered using a pharmacologically derived schedule is associated with marked clinical efficacy in refractory, genetically high-risk chronic lymphocytic leukemia. *Blood*, **109**, 399–404.

Calin GA, *et al.* (2002). Frequent deletions and down-regulation of micro-RNA genes miR15 and miR16 at 13q14 in chronic lymphocytic leukemia. *Proc Natl Acad Sci U S A*, **99**, 15 524–9.

Catovsky D, *et al.* (2007). Assessment of fludarabine plus cyclophosphamide for patients with chronic lymphocytic leukaemia (the LRF CLL4 Trial): a randomised controlled trial. *Lancet*, **370**, 230–9.

Chanan-Khan A, *et al.* (2006). Clinical efficacy of lenalidomide in patients with relapsed or refractory chronic lymphocytic leukemia: results of a phase II study. *J Clin Oncol*, **24**, 5343–9.

Cheson BD, *et al.* (1996). National Cancer Institute-Sponsored Working Group guidelines for chronic lymphocytic leukemia: revised guidelines for diagnosis and treatment. *Blood*, **87**, 4990–7.

Crespo M, *et al.* (2003). ZAP-70 expression as a surrogate for immunoglobulin-variable-region mutations in chronic lymphocytic leukemia. *N Engl J Med*, **348**, 1764–75.

Damle RN, *et al.* (1999). Ig V gene mutation status and CD38 expression as novel prognostic indicators in chronic lymphocytic leukemia. *Blood*, **94**, 1840–7.

Dighiero G, Hamblin TJ (2008). Chronic lymphocytic leukaemia. *Lancet*, **371**, 1017–29.

Ding W, Zent CS (2007). Diagnosis and management of autoimmune complications of chronic lymphocytic leukemia/ small lymphocytic lymphoma. *Clin Adv Hematol Oncol*, **5**, 257–61.

Dores GM, *et al.* (2007). Chronic lymphocytic leukaemia and small lymphocytic lymphoma: overview of the descriptive epidemiology. *Br J Haematol*, **139**, 809–19.

Eichhorst BF, *et al.* (2006). Fludarabine plus cyclophosphamide versus fludarabine alone in first-line therapy of younger patients with chronic lymphocytic leukemia. *Blood*, **107**, 885–91.

Faderl S, *et al.* (2003). Experience with alemtuzumab plus rituximab in patients with relapsed and refractory lymphoid malignancies. *Blood*, **101**, 3413–15.

Flinn IW, *et al.* (2007). Phase III trial of fludarabine plus cyclophosphamide compared with fludarabine for patients with previously untreated chronic lymphocytic leukemia: US Intergroup Trial E2997. *J Clin Oncol*, **25**, 793–8.

Ghia P, *et al.* (2004). Monoclonal CD5+ and CD5- B-lymphocyte expansions are frequent in the peripheral blood of the elderly. *Blood*, **103**, 2337–42.

Grever MR, *et al.* (2007). Comprehensive assessment of genetic and molecular features predicting outcome in patients with chronic lymphocytic leukemia: results from the US Intergroup Phase III Trial E2997. *J Clin Oncol*, **25**, 799–804.

Gribben JG (2005). Salvage therapy for CLL and the role of stem cell transplantation. *Hematology Am Soc Hematol Educ Program*, 292–8.

Hallek M, *et al.* (2008). Guidelines for the diagnosis and treatment of chronic lymphocytic leukemia: a report from the International Workshop on Chronic Lymphocytic Leukemia (IWCLL) updating the National Cancer Institute-Working Group (NCI-WG) 1996 guidelines. *Blood*, **111**, 5446–56.

Hamblin T (2001). Autoimmune disease and its management in chronic lymphocytic leukemia. In: Cheson B (ed) *Chronic lymphocytic leukemias*, pp. 435–58. Marcel Dekker, New York.

Hamblin T, *et al.* (1999). Unmutated Ig V(H) genes are associated with a more aggressive form of chronic lymphocytic leukemia. *Blood*, **94**, 1848–54.

Harris N, *et al.* (1994). A revised European-American classification of lymphoid neoplasms: a proposal from the International Lymphoma Study Group. *Blood*, **84**, 1361–92.

Kay NE, *et al.* (2007). Combination chemoimmunotherapy with pentostatin, cyclophosphamide and rituximab shows significant clinical activity with low accompanying toxicity in previously untreated B-chronic lymphocytic leukemia. *Blood*, **109**, 405–11.

Keating MJ, *et al.* (2002). Therapeutic role of alemtuzumab (Campath-1H) in patients who have failed fludarabine: results of a large international study. *Blood*, **99**, 3554–61.

Keating MJ, *et al.* (2005). Early results of a chemoimmunotherapy regimen of fludarabine, cyclophosphamide, and rituximab as initial therapy for chronic lymphocytic leukemia. *J Clin Oncol*, **23**, 4079–88.

Lundin J, *et al.* (2002). Phase II trial of subcutaneous anti-CD52 monoclonal antibody alemtuzumab (Campath-1H) as first-line treatment for patients with B-cell chronic lymphocytic leukemia (B-CLL). *Blood*, **100**, 768–73.

Marti G, *et al.* (2007). Overview of monoclonal B-cell lymphocytosis. *Br J Haematol*, **139**, 701–8.

Messmer BT, *et al.* (2005). In vivo measurements document the dynamic cellular kinetics of chronic lymphocytic leukemia B cells. *J Clin Invest*, **115**, 755–64.

Muller-Hermelink HK, *et al.* (2001). Chronic lymphocytic leukemia/ small lymphocytic lymphoma. In: Jaffe E, *et al.* (eds) *Tumours of haematopoietic and lymphoid tissues*, pp. 127–30. IARC Press, Lyon.

Nowakowski GS, *et al.* (2005). Interphase fluorescence in situ hybridization with an IGH probe is important in the evaluation of patients with a clinical diagnosis of chronic lymphocytic leukaemia. *Br J Haematol*, **130**, 36–42.

Nowakowski GS, *et al.* (2007). Using smudge cells on routine blood smears to predict clinical outcome in chronic lymphocytic leukemia: a universally available prognostic test. *Mayo Clin Proc*, **82**, 449–53.

Rai KR, *et al.* (1975). Clinical staging of chronic lymphocytic leukemia. *Blood*, **46**, 219–34.

Rai KR, *et al.* (2000). Fludarabine compared with chlorambucil as primary therapy for chronic lymphocytic leukemia. *N Engl J Med*, **343**, 1750–7.

Rawstron AC, *et al.* (2002). Monoclonal B lymphocytes with the characteristics of "indolent" chronic lymphocytic leukemia are present in 3.5% of adults with normal blood counts. *Blood*, **100**, 635–9.

Shanafelt TD, Kay NE (2007). Comprehensive management of the CLL patient: a holistic approach. *Hematology Am Soc Hematol Educ Program*, **2007**, 324–31.

Shanafelt TD, *et al.* (2006). Narrative review: initial management of newly diagnosed, early-stage chronic lymphocytic leukemia. *Ann Intern Med*, **145**, 435–47.

Shanafelt TD, *et al.* (2006). Prospective evaluation of clonal evolution during long-term follow-up of patients with untreated early-stage chronic lymphocytic leukemia. *J Clin Oncol*, **24**, 4634–41.

Zent CS, *et al.* (2001). Chronic lymphocytic leukemia incidence is substantially higher than estimated from tumor registry data. *Cancer*, **92**, 1325–30.

Zent CS, *et al.* (2006). Update on risk-stratified management for chronic lymphocytic leukemia. *Leuk Lymphoma*, **47**, 1738–46.

Zent CS, *et al.* (2008). The prognostic significance of cytopenia in chronic lymphocytic leukemia/small lymphocytic lymphoma. *Br J Haematol*, **141**, 615–21.

22.3.6 Chronic myeloid leukaemia

Tariq I. Mughal and John M. Goldman

Essentials

Chronic myeloid leukaemia has a worldwide incidence of 1 to 2 per 100 000 population. Most cases are caused by translocation of the distal end of chromosome 9 on to chromosome 22 (known as a Philadelphia chromosome), which leads to the creation of a fusion protein from the *BCR* (break-point cluster region) and *ABL* genes that is a constitutive tyrosine kinase and appears to operate as an initiator for the development of the leukaemia. Why this translocation occurs is not known.

Clinical features, diagnosis, and (historical) prognosis

Clinical features—many patients are asymptomatic at diagnosis, which is made following a routine blood test. Others present with signs and symptoms including fatigue, sweats, fever, weight loss, haemorrhagic manifestations, and abdominal discomfort (due to splenomegaly).

Diagnosis—this is typically made by the examination of a peripheral blood film (revealing features including increased numbers of myelocytes) and the demonstration of the Philadelphia chromosome by conventional cytogenetics on a bone marrow aspirate sample. PCR analysis of peripheral blood or marrow confirms the presence of a *BCR-ABL1* gene and characterizes the *BCR-ABL1* junction.

Prognosis—before the introduction of tyrosine kinase inhibitors (see below) the condition, having usually been diagnosed in the chronic phase, then spontaneously progressed after (typically) 3 to 6 years to myeloid (or less commonly lymphoid) blast transformation, which had very poor prognosis.

Treatment

Aside from supportive care, first line management is with the tyrosine kinase inhibitor imatinib, which induces complete haematological remission in 98% of all previously untreated patients and prolongs overall survival very substantially, although it does not totally eradicate disease in most cases. Patients with sub-optimal responses to imatinib can be offered (1) newer tyrosine kinase inhibitors—e.g. dasatinib, nilotinib, and bosutinib; and (2) allogeneic stem cell transplantation—for patients less than 50 years of age and with a suitable donor.

Introduction

Patients with the rare malignancy, chronic myeloid leukaemia (CML), have been well served by translational research over the past half century. Though the disease was first described in 1845 and characterized by the 1920s, it was 60 years before the unravelling of initiating molecular events paved the way to define specific targets for treatment. CML is a clonal disease that results from an acquired molecular change in a pluripotential haematopoietic stem cell. The leukaemia cells have a consistent cytogenetic abnormality, the Philadelphia (Ph) chromosome, which carries a *BCR-ABL1* fusion gene (Fig. 22.3.6.1). This gene encodes a Bcr-Abl1 oncoprotein with enhanced tyrosine kinase activity, which is generally considered to be the 'initiating event' in the chronic phase of CML, though there remains debate as to whether this is the first molecular event in all cases.

Imatinib mesylate can inhibit the enzymatic activity of this dysregulated tyrosine kinase of the Bcr-Abl1 oncoprotein and has now become the preferred treatment for all newly diagnosed patients with CML, except perhaps for some children. Imatinib substantially reduces the number of leukaemia cells in a patient's body, and comparison with historical data confirms the notion that it prolongs overall survival very substantially. However, complete molecular responses occur only in a minority of patients, and allogeneic stem cell transplantation (allo-SCT) remains the only treatment that can reliably produce complete and durable molecular remission due presumably to eradication of all residual leukaemia stem cells. The second-generation ABL-kinase inhibitors, notably dasatinib and nilotinib, are now firmly established in clinical use for the treatment of imatinib-resistant/refractory CML and Ph-positive acute lymphoblastic leukaemia. Both drugs are now being tested as potential first-line therapies.

Epidemiology

The annual incidence of CML is constant worldwide at about 1.0 to 2.0 per 100 000 of population per annum. In the Western world, it represents approximately 15% of all adult leukaemias and less than 5% of all childhood leukaemias, but it is higher as a percentage of all leukaemias in China and India, where chronic lymphocytic leukaemia is very rare. In the Western world, the median age of onset is about 50 years, and there is a slight male excess.

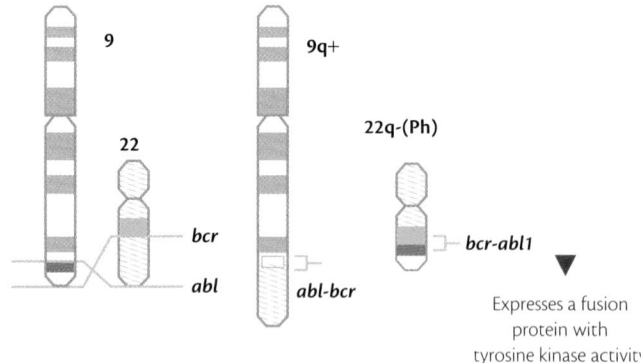

Fig. 22.3.6.1 A schematic representation of how the t(9;22) translocation produces the Philadelphia (Ph) chromosome.

In contrast, the median age of onset may be considerably younger, around 36 years, in some countries such as India.

Aetiology

For most patients with CML, possibly for all, there appear to be no obvious predisposing factors, and the disease arises sporadically. Epidemiology studies have suggested a marginal increment in the number of cases of CML following exposure to high doses of irradiation as occurred in survivors of the Hiroshima and Nagasaki atomic bombs in 1945. A small number of families with a high incidence of the disease have also been reported, though no specific HLA genotypes have been identified. One convincing case has been reported of CML recurring in cells of donor origin following related allo-SCT.

Natural history

CML is a remarkably heterogeneous disease. Before the introduction of tyrosine kinase inhibitors, it typically ran a biphasic or triphasic course. It was usually diagnosed in the chronic phase, which lasted typically 3 to 6 years; the leukaemia then spontaneously progressed to blast transformation. About 70 to 80% of patients had a myeloid blast transformation, and they usually survived 2 and 6 months; the 20 to 30% of patients with a lymphoid blast transformation had a slightly better survival. About half the patients in

the chronic phase transformed directly into blast transformation, and the remainder did so following a period of accelerated phase.

Soon after the introduction of imatinib mesylate, it was observed that the natural history for most patients with CML who received this drug as initial therapy, particularly for patients who remain in complete cytogenetic response beyond the fourth year of therapy, was very greatly improved. The recent follow-up of the phase III prospective trial (IRIS) which compared imatinib to the previous best nontransplant therapy, interferon-α (IFN-α) and cytarabine, showed that about 60% of the original cohort randomized to receive the drug were still taking imatinib and were still in complete cytogenetic remission 6 years after starting the drug; none of these patients had entered the more advanced phases of the disease (Figs. 22.3.6.2 and 22.3.6.3). Patients presenting in the late chronic phase appear to fare less well, and those in the advanced phases, particularly the blast phase, generally do poorly, including those who did initially respond to imatinib mesylate. In patients with lymphoid blast phase CML, there appear to be no durable responses beyond 6 months.

For patients who receive an allo-SCT, most remain in a complete cytogenetic and molecular remission for 10 years or more. Many of these patients are probably completely cured, if one defines cure as the complete eradication of all molecular evidence of the disease. It is of interest, however, that some of these patients do become intermittently positive for Bcr-Abl1 transcripts, albeit at low levels, but the rare patient with a persisting high transcript level is at a high risk of relapse. A very small minority appear to relapse directly into the advanced phases of the disease.

Clinical features and diagnosis

Current estimates suggest that one-third to one-half of patients with CML are totally asymptomatic at diagnosis, which is made following a routine blood test. The remainder present with signs and symptoms often of about 3 months' duration and related to altered haematopoiesis, particularly anaemia and platelet dysfunction and increasing disease burden, resulting in splenomegaly. Most patients will have leucocytosis due to increased numbers of myelocytes and segmented neutrophils; basophilia is almost universal, and some patients have a eosinophilia. The anaemia tends to be mild and normochromic normocytic in nature; some patients have a degree

Fig. 22.3.6.2 IRIS study following a 6-year follow-up: annual events in all patients. AP, accelerated-phase; BC, blast crisis; CHR, complete haematologic response; MCyR, major cytogenetic response.
(Adapted from Hochhaus A, *et al.*; (2007). IRIS 6-year follow-up: sustained survival and declining annual rate of transformation in patients with newly diagnosed chronic myeloid leukemia in chronic phase (CML-CP) treated with imatinib. *Blood* (ASH Annual Meeting Abstracts), **110**, Abstract 25.)

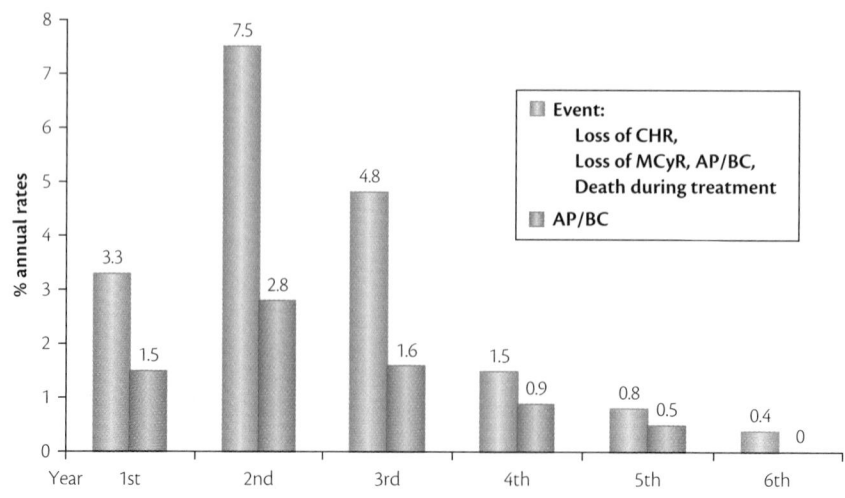

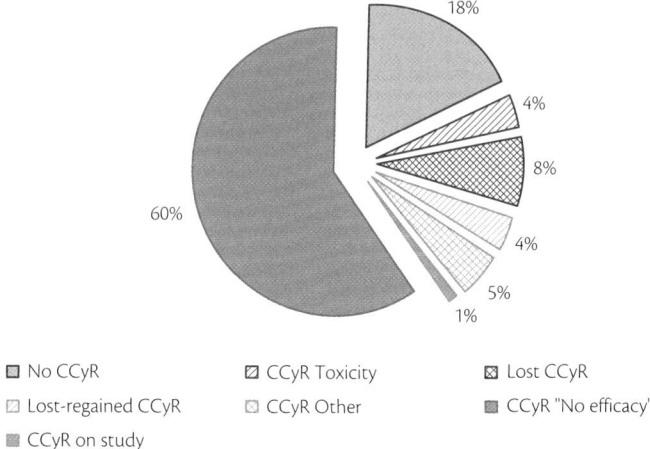

Fig. 22.3.6.3 IRIS study following a 6-year follow-up post imatinib mesylate (IM) treatment: outcomes. CCyR, complete cytogenetic response.
(Adapted from Hochhaus A, et al. (2007). IRIS 6-year follow-up: sustained survival and declining annual rate of transformation in patients with newly diagnosed chronic myeloid leukemia in chronic phase (CML-CP) treated with imatinib. *Blood* (ASH Annual Meeting Abstracts), **110**, Abstract 25.)

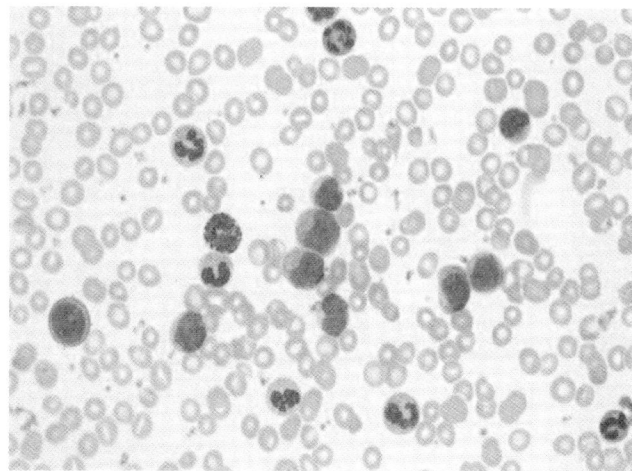

Fig. 22.3.6.4 A peripheral blood film from a patient with CML in chronic phase.

of thrombocytosis. Nearly all patients diagnosed in the advanced phases of CML are symptomatic. Occasionally patients may present with an extramedullary event, such as a chloroma.

Classical clinical features include sweats, weight loss, haemorrhagic manifestations such as spontaneous bruising and retinal haemorrhages, abdominal discomfort due to splenomegaly, fatigue often, but not always, related to anaemia and fever (Box 22.3.6.1). The diagnosis is typically made by the examination of a peripheral blood film and the demonstration of the Ph chromosome by conventional cytogenetics on a bone marrow aspirate sample. Most haematologists carry out a bone marrow trephine examination also; this is often hypercellular with complete or near complete loss of fat spaces and a high myeloid to erythroid ratio. There may be up to 10% of blast cells (Fig. 22.3.6.4).

Sometimes the diagnosis is made by demonstrating the presence of a *BCR-ABL1* gene by fluorescence *in situ* hybridization (FISH) on a peripheral blood sample. Modern practice dictates

Box 22.3.6.1 Clinical features of patients with chronic phase CML seen at the Hammersmith Hospital, London

- Fatigue 33.5%
- Bleeding 21.3%
- Weight loss 20.0%
- Abdominal discomfort (left upper quadrant) 18.6%
- Sweats 14.6%
- Bone pain 7.4%
- Splenomegaly 75.8%
- Hepatomegaly 2.2%

(Adapted with permission from Savage D, et al. (1997). Clinical features at diagnosis in 430 patients with chronic myeloid leukaemia seen at a referral centre over a 16-year period. *Br J Haematol*, **96**, 111–16.)

the use of a baseline real-time quantitative polymerase chain reaction (RQ-PCR) analysis of peripheral blood or marrow to confirm the presence of a *BCR-ABL1* gene and characterize the *BCR-ABL1* junction. Such an analysis is particularly useful in the subsequent monitoring of patients.

Molecular biology

The Ph chromosome is an acquired cytogenetic abnormality present in all leukaemic cells of the myeloid lineage and in some B cells and T cells. It is formed as a result of a reciprocal translocation of DNA from chromosomes 9 and 22, t(9; 22)(q34;q11) (Fig. 22.3.6.1). The classical Ph chromosome is easily identified in about 90% of CML patients. A further 5% of patients have variant translocations which may be 'simple' involving chromosome 22 and a chromosome other than chromosome 9, or 'complex', where chromosome 9, 22, and other additional chromosomes are involved. About 5% of patients with clinical and haematological features typical of CML lack the Ph chromosome and are referred to as having 'Ph-negative' CML. About half of these patients have a *BCR-ABL1* chimeric gene and are referred to as Ph-negative, *BCR-ABL1*-positive cases; the remainder are *BCR-ABL1*-negative, and some of these have mutations in the *RAS* gene. These *BCR-ABL1*-negative patients have a more aggressive clinical course. Some patients acquire additional clonal cytogenetic abnormalities, in particular +8, +Ph, iso17q–, and +19, as their disease progresses. The emergence of such clones may herald the onset of blastic transformation.

The various genetic events have now been elucidated, and the chimeric *BCR-ABL1* gene is believed to play a central role in the pathogenesis of CML, though the precise mechanism(s) are still not fully understood. Three distinct breakpoint locations in the BCR gene in chromosome 22 have been identified (Fig. 22.3.6.5). The break in the major breakpoint cluster region (M-bcr) occurs in the intron between exon e13 and e14 or in the intron between exon e14 and e15 (toward the telomere). By contrast, the position of the breakpoint in the *ABL1* gene on chromosome 9 is highly variable and may occur at almost any position upstream of exon a2. The Ph translocation results in the juxtaposition of 5′ sequences from the *BCR* gene with 3′ sequences from the *ABL1* gene. This event results in the generation of the chimeric *BCR-ABL1* fusion gene

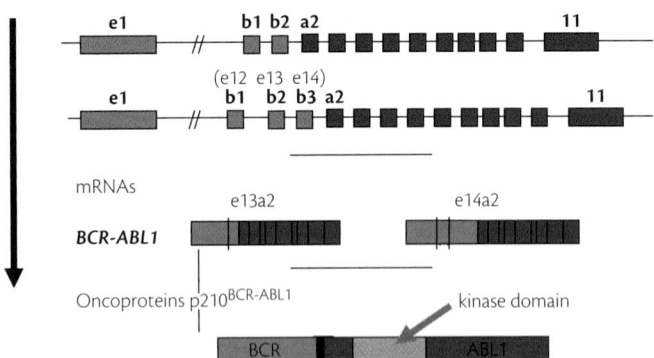

Alternative fusion genes in CML (+/− BCR exon e13 or b3)

Fig. 22.3.6.5 The various breakpoints identified so far in the Ph-positive leukaemias.

transcribed as an 8.5-kbp mRNA. This mRNA encodes a protein of 210 kDa (p210$^{BCR-ABL1}$) that has a greater tyrosine kinase activity compared with the normal ABL protein. The different breakpoints in the M-bcr result in two slightly different chimeric *BCR-ABL1* genes, resulting in either an e13a2 or an e14a2 transcript. The type of *BCR-ABL1* transcript has no important prognostic significance.

The second breakpoint location in the *BCR* gene occurs between exons e1 and e2 in an area designated the minor breakpoint cluster region (m-bcr) and forms a smaller *BCR-ABL1* fusion gene. This is transcribed as an e1a2 mRNA which encodes a p190$^{BCR-ABL1}$ oncoprotein. This protein characterizes about two-thirds of patients with Ph-positive acute lymphoblastic leukaemia (ALL). A third breakpoint location is found in patients with the very rare Ph-positive chronic neutrophilic leukaemia. This has been designated as a micro breakpoint cluster region (μ-bcr) and results in e19a2 mRNA, which encodes a larger protein of 230 kDa (p230$^{BCR-ABL1}$).

The recognition of several features in the Bcr-Abl1 oncoprotein that are essential for cellular transformation led to the identification of signal transduction pathways activated in *BCR-ABL1*-positive cells (Fig. 22.3.6.6). Much attention has since focused on

determining the precise role played by the various Bcr-Abl1 proteins in the pathogenesis of CML. A number of possible mechanisms of *BCR-ABL1*-mediated malignant transformation have been implicated, which are not necessarily mutually exclusive. These include constitutive activation of mitogenic signalling, reduced apoptosis, impaired adhesion of cells to the stroma and extracellular matrix, and proteasome-mediated degradation of Abl inhibitory proteins. The deregulation of the Abl tyrosine kinase facilitates autophosphorylation, resulting in a marked increase of phosphotyrosine on Bcr-Abl1 itself, which creates binding sites for the SH2 domains of other proteins. A variety of such substrates, which can be tyrosine phosphorylated, have now been identified. Although much is known of the abnormal interactions between the Bcr-Abl1 oncoprotein and other cytoplasmic molecules, the finer details of the pathways through which the 'rogue' proliferative signal is mediated, such as the RAS-MAP kinase, JAK-STAT, and the PI3 kinase pathways, are incomplete, and the relative contributions to the leukaemic 'phenotype' are still unknown. Moreover, the multiple signals initiated by the Bcr-Abl1 have both proliferative and antiapoptotic qualities, which are often difficult to separate. Much remains to be learned about the significance of tyrosine phosphatases in the transformation process.

It is generally believed that the some CML stem cells, at a cytokinetic level, are in a 'quiescent' or 'dormant' (G$_0$) phase. These quiescent CML cells appear to be able to exchange between a quiescent and a cycling status, allowing them to proliferate under certain circumstances. This provides some rationale for autografting as treatment for CML. There is also evidence that some Ph-positive cells are quiescent and cannot be eradicated by cycle-dependent cytotoxic drugs, even at high doses, or indeed by imatinib mesylate.

It is likely that the acquisition of a *BCR-ABL1* fusion gene by a haematopoietic stem cell and the ensuing expansion of the Ph-positive clone set the scene for acquisition and expansion of one or more Ph-positive subclones that are genetically more aggressive than the original Ph-positive population. The propensity of the Ph-positive clone to acquire such additional genetic changes is an example of 'genomic instability', but the molecular mechanisms underlying this instability are poorly defined. Such new events

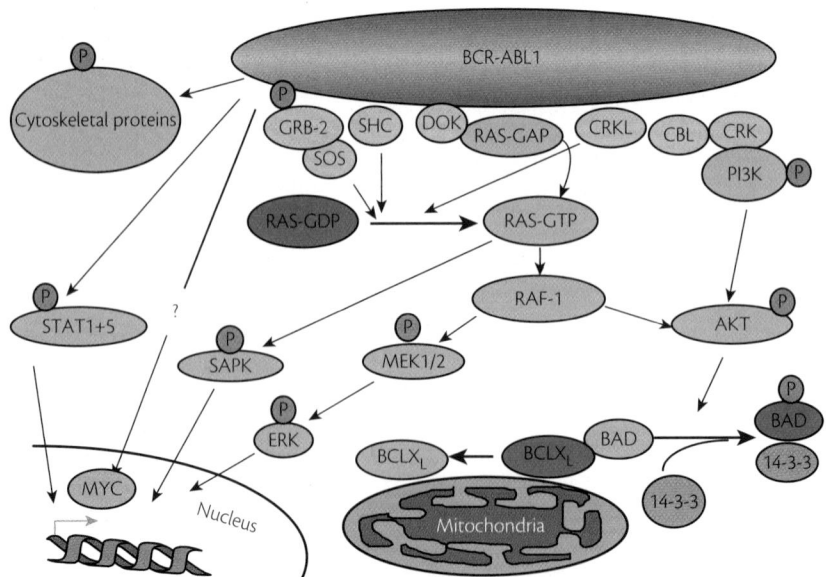

Fig. 22.3.6.6 The various signal transduction pathways identified in patients with CML.

may occur in the *BCR-ABL1* fusion gene or indeed in other genes in the Ph-positive population of cells and presumably underlie the progression to advanced phases of the disease. The average length of chromosomal telomeres in the Ph-positive cells is generally less than that in corresponding normal cells, and the enzyme telomerase, which is required to maintain the length of telomere, is up-regulated as the patient's disease enters the advanced phases. About 25% of patients with CML in myeloid transformation have point mutations or deletions in the p53 gene, and about half of all patients in lymphoid transformation show homozygous deletion in the p16 gene. There is also evidence supporting the role of the *RB* (retinoblastoma) and the *MYC* genes in disease progression.

Prognostic factors

Various efforts have been made to establish criteria definable at diagnosis, both prognostic (disease-related) and predictive (treatment-related), that may help to predict survival for individual patients. The most frequently used method is that proposed by Sokal in 1984, whereby patients can be divided into various risk categories based on a mathematical formula that takes into account the patient's age, blast cell count, spleen size, and platelet count at diagnosis. The Euro or Hasford system is an updated Sokal index, which includes consideration of basophil and eosinophil numbers. Stratifying patients into good-, intermediate-, and poor-risk categories may assist in the decision-making process regarding appropriate treatment options. Recent observations, however, suggest that age *per se* might not influence the biology of the disease, but rather increases the probability of treatment-related adverse effects by virtue of potential comorbid conditions.

More recent efforts have identified other possible risk-stratification factors. Green and colleagues from Cambridge, United Kingdom, described the presence of small deletions in the region of the reciprocal *ABL-BCR1* fusion gene on the derivative 9q+ chromosome arm, which were associated with poor prognosis, at least in the IFN-α era, though not necessarily in the imatinib era. It is of interest that a number of imatinib mesylate–specific parameters, which may carry a prognostic significance, such as the degree of myelosuppression associated with treatment with imatinib and the plasma levels of the agent at a specific time, are now being described. There is also evidence that the depth and quality of the cytogenetic and molecular responses may be influenced by the actual dose of imatinib mesylate, with patients who receive higher doses of imatinib mesylate achieving a complete cytogenetic remission and a major molecular response much earlier than those treated with conventional doses, and there is a trend for an improved event-free survival.

Gene expression changes associated with progression and response in CML have also been introduced and are currently being validated (Fig. 22.3.6.7). Other candidate biomarkers include the polycomb group *BMI1* gene, which regulates both normal and leukaemic stem cells, and the rate of shortening of telomeres in the leukaemia clone.

Management

A decade ago, it was standard practice to recommend an allo-SCT to all patients younger than 50 years of age with newly diagnosed CML in the chronic phase, provided they had suitable HLA-identical

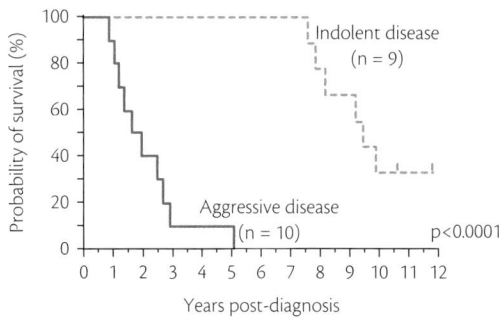

Fig. 22.3.6.7 Risk stratification of patients with CML in chronic phase by molecular profiling of CD38⁺ cells. Survival in accordance with molecular profiling of CD38⁺ cells in chronic-phase (CP) CML.
(Adapted with permission from Yong A, *et al.* (2006). Molecular profiling of CD34+ cells identifies low expression of CD7, along with high expression of proteinase 3 or elastase, as predictors of longer survival in patients with CML. *Blood*, **107**, 205–12.)

sibling or 'matched' unrelated donors. Patients presenting in the advanced phases of CML usually received combination chemotherapy, often followed by an allo-SCT if a 'second' chronic phase could be achieved. The treatment algorithm for newly diagnosed patients changed dramatically once the impressive success of imatinib mesylate in inducing durable complete cytogenetic remissions in the majority of newly diagnosed patients with CML in the chronic phase was recognized. Imatinib mesylate is now the preferred treatment for most, if not all, newly diagnosed patients with CML in the chronic phase, and is also useful in the management of patients presenting in the advanced phase.

Imatinib mesylate inhibits the enzymatic action of the activated Bcr-Abl1 tyrosine kinase by occupying the ATP-binding pocket of the kinase component of the Bcr-Abl1 oncoprotein, thereby blocking the capacity of the enzyme to phosphorylate and activate downstream effector molecules that cause the leukaemic phenotype. It also binds to an adjacent part of the kinase domain in a manner than holds the Abl–activation loop of the oncoprotein in an inactive configuration.

Imatinib mesylate induces 'cumulative best' complete haematological remissions in 98% of all previously untreated patients with CML in the chronic phase and 'cumulative best' complete cytogenetic remission in about 85% of such patients. About 2% of all patients in the chronic phase, progress to advanced-phase disease each year, which contrasts with estimated annual progression rates of >15% for patients treated with hydroxycarbamide and about 10% for patients receiving IFN-α, either with or without cytarabine. Indeed, preliminary evidence suggests that this annual rate of progression, about 2%, might actually be diminishing as the years pass. Complete molecular responses are, however, less common, and imatinib mesylate will probably not eradicate residual CML in most patients.

Nevertheless, the drug prolongs overall survival very substantially compared with historical patients who received IFN-α or hydroxycarbamide. Furthermore, the majority of patients who achieve a ≥3-log reduction in Bcr-Abl1 transcripts remain alive in complete cytogenetic remission at 6 years after initiation of treatment with imatinib. Therefore, a current topical issue is whether total eradication of all residual leukaemia stem cells is actually necessary, since the survival of small numbers of residual leukaemia stem cells might well be compatible with an individual patient's long-term survival. Conversely, if such a population of cells remained a possible source for progression of the leukaemia, the notion of two contrasting therapeutic algorithms for patients based on prognostic factors—both disease-related, such as the Sokal risk score, and treatment-related, such as the European Group for Blood and Marrow Transplantation (EBMT) risk score—can be considered.

For most patients with CML in the chronic phase, imatinib mesylate at a standard starting dosage of 400 mg/day is the first-line treatment of choice, although several studies suggest that higher doses, up to 800 mg daily, might give better results with a greater proportion of patients achieving a complete molecular response. Such studies also suggest better progression-free and transformation-free survivals, but with potentially more adverse effects, particularly myelosuppression. The higher-dose studies are still ongoing, and until the longer term results are available, it is reasonable to start newly diagnosed patients in the chronic phase on imatinib mesylate at 400 mg/day.

Adverse effects of imatinib mesylate, which appear to be dose-related, include nausea, headache, rashes, bone pains, various skin reactions, and fluid retention. Significant cytopenias and hepato-toxicity occur less commonly and usually in the first 6 to 12 months of therapy. Very rare cases of severe or fatal cerebral oedema have been reported, and there have been some concerns about potential cardiomyopathy, though the recent 6-year IRIS study analysis reassures us that this might not be a major problem, except for older patients, who might have other predisposing cardiac risks and have anaemia. Another potential issue of concern is the potential tera-togenicity of imatinib mesylate. A recent study assessing outcomes in 125 of 180 study patients exposed to the agent during pregnancy concluded that about half of the offspring born were normal; 28% of the study cohort elected to undergo termination of pregnancy, including three postidentification of fetal abnormalities. In sum there were 12 infants in whom abnormalities were identified, including 3 who had strikingly similar complex malformations. It would therefore appear sensible to avoid imatinib mesylate exposure during pregnancy.

The alternative treatment option should involve an early allo-SCT for the small minority of patients who would clearly benefit from an immediate transplant compared with continuing imatinib irre-spective of its outcome. A retrospective analysis from the Center for International Blood and Marrow Transplant Research (CIBMTR) and the EBMT suggests that for adult patients, including those who are at low risk for transplant-related mortality by EBMT criteria, it is not possible to identify a cohort who would clearly benefit from an immediate stem cell transplant vs continuing imatinib mesylate irrespective of the outcome. The best initial treatment for children, for adults with a potential syngeneic donor, and possibly for adults with high-risk disease by Sokal or Hasford criteria is still uncertain. The current EBMT experience, however, suggests that patients with high-risk disease and a low-transplant risk should probably still be considered for an early transplant. Such a cohort, if treated with imatinib in the first instance should probably not receive a second tyrosine kinase inhibitor on relapse (see below) and rather proceed to stem cell transplantation. For children, many paediatric hae-matologists recommend initial treatment by allo-SCT for patients under the age of 16 years who have HLA-identical siblings, largely because of a lack of adequate long-term data on the use of imatinib mesylate as first-line therapy in children.

	3 mos	6 mos	12 mos	18 mos
Conservative goals	CHR	<95% Ph+	<35% Ph+	0% Ph+
Aggressive goals	<95% Ph+	<35% Ph+	0% Ph+ or MMR	MMR

Suboptimal response: Failure to achieve aggressive goals → continuation of imatinib may be justified

Imatinib failure: Failure to achieve conservative goals OR loss of response → change of strategy needed

Warning signs: Clonal cytogenetic evolution, low level resistance mutations → intensify monitoring

Fig. 22.3.6.8 Therapeutic milestones: definitions of failure, suboptimal responses and warning signs for patients with chronic-phase CMP treated with imatinib mesylate; MMR [Major molecular response].
(Adapted with permission from Baccarani M, et al. (2006). Evolving concepts in the management of chronic myeloid leukemia: recommendations from an expert panel on behalf of the European LeukemiaNet. *Blood*, **108**, 1809–20.)

Second line-therapy and issues regarding resistance to imatinib mesylate

Various efforts to define 'failure' and 'suboptimal responses' to imat-inib have resulted in two principal consensus panels (Fig. 22.3.6.8). Primary resistance or refractoriness to the drug appears to be very rare and when seen may be related to poor drug compliance, poor gastrointestinal absorption, p450 cytochrome polymorphisms, interactions with other medications, and abnormal drug efflux and influx at the cellular level. In a small cohort of patients, a correla-tion between the transcription factor OCT-1 expression and response has been observed: the higher the levels of OCT-1, the better the molecular responses (Fig. 22.3.6.9).

A somewhat larger proportion of patients, about 20% in the chronic phase, respond initially to imatinib mesylate and then lose their response. This acquired or 'secondary' resistance results from a variety of mechanisms, including amplification of the *BCR-ABL1* fusion gene, relative overexpression of Bcr-Abl1 protein, and expansion of subclones with point mutations in the *BCR-ABL1*

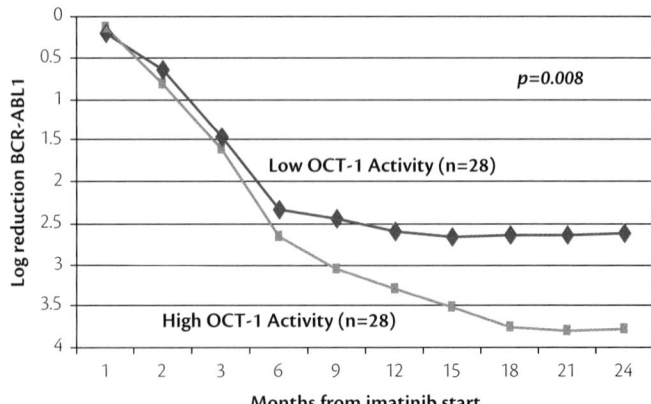

Fig. 22.3.6.9 Correlation of molecular response with levels of OCT-1 activity in CML.
(Adapted with permission from White DL, et al. (2006). OCT-1–mediated influx is a key determinant of the intracellular uptake of imatinib but not nilotinib (AMN107): reduced OCT-1 activity is the cause of low in vitro sensitivity to imatinib. *Blood*, **108**, 697–704.)

kinase domain (KD). Such point mutations code for amino acid substitutions that may impede binding of imatinib but do not impair phosphorylation of downstream substrates that mediate the leukaemia signal. The precise position of the mutation appears to dictate the degree of resistance to imatinib; some mutations are associated with minor degrees of drug resistance, whereas one notorious mutation, the replacement of isoleucine by threonine at position 315 (T315I), is associated with near-total nonresponsiveness to imatinib, as well as with resistance to the newer tyrosine kinase inhibitors, namely dasatinib, nilotinib, and bosutinib. The precise significance and indeed the kinetics of the over 70 currently well-characterized mutations remain largely unknown.

The majority of patients who are resistant/intolerant to imatinib mesylate should receive dasatinib or nilotinib. Dasatinib is a thiazole-carboxamide structurally unrelated to imatinib. Furthermore, it binds to the ABL KD regardless of the conformation of the activation loop—whether open or closed. It also inhibits some of the Src family kinases. Preclinical studies showed that dasatinib was 300-fold more potent than imatinib and is active against 18 of 19 tested imatinib-resistant KD mutant subclones, with the notable exception of the T315I mutant.

Current experience with dasatinib in patients with chronic-phase CML resistant/refractory to imatinib suggest that about 90% of the patients have a complete haematological response and 52% have a complete cytogenetic remission. About 25% of patients with the more advanced phases of CML and Ph-positive ALL also achieve reasonable responses. Responses are seen in patients with most of the currently known ABL-kinase mutations, except the T315I mutation. Haematological toxicity is common, particularly in those with advanced phases of CML and Ph-positive ALL. These include neutropenia (49%), thrombocytopenia (48%), and anaemia (20%). Nonhaematological toxicity includes diarrhoea, headaches, superficial oedema, pleural effusions, and occasional pericardial effusions. Grade 3/4 side effects are rare, and grade 3/4 pleural effusions occurred in 6% of patients.

Dasatinib is also being assessed as a potential first-line treatment, and studies involving patients in the chronic phase, following at least 3 months of dasatinib therapy, show 89% complete haematological response and 79% cytogenetic remission rates. These data compare well with first-line responses to imatinib. The toxicity profile appears to be similar to that seen in the drug-resistance studies, but the number of patients entered so far is quite small. The drug has also been tested in patients with CML in advanced phases whose disease was resistant to both imatinib and nilotinib; remarkably, 57% haematological responses, including 43% complete haematological remission, were observed. Among those patients who had a haematological response, 32% had a cytogenetic response, including 2 patients who achieved cytogenetic remission.

Nilotinib, like imatinib, acts by binding to the closed (inactive) conformation of the Abl-KD, but with a much higher affinity. Like imatinib, it inhibits the dysregulated tyrosine kinase activity of the Abl kinase by occupying the ATP-binding pocket of the oncoprotein and blocking the capacity of the enzyme to phosphorylate downstream effector molecules. *In vitro* studies suggest that nilotinib is about 30- to 50-fold more potent than imatinib mesylate. Nilotinib is also active in 32 of the currently 33 imatinib-resistant cell lines with mutant Abl kinases, but like imatinib and dasatinib has no activity against the Bcr-Abl1^{T315I} mutation. Phase II studies in patients who are resistant or intolerant to imatinib mesylate are still in progress, and preliminary results suggest a complete haematological response in about 70% or a third of these patients who show a complete cytogenetic remission. Patients in the advanced phases of CML also respond, but to a lesser degree. The most common treatment-related toxicity is myelosuppression, followed by headaches, pruritus, and rashes. Overall, 22% of the patients in the chronic phase experienced thrombocytopenia, with 19% having either grade 3/4 severity; 16% had neutropenia and a further 16% had anemia. Most of the nonhaematological adverse effects were of a grade 1/2 severity. All, including the haematological effects, were fully reversible. About 19% of all patients experience arthralgias, and about 14% experience fluid retention, particularly pleural and pericardial effusions. Importantly, patients with the acquired Bcr-Abl1^{T315I} mutation appear to be refractory to nilotinib.

As discussed earlier, based on current EBMT experience, it is reasonable to consider an early allogeneic transplantation for those patients who are resistant to imatinib and have high-risk disease, by Sokal and Hasford risk stratification, and a low transplant risk, by EBMT criteria, and wish to be transplanted, rather than subjecting them to the next generation tyrosine kinase inhibitors. An alternative would be to prescribe a second tyrosine kinase inhibitor for a defined period and then to proceed to an allo-SCT if the response is suboptimal. In practice, however, many patients will opt to receive a trial of a next generation of the tyrosine inhibitor drugs.

Third-line therapy

For patients who are resistant/refractory to the current generation of inhibitors, and are under the age of 50 years, it is probably best to consider an allo-SCT, provided a suitable donor is identified and the patient remains in the chronic phase of the disease. For those with advanced-phase disease, one could offer combination chemotherapy or an appropriate clinical trial assessing one of the newer drugs and then consider allo-SCT if a second chronic phase is achieved. Clearly, this is an area which is evolving rapidly, so it is difficult to make firm recommendations at present.

Patients who proceed to a transplant after treatment with imatinib appear to have a higher relapse incidence than those who have not previously received the drug (Fig. 22.3.6.10). This most probably represents a selection bias for relatively resistant disease. Preliminary data based on small patient series do not, however, suggest that prior treatment with imatinib increases the probability of transplant-related mortality. Moreover, patients with kinase domain mutations appear to fare as well post-transplant as those lacking such mutations. The experience with allo-SCT after initial treatment of advanced-phase disease with imatinib mesylate is still limited.

Investigational approaches

Immunotherapy

Following the realization that a molecular remission and 'cure' might not be possible with imatinib alone, many efforts were directed to exploring the potential of developing an active specific immunotherapy strategy for patients with CML by inducing an immune response to a tumour-specific or tumour-associated antigen (Fig. 22.3.6.11). The principle involves generating an immune response to the unique amino acid sequence of p210 at the fusion point. Clinical responses to the Bcr-Abl1 peptide vaccination, including complete cytogenetic remissions, have been

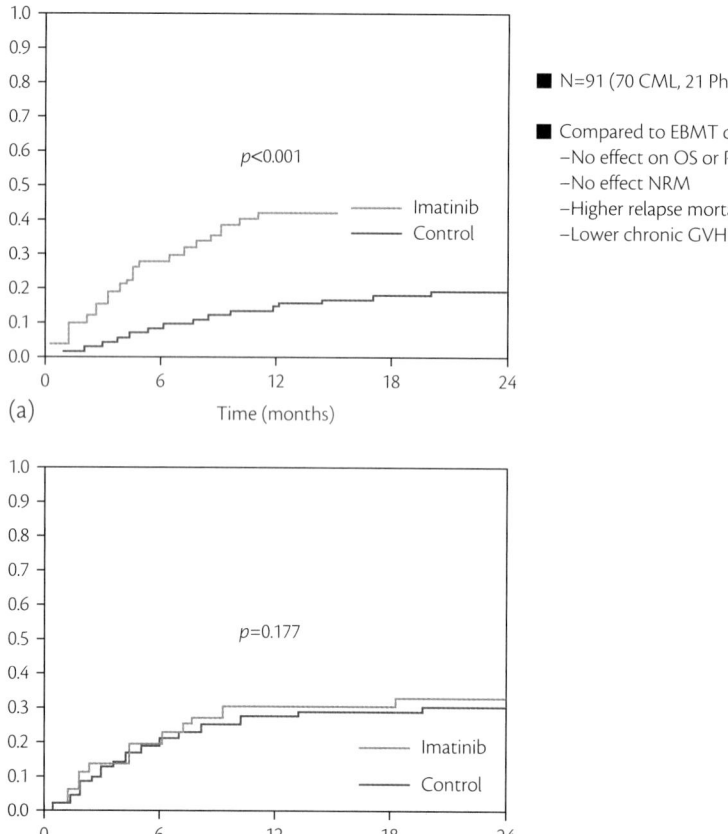

- N=91 (70 CML, 21 Ph+ ALL)

- Compared to EBMT controls
  - No effect on OS or PFS
  - No effect NRM
  - Higher relapse mortality
  - Lower chronic GVHD

Fig. 22.3.6.10 Effect of prior imatinib treatment in patients subjected to an allogeneic stem cell transplant, with regard to relapse (A) and nonrelapse (B) mortality. EBMT, European Group for Blood and Marrow Transplantation; GVHD, graft-vs-host disease; NRM, OS, PFS, .
(Adapted with permission from Deininger M, et al. (2006). The effect of prior exposure to imatinib on transplant-related mortality. *Haematologica*, **91**, 452–9.)

reported in a small series. In contrast to previous earlier unsuccessful attempts, the current series included administration of granulocyte–macrophage colony-stimulating factor as an immune adjuvant, and patients were only enrolled if they had measurable residual disease and human leucocyte antigene known to which the selected fusion peptides were predicted to bind avidly. If these results can be confirmed, vaccine development against Bcr-Abl1 and other CML-specific antigens could become an attractive treatment for patients who have a minimal residual disease status with imatinib mesylate. Other targets for vaccine therapy now being studied include peptides derived from the Wilms tumor 1 protein, proteinase 3, and elastase, all of which are overexpressed in CML cells.

Investigational drugs

Bosutinib (SKI-606, Wyeth) is an emerging oral dual Abl/Src kinase inhibitor currently in phase I/II study (Fig. 22.3.6.12). This drug appears to be about 200 times more potent than imatinib, and unlike imatinib and dasatinib, does not inhibit other targets such as KIT or platelet-derived growth factor receptor. The preliminary results of treating patients with CML in chronic and advanced phase, as well as Ph-positive ALL, appear encouraging, and the toxicity profile appears reasonable, with gastrointestinal cutaneous toxicity being the major grade 3/4 adverse effects.

Other specific inhibitors of signal transduction pathways downstream of Bcr-Abl1 have been tested alone and in combination with

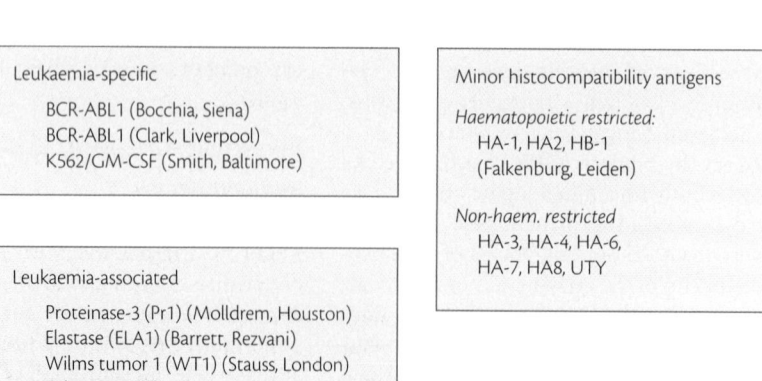

Fig. 22.3.6.11 Possible antigens that can be targeted in patients with CML. Principal researchers and their locations are given in parentheses.

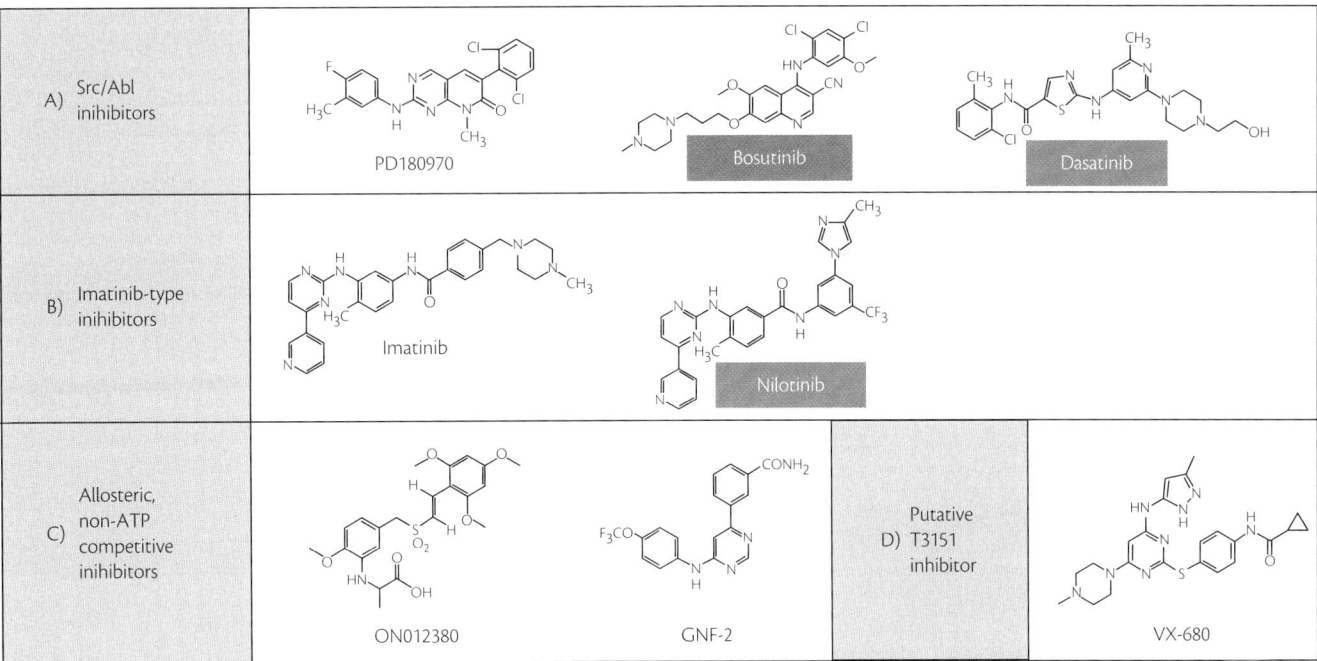

Fig. 22.3.6.12 Alternative Abl tyrosine kinase inhibitors.
(Adapted with permission from O'Hare T, Eide CA, Deininger MW (2007). Bcr-Abl1 kinase domain mutations and the unsettled problem of Bcr-AblT315I: looking into the future of controlling drug resistance in chronic myeloid leukemia. *Clin Lymphoma Myeloma*, **7** Suppl 3, S120–30.)

imatinib mesylate. Some of these agents, such as 17-allylamino-geldanamycin (17-AAG), are just entering formal clinical trials or might do so in the near future. 17-AAG, a drug which degrades the Bcr-Abl1 oncoprotein by inhibiting the heat shock protein 90, a molecular chaperone required for stabilization of Bcr-Abl1, has just entered phase I studies. 17-AAG appears to have activity in patients with the E255K and T315I mutations. It also down-regulates *BCR-ABL1* mRNA, though the precise mechanism remains unclear. Another novel tyrosine kinase inhibitor, PD166 326, also appears to have significant activity in patients with the H396P and M351T mutations. This agent also appears to be superior to imatinib in murine models. Other potential agents include rapamycin, an mTOR inhibitor, and wortmannin, which is a PI3K inhibitor not currently available in a formulation suitable for clinical use. Rapamycin synergizes with imatinib mesylate in inhibiting Bcr-Abl1–transformed cells, including those that are imatinib mesylate resistant.

Recently, there has been considerable interest in combining imatinib mesylate with diverse agents, including hypomethylating agents, farnesyl transferase inhibitors, pegylated IFN-α, arsenic trioxide, bortezomib, and other cytotoxic drugs, such as homoharringtonine. Homoharringtonine is a semisynthetic plant alkaloid that enhances apoptosis of CML cells, is active in combination with imatinib in drug-resistant/refractory patients.

Conclusions

The substantial understanding of the molecular features and pathogenesis of CML has provided important insights into targeting treatment to specific molecular defects. The successful introduction of imatinib mesylate as targeted therapy for CML has made the approach to management of the newly diagnosed patient fairly complex. The second generation of tyrosine kinase inhibitors,

dasatinib and nilotinib, have significant activity in selected patients in both chronic and the more advanced phases of the disease, who are resistant to imatinib. Efforts are also in progress to assess the potential first-line role of both these drugs. The notion that the graft-vs-leukaemia effect is the principal reason for success in patients with CML subjected to an allograft transplant has renewed interest in immunotherapy. The use of kinase inhibitors in conjunction with various immunotherapeutic strategies is now being studied.

For the moment, the various treatment options should be assessed carefully in terms of the relative risk–benefit ratios, and a management strategy should be developed accordingly. For a small minority of patients, namely children or adults in whom the risk of transplant-related mortality is relatively low but with high Sokal risk stratification, it appears reasonable to recommend an early allo-SCT. It would also be reasonable to contemplate an early transplant procedure for patients who have an identical twin donor. For all other patients (who constitute the majority), it is best to commence imatinib mesylate at 400 mg/day, increasing to a maximum of 800 mg/day in patients with a suboptimal response.

Patients who are resistant/refractory to imatinib should receive dasatinib or nilotinib. For those who are resistant/refractory to these drugs, it is best to consider an allo-SCT, provided that a suitable donor is identified or after an appropriate clinical trial assessing emerging drugs, for those with a T315I mutation. Clearly, this is an area which is evolving rapidly; it is difficult to make firm recommendations at present.

Finally efforts in improving the technology of allo-SCT, such as the ability to prevent graft-vs-host disease without abrogation of graft-vs-leukaemia, are also in progress. If successful, they might restore allo-SCT as an alternative treatment option for some newly diagnosed patient, who might otherwise have to continue lifelong therapy with a tyrosine kinase inhibitor at considerable expense, both financial and perhaps personal.

Further reading

Baccarani M, *et al.* (2006). Evolving concepts in the management of chronic myeloid leukemia: recommendations from an expert panel on behalf of the European LeukemiaNet. *Blood*, **108**, 1809–20.

Baccarani M *et al.* (2009). Chronic myeloid leukemia: An update of concepts and management recommendations of European LeukemiaNet. *J Clin Oncol*, **27**, 6041–51.

Bocchia M, *et al.* (2005). Effect of a p210 multipeptide vaccine associated with imatinib or interferon in patients with chronic myeloid leukaemia and persistent residual disease: a multicentre observational trial. *Lancet*, **365**, 657–9.

Daley GQ, *et al.* (1990). Induction of chronic myelogenous leukemia in mice by the p210 bcr/abl gene of the Philadelphia chromosome. *Science*, **24**, 824–30.

Deininger MW, *et al.* (2000). The molecular biology of chronic myeloid leukemia. *Blood*, **96**, 3343–56.

Druker BJ, *et al.* (2000). Effects of a selective inhibitor of the Abl tyrosine kinase on the growth of the BCR-ABL positive cells. *Nat Med*, **2**, 561–6.

Druker BJ, *et al.* (2006). Five-year follow-up of patients receiving imatinib for chronic myeloid leukemia. *N Engl J Med*, **355**, 2408–17.

Fialkow PJ (1981). Evidence for a multistep origin of chronic myeloid leukemia. *Blood*, **58**, 158–63.

Goldman JM (2007). How I treat chronic myeloid leukemia in the imatinib era. *Blood*, **110**, 2828–37.

Goldman JM, *et al.* (1986). Bone marrow transplantation for patients with chronic myeloid leukemia. *N Engl J Med*, **314**, 202–7.

Gratwohl A, *et al.* (1998). Risk assessment for patients with chronic myeloid leukaemia before allogeneic blood or marrow transplantation. *Lancet*, **352**, 1078–92.

Hasford J, *et al.* (1998). A new prognostic score for survival of patients with chronic myeloid leukemia treated with interferon alfa. *J Natl Cancer Inst*, **90**, 850–8.

Hughes T, Hoomissen I, Goldman JM, Radich JP (2003). Frequency of major molecular responses to imatinib or interferon alfa plus cytarabine in newly diagnosed chronic myeloid leukemia. *N Engl J Med*, **349**, 1421–30.

Hughes T, *et al.* (2006). Monitoring CML patients responding to treatment with tyrosine kinase inhibitors: recommendations for 'harmonizing' current methodology for detecting BCR-ABL transcripts and kinase domain mutations and for expressing results. *Blood*, **108**, 28–37.

Huntly BJ, *et al.* (2001). Deletions of the derivative chromosome 9 occur at the time of the Philadelphia translocation and provide a powerful and independent prognostic indicator in chronic myeloid leukemia. *Blood*, **98**, 1732–8.

Ichimaru M, Ishimaru T, Belsky JL (1978). Incidence of leukemia in atomic bomb survivors belonging to a fixed cohort in Hiroshima and Nagasaki, 1950–1971: radiation dose, years after exposure, age at exposure, and type of leukemia. *J Radiat Res (Tokyo)*, **19**, 262–82.

Kantarjian H, *et al.* (2008). Monitoring the response and course of chronic myeloid leukemia in the era of Bcr-Abl tyrosine kinase inhibitors: practical advice on the use and interpretation of monitoring methods. *Blood*, **111**, 1774–80.

Marmont A, *et al.* (1984). Recurrence of Ph'-leukemia in donor cells after marrow transplantation for chronic myelogenous leukemia. *N Engl J Med*, **310**, 903–6.

Melo JV (1996). The diversity of the BCR–ABL fusion proteins and their relationship to leukemia phenotype. *Blood*, **88**, 2375–84.

Mughal TI, Goldman JM (1995). Chronic myeloid leukaemia: a therapeutic challenge. *Ann Oncol*, **6**, 637–44.

Mughal TI, Goldman JM (2006). Molecularly targeted treatment of chronic myeloid leukemia: beyond the imatinib era. *Front Biosci*, **1**, 209–20.

Mughal TI, *et al.* (2001). Molecular studies in patients with chronic myeloid leukaemia in remission 5 years after allogeneic stem cell transplant define the risk of subsequent relapse. *Br J Haematol*, **115**, 569–74.

Nowell PC, Hungerford DA (1960). A minute chromosome in human chronic granulocytic leukemia. *Science*, **132**, 1497.

Pane F, *et al.* (1996). Neutrophilic-chronic myeloid leukemia: a distinct disease with a specific molecular marker. *Blood*, **88**, 2410–14.

Radich J, *et al.* (2006). Gene expression changes associated with progression and response in CML. *Proc Natl Acad Sci U S A*, **103**, 2794–9.

Sawyers CL (1999). Chronic myeloid leukemia. *N Engl J Med*, **340**, 1330–8.

Sokal JE, *et al.* (1984). Prognostic discrimination in 'good-risk' chronic granulocytic leukemia. *Blood*, **63**, 789–99.

Srivastava PK (2000). Immunotherapy of human cancer: lessons from mice. *Nat Immunol*, **1**, 363–6.

22.3.7 Myelodysplasia

Lawrence B. Gardner and Chi V. Dang

Essentials

Myelodysplasia is a common haematological disorder that may occur at any age, although prevalence increases with age and most patients are over 60 years old. It is associated with a wide variety of acquired clonal abnormalities that may affect all lineages of blood cells and frequently lead to the development of leukaemia. Some particular chromosomal abnormalities are characteristic, and in a few cases functional studies of candidate genes implicated in the chromosomal abnormalities suggest cause–effect relationships, e.g. an activating mutation in the JAK2 kinase.

Clinical features, diagnosis, and classification

Most patients present with features of chronic anaemia or manifestations related to thrombocytopenia (bleeding and bruising) or infection (usually when the absolute neutrophil count is $<0.5 \times 10^9$/litre).

Diagnosis—this may be suggested by the presence of normocytic or macrocytic anaemia, with the peripheral blood smear showing dysplastic changes in red blood cells and/or neutrophils. Bone marrow aspirate and biopsy confirms these findings and permits detailed cytogenetic study, which is critical for diagnostic classification and prognosis

Classification—based on the morphological appearance of the peripheral blood and bone marrow, the following are recognized in the World Health Organization (WHO) classification: (1) refractory anaemia; (2) refractory anaemia with ringed sideroblasts; (3) refractory cytopenias with multilineage dysplasia; (4) refractory cytopenias with multilineage dysplasia and ringed sideroblasts; (5) refractory anemia with excess blasts-1; (6) refractory anemia with excess blasts-2; (7) 5q– syndrome; and (8) other subtypes—including chronic myelomonocytic leukaemia, refractory anaemia with thrombocytosis, and secondary myelodysplastic syndrome.

Treatment and prognosis

Treatment is symptomatic in most cases. The only potentially curative treatment is allogeneic bone marrow transplantation, but this is not usually an option for the elderly. Some patients, particularly those with a hypocellular marrow, may show a response to immunosuppression with ciclosporin. Many of the few patients with isolated 5q– deletions respond dramatically to lenalidomide, an immunomodulatory and antiangiogenic drug.

Prognosis—mean survival is 12 to 28 months from the time of diagnosis, but prognosis varies widely according to particular subtype. Most patients die as a result of either bleeding or infection, but in some transformation to leukaemia proves fatal.

Definition

The myelodysplastic syndromes (MDS) are a collection of acquired, clonal, haemopoietic disorders characterized by cytopenias and abnormal cellular morphologies. The vast majority of MDS are marked by progressive, multilineage cytopenias, ineffective maturation of cells with dysplastic appearances and chromosomal abnormalities, and a tendency to degenerate into poorly responsive leukaemias. Historically, these syndromes have been referred to as preleukaemias, smouldering leukaemias, and refractory anaemias. In 1976 the French-American-British (FAB) Cooperative Group proposed a classification system of these heterogeneous disorders based on the histological appearance of the peripheral blood and bone marrow, with primary emphasis placed on the percentage of immature cells, or myeloblasts, present. More recently the World Health Organization (WHO) has modified this classification in an attempt to better separate those patients who are better thought of as having early leukaemia or a myeloproliferative disorder. While these artificial classification systems have provided a helpful outline for physician communication and research, the presentation and prognosis of individuals with MDS vary greatly, depending on the biological impact of the genetic mutation(s) present in an individual's clone. MDS is more common in adults than any acute or chronic leukaemia. While MDS can occur at any age, it is primarily a disease of the old; over 80% of those affected are older than 60 years, and after age 70 there is a prevalence of approximately 33 in 100 000. The incidence of the disease appears to be increasing, probably in part due to more common screening with complete blood counts, and an increase in secondary, treatment-related MDS. There is currently no effective cure for MDS, except for allogeneic bone marrow transplantation, which is often not an option for the older patient with MDS. Treatment therefore remains supportive, consisting of transfusion and antibiotic treatment for documented infections, although recent data suggest that some agents may be altering the natural course of the disease. Patients often die as a result of their cytopenias (e.g. from bleeding or infection) or transformation to leukaemia.

Pathogenesis and pathophysiology

The biology of MDS is difficult to study, since disorders grouped under MDS probably include diagnoses of disparate aetiologies. It is clear from karyotypic analysis, including chromosomal studies, and X-linked inactivation of genetic markers, that MDS is a clonal disorder involving a defect in an early haemopoietic progenitor cell. Thus erythrocytes, platelets, neutrophils, and monocytes may all be affected in MDS. The ability of progenitor cells from patients with MDS to form colonies in vitro is markedly diminished. Haemopoietic growth factor production by lymphocytes from these patients is often decreased, and growth-inhibitory cytokines may be increased. In addition to the abnormal growth characteristics found in MDS progenitor cells in culture, there appears to be a higher rate of programmed cell death, or apoptosis, in such cells, which may contribute to the peripheral cytopenias and ineffective haemopoiesis noted on bone marrow examination. This increased rate of apoptosis has been particularly noted in low-grade MDS, which may be related to deregulated expression of the proapoptotic mediators tumour necrosis factor-α (TNFα), TRAIL ligand, and nuclear factor κB (NFκB), among others. In later stages of MDS, when evolution to acute myeloid leukaemia (AML) may be occurring, an inhibition of apoptosis in the leukaemia clone may be evident.

Chromosomes are often abnormal in MDS. In both therapy-related and de novo–acquired MDS. As opposed to AML, where cytogenetic abnormalities are often simple translocations modifying the activity of transcription factors, in MDS, deletions of chromosomes and complex cytogenetics are common. High-density single nucleotide polymorphism (SNP) analysis has demonstrated that even when chromosomes appear normal by classic banding techniques, subtle deletions and duplications are often present. Specific chromosomal abnormalities (including deletions of chromosomes 5 and 7, and trisomy 8) are relatively common. While the regions of chromosome 5 and 7 often deleted in MDS contain several genes important for haemopoiesis, including granulocyte–macrophage colony-stimulating factor (GM-CSF), erythropoietin, interleukin 6 (IL-6), and the receptors for several haemopoietic growth factors, no single gene or group of genes has been found to be consistently mutated in MDS. Although the pathogenic importance of specific deletions has not been well established, a recent functional study of candidate genes commonly deleted in chromosome arm 5q suggests that loss of function of the small subunit ribosomal protein RPS14 gene results in dyserythropoiesis as seen clinically in patients with the 5q– MDS. In this regard, the 5q– MDS is similar to the bone marrow failure Diamond–Blackfan syndrome, in which a significant fraction of patients have mutations in the RPS19 ribosomal protein. While a number of mouse models for MDS have been generated by the manipulation of expression levels of a number of genes (e.g. the haematopoietic transcription factor GATA-1), there is scant evidence of the relevance of these genes in human MDS. A number of genes important for proliferation and apoptosis have been described to be abnormally expressed in MDS, including the mutated ras oncogene which is present in up to 30% of cases, but again the importance of these abnormalities in the causation of MDS is unclear. Progression of MDS is often associated with the accumulation of additional chromosomal abnormalities. This stepwise accumulation of mutations, often found in many types of cancers, suggests the dominance of new clones with a proliferation and/or survival advantage.

Primary acquired sideroblastic anaemia is a unique subset of MDS. Other causes of an anaemia with the morphological appearance of ringed sideroblasts include an X-linked inherited form, and a secondary toxic form. Inherited and secondary sideroblastic anaemias are believed to result from a disruption in haem synthesis, producing ineffective haemopoiesis and iron overload. Alcohol, isoniazid, and pyrazinamide are among the common medications that can cause acquired sideroblastic anaemia. More recently, a form of refractory anaemia with thrombocytosis has been associated with an activating mutation in the JAK2 kinase, the kinase also affected in polycythaemia vera and other myeloproliferative disorders. Less commonly, a specific chromosomal translocation resulting in an oncogenic fusion protein is found in chronic myelomonocytic leukaemia (CMMoL).

Clinical features

While MDS has been described in children, it is uncommon, and other congenital haemopoietic diseases should be strongly considered. And, while secondary MDS may occur in younger adults, MDS is primarily a disease of the older adult. The clinical presentation of a patient with MDS depends on the specific cytopenias present, and the extent to which a lineage is depressed. Most commonly, patients present due to a symptomatic anaemia. Because the onset of MDS is gradual and progressive, patients typically present with signs and symptoms of chronic, not acute, anaemia, including fatigue and exertional dyspnoea. If the platelet count is low, petechiae or other forms of bleeding, typically mucosal or gastrointestinal, may be present. Infections occur with suppressed numbers of white cells, particularly when the absolute neutrophil count is below 500/ml. CMMoL, which has been historically classified as a myelodysplastic disorder, shares many characteristics with myeloproliferative diseases. In CMMoL, the monocyte count can be quite high, resulting in pleural, pericardial, and peritoneal effusions, as well as splenomegaly. Rheumatological and autoimmune processes have been noted to occur with MDS, sometimes leading to haemolytic anaemia and/or immune thrombocytopenia.

Laboratory diagnosis

Because MDS is a chronic disease, obtaining old laboratory data documenting a progressive, often macrocytic anaemia, thrombocytopenia, and leucopenia, can be invaluable in making the diagnosis. All patients diagnosed with MDS have an anaemia, which is typically either normocytic or macrocytic, although extreme macrocytosis (mean corpuscular volume (MCV) >120 fl) is not common. Anaemia and leucopenia in the setting of a normal or elevated platelet count should lead one to consider a subtype of MDS, the 5q– syndrome. The hallmark of MDS is dysplasia, which is often noted on a peripheral blood smear (Fig. 22.3.7.1a). Erythrocytes may show anisocytosis (varying sizes), poikilocytosis (abnormal morphology) with bizarre shapes, and basophilic stippling. Polymorphonuclear neutrophils may be hyperlobulated or, more commonly, hypolobulated, sometimes showing the characteristic bilobed appearance of pseudo-Pelger–Huët cells. Hypogranulation may be present, and chromatin may be abnormally clumped. Myeloblasts may be seen in the periphery and are a poor prognostic sign.

A bone marrow aspirate and biopsy, along with cytogenetics, are crucial for the diagnosis of MDS (Fig. 22.3.7.1b). Although the bone marrow biopsy may reveal a hypocellular bone marrow, this is rare, and should lead one to question the diagnosis and consider aplastic anaemia as the cause of a cytopenia. Typically, the bone marrow biopsy reveals a hypercellular marrow, consistent with the ineffective haemopoiesis common in MDS. The morphology of early progenitor cells shows a lack of maturation, with abnormal forms. Dyserythropoiesis, with multilobed erythroid progenitors, may be present. Megaloblastoid erythropoiesis is common; this is evidenced by an asynchrony of nuclear/cytoplasmic maturation, so that haemoglobin synthesis occurs while the erythroid nucleus is large and young. Megakaryocytes may be diminished and/or be small and hypolobulated. The bone marrow biopsy may show an abnormal localization of immature myeloid precursors; typically granulopoiesis occurs in a paratrabecular location, but in MDS there may be a shift to a central intratrabecular site. Depending on the stage of MDS, the number of blasts may be elevated. According to the FAB classification scheme, more than 30% blasts in the marrow defines acute leukaemia, while less than 30% are consistent with MDS. More recently, the WHO has defined acute leukaemia as greater than 20% blasts (see classification, below).

Chromosomal abnormalities (deletions, additions, or translocations) are very common in MDS. In MDS as a whole, chromosomal abnormalities are found 40% of the time. While MDS may be associated with a normal karyotype, especially in an early stage with few blasts, some chromosomal abnormalities are so typical that their presence strongly suggests the diagnosis. Similarly, multiple complex chromosomal abnormalities leads one to strongly consider a diagnosis of MDS. Typically, the longer a patient has MDS, the more chromosomal abnormalities may occur, leading to a more aggressive clone. The most common abnormalities include monosomy 7, 7q–, monosomy 5, 5q–, trisomy 8, and 20q–.

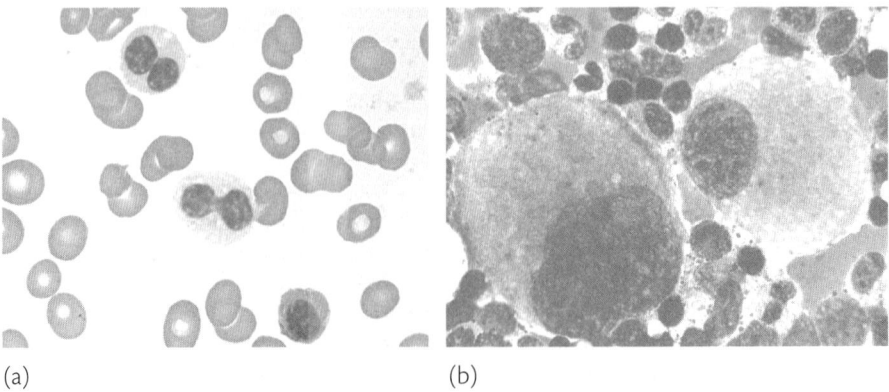

Fig. 22.3.7.1 (a) Peripheral blood smear in MDS showing several dysplastic neutrophils, including a pseudo-Pelger–Huët neutrophil with a bilobed nucleus. The chromatin in the neutrophils is clumped, and the red cells show a range of sizes and appearances. (b) A bone marrow aspirate with a small, monolobed megakaryocyte, typical in MDS.

(a)   (b)

Abnormalities in 11q23 are commonly found in secondary MDS due to treatment with topoisomerase II inhibitors, such as the epipodophyllotoxin, VP16 (etoposide). As discussed below, chromosomal abnormalities are important not only in suggesting the diagnosis of MDS, but also in its prognosis. Other diagnostic tests, such as abnormal growth of progenitor colonies in *in vitro* assays, are not widely utilized.

Differential diagnosis

When working up the possible aetiologies of a mild asymptomatic anaemia or pancytopenia in the older patient, where making a diagnosis may not change management, the extent of the work-up should depend on the patient's wishes. However, certain reversible diseases, several of which may be significant to the patient's overall health, must be ruled out. Aplastic anaemia also presents with pancytopenia; however, in contrast to MDS, the bone marrow is hypocellular, CD34$^+$ early progenitor stem cells in the bone marrow are relatively diminished, and there is little evidence of dysplasia. Multiple cytogenetic abnormalities are also more common in MDS than in aplastic anaemia, although recurrent chromosomal deletions have been noted in aplastic anaemia. To complicate matters, many patients with 'hypocellular MDS' may respond to treatments that are standardly used to treat aplastic anaemia (see below). In paroxysmal nocturnal haemoglobinuria the absence of the marker CD59 on the surface of cells, a lack of dysplasia, and low iron stores should differentiate this disease from MDS. Macrocytic, megaloblastoid anaemias as well as pancytopenias are common in patients with vitamin B$_{12}$ and folate deficiency. These may be ruled out with simple blood tests. Additionally, these defects should respond rapidly to replacement therapy. Copper deficiency may also give a similar picture. The anaemia of chronic disease is primarily a clinical diagnosis, but little dysplasia should be present. Alcoholism and/or hypersplenism can result in a mild pancytopenia, and an abnormal physical examination and normal bone marrow biopsy will rule these out. Bone marrow infiltration by a tumour or fibrosis usually presents with a myelophthisic blood smear consisting of nucleated red cells, teardrop red-cell forms, and a left-shifted myeloid series. Although both MDS and myeloproliferative diseases may present with a hypercellular marrow, it should not be difficult to delineate these two. Myeloproliferative disorders are not marked by dysplasia and bone marrow failure, but by increased proliferation and usually elevated cell counts.

Classification

The 1976 FAB classification divided MDS into five subgroups based on the morphological appearance of the peripheral blood and bone marrow. These subgroups consisted of refractory anaemia, refractory anaemia with ringed sideroblasts, refractory anaemia with excess blasts (10–20% blasts in the bone marrow), refractory anaemia with excess blasts in transformation (20–30% blasts in the bone marrow), and CMMoL (greater than 1000 monocytes/µl). Although this classification system remains helpful clinically and is the basis of patient stratification in most recent MDS research, dissatisfaction has arisen over the inclusion of CMMoL, which although it is marked by dysplasia also has many characteristics of a myeloproliferative disorder. The arbitrary cut-off of 30% blasts as demarcating MDS from AML, even though there is little clinical difference between MDS patients with greater than 20% blasts and patients with AML, and the desire to separate those with evolving *de novo* AML with low blast counts, from those who have high-grade MDS, from those who have AML which has arisen from MDS, has lead to a modification of the FAB classification system. In an attempt to better delineate these disorders in a clinically and biologically relevant fashion, the WHO has proposed a classification system for myeloid disorders. The proposed WHO classification for MDS contains eight categories (Table 22.3.7.1). It separates those with refractory anaemias, and those with refractory cytopenias with dysplasia, and defines those with greater than 20% blasts as having AML (and new category of AML with multilineage dysplasia). This WHO classification has been prospectively validated as dividing patients into groups with different likelihood of cytogenetic abnormality and survival. As in the FAB system, in many patients there is a gradual progression through the subgroups, eventually leading to acute leukaemia, although patients with lower grade MDS may do well for long periods of time.

Refractory anaemia

Refractory anaemia (RA) accounts for approximately 10% of all cases of MDS. By definition, less than 5% blasts are present in the bone marrow, and less than 15% ringed sideroblasts are seen with iron staining. Dysplasia in the peripheral blood and bone marrow are minimal, and there are few chromosomal abnormalities. These patients have a relatively low risk of progressing to leukaemia, and may do well for prolonged periods of time.

Refractory anaemia with ringed sideroblasts

Ringed sideroblasts are erythroblasts with iron-laden mitochondria encircling more than one-third of the nucleus. More than six Prussian Blue–stained iron granules must be noted, in more than 15% of the cells to make the diagnosis of refractory anaemia with ringed sideroblasts (RARS). In addition, fewer than 5% blasts must be found in the bone marrow. As alluded to above, several drug-induced and hereditary syndromes may also present with ringed sideroblasts: for example, alcohol- and isoniazid-induced and X-linked disease, respectively. It is important to differentiate these states, as their prognosis and treatment may be different than for RARS. For example, inherited RARS may sometimes be successfully treated with pyridoxine, and the most common complication is usually iron overload. RARS, like refractory anaemia, has a relatively low risk of progression to acute leukaemia (approximately 10%), especially when only the erythroid series is suppressed. Median survival is almost 6 years. RARS and perhaps other low-grade MDS are particularly responsive to combinations of growth factors, as discussed later.

Refractory cytopenias with multilineage dysplasia

Refractory cytopenias with multilineage dysplasia (RCMD) patients have fewer than 5% of blasts in their bone marrow, and rare or no blasts in peripheral blood. If present, these peripheral blood blasts do not contain Auer rods. As opposed to RA, where there is isolated anaemia with only erythroid dysplasia, patients with RCMD have bicytopenias and dysplasia in two or more myeloid cell lines. Cytogenetic abnormalities are more common than in RA or RARS, and while these patients may still do well for long periods of time, survival is decreased over control populations.

Table 22.3.7.1 General characteristics of MDS subtypes

	%	Peripheral blood	Ringed sideroblasts (%)	Dysplasia	Peripheral monocytes	% blast bone marrows	% blasts peripheral blood	Abnormal cytogenetic	Median survival (months)	5-year survival (%)	AML progression (%)
RA	8.5	Anaemia	<15	Erythroid only	<1.000/µl	<5	Rare	8.5%	69	91	7.5
RARS	11	Anaemia	>15	Erythroid only	<1.000/µl	<5	None	11%	69		1.4
RCMD	24	Bi- or pan-cytopenia	<15	In >10% cells in >2 myeloid cell lines	<1.000/µl	<5	None or rare	24%	33	65	10
RCMD-RS	15	Bi- or pan-cytopenias	>15	In >10% cells in >2 myeloid cell lines	<1.000/µl	<5	None or rare	15%	32	58	13
RAEB-1	21	Cytopenias		Unilineage or multilineage		5–9	>5 + Auer rods	21%	18	24	21
RAEB-2	18.5	Cytopenias				10–20	>5 + Auer rods	18.5%	10	24	34
Del 5q	2.2	Anaemia, platelets normal or increased		<5%				2.2%	116	85	8
MDS U		Cytopenias		Unilineage in megakaryocytes or myeloids		<5, hypolobulated megakaryocytes	None or rare	4%		85	28

RA, refractory anaemia; RARS, refractory anaemia with ringed sideroblasts; RCMD, refractory cytopenias with multilineage dysplasia; RCMD-RS, refractory cytopenias with multilineage dysplasia and ringed sideroblasts; RAEB, refractory anaemia with excess blasts; MDS-U, myelodysplastic syndrome unclassified.

Data from Germing U, et al. (2000). Validation of the WHO proposals for a new classification of primary myelodysplastic syndromes: a retrospective analysis of 1600 patients. *Leuk Res*, **24**, 983–92; and Bernasconi P, et al. (2007). World Health Organization classification in combination with cytogenetic markers improves the prognostic stratification of patients with *de novo* primary myelodysplastic syndromes. *Br J Haematol*, **137**, 1365–2141.

Refractory cytopenias with multilineage dysplasia and ringed sideroblasts

Refractory cytopenias with multilineage dysplasia and ringed sideroblasts (RCMD-RS) is similar to RCMD except that the bone marrow contains >15% of ringed sideroblasts. Cytogenetic abnormalities, transformation to acute leukaemia, and overall survival are similar to that of RCMD.

Refractory anaemia with excess blasts-1

Whereas in the FAB classification, patients with 5 to 10% blasts in their bone marrow were categorized with refractory anaemia, in the WHO classification these patients are categorized as having refractory anaemia with excess blasts-1 (RAEB-1). These patients have cytopenias in multiple cell lines and unilineage or multilineage dysplasia in their bone marrow, but blasts do not contain Auer rods. There is a significant risk of progression to AML and/or decreased survival.

Refractory anaemia with excess blasts-2

These patients have 10 to 19% blasts in their bone marrow, and these blasts may contain Auer rods. Multilineages are affected with both cytopenias and dysplasia. These patients have the highest risk of progression to AML.

5q–syndrome

The 5q– syndrome is a unique subtype of MDS with specific morphological, laboratory, and clinical characteristics. Platelet counts are typically normal, or even elevated. Megakaryocytes are small and hypolobulated. When the only chromosomal abnormality is a deletion of 5, patients have an excellent prognosis with a low risk of transforming to a leukaemic state. As discussed below, recent data suggest that patients with 5q– syndrome, when they need treatment, respond excellently to lenalidomide.

Other subtypes of MDS—CMMoL, RARS with thrombocytosis (RARSt), and secondary MDS

While not part of the WHO classification, CMMoL was part of the FAB classification of MDS. CMMoL, characterized by fewer than 20% bone marrow blasts and a peripheral monocytosis of more than 1000 monocytes/µl, has many similarities to myeloproliferative diseases such as chronic myelogenous leukaemia. The white blood cell count is typically very elevated, marrow fibrosis can occur, and extramedullary diseases (hepatosplenomegaly, skin) and serositis are common. Splenomegaly is found in approximately 20% of cases. However, similar to other MDS types, trilineage dysplasia is typically evident. Prognosis best correlates with the percentage of bone marrow blasts, not with the degree of peripheral monocytosis. Approximately 25% of patients progress to acute leukaemia, and death due to cytopenia is common.

Up to 1% of patients with MDS have a subtype of refractory anaemia with at least 15% ringed sideroblasts and also a platelet count of greater than 600×10^9/litre. These patients have been defined as having refractory anaemia with ringed sideroblasts associated with marked thrombocytosis (RARS-T), which has been associated with the JAK2 mutation.

Secondary, or treatment-related MDS, is becoming more prevalent. This is probably due to several factors. Patients with solid malignancies are being treated with more aggressive chemotherapeutic regimens, and they are living longer after these treatments. In addition, it has been postulated that haemopoietic growth factor support during intensive chemotherapy may be a contributing factor to the development of MDS. Most cases of secondary MDS present within the first decade after treatment. Chromosomal abnormalities are common, occurring more than 90% of the time. Chromosomes 5 or 7, are typically involved, with monosomy 7 occurring in 60% of cases. Alkylating agents and topoisomerase II inhibitors are the most commonly implicated in causing secondary MDS.

Treatment

With the exception of allogeneic transplant, there is no curative treatment for MDS. In addition, once acute leukaemia has evolved from MDS, treatment with aggressive chemotherapy does not usually result in long-term, curative remission. Although there are several treatments for MDS, only recently have there been data to suggest that therapy may prolong survival over that of standard, supportive care. However, many treatments can improve quality of life, and new treatments are being explored.

Because of the limits of therapy, there is no need to treat asymptomatic patients, except when an allogeneic bone marrow transplant is clinically possible and the patient wishes to undergo such a procedure. Thus, mild anaemia and thrombocytopenia without bleeding do not necessitate transfusion. There is no evidence that prophylactic antibiotics are beneficial. However, for symptomatic anaemia, or anaemia in the older patient with cardiovascular disease, and for severely thrombocytopenic patients with episodes of bleeding or who are at high risk for significant bleeds, supportive transfusions are the mainstay of care. Patients may need regular transfusions. It is important to recognize patients who will live for long periods with red-cell transfusion; such patients should have their iron status followed and be initiated on iron chelation therapy to avoid the side effects of haemosiderosis. This has become more practical with the introduction of oral chelating agents. There are reports that effective chelation may improve haematopoiesis in some patients.

A wide range of myeloablative chemotherapeutic regimens have been explored; for instance, regimens commonly used to treat AML, including aplasia-inducing doses of cytosine arabinoside (Ara-C), anthracyclines, cyclophosphamide, and topotecan. A few studies have suggested that selected patients with good risk characteristics may do as well with such regimens as patients with AML, particularly if the MDS patients have normal cytogenetics, but the results have usually been disappointing. Complete responses have ranged from 10 to 50%, but these are generally of short duration and accompanied by significant morbidity and mortality. This is probably due to several factors, including the relatively older age of most patients with MDS, the drug resistance of MDS due to the increased expression of multidrug resistance proteins, and limited reserves of normal, healthy marrow for recovery. Low-dose chemotherapy has also been used. While initially explored because these dosing regimens are better tolerated in the older MDS population, many of these agents may have differentiating as well as cytotoxic effects. These have resulted in complete responses from 10 to 40%, but again these responses are not durable. For CMMoL, hydroxycarbamide (hydroxyurea) and the control of peripheral monocytosis has been shown to be as effective as aggressive chemotherapy.

Although most patients with MDS are ineligible for an allogeneic stem cell transplant (either because of their age, comorbid disease, or lack of suitable donor), for some, this remains a viable option and hope for cure. Bone marrow transplantation has been successively carried out in highly selected 55- to 66-year-old patients with MDS. The 5-year survival rate for all patients undergoing a transplant ranges from 30 to 70%, but early mortality is common. Patients with refractory anaemia and RARS and younger patients have the best outcomes with transplantation. Normal or good chromosomal abnormalities are also predictive of a better response with a transplant. All high-risk (see next section) young patients should be considered for allogeneic bone marrow transplantation.

Multiple trials have utilized haemopoietic growth factors, such as recombinant human erythropoietin and granulocyte colony-stimulating factor (G-CSF) or GM-CSF, sometimes in combination. Short-term (1–2 weeks) and prolonged treatment with recombinant human erythropoietin and G-CSF or GM-CSF do not appear to increase the progression to acute leukaemia. In a majority of patients, neutrophil counts increase, sometimes with a documented decrease in infection, and there are often improvements in red-cell and platelet counts with decreased transfusion requirements. Some patients may actually respond with a decreased platelet count, and some patients may not tolerate some of the side effects of the injections. Current evidence suggests that overall survival does not appear to be improved. Generally higher dosages of recombinant human erythropoietin (>200 U/kg per day) may be necessary, and patients with lower serum erythropoietin levels (<500 mU/ml) tend to have better responses. Laboratory data have suggested that the combination of recombinant human erythropoietin and G-CSF may be synergistic in promoting the growth of haemopoietic progenitor colonies. Several clinical studies have suggested that the combination of recombinant human erythropoietin and G-CSF is more effective than either alone, especially in patients with low serum erythropoietin levels and in those with ringed sideroblasts.

Over the past few decades there has been significant scientific enthusiasm for exploring other uses of differentiating agents, alone or in combination with growth factors and cytotoxic agents, in the treatment of MDS. 5-Azacitidine has been demonstrated to have *in vitro* activity in inhibiting DNA methyltransferases, reactivating genes that had been silenced by DNA methylation in their promoter regions, and promoting differentiation. Several studies have demonstrated haematological remissions, decreased progression to AML, and improved survival for patients treated with 5-azacitidine over supportive care. Although it has been postulated that 5-azacitidine may be functioning *in vivo* by reactivating genes either important for tumour suppression or differentiation, to date it has been difficult to prove a correlation between the reactivation of gene(s) and clinical outcome, let along causality. Other demethylating agents also have activity in MDS, and studies are ongoing to combine these with other drugs including histone acetylator inhibitors which can also regulate gene expression through epigenetic modification.

Lenalidomide has a dramatic response rate in patients with isolated 5q– deletions, leading to complete haematological and even cytogenetic responses in a large proportion of patients. Patients with 5q– and other cytogenetic responses still have a good response rate, better than those who do not have a 5q deletion. While

Table 22.3.7.2 The International Prognostic Scoring System (IPSS)

Prognostic	Score				
Variable	**0**	**0.5**	**1.0**	**1.5**	**2**
Marrow blasts (%)	<5	5–10	–	11–20	21–30
Cytogenetics	Good	Intermediate	Poor		
Cytopenias	0–1	2–3			
Combined score	0	0.5–1.0		1.5–2.0	≥2.5
Risk category	Low	Intermediate-1		Intermediate-2	High

Cytogenetics: 'good', normal, -Y, del(5q), del(20q); 'intermediate', all others; 'poor', complex, chromosome 7 abnormalities. Cytopenias: neutrophils $<1.8 \times 10^3/\mu l$; platelets $<10^5/\mu l$; haemoglobin $<10\,g/dl$.

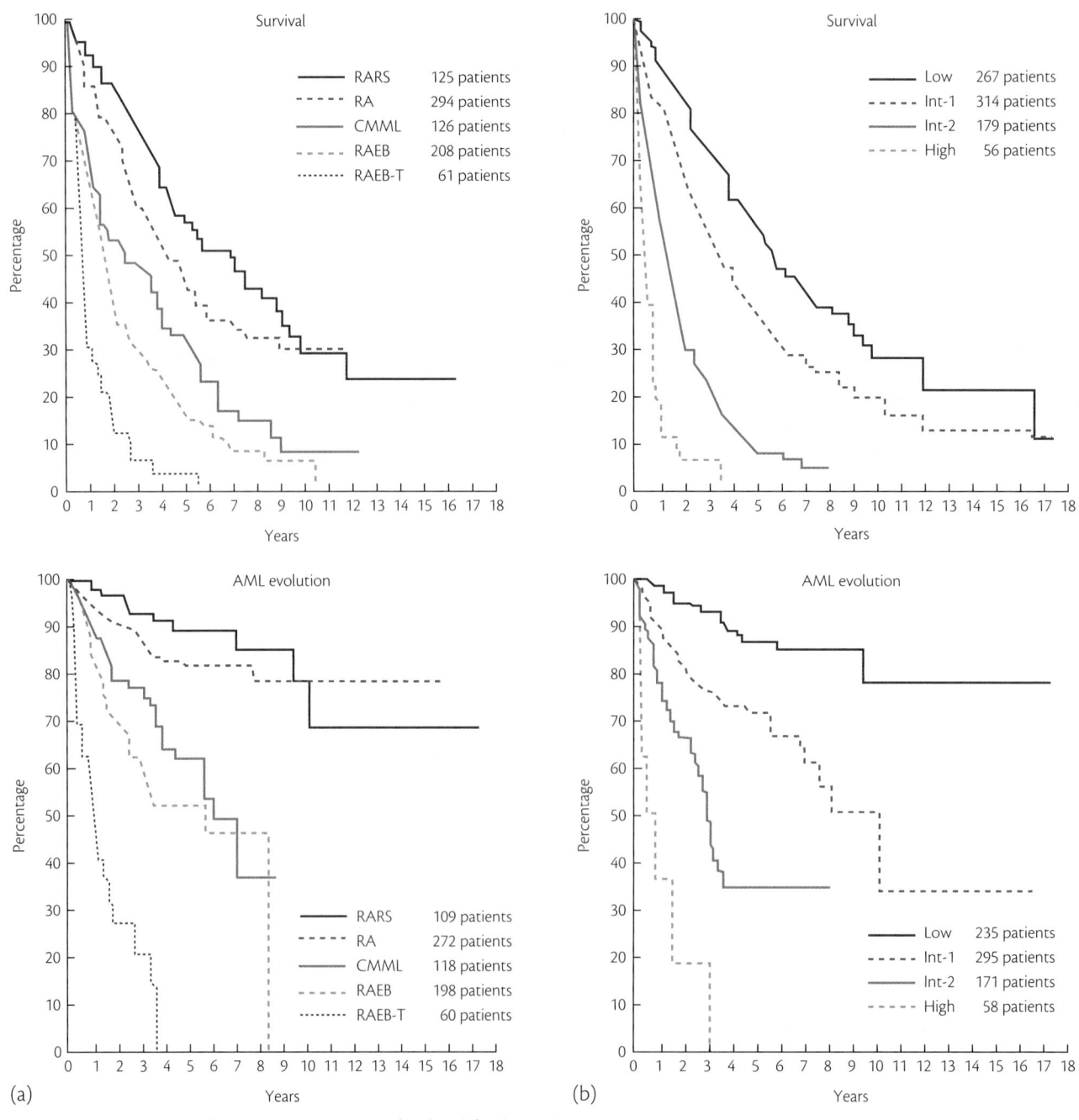

Fig. 22.3.7.2 Survival International Prognostic Scoring System (IPSS) as defined in Table 22.3.7.2.
(From Greenberg P, *et al.* (1997). International scoring system for evaluating prognosis in myelodysplastic syndromes. *Blood*, **89**, 2079–88, with permission from the publisher.)

lenalidomide has been demonstrated to have both immunomodulatory and antiangiogenic activity, and there is evidence that both the immune system and angiogenesis may be aberrant in MDS, the mechanisms by which this drug is active and why its activity appears to be greatest in those missing a portion of chromosome 5 is unknown. Ciclosporin, an immunosuppressant, has also recently been reported as effective in MDS, especially when the marrow is hypocellular. In general, treatment choices should be based on the patient's performance status and age, the prognosis of the disease, and, whenever possible, in the setting of a clinical research protocol.

Prognosis

The median survival of all those with MDS has been reported to be between 12 and 28 months. However, since MDS consists of a variety of diseases, prognosis varies widely. A number of prognostic factors have been studied. Many of the factors which have proven to be predictive in prospective and retrospective studies are intuitive. Because the most common causes of death in patients with MDS are transformation to leukaemia or symptomatic cytopenias, a poorer prognosis is seen in those with increased bone marrow blasts and with more severe cytopenias. Other important prognostic factors include age and specific karyotypic abnormalities.

Because both the FAB classification and the WHO classification systems are heavily reliant on the percentage of bone marrow blasts, these defined subtypes closely correlate with both overall survival and evolution to acute leukaemia. Those with RA and RARS have a low incidence of leukaemia, both within the first 2 years and overall, and an improved survival rate. Patients with increased blasts, as seen in RAEB, do worse, Univariate analysis has also indicated that those with two or three cytopenias do worse than those with none or just one cytopenia, probably because those with more cytopenias have increased blasts, and are more prone to bleeding and infection. Marrow cytogenetics have also been found to be important. A relatively good prognosis is found in deletions of 5q, 20q, -Y in men, or normal cytogenetics. Of note, when these deletions are accompanied with other chromosomal abnormalities, they do not connote a good prognosis. Those with complex chromosomal abnormalities or deletions of 7 do particularly poorly, with a high progression to acute leukaemia.

Several of these prognostic indicators have been combined in various scoring systems to predict the survival of patients with MDS. One of the most accurate, and most widely used, is the International Prognostic Scoring System (IPSS) (Table 22.3.7.2). The IPSS assigns points for unfavourable characteristics, such as unbalanced chromosomal translocations, percentage of blasts in the bone marrow, and lineages affected by the MDS (Fig. 22.3.7.2). Although the IPSS is somewhat cumbersome to use for clinicians, and no scoring system is perfect for individual patients, the IPSS is useful for investigators and for making general decisions regarding the aggressiveness of treatment.

Further research

Increasing information on normal stem cell biology and haemopoiesis will clearly lead to increased understanding of the abnormal haemopoietic development seen in MDS. Particular areas of research being explored include the role of apoptosis in MDS, and specific genetic mutations (or groups of mutations) that are necessary for the development of MDS. The importance of individual mutations or chromosomal abnormalities for prognosis is still being explored. A major emphasis in the stem cell transplantation field is on increasing the availability of transplants. This includes making transplantation less toxic through nonmyeloablative induction strategies, capitalizing on the graft-versus-tumour phenomena, and increasing the number of potential donors with international registries and by minimizing the importance of HLA barriers. Clearly these improvements will aid in the treatment of MDS. The most active area of research in the specific treatment of MDS is in the role of nontoxic differentiating agents.

Further reading

Bennett JM, *et al.* (1982). Proposal for the classification of the myelodysplastic syndromes. *Br J Haematol*, **51**, 189–99.

Bernasconi P, *et al.* (2007). World Health Organization classification in combination with cytogenetic markers improves the prognostic stratification of patients with *de novo* primary myelodysplastic syndromes. *Br J Haematol*, **137**, 1365–2141.

Cheson BD (1998). Standard and low-dose chemotherapy for the treatment of myelodysplastic syndromes. *Leuk Res*, **22** Suppl 1, S17–21.

Deeg HJ, Appelbaum FR (2000). Hematopoietic stem cell transplantation for myelodysplastic syndrome. *Curr Opin Oncol*, **12**, 116–20.

Eillman CL (1998). Molecular genetic features of myelodysplastic syndromes. *Leukaemia*, **12** Suppl 1, S2–6.

Estey EH (1998). Prognosis and therapy of secondary myelodysplastic syndromes. *Haematologica*, **83**, 543–9.

Germing U, *et al.* (2000). Validation of the WHO proposals for a new classification of primary myelodysplastic syndromes: a retrospective analysis of 1600 patients. *Leuk Res*, **24**, 983–92.

Germing U, *et al.* (2006). Prospective validation of the WHO proposals for the classification of myelodysplastic syndromes. *Hematologica*, **91**, 1596–1604.

Greenberg P, *et al.* (1997). International scoring system for evaluating prognosis in myelodysplastic syndromes. *Blood*, **89**, 2079–88.

Kerbauy DB, Deeg HJ (2007). Apoptosis and antiapoptotic mechanisms in the progression of myelodysplastic syndrome. *Exp Hematol*, **35**, 1739–46.

Sole F, *et al.* (2000). Incidence, characterization and prognostic significance of chromosomal abnormalities in 640 patients with primary myelodysplastic syndromes. Grups Cooperativo Espanol de Citogenetica Hematologica. *Br J Haematol*, **108**, 346–56.

Van Etten RA, Shannon KM (2004). Focus on myeloproliferative diseases and myelodysplastic syndromes. *Cancer Cell*, **6**, 547–52.

Yoshida Y, Mufti GJ (1999). Apoptosis and its significance in MDS: controversies revisited. *Leuk Res*, **23**, 777–85.

22.3.8 The polycythaemias

Stefan O. Ciurea and Ronald Hoffman

Essentials

Polycythaemia or erythrocytosis is characterized by an abnormal increase in the numbers of red blood cells, leading to an elevation in the haemoglobin concentration and haematocrit (>52% in men and >48% in women). The cause may be either (1) primary—due to an intrinsic defect of haemopoietic stem cells; or (2) secondary—due to extrinsic stimulation of progenitor erythroid cells by circulating growth factors; and the condition needs to be distinguished from (3) pseudopolycythaemia—in which haematocrit is raised because the plasma volume is decreased.

Normal erythropoiesis

The primary controlling factor for erythropoiesis is the glycoprotein hormone erythropoietin. This is produced by the kidney in response to hypoxia, which leads to the accumulation of a transcriptional factor, hypoxia-inducible factor-1 (HIF-1), the principal regulator of numerous genes that participate in the hypoxic response. Mutation in genes encoding for proteins involved in the oxygen sensing mechanism, in the erythropoietin receptor, or in pathways downstream of the receptor, can all (rarely) lead to polycythaemia.

Secondary polycythaemias

Associated with appropriate erythropoietin secretion—conditions that are ultimately the result of tissue hypoxia and subsequent excessive erythropoietin production include (1) living at high altitude, (2) chronic lung disease, (3) cyanotic congenital heart disease with right-to-left shunting, (4) carbon monoxide intoxication—as occurs in heavy smokers, (5) haemoglobin variants with increased oxygen affinity, (6) mutations in genes involved in the oxygen sensing pathway—e.g. von Hippel–Lindau gene (Chuvash polycythaemia), prolyl hydroxylases.

Associated with inappropriate erythropoietin secretion—in the absence of tissue hypoxia, inappropriate erythropoietin production commonly originates from the kidney and many renal disorders are associated with erythrocytosis, e.g. renal artery stenosis, polycystic kidney disease, tumours. Tumour-associated polycythaemia may also result from cerebellar haemangioblastoma, hepatocellular carcinoma, phaeochromocytoma, and other adrenal tumours.

Primary polycythaemia—polycythaemia vera

This is a clonal, chronic progressive haematological malignancy characterized by excessive proliferation of erythroid, myeloid, and megakaryocytic elements in the bone marrow.

Aetiology—up to 95% of cases are caused by somatic mutation in the pluripotential haemopoietic stem cells leading to replacement of a key valine residue by phenylalanine at position 617 of the JAK2 kinase (V617F), which releases it from autoinhibition.

Clinical features—may be detected on a 'routine' full blood count in asymptomatic patients, or present with a wide range of non-specific symptoms (notably including pruritus). Signs include those directly related to polycythaemia (e.g. ruddy complexion),

also splenomegaly and hepatomegaly. Complications of particular note include (1) thrombotic tendency—deep venous thrombosis/pulmonary embolism, hepatic or portal venous thrombosis, venous thrombosis in unusual sites, transient ischaemic attack/stroke; (2) other neurological syndromes—a wide variety are described; (3) haemorrhagic tendency—due to abnormalities of platelet function; (4) gout—associated with hyperuricaemia. Myelofibrosis with marrow failure develops in about half with polycythaemia vera for 20 years.

Diagnosis—major criteria are (1) evidence of elevated red blood cell mass, and (2) presence of JAK2(V617F) or similar mutation. Minor criteria are (1) trilineage myeloproliferation in the bone marrow, (2) a low serum erythropoietin level, and (3) abnormal marrow proliferative capacity as manifested by the formation of erythroid colonies in the absence of exogenous erythropoietin. Diagnosis requires the presence of both major criteria and one minor criterion, or the first major criterion and two minor criteria.

Treatment—patients should be strongly advised to stop smoking. Phlebotomy should be initiated as soon as the diagnosis is established to reduce and maintain the haematocrit to at less than 45% in men and less than 42% in women. Low-dose aspirin should be given. Myelosuppressive therapy with hydroxycarbamide (hydroxyurea) or other agents should be considered in older patients intolerant of phlebotomies and in those with repeated thrombotic episodes and/or high platelet counts. Haematopoietic stem-cell transplantation is a potentially curative option for myelofibrosis. The use of tyrosine kinase inhibitors to control the downstream effects of the mutant JAK-2 protein hold much promise for future management.

Prognosis—survival is about 18 months in untreated patients, whereas with appropriate management survival of over 10 years is now common. Patients previously treated with alkylating agents and/or radioactive phosphorous have an increased long-term risk of leukaemia.

Rare causes of primary polycythaemia

These include primary familial and congenital polycythaemia—caused by germ-line mutations in the erythropoietin receptor gene and genes encoding components of the JAK2-STAT pathway; may be suggested by family history (autosomal dominant).

Introduction

Erythropoiesis is the process responsible for maintaining a normal red blood cell mass. This is a tightly regulated process, which maintains a balance between the production and destruction of erythrocytes. Polycythaemia or erythrocytosis is a distinct group of disorders characterized by an abnormal increase in the numbers of red blood cells, leading to an elevation in the haemoglobin concentration and haematocrit. Absolute polycythaemias (increased red-cell mass) can be attributed to either an intrinsic defect of haemopoietic stem cells (primary) or to the stimulation of progenitor cells by excessive levels of circulating growth factors (secondary). A pathophysiological classification of polycythaemia is provided in Box 22.3.8.1. Patients with absolute polycythaemias should be distinguished from individuals in whom a minimally elevated haematocrit is not accompanied by a corresponding absolute increase in

Relative polycythaemias

◆ Associated with volume loss or contraction:

   • Gastrointestinal losses: diarrhoea, vomiting, ileostomy

   • Renal losses: osmotic diuresis, therapeutic diuresis, Addison's disease, hypercalcemia

   • Insensible losses: profuse sweating, fever

   • Stress or Gaisbock's polycythaemia

Absolute polycythaemias

Primary polycythaemias

◆ Primary familial and congenital polycythaemia

◆ Polycythaemia vera

Secondary polycythaemias associated with appropriate secretion of EPO

◆ Smokers' polycythaemia

◆ Hypobaric hypoxia

◆ Chronic pulmonary disease

◆ Alveolar hypoventilation

◆ Congenital heart diseases associated with right-to-left shunts

◆ High-affinity haemoglobins

◆ 2,3-DPG deficiency

◆ Methaemoglobinaemias

◆ Chuvash polycythaemia

◆ Prolyl hydroxylase mutations

Secondary polycythaemias associated with inappropriate secretion of EPO

◆ Polycythaemia of renal disease

◆ Tumour-associated polycythaemia

◆ Endocrine disorders—phaeochromocytomas, aldosterone-producing adenomas, Cushing's, syndrome

the red-cell mass (spurious polycythaemia, stress erythrocytosis, Gaisbock's syndrome), but rather by a contraction of plasma volume. Haematocrit levels above 52% in men and 48% in women are abnormal and require further evaluation to determine the cause of the polycythaemia.

Normal erythropoiesis

Erythropoietin (EPO), a 34.4-kDa glycoprotein hormone, is the primary humoral regulator of erythropoiesis. Alterations in its production are accompanied by adjustments in the rate of red-cell production. Production of EPO is controlled by the relative supply of oxygen to the kidney and can increase by 1000-fold in states of severe hypoxia. Under normal conditions EPO production is mediated by decreased oxygen content of haemoglobin within red cells, termed hypoxemia, which leads to decreased oxygen delivery to tissues.

Decreased tissue oxygenation (partial pressure of oxygen (Po_2) <60 mmHg) is associated with accumulation of hypoxia-inducible factor-1 (HIF-1), the major transcriptional factor responsible for activation of the EPO gene. The HIF transcriptional system is a master regulator of the hypoxic response controlling a large number of genes including phosphoglycerate kinase, glucose transporter-1,vascular endothelial growth factor, and EPO. HIF-1α is continuously synthesized irrespective of oxygen availability. It is barely detected in steady-state cells because of its rapid degradation by the ubiquitin proteasome pathway. During hypoxic conditions, a rapid accumulation of HIF-1α occurs due to a blockade of its degradation. This pathway permits a rapid response to hypoxia without activating transcriptional/translational machinery. Increased. HIF-1α mRNA and protein levels are induced by hypoxia while protein levels rapidly decay during normoxia. The degradation of HIF-1α requires the von Hippel–Lindau (VHL) protein, oxygen, and three different iron requiring proline hydroxylase (PH) enzymes. The *VHL* gene is a tumor suppressor gene, which participates in the hypoxia-sensing pathway by binding HIF-1α facilitating its degradation by the proteasome. The PH enzymes, which hydroxylate HIF, are required for HIF proteloytic degradation by promoting the interaction between HIF and VHL. As oxygen levels decrease, hydroxylation of HIF decreases and HIF-1α is no longer able to bind VHL and becomes stabilized. In normal individuals, VHL protein binds to hydroxylated HIF-1α and causes its ubiquitination and proteosomal degradation. Genetic mutations in VHL or PH are frequently capable of leading to inherited forms of erythrocytosis by causing alterations in the binding of the VHL to HIF-1α, leading to its accumulation and activation of hypoxia-related genes including EPO and vascular endothelial growth factor (VEGF). EPO binds to its receptor, and initiates downstream effects via the Janus tyrosine kinase 2 (JAK2)and signal transducer and activator of transcription (STAT) intracellular signalling pathways. Binding of EPO causes dimerization of the EPO receptor, phosphorylation of intracytoplasmic residues, and activation of STAT, which shuttles from the cytoplasm into the nucleus and initiates protein transcription. JAK2–STAT activation promotes erythroid cell division, differentiation, proliferation, and prevention of precursor cell apoptosis. Mutations in EPO receptor gene leading to its constitutive activation have been observed in some patients with familial and congenital forms of polycythaemia.

Oxygen transport is a complex process dependent on a number of variables, including ambient oxygen levels, minute ventilation rates, lung diffusion capacity, cardiac output, red-cell mass, regional blood flow, tissue capillary density, and haemoglobin–oxygen affinity. Acute changes in tissue oxygen demands or in environmental oxygen levels are compensated not only by increased EPO production but also increased ventilation rates, cardiac output, blood flow distribution, and haemoglobin–oxygen affinity (through the modulation of 2,3-disphosphoglycerate (2,3-DPG) production). Sustained hypoxia is required for polycythaemia to occur as a compensatory mechanism.

Relative polycythaemias

These disorders are characterized by an elevated haemoglobin or haematocrit level, which occurs as the result of contraction in plasma volume. The red-cell mass remains normal. There are two major groups of patients with relative forms of polycythaemia. The first includes patients with more acute conditions associated with significant degrees of dehydration, with a consequential decrease in plasma volume: e.g. gastrointestinal fluid losses, therapeutic diuresis, endocrine disorders such as Addison's disease, and hypercalcaemia. In most cases, the consequences of volume contraction are clinically obvious. The aetiology of the increase in haematocrit does not usually present a diagnostic challenge.

The second group is associated with a slight but sustained increase in the haematocrit. These patients are frequently active, middle-aged, mildly hypertensive, obese men subjected to considerable stress who present with persistent polycythaemia. Characteristically, they appear plethoric but without any of the other typical features of polycythaemia vera. The cause for the contraction in the plasma volume is poorly understood, but autonomic dysregulation with changes in venous capacitance may be responsible.

The usual range of haemoglobin levels in these individuals is between 18 and 20 g/dl with haematocrits ranging from 49 to 55%. Most of these patients seek medical evaluation for an unrelated condition, and are incidentally found to have increased haemoglobin and haematocrit values. Suitable advice regarding weight reduction, control of hypertension, and smoking cessation is usually provided to these patients. The optimal therapy is unknown but is generally directed to correcting the patient's underlying cardiovascular risk factors.

Overfilling blood collection tubes can cause the artefact of pseudopolycythaemia due to inadequate sample collection. Attention to this error can frequently avoid unnecessary investigation.

Absolute polycythaemia

Absolute polycythaemias may be classified as being primarily due to autonomous cell growth or to an enhanced response to growth factors that promotes the proliferation of developing erythroid cells, or secondary, due to excessive production of EPO in response to a variety of stimuli. Primary polycythaemia, caused by defects in haemopoietic stem cells, is accompanied, in general, by low levels of circulating EPO. Germ-line mutations of the EPO receptor that lead to enhanced erythropoiesis cause primary familial congenital polycythaemias. Polycythaemia vera, the most common primary polycythaemia, is caused by an acquired defect in haemopoietic stem cells resulting in an excessive proliferation of myeloid cells. Recently, a mutation in the autoinhibitory domain of JAK2 tyrosine kinase (V617F) has been associated with polycythaemia vera in up to 95% of the cases. By contrast, secondary polycythaemia is generally caused by elevated EPO production and is not associated with mutation in the JAK2 tyrosine kinase. Elevated levels of plasma EPO can accompany systemic hypoxaemia, certain neoplasms, and disorders that impair oxygen delivery to tissues (see Box 22.3.8.1).

Absolute polycythaemias are accompanied by an increased red-cell mass. Documentation of such an increased red-cell mass may require a blood volume study with direct determination of both the red-cell mass and plasma volume. This test is presently available in select referral centres and the need for its performance is limited to special situations due to the availability of JAK2 V617F testing. A haematocrit greater than 60% in men and greater than 55% in women, however, is almost always associated with absolute erythrocytosis. In such cases it is usually unnecessary

to do blood volume studies to be assured that the patient has an absolute polycythaemia.

Secondary polycythaemias associated with appropriate EPO secretion

This group of polycythaemias encompasses a number of conditions that are ultimately the result of tissue hypoxia and subsequent excessive EPO production leading to erythrocytosis. These disorders are collectively regarded as hypoxic erythrocytoses.

Hypobaric hypoxia

At high altitudes the barometric pressure and, consequently, the ambient oxygen tension are reduced, resulting in alveolar and arterial hypoxia. Natives of the Andes (South America) who live above 4200 m have been reported to have haematocrits 30% higher than individuals who live at sea level. Acutely, changes in minute ventilation, heart rate, blood flow, and haemoglobin–oxygen affinity occur as an individual reaches a high altitude. Serum EPO is elevated initially, but eventually returns to the normal range in the absence of extreme hypoxia. This decline will not prevent the increase in red-cell mass, which will be sustained, because early unsustained elevations of EPO promote expansion of the erythroid progenitor pool. Only very small quantities of the hormone are subsequently required to sustain the red-cell mass under normal circumstances. Healthy highlanders develop pulmonary hypertension, right ventricular hypertrophy, and increased amounts of smooth muscle cells in distal pulmonary arterial branches, which leads to increased pulmonary vascular resistance and pulmonary artery pressures as compared to individuals who live at sea level. Due to these adaptive changes healthy highlanders are able to perform physical activities similar to or often even more strenuous than those living at sea level.

Chronic mountain sickness is a pathological loss of adaptation to high altitude by highlanders that occurs in native or lifelong residents living above 2500 m. They suffer from headaches, fatigue, impaired exercise tolerance, cyanosis, clubbing, right heart failure, and absolute polycythaemia. These symptoms frequently resolve with descent to lower altitudes. The prevalence of chronic mountain sickness is higher in men than in women and increases with altitude, ageing, associated lung disease history of smoking, and air pollution. The chronic response to high altitudes is probably determined by poorly defined genetic factors, which likely contribute to the development of chronic mountain sickness. The major mechanism underlying chronic mountain sickness is relative hypoventilation, since healthy highlanders characteristically hyperventilate. Chronic mountain sickness is a common problem, affecting 6–8% of males in La Paz (Peru), for instance. The definitive treatment of chronic mountain sickness is descent to lower altitudes or sea level. Phlebotomy and acetazolamide therapy are recommended for affected individuals who must remain at high altitudes.

Chronic pulmonary disease

Pulmonary diseases are a common cause of secondary polycythaemia. Defects in gas exchange result in hypoxia, with consequent increases in EPO and red-cell mass. Not every patient with hypoxia secondary to respiratory disease develops polycythaemia. The presence of concurrent inflammation or infection may blunt the marrow response to hypoxia. It is important to be aware that smoking itself may also contribute significantly to the polycythaemia associated with chronic respiratory disease. Phlebotomy may be indicated in patients with relatively high haematocrits (55–60%), given the known deleterious of hyperviscosity. Chronic oxygen therapy in patients with severe chronic obstructive pulmonary disease has resulted in relief of hypoxia and modest reductions of haematocrit levels.

Alveolar hypoventilation

Hypoventilation may lead to hypoxia and an EPO-mediated increase in red-cell mass. These disorders include the sleep apnoea syndrome and supine hypoventilation. Up to 25% of patients with unexplained polycythaemia are subsequently found to have sleep apnoea. Common symptoms include loud snoring, breathing pauses, feelings of nonrefreshing sleep and excessive daytime sleeping. In these conditions, significant degrees of hypoxia may occur without evident parenchymal pulmonary disease. Decreases in blood oxygen content may occur intermittently; consequently EPO levels and arterial blood gas values may be normal. Diseases affecting the central nervous system may also impair respiratory centre function and trigger hypoventilation. These defects have been described in association with encephalitis, cerebrovascular accidents, and drug intoxication (i.e. barbiturates). Impaired skeletal muscle function of the chest wall or diaphragm may also sufficiently compromise alveolar ventilation to trigger polycythaemia. In these cases, correction of hypoxia is warranted. The role of phlebotomy is unclear, but not unreasonable in patients with significant elevations in haematocrit and associated cardiovascular or cerebrovascular disease. The obesity–hypoventilation syndrome seen in morbidly obese individuals is characterized by chronic hypoxia and hypercapia due to alveolar hypoventilation with a resultant increase in EPO production, polycythaemia and cor pulmonale. Effective treatment includes surgically induced weight loss, nasal continuous positive airway pressure ventilation, and occasionally the use of respiratory stimulants.

Cardiovascular disease

Cyanotic congenital heart diseases with an associated right-to-left shunt result in oxygen desaturation and an elevation of EPO, causing secondary polycythaemia. After compensatory erythrocytosis in response to oxygen desaturation occurs, serum EPO levels may return to normal levels. An extremely elevated haematocrit may be detrimental to optimal oxygen delivery. Some children with congenital heart disease may develop extreme haematocrit values (≥80%), which leads to a significant risk of a thrombotic event, especially during periods of dehydration due to hyperviscosity and sludging within the microcirculation. The treatment of erythrocytosis in patients with cyanotic congenital heart disease is controversial. Phlebotomy may be indicated in some instances where it has been shown to improve cerebral blood flow and neurological symptoms and to increase exercise capacity. To date there is no consensus which defines the precise target haematocrit values for therapeutic phlebotomy in the management of patients with these disorders.

Carbon monoxide intoxication

Chronic carbon monoxide intoxication most commonly occurs as a consequence of smoking. Elevated haematocrits have been reported in 3% of all smokers. Other less common causes include work-related exposures such as those seen in caisson workers or tunnel toll-collectors. Carbon monoxide has a much higher affinity for haemoglobin than oxygen does, thereby reducing the amount of oxygen that can be bound and transported by haemo-

globin. It also shifts the oxygen–haemoglobin dissociation curve to the left, decreasing the ability of haemoglobin to release oxygen to peripheral tissues. Furthermore, carbon monoxide impairs normal compensatory mechanisms; carboxyhaemoglobin is known to decrease 2,3-DPG production by red cells and to reduce the affinity of haemoglobin for 2,3-DPG. Polycythaemia due to chronic carbon monoxide intoxication may be associated with an increased risk of thromboembolic phenomena. Phlebotomy may be indicated in patients with very high haematocrits (>55–60%).

The decreased oxygen-carrying capacity associated with carbon monoxide intoxication is not detected by standard blood gas measurements; therefore, a direct measure of carboxyhaemoglobin levels is required. Morning carboxyhaemoglobin levels ranging from 4% to 20% have been reported. Individuals with chronic carbon monoxide poisoning may experience neuropsychiatric and cardiac abnormalities. The treatment is smoking cessation or removal of the patient from the source of carbon monoxide.

High-affinity haemoglobins

At least 50 haemoglobin variants exhibit increased avidity for oxygen. These mutations are transmitted as autosomal dominants. Oxygen transport by haemoglobin occurs as a function of the oxygen–haemoglobin affinity curve. This function is represented by a sigmoid curve and is a reflection of the initial binding of oxygen by deoxygenated haemoglobin occurring with significant difficulty. As oxygen molecules are bound to normal haemoglobin, further binding is facilitated by structural changes that occur in the haemoglobin molecule. High-affinity haemoglobin variants arise when mutations alter key amino acid residues in regions of haemoglobin that affect these rearrangements, or at the interface between α and β chains. Another group of mutations induces changes in oxygen affinity indirectly, by causing structural changes in haemoglobin regions that are critical for the binding of 2,3-DPG.

Increases in oxygen affinity result in a shift of the oxygen dissociation curve to the left. Consequently, haemoglobin binds oxygen more readily and retains more oxygen at lower Po_2 levels. This ultimately results in decreased delivery of oxygen to tissues where capillary Po_2 is low (35–45 mmHg). Mild tissue hypoxia then triggers an increase in the production of EPO with consequent polycythaemia.

Oxygen affinity by variant haemoglobin is usually measured as the $P_{50}O_2$, which represents the partial oxygen pressure at which 50% of haemoglobin is saturated with oxygen. This analysis is necessary for the identification of patients with high-affinity haemoglobins. High-affinity haemoglobins are associated with lower than normal values of $P_{50}O_2$; values below 17 mmHg are usually diagnostic of such an abnormal haemoglobin. Haemoglobin electrophoresis may, on occasion, aid in the recognition of an abnormal haemoglobin, but many high-affinity haemoglobins display normal electrophoretic mobility. Conversely, the presence of an abnormal band per se does not provide information regarding oxygen affinity. A study of family members is important, but a negative family history does not negate the diagnosis since there is a high rate of spontaneous mutations.

Most patients with high-affinity haemoglobins have mild polycythaemia and are asymptomatic since the compensatory polycythaemia results in normal oxygen delivery to tissues. Phlebotomy therapy of such patients has been reported to be of no value and has been shown to reduce exercise tolerance.

Methaemoglobinaemias

Hereditary methaemoglobinaemia may be associated with a mild polycythaemia. Methaemoglobin results from the oxidation of ferrous ions (Fe^{2+}) to the ferric state (Fe^{3+}). Oxygen does not bind reversibly to methaemoglobin, resulting in a left shift of the oxygen dissociation curve, impaired oxygen delivery, and chronic tissue hypoxia.

2, 3-DPG deficiency

This rare familial form of polycythaemia is due to a deficiency of the enzyme biphosphoglycerate mutase. Deficiency leads to a decrease in 2,3-DPG, resulting in the increased affinity of oxygen to haemoglobin, peripheral tissue hypoxia, and hypoxic erythrocytosis. This disorder should be suspected in patients with familial polycythaemia with a low $P_{50}O_2$ in the absence of a mutant haemoglobin. Measurements of 2,3-DPG in fresh red cell reveals reduced levels.

Chuvash polycythaemia

Chuvash polycythaemia is a recognized form of congenital and familial polycythaemia endemic to the Chuvash population of the Russian Federation, which has also been reported to occur in a variety of other racial and ethnic groups. The extreme elevations of haemoglobin in this autosomal recessive disorder are accompanied by increased EPO levels. Chuvash polycythaemia is caused by germ-line mutations in the von Hippel–Lindau gene, most common being the 598 C→T mutation. Stimulated EPO production is caused by the inability of the mutated von Hippel–Lindau gene to bind to HIF-1α, which escapes degradation and accumulates. These patients present with isolated erythrocytosis without elevations of white cells or platelets, have low blood pressure, varicose veins, and vertebral haemangiomas probably due to increased levels of VEGF. Death frequently occurs before the age of 40 due to thrombotic and haemorrhagic complications. Cerebral vascular events are especially common causes of death.

Prolyl hydroxylase mu tations

Mutations in the prolyl hydroxylases are inherited as an autosomal dominant and are associated with failure of hydroxylation of prolyl residues of HIF-1α, increased hypoxia-inducible factor levels, and EPO production leading to the development of erythrocytosis. In contrast to the patients with Chuvash polycythaemia, patients with mutations of prolyl hydroxylases do not have the clinical consequences described above.

Secondary polycythaemias associated with the inappropriate secretion of EPO

Enhanced EPO levels and secretion occur in the absence of tissue hypoxia in this group of disorders. The EPO response is therefore inappropriate to systemic oxygen requirements.

Polycythaemia of renal disease

As the kidney is the principal site of EPO production, it is not surprising that renal disorders may be associated with erythrocytosis or anaemia. Patients with hypertension and renal artery stenosis have a higher incidence of erythrocytosis than similarly hypertensive patients without renal artery disease. Other benign kidney diseases associated with an increase in EPO production and erythrocytosis include polycystic kidney disease (acquired or familial) and renal cysts. Unusual patients with glomerulonephritis may also occasionally present with an elevated haematocrit. An uncommon cause of polycythaemia is Bartter's syndrome, a hereditary tubular disorder characterized by hypokalaemia secondary to renal potassium loss in association with elevated plasma renin activity and aldosterone secretion. Post-renal-transplant polycythaemia is defined as a persistently elevated haematocrit greater than 51% after renal transplantation without an elevation of the white blood cell or platelet count. Between 5 and 13% of patients have been reported to develop erythrocytosis 8 to 24 months after renal transplantation. It has been postulated that the excessive response to EPO from the donor kidney in a patient with previously low EPO levels could cause this elevation in haematocrit in these patients. Approximately 60% of patients with post-transplant erythrocytosis experience headaches, plethora, lethargy, and dizziness and approximately 10 to 20% develop thromboembolic complications. Retention of the native kidney is essential for the development of post-transplant erythrocytosis with the native kidney overproducing EPO leading to the development of erythrocytosis. Frequently the erythrocytosis resolves with the removal of the kidney. Angiotensin-converting enzyme (ACE) inhibitors have proved useful in controlling post-transplant polycythaemia, but phlebotomy may still be required in patients with haematocrit levels over 55 to 60% to rapidly decrease the risk of thrombotic complications.

Tumour-associated polycythaemia

A number of tumours are associated with an inappropriately increased production of EPO, including benign and malignant tumours of the kidney, hepatomas, cerebellar haemangioblastomas, and phaeochromocytomas. Polycythaemia occurs in 1% of patients with renal carcinomas, 9 to 20% of patients with cerebellar haemangioblastomas, and 10% of patients with hepatomas. Resection of the tumour, if feasible, may be associated with regression of the polycythaemia. Therapeutic phlebotomy is recommended in patients with extreme increases in the haematocrit.

Endocrine disorders

Phaeochromocytomas and aldosterone-producing adenomas have been associated with increased levels of EPO. Mild forms of polycythaemia have also been observed in some patients with Cushing's syndrome, probably related to marrow stimulation by steroid hormones. Recombinant human EPO has been abused by athletes and its use can lead to erythrocytosis. The recombinant form of EPO can be distinguished from native EPO by its electrophoretic mobility.

Primary polycythaemia

Primary familial and congenital polycythaemia

Primary familial and congenital polycythaemia is an inherited form of polycythaemia caused by mutations in the EPO receptor, thereby resulting in the hypersensitivity of erythroid progenitor cells to EPO and low serum EPO levels. Most of the disease-causing mutations result in truncation of the cytoplasmic C-terminal portion of the EPO receptor, which leads to constitutive activation of the receptor due to loss of its negative regulatory domain. In the autosomal dominant form of the disease, family members have plethora, headaches, dizziness, nosebleeds, and exertional dyspnoea. These symptoms resolve with phlebotomy and reduction of the haematocrit. Unlike those with polycythaemia vera, primary familial and congenital polycythaemia patients have normal platelet counts, are

JAK2 V617F negative, lack splenomegaly, and do not progress to acute leukaemia. Not all cases of primary familial and congenital polycythaemia can be attributed to the mutations of the EPO receptor (which occur in c.10–20% of cases), suggesting that other genetic defects can lead to a similar phenotype.

Polycythaemia vera

Polycythaemia vera is a clonal, chronic progressive haematological malignancy characterized by excessive proliferation of erythroid, myeloid, and megakaryocytic elements in the bone marrow. The other myeloproliferative neoplasms include essential thrombocythaemia and primary myelofibrosis. The hallmark of polycythaemia vera is an absolute form of erythrocytosis usually associated with leucocytosis, thrombocytosis, splenomegaly, hypersensitivity of haematopoietic progenitor cells and the JAK2 V617F mutation. This mutation accounts for the cytokine hypersensitivity, which characterizes hematopoietic progenitors from patients with this disorder. The use of recently developed molecular tools to detect JAK2 V617F has already revolutionized the diagnosis of polycythaemia vera (Table 22.3.8.1). This mutation is a recognized molecular target for future therapies. In contrast to those with other haematological malignancies, patients suffering from polycythaemia vera may enjoy prolonged survival, provided that the excessive production of red cells and platelets is controlled. This prolonged survival is occasionally punctuated by the development of myelofibrosis and/or acute leukaemia.

Epidemiology

Polycythaemia vera was thought to be a rare disorder, with an estimated yearly incidence in the Western world between 5 and 17 cases per million population. Recent data suggests that its prevalence might be higher than previously expected with rates of at least 300 cases per million population being reported. The very high association between JAK2 V617F and polycythaemia vera will probably have an impact on future studies of the incidence and prevalence of

Table 22.3.8.1 The 2008 WHO diagnostic criteria for polycythaemia vera

Major criteria
1   Evidence of elevated red-cell mass: Hgb >18.5 g/dl (men), >16 g/dl (women), or Hgb or Hct >99th percentile of reference range for age, sex, altitude of residence, or Hgb > 17 g/dl (men), or >15 g/dl (women) if associated with a sustained increase of ≥2 g/dl from baseline that cannot be attributed to correction of iron deficiency, or Elevated red-cell mass >25% above mean normal predicted value
2   Presence of JAK2 V617F or similar mutation

Minor criteria
1   BM trilineage myeloproliferation
2   Low serum EPO levels (<4.0 U/litre)
3   Abnormal marrow proliferative capacity as manifested by the formation of erythroid colonies in the absence of exogenous EPO

BM, bone marrow; EPO, erythropoietin; Hct, haematocrit; Hgb, haemoglobin.
The diagnosis of polycythaemia vera is made in the presence of both major criteria and one minor criterion or the first major criterion and two minor criteria.
(Adapted from Tefferi A, Vardiman JW (2008). Classification and diagnosis of myeloproliferative neoplasms: the 2008 World Heath Organization criteria and point-of-care diagnostic algorithms. *Leukemia*, **22**, 14–22.)

this disease, and could change our knowledge of the average age of diagnosis. A very low incidence of 2 cases per year per million population has been reported in Japan. These differences suggest that environmental as well as genetic factors might be important.

Polycythaemia vera is slightly more common in men than in women, with a male/female ratio of 1.2:1. The average age at diagnosis is 60 years; it is very rare in individuals younger than 30 years of age. Only a handful of cases have been reported during childhood.

Biological and molecular aspects

The exaggerated production of red cells, granulocytes, and platelets in polycythaemia vera suggests that the fundamental defect occurs at the level of the pluripotent haemopoietic stem cell. The clonal, and thereby malignant, nature of polycythaemia vera was first established by the cellular analysis of blood cell production in Afro-American women heterozygous for X-linked glucose-6-phosphate dehydrogenase isoenzymes. These results have been confirmed using restriction fragment length polymorphisms of the active X chromosomes.

In patients with polycythaemia vera, EPO concentrations often fall below the levels observed in normal individuals. These low levels persist even after repeated phlebotomies, suggesting that excessive production of EPO is not a critical component in the pathogenesis of this disorder. Using *in vitro* cell-culture systems, polycythaemia vera bone marrow cells can form erythroid colonies in the absence of EPO and are hypersensitive to EPO (endogenous colony formation). Polycythaemia vera progenitor cells are also hypersensitive to other cytokines such as stem-cell factor, interleukin-3, and granulocyte macrophage colony-stimulating factor (GM-CSF). The presence of JAK2 V617F mutation can now explain both the hypersensitivity to EPO and to multiple other growth factors which use the JAK2–STAT5 signalling pathway. A valine to phenylalanine substitution occurs within exon 14 of the JH2 domain of the *JAK2* tyrosine kinase gene. In the normal kinase, this domain has an inhibitory effect over the catalytic domain, JH1. A mutation in the JH2 domain disrupts this autoinhibitory effect and renders the kinase constitutively active, leading to a constant downstream phosphorylation and substrate activation. STATs are intracytoplasmic molecules that initiate gene transcription. One of the target genes of STATs is *BCL2L1*, which expresses an antiapoptotic protein, overexpressed in polycythaemia vera and believed to play an important role in increased survival of erythroid precursors and megakaryocytes. Overexpression of JAK2 V617F in cell lines is associated with increased cellular proliferation and cytokine hypersensitivity and its transfection into marrow cells which are then transplanted into mice is associated with the development of a clinical phenotype similar to polycythaemia vera. Progression of the disease has been also shown to correlate with the level of allele chimerism. Retrospective analyses have revealed that patients with a low burden of the mutated allele can evolve over time to a higher burden of the mutated allele. Loss of heterozygosity on the short arm of chromosome 9 (the location of the *JAK2* gene) is a consequence not of gene deletion but rather uniparental disomy or mitotic recombinantion. Even in patients with a low burden of JAK2 V617F, erythroid progenitors that are homozygous for JAK2 V6717F are usually present. This finding is characteristic of polycythemia vera but occurs less frequently in primary myelofibrosis and rarely in essential thrombocythaemia. The burden of JAK2 V617F is correlated with disease progression and the development of complications in polycythaemia vera patients. Additional mutations of *JAK2* that are associated with erythrocytosis have also been identified. Somatic gain-of-function mutations involving exon 12 rather than exon 14 has been identified in patients with isolated erythrocytosis and low serum EPO levels. All erythroid colonies cloned from the hematopoietic cells of such patients are heterozygous for this mutation. *JAK2* exon 12 mutations could therefore identify a distinctive myeloprolioiferative disorder that affects patients who currently carry a diagnosis of idiopathic erythrocytosis.

Pathobiology

Patients with polycythaemia vera have an increased thrombotic tendency resulting from the expansion of the red-cell mass which represents the main cause of mortality in these patients. There is a direct relationship between the risk of thrombosis and age, incidence of cardiovascular complications being higher in patients over 65 years of age. Younger individuals are also at risk for thrombotic episodes, many of them life threatening, such as Budd–Chiari syndrome, cerebrovascular thrombosis, acute myocardial infarction, or pulmonary embolism. The main rheological abnormality is elevation of the total blood viscosity. Cerebral blood flow is reduced in patients with polycythaemia vera and a haematocrit of 53 to 62%. Reductions in blood flow are correctable by phlebotomy. Even small reductions in the haematocrit result in significant reductions in blood viscosity and increased cerebral blood flow, thereby reducing the likelihood of thrombus development. Thrombocytosis and functional platelet abnormalities and increased white blood cell count (found in 50% of the patients) are frequently present, and may play a role in the development of thrombosis.

Patients with polycythaemia vera are also at an increased risk of developing life-threatening haemorrhagic complications. Abnormalities in platelet function and number have been implicated. Qualitative platelet abnormalities include defective platelet aggregation *in vitro*, acquired storage pool disease, and dysregulated thromboxane A_2 metabolism. Acquired von Willebrand disease has been described in patients who have very high platelet counts (>1000 × 10^6/litre), in association with life-threatening bleeding episodes. No laboratory test has proven useful for the *a priori* identification of patients at an increased risk of developing haemorrhagic or thrombotic events.

The progression to a post-polycythaemic related myelofibrosis phase of the disease is a common cause of morbidity. This stage is characterized by cytopenias, marrow fibrosis, and extramedullary haemopoiesis. There is conflicting data on the incidence of this complication. Some studies found a very low incidence after 10–20 years, others reported that up to 25–50% of patients with polycythemia vera may develop polycythemia vera-related myelofibrosis. The fibroblastic component represents a reactive event, and may be due to the local release of growth factors, particularly TGFβ, by haematopoietic cells. The association between the treatment modality and the development of myelofibrosis is as yet unclear. There is, however, an established association between the treatment type (alkylating agents and radioactive phosphorus (^{32}P)), and the development of acute leukaemia. It must be emphasized, however, that even those patients treated with phlebotomy alone have a leukaemogenic risk significantly higher than that expected in the general population.

Clinical manifestations

The clinical manifestations of polycythaemia vera are the direct consequence of the excessive production of cellular elements of the various haemopoietic cell lineages.

The routine and widespread use of laboratory screening tests during medical evaluations has led to an increased detection of asymptomatic patients. In contrast, symptomatic patients may present to their physician with a large array of nonspecific complaints including headache, weakness, pruritus, dizziness, excessive sweating, visual disturbances, paraesthesias, joint symptoms, and epigastric distress. Some one-third of patients will have lost 10% of their body weight by the time they present, presumably due to the associated hypermetabolism. Joint disease is usually the manifestation of gout, due to the increased production of uric acid. The most important signs on physical examination include ruddy cyanosis, conjunctival plethora, splenomegaly, hepatomegaly, and hypertension.

Patients left without appropriate treatment are at a particularly high risk of developing thrombotic or haemorrhagic events. In fact, thrombosis may be the cause of death in up to 30 to 40% of patients. Thrombosis may occur in the deep venous system of the lower extremities, or present as a pulmonary embolism. Cerebrovascular, coronary, and peripheral vascular occlusions are not rare. Thromboses at unusual sites are also characteristic of polycythaemia vera. They include occlusion of the splenic, portal, hepatic, and mesenteric veins. Cardiac valve abnormalities affecting the aortic or the mitral valves are commonly seen, frequently in the form of leaflet thickening or frank vegetations. These lesions are associated with the occurrence of arterial thromboembolism. Hepatic venous or inferior vena caval thrombosis is known as Budd–Chiari syndrome and is characterized by hepatosplenomegaly, ascites, oedema of the peripheral extremities, jaundice, abdominal pain, and distension of superficial abdominal veins as a result of portal hypertension. The prevalence of myeloproloferative neoplasms in patients with splanchnic vein thrombosis was estimated to be as high as 49% for hepatic vein thrombosis and 23% for portal vein thrombosis. Often these patients will present with normal haemoglobin and haematocrit levels. This phenomenon is regarded as 'inapparent polycythaemia vera' and requires a full evaluation for the presence of a myeloproliferative neoplasms. Detection of the JAK2 V617F mutation will help identify and appropriately treat these patients earlier. Up to 34% of patients with portal vein thrombosis and up to 58% of patients with Budd–Chiari syndrome may have a myeloproliferative neoplasms, identified by the presence of JAK2 V617F. Iron deficiency may also mask the expected erythrocytosis in some patients with polycythaemia vera. Leucocytosis, thrombocytosis, and splenomegaly are usually present.

Neurological abnormalities are also common and occur in up to 60 to 80% of patients. They include transient ischaemic attacks, cerebral infarction, cerebral haemorrhage, confusional states, fluctuating dementia, and involuntary movement syndromes. Dizziness, paraesthesias, tinnitus, visual problems, and headaches are common symptoms attributed to the hyperviscosity state. Small infarcts in the basal ganglia region, also known as lacunae, might be related to some of the transient neurological manifestations. Symptoms of carotid, vertebral, or basilar artery insufficiency occur frequently. Peripheral vascular insufficiency may be manifested by intense redness or cyanosis of the digits, burning, classical erythromelalgia, digital ischaemia with palpable pulses, or thrombophlebitis. Erythromelalgia consists of a burning pain in the digits of either the lower and/or upper extremities, an objective sensation of increased temperature, and relief by cooling. If left untreated it may evolve into gangrene. Antiplatelet aggregation therapy rapidly reverses the symptoms. Peripheral pulses are usually normal in these patients, as this phenomenon is due to changes in the microcirculation related to arteriolar activation and aggregation of platelets *in vivo*.

Haemorrhagic complications are the cause of death in 2 to 10% of patients with polycythaemia vera; 30 to 40% of patients will experience a haemorrhagic event sometime during the course of their disease. Peptic ulcer disease occurs frequently and contributes to the gastrointestinal tract being the most common source of bleeding. Oesophogeal varices are another common site of bleeding in patients with intra-abdominal thromboses The bleeding diathesis may relate to abnormalities in platelet function, and thus occurs frequently after the ingestion of anti-inflammatory agents. Spontaneous bleeding is rare. Recent data suggests that low-dose aspirin might not increase the frequency of life-threatening haemorrhages.

Generalized pruritus affects 50% of all patients, but its aetiology is unknown. Increased blood and urine histamine levels have been implicated by some. Pruritus triggered by water contact is characteristic, and very poorly tolerated. There is no relationship between the severity of the disease and the intensity of the pruritus. Up to 20% of patients experience persistent pruritus even after normalization of their counts.

The risk of postoperative complications is high in patients with polycythaemia vera. Bleeding, thrombosis, or a combination of both can occur. The risk is higher for those patients who undergo surgery with uncontrolled erythrocytosis. Inadequately controlled disease may be associated with almost 80% risk of complications. The duration of controlled blood counts is also important, the longer this duration is the lesser risks of complications (as low as 5%).

Polycythaemia vera evolves to polcthemia vera-related myelofibosis in up to 50% of the patients 10 to 20 years after the initial diagnosis. It is characterized by increased splenomegaly, tear-drop red cells, a leucoerythroblastic blood picture, marrow fibrosis, and a normal or decreasing red-cell mass. Fatigue, dizziness, weight loss, anorexia, progressive anaemia, and thrombocytopenia associated with bleeding are common. Patients with progressive anaemia should be evaluated for folate and iron deficiency. Occasional patients will respond to iron supplementation with resurgence of erythropoiesis. Severe hyperuricaemia may induce gout or uric acid nephropathy. Polycythemia vera-related myelofibrosis portends a grave prognosis, with over two-thirds of patients dying within 3 years. In the appropriate setting, strong consideration should be given to allogeneic stem cell transplantation, which offers an opportunity for cure.

The evolution to acute leukaemia is probably the natural consequence of the malignant nature of polycythaemia vera, which can be accentuated by therapeutic interventions commonly used for its treatment, such as alkylating agent or radioactive phosphorus. In a recent study, older age, prior exposure to radioactive phosphorus and busulfan but not hydroxyurea therapy was associated with increased risk of leukaemia. Between 30 and 50% of patients who develop leukaemia have previously developed myelofibrosis whereas 50% progress directly from the erythrocytotic phase. A significant number of patients experience a myelodysplastic interval

before transforming to acute leukaemia. The acute leukaemias occurring in such patients are almost always refractory to induction regimens currently used to treat patients with acute myeloid leukaemia.

Laboratory evaluation

Laboratory evaluation of patents with erythrocytosis involves the careful use of a battery of diagnostic tests. The diagnosis of polycythaemia vera has been dramatically simplified with the advent of the molecular tests for the JAK2 V617F mutation. The use of analyses for the JAK2 V617F and JAK2 exon 12 mutations has proven particularly useful in diagnostically challenging cases and in patients with inapparent erythrocytosis and a serious thrombotic event occurring at especially at a younger age. Allele-specific polymerase chain reaction methods can be used to detect JAK2 V617F in at least 95% of patients with polycythemia vera. Those patients who fulfil clinical criteria for polycythemia vera but are JAK2 V617F negative should be evaluated for JAK2 exon 12 mutations. Approximately 10% of such patients who are negative for JAK2 V617F harbour an exon12 JAK2 mutation. Quantitation of the red-cell mass to document absolute erythrocytosis remains a useful diagnostic test in characterizing patients without JAK2 mutations or erythrocytosis. Approximately two-thirds of the patients present with leukocytosis and approximately 50% have thrombocytosis. Red-cell morphology usually reflects an underlying iron-deficiency state present in the great majority of patients: microcytosis, hypochromia, polychromatophilia, poikilocytosis, and anisocytosis are frequently seen. White blood cell morphology is usually normal. Increased numbers of basophils, eosinophils, and immature myeloid cells are observed. Megathrombocytes are often seen in the peripheral blood smear. Platelet counts are usually under 1000×10^9/litre, but higher counts may be seen. The progression to polycythemia vera related myelofibrosis is characterized by the appearance of a leucoeryth roblastic blood picture with the presence in the peripheral blood of tear-drop red cells (dacrocytes), immature myeloid cells, megathrombocytes and nucleated red blood cells. Bleeding time and platelet aggregation studies are frequently, but not always, abnormal. Prolongation of prothrombin and partial thromboplastin times are frequently encountered, usually reflecting a laboratory artefact due to erythrocytosis (the volume of plasma in the collection tube might be too small relative to the amount of anticoagulant (citrate) present in these tubes).

In patients with extreme thrombocytosis, acquired von Willebrand disease occurs, characterized by a significant decrease in large von Willebrand factor multimers due to their adsorption to platelets and megakaryocytes. This acquired defect occurs mainly in patients with very high platelet counts ($>1000 \times 10^9$/litre) and resembles type II von Willebrand disease. The defect is corrected by normalization of the thrombocytosis. Elevations in leucocyte alkaline phosphatase (70%), serum vitamin B_{12} levels (40%), and serum vitamin B_{12} binding proteins (70%) are common, as are hyperuricaemia and increased histamine levels.

Bone marrow examination reveals a hypercellular marrow with an increased number of megakaryocytes. The cellular elements are morphologically normal. Iron stores are usually absent prior to treatment. Reticulin is often seen, but is not predictive of evolution into the myelofibrotic phase. At diagnosis, EPO levels are either reduced or within the lower limits of normal. Low levels persist in two-thirds of patients after normalization of the haematocrit.

Cytogenetic abnormalities have been observed in 25% of patients, but none are characteristic. A recent study using fluorescence *in situ* hybridization (FISH) analyses has shown that abnormalities involving chromosome 9 rearrangements are common, being present in up to 53% of PV patients. A gain in 9p is the most frequent genomic abnormality in polycythemia vera. JAK2 is located on 9p and the duplication of 9p in ploycythemia vera is thought to be the consequence of homologous recombination. Other chromosomal abnormalities involving chromosomes 1, 5, 7, 8, 12, and 13 have been associated with disease progression.

Diagnostic criteria for polycythaemia vera

The diagnosis of polycythaemia vera has been greatly simplified by the recent discovery of the JAK2 V617F mutation. Tests for this molecular defect have now been incorporated as a major criterion for diagnosis of polycythemia vera in the recently revised WHO diagnostic criteria (see Table 22.3.8.1).

Approach to the patient with polycythaemia

It is wise to avoid the temptation of diagnosing polycythaemia on the basis of a single blood count unless extremely high haematocrit levels should be observed. A rational diagnostic approach is required to avoid unnecessary emotional distress to the patient as well as expensive and unnecessary evaluations (Fig. 22.3.8.1).

Dehydration from any cause can produce a spurious elevation in the blood counts. Heavy smokers with mild polycythaemias should be asked to stop smoking and their counts repeated after a few weeks. Once a genuine elevation of haemoglobin or haematocrit has been established, the next step is to decide whether this represents an absolute increase in total red-cell mass, or merely a relative phenomenon. A blood volume study with direct quantitation of both

red-cell mass and plasma volume can be helpful in making this distinction if available. In patients with extreme degrees of erythrocytosis (>60% in men and >55% in women) one can be assured that the red-cell mass is elevated. If absolute polycythaemia is confirmed, it is essential to elucidate whether it is the consequence of a primary myeloproliferative disorder such as polycythaemia vera or a secondary condition.

The determination of EPO levels may be useful in differentiating between polycythaemia vera and secondary polycythaemia. An elevated serum EPO level is indicative of the presence of a secondary polycythaemia and a low level supports the diagnosis of polycythaemia vera, but a normal EPO value does not exclude hypoxia-induced causes of erythrocytosis or the autonomous production of EPO leading to erythrocytosis Normal values may also be encountered in some cases of polycythaemia vera.

The presence of leucocytosis, thrombocytosis, or splenomegaly is suggestive of polycythaemia vera as the cause for the elevated red-cell mass. Arterial blood gases and the direct determination of oxygen saturation in arterial blood, if decreased, may aid in the recognition of a chronic pulmonary or congenital cardiovascular abnormality. If blood oxygen saturation is normal, the quantification of haemoglobin's oxygen affinity ($P_{50}O_2$) may indicate the presence of high-affinity haemoglobin variant. Otherwise, causes for a physiologically inappropriate polycythaemia should be sought.

Molecular methods to detect JAK2 V617F and exon 12 JAK2 mutations provide new diagnostic tools for the evaluation of patients suspected of having polycythaemia vera.If one does not have access to blood volume studies, a JAK2 mutant analysis provides a direct means of identifying the overwhelming number of patients with polycythemia vera. There is a small but definite group of patients in whom a specific cause for polycythaemia remains elusive, despite appropriate diagnostic testing. Examining close

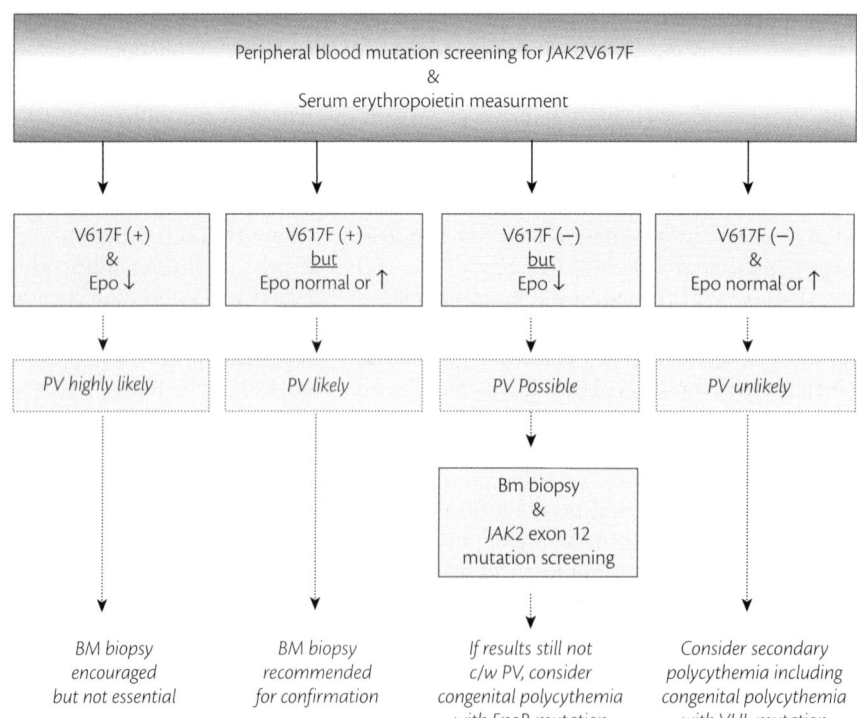

Fig. 22.3.8.1 Diagnostic algorithm for patients with polycythemia. (From Tefferi A, Vardiman JW (20078). Classification and diagnosis of myeloproliferative neoplasms: the 2008 World Heath Organization criteria and point-of-care diagnostic algorithms. *Leukemia*, **22**, 14–22, with permission.).

relatives might disclose the presence of a familial form of poly-cythaemia, a rare condition caused by an abnormality in EPO receptor or defects in hypoxia sensing (Chuvash polycythemia). Regular, continued surveillance is recommended for all noncate-gorized patients, as some of them develop polycythaemia vera in the future.

Management of polycythaemia

The two main goals in the management of patients with poly-cythaemia vera involve the confirmation of the diagnosis and reduction of the red-cell mass. The untoward effects of an increased red-cell mass on tissue blood flow occur independently from the specific cause of the polycythaemia. It is thus reasonable to rec-ommend that all patients with uncorrectable erythrocytosis be offered phlebotomy.

The main therapeutic goals are the maintenance of well-being and the prevention of complications for as long as possible. Several therapeutic strategies have resulted in dramatic increases in the sur-vival of patients. Historical evidence suggests a median survival of approximately 18 months in untreated patients with polycythae-mia vera, whereas with appropriate management survival of over 10 years is now common. The main therapeutic objective is the reduction of the haematocrit to a normal level. This is usually accomplished by the implementation of repeated phlebotomies. Every possible effort should be made to discourage patients with polycythaemia vera from smoking. A regimen of phlebotomies should be prescribed as soon as the diagnosis has been clearly established. It is often feasible to remove between 350 and 500 ml of blood every other day until the desired haematocrit level is attained. Haematocrit levels of less than 45% in men and 42% in women are desirable, although the optimal target haematocrit level remains unknown. The removal of smaller aliquots might be necessary in older patients.

Once the target haematocrit level is achieved, a maintenance regimen should be instituted. Venesection is preferred in those younger individuals without critical elevations in their platelet counts. Myelosuppressive therapy should be considered in eld-erly patients who are intolerant of phlebotomies, and in younger individuals with repeated thrombotic episodes and extremely high platelet counts. There is controversy regarding what represents the optimal myelosuppressive agent. A major concern has been the growing evidence that supports the association between exposure to some of these agents and the development of leukaemia.

Hydroxycarbamide (hydroxyurea) is useful for the management of patients with polycythaemia vera and represents the first-line therapy in especially older patients in which phlebotomy alone is insufficient or intolerable, due to its minimal leukaemogenic potential. It should, however, be used with great caution in patients formerly treated with radioactive phosphorus or alkylating agents as the risk of leukaemia is higher.

Low-dose aspirin (81–100 mg/day) administered to polycythaemia vera patients has been shown to decrease the risk of arterial and venous events. Although there is no overall survival benefit, no significant increased risk of bleeding was reported.

In younger patients, given their potential long-term survival, strong consideration should be given to the use of phlebotomy therapy in combination with low-dose aspirin, as well as with other apparently nonleukaemogenic interventions such as interferon-α

and anagrelide. In two recent studies, one in polycythaemia vera patients and another in essential thrombocythaemia patients, hydroxyurea has been shown to be nonleukaemogenic, and can be use as alternative to phlebotomy or in combination with it. Interferon-α2a and pegylated forms of interferon have been shown to be effective in controlling the blood counts and symptoms (especially pruritus). The use of pegylated forms of interferon has been reported to be associated with a reduction of the percentage of cells bearing the JAK2 V617F mutation, suggesting its activity at the level of an early haematopoietic stem cell/progenitor cell. In patients with a history of thrombosis where uncontrolled thrombo-cytosis is a problem, anagrelide, an inhibitor of megakaryocytic mat-uration, has proven effective. Refractory pruritus can be managed in the majority of cases, in addition to interferon, with cyproheptadine or selective serotonin reuptake inhibitors.

At present, radioactive phosphorus should be used only patients who are incapable of complying with the other forms of therapy or are unwilling or unable to return for follow-up.

Elective surgery should only be undertaken after adequate and sustained control of the blood counts has been achieved. When emergency surgery is required the patient should be phlebot-omized rapidly until a normal haematocrit is achieved, and plate-lets should be available in case excessive operative bleeding occurs. Patients should be mobilized promptly, and the use of prophylac-tic doses of low molecular weight heparin should be considered unless contraindicated. Dental extractions are associated with an increased bleeding risk and should only be pursued in patients with good haematological control. A particularly high-risk intervention is splenectomy, which has an operative mortality rate of approxi-mately 9%. The haematocrit should be normalized and platelet count maintained below 400×10^9/litre before splenctomy. After splenectomy there is a particular risk of extreme thrombocytosis. Although no prospective studies have been done, prophylactic low-molecular-weight heparin is probably warranted in all patients undergoing splenctomy during the perioperative period. Because of the high probability of expanding extramedullary hematopoiesis with rapid development of liver enlargement after splenectomy, patients should receive hydroxyurea therapy postoperatively.

In patients with polycythaemia-related myelofibrosis, the management is quite similar to that for primary myelofibrosis. Allogeneic stem cell transplantation is now a curative option for patients with myelofibrosis, both primary and secondary to other myeloproliferative neoplasms, and should be considered in appro-priately selected patients.

Pregnant patients with polycythaemia vera experience an increased incidence of fetal loss, with 30% of pregnancies culminat-ing in spontaneous abortions. Unexpectedly, pregnancy in patients with polycythaemia vera is frequently associated with a gradual normalization of blood values, and it is not unusual for a woman who has required extensive therapy for control of her disease to no longer require phlebotomies during pregnancy. Delivery appears not to be complicated by excessive haemorrhage or by an increased risk of venous thrombosis. Treatment with low-dose aspirin should be continued and, if needed, phlebotomy (to maintain a haematocrit <45%) or interferon therapy (for a platelet count >1000–1500 × 10^9/litre) should be used as cytoreductive methods of therapy.

Innovative therapies based on JAK2 inhibition are in develop-ment and this approach might change the way we currently treat polycythaemia vera dramatically.

Prognosis

The outcome of patients with secondary polycythaemia is usually related to the prognosis of the underlying disorder. In polycythaemia vera, the nature and severity of the complications during the clinical course of the disease are the most important determinants of outcome. Disease duration is also important, as long-term survival is strongly associated with progression to myelofibrosis or acute leukaemia. As previously emphasized, prompt and appropriate therapy results in dramatic improvements in survival. Young patients should be initially managed with phlebotomy and low doses of aspirin. Supplemental therapy with interferon, anagrelide, or hydroxyurea might be required in patients with serious haemorrhagic or thrombotic episodes. The use of either hydroxyurea or radioactive phosphorus appears warranted in the treatment of elderly patients who, because of their age, have a limited survival.

Further reading

Falanga A, *et al.* (2005). Pathogenesis of thrombosis in essential thrombocythemia and polycythemia vera: the role of neutrophils. *Semin Hematol*, **42**, 239–47.

Finazzi G, Barbui T (2007). How do I treat patients with polycythemia vera. *Blood*, **109**, 5104–11.

Hoffman R, *et al.* (2005). The polycythemias. In: Hoffman R, *et al.* (eds) *Hematology: basic principles and practice*, pp 1209–1245. Churchill Livingstone, Philadelphia.

Hoffman R, *et al.* (2007). Philadelphia chromosome-negative myeloproliferative disorsers: biology and treatment. *Biol Blood Marrow Transplant*, **13** (suppl 1), 64–72.

James C *et al.* (2005). A unique clonal JAK2 mutation leading to constitutive signalling causes polycythemia vera. *Nature*, **434**, 1144–8.

James C, *et al.* (2005). A JAK2 mutation in myeloproliferative disorders: pathogenesis and therapeutic and scientific prospects. *Trends Mol Med*, **11**, 546–54.

Landolfi R, *et al.* (2004). Efficacy and safety of low-dose aspirin in polycythemia vera. *N Engl J Med*, **350**, 114–24.

Levine RL, *et al.* (2007). Role of JAK2 in the pathogenesis and treatment of myeloproliferative disorders. *Nat Rev Cancer*, **7**, 673–83.

Papayannopoulou T, *et al.* (2005). Biology of erythropoiesis, erythroid differentiation, and maturation. In: Hoffman R, *et al.* (eds) *Hematology: basic principles and practice*, pp 267–288. Churchill Livingstone, Philadelphia.

Prchal JT (2005). Polycythemia vera and other primary polycythemias. *Curr Opin Hematol*, **12**, 112–16.

Scott LM, *et al.* (2007). JAK2 exon 12 mutations in polycythemia vera and idiopathic erythrocytosis. *N Engl J Med*, **356**, 459–68.

Silver RT (2006). Treatment of polycythemia vera. *Semin Thromb Hemost*, **32**, 437–42.

Skoda R, Prchal JT (2005). Lessons from familial myeloproliferative disorders. *Semin Hematol*, **42**, 266–73.

Tefferi A, Spivak JL. Polycythemia vera: scientific advances and current practice. *Semin Hematol*, **42**, 206–20.

Tefferi A, Vardiman JW (2008). Classification and diagnosis of myeloproliferative neoplasms: The 2008 World Health Organization criteria and point-of-care diagnostic algorithms. *Leukemia*, **22**, 14–22.

Tefferi A, *et al.* (2007). Proposals and rationale for revision of the World Health Organization diagnostic criteria for polycythemia vera, essential thrombocythemia, and primary myelofibrosis: recommendations from an ad hoc international expert panel. *Blood*, **110**, 1092–7.

Villeval JL, *et al.* (2006). New insights into the pathogenesis of JAK2 V617F-positive myeloproliferative disorders and consequences for the management of patients. *Semin Thromb Hemost*, **32**, 341–51.

Zhao ZJ, *et al.* (2005). Role of tyrosine kinases and phosphatases in polycythemia vera. *Semin Hematol*, **42**, 221–9.

22.3.9 Idiopathic myelofibrosis

Jerry L. Spivak

Essentials

Myelofibrosis is a reactive process common to many malignant and benign disorders. Idiopathic myelofibrosis is a chronic myeloproliferative disorder of unknown aetiology that involves a multipotent haemopoietic progenitor cell and results in abnormalities in red cell, white cell, and platelet production in association with marrow fibrosis and extramedullary haemopoiesis.

Aetiology

This is unknown. Many chromosomal abnormalities have been found, and in about 50% of cases there is expression of the JAK2 V617F missense mutation typical of polycythaemia vera (see Chapter 22.3.8), but the mutation is not specific for idiopathic myelofibrosis.

Clinical features and prognosis

Many patients are asymptomatic at the time of diagnosis, but common presenting manifestations include fatigue, weight loss, night sweats, fever, dyspnoea, and abdominal discomfort due to splenomegaly (which may be massive). The major complications are the consequences of bone marrow failure and extramedullary haemopoiesis, which most commonly occurs in the spleen and liver, but can occur at any site and compromise organ or tissue function. About 20% of patients develop acute leukaemia as a terminal event.

Investigation and diagnosis

Anaemia is the most consistent abnormality, with the blood film showing evidence of a leucoerythroblastic reaction (presence of metamyelocytes, myelocytes, promyelocytes, myeloblasts, nucleated red cells, and tear drop-shaped red cells) due to extramedullary haemopoiesis. The presence of marrow fibrosis is essential for diagnosis and usually results in the inability to aspirate marrow from a properly placed needle ('dry tap').

Treatment

There is no specific treatment. Aside from supportive care, oral administration of folic acid and a trial of oral pyridoxine are reasonable, and hyperuricaemia should be treated with allopurinol. The few patients under 45 years of age who have a matched, related donor should be considered for allogeneic bone marrow transplantation, in the absence of which a variety of other treatments (e.g. thalidomide and prednisolone) have been tried, often more in hope than expectation of benefit. Splenomegaly is the most distressing complication: reduction in splenic size can be achieved with interferon, thalidomide, alkylating agents, hydroxycarbamide, splenectomy, or splenic irradiation. JAK2 inhibitors, currently in clinical trials, have proved effective in reducing splenomegaly and constitutional symptoms.

Introduction

Idiopathic myelofibrosis (also called primary myelofibrosis, myelofibrosis with myeloid metaplasia, agnogenic myeloid metaplasia, or primary myelosclerosis) is a chronic myeloproliferative disorder of unknown aetiology, involving a multipotent haemopoietic progenitor cell that results in abnormalities in red cell, white cell, and platelet production in association with marrow fibrosis and extramedullary haemopoiesis. Although myelofibrosis in association with leucoerythroblastosis and splenomegaly are the clinical hallmarks of idiopathic myelofibrosis, these abnormalities can also be seen in other chronic myeloproliferative disorders such as polycythaemia vera and chronic myelogenous leukaemia, as well as in a variety of benign and malignant disorders that involve the bone marrow (Box 22.3.9.1). Since there is no specific clonal marker for

---

Box 22.3.9.1 Causes of marrow fibrosis

- ◆ Malignant
  - Acute lymphocytic leukaemia
  - Acute myelogenous leukaemia
  - Acute megakaryocytic leukaemia
  - Chronic myelogenous leukaemia
  - Hairy-cell leukaemia
  - Hodgkin's disease
  - Idiopathic myelofibrosis
  - Lymphoma
  - Multiple myeloma
  - Metastatic carcinoma
  - Polycythaemia vera
  - Systemic mastocytosis
- ◆ Nonmalignant
  - HIV infection
  - Hyperparathyroidism
  - Renal osteodystrophy
  - Systemic lupus erythematosus
  - Thorium dioxide exposure
  - Tuberculosis
  - Vitamin D deficiency

---

idiopathic myelofibrosis, and since many of the disorders listed in Box 22.3.9.1 are responsive to specific therapies not effective in idiopathic myelofibrosis, the diagnosis of this disorder is one of exclusion.

Aetiology

The aetiology of idiopathic myelofibrosis is unknown. Analysis of glucose-6-phosphate dehydrogenase (G6DP) isoenzyme expression, X-linked gene inactivation patterns in informative women, and a mutation in the *N-ras* proto-oncogene mutation have established that idiopathic myelofibrosis is a clonal disorder with origin in a multipotent haemopoietic progenitor cell. In some patients, T lymphocytes express the same clonal marker as B lymphocytes and myeloid cells, indicating involvement at the level of the pluripotent stem cell. Nonrandom chromosome abnormalities primarily involving chromosomes 13 (del .13q), 20 (del .20q), 8 (trisomy 8), 1, 7, and 9 are found in approximately 50% of patients using conventional cytogenetics. With comparative genomic hybridization, additional abnormalities have been identified; most commonly gains on 9p and losses on 17q. No abnormalities of the known tumour suppressor genes associated with these chromosomes have yet been identified, but recently a mutation in the gene for the tyrosine kinase JAK2 (V617F), which is located on 9p, and several mutations in the thrombopoietin receptor gene, *MPL* (W515K/L), located on 1p, have been identified in approximately 50% and 5% of idiopathic myelofibrosis patients respectively, and rarely both mutations have been observed in the same patient. JAK2 V617F is also present in over 90% of polycythemia vera patients and 50% of essential thrombocytosis patients, but the role of this mutation and those involving MPL in the pathogenesis of idiopathic myelofibrosis or the other chronic myeloproliferative disorders has not been established.

Marrow fibroblasts in idiopathic myelofibrosis, in contrast to the hematopoietic stem cells, are polyclonal, suggesting that the marrow fibrosis is a reactive process initiated by expansion of the malignant clone. Marrow collagen is argyrophilic, so that changes in its distribution and content can be analysed histochemically by silver staining. Under normal circumstances, the connective tissue stroma of the bone marrow is composed of collagen types I, III, IV, and V together with noncollagen proteins such as fibronectin, laminin, vitronectin, and the proteoglycans. Collagen types I, III, and V form a delicate and usually noncontinuous supporting network for haemopoietic cells, while type IV collagen, laminin, and fibronectin are localized in the basement membranes of arteries in a continuous fashion and along marrow sinusoids in a discontinuous fashion. With increasing marrow cellularity, the collagenous supporting network also increases. With myelofibrosis, however, there is both an increase in the collagen network and a change in its physical characteristics. Condensation of the interstitial fibres results in the formation of thick, continuous and often wavy bundles in association with an increase in reticular or fibroblastic cells. Sinusoidal basement membrane collagen becomes continuous, leading to sinusoidal dilatation and obliteration with an associated capillary neovascularization. The content of basement membrane fibronectin as well as stromal fibronectin and vitronectin also increases. Although best studied in idiopathic myelofibrosis, the types of collagen involved in marrow fibrosis in this condition do not appear to differ from those involved in the marrow fibrosis associated with the other disorders listed in Box 22.3.9.1.

The commonality of the types of collagen involved and the similarity of the histological process, regardless of disease association, implies that marrow fibrosis *per se* represents a final common pathway involved in the response to diverse immunological, metabolic, toxic, or infectious stimuli (Box 22.3.9.1). Megakaryocytic hyperplasia, dysplasia, and clustering are characteristic features of idiopathic myelofibrosis. These cells produce cytokines such as platelet-derived growth factor (PDGF) and transforming growth factors (TGFβ) that promote fibroblast proliferation, and platelet factor 4 (PF4), which, like TGFβ, inhibits collagenase. These findings suggest that inappropriate release of these fibrogenic proteins by dysfunctional megakaryocytes is the stimulus for myelofibrosis. In support of this contention, increased concentrations of PDGF and TGFβ as well as basic fibroblast growth factor have been observed in the platelets and megakaryocytes from idiopathic myelofibrosis patients. Circulating levels of TGFβ are also increased in idiopathic myelofibrosis, as is the urinary excretion of basic fibroblast growth factor and calmodulin, another potential fibroblast stimulant present in platelets. Finally, TGFβ promotes the synthesis of osteoprotegerin, which impairs osteoclast proliferation and promotes osteosclerosis. The observation that thrombopoietin overexpression in mice recapitulates the histological features of idiopathic myelofibrosis supports the contention that megakaryocytes are integrally involved in the development of marrow fibrosis in idiopathic myelofibrosis, as does the development of marrow fibrosis in the grey platelet syndrome, in which impaired megakaryocyte α granule synthesis results in release of cytokines and growth factors into the marrow extracellular matrix.

Additional distinct histologic abnormalities in idiopathic myelofibrosis include increased marrow angiogenesis due to an increase in vascular endothelial growth factor (VEGF) production, marrow sinusoidal dilatation, and intravascular haemopoiesis with an increase in circulating CD34+ cells. Increased angiogenesis appears to be an early feature of the disease and correlates better with increased marrow cellularity than with marrow fibrosis. The increase in circulating CD34+ cells appears to be a consequence of elevations in neutrophil elastase and matrix metalloproteinases with cleavage of the endothelial cell adhesion molecule VCAM-1 and down regulation of the chemokine receptor CXCR4 on the CD34+ cells.

Clinical features

Although considered to be an uncommon disorder with an incidence of approximately 1/100 000 person-years, clinical studies of more than 1000 patients have been reported over the last 50 years. In contrast to the other chronic myeloproliferative disorders, the median age at diagnosis of myelofibrosis, 61 years (range 15–94), is much older. No gender differences exist and familial clustering is sufficiently unusual that another myeloproliferative disorder such as polycythaemia vera should be considered when this occurs. The presenting manifestations depend on the stage of the illness but are often bland. Many patients are asymptomatic at the time of discovery. Fatigue is the commonest presenting complaint, followed by weight loss, night sweats, fever, dyspnoea, and abdominal discomfort due to splenomegaly. Hearing loss due to otosclerosis is

an interesting but often nonelicited symptom. Easy bruising or bleeding and acute gout or renal stones are other presenting manifestations that are reasonably common and directly related to the underlying disease process. Rarely, periostitis may occur. In 10 to 15% of patients, isolated thrombocytosis is the presenting manifestation in the absence of marrow fibrosis or splenomegaly and such patients may or may not produce JAK2 V617F.

Splenomegaly is present in virtually every patient with idiopathic myelofibrosis at diagnosis. When it is absent, one should consider other causes for the clinical abnormalities. The degree of splenomegaly varies but is frequently substantial. Moreover, since the rate of splenic enlargement is variable, spleen size cannot be used as an indication of disease duration. Hepatomegaly, invariably of a lesser extent than the splenomegaly, is present initially in approximately 50% of patients and is usually proportional to the degree of splenomegaly. Lymphadenopathy is uncommon. With substantial splenomegaly, wasting may be prominent.

Laboratory studies

Because of its origin in a multipotent haemopoietic progenitor cell, idiopathic myelofibrosis affects all blood cell types but not in a predictable manner. Anaemia, usually mild, is the most consistent abnormality. Indeed, a normal haemoglobin or haematocrit in the presence of substantial splenomegaly should lead to immediate consideration of polycythaemia vera, since the expanded plasma volume associated with splenomegaly can mask a substantial increase in the red-cell mass. The leucocyte and platelet counts can be low, normal, or high without reference to spleen size. Inevitably, due to extramedullary haemopoiesis, metamyelocytes, myelocytes, promyelocytes, myeloblasts, and nucleated red cells will be present in the circulation together with the tear drop-shaped red cells characteristic of this situation (Fig. 22.3.9.1). Although this so-called leucoerythroblastic reaction is not specific for idiopathic myelofibrosis, its absence should challenge the clinical impression.

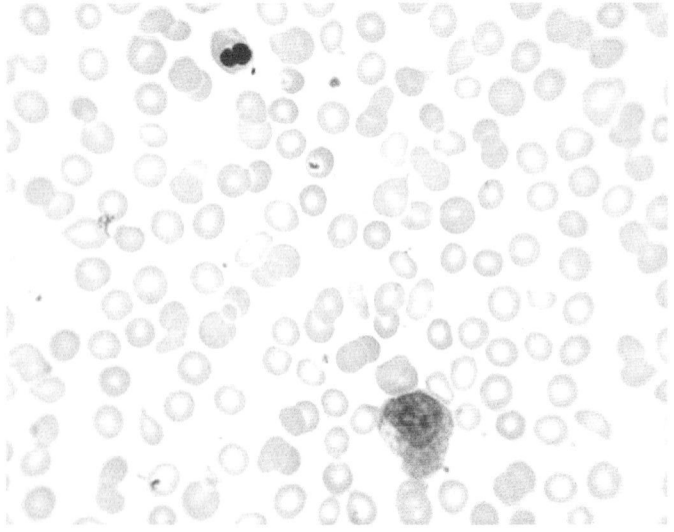

Fig. 22.3.9.1 Peripheral smear showing tear drop cells with leuko erythroblastic picture.
Copyright ©2009 American Society of Hematology.

Abnormalities in liver function tests are not uncommon but are usually mild and most often involve a reduction in serum albumin and an elevation of liver alkaline phosphatase, an abnormality that is magnified by splenectomy. The lactate dehydrogenase (LDH) level is usually mildly increased and correlates best with the leucocyte count. Hyperuricaemia is not infrequent. The leucocyte alkaline phosphatase concentration can be low, normal, or high and cannot be recommended as a diagnostic test. As mentioned, the JAK2 V617F mutation and much less commonly, MPL mutations, are present in some patients but their absence does not exclude the diagnosis. Cytogenetic abnormalities include 13q-, 20q-, trisomy 9, trisomy 8, 12p-, and abnormalities of chromosomes 1 and 7. An increase in circulating CD34+ cells is also characteristic but none of these abnormalities is diagnostic for idiopathic myelofibrosis or present in a majority of patients.

Perhaps the most intriguing laboratory abnormalities in idiopathic myelofibrosis are those linked to autoreactivity, such as circulating immune complexes, complement activation, elevations in antinuclear antibody (ANA) and rheumatoid factor titres, and a positive Coombs' test in the absence of an overt connective tissue disorder. Although marrow fibrosis has been documented in patients with systemic lupus erythematosus, the linkage between autoimmune abnormalities and marrow fibrosis is unclear. It does, however, provide another therapeutic option as discussed below.

The presence of marrow fibrosis is essential for a diagnosis of idiopathic myelofibrosis and usually results in a 'dry tap' or the inability to aspirate marrow from a properly placed needle. A prefibrotic phase of idiopathic myelofibrosis has been described retrospectively. However, given the similarity of the histopathology of polycythaemia vera, essential thrombocytosis, and prefibrotic idiopathic myelofibrosis, prospective substantiation of the latter is not possible in the absence of a specific clonal marker for the disease. Even the presence of myelofibrosis, although mandatory, is not in itself sufficient for diagnosis. This is because polycythaemia vera and chronic myelogenous leukaemia and other disorders such as hairy-cell leukaemia, myelodysplasia, and acute leukaemia can present with myelofibrosis. Thus, it is essential to employ the appropriate diagnostic tests (cytogenetics, *BCR-ABL1* FISH, flow cytometry, and immunohistochemistry) to exclude these and the other disorders listed in Table 22.3.9.1 that can cause myelofibrosis.

Marrow cellularity in idiopathic myelofibrosis may be increased with trilineage hyperplasia and erythroblastic and megakaryocytic islands, decreased with scattered areas of hyperplastic marrow embedded in a collagenous matrix, or hypoplastic with intense osteomyelosclerosis and residual megakaryocytic islands (Fig. 22.3.9.2). While there is a correlation between the degree of fibrosis and osteosclerosis, there is no correlation between bone marrow histology and disease duration, platelet count, or splenomegaly; marrow fibrosis does, however, appear to correlate with the leucocyte count. In general, marrow fibrosis and extramedullary haemopoiesis with myeloid metaplasia appear unrelated, and the latter abnormalities cannot be considered as compensation for the former. Increased marrow angiogenesis is a recently recognized feature of idiopathic myelofibrosis that correlates with increased cellularity and extramedullary haematopoiesis independently of the marrow fibrosis.

Table 22.3.9.1 Two scoring systems for predicting survival in patients with idiopathic myelofibrosis

(a) Prognostic factors:

HgB	<10 g/dl
WBC	<4 or >30 × 10^6/ml

Number of prognostic factors	Risk group	Median survival (months)
0	Low	93
1–2	High	17

(b) Prognostic factors:

HgB	<10 g/dl
Constitutional symptoms	
Blast cells	>1%

Number of prognostic factors	Risk group	Median survival (months)
0–1	Low	99
2–3	High	21

(a) from Dupriez B, *et al.* (1996). Prognostic factors in agnogenic myeloid metaplasia: a report on 195 cases with a new scoring system. *Blood*, **88**, 1013–18, with permission; (b) from Cervantes F, *et al.* (1997). Identification of 'short-lived' and 'long-lived' patients at presentation of idiopathic myelofibrosis. *Br J Haematol*, **97**, 635–40, with permission.

In conjunction with the most severe degree of marrow fibrosis, osteosclerosis develops, with characteristic radiographic abnormalities. These primarily involve the axial skeleton but can include the skull, with thickening of the bony trabeculae and patchy or coalescent sclerosis. With obliteration of the axial marrow cavities, extension of the marrow into the long bones occurs. Interestingly, the increase in trabecular bone in idiopathic myelofibrosis is not accompanied by an increase in either osteoblastic or osteoclastic activity. This feature distinguishes the osteosclerosis of idiopathic myelofibrosis from that associated with metabolic causes of osteosclerosis.

Course and prognosis

Idiopathic myelofibrosis is a chronic progressive disorder with a median lifespan (5.5 years) that is much shorter than for polycythaemia vera and essential thrombocytosis. However, the heterogeneity characterizing the initial clinical presentation is also evident with respect to survival, which can range from less than a year to more than 30 years. Death is usually a consequence of bone marrow failure (haemorrhage, anaemia, or infection), transformation to acute leukaemia, portal hypertension, heart failure, cachexia, or myeloid metaplasia with organ failure. Retrospective analysis of the adverse prognostic value of presenting manifestations has identified a number of factors that may be useful for both prognostic and therapeutic purposes. These include age at onset (>64 years), anaemia (haemoglobin <10 g/dl), constitutional symptoms, white cell count abnormalities (<4000/µl or >12 000/µl), thrombocytopenia, circulating blast cells (>1%), and certain cytogenetic abnormalities (trisomy 8, 12p–). A number of scoring systems have been devised for identifying long- and short-term survivors based on the

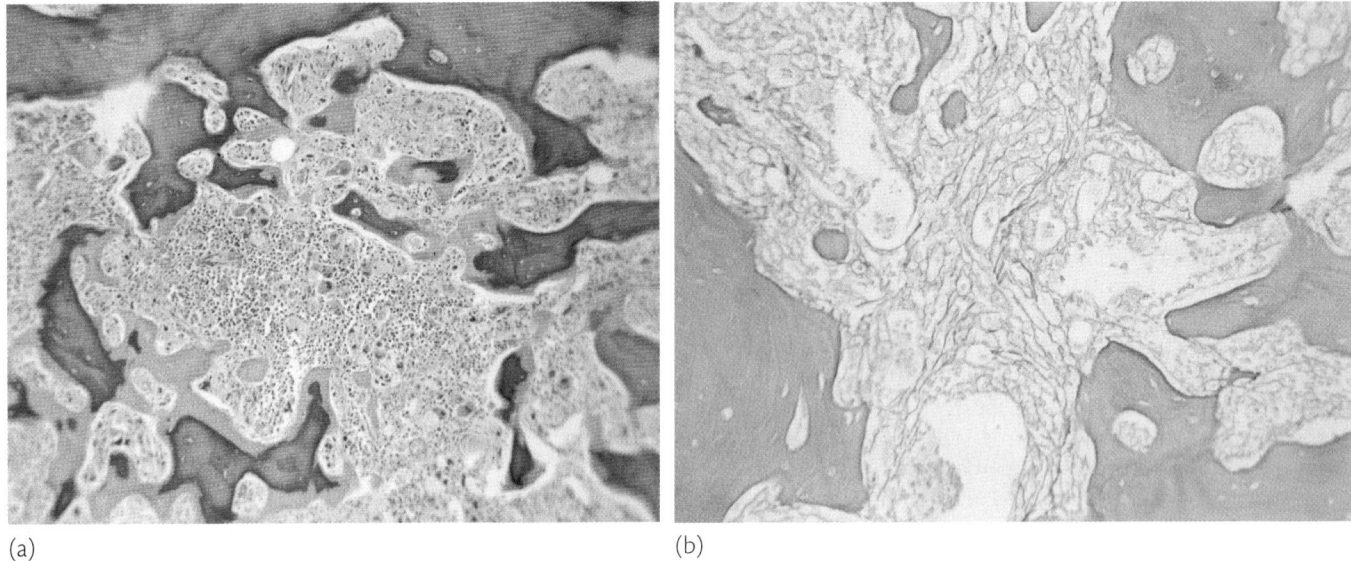

(a)   (b)

Fig. 22.3.9.2   (a) Bone marrow biopsy: showing thick irregular bone trabeculae with new bone formation, hypercellular marrow with increased megakaryocytes.
(b) Bone marrow trephine biopsy: showing thick coarse reticulin fibres (Grade 4 fibrosis).
Copyright ©2009 American Society of Hematology.

presence of more than one adverse presenting manifestation. Two such scoring systems that are useful in separating patients of any age with myelofibrosis into low- and high-risk groups with respect to survival are shown in Table 22.3.9.1, but these should also be coupled with cytogenetic abnormalities for a more complete perspective. More complex scoring systems have been proposed but whether they are more useful has not yet been established.

Complications

The major complications of idiopathic myelofibrosis are the consequences of bone marrow failure and extramedullary haemopoiesis. Anaemia may be the result of ineffective erythropoiesis, but haemodilution due to an expanded plasma volume associated with splenomegaly, iron deficiency due to gastrointestinal blood loss, folic acid deficiency due to the increased demands of haemopoiesis, haemolysis due to autoimmune phenomena or hypersplenism, and, rarely, pyridoxine deficiency are also considerations. In some patients, erythropoietin production may be inappropriately low for the degree of anaemia but in this instance haemodilution also needs to be excluded. Red cell survival and splenic sequestration studies can be useful in determining the splenic contribution to anaemia.

Hyperuricaemia is a consequence of increased cell turnover and can provoke acute gout or renal stone formation if left untreated. Splenic enlargement is inevitable and can lead to splenic infarction, malnutrition due to easy satiety, plasma volume expansion, hypersplenism, portal hypertension, splanchnic vein thrombosis, extreme discomfort due to its mass, and eventually cachexia (Fig. 22.3.9.3). Hepatomegaly is associated with splenomegaly. Impaired hepatic function is usually a consequence of extramedullary haemopoiesis, which can lead to hepatic fibrosis and portal hypertension.

Although myeloid metaplasia due to exuberant extramedullary haemopoiesis is most common in the spleen and liver, it can occur at any site and compromise organ or tissue function. For example, peritoneal involvement can lead to ascites; epidural involvement to

spinal cord compression; retroperitoneal involvement to obstructive uropathy or portal hypertension; and pulmonary extramedullary haemopoiesis to pulmonary hypertension. The reason why myeloid metaplasia is more aggressive in some patients than in others is unclear.

Approximately 20% of patients with idiopathic myelofibrosis develop acute leukaemia as a terminal event. Although some clinicians do not distinguish acute leukaemia presenting with myelofibrosis (malignant myelosclerosis) from idiopathic myelofibrosis, they are clinically distinct entities. The extent to which therapeutic intervention with mutagenic drugs such as hydroxycarbamide (hydroxyurea), alkylating agents, or irradiation predisposes patients with idiopathic myelofibrosis to progress to acute leukaemia (as it does in patients with polycythaemia vera or essential thrombocytosis) is unknown. Again for unknown reasons, splenectomy also appears to be a predisposing factor for the development of acute leukaemia.

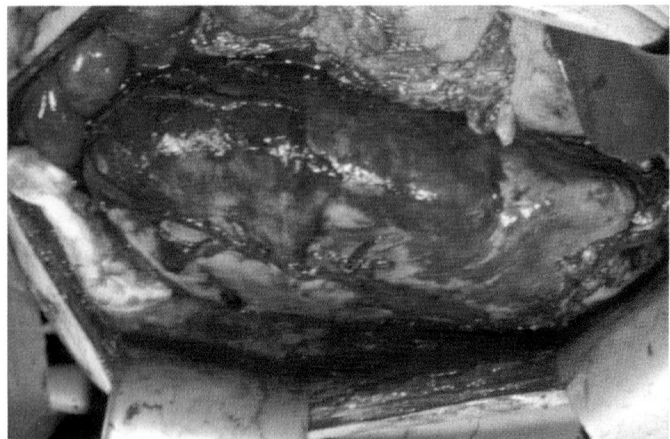

Fig. 22.3.9.3   Patient with AMM and massive splenomegaly who underwent splenectomy.
Copyright ©2002 American Society of Hematology.

Platelet dysfunction is a common feature of the chronic myelo-proliferative disorders and can lead to spontaneous haemorrhage as well as increased bleeding during surgical procedures. Although abnormalities in platelet morphology, prolongation of the bleeding time, and abnormal platelet aggregation are frequently observed in patients with idiopathic myelofibrosis, no consistent biochemical abnormality has been identified and no platelet function test is predictive for the risk of haemorrhage.

Therapy

There is no specific therapy for idiopathic myelofibrosis. Treatment should be individualized, based on the patient's risk group and age. Asymptomatic, low-risk patients without hyperuricaemia or a remedial cause of anaemia require no therapy, although the oral administration of folic acid (1 mg/day) and a trial of oral pyridoxine (250mg/day for 3 months) appears reasonable. Anaemia associated with an inappropriately low endogenous erythropoietin level (<100 mU/ml) may respond to recombinant erythropoietin therapy, but the hormone can cause an increase in splenomegaly or hepatomegaly. Patients most likely to respond are those with a low transfusion requirement. Hyperuricaemia should be treated with allopurinol. Asymptomatic leucocytosis or thrombocytosis requires no therapy. Patients less than 45years of age who have a matched, related donor should be considered for allogeneic bone marrow transplantation. Unfortunately, the best results have been obtained in patients with good prognosis disease and the transplantation-related mortality was as high as 32% with a 5-year survival of 60%. Recently, reduced-intensity conditioning was found to decrease transplant-related mortality and achieve remission rates of more than 70%. However, prospective studies will be required to establish the most effective conditioning regimen, the optimal timing for transplantation and which patients will benefit most from this procedure.

In the absence of a suitable donor, a variety of therapies can be considered, none of which is uniformly effective or without side effects. Danazol has been employed to treat anaemia but it is unclear whether its apparent effect is a consequence of plasma volume shrinkage as opposed to an actual increment in the red-cell mass. Thalidomide at low doses (50–100 mg/day) in combination with prednisone has proved to be effective in ameliorating anaemia as well as thrombocytopenia in approximately 60% of idiopathic myelofibrosis patients, and reducing spleen size in approximately 20%. Lenalidomide has not proved to be more effective than thalidomide in small phase II trials. Recombinant interferon-α has had a low rate of success in idiopathic myelofibrosis, in part due to poor toleration in elderly patients, and therapy can also be limited by its induction of leucopenia or thrombocytopenia. Nevertheless, given the lack of available remedies in this disease, it is worth considering to reduce splenomegaly.

Chemotherapeutic agents or irradiation therapy should be used judiciously in the treatment of idiopathic myelofibrosis. Hydroxycarbamide, while easy to use and with a low incidence of acute toxicity, can cause marrow depression and is potentially leukaemogenic. Low-dose alkylating agent therapy has been demonstrated to reduce organomegaly, reverse marrow fibrosis, and improve blood counts in idiopathic myelofibrosis, occasionally in a durable fashion. However, alkylating agents can cause severe bone marrow depression and are leukaemogenic.

Splenomegaly is the most distressing complication of idiopathic myelofibrosis, leading to mechanical discomfort, inanition, splenic infarction, portal and pulmonary hypertension, and blood cell sequestration. Reduction in splenic size can be achieved with interferon, thalidomide, alkylating agents, hydroxycarbamide, splenectomy, or splenic irradiation. Thalidomide is the initial treatment of choice, followed by interferon and then chemotherapy with either hydroxycarbamide or low-dose busulfan. Splenic irradiation can be effective at alleviating splenic pain and temporarily reducing spleen size. However, its use should be restricted to inoperable patients since there is an unpredictable risk of severe cytopenias as well as an increased risk of haemorrhage, if irradiation precedes splenectomy. Local irradiation is, of course, appropriate for the management of symptomatic extramedullary haemopoiesis in tissues and organs other than the spleen.

Splenectomy in idiopathic myelofibrosis is a prodigious procedure, given the large size of the spleen and its vessels, the inevitable presence of adhesions, the haemorrhagic tendency of idiopathic myelofibrosis patients, and their often poor nutritional status. Evaluation for portal hypertension should precede surgery and, if necessary, parental hyperalimentation should be employed to avoid postoperative complications. ε-Aminocaproic acid can be used if bleeding is a problem.

Leucocytosis, thrombocytosis, and postoperative hepatic enlargement are the usual consequences of splenectomy, as is elevation of liver alkaline phosphatase. Postoperative splenic and portal vein thrombosis occur in approximately 10% of patients, most often in the first few weeks after surgery and presumably due to the size of the splenic vein remnant. However, there is no correlation between splenic or portal vein thrombosis and the platelet count. Surveillance by ultrasonography or CT may useful in identifying this complication with the intent of administering anticoagulants or thrombolytic agents. Although most patients tolerate splenectomy well, for unknown reasons the incidence of the transformation of idiopathic myelofibrosis to acute leukaemia is increased postsplenectomy. Postoperative ventral hernia can be a source of distress, particularly in women.

Finally, as mentioned earlier, autoimmune phenomena are features of idiopathic myelofibrosis. Corticosteroids may be beneficial if autoimmune phenomena are clinically significant, if there are associated constitutional symptoms and for the amelioration of anaemia. Tuberculosis was once a frequent complication of idiopathic myelofibrosis and, thus, constitutional symptoms in these patients should not be attributed to the myeloproliferative disease without first excluding an infectious process.

Recent phase II clinical trials have shown that JAK2 inhibitors can rapidly reduce spleen size and alleviate constitutional symptoms in idiopathic myelofibrosis patients, supporting a role for inflammatory cytokines in this disorder. They may be also effective in JAK2 V6127F-negative patients but their effects are reversible and to date there has been little effect on malignant stem cell pool.

Further reading

Cervantes F, et al. (1997). Identification of 'short-lived' and 'long-lived' patients at presentation of idiopathic myelofibrosis. Br J Haematol, **97**, 635–40.

Cervantes F, Dupriez B, Pereira A et al. (2009). New prognostic scoring system for primary myelofibrosis based on a study of the International

Working Group for Myelofibrosis Research and Treatment. *Blood*. **113**, 2895–2901.

Chagraoui H, Wendling F, Vainchenker W. (2006). Pathogenesis of myelofibrosis with myeloid metaplasia: Insight form mouse models. *Best Pract Res Clin Haematol*, **19**, 399–412.

Dupriez B, *el al.* (1996). Prognostic factors in agnogenic myeloid metaplasia: a report on 195 cases with a new scoring system.*Blood*, **88**, 1013–18.

Elliott MA, *et al.* (1998). Splenic irradiation for symptomatic splenomegaly associated with myelofibrosis with myeloid metaplasia. *Br J Haematol*, **103**, 505–1 1.

Glew RH, Wolfgang HH, Mclntrye PA (1973). Myeloid metaplasia with myelofibrosis. The clinical spectrum of extrainedullaty hematopoiesis and tumor formation. *Johns Hopkins Med J*, **132**, 253–70.

Kroger N, Holler E, Kobbe G *et al.* (2009). Allogeneic stem cell transplantation after reduced-intensity conditioning in patients with myelofibrosis: a prospective, multicenter study of the Chronic Leukemia Working Party of the European Group for Blood and Marrow Transplantation. *Blood*, **114**, 5264–5270.

Mesa RA, *et al.* (2000). Evaluation and clinical correlations of bone marrow angiogenesis in myelofibrosis and myeloid metaplasia. *Blood*, **96**, 3374–80.

Mesa R, *et al.* (2006). Myelofibrosis with myeloid metaplasia: disease overview and non-transplant options. *Best Pract Res Clin Haematol*, **19**, 495–517.

Mesa R, *et al.* (2006). Pallative goals, patient selection, and perioperative platelet management. *Cancer*, **107**, 361–70.

Pardanani AD, *et al.* (2006). MPL515 mutations in myeloproliferative and other myeloid disorders: a study of 1182 patients. *Blood*, **108**, 3472–76.

Passamonti F, Cervantes F, Vannucchi AM *et al.* (2009). A dynamic prognostic model to predict survival in primary myelofibrosis: a study by the IWG-MRT (International Working Group for Myeloproliferative Neoplasms Research and Treatment). Blood. ePub ahead of print.

Reilly JT (2006). Idiopathic myelofibrosis: pathogenesis to treatment. *Hematol Oncol*, **24**, 56–63.

Rondelli D, *et al.* (2005). Allogeneic hematopoietic stem-cell transplantation with reduced-intensity conditioning in intermediate- or high-risk patients with myelofibrosis with myeloid metaplasia. *Blood*, **105**, 4115.

Tefferi A, *et al.* (2005). The JAK2(V617) tryosine kinase mutation in myelofibrosis with myeloid metaplasia: lineage specificity and clinical correlates. *Br J Haematol*, **131**, 320–8.

Truong LD, Saleem A, Schwartz MR (1984). Acute myelofibrosis. a report of four cases and review of the literature. *Medicine*, **63**, 182–7.

Tsiara SN, *et al.* (2007). Recombinant erythropoietin for the treatment of anaemia in patients with chronic idiopathic myelofibrosis. *Acta Haematol*, **117**, 156–61.

Verstovsek S. (2009). Therapeutic potential of JAK2 inhibitors. Hematology Am Soc Hematol Educ Program,636–642.

22.3.10 **Thrombocytosis**

Stefan O. Ciurea and Ronald Hoffman

Essentials

Thrombocytosis describes a platelet count elevated above 450×10^9/litre, which can be (1) primary—including essential thrombocythaemia, chronic myeloid leukaemia, polycythaemia vera and myelodysplastic syndromes; or (2) secondary—including iron deficiency, infection, blood loss, malignancy.

Normal megakaryocytopoiesis

Platelets are released from megakaryocytes, whose development is principally regulated by thrombopoietin. This is chiefly produced in the liver and binds to its receptor (c-Mpl) to cause activation via the JAK-STAT signalling pathway at different levels of the platelet production pathway, ranging from the proliferation and survival of haematopoietic stem cell/progenitor cells to megakaryocyte maturation. Thrombopoietin production is increased by a wide variety of stimuli, which explains the many causes of secondary thrombocytosis.

Essential thrombocythaemia

Aetiology—the JAK2 V617F missense mutation typical of polycythaemia vera (see Chapter 22.3.8) is found in about 50% of cases.

Clinical features—many patients (usually in late middle age) are asymptomatic at diagnosis, but common manifestations include (1) thrombotic episodes—(a) venous thromboses, including of the hepatic veins; (b) arterial thromboses, including stroke, erythromelalgia (redness and burning pain in the extremities), and (occasionally) frank arterial thrombosis with gangrene; (2) bleeding episodes; (3) splenic enlargement—splenectomy, which is not recommended but may be performed in ignorance of the diagnosis, causes extreme elevation of the platelet count with a greatly increased risk of thrombosis and/or bleeding.

Diagnosis—this requires all of the following four criteria: (1) platelet count >450×10^9/litre, (2) megakaryocyte proliferation with large and mature morphology, and no or little granulocyte or erythroid proliferation, (3) not meeting criteria for other specified haematological disorders, and (4) presence of JAK2(V617F) or similar mutation, or no evidence of reactive thrombocytosis.

Treatment—this requires risk stratification based on the age of the patient and any prior history of thrombosis, with treatment being reserved for those at a high risk of developing complications and not introduced simply on the basis of platelet counts alone unless there is extreme thrombocytosis (>1500×10^9/litre). Therapies include: (1) low dose aspirin—should be considered in patients with platelet counts <1000×10^9/litre and without evidence of acquired von Willebrand disease; (2) cytoreduction—hydroxyurea effectively reduces platelet counts and thrombotic episodes in high-risk patients; interferon-α, anagrelide, and other agents are also used.

Prognosis—most patients will survive more than 10 years from diagnosis. Most deaths result from thrombotic complications.

Introduction

Thrombocytosis refers to a platelet count elevated above the accepted normal range ($>450 \times 10^9$/litre). The widespread use of automated cell counters has made the identification of platelet count abnormalities a relatively common event. The clinical consequences of elevated platelet counts are usually determined by the cause of the thrombocytosis, ranging from the uneventful recognition of a laboratory abnormality, to medical emergencies such as life threatening thrombosis or haemorrhage.

Normal megakaryocytopoiesis

An understanding of disorders of platelet production requires knowledge of the regulatory events that occur during normal megakaryocytopoiesis. Megakaryocyte development is a complex process in which a wide variety of regulatory signals work in concert to direct a highly specific response to thrombopoietic demand. A large number of cytokines including interleukins (IL-3, IL-6, and IL-11), stem cell factor, granulocyte–macrophage colony stimulating factor (GM-CSF), thrombopoietin, and, possibly, erythropoietin have been shown to stimulate megakaryocyte development. Thrombopoietin and its receptor, c-Mpl, are the primary physiological regulators of *in vivo* magakaryocytopoiesis. Thrombopoietin is produced primarily by the liver, but its mRNA has also been found in the kidney, muscle, and bone marrow. Thrombopoietin acts at different levels of megakaryocyte maturation ranging from the proliferation and survival of haematopoietic stem cells/progenitor cells to megakaryocyte maturation, but does not significantly affect the release of platelets from megakaryocytes; thrombopoietin levels are regulated by the total mass of platelets and megakaryocytes, and thrombopoietin is cleared by binding to receptors on the surface of these cells. Like erythropoietin, thrombopoietin uses the JAK-STAT signalling pathway (see Chapter 22.3.8). Activation of the receptor c-Mpl by thrombopoietin provokes a conformational change of the JAK2 tyrosine kinase, phosphorylation of intracytoplasmic residues, and downstream activation of the genes controlling cell cycle status, differentiation, and apoptosis. A mutation in the 617 position of the *JAK2* gene replacing the amino acid phenylalanine with valine disrupts the autoinhibitory domain of JAK2 and renders the kinase constitutively active. This mutation, JAK2 V617F, is present in the vast majority of patients with polycythaemia vera and in approximately 50% of patients with essential thrombocythaemia.

During times of thrombopoietic stress, there is increased production of thrombopoietin by the spleen and bone marrow. Inappropriately elevated levels of thrombopoietin may be observed in essential thrombocythaemia. This is probably not due to excessive production but rather impaired thrombopoietin clearance associated with decreased expression of the thrombopoietin receptor by megakaryocytes and platelets. Molecular abnormalities in the thrombopoietin gene, however, have been recently identified in several families with an autosomal dominant form of hereditary thrombocytosis where serum thrombopoietin levels are significantly elevated. This syndrome has been shown to be due to a mutation in a portion of the thrombopoietin gene, which plays a crucial role in regulating its expression.

Pathophysiology and classification of thrombocytosis

Thrombocytosis can occur in response to many underlying clinical conditions (secondary or reactive), or as a consequence of a primary abnormality in bone marrow function (primary). A classification of the causes of thrombocytosis is provided in Box 22.3.10.1. Reactive or secondary thrombocytosis accounts for over 80% of all recognized cases of thrombocytosis, iron deficiency being the most common cause. Short-lived, secondary thrombocytosis may be observed in situations such as trauma, acute bleeding, major surgery, or after strenuous physical exercise. Longer-term thrombocytosis is associated with the presence of chronic disorders such as malignancy, inflammation, chronic infections, and iron-deficiency anaemia. The pathophysiology underlying reactive thrombocytosis is not fully understood but probably involves the increased generation of inflammatory cytokines such as IL-6, which appear to mediate increased transcription of thrombopoietin by the liver. Primary thrombocytosis by contrast is associated with a group of bone marrow disorders including chronic myeloid leukaemia, essential thrombocythaemia, polycythaemia vera, primary myelofibrosis, and the myelodysplastic syndromes. The level of elevation of platelet numbers is not helpful in differentiating a reactive from a primary process.

An abnormality of thrombopoietin production or of the thrombopoietin receptor has been suggested as the basis of several familial disorders associated with thrombocytosis. In several families a point mutation of the thrombopoietin gene leads to overproduction of thrombopoietin resulting in elevated levels of thrombopoietin and thrombocytosis. Patients with this autosomal dominant form of familial thrombocytosis have a benign course which is not complicated by thrombosis or haemorrhage or the development of acute leukaemia or myelofibrosis. A second familial form of thrombocytosis has been attributed to a mutation in the transmembrane mutation of cMpl leading to its constitutive activation. These familial forms of thrombocytosis are the consequence of germ-line mutations while the myeloproliferative disorders are the consequence of acquired somatic mutations.

For the most part, the underlying medical disorder leading to reactive thrombocytosis can be identified by clinical criteria. A number of laboratory tests can be useful in distinguishing primary from secondary thrombocytosis. C-reactive protein synthesis in the liver is mediated by IL-6, with C-reactive protein levels being high in those patients with elevated IL-6 levels. Elevated levels of both IL-6 and C-reactive protein are strongly indicative of the elevated platelet count being reactive in origin. The presence of 'endogenous erythroid colonies' (erythroid progenitor cells that proliferate *in vitro* without the addition of erythropoietin) and of megakaryocyte progenitor cells that are hypersensitive to certain stimulatory cytokines *in vitro* may be helpful in the identification of myeloproliferative disorders. Cytogenetic analyses and use of the polymerase chain reaction for the *BCR-ABL1* translocation are useful to exclude the presence of a Philadelphia chromosome and a diagnosis of chronic myeloid leukaemia in a patient with thrombocytosis. Assays using probes for restriction fragment polymorphisms of genes located on the X chromosome are helpful in identifying clonal haematopoiesis in females with

---

Box 22.3.10.1 Classification of the causes of thrombocytosis

- Autosomal dominant thrombocytosis
- Secondary thrombocytosis (reactive)
  - Iron deficiency
  - Infection
  - Postsplenectomy (or hyposplenism)
  - Malignancy
  - Trauma
  - Inflammation (non-infectious)
  - Blood loss
  - Major surgery
  - Exercise
  - Rebound from myelosupression
- Primary thrombocytosis (nonreactive)
  - Essential thrombocythaemia
  - Chronic myelogenous leukaemia
  - Polycythaemia vera
  - Agnogenic myeloid metaplasia with myelofibrosis
  - Unclassified myeloproliferative disorders
  - Myelodysplastic syndromes
- Uncertain aetiology

Modified from Buss DH, *et al.* (1994). Occurrence, etiology and clinical significance of extreme thrombocytosis: a study of 280 cases. *Am J Med*, **96**, 247–53.

---

thrombocytosis. Clonal haematopiesis occurs in patients with myeloid malignancies such as essential thromocythaemia but not in cells of patients with secondary forms of thrombocytosis. More recently, the presence or absence of the JAK2 V617F mutation and/or *MPL* mutations (MPL W515L, MPL W515K, and MPL W515N) has been used to differentiate secondary cases of thrombocytosis from a Philadelphia-negative myeloproliferative neoplasm leading to elevated platelet numbers. The presence of these mutations in a patient with thrombocytosis is diagnostic of a myeloproliferative neoplasm.

The natural history and prognosis of reactive thrombocytosis is defined by its underlying cause. The thrombocytosis *per se* is probably inconsequential and does not require specific therapy; it usually resolves after the treatment of the underlying cause. In contrast, the thrombocytosis due to underlying myeloproliferative neoplasm can cause life-threatening thromboembolic phenomena and bleeding episodes, and frequently requires specific cytoreductive therapy, emphasizing the need for accurate recognition.

Essential thrombocythaemia

Essential thrombocythaemia is a chronic myeloproliferative disease characterized by marked bone marrow megakaryocytic hyperplasia

and peripheral blood thrombocytosis. The clinical course is punctuated by episodes of thrombosis and/or bleeding. In 1951, Dameshek suggested that essential thrombocythaemia represented a myeloproliferative disease and hypothesized its clonal nature. The myeloproliferative diseases are currently thought to represent malignant stem cell disorders.

Aetiology and pathogenesis

The causative factors which lead to essential thrombocythaemia are poorly understood. Its pathogenesis involves the abnormal proliferation of a blood cell precursor that differentiates mainly towards the megakaryocytic/platelet lineage. Current evidence suggests that hypersensitivity to stimulatory cytokines such as IL-3, IL-6, thrombopoietin, and GM-CSF might provoke the expansion of the megakaryocytic progenitor pool. The clonal origin of haematopoiesis in patients with myeloproferative disorders was initially established through biochemical isoenzyme characterization of the blood cells of affected women who were heterozygous for glucose-6-phosphate dehydrogenase. Analysis of X-linked restriction fragment length polymorphisms (RFLPs) in affected women has confirmed a clonal pattern in some cases. There are however, a significant number of patients with polyclonal myelopoiesis. These nonclonal cases may have a decreased risk for thrombosis. The recent finding of the JAK2 V617F mutation in Philadelphia-chromosome negative myeloproliferative neoplasms has provided new insight into the pathogenesis of this disease. Approximately 50% of patients with essential thombocythaemia are JAK2 V617F positive. The patients who are positive for the mutation almost uniformly have a low burden of JAK2 V617F (<50%) as compared with polycythaemia vera. Essential thrombocythaemia patients with a high allele burden are older, have more symptoms (especially aquagenic pruritus), a larger spleen volume, and significantly higher rate of cardiovascular complications. Although polycythaemia vera patients almost always have haematopoietic progenitors that are homozygous for the JAK2 V617F mutation, such homozygous progenitor cells are only occasionally observed in essential thrombocythaemia patients. These data indicate that the homologous recombination step which leads to mutational homozygosity in polycythaemia vera rarely occurs in essential thrombocythaemia. Furthermore the degree of mutant allelic chimerism remains constant over time. Patients with JAK2 V617F-positive essential thrombocythaemia have a higher haematocrit, higher white blood cell count, and higher rate of transformation to polycythaemia vera than patients who are JAK2 V617F negative. These findings have led some investigators to suggest that JAK2 V617F-positive essential thrombocythaemia represents a *forme fruste* of polycythaemia vera. Acquired mutations of the thrombopoietin receptor, MPL at position 515 have been observed in 4 to 5% of patients with essential thrombocythaemia and 9% of patients with JAK2 V617F-negative essential thrombocythaemia. A number of patients have been shown to possess both the MPL and JAK2 V617F mutations. Although the MPL mutations were first observed in patients with primary myelofibrosis they are now known to also occur in patients with essential thrombocythaemia. MPL mutant-positive patients have lower haemoglobin levels but higher platelet counts than essential thermbocythaemia patients who do not have a mutation of the thrombopoietin receptor. A recent study of essential thrombocythaemia patients in a paediatric population revealed that haematopoiesis was more often polyclonal and JAK2 V617F negative. As compared with the adult population, about 20% of such paediatric cases had monoclonal haematopoiesis and JAK2 V617F positivity was significantly less frequent than in adults (20% vs 50–60%). Although one may hypothesize that clonal haematopoiesis in nonclonal essential thrombocythaemia patients may become more apparent with age, no significant evidence has been provided so far to support the transition from nonclonal to clonal haematopoiesis. Furthermore, patients who are negative for JAK2 V617F or MPL mutation at presentation have not been observed to acquire the mutation over time.

Epidemiology

The true incidence of essential thrombocythaemia is unknown due to the lack of large epidemiologic studies. Several smaller studies estimated the incidence of essential thrombocythaemia to be 1.5 to 2.4 patients per 100 000 population annually. Approximately 6000 new cases are identified each year in the United States of America. There seems to be a slight female predominance and the usual age at onset is between 50 and 60 years. Approximately 20% of all cases occur in individuals younger than 40, but it is very rarely seen during childhood.

Pathobiology

The characteristic clinical features are dominated by the thrombocytosis and abnormalities in platelet function. The association between increased numbers of circulating platelets and ischaemic episodes remains unclear, but the duration of thrombocytosis may play a role. Microvascular thrombosis results in a variety of clinical syndromes associated with digital and cerebrovascular ischaemia. Abnormalities in platelet aggregation occur in 35% to 100% of patients, and prolongation of the bleeding time occurs in 7% to 19%. Despite being common, these abnormalities are poor predictors of bleeding and/or thrombotic risk. This is in contrast to the acquired von Willebrand disease and erythromelalgia, clinical entities not infrequently seen in association with essential thrombocythaemia. In acquired von Willebrand disease, extreme thrombocytosis ($>1000 \times 10^9$/litre) induces the adsorption of larger von Willebrand multimers on to platelet membranes and their subsequent degradation, triggering a haemostatic defect causing a bleeding diathesis quite similar to that observed in type II von Willebrand disease. Erythromelalgia occurs commonly in patients with essential thrombocythaemia. Erythromelalgia refers to a syndrome characterized by redness and burning pain in the extremities which results from platelet-mediated thrombosis of the arterial microvasculature. If left untreated it may progress to frank gangrene. The exquisite platelet response to cyclooxygenase inhibitors such as aspirin and indomethacin suggests that prostaglandin endoperoxides produced by the metabolism of arachidonic acid might play a major role in the generation of platelet-associated thrombosis.

Increased frequency of venous thrombosis in uncommon sites such as the splanchnic vasculature leading to catastrophic intra-abdominal thromboses such as Budd–Chiari syndrome have recently reported in JAK2 V617F-positive patients who subsequently go on to develop essential thrombocythaemia. Although the increased thrombotic risk cannot be explained exclusively by the presence of JAK2 V617F mutation, it appears to contribute to the increased risk of thrombosis in these patients.

Clinical manifestations

As many as two-thirds of patients with essential thrombocythaemia are asymptomatic at diagnosis. Most symptomatic patients present with either a thrombotic episode or a minor bleeding episode. Bleeding can occur spontaneously but is frequently associated with the recent use of a nonsteroidal anti-inflammatory drug (NSAID). Common sites of haemorrhage include the gastrointestinal and the genitourinary tracts as well as easy bruisability of the skin. Thrombosis leads to the most common presenting symptoms and can occur in arteries and veins, large or small. Occlusion of the splanchnic vessels and of the superficial and deep veins of the lower extremities is common. Pulmonary emboli may also occur. An occasional patient presents with thrombosis of the hepatic veins causing the Budd–Chiari syndrome or with occlusion of the renal veins manifesting clinically as nephrotic syndrome.

When the microcirculation is involved, a number of clinical syndromes may occur. Palpable lesions with small areas of gangrene indistinguishable from vasculitic lesions of rheumatoid arthritis or systemic lupus erythematosus may be observed. Erythromelalgia may occur in association with transient ischaemic attacks or acute episodes of cardiac angina. Peripheral pulses are usually preserved; this helps differentiate erythromelalgia from atherosclerotic-related ischaemia. Neurological symptoms are common and include headaches and paresthesias of the extremities. Transient ischaemic attacks may present with symptoms of unsteadiness, dysarthria, dysphoria, motor hemiparesis, scintillating scotomas, amaurosis fugax, vertigo, dizziness, migraine headaches, and seizures. On occasion, transient ischaemic attacks may progress to established infarcts. Myocardial ischaemia with normal angiograms occurs occasionally. Thrombotic nonbacterial endocarditis, usually affecting the mitral or aortic valves, may manifest with findings of distal emboli. Splenic enlargement is observed in 40 to 50% of individuals and 20% have hepatic enlargement. Patients unaware of their diagnosis who have undergone splenectomy as part of the diagnostic work-up for splenomegaly will predictably develop extreme elevations in their platelet counts, with a consequent increased risk for bleeding and/or thrombosis.

Laboratory evaluation

Elevated platelet count, often above 450 to 1000×10^9/litre, is characteristic. The absolute number of platelets, even if higher than 1000×10^9/litre, is not diagnostic of essential thrombocythaemia. Extreme elevations in platelet numbers have been observed in reactive thrombocytosis. Marked changes in platelet morphology, which include large and bizarre-looking platelets sometimes forming aggregates, are also characteristic and may be more useful in helping distinguishing primary from reactive thrombocytosis. The bone marrow is hypercellular with megakaryocytic hyperplasia. Clusters of hyperlobulated megakaryocytes are often observed within the marrow. Absent or diminished iron stores are seen frequently. This may be an epiphenomenon of an underlying myeloproliferative neoplasm or a true expression of iron depletion in patients with chronic bleeding. Reticulin fibrosis is present in one-quarter of bone marrow specimens but collagen is usually absent. Mild leucocytosis is common.

JAK2 V617F and the MPL mutations are important new diagnostic tools useful in identifying patients with a myeloproliferative neoplasms. If thrombocytosis associated with megakaryocytic hyperplasia, and a JAK2 V617F or MPL mutation is observed in the absence of the clinical or laboratory features of one of the other myeloproliferative neoplasms such as polycythaemia vera or primary myelofibrosis, a diagnosis of essential thrombocythaemia is certain. Unfortunately, for the other 50% of the patients with essential thrombocythaemia who lack the above-mentioned mutations the diagnosis remains one of exclusion, although haematopoitic cell clonality assays are frequently useful in women.

Platelet function abnormalities are commonly found and include defective platelet aggregation in response to adrenaline, ADP, and collagen. Aggregation in response to arachidonic acid and ristocetin is often normal. An acquired platelet storage pool disease also occurs due to abnormalities in the content and release of α granules associated with a state of increased platelet activation. The bleeding time is occasionally prolonged but does not predict bleeding risk. Cytogenetic evidence for a Philadelphia-chromosome and/or the molecular identification of the *BCR-ABL1* fusion gene aids in distinguishing essential thrombocythaemia from chronic myeloid leukaemia. The presence of dyspoietic changes in bone marrow precursor cells and of characteristic chromosomal abnormalities suggests the diagnosis of myelodysplasia. In particular, the 5q–syndrome is associated with thrombocytosis. The diagnostic criteria and management of the other myeloproliferative neoplasms associated with thrombocytosis are outlined in other chapters. Cytogenetic abnormalities occur in approximately 5% of patients with essential thrombocythaemia, and the most common are 1q–, 20q–, 21q–, and 1q+. Elevated vitamin B_{12} levels occur in 25% of patients.

Diagnostic criteria and differential diagnosis

The revised World Health Organization (WHO) diagnostic criteria for essential thrombocthaemia are given in Box 22.3.10.2. Essential thrombocythaemia was previously a diagnosis of exclusion, but the advent of JAK2 V617F and MPL mutational analyses have greatly facilitated the diagnosis in approximately 50% of cases. The presence of these mutations in the setting of thrombocytosis without evidence of polycythaemia vera is virtually diagnostic of essential thrombocythaemia. These diagnostic criteria are, however, of less use in paediatric patients since many of these individuals are JAK2 V617F negative. Recently a group of patients with refractory anaemia with ringed sideroblasts and extreme thrombocytosis have been reported who are JAK2 V617F positive and occasionally possess exon 12 *JAK2* mutations or *MPL* mutations. This syndrome represents a myelodsplastic/myeloproliferative neoplasm variant. Any condition associated with elevations in circulating platelets is part of the differential diagnosis of essential thrombocythaemia. Thrombocytosis may be the consequence of primary bone marrow disorders associated with increased platelet production (nonreactive thrombocytosis), or a secondary response to an underlying disorder (reactive thrombocytosis). Box 22.3.10.1 summarizes the most important causes of thrombocytosis: iron-deficiency anemia, infection/inflammation, malignancy, trauma, and hyposplenism, are the most commonly encountered disorders. The exclusion of an identifiable cause for reactive thrombocytosis, in particular iron deficiency, is a necessary step.

Risk assessment

Essential thrombocythaemia is a heterogeneous disorder associated with patients encountering a varied risk of developing life-threatening complications. Many patients enjoy survival fairly similar to that of their unaffected peers but a subset of patients is at a high risk of developing additional thromboses. Myelosuppressive therapy should be reserved for patients at a high risk of developing such complications. A risk-based decision approach to therapy is outlined in Box 22.3.10.2 to identify such patients. Advanced age (≥60 years) and a previous history of thrombosis clearly defines a group at high risk for the development of life-threatening complications. The degree of thrombocytosis and the presence of associated cardiovascular risk factors, particularly smoking and obesity, are also taken into consideration when making treatment decisions. Isolated thrombocytosis *per se* is not an indication for therapy; however, it is common practice to treat extreme thrombocytosis (platelet count >1500 × 10⁹/litre) because of the increased risk of complications.

Treatment

The goal of therapy in essential thrombocythaemia is to control symptoms and prevent complications, the most feared being thrombotic events. Should a decision be made to treat the patient based on risk assessment, the platelet count should be reduced to about 400 × 10⁹/litre. Although this threshold has not been determined to be optimal to reduce the incidence of thrombotic episodes in rigorous clinical trials, it is considered a safe level by most practising physicians in the field.

A number of agents can lower the platelet count in patients with essential thrombocythaemia. Low-dose aspirin (81–100 mg/day) has been shown to be safe and may decrease the recurrence of microcirculatory events (erythromelalgia/transient ischaemic attacks) and prevent the development of other thrombotic phenomena, especially in combination with myelosuppressive agents. In order to minimize the risk of iatrogenic bleeding, only patients

---

Box 22.3.10.2 Revised WHO criteria for the diagnosis of essential thrombocythaemia

Diagnosis of essential thrombocythaemia requires all four of the following major criteria:

1 Platelet count ≥450 × 10⁹/litre

2 Megakaryocyte proliferation with large and mature morphology; no or little granulocyte or erythroid proliferation.

3 Not meeting WHO criteria for CML, PV, PMF, MDS or other myeloid neoplasm

4 Demonstration of JAK2 V617F or other clonal marker, *or* no evidence of reactive thrombocytosis

CML, chronic myeloid leukaemia; MDS, myelodysplastic syndrome; PMF, primary myelofibrosis; PV, polycythaemia vera.

Adapted with permission from Tefferi A, Vardiman JW (2008). Classification and diagnosis of myeloproliferative neoplasms: the 2008 World Health Organization criteria and point-of-care diagnostic algorithms. *Leukemia*, **22**, 14–22.

with platelet counts less than 1000×10^9/litre and without evidence of an acquired von Willebrand disease should be considered for low-dose aspirin administration.

There is evidence that cytoreduction using hydroxyurea, at least in high-risk patients, results in a significant reduction in the number of thrombotic episodes. The use of hydroxyurea, an antimetabolite that interferes with DNA repair, decreased the number of thrombotic events in a randomized study of high risk patients when given at 15 mg/kg initially, with subsequent adjustments based on initial response. In this study, the target was a platelet count of less than 600×10^9/litre, but it is possible that tighter control ($<350–400 \times 10^9$/litre) may be more effective. Onset of action is usually 3 to 5 days. Frequent side effects include dose-related neutropenia, nausea, stomatitis, hyperpigmentation, rash, nail changes, leg ulcers, and hair loss. The leukaemogenic potential of hydroxyurea when given as a single agent is still a subject of controversy although it is clearly less leukaemogenic than alkylating agents or radioactive phosphorus. Recent data from at least two large studies, one in polycythaemia vera and the other one in essential thrombocythaemia patients, failed to show an increased incidence of acute leukaemia in patients treated with hydroxyurea.

Interferon-α, a biological response modifier, is also useful in treating patients with essential thrombocythaemia. Ninety per cent response rates with median times to response of approximately 3 months are seen when 3 to 5 million units are administered subcutaneously 3 to 5 days per week. It is nonmutagenic and does not cross the placenta. Frequent side-effects include influenza-like symptoms, fatigue, lethargy, and depression. The long-term use of interferon is associated with mild weight loss, alopecia, autoimmune thyroiditis, and autoimmune haemolytic anaemia. Its extensive toxicity profile and the need for parenteral administration limit its use as initial therapy, particularly in elderly patients. Pegylated forms of interferon have a prolonged half-life, can be administered weekly, and are often better tolerated.

Anagrelide is another treatment option for patients with essential thrombocythaemia. This drug acts by selectively inhibiting megakaryocytic maturation. Responses have been documented in over 90% of treated patients with a median time to response of 2.5 to 4 weeks and an onset of action of 6 to 10 days. Anagrelide is nonmutagenic and its use has not been associated with the development of acute leukaemia. A recent large randomized study (UKMRC PT-1) comparing hydroxyurea with anagrelide in addition to aspirin therapy found that patients treated with anagrelide plus aspirin had an increased rate of arterial thrombotic events, haemorrhage, and transformation to myelofibrosis as compared to the hydroxyurea plus aspirin arm. There was no increase in the incidence of acute leukaemia in the hydroxyurea arm. These findings strongly suggest that hydroxyurea plus aspirin therapy should remain the first-line treatment for high-risk patients with this disease. Anagrelide is a good second-line treatment option for patients intolerant to hydroxyurea. Common side effects of anagrelide therapy include headaches, dizziness, fluid retention, palpitations, nausea, abdominal pain, and diarrhoea, and it triggers episodes of tachyarrhythmias and heart failure. For this reason, it should be used carefully in older people and avoided in patients with known heart disease.

Alkylating agents have been extensively used in the past to treat essential thrombocythaemia. Within this group of agents, busulfan has been shown to be quite effective and relatively nontoxic, with predictable cytopenias as its major untoward effect. It is usually prescribed at 4 mg/day until a platelet count of 400×10^9/litre is reached. Additional 2-week courses are given if and when the platelet count rises over 400×10^9/litre. Extensive experience has also accumulated with radioactive phosphorus (^{32}P), but its use is now limited to selected cases. Alkylating agents and radioactive phosphorus have been associated with significant increases in the risk of leukaemic transformation.

Given the number of available therapeutic options and their different toxicity profiles, the choice of the appropriate cytoreductive drug for a given individual requires the consideration of a number of variables. These include age, childbearing potential, projected life expectancy, comorbidities, and cost of treatment. Furthermore, the overall low risk for the development of life-threatening complications that affects patients with essential thrombocythaemia highlights the need for systematic, risk-based approaches to therapeutic decision-making (Table 22.3.10.1). All patients should stop smoking. Indiscriminate use of high doses of NSAIDs should be avoided; their excessive use is clearly associated with bleeding episodes.

Low-risk patients have a risk of thrombosis similar to that of an age and sex-matched control population and a very low risk of life-threatening bleeding. These observations support close observation without cytoreductive therapy as the most sensible approach. High-risk patients are those more than 60 years of age and with prior history of thrombosis. According to the results presented in the PT-1 trial, these patients should be treated with hydroxyurea as the cytoreducive agent of choice, in addition to aspirin. Anagrelide should be offered to patients who are intolerant or developed adverse effects to hydroxyurea. For elderly patients with limited projected survival (<10 years) and who either have

Table 22.3.10.1 Risk stratification-based treatment of essential thrombocythaemia

Risk category[a]	Treatment
Low risk	Observation
Age < 60 years, and	
No history of thrombosis, and	
Platelet count < 1000×10^9/litre, and	
No cardiovascular risk factors (smoking, obesity)	
High risk	Treatment
Age ≥ 60 years, or	
Previous history of thrombosis	
Intermediate risk	Treatment[b]
Age < 60 years, and	
Platelet count > $1000–1500 \times 10^9$/litre, or	
Cardiovascular risk factors (smoking, obesity)	

[a] Leukocytosis and JAK2 V617F mutation appear to confer a higher risk of thrombosis, but no established treatment guidelines exist for these patients.

[b] The decision to treat is at the discretion of the clinician. We offer treatment to most of our patients with platelets more than $1000–1500 \times 10^9$/litre. Risk modification is strongly encouraged.

Adapted from Finazzi G, Barbui T (2005). Risk-adapted therapy in essential thrombocythemia and polycythemia vera. *Blood Rev*, **19**, 243–52.

problems with drug compliance or are too ill to comply with the minimum follow-up requirements during cytoreductive therapy, administration of radioactive phosphorus might be appropriate. α-Interferon may be an acceptable option in younger patients. Alkylating agents and radioactive phosphorus are usually avoided, given their known leukaemogenic potential, unless the patient needs a third- or fourth-line agent to control blood counts. In patients at intermediate risk based on platelet numbers at or more than 1000 to 1500 × 10⁹/litre and/or patients who have acquired von Willebrand disease, platelet reduction therapy is indicated to avoid the higher risk of complications.

Smokers and obese individuals, unless symptomatic, should be managed by risk modification. Smoking has been proved to be an independent risk factor for developing arterial thrombotic complications. Patients with essential thrombocytopenia should be strongly encouraged to stop smoking to decrease their thromboembolic risk.

In severe, life-threatening episodes, rapid cytoreduction may be achieved by plateletpheresis or by the administration of high doses of hydrxyurea. In patients who present with a life-threatening episode of acute bleeding, the site of bleeding should be promptly identified and any antiplatelet agent should be stopped. Those suffering from an acquired von Willebrand's disease can be treated with desmopressin and factor VIII concentrates that contain high concentrations of von Willebrand factor. Cytoreductive therapy with hydroxyurea must be promptly initiated. In bleeding patients who fail to respond to desmopressin and factor VIII administration, the bleeding frequently resolves following platelet transfusions.

Up to 10% of patients with essential thrombocythaemia will evolve to secondary myelofibrosis, recognized by the development of cytopenias, leukoerythroblastic blood picture, and worsening splenomegaly. These patients have a very poor prognosis and should undergo evaluation for allogeneic stem cell transplantation. The use of reduced-intensity conditioning regimens for allogeneic stem cell transplantation has been shown recently to improve the outcome of such patients with a relatively low mortality rate.

New kinase inhibitors targeting the JAK2 V617F mutation are being developed, with the hope that at least half of the patients with essential thrombocythaemia will benefit from these new therapeutic options.

The management of patients who are or want to become pregnant requires special consideration. The risk of fetal loss is quite high (c.40%). High-risk pregnancy is defined as one occurring in an individual with a previous thrombosis or major bleeding episode, platelet count more than 1500 × 10⁹/litre, and previous severe complications such as fetal loss or placental abruption. Patients with low or intermediate disease risk should be managed with careful observation. Specific treatment should be considered for high-risk pregnancies as follows. (1) If previous thrombosis or major complications during prior pregnancies have occurred, patients should receive low-molecular-weight heparin throughout pregnancy until 6 weeks postpartum. (2) If there is a history of major bleeding, or platelet count is above 1500 × 10⁹/litre, aspirin should be avoided and consideration should be given to cytoreduction with interferon to decrease the platelet count to normal levels. Despite the lack of endorsement by the manufacturers of α-interferon, it is the drug of choice during pregnancy given its lack of mutagenic potential and its inability to cross the placenta. Hydroxyurea, given

its mechanism of action, could theoretically cause fetal malformations, and anagrelide, because of its small molecular size, probably crosses the placenta and may cause life-threatening thrombocytopenia and haemorrhage in the fetus. Despite these concerns, recent reports have described first-trimester exposures to these two drugs resulting in the delivery of normal newborns. We therefore do not consider unintended exposures to hydroxyurea or anagrelide as absolute indications for the termination of a pregnancy. Recently, JAK2 V617F-positive essential thrombocthaemia has been found to be an independent adverse predictor of pregnancy outcome. These pregnancy-associated complications in patients with JAK2 mutations were not prevented by the use of aspirin therapy raising the question of whether prophylactic anticoagulant therapy is warranted for JAK2 V617F positive patients.

Prognosis

The probability that a patient with essential thrombocythaemia will survive 10 years is 64 to 80%, not substantially different from that of a control age- and sex-matched population. The actual risk for the development of a catastrophic thrombotic or haemorrhagic event in an asymptomatic patient is quite low. Most deaths come from thrombotic complications. Transformation to myelofibrosis and/or acute leukaemia has been reported with increasing frequency at a rate of transformation of 3 to 10%. Prior administration of cytotoxic therapy is the strongest predictor of evolution to leukaemia, but spontaneous transformations also occur, as in other myeloproliferative disorders. JAK2 V617F-positive essential thrombocythaemia not infrequently evolves into the clinical picture of polycythaemia vera.

Future directions

A better understanding of the mechanisms involved in the regulation of platelet production and of the molecular abnormalities specifically associated with essential thrombocythaemia will potentially offer rational targets against which new and more specific therapies can be developed. The discovery of the JAK2 V617F mutation has revolutionized the field of Philadelphia-negative myeloproliferative diseases, but its presence in only about 50% of patients with essential thrombocythaemia has raised the necessity to evaluate the role of this mutation in the pathobiology of patients with essential thrombocythaemia and to search for additional mutations in the patients who lack JAK2 or MPL mutations.

Further reading

Barbui T, Finazzi G (2007). Therapy for polycythemia vera and essential thrombocythemia is driven by the cardiovascular risk. *Semin Thromb Hemost*, **33**, 321–9.

Barbui T (2004). The leukemia controversy in myeloproliferative disorders: is it a natural progression of disease, a secondary sequela of therapy, or a combination of both? *Semin Hematol*, **41**(2 Suppl 3), 15–17.

Ding J, et al.(2004). Familial essential thrombocythemia associated with a dominant-positive activating mutation of the c-MPL gene, which encodes for the receptor for thrombopoietin. *Blood*, **103**, 4198–200.

Dingli D, Tefferi A (2005). A critical review of anagrelide therapy in essential thrombocythemia and related disorders. *Leukemia Lymphoma*, **46**, 641–50.

Elliott MA, Tefferi A (2005). Thrombosis and haemorrhage in polycythaemia vera and essential thrombocythaemia. *Br J Haematol*, **128**, 275–90.

Finazzi G, Barbui T (2005). Risk-adapted therapy in essential thrombocythemia and polycythemia vera. *Blood Rev*, **19**, 243–52.

Finazzi G, Harrison C (2006). Essential thrombocythemia. *Semin Hematol*, **42**, 230–8.

Fruchtman SM, Hoffman R (2005). Essential thrombocythemia. In: Hoffman R, *et al.* (eds) *Hematology: basic principles and practice*, pp. 1177–296. Churchill Livingston, Philadelphia.

Gisslinger H (2006). Update on diagnosis and management of essential thrombocythemia. *Semin Thromb Hemost*, **32**, 430–6.

Harrison CN, *et al.* (2005). Hydroxyurea compared with anagrelide in high-risk essential thrombocythemia. *N Engl J Med*, **353**, 33–45.

Harrison C (2005). Pregnancy and its management in the Philadelphia negative myeloproliferative diseases. *Br J Haematol*, **129**, 293–306.

Kaushansky K (2005). The molecular mechanisms that control thrombopoiesis. *J Clin Invest*, **115**, 3339–47.

Levine RL, *et al.* (2007). Role of JAK2 in the pathogenesis and treatment of myeloproliferative disorders. *Nat Rev Cancer*, **7**, 673–83.

Long MW, Hoffman R (2005). Thrombocytopoiesis. In: Hoffman R, *et al.* (eds) *Hematology: Basic Principles and Practice*, pp. 303–20. Churchill Livingston, Philadelphia.

McIntyre CJ, *et al.* (1991). Essential thrombocythaemia in young adults. *Mayo Clin Proc*, **66**, 149–54.

Pardanani AD, *et al* (2006). MPL515 mutations in myeloproliferative and other myeloid disorders: a study of 1182 patients. *Blood*, **108**, 3472–6.

Tefferi A, Vardiman JW (2008). Classification and diagnosis of myeloproliferative neoplasms: The 2008 World Health Organization criteria and point-of-care diagnostic algorithms. *Leukemia*, **22**, 14–22.

Tefferi A, *et al.* (2007). Proposals and rationale for revision of the World Health Organization diagnostic criteria for polycythemia vera, essential thrombocythemia, and primary myelofibrosis: recommendations from an ad hoc international expert panel. *Blood*, **110**, 1092–7.

Van Genderen PJJ, *et al.* (1996). Acquired von Willebrand disease in myeloproliferative disorders. *Leukemia Lymphoma*, **22** (Suppl 1), 79–82.

Van Genderen PJJ, *et al.* (1997). Prevention and treatment of thrombotic complications in essential thrombocythemia: efficacy and safety of aspirin. *Br Jo Haematol*, **97**, 179–84.

Wagstaff AJ, Keating GM (2006). Anagrelide: a review of its use in the management of essential thrombocythaemia. *Drugs*, **66**, 111–31.

22.3.11 Aplastic anaemia and other causes of bone marrow failure

Judith C.W. Marsh and E.C. Gordon-Smith

Essentials

Bone marrow failure implies a deficiency of one or more circulating blood cell lineages caused by primary proliferative failure of haemopoietic progenitor cells in the marrow. Several conditions both acquired and inherited result in marrow failure. Differential distinction is important for planning treatment.

Aplastic anaemia

Aetiology—this may be (1) idiosyncratic—the commonest type (70–80% of cases); most often of unknown cause ('idiopathic'), but sometimes a drug or chemical or a virus infection is implicated; believed to have an autoimmune basis; (2) inevitable—e.g. after treatment with cytotoxic drugs or radiation; (3) immune—e.g. associated with systemic lupus erythematosus (SLE); (4) malignant—e.g. in association with childhood acute lymphoblastic leukaemia; (5) inherited—e.g. Fanconi anaemia, dyskeratosis congenita, Shwachman–Diamond syndrome.

Clinical features—the commonest presenting manifestations are those of (1) anaemia, (2) bleeding—skin or mucosal haemorrhage, or visual disturbance due to retinal haemorrhage, and (less commonly) (3) infection—particularly sore throat or failure of minor infections to clear.

Diagnosis—this requires at least two of the following: (1) haemoglobin less than 10 g/dl, (2) platelet count less than 50×10^9/litre, and (3) neutrophil count less than 1.5×10^9/litre. The bone marrow is hypocellular with prominent fat spaces and variable amounts of residual haemopoietic cells.

Treatment and prognosis—aside from supportive care, this depends on severity of disease: (1) Nonsevere—depends on requirement for red cell and/or platelet transfusion: (a) no requirement—observe; (b) required—first-line treatment is with antithymocyte globulin (ATG) and ciclosporin. (2) Severe—depends on patient's age and whether they have an HLA-identical sibling: (a) aged under 40 years with HLA-identical sibling—bone marrow transplant; (b) others—first-line treatment is with ATG and ciclosporin. For patients who lack an HLA-identical bone marrow donor, the outlook is poor.

Pure red cell aplasia

In this condition there is defective maturation of red cell precursors, with failure to produce reticulocytes and hence mature red cells. Causes include most commonly (1) acquired, idiopathic—usually immune in origin; associations include autoimmune diseases (e.g. SLE), thymoma, drugs (e.g. phenytoin, erythropoietin), lymphoproliferative disorders, parvovirus B19 infection; and rarely (2) congenital—e.g. Diamond–Blackfan, and (3) transient erythroblastopenia of childhood, which often follows a viral illness.

Clinical presentation is with features of severe anaemia. Aside from supportive care, treatment of acquired, idiopathic disease depends on the associated cause, e.g. stopping any relevant drug, intravenous immunoglobulin for parvovirus-induced disease. For other patients first-line treatment is with prednisolone, with refractory disease being treated with other immunosuppressive agents, e.g. ciclosporin, ATG.

Introduction—the concept of bone marrow failure

Bone marrow failure describes conditions where there is failure of production of circulating blood cells by the bone marrow, resulting in single cytopenias or pancytopenia. Most often they are acquired, but there are also rare congenital disorders (Table 22.3.11.1). Bone marrow failure may occur because of failure within the haemopoietic stem cell compartment giving rise to aplastic anaemia. Examples of congenital aplastic anaemia include Fanconi's anaemia and dyskeratosis congenita. Alternatively, failure of a single haemopoietic cell lineage occurs in pure red cell aplasia (the congenital form is Diamond–Blackfan anaemia OMIM 105 656), amegakayocytic thrombocytopenia (acquired and congenital) and Kostmann's syndrome (autosomal recessive form of severe congenital neutropenia, OMIM 610 738)

Other causes of bone marrow failure include (1) proliferative bone marrow failure which occurs in myelodysplastic syndromes where there is ineffective haemopoiesis with abnormal differentiation, and also in the congenital dyserythropoietic anaemias; (2) an abnormal bone marrow microenvironment as in myelofibrosis; (3) bone marrow infiltrations such as leukaemia, lymphoma, and lipid storage disease such as Gaucher's disease; (4) infections such as HIV, parvovirus B19, and other viral and mycobacterial infections; and (5) bone marrow necrosis from prolonged starvation and malignant infiltration.

This chapter focuses on the first two entities of bone marrow failure resulting from failure at the level of the haemopoietic stem cell resulting in pancytopenia or affecting the erythroid lineage giving rise to pure red-cell aplasia. Thrombocytopenia and neutropenia are discussed in Chapters 22.6.3 and 22.4.1 respectively.

Aplastic anaemia

Classification and definition of aplastic anaemia

Aplastic anaemia is characterized by pancytopenia with a hypocellular bone marrow in the absence of an abnormal infiltrate and with no increase in reticulin. The term aplastic anaemia encompasses different entities, including the following.

- Idiosyncratic aplastic anaemia is the disease to which 'aplastic anaemia' usually refers. It is most often idiopathic but sometimes a drug or chemical or a virus infection is implicated. It has a prolonged course with unpredictable recovery and a risk of later clonal evolution to myelodysplastic syndrome, acute myeloid leukaemia and paroxysmal nocturnal haemoglobinuria.

- Inevitable aplastic anaemia occurs after treatment with cytotoxic drugs or radiation. It is dose dependent and recovery is usually predictable.

- Immune aplastic anaemia occurs rarely after Epstein–Barr virus (EBV) infection or in association with systemic lupus erythematosus. It usually recovers spontaneously or with treatment of the primary disorder.

- Malignant aplastic anaemia may occur in association with childhood acute lymphoblastic leukaemia. Hypocellular MDS shares many characteristics with idiosyncratic aplastic anaemia (overlap syndrome) but remaining haemopoietic cells have dysplastic features.

- Inherited aplastic anaemias are usually progressive with an increased risk of leukaemia and mucosal malignancy.

Acquired aplastic anaemia

Definition

To define aplastic anaemia there must be at least two of the following findings: (1) haemoglobin below 10 g/dl; (2) platelet count $<50 \times 10^9$/litre; (3) neutrophil count $<1.5 \times 10^9$/litre. The severity of the

Table 22.3.11.1 Defining aplastic anaemia

		Confirmation of diagnosis
1	**Traditional definition**	
	Pancytopenia with hypocellular BM, haemopoietic tissue replaced by fat cells, in absence of abnormal infiltrate or increase in reticulin At least 2 of the following required: Hb <10 g/dl; platelet count < 100 × 10⁹/litre; and neutrophil count < 1.5 × 10⁹/litre	FBC, reticulocyte count, blood film examination, BM aspirate and trephine
2	**Is the diagnosis really AA?**	
	Or is there another cause for pancytopenia and hypocellular BM ?	Exclude hypocellular MDS/AML, myelofibrosis, lymphoma, atypical mycobacterial infection, anorexia nervosa
3	**Is the disease an inherited bone marrow failure syndrome?**	Clues in medical history and clinical examination and diagnostic tests:
	Fanconi anaemia	Presence of café-au-lait spots, short stature, anomalies of upper extremities etc. Increased chromosome breakages of peripheral blood lymphocytes with DEB/MMC
	Dyskeratosis congenita	Nail dystrophy, leukoplakia and skin pigmentation, but also pulmonary fibrosis, osteoporosis, liver function abnormality. *DKC1* (X-linked), *TERC* (autosomal dominant), *TERT* gene mutation analysis
	Shwachman–Diamond syndrome	History of pancreatic insufficiency, neutropenia prior to AA, short stature. *SBDS* gene mutation analysis
4	**What is the aetiology?**	
	Idiopathic	70–80% of cases
	Posthepatitic	Liver function tests, viral studies (hepatitis A, B, C, G, usually negative, EBV rarely)
	Drugs and chemicals; environmental/occupational exposures	Careful drug and exposure history, but no tests available to prove association
	PNH	Flow cytometry of GPI-anchored proteins on red cells, neutrophils, and monocytes
	Rarely: pregnancy, SLE, thymoma, eosinophilic fasciitis	
5	**Are there abnormal clones present?**	
	PNH	Flow cytometry as above
	Cytogenetic clone	BM cytogenetics ± FISH

Table 22.3.11.1 *(Cont'd)* Defining aplastic anaemia

	Confirmation of diagnosis
6 How severe is the disease ?	
Severe AA	Criteria: BM cellularity <25% or 25–50% with <30% residual hematopoietic cells, with 2 out of 3 of the following: neutrophils <0.5 × 10^9/litre, platelets <20 × 10^9/litre, reticulocytes <20 × 10^9/litre
Very severe AA	Same as for severe AA, except neutrophil count < 0.2 instead of < 0.5 × 10^9/litre

AA, aplastic amaemia; BM, bone marrow; DEB, diepoxybutane; EBV, Epstein–Barr virus; FBC, full blood count; FISH, fluorescence *in situ* hybridization' Hb, haemoglobin; MDS/AML, myelodysplastic syndrome/acute myeloid leukemia; MMC, mitomycin C; PNH, paroxysmal nocturnal haemoglobinuria.

disease is graded according to the blood count parameters and bone marrow findings, as summarized in Table 22.3.11.1. The assessment of disease severity is important in treatment decisions and has prognostic significance. Patients with bi-or trilineage cytopenias which are less severe than this are not classified as aplastic anaemia. However, they should have their blood counts monitored to determine whether they will later develop aplastic anaemia.

Aetiology and incidence

Most cases (70–80%) of acquired aplastic anaemia are considered to be idiopathic. There is a biphasic age distribution with peaks from 10–25 years and >60 years. There is no significant difference in incidence between males and females. Because aplastic anaemia is a rare disease, only large national and international prospective studies will provide meaningful data on the aetiology of this condition. The incidence in the West is about 1 to 2 per million per year, but it occurs more commonly in eastern Asia, with a two- to four-fold higher incidence. Reasons for this difference in incidence are not known but may include infections and genetic factors. In rural areas of Thailand, the use of nonbottled water, agricultural pesticides, nonmedical needle exposures, and exposure of farmers to ducks and geese are significant environmental risk factors for developing aplastic anaemia.

Many drugs and chemicals have been implicated in the aetiology of aplastic anaemia, but for only a few is there strong evidence for an association, and even then it is usually impossible to prove causality (Table 22.3.11.2). A careful drug history must be obtained. Drug exposure in the year preceding presentation should be detailed. Earlier exposures should be recorded but are not likely to be relevant unless the particular drug or drug group has been taken again during the presumed critical period. If the patient is taking several drugs which may have been implicated in aplastic anaemia, even if the evidence is based on case report(s) alone, then all the putative drugs should be discontinued and the patient should not be rechallenged with the drugs at a later stage after recovery of the blood count. Drugs most commonly implicated include antibiotics and nonsteroidal anti-inflammatory drugs. Posthepatitic aplastic anaemia accounts for about 5% of all cases, in most cases being non-A, non-B, non-C, non-G. Patients usually present

with jaundice and hepatic symptoms, then, on average 6 weeks later, develop pancytopenia when the liver function has usually improved. Rarely aplastic anaemia follows EBV infection. Aplastic anaemia later develops in 10% of patients with haemolytic paroxysmal nocturnal haemoglobinuria. A careful occupational history may reveal exposure to chemicals or pesticides that have been associated with aplastic anaemia (see Table 22.3.11.2).

Pathogenesis

Aplastic anaemia is characterized by both a quantitative and qualitative defect in the haemopoietic stem cell compartment, while the bone marrow microenvironment functions normally in most patients, as assessed by long-term bone marrow cultures. The primitive long term culture-initiating cells and more mature haemopoietic progenitors in the bone marrow (colony-forming cells) of all cell lineages are reduced or absent. There is a reduction in the percentage of CD34+ bone marrow cells, and they are more apoptotic than normal CD34+ cells. Aplastic anaemia bone marrow cells also have shortened telomere length compared with normal bone marrow cells.

Table 22.3.11.2 Currently licensed drugs and occupational exposures reported as a probable cause of aplastic anaemia

(a) Currently licensed drugs	
Antibiotics	Chloramphenicol[a], sulphonamides, co-trimoxazole, linezolid
Anti-inflammatories	Phenylbutazone, indomethacin, diclofenac, naproxen, piroxicam, gold, penicillamine
Anticonvulsants	Phenytoin, carbamazepine
Antithyroid	Carbimazole[b], thiouracil
Antidepressants	Dothiepin, phenothiazides
Antidiabetic	Chlorpropamide, tolbutamide
Antimalarial	Chloroquine
Others	Mebendazole, thiazides[c], allopurinol

(b) Occupational and environmental exposures	
Evidence base	**Agent**
Benzene	Large industrial studies, case–control study from Thailand
Pesticides: organochlorines e.g. lindane; organophosphates; pentachlorophenol	Literature review of case reports and UK case–control study
Cutting oils and lubricating agents	UK case control study
Recreational drugs e.g. methylenedioxymethamphetamine (MDMA, ecstasy)	Case reports

[a] No association with chloramphenicol tablets was observed in case control study from Thailand. There is no evidence for an association between chloramphenicol eye drops and aplastic anaemia.
[b] More likely to cause neutropenia;
[c] From case–control study in Thailand.

Observations which support an autoimmune basis for the disease are: (1) there is evidence of HLA restriction with over-representation of HLA DR15; (2) stem cell transplants from identical twins fail to correct the defect unless prior immunosuppression is given; (3) 60 to 80% of patients respond to immunosuppressive therapy with antithymocyte globulin ± ciclosporin; (4) increased levels of interferon-γ and tumour necrosis factor-α, cytokines that inhibit haemopoiesis, are produced by mononuclear cells in aplastic anaemia; (5) there is increased Fas-antigen expression on bone marrow CD34+ cells, indicating increased apoptosis; (6) activated autoreactive cytotoxic T-cells are present in blood and bone marrow; (7) T-cell repertoire analysis shows oligoclonal expansion of CD8 T-cells; and (8) there is upregulation of apoptosis and immune response genes. See Fig. 22.3.11.1 for a summary of current knowledge on the proposed mechanism for immune destruction of haemopoiesis. However, specific target antigens have not been identified. Potential candidates, identified by screening antibodies in patients' serum against a peptide library, include kinectin, diazepam-binding inhibitor-related protein-1 (DRS-1), postmeiotic segregation increased 1 (PMS1), and moesin.

Clinical features

Patients with aplastic anaemia most commonly present with symptoms of anaemia and skin or mucosal haemorrhage (ecchymoses or petechiae), or visual disturbance due to retinal haemorrhage. Infection, particularly sore throat or failure of minor infections to clear, may be a presenting feature, but is less common. There is no lymphadenopathy or hepatosplenomegaly (in the absence of infection) and these findings strongly suggest another diagnosis. In children and young adults, the findings of inherited bone marrow failure disorders are listed in Table 22.3.11.3, but some affected patients may have none of these clinical features and the diagnosis is often made later after failure to respond to immunosuppressive therapy. A preceding history of jaundice, usually 2 to 3 months before, may indicate a posthepatitic aplastic anaemia.

Differential diagnosis

The following disorders may sometimes present with pancytopenia and a hypocellular bone marrow:

◆ Hypocellular MDS/acute myeloid leukaemia (AML); the presence of dysplastic granulocytic and megakaryocytic cells and blasts are not seen in aplastic anaemia.

◆ Hypocellular acute lymphoblastic leukaemia (ALL) occurs in 1–2% of cases of childhood ALL.

◆ Hairy-cell leukaemia classically presents with pancytopenia, monocytopenia., an interstitial infiltrate of hairy cells and increased bone marrow reticulin. Splenomegaly is a common finding.

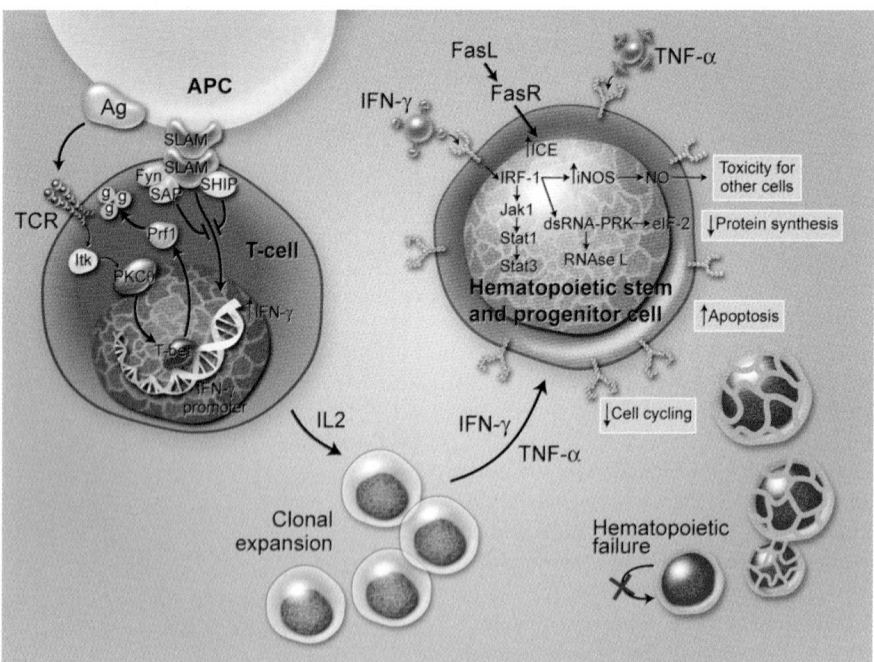

Fig. 22.3.11.1 Immune destruction of haemopoiesis. Antigens are presented to T-lymphocytes by antigen presenting cells (APCs), which trigger T-cells to activate and proliferate. T-bet, a transcription factor, binds to the interferon-γ (INF-γ) promoter region and induces gene expression. SAP binds to Fyn and modulates SLAM activity on IFN-γ expression, diminishing gene transcription. Patients with aplastic anaemia show constitutive T-bet expression and low SAP levels. IFN-γ and TNF-α up-regulate other T-cells' cellular receptors and also the Fas receptor. Increased production of interleukin-2 (IL-2) leads to polyclonal expansion of T-cells. Activation of Fas receptor by the Fas ligand leads to apoptosis of target cells. Some effects of IFN-γ are mediated through interferon regulatory factor 1 (IRF-1), which inhibits the transcription of cellular genes and entry into the cell cycle. IFN-γ is a potent inducer of many cellular genes, including inducible nitric oxide synthase (NOS), and production of the toxic gas nitric oxide (NO) may further diffuse toxic effects. These events ultimately lead to reduced cell cycling and cell death by apoptosis.
(This research was originally published in Young NS, Calado RT, Scheinberg P (2006). Current concepts in the pathophysiology and treatment of aplastic anaemia. *Blood*, **108**, 2509–19, © the American Society of Hematology.)

Table 22.3.11.3 Abnormalities associated with inherited bone marrow failure disorders

Abnormality	% of patients
Fanconi's anaemia	
Skeletal, e.g. aplasia/hypoplasia of thumb, radii, syndactyly, scoliosis	71
Skin—café-au-lait spots, hypopigmentation	64
Short stature	63
Microphthalmia	38
Renal—absent or misplaced kidney, horseshoe kidney	34
Cryptorchidism	20
Mental retardation	16
Gastrointestinal, e.g. anorectal and duodenal atresia	14
Cardiac	13
Deafness	11
No abnormalities	30
Shwachman–Diamond syndrome	
Exocrine pancreatic dysfunction	100
Skeletal—metaphysel dysostosis, osteoporosis	75, 80
Short stature	70
Icthyotic rash	60
Dental caries, dysplastic teeth	38, 14
Behavioural, developmental delay	common
Others—cleft palate, dysmorphic facial features, cardiac	
Dyskeratosis congenita	
Reticulate skin pigmentation	89
Nail dystrophy	88
Leukoplakia	78
Epiphora	30
Mental retardation/developmental delay	25
Pulmonary fibrosis	20
Short stature	20
Extensive dental caries/dental loss	17
Oesophageal stricture	17
Premature hair loss/greying/sparse eyelashes	16
Hyperhydrosis	15
Others—liver disease, peptic ulcer, enteropathy, osteoporosis, avascular necrosis, male genital, cerebellar hypoplasia	
Diamond—Blackfan anaemia	
Craniofacial dysmorphism, e.g. cleft palate, high arch palate, flat nasal bridge, hypertelorism	37
Short stature	28
Thumb anomalies	18
Others—cardiac, urogenital anomalies	
Congenital amegakaryocytic thrombocytopenia	See text
Thrombocytopenia with absent radii (TAR)	See text

Data obtained from the International Fanconi Anemia Registry, the Dyskeratosis Congenita Registry at Hammersmith Hospital, the UK Diamond–Blackfan Anaemia Registry, and a review on Shwachman–Diamond syndrome by Dror and Freedman (2002).

• Lymphomas, either Hodgkin's disease or non-Hodgkin's lymphoma, and myelofibrosis. Myelofibrosis is usually accompanied by splenomegaly.

• Mycobacterial infections, especially atypical infection. Other bone marrow abnormalities include granulomas, fibrosis, marrow necrosis, haemophagocytosis, and demonstrable acid–alcohol-fast bacilli.

• Anorexia nervosa or prolonged starvation. The bone marrow may show hypocellularity and gelatinous transformation (serous degeneration/atrophy) with loss of fat cells as well as haemopoietic cells, and increased ground substance.

Clinical investigation

The following investigations are required for the diagnosis.

Full blood count

This typically shows pancytopenia. In the early stages isolated cytopenia, particularly thrombocytopenia, may occur. Anaemia is accompanied by reticulocytopenia, and macrocytosis is common. Careful examination of the blood film is essential to exclude the presence of dysplastic neutrophils and platelets, blasts, and other abnormal cells such as hairy cells.

Bone marrow aspirate and trephine biopsy

The bone marrow is hypocellular with prominent fat spaces and variable amounts of residual haemopoietic cells. Erythroid precursors, megakaryocytes, and granulocytic precursors are reduced or absent. Lymphocytes, macrophages, plasma cells, and mast cells appear prominent. A trephine is crucial to assess overall cellularity and to exclude an abnormal infiltrate. Sometimes the bone marrow is patchy, with hypocellular and cellular areas (Fig. 22.3.11.2).

Liver function tests and virology

In posthepatitic aplastic anaemia the serology is usually negative for all the known hepatitis viruses. Blood should be sent to testing for hepatitis A antibody, hepatitis B surface antigen, hepatitis C antibody, and EBV. Parvovirus causes red cell aplasia but not aplastic anaemia. The CMV status of the patient should be determined.

Vitamin B_{12} and folate levels

These should be tested to exclude megaloblastic anaemia, which when severe can present with pancytopenia.

Antinuclear antibody and anti-DNA antibody

These should be tested to exclude systemic lupus erythematosus, a rare cause of aplastic anaemia.

Paroxysmal nocturnal haemoglobinuria (PNH) screen

The Ham test has been replaced as the diagnostic test for PNH by flow cytometry to identify clones of cells that lack glycosylphosphatidylinositol (GPI)-anchored proteins, such as CD55 and CD59. This is a sensitive and quantitative test for analysis of PNH populations.

Bone marrow cytogenetics

This should be done in all new cases. Abnormal cytogenetic clones may be present in up to 11% of patients with otherwise typical aplastic anaemia, and do not necessarily indicate myelodysplasia or leukaemia, but do require following carefully.

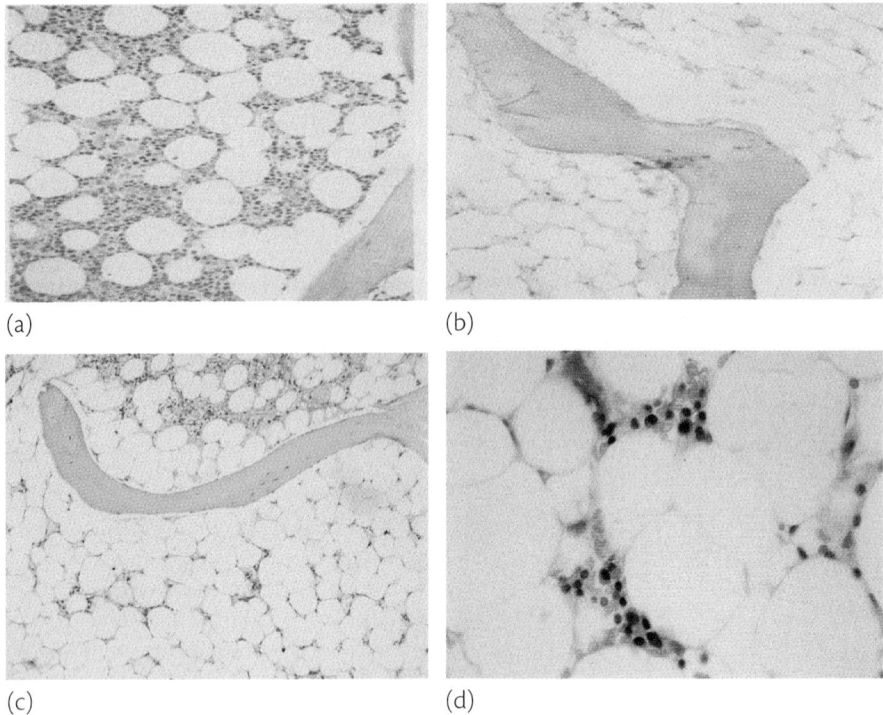

Fig. 22.3.11.2 Bone marrow trephine biopsy sections. A, normal bone, showing normal distribution of haemopoietic cells and fat cells within the bone trabeculum; B, severe aplastic anaemia showing replacement of haemopoietic cells by fat cells; C, nonsevere aplastic anaemia showing patchy distribution of remaining haemopoietic cells; D, high-power view of severe aplastic anaemia showing fat cells interspersed by lymphocytes andmacrophages.

Screen for inherited disorders

Peripheral blood lymphocytes, from all patients under the age of 35 years and older patients who are potential candidates for bone marrow transplanation, should be tested for chromosomal instability to identify or exclude Fanconi's anaemia (see later). Dyskeratosis congenita may be excluded by identifying a known mutation but there are probably many mutations yet to be identified. Screening for abnormally short telomeres in blood cells may become a practical possibility in the near future, a more reliable screening test for dyskeratosis congenita.

Chest radiograph and abdominal ultrasonography

These should be done to exclude infection and an enlarged spleen and/or enlarged lymph nodes, respectively. In younger patients, abnormal or anatomically displaced kidneys are features of Fanconi's anaemia.

Treatment and prognosis

Once the diagnosis is firmly established and the severity of the bone marrow suppression has been determined, the treatment plan for the patient should be mapped out and discussed. Treatment is influenced by age of the patient, disease severity, and the availability of a suitable stem cell donor.

Supportive care

Transfusions Initial treatment involves stabilizing the patient clinically with red-cell and platelet transfusions (and to treat infection or fevers with broad-spectrum intravenous antibiotics). Many centres give prophylactic platelet transfusions when the platelet count is below 10×10^9/litre (or higher in the presence of fever or bleeding). Purpura, menorrhagia, and spontaneous bleeding, mostly from the gums and buccal mucosa, usually develop below this level but there is also a risk of life-threatening haemorrhage, particularly in the presence of infection.

Transfusions may induce alloimmunization to leucocytes present in red-cell and platelet transfusions by generating human leucocyte antigen (HLA) or non-HLA (minor histocompatibility) antibodies or platelet specific antibodies which cause refractoriness to platelet transfusions. The use of leucocyte-depleted blood may reduce the risk of inducing HLA antibodies. If the patient does develop HLA antibodies, HLA-compatible platelets may be needed. Other important practical measures to help prevent bleeding include good dental hygiene, the use of oral tranexamic acid, and control of menorrhagia with appropriate hormone therapy.

Infections Patients with aplastic anaemia are at risk of bacterial and fungal infections, the level of risk depending on the degree of neutropenia. Severe neutropenia (neutrophils $<0.2 \times 10^9$/litre) carries a high risk of systemic infection arising from endogenous organisms. These include Gram-negative bacteria, *Pseudomonas aeruginosa*, enterobacteria, and Gram-positive *Staphylococcus epidermidis*. At neutrophil counts between 0.2 and 0.5×10^9/litre the risk of endogenous infection is less but acquired infection cannot be readily counteracted. Above 0.5×10^9/litre, response to infection is adequate though acquired infections should be promptly treated with appropriate antimicrobial drugs. Fungal infections, particularly aspergillus, occur in severe neutropenia.

If there is severe neutropenia, nonabsorbable antibiotics are usually given to reduce the potential pathogenic load from the gastrointestinal tract. Oral hygiene is important. Entry sites for venous access are potential sources of systemic infection. Fever should be treated with broad-spectrum antibiotics, without waiting for laboratory identification of organisms. Failure to respond is a strong indication of fungal infection. Granulocyte colony-stimulating factor (G-CSF) is usually ineffective in severe aplastic anaemia because of a severe reduction or absence of myeloid progenitor cells. G-CSF, erythropoietin, and other haemopoietic growth factors should not be used on their own in an attempt to treat aplastic anaemia, as the disorder is not caused by a deficiency of any known growth factors.

Psychological support Psychological support for the patient, family, and close friends is of great importance. Aplastic anaemia is a rare disease and requires careful explanation of its nature and prognosis. Patients should be given the opportunity to be referred to a centre that specializes in the management of aplastic anaemia. The chronic nature and slow response to treatment should be stressed early in the disease. There is an excellent patient support group based in the United Kingdom (http://www.theaat.org.uk).

Specific treatment
Algorithms for treatment of severe and nonsevere aplastic anaemia are shown in Fig. 22.3.11.3.

Bone marrow transplantation Bone marrow transplantation from an HLA-identical sibling donor is indicated as first-line treatment for patients with severe or very severe aplastic anaemia who are <40 years of age. Overall survival is 70 to 90% (Fig. 22.3.11.4). Results are less successful for patients >40 years of age and these patients should therefore receive immunosuppressive therapy with antithymocyte globulin (ATG) and ciclosporin as first-line treatment.

An immunosuppressive, nonmyeloablative conditioning regimen is employed, using cyclophosphamide 200 mg/kg body weight with or without ATG. Ciclosporin (usually with methotrexate) is given to suppress graft-vs-host disease (GVHD) and to aid engraftment. Irradiation should not be given. Children grow and develop normally and fertility is well preserved post transplant. Chronic GVHD and infection are the main causes of transplant related morbidity and mortality.

Graft rejection may be (1) early, with failure of engraftment of host cells, or (2) late, after initial engraftment. It occurs in 10 to 14% of patients. Mixed chimerism may occur in up to 25% of patients; low levels (<10% recipient cells) are associated with excellent survival and a low incidence of chronic GVHD.

It is recommended that bone marrow stem cells, and not G-CSF-mobilized peripheral blood stem cells, should be used for transplantation in aplastic anaemia. Although engraftment occurs earlier with peripheral blood stem cells, their use is associated with worse outcome, more chronic GVHD, and no reduction in risk of graft rejection. It is important to give at least 3×10^8 nucleated marrow cells/kg body weight to reduce the risk of graft rejection.

Unrelated donor bone marrow transplantation may be considered for young patients who have no HLA-compatible donor and who have failed treatment with immunosuppressive therapy. Patients should have a fully matched donor at both HLA class I and II antigens, and should receive a reduced intensity conditioning regimen. Unrelated donor bone marrow transplantation is not as successful as HLA identical sibling transplantation, but results show improvement in overall survival from 30 to 40% before 1999 to 60 to 70% in 2000–2005.

Immunosuppressive therapy (ATG and ciclosporin) ATG is a polyclonal IgG antibody preparation prepared by immunizing horses or rabbits with human thymocytes. Its mechanism of action in aplastic anaemia is not entirely clear, but may be partly due to depletion of autoreactive cytotoxic T-cells, in addition to direct stimulation of residual bone marrow CD34+ cells and a reduction in their degree of apoptosis. The response rate to ATG in severe aplastic anaemia is increased when it is combined with ciclosporin.

ATG and ciclosporin are indicated for patients who are ineligible for bone marrow transplantation or whose disease is not severe enough to warrant a transplant. This includes all patients >40 years of age, patients with nonsevere aplastic anaemia, and younger patients who have severe disease but who lack an HLA-identical sibling donor.

ATG is highly immunosuppressive and must be given as an inpatient treatment, preferably with patients nursed in isolation facilities. Response is delayed, rarely occurring before 3 to 4 months. Between 60 and 80% will respond and achieve normal or near-normal blood counts, but recovery is unstable. Relapse occurs in up to 30%, necessitating further treatment with ATG. Late clonal disorders such as paroxysmal nocturnal haemoglobinuria (PNH; see Chapter 22.3.12) or myelodysplastic syndrome/acute myeloid leukaemia may occur. Almost all patients with acquired aplastic anaemia have one or more small clones of PNH cells, but the proportion of cells is too low to produce symptoms. Retreatment with a second course of immunosuppression results in response rates of 30 to 60% for nonresponse and 50 to 60% for relapse after the first course. Good survival and quality of life is possible for most patients after ATG treatment (Fig. 22.3.11.5).

Patients with nonsevere aplastic anaemia who are not dependent on red-cell or platelet transfusions may remain stable for months or years without definitive treatment. They should have their blood count monitored regularly, and if it worsens such they require transfusions, they should then be treated with ATG and ciclosporin. Oral ciclosporin may be used on its own, although the response rate is lower than with the combination of ATG and ciclosporin.

Oxymetholone and corticosteroids Oxymetholone is still sometimes used in severe and nonsevere aplastic anaemia. Up to 25% of patients with severe refractory aplastic anaemia will respond to this drug. Response to androgens, particularly if no PNH clone is present, raises the possibility of a congenital cause for marrow failure. The hepatotoxicity and virilizing side effects often restrict their use. Corticosteroids have no role in the treatment of aplastic anaemia, other than helping to prevent serum sickness after treatment with ATG. Corticosteroids are not effective in treating the disease and merely increase the risk of infections and later complications such as avascular necrosis and osteoporosis.

Cyclophosphamide High dose cyclophosphamide (200 mg/kg body weight) without haemopoietic stem cell support has been proposed as another treatment for refractory aplastic anaemia. However, a prospective randomized study comparing cyclophosphamide and ciclosporin with ATG and ciclosporin was terminated prematurely because of a high incidence of systemic fungal infections and early deaths after cyclophosphamide. Because of the predictably prolonged period of neutropenia and thrombocytopenia, the use of cyclophosphamide in this way has not been met with much enthusiasm.

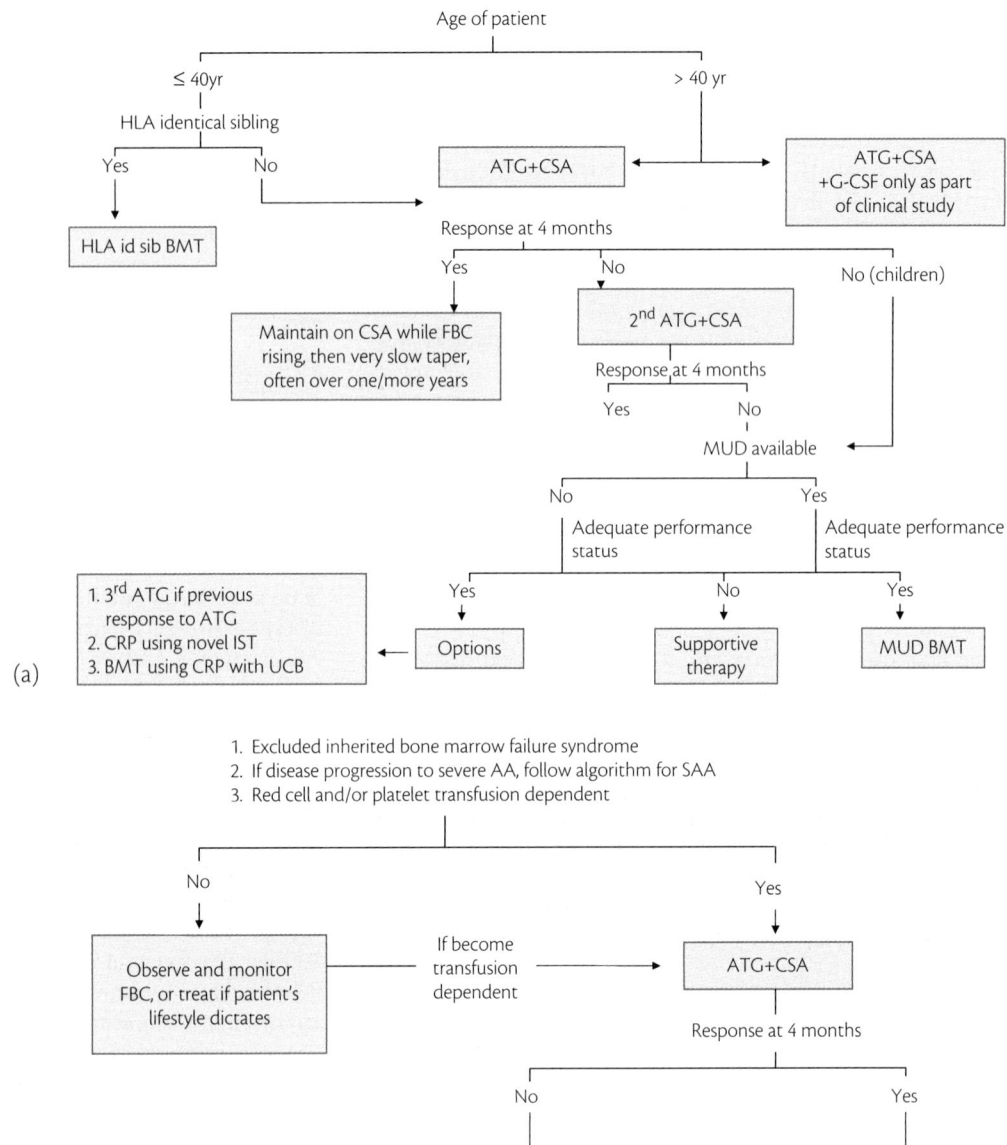

Fig. 22.3.11.3 Algorithms for treatment of acquired (a) severe and (b) nonsevere aplastic anaemia. ATG, antithymocyte globulin; CRP, clinical research protocol;CSA, ciclosporin; FBC, full blood count;G-CSF, granulocyte colony stimulating factor; HLA id sib, HLA-identical sibling; IST, immunosuppressive therapy; MUDBMT, matched unrelated donor bone marrow transplantation; SAA, severe aplastic anaemia; UCB, umbilical cord blood.

Congenital aplastic anaemia

The most common form of congenital aplastic anaemia is Fanconi's anaemia. Other examples are summarized in Table 22.3.11.3. Subclinical presentation of Fanconi's anaemia or dyskeratosis congenita, without the typical somatic anomalies of the disease, may result in delayed diagnosis in adult patients with apparent acquired aplastic anaemia.

Fanconi's anaemia

Genetics, incidence, and epidemiology

Fanconi's anaemia is an autosomal recessive (OMIM 227 650), or very rarely an X-linked (FA-B group) disorder and is characterized by somatic anomalies (Table 22.3.11.3). The prevalence of Fanconi's anaemia is estimated to be 1–5 per million and the overall frequency of the heterozygote is 1 in 300, but higher in South African Afrikaaners and Ashkenasy Jews.

Clinical features

The skin often shows café-au-lait spots or areas of hyper- or depigmentation. Other anomalies include skeletal (absent thumbs, radii), genitourinary,and renal anomalies. The blood count at birth is usually normal, but infants are often of low birth weight and retain short stature in later life. Most patients present between 5 and 10 years of age with pancytopenia, although some present later in adolescence or early adulthood, and occasionally in the fourth or fifth decade.

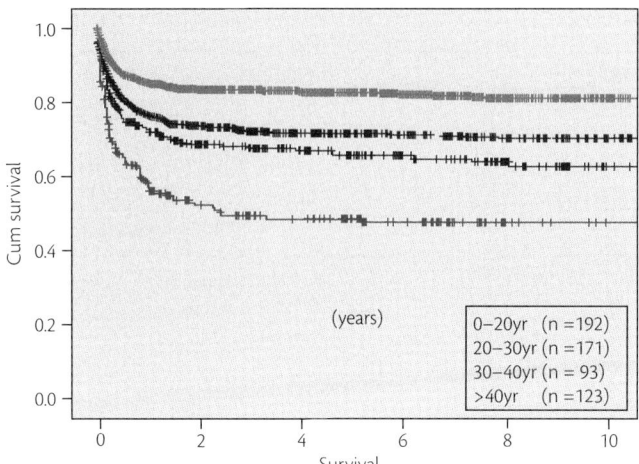

Fig. 22.3.11.4 Overall survival after bone marrow transplantation for acquired severe aplastic anaemia, from HLA-identical sibling donors.
(Data for HLA-identical sibling transplants obtained with permission from the European Blood and Marrow Transplant (EBMT) Severe Aplastic Anaemia Working Party, 2006.)

Patients commonly present with bleeding due to thrombocytopenia and anaemia with relative preservation of the neutrophil count. The bone marrow becomes progressively more hypocellular, often with evidence of haemophagocytosis. There is an increased risk of malignancy, especially acute myeloid leukaemia, and also solid tumours, particularly hepatocellular carcinoma and squamous cell carcinoma of the head and neck, vulva, and oesophagus. The risk of liver tumours is increased further in Fanconi's anaemia patients treated with anabolic steroids. By the age of 40 years, the cumulative incidences of bone marrow failure, haematological malignancy, or a solid tumour are 90%, 33%, and 28%, respectively.

Laboratory diagnosis
Fanconi's anaemia is a chromosome instability syndrome due to failure of DNA repair, accounting for the ineffective haemopoiesis and increased risk of malignancy. Fanconi's anaemia cells are

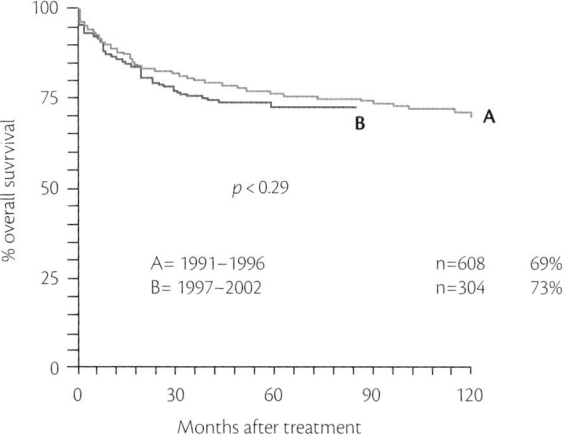

Fig. 22.3.11.5 Survival curves for treatment of aplastic anaemia with immunosuppression in two time periods: 1991–1996 and 1997–2003.
(Data from the EBMT Severe Aplastic Anaemia Register 2007. Reproduced from Locasciulli A, et al. (2007). Outcome of patients with acquired aplastic anemia given first line bone marrow transplantation or immunosuppressive treatment in the last decade: a report from the European Group for Blood and Marrow Transplantation (EBMT). Haematologica, **92**, 11–18.)

hypersensitive to cross-linking agents such as diepoxybutane (DEB) and mitomycin C. This forms the basis of the diagnostic test for Fanconi's anaemia (the DEB stress test). Chromosome breakages and aberrations are increased, especially on exposure to low concentrations of DEB (or mitomycin C). This test is usually performed on cultured peripheral blood lymphocytes.

Molecular biology
Complementation analysis of somatic cell hybrids has revealed 12 complementation groups, and so far genes for 11 complementation groups have been cloned. These genes are involved in the DNA repair process. Of interest, the D1 (*FANCD1*) gene is identical to *BRCA2*, the gene for breast cancer susceptibility. Fanconi's anaemia subtype based on complementation group shows some correlation with phenotype although there is variation within a specific group.

Treatment and prognosis
Supportive care, with blood and platelet transfusions, antibiotic therapy, anabolic steroids, and haemopoietic growth factors, is important for the survival of patients. Oxymetholone induces a trilineage haematological response in approximately 60% of patients. Most patients who respond later relapse, but it is a useful drug to help maintain blood counts while planning for bone marrow transplantation. Regular monitoring of liver function and liver ultrasonography is important for early detection of liver complications of oxymetholone, i.e. peliosis hepatis and liver tumours. The virilizing side effects in female patients and behavioural problems in children often restrict the use of oxymetholone. Bone marrow transplantation is the only treatment option that can restore normal haemopoiesis. Genetic counselling is of major importance to identify the familial nature of the disease, and particularly to screen siblings who may be potential bone marrow donors.

The actuarial survival after HLA-identical sibling bone marrow transplantation is 70 to 80%. The conditioning regimen employs a reduced dose of cyclophosphamide and total body irradiation (or fludarabine) compared to patients transplanted with acquired aplastic anaemia, due to hypersensitivity to these agents. If there is no compatible sibling donor, a search is made for a volunteer unrelated donor. The results of unrelated donor bone marrow transplantation are less good, with survival of around 20 to 40%. The outlook is poor for those patients who lack an HLA-identical bone marrow donor.

Dyskeratosis congenita
Clinical features
Dyskeratosis congenita is a disorder of telomerase. Most cases are diagnosed in adulthood with the classical clinical features of this syndrome (leukoplakia, nail dystrophy, and reticulated skin pigmentation), although other features, for example, osteoporosis or pulmonary fibrosis, may occur (see Table 22.3.11.3).

Genetics and molecular biology
DKC1 gene mutations occur in X-linked dyskeratosis congenita (OMIM 305000) and *TERC* gene (encodes the RNA component of telomerase) mutations in autosomal dominant dyskeratosis congenita (OMIM 127550). The genetic basis for the autosomal recessive form of dyskeratosis congenita is unknown. *TERC* or *TERT* (reverse transcriptase component of telomerase) gene mutations have recently been detected in 1 to 5% of adults with apparent

acquired aplastic anaemia who lack clinical features of dyskeratosis congenita (subclinical dyskeratosis congenita).

Treatment

Oxymetholone often induces a remission of variable duration, and transient responses may be seen with G-CSF or erythropoietin. Allogeneic bone marrow transplantation is indicated for severe bone marrow failure but late pulmonary and vascular complications contribute to transplant-related mortality, despite the use of reduced-intensity conditioning regimens.

Shwachman–Diamond syndrome

Shwachman–Diamond syndrome (OMIM 260 400) is an autosomal recessive disorder associated with exocrine pancreatic dysfunction and bone marrow dysfunction and other features (see Table 22.11.3.3). Neutropenia occurs commonly (with defects in neutrophil chemotaxis), but about 40% develop additional cytopenias, including aplastic anaemia. Patients are also at risk of myelodysplasia or acute myeloid leukaemia. *SBDS* gene mutations are found in about 80% of patients. The gene codes for a protein which may function in RNA metabolism and translation. G-CSF often improves the neutropenia, and oxymetholone may induce temporary remission of aplastic anaemia. Bone marrow transplantation may be considered for severe bone marrow failure or acute leukaemia.

Bone marrow failure affecting the erythroid cell lineage: pure red-cell aplasia

Criteria for diagnosis

There is defective maturation of red-cell precursors in pure red-cell aplasia, with failure to produce reticulocytes and hence mature red cells. The block in maturation may occur at the level of early (burst-forming unit, BFU-e) or late (colony-forming unit, CFU-e) erythroid progenitors, resulting in an absence of erythroid precursors in the bone marrow, or at the early normoblast stage producing a maturation arrest in the bone marrow with absence of late normoblasts. This results in a normocytic, normochromic anaemia with severe reticulocytopenia. The neutrophil and platelet counts are normal.

Aetiology and pathogenesis

Conditions associated with pure red cell aplasia are listed in Table 22.3.11.4. Diamond–Blackfan anaemia (DBA) is a rare, congenital form of pure red-cell aplasia usually presenting in infancy with normochromic macrocytic anaemia, reticulocytopenia, and reduced bone marrow erythroid precursors. Most cases are sporadic, but some families show a dominant or recessive inheritance. It is often associated with short stature and various skeletal anomalies (see Table 22.3.11.3). The red-cell adenine deaminase concentration is elevated in affected subjects and may be elevated in family members who have no anaemia but who none the less have defective erythropoiesis. Hb F level is raised. Mutations in the ribosomal protein S19 gene (*RPS19*) are found in 25% of affected individuals and the *RPS24* gene in 2%. Another DBA gene is linked to chromosome 8p23.3-22.

Transient erythroblastopenia of childhood describes the sudden onset of anaemia with reticulocytopenia and absent erythroid

Table 22.3.11.4 Conditions associated with pure red-cell aplasia

Condition	Comments
Congenital	
Diamond–Blackfan anaemia	Most cases are sporadic, dominant and recessive inheritance also reported
Transient erythroblastopenia of childhood	Often follows an acute viral illness
Acquired idiopathic	Immune-mediated; account for majority of cases
Systemic lupus erythematosus, rheumatoid arthritis, Sjögren's disease	Immune-mediated
Thymoma (often associated with myasthenia gravis and hypogammaglobulinaemia	Immune-mediated
Drugs, e.g. phenytoin, isoniazid, procainamide, azathioprine	Direct marrow toxicity, drug-dependent antibodies
Erythropoietin in chronic kidney disease	Antierythropoietin antibodies
B-cell lymphoproliferative disorders, e.g. lymphoma, chronic lymphocytic leukaemia	Immune-mediated: suppression of erythropoiesis by T-large granular lymphocytes
T-LGL/TCUS	Mechanism? Release of inhibitory cytokines; direct cytotoxicity of erythroid cells
Myelodysplastic syndrome	Mechanism? Extreme apoptosis of red cell progenitors
Parvovirus B19 infection; CMV, EBV infection rarely	Lysis of late erythroid progenitors (CFU-e) and red cell precursors by B19 virus (receptor is P blood group antigen)
ABO-incompatible haemopoietic stem cell transplantation	Recipient antibody against incompatible donor ABO blood group antigens may inhibit red cell regeneration
Rarely, pregnancy	Mechanism unknown

CMV, cytomegalovirus; DEB, diepoxybutane; EBV, Epstein–Barr virus; FISH, fluorescence *in situ* hybridization; MMC, mitomycin C; TCUS, T-cell clonopathy of uncertain significance; T-LGL, T-cell large granular lymphocyte proliferative disease.

precursors in the bone marrow of children, often following an acute viral illness. There are no associated somatic anomalies.

Many cases of acquired pure red cell aplasia are idiopathic and immune in origin (Table 22.3.11.4). A thymoma occurs in up to 10% of patients with pure red-cell aplasia and up to 5% of patients with thymoma have red-cell aplasia. The red-cell aplasia may precede, accompany, or follow the development of the thymoma. Associated findings with thymoma are myasthenia gravis and hypo-γ-globulinaemia. A long list of drugs has been incriminated in the aetiology of red-cell aplasia, but the association is very rare and mostly there is only a single case for each drug. Exceptions are azathioprine, phenytoin, procainamide, and isoniazid, for which several cases each have been reported. Severe and sudden onset of red-cell aplasia due to recombinant human erythropoietin was previously reported. This was associated with antierythropoietin antibodies, and in most cases, with use of epoetin-α (Eprex) when given subcutaneously in chronic kidney disease. It was most likely due to changes in the formulation of the drug.

Pure red-cell aplasia may occur in association with other systemic autoimmune disorders, and with other haematological disorders including B-cell lymphoproliferative disorders, namely lymphoma and chronic lymphocytic leukaemia (CLL). In T-cell clonopathy of uncertain significance (TCUS), a variant of T-cell large granular lymphocyte proliferative disorders, T-cell gene rearrangement can be demonstrated but in the absence of malignancy. In such cases the red-cell aplasia often responds well to immunosuppressive therapy. Transient red-cell aplasia is seen with acute parvovirus B19 infection in patients with haemolytic anaemias (so called 'aplastic crisis'). The receptor for the virus is the blood group P antigen expressed on CFU-e, red-cell progenitors, and mature red cells. The virus invades and destroys the cells, resulting in sudden and severe anaemia with reticulocytopenia.

Clinical investigation

See Box 22.3.11.1.

Treatment and prognosis

Transient erythroblastopenia of childhood recovers spontaneously, usually after a few weeks, although the patient may require blood transfusions support during this time.

The first line of treatment for Diamond–Blackfan anaemia is blood transfusions followed by corticosteroids; 20% respond, requiring no further transfusions or steroids, and 40% become transfusion independent but needing continuous corticosteroids. Some patients develop major side effects if the condition is steroid dependent. The remaining patients are refractory or later become refractory to steroids and require long-term transfusions, along with iron chelation therapy to help prevent complications of transfusional haemosiderosis. Splenectomy may be required, as the spleen may later enlarge and result in increased transfusional requirements due to hypersplenism. Haemopoietic stem cell transplantation has been performed in some patients with transfusion-dependent DBA who have an HLA-identical sibling donor, as this is potentially curative but is still associated with significant transplant-related mortality and morbidity.

For acquired pure red-cell aplasia, blood transfusions are required until recovery occurs. Any drugs that have been implicated in the disease should be discontinued. Thymectomy should be considered in patients with a thymoma, although recent

studies report variable response rates of 0 to 25%. Immunosupression with ciclosporin or ATG is often effective but may be complicated by infections. Intravenous immunoglobulin (IVIG) is indicated for parvovirus-induced red-cell aplasia. For other patients, prednisolone starting at 1 mg/kg body weight per day is used as first-line therapy, given for 4 weeks then slowly tapering the dose. Approximately 50% of patients respond to prednisolone. For nonresponders, remission may be induced by azathioprine or ciclosporin (with or without ATG), and there have been reports of response to cyclophosphamide and vincristine. There are anecdotal reports on the use of monoclonal antibody therapy with alemtuzumab (anti-CD52) and rituximab (anti-CD20) for treatment of refractory red-cell aplasia and other autoimmune cytopenias. The optimal treatment of pure red-cell aplasia is restricted by the rarity of the condition.

Likely future developments

It is likely that pathogenetic mechanisms other than autoimmunity occur in patients with aplastic anaemia, particularly those who fail to respond to immunosuppressive therapy. Genetic predisposition to developing aplastic anaemia has already identified in 1 to 5% of patients who have *TERC* or *TERT* gene mutations, and other genes may be involved in the telomerase repair process and genes of the immune response, which may in future help to select specific treatment options.

Identification of potential antigenic targets on aplastic anaemia haemopoietic stem cells for autoimmune attack is under investigation. Early screening for clonal evolution may guide management decisions.

Novel transplant approaches are needed for those patients who lack an HLA-matched bone marrow donor. Double umbilical cord blood transplantation and haploidentical haemopoietic stem cell transplantation are showing promise for haematological malignancies, but it is, as yet, uncertain if they will overcome the major problem of graft rejection in transplantation for aplastic anaemia.

Further reading

Bacigalupo A, *et al.* (2000). Treatment of acquired severe aplastic anemia: Bone marrow transplantation compared with immunosuppressive therapy—The European Group for blood and marrow transplantation experience. *Semin Haematol*, **37**, 69–80. [European registry data comparing treatment options.]

Bacigalupo, *et al.* (2005). Fludarabine, cyclophosphamide and ATG for alternative donor transplants in acquired severe aplastic anaemia—a report of the EBMT SAA Working Party. *Bone Marrow Transplant*, **36**, 947–50. [Multicentre study showing recent improvement in outcome.]

Ball SE, *et al.* (1996). Diamond–Blackfan anaemia in the UK—analysis of 80 cases from a 20-year birth cohort. *Br J Haematol*, **94**, 645–53. [This UK registry summarizes the clinical features.]

Bennett CL, *et al.* (2004). Pure red-cell aplasia and epoetin therapy. *N Engl J Med*, **351**, 1403–8. [Summary of the significance of this problem.]

Calado RT, Young NS (2009). Telomere diseases. *New Engl J Med*, **361**, 2353–65. [Authoritative review of role of telomeres in bone marrow failure.]

Camitta BM (2000). What is the definition of cure for aplastic anemia? *Acta Hematol*, **103**, 16–18. [Key report from an international working group summarizing diagnostic criteria and response criteria to immunosuppressive therapy.]

Box 22.3.11.1   Clinical investigation of red-cell aplasia

- Full blood count and blood film show normocytic, normochromic anaemia

- Reticulocyte count shows a severe reticulocytopenia

- Bone marrow aspirate and trephine biopsy—examine for a secondary cause of red-cell aplasia

- Immunophenotyping and gene rearrangement studies for heavy chain and T-cell receptor monoclonal expansion

- Chest radiograph and CT of thorax to exclude thymoma

- Autoimmune profile

- Parvovirus B19, cytomegalovirus, and EBV serology

- Red-cell adenine deaminase and Hb F level (both increased in Diamond–Blackfan anaemia)

Champlin R, *et al.* (2007). Bone marrow transplantation for severe aplastic anemia: a randomized controlled study of conditioning regimens. *Blood*, **109**, 4582–5. [Trial showing no difference in outcome comparing conditioning using cyclophosphamide and ATG with cyclophosphamide alone.]

Davies JK, Guinan EC (2007). An update on the management of severe idiopathic aplastic anaemia in children. *Br J Haematol*, **136**, 549–64. [A key review.]

De Winter JP, Joenje H (2009). The genetic and molecular basis of Fanconi Anemia. *Mutation Research*, **668**,11–19 (Review of FA genes in DNA repair).

Dokal I (2000). Dyskeratosis congenita in all its forms. *Br J Haematol*, **110**, 768–79. [Key summary including clinical data from the UK Dyskeratosis congenita register. See also reference by Walne and Dokal.]

Dror Y, Freedman M (2002). Shwachman–Diamond syndrome. *Br J Haematol*, **118**, 701–13. [A key review of clinical features and management.]

Fisch P, Handgretinger R, Schaefer H-E (2000). Pure red cell aplasia. *Br J Haematol*, **111**, 1010–22. [Useful overview of the condition.]

Flygare J, Karlsson S (2007). Diamond-Blackfan anemia: erythropoiesis lost in translation. *Blood*, **109**, 3152–60. [Comprehensive review of recent advances in pathogenesis and molecular basis of this condition.]

Frickhofen N, *et al.* (2003). Antithymocyte globulin with or without cyclosporin A: 11-year follow-up of a randomized trial comparing treatments of aplastic anemia. *Blood*, **101**, 1236–42. [Trial showing superiority of combination of ATG and ciclosporin over ATG alone.]

Georges GE, Storb R (2004). Allogeneic hematopoietic stem cell transplantation for aplastic anaemia. In: Blume KG, Forma SJ, Appelbaum FR (eds) Thomas' hematopoietic cell transplantation, pp 981–1001. Blackwell, Oxford. [Comprehensive review including historical evolution of advances in transplantation for aplastic anaemia.]

Gluckman E, *et al.* (2002). Results and follow-up of a phase III randomized study of recombinant human-granulocyte stimulating factor as support for immunosuppressive therapy in patients with severe aplastic anaemia. *Br J Haematol*, **119**, 1075–82. [Multicentre European trial showing no difference in response or survival using G-CSF.]

Gupta V, *et al.* (2004). Favourable effect on acute and chronic graft-versus-host disease with cyclophosphamide and in vivo anti-CD52 monoclonal antibodies for marrow transplantation from HLA-identical sibling donors for acquired aplastic anemia. *Biol Blood Marrow Transplant*, **10**, 867–76. [Only study to date showing a major reduction in incidence of chronic graft versus host disease.]

Issaragrisil S, *et al.* (2006). The epidemiology of aplastic anemia in Thailand. *Blood*, **107**, 1299–307. [Largest case–control study on the epidemiology of aplastic anaemia.]

Kuijpers T, *et al.* (2005). Hematologic abnormalities in Shwachman Diamond syndrome: lack of genotype-phenotype relationship. *Blood*, **106**, 356–61. [Useful summary of this condition.]

Kutler D, *et al.* (2003). A 20-year perspective on the International Fanconi Anemia Registry (IFAR). *Blood*, **101**, 1249–56. [Key summary of clinical features and long-term disease outcome.]

Marsh J, *et al.* (1999). Prospective randomised multicentre study comparing cyclosporine alone versus the combination of antithymocyte globulin and cyclodporin for treatment of patients with non-severe aplastic anaemia: a report from the European Blood and Marrow Transplant (EBMT) Severe Aplastic Anaemia Working Party. *Blood*, **93**, 2191–5. [Important trial showing superiority of combination of ATG and ciclosporin over ciclosporin alone.]

Marsh JC, *et al.* (2004). Guidelines for the diagnosis and management of acquired aplastic anaemia. *Br J Haematol*, **123**, 782–801. [Key national guidelines.]

Schrezenemeir H, *et al.* (2007). Worse outcome and more chronic GVHD using peripheral blood stem cells compared with bone marrow in HLA-matched sibling donor transplants for young patients with severe acquired aplastic anemia. *Blood*, 110, 1397–400. [First study to show the impact of the source of stem cells on outcome after transplantation for aplastic anaemia.]

Socie G, *et al.* (2007). Granulocyte-stimulating factor and severe aplastic anemia: a survey by the European Group for Blood and Marrow Transplantation (EBMT). *Blood*, **109**, 2794–6. [Large study highlighting the risk of myelodysplastic syndrome and acute myeloid leukaemia when using G-CSF with immunosuppressive therapy.]

Taniguchi T, D'Andrea AD (2006). Molecular pathogenesis of Fanconi anemia: recent progress. *Blood*, **107**, 4223–3. [Major review of this condition.]

Thompson CA, Steensma DP (2006). Pure red cell aplasia associated with thymoma: clinical insights from a 50-year single institutional experience. *Br J Haematol*, **135**, 405–7. [Invaluable experience of this rare association, particularly relating to therapeutic outcomes.]

Tisdale JF, *et al.* (2000). High dose cyclophosphamide in severe aplastic anemia: a randomised trial. *Lancet*, **356**, 1554–9. [Important trial demonstrating high mortality and morbidity using high dose cyclophosphamide without stem cell support.]

Walne AJ, Dokal I (2009). Advances in the understanding of dyskeratosis congenita. *Br J Haematol*, **145**, 164–172 (Definitive review).

Young NS, Calado RT, Scheinberg P (2006). Current concepts in the pathophysiology and treatment of aplastic anaemia. *Blood*, **108**, 2509–19. [A key review.]

22.3.12 **Paroxysmal nocturnal haemoglobinuria**

Lucio Luzzatto

Essentials

Paroxysmal nocturnal haemoglobinuria (PNH) is a unique disorder in which a substantial proportion of the patient's red cells have an abnormal susceptibility to activated complement. This results from the presence of a clone that originates from a haematopoietic stem cell bearing an acquired somatic mutation in the X-linked gene *PIGA* , required for the biosynthesis of the glycanphosphatidylinositol molecule which anchors many proteins to the cell membrane, including the complement regulators CD59 and CD55. Clinical features and diagnosis—the 'classical' presentation is with 'passing blood instead of urine' (haemoglobinuria). Sometimes the patient presents with the full triad of (1) haemolytic anaemia, (2) pancytopenia, and (3) thrombosis—most commonly of intra-abdominal veins. An element of bone marrow failure is always present; and sometimes the disease may be preceded by or may evolve to bone marrow aplasia indistinguishable from acquired aplastic anaemia. Definitive diagnosis is based on demonstrating the presence of a discrete population of 'PNH red blood cells' by flow cytometry using anti-CD59.

Definition

Paroxysmal nocturnal haemoglobinuria (PNH) is an acquired chronic disorder characterized by persistent intravascular haemolysis, subject to recurrent exacerbations, often associated with pancytopenia, and with a distinct tendency to venous thrombosis. The triad of haemolytic anaemia, pancytopenia, and thrombosis makes PNH a truly unique clinical condition: however, even in the absence of one or more of these manifestations a conclusive diagnosis can be made by appropriate laboratory investigations (see below).

Epidemiology

PNH is encountered in all populations throughout the world, and it can affect people of all socioeconomic groups. The prevalence of PNH is not accurately known: however, it is more rare than the related disorder, acquired aplastic anaemia (AAA). A rough estimate of the frequency of PNH is between 1 in 100 000 and 1 in 1 million. Like AAA, PNH may be somewhat less rare in south-east and east Asia. Most patients present as young adults, but we have seen PNH in a 2-year-old child and in people in their seventies. PNH has never been reported as a congenital disease, and there is no reported evidence of inherited susceptibility. The sex ratio is not far from even.

Clinical features

The patient may seek medical attention because, one morning, he or she has 'passed blood instead of urine'. This distressing or frightening event—the direct evidence of haemoglobinuria—may be regarded as the classical presentation; however, not infrequently the patient presents as a problem in the differential diagnosis of anaemia, whether symptomatic or discovered incidentally. The anaemia may be associated with jaundice (suggesting haemolytic anaemia), and/ or with neutropenia, thrombocytopenia, or both. Venous thrombosis may be the first clinical manifestation in other patients. Although any vein may be affected, the most common localization is intra-abdominal: indeed, recurrent attacks of severe abdominal pain defying a specific diagnosis, and sometimes eventually found to be related to thrombosis, have given to PNH the attribute of being a great impostor. On the other hand, when thrombosis affects the hepatic veins it may produce acute hepatomegaly and ascites—i.e. a fully fledged Budd–Chiari syndrome.

The natural history of PNH can extend over decades. Without treatment the median survival is estimated to be about 8 to 10 years (see Fig. 22.3.12.1) but now several forms of treatment are possible in the past the most common causes of death have been thrombosis, or infection associated with severe neutropenia, or haemorrhage associated with severe thrombocytopenia. PNH may evolve to bone marrow aplasia undistinguishable from AAA; and more frequently PNH may manifest itself in patients who previously had AAA. Rarely (estimated 1–2% of all cases), PNH may terminate in acute myeloid leukaemia. On the other hand, full spontaneous recovery from PNH has been also well documented.

Laboratory investigations and diagnosis

The most consistent blood finding is anaemia, which may range from mild to moderate to very severe. The anaemia is usually normomacrocytic; a high mean cell volume (MCV) is usually largely accounted for by reticulocytosis, which may be quite

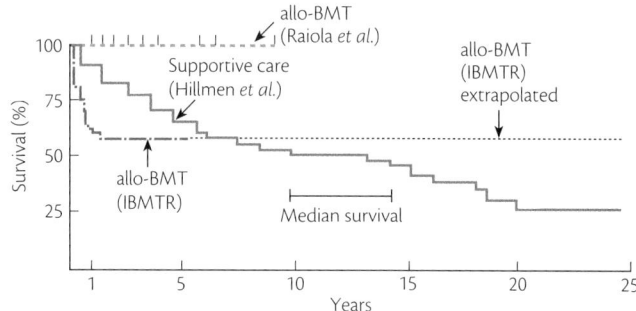

Fig. 22.3.12.1 PNH is a chronic disorder, the time course of which is often measured in decades. From a series of 80 patients who received only minimal supportive treatment we estimate a median survival of about 10 years. Allogeneic bone marrow reansplanation has still been associated with significant mortality, and therefore may have reduced the survival of some patients; but more encouraging results have been reported on a small series from a single centre.

marked—up to 20%. The anaemia may become microcytic if the patient is allowed to become iron-deficient as a result of chronic urinary blood loss through haemoglobinuria. The red cell morphology is otherwise usually normal. There may be neutropenia and/or thrombocytopenia. Unconjugated bilirubin is mildly or moderately elevated; lactate dehydrogenase (LDH) is typically markedly elevated; haptoglobin is usually undetectable. All these findings make the diagnosis of haemolytic anaemia compelling. Haemoglobinuria may be overt in a random urine sample: if it is not, it may be helpful to obtain serial urine samples, since haemoglobinuria can vary dramatically from day to day, and even from hour to hour (it is more common, but not always, in the early morning: hence the adjective 'nocturnal'). Obviously, haemoglobinuria must be distinguished from haematuria. Surprisingly, even today a patient may undergo extensive urological investigations before it is realized that the patient has PNH. There may be free haemoglobin in the serum, and sometimes this is so high as to interfere with clinical chemistry. These findings clearly indicate intravascular haemolysis, thus increasing, by an order of magnitude, the likelihood that the haemolytic anaemia is in fact PNH (see Table 22.3.12.1). The bone marrow is usually cellular, with marked to massive erythroid hyperplasia, often with mild to moderate dyserythropoietic features. However, at some stage of the disease the marrow may become hypocellular or even frankly aplastic (see below).

The definitive diagnosis of PNH must be based on the demonstration that a substantial proportion of the patient's red cells have an increased susceptibility to complement, due to the deficiency on their surface of proteins that normally protect the red cells from activated complement. For decades this has been done reliably b using the acidified serum (Ham–Dacie) test. Nowadays the gold standard is the demonstration of a discrete population of 'PNH red blood cells' by flow cytometry, using anti-CD59 or anti-CD48. This analysis is quantitative, and it has a higher sensitivity when applied to granulocytes (see Fig. 22.3.12.2).

Pathophysiology

Haemolysis

Haemolysis in PNH is due to an intrinsic abnormality of the red cell, which makes it exquisitely sensitive to activated complement, whether it is activated through the alternative pathway or through

Table 22.3.12.1 Differential diagnosis of dark urine

Different sorts of dark urine	Causes	Additional tests	Possible diagnosis
Haematuria	Many	Clears on centrifugation	Mostly urinary tract pathology
Myoglobinuria	Rhabdomyolysis	Ultrafiltration; spectroscopy	March myoglobinuria
Haemoglobinuria	Intravascular haemolysis	Serology after blood transfusion	Incompatible blood transfusion
		Donath–Landsteiner antibody	Paroxysmal cold haemoglobinuria
		G6PD activity	G6PD deficiency
		Blood film for malaria parasites	'Blackwater fever'
		Ham; flow cytometry for CD59	PNH

G6PD, glucose-6-phosphate dehydrogenase; PNH, paroxysmal nocturnal haemoglobinuria.

an antigen–antibody reaction. The former mechanism is probably the reason why there is chronic intravascular haemolysis in PNH. The latter mechanism explains why the haemolysis can be dramatically exacerbated in the course of a viral or bacterial infection. Hypersusceptibility to complement is due to the deficiency of several protective membrane proteins, of which CD59 is the most important, because it hinders the insertion into the membrane of C9 polymers.

The molecular basis for the deficiency of these proteins has been pinpointed not to a defect in any of the respective genes,

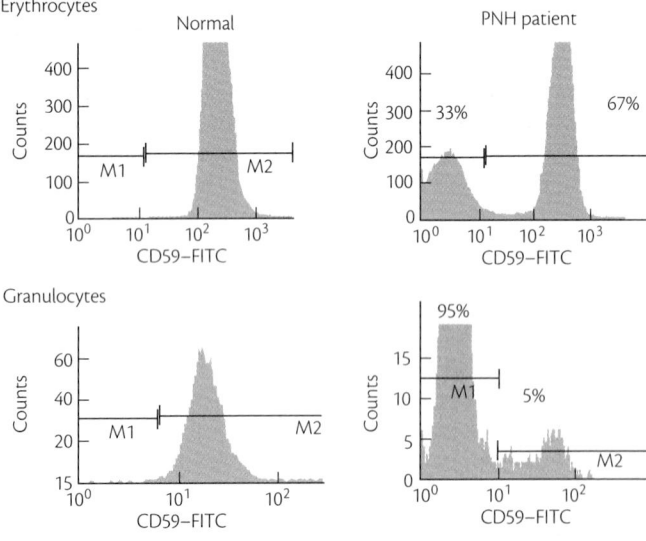

Fig. 22.3.12.2 Flow cytometry analysis of blood cells in a patient with PNH. On the left, red cells and granulocytes from a normal person display a unimodal distribution of surface expression of the GPI-linked protein CD59, which protects red cells against complement-mediated lysis. On the right, a similar analysis reveals, in a patient with PNH, a clearly bimodal distribution: from this analysis the size of the PNH cell population can be quantified. (Courtesy of Dr David Araten.)

but rather to the shortage of a unique glycolipid molecule, glycosyl phosphatidyl inositol (GPI), which, through a peptide bond, anchors these proteins to the surface membrane of cells. The shortage of GPI is due in turn to a mutation in an X-linked gene, called *PIGA*, required for an early step in GPI biosynthesis. In virtually each patient the *PIGA* mutation is different. This is not surprising, since these mutations are not inherited: rather, each one takes place *de novo* in a haemopoietic stem cell (in other words, they are somatic mutations). As a result, the patient's bone marrow is a mosaic of mutant and nonmutant cells, and the peripheral blood always contains both GPI-negative PNH cells and GPI-positive cells (see Fig. 22.3.12.2).

Thrombosis

This is one of the most immediately life-threatening complications of PNH, and yet one of the least understood pathogenetically. It could be due to impaired fibrinolysis, because the urokinase plasminogen Activator Receptor (uPAR) is a GPI-linked protein; more likely, complement activation could cause hypercoagulability, or hyperactivity of platelets, or both.

Bone marrow failure and the relationship between PNH and AAA

PNH has an intimate link with AAA, which manifests in several ways. (1) As stated above, sometimes a patient with PNH becomes 'less haemolytic' and 'more pancytopenic' and ultimately evolves to frank AAA. (2) In terms of pathogenesis, AAA is regarded as an organ-specific autoimmune disease mediated by 'activated' cytotoxic (CD8+) T lymphocytes, which are able to inhibit haemopoietic stem cells. Recently, skewing of the T-cell repertoire, indicating the presence of abnormally expanded T-cell clones, has also been observed in patients with PNH. (3) Most important, intensive immunosuppressive treatment is the standard of care in those with AAA, and a beneficial response to the same treatment can be seen also in patients with PNH (see below).

Thus, it seems that an element of bone marrow failure in PNH is the rule rather than the exception: an extreme view is that PNH is a form of AAA, in which bone marrow failure is masked by the enormous expansion of the PNH clone that populates the patient's bone marrow. In other words, it appears that two different mechanisms co-operate in producing PNH (see Fig. 22.3.12.3): autoimmune damage to stem cells, and a somatic mutation in the *PIGA* gene. This notion is supported by two further lines of evidence. (1) By targeted inactivation of the *Piga* gene in mouse embryonic stem cells one can produce mice with a PNH cell population. However, this population does not grow further, as it does in patients with PNH. (2) By using refined flow cytometry technology, PNH cells harbouring *PIGA* mutations can be demonstrated in normal people at a frequency in the order of 10 per million. Both these findings indicate that some other factor is required, in addition to a somatic mutation in the *PIGA* gene, in order to cause PNH. Most likely, the same cytotoxic damage to stem cells that would otherwise cause AAA spares the PNH stem cells, thus allowing the PNH clone to grow to the size when it gives clinical PNH. The mechanism whereby the PNH cells escape damage is not yet known.

Complications

The most important complication is thrombosis, which is nearly always venous, and can be life-threatening especially if it affects

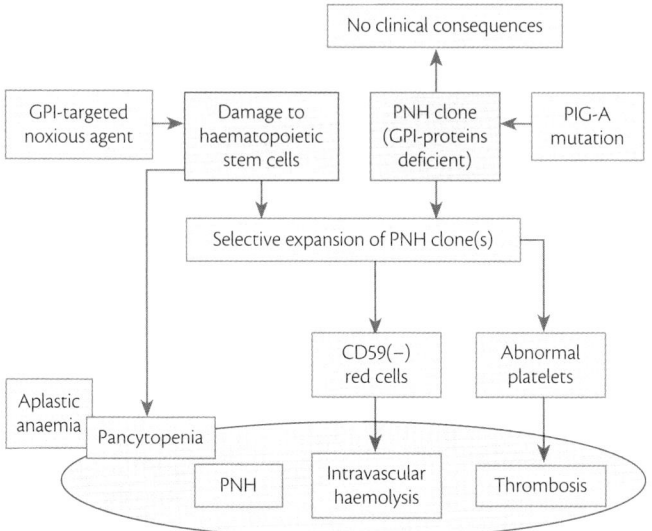

Fig. 22.3.12.3 The role of somatic mutation and bone marrow failure in causing PNH. This diagram aims to emphasize that two separate factors are required to bring about PNH as a clinical disease. On the one hand, a *PIGA* mutation on its own will produce a PNH clone, but there will be no basis for it to expand; on the other hand, damage to haemopoietic stem cells (HSC) can cause aplastic anaemia without PNH. When both factors co-operate, and if the damage to HSC is GPI-mediated, then there will be selective expansion of the PNH clone.

either the abdominal veins (see Fig. 22.3.12.4) or the intracranial veins. The Budd–Chiari syndrome has already been mentioned: because of its characteristic clinical picture it is usually easy to recognize. However, in PNH it is sometimes associated with portal vein thrombosis, and this may limit the extent of liver enlargement. Thrombosis of the splenic vein should be suspected whenever a patient with PNH has, or develops, splenomegaly. Thrombosis of one of the mesenteric veins is much more difficult to diagnose clinically. Appropriate investigations include Doppler ultrasonography, contrast-enhanced CT, and MRI: in our experience, the most sensitive methodology is magnetic resonance (MR) venography. Recognizing venous thrombosis is of great practical importance, because thrombolytic therapy with tissue plasminogen activator (Fig. 22.3.12.4) has been carried out successfully even after 6 weeks from the onset of signs and symptoms.

Treatment

Unlike other acquired haemolytic anaemias, PNH may be lifelong, and this is important in our approach to management. Until recently, there were essentially two options. On hand, allogeneic bone marrow transplantation is the only form of treatment that can provide a cure for PNH: therefore, it should be offered for consideration to any young patient with PNH for whom a human leucocyte antigen (HLA)-identical sibling is available. Results similar to those for AAA can be expected, with long-term disease-free survival ranging from 60 to 100% in the few series that have been published (see Fig. 22.3.12.1: by contrast, the past record of bone marrow transplantation from unrelated donors in PNH is poor). On the other hand, supportive management supervised by somebody who has previous experience of PNH can help the patient to 'live with PNH' for years, sometimes for decades, and sometimes with a good quality of life. The mainstay of support is the transfusion of filtered red cells whenever necessary. Folic acid supplements (≥3 mg/day) are mandatory; the serum iron concentration should be checked periodically and iron supplements added as indicated. There is no evidence that prednisone (which used to be administered at a dose of 15–30 mg on alternate days) decreases the rate of haemolysis, and long-term administration of prednisone, even at a low dosage, is contraindicated, in view of its well known serious potential side effects (a short course of prednisone may sometimes appear helpful in dealing with an episode of massive haemoglobinuria associated with intercurrent infection). Any patient who has had a deep vein thrombosis should be given anticoagulant prophylaxis.

A major advance in the management of PNH has been the introduction of complement blockade by the use of a humanized monoclonal antibody, eculizumab, specific for the C5 component of complement. In an international double-blind placebo-controlled trial carried out on patients with severe haemolytic PNH who were dependent on periodic red cell transfusions, eculizumab has proven effective in controlling intravascular haemolysis: so much so, that haemoglobinuria disappears, about one-half of the patients are no longer transfusion-dependent (see Fig. 22.3.12.5), and in the other half the number of transfusions required is generally decreased. Thus, the quality of life is markedly improved. Why not all patients improve as dramatically as others is currently under investigation. It is already known that in treated patients a proportion of PNH red

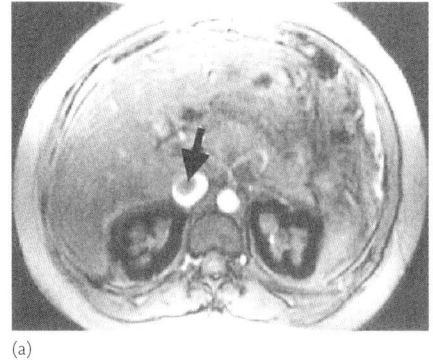
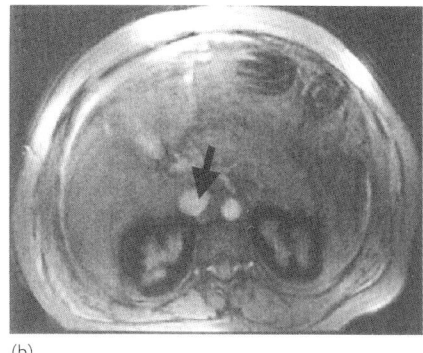

(a)   (b)

Fig. 22.3.12.4 Abdominal vein thrombosis in PNH can resolve with thrombolytic therapy. (a) Extensive thrombus in the inferior vena cava in a patient with known PNH who had developed Budd–Chiari syndrome a few days earlier: it is not infrequent in PNH for thrombosis to involve multiple veins in the abdomen all at once. (b) A thrombus-free vena cava 2 days after an intravenous infusion of tissue plasminogen activator. (Courtesy of Dr Raymond Thertulien.)

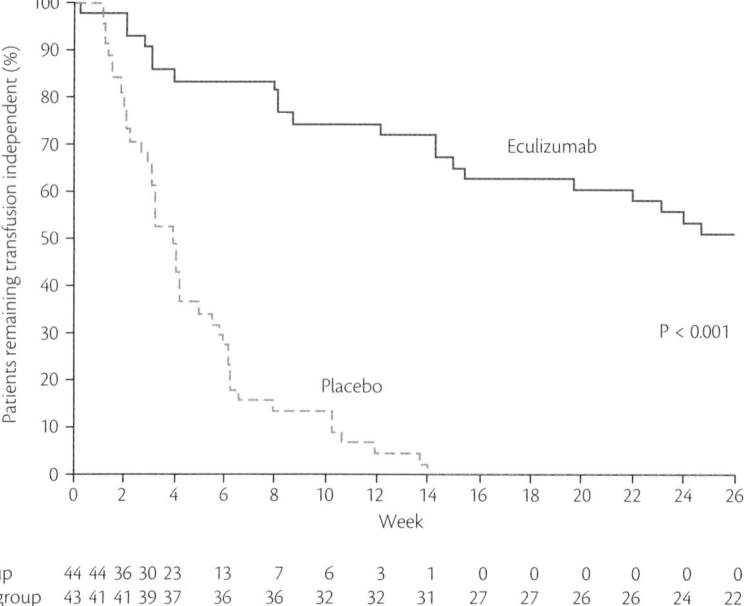

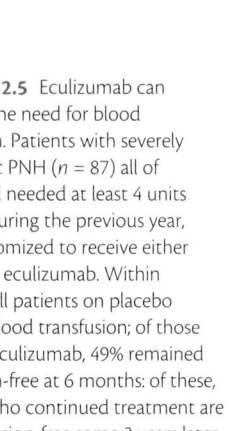

Fig. 22.3.12.5 Eculizumab can abrogate the need for blood transfusion. Patients with severely haemolytic PNH (*n* = 87) all of whom had needed at least 4 units of blood during the previous year, were randomized to receive either placebo or eculizumab. Within 14 weeks all patients on placebo required blood transfusion; of those receiving eculizumab, 49% remained transfusion-free at 6 months: of these, all those who continued treatment are still transfusion-free some 3 years later.

cells become coated with C3 fragments and these may be susceptible to extravascular haemolysis. Given its mechanism of action, eculizumab is clearly not a curative treatment: its benefits will last as long as the agent is administered, through an intravenous infusion, at fortnightly intervals. Because the distal complement pathway is blocked in patients on eculizumab, they are at an increased risk for infection by meningococcus: thus, immunization against this organism is mandatory before starting eculizumab. In most patients this treatment has been remarkably free of serious side effects: however, there have been a few instances of severe infection which have responded to antibiotics.

Eculizumab will have clearly no effect on the bone marrow failure component of PNH. When the manifestations of bone marrow failure predominate, the approach to treating PNH becomes similar to that indicated for AAA: accordingly, a logical option is intensive immunosuppressive treatment with antilymphocyte globulin (ALG) and ciclosporin. Although no formal trial has ever been conducted, this approach has particularly helped to relieve severe thrombocytopenia and/or neutropenia in patients in whom these were the main problem(s): by contrast, there is often little beneficial effect on the haemolysis itself. Thus, the therapeutic effects of ALG and eculizumab are in a sense complementary.

From recent data, it appears that administration of eculizumab, in addition to abrogating intravascular haemolysis, also decreases the risk of thrombosis: this is especially important, since patients with PNH are not fully protected from thrombosis even by painstaking anticoagulant treatment. Thus, it is clear that the availability of eculizumab, though very expensive, will influence significantly therapeutic choices, including bone marrow transplantation.

Further reading

Araten D, *et al.* (1999). Clonal populations of hematopoietic cells with paroxysmal nocturnal hemoglobinuria genotype and phenotype are present in normal individuals. *Proc Natl Acad Sci U S A*, **96**, 5209–14.

Dacie JV (1999). *The haemolytic anaemias*, 3rd edition, Vol. 5. Churchill Livingstone, London.

Gargiulo L, *et al.* (2007). Highly homologous T-cell receptor beta sequences support a common target for auto-reactive T cells in most patients with paroxysmal nocturnal hemoglobinuria.*Blood*, **109**, 5036–5042.

Hillmen P, *et al.* (1995). Natural history of paroxysmal nocturnal hemoglobinuria. *N Engl J Med*, **333**, 1253–8.

Hillmen P, *et al.* (2006). The complement inhibitor eculizumab in paroxysmal nocturnal hemoglobinuria. *New Engl J Med*, **355**, 1233–43.

Karadimitris A, Luzzatto L (2001). The cellular pathogenesis of paroxysmal nocturnal haemoglobinuria. *Leukemia*, **15**, 1148–52.

Luzzatto L, Bessler M, Rotoli B (1997). Somatic mutations in paroxysmal nocturnal hemoglobinuria: a blessing in disguise? *Cell*, **88**, 1–4.

Luzzatto L, Notaro R (2006). Paroxysmal nocturnal hemoglobinuria. In: Young N, Gerson SL, High KA (eds) *Clinical hematology*, pp. 726–38. Mosby, New York.

Raiola AM, *et al.* (2000). Bone marrow transplantation for paroxysmal nocturnal hemoglobinuria. *Haematologica*, **85**, 59–62.

Rosse WF (1997). Paroxysmal nocturnal hemoglobinuria as a molecular disease. *Medicine (Baltimore)*, **76**, 63–93.

Rotoli B, Luzzatto L (1989). Paroxysmal nocturnal hemoglobinuria. *Seminars in Haematology*, **26**, 201–7.

Takeda J, *et al.* (1993). Deficiency of the GPI anchor caused by a somatic mutation of the PIG-A gene in paroxysmal nocturnal hemoglobinuria. *Cell*, **73**, 703–11.

22.4

The white cells and lymphoproliferative disorders

Contents

22.4.1 Leucocytes in health and disease

Joseph Sinning and Nancy Berliner

Essentials

White cells (leucocytes) mediate inflammatory and immune responses and are key to the defence of the host against microbial pathogens. Subpopulations of leucocytes include (1) granulocytes—neutrophils, eosinophils (see Chapter 22.4.6) and basophils, (2) monocytes, and (3) lymphocytes (see Section 5 and Chapter 22.4.2).

Neutrophils and their disorders

Neutrophils comprise half the peripheral circulating leucocytes and are characterized by (1) heterogeneous primary and second-ary granules—with contents including a variety of degradative enzymes, and (2) a segmented nucleus. Maturation from the haematopoietic stem cell occurs in the bone marrow and takes 10 to 14 days, after which neutrophils circulate in the intravascular space for 4 to 12 h before migrating through the vascular endothelium into the extravascular space, where they survive for 1 to 3 days.

Neutrophilia—defined as an increase in the circulating neutrophil count to $>7.5 \times 10^6/\mu l$, usually occurs as an acquired reactive response to underlying disease. Causes include (1) infection, particularly bacterial—the commonest cause of an elevated leucocyte count; (2) drugs—e.g. steroids; (3) malignancies—including myeloproliferative disorders and nonhaematological cancers; and (much less commonly) (4) hereditary conditions—including hereditary neutrophilia, leucocyte adhesion deficiency, chronic idiopathic neutrophilia.

Neutropenia—defined as a reduction in the absolute neutrophil count to $<1.5 \times 10^6/\mu l$, is of particular importance because, when severe ($<0.5 \times 10^6/\mu l$), it markedly increases the risk of life-threatening infection. Causes include (1) drugs and toxins. Mechanisms of drug-induced neutropenia include (a) direct marrow suppression, (b) immune destruction with antibody- or complement-mediated damage of myeloid precursors, and (c) peripheral destruction of neutrophils; common offending drugs that cause dose-dependent neutropenia include cancer chemotherapeutic agents, phenothiazines, anticonvulsants and ganciclovir; (2) postinfectious—particularly after viral infections; (3) nutritional deficiencies—e.g. vitamins B_{12}, folic acid; (4) autoimmune—usually attributable in adults to disorders such as systemic lupus erythematosus (SLE) and rheumatoid arthritis; (5) large granular lymphcytosis; (6) congenital—including severe congenital neutropenia, cyclic neutropenia.

Disorders of neutrophil function include (1) chronic granulomatous disease—a heterogeneous group of rare disorders (most X-linked) characterized by defective production of superoxide by neutrophils, monocytes and eosinophils; patients usually present in childhood with severe infections, often with catalase-negative pathogens; (2) leucocyte adhesion deficiency, (3) myeloperoxidase deficiency, and (4) Chediak–Higashi syndrome.

Monocytes and their disorders

Monocytes share a common myeloid precursor with granulocytes, present antigens to T cells, produce several important cytokines with immunomodulatory and inflammatory functions, and are the precursors to resident tissue macrophages. They are especially important in defence against intracellular pathogens.

Causes of monocytosis (>0.9 × 10^6/μl) include (1) chronic infection—e.g. tuberculosis, endocarditis; (2) autoimmune diseases—e.g. SLE; (3) malignancy—e.g. primary malignancies of the marrow or marrow infiltration with solid tumours.

Basophils and their disorders

Basophils are nonphagocytic granulocytes that function in immediate-type hypersensitivity. Basophilia (> 0.2 × 10^6/μl) is seen in myeloproliferative disorders, hypersensitivity reactions, and with some viral infections.

Introduction

Leucocytes perform a critical role in the host defence against pathogens. They mediate inflammation and modulate the immune response. Leucocytes can be divided into granulocytes (neutrophils, eosinophils, and basophils), monocytes, and lymphocytes. This chapter will focus on the role of granulocytes and monocytes in the normal host response and pathological manifestations of abnormalities of their number and/or function. Lymphocytes are discussed elsewhere.

Neutrophils

Morphology

Under normal conditions neutrophils make up over one-half of the leucocytes in the peripheral blood. The morphological hallmarks of these cells include heterogeneous granules and a multilobated or segmented nucleus. The two predominant types of granules in the neutrophil's cytoplasm are the azurophilic (or primary) granules and the specific (or secondary) granules. Azurophilic granules arise at the promyelocytic stage of differentiation. They contain myeloperoxidase, proteases, acid hydrolases, and microbicidal proteins. Specific granules and their content proteins are synthesized at the myelocytic stage of differentiation. Their contents include lactoferrin, lysozyme, vitamin B$_{12}$-binding protein, gelatinase, and neutrophil collagenase. The specific granules are not a uniform population, and their variable content is determined mainly by the timing of their formation. Those formed early in the myelocyte stage contain abundant lactoferrin, while those formed later are enriched for gelatinase, and are often referred to as 'tertiary' granules or gelatinase granules. The specific granule membrane contains the cytochrome *b*-558 component of the respiratory burst oxidase, as well as chemotactic and opsonic receptors, which are transferred to the plasma membrane upon activation of the neutrophil. Finally, the neutrophil cytoplasm also contains secretory vesicles that are endocytic vesicles containing primarily plasma proteins, and are the most rapidly mobilized fraction of cytoplasmic granules in the neutrophil. The membrane of secretory vesicles is rich in receptors and cytochrome *b*, and the vesicles contribute these proteins to the plasma membrane upon neutrophil activation.

Common variants of neutrophil morphology include the Pelger–Huet anomaly, hypersegmentation of the nucleus, Dohle bodies,

and toxic granulations. The Pelger–Huet anomaly is a dominantly inherited defect in nuclear segmentation that results in a dumb-bell- or rod-shaped nucleus. Neutrophils with nuclei similar to this ('pseudo-Pelger–Huet anomaly') may be seen in acquired myelodysplastic syndromes. Hypersegmented nuclei (containing five or more segments) are characteristic of megaloblastic haematopoiesis due to folic acid or vitamin B$_{12}$ deficiency. Dohle bodies are large basophilic inclusions that may be seen in sepsis, pregnancy, and following cytotoxic chemotherapy. Toxic granulations are abnormally staining primary granules that arise when neutrophils are released prematurely from the marrow, as in severe bacterial infections.

Maturation

There are three cellular compartments that contain myeloid cells: the marrow, the intravascular compartment, and the extravascular space. Maturation from the haematopoietic stem cell occurs in the bone marrow and takes from 10 to 14 days. The marrow compartment can be subdivided into the mitotic compartment and the postmitotic and storage compartment. In the marrow mitotic compartment neutrophils arise through serial division of myeloid precursors. The mitotic compartment contains myeloid cells with the ability to replicate: myeloblasts, promyelocytes, and myelocytes. The marrow postmitotic and storage compartment contains myeloid elements that have lost the ability to divide, including metamyelocytes, bands, and segmented neutrophils. Neutrophils are released from the storage pool into the intravascular space, where they remain for 4 to 12 h. Within this space approximately one-half of the neutrophils circulate freely in the peripheral blood while the other half remain 'marginated' along the vascular endothelium. The marginated and circulating cells are in dynamic equilibrium with one another. Neutrophils then migrate through the vascular endothelium into the extravascular space, where they survive for 1 to 3 days. At any given time approximately 90% of neutrophils are in the marrow compartment and 2 to 3% are in the intravascular space, with the remainder in the extravascular space.

Neutrophilia

Neutrophilia is defined as an elevation of the circulating neutrophil count (>7.5 × 10^6/μl). Although it may reflect a primary haematological process, it usually occurs as a secondary manifestation of an underlying disease process or drug. The causes of an elevated neutrophil count are summarized in Box 22.4.1.1.

Hereditary neutrophilias

Hereditary neutrophilia

This is a dominantly inherited syndrome manifested by leucocytosis, splenomegaly, and widened diploë of the skull. Laboratory evaluation reveals a white blood count of 20 000 to 70 000/μl with a neutrophilic predominance, and an elevated leucocyte alkaline phosphatase. Its clinical course is benign.

Chronic idiopathic neutrophilia

This is a sporadically occurring condition manifest as a white blood count of 11 000 to 40 000/μl with a neutrophilic predominance. Patients are otherwise well and have been followed for up to 20 years without the development of significant pathology.

Leucocyte adhesion deficiency

This is a rare inherited disorder characterized by recurrent life-threatening bacterial and fungal infections, cutaneous abscesses, gingivitis, or periodontal infections. Expression of the CD11b/CD18 integrin is deficient, resulting in the inability of neutrophils to migrate to sites of infection (see below under disorders of neutrophil function for further discussion).

Acquired neutrophilias

Infection

The most common cause of an elevated leucocyte count is infection. Acute infection often causes a modest rise in the white blood count, which may be accompanied by an increase in circulating immature precursors ('left shift'). This occurs more commonly with bacterial infection but can also occur with viral processes. Along with a left shift, morphological changes in the neutrophil may be seen with bacterial infection, including toxic granulation, Dohle bodies, and cytoplasmic vacuoles. Neutrophilia resolves with treatment or resolution of the infectious process. In chronic inflammation, marrow granulocyte production is stimulated, resulting in moderate neutrophilia, sometimes with monocytosis. Chronic infections such as osteomyelitis, empyema, and tuberculosis can also give rise to a leukaemoid reaction with white blood counts markedly elevated (>50 000/μl), usually associated with a marked left shift.

Drugs

Drugs can cause leucocytosis by several different mechanisms. Steroids increase the release of mature neutrophils from the marrow and should not cause a left shift. β-Agonists acutely raise the neutrophil count by inducing the demargination of neutrophils adherent to the vascular endothelium, and may result in a neutrophil count twice that of baseline. Acute stress also results in demargination of neutrophils, which is probably mediated by adrenergic stimulation. Stresses that can cause this include exercise, surgery, seizure, and myocardial infarction. The cytokines granulocyte colony-stimulating factor (G-CSF) and granulocyte–macrophage colony-stimulating factor (GM-CSF) stimulate marrow production of neutrophils and can cause dramatic elevations in the white blood count. The majority of white cells formed are neutrophils and a left shift is often seen. The use of these cytokines therefore requires careful monitoring.

Primary haematological conditions

In other situations, neutrophilia may reflect a primary haematological condition. Marrow hyperstimulation in the setting of autoimmune haemolytic anaemia, immune thrombocytopenia, or recovery following chemotherapy or toxic insult to the marrow may result in a reactive leucocytosis. In autoimmune haemolytic anaemia and immune thrombocytopenia, neutrophilia may reflect disease activity, but steroid therapy or splenectomy may contribute. Splenectomy or hyposplenic states (e.g. sickle cell disease) may also result in modest neutrophilia at baseline with more marked neutrophilia at times of stress or infection, reflective of the loss of the spleen as a site of margination and sequestration of leucocytes.

Myeloproliferative disorders

Neutrophilia is a common feature of the myeloproliferative disorders chronic myelogenous leukaemia, polycythaemia vera, and agnogenic myeloid metaplasia, as well as familial myeloproliferative disorders. Elevated eosinophil and basophil counts are also often seen in these disorders. Leucocyte alkaline phosphatase may be low or undetectable in chronic myelogenous leukaemia. The myeloproliferative disorders are discussed in further detail elsewhere.

Nonhaematological malignancies

Various nonhaematological malignancies including lung and breast tumours may also cause neutrophilia. Tumours may secrete colony-stimulating factors or may cause a leukaemoid reaction. Tumour metastatic to the bone marrow may cause leucoerythroblastic changes, characterized by fragmented erythrocytes, teardrops, and nucleated red cells (myelophthysic changes), as well as leucocytosis with a left shift.

Evaluation of neutrophilia

The evaluation of neutrophilia should take account of the fact that leucocytosis is usually reactive, and that primary haematological aetiologies are relatively rare. The abnormal laboratory value should be verified to rule out laboratory error or a transient unexplained leucocytosis that resolves spontaneously. A careful history and physical examination are essential to evaluate for potential infectious processes, and to obtain a history of medication use. Examination of the bone marrow is usually not necessary for the evaluation of neutrophilia, but examination of a peripheral smear may be very helpful. Evidence of leucoerythroblastic changes warrants examination of the bone marrow to rule out granulomatous disease or tumour infiltration of the marrow. If a bone marrow aspirate and biopsy are performed, evaluation should include culture of the marrow for fungus or mycobacteria.

Features that raise the question of myeloproliferative disease include concomitant elevation of platelets and haematocrit, basophilia and/or eosinophilia, and splenomegaly. In that setting, evaluation should include cytogenetics or FISH examination for *BCR-ABL1* (diagnostic of chronic myelogenous leukemia), and assay for mutations in JAK2 (for diagnosis of polycythemia vera and other myeloproliferative syndromes). Stem cell culture of the peripheral blood or bone marrow to assay for cytokine-independent colony growth was formerly the gold standard for the diagnosis of myeloproliferative syndromes. Although it has been largely supplanted by evaluation for JAK2 mutations, it may still have a role in defining myeloproliferative syndromes in patients with normal JAK2. Evaluation for myeloproliferative disease is discussed in detail elsewhere.

Neutropenia

Neutropenia is defined as an absolute neutrophil count (ANC) of less than $1.5 \times 10^6/\mu l$. In some populations, such as Africans and Yemeni Jews, normal absolute neutrophil counts are lower, with a lower limit of normal of $1.2 \times 10^6/\mu l$. Neutropenia may pose a risk of serious bacterial infection, and this risk is directly related to the degree of neutropenia. In mild neutropenia (ANC 1000–1500 × $10^6/\mu l$) the risk of life-threatening infection is not increased, and in moderate neutropenia (ANC 500–1000 × $10^6/\mu l$) the risk of severe infection is only mildly elevated. Severe neutropenia (ANC <500 × $10^6/\mu l$) markedly increases the risk of life-threatening infection. The duration and acuity of neutropenia may also be important, as the acute onset of severe neutropenia is associated with a higher risk of serious infection than is chronic neutropenia of similar severity. Neutropenia in the setting of marrow failure is more threatening than neutropenia with an intact marrow, as the marrow reserve pool may afford protection. Fever of new onset in the setting of severe neutropenia is a medical emergency requiring immediate evaluation and treatment. Common causes of infection in these patients include Gram-negative enteric pathogens such as *Escherichia coli*, pseudomonas, and *Klebsiella pneumoniae*, as well as *Staphylococcus aureus*. The causes of neutropenia are summarized in Box 22.4.1.2.

Hypersplenism/sequestration

Congenital neutropenia
Severe congenital neutropenia
Severe congenital neutropenia (SCN), originally characterized by Rolf Kostmann as an autosomal recessive disorder (Kostmann's

---

Box 22.4.1.2 Differential diagnosis of neutropenia

Decreased production of neutrophils
- Constitutional neutropenia
- Congenital neutropenias:
  - Severe congenital neutropenia (incl. Kostmann's syndrome)
  - Schwachman–Diamond–Oski syndrome
  - Chediak–Higashi syndrome
  - Reticular dysgenesis
  - Dyskeratosis congenital
- Cyclic neutropenia
- Postinfectious
- Nutritional deficiency:
  - Vitamin B12
  - Folic acid
  - Copper
- Anorexia nervosa
- Drug or toxin induced
- Primary marrow failure:
  - Aplastic anaemia
  - Myelodysplastic syndromes
  - Acute leukaemia
  - Paroxysmal nocturnal haemoglobinuria
  - Pure white-cell aplasis
  - Schwachman–Diamond–Oski syndrome
  - Chediak–Higashi syndrome
  - Reticular dysgenesis
  - Dyskeratosis congenita
  - Large granular lymphocytosis

Increased peripheral destruction of neutrophils
- Overwhelming infection
- Immune destruction:
  - Drug-related
  - Collagen vascular disease-associated
  - Large granular lymphocytosis
  - Felty's syndrome
  - Isoimmune

syndrome), is characterized by severe persistent neutropenia, and the early onset of frequent, life-threatening infections. Bone marrow aspirate reveals a maturation arrest at the promyelocyte stage. This syndrome was originally described as an autosomal recessive disorder, but recent evidence suggests that SCN is a heterogeneous disorder with autosomal dominant, autosomal recessive, X-linked, and sporadic forms. Autosomal dominant SCN has been linked to mutations in the gene encoding neutrophil elastase (*ELANE*), a primary granule protein gene expressed at high levels at the promyelocyte stage of differentiation. Current evidence suggests that the impact of the mutations is not related to the enzymatic function of elastase, but rather reflects the failure of the protein to fold properly. This induces the 'unfolded protein response', a protective response to cellular stress that leads to decreased protein synthesis, degradation of unfolded proteins in the endoplasmic reticulum, and increased apoptosis. Autosomal recessive SCN (Kostmann's syndrome) is caused by mutations in HAX-1, a mitochondrial protein that is important for stabilizing the inner mitochondrial membrane. Homozygous loss of HAX-1 leads to loss of mitochondrial membrane potential, and also leads to apoptosis. Other rare cases of SCN are linked to mutations in G6PC3, the Wiskott–Aldrich protein (WASp) and the transcription factor Gfi-1.

Most patients with SCN respond to G-CSF with increases in their absolute neutrophil count and decreased incidence of infection. Haematopoietic stem cell transplantation is another viable treatment option. With the prolongation of life offered by G-CSF therapy, it has become apparent that patients with SCN have an increased incidence of myelodysplastic syndrome (MDS) and acute myeloblastic leukaemia (AML). These malignancies often develop in association with an acquired mutation in the G-CSF receptor. A relationship has been speculated to exist between G-CSF therapy and the development of these mutations in the G-CSF receptor, but this connection remains unproven, as has the pathogenetic role of the mutations in G6PC3 the subsequent development of MDS/AML.

Cyclic neutropenia (cyclic haematopoiesis)

This is a rare, dominantly inherited, marrow disorder characterized by cyclic fluctuations in neutrophil counts approximately every 21 days and lasting 3 to 7 days. Along with the neutropenia, cyclic drops in the reticulocyte and monocyte counts are also observed. Episodes of neutropenia may be severe, often with an absolute neutrophil count less than $200 \times 10^6/\mu l$, and may be accompanied by fevers, pharyngitis, stomatitis, and other bacterial infections. Cyclic neutropenia has also been linked to mutations in the neutrophil elastase gene. Why some mutations give rise to cyclic haematopoiesis and others to SCN is still a matter of speculation. For the most part, different mutations are associated with different phenotypes and it is rare for the same *ELANE* mutation to give rise to both SCN and cyclic neutropenia. This has led to the hypothesis that the severity of the phenotype is related to the degree of abnormal protein folding and induction of the unfolded protein response associated with different *ELANE* mutations. Cyclic neutropenia can be treated safely and effectively with G-CSF. Unlike Kostmann' s syndrome, cyclic haematopoiesis is not associated with an increased incidence of AML and MDS.

Acquired neutropenias
Postinfectious neutropenia

This is commonly seen following viral infections. It usually occurs several days after the onset of infection and may last several weeks. Varicella zoster, measles, Epstein–Barr, cytomegalovirus, influenza A and B, and hepatitis A and B are some of the viruses most commonly associated with postinfectious neutropenia. The neutropenia resolves spontaneously. Transient neutropenia may also be seen with parvovirus infection. Neutropenia occurs commonly in

patients with HIV. The causes are multifactorial and may be related directly to the viral infection, to opportunistic infections or associated conditions, or to the treatment of the virus or its complications.

Several bacterial infections can cause neutropenia, including rickettsial infections, typhoid fever, brucellosis, and tularaemia. Bacterial sepsis of any cause can result in acute neutropenia. This occurs both as a result of marrow suppression and increased destruction of neutrophils. Acute neutropenia in bacterial infections suggest that egress to tissue exceeds the capacity of the marrow reserve pool. The neutropenia may be severe and it portends a poor prognosis. Fungal infections, such as disseminated histoplasmosis, and mycobacterial diseases may also cause neutropenia.

Nutritional deficiencies

Nutritional deficiencies of vitamins B_{12} and folic acid result in megaloblastic haematopoiesis with ineffective myelopoiesis. Deficiency of copper is a rare nutritional cause of neutropenia seen in the setting of severe malnutrition or long-term parenteral alimentation. Mild neutropenia may also be seen with anorexia nervosa.

Drugs and toxins

Numerous drugs and toxins are known to cause neutropenia. Mechanisms of drug-induced neutropenia include: (1) direct marrow suppression, (2) immune destruction with antibody- or complement-mediated damage of myeloid precursors, and (3) peripheral destruction of neutrophils. In most cases direct marrow suppression is dose dependent. Common offending drugs that cause dose-dependent neutropenia include cancer chemotherapeutic agents, phenothiazines, anticonvulsants, and ganciclovir. Alcohol can also cause neutropenia by marrow suppression. If a drug is suspected of causing dose-dependent neutropenia, it is best to stop the suspected offending agent when possible. However, if it is not possible to stop the drug and the neutropenia is not severe, the drug may be continued with careful monitoring. Neutropenia is often related to the dose and duration of therapy. In contrast, those drugs that cause immune neutropenia usually cause profound agranulocytosis, resulting from both intramedullary destruction of myeloid precursors and peripheral destruction of mature neutrophils. Such drugs include antithyroid medications, sulfonamides, and semisynthetic penicillins. Examination of the bone marrow shows a maturation arrest of the myeloid lineage, reflecting immune destruction of myeloid precursors. The offending agent must be stopped. Recovery of the neutrophil count can be accelerated by the administration of G-CSF.

Autoimmune neutropenia

Primary autoimmune neutropenia is a disease of childhood, with an average age of onset of 6 to 12 months. Patients present with moderate to severe neutropenia that spontaneously remits within 2 years in 95% of patients. Treatment with prophylactic antibiotics prevents most serious complications, and G-CSF therapy is recommended only in the setting of severe or recurrent infections.

Secondary autoimmune neutropenia is seen primarily in adults, and may occur in association with collagen vascular disorders such as systemic lupus erythematosus and rheumatoid arthritis, as well as with immune thrombocytopenia and autoimmune haemolytic anaemia. Destruction may be mediated by IgG or IgM antibodies. The neutropenia may be severe but the degree of neutropenia frequently does not correlate as well with the risk of infection as in other conditions. The marrow typically is hypercellular with a late myeloid maturation arrest. Treatment is indicated in the setting of severe, recurrent infections.

Treatment options include intravenous immunoglobulin, splenectomy, and other therapies directed at the underlying collagen vascular disorder. In Felty's syndrome, neutropenia accompanies rheumatoid arthritis and splenomegaly and neutropenia probably reflects both immune destruction and splenic sequestration. Granulopoiesis is inhibited by either antibodies or T cells. This can lead to severe and recurrent infections. It may be managed with G-CSF. Splenectomy relieves the neutropenia in the majority of cases. However, given its close association with large granular lymphocytosis (see below), treatment with low-dose methotrexate is the chosen approach in many patients.

Large granular lymphocytosis

Large granular lymphocytosis (LGL) occurs in an older population, and is frequently seen in association with rheumatological diseases such as rheumatoid arthritis. Because of the association with systemic inflammatory disease, large granular lymphocytosis was originally hypothesized to be a polyclonal abnormal immune response. However, gene rearrangement studies have confirmed that large granular lymphocytosis is frequently a clonal disease representing a form of T-cell lymphoma. There are two distinct subtypes, with cells expressing either an unusual Tγ phenotype (CD3+,CD8+, CD56–) or a natural killer (NK) phenotype (CD56+). When seen in association with rheumatoid arthritis, the disease has significant overlap with Felty's syndrome. Both LGL and Felty's syndrome are associated with a very high frequency (80–90%) of HLA D4, and investigators now believe that these diseases represent a spectrum of a single disease. Neutropenia related to large granular lymphocytosis is associated with a myeloid maturation arrest in the marrow, consistent with immune-mediated neutrophil destruction. Surprisingly, however, the neutrophil count will often respond to G-CSF. The neutropenia responds well to low-dose methotrexate in 50% of patients, and other immunosuppressive agents also have activity in restoring neutrophil counts. The course of lymphoma in large granular lymphocytosis varies from indolent to rapidly progressive.

Other causes

Aplastic anaemia reflects a primary failure of haematopoiesis with neutropenia, anaemia, and thrombocytopenia. In the myelodysplastic syndromes and acute leukaemias the marrow does not produce adequate numbers of neutrophils.

Isoimmune neutropenia occurs in 1 in 500 babies born alive. It is caused by placental transfer of maternal IgG directed against fetal neutrophils, and it presents in the first days of life.

Hypersplenism usually causes mild or moderate neutropenia along with anaemia and thrombocytopenia. Normal myeloid maturation is seen in the marrow. The neutropenia is rarely severe.

Evaluation of neutropenia

In contrast to the evaluation of neutrophilia, most patients with confirmed neutropenia require bone marrow examination. A comprehensive history and physical examination may identify the occasional patient with mild neutropenia and no other evidence of disease that may warrant close observation only. However, recurrent infections, including oral and mucosal infections, abnormalities observed in a peripheral blood smear, or severe neutropenia increase the likelihood of significant marrow pathology and marrow

aspiration and biopsy is indicated. If neutropenia is accompanied by anaemia or thrombocytopenia, marrow examination is required to rule out aplasia, leukaemia, myelodysplasia, or other primary marrow malignancy. A marrow that shows hyperplastic myeloid precursors and a maturation arrest supports a diagnosis of peripheral neutrophil destruction and/or immune neutropenia, which should lead to a search for an underlying collagen vascular disorder or drug-induced neutropenia.

Management of neutropenia

Fever of new onset in the setting of severe neutropenia (ANC $<500 \times 10^6/\mu l$) is a medical emergency. A careful history and physical examination should be performed in a timely fashion. Because of the lack of neutrophils, sites of infection may be difficult to find as significant inflammation or tissue infiltration by neutrophils may not occur. Blood and bodily fluids should be cultured. Empirical broad-spectrum antibiotics should be initiated without delay. In patients with fever in the setting of neutropenia that is expected to resolve (usually neutropenia induced by chemotherapy or drug reaction), antibiotics should be continued until the neutrophil count recovers to over $500/\mu l$. In patients with chronic neutropenia that is expected to persist indefinitely, antibiotics should be continued for several days past the resolution of fever. If fever persists for more than 1 week despite antibiotic therapy, empirical antifungal therapy should be given. Granulocyte transfusion should be considered in culture-positive Gram-negative sepsis not responsive to antibiotics in the setting of continued neutropenia.

Granulocyte colony-stimulating factor (G-CSF)

G-CSF (filgrastim) is a haematopoietic growth factor that has effects primarily on the neutrophilic myeloid lineage. G-CSF reduces the time of maturation of committed neutrophil precursors, prolongs the lifespan of mature neutrophils, and primes them for enhanced function of the respiratory burst, phagocytosis, and chemotaxis. Clinically, G-CSF is used in the treatment and prevention of neutropenia. When used in conjunction with myelosuppressive chemotherapy, G-CSF has been shown to reduce the severity of neutropenia, shorten the duration of neutropenia, reduce the risk of developing neutropenic fever, and reduce the length of stay in hospital. G-CSF has also been utilized successfully in the treatment of severe neutropenia secondary to congenital disorders such as cyclic neutropenia and SCN, and may be useful in the treatment of autoimmune neutropenia as seen in Felty's syndrome and systemic lupus erythematosus. The neutropenia of marrow failure states, such as the myelodysplastic syndromes, may respond to G-CSF.

Neutropenia secondary to the treatment of HIV infection can also be controlled with G-CSF. The other major use of G-CSF is in the mobilization of haematopoietic progenitor cells from the bone marrow to the peripheral blood. While in the peripheral blood, these cells can be collected by cytopheresis for use in haematopoietic cell transplantation.

Disorders of neutrophil function

Chronic granulomatous disease

Chronic granulomatous disease is a heterogeneous group of rare disorders characterized by defective production of superoxide (O_2^-) by neutrophils, monocytes, and eosinophils. The majority of cases are inherited in an X-linked fashion, but autosomal recessive inheritance also occurs. The genetic lesions causing chronic granulomatous disease have been characterized, and involve mutations in any of four genes encoding the proteins of the respiratory burst oxidase. These include the 91-kDa (X-linked) and 22-kDa (autosomal) components of the membrane cytochrome *b*-558 complex, and the 47- and 67-kDa soluble components (autosomal) of the oxidase complex. Patients usually present in childhood with severe infections, often with catalase-negative pathogens. The most common infection in patients with chronic granulomatous disease is pneumonia, with *Staphylococcus aureus*, *Burkholderia cepacia*, aspergillus, and enteric Gram-negative bacteria often implicated. Other common infections in chronic granulomatous disease include lymphadenitis, cutaneous infections, hepatic abscesses, and osteomyelitis. Aphthous ulceration of the oral mucosa is common, as are chronic mucosal inflammation, perirectal abscesses or fissures, and granulomas of the gastrointestinal and genitourinary tract. The diagnosis of chronic granulomatous disease should be considered in an individual with a history of multiple severe bacterial and fungal infections or a family history of the disorder. The diagnosis is established by confirming abnormal neutrophil oxidative metabolism with tests such as the nitroblue tetrazolium (NBT) slide test or measurements of superoxide or peroxide production. The management of chronic granulomatous disease is based on aggressive prophylaxis and prompt treatment of infection. Prophylactic trimethoprim–sulphamethoxazole or dicloxacillin can significantly decrease the number of bacterial infections in patients with chronic granulomatous disease. Potentially serious infections require the prompt initiation of parenteral antibiotics. Surgical interventions including drainage of abscesses and resection of infected tissue are in important adjunct to antimicrobial chemotherapy. Prophylaxis with recombinant human interferon-γ was shown in a phase III trial to decrease substantially the number of serious infections in patients with chronic granulomatous disease, although oxidase activity was unaffected. Chronic granulomatous disease has also been a target of early gene therapy trials.

Leucocyte adhesion deficiency

Leucocyte adhesion deficiency is an inherited disorder of neutrophil function. Two types of leucocyte adhesion deficiency have been characterized. Type 1 deficiency is a rare autosomal recessive disorder resulting from mutations in CD18, the gene encoding for the β-chain of leucocyte function antigen-1 (LFA-1, CD11a/CD18), Mac-1 (CD 11b/CD18, CR3, the receptor for the opsonin C3Bi), and gp150,95 (CD11c/CD18). Deficient expression of these three integrin complexes on the neutrophil cell surface results in decreased neutrophil adhesion to the endothelium, impaired chemotaxis, and defective C3Bi-mediated pathogen ingestion, degranulation, and respiratory burst activation. Patients with leucocyte adhesion deficiency typically present in early childhood with recurrent pyogenic infections of the skin, respiratory and digestive tracts, and mucosal membranes. A history of delayed umbilical cord separation is also often noted. Common pathogens in patients with type 1 leucocyte adhesion deficiency include *S. aureus* and Gram-negative enterics. Foci of infection notably lack neutrophil infiltration. A mild leucocytosis persists due to impaired margination. The diagnosis is confirmed by flow cytometric measurement of neutrophil CD11b/CD18 expression. The treatment of type 1 leucocyte adhesion deficiency includes aggressive use of parenteral antibiotics for pyogenic infections. Prophylactic trimethoprim–sulphamethoxazole may

benefit some patients. Patients with a severe phenotype often die in the first 2 years of life, but patients with mild disease may survive to early adulthood. Type 2 leucocyte adhesion deficiency is caused by a deficiency of sialyl–Lewis X moieties on neutrophil selectins. In addition to neutrophil function abnormalities, this extremely rare syndrome also is characterized by mental retardation, short stature, and the rare Bombay erythrocyte phenotype.

Myeloperoxidase deficiency

Myeloperoxidase deficiency is a relatively common, autosomal recessively inherited, disorder of neutrophil function. Complete deficiency occurs in 1 in 2000 individuals and partial deficiency occurs twice as frequently. Myeloperoxidase catalyses the production of hypochlorous acid, which is an antimicrobial agent. Myeloperoxidase deficiency is often of no clinical consequence because other host defence mechanisms can adequately compensate for the defective myeloperoxidase; however, when myeloperoxidase deficiency coexists with another defect in host defence, such as diabetes mellitus, disseminated candidal or fungal infections may occur. The diagnosis of myeloperoxidase deficiency is made by histochemical staining of neutrophils and monocytes. Therapy consists of aggressive treatment of fungal infections as well as careful control of glucose levels in patients with diabetes. An acquired form of myeloperoxidase deficiency occurs in some myeloid leukaemias.

Chediak–Higashi syndrome

Chediak–Higashi syndrome (OMIM 214500) is a rare disorder of neutrophil function. Neutrophils and monocytes contain giant primary granules and demonstrate impaired degranulation and fusion with phagosomes. Chemotaxis is also defective. Neutropenia results from defective granulopoiesis. Chediak–Higashi syndrome is inherited in an autosomal recessive manner. The gene responsible has been cloned, and is homologous to a murine lysosomal trafficking protein. Chediak–Higashi syndrome manifests in childhood or infancy with infections of the skin, lungs, and mucous membranes. *S. aureus*, Gram-negative enterics, candida, and aspergillus species are responsible for most infections in this syndrome. Nonhaematological manifestations of Chediak–Higashi syndrome include partial oculocutaneous albinism, progressive peripheral and cranial neuropathies, and in some cases, mental disability. The majority of patients will develop an accelerated phase of the syndrome, manifested by lymphohistiocytic proliferation in the liver, spleen, bone marrow, and lymphatics. The diagnosis of Chediak–Higashi syndrome is made by the demonstration of giant

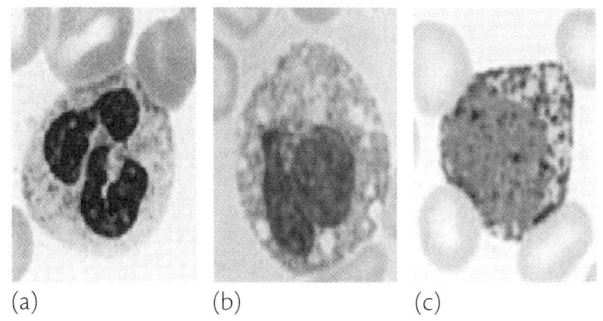

(a) (b) (c)

Fig. 22.4.1.1 Peripheral blood granulocytes: (a) polymorphonuclear leucocyte (neutrophil), (b) eosinophil, (c) basophil.

peroxidase-containing granules in peripheral blood or bone marrow myeloid cells, outside of the setting of myelogenous leukaemia. Chediak–Higashi syndrome is treated in the early or stable phase with prophylactic antibiotics and aggressive parenteral antibiotics for infections. Ascorbic acid may also be of benefit. The accelerated phase is treated with vinca alkaloids and glucocorticoids, but often responds poorly to these measures. Allogeneic haematopoietic cell transplantation from HLA-compatible donors is the only potentially curative therapy for Chediak–Higashi syndrome.

Specific granule deficiency

An extremely rare disorder, neutrophil specific granule deficiency is characterized by absent or empty neutrophil specific granules. Specific granule deficiency is manifested clinically as recurrent skin and pulmonary infections resulting from the absence of antimicrobial neutrophil granule proteins such as lactoferrin and defensins. An inability to upregulate the expression of integrins stored on the specific granule membrane may also be responsible for the impairment of host defence. The diagnosis of specific granule deficiency is made by microscopic examination of neutrophils. With appropriate antibiotic prophylaxis and aggressive treatment of infections, patients may live to adulthood. A truncation mutation in the transcription factor C/EBPε has been demonstrated to be responsible for some, but not all, cases of specific granule deficiency.

Monocytes

Monocytes are large circulating cells with a nonsegmented nucleus and cytoplasmic granules. They function as phagocytes both in antimicrobial defence and in clearing cellular debris. Their granules are essentially identical to neutrophil azurophilic granules, and contain acid hydrolases and myeloperoxidase. Monocytes are also capable of producing reactive oxygen and nitrogen compounds with microbicidal activity. Monocytes play a critical role in the immune response as they present antigens in the context of MHC to T cells. They also produce a variety of immunomodulatory cytokines including interleukins 1 and 6, tumour necrosis factor-α, and interferon-β.

Monocytes arise from bone marrow stem cells. They share a common myeloid precursor with granulocytes. The differentiation to the monocyte is modulated by several cytokines, most importantly monocyte CSF and granulocyte–monocyte CSF. The majority of monocytes are marginated to the vascular endothelium. Upon stimulation, they migrate to the tissue where they develop into macrophages. In the tissue they kill bacteria, mycobacteria, fungi, and protozoa. They are especially important in defence against intracellular pathogens. Specialized resident tissue macrophages include the Langerhans' cells of the skin, dendritic cells of lymph nodes, Kupffer's cells of the liver, and alveolar macrophages.

Monocytosis is defined as a monocyte count of greater than $0.9 \times 10^6/\mu l$. Disorders causing monocytosis are heterogeneous. Recovery of the marrow following chemotherapy or agranulocytosis is heralded by monocytosis prior to the return of neutrophils. Monocytosis is also seen in syndromes such as cyclic neutropenia, SCN, and idiopathic neutropenia.

The most common causes of monocytosis include chronic infection, inflammation, or tumour, as well as some primary haematological disorders (Box 22.4.1.3). Chronic infections leading to

monocytosis include subacute bacterial endocarditis and mycobacterial diseases. Monocytosis is typically moderate and resolves with treatment of the infection. Autoimmune processes such as systemic lupus erythematosus, rheumatoid arthritis, and vasculitis also cause moderate monocytosis. Monocytosis may arise from primary malignancies of the marrow or in the setting of marrow infiltration with solid tumours (myelophthysis).

Primary marrow disorders causing monocytosis include acute monocytic leukaemia, chronic myelogenous leukaemia and other myeloproliferative disorders, and chronic myelomonocytic leukaemia, which has features of both myelodysplastic and myeloproliferative disorders. Juvenile chronic myelogenous leukaemia is a rare disorder occurring in children less than 4 years of age. Lymphadenopathy and splenomegaly are also prominent features.

Monocytopenia in isolation is uncommon. Monocytopenia is sometimes seen following steroid administration, endotoxaemia, or in marrow failure syndromes such as aplastic anaemia.

Box 22.4.1.3 Causes of monocytosis

Inflammatory diseases
- Infectious diseases:
  - Tuberculosis
  - Syphilis
  - Subacute bacterial endocarditis
  - Fungal infections
  - Kala-azar
  - Brucellosis
- Autoimmune processes:
  - Systemic lupus erythromatosis
  - Rheumatoid arthritis
  - Polyarteritis
  - Inflammatory bowel disease
  - Sarcoidosis

Malignancy
- Acute myelogenous leukaemia
- Chronic myelogenous leukaemia
- Chronic myelomonocytic leukaemia
- Juvenile chronic myelogenous leukaemia
- Hodgkin's disease
- Non-Hodgkin's lymphoma
- Histiocytoses
- Solid tumours

Miscellaneous
- Chronic neutropenia
- Postsplenectomy
- Marrow recovery

Eosinophils

Morphology

Eosinophils have a bilobate nucleus and contain characteristic elliptical granules that stain with eosin. There are three types of eosinophil granules. Primary granules are round in shape. Secondary granules are abundant and contain crystalloid material, and account for the eosinophil's staining properties. The third type of granule is small and contains lysosomal enzymes. Granules contain high concentrations of eosinophil major basic protein, histaminase, eosinophil cationic protein, hydrolases, and peroxidase. Eosinophils are capable of phagocytic function but more commonly release their granule contents to the environment. Eosinophils are also capable of producing reactive oxygen species, and produce prostaglandins, thromboxane A_2, and leukotriene C_4. Eosinophils play a prominent role in defence against helminths and parasites. They arise in the marrow from a common myeloid precursor, and their production is dependent on GM-CSF, IL-3, and IL-5. Disorders associated with eosinophilia are discussed elsewhere (see Chapter 22.4.6); causes of eosinophilia are listed in Box 22.4.1.4.

Basophils

Basophils are rare circulating cells, accounting for less than 0.1% of white blood cells. They are nonphagocytic granulocytes. Their large heterogeneous granules account for their purple–black staining. Their granules contain histamine, heparin, tryptase, chemotactic factors for neutrophils and eosinophils, leukotrienes, prostaglandins, and platelet-activating factor. They arise in the marrow from the same myeloid precursor as eosinophils. Basophils function in immediate-type hypersensitivity. They are structurally similar to mast cells but the exact relationship between these cell types is not clear. Basophilia ($> 0.2 \times 10^6/\mu l$) is seen in myeloproliferative disorders such as chronic myelogenous leukaemia and polycythaemia vera, hypersensitivity reactions, and with some viral infections including varicella and influenza. Mast cell leukaemia is a rare disorder with a poor prognosis.

Further reading

Baehner RL (2000). Normal neutrophil structure and function. In: Hoffman R, *et al.* (eds.) *Hematology: basic principles and practice*, pp. 667–86. Churchill Livingstone, Philadelphia.

Berliner N, Horwitz M, Loughran TP (2004). Congenital and acquired neutropenia. *Hematology Am Soc Hematol Educ Program*, 63–79.

Curnutte IT, Coates TD (2000). Disorders of phagocyte function and number. In: Hoffman R, *et al.* (eds.) *Hematology: basic principles and practice*, pp. 720–62. Churchill Livingstone, Philadelphia.

Dale DC, *et al.* (2000). Mutations in the gene encoding neutrophil elastase in congenital and cyclic neutropenia. *Blood*, **96**, 2317.

Malech HL, Gallin JI (1987). Current concepts: immunology. Neutrophils in human disease. *N Engl J Med*, **317**, 687.

Pizzo PA (1993). Drug therapy: management of fever in patients with cancer and treatment-induced neutropenia. *N Engl J Med*, **328**, 1323.

Rothberg ME (1998). Mechanisms of disease: eosinophilia. *N Engl J Med*, **338**, 1592.

Stock W, Hoffman R (2000). White blood cells 1: non-malignant disorders. *Lancet*, **355**, 1351.

Winkelstein JA, *et al.* (2000). Chronic granulomatous disease: report on a national registry of 368 patients. *Medicine (Baltimore)*, **79**, 155.

22.4.2 Introduction to the lymphoproliferative disorders

Barbara A. Degar and Nancy Berliner

Essentials

Lymphoproliferative disorders occur when the normal mechanisms of control of proliferation of lymphocytes break down, resulting in autonomous, uncontrolled proliferation of lymphoid cells and typically leading to lymphocytosis and/or lymphadenopathy, and sometimes to involvement of extranodal sites, e.g. bone marrow.

Causes of lymphoproliferative disorder

These include (1) malignant—clonal in nature, resulting from the uncontrolled proliferation of a single transformed cell, e.g. lymphoma; (2) nonmalignant—polyclonal lymphoproliferative disorders may result from conditions including (a) infections—lymphocytosis is commonly caused by viral infections, e.g. Epstein–Barr virus (EBV); lymphadenopathy is a common feature of a very wide variety of infections, (b) reactive—conditions such as systemic lupous erythematosus (SLE) and sarcoidosis frequently cause lymphadenopathy.

Clinical approach

Distinguishing among the lymphoproliferative disorders clinically and pathologically is not always easy.

Box 22.4.1.4 Causes of eosinophilia

- ◆ Allergies
- ◆ Atopy
- ◆ Inflammation
  - • Collagen vascular diseases (rheumatoid arthritis, polyarteritis nodosa, eosinophilic fasciitis
- ◆ Infection:
  - • Helminths
  - • Parasites
- ◆ Neoplasms
  - • Hodgkin's disease, non-Hodgkin's lymphoma
  - • Chronic myelogenous leukaemia
  - • Eosinophilic leukaemia
- ◆ Job's syndrome
- ◆ Idiopathic hypereosinophilic syndromes
- ◆ Addison's disease

Clinical assessment—when eliciting the history of a patient with suspected lymphoproliferation, particular note should be taken of their general health, the type and duration of any constitutional symptoms, and any episodes of recent infection/exposure to drugs/travel. Thorough examination of all lymph node sites is required, as is careful examination of the oropharynx, tonsils, skin, spleen, and liver.

Investigation—whenever a lymphoproliferative disorder is suspected, the key initial investigation is the full blood count and examination of the blood film, sometimes augmented by immunocytochemistry and flow cytometry. Depending on clinical context, other investigations may include (1) serological studies for viral pathogens; (2) serological studies for rheumatological disease; (3) imaging for mediastinal and intra-abdominal lymphadenopathy; (4) bone marrow examination; and—if no diagnosis is apparent—(5) lymph node biopsy. However, there are many pitfalls in morphological interpretation of lymph node histology, which is a matter for the specialist, who will often draw on supplementary information from flow cytometry, cytogenetics, and immunoglobulin/TCR gene rearrangement studies to demonstrate the clonal nature of malignant disease and provide data with prognostic and therapeutic significance, or to identify the presence of specific viruses such as EBV and human herpes virus 8.

The human immune system has the capacity to identify and respond specifically to invading pathogens. It can also 'remember' the exposure, such that subsequent exposure to the same pathogen results in a more rapid and potent immune response. Lymphocytes play the key role in the adaptive immune response, mediating both specificity and memory.

Lymphocytes

The lymphocytes can be divided into two morphologically indistinguishable types, which play different and complementary roles in the immune system. Both are derived from lymphohaemopoietic stem cells that reside in fetal liver and in adult bone marrow. B cells develop in the marrow (the human equivalent of the avian bursa of Fabricius) and their principal role is to generate immunoglobulin (antibodies). B cells represent about 20% of the lymphocyte population in peripheral blood. T cells,which mature within the thymus, orchestrate the immune response: they are capable of cell-mediated cytotoxicity, they generate inflammatory cytokines, and they provide help for B-cell function. T cells account for approximately 80% of the lymphocytes in the peripheral circulation. A much smaller population of lymphoid-appearing cells express neither B-cell nor T-cell markers. These null cells, also known as natural killer (NK) cells and large granular lymphocytes (LGLs), are capable of cell-mediated cytotoxicity, especially against tumour cells and virally infected cells. NK cells are a component of the innate immune response, as they do not demonstrate immunological memory.

Lymph nodes

In their role in infection surveillance, lymphocytes circulate through the body via a network of lymphatic and blood vessels. At strategic locations, lymphoid cells are organized to allow direct interaction among lymphocytes and other specialized cells of the immune system.

These interactions permit the production of specific, functional effector cells. The network includes approximately 500 to 600 discrete lymph nodes, lymphoid populations in the oropharynx (Waldeyer's ring), bronchial tree, and gut, as well as in the thymus, the bone marrow, and the spleen.

Within lymph nodes, lymphocytes are arranged in a central medulla surrounded by an outer cortex contained within a connective tissue capsule (Fig. 22.4.2.1). Afferent lymphatics penetrate the cortex and lymphocyte-rich fluid filters toward the medullary sinusoids and the efferent lymphatics at the hilum of the node. The vascular supply to the lymph node includes specialized postcapillary venules that allow the passage of peripheral blood lymphocytes into the node. Lymphocytes are ultimately returned to the bloodstream via the thoracic duct.

Roughly spherical follicles are found in the lymph node cortex and predominantly comprise B cells. Primary follicles contain clusters of naive, unstimulated B cells. Secondary follicles, with pale 'germinal centres' surrounded by a darker 'mantle' zone, represent foci of B cells proliferating and differentiating in the presence of antigen-bearing dendritic cells and activated 'helper' T cells (Th cells). The interfollicular and paracortical zones of the lymph node are densely populated by T cells. Macrophages, follicular dendritic cells, and interdigitating reticulum cells all process and present antigen to the lymphocytes within the node.

The design of the lymph node facilitates the process whereby the subpopulation of lymphocytes capable of responding to a specific antigen is expanded. Antigens are delivered to the subcapsular sinus of the node via afferent lymphatics, and are taken up by reticulum cells and presented on their surface in the context of the major histocompatibility complex (MHC) proteins. Specific T-lymphocyte responses require that peptide antigens, which are derived from 'foreign' proteins, appear on the surface of antigen-presenting cells in close association with a 'self' MHC molecule. B cells, on the other hand, are capable of responding to some antigens in solution. Optimal B-cell responses require the 'help' of T cells both via direct cell–cell contact and in response to cytokines

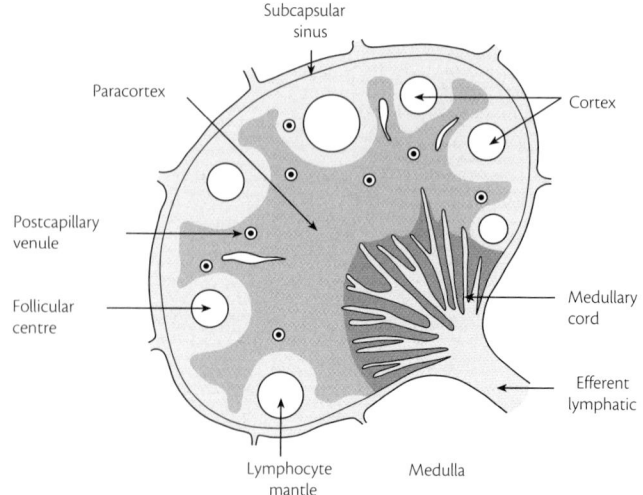

Fig. 22.4.2.1 Functional architecture of a normal lymph node.
(From Arno J (1980). *Atlas of lymph node pathology*, with permission.)

secreted by T cells. Only those T cells and B cells that have been genetically preprogrammed to interact with a specific antigen will proliferate and differentiate in response to it.

Antigen receptors

Both B and T cells express transmembrane receptors on their cell surfaces. These proteins bind antigen and define the antigenic specificity of the cell. In the case of B cells, the immunoglobulin molecule serves as the B-cell receptor (Fig. 22.4.2.2). Each immunoglobulin molecule is a bivalent tetramer comprising a pair of heavy chains bound to two light chains (of either κ or λ type). Genetic recombination of approximately 400 immunoglobulin gene segments (located on chromosomes 2, 14, and 22), generates about 1015 distinct antibody specificities. The expression of recombination activating genes (*RAG1* and *RAG2*) early in B-cell development mediates the random rearrangement of variable (V), diversity (D), and joining (J) gene segments. Terminal deoxyribonucleotidyl transferase (TdT) contributes to the diversity of immunoglobulin molecules by inserting additional nucleotides during the splicing of gene segments. This process gives rise to a vast repertoire of antibody molecules, each with a unique antigen-binding cleft. All of the progeny cells of a B cell that has rearranged its immunoglobulin genes have the same antigenic specificity and are referred to as a clone. Most protein antigens are complex and contain many different epitopes (structures capable of binding an antigen receptor). Therefore, most pathogens stimulate many lymphocyte clones to proliferate: that is to say, they result in polyclonal responses. As B-cell clones mature, the isotype of the antibodies they produce 'switches' from IgM/IgD to IgG, IgA, or IgE.

In an analogous fashion, T-cell precursors rearrange the T-cell receptor (TCR) genes. The TCR consists of a heterodimer of α and β chains, or γ and δ chains in a minority of T cells. The α and

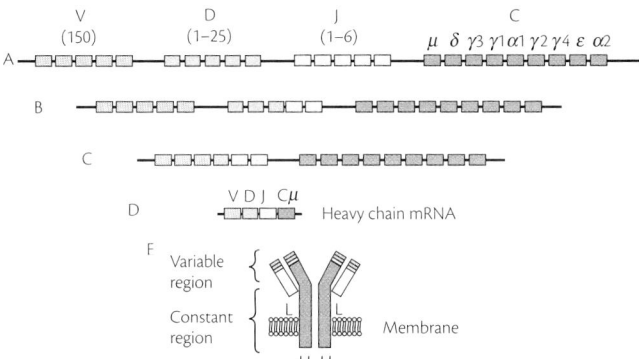

Fig. 22.4.2.2 Immunoglobulin gene rearrangement. The top line (A) represents the germ-line pattern of the immunoglobulin heavy chain locus found on human chromosome 14. B-cell progenitors express recombination activating genes that mediate the random, sequential rearrangement of gene modules (lines B and C) such that only one of several variable (V), diversity (D), and joining (J) segments is expressed by a B-cell clone (line D). As the gene components are spliced, terminal deoxynucleotidyl transferase (TdT) randomly inserts additional nucleotides at splice junctions. Diverse antigenic specificity is thus somatically generated from a relatively small amount of genetic material. The immunoglobulin molecule (line E) is a tetramer of two heavy and two light chains that may be cell-associated (as shown) or secreted. The region of the molecule that interacts specifically with antigen is the variable region. The constant region of the light chain is of either the κ or λ type. The constant region of the heavy chain determines the isotype of the antibody (IgM, IgD, IgG, IgA, IgE).

β genes are encoded on chromosomes 14 and 7, respectively, while the γ and δ chains are on chromosomes 7 and 14, respectively. T-cell precursors randomly assemble variable, joining, and diversity gene segments to generate a vastly diverse array of antigen-specific T-cell clones. When the T cell encounters antigen to which it can productively bind, the cell undergoes clonal expansion, and generates both activated effector cells and long-lived memory cells.

Lymphocyte ontogeny

As lymphocytes develop and mature from multipotent progenitors to terminally differentiated effector cells, they express a sequential pattern of surface proteins. Some of these cell-surface molecules subserve known, critical functions in the cells that bear them. Others are of less clear biological significance, but are useful markers of cell type and status of differentiation and activation. Malignant lymphomas and lymphoid leukaemias are frequently classified and understood on the basis of their expression of cell-surface markers (Fig. 22.4.2.3) In some cases, the stage of differentiation at which malignant transformation occurred can be inferred from the pattern of the surface antigens expressed by the malignant cells.

Lymphocytes develop from bone marrow-derived haemopoietic stem cells. Although the surface characteristics of these elusive cells are not well understood, it is likely that human stem cells express the cell-surface glycoprotein CD34. The first recognizable sign of commitment to the B-lymphoid lineage is the expression of TdT and the rearrangement of the immunoglobulin heavy chain. As differentiation progresses, B-cell progenitors turn on the expression of class II MHC molecules (HLA DR) as well as CD19 and then CD10 (the latter is also known as the 'common acute lymphoblastic leukaemia antigen', CALLA). The immunoglobulin light chain is rearranged and the cells (now termed pre-B cells) express the μ heavy chain within their cytoplasm. As the cells progress to the early B-cell stage, CD34, TdT, and CD10 expression are extinguished, and CD19, CD20, and CD21, as well as IgM, are expressed on the cells' surface. Mature B cells express surface IgM and/or IgD, in addition to CD19 and CD20. Plasma cells, the end result of B-cell differentiation, produce cytoplasmic as well as secreted immunoglobulin, but do not express surface immunoglobulin. They lack CD19 and CD20 expression.

Similarly, as T cells mature they progress through an orderly cascade of genetic and cell-surface events. CD34-positive progenitors that are destined for a T-lymphoid fate migrate from the marrow to the thymus and express TdT as well as CD7. Next, the cells express the CD2 molecule, which, among other things, mediates the binding of T cells to sheep erythrocytes. The T-cell receptor genes are then rearranged and subsequently expressed on the surface of the thymocyte in association with the CD3 molecule. Distinct populations of mature thymocytes emerge: those that express CD4 and function as cytokine-secreting 'helper' cells and those that express CD8 and function as cytotoxic 'killer' cells. Rare 'double-positives' (CD4+CD8+) and 'double-negatives' (CD4−CD8−) also exist. The CD4 molecule mediates the binding of T cells to MHC class II molecules, whereas CD8 binds MHC class I proteins.

The third descendant of the lymphoid stem cell, the NK cell, is characterized by its expression of CD7, CD2, CD16, and CD56, in addition to other surface proteins. NK cells are distinguished from T cells by the fact they do not express CD3 (and therefore the T-cell receptor).

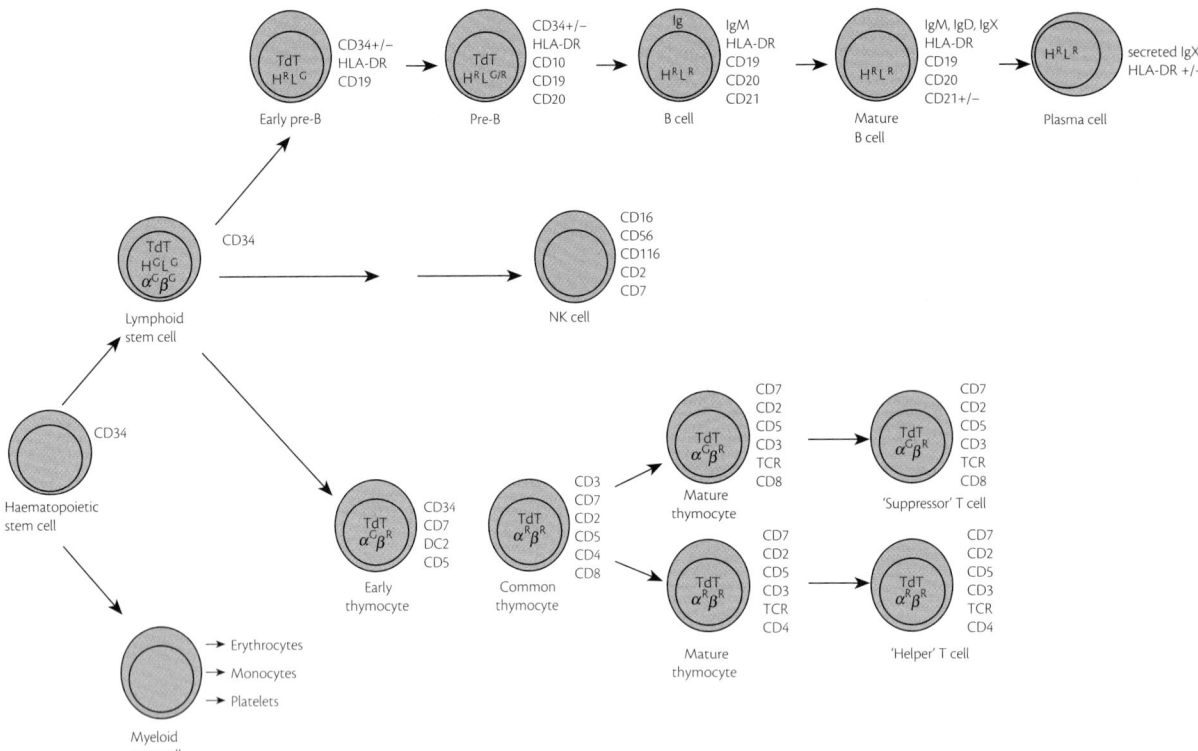

Fig. 22.4.2.3 Simplified depiction of lymphocyte ontogeny. Lymphocytes derive from lymphoid progenitors in the bone marrow, which in turn are derived from multipotent haemopoietic stem cells. B-lymphoid progenitors are recognized by their expression of terminal deoxynucleotidyl transferase (TdT) and the rearrangement of the immunoglobulin heavy chain locus. As B cells mature, the light chain is rearranged and immunoglobulin is expressed first within the cell cytoplasm, then on the cell surface, and is ultimately secreted. T-lymphoid progenitors migrate to the thymus where they express TdT and rearrange the β-subunit followed by the α-subunit of the T-cell receptor (TCR). An overlapping sequence of cell-surface proteins are expressed as the cells differentiate, these have been numerically classified using cluster of differentiation (CD) designations. The status of the immunoglobulin and *TCR* genes are represented as follows: α, TCR-α; β, TCR-β; G, germline; H, immunoglobulin heavy chain; L, light chain; R, rearranged.

Lymphoproliferative disorders

A variety of conditions spanning the spectrum of benign, reactive processes to frank malignant transformation results in the expansion of lymphocyte populations. The lymphoproliferative disorders are a loosely defined group of malignant and nonmalignant entities characterized by the autonomous, poorly controlled proliferation of lymphoid cells. Lymphoproliferation is typically manifested by lymphocytosis and/or lymphadenopathy. In addition, lymphoproliferation may involve extranodal sites, including bone marrow, liver, skin and soft tissues. Distinguishing among the lymphoproliferative disorders clinically and pathologically is not always easy. Malignant tumours are clonal in nature; they result from the uncontrolled proliferation of a single transformed cell. In contrast, nonmalignant lymphoproliferation contains polyclonal lymphocyte populations. Lymphoproliferative disorders may result from chronic antigenic stimulation, certain viral infections, or from an imbalance among interacting lymphocyte populations, as may occur in congenital or acquired immunodeficiency syndromes. In addition, lymphocytes are prone to the acquisition of chromosomal translocations, particularly involving the immunoglobulin and T-cell receptor genes, and such changes may contribute to malignant transformation (see Table 22.4.2.1).

Lymphocytosis

Normal peripheral blood usually contains approximately 1000 to 5000 lymphocytes/μl, accounting for approximately 40% of the circulating leucocytes. Infants and young children typically have higher absolute lymphocyte counts. Increased numbers of circulating lymphocytes (lymphocytosis) and/or the appearance of abnormal (or atypical) lymphocytes in the blood are usually caused by either viral infection or lymphoid malignancy. The appearance of the circulating lymphocytes on a peripheral blood smear may provide clues to the pathogenesis of the elevated lymphocyte count. For example, infectious mononucleosis results from primary infection with the Epstein–Barr virus (EBV), and gives rise to large numbers of 'atypical' lymphocytes with abundant cytoplasm in the peripheral blood. Chronic lymphocytic leukaemia (CLL) leads to an increase in circulating normal-appearing 'mature' lymphocytes. CLL is also frequently associated with the appearance of 'smudge' cells in the peripheral smear, a preparation artefact caused by the destruction of the fragile CLL cells. Follicular lymphoma may be associated with the circulation of characteristic cells with a cleaved nucleus.

Lymphadenopathy

Enlargement of one or more lymph nodes (lymphadenopathy) is an extremely common clinical finding. With the exception of inguinal nodes, normal lymph nodes are non-palpable. Nodes that are palpable and/or exceed approximately 1 × 1 cm on imaging studies are considered pathological. Lymph node enlargement often results from the body's normal and adaptive response to an immunological challenge; however, it may signify a pathological inflammatory or malignant disease. The causes of lymphadenopathy

Table 22.4.2.1 Causes of lymphadenopathy

	Clinical features	Histological characteristics
Infectious		
Bacterial	Regional, often tender	Suppurative
Mycobacterial (tuberculosis, leprosy)	Regional or generalized	Suppurative granulomas
Viral (EBV, CMV, HIV)	Often generalized	Follicular hyperplasia
Fungal (*Histoplasma, Coccidioides* spp.)	Often hilar	Suppurative granulomas
Parasitic (*Toxoplasma, Chlamydia* spp.)	Usually regional (cervical, inguinal)	Suppurative granulomas
Reactive		
Rheumatological conditions (SLE, RA)	Often generalized	Follicular hyperplasia
Sarcoidosis	Especially hilar	Epithelioid granulomas
Drugs (e.g. phenytoin)	Generalized	Paracortical expansion
Castleman's disease	Localized/multicentric	Follicular hyperplasia (hyaline vascular or plasma cell)
Rosai–Dorfman disease	Usually cervical	Sinus hyperplasia
Neoplastic		
Leukaemia/lymphoma	Often generalized, 'rubbery'	Effacement of nodal architecture
Metastatic(carcinoma, melanoma)	Regional, rock hard	Subcapsular expansion, effacement of nodal architecture
Other		
Storage diseases(e.g. Gaucher's)	Generalized	Paracortical or sinusoidal lipogranulomas

EBV, Epstein–Barr virus; CMV, cytomegalovirus; HIV, human immunodeficiency virus; SLE, systemic lupus erythematosus; RA, rheumatoid arthritis.

fall into three main categories: infectious, inflammatory (reactive), and neoplastic (see Table 22.4.2.1) Younger patients, especially children, are more likely to develop adenopathy as a result of infection, while the likelihood of haematological or metastatic malignancy increases with age.

Approach to the patient with suspected lymphoproliferation

The evaluation of the patient with a suspected lymphoproliferative disorder should take into account the age and general health of the patient, the duration of the adenopathy, the coexistence of fever, weight loss, night sweats, pruritus, and cough, as well as any recent infections, medications, travel, and animal exposures. The physical examination should make note of the location (generalized vs regional), the texture (hard vs rubbery), and the mobility (fixed vs mobile) of the lymph nodes, and the presence or absence of associated signs of inflammation (warmth, tenderness, erythema). The skin and oropharynx should be examined and the size of the liver and spleen should be assessed. Additional screening studies may include a complete blood count, measurement of the erythrocyte sedimentation rate (ESR) and/or C-reactive protein (CRP). The level of lactate dehydrogenase (LDH) may be elevated. Serological studies for certain viral pathogens and for rheumatological diseases can be helpful. Radiographs of the chest should be obtained if mediastinal adenopathy is suspected. Ultrasound of enlarged nodes may demonstrate central suppuration, which is characteristic

of acute lymphadenitis. Axial imaging, e.g. CT, is required to diagnose intra-abdominal adenopathy.

Biopsy

When a lymphoproliferative disorder is suspected, pathologic analysis of involved tissue is necessary to determine the specific diagnosis. In some cases, analysis of peripheral blood and/or bone marrow may yield a diagnosis. However, lymph node biopsy is often needed. Before proceeding to biopsy, a trial of observation with or without empirical antibiotics (usually an antistaphylococcal agent) may be appropriate in some patients with lymphadenopathy. However, empirical treatment with steroids should be avoided because it may undermine the diagnosis and proper therapy of lymphoid malignancy. If the lymphadenopathy does not improve within 2 weeks, then a lymph node biopsy should be strongly considered. The largest accessible node is most often selected for biopsy. A fine-needle aspiration of lymph nodes is adequate for diagnosis in a restricted set of clinical circumstances: for example, diagnosis of recurrent disease or metastatic carcinoma or melanoma. Culture of a lymph node aspirate may yield a microbiological diagnosis in infective lymphadenitis. Most pathologists prefer an excisional biopsy, when possible, because nodal architecture is preserved. A portion of the sample should be reserved fresh (i.e. not fixed in formalin) for flow cytometry and cytogenetic studies, if indicated.

Histological examination of lymph nodes is the mainstay of diagnostic studies, however nondiagnostic or nonspecific inflammatory findings are frequently encountered. Reactive lymph nodes demonstrate characteristic, but by no means specific, histological patterns that involve the three functional domains of the lymph node: the follicles, the paracortex, and the medullary sinuses.

An increase in the size and/or number of lymphoid follicles (which contain proliferating B cells,) is termed 'follicular hyperplasia'. The specific cause is rarely identified. This pattern of lymph node reactivity is characteristic of rheumatological conditions and of HIV infection and Castleman's disease. Castleman's disease is a rare and poorly understood non-neoplastic cause of lymphadenopathy that occurs in localized and multicentric forms. The multicentric form is a systemic illness without defined therapy that is associated with infection with human herpesvirus-8 (HHV-8, also known as Kaposi's sarcoma herpesvirus).

Paracortical expansion accompanies T-cell proliferation and is characteristic of certain viral causes of lymphadenopathy, such as EBV infection. Paracortical expansion with granuloma formation is typical of mycobacterial infections and sarcoidosis. In Kikuchi's disease and Kawasaki's disease (mucocutaneous lymph node syndrome), paracortical necrosis is seen in involved lymph nodes.

Sinus hyperplasia is caused by an increased number of histiocytes in the medullary sinuses. This pattern of lymph node reactivity is seen in the histiocytic syndromes and in storage diseases. A rare condition known as sinus histiocytosis with massive lymphadenopathy or Rosai–Dorfman disease is characterized by an extreme polyclonal proliferation of macrophages. This entity often involves the cervical lymph nodes, but may occur in virtually any nodal or extranodal site and is usually, but not always, self-limited.

Involvement by a malignant lymphoma leads to effacement of the lymph node structure to a greater or lesser degree. Histology correlates with clinical behaviour and will be described in subsequent sections focused on the classification of lymphoma. Histology alone may be inadequate to distinguish the malignant from the non-malignant lymphoproliferative disorders. Supplemental information from flow cytometry, cytogenetics, and immunoglobulin/TCR gene rearrangement studies demonstrate the clonal nature of malignant disease and provide data with prognostic and therapeutic significance.

Immunohistochemistry and flow cytometry

Immunohistochemistry is used to characterize the pattern of surface marker expression in fixed or frozen tissue samples. Flow cytometry is performed on cells in suspension, such as peripheral blood or bone marrow, or on cell suspensions prepared from a lymph node or other solid tumour. For flow cytometry, solid specimens should not be fixed or frozen but kept refrigerated until processing. Both techniques detect the binding of monoclonal antibodies of known specificity to the clinical sample. Using a panel of antibodies, these studies demonstrate the types of cells present in the sample. Nonhaemopoietic metastatic tumours can be identified. The lineage of lymphoid malignancies can be revealed, e.g. B cell vs T cell vs NK cell. In the case of B-cell lymphoproliferation, the relative expression of κ and λ light chains can be measured. As described above, B cells express either the κ or the λ light chain, but not both. Predominant expression of either the κ or λ light chain by a population of B cells, a phenomenon known as light-chain restriction, suggests a clonal process. Using flow cytometry, lymphoid neoplasms can be placed within the hierarchy of normal lymphocyte ontogeny, and clinical behaviour, such as response to cytotoxic therapy, can often be predicted. These studies may be used to demonstrate the presence of a surface antigen to which monoclonal antibody-based therapy has been developed (e.g. CD20 and rituxumab). Sometimes, malignant cells demonstrate lineage infidelity, with expression of a pattern of surface markers that does not correspond to a normal cellular counterpart. This may fortuitously provide an immunophenotypical fingerprint to detect small amounts of disease, early relapse, or minimal residual disease after therapy.

Genetic studies

The high proliferative rate of lymphocytes and the genetic events that occur within them, set the stage for the development of chromosomal translocations that are aetiologically linked to malignant transformation. Increasingly, haemopoietic cancers are being defined genetically by the presence of specific, nonrandom chromosomal translocations. The detection and study of these translocations has increased diagnostic precision, has provided insights into the molecular mechanisms of oncogenesis, and has revealed molecular targets for rational therapeutic design. Chromosomal translocations can be demonstrated using classical cytogenetic techniques. Additionally, specific gene rearrangements may be detected using the polymerase chain reaction (PCR) and/or fluorescence *in situ* hybridization (FISH). As experience with these specialized studies in lymphoproliferative disorders has accumulated, certain genetic abnormalities have become highly associated with specific clinical entities. For example, rearrangement of the c-*MYC* oncogene on chromosome 8 is detected in the majority of patients with Burkitt's lymphoma and its presence may be used to support this diagnosis. Other examples are discussed in detail in subsequent chapters in this text. In some circumstances, these techniques are applied to the detection of minimal residual disease during and after therapy. In addition, molecular methods may be used to identify the presence of specific viral sequences, such as those encoded by EBV and HHV-8.

As described above, the hallmark of lymphocyte differentiation is the somatic rearrangement of the antigen-receptor genes, immunoglobulin in the case of B cells and the TCR in the case of T cells. Each lymphocyte clone has a unique arrangement of the components of the antigen-receptor genes, while cells of non-lymphocyte lineage preserve the germ-line structure of these genes. Lymphoproliferative malignancies are composed of clonal proliferations arising from a single cell with a rearranged antigen-receptor locus. The pattern of gene rearrangement helps to characterize the lineage and stage of differentiation of the tumour. For example, pre-B-cell acute lymphoblastic leukaemia cells usually contain rearranged heavy-chain genes with germ-line light-chain genes, whereas B-CLL cells usually have a rearrangement of both heavy- and light-chain genes and express surface immunoglobulin. Furthermore, since clonal populations of lymphocytes all contain the same antigen–receptor rearrangement, these cells possess a 'molecular signature' that is unique to the malignant clone.

Consequently, antigen-receptor rearrangements have become the target of DNA diagnostic techniques for diagnosing and following lymphoproliferative malignancies. Antigen–receptor rearrangements can be detected by several methods including Southern blot and PCR-based techniques. The genetic detection of clonal B-cell populations was first achieved using Southern blotting. While Southern blotting is still the 'gold standard' for determining B-lymphoid clonality of confusing lymphoproliferations, PCR-based techniques have largely supplanted it for the detection of MRD. For these studies, PCR is performed using oligonucleotide primers based on conserved sequences within the immunoglobulin heavy-chain locus; approximately 70 to 90% of rearrangements can be detected by this approach. To detect MRD with maximal sensitivity, such rearrangements are then subjected to sequence analysis to determine the antigen-specific sequences unique to the tumour rearrangement. An allele-specific oligonucleotide can then be synthesized and used in a PCR analysis that can detect residual clonal populations representing as few as 1 in 10^5 cells.

Further reading

Berliner N, Smith BR (1994). Pathobiology of lymphoproliferative disease. In Benz EJ *et al.* (eds) *Hematology, Basic Principles and Practice*. Churchill Livingstone, New York, p.1193.

Cooper MA, *et al.* (2006). Lymphocyte Biology. In Young, Gerson, and High (eds) *Clinical Hematology*, pp. 71–88, Elsevier, Philadelphia.

Delves P, Roitt I (2000). Advances in immunology 1. *N Engl J Med*, **343**, 37–49.

Delves P, Roitt I (2000). Advances in immunology 2. *N Engl J Med*, **343**, 108–17.

Foon KA, Todd RF 3rd (1986). Immunologic classification of leukemia and lymphoma. *Blood*, **68**, 1–31.

Look A (1997). Oncogenic transcription factors in human acute leukemias. *Science*, **278**, 1059–64.

Macintyre EA, Delabesse E (1999). Molecular approaches to the diagnosis and evaluation of lymphoid malignancies. *Semin Hematol*, **36**, 373–89.

Rose MG, Degar BA, Berliner N. (2004). Molecular Diagnostics of Malignant Disorders. *Clinical Advances in Hematology & Oncology*, **2**, 650–660.

Sell S (1996). *Immunology, immunopathology, and immunity*. Appleton & Lange, Stamford, CT.

Strauchen J (1998). *Diagnostic histopathology of the lymph node*. Oxford University Press, New York.

Wickremasinghe R, Hoftbrand A (1999). Biochemical and genetic control of apoptosis: relevance to normal hematopoiesis and hematological malignancies. *Blood*, **93**, 3587–600.

22.4.3 Lymphoma

James O. Armitage

Essentials

Lymphomas are malignancies of lymphoid cells. Genetic abnormalities determine the nature of a lymphoma by leading to the overexpression, underexpression, or abnormal expression of specific genes ('oncogenes'), which are typically those that regulate cell cycle differentiation, rate of proliferation, and apoptosis.

Clinical features—the usual manifestation is with palpable nontender lymphadenopathy. Symptoms from a large mediastinal mass are a common initial presentation. A significant minority of patients present with fevers, night sweats and/or weight loss. Manifestations due to bone marrow or gastrointestinal tract involvement are seen frequently in some subtypes of disease.

Diagnosis—this should always be based on evaluation by an expert haematopathologist of (preferably) an adequate biopsy of a lymph node, or of an extranodal tumor mass if lymph nodes are unavailable. Expression of surface proteins involved in cell recognition and intracellular signalling are important in diagnosis, predicting clinical course, and therapy, as are the presence or absence of specific chromosomal translocations. Various types of lymphoma are recognized, with initial division into Hodgkin's disease and non-Hodgkin's lymphomas.

Clinical approach to the patient—after the diagnosis of lymphoma is established, studies should be carried out to determine the extent of disease. The Ann Arbor Staging system defines (1) Stage I—one nodal site involved (IE if one site of localized extranodal involvement); (2) Stage II—two or more nodal sites involved, but only on one side of the diaphragm (IIE if one site of localized extranodal involvement plus regional nodes involved, but all on one side of the diaphragm); (3) Stage III—nodal involvement (including spleen) on both sides of the diaphragm; (4) Stage IV—bone marrow, liver, or other extensive extranodal involvement; with each stage being classified A (absence) or B (presence) of unexplained fever (i.e. >38 °C), drenching night sweats, or weight loss (≥10% in 6 months). The Ann Arbor staging, along with other factors, is used to determine a prognostic index for each patient, which informs decisions about management.

General approach to treatment—for most patients, the goal of therapy is to achieve a complete remission. Most cases are treated with cytotoxic chemotherapy, often in association with therapeutic antibodies, sometimes with radiotherapy, and sometimes with bone marrow transplantation. Decisions should be made in conjunction with the patient, and require good judgement in addition to technical knowledge.

Hodgkin's disease

The incidence of Hodgkin's disease is about 3 per 100 000 per year in Western countries. Its cause is unknown.

Diagnosis and classification—this requires the identification of Reed–Sternberg cells (which are of B-cell origin and typically CD15 and CD30 positive, but CD20 negative) in a characteristic cellular background, with subclassification into (1) classical Hodgkin's disease—95% of cases; subdivided into (a) nodular sclerosis, (b) mixed cellularity, (c) lymphocyte depletion, and (very rarely) (d) lymphocyte-rich/predominant; (2) nodular lymphocyte predominant Hodgkin's disease—5% of cases.

Prognostic factors—adverse prognostic factors at presentation include age over 45 years, Ann Arbor stage IV disease, male gender, white cell count over 15×10^9/litre, lymphocyte count less than 0.6×10^9/litre or less than 8% of all white cells, albumin less than 40 g/litre, and haemoglobin less than 10.5 g/dl. Patients with no adverse factors have a 5-year freedom from progression of over 80%, compared with about 40% for those with four or five factors. However, the most important factor in predicting outcome is response to therapy.

Treatment—(1) Primary therapy—patients with localized Hodgkin's disease (i.e. stage I or nonbulky stage II) can be cured with radiotherapy, chemotherapy, or combined modality therapy. Patients who present with B-symptoms or stage III or IV disease are best treated initially with a combination-chemotherapy regimen, with the most popular currently being ABVD (doxorubicin [Adriamycin], bleomycin, vinblastine, dacarbazine). (2) Relapse—25 to 35% of patients treated with chemotherapy for stage III or IV Hodgkin's disease will suffer relapse after achieving a remission, and a few patients will fail to enter initial complete remission; autologous bone marrow transplantation can be curative in 25 to 50% of such patients.

Complications of treatment—(1) Short-term complications—these include hair loss, emesis, fatigue, anaemia, and infection due to chemotherapy-induced neutropenia. (2) Longer term complications—these are a major problem for young patients who are cured of their lymphoma; indeed, for patients with good-prognosis Hodgkin's disease they might lead to a higher mortality rate than the Hodgkin's disease itself. Radiotherapy can cause delayed pulmonary fibrosis, accelerated coronary artery disease, and the development of secondary cancers (particularly lung and breast). Complications of chemotherapy include treatment-related leukaemia, infertility, and aseptic necrosis of bone.

Non-Hodgkin's lymphoma

The incidence of non-Hodgkin's lymphoma varies from about 2 cases per 100 000 per year in EastAsia to more than 15 per 100 000 per year in the United States of America. The aetiology of most cases is unknown, but increased risk is associated with immune deficiencies (e.g. immunosuppression following organ transplantation, various hereditary immune deficiencies), agricultural chemicals, autoimmune disorders, treated Hodgkin's disease, and some infectious agents (e.g. *Helicobacter pylori*, HTLV-1, HIV, EBV, HHV-8).

Classification—the World Health Organization (WHO) histological classification divides non-Hodgkin's lymphomas into the following subtypes: (1) precursor B-cell and T-cell neoplasms; (2) mature B-cell neoplasms—including chronic lymphocytic leukaemia, extranodal marginal zone B-cell lymphoma of mucosa-associated lymphoid tissue (MALT lymphoma), mantle cell lymphoma, follicular lymphoma (22% of all cases), diffuse large B-cell lymphoma (31% of all cases); (3) mature T-cell and NK-cell neoplasms—including leukaemic/disseminated, cutaneous (e.g. mycosis fungoides, Sezary syndrome), other extranodal, nodal, and neoplasms of uncertain lineage and stage of differentiation.

Prognostic factors—these include the specific subtype of non-Hodgkin's lymphoma and individual patient characteristics, with adverse factors including age over 60 years, Ann Arbor stage III/IV disease, serum lactate dehydrogenase level greater than normal, reduced performance status, and multiple extranodal sites of involvement by lymphoma.

Treatment—(1) Diffuse large B-cell lymphoma—all regimens will include rituximab unless the particular patient's tumor has been shown to be CD20 negative; the most popular regimen is CHOP (cyclophosphamide, doxorubicin, vincristine [Oncovin], and prednisone) plus rituximab, but other regimens including ACVBP (doxorubicin, cyclophosphamide, vindesine, bleomycin, and prednisone) are at least as efficacious. Local radiotherapy is sometimes added to very bulky (i.e. >10 cm) sites of disease. About 80% of patients with localized disease and 50% of those with disseminated disease can be cured, and those who relapse from complete remission can sometimes be cured with autologous haematopoietic stem cell transplantation. (2) Follicular lymphoma—asymptomatic patients may initially be managed by 'watchful waiting', but almost all patients will progress and require therapy. There is no 'standard' treatment: the most often utilized initial treatments are single-agent chemotherapy, CVP (cyclophosphamide, vincristine, and prednisone), CHOP, and fludarabine-containing regimens, each usually combined with rituximab. An increasingly popular approach, and one that is sometimes utilized instead of watchful waiting, is single-agent therapy with rituximab. Most patients will eventually fail their initial treatment regimen, in which case a wide variety of treatments are used, including autologous and allogeneic haematopoietic stem cell transplantation. (3) Other subtypes of lymphoma—a wide variety of chemotherapeutic regimen are employed, depending on subtype of disease and the patient's performance status. Eradication of *Helicobacter pylori* can cure some patients with MALT lymphoma.

Introduction

Lymphomas are malignancies of lymphoid cells and almost always present as solid tumours, ranging from among the least to among the most aggressive of human cancers. They frequently respond to available therapies, and a significant subset of patients who develop lymphomas can be cured.

Lymphomas are usually divided into Hodgkin's disease and non-Hodgkin's lymphomas (NHL). NHL is much more frequent, with more than 60 000 new cases being diagnosed in the United States of America each year, and about 8000 in the United Kingdom. NHL increased in incidence at a higher rate than almost all other malignancies from 1950 to 2000, but recent data suggests that the incidence is stabilizing. In contrast, the incidence of Hodgkin's disease has been stable over the same time period, with approximately 7500 new cases diagnosed each year in the United States of America and 1200 in the United Kingdom.

Presenting manifestation

Patients with lymphoma most commonly present with lymphadenopathy, but a variety of presentations are possible. These include systemic symptoms such as fevers, night sweats, weight loss, and pruritus, which are believed to be the result of the release of cytokines by normal or malignant cells. Patients can present with symptoms secondary to a mediastinal or retroperitoneal mass such as superior vena cava obstruction, pleural effusion, pericardial tamponade, abdominal or back pain, intestinal obstruction or perforation, gastrointestinal bleeding, or renal failure from urethral obstruction. Central nervous system presentations include primary brain tumours, signs of meningeal involvement and spinal cord compression. Patients might present with cytopenia secondary to either bone marrow involvement or autoimmune destruction of the formed elements of the blood. Symptoms secondary to the overproduction of a monoclonal immunoglobulin or hypogammaglobulinaemia can be seen. In short, the possible presentations of lymphomas are so varied that the diagnosis should be considered in many patients, and not just those presenting with lymphadenopathy or splenomegaly.

Establishing a diagnosis

The diagnosis of lymphoma should always be based on evaluation by an expert haematopathologist of (preferably) an adequate biopsy of a lymph node, or of an extranodal tumour mass if lymph nodes are unavailable. As one of the major challenges that pathologists face is the diagnosis of lymphoma, it is important not to handicap the haematopathologist by providing inadequate material. Needle aspirates or small biopsies should be avoided as the basis for diagnosing lymphoma whenever possible. The differential diagnosis that the pathologist considers when diagnosing a lymphoma includes benign proliferations of lymphoid tissue, malignancies of myeloid cells, nonhaemopoietic malignancies, viral infections, and unusual disorders such as Castleman's disease and giant lymph node hyperplasia. Having tissue available for immunological studies and/or genetic studies will frequently help to confirm the diagnosis.

Patient evaluation

Once the diagnosis of a type of lymphoma has been established, a series of studies should be carried out to determine the extent of disease. The anatomical spread of disease is usually expressed as an Ann Arbor stage (Table 22.4.3.1). This staging system was originally developed for Hodgkin's disease and divides patients into those with disease confined to one lymphatic site, multiple lymphatic sites on one side of the diaphragm, lymphatic involvement on both sides of the diaphragm, and those with bone marrow involvement, liver involvement, or other extensive extranodal disease. The Ann Arbor stage also includes a suffix A or B indicating the absence (A) or presence (B) of unexplained fevers above 38 °C, weight loss of more than 10% of the body weight in the preceding 6 months, or drenching night sweats. Additional factors can also have an impact on a patient's response to therapy and survival. For NHL, these factors are incorporated into the International Prognostic Index. In this system, the Ann Arbor stage represents one factor with an adverse risk associated with stage III or IV. Other adverse risk factors include an elevated serum lactate dehydrogenase (LDH) level, age of 60 years or greater, multiple sites of extranodal disease, and a reduced performance status.

Table 22.4.3.1 The Ann Arbor Staging system

Stage	Characteristics
I	1 nodal site involved
IE	1 site of localized extranodal involvement
II	2 or more nodal sites involved, but only on 1 side of the diaphragm
IIE	1 site of localized extranodal involvement plus regional nodes involved—all on 1 side of the diaphragm
III	Nodal involvement (i.e. spleen counts as a nodal site) on both sides of the diaphragm
IV	Bone marrow, liver, or other extensive extranodal involvement (e.g. multiple pulmonary nodules)
A	Absence of unexplained fever (i.e. >38 C), drenching night sweats, or weight loss (i.e. ≥10% in 6 months)
B	Presence of unexplained fever (i.e. >38 C), drenching night sweats, or weight loss (i.e. ≥10% in 6 months)

The International Prognostic Index score is determined by adding the number of adverse risk factors. (Table 22.4.3.2).

The laboratory and radiological evaluation of patients with lymphoma typically involves a standardized series of tests, such as a complete blood count, erythrocyte sedimentation rate (ESR) determination, chemistry studies reflecting major organ function, CT of the chest, abdomen, and pelvis, and a bone marrow biopsy (Box 22.4.3.1). In patients with NHL, serum LDH, serum β_2-macroglobulin, and serum protein electrophoresis are often useful adjuncts. Functional images, today obtained using fluorodeoxyglucose positron emission tomographic (FDG-PET) scans, identify areas of abnormal glucose metabolism that is present in most lymphomas. Thus, PET complements CT. The staging of a patient with a newly diagnosed lymphoma should involve CT of the chest, abdomen, and pelvis, and, in many instances, a PET scan. At the completion of therapy, repeat CT will often show partial regression of mediastinal or retroperitoneal masses because of a sclerotic reaction to the tumour. In these patients reversion of a previously abnormal PET scan to normal can confirm a complete response to therapy.

Other studies can be useful in particular situations. Most patients will be given a chest radiograph. This offers an easy way to follow mediastinal or pulmonary involvement. MRI studies are particularly

Table 22.4.3.2 International Prognostic Index

Full index	Age adjusted (i.e. for patients < 60 years)
Prognostic factors (APLES)	**Prognostic factors (PLS)**
Age >60 years	Performance status >1
Performance status ≥ 2	LDH >1 × normal
LDH >1 × normal	Stage III or IV
Extranodal sites ≥ 2	
Stage III or IV	
Risk category factors	**Risk category factor**
Low 0 or 1	Low 0
Low–intermediate 2	Low–intermediate 1
High–intermediate 3	
High 4 or 5	

Box 22.4.3.1 Staging evaluation for a new patient with lymphoma

- Complete history and physical examination
- Haematological studies
  - complete blood count, sedimentation rate (for Hodgkin's disease)
- Chemistry studies to predict prognosis
  - Serum (LDH) and β_2-microglobulin (both for NHL)
- Chemistry studies to measure normal organ function:
  - Serum creatinine, liver function studies
- Miscellaneous chemistry studies
  - Serum protein electrophoresis
- Imaging studies
  - Chest radiograph[a]
  - CT of the chest, abdomen, and pelvis
  - PET scan[a]
- Bone marrow biopsy
- Other studies as appropriate to evaluate specific complaints and to follow up abnormal results found from the studies listed above

[a] Not appropriate in all patients.

useful in evaluating suspected bone or central nervous system sites of involvement by a lymphoma. Technetium scans of bone or the liver and spleen are occasionally valuable in detecting occult sites of involvement by a lymphoma. In some patients, abdominal ultrasonography will provide a more economical way to follow intra-abdominal disease.

Bilateral lower limb lymphangiography and staging laparotomy were once performed in most patients with newly diagnosed Hodgkin's disease. With rare exceptions, there is no reason for either of these investigations to be performed today. Effective systemic therapies have reduced the use of radiotherapy in Hodgkin's disease and made clinical, as opposed to surgical, staging appropriate for essentially all patients.

Pathobiology of lymphoma

Increased understanding of the biology of the immune system has allowed the improved classification of lymphomas, and provided new prognostic information and new potential targets for therapy. Lymphomas are malignancies of lymphocytes in which the surface proteins involved in cell recognition and intracellular signalling are important in diagnosis, predicting clinical course, and therapy. Although the genetics of lymphomas are complicated, they too are beginning to be unravelled. Information gleaned from all these studies is likely to further change both the classification and therapy of the lymphomas.

Immunology

The recognition of new surface antigens has improved the ability to recognize specific subtypes of lymphoma. For example, discovery of the Ki-1 (CD30) antigen by investigators in Germany provided a marker for the Reed–Sternberg cells in classical Hodgkin's disease. However, it was soon discovered that this antigen was found on the surface of cancers that were previously felt to be undifferentiated carcinomas and malignant histiocytosis. This observation allowed the description of anaplastic large T/null-cell lymphoma as a diagnostic entity and, more importantly, allowed some patients with lymphoma to receive appropriate therapy.

For B-cell NHL it is possible to use immunophenotyping to help identify the cell of origin of the lymphoma. For example, Burkitt's lymphoma, follicular lymphoma, and some diffuse large B-cell lymphomas arise from germinal centre B cells. Other diffuse large B-cell lymphomas arise from post-germinal centre B-cells, demonstrating the biological variability of tumours that can be morphologically similar. Further insights into such phenomena are presented in the section below on genetics of lymphomas.

The recognition of specific antigens by standardized antibodies has improved the accuracy of diagnosis. Some of the more commonly recognized antigens are presented in Table 22.4.3.3. A characteristic pattern of occurrence can be a key factor in making an accurate diagnosis. Some types of lymphoma, such as follicular lymphoma and nodular sclerosing Hodgkin's disease, can be diagnosed accurately without immunological studies. Others such as all T-cell

lymphomas, diffuse large B-cell lymphoma, and mantle-cell lymphoma can only be accurately diagnosed with immune markers.

Genetics

A theme common to malignant disorders is the abnormal expression of specific genes. The search for these genes was facilitated by the frequent occurrence of chromosomal abnormalities detectable by cytogenetic studies. These abnormalities include chromosomal deletions or deletions of parts of a chromosome, chromosomal duplications, and translocation of genetic material from one chromosome to another. Chromosomal translocations, through studying the sites of chromosome breakage, led to the discovery of a number of genes that appear to be important in lymphomagenesis or in determining the character of a particular lymphoma. The best-documented chromosomal abnormalities associated with lymphomas, along with the involved oncogenes, are presented in Table 22.4.3.4.

Specific chromosomal translocations are highly associated with certain subtypes of lymphoma and thus are useful in diagnosis. These include the t(2;5) and anaplastic large T/null-cell lymphoma; the t(14;18) in follicular lymphoma; the t(8;14), t(2;8), and t(8;22) in Burkitt's lymphoma; and the t(11;14) in mantle-cell lymphoma. Cytogenetic studies in most patients with NHL display a large number of chromosomal abnormalities. However, only a few have been shown to be of diagnostic or prognostic significance. No such abnormalities have been consistently identified in patient's with Hodgkin's disease.

Genetic abnormalities determine the nature of a lymphoma by leading to the overexpression, underexpression, or abnormal expression of specific genes. The genes involved, frequently termed 'oncogenes', are typically those that regulate the cell cycle differentiation, rate of proliferation, and apoptosis. Since the work of genes is done by the proteins for which they code, the under-, over-, or abnormal translation of specific proteins is an increasing subject for study. In some cases, protein translations might be abnormal despite no obvious translocation. For example, diffuse large B-cell lymphoma displays the t(14;18) in approximately 30%

Table 22.4.3.3 (a) Immunological markers and their target useful in the diagnosis or management of lymphomas

Marker	Target
CD3	T cells
CD4	Helper/inducer T cells
CD5	T cells, early B cells
CD8	Cytotoxic/suppressor T cells and NK cells
CD10	CALLA
CD15	Lewis-X
CD19	B4(leuk 12)
CD20	B cells
CD23	IgE receptor
CD25	IL-2 receptor
CD30	Ki-1
CD57	HNK-1

CALLA, common acute lymphoblastic leukemia antigen; IL-2, interleukin-2; NK, natural killer.

(b) Characteristic immunophenotype of selected lymphoma[a]

Subtype	Characteristic immunophenotype
Diffuse large B-cell	CD5−, CD10+/−, CD20+, CD23+/−
Follicular	CD5−, CD10+, CD20+, CD23+/−, Bcl6+
Small lymphocytic/CLL	CD5+,CD10−,CD20+ (dim), CD23+
Mantle cell	CD5+, CD10−, CD20+, CD23−, cyclic D1+
Classical Hodgkin's	CD15+,CD20−, CD30+
Nodular lymphocyte-predominant Hodgkin's	CD15−, CD20+, CD30−

[a]It is important to remember that not all cases of a particular type of lymphoma will have exactly the characteristic immunophenotype, and this does not invalidate the diagnosis.

Table 22.4.3.4 Chromosomal translocations characteristic of non-Hodgkin's lymphoma

NHL subtype	Translocation	Genes involved	Frequency
Diffuse large B-cell	t(3q27)	BCL-6	35%
	t(14;18)(q32;q21)	IgH, BCL-2	15–20%
	t(18;14)(q24;q32)	C-Myc, IgH	<5%
Burkitt's	t(8;14)(q24;q32)	C-Myc, IgH	100% have one of these; most commonly t(8;14)
	t(8;22)(q24;q11)	C-Myc,IgL	
	t(2;8)(p12;q24)	IgK, C-myc	
Follicular	t(14;18)(q32;q21)	IgH, BCL-2	90%
Mantle cell	t(11;14)(q13;q32)	BCL-1, IgH	>90%
ALCL	t(2;5)(p23;q35)	ALK, NPM	>80% of ALK + ALCLs
MALT	t(11;18)(q21;q21)	API 2, MALT 1	35%
	t(14;18)(q21;q32)	IgH, MALT 1	20%
	t(1;14)(p22;q32)	BCL-10, IgH	10%

of patients. This translocation involves the *BCL2* gene on chromosome 18, whose protein product is involved in suppressing apoptosis (i.e. the mechanism of cell death usually triggered by chemotherapeutic agents). Tumours can overproduce the BCL-2 protein with or without the t(14;18). Overproduction of BCL-2 protein might be expected to lead to the increased survival of lymphoma cells when they are exposed to therapeutic agents. In patients with diffuse large B-cell lymphoma, poorer outcome has been associated with overproduction of the BCL-2 protein, rather than with the t(14;18).

The discovery of genetic abnormalities in lymphomas can be accomplished with cytogenetic analysis, fluorescent *in situ* hyberdization (FISH), and—more recently—by gene arrays. Cytogenetic studies require fresh tissue. FISH studies can be done on fixed tissue, but only specific abnormalities for which probes are available can be investigated. Gene array studies are currently a research technique that allows identification of genes that are over- or underexpressed in specific specimens. They allow the analysis of thousands of genes simultaneously and have shown that histologically identical groups of lymphomas can be subdivided into clinically relevant subgroups on the basis of their gene expression patterns. For example, diffuse large B-cell lymphoma can be subdivided into at least three subgroups using gene expression patterns that have different clinical characteristics and/or treatment outcome. Similar studies have been done in other subtypes of lymphoma. At least one report of patients with follicular lymphoma suggested that survival might be more affected by the gene expression pattern of infiltrating normal immune cells (i.e. a pattern characteristic of T lymphocytes versus one characteristic of macrophage/dendridic cells) than by the gene expression pattern in the tumour cells themselves. Future studies using this technology are likely to provide more insights into the biology of lymphomas, improve classification, affect choice of therapy, and—perhaps—provide targets for the development of new treatments.

General principles of lymphoma treatment

Types of treatment

Those treatments effective in the management of patients with cancer include surgery, radiotherapy, cytotoxic chemotherapy, and a variety of new approaches developed through increasing understanding of the biology of the immune system. The latter include cytokines, antibodies, and attempts to direct an immune reaction against cancer.

Because few patients with lymphoma have truly localized disease, surgery has not been a major treatment modality, except for selected patients with extranodal MALT lymphomas. Since its utilization in medicine in the first part of the 20th century radiotherapy has been a major treatment modality for patients with lymphoma, but is limited in its application by toxicity. Its curative potential depends upon being able to achieve a tumoricidal dose (typically 3000–4000 cGy) without irreversibly injuring normal organs. Thus, the site of involvement by a lymphoma, as well as the number of sites involved, can limit the effectiveness of this treatment, since toxicity increases with the volume of tissue irradiated. If a lymphoma is truly localized, radiotherapy is often curative. However, most patients have occult metastatic disease and cure rates are often higher when a brief course of chemotherapy precedes the radiation. Two approaches have been utilized to

make radiotherapy a 'systemic' treatment. One involves radiation of the total body. When this is part of a bone marrow transplant regimen, a total dose of 1000 to 1200 cGy can be administered. More recently, it has been demonstrated that it is possible to give higher doses of radiotherapy to multiple areas by attaching radioactive molecules to antibodies that home to sites of involvement by lymphoma.

Cytotoxic chemotherapeutic agents were first discovered in the 1940s when mechlorethamine (i.e. the nitrogen mustard gas used in warfare), and subsequently methotrexate, were found to cause regressions in immune-system malignancies. A wide variety of agents have since been shown to be able to cause disease regression in many patients with lymphomas. Unfortunately, early studies showed that regressions induced by single agents were almost invariably followed by regrowth of the tumour and eventual death of the patient. In an attempt to circumvent this, combinations of chemotherapeutic agents were first utilized in the 1960s and early 1970s. The drugs were combined by attempting to choose agents with different mechanisms of action and nonoverlapping toxicities to allow the administration of doses that were near to the maximum tolerated dose with an individual agent. In both childhood acute leukaemia and Hodgkin's disease this approach was validated by the cure of a significant number of patients. Today, several combination chemotherapy regimens with acceptable toxicity have been shown to be effective and are widely used worldwide (Table 22.4.3.5). All regimens are not equally good for treating all types of lymphoma.

Increasing knowledge of the immune system has further led to the recognition that a number of biologically active molecules

Table 22.4.3.5 Popular combination chemotherapy regimens used in treating patients with lymphoma

Regimen	Drug	Dose (mg/m²)	Route	Schedule
Hodgkin's disease				
ABVD	Doxorubicin	25	IV	D1 and 15
28-day cycles	Bleomycin	10	IV	D1 and 15
	Vinblastine	6	IV	D1 and 15
	Dacarbazine	375	IV	D1 and 15
Non-Hodgkin's lymphoma				
CVP-R	Cyclophosphamide	750–1200	IV	D1
21-day cycles	Vincristine	1.4 (max. 2)	IV	D1
	Predinsone	100 total dose (not by m²)	PO	D1–5
	Rituximab	375	IV	D1
CHOP-R	Cyclophosphamide	750	IV	D1
21-day cycles	Doxorubicin	50	IV	D1
	Vincristine	1.4 (max. 2)	IV	D1
	Prednisone	100 total (not by m²)	PO	D1–5
	Rituximab	375	IV	D1

can cause regression of lymphomas and, in some cases, impact on survival. The first such agent to be widely used was interferon-α, which has some activity in both NHL and Hodgkin's disease. When administered at an adequate dose, it has been shown to prolong survival in patients with poor-prognosis follicular lymphoma who received an anthracycline-containing chemotherapy regimen as their initial treatment.

The ability to produce monoclonal antibodies has provided new therapeutic molecules. In B-cell NHL, antibodies directed against the CD20 molecule have been incorporated into clinical practice. Rituximab has been shown to be active in a variety of B-cell lymphomas. An antibody directed against CD52 (i.e. alemtuzumab) has become widely used for the treatment of patients with small lymphocytic lymphoma/chronic lymphocytic leukaemia.

Very high doses of cytotoxic chemotherapeutic agents with or without radiotherapy and biologically active molecules have been utilized in the treatment of patients with lymphomas as part of the bone marrow transplantation procedure. This involves the administration of very high doses of antilymphoma therapy in an attempt to overcome presumed treatment resistance. Patients are rescued from the toxicity of treatment by the reinfusion of haemopoietic stem cells. The patient's own haemopoietic stem cells (an autologous transplant) or those from another individual with identical HLA genes (an allogeneic transplant) can be utilized. Cells for this procedure can be obtained from either bone marrow or peripheral blood. Autologous transplantation has been widely used for patients with lymphoma and shown to be able to cure patients with relapsed Hodgkin's disease and aggressive NHL. In aggressive NHL, a possible increased cure rate has been demonstrated by utilizing adjuvant transplantation following initially effective standard chemotherapy in patients with a poor prognosis. Transplantation is utilized in patients with follicular lymphoma, although allogeneic transplantation, while apparently curative, has a high mortality rate.

Various new treatments are being studied for patients with lymphoma. These include attempts to stimulate the patient's endogenous immune system to develop antibodies against lymphomas; such 'tumour vaccines' are in clinical trials. Another approach, which has been called 'antisense therapy', involves the use of antisense oligonucleotides aimed at interrupting the transcription and expression of key genes.

General strategy of treatment

A number of factors need to be taken into account when formulating a treatment recommendation for a patient with lymphoma (Box 22.4.3.2). These include the patient's age, general health, extent of disease, likelihood of cure, coexisting illnesses, long-term goals, and concerns about treatment toxicity. This decision should be made in conjunction with the patient, and requires good judgement in addition to technical knowledge. The aggressiveness of the treatment that is finally chosen will often depend upon the physician's interpretation of the chances for cure. It is obvious that more toxicity will be acceptable if the goal is cure rather than palliation. For this reason, patients with definitely curable lymphomas, such as diffuse large B-cell lymphoma and Burkitt's lymphoma, are almost always treated promptly with intensive regimens. By contrast, the best treatment for patients with follicular lymphoma remains a point for intense debate. Since the curability of this disease is less clear, many physicians would favour no initial therapy

---

Box 22.4.3.2 Factors to consider in therapy for a patient with lymphoma

- Specific type of lymphoma
- Age
- Performance status
- Presence of other diseases
- Stage
- Systemic symptoms
- Pace of disease
- Potential side-effects
- Is there a chance of cure?
- Patient's concerns about specific treatments
- Convenience
- Patient's immediate and long-term goals
- Quality of life

---

in an asymptomatic patient, but—as discussed below—this is not a simple decision.

For most patients, the goal of therapy is to achieve a complete remission. This implies the disappearance of all symptoms and objective evidence of lymphoma. In practice, a complete remission is documented by repeating all abnormal staging studies after several cycles of therapy or at the completion of the planned therapy. Sometimes, persisting masses visualized on CT scans represent residual fibrosis rather than persisting tumour. In this setting, PET scans are extremely helpful. A PET scan that reverts to normal is strong evidence of complete remission. Documentation of complete remission is important. Patients who achieve a complete remission have a chance for cure; those who do not achieve a complete remission with initial therapy will often go directly to second-line treatments.

Patients who fail to be cured with initial therapy, either because they do not achieve an initial remission or because they relapse from remission, are candidates for what has been termed 'salvage therapy.' These second-line regimens can regularly cause tumour regression in most patients with lymphoma and can occasionally produce long-term, disease-free survival. However, for most patients, the only curative approach in this setting is bone marrow transplantation. The toxicity of bone marrow transplantation limits its use to patients under 70 years of age for autologous transplantation and under 55 years for allogeneic transplantation, who have a good performance status, without serious compromise of major organ function; and to patients who do not have bulky/chemotherapy-refractory disease.

Hodgkin's disease

In 1832, Thomas Hodgkin of Guy's Hospital, London, reported seven patients who died from a disorder involving lymph node and spleen enlargement. Then, early in the 20th century, Sternberg and Reed independently described the characteristic giant cells that now bear their name. This made it possible for pathologists to separate the disorder we now know as Hodgkin's disease from other lymphomas.

Incidence and epidemiology

Unlike that of NHL, the incidence of Hodgkin's disease appears to be stable, with about 3 new cases per 100 000 per year in Western countries. The condition displays a peculiar bimodal distribution of occurrence, with peaks in young adulthood and older age (Fig. 22.4.3.1). This dual peak has led some to propose that Hodgkin's disease actually represents two illnesses, with the earlier peak being related to an infectious aetiology and the latter representing a true malignancy, but there is little evidence to support this hypothesis.

An association has been demonstrated between the occurrence of Hodgkin's disease and infection by the Epstein–Barr virus (EBV). Monoclonal or oligoclonal proliferation of EBV-infected cells is found in 20 to 40% of patients with Hodgkin's disease. Patients infected by HIV are at an increased risk for Hodgkin's disease in addition to NHL.

The subtypes of Hodgkin's disease vary geographically and by age group. Patients in Western countries who develop Hodgkin's disease in young adulthood usually have the nodular sclerosis subtype. Patients from developing countries, elderly patients, and those infected with HIV, frequently have mixed-cellularity or lymphocyte-depleted classical Hodgkin's disease.

Hodgkin's disease is approximately 100 times more likely in an identical twin of an infected patient. Numerous instances of case-clustering have been described. Although these might be taken as evidence of a genetic or infectious aetiology, the cause of Hodgkin's disease remains unknown.

Pathology

The diagnosis of Hodgkin's disease requires the identification of Reed–Sternberg cells in a characteristic cellular background. The World Health Organization (WHO) classification for Hodgkin's disease is presented in Table 22.4.3.3. The diagnosis requires

review of an adequate biopsy by an expert haematolopathologist. Fine needle aspiration should not be utilized and is not accurate. Hodgkin's disease is unique in that the tumour cells constitute a minority of the total cellular population of involved lymph nodes. The tumour cell, i.e. the Reed–Sternberg cell, has been shown to be of B-cell origin. In the WHO classification Hodgkin's disease is divided into classical Hodgkin's diseases (95% of cases), and nodular lymphocyte predominant Hodgkin's disease (5% of cases). Classical Hodgkin's disease is subdivided into nodular sclerosis, which is characterized by bands of fibrosis that are often visible to the naked eye; mixed cellularity, where a larger number of Reed–Sternberg cells in a mixed cellular background are typical; and lymphocyte-depletion Hodgkin's disease, which has either a large number of Reed–Sternberg cells and atypical mononuclear cells, or a background of diffuse fibrosis with occasional Reed–Sternberg cells. The diagnosis of lymphocyte-depletion Hodgkin's disease should always raise the possibility that an unusual diffuse large B-cell lymphoma is being confused with Hodgkin's disease.

Although diffuse lymphocyte-rich (or predominant) Hodgkin's disease is listed as a diagnosis, in practice this is exceedingly rare. Almost all patients with lymphocyte-predominant Hodgkin's disease have the entity nodular lymphocyte predominant Hodgkin's disease, which is a different illness that in many ways is more like an indolent B-cell NHL. The Reed–Sternberg cells in nodular lymphocyte-predominant Hodgkin's disease express the leucocyte common antigen and other B-cell markers including CD20: typical Reed–Sternberg cells are CD20 negative but do express CD15 and CD30.

Clinical features and evaluation

Patients with classical Hodgkin's disease usually present with palpable nontender lymphadenopathy. In most patients, lymph nodes are discovered in the cervical, supraclavicular, and axillary regions. More than half the patients have mediastinal lymphadenopathy at diagnosis, and symptoms from a large mediastinal mass are often the initial presentation. Subdiaphragmatic presentation of Hodgkin's disease is unusual, and more common in older men. Approximately one-third of patients with classical Hodgkin's disease present with fevers, night sweats, and/or weight loss.

Hodgkin's disease can present as a fever of unknown origin. This is more likely in older patients, those with mixed-cellularity or lymphocyte-depletion subtypes, and those who present with disease below the diaphragm. Fevers associated with Hodgkin's disease occasionally persist for days to weeks, followed by afebrile

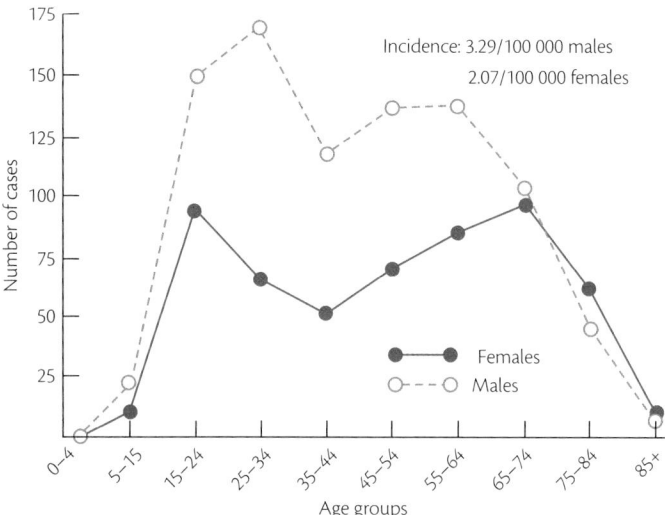

Fig. 22.4.3.1 Age distribution of Hodgkin's disease expressed as new cases registered in England and Wales in 1973.

Incidence: 3.29/100 000 males
2.07/100 000 females

Box 22.4.3.3 World Health Organization classification of Hodgkin's lymphoma

♦ Nodular lymphocyte predominance (5%)

♦ Classical Hodgkin's disease (95%):
  • Nodular sclerosis
  • Mixed cellularity
  • Lymphocyte depletion
  • Lymphocyte rich

periods, with subsequent reoccurrence of the fever. This pattern is known as Pel–Ebstein fever. Unusual presentations of Hodgkin's disease include severe and unexplained pruritus, paraneoplastic cerebellar degeneration, nephrotic syndrome, immune haemolytic anaemia and/or thrombocytopenia, hypercalcaemia, and pain in lymph nodes with alcohol ingestion.

The diagnosis of Hodgkin's disease is based on a review of an adequate biopsy by an expert haematopathologist. Subsequent evaluation should include a careful history and physical examination, complete blood count, ESR determination, serum chemistry studies including serum lactate dehydrogenase, chest radiograph, CT of the chest, abdomen, and pelvis, and bone marrow biopsy. PET scans are consistently abnormal in patients with Hodgkin's disease. They are particularly useful when performed at the end of therapy for documenting complete remission. At one time both bipedal lymphangiography and staging laparotomy were popular studies in evaluating new patients with Hodgkin's disease, but they are now rarely—if ever—indicated.

Nodular lymphocyte-predominant Hodgkin's disease, as noted above, is a different clinical entity from classical Hodgkin's disease. These patients represent less than 5% of all patients found to have Hodgkin's disease. The evaluation of such patients is carried out in a similar way to that for classical Hodgkin's disease. However, nodular lymphocyte-predominant Hodgkin's disease tends to follow a chronic, relapsing course and sometimes transforms to diffuse large B-cell lymphoma.

Prognostic factors

The major factors determining treatment outcome for patients with Hodgkin's disease include the Ann Arbor stage, the presence or absence of systemic symptoms, age, and gender. Patients with asymptomatic, localized disease who are young and female have the best outlook. Histological subtypes do not appear to have major independent prognostic significance. Patients with nodular sclerosing Hodgkin's disease are less likely to have adverse prognostic factors than those with mixed-cellularity or lymphocyte-depleted subtypes. The results of several laboratory studies can predict outcome in patients with Hodgkin's disease. Adverse results include anaemia, a greatly elevated ESR, a low albumin level, and a low lymphocyte count. The ESR is sometimes used to follow the course of patients with Hodgkin's disease as it reverts to normal with successful treatment.

An International Prognostic Index for Hodgkin's disease has been developed (Table 22.4.3.6). This index uses seven adverse prognostic factors that determine the treatment outcome. These include age >45 years, stage IV, male sex, white count $>15 \times 10^9$/litre, lymphocyte count $<0.6 \times 10^9$/litre or less than 8% of all white cells, albumin <4 g/dl, and haemoglobin <10.5 g/dl. The adverse prognostic factors present in an individual patient are summed. In a large study, patients with no adverse prognostic factors had a 5-year freedom from progression of 84%, whereas for patients with five or four factors it was only 42%.

The most important factor in predicting outcome for patients with Hodgkin's disease is their response to therapy. Patients who have a prompt, complete response to chemotherapy and/or radiotherapy have the best outlook and are most likely to be cured. It is important to note that residual masses do not always represent persisting disease. This is particularly true for residual mediastinal and retroperitoneal masses. These sites tend to be associated with

Table 22.4.3.6 Prognostic factors for advanced Hodgkin's lymphoma

Adverse prognostic factors	
Age	≥45 years
Stage	IV
gender	Male
White blood count	≥15 000 cells/µl
Lymphocyte count	<600 cells /µl or <8% of all white cells
Albumin	<40 g/litre
Hemoglobin	<10.5 g/dl

Outcome according to prognostic score

Number of factors	5-year freedom from progression (%)	5-year overall survival (%)
0	84	89
1	77	90
2	67	81
3	60	78
4	51	61
>5	42	56

a considerable amount of fibrosis that can persist after effective therapy. Normalization of a PET scan can be used to document remission.

Patients who relapse after initial successful treatment for Hodgkin's disease can sometimes be effectively treated with further chemotherapy or radiotherapy. The chances for successful treatment depend, in part, on the duration of initial remission in addition to other prognostic factors present at relapse. Patients with a longer initial remission are more likely to be successfully retreated.

Primary therapy

Patients with localized Hodgkin's disease (i.e. stage I or nonbulky stage II) can be cured with radiotherapy, chemotherapy, or combined modality therapy. When radiotherapy alone is utilized, a dose of 3500 to 4400 cGy is usually administered in fractions of 175 to 200 cGy daily to known sites of involvement and adjacent lymph node-bearing areas. However, it is increasingly popular to treat patients with an abbreviated course of a standard chemotherapy regimen, e.g. doxorubicin (Adriamycin), bleomycin, vinblastine, dacarbazine (ABVD), followed by involved-field radiotherapy to limit radiotherapy toxicity. It is possible that chemotherapy alone will become standard for patients with localized Hodgkin's disease who have a prompt and complete response to therapy, although most patients currently still receive radiation.

Patients with otherwise localized Hodgkin's disease who present with a large mediastinal mass pose special therapeutic problems. A large mediastinal mass is often defined as one whose maximum diameter is greater than one-third of the maximum thoracic diameter. Treatment with radiotherapy alone, or chemotherapy alone, is associated with a high relapse rate. Large mediastinal masses are one definite indication for combined-modality therapy, although not irradiating patients who achieve a complete remission as documented by a PET scan after chemotherapy alone is under study.

Patients who present with B-symptoms or stage III or IV disease are best treated initially with a combination chemotherapy regimen. If complete remission is documented after completing a course of chemotherapy, the majority of patients will be cured. Patients who have large masses often receive adjuvant radiotherapy to the sites of previous bulky disease after completing the chemotherapy regimen. The most popular regimen for treating Hodgkin's disease is currently ABVD (Table 22.4.3.5). ABVD has been shown to be equivalent to more complicated regimens that include the same drugs plus alkylating agents, and superior to alkylator-based regimens alone. New treatment regimens that are being studied include BEACOPP (bleomycin, etoposide, doxorubicin, cyclophosphamide, vincristine, procarbazine, and prednisone) and Stanford V (bleomycin, etoposide, doxorubicin, mechlorethamine, vinblastine, vincristine and prednisone plus radiotherapy). BEACOPP involves higher doses of drugs given in a very dose intensive fashion, while the drugs are administered weekly for 12 weeks in the Stanford V regimen. Excellent results have been reported with both of these new approaches and comparative trials are under way to determine subgroups of patients in which they might provide an advantage over ABVD.

Elderly and pregnant patients pose special therapeutic problems. In Hodgkin's disease, elderly patients have a much worse prognosis than younger ones: patients over 60 years of age at the time of diagnosis have a survival rate less than half that of younger patients. Elderly patients with localized disease seem to benefit from radiotherapy in a manner comparable to younger patients. However, older patients tolerate aggressive chemotherapy regimens much less well and, even if the drugs can be administered, have a higher relapse rate.

Since it occurs frequently in young adults, Hodgkin's disease is sometimes diagnosed in pregnant women. It is now clear that Hodgkin's disease can be treated with chemotherapy at any point during pregnancy with a chance of a good treatment outcome and a surviving infant. However, the risks are higher in the first trimester. Most physicians would favour delaying therapy past the first trimester, if possible, and would discuss the possibility of a therapeutic abortion with the patient. Some patients can be treated with intermittent vinblastine to control the disease until delivery, after which the patient can receive standard therapy. Pregnant patients should not be treated with radiotherapy. If the decision is made to treat a pregnant patient with chemotherapy, it must be remembered that the fetus will be myelosuppressed in a manner similar to the mother, and this must be taken into account when planning delivery of the baby.

The optimal treatment for nodular lymphocyte predominant Hodgkin's disease is unclear. Some clinicians favour no initial therapy in asymptomatic patients. However, involved-field radiotherapy, or a brief course of chemotherapy plus radiation, can produce durable remissions in some patients with this subtype of Hodgkin's disease. Rituximab is an active agent in nodular lymphocyte predominant Hodgkin's disease. The clinician must be alert for transformation to diffuse, large B-cell lymphoma.

Treatment of relapse

Approximately 25 to 35% of patients treated with chemotherapy for stage III or IV Hodgkin's disease will suffer relapse after achieving a remission, and a few patients will fail to enter initial complete remission. Patients who fail to enter complete remission or relapse within 1 year of completing therapy have a poor prognosis with further standard chemotherapy. Autologous bone marrow transplantation can be curative in 25 to 50% of such patients, and is the treatment of choice. Patients who have an initial remission of longer than 1 year pose a more complicated therapeutic problem. These patients are likely to achieve a second remission with a standard chemotherapy regimen. However, long-term follow-up has demonstrated that most of these remissions are not durable, and many physicians would recommend autologous transplantation to such patients. The occasional patient with a localized relapse after chemotherapy can sometimes be cured with radiotherapy. Patients who relapse after treatment with initial radiotherapy have an excellent result with standard chemotherapy regimens and a high likelihood of cure.

Treatment complications

The treatment of Hodgkin's disease is associated with both short-term and long-term complications. Prominent short-term complications include hair loss, emesis, fatigue, anaemia, and infection due to chemotherapy-induced neutropenia. Hair loss is usually transient. Emesis can be prevented in almost all patients by using 5-hydroxytryptamine antagonists. Anaemia and fatigue do not usually limit the administration of therapy. Chemotherapy-induced neutropenia is a major problem, and neutropenic fever needs to be managed aggressively with intravenous antibiotics after cultures are obtained. Even so, treatment for Hodgkin's disease is administered entirely on an outpatient basis.

Delayed toxicity from the treatment of Hodgkin's disease has become a major problem for young patients who are cured of the disease and have been followed for extended periods. In fact, for patients with good-prognosis Hodgkin's disease, long-term complications might lead to a higher mortality rate than the Hodgkin's disease itself.

Most of the serious complications of radiotherapy appear after long follow-up. In the first few months after treatment, some patients will develop an electric shock sensation down the spine and into the legs on flexion of the neck. This represents Lhermitte's syndrome and needs to be recognized so that further evaluation can be avoided. It is usually transient. In some patients, delayed pulmonary fibrosis or cardiac injuries are associated with thoracic radiotherapy. Modern radiotherapy techniques have minimized the risk of these problems, but accelerated coronary artery disease is a significant problem and leads to a number of treatment-related deaths. Follow-up of these patients should emphasize reducing risk factors for coronary artery disease. The major delayed problem with radiotherapy is the development of secondary cancers. This risk begins to appear beyond 10 years after therapy, and by 20 years after therapy leads to a significant number of deaths. Patients treated with thoracic radiotherapy for Hodgkin's disease should be strongly encouraged not to smoke, to reduce the risk of lung cancer. Young women should have screening mammography instituted 5 to 10 years earlier than for women not irradiated, or by 10 years after completing treatment.

Patients who receive radiotherapy to the neck have a high risk of developing subsequent hypothyroidism. Follow-up in such patients should include periodic quantitation of their thyrotropin levels to anticipate this problem. Some patients treated with either radiotherapy or chemotherapy will develop herpes zoster. This diagnosis does not necessarily signify a relapse of Hodgkin's disease.

Long-term problems associated with chemotherapy include treatment-related leukaemia, infertility, and aseptic necrosis of bone. Infertility is most likely in patients who receive alkylating agent-containing regimens. In women, the risks of infertility are age-related. Women over 30 years of age are much more likely to be permanently infertile than those under 30 years. However, in any patient, resumption of fertility is possible and the patient should be aware of this. Infertility is less of a problem in patients who receive the ABVD regimen. Men who are very anxious to retain fertility can be offered semen storage and women, in extraordinary cases, can be offered egg storage.

Treatment-related leukaemia is most frequent in patients who receive chemotherapy regimens containing alkylating agents and who are treated on more than one occasion. Young patients treated with only one chemotherapy sequence are unlikely to develop leukaemia. The incidence of leukaemia rises dramatically in patients over 40 years of age, and in those who receive alkylating agents on more than one occasion. Leukaemia is unusual in patients treated with ABVD. The combination of chemotherapy and radiotherapy seems to increase the risk of leukaemia. The leukaemias that occur in this setting usually present with myelodysplasia and typically have genetic abnormalities involving chromosomes 5, 7, and 8. Etoposide can lead to the development of acute leukaemia that involves abnormalities on chromosome 11 without a preceding myelodysplasia.

Patients who receive corticosteroid treatment as part of a combination therapy are at risk for aseptic necrosis of the femoral heads, and those who develop hip pain on follow-up should be evaluated for this possibility.

Non-Hodgkin's lymphoma (NHL)

Incidence

In much of the world, it appears that the incidence of NHL is increasing, but the incidence still varies widely between countries. The incidence appears to be approximately 2 cases per 100 000 per year in east Asia, 10 per 100 000 per year in the United Kingdom, and more than 15 per 100 000 per year in the United States od America. In the United States, the disease increased in frequency in patients of all ages, but more strikingly in elderly people, by approximately 4% per year between 1950 and the mid-1990s, although recent data suggest that the rate of increase may be stabilizing.

The specific types of NHL vary in occurrence between countries. For example, follicular lymphoma is more common in North America than in Europe or Asia. T-cell lymphomas have been seen more frequently in Asia, and certain types of T/NK-cell lymphomas (NK, natural killer) such as angiocentric nasal lymphomas are common only in a few countries in Asia and Latin America. The explanation for this geographical difference is unclear.

Aetiology

The aetiology of most NHL is unknown. Various aetiological factors, either proven or suggested to be associated with the development of NHL, are listed in Table 10. It is now clear that exposure to certain agriculture chemicals does increase the risk of this disease. A variety of immune deficiencies, such as those associated with immunosuppression following organ transplantation and various hereditary immune deficiencies, are also associated with an increased risk of developing NHL. Patients with disorders of the immune system such as rheumatoid arthritis and systemic lupus erythematosus also appear to be at increased risk.

A variety of infectious agents have been shown to be associated with the development of NHL. Gastric *Helicobacter pylori* infection is associated with the development of gastric mucosa-associated lymphoid tissue (MALT) lymphoma, and eradication of the infection by antibiotics can lead to regression of the lymphoma. Human T-cell lymphoma/leukaemia virus-1 (HTLV-1) appears to be the cause of a specific type of NHL, seen predominantly in southern Japan and the Caribbean, called adult T-cell lymphoma/leukaemia. EBV has been associated with Burkitt's lymphoma in Africa, the development of aggressive B-cell lymphomas in immunosuppressed patients, Hodgkin's disease, and certain aggressive T-cell lymphomas. Human herpesvirus-8 (HHV-8) has been closely associated with a rare, diffuse, large B-cell lymphoma called effusion lymphoma that is most frequently seen in immunosuppressed patients. HIV infection can lead to the development of aggressive B-cell lymphomas that are often EBV-positive. An association between hepatitis C virus (HCV) infection and the development of splenic or large B-cell lymphomas has been suggested. Similarly, the association of *Chlamydia psittaci* and ocular adenexal lymphomas has been reported. Other bacteria that have been associated with MALT lymphomas include *Campylobacter jejuni* (i.e. small bowel) and *Borrelia borgdorferi* (skin).

REAL/WHO classification

The classification of NHL changed several times during the 20th century. The first popular classification proposed by Gall and Mallory divided lymphomas into giant follicular lymphoma, reticulum-cell sarcoma, and lymphosarcoma. Both the lack of adequate clinical correlation and clear definitions of the entities led to further proposals. Henry Rappaport recognized the importance of growth pattern in the prognosis of NHL, and put forward his system that divided patients into those with nodular (i.e. follicular) or diffuse lymphomas and those with large- or small-cell lymphomas. However, this system was proposed before the recognition that lymphomas were all malignancies of lymphocytes and before the discovery of the existence of subtypes of lymphocytes. The advent of modern immunology led to new classification systems proposed by Lennert and colleagues in Europe and Lukes and Collins in the United States of America. The Kiel classification proposed by Lennert and colleagues became the most widely used system in Europe. An attempt to unify the classifications of lymphomas led to the development of the Working Formulation. This is a compromise system taking major elements from the Rappaport classification, the Kiel classification, and the Lukes/Collins classification. It became widely used in the United States of America but less so in Europe.

In the 1990s a group of haematopathologists from Europe, North America, and other parts of the world proposed a new system not just based on morphology and immunophenotyping, but taking into account other genetic and biological information that had become available. In the 1990s, a number of 'new' lymphomas were discovered that did not fit into previous classification systems. These included mantle-cell lymphoma, anaplastic large T/null-cell lymphoma, and MALT lymphomas. The Revised European/American Lymphoma (REAL) classification classified lymphomas based on clinical pathological syndromes (in other words, 'real' diseases) rather than simply morphology. This system was tested

Box 22.4.3.4 Factors predisposing to the development of NHL

- Immune deficiencies:
  - Organ transplantation
  - Inherited immune deficiencies
  - AIDS
- Agricultural chemicals
- Autoimmune disorders:
  - Rheumatoid arthritis
  - Lupus erythematosus
- Treated Hodgkin's disease
- Infectious agents:
  - Viruses: EBV, HTLV-1, HIV, HHV-8, HCV
  - Bacteria: *Helicobacter pylori, Chlamydia psittaci, Borelia borgdorferi, Campylobacter jejuni*

EBV, Epstein–Barr virus; HCV, hepatitis C virus; HHV-8, human herpesvirus-8; HTLV-1, human T-cell leukaemia virus-1.

Box 22.4.3.5 WHO Classification of NHL (2008)

- Precursor lymphoid neoplasms
  - B-lymphoblastic leukaemia/lymphoma
  - T-lymphoblastic leukaemia/lymphoma
- Mature B-cell neoplasms
  - Chronic lymphocytic leukaemia/small lymphocytic lymphoma
  - Splenic marginal zone lymphoma
  - Lymphoplasmacytic lymphoma
  - Extranodal marginal zone lymphoma of MALT (lymphoma)
  - Nodal marginal zone lymphoma
  - Follicular lymphoma
  - Primary cutaneous follicle centre lymphoma
  - Mantle cell lymphoma
  - Diffuse large B-cell lymphoma (DLBCL), NOS
    - T-cell rich DLBCL
    - Primary cutaneous DLBCL leg type
    - Intravascular DLBCL
    - Plasmablastic lymphoma
    - Primary effusion lymphoma
  - Primary mediastinal DLBCL
  - Burkitt lymphoma
- Mature T-cell neoplasms
  - Adult T-cell leukaemia/lymphoma
  - Extranodal NK/T cell lymphoma, nasal type
  - Enteropathy associated T-cell lymphoma
  - Hepatosplenic T-cell lymphoma
  - Subcutaneous panniculitis-like T-cell lymphoma
  - Mycosis fungoides
  - Sezary syndrome
  - Primary cutaneous CD30 positive T-cell lymphoproliferative disorders
  - Peripheral T-cell lymphoma, NOS
  - Angioimmunoblastic T-cell lymphoma
  - Anaplastic large cell lymphoma, ALK positive
  - Anaplastic large cell lymphoma, ALK negative

in a large international study and shown to be more accurate than previous systems and to have high clinical relevance. Leaders in the fields of both haematopathology and clinical haematology/oncology agreed on a modified REAL classification to be endorsed by the WHO and published as the WHO classification (Box 22.4.3.5). This, with modifications, is likely to be the major lymphoma classification for at least the next decade. The incidence of major lymphoma subtypes according to the WHO classification is listed in Table 22.4.3.7. Knowledge of 10 to 12 specific subtypes of NHL and the 2 major subtypes of Hodgkin's disease will allow a clinician to care for almost all patients with lymphoma.

International Prognostic Index

Knowledge of the specific subtype of NHL is only one of two pieces of information necessary to plan the intelligent management of patients with these disorders. The other that must be available involves the delineation of the prognostic characteristics of the individual patient. Although it is true that follicular lymphoma has a higher median overall survival than diffuse large B-cell lymphoma, individual patients with follicular lymphoma might have a much worse survival because of adverse prognostic characteristics than an individual patient with diffuse large B-cell lymphoma who has good prognostic characteristics. Codification of these prognostic characteristics into a practical clinical tool was accomplished by a large international study that yielded the International Prognostic Index (IPI) (Table 22.4.3.2). The IPI is a summation of a number of specific adverse prognostic factors in an individual patient. The important factors include age greater than 60 years, Ann Arbor stage III/IV, serum LDH level greater than normal, reduced performance status, and multiple extranodal sites of involvement by lymphoma. The IPI is useful in essentially all types of NHL, although it was developed using patients with diffuse large cell lymphoma of both T- and B-cell origin. A new index for use in patients with follicular lymphoma has been developed and referred to as the FLIPI (i.e. follicular lymphoma International

Table 22.4.3.7 Relative frequency of occurrence of major subtypes of NHL

Type of NHL	Percentage of all NHL
Diffuse large B-cell	31
Follicular	22
Small lymphocytic/LLL	6
Mantle-cell	6
Peripheral T-cell	6
MALT	5
Anaplastic large T/null-cell	2
Lymphoblastic	2
Burkitt's	<1

LLL, large lymphocytic leukaemia; MALT, mucosa-associated lymphoid tissue.

Prognostic Index), but this has not been as widely used as the IPI. The treatment plan for any individual patient with lymphoma must always include knowledge of the specific subtype of lymphoma and the patient's prognostic characteristics.

Precursor B- and T-cell lymphomas

Lymphoblastic lymphoma of B-cell and T-cell origin

Lymphoblastic lymphoma is a tumour of the precursor cells of T- and B-lymphocytes. It is intimately related to the acute lymphoid leukaemias, with the difference being the method of presentation. Sometimes it is difficult to determine when a patient should be said to have acute lymphoid leukaemia or lymphoblastic lymphoma, since bone marrow involvement is frequent with a lymphomatous presentation and lymphadenopathy and mediastinal mass are common in patients who present with leukaemia.

Most patients with lymphoblastic lymphoma have tumours derived from T-lymphoblasts, but approximately 10% are B-cell in origin. The differential diagnosis of lymphoblastic lymphoma includes a blastic variant of mantle-cell lymphoma, acute myeloid leukaemia, and peripheral T-cell lymphoma in children and young adults.

The median age of patients with lymphoblastic lymphoma is the late twenties; most patients are male with widely disseminated disease and an elevated serum LDH level, and about 50% will have bone marrow involvement. Patients with lymphoblastic lymphoma who present with stage IV disease, elevated LDH levels, and bone marrow or central nervous system involvement have a poorer prognosis than adult patients who do not have these adverse characteristics. Patients with none of these adverse characteristics have a high cure rate with regimens such as those used for adult acute lymphoblastic leukaemia. Some patients with stage IV disease, elevated LDH levels, and bone marrow and central nervous system involvement can also be cured, but this is less likely. Treatment in both groups of patients should include central nervous system prophylaxis and either maintenance or consolidation treatment. Patients with high risk characteristics, or those who relapse after initial therapy, are candidates for allogeneic or autologous haematopoietic stem cell transplantation.

Mature B-cell lymphomas

Diffuse large B-cell lymphoma

Diffuse large B-cell lymphoma is the most common type of NHL, representing approximately one-third of all patients. It most

Table 22.4.3.8 Recognized molecular subtypes of diffuse large B-cell lymphoma

Characteristics	Germinal centre B-cell type	Activated B-cell type	Mediastinal large B-cell lymphoma
% of all patients with diffuse large B-cell lymphoma	~50	~30	7
Median age (years)	58	66	37
% female	50	40	70
% 5-year survival (i.e. with rituximab)	70–90	60–65	>70

commonly presents *de novo*, but can also develop after histological transformation of a small-cell lymphoma such as follicular, small lymphocytic, or MALT lymphoma. This tumour can arise in lymph nodes or essentially in any extranodal site, including the central nervous system. Rare presentations include pleural effusions from involvement of serosal surfaces (effusion lymphoma) and multiple organ system dysfunction secondary to endothelial involvement (intravascular lymphomatosis).

Almost all diffuse large B-cell lymphomas display the CD20 antigen, and several cytogenetic abnormalities are frequently associated (Table 22.4.3.4). The condition can be subdivided using gene microarrays into the germinal centre B-cell type, the activated B-cell type, and the mediastinal large B-cell type. These have different clinical characteristics and response to therapy (Table 22.4.3.8 and Fig. 22.4.3.2).

The differential diagnosis of diffuse large B-cell lymphoma includes undifferentiated carcinoma, acute myeloid leukaemia, Hodgkin's disease, and extramedullary plasmacytoma. Occasional patients with diffuse large B-cell lymphoma have a large number of infiltrating T cells, and can be confused with a peripheral T-cell lymphoma. Appropriate immunological studies and genetic studies can usually resolve any confusion.

The clinical characteristics of patients with diffuse large B-cell lymphoma are presented in Table 22.4.3.9. The median age at presentation of patients with diffuse large B-cell lymphoma is approximately 64 years and there is a slight male predominance. About one-half of the patients will have stage I or II disease and about one-half will have a more widely disseminated lymphoma: approximately two-thirds will have some sign of extranodal involvement,

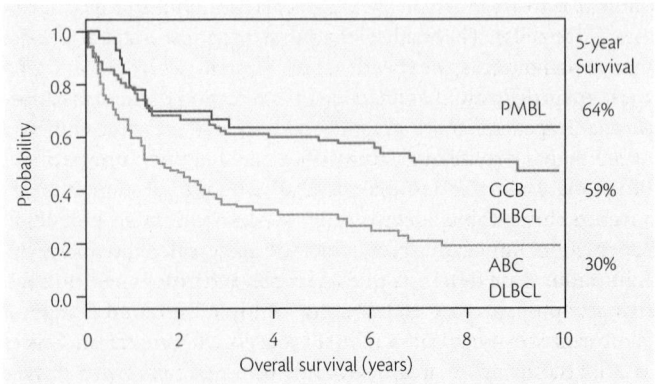

Fig. 22.4.3.2 Survival of patients with subtypes of diffuse large B-cell lymphoma (DLBCL) treated largely in the pre-rituximab era. ABC, activated B-cell; GCB, germinal centre B cell; PMBL, primary mediastinal B-cell lymphoma.

one-third will have B-symptoms at presentation, and one-half have an elevated LDH. Bone marrow involvement is seen in approximately 15% of cases.

Since the early 1970s it has been known that patients with diffuse large B-cell lymphoma could sometimes be cured with combination chemotherapy regimens alone—even those with disseminated disease. The most popular regimen in use today is CHOP (cyclophosphamide, doxorubicin, vincristine (Oncovin), and prednisone) plus the antibody rituximab. However, a large number of other regimens including ACVBP (doxorubicin, cyclophosphamide, vindesine, bleomycin, and prednisone) are at least as active. Today all regimens used to treat diffuse large B-cell lymphoma will include the antibody rituximab unless the patient's individual tumour has been shown to be CD20 negative. When a staging evaluation shows disease confined to one site (i.e. stage I) or two nearby sites (i.e. minimal stage II) a brief course of chemotherapy followed by radiotherapy has been the most popular treatment approach, although a complete course of CHOP plus rituximab might be equally effective. In patients with disseminated disease, a complete course of CHOP plus rituximab, or another active regimen plus rituximab, is standard therapy. Local radiotherapy is sometimes added to very bulky (i.e. >10 cm) sites of disease. In patients who present with the multiple adverse risk factors listed in the IPI, adjuvant autologous haemopoietic stem-cell transplantation after achieving an initial remission might benefit selected patients.

Approximately 75–85% of patients with localized disease can be cured with CHOP plus rituximab plus/minus radiotherapy. Approximately 50% of patients with more disseminated disease can be cured with combination chemotherapy regimens including rituximab. Patients who relapse from complete remission can sometimes be cured with autologous hematopoietic stem cell transplantation. Patients who remain chemotherapy-sensitive after relapse have been cured approximately 40% of the time while chemotherapy resistant patients are cured only about 10% of the time.

Follicular lymphoma

The second most common type of NHL is follicular lymphoma. The clinical characteristics of patients with this disease are listed in Table 22.4.3.9. The differential diagnosis of follicular lymphoma includes benign follicular hyperplasia and follicular variants of other NHLs.

Patients with follicular lymphoma are subdivided based on the number of large cells in the tumour into grade 1 (i.e. those with the least large cells), grade 2 and grade 3 (i.e. those with the most large cells). The method for assigning grade is controversial among pathologists, whose ability to reproduce grading is much lower than their ability to reproducibly diagnose follicular lymphoma. In general, a higher proportion of large cells is associated with a higher proliferative rate, more rapid tumour progression, and perhaps a better response to anthracycline-containing combination chemotherapy regimens. The natural history of follicular lymphoma involves a reduction in the degree of follicularity in the tumour over time and an increase in the proportion of large cells. At autopsy, most tumours will be found to have undergone transformation—usually to diffuse large B-cell lymphoma. This is recognized during life in approximately 50% of patients and associated with a poor prognosis in most cases.

Follicular lymphomas regularly display the CD20 antigen. Most tumours will have the t(14;18) translocation and oversecrete the

Box 22.4.3.6 Treatment regimens used for patients with follicular lymphoma

- Close observation and no initial therapy
- Radiotherapy
- Single-agent therapy: chlorambucil, cyclophosphamide, fludarabine, bendamustine—all with rituximab—or rituximab alone
- Combination chemotherapy: CHOP-R, CVP-R, FND-R
- Interferon-α
- Radioantibodies, tositumomab, ibritumomab
- Haemopoieteic stem-cell transplantation: autologous, allogeneic

CHOP, cyclophosphamide, doxorubicin, vincristine, prednisone; CVP, cyclophosphamide, vincristine, prednisone; FND, fludarabine, mitoxantrone, dexamethasone.

bcl-2 protein. Transformation to diffuse large B-cell lymphoma is frequently associated with additional cytogenetic abnormalities

Treatment approaches commonly utilized in the management of patients with follicular lymphoma are presented in Box 22.4.3.6. Asymptomatic patients with nonbulky disease and no organ compromise are often managed with no initial therapy—a strategy that is sometimes called 'watchful waiting'. When followed in this manner, approximately 25% of patients will undergo at least a partial spontaneous regression (i.e. what would be called a partial response if a treatment had been utilized), although these regressions are not durable. Over time, almost all patients will progress and require therapy. There is no 'standard' treatment for patients with follicular lymphoma. The most often utilized initial treatments are single-agent chemotherapy including bendamustine, CVP (cyclophosphamide, vincristine, and prednisone), CHOP, and fludarabine-containing regimens. With few exceptions, each of these regimens will be combined with the antibody rituximab. An increasingly popular treatment approach, and one that is sometimes utilized instead of watchful waiting, is single-agent therapy with rituximab. Most patients respond, although less than one-half will achieve a complete remission. When ongoing or 'maintenance' treatment with the antibody is continued after the initial induction therapy, the duration of remissions is prolonged. It is now clear that when combinations of traditional chemotherapeutic agents are combined with rituximab as initial therapy, then patients have a longer survival than when combination chemotherapy alone is utilized.

Particular treatment approaches are more appropriate for certain subsets of patients with follicular lymphoma. The rare patients with localized follicular lymphoma can be managed with radiotherapy alone. These patients have an excellent outlook with a 10-year survival of 70 to 90% in most series, and approximately 40 to 50% of patients not relapsing after 10 years of follow-up. Patients with grade 3 follicular lymphoma often respond to treatments used for diffuse large B-cell lymphoma, and many physicians would favour CHOP plus rituximab (CHOP-R) as the initial treatment for these patients.

Bone marrow specimens from patients with follicular lymphoma frequently test positive for the BCL2 gene rearrangement using polymerized chain reaction (PCR) technology. Some but not all patients who achieve a complete remission will revert to a BCL-2 negative status. This test has not been widely utilized clinically since some patients who remain positive do not relapse, some patients who become negative do relapse, and circulating lymphoid cells in normal patients occasionally have the *BCL2* gene rearrangement. This presumably reflects that rearrangement of the *BCL2* gene is a very early step in lymphomagenesis.

Most patients with follicular lymphoma will eventually fail their initial treatment regimen, with this especially true for patients with follicular lymphoma grade 1 and grade 2. Subsequent treatments have included single drugs such as chlorambucil or fludarabine, a variety of combination chemotherapy regimens, and new drugs such as bortezomib, interferon, unlabelled antibodies (e.g. rituximab), radiolabelled antibodies, and both allogeneic and autologous haematopoietic stem cell transplantation. Both autologous and allogeneic haematopoietic stem cell transplantation can produce long-term disease-free survival in a proportion of patients with follicular lymphoma. Autologous haematopoietic stem cell transplantation is more effective when utilized at first relapse. Allogeneic transplantation has a much lower relapse rate than autologous transplantation, but is associated with a higher mortality rate.

The median survival of patients treated for follicular lymphoma in most series has been approximately 10 years. The improvement in average survival in a variety of studies utilizing the addition of rituximab to standard chemotherapeutic agents suggests that this is likely to improve. Some patients survive free of disease for extended periods of time, and hopefully this proportion will increase with new treatments

MALT lymphoma

This lymphoma, also known as the extranodal marginal-zone B-cell lymphoma of MALT type, always presents in extranodal sites.

A nodal presentation of a similar lymphoma is referred to as nodal marginal-zone lymphoma or monocytoid B-cell lymphoma (see below). Before the recognition of the existence of MALT lymphomas, orbital, pulmonary, and gastric presentations were sometimes referred to by pathologists as pseudolymphoma. The differential diagnosis of MALT lymphoma includes benign lymphocytic infiltration of extranodal organs and other small-cell B-cell lymphomas.

MALT lymphomas are tumours of CD5 negative and CD23 negative B cells that express CD20. The commonly seen cytogenetic abnormalities are listed in Table 22.4.3.4. Gastric MALT lymphomas are associated with infection by *Helicobacter pylori*, thyroid MALT lymphomas are frequently associated with Hashimoto's thyroiditis, and orbital MALT lymphomas are sometimes associated with Sjögren's syndrome. MALT lymphomas can undergo histological transformation to diffuse large B-cell lymphomas. After this transformation, the patient should be treated for diffuse large B-cell lymphoma.

MALT lymphomas have a slight female predominance with a median age at presentation of approximately 60 years. The symptoms of the disorder are those associated with involvement of the extranodal site. The disease is usually localized and the presence of systemic symptoms or elevated LDH is unusual. The characteristics of patients with this lymphoma are listed in Table 22.4.3.9.

Gastric MALT lymphomas are the first example of a lymphoma that can be treated by eliminating a chronic infection. If the tumour does not transform to a large-cell lymphoma, and has not deeply invaded the stomach, then most patients will have their tumour regress with the eradication of *Helicobacter pylori* using antibiotics, proton pump inhibitors, and bismuth. It appears that in some patients this treatment might be curative. Other local

Table 22.4.3.9 Clinical characteristics of the major subtypes of B-cell NHL

	Diffuse large B-cell lymphoma	Follicular lymphoma	MALT lymphoma	Small lymphocytic lymphoma	Mantle-cell lymphoma
Median age (years)	64	59	60	65	63
Percentage male	55	42	48	53	74
Stage (%):					
I	25	18	39	4	13
II	19	15	28	5	7
III	13	16	2	8	9
IV	33	51	31	83	71
B-symptoms (%)	33	28	19	33	28
Elevated LDH (%)	53	30	27	41	40
Reduced performance status (%)	24	9	15	11	21
Tumour mass >10 cm (%)	30	28	8	13	81
Bone marrow involvement (%)	16	47	14	72	64
Gastrointestinal tract involvement (%)	18	4	50	3	9
IPI score (%)					
0–1	35	45	44	23	23
2–3	46	48	48	64	54
4–5	19	7	8	13	23

IPI, International Prognostic Index.

therapies are also effective. Patients with localized MALT lymphomas can be effectively treated with local radiotherapy or, in some cases, surgery. These lymphomas also respond to rituximab, single-agent chemotherapy, and combination chemotherapy. Patients with disseminated MALT lymphomas usually respond to therapy, but are rarely curable.

Most patients with localized MALT lymphoma can be cured, and the 5-year survival in such patients is approximately 90%. However, patients with disseminated disease have a more serious illness and those with a high International Prognostic Index score have a 5-year survival of only 50%.

Small lymphocytic lymphoma/chronic lymphocytic leukaemia

Small lymphocytic lymphoma is the tissue manifestation of chronic lymphocytic leukaemia. Patients who present predominantly with blood and bone marrow involvement will be diagnosed with chronic lymphocytic leukaemia, and those who present with lymphadenopathy as having small lymphocytic lymphoma, although the WHO classification suggests that all these patients might be called chronic lymphocytic leukaemia. Patients with plasmacytoid differentiation and monoclonal IgM protein in the serum can present the syndrome of Waldenström's macroglobulinaemia (see 'Less common B-cell lymphomas', below).

Small lymphocytic lymphoma makes up approximately 7% of NHL worldwide, although is more often seen in Western countries. The differential diagnosis includes other small B-cell lymphomas, and patients with small lymphocytic lymphoma can undergo histological transformation to diffuse large B-cell lymphoma. This syndrome is seen in approximately 3%–10% of patients and is called Richter's syndrome. It is associated with a poor prognosis.

The lymphoma cells are B-cells that are CD5, CD20, and CD23 positive, although the concentration of CD20 on the surface of the tumour cells is less than in most other B-cell lymphomas. Common cytogenetic abnormalities seen in chronic lymphomcytic leukemia/small lymphocytic lymphoma include trisomy 12, del(11q), and del(17p), and del (13q), with del (17p) being particularly associated with a very poor prognosis. Other biological measurements to predict outcome in patients with chronic lymhocytic/small lymphocytic lymphoma have included the proportion of cells that express CD38, those that express ZAP70, and those with unmutated IgVH genes. As a practical issue for therapy, del(17p) is seen in only approximately 3% of patients, and other biological measurements are not sufficiently standardized for wide use. Patients with lymphoplasmacytic lymphoma can have the t(9;14) cytogenetic abnormality.

The clinical characteristics of patients with small lymphocytic lymphoma are listed in Table 22.4.3.9. Patients with chronic lymphocytic leukaemia/small lymphocytic lymphoma sometimes have acquired immunological abnormalities including hypogammaglobulinaemia, autoimmune thrombocytopenia, and autoimmune haemolytic anaemia. When present, these immune abnormalities should be treated specifically, in addition to any treatment given for the lymphoma. Hypogammaglobulinaemia should be treated with intermittent immunoglobulin interfusions.

Patients with chronic lymphocytic leukaemia/small lymphocytic lymphoma can be followed without therapy when they present with no systemic symptoms or organ compromise. However, most patients will require treatment within the first few years of follow-up. Currently, the most popular treatments for patients with chronic lymphocytic leukaema/small lymphocytic lymphoma contain fludarabine, the related drug pentostatin, or bendamustine. Combinations of fludarabine (or penostatin) and rituximab plus/minus cyclophosphamide have a high complete response rate. Patients who cannot tolerate these treatment approaches are often treated with oral chlorambucil. However, most patients treated with any of these approaches will eventually progress and require further treatment. Only a few patients are candidates for allogeneic haematopoietic stem cell transplantation, but this can achieve long-term disease-free survival in some cases.

Mantle-cell lymphoma

The clinical characteristics of patients with mantle-cell lymphoma are listed in Table 22.4.3.9. This lymphoma was recognized as a specific entity because of its characteristic cytogenetic abnormality, these tumours regularly manifesting the t(11;14) translocation that involves the BCL1 gene on chromosome 11 and leads to overproduction of the BCL-1 protein, which can be useful in diagnosis. Indeed, before the recognition of this disorder, patients with mantle-cell lymphoma were placed in many other histological categories, usually being termed centrocytic lymphoma under the Kiel classification. An expert haematopathologist is important in making the diagnosis, since this lymphoma can be confused with small lymphocytic lymphoma, follicular lymphoma, and lymphoblastic lymphoma.

Extranodal sites of involvement by mantle-cell lymphoma are not unusual. Large-bowel involvement can present as the syndrome of lymphomatous polyposis, and patients without this syndrome will usually have mantle cell lymphoma discovered on blind biopsies of the colon. Patients with distal gastrointestinal tract lymphoma often have Waldeyer's ring involvement in addition.

Mantle-cell lymphoma has been among the most difficult types of NHL to treat. Using standard chemotherapy regimens such as CHOP, the remission duration has been brief and the median overall survival approximately 3–5 years. The addition of the antibody rituximab and the use of very intensive chemotherapy regimens has improved the response rate and remission duration. However, the cure of these patients with standard chemotherapy regimens is still uncertain, hence many patients receive autologous or allogeneic transplantation in first remission. Allogeneic transplantation can occasionally cure patients who have failed their primary regimen. Because most patients with mantle cell lymphoma are elderly, these more aggressive treatment approaches are often inappropriate or impractical.

Less common B-cell lymphomas

Burkitt's lymphoma was originally described by Dennis Burkitt while studying an aggressive lymphoma that occurred in the jaw of children in Central Africa; the disease can also present as acute leukaemia. An association has been demonstrated between EBV infection and this lymphoma, which is much more frequent in children and young adults and in patients infected by HIV. The condition is associated with specific chromosomal translocations involving the heavy-chain immunoglobulin gene on chromosome 14 or the light-chain immunoglobulin genes on chromosomes 2 and 22. In each case, the associated oncogene is the c-myc gene on chromosome 8 (namely, t(8;14), t(2;8), and t(8;22)). The condition can frequently be cured utilizing short courses of very intensive regimens that incorporate high doses of cyclophosphamide, hence distinction between Burkitt's lymphoma and diffuse large B-cell lymphoma is extremely important.

Nodal marginal-zone lymphoma or monocytoid B-cell lymphoma is immunologically related to MALT lymphoma (see above), but presents in a manner similar to follicular lymphoma. These patients respond to therapy and have an overall survival similar to those with follicular lymphoma.

Splenic marginal-zone lymphoma is a rare disorder, also known as splenic lymphoma with villous lymphocytes. It is an indolent condition that often responds dramatically to rituximab.

Primary mediastinal diffuse large B-cell lymphoma varies from other diffuse large B-cell lymphomas in that it occurs at a younger age and has a striking female predominance. Gene expression profiling has shown that these tumours are genetically distinct and have some similarities to nodular sclerosing Hodgkin's disease. However, the treatment and response to therapy are similar to that seen in the germinal centre B-cell type of diffuse large B-cell lymphomas (Table 22.4.3.8 and Fig. 22.4.3.2).

Lymphoplasmacytic lymphoma, a subtype of small lymphocytic lymphoma (see above), is the histological subtype of lymphoma seen in lymph nodes biopsied in patients with Waldenström's macroglobulinaemia. All patients with Waldenstrom's macroglobulinaemia have a lymphoplasmacytic lymphoma, but all patients with lymphoplasmacytic lymphoma will not manifest the syndrome of Waldenstrom's macroglobulinaemia. Treatment often includes alkylator or fludarabine-based regimens, frequently combined with rituximab, or rituximab as a single agent. Patients with symptoms from a very high IgM level will require plasmapheresis

Mature T-cell lymphomas

T-cell lymphomas are much less common than their B-cell counterparts, accounting for about 10% of NHL in Western countries. Mature T-cell lymphomas are frequently called 'peripheral T-cell lymphoma'. This refers not to the site of origin of the disease, but to the mature T-cell immunophenotype. Pathologists have been less accurate in diagnosing T-cell lymphomas than B-cell lymphomas, which in part might relate to the absence of a characteristic immunophenotype for most diseases, and only a few subtypes having consistent genetic abnormalities. For T-cell lymphomas, but not for NK-cell lymphomas, demonstration of rearrangements of the T-cell receptor gene will sometimes help solve difficult diagnostic dilemmas.

The differential diagnosis of peripheral T-cell lymphomas includes diffuse large B-cell lymphoma and T-cell hyperplasias, such as are seen in viral infections and drug reactions. The characteristics of the mature T-cell lymphoma are presented in Table 22.4.3.10.

Nodal T-cell lymphomas

The nodal T-cell lymphomas recognized in the WHO classification include peripheral T-cell lymphoma unspecified, angioimmunoblastic T-cell lymphoma, and anaplastic large T/null cell lymphoma. Patients with peripheral T-cell lymphoma unspecified represent a heterogenous group of NHL and are the largest subgroup of peripheral T-cell lymphomas. These tumours are generally CD3 and CD4 positive, although a few will be CD8 positive. Although cytogenetic abnormalities are frequent, there is no consistent abnormality. Most patients have widespread disease and systemic symptoms are frequent.

Angioimmunoblastic T-cell lymphoma is the second most common subtype. These patients typically present with widespread disease, systemic symptoms, and frequently skin rashes and polyclonal hypergammaglubulinaemia. This type of peripheral T-cell lymphoma seems somewhat more frequent in northern Europe.

Anaplastic large T/null cell lymphoma has a characteristic histological appearance and consistently overexpresses the CD30 antigen. Many of the tumours have the t(2;5) translocation and overproduction of the ALK protein (in ~50% of cases). Patients whose tumours are ALK positive are younger, predominantly male, and might have a better outlook than those whose tumours are ALK negative. Some patients have lymphoma with the histological

Table 22.4.3.10 Clinical characteristics of T-cell lymphomas

	PTCL-unspecified	ATL	Angioimmunoblastic	ALCL Alk +	ALCL Alk −	Nasa NK/T l	Sub-Q Panniculitis-like	Hepatosplenic	Enteropathy associated
Median age (years)	60	62	65	33	58	49	33	34	61
Percentage male	66	55	56	63	61	65	75	68	53
ıge (%):									
I	13	5	1	12	19	48	17	5	10
II	17	5	10	23	22	20	0	0	21
III	26	18	41	29	21	4	0	0	5
IV	43	73	48	36	38	33	83	95	64
B-symptoms (%)	35	31	69	60	57	46	67	84	63
Elevated LDH (%)	47	40	62	36	44	49	75	84	32
IPI (%):									
0/1	27	19	13	49	41	44	42	5	25
2/3	57	64	58	37	44	50	42	47	62
4/5	15	16	28	14	14	6	17	47	12
% 5-year survival	31	14	32	70	49	32	64	7	20

ALCL, anaplastic large T/null cell lymphoma; Alk +/−, ALK protein positive/negative; ATL, angioimmunoblastic T-cell lymphoma; IPI, International Prognostic Index; PTCL, peripheral T-cell lymphoma; nasal NK/T, angiocentric nasal NK-cell lymphoma.

appearance of anaplastic large T/null cell lymphoma, but with the disease confined to the skin: these are one part of an entity that has been referred to as CD30-positive cutaneous lymphoproliferative disorders.

The treatment of patients with nodal peripheral T-cell lymphomas has been largely unsatisfactory. Localized disease is unusual and patients with disseminated disease are treated with combination chemotherapy regimens. There is no consistently effective approach for patients with peripheral T-cell lymphoma unspecified and angioimmunoblastic T-cell lymphomas. Patients with anaplastic large T/null cell lymphoma seem more likely to respond to anthracycline containing combination chemotherapy regimens. Young patients whose tumours overexpress the ALK protein are cured more than 50% of the time. Patients with cutaneous anaplastic large T/null cell lymphoma have a particularly indolent course and often do not need to be treated aggressively.

Extranodal peripheral T-cell lymphomas
Mycosis fungoides or cutaneous T-cell lymphoma is an indolent lymphoma of mature T cells predominantly involving the skin. Patients who present with circulating, atypical (that is, Sezary) cells and erythroderma are said to have Sezary syndrome. The median age is approximately 50 years and the disease is more common in males and blacks.

Mycosis fungoides often presents with eczematous or dermatitic skin lesions for many years, and patients will often have several skin biopsies before the diagnosis is confirmed. Lymphoma first manifests itself as superficial lesions in the skin that thicken and eventually ulcerate. In the late stages of the illness, lymphoma can metastasize to lymph nodes and visceral organs.

Treatments utilized for mycosis fungoides include topical corticosteroids, topical nitrogen mustard, phototherapy, psoralen ultraviolet A-range (PUVA) therapy, electron-beam radiation, interferon, vorinostat, bexarotene and systemic cytotoxic therapy among others. Some patients with localized mycosis fungoides can be cured with radiotherapy, but most will progress. In the endstages of this disease, management is difficult and the ulcerating cutaneous lesions present unpleasant problems for both the patient and the physician. The median survival from diagnosis averages over 10 years.

A number of distinctive but unusual clinical syndromes are grouped in the category of extranodal peripheral T-cell lymphomas. These include angiocentric nasal NK-cell lymphoma, which often presents with necrotic nasal or facial lesions. These patients are most often seen in South-East Asia and certain parts of Latin America. Radiotherapy is often an important part of the management of this disease. Enteropathy-type T-cell lymphoma is a rare disorder that occurs in patients with gluten enteropathy. Patients are frequently wasted, sometimes present with intestinal perforation, and have a particularly poor outlook. Hepatosplenic γδ T-cell lymphoma presents as a systemic illness with sinusoidal infiltration of the liver, spleen, and bone marrow by malignant T-cells. These patients often present a diagnostic dilemma, and treatment results have been poor. Subcutaneous panniculitis-like T-cell lymphoma is a rare disorder that presents with subcutaneous nodules and is frequently confused with panniculitis. This is true even on biopsy if the slides are not reviewed by an expert haematopathologist. This frequently has a more indolent course than some other types of extranodal peripheral T-cell lymphoma.

Adult T-cell lymphoma/leukaemia
The two major manifestations of infection by HTLV-1 are tropical spastic paraparesis and adult T-cell lymphoma/leukaemia. Patients can be infected with HTLV-1 through sexual transmission, blood transmission, or transplacentally. The risk of developing lymphoma in a patient infected with HTLV-1 is between 1% and 7% according to various studies. The latency between infection and the development of lymphoma averages approximately 20 years. The diagnosis is established by review of an adequate biopsy by an expert haematopathologist, demonstration of a T-cell immunophenotype, and demonstration of antibodies to HTLV-1. Most patients will have circulating tumour cells with a characteristic pleomorphic histology.

Adult T-cell lymphoma/leukaemia is most frequently seen in the southern islands of Japan and in the Caribbean. Most patients seen in Europe and North America are immigrants from those regions. Blood transfusion provides a possible source for infection, but screening for HTLV-1 has reduced the risk.

The clinical characteristics of patients with adult T-cell lymphoma/leukaemia vary considerably. Some patients present with an indolent disease manifested by lymphadenopathy and skin lesions and survive for extended times without specific therapy. Others present with progressive lymphadenopathy, hepatosplenomegaly, skin infiltration, hypercalcaemia, lytic bone lesions, and elevated LDH levels. Although patients sometimes respond to combination chemotherapy regimens, complete remissions are unusual and survival is poor. Patients frequently respond to newer combination chemotherapy regimens and survival seems to be improving, but cure is still unusual.

Lymphoma-like disorders (see Chapter 22.4.2)
Lymphadenopathy caused by infectious mononucleosis; drug reactions to diphenylhydantoin or carbamazepine; autoimmune disorders such as rheumatoid arthritis and systemic lupus erythematosus; and bacterial infections such as cat-scratch disease, can all be confused on biopsy with lymphoma.

Castleman's disease is a specific condition that can present with localized or disseminated lymphadenopathy and systemic symptoms. The disease appears to be related to an overproduction of interleukin-6 (IL-6) and is frequently associated with infection by HHV-8. The disseminated form of Castleman's disease is frequently accompanied by anaemia and polyclonal hypergammaglobulinaemia. Patients with localized disease can frequently be treated with local therapy, while systemic disease sometimes responds to systemic glucocorticoids, combination chemotherapy regimens, autologous or allogeneic bone marrow transplantation, rituximab, and antibodies against IL-6.

Sinus histiocytosis with massive lymphadenopathy (Rosai–Dorfman disease) typically presents with bulky lymphadenopathy in children or young adults. The disease is usually nonprogressive and self-limited. Lymphomatoid papulosis is a cutaneous lymphoproliferative disorder that can be confused with T-cell lymphoma in the skin. It is one of the CD30-positive cutaneous lymphoproliferative disorders. The cells in lymphomatoid papulosis stain for CD30 and have a monoclonal T-cell receptor gene rearrangement. The condition is characterized by waxing and waning skin lesions that usually heal leaving small scars. Although these patients have an increased risk of developing lymphoma, aggressive therapy is inappropriate.

Further reading

Armitage JO, *et al.* (2009). Non-Hodgkin Lymphomas. Wolters Kluwer/ Lippincott Williams, Wilkins (Philadelphia).

Armitage JO, Vose JM, Weisenburger D (2008). International peripheral T-cell and natural killer/T-cell lymphoma study: pathology findings and clinical outcomes. *J Clin Oncol*, **26**, 4124–130.

Chan WC, Armitage JO (2010). Economic analysis of lymphoma: potential for clinical applications. JNCCN.

Cheson BD, *et al.* (2007). Revised response criteria for malignant lymphoma. *J Clin Oncol*, **25**, 59–86.

Hasenclever D, Diehl V (1998). A prognostic score for advanced Hodgkin's disease. International Prognostic Factors Project on Advanced Hodgkin's Disease. *N Engl J Med*, **339**, 1506–14.

Hoppe R, *et al.* (eds) (2007). *Hodgkin's disease*. Lippincott Williams & Wilkins, Philadelphia.

Juweid ME, *et al.* (2007). Use of positron emission tomography for response assessment of lymphoma: consensus of the Imaging Subcommittee of International Harmonization Project in Lymphoma. *J Clin Oncol*, **25**, 571–8.

Pfreundschuh M, *et al.* (2006). CHOP-like chemotherapy plus rituximab versus CHOP-like chemotherapy alone in young patients with good-prognosis diffuse large B-cell lymphoma: a randomized controlled trial by the MabThera International Trial (MInT) Group. *Lancet Oncol*, **7**, 379–91.

Swerdlow SH, Campo E, Harris NL, *et al.* (2008). Classifications of tumours of haemopoietic and lymphoid tissues, 4th ed. Lyon, France, International agency for research on cancer.

22.4.4 The spleen and its disorders

D. Swirsky

Essentials

The spleen is the single largest lymphoid organ in the body, performing important immune functions. Intrinsic disorders of the spleen are very rare: its importance in clinical practice relate to the causes of its enlargement, its hyperfunction (hypersplenism), acute rupture, and the consequences of its physical or physiological absence.

Splenomegaly

Causes can broadly be divided into (1) infective—acute and chronic, with the prevalence of particular disorders being very dependent on geography; globally, most cases of splenomegaly are caused by parasitic infections, particularly malaria, leishmaniasis, and schistosomiasis; (2) congestive—most commonly portal hypertension; (3) haemolytic anaemias—both hereditary (including structural haemoglobinopathies and some thalassaemias) and acquired; (4) primary blood disorders—causes of massive splenomegaly include chronic myeloid leukaemia, chronic lymphocytic leukaemia, hairy cell leukaemia, and myelofibrosis; (5) malignant lymphomas; (6) connective tissue disorders—e.g. systemic lupus erythematosus (SLE), Felty's syndrome; (7) others—including storage diseases, e.g. type I Gaucher's disease.

Hypersplenism

Any cause of splenomegaly may give rise to hypersplenism, manifest as (1) variable peripheral blood cytopenias; (2) a cellular or hypercellular bone marrow; (3) premature release of cells into the peripheral blood, resulting in a mild reticulocytosis with nucleated red cells and occasional immature granulocytes. Other features include decreased red cell and platelet survival, and hypervolaemia.

Deficient splenic function

The most serious consequence of splenectomy or hyposplenism/ asplenia is vulnerability to overwhelming infection, which carries a very high mortality rate and is most frequently caused by *Streptococcus pneumoniae*.

All patients without a functioning spleen require vaccination against *S. pneumoniae*, haemophilus, and *Neisseria meningitides*, with additional lifelong antibiotic prophylaxis in some situations. Special warnings, advice about avoidance, and prophylaxis are required for those in or travelling to areas endemic for malaria and babesiosis.

Historical introduction

Since Hippocratic times the role of the spleen has been controversial. Galen called it an organ of mystery. Its structure was described during the 17th and early 18th centuries by Harvey, Glisson, Wharton, Malpighi, and van Leeuwenhoek. In 1777 William Hewson recognized an association with the lymphatic system, and in 1846 Virchow demonstrated that the Malpighian follicles are associated with the formation of white blood cells. In 1885 Ponfick showed that the spleen can remove particles from the blood and might be involved in the destruction of blood cells. Two years later Spencer Wells performed a laparotomy on a 27-year-old woman with a lifelong history of passing dark urine with attacks of jaundice and who had an abdominal tumour thought to be a fibroid. This turned out to be a large spleen, and its removal was followed by a complete remission. The retrospective diagnosis of hereditary spherocytosis was made by Lord Dawson of Penn some 40 years later, by which time splenectomy was being performed quite frequently for the treatment of leukaemia, Hodgkin's disease, Banti's haemolytic jaundice, Gaucher's disease, polycythaemia, and thrombocytopenic purpura. The frequent success of the operation led Doan and Dameshek to engage in a lively argument on the mechanisms by which the spleen might destroy blood cells or suppress their formation, a process which Chauffard had earlier called 'hypersplenism'.

There is now a greater understanding of the splenic function in health and of the spleen's involvement in disease. Methods have been developed by which the various functions of the spleen can be defined and measured, sometimes with important clinical application.

Structure of the spleen

At birth the spleen has a mean weight of 11 g. By the age of 1 year the weight is 15 to 25 g; by 5 years it is 40 to 70 g, and by 10 years it is 80 to 100 g. It reaches a maximum weight of 200 to 300 g soon after puberty, and is slightly lighter throughout adult life until the age of about 65 years, when it decreases to 100 to 150 g or less. These figures have been derived from autopsy studies and are probably underestimates. This is mainly due to the splenic red-cell pool which will be described later. Ultrasonography, CT, MRI, and scintigraphic radionuclide scans have shown that, *in vivo*, the normal adult spleen has a length of 8 to 13 cm, a width of 4.5 to 7 cm, a surface area of the order of 45 to 80 cm^2, and a volume less than 275 cm^3. A spleen more than 14 cm long is usually palpable.

The spleen has a complicated structure (Fig. 22.4.4.1). It consists of a connective tissue framework, vascular channels, lymphatic tissue, lymph drainage channels, and cellular components of the haemopoietic and mononuclear phagocyte systems. There are two main components: (1) the red pulp and (2) the white pulp. The red pulp consists of sinuses and pulp cords. The sinuses, 20 to 40 μm in diameter, are lined by endothelial macrophages. The white pulp consists of a periarteriolar lymphoid sheath and the adjoining lymphoid follicles (malpighian bodies), which contain a germinal centre and are structurally similar to lymphoid follicles. From the capsule many lace-like trabeculae extend into the pulp, carrying blood vessels and autonomic nerve fibres. Within the spleen the trabeculae are in direct continuity with a mesh of reticular fibres that supports the pulp vessels and forms the basement membranes of arterial capillaries and the splenic sinuses. Along the reticular fibres lie adventitial reticular cells. These cells have an important role in regulating blood flow through the interendothelial slits of the vascular sinuses.

Blood is supplied by the splenic artery and passes through the trabecular arteries, into the central arteries, which are sited in the white pulp. The central arteries run into the central axis of the periarteriolar lymphatic sheaths; they give off many arterioles and capillaries, some of which terminate in the white pulp whilst others go on to the red pulp. There they either connect directly with the sinuses and thence, via the collecting vein, to the trabecular vein (closed system), or they first pass into the cord spaces before joining up with the sinuses (open system).

Thus, as blood flows through the spleen it will come into contact with the reticular fibres, and also with endothelial macrophages, which line the interstices of the reticular mesh.

Blood flow in the spleen

Because the spleen has two vascular systems (open and closed) as described above, there are both rapid- and slow-transit components in the splenic circulation. The rapid transit (closed system) is of the order of 1 to 2 min and the slow transit (open system) about 30 to 60 min. In normal subjects the open system has a minor role and the blood flows through the spleen as rapidly as through organs possessing a conventional vasculature, at a rate of 5 to 10% of the blood volume per minute, so that each day the circulating blood has repeated passages through the spleen. When the spleen is enlarged, blood flow increases up to 20% or more of the blood volume per minute. At the same time, a proportion of the blood may be pooled in the cord spaces (see below). As blood traverses the spleen, the plasma and leucocytes pass preferentially to the white pulp by a process of plasma skimming, and the plasma rapidly reaches the venous system, whilst blood with a relatively high packed-cell volume remains in the axial stream of the central artery. Some of this blood flows directly through the sinusoids to the venous system, while the remainder passes into the cords of the red pulp. The normally flexible red cells squeeze through the endothelial slits into the sinuses, while inflexible cells with fixed membranes or with inclusions remain in the cords where they either become conditioned for later transit or are destroyed.

Functions of the spleen

Haemopoiesis

In the fetus and compared with the liver, the spleen is a minor haemopoietic organ. There is, however, some erythropoiesis and granulopoiesis in the spleen from the 12th week of gestation; this continues until birth, after which there is normally no demonstrable haemopoiesis. However, the potential remains, and under severe haematological stress, e.g. in thalassaemia and in chronic haemolytic anaemias, extramedullary haemopoiesis may occur together with intense erythroid hyperplasia of the bone marrow. This must be distinguished from myeloid metaplasia occurring in myelofibrosis, chronic myeloid leukaemia, and occasionally other leukaemias and secondary carcinomas. In these conditions, foci of haemopoietic tissue become established in the spleen and elsewhere outside the bone marrow. They represent an abnormal proliferation which is distinct from compensatory haemopoiesis.

Cell sequestration, phagocytosis, and pooling

The spleen has a remarkable ability to 'cleanse' or 'recondition' red cells for recirculation and also to remove from the circulation effete or damaged cells as well as foreign matter. Of particular importance is the trapping of encapsulated blood-borne bacteria. It is important to distinguish between the three mechanisms involved. (1) Sequestration is a temporary (reversible) process whereby cells are held in the spleen before returning to the circulation; (2) phagocytosis represents the irreversible uptake of nonviable cells by macrophages, or the destruction of viable cells that have been damaged; (3) pooling is the presence in the spleen of an increased amount of blood (or some of its component parts). In contrast to sequestration, pooled cells are in continuous exchange with the circulation.

As blood flows through the sinuses and cords, effete and damaged cells and particulate foreign matter are promptly phagocytosed by the endothelial macrophages. Intact red cells are held up temporarily, during which time siderotic granules, Howell–Jolly bodies, and Heinz bodies are removed. After the inclusions have been removed, the red cells return to the circulation. Sequestration of reticulocytes also occurs, and they are retained in the splenic cords for part of their last 2 or 3 days of maturation while they lose their

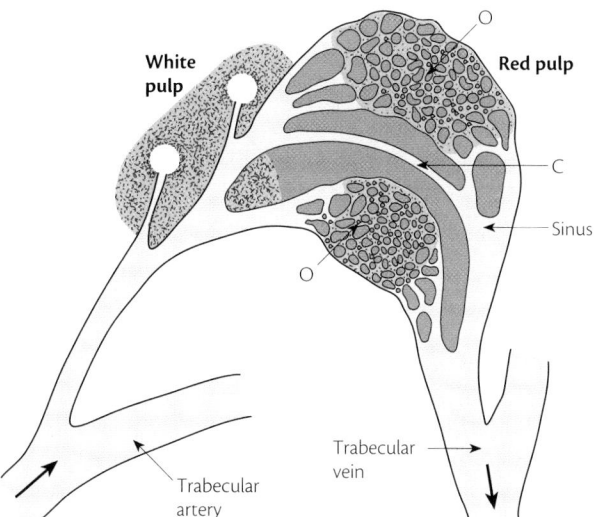

Fig. 22.4.4.1 Diagrammatic illustration of the spleen. The blood passes either directly into a sinus (C, closed system) or first into the cord space in the red pulp (O, open system).

intracellular inclusions, alter their surface membrane composition, and become smaller. The spleen normally sequesters 30 to 45% of the total circulating platelet content of the blood. This platelet pool is rapidly mobilized under conditions of stress, and normally there is a constant transit between the spleen and vascular pools.

As the blood becomes more viscous in the spleen, red cells are subjected to a further hazard. Because they are packed together in the presence of metabolically active macrophages, they are depleted of glucose and oxygen. This increases their membrane rigidity and reduces their deformability. Cells may become inflexible if: (1) they are metabolically abnormal (as in some congenital haemolytic anaemias) and thus unduly sensitive to the unfavourable environment of the spleen; (2) if they are held up in the spleen for a prolonged period and are thus rendered metabolically abnormal; and (3) if they are already spherical (as in hereditary spherocytosis), fragmented (as in microangiopathic haemolytic anaemia), or misshapen in some other way. This results in their being trapped in the cord spaces where they subsequently undergo phagocytosis.

Immune function

The spleen contains the largest single accumulation of lymphoid tissue in the body; about 25% of the total T-lymphocyte pool and 10 to 15% of the B-lymphocyte pool, with very marked exchange between circulating and splenic lymphocytes. Splenic macrophages are instrumental in antigen presentation to lymphocytes. The spleen is a major, but not unique, site for the conversion of naive circulating B cells into plasma cells which migrate to the bone marrow and into long-lived memory cells.

Microorganisms or other antigens that find their way to the spleen are taken up and processed by cord macrophages and are presented to immunocompetent cells in the lymphoid tissue. This stimulates antibody production and an increase in size of the lymphoid germinal centres of the spleen. Secondary stimulation with the antigen enhances antibody production, usually IgG.

Antibody-coated red cells lose pieces of their membrane as they come in contact with the Fc receptors on macrophages, and become spherical and less flexible each time they pass through the sinus vasculature, until finally they become too rigid to traverse the endothelial pores and are trapped and destroyed. Red cells sensitized by IgG do not, as a rule, agglutinate in the peripheral blood, but the environment in the spleen promotes local agglutination with consequent sequestration and destruction (autoimmune haemolysis). Antibody-coated neutrophils and platelets are similarly destroyed by splenic macrophages.

Blood pool

The normal red cell content of the spleen is less than 80 ml of red cells, and always less than 5% of the total red cell mass. There is no significant red cell pool in human spleens. However, enlarged spleens are capable of developing remarkably large pools with a relatively slow exchange of red cells with the general circulation. In the myeloproliferative disorders, as much as 40% of the blood volume may be present in the spleen. Increased pools also occur in lymphoproliferative disorders, especially hairy-cell leukaemia and prolymphocytic leukaemia.

In health there is a good correlation between the amount of blood in the spleen and its size. In lymphomas, however, the splenomegaly is greater than can be accounted for by the pool alone; in such cases the increase in spleen size is due primarily to an expansion of the lymphoid components with replacement of splenic sinuses by tumour. In myelofibrosis there is an increase in the reticular element with expansion of the closed system in the red pulp. A similar effect occurs in hairy-cell leukaemia.

Not unexpectedly, the red-cell content of the spleen increases with increasing body haematocrit. There is a disproportionately increased pool in primary proliferative polycythaemia compared with secondary polycythaemia, where the pool remains small irrespective of the haematocrit level. Increased pools are also found in patients with hepatic cirrhosis. Here it is the increased portal pressure that leads to an increased splenic blood flow: the splenic arteries are dilated and the splenic pulp becomes expanded with prominent dilated sinuses. Portal hypertension may result from myeloproliferative disorders associated with splenomegaly.

In myeloproliferative disorders and some other conditions an enlarged splenic blood pool may contribute significantly to anaemia. A low venous haematocrit can be present despite a normal red-cell mass (pseudoanaemia). Direct measurement of the splenic red-cell volume makes it possible to predict the extent to which splenectomy will improve anaemia and reduce transfusion requirements.

There is also a significant reservoir of platelets in the spleen, which is rapidly interchangeable with the circulation. In some cases of thrombocytopenia, destruction occurs mainly in the spleen and it is essential to distinguish this from pooling. As far as granulocytes are concerned, no pool is demonstrable in the normal spleen, but an abnormally large marginal pool has been found in cases of splenomegaly associated with neutropenia.

Plasma volume

Splenomegaly is frequently associated with an increased plasma volume, which may lead to an apparent anaemia (pseudoanaemia or dilutional anaemia), when a reduced venous haematocrit is the result of an expanded plasma volume in the presence of a normal or slightly reduced red-cell mass.

Splenomegaly

A palpable spleen is usually enlarged. Occasionally a normal spleen is palpable if it is displaced downwards, by a pleural effusion for example. The spleen has to be 1.5 to 2 times its normal size to be palpable. Ultrasonography, CT, and MRI provide reliable methods for measuring the actual spleen size.

Investigation of splenomegaly

The clinical history should include a relevant travel history (e.g. to tropical areas) and family history (e.g. Gaucher's disease, hereditary spherocytosis). Physical examination should specifically include assessment for hepatomegaly and lymphadenopathy. Laboratory investigations should include a full blood count, liver function tests and hepatitis serology, serum protein electrophoresis, total cholesterol, triglyceride and lipoprotein determinations, and immunoglobulin measurements. A bone marrow aspirate and trephine biopsy, and/or lymph node biopsy, with appropriate cytogenetic and immunophenotyping studies, should be done as indicated. These investigations will reveal the diagnosis in most haematological disorders and many chronic infections. CT or ultrasound scanning, with liver biopsy as required, will reveal hepatic or thrombotic causes of portal hypertension. HIV serology should always be done in puzzling cases of splenomegaly; in patients of Ashkenazi Jewish ancestry, Gaucher's disease or Niemann–Pick disease may be reasonably excluded by determining lysosomal hydrolase activity in leucocytes. If all investigations are negative, diagnostic splenectomy may be necessary, and in non-tropical areas the diagnosis will usually be non-Hodgkin's lymphoma or Hodgkin's disease.

Causes of splenomegaly

So many conditions are associated with splenomegaly that it is impossible to give a comprehensive list. It is even more difficult to list the 'common' causes, as these depend on geographical pathology. In western Europe and the United States of America viral infections and portal hypertension are the most common causes of splenomegaly, and these together with leukaemias, malignant lymphomas, myeloproliferative disorders, haemolytic anaemias, and other infections account for most cases. Isolated splenomegaly is a common manifestation of type I Gaucher's disease. Globally, however, the incidence of these haematological causes of splenomegaly is swamped by the great preponderance of splenic enlargement caused by parasitic infections, particularly malaria, leishmaniasis, and schistosomiasis. HIV infection, particularly in the later stages of the disease, is an increasing cause of mild to moderate splenomegaly. Haemoglobinopathies head the list in some countries. Portal hypertension is an important cause of splenomegaly in most tropical countries but it is especially prevalent in north-eastern India and southern China. The 'tropical splenomegaly syndrome' associated with malaria is seen commonly in New Guinea and Central Africa.

Some of the causes of splenomegaly are listed in Box 22.4.4.1. The conditions which commonly give rise to massive splenomegaly are indicated. The spleen sizes indicated are only a rough guide. Most of the conditions listed are described in other chapters.

Hypersplenism

Hypersplenism is a clinical syndrome of varied aetiology. It is characterized by:

* splenomegaly, although this may only be moderate
* cytopenias—pancytopenia, single cytopenias, or any combination of anaemia, neutropenia, and thrombocytopenia

---

Box 22.4.4.1 Some causes of enlargement of the spleen

Infections
* Acute viral and bacterial infections
* Chronic bacterial infections: mycobacterial and brucellosis
* Chronic parasitic infections: malaria, kala azar, schistosomiasis[a]
* Histoplasmosis

Splenomegaly
* Idiopathic non-tropical splenomegaly[a]
* Tropical splenomegaly[a]

'Congestive'
* Portal and biliary cirrhosis, portal vein obstruction, splenic vein obstruction, Budd–Chiari syndrome, cardiac failure

Inherited haemolytic anaemias
* Hereditary spherocytosis
* Haemolytic hereditary elliptocytosis
* Structural haemoglobinopathies
* Thalassaemia major and intermedia
* Red-cell enzyme defects

Acquired haemolytic anaemias
* Warm-antibody immune haemolytic anaemia
* Cold-agglutinin disease

Primary blood disorders
* Chronic myeloid leukaemia[a]
* Chronic lymphocytic leukaemia[a]
* Prolymphocytic leukaemia[a]
* Hairy-cell leukaemia[a]
* Acute leukaemia
* Myelofibrosis[a]
* Polycythaemia vera
* Megaloblastic anaemia

Malignant lymphoma
* Hodgkin's disease
* Non-Hodgkin's lymphoma

HIV infection
* Acute seroconversion
* Advancing disease, pre-AIDS
* AIDS
* AIDS-related lymphoma
* AIDS-related opportunistic infection

Connective tissue disorders
* Systemic lupus erythematosis
* Felty's syndrome

Miscellaneous
* Amyloid
* Sarcoidosis
* Castleman's disease
* Storage diseases[a]
* Cysts
* Haemangiomas
* Littoral-cell angioma

[a] May be associated with massive splenomegaly.

- a cellular or hypercellular bone marrow, sometimes showing a paucity of mature granulocytes
- a premature release of cells into the peripheral blood, resulting in a mild reticulocytosis with nucleated red cells and occasional immature granulocytes

Other features are:

- decreased red-cell survival
- decreased platelet survival
- hypervolaemia (i.e. increased plasma volume) if splenomegaly is marked

The haematological features may be obscured or dominated by the primary disease, especially if it involves the marrow. The diagnosis of hypersplenism is ultimately confirmed by the response to treatment of the underlying cause or of splenectomy, although an immediate remission may be followed in the longer term by relapse with a return of cytopenia.

Tropical splenomegaly syndrome—'big spleen disease'

In areas where malaria is endemic, adults may present with moderate to massive splenomegaly, no obvious signs of active malaria, but all the features of hypersplenism including pancytopenia, expanded plasma volume, and haemolysis. The serum IgM level is usually high, and malarial antibody titres are raised. The spleen shows diffuse proliferation of macrophages. The relationship to malaria is evident by the response to long-term antimalarial treatment, which produces a sustained reduction in spleen size and reversal of the cytopenias. It is unclear why this effect is only seen in a proportion of individuals in areas of the world where malaria is endemic.

A similar degree of splenomegaly occurs in schistosomiasis (see Chapter 7.11.1). However, in this condition there is the further complication that the eggs (especially of *Schistosoma mansoni*) have a direct effect on the liver, resulting in hepatic fibrosis and leading to portal hypertension, which may be further exacerbated by splenic vein thrombosis.

Nontropical idiopathic splenomegaly

Rare patients present with marked splenomegaly and the haematological features of hypersplenism but without exposure to malaria or other parasitic disorders. There may be a positive antiglobulin test and other evidence of autoantibody production. Some of these patients have a malignant lymphoma at the time of presentation, but in others the essential feature is non-neoplastic lymphoid hyperplasia, which probably represents an immunological reaction to as yet unidentified stimuli. The chances of long-term cure after splenectomy appear to be good. However, a lymphoma may appear from months to years after splenectomy. The disorder is diagnosed by the finding of massive splenomegaly in the absence of any other cause and by the non-specific histological appearances in the spleen.

Storage disease

The storage diseases are described in detail in Section 12. Some of them, notably Gaucher's disease and Niemann–Pick disease, may be complicated by marked splenomegaly. This may lead to hypersplenism, particularly in Gaucher's disease. The advent of specific enzyme therapy for Gaucher's disease has largely removed the need to consider splenectomy. The clinical picture of Niemann–Pick disease is dominated by hepatosplenomegaly and mental disability. The disorder presents in infancy, and death often occurs between the second and third years of age, but, as with Gaucher's disease, it may present later in life. Hypersplenism becomes a feature in the older age groups, but anaemia and thrombocytopenia are uncommon in the childhood cases, and, if present, are mild. Several other lipid storage diseases may cause hypersplenism. They include Tangier's disease, in which cholesterol esters fill the histiocytes, and Wolman's disease, which is associated with an accumulation of triglycerides and cholesterol esters. Sea-blue histiocytosis is characterized by splenomegaly, hepatomegaly, thrombocytopenia, and, occasionally, neurological damage in this case the storage cells may be due to Niemann-Pick disease type C. The bone marrow and spleen contain cells that have an accumulation of glycosphingolipids, phospholipids, and mucopolysaccharides.

Rarely, histiocytosis X (including Hand–Schuller–Christian disease, eosinophilic granuloma, Letterer–Siwe disease, and Langerhans' cell histiocytosis) cause splenomegaly. This is usually moderate, but occasionally it is more marked and may be associated with hypersplenism.

Space-occupying lesions and injury of the spleen

The most common causes of splenic masses are trauma leading to haematoma or rupture, abscesses, tumours, and cysts.

Splenic injury

The spleen is relatively unprotected and easily injured. Spontaneous rupture has been reported in a number of conditions in which the spleen is enlarged: these include typhoid, malaria, Epstein–Barr virus infection, leukaemia, Gaucher's disease, and polycythaemia. This may be restricted to a subcapsular haematoma or there may be rupture into the peritoneal cavity.

The diagnosis is suggested by the symptoms of shock, left upper quadrant tenderness, guarding, pain referred to the left shoulder, and clinical and laboratory evidence of bleeding. Plain abdominal radiography is not, as a rule, helpful in diagnosis but CT scanning, ultrasound examination, and splenic arteriography are more useful.

Abscess

Although the spleen is frequently enlarged in association with systemic infection, splenic abscesses are rare. They result from direct or haematogenous spread, or when a haematoma becomes infected. Conditions associated with splenic infarction, such as sickle cell disease, are particularly likely to give rise to splenic abscesses. Almost any organism can be involved.

Tumours

The spleen may be affected by benign tumours such as hamartomas. The very rare littoral cell angioma is the only tumour confined to the spleen. Metastases in the spleen are uncommon by comparison to other organs, possibly because the spleen, unlike lymph nodes, lacks an afferent lymphatic system. They occur late in the course of carcinoma and are not found in the absence of metastases elsewhere. Metastases in the spleen are most frequently derived from malignant lymphomas, especially Hodgkin's disease. Lung, breast, prostate, colon, and stomach are the primary sites from which carcinoma is most likely to disseminate to the spleen. Melanoma is also a relatively frequent primary source.

Cysts

Splenic cysts are rare. The most frequent cause is *Echinococcus granulosum* (hydatid); other causes include haemangiomas, lymphangiomas, and dermoids. Cysts may also develop in areas of haemorrhage or infarction.

Loss of spleen function and splenic infarction

Splenic hypoplasia or atrophy

Congenital hypoplasia is rare; in some cases it is associated with extensive developmental abnormalities of the heart and gut. Splenic atrophy may occur in a number of conditions—sickle cell disease, coeliac disease, dermatitis herpetiformis, ulcerative colitis, Crohn's disease, amyloidosis, selective IgA deficiency, and Fanconi's anaemia. There is evidence of reduced splenic reticuloendothelial function in alcoholics. The spleen shrinks in size in old age. Vascular blockade and repeated infarction is the basis for splenic atrophy in sickle cell disease, and occurs in early childhood. The peripheral blood changes of hyposplenism, when present, are proportional to disease activity in gut diseases. In coeliac disease, withdrawal of gluten from the diet reverses the changes unless splenic atrophy has occurred. The mechanism of the splenic atrophy is unknown.

Splenic hypofunction and atrophy are characterized by changes in the blood film appearances; the main features are the presence of Howell–Jolly bodies and siderotic granules in some of the red cells. This is due to the loss of the spleen's macrophage 'pitting' function. Reduced sequestration (pooling) of red cells also occurs.

Splenic infarction

Splenic infarction occurs quite frequently in patients who have very large spleens from any cause. It is particularly common in association with myelosclerosis and chronic myeloid leukaemia. It also occurs in most patients with sickle cell anaemia. In this disorder, splenic infarction occurs early in life and repeated episodes result in an autosplenectomy. Occasionally, when there is rapid growth of the spleen in association with an aggressive form of non-Hodgkin's lymphoma there may be multiple infarctions and spontaneous rupture of the spleen. Splenic infarcts are one of the presenting features of chronic myeloid leukaemia.

Splenic infarction causes pain in the left upper quadrant. If the diaphragmatic surface of the spleen is involved, the pain may be referred to the left shoulder tip. The physical signs include tenderness over the spleen, and sometimes a loud splenic rub is heard. Treatment is by rest and analgesia. The occurrence of repeated splenic infarction may be an indication for splenectomy, which may be complicated by adhesions between the spleen and the overlying peritoneum.

Specialized investigation of splenic function

Assessment of splenic function may be helpful, particularly in assessing the likely effect of splenectomy in haematological disorders. In many conditions it is sufficient to assess the spleen size, examine the peripheral blood for evidence of pancytopenia or a reduction in the number of neutrophils and platelets, and examine the bone marrow to determine whether haemopoiesis is normal. Often this simple approach, combined with a knowledge of the likely effects of splenectomy for a particular haematological disorder, will be all that is necessary to make a decision about whether to proceed to surgery.

Studies with radionuclides provide information about the extent of splenic involvement in a disease process, the role of the spleen in producing anaemia, and the likely benefits of splenectomy. Details of the methods used and analysis of the results obtained in various conditions are to be found in specialized textbooks.

The following list summarizes the various *in vivo* tests useful for investigating splenic function:

- Delineation of functional splenic tissue—The spleen can be visualized and its size estimated by scintillation scanning following injection of isotope-labelled, autologous, heat-damaged red cells, which are selectively removed by functional splenic tissue. A gamma camera or rectilinear scanner visualizes splenic tissue (Fig. 22.4.4.2). The technique is most useful for identifying accessory spleens (splenunculi) associated with a postsplenectomy relapse of immune thrombocytopenia. The rate at which heat-damaged red cells are cleared from the circulation provides a rough guide to the competence of splenic function. A slow clearance may identify splenic hypofunction before the blood film shows Howell–Jolly bodies and other morphological changes.

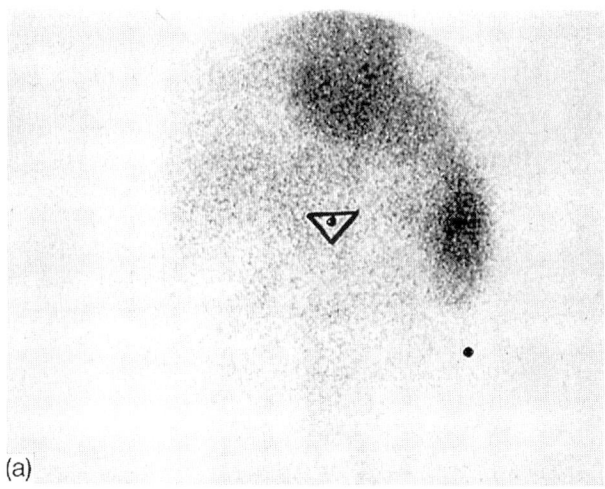

(a)

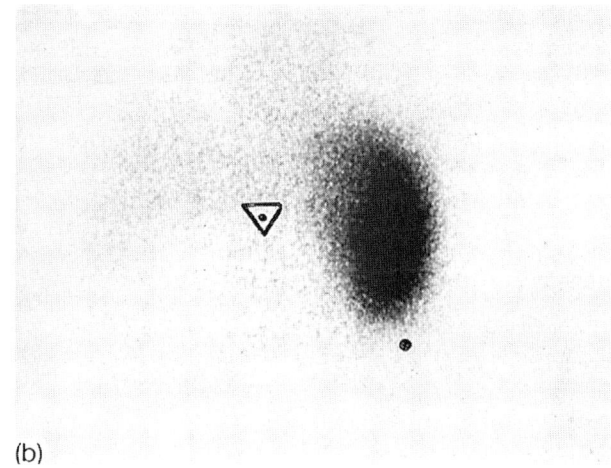

(b)

Fig. 22.4.4.2 Images obtained by scintillation camera following administration of (a) technetium-99 labelled red cells and (b) indium-111 labelled, heat-damaged red cells.

- Measurement of splenic red-cell pool—Quantitative scanning of the spleen after injection of undamaged, isotope-labelled, autologous red cells allows measurement of the splenic red-cell pool. The size of the splenic red-cell pool should be taken into account when assessing the significance of anaemia in the presence of splenomegaly. Measuring the pool is particularly useful for distinguishing polycythaemia vera (increased pool) from secondary polycythaemia (normal pool) and assessing the (useless) spleen pool in massive splenomegaly (Fig. 22.4.4.3).

- Identification of sites of red-cell destruction and quantification of splenic red-cell destruction—Surface counting over the spleen, heart, and liver following injection of autologous chromium-51 labelled erythrocytes provides a qualitative indication of splenic red-cell destruction in various haemolytic anaemias; quantitative scanning provides a more accurate measurement of the actual proportion of the cells that are destroyed in the spleen and elsewhere. These studies are moderately predictive of the outcome of splenectomy.

- Identification and quantification of splenic extramedullary erythropoiesis—Normally, transferrin-bound iron passes to the bone marrow, where the iron is released and enters erythroblasts for incorporation into the haemoglobin of developing erythrocytes. In the normal spleen, iron does not dissociate from transferrin. Hence, the uptake of iron demonstrable by surface counts shortly after administration of radioactive iron (59Fe or 52Fe), indicates that there is erythropoiesis in the spleen. Extramedullary erythropoiesis in the spleen occurs in the majority of patients with myelofibrosis (Fig. 22.4.4.4), and some patients with essential thrombocythaemia, but not in patients with polycythaemia vera. Iron-52 studies are useful for detecting early stages of transition from polycythaemia vera to myelofibrosis and for diagnosing the syndrome of transitional myeloproliferative

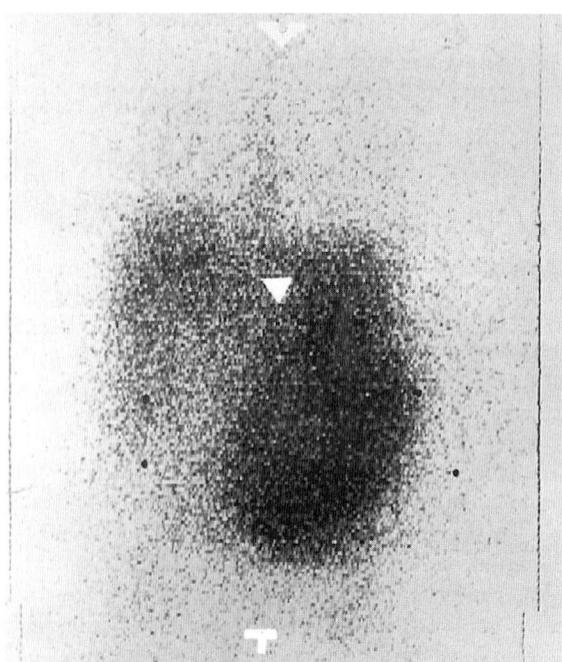

Fig. 22.4.4.4 Iron-52 scan in a patient with myelofibrosis showing the extent of splenic erythropoiesis. Vertebral erythropoiesis is markedly reduced.

disorder. Extramedullary haemopoiesis can be accurately identified in thalassaemia major or intermedia and sickle-cell disease by positron emission tomography (PET) after iron-52 administration, e.g. paraspinal, mediastinal, or in lymph nodes.

- Role of the spleen in platelet destruction—About one-third of an injection of chromium-51 labelled platelets disappears from the circulation during their lifespan, mainly in the spleen pool. Splenomegaly is associated with a marked increase in pooling: by contrast, in asplenia, nearly 100% of the labelled platelets are recovered in the circulating blood. Surface counting and quantitative scanning have been used to assess the role of the spleen in thrombocytopenia, but are less reliable in predicting the response to splenectomy than in autoimmune haemolytic anaemia.

The combinations of investigations used depends on the particular clinical problem. In many conditions associated with splenomegaly, it is important to distinguish increased macrophage activity causing cell destruction from increased red-cell accumulation in a large pool, and to determine to what extent enlargement of the spleen is due to tumour infiltration. In myelofibrosis and hypersplenism, it may be helpful to ascertain the relative importance of the splenic red-cell pool, red-cell destruction, and extramedullary erythropoiesis, if present.

Indications for splenectomy

The main indications for splenectomy are summarized in Box 22.4.4.2. Splenectomy should not be undertaken lightly. Where traumatic damage, usually from a blunt injury, has occurred, every effort should be made to preserve the spleen in whole or in part. Ultrasonography and CT are vital in assessing the damage, as rupture and haematoma can be confused clinically. Surgical techniques for repairing or partially preserving the spleen have improved and should be encouraged. The use of diagnostic laparotomy and

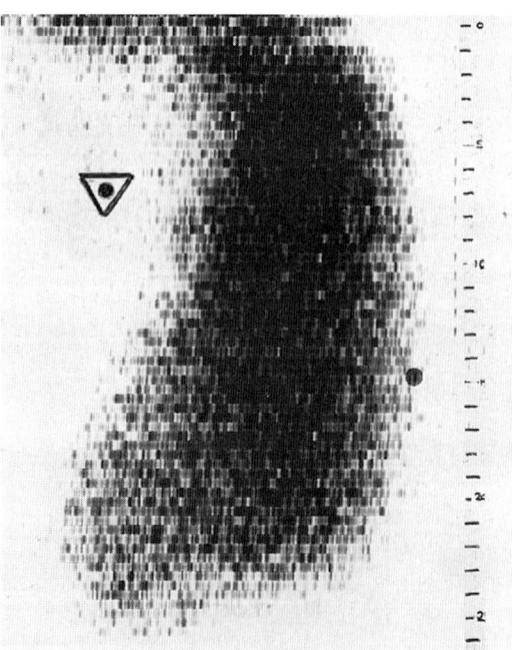

Fig. 22.4.4.3 Splenic enlargement and increased red-cell pool in a patient with myelofibrosis. Demonstrated by scanning after the administration of indium-113m labelled red cells. The markings indicate the costal margin. The upper pole of the spleen merges with the image produced by labelled blood in the heart.

splenectomy in Hodgkin's disease has fallen into disuse, partly as a result of improved imaging in the CT and MRI scans, and partly because of the absence of therapeutic advantage, combined with the long-term dangers of splenectomy. In primary haematological disorders, splenectomy is indicated to alleviate complications—e.g. repeated infarction, massive red-cell pooling, and hypersplenism. The decision is usually based on clinical assessment, but radioisotope studies to measure the splenic red-cell pool, splenic erythropoiesis, and red-cell survival may be helpful in difficult cases. Diagnostic splenectomy may still be required for splenic lymphomas where no other organ is affected. Increasingly, diagnostic splenectomy may be required in HIV-related diseases, particularly for a suspected lymphoma or opportunistic infection. The course of HIV disease is not influenced by splenectomy.

Clinical and haematological effects of splenectomy

Removal of the spleen is associated with certain immediate and delayed clinical complications, and with the presence of permanent changes in the peripheral blood picture.

Clinical complications

Early

In some splenectomies, particularly when the spleen is bound down by adhesions following a previous splenic infarction, there may be difficulty in achieving haemostasis, particularly if the preoperative platelet count is less than 50×10^9/litre. Platelets should be infused as soon as the splenic pedicle has been ligated. Subphrenic abscess is a significant complication and may occasionally be fatal. Because the platelet count tends to rise immediately after the operation, there is an increased risk of thromboembolic disease in the first 2 or 3 weeks after splenectomy.

Subcutaneous heparin can be used if the preoperative platelet count is 50×10^9/litre or greater. After wound healing, aspirin 75 mg daily should be given if the platelet count is elevated above 500×10^9/litre, and continued until this normalizes. There is a small, long-term increase in myocardial infarction in splenectomized

patients with persistently raised platelet counts, and in these patients aspirin should be given indefinitely.

Mortality depends on the clinical condition of the patient and the size of the spleen. Laparoscopic techniques for splenectomy are safer and reduce morbidity for small or moderately enlarged spleens. In patients with massive splenomegaly, usually myeloproliferative disorders, the mortality rate is up to 15% in those patients thought fit for surgery.

Long term

All patients, whatever the reason for splenectomy, are at risk of overwhelming postsplenectomy infection (OPSI). Classically, OPSI presents with a vague general prodrome, followed by prostration, bacteraemic shock, and frequently disseminated intravascular coagulation. Death may occur within 6h of the onset. The mortality rate in patients reaching hospital alive is in excess of 30%. By far the most important causative organism is the pneumococcus (*Streptococcus pneumoniae*), but *Haemophilus influenzae*, *Neisseria meningitidis*, *Escherichia coli*, and pseudomonas have all been implicated.

In endemic areas, plasmodium and babesia infections are of increased severity in nonimmune individuals. Special warnings should be given to splenectomized patients travelling to malarial areas. Viral illnesses may also be of increased severity postsplenectomy.

The risk of OPSI does not decline significantly in the years after splenectomy. Children are at the greatest risk, followed by adults splenectomized for an underlying disorder that itself is immunosuppressive, or who require immunosuppressive treatment. Adults splenectomized for trauma are at least risk, but they still carry a lifelong susceptibility. OPSI has been recorded more than 40 years after splenectomy. The relative risk of severe infection compared with the non-splenectomized population is about 10-fold for traumatic splenectomy and as much as 100-fold for small children and patients with Hodgkin's disease.

Infections indistinguishable from OPSI also occur in nonsplenectomized individuals who have hypofunctional spleens. It is well recognized as a cause of death in patients with sickle cell disease, particularly in children. Fatal overwhelming pneumococcal sepsis has been reported in patients with coeliac disease and primary amyloidosis affecting the spleen. Dermatitis herpetiformis and inflammatory bowel disease are also associated with splenic hypofunction. Bone marrow transplant recipients, particularly in the presence of chronic graft-vs-host disease are hyposplenic and have an increased risk of pneumococcal disease. Patients with lymphoproliferative disorders, particularly myeloma, are at increased risk of sepsis with encapsulated bacteria and should be considered for prophylaxis.

Strategies for preventing OPSI

All patients undergoing elective splenectomy should be immunized with polyvalent pneumococcal vaccine (Pneumovax), which currently gives variable protection against 23 strains of *S. pneumoniae*. Where possible, it should be given at least 1 month before splenectomy to allow IgG antibody production. Antibody responses may be suboptimal in patients with immunosuppressive diseases or in those receiving immunosuppressive treatment, or when it the vaccine is given perioperatively in an emergency. Patients should also be immunized against *H. influenzae* type b. Protection against *N. meningitidis* is of relatively short duration, and vaccination should be reserved for patients travelling to high incidence areas. Pneumovax is not fully protective, and a small proportion of patients fail to make detectable antibodies after vaccination. There are reports of OPSI occurring with strains of *S. pneumoniae* covered by the type of vaccine given, and therefore it should always be combined with life-long prophylactic antibiotics. Some authorities recommend the Pneumococcal conjugate vaccine, which may provide better protection because of its dependence on T cell immunity. Revacci-nation with Pneumovax every 5 to 10 years is recommended. Splenectomized individuals should always carry a card or wear a bracelet stating they have no spleen. At the onset of any febrile illness, particularly upper and lower respiratory infections, penicillin V should be stopped and therapeutic doses of a broad-spectrum antibiotic started. The penicillin V is resumed at the end of the course of antibiotics.

Prophylactic penicillin V, 250 mg twice daily, should be started postoperatively. Erythromycin can be substituted in penicillin-sensitive patients. The lifesaving value of prophylactic penicillin V in children with sickle cell disease (i.e. functional asplenia) has been proven beyond doubt, and there are only rare reports of OPSI in splenectomized patients regularly taking penicillin V. Surveys of patients dying of OPSI have identified the failure to follow the above guidelines as the greatest risk factor. Although the penicillin does not prevent infection, it prevents the rapid onset of the OPSI syndrome. There is controversy as to the effectiveness of penicillin V in areas where resistant strains of pneumococci are common and it has no protective role against Neisseria or Haemophilus influenzae.

After spleen rupture, splenic tissue may seed into the peritoneum, giving rise to nodules of recognizable splenic tissue (splenosis). These nodules have been shown to have some phagocytic function. This has led to the deliberate autotransplantation of splenic tissue at the time of splenectomy where partial splenic preservation has not been possible. Although such nodules of splenic tissue can phagocytose damaged red cells and reduce hyposplenic changes on the blood film, their protective capacity from infection is not established. The presence of demonstrable splenosis should not be relied upon to replace vaccination and penicillin prophylaxis.

The safest course is to immunize all patients, counsel them carefully about the dangers of infection, and impress upon them the need for lifelong penicillin prophylaxis. This should be reinforced at outpatient follow-up visits, and every effort should be made to maintain good compliance.

Further reading

Anon (1996). Guidelines for the prevention and treatment of infection in patients with an absent or dysfunctional spleen. *BMJ*, **312**, 430–4.
Berman RS, *et al.* (1999). Laparoscopic splenectomy in patients with hematologic malignancies. *Am J Surg*, **178**, 530–6.
Bowdler AJ (ed.) (1990). *The spleen. Structure, function and clinical significance.* Chapman & Hall, London.
Crane CG (1981). Tropical splenomegaly. Part 2: Oceanian. *Clin Haematol*, **10**, 976–82.
Dacie JV, Lewis SM (1995). *Practical haematology*, 8th edition. Churchill Livingstone, Edinburgh.
Fakunle YM (1981). Tropical splenomegaly. Part 1: Tropical Africa. *Clin Haematol*, **10**, 963–75.
Frank JM, Palomino NJ (1987). Primary amyloidosis with diffuse splenic infiltration presenting as fulminant pneumococcal sepsis. *Am J Clin Pathol*, **87**, 405–7.
Gaston M, *et al.* (1986). Prophylaxis with oral penicillin in children with sickle cell anemia. *N Engl J Med*, **314**, 1593–9.
Imbert P, *et al.* (2009).Pathological rupture of the spleen in malaria: analysis of 55 cases (1958-2008). *Travel Med Infect Diseases*, **7**, 147–59.
Lucas CE (1991). Splenic trauma. Choice of management. *Ann Surg*, **213**, 98–112.
O'Donoghue DJ (1986). Fatal pneumococcal septicaemia in coeliac disease. *Postgrad Med J*, **62**, 229–30.
Oksenhendler E, *et al.* (1993). Splenectomy is safe and effective in human immunodeficiency virus-related immune thrombocytopenia. *Blood*, **82**, 29–32.
Spickett GP, *et al.* (1999). Northern region asplenia register—analysis of first two years. *J Clin Pathol*, **52**, 424–9.
Tefferi A, *et al.* (2000). Splenectomy in myelofibrosis with myeloid metaplasia: a single-institution experience with 223 patients. *Blood*, **95**, 2226–33.
Traub A, *et al.* (1987). Splenic reticuloendothelial function after splenectomy; spleen repair and spleen autotransplantation. *N Engl J Med*, **317**, 1559–64.
Waghorn DJ, Mayon-White RT (1997). A study of 42 episodes of overwhelming post-splenectomy infection: is current guidance for asplenic individuals being followed? *J Infect*, **35**, 289–94.
William BM, Corazza GR (2007). Hyposplenism: a comprehensive review. Part I: basic concepts and causes. *Hematology*, **12**, 1–13.

22.4.5 Myeloma and paraproteinaemias

Robert A. Kyle and S. Vincent Rajkumar

Essentials

The paraproteinaemias are a group of neoplastic (or potentially neoplastic) diseases associated with the proliferation of a single clone of immunoglobulin-secreting plasma cells.

Monoclonal gammopathy of undetermined significance (MGUS)

This asymptomatic condition of unknown cause is characterized by a serum paraprotein concentration under 30 g/l, less than 10% plasma cells in the bone marrow, and no evidence of end-organ damage related to the plasma cell proliferative process.

Epidemiology and prognosis—MGUS is found in 3% of people aged over 50 years and in 5% of those over 70 years. The risk of progression to multiple myeloma or a related disorder is about 1% per year, with factors increasing the risk being higher concentration of the monoclonal protein, some particular types of monoclonal protein (IgA and IgM > IgG), or an abnormal serum-free light chain ratio.

Management—the monoclonal protein in the serum and urine should be monitored, together with re-evaluation of clinical and laboratory tests, to determine whether multiple myeloma or a related disorder has developed.

Multiple myeloma

Multiple myeloma accounts for about 10% of haematological malignancies, with the clonogenic cell appearing to arise from the germinal centre, circulate in the peripheral blood, and home to the bone marrow by means of adhesion molecules. The cause is unknown, but conventional cytogenetics reveals an abnormal karyotype in 35% of patients, and fluorescence *in situ* hybridization (FISH) reveals specific primary translocations or chromosomal deletions (some of which are predictors of poor outcome) in many cases.

Clinical features—the commonest symptoms are weakness and fatigue, and bone pain is present at diagnosis in almost two-thirds of cases. Other presentations include acute infection, renal failure, hypercalcaemia and amyloidosis.

Investigations—a paraprotein (usually >30 g/litre) is found in the serum or urine at diagnosis in 97% of cases. The bone marrow usually contains more than 10% plasma cells, with the presence of monoclonal κ or λ in their cytoplasm being useful for differentiating monoclonal from reactive (polyclonal) plasmacytosis. Conventional radiographs show lytic lesions, osteoporosis or fractures in almost 80% of patients at diagnosis.

Treatment and prognosis—some patients are asymptomatic and should not be treated, but most have symptomatic disease at diagnosis and require treatment, for which first-line options—aside from supportive care—are: (1) Autologous peripheral stem-cell transplantation—this comprises (a) 3 to 4 months of induction therapy (e.g. dexamethasone plus lenalidomide), (b) collection of peripheral stem cells utilizing granulocyte colony-stimulating factor (G-CSF), (c) preparative or conditioning treatment (e.g. high-dose melphalan), (d) infusion of the previously collected peripheral blood stem cells. (2) Chemotherapy—for patients who are not eligible for stem cell transplantation (on account of excessive risk), the standard of therapy has been melphalan and prednisone (or combinations of alkylating agents) for the past four decades, but the addition of thalidomide has produced better results. Patients with relapsed refractory disease are usually treated with dexamethasone, with or without thalidomide, bortezomib or lenalidomide. The median duration of survival is about 3 to 4 years.

Waldenstrom's macroglobulinaemia

Waldenstrom's macroglobulinaemia is characterized by a high concentration of serum immunoglobulin M (IgM) paraprotein. Characteristic symptoms include chronic nasal bleeding or oozing from the gums, and blurring or loss of vision, with retinal vein engorgement and flame-shaped haemorrhages commonly seen and typical of symptomatic hyperviscosity syndrome. Symptoms and findings of hyperviscosity are quickly controlled by plasmapheresis. Chlorambucil, given continuously or intermittently, has been a standard therapy for more than 40 years. Rituximab, a monoclonal antibody directed against the CD20 antigenic determinant, produces a response in about 50% of patients with refractory disease. The median duration of survival is about 5 years.

Primary amyloidosis

Primary amyloidosis is characterized by tissue deposition of fibrils consisting of monoclonal κ or λ light chains. Weakness, fatigue, and weight loss are the commonest initial symptoms. Characteristic findings include periorbital purpura (15% of cases), macroglossia (10%), nephrotic syndrome/renal failure (>25%), and congestive heart failure (20%), but virtually any organ system can be affected.

Standard treatment is with alkylating agents, but prognosis is poor (median survival 13 months, although this varies greatly depending on the associated syndrome). Autologous peripheral blood stem cell transplantation has been used with encouraging results, although treatment-related mortality is high.

Other conditions

Rare paraprotein disorders include (1) plasma cell leukaemia; (2) nonsecretory myeloma; (3) POEMS syndrome—characterized by polyneuropathy, organomegaly, endocrinopathy, M-protein, and skin changes (osteosclerotic myeloma); (4) solitary plasmacytoma of bone; (5) extramedullary plasmacytoma; and (6) heavy chain diseases.

Introduction

The paraproteinaemias are a group of neoplastic, or potentially neoplastic, diseases associated with the proliferation of a single clone of immunoglobulin-secreting plasma cells. They include multiple myeloma (MM); smouldering multiple myeloma (SMM); Waldenström's macroglobulinaemia (WM); heavy-chain diseases (HCD)—solitary plasmacytoma of bone, extramedullary plasmacytoma, plasma-cell leukaemia, POEMS syndrome (osteosclerotic myeloma); monoclonal gammopathy of undetermined significance (MGUS); and primary systemic amyloidosis (AL).

The paraproteinaemias are characterized by the secretion of electrophoretically and immunologically homogeneous (monoclonal) (M) proteins (Box 22.4.5.1). Each M-protein consists of two heavy (H) polypeptide chains of the same class and subclass and two light (L) polypeptide chains of the same type. The heavy polypeptide chains are designated by Greek letters: γ in IgG, α in IgA, μ in IgM, δ in IgD, and ε in IgE. The light-chain types are κ (kappa) or λ (lambda).

Recognition of M-proteins

Agarose gel electrophoresis is preferred for the detection of M-proteins. Immunofixation should be used to confirm the presence of an M-protein and distinguish the immunoglobulin class and its light-chain type.

Serum protein electrophoresis should be done when MM, WM, or AL amyloidosis is suspected. A paraprotein is characterized by a narrow peak or spike in the densitometer tracing, or as a dense, discrete band on agarose gel (Fig. 22.4.5.1). In contrast, an excess of polyclonal immunoglobulins (having one or more heavy-chain types and both κ and λ light chains) produces a broad-based peak or broad band. It is important to differentiate an M-protein from a polyclonal increase because the former is associated with a malignant process or a potentially neoplastic condition, whereas a polyclonal increase in immunoglobulins is associated with a reactive or inflammatory process. Immunofixation is the preferred technique for identifying an M-protein. Diseases associated with a paraprotein, as found recently in the authors' practice, are shown in Fig. 22.4.5.2. Immunofixation of an adequately concentrated 24-h urine specimen is best for detection of a monoclonal light chain (Bence Jones protein). The presence of a monoclonal light chain in nephrotic urine is strongly suggestive of AL or light-chain deposition disease.

Box 22.4.5.1 Classification of plasma-cell proliferative disorders

I Monoclonal gammopathies of undetermined significance (MGUS)

  A Benign (IgG, IgA, IgD, IgM, and, rarely, free light chains)

  B Associated neoplasms or other diseases not known to produce monoclonal proteins

  C Biclonal and triclonal gammopathies

  D Idiopathic Bence Jones proteinuria

II Malignant monoclonal gammopathies

  A Multiple myeloma (IgG, IgA, IgD, IgE, and free light chains)

    1 Symptomatic multiple myeloma

    2 Smouldering multiple myeloma

    3 Plasma cell leukaemia

    4 Non-secretory myeloma

    5 IgD myeloma

    6 POEMS syndrome (osteosclerotic myeloma)

    7 Solitary plasmacytoma of bone

    8 Extramedullary plasmacytoma

  B Malignant lymphoproliferative disorders

    1 Waldenström's macroglobulinaemia

    2 Malignant lymphoma

    3 Chronic lymphocytic leukaemia

III Heavy-chain diseases (HCD)

  A γ-HCD

  B α-HCD

  C μ-HCD

IV Cryoglobulinaemia

V Primary amyloidosis (AL)

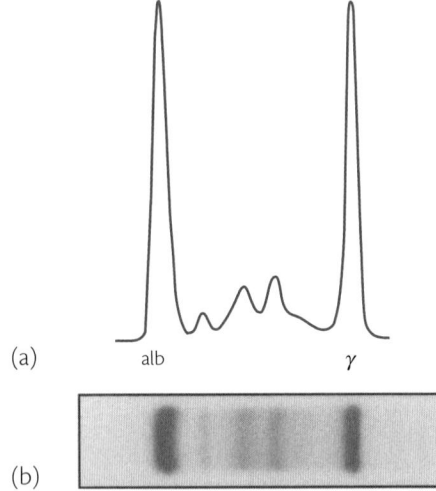

Fig. 22.4.5.1 (a) Monoclonal pattern of serum protein as traced by a densitometer after electrophoresis on agarose gel; tall, narrow-based peak of γ mobility. (b) Monoclonal pattern from electrophoresis of serum on agarose gel (anode on left); dense, localized band representing monoclonal protein of γ mobility.
(From Kyle RA, Katzmann JA (1997). Immunochemical characterization of immunoglobulins. In: Rose NR, et al. (eds) *Manual of clinical laboratory immunology*, 5th edition, pp 156–76. ASM Press, Washington, DC. By permission of the *American Society for Microbiology.*)

of IgG (73%), IgA (11%), IgM (14%), or biclonal (2%). The bone marrow plasma cells ranged from 1% to 10% (median, 3.0%).

After 3579 person-years of follow-up, the 241 patients were classified into four groups (Table 22.4.5.1). Of these patients, 6% have remained stable and could be classified as having 'benign' monoclonal gammopathy, but they must continue to be observed because serious disease may still develop. More than half of the patients died of unrelated causes without developing MM or a related disorder. In 27%, MM (69%), WM (11%), AL (12%), or related disorders (8%) developed; the actuarial rate was 17% at 10 years, 34% at 20 years, and 39% at 25 years, a rate of approximately 1.5% per year. The interval from the time of recognition of the paraprotein to the diagnosis of serious disease ranged from 1 to 32 years (median, 10.4 years). In 10 patients, MM was diagnosed more than 20 years after detection of the paraprotein.

Monoclonal gammopathy of undetermined significance

The term 'monoclonal gammopathy of undetermined significance' (MGUS) (benign monoclonal gammopathy) denotes the presence of a paraprotein in persons without evidence of MM, WM, AL, or related disorders. MGUS is characterized by a serum paraprotein concentration of less than 30 g/litre; fewer than 10% plasma cells in the bone marrow and no evidence of end-organ damage (hypercalcaemia, renal insufficiency, anaemia or bone lesions) related to the plasma cell proliferative process. The prevalence of MGUS is 3% in patients 50 years or older, 5% in those over 70 years of age, and is higher in men than women (Fig. 22.4.5.3).

In a series of 241 patients with MGUS seen at Mayo Clinic from 1956 to 1970 and followed for up to 39 years, 27% developed MM, WM, or AL. The median age at diagnosis was 64 years. Laboratory abnormalities such as anaemia or renal insufficiency were the result of unrelated disorders. The paraprotein concentration ranged from 3 to 30 g/litre (median, 17 g/litre). The paraproteins consisted

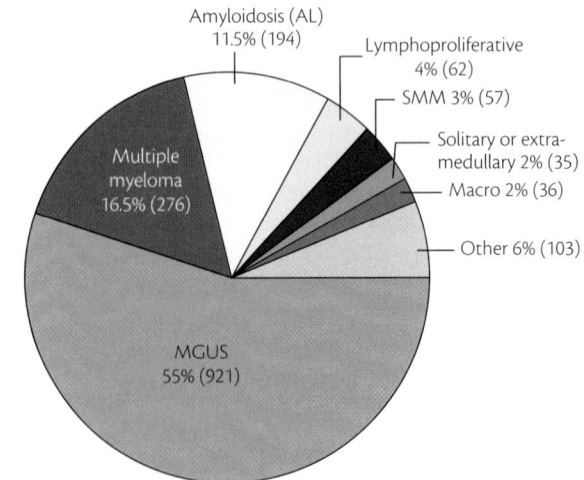

Fig. 22.4.5.2 Types of monoclonal gammopathies in 1684 Mayo Clinic cases in 2006.

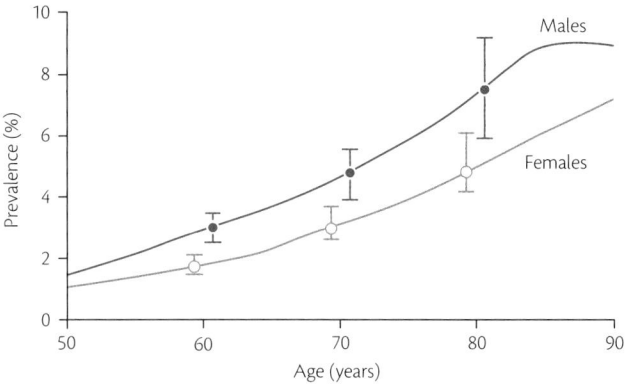

Fig. 22.4.5.3 Prevalence of MGUS according to age. The I-bars represent 95% confidence intervals. Years of age greater than 90 have been collapsed to 90 years of age.
(From Kyle RA (2006). Prevalence of monoclonal gammopathy of undetermined significance. *N Engl J Med*, **354**, 1362–9.)

To confirm the findings of the 241 Mayo Clinic patients from the United States of America and other countries, which may be subject to referral bias, we conducted a study of 1384 patients with MGUS from the 11 counties of southeastern Minnesota evaluated at Mayo Clinic from 1960 to 1994. The median age at diagnosis was 72 years, which is 8 years older than the 241 cohort; 2% were younger than 40 years at diagnosis and 59% were 70 years or older. The monoclonal protein ranged from unmeasurable to 30 g/litre. The IgM protein was IgG in 70%, IgM in 15%, IgA in 12%, and biclonal in 3%. A reduction of uninvolved (normal or background) immunoglobulins was found in 38% of 840 patients who were evaluated. Of the 418 patients who had immunofixation of urine, 31% had a monoclonal light chain. The bone marrow contained 0 to 10% plasma cells (median 3%). In this study 1384 patients were followed for a total of 11 009 person-years (median 15.4 years; range 0–35 years) and 963 (70%) died. During follow-up, 115 patients (8%) developed MM, AL, lymphoma with an IgM serum protein, WM, plasmacytoma, or chronic lymphocytic leukaemia (CLL). The rate of progression was 10% at 10 years, 21% at 20 years, and 26% at 25 years, which is approximately 1% per year (Fig. 22.4.5.4).

Table 22.4.5.1 Course of 241 patients with MGUS*

Patient group[a]	Description	No. (%) of patients at follow-up[b]
1	Living patients with no substantial increase of monoclonal protein	14 (6)
2	Monoclonal protein value ≥3.0 g/dL but no myeloma or related disorder	25 (10)
3	Died of unrelated causes	138 (57)
4	Developed multiple myeloma, macroglobulinaemia, amyloidosis, or related disorder	64 (27)
Total		241 (100)

MGUS, monoclonal gammopathy of undetermined significance.
[a] The patient groups are described in the text.
[b] Person-year follow-up = 3579 (median 13.7 year per patient; range 0–39 years).
(From Kyle RA (2004). Monoclonal gammopathy of undetermined significance. *Mayo Clin Proc*, **79**, 859–66.)

For 32 additional patients symptomatic MM or WM did not develop although the serum monoclonal protein value increased to more than 30 g/litre or the percentage of bone marrow plasma cells increased to more than 10%. The number of individuals with progression to a plasma cell disorder (115 patients) was 7.3 times the number expected (Box 22.4.5.2). The risk of developing MM was increased 25-fold, WM 46-fold, and AL 8.4-fold. The 75 patients in whom MM developed accounted for 65% of the 115 patients who progressed to a plasma cell disorder. The characteristics of these 75 MM patients were comparable with those of the 1027 patients with newly diagnosed MM who were referred to Mayo Clinic between 1985 and 1998, except that the southeastern Minnesota population was older (median 72 years vs 66 years) and had a smaller percentage of men (46% vs 60%).

Pathophysiology

MGUS represents a limited, initially nonmalignant, expansion of monoclonal plasma cells. The cause of MGUS is unknown. It is postulated that infection, inflammation, or other antigenic stimuli in addition to primary translocations of the immunoglobulin heavy chain locus on chromosome 14q32 may be the initiating pathogenic event. The most common primary translocations have been identified at t(11;14) (which results in upregulation of the cyclin D1 oncogene), t(4;14) (up-regulation of FGFR3 and MM SET oncogenes), and t(14;16) (up-regulation of the C-MAF oncogenes).

Smouldering (asymptomatic) multiple myeloma

SMM is characterized by a serum monoclonal protein 30 g/litre or more and/or bone marrow clonal plasma cells 10% or more

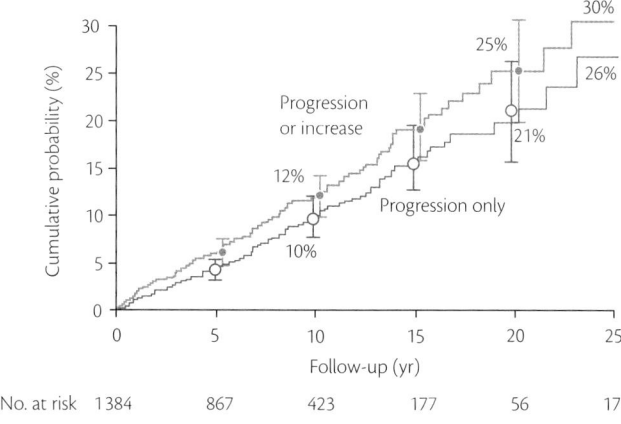

Fig. 22.4.5.4 Probability of progression among 1384 residents of southeastern Minnesota in whom monoclonal gammopathy of undetermined significance (MGUS) was diagnosed, 1960–1994. The top curve shows the probability of progression to a plasma-cell cancer (115 patients) or of an increase in the monoclonal protein concentration to more than 30 g/litre or the proportion of plasma cells in bone marrow to more than 10% (32 patients). The bottom curve shows only the probability of progression of MGUS to multiple myeloma, IgM lymphoma, primary amyloidosis, macroglobulinaemia, chronic lymphocytic leukaemia, or plasmacytoma (115 patients). The bars show 95% confidence intervals.
(From Kyle RA (2002). Prognosis in monoclonal gammopathy of undetermined significance. *N Engl J Med*, **346**, 564–9.)

and no end-organ damage. Risk of progression to MM or AL is almost 10% per year for the first 5 years, approximately 3% per year for the next 5 years, and then 1–2% per year for the following 10 years.

Differential diagnosis of MGUS from MM and WM

The magnitude of the paraprotein in the serum or urine may assist. SMM is characterized by the presence of a paraprotein concentration of more than 30 g/litre or more than 10% plasma cells in the bone marrow, but no anaemia, renal insufficiency, or skeletal lesions. Affected patients should be identified for monitoring because they may remain stable for years and not require therapy. The presence of a urinary paraprotein suggests MM, but small amounts of κ or λ paraprotein may persist in the urine and remain stable for years. Large numbers of plasma cells in the bone marrow suggest MM, but some patients may have a plasmacytosis of more than 10% and remain stable. The presence of osteolytic lesions strongly suggests MM, but metastatic carcinoma must be excluded. The plasma-cell labelling index measures the synthesis of DNA, and when increased it is good evidence that the patient has MM. The presence of circulating plasma cells in the peripheral blood usually indicates MM rather than MGUS. No single test will distinguish the patient with MGUS who remains stable from those who develop MM or related disorders. The paraprotein level in the serum and urine should be serially measured, along with periodic re-evaluation of clinical and other features to determine whether MM or a similar disorder is present. The cytogenetic changes found with fluorescence *in situ* hybridization (FISH) are similar to those of MM.

Serum-free light chains (FLC) can be measured by an automated nephelometric assay. It is helpful in detection of a monoclonal gammopathy and it is of prognostic value in MGUS. MGUS may be associated with lymphoproliferative disorders, leukaemia, other haematological diseases, neurological disorders, connective tissue diseases, peripheral nerves, skin disease, endocrine disorders, liver disease, and immunosuppression following bone marrow, peripheral blood, liver, kidney, or heart transplantation.

Prognosis and treatment

Patients with MGUS should not be treated. The monoclonal protein in the serum and urine should be monitored together with re-evaluation of clinical and laboratory tests to determine whether multiple myeloma or a related disorder has developed. In general, serum protein electrophoresis should be repeated in 6 months and, if stable, annually thereafter. Patients who meet the criteria for low-risk MGUS (serum monoclonal protein <15 g/litre, IgG subtype, normal FLC ratio) can be followed less often. Routine skeletal radiography, bone marrow examination, and a 24-h urine collection for immunofixation are rarely necessary in patients with low-risk MGUS. Bone marrow examination and a metastatic bone survey should be performed initially if the serum monoclonal protein is at least 15 g/litre, IgA or IgM MGUS, or an abnormal FLC ratio. Bone marrow examination should also be performed in patients with unexplained anaemia, renal insufficiency, hypercalcaemia, or bone lesions.

Biclonal gammopathies

Biclonal gammopathies consist of two different monoclonal proteins and occur in approximately 5% of patients with monoclonal gammopathies. Approximately two-thirds of patients have biclonal gammopathy of undetermined significance, with the remainder representing MM, WM, or another malignant lymphoproliferative disorder. Triclonal gammopathies may also occur.

Idiopathic Bence Jones proteinuria

Although Bence Jones proteinuria occurs in MM, AL, and WM, occasionally patients may produce large amounts of Bence Jones protein (monoclonal light chain) in the absence of end-organ damage. They should be recognized as such and not treated because patients with idiopathic Bence Jones proteinuria may remain stable for many years.

Multiple myeloma

MM (myelomatosis, Kahler's disease) is characterized by the neoplastic proliferation of a single clone of plasma cells producing a paraprotein. Proliferation of the plasma cells in the bone marrow produces skeletal destruction that leads to bone pain and pathological fractures. The paraprotein can lead to renal failure, recurrent bacterial infections, or hyperviscosity syndrome.

History

MM was documented by the description of Sarah Newbury which was followed by that of Thomas Alexander McBean a few years later. The physician and clinical pathologist, Henry Bence Jones described the unusual protein excreted by McBean in the mid 19th century. Although Jones erroneously described the protein as 'hydrated deuteroxide of albumen', he correctly emphasized that the protein should be sought in other cases of mollities ossium. The term 'multiple myeloma' was introduced by J Von Rustizky in 1873. It was the case report of Dr Loos, published by Professor Otto Kahler in 1889, that introduced MM to clinical practice. Only 3 years after Röentgen's discovery of X-rays, Wright reported that radiographs showed changes in the ribs. In 1956, Korngold and Lipari demonstrated that there were two main classes of light-chain proteins which were known as Bence Jones protein. Six years later, Edelman and Gally demonstrated that the Bence Jones protein was identical to the light chains of the intact serum immunoglobulin in the same MM patient.

Urethane was introduced in 1947 as a treatment for MM. Almost 20 years later, a randomized study showed no difference in survival among patients who were randomized to urethane or to a placebo. The introduction of melphalan in the late 1950s was a major step forward. Autologous stem cell transplantation was introduced in the 1980s and refined in the 1990s. During the last decade thalidomide, bortezomib, and lenalidomide have been developed and became important agents for treatment of MM.

Epidemiology and aetiology

MM accounts for 1% of all malignant diseases and slightly more than 10% of haematological malignancies in the United States of America. The annual incidence is 5 per 100 000. The apparent increase during the past few decades is probably related to the increased availability and use of medical facilities, especially in older persons. The incidence in African Americans is twice that in whites, but rates are lower in Asian populations. The median age at diagnosis is 66 years. Only 10% of patients are younger than 50 years, and 2% are younger than 40 years. The cause of MM is unknown, but radiation, benzene and other organic solvents, herbicides, and insecticides may play a role. MM has been reported in two or more first-degree relatives and in identical twins, suggesting a genetic element.

Biological aspects

The plasma cells are phenotypically CIg+, CD38+, PCA-1+, and CD56+, with only a minority expressing CD10, CD20, and HLA DR. Although still unknown, the clonogenic cell in MM appears to arise from the germinal centre, circulates in the peripheral blood, and may home to the bone marrow by means of adhesion molecules. Interleukin-6 (IL-6) is a potent plasma-cell growth factor and may be increased in MM, in contrast to MGUS. Overproduction of interleukin-1 (IL-1), macrophage inflammatory protein α (MIP-1α) and tumour necrosis factor, which have bone-resorbing activity, have been found in MM.

Conventional cytogenetic studies reveal an abnormal karyotype in only 35% of patients because of the low proliferative rate of plasma cells. FISH using chromosome-specific probes identifies abnormalities in more than 90% of patients with MM. Primary translocations involving the immunoglobulin heavy-chain loci (chromosome 14q32) are seen in approximately 70% of patients with MM. Deletions of chromosome 13 occur in 15% of patients by conventional cytogenetic studies and in 50% of patients with FISH studies. Flow cytometry reveals hyperdiploidy in 70% and hypodiploidy in 10%.

Clinical manifestations

Bone pain, frequently in the back or chest, is present at diagnosis in almost two-thirds of patients. Loss of height from multiple vertebral collapses may occur. The most common symptoms are weakness and fatigue, which are often due to anaemia. Fever is rare and, when present, is usually due to an infection. An acute infection, renal failure, hypercalcaemia, or amyloidosis may be the presenting feature. The liver is palpable in about 5% of patients, and the spleen in 1%. Extramedullary plasmacytomas are uncommon and are usually observed late in the course of the disease as large, purplish, subcutaneous masses.

Laboratory findings

If MM is suspected, the laboratory tests listed in Table 22.4.5.1 should be performed. Anaemia is initially present in 70% of patients but eventually is found in almost all. The serum protein electrophoretic pattern shows a spike or localized band in 80% of cases, hypogammaglobulinaemia is present in almost 10%, and no apparent abnormality is found in the remainder. The paraprotein is IgG in about 50% of patients, IgA in 20%, and Bence Jones proteinaemia in almost 20%. IgD occurs in 2%, and biclonal paraproteinaemias are found in 2%, whereas the remainder of the patients have no serum M-protein at diagnosis. Immunofixation of the urine shows a paraprotein in approximately 75% of cases. The κ/λ ratio is 2:1. A paraprotein is found in the serum or urine at diagnosis in 97% of cases. Hypercalcaemia (≥11 mg/dL) is initially present in almost 15%; about one-fifth have a serum creatinine value of 20 mg/litre or more.

The bone marrow usually contains more than 10% plasma cells, but involvement may be focal, and repeat bone marrow examination may be necessary for diagnosis. The presence of monoclonal κ or λ in the cytoplasm of plasma cells, identified by immunoperoxidase staining, is useful for differentiating monoclonal from reactive plasmacytosis (polyclonal) due to connective tissue disorders, metastatic carcinoma, liver disease, or chronic infections.

Conventional radiographs show abnormalities consisting of lytic lesions, osteoporosis, or fractures in almost 80% of patients at diagnosis. The vertebrae, skull, thoracic cage, pelvis, and humeri and femurs are the most commonly involved sites. Osteoblastic lesions are rare. Technetium-99m bone scanning is inferior to conventional radiography and should not be used. MRI reveals abnormalities in 90% of patients with MM. It is particularly helpful in patients who have back pain but no abnormalities on radiography, in whom spinal cord compression must be considered.

Organ involvement

Renal

The serum creatinine value is 20 mg/litre or more in 20% of patients at diagnosis. Bence Jones proteinuria is present in 75%. The two major causes of renal failure are myeloma kidney and hypercalcaemia. Myeloma kidney is characterized by the presence of dense, waxy, laminated casts in the distal and collecting tubules. The casts consist mainly of monoclonal light chains. Dilatation and atrophy of the tubules occur, and the entire nephron becomes nonfunctional. Dehydration contributes to acute renal failure and must be avoided. Hypercalcaemia, present in 15% of patients initially, is a major and treatable cause of renal insufficiency. Amyloidosis occurs in about 10% of patients and may produce nephrotic syndrome and renal insufficiency. Hyperuricaemia, contrast media, antibiotics, and dehydration may contribute to renal failure.

Neurological

Radiculopathy is the most frequent neurological complication and usually involves the thoracic or lumbosacral areas. Compression of the spinal cord from extradural myeloma occurs in 5% of patients. Leptomeningeal involvement is uncommon but is being recognized more frequently.

Other organ systems

The incidence of bacterial infection is increased in MM. Impairment of antibody response, neutropenia, treatment with glucocorticoids, and reduction of normal immunoglobulins increase the likelihood of infection. Coating of platelets by paraprotein may cause bleeding. Occasionally, a tendency to thrombosis is present.

Diagnosis

The diagnosis of MM depends on the presence of an increased number of plasma cells in the bone marrow (usually >10%), a paraprotein in the serum (usually >30 g/litre), Bence Jones proteinuria, and end-organ damage (hypercalcaemia, renal insufficiency, anaemia, and bone lesions). The clinical features of MM must also be present for diagnosis. Metastatic carcinoma, connective tissue disorders, lymphoma, or chronic infections must be considered in the differential diagnosis.

MGUS, SMM, primary systemic AL, and metastatic carcinoma are the main conditions considered in the differential diagnosis. In MGUS, the paraprotein value is less than 30 g/litre, and the bone marrow contains fewer than 10% plasma cells. There are no osteolytic lesions, anaemia, hypercalcaemia, or renal insufficiency. SMM is characterized by the presence of a paraprotein value of 30 g/litre or more and/or 10% or more plasma cells in the bone marrow but no other findings or symptoms of MM. An increased plasma-cell labelling index strongly suggests that the patient has or soon will have symptomatic MM. However, it must be kept in mind that this value is normal in one-third of patients with symptomatic MM. Monoclonal plasma cells of the same isotype are present in the peripheral blood in 75% of patients with active MM, but patients with MGUS or SMM have few or no circulating plasma cells.

The differentiation of AL and MM is arbitrary because both diseases are plasma-cell proliferative disorders with different manifestations. In AL, the bone marrow plasma-cell content is usually less than 20%, there are no osteolytic lesions, and the amount of Bence Jones proteinuria is modest. Obviously, there is considerable overlap between AL and MM.

Prognostic features

The median duration of survival in MM is approximately 3 to 4 years, but there is a great deal of variability from one patient to another. Cytogenetic abnormalities are an important prognostic factor. The deletion of chromosome 13 by cytogenetics and the presence of t(4;14), t(14;16) or –17P13 are predictors of poor outcome. An International Staging System (ISS) consisting of serum albumin and serum β-2 microglobulin is a useful simple measure of survival. Patients with a serum albumin 35 g/litre or more and serum β-2 microglobulin less than 3.5 µg/ml have a median survival of 62 months, while those with a serum β-2 microglobulin value 5.5 µg/ml or more have a median survival of

29 months. An elevated plasma-cell labelling index, plasmablastic morphology, or circulating plasma cells in the peripheral blood are all associated with more aggressive disease. Hypodiploidy, age, levels of creatinine and calcium, and immunoglobulin class also have prognostic value. The Durie–Salmon clinical staging system, in use for over 30 years, has been superseded by these newer parameters.

Treatment

Although most patients with MM have symptomatic disease at diagnosis and require therapy, some are asymptomatic and should not be treated. There is no evidence that early treatment of patients with SMM or asymptomatic MM prolongs survival compared with therapy at the time of onset of symptoms. All symptoms, physical findings, and laboratory data must be considered in making the decision to begin therapy. An increasing level of the paraprotein in the serum or urine requires evaluation and consideration of therapy. The development of anaemia, hypercalcaemia, or renal insufficiency, or the occurrence of lytic lesions or extramedullary plasmacytomas, are all indications for therapy. If there is doubt about beginning treatment, the most reasonable approach is to re-evaluate the patient in 2 months and to delay therapy until progressive disease is evident.

Patients eligible for autologous stem cell transplantation

If patients are considered eligible for stem cell transplantation, it is important to avoid alkylators such as melphalan which can damage the stem cells. Autologous peripheral stem cell transplantation has virtually replaced autologous bone marrow transplantation, because engraftment is more rapid and there is less contamination by myeloma cells. Autologous peripheral stem cell transplantation is applicable for more than half the patients with MM. The two major shortcomings are that (1) the myeloma is not eradicated even with large doses of chemotherapy, and (2) autologous peripheral stem cells are contaminated by myeloma cells and their precursors. Fortunately, the mortality from autologous transplantation is currently 1% if patients are appropriately selected.

Induction therapy is utilized for approximately 4 months to alleviate symptoms, decrease or reverse end-organ damage, and reduce tumour cells before stem cell harvest. We prefer lenalidomide plus dexamethasone which are given orally and produce a response rate of approximately 90%. Dexamethasone plus thalidomide, dexamethasone plus bortezomib, or dexamethasone alone are other options. There have been no studies comparing these regimens. Deep venous thrombosis occurs in 15 to 20% of patients given thalidomide or lenalidomide with high-dose dexamethasone. Consequently, patients should be given aspirin or, if at high-risk for thromboembolic phenomena, full anticoagulation with warfarin or low-dose heparin. Vincristine, doxorubicin, and dexamethasone (VAD) is infrequently used because of its inconvenience. Following 3 to 4 months of induction therapy, peripheral stem cells are collected utilizing granulocyte colony-stimulating factor (G-CSF). There are no data suggesting that the degree of response before transplantation affects overall survival. Patients in whom objective response is not achieved with induction therapy still obtain similar benefit from transplantation.

Following recovery from stem cell collection, we proceed with melphalan 200 mg/m^2 as the preparative or conditioning regimen for transplantation. It is superior to melphalan 140 mg/m^2 and total body radiation. The other choice is to treat the patient with alkylating agents after stem cell collection until a plateau state is reached, and then proceed with high-dose melphalan followed by infusion of the previously collected peripheral blood stem cells when the patient relapses. There is no difference in survival between early and late stem cell transplantation, but we prefer an early transplant because the patient can avoid continued chemotherapy.

A randomized trial performed by the French Myeloma Group compared high-dose chemotherapy and autologous bone marrow transplantation with conventional chemotherapy in 200 previously untreated patients under 65 years of age. The rates of response (81% vs 57%) and complete responses (20% vs 5%) were superior in the transplant group. The transplant group had a higher rate of 5-year, event-free survival (28% vs 10%) and overall survival (52% vs 12%). The Medical Research Council compared conventional-dose chemotherapy consisting of ABCM (adriamycin, BCNU, melphalan, and prednisone) with high-dose therapy and autologous stem cell transplantation in 401 previously untreated patients with myeloma under 65 years of age. At a median follow-up of 42 months, intent-to-treat analysis showed that high-dose therapy followed by autologous stem cell transplantation increased median survival by 1 year (54 vs 42 months). It has been suggested that better results could be obtained with two (tandem) autologous peripheral stem cell transplants. A randomized trial of 399 previously untreated MM patients under 60 years of age from France found significantly improved 7-year event-free survival (20% vs 10%) and overall survival (42% vs 21%) in recipients of double vs single autologous transplantation. Patients who received a complete response or a very good partial response from the first transplant did not benefit significantly from a second transplant. Those patients who did not have at least a very good partial response to the first transplant had a significant benefit from the second transplant. Overall survival at 7 years was 11% vs 43% for those in the single or tandem transplant groups, respectively.

A major hurdle is improvement of the preparative regimen because residual myeloma is the likely source of relapse in most patients. Investigational studies utilizing samarium-153 ethylenediamine tetramethylene phosphonate (EDTMP) are being done to determine if an improved conditioning regimen is beneficial. The other major shortcoming of autologous stem cell transplantation is the presence of myeloma cells and their precursors in the blood. Collection of CD34+ cells produces a lower number of tumour cells, but this does not result in delay of time to progression or overall survival indicating that residual myeloma is the likely cause of relapse.

Autologous stem cell transplantation is possible in patients with renal failure, but the morbidity and mortality are higher.

Allogeneic bone marrow transplantation

This is advantageous because the graft contains no tumour cells that can lead to relapse. Unfortunately, the mortality rate is approximately 25% within 3 months. Furthermore, more than 90% of patients with MM are ineligible for an allogeneic transplant because of their age, lack of an human leucocyte antigen (HLA)-matched sibling donor, or inadequate renal, pulmonary, or cardiac function.

The mortality rate for allogeneic transplantation must be reduced before it can assume an important role in the treatment of MM. An experimental alternative is autologous stem cell transplantation followed by a nonmyeloablative ('mini' allogeneic transplantation), but treatment-related mortality is still 10 to 15%. There is also a high risk of acute and chronic graft vs host disease (GVHD), but the occurrence of GVHD appears necessary for disease control. Currently, this approach is investigational and should be performed only in the context of clinical trials.

The use of donor leucocyte infusions for relapses after allogeneic transplantation produces benefit in about one-half of patients. However, allogeneic transplantation is currently associated with a high mortality and cannot be recommended as a routine procedure except in carefully selected younger patients with high-risk disease.

Maintenance therapy

It would be desirable to keep the patient in a plateau state indefinitely, but this is not possible. An overview by the Myeloma Trialists' Group revealed relapse-free survival at 5 years in 23% of patients receiving interferon (IFN)-α_2 and 16% without IFN-α_2 ($p <0.001$). The overall survival at 5 years was only slightly prolonged. Consequently, IFN-α_2 cannot be recommended for maintenance therapy. Another study reported that prednisone in a dosage of 50 mg vs 10 mg taken orally every other day resulted in a superior progression-free survival and overall survival. However, this comparison included only patients who responded initially to corticosteroid-based therapy and they did not receive stem cell transplantation. Generalization of these results to current practice is not possible. A French randomized trial showed improvement in event-free survival and overall survival comparing thalidomide with no maintenance. However, side effects of long-term thalidomide usage are troublesome.

Patients should be monitored closely during the plateau phase, and the same therapy should be reinstituted if relapse occurs more than 6 months after the plateau state has begun. Patients who have relapsed more than 2 years following an autologous stem cell transplant are candidates for a second transplant.

Patients not eligible for stem cell transplantation

Chemotherapy is the preferred initial therapy for overt symptomatic MM in persons who are not eligible for an autologous stem cell transplant because of age, performance status, or comorbidities. The standard regimen for the past four decades has been melphalan and prednisone which produces an objective response in 50 to 60% of patients. Melphalan should be given when the patient is fasting. Leucocytes and platelet counts must be determined at 3-week intervals and the melphalan dosage altered until mid-cycle neutropenia or thrombocytopenia occurs. Melphalan and prednisone therapy should be repeated every 6 weeks and the dosage altered depending on the blood counts. Unless the disease progresses rapidly, at least three courses of melphalan and prednisone should be given before therapy is discontinued. An objective response may not be achieved for 6 to 12 months, or even longer in some patients. Chemotherapy should be continued until the patient is in a plateau state, or for at least 1 year. A plateau state is defined as stable serum and urine paraprotein levels and no evidence of progression. Chemotherapy should be discontinued when a plateau state occurs, because continued therapy may lead to the development of a myelodysplastic syndrome or acute leukaemia.

Because of the obvious shortcomings of melphalan and prednisone, various combinations of therapeutic agents have been tried.

In an overview of individual data in 4930 patients from 20 randomized trials comparing melphalan and prednisone with various combinations of therapeutic agents, the response rates were significantly higher with combination chemotherapy (60%) than with melphalan and prednisone (53%) ($p <0.00001$). There was no difference in survival and no evidence that any subset of patients benefited from receiving combination therapy.

Recently two randomized studies showed superior response rates and progression-free survival using melphalan, prednisone, and thalidomide compared to melphalan and prednisone. In an Italian study, patients were randomized for 6 months to standard dose melphalan–prednisone (MP) or melphalan, prednisone, and thalidomide (MPT). Response rates were significantly higher with MPT than MP (76% vs 48%) as were the complete CR rates (28% vs 7%) and 2-year event-free survival rates (54% vs 27%). However, thromboembolic phenomena, infections, and peripheral neuropathy were more common in the MPT regimen. In a French study, patients were randomized to MPT or MP for 12 months which resulted in superior progression-free survival (28% vs 17%) and overall survival (>55 months vs 30 months), respectively. Other novel combinations utilizing bortezomib and lenalidomide are being tested.

Refractory MM

Almost all patients with MM eventually relapse. Patients who have a slow relapse can often be treated with melphalan and prednisone. These patients present with asymptomatic increases in serum and urine M-protein, mild anaemia, or a few new small lytic bone lesions. Patients who experience more aggressive relapse usually require therapy with a combination of active agents.

Corticosteroids and alkylating agents

Dexamethasone (40 mg daily on days 1–4, 9–12, and 17–20) or IV methylprednisone (2 g 3 times weekly and then tapered) are reasonable options for treatment of relapsed MM. VAD, which was the standard for almost 20 years, is now rarely used. Combination chemotherapy regimens such as VBMCP (vincristin, carmustine, and doxorubicin plus prednisone) may be helpful but are infrequently used today.

Thalidomide

Thalidomide produces an objective response in about one-third of patients with relapsed or refractory MM. The median duration of response is approximately 1 year. It is usually given in a dosage of 200 mg/day, but some patients respond to 50 or 100 mg/day. It has been shown that 100 mg/day is not inferior to 400 mg/day. The median duration of response is approximately 1 year. Following response, the dose should be reduced to the lowest level because of long-term toxicity. Thalidomide plus dexamethasone produces an objective response in about one-half of patients. Thalidomide has been combined with cisplatin, doxorubicin, cyclophosphamide, etoposide, clarithromycin, or melphalan. Thalidomide is absolutely contraindicated in pregnancy and the System for Thalidomide Education and Prescribing Safety (STEPS) programme must be followed to prevent teratogenicity. The incidence of deep venous thrombosis is 1 to 3% in patients receiving thalidomide alone but increases to 10 to 15% in patients who receive thalidomide in combination with dexamethasone and to approximately 25% in patients who receive thalidomide and doxorubicin. Anticoagulation is required in this setting.

Bortezomib

Bortezomib is a proteasome inhibitor that has been approved for relapsed and refractory MM. One-third of 202 patients with relapsed and/or refractory MM responded to bortezomib with a response duration of approximately 1 year. In a randomized trial, progression-free survival was superior with bortezomib compared to dexamethasone alone in patients with relapsed, refractory MM (6.2 vs 3.5 months). The beginning dose of bortezomib is 1.3 mg/m^2 given on days 1, 4, 8, and 11, and repeated every 21 days. Bortezomib with or without dexamethasone is an active regimen for treatment of aggressive relapse.

Lenalidomide

Lenalidomide is an immunomodulatory analogue of thalidomide. As a single agent, it produces an objective response in about 30% of patients with relapsed, refractory MM. Two large randomized trials of lenalidomide plus dexamethasone vs placebo plus dexamethasone showed a superior response (59 vs 22.5% and time to progression 12 months vs 5 months). Neutropenia and thrombocytopenia are the most common side effects. The usual dose of lenalidomide is 25 mg on days 1 to 21 and repeated every 28 days.

New agents being tested included vorinostat, a histone deacytylase inhibitor and tanespimycin, a heat shock protein 90 inhibitor, as well as VEGF inhibitors, farnesyl transferase inhibitors, oral proteasome inhibitor (salinosporamide A, NPI-0052), and an inhibitor of FGFR3 (CHIR-258).

Supportive care

Skeletal complications

Skeletal involvement often leads to pathological fractures, spinal cord compression, pain, or hypercalcaemia. These complications result from increased osteoclastic induced bone resorption. Bisphosphonates are important for the treatment of patients with multiple myeloma and associated bony disease. Patients who have destruction of bone or compression fractures of the spine from osteopenia demonstrated by plain radiographs or imaging should be treated with intravenous bisphosphonates. Pamidronate 90 mg intravenously over at least 2 h or zoledronic acid 4 mg over at least 15 min every 3 to 4 weeks are recommended. Because of the apparent greater risk for the development of osteonecrosis of the jaw with zoledronic acid, pamidronate may be preferred. Clodronate is an alternative bisphosphonate approved worldwide except in the United States of America for either oral or intravenous administration. Intravenous bisphosphonates should be continued for 1–2 years and if the patient has stable disease, bisphosphonates should be discontinued. Bisphosphonates should be resumed upon relapse with new skeletal-related events. Other potential side effects of intravenous bisphosphonates are the development of proteinuria or, rarely, acute renal failure.

Both vertebroplasty (injection of methylmethacrylate into a collapsed vertebral body) and kyphoplasty (introduction of an inflatable bone tamp into the vertebral body and after inflation, the injection of methylmethacrylate into the cavity) have been used successfully to decrease pain and help restore vertebral height. Pain relief is generally rapid and may be long-lasting.

Patients should be encouraged to be as active as possible, but they must avoid undue trauma. Fixation of fractures or pending fractures with an intramedullary rod and methylmethacrylate has produced good results. Bone pain should be treated with analgesics or narcotics as necessary.

Hypercalcaemia

This is present in 15% of patients at diagnosis and should be suspected in the presence of anorexia, nausea, vomiting, polyuria, polydipsia, increased constipation, weakness, confusion, or stupor. If untreated, renal insufficiency develops. Hydration with saline plus prednisone (25 mg four times a day until the serum calcium level decreases) is effective in most cases. If these measures fail, zoledronic acid or pamidronate is effective.

Renal failure

Two main causes of renal insufficiency are 'myeloma kidney' and hypercalcaemia. Maintenance of a high urine output (3 litres/day) is important for preventing renal failure in patients with Bence Jones proteinuria. Nonsteroidal anti-inflammatory agents, dehydration, infections, or radiographic contrast media may contribute to acute renal failure. Patients with acute or subacute renal failure should be treated with thalidomide and dexamethasone or high-dose dexamethasone to reduce the tumour mass as quickly as possible. Plasmapheresis may be useful in acute renal failure, but patients with severe myeloma cast formation or other irreversible changes are unlikely to benefit. Allopurinol should be administered if hyperuricaemia is present. Haemodialysis or peritoneal dialysis is necessary in the event of symptomatic azotaemia.

Infection

Appropriate antibiotic therapy for bacterial infections is essential. Patients should receive pneumococcal and influenza vaccination despite their suboptimal antibody response. Because many infections occur in the first 2 months after instituting therapy, trimethoprim–sulfamethoxazole may be useful. Prophylaxis against pneumocystis pneumonia should be considered in all patients receiving high-dose corticosteroids. Intravenously administered gammaglobulin can be used for severe recurrent infections, but it is very expensive.

Neurological

Spinal cord compression should be suspected in patients with back pain who develop weakness or paraesthesias of the lower extremities or bladder or bowel dysfunction. Imaging by MRI or CT must be done immediately. Radiation therapy and dexamethasone are usually effective, and surgical decompression is rarely necessary.

Hyperviscosity

This is characterized by oral or nasal bleeding, blurred vision, paraesthesias, headache, reduced cerebration, or congestive heart failure. Serum viscosity levels do not correlate well with the symptoms or clinical findings. A decision to perform plasmapheresis depends on the symptoms and changes in the ocular fundus. Plasmapheresis promptly relieves the symptoms and should be done regardless of the viscosity level if the patient has signs or symptoms of hyperviscosity.

Anaemia

Anaemia occurs in almost all patients during the course of MM. Erythropoietin (40 000 U subcutaneously weekly) or darbepoetin (200 µg subcutaneously every 2 weeks) is beneficial. Blood transfusions are indicated for patients with symptomatic anaemia who do not benefit from other therapy. Iron, folate, or vitamin B_{12} deficiency may be responsible for anaemia and must be recognized and treated.

Emotional support

All patients with MM need substantial and continuing emotional support. The physician's approach must be positive and emphasize the potential benefits of therapy. It is reassuring for patients to know that some survive for 10 years or more. It is vital that the physician caring for patients with MM has the interest and capacity to deal with an incurable disease over the space of years with assurance, sympathy, and resourcefulness.

Variant forms of multiple myeloma

Smouldering multiple myeloma
See above.

Plasma-cell leukaemia

Plasma-cell leukaemia is defined as the presence of more than 20% plasma cells in the peripheral blood and an absolute plasma-cell count of more than 2×10^9/litre. It is classified as primary when it presents *de novo* (60% of cases) and as secondary when it is a leukaemia transformation of a previously recognized myeloma (40%). Patients with primary plasma-cell leukaemia are younger and have a higher platelet count, fewer bone lesions, a smaller serum paraprotein, a greater incidence of hepatosplenomegaly and lymphadenopathy, and a longer duration of survival than patients with secondary plasma-cell leukaemia. Cytogenetic abnormalities are more common than in patients with MM. Although therapy of plasma cell leukaemia is unsatisfactory, partial responses may occur with dexamethasone, thalidomide or bortezomib plus dexamethasone, or alkylating agents. Autologous stem cell transplantation after high-dose chemotherapy is beneficial for some patients. Those with secondary plasma-cell leukaemia rarely respond to chemotherapy because they already received treatment and are resistant.

Nonsecretory myeloma

These patients have no paraprotein in either the serum or the urine and account for only 3% of patients with MM at diagnosis. The serum-free light chain assay is abnormal in about two-thirds of patients and can be used to monitor the response to therapy. The diagnosis is established by identification of an M-protein in the cytoplasm of the plasma cells by immunoperoxidase or immunofluorescence staining. Response to therapy and survival is similar to those in patients who have myeloma with a monoclonal protein in the serum or urine. Renal insufficiency is less common.

POEMS syndrome (osteosclerotic myeloma)

This is characterized by polyneuropathy (P), organomegaly (O), endocrinopathy (E), M-protein (M), and skin changes (S). The major clinical finding is a chronic inflammatory–demyelinating neuropathy with predominantly motor disability. Sclerotic bone lesions are found in most patients. The cranial nerves are not involved except for the presence of papilloedema. Hepatomegaly occurs in almost half of patients, but splenomegaly and lymphadenopathy occur in a minority. Hyperpigmentation and hypertrichosis are frequent but may be easily overlooked. Gynaecomastia and atrophic testes as well as clubbing of the fingers and toes may be present. Angiomatous lesions of the trunk are often prominent. Pulmonary hypertension has been recognized in several instances. Ascites, pleural effusion, and peripheral oedema may be present.

In contrast to MM, the haemoglobin level is usually normal or increased, and thrombocytosis is common. The bone marrow usually contains fewer than 5% plasma cells, and hypercalcaemia and renal insufficiency rarely occur. Most patients have a λ light chain, and IgA is the most common heavy-chain type. Castleman's disease may be present. The diagnosis is confirmed by the identification of monoclonal plasma cells obtained from an osteosclerotic lesion. If the skeletal lesions are in a limited area, radiation almost always produces a substantial improvement of the neuropathy. If widespread osteosclerotic lesions exist, an autologous stem cell transplant should be considered for therapy. Chemotherapy similar to that used in myeloma may be helpful. The median survival is 14 years.

Solitary plasmacytoma (solitary myeloma) of bone

The diagnosis depends on histological evidence of a plasma-cell tumour but no evidence of MM. Complete skeletal radiographs, bone marrow aspiration and biopsy, and immunofixation of the serum and urine should reveal no evidence of MM. Occasionally, a small paraprotein may be found in the serum or urine, but it usually disappears after radiation of a solitary lesion. In a study of 116 patients with solitary plasmacytoma of bone, the persistence of a serum monoclonal protein level of 5 g/litre or more 1 to 2 years after diagnosis and an abnormal free light-chain ratio at the time of diagnosis are predictive of disease progression. Treatment consists of tumoricidal radiation (40–50 Gy). Overt MM develops in approximately 55% of patients, and new solitary lesions or local recurrence develop in about 10%. MRI scans may be helpful for identifying patients in whom MM will develop in the near future. There is little evidence that adjuvant chemotherapy decreases the rate of conversion to multiple myeloma.

Extramedullary plasmacytoma

This is a plasma-cell tumour that arises outside the bone marrow. It is located in the upper respiratory tract in approximately 80% of cases, and the nasal cavity and sinuses, nasopharynx, and larynx are most often involved. The gastrointestinal tract, central nervous system, urinary bladder, thyroid, breast, testes, parotid gland, and lymph nodes have all been reported as the initial site of an extramedullary plasmacytoma. There is a predominance of IgA M-protein in extramedullary plasmacytomas. The diagnosis depends on the finding of a plasma-cell tumour in an extramedullary location and the absence of MM on bone marrow examination, radiography, and appropriate studies of serum and urine. Treatment consists of tumoricidal radiation (40–50 Gy). Regional occurrences develop in approximately 10% of patients, while development of typical MM occurs in 10 to 15%.

Waldenström's macroglobulinaemia

This malignant plasma-cell proliferative disorder produces a high concentration of immunoglobulin M (IgM) paraprotein. It bears similarities to MM, lymphoma, and chronic lymphocytic leukaemia. The incidence rate is 0.5/100 000, and in our practice it is one-seventh as common as MM. The median age is approximately 65 years, and 60% of patients are male.

Clinical findings

Weakness and fatigue are the most common symptoms of WM. Chronic nasal bleeding or oozing from the gums is characteristic, but postsurgical or gastrointestinal bleeding may occur. Blurring or loss of vision may be prominent. Dyspnoea and congestive heart failure may develop. Dizziness, headaches, vertigo, nystagmus, ataxia, and diplopia have been seen. Constitutional symptoms including fever, night sweats, and loss of weight may be present. Bone pain is rare. Hepatomegaly occurs in about 25% of patients at diagnosis, and splenomegaly and lymphadenopathy are slightly less common. Retinal vein engorgement and flame-shaped haemorrhages are common and are a better measure of symptomatic hyperviscosity syndrome than is the measurement of serum viscosity.

Pulmonary involvement may be manifested by diffuse pulmonary infiltrates, isolated masses, or pleural effusion. Retroperitoneal and mesenteric lymphadenopathy are common, but they are usually asymptomatic. The most common neurological manifestation is sensorimotor peripheral neuropathy. It is related to amyloid deposition in some instances.

Laboratory findings

Anaemia is found in most patients with symptomatic WM. Spuriously low haemoglobin and haematocrit levels may result from an increased plasma volume due to the large amount of paraprotein.

Serum protein electrophoresis reveals a tall, narrow spike or dense band usually migrating in the γ area. About 75% of the IgM paraproteins are κ. The IgM level obtained by nephelometry is often 10 to 30 g/litre more than that found with serum protein electrophoresis. A reduction of uninvolved IgG and IgA immunoglobulins is less striking than in MM. About 10% of macroglobulins precipitate in the cold (cryoglobulin) but are usually asymptomatic. A monoclonal light chain detected by immunofixation is present in the urine in 75% of patients, but it is usually small.

Fewer than 5% of patients with WM have lytic bone lesions. The bone marrow aspirate is often hypocellular, but the biopsy specimen is usually hypercellular and extensively infiltrated with lymphoid or plasmacytoid cells. Increased mast cells are frequently present.

Diagnosis

The diagnosis of WM depends on the presence of an IgM paraprotein and a 10% or greater monoclonal lymphocyte–plasma cell infiltration of the bone marrow producing symptoms and physical findings consistent with WM. The lymphoplasmacytic cells express CD19, CD20, and CD22. The differential diagnosis includes MM, MGUS of the IgM type, chronic lymphocytic leukaemia, lymphoma, and undifferentiated lymphoplasma-cell proliferative disorders.

Treatment

Patients with WM should not be treated unless they are symptomatic. Symptoms and findings of hyperviscosity are quickly controlled by plasmapheresis with a cell separator. Therapy must be directed against the proliferating lymphocytes and plasma cells because symptoms will recur quickly.

Rituximab, a monoclonal antibody directed against the CD20 antigenic determinant, produces a response in approximately one-half of patients with refractory disease. It may also be given with cyclophosphamide or CHOP (cyclophosphamide, doxorubicin, vincristine and prednisone). The IgM levels temporarily increase following therapy. The response may be delayed and not occur until 2 or 3 months after therapy. Chlorambucil, given continuously or intermittently, has been a standard therapy for more than 50 years. It is usually given orally in an initial dosage of 6 to 8 mg daily and is reduced when the leucocytes or platelets decrease. It also may be given intermittently at 4- to 6-week intervals. Patients should be treated until the disease has reached a plateau state, which occurs in about 70% of patients. Patients should be treated for at least 6 months before chlorambucil therapy is abandoned because of a slow response. Cyclophosphamide or combinations of alkylating agents such as the M2 protocol (vincristine, BCNU, melphalan, cyclophosphamide, and prednisone) have also been beneficial. Patients must be followed closely, and chemotherapy of the same type should be reinstituted when the disease relapses. Purine nucleoside analogues, fludarabine or cladribine (2-chlorodeoxyadenosine [2CDA]), produce responses in approximately one-half of patients. IFN-α_2 has also been used for therapy. Use of thalidomide has been disappointing. Autologous stem cell transplantation is another option.

Packed red cells should be transfused into patients with symptomatic anaemia. Erythropoietin may be of help. The median duration of survival for patients with macroglobulinaemia is approximately 5 years.

Heavy-chain diseases

γ-Heavy-chain diseases

The paraprotein consists of a monoclonal γ chain with significant amino acid deletions. The median age of patients is approximately 60 years, but the disease has been recognized in individuals under 20 years of age. The initial presentation is often a lymphoma-like illness, but the symptoms and clinical findings are diverse and range from an aggressive lymphoproliferative process to an asymptomatic state. Weakness, fatigue, and fever are the most common presenting symptoms. Hepatosplenomegaly and lymphadenopathy are found in about 60% of patients. Anaemia is present in 80%. The serum protein electrophoretic pattern usually shows a broad-based band more suggestive of a polyclonal than an M-protein. The urinary heavy-chain protein value is usually less than 1 g/24 h. Bence Jones proteinuria is not found. The bone marrow and lymph nodes contain an increased number of monoclonal plasma cells, lymphocytes, and lymphoplasmacytoid cells.

Only symptomatic patients should be treated. Therapy with cyclophosphamide, vincristine, and prednisone is a reasonable choice. If there is no response, a doxorubicin-containing regimen should be used. Melphalan plus prednisone is another option for therapy. The median duration of survival in a series of 23 patients was 7.4 years (range 1 month to 21 years).

α-Heavy-chain diseases

α-HCD is the most common type of heavy-chain disease, with more than 400 reported patients since its recognition. It usually occurs in the second or third decade of life, and about 60% of patients are male. Most patients have been from relatively poor countries in the Mediterranean region and Middle East. Gastrointestinal tract involvement is most common and is manifested by malabsorption with loss of weight, diarrhoea, and steatorrhoea. It is similar to 'immunoproliferative small intestinal disease' (IPSID), but patients with IPSID do not synthesize α heavy chains. The serum protein electrophoretic pattern shows no spike. The diagnosis depends on recognition of a monoclonal α heavy chain in the serum or jejunal fluid. Bence Jones proteinuria never appears. The bone marrow is not infiltrated with lymphocytes. α-HCD is progressive and fatal without therapy. Surprisingly, antibiotics may produce remission, particularly if given early in the course of the disease. Patients who have advanced disease or who do not respond to antibiotics should be treated with a combination of chemotherapy consisting of cyclophosphamide, doxorubicin, vincristine, and prednisone.

μ-Heavy-chain diseases

μ-HCD is characterized by the presence of a monoclonal μ-chain fragment in the serum. Most patients have a chronic lymphoproliferative process resembling chronic lymphocytic leukaemia or lymphoma. Fewer than 40 cases have been reported. The serum protein electrophoretic pattern contains a spike or localized band in about 40% of patients. Bence Jones proteinuria, which is usually κ, has been recognized in two-thirds of cases. Vacuolization of the plasma cells in the marrow is an important clue for the diagnosis of μ-HCD. There is an increase in lymphocytes, plasma cells, and lymphocytoid cells in the marrow. The course of μ-HCD is variable, with a median survival of approximately 2 years. A combination of cyclophosphamide, vincristin, and prednisone with or without doxorubicin is a reasonable choice. Treatment with corticosteroids and alkylating agents has also produced benefit.

Primary amyloidosis

Amyloid is a substance consisting of fibrils that appear homogeneous and amorphous under the light microscope and stain pink with haematoxylin–eosin. With polarized light, amyloid stained with Congo red produces an apple-green birefringence. Linear, non-branching, aggregated fibrils 7.5 to 10 nm wide and of indefinite length are seen with electron microscopy. These fibrils consist of various proteins such as monoclonal κ or λ light chains in AL, protein A in secondary amyloidosis, transthyretin (prealbumin) in familial or senile systemic amyloidosis, and β_2-microglobulin in dialysis-associated amyloidosis. Because paraproteins are associated only with primary amyloidosis, the other types are not discussed here.

Aetiology and epidemiology

The annual incidence of AL is 0.9/100 000. The median age at diagnosis is 64 years, and only 1% of patients are younger than 40 years. The cause of AL is unknown.

Clinical features

Weakness, fatigue, and weight loss are the most common initial symptoms. Light-headedness, syncope, change in the tongue or voice, jaw or hip claudication, paraesthesias, dyspnoea, and oedema are the most frequent symptoms. Macroglossia is present in 10% of patients, and purpura, particularly in the periorbital and facial areas, is found in 15%. The liver is palpable in 25% of patients, but splenomegaly occurs in only 5%. Nephrotic syndrome or renal failure is found in more than 25% of patients at diagnosis (Fig. 22.4.5.5). Congestive heart failure, carpal tunnel syndrome, sensorimotor peripheral neuropathy, and orthostatic hypotension are other important features. The presence of one of these syndromes and a paraprotein in the serum or urine are strong indications of AL, for which appropriate biopsy specimens must be taken for diagnosis.

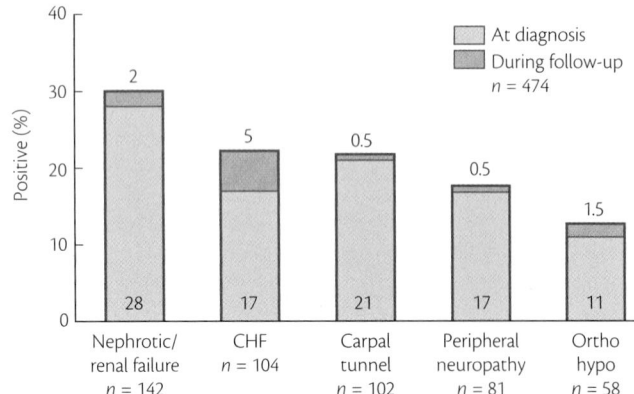

Fig. 22.4.5.5 Frequency of amyloid syndromes at diagnosis of primary systemic amyloidosis. CHF, congestive heart failure; Ortho hypo, orthostatic hypotension. (From Kyle RA, Gertz MA (1995). Primary systemic amyloidosis: clinical and laboratory features in 474 cases. *Semin Hematol*, **32**, 45–59. By permission of W B Saunders Company.)

Laboratory findings

Anaemia is not a prominent feature of AL and, when present, is usually the result of MM, renal insufficiency, or gastrointestinal bleeding. Thrombocytosis (platelets $>500 \times 10^9$/litre) is present in about 10% of cases. Renal insufficiency is present in almost half of patients at diagnosis; 20% have a serum creatinine value of 20 mg/litre or more. The serum protein electrophoretic pattern shows a modest localized band or spike in about half of the patients (median 14 g/litre). A paraprotein is found in the serum or urine in 90% of patients, and λ light chains are twice as common as κ. The bone marrow contains 5% or less monoclonal plasma cells in almost half of patients. Only one-fifth of patients have more than 20% plasma cells in the bone marrow, but they usually do not have the other features of MM.

An increased serum alkaline phosphatase level is not uncommon. Hyperbilirubinaemia is infrequent, but when present it is an ominous sign. The coagulation factor X concentration is decreased in more than 10% of patients but is rarely the cause of bleeding.

Congestive heart failure is present in about 20% of patients at diagnosis. Electrocardiography frequently reveals low voltage in the limb leads or characteristics consistent with anteroseptal infarction (loss of anterior forces). Arrhythmias, including atrial fibrillation or heart block, are common. Almost two-thirds of patients have an abnormal echocardiogram at diagnosis. Early cardiac involvement is characterized by abnormal relaxation followed by the features

of constrictive cardiomyopathy. Amyloid heart disease may closely resemble constrictive pericarditis or hypertrophic obstructive cardiomyopathy. A sensorimotor peripheral neuropathy is present in about 15% of patients at diagnosis. Autonomic dysfunction may be a prominent feature and is often manifested by orthostatic hypotension, diarrhoea, and impotence.

Diagnosis

The diagnosis depends on the demonstration of amyloid deposits. The possibility of AL must be considered in every patient who has a paraprotein in the serum or urine and who has a nephrotic syndrome, congestive heart failure, sensorimotor peripheral neuropathy, carpal tunnel syndrome, giant hepatomegaly, or idiopathic malabsorption syndrome. A paraprotein in the serum or urine or a monoclonal proliferation of plasma cells in the bone marrow occurs in 98% of patients with AL.

The initial diagnostic procedure should be an abdominal fat aspiration, which is positive in about 75% of patients (Fig. 22.4.5.6). A bone marrow aspiration and biopsy should be done to determine the degree of plasmacytosis, and amyloid stains will be positive in more than half of patients. The abdominal fat or bone marrow biopsy is positive in 90% of cases; if negative, a rectal biopsy (including submucosa) or biopsy of a suspected involved organ such as the kidney, liver, heart, or sural nerve is indicated. Immunohistochemical staining using antisera to κ, λ, protein A, transthyretin, and β_2-microglobulin is needed for identifying the type of systemic amyloidosis. Iodine-123 labelled human serum amyloid-P component is helpful for detecting amyloid deposition.

Prognosis

The median duration of survival for patients with AL is approximately 13 months. Survival varies greatly depending on the associated syndrome. It is only 6 months after the onset of congestive heart failure but more than 2 years in patients presenting with peripheral neuropathy. Almost one-half of the deaths are due to cardiac involvement.

Treatment

Because amyloid fibrils consist of a monoclonal light chain, treatment with alkylating agents has been a common approach. In a randomized trial, survival of patients receiving the two

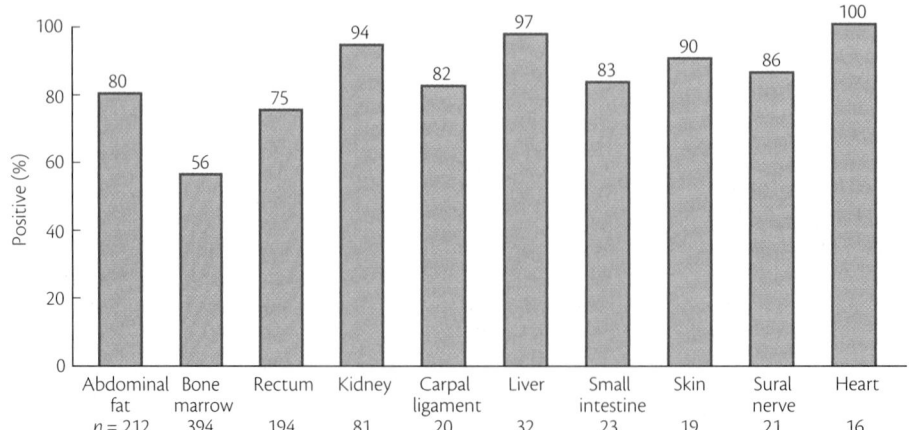

Fig. 22.4.5.6 Diagnosis of amyloidosis on the basis of deposits in tissues. (From Kyle RA, Gertz MA (1995). Primary systemic amyloidosis: clinical and laboratory features in 474 cases. *Semin Hematol*, **32**, 45–59. By permission of W B Saunders Company.)

melphalan–prednisone containing regimens (17–18 months) was superior to that of patients receiving colchicine (8.5 months). Patients were initially reported to have clinical improvement after the administration of 4′-iodo-4′-deoxyrubicin (I-DOX), but further experience has shown negligible benefit. Thalidomide, which has been used successfully in MM, is poorly tolerated in patients with AL and the results have been disappointing. Lenalidomide and dexamethasone produce responses, but experience is limited.

Autologous peripheral blood stem cell transplantation has been used with encouraging results. Patients must be carefully selected to eliminate those with significant cardiac involvement or with more than three involved organs. Even with careful selection, the 100-day treatment related mortality is 10 to 15%, in contrast to 1 to 2% for multiple myeloma.

Future developments

Despite the introduction of new agents for the treatment of MM during the past decade, much remains to be done. Gene expression profiling and refinement of FISH studies in MGUS and MM may lead to better understanding and consequently improved therapy. Identification and testing of new agents for treatment are needed. Better methods for identifying high-risk myeloma patients and improved therapy for these patients are needed. New agents may well be used in conjunction with current drugs. Efforts must be made to determine the role of maintenance therapy following transplantation or containment of response with chemotherapy. The development of interventions to delay progression of SMM is a laudable goal. Prediction of response to therapy may lead to more personalized care and is a major goal for the future.

Further reading

Attal M, et al. (1996). A prospective, randomized trial of autologous bone marrow transplantation and chemotherapy in multiple myeloma. Intergroupe Francais du Myelome. N Engl J Med, 335, 91–7.

Attal M, et al. (2006). Maintenance therapy with thalidomide improves survival in patients with multiple myeloma. Blood, 108, 3289–94.

Bruno B, et al. (2007). A comparison of allografting with autografting for newly diagnosed myeloma. N Engl J Med, 356, 1110–20.

Child JA, et al. (2003). High-dose chemotherapy with hematopoietic stem-cell rescue for multiple myeloma [see comment]. N Engl J Med, 348, 1875–83.

Dingli D, et al. (2006). Immunoglobulin free light chains and solitary plasmacytoma of bone. Blood, 108, 1979–83.

Dispenzieri A, et al. (2003). POEMS syndrome: definitions and long-term outcome. Blood, 101, 2496–506.

Dispenzieri A, et al. (2007). Treatment of newly diagnosed multiple myeloma based on Mayo stratification of myeloma and risk-adapted therapy (mSMART): consensus statement. Mayo Clin Proc, 82, 323–41.

Facon T, et al. (2005). Major superiority of melphalan and prednisone (MP) plus thalidomide (THAL) over MP and autologous stem cell transplantation in the treatment of newly diagnosed elderly patients with multiple myeloma. Blood, 106, A780 (abst).

Falk RH, Comenzo RL, Skinner M (1997). The systemic amyloidoses. N Engl J Med, 337, 898–909.

Garcia-Sanz R, et al. (1999). Primary plasma cell leukaemia: clinical, immunophenotypic, DNA ploidy, and cytogenetic characteristics. Blood, 93, 1032–7.

Gertz MA, Kyle RA (1995). Hyperviscosity syndrome. [Review] [138 refs]. J Intensive Care Med, 10, 128–41.

Ghobrial IM, et al. (2006). Prognostic model for disease-specific and overall mortality in newly diagnosed symptomatic patients with Waldenstrom macroglobulinaemia. Br J Haematol, 133, 158–64.

Hideshima T, et al. (2004). Advances in biology of multiple myeloma: clinical applications. Blood, 104, 607–18.

International Myeloma Working Group (2003). Criteria for the classification of monoclonal gammopathies, multiple myeloma and related disorders: a report of the International Myeloma Working Group. Br J Haematol, 121, 749–57.

Katzmann JA, Kyle RA (2006). Immunochemical characterization of immunoglobulins in serum, urine, and cerebrospinal fluid. In: Detrick B, Hamilton R, Folds J (eds) Manual of molecular and clinical laboratory immunology, pp. 88–100. ASM Press, Washington, DC.

Kyle RA (2000). Multiple myeloma: an odyssey of discovery. Br J Haematol, 111, 1035–44.

Kyle RA, Garton JP (1987). The spectrum of IgM monoclonal gammopathy in 430 cases. Mayo Clin Proc, 62, 719–31.

Kyle RA, Gertz MA (1995). Primary systemic amyloidosis: clinical and laboratory features in 474 cases. Semin Hematol, 32, 45–59.

Kyle RA, Rajkumar SV (2004). Multiple myeloma: drug therapy (review article). N Engl J Med, 351, 1860–73.

Kyle RA, Rajkumar SV (2006). Monoclonal gammopathy of undetermined significance. Br J Haematol, 134, 573–589.

Kyle RA, et al. (1997). A trial of three regimens for primary amyloidosis: colchicine alone, melphalan and prednisone, and melphalan, prednisone, and colchicine [see comment]. N Engl J Med, 336, 1202–7.

Kyle RA, et al. (2002). A long-term study of prognosis in monoclonal gammopathy of undetermined significance [see comment]. N Engl J Med, 346, 564–9.

Kyle RA, et al. (2003). Review of 1027 patients with newly diagnosed multiple myeloma [see comment]. Mayo Clin Proc, 78, 21–33.

Kyle RA, et al. (2004). Long-term follow-up of 241 patients with monoclonal gammopathy of undetermined significance: the original Mayo Clinic series 25 years later [see comment]. Mayo Clin Proc, 79, 859–66.

Kyle RA, et al. (2006). Prevalence of monoclonal gammopathy of undetermined significance. N Engl J Med, 354, 1362–69.

Liebross RH, et al. (1998). Solitary bone plasmacytoma: outcome and prognostic factors following radiotherapy. Int J Radiat Oncol Biol Phys, 41, 1063–7.

Myeloma Trialists' Collaborative Group (1998). Combination chemotherapy versus melphalan plus prednisone as treatment for multiple myeloma: an overview of 6,633 patients from 27 randomized trials. J Clin Oncol, 16, 3832–42.

Palumbo A, et al. (2006). Oral melphalan and prednisone chemotherapy plus thalidomide compared with melphalan and prednisone alone in elderly patients with multiple myeloma: randomised controlled trial. Lancet, 367, 825–31.

Rajkumar SV, et al. (2005). Combination therapy with lenalidomide plus dexamethasone (Rev/Dex) for newly diagnosed myeloma. Blood, 106, 4050–3.

Rajkumar SV, et al. (2005). Serum free light chain ratio is an independent risk factor for progression in monoclonal gammopathy of undetermined significance. Blood, 106, 812–7.

Richardson PG, et al. (2003). A phase 2 study of bortezomib in relapsed, refractory myeloma [see comment]. N Engl J Med, 348, 2609–17.

Singhal S, et al. (1999). Antitumor activity of thalidomide in refractory multiple myeloma [see comment]. N Engl J Med, 341, 1565–71 (erratum in N Engl J Med 2000, 342, 364).

Susnerwala SS, et al. (1997). Extramedullary plasmacytoma of the head and neck region: clinicopathological correlation in 25 cases. Br J Cancer, 75, 921–7.

Wahner-Roedler DL, et al. (2003). Gamma-heavy chain disease: review of 23 cases. Medicine, 82, 236–50.

22.4.6 Eosinophilia

Peter F. Weller

Essentials

Eosinophilia (eosinophil count >0.45 × 10^9/litre) is associated with some infections, some allergic diseases, and a variety of other conditions, often neoplastic.

Infectious diseases

Parasitic diseases—eosinophilia is a characteristic feature of infection by multicellular helminth parasites, e.g. *Strongyloides stercoralis*, with diagnosis typically based on geographical/dietary history and examination of stool for ova and larvae.

Other diseases—eosinophilia can be caused by the fungal disease coccidioidomycosis, and modest eosinophilia (0.45–1.5 × 10^9/litre) may accompany viral infections such as HIV and HTLV-1.

Allergic, immunological, neoplastic, and other disorders

Common allergic diseases—asthma, rhinitis, and atopic dermatitis are associated with modest eosinophilia.

Drug reactions—these are a frequent cause of eosinophilia, often in reactions characterized by rashes and pyrexia. More severe reactions may also manifest with (1) pulmonary eosinophilia and lung infiltrates; (2) interstitial nephritis; (3) hepatitis; (4) myocarditis; (5) drug-induced hypersensitivity vasculitis; (6) gastroenterocolitis; and (7) drug-induced rash, eosinophilia and systemic symptoms (DRESS syndrome).

Other conditions—these include (1) Churg–Strauss syndrome; (2) hyper-IgE syndrome—comprising recurrent staphylococcal abscesses, dermatitis, hyperimmunoglobulinaemia E, and eosinophilia; (3) chronic myeloid leukaemia, acute myeloblastic leukaemia (some types), Hodgkin's disease (some types); (4) a variety of pulmonary, skin, gastrointestinal and endocrine diseases.

Hypereosinophilic syndromes

These are defined by (1) sustained eosinophilia (>1.5 × 10^9/litre), (2) lack of an identifiable cause precipitating a secondary eosinophilia, and (3) symptoms and signs of organ involvement. About 30% of patients will have either a myeloproliferative condition (chronic eosinophilic leukaemia) or hypereosinophilia mediated by clonal expansion of specific T cells producing interleukin 5 (IL-5).

Clinical features—common manifestations are (1) cardiac—endomyocardial damage typically leads to a restrictive cardiomyopathy; (2) neurological—strokes related to thromboemboli, encephalopathy, and polyneuropathy; (3) dermatological—e.g. angiooedema, urticarial lesions; (4) pulmonary—infiltrates of eosinophils may be seen in any part of the lung, sometimes leading to pulmonary fibrosis.

Treatment—patients without organ damage do not require treatment. Aside from supportive care (1) chronic eosinophilic leukaemia—may respond to tyrosine kinase inhibitors, e.g. imatinib; (2) nonmyeloproliferative hypereosinophilic syndrome—may respond to high-dose corticosteroids, with hydroxyurea, interferon-α and anti-IL-5 monoclonal antibody (mepolizumab) used in refractory cases.

Introduction

Eosinophilia is associated with distinct diseases that include helminth parasitic infections, allergic diseases, and varied diseases of often ill-defined cause.

In comparison with other leucocytes, eosinophils are distinguished by their morphologies, constituents, products, and associations with specific diseases. The cytokine interleukin 5 (IL-5), specific in promoting the development, differentiation, and release of bone marrow-derived eosinophils, is principally responsible for increases in eosinophilopoiesis. Eosinophils are normally tissue-dwelling cells primarily distributed in those tissues with an epithelial interface with the environment, including the gastrointestinal and lower genitourinary tracts. Eosinophils are distinguished morphologically from neutrophils by their cytoplasmic granules, which uniquely contain crystalloid cores visible by electron microscopy. Within these granules are four specific cationic proteins: major basic protein, eosinophil peroxidase, eosinophil cationic protein, and eosinophil-derived neurotoxin. The heavy content of these cationic granule proteins, which bind acidic dyes such as eosin, are responsible both for the identifying tinctorial properties of eosinophils and for many of the functional properties of eosinophils. Eosinophils are sources of over three dozen cytokines; and many, if not all, of these are stored preformed within eosinophil granules and cytoplasmic vesicles. In addition to their content of preformed proteins, eosinophils synthesize lipid mediators, including the 5-lipoxygenase pathway-derived eicosanoid, leukotriene C_4. The potential functional roles of eosinophils in parasite–host defence, in the pathogenesis of allergic diseases, and in other immunological responses remain uncertain, due to varied and at times conflicting experimental findings, but are subjects of active ongoing investigations.

Eosinophils normally number less than 450/μlitre in the blood with a mild diurnal variation, being higher in the morning and falling as endogenous glucocorticosteroid levels rise. Blood eosinophil numbers do not, however, always reflect the extent of eosinophil involvement in affected tissues in various diseases; and at times, as in eosinophilic pneumonias, eosinophils may be recruited into involved tissues without a concomitant increase in enumerable blood eosinophils. Eosinopenia, diminished blood eosinophil levels, occurs with corticosteroid administration and is frequent with active bacterial and viral infections. Thus, even normal blood eosinophil numbers in a febrile patient suggest that an illness is not simply due to a bacterial or viral infection.

Some, but not necessarily all, patients with sustained blood eosinophilia can develop organ damage, especially cardiac, as found in hypereosinophilic syndromes, and patients with sustained eosinophilia should be monitored for evidence of cardiac disease.

Diseases associated with eosinophilia

Infectious diseases

Parasitic diseases

Eosinophilia is not elicited by infections with protozoan parasites (with the exceptions of the intestinal parasites *Isospora belli* and *Dientamoeba fragilis*), but rather characteristically by multicellular helminth parasites. Magnitudes of eosinophilia tend to parallel the extent of tissue invasion, especially by helminth larvae. Eosinophilia may be absent in established infections which are well-contained within tissues or are solely intraluminal within the gastrointestinal tract (e.g. ascaris, tapeworms). Even with helminth diseases, superimposed bacterial infections (e.g. in disseminated strongyloidiasis) can suppress expected eosinophilia. In patients with eosinophilia, geographical and dietary histories are pertinent in suggesting potential exposures to helminth parasites. Stool examinations for diagnostic ova and larvae should be obtained. In addition, for several helminth parasites that cause eosinophilia, diagnostic parasite stages are never present in faeces. Hence, negative stool specimens do not necessarily exclude a helminth aetiology for eosinophilia; and examination of appropriate blood or tissue biopsies and/or serologic tests, as guided by clinical findings and exposure histories, may be needed to diagnose specific tissue- or blood-dwelling infections, including trichinellosis and filarial infections.

Other infectious diseases

The characteristic response in acute bacterial and viral infections is eosinopenia. The fungal disease, coccidioidomycosis, either following primary infection, at times with progressive disseminated disease, or with central nervous system infection (with cerebrospinal fluid eosinophilia), may be associated with eosinophilia.

HIV and retroviral infections

Eosinophilia may be associated with HIV infections as a result of adverse reactions to medications or adrenal insufficiency in patients with AIDS from cytomegalovirus and other infections. In addition, eosinophilia, often modest, is observed in some HIV-infected patients and may accompany eosinophilic folliculitis in HIV infection. Eosinophilia frequently develops with HTLV-1 infections.

Allergic and immunological disorders

Common allergic diseases, including allergic rhinitis, asthma, and atopic dermatitis, are accompanied by tissue eosinophil infiltration and usually modest blood eosinophilia. The occurrence of marked blood eosinophilia suggests the presence of other diseases, such as Churg–Strauss vasculitis.

Medication-related eosinophilias

Therapeutic agents, including herbal or 'natural' therapies, can elicit eosinophilia. Eosinophilia may develop without other manifestations of adverse drug reactions, such as rashes or drug fevers. In the absence of organ involvement, blood eosinophilia by itself need not mandate cessation of drug therapy, if such is medically indicated. Drug-induced blood eosinophilia, however, should prompt an evaluation of whether organs, including the lungs, kidneys, and heart, are involved in the eosinophil-associated drug reaction. If organ involvement develops, cessation of drug administration is necessary.

Some cytokines are potential causes of eosinophilia. Granulocyte–macrophage colony-stimulating factor (GM-CSF) and IL-2 can cause prominent blood and tissue eosinophilia and, less commonly, eosinophil-associated diseases, including eosinophilic pneumonia and eosinophilic endomyocardial fibrosis. Diverse agents, including many antimicrobial agents and nonsteroidal anti-inflammatory agents (NSAIDs), may elicit pulmonary eosinophilia. Blood eosinophilia is usually, but not always, present; and if blood eosinophilia is absent, sputum or bronchoalveolar lavage eosinophilia is necessary to help make the diagnosis.

In drug-induced acute interstitial nephritis, eosinophilia is common in the involved kidneys, urine, and at times, the blood. In addition to eosinophilia, fever, rash, and arthralgia support the diagnosis, but these are commonly absent in cases of drug-induced acute interstitial nephritis. Eosinophiluria is not uniformly present in all with drug-induced interstitial nephritis.

Acute necrotizing eosinophilic myocarditis is a serious but uncommon type of hypersensitivity myocarditis, with reactions to medications, responsible in some cases. A syndrome of hepatitis with eosinophilia can be a manifestation of drug reactions, Other medication-related eosinophilic responses include drug-induced hypersensitivity vasculitis, the DRESS syndrome (drug-induced rash, eosinophilia, and systemic symptoms), and forms of gastro-enterocolitis.

Immunological disorders

The hyper-IgE syndrome is characterized by recurrent staphylococcal abscesses of the skin, lungs, and other sites, pruritic dermatitis, hyperimmunoglobulinaemia E, and blood, sputum, and tissue eosinophilia. Eosinophilia is characteristic of Omenn's syndrome, combined immunodeficiency with hypereosinophilia.

Eosinophil infiltration accompanies rejection of lung, kidney, and liver allografts. Tissue and blood eosinophilia occur early in the rejection process.

Myeloproliferative and neoplastic diseases

The hypereosinophilic syndromes are considered below. Eosinophilia may accompany chronic myelogenous leukaemia and the M4Eo subtype of acute myelogenous leukaemia. Blood eosinophils may be elevated in the nodular sclerosing form of Hodgkin's disease. Some patients with carcinomas, especially of mucin-producing epithelial cell origins, have blood eosinophilia. Eosinophilia may accompany angio-immunoblastic lymphadenopathy, mycosis fungoides, Sézary's syndrome, lymphomatoid papulosis, and systemic mastocytosis.

Pulmonary syndromes

Diverse eosinophilic pulmonary syndromes are noted in Box 22.4.6.1.

Skin and subcutaneous diseases

Various cutaneous diseases can be associated with a heightened level of blood eosinophils (Box 22.4.6.1). In episodic angiooedema with eosinophilia, recurrences are marked by prominent blood eosinophilia, significant angiooedema, at times with excessive weight gain due to fluid retention, and less frequently by fever.

Gastrointestinal diseases

Eosinophilia is common with eosinophilic gastroenteritis and eosinophilic oesophagitis, and tissue eosinophils are found in inflammatory bowel diseases and collagenous colitis.

Box 22.4.6.1 Diseases and disorders associated with eosinophilia

Infectious diseases

- Helminth parasites
- Coccidioidomycosis
- Other infections—infrequent, but includes HIV-1 and HTLV-1

Allergic and immunological disorders

- Allergic rhinitis, asthma
- Medication-related eosinophilias
- Immunodeficiency diseases: Job's syndrome and Ommen's syndrome
- Transplant rejections

Myeloproliferative and neoplastic disorders

- Hypereosinophilic syndromes
- Leukaemia, notably M4Eo subtype of acute myelogenous leukaemia
- Lymphoma- and tumour-associated, notably with nodular sclerosing Hodgkin's disease
- Mastocytosis

Pulmonary syndromes

- Parasite-induced eosinophilic lung diseases:

  - Transpulmonary passage of developing larvae (Löffler's syndrome): patchy migratory infiltrates, especially ascaris

  - Tropical pulmonary eosinophilia: miliary lesions and fibrosis; heightened immune responses to lymphatic filariae with increased IgE and antifilarial antibodies

  - Pulmonary parenchymal invasion: paragonimiasis

  - Heavy haematogenous seeding with helminths: disseminated strongyloidiasis, trichinellosis, schistosomiasis, larva migrans

  - Allergic bronchopulmonary aspergillosis

- Chronic eosinophilic pneumonia: dense peripheral infiltrates, fever; blood eosinophilia may be absent; steroid responsive

- Acute eosinophilic pneumonia—acute presentation, often without blood eosinophilia; diagnosed by bronchoalveolar lavage or biopsy

- Churg–Strauss vasculitis: small and medium-sized arteries; perivascular eosinophilia early and granulomas and necrosis later; asthma often antecedent; extrapulmonary, e.g. neurological,

cutaneous, cardiac, or gastrointestinal, vasculitic involvement likely

- Drug- and toxin-induced eosinophilic lung diseases
- Other: neoplasia, hypereosinophilic syndromes, bronchocentric granulomatosis

Skin and subcutaneous diseases

- Skin diseases—atopic dermatitis, blistering diseases, including bullous pemphigoid, urticarias, drug reactions
- Diseases of pregnancy: pruritic urticarial papules and plaques syndrome, herpes gestationis
- Eosinophilic pustular folliculitis
- Eosinophilic cellulitis (Wells' syndrome)
- Kimura's disease and angiolymphoid hyperplasia with eosinophilia
- Shulman's syndrome (eosinophilic fasciitis)
- Episodic angio-oedema with eosinophilia—recurrent periodic episodes with fever, angio-oedema, and secondary weight gain; may be long-standing without untoward cardiac dysfunction

Gastrointestinal diseases

- Eosinophilic gastroenteritis—(1) blood eosinophilia; (2) eosinophil cell infiltrates in the mucosa, muscularis, or serosa; (3) oedema of stomach or intestines; and (4) absence of extraintestinal involvement
- Inflammatory bowel disease and collagenous colitis—eosinophils in tissue lesions

Rheumatological diseases

- Churg–Strauss vasculitis
- Cutaneous necrotizing eosinophilic vasculitis

Endocrine disease

- Hypoadrenalism: Addison's disease, adrenal haemorrhage, hypopituitarism

Other causes of eosinophilia

- Atheromatous cholesterol embolization
- Hereditary
- Serosal surface irritation, including peritoneal dialysis and pleural eosinophilia

Rheumatological diseases

The principal eosinophil-related vasculitis is the Churg–Strauss syndrome. Cutaneous necrotizing eosinophilic vasculitis with hypocomplementaemia and eosinophilia, a distinct vasculitis of small dermal vessels which are extensively infiltrated with eosinophils, may occur in patients with connective tissue diseases. Eosinophilia may uncommonly accompany rheumatoid arthritis itself but is more commonly due to adverse reactions to medications or concomitant vasculitis.

Endocrine diseases

Loss of normal adrenoglucocorticosteroid production causes increased blood eosinophilia.

Other disorders

The syndrome of atheromatous cholesterol embolization can be associated with eosinophilia and eosinophiluria. Rare kindreds with hereditary eosinophilia have been recognized. Irritation of serosal surfaces, as in eosinophilic pleural effusions and peritoneal, and at times blood, eosinophilia developing during chronic peritoneal dialysis, can be associated with eosinophilia.

Hypereosinophilic syndromes

Patients with pronounced and prolonged eosinophilia not associated with other clinical diseases noted above had been classified previously as having the idiopathic hypereosinophilic syndrome. More recently, it has become clear that the hypereosinophilic syndromes (HES) include a clinically heterogeneous diverse group of eosinophilic disorders. For myeloproliferative and lymphocytic variants of HES, aetiologies are now known, yet for many others with HES underlying aetiologies remain to be delineated.

Definition

Chusid and collaeagues proposed three defining criteria for HES that may can now be modified and updated. Contemporary criteria include the following.

◆ Eosinophilia in excess of 1500/µl of blood. Although the initial criterion stipulated that the eosinophilia persist for longer than 6 months, in current practice the eosinophilia needs to be sustained, but does not require a 6-month period, especially if therapies are needed.

◆ Lack of an identifiable parasitic, allergic, or other aetiology for eosinophilia. Amongst parasitic aetiologies of eosinophilia, it is especially important to exclude *Strongyloides stercoralis*, which may persist for decades and be difficult to diagnose solely by stool examinations, not only because of its capacity to cause marked eosinophilia mimicking HES, but also because it, unlike other helminthic causes of marked eosinophilia, can develop into a disseminated, often fatal, disease (hyperinfection syndrome) in patients given immunosuppressive corticosteroids. Moreover, as noted below, some forms of HES now have identified aetiologies.

◆ Evidence by symptoms and signs of organ involvement. Not all patients with prolonged eosinophilia develop organ involvement and many have benign courses. These patients are often not reported or subjected to evaluation at referral centres due to the absence of eosinophil-associated disease. Blood eosinophilia *per se* does not warrant therapy in the absence of evidence of concomitant organ involvement.

Aetiologies

HES encompasses a spectrum of hypereosinophilic disorders, for which aetiologies are now recognized for a couple of HES variants:

◆ Myeloproliferative variants—These represent forms of chronic eosinophilic leukaemia. The most common form arises from an interstitial deletion on chromosome 4q12 that leads to fusion of the *FIPL1* (FIP1-like 1) and *PDGFRA* genes that generates a protein with constitutively active receptor tyrosine kinase activity. Rearrangements of the *PDGFRB* and *FGFR1* genes are additional causes of chronic eosinophilic leukaemia. In addition, clonal abnormalities in the eosinophil lineage have been detected uncommonly based on analyses of X-linked polymorphisms and hence applicable only to the minority of women with HES.

◆ Lymphocytic variants—These represent causes of HES mediated by clonal expansions of specific T cells. The most common are due to CD3– CD4+ T-cell subsets and less frequently CD3+ CD4– CD8– or other T-cell subsets. These clonal T cells elaborate eosinophil-stimulating IL-5 and often other Th2-associated cytokines, including IL-4.

◆ Other—While the recognition of the above aetiologies for some variants of HES is recent, over half of patients with HES currently have undefined aetiologies for their eosinophilia.

Clinical features

With the evolving recognition of variant forms of HES, some clinical features are more common with myeloproliferative, lymphocytic or other variants of HES, but these have not been fully delineated as yet. Myeloproliferative HES is more common in men than women (9:1); whereas other variants of HES have no gender bias. HES tends to occur between the ages of 20 and 50, although cases have developed in children. Initial manifestations may be due to sudden cardiac or neurological complications, but tend to be more insidious and present over months or longer. Eosinophilia may be detected only incidentally. Other frequent presenting symptoms include tiredness, cough, breathlessness, muscle pains, angioedema, rash, sweating, pruritus, or retinal lesions. Patients with HES do not exhibit a propensity to bacterial or other infections.

Haematological manifestations

The defining haematological abnormality is sustained eosinophilia. Total leucocyte counts are usually less than 25 000/µl, with between 30 and 70% eosinophils, but extremely high leucocyte counts (>90 000/µl) develop in some patients and are associated with a poor prognosis. Eosinophils in the blood may be mature or less commonly can include numbers of eosinophilic myeloid precursors. Eosinophils often exhibit morphological abnormalities including diminished granule numbers, cytoplasmic vacuolization, and nuclear hypersegmentation.

Many patients with HES will have an absolute neutrophilia along with their eosinophilia, further contributing to elevations in the white blood cell count. Band forms and less mature neutrophilic precursors may be present in the peripheral blood. Serum vitamin B_{12} and tryptase levels are often elevated in myeloproliferative variant HES. Anaemia is present in some patients.

Bone marrow findings demonstrate increased numbers of eosinophils, often 30 to 60%, with a shift to the left in eosinophil maturation. Increased numbers of myeloblasts are not usually seen. Myelofibrosis and splenomegaly are more frequent in myeloproliferative variant HES.

Cardiac manifestations

In HES, the heart is a commonly affected organ due to the development of endomyocardial damage leading to a restrictive cardiomyopathy. This distinct form of cardiac involvement may also complicate other varied diseases marked by sustained eosinophilia, including Churg–Strauss vasculitis, eosinophilic leukaemia, eosinophilia with carcinomas or lymphomas, eosinophilia from GM-CSF or IL-2 administration or drug reactions, and eosinophilia from helminthic infections such as trichinellosis, visceral larva migrans, and filariasis. However, many patients with eosinophilia do not develop any evidence of endomyocardial damage; hence in addition to increased numbers of eosinophils, the pathogenesis of eosinophil-mediated cardiac damage probably involves some, as yet ill-defined, activating events that promote eosinophil-mediated endomyocardial damage. Patients with sustained eosinophilia should be monitored by troponin assays, echocardiography or cardiac MRI for evidence of cardiac disease.

Cardiac damage progresses through three stages, the first involving acute necrosis in the early weeks, the second involving the development of endocardial thrombi over many months, and the final stage being the fibrotic stage after a couple of years of disease.

The risks of developing cardiac disease in two series of patients with HES were not related to the extent of eosinophilia or duration of disease. Those who developed evident cardiac disease were more likely to be male and to have splenomegaly, thrombocytopenia, elevated levels of vitamin B_{12}, hypogranular or vacuolated eosinophils, and abnormal early myeloid precursors in their blood. Cardiac involvement is likely more common in the myeloproliferative than the lymphocytic variants of HES.

Neurological manifestations

Neurological complications may be of three types. The first type is due to thromboemboli originating from the left ventricle, which may occur before cardiac disease is demonstrable by echocardiography and can be the presenting manifestation of HES. The second type of neurological disease is primary central nervous system dysfunction, presenting as an encephalopathy including changes in behaviour, confusion, ataxia, and memory loss, and exhibiting upper motor neuron signs with increased muscle tone, deep tendon reflexes, and a positive Babinski. Impaired cognitive abilities may persist for months. The pathological basis for this form of diffuse central nervous system disease remains unknown. Peripheral neuropathies constitute the third type of neurological dysfunction. Symmetric or asymmetric polyneuropathies manifest by sensory deficits, painful paraesthesiae, or mixed sensory and motor deficits are most common, but mononeuritis multiplex occurs with HES, as do radiculopathies and muscle atrophy due to denervation. Biopsies of affected nerves generally show an axonal neuropathy with varying degrees of axonal loss and no evidence of vasculitis or contiguous eosinophil infiltration.

Cutaneous manifestations

The skin is one of the most frequently involved organs, especially with lymphocytic variant HES. The most common skin manifestations are of two types, either angio-oedematous and urticarial lesions, or erythematous, pruritic papules and nodules. Some patients with angio-oedema and eosinophilia have a syndrome of episodic angiooedema and eosinophilia,. Particularly incapacitating mucocutaneous manifestations of HES are mucosal ulcers that may occur in the mouth, nose, pharynx, penis, oesophagus, stomach, and anus.

Pulmonary manifestations

Pulmonary involvement is reported in about 40% of HES patients, the commonest respiratory symptom being a chronic, persistent, generally nonproductive cough. The basis for this may be sequestration of eosinophils in pulmonary tissues, although most symptomatic individuals have clear chest radiographs. Pulmonary involvement in HES may also be secondary to congestive heart failure, pulmonary emboli originating from right ventricular thrombi, or primary infiltration of the lungs by eosinophils. Infiltrates may be diffuse or focal without a predilection for any region of the lungs, in contrast to the often peripheral infiltrates in chronic eosinophilic pneumonia (see Chapter 18.14.2). Pulmonary fibrosis may develop over time, especially in those with cardiac fibrosis.

Other manifestations

Arthralgias, large joint effusions, cold-induced Raynaud's phenomenon, and digital necrosis of fingers or toes can occur with HES. Although myalgias are frequent, focal myositis or polymyositis occur only uncommonly. Gastrointestinal tract involvement can accompany HES, and 20% of patients at some time may have diarrhoea. Eosinophilic gastritis, enterocolitis, or colitis may be present. Pancreatitis and sclerosing cholangitis occur rarely. Hepatic involvement with HES includes chronic active hepatitis and the Budd–Chiari syndrome from hepatic vein obstruction.

Diagnosis

Patients with myeloproliferative HES due to the *FIP1L1-PDGFRA* fusion can be identified by polymerase chain reaction or by evaluating the associated deletion of the CHIC2 gene by fluorescence *in situ* hybridization (FISH). Bone marrow biopsy with cytogenetics may identify less common myeloproliferative variants. Lymphocytic variants of HES are diagnosed based on both peripheral T-cell phenotyping by flow cytometry and assessments of clonal T-cell receptor rearrangements. For others with HES, additional specific diagnostic tests are not available.

Treatment

For patients with myeloproliferative HES, therapy for chronic eosinophilic leukaemia is with imatinib or related tyrosine kinase inhibitors. For those eosinophilic patients without organ damage, no therapy need be administered. There is no clear threshold value of blood eosinophilia that predicts organ involvement or damage. For HES patients without myeloproliferative variants requiring therapy, prednisolone is the initial agent, administered at 60 mg/day in adults. For those not responsive to prednisolone or needing a steroid-sparing regimen, daily hydroxyurea or interferon-α (1–10 million units/day or 3 times a week) are options. Anti-IL-5 monoclonal antibody (mepolizumab) may also prove to be an additional therapy for HES.

Medical management of cardiac complications, including arrhythmias and congestive heart failure, is important and effective in the longer-term management of HES, as is surgical replacement of damaged valves. Although early reports emphasized the mortality due to this disorder, many of the deaths were due to congestive heart failure and complications of endomyocardial damage. If the sequelae of organ damage, especially to the heart, can be managed, many patients with HES can have a prolonged course.

Further reading

Klion AD (ed.) (2007). Hypereosinophilic syndromes. *Immunol Allergy Clin N Am*, **27**, 1–560. [A multi-chapter monograph providing a thorough contemporary consideration of the forms, manifestations, diagnoses and therapies of the hypereosinophilic syndromes.]

Ogbogu PU, *et al.* (2009). Hypereosinophilic syndrome: a multicenter, retrospective analysis of clinical characteristics and response to therapy. *J Allergy Clin Immunol*, **124**, 1319-1325. [An analysis of 188 patients seen from 2001 to 2006 at 11 institutions in the United States and Europe.]

Roufosse F, *et al.* (2007). Lymphocytic variant hypereosinophilic syndromes. *Immunol Allergy Clin N Am*, **27**, 389–413. [A current consideration of the lymphocytic variants of HES.]

Sade K, *et al.* (2007). Eosinophilia: A study of 100 hospitalized patients. *Eur J Intern Med*, **18**, 196–201. [A review of the varied aetiologies of eosinophilia encountered in hospitalized patients.]

Tefferi A, Gotlib J, Pardanni A (2010). Hypereosinophilic syndrome and clonal eosinophilia: Point-of-care diagnostic alogorithm and treatment update. *Mayo Clin Proc*, **85**, 158-164.

Weller PF (2007). Eosinophilia and eosinophil-related disorders. In: Adkinson NF, Jr *et al.* (eds) *Allergy: principles and practice*, 7th edition. Mosby, St. Louis. [A thorough review of the clinical disorders associated with eosinophilia.]

Wilson ME, Weller PF (2006). Eosinophilia. In: Guerrant RL, Walker DH, Weller PF (eds) *Tropical infectious diseases: principles, pathogens and practice*, 2nd edition. pp 1478–98. Elsevier, Philadelphia. [Considerations of the aetiologies of eosinophilia with special emphasis on helminth infections.]

22.4.7 Histiocytoses

D.K.H. Webb

Essentials

The histiocytoses are characterized by the infiltration of affected tissues with cells of monocyte/macrophage lineage.

Disorders of dendritic cells

Langerhans' cell histiocytosis—may present with (1) disease affecting a single organ—typically skin (rash) or bone (pain and soft tissue swelling, or asymptomatic radiographic lesions); or (2) multisystem disease—characteristic features include ear discharge, diabetes insipidus, and lung involvement (diffuse micronodular shadowing on chest radiography, with progression to cyst formation and a honeycomb lung appearance). Diagnosis requires identification of Langerhans' cells within lesional inflammatory cell infiltrate, with demonstration of either the CD1a surface antigen on immunohistochemistry or the presence of Birbeck granules on electron microscopy. Most cases eventually resolve spontaneously. Immunosuppressive and/or cytotoxic drugs are given when there is progressive organ injury, but the most effective and least toxic approach to treatment is not known.

Disorders of macrophages

Haemophagocytic lymphohistiocytosis—this may be (1) primary—an autosomal recessive disorder, caused in some cases by mutation in one of several genes involved in down-regulation of the T-cell response via apoptosis; or (2) secondary—the condition may be associated with a range of infectious, malignant and other disorders. Manifestations include fever, a variety of neurological conditions, splenomegaly, hepatomegaly, lymphadenopathy, pancytopenia, abnormal liver function, and coagulopathy. Diagnosis requires histopathological demonstration of haemophagocytosis in an appropriate clinical context. Aside from supportive care, standard treatment of primary disease is with (1) etoposide and corticosteroids, or (2) antithymocyte globulin, corticosteroids, and ciclosporin.

Malignant histiocyte disorders

Acute myelomonocytic and acute monocytic leukaemia—see Chapter 22.3.4.

Introduction

The histiocytoses are characterized by the infiltration of affected tissues with cells of monocyte/macrophage lineage. A classification subdividing the disorders into three classes has been proposed (Box 22.4.7.1). However, the boundaries between classes I and II may be blurred, and more than one class of disorder may be present in the same patient.

Aetiology and epidemiology

Histiocytes are of bone marrow origin, derived by the migration and differentiation of blood monocytes, although local proliferation in the tissues may occur following contact with antigen, and in disease states. Growth and differentiation are controlled by haemopoietic growth factors produced by bone marrow stromal cells, fibroblasts, macrophages, and lymphocytes.

Normal histiocytes are divided into two subgroups: (1) dendritic cells (Langerhans' cells, dendritic reticulum cells, and interdigitating reticulum cells); and (2) macrophages. Langerhans' cells are normally found in the epidermis, the mucosa of the bronchial tree, lymph nodes, and thymus. Characteristic features include the expression of the CD1a surface antigen, and the presence of specific

> **Box 22.4.7.1** Classification of the histiocytosis syndromes
>
> **Class I—disorders of dendritic cells**
> a Langerhans' cell histiocytosis (formerly histiocytosis X)
> b Juvenile xanthogranuloma
> c Solitary dendritic-cell histiocytomas
>
> **Class II—disorders of macrophages**
> a Haemophagocytic lymphohistiocytosis
>   i Primary (genetic)
>   ii Sporadic
> b Sinus histiocytosis with massive lymphadenopathy
> c Solitary macrophage histiocytomas
>
> **Class III—malignant histiocyte disorders**
> a i Acute monocytic leukaemias (AML FAB types M4/M5)
>   ii Extramedullary monocytic tumours
> b Malignant histiocytosis
> c Disseminated or localized malignancies with dendritic-cell phenotype
> d Disseminated or localized malignancies with macrophage phenotype

cytoplasmic organelles (Birbeck granules). These arise either by invagination of the surface membrane during endocytosis of antigen, or as secretory organelles derived from the Golgi apparatus. CD1a has considerable homology with human leucocyte antigen (HLA) class I molecules and may have a role in antigen presentation to T cells. Following stimulation by antigen, Langerhans' cells migrate to lymph nodes, where they present antigen to T cells. Dendritic and interdigitating reticulum cells are localized to lymph nodes, where they present antigen to B and T cells, respectively.

Macrophages occur widely throughout the tissues where they have multiple functions in the immune response, wound healing, bone remodelling, haemopoiesis, haemostasis, the secretion of inflammatory cytokines, phagocytosis of particulate matter/antigens, and the release of proteases, antiproteases, and arachidonate metabolites.

Classification

Class I disorders

Langerhans' cell histiocytosis (LCH)

The term 'Langerhans' cell histiocytosis' has been widely adopted to replace the diagnosis 'histiocytosis X', following the recognition that the presence of Langerhans' cells is characteristic of lesions in the disorder. LCH is rare and can occur at any age, although there are few epidemiological data regarding the disease in adults. It affects 4 per million children each year, with a peak incidence between 1 and 3 years of age, and is considered to be a reactive disorder resulting from immune activation. Searches for potential triggers have been unsuccessful. There is no evidence of a viral aetiology. High levels of cytokines have been demonstrated both in lesions and in the serum of children with multisystem disease. Two studies of X-linked DNA polymorphisms have demonstrated clonality in lesional Langerhans' cells, but these data do not define LCH as a neoplastic disorder. Clonality has been demonstrated in a variety of non-neoplastic disorders. There is a recognized association between LCH and malignancy. A literature review revealed details of 87 LCH-associated malignancies—39 lymphomas, 22 acute leukaemias, and the remainder solid tumours, including secondary tumours arising within fields of previous irradiation. Amongst 341 children registered with Langerhans' cell histiocytosis, in two large international treatment trials, the incidence of secondary malignancy was 1%.

Juvenile xanthogranuloma

Juvenile xanthogranuloma usually presents with single or multiple yellow–red skin lesions in newborns and infants—in one series, the median age at presentation in 36 children was 0.3 years (range from birth to 12 years). Histology shows a cutaneous accumulation of lipid-filled macrophages, Touton giant cells, and fibroblasts. Extracutaneous disease may occur in about 10% of patients involving the central nervous system, liver, spleen, lung, eye, oropharynx, and muscles.

Class II disorders

Haemophagocytic lymphohistiocytosis (HLH)

The disease is due to disordered T cell activation, and clinical features are largely due to the dysregulated secretion of cytokines. It is a rare disorder with typical histology showing tissue infiltration by lymphocytes and macrophages, some manifesting haemophagocytosis (Fig. 22.4.7.1). The disorder occurs in primary and secondary

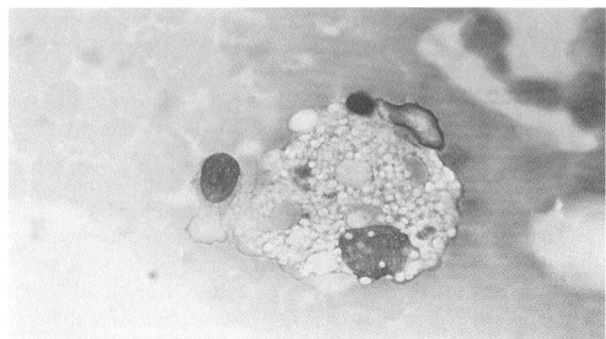

Fig. 22.4.7.1 Macrophage exhibiting haemophagocytosis in the bone marrow of a child with haemophagocytic lymphohistiocytosis.

forms. Primary HLH is an autosomal recessive disorder with an incidence of between 1 and 2 cases per million children each year in the United Kingdom and Sweden. Mutations in several genes (perforin, munc, syntaxin) involved in the downregulation of the T cell response via apoptosis have been identified in primary HLH. However, up to half of primary cases have no as yet identifiable mutation. In about 20% of cases there is a history of previously affected siblings (familial HLH). Parental consanguinity or onset in early infancy are further supportive features.

Secondary HLH is at least as common as primary disease. Precipitants include viral, bacterial, fungal, or protozoan infections, often in an immunocompromised host. Other precipitants include malignancy, particularly T-cell lymphoproliferative states, autoimmune diseases, and lipid infusions. HLH may be a feature of X linked lymphoproliferative syndrome, Chediak–Higashi syndrome, and Griscelli syndrome, each of which may be suspected from clinical and laboratory features, and confirmed by appropriate testing.

Criteria for the diagnosis of HLH are shown in Box 22.4.7.2, although not all features are present in every case. The tissues which are most frequently sampled to substantiate the diagnosis are bone marrow, lymph node, and liver, although fine-needle aspiration of the spleen is reported to have a high diagnostic yield. Diagnostic changes may be difficult to demonstrate, and the bone marrow in particular is hypercellular and reactive in the early stages of the disease. Haemophagocytosis may not be a feature on liver biopsy, but there may be prominent sinusoidal Kupffer cells and lymphoid portal infiltrates similar to those seen in chronic persistent hepatitis.

Sinus histiocytosis with massive lymphadenopathy

This disease was described in 1969 by Rosai and Dorfman as a syndrome of cervical lymphadenopathy with typical histology showing preserved lymph node structure, dilated lymph node sinuses containing mixed inflammatory cells, with vacuolated macrophages manifesting haemophagocytosis and emperipolesis of lymphocytes (i.e. a process whereby lymphocytes move straight through the cytoplasm of cells). Fibrosis may be marked. Although most cases are isolated, it has occurred in individuals with malignancy, autoimmune diseases, or other histiocyte disorders, especially LCH.

Class III disorders

Acute myelomonocytic and acute monocytic leukaemia account for 30% of cases of acute myeloid leukaemia. Considerable controversy exists regarding other malignancies of the monocyte/macrophage

Box 22.4.7.2 Diagnostic guidelines for haemophagocytic lymphohistiocytosis

- ◆ Clinical criteria
  - Fever
  - Splenomegaly
- ◆ Laboratory criteria
  - Cytopenias (affecting >2 of 3 lineages in the peripheral blood)
  - Haemoglobin (<9 g/dl)
  - Platelets (<100 × 10⁹/litre)
  - Neutrophils (<1.0 × 10⁹/litre)
  - Hypertriglyceridaemia and/or hypofibrinogenaemia fasting triglycerides >2 mmol/l, fibrinogen <1.5 g/litre
  - Ferritin >500 μg/litre
  - Absent or reduced natural killer (NK) cell function
  - Soluble CD25 >2400 u/ml
- ◆ Histopathological criteria
  - Haemophagocytosis in bone marrow, spleen, or lymph nodes
  - No evidence of malignancy

Five criteria are required for the diagnosis of HLH. The presence of an HLH-causing gene mutation is absolute evidence of HLH. The diagnosis of familial HLH is justified by a positive family history or gene mutation, and parental consanguinity is suggestive. The following findings may provide strong supportive evidence for the diagnosis:

- ◆ Spinal fluid pleocytosis (mononuclear cells)
- ◆ Histological picture in the liver resembling chronic persistent hepatitis
- ◆ Low NK cell activity
- ◆ High serum ferritin

system, owing to difficulties in nosology. Malignant histiocytosis was described as a clinical picture of lymphadenopathy, hepatosplenomegaly, fever, wasting, and pancytopenia, with histology showing tissue infiltration by large cells with copious cytoplasm and irregular nuclei. However, recent studies of cell lineage in such cases indicate that the majority of these tumours are in fact of lymphoid origin, and reclassifiable as anaplastic large-cell (Ki 1-positive) lymphomas. Accordingly, true 'malignant histiocytosis' is an extremely rare entity, requiring careful pathological assessment to substantiate the diagnosis. Both localized and disseminated malignancies of dendritic cells occur, although these are extremely rare.

Clinical features

Langerhans' cell histiocytosis

Some 60% of children with LCH have single-system disease of skin or bone. The remaining 40% have multisystem disease affecting two or more organ systems. There are inadequate data regarding the patterns of disease in adults, although lung involvement appears common, perhaps due to the association with smoking (see below). However, it is clear that adults may manifest a similar pattern of disease to that seen in childhood.

Skin

The skin eruption comprises red or yellow-brown papules on the trunk, erythema in skin folds and behind the ears, and scaling, particularly affecting the scalp. Rarely, young infants manifest a vesicular rash, similar to varicella, which may be present at birth.

Ears

Ear discharge is a classic sign, and may be due either to skin involvement in the external auditory canal, or bone destruction around and in the middle ear, with polyp formation. Such destructive lesions may result in hearing loss, and formal ear, nose, and throat assessment is essential.

Bone

Bone lesions may be occult, but present clinically with pain and soft tissue swelling. They are best seen on plain radiographs as irregular lytic areas, sometimes with marked periosteal reaction, most commonly affecting the skull and long bones (Fig. 22.4.7.2). There may be pathological fractures. Involvement of the axial skeleton may result in vertebral collapse and vertebral plana, although spinal cord compression is rare. Orbital disease may cause proptosis, a classical feature, but visual impairment is unusual.

Diabetes insipidus

Diabetes insipidus due to involvement of the hypothalamus and pituitary stalk is most common in multisystem disease, occurring in 40% of patients in some series. Other risk factors include skull lesions, especially of the orbits or parietal bones. MRI may demonstrate thickening of the pituitary stalk, a suprasellar mass, and/or loss of the posterior pituitary bright signal on T_2-weighted images. Once true diabetes insipidus is established it is irreversible.

Lungs

Lung disease occurs in one-third of children with multisystem disease but is very rare as a single site; it is characterized by cough, chest pain, and tachypnoea, with diffuse micronodular shadowing on chest radiograph. Progression to cyst formation and a honeycomb lung appearance occurs, and hypoxia, pleural effusions, and pneumothorax may occur in advanced disease. Among adults, tobacco smoking is a risk factor for pulmonary disease. There may be doubt as to the cause of pulmonary signs, but the diagnosis can be confirmed, and infection excluded, by bronchoalveolar lavage or lung biopsy. As Langerhans' cells are normally present in the bronchial tree, more than 5% CD1a-positive cells should be present in lavage fluid to support the diagnosis.

Liver

Hepatomegaly and elevated transaminases may occur without evidence of liver infiltration on biopsy. Jaundice may result from obstruction of the biliary tract by enlarged portal nodes, and therefore is not necessarily diagnostic of liver dysfunction. These provisos emphasize the need for careful assessment of the methods used for clinical findings and of the investigation results in the initial evaluation. Severe liver disease may result in fibrosis, sclerosing cholangitis, and hepatic failure.

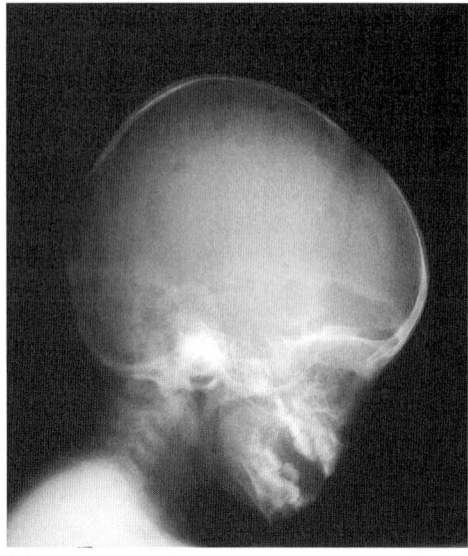

(a)

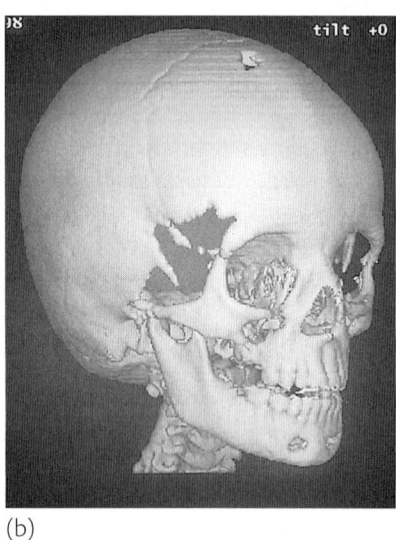

(b)

Fig. 22.4.7.2 Plain radiograph and three-dimensional CT showing bone lesions of Langerhans' cell histiocytosis in the skull.

Bone marrow and blood

Anaemia of chronic disease is a common finding in active disease. Iron deficiency should be excluded in children with microcytosis and hypochromia. Pancytopenia due to secondary bone marrow infiltration by macrophages and haemophagocytosis may occur, and is associated with severe disease, liver involvement, and splenomegaly; it carries a poor prognosis. CD1a-positive cells may be demonstrated with monoclonal antibodies by flow cytometry or by the alkaline phosphatase/antialkaline phosphatase technique on slides, but their significance is unclear.

Gut

Gut involvement with vomiting, diarrhoea, malabsorption, and protein-losing enteropathy occurs in less than 5% of children, and requires full investigation, including adequate biopsy. Although infiltrates may be seen in the mucosa and submucosa, biopsy of the muscle wall may be required. Barium studies may reveal alternate dilated and stenotic segments throughout the intestine. Mandibular and maxillary disease may result in floating teeth, and there may be gingivitis and buccal ulceration.

Central nervous system

Disease in the central nervous system (CNS), excluding diabetes insipidus, occurs in around 4% of cases, and typically affects the cerebellar and cerebral white matter, with ataxia, dysarthria, nystagmus, and cranial nerve palsies. CNS disease usually develops around 5 years from the original presentation. The mechanism of CNS disease is unknown. Most cases occur in individuals with multisystem disease, but also in the setting of single-system bone disease especially of the skull, and in children with diabetes insipidus. On imaging, several patterns are seen:

- poorly defined changes in the white matter of the cerebellum, cerebrum, and basal ganglia—biopsy in these cases shows perivascular and parenchymal infiltrates of macrophages and lymphocytes associated with oedema and demyelination
- well-defined lesions in the white and grey matter
- hypothalamic–pituitary involvement including suprasellar masses
- extraparenchymal masses, generally not in continuity with skull lesions, which on biopsy comprise xanthomatous histiocytes, lymphocytes and Touton giant cells similar to those found in juvenile xanthogranuloma

Lymph nodes

Lymphadenopathy occurs in both single- and multisystem disease, and may be gross. Local pressure effects may cause obstruction of the airways, vasculature, or biliary tree, and discharging sinuses may form to the overlying skin. Involvement of the thymus may be detected on chest radiography, and may be present on tissue examination even without enlargement of the organ.

Haemophagocytic lymphohistiocytosis

Clinical manifestations include fever, splenomegaly, hepatomegaly, lymphadenopathy, pancytopenia, abnormal liver function, coagulopathy, and signs and symptoms referable to the CNS. Occasionally CNS involvement has been the only evidence of disease at presentation. Initial blood changes may show anaemia or thrombocytopenia, with the development of pancytopenia as the disease progresses. Other features include high fasting triglyceride levels, low fibrinogen, mononuclear pleocytosis and increased protein in the cerebrospinal fluid, high serum ferritin, and reduced or absent natural killer cell function. Many of these changes result from immune activation with cytokine production. Involvement of the CNS varies from asymptomatic cerebrospinal fluid pleocytosis (usually to moderate levels comprising lymphocytes and macrophages) to symptomatic disease with encephalitis, abnormal head movements, fits, cranial nerve palsies, ataxia, regression of developmental milestones, and coma. In children who have died with CNS disease, histology of the brain shows oedema, softening and destruction of tissue, perivascular, parenchymal, and leptomeningeal infiltrates, with necrosis and destruction, especially of white matter.

Sinus histiocytosis with massive lymphadenopathy (SHML)

The lymphadenopathy may be gross. It is often painless, and may wax and wane with time. Involvement of cervical lymph nodes is present in most cases, but other groups are affected, either jointly or alone. Extranodal disease of the head and neck or a variety of other sites is present in almost half of cases, either alone or in association with lymphoid masses. Other features of SHML include systemic ill health with fever and weight loss; destructive infiltrates in skin, bone, and other extranodal sites; hypergammaglobulinaemia; an elevated erythrocyte sedimentation rate; reactive leucocytosis; and immune dysfunction including autoimmune anaemia and neutropenia.

Management of histiocyte disorders

Langerhans' cell histiocytosis

Initial work-up requires confirmatory biopsy and an accurate assessment of the extent of disease. Identification of Langerhans' cells within the lesional inflammatory cell infiltrate, with demonstration of either the CD1a surface antigen on immunohistochemistry or the presence of Birbeck granules on electron microscopy, is recommended. Thorough physical examination and investigations are required to determine the extent of disease, and investigations must include a full blood count, liver function tests, serum albumin, a coagulation screen, paired urine and plasma osmolalities, and skeletal survey by plain radiographs. Further investigations should be guided by the need to explain specific symptoms and signs. It is important to carefully assess the function of affected organs, as dysfunction carries prognostic significance (see below).

Most cases of LCH eventually resolve spontaneously. No therapy is uniformly effective. Approaches to treatment have varied, with particular controversy regarding the role of chemotherapy for children with multisystem disease. Deaths occur in 10 to 15% of cases, and are largely restricted to children with organ dysfunction. For most cases the primary objectives are control of symptoms, and limitation of long-term disability, which affects 50% of those with extensive disease. For children with skin disease requiring therapy, topical application of corticosteroids may prove beneficial. For those with more severe skin involvement, topical mustine has proved highly effective—in one study rapid improvement within 10 days occurred in each of 16 children, with complete healing in 14. Some children require systemic therapy. Oral corticosteroids result in improvement in over half of cases. Bone lesions may resolve following biopsy, but further local therapies include curettage or injected steroids. Radiotherapy is now uncommon because of concerns over late effects—in particular, secondary malignancies have been described within the radiation field. Systemic therapy is indicated for children with multifocal bone disease (30% of all children with bone disease), or single, symptomatic lesions unsuitable for local therapy. Indomethacin may be effective, but it is unclear whether the drug provides more than symptomatic relief. Further lesions and reactivations of initially responding lesions develop in up to one-third of patients.

Children with multisystem disease may be managed conservatively, with systemic therapy reserved for those who have organ dysfunction, pain, systemic upset, or failure to thrive. This issue is controversial. There are claims for better results if initial treatment employs relatively intensive chemotherapy, especially in regard to response rates and late effects. There is no evidence that a more-intensive therapy reduces the 40% mortality rate in children with organ dysfunction. For children who require systemic treatment, the accepted agents are prednisolone, vinblastine, and etoposide in varying combinations. The uncertainty regarding the most effective and least toxic approach to treatment, together with the

rarity of LCH, emphasizes the need for international collaborative randomized studies. Hepatic failure due to LCH has been successfully treated by orthoptic liver transplantation—80% of children reported in the literature were alive at a median follow-up of 3 years. For children who fail first-line treatment, further options are limited. There is little evidence that immune modulation with ciclosporin or antilymphocyte globulin is effective. Responses have been obtained with cladribine (2-chlorodeoxyadenosine), especially in children with single-system disease. There is some evidence that cladribine combined with cytarabine may be effective for children with bone marrow involvement and haemophagocytosis. Bone marrow transplantation experience is limited, but has been associated with a high treatment related mortality rate. This is partly because bone marrow transplantation is used for endstage patients, and because earlier intervention and the use of reduced intensity conditioning may improve outcome.

LCH is associated with a wide range of potential late effects, particularly skeletal deformity and dysfunction, diabetes insipidus, growth hormone deficiency, ataxia, intellectual impairment, and lung and liver fibrosis. These data stress the need for therapeutic trials to include standardized assessments for late effects which can be compared between treatments.

Juvenile xanthogranuloma

Spontaneous resolution is usual, and no treatment has been proven to be undoubtedly beneficial. Excision may be indicated for lesions resulting in complications.

Class II disorders

Haemophagocytic lymphohistiocytosis

In the absence of a gene mutation or family history of the disease, it can be difficult to determine whether a patient has primary or secondary HLH, particularly in children with evidence of recent viral infection. Among 93 children with HLH reported to the Histiocyte Society registry, there was no difference in outcome between 40 children with and 53 children without evidence of viral infection. These data emphasize the overlap between these disorders, and the need for circumspection in determining the best approach to therapy in each case.

There are two standard approaches to treatment for primary HLH, one using etoposide and corticosteroids, and the other antithymocyte globulin, corticosteroids, and ciclosporin. Around 80% of patients respond, but eventual disease recurrence is usual in primary HLH unless the child receives an allogeneic bone marrow transplant. Inadequate disease control, or reactivation, may also occur in some secondary cases. These children should then be treated in line with strategies for primary disease. Adequate control of CNS involvement is very important, but the role of routine intrathecal methotrexate in the control of CNS disease is controversial. Experience with bone marrow transplantation is greatest using matched sibling donors, with around 80% of children remaining disease-free. Increasing use of alternative donors, including matched and mismatched unrelated donors, has demonstrated that similar results may be achieved by this approach. Haploidentical bone marrow transplantation carries a higher risk of treatment failure. Full engraftment following transplantation is not a prerequisite for cure, as low levels of donor T cells provide adequate disease control. A particular worry regarding the use of a sibling donor is that in familial disease there is a 25% risk that the donor will also develop HLH. Where a genetic mutation is identified, screening of the donor is practical. Continued improvement in the results of alternative donor procedures may make these the treatment of choice. It must also be remembered that some children, usually sporadic cases aged over 2 years at diagnosis, remain well following initial therapy. Bone marrow transplantation is not indicated for this group.

Case reports regarding the prognosis for secondary HLH are conflicting. The appropriate approach for these patients is treatment of the associated condition or removal of immunosuppression where possible, with specific HLH therapy as for primary disease for individuals who fail to improve. Etoposide may be useful in severe virus-associated cases.

Sinus histiocytosis with massive lymphadenopathy

The natural history of the disorder is chronic, with spontaneous resolution over months or years in many cases, although approximately 5% of patients have died as a result of immune-mediated organ dysfunction, amyloidosis, or infection. Few individuals have died directly as a result of lymphohistiocytic infiltrates. Therapy with steroids, cytotoxic drugs, particularly vincristine and alkylating agents, or radiotherapy has been variably effective, and is unnecessary in most cases.

Class III disorders

The outlook for monocytic variants of acute myeloid leukaemia has improved considerably over recent years, with around a 50% survival at 5 years from diagnosis in children and young adults following standard chemotherapy regimens. The uncertainty over the pathology of reported cases of malignant histiocytosis clouds the issues regarding therapy. It appears appropriate to treat malignancies of macrophages with acute myeloid leukaemia chemotherapy. Because of the rarity of dendritic-cell malignancies, treatment recommendations are anecdotal, but based on excision with or without adjuvant therapy.

Further reading

Egeler RM, D'Angio G (1998). The histiocytoses (editorial). *Hematol Oncol Clin N Am*, **12**, 2.

Favara BE, *et al.* (1997). Contemporary classification of histiocytic disorders. The WHO committee on histiocytic/reticulum cell proliferations. Reclassification working group of the Histiocyte Society. *Med Pediatr Oncol*, **29**, 157–66.

Henter J-I, *et al.* (1991). Incidence and clinical features of familial hemophagocytic lymphohistiocytosis. *Acta Paediatr Scand*, **80**, 428–35.

Henter JI, *et al.* (2002). Treatment of hemophagocytic lymphohistiocytosis with HLH-94 immunochemotherapy and bone marrow transplantation. *Blood*, **100**, 2367–73.

Henter JI, *et al.* (2007). Diagnostic and therapeutic guidelines for HLH. *Pediatr Blood Cancer*, **48**, 124–31.

Ladisch S, Gadner H (1994). Treatment of Langerhans' cell histiocytosis—evolution and current approaches. *Br J Cancer*, **70** (suppl xxiii), S41–S46.

Schmidt D (1994). Monocyte/macrophage system and malignancies. *Med Pediatr Oncol*, **23**, 444–51.

22.5

The red cell

Contents

22.5.1 Erythropoiesis and the normal red cell

Anna Rita Migliaccio and Thalia Papayannopoulou

Essentials

Biological mechanisms of erythropoiesis

Erythropoiesis is a highly regulated, multistep process in which stem cells, after a series of amplification divisions, generate multipotential progenitor cells, then oligo- and finally unilineage erythroid progenitors, and then morphologically recognizable erythroid precursors and mature red cells.

Ontogeny of erythropoiesis—this involves a series of well-coordinated events during embryonic and early fetal life: (1) embryo—the fetal yolk sac makes embryonic haemoglobins; (2) fetus—the main site of erythopoiesis is the liver, which initially produces mainly fetal haemoglobin (Hb F, $\alpha_2\gamma_2$) and a small component (10–15%) of adult haemoglobin (Hb A, $\alpha_2\beta_2$), with the fraction of HbA rising to about 50% at birth; (3) after birth—the site of erythroid cell production maintained throughout life is the bone marrow, with the final adult erythroid pattern (adult Hb with <1% fetal Hb) being reached a few months after birth.

Regulation of erythropoiesis—the main regulator is erythropoietin, a 33- to 38-kDa sialoglycoprotein that is produced by interstitial cells in the kidney in response to tissue hypoxia and exerts its biological effect by binding to a specific receptor on burst-forming units-erythroid (BFU-e), colony-forming units-erythroid (CFU-e) and proerythroblasts.

Abnormalities of erythroid production

Acquired and congenital defects in erythropoietin production—causes include (1) kidney disease—the main cause of anaemia in chronic kidney disease is deficiency of erythropoietin; some kidney cancers increase erythropoietin production and hence cause secondary erythrocytosis; (2) impaired tissue oxygen delivery—tissue hypoxia is a common cause of secondary erythrocytosis, often caused by chronic lung disease, sometimes by congenital heart anomalies, and rarely by haemoglobin mutations.

Other causes of abnormal erythroid production—these include (1) acquired and congenital defects in erythropoietin signalling; (2) acquired and congenital defects in the transcription factor GATA1, which is required for activation of all erythroid genes; (3) factors that lead to premature red cell destruction, including inherited defects in protein structure (e.g. hereditary spherocytosis), enzyme defects in metabolic pathways (e.g. pyruvate kinase) and haemoglobin defects (e.g. sickle cell anaemia).

Introduction

Mature circulating red cells are specialized cellular elements of the blood responsible for both the delivery of oxygen to and for the removal of CO_2 from all tissues of the body. In the adult, their number is constantly maintained by the balance of two ongoing processes: the destruction of old red cells, mainly in the spleen; and the generation of new red cells within the bone marrow by a process referred to as erythropoiesis.

The generation of new red cells, like other cellular elements, is accomplished through a complex interplay between haemopoietic cells, stromal cells, and the extracellular matrix within the bone marrow microenvironment. Unique to the erythropoietic process is its regulation not only by growth factors produced *in situ* in the bone marrow, but also circulating erythropoietin (EPO), a true 'hormone' produced by the kidneys in the adult. Positive or negative alterations of EPO production, whether acquired or congenital, and/or of its signalling pathway, result in quantitative changes in red cell production—i.e. anaemia or erythrocytosis.

The erythroid compartment

Erythropoiesis is a highly regulated, multistep process through which 10^{11} functional red cells are generated daily from very few haemopoietic stem cells (1 in 10^4–10^5 marrow cells). Stem cells, after a series of amplification divisions, generate multipotential progenitor cells, then oligo- and finally unilineage erythroid progenitors,

which give rise to morphologically recognizable erythroid precursors and mature red cells (Fig. 22.5.1.1).

Erythroid progenitors

Progenitor cells committed to a specific lineage are defined by their ability to generate colonies of differentiated cells *in vitro*. In these assays, multipotential progenitors generate colonies consisting of cells of several lineages, whereas unilineage cells give rise to colonies of only one lineage. The earliest erythroid progenitor is the burst-forming unit-erythroid (BFU-e), which generates colonies containing several thousand erythroid cells. The colony-forming unit-erythroid (CFU-e) generates smaller colonies that mature early in culture. Between these two extremes, there exist intermediate classes of BFU-e with less proliferative potential and shorter maturation time in culture. BFU-e tend to have an antigenic profile similar to progenitor cells of other lineages with few exceptions (i.e. they are negative for CD45 RA, CD33, and AC133, but express higher levels, or possibly specific isoforms, of the transferrin receptor). CFU-e, in contrast, begin to express more of the markers found specifically in mature erythroid cells (i.e. glycophorin A and blood group antigens). The first blood group antigen to be expressed at the BFU-e level is the glycoprotein (gp) Kell, followed by the orderly activation of the expression of Rh gp, Landersteiner–Wiener (LW) gp, glycophorin A, Band 3, Lutheran gp, and finally, at the erythroblast level, Duffy gp.

Progression of progenitor cells to terminal differentiation is marked not only by the acquisition of phenotypic markers, but also by the acquisition of specific responses to growth factors. The most active of these on early progenitors are stem-cell factor (SCF, or Steel factor, or kit ligand), interleukin-3 (IL-3), granulocyte/macrophage colony-stimulating factor (GM-CSF), and EPO and thrombopoietin (TPO) on later progenitors.

The special importance of SCF in erythropoiesis is shown by genetic mutations of SCF (such as *Sl/Sld*), or of its receptor, kit (such as *W/Wv*), that result in mice with anaemia, the severity of which correlates with impairment in kit kinase activity. In humans, heterozygotes with c-*kit* mutations have been reported in individuals with piebaldism, but no homozygotes have been described. Furthermore, mice treated with anti-kit antibodies became anaemic, whereas human kit-antisense containing cultures did not expand the BFU-e compartment.

Erythroid precursors

Erythroid precursors, in contrast to progenitor cells, are morphologically recognizable and include cells at different maturation

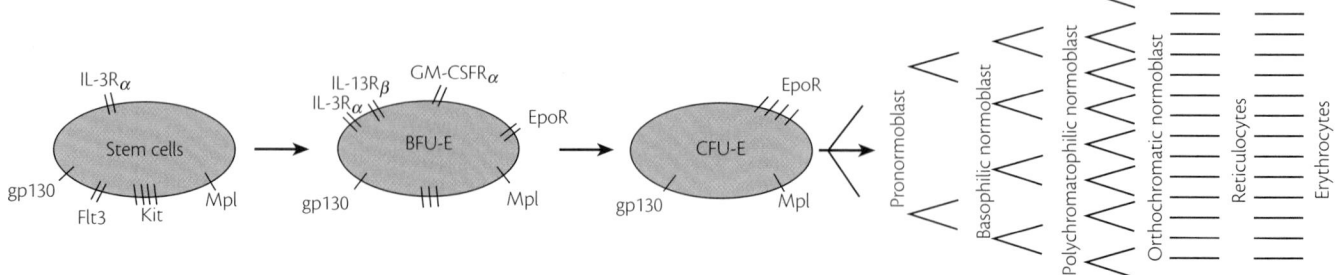

Fig. 22.5.1.1 Adult erythroid progenitor- and precursor-cell compartments. The number of bars on the cell surface is an estimate of the growth factor-receptor concentration/cell responsiveness during erythroid differentiation. A complex of IL-6 and its soluble receptor (or a fusion molecule called hyper IL-6) may induce growth of BFU-e and erythroid maturation in the absence of exogenously added EPO through activation of an autocrine EPO loop. BFU-e, burst-forming units-erythroid; EPO, erythropoietin; IL-6, interleukin-6.

stages (Fig. 22.5.1.1). The earlier cell is the proerythroblast which, after around 7 days of proliferation and further maturation, gives rise to mature red cells. The maturation process includes haemoglobin synthesis, chromatin condensation (orthochromatic normoblast), and, finally, extrusion of the nucleus and a reduction in cell size (reticulocytes). Influence on late-stage erythropoiesis is exerted by a stromal macrophage surrounded by adherent erythroblasts in an unit termed the erythroblastic island. Four specific proteins (VCAM1, αVβ1, EMP, and CD163) on the surface of the macrophage mediate the adherence of erythroblasts and facilitate the subsequent phagocytosis of nuclei extruded from erythroblasts. Morphological maturation changes are paralleled by the accumulation of haemoglobin and by several biochemical changes in the cytoskeleton, which guarantee maximum resistance to stress and flexibility during capillary passage. It has been estimated that about 64 reticulocytes are generated from each pronormoblast, 90 to 95% of which emerge into the bloodstream. Within a day or two in the peripheral circulation, the reticulocytes mature further into red cells.

Ontogeny of erythropoiesis

The ontogenetic development of the erythroid system encompasses a series of well-coordinated events during embryonic and early fetal life, the timing of which is distinct for each mammal species. Erythroid cells are the first differentiated haemopoietic cells to appear during ontogeny, initially in the blood islands of the yolk sac and later in the fetal liver. The recruitment of new erythropoietic sites during ontogeny (from yolk sac to fetal liver to bone marrow) is accompanied by profound differences in the stem-cell differentiation programme and the phenotypic/functional properties of the erythroid cells being developed in each site. Haemopoietic cytokines, specifically expressed and/or sequestered by each microenvironment, may probably mediate these changes in concert with a regime of cell intrinsic transcriptional factors. Furthermore, adhesion receptors on haemopoietic cells and their counter-receptors in the microenvironment ensure patterns of firm adherence, migration, and colonization of the successive haemopoietic sites.

Yolk sac erythropoiesis

In humans, the first erythroid cells (the primitive nucleated erythroblasts) are detected in the yolk sac at 3 to 4 weeks and are the only red cells circulating until week 8 of gestation. They synthesize mainly embryonic haemoglobins, such as Gower I ($\zeta_2\epsilon_2$), Gower II ($\alpha_2\epsilon_2$), and Portland ($\zeta_2\gamma_2$).

In addition to differentiated primitive erythroid cells, the yolk sac contains progenitor cells of definitive lineage that do not differentiate in the yolk sac but generate BFU-e-like colonies *in vitro*, which are composed of definitive erythroblasts. It is currently undecided whether primitive and definitive progenitor cells derive from the same stem cell although the weight of recent evidence would suggest a common progenitor, the haemangioblast.

Gene ablation studies indicate that yolk sac and fetal liver/bone marrow erythropoiesis have clearly distinct growth factor and molecular requirements. Primitive erythropoiesis is not significantly affected by the ablation of several transcription factors (GATA1, AML-1, Rb, Myb, etc.) that affect definitive cells. Also, primitive erythropoiesis *in vivo* is SCF- and EPO-independent, whereas TPO, but not EPO, is produced *in situ* and may be important for cell survival and partial differentiation. Within the yolk sac, erythroid cells are found in close proximity to endothelial

cells and macrophages. Therefore, they are most probably exposed to growth factors produced by these cells, including vascular endothelial growth factor (VEGF) and M-CSF. In this regard, yolk-sac-derived endothelial cell lines *in vitro* produce leucocyte inhibiting factor (LIF), IL-6, flt-3 ligand, SCF, and M-CSF, but not G-CSF, GM-CSF, IL-3, IL-1, EPO, and TPO. The exchange of trophic signals between endothelial and haemopoietic cells is also mutual at these early stages.

Fetal liver haemopoiesis

The major anatomical site of erythropoiesis in fetal life is the liver, in which newly formed definitive erythroblasts appear at 7 to 8 weeks gestation within the sinusoidal walls of its parenchyma. Definitive erythroblasts are released into the blood after week 8 and remain the main circulating erythroid cells until birth.

The haemoglobin (Hb) patterns expressed by erythroid cells during ontogeny represent one of the best-studied developmental differences in gene expression. In contrast to primitive erythroblasts, the definitive cells synthesize mainly fetal haemoglobin (HbF, $\alpha_2\gamma_2$), together with a small component (10–15%) of adult haemoglobin (HbA, $\alpha_2\beta_2$). The fetal pattern of haemoglobin expression remains stable until 30 weeks gestation, when a progressive increase in HbA and a parallel slow decline in HbF begins. At birth, approximately equal amounts of HbA and HbF are synthesized, with the final adult erythroid pattern (adult Hb with <1% fetal Hb) being reached a few months after birth. The fetal to adult Hb switch is strictly related to gestational age and occurs within the same population of cells that undergo an intrinsic modification of its gene expression programme. Its molecular mechanism involves the formation and activation of specific transcriptional complexes within cells at specific stages of ontogeny, but details remain elusive.

Fetal erythroid progenitor cells display a unique phenotypic and functional profile, including higher cell-cycling rates (>30% vs the adult rate of 10%), a lower doubling time (20 h vs the 32 h for the adult cells), and faster kinetics of *in vitro* differentiation (10 days vs 16 days). The average telomeric length is also different (12.8 ± 0.35 kb vs 8.4 ± 0.3 kb). Human fetal BFU-e are exquisitely sensitive to EPO, which is sufficient to sustain their maximal differentiation, whereas SCF complemented by IL-6 alone is sufficient for their maximal *ex vivo* expansion. Whether fetal progenitors do not truly require any other factors, or whether they, unlike adult cells, do not produce autocrine growth inhibitors (transforming growth factor-β (TGFβ)) or are insensitive to them, is unclear.

Unique to the fetal liver stage of haemopoiesis is its almost exclusive erythroid output, whereas its microenvironment is less conducive to myelomonocytic cell differentiation despite the abundant presence of their progenitors.

At the end of fetal development, liver erythropoiesis is suppressed and the organ enters the adult hepatic phase. Oncostatin-M, produced in the liver by haemopoietic CD45+ cells, may facilitate this transition by inhibiting the growth of haemopoietic progenitors while promoting the growth of the hepatocytes expressing its receptor. Increasing glucocorticoid concentrations in fetal liver near term may also contribute to the suppression of liver erythropoiesis.

Bone marrow erythropoiesis

The final site of erythroid cell production maintained throughout life is the bone marrow. Haemopoiesis in the marrow appears between 6.6 and 8.5 weeks after the establishment of a rudimental stroma of cartilagenous and endothelial cells, and is accomplished in four separate phases. Within the bone marrow, granulopoiesis predominates during all the stages of development (fetal and adult).

Erythropoietin and the regulation of erythropoiesis

EPO was the first haemopoietic growth factor to be identified. Its existence was hypothesized in 1906 by Carnot and Deflandre, and formal proof was obtained by Reissman in 1950 and Stohlman *et al.* in 1954. Human EPO, a 33- to 38-kDa sialoglycoprotein, was purified to homogeneity in 1977 and its gene, localized on chromosome 7q11, was cloned in 1984. EPO was also the first growth factor to be used in the treatment of patients because of the clear-cut relationship between its concentration in the blood and the numbers of red cells in the circulation.

EPO has a short half-life (<5 h; 90% of EPO is rapidly degraded by the liver and 10% secreted in urine), but its blood concentration (0.02 units/ml) is kept constant by continuous production. EPO levels are exquisitely regulated by changes in oxygen tension, and the kidney is in the ideal anatomical position for sensing these changes (Fig. 22.5.1.2). The kidney is the major producer of EPO, although the liver, which is the main source of EPO in the fetus, retains some capacity of low hypoxia sensitivity in the adult. Low levels of EPO are also produced in the marrow by the erythroid progenitors themselves.

Several EPO-mimetic molecules have been recently developed. These molecules include small polypeptides restricted to the growth factor domain involved in receptor binding, molecularly engineered forms of EPO that allow higher glycosilation or constitutive dimerization, and nonpeptide molecules with similar shape and electrical properties to the receptor-binding domain of EPO. It has been suggested that these EPO-mimetics might have a biological activity partially different from, and possible more effective than, the native protein, especially in the stimulation of nonhematopoietic tissues.

EPO triggers its biological effect by binding to a specific 64- to 78-kDa (depending on its glycosylation degree) receptor, EPO-R, encoded by a gene on human chromosome 19p. This gene is expressed in erythroid, megakaryocytic, and endothelial cells. Also, marrow cells express high levels of soluble EPO-R species. These may be involved in the fine tuning of EPO concentrations in specific marrow niches, thus allowing erythroid vs myeloid development. In addition to the full-length EPO-R (EPO-RF), immature erythroid cells express a truncated form of the receptor (EPO-RT) that acts as a dominant negative regulator of the EPO-RF mediated signals in mice.

The concentration of EPO-R on the surface of erythroid cells is roughly proportional to their EPO responsiveness *in vitro* (Fig. 22.5.1.1). EPO-R is first detected on BFU-e (*c.*300 high-affinity EPO binding sites per cell). Its expression increases as the cells progress to CFU-e and proerythroblasts (*c.*1100 high-affinity sites), but is virtually absent on late normoblasts and reticulocytes. The increase in EPO-R expression observed during erythroid differentiation is also accompanied by a decreased expression of receptors for early-acting growth factors, such as SCF and IL-3 (Fig. 22.5.1.1).

The rapid dimerization induced by EPO binding to its receptor triggers a conformational change that results in autophosphorylation and activation of the kinase catalytic domain of JAK2, a member of the Janus kinase family (Fig. 22.5.1.2). JAK2 phosphorylates and activates several proteins, some of which are responsible for

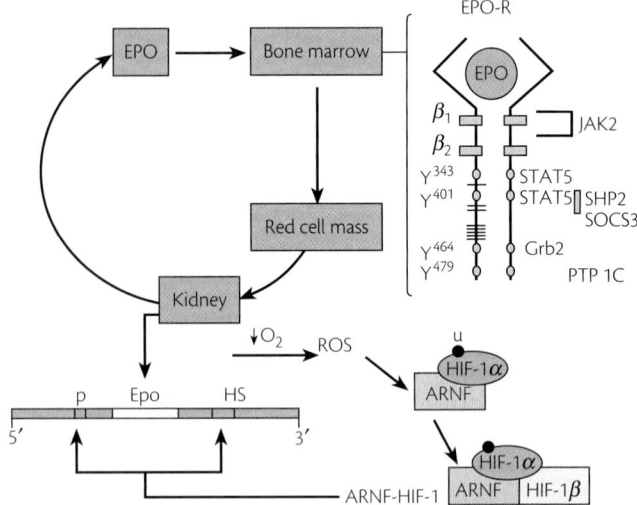

Fig. 22.5.1.2 The regulation of erythroid cell mass. The number of circulating red cells is regulated by the levels of erythropoietin (EPO) produced by the kidney under the exquisite control of the hypoxia-sensing machinery. Several pathways are involved in hypoxic recognition and respond by producing reactive oxygen species (ROS). The purpose is to rescue (by ubiquitination) hypoxia-induced factor-1α (HIF-1α) from degradation, to facilitate its complex formation with aryl-hydrocarbon nuclear translocator (ARNF) and with the ubiquitously expressed β subunit of HIF-1. ARNF–HIF-1 activates the expression of several hypoxia-responsive genes such as *EPO*, glucose transporters, glycolytic enzymes, platelet-derived growth factor (*PDGF*), and vascular endothelial factor (*VEFG*) (*ARNF* ablation results in embryonic lethality attributed to the loss of induction of *VEGF*). ARNF–HIF-1 activates the expression of hypoxia-inducible genes by binding to specific cognate sequences, that, in the case of *EPO*, are present both in its promoter (indicated as p, a typical TATA less promoter) and in its DNA-hypersensitive site (HS), which has the function of a hypoxia-inducible enhancer. The enhancer is activated by the binding of a protein complex formed by HIF-1 itself, by the constitutively expressed hepatic nuclear factor-4 (HNF-4), and by the general transcriptional activator p300. Of note, the EPO promoter and enhancer also contain binding sites for the steroid hormone receptor, closing the bridge between activation of these receptors and control of the haematocrit level. Another link between a response to stress and EPO expression is provided by p38α, a member of the mitogen-activated protein (MAP) family that may be involved in cobalt-induced stabilization of HIF-1α and induction of EPO expression, at least in the fetal liver. EPO induces its effects in the marrow by binding to a specific receptor (EPO-R) present on erythroid cells. EPO/EPO-R binding induces tyrosine autophosphorylation and the activation of JAK2 (Janus kinase-2) which is physically associated to its cytoplasmic Box 1 (β1) domain. The activation of the JAK2 catalytic domain is responsible for the phosphorylation of several other proteins, including the EPO-R itself (phosphotyrosine residues involved in docking EPO-R with its transducer proteins are indicated as filled circle, not to scale), STAT5 (signal transducer and activator of transcription-5), and proteins involved in the Ras and PKC (protein kinase C) signal-transduction pathways. On the other hand, at least three other pathways are involved in bringing the receptor complex back to its resting configuration after activation: the phosphatase PTP-1C (protein tyrosine phosphatase-1C) /SHP2 (Src-homology-phosphatase 2), SOCS3 (suppressor of cytokine signalling-3) (overexpression of SOCS3 in transgenic mice results in embryonically lethal anaemia), and the proteasomes, which downregulate the number of activated receptors on the cell surface. PTP-1C becomes physically associated through its SH2 domains with Y479 after EPO stimulation, and SOCS3 becomes associated with the Y401 of EPO-R and with JAK2. The narrow bars on the left side of the EPO-R diagram indicate mutations identified in humans that result in familial erythrocytosis.

further transmitting the signal to the nucleus, while others, such as the protein tyrosine phosphatases (PTP)-1C (also called HCP or SHP) and -1D (or Syp), dephosphorylate the receptor complex, bringing it back to its resting configuration (Fig. 22.5.1.2).

Signalling through EPO-R triggers several cellular responses, including inhibition of apoptosis, stimulation of cell proliferation, and the induction of expression of erythroid specific genes—i.e. the globin genes. The best-studied effect of EPO on erythroid cells is suppression of apoptosis. EPO/EPO-R signalling inhibits apoptosis through suppression of caspases (cysteine proteases with aspartate specificity). In erythroid cells, these degrade the erythroid-specific transcription factor GATA1, which is responsible for the activation of all the erythroid-specific genes analysed so far and for activation of the gene that encodes the antiapoptotic protein Bcl-xL.

Perturbations in erythroid production and molecular defects in humans

Anaemia and polycythaemia are relatively common conditions that may result from either acquired of congenital abnormalities of the erythroblast producing machinery. The three elements most often involved in erythroid perturbations are EPO, the EPO receptor and its signal transduction pathway, and the transcription factor GATA1.

Acquired and congenital defects in EPO production

As the kidney is the primary site of EPO production, it is not surprising that irreversible damage to this organ results in low or no EPO production and consequently results in anaemia. At the other extreme, some kidney cancers, by increasing the number of EPO-producing cells, also increase EPO production and then lead to secondary erythrocytosis. Additionally, renal and neuronal cancers associated with mutations in the von Hippel–Lindau(VHL) gene also impair the hypoxia-sensing mechanism and induce acquired polycythaemias. The product of VHL, in fact, is a member of the protein complex responsible for the stabilization/degradation of HIF-1α and mutations in this gene result in overexpression of VEGF and of other oxygen-regulated genes. Furthermore, disorders that impair oxygen delivery to the tissue are sensed by the kidney as hypoxia and result in increased EPO production leading to secondary erythrocytosis (e.g. in chronic lung diseases and congenital heart anomalies). In haemoglobin mutations, because there is inefficient oxygen delivery to the tissues due to altered Hb/oxygen affinity, hypoxia is sensed and causes increased EPO serum levels and secondary erythrocytosis. There are more than 50 different mutations in which changes in either the α- or β-globin gene result in increased Hb/oxygen affinity. Secondary autosomal recessive erythrocytosis (polycythaemias) can also be caused by abnormalities in enzymes such as 2,3-diphosphoglycerate (2,3-DPG) mutase, involved in the regulation of tissue oxygen delivery (familial 2,3-DPG deficiency). Secondary asymptomatic polycythaemias are also seen in methaemoglobinaemias. Methaemoglobin is a derivative of haemoglobin in which Fe^{2+}, which binds oxygen reversibly, is replaced by its oxidized form (Fe^{3+}), which binds oxygen irreversibly.

A genetic abnormality in the oxygen-sensing system (summarized briefly in Fig. 22.5.1.2) has recently been associated with the congenital polycythaemia common in the Chuvashia region of Russia and in the small island of Ischia, in Italy. The genetic lesion involved in this disease is represented by a point mutation (C598T) in the oxygen-sensing VHL gene and induces increased EPO responsiveness of the erythroid cells and increased EPO concentration in serum.

Anaemia in chronic inflammatory states, such as rheumatoid arthritis, is due instead to the fact that proinflammatory cytokines, such as IL-1 and tumour necrosis factor (TNF), inhibit erythropoiesis both directly (by inhibiting the proliferation of the progenitor cells and proper iron recycling) and indirectly (by inhibiting EPO synthesis by the kidney).

Acquired and congenital defects in EPO signalling

The C-terminal domain of EPO-R, a region that is physically associated with PTP-1C, is deleted in all of the different mutations (>8) of EPOR found to be associated with congenital erythrocytosis. 32D cells transfected with one such mutant receptor required EPO to activate the JAK2/STAT5 pathway, but in these cells the activation lasted longer than in cells transfected with the normal receptor. This may explain why congenital polycythaemia/erythrocytosis is characterized by hyper-responsive, EPO-dependent, CFU-e growth. Not all mutations of EPOR cause polycythaemia, however. Two additionally described single-point EPOR mutations are not accompanied by functional consequences or changes in hematocrit.

On the other hand, polycythaemia vera (PV) is a human myeloproliferative disorder caused by an acquired mutation, presumed to be at the stem-cell level, that results in the formation of CFU-e-derived colonies in the absence of EPO. A familiar autosomal dominant predisposition towards acquiring polycythaemia vera between the ages of 50 and 60 years of age has been described. In contrast to familial polycythaemia, PV may evolve into leukaemia. It is therefore possible that its defect involves alterations in the proliferative control of erythroid cells. Several investigators have recently reported a mutation in the Jak2 gene resulting in a valine phenylalanine substitution at position 617 of the protein (the ^{V617F}JAK2 mutation) in patients with Ph-negative chronic proliferative disorders, including PV. Depending on the study, the frequency of the ^{V617F}JAK2 mutation in PV patients has been reported to be 60 to 90%. The mutation is also present in some of the patients with other Ph-negative myeloproliferative neoplasm such as essential thrombocythemia and primary myelofibrosis. The mutation is harboured either at the heterozygous stage or, by somatic recombination, at the homozygous stage, and is detectable in all myeloid cells up to the clonal hematopoietic stem cells. This mutation affects a domain of the protein not directly involved in signal transduction but necessary to return the protein to its resting configuration after signalling. As JAK2 is the earliest element of the EPO-R pathway, it is conceivable that the high red-cell numbers found in PV patients are a direct consequence of constitutive EPO signalling in erythroid cells. The biochemistry of the ^{V617F}JAK2 mutation is currently being explored by structural and computer modelling approaches, in the hope of identifying chemical inhibitors that would target the ^{V617F}JAK2 mutation for therapeutic reasons. A first series of Jak2 inhibitors have been already tested in clinical trials. However, the beneficial effects of the majority of drugs which inhibit JAK2 either directly (INCB018424, XL019 and TG101348) or as off-target kinase-inhibitors (MKS-0457, CEP-701 and AT9283) tested in PMF patients to date are modest. More recent studies, in fact suggest that Jak2 mutations do not represent the primary genetic lesion of myeloproliferative neoplasms but rather intermediate steps of a multistep transformation process.

Acquired and congenital defects in the transcription factor GATA1

GATA1 is a member of the zinc-finger transcription factor family and is required for activation of all the erythroid genes. It activates gene expression by binding to specific DNA cognate sequences either directly or as heterodimer with an obligatory partner, FOG-1. Mutations either in the FOG1- or in the DNA-binding domain of the N-terminal zinc finger of GATA1 cause anaemia and/or thrombocytopenia. As *GATA1* is on the X chromosome, these mutations have been detected in inherited dysfunctions of the erythroid and megakaryocytic lineage that show an X-linked transmission pattern in humans (X-linked familial dyserythropoietic anaemia, thrombocytopenia, dyserythropoietic anaemia with macrothrombocytopenia, thalassaemia, grey platelet syndrome, and congenital erythropoietic porphyria). Frameshift and splice mutations encoding Gata1s, a protein lacking the N-terminal domain, have been instead found in one family with impaired inherited erythropoiesis and in patients with the acquired megakaryocytic leukemia in Down's syndrome, with transient myeloproliferative syndrome of the neonates, and in one patient with megakaryocytic leukaemia.

Red cell homeostasis and premature red cell destruction

Normal red cells have a finite lifespan of 120 ± 20 days. With red-cell ageing, metabolic changes decrease their flexibility as they traverse through the microvasculature and promote their lysis or phagocytosis. Thus, the red cell's longevity and ability to carry out its proper function is critically dependent on cell-membrane structure and metabolism (see Chapter 22.5.10). The red-cell membrane consists of a lipid bilayer and structural and integral membrane proteins which provide a lattice network under the bilayer and create the red cell cytoskeleton. Inherited defects in protein structure (hereditary spherocytosis, HS; hereditary elliptocytosis, HE; hereditary pyropoikilocytosis, HPP; etc.) lead to enhanced red-cell destruction and haemolytic anaemias. A number of specific receptors and enzymes are also associated with membrane proteins, several of which are important for the maintenance of its structural integrity or for nutrient and ion transport. Enzyme defects in metabolic pathways (pyruvate kinase, PK; hexokinase, G6PD; see Chapter 22.5.12), or haemoglobin defects (sickle cell anaemia) can also increase the haemolytic potential of the red cell.

Proper red-cell functioning is dependent on high concentrations of haemoglobin within the cells. It is not surprising that anaemia represents one of the first manifestations of genetic defects that impair the mRNA translational machinery. Diamond-Blackfan anaemia is a rare congenital red-cell aplasia characterized by anaemia, bone-marrow erythroblastopenia, and congenital anomalies. Although in many cases the genetic defect inducing the disease is still unknown, in large cohorts of families the disease is associated with heterozygous mutations affecting either the coding sequence or spicing sites of the ribosomal protein (RP) S19 gene (*RPS19*). Additionally, *de novo* nonsense and splice-site mutations in another ribosomal protein, RPS24, were identified in approximately 2% of RPS19 mutation-negative probands. The essential role played by RPS19 in the biogenesis and maturation of the 40S small ribosomal subunit in human cells suggests that the pathogenesis of the anaemia in Diamond-Blackfan disease is a direct consequence of poor ribosome organization.

The character of the external red cell surface is defined by its antigenic structure. Over 300 antigens have been identified and many of these contribute to 15 genetic blood group systems. The latter are composed of oligosaccharide prosthetic groups of the integral membrane proteins and complex glycolipids. Nearly all (the Lewis system is an exception) are intrinsic components of the membrane and appear early in the differentiation process. Coating of red-cell surface antigens with antibodies in cases of acquired autoimmunity interferes with the membrane functional integrity and allows rapid phagocytosis.

The transport of oxygen by red cells is dependent on their number, their haemoglobin content, and the ability to release oxygen or to increase 2,3-DPG, according to tissue needs. However, oxygen transport by red cells is but one of the elements in a multicomponent, highly integrated process that is responsible for appropriate oxygen supply to the tissues. A number of other physiological parameters, such as pulmonary function (sufficient oxygen loading in the lungs), and haemodynamic factors (cardiac output, blood volume, and viscosity) must be incorporated in an integrated fashion. When anaemia is present, restoration of red-cell number is dependent on the degree of EPO stimulation, the ability to increase erythroid proliferation (adequate folic acid, vitamin B_{12} levels, etc.) within the bone marrow, and on the circulating levels and a normal erythroid cell response to iron. Several of these issues are addressed in more details in other chapters.

Finally, several hormones involved in the control of the cellular metabolism, such as corticosteroids, androgens, growth hormone, thyroxine, β-adrenergic agonists, and certain prostaglandins, stimulate erythroid differentiation *in vitro* in synergy with EPO, or can alter hematocrit levels *in vivo*. A direct involvement of glucocorticoids in the control of the red cell mass has recently been provided by the observation that mice lacking the glucocorticoid receptor recover very poorly from haemolytic anaemia caused by phenylhydrazine treatment.

Further reading

Adamson JW (1968). The erythropoietin–hematocrit relationship in normal and polycythemic man: implications of marrow regulation. *Blood*, **32**, 597–609.

Ang S, Chen H, Hirota K (2002). Disruption of oxygen homeostasis underlies congenital Chuvash polycythemia. *Nat Genet*, **32**, 614–21.

Arcasoy MO, Harris KW, Forget BG (1999). A human erythropoietin receptor gene mutant causing familial erythrocytosis is associated with deregulation of the rates of Jak2 and Stat5 inactivation. *Exp Hematol*, **27**, 63–74.

Bauer A, *et al.* (1999). The glucocorticoid receptor is required for stress erythropoiesis. *Genes Devel*, **13**, 2996.

Baxter EJ, *et al.* (2005). Acquired mutation of the tyrosine kinase JAK2 in human myeloproliferative disorders. *Lancet*, **365**, 1054–61.

Broudy VC, *et al.* (1996). Interaction of stem cell factor and its receptor c-kit mediates lodgment and acute expansion of hematopoietic cells in the murine spleen. *Blood*, **88**, 75–81.

Bunn HF (2007). New agents that stimulate erythropoiesis. *Blood*, **109**, 868–73.

Carnot P, Deflandre C (1906). Sur l'activité hématopoétique du serum au cours de la régénération du sang. *Acad Sci Med*, **3**, 384.

Charbord P, *et al.* (1996). Early ontogeny of the human marrow from long bones: an immunohistochemical study of hematopoiesis and its microenvironment. *Blood*, **87**, 4109–19.

Chasis JA, (2006). Erythroblastic islands: specialized microenvironmental niches for erythropoiesis. *Curr Opin Hematol*, **13**, 137–41.

Choesmel V, *et al.* (2007). Impaired ribosome biogenesis in Diamond-Blackfan anemia. *Blood*, **109**, 1275–83.

Coleman TR, *et al.* (2006). Cytoprotective doses of erythropoietin or carbamylated erythropoietin have markedly different procoagulant and vasoactive activities. *Proc Natl Acad Sci U S A*, **103**, 5965–70.

Draptchinskaia N, *et al.* (1999). The gene encoding ribosomal protein S19 is mutated in Diamond-Blackfan anaemia. *Nat Genet*, **21**, 169–75.

Dybedal I, Jacobsen SE (1995). Transforming growth factor beta (TGF-beta), a potent inhibitor of erythropoiesis: neutralizing TGF-beta antibodies show erythropoietin as a potent stimulator of murine burst-forming unit erythroid colony formation in the absence of a burst-promoting activity. *Blood*, **86**, 949–57.

Ebert BL, Bunn HF (1999). Regulation of the erythropoietin gene. *Blood*, **94**, 1864–77.

Era T, *et al.* (1997). Thrombopoietin enhances proliferation and differentiation of murine yolk sac erythroid progenitors. *Blood*, **89**, 1207–13.

Eschbach J, *et al.* (1987). Correction of the anemia of endstage renal disease with recombinant human erythropoietin. *N Engl J Med*, **316**, 73.

Fennie C, *et al.* (1995). CD34+ endothelial cell lines derived from murine yolk sac induce the proliferation and differentiation of yolk sac CD34+ hematopoietic progenitors. *Blood*, **86**, 4454–67.

Fleischman RA, Gallardo T, Mi X (1996). Mutations in the ligand-binding domain of the kit receptor: an uncommon site in human piebaldism. *J Invest Dermatol*, **107**, 703–6.

Flygare J, *et al.* (2007). Human RPS19, the gene mutated in Diamond-Blackfan anemia, encodes a ribosomal protein required for the maturation of 40S ribosomal subunits. *Blood*, **109**, 980–6.

Freson K, *et al.* (2001). Platelet characteristics in patients with X-linked macrothrombocytopenia because of a novel GATA1 mutation. *Blood*, **98**, 85–92.

Furukawa T, *et al.* (1997). Primary familial polycythaemia associated with a novel point mutation in the erythropoietin receptor. *Br J Haematol*, **99**, 222–7.

Gallagher PG, Benz EJ, Jr (2001). The erythrocyte membrane and cytoskeleton: structure, function and disorders. In: Stamatoyannopoulos G, *et al.* (eds) *The molecular basis of blood diseases*, 3rd edition, pp. 275–305. W B Saunders, Philadelphia.

Gazda HT *et al.* (2006). Ribosomal protein S24 gene is mutated in Diamond-Blackfan anemia. *Am J Hum Genet*, **79**, 1110–18.

Gazda HT, *et al.* (2006). Defective ribosomal protein gene expression alters transcription, translation, apoptosis, and oncogenic pathways in Diamond-Blackfan anemia. *Stem Cells*, **24**, 2034–44.

Hiyake T, Kung CK-H, Goldwasser E (1977). Purification of human erythropoietin. *J Biol Chem*, **252**, 5558.

Hollanda LM, *et al.* (2006). An inherited mutation leading to production of only the short isoform of GATA-1 is associated with impaired erythropoiesis. *Nat Genet*, **38**, 807–12.

Huang LJ, *et al.* (2001). The N-terminal domain of Janus kinase 2 is required for Golgi processing and cell surface expression of erythropoietin receptor. *Mol Cell*, **8**, 1327–38.

Huang X, Cho S, Spangrude GJ (2007). Hematopoietic stem cells: generation and self-renewal. *Cell Death Differ*, 14, 1851–9.

Huehns ER, *et al.* (1964). Human embryonic haemoglobins. *Nature*, **201**, 1095.

Ihle JN (2001). Signal transduction in the regulation of hematopoiesis. In: Stamatoyannopoulos G, *et al.* (eds) *The molecular basis of blood diseases*, 3rd edition, pp. 103–25. W B Saunders, Philadelphia.

Iliopoulos O, *et al.* (1996). Negative regulation of hypoxia-inducible genes by the von Hippel-Lindau protein. *Proc Natl Acad Sci U S A*, **93**, 10 595.

Jacobs K, *et al.* (1985). Isolation and characterization of genomic and cDNA clones of human erythropoietin. *Nature*, **313**, 806.

James C, *et al.* (2005). A unique clonal JAK2 mutation leading to constitutive signalling causes polycythaemia vera. *Nature*, **434**, 1144–8.

Jamieson CH, *et al.* (2006). The JAK2 V617F mutation occurs in hematopoietic stem cells in polycythemia vera and predisposes toward erythroid differentiation. *Proc Natl Acad Sci U S A*, **103**, 6224–9.

Kaushansky K, (2005). On the molecular origins of the chronic myeloproliferative disorders: it all makes sense. *Blood*, **105**, 4187–90.

Kaushansky K, (2006). Lineage-specific hematopoietic growth factors. *New Engl J Med*, **354**, 2034–45.

Kelemen E, Calvo W, Fliedner TM (1979). *Atlas of human hemopoietic development*. Springer, Berlin.

Koury MJ, Bondurant MC (1990). Erythropoietin retards DNA breakdown and prevents programmed death in erythroid progenitor cells. *Science*, **248**, 378–81.

Kralovics R, *et al.* (1997). Two new EPO receptor mutations: truncated EPO receptors are most frequently associated with primary familial and congenital polycythemias. *Blood*, **90**, 2057–61.

Kralovics R, *et al.* (1998). Absence of polycythemia in a child with a unique erythropoietin receptor mutation in a family with autosomal dominant primary polycythemia. *J Clin Invest*, **102**, 124–9.

Kralovics R, *et al.* (2005). A gain-of-function mutation of JAK2 in myeloproliferative disorders. *N Engl J Med*, **352**, 1179–90.

Kralovics R, Prchal JT (2000). Congenital and inherited polycythemia. *Curr Opin Pediatr*, **12**, 29–34.

Leist M, *et al.* (2004). Derivatives of erythropoietin that are tissue protective but not erythropoietic. *Science*, **305**, 239–42.

Levine RL, *et al.* (2005). Activating mutation in the tyrosine kinase JAK2 in polycythemia vera, essential thrombocythemia, and myeloid metaplasia with myelofibrosis. *Cancer Cell*, **7**, 387–97.

Lin CS, *et al.* (1996). Differential effects of an erythropoietin receptor gene disruption on primitive and definitive erythropoiesis. *Genes Dev*, **10**, 154–64.

Maltepe E, *et al.* (1997). Abnormal angiogenesis and responses to glucose and oxygen deprivation in mice lacking the protein ARNT. *Nature*, **386**, 403–7.

Marcus D (ed.) (1981). Blood group immunochemistry and genetics. *Semin Hematol*, **18**(1).

Marine JC, *et al.* (1999). SOCS3 is essential in the regulation of fetal liver erythropoiesis. *Cell*, **98**, 617–27.

Mehaffey MG, *et al.* (2001). X-linked thrombocytopenia caused by a novel mutation of GATA-1. *Blood*, **98**, 2681–8.

Migliaccio AR, Papayannopoulou T (2001). Erythropoiesis. In: Steinberg MH, *et al.* (eds) *Disorders of hemoglobin, genetics, pathophysiology, clinical management*, pp. 52–71. Cambridge University Press, Cambridge.

Mohandas N, Narla A (2005). Blood group antigens in health and disease. *Curr Opin Hematol*, **12**, 135–40.

Moore MA, Metcalf D (1970). Ontogeny of the haemopoietic system: yolk sac origin of *in vivo* and *in vitro* colony forming cells in the developing mouse embryo. *Br J Haematol*, **18**, 279–96.

Moritz KM, Lim GB, Wintour EM (1997). Developmental regulation of erythropoietin and erythropoiesis. *Am J Physiol*, **273**, 1829–44.

Nakamura Y, *et al.* (1998). Impaired erythropoiesis in transgenic mice overexpressing a truncated erythropoietin receptor. *Exp Hematol*, **26**, 1105–10.

Nichols KE, *et al.* (2000). Familial dyserythropoietic anaemia and thrombocytopenia due to an inherited mutation in GATA1. *Nat Genet*, **24**, 266–70.

Orkin SH (2001). Transcription factors that regulate lineage decisions. In: Stamatoyannopoulos G, *et al.* (eds) *The molecular basis of blood diseases*, 3rd edition, pp. 80–94. W B Saunders, Philadelphia.

Orkin SH, Zon LI (2008).Hematopoiesis: an evolving paradigm for stem cell biology. *Cell*, **132**, 631–44.

Orru S, *et al.* (2007). Analysis of the ribosomal protein S19 interactome. *Mol Cell Proteomics*, **6**, 382–93.

Pallis J (2008). Ontogeny of erythropoiesis. *Curr Opin Hematol*, **15**, 155–61.

Papayannopoulou T, *et al.* (2009). Biology of erythropoiesis, erythroid differentiation, and maturation. In: Hoffman R, *et al.* (eds) *Hematology. Basic principles and practice*, 5th edition, Chapter 25, 276–294. Churchill Livingstone, New York.

Pardanani A (2008). JAK2 inhibitor therapy in myeloproliferative disorders: rationale, preclinical studies and ongoing clinical trials. *Leukemia*, **22**, 23–30.

Pastore YD, Jelinek J, Ang S (2003). Mutations in the VHL gene in sporadic apparently congenital polycythemia. *Blood*, **101**, 1591–5.

Perrotta S, *et al.* (2006). Von Hippel-Lindau-dependent polycythemia is endemic on the island of Ischia: identification of a novel cluster. *Blood*, **107**, 514–19.

Philips JD, *et al.* (2007). Congenital erythropoietic porphyria due to a mutation in GATA1: the first trans-acting mutation causative for a human porphyria. *Blood*, **109**, 2618–21.

Ponka P (1997). Tissue-specific regulation of iron metabolism and heme synthesis: distinct control mechanisms in erythroid cells. *Blood*, **89**, 1–25.

Raskind WH, *et al.* (2000). Mapping of a syndrome of X-linked thrombocytopenia and thalassemia to band Xp11–12: further evidence of genetic heterogeneity of X-linked thrombocytopenia. *Blood*, **95**, 2262.

Reissmann KR (1950). Studies on the mechanism of erythropoietic stimulation in parabiotic rats during hypoxia. *Blood*, **5**, 372.

Rico-Vargas SA, *et al.* (1994). c-kit expression by B cell precursors in mouse bone marrow. Stimulation of B cell genesis by *in vivo* treatment with anti-c-kit antibody. *J Immunol*, **152**, 2845–52.

Royer Y, *et al.* (2005). Janus kinases affect thrombopoietin receptor cell surface localization and stability. *J Biol Chem*, **280**, 27 251–61.

Russell ES (1979). Hereditary anemias of the mouse: a review for geneticists. *Adv Genet*, **20**, 357–459.

Sasaki A, *et al.* (2000). CIS3/SOCS3 suppresses erythropoietin signaling by binding the EPO receptor and JAK2. *J Biol Chem*, **275**, 29 338–47.

Sato T, *et al.* (2000). Erythroid progenitors differentiate and mature in response to endogenous erythropoietin. *J Clin Invest*, **106**, 263–70.

Semenza GL (1999). Perspectives on oxygen sensing. *Cell*, **98**, 281–4.

Shimizu R, Komatsu N, Miura Y (1999). Dominant negative effect of a truncated erythropoietin receptor (EPOR-T) on erythropoietin-induced erythroid differentiation: possible involvement of EPOR-T in ineffective erythropoiesis of myelodysplastic syndrome. *Exp Hematol*, **27**, 229–33.

Skoda R, Prchal JT (2005). Lessons from familial myeloproliferative disorders. *Semin Hematol*, **42**. 266–73

Southcott MJ, Tanner MJ, Anstee DJ (1999). The expression of human blood group antigens during erythropoiesis in a cell culture system. *Blood*, **93**, 4425–35.

Spivak JL (2000). The blood in systemic disorders. *Lancet*, **355**, 1707–12.

Spritz RA, Beighton P (1998). Piebaldism with deafness: molecular evidence for an expanded syndrome. *Am J Med Genet*, **75**, 101–3.

Stamatoyannopoulos G, Grosveld F (2001). Hemoglobin switching. In: Stamatoyannopoulos G, *et al.* (eds) *The molecular basis of blood diseases*, 3rd edition, pp. 135–65. W B Saunders, Philadelphia.

Stohlman K Jr, Rath CE, Rose JC (1954). Evidence for a humoral regulation of erythropoiesis: studies on a patient with polycythemia secondary to regional exposure to hypoxia. *Blood*, **9**, 721.

Stopka T, *et al.* (1998). Human hematopoietic progenitors express erythropoietin. *Blood*, **91**, 3766–72.

Takakura N, *et al.* (2000). A role for hematopoietic stem cells in promoting angiogenesis. *Cell*, **102**, 199–209.

Tamura K, *et al.* (2000). Requirement for p38α in erythropoietin expression: a role for stress kinases in erythropoiesis. *Cell*, **102**, 221–31.

Tefferi A, Skoda R, Vardiman JW (2009). Myeloproliferative neoplasms: contemporary diagnosis using histology and genetics. *Nat Rev Clin Oncol*, **6**, 627–37.

Tubman VN, *et al.* (2007). X-linked gray platelet syndrome due to a GATA1 Arg216Gln mutation. *Blood*, **109**, 3297–9.

Vaziri H, *et al.* (1994). Evidence for a mitotic clock in human hematopoietic stem cells: loss of telomeric DNA with age. *Proc Natl Acad Sci U S A*, **91**, 9857–60.

Verdier F, *et al.* (2000). Proteasomes regulate the duration of erythropoietin receptor activation by controlling down-regulation of cell surface receptors. *J Biol Chem*, **275**, 18 375–81.

Verfaillie CM (2000). Anatomy and physiology of hematopoiesis. In: Hoffman R, *et al.* (eds) *Hematology. Basic principles and practice*, pp 139–54. Churchill Livingstone, New York.

Watowich SS, *et al.* (1999). Erythropoietin receptor mutations associated with familial erythrocytosis cause hypersensitivity to erythropoietin in the heterozygous state. *Blood*, **94**, 2530–2.

Willig TN, *et al.* (1999). Mutations in ribosomal protein S19 gene and diamond blackfan anemia: wide variations in phenotypic expression. *Blood*, **94**, 4294–306.

Winearls C, *et al.* (1986). Effects of human erythropoietin derived from recombinant DNA on the anemia of patients maintained on chronic hemodialysis. *Lancet*, **ii**, 1175.

Wu H, *et al.* (1995). Generation of committed erythroid BFU-E and CFU-E progenitors does not require erythropoietin or the erythropoietin receptor. *Cell*, **83**, 59–67.

Yu AY, *et al.* (1999). Impaired physiological responses to chronic hypoxia in mice partially deficient for hypoxia-inducible factor 1α. *J Clin Invest*, **103**, 691–6.

Yu C, *et al.* (2002). X-linked thrombocytopenia with thalassemia from a mutation in the amino finger of GATA-1 affecting DNA binding rather than FOG-1 interaction. *Blood*, **100**, 2040–5.

Zucali JR, Stevens V, Mirand EA (1975). *In vitro* production of erythropoietin by mouse fetal liver. *Blood*, **46**, 85–90.

22.5.2 Anaemia: pathophysiology, classification, and clinical features

D.J. Weatherall

Essentials

Anaemia is usually defined clinically as a reduction of the haemoglobin concentration to less than 13 g/dl (males) or less than 12 g/dl (females). It is a common problem, with prevalence around 3% for middle-aged men and 14% for middle-aged women in the United Kingdom, and much greater prevalence in the developing world.

Adaptation to anaemia

Reduction in delivery of oxygen to the tissues triggers a variety of compensatory mechanisms, including (1) modulation of oxygen affinity—largely mediated by an increase in red blood cell 2,3-biphosphoglycerate; (2) increased production of erythropoietin—the main growth factor for red blood cell production; (3) redistribution of flow to benefit the myocardium, brain, and muscle; (4) increase in cardiac output; and (5) reduction of mixed venous oxygen tension to increase the arteriovenous oxygen difference.

Clinical manifestations

The clinical picture depends on whether anaemia is of rapid or insidious onset. Acute blood loss presents with features of intravascular volume depletion (see Chapter 17.3). Anaemia of gradual onset may (if mild) be asymptomatic or simply manifest as slight fatigue and pallor, or (if more severe) present with features including exertional dyspnoea, tachycardia, palpitations, angina, light-headedness, faintness, and signs of 'cardiac failure'.

Causes and classification

Anaemia can be caused by the defective production of red cells or an increased rate of loss of cells, either by bleeding or premature destruction (haemolysis).

Defective production of red cells—causes include (1) deficiency of iron, vitamin B_{12} or folate; (2) anaemia of chronic disorders; (3) reduced erythropoietin production—chronic kidney disease; (4) primary diseases of the bone marrow.

Haemolytic anaemias—causes are (1) genetic—including membrane defects, haemoglobin disorders, and enzyme deficiencies; or (2) acquired—including autoimmune and nonimmune disorders.

Clinical approach

The key issues are to determine (1) the degree of disability caused by the anaemia and hence how quickly treatment must be started, a key question being 'is blood transfusion required?', and (2) cause of the anaemia.

The main causes of anaemia can be usefully classified according to the associated red cell changes: (1) hypochromic, microcytic—including iron deficiency (the commonest cause of anaemia), thalassaemia (common in some populations); (2) normochromic, macrocytic—vitamin B_{12} or folate deficiency, alcohol, myelodysplasia; (3) polychromatophilic, macrocytic—haemolysis; (4) normochromic, normocytic—chronic disorders, renal failure, diseases of the bone marrow; (5) leucoerythroblastic—myelosclerosis, leukaemia, metastatic carcinoma.

Definition of anaemia

The main function of the red blood cells is oxygen transport. Hence a functional definition of anaemia is 'a state in which the circulating red-cell mass is insufficient to meet the oxygen requirements of the tissues'. However, many compensatory mechanisms can be brought into play to restore the oxygen supply to the vital centres, and therefore in clinical practice this definition is of limited value. For this reason anaemia is usually defined as 'a reduction of the haemoglobin concentration, red-cell count, or packed cell volume to below normal levels'.

It has been extremely difficult to establish a normal range of haematological values, and hence the definition of anaemia usually involves the adoption of rather arbitrary criteria. For example, the World Health Organization recommends that anaemia should be considered to exist in adults whose haemoglobin levels are lower than 13 g/dl (men) or 12 g/dl (women). Children aged 6 months to 6 years are considered anaemic at haemoglobin levels below 11 g/dl, and those aged 6 to 14 years below 12 g/dl. The disadvantage of such arbitrary criteria for defining anaemia is that there may be many apparently normal individuals whose haemoglobin concentration is below their optimal level. Furthermore, the published 'normal values' for adults (see Chapter 22.1) indicate that there is such a large standard deviation that many women must be considered 'normal' even though they have haemoglobin levels below 12 g/dl.

Prevalence of anaemia

Anaemia is a major world health problem and its distribution and prevalence in the developing world are considered in detail in the next chapter.

The prevalence of anaemia has been studied in many populations, but it is difficult to compare data from different sources because of variations in methodology and criteria. Certain patterns emerge, however. An early survey carried out in the United Kingdom established that haemoglobin levels were low in a significant proportion of the population, particularly susceptible groups being children under the age of 5 years, pregnant women, and those in social classes IV and V. A later random population study, also in the United Kingdom, reported a prevalence of anaemia of 14% for women aged 55 to 64 years and 3% for men aged 35 to 64 years. These and similar studies have shown that anaemia is most common in women between the ages of 15 and 44 years and that it then becomes relatively less frequent, although the prevalence increases again in the 75-and-over age group. Interestingly, it is only in the last group that the prevalence in men and women is almost the same. Where the cause of the anaemia has been analysed in these surveys, most cases have been due to iron deficiency. No doubt these prevalence data vary considerably between the developed countries, but it is clear that nutritional anaemia is relatively common in most populations at certain periods during development and late in life.

Adaptation to anaemia

The function of the red cell is to carry oxygen between the lungs and the tissues. However, tissue oxygenation is the result of a complex series of interactions of different organ systems, of which the red cell is only one (Table 22.5.2.1). Obviously the cardiac output, ventilatory function, and state of the capillaries are of great importance as well. Each of these oxygen supply systems is regulated differently. Ventilation responds to changes in pH, CO_2, and hypoxia. Cardiac output responds to the amount of blood entering the heart, and this is regulated mainly by the effects of tissue metabolism as it modifies the resistance to blood flow in the microvasculature. The erythron itself responds to changes in haemoglobin concentration, arterial oxygen saturation, and the oxygen affinity of the circulating haemoglobin. Thus a decreased capacity of any of these components may be compensated for by increased activity of the others in an attempt to maintain tissue oxygenation.

Oxygen diffuses across the alveolar membrane and into the blood, which equilibrates with the alveolar gas; the approximate oxygen tension is 100 mmHg, at which the blood is fully saturated with an oxygen content of 20 vol%. As blood is pumped through the tissue capillaries, oxygen diffuses out. Although the venous oxygen tension varies between organs, the oxygen tension of the pooled venous blood in the pulmonary artery, the 'mixed venous oxygen tension', is remarkably constant at 40 mmHg. At this oxygen

Table 22.5.2.1 The steps involved in the transport of oxygen to the tissues

Steps	Factors involved
Ambient O_2 tension ↓	Altitude
Ventilation ↓	Alveolar ventilation
	Gas-to-blood diffusion
	Ventilation/perfusion ratio
	Anatomical shunt
Circulation ↓	Cardiac output
	Blood: haemoglobin concentration, oxygen dissociation curve
Tissue diffusion	Intercapillary distance

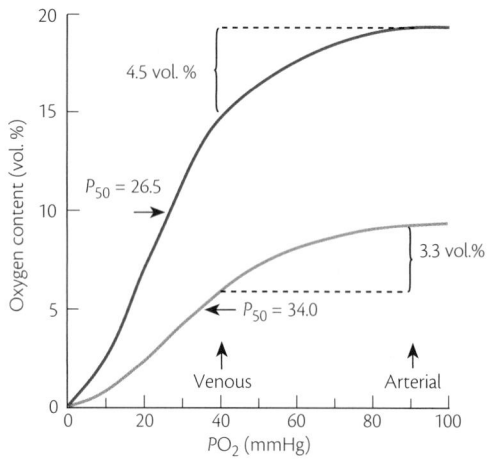

Fig. 22.5.2.1 Enhancement of oxygen loading by decreased red-cell oxygen affinity in a patient with anaemia. An anaemic patient with a 50% reduction in haemoglobin concentration has only a 27% reduction in oxygen unloading. (Based on Klocke RA (1972). Oxygen transport and 2,3-diphosphoglycerate (DPG). *Chest*, **62** 5 Suppl, 795–855.)

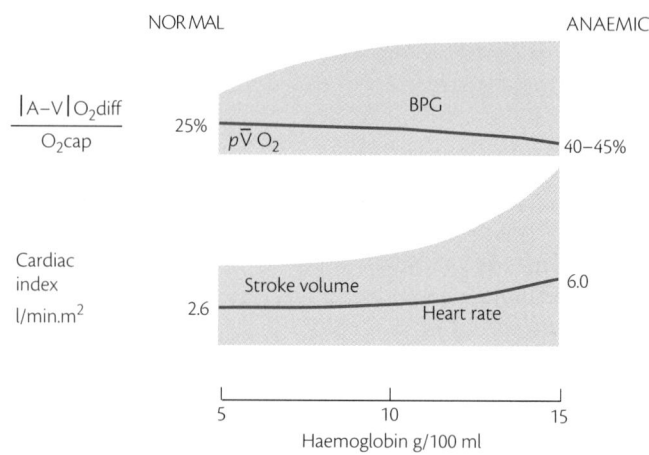

Fig. 22.5.2.2 The changes in factors involved in oxygen delivery with progressive anaemia. As anaemia becomes more severe, cardiac compensation becomes more significant ($P(V)o_2$, mixed venous oxygen tension). (From Bellingham AJ (1974). The red cell in adaptation to anaemic anoxia. *Clin Haematol*, **3**, 577–94.)

tension the oxygen content is 15 vol%. Hence, oxygen delivery, as measured by the arteriovenous oxygen difference, is normally 5 vol%. By reducing the oxygen-carrying capacity of blood, anaemia tends to reduce the arteriovenous oxygen difference, and this may be compensated for by the following mechanisms: (1) modulation of oxygen affinity; (2) increased production of erythropoietin; (3) redistribution of flow between different organs; (4) increase in cardiac output; and (5) reduction of mixed venous oxygen tension to increase the arteriovenous oxygen difference.

Intrinsic red-cell adaptation

The consequences of anaemia on the normal oxygen-binding curve of blood are shown in Fig. 22.5.2.1. Anaemia, by lowering the haemoglobin concentration, proportionally reduces the oxygen-carrying capacity of the blood. As a response to this there is an increase in the 2,3-diphosphoglycerate (2,3-BPG) concentration in the red cell, shifting the dissociation curve to the right, so significantly enhancing tissue oxygen delivery (Fig. 22.5.2.1).

With increasing severity of anaemia there is a progressive increase in 2,3-BPG, which may increase oxygen delivery by as much as 40% for the same haemoglobin concentration. It should be noted, however, that a consequence of this adaptation is a lower venous oxygen content and hence a lower reserve of oxygen available for a further increase in oxygen demand, as might occur on exercise for example. Hence the increase in 2,3-BPG in anaemia tends to ameliorate the effects of the diminished oxygen-carrying capacity of the blood, so reducing the adaptation required by other steps involved in tissue oxygen delivery (Fig. 22.5.2.2). 2,3-BPG levels vary in a variety of other clinical conditions, some of which are summarized in Box 22.5.2.1.

Erythropoietin

Erythropoietin (EPO) is the major hormone involved in the regulation of erythropoiesis. Interaction of EPO with its receptor on red cell precursors results in the stimulation of erythroid-cell division, differentiation, and the prevention of the apoptosis of erythroid progenitors. The hormone is produced in the kidney in

adult life and in the liver during fetal development. Erythropoietin production is increased by a hypoxic stimulus secondary to anaemia.

Much has been learnt in recent years about the way in which EPO production is regulated. A nucleotide sequence close to the EPO gene, called the hypoxia regulatory element, is responsible for hypoxic regulation of the EPO gene transcription. This, in turn, is controlled by a transcription factor called hypoxia inducible factor-1 (HIF-1). HIF-1 is part of a widespread oxygen-sensing

---

Box 22.5.2.1 Some conditions in which there is a change in red-cell 2,3-BPG levels leading to modification of oxygen transport

Increased 2,3-BPG; increased p50, reduced whole-blood oxygen affinity

◆ Anaemia

◆ Alkalosis

◆ Hyperphosphataemia

◆ Renal failure

◆ Hypoxia

◆ Pregnancy

◆ Cyanotic congenital heart disease

◆ Thyrotoxicosis

◆ Some red-cell enzyme deficiencies

Decreased 2,3-BPG; decreased p50, increased whole-blood oxygen affinity

◆ Acidosis

◆ Cardiogenic or septicaemic shock

◆ Hypophosphataemia

◆ Hypothyroidism

◆ Hypopituitarism

◆ Following replacement with stored blood

mechanism and is found in many cell types that do not express EPO. It is made up of two subunits, HIF-1α and HIF-1β; only the former is regulated by hypoxia. HIF-1 protein levels are increased by hypoxia and return to normal with adequate oxygenation. In the presence of oxygen HIF-1α is hydroxylated by an oxygen-sensitive proline hydroxylase. Hydroxylated HIF-1α becomes a target for interaction with the von Hippel–Lindau protein that initiates the rapid destruction of HIF-1α. In essence, this complex constitutes the oxygen sensor.

Thus, variation in the production of EPO in various conditions, particularly renal disease, may have profound effects on adaptation to anaemia.

Local changes in tissue perfusion

The total blood volume does not change greatly in anaemia and therefore increased tissue perfusion has to be achieved by shunting blood from less to more vital organs. There is vasoconstriction of the vessels of the skin and kidney; this mechanism has little effect on renal function. The organs that gain from the redistribution seem to be mainly the myocardium, brain, and muscle.

Cardiovascular changes

It seems likely that mild anaemia is compensated for by shifts in the oxygen dissociation curve. Overall, oxygen consumption is unchanged in anaemia. However, when the haemoglobin level falls below 7 to 8 g/dl, there is an increase in cardiac output, both at rest and after exercise (Fig. 22.5.2.2). The stroke rate increases and a hyperkinetic circulation develops, characterized by tachycardia, arterial and capillary pulsation, a wide pulse pressure, and haemic murmurs. The circulation time is shortened, left ventricular stroke work is increased, and coronary flow increased in proportion to the increased cardiac output. It has been found that there is an acute reversal of the high-output state of chronic anaemia in response to orthostatic stress or pressor amines. This suggests that redistribution of blood volume and vasodilatation with reduced afterload play a dominant role in the hyperkinetic circulatory responses to chronic anaemia. The mechanism of the vasodilatation is not known; it may be a direct result of tissue hypoxia. An additional factor that may be of some importance in increasing cardiac output is the reduction in blood viscosity produced by a relatively low red-cell mass.

Although the normal myocardium may tolerate sustained hyperactivity of this type indefinitely, patients with coronary artery disease or those with extreme anaemia may have impaired oxygenation of the myocardium. In such cases, cardiomegaly, pulmonary oedema, ascites, and peripheral oedema may occur, and a state of high-output cardiac failure is established. At this stage the plasma volume is almost always increased.

Pulmonary function

As blood, regardless of its oxygen-carrying capacity, is almost completely oxygenated in the lungs, the oxygen pressure of arterial blood in an anaemic patient should be the same as that in a normal individual, and hence an increase in respiratory rate should not improve the oxygenation of the tissues. Curiously, however, severe anaemia is associated with dyspnoea. Although in some patients this may be related to incipient cardiac failure, in most cases it appears to be an inappropriate response to hypoxia which is centrally mediated.

Clinical manifestations and classification of anaemia

Clinical effects of anaemia

Because anaemia reduces tissue oxygenation it is not surprising that it is associated with widespread organ dysfunction and hence an extremely varied clinical picture. The picture depends, of course, on whether the anaemia is of rapid or more insidious onset.

After acute blood loss the red-cell mass and plasma volume are reduced proportionately and the symptoms are mainly of volume depletion. Depending on the amount of fluid replacement there may be a small fall in the packed cell volume (PCV) during the first 10 h; volume replacement by the influx of albumin from the extravascular compartment takes between 60 and 90 h. Hence the picture of rapid blood loss is characterized by the typical syndrome of shock, with collapse, dyspnoea, tachycardia, a poor volume pulse, reduced blood pressure, and marked peripheral vasoconstriction.

With anaemia of a more insidious onset, the compensatory mechanisms outlined above have time to come into play. In mild anaemia there may be no symptoms or simply increased fatigue and a slight pallor. As the anaemia becomes more marked the symptoms and signs gradually appear. Pallor is best discerned in the mucous membranes; the nail beds and palmar creases, although often said to be useful sites for detecting anaemia, are relatively insensitive for this purpose. Cardiorespiratory symptoms and signs include exertional dyspnoea, tachycardia, palpitations, angina or claudication, night cramps, increased arterial pulsation, capillary pulsation, a variety of cardiac bruits, reversible cardiac enlargement, and, if cardiac failure occurs, basal crepitations, peripheral oedema, and ascites. Neuromuscular involvement is reflected by headache, vertigo, light-headedness, faintness, tinnitus, roaring in the ears, cramps, increased cold sensitivity, and haemorrhages in the retina. Acute anaemia may occasionally give rise to papilloedema. Gastrointestinal symptoms include loss of appetite, nausea, constipation, and diarrhoea. Genitourinary involvement causes menstrual irregularities, urinary frequency, and loss of libido. There may be a low-grade fever.

In older people, in whom associated degenerative arterial disease is common, anaemia may present with the onset of cardiac failure. Alternatively, previously undiagnosed coronary narrowing may be unmasked by the onset of angina. Other symptoms of arterial degenerative disease may be also exacerbated or unmasked, e.g. intermittent claudication and a variety of neurological pictures associated with cerebral arteriosclerosis. It is important that anaemia is recognized as a contributing factor to the symptoms of these degenerative diseases as its correction may frequently bring about considerable symptomatic improvement.

Causes and classification of anaemia

A reduction in the red-cell mass can result from either the defective production of red cells or an increased rate of loss of cells, by either premature destruction or bleeding. Decreased production of red cells may result from a reduced rate of proliferation of precursors in the bone marrow or from failure of maturation leading to their intramedullary destruction: i.e. ineffective erythropoiesis. Based on this approach we can derive a very simple pathophysiological classification of anaemia, as shown in Box 22.5.2.2, in which the

Box 22.5.2.2 The main groups of anaemias classified according to the underlying cause

- Reduced red-cell production:
  - Defective precursor proliferation
  - Defective precursor maturation
  - Defective proliferation and maturation
- Increased rate of red-cell destruction:
  - Haemolysis
- Loss of red cells from the circulation:
  - Bleeding

Box 22.5.2.3 Main causes of anaemia due to defective production of red cells

Reduced proliferation of precursors

- Iron deficiency anaemia
- Anaemia of chronic disorders:
  - Infections, malignancy, collagen disease, etc.
- Reduced erythropoietin production:
  - Renal disease
- Reduced oxygen requirements:
  - Hypothyroidism
  - Hypopituitarism
- Reduced oxygen affinity of haemoglobin
- Primary disease of the bone marrow:
  Aplastic anaemia:
    - primary
    - secondary to drugs, irradiation, chemicals, toxins, etc.
- Pure red-cell hypoplasia
- Infiltrative disorders:
  - Leukaemia
  - Lymphoma
  - Secondary carcinoma
  - Myelofibrosis

Defective maturation of precursors

- Nuclear maturation:
  - Vitamin B_{12} deficiency
  - Folate deficiency
  - Erythroleukaemia
- Cytoplasmic maturation:
  - Iron deficiency
  - Disorders of globin synthesis
  - Disorders of haem and/or iron metabolism
  - Disorders of porphyrin metabolism
- Other mechanisms:
  - Congenital dyserythropoietic anaemias
  - Myelodysplastic syndrome
  - Infection
  - Toxins and chemicals

causes are divided into failure of red-cell proliferation, defective maturation, haemolysis, and blood loss.

Anaemia due to defective proliferation of red-cell precursors

The major causes of this group of anaemias are an inadequate supply of iron, primary diseases of the bone marrow that involve stem cells or later erythroid precursors, and a reduction in the amount of erythropoietin reaching the red-cell precursors (Box 22.5.2.3).

Iron deficiency results in defective erythroid proliferation and also in abnormal maturation of the red-cell precursors as a result of defective haemoglobin synthesis. Red-cell precursors require adequate iron supplies for normal proliferation, and the anaemia of iron deficiency tends to be hypoproliferative as well as dyserythropoietic. Chronic inflammatory disorders and related conditions also interfere with the iron supply to precursors, probably by blocking the release of catabolized red-cell iron from reticuloendothelial cells. The basic defect in iron-deficiency anaemia and that due to inflammation is similar, therefore, in that the supply of iron is inadequate to meet the requirements for erythropoiesis.

Defective proliferation of red-cell precursors can result from any of the causes of bone marrow failure, including infiltration with leukaemic or other neoplastic cells, damage due to ionizing radiation, drugs, or infection, and various intrinsic lesions of the stem cells or red-cell precursors. The intrinsic disorders include the congenital hypoplastic anaemias, involving either all the formed elements or the red-cell precursors alone.

Finally, decreased proliferation of the red-cell precursors may result from erythropoietin deficiency. The most common cause is chronic renal failure. A similar mechanism may be involved in conditions in which the tissue requirement for oxygen is reduced. These include various endocrine disorders such as hypothyroidism and hypopituitarism. It may also explain the mild anaemia associated with haemoglobin variants with decreased oxygen affinity.

As a group, the hypoproliferative anaemias are associated with a low reticulocyte count and defective proliferation of the bone marrow precursors. The red cells are usually normochromic and normocytic, although there may be a mild macrocytosis. If the anaemia is due to iron deficiency, the cells are hypochromic. If granulopoiesis is normal, the defect in red-cell proliferation is reflected by an increase in the myeloid:erythroid (M/E) ratio.

Defective red-cell maturation

Defects of red-cell maturation may involve primarily nuclear or cytoplasmic maturation (Box 22.5.2.3). Those involving nuclear maturation include vitamin B_{12} and folic acid deficiency and other causes of megaloblastic anaemia, and some of the primary marrow disorders including erythroleukaemia. The important causes of defective cytoplasmic maturation include the inherited disorders of globin synthesis, the thalassaemia syndromes, and the genetic and acquired defects of iron metabolism that characterize the sideroblastic anaemias. There are other genetic defects of red-cell maturation, the congenital dyserythropoietic anaemias, in which the aetiology is unknown. Furthermore, agents such as drugs, chemicals, and infections may interfere with erythroid maturation.

The main pathological mechanism common to all the anaemias that result from maturation abnormalities is ineffective erythropoiesis. In other words, there is marked erythroid proliferation but many of the precursors are destroyed in the bone marrow before they enter the circulation. Hence, the characteristic finding is marked erythroid hyperplasia with a reduction in the M/E ratio, associated with a low reticulocyte count. Because of the significant intramedullary destruction of precursors there is usually an elevated level of bilirubin and lactate dehydrogenase. Furthermore, there are nearly always morphological abnormalities of the red-cell precursors. The anaemias that are associated with abnormal nuclear maturation, such as those due to vitamin B$_{12}$ and folic acid deficiency, are characterized by megaloblastic erythropoiesis and macrocytic red cells, while those caused by abnormal cytoplasmic maturation are characterized by normoblastic hyperplasia and hypochromic and microcytic red cells. However, even in these last conditions, there is marked anisocytosis and there may be a proportion of macrocytes in the peripheral circulation.

Blood loss

As mentioned earlier, the clinical picture associated with an acute loss of a large volume of blood is that of hypovolaemic shock.

Anaemias due to chronic blood loss may develop very insidiously and cause considerable diagnostic problems. Chronic blood loss from the gastrointestinal tract or uterus of more than 15 to 20 ml/day produces a state of negative iron balance. Assuming that the patient starts with a normal body store of iron, which is usually in the region of 1 g, the bone marrow will be able to maintain a normal haemoglobin level until the iron stores are totally depleted. At this stage there is no demonstrable iron in the bone marrow and the plasma iron level starts to fall, but the patient is not anaemic. With a further fall in the plasma iron level, the haemoglobin level starts to fall, although at this stage the erythrocyte morphology may be relatively normal, as are the red-cell indices. It is only when iron-deficiency anaemia is well established that the typical morphological appearances of the red cells develop, and only after extreme periods of iron depletion that the tissue changes of iron deficiency become manifest.

From these considerations it is apparent that there may be prolonged blood loss before a patient presents with the symptoms and signs of anaemia. During the earlier stages the peripheral blood film may not be helpful in diagnosis, even though the serum iron level may be extremely low. Indeed, sometimes a dimorphic blood picture with normochromic and hypochromic cell populations may be seen. With chronic blood loss there is quite often a persistent thrombocytosis, and a hypochromic blood picture with thrombocytosis should always raise the possibility of chronic bleeding. In practice, the most common sites of such bleeding are a hiatus hernia, peptic ulcer, and tumour of the large bowel or the uterus.

Haemolytic anaemia

When the lifespan of red cells is shortened there is a reduction in the circulating red-cell mass, which leads to relative tissue hypoxia.

This causes an increased output of erythropoietin with stimulation of the bone marrow and an increased rate of red-cell production. This is reflected by a raised reticulocyte count and a macrocytosis due to the presence of young cells in the peripheral circulation. Because of the increased rate of red-cell destruction, there is an increased production of bilirubin, which leads to mild icterus and the presence of increased amounts of urobilinogen in the urine and stool. Thus the haemolytic anaemias (Box 22.5.2.4) are characterized by a variable degree of anaemia, a reticulocytosis, and hyperbilirubinaemia. Their pathophysiology is considered in detail elsewhere.

Red cells are prematurely destroyed either because of an intrinsic lesion or as a result of the action of an extrinsic agent. The intrinsic abnormalities of the red cells that lead to their premature removal are nearly all genetic defects of either the membrane, haemoglobin, or metabolic pathways. The extrinsic agents that may cause premature destruction of the cells include a variety of antibodies, chemicals, drugs, and toxins, or bacteria and parasites. In addition, red cells may be damaged by direct trauma in the microcirculation or on body surfaces.

Premature destruction of red cells may take place either intravascularly or extravascularly, or, as occurs more commonly, in both sites. The site of destruction depends on the type and degree of damage to the red cell. For example, complement-damaged cells develop large holes in the membrane and are destroyed in the circulation, whereas IgG-coated cells are removed mainly in the reticuloendothelial system.

Clearly, there are numerous causes of premature destruction of red cells. These will be considered in detail later in this section. Usually it is easy to recognize that a particular anaemia has a haemolytic basis, by virtue of the reticulocytosis and macrocytosis associated with erythroid hyperplasia of the bone marrow, hyperbilirubinaemia, and increased urinary urobilinogen. However, it should be remembered that many anaemias associated with the abnormal proliferation or maturation of red cells have a haemolytic component. For example, there may be a slightly shortened red-cell

---

Box 22.5.2.4 General classification of haemolytic anaemia

- ◆ Genetically determined:
  - Defects involving the structure and/or metabolism of the membrane
  - Haemoglobin disorders
  - Enzyme deficiencies involving the main metabolic pathways
- ◆ Acquired:
  - Immune (iso- or auto-)
  - Nonimmune:
  - Trauma
  - Membrane defects
  - Drugs, chemicals, toxins
  - Bacteria, parasites
  - Hypersplenism

A more detailed classification is given in Chapter 22.5.9.

survival in patients with pernicious anaemia or thalassaemia and yet there may be a very poor reticulocyte response. Similarly, there is a haemolytic component in the anaemia due to inflammation or malignancy but again the marrow response is poor. In such cases it may be necessary to measure the lifespan of the red cells directly in order to determine the magnitude of the haemolytic component as compared with defective proliferation or maturation.

General approach to the anaemic patient

Clinical assessment

The clinical assessment of patients with anaemia has two main objectives. First, it is essential to determine the degree of disability caused by the anaemia and hence how quickly treatment must be started. Second, as much information as possible about the likely cause of the anaemia must be obtained from a detailed clinical history and physical examination. There is no place for the 'blind' treatment of anaemia without first establishing the cause.

In assessing the severity of the anaemia and how urgently treatment should be instituted, a detailed history of the patient's exercise tolerance must be obtained. This should include a specific enquiry of symptoms suggestive of cardiac complications including angina, dysrhythmias, positional dyspnoea, cough, or ankle swelling. The clinical examination should include a careful assessment of the degree of pallor, the position of the neck veins, whether there are warm extremities and a bounding pulse with a large pulse pressure, the presence of ankle or sacral oedema, and whether there are basal crepitations. The finding of profound anaemia with signs of cardiac failure indicates that urgent treatment is required. If the anaemia is associated with marked splenomegaly there will almost certainly be an increased blood volume and, particularly if there are already signs of cardiac failure, the patient may well go into acute left ventricular failure if transfused. Severely ill patients with profound anaemia require immediate treatment in an environment where they can be under constant observation, have regular measurements of their central venous pressure, and be managed by experienced clinical and nursing staff.

An account of history taking and clinical examination in patients with haematological disorders was given earlier in this section (Chapter 22.1). It cannot be emphasized too strongly that in many cases the anaemia is a symptom of a nonhaematological disorder. A detailed history and clinical examination will often provide a clue as to the likely cause of the anaemia, and which laboratory investigations are likely to be most productive for confirming the diagnosis.

Haematological investigation

A preliminary blood count and blood film examination should classify anaemia into hypochromic-microcytic, and macrocytic or normochromic, normocytic varieties (Box 22.5.2.5). In middle-aged women with a history of several pregnancies or heavy menstrual loss it is reasonable to assume that a hypochromic anaemia is due to iron deficiency, and to treat them with iron without further investigation. However, hypochromic anaemia in men or young or postmenopausal women always suggests blood loss and should be investigated accordingly. If there is any doubt about a hypochromic anaemia being due to iron deficiency, the serum iron level and total iron-binding capacity should be established. Hypochromic anaemia with a normal serum iron suggests a genetic or acquired defect in haemoglobin synthesis, common causes being thalassaemia

---

> **Box 22.5.2.5** The main causes of anaemia classified according to the associated red-cell changes
>
> **Hypochromic–microcytic (reduced MCV, MCH, and MCHC)**
> - Genetic:
>   - Thalassaemia
>   - Sideroblastic anaemia
> - Acquired:
>   - Iron deficiency
>   - Sideroblastic anaemia
>   - Chronic disorders (mildly hypochromic, occasionally)
>
> **Normochromic–macrocytic (increased MCV)**
> - With megaloblastic marrow:
>   - Vitamin B$_{12}$ or folate deficiency
> - With normoblastic marrow:
>   - Alcohol, myelodysplasia
>
> **Polychromatophilic–macrocytic (increased MCV)**
> - Haemolysis
>
> **Normochromic–normocytic (normal indices)**
> - Chronic disorders:
>   - Infection, malignancy, collagen disease, rheumatoid arthritis
> - Renal failure
> - Hypothyroidism, hypopituitarism
> - Aplastic anaemia or primary red-cell hypoplasia
> - Primary disease of bone marrow, leukaemia, myelosclerosis, infiltration with other tumours
>
> **Leucoerythroblastic (indices usually normal)**
> - Myelosclerosis
> - Leukaemia
> - Metastatic carcinoma
>
> MCH, mean cell haemoglobin; MCHC, mean cell haemoglobin concentration; MCV, mean cell volume.

---

and sideroblastic anaemia. The diagnosis of a macrocytic anaemia always requires further investigation and should be followed up with a bone marrow examination. A macrocytosis with a normoblastic bone marrow may result from alcohol abuse, haemolysis, or, occasionally, one of the refractory anaemias with hyperplastic bone marrow (see Chapter 22.5.8). Macrocytic anaemias with megaloblastic bone marrows are usually due to vitamin B$_{12}$ or folate deficiency and should be investigated accordingly. If there is macrocytosis with a reticulocytosis, hyperbilirubinaemia, and a normoblastic marrow, a haemolytic anaemia is likely; an approach to the further investigation of haemolysis is described in Chapter 22.5.9.

The normochromic, normocytic anaemias often cause more diagnostic difficulty. Some help can be gained from a determination of whether the white-cell and platelet counts are normal. If there is associated neutropenia and thrombocytopenia, a primary disease of the bone marrow is likely; hence, bone marrow examination should be made to determine whether there is hypoplasia of the various precursor forms, hypoplastic or aplastic anaemia, or whether the pancytopenia results from infiltration of the bone marrow as occurs in the various forms of leukaemia. If there are nucleated red cells or young white cells on the peripheral film (i.e. a leucoerythroblastic picture), a bone marrow examination is essential, as this type of reaction usually indicates infiltration of the bone marrow with abnormal cells, either as part of a primary marrow disease such as leukaemia, or metastatic carcinoma. In the normochromic, normocytic anaemias in which the white-cell count and platelet count are normal, it is also helpful to make a bone marrow analysis. The most common cause is anaemia of chronic disorders, the diagnosis of which is described in detail below. Another particularly common cause is chronic renal failure. After these conditions have been excluded, there remain the chronic anaemias associated with endocrine deficiencies (see Chapter 22.7) or the primary red-cell hypoplasias (Chapter 22.3.11).

The management of anaemia

The management of specific forms of anaemia is described in detail in subsequent chapters. However, a few principles can be outlined here. In general, a cause should always be sought before treatment is instituted. There is no place whatever for treating anaemia 'blind' with multihaematinic preparations. As mentioned above, most cases of iron-deficiency anaemia require further investigation for a source of blood loss. If there is a clear-cut history of poor diet, multiple pregnancies, or obvious uterine bleeding, it is reasonable to start iron therapy and observe the haemoglobin level both during the period of treatment and for some months after iron therapy has been stopped. A rise in the haemoglobin level of approximately 1 g/dl per week indicates a full haematological response. For the megaloblastic anaemias it is quite reasonable to start treatment with vitamin B_{12} and folic acid once a diagnosis has been established and blood samples have been obtained for serum folate and vitamin B_{12} levels. The precise cause of the megaloblastic anaemia can be established at leisure once these samples have been obtained. A brisk reticulocyte response 5 to 7 days after initiating therapy suggests that there will be a full restoration of the haemoglobin level to normal. Failure of response of a hypochromic anaemia to adequate iron therapy should be managed by first finding out whether the iron is being taken by the patient and, if so, by determining the serum iron level. If it is normal, causes of hypochromic anaemia that are not associated with iron deficiency, e.g. thalassaemia and sideroblastic anaemia, should be sought. Similarly, refractory macrocytic anaemias require detailed analysis of the bone marrow morphology as there may be an underlying preleukaemic state.

Blood transfusion should always be avoided unless the haemoglobin level is dangerously low, in which case it is reasonable to transfuse the patient up to a safe level and then allow the haemoglobin to return to normal following appropriate treatment of the underlying cause. The decision whether to transfuse an anaemic patient depends mainly on the severity of the anaemia and its cause. For example, a young patient with a haemoglobin of 5 g/dl who is shown to have an active duodenal ulcer should probably be transfused because they would be at severe risk from a further brisk bleed from the ulcer. On the other hand, a patient of similar age with a similar haemoglobin level due to chronic nutritional iron deficiency might well be allowed to restore their haemoglobin level by oral iron therapy.

Occasionally, patients present in gross congestive cardiac failure with profound anaemia. This picture is usually seen in elderly patients with long-standing pernicious anaemia or iron deficiency. This type of condition still carries a high mortality and requires urgent treatment. Such profoundly anaemic patients require transfusing up to a safe level, that is a haemoglobin value of 6 to 8 g/dl. This can usually be achieved by the slow transfusion of two or three units of red cells with the intravenous administration of a potent diuretic such as furosemide (frusemide) with each unit; the diuretic should never be mixed directly with the blood. A very careful check on the neck veins and lung bases should be made throughout the period of transfusion. Ideally, a central venous pressure line should be inserted before the transfusion is started. Occasionally, patients are encountered in such gross heart failure that the administration of packed cells and diuretics worsens the failure. In this situation it is possible to raise the circulating red-cell mass by infusing packed cells or whole blood through one arm while removing an equal volume of blood from the other. By carrying out a two-to-three unit exchange transfusion of this type it may be possible to tide the patient over while treating the heart failure by conventional means.

Further reading

Koury MJ (2005). Erythropoietin: the story of hypoxia and a finely regulated hematopoietic hormone. *Exp Hematol*, **33**, 1263–70.

Prchal JT (2006). Clinical manifestations and classification of erythrocyte disorders. In: Lichtman MA, *et al.* (eds) *Williams' hematology*, 7th edition, pp. 417–18. McGraw-Hill Medical, New York.

22.5.3 Anaemia as a challenge to world health

D.J. Weatherall

Essentials

Anaemia is a very common problem in the developing world: 47% of women aged 15 to 49 years have haemoglobin less than 12 g/dl; 59% of pregnant women have haemoglobin less than 11 g/dl; 26% of men aged 15 to 49 years have haemoglobin less than 13 g/dl. About 20% of perinatal mortality and 10% of maternal mortality in developing countries is attributable to iron deficiency.

Causes of anaemia in developing countries—this is often multifactorial, with causes including (1) nutritional deficiencies—iron, folate, vitamin B_{12}; (2) chronic infection—including malaria, tuberculosis, AIDS; (3) blood loss—hookworm, schistosomiasis; (4) protein–energy malnutrition; (5) malabsorption—e.g. tropical sprue;

(6) hereditary—e.g. thalassaemias, haemoglobin variants, glucose-6-phosphate dehydrogenase deficiency.

A series of vicious cycles in the developing world—maternal anaemia due to iron or folate deficiency and chronic malaria is associated with the birth of underweight infants who frequently have low iron stores, may also be folate deplete, and are usually anaemic from about 6 months of age. Such infants are prone to infection, particularly gastrointestinal, and may be further depleted of iron or folate by inappropriately prolonged breastfeeding or weaning onto an inadequate diet. They are exposed to hookworm infection as soon as they start to crawl, malaria becomes an important problem after 6 months, and in many populations the increasingly common haemoglobinopathies are a further cause of anaemia after the first few months of life.

Introduction

Despite improvements in nutrition and hygiene, which have reduced childhood mortality in many developing countries, anaemia continues to be an important problem in the health of the world's population. It is not, of course, a disease in its own right but simply a by-product of a wide variety of different disorders, most of which are described in detail elsewhere. However, because of its importance as a source of chronic ill health in many populations, the global aspects of the aetiology and manifestations of anaemia are summarized briefly in this chapter. Readers who wish to learn more of the complex literature on this important topic are referred to the extensive reviews cited at the end of the chapter.

Definition and prevalence

It has been very difficult to produce an adequate definition of anaemia. 'Normal' haematological values vary with age, between sexes, at different altitudes, and, possibly, between races. On the other hand, it is helpful to have a standard set of haemoglobin levels at different ages below which 'anaemia' is defined. The World Health Organization (WHO) have attempted to set out criteria of these kind, summarized in Table 22.5.3.1. Despite their many shortcomings, including methodological vagaries, they at least provide a way of obtaining an approximate comparison of the distribution and frequency of anaemia among the different countries of the world.

The global prevalence of anaemia, based on WHO criteria, was estimated in the 1980s. A review of the epidemiological data available at this time suggested that about 1.3 billion people were affected by anaemia, particularly in the developing countries. Infants, young children, menstruating, and, especially, pregnant women were the most severely affected groups (Table 22.5.3.2). More recent estimations of the prevalence of anaemia suggest that there has been little improvement. For example it is now estimated that some 2 billion people worldwide are affected by iron-deficiency anaemia. About one-fifth of perinatal mortality and one-tenth of maternal mortality in developing countries is attributable to iron deficiency. In total, 0.8 million deaths worldwide are now attributable to iron deficiency, i.e. about 1.3% of all male deaths and 1.8% of all female deaths. Attributable disability-adjusted life years (DALYs) are even greater, accounting for the loss of about 35 million healthy life years, again the bulk of which are in the developing countries.

Table 22.5.3.1 Definition of haemoglobin levels below which anaemia is said to exist in populations at sea level (WHO 1968)

	Haemoglobin (g/dl) below
Children, 6 months–6 years	11.0
Children, 6–14 years	12.0
Adult males	13.0
Adult females (nonpregnant)	12.0
Adult females (pregnant)	11.0

The complex and multiple aetiology of anaemia in developing countries

The main causes of anaemia in developing countries are summarized in Box 22.5.3.1. It is very difficult to determine their relative importance, particularly in tropical countries. Most surveys have focused on one particular mechanism, e.g. iron or folate deficiency. To obtain a true picture of the cause of anaemia in a particular population it is essential to obtain consecutive data over a long period. For example, work in the Gambia has shown that the haemoglobin levels in children vary significantly at different times of the year; anaemia is much more common in the wet season when malaria transmission is at its highest. To complicate matters, this is also the time when diarrhoea and malnutrition are most common. Heavy rains after many dry months have profound effects on the community; sanitation measures are disrupted and food stores are at the lowest level in the annual cycle (Fig. 22.5.3.1).

These observations underline the multifactorial aetiology of anaemia in the developing world. Nonetheless it is clear that iron deficiency, which probably affects at least 20% of the world's population, is the most important factor; the many other diseases that can exacerbate anaemia are often operating in the background of low body-iron stores.

Iron deficiency

The causes of iron-deficiency anaemia are extremely complex and vary widely among different populations. The absorption of non-haem iron, except from breast milk, is comparatively restricted, and the content of iron in breast milk is very low. Iron deficiency is particularly common in communities in which food is predominantly of vegetable origin. The three great staples in these populations are rice, wheat, and maize. Sorghum and millet are also important in parts of Africa and Asia. Soy and similar legumes are an important

Table 22.5.3.2 Estimated prevalence of anaemia by region and sex

Region	Percentage anaemic				
	Children		Women 15–49 years		Men
	0–4 years	5–12 years	Pregnant	All	15–59 years
Developing	51	46	59	47	26
Developed	12	7	14	11	3
World	43	37	51	35	18

Data from DeMaeyer EM, Adiels-Tegman M (1985). The prevalence of anemia in the world. *World Health Statist Quart*, **38**, 302–16.

Box 22.5.3.1 Important causes of anaemia in the developing countries

Acquired

- Nutritional
  - Iron, folate, vitamin B$_{12}$
- Chronic infection
  - Malaria, leishmaniasis, schistosomiasis, tuberculosis, AIDS
- Blood loss
  - Hookworm
  - Schistosomiasis
- Protein–energy malnutrition
- Malabsorption
  - Tropical sprue and related disorders

Hereditary

- Thalassaemias
- Haemoglobin variants
- Glucose-6-phosphate dehydrogenase deficiency
- Ovalocytosis

source of protein in many countries. The iron content of these diets is generally low, and, furthermore, absorption is inhibited by fibre, phytates, phosphates, and polyphenols, all of which occur in high levels in vegetarian diets. Populations who have remained as hunter-gatherers, and pastoralists who eat blood and meat, appear to have a lower frequency of iron-deficiency anaemia.

Against this background of deficient or borderline dietary iron intake, there are several other factors which may exacerbate iron deficiency. Iron requirements are greatly increased during pregnancy because of the expansion of the maternal red-cell mass (c.500 mg), iron transport to the fetus (c.300 mg), and the constitution of the placenta (c.25 mg), together with any blood loss at birth.

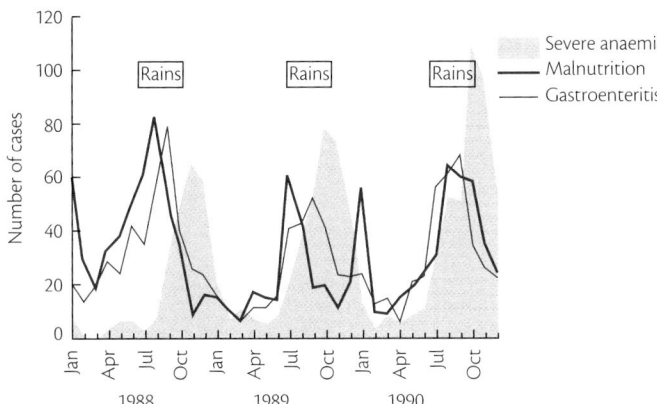

Fig. 22.5.3.1 Admissions to the children's ward in a hospital in the Gambia over dry and rainy seasons.
(Data from Brewster DR, Greenwood BM (1993). Season variation of paediatric disease in The Gambia, West Africa. *Ann Trop Paediatr*, **13**, 133.)

Although there is some compensation by the cessation of iron loss due to menstruation (c.200 mg), the total requirements for a single pregnancy are more than 1 g. Iron is also excreted in breast milk and although the concentration is low this loss, particularly with prolonged breastfeeding, places a further burden on maternal iron stores.

In many tropical countries, there are important sources of pathological iron loss due to parasitic infection. Hookworm infestation affects millions of people worldwide. These parasites attach themselves to the mucosa of the intestinal tract. With a worm load of 1000 eggs/g faeces, the intestinal blood loss averages about 2.5 ml/day, representing 1 mg of iron. Although some of this is reabsorbed, perhaps up to 40%, hookworm infestation is an important source of iron imbalance. Infection with *Schistosoma mansoni* results in intestinal blood loss, while *S. haematobium* results in chronic haematuria. In Kenyan children, for example, mean iron losses in those infected with *S. haematobium* varied from 149 to 652 µg/day, according to the magnitude of the egg counts.

Finally, it should be remembered that chronic ill health due to protein–calorie malnutrition or chronic infection may, by its effect on a patient's appetite, result in further depletion of iron intake.

It must be emphasized that many surveys for assessing body iron stores have used methods which are confounded by associated inflammatory disease or other disorders. These problems are particularly germane to surveys which have been based on serum iron or ferritin levels. More recently, screening methods based on estimation of transferrin receptor levels have been developed but their application to large populations is, as yet, limited.

Folate deficiency

Folate deficiency is thought to be the second most frequent cause of nutritional anaemia in the world population. The mechanisms are complex and differ widely between different populations depending in the way in which food is prepared, in particular the temperature at which it is cooked. It is also clear that dietary folate deficiency is not the whole story. Research in Africa suggests that the continuous anorexia which accompanies recurrent infections such as malaria or tuberculosis is a major cause of folate deficiency in children. Postinfective malabsorption and the tropical sprue syndrome are also important causes of folate deficiency, particularly in the Indian subcontinent. Folate requirements may be increased in patients with erythroid hyperplasia secondary to chronic haemolytic anaemia, e.g. sickle cell anaemia, or chronic malarial infection. They also increase markedly during pregnancy. In women with low baseline folate stores, megaloblastic anaemia in pregnancy or the puerperium is particularly common.

Vitamin B$_{12}$ deficiency

Nutritional vitamin B$_{12}$ deficiency is uncommon, although it is observed in true vegans, particularly in the Indian subcontinent. Infants born of mothers with sprue or postinfective malabsorption who are fed on breast milk or goat's milk containing insufficient vitamin B$_{12}$ may develop megaloblastic anaemia with locomotor complications during the early months of life.

Infection

Almost any chronic infection may produce anaemia. Globally, the most important are the parasitic disorders, malaria, visceral leishmaniasis (kala-azar), schistosomiasis, and some forms of trypanosomiasis. The anaemias due to chronic hookworm infestation are considered in Chapter 22.5.2.

Malaria is still the most important parasitic illness of humans. Currently it is estimated that it has a global incidence of about 200 million cases per year, with over 1 million deaths. Its transmission and clinical manifestations are considered in Section 7. Profound anaemia is a major cause of mortality and morbidity during acute attacks of *P. falciparum* malaria in nonimmune individuals, but, from the perspective of health in the developing world, chronic infection with this organism in childhood is an extremely common cause of anaemia. This is most commonly seen in areas of high malarial transmission and is also a growing problem in regions of lower transmission because the rise in antimalarial drug resistance prolongs the average duration of infection. The anaemia of chronic malaria has a complex basis involving haemolysis, hypersplenism, and a suboptimal bone marrow response, often set against a background of iron or folate deficiency. In some populations, notably those of Africa, India, and parts of South-East Asia, chronic malarial infection may be complicated by the hyper-reactive malarial splenomegaly syndrome, in which hypersplenism plays a major role in the generation of chronic anaemia.

The haematological manifestations of the other common parasitic illnesses in the tropics are considered elsewhere.

Malabsorption

Many people in tropical climates, both indigenous populations and expatriates who have worked in rural areas, have abnormalities of the intestinal mucosa, often associated with impairment of absorption. These structural and functional alterations of the gut have been called 'tropical enteropathies' (see Chapter 15.10.8). It is likely that they result from adaptation to life in the contaminated environment of the tropics, with frequent gastrointestinal infections and differences of diet.

More severe malabsorption syndromes, called sprue and postinfective malabsorption, are associated with chronic diarrhoea, wasting, and a variable degree of anaemia. The pathophysiology and world distribution of these syndromes are considered in Section 15. They are nearly all associated with anaemia, which has a complex aetiology including folate deficiency and, in some cases, iron deficiency.

It should also be remembered that in a tropical setting malabsorption can also result from colonization of the small bowel by specific parasites, including *Giardia lamblia*, *Strongyloides stercalis*, cryptosporidium, and others. Abdominal tuberculosis with malabsorption is also common. In Africa, HIV infection is now an important cause of malabsorption.

Inherited anaemias

The inherited haemoglobin disorders are becoming an increasingly common cause of anaemia, particularly in tropical countries. They are described in detail in Chapter 22.5.7.

Because of heterozygote advantage against *P. falciparum* malaria, the important inherited haemoglobin disorders, notably sickle cell anaemia and the thalassaemias, have a high frequency throughout tropical populations of the Old World. Sickle cell anaemia and its variants are particularly common in Africa, some Mediterranean populations, and throughout the Middle East and parts of India.

They also occur at a high frequency in the Caribbean and in other regions with large African populations. The thalassaemias occur at a high frequency in parts of Africa, the Mediterranean, the Middle East, the Indian subcontinent, and throughout South-East Asia. There is now clear evidence that these conditions will produce a major public health problem in these countries in the future. As poorer countries go through the demographic transition, resulting from better hygiene and control of infectious illness, infants with these genetic anaemias are now surviving long enough to present for diagnosis and treatment. Some estimated figures for the annual numbers of new births of babies with sickle cell anaemia or β-thalassaemia are shown in Fig. 22.5.3.2.

The effect that a high frequency of a disease such as thalassaemia can have on the health economy of an emerging country was shown graphically in the case of Cyprus after it passed through the demographic transition in the 1950s. It was estimated that if every patient with this disease was treated with regular blood transfusion and appropriate medication, within 15 years the management of this one condition would consume up to 40% of the island's health budget. Recent studies in Indonesia indicate that, at a minimum estimate, approximately 1.25 million units of blood will be required each year to treat a proportion of the thalassaemic population in future years.

In many populations, there are hundreds of thousands of carriers for β-thalassaemia or the more common severe forms of α-thalassaemia. Although they are asymptomatic they have haemoglobin values which are, on average, 1 to 1.5 g/dl below normal. During pregnancy they retain this difference so that in the midtrimester they have haemoglobin values of approximately 8 g/dl or less. They have increased folate requirements and, in some populations, there appears to be an increased frequency of folate deficiency in pregnancy.

It should be remembered that the inherited anaemias may be exacerbated by other illnesses which are widespread in tropical

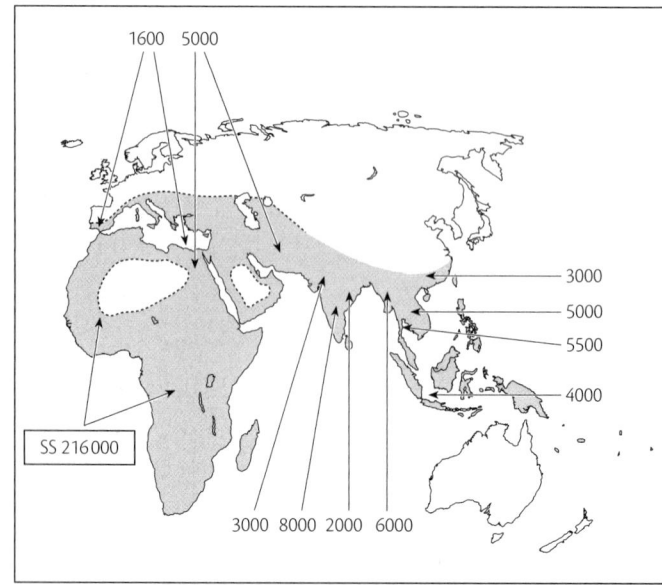

Fig. 22.5.3.2 Estimated annual numbers of births of babies with β-thalassaemia and sickle cell anaemia (SS).
(Original data in Weatherall DJ, Clegg JB (2001). *The thalassaemic syndromes*, 4th edition, p. 599. Blackwell, Oxford.)

countries. Folate requirements are increased in all these conditions and secondary folate deficiency is extremely common. They may also be exacerbated by malaria; children may develop malarial infection from infected blood donors. There is also a high frequency of other blood-borne infections, particularly hepatitis C and, in some populations, HIV. Furthermore, there is clear evidence that sickle cell anaemia and thalassaemia can render children more prone to infection. In short, like all forms of anaemia in the tropical world, the inherited disorders of haemoglobin may present with a complex series of complications due to a background of nutritional deficiency and a wide variety of infections.

These complex interactions have a dominant effect on the prognosis for the important inherited haemoglobin disorders. Early studies in Africa reported a marked paucity of patients with sickle cell anaemia despite a very high carrier frequency, indicating that very few patients with this disorder were surviving beyond early childhood. This may still be the case in parts of rural Africa. On the other hand, in more developed countries, and with a high quality of medical care, patients with this disease are regularly surviving into adult life; the mean survival time in the United States of America is now approximately 42 years, with many patients surviving to old age. A similar situation exists for β-thalassaemia. In poorer countries, supplies of blood may be limited, there may be difficulties in screening blood for agents such as hepatitis C and HIV, and the prohibitive cost of iron-chelating agents means that even children who receive transfusion die from iron loading before they reach the age of 20 years.

There are other inherited anaemias which are particularly common on tropical countries due to heterozygote advantage against malaria. Glucose-6-phosphate dehydrogenase deficiency is estimated to occur in some 100 million individuals world-wide. Its clinical and haematological manifestations are discussed in Chapter 22.5.12. They include haemolytic reactions to a wide variety of drugs, and, of particular public health significance, to certain foods (favism). There is a form of ovalocytosis, particularly common in Melanesia, which is associated with a mild and well compensated haemolytic anaemia. Recent studies have shown that carriers of Melanesian ovalocytosis are completely protected against cerebral malaria.

Consequences of anaemia

The results of many studies directed at determining the functional consequences of anaemia are still controversial. It is often difficult to distinguish between the effects of anaemia *per se* and the consequences of iron or folate deficiency on other physiological functions. Whatever the mechanism, chronic anaemia is associated with diminished function.

Many studies have suggested that even mild anaemia may reduce near-maximal work capacity. WHO has recently stressed the increasing evidence that iron deficiency in children may reduce intelligence and, in extreme cases, may lead to intellectual disability. There is no doubt that anaemia increases maternal mortality and morbidity. There is a very large literature on the effect of iron deficiency on resistance to infection, as mediated through either immune function or the bacteriostatic and bacteriocidal roles of iron-containing proteins such as transferrin and lactoferrin. The complex relationship between iron status and susceptibility of infection requires further work. It is clear that folate deficiency is associated with an increased prevalence of obstetric complications and fetal malformation, although its effect on intellectual and immune function is less clear.

In short, because of the remarkable ability of otherwise healthy individuals to adapt to moderate anaemia it seems likely that many of the associated manifestations which have been observed result from the effects of different deficiency states on other physiological functions rather than the anaemia *per se*. On the other hand, chronic severe anaemia, particularly in childhood, results in a wide variety of complications including failure of growth and development and, possibly, proneness to infection.

Prevention

It is beyond the scope of this brief review to discuss the protean aspects of the prevention of anaemia, particularly in poorer countries. Its high prevalence is a reflection of gross poverty, particularly as manifested by nutritional deficiency, infection, and malabsorption. Its control requires action on many different fronts, including improvements in diet, fortification of commonly eaten foods with iron, the use of modified milk formulae for infants, malaria and hookworm control, iron and folate supplementation in pregnancy, and all-round improvements in hygiene. The problem of the population control of sickle cell anaemia and thalassaemia is discussed in Chapter 22.5.7. Good antenatal care helps to prevent anaemia in childhood by reducing prematurity, increasing average birth weight, and improving the nutritional status of the newborn.

Further reading

Beales PF (1997). Anaemia in malaria control: a practical approach. *Ann Trop Med Parasitol*, **91**, 713–18.

DeMaeyer EM, Adiels-Tegman M (1985). The prevalence of anemia in the world. *World Health Statist Quart*, **38**, 302–16.

DeMaeyer EM, *et al.* (1989). *Preventing and controlling iron-deficiency anaemia through primary health care*. World Health Organization, Geneva.

Fleming AF (1989). Tropical obstetrics and gynaecology. 1. Anaemia in pregnancy in tropical Africa. *Trans R Soc Trop Med Hyg*, **83**, 441–8.

Gallacher PG, Ehrenkranz RA (1995). Nutritional anaemias in infancy. *Clin Perinatol*, **22**, 671–92.

Hercberg S, Galan P (1992). Nutritional anaemias. *Clin Haematol*, **5**, 143–68.

Khusun H, *et al.* (1999). World Health Organization hemoglobin cut-off points for the detection of anemia are valid for an Indonesian population. *J Nutr*, **129**, 1669–74.

Weatherall DJ, Kwiatkowski D, Roberts D (2009). Hematologic manifestations of systemic diseases in children of the developing world. In: Orkin, S.H. *et al.* (eds) *Nathan & Oski's Hematology of Infancy and Childhood*, 7th ed, pp. 1741–1768, W.B. Saunders, Philadelphia.

WHO (1968). *Nutritional anaemias*. Technical Report Series No. 405. World Health Organization, Geneva.

WHO (2002). *The world health report 2002—reducing risks, promoting healthy life*. World Health Organization, Geneva.

22.5.4 Iron metabolism and its disorders

Timothy M. Cox

Essentials

Iron is a component of haem proteins and nonhaem enzyme systems required for oxygen transport, mitochondrial respiration, and other key metabolic reactions. The metal exists in two readily interconvertible redox states (divalent ferrous and trivalent ferric iron) that are highly reactive and toxic to tissues. High-affinity iron-binding proteins, which form stable ferric complexes, have evolved to facilitate iron transport and delivery to sites of storage and utilization, including haem biosynthesis.

Iron homeostasis

Iron is an essential constituent of the diet, with the recommended daily allowance being 10 to 20 mg depending on the bioavailability of food iron components: haem iron may be more readily absorbed than inorganic iron; dietary phytates and some medications (e.g. antacids, proton pump inhibitors, H_2 antagonists) reduce iron absorption. The requirement for iron is greater in patients with recurrent bleeding, during pregnancy, and during periods of growth in childhood and adolescence.

Iron absorption—this occurs in the duodenum and upper jejunum. The processes are complex, but the following are involved: (1) divalent metal transporter protein (DMT1)—essential for uptake of ferrous ions; (2) ferrireductase—expression in the apical microvillous membrane of the intestinal mucosa appears to be induced in response to nutritional iron deficiency; (3) uptake of haem by enterocytes—probably mediated principally by an as-yet-unknown membrane protein; (4) ferroportin—mediates egress of ferric ions from enterocytes.

Body iron composition—most iron in the body is coordinated in protoporphyrin IX as haem. Small amounts of iron circulate in the plasma, bound in the ferric form to the glycoprotein transferrin. Iron is stored in the mononuclear phagocyte (reticuloendothelial) system principally as intracellular ferritin and its proteolytic degradation product, haemosiderin.

Iron homeostasis—this is maintained by rigorous control of absorption from the diet, which appears to be orchestrated principally by the actions of the peptide hormone, hepcidin, which is synthesized by the liver and regulates the process by inhibiting efflux of iron from enterocytes. The capacity for safe storage of iron in intracellular deposits (mainly in tissue macrophages) is limited, as is the physiological capacity for disposal of iron by excretion from the body.

Iron deficiency

Clinical features—the commonest manifestations are pallor, angular cheilosis, atrophic glossitis, and dystrophy of the nails with longitudinal ridging and koilionychia.

Investigation and diagnosis—iron deficiency results in a microcytic anaemia, usually in association with an unequivocal reduction in serum transferrin saturation (<16%) and a reduced serum ferritin concentration (<12 µg/litre). In many cases the cause will be obvious, e.g. menorrhagia in a young woman, but in other cases diligent investigation will be required, e.g. to diagnose or exclude colonic carcinoma.

Causes—iron-poor diets rarely cause iron-deficiency anaemia, except in growing children, and the following require consideration: (1) loss of iron—common causes include menstruation, pregnancy, from the gastrointestinal tract (hookworms, ulcerating lesions); (2) malabsorption of iron—e.g. coeliac disease.

Treatment—aside from dealing with the underlying cause, this involves iron-replacement therapy, which should normally be administered orally, although parenteral preparations are occasionally necessary.

Iron storage disease

Ferrous and ferric ions are chemically reactive so that excess of iron is toxic; tissues with elevated concentrations of the metal show functional impairment and structural injury leading to 'iron storage disease' (haemochromatosis).

Clinical features—these include (1) heart disease—cardiomyopathy leading to cardiac failure and/or (sometimes fatal) arrhythmia, which are a leading cause of death in refractory anaemias such as β-thalassaemia; (2) fibrotic liver disease; (3) endocrine failure—e.g. hypogonadotrophic hypogonadism, diabetes mellitus; and (4) skin and joint manifestations.

Investigation and diagnosis—iron storage disease is usually suspected on the basis of (1) raised serum ferritin measurements, and (2) when the saturation of serum transferrin is over 60%. Definitive diagnosis may require tissue biopsy and specific elemental analysis or histochemical staining for iron.

Causes—these are (1) genetic, hereditary, or primary haemochromatosis—see Chapter 12.7.1); or (2) secondary—including (a) diseases characterized by dyserythropoiesis—e.g. thalassaemia, sideroblastic anaemia—which are associated with increased dietary iron absorption by the intestine; (2) repeated blood transfusion.

Treatment—in the early stages, potentially fatal sequelae of iron toxicity can be prevented by prompt institution of measures to deplete iron: (1) where the bone marrow is normal—repeated venesection; (2) with disordered haematopoiesis—iron chelators; daily administration of parenteral desferrioxamine has provided the best standard of care, but this treatment is challenging for lifelong use, and powerful orally active chelators hold promise for improved acceptability in patients with better therapeutic efficacy overall.

Homeostasis, transport, and storage of iron

As a component of metalloenzymes and complexed to form haem, iron participates in the transport of oxygen by haemoglobin and myoglobin and in the harnessing of metabolic energy by cytochromes of the electron transport chain.

Iron is abundant in the environment and is a common element in the Earth's crust, but its electrochemistry poses exceptional problems for living organisms. The metal exists in two readily interconvertible redox states (divalent ferrous iron, Fe^{2+}, and trivalent ferric iron, Fe^{3+}) which are highly reactive. In the environment, most iron is oxidized to the trivalent state which, under neutral conditions, is then rapidly hydrolysed to insoluble polyhydroxide complexes which cannot be assimilated. High-affinity iron-binding proteins, which form stable ferric complexes, have evolved to facilitate iron transport and delivery to sites of storage and utilization, including haem biosynthesis. Free iron promotes formation of damaging oxygen free radicals, which mediate the injury to cells and tissues that characterizes iron storage disease. Iron is highly electroreactive, and readily catalyses formation of hydroxyl radicals as a result of interactions between superoxide and ferric ions. Tissues with significant iron storage show peroxidative injury in membrane lipid fractions; and, whatever their physiochemical basis, common mechanisms of iron toxicity clearly exist, since the pathological and clinical manifestations of all iron-storage syndromes, including secondary haemochromatosis associated with blood transfusion and the iron-loading anaemias, are almost identical. In disorders of iron overload the iron-binding capacity of plasma transferrin may be exceeded so that a proportion of the iron present in the blood remains reactive as a low-molecular-weight species only loosely attached to plasma proteins. Nontransferrin iron in human plasma stimulates the peroxidation of unsaturated lipids and can form reactive complexes that damage DNA—thus suggesting a mechanism for genome toxicity and carcinogenesis related to iron overload.

In humans, iron deficiency is probably the most frequent organic illness worldwide. It affects infants, children, young adults, and older people in many populations. Iron deficiency is associated with anaemia and nonhaematopoietic disturbances that impair work efficiency and contribute to chronic ill health as well as loss of mucosal integrity; iron-deficiency anaemia is frequently associated with pica, which has important environmental and behavioural associations with hookworm infection. In any event, the prevalence of iron deficiency provides strong evidence of the critical availability of iron as a key nutrient. The harmful effects of iron result directly from its electrochemical properties and potential to generate reactive oxygen and nitrogen species which injure cell structures—including DNA. There are many causes of excess iron in the tissues, but all represent disturbances of iron homeostasis that overwhelm the mechanisms which the body uses to acquire, transport, and store iron safely.

Body iron composition

The total amount of iron in the adult body is between 3 and 4 g, most of which is coordinated in protoporphyrin IX as haem (Fig. 22.5.4.1). Haem is found principally as haemoglobin and myoglobin, although appreciable quantities are found in the viscera, especially the liver, kidney, and intestine. Cytochromes of the electron transport chain and of the P450 system for the metabolism of xenobiotics are abundant in these organs and remarkably selective regions of the brain. In an adult, about 2.5 g of iron is complexed in haemoglobin with an additional 0.5 g as myoglobin in the muscles. In the plasma compartment, very small amounts of iron circulate, bound in the ferric form to the glycoprotein transferrin—this protein is normally only one-third saturated with iron, so that with a mean concentration of 3 g/litre for a protein of molecular weight

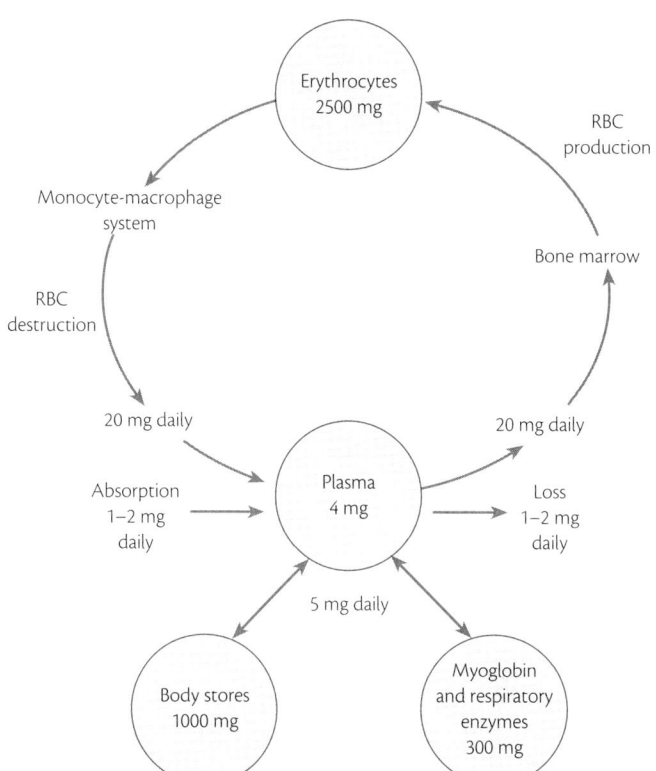

Fig. 22.5.4.1 Daily flux of iron through storage and transport compartments.

80 000, it represents less than 2 mg of elemental iron. The normal concentration of ferritin in the serum does not exceed about 250μg/litre; and like transferrin, this does not itself contain appreciable iron—nonetheless, serum ferritin faithfully reflects the stores of iron in the body. Iron is stored in the mononuclear phagocyte system (previously known as the reticuloendothelial system) principally as intracellular ferritin and its proteolytic degradation product, haemosiderin. Body iron stores do not exceed 1.5 g in men and are usually 0.5 g or less in adult women. Nonhaem deposits of iron that serve as stores in the iron-rich tissues may be visualized by staining with Perls's reagent (acid potassium ferrocyanide) with which they give a strong Prussian blue reaction. Faint staining with Perls's reagent may be observed in normal parenchymal liver cells, but in health the principal deposits of storage iron are observed in bone marrow and spleen macrophages as well as in Kupffer cells of the liver.

Erythropoiesis and iron balance

The mean lifespan of the red cell is 120 days and thus approximately 1% of the steady-state haemoglobin pool is turned over daily—this requires de novo synthesis of approximately 6 g of haemoglobin into which 20 mg of iron is incorporated. The principal fraction of the iron required for daily haemoglobin production in the basal state is recycled from senescent red cells after their destruction by macrophages; the iron is delivered to the erythron in the plasma by transferrin that binds to cell surface transferrin receptors on erythroid precursors (Fig. 22.5.4.1). The transferrin–receptor complex is internalized and, after acidification in endosomes, the iron is released leaving the apotransferrin to be recycled to the surface and reutilized. Transferrin is the principal mediator of iron delivery and transport about the body.

Under circumstances in which erythropoiesis is stimulated, e.g. under conditions of reduced oxygen saturation, after bleeding and haemolysis, as well as in dyserythropoietic conditions (including thalassaemia and megaloblastic anaemia), uptake and delivery of iron are greatly increased. Increased delivery of iron occurs in association with an expansion in the number of erythroid precursors that express cell surface transferrin receptors under the influence of the hepatorenal hormone, erythropoietin.

Iron homeostasis

Iron, an essential nutrient, is fastidiously conserved by the body and only a fraction of that which is utilized in the bone marrow is subject to obligatory daily losses through the exfoliation of epithelia and intercurrent blood loss, such as that incurred in trauma or menstruation. These requirements are met from the diet by the specific absorption of iron in the upper small intestine. The amount of iron available in the diet varies greatly, and even under optimal circumstances only a fraction is normally absorbed: in adult men the daily requirement is on average 0.8 mg, whereas in adult women of the reproductive age group, the requirement is usually more than 2 mg daily—the recommended daily allowance in the diet is 10 to 20 mg depending on the bioavailability of food iron components. Inorganic and haem iron complexes are released by digestion; there is a belief that haem iron may be more readily absorbed than inorganic iron in the human intestine and, depending principally on the content in meat, may constitute an important source of iron in nonvegetarians. Dietary phytates and medication including antacids and tetracycline antibiotics, as well as proton pump inhibitors, H_2 antagonists, and prior upper gastrointestinal surgery, strongly influence the intraluminal bioavailability and hence absorption of food iron. The requirement for iron is greater in patients with recurrent bleeding, or in those who are blood donors; iron requirements are also increased during periods of growth in childhood and adolescence. In pregnancy, the daily requirement may be as much as 5 mg and the maternal investment of iron, depending in part on peripartum blood losses, may be as much as 1.5 g—this greatly exceeds the savings due to the cessation of menstruation. Given its iron content, the exsanguination of 1 ml of blood constitutes a loss of approximately 0.5 mg of iron; this relationship facilitates estimates of iron requirements as a result of blood losses, e.g. those incurred by menorrhagia (>80 ml/month) or from other sources.

Iron absorption

In health, iron absorption in the duodenum and upper jejunum is a finely regulated process which matches the acquisition of iron from the diet to body requirements for erythropoiesis and to replace obligatory losses. Genetic studies of mutant strains of mice with abnormalities of iron metabolism have shed light on the iron-absorption mechanism. The divalent metal transporter protein, DMT 1, which is expressed in the upper small intestine and cells of the erythron, is essential for uptake of ferrous ions. The human *DMT1* gene maps to the long arm of chromosome 12 and encodes a 12 membrane-spanning protein that is expressed in the apical membrane of the upper intestine. DMT 1 is also produced in developing erythroid cells, in which it is responsible for the intracellular delivery of iron derived from transferrin for haemoglobin synthesis. Contemporaneous studies in experimental animals have identified a ferrireductase localized also to the intestinal brush-border membrane. Expression of mucosal ferrireductase is specific to the apical microvillous membrane of mammalian intestinal mucosa and appears to be induced in response to nutritional iron deficiency. Dietary iron is often present as a complex in haem—a component of haemoglobin, myoglobin, and tissue cytochromes. Haem iron occurs principally, but not exclusively in meat, which represents an important facultative source of iron in the diet of many humans. The uptake of haem by enterocytes is probably mediated principally by a membrane protein, but the molecular identity of this putative carrier entity has yet to be clarified. Egress of ferric ions from macrophages and enterocytes is mediated by a protein, ferroportin, which is localized to the basolateral membrane of intestinal epithelial cells; heterozygous deficiency of ferroportin gives rise to excess storage of iron in the macrophages. A putative copper protein, hephaestin, which maps to the X chromosome and has sequence similarity to caeruloplasmin, apparently mediates oxidation of ferrous iron and cooperates functionally with ferroportin in promoting the transepithelial transport of iron in enterocytes.

Under conditions of iron deficiency or on depletion of body iron stores, a greater proportion of the bioavailable iron is assimilated by the intestine. Hypoxia similarly increases the absorptive capacity of the small intestine. For reasons that are not fully understood, certain anaemias, particularly those associated with ineffective erythropoiesis and dyserythropoiesis, are also associated with enhanced absorption of iron in the intestine. Where the anaemia is long-standing, e.g. congenital or acquired sideroblastic anaemia, or in haemoglobinopathies such as β thalassaemia, inappropriate intestinal absorption of iron which accompanies massive expansion of the erythropoietic marrow, may be such as to cause iron overload leading to tissue injury—secondary haemochromatosis—even in the absence of iron loading from multiple transfusions of red cells.

The regulation of iron balance by the intestine normally protects the body from iron-rich diets; only under exceptional circumstances, such as the ingestion of alcoholic beverages containing abundant iron as a result of toxic manufacturing processes (e.g. the kaffir beers that are fermented in iron pots by the South African Bantu), does excess dietary iron lead to iron storage disease. It seems probable that those individuals who develop iron storage disease because of long-standing excessive ingestion of highly available iron, do so as a result of the operation of genetic cofactors such as mutant alleles of the adult haemochromatosis gene product, *HFE*, or because of an underlying haematological disorder such as α- or β thalassaemia trait.

Hepcidin, a member of a family of cysteine-rich peptides with antimicrobial activities, is an 'iron hormone' which regulates iron metabolism by inhibiting efflux of iron from macrophages and enterocytes. Deficiency of hepcidin is associated with iron overload, while excess release of hepcidin inhibits the release of iron from the storage compartment and reduces the net absorption of iron. One action of hepcidin appears to be mediated by binding to the ferric ion transporter ferroportin; hepcidin induces the endocytosis and intracellular breakdown of ferroportin and thus diminishes efflux of iron from enterocytes and macrophages into the bloodstream. In hepcidin-deficient humans (with juvenile haemochromatosis) and mice, intestinal absorption of iron proceeds in an unrestrained manner and marked storage excess with parenchymal injury results. Lattely it has been shown that bone morphogenetic protein (BMP) signalling induces hepcidin expression as a result of activation of serine/threonine kinases present on the surface of liver parenchymal cells: this effect is apparently mediated by phosphorylation of several of a group of intracellular transducing molecules (receptor-regulated or R-Smads), which then form heteromeric molecular complexes with the mediator Smad 4. After translocation to the cell nucleus, R-Smad—Smad 4 complexes appear to promote transcription of specific genes including hepcidin. The large multidomain molecule haemojuvelin—mutations in the gene for which, as with hepcidin, induce early-onset or juvenile haemochromatosis in humans—appears also to be a coreceptor for bone morphogenetic protein signalling in the regulation of hepcidin expression. At the time of writing however, all the molecules that interact with haemojuvelin in this pathway, including the range of bone morphogenetic protein ligands, have yet to be identified.

Recently several members of a Sardinian family have been reported with microcytic anaemia due to defective iron absorption and utilization: iron-deficiency anaemia unresponsive to oral iron and only partially responsive to parenteral iron administration was inherited as a recessive trait. After excluding the involvement of known genes implicated in iron metabolism, a genome-wide search identified a locus encompassing the matriptase-2 gene *TMPRSS6* (also known as transmembrane protease, serine 6), which was shown to harbour a homozygous splicing mutation, predicted partially to inactivate protease function. Plasma and urinary hepcidin concentrations were later shown to be inappropriately elevated. The corresponding murine gene (*Tmprss6*) has been shown to be an essential component of a pathway that is sensitive to iron lack and suppresses the release of hepcidin. Finally, there is considerable research activity in the field of iron sensing; although little is known about the means by which cells detect hypoxia and iron requirements, complex molecular interactions between the HFE protein (mutations in which predispose to adult haemochromatosis) and transferrin–transferrin receptors 1 and 2 have been strongly implicated in this process. At the time of writing, however, these putative interactions are based largely on inferences from structural analysis of soluble protein complexes *in vitro* and confocal microscopy.

Evaluation of body iron status

Clinical features

The most useful clinical measures of iron status include the detection of pallor and nonerythropoietic manifestations of disease including angular cheilosis, atrophic glossitis, and dystrophy of the nails with longitudinal ridging and koilonychia; moderate hair loss may also be a feature of integumental iron deficiency. Iron deficiency induces behavioural changes in experimental animals. In humans, unusual syndromes of food craving (pica) have long been recognized and usually respond to iron supplementation: this includes craving for soils and the ingestion of silica-rich earths as a cult practice in black populations of the southern United States of America—geophagia. Pagophagia (ice-craving) combined with the abnormal taste preferences of pregnancy may account for the bizarre food craving that constitutes part of the folklore of pregnancy. Severe iron deficiency may occasionally be associated with splenomegaly and the signs of underlying disease include peripheral oedema (hypoalbuminaemia associated with massive hookworm infection) and oronasal and palatal telangiectasia associated with Osler–Rendu–Weber disease (hereditary haemorrhagic telangiectasia).

Laboratory findings

The most useful measurements, apart from those identifying the hypochromic microcytic anaemia accompanied by abnormal blood cell indices and confirmed by microscopy of the blood film, involve surrogate measures of body iron stores. A raised platelet count suggests a haemorrhagic cause of the iron-deficiency anaemia. Iron-deficient erythropoiesis is associated with failure to utilize free protoporphyrin in red cell precursors and thus a raised free erythrocyte protoporphyrin concentration in the peripheral blood; this may be easily identified by the use of portable fluorimeters using only a few microlitres of blood drawn, for example, as part of population screening.

In iron-deficiency anaemia, the absolute concentration of transferrin is raised: there is an increase in transferrin iron-binding capacity (TIBC), which is reflected by a decrease in serum iron and serum iron transferrin saturation. Such measurements may often serve to discriminate the hypochromic microcytic anaemias of thalassaemia and sideroblastic anaemia from true iron-deficiency anaemia. Such discrimination is vital before a commitment to treatment by iron supplementation is undertaken.

Measurement of the serum ferritin is often helpful in iron deficiency; serum ferritin concentrations are low, reflecting reduced or absent body iron stores. Neither the serum transferrin saturation nor serum ferritin, however, are absolutely infallible measures of iron deficiency: serum transferrin iron saturation may be artificially elevated with a low transferrin and low serum iron in chronic inflammatory states associated with the anaemias of chronic disorders. Likewise, serum ferritin serves as an acute-phase reactant and may be elevated in malignant disease (especially lymphomas including Hodgkin's disease), or released from the liver in hepatitis and in chronic inflammatory states. Recently there are advocates for the measurement of free circulating transferrin receptors which may be determined by immunoassay. Expression of soluble transferrin receptor protein is enhanced under conditions of iron deficiency and plasma concentrations are elevated in the presence of functionally iron-deficient erythropoiesis; however, greatly increased serum transferrin receptor concentrations are found under conditions of erythroid hyperplasia in the bone marrow and especially when ineffective erythropoiesis occurs (megaloblastic anaemia, haemoglobinopathies, sideroblastic anaemia).

Staining of iron stores in the bone marrow with Perls's reagent is a robust and relatively simple method for resolving difficulties that arise in the investigation of patients with suspected iron-deficiency anaemia. Although an examination of the amount of iron (usually graded semiquantitatively on a scale from 0 to 4, reflecting the strength of Prussian blue staining) does not provide any information as to the availability of the iron for haemoglobin formation, it does provide useful information as to the appropriateness of iron therapy for hypochromic anaemia. Bone marrow examination, moreover, may be diagnostic in patients suffering from hypochromic anaemias due to primary or sideroblastic change in the marrow, since the characteristic ring sideroblasts with or without other myeloblastic changes will be apparent.

In summary, the laboratory evaluation of patients with suspected iron deficiency should include a full examination of haematological parameters including microscopy of the blood film. Quantification of serum iron, serum transferrin, and transferrin saturation (TIBC) may be valuable in establishing the cause of the hypochromic or microcytic anaemia. Serum ferritin measurements are often confirmatory in the absence of malignant, hepatitic, or other inflammatory diseases—as may fluorimetric red-cell zinc protoporphyrin assays. Determinations of serum transferrin receptor concentration may provide evidence of increased demands for iron by the marrow or indeed expansion of the erythron, but this test is not universally available. Microscopic examination of a bone marrow aspirate, including staining with Perls's reagent, may provide valuable information about iron stores in macrophages and the need for iron supplementation.

Disturbances of iron metabolism

Disorders of iron metabolism are common contributory factors in disease: iron deficiency is rife, particularly among those living in poverty, others whose access to meat is limited, and those in whom hookworm infestation occurs. At the same time, the prevalence of haemoglobinopathies and other anaemias such as myelodysplasia and sideroblastic syndromes that require transfusion and cause hyperabsorption of iron associated with ineffective erythropoiesis mean that iron storage disease also represents a major world health problem. In addition, as discussed in Chapter 11.7.1, hereditary haemochromatosis occurs at a high gene frequency in certain populations: this includes peoples of north European descent (adult haemochromatosis, due to mutations in *HFE*) and those of sub-Saharan African origin (African iron overload), in whom the nature of the predisposing gene is unknown.

Iron deficiency

About 30% of the world's population—nearly 2 billion people—is anaemic, and at least half of these are believed to have iron-deficiency anaemia. Even in rich countries, such as the United States of America and Europe, up to 20% of menstruating women have signs of iron deficiency. In children and young adults, there is a frequency of between 5 and 10% of iron-deficiency anaemia—particularly in deprived socioeconomic groups.

Many population studies have in the past been based on erroneous attribution of anaemia solely to iron deficiency: there are many conditions, including the anaemia of chronic disorders and haemoglobinopathies such as β thalassaemia trait,that lead to hypochromic or microcytic red-cell indices. Population surveys based on the detection of iron-deficient erythropoiesis, especially those using determination of free red-cell zinc protoporphyrin concentrations by fluorimetry, may enhance the detection of true iron-deficiency anaemia; determinations of serum ferritin concentrations also facilitate discrimination between the anaemia of chronic disease and true iron deficiency.

Causative factors

Iron-deficiency anaemia in populations is often attributed solely to an iron-poor diet, but in the absence of significant blood loss or intestinal parasites including hookworm, even the most iron-poor diets rarely cause iron-deficiency anaemia, except in growing children. The amount of iron required to repair obligatory losses is very small, so that at least 90% of the iron required for *de novo*

haemoglobin formation in erythropoiesis is retrieved from senescent erythrocytes broken down by the mononuclear phagocyte system. Furthermore, once iron deficiency develops, striking adaptive changes occur in the absorptive mechanism for iron in the upper small intestine. In experimental animals with iron deficiency, mucosal expression of the divalent metal transporter 1 (DMT 1), on the brush border membrane of the intestinal epithelium, is induced. Iron-deficiency anaemia is also associated with enhanced intestinal expression of mucosal ferrireductase activity.

These changes do not represent the complete portfolio of adaptive changes that occur in response to iron deficiency. There is evidence that iron deficiency is associated with the recruitment of a greater length of mucosal surface in the upper small intestine for participation in the absorption of luminal iron. Iron deficiency, and the response to the removal of a unit of blood, may increase the overall absorptive efficiency of the intestine for iron up to tenfold—thus greatly enhancing the bioavailability of dietary iron.

Alcoholic beverages may provide a source of iron, and the absorption of haem iron present in red meat, poultry, and fish is usually between 15 and 35%. Between 2 and 20% of nonhaem iron present in fruit and vegetable sources is absorbed. Natural enhancers of iron absorption such as ascorbic acid, which maintains ferrous iron in its reduced form in the intestinal lumen, promote direct uptake by DMT 1. Fructose and other organic compounds of low molecular weight also form soluble and reduced complexes with iron released from nonhaem sources in food. In the West, normal individuals ingest between about 10 and 15 mg of iron daily. Adult men with normal iron stores absorb approximately 2% of the nonhaem iron ingested, whereas men with iron deficiency absorb more than 20% of iron from this source in the diet; the comparable figures for haem iron are 26 and 47%, respectively.

Many compounds present in the diet also inhibit or impede the absorption of iron released by digestion in the lumen. These compounds include tannin, especially present in tea, phytates present in bran and nuts, dietary fibre, and other inhibitory factors such as drugs, including tetracycline and alkalis. Some vegetarians of Asian origin ingest large amounts of phosphate and phytates which inhibit the absorption of iron provided in diets that may contain up to 30 mg of assayable total iron each day. A typical example is spinach which, although rich in iron, leads to the appearance of black stools when consumed in small or moderate amounts; these stools are black because of the passage of iron through the small intestine and its delivery to the colon where it forms insoluble ferrous sulphide complexes through the action of colonic sulphur-reducing bacteria.

Malabsorption of iron

The inability to release and absorb adequate amounts of iron from the diet is an important but unusual cause of iron deficiency. Disease of the stomach, duodenum, and upper jejunum may be responsible for the malabsorption of food iron, which may not be readily detected by studies involving the use of simple radioactive tracer measurements. On the other hand, properly conducted radioactive food labelling studies show that after gastric bypass surgery and after intestinal resection, there is malabsorption of nonhaem and haem food iron sources. Rarely, iron deficiency may result from inflammatory disease of the upper intestine that causes malabsorption: coeliac disease in infants and adults may be responsible, and the iron deficiency may be combined with deficiency of folic acid. Sometimes large pharmacological doses of iron with or without folic acid may overcome the anaemia caused by coeliac disease, but unless a strict gluten-free diet is instituted the anaemia recurs rapidly after iron therapy is stopped. Although malabsorption of food iron is an important aspect of the iron deficiency associated with coeliac disease, loss of iron exacerbates the effects of malabsorption. In coeliac disease this results from increased exfoliation of the epithelium in association with crypt hyperplasia and bleeding due to ulceration. The abnormal motility and maldigestion associated with upper gastrointestinal surgery compounded by anacidity caused by gastritis, or acid-suppressing agents, also impair the absorption of food iron. Bariatric surgery, which leads to diminished gastric acid secretion and bypasses the duodenum, is frequently complicated by iron-deficiency anaemia; prophylactic supplementation is thus recommended after this procedure, particularly in menstruating women.

Loss of iron

Women in the reproductive age group lose iron regularly at menstruation. An increased recommended daily allowance for women is higher than in all other groups: the average requirement for healthy menstruating women is approximately 1.4 mg of iron daily to replace losses, compared with normal men who lose about 0.8 to 0.9 mg of iron per day. Pregnancy is often associated with iron deficiency when growth of the fetus is rapid. Twin pregnancies and frequent childbirth, especially in women of low socioeconomic groups, are associated with iron-deficiency anaemia. Although anaemia is important, a very large study has been conducted that shows no reliable association between maternal anaemia and the complications of pregnancy, including preterm labour. Pregnancy itself is associated with the development of adaptive responses in the intestine and iron transport proteins that enhance the avidity of the gastrointestinal tract for bioavailable food iron. Clearly socioeconomic and sociopolitical considerations are likely to influence the population occurrence of iron deficiency in women of the reproductive age group, particularly since the investment of about 1 to 1.5 g of iron occurs with each pregnancy carried to term. This estimate includes blood loss associated with the birth and the investment of iron placed in human milk, which contains up to 0.5 mg/litre of iron bound to a whey protein, lactoferrin.

Other sources of iron loss

Intestinal parasites

Several hundred million people are heavily infested with hookworms. The two common hookworms of humans are *Anclyostoma duodenale* and *Necator americanus*. These helminths attach themselves to the lining of the small intestine by their buccal capsules and cause chronic blood loss by sucking blood from the intestinal villi. Hookworm infestation may be light, so that iron loss is not sufficient to cause iron deficiency. In hookworm disease, involving Old World and New World hookworms, heavy infestation occurs as a result of repeated exposure of the skin to contaminated soil. Mucosal immunity may also be reduced in the susceptible host. Although it is not known exactly what hookworms abstract from human blood, microscopic preparations show red cells expelled from the worm: each *Anclyostoma* induces the loss of up to 300 μl of blood daily, whereas each *Necator* causes the loss of up to 50 μl of blood. Clearly the occurrence of anaemia is dependent on the iron content of the diet, the extent of tissue iron stores, and the duration and intensity of the mucosal helminth infestation itself.

Since up to two-thirds of the haemoglobin iron released by the worms can be reabsorbed in the intestine, significant anaemia requires a very heavy parasite load; nonetheless, extremely severe anaemia may develop in patients with hookworm disease with all the attendant symptoms of fatigue, dyspnoea, palpitations, and mental changes—including pica. Nonspecific abdominal pain may occur and radiographic examination of the intestine or endoscopy may reveal duodenitis with a punctate inflammation associated with partial villus atrophy of the duodenojejunal mucosa. Oedema may result from cardiac failure in severe cases and also in association with hypoalbuminaemia, since heavy infestation may lead to significant protein-losing enteropathy. Hookworm disease may be associated with other helminth infections such as strongyloidiasis and ascariasis and itself may contribute to poor socioeconomic circumstances as a result of incapacity for work due to illness.

Hookworm parasites are widely distributed in southern Europe, Africa, the Middle East the Indian subcontinent, eastern Asia, and the New World, including southern United States of America. The heaviest infections usually affect rural workers in agricultural communities where repeated exposure occurs in isolated locations and where crops are harvested under conditions of poor sanitation. The iron-deficiency anaemia of hookworm disease may present difficulties for diagnosis when the mucosal inflammation that accompanies heavy infestation is associated with reduction in serum proteins such as albumin and transferrin; this, combined with an acute-phase response, may at first lead to a mistaken diagnosis of the anaemia of chronic disorders. Hookworm infestation as a cause of maternal anaemia is under-recognized, and this has inhibited the use of anthelmintic treatment in health provision for pregnant women. A recent study in sub-Saharan Africa estimated that nearly 40 million women of reproductive age are infected with hookworm; of these, about 7 million were pregnant in 2005. As expected, increasing intensity of infestation was associated with lower haemoglobin concentrations in pregnant women in poor countries. Given the number of pregnant women with hookworm and at risk of preventable hookworm-related anaemia, more studies on the potential benefit of anthelmintic treatment are warranted.

Other sources of blood loss

The gastrointestinal tract represents an important source of blood loss which should always be considered in patients with iron-deficiency anaemia. Ulcerating lesions of the small and large intestine, including cancers, are frequent causes of iron-deficiency anaemia. However, chronic intermittent bleeding can arise from unusual sources such as Meckel's diverticula, angiodysplastic lesions, hamartomas, and other benign ulcerating tumours such as leiomyomas. Gastric ulcers may be associated with chronic intermittent bleeding, but duodenal ulcers rarely cause chronic gastrointestinal blood loss.

Oesophageal ulceration and inflammatory lesions can cause iron-deficiency anaemia, but precaution is needed in attributing blood loss sufficient to cause iron deficiency to such a source unless other potential sites of bleeding have been excluded. Other unusual sources of gastrointestinal bleeding include multiple telangiectatic lesions of Osler–Rendu–Weber disease (hereditary haemorrhagic telangiectasia)—in which bleeding may occur anywhere from the nasal or oropharynx down to the stomach and upper intestine. The blue bleb naevus syndrome, the Peutz–Jeghers syndrome, and other hereditary gut polyposes are rare causes of chronic gastrointestinal bleeding. Inflammatory disease of the lower small intestine and colon such as Crohn's disease and ulcerative colitis, usually associated with chronic intestinal blood loss, may present with an abdominal history in which iron-deficiency anaemia is prominent. Very occasionally, artefactual iron-deficiency anaemia due to self-bleeding may occur; blood may be removed from any source but bizarre methods may be adopted to conceal it, thus requiring considerable ingenuity, and often detective work, to identify the cause. Because of the striking appearance of expectorated blood, iron-deficiency anaemia associated with frank haemoptosis requires little diagnostic skill, but occasionally recurrent intra-alveolar lung haemorrhage causes unexplained illness and anaemia. Occasionally, iron may be lost in the urine through the kidney in conditions where chronic intravascular haemolysis occurs. Losses may be sufficient to induce iron deficiency in the absence of marked changes in urine colour. Patients with haemolysis due to prosthetic or paraprosthetic cardiac valve malfunction may be revealed by the presence of characteristic red-cell changes; likewise in paroxysmal nocturnal haemoglobinuria, chronic intravascular haemolysis causes chronic urinary iron loss with or without visible haemoglobinuria. In these circumstances, free haemoglobin is released which quickly saturates the capacity of the plasma protein haemopexin to bind it; free haemoglobin spills into the glomerular filtrate where it is taken up by the proximal tubular cells and degraded. After degradation to haemosiderin, iron is lost in the urine when the iron-loaded epithelial cells are exfoliated.

Clinical and laboratory features of iron deficiency

Symptoms of iron deficiency include fatigue, pallor, palpitations, irritability, and little-recognized mental changes, such as pica. The patient may complain of a sore tongue, deleterious changes in the appearance of hair or hair loss, and angular cheilosis. Examination of the nails may reveal longitudinal ridging and, most often in elderly women with chronic iron deficiency for many years, koilionychia. There may be a complaint of dysphagia associated with the development of an oesophageal web (Patterson–Brown–Kelly or Plummer–Vinson syndrome). This again usually occurs in elderly or middle-aged women with chronic iron deficiency. A small proportion of patients with iron-deficiency anaemia have detectable but modest splenomegaly.

Diagnosis

Blood parameters will reveal microcytic anaemia usually in association with an unequivocal reduction in serum transferrin saturation (<16%) and a reduced serum ferritin concentration (<12 µg/litre). The absence of these features and of an acute-phase reactive response may suggest dyserythropoietic or sideroblastic anaemia or β thalassaemia trait. Lead poisoning may be associated with iron-deficient indices, with or without full-blown sideroblastic changes. A bone marrow aspirate stained with Perls's reagent for iron in marrow macrophages will rapidly confirm reduced or absent stainable iron in the storage compartment and may also be revealing about other aspects of the anaemia, such as the presence of ring sideroblasts, dyserythropoietic features, and/or megaloblastic change.

The presence of immunoreactive serum transferrin receptors may provide additional evidence in favour of iron-deficiency anaemia, but because increased serum concentration of these receptors may be observed in several disorders of the bone marrow and the ELISA tests are relatively expensive, the role of this determination in the routine diagnosis of iron deficiency is not as yet established. Red-cell zinc protoporphyrin concentrations greater than 35 µg/dl of whole blood are usually observed in patients with iron deficiency; values greater than 100 µg/dl are generally associated with lead toxicity. Extremely high values may indicate the presence of erythropoietic protoporphyria or lead poisoning in the latter, free, rather than zinc protoporphyrin IX accumulates. Modest elevations in erythrocyte protoporphyrin can be observed in patients with haemolytic anaemias, sideroblastic anaemia, and occasionally, the anaemia of chronic disorders.

Investigations and management

The identification of iron-deficiency anaemia should be regarded in a sense as a symptom rather than a diagnosis of a patient's malady: the management of those affected should always include an attempt to determine the cause. Common errors occur when, in elderly patients, iron deficiency is cynically ascribed to the presence of mild oesophagitis or gastritis observed at endoscopy, when the underlying cause is bleeding due to a coincidental but sinister gastrointestinal cancer elsewhere—and for which a diligent search is often required.

A full evaluation of the patient with iron deficiency should include an adequate dietary history including the consumption of drugs, such as aspirin and nonsteroidal anti-inflammatory drugs, which may be responsible for gastrointestinal bleeding. An enquiry should be made about additional gastrointestinal symptoms and other signs of blood loss; reasonable attempts should be made to evaluate the extent of menstrual loss, if the bleeding is to be ascribed to menorrhagia in women of reproductive age. Attention should be paid to the family history and a travel history to exclude causes such as hereditary haemorrhagic telangiectasia or hookworm disease.

Clinical examination should extend from an enquiry about previous gastrointestinal disease or surgery to an examination for visceral enlargement, abdominal lymphadenopathy, splenomegaly, and other features suggestive of intra-abdominal pathology such as portal hypertension and abdominal cancer. Hereditary haemorrhagic telangiectasia may be detected by the presence of the most subtle oronasal or palatal lesions.

With patients in whom the cause of the iron deficiency is not apparent, further studies may be needed to search for gastrointestinal bleeding, including detection of occult faecal blood on several samples taken consecutively. Endoscopic and radiographic studies of the gastrointestinal tract and serological studies for the presence of coeliac disease may be required and occasionally there is a need to quantify the amount of blood loss daily in the faeces or during menstrual flow by using radiolabelled chromium red-cell studies. In difficult cases, percutaneous visceral angiography of the coeliac and mesenteric arteries has proved invaluable for detecting sites of active gastrointestinal bleeding that are beyond the reach of conventional endoscopic procedures; in those patients who are actively bleeding, such a procedure can identify local sites of blood loss greater than 0.5 to 1.0 ml/min. The recent introduction of fibre optic double-balloon enteroscopy and wireless capsule endoscopy now offers powerful means to examine the entire small-intestinal mucosa extensively for the presence of bleeding lesions.

Meckel's diverticulum is a potential cause of obscure gastrointestinal bleeding in young adults and children. Some Meckel's diverticula can be diagnosed by scintigraphic studies using technetium-99m labelled pertechnetate which may be concentrated in the ectopic gastric mucosa. Meckel's diverticulum and intestinal strictures, particularly in the ileum, may be occasionally revealed by retrograde colonic contrast radiographic studies. Other diagnostic tests include searching for endomysial (transglutaminase) antibodies, with confirmatory duodenojejunal biopsy to detect coeliac disease. Examination of the urine and sometimes sputum may be required to detect occult iron loss in exfoliated macrophages or proximal tubular cells, respectively, where intrapulmonary haemorrhage or renal iron loss is suspected.

Sometimes extensive diagnostic procedures fail to identify the cause of iron deficiency when occult gastrointestinal bleeding is responsible. Under these circumstances, it remains appropriate to conduct a diagnostic laparotomy, after consultation with an experienced surgeon, to identify the bleeding lesion. In adults of any age, an appreciable number of obscure gastrointestinal malignancies or treatable benign tumours can be identified by such a procedure which, when combined with angiography with or without enteroscopy, may permit identification of angiodysplastic lesions at remote sites. In younger adults and children, diagnostic laparotomy may be indicated to identify Meckel's diverticula, intestinal stricture, and congenital abnormalities such as duplications that serve as occult sources of blood loss.

It is not unusual for the patient with recurrent chronic iron-deficiency anaemia to present a challenge for diagnosis. Even the most experienced physician would be well advised to consult widely with colleagues with expertise in radiology, nuclear medicine, and surgery before either prematurely abandoning the search for the causal lesion or for an ill-considered laparotomy without a thorough appreciation of the further difficulties it may pose.

Replenishing iron stores is but one aspect of the treatment of iron-deficiency anaemia. Iron should be replaced not only to restore the normal haemoglobin concentration but to replenish body iron stores. It is necessary to replace iron depleted in systemic tissues such as the muscles, where it is an essential component of cytochromes and other enzymes critical for optimal aerobic metabolism. Occasionally a therapeutic trial of oral iron for a defined period may be used to verify the suspected diagnosis of iron-deficiency anaemia. Adequate replacement of iron should be monitored for its effects: a reticulocyte response should be observed in peripheral blood maximally between the 7th and 10th days after initiating treatment and significant increases in blood haemoglobin concentration should be apparent within 2 to 4 weeks. If there is no evidence of continued blood loss, the haemoglobin concentration should come within the normal range within 2 months. Failure to meet these expectations suggests either that the anaemia is not caused by iron deficiency or that there is continued depression of bone marrow function—or that there is bleeding for which further investigation is needed.

Therapeutic preparations of iron

Iron salts should be administered by mouth unless there are overwhelming reasons for using the parenteral route—parenteral preparations of iron are associated with a greatly increased risk of toxicity. Iron–dextran complex and the newer iron–sucrose preparation are associated with hypersensitivity, including severe anaphylactoid reactions. Oral ferrous salts are better absorbed than ferric salts and show little difference amongst preparations in terms of rate of repair of anaemia at a given dosage of elemental iron.

It is usual to treat iron-deficiency anaemia with at least 100 to 200 mg of elemental iron daily. For full-blown iron-deficiency anaemia, ferrous sulphate is administered three times daily (equivalent to 3×65 mg of elemental iron). Some patients are unable to tolerate such a dose of iron because of constipation, diarrhoea, or abdominal pain; the presence of tarry, black stools may interfere with personal hygiene and thus lead to ultimate rejection of iron therapy by the patient. Under these circumstances the dose of iron may be reduced and this, rather than a change of iron salt preparation, usually improves tolerability. The frequency of unwanted effects with ferrous sulphate is the same as that of other iron salts when compared with the amount of elemental iron ingested. Once established, the optimal therapeutic response to oral iron increases the blood haemoglobin concentration by 0.1 to 0.2 g/dl per day. Replenishment of iron has a slow effect on the epithelial changes of iron deficiency and the atrophic glossitis may take several months to improve as iron stores are replenished.

Slow-release oral preparations of iron are available, which the manufacturers often claim release sufficient iron over a 24-h period for optimal haematological responses after once daily dosages. However, these preparations are likely to distribute the iron beyond the upper jejunum and thereby bypass those regions of the intestine in which iron absorption is most avid. Compound preparations of iron including B vitamins and folic acid are available, but there is little justification for prescribing these except for prophylactic use in pregnancy (see below). In infants and children, sugar-free preparations of iron complexes are available in the form of polysaccharide iron or iron–sodium EDTA (sodium ironedetate) complexes, which can be used as recommended by the manufacturer. In premature infants, up to 2.5 ml of syrup containing approximately 5 mg/ml may be used twice daily; up to 5 ml three times daily may be given to children aged 6 to 12 years.

Pregnancy

Prophylactic iron preparations are recommended in pregnant women who have risk factors for iron deficiency such as poor diet or prior menorrhagia, or those in whom gastric surgery has been carried out. Prophylactic iron may also be used in the management of infants of low birth weight including premature babies, twins, and infants delivered by caesarean section. Compound preparations of iron with folic acid may be used for the treatment of iron and folic acid deficiencies in pregnancy. For the prevention of neural tube defects in women planning a pregnancy, the United Kingdom Department of Health advises that a medicinal or food supplement of 400 µg/day of folic acid be taken before conception and during the first 12 weeks of pregnancy. Lone or combined iron compound preparations are not routinely indicated for prophylaxis in patients with chronic haemolysis or in renal dialysis since they may lead, in the circumstances of dyserythropoiesis, to chronic iron overload and secondary haemochromatosis.

Parenteral preparations of therapeutic iron

Given its potential toxicity, the only justification for the use of parenteral iron is in patients who are unable to cooperate with or tolerate oral iron therapy, or those with severe gastrointestinal disease that causes malabsorption or continuing severe blood loss.

Provision of iron by the parenteral route does not normally lead to more rapid repair of anaemia than when adequate oral iron preparations are administered. Some patients with renal failure who receive haemodialysis have obligatory blood losses which cannot be treated adequately with oral iron preparations. These patients, and occasional patients receiving peritoneal dialysis, may require intravenous iron regularly. Two parenteral preparations of iron are now available in the United Kingdom: a ferric hydroxide–sucrose complex containing 20 mg/ml of iron (2%) and ferric hydroxide with dextran that consists of a colloidal stabilized preparation of iron containing 50 mg/ml. Severe sensitivity reactions to these agents may occur and facilities for cardiopulmonary resuscitation should be at hand with the use of either therapeutic iron preparation.

A very small test dose is recommended. Administration of these preparations should not be followed by oral iron therapy until at least 5 days after the last injection.

Unwanted and toxic effects of parenteral iron preparations

A history of allergic disorders including asthma, eczema, and prior anaphylaxis are regarded as contraindications to the use of parenteral iron, as is liver disease and concurrent infection. Moreover, these drugs are not recommended for children. Side effects include nausea, vomiting, taste disturbances, hypotension, parasthesias, abdominal disorders, fever, flushing, anaphylactoid reactions, and the reactivation of inflammatory arthropathy. Injection site reactions, including phlebitis, have been reported. Parenteral iron should probably be avoided in patients with pre-existing cardiac disease including arrythmias or angina. Parenteral iron is contraindicated in children below the age of 14 years.

Administration

Iron–dextran may be given by deep intramuscular injection into the gluteal region, as well as by slow intravenous injection. Iron–sucrose complex may be given slowly intravenously or by intravenous infusion. In both instances the total dose is calculated according to body weight and the presumed iron deficit set out in the manufacturer's product literature. At least 15 min, with close observation, should elapse after the test dose before the therapeutic dose is administered.

General aspects of iron therapy

Treatment of causes of anaemia, including bleeding, is clearly a critical aspect of the management of iron-deficiency anaemia and its diagnosis. Coeliac disease should be treated with a gluten-free diet; bleeding lesions in the gastrointestinal tract may require definitive surgery directed to their healing. Occasionally, patients with a chronic bleeding disorder for which surgery is not indicated, such as hereditary haemorrhagic telangiectasia, may require long-term iron supplementation at doses less than that required to treat the acute iron-deficiency state. Periodic monitoring is required to ensure that the level of iron replacement is adequate to meet the demands of the bone marrow for *de novo* haem synthesis and that iron overload is not occurring. It should be recognized that relief of iron deficiency will improve many symptoms suffered by a patient even though they may suffer from an incurable underlying disease.

Treatment with iron should be continued until iron stores are replenished: there is no excuse for inadequate therapy, especially in those patients who are likely to suffer recurrent bleeding.

Particular attention is needed for iron-deficient patients who have had episodes of acute bleeding treated by blood transfusion and who at the time of therapy are not anaemic. These patients require appropriate iron replacement to replenish iron stores for their long-term restitution of health. Because iron therapy leads to a reduction in the avidity of the transport system of the intestine for iron, it should be continued for several months after the anaemia has been corrected to re-establish appropriate iron stores, ideally as reflected by a serum ferritin determination within the normal range.

Unusual syndromes with iron-deficient erythropoiesis

Congenital deficiency of serum transferrin

There are a few reports of deficiency or virtual absence of serum transferrin in infants with disturbed growth, marked hypochromic anaemia, and disordered iron metabolism associated with systemic iron storage leading to tissue injury. This disease is extremely rare but holds great fascination for those investigators with an interest in the pathophysiology of iron metabolism. Profound deficiency of serum transferrin disturbs the normal ligand–receptor signalling mechanisms indicated in the overall control of body iron balance and absorption in the intestine. Hypo- or atransferrinaemia in humans appears to be inherited as an autosomal recessive trait; the gene encoding human serum transferrin maps to chromosome 3.

Studies of a naturally occurring mutant mouse, the *hpx* mouse, that also has deficiency of serum transferrin associated with runting and hypochromic anaemia due to iron-deficient erythropoiesis, indicate that the disorder responds to infusions of serum transferrin or plasma. These infusions restore normal growth and improve the abnormalities of iron homeostasis; iron-deficient erythropoiesis is also corrected, with resolution of the anaemia. The half-life of transferrin in the plasma is 5 to 10 days and so infusions of plasma or purified preparations enriched with transferrin can be administered at intervals. Since most individuals with transferrin deficiency produce limited amounts of the protein antigen, immune reactions to exogenous human transferrin appear to be either mild or rare. Absolute deficiency of transferrin receptors, e.g. as occurs in mouse embryos generated as a result of gene disruption technology in embryonic stem cells, is incompatible with normal development beyond the late embryo stage.

Other causes of refractory iron-deficient erythropoiesis

There are sporadic reports of iron deficiency occurring in children and adults for which no cause can be established after intensive investigation. In some instances the expected parameters of iron deficiency associated with iron-deficient erythropoiesis can be demonstrated in individuals who fail to respond to generous oral supplementation with iron salts; administration of parenteral iron, however, leads to an improvement in reticulocytosis with resolution of iron-deficient red-cell indices. Although at the time of writing no molecular lesions have been identified in any of the implicated iron and transport proteins, it is not impossible that disturbed function of DMT1, ferroportin, hephaestin, or as yet uncharacterized moieties involved in the transport of iron across the intestine will be found in these disorders.

Occurrence of iron-deficient erythropoiesis in both females and males that responds only to parenteral iron supplementation is unlikely to be caused by hephaestin mutations, since this gene maps to the long arm of the X chromosome in humans. It is possible that acquired defects of the intestinal mucosa other than inflammatory disorders may contribute to malabsorption of therapeutic iron. Several young children have been reported with iron-deficiency anaemia refractory to oral therapy but which was corrected by parenteral supplementation. Careful investigation revealed an absorptive defect for iron which was corrected itself by systemic iron supplementation, and raises the possibility that severe iron deficiency itself prejudices the ability of the mucosal epithelium in the upper small intestine to carry out its normal absorptive function. However, no further investigations to identify the nature of this acquired metabolic defect have been provided. There is at least one well-documented instance of an acquired defect of iron delivery associated with signs of iron-deficient erythropoiesis caused by loss of human transferrin receptor function. This condition was associated with the development of antinuclear factor and other autoantibodies as part of an autoimmune illness in an adult woman with hypochromic anaemia. Autoantibodies directed against the transferrin receptor were identified in the serum of the patient, but the anaemia with its attendant sideropenia ultimately responded to a combination of steroids and azathioprine therapy; the titre of transferrin receptor autoantibodies of peripheral blood cells diminished. The extent to which this phenomenon occurs generally during the course of autoimmune disorders associated with anaemia is unknown.

Secondary iron storage disease (secondary haemochromatosis)

This is a worldwide problem. It occurs when excess iron is absorbed from the intestine or obtained by the breakdown of transfused red cells in the mononuclear phagocyte system. Each transfused unit of blood contains 200 to 250 mg of iron as haemoglobin. There are instances of iron storage disease occurring in patients who have received oral iron therapy over many years as medicinal tonics or as treatment for refractory anaemia. However, it is unknown if this would occur in the absence of another disorder, such as homozygosity for mutant alleles of the *HFE* gene that predisposes to iron storage disease, or underlying bone marrow disease. Conversely, iron excess may develop spontaneously in patients with haemolytic (and especially dyserythropoietic) anaemias alone, although it most commonly results from transfusion with or without underlying bone marrow disease (Table 22.5.4.1).

Table 22.5.4.1 Anaemias associated with iron storage disease

Congenital dyserythropoietic anaemia types I and II
β-Thalassaemia including the intermediate phenotype (non-transfusion dependent)
Sideroblastic anaemia (congenital or acquired)
Hereditary spherocytosis (in association with one or more mutant alleles of the *HFE* gene)
Megaloblastic anaemia (especially pernicious anaemia)
α-Thalassaemia (haemoglobin H disease)

Each millilitre of human blood contains the equivalent of 0.5 mg of elemental iron complexed with protoporphyrin. Iron present in transfused red cells is eventually retrieved after their breakdown in the macrophage system as a result of the actions of haem oxygenase, which releases bilirubin, carbon monoxide, and one atom of iron per haem molecule; thus each molecule of haemoglobin A yields four iron atoms. Although it is the mononuclear phagocyte system in which significant iron storage is first detected in transfused individuals, continued delivery of iron by this route leads to the excess of iron-loaded ferritin and its breakdown product, haemosiderin, in parenchymal cells throughout the body, with ensuing tissue injury and functional impairment. After the transfusion of 15 to 20 units of blood (representing about 5 g of elemental iron), iron toxicity occurs.

In dyserythropoietic anaemias such as thalassaemia and sideroblastic anaemia, symptoms and signs of iron storage disease may develop early in life and are related to increased dietary iron absorption by the intestine. Although some patients with β thalassaemia intermedia are treated by occasional transfusion, much of the excess iron stored in the body originates from ingested rather than transfused iron. Iron absorption in healthy adults amounts to 1 to 2 mg/day, but in β thalassaemia intermedia this may be increased more than fivefold. In regularly transfused patients with β thalassaemia major, the massive expansion of the erythropoietic marrow may be suppressed to render absorption of iron normal or near normal. However, in patients with thalassaemia who are transfused only intermittently, erythroid hyperplasia persists and excessive absorption of iron from the diet contributes significantly to the iron storage derived from transfused cells; several grams of additional iron may thus be acquired each year.

Patients with hypochromic anaemias due to sideroblastic change in the marrow are particularly at risk because they may be misdiagnosed as suffering from chronic or recurrent iron-deficiency anaemia; they thus receive long-term supplementation with oral iron that serves merely to exacerbate the iron-loading state. It is noteworthy, however, that patients with haemolytic anaemia due to sickle cell haemoglobin C disease do not commonly develop iron overload as a result of enhanced iron absorption: iron storage disease is thus generally restricted to transfused patients with chronic anaemias. Particular difficulties arise in refractory anaemias in which there is a hyperplastic bone marrow with ineffective erythropoiesis which appears to drive the inappropriate absorption of iron by the intestine.

In the South African Bantu people, the excess iron is ingested in an unusually bioavailable form in beers and other alcoholic drinks prepared by fermentation in iron pots (kaffir beers). Soluble complexes of readily bioavailable iron in these drinks contribute to secondary haemochromatosis, which is common in men in this population and other related sub-Saharan African populations. Although much of the iron is at first detected in the mononuclear phagocyte system (and is seen particularly in Kupffer's cells on liver biopsy), associated hypogonadism and vitamin C deficiency later induce scurvy and osteoporosis. Dietary adjustment and iron chelation therapy may relieve the disorder, which is becoming less common after its recognition in the early 1950s. It is of interest that family studies point to a genetic component which predisposes individuals to this secondary iron storage disease within given pedigrees.

The nature of the stimulus leading from the excess iron turnover that accompanies hyperplastic bone marrow to the intestinal disturbance is unknown. The degree of excess iron absorption is however related to the extent of expansion of the red-cell precursor population: blood transfusions, which suppress the marrow, decrease the absorption of food iron. The toxic properties of iron appear to be related to its capacity to participate in free-radical-generating reactions that form reactive oxygen and nitrogen intermediates implicated in cellular and tissue injury.

Clinical features

The clinical features of secondary iron storage disease in children with chronic anaemias closely resemble hereditary forms of juvenile haemochromatosis (see Chapter 11.7.1). Iron accumulates rapidly in the liver and in the endocrine glands. The several hundred gonadotrophs present within the anterior pituitary gland appear to be particularly susceptible to iron toxicity and hypogonadotrophic hypogonadism results. Iron also accumulates in the β-cells of pancreatic islets, leading to diabetes; in the zona glomerulosa of the adrenal glands, with adrenal failure and mineralocorticoid deficiency; and in the parathyroid glands, ultimately causing hypoparathyroidism. Secondary iron storage disease also has a predilection for the myocardium. This causes sudden death as a result of tachyarrythmias and injury to cardiac conducting tissue or cardiomyopathy with intractable cardiac failure. Secondary iron storage disease in β thalassaemia and congenital dyserythropoietic anaemias is thus characterized by progressive myocardial disease, endocrine failure, and infantilism.

Untreated iron storage disease is the most common cause of death in these disorders. Similar manifestations of iron toxicity are observed in other patients with secondary iron storage in which the accumulation of iron is less rapid. A picture resembling full-blown adult haemochromatosis ultimately supervenes with diabetes and cirrhosis (sometimes complicated by transfusion-related viral hepatitis and the formation of hepatocellular carcinomas) in the presence of deep skin pigmentation. Secondary iron storage disease represents a significant threat to well-being and prognosis in the chronic anaemias. Once cardiac arrythmias have developed, the outlook is usually bleak and urgent chelation therapy with parenteral desferrioxamine is indicated.

Diagnosis

Secondary iron storage disease should be suspected when the saturation of serum transferrin is greater than 60%. In established secondary iron storage disease, there is a raised nontransferrin iron-binding fraction which may contribute to the tissue injury, since the amount of circulating iron may exceed the binding capacity of circulating transferrin. Under these circumstances, transferrin saturation is usually measured at greater than 90 to 95% and is accompanied by an elevation of serum ferritin which, in the absence of active liver disease, faithfully reflects the extent of iron storage disease and the risks of iron-mediated damage.

Iron chelation therapy should probably be introduced at serum ferritin concentrations greater than 1000 μg/litre or if there is biopsy evidence of excess iron storage or a transfusion load of more than 15 units of exogenous red blood cells. Diagnostic evidence of iron storage may be obtained from biopsies of the liver or myocardium; skin biopsy shows excess iron in the sweat gland acini and perifollicular apocrine glands together with increased melanin deposition. In biopsy samples of the liver and heart, histochemical iron storage can be quantified by chemical iron estimations: often the liver iron content exceeds 2% of tissue dry weight (normally less than 0.14% or approximately 7 mg of iron per gram dry weight). Iron concentrations may exceed 5% in affected tissues such as endocrine glands and the pancreas. Liver biopsy may facilitate staging of the disease, particularly in relation to coincidental viral hepatitis where the presence of fibrosis and cirrhosis combined with iron deposits in the parenchymal cell may contribute useful prognostic information. In patients in whom tissue biopsy determinations are not possible, an estimate of body iron overload may be gained by injection of a single dose of 500 mg of desferrioxamine intramuscularly and collection of urine for 24 h in an iron-free plastic container; the daily excretion of more than 2 mg of the coloured ferrioxamine–iron complex indicates iron excess.

Although serum ferritin concentrations generally reflect the amount of iron stored in the tissues, there is a poor correlation between the levels of ferritin in iron-overloaded subjects and clinical outcome. Ferritin concentrations in serum are subject to wide variations; as a result of infection or inflammation (when as an acute reaction it is spuriously elevated), and ferritin concentrations may be reduced when vitamin C is deficient. In contrast, since the liver is the principal site of the iron storage, hepatic iron concentrations provide useful guidance as to prognosis overall, including outcomes from iron-induced cardiac injury, fatal complications of which are usually observed in patients when tissue iron exceeds 1.5% of dry liver weight. In specialized centres, noninvasive methods have been developed to measure liver iron concentrations, including whole-body magnetic susceptibility techniques but neither this nor sophisticated T_2-weighted MRI of the heart or liver has been so far generally accepted in practice. Conventional T_2-weighted imaging may provide a crude assurance that iron storage is either present or under control but is too insensitive to contribute to serial monitoring of secondary iron storage disease—except for the investigation of potential complications such as hepatocellular carcinoma.

Treatment

Patients with homozygous β thalassaemia, sickle cell disease, and related conditions such as myelodysplasia, who are transfusion dependent require adequate blood transfusion to maintain a normal or near normal haemoglobin concentration combined with an iron-chelating agent. Long-term studies provide compelling evidence over 30 years that survival in iron-loaded β thalassaemic subjects is greatly enhanced by treatment with subcutaneous desferrioxamine, which prevents and reverses the cardiac manifestations of iron storage disease. It must be noted, however, that full compliance with this demanding treatment is required for benefit to accrue, which requires equal commitment from the patient and attending medical and nursing personnel alike. Splenectomy or bone marrow transplantation may be considered in certain cases but is beyond the scope of this chapter (see Chapter 22.5.7). The overall outcome and prognosis for β thalassaemia has also been improved by screening donor blood for HIV and hepatitis B and C viruses, as well as other pathogens. These factors are ancillary but may potentiate the development and complications of secondary iron storage disease.

The primary goal of chelation therapy is to remove iron at the rate that it is accumulating, but the effectiveness of this approach is limited because, with the exception of the liver, only a fraction of the tissue iron pool is accessible to chelating agents. This applies particularly to iron in the key organs such as the heart, from which tissue iron extraction is slow. In general the most efficient regimens for removing iron depend on continuous provision of the chelating agent. This can only be achieved with difficulty in the case of desferrioxamine, since the drug has a short plasma half-life. A new orally active chelator, deferasirox, is able to achieve continuous removal of iron after a single daily dose. This agent is able to attain trough concentrations which decrease labile iron species in the plasma persistently over time. Another agent, deferiprone, is also orally active but neither it nor desferrioxamine appears to be as effective as deferasirox.

The preferred route for desferrioxamine mesilate administration is by slow subcutaneous infusion over 12 to 16 h for up to 7 days/week; this is usually done on an ambulatory basis in adults but nocturnal administration is used particularly in children. Nocturnal administration relies on the use of slow clockwork or battery-operated infusion devices. Although electrical syringe pumps are in common use (such as the Graseby driver device), smaller quieter infusion devices (such as the Cronoject) are now available. Light precharged balloon pumps manufactured by Baxter, though expensive, are also in use. The total daily dose of desferrioxamine is usually set at 20 to 30 mg/kg of body weight in children with the maximum usually determined by the extent to which near-saturated solutions of the drug can be tolerated by the patient; in established iron overload the daily dose is usually 20–50 mg/kg. Additional benefit has been suggested from the intravenous administration of up to 2 g desferrioxamine with each unit at the time of blood transfusion: it is important that the drug is not added to the blood but it may be coadministered through a separate intravenous line given through the same cannula. In patients without cardiac disease it has been shown that the daily oral administration of ascorbic acid at 2 to 3 mg/kg increases the amount of iron that can be chelated by desferrioxamine. Serial determinations of serum ferritin concentrations, combined with regular clinical monitoring and assessment of cardiac, hepatic, and endocrine function assist in the assessment of iron storage disease and the efficacy of iron chelation therapy. Periodic echocardiograms and electrocardiography, with 24-h ECG monitoring, are desirable aspects of management. Urinary excretion of the coloured ferrioxamine complex can be easily measured by light spectroscopy. Desferrioxamine promotes not only urinary excretion of iron but also chelates iron from the body stores, which is excreted into the faeces via the biliary system.

Several studies show that patients with β thalassaemia maintained on adequate transfusion regimes who are able to tolerate their infusions of subcutaneous desferrioxamine grow and develop normally and have a better prognosis than those who either default from or do not comply fully with the chelation regimen. When treatment is initiated, careful monitoring is needed using 24-h urine collections for iron measurements to judge the excretion of iron as the dose of desferrioxamine is escalated. Recently, the use of T_2^*-weighted cardiac MRI studies to monitor iron overload in heart tissue has proved to be particularly valuable and allows for intensification of chelation regimens in high-risk patients. Daily doses of desferrioxamine may be increased to about 50 mg/kg of body weight; this usually represents the maximum that can be tolerated. In infants and growing children, unless severe cardiac disease or iron overload is present, the dose should not exceed 35 mg/kg per day over 5 nights each week. Thereafter, most well-transfused patients with β thalassaemia can be maintained in negative iron balance by the use of not more than 40 mg/kg. For patients who receive blood transfusions, a single intravenous infusion of desferrioxamine given separately from but at the same time as each blood transfusion, at a dose of approximately 150 mg/kg of body weight, also contributes to the control of iron storage disease. In patients who develop endocrine failure, prompt replacement of deficient hormones should be introduced. Sex-steroid hormone replacement may relieve infantilism and improve self-esteem in developmentally arrested adolescents and children.

Desferrioxamine is usually well tolerated and, apart from minor skin reactions, is remarkably nontoxic. These reactions can usually be controlled by lowering the concentration of the drug in the infusion and by alternating sites of infusion; hydrocortisone in doses of up to 10 mg has been reported to reduce severe cutaneous reactions. Very high doses of desferrioxamine, particularly those used for treatment of life-threatening cardiac iron overload and given by intravenous rather than subcutaneous infusion (see below), have been associated with retinal injury and lens opacities as well as hearing loss. Since high-tone hearing loss may occur also, it may be prudent to monitor visual acuity and auditory function at intervals during treatment over the years for which desferrioxamine is required. Minor gastroenterological disturbances, myalgia, and very rarely anaphylaxis may occur; rapid administration of desferrioxamine may be associated with hypotension, especially when given intravenously. Desferrioxamine interacts unfavourably with phenothiazines and coma may result from its use in patients receiving these agents. Some patients receiving desferrioxamine develop infections with microorganisms such as yersinia and fungi such as mucor that have fastidious requirements for iron. Iron-overloaded patients may also develop other systemic microbial infections and are particularly susceptible to infections with the marine vibrio, *V. vulnificus*. It seems likely that under these circumstances the desferrioxamine may serve, as nature intended, as a source of iron for uptake by microbial siderophore systems. In patients with acute or subacute cardiac manifestations of iron overload, there are encouraging reports of the effects of high-dose intravenous desferrioxamine: desferrioxamine may reverse cardiac failure and life-threatening tachyarrythmias.

For many patients the emerging orally active tridentate ferric iron chelator deferasirox offers an attractive option for once-daily therapy without the discomfort and limitations of continuous subcutaneous infusions. Deferasirox is now licensed in many countries including the United States of America and Europe. In Europe it is recommended for the treatment of chronic iron overload in adults and children over the age of 6 years with thalassaemia major who receive frequent blood transfusions (>7 ml packed red cells/kg per month). Deferasirox is also licensed for chronic iron overload where desferrioxamine is contraindicated or inadequate in thalassaemia major requiring less frequent transfusions, in patients with other anaemias, and in children aged 2–5 years. The dose is 20–30 mg/kg once daily according to the extent of iron overload (as judged by transfusion history and serum ferritin concentrations). Dosage adjustments should be made every 3–6 months. The drug is a very powerful chelator, and annual ear and eye examinations are required as well as height and sexual development in children. Monitoring of baseline and monthly hepatic and renal function (including tests for proteinuria) is required; at the start of therapy, weekly monitoring is recommended. Although deferasirox may cause proteinuria and headache as well as gastrointestinal effects, and less commonly visual and hearing disturbances occur as well as acute renal failure, these unwanted effects appear to be only rarely encountered. Deferasirox 20 or 30 mg/kg per day has been shown to have a beneficial effect on liver iron concentrations and serum ferritin concentrations, and there are several reports of acceptable tolerability with regular patient monitoring. At the time of writing, longer-term efficacy and safety data are required but as an oral iron chelator the agent appears to offer unique advantages for the management of secondary iron storage disease.

Deferiprone, a novel bidentate an oral iron chelator of a different chemical class from the naturally occurring bacterial agent desferrioxamine, has recently been licensed in Europe for treatment of iron overload in patients unable to tolerate desferrioxamine or in whom it is contraindicated. This drug, of the hydroxpyridone class, is used at a dose of 25 to 100 mg/kg of body weight daily in three divided doses; it is not recommended for children under the age of 6 years. Deferiprone appears to induce overall negative body iron balance in patients with severe homozygous β thalassaemia, with attendant reductions in serum ferritin concentrations, and clearly represents the first newly licensed oral drug with this important indication. In a proportion of patients, however, negative iron balance does not appear to be maintained and the drug may cause serious toxicity including neutropenia and the occasional incidence of agranulocytosis which appears to be mediated by an immune mechanism.

The use of deferiprone remains somewhat controversial following a report that its continued administration may be associated with progressive hepatic fibrosis. Conversely, despite the inconvenience of its use, long-term studies of patients receiving desferrioxamine for iron storage disease in homozygous β thalassaemia show that it is largely safe; moreover, desferrioxamine improves cardiac function and life expectancy and arrests hepatic fibrosis in secondary haemochromatosis. Recently, a randomized, placebo-controlled, double-blind trial of the effect of combined therapy with desferioxamine and deferiprone on myocardial iron in thalassemia major using cardiovascular MRI has been reported. This study shows that the combination of deferiprone and desferioxamine improved cardiac iron deposition more than monotherapy. However, direct comparisons between deferiprone and deferasirox have yet to be undertaken. Safety information and a side-effect profile on the use of deferiprone at a daily dose of 75 mg/kg is available; at the time of writing the drug is not approved by the United States Food and Drug Administration.

Other aspects of care

The single most important aspect of care is compliance with iron chelation therapy and monitoring, especially for infants and other young patients with iron-loading anaemias such as thalassaemia. Regular attendance of special clinics is advisable so that wide-ranging professional support from familiar personnel can be given to reinforce medical care delivered with attention to continuity and the nurturing of independence.

Patients with secondary iron overload should be monitored not only for the progression of their iron storage as determined by parameters of iron metabolism, but also clinically for the presence of iron-mediated tissue injury. Regular echocardiography, electrocardiography, hormone measurements, and physical examinations are required to search for the presence of endocrine failure, including hypoparathyroidism and adrenocortical failure, both of which may be very difficult to detect. Patients with evidence of hypogonadism should be treated with hormone supplementation to ensure normal sexual characteristics, and vigilance should be maintained for the development of diabetes mellitus. Psychological difficulties are prevalent in children and adolescents receiving iron-chelation therapy and transfusion for chronic anaemias and appropriate counselling is often needed over long periods to build up trust with them and their families and to maintain compliance with treatment. Patients with established infantilism and stunted growth frequently develop skeletal disease in addition to that related to their marrow disorder, and investigations should be carried out to search for osteopenia and osteoporosis for which additional therapy will be needed. Bone disease and growth arrest may be caused by the overenthusiastic use of desferrioxamine in young infants, and in these patients the daily dose of desferrioxamine should be reduced to below 40 mg/kg, which usually restores growth velocity to normal.

Finally, patients with secondary iron storage disease should be advised to moderate their dietary intake of iron-rich foods such as meat: some investigators advocate the drinking of strong tea at meal times, especially in patients with thalassaemia intermedia. This tannin-rich drink has been shown to decrease bioavailability of dietary iron and should improve overall iron balance in this at-risk group. As far as possible, the blood haemoglobin concentration should be maintained in the normal range to ensure growth and responsiveness to hormone supplements; patients with significant transfusion requirements should be considered for splenectomy when they reach an age of over 5 years. As with patients who are not iron overloaded, splenectomized individuals should be treated appropriately by immunization and antimicrobial prophylactic therapy as far as possible to reduce the risk of intercurrent bacterial infection. This risk is potentiated by systemic iron storage.

Treatment of severe cardiac manifestations of iron storage disease

Continuous intravenous infusions of desferrioxamine not exceeding 50 to 60 mg/kg daily are now recommended for life-threatening heart disease. High-dose intravenous infusions may cause unacceptable toxic injury, especially in the retina and inner ear. Desferrioxamine given continuously through a permanent indwelling portable catheter within the superior vena cava, with careful attention to sepsis, is a satisfactory method for securing reversal of cardiac disease in high-risk patients with serum ferritin concentrations that persist at greater than 2500 µg/litre or who have hepatic iron concentrations that exceed 1.5% of dry liver weight. Improved outcomes have been reported with the use of anticoagulation induced by warfarin, and scrupulous attention to cutaneous needle resiting and skin care to reduce the risk of thrombosis and complicating infections.

Pregnancy

Desferrioxamine therapy is not recommended by the manufacturer during pregnancy but, despite this, many successful pregnancies have been reported without fetal injury. The drug should probably be avoided during the middle trimester and should almost certainly be avoided, because of unknown teratogenicity, in early pregnancy or at the time of any planned conception. None the less, it may be reasonable to restart desferrioxamine therapy in the final trimester of pregnancy if the risks to the mother from iron storage disease are high. No information is available on deferasirox or deferiprone in pregnancy and these drugs should probably not be used until more experience is forthcoming.

Prognosis and outcome

The principal causes of death in secondary iron storage disease include cardiac failure and arrythmias, endocrine failure and the consequences of diabetes mellitus, infection, and hepatocellular carcinoma. Unless treated, secondary haemochromatosis is a rapidly fatal disease when associated with transfusion therapy and intestinal hyperabsorption of iron in the chronic anaemias. Less than one-third of those unable to comply with iron chelation therapy survive with β thalassaemia major to the age of 25 years. However, the outcome of iron storage disease in patients with chronic anaemia is now greatly improving, with enhanced life quality and duration. One study has indicated that 95% of patients with β thalassaemia who administer desferrioxamine subcutaneously more than 250 times each year will survive to 30 years; whereas only 12% of those who do not will survive to this age. In the United Kingdom the overall survival is 50% at 35 years, but at one specialist centre the actuarial survival in more than 100 patients was 80% at 40 ears. Continuous intravenous desferrioxamine can be claimed to reverse life-threatening arrythmias in cardiac iron overload and also improve or reverse left ventricular or biventrical heart failure in a majority of cases. One report describes the actuarial survival of more than 60% at 13 years of patients with life-threatening disease and β thalassaemia so treated; this outcome appears to be accompanied by improved cardiac tissue iron signals on MRI.

This again emphasizes the benefits of care administered at a dedicated treatment centre. From 1980 to 1999 there were 12.7 deaths from all causes per 1000 patient years. In 2000–2003, the death rate from all causes fell significantly to 4.3 per 1000 patient years. This was mainly accounted for by the reduced death rate from iron overload, which fell from 7.9 to 2.3 deaths per 1000 patient years. Several reports also show that the frequency of hypogonadism, diabetes, and growth retardation is significantly reduced by effective iron chelation.

Further reading

Adamkiewicz TV et al. (1998). Infection due to Yersinia enterocolitica in a series of patients with β-thalassaemia: incidence and predisposing factors. Clin Infect Dis, 27, 1362–6.

Anderson GJ, et al. (2005). Mechanisms of haem and non-haem iron absorption: lessons from inherited disorders of iron metabolism. Biometals, 18, 339–48.

Andrews NC, Schmidt PJ (2007). Iron homeostasis. Annu Rev Physiol, 69, 69–85.

Babitt JL, et al. (2006). Bone morphogenetic protein signaling by hemojuvelin regulates hepcidin expression. Nat Genet, 38, 531–9.

Bothwell T, et al. (1989). Nutritional iron requirements and good iron absorption. J Intern Med, 226, 357–65.

Brooker S, Hotez PJ, Bundy DA (2008). Hookworm-related anaemia among pregnant women: a systematic review. PLoS Neglected Trop Dis, 2, e291.

Calis JC, et al. (2008). Severe anemia in Malawian children. N Engl J Med, 358, 888–99.

Chen FE, et al. (2000). Genetic and clinical features of haemoglobin H disease in Chinese patients. N Engl J Med, 343, 544–50.

Cohen AR, et al. (2000). Safety profile of the oral iron chelator Deferiprone: a multi-centre study. Br J Haematol, 108, 305–12.

Cox TM (1998). Iron salts, iron–dextran complex and iron–sorbitol citrate. In: Dollery CT (ed.) Therapeutic drugs: a clinical pharmacopoeia, 2nd edition, Vol 2, pp. 178–83. Baillière Tindall, Edinburgh.

Dallman PR (1989). Iron deficiency: does it matter? J Intern Med, 226, 367–72.

De Maeyer EM (1989). Preventing and controlling iron-deficiency anaemia through primary health care. World Health Organization, Geneva.

Enns CA, Zhang AS (2009). Iron homeostasis: recently identified proteins provide insight into novel control mechanisms. J Biol Chem, 284, 711–15.

Finch C (1994). Regulations of iron balance in humans. Blood, 84, 1697–702.

Hurrell RF (2007). Iron fortification: its efficacy and safety in relation to infections. Food Nutr Bull, 28 (4 Suppl), S585–94.

Gordeuk VR, Boyd D, Brittenham G (1986). Dietary iron overload persists in rural sub-Saharan Africa. Lancet, i, 1310–13.

Kent S (2000). Iron deficiency and anaemia of chronic disease. In: Kiple KF, Ornelas KC (eds) The Cambridge world history of food, pp 919–39. Cambridge University Press, Cambridge.

Magio A (2007), Light and shadows in the chelation treatment of haematological diseases. Br J Haematol, 138, 407–421. [A comprehensive, balanced and contemporary review of evidence and practice.]

McCance RA, Widdowson EM (1937). Absorption and excretion of iron. Lancet, ii, 680–4.

McCann JC, Ames BN (2007). An overview of evidence for a causal relation between iron deficiency during development and deficits in cognitive or behavioral function. Am J Clin Nutr, 85, 931–45. [An authoritative review of the evidence (suggestive but not definitive) of the (often-stated assertion) that that iron deficiency, with or without anaemia, is independently associated with developmental delay or cognitive defects in children.]

McCleod C et al. (2009). Deferasirox for the treatment of iron overload associated with regular transfusions (transfusional haemosiderosis) in patients suffering with chronic anaemia: a systemic review and economic evaluation. Health Technology Assessment, 13, iii–iv, ix–xi, 1–121.

Melis MA, et al. (2008). A mutation in the TMPRSS6 gene, encoding a transmembrane serine protease that suppresses hepcidin production, in familial iron deficiency anemia refractory to oral iron. Haematologica, 93, 1473–9.

Modell B, et al. (1982). Survival and desferrioxamine in thalassaemia major. BMJ, 284, 1081–4.

Modell B, et al. (2008). Improved survival of thalassaemia major in the UK and relation to T2* cardiovascular magnetic resonance. J Cardiovasc Magn Res, 10, 42.

Moore DF, Sears DA (1994). Pica, iron deficiency and the medical history. Am J Med, 97, 390–3.

Neufeld E (2006). Oral chelators deferasirox and deferiprone for transfusional iron overload in thalassemia major: new data, new questions. Blood, 107, 3436–41.

Olivieri NF, et al. (1994). Survival in medically treated patients with homozygous β-thalassaemia. N Engl J Med, 331, 574–8.

Olivieri NF, et al. (1998). Long-term safety and effectiveness of iron-chelation therapy with deferiprone for thalassemia major. N Engl J Med, 339, 417–23.

Pippard MJ, Weatherall DJ (1984). Iron absorption in iron-loading anaemias. Haematologia, 17, 407–14.

Pippard MJ, Weatherall DJ (2000). Oral iron chelation therapy for thalassaemia: an uncertain scene. Br J Haematol, 111, 2–5. [A useful review of iron chelation and a dispassionate evaluation of the emerging role of deferiprone.]

Porter JB (2001). Practical management of iron overload. Br J Haematol, 115, 239–52. [An excellent contemporary review with abundant practical as well as theoretical and scientific information.]

Porter JB (2006). Deferasirox: An effective once-daily orally active iron chelator. Drugs Today, 42, 623–37.

Porter JB (2007). Concepts and goals in the management of transfusional iron overload. Am J Hematol, 82(12 Suppl), 1136–9. [A useful update including the beneficial effects of new chelators such as the orally active deferasirox.]

Roche M, Layrisse M (1966). The nature and cause of hookworm anaemia. Am J Trop Med, 15, 1029–102.

Shaker M, *et al.* (2009). An economic analysis of anemia prevention during infancy. *J Pediatr*, **154**, 44–9. [A valuable contemporary evaluation of the usefulness and economic success of detecting iron-deficiency anaemia and treating it in infants—with comments on the benefits to neurocognitive outcomes.]

Tanner MA, *et al.* (2007). A randomized, placebo-controlled, double-blind trial of the effect of combined therapy with deferoxamine and deferiprone on myocardial iron in thalassemia major using cardiovascular magnetic resonance. *Circulation*, **115**, 1876–84.

Upchurch BR, Vargo JJ (2008). Small bowel enteroscopy. *Rev Gastroenterol Disord*, **8**, 169–77. [A contemporary review of a useful technique for definitive diagnosis of bleeding from the small intestine.]

22.5.5 Normochromic, normocytic anaemia

D.J. Weatherall

Essentials

A mild normochromic, normocytic anaemia is a common finding and usually a consequence of other diseases, including (1) anaemia of chronic disorders—associated with chronic infection, all forms of inflammatory diseases, and malignant disease; mechanism unknown but likely to involve multiple factors; typically leads to a reduction in the serum iron concentration with concurrent reduction in the level of transferrin, hence saturation of the iron binding capacity is usually normal or only slightly reduced; (2) other disorders—including renal failure, hypothyroidism, hypopituitarism, marrow failure (aplastic anaemia, infiltration, pure red-cell aplasia), acute blood loss, and polymyalgia rheumatica. Treatment is that of the underlying condition, with a therapeutic trial of corticosteroids justified—after exclusion of underlying blood dyscrasias and paraproteinaemias—in elderly patients with anaemia in association with a very high sedimentation rate.

Introduction

A mild normochromic anaemia is one of the most frequent findings in every branch of clinical practice. It is important to decide whether the anaemia is of significance and how far it should be investigated.

The first decision to be made is whether the blood findings represent 'anaemia' for the particular patient. The haemoglobin concentration varies considerably at different ages and there is a wide range of 'normal' values. Knowledge of any previous blood count is particularly useful since a haemoglobin value in the lower range of normal may represent anaemia in a patient previously known to have a higher haemoglobin when in good health.

Most of the normochromic, normocytic anaemias are a consequence of other diseases; a minority reflect a primary disorder of the blood. The most common causes are summarized in Box 22.5.5.1.

Box 22.5.5.1 Some normochromic, normocytic anaemias

- Anaemia of chronic disorders
  - Inflammation
  - Neoplasia
- Renal failure
- Endocrine failure
  - Hypothyroidism
  - Hypopuitarism
- Marrow failure
  - Pure red-cell aplasia
  - Aplastic anaemia
  - Infiltration
- Acute blood loss
- Polymyalgia rheumatica

Anaemia of chronic disorders (ACD)

This is the rather unsatisfactory phrase used to describe the most common of the normochromic, normocytic anaemias, i.e. those found in association with chronic infection, all forms of inflammatory diseases, and malignant disease. It is important for clinicians to be able to identify the main features of this type of anaemia. Although it may be mild and asymptomatic, the presence of this blood picture should always alert the clinician to the possibility of there being a serious underlying disease.

Pathogenesis

The precise mechanism of the anaemia of chronic disorders is still not understood. Several different pathological processes that occur in response to inflammation conspire to cause a defective proliferation of red cell progenitors. In addition, at least in some cases, there may be a mild haemolytic component.

The most constant feature of ACD is a low serum iron level despite adequate iron stores in the reticuloendothelial elements of the bone marrow. This abnormal accumulation of iron in the storage cells, together with a low serum iron level in the blood, suggests that there is a block in the release of iron to the developing red cell precursors. There is also a reduced concentration of transferrin, and turnover studies suggest that this reflects a decreased rate of production. Recent studies in mice and in patients with liver tumours secreting the iron-regulatory hormone hepcidin suggest that increased levels of this peptide, which occur in many inflammatory conditions, can result in many of the abnormalities of iron metabolism seen in ACD.

Several studies have found a mild shortening of the red-cell lifespan in ACD, which appears to be due to an extracorpuscular factor and not to an intrinsic abnormality of the red cells. The red-cell survival is not markedly shortened; if marrow function were normal it should be able to compensate for the reduced survival. However, there is a defect in the proliferation of red-cell progenitors in ACD. This may reflect inadequate iron delivery or the effect of cytokines produced as a response to infection, or both. There also seems to be a subnormal erythropoietin response for the degree of anaemia, possibly arising from the action of various cytokines.

Recent studies have identified a number of cytokines that inhibit haemopoiesis in bone marrow culture and reduce the output of erythropoietin in hepatoma cell lines. The relevance of these *in vitro* studies to the generation of ACD in patients with such a diversity of associated disorders is uncertain. It is very unlikely that one mechanism will be found to account for such diverse abnormalities. Rather, it appears that ACD is a by-product of the acute phase reaction, probably augmented by a variety of different cytokine responses.

Clinical and laboratory findings

The anaemia of chronic disorders is usually mild. In patients with severe inflammation the haematocrit may fall to levels at which symptoms are experienced. Although the anaemia is usually normocytic and normochromic there may be mild hypochromia with a slight reduction in the mean corpuscular haemoglobin (MCH) and mean corpuscular volume (MCV), particularly in children. Occasionally there may be marked microcytosis. Microcytosis should prompt consideration of concomitant iron deficiency, especially in patients who might have gastrointestinal bleeding, e.g. individuals with inflammatory bowel disease or rheumatoid arthritis on aspirin. The reticulocyte count is in the normal range.

The most important finding is a reduction in the serum iron concentration. Because there is a concurrent reduction in the level of transferrin, the per cent saturation of the iron binding capacity is usually normal or only slightly reduced. This observation clearly distinguishes ACD from true iron deficiency anaemia (Table 22.5.5.1). This distinction can also be confirmed by measuring the serum ferritin level, which is usually in the normal range or slightly elevated in patients with ACD while it is low in those who are iron deficient.

The bone marrow appearance is unremarkable. There may be a slight deficiency of red cell progenitors. Iron staining shows a paucity of iron in the red cell precursors and an accumulation of iron in the storage elements of the marrow. Again, this distinguishes ACD from true iron deficiency in which there is an absence of both sideroblasts and storage iron. The abnormal distribution of iron in an adequately stained sample, together with the low serum iron level, is the true hallmark of ACD and a finding that should always

Table 22.5.5.1 Distinction between iron-deficiency anaemia and anaemia of chronic disorders

	Iron deficiency	Anaemia of chronic disorders
Red cells	Hypochromic microcytic	Normochromic or slightly microcytic
Bone marrow		
Sideroblasts	Absent	Absent
Storage iron	Absent	Present or increased
Serum iron	Low	Low
Total iron-binding capacity	Normal or high	Low or normal
Percentage saturation	Low	Normal
Serum ferritin	Low	Normal

be followed up by a search for an underlying inflammatory or neoplastic condition.

Other forms of normochromic, normocytic anaemia

Other causes of this type of blood picture are summarized in Box 22.5.5.1.

Renal failure

Normochromic, normocytic anaemia is a common presenting feature of renal disease. The features of the anaemia of renal failure are discussed in more detail in the section on blood changes in systemic disease.

Endocrine disease

The hypometabolism observed in hypopituitary and hypothyroid states reduces demand for oxygen in the tissues and, therefore, output of erythropoietin. This is probably the principal factor in the development of the mild normochromic, normocytic anaemia which is observed in some patients with these conditions.

Bone marrow failure

Nonspecific anaemia is a common feature of bone marrow failure. It may occur in the pure red cell aplasias or as part of aplastic anaemia.

Acute blood loss and early iron deficiency

Blood loss from the gastrointestinal or genitourinary tract may be sufficient to cause anaemia but as long as the iron stores are sufficient to maintain an output of normal red cells the anaemia is normochromic and normocytic. This picture is seen in early cases of bleeding or intermittent bleeding. There is usually a slight increase in the reticulocyte count, reflecting an increased rate of proliferation of red cell progenitors.

Polymyalgia rheumatica and giant cell arteritis

Polymyalgia rheumatica (see Chapter 18.10.4) is nearly always associated with a moderate normochromic, normocytic anaemia together with a marked increase in the erythrocyte sedimentation rate. However, particularly in elderly patients, anaemia may be the presenting feature. The symptoms of polymyalgia or cranial arteritis may be minimal or even absent. This common variant of the polymyalgia syndrome should always be considered in old people with anaemia and a very high sedimentation rate who do not have paraprotein in the blood. The anaemia responds quite dramatically to corticosteroids.

Management

Mild, nonspecific anaemias should always be investigated because they may be the first indication of a serious underlying disease. It is important to try to distinguish ACD from iron deficiency or other nonspecific normochromic, normocytic anaemias. In ACD, the serum iron level is low and there is a normal saturation of the iron binding capacity. It is worth carrying out a bone marrow examination to study the distribution of iron between the red cell precursors and the storage cells. If the pattern of ACD is observed, it is important to carry out a careful search for chronic inflammation or neoplastic disease. The most common causes of ACD which give rise to diagnostic problems are low-grade urinary infections, chronic sinus infection, and occult malignancy.

The treatment of anaemias of this type is essentially that of the underlying disease. In the subgroup of elderly patients presenting with this type of anaemia in association with a very high sedimentation rate, in whom underlying blood dyscrasias and paraproteinaemias have been excluded, it is justifiable to give a therapeutic trial of corticosteroids, and to proceed to further investigations only if there is no immediate and dramatic response characteristic of the polymyalgia syndromes. Early recognition of the true diagnosis may save weeks of fruitless investigation for a nonexistent neoplasm.

The principal difficulty in the management of this condition is encountered in those case in which it is impossible to correct the underlying disorder, e.g. patients with advanced malignant disease or intractable rheumatoid arthritis. It has been found that the quality of life is undoubtedly improved for many patients of this type if the haemoglobin concentration is raised. This may be achieved by instituting a regular blood transfusion regimen. As an alternative approach, a number of disorders of this type have been treated with erythropoietin at varying doses. A limited number of trials, some of which were placebo-controlled, have suggested that at least some patients with malignant disease, rheumatoid arthritis, or AIDS experience a useful rise in the haemoglobin concentration using this approach. A full response may be delayed for up to 2 months.

Further reading

Gardner LB, Benz EJ (2005). Anemia of chronic diseases. In: Hoffman R, *et al.* (eds) *Hematology, basic principles and practice*, 4th edn, pp. 465–71. Churchill Livingstone, New York.

22.5.6 Megaloblastic anaemia and miscellaneous deficiency anaemias

A.V. Hoffbrand

Essentials

Megaloblastic anaemias are characterized by red blood cell macrocytosis. They arise because of inhibition of DNA synthesis in the bone marrow, usually due to deficiency of one or other of vitamin B_{12} (cobalamin) or folate, but sometimes as a consequence of a drug or a congenital or acquired biochemical defect that disturbs their metabolism, or affects DNA synthesis independent of vitamin B_{12} or folate.

Biochemical and nutritional aspects of vitamin B_{12} and folate

Vitamin B_{12}—synthesized by bacteria; in humans the daily requirement of 1 to 2 µg is acquired from secondary animal sources including fish, eggs, milk, and meat. Processing within the body occurs as

follows: (1) proteolysis of food releases dietary vitamin B_{12} for binding to a glycoprotein haptocorrin; (2) pancreatic trypsin degrades the glycoprotein, releasing vitamin B_{12} for attachment to intrinsic factor; (3) the B_{12}–intrinsic factor complex binds to a specific receptor—cubilin amnion—expressed on the luminal brush border of the mucosal cells of the ileum, and is endocytosed; (4) after lysosomal degradation, vitamin B_{12} is complexed with transcobalamin (TC)II and secreted into the circulation; (5) the TCII–B_{12} complex is incorporated by cellular endocytosis in peripheral tissues and vitamin B_{12} released by digestion in the lysosomal compartment.

Folic acid—natural folate occurs principally in leaves and vegetables, but is destroyed by cooking. The daily requirement is about 100 µg, with absorption occurring through a proton-coupled folate transporter in the proximal small intestine and duodenum. Attached glutamate residues are cleaved, releasing methyl tetrahydrofolate into the portal plasma.

Biochemical basis of megaloblastic anaemia—(1) Folate deficiency reduces the availability of 5,10-methylene tetrahydrofolate, thus inhibiting synthesis of thymidylate, which is the rate-limiting precursor for DNA synthesis. (2) Vitamin B_{12} deficiency impairs DNA synthesis indirectly because it is an acceptor for single-carbon moieties required for conversion of methyltetrahydrofolate to tetrahydrofolate, the source of active folate. It also appears to be critical for function of the enzyme methionine synthase, inhibition of which appears to be the principal cause of the neuropathy and spinal cord disease characteristic of severe vitamin B_{12} deficiency

Causes of megaloblastic anaemia

Vitamin B_{12} deficiency—(1) malabsorption—including (a) gastric causes—e.g. acquired (addisonian) pernicious anaemia, gastrectomy; (b) intestinal causes—e.g. bacterial overgrowth, ileal resection, Crohn's disease; (2) nutritional—e.g. vegans.

Folate deficiency—(1) poor diet—e.g. poverty, alcoholism; (2) malabsorption—e.g. coeliac disease, tropical sprue; (3) excessive requirements—e.g. pregnancy, haemolytic anaemia; (4) excess excretion—e.g. chronic haemodialysis; (5) drugs—e.g. anticonvulsants; (6) liver disease.

Not due to vitamin B_{12} or folate deficiency—(1) abnormalities of vitamin B_{12} or folate metabolism—including (a) congenital—e.g. TCII deficiency; (b) acquired—e.g. dihydrofolate reductase inhibitors; (2) independent of vitamin B_{12} or folate—including (a) congenital—e.g. orotic aciduria; (b) acquired—e.g. various myeloid leukaemias; (c) drugs—e.g. antimetabolites.

Laboratory investigation

This consists of three stages: (1) Recognition that megaloblastic anaemia is present—the mean corpuscle volume (MCV) is raised to 100 to 140 fl, and the peripheral blood shows hypersegmented neutrophils, with the leucocyte count often moderately reduced. The bone marrow is hypercellular, with the myeloid/erythroid ratio often reduced or reversed. (2) Distinction between vitamin B_{12} or folate deficiency (or rarely some other factor) as the cause of the anaemia—usually achieved by assay of serum vitamin B_{12} and serum folate. (3) Diagnosis of the underlying disease causing the deficiency—depends on taking a dietary history, measurement of parietal-cell and intrinsic factor antibodies (see below), and pursuing clinical clues to other possible causes.

Acquired (addisonian) pernicious anaemia

Antibodies in serum and gastric juice directed against parietal cells (85–90% of cases) and intrinsic factor (50%), and cell-mediated immunity to intrinsic factor, are associated with gastritis and failure of absorption of vitamin B_{12}.

Clinical features—anaemia usually develops gradually, and symptoms may not occur until it is severe. Aside from pallor, other manifestations can include (1) mild jaundice; (2) mild pyrexia; (3) psychiatric disturbance; (4) glossitis and angular cheilosis; (5) features of an associated disorder—e.g. vitiligo, thyroid disease. Complications include (1) peripheral sensorimotor neuropathy; (2) subacute combined degeneration of the spinal cord—manifest as loss of proprioception and pyramidal weakness; (3) psychiatric disturbance.

Treatment and prevention of megaloblastic anaemia

Vitamin B_{12} deficiency—may be treated with intramuscular hydroxocobalamin (1-mg doses, given frequently at initiation of treatment, then every 3 months) or (provided malabsorption is not responsible) oral hydroxocobalamin. Neurological complications are irreversible unless treated early.

Folate deficiency—high-dose oral folic acid (1–5 mg daily) usually overcomes folate malabsorption, but this should not be given alone where vitamin B_{12} deficiency coexists because neurological disease may be precipitated or exacerbated (although the haematological abnormalities improve). Where folate metabolism is disturbed, oral or parenteral folinic acid may restore pyrimidine synthesis.

Prevention—the role of dietary folate supplementation is an accepted and highly effective public health measure in many countries for preventing neural tube birth defects. Deficiency of folic acid may influence the development of cardiovascular disease, but the role of folate supplementation in the prevention of cardiovascular disease remains controversial.

Introduction

The megaloblastic anaemias are a group of disorders characterized by a macrocytic anaemia and distinctive morphological abnormalities of the developing haemopoietic cells in the bone marrow. In severe cases, the anaemia may be associated with leucopenia and thrombocytopenia. Megaloblastic anaemia arises because of inhibition of DNA synthesis in the bone marrow, usually due to deficiency of one or other of two water-soluble B vitamins: vitamin B_{12} (cobalamin) or folate. Vitamin B_{12} deficiency may also cause a severe neuropathy. In a minority of cases, megaloblastic anaemia arises because of a disturbance of DNA synthesis due to a drug or a congenital or acquired biochemical defect that causes a disturbance of vitamin B_{12} or folate metabolism or affects DNA synthesis independent of vitamin B_{12} or folate. Vitamin B_{12} and folate are discussed first and the other rare megaloblastic anaemias are mentioned later in this chapter.

Much current interest concerns general systemic effects of folate deficiency and whether folic acid supplements or food fortification with folic acid aimed at preventing neural tube defects will affect the incidence of cardiovascular or malignant diseases or cognitive defects in older people. These aspects are also discussed.

Biochemical and nutritional aspects of vitamin B_{12} and folate

Vitamin B_{12}

Biochemistry

Four major forms of the vitamin exist in humans, all with the same cobalamin nucleus, which consists of a planar corrin ring (hence the term 'corrinoids' for vitamin B_{12} compounds) attached at right angles to a nucleotide portion, 5,6-dimethylbenzimidazole joined to ribose-phosphate (Fig. 22.5.6.1; Table 22.5.6.1). 5'-Deoxyadenosyclobalamin (adocobalamin) accounts for about 80% of vitamin B_{12} inside mammalian cells and is located mainly in mitochondria; methylcobalamin is a minor cellular component but the main form in plasma. Both are extremely light-sensitive and are rapidly photolysed to hydroxocobalamin by daylight; hydroxocobalamin is present in small amounts in tissues and plasma and is available commercially for therapeutic use. The fourth form, cyanocobalamin, is found only in trace amounts naturally, but is stable and after radioactive labelling with cobalt-57 or cobalt-58 is used to study vitamin B_{12} metabolism. Hydroxo- and cyanocobalamins are converted to the two biochemically active forms. The fully reduced compounds are termed Cob(I)alamins, and the oxidized compounds Cob(III)alamins. Analogues of vitamin B_{12} (pseudo-vitamin B_{12}s) exist in nature, endogenous production of which in humans is suggested by their presence in all sera (including fetal serum) and their fall in parallel with physiologically active vitamin B_{12} in vitamin B_{12} deficiency.

Vitamin B_{12} is known to be involved in only three reactions in human tissues: as adocobalamin in the isomerization of methylmalonyl CoA to succinyl CoA and of α-leucine to β-leucine, and as

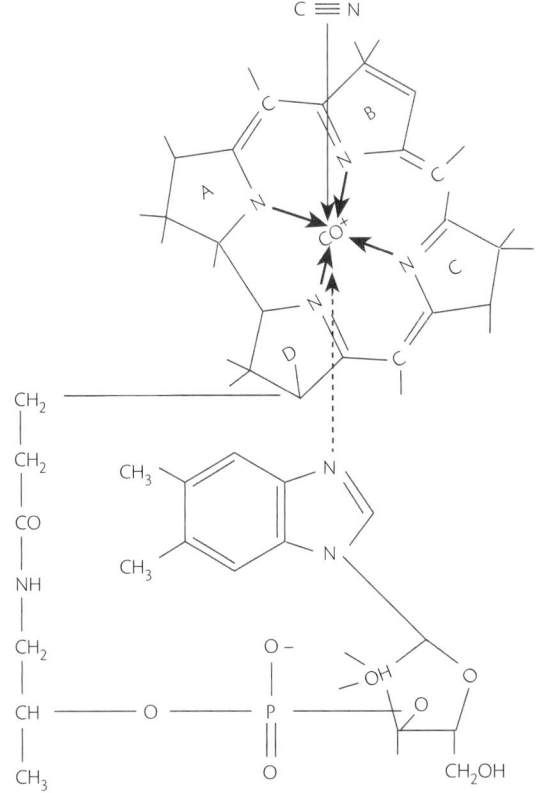

Fig. 22.5.6.1 The structure of cyanocobalamin.

Table 22.5.6.1 Vitamin B$_{12}$ and folate

	Vitamin B$_{12}$	Folate
Parent form	Cyanocobalamin (cyano-B$_{12}$), mol. wt. 1355	Folic acid (pteroyglutamic acid), mol. wt. 441.4
Crystals	Dark-red needles	Yellow, spear-shaped
Natural forms	Deoxyadenosylcobalamin	Reduced (di- or tetrahydro-), methylated, formylated, other single carbon additions; mono- and polyglutamates
	Methylcobalamin	
	Hydroxocobalamin	
Foods	Animal produce (especially liver) only	All, especially liver, kidney, yeast, greens, nuts
Adult daily requirements	2 µg	100 µg
Adult body stores	2–5 mg	6–20 mg
Length of time to deficiency	2–4 years	4 months
Daily diet content	5–30 µg	About 200–250 µg
Cooking	Little effect	Easily destroyed
Absorption	Intrinsic factor (+ neutral pH + Ca^{2+}) via ileum	Deconjugated, reduction, and methylation via duodenum and jejunum
Plasma transport	Tightly and specifically bound to transcobalamins	One-third loosely bound albumin, other proteins; ?specific protein
Enterohepatic circulation	3–9 µg/day	60–90 µg/day

methylcobalamin in the methylation of homocysteine to methionine, a reaction that also requires methyltetrahydrofolate (Fig. 22.5.6.2). In some bacteria, but not in humans, vitamin B$_{12}$ has a direct role in DNA synthesis by virtue of its involvement in ribonucleotide reductase.

Nutrition

Vitamin B$_{12}$ is synthesized by microorganisms; animals obtain it by consuming the flesh of other animals or their produce (milk, cheese, eggs, etc.)—or vegetable foods containing yeast extract, and those contaminated by bacteria. A healthy mixed diet contains between 5 and 30 µg daily. In some species, but not in humans, vitamin B$_{12}$ is absorbed after synthesis by bacteria in the large intestine. The vitamin B$_{12}$ content in humans is about 3 to 5 mg; it is found mainly in the liver (c.0.7–1.1 µg/g). Adult daily losses are related to body stores; to maintain normal body stores, daily requirements are of the order of 1–2 µg. It takes 3 to 4 years, on average, for deficiency to develop if supplies are totally cut off by malabsorption. There is an enterohepatic circulation for vitamin B$_{12}$, variously estimated at 3 to 9 µg daily, which is intact in vegans, which may partly account for their tendency to maintain low body stores without incurring severe deficiency. The body is unable to degrade vitamin B$_{12}$ and deficiency has not been shown to be due to excess utilization or loss.

Absorption

About 15% of dietary vitamin B$_{12}$ is available for absorption. It is released from protein binding in food by proteolytic enzymes, heat, and acid, and combines one molecule to one molecule with a glycoprotein R vitamin B$_{12}$-binding protein (also called haptocorrin) in gastric juice. The glycoprotein binds dietary forms of vitamin B$_{12}$ but does not facilitate its absorption. Pancreatic trypsin degrades this protein and so releases vitamin B$_{12}$ for attachment to intrinsic factor (IF) and subsequent absorption. IF is a glycoprotein produced mainly by the parietal cells (Table 22.5.6.2). The normal stomach produces a vast excess of IF, measured in units (1 unit binds 1 ng vitamin B$_{12}$). Vitamin B$_{12}$ in bile is also attached

to IF and reabsorbed through the ileum. At neutral pH, in the presence of calcium ions, the vitamin B$_{12}$–IF complex attaches passively to a complex specific IF receptor, cubilin amnion, on the brush border of the mucosal cells of the terminal ileum. Cubulin is a 640-kDa peripheral membrane protein present in the epithelium of intestine and kidney. Amnionless (AMN) (50 kDa) binds to cubilin and is essential for production of mature cubilin and its transport to the apical brush border. AMN directs sublocalization and endocytosis of cubilin and the IF–vitamin B$_{12}$ complex. Mutations of cubilin or AMN underlie hereditary malabsorption of vitamin B$_{12}$ (discussed later in this chapter).

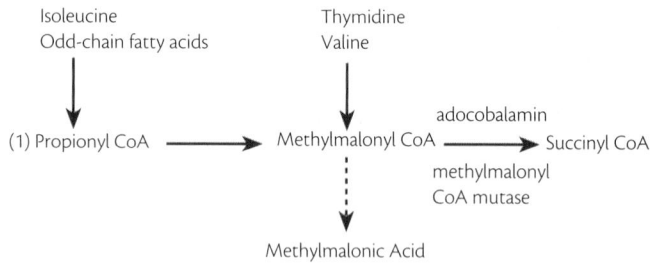
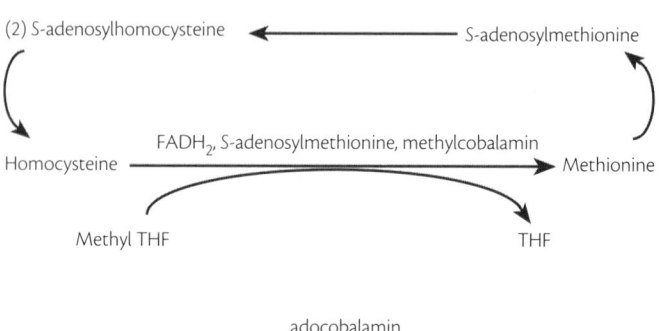

Fig. 22.5.6.2 Biochemical reactions of vitamin B$_{12}$ (cobalamin) in human tissues.

Table 22.5.6.2 Vitamin B$_{12}$-binding proteins

	Intrinsic factor	Transcobalamin I and III[1]	Transcobalamin II
Present in	Gastric juice	Plasma	Plasma, cerebrospinal fluid
Source	Gastric parietal cell	Granulocytes? other organs	Macrophages, liver parenchyma, ileum
Molecular weight	45 000	60 000	45 500
Structure	Glycoprotein (15% sugar)	Glycoprotein	Polypeptide
Normal total binding capacity	30–110 µg/l	700–800 ng/l	900–1000 ng/l
B$_{12}$ content	No B$_{12}$	300–400 ng/l B$_{12}$	30–60 ng/l B$_{12}$
Function	B$_{12}$ absorption (not itself absorbed)	? storage of B$_{12}$ / ? protection of B$_{12}$ / Binding of B$_{12}$ analogues	B$_{12}$ delivery to marrow, placenta, brain, and other tissues, B$_{12}$ absorption

[1] Related 'R' binders (haptocorrins) occur in other tissues and secretions, e.g. milk, gastric juice, saliva, and tears.

After cubilin–AMN-mediated endocytosis, IF undergoes lysosomal degradation. After a delay of 3 to 5 h, vitamin B$_{12}$ appears in portal blood, with a peak concentration 8 h after ingestion, complexed with transcobalamin II (TCII) secreted into the circulation from the basolateral side of the intestinal cells. Ileal absorption of vitamin B$_{12}$ is limited by the number of cubilin receptors to a few micrograms daily, and although 80% of a single dose of 1 to 2 µg may be absorbed, the proportion diminishes steeply at higher doses. A small (<1%) trace of a large (≥1 mg) dose of vitamin B$_{12}$ can be absorbed passively and rapidly through the buccal, gastric, and duodenal mucosae without the involvement of the IF pathway.

Transport

Vitamin B$_{12}$ in plasma is 70 to 90% attached to a glycoprotein, transcobalamin I (TCI), and 0–10% to transcobalamin III (TCIII) which does not enhance cell uptake of vitamin B$_{12}$ (see Table 22.5.6.2). TCI and III belong to a group of glycoproteins, the R binders or haptocorrins (see above), that are present in many tissues and fluids; these molecules have the same amino acid composition but differ in the carbohydrate moiety. The haptocorrins may have the role of binding analogues of vitamin B$_{12}$ derived from food or intestinal organisms and transporting them to the liver for excretion in the bile.

The most important plasma vitamin B$_{12}$-binding protein, TCII, is synthesized in macrophages, liver, the ileum and possibly endothelium. TCII is loaded with vitamin B$_{12}$ from the ileum and by release of free vitamin B$_{12}$ from the liver and other organs. It is normally almost completely unsaturated because it actively enhances uptake of vitamin B$_{12}$ by bone marrow, placenta, and other tissues of the body that contain TCII receptors. TCII–vitamin B$_{12}$ is internalized by endocytotosis; vitamin B$_{12}$ is released by proteolytic cleavage in lysosomes but TCII is not reutilized (Table 22.5.6.1). TCII has a 20% amino acid homology and greater than 50% nucleotide homology with human TCI and with rat IF. It shows at least five genetic variants. Serum TCII is normally higher in women than men and in black populations compared with white. The concentration of vitamin B$_{12}$ in cerebrospinal fluid is low, with a mean of 10 ng/litre in normal subjects. Most of this is attached to TCII. There is virtually no vitamin B$_{12}$ in normal urine.

Folate

Biochemistry

This vitamin exists in nature in over 100 forms, all of which are derivatives of folic acid (pteroylglutamic acid), which consists of a pteridine, a *para*-aminobenzoic acid moiety and L-glutamic acid (Fig. 22.5.6.3). Natural folates differ from folic acid by:

- being reduced in the pteridine ring to di- or tetrahydo- forms
- having a single carbon moiety attached at positions N$_5$ or N$_{10}$ (e.g. methyl, formyl, etc.)
- having a chain of glutamate moieties attached by γ-peptide bonds to the L-glutamate moiety

In human and other mammalian cells, the number of glutamates is mainly four, five, or six. Polyglutamate forms of folate are the active coenzymes; these show increased affinity or lowered K_m values for most of the enzymes of one-carbon metabolism. In body fluids however, folates are monoglutamate derivatives. In plasma, 5-methyltetrahydrofolate (methyl-THF) predominates.

The biochemical reactions of folates are shown in Table 22.5.6.3. In each there is transfer of a single carbon group, methyl (–CH$_3$), formyl (–CHOH), methenyl (≡CH), methylene (=CH$_2$), or formimino (=CHNH), from one compound to another. Three of the reactions are concerned with synthesis of DNA precursors (two purine and one pyrimidine). During thymidylate synthesis, oxidation of folate to the dihydro state occurs; the enzyme dihydrofolate reductase, the principal target for the antifolates methotrexate and pyrimethamine, returns folate to the active tetrahydro state (Fig. 22.5.6.4). During its reactions, folate is not completely reutilized, some degradation at the C$_9$–N$_{10}$ bond occurs to nonfolate compounds. Thus, folate utilization is increased and folate

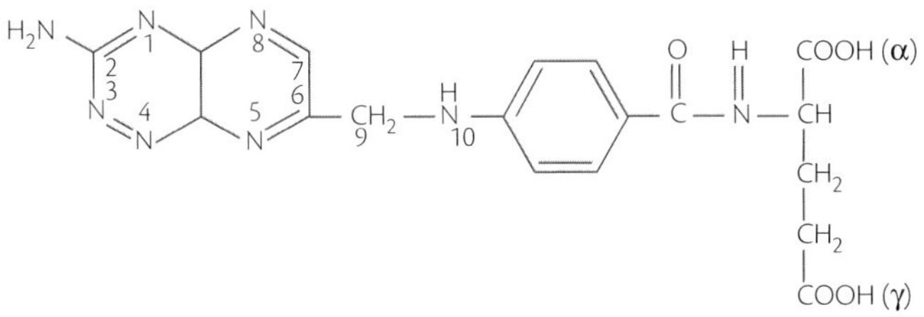

Fig. 22.5.6.3 The structure of pteroylglutamic (folic) acid.

Table 22.5.6.3 Biochemical reactions of folates

Reaction	Enzyme
1. Conjugation or deconjugation	
Hydrolysis of poly- to monoglutamates	Folate 'conjugase' (α-glutamylcarboxypeptidase; pteroylpolyglutamate hydrolase)
Conjugation of monoglutamates to polyglutamates	Folate-polyglutamate synthetase
2. Oxidation–reduction	
Oxidized or dihydrofolates, converted to tetrahydrofolates	Dihydrofolate reductase
3. Amino acid interconversions	
(a) homocysteine → methionine[1]	+ +
+ +	5-Methyl THF methyltransferase
methyl THF →THF	
(b) 5-formiminoglutamic acid → glutamic acid (Figlu)	Figlu transferase
+ +	
THF → formimino THF	Serine–hydroxymethyltransferase
(c) serine → glycine	
++	
THF → 5,10-methylene THF	
4. DNA synthesis	
Purine synthesis:	
(a) GAR → formyl GAR	GAR transformylase
+ +	
5,10 methenyl THF →THF	
(b) AICAR → inosinic acid	AICAR transformylase
+ +	
10-formyl THF →THF	
Pyrimidine synthesis:	
Deoxyuridine monophosphate (dUMP) → thymidine monophosphate (TMP)	Thymidylate synthetase
5,10-methylene THF → THF	
5. Formate fixation	
Formic acid + ATP + THF → 10-formyl-THF + ADP	THF formylase
6. ? Methylation of biogenic amines	
e.g. dopamine → epinine	? dopamine methyltransferase
++	
methyl THF → THF	

[1] See Figs. 2 and 4.
THF, tetrahydrofolate; DHF, dihydrofolate; GAR, glycinamide ribotide; AICAR, 5-amino-4-imidazolecarboxamide ribotide.
Reaction (6) has been demonstrated only *in vitro* and may not take place *in vivo*.

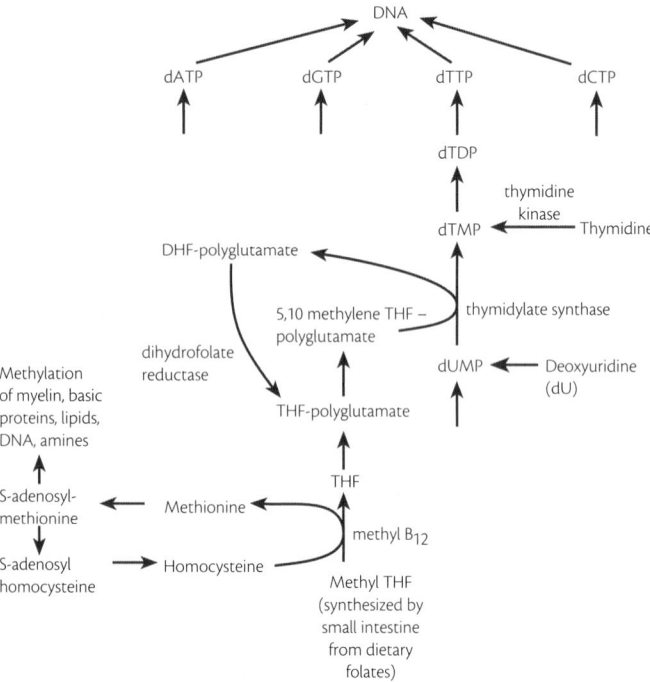

Fig. 22.5.6.4 Suggested mechanisms by which vitamin B_{12} deficiency affects folate metabolism and interferes with DNA synthesis. Indirect involvement of vitamin B_{12}, as methylcobalamin, in DNA synthesis is suggested by the 'methylfolate' trap ('tetrahydrofolate starvation') hypothesis. Methylcobalamin is involved in formation of intracellular THF from plasma methyl-THF. THF and/or its formyl derivative, but not methyl-THF, are the 'ground substances' from which all folate coenzymes are made by glutamate addition and single carbon unit transfer. 5,10-Methylene-THF polyglutamate is involved in thymidylate synthesis. A, adenine; C, cytosine; D, deoxyribose; DP, diphosphate; G, guanine; T, thymine; THF, tetrahydrofolate; TP, triphosphate; U, uridine.

deficiency likely when cell turnover and DNA synthesis are increased.

Nutrition

Folate occurs in most foods, the highest concentrations (more than 30 μg/100 g wet weight) in liver (in which it is easily destroyed by cooking). Vitamin C protects folate from oxidative destruction. An average Western daily intake is about 250 μg, with 50% or more in the polyglutamate form. Body stores are about 10 to 12 mg, with a mean liver concentration of about 7 μg/g. Primitive or rapidly growing tissues have higher folate concentrations than corresponding mature tissues. Daily adult requirements are about 100 μg.

Absorption

Folates are absorbed rapidly, mainly through the duodenum and jejunum. Polyglutamates are deconjugated in the intestinal lumen, at the brush border, and possibly in lysosomes of intestinal cells by an enzyme known as folate conjugase (γ-glutamylcarboxypeptidase, pteroylpolyglutamate hydrolase). They are reduced to the tetrahydro state and methylated at the N_5 position so that methyl-THF enters portal plasma whatever food folate is ingested (Table 22.5.6.1). Folic (pteroylglutamic) acid itself, which is not present in food, but is used therapeutically, enters the portal blood largely unchanged at doses of more than 100 to 200 μg, as it is a poor substrate for reduction by dihydrofolate reductase. A proton-coupled folate transporter (PCFT) with high affinity and a low pH optimum is essential for absorption of reduced folates and folic acid. It is expressed particularly in the apical brush border of the enterocytes of the duodenum and jejunum. Various mutations have been found in this transporter in patients with a specific hereditary malabsorption of folate. The protein is expressed in other tissues and may be involved in intracellular transportation of folates from endocytic vesicles. As it is also active at neutral pH for methyl THF, it may play a role in delivering this folate to systemic cells, e.g. the liver. It may also transport antifolates, e.g. methotrexate and pemetrexed, into the acid interior of solid tumours. The small intestine has a large capacity to absorb folate; on average 50% of natural folate is absorbed whatever the dose. If excessive amounts are fed, the excess is largely excreted in urine as folates or their breakdown products after cleavage of the $C_9–N_{10}$ bond. There is a substantial enterohepatic circulation for folate, estimated at up to 90 µg folate daily; if this is interrupted, plasma folate concentrations decrease to about one-third within 24 h.

Transport

Folate is transported in plasma, two-thirds unbound and about one-third loosely bound to albumin and possible other proteins. There are two highly specific mammalian folate transporters. SLC19A1 is a facilitative transporter with the characteristics of an anion exchanger. The gene is located at chromosome 21q 22.2. The protein has 12 transmembrane domains and both N- and C-termini are directed to the cytoplasm. It is ubiquitously expressed on normal tissues and tumours. Its affinity for folic acid and methotrexate is one to two orders less than for reduced folates. The second is a group of high affinity binding proteins (FRs) encoded by three genes, designated α, β, and γ, localized to chromosome 11q 13.3-q 13.5. FRα and FRβ are both glycosylphosphatidylinositol (GPI) anchored proteins. The physiological role of the FRs is not clear. They are expressed in the apical brush border of the renal tubular epithelial cells so may have a role in renal reabsorption of folates.

Folate taken up by membrane-bound FRs is thought to enter endocytic vesicles. FRα (but not FRβ) knockout mice show fatal morphological abnormalities, suggesting a critical role in mouse development. The FRs have enhanced expression on certain tumour cells and this has prompted studies aimed at developing tumour-specific antifolates or folate-conjugated radiopharmaceuticals or other molecules.

Plasma folate is filtered by the glomerulus and mostly reabsorbed unless the renal tubular maximum is exceeded. Normal urine folate is 0 to 13 µg in 24 h. Folate is secreted into cerebrospinal fluid (which has a mean concentration of 24 µg/litre) and is present in bile. Human milk has a folate concentration of 50 µg/litre. Prostate-specific membrane antigen is a folate hydrolase carboxypeptidase which can release glutamates in either α or γ linkages. The physiological significance of this is unknown.

Biochemical basis of megaloblastic anaemia

All known causes of megaloblastic anaemia, whether drugs, deficiencies, or inborn errors of metabolism, inhibit DNA synthesis by reducing the activity of one of the many enzymes concerned in purine or pyrimidine synthesis or by inhibiting DNA polymerization from its precursors. Folate deficiency, by reducing supply of the active coenzyme form, 5,10-methylene-THF, inhibits thymidylate synthesis, a rate-limiting reaction in DNA synthesis.

Vitamin B_{12} does not have a direct role in this or any other reaction in mammalian DNA synthesis. Vitamin B_{12} deficiency inhibits DNA synthesis indirectly because of the requirement for methylcobalamin in the conversion of methyl-THF that has entered cells from the plasma to THF. Deficiency of vitamin B_{12} is considered to decrease the intracellular supply of THF, from which the natural folate coenzymes, folate polyglutamates, are made. Methyl-THF cannot act as a substrate for synthesis of folate polyglutamates in human cells. When vitamin B_{12} is deficient there is reduced activity of all reactions requiring folate coenzymes, including those involved in DNA synthesis (Fig. 22.5.6.4). Misincorporation of the base uracil, because of the accumulation of dUMP (Fig. 22.5.6.1), and hence of dUTP, has been proposed to contribute to the DNA abnormality.

Clinical features and causes of megaloblastic anaemia

Although pernicious anaemia (PA) is only one of the many causes of megaloblastic anaemia (Tables 22.5.6.4–22.5.6.6), it is convenient to describe the general clinical features of the anaemia under this

Table 22.5.6. 4 Causes of B_{12} deficiency and malabsorption of B_{12}

1. Causes of severe B_{12} deficiency
(a) Nutritional:
vegans
long-continued extremely poor diet (rarely)
(b) Malabsorption:
gastric causes
acquired (addisonian) pernicious anaemia
congenital intrinsic-factor deficiency or abnormality
total and partial gastrectomy
destructive lesions of stomach
intestinal causes
gut flora associated with (jejunal diverticulosis, ileocolic, fistula, anatomical blind loop, stricture, Whipple's disease, scleroderma, HIV disease)
ileal resection and Crohn's disease
chronic tropical sprue
selective malabsorption with proteinuria
irradiation to cervix
HIV disease
fish tapeworm
transcobalamin II deficiency

2. Causes of malabsorption of B_{12} usually without severe B_{12} deficiency
Simple atrophic gastritis, gastric bypass, severe chronic pancreatitis
Zollinger–Ellison syndrome, adult gluten-induced enteropathy, giardiasis
Drugs:
PAS, colchicine, neomycin, slow K, ethanol, metformin, phenformin, anticonvulsants
Deficiencies of folate, B_{12}, protein

Table 22.5.6.5 Causes of folate deficiency

1. Poor diet

Especially poverty, psychiatric disturbance, alcoholism, dietary fads, scurvy, kwashiorkor, goat's milk anaemia, partial gastrectomy, other gastrointestinal disease

2. Malabsorption

Gluten-induced enteropathy (child or adult or associated with dermatitis herpetiformis)

Tropical sprue

Congenital specific malabsorption

Minor factor: partial gastrectomy, jejunal resection, inflammatory bowel disease, lymphoma, systemic infections

Drugs: cholestyramine, sulphasalazine, methotrexate, ? others (see (5) below).

3. Excessive requirements

Physiological

Pregnancy

Prematurity and infancy

Pathological:

(a) Malignancies—leukaemia, carcinoma, lymphoma, myeloma, sarcoma, etc.

(b) Blood disorders—haemolytic anaemia (especially sickle-cell anaemia, thalassaemia major), primary myelofibrosis

(c) Inflammatory—tuberculosis, malaria, Crohn's diseases, psoriasis, exfoliative dermatitis, rheumatoid arthritis, etc.

(d) Metabolic—homocystinuria (some cases)

4. Excess urinary excretion

Congestive heart failure, acute liver damage, chronic dialysis

5. Drugs

Mechanism uncertain

Anticonvulsants (diphenylhydantoin, primidone, barbiturates)

? nitrofurantoin

? alcohol

Also drugs causing malabsorption of folate (see (2) above)

6. Liver disease

Mixed causes above, and poor storage

Table 22.5.6.6 Megaloblastic anaemia not due to vitamin B_{12} or folate deficiency

1. Abnormalities of B_{12} or folate metabolism

Congenital

Transcobalamin II deficiency or functional abnormality

Inborn errors of folate metabolism e.g. methylfolate transferase deficiency

Homocystinuria and methylmalonic aciduria (some cases)

Acquired

Nitrous oxide

Dihydrofolate reductase inhibitors: methotrexate, pyrimethamine, trimethoprim, ?pentamidine, triamterene

2. Independent of B_{12} or folate

Congenital

Orotic aciduria, (responds to uridine)

Lesch–Nyhan syndrome, ? responds to adenine

Thiamine-responsive

Some cases of congenital dyserythropoietic anaemia

Acquired

AML FAB M_6, other myeloid leukaemias (some cases)

Myelodysplasia

Drugs

Antimetabolites: 6-mercaptopurine, cytosine arabinoside, hydroxyurea, 5-fluorouracil, azathioprine, etc.

heading; PA is the most frequent cause of megaloblastic anaemia in Western countries. The laboratory findings and treatment of PA and other megaloblastic anaemias are discussed later.

Acquired pernicious anaemia (Addisonian pernicious anaemia, Biermer's anaemia, pernicious anaemia)

Definition

An autoimmune disease in which there is atrophy of the stomach with severely reduced or absent IF and acid secretion with consequent malabsorption of vitamin B_{12} and vitamin B_{12} deficiency.

Aetiology

PA is a disease of older people: less than 10% of patients are under the age of 40 years. There is a female:male ratio in most (but not all) series of about 1.6:1. There is a slightly higher prevalence

(c.44% vs 40%) of blood group A in patients with PA compared with controls in the United Kingdom. No overall association between PA and HLA type has been found, but those with an endocrine disease have a greater incidence of HLA B8, B_{12}, and BW15. Contrary to previous opinions, PA occurs in all ethnic groups including African, Indian, Native American, and Chinese, as well as white Europeans. There is a higher incidence in close relatives, of either sex, of an affected person.

DNA sequence variants of a gene *NLRP1*, located at chromosome 17p13, encoding NACHT, a leucine-rich repeat protein which is a regulator of the innate immune response, have been associated with vitiligo and its associated diseases including PA.

About 55% of patients have serum thyroid antibodies and 33% with primary myxoedema have parietal-cell antibody. There is probably no association with diabetes mellitus. Other evidence for an immune aetiology of the gastritis of PA is the improvement in mucosal appearance and function with corticosteroid therapy, the presence of antibodies in serum and gastric juice directed against parietal cells and IF, and of cell-mediated immunity to IF (see Chapter 5.2). Parietal-cell antibody is present in the serum of 85 to 90% of patients. The autoantigens are the α- and β-subunit of the gastrin proton pump (H^+,K^+ ATPase). Two antibodies to IF exist in serum. Type I ('blocking') occurs in about 50% of patients and is directed against the vitamin B_{12}-binding site. Type II (to the ileal binding site) occurs in 30 to 35% but only if type I antibody is also present. Antibodies to IF exist in gastric juice and here they may neutralize the action of remaining IF. The incidence of parietal-cell and IF antibodies in serum in PA may be different in different groups of patients, younger patients having a lower incidence of parietal-cell antibody while blacks and Hispanics may have a higher incidence of IF antibodies. The antibodies to IF are virtually specific for PA but parietal-cell antibody occurs in many subjects with atrophic gastritis without PA. An autoantibody to the gastrin receptor may also occur in serum in PA.

PA may be associated with hypgogammaglobulinaemia or with selective IgA deficiency when it tends to present at an early age. Serum gastrin concentrations are raised (>200 μg/litre) in 90% of patients with PA, and serum pepsinogen (PG) concentrations are less than 30 μg/litre in 92% of such patients with a low PGI/PGII ratio.

The relationship of PA, auto immune gastritis, and *Helicobacter pylori* infection is not clear. Young subjects (<40 years) with gastritis, hypergastrinaemia, and positive antiparietal cell antibody in serum will usually show iron deficiency anaemia whereas older (>60 years) with these features more frequently have macrocytic red cells and low serum vitamin B_{12} levels. *H. pylori* infection occurs in up to 40% of such subjects less than 20 years old but in only 10% of those older than 60 years.

Pathology

There is a gastritis in which all layers of the body and fundus of the stomach are atrophied with loss of normal gastric glands, mucosal architecture, and absence of parietal and chief cells, but mucous cells lining the gastric pits are well preserved. An infiltrate of plasma cells and lymphocytes with an excess of CD8 cells occurs and intestinal metaplasia may be present. The antral mucosa is well preserved except in hypogammaglobulinaemia, and, like the fundus, shows an increased number of gastrin-secreting cells.

Clinical features

The general features of megaloblastic anaemia are similar, whatever the underlying cause. Particular clinical features may point to the underlying disease, whether PA or some other cause. In PA, the anaemia usually develops gradually, perhaps over several years, and symptoms may not occur until it is severe. The most common complaints are due to the anaemia, but loss of mental and physical drive, numbness, or difficulty in walking suggest neurological complications. Psychiatric disturbances are common and range from mild neurosis to severe organic dementia. They may occur in the absence of anaemia or macrocytosis. Mild jaundice, loss of appetite and weight, indigestion, and episodic diarrhoea are frequent. An intercurrent infection may precipitate severe anaemia and thus symptoms. Older patients may present with congestive heart failure. In a few patients, bruising due to thrombocytopenia is marked. Many symptomless patients are diagnosed because a routine blood test is made.

Physical signs, if present, are those of anaemia, perhaps with mild jaundice, giving the patient a so-called lemon-yellow tint. A few patients with deficiency of either vitamin B_{12} or folate develop a widespread brown pigmentation, affecting nail beds and skin creases particularly, but not mucous membranes. This is reversible with the appropriate therapy. The tongue may be red, smooth, and shiny, occasionally with ulcers. A mild pyrexia up to 38°C is common in patients with moderate to severe anaemia. The liver may be enlarged while the cardiovascular system shows changes due to anaemia. Patients with PA may also have features of an associated disorder on presentation, most commonly myxoedema. Other thyroid disorders, vitiligo, carcinoma of the stomach (incidence three times controls), Addison's disease, and hypoparathyroidism,

may precede, occur simultaneously with, or follow the onset of the anaemia.

Neurological complications of vitamin B_{12} deficiency

Vitamin B_{12} deficiency may cause a symmetrical neuropathy affecting the lower limbs more than the upper (Chapter 24.13), which usually presents with paraesthesiae or with ataxia, particularly in the dark. In some cases, loss of cutaneous sensation, spastic paraparesis, muscle weakness, urinary or faecal incontinence, an optic neuropathy, or psychiatric disturbance dominates. The nervous system disease is due to severe deficiency judged by serum vitamin B_{12} levels or methylmalonic acid (MMA) excretion, but may occur with mild or no anaemia. A similar neurological syndrome with paraparesis has been described in dentists and others repeatedly exposed to nitrous oxide (N_2O), which inactivates methionine synthase. The biochemical explanation for the neurological disease is not clear. A defect in fatty acid metabolism in myelin tissue has been suggested. Studies in N_2O-treated monkeys have also suggested that the neuropathy results from accumulation of *S*-adenosyl homocysteine (caused by the block in conversion of homocysteine to methionine) with inhibition of transmethylation biogenic amines, proteins, phospholipids, and neurotransmitters in the spinal cord and brain. Methionine has been shown to prevent the neurotoxicity caused by N_2O in experimental animals. There is a more rapid decline in cognitive function in subjects with low serum holotranscobalamin and raised serum MMA concentrations. In some studies, subjects with low folate concentrations have, on long-term follow-up, a higher incidence of Alzheimer's disease and decreased cognitive function than those with serum folate in the healthy reference range. There are conflicting reports on whether administration of folic acid or vitamin B_{12} improve cognitive function in older people with or without low serum vitamin B_{12} or folate concentrations.

General tissue effects of vitamin B_{12} and folate deficiencies: the effects of folic acid supplementation

Both deficiencies cause macrocytosis and related cytopathic effects on proliferating epithelial cells throughout the body (e.g. bronchial, bladder, buccal, and uterine cervix), with glossitis and angular cheilosis, a mild malabsorption syndrome, and reduced regeneration of damaged liver cells. In both sexes, sterility (reversible with vitamin B_{12} or folate therapy) may result from effects on the gonads. It is possible that the deficiencies in children affect overall body growth. Nutritional vitamin B_{12} deficiency in infants long term causes failure to thrive and poor brain growth with poor intellectual outcome.

Generalized, reversible melanin pigmentation occurs in a few patients with vitamin B_{12} or folate deficiency, the cause of which is uncertain. Defective bactericidal activity of phagocytes due to impaired intracellular killing has been described in vitamin B_{12} deficiency but not in folate deficiency. Vitamin B_{12} deficiency reduces serum concentrations of the osteoblast-related proteins alkaline phosphatase and osteocalcin, but whether clinically important bone disease occurs is unknown.

Neural tube defects (NTD)

Folic acid supplements at the time of conception and in early (first weeks) of pregnancy reduce the incidence of NTD (anencephaly, encephalocele, and spina bifida) in the first pregnancy and in subsequent pregnancies where such a malformation has occurred previously.

Folic acid fortification of the diet has led to a substantial reduction of incidence of NTD, e.g. in the North America. The explanation for the effect of folic acid on NTD is not certain. Women carrying affected fetuses have lower serum folate and vitamin B_{12} concentrations and higher serum homocysteine levels than matched controls. There is a linear relationship when plotted on logarithmic scales between the birth incidence of NTD and maternal red-cell folate, indicating that an increase in red-cell folate even within normal range is associated with a constant, proportional decrease in the birth frequency of NTD. Folic acid prevention of NTD (and in some studies cleft lip and palate), despite apparently normal serum and red cell folate concentrations, suggests that folic acid is overcoming a metabolic abnormality in folate metabolism. Only one such defect, a mutated tetrahydofolate reductase, has been identified so far.

Mutated 5,10 methylene tetrahydrofolate reductase (MHTFR), a common thermolabile variant (677C→T) (Ala225Val) of the enzyme MHTFR is associated with lower serum and red-cell folate concentrations and with higher plasma homocysteine than in control subjects in the general population. The prevalence of the homozygous state in the population is approximately 5% and in parents of fetuses with NTD the prevalence is approximately 13%. The presence of this mutation can therefore account for only a small proportion of NTDs. Mutations of other genes, e.g. *VANGL1*, not related to folate metabolism, have been found in NTD families.

Cardiovascular disease

McCully (1969) first implicated homocysteine as a cause of atherosclerosis. This was based on pathological studies of children or young adults with congenital homocystinuria, whether due to a defect of cystathionine synthase, methionine synthase, or MHTFR (Fig. 22.5.6.5). In these children, plasma homocysteine concentrations are raised to 10 to 100 times normal. It is now apparent that even mild rises in plasma homocysteine are associated with coronary or peripheral arterial disease, stroke, and deep vein thrombosis. Homocysteine can directly injure endothelial cells, activate platelets and leucocytes, stimulate vascular smooth muscle proliferation, oxidize low-density lipoprotein (LDL) and disturb collagen and extracellular matrix formation. Determinants of

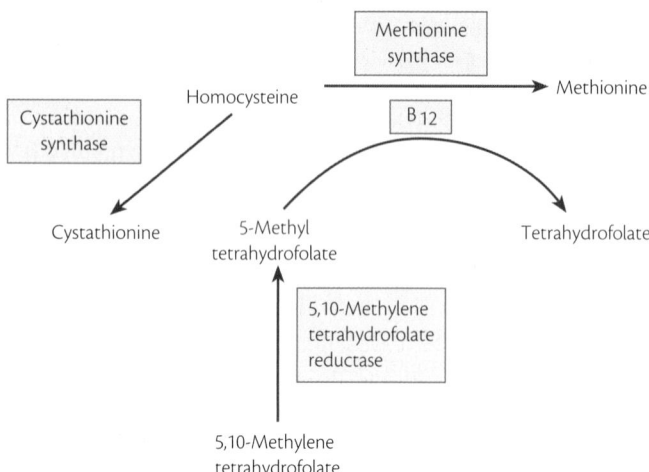

Fig. 22.5.6.5 The role of three enzymes (cystathione synthase, methionine synthase, and MHTFR) and three vitamins (vitamin B_{12}, vitamin B_6, and folate) in homocysteine metabolism.

plasma homocysteine include age, sex, renal function, protein intake, vitamin B_6, folate, and vitamin B_{12} status, the presence of the thermolabile variant MHTFR, smoking, and alcohol consumption, as well as intake of various drugs.

Folate deficiency assessed by serum or red-cell folate or by dietary folate intake is also associated with coronary vascular disease, myocardial infarct, and peripheral vascular disease. Meta-analysis of prospective trials shows that a 25% lower starting homocysteine level is associated with 11% lower coronary heart disease risk (and 19% lower stroke risk). There is also an association of the MTHFR homozygous state TT, a 3 µmol average higher homocysteine and a 10–15% higher risk of coronary heart disease and 20–25% stroke risk compared to subjects homozygous for the wild CC genotype.

It remains controversial whether homocysteine is a cause of vascular disease rather than an associated abnormality. Folic acid fortification of the diet reduces plasma homocysteine levels. It has been estimated that fortification of the British diet with folic acid will result in 10 000 fewer annual deaths from myocardial infarct. Preliminary results of electrocardiographic studies and of coronary restenosis after coronary angioplasty in patients with coronary arterial disease receiving folic acid are encouraging.

However, randomized prospective trials of homocysteine-lowering vitamins including folic acid, in contrast to the results with stroke prevention, have not shown a benefit for myocardial infarct or coronary heart disease. The results of much larger trials including many thousands of patients subjects, show no consistent benefits from folate supplementation on cardiovascular disease. Small studies have shown decreased risk of stenosis in those treated by balloon angioplasty but increased risk in those with stents.

Stroke

The results of eight randomized trials of folic acid supplementation have been analysed by Wang *et al.* (2007). They concluded that folic acid significantly reduced the risk of stroke by 18%, the greater benefit occurring in trials longer than 3 years, in those with a lowering of homocysteine more than 20%, in those in countries with no orally fortified grain, and in those with no history of a stroke. Moreover, a reduction in evidence of stroke occurred in the United States of America and Canada coinciding with the introduction of dietary folic acid fortification, whereas no reduction in incidence occurred over the same period (1998–2002) in England and Wales without fortification. In some trials, patients with previous strokes have been included, and the period of follow-up has been less than 36 months, which may explain discrepancies in conclusions between individual trials.

Malignancy

Positive and negative associations between the occurrence of various types if lymphoblastic or myeloblastic leukaemias in infancy and childhood and polymorphisms of folate-metabolizing enzymes including MHTFR have been reported. Folic acid prophylactically in pregnancy has been reported to reduce the incidence of a subsequent childhood acute lymphoblastic leukaemia and of brain tumours. In Canada, food fortification with folic acid has been associated with a 60% reduction in incidence of neuroblastoma.

Epidemiological studies show an inverse risk of colorectal cancer or adenoma and folate status and a less clear-cut relation exists with other gastrointestinal, lung, breast, ovary, and cervical carcinomas. Also small randomized and nonrandomised trials suggest a benefit of supplemental folic acid on incidence of colorectal cancer. A large randomized trial has shown no difference in overall incidence of colonic adenomas between controls and folic acid and aspirin-supplemented groups but secondary analysis showed a higher incidence of more than three adenomas in the supplemented group. This result might have arisen by chance, since a similar trial in which aspirin and folic acid were both given showed no excess of adenomas in association with administration of supplemental folic acid.

It has also been suggested that an increased incidence of colorectal cancer in the United States of America and Canada is associated with the fortification of the diet with folic acid, but the temporal disassociation between fortification and risk in colorectal cancer incidence makes this unlikely—increased detection by screening endoscopy is a more likely explanation. There has been no increase in mortality rate from colorectal cancer in the United States or Canada since fortification started.

Soon after its discovery, folic acid in large doses was found to promote the growth of existing cancers. Antifolate drugs were developed as a result of these observations. Recent studies suggest that dietary folic acid fortification may overall be of benefit to the population in reducing the incidence of malignancies but prospective randomized trials will help to resolve these issues. Secondary analysis of cardiovascular prevention trials have not shown a significant effect of folic acid supplementation on cancer incidence.

Other effects
High folate status may increase the risk of multiple births after in vitro fertilisation.

Other causes of vitamin B$_{12}$ deficiency

Juvenile PA
A few cases of PA with gastric atrophy, achlorhydria, and IF antibodies have occurred in children. They may show associated ('autoimmune') conditions, e.g. myxoedema, hypoparathyroidism, Addison's disease, or chronic mucocutaneous candidiasis.

Congenital deficiency or structural abnormality of intrinsic factor
Fewer than 100 cases have been reported of a child being born with absent or nonfunctioning IF due to a mutation of the IF gene. There is an otherwise normal stomach on biopsy and normal secretion of acid. Inheritance is autosomal recessive. In different cases, IF may be present in the gastric juice but susceptible to acid degradation or cannot bind vitamin B$_{12}$, or binds it but cannot attach it to ileal receptors. These children tend to present with irritability, vomiting, diarrhoea, and loss of weight, and are found to have megaloblastic anaemia. The usual age of diagnosis is about 2 years, although a few have been diagnosed as early as 4 months and others only in their teens.

Total gastrectomy
All patients who have this operation will develop vitamin B$_{12}$ deficiency, which usually presents between 2 and 6 years postoperatively. They should be treated with prophylactic vitamin B$_{12}$ injections from the time of the operation.

Partial gastrectomy
Iron deficiency usually accounts for the anaemia that occurs after this operation. About 6% develop megaloblastic anaemia due to

vitamin B$_{12}$ deficiency. In most of these patients, malabsorption of vitamin B$_{12}$ is due to an abnormal jejunal flora. The exact incidence of vitamin B$_{12}$ deficiency depends mainly on the size of the gastric remnant.

Small-intestinal lesions
Colonization of the upper small intestine with colonic bacteria, if sufficiently heavy as in the stagnant-loop syndrome, leads to malabsorption of vitamin B$_{12}$. The most common causes are listed in Table 22.5.6.4. It appears that the bacteria destroy IF. Infestation with the fish tapeworm (*Diphyllobothrium latum*) has a similar effect but is now almost completely eradicated; infestation is only sufficiently marked in Finland and Russian lake regions to represent a likely cause of megaloblastic anaemia.

HIV infection
Serum vitamin B$_{12}$ concentrations fall progressively in HIV-infected patients and subnormal serum values occur in 10 to 35% of individuals with AIDS. Increased concentrations of TCII are usual and malabsorption of vitamin B$_{12}$, not corrected by IF, has been found in some of these patients. An abnormal small-intestinal flora is the most likely cause of vitamin B$_{12}$ malabsorption. Megaloblastic anaemia due to vitamin B$_{12}$ deficiency is, however, rare.

Resection of 1 m or more of terminal ileum
This causes severe malabsorption of vitamin B$_{12}$. Other diseases that may affect ileal structure and function include: tropical sprue, in which severe vitamin B$_{12}$ deficiency with anaemia or, rarely, neuropathy is a manifestation only in the chronic phase; gluten-induced enteropathy in which megaloblastic anaemia, if it occurs, is always due to folate deficiency (and vitamin B$_{12}$ deficiency, if it occurs, is mild); in Crohn's disease malabsorption of vitamin B$_{12}$ is frequent but severe vitamin B$_{12}$ deficiency is unusual unless an ileal resection, fistula, or stagnant loop occurs.

Selective malabsorption of vitamin B$_{12}$ with proteinuria (Imerslund's disease, Imerslund–Gräsbeck syndrome, recessive megaloblastic anaemia, MGA1) (OMIM 261100)
This congenital disorder with autosomal recessive inheritance is the most common cause of megaloblastic anaemia due to vitamin B$_{12}$ deficiency in nonvegan children. The child secretes IF normally but is unable to transport vitamin B$_{12}$ across the ileum to portal blood. Most Finnish patients with MGA1 carry the disease-specific mutation P1297L (FM1) in cublin. A second less frequent mutation (FM2) activates a cryptic splice site with insertion of multiple stop codons in the CUB6 domain. In Norway at least six different mutations of the *AMN* gene have been reported in affected families. The proteinuria, present in over 90% of cases, is benign, non-specific, and persists after vitamin B$_{12}$ therapy. The clinical presentation of the disease is identical to that of congenital IF deficiency.

Other causes of malabsorption of vitamin B$_{12}$
Several other conditions and drugs may cause malabsorption of vitamin B$_{12}$ but rarely cause deficiency of clinical severity. *p*-Aminosalicylate, colchicine, neomycin, 'slow' potassium tablets, metformin, phenformin and sunitinib, a tyrosine kinase inhibitor used to treat renal cell carcinoma, have all been reported to cause malabsorption of vitamin B$_{12}$. In chronic pancreatitis and the Zollinger–Ellison syndrome, there is failure to release vitamin B$_{12}$

from haptocorrin due to absence or inactivation of pancreatic trypsin. Malabsorption of vitamin B_{12} also occurs in inherited TCII deficiency.

Malabsorption of vitamin B_{12} occurs temporarily after total-body irradiation before stem cell transplantation. In chronic graft vs host disease affecting the gut malabsorption of vitamin B_{12} is usual, due to the abnormal gut flora as well as any ileal defect. Irradiation to the ileum during radiotherapy treatment for carcinoma of the cervix has also been reported to cause vitamin B_{12} malabsorption.

Dietary vitamin B_{12} deficiency

This occurs most commonly in Hindus who omit all animal produce from their diet. The incidence of overt megaloblastic anaemia is much lower than the incidence of subclinical deficiency assessed by the serum vitamin B_{12} assay. These individuals have low vitamin B_{12} stores. In India, babies have been born vitamin B_{12} deficient with megaloblastic anaemia caused by severe vitamin B_{12} deficiency (due to poor diet or tropical sprue) in the mother. Dietary deficiency of vitamin B_{12} also occurs in non-Hindu vegans, and rarely in nonvegetarian people living on inadequate diets because of poverty.

Folate deficiency

Clinical features

The main clinical features of megaloblastic anaemia due to folate deficiency are similar to those when the anaemia is due to vitamin B_{12} deficiency, except that a severe neuropathy does not occur and the underlying aetiology tends to be different. Cognitive changes and depression may be caused by the deficiency. Neurological abnormalities do occur with inborn errors of folate metabolism and may be precipitated by antifolate drugs. Folate deficiency may develop rapidly, and although many mildly deficient patients do not progress for months or years, in some patients the deficiency may lead to a severe pancytopenia ('arrest of haemopoiesis') over a short period, particularly if an infection supervenes.

Nutritional folate deficiency

Minor degrees of nutritional folate deficiency are frequent in most countries, but severe folate deficiency may account for about 17% of all cases of megaloblastic anaemia in the United Kingdom. It occurs mainly in people who are old, poor, and psychiatrically disturbed, living alone on an inadequate diet from which liver, fruit, and fresh vegetables are omitted; in some, barbiturates or consumption of spirits or cough mixtures or a physical abnormality such as rheumatoid arthritis, or tuberculosis may aggravate the effect of a poor diet. A few cases have developed because a special diet is taken, such as for phenylketonuria or for slimming. Scurvy is usually accompanied by severe folate deficiency. Goat's milk anaemia is a nutritional folate deficiency due to the low (6 µg/litre) folate content of goat's milk. In some countries (e.g. Burma, Malaysia, Africa, or India), nutritional folate deficiency is the main cause of megaloblastic anaemia, often presenting in pregnancy. Among Hindus, nutritional vitamin B_{12} deficiency is also common, however, and in many countries—e.g. Caribbean islands, Sri Lanka, and South-East Asia—tropical sprue (see Chapter 15.10.8) is an important cause of both deficiencies and is difficult to distinguish from 'pure' nutritional deficiency.

Malabsorption (see Section 15)
Gluten-induced enteropathy

Folate deficiency due to malabsorption of folates occurs in virtually all untreated patients, the serum folate being subnormal in virtually 100% and red-cell folate subnormal in 80% or more. Anaemia occurs in about 90% of adult cases, due to folate deficiency alone in 30 to 50% and to mixed iron and folate deficiency in the remainder. Mild vitamin B_{12} deficiency may also occur, but it is not a cause of anaemia in uncomplicated cases. Spontaneous atrophy of the spleen occurs in most of the patients; in about 10 to 15% of cases; the blood film shows the presence of Howell–Jolly bodies, and other features of hyposplenism. A gluten-free diet produces a spontaneous rise in serum and red-cell folate in those patients who respond. In children with gluten-induced enteropathy, anaemia is most often due to combined iron and folate deficiency.

Patients with dermatitis herpetiformis almost all show some degree of gluten-induced duodenal and jejunal abnormality; the severity of folate malabsorption and deficiency correlates with the severity of the intestinal lesion.

Tropical sprue (see Chapter 15.10.8)

Malabsorption of folate occurs in all severe, untreated patients in the acute phase and megaloblastic anaemia due to folate deficiency may develop within a few months. Not only does the anaemia respond to folate therapy but in many patients all the clinical features, and malabsorption of fat, vitamin B_{12}, and other substances, improves on folate therapy alone. In the first year about 60% of patients appear to be cured by folic acid alone. Long-standing cases are more likely to be vitamin B_{12} deficient and thus to require vitamin B_{12} as well as folate and antibiotic therapy.

Congenital specific malabsorption of folate

This is a rare, autosomal recessive abnormality. Affected children show features of damage to the central nervous system (mental retardation, fits, athetotic movements) and present with megaloblastic anaemia responding to physiological doses of folic acid given parenterally but not orally. Folate levels in cerebrospinal fluid are low. It is due to inherited mutations of the proton-coupled folate transporter (PCFT) affecting protein stability or its membrane trafficking.

Other causes

Absorption of folate is impaired by systemic infections. Mild degrees of folate malabsorption have also been reported after jejunal resection or partial gastrectomy, with Crohn's disease, and with lymphoma. In the intestinal stagnant-loop syndrome, folate levels tend to be high due to absorption of bacterially produced folate. Alcohol, anticonvulsants, oral contraceptives, antituberculous drugs, nitrofurantoin, and sulphasalazine have been suggested, on variable evidence, to cause malabsorption of folate in some subjects but none is definitely established except sulphasalazine.

Increased folate utilization

A general mechanism of increased folate utilization in conditions of increased cell turnover has emerged. This consists of partial degradation of folate at the C_9–N_{10} bond rather than complete recycling of the folate coenzymes required in DNA synthesis.

Pregnancy (see also Section 14)

This, associated with poor nutrition, is probably the most common cause of megaloblastic anaemia world-wide, unless folic acid supplements are taken. The frequency of the anaemia was about 0.5% in most Western cities and up to 50% in some areas of Asia and Africa until the introduction of prophylactic folic acid. The incidence increases with parity and is higher in twin pregnancies. Folate requirements in a normal pregnancy are increased to about 300 to 400 μg daily. Serum and red-cell folate tend to fall as pregnancy progresses, and to rise spontaneously about 6 weeks after delivery. Lactation may prove an additional cause of folate deficiency, however, which may precipitate megaloblastic anaemia postpartum.

The cause of the deficiency in pregnancy is increased degradation of folate. Folate transfer to the fetus may play a minor part; in a few, megaloblastic anaemia of pregnancy is the first sign of gluten induced enteropathy. The statistical association of iron and folate deficiencies in pregnancy is probably due to a poor quality of the diet in certain women.

Prophylactic folic acid should now be given routinely in pregnancy; 400 μg/day is recommended (see earlier) and intake in women who may become pregnant should be at least this amount daily from food or supplements. Larger doses (4–5 mg/day) should be used if there has been a previous infant with an NTD.

Prematurity
Newborn infants have higher serum and red-cell folate concentrations than adults. These fall to a lowest value at about 6 weeks of age. In premature infants, the decline is particularly steep and megaloblastic anaemia may develop, particularly if infections, feeding difficulties, or haemolytic disease with exchange transfusion have occurred. Prophylactic folic acid (e.g. 1 mg/week for the first 3–4 weeks of life) may be given, particularly to those babies weighing less than 1.5 to 1.8 kg at birth.

Malignant diseases
Mild folate deficiency is frequent in patients with cancer (Table 22.5.6.5). In general, the severity correlates with the extent and degree of dissemination of the underlying disease. Patients with megaloblastic anaemia due to folate deficiency are unusual and, as folic acid might 'feed the tumour', it should be withheld unless there is a real indication for its use, e.g. gross megaloblastosis causing severe anaemia, leucopenia, or thrombocytopenia. The potential effects of food fortification with folic acid on malignant disease were discussed earlier.

Blood disorders
Chronic haemolytic anaemia Requirements for folate are increased in patients with increased erythropoiesis, particularly when there is ineffective erythropoiesis with a high turnover of primitive cells. Occasional patients, presumably those with a poor folate intake, develop megaloblastic anaemia, particularly in sickle cell anaemia, thalassaemia major, hereditary spherocytosis, and warm-type autoimmune haemolytic anaemia; prophylactic folic acid is usually given in these disorders.

Primary myelofibrosis Megaloblastic haemopoiesis was reported in as many as one-third of patients. Circulating megaloblasts, increased transfusion requirements, severe thrombocytopenia, or pancytopenia may be the first indication that folate deficiency has developed. Polycythaemia vera is not a cause of folate deficiency.

Sideroblastic anaemia Folate deficiency, usually mild, may occur in about half of acquired cases. Megaloblastosis, refractory to folate

or vitamin B_{12}, also occurs in the acquired form as in other myelodysplastic diseases.

Inflammatory diseases
Folate deficiency has been described in patients with tuberculosis, malaria, Crohn's disease, psoriasis, widespread eczema, and rheumatoid arthritis. The degree of deficiency is related to the extent and severity of the underlying disorder. Increased demand for folate probably is a factor but reduced appetite is also important in those who develop megaloblastic anaemia.

Metabolic
Homocystinuria (see Chapter 12.2) Patients with the most common form of this disorder, due to cystathionase deficiency, may show folate deficiency, possibly due to excess conversion of homocysteine to methionine and thus excess utilization of the folate coenzyme concerned.

Excess urinary loss of folate
Urine folate excretion of 100 μg a day or more occurs in some patients with congestive cardiac failure or active liver disease causing necrosis of liver cells. It is presumed that losses are due to release of folate from damaged liver cells. Haemodialysis and peritoneal dialysis remove folate from plasma. Folic acid (e.g. 5 mg/week) is now usually given prophylactically to patients with renal failure who require long-term dialysis.

Drugs

Dihydrofolate reductase (DHFR) inhibitors
Methotrexate, aminopterin, pyrimethamine, and trimethoprim all inhibit DHFR but have different relative activities against the human, malarial, and bacterial enzymes. Methotrexate is converted to polyglutamate forms, which increases its activity against DHFR and also increases its retention in cells. These methotrexate derivatives invariably impair human folate metabolism. Trimethoprim, used as an antibacterial agent, may aggravate pre-existing folate or vitamin B_{12} deficiency but does not in itself cause megaloblastic anaemia.

Alcohol
Folate deficiency may occur in spirit-drinking alcoholics. The main factor is poor nutrition and it is likely that alcohol interrupts the enterohepatic circulation for folate. It also has a direct effect on haemopoiesis, causing vacuolation of normoblasts, impaired iron utilization, sideroblastic changes, macrocytosis, megaloblastosis, and thrombocytopenia, even in the absence of folate deficiency. Beer drinkers usually appear to avoid folate deficiency because of the high folate content of beer. The usual macrocytosis in nonanaemic alcoholics is not related to folate deficiency.

Anticonvulsants, barbiturates
Diphenylhydantoin, primidone, and barbiturate therapy may be associated with folate deficiency. The more severe deficiency is associated with poor dietary intake of folate and prolonged drug therapy at high doses. The mechanism of the deficiency is unknown and double-blind trials have shown no effect of folic acid supplementation on the frequency of seizures.

Other drugs
Nitrofurantoin, triamterene, proguanil, and pentamidine have been reported to cause folate deficiency.

Liver disease

Folate deficiency occurs most commonly in alcoholic cirrhosis where alcohol, poor nutrition, release of stored folate with excess urine losses may all be important. The deficiency is less frequent in other types of liver disease.

Laboratory investigation of megaloblastic anaemia

This consists of three stages: (1) recognition that megaloblastic anaemia is present; (2) distinction between vitamin B_{12} or folate deficiency (or rarely some other factor) as the cause of the anaemia; (3) diagnosis of the underlying disease causing the deficiency (Table 22.5.6.7).

Recognition of megaloblastic anaemia

Peripheral blood

The mean corpuscle volume (MCV) is raised to between 100 and 140 fl. Oval macrocytes are seen in the blood film. In mild cases, macrocytosis is present before anaemia has developed. Cabot rings (composed of arginine-rich histone and nonhaemoglobin iron) and occasional Howell–Jolly bodies (DNA fragments) may occur due to extramedullary haemopoiesis in the liver and spleen. The MCV may be normal if there is associated iron deficiency, when the blood film appears dimorphic, or if the anaemia (usually due to folate deficiency or antimetabolite drug therapy) develops acutely

Table 22.5.6.7 Laboratory diagnosis of megaloblastic anaemia

1. **General tests**
Peripheral blood film and count
Bone marrow
Serum bilirubin, iron, LDH
2. **Tests for B_{12} or folate deficiency**
Serum B_{12} and folate; red-cell folate
Serum homocysteine and methylmalonic acid levels
3. **Tests for cause of B_{12} or folate deficiency**
B_{12} deficiency:
Serum antibodies to parietal cell, intrinsic factor
Serum immunoglobulins
Gastric secretion; intrinsic factor, acid, serum gastrin
Endoscopy, gastric biopsy
Barium meal + follow-through
Proteinuria, fish tapeworm ova, intestinal flora, etc.
Folate deficiency:
Small-intestinal function
Xylose, glucose, vitamin A, fat, B_{12} absorption
Duodenal or jejunal biopsy
Barium follow-through
Tests for many underlying conditions

over the course of a few weeks. The MCV is also normal in some severely anaemic cases involving excess red-cell fragmentation. The reticulocyte count is low for the degree of anaemia, usually of the order of 1 to 3%.

The peripheral blood also shows hypersegmented neutrophils (which have nuclei with more than five lobes; Fig. 22.5.6.6) and the leucocyte count is often moderately reduced in both neutrophils and lymphocytes, although the total leucocyte count rarely falls to less than 1.5×10^9/litre. The lymphocyte CD4/CD8 ratio is reduced. The platelet count may be moderately reduced but rarely falls below 40×10^9/litre.

Biochemical changes

These are confined to the anaemic patient and include a mild rise in serum bilirubin (up to $50\,\mu$mol/litre), mainly unconjugated, a rise in serum lactic dehydrogenase of up to $10\,000$ IU/litre. The serum iron and ferritin are also raised and fall with effective treatment. The serum cholesterol is low and alkaline phosphatase mildly reduced. Absence of haptoglobins is usual. In severe cases, free haemoglobin may be present in plasma, Schumm's test for methaemalbumin in serum is positive, and haemosiderin and fibrin degradation products are present in urine. The direct antiglobulin test is weakly positive in some patients, due to complement.

Bone marrow

The bone marrow is hypercellular in moderate or severely anaemic cases. The myeloid–erythroid ratio is often reduced or reversed. The erythroblasts are larger than normal and show asynchronous maturation of nucleus and cytoplasm, nuclear chromatin remaining primitive with an open, lacy, fine granular pattern despite normal maturation and haemoglobinization of the cytoplasm. Excessive numbers of dying cells, and nuclear remnants including Howell–Jolly bodies, mitoses, and multinucleate cells may be present. Because of death (by apoptosis) of later cells, there is a disproportionate accumulation of early cells. Giant and abnormally shaped metamyelocytes and megakaryocytes with hypersegmented nuclear lobes are also usually present (Fig. 22.5.6.7).

The severity of these changes parallels the degree of anaemia. In milder cases, changes, described as 'intermediate', 'transitional', or 'moderate', are principally in the size and nuclear chromatin pattern of the erythroblasts, with giant metamyelocytes present; hypercellularity and gross dyserythropoiesis may be absent. In very

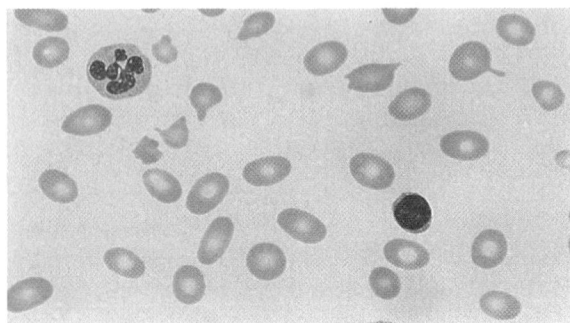

Fig. 22.5.6.6 Megaloblastic anaemia. Hb 4.0 g/dl, MCV 120 fl. Hypersegmented neutrophil, oval macrocytes, and a small lymphocyte to show size of macrocytes. The fragmentation of advanced megaloblastosis is present. Thrombocytopenia is marked.

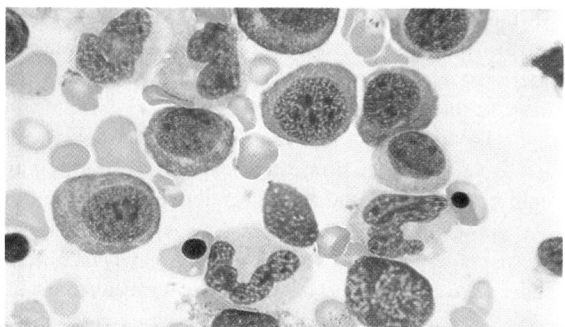

Fig. 22.5.6.7 Megaloblastic anaemia. Bone marrow aspirate showing megaloblasts at different stages and giant metamyelocytes.

mild cases, megaloblastic changes are difficult to recognize. In patients with severe anaemia but only mild megaloblastic changes, some additional cause for the anaemia should be sought.

Chromosomes

Changes found in marrow and other proliferating cells include: (1) random chromatin breaks; (2) exaggeration of centromere constriction; and (3) thin, elongated, uncoiled chromosomes.

Ineffective haemopoiesis

The increased cellularity of the marrow with degenerate forms, and the low reticulocyte count suggest that many developing cells are dying in the marrow. This occurs by apoptosis, especially of late erythroblasts. The raised unconjugated serum bilirubin, lactic dehydrogenase, and lysosyme are all due to ineffective haemopoiesis.

Differential diagnosis

Other causes of macrocytosis include a high reticulocytosis (e.g. haemolytic anaemia or regeneration of blood after haemorrhage), aplastic anaemia, red-cell aplasia, liver disease, alcoholism and myxoedema, the myelodyplastic syndromes, myeloid leukaemias, cytotoxic drug therapy, chronic respiratory failure, myelomatosis, and other paraproteinemia. Once a bone marrow biopsy has been done, the principal differentiation is from other causes of megaloblastosis, particularly myelodysplasia. Other causes of megaloblastic anaemia not due to vitamin B_{12} or folate deficiency are listed in Table 22.5.6.6.

Some patients with rapidly developing megaloblastic anaemia, particularly due to folate deficiency, may develop almost complete aplasia of the red-cell series, and the peripheral blood and bone marrow may resemble that of acute myeloid leukaemia.

Diagnosis of vitamin B_{12} or folate deficiency

The peripheral blood and bone marrow appearances are identical in folate or vitamin B_{12} deficiency. Special tests are, therefore, needed to distinguish between the two deficiencies.

Vitamin B_{12} deficiency

The assay of serum vitamin B_{12} content of serum is now by immunoassay. The reference range, depending on the assay, is from 160–200 to 960–1200 ng/litre. The concentrations are low in vitamin B_{12} deficiency, being extremely low in patients with neurological disease. Subnormal serum vitamin B_{12} concentrations in the absence of tissue vitamin B_{12} deficiency have been reported in

pregnancy, in inherited mutations of TCI (haptocorrin), in severe nutritional folate deficiency, in subjects taking large doses of vitamin C, and occasionally in iron deficiency. In the elderly, low serum vitamin B_{12} concentrations usually in the range 100–160 ng/litre may occur in the absence of anaemia or macrocytosis. In some research studies serum holo TCII levels have been measured to diagnose vitamin B_{12} deficiency.

Raised serum vitamin B_{12} concentrations, if not due to therapy, are most commonly caused by a rise in TCI as in a leucocytosis due to a myeloproliferative disease. Raised haptocorrin also occur in association with some tumours, especially hepatoma and fibrolamellar tumour of the liver. In benign leucocytosis, the rise is mainly of TCIII and this is often not accompanied by a high serum vitamin B_{12}. Raised serum TCII concentrations occur in conditions where macrophages are stimulated, e.g. autoimmune diseases such as systemic lupus erythematosus, rheumatoid arthritis, in Gaucher's disease and in some monocytic or monoblastic leukaemias, in histiocytic lymphomas, and inflammatory bowel disease. In active liver diseases, serum vitamin B_{12} leaks from the liver with saturation of the serum vitamin B_{12} binders.

A second and less widely used test for vitamin B_{12} deficiency is serum methylmalonic acid (MMA). Serum MMA levels are raised in vitamin B_{12} deficiency but not in folate deficiency but raised levels may occur in renal failure. Rare cases of congenital methylmalonicaciduria have been described, owing to a variety of enzyme defects.

A sensitive method of measuring MMA in serum has been introduced and combined with serum homocysteine assay for the diagnosis of vitamin B_{12} or folate deficiency. The significance of minor rises in serum MMA concentration found particularly in older people in the absence of macrocytes or anaemia with or without borderline vitamin B_{12} concentrations suggests 'biochemical' vitamin B_{12} deficiency which does not progress to megaloblastic anaemia. Randomized trials are needed to assess the value of preventing or treating disease due to putative vitamin B_{12} deficiency in these subjects.

Folate deficiency

Direct tests include the serum and red-cell folate assay. The serum folate is always low in folate deficiency (and is normal or raised in vitamin B_{12} deficiency unless folate deficiency is also present). Raised levels occur after folate therapy and also in vitamin B_{12} deficiency and in the stagnant-loop syndrome. Red-cell folate is a better guide than the serum folate to tissue folate stores but is low in a proportion of patients with megaloblastic anaemia solely due to vitamin B_{12} deficiency. Serum homocysteine levels are usually raised in folate and vitamin B_{12} deficiency and many other situations (see Chapter 12.2).

Diagnosis of the cause of vitamin B_{12} deficiency

Although the clinical and family history and the clinical findings may point to PA or some other cause of vitamin B_{12} deficiency, it is important to establish this for certain. A brief dietary history will rapidly establish whether or not the patient is a vegan or takes a very inadequate diet. Radioactive vitamin B_{12} absorption tests were valuable to demonstrate malabsorption of vitamin B_{12} and to differentiate gastric from small-intestinal lesions as the cause. These tests are now obsolete because of lack of availability of radioactive B12 and of intrinsic factor.

Endoscopy and gastric biopsy will show features of gastric atrophy and help to exclude gastric carcinoma. Follow-through radiographic examination of the small intestine will help to exclude a small-intestinal lesion, e.g. duodenal or jejunal diverticulosis.

The serum gastrin concentration is raised in most patients with PA and gastric atrophy and the serum is tested for antibodies to IF, parietal cells, and thyroid; serum immunoglobulins are measured in view of the association with hypogammaglobulinaemia.

Diagnosis of the cause of folate deficiency

An inadequate diet is usually at least partly implicated, but an exact estimate of dietary intake from the clinical history is impossible because of variation in folate content of foods, losses in cooking, and size of portions. Often it is the general social circumstances that suggest a poor intake. Drug intake, particularly of barbiturates, is important. Many underlying inflammatory or malignant diseases may exaggerate the tendency to folate deficiency in patients with inadequate diets. The main cause of malabsorption of folate is gluten-induced enteropathy; in patients with severe folate deficiency, tests for transglutaminase and antigliadin antibodies and a duodenal biopsy are usually necessary. In certain tropical countries, sprue may cause a generalized malabsorption syndrome in which folate deficiency commonly occurs.

Treatment of megaloblastic anaemia

Therapy is aimed at correcting the anaemia, completely replenishing the body of whichever vitamin is deficient, treatment of the underlying disorder, and prevention of relapse. In most cases, it is possible to diagnose which deficiency is present before starting therapy.

Vitamin B$_{12}$ deficiency

Hydroxocobalamin 1000 μg intramuscularly given six times at several days' interval over the first few weeks will restore normal vitamin B$_{12}$ stores. There is no evidence that patients with vitamin B$_{12}$ neuropathy derive greater benefit from more frequent doses, although many physicians use these for 6 months or so.

Response to therapy

The patient feels better within 24 to 48 h, and the mild fever, if not due to infection, abates. A painful tongue and uncooperative, disorientated state may also be improved in 48 h. The white-cell count becomes normal by 3 to 7 days and the platelet count rises and may reach levels of 500 to 1000 × 10^9/litre before falling to normal at about 10 to 14 days. The bone marrow reverts to normoblastic by 36 to 48 h, although giant metamyelocytes persist for 10 to 12 days.

The neuropathy always improves with therapy but residual deficits remain in some patients; this applies usually to those with the longest histories or the most severe manifestations, particularly where there is subacute combined degeneration of the spinal cord and spastic paraparesis.

Maintenance

Hydroxocobalamin, 1000 μg intramuscularly, is given once every 3 months for life in PA and most other causes of vitamin B$_{12}$ deficiency to prevent relapse. The life expectancy in PA once treated, is as good as that in the general population in women, and slightly lower in men, probably due to the increased incidence of carcinoma of the stomach. In a few patients with vitamin B$_{12}$ deficiency, the underlying cause can be reversed; e.g. expulsion of the fish tapeworm, improvement of vegan diet, surgical correction of an intestinal stagnant loop. A few micrograms of vitamin B$_{12}$ can be absorbed each day in PA from oral doses of 1000 μg or more by passive diffusion, but this maintenance therapy is usually reserved for those who cannot have injections—e.g. those with a bleeding disorder, or who refuse them—and for the extremely rare individual who is allergic to all injectable forms of vitamin B$_{12}$. Vegans may be maintained on much smaller oral doses of vitamin B$_{12}$ each day, such as 50 μg as a tablet or syrup.

Prophylaxis

Vitamin B$_{12}$ therapy should be given from the time of operation after total gastrectomy or ileal resection. Patients with PA tend to develop iron-deficiency anaemia and they may also develop thyroid disorders or carcinoma of the stomach. It is advisable that a regular blood count be made once a year. Routine endoscopy is not warranted but these diseases must be particularly borne in mind if relevant symptoms or signs develop.

It is unclear whether vitamin B$_{12}$ should be given orally or parenterally to those with biochemical vitamin B$_{12}$ deficiency (see Chapter 11.2) without anaemia or macrocytosis or clinical symptoms. Trials are needed.

Folate deficiency

This is corrected by giving 5 mg folic acid by mouth daily. It is essential to first exclude vitamin B$_{12}$ deficiency so that precipitation of a neuropathy is avoided. It is usual to continue for at least 4 months until there is a completely new set of red cells, although body stores will theoretically be normal within a few days of therapy. In patients with severe malabsorption of folate, larger oral doses of folic acid (e.g. 5 mg three times a day) may be used but it is not necessary to give parenteral folate except for those unable to swallow tablets. The response to therapy is as described for vitamin B$_{12}$. The decision whether or not to continue folic acid beyond 4 months depends on whether or not the cause can be corrected. In practice, long-term folic acid is usually needed only in patients with severe haemolytic anaemias (e.g. sickle cell anaemia and thalassaemia major), myelofibrosis, and in gluten-induced enteropathy when a gluten-free diet is either unsuccessful or not feasible.

Prophylactic folic acid

This should be given to all pregnant women to prevent megaloblastic anaemia and reduce the incidence of neural tube defects (doses of 300 to 400 μg/day are used). Doses of 5 mg/day would have a greater effect but currently need a medical prescription in the United Kingdom. They are given if there has been a previous infant with an NTD. Folic acid is given to patients undergoing regular haemodialysis or peritoneal dialysis, to premature infants weighing less than 1.5 kg at birth, and to selected patients in intensive care units or receiving parenteral nutrition. In young children exposed to a high risk of malaria combined iron and folic acid supplements may be harmful and should be avoided.

Folate therapy has been shown to improve chromosomal stability in the fragile X syndrome, even though these patients do not have folate deficiency or a demonstrable defect of folate metabolism.

Food fortification

Mandatory fortification of cereals and grains with folic acid ($140\,\mu g/100\,g$ cereal grain) aimed at reducing the incidence of NTDs began in the United States of America in 1997 and is now also practised in Canada, Chile, and other countries. Median serum folate in clinical specimens in United States rose from 12.6 to $18.7\,\mu g/litre$ between 1997 and 1998. There was also a fall in serum homocysteine levels. The theoretical side effects of fortification are largely in patients with unsuspected vitamin B_{12} deficiency who, it has been suggested, might present with neuropathy if the extra folate consumed prevents the development of anaemia due to vitamin B_{12} deficiency. There is, however, no evidence for an increased incidence of nonanaemic subjects with low serum vitamin B_{12} levels in the United States since fortification. In the United Kingdom fortification of flour with folic acid ($240\,\mu g/100\,g$ flour) has been recommended but not implemented. The possible effects of fortification on cardiovascular disease and cancer have been discussed.

Folinic acid (5-formyl-THF)

This reduced folate is used to prevent or treat toxicity due to methotrexate or other dihydrofolate reductase inhibitors.

Severely ill patients

Some patients, usually elderly, are admitted to hospital severely ill with megaloblastic anaemia, perhaps in congestive heart failure or with pneumonia. In this case, it is necessary to commence therapy immediately after obtaining blood for vitamin B_{12} and folate assay, before it is known which deficiency is present. Both vitamins should be given simultaneously in large doses. Heart failure and infection should be treated in conventional fashion but blood transfusion should be avoided, except in cases of extreme anaemia, when 1 to 2 units of packed cells may be given slowly, accompanied by removal of a similar volume of blood from the other arm, and diuretic therapy.

Other therapy

Hypokalaemia has been reported to occur during initial therapy but is, rarely, if ever, clinically important. An attack of gout has been reported on the days 6 to 7 of therapy. Most patients develop hyperuricaemia at this stage but the clinical disease probably only occurs in those with a strong gouty tendency. Iron deficiency commonly develops in the first few weeks of therapy and this should be treated initially with oral ferrous sulphate in the usual way.

Megaloblastic anaemia due to inborn errors of folate or vitamin B_{12} metabolism

Folate

A number of babies have been described with congenital deficiency of one or other enzyme concerned in folate metabolism: 5-methyltetrahydro-folate, methylene THF-reductase, FIGLU-transferase, methenyl-THF cyclohydrolase. Some of the babies had multiple congenital defects including the heart and cerebral ventricles and nearly all showed impaired mental development. In the methylfolate transferase deficiency, megaloblastic anaemia was present.

Vitamin B_{12}

Congenital deficiency of TCII was first reported as an autosomally recessive disease in 1971 in two siblings who developed megaloblastic anaemia requiring therapy with large daily doses of vitamin B_{12} at 3 and 5 weeks of age. Similarly affected families have been described. A spectrum of mutations in the gene for TCII have been detected, in some cases, TCII is undetected; in others, functionally inactive TCII has been detected often presenting later in life. The serum vitamin B_{12} concentration is normal, vitamin B_{12} being bound to TCI. Absorption of vitamin B_{12} is impaired. Treatment is with massive doses of vitamin B_{12} (e.g. $1000\,\mu g$ intramuscularly three times each week). Delay in treatment may allow a neuropathy to occur. In contrast, in subjects with rare, inherited, mutations of TCI, low serum vitamin B_{12} concentrations occur, but haemopoiesis is normal.

Children with one form of congenital methylmalonicaciduria, which responds to vitamin B_{12} therapy in large doses, have been shown to have a defect in conversion of hydroxocobalamin to adocobalamin. They do not show megaloblastic anaemia. In a few, this defect has been associated with a defect of formation of methylcobalamin and with homocystinuria, but some of the children have also surprisingly not shown megaloblastic anaemia. Neurological abnormalities are usual. Homocystinuria and megaloblastic anaemia without methymalonicaciduria have also been reported. In some cases, the defect appears to be in maintaining vitamin B_{12} bound to methionine synthase in the reduced state.

Megaloblastic anaemia due to acquired disturbances of folate or vitamin B_{12} metabolism

Folate

Therapy with dihydrofolate reductase inhibitors may cause megaloblastic anaemia. This is usual with methotrexate and less likely with pyrimethamine unless high doses are used or the patient is already folate deficient. Trimethoprim and triamterene are very weak folate antagonists in man, but may precipitate megaloblastic anaemia in patients already vitamin B_{12} or folate deficient (see earlier).

Vitamin B_{12}

Nitrous oxide (N_2O)

This anaesthetic gas oxidizes vitamin B_{12} from the active fully reduce cob(I)alamin form to the inactive cob(II)alamin and cob(III)alamin forms, inactivating methylcobalamin and hence methionine synthase. Megaloblastosis develops within several hours in humans. This recovers over several days when exposure to N_2O is discontinued. After many weeks exposure to N_2O, monkeys develop a neuropathy resembling vitamin B_{12} neuropathy in humans; peripheral neuropathies and more severe neurological disease have also been described in humans (e.g. dentists and anaesthetists) repeatedly exposed to the gas. When N_2O is used as anaesthetic for patients with low vitamin B_{12} stores, megaloblastic anaemia or neuropathy may be precipitated months later, due to failure to replenish vitamin B_{12} stores by absorption. Recovery from N_2O exposure needs new cobalamin and also synthesis of new apoenzyme (methionine synthase) because this protein is also damaged by active oxygen derived from the N_2O–cobalamin reaction. Methylmalonicaciduria has not been found in animals or humans exposed for short periods to N_2O, as methylmalonic CoA mutase does not need reduced vitamin B_{12}.

Megaloblastic anaemia not due to folate or vitamin B_{12} deficiency or metabolic defect

Congenital

Orotic aciduria

This is a very rare, recessive disorder involving two consecutive enzymes (orotidsylic pyrophosphatase and orotidylic decarboxylase) in pyrimidine synthesis and presents with megaloblastic anaemia in the first few months of life. The diagnosis is made if needle-shaped, colourless crystals of orotic acid are found in the urine, daily excretion ranging from 0.5 to 1.5 g. Heterozygotes excrete slightly raised amounts of orotic acid but show no haematological disorder. Treatment with uridine (1–1.5 g/day) leads to a haematological response, restoration of normal haemopoiesis and growth, and reduction in orotic acid excretion.

Lesch–Nyhan syndrome

A few patients with this rare disorder of purine synthesis have shown megaloblastic change but whether this was due to associated folate deficiency or a direct result of reduced purine synthesis is not certain (see Chapter 12.2).

Vitamin E deficiency

This has been reported to cause megaloblastosis in a group of children with kwashiorkor. However, many were also folate deficient.

Vitamin C deficiency

Megaloblastic appears to be due to associated folate deficiency.

Thiamine responsive

About 12 cases have been well documented. They have also shown sideroblastic change and a defect in phosphorylation of thiamine has been implicated. Diabetes mellitus and sensineural deafness are additional features. There is a fault in thiamine phosphorylation due to a genetic defect of the phosphorylase enzyme.

Responding to large doses of vitamin B_{12} and folate

A single patient has been reported who needed both vitamins in large doses, but the site of the defect was not elucidated.

Congenital dyserythropoietic anaemia

Some cases of congenital dyserythropoietic anaemia show megaloblastic changes not due to vitamin B_{12} or folate deficiency.

Acquired

Megaloblastic changes are often marked in acute myeloid leukaemia and less commonly in other forms of acute myeloid leukaemia. They also occur in the myelodysplastic syndromes. The exact site of block in DNA synthesis in these syndromes is unknown.

Drugs that directly inhibit purine or pyrimidine synthesis (e.g. cytosine arabinoside, 5-fluorouracil, hydroxyurea, 6-mercaptopurine,

or azathioprine and azidothymidine (AZT)) may cause megaloblastic anaemia. Alcohol has also been found to have a direct effect on the bone marrow, causing megaloblastosis in some cases even in the absence of vitamin B_{12} or folate deficiency. On the other hand, drugs that inhibit mitosis (e.g. colchicine or daunorubicin) or alkylate preformed DNA (e.g. cyclophosphamide, chlorambucil, or busulfan) do not cause megaloblastosis.

Other deficiency anaemias

Vitamin C

Anaemia is usual in scurvy but the pathogenesis is complicated. It is likely that vitamin C has a direct effect on erythropoiesis but folate and iron deficiencies, haemorrhage, or haemolysis often complicate the picture.

Biochemical and nutritional aspects

Vitamin C is needed for collagen synthesis by its involvement in the hydroxylation of protein and for maintenance of intercellular substance of skin, cartilage, periosteum, and bone. It may also have a general role in oxidation–reduction systems, e.g. glutathione, cytochromes, pyridine, and flavin nucleotides. Although vitamin C is also thought to be needed for maintaining body folates in the reduced active state, the exact reactions involved are unclear. Vitamin C has a particular role in iron metabolism, iron excess causing increased utilization of vitamin C and in extreme cases clinical scurvy, whereas iron deficiency is associated with a raised leucocyte ascorbate concentration. Vitamin C is needed for incorporation of iron from transferrin into ferritin and for iron mobilization from ferritin. Vitamin C therapy increases iron excretion in patients receiving subcutaneous desferrioxamine infusions and also, at least in experimental animals, affects iron distribution by increasing parenchymal relative to reticuloendothelial iron. Minimum adult daily requirements for vitamin C are about 10 mg but 30 to 70 mg is recommended; utilization, and therefore requirement, are relatively higher in infants, children, and pregnant and lactating women. Vitamin C may be excreted as such but is also broken down to oxalate.

Vitamin C is present in food as its reduced (ascorbic acid) and oxidized (dehydroascorbic acid) forms, the highest concentrations occurring in green vegetables, fruits, tomatoes, liver, and kidney. Potatoes are not a rich source but provide a substantial proportion of normal dietary intake. Cooking, particularly in alkaline conditions with large volumes of water, destroys the vitamin, which is also lost on storage with exposure to the air. Absorption occurs through the length of the small intestine and deficiency is never solely due to malabsorption.

The anaemia of scurvy is typically normochromic, normocytic with a slightly raised reticulocyte count (to 5 to 10%) and a normoblastic marrow with erythroid hyperplasia. This suggests a direct role for vitamin C in erythropoiesis but not all patients with clinical scurvy are anaemic. Extravascular haemolysis with mild jaundice and increased urobilinogen excretion occurs in many of the patients. Moreover, in many the anaemia is complicated by folate deficiency (due to inadequate folate intake) with a megaloblastic marrow, or in a few by iron deficiency due to external haemorrhage, reduced diet intake, and possibly reduced iron absorption. In a few patients placed on a low-folate diet, response of megaloblastic haemopoiesis to vitamin C alone has been described. In others, response of the megaloblastic anaemia to folic acid alone on a diet low in vitamin C has occurred but in most such cases, both vitamin C and folic acid have been found necessary.

Vitamin B$_6$

This, as its coenzyme form pyridoxal-5-phosphate, is involved in many reactions of the body, especially transaminases and decarboxylases. It is also a cofactor in the important rate-limiting reaction in haem synthesis, δ-aminolaevulinic acid (ALA)-synthase (see Section 12). It occurs in natural tissues in three major forms: pyridoxine, pyridoxamine, and pyridoxal phosphate. Red cells are capable of interconverting them. Anaemia due purely to vitamin B$_6$ deficiency has been produced in animals. It is hypochromic and microcytic with a raised serum iron and increased iron in erythroblasts, with some partial or complete ring sideroblasts. A similar anaemia has occurred in humans with malabsorption, pregnancy, or haemolysis but has not been fully documented to respond to physiological doses of vitamin B$_6$ alone. Vitamin B$_6$-responsive anaemia is, however, well documented among patients with sideroblastic anaemia of all types. Pyridoxine responses occur particularly in the inherited form (when it is assumed that a fault in one or other enzyme of haem synthesis, e.g. ALA-synthase, increases the need for pyridoxal phosphate as cofactor) and when sideroblastic anaemia occurs in patients receiving pyridoxine antagonists, such as antituberculous drugs. The value of pyridoxine dietary supplements in lowering serum homocysteine and reducing the incidence of cardiovascular disease has yet to be proven.

Riboflavin

On the basis of studies in experimental animals and humans fed a deficient diet together with a riboflavin antagonist, deficiency of this vitamin is known to cause a normochromic, normocytic anaemia associated with a low reticulocyte count and red-cell aplasia in the marrow, sometimes with vacuolated normoblasts. The exact biochemical basis is undecided. Clinically, a similar anaemia may occur in pure form but is usually associated with the anaemia due to protein deficiency, as in kwashiorkor or marasmus. Other clinical features of riboflavin deficiency—dermatitis, angular cheilosis, and glossitis for example—may be present.

Thiamine

For discussion, see under megaloblastic anaemia not due to folate or vitamin B$_{12}$ deficiency or metabolic defect.

Nicotinic acid, pantothenic acid, and niacin

Deficiencies of these vitamins cause anaemia in experimental animals, but anaemia purely due to one or other of these deficiencies has not been established to occur in humans.

Vitamin E

This vitamin is needed for preventing peroxidation of cell membranes. A haemolytic anaemia responding to vitamin E has been reported in premature infants. Less well documented is a macrocytic anaemia due to vitamin E deficiency in protein–calorie-deficient infants and aggravation of anaemia in patients with thalassaemia major because of vitamin E deficiency.

Protein deficiency (see Chapter 11.3)

Anaemia is usual in both 'pure' protein deficiency (kwashiorkor) and in protein–calorie malnutrition (marasmus). It has been reported in many parts of the world where malnutrition, especially in children and pregnant women, is common. The anaemia also occurs in patients with gastrointestinal disease and severe malabsorption. The anaemia is typically normochromic, normocytic, and of the order of 8.0 to 9.0 g/dl. The reticulocyte count is usually reduced and the marrow may show a selective reduction in erythropoiesis. Experimental studies in animals suggest that the anaemia is largely due to reduced serum erythropoietin levels consequent on a lack of stimulus for erythropoietin secretion. Lack of amino acids for synthesis of erythropoietin or globin is not the cause. In many patients, the anaemia is complicated by infection, folate or iron deficiency, and possibly other vitamin deficiencies (e.g. riboflavin, vitamin E) and then it may be more severe and show additional morphological abnormalities in the blood and marrow.

Further reading

General

Lewerin C (2008). Serum biomarkers for atrophic gastritis and antibodies against Helicobacter pyloric in the elderly: Implications for vitamin B12, folic acid and iron status and response to oral vitamin therapy. *Scand J Gast*, **143**, 1502–08.

Whitehead VM (2006). Acquired and inherited disorders of cobalamin and folate in children. *J Haematol*, **134**, 125–36.

Wickramasinghe SN (ed.) (1995). Megaloblastic anaemia. *Baillière's Clin Haematol*, **8**, 441–703. [A volume containing 12 major articles reviewing different aspects of vitamin B$_{12}$ and folate; also contains reviews of different aspects of vitamin B$_{12}$ and folate.]

Wickramasinghe SN (1999). The wide spectrum and unresolved issues of megaloblastic anemia. *Semin Haematol*, **36**, 3–18. [An excellent general update on megaloblastic anaemia.]

Vitamin B$_{12}$

Chanarin I, Metz J (1997). Diagnosis of cobalamin deficiency: the old and the new. *Br J Haematol*, **97**, 695–700. [Discusses whether vitamin assays or measurement of serum methylmalonic acid or homocysteine should be used to diagnose the deficiencies.]

Clarke R, et al. (2007). Low B$_{12}$ status and risk of cognitive decline in older adults. *Am J Clin Nutr*, **86**, 1384–91.

Dali-Youcef N, Andres E (2009). An update on cobalamin deficiency in adults. *QJM*, **102**, 17–28.

Hershko C, et al. (2006). Variable hematological presentation of autoimmune gastritis: age related progression from iron deficiency to cobalamin depletion. *Blood*, **107**, 1673–9.

Quandros EV (2009). Advances in the understanding of cobalamin assimilation and metabolism. *Brit J Haematol*, **148**, 195–204.

Weir DG, Scott JM (1997). Brain function in the elderly: role of B$_{12}$ and folate. *Br Med Bull*, **55**, 669–82. [A large review of this important topic.]

Yin Y, et al. (2007). NALPI in vitiligo-associated multiple auto immune disease. *N Engl J Med*, **356**, 1216–25.

Folate

Clarke R, et al. (2008). Folate and vitamin B$_{12}$ status in relation to cognitive impairment and anaemia in the selling of voluntary fortification in the United Kingdom. *Br J Nutr*, **100**, 1054–9.

Eichholzer M, Tonz O, Zimmermann R (2006). Folic acid: a public health challenge. *Lancet*, **367**, 1352–61.

English M, Snow RW (2006). Iron and folic acid supplements and malaria risk. *Lancet*, **367**, 90–1.

Hoffbrand AV, Weir DG (2001). The history of folic acid. *Br J Haematol*, **113**, 579–89.

Kibar Z, *et al.* (2007). Mutations in VANGLI associated with neural tube defects. *N Engl J Med*, **356**, 1432–7.

Matherly LH, Goldman ID (2003). Membrane transport of folates. *Vitam Horm*, **66**, 403–56.

McMahon JA, *et al.* (2006). A controlled trial of homocysteine lowering and cognitive performance. *N Engl J Med*, **354**, 2764–72.

Mills JH, *et al.* (2003). Low B_{12} concentrations in patients without anemia: the effect of folic acid fortification of grain. *Am J Clin Nutr*,**77**, 1474–7.

Qui A, *et al.* (2006). Identification of an intestinal folate transporter and the molecular basis for hereditary folate malabsorption. *Cell*, **127**, 917–28.

Wright AJA, Dainty JR, Finglas PM (2007). Folic acid metabolism in human subjects revisited: potential implications for proposed mandatory folic acid fortification in the U.K. *Br J Nutr*, **98**, 667–75.

Zhao R, *et al.* (2007). The spectrum of mutations in the PCFT gene, coding for an intestinal folate transporter that are the basis for hereditary folate malabsorption. *Blood*, **110**, 1147–52.

Neural tube defects

Botto L, *et al.* (1999). Neural-tube defects. *N Engl J Med*, **341**, 1509–18. [A major review of all aspects of NTD.]

De Wals P, *et al.* (2007). Reduction in neural tube defects after folic acid fortification in Canada. *N Engl J Med*, **357**, 135–42.

Cardiovascular disease

B Vitamin Treatment Trialists' Collaboration (2007). Homocysteine lowering trials for prevention of vascular disease: protocol for a collaborative meta-analysis. *Clin Chem Lab Med*, **45**, 1575–81.

Bazzano LA, *et al.* (2006). Effect of folic acid supplementation on risk of cardiovascular disease. A meta-analysis of randomized controlled trials. *JAMA*, **296**, 2720–6.

Bazzano LA. (2009). Folic acid supplementation and cardiovascular disease: the state of the art. *Am J Med Sci*. **338**, 48–9.

Bonaa KH, *et al.* (2006). Homocysteine lowering and cardiovascular events after acute myocardial infarction. *N Engl J Med*, **354**, 1578–88.

Lonn B, *et al.* (2006). Homocysteine lowering with folic acid and B vitamins in vascular disease. *N Engl J Med*, **354**, 1567–77.

Took JF, *et al.* (2004). Lowering homocysteine in patients with ischemic stroke to prevent recurrent stroke, myocardial infarction and death: the Vitamin Intervention for Stroke Prevention (VISP) randomised control trial. *JAMA*, **291**, 565–75.

Wald DS, Law M, Morris JK (2002). Homocysteine and cardiovascular disease: evidence on causality from a meta-analysis. *BMJ*, **325**, 1202–6.

Wald DS, *et al.* (2006). Folic acid, homocysteine and cardiovascular disease: judging causality in the face of inconclusive trial evidence. *BMJ*, **333**, 114–17.

Wang X, *et al.* (2007). Efficacy of folic acid supplementation in stroke prevention: a meta-analysis. *Lancet*, **369**, 1876–82.

Cancer

Cole BF, *et al.* (2007). Folic acid for the prevention of colorectal adenomas: a randomized clinical trial. *JAMA*, **297**, 2351–9.

Giovannucci E, *et al.* (1998). Multivitamin use, folate and colon cancer in women in the nurses' health study. *Ann Intern Med*, **129**, 517–24. [A large study implying but not proving that folate deficiency predisposes to colon cancer.]

Kim YI (2007). Folate and colorectal cancer: an evidence based critical review. *Mol Nutr Food Res*, **51**, 267–92.

Logan RFA, *et al.* (2007). Aspirin and folic acid for the prevention of recurrent colorectal adenomas. *Gastroenterology*, **134**, 29–38.

Miscellaneous

Adams EB (1970). Anemia associated with protein deficiency. *Semin Haematol*, **7**, 55–66. [An excellent review of the role of protein deficiency in causing anaemia.]

Cox EV (1968). The anaemia of scurvy. *Vitam Horm*, **26**, 635–52. [An excellent review of the role of vitamin C in haemopoiesis.]

Rindi G, *et al.* (1994). Further studies of erythrocyte thiamin transport and phosphorylation in seven patients with thiamin-responsive megaloblastic anaemia. *J Inher Metabol Dis*, **17**, 667–77. [Shows the mechanism of thiamine responsive anaemia.]

22.5.7 Disorders of the synthesis or function of haemoglobin

D.J. Weatherall

Essentials

The inherited disorders of haemoglobin are the commonest single-gene disorders in the world. They cause much morbidity and mortality in those individuals who are severely affected, and place a major burden on health services in some places, in particular the Mediterranean region and South-East Asia, when economic conditions improve and infant and childhood death rates fall. Mass migrations of populations from high-incidence areas for the haemoglobin disorders, together with the general ease of international travel, means that these conditions are being seen with increasing frequency in parts of the world where they have not been recognized previously.

Structure, function, and genetic control of the synthesis of haemoglobin

Structure—human haemoglobins have a tetrameric structure made up of two different pairs of globin chains, each attached to one haem molecule. Adult and fetal haemoglobins have α chains combined with β chains (Hb A, $\alpha_2\beta_2$), δ chains (Hb A_2, $\alpha_2\delta_2$), or γ chains (Hb F, $\alpha_2\gamma_2$); other forms of haemoglobin are found in embryos.

Function—the sigmoid shape of the oxygen dissociation curve ensures that oxygen is rapidly taken up at high oxygen tension in the lungs, and that it is released readily at the lower tensions encountered in the tissues.

Genetic control—there are linked clusters of β-like globin genes on chromosome 11, and of α-like globin genes on chromosome 16; various regulatory elements interact to promote erythroid-specific gene expression and to coordinate changes in globin gene activity during development.

Classification of the disorders of haemoglobin

These can be (1) genetic—including thalassaemia, structural variants, hereditary persistence of fetal haemoglobin; or (2) acquired—including methaemoglobin, carbonmonoxyhaemoglobin, sulphaemoglobin, defective synthesis (e.g. haemoglobin H/leukaemia, other neoplastic disorders).

Thalassaemias—general considerations

This heterogeneous group of genetic disorders all result from a reduced rate of production of one or more of the globin chains of haemoglobin: they are divided into the α, β, $\delta\beta$, or $\varepsilon\gamma\delta\beta$ thalassaemias, according to which globin chain is produced in reduced amounts. They are inherited in a simple mendelian fashion. Heterozygotes are usually symptomless; more severely affected patients are either homozygotes for α or β thalassaemia, compound heterozygotes for different molecular forms of α or β thalassaemia, or compound heterozygotes for thalassaemia and a structural haemoglobin variant. They are clinically classified into major, intermediate, and minor forms according to severity.

β Thalassaemias

These are most important types of thalassaemia because they are very common and produce severe anaemia in their homozygous and compound heterozygous states. They occur widely in a broad belt ranging from the Mediterranean and parts of North and West Africa, through the Middle East and Indian subcontinent, to South-East Asia.

Molecular pathology and pathophysiology—can be caused by more than 200 different mutations in the β globin gene, most of which are single base changes or small deletions or insertions of one or two bases, resulting in absent or reduced β chain production. In the absence of their partner chains the excess α chains are unstable and precipitate in the red cell precursors, leading to both ineffective erythropoiesis and shortened red-cell survival. The anaemia acts as a stimulus to increased erythropoietin production, causing massive expansion of the bone marrow which may lead to serious deformities of the skull and long bones, and splenic uptake of abnormal red cells leads to splenomegaly.

Clinical features—(1) Severe homozygous or compound heterozygous forms—usually present within the first year of life with failure to thrive, poor feeding, intermittent bouts of fever, or failure to improve after an intercurrent infection. Progress then depends on management: (a) well transfused—early growth and development is normal, but without adequate iron chelation complications due to iron overloading arise, most notably progressive cardiac damage that is eventually fatal; (b) inadequately transfused—growth and development are markedly retarded; there is progressive splenomegaly, with hypersplenism sometimes causing a worsening of anaemia; other complications include bone marrow expansion that leads to deformities of the skull with marked bossing and overgrowth of the zygomata. (2) Carriers for β thalassaemia—are usually well except from symptoms of mild anaemia.

Investigation—(1) Severe homozygous or compound heterozygous forms—haemoglobin values on presentation range from 2 to 8 g/dl, with the red cells showing marked hypochromia and variation in shape and size. In β° thalassaemia there is no haemoglobin A and the haemoglobin consists of F and A_2 only; in β^+ thalassaemia the level of haemoglobin F ranges from 30 to 90% of the total haemoglobin. (2) Carriers for β thalassaemia—haemoglobin values are typically 9 to 11 g/dl, with the red cells showing hypochromia and microcytosis. Haemoglobin A_2 is elevated to 4 to 6%.

β thalassaemia in association with other haemoglobin variants—in many populations it is common for an individual to inherit a β thalassaemia gene from one parent and a gene for a structural haemoglobin variant from the other, with clinically important conditions being sickle cell β thalassaemia, haemoglobin C β thalassaemia, and haemoglobin E β thalassaemia.

α Thalassaemias

These are commoner than the β thalassaemias, but pose less of a public health problem because their severe forms only occur in a few regions. They occur widely through the Mediterranean region, parts of West Africa, the Middle East, parts of the Indian subcontinent, and throughout South-East Asia in a line stretching from southern China through Thailand, the Malay peninsula, and Indonesia to the Pacific island populations.

Molecular pathology and pathophysiology—normal individuals receive two linked α globin genes from each of their parents (genotype $\alpha\alpha/\alpha\alpha$), with loss of both copies on an affected chromosome (genotype $--$) causing more severe disease than loss or mutation of one (genotype $-\alpha$ or $\alpha^T\alpha$). Deficiency of α chains leads to the production of excess γ chains in the fetus, which form $\gamma4$ tetramers (haemoglobin Bart's), and excess of β chains in the adult, which form β_4 tetramers (haemoglobin H). These both have very high oxygen affinity and are physiologically useless, and haemoglobin H is unstable and precipitates in red cells as they age leading to a shortened red-cell survival.

Clinical features and investigation—(1) haemoglobin Bart's hydrops syndrome ($--/--$)—infants are usually stillborn at 28 to 40 weeks; (2) haemoglobin H disease (usually $-\alpha/--$ or $\alpha^T\alpha/--$)—there is variable anaemia and splenomegaly; haemoglobin values range from 7 to 10 g/dl, with the blood film showing typical thalassaemic changes; patients usually survive into adult life.

α Thalassaemia and mental retardation—also characterized by dysmorphic features, these conditions are usually caused by mutations that involve the α globin gene cluster on chromosome 16 (ATR-16) or mutations on the X chromosome (ATR-X).

Thalassaemias—prevention and treatment

Prevention—since there is no definitive treatment, most countries in which the disease is common are putting a major effort into programmes for its prevention, most often by offering prenatal diagnosis to couples at risk for having children with severe forms of β thalassaemia.

Treatment—symptomatic management of severe β thalassaemia requires regular blood transfusion, the judicious use of splenectomy if hypersplenism develops, and the administration of chelating agents to reduce iron overload.

Structural haemoglobin variants—general considerations

There are more than 400 structural haemoglobin variants, most of which result from single amino acid substitutions and cause clinical disorders only if they alter the stability or functional properties of the haemoglobin molecule. Manifestations include (1) haemolysis and tissue damage—haemoglobin S (sickling disorders); (2) drug-induced and chronic haemolysis—various haemoglobins; (3) congenital polycythaemia—high affinity variants; (4) congenital cyanosis—haemoglobin(s) M, low affinity variants; (5) hypochromic thalassaemic phenotypes.

Sickling disorders

These occur very frequently in African populations and, sporadically, throughout the Mediterranean region, the Middle East, and in India. The high frequency of the sickle cell gene occurs because carriers are more resistant than normal individuals to *Plasmodium falciparum* malaria.

Molecular pathology and pathophysiology—haemoglobin S differs from haemoglobin A by the substitution of valine for glutamic acid at position 6 in the β chain. Sickling disorders are caused by the heterozygous state for haemoglobin S (sickle cell trait, AS), the homozygous state (sickle cell disease, SS), and the compound heterozygous state for haemoglobin S together with haemoglobins C, D, E, or other structural variants. The sickling phenomenon appears to be due to the unusual solubility characteristics of haemoglobin S, which undergoes liquid crystal (tactoid) formation as it becomes deoxygenated.

Clinical features and investigation—(1) Sickle cell trait—causes no clinical disability except in conditions of extreme hypoxia. Diagnosed by the finding of a positive sickling test together with haemoglobins A and S on electrophoresis. (2) Sickle cell disease—typical presentations in infancy include symptoms related to anaemia or infection, and infarction of bones in the hands or feet causes dactylitis ('hand and foot' syndrome). The haemoglobin level is typically 6 to 8 g/dl with a reticulocyte count of 10 to 20%, and examination of the peripheral blood film shows anisochromia and poikilocytosis with a variable number of sickled erythrocytes, with diagnosis confirmed by a positive sickling test and typical appearances on haemoglobin electrophoresis. Acute exacerbations ('crises') can be (1) thrombotic—generalized or localized bone pain, abdominal, pulmonary, neurological; (2) aplastic; (3) haemolytic; (4) sequestration—spleen, liver, lung; (5) various combinations of (1) to (4). Chronic complications include (1) aseptic necrosis of bone; (2) chronic leg ulceration; (3) chronic kidney disease; (4) recurrent priapism.

Treatment—babies of 'at risk' pregnancies should be screened at birth to establish the diagnosis as early as possible because early deaths due to infection and the frequency of crises may be reduced by oral penicillin. Patients should be given folate supplements. Painful crises require adequate rehydration, oxygen, antibiotics where appropriate, and—in particular—analgesia. Patients with sequestration crises can be extremely ill, requiring intensive support including oxygen and exchange or top-up transfusion. Hydroxyurea can reduce infarction crises, possibly by favouring release of erythrocytes with a greater content of fetal haemoglobin which inhibits the sickling tendency.

Introduction

Disorders of the synthesis or structure of haemoglobin may be either inherited or acquired. The inherited disorders of haemoglobin are the commonest single gene disorders in the world population. Figures compiled by the World Health Organization suggest that there are hundreds of millions of carriers. Each year 200 000 to 300 000 severely affected homozygotes or compound heterozygotes are born. In many developing countries, the very high mortality from infection and malnutrition in the first year of life causes these conditions to be underappreciated as an important public health problem. However, once economic conditions improve and infant and childhood death rates fall, the genetic disorders of haemoglobin start to place a major burden on the health services. This phenomenon has already been observed in parts of the Mediterranean region and South-East Asia.

As a result of mass migrations of populations from high incidence areas for the haemoglobin disorders, these conditions are being seen with increasing frequency in parts of the world where they have not been recognized previously. Some of them, particularly sickle cell anaemia and the more severe forms of thalassaemia, can produce life-threatening medical emergencies. It is thus important for clinicians to have a working knowledge of their clinical features, management, and prevention.

Haemoglobin disorders have also become of particular interest in recent years because they were the first group of diseases to be analysed by the methods of recombinant DNA technology. More is known about their molecular pathology than any other genetic disorders. Their study has given us a good idea of the repertoire of mutations that underlie inherited diseases in humans.

Before describing the haemoglobin disorders it is necessary to discuss briefly the structure, function, and synthesis of haemoglobin and the way that it is genetically determined.

The structure, function, genetic control, and synthesis of haemoglobin

Structure

Human haemoglobin is heterogeneous at all stages of development; different haemoglobins are synthesized in the embryo, fetus, and adult, each adapted to the particular oxygen requirements.

Each human haemoglobin has a tetrameric structure made up of two different pairs of globin chains, each attached to one haem molecule (Fig. 22.5.7.1). Adult and fetal haemoglobins have α chains combined with β chains (Hb A, $\alpha_2\beta_2$), δ chains (Hb A$_2$, $\alpha_2\delta_2$), or γ chains (Hb F, $\alpha_2\gamma_2$). In embryos, α-like chains, called ζ chains, combine with γ chains to produce Hb Portland ($\zeta_2\gamma_2$), or with ε chains to make Hb Gower 1 ($\zeta_2\varepsilon_2$), and α and ε chains combine to form Hb Gower 2 ($\alpha_2\varepsilon_2$). Fetal haemoglobin is itself heterogeneous; there are two kinds of γ chains which differ in their amino acid composition at position 136, where they have either glycine (Gγ) or alanine (Aγ). The Gγ and Aγ chains are the products of separate (Gγ and Aγ) loci.

Function

The well-known sigmoid shape of the oxygen dissociation curve, which reflects the allosteric properties of haemoglobin, ensures that oxygen is rapidly taken up at high oxygen tensions in the lungs, and that it is released readily at the lower tensions encountered in the tissues. The shape of the curve is due to cooperativity between the four haem molecules. When one takes on oxygen, the affinity for oxygen of the remaining haems of the tetramer increased dramatically. This is because haemoglobin can exist in two configurations, deoxy (T) and oxy (R) (T and R stand for tight and relaxed states, respectively). The T form has a lower affinity than the R form for ligands such as oxygen. During the sequential addition of oxygen to the four haems, transition from the T to R configuration occurs and the oxygen affinity of the partially liganded molecule increases rapidly.

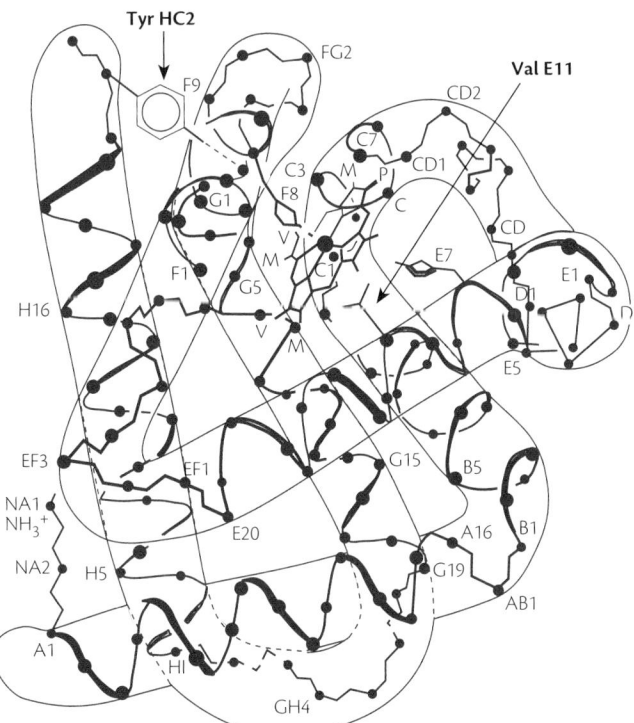

Fig. 22.5.7.1 The α chain subunit of human haemoglobin showing the position of the haem molecule in a cleft formed by the globin chain. The helical parts of the chain are given letters of the alphabet and each amino acid residue in each helical region has a specific number, e.g. Val E11 is the eleventh amino acid in the E helical region. The nonhelical regions of the N- and C-terminal ends of the chains are labelled NA and HC respectively.
(Reproduced by permission of Dr M F Perutz and the editors of the Cold Spring Harbor Symposia for Quantitative Biology.)

The position of the oxygen dissociation curve can be modified in many ways. First, oxygen affinity is decreased with increasing CO_2 tensions, the Bohr effect. This facilitates oxygen delivery to the tissues, where a drop in pH due to CO_2 influx lowers oxygen affinity. The opposite effect occurs in the lungs. Oxygen affinity is also modified by the level of 2,3-biphosophoglycerate (2,3-BPG) in the red cell. Increasing concentrations move the curve to the right, reducing oxygen affinity. Diminishing concentrations have the opposite effect. The 2,3-DPG mechanism plays an important role in response to hypoxia (see Chapter 22.5.2).

Genetic control

The arrangement of the two main families of globin genes is illustrated in Fig. 22.5.7.2. The β-like globin genes form a linked cluster on chromosome 11 that spans about 60 kb; they are arranged in the order 5′-ε-Gγ-Aγ-ψβ-δ-β-3′. The α-like globin genes form a linked cluster on chromosome 16, in the order 5′-ζ-ψζ-ψα-α2-α1-3′. The ψβ, ψζ, and ψα genes are pseudogenes; their sequences resemble the β, ζ, or α genes but contain mutations which prevent them from functioning as structural genes. They may be 'burnt out' remnants of genes which were functional at an earlier stage of evolution.

Some of the important structural aspects of the globin genes and their flanking sequences are illustrated in Figs. 22.2.7.2 and 22.2.7.3. Like most mammalian genes, the globin genes are interrupted by one or more noncoding regions called introns. The non-α globin genes contain two introns of 122 to 130 and 850 to 900 bp between codons 30 and 31 and 104 and 105, respectively. Similar though smaller introns are found in the α and ζ globin genes. In the 5′ flanking regions of the globin genes there are blocks of nucleotide homology which are found in analagous positions in many species. The first, the ATA box, is about 30 bases upstream (to the left) of the initiation codon. The second, called the CCAAT box, is found about 70 bp upstream from the 5′ end of the genes. There is a third region of this kind, about 100 bp upstream. These regions, called promoters, are involved in the initiation of transcription and hence play an important role in the regulation of the structural genes. As we shall see later, mutations which involve them can reduce the output of the related genes. In the 3′ noncoding regions of all the globin genes there is a sequence AATAAA (Fig. 22.5.7.3) which is the signal for polyA addition to RNA transcripts; we shall discuss the significance of this when we consider the disorders of globin chain synthesis.

The globin gene clusters also contain other types of regulatory elements that interact to promote erythroid-specific gene expression and to coordinate changes in globin gene activity during development. They include enhancers, regulatory elements that increase gene expression despite being located at a variable distance from the genes, and master sequences upstream from the clusters which render them transcriptionally active. All these regulatory regions contain sequences to which an array of regulatory molecules called transcription factors are able to bind, some of which are specific for erythropoiesis, while others are ubiquitous in their tissue distribution.

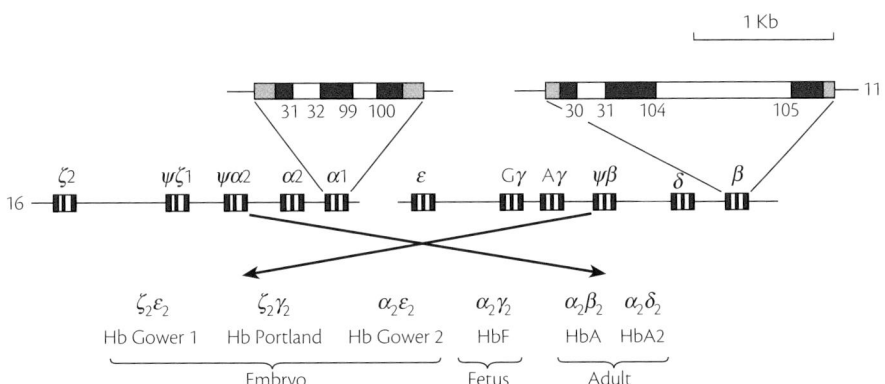

Fig. 22.5.7.2 The genetic control of human haemoglobin. Two of the genes are enlarged to show the introns (unshaded) and exons (dark staining). 1 kb = 1000 nucleotide bases.

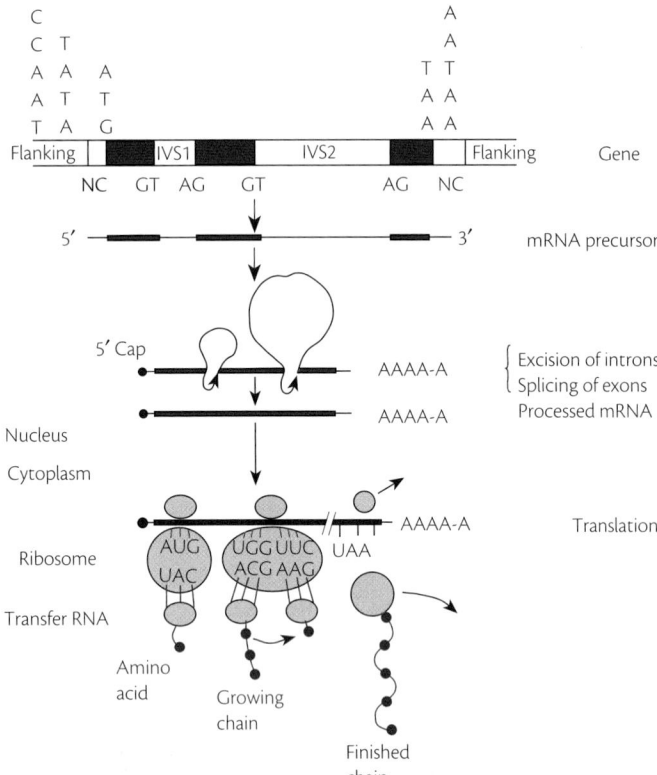

Fig. 22.5.7.3 Globin gene structure, mRNA processing, and globin synthesis. Each of the structures and steps illustrated is described in the text and in Section 5.

Synthesis

When a globin gene is transcribed a messenger RNA (mRNA) molecule is synthesized from one of its strands by the action of an enzyme called RNA polymerase. The primary transcript of the globin genes is the large mRNA precursor molecule which contains both introns and the coding regions or exons. While in the nucleus, this molecule undergoes a number of modifications (Fig. 22.5.7.3). First, the introns are removed and the exons are joined together, a process called splicing. The exon/intron junctions always have the sequence GT at their 5′ end, and AG at their 3′ end. This appears to be essential for accurate splicing and if there is a mutation in these sites normal splicing cannot occur. The mRNAs are chemically modified (capped) at their 5′ end, and at their 3′ end a string of adenylic acid residues (polyA) is added. The processed mRNA now moves into the cytoplasm to act as a template for globin chain production.

Globin mRNA is transported from the nucleus to the cytoplasm where it associates with ribosomes, tRNA, and translation factors. These complexes, called polyribosomes, translate the information encoded in the globin mRNA into the primary amino acid sequence of each globin chain. Individual globin chains combine with haem, which is synthesized through a separate pathway, and with themselves, to form definitive haemoglobin molecules.

Classification of the disorders of haemoglobin

The main groups of disorders of haemoglobin are shown in Box 22.5.7.1. The genetic disorders are divided into those in which

---

Box 22.5.7.1 Disorders of haemoglobin

Genetic

- Thalassaemia
- Structural variants
- Hereditary persistence of fetal haemoglobin

Acquired

- Methaemoglobin
- Carbonmonoxyhaemoglobin
- Sulphaemoglobin
- Defective synthesis
- Haemoglobin H/leukaemia
- Other neoplastic disorders

---

there is a reduced rate of production of one or more of the globin chains, the thalassaemias, and those in which a structural change in a globin chain leads to instability or to abnormal oxygen transport. In addition, there is a harmless group of mutations, known collectively as hereditary persistence of fetal haemoglobin, that interfere with the normal switching of fetal to adult haemoglobin production. The acquired disorders of haemoglobin can also be subdivided into those characterized by defective synthesis of the globin chains and those in which the structure of the haem molecules is altered, leading to inefficient oxygen transport.

Like all biological classifications, this way of splitting up the haemoglobin disorders is not entirely satisfactory. For example, some structural variants are synthesized in reduced amounts and hence produce the clinical picture of thalassaemia.

The thalassaemias
Historical introduction

The thalassaemias are the commonest of the inherited haematological disorders and, indeed, are the commonest single gene disorders in the world population. The condition was first recognized in 1925 by a Detroit physician called Thomas B Cooley who described a series of infants who became profoundly anaemic and developed splenomegaly over the first year of life. A milder form was described independently in the same year by an Italian physician, Fernando Rietti. Subsequently, further cases were identified and the disorder was variously called von Jaksch's anaemia, splenic anaemia, erythroblastosis, Mediterranean anaemia, or Cooley's anaemia. In 1936, George Whipple and Lesley Bradford recognized that many of their patients came from the Mediterranean region and hence they invented the word 'thalassaemia' from a Greek word meaning 'the sea'. Although it was realized later that the disorder occurs throughout the world and is not localized to the Mediterranean region, the name has stuck.

Thalassaemia is extremely heterogeneous. Its clinical picture can result from the interaction of many different genetic defects. This chapter concentrates mainly on the clinical and haematological aspects; readers who wish to learn more about the molecular pathology and population genetics of thalassaemia are referred to several reviews and monographs which are listed at the end of this chapter.

Box 22.5.7.2   The thalassaemias

α Thalassaemia

- α°
- α⁺

β Thalassaemia

- β°
- β⁺

δβ Thalassaemia

- (δβ)°
- Haemoglobin Lepore (δβ)⁺
- (εγδβ)° Thalassaemia
- δ Thalassaemia

Table 22.5.7.1   The β, δβ, and γδβ thalassaemias

Type of thalassaemia	Findings in homozygote	Findings in heterozygote
β°	Thalassaemia major[a,b]	Thalassaemia minor
	Hbs F and A₂	Raised Hb A₂
β⁺	Thalassaemia major[a,b]	Thalassaemia minor
	Hbs F, A, and A₂	Raised Hb A₂
δβ	Thalassaemia intermedia	Thalassaemia minor
	Hb F only	Hb F 5–15%; Hb A₂ normal
(δβ)⁺	Thalassaemia major or intermedia	Thalassaemia minor
(Lepore)	Hbs F and Lepore	Hb Lepore 5–15%; Hb A₂ normal
εγδβ	Not viable	Neonatal haemolysis
		Thalassaemia minor in adults, with normal Hbs F and A₂

[a]Occasionally have thalassaemia intermedia phenotype.
[b]Many patients with thalassaemia are compound heterozygotes for different molecular forms of β° or β⁺ thalassaemia.

Definition and classification

The thalassaemias are a heterogeneous group of genetic disorders of haemoglobin synthesis, all of which result from a reduced rate of production of one or more of the globin chains of haemoglobin. They are divided into the α, β, δβ, or εγδβ thalassaemias, according to which globin chain is produced in reduced amounts (Box 22.5.7.2). In some thalassaemias, no globin chain is synthesized at all, they are called α° or β° thalassaemias. In others, the α⁺ or β⁺ thalassaemias, globin chain is produced but at a reduced rate. Thalassaemia occurs in populations in which structural haemoglobin variants are common. It is not at all unusual for an individual to inherit a thalassaemia gene from one parent and a gene for a structural haemoglobin variant from the other. Both α and β thalassaemia occur commonly in some countries and hence individuals may receive genes for both types. These different interactions produce an extremely complex and clinically diverse series of genetic disorders which range in severity from death *in utero* to extremely mild, symptomless hypochromic anaemias.

The thalassaemias are inherited in a simple mendelian fashion. Heterozygotes are usually symptomless, although they can be easily recognized by simple haematological analysis. More severely affected patients are either homozygotes for α or β thalassaemia, compound heterozygotes for different molecular forms of α or β thalassaemia, or compound heterozygotes for thalassaemia and a structural haemoglobin variant. Clinically, the thalassaemias are classified according to their severity in major, intermediate, and minor forms. Thalassaemia major is a severe transfusion-dependent disorder. Thalassaemia intermedia is characterized by anaemia and splenomegaly though not of such severity as to require regular transfusion. Thalassaemia minor is the symptomless carrier state. While these descriptive terms do not have a precise genetic meaning, they remain useful in clinical practice.

β Thalassaemias

The β thalassaemias are the most important types of thalassaemia because they are very common and produce severe anaemia in their homozygous and compound heterozygous states (Table 22.5.7.1).

Distribution

The β thalassaemias occur widely in a broad belt ranging from the Mediterranean and parts of north and west Africa through the Middle East and Indian subcontinent to South-East Asia (Fig. 22.5.7.4). The high incidence zone stretches north through Yugoslavia and Romania and the southern parts of the former Soviet Union and includes the southern regions of the People's Republic of China. The disease is particularly common in South-East Asia where it occurs in a line starting in southern China and stretching down through Thailand and the Malay peninsula

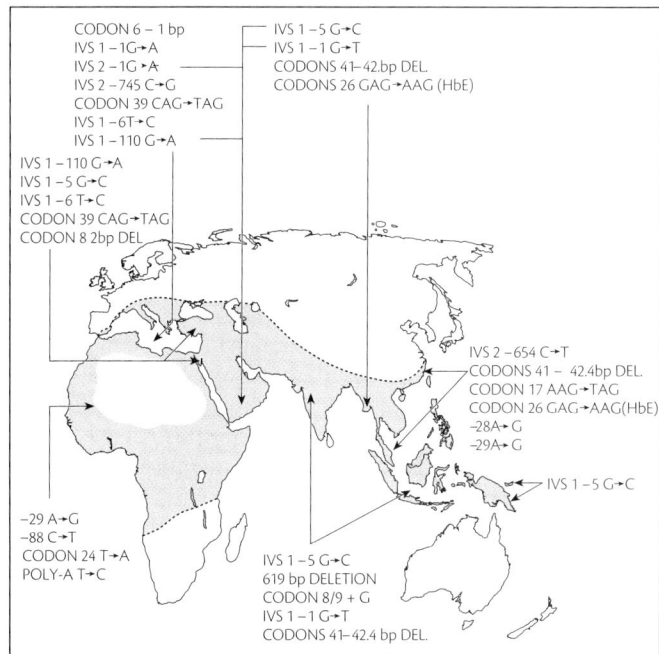

Fig. 22.5.7.4   World map showing the distribution of the different β thalassaemia mutations.

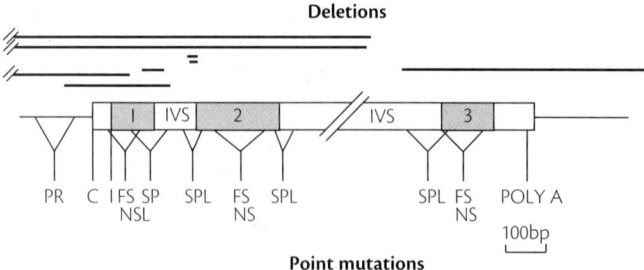

Deletions

Point mutations

Fig. 22.5.7.5 Some of the mutations that produce β thalassaemia. The β globin gene is divided into three exons (hatched) and two introns (IVS; unshaded). The different deletions are shown at the top of the figure while below the general position of the different point mutations is represented. C, CAP site; FS, frameshift; I, initiation site; NS, nonsense; polyA, RNA cleavage and polyA addition site; PR, promoter; SPL, splice-site mutation.

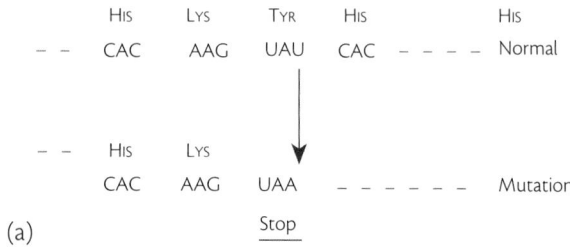

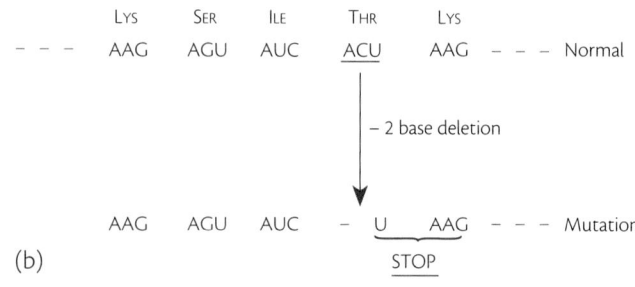

Fig. 22.5.7.6 Point mutations that cause β° thalassaemia: (a) premature stop codon (nonsense mutation); (b) frameshift mutation. See text for further details.

through Indonesia to some of the Pacific islands. In these populations, and in some of the Mediterranean island and mainland countries, gene frequencies for the various forms of β thalassaemia range between 2% and 20%. It should be remembered that β thalassaemia is not entirely confined to these high incidence regions; it occurs sporadically in every racial group.

Molecular pathology

The precise molecular lesions responsible for the defective synthesis of the β globin chains have been determined for many patients with β thalassaemia. The disease is extremely heterogeneous. Over 200 different mutations can produce the clinical phenotype of β thalassaemia. Some completely inactivate the β globin genes leading to β° thalassaemia; others cause a reduced output from the genes and hence the picture of β⁺ thalassaemia.

The main classes of mutations that cause β thalassaemia are summarized in Fig. 22.5.7.5. With the exception of a deletion of about 600 bases at the 3' end of the β globin gene, which is only found in certain populations of northern India, deletions are an uncommon cause of β thalassaemia. Most of the mutations are single base changes or small deletions and insertions of one or two bases. As shown in Fig. 22.5.7.5, they occur in both introns and exons, and also outside the coding regions.

Many of the exon mutations are nonsense mutations, i.e. the substitution of a single base in a codon produces a stop codon in the middle of the coding part of the mRNA (Fig. 22.5.7.6). Some mutations result in frame shifts; because the information carried by mRNA is in the form of a triplet code, the loss of one, two, or four bases throws the reading frame out of phase (Fig. 22.5.7.6). Another important class interfere with splicing. They may alter the invariate GC/AG dinucleotides at the intron/exon junctions, in which case they usually cause β° thalassaemia. Alternatively, they may activate so-called cryptic splice sites, providing an alternate splice site so that both normal and abnormal mRNA species are produced (Fig. 22.5.7.7). These lesions cause a β⁺ thalassaemia, the severity of which depends on the relative usage of the normal and abnormal splice site and hence the quantity of normal and abnormal β globin mRNA that is produced.

Many single base substitutions have also been found in the flanking regions of the β globin genes. They alter either the proximal promoter regions or adjacent sequences, causing down regulation of β globin gene transcription to a varying degree. They are usually associated with milder forms of β⁺ thalassaemia.

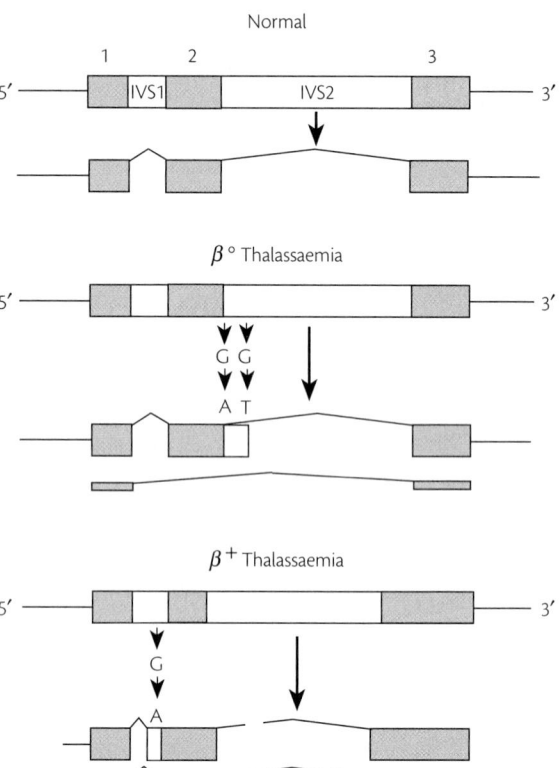

Fig. 22.5.7.7 The consequences of different splice-site mutations. In β° thalassaemia two different mutations are shown, one that inactivates the normal splice site, and another that produces a new splice site. Two abnormal mRNA molecules are produced. In the β⁺ thalassaemia case a new splice site is produced in the first intron. Both normal and abnormal mRNAs are produced, the latter in greater amounts.

Because there are so many different β thalassaemia mutations it follows that many patients who are apparently homozygous for β thalassaemia are, in fact, compound heterozygotes for two different molecular lesions.

Pathophysiology

The mutations that cause β thalassaemia result in absent or reduced β chain production. The synthesis of α chains proceeds at a normal rate and hence there is imbalanced globin chain synthesis (Fig. 22.5.7.8). In the absence of their partner chains the excess α chains are unstable and precipitate in the red-cell precursors, forming large intracellular inclusions. These interfere with red-cell maturation, and hence there is a variable degree of intramedullary destruction of red-cell precursors, that is ineffective erythropoiesis. Those red cells which mature and enter the circulation contain α chain inclusions which interfere with their passage through the microcirculation, particularly in the spleen. These cells are prematurely destroyed. Thus the anaemia of β thalassaemia results from both ineffective erythropoiesis and a shortened red-cell survival. The mechanisms of the destruction of red-cell precursors and their progeny are extremely complex and are not simply a reflection of mechanical damage to the red cells. Free α chains and their degradation products, particularly haem and iron, cause severe oxidative damage to the red-cell membrane proteins. The end result is a dehydrated, rigid erythrocyte with a markedly shortened survival.

The anaemia acts as a stimulus to increased erythropoietin production, causing massive expansion of the bone marrow which may lead to serious deformities of the skull and long bones. Because the spleen is being constantly bombarded with abnormal red cells, it hypertrophies. The resulting splenomegaly and bone marrow expansion gives rise to an increase in the plasma volume which, together with pooling of the red cells in the enlarged spleen, causes an exacerbation of an already severe degree of anaemia.

As mentioned previously, fetal haemoglobin production largely ceases after birth. However, some adult red-cell precursors (F cells) retain the ability to produce a small number of γ chains. Because the latter can combine with excess α chains to form haemoglobin F, cells which make relatively more γ chains in the bone marrow of β thalassaemics are partly protected against the deleterious effect of α chain precipitation. Red-cell precursors which produce haemoglobin F are selected in the marrow and peripheral blood of these patients. Thus, they have relatively large amounts of haemoglobin F in their red cells. Furthermore, because δ chain synthesis is unaffected, the disorder is characterized by a relative or absolute increase in haemoglobin A_2 ($\alpha_2\delta_2$) production. These interactions are summarized in Fig. 22.5.7.7.

If the anaemia is corrected with blood transfusion the erythropoietic drive is reduced, growth and development are improved, and bone deformities do not occur. On the other hand, each unit of blood contains 200 mg of iron; with regular transfusion there is steady accumulation of iron in the liver, endocrine glands, and myocardium. Even though well-transfused thalassaemic children grow and develop normally, they die of iron overload unless steps are taken to remove iron.

The severe homozygous or compound heterozygous forms of β thalassaemia

These are the commonest and most important forms of thalassaemia and give rise to a major public health problem in many parts of the world.

Clinical features

Most severe forms of β thalassaemia present within the first year of life, as fetal haemoglobin production declines, with failure to thrive, poor feeding, intermittent bouts of fever, or failure to improve after an intercurrent infection. At this stage the affected infant looks pale. In many cases splenomegaly is already present. There are no other specific clinical signs. Diagnosis depends on the haematological changes outlined below. If the infant is established on a regular transfusion regimen at this stage, early development is normal. Further symptoms do not occur until puberty, when the effects of iron loading start to appear. If, on the other hand, the infant is not adequately transfused, the typical clinical picture of homozygous β thalassaemia develops. Thus the clinical manifestations of the severe forms of β thalassaemia have to be described in two contexts: (1) the well-transfused child and (2) the child with chronic anaemia throughout early life.

In the well-transfused thalassaemic child, early growth and development is normal. Splenomegaly is minimal. However, there

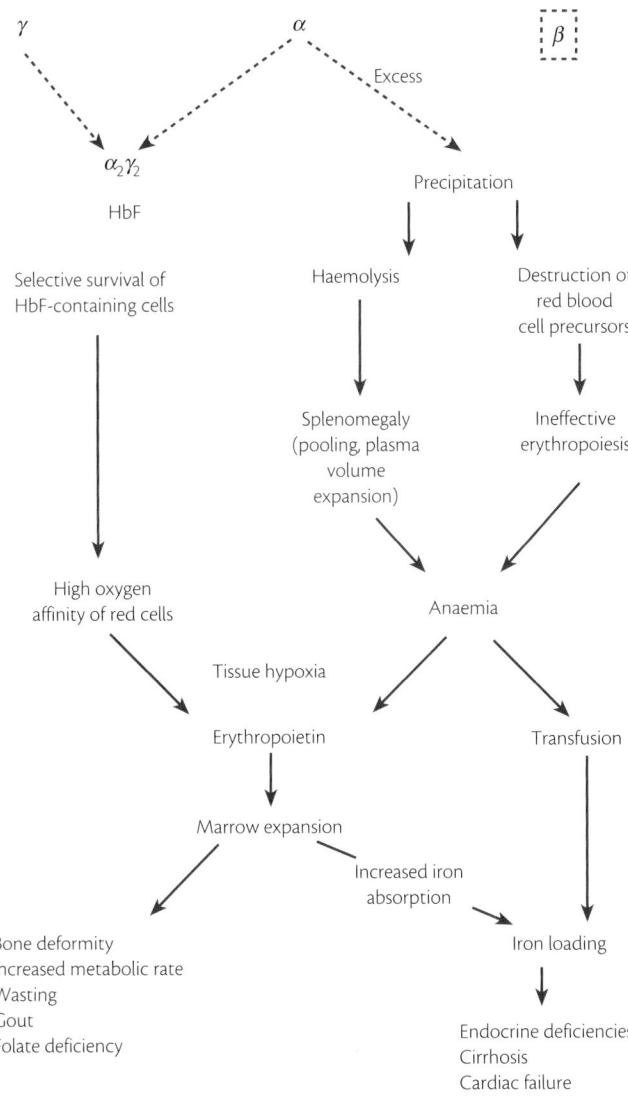

Fig. 22.5.7.8 The pathophysiology of β thalassaemia.

is a gradual accumulation of iron. The effects of tissue siderosis start to appear by the end of the first decade. The normal adolescent growth spurt fails to occur. Hepatic, endocrine, and cardiac complications of iron overloading produce a variety of problems including diabetes, hyopoparathyroidism, adrenal insufficiency, and progressive liver failure. Secondary sexual development is delayed or does not occur at all. Short stature and lack of sexual development may lead to serious psychological problems. By f ar the commonest cause of death, which usually occurs toward the end of the second or early in the third decade, is progressive cardiac damage. Ultimately these patients die either as a result of protracted cardiac failure or suddenly, as the result of an acute arrhythmia.

There is now good evidence that children who have been both adequately transfused and chelated may grow and develop normally, pass through a normal puberty, and survive to adult life in excellent condition. However, it is becoming apparent that even children who have been well managed in this way still tend to suffer from complications as they get older, particularly delayed sexual maturation, growth disturbances, and osteoporosis. It seems likely that many of these problems are due to subtle damage to the hypothalamic–pituitary axis with secondary hypogonadism. In addition, some of the growth disturbances may reflect toxicity of the chelating agents used to remove iron (see below).

The clinical picture in children who are inadequately transfused is quite different. Early childhood is interspersed with a series of distressing complications. The overall rates of growth and development are markedly retarded. There is progressive splenomegaly; hypersplenism may cause a worsening of the anaemia, sometimes associated with thrombocytopenia and a bleeding tendency. Because of the bone marrow expansion there may be deformities of the skull with marked bossing and overgrowth of the zygomata giving rise to the classical mongoloid facial appearance of β thalassaemia (Fig. 22.5.7.9a, b). These findings are reflected by radiological changes which include a lacy, trabecular pattern of the long bones and phalanges and a typical 'hair on end' appearance of the skull (Fig. 22.5.7.10). These bone changes may be associated with recurrent fractures. There is increased susceptibility to infection which may cause a catastrophic drop in the haemoglobin level. Because of the massive marrow expansion, these children are hypermetabolic, run intermittent fevers, lose weight (Fig. 22.5.7.8b), have increased requirements for folic acid, and may become acutely folate depleted with worsening of their anaemia. Increased turnover of red-cell precursors occasionally gives rise to hyperuricaemia and secondary gout. There is a bleeding tendency which, partly due to thrombocytopenia secondary to hypersplenism, may be exacerbated by liver damage associated with iron loading and extramedullary haemopoiesis. There is also an increased risk of thrombotic complications, reflecting procoagulant properties of the abnormal red-cell membranes. The bone deformities of the skull can cause distressing dental complications with poorly formed teeth and malocclusion, and inadequate drainage of the sinuses and middle ear which may lead to chronic sinus infection and deafness. If these unfortunate children survive to puberty, they develop the same complications of iron loading as the well-transfused patients. In this case, some of the iron accumulation results from an increased rate of gastrointestinal absorption as well as that derived from the inadequate transfusion regimen.

Haematological changes

There is always a severe anaemia. The haemoglobin values on presentation range from 2 to 8 g/dl. The appearance of the stained peripheral blood film is grossly abnormal (Fig. 22.5.7.11). The red cells show marked hypochromia and variation in shape and size. There are many hypochromic macrocytes and misshapen microcytes, some of which are mere fragments of cells. There is a moderate degree of anisochromia and basophilic stippling. There are always some nucleated red cells in the peripheral blood. After splenectomy,

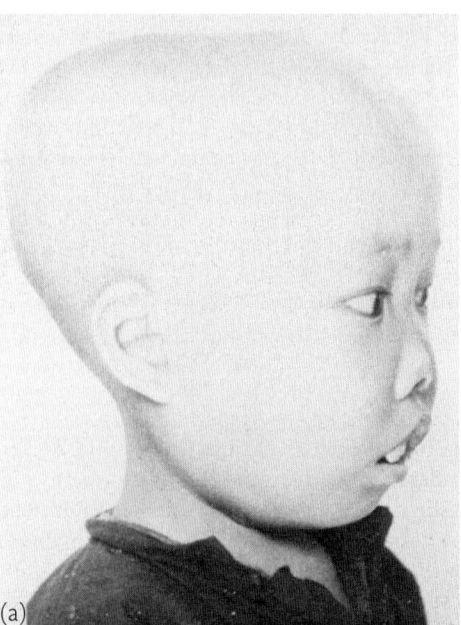

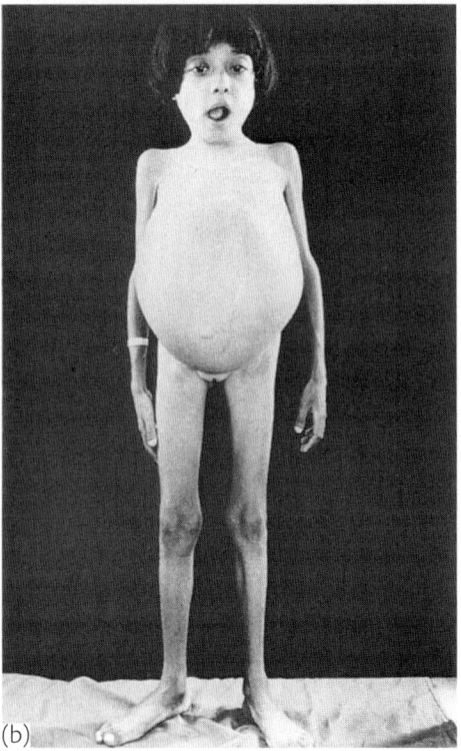

Fig. 22.5.7.9 Homozygous β thalassaemia: (a) skull and facial deformity due to bone marrow expansion; (b) gross wasting of the limbs and hepatomegaly in an undertransfused child.

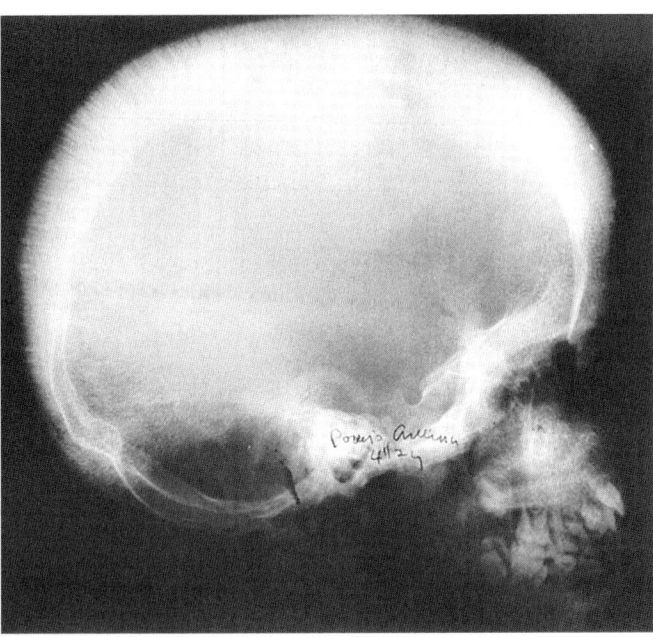

Fig. 22.5.7.10 Radiological changes of the skull in homozygous β thalassaemia.

these are found in large numbers. In the postsplenectomy film, many of the nucleated cells and mature erythrocytes show ragged inclusions after incubation of the blood with methyl violet. There is usually a slight elevation in the reticulocyte count. The white cell and platelet counts are normal unless there is hypersplenism in which case they are reduced. The bone marrow shows marked erythroid hyperplasia, with a myeloid/erythroid (M/E) ratio of 1 or less. Many of the red-cell precursors show ragged inclusions after incubation with methyl violet.

There are biochemical changes of increased haemolysis and progressive iron loading. The bilirubin level is usually elevated and haptoglobins are absent. The ^{51}Cr red-cell survival is shortened. The serum iron rises progressively. Most transfusion-dependent children have a totally saturated iron-binding capacity. This change is mirrored by a high plasma ferritin level. Liver biopsies show a marked increase in hepatic iron, which may be distributed both in the reticuloendothelial and parenchymal cells (Fig. 22.5.7.12).

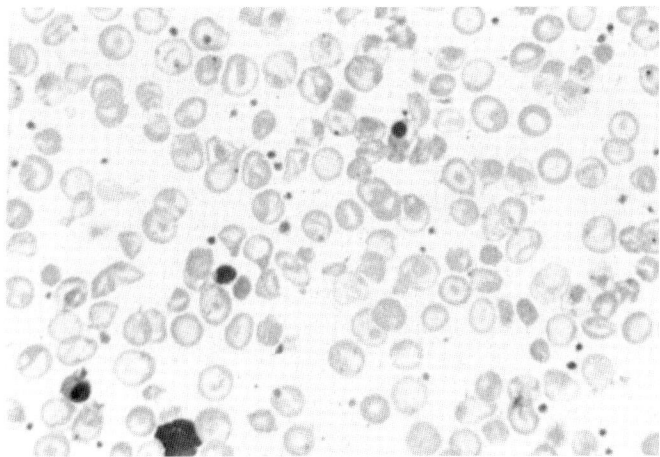

Fig. 22.5.7.11 Peripheral blood film in homozygous β thalassaemia (×630, Leishman stain).

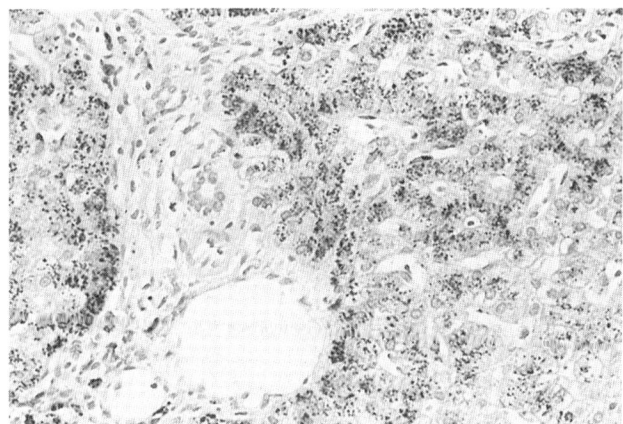

Fig. 22.5.7.12 Histological appearances of the liver in homozygous β thalassaemia showing gross iron deposition (×270, iron stain).

Other biochemical changes

Many thalassaemic children are depleted in vitamin E and ascorbate. Folic acid deficiency has already been mentioned. Frank diabetes may develop and endocrine function tests may reveal parathyroid or adrenal insufficiency, or inappropriate response by the pituitary to various release hormones; growth hormone levels are usually normal.

Haemoglobin changes (Table 22.5.7.1)

The haemoglobin F level is always elevated. In β° thalassaemia there is no haemoglobin A and the haemoglobin consists of F and A_2 only. In β+ thalassaemia the level of haemoglobin F ranges from 30 to 90% of the total haemoglobin. The haemoglobin A_2 level is usually normal and is of no diagnostic value.

Heterozygous β thalassaemia

Carriers for β thalassaemia, apart from symptoms of mild anaemia, are usually well except in periods of stress such as pregnancy, when they may become more anaemic. Splenomegaly is rarely present.

Haematological changes

There is a mild degree of anaemia with haemoglobin values in the 9 to 11 g/dl range. The red cells show hypochromia and microcytosis with characteristically low MCH and MCV values. The reticulocyte count is usually normal. The bone marrow shows moderate erythroid hyperplasia.

Haemoglobin changes

The characteristic finding is an elevated haemoglobin A_2 level in the 4 to 6% range. There is a slight elevation of haemoglobin F in the 1 to 3% range in about 50% of cases. A less common form occurs in which the haemoglobin A_2 is not elevated.

β Thalassaemia in association with haemoglobin variants

In many populations where there is a high incidence of both β thalassaemia and various haemoglobin variants it is common for an individual to inherit a β thalassaemia gene from one parent and a gene for a structural haemoglobin variant from the other. Although numerous interactions of this type have been described, in clinical practice only three are of importance: sickle cell β thalassaemia, haemoglobin C β thalassaemia, and haemoglobin E β thalassaemia.

Sickle cell β thalassaemia

The clinical manifestations which result from the interaction of the β thalassaemia and sickle cell genes vary considerably from race to race. In African populations there are mild forms of β^+ thalassaemia which, when they interact with the sickle cell gene, produce a condition characterized by mild anaemia and few sickling crises; it is compatible with normal survival and is often ascertained by chance haematological examination. On the other hand, in Mediterranean populations it is quite common for an individual to inherit a β° or severe β^+ thalassaemia determinant from one parent and a sickle cell gene from the other. These interactions are often associated with a clinical picture which is indistinguishable from sickle cell anaemia.

The diagnosis of sickle cell thalassaemia rests on the clinical features of a sickling disorder found in association with a peripheral blood picture with typical thalassaemic red-cell changes, i.e. a low MCH and MCV. In the more severe forms of sickle cell β° thalassaemia, there may be an elevated reticulocyte count and sickled red cells are found on the peripheral blood film. The diagnosis can be confirmed by haemoglobin electrophoresis, which in sickle cell β^+ thalassaemia shows haemoglobin S together with 10 to 30% haemoglobin A and an elevated haemoglobin A_2 value. In sickle cell β° thalassaemia, the haemoglobin consists mainly of haemoglobin S with an elevated level of haemoglobins F and A_2. To confirm the diagnosis it is necessary to examine the parents; one should have the sickle cell trait and the other the β thalassaemia trait.

Haemoglobin C thalassaemia

This disorder is restricted to West Africans and some North African and southern Mediterranean populations. It is characterized by a mild haemolytic anaemia associated with splenomegaly. The peripheral blood film shows numerous target cells and thalassaemic red-cell changes with a moderately elevated reticulocyte count. Haemoglobin electrophoresis shows a preponderance of haemoglobin C. The diagnosis is confirmed by finding the haemoglobin C trait in one parent and the β thalassaemia trait in the other.

Haemoglobin E β thalassaemia

This is the commonest form of severe thalassaemia in many Asian countries, where it is leading to an increasingly serious public health burden. The mutation that underlies haemoglobin E causes a frameshift and therefore the production of a haemoglobin variant at a much lower rate than haemoglobin A. Thus, when a haemoglobin E gene is inherited together with a severe β thalassaemia mutation there is a marked efficiency of β chain production. One of the major characteristics of haemoglobin E β thalassaemia, which causes particular difficulties for its management, is its extraordinary clinical heterogeneity. At one end of the spectrum it is indistinguishable from β thalassaemia major, while at the other end there are patients who grow and develop normally without the need for transfusion. Many patients are encountered whose clinical course lies between these extremes. While some of this phenotypic variability can be ascribed to the inheritance of β thalassaemia alleles of varying severity, or the coinheritance of various modifier genes, much of it still remains unexplained. Recently, factors such as variability of adaptation to anaemia and the role of environmental factors such as malaria have been found to be of considerable importance.

In the more severe forms of this condition the findings are very similar to those in severe β thalassaemia (Fig. 22.5.7.13), while in the milder forms they resemble those of β thalassaemia intermedia, as described later in this chapter. Complications include a marked susceptibility to infection, hypersplenism, progressive iron

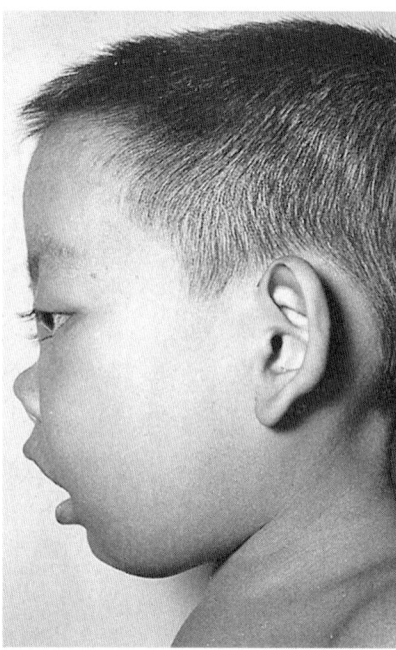

Fig. 22.5.7.13 Bossing of the skull in haemoglobin E thalassaemia.

loading, neurological lesions due to tumours caused by extramedullary erythropoiesis extending inwards from the inner tables of the skull or vertebrae, folate deficiency, and recurrent pathological fractures. From the limited data that are available, it seems that patients at the milder end of the clinical spectrum, though often quite anaemic, survive in good health well into adult life, at which time they do not appear to develop cardiac complications unless they have become particularly iron loaded due to intestinal absorption.

The diagnosis of haemoglobin E thalassaemia is confirmed by finding haemoglobins E and F and little or no haemoglobin A on haemoglobin electrophoresis and by demonstrating the haemoglobin E trait in one parent and the β thalassaemia trait in the other.

Other β thalassaemia variants

It is not uncommon to encounter patients with the clinical and haematological features of heterozygous β thalassaemia who do not have an elevated haemoglobin A_2 level. Many of these individuals are heterozygotes for both β and δ thalassaemia. It is important to recognize this interaction because, if it is inherited together with a typical β thalassaemia gene, it can produce a severe transfusion-dependent disorder. Hence this variant is important in antenatal screening programmes. It can only be identified for certain by globin chain synthesis or gene analysis in a specialized laboratory. Families are encountered occasionally in which there is a more severe form of heterozygous β thalassaemia associated with anaemia, jaundice, and splenomegaly. In some of these families it is apparent that the affected individuals are in fact compound heterozygotes for β thalassaemia and the so-called 'silent' β thalassaemia gene, i.e. a determinant which cannot be identified haematologically in heterozygotes. In other families, a severe form of β thalassaemia behaves as a single gene disorder with full expression in heterozygotes, that is it follows a dominant form of inheritance. In most of these families, the disorder results from the synthesis of a highly unstable β globin chain.

The δβ thalassaemias (Table 22.5.7.1)

Molecular genetics and classification

Disorders due to reduced β and δ chain synthesis are much less common than those due to defective β chain production. They are remarkably heterogeneous at the molecular level. In some cases they result from deletions of the β and δ globin genes, while in others there appears to have been mispaired synapsis and unequal crossing over between the δ and β globin gene loci with the production of δβ fusion genes. The latter produce δβ fusion chains which combine with α chains to form haemoglobin variants called the Lepore haemoglobins (Lepore was the family name of the first patient to be recognized with this disorder). Hence it is usual to classify this group of conditions into the (δβ)° thalassaemias and the haemoglobin Lepore or (δβ)+ thalassaemias.

Clinical and haematological changes

The (δβ)° thalassaemias have been reported in many populations, although there are no high-frequency areas. In the homozygous state there is a mild degree of anaemia with haemoglobin values of 8 to 10 g/dl. There is often a moderate degree of splenomegaly but these patients are usually symptomless except during periods of stress such as infection or pregnancy. Haemoglobin analysis shows 100% haemoglobin F. Heterozygous carriers have thalassaemic blood pictures, elevated levels of haemoglobin F of 5 to 20%, and normal levels of haemoglobin A_2. The homozygous state for haemoglobin Lepore is characterized by a clinical picture which is usually similar to that of homozygous β thalassaemia although in some cases it may be milder and nontransfusion dependent. The haematological findings are similar to those of β thalassaemia. The haemoglobin consists of F and Lepore only. Heterozygous carriers have thalassaemic blood pictures associated with about 5 to 15% haemoglobin Lepore.

The (εγδβ)° thalassaemias

There are several rare forms of thalassaemia which result from long deletions of the β globin gene cluster which, as well as removing or inactivating the β genes, involve the δ, γ, and embryonic ε genes. They also involve the main regulatory sequence upstream of the β globin gene cluster, the locus control region. This means that there is no output of globin chains from this gene cluster at all. Clearly, the homozygous state for these disorders would not be compatible with survival. Heterozygotes often have severe haemolytic disease of the newborn with anaemia and hyperbilirubinaemia. If they survive the neonatal period they grow and develop normally; in adult life they have the haematological picture of heterozygous β thalassaemia with mild anaemia, hypochromic microcytic red cells, and a haemoglobin pattern consisting of haemoglobin A, no elevation of haemoglobin F, and a normal level of haemoglobin A_2.

Hereditary persistence of fetal haemoglobin

There is a complex family of conditions characterized by persistent fetal haemoglobin synthesis into adult life associated with no major haematological abnormalities. In some cases they result from long deletions of the β globin gene cluster, similar to those that cause δβ thalassaemia. Indeed, they form a continuum with this condition; homozygotes have 100% fetal haemoglobin, elevated haemoglobin levels, and no clinical findings. Other forms result from point mutations in the promoter regions of the γ globin genes. In this case there is increased γ chain production together with reduced

β chain production on the affected chromosome. Hence, homozygotes have markedly elevated levels of haemoglobin F but also produce some haemoglobin A. Finally, there is a group in which persistent low levels of haemoglobin F, in the 3 to 10% range, are observed. They result from mutations either within the β globin gene cluster or on other chromosomes.

The only clinical importance of this complex group of conditions is that they may interact with the thalassaemias or structural haemoglobin variants and reduce the severity of different phenotypes by increasing the amount of haemoglobin F that is produced.

The α thalassaemias

Although the α thalassaemias are commoner on a global basis than the β thalassaemias, they pose less of a public health problem because their severe forms only occur in a few regions.

Distribution

The α thalassaemias occur widely through the Mediterranean region, parts of West Africa, the Middle East, parts of the Indian subcontinent, and throughout South-East Asia in a line stretching from southern China through Thailand, the Malay peninsula, and Indonesia to the Pacific island populations (Fig. 22.5.7.14). For reasons which will become apparent when we consider the molecular pathology of these disorders, the serious forms of α thalassaemia are restricted to some of the Mediterranean island populations and South-East Asia.

Inheritance and molecular pathology

Because both haemoglobins A and F have α chains, genetic disorders of α chain synthesis result in defective fetal and adult haemoglobin production. In the fetus, deficiency of α chains leads to the production of excess γ chains which form γ_4 tetramers, or haemoglobin Bart's (Fig. 22.5.7.15). In adults, a deficiency of α chains leads to an excess of β chains which form β_4 tetramers, or haemoglobin H, the adult counterpart of haemoglobin Bart's. Thus, the presence of haemoglobins Bart's or H in red cells is the hallmark of α thalassaemia. For reasons which are not yet clear, a critical level of globin chain imbalance is required before detectable amounts of haemoglobins Bart's or H appear in the red cells. Unfortunately for clinicians, in individuals with mild forms of α thalassaemia this

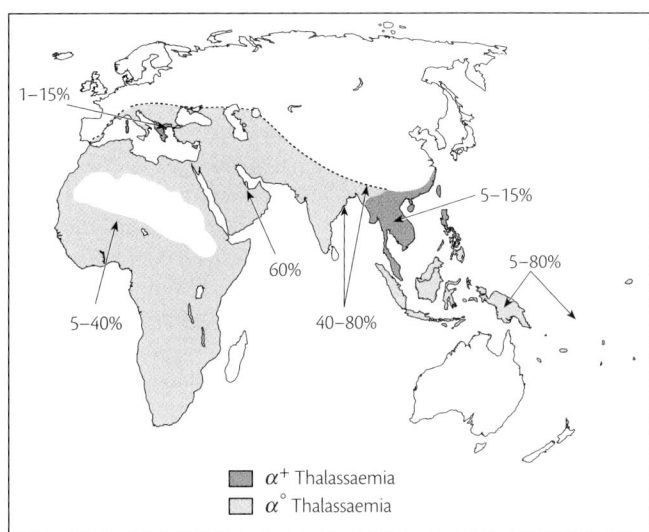

Fig. 22.5.7.14 World map showing the distribution of the α thalassaemias.

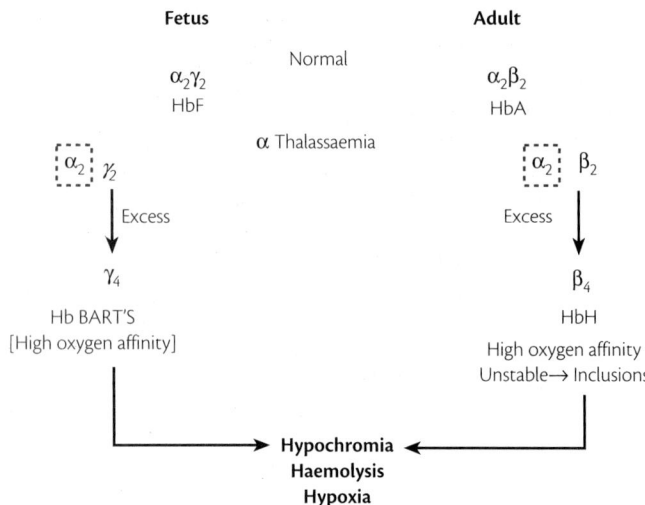

Fig. 22.5.7.15 The pathophysiology of α thalassaemia.

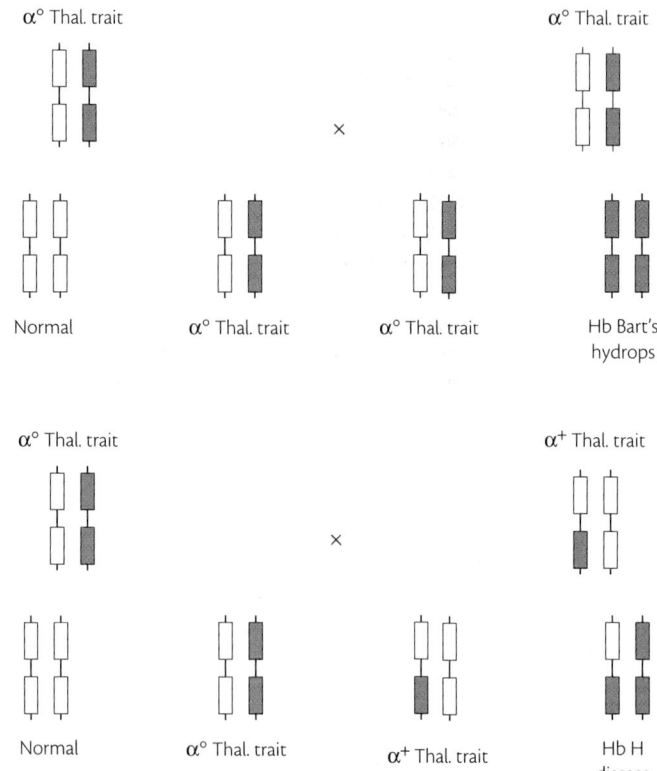

Fig. 22.5.7.16 The genetics of α thalassaemia. The blue α genes represent gene deletions or otherwise inactivated genes. The open α genes represent normal genes. α° Thalassaemia and α+ thalassaemia are defined in the text.

level is not reached; significant amounts of these variants occur only in the red cells of patients who have a severe degree of α chain deficiency. This means that the carrier states for different forms of α thalassaemia are difficult to diagnose.

Because normal individuals receive two α globin genes from each of their parents, αα/αα, the genetics of the α thalassaemias is more complicated than that of the β thalassaemia. It is useful to define these conditions in heterozygotes. First, there is a more severe form which is called α° thalassaemia, which results from loss of both of the linked α globin genes, – –/αα. The second type is almost completely silent in carriers; their red cells are normal or are only slightly hypochromic. This condition is due to the deletion, –α/αα, or reduced activity due to a mutation, $α^Tα/αα$, of one of the linked α globin genes. Because there is still some output of α globin from the affected chromosome this is called α⁺thalassaemia. To put it in another way, the terms α° and $α^T$ thalassaemia describe haplotypes, i.e. the products of two linked α globin genes on one of a pair of homologous chromosomes 16.

In clinical practice we encounter two symptomatic types of α thalassaemia, the haemoglobin Bart's hydrops syndrome and haemoglobin H disease (Table 22.7.5.2). The former results from the homozygous inheritance of α° thalassaemia. On the other hand, haemoglobin H disease usually results from the coinheritance of both α° and α⁺ thalassaemia. We now know that there are many different molecular types of both α° and α⁺ thalassaemia. These genetic interactions are summarized in Fig. 22.5.7.16.

Like the β thalassaemias, the α thalassaemias are extremely heterogeneous at the molecular level. Many different-sized deletions can remove either both the α globin genes or the main regulatory regions of the α globin gene cluster and cause α° thalassaemia, but there are only two that are common. One is found in South-East Asia. The other occurs mainly in Mediterranean populations (Fig. 22.5.7.17). Similarly, there are several different-sized deletions that remove a single α globin gene to produce the deletion forms of α⁺ thalassaemia; the commonest are those that remove either 3.7 kb or 4.2 kb of the α gene cluster. There are also many different mutations that can produce the nondeletion forms of α⁺ thalassaemia. Many of them are similar to those that produce β thalassaemia. A particularly common form of nondeletion α+ thalassaemia, found in up to 5% or more of some South-East Asian populations, results

from a single base change in the α globin chain termination codon UAA, which changes to CAA. The latter is the code for the amino acid glutamine. When the ribosomes reach this point, instead of the chain terminating, they read through mRNA that is not normally translated until another stop codon is reached. An elongated α chain variant is synthesized, but the mRNA is destabilized by read-through of sequences which are not normally translated and so the variant is also produced at a reduced rate. It is called haemoglobin Constant Spring after the name of the town in Jamaica in which it was first discovered.

Genotype–phenotype relationships

Molecular studies explain much of the clinical variability of α thalassaemia in different populations. Since the haemoglobin Bart's hydrops syndrome requires the homozygous inheritance of α° thalassaemia (– –/– –), this condition only occurs in populations in which α° thalassaemia is common. It is mainly confined to South-East Asia and the Mediterranean islands, populations in which the haemoglobin Bart's hydrops syndrome causes a public health problem. Most forms of haemoglobin H disease are due to the inheritance of α° thalassaemia from one parent and α⁺ thalassaemia from the other (–α/– – or $α^T$/– –). Thus, haemoglobin H disease is also restricted mainly to Mediterranean and Asian populations. On the other hand, α⁺ thalassaemia occurs very commonly throughout parts of West Africa, the Indian subcontinent, and the Pacific island populations. α° Thalassaemia does not occur in these regions, so that the haemoglobin Bart's hydrops syndrome and haemoglobin H disease are not seen. The homozygous state for α⁺ thalassaemia (–α/–α) is characterized by a mild hypochromic

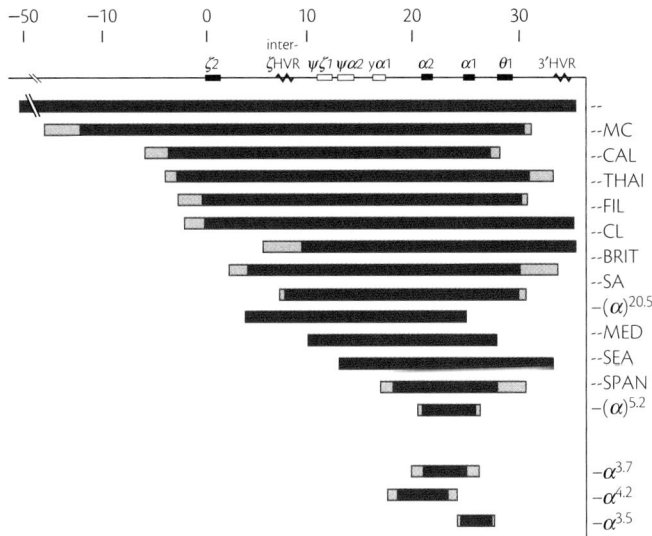

Fig. 22.5.7.17 The different-sized deletions responsible for some forms of α° or $\alpha+$ thalassaemia. The α globin gene cluster is shown at the top of the figure. Two highly variable regions (HVR) are shown. The abbreviations on the right-hand side indicate the source of origin of patients with the deletions: MED, Mediterranean; SEA, South-East Asia. The three smaller deletions at the bottom of the figure show some of the main classes of α^+ thalassaemia. The superscripts 3.7, 4.2, and 3.5 indicate the size of the deletions.

anaemia, very similar to the heterozygous state for α° thalassaemia; the results of having only two out of the normal four α genes seem to be the same whether the two genes are missing from the same chromosome or opposite pairs of homologous chromosomes. To complicate matters, sometimes the homozygous state for the nondeletion forms of α^+ thalassaemia, $\alpha^T\alpha/\alpha^T\alpha$, are more severe and cause haemoglobin H disease.

Pathophysiology

The pathophysiology of α thalassaemia is different from that of β thalassaemia. A deficiency of α chains leads to the production of excess γ chains or β chains which form haemoglobins Bart's and H respectively (Fig. 22.5.7.15). These more soluble tetramers do not precipitate to any great extent in the bone marrow. Erythropoiesis is thus more effective than in β thalassaemia, that is there is less intramedullary destruction of red-cell precursors. However, haemoglobin H is unstable and precipitates in red cells as they age. The large inclusion bodies produced in this way are trapped in the spleen and other parts of the microcirculation leading to a shortened red-cell survival. Furthermore, both haemoglobins Bart's and H have a very high oxygen affinity; because they have no α chains there is no haem–haem interaction and their oxygen dissociation curves resemble that of myoglobin. Thus the pathophysiology of severe forms of α thalassaemia is based on defective haemoglobin production, the synthesis of homotetramers which are physiologically useless, and a haemolytic component due to their precipitation in older red cells. Furthermore, excess β chains cause a different pattern of damage to red-cell membrane proteins than free α chains; the red cells tend to be overhydrated in α thalassaemia.

Haemoglobin Bart's hydrops syndrome

This condition is a common cause of fetal loss throughout South-East Asia and in Greece and Cyprus. Affected infants produce no α chains and hence can make neither fetal nor adult haemoglobin.

The clinical picture is very characteristic (Fig. 22.5.7.18). Infants are usually stillborn between 28 and 40 weeks. Liveborn infants take a few gasping respirations and then expire within the first hour after birth. They show the typical picture of hydrops fetalis with gross pallor, generalized oedema, and massive hepatosplenomegaly. There is a high frequency of other congenital abnormalities, and a very large, friable placenta, all due to severe intrauterine anaemia. The haemoglobin values are in the 6 to 8 g/dl range and there are gross thalassaemic changes of the peripheral blood film with many nucleated red cells. The haemoglobin consists of approximately 80% haemoglobin Bart's and 20% of the embryonic haemoglobin Portland ($\zeta_2\gamma_2$). It is

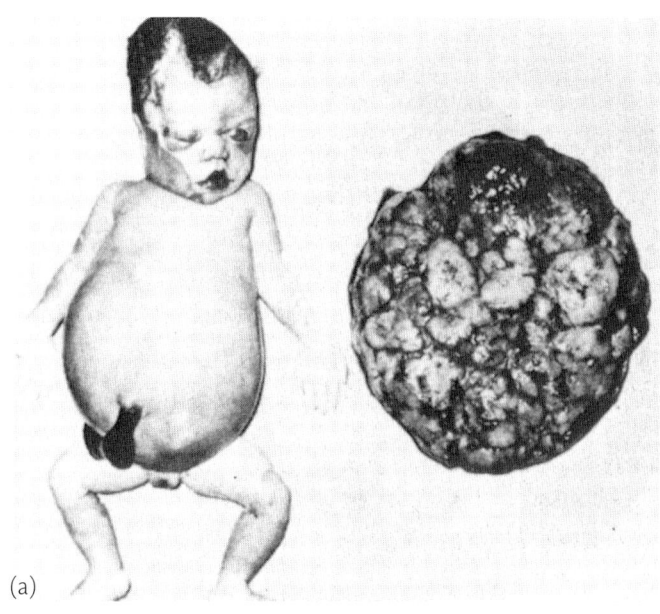

(a)

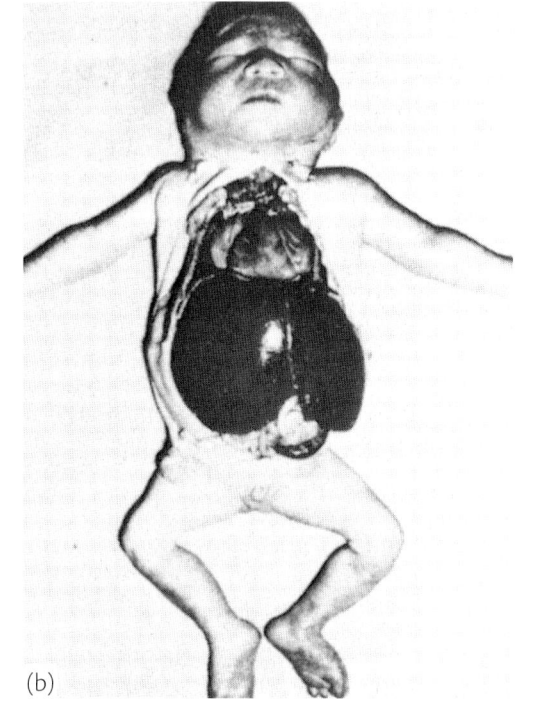

(b)

Fig. 22.5.7.18 The haemoglobin Bart's hydrops syndrome: (a) a hydropic infant with massively enlarged placenta; (b) autopsy findings with an enlarged liver. (By permission of Professor P Wasi.)

believed that these infants survive to term because they continue to produce embryonic haemoglobin at this level; haemoglobin Bart's is, as mentioned above, useless as an oxygen carrier.

This syndrome is also characterized by a high incidence of maternal toxaemia of pregnancy and considerable obstetric difficulties due to the presence of the large, friable placenta. Both parents have thalassaemic red-cell changes with normal haemoglobin A_2 values, i.e. the characteristic finding of the heterozygous state for α° thalassaemia.

Haemoglobin H disease

As mentioned earlier, haemoglobin H is a tetramer of normal β chains with the formula β_4. It is produced when there is a marked reduction of α chain synthesis. Haemoglobin H disease usually results from the inheritance of α° thalassaemia from one parent and α^+ from the other. It may also result from the inheritance of α° thalassaemia and haemoglobin Constant Spring or from the homozygous state for a severe, nondeletion form of α thalassaemia. The latter form of inheritance is particularly common in Saudi Arabia.

There is a variable degree of anaemia and splenomegaly but it is most unusual to see severe thalassaemic bone changes or the growth retardation characteristic of homozygous β thalassaemia. Patients usually survive into adult life although the course may be interspersed with severe episodes of haemolysis associated with infection, or worsening of the anaemia due to progressive hypersplenism. Oxidant drugs such as sulphonamides may increase the rate of precipitation of haemoglobin H and therefore exacerbate the anaemia.

Haemoglobin values range from 7 to $10 \, g/dl$. The blood film shows typical thalassaemic changes. There is a moderate reticulocytosis. Incubation of the red cells with brilliant cresyl blue generates numerous inclusion bodies by precipitation of the haemoglobin H under the redox action of the dye. After splenectomy large, preformed inclusions can be demonstrated on incubation of blood with methyl violet. The haemoglobin consists of from 5 to 40% haemoglobin H together with haemoglobin A and a normal or reduced level of haemoglobin A_2.

Usually one parent is heterozygous for α° thalassaemia and the other for α^+ thalassaemia, the deletion or nondeletion varieties. Less commonly, both parents are heterozygous for a nondeletion form of α^+ thalassaemia.

The haematological findings in the α° and α^+ thalassaemia traits are summarized in Table 22.5.7.2. They can only be identified with certainty by analysis of the α globin genes.

α Thalassaemia and intellectual disability or myelodysplasia

There is an increasingly important group of α thalassaemias which are not restricted to individuals from tropical backgrounds. They are observed in all racial groups and have been best characterized in those of northern European origin. These conditions are charac-

Table 22.5.7.2 The α thalassaemias

Type	Homozygotes	Heterozygotes
α°	Hb Bart's hydrops	Thalassaemia minor
α^+(deletion)	Thalassaemia minor	Normal blood picture[b]
α^+(nondeletion)	Hb H disease[a]	Normal blood picture[b]

[a]Haemoglobin H disease more commonly results from the compound heterozygous inheritance of α° and either variety of α^+ thalassaemia.
[b]There may be very mild red-cell hypochromia.

terized by variable degrees of intellectual disability, dysmorphic features, and α thalassaemic blood pictures. They follow a completely different form of inheritance from the commoner genetic forms of α thalassaemia and constitute a increasingly heterogeneous group of disorders. There are two major varieties of this condition. The first is due to lesions that involve the α globin gene cluster on chromosome 16, ATR-16. There is another group resulting from mutations on the X chromosome, ATR-X.

The ATR-16 disorders are characterized by a very variable degree of intellectual disability and equally variable dysmorphic features. The blood film shows mild α thalassaemic changes and some cells which contain typical haemoglobin H inclusion bodies. It is now clear that they have a heterogeneous molecular pathology. In some cases the condition results from long deletions which remove the end of the short arm of chromosome 16 and extend for 1 to $2 \, Mb$. Occasionally they also include the genes that are involved in tuberous sclerosis and adult polycystic disease of the kidney. In other cases, the loss of the end of the short arm of chromosome 16 is the result of an inherited cytogenetic abnormality, including translocations and other rearrangements.

The ATR-X syndrome is characterized by a much more consistent series of dysmorphic features and more severe intellectual disability. These infants often suffer from convulsions after birth. They develop typical facial features, genital abnormalities, and a very mild form of haemoglobin H disease. This condition is inherited as a typical sex-linked disorder which affects males. It results from mutations of a gene on the X chromosome called *ATR-X* which is now known to act as a regulator of transcription via an effect on the structure of chromatin. Female carriers may show a very small proportion of red cells containing haemoglobin H bodies. Mutations of *ATR-X* are sometimes found in elderly patients who have a mild form of haemoglobin H disease associated with myelodysplasia. The relationship between the mutations and the disease of the bone marrow is still not clear.

Thalassaemia intermedia

Definition and pathogenesis

The term 'thalassaemia intermedia' is used to describe patients with the clinical picture of thalassaemia which, although not transfusion dependent, is associated with a much more severe degree of anaemia than that found in carriers for α or β thalassaemia. Many of the conditions which have been described previously in this section follow this clinical course, for example haemoglobin C or E thalassaemia, the various $\delta\beta$ thalassaemias and haemoglobin Lepore disorders, and the wide variety of conditions which can result from the interactions of the different β and $\delta\beta$ thalassaemia determinants. However, some children with this condition have parents with typical heterozygous β thalassaemia blood pictures and elevated haemoglobin A_2 levels. These patients appear to be homozygous for β thalassaemia, yet they run a much milder course than is usually the case with this condition. Some of them have inherited an α thalassaemia determinant as well as being homozygous for β thalassaemia. This reduces the overall degree of globin chain imbalance and consequently the severity of the dyserythropoiesis which usually accompanies homozygous β thalassaemia; hence these children run a milder clinical course. In other cases, particularly in Africans, relatively mild forms of homozygous β thalassaemia seem to reflect the action of less severe β thalassaemia mutations. Finally, some intermediate forms of β thalassaemia seem to result from the coinheritance of a gene for unusually effective haemoglobin F production.

Clinical and haematological changes

The clinical features of the intermediate forms of thalassaemia are extremely variable. At one end of the spectrum are patients who are virtually symptom free except for moderate anaemia. At the other end there are patients who have haemoglobin values in the 5 to 7 g/dl range and who develop marked splenomegaly, severe skeletal deformities due to expansion of bone marrow, and, as they get older, become heavily iron loaded because of increased intestinal absorption of iron. Recurrent leg ulceration, folate deficiency, symptoms due to extramedullary haemopoietic tumour masses in the chest and skull (Fig. 22.5.7.19), gallstones, and a marked proneness to infection are particularly characteristic of this group of thalassaemias.

Because of the heterogeneity of these disorders, it is only possible to determine the course that is likely to evolve in any individual patient by following the disorder very carefully from early childhood.

Differential diagnosis of the thalassaemias

There are few conditions that are likely to be confused with the more severe forms of homozygous β thalassaemia or haemoglobin H disease. The ethnic background of the patient, the presence of anaemia from early life, and the characteristic haematological changes make the diagnosis relatively easy. Once thalassaemia is suspected, the parents and near relatives should be examined for the carrier states for α or β thalassaemia. Both disorders can be

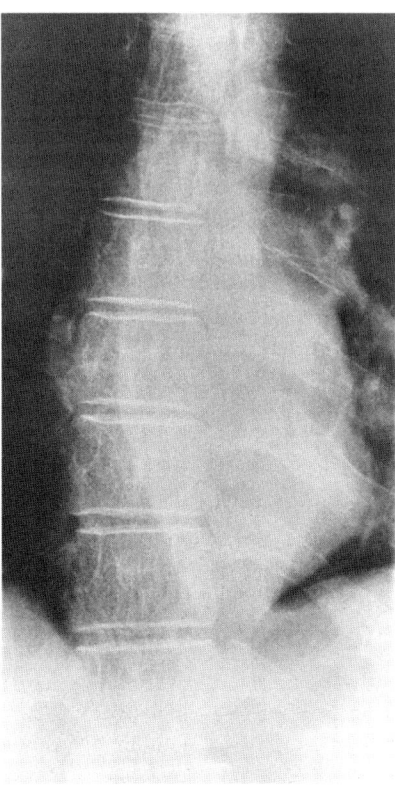

Fig. 22.5.7.19 An extramedullary haemopoietic mass in a patient with β thalassaemia intermedia.

distinguished from simple iron deficiency by the finding of a normal serum iron or ferritin level and by the associated changes in the haemoglobin pattern. It should be remembered, however, that in some groups iron deficiency and heterozygous thalassaemia frequently occur together in the same person, particularly during pregnancy. The sideroblastic anaemias can be easily distinguished from thalassaemia by the morphological appearances of the red cells and the presence of ring sideroblasts in the bone marrow. It should be remembered that there are some rare forms of acquired haemoglobin H disease in elderly patients with myelodysplasia.

Laboratory diagnosis of thalassaemia

The homozygous states for the severe forms of β thalassaemia are easily recognized by the haematological changes associated with very high levels of haemoglobin F; haemoglobin A_2 values vary so much that they are of no diagnostic help. The heterozygous states are recognized by microcytic hypochromic red cells and an elevated level of haemoglobin A_2. The δβ thalassaemias are characterized by the finding of 100% haemoglobin F in homozygotes and 5 to 15% haemoglobin F together with a normal level of haemoglobin A_2 in heterozygotes (see Table 22.5.7.1).

When β thalassaemia is diagnosed, a quantitative haemoglobin electrophoresis should be carried out to exclude the presence of an abnormal haemoglobin variant such as haemoglobin E or Lepore.

The haemoglobin Bart's hydrops syndrome is recognized by the finding of a hydropic infant with a severe anaemia, a thalassaemic blood picture, and 80% or more haemoglobin Bart's on haemoglobin electrophoresis. Haemoglobin H disease is identified by the finding of a typical thalassaemic blood picture with an elevated reticulocyte count, generation of multiple inclusion bodies in the red cells after incubation with brilliant cresyl blue, and the finding of variable amounts of haemoglobin H on haemoglobin electrophoresis. There are no really useful, simple diagnostic tests for the different α thalassaemic carrier states although α° thalassaemia heterozygotes usually have typical thalassaemic red-cell changes with a normal haemoglobin A_2 value. It is essential for counselling purposes to diagnose the different carrier states for α thalassaemia, blood samples should be referred to a laboratory that can carry out DNA analysis of the globin genes.

Prevention and treatment

Thalassaemia produces a severe public health problem and a serious drain on medical resources in many populations. Since there is no definitive treatment, most countries in which the disease is common are putting a major effort into programmes for its prevention.

Prevention

There are two major approaches to the prevention of the thalassaemias. Since the carrier states for the β thalassaemias can be easily recognized, it is at least theoretically possible to screen populations and provide genetic counselling about the choice of marriage partners. If β thalassaemia heterozygotes marry other carriers, one in four of their children will have the severe, transfusion-dependent homozygous disorder. Large-scale programmes of this type have been set up in Italy, but the results are not yet available, and in smaller pilot studies in Greece the outcome has not been encouraging. Until more is known about the usefulness of this form of prospective genetic counselling, most countries are developing screening programmes at antenatal clinics. When heterozygous carrier mothers are found, the husbands are tested and if they are also carriers the couple are offered the possibility of prenatal diagnosis and termination of pregnancies carrying fetuses with severe forms of thalassaemia.

Prenatal diagnosis

Prenatal diagnosis can be offered to couples at risk for having children with severe forms of β thalassaemia. Because of the serious obstetric complications and the trauma of carrying a hydropic fetus to term there is also a good case for prenatal diagnosis for the haemoglobin Bart's hydrops syndrome. Termination of pregnancies at risk for milder forms of thalassaemia is also undertaken, but should only be considered after very careful counselling of the parents. Some children with intermediate forms of thalassaemia are symptom free and develop normally; others have more severe anaemia and bone deformity. There has been some success in determining which particular molecular defects and interactions are associated with these different clinical courses. When in doubt, parents should be referred for expert analysis of their variety of thalassaemia and appropriate counselling.

Prenatal diagnosis of thalassaemia can be carried out in several ways. The diagnosis can be made by globin chain synthesis studies of fetal blood samples obtained by fetoscopy at 18 to 20 weeks gestation. The diagnosis can also be made by fetal DNA analysis on amniotic fluid cells obtained by amniocentesis earlier in the second trimester. Currently, it is usual to carry out prenatal diagnosis of thalassaemia and sickle cell anaemia by direct analysis of fetal DNA obtained by chorion biopsy at about the 12th week of gestation. This approach has largely replaced fetal blood sampling or amniocentesis for the prenatal diagnosis of the thalassaemias. First-trimester diagnosis is much more acceptable to many women, because it reduces the long period of uncertainty during which the fetus is growing and the mother and her relatives and friends are coming to accept that she is to have a child, and because late second-trimester terminations are often difficult. Prenatal diagnosis of thalassaemia is now carried out in many countries, and has significantly reduced the number of new cases of thalassaemia in the community.

Because prenatal diagnosis of thalassaemia is now well established it is very important to discuss the genetic implications of the condition when carriers are detected by chance, regardless of the individual's ethnic background. They should also be given a letter explaining, in simple terms, the pattern of inheritance and the dangers for their children. This approach should always be followed, even for sporadic cases in low-incidence regions, such as northern Europe. Because of the increasing movements of populations they might still marry another carrier and have severely affected children.

Symptomatic treatment

The symptomatic management of severe β thalassaemia requires regular blood transfusion, the judicious use of splenectomy if hypersplenism develops, and the administration of chelating agents to reduce iron overload. When the diagnosis of severe β thalassaemia is suspected during the first year of life, the infant should be followed for several weeks to make sure that the haemoglobin has fallen to a level at which regular transfusion will be necessary. It is difficult to be dogmatic about exactly when transfusions should be started. A severely anaemic infant who is feeding poorly, inactive, or otherwise failing to thrive, will almost certainly need to be transfused. The object is to maintain the pretransfusion haemoglobin level at about 9.5 g/dl. This usually requires transfusion of 10 to 15 mg/kg red cells every 4 weeks. Washed red cells should be used. Whole blood should be avoided because of the danger of sensitization to serum or white cell components. The rate of transfusion should not exceed 4 to 5 ml/kg per h. In patients who are profoundly anaemic or show evidence of cardiac insufficiency, the rate should be no more than 2 ml/kg per h. It is important to calculate the annual blood consumption by dividing the total volume of blood transfused over 12 months by the patients weight in the middle of the year. If it is higher than 200 ml/kg body weight, splenectomy should be considered. All blood should be screened for hepatitis B and C, and for HIV.

Hypersplenism is becoming much less common if children are maintained on an adequate transfusion regimen. Increasingly blood requirements, or evidence of hypersplenism, pancytopenia for example, should prompt one to consider splenectomy. It should be avoided before the age of 6 years because of the particularly high incidence of infection in asplenic children. Two to three weeks before splenectomy the child should be given: (1) pneumococcal vaccine; (2) *Haemophilus influenzae* type B vaccine; (3) meningococcal A and C vaccine. After the operation the children should be maintained on oral penicillin V, 125 mg twice daily, increasing to 250 mg twice daily for older children. For those who are allergic to penicillin, erythromycin should be given.

The only effective chelating agent for the prevention or treatment of iron overload in thalassaemia is desferrioxamine (deferoxamine). It is now clear that this drug should not be given too soon because toxic effects are observed at low body iron loads. Ideally, the hepatic iron concentration should be measured at about 1 year after regular transfusion has started. Chelation should be initiated in patients with hepatic iron concentrations of above 7 mg/g liver dry weight. Where this investigation is not possible, the drug should be given when the serum ferritin value has reached or exceeded 1000 µg/litre, although it is becoming increasingly clear that the serum ferritin level is a very imprecise estimate of body iron load. The initial dose should not exceed 25 to 35 mg/kg body weight per 24 h. Iron excretion is potentiated if children receive 100 mg vitamin C by mouth on the days of the infusion. Ideally, progress should be monitored by regular estimates of the hepatic iron concentration by MRI or liver biopsy but if this is not possible the serum ferritin level should be maintained below 1500 µg/litre. In patients who become iron loaded, it is possible to increase the rate of iron excretion considerably but the daily dose of desferrioxamine should normally not exceed 50 mg/kg body weight. Patients should be monitored continuously for side effects of desferrioxamine; these include retinal damage, ototoxicity, and interference with growth.

There is now extensive evidence that patients who have been maintained at a safe body iron level with desferrioxamine can grow and develop normally and live well into adult life. The major problem is difficulties with compliance and the expense of the drug in the developing countries. An effective oral chelating agent would be a major advance. The most widely studied, deferiprone does not appear to be as effective in maintaining body iron in a proportion of patients as desferrioxamine and is also associated with agranulocytosis, arthritis, and a reversible neurological syndrome. Reports that it may be more effective in removing cardiac iron require prospective controlled studies. Preliminary studies with a new oral chelator, deferasirox, have shown promising results but a great deal more experience of this agent will be required before it could replace the use of desferrioxamine.

It is very important to monitor transfusion-dependent patients for hepatitis B and C and HIV infection. The management of these conditions is considered elsewhere in this book. Other complications relating to iron load, including hypoparathyroidism, diabetes, and delayed puberty and hypogonadism, require expert endocrinological assessment with appropriate replacement therapy.

Increasing experience with bone marrow transplantation indicates that, if done early with adequate HLA matching, the results are extremely good. Patients who have become iron loaded and who have liver damage have a less good prognosis but, as more experience has been gained, there appears to be a place for transplantation in older patients.

The intermediate forms of thalassaemia should be treated by careful observation, folic acid supplementation, and, in the face of a falling haemoglobin and increasing spleen size, the judicious use of splenectomy. It is important to monitor the iron status regularly because some of these patients become iron loaded due to increased intestinal absorption later in life and chelation therapy may be necessary.

Currently, a number of experimental approaches to the treatment of the thalassaemias are being pursued, including the stimulation of fetal haemoglobin production or somatic gene therapy.

Structural haemoglobin variants

Over 400 structural haemoglobin variants have been described, most of which result from single amino acid substitutions. Many of them are harmless and have been discovered during surveys of the electrophoretic patterns of human haemoglobin. Of course, this approach underestimates the number of variants because it only identifies those in which the amino acid substitution alters the charge of the haemoglobin molecule.

Single amino acid substitutions cause clinical disorders only if they alter the stability or functional properties of the haemoglobin molecule. A classification of these diseases is shown in Table 22.5.7.3. They include the sickling disorders, chronic or drug-induced haemolytic anaemia associated with unstable

haemoglobins, and polycythaemia or congenital cyanosis, associated with high and low oxygen affinity haemoglobin variants, respectively. There is a rare group of haemoglobin variants that produce methaemoglobinaemia.

Nomenclature

Originally, the structural haemoglobin variants were named by letters of the alphabet. By the late 1950s there were none left; it was decided to designate new haemoglobin variants by the place of origin of the first patient in whom they were characterized. It is customary to call the heterozygous carrier state the 'trait' and the homozygous condition the 'disease'. For example, haemoglobin S heterozygotes (genotype AS) are said to have the sickle cell trait, while those homozygous for the sickle cell mutation (genotype SS) are said to have sickle cell disease. In practice it is very important to distinguish between the carrier state and the homozygous or compound heterozygous state for a haemoglobin variant; carriers are usually asymptomatic.

The sickling disorders

Sickling disorders (Table 22.5.7.4) consist of the heterozygous state for haemoglobin S, sickle cell trait (AS), the homozygous state or sickle cell disease (SS), and the compound heterozygous state for haemoglobin S together with haemoglobins C, D, E, or other structural variants. Several disorders result from the inheritance of the sickle cell gene together with different forms of thalassaemia (see earlier section).

Pathogenesis

Haemoglobin S differs from haemoglobin A by the substitution of valine for glutamic acid at position 6 in the β chain. Although this has been known for nearly half a century, it is still not absolutely clear how it gives rise to the sickling phenomenon. The latter appears to be due to the unusual solubility characteristics of haemoglobin S which undergoes liquid crystal (tactoid) formation as it becomes deoxygenated. In this state, aggregates of sickled haemoglobin molecules arrange themselves in parallel, rod-like fibres, made up of a complex solid core about 21 nm in diameter, composed of 14 filaments arranged as 7 pairs of double filaments. Much is now known about the complex interactions whereby the $\beta6$ valine substitution stabilizes the molecular stacks in the deoxy configuration of haemoglobin. There is considerable variation in the extent to which different haemoglobins are able to participate with

Table 22.5.7.3 Clinical disorders due to structural haemoglobin variants

Disorder	Variants
Haemolysis and tissue damage	Haemoglobin S
Drug-induced haemolysis	Haemoglobin Zürich and other unstable haemoglobins
Chronic haemolysis	Unstable haemoglobin variants
	Haemoglobin C
Congenital polycythaemia	High-affinity variants
Congenital cyanosis	Haemoglobin(s) M
	Low-affinity variants
Hypochromia: thalassaemic phenotype	Haemoglobin E
	Haemoglobin Constant Spring

Table 22.5.7.4 The major sickling disorders

Disorder	Genotype	
	(normal = $\alpha\alpha/\alpha\alpha.\beta/\beta$)	
SS disease	$\alpha\alpha/\alpha\alpha$	β^S/β^S
SC disease	$\alpha\alpha/\alpha\alpha$	β^S/β^C
SD disease	$\alpha\alpha/\alpha\alpha$	β^S/β^D
S–β thalassaemia	$\alpha\alpha/\alpha\alpha$	$\beta^S\beta^0$ or β^S/β^+
S–hereditary persistence of fetal Hb	$\alpha\alpha/\alpha\alpha$	$\beta^S/-^a$
S–α thalassaemia	$\alpha-/\alpha\alpha$ or $\alpha-/\alpha-$	β^S/β^S

SS, sickle cell anaemia. See text for details of other conditions.
[a] Indicates β gene deletion.

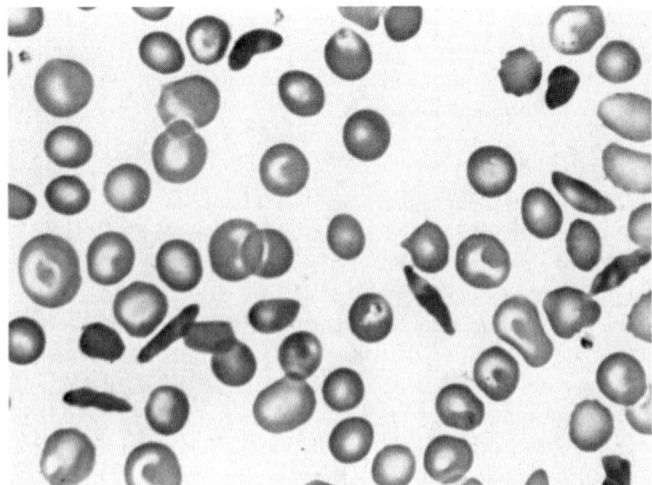

Fig. 22.5.7.20 Irreversibly sickled cells in the peripheral blood (×1000, Leishman stain).

haemoglobin S in the sickling process. This accounts for some of the clinical variability of the different sickling conditions. For example, haemoglobin F is almost completely excluded from the sickling process; increasing concentrations in the red cell reduce the rate of sickling.

The pathophysiology of sickling is an extremely dynamic process. Red cells containing sickle haemoglobin at a high concentration endure a series of cycles of sickling and desickling with progressive membrane damage and loss of plasticity. Finally these dry, rigid cells become irreversibly sickled (Fig. 22.5.7.20). Sickling of this type has two main effects. First, sickled erythrocytes have a shortened survival, leading to a chronic haemolytic anaemia. Second, and more importantly, these abnormal red cells tend to adhere to the various receptors on the walls of small blood vessels with the production of aggregates, blockage of the vessels, vascular stasis, and, ultimately, tissue damage. Changes in nitric oxide-induced vascular relaxation may also contribute to these complex interactions.

Distribution

The sickling disorders occur very frequently in African populations and, sporadically, throughout the Mediterranean region and the Middle East. There are extensive pockets in India but the disease has not been seen in South-East Asia. The high frequency of the sickle cell gene occurs because carriers are more resistant than normal individuals to *Plasmodium falciparum* malaria.

Clinical features

Except in conditions of extreme hypoxia, such as flying in an unpressurized aircraft, the sickle cell trait causes no clinical disability. However, it is possible for individuals to suffer vaso-occlusive episodes if they become oxygen deprived under anaesthesia. Therefore all individuals of the appropriate racial background should have a sickling test (see below) before receiving an anaesthetic. If the test is positive, the anaesthetic should be given with adequate oxygenation and special care should be taken to avoid postoperative dehydration.

Sickle cell anaemia runs an extremely variable clinical course. At one end of the spectrum it is characterized by a crippling haemolytic anaemia interspersed with severe exacerbations, or crises. On the other hand, it may be extremely mild and only found by chance on routine haematological examination. The reason for these remarkable differences in phenotypic expression, which are only partly understood, include the level of haemoglobin F, coinheritance of α thalassaemia, climate, and, probably most important, socioeconomic factors such as availability of early treatment of infection.

Typically, sickle cell anaemia presents in infancy with symptoms related to anaemia or infection. A common presenting symptom is the hand and foot syndrome. It occurs early in infancy and is characterized by a painful dactylitis with swelling of the fingers or feet. Epiphyseal damage during one of these episodes may lead to chronic shortening of a digit. Infants are anaemic from about the third month of life. During early development they often have significant splenomegaly that gradually resolves due to repeated infarction. Indeed, it is most unusual to feel the spleen after the end of the first decade. Typically, the haemoglobin levels are in the 6 to 8 g/dl range with a reticulocyte count of 10 to 20%. There is chronic, mild icterus with an elevated bilirubin level. Examination of the peripheral blood film shows anisochromia and poikilocytosis with a variable number of sickled erythrocytes (Fig. 22.5.7.20). As the children grow older the haematological changes of hyposplenism develop with the appearance of pits on the surface of the red cells, Howell–Jolly bodies, and distorted red cells. The white cell and platelet counts are usually normal or slightly elevated.

Growth and development are usually otherwise normal although there may be some skeletal deformities, including frontal bossing of the skull due to expansion of the bone marrow. In some series, children have tended to be short for their age, while postadolescents were usually tall. Inequalities between upper and lower segments, stressed in the early literature, are unusual. The only other physical finding is chronic leg ulceration; this is discussed below.

Complications

The chronic haemolysis of sickle cell disease is interspersed with acute exacerbations of the illness called sickling crises. Furthermore, there are a series of serious and life-threatening long-term complications which develop in many patients with sickle cell anaemia.

Box 22.5.7.3 Acute exacerbations ('crises') in sickle cell disease

◆ Thrombotic
- Generalized or localized bone pain
- Abdominal
- Pulmonary
- Neurological
◆ Aplastic
◆ Haemolytic
◆ Sequestration
- Spleen
- Liver
- ?Lung
◆ Various combinations of above

The different forms of sickle cell crises are summarized in Table 22.5.7.7. The commonest is the painful crisis. This is sometimes precipitated by infection, dehydration, or exposure to cold, although quite often no underlying cause can be found. The episode starts with vague pain, often in the back or bones of the limbs. The pain gradually worsens and its bizarre distribution may cause a major diagnostic puzzle. The pain is almost certainly due to blockage of small vessels with sickled erythrocytes; aspiration over areas of bone tenderness has shown infarction of marrow tissue. Occasionally, abdominal pain is the major symptom and this may be associated with distension and rigidity, a picture very similar to an acute abdominal emergency. The diagnostic difficulties in distinguishing between an abdominal crisis and a surgical abdomen are compounded by the fact that the bowel sounds are often diminished during abdominal crises. Two other serious forms of thrombotic crisis are known as the 'chest' and 'brain' syndromes. The 'chest' syndrome, characterized by acute dyspnoea and pleuritic pain together with infiltrates on the chest radiograph, is due to sequestration of sickle cells in the pulmonary circulation. It is sometimes accompanied by a fall in the PCV and platelet count which also may reflect sequestration of sickled cells in the pulmonary vessels. Neurological complications may present in a variety of ways. Stroke is particularly common and appears to follow damage to the intima of the vessels that comprise the circle of Willis; infarctive strokes probably arise in this region while haemorrhagic strokes are thought to be caused by rupture of aneurysms formed in these vessels. MRI studies show a high frequency of silent infarcts, even within the first few years of life. Priapism, often recurrent, is also a common and distressing acute complication.

During painful crises there may be a marked increase in the rate of haemolysis with a fall in the haemoglobin level. Such haemolytic episodes are uncommon. Much more serious are periods of transient bone marrow aplasia called aplastic crises. These seem to result from intercurrent infection, particularly due to parvovirus, and frequently affect more than one sibling in the same family.

Finally, and most serious, are the sequestration crises. Occurring mainly in babies and young children, they are characterized by a rapid enlargement of the spleen or liver, which become engorged with sickled erythrocytes. As the crisis progresses a large proportion of the total red-cell mass may be trapped in the spleen or liver. Death may occur due to profound anaemia. These episodes show a tendency to recur in the same individual. Hepatic sequestration, which may occur in adults, is easily overlooked if the liver size is not monitored carefully.

The commonest cause of death in sickle cell anaemia appears to be a sequestration crisis or acute infection, or both. It is not absolutely clear why patients with this disorder are so prone to infection, although reduced splenic function may play a role. Abnormalities of the alternate pathway of complement activation have also been described. A variety of organisms are involved, particularly the pneumococcus, and, mainly in tropical countries, typhoid infection of bone infarcts leads to typhoid osteomyelitis. The long held belief that children in Africa with sickle cell anaemia are particularly likely to die from *P. falciparum* infection has recently been disproved.

Pregnancy may be uneventful, or associated with an increased incidence of painful crises. There is slightly increased incidence of maternal mortality and a definite increase in the rate of fetal loss.

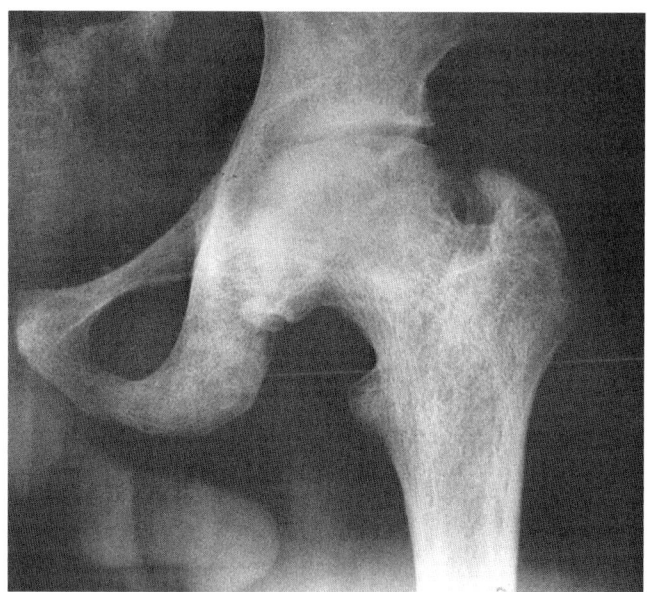

Fig. 22.5.7.21 Aseptic necrosis of the left femoral head in sickle-cell thalassaemia. (Courtesy of Dr Graham Serjeant.)

Chronic complications

Many of the chronic complications of sickle cell anaemia result largely from infarcts following repeated episodes of vascular occlusion. Almost any organ can be involved. Those at particular risk are areas which rely largely on small vessels for their blood supply. The bones are particularly prone to infarction. Aseptic necrosis of the humeral or femoral heads may lead to gross deformity of the shoulder and hip joints (Fig. 22.5.7.21). Bone infarcts may result in chronic sequestra formation which may become secondarily infected with the production of osteomyelitis. Recent studies have demonstrated a high frequency of 'silent' infarcts of the brain and these together with strokes, are associated with a variable degree of long-term intellectual impairment.

Another organ at particular risk is the kidney. During early childhood renal function may be impaired but this can be corrected by blood transfusion, suggesting that it is due to reversible changes in the renal vasculature. These alterations in renal function are not reversible in later life. Chronic renal failure due to damage of the renal vessels is one of the commonest causes of death in adults with sickle cell anaemia. A typical nephrotic syndrome may develop at some stage during the illness. Pulmonary infarction occurs quite frequently, but repeated episodes leading to severe pulmonary hypertension and right heart failure are unusual, although this complication has been well documented.

There is usually some degree of cardiomegaly. A variety of flow murmurs may be heard but most of these signs seem to be the result of chronic anaemia. Myocardial infarction or fibrosis is not a feature of the disease. Recurrent attacks of painful priapism may lead to permanent deformity of the penis. Ocular manifestations are also relatively common in sickle cell anaemia although they tend to be more serious in haemoglobin SC disease; they will be considered with the later disorder in a later section. Other important chronic complications include defective growth and maturation and a greatly increased susceptibility to gallstone formation and gallbladder disease.

Course and prognosis

There are still large gaps in our knowledge about the natural history of sickle cell anaemia. Prognosis seems to depend on the racial background of the patient, socioeconomic and ill-defined genetic factors, and, especially, the availability of good paediatric care in the early years.

In rural East Africa, the disease still has a high mortality in the first year or two of life. In Jamaica there appears to be a 10% mortality in the early years although survival into adult life and old age is common. This is also the case in some urban parts of Africa and in the United States of America and Europe. Data from the United States Cooperative Study of Sickle Cell Disease suggest that the median age at death for males is 42 years and for females 48 years. In Saudi Arabia and India, a particularly mild form of the condition occurs. Mortality is extremely low in childhood and a normal survival seems to be common. It is becoming increasingly apparent that the commonest cause of death in the first year or two of life is infection, often associated with splenic sequestration. Later in life infection is still a frequent cause of death, although studies in Jamaica indicate that chronic, progressive renal failure may be responsible for a significant number of deaths. The introduction of prophylactic penicillin has made a major inroad into early deaths from infection (see below).

Laboratory diagnosis

Sickle cell trait causes no haematological changes and is diagnosed by the finding of a positive sickling test together with haemoglobins A and S on electrophoresis (Fig. 22.5.7.22). Sickle cell anaemia is diagnosed by the finding of a variable degree of anaemia, an elevated reticulocyte count, sickled erythrocytes on the peripheral blood film, a positive sickling test, and a haemoglobin electrophoresis pattern characterized by the absence of haemoglobin A

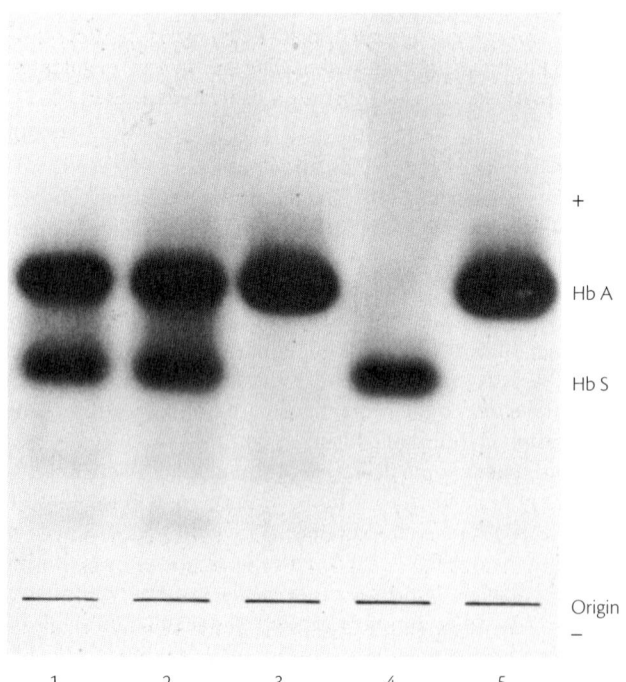

Fig. 22.5.7.22 The haemoglobin pattern in the sickling disorders (starch gel electrophoresis, protein stain, pH 8.5). The following are shown (left to right): (1 and 2) the sickle cell trait; (3) normal; (4) sickle cell anaemia; (5) normal.

and a preponderance of haemoglobin S with a variable amount of haemoglobin F (Fig. 22.5.7.22). The diagnosis is confirmed by finding sickle cell trait in both parents.

A variety of simple sickling tests is available. For ward laboratories the simplest it to take a drop of blood, mix it with two volumes of freshly prepared 2% sodium metabisulphite, place a coverslip over the mixture, seal the edges with vaseline, and examine the slide for sickling after 1 h.

Control and management

There is very little experience of prospective genetic counselling and education of communities as an approach to reducing the number of patients with sickle cell disease. Although prenatal diagnosis of sickle cell disease can be carried out by DNA analysis following chorionic villus sampling, it has not been taken up as extensively as it has for the thalassaemias. We need to know a great deal more about the factors which modify the clinical prognosis before the place of prenatal diagnosis is clarified.

It is very important that the babies of 'at risk' pregnancies are screened at birth and that the diagnosis is made as early as possible. This is because early deaths due to infection and the frequency of crises may be reduced by the administration of oral penicillin. This should be given to all affected babies at a dosage of 62.5 mg three times a day, up to 1 year of age, 125 mg twice a day from the age of 1 to 3 years, and 250 mg twice a day thereafter. It is also now standard practice for these babies to receive pneumococcal vaccine; in many centres they also receive vaccines against meningococcus and *H. influenzae*.

Patients with sickle cell anaemia adapt well to their low haemoglobin levels and regular blood transfusion is not required. Particularly in populations in which the diet is low in folate, regular folate supplements should be given. Patients should be given access to a centre that has expertise in the management of this disorder and advised to present at the first sign of a painful crisis. They should also be given a card to carry which states their haemoglobin genotype.

All but the mildest painful crisis should be managed in hospital. Patients should be examined in detail at regular intervals for evidence of underlying infection and given adequate rehydration, oxygen, antibiotics where appropriate, and, in particular, analgesia. The haemoglobin level and reticulocyte count should be estimated at frequent intervals to anticipate an aplastic crisis or pulmonary sequestration episode. Although a mild crisis may be managed with first-line analgesics, stronger pain relief is often necessary. There has been concern about the possible dangers of the use of pethedine; it has become fashionable to administer diamorphine by slow, titratrated intravenous infusion. This has to be done under constant surveillance with regular monitoring of respiration and blood gases. It is very unusual for a painful crisis to last more than a few days.

Pulmonary sequestration requires urgent treatment in an intensive care unit. Oxygen should be administered and the blood gases monitored. An exchange transfusion should be initiated unless the haemoglobin level is lower than 4 to 5 g/dl, when the same result can be achieved by rapid transfusion up to 10 to 12 g/dl. Similarly, cerebral complications should be treated by exchange or top-up transfusion. There is evidence that this complication may be prevented by regular Doppler analysis of cerebral blood flow followed, where appropriate, by regular transfusion. Transfusion therapy also prevents recurrence of the cerebral episodes. Hypertransfusion or exchange transfusion should also be used to cover major surgical emergencies or for patients who are having recurrent crises. Occasionally, and most often in young children, the spleen may enlarge to such a degree that secondary hypersplenism develops and splenectomy is required. Splenic sequestration crises require urgent transfusion. Because they tend to recur, they may require splenectomy.

No special management is required during pregnancy. Occasionally, if the haemoglobin level falls to a value at which symptoms of anaemia occur, or if there are recurrent crises, a regular transfusion regimen should be started to cover pregnancy and delivery.

Ocular manifestations, particularly proliferative retinopathy, require expert ophthalmological treatment. The current place for prophylactic zenon arc or argon laser therapy remains uncertain. Chronic disability due to aseptic necrosis of the femoral head may require hip replacement, although results are often disappointing and this complication requires a great deal more study. Surgical procedures should be undertaken with great caution. It is vital to maintain adequate oxygenation and hydration; limb tourniquets should be avoided. Major procedures are best carried out after exchange transfusion. Haematuria usually resolves without treatment. Terminal renal failure should be managed as for any other form of renal insufficiency; renal transplantation has been shown to be successful in several studies.

Recurrent priapism is a particular problem. Nearly two-thirds of major episodes are preceded by stuttering attacks and therefore it has been suggested that effective therapy at this stage may reduce the risk of sustaining a major attack, with danger of permanent deformity of the penis. Several forms of management have been suggested although none have been studied in sufficient detail. One approach has been to commence stilboestrol, 5 mg daily, during the stuttering phase. Other forms of treatment at this stage that have been reported to give benefit are the use of opioid analgesics with benzodiazepine or pseudoephedrine hydrochloride. As well as these approaches, the patient should be hydrated, given analgesia, and, possibly, exchange transfusion. Centres with experience of this complication suggest that conservative treatment should be restricted to 24 h at the most. If there is no improvement, surgical correction is recommended, with a cavernosus–spongiosum shunt, a relatively minor procedure that may produce a good cosmetic result.

The management of leg ulcers is unsatisfactory. They may heal with bed rest and debridement but often relapse. Skin grafting does not always give good results and controlled trials have shown that transfusion does not appear to increase the rate of healing.

Experimental forms of treatment have shown some promise. Bone marrow transplantation has been carried out with reasonably good results. However, because of the inherent risks, and the uncertainty of the prognosis, the precise indications are not yet clear. Other studies have been directed at trying to elevate fetal haemoglobin. In a placebo-controlled trial involving adult patients it was found that the administration of hydroxyurea caused a significant reduction in the number of painful crises. This may have resulted from the modest elevation in fetal haemoglobin in response to the drug but other factors such as the reduced white count and increased red-cell volume may have played a role. Currently, this drug is licensed by the United States Food and Drug Administration for treatment of adult patients. It has also been used effectively in children, but because of its possible leukaemogenic effects its use earlier in life is still restricted to clinical trials.

Other sickling disorders

The other sickling disorders include the interaction of haemoglobin S with haemoglobins C, D, and some of the rarer haemoglobin variants. The interactions with the different forms of β thalassaemia were described above. In many of these conditions, the clinical manifestations are little different from the sickle cell trait, but haemoglobin SC disease and SD disease more closely resemble sickle cell anaemia.

Haemoglobin SC disease

This disease is found in West Africa and less frequently in North Africa. Characterized by a milder anaemia than sickle cell disease, it often goes unrecognized until adult life. It may present with a complication resulting from damage to the microvasculature, probably because of the relatively high haemoglobin level and the combined effects of sickling and red-cell rigidity caused by haemoglobin C (see below). Aseptic necrosis of the femoral or humeral heads and unexplained haematuria are the most common complications. Widespread thrombotic episodes, particularly involving the lungs, may occur during intercurrent infection or in pregnancy or the puerperium. Repeated blockage of the retinal vessels may lead to retinitis proliferans, retinal detachment, and permanent blindness.

Haemoglobin SC disease is diagnosed by finding a mild anaemia with splenomegaly and characteristic morphological changes of the red cells, including many target forms, intracellular crystals, and sickle cells. The sickling test is positive and haemoglobin electrophoresis shows haemoglobins S and C in about equal proportions. One parent shows the sickle cell trait and the other the haemoglobin C trait.

Severe thrombotic episodes, particularly in pregnancy, should be treated by exchange transfusion. The role of anticoagulants has never been established. Retinal disease is treated by laser.

Haemolysis due to other common haemoglobin variants

After haemoglobin S the second commonest variant in West Africa is haemoglobin C. Because of its relatively low solubility haemoglobin C appears to exist in a precrystalline state in red cells, causing their rigidity and premature destruction in the microcirculation. The homozygous state, haemoglobin C disease, is characterized by a mild haemolytic anaemia with splenomegaly, and 100% target cells on the blood film. Haemoglobin analysis shows haemoglobin C with small amounts of haemoglobin F. This is a mild disorder and no specific treatment is required.

The commonest haemoglobin variant throughout South-East Asia and the Indian subcontinent is haemoglobin E. The homozygous state for this variant, haemoglobin E disease, is characterized by a very mild degree of anaemia with a slight reticulocytosis. The blood film shows mild morphological changes of the red cells which are hypochromic and microcytic, resembling the changes seen in β thalassaemia. No treatment is required.

Haemoglobin variants which migrate in the position of haemoglobin S but which do not sickle have been given the general title of haemoglobin D. There are several different molecular varieties of this variant; the commonest is haemoglobin D Los Angeles. The homozygous state is associated with moderate anaemia, splenomegaly, and a mild degree of haemolysis. The compound heterozygous state with haemoglobin S produces a disorder very similar to sickle cell anaemia. It is diagnosed by finding one parent with the haemoglobin D trait and the other with the sickle cell trait.

The unstable haemoglobin disorders

The unstable haemoglobin disorders are a rare group of inherited haemolytic anaemias which result from structural changes in the haemoglobin molecule that cause intracellular precipitation with the formation of Heinz bodies. Their true incidence is not known. There have been several well-documented families in which patients with one of these haemoglobin variants have had no affected relatives, suggesting that the condition has arisen by a new mutation.

Aetiology and pathogenesis

Most of the unstable haemoglobin variants result from single amino acid substitutions at critical areas of the molecule. For example, substitutions in or around the haem pocket can disrupt the normal anatomy and allow in water, with subsequent oxidative damage to haem which leads to precipitation of the haemoglobin. Some substitutions, such as those involving proline residues, cause a marked disruption of the secondary structure of a globin chain. A few of these variants result from deletions of either single or several amino acid residues. For example, in haemoglobin Gun Hill five amino acids are missing including the haem binding site. As the unstable haemoglobins precipitate in the red cells or their precursors, they produce intracellular inclusions, or Heinz bodies, which make the cells more rigid causing their premature destruction in the microcirculation (Fig. 22.5.7.23). The degradation products of the precipitated haemoglobin, notably haem and iron, cause oxidative damage to the red-cell membrane proteins in much the same way as the excess α and β chains produced in the thalassaemias.

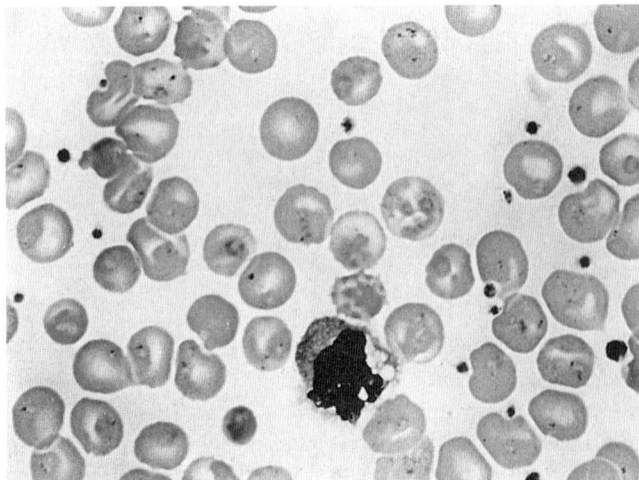

Fig. 22.5.7.23 The peripheral blood film of a patient with an unstable haemoglobin disorder, haemoglobin Hammersmith. This is a postsplenectomy film, which shows small inclusions in many of the red cells (×1000, Leishman stain).

Clinical features

All these conditions are characterized by a haemolytic anaemia of varying severity and splenomegaly. There may be a history of the passage of dark urine, particularly during episodes of infection. As in all chronic haemolytic anaemias, there is an increased incidence of pigment gallstones. The condition may become worse during periods of intercurrent infection. In the more severe forms, such episodes are associated with life-threatening anaemia. Patients with unstable haemoglobins are at particular risk of haemolytic episodes following the administration of oxidant drugs. Apart from intermittent icterus and splenomegaly there are no characteristic physical findings.

Laboratory diagnosis

This condition should be thought of in any familial haemolytic anaemia, particularly if a red-cell enzyme deficiency cannot be demonstrated. The peripheral blood film shows the features of haemolysis but the red-cell morphology may be relatively normal. Occasionally there is a mild degree of hypochromia and microcytosis. Unless splenectomy has been carried out, Heinz bodies are not seen in the peripheral blood (Fig. 22.5.7.23).

The most characteristic feature of the unstable haemoglobins is their heat instability. If a dilute haemoglobin solution is heated at 50 °C for 15 min, most of the unstable haemoglobins precipitate as a dense cloud. A similar phenomenon can be induced by isopropanol. Some variants can be identified by haemoglobin electrophoresis but others, because they result from the substitution of a neutral amino acid, produce no electrophoretic changes, and can only be demonstrated by the heat precipitation test.

Treatment

Because these conditions are so rare, there has been very little experience of the effects of splenectomy. From the information that is available, and from the author's personal experience, it appears that if a child has had several life-threatening episodes of anaemia or is running a steady-state haemoglobin level which is impairing development or well-being, splenectomy should be undertaken. It is interesting to note that some of these haemoglobin variants produce a 'right shift' in the oxygen dissociation curve, and a measurement of the P_{50} as part of the presplenectomy assessment may help to decide whether to proceed to surgery; a marked right shift, i.e. an increased P_{50}, indicates that the anaemia should be more easily tolerated than if the oxygen dissociation curve is moved in the opposite direction with a low P_{50}. An accurate history from the child or its parents is probably more helpful, however.

Haemoglobin variants which cause abnormal oxygen binding

In 1966, an 81-year-old man presented at Johns Hopkins Hospital, Baltimore with mild angina and a haemoglobin value of 19.9 g/dl. No cause could be found for his polycythaemia but it was noted that he had an abnormal haemoglobin (Chesapeake). The oxygen dissociation curve of his blood was found to be displaced to the left. This suggested that the abnormal haemoglobin might have a high oxygen affinity and that the patient's increased red-cell count might be compensating for a primary defect in oxygen unloading. Further studies showed that this was the case, documenting a new cause for secondary polycythaemia. Since then over

40 haemoglobin variants of this type have been defined, all associated with familial polycythaemia.

Aetiology

The high-oxygen-affinity haemoglobin variants result from single amino acid substitutions at critical parts of the haemoglobin molecule which are involved in the configuration changes that underlie haem–haem interaction and the production of a sigmoid oxygen dissociation curve. Many occur at the junctions between the α and β subunits. Others involve the amino acids which are involved with the binding of 2,3-biphosphoglycerate (2,3-BPG) to haemoglobin. As mentioned earlier, increasing concentrations of 2,3-BPG tend to push the oxygen dissociation curve to the right; fetal haemoglobin has a high oxygen affinity (left-shifted curve) because it cannot interact with 2,3-DPG; mutations of the DPG binding sites have a similar effect.

Pathophysiology

The high-oxygen-affinity variants have a left-shifted oxygen dissociation curve with a reduced P_{50}. Thus the variant haemoglobin holds on to oxygen more avidly than normal haemoglobin. This leads to tissue hypoxia. This in turn causes an increased output of erythropoietin and an elevated red-cell mass.

Clinical features

Many patients with high-oxygen-affinity variants are completely healthy and are only found to carry the variant when a routine haematological examination shows an unusually high haemoglobin level or packed cell volume. There have been one or two reports of arterial or venous occlusive disease in these patients. However, this is uncommon. Most patients are asymptomatic. There is no splenomegaly and no other associated haematological findings. Although it might be expected that a high-oxygen-affinity haemoglobin would cause defective oxygenation of the fetus, none of the reported families has had a history of frequent stillbirths.

Diagnosis

The condition should be suspected in any patient with a pure red-cell polycythaemia associated with a left-shifted oxygen dissociation curve. The diagnosis can be confirmed by haemoglobin analysis.

Treatment

In asymptomatic patients with high-oxygen-affinity haemoglobin variants no treatment is necessary. The difficulty arises if the patient has associated vascular disease with symptoms of coronary or cerebral artery insufficiency. There is insufficient published information to make any dogmatic statements about how this complication should be managed. The author has seen several patients of this type who seem to have responded to venesection, but more experience is required before this form of treatment can be recommended. These patients require a high haemoglobin level for oxygen transport; half their haemoglobin is physiologically useless.

Low-oxygen-affinity variants

At least six haemoglobin variants with reduced oxygen affinity have been reported. The first to be described, haemoglobin Kansas, was found in a mother and son with unexplained cyanosis. The subjects were asymptomatic and had normal haemoglobin levels without any evidence of haemolysis. Like many of the high-affinity variants, the amino acid substitution in this variant was at the interface between the α and β globin chains. For reasons which are not clear, some substitutions in this region give rise to variants with a relatively low oxygen affinity. This condition should be thought of in any patient with an unexplained congenital cyanosis; the differential diagnosis is considered below.

Methaemoglobinaemia, carboxyhaemoglobinaemia, and sulphaemoglobinaemia

Methaemoglobinaemia is a condition characterized by increased quantities of haemoglobin in which the iron of haem is oxidized to the ferric (Fe^{3+}) form. Carboxyhaemoglobinaemia (carbonmonoxyhaemoglobinaemia) results from the binding of carbon monoxide to the haem molecules. Sulphaemoglobinaemia is a rare condition in which there is a mixture of haemoglobin derivatives whose structure is poorly characterized but which can be defined by their specific spectral characteristics.

Pathogenesis

As mentioned earlier, each haemoglobin molecule has four haem moieties. At first sight it is not clear why the oxidation of a proportion of the iron atoms, or the fact that they are liganded to carbon monoxide, should cause such profound changes in oxygen transport. However, oxidation of 30% of the haem molecules has a much more serious effect on tissue oxygenation than a reduction of the haemoglobin level by the same amount. This is because, if a single haem is oxidized, it so alters the conformation of the haemoglobin molecule that the oxygen affinity of the other three haems is increased. Thus methaemoglobin, carboxyhaemoglobin, and cyanmethaemoglobin all have very high oxygen affinities with left-shifted oxygen dissociation curves, and hence are associated with impaired unloading of oxygen to the tissues.

Methaemoglobinaemia

Methaemoglobin causes a variable degree of cyanosis. It should be suspected in any patient with significant central cyanosis in whom there is no evidence of cardiorespiratory disease. The degree of cyanosis produced by 5 g/dl of deoxygenated haemoglobin can be produced by 1.5 g/dl methaemoglobin and 0.5 g/dl of sulphaemoglobin. Methaemoglobin concentrations of 10 to 20% are tolerated quite well. It is useless as an oxygen carrier; levels above this are thus often associated with dyspnoea and headache. Much depends on the rapidity at which it is formed. Many patients with lifelong methaemoglobinaemia are asymptomatic, while individuals who have accumulated a similar level of methaemoglobin acutely may be acutely dyspnoeic. For reasons that are not clear, it is unusual for patients with chronic methaemoglobinaemia to have an increased haemoglobin level or red-cell count.

Methaemoglobinaemia may arise as a result of a genetic defect in red-cell metabolism or haemoglobin structure, or may be acquired following the ingestion of various oxidant drugs and toxic agents.

Genetic methaemoglobinaemia

There are two forms of inherited methaemoglobinaemia. The first results from a deficiency of red-cell NADH-cytochrome b_5 reductase, the second from a structural alteration in either the α or β globin chains of haemoglobin.

NADH-diaphorase catalyses a step in the major pathway for methaemoglobin reduction. The enzyme reduces cytochrome b_5

using NADH as a hydrogen donor. The reduced cytochrome b_5, in turn, reduces methaemoglobin to haemoglobin. There are several different molecular forms of NADH-cytochrome b_5 reductase deficiency which have been identified by electrophoretic analysis of NADH-cytochrome b_5 reductase in the red cells of affected patients. The condition is inherited as an autosomal recessive. Homozygotes have elevated levels of methaemoglobin and are cyanotic from birth. Heterozygotes do not have elevated levels of methaemoglobin but seem to be unusually susceptible to the oxidant action of drugs. For example, severe cyanosis has been precipitated by the use of antimalarial drugs.

There are several abnormal haemoglobin variants which are associated with genetic methaemoglobinaemia, all of which are designated haemoglobin M, and further identified by their place of discovery, e.g. haemoglobin M Boston, M Milwaukee. These variants usually result from amino acid substitutions near the haem pocket. Normally, haem lies between two histidine residues, one called the proximal histidine to which it is attached, and the other called the distal histidine. Oxygen is bound to haem at a site opposite to the distal histidine. If the latter is substituted by tyrosine, as occurs in the α chain variant haemoglobin M Boston and in the β chain variant M Saskatoon, a stable bond is formed between the haem iron and the phenolic ring of the tyrosine. The iron atom is 'fixed' in the Fe^{3+} state. These variants are associated with cyanosis which is present from early life. In the case of the α chain variants it is present from birth, while the β chain haemoglobin variants only produce cyanosis after the first few months of life as adult haemoglobin synthesis becomes established. Unlike NADH diaphorase deficiency, which is inherited as a recessive trait, the haemoglobin Ms have a dominant form of inheritance. Thus it is very simple to make the diagnosis of genetic methaemoglobinaemia and to determine the likely molecular basis by taking a good history; even the affected globin chain can be ascertained!

The diagnosis is confirmed by spectroscopic examination of the blood and by determination of methaemoglobin levels. The precise cause can be established by an assay of NADH-diaphorase or by haemoglobin analysis under appropriate conditions.

Genetic methaemoglobinaemia due to NADH-diaphorase deficiency is readily treated by the administration of ascorbic acid, 300 to 600 mg daily by mouth in divided doses, or by the administration of methylene blue, either intravenously (1 mg/kg body weight) or by mouth 60 mg three to four times daily. On the other hand, the genetic methaemoglobinaemias due to structural haemoglobin variants do not respond to ascorbic acid, methylene blue, or any other treatment. Most affected individuals go through life asymptomatic and require no treatment.

Acquired methaemoglobinaemia

Acquired methaemoglobinaemia usually results from the administration of drugs or exposure to chemicals which cause oxidation of haemoglobin. There are many agents which are capable of exceeding the red cells' ability to reduce methaemoglobin. They include ferricyanide, bivalent copper, chromate, chlorate, quinones, and certain dyes with a high oxidation–reduction potential. Nitrite, often used as a preservative, is one of the most common methaemoglobin-forming agents. Nitrates, after conversion to nitrites in the gut, may cause serious methaemoglobinaemia in infants. Other agents which commonly cause methaemoglobinaemia

include phenacatin, primaquine, sulfonamides, and various analine dye derivatives.

If any of the agents listed above is given in low dose over a long period of time it may lead to chronic methaemoglobinaemia with or without a haemolytic anaemia. However, after exposure to a large amount of these agents, and the development of in excess of 50 to 60% methaemoglobin, the symptoms of acute anaemia develop because methaemoglobin lacks the capacity to transport oxygen. Thus the clinical picture may be characterized by vascular collapse, coma, and death.

Methaemoglobinaemia with haemolytic anaemia

The haemolytic action of oxidant drugs is described elsewhere. Chronic methaemoglobinaemia with haemolytic anaemia, characterized by Heinz body formation and fragmented red cells, occurs commonly in patients receiving dapsone, salazopyrine, or phenacatin. This condition is usually innocuous and can be modified by adjusting the dose of the drug.

Occasionally, acute intravascular haemolysis associated with methaemoglobinaemia and intravascular coagulation occurs. It usually follows the ingestion or infusion of a strong oxidizing agent such as chlorate or arsine. There is gross intravascular haemolysis and methaemoglobinaemia together with evidence of disseminated intravascular coagulation. The haemoglobin level may fall very rapidly and may be complicated by renal failure.

Treatment

In cases of chronic acquired methaemoglobinaemia, the drug or chemical agent should be removed where possible. If continued therapy is required, it should be administered at a lower dose.

Acute toxic methaemoglobinaemia presents a serious medical emergency. Methylene blue should be administered in a dose of 1 to 2 mg/kg intravenously over a 5-min period. Repeated doses may be needed. Toxicity is uncommon, although doses of over 15 mg/kg may cause haemolysis in young infants. The drug should not be used if the methaemoglobinaemia is due to chlorate poisoning, as it may convert the chlorate to hypochlorite which is an even more toxic compound. In cases of acute methaemoglobinaemia with intravascular haemolysis, haemodialysis with exchange transfusion is the treatment of choice.

Carboxyhaemoglobinaemia

Carbon monoxide has an affinity for haemoglobin approximately 210 times that of oxygen. Following acute exposure it is so tightly bound that it takes about 4 h for an individual with normal ventilation to expel half of it. At levels of 5 to 10% there may be no symptoms, but above 20% there is usually headache and weakness. Levels of 40 to 60% or more lead to unconsciousness and death.

Carbon monoxide poisoning is discussed in Chapter 8.1 and secondary polycythaemia due to chronic exposure is considered elsewhere in this chapter.

Sulphaemoglobinaemia

This poorly defined condition derives its name from the fact that it can be produced in vitro by the action of hydrogen sulphide on haemoglobin. It has not been reported as a genetic disorder. It is usually associated with the administration of drugs, particularly sulfonamides or phenacetin. It has also been reported in patients with chronic constipation or malabsorption syndromes (enterogenous cyanosis) although its relationship to these disorders is far from clear.

Other acquired abnormalities of the structure or synthesis of haemoglobin

Glycosylated haemoglobin, haemoglobin AIc

Haemoglobin may undergo post-translational modification in patients with diabetes. The abnormal haemoglobin, haemoglobin AIc, is formed by the nonenzymic combination of glucose with the N-terminus of the β chain, first forming a Schiff base which then undergoes a rearrangement to form a stable ketoamine. The level of haemoglobin AIc is raised in diabetics and is related to the blood sugar level over the previous weeks. The value of the estimation of haemoglobin AIc as an index of the control of diabetes is considered elsewhere.

Haemoglobin Pb

Some children with lead poisoning develop a modified haemoglobin which migrates rapidly on alkaline electrophoresis. The precise structural alteration is not known but, if present, this variant is a useful indicator of severe lead poisoning.

Fetal haemoglobin production in adult life

A number of haematological disorders are associated with a reversion to fetal haemoglobin production after the neonatal period. These include juvenile myeloid leukaemia, other forms of leukaemia, and congenital hypoplastic anaemias. Haemoglobin F may also appear transitorily during rapid regeneration of the bone marrow after drug induced hypoplasia, virus infection, or bone marrow transplantation.

Further reading

Ballas SK (1998). Sickle cell disease: clinical management. *Clin Haematol*, **11**, 185–214.

Cao A, Galanello R, Rosatelli MC (1998). Prenatal diagnosis and screening of the haemoglobinopathies. *Clin Haematol*, **11**, 215–38.

Heeney M, Dover GJ (2009). Sickle cell disease. In: Orkin SH, *et al.* (eds) *Nathan & Oski's hematology in infancy and childhood*, 7th edition, pp. 949–1014. W B Saunders, Philadelphia.

Higgs DR, Weatherall DJ (2009). The alpha thalassaemias. *Cell. Mol. Life Sci.* **66**, 1154–1162.

Olivieri N (1998). Thalassaemia: clinical management. *Clin Haematol*, **11**, 147–62.

Steinberg MH, *et al.* (eds) (2010). *Disorders of hemoglobin*, 2nd edition. Cambridge University Press, New York.

Weatherall DJ, Clegg JB (2001). *The thalassaemia syndromes*, 4th edition. Blackwell Science, Oxford.

Weatherall DJ, *et al.* (2001). The haemoglobinopathies. In: Scriver CR, *et al.* (eds) *The metabolic basis of inherited disease*, 8th edition, pp. 3417–84. McGraw-Hill, New York.

Weatherall DJ, *et al.* (2006). Inherited disorders of hemoglobin. In: Jamieson D, *et al. Disease Control priorities in developing countries.* 2nd edition, pp. 6636–80. Oxford University Press, New York and The World Bank, Washington, DC.

22.5.8 Anaemias resulting from defective maturation of red cells

James S. Wiley

Essentials

Defective maturation of red cells leads to premature destruction of nucleated red cell precursors before they leave the haematopoietic bone marrow, which results in expansion of the marrow, haemolytic jaundice, peripheral signs of increased erythroid turnover on blood films, and (in long-standing disorders) iron overload due to enhanced absorption.

Causes of ineffective erythropoiesis

These include (1) inhibition of erythroid DNA synthesis—e.g. megaloblastic anaemias (vitamin B_{12} or folate deficiency), drugs blocking DNA synthesis; (2) clonal disorders of erythropoiesis—e.g. refractory anaemia, acquired idiopathic sideroblastic anaemia, acute erythroleukaemia; (3) genetic disorders of erythropoiesis—e.g. thalassaemia syndromes, hereditary sideroblastic anaemia, congenital dyserythropoietic anaemia; (4) other causes—e.g. alcohol.

Sideroblastic anaemias

These result from defects in haem biosynthesis, with most cases being acquired as a clonal disorder of erythropoiesis, with varying degrees of myelodysplasia. Other causes are (1) hereditary—e.g. inherited deficiency of the erythroid-specific 5-aminolaevulinic acid synthase 2 gene on the X-chromosome causes congenital sideroblastic anaemia; (2) acquired—e.g. due to drugs or toxins such as ethanol, isoniazid, or lead; following chemotherapy or irradiation; or of unknown cause (idiopathic).

Diagnosis, treatment and prognosis—diagnosis is achieved by finding ring sideroblasts (erythroblasts containing iron-positive granules arranged in a perinuclear location around one-third or more of the nucleus) on bone marrow aspirate stained with Prussian blue iron reagent. Aside from supportive care with blood transfusion and iron chelation, a trial of pyridoxine is generally indicated (25% of hereditary cases—but few acquired cases—show some response). Acquired idiopathic sideroblastic anaemia has a median survival of 42 to 76 months, with 3 to 12% progressing to acute leukaemia.

Introduction

Erythroid cell maturation is specialized towards the coordinated synthesis of large amounts of haem and globin necessary to attain the high concentration of haemoglobin found in the mature red cell. Hereditary or acquired defects in the production of either of these cause a maturation block, which leads to ineffective erythropoiesis in which many of the developing nucleated erythroblasts are destroyed in the marrow before they can reach the circulation. Thus in thalassaemia, defective synthesis of either α or β globin leads to unbalanced production of the other chain, which precipitates and leads to destruction of the precursor erythroblast. Defective haem synthesis in the sideroblastic anaemias also leads to an anaemia which is characterized by ineffective erythropoiesis (Box 22.5.8.1). Abnormalities of DNA synthesis in the developing erythroid cells, produced e.g. by vitamin B_{12} or folic acid deficiency, blocks cell division required for erythroid maturation and produces morphological and biochemical evidence of ineffective erythropoiesis.

Ineffective erythropoiesis may be recognized by the characteristic erythroid hyperplasia of the bone marrow with normal or only slight increase in reticulocyte numbers. Some other features of ineffective erythropoiesis may be variably present: a mild increase in bilirubin, decrease in haptoglobin, and increased serum lactic dehydrogenase activity. As a result, iron absorption is increased, serum iron and ferritin become elevated, and, after many years, iron overload develops which is indistinguishable from idiopathic haemochromatosis. However, the degree of iron overload does not depend on either the severity of the anaemia or the presence of the characteristic mutation (Cys282Tyr) of the *HFE* gene associated with genetic haemochromatosis.

Sideroblastic anaemias

The sideroblastic anaemias are a group of hereditary or acquired anaemias of varying severity diagnosed by the finding of ring sideroblasts in the bone marrow aspirate. The peripheral blood film shows hypochromic red cells which are microcytic in the hereditary form (Fig. 22.5.8.1), but are often macrocytic in the acquired forms of the disease. Normochromic and normocytic red cells are also present which gives the film a dimorphic distribution of red cell sizes. The diagnostic procedure is bone marrow aspirate followed by staining of the smear with Prussian Blue iron reagent. Ring sideroblasts are diagnostic (Fig. 22.5.8.2) and are defined as

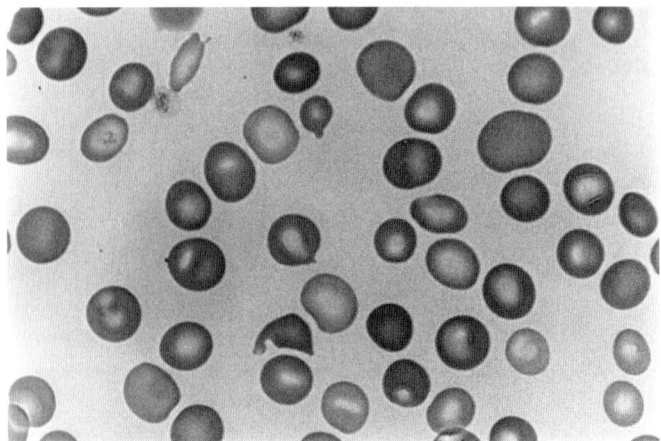

Fig. 22.5.8.1 Peripheral blood smear in hereditary sideroblastic anaemia showing a population of hypochromic and microcytic erythrocytes.
(Courtesy of Gillian Rozenberg.)

erythroblasts containing iron-positive granules arranged in a perinuclear location around one-third or more of the nucleus. Electron microscopy reveals that the iron-containing granules are mitochondria containing precipitated ferric phosphate and ferric hydroxide. The sideroblastic anaemias have diverse aetiologies (Table 22.5.8.2) but have in common an impaired biosynthesis of haem in the erythroid cells of the marrow. Most sideroblastic anaemias are acquired as a clonal disorder of erythropoiesis, with varying degrees of myelodysplasia. The hereditary forms are uncommon. Most are found in males with an X-linked pattern of inheritance. A number of drugs have been associated with reversible sideroblastic anaemia, chiefly in patients with alcohol abuse (Box 22.5.8.2).

Hereditary sideroblastic anaemias

Aetiology and pathogenesis

Haem biosynthesis occurs by a cascade of eight enzymes (Fig. 22.5.8.3). In humans, mutations affecting the first enzyme of this pathway produce hereditary sideroblastic anaemia. Inborn errors that occur in later enzymes in this pathway result in metabolic disorders known as the porphyrias (Fig. 22.5.8.3). The pathway begins with the condensation of glycine with succinyl CoA to form 5-aminolaevulinic acid (ALA), a step which is under the control of

---

Box 22.5.8.1 Anaemias with defective red cell maturation and ineffective erythropoiesis as a major cause

- Inhibition of erythroid DNA synthesis
  - Megaloblastic anaemias (vitamin B_{12} or folate deficiency)
  - Drugs blocking DNA synthesis (e.g. hydroxyurea, 6-mercaptopurine)
- Clonal disorders of erythropoiesis
  - Refractory anaemia
  - Acquired idiopathic sideroblastic anaemia (refractory anaemia with ring sideroblasts)
  - Acute erythroleukaemia (acute myeloid leukaemia: FAB-M6)
- Genetic disorders of erythropoiesis
  - Thalassaemia syndromes
  - Hereditary sideroblastic anaemias
  - Congenital dyserythropoietic anaemias (CDA)
- Miscellaneous
  - Alcohol
  - Drugs
  - Heavy metal poisoning (e.g. arsenic)
  - Falciparum malaria

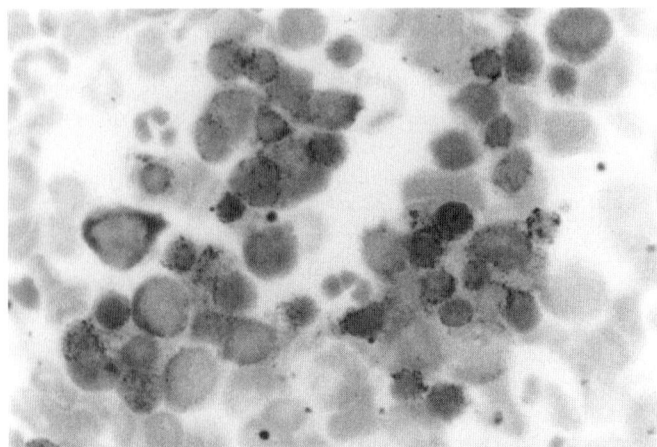

Fig. 22.5.8.2 Bone marrow smear stained with Prussian blue, showing the ring sideroblasts (arrow).
(Courtesy of Gillian Rozenberg.)

- Hereditary
  - X-linked[a]
  - Autosomal dominant or recessive[a]
- Acquired
  - Refractory anaemia with ring sideroblasts[a] (acquired idiopathic sideroblastic anaemia)
  - Associated with previous chemotherapy, irradiation
  - Overlap myelodysplasia/ myeloproliferative diseases
- Drugs
  - Alcohol
  - Isoniazid, cycloserine, pyrazinamide
  - Chloramphenicol
- Rare causes
  - Erythropoietic protoporphyria
  - Pearson's syndrome
  - Copper deficiency or zinc overload
  - Hypothermia

[a] Trial of pyridoxine indicated.

the mitochondrial enzyme ALA synthase. This enzyme requires pyridoxal phosphate as a cofactor. Two isoenzymes of ALA synthase have been identified. One is found in liver and other tissues (ALAS 1); the other is confined to erythroid cells of the bone marrow (ALAS 2). The gene for the erythroid-specific ALAS 2 isoenzyme resides on the X chromosome and is now known to be the site of most mutations giving rise to X-linked hereditary sideroblastic anaemia. Several dozen different mutations have been described in different families. All result from a single amino acid alteration arising from a point mutation in the ALAS 2 coding region of DNA. In nearly half the families with hereditary sideroblastic anaemia, the structure of the *ALAS2* gene is normal, and a significant proportion of these families had a defect in an erythroid specific mitochondrial transporter, SLC25A38, which is thought to transport glycine into the mitochondrion. In most families, males are affected with an X-linked pattern of inheritance consistent with a mutation on the X chromosome (Fig. 22.5.8.4). However, occasionally the disease is transmitted as an autosomal dominant; there are even well-documented families in which only females are affected.

Clinical and laboratory features

Typically the anaemia presents in infancy or childhood, but when the condition is mild the diagnosis may not be made until adult life. Occasionally, such patients may present with features of iron overload such as diabetes or cardiac failure. Others may be found in family surveys, which should be undertaken when this anaemia is diagnosed. Slight enlargement of the liver or spleen may occur. The degree of anaemia is variable, ranging from severe (<80 g/litre haemoglobin) to mild (>100 g/litre haemoglobin) but even with mild or no anaemia the mean corpuscular volume (MCV) is below the normal range. Blood film shows a population of cells with hypochromic, microcytic morphology. Female carriers may show

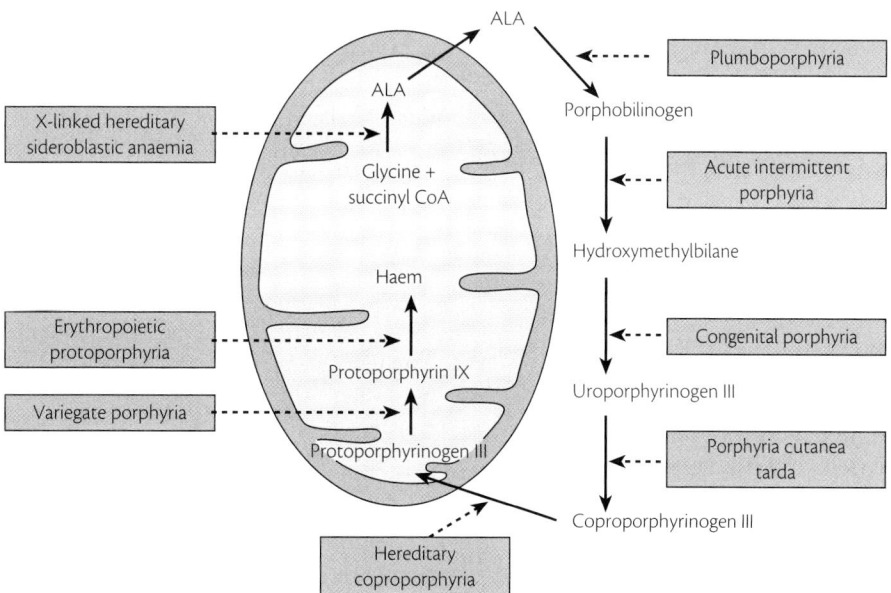

Fig. 22.5.8.3 Pathway of haem biosynthesis in mammalian cells. The first step in the pathway is catalysed by ALAS and occurs within the mitochondrion using pyridoxal 5′-phosphate as a cofactor. ALA then leaves the mitochondrion and is converted by ALA dehydratase to give a monopyrrole, porphobilinogen. Four molecules of this are converted by porphobilinogen deaminase to a linear tetrapyrrole, hydroxymethylbilane. This molecule is then cyclized by uroporphyrinogen III synthase to uroporphyrinogen III, which is then decarboxylated to coproporphyrinogen III. This molecule enters the mitochondrion and is oxidized in succession by coproporphyrinogen III oxidase and protoporphyrinogen III oxidase. The product is protoporphyrin IX, a substrate for ferrochelatase, which catalyses the insertion of Fe²⁺ to form haem. The defective steps associated with specific porphyrias and X-linked hereditary sideroblastic anaemias are shown.
(From Hoffman R, *et al.* (eds) (1999). *Hematology: basic principles and practice*, 3rd edition. W B Saunders, Philadelphia, with permission.)

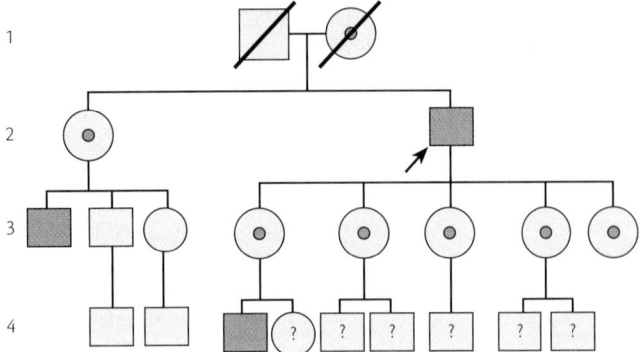

Fig. 22.5.8.4 Pedigree of a family with pyridoxine-responsive sideroblastic anaemia showing X-linked recessive inheritance. ▪ affected; ○carrier;? unknown status. Diagonal lines indicate deceased members. The pedigree has been abbreviated to show only the affected branches of the family. The arrow indicates the proband.
(Copyright 1994 Massachusetts Medical Society. All rights reserved. Reproduced from Cox *et al.* (1994)).

the characteristic red cell dimorphism. White cell counts are normal, while platelet counts are normal or slightly elevated. Serum iron and ferritin concentrations are invariably increased and transferrin shows an increased percentage saturation with iron. The differential diagnosis includes idiopathic haemochromatosis, since both diseases have evidence of iron overload. Examination of the blood film, the MCV, and the bone marrow should establish the diagnosis.

Treatment and prognosis

A trial of pyridoxine, 100 to 200 mg/day taken orally, is indicated for 3 months in all patients with proven or suspected hereditary sideroblastic anaemia. About 25% of patients experience a full or partial correction. This vitamin should be continued lifelong in responders but at a lower maintenance dosage. Regular transfusions of packed red cells are the mainstay of treatment of severe anaemia. These should be given to relieve symptoms and allow normal childhood development. Splenectomy is contraindicated in this condition. Iron overload progresses rapidly once transfusions begin. Chelation therapy with desferrioxamine or oral iron chelators should thus be commenced after the first 10 to 20 transfusions. Iron removal may greatly benefit patients with mild or moderate anaemia and evidence of iron overload. Intermittent phlebotomy of 100 to 200 ml blood should be attempted as this is more effective than chelation therapy in removing iron and should be continued if symptoms allow until the serum ferritin becomes normal. Finally, patients should avoid alcohol and ascorbic acid supplements, both of which enhance iron absorption.

Acquired idiopathic sideroblastic anaemia (refractory anaemia with ring sideroblasts)

Acquired idiopathic sideroblastic anaemia is a refractory anaemia with a hypercellular marrow containing ring sideroblasts which may either be idiopathic or develop following chemotherapy or irradiation (Table 22.5.8.2). Since nearly all cases also show evidence of dyserythropoiesis, this anaemia was classified as one of the myelodysplastic syndromes and termed 'refractory anaemia with ring sideroblasts' by the French–American–British Group. This classification is supported by the demonstration that the defective haematopoiesis is clonal, both in acquired idiopathic sideroblastic anaemia and the other myelodysplastic syndromes.

Clonal haematopoiesis has also been shown in acute erythroleukaemia, in which bizarre dysplastic changes and ineffective erythropoiesis are seen in the developing erythroblasts. These comprise a majority (>50%) of all nucleated marrow cells. The fact that more than 20% of the myeloid cells are blasts distinguishes acute erythroleukaemia from one of the myelodysplastic syndromes.

Aetiology and pathogenesis

The cause of the defective haem synthesis in acquired sideroblastic anaemia is unclear. Recent reports indicate that levels of ALAS in bone marrow are normal. Indirect evidence points to an acquired defect in the mitochondrial respiratory chain that impairs the reduction of Fe^{3+} to Fe^{2+} since ferrous iron is essential for the terminal ferrochelatase reaction (Fig. 22.5.8.3). Clonal haematopoiesis has been demonstrated in this anaemia by both molecular and karyotypic analysis. Thus a single glucose-6-phosphate dehydrogenase (G6PD) isoenzyme was found in erythrocytes of a woman heterozygous for G6PD who expressed two isoenzymes in her somatic tissues. Clonal chromosome changes are also found in bone marrow cells in many patients with acquired sideroblastic anaemia. Characteristic changes include monosomy 7, trisomy 8, deletions involving chromosomes 5, 7, 11, 13, or 20, and a number of translocations. When sideroblastic anaemia is acquired secondary to chemotherapy or irradiation, chromosomal changes are nearly always found and tend to be multiple. However, they are probably a late event in the course of this anaemia and may be preceded by the expansion of a clone of genetically unstable stem cells. Some patients with acquired sideroblastic anaemia with high platelet counts carry the JAK2-V617F mutation.

Clinical and laboratory features

Acquired sideroblastic anaemia typically has an insidious onset. Most patients are middle aged or older, but young adults can be affected. Mild splenomegaly may be present. White cell and platelet counts are usually normal; some patients may have thrombocytosis. The bone marrow shows erythroid hyperplasia with varying degrees of dyserythropoiesis, including irregular nuclear contour, nuclear fragmentation (karyorrhexis), bi- or trilobed nuclei, and internuclear bridges. Iron stain of the aspirate shows ring sideroblasts which should total more than 15% of the nucleated erythroid cells to make the diagnosis. Dysplasia of myeloid precursors or megakaryocytes may be present. When associated with leucopenia and/or thrombocytopenia the more descriptive term 'refractory cytopenia' is sometimes used. If the overall blast count exceeds 5% or the peripheral blood monocyte count exceeds 1.0×10^9/litre, the condition falls within a different category of the myelodysplastic syndrome. Thus, ring sideroblasts may be seen in other myelodysplastic conditions such as refractory anaemia with excess blasts. Distinguishing acquired idiopathic sideroblastic anaemia from a mild hereditary sideroblastic anaemia presenting in adult life can be difficult. However, careful examination of the marrow for dysplastic changes, the MCV, possible response to pyridoxine, and a family survey all help to distinguish these two entities.

Treatment and prognosis

Transfusions of packed red cells should be given for relief of symptomatic anaemia. A trial of pyridoxine, 100 to 200 mg/day for 3 months, is worthwhile but few patients respond to this vitamin. Acquired idiopathic sideroblastic anaemia and the closely related refractory anaemia have the most favourable outlook among the myelodysplastic syndromes, with a median survival of 42 to 76 months and a 3 to 12% incidence of progression to acute leukaemia. A simple prognostic scoring system has been developed in which two or more of the following place the patient in a poor prognostic category:

◆ haemoglobin less than 100 g/litre

◆ neutrophils less than 1.5×10^9/litre

◆ platelets less than 100×10^9/litre

◆ blasts more than 5%

Karyotypic analysis of marrow aspirates is valuable since a normal karyotype confers a favourable prognosis. In contrast, certain recurring chromosomal abnormalities are considered as presumptive evidence of myelodysplasia in the absence of definitive morphological features.

Defective red-cell maturation secondary to alcohol and drugs

Alcohol has a direct toxic effect on erythropoiesis, manifested by the macrocytosis that characterizes the red cells of subjects chronically ingesting alcohol in excess. Malnourished and anaemic alcoholics may exhibit ring sideroblasts in the bone marrow as well as vacuolation of erythroblasts. These manifestations gradually disappear over 4 to 12 days when alcohol is withdrawn, although the macrocytosis may take several months to normalize. The antibiotic chloramphenicol when given in dosages greater than 2 g/day produces a reversible inhibition of erythropoiesis associated with ring sideroblasts and vacuolation of erythroblasts. This effect, due to inhibition of mitochondrial protein synthesis, is quite separate from the rare idiosyncratic side effect of aplastic anaemia. Protracted exposure to the antituberculous drug isoniazid has been occasionally associated with development of a sideroblastic anaemia.

Defective red-cell maturation secondary to lead, arsenic, or zinc ingestion or copper deficiency

Patients suffering lead poisoning show clinical and laboratory evidence of reduced haem biosynthesis. Basophilic stippling of red cells is prominent. Mild hypochromic, microcytic anaemia may develop. Red-cell protoporphyrin, increased due to inhibition of the terminal step in the haem pathway, provides a sensitive measure of lead exposure. The peripheral neuropathy of lead poisoning may be a result of reduced haem biosynthesis, as in the porphyrias. Acute or chronic arsenic ingestion can cause anaemia with marked dyserythropoiesis. Basophilic stippling of red cells is characteristic while neutropenia and thrombocytopenia may be present. Copper deficiency has been described only in malnourished premature infants or in patients receiving long-term parenteral hyperalimentation. This syndrome consists of anaemia and neutropenia associated with marrow findings of ring sideroblasts and vacuolated erythroid and myeloid precursors. Large quantities of ingested zinc interfere with copper absorption and reproduce the sideroblastic anaemia and neutropenia characteristic of copper deficiency.

Congenital dyserythropoietic anaemias (CDA)

This rare group of inherited refractory anaemias is characterized by gross multinuclearity of erythroid precursors in the marrow,

ineffective erythropoiesis, and associated iron overload. Three types have been described based on morphology of the bone marrow and serological features. The most common, type II (OMIM 224 100), is also known as HEMPAS (hereditary erythroblast multinuclearity with positive acidified serum test) since red cells are lysed by acidified (pH 6.8) serum from about 30% of normal subjects. In CDA type II, a defect in glycosylation of erythroblast membrane proteins has been identified. Most patients are diagnosed in late childhood or adolescence with mild to moderate anaemia, with intermittent jaundice or in older patients with manifestations of iron overload. Splenomegaly or hepatomegaly may be variably present. CDA carries a good prognosis with few patients requiring transfusions. The degree of iron overload should be monitored and treated when appropriate.

Further reading

Aivado M, et al. (2006). X-linked sideroblastic anemia associated with a novel ALAS2' mutation and unfortunate skewed X-chromosome inactivation patterns. *Blood Cells Mol Dis*, **37**, 40–5.

Bergmann, AK, et al. (2010). Systematic Molecular Genetic Analysis of Congenital Sideroblastic Anemia: Evidence for Genetic Heterogeneity and Identification of Novel Mutations. *Pediatric Blood Cancer*, **54**, 273–278.

Boissinot M, et al. (2006). The JAK2-V617F mutation and essential thrombocythemia features in a subset of patients with refractory anemia with ring sideroblasts (RARS). *Blood*, **108**, 1781–82.

Bottomley, SS. Sideroblastic anemias. In: Wintrobe's Clinical Hematology, 12th ed, Greer, JP, Foerster, J, Lukens, J, et al. (Eds), Lippincott, Williams and Wilkins, Philadelphia 2008. p.835.

Camaschella, C (2008). Recent advances in the understanding of inherited sideroblastic anaemia. *Br J Haematol*, **143**, 27–38.

Cotter PD, et al. (1995). Late-onset X-linked sideroblastic anemia. Missense mutations in the erythroid δ-aminolevulinate synthase (*ALAS2*) gene in two pyridoxine-responsive patients initially diagnosed with acquired refractory anemia and ringed sideroblasts. *J Clin Invest*, **96**, 2090–6.

Cox TC, et al. (1994). X-linked pyridoxine-responsive sideroblastic anemia due to a THR[388]- to -SER substitution in erythroid 5-aminolevulinate synthase. *N Engl J Med*, **330**, 675–9. [Shows a typical response of hereditary sideroblastic anaemia to pyridoxine.]

Greenberg P, et al. (1997). International scoring system for evaluating prognosis in myelodysplastic syndromes. *Blood*, **89**, 2079–88.

Guernsey, DL, et al. (2009). Mutations in mitochondrial carrier family gene SLC25A38 cause nonsyndromic autosomal recessive congenital sideroblastic anemia. *Nat Genet*, **41**, 651–653.

Haas D, et al. (2007). New insights into the prognostic impact of the karyotype in MDS and correlation with subtypes. Evidence from a core dataset of 2124 patients. *Blood*, **110**, 4385–95.

Hasserjian RP, et al. (2008). Refractory anemia with ring sideroblasts in WHO classification of Tumours of Haemopoietic and Lymphoid Tissues, Fourth Ed. *Lyon: IARC Press*, pp. 96–97.

Raskin WH, et al. (1984). Evidence for a multistep pathogenesis of a myelodysplastic syndrome. *Blood*, **63**, 1318–23.

Savage D, Lindenbaum J (1986). Anemia in alcoholics. *Medicine*, **65**, 322–38.

Steensma DP. (2009). The changing classification of myelodysplastic syndromes: what's in a name? *Hematology Am Soc Hematol Educ Program*, 645–655.

Szpurka H, et al. (2006). Refractory anemia with ringed sideroblasts associated with marked thrombocytosis (RARS-T) another myeloproliferative condition characterized by JAK2 V617F mutation. *Blood*, **108**, 2173–2181.

Wiley JS, Moore MR (2009). Heme biosynthesis and it disorders: porphyrias and sideroblastic anemias. In: Hoffman R, et al. (eds) *Hematology: basic principles and practice*, pp. 475–89. Churchill Livingstone, Elsevier. Philadelphia 5th Ed.

22.5.9 Haemolytic anaemia—congenital and acquired

Amy Powers, Leslie Silberstein, and Frank J. Strobl

Essentials

Premature destruction of red cells occurs through two primary mechanisms: (1) decreased erythrocyte deformability that leads to red-cell sequestration and extravascular haemolysis in the spleen and other components of the reticuloendothelial system—may be caused by membrane defects, metabolic abnormalities, exogenous oxidizing agents, or pathological antibodies; (2) red-cell membrane damage and intravascular haemolysis—may be caused by exposure to pathological antibodies, activated complement, mechanical forces, chemicals, and infectious agents.

Clinical features—general aspects

These include (1) increased red cell production—manifestations include reticulocytosis, polychromasia, macrocytosis, erythroid hyperplasia, and bone changes; (2) increased red-cell destruction—features include decreased haemoglobin levels, fragmented red cells, decreased haptoglobin levels, increased unconjugated bilirubin levels, increased plasma LDH levels, haemoglobinaemia, haemoglobinuria, haemosiderinuria, splenomegaly.

Congenital disorders of the red-cell membrane

Hereditary spherocytosis—usually an autosomal dominant condition due to defects in α- or β-spectrin, or the proteins that bind spectrin to the plasma membrane. Presentation is typically in childhood with anaemia, jaundice, and splenomegaly, with red cells demonstrating increased osmotic fragility. Anaemia can be corrected in almost all cases by splenectomy. See also Chapter 22.5.10.

Hereditary elliptocytosis—a genetically heterogeneous disorder caused in most cases by defects in both α-spectrin and β-spectrin that interfere with spectrin self-association. Less than 10% of cases exhibit significant haemolysis, but the peripheral blood smear contains elliptocytes, 'pencil cells', and other abnormally shaped red cells. Asymptomatic individuals require no treatment; patients who are symptomatic often obtain some benefit from splenectomy. See also Chapter 22.5.10.

Other disorders—these include hereditary pyropoikilocytosis, hereditary spherocytic elliptocytosis, hereditary stomatocytosis, and hereditary xerocytosis.

Congenital disorders of red-cell enzymes

Glucose-6-phosphate dehydrogenase (G6PD) deficiency—an X-linked, recessive disorder that is maintained in populations because it confers some resistance to *Plasmodium falciparum* infection. Causes little to no haematological abnormality under normal circumstances, but severe haemolysis and anaemia occur during periods of oxidant stress that may be caused by chemicals, drugs, infectious agents, and the bean *Vicia faba* (favism). Diagnosis depends on the demonstration of decreased red-cell G6PD activity, for which there is a rapid fluorescent screening assay. Management involves avoidance of precipitants, with blood transfusion required during severe haemolytic episodes. See also Chapter 22.5.12.

Pyruvate kinase deficiency—an autosomal recessive condition, with severe deficiency causing haemolysis, anaemia and jaundice throughout life, eventually resulting in splenomegaly, gallstones, and aplastic anaemia. See Chapter 22.5.11 for further discussion.

Acquired immune haemolytic anaemias

Immune haemolysis may occur when IgG, IgM, or IgA antibodies and/or complement bind to the erythrocyte surface. The direct antiglobulin test (DAT) or direct Coombs' test detects the presence of IgG antibody or complement on the red-cell surface: IgM and IgA antibodies are not directly detectable with standard testing reagents.

Autoimmune haemolytic anaemias (HA)—these are best classified according to the temperature at which the antibody optimally binds to the erythrocyte. (1) Warm autoimmune HA—typically IgG; symptomatic patients present with anaemia, jaundice, and splenomegaly; associated with lymphoid malignancies; first-line treatment is with corticosteroids. (2) Cold agglutinin syndrome—autoantibodies are typically IgM and are most active at low temperatures; seen in younger patients following infection with *Mycoplasma pneumoniae* or infectious mononucleosis and in older patients in association with lymphoma, chronic lymphocytic leukaemia, or Waldenström macroglobulinaemia. (3) Paroxysmal cold haemoglobinuria. (4) Mixed type autoimmune HA—both IgG and complement are present on the red cells; may be idiopathic or secondary (most often to systemic lupus erythematosus). (5) Drug induced—haemolysis can be caused by drugs that induce a positive direct antiglobulin test by (a) acting as a drug hapten, (b) immune complex formation, (c) autoantibody production.

Alloimmune HA—these include (1) acute haemolytic transfusion reactions—may begin after the infusion of as little as 10 ml of incompatible blood, with symptoms and signs including chest or flank pain, nausea, vomiting, fever, chills, hypotension, respiratory distress, and haemoglobinuria. Despite immediate stopping of the transfusion and optimal supportive care, patients can develop renal failure, disseminated intravascular coagulation, and even die. (2) Other conditions—these include delayed haemolytic transfusion reactions, passenger lymphocyte haemolysis, haemolytic disease of the newborn (caused by rhesus (Rh) D incompatibility or ABO incompatibility).

Acquired nonimmune haemolytic anaemias

Common or important causes include (1) infections—e.g. malaria, babesiosis; (2) drugs and chemicals—e.g. nitrofurantoin; (3) mechanical—e.g. incompetent prosthetic heart valves; microangiopathic haemolytic anaemia (MAHA), which describes a spectrum of disorders including haemolytic uraemic syndrome and thrombotic thrombocytopenic purpura that are characterized by mechanical destruction of red cells resulting from thrombi that occlude the microvasculature.

Introduction

Mechanisms of haemolysis

After release into the circulation, normal red cells survive for approximately 120 days. As the circulating red-cell mass decreases (anaemia), less oxygen is transported from the lungs to other tissues. In response, the kidneys increase their synthesis and secretion of erythropoietin, which stimulates erythropoiesis, in order to restore normal red-cell mass and oxygen delivery. A deficient red-cell mass results from inadequate production (hypoplasia), loss (haemorrhage), or premature destruction (haemolysis) of the red cells. In cases where red-cell survival is reduced to such an extent that normal bone marrow cannot compensate, a haemolytic anaemia results. The haemolytic anaemias are either genetically determined or acquired.

Consequences of haemolysis

The clinical and laboratory changes associated with haemolysis reflect the physiological mechanisms responsible for restoring red-cell mass and removing free haemoglobin from the plasma. These changes are outlined in Box 22.5.9.1. Within several days of the onset of haemolysis and the development of anaemia, increased erythropoiesis results in erythroid hyperplasia (decreased myeloid/erythroid ratio) in the bone marrow and reticulocytosis (polychromasia and macrocytosis) in the peripheral blood. The peripheral blood film will also often exhibit microspherocytes, fragmented red blood cells, and nucleated red blood cells. If the haemolysis and anaemia begin early in life and persist, extramedullary erythropoiesis can develop in the spleen, liver, and lymph nodes. Chronic anaemia

and the resulting marrow hyperplasia can also result in long-bone deformities. Free haemoglobin in the circulation binds to the serum protein haptoglobin. Haptoglobin–haemoglobin complexes are removed from the intravascular space by the reticuloendothelial system. If the rate of haemolysis is greater than the liver's ability to synthesize haptoglobin, serum haptoglobin levels fall. In patients with severe haemolysis, haemoglobinaemia and haemoglobinuria may develop. At low plasma haemoglobin levels, much of the free haemoglobin is reabsorbed in the proximal renal tubules. The renal tubular cells catabolize the haemoglobin, converting iron into haemosiderin, which is eventually shed along with renal tubular cells into the urine resulting in haemosiderinuria. Haemosiderinuria is a reliable indicator of chronic intravascular haemolysis. At higher levels, free haemoglobin is found in the urine. Within the reticuloendothelial system, haemoglobin is metabolized and released into the serum as unconjugated bilirubin. The bilirubin is conjugated in the liver, excreted in the gut, converted to faecal urobilinogen, partially reabsorbed, and excreted by the kidneys as urinary urobilinogen. The intracellular enzyme lactate dehydrogenase is released from lysed red cells into the plasma.

Congenital anaemias

Congenital anaemias result from inherited defects in the red-cell membrane, red-cell enzymes, or haemoglobin. The haemoglobinopathies and thalassaemias are discussed elsewhere.

Disorders of the red-cell membrane

The strength and flexibility required of the red-cell membrane is provided by the lipid bilayer and a proteinaceous, membrane-bound cytoskeleton. The membrane skeleton forms an underlying lattice which both supports and stabilizes the plasma membrane. Figure 22.5.9.1 provides a schematic model of the erythrocyte membrane and membrane-skeleton. The major, integral membrane proteins are Band 3 and the glycophorins. Band 3 functions as a transmembrane channel for the diffusion of anions and glucose. The physiological role of the glycophorins is unknown. Cytoplasmic proteins located adjacent to the plasma membrane include spectrin, actin, Band 4.1, ankyrin, and Band 4.2. Spectrin,

---

Box 22.5.9.1 The main features of haemolytic anaemia

Increased red cell production

- Reticulocytosis
- Polychromasia
- Macrocytosis
- Erythroid hyperplasia
- Bone changes

Increased red cell destruction

- Decreased haemoglobin levels
- Increased unconjugated bilirubin levels
- Decreased haptoglobin levels
- Increased faecal and urinary urobilinogen
- Haemoglobinaemia
- Haemoglobinuria
- Haemosiderinuria
- Splenomegaly
- Increased plasma LDH levels
- Microspherocytes
- Fragmented red blood cells
- Nucleated red blood cells

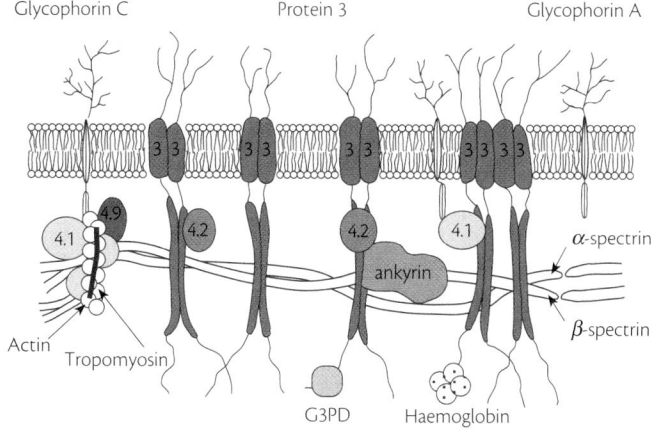

Fig. 22.5.9.1 Schematic illustration of the major components of the red-cell membrane and membrane skeleton.
(Reproduced from Lux SE (1989). Hereditary disorders of the red-cell membrane skeleton. *Trends Genet,* **5**, 222–7, with permission.)

a heterodimeric protein composed of α and β subunits, is the principal component of the membrane-skeleton. The heterodimers of spectrin are bound to each other, head-to-head, to form heterotetramers and larger oligomers. The spectrin tetramers are cross-linked at their ends by actin. This interaction is strengthened by Band 4.1. Band 4.1 also binds the cytoplasmic domain of glycophorin to spectrin. Ankyrin binds Band 3 to the β chain of spectrin. Band 4.2 probably strengthens this interaction. A deficiency in any of these cytoskeletal proteins would be expected to result in defects in erythrocyte shape and deformability.

Hereditary spherocytosis

Hereditary spherocytosis is inherited primarily in an autosomal dominant manner. Up to a quarter of cases, however, exhibit a nondominant or recessive pattern of inheritance. The disorder is characterized by small spherocytic red cells with reduced deformability. The increased rigidity results in entrapment of the spherocytes, primarily in the microcirculation of the spleen. For a full description of this disorder, see Chapter 22.5.10.

Hereditary elliptocytosis

Hereditary elliptocytosis is a genetically heterogeneous disorder characterized by elliptical red cells and haemolysis. Autosomal dominant and rare autosomal recessive forms of the disease have been identified. The clinical severity ranges from an asymptomatic condition to a severe haemolytic anaemia. For a full description of this disorder, see Chapter 22.5.10.

Hereditary pyropoikilocytosis

Hereditary pyropoikilocytosis is inherited in an autosomal recessive fashion. There is marked red-cell fragmentation, microcytosis, poikilocytosis, and spherocytosis (Fig. 22.5.9.2). For a full description of this disorder, see Chapter 22.5.10.

Hereditary spherocytic elliptocytosis

This form of hereditary elliptocytosis is characterized by mild to moderate haemolytic anaemia with both elliptocytes and spherocytes. The molecular basis of this disorder has yet to be identified. The osmotic fragility is increased. Splenectomy may be useful in symptomatic individuals.

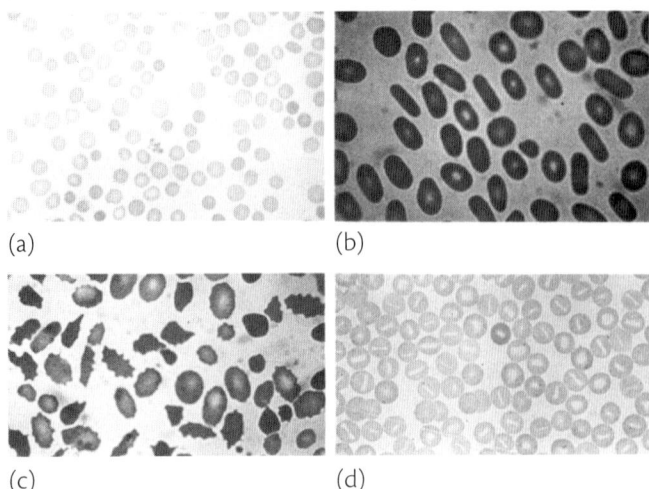

Fig. 22.5.9.2 Altered red-cell morphology: (a) spherocytes; (b) elliptocytes; (c) poikilocytes; (d) stomatocytes.

Hereditary stomatocytosis

Several families have been identified with members exhibiting moderate to severe anaemia and circulating stomatocytes (Fig. 22.5.9.2). For a full description of this disorder, see Chapter 22.5.10.

Hereditary xerocytosis

Hereditary xerocytosis is a rare, autosomal dominant disorder characterized by red-cell dehydration and decreased osmotic fragility. The cellular dehydration appears to be caused by a defect in membrane K^+ permeability that leads to intracellular K^+ and H_2O loss. The crenated cells are cleared by the reticuloendothelial system resulting in moderate to severe haemolysis. Splenectomy may provide therapeutic benefit. As with hereditary stomatocytosis, the risk of hypercoagulability and thrombosis are increased following splenectomy in patients with xerocytosis.

Acanthocytosis

Acanthocytes or spur cells are red cells with many thorn-like projections of the membrane surface. Changes in the composition of membrane lipids within the membrane lipid bilayer appear to be responsible for the development of acanthocytosis. Acanthocytosis and haemolytic anaemia are seen in severe liver disease, abetalipoproteinaemia, and the McLeod syndrome. Infrequently, patients with severe liver disease accumulate free cholesterol in the outer leaflet of the red-cell membrane resulting in spur cell shape, trapping of the acanthocytes in the spleen, and rapidly progressive anaemia. For a full description of this disorder, see Chapter 22.5.10.

Disorders of red-cell enzymes

Erythrocytes circulate throughout the body for approximately 4 months lacking a nucleus, mitochondria, and ribosomes. As a result, red cells cannot synthesize protein nor take advantage of oxidative metabolism. Glucose metabolism is necessary to maintain the integrity of both the erythrocyte membrane and haemoglobin. In red cells, glucose is metabolized to lactate primarily through the anaerobic Embden–Meyerhof pathway (Fig. 22.5.9.3). Eleven enzymes are required to break glucose down to lactate, generating 2 moles of ATP and reducing 2 moles of NAD^+ to NADH. ATP is used primarily by membrane-associated ATPases which pump Na^+ and K^+ against their concentration gradients. NADH prevents the oxidation of iron in haemoglobin. 2,3-diphosphoglycerate (2,3-DPG) which binds to the β-subunits of haemoglobin and facilitates the release of oxygen is also a product of the Embden–Meyerhof pathway. In red cells, the production of 2,3-DPG is exaggerated in order to maintain intracellular concentrations equimolar with the concentration of haemoglobin. The production of 2,3-DPG occurs in a side pathway referred to as the Rapaport–Luebering shunt that branches from the main glycolytic pathway after the formation of 1,3-DPG. The other major red-cell energy pathway is the hexose–monophosphate shunt, which results in the reduction of $NADP^+$ to NADPH (Fig. 22.5.9.4). NADPH maintains adequate levels of reduced glutathione, which protects the red cells against oxidative damage.

Many enzyme deficiencies are associated with haemolytic anaemia. Most of these enzyme deficiencies are not limited to the erythrocyte and, thus, are associated with multisystem disease (Table 22.5.9.1). The remaining enzyme deficiencies associated with haemolytic anaemia are clinically specific to the red cell. The majority of these enzyme deficiencies are rare, having been found in only a few

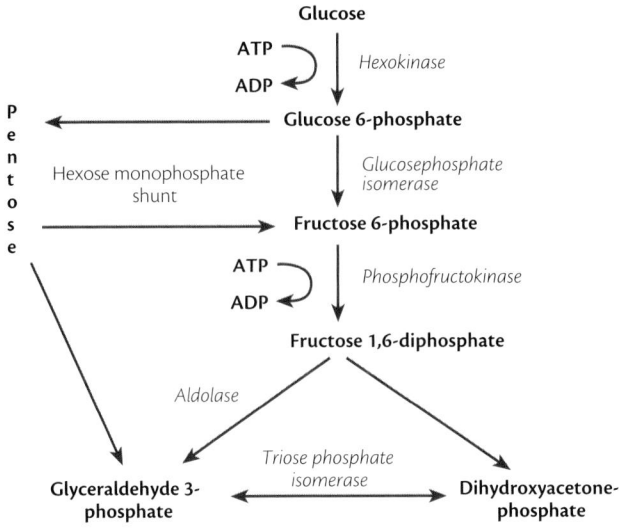

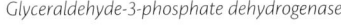

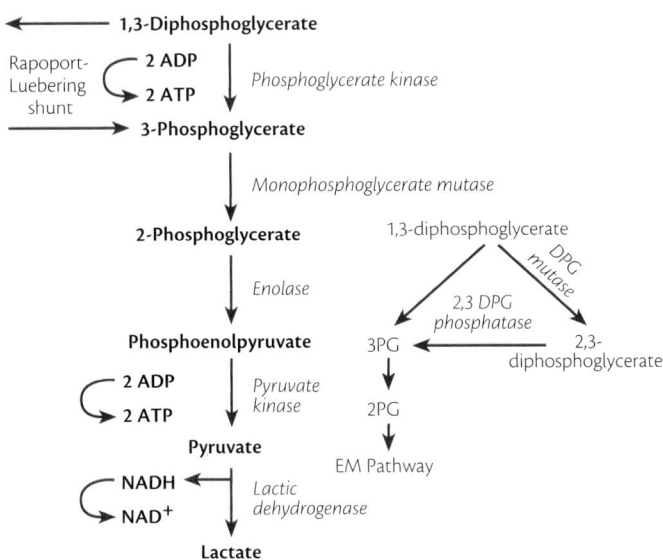

Fig. 22.5.9.3 The relationship between the main red-cell glycolytic pathway (Embden–Meyerhof) and the other metabolic pathways. The insert shows the production of 2,3-DPG in the Rapoport–Luebering shunt.

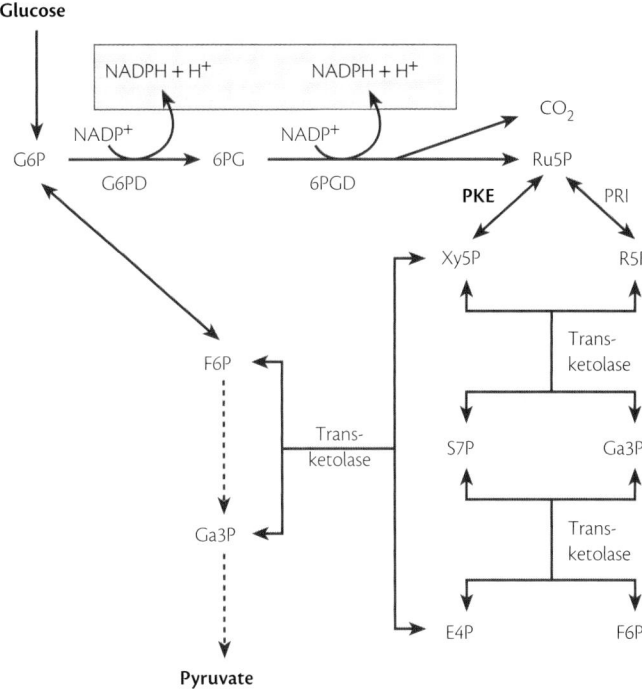

Fig. 22.5.9.4 The hexose monophosphate pathway. Intermediates: G6P, glucose 6-phosphate; F6P, fructose 6-phosphate; Ga3P, glyceraldehyde 3-phosphate; 6PG, 6-phosphogluconate; Ru5P, ribulose 5-phosphate; R5P, ribose 5-phosphate; Xy5P, xylulose 5-phosphate; S7P, sedoheptulose 7-phosphate; E4P, erythrose 4-phosphate. Enzymes: G6PD, glucose 6-phosphate dehydrogenease; 6PGD, 6-phosphogluconate dehydrogenase; PKE, epimerase; PRI, phosphoribose isomerase. Cosubstrates: $NADP^+$ and $NADPH + H^+$, oxidized and reduced forms of nicotinamide-adenine dinucleotide phosphate.

faba (favism). G6PD deficiency is the most common hereditary enzyme deficiency in humans, affecting hundreds of millions of people worldwide. For a full description of this disorder, see Chapter 22.3.12.

Pyruvate kinase deficiency
Aetiology
Pyruvate kinase converts phosphoenol pyruvate to lactate and in the process generates ATP (see Fig. 22.5.9.3). a deficiency in pyruvate kinase therefore impairs the glycolytic pathway, resulting in

families (Table 22.5.9.2). The two most common red-cell enzyme deficiencies—glucose-6-phosphate dehydrogenase deficiency and pyruvate kinase deficiency—are described below.

Glucose-6-phosphate dehydrogenase (G6PD) deficiency
G6PD catalyses the first step in the hexose-monophosphate shunt, which is responsible for reducing $NADP^+$ to NADPH. NADPH along with glutathione reductase maintains adequate supplies of reduced glutathione. Reduced glutathione is used by catalase and glutathione peroxidase to convert hydrogen peroxide to water. Oxygen radicals generated either through normal metabolism or by external oxidizing agents are converted to hydrogen peroxide, a highly oxidative agent. Therefore, through this series of enzyme reactions (Fig. 22.5.9.5) haemoglobin and other red-cell proteins are protected from oxidative damage. On the other hand, red cells deficient in G6PD are extremely sensitive to the oxidative actions of chemicals, drugs, infectious agents, and the bean *Vicia*

Table 22.5.9.1 Red-cell enzyme deficiencies associated with multisystem disease

Pathway	Enzyme	Clinical features
Embden–Meyerhof	Phosphofructokinase	Mild HA; myopathy; gout
	Triosephosphate isomerase	Moderate HA; neurological abnormalities
	Phosphoglycerokinase	Severe HA; mental retardation
	Aldolase	Mild HA; mental retardation
Hexose monophosphate shunt	Glutathione synthetase	HA; ± metabolic acidosis; ± neutropenia
	Glutamyl cysteine synthetase	HA; ± neurological abnormalities

HA, haemolytic anaemia.

Table 22.5.9.2 Other rare red-cell enzyme deficiencies

Pathway	Enzyme	Type of haemolytic anaemia
Embden–Meyerhof	Hexokinase	Mild to severe
	Glucose phosphate isomerase	Mild to severe
Hexose monophosphate shunt	Glutathione peroxidase	Oxidant-sensitive
	Glutathione reductase	Oxidant-sensitive
Nucleotide metabolism	Pyrimidine-5-nucleotidase	Mild to moderate (basophilic stippling)
	Adenylate kinase	Mild

decreased production of ATP and inadequate energy supply. Pyruvate kinase deficiency is inherited in an autosomal recessive fashion; homozygotes have little to no pyruvate kinase activity and exhibit haemolytic anaemia and splenomegaly. A further description of this disorder and other enzymopathies of the red cell is to be found in Chapter 22.5.11.

Acquired haemolytic anaemias

Immune haemolytic anaemias

Immune haemolysis may occur when IgG, IgM, or IgA antibodies and/or complement bind to the erythrocyte surface. The red-cell-bound antibodies may induce extravascular haemolysis, intravascular haemolysis, or both. Red cells coated with IgG typically undergo extravascular haemolysis during their transport through the reticuloendothelial system. Interactions between the Fc portion of IgG and surface Fc receptors allow the macrophages to phagocytose the coated erythrocytes. IgM, IgA, and, occasionally, IgG activate and fix complement to the erythrocyte surface. Macrophages also have receptors for the activated complement component C3b and likely phagocytose red cells through this pathway. The fixed complement can also induce intravascular haemolysis through activated membrane complex-mediated lysis.

The direct antiglobulin test (DAT) or direct Coombs' test detects the presence of IgG antibody or complement on the red-cell surface. IgM and IgA antibodies are not directly detectable with standard testing reagents. Rather, their presence may be indirectly demonstrated by the detection of complement on the erythrocyte. In rare cases, the haemolytic anaemia is due to non-complement-fixing IgM or IgA antibodies. In this situation the

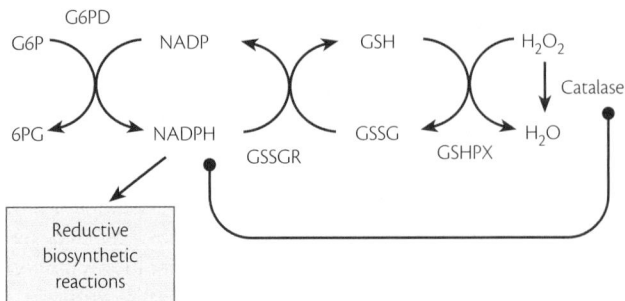

Fig. 22.5.9.5 The role of G6PD in red-cell metabolism: NADPH plays a dual role in (1) regeneration of glutathione (GSH) and (2) stabilization of catalase.

direct antiglobulin test will be falsely negative. Eluates can be obtained from the antibody-coated red cells to determine the specificity of the antibody. Alternatively, the antibody may be free in the serum and its specificity determined by the indirect antiglobulin test or indirect Coombs' test. The presence of antibody or complement on the red cell, however, need not reflect ongoing haemolysis. Rather, the diagnosis of haemolytic anaemia rests on clinical findings and other laboratory data, such as red-cell morphology, haemoglobin, bilirubin, haptoglobin, LDH levels, reticulocyte count, and the presence or absence of haemoglobinaemia, haemoglobinuria, or haemosiderinuria. The serological findings provide information as to whether an immune basis exists and what type of immune haemolytic anaemia may be present. Autoantibodies, alloantibodies, and drugs may induce immune haemolytic anaemias.

Autoimmune haemolytic anaemia

Haemolytic antibodies directed against the individual's own red cells may arise as a primary/idiopathic event or may be secondary to lymphoid malignancies, connective tissue disorders, and infection. Autoimmune haemolytic anaemia is best classified according to the temperature at which the antibody optimally binds to the erythrocyte. The four major types of autoimmune haemolytic anaemia are warm autoimmune haemolytic anaemia, cold agglutinin syndrome, paroxysmal cold haemoglobinuria, and mixed-type autoimmune haemolytic anaemia.

Warm autoimmune haemolytic anaemia

Aetiology The offending antibody in warm autoimmune haemolytic anaemia is typically IgG and can be found on the red cell, in the serum, or both. The exact specificity of the antibody is often difficult to determine. With very rare exception, warm-reactive autoantibodies bind to all red cells tested, while others appear to have broad specificity within the Rh system. Occasionally, warm reactive autoantibodies will have relative specificity against an individual antigen such as Rh(D), Rh(C), or Kell.

Clinical features Warm autoimmune haemolytic anaemia can arise at any age but is more common in older individuals, probably because of its association with lymphoid malignancies. Women are affected slightly more often than men. The direct antiglobulin test is positive for IgG and/or complement. In its mildest form the direct antiglobulin test is positive but red-cell survival is not significantly affected. Symptomatic patients present with anaemia, jaundice, and splenomegaly. Most patients with warm autoimmune haemolytic anaemia have a chronic, stable anaemia (haemoglobin <8 g/dl). In its severest form, patients present with fulminant intravascular haemolysis, progressive anaemia, congestive heart failure, respiratory distress, and neurological abnormalities. As with other haemolytic anaemias, the peripheral smear often demonstrates anisocytosis and reticulocytosis with spherocytes and macrocytes (Fig. 22.5.9.6). The platelet count is usually normal except in patients with Evans' syndrome where the autoantibody destroys both red cells and platelets. Rarely, patients with clinical and laboratory findings consistent with a warm autoimmune haemolytic anaemia may have a negative DAT. These cases have been attributed to IgA, IgM, or low affinity IgG antibodies. Alternatively, bound IgG has been reported below the level of routine DAT detection.

Treatment Corticosteroids, which presumably block macrophage Fc receptor activity and inhibit antibody production, are the primary

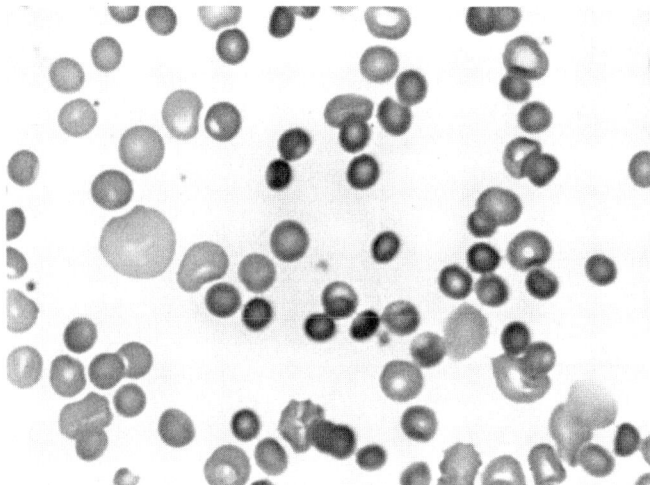

Fig. 22.5.9.6 The peripheral blood changes in autoimmune haemolytic anaemia. There is marked anisocytosis and anisochromia with many macrocytes and microspherocytes. The macrocytes reflect the reticulocytosis (×1000, Leishman stain).

therapy for autoimmune haemolytic anaemia. Prednisone at a dose of approximately 1 to 2 mg/kg body weight in divided doses is effective in most patients. Higher doses rarely provide additional benefit, but do increase the number and severity of side-effects. Treatment continues until the haemoglobin levels stabilize. The initial dose of prednisone can then be tapered at a rate of 5 to 10 mg/week. Once a dose of 10 mg/day is reached, the steroid taper should progress more slowly in order to determine the minimum controlling dose. Side effects may be reduced by using an alternate-day schedule. Splenectomy should be performed only in steroid-refractory patients or patients requiring unacceptably high doses of prednisone to maintain remission. Alternative therapies include azathioprine, cyclophosphamide, intravenous immunoglobulin (IVIG), danazol, and plasma exchange. These therapeutic options should be reserved for patients unfit for splenectomy or who have failed to respond to steroids and surgery. Recently, rituximab (chimeric anti-CD20 monoclonal antibody) has been demonstrated to have a favourable response rate and safety profile in patients with autoimmune haemolytic anaemia, prompting some experts to attempt a trial of rituximab prior to consideration of splenectomy.

The decision to transfuse patients with warm autoimmune haemolytic anaemia requires careful consideration. Due to the panreactive nature of most warm RBC autoantibodies, all crossmatched RBCs for transfusion will appear incompatible. Transfusion of ABO- and Rh-compatible blood should not be withheld because of this serological incompatibility if clinically indicated for a patient with symptomatic anaemia. Active serum autoantibodies can, however, mask the presence of clinically significant alloantibodies. Therefore, the most important consideration before transfusion is to confirm the presence or absence of alloantibodies in the patient's serum. Various autologous and allogeneic red-cell absorption techniques exist to remove the autoantibody from a sample of the patient's serum and allow identification of any existing alloantibodies. If clinically significant alloantibodies are present, red cells lacking the corresponding antigen(s) should be selected for transfusion. If possible, it is recommended that patients be antigen typed and provided with RBCs which are matched for all clinically significant antigens in order to prevent subsequent alloimmunization and delayed haemolytic transfusion reactions. Transfusions in life-threatening situations should not be delayed, however, if the above tests are not readily available or completed.

Cold agglutinin syndrome

Aetiology Cold agglutinin syndrome accounts for approximately one-quarter of all cases of autoimmune haemolytic anaemia. The disorder occurs as an acute or chronic condition. In cold autoimmune disorders the signs and symptoms of disease result from either the agglutination of red cells or from haemolysis. The autoantibodies are typically IgM and are most active at low temperatures. Rare examples of IgG and IgA cold-reactive autoantibodies have been reported. In the lower temperatures of the peripheral circulation, the IgM autoantibodies bind to red cells and activate complement. In warmer areas of the circulation, the IgM dissociates from the erythrocyte leaving activated complement fixed to the red-cell surface. The autoantibody specificity in cold agglutinin syndrome is usually anti-I. Anti-i specificity is associated with infectious mononucleosis.

Clinical features Acute cold autoimmune haemolytic anaemia is commonly seen in adolescents and young adults following infection with *Mycoplasma pneumoniae* or infectious mononucleosis. Haemolysis occurs approximately 1 to 2 weeks after infection and is most commonly associated with a rise in polyclonal anti-I IgM antibody with *Mycoplasma pneumonia* or polyclonal anti-i IgM antibody with infectious mononucleosis. Chronic cold autoimmune haemolytic anaemia occurs most commonly in older people, either idiopathically or associated with lymphoma, chronic lymphocytic leukaemia, or Waldenström's macroglobulinaemia. Patients may experience chronic intravascular haemolysis and anaemia that are exacerbated by cold temperature. Patients are often also plagued by episodes of Raynaud's phenomenon. Monoclonal IgM antibodies with κ light chains and anti-I specificity usually cause the red-cell agglutination and haemolysis in this condition. In typical cases of chronic cold agglutinin disease, the cold agglutinin titre is very high ($>1:10^5$). The thermal amplitude of the cold agglutinin, not the titre of the antibody, most accurately predicts the severity of the disease. Examination of the peripheral smear shows red-cell agglutination. The direct antiglobulin test is positive for complement.

Treatment Acute cold agglutinin disease is a rare form that is always self-limited. Supportive measures, including transfusions and avoidance of cold, may suffice. Treatment of the mycoplasma infection, if detected, shortens the duration and severity of the haemolysis. Corticosteroids are usually not helpful, and splenectomy is almost never indicated.

Severe cold autoimmune haemolytic anaemia secondary to a B-cell neoplasm can be treated with chlorambucil, cyclophosphamide, or α-interferon. Blood transfusion should be avoided. In situations of life-threatening anaemia, the blood should be given slowly through a blood warmer. Hypothermia must be avoided during surgery (especially surgical procedures involving extracorporeal circuits) in patients with cold autoimmune haemolytic anaemia. Plasma exchange may be helpful as a temporizing measure in acute situations due to the primarily intravascular location of IgM. Corticosteroids and splenectomy are rarely effective. Rituximab, anti-CD-20 monoclonal antibody, has demonstrated some clinical effectiveness in published cases of cold agglutinin disease.

Paroxysmal cold haemoglobinuria

Aetiology Paroxysmal cold haemoglobinuria is the rarest form of autoimmune haemolytic anaemia. The disorder is caused by the complement-fixing Donath–Landsteiner IgG antibody. In the cold, this antibody binds to, and irreversibly fixes, complement to the red-cell membrane. Upon return to warmer temperatures, the antibody dissociates from the red cell leaving activated complement to lyse the cell. The Donath–Landsteiner antibody appears to have an anti-P specificity allowing it to bind to practically all red cells.

Clinical features Patients present with acute intravascular haemolysis, abdominal pain, peripheral cyanosis, Raynaud's phenomenon, haemoglobinaemia, and haemoglobinuria after exposure to cold. In the past, paroxysmal cold haemoglobinuria was commonly associated with congenital syphilis but most cases are now associated with viral infections in children or are idiopathic in adults. During or shortly after a haemolytic episode, the direct antiglobulin test may be positive for complement but will be negative for IgG.

Treatment No specific therapy for paroxysmal cold haemoglobinuria exists; steroids are not useful. Most postinfectious cases of paroxysmal cold haemoglobinuria are self-limited and require only supportive care. Avoidance of cold ambient temperatures can help prevent recurrent attacks in patients with chronic paroxysmal cold haemoglobinuria. Transfusion is indicated only for severe haemolysis and life-threatening anaemia. Since the Donath–Landsteiner antibody rarely causes agglutination, most random donor blood units will be compatible with patient sera. Transfusions with extremely rare P-antigen-negative blood should be reserved only for those patients who do not respond to random donor blood. The use of a blood warmer should be considered.

Mixed-type autoimmune haemolytic anaemia

Aetiology Approximately 8% of all autoimmune haemolytic anaemias are of the mixed type. Both IgG and complement are present on the red cells. Both warm-reactive IgG autoantibodies and cold-reactive agglutinating IgM autoantibodies are present in the serum. The warm-reactive IgG autoantibodies are indistinguishable from antibodies encountered in warm autoimmune haemolytic anaemia. The IgM autoantibodies are unlike those in cold-agglutinin syndrome in that they generally have low titres at 4°C and have high thermal amplitudes, reacting at 30°C or above. These IgM autoantibodies usually have no distinguishable specificity, but on occasion have I or i specificities.

Clinical features Mixed-type autoimmune haemolytic anaemia may be idiopathic or secondary, most commonly associated with systemic lupus erythematosus. The haemolytic anaemia is often severe and chronic with intermittent exacerbations. Exposure to cold does not increase the haemolysis.

Treatment Steroids, splenectomy, or cytotoxic agents often provide therapeutic benefit in mixed-type autoimmune haemolytic anaemia. If blood transfusions are necessary, selection of blood should adhere to transfusion guidelines outlined earlier for warm autoimmune haemolytic anaemia. Administration of blood through a warmer should be considered.

Drug-induced haemolytic anaemia

Drugs may induce antibodies to bind to the erythrocyte surface resulting in a positive direct antiglobulin test or haemolysis. There are four mechanisms by which drugs can cause a positive direct antiglobulin test: (1) drug hapten, (2) immune complex formation, (3) autoantibody production, and (4) nonspecific adsorption. Only the first three mechanisms are associated with haemolysis. Treatment and prevention are as straightforward as drug avoidance.

Drug hapten Certain drugs bind to the red-cell membrane with a high affinity. Association of the drug with the membrane constituents allows the drug to act as a hapten. The antibodies produced are commonly IgG and are directed predominantly against the drug. Extravascular haemolysis develops gradually, but may be life-threatening if left untreated. After the offending drug is identified and withdrawn, the positive direct antiglobulin test and the haemolysis may persist for several weeks. Serum from these patients will not react with other red cells unless the drug is also present. Penicillin and the cephalosporins are the most notorious examples of this phenomenon. Approximately 3% of patients receiving large doses of penicillin (millions of unit per day) intravenously will develop a positive direct antiglobulin test. Only the rare patient develops haemolytic anaemia.

Immune complex Other drugs induce the binding of IgM or IgG antibodies that activate complement and cause intravascular haemolysis. The antibodies appear to recognize both the drug and a component of the red-cell membrane. The direct antiglobulin test is often positive for complement but not antibody. Haemoglobinaemia and haemoglobinuria are common. Renal failure occurs in about half of the cases. Once the offending drug is withdrawn, the haemolysis stops. Serum from these patients will lyse normal red cells only in the presence of the drug. Quinine, quinidine, phenacetin, chlorpropamide, and sulfonylureas are examples.

Autoantibodies Some drugs stimulate the synthesis of red-cell autoantibodies. Patient serum and red-cell eluates react with normal red cells in the absence of the drug. The autoantibodies are indistinguishable from those found in warm autoimmune haemolytic anaemia. The direct antiglobulin test usually becomes positive after 3 to 6 months of drug administration. The haemolysis typically ceases within 2 weeks after the withdrawal of the drug, but the direct antiglobulin test can remain positive for up to 2 years. α-methyldopa, L-dopa, procainamide, mefenamic acid, and sulindac are examples of drugs that can stimulate the production of red cell autoantibodies.

Nonspecific protein adsorption Often a drug-induced positive direct antiglobulin test reflects nonimmunological adsorption of protein, including immunoglobulins. First-generation cephalosporins were originally associated with this phenomenon. More recently, other drugs, including suramin, cisplatin, and sulbactam, have also been implicated. This mechanism is not associated with reduced red-cell survival.

Alloimmune haemolytic anaemias
Acute haemolytic transfusion reactions

Aetiology The most catastrophic cases of alloimmune haemolysis occur following the transfusion of ABO-incompatible red cells. Naturally occurring IgM anti-A and anti-B antibodies bind to the incompatible red cells and activate complement resulting in intravascular haemolysis. Human error leading to the misidentification of patients, their blood samples, or the units of red cells to be transfused is responsible for virtually all cases of ABO incompatibility.

Only rarely do other non-ABO IgG alloantibodies cause acute, severe haemolysis.

Clinical features Symptoms of an acute haemolytic transfusion reaction may begin after the infusion of as little as 10 ml of incompatible blood. The signs and symptoms include fever, chills, nausea, vomiting, hypotension, respiratory distress, haemoglobinuria, and chest or flank pain. Despite treatment, acute haemolytic transfusions reactions can result in renal failure, disseminated intravascular coagulation, and even death.

Treatment Once an acute haemolytic transfusion reaction is suspected, the blood transfusion should be stopped immediately. Intravenous access should be maintained for aggressive treatment of hypotension with intravenous fluids. Pressor agents (low-dose dopamine) are crucial for mitigation of renal complications. Other critical measures include monitoring the urine output and promoting renal blood flow with diuretics (furosemide or mannitol). Transfusion of platelets, plasma, or cryoprecipitate may be necessary for the treatment of life threatening bleeding secondary to disseminated intravascular coagulation.

Delayed haemolytic transfusion reactions

Aetiology Delayed haemolytic transfusion reactions typically occur in patients who have been alloimmunized to RBC antigens by previous transfusions or pregnancies. Approximately 2 to 3% of transfusion recipients become alloimmunized to non-ABO red-cell antigens. Haemolysis is not generally seen during the primary immune response since the transfused red cells often disappear from the circulation before antibody titres reach clinically significant levels. In the absence of further antigenic stimuli antibody titres may diminish to undetectable levels. Subsequent transfusion of red cells possessing the offending antigen, however, will induce an anamnestic response with reappearance of the IgG antibodies within hours to days. Binding of the IgG antibody to the transfused antigen-positive red cells results in a positive direct antiglobulin test and possibly mild to moderate extravascular haemolysis. Although numerous specificities are described, antibodies against the Rh and Kidd system antigens are the most commonly implicated in delayed haemolytic transfusion reactions.

Clinical features Most patients experiencing a delayed haemolytic transfusion reaction present with fever, jaundice, and decreasing haemoglobin levels 1 to 2 weeks after the transfusion of incompatible red cells. Delayed haemolytic transfusion reactions are often discovered during evaluation for fever of unknown origin or when the haemoglobin level fails to increase following transfusion.

Treatment Treatment is rarely necessary; acute renal failure or disseminated intravascular coagulation is uncommon. If a delayed haemolytic transfusion reaction is suspected, both the patient's serum and an eluate from the circulating red cells should be tested for alloantibodies. If alloantibodies are present, their specificities should be determined. Donor red-cell units lacking the offending antigen should be selected for all subsequent transfusions, even if the antibody is no longer detectable on routine antibody screens.

Passenger lymphocyte haemolysis

Aetiology Recipients of a haematopoietic or a solid-organ transplant may experience delayed extravascular haemolysis. In this circumstance, lymphocytes of donor origin produce haemolytic antibodies against ABO or other red-cell antigens possessed by the recipient.

Clinical features Haemolysis due to passenger lymphocytes is most commonly seen in out-of-group yet ABO-compatible liver and bone marrow transplants (group A or group B recipients of group O tissue) but can also occur in recipients of lung, heart, and kidney transplants. A positive DAT and haemolysis can begin within several days after the transplant and continue for several months.

Treatment If significant ABO haemolysis occurs, patients should be transfused with group O red cells. If non-ABO haemolysis is present, elution of the patient's red cells may help to identify the antibody specificity and allow transfusion of antigen-negative red cells.

Haemolytic disease of the newborn (HDN)
Haemolytic disease of the newborn occurs when maternal IgG antibodies cross the placenta and bind to fetal red cells resulting in extravascular haemolysis. Usually these antibodies possess specificities within the Rh or ABO blood group systems. Occasionally the antibodies are directed against other red-cell antigens such as the Kell, Kidd, and Duffy. In the mildest cases, anaemia develops after birth and is of little clinical consequence. In more severe cases the neonate develops progressive anaemia and jaundice within the first week of life. If left untreated, bilirubin may reach levels associated with kernicterus causing brain damage and death. In the most severe cases, the fetus develops profound anaemia during gestation and may be stillborn or delivered grossly oedematous (hydrops fetalis). An infant with hydrops fetalis also has ascites, hepatosplenomegaly, and erythroblastosis and usually dies shortly after birth.

Rhesus incompatibility
Although incompatibility for the A and B blood group antigens is now the most common cause of haemolytic disease of the newborn, the most severe cases are still attributed to the anti-Rh(D) antibody. In the majority of these cases, haemolytic disease of the newborn occurs in Rh(D)-negative women carrying a Rh(D)-positive fetus. The mother develops anti-D IgG antibodies following exposure to the D antigen during a previous pregnancy, or as a result of the transfusion of D-antigen-positive red cells. One half of all cases of Rh(D) alloimmunization are due to transplacental haemorrhage from the fetus at the time of delivery. Spontaneous transplacental haemorrhage can also occur during gestation, particularly during the third trimester. The risk of transplacental haemorrhage increases with ectopic pregnancy, spontaneous or therapeutic abortion, chorionic villus sampling, amniocentesis, caesarean section, and trauma. Approximately 16% of untreated Rh(D)-negative women who deliver a Rh(D)-positive child will become alloimmunized to the D antigen. Exposure of a Rh(D)-negative mother to as little as 0.1 ml of fetal D-positive blood can result in sensitization.

It is essential to identify pregnant women at risk for Rh(D) haemolytic disease of the newborn to prevent sensitization. All pregnant women should have their ABO and Rh types identified as early as possible. Their serum should be screened for alloantibodies against the D antigen and other red-cell antigens. Pregnant women who are D-antigen-negative and have an initial negative antibody screen should have their serum retested for alloantibodies at 28 weeks gestation. If the initial antibody screen is found positive, antibody titres should be followed at 2- to 4-week intervals to determine whether further sensitization is occurring. The presence of an antibody, however, does not indicate ongoing haemolysis in all cases.

Naturally occurring IgM antibodies are common during pregnancy but do not cross the placenta. Furthermore, fetal red cells may lack the antigen corresponding to the mother's antibody. Molecular typing of the father's DNA or even fetal DNA is available for several red-cell antigens including D, E/e, C/c, Jka/Jkb, and K1/K2. A rising titre of anti-D antibody or other clinically significant red-cell alloantibodies indicates ongoing sensitization and possible haemolytic disease of the newborn.

Middle cerebral artery peak systolic velocity measured by Doppler ultrasonography is a noninvasive and accurate tool which can be used to monitor and assess the severity of haemolysis. If the fetus is experiencing significant haemolysis and anaemia, clinical intervention must be prompt. Before 34 weeks of gestation, intrauterine transfusion with leucoreduced and irradiated blood lacking the offending antigen should be performed. After 36 weeks gestation, induced labour should be considered. Upon birth of an 'at risk' fetus a sample of cord blood should undergo a direct antiglobulin test and have measurements of haemoglobin and bilirubin performed. If the direct antiglobulin test on the cord blood sample is positive and the mother's antibody screen remains negative, haemolytic disease secondary to ABO incompatibility or antibodies against low-incidence red-cell antigens should be considered.

Infants with severe anaemia or severe jaundice should undergo exchange transfusion. Phototherapy can also be used to decrease bilirubin levels. A nonsensitized Rh(D)-antigen-negative mother's blood should also be tested to determine the amount of fetomaternal haemorrhage at delivery. Administration of 300 µg of IgG anti-D (RhIg) within 72 h of delivery will protect 99% of D-antigen-negative mothers from developing anti-D antibodies. Prophylactic administration of RhIg at 28 weeks gestation and following invasive procedures or traumatic events will virtually eliminate the chance of alloimmunization. Patients with large transplacental haemorrhages quantitated by the Kleihauer–Betke acid-elution technique should receive additional RhIg at a dose equivalent to 300 µg for every 15 ml of fetal red blood cells or 30 ml of fetal blood.

ABO incompatibility

Although 20% of pregnancies are ABO incompatible, severe haemolytic disease of the newborn due to ABO incompatibility is rare. Group A and group B infants of group O mothers are at greatest risk, due to the IgG antibody anti-A,B made by group O individuals. Unlike with the Rh(D) antigen, ABO-haemolytic disease of the newborn occurs during the first pregnancy as often as subsequent pregnancies. Most cases are asymptomatic to mild and exchange transfusion with group O red cells is rarely required. The decrease in severity observed in cases due to ABO incompatibility may be due to decreased surface expression of the A and B antigens on fetal cells, and the presence of A and B antigens on many tissues leading to dilution of the antibody effect.

Nonimmune acquired haemolytic anaemias

Red-cell survival may also be reduced by a number of noninherited, nonimmune mechanisms. As red cells circulate they are vulnerable to a variety of insults that may cause structural or metabolic alterations. These changes generally result in reduced red-cell deformability leading ultimately to extravascular haemolysis.

These insults include infection, mechanical trauma, and exposure to chemicals, heat, or venom. They often also cause intravascular haemolysis by directly lysing the red-cell membrane. Other less-understood causes of acquired nonimmune haemolytic anaemias are listed in Box 22.5.9.2.

Infection

Infectious causes of haemolysis are primarily parasites and bacteria. Direct parasitization of red cells by *Plasmodium falciparum*, *P. vivax*, and *P. malariae* causes both intravascular haemolysis due to direct membrane destruction and extravascular haemolysis due to membrane alteration and activation of the reticuloendothelial system. Infrequently, *in utero* infection of the fetus with *Toxoplasma gondii* resembles severe haemolytic disease of the newborn. Infants are born hydropic and severely anaemic. Premature delivery and stillbirth are common. *Babesia microti*, endemic in areas of the North American north-east and midwest, is transmitted by ticks and causes severe haemolysis during the erythrocytic phase of its life cycle. Bacterial infections, particularly Gram-negative organisms which produce endotoxin or proteolytic enzymes, may produce mechanical haemolysis by inducing disseminated intravascular haemolysis or red-cell membrane damage via degradation of membrane phospholipids and proteins. *Bartonella bacilliformis* endemic to western South America causes Oroya fever characterized by fever, chills, musculoskeletal pain, and acute intravascular haemolysis.

Chemical

Drugs and chemicals known to cause haemolysis through direct oxidative damage are summarized in Tables 22.5.9.3 and 22.5.9.4. In most cases the strong oxidant activity of these chemicals overwhelm normally functioning reduction mechanisms responsible for protecting haemoglobin and the red-cell membrane. Variability in

---

Box 22.5.9.2 Other causes of acquired haemolytic anaemia

- Paroxysmal nocturnal haemoglobinuria
- Lipid disorders
- Liver disease
  - Hepatitis
  - Cirrhosis
  - Gilbert's disease

Chronic alcoholism (Zieve's syndrome)

- Wilson's disease
- Vitamin E deficiency
- Hypersplenism
- Hyperbaric oxygen therapy
- Total body irradiation
- Chronic large granular lymphocytic leukaemia
- Renal disease
- Cardiopulmonary bypass
- Freshwater/saltwater drowning

Table 22.5.9.3 Some drugs that may induce haemolysis in G6PD-deficient individuals

Antimalarials	Sulfones
Primaquine	Thiazolesulfone
Pamaquine	Dapsone
Pentaquine	Nitrofurans
Chloroquine	Nitrofurantoin
Quinidine	Nitrofurazone
Quinine	Furazolidone
Quinacrine	**Antipyretics/analgesics**
Sulfonamides	Acetanilide
Sulfanilamide	Aspirin
Sulfacetamide	Paracetamol (acetominophen)
Sulfapyridine	Phenacetin
Sulfamethoxazole	Aminopyrine
Sulfafurazole	**Other drugs**
Sulfamethoxypyridazine	Methylene blue
Sulfoxone	Nalidixic acid
Sulfadiazine	Chloramphenicol
Sulfamerizine	Doxorubicin
Sulfisoxazole	Dimercaprol
Sulfadimidine	Probenecid
Other chemicals	Vitamin K analogues
Napthalene	Phenazopyridine
Trinitrotoluene	*p*-Aminosalicylic acid
Toluidine blue	Ciprofloxacin
	Norfloxacin

the absorption of the chemical or its metabolism determine whether a particular individual will develop chemical-induced haemolytic anaemia. Often it is the chemical's metabolite that is responsible for inducing haemolysis. The red cells of newborns do not have functional reduction mechanisms and thus are more sensitive to oxidant activity.

Table 22.5.9.4 Chemicals that cause haemolysis

Oxidative haemolysis	
Nitrofurantoin	Arsine gas
Sulfonamides	Chlorate
Sulfones (dapsone)	*p*-Aminosalicylic acid
Phenazopyridine	*p*-Nitroaniline
Phenacetin	Nitrobenzene derivatives
Phenylhydrazine	Vitamin K analogues
Phenothiazine	Paraquat
Isobutyl nitrate	Naphthalene (mothballs)
Amyl nitrite	Hydrogen peroxide
Nonoxidative haemolysis	
Copper	Lead

Mechanical

Mechanical fragmentation of erythrocytes can occur when foreign material is placed within the vasculature, when fibrin strands or platelet thrombi obstruct small blood vessels, or when direct physical forces compress superficial blood vessels.

Foreign material

Mechanical haemolysis occurs most commonly with artificial valvular prostheses, particularly when accompanied by turbulent blood flow. Bacterial endocarditis and associated valvular vegetations can also cause fragmentation of red cells. Haemolysis also occurs in up to 10% of patients with transjugular intrahepatic portosystemic shunts (TIPS). Increased cardiac output as a result of anaemia, exercise, or medications can increase the rate of red-cell fragmentation. The peripheral smear usually demonstrates schistocytes and microspherocytes. Severe haemolysis usually requires surgical repair.

Microangiopathic haemolytic anaemia (MAHA)

MAHA describes a spectrum of disorders characterized by mechanical destruction of red cells resulting from thrombi that occlude the microvasculature. The red cells are probably fragmented during their forced passage through the meshwork of fibrin strands that make up the microthrombi. The degree of anaemia is variable. The peripheral smear reveals findings typical of mechanical haemolysis including schistocytes, microspherocytes, and a reticulocytosis (Fig. 22.5.9.7). The absence of a positive direct antiglobulin test along with significant thrombocytopenia helps to confirm the diagnosis. Two other major forms of MAHA are haemolytic uraemic syndrome and thrombotic thrombocytopenic purpura (TTP).

Haemolytic uraemic syndrome Haemolytic uraemic syndrome is primarily, but not exclusively, a disease of childhood. The disorder consists of widespread damage to the vascular endothelium and fibrin deposition. These pathological changes are frequently most severe in the renal arterioles and glomerular capillaries. The disorder usually develops following a febrile illness. Numerous reports have documented the development of haemolytic uraemic syndrome following infections with toxin-secreting strains of *Escherichia coli*

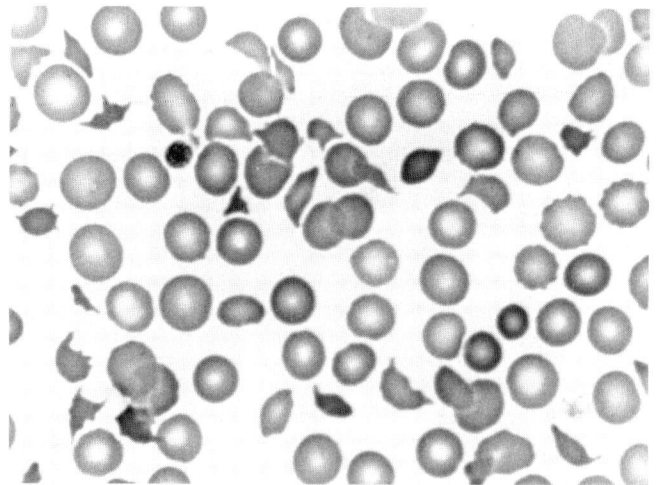

Fig. 22.5.9.7 The peripheral blood changes in microangiopathic haemolytic anaemia. This patient had recurrent thrombocytopenic purpura and the marked fragmentation of the red cells together with microspherocytosis is evident on the blood film (× 1000, Leishman stain).

(strain O157:H7) or shigella. Initial nausea, vomiting, and diarrhoea can develop into severe abdominal pain and bloody diarrhoea. Acutely, the child may develop hypertension, oliguria, purpura, bleeding, and anaemia. If left untreated, convulsions, coma, and death may occur. Mortality rates as high as 10% have been associated with haemolytic uraemic syndrome. The peripheral smear exhibits schistocytosis and thrombocytopenia. Therapy consists mainly of supportive care, transfusion, control of blood pressure, and dialysis.

Thrombotic thrombocytopenic purpura (TTP) TTP is caused by either a congenital deficiency of, or an acquired inhibitor to, a serum metalloprotease (ADAMTS 13) which is responsible for cleaving unusually large multimers of von Willebrand factor. Left uncleaved, the large von Willebrand factor multimers induce TTP by causing the agglutination of circulating platelets. Most episodes of TTP occur without an obvious inciting event. However, TTP has been associated with infection, pregnancy, transplantation, AIDS, and drugs such as mitomycin C, ticlopidine, ciclosporin, and tacrolimus. TTP occurs mainly in adults and more commonly involves the central nervous system, although renal abnormalities can occur. The onset is often sudden with fever, purpura, petechiae, anaemia, thrombocytopenia, and neurological abnormalities. The neurological sequelae include convulsions, coma, paralysis, delirium, and stroke. The peripheral smear demonstrates schistocytes, thrombocytopenia, and a reticulocytosis. During acute episodes front-line therapy includes steroids and daily plasma exchange with fresh frozen plasma or virally-inactivated solvent-detergent plasma (SD plasma). Plasma exchange probably accomplishes one or more of the following: (1) removal of the antibody to the protease; (2) removal of large multimers of von Willebrand factor; (3) replenishment of normal protease.

In patients who do not initially respond to plasma exchange with fresh frozen plasma, cryopoor-supernatant is often used as the replacement fluid. Cryopoor-supernatant contains markedly reduced levels of normal von Willebrand factor which is believed to enhance the formation of microthrombi in some patients. Individuals with drug-induced TTP appear to be less responsive to therapy. Additional therapies in refractory or relapsing patients include rituximab, cytoxan, ciclosporin, vincristine, and splenectomy. Anecdotal evidence suggests that platelet transfusion can exacerbate the disorder. Therefore, platelet transfusions should be avoided unless absolutely necessary to treat haemorrhage.

March haemoglobinuria
Haemoglobinuria can occur in soldiers or joggers following extended periods of marching or running on a hard surface, or in karate or conga drummer enthusiasts following practice. This mechanical haemolysis appears to be the result of red-cell compression in superficial blood vessels during the period of contact between the extremity and the hard surface. The peripheral smear is normal. Treatment is unnecessary as the syndrome is otherwise symptomless and lacks significant clinical sequelae.

Thermal haemolysis
Normal red cells undergo fragmentation and lysis when heated to temperatures of 49°C or higher. The two most common clinical situations associated with heat-induced red-cell lysis are the use of faulty blood warmers during transfusion or patients who have sustained extensive burns.

Venom
Haemolysis has been observed following bee and wasp stings, spider bites, and snake bites. The haemolysis occurs secondary to disseminated intravascular coagulation or as a result of proteolytic enzymes contained within the venom.

Further reading
Agre P, *et al.* (1985). Partial deficiency of erythrocyte spectrin in hereditary spherocytosis. *Nature*, **314**, 380–3.

Bretcher ME (ed.) (2005). *Technical manual*, 15th edn. American Association of Blood Banks, Bethesda, MD.

Conboy JG, *et al.* (1993). An isoform specific mutation in the protein 4.1 gene results in hereditary elliptocytosis and complete deficiency of protein 4.1 in erythrocytes but not in nonerythroid cells. *J Clin Invest*, **91**, 77–82.

Davidson RJL (1969). March or exertional hemoglobinuria. *Semin Hematol*, **6**, 150.

Freedman J (1987). The significance of complement on the red cell surface. *Transfus Med Rev*, **1**, 58–70.

Furlan M, *et al.* (1998). Von Willebrand factor-cleaving protease in thrombotic thrombocytopenic purpura and the hemolytic-uremic syndrome. *N Engl J Med*, **399**, 1578–84.

Garratty G (1987). The significance of IgG on the red cell surface. *Transfus Med Rev*, **1**, 47–57.

Hows J (1986). Donor-derived red blood cell antibodies and immune hemolysis after allogeneic bone marrow transplantation. *Blood*, **67**, 177–81.

Judd WJ. (2001). Practice guidelines for prenatal and perinatal immunohematology, revisited. *Transfusion*, **41**, 1445–52.

Leger RM, Garratty G (1999). Evaluation of methods for detecting alloantibodies underlying warm autoantibodies. *Transfusion*, **39**, 11–16.

Liu SC, Palek J, Prchal J (1982). Defective spectrin dimer-dimer association in hereditary elliptocytosis. *Proc Nat Acad Sci U S A*, **79**, 2072–6.

Marsh GW, Lewis SM (1969). Cardiac hemolytic anemia. *Semin Hematol*, **6**, 133–45.

Moake, JL. (2002). Thrombotic microangiopathies. *N Engl J Med*, **347**, 589–600.

Petz LD, Garratty G (2004). *Immune hemolytic anemias*. Churchill Livingstone, Philadelphia.

Prchal JT, Gregg XT (2000). Red cell enzymopathies. In: Hoffman R, *et al.* (eds) *Hematology: basic principles and practice*, pp. 561–76. Churchill Livingstone, Philadelphia.

Ramsey G (1991). Red cell antibodies arising from solid organ transplants. *Transfusion*, **31**, 76–86.

Savvides P, *et al.* (1993). Combined spectrin and ankyrin deficiency is common in autosomal dominant hereditary spherocytosis. *Blood*, **82**, 2953–60.

Schrier SL (2000). Extrinsic nonimmune haemolytic anemias. In: Hoffman R, *et al.* (eds) *Hematology: basic principles and practice*, pp. 630–8. Churchill Livingstone, Philadelphia.

Shepard KV, Bukowski RM (1987). The treatment of thrombotic thrombocytopenic purpura with exchange transfusions, plasma infusions, and plasma exchange. *Semin Hematol*, **24**, 178–93.

Shirey RS, *et al.* (2002). Prophylactic antigen-matched donor blood for patients with warm autoantibodies: an algorithm for transfusion management. *Transfusion*, **41**, 1435–41.

Shirey RS, *et al.* (2007). Hemolytic transfusion reactions: acute and delayed. In: Hillyer C, *et al.* (eds) *Blood banking and transfusion medicine: basic principles and practice*, pp. 668–676. Churchill Livingstone, Philadelphia.

Shulman NR, Reid DM (1993). Mechanisms of drug-induced immunologically mediated cytopenias. *Transfus Med Rev*, **7**, 215–29.

Tsai H-M, Lian EC-Y (1998). Antibodies to von Willebrand factor-cleaving protease in acute thrombotic thrombocytopenic purpura. *N Engl J Med*, **399**, 1585–94.

Vulliamy TJ, Beutler E, Luzzatto L (1993). Variants of glucose 6-phosphate dehydrogenase are due to missense mutations spread throughout the coding region of the gene. *Hum Mut*, **2**, 159–67.

22.5.10 Disorders of the red cell membrane

Patrick G. Gallagher

Essentials

The integrity of the red-cell membrane depends on molecular inter-actions between proteins and protein–lipid interactions: vertical interactions stabilize the membrane lipid bilayer; horizontal interactions provide resistance against shear stress.

Hereditary spherocytosis

This disorder affects 1 in 25 000 individuals of northern European descent. There is typically a dominant family history, but the condition is genetically heterogeneous: combined spectrin and ankyrin deficiency is the most common defect observed, followed by band 3 deficiency, isolated spectrin deficiency, and protein 4.2 deficiency. These affect vertical membrane interactions with loss of surface area relative to red-cell volume.

Clinical features and diagnosis—the key clinical manifestations are anaemia and signs of persistent haemolysis, with jaundice and a marked propensity to gallstones. The best diagnostic test is probably the incubated osmotic fragility test, in which spherocytes burst at higher saline concentrations than normal.

Complications and treatment—parvovirus B19 infection of eryth-ropoietic precursors may cause acute aplastic crises. Megaloblastic anaemia due to folate deficiency occurs in response to increased requirements during growth and pregnancy, but is preventable with supplementation. Splenectomy cures or alleviates the anaemia in most patients and reduces the risk of gallstones.

Hereditary elliptocytosis

This disorder occurs with a frequency of 1 in 2000 to 1 in 4000 worldwide, and is more frequent in parts of Africa. The inheritance is usually dominant, with defects in red-cell proteins such as α and β spectrin causing disturbances in horizontal interactions in the erythrocyte membrane

Clinical features, diagnosis, and treatment—most patients are asymptomatic and are typically diagnosed incidentally during testing for unrelated conditions, but about 10% experience haemo-lysis, anaemia, splenomegaly, and intermittent jaundice. Diagnosis is based on the presence of elliptocytes on peripheral blood smear. Treatment is rarely required.

Other conditions

These include (1) Hereditary pyropoikilocytosis—a rare cause of severe haemolytic anaemia, usually seen in patients of African descent. (2) South-East Asian (or Melanesian) ovalocytosis—an asymptomatic autosomal dominant condition due to band 3 protein abnormalities that confer resistance to invasion by malaria parasites. (3) Stomatocytosis—characterized by mouth-shaped red cells; a heterogeneous group of disorders that are often asympto-matic but may cause haemolysis and anaemia; may be hereditary (e.g. missense mutations in band 3) or acquired (e.g. cholestatic liver disease, alcoholism, vinca alkaloids). (4) Acanthocytosis—characterized by contracted red cells with spiky projections; may be hereditary (e.g. neuroacanthocytosis syndromes, abetalipoprotein-aemia) or acquired (e.g. severe hepatic disease).

The red cell membrane

Composition and function

Although the primary structure and a number of the important functions of the red cell membrane have been known for many years, its study continues to yield important insights into our understanding of membrane structure and function. The red cell membrane is composed of three major structural elements: a lipid bilayer primarily composed of phospholipids and cholesterol; inte-gral proteins embedded in the lipid bilayer that span the mem-brane; and a membrane skeleton on the internal side of the red cell membrane.

The membrane and its skeleton provide the erythrocyte with the ability to undergo significant deformation without fragmentation or loss of integrity during its travel through the microcirculation. The membrane also assembles and organizes the proteins of the lipid bilayer and the membrane skeleton, allowing the red cell to participate in a wide range of functions. These include influenc-ing cellular metabolism by selectively and reversibly binding and inactivating glycolytic enzymes, retaining organic phosphates and other vital compounds, removing metabolic waste, and seques-tering the reductants required to prevent corrosion by oxygen. During erythropoiesis, the membrane responds to erythropoietin and imports the iron required for the synthesis of haemoglobin. The lipid bilayer provides an impermeable barrier between the cytoplasm and the external environment and helps maintain a slippery exterior so that erythrocytes do not adhere to endothe-lial cells or aggregate in the microcirculation. The membrane also participates in erythrocyte biogenesis and ageing. Finally, the membrane participates in the maintenance of pH homeostasis by participating in chloride–bicarbonate exchange.

Interactions of membrane proteins and disorders of red cell shape

Membrane protein–protein and protein–lipid interactions have been classified into two categories, vertical and horizontal interac-tions (Fig. 22.5.10.1). Vertical interactions stabilize the lipid bilayer membrane while horizontal interactions support the structural integrity of erythrocytes after their exposure to shear stress. The interactions between proteins and lipids of the erythrocyte mem-brane are more complex than this simplistic model, but it serves as a useful starting point for understanding red cell membrane inter-actions, particularly in membrane-related disorders. According to this model, hereditary spherocytosis (HS) is a disorder of vertical interactions. Although the primary molecular defects in HS are heterogeneous (see below), one common feature of HS erythro-cytes is a weakening of the vertical contacts between the skeleton

Acknowledgement: Supported in part by grants from the National Institutes of Health, NIDDK, and NHLBI.

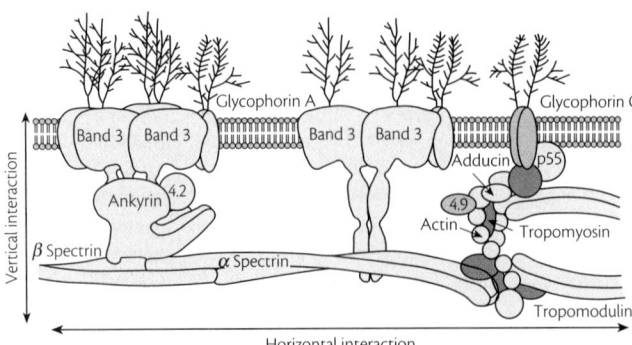

Fig. 22.5.10.1 Schematic diagram of the red cell membrane (not to scale). Membrane–protein and membrane–lipid interactions can be divided into two categories: (1) vertical interactions, which are perpendicular to the plane of the membrane and involve spectrin–ankyrin–Band 3 interactions, spectrin–Protein 4.1–glycophorin C interactions, and weak interactions between spectrin and the lipid bilayer, and (2) horizontal interactions, which are parallel to the plane of the membrane.

(From Tse WT, Lux SE (1999). Red blood cell membrane disorders. *Br J Haematol,* **104**, 2–13, with permission.)

and the lipid bilayer. As a result, the lipid bilayer membrane is destabilized, leading to release of lipids in the form of skeleton-free lipid vesicles, which in turn results in membrane surface area deficiency and spherocytosis. In this model, hereditary elliptocytosis is a defect of horizontal interactions, primarily those involving spectrin dimer self-association. Defects of horizontal interactions disrupt the membrane skeletal lattice leading to elliptocytic shape in mild cases and skeletal instability and cell fragmentation in severe cases.

Hereditary spherocytosis (HS)

This group of inherited disorders is characterized by the presence of spheroidal erythrocytes on peripheral blood smear. HS occurs in all racial and ethnic groups. It is the most common inherited anaemia in individuals of northern European descent, affecting approximately 1 in 2500 individuals in the United States of America and England. It is much more common in whites than in individuals of African descent. Clinical, laboratory, biochemical, and genetic heterogeneity characterize the spherocytosis syndromes.

Aetiology and pathogenesis

The primary defect in HS is loss of membrane surface area relative to intracellular volume, accounting for the spheroidal shape and decreased deformability of the red cell. This loss of surface area results from increased membrane fragility due to defects in erythrocyte membrane proteins. Increased fragility leads to membrane vesiculation and membrane loss. Splenic destruction of these non-deformable erythrocytes is the primary cause of haemolysis experienced by HS patients. Physical entrapment of erythrocytes in the splenic microcirculation and ingestion by phagocytes have been proposed as mechanisms of destruction. Furthermore, the splenic environment is hostile to erythrocytes. Low pH, glucose, and ATP concentrations, and high local concentrations of toxic free radicals produced by adjacent phagocytes, all contribute to membrane damage.

Membrane loss is due to defects in several membrane proteins, including ankyrin, band 3, α-spectrin, β-spectrin, and protein 4.2.

Combined spectrin and ankyrin deficiency is the most common defect observed, followed by band 3 deficiency, isolated spectrin deficiency, and protein 4.2 deficiency. The genetic defects underlying HS are heterogeneous. Multiple genetic loci are implicated and various abnormalities, including point mutations, defects in mRNA processing, and gene deletions, have been described. Except for a few rare exceptions, HS mutations are private, i.e. each individual kindred has a unique mutation.

Clinical features

The clinical manifestations of the spherocytosis syndromes vary widely. The typical picture of HS combines evidence of haemolysis (anaemia, jaundice, reticulocytosis, gallstones, and splenomegaly) with spherocytosis (spherocytes on peripheral blood smear, positive osmotic fragility) and a positive family history (Box 22.5.10.1). Mild, moderate, and severe forms of HS have been defined according to differences in haemoglobin, bilirubin, and reticulocyte counts correlated with the degree of compensation for the haemolysis (Table 22.5.10.1). Initial assessment of a patient with suspected HS should include a family history and questions about history of anaemia, jaundice, gallstones,

---

Box 22.5.10.1 Characteristics of hereditary spherocytosis

Clinical manifestations

- Anaemia
- Splenomegaly
- Intermittent jaundice:
  - from haemolysis
  - from biliary obstruction
- Haemolytic, aplastic, and megaloblastic crises
- Inheritance
  - dominant *c.*75%
  - nondominant *c.*25% *de novo* or recessive
- Rare manifestations
  - leg ulcers, gout, chronic dermatitis
  - extramedullary haematopoietic tumours
  - thrombosis
  - neuromuscular disorders
  - cardiomyopathy
  - spinocerebellar abnormalities
- Excellent response to splenectomy

Laboratory characteristics

- Reticulocytosis
- Spherocytosis
- Elevated mean corpuscular haemoglobin concentration
- Increased osmotic fragility
- Normal direct antiglobulin test

Table 22.5.10.1 Clinical classification of hereditary spherocytosis

	Trait	Mild spherocytosis	Moderate spherocytosis[a]	Severe spherocytosis
Haemoglobin (g/dl)	Normal	11–15	8–12	≤ 8
Reticulocytes (%)	1–3	3–8	≥ 8	≥ 10
Bilirubin (mg/dl)	0–1	1–2	> 2	> 3
Spectrin content[b] (% of normal)	100	80–100	50–80	20–80
Peripheral smear	Normal	Mild spherocytosis	Spherocytosis	Spherocytosis and poikilocytosis
Osmotic fragility				
Fresh	Normal	Slightly increased	Distinctly increased	Distinctly increased
Incubated	Slightly increased	Distinctly increased	Distinctly increased	Markedly increased

[a] Values in untransfused patients.

[b] In most patients ankyrin content is decreased to a comparable degree. A minority of hereditary spherocytosis patients lack band 3 or protein 4.2 and may have mild to moderate spherocytosis with normal amounts of spectrin and ankyrin.

and splenectomy. Physical examination should seek signs such as scleral icterus, jaundice, and splenomegaly. After diagnosing a patient with HS, family members should be examined for the presence of HS.

HS typically presents in childhood, but may present at any age. In children, anaemia is the most frequent presenting complaint (50%), followed by splenomegaly, jaundice, or a positive family history. Two-thirds to three-quarters of HS patients have incompletely compensated haemolysis and mild to moderate anaemia. The anaemia is often asymptomatic except for fatigue and mild pallor. Jaundice is seen at some time in about 50% of patients, usually in association with viral infections. When present, it is acholuric, that is there is unconjugated hyperbilirubinaemia without detectable bilirubinuria. Palpable splenomegaly is detectable in most (75–95%) older children and adults. Typically, the spleen is modestly enlarged but it may be massive.

About 20–30% of HS patients have 'compensated haemolysis,' i.e. erythrocyte production and destruction are balanced. Although the erythrocyte lifespan may only be about 20–30 days, these patients adequately compensate for their haemolysis with increased marrow erythropoiesis. They are not anaemic and are usually asymptomatic. Many of these individuals escape detection until adulthood, when they are being evaluated for unrelated disorders or when complications related to anaemia or chronic haemolysis occur. Haemolysis may become severe with illnesses that cause splenomegaly, such as infectious mononucleosis, or may be exacerbated by other factors such as pregnancy. Because of the asymptomatic course of HS in these patients, diagnosis of HS should be considered during evaluation of splenomegaly, gallstones at a young age, or anaemia from viral infection.

Approximately 5 to 10% of HS patients have moderate to severe anaemia. Patients with 'moderately severe' disease typically have a haemoglobin of 6 to 8 g/dl, reticulocytes about 10%, bilirubin 2 to 3 mg/dl, and 40 to 80% of the normal red cell spectrin content. This category includes patients with both dominant and recessive HS and a variety of molecular defects. Patients with 'severe' disease, by definition, have life-threatening anaemia and are transfusion-dependent. They almost always have recessive HS. Most have isolated severe spectrin deficiency. In addition to the risks of recurrent transfusions, these patients often suffer from haemolytic and aplastic crises and may develop complications of severe uncompensated

anaemia including growth retardation, delayed sexual maturation, or aspects of thalassaemic faces.

The parents of patients with recessive HS are clinically asymptomatic and do not have anaemia, splenomegaly, hyperbilirubinaemia, or spherocytosis on peripheral blood smears ('Trait', Table 22.5.10.1). Most have subtle laboratory signs of HS including: slight reticulocytosis and slightly elevated osmotic fragility. The incubated osmotic fragility test is probably the most sensitive measure of this condition, particularly the 100% lysis point (0.43 ± 0.05 g NaCl/dl compared to control 0.23 ± 0.07). It has been estimated that at least 1.4% of the population are silent carriers.

Inheritance

The genes responsible for HS include ankyrin, β-spectrin, band 3 protein, α-spectrin, and protein 4.2. In approximately two-thirds to three-quarter of HS patients, inheritance is autosomal dominant. In the remaining patients, inheritance is nondominant due to autosomal recessive inheritance or a *de novo* mutation. Cases with autosomal recessive inheritance are due to defects in either α-spectrin or protein 4.2. A surprising number of *de novo* mutations have been reported in the HS genes. A few cases of 'double dominant' HS due to defects in band 3 or spectrin that result in fetal death or severe haemolytic anaemia presenting in the neonatal period have been reported. In general, affected individuals of the same kindred experience similar degrees of haemolysis.

Complications

Gallbladder disease

Chronic haemolysis leads to the formation of bilirubinate gallstones, the most frequently reported complication in HS patients. Although gallstones have been detected in infancy, most occur between 10 and 30 years of age. Management should include interval ultrasonography to detect gallstones, as many patients with cholelithiasis and HS are asymptomatic. Timely diagnosis and treatment will help prevent complications of symptomatic biliary tract disease including biliary obstruction, cholecystitis, and cholangitis.

Haemolytic, aplastic, and megaloblastic crises

Haemolytic crises are usually associated with viral illnesses and typically occur in childhood. They are generally mild and are characterized by jaundice, increased splenomegaly, decreased haematocrit, and reticulocytosis. Intervention is rarely necessary. When severe haemolytic crises occur, there is marked jaundice, anaemia, lethargy, abdominal pain, and tender splenomegaly. Hospitalization and erythrocyte transfusion may be required.

Aplastic crises following virally induced bone-marrow suppression are uncommon, but may result in severe anaemia with serious complications including congestive heart failure or even death. The most common aetiological agent in these cases is parvovirus B19. Parvovirus selectively infects erythropoietic progenitor cells and inhibits their growth. Parvovirus infections are frequently associated with mild neutropenia, thrombocytopenia, or even pancytopenia. During the aplastic phase, the haemoglobin and the production of new red cells fall, the cells that remain age, and microspherocytosis and osmotic fragility increase. Aplastic crises usually last 10 to 14 days (about half the lifespan of HS red cells), and the haemoglobin typically falls to half its usual level before recovery occurs. In patients with severe HS, the anaemia may be profound, requiring hospitalization and transfusion. As the marrow recovers, granulocytes, platelets, and, finally, reticulocytes return to the peripheral blood. Aplastic crisis brings many patients to medical attention, particularly asymptomatic HS patients with normally compensated haemolysis. Because parvovirus may infect several members of a family simultaneously, leading to aplastic crises, there have been reports of 'outbreaks' of HS.

Megaloblastic crisis occurs in HS patients with increased folate demands, for example the pregnant patient, growing children, or patients recovering from an aplastic crisis. With appropriate folate supplementation, this complication is preventable.

Diagnosis

The laboratory findings in HS are heterogeneous. Initial laboratory investigation should include a complete blood count with peripheral smear, reticulocyte count, Coombs' test, and serum bilirubin. When the peripheral smear or family history is suggestive of HS, an incubated osmotic fragility should be obtained. Rarely, additional, specialized testing is required to confirm the diagnosis.

Peripheral blood smear

Erythrocyte morphology is quite variable. Typical HS patients have blood smears with obvious spherocytes lacking central pallor (Fig. 22.5.10.2a). Less commonly, patients present with only a few spherocytes on peripheral smear or, at the other end of the spectrum, with numerous small, dense spherocytes and bizarre erythrocyte morphology with anisocytosis and poikilocytosis (Fig. 22.5.10.2b). Specific morphological findings have been identified in patients with certain membrane protein defects such as pincered erythrocytes (band 3) or spherocytic acanthocytes (β-spectrin).

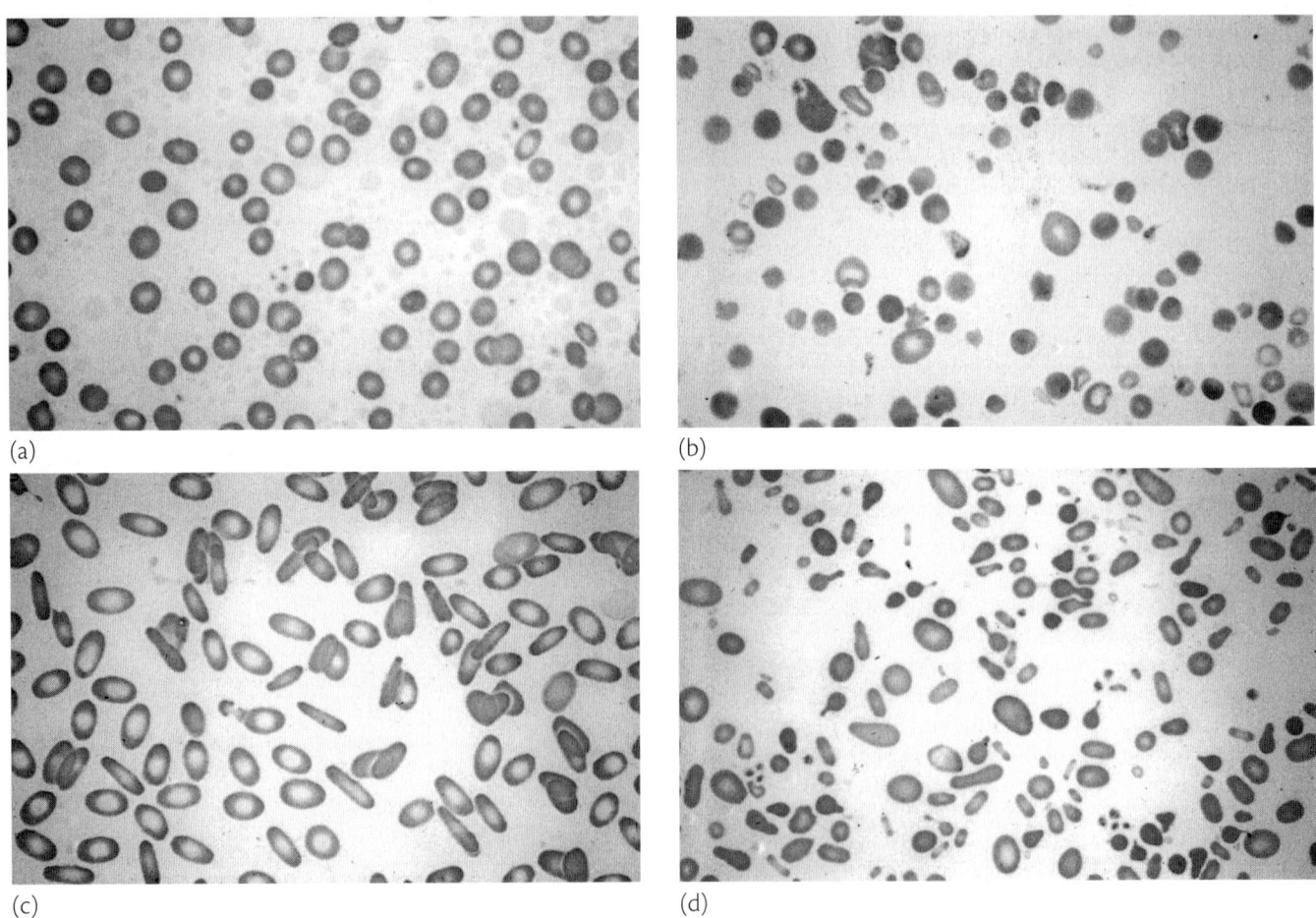

Fig. 22.5.10.2 Peripheral blood smears: (a) typical hereditary spherocytosis; (b) severe, recessively-inherited spherocytosis; (c) hereditary elliptocytosis; (d) hereditary pyropoikilocytosis.

Erythrocyte indices

Most patients have mild to moderate anaemia. The mean corpuscular volume (MCV) is normal except in severe HS cases, when it is slightly decreased despite reticulocytosis, reflecting membrane loss and cellular dehydration. The mean corpuscular haemoglobin concentration (MCHC) is increased (≥35 g/dl) due to relative cellular dehydration in around 50% of patients. Strategies using erythrocyte indices have combined MCHC and red cell distribution width (>35.4 g/dl and >14, respectively) or utilized histograms of hyperdense erythrocytes (MCHC>40 g/dl) obtained from laser-based cell counters, sometimes combined with elevated MCHC, in attempts to rapidly identify HS patients.

Osmotic fragility

In the normal erythrocyte, membrane redundancy gives the cell its characteristic discoid shape and provides it with abundant surface area. In spherocytes, there is a decrease in surface area relative to cell volume, resulting in their abnormal shape. This change is reflected in the increased osmotic fragility found in these cells (Fig. 22.5.10.3). Osmotic fragility is tested by adding increasingly hypotonic concentrations of saline to red cells. The normal erythrocyte is able to increase its volume by swelling, but spherocytes, which are already at maximum volume for surface area, burst at higher saline concentrations than normal. Approximately 25% of HS individuals will have a normal osmotic fragility on freshly drawn red cells, with the osmotic fragility curve approximating the number of spherocytes seen on peripheral smear. However, after incubation at 37°C for 24 h, HS red cells lose membrane surface area more readily than normal because their membranes are leaky and unstable. Thus incubation accentuates the defect in HS erythrocytes and brings out the defect in osmotic fragility, making incubated osmotic fragility the standard test for diagnosing HS. When the spleen is present, a subpopulation of very fragile erythrocytes, which have been conditioned by the spleen, form the 'tail' of the osmotic fragility curve; this disappears after splenectomy (Fig. 22.5.10.3). Osmotic fragility testing suffers from poor sensitivity as about 20% of mild cases of HS are missed after incubation. It is unreliable in patients with small numbers of spherocytes, including those who have been recently transfused. It is abnormal in other conditions where spherocytes are present.

Additional testing

Other investigations, such as the autohaemolysis test and the acidified glycerol test, suffer from lack of specificity and are not widely used. Flow cytometry analysis of the relative amounts of eosin-5-maleimide binding to band 3 and Rh-related proteins in the erythrocyte membrane has recently been developed for the diagnosis of HS. Although utilization has been limited, it appears to have high predictive value, but suffers from some lack of specificity, as other erythrocyte abnormalities such as congenital dyserythropoietic anaemia, sickle cell disease, and abnormalities of erythrocyte hydration may yield positive results. Because it is a flow-based technique, it may become a rapid, reproducible strategy for HS screening. Specialized testing, such as ektacytometry, membrane protein quantitation, and genetic analyses, are available for studying difficult cases or cases where additional information is desired.

Other laboratory manifestations in HS are markers of ongoing haemolysis. Reticulocytosis, increased bilirubin, increased lactate dehydrogenase, increased urinary and faecal urobilinogen, and decreased haptoglobin reflect increased erythrocyte production or destruction.

Differential diagnosis

HS should be able to be distinguished from other haemolytic anaemias by additional diagnostic testing, such as autoimmune haemolytic anaemia via a Coombs' test. Other causes of haemolytic anaemia (with spherocytes on peripheral smear) (Table 22.5.10.2) should be viewed in the appropriate clinical context. Occasional spherocytes are also seen in patients with a large spleen (such as in cirrhosis, myelofibrosis) or in patients with microangiopathic anaemias, but the differentiation of these conditions from HS is not usually difficult.

Treatment

Splenectomy

Splenic sequestration is the primary determinant of erythrocyte survival in HS patients. Thus splenectomy cures or alleviates the anaemia in the overwhelming majority of patients, reducing or

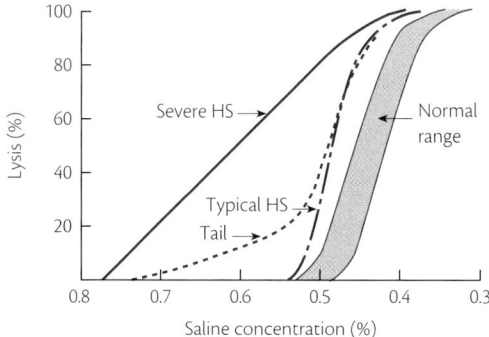

Fig. 22.5.10.3 Osmotic fragility curves in hereditary spherocytosis. The shaded region is the normal range. Results representative of both typical and severe spherocytosis are shown. A tail, representing very fragile erythrocytes that have been conditioned by the spleen, is common in many spherocytosis patients prior to splenectomy.

Table 22.5.10.2 Conditions with spherocytes on peripheral blood smear

Hereditary spherocytosis
Autoimmune haemolytic anaemia
Liver disease
Thermal injury
Microangiopathic and macroangiopathic haemolytic anaemias
Transfusion reaction with haemolysis
Clostridial sepsis
Severe hypophosphataemia
Poisoning from certain snake, spider, bee, and wasp venoms
Heinz body anaemias
Hypersplenism
ABO incompatibility (neonates)

eliminating the need for transfusions and decreasing the incidence of cholelithiasis. Postsplenectomy, spherocytosis and altered osmotic fragility persist, erythrocyte lifespan nearly normalizes, and reticulocyte counts fall to normal or near normal levels. Typical postsplenectomy changes, including Howell–Jolly bodies, target cells, and acanthocytes, become evident on peripheral smear. Postsplenectomy, patients with the most severe forms of HS still suffer from shortened erythrocyte survival and haemolysis, but their clinical improvement is striking.

Early complications of splenectomy include local infection, bleeding, and pancreatitis due to injury to the tail of the pancreas incurred during surgery. Overwhelming postsplenectomy infection (OPSI), typically from encapsulated organisms, is an uncommon but significant late complication of splenectomy, especially in the first few years of life. The introduction of pneumococcal vaccines and the promotion of early antibiotic therapy for febrile children who have had a splenectomy have led to decreases in the incidence of OPSI. Increasing rates of penicillin-resistant pneumococci has raised concerns about the potential increases in this feared complication. Another postsplenectomy complication is the increased risk of cardiovascular disease, particularly thrombosis and pulmonary hypertension. Finally, as global travel increases, increasing importance has been placed on the critical role of the spleen in protection from parasitic diseases such as malaria or babesiosis.

Indications for splenectomy

In the past, splenectomy was considered routine in HS patients. However, the risk of OPSI with penicillin-resistant pneumococci, increased recognition of postsplenectomy cardiovascular disease, and increased international travel, have led to a re-evaluation of the role of splenectomy in the treatment of HS. The risks and benefits of splenectomy should be reviewed and discussed between health care providers, patient, and family when splenectomy is considered. Considering the risks and benefits, a reasonable approach would be to splenectomize all patients with severe spherocytosis and all patients who suffer from significant signs or symptoms of anaemia including growth failure, skeletal changes, leg ulcers, and extramedullary haematopoietic tumours. Other candidates for splenectomy are older HS patients who suffer vascular compromise of vital organs.

Whether patients with moderate HS and compensated asymptomatic anaemia should have a splenectomy remains controversial. Patients with mild HS and compensated haemolysis can be followed and referred for splenectomy if clinically indicated. The treatment of patients with mild to moderate HS and gallstones is also debatable, particularly since new treatments for cholelithiasis, including laparoscopic cholecystectomy, endoscopic sphincterotomy, and extracorporal choletripsy, lower the risk of this complication.

When splenectomy is warranted, laparoscopic splenectomy is the method of choice as it results in less postoperative discomfort, shorter hospitalization, and decreased costs. Partial splenectomy has been advocated for infants and young children with significant anaemia associated with HS and it may be of benefit in typical HS patients. The goals of this procedure are to allow for the palliation of haemolysis and anaemia while maintaining some residual splenic immune function. Long-term follow-up data for this procedure are lacking.

Before splenectomy, preferably several weeks preoperatively, patients should be immunized with vaccines against pneumococcus, *Haemophilus influenzae* type b, and meningococcus. The use and duration of prophylactic antibiotics postsplenectomy is controversial. Presplenectomy, and in severe cases, postsplenectomy, HS patients should take folic acid to prevent folate deficiency.

Elliptocytosis, pyropoikilocytosis, and related disorders

Hereditary elliptocytosis (HE) is characterized by the presence of elliptical or cigar-shaped erythrocytes on peripheral blood smears of affected individuals. The worldwide incidence of HE has been estimated to be 1 in 2000 to 1 in 4000 individuals. The true incidence of HE is unknown because most patients are asymptomatic. It is common in individuals of African and Mediterranean ancestry, presumably because elliptocytes confer some resistance to malaria. In parts of Africa, the incidence of HE approaches 1 in 100. HE is typically inherited in an autosomal dominant pattern. Rare cases of *de novo* mutations have been described.

Hereditary pyropoikilocytosis (HPP) is a rare cause of severe haemolytic anaemia with erythrocyte morphology reminiscent of that seen in severe burns. Initial studies of erythrocytes from these patients revealed abnormal thermal sensitivity compared to normal erythrocytes. HPP occurs predominantly in patients of African descent. There is a strong relationship between HPP and HE. Approximately one-third of parents or siblings of patients with HPP have typical HE. Many patients with HPP experience severe haemolysis and anaemia in infancy that gradually improves, evolving toward typical HE later in life.

Aetiology and pathogenesis

The principle defect in HE/HPP erythrocytes is an intrinsic mechanical weakness or fragility of the erythrocyte membrane skeleton due to a defect of horizontal interactions (see above). This is due to defects in the red cell membrane proteins α-spectrin, β-spectrin, protein 4.1, or glycophorin C. The majority of defects occur in spectrin, the principal structural protein of the membrane skeleton. A variety of mutations in the genes encoding these proteins have been described, with several mutations identified in a number of individuals on the same genetic background, suggesting a 'founder effect' for these mutations.

Clinical features

The clinical presentation of HE is heterogeneous, ranging from asymptomatic carriers to patients with severe, transfusion-dependent anaemia. Most patients with HE are asymptomatic and are typically diagnosed incidentally during testing for unrelated conditions. The erythrocyte lifespan is normal in most patients. The 10% of patients with decreased red-cell lifespan are the ones who experience haemolysis, anaemia, splenomegaly, and intermittent jaundice. Many of these symptomatic patients have parents with typical HE and thus are homozygotes or compound heterozygotes for defects inherited from each of the parents. Symptomatology may vary between members of the same family, indeed, it may vary in the same individual at different times. To explain these observations, modifier alleles have been hypothesized to influence spectrin expression and clinical severity. One such allele, αLELY (low expression Lyon), has been identified and characterized.

Diagnosis

The hallmark of HE is the presence of elliptocytes on peripheral blood smear (Fig. 22.5.10.2c). These normochromic, normocytic elliptocytes number from a few to 100%. The degree of haemolysis and anaemia do not correlate with the number of elliptocytes present. A few ovalocytes, spherocytes, stomatocytes, and fragmented cells may also be seen. Elliptocytes may be seen in association with several disorders including megaloblastic anaemias, hypochromic microcytic anaemias (iron deficiency anaemia and thalassaemia), myleodysplasic syndromes, and myelofibrosis; however, elliptocytes generally make up less than one-third of red cells in these conditions. History and additional laboratory testing usually clarify the diagnosis of these disorders. In addition to the peripheral blood smear findings found in HE, HPP erythrocytes are bizarre-shaped with fragmentation and budding (Fig. 22.5.10.2d). Microspherocytosis is common and the MCV is frequently decreased (50–65 mm³).

The osmotic fragility is abnormal in severe HE and HPP. Other laboratory findings in HE are similar to those found in other haemolytic anaemias and are nonspecific markers of increased erythrocyte production and destruction. When indicated, specialized testing, such as membrane protein quantitation, ektacytometry, spectrin analyses, and genetic studies can be performed.

Treatment

Therapy is rarely necessary. In rare cases, occasional red blood cell transfusions may be required. In cases of severe HE and HPP, splenectomy has been palliative. The same indications for splenectomy in HS can be applied to patients with symptomatic HE or HPP. Postsplenectomy, patients with HE or HPP experience increased haemoglobin, decreased haemolysis, and improvement in clinical symptoms.

During acute illnesses, patients should be followed for signs of haematological decompensation. Ultrasonography at regular intervals to detect gallstones should be performed. In patients with significant haemolysis, folate should be administered daily.

South-East Asian ovalocytosis (SAO)

SAO is characterized by the presence of oval erythrocytes with a central longitudinal slit or transverse bar on peripheral blood smears of affected individuals. It is common in parts of the Philippines, Indonesia, Malaysia, and New Guinea and is inherited in an autosomal dominant fashion. Incredibly rigid, SAO erythrocytes are resistant to invasion by malaria parasites. The underlying defect is a mutation in a critical region of band 3. Haematologically, patients with SAO are asymptomatic, with little or no evidence of haemolysis or anaemia. Osmotic fragility is normal. The finding of characteristic ovalocytes in the peripheral blood of an asymptomatic individual from one of the above mentioned ethnic backgrounds is highly suggestive of the diagnosis. Biochemical and DNA diagnostic techniques are available to detect this condition.

Stomatocytosis

The hereditary stomatocytosis syndromes are a heterogeneous group of disorders characterized by mouth-shaped (stomatocytic) erythrocyte morphology on peripheral blood smear (Fig. 22.5.10.4). The clinical severity of stomatocytosis patients is variable; some patients experience haemolysis and anaemia, while others are asymptomatic. An unusual feature of the stomatocytosis syndromes

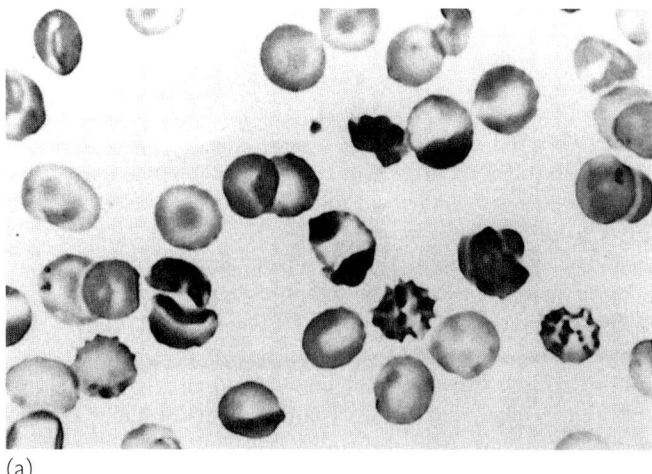

(a)

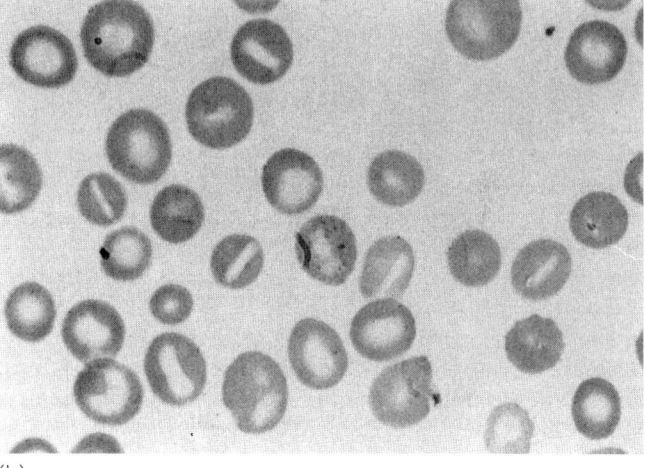

(b)

Fig. 22.5.10.4 Peripheral blood smears: (a) dehydrated stomatocytosis. (b) overhydrated stomatocytosis.
(From Lande WM, Mentzer WC (1985). Haemolytic anaemia associated with increased cation permeability. *Clin Haematol*, **14**, 89–103, with permission.)

is a dramatically increased predisposition to thrombosis or pulmonary hypertension post splenectomy. Fortunately, anaemia is well compensated in most patients and splenectomy is not required.

The red blood cell membranes of stomatocytosis patients usually exhibit abnormal permeability to the cations sodium and potassium, with consequent modification of intracellular water content, ranging from dehydrated (xerocytosis) to overhydrated (hydrocytosis) erythrocytes. The molecular basis of stomatocytosis is poorly understood. The variable clinical, laboratory, and pathophysiologic findings associated with the stomatocytosis syndromes suggest these are a complex collection of syndromes caused by various molecular defects. A locus for both hereditary xerocytosis maps to a region of chromosome 16, but the causative gene has not been identified. In one subgroup of stomatocytosis patients, some with a spherocytic phenotype, missense mutations in band 3 have been identified that convert it from an anion exchanger to a nonselective cation leak channel. In some hydrocytosis patients, mutations in the *RHAG* gene have been found.

Other conditions

Other conditions associated with hereditary stomatocytosis include the Rh deficiency syndromes, sitosterolemia, and familial deficiency of high-density lipoproteins. The rare Rh deficiency syndromes are associated with mild to moderate haemolytic anaemia and absent

(Rh_{null}) to decreased (Rh_{mod}) erythrocyte expression of Rh antigens associated with mutation in the *RHD* and *RHAG* genes. Sitosterolemia is associated with early onset atheroscleosis, anaemia, and macrothrombocytopenia associated with mutation of the ABCG5/ABCG8 cotransporters, leading to increased intestinal absorption and decreased biliary elimination of sterols, particularly those derived from plants. Familial deficiency of high-density lipoproteins (Tangier disease, OMIM 205 400) is due to mutation of ABCA1, a protein critical for cellular cholesterol export, leading to accumulation of tissue cholesterol esters manifest as enlarged orange-yellow tonsils, hepatosplenomegaly, cloudy corneas, neuropathy, and premature atherosclerosis. Affected patients exhibit mild to moderate haemolytic anaemia.

Acquired stomatocytosis has been observed in a large number of conditions, particularly hepatobiliary disease and acute alcoholism. Acquired stomatocytosis has also been seen in patients with various malignant neoplasms, cardiovascular disease, and after the administration of vinca alkaloids.

Acanthocytosis

Acanthocytes are dense, contracted erythrocytes with irregular 'thorny' projections. Acanthocytes may also been found on the peripheral smears of patients with abetalipoproteinemia, the McLeod phenotype, or one of the neuroacanthocytosis syndromes. Abetalipoproteinemia (OMIM 200 100) is associated with hypolipidemia, fat malabsorption, progressive ataxia, retinitis pigmentosa, and poor growth in childhood due to the inability to produce or secrete the B apoproteins B100 and B48, or defects in the microsomal triglyceride transfer protein (MTTP), required for production of apoprotein B-containing β-lipoproteins. The X-linked McLeod phenotype (OMIM 314 850) is due to mutation of XK, necessary for Kell antigen expression. Affected individuals experience compensated anaemia, susceptibility to Kell D antigen alloimmunization, and late-onset myopathy and nervous system abnormalities.

The neuroacanthocytosis syndromes are a heterogeneous group of neurodegenerative disorders including the McLeod syndrome, chorea-acanthocytosis due to mutation of chorein or VPS13A, Huntington's Disease Like 2 due to mutation of junctophilin-3, and pantothenate kinase-associated neurodegeneration (formerly known as Hallervorden–Spatz syndrome and its allelic variant HARP syndrome–hypobetalipoproteinemia, acanthocytosis, retinitis pigmentosa, pallidal degeneration) due to mutations of pantothenate kinase 2. The cause of the acanthocytosis in these disorders is unknown.

Acquired acanthocytosis may be seen in patients with severe hepatic disease (commonly known as spur cell anaemia), hypothyroidism, malnutrition, and after splenectomy.

Further reading

An X, Mohandas N (2008). Disorders of red cell membrane. *Br J Haematol*, **141**, 367–75.

Bennett V, Healy J (2008). Organizing the fluid membrane bilayer: diseases linked to spectrin and ankyrin. *Trends Mol Med*, **14**, 28–36.

Bolton-Maggs PH, *et al.* (2004). Guidelines for the diagnosis and management of hereditary spherocytosis. *Br J Haematol*, **126**, 455–74.

Bonderman D, *et al.* (2005). Medical conditions increasing the risk of chronic thromboembolic pulmonary hypertension. *Thromb Haemost*, **93**, 512–6.

Bruce LJ, *et al.* (2009). The monovalent cation leak in overhydrated stomatocytic red blood cells results from amino acid substitutions in the Rh-associated glycoprotein. *Blood*, **113**, 1350–57.

Delaunay J (2004). The hereditary stomatocytoses: genetic disorders of the red cell membrane permeability to monovalent cations. *Semin Hematol*, **41**, 165–72.

Delaunay J (2007). The molecular basis of hereditary red cell membrane disorders. *Blood Rev*, **21**, 1–20.

Dhermy D, *et al.* (2007). Spectrin-based skeleton in red blood cells and malaria. *Curr Opin Hematol*, **14**, 198–202.

Eber S, Lux SE (2004). Hereditary spherocytosis—defects in proteins that connect the membrane skeleton to the lipid bilayer. *Semin Hematol*, **41**, 118–41.

Gallagher PG (2004). Hereditary elliptocytosis: spectrin and protein 4.1R. *Semin Hematol*, **41**, 142–64.

Johnson CP, *et al.* (2007). Pathogenic proline mutation in the linker between spectrin repeats: disease caused by spectrin unfolding. *Blood*, **109**, 3538–43.

Lusher JM, Barnhart MI (1980). The role of the spleen in the pathoophysiology of hereditary spherocytosis and hereditary elliptocytosis. *Am J Pediatr Hematol Oncol*, **2**, 31.

Nicolas V, *et al.* (2006). Functional interaction between Rh proteins and the spectrin-based skeleton in erythroid and epithelial cells. *Transfus Clin Biol*, **13**, 23–8.

Pasini EM, *et al.* (2006). In-depth analysis of the membrane and cytosolic proteome of red blood cells. *Blood*, **108**, 791–801.

Perrotta S, *et al.* (2008). Hereditary spherocytosis. *Lancet*, **372**, 1411–26.

Rees DC, *et al.* (2005). Stomatocytic haemolysis and macrothrombocytopenia (Mediterranean stomatocytosis/macrothrombocytopenia) is the haematological presentation of phytosterolaemia. *Br J Haematol*, **130**, 297–309.

Schilling RF. (2009). Risks and benefits of splenectomy versus no splenectomy for hereditary spherocytosis--a personal view. *Br J Haematol*, **145**, 728–32.

Tracy ET, Rice HE (2008). Partial splenectomy for hereditary spherocytosis. *Pediatr Clin North Am*, **55**, 503–19.

Walker RH, *et al.* (2007). Neurologic phenotypes associated with acanthocytosis. *Neurology*, **68**, 92–8.

Yawata Y, *et al.* (2000). Characteristic features of the genotype and phenotype of hereditary spherocytosis in the Japanese population. *Int J Hematol*, **71**, 118–35.

Young NS (2006). Hematologic manifestations and diagnosis of parvovirus B19 infections. *Clin Adv Hematol Oncol*, **4**, 908–10.

22.5.11 **Erythrocyte enzymopathies**

Ernest Beutler[†]

Essentials

Numerous enzymes, including those of the hexose monophosphate pathway and glycolysis, are active in the red cell. They are required for the generation of ATP (needed to supply energy for sodium extrusion) and the reductants NADH and NADPH, necessary to maintain haemoglobin in its active ferrous atomic state, as well as for the integrity of sulphydryl groups present on essential proteins. 2,3-diphosphoglycerate (2,3-DPG), an intermediate of

---

† It is with regret that we report the death of Professor Ernest Beutler during the preparation of this edition of the textbook.

Acknowledgements: This is manuscript 18838-MEM from The Scripps Research Institute. Supported by the Stein Endowment Fund.

glucose metabolism, is a key regulator of the affinity of haemoglobin for oxygen, and accessory enzymes are also active for the synthesis of glutathione, disposal of oxygen free radicals, and nucleotide and nucleotide metabolism.

Clinical features—general considerations

With the exception of heavy metal poisoning, most red-cell enzyme deficiency disorders are inherited conditions, which may (1) cause haematological disorders, including most commonly haemolytic anaemias, but rarely polycythaemia or methaemoglobinaemia; (2) mirror important metabolic disorders, without producing haematological problems, making them of diagnostic value, e.g. galactosaemia; (3) be of no known consequence.

Genetics—one-half of the normal activity of red-cell enzymes is generally sufficient for normal function, hence most haemolytic anaemias due to red-cell enzyme deficiencies occur as autosomal recessive or sex-linked disorders.

Diagnosis of red-cell enzymopathies

With rare exceptions it is impossible to differentiate the enzymatic defects from one another by clinical or routine laboratory methods. Diagnosis depends on the combination of (1) accurate ascertainment of the family history; (2) morphological observations—these can determine whether haemolysis is present, rule out some causes of haemolysis (e.g. hereditary spherocytosis), and diagnose pyrimidine 5′-nucleotidase deficiency (prominent red cell stippling); (3) estimation of red-cell enzyme activity; and (4) DNA analysis.

Specific red-cell abnormalities that may cause haemolytic anaemia

These include (1) glucose-6-phosphate dehydrogenase (G6PD) deficiency—see Chapter 22.5.12; (2) pyruvate kinase deficiency; (3) glucosephosphate isomerase deficiency; (4) pyrimidine 5′-nucleotidase deficiency—which may also induced by exposure to environmental lead; (5) triosephosphate isomerase deficiency.

Introduction

Erythrocytes are living cells that contain a large number of enzymes required to carry out a variety of metabolic processes. Some inherited deficiencies of these enzymes are designated red-cell enzymopathies. They may cause haematological disorders, including haemolytic anaemias, polycythaemia, and methaemoglobinaemia. Other deficiencies do not produce haematological disorders, but instead mirror important metabolic disorders such as galactosaemia and are therefore of diagnostic value. Some deficiencies, for example those of lactate dehydrogenase or inosine triphosphatase (ITPase) are, as far as has been determined, 'nondiseases'.

This section deals with those red-cell enzyme defects that cause haemolytic anaemia. Many have been described; most are rare but some are sufficiently common that several hundred or even thousands of cases have been documented. Although the enzymatic bases of these defects are very different, the clinical presentation is similar and relatively nondescript. Except for pyrimidine 5′-nucleotidase deficiency, in which red cell stippling is a prominent feature, it is impossible to differentiate the enzymatic defects from one another by clinical or routine laboratory methods.

Red-cell metabolism

The two major pathways of red-cell glucose metabolism are illustrated in Fig. 22.5.11.1. Glucose is phosphorylated to glucose 6-phosphate in the hexokinase reaction. It is then either metabolized in the anaerobic Embden–Meyerhof pathway or is oxidized in the glucose 6-phosphate dehydrogenase (G6PD) reaction, entering the hexose monophosphate pathway.

Anaerobic metabolism of glucose phosphorylates ADP to ATP, providing energy to maintain erythrocyte shape and to transport molecules into and out of erythrocyte. It also reduces NAD to NADH, which serves to reduce methaemoglobin to haemoglobin. The hexose monophosphate pathway, reduces NADP to the NADPH and thus serves to maintain glutathione and protein sulphydryl groups in the reduced state. These pathways are similar in red cells, other tissues and in lower organisms. However, the 2,3-diphosphoglycerate (2,3-DPG) shunt is a unique feature of the

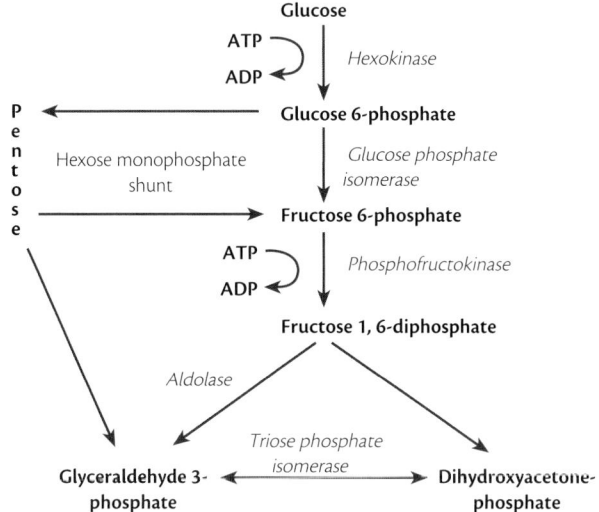

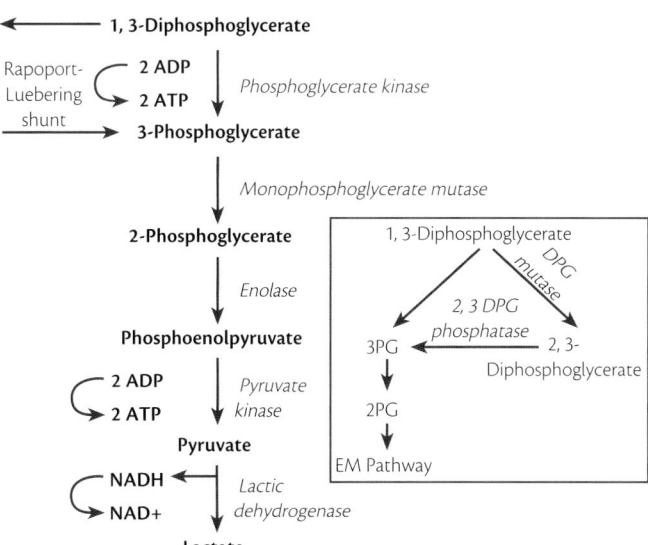

Fig. 22.5.11.1 The relationship between the main red-cell glycolytic pathway EM, (Embden–Meyerhof) and the other metabolic pathways. The insert shows the production of 2,3-DPG in the Rapoport–Luebering shunt (DPG, diphosphoglycerate; PG, phosphoglycerate).

Embden–Meyerhof pathway in erythrocytes. This 'energy clutch' of erythrocyte metabolism not only allows flexibility in the amount of ATP that is generated in glycolysis, but also provides a source of 2,3-DPG, the key modulator of haemoglobin oxygen affinity.

There are, in addition, many other metabolic functions that the erythrocyte must carry out. Among these are the synthesis of glutathione, the synthesis and degradation of nucleotides and nucleosides, the detoxification of active oxygen radicals, and the transport of small molecules into and out of the cell.

Genetics

Half of the normal activity of red-cell enzymes is generally sufficient for normal function. Thus, most haemolytic anaemias due to red-cell enzyme deficiencies occur as autosomal recessive or sex-linked disorders. The only exception is the haemolytic anaemia associated with elevated adenosine deaminase activity, which is

inherited as an autosomal dominant disorder. Only two of the deficiencies, those of G6PD and phosphoglycerate kinase, are encoded by genes on the X chromosome; all of the others are autosomal. Extensive mutation analysis at the DNA level has been carried out on patients with most of the enzyme defects. Most mutations of the genes encoding these enzymes are missense mutations or nonsense mutations, but a few deletions, insertions, and splicing mutations have been described. Very few regulatory mutations have been documented. DNA-based diagnosis has assumed an increasingly valuable role in the diagnosis of these disorders.

Specific red-cell abnormalities that may cause haemolytic anaemia

Table 22.5.11.1 summarizes some of the clinical and genetic characteristics of red-cell enzyme deficiencies.

Table 22.5.11.1 Red-cell enzyme abnormalities leading to haematological disease

Enzyme	OMIM	Clinical features	Inheritance	Red cell morphology	Response to splenectomy[a]	Prevalence[b]
Hexokinase	235 700	HNSHA[d]	AR	Unremarkable	++	Rare
Glucose-6-phosphate isomerase	172 400	HNSHA	AR	Unremarkable	+++	Unusual
		Neurological abnormalities (?)				
Phosphofructokinase	232 800	HNSHA and/or muscle glycogen storage disease	AR	Unremarkable	0	Rare
Aldolase	103 850	HNSHA and mild liver glycogen storage; ? mental retardation	AR	Unremarkable	?	Very rare
Triosephosphate isomerase	190 450	HNSHA and severe neuromuscular	AR	Unremarkable		Rare
		Disease				
Phosphoglycerate kinase	300 653	HNSHA; myoglobinuria; behavioural disturbances	SL	Unremarkable	++	Rare
Disphosphoglycerate mutase	222 800	HNSHA; polycythaemia	AR	Unremarkable		Rare
Pyruvate kinase	266 200	HNSHA	AR	Usually unremarkable; occasional contracted echinocytes	++	Unusual
Glucose-6-phosphate dehydrogenase	305 900	HNSHA; drug or infection-induced haemolysis; favism	SL	Usually unremarkable; rarely 'bite cells'	±	Very common
Glutathione reductase (complete)	138 300	Drug sensitive haemolytic anaemia and favism	AR	Unremarkable	?	Very rare
γ-Glutamyl cysteine synthetase	230 450	HNSHA; drug- or infection-induced haemolysis; spinocerebellar degeneration (?)	AR	Unremarkable	?	Very rare
Glutathione synthetase	231 900	HNSHA; drug- or infection-induced haemolysis; neurological defect and 5-oxoprolinuria in some cases	AR	Usually unremarkable	0	Rare
Pyrimidine-5′-nucleotidase	606 224	HNSHA; ? mental retardation in some cases	AR	Prominent stippling	0	Rare
Adenosine deaminase (increased activity)	102 730	HNSHA	AD	Unremarkable		Rare
Adenosine deaminase (decreased activity)	102 700	Immunodeficiency	AR	Unremarkable		Rare
NADH-diaphorase (cytochrome b_5 reductase)	250 800	Methaemoglobinaemia; sometimes with mental retardation	AR	Unremarkable		Unusual

AD, autosomal dominant; AR, autosomal recessive; HNSA, hereditary non-spherocytic haemolytic anaemia; SL, sex linked.

[a] On a scale of 0 to 4+ where 4+ is a complete response. In many cases data are meagre.

[b] Very common, incidence >5%; Unusual, >100 cases reported; Rare, 10 to 100 cases reported; Very rare, <10 cases reported.

The more common red-cell enzyme abnormalities

G6PD deficiency

This enzymopathy is described in Chapter 22.5.12.

Pyruvate kinase deficiency

Pyruvate kinase deficiency can be considered the clinical prototype of the nonspherocytic haemolytic anaemias caused by red-cell enzymopathies. The severity of the anaemia varies greatly from patient to patient. At one extreme, the anaemia can be quite mild; at the other, the patient may be entirely transfusion-dependent. Indeed, the circulating red cells in such patients may have normal pyruvate kinase activity because there are scarcely any of the patient's own cells present; it appears that most of the patient's cells are destroyed before they leave the marrow and it may be only the transfused cells that are sampled and sent to the laboratory for diagnosis. Pyruvate-kinase-deficient patients have the usual stigmata of haemolytic anaemia; i.e. pallor, lack of energy, jaundice, and sometimes gallstones. In those patients who are transfusion-dependent, haemochromatosis occurs commonly, probably more so than in patients with many other types of haemolytic anaemia. Patients with pyruvate kinase deficiency usually enjoy a fairly good response to splenectomy, but this is less complete than is observed in hereditary spherocytosis, although it may be clinically quite helpful, particularly in reducing the requirement for transfusions.

Pyruvate kinase deficiency is one of the more difficult red-cell enzymopathies to diagnose, because the enzyme is a complex one with allosteric properties. The residual enzyme activity is not always greatly reduced. Cases have been described in which the residual pyruvate kinase activity is actually higher than is found in normal individuals. In such cases, establishing the diagnosis may depend upon showing that the level of 2,3-DPG or of 3-phosphoglyceric acid in the erythrocytes is greatly elevated, a finding that is characteristic of pyruvate kinase deficiency. It is also useful to measure the thermal stability of the residual enzyme; mutant enzymes are very often unstable on heating. Many different mutations have been documented in patients with pyruvate kinase deficiency. In European populations, the most common of these is a $c.1529\,G{>}A$ (A510G) mutation. This mutation has not been detected among Asians with pyruvate kinase deficiency; among Gypsies the characteristic mutation is a deletion of exon 11.

The less common red-cell enzyme abnormalities

Glucose-6-phosphate isomerase deficiency

Patients with glucose-6-phosphate isomerase deficiency generally have a milder haemolytic disorder than patients with pyruvate kinase deficiency. The response to splenectomy is usually satisfactory. Although milder in general, this enzymopathy seems to be associated with hydrops fetalis more frequently than the other red-cell enzyme defects. Diagnosis is generally straightforward. A fluorescent screening test can be used to detect the deficiency.

Pyrimidine 5′-nucleotidase deficiency

Basophilic stippling is the hallmark of pyrimidine 5′-nucleotidase deficiency. Interestingly, this enzyme is very sensitive to inhibition by lead. The stippling that is so characteristic of lead poisoning may be the consequence of inhibition of this enzyme. Pyrimidine 5′-nucleotidase is the most age-sensitive all of the red-cell enzymes; this one alone is decreased in activity in aplastic anaemia or other disorders, such as transient erythroblastopenia of childhood, in which the mean red-cell age is greatly increased. This can lead to misdiagnosis; while it is not uncommon to encounter enzyme activities of one-half normal in patients with decreased erythropoiesis, these patients do not suffer from clinically significant pyrimidine 5′-nucleotidase deficiency. Accumulation of pyrimidine nucleotides, which can be documented by measuring the ultraviolet absorption spectrum, does not occur in such patients.

Triosephosphate isomerase deficiency

Triosephosphate isomerase deficiency is the most devastating all of the red-cell enzymopathies. With few exceptions, patients with this abnormality die by the time they are 4 years of age. All tissues are affected, and death is usually due to cardiopulmonary complications. Many different mutations have been detected in patients with triosephosphate isomerase deficiency; one, at genomic nucleotide 1591, accounts for approximately 50% of the patients with this disorder. Polymorphic changes occur in the promoter region of the triosephosphate isomerase gene, but the significance of these mutations is not yet clear. No treatment has been effective.

The rare red-cell enzyme deficiencies

Hexokinase deficiency

Hexokinase deficiency is one of the more difficult red-cell enzymopathies to diagnose, because the activity of this enzyme is much higher in young red cells than in older erythrocytes. As a result, red-cell hexokinase activity is usually increased in patients with haemolytic anaemia of any type. In patients with hexokinase deficiency, this often gives rise to the anomalous finding that the red-cell hexokinase activity in the affected patient is normal, usually higher than that found in the heterozygous parents. The diagnostic hallmark is normal, rather than elevated, hexokinase activity in the face of a high reticulocyte count and high levels of other red-cell enzymes.

Enzymes of glutathione synthesis

Erythrocytes synthesize glutathione from the amino acids glutamate, cysteine, and glycine in two consecutive enzymatic reactions, each of which utilizes ATP. In the first step, catalysed by γ-glutamylcysteine synthetase, a peptide bond is formed between the γ-carboxyl group of glutamic acid and cysteine. Several patients deficient in this enzyme have been found. In addition to haemolytic anaemia, spinocerebellar degeneration was documented in the initial patient described, but neurological symptoms have not been present in subsequent patients. Defects of the second step of glutathione synthesis, the formation of a peptide link between γ-glutamylcysteine and glycine, catalysed by the enzyme glutathione synthetase, appear in two clinical forms. In some patients, the deficiency is limited to the erythrocytes. Haemolytic anaemia appears to be the sole clinical manifestation. In other patients, the deficiency is generalized. These patients excrete large amounts of pyroglutamic acid (5-oxyproline); this product of γ-glutamylcysteine degradation is overproduced in the absence of the feedback inhibition of γ-glutamylcysteine synthetase by glutathione. Patients with the generalized defect have severe neuromuscular manifestations in addition to haemolytic anaemia.

Glutathione reductase deficiency

Only a single family with a severe, hereditary deficiency of glutathione reductase has been described. No haemolysis was present except after the ingestion of fava beans. Low activity of red-cell glutathione reductase, a flavin enzyme, are found when the intake of riboflavin is suboptimal, but this mild or moderate enzyme deficiency has no clinical consequences.

Phosphofructokinase deficiency

Erythrocytes contain two types of genetically distinct phosphofructokinase subunits, L (liver) and M (muscle). Deficiency of the M subunit causes haemolysis, but the haemoglobin level in the blood is often normal or even higher than normal because of the diminished 2,3-DPG levels that are characteristic of this disorder. Muscle enzyme activity is also compromised and a myopathy results. This disorder is sometimes designated Tarui disease or type VII glycogenosis. Deficiency of the L subunit of phosphofructokinase has also been reported, but did not have any clinical consequences.

Aldolase deficiency

A few cases of aldolase deficiency been reported. An association with mental retardation was noted in one case, but it is not clear whether a cause-and-effect relationship exists.

Phosphoglycerate kinase deficiency

Phosphoglycerate kinase shares with G6PD deficiency the distinction of being an X-linked enzymopathy. In addition to haemolytic anaemia, behavioural disturbances, and myopathies have been documented. The latter may occur without anaemia being present.

Diphosphoglycerate mutase deficiency

The result of diphosphoglycerate mutase deficiency is more frequently erythrocytosis than haemolytic anaemia, because a lack of this enzyme prevents the formation of 2,3-DPG. Consequently, the oxygen affinity of the red cells is increased, stimulating erythropoiesis.

High adenosine deaminase activity

Haemolytic anaemia, inherited as an autosomal dominant disorder, has rarely been found to be associated with greatly elevated red-cell adenosine deaminase levels. The adenosine deaminase that is formed appears to be normal. The abnormality that causes this tissue-specific increase in enzyme activity has not yet been discovered.

Adenylate kinase deficiency

A number of patients with familial haemolytic anaemia have been documented to have markedly decreased levels of red-cell adenylate kinase. However, one very well-studied patient with virtually absent enzyme activity had no clinical disorder. The relationship between this enzyme deficiency and haemolytic anaemia remains unclear.

Specific red-cell abnormalities that do not cause haemolytic anaemia

Severe deficiencies of many red-cell enzymes do not produce haematological abnormality or, indeed, in many cases, any clinical abnormality at all. Included are deficiencies of 6-phosphogluconate dehydrogenase, δ-aminolaevulinic acid dehydrase, acetylcholinesterase, AMP deaminase, carbonic anhydrase, catalase, galactokinase, galactose-1-phosphate uridyltransferase, glutathione peroxidase, hypoxanthine-guanine phosphoribosyltransferase, ITPase, and phosphoglucomutase. Discussion of these enzyme deficiencies is beyond the scope of this chapter.

Diagnosis

The diagnosis of red-cell enzymopathies has been carried out at three levels: morphological observations, estimation of red-cell enzyme activity, and DNA analysis.

Morphological observations

The appearance of erythrocytes on a stained blood film may be useful in determining whether haemolytic anaemia is present and in ruling out some causes of haemolysis, such as hereditary spherocytosis, ovalocytosis, or microangiopathic haemolytic anaemia. The presence of prominent red-cell stippling suggests a diagnosis of pyrimidine 5′-nucleotidase deficiency.

Qualitative and quantitative estimations of red-cell enzyme activity

The most generally useful means for differentiating red-cell enzyme defects from one another and from defects other than known enzyme deficiencies is to semiquantitate or quantitate the red-cell enzyme activities. Fluorescent screening tests have been developed that allow nonspecialized laboratories to detect decreases in the activity of enzymes such as G6PD, pyruvate kinase, glucosephosphate isomerase, or triosephosphate isomerase with a high degree of reliability. The accumulation of pyrimidine nucleotides can be detected by measuring the ultraviolet spectrum of a perchloric acid extract of red cells. This can be used by nonspecialized laboratories to detect this abnormality.

Quantification of red-cell enzyme activities is a more specialized task that can be accomplished by the use of standardized techniques in an experienced laboratory. There are a number of caveats that must be taken into account, both with respect to the performance of red-cell enzyme assays and the interpretation of the results. Leucocyte pyruvate kinase and red-cell pyruvate kinase are encoded by different genes. Moreover, the activity of the white cell enzyme is very high. Thus, contamination of a red-cell suspension with a relatively small number of white cells may obscure the diagnosis of red-cell pyruvate kinase deficiency. The interpretation of the results of red-cell enzyme assays may also be confounded by the fact that the blood of patients with haemolytic anaemia is enriched with reticulocytes and young erythrocytes. Since many of the mutations that cause red-cell enzymopathies result in the production of unstable enzymes, the young erythrocytes that circulate may actually contain normal or near-normal levels of enzyme. It is therefore essential to take into account the age of the circulating cells. It may be helpful to obtain blood samples from parents or children of the patient to determine whether half-normal activities can be documented.

Problems in interpretation may also arise when the activity of an enzyme as measured *in vitro* does not accurately reflect its intracellular *in vivo* activity. This comes about because of the necessity of using unphysiologically high substrate concentrations for *in vitro* assays. This difficulty is particularly prone to arise in the case of pyruvate kinase deficiency, because this is a complex allosteric enzyme that not only has binding sites for two substrates, ADP and phosphoenolpyruvate, but also for fructose diphosphate, an allosteric effector.

Finally, there is the confounding effect of red-cell transfusions. It is clearly best to wait until just before a transfusion to draw blood for testing. When this is not possible, family studies can be very useful, since the enzyme activity of the red cells of heterozygotes tends to be about one-half normal.

DNA-based diagnosis

With the development of PCR-based technologies for the detection of mutations, and for the sequencing of DNA, mutation analysis at the DNA level now plays an increasing role in the diagnosis of red-cell enzyme defects. DNA is extracted from peripheral blood leucocytes and the exons of the gene of interest are amplified. Although mRNA may be reverse transcribed and the cDNA amplified, in some cases the abundance of mRNAs in reticulocytes is very low. Moreover the stability of DNA is greater than that of RNA, and samples may need to be transported to distant specialized laboratories. Direct DNA amplification of genomic DNA is generally the preferred technology. For laboratories experienced with the techniques involved, DNA-based diagnosis is not particularly difficult. It has some advantages over enzyme assay-based diagnosis. First of all, DNA is very stable, even before it is purified, so shipping of blood is less of a logistical problem. Transfused red cells do not pose a problem in performing DNA-based diagnosis, since transfused leucocytes do not persist in the circulation. Once the mutation has been established, family studies are more readily performed; heterozygote detection using quantitative enzyme levels is often of dubious reliability. Prenatal diagnosis, too, is more readily accomplished utilizing DNA-based diagnosis.

However, there are some major problems in DNA-based diagnosis of red-cell enzymopathies. While it is quite straightforward to identify a known mutation in the coding region of the gene encoding any one of the red-cell enzymes, doing so by examining the genes that encode all of the enzymes that may cause haemolytic anaemia would be a daunting task. Moreover, even if the entire coding region of the enzyme is sequenced, one cannot be certain that the mutation was not in a promoter, an enhancer, or a splice site.

General approach to diagnosis of red-cell enzymopathies

The first step is to make certain that the patient has a haemolytic anaemia. The reticulocyte count should be elevated, unless it has been temporarily suppressed by infection. If the patient's history suggests that the anaemia is chronic in nature, a positive family history can be very helpful. Dominant inheritance suggests that an enzymopathy is not the cause; only the very rare anaemia caused by elevated adenosine deaminase levels falls into this category. Instead, dominant inheritance suggests that the patient either has an unstable haemoglobin or hereditary spherocytosis. Sex-linked inheritance may also appear as though it is dominant, but is excluded if there is father-to-son transmission. G6PD deficiency and phosphoglycerate kinase deficiency are the only red-cell enzymopathies that are sex-linked. Often there is no clear-cut family history. Before attempting to establish whether or not a red-cell enzymopathy is present, hereditary spherocytosis and related erythrocyte membrane defects, haemoglobinopathies, and other disorders, such as a paroxysmal nocturnal haemoglobinuria, should be excluded.

Fluorescent screening tests are appropriate starting points for the diagnosis of the red-cell enzymopathies. Screening tests for G6PD deficiency, pyruvate kinase deficiency, and glucose-6-phosphate isomerase deficiency should be carried out. If the patient is a child with neuromuscular disease, a fluorescent test for triosephosphate isomerase deficiency is also indicated. Stippling of the red cells suggests that the patient may have pyrimidine 5′-nucleotidase deficiency. In this instance the ultraviolet spectrum of a perchloric acid of extract of the red cells should be examined. A clear-cut positive screening test for one of the red-cell enzymopathies, carried out with appropriate controls, is adequate for diagnosis. Quantitative assays for red-cell enzymes can be performed by specialized laboratories, and these may include those enzymes for which no screening tests have been developed.

When a diagnosis has been established, either by performing a screening test or by quantitative assay, it is sometimes useful to identify the mutation at the DNA level. This need not be done in every case, but is particularly useful in the case of young couples who hope to have more children and desire genetic counselling and prenatal diagnosis.

Further reading

Beutler E, *et al.* (1977). International committee for standardization in haematology: Recommended methods for red-cell enzyme analysis. *Br J Haematol*, **35**, 331–40.

Beutler E (1984). *Red cell metabolism: a manual of biochemical methods*, 3rd edition. Grune & Stratton, New York.

Beutler E (2006). The clinician's approach to the diagnosis of enzyme deficiencies of red blood cells. *11th Congress of the European Hematology Association, Amsterdam, the Netherlands, 15–18 June 2006*, **2**, 50–4.

Beutler E (2007). PGK deficiency. *Br J Haematol*, **136**, 3–11.

Van Wijk R, van Solinge WW (2005). The energy-less red blood cell is lost: erythrocyte enzyme abnormalities of glycolysis. *Blood*, **106**, 4034–42.

Zanella A, *et al.* (2005). Red cell pyruvate kinase deficiency: molecular and clinical aspects. *Br J Haematol*, **130**, 11–25.

Zanella A, Fermo E, Valentini G (2006). Hereditary pyrimidine 5′-nucleotidase deficiency: from genetics to clinical manifestations. *Br J Haematol*, **133**, 113–23.

Zanella A, Bianchi P, Fermo E (2007). Pyruvate kinase deficiency. *Haematologica*, **92**, 721–3.

22.5.12 Glucose-6-phosphate dehydrogenase (G6PD) deficiency

Lucio Luzzatto

Essentials

Deficiency of the enzyme glucose 6-phosphate dehydrogenase (G6PD) in red blood cells is an inherited abnormality due to mutations of the G6PD gene on the X chromosome that renders the cells vulnerable to oxidative damage. The condition is widespread in many populations living in or originating from tropical and subtropical areas of the world because it confers a selective advantage against *Plasmodium falciparum* malaria.

Clinical features

G6PD deficiency is mostly an asymptomatic trait, but it predisposes to acute haemolytic anaemia in response to exogenous triggers, including (1) ingestion of fava beans—favism, the most spectacular manifestation of the condition; (2) certain bacterial and viral infections; and (3) some drugs—notably some antimalarials (e.g. primaquine), some antibiotics (e.g. sulphanilamide, dapsone, nitrofurantoin), and even aspirin in high doses. Other manifestations include (1) severe neonatal jaundice; (2) chronic nonspherocytic haemolytic anaemia.

The acute haemolytic attack—this typically starts with malaise, weakness, and abdominal or lumbar pain, followed by the development of jaundice and passage of dark urine (haemoglobinuria). Most episodes resolve spontaneously.

Diagnosis, prevention, and treatment

Diagnosis relies on the direct demonstration of decreased activity of G6PD in red cells: a variety of screening tests are available, with (ideally) subsequent confirmation by quantitative assay. Prevention is by avoiding exposure to triggering factors of previously screened subjects. Prompt blood transfusion is indicated in severe acute haemolytic anaemia and may be life-saving.

Definition

Glucose-6-phosphate dehydrogenase (G6PD) is a key enzyme in redox metabolism. G6PD deficiency (OMIM 305 900) is an inherited condition in which red cells have a markedly decreased activity of G6PD, which predisposes to haemolytic anaemia.

Epidemiology

G6PD deficiency is distributed worldwide (see Fig. 22.5.12.5). Areas of high prevalence (up to 10–20% or more) are in Africa, southern Europe, the Middle East, South-East Asia, and Oceania. In the Americas and in parts of northern Europe, G6PD deficiency is also quite prevalent as a result of migrations that have taken place in relatively recent historical times.

Genetics

G6PD deficiency is inherited as an X-linked Mendelian trait, and the gene encoding G6PD is in the telomeric region of the long arm of the X-chromosome (band Xq28), physically very close to the genes for haemophilia A, dyskeratosis congenita, and colour blindness. At the genomic level, the G6PD gene consists of 13 exons and spans some 18.5 kb. Structural and functional studies have revealed features of a 'housekeeping gene'; this is in accord with the fact that G6PD is found in all cells.

The X-linkage of the G6PD gene has important implications. First, as males have only one G6PD gene (i.e. they are hemizygous for this gene), they must be either normal or G6PD deficient. By contrast, females, having two G6PD genes, can be either normal, or deficient (homozygous), or intermediate (heterozygous).

Moreover, as a result of the phenomenon of X-chromosome inactivation, heterozygous females are genetic mosaics, and this in turn has clinical implications. Indeed, in most other (autosomal) enzyme deficiencies, heterozygotes are asymptomatic because cells with an enzyme level close to 50% of normal are biochemically normal. But in the case of G6PD, as a result of X-inactivation, the abnormal cells of a woman heterozygous for G6PD deficiency are just as deficient as those of a hemizygous deficient man, and therefore just as susceptible to pathology. Thus, although G6PD deficiency is still often referred to as an X-linked recessive trait, this is a misnomer because a recessive trait is, by definition, not expressed in a heterozygote: instead, G6PD deficiency is expressed in heterozygotes both biochemically and clinically—although it is true that heterozygotes are generally less severely affected.

Clinical manifestations

Acute haemolytic anaemia

In view of the large number of people who carry a G6PD deficiency gene, it is fortunate that the vast majority of them remain clinically asymptomatic throughout their lifetime. However, they are all at risk of developing acute haemolytic anaemia in response to three types of trigger: (1) drugs (see Table 22.5.12.1), (2) infections, and (3) fava beans. Typically, a haemolytic attack starts with malaise, sometimes associated with more or less profound weakness, and abdominal or lumbar pain. After an interval of several hours to 2 to 3 days the patient develops jaundice and may pass dark urine (haemoglobinuria). In the majority of cases the haemolytic attack, even if severe, is self-limiting and tends to resolve spontaneously. In the absence of additional or pre-existing pathology the bone marrow response is prompt and effective. Depending on the proportion of red cells that have been destroyed (reflected in the severity of the

Table 22.5.12.1 Drugs that can trigger haemolysis in children with G6PD[a]

Category of drug	Definite risk	Possible risk
Antimalarials	Primaquine Dapsone-containing combinations[b]	Chloroquine Quinine
Analgesics	Acetanilid	Aspirin
Sulfonamides/ sulfones	Sulfamethoxazole/co-trimoxazole Dapsone[b]	Sulfasalazine Sulfadiazine
Quinolones	Nalidixic acid Ciprofloxacin Norfloxacin Moxifloxacin Ofloxacin	
Other antimicrobials	Nitrofurantoin Methylene blue	Chloramphenicol
Other	Niridazole	Vitamin K Rasburicase Ascorbic acid Glibenclamide

[a] For all drugs the risk of haemolysis is dose-related, and so is the severity of haemolysis. For instance, aspirin up to 20 mg/kg is probably safe; three times that dose will almost certainly cause some haemolysis.

[b] Dapsone can cause hemolysis even in non-G6PD deficient subjects.

Table modified from *British National Formulary*, 55th edition, March 2008.

anaemia), the haemoglobin level may be back to normal in 3 to 6 weeks. The most serious threat in adults is the development of acute renal failure (this is exceedingly rare in children). The anaemia is usually normocytic and normochromic, and it varies from moderate to extremely severe (haemoglobin levels of 4 g/dl or less have been recorded); it is due largely to intravascular haemolysis, and hence it is associated with haemoglobinaemia, haemoglobinuria and low or absent plasma haptoglobin. The blood film shows anisocytosis, polychromasia, and other features associated with acute haemolysis, including spherocytes (Fig. 22.5.12.1a); in severe cases the poikilocytosis is very marked, with bizarre forms, numerous red cells that appear to have unevenly distributed haemoglobin ('hemighosts'), and red cells that appear to have had parts of them bitten away ('bite cells' or 'blister cells'). Supravital staining with methyl violet, if done promptly, reveals the presence of 'Heinz bodies', consisting of precipitates of denatured haemoglobin (Fig. 22.5.12.1b: apart from the rare cases when they are formed because of a genetic abnormality of haemoglobin, Heinz bodies can be regarded as a signature of oxidative damage to red cells). The white blood-cell count may be elevated, with predominance of granulocytes. The platelet count may be normal, increased, or moderately decreased. The unconjugated bilirubin is elevated but the 'liver enzymes' are usually normal.

Bacterial infection has been underestimated as a trigger of haemolytic anaemia in G6PD deficient subjects. Recently a higher rate of infectious complications and a more marked degree of anaemia have been observed in these subjects after major trauma.

Favism

This is perhaps the most spectacular form of acute haemolytic anaemia associated with G6PD deficiency: it can occur at any age, but far more commonly in children. The clinical picture is similar to that described above: but particularly prominent is haemoglobinuria, that often develops within 6 to 24 h from the onset of symptoms; there may be evidence of hypovolaemic shock or, more rarely, of high-output heart failure: either can be life-threatening. The cause of favism is the presence in fava beans (or broad beans *Vicia faba*) of vicine and convicine, two β-glycosides having as aglycones the substituted pyrimidines divicine and isouramil, which produce free radicals in the course of their auto-oxidation. Thus, haemolysis is highly specific for fava beans; other beans are safe. G6PD-deficient subjects (especially when they are adults) do not develop an acute attack of favism every time they eat fava beans: the reasons for this are not yet clear, but important factors are the quantity and quality of fava beans consumed. On the other hand, the widespread notion that favism occurs only with some G6PD-deficient variants and not with others is incorrect. For instance, favism has been well documented even with G6PD Seattle, a variant associated with rather mild enzyme deficiency (c.25% of normal). Favism is a paradigm of gene–environment interaction: it is practically nonexistent in parts of Africa where G6PD deficiency is common but fava beans are not eaten; and if fava beans are consumed it can occur in areas (including the United Kingdom) where G6PD deficiency is rare.

Neonatal jaundice

Not every G6PD-deficient baby becomes jaundiced after birth; however, the risk of developing neonatal jaundice (NNJ) is much greater in G6PD-deficient than in G6PD-normal newborns.

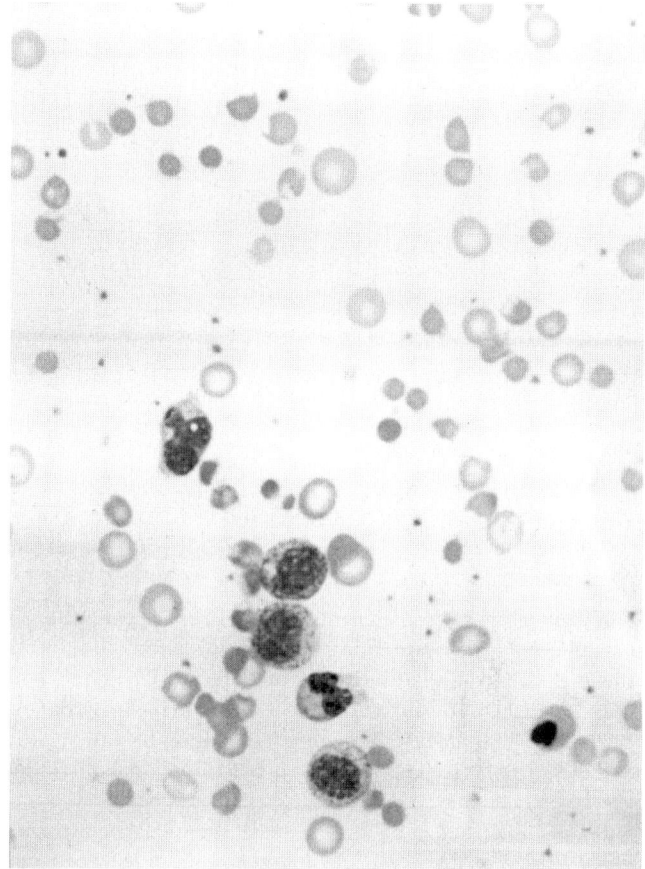

(a)

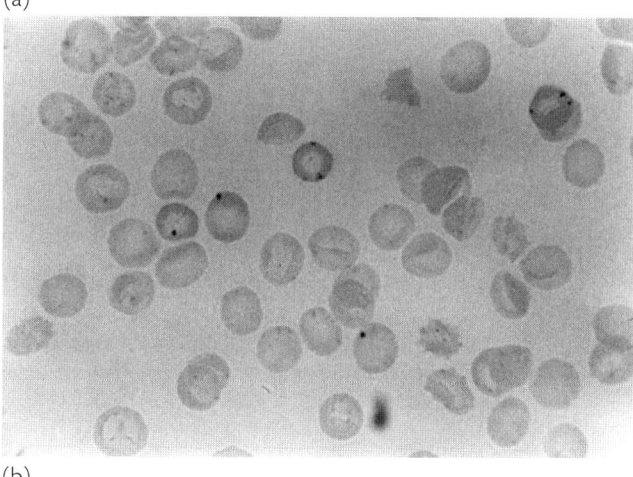

(b)

Fig. 22.5.12.1 Blood film in a case of acute haemolytic anaemia in a G6PD-deficient patient (favism). (a) Romanovsky stain, showing marked poikilocytosis, polychromatic macrocytes, bite cells, nucleated red cells, and a shift to the left in the granulocytic series. (b) Supravital stain with methyl violet, showing the characteristic Heinz bodies.

The extent of the association between G6PD deficiency and NNJ appears to vary greatly in different populations. The clinical picture of neonatal jaundice related to G6PD deficiency differs from the 'classical' rhesus-related neonatal jaundice in two main respects: (1) it is very rarely present at birth, with the peak incidence of clinical onset being between day 2 and day 3; (2) there is more jaundice than anaemia, and the anaemia is very rarely severe.

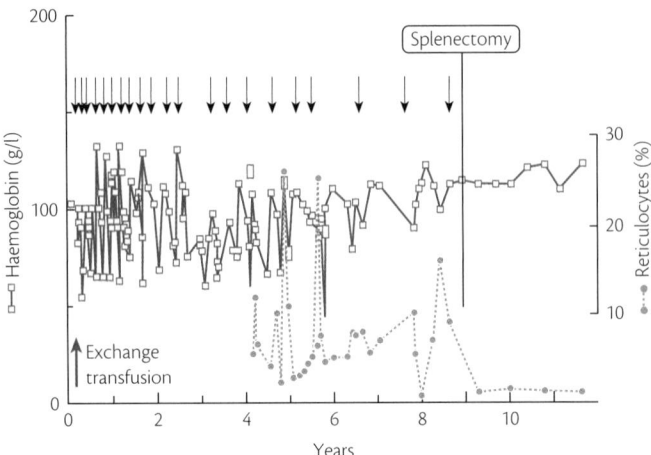

Fig. 22.5.12.2 Clinical course of a patient with chronic non-spherocytic haemolytic anaemia caused by severe G6PD deficiency, illustrating the high transfusion requirement, which was alleviated after splenectomy.

The severity of G6PD-related neonatal jaundice varies enormously, from subclinical, to overlapping with 'physiological jaundice', to imposing the threat of kernicterus if not treated. The reasons for this are not clear, but prematurity, infection, and environmental factors, e.g. naphthalene (camphor balls) used in babies' bedding and clothing, certainly play a part in making neonatal jaundice more severe and more dangerous. Other things being equal, the risk of NNJ is higher in babies who have the *UDP1A1* mutation characteristic of Gilbert disease. From the point of view of public health, it is important to realize that in some parts of the world G6PD deficiency is the commonest cause of severe NNJ; in addition, if not correctly managed, severe NNJ can produce permanent neurological damage.

Chronic nonsperocytic haemolytic anaemia

In contrast to the large majority of G6PD-deficient subjects who have no appreciable haemolysis in the steady state, a very small minority have chronic anaemia of very variable severity. The patient is virtually always a male, and in general he presents because of unexplained jaundice. Frequently the onset is at birth, and a diagnosis is made of neonatal jaundice (see Fig. 22.5.12.2) which may be severe enough to require exchange transfusion. Subsequently the anaemia recurs and the jaundice fails to clear completely; or the patients is only reinvestigated much later in life, perhaps because of gallstones in a child or in a young adult. The spleen is usually moderately enlarged, but it may increase in size sufficiently to cause mechanical discomfort, or hypersplenism, or both. The severity of anaemia ranges in different patients from borderline to transfusion dependent. The anaemia is usually normochromic but somewhat macrocytic; because a large proportion of reticulocytes (up to 20% or more) will cause an increased mean corpuscle volume and a shifted, wider than normal, size-distribution curve. The red-cell morphology is not characteristic, and for this reason it is referred to in the negative as being 'nonspherocytic'. The bone marrow is normoblastic, unless the increased requirement of folic acid associated with the high red-cell turnover has caused it to become megaloblastic. There is chronic hyperbilirubinaemia, decreased haptoglobin and increased lactate dehydrogenase. In this condition, unlike in the acute haemolytic anaemia described above,

haemolysis is mainly extravascular. However, the red cells of these patients are naturally also vulnerable to acute oxidative damage, and therefore the same agents (see Table 22.5.12.1) that can cause acute haemolytic anaemia in people with the ordinary type of G6PD deficiency will cause severe exacerbations with (sometimes massive) haemoglobinuria in people with the severe form of G6PD deficiency.

Laboratory diagnosis

Although the clinical picture of favism and of other forms of acute haemolytic anaemia associated with G6PD deficiency is quite characteristic, the final diagnosis must rely on the direct demonstration of decreased activity of this enzyme in red cells. With neonatal jaundice and chronic nonspherocytic haemolytic anaemia the differential diagnosis is much wider, and therefore this test is even more important. The most popular screening tests are the dye decolorization test, the methaemoglobin reduction test, and the fluorescence spot test. Any of these, provided it is properly standardized and subjected to quality control, is perfectly adequate for diagnostic purposes in patients who are in the steady state; but these semiquantitative tests are not adequate for patients in the acute haemolytic or in the posthaemolytic period, or with other complications; nor can they be expected to identify all heterozygotes. Ideally, every patient found to be G6PD deficient by screening should then be retested for confirmation by a quantitative assay. In normal red cells the range of G6PD activity, measured at 30 °C, is 7 to 10 IU/g Hb. In G6PD-deficient males (or homozygous females) the level of G6PD in the steady state is, by definition, less than 50% of normal; but with most variants it is less than 20% and with some it is almost undetectable. In heterozygous females the level is intermediate and extremely variable; in some cases the diagnosis may be therefore difficult without family studies or DNA analysis. However, for practical purposes it is most unlikely that a woman will have clinical manifestations if her G6PD level is more than 70% of normal.

Biochemistry and pathophysiology

Red cells are very vulnerable to oxidative damage for two reasons. First, oxygen radicals are generated continuously from within the red cells as haemoglobin cycles from its deoxygenated to its oxygenated form. Second, red cells are directly exposed to a variety of exogenous oxidizing agent. Oxygen radicals produced by such compounds are converted by superoxide dismutase to hydrogen peroxide, which is itself highly toxic. G6PD, the first enzyme of the pentose phosphate pathway (see Fig. 22.5.12.3), catalyses the conversion of glucose 6-phosphate (G6P) and NADP to 6-phosphogluconolactone and NADPH. The most important product of the G6PD reaction, certainly in red cells, is NADPH because, by producing glutathione (GSH) via GSH reductase, it is crucial for the operation of GSH peroxidase; on the other hand, it stabilizes catalase: these are the two enzymes able to detoxify hydrogen peroxide (by converting it to water). Normally, G6PD activity in red cells is such that NADPH is maintained at a high level and there is practically no NADP: the NADPH/NADP ratio plays a large part in the intracellular regulation of G6PD activity.

The enzymatically active form of G6PD is either a dimer or a tetramer of a single protein subunit of 514 amino acids with a molecular mass of 59 096 Da. Some regions of the molecule critical for its functions have been identified because they are highly

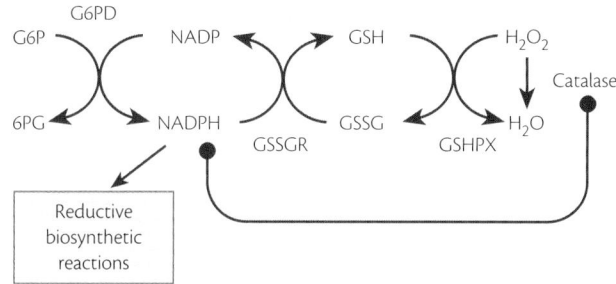

Fig. 22.5.12.3 The role of G6PD in red cell metabolism: NADPH plays a dual role in (i) regeneration of glutathione (GSH) and (ii) stabilization of catalase.

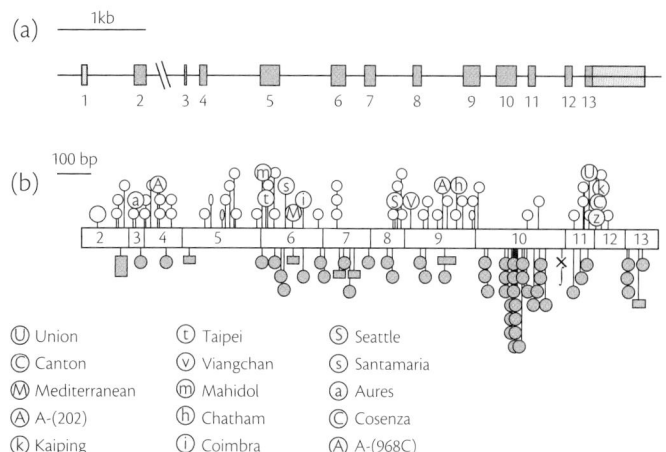

Symbol	Name	Symbol	Name	Symbol	Name
Ⓤ	Union	Ⓣ	Taipei	Ⓢ	Seattle
Ⓒ	Canton	Ⓥ	Viangchan	Ⓢ	Santamaria
Ⓜ	Mediterranean	Ⓜ	Mahidol	Ⓐ	Aures
Ⓐ	A-(202)	Ⓗ	Chatham	Ⓒ	Cosenza
Ⓚ	Kaiping	Ⓘ	Coimbra	Ⓐ	A-(968C)

Fig. 22.5.12.4 Hetereogeneity of G6PD deficiency. The 13 exons of the *G6PD* gene are drawn approximately to scale; the introns (not drawn to scale) are shown by thin lines connecting the exons. The location of the mutations for the variants listed in Table 2 are shown; plus that of G6PD Sunderland, as example of an English sporadic variant associated with chronic non-spherocytic haemolytic anaemia and due to a deletion of a triplet of bases, corresponding to codon 35.

conserved in evolution. The G6P-binding site and the active centre of the enzyme are located near lysine 205. Recently the three dimensional structure of G6PD has been solved. In the dimer structure the two subunits are symmetrically located across a complex interface of β-sheets. The NADP binding site is near the N-terminus, and bound NADP is important for the stability of G6PD.

Acute haemolytic anaemia associated with G6PD deficiency clearly results from the action of an exogenous factor on intrinsically abnormal red cells. Although the sequence of events ending in haemolysis is not completely understood, we know that oxidative agents cause glutathione depletion in G6PD-deficient red cells. This is followed by oxidation of sulphydryl groups and consequent denaturation of haemoglobin (hence the Heinz bodies) and probably of other proteins, which eventually causes irreversible damage to the membrane of red cells and hence their destruction, partly in the bloodstream and partly through phagocytosis by macrophages. An important feature of haemolysis in G6PD-deficient patients depends on the fact that G6PD decays gradually during red-cell ageing (e.g. in normal blood, reticulocytes have about five times more activity than the 10% oldest red cells), and this loss of enzyme activity is accelerated with many G6PD variants. Thus, a haemolytic attack selectively destroys older red cells because they have a more severe shortage of G6PD. This is why in the post-haemolytic state there is a significant increase in G6PD activity (hence the risk of misdiagnosis). By contrast, with some other variants the steady-state level of G6PD is so low that, even in the absence of any oxidant challenge, it becomes limiting for red-cell survival: this is the case in the patients with chronic nonsperocytic haemolytic anaemia, who may have a red-cell lifespan of between 10 and 50 days.

Molecular basis of G6PD deficiency

Characterization of G6PD from patients has often demonstrated that there is not only a quantitative abnormality of the enzyme (G6PD deficiency), but qualitative abnormalities as well. By sequencing G6PD from G6PD deficient subjects it has been verified that of some 150 mutations known, all are indeed in the coding sequence (except for one that affects splicing) (Fig. 22.5.12.4). Nearly all are missense point mutations producing single amino acid replacements in the G6PD protein. The exceptions are small deletions of one to eight amino acids, and in a few instances there are two point mutations rather than one (for instance, in G6PD A–, the variant most commonly encountered in Africa). Amino acid replacements can cause G6PD deficiency either by affecting its catalytic function or by decreasing the *in vivo* stability of the protein: the

latter is by far the most common mechanism (see Table 22.5.12.2). The molecular basis of chronic nonsperocytic haemolytic anaemia associated with G6PD deficiency is highly specific, in the sense that the underlying mutations are not the same as those underlying asymptomatic G6PD deficiency. The more severe clinical phenotype can be ascribed in most cases to extreme instability of the enzyme; e.g. a cluster of mutations that map to the dimer interface severely compromise the formation of the dimer, and the result is chronic nonsperocytic haemolytic anaemia.

Because the G6PD gene is X-linked, frequencies of G6PD deficiency in males are identical to gene frequencies, and they are as high as 20% or more in some parts of the world (see Fig. 22.5.12.5). The frequency of homozygous females is of course lower, but the frequency of heterozygous females is higher (according to the Hardy–Weinberg rule) than that of G6PD-deficient males. Different G6PD variants underlie G6PD deficiency in different parts of the world: e.g. G6PD Mediterranean on the shores of that sea, in the Middle East and in India; G6PD A– in Africa and in southern Europe; G6PD Viangchan in South-East Asia; G6PD Canton in China; and G6PD Union worldwide. It is also important to realize that in some populations several different polymorphic variants coexist. The overall geographical distribution of G6PD deficiency and its heterogeneity, together with findings from clinical field studies and *in vitro* experiments, strongly support the view that this common genetic trait has been selected by *Plasmodium falciparum* malaria, by virtue of the fact that it confers a relative resistance against this highly lethal infection.

Management

Prevention

The acute haemolytic anaemia of G6PD deficiency is largely preventable by avoiding exposure to triggering factors of previously screened subjects. Of course, the practicability and cost-effectiveness of screening depends on the prevalence of G6PD deficiency in each individual community. Favism is entirely preventable by not eating

Table 22.5.12.2 Genetic heterogeneity of G6PD deficiency

Variant class	Clinical expression	Degree of enzyme deficiency	Examples	Amino acid replacements	Populations where prevalent	Mechanism of enzyme deficiency
I	Chronic non-spherocytic haemolytic anaemia	Usually less than 10% of normal	Harilaou	216 Phe→Leu	All class I variants are sporadic	Unstable
			Barcelona	Not yet known		Abnormal kinetics
II	Acute haemolytic anaemia triggered by broad beans or infection or drugs	Less than 10% of normal	Mediterranean	188 Ser→Phe	Mediterranean, Middle East, India	Unstable
			Mahidol	163 Gly→Ser	South-East Asia	Unstable
			Canton	459 Arg→Leu	China	Unstable
			Union	454 Arg→Cys	Worldwide	?
III	As for class II	10 to 50% of normal	A–	68 Val→Met	Africa,	Unstable
				126 Asn→Asp	Southern Europe	
			Seattle	282 Asp→His	Europe	?
IV	None	More than 60% of normal	A	126 Asn→Asp	Africa	None

fava beans. Prevention of drug-induced haemolysis is possible in most cases by choosing alternative drugs. A common practical problem is the need to give primaquine for eradication of malaria due to *P. vivax* or *P. malariae*; in these cases the administration of a lower dose of the drug for a longer time is the recommended approach: this will still cause haemolysis, but of an acceptably mild degree.

Treatment of acute haemolytic anaemia and favism

A patient with acute haemolytic anaemia may be a diagnostic problem, that once solved, does not require any specific treatment at all; or the patient may be a medical emergency requiring immediate action, With severe anaemia, prompt blood transfusion is definitely indicated and may be life-saving. If there is acute renal failure, haemodialysis may be necessary. Recovery is the rule.

Management of neonatal jaundice

This does not differ from that of neonatal jaundice due to other causes than G6PD deficiency. In most cases, prompt phototherapy is highly effective and sufficient; but with bilirubin levels above 300 µmol/1litre (or even less in babies who are premature, or who have acidosis or infection), exchange blood transfusion is imperative to prevent neurological damage.

Management of chronic nonsperocytic haemolytic anaemia

In general terms, this does not differ from that of chronic nonspherocytic haemolytic anaemia due to other causes, e.g. pyruvate kinase deficiency. If the anaemia is not severe, regular folic acid supplements and regular haematological surveillance will suffice.

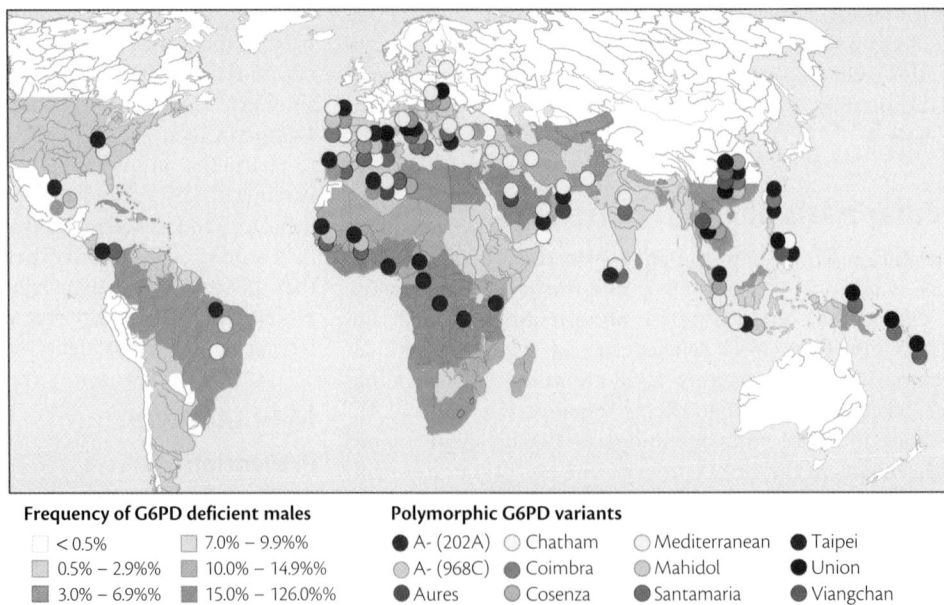

Frequency of G6PD deficient males

< 0.5%	7.0% – 9.9%%
0.5% – 2.9%%	10.0% – 14.9%%
3.0% – 6.9%%	15.0% – 126.0%%

Polymorphic G6PD variants

- A- (202A)
- ○ Chatham
- ○ Mediterranean
- Taipei
- A- (968C)
- Coimbra
- ○ Mahidol
- Union
- Aures
- Cosenza
- Santamaria
- Viangchan
- Canton
- Kaiping
- Seattle
- Local variant

Fig. 22.5.12.5 Frequency of G6PD-deficient males and polymorphic G6PD variants.

It will be important to avoid exposure to potentially haemolytic drugs, and blood transfusion may be indicated when exacerbations occur, mostly in concomitance with intercurrent infection. In rare patients the anaemia is so severe that it must be regarded as transfusion dependent. In these cases, blood transfusion will be probably needed at approximately 2-month intervals, in order to keep the haemoglobin in the 8 to 10 g/dl range. A hypertransfusion regimen aiming to maintain a normal haemoglobin level is not indicated (as there is no ineffective erythropoiesis in the bone marrow). However, in patients requiring regular transfusions, appropriate iron chelation should be instituted by the age of 2 years, and must be continued as long as transfusion treatment is necessary; sometimes the transfusion requirement may decrease after puberty. Although, unlike in hereditary spherocytosis, there is no evidence of selective red-cell destruction in the spleen, splenectomy has proven beneficial in severe cases. When a diagnosis of chronic non-spherocytic haemolytic anaemia is made, the family must be given genetic counselling, and an effort should be made to establish whether the mother is a heterozygote; if she is, the chance of recurrence is 1:2 for every subsequent male pregnancy. Prenatal diagnosis can be made by DNA analysis if the mutation is first identified in an affected relative. In principle, since the clinical manifestations of severe G6PD deficiency are confined to the blood, *i.e.* chronic non-spherocytic haemolytic anaemia, this condition could be cured by allogeneic bone marrow transplantation, but this has never been reported. For the same reason the condition ought to be amenable to correction by gene transfer into haematopoietic stem cells (gene therapy): this has been done in a pre-clinical mouse model.

Further reading

Beutler E (1991). Glucose 6-phosphate dehydrogenase deficiency. *N Engl J Med*, **324**, 169–74.

Cappellini MD, Fiorelli G (2008). Glucose-6-phosphate dehydrogenase deficiency. *Lancet*, **371**, 64–74.

Dacie JV (1985). Hereditary enzyme deficiency haemolytic anaemias. III: Deficiency of glucose-6-phosphate dehydrogenase. In: *Haemolytic anaemias*, Vol. 3, pp. 364–418. Churchill Livingstone, London.

Luzzatto L, Notaro R (2001). Malaria. Protecting against bad air. *Science*, **293**, 442–3.

Luzzatto L, Poggi V (2008). Glucose 6-phosphate dehydrogenase deficiency and hemolytic anemia. In: Orkin S, Nathan DG, Lux S (eds) *Hematology of infancy and childhood*, 7th edition, Chapter 17. W B Saunders, Philadelphia.

Mason PJ, Bautista JM, Gilsanz F (2007). G6PD deficiency: the genotype-phenotype association. *Blood Rev*, **21**, 267–83.

Rovira A, De Angioletti M, Camacho-Vanegas O, *et al.* (2000). Stable in vivo expression of glucose-6-phosphate dehydrogenase (G6PD) and rescue of G6PD deficiency in stem cells by gene transfer. *Blood*, **96**(13), 4111–7.

Spolarics Z, *et al.* (2001). Increased incidence of sepsis and altered monocyte functions in severely injured type A– glucose-6-phosphate dehydrogenase-deficient African American trauma patients. *Critical Care Med*, **29**, 728–36.

Haemostasis and thrombosis

Contents

22.6.1 The biology of haemostasis and thrombosis

Harold R. Roberts and Gilbert C. White

Essentials

Haemostasis—a component of the wound defence mechanism—is a process by which vessel wall components and platelets act in concert with procoagulant and anticoagulant proteins to form a plug of cells and cross-linked fibrin. The plug is later remodelled and replaced by new tissue as part of wound healing. These processes are very complex and involve highly controlled pathways of interaction between cells, glycans, and membrane-bound and soluble proteins of coagulation and fibrinolysis, as well as their cognate inhibitors.

Thrombosis—this is an abnormal state leading to formation of a clot obstructing blood vessel flow; dislodgement leads to thromboembolism.

Blood-vessel wall

Endothelial cells—these make many contributions to haemostasis: (1) vascular tone—by production of (a) vasodilators, most notably nitric oxide (NO) and prostacyclin (PGI_2), and (b) vasoconstrictors, particularly endothelin and angiotensin 2; (2) anticoagulant effects—by production of PGI_2, NO, thrombomodulin, tissue factor pathway inhibitor, glycosaminoglycans, CD39, tissue plasminogen activator; (3) procoagulant effects—the dominant effect of endothelial cells is anticoagulant, but they store/produce Von Willebrand factor and tissue factor (TF); (4) expression of receptors—including thrombin receptors, endothelial cell protein C receptor, and a number of adhesive receptors that are important for the interaction of leucocytes and the vessel wall.

Other elements—these include (1) extracellular matrix—promotes platelet adhesion, cellular migration, cell proliferation, and endothelial and smooth muscle cell interactions; (2) smooth muscle cells; (3) adventitia.

Platelets

Platelets are key components of the haemostatic plug. They adhere to damaged vessels where subendothelial matrix is exposed, aggregating to form an initial plug that prevents blood loss by occluding the breach in the vessel wall. Their involvement in haemostasis can broadly be divided into the following processes: (1) platelet adhesion—accomplished by a number of glycoprotein and other adhesion receptors on the platelet surface; (2) platelet activation—following adhesion and in response to soluble agonists, platelets undergo reactions (including changes in metabolism of membrane inositol phospholipids) that lead to generation of platelet coagulant activity, thrombin, and release of ADP, which lead to activation of additional platelets; (3) platelet aggregation—mediated by binding of activated platelet surface glycoprotein GPIIb–IIIa to fibrinogen or fibrin, which by virtue of its dimeric structure can bind to more than one platelet and thereby facilitate their aggregation, which serves to localize the haemostatic plug at the site of injury.

Blood coagulation

Blood coagulation depends on the presence of serial proenzymes that are sequentially activated in the presence of activators and cofactors, with key elements being (1) TF—this is constitutively produced in several extravascular tissues such as fibroblasts and smooth muscle cells, but not in cells exposed to the circulating blood; it functions as a receptor for factor VII and initiates the blood coagulation pathway after it binds to and activates factor VII; (2) TF–VIIa complex—this activates factors IX and X which, in the presence of their respective cofactors (VIII and V), rapidly convert prothrombin (factor II) to thrombin; (3) thrombin converts soluble fibrinogen to fibrin; (4) fibrin undergoes cross-linking by activated factor XIII to form the stable haemostatic plug.

Important aspects of the system include: (1) platelets are essential in several steps of the clotting mechanism and form the surface for activated clotting factors, which lead to the explosive generation of thrombin and subsequent clot formation; (2) the initial generation of relatively small amounts of thrombin is essential for feedback activation of factors V, VIII, XI, and XIII, as well as of platelets.

Inhibitors of the coagulation reactions—there are numerous inhibitors of the reactions involved in blood coagulation, which are essential for the time control and safety of the process. These include (1) TF pathway inhibitor—occurs in forms free within the circulation and anchored to cell surfaces; inhibits the VIIa–TF–Xa complex; (2) antithrombin—a serpin inhibitor of thrombin, factor X, and other proteases; (3) other inhibitors—these include α_1-antitrypsin, C-1 esterase inhibitor, and protein Z-dependent protease inhibitor.

The fibrinolytic system

The fibrinolytic system depends on the activation of plasminogen in the circulation by tissue plasminogen activator to form plasmin, which degrades (1) fibrinogen and fibrin to form specific fibrin degradation products, and also (2) factors VIII and V, and von Willebrand factor.

Important aspects of the system include: (1) free plasmin in the circulation is inhibited by α_2-antiplasmin; (2) plasminogen and tissue plasminogen activator associate in the circulation with fibrinogen, hence when fibrinogen is converted to fibrin, the clot is rich in both of these proteins, which are protected from the inhibitory action of antiplasmin, hence clots can be lysed without interference from inhibitors; (3) many other regulatory mechanisms, including plasminogen activator inhibitor I, urokinase plasminogen activator, and thrombin-activatable fibrinolytic inhibitor.

The balance of fibrinolysis and coagulation

Fibrinolysis and coagulation are interrelated: fibrin clots are normally lysed by plasmin locally released from plasminogen by the action of tissue plasminogen activator, and this process is enhanced by some procoagulant factors, e.g. activated factors XI and XII, protein C. This system, so delicately controlled and normally maintained in a dynamic equilibrium, is strongly influenced by components involved in inflammatory and other defence mechanisms in the host. An integrated understanding of these processes offers the potential for improved means to predict the adverse complications of many diseases and ultimately to prevent their occurrence.

Introduction

Fluid blood is contained within the vascular tree, but as a result of minor trauma that occurs during the wear and tear of everyday living, leaks occur in the blood vessel wall that must be sealed by a solid impermeable fibrin clot in order to prevent significant

blood loss. The clot is formed from factors in flowing blood and is located and restricted to the site of the leak without dissemination throughout the vascular tree. This is the process of haemostasis, an exquisitely controlled mechanism that requires components of the vessel wall, blood platelets, and soluble procoagulant and anticoagulant proteins. The haemostatic plug consists of a mass of platelets, red blood cells, and leucocytes enmeshed in interlocking strands of insoluble and cross-linked fibrin fibres that plug the leak.

Once formed, the haemostatic plug is gradually replaced by new tissue that results in wound healing. This process requires lysis of the blood clot by the fibrinolytic system and subsequent ingrowth of new cells. Thus, haemostasis is not an isolated phenomenon, but is one component of the defence mechanisms that lead to eventual wound healing.

Thrombosis, as opposed to haemostasis, is a pathological state in which normal haemostasis is disturbed to the extent that a clot is formed that partially or completely obstructs the flow of blood within the blood vessel and sometimes dislodges to become an embolus.

To understand the biology of haemostasis and thrombosis, it is necessary to know the roles of the vessel wall, the platelets, the coagulation and fibrinolytic systems, and their respective inhibitors.

Blood vessel wall

The anatomy of the wall of both an artery and a vein is shown schematically in Fig. 22.6.1.1. All blood vessels are lined by an intima consisting of a monolayer of endothelial cells that rest upon a loose network of tissue called the extracellular matrix. In addition to the intima, larger and intermediate arteries contain two other layers: the media, composed mostly of smooth muscle cells, and the adventitia, consisting largely of connective tissue, nerves, and nutrient vessels. These three layers also exist in veins, but the media and adventitia are much less distinct and are not visible in the smaller arterioles, venules, and capillaries.

Endothelial cells

Endothelial cells form the basis of vascular development and are derived from embryonic mesoderm. Embryonic endothelial cells

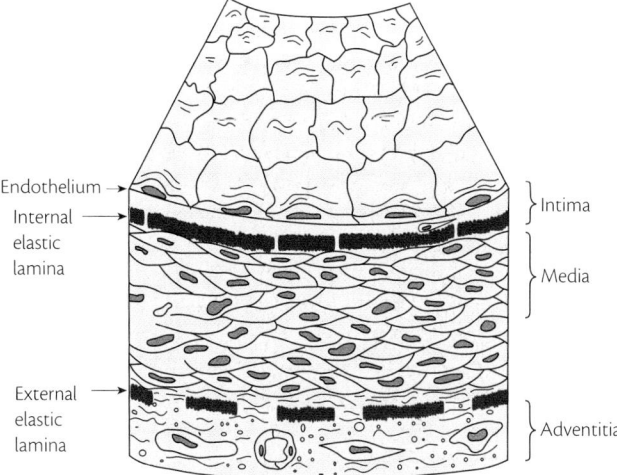

Fig. 22.6.1.1 Schematic diagram of a vessel wall consisting of the intima, the media (smooth muscle cells), and the adventitia. The intima consists of a layer of endothelium that is exposed to the circulating blood. The subendothelial matrix lies below the endothelium and is separated from the media by the internal elastic membrane. See text for detailed description of each layer.

(angioblasts) develop under the influence of growth hormones including basic fibroblast growth factor (b-FGF) and vascular endothelial growth factor (VEGF), both of which interact with receptors on the cell membrane termed receptor tyrosine kinases. These early blood vessels expand into a vascular tree under the influence of two major hormones, angiopoietin 1 and 2, that bind to a family of tyrosine kinase receptors called tie-1 and tie-2 (tyrosine kinase plus Ig and epidermal growth factor-like domains) on endothelial cells. To fully develop into an intact vascular tree, endothelial cells must interact with the extracellular matrix and other cells, a process that requires cell-cell adhesion that is dependent upon cell surface cytoadhesive molecules (CAMs) such as platelet-endothelial cell adhesion molecule-1 (PECAM-1), and vascular endothelial cell cadherin (VE-cadherin). Endothelial cell structure is also dependent upon the integrin family of molecules and interactions with the extracellular matrix.

Endothelial cells are heterogeneous in appearance, function, and genetic regulation. In the brain, endothelial cells form very tight junctions with one another to preserve the blood–brain barrier; in the spleen and liver, the interendothelial gaps are wide, permitting soluble and cellular trafficking between blood and the extravascular space. Not all endothelial cells synthesize the same proteins. Tissue plasminogen activator is synthesized by only about 3% of cells. Even von Willebrand factor (VWF), often regarded as a specific marker for endothelial cells, is not expressed in all cells. The microenvironment also plays an important role in regulating endothelial cell function. Haemodynamic forces, including hydrostatic pressure, and shear stresses and strains can influence endothelial cell structure and function. Haemodynamic forces can even regulate endothelial cell gene expression. For example, there is a shear-stress response element in the gene governing the synthesis of the β chain of the platelet-derived growth factor (PDGF). Other endothelial cell genes responsive to shear forces include those for tissue plasminogen activator, intercellular adhesion molecule (ICAM), and vascular cell adhesion molecule-1 (VCAM-1).

Endothelial cells contribute to haemostasis by their contributions to vascular tone, procoagulant, anticoagulant, fibrinolytic, and antifibrinolytic activities.

Vascular tone

Vasoregulatory substances produced by endothelial cells are shown in Table 22.6.1.1. The most important vasoregulators are nitric

Table 22.6.1.1 Vasoregulatory substances produced by endothelial cells

Vasoregulatory substance	Action
Vasodilators	
Nitric oxide (NO)	↑cGMP in SMC
Prostacyclin (PGI$_2$)	↑cyclic AMP in platelets
Monoamine oxidase (MAO)	↓catecholamines
Vasoconstrictors	
Endothelin	activates Ca^{++} channels in SMC
Angiotensin 2	converts angiotensin 1 to 2 by ACE
Prostaglandin G$_2$H$_2$(PGG$_2$, PGH$_2$)	acts on SMC

SMC = smooth muscle cells; AMP = adenosine-monophosphate (converted to adenosine); ACE = angiotensin-converting enzyme on endothelial cells.

Table 22.6.1.2 Procoagulant and anticoagulant properties of endothelial cells

Procoagulant and anticoagulant	Synthesis	Action
Procoagulants		
von Willebrand Factor (vWF)	Constitutive	Carrier of Factor VIII; platelet adhesion to vessel wall
Tissue Factor (TF)	Inducible	Receptor for Factor VII
Anticoagulants		
Prostacyclin (PGI2)	Constitutive	Inhibits platelet aggregation
Nitric oxide (NO)	Constitutive	Vasodilation
Thrombomodulin (TM)	Constitutive	TM/thrombin complex, activates protein C
Tissue factor pathway inhibitor (TFPI)	Constitutive	Inhibits TF–VIIa–Xa complex
Glycosoaminoglycans (GAG)	Constitutive	Antithrombins
CD 39	Constitutive	Inhibits platelet aggregation
Tissue plasminogen activator (t-PA)	Constitutive	Converts plasminogen to plasmin

oxide, previously known as endothelial cell-derived relaxation factor (EDRF), and prostacyclin. Nitric oxide and prostacyclin are also important antiplatelet agents. On the other hand, the most important vasoconstrictors are endothelin and angiotensin 2. Endothelin is also a mitogen for smooth muscle cells.

Anticoagulant properties

The anticoagulant properties of the endothelial cells are shown in Table 22.6.1.2. Prostacyclin not only causes vasodilation, but it is a potent inhibitor of platelet aggregation. Nitric oxide has a similar effect. An important anticoagulant function of endothelial cells is due to the expression of thrombomodulin, a transmembrane-bound protein that acts as a receptor for thrombin. The thrombomodulin–thrombin complex is the physiologic activator of protein C, which inactivates clotting factors Va and VIIIa to turn off coagulation. The action of the thrombin–thrombomodulin complex is enhanced when protein C occupies the endothelial cell protein C receptor (see below).

Endothelial cells contribute to the control of coagulation by synthesizing tissue factor pathway inhibitor (TFPI), which inhibits the tissue factor-mediated initiation of the clotting reactions. They also secrete glycosaminoglycans such as heparan sulphate and other proteoglycans that inhibit thrombin. In addition, they express vascular ATP diphosphohydrolase, otherwise known as CD39, on their surface. CD39 acts in concert with 5′ ectonucleotidase to convert ATP/ADP to AMP and then to adenosine, which inhibits platelet aggregation. Endothelial cells also secrete fibrinolytic factors including prostacyclin and tissue plasminogen activator, among others.

Procoagulant properties

Although the overall effect of endothelial cells is anticoagulant, these cells do participate in coagulation by storing proteins like VWF and by synthesizing tissue factor (TF) under certain conditions. Procoagulant properties of the endothelial cell are also listed

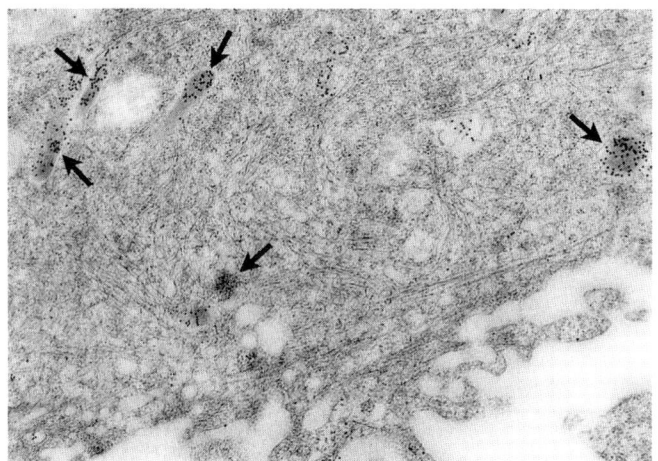

Fig. 22.6.1.2 Electron micrograph of an endothelial cell. Weibel–Palade bodies containing multimers of vWF are depicted by the arrows.

in Table 22.6.1.2. VWF is synthesized constitutively by endothelial cells and is essential for platelet adhesion to the vessel wall and as a carrier for blood clotting factor VIII. VWF is stored in Weibel–Palade bodies as depicted in Fig. 22.6.1.2. It is released into the circulation in multimers of heterogeneous molecular mass ranging from 1000 kDa to about 20 000 kDa. Endothelial cells also secrete very large VWF multimers abluminally into the extracellular matrix.

TF acts as a binding protein for factor VII and is essential for the initiation of coagulation. It is not constitutively produced by endothelial cells, but it can be induced by tissue necrosis factor (TNF), endotoxin, and other inflammatory substances.

Receptors

The receptor function of endothelial cells plays an important role in haemostasis and thrombosis (Table 22.6.1.3). They express thrombin receptors such as protease-activated receptor (PAR)-1, -2, and -4. Thrombin cleaves the C-terminal end of the receptor, which then binds to the remaining cell-associated protein (a so-called tethered ligand) and triggers intracellular signalling through G proteins, resulting in activation of endothelial cells. PARs influence vascular tone but do so through different intracellular signalling mechanisms.

The thrombin–thrombomodulin complex not only activates protein C, but also activates a protein known as the thrombin-activatable

Table 22.6.1.3 Receptor function of endothelial cells

Receptor	Ligand
Protease activated receptor 1 (PAR-1)	Thrombin
Thrombomodulin	Thrombin
Protein C receptor	Protein C
Urokinase plasminogen activator receptor (u-PAR)	Urokinase
Adhesive receptors	
Intercellular cytoadhesive molecule (ICAM) 1, 2	Integrins $\alpha_1\beta_2$; $\alpha_m\beta_2$
Vascular cytoadhesive molecule (VCAM)	$\alpha_1\beta_2$; $\alpha_4\beta_1$
P-selectin	Sialyl–Lewis antigen
E-selectin	

fibrinolytic inhibitor (TAFI), a procarboxypeptidase that functions to inhibit fibrinolysis. Endothelial cells also express endothelial cell protein C receptor (EPCR) that acts to modulate the activity of activated protein C. EPCR resides on the endothelial cell and enhances protein C activation by about 20-fold *in vivo*. EPCR binds protein C or activated protein C and presents it to the thrombin–thrombomodulin complex. Binding of APC to EPRC is also important in the inflammatory process in that through cell signalling mechanisms it decreases inflammatory cytokines and other molecules involved in inflammation. In addition, EPCR acts as a receptor for coagulation factor VII which binds to EPCR with an affinity similar to that of protein C.

Urokinase plasminogen activator receptors (u-PARS) are not found on resting endothelial cells, but are found on those involved in angiogenesis. There are a number of adhesive receptors on the surface of endothelial cells, as shown in Table 22.6.1.3. The adhesion of neutrophils is dependent upon the expression of P-selectin. P-selectin is rapidly internalized by the endothelial cell, but this is followed by expression of another cytoadhesive molecule, E-selectin, which is necessary for continued adherence and rolling of neutrophils along the endothelial cell surface. ICAM and VCAM are receptors for leucocytes and are important for the interaction of leucocytes and the vessel wall.

Extracellular matrix

The extracellular matrix is a complex, heterogeneous structure beneath the endothelium with a number of constituents that contribute to haemostasis and thrombosis. The matrix consists of a network of collagens, elastins, proteoglycans, and glycoproteins, including fibronectin, vitronectin, laminin, tenascin, thrombospondin, VWF, and osteopontin, as shown in Table 22.6.1.4. The matrix

Table 22.6.1.4 The extracellular matrix

Structural proteins
Collagens
I, III, IV, V, VI, VII
Elastin
Adhesive proteins
fibronectin
vitronectin
laminin
Von Willebrand factor
Antiadhesive
tenascin
thrombospondin
Ground substance
hyaluronic acid
proteoglycans
chondroitin sulphate
dermatan sulphate
heparan sulphate
others
Degradation and repair
matrix metalloproteinases

proteins promote platelet adhesion, cellular migration, cell proliferation, and endothelial and smooth muscle cell interactions.

Collagens are the most abundant proteins in subendothelial connective tissue. Collagen types I, II, III, IV, V, VI, and VII have been identified in various matrix tissues. The collagens are synthesized by endothelial cells, smooth muscle cells, and adventitial fibroblasts. The various collagens contribute to the integrity of the vessel wall, but they also play a role in platelet activation and, in some instances, coagulation. For example, collagen IV has been shown to be a specific high-affinity binding protein for blood coagulation factor IX, although the function of this complex is not yet known.

The proteoglycans constitute a heterogeneous group of molecules composed of a core protein attached to a glycosoaminoglycan. These include decorin, biglycan, heparan sulphate, dermatan sulphate, and others. Heparan sulphate, for example, can combine with antithrombin and inhibit thrombin. The precise role of all of the protoglycans is not known, but some attach to collagen and are necessary for maintaining the structure of the vessel wall.

The matrix also contains elastin, which is secreted by endothelial and smooth muscle cells as tropoelastin that is converted to mature elastin in the matrix where it is assembled into fibres. One function of elastin is simply to maintain the elastic structure of the vessel wall. This substance is found interspersed between smooth muscle cells as well as the matrix. It may also function in cell migration from the vessel wall to the extravascular space.

Fibronectin, vitronectin, and laminins are also components of the extracellular matrix which function in fibrinolysis and platelet adhesion.

Within the extracellular matrix there are a number of matrix metalloproteinases (MMP), a group of enzymes useful in matrix degradation and repair. They are secreted as proenzymes and converted to active enzymes that require zinc or calcium as cofactors. They have several functions as listed in Table 22.6.1.5. Their activities in matrix degradation and repair are controlled by tissue inhibitors of metalloproteinases.

Smooth muscle cells

The smooth muscle cell layer, found in medium and larger-sized vessels and more prominently in arteries, has several functions related to the biology of haemostasis and thrombosis. Smooth muscle

Table 22.6.1.5 Matrix metalloproteinases (MMP)

MMP number	Activity	Substrate
MMP-1	collagenase	collagen I, II, III, VII, VIII, X
MMP-2	gelatinase	collagen IV, V, VII, X
MMP-3	stromelysin	microglycans
MMP-8	collagenase	–
MMP-7	matrilysin	fibronectin, laminin, collagen IV
MMP-9	gelatinase	elastin, fibronectin
MMP-10	stromelysin	fibronectin, laminin, elastin, various collagens
MMP-11	stromelysin	fibrinogen, fibrin
MMP-12	elastase	elastin
MMP-14	–	collagen IV, progelatinase A
MMP-15	–	gelatin

Modified from Plow EF, Ugarova T, Miles LA (1998). In: Localzo J, Shafer AI, eds. *Thrombosis and hemorrhage*, 2nd edn, ch. 18, p. 381. Williams and Wilkins, Baltimore.

cells possess contractile, biosynthetic, and proliferative functions. Contractile properties governed by such substances as nitric oxide, prostacyclin, and endothelin play important roles in vasodilation and vasoconstriction, respectively. Smooth muscle cells, like endothelial cells, synthesize growth factors such as VEGF, insulin-like growth factors (IGF), epidermal growth factors (EGF), activins, and others that are important in smooth muscle cell generation. Smooth muscle cell proliferation is a hallmark of the atherosclerotic lesion. Biosynthetic products of the smooth muscle cells include various types of collagens, elastin, glycoproteins, and proteoglycans. When exposed to injury, smooth muscle cells can also produce TF, contributing to the initiation of blood coagulation.

Adventitia

The adventitia is composed of a loose network of cells consisting of fibroblasts, adipocytes, and mast cells. Collagens I and III, glycoproteins, and elastin are synthesized by fibroblasts. Fibroblasts also contain TF. Adipocytes secrete collagen I and III and synthesize lipids.

Platelets

Platelets are the smallest of the circulating blood cells, about 0.5 μm in diameter. They are essential components of the haemostatic plug and are derived from bone marrow megakaryocytes. Although platelets are anucleate and appear to be simple cells composed of cytoplasm, a surface canalicular system, and storage granules (δ or dense granules and α-granules); they are, nevertheless, complicated cells with a variety of very important functions essential for normal haemostasis. These can be broadly divided into the following: (1) platelet adhesion, defined as platelets adhering to the damaged area of the vessel wall where subendothelial matrix tissue is exposed; (2) platelet activation, both by agents within the matrix as well as by soluble agonists; (3) platelet secretion of granule contents; (4) platelet aggregation, defined as platelets sticking to one another in an aggregated mass, forming a platelet plug. The following sections describe each of these broad areas of platelet function in more detail.

Platelet adhesion

The initial platelet response to vascular injury is adhesion to the vessel wall. Resting, nonactivated platelets are not attracted to the vessel wall. However, following vascular damage, platelets rolling along the endothelium rapidly adhere to the subendothelial interstitial matrix exposed by injury. A number of matrix proteins, such as VWF, fibronectin, fibrinogen, and thrombospondin, are also present in platelet granules as well as the circulating blood.

Platelets possess numerous mechanisms for adhering to the subendothelial matrix (Fig. 22.6.1.3). Adhesion is accomplished by a number of protein receptors on the surface of platelets as described below.

Glycoprotein Ib–IX–V (CD42a–d)

The main function of the platelet membrane glycoprotein (GP) Ib–IX–V complex is to act as a receptor that mediates VWF-dependent binding of platelets to collagen, resulting in adhesion of platelets to the vessel wall. Glycoproteins Ibα, Ibβ, IX, and V are members of the leucine-rich glycoprotein family and are characterized by the presence of a common structural motif in the extracellular

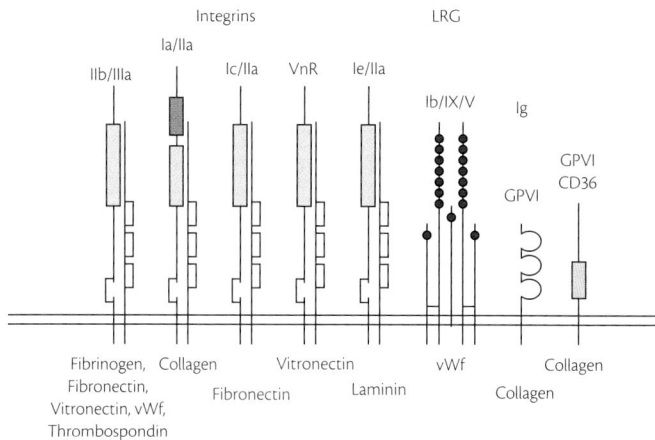

Fig. 22.6.1.3 Receptors mediating the interaction of platelets with subendothelial matrix proteins. Adhesion receptors on platelets include members of the integrin family, leucine-rich glycoproteins (LRG), members of the immunoglobulin (Ig) family, and others. Integrins on the surface of platelets are glycoproteins (GP) IIb–IIIa, which binds multiple ligands; GPIa–IIa, a collagen receptor, GPIc–IIa, which binds fibronectin; VnR, which is a receptor for vitronectin; and GPIc′–IIa, a laminin binding site. Glycoproteins Ib/IX/V are leucine-rich glycoproteins. Glycoprotein VI (GPVI) is a member of the immunoglobulin family and a collagen receptor. Glycoprotein IV (GPIV, CD36) is also a collagen receptor.

domain composed of a leucine-rich sequence. GPIbα contains seven leucine-rich repeats; GPV contains 15 leucine-rich repeats while GPIbβ and GPIX each contain a single leucine-rich repeat, all in the extracellular domains. GPIbα, GPIbβ, GPIX, and GPV are synthesized as separate gene products which coassociate in a ratio of 2:2:2:1 during transit through the endoplasmic reticulum. Coassociation of GPIbα, GPIbβ, and GPIX, but not GPV, is required for the complex to be expressed on the surface of cells. The role of GPV, a substrate for thrombin, in the function of the complex is uncertain, and mice deficient in GPV bind VWF normally and have normal platelet adhesion.

Adhesion to VWF-coated surfaces through GPIb–IX–V is increased by shear, which is thought to induce a structural change in the receptor that enhances the interaction with VWF. The A1 domain of VWF forms the principal site that interacts with GPIb. The site in GPIb that binds VWF is less well defined. Binding occurs in the N-terminal 45-kDa tryptic fragment from GPIbα. Within this region of GPIbα, an anionic site, [276]YDYYPEE[282], containing two sulphated tyrosine residues at tyrosines 278 and 279, has been further implicated in VWF binding. The A3 domain of VWF mediates the interaction with collagens type I and III. A model derived from the crystal structure of the VWF A3 domain suggests that the VWF–collagen interaction is primarily between negatively charged residues in the A3 domain and positively charged residues in collagen. Plasma VWF does not interact with unstimulated circulating platelets. For binding to occur, platelets have to be activated and plasma VWF must undergo a conformational change. After secretion by endothelial cells, VWF binds to underlying connective tissue matrix, providing an active surface for platelet attachment after the vessel wall is damaged.

Glycoprotein IIb–IIIa (αIIb/β3)

Under conditions of low shear, platelets can adhere to matrix-bound VWF through a mechanism that involves platelet GPIIb–

IIIa. GPIIb and IIIa are members of the integrin superfamily, a conserved family of heterodimeric surface receptors, each composed of a larger two-chain α subunit and a smaller β subunit, bound noncovalently. Integrins were initially identified by an ability to bind adhesive glycoproteins containing a tripeptide sequence, arginine–glycine–aspartic acid (RGD), although subsequent work has identified other ligand sequences recognized by integrins. The interaction of VWF with GPIIb–IIIa is mediated by an RGD sequence in the C1 domain of VWF. GPIIb–IIIa is also able to bind fibronectin, thrombospondin, and vitronectin and may therefore represent an adhesion receptor with broad specificity.

Glycoprotein Ia–IIa (α2β1)

GPIa–IIa is a receptor for types I and IV collagen and mediates platelet adhesion to the vessel wall independent of VWF. The integrin sequences that mediate the interaction with collagen reside in a broad sequence called the I domain in the extracellular portion of the molecule. GPIa–IIa is constitutively active and does not require activation to interact with collagen.

Glycoprotein VI–Fc receptor α-chain complex

GPVI–FcRα is the major platelet receptor mediating collagen-induced activation of platelets. GPVI is a member of the immunoglobulin superfamily and is characterized by immunoglobulin domains, a transmembrane domain, and a short cytoplasmic tail that lacks known signalling components. GPVI is associated on the platelet surface with FcRα, apparently in a 1:1 stoichiometry. The complex binds collagen and mediates collagen-generated signals, presumably through the immunoglobulin receptor tyrosine-based activation motif (ITAM) of FcRα. Cross-linking of the GPVI–FcRα leads to tyrosine phosphorylation of the ITAM sequence by Src kinase. Syk, another tyrosine kinase, binds to the phosphorylated ITAM sequence through Syk sulphydryl domains, initiating a signal that leads to tyrosine phosphorylation of phospholipase Cα2 and the generation of inositol phospholipids.

Glycoprotein IV (CD36)

CD 36 is a highly glycosylated transmembrane protein present on platelets, monocytes, endothelial cells, and nucleated erythrocytes which binds thrombospondin and collagen. The thrombospondin-binding site has been mapped to a single disulphide loop in the extracellular domain of GPIV, but the collagen-binding site is unknown. Although GPIV is a receptor for collagen *in vitro*, individuals with a deficiency of GPIV have no apparent defect in platelet function.

Other adhesion receptors

Platelets can also adhere to subendothelial matrix through glycoprotein Ic–IIa (VLA-5, α5β1), glycoprotein Ic′–IIa (VLA-6, α6β1), or the vitronectin receptor (αvβ3, VnR). GPIc–IIa is a constitutively active receptor for fibronectin that does not require cell activation. There are two sequences in fibronectin which interact with GPIc–IIa: an RGD sequence in the tenth type III repeat which interacts primarily with the GPIIa (β1) subunit and a synergy sequence in the adjacent ninth type III repeat which interacts primarily with the GPIc (α5) subunit. GPIc′–IIa is a laminin receptor which is expressed on platelets. Immunoprecipitation studies suggest that GPIc′–IIa may exist on the cell surface in a complex with proteins with four transmembrane domains, so-called tetrapanins, such as CD9, CD81, and NAG-2. The nature of these interactions is presently unclear. GPIc′–IIa recognizes a sequence in the long arm E8 fragment of laminin obtained after elastin digestion. The binding requires the presence of divalent cations which bind to specific sites on the integrin α subunit. Small numbers of the vitronectin receptor are expressed on platelets.

Current evidence indicates that all of these adhesion mechanisms may be important. The redundancy in adhesion receptors may (1) provide backup mechanisms to protect against blood loss; (2) generate different signals in response to interaction with different matrix proteins; or (3) represent different systems at work in different parts of the vascular tree. An example of the latter might be the relative roles of GPIb–IX–V and GPIIb–IIIa in the VWF-mediated adhesion of platelets to collagen. Under high shear conditions, like those found in capillaries and small arterioles, GPIb–IX–V may be the predominant mechanism mediating platelet adhesion to collagen and VWF-dependent adherence; whereas under low shear conditions, like those found in large veins and in arteries, GPIb–IX–V may be less effective and other mechanisms that require a shorter residence time of platelets on the subendothelial matrix, including GPIc–IIa interaction with fibronectin and GPIa–IIa interaction with collagen, may be important. The presence of multiple receptors for collagen on the platelet surface, including GPIb–IX–V, GPIIb–IIIa, GPIa–IIa, GPIV, and GPVI is interesting and raises the possibility of different collagen responses. Vitronectin also appears to be important for adhesion at high shear, and can bind to both GPIIb–IIIa and specific vitronectin receptors. Recent evidence suggests that platelet adhesion to collagen types I and III in flowing blood is dependent on both VWF and fibronectin. Collagen types I, II, and III have been shown to bind VWF.

Platelet activation

Following adhesion and in response to soluble agonists such as thrombin, platelets undergo a series of complex biochemical reactions leading to cell activation. As a result, platelets undergo changes in shape, alterations in surface lipid composition leading to the generation of platelet coagulant activity and thrombin generation, and secretion of the contents of intracellular granules leading to the release of ADP. The thrombin generated at the platelet surface and ADP secreted from platelet granules lead to activation of additional platelets. These reactions involve the metabolism of membrane inositol phospholipids, changes in cellular levels of calcium, activation of contractile proteins, stimulation of heterotrimeric and low-molecular-weight GTP-binding proteins, and tyrosine and serine-threonine phosphorylation of proteins, among other events. These biochemical reactions initiate second messenger signals that drive the functional changes that occur in platelets which transform them from the resting state to an activated one, and which play a crucial role in haemostasis. Some of these signalling pathways are described in the following sections (see Fig. 22.6.1.4).

Phospholipid metabolism

Metabolism of membrane phospholipids is one of the first signalling pathways identified in platelets and remains one of the most important. Platelet stimulation by a variety of agonists results in activation of membrane-associated phospholipases, including phospholipases C, A2, and D, which cleave fatty acids from the phospholipid. The lipid products generated by these pathways are signalling compounds which are important for changes in cytoplasmic calcium and activation of kinases and phosphatases.

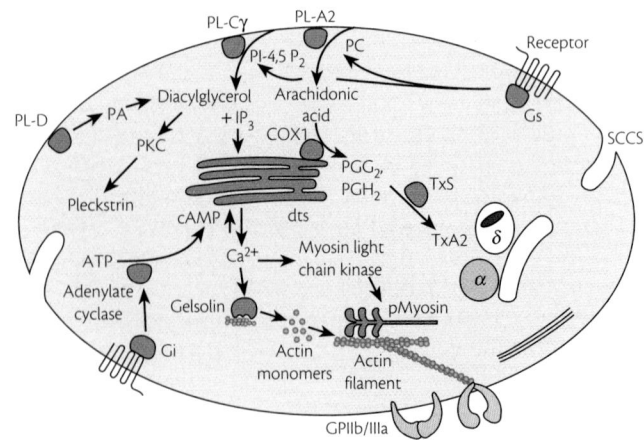

Fig. 22.6.1.4 Signalling pathways involved in platelet activation. Following the interaction of agonist with receptor, there is G protein (Gs) coupled activation of phospholipid metabolic pathways through phospholipase A2 (PL-A2), phospholipase Cγ (PL-Cγ), and phospholipase D (PL-D) leading to generation of thromboxane A2 (TxA2), inositol trisphosphate (IP$_3$), diacylglycerol, and phosphatidic acid (PA). Arachidonic acid generated by the action of phospholipase A2 is converted by cyclooxygenase-1 (COX-1) to prostaglandin endoperoxides G$_2$ (PGG$_2$) and H$_2$ (PGH$_2$) which are, in turn, converted to thromboxane A2 through the action of thromboxane synthase (TxS). Thromboxane generated through arachidonate metabolism is thought to play a role in secretion, through the fusion of α-granule (α) and dense granule (δ) membranes with the membrane of the surface-connected canalicular system (SCCS). Granule contents, including adenosine diphosphate, are emptied into the SCCS and make their way to the outside of the cell. Diacylglycerol stimulates activation of protein kinase C (PKC), resulting in serine-threonine phosphorylation of proteins such as pleckstrin. Inositol trisphosphate stimulates calcium release from storage sites in the dense tubular system (dts). The release of calcium from the dense tubular system is antagonized by cyclic AMP, generated through G protein (Gi) coupled inhibitory receptor activation of adenylate cyclase. Calcium, released in response to IP$_3$, activates gelsolin, an actin-capping and -severing protein, which generates actin monomers that then serve as nucleation sites for formation of actin filaments and assembly of the activation-dependent cytoskeleton. Assembly of the cytoskeleton and interaction of the cytoskeleton with surface integrins such as glycoproteins IIb and IIIa (GPIIb–IIIa) may be involved in integrin activation. Calcium also activates myosin light chain kinase which phosphorylates myosin light chain-generating actinomyosin contraction, important for changes in platelet shape and the secretion process.

The most intensively studied of these pathways is the metabolism of inositol phospholipids through phospholipase C. Membrane phosphatidylinositol (PI) exists in multiple phosphorylation states: PI, PI–P, PI–P2 which is phosphorylated in the 3,4 or 4,5 positions, and PI–P3 which is phosphorylated in the 3,4,5 positions. Phosphatidylinositol-specific kinases and phosphatases maintain pools of phosphorylated phosphoinositides in a proper concentration range. Platelets contain several isoforms of phospholipase C which are activated by different mechanisms. All cleave phosphatidylinositol 4,5-bisphosphate (PI 4,5–P2) and, later, phosphatidylinositol, as well as phosphatidylinositol 4-phosphate (PI 4–P), to yield diglyceride and inositol trisphosphate (IP3). Phospholipase Cα and Cβ are coupled to heterotrimeric G proteins where phospholipase Cα is coupled to growth factor receptors. IP3 generated by phospholipase C cleavage of inositol phospholipids has been implicated in the release of calcium from intracellular storage sites in the platelet-dense tubular system. The other product of phospholipase C cleavage, diacylglycerol, activates protein kinase C, which phosphorylates pleckstrin, a 47-kDa protein, and other proteins.

Phospholipase A2 is linked to G-protein coupled receptors and cleaves fatty acids in the *sn-2* position in membrane phospholipids, primarily phosphatidylcholine. In most individuals in developed countries, the fatty acid in this position is arachidonic acid. Arachidonic acid, liberated by the action of phospholipase A2, is converted to a variety of possible products by the microsomal enzymes, cyclooxygenase, and lipoxygenase. Cyclooxygenase converts arachidonic acid to prostaglandin endoperoxides, prostaglandins F_2, E_2, and D_2, whose main fate in platelets is rapid conversion to thromboxane A_2 by thromboxane synthase. Thromboxane A_2 is believed to play an important role in the release of intracellular granules by acting as a membrane fusogen, fusing granule membranes with the membrane of the surface connected canalicular system and permitting secretion of the granule contents to the outside of the cell. Thromboxane A_2 is also an exceptionally potent constrictor of vascular smooth muscle and a strong platelet-aggregating agent.

Inhibition of the arachidonate pathway has been a primary target for platelet inhibition. Cyclooxygenase is irreversibly inhibited by aspirin, which acetylates serine 340, and reversibly inhibited by nonsteroidal anti-inflammatory agents. Inhibition of cyclooxygenase inhibits thromboxane formation and results in inhibition of the release of intracellular granules. The mechanism by which aspirin is thought to act as an anti-atherosclerosis agent is by inhibition of the release of PDGF.

Phospholipase D acts primarily on phosphatidylcholine to produce choline and phosphatic acid. Protein kinase C and PI–P2 play an important role in activation of phospholipase D. Phosphatidic acid is an intracellular messenger which is proposed to play a role in platelet activation. In addition, phosphatidic acid can be converted to lysophosphatidic acid through the action of phospholipase A2. Like phosphatidic acid, lysophosphatidic acid is an intracellular messenger which is involved in phospholipase activation, signalling by low-molecular-weight G proteins, and cytoskeleton reorganization.

Calcium metabolism

Calcium ions are extremely important in platelet function, as described below. In resting platelets, the cytoplasmic concentration of calcium is maintained at a low level by active transport of calcium both inside and outside the cell and into the dense tubular system (DTS), a sarcoplasmic reticulum-like fraction in platelets. Calcium transport in the platelet is accomplished by a plasma membrane sarcoplasmic–endoplasmic reticulum-like calcium ATPase (SERCA2-b), a dense tubular system SERCA3, a sodium-calcium exchange pump in the plasma membrane, and passive calcium fluxes. During platelet activation, IP3, generated by metabolism of membrane inositol phospholipids, induces the rapid release of calcium stored in the dense tubular system. This increase in cytoplasmic calcium is essential for platelet activation, and agents that cause decreases in cytoplasmic calcium inhibit platelet activation while agents that increase cytoplasmic calcium stimulate platelet activation.

Calcium functions as a major intracellular messenger in platelets, mediating calcium-dependent reactions important in almost all phases of platelet activation. An increase in the concentration of cytoplasmic free calcium activates gelsolin, the calcium-dependent actin capping and severing protein, which plays an important role in reorganization of the cytoskeleton. Calcium also activates the

calcium and calmodulin-dependent myosin light chain kinase, leading to phosphorylation of myosin light chains, activation of actin-stimulated myosin ATPase activity, and the development of contractile forces. The contraction generated by actin and myosin mediates changes in platelet shape and is important for events leading to platelet secretion. In the absence of calcium ions, tropomyosin inhibits the interaction of myosin with actin, and this may be an additional regulatory role of calcium in platelets. Calpain, a calcium-dependent thiol protease, hydrolyses numerous proteins involved in platelet signalling. Activation of calpain is believed to be important both for regulation of cytoskeletal events and integrin-mediated signalling.

Cytoskeletal reorganization

Resting platelets are discoid in shape and feature a cellular cytoskeleton that consists of a network of actin filaments that fill and shape the cytoplasm of the cell and a single microtubule coil at the margin of the disc. Upon activation, platelets undergo remarkable morphological changes (Fig. 22.6.1.5). There is an initial change from the normal discoid shape of the resting platelet to a sphere as calcium levels in the cell increase. Filamentous actin appears in the form of stress fibres, and the cellular content of filamentous actin increases. Membrane ruffles form as long cellular projections called pseudopodia, processes that also involve the low-molecular-weight GTPases rac, rho, and cdc 42. Actin cables are present in these pseudopodia, extending to the end of the projections. Also during activation, microtubules contract and 'squeeze' granules toward the centre of the cell.

The energy for contraction is provided by a magnesium ion-dependent ATPase present in myosin and stimulated by actin. Contraction occurs by actin filaments and myosin rods sliding over one another. Myosin light-chain phosphatase may switch off myosin. Membrane glycoproteins GPIIb–IIIa, GPIb–IX–V, and other membrane proteins are associated with the cytoskeleton and provide direction for the contractile process. This activation-dependent cytoskeleton is more than just a structural scaffold for platelet shape changes. Numerous signalling proteins are incorporated into the cytoskeleton and may function in specialized compartments by virtue of their association with the cytoskeleton.

Platelet coagulant activity (platelet factor 3)

Platelet membranes have an asymmetrical distribution of phospholipids, with almost all of the acidic (negatively charged) phospholipids such as phosphatidylserine and phosphatidylinositol located in the inner leaflet of the plasma membrane. After platelet activation, the acidic phospholipids are translocated to the outer half of the membrane, while phosphatidylcholine moves to the inner half, in a phenomenon known as a 'flip-flop' reaction. This transbilayer movement of phospholipids in the platelet membrane is not well understood, but evidence for a 'flipase' which enzymatically contributes to it has been presented. There is also a translocase enzyme that works in the opposite way and is capable of restoring the acidic phospholipids to the inner leaflet of the membrane bilayer.

The exposed phosphatidylserine and other negatively charged phospholipids account for some of the activity traditionally known as platelet factor 3 (PF3) by contributing to surface properties for binding of factor X and prothombin activation complexes. This interaction with platelet phospholipids increases the rate of factor

Surface-connected
canalicular system
Microtubules
Alpha granule
Dense granule
Glycogen
Mitochondrion

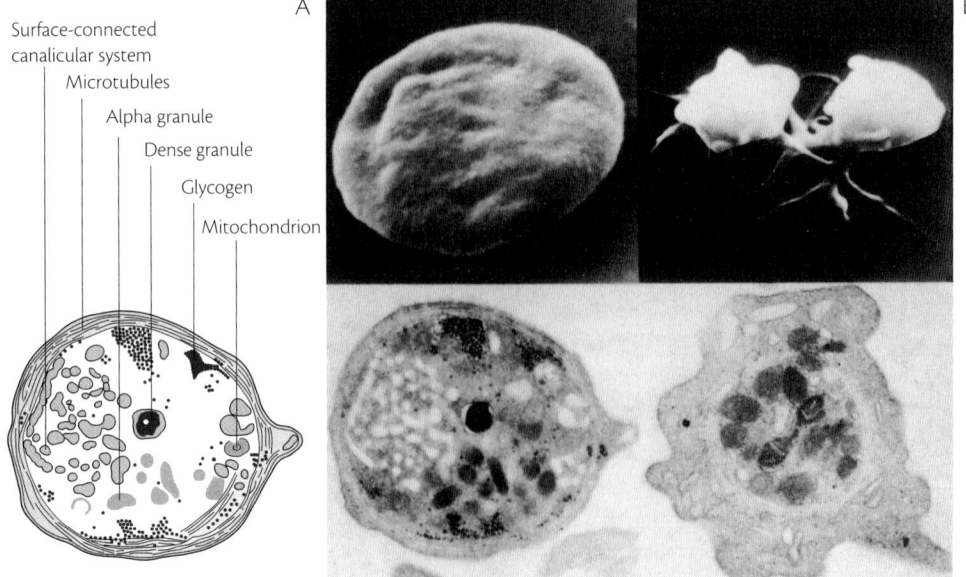

Fig. 22.6.1.5 Platelet morphology. Platelets are small, anucleate cells. In the resting state (A), platelets are ducoid shaped and contain a marginal rim of microtubules. After activation (B), platelets undergo changes in shape, becoming more rounded and extending cytoplasmic projections, called pseudopods, outward.

X activation and prothrombin activation nearly a thousand fold. In addition to phospholipids on the platelet membrane, there appear to be other specific binding proteins for blood clotting factors.

cAMP pathway

The major mechanism for down-regulation of platelet function is the stimulation of adenylate cyclase, which increases cAMP concentrations. Adenylate cyclase is mainly localized in microsomal fractions and is stimulated by adenosine, prostacyclin, and prostaglandin E_1 through activation of Gs, a heterotrimeric GTPase associated with the prostaglandin receptor on the platelet surface. cAMP inhibits platelet aggregation, platelet secretion, and platelet adhesion to the vessel wall. These effects are probably exerted by inhibiting calcium flux and/or promoting calcium reuptake.

Activation by soluble agonists

In addition to activation through interaction with subendothelial connective tissues, platelets may also be activated by soluble agonists. These include ADP, adrenaline, and thrombin. In general, this activation occurs through the interaction between soluble agonist and specific receptors on the platelet surface.

Thrombin is one of the most powerful of platelet agonists. Generated during blood coagulation, thrombin activation of platelets occurs through a novel family of receptors called protease-activated receptors (PARs). These are G protein-coupled, seven-membrane-spanning molecules which are activated by proteolysis. Thrombin cleaves the N-terminal exo-domain, unmasking a new N-terminal, which functions as a tethered peptide agonist. The tethered peptide binds intramolecularly to the remainder of the receptor to trigger activation. Four members of the PAR family of receptors have been identified, but only PAR 1 and PAR 4 mediate activation of human platelets by thrombin.

Thrombin interacts with other proteins on the surface of platelets, but the nature of these interactions is uncertain. Glycoprotein V, part of the GPIb–IX–V complex, is a substrate for thrombin although the absence of GPV does not appear to inhibit thrombin activation of platelets. GPIb is an equilibrium binding site for thrombin. Patients with a deficiency of GPIb have been reported

to have changes in the rate of activation of platelets by thrombin which is overcome at higher concentrations of agonist.

There are at least three receptors for ADP on platelets, all members of the seven-transmembrane-spanning members of the purinergic (P2) receptor family, either P2Y (G-protein-coupled purinergic receptors) or P2X (ligand-gated channel receptors). One receptor, designated P2Y1, is coupled to phospholipase Cβ, probably through Gq. A second receptor, P2Y12, is coupled to adenylate cyclase through Gi2. The third receptor, P2X1, is coupled to rapid calcium influx and is a member of the intrinsic ion channel family. Full platelet activation by ADP likely involves an interaction of ADP with all three receptors. ADP-induced activation of the GPIIb–IIIa on platelets requires both P2Y1 and P2Y12 and concomitant signalling through GTP-binding proteins, Gq and Gi2.

Platelet secretion

A primary endpoint of platelet activation is the secretion of platelet granule contents to the outside of the cell. During platelet activation, the granules are 'squeezed' to the centre of the cell where the granules fuse with the surface-connected canalicular system, a series of intracellular canals that are connected to the cell surface. The contents of the granules make their way to the outside of the cell. Secretion requires prostaglandin metabolism and is dependent on contractile events. Products of prostaglandin metabolism, primarily thromboxane A2, may act in the fusion of the granule membrane with that of the surface-connected canalicular system.

Platelets possess two types of storage granules (Table 22.6.1.6), both of which are involved in secretion of active ingredients that modulate platelet function. One type is the dense granule, so called because it is dense by electron microscopy. The other type is the α-granule.

Dense granules contain adenine nucleotides, calcium, and serotonin. Adenine nucleotides are sequestered in the dense granules mainly as ADP and ATP in a complex with calcium ions and pyrophosphate, and are not interchangeable with the nucleotides involved in general cell metabolism. ADP released from platelet-dense granules activates additional platelets and recruits them to the growing platelet thrombus. Serotonin, a potent modulator of vascular tone and integrity, is also a constituent of dense granules.

Table 22.6.1.6 Platelet granule contents

α Granules

α_2-Antiplasmin	Immunoglobulin
Albumin	Multimerin
β-Amyloid precursor	Plasminogen activator
β-Thromboglobulin (β-TG)	Platelet-derived growth factor (PDGF)
Clusterin	Platelet factor 4 (PF4)
Endothelial cell growth factor (ECGF)	P-selectin (GMP-140)
Factor V	Transforming growth factor (TGF)-α
Fibrinogen	Transforming growth factor(TGF)-β1
Fibronectin	Vitronectin
Granule membrane protein (GMP) 33	von Willebrand factor

Dense (δ) granules

Adenosine diphosphate (ADP)	Granulophysin
Adenosine triphosphate (ATP)	Pyrophosphate (PPi)
Calcium	Magnesium
Guanosine diphosphate (GDP)	Serotonin (5-hydroxytryptamine)
Guanosine triphosphate (GTP)	

Lysosomal (γ) granules

β-Galactosidase	Elastase
β-Glucuronidase	Endoglucosidase
β-Glycerophosphatase	LAMP-1
β-Hexosaminidase	LAMP-2
Cathepsins	LIMP-CD63
Collagenase	N-acetylglucosaminidase

α-Granules contain PDGF, β-thromboglobulin, PF4, fibrinogen, factor V, VWF, and thrombospondin. PDGF is mitogenic for smooth-muscle cells and when released from platelets at a site where the vessel wall is damaged, it stimulates proliferation and migration of smooth-muscle cells in the intima, contributing to the atherosclerotic process. β-Thromboglobulin and PF4 are basic, lysine-rich proteins that interact with glycosaminoglycans such as heparan sulphate, dermatan sulphate, and chondroitin sulphate, which are components of the endothelial cell surface. PF4 has a strong heparin-neutralizing activity and has been implicated in the aetiology of heparin-induced thrombocytopenia. Thrombospondin is a major α-granule glycoprotein, but it is also secreted by fibroblasts, endothelial and smooth-muscle cells. Thrombospondin is a high-molecular-weight adhesive protein which binds to glycosaminoglycans, fibrinogen, plasminogen, histidine-rich glycoprotein, type V collagen, and calcium ions. It associates with cell surfaces and extracellular matrices and facilitates cell–cell and cell–matrix interactions.

Platelet aggregation

Platelet aggregation, the interaction of one platelet with another, is a major function of platelets and is very important in the haemostatic process. The formation of an aggregated platelet mass at the site of injury provides a physical plug that occludes the defect in the vessel wall and prevents blood loss.

Aggregation is mediated by two glycoproteins on the platelet surface, GPIIb–IIIa, which constitute a receptor for fibrinogen/fibrin. Thus, GPIIb–IIIa on one platelet binds fibrinogen or fibrin which, by virtue of its dimeric structure, interacts with GPIIb–IIIa on another platelet. On resting platelets, GPIIb–IIIa is in an inactive state and is unable to bind fibrinogen. Following platelet activation, GPIIb–IIIa becomes activated through a process that involves calcium, protein kinase C, and heterotrimeric G proteins. Activation of GPIIb–IIIa requires energy and is a multistep process. Fibrinogen binding to GPIIb–IIIa occurs through a C-terminal dodecapeptide sequence, HHLGGAKQAGDV (His, his, leu, gly, gly, ala, lys, glutamine, ala, gly), in the α chain of fibrinogen where the AGDV (aspartic acid, val) sequence has been suggested to have structural similarity to the RGD (arginine, glycine, asparic acid) sequence.

Blood coagulation

The blood coagulation system consists of a number of zymogens (proenzymes) that are proteolytically converted to active enzymes in a series of steps involving activators and cofactors. The coagulation reactions are initiated by TF in complex with activated factor VII (VIIa). The TF–VIIa complex then activates both factor IX and factor X, which, in the presence of their respective cofactors (factors VIII and V), lead to the rapid conversion of prothrombin to thrombin. Thrombin converts fibrinogen into a solid fibrin clot that finally undergoes cross-linking by activated factor XIII to become a stable haemostatic plug. Platelets are essential in several steps of the clotting mechanism and form the surface for activated clotting factors, which lead to the explosive generation of thrombin and subsequent clot formation. The initial generation of relatively small amounts of thrombin is essential for feedback activation of factors V, VIII, XI, and XIII as well as platelets. Activated platelets aggregate and localize the haemostatic plug at the site of injury.

Understanding the modern concept of the clotting reactions requires a detailed knowledge of each of the clotting factors. Table 22.6.1.7 depicts the clotting factors and their inhibitors, including the vitamin K-dependent clotting proenzymes, the non-vitamin K-dependent zymogens, the cofactors, the inhibitors of the clotting factors, and the structural proteins.

Vitamin K-dependent zymogens

The vitamin K-dependent blood clotting zymogens include prothrombin, factor VII, factor IX, factor X, and protein C; their characteristics are listed in Table 22.6.1.7 and their schematic structures in Fig. 22.6.1.6. A common feature of all these clotting factors is the presence of γ-carboxyglutamic acid (Gla) domains in the N-terminal region of the molecules. Glutamic acid residues in these proteins undergo carboxylation, a post-translational event that is affected by hepatic carboxylase that requires reduced vitamin K as a cofactor. The vitamin K-dependent factors are highly homologous in terms of amino acid sequence. Factors VII, IX, X, and protein C have a similar domain structure with a Gla domain, two EGF domains, and a catalytic domain (Fig. 22.6.1.6). Prothrombin differs from other vitamin K-dependent factors in that it has two kringle domains (Fig. 22.6.1.6). Both factor X and protein C are secreted as two-chain zymogens while the others are secreted as single-chain proteins.

Table 22.6.1.7 Characteristics of coagulation proteins

Protein	Plasma concentration (μg/ml)	Biological half-life (hours)	Chromosome
Vitamin K- dependent zymogens			
Prothrombin	100–150	60–70	11p11–q12
Factor VII	0.5	3–6	13q34
Factor IX	4–5	18–24	Xq27.1–q27.2
Factor X	8–10	30–40	13q34
Protein C	4–5	6	2q13–q14
Non-vitamin K dependent zymogens			
Factor XI	5	72	4q32–q35
Factor XII	30	60	5q33
Prekallikrein	50	35	4q35
Factor XIII-A chain[1,2]	10	240	6p24–p25
Soluble cofactors			
Factor V[2]	5–10	12	1q21–q25
Factor VIII	0.1–0.2	8–12	Xq28
von Willebrand factor	10	12	12p13.2
Protein S[3]	25	42	3p11.1–q11.2
Protein Z	2.9	?	13q34
High molecular weight kininogen	70	150	3q26
Factor XIII-B chain[1]			1q31–q32.1
Cellular cofactors			
Tissue factor	–	–	1p21–p22
Thrombomodulin	–	–	20p12–cen
Structural protein			
Fibrinogen	2000–4000	72–120	
Aα chain			4q23–32
Bβ chain			4q23–q32
γ chain			4q23–q32
Inhibitors			
Antithrombin	150–400	72	1q23–q25
Tissue factor pathway inhibitor	0.1		2q31–q32.1
Protein Z-dependent protease inhibitor (ZPI)			

[1] All of the plasma factor XIII-A chain is in complex with factor XIII-B chain; only half of factor XIII-B chain is in complex with factor XIII-A chain, the rest is free in plasma.
[2] Platelets carry significant amounts of factor XIIIA (roughly half of the total factor XIII activity) and factor V (20 per cent of circulating factor V). The B chain of factor XIII is not in platelets.
[3] Some protein S is in complex with C4b binding protein.
(Reprinted by permission of McGraw-Hill Companies from Roberts HR *et al.* (2001). Molecular biology and biochemistry of the coagulation factors. *Williams Hematology*, 6th edn, p.1460.)

The Gla domains of these factors are necessary for binding to phospholipid membranes, such as the surface of activated platelets. Calcium ions occupy the Gla domain to result in a conformational change in the protein that favours binding to platelet membrane surfaces. Phosphatidylserine is the major phospholipid in these reactions.

The vitamin K zymogens are all serine proteases with the typical active site: a serine/histidine/aspartic acid triad. Exposure of the active site requires that the zymogen be activated by cleavage of specific arginyl residues. As a result, all the activated vitamin K-dependent zymogens become two-chain enzymes linked by disulphide bonds as depicted in Fig. 22.6.1.6. Despite the high degree of sequence homology of these proteins, they are highly specific in their interaction with their cofactors and substrates.

Prothrombin

Prothrombin is synthesized in the liver and has a molecular mass of about 72 kDa. The molecule has 10 Gla residues that play a role in the binding of prothrombin to the surface of activated platelets where it is converted to the active enzyme, thrombin, by the so-called 'prothrombinase complex' consisting of factors Xa/Va/Ca^{2+} on the platelet surface. Thrombin is a potent enzyme with a molecular mass of about 38 kDa that rapidly converts fibrinogen to a fibrin clot. Thrombin also has many other actions including its role as: a potent activator of platelets; an activator of smooth muscle cells; an activator of factor V, VIII, and XIII; an activator of protein C in the presence of its cofactor thrombomodulin; an activator of procarboxypeptidase to form a TAFI; and as a growth factor. The primary inhibitor of thrombin is antithrombin (AT).

Factor VII

Factor VII is synthesized in the liver and has a molecular mass of about 50 kDa. It has a very short half-life of 3.5 h. The specific receptor for factor VII is TF, found on the surface of many cells such as pericytes that surround small vessels, fibroblasts, activated monocytes, and many other cell types. The EPCR is also a specific receptor for factor VII, although the function of this relationship is not known.

Once bound to TF, factor VII must be activated for the complex to be functional. The physiologic activator of factor VII is unknown, although it has been suggested that it might be activated factor X. The factor VIIa–TF complex activates both factors IX and X. The factor VIIa–TF–Xa complex is inhibited by TFPI. Factor VIIa is not appreciably inhibited by AT except in the presence of heparin.

Factor IX

Factor IX is synthesized by hepatocytes and has a molecular mass of about 57 kDa. Its plasma half-life is 18 to 24 h. The molecule has 12 Gla residues. About 40% of the factor IX molecules carry a β-hydroxyaspartic acid at position 64 of the molecule. Factor IX is activated by factor VIIa–TF and by activated factor XI, both of which cleave an arginyl bond at position 145 and 180 of the molecule to release an activation peptide of about 10 kDa. Factor IXa, in complex with its cofactor (activated factor VIII), cleaves factor X to Xa. Antithrombin will inhibit factor IXa, but the inhibition is not as rapid as the AT inhibition of thrombin or factor Xa.

Factor X

Factor X is also synthesized by hepatocytes and has a molecular mass of 59 kDa. It is secreted as a two-chain molecule linked by

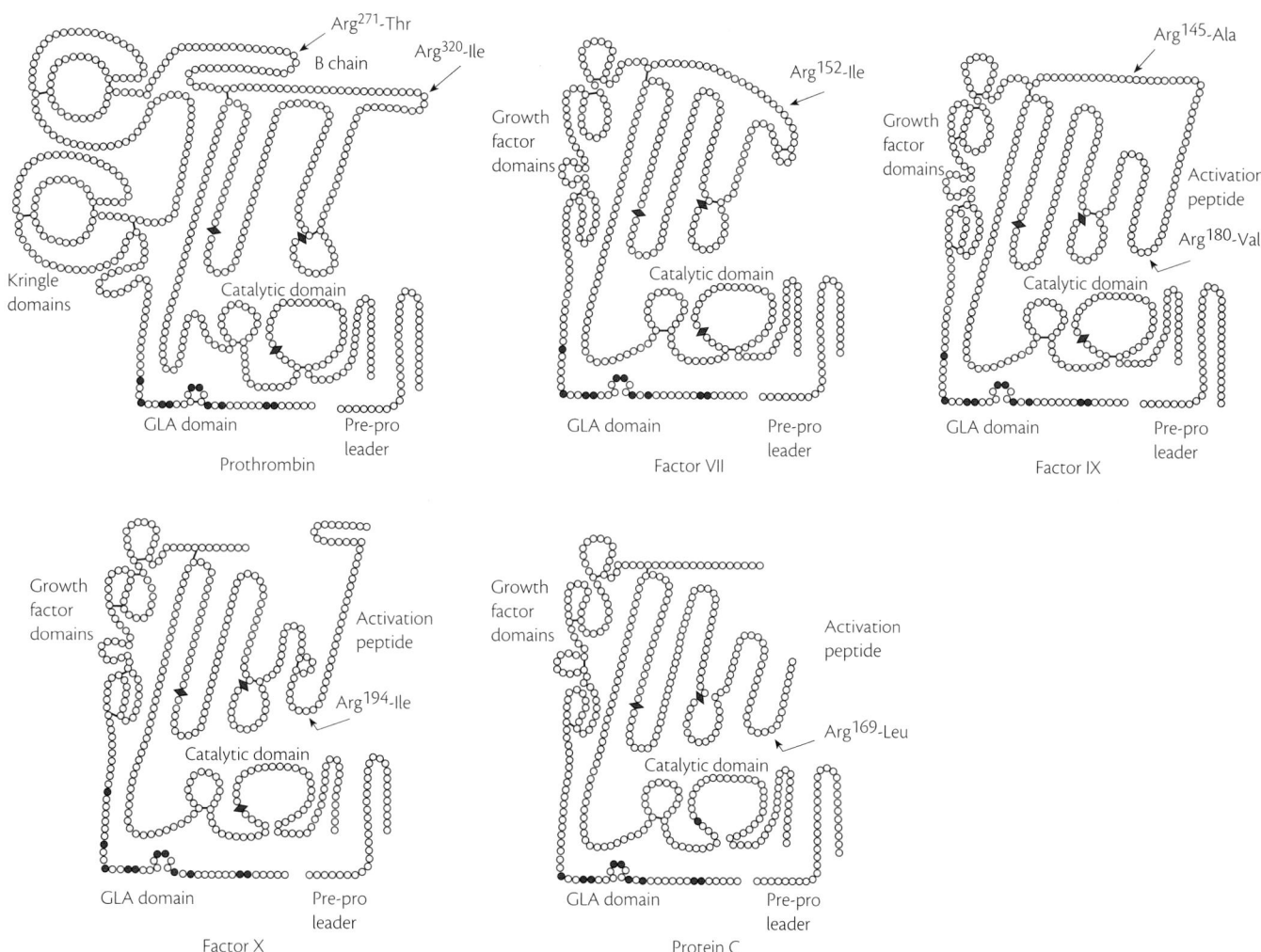

Fig. 22.6.1.6 Schematic diagram of the vitamin K-dependent factors, prothrombin and factors VII, IX, X, and protein C. •, γ-carboxyglutamic acid residues; ♦, active site triad of serine, histidine, and aspartic acid; arrows denote cleavage site.

disulphide bonds and has 11 Gla residues. When activated by factor IXa or factor VIIa–TF, an activation peptide is cleaved from the heavy chain to expose the serine-active site on the heavy chain. Factor Xa, in the presence of its cofactor (factor Va), rapidly converts prothrombin to thrombin. The primary inhibitor of factor Xa is AT.

Protein C

Unlike the other vitamin K-dependent zymogens, protein C is not a procoagulant, but, when activated by the thrombin–thrombo-modulin complex on the surface of endothelial cells, it becomes an anticoagulant by proteolysis of factors Va and VIIIa, thus inhibiting coagulation. To function in this way as an anticoagulant, activated protein C (APC) requires a nonenzymatic cofactor, protein S, which also contain vitamin K-dependent Gla residues. Protein C is synthesized in the liver and has a very short half-life of about 6 h. It contains nine Gla residues and has a molecular mass of 59 kDa. The primary inhibitor of APC is the protein C inhibitor (PCI).

Non-vitamin-K-dependent zymogens

Factor XI

Factor XI is synthesized in the liver as a dimeric protein composed of identical subunits. It has a molecular mass of 160 kDa and

a plasma half-life of about 72 h (Table 22.6.1.7). In plasma, factor XI circulates in complex with high-molecular-weight kininogen (HK), a nonenzymatic cofactor. The physiologic activator of factor XI is thought to be thrombin, although *in vitro*, this factor can be activated by factor XIIa. The main function of factor XIa is to boost thrombin generation by activating factor IX on the surface of platelets, over and above the factor IX activated by the VIIa–TF complex. A few patients with factor XI deficiency have virtually no bleeding tendency, and those who do usually exhibit mild bleeding when compared to severely affected haemophilic patients.

Factor XII and prekallikrein (PK) (Table 22.6.1.7)

These factors have been collectively referred to as contact factors since it appears that activation of factor XII is enhanced by contact with a surface. Factor XII and PK are zymogens, which, when activated, expose a serine-active site. High-molecular-weight kininogen (HK) is a nonenzymatic protein cofactor that circulates in complex with factor XI and PK. All of these factors are synthesized in the liver. Unlike the vitamin K-dependent proteins, factors XI, XII, and prekallikrein all possess so-called 'apple domains' that have specific functional characteristics. Deficiencies of factor XII and PK are not associated with bleeding tendencies in patients with complete deficiency of these factors. However, deficiency of each factor is associated with a marked prolongation of the partial thromboplastin time (PTT). In this test and in the presence of glass, ellagic acid, or some inert earth material, factor XII is activated and in the active conformation it can activate factor XI. Factor XII, PK, and HK may not play a major physiological role in haemostasis, but there is evidence that they participate in inflammatory responses that involve blood coagulation, fibrinolysis, and kinin generation. The precise role of factor XII in coagulation reactions *in vivo* is not known. Despite the fact that patients with factor XII deficiency do not exhibit bleeding symptoms, the factor is considered to be part of the 'intrinsic system' of coagulation and in some instances it may contribute to coagulation by virtue of exposure to collagen or other surfaces. Studies in animals lacking factor XII suggest that the protease may play a role in formation of pathological thrombi.

Factor XIII (Table 22.6.1.7)

Factor XIII is a proenzyme which circulates in the plasma as a heterotetramer composed of two A chains and two B chains. Factor XIII has a molecular mass of 320 kDa and a half-life of about 10 days. It circulates in plasma in association with fibrinogen. The A chain contains the active site cysteine, while the B chain is enzymatically inactive and serves as a carrier for the A chain. The A chain is found in platelets where it is not associated with the B chain. Upon activation by thrombin, the A and B chains are separated. In addition, thrombin cleaves the A chain so as to expose the active site cysteine. The activated A chain then cross-links the α and γ chains of fibrin to form a stable, impermeable fibrin clot that is more resistant to lysis by plasmin than non-cross-linked fibrin.

Cofactors

Some of the cofactors are soluble and exist in circulation, namely protein S, protein Z, factors V and VIII, HK, and VWF. Others are cell-bound, such as TF and thrombomodulin. (Table 22.6.1.7)

Protein S

Protein S is synthesized in the liver and endothelial cells and is dependent on vitamin K for complete synthesis. It circulates in plasma and is also found in platelets. It has a molecular mass of 75 kDa and a plasma half-life of about 42 h. It contains 11 Gla residues in the N-terminal region. In structure, protein S differs dramatically from the other vitamin K clotting factors in that the C-terminal end is homologous to growth hormone. Protein S acts as a cofactor for activated protein C. Protein S exists in two forms: one form is bound to C4b-binding protein and the other exists as a free form in the circulation. It is the free form of protein S that acts as a cofactor for protein C and is in equilibrium with the bound form.

Protein Z

Protein Z is synthesized in the liver and has a molecular mass of 62 kDa. There is now convincing evidence that when protein Z is incubated with factor Xa, the activity of the latter is reduced. The inhibition of factor Xa activity is due to the presence of a protease inhibitor that requires protein Z as a cofactor. Whether protein Z has other functions is unknown.

Factor V

Factor V is synthesized in the liver and has a biological half-life of between 12 and 36 h. It is a large glycoprotein with a molecular mass of 330 kDa. Factor V is highly homologous to factor VIII, and

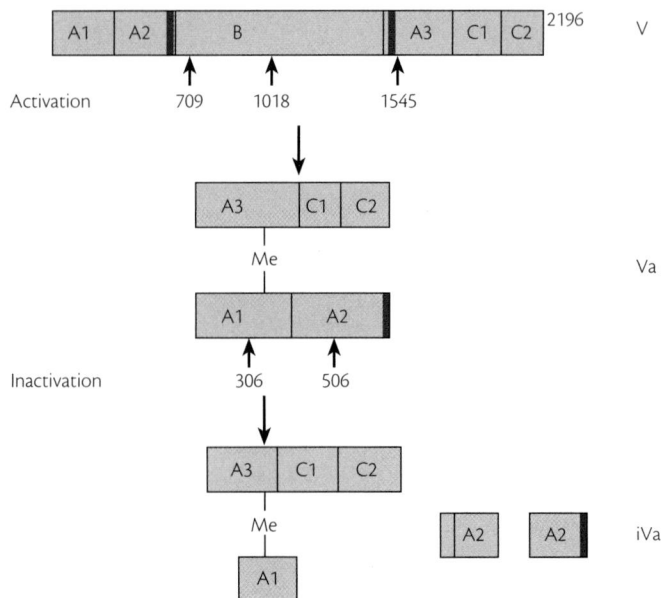

Fig. 22.6.1.7 Schematic diagram of factor V. Factor V is activated by thrombin to factor Va. Factor Va is inactivated by activated protein C (iVa). Activation of factor V by thrombin results in loss of the B chain and formation of a heterodimeric molecule covalently linked by metal ions (Me). Inactivation is by activated protein C that cleaves arginyl bonds at positions 306 and 506.

is composed of A, B, and C domains. A schematic diagram of the structure is shown in Fig. 22.6.1.7. The A domains are homologous to the copper-binding protein ceruloplasmin, so it is not surprising that this domain of factor V is involved in binding to calcium and copper. The C domains are homologous to fat-globule proteins and are involved in the binding of factor V to phospholipid-rich platelet membranes. The A and C domains are homologous to similar domains in factor VIII, but the B domain is completely different from that of factor VIII. For factor V to act as a cofactor for factor Xa, it must be activated by thrombin with cleavage of arginyl bonds at positions 708, 1018, and 1545 as shown in Fig. 22.6.1.7. It is inactivated by APC, which cleaves bonds at 306 (slow) and 506 (fast).

Factor VIII

Like factor V, factor VIII is synthesized in the liver. Factor VIII mRNA is found largely in sinusoidal endothelial cells and Kupfer cells, though low but significant factor VIII mRNA may also be found in hepatocytes. It is a large glycoprotein, similar in size to factor V. Again, like factor V, factor VIII has A, B, and C domains with the A domains homologous to ceruloplasmin and the C domains homologous to fat globule proteins (Fig. 22.6.1.8). The C domains of factor VIII are essential for binding to phospholipid membranes. The B domain of factor VIII is cleaved in the circulation and has no change. To act as a cofactor for factor IXa, factor VIII must be activated by thrombin or factor Xa. Unlike activated factor V, activated factor VIII exists as a heterotrimer composed of A1, A2, and A3-C1-C2 domains linked by calcium ions. Factor VIII circulates in a noncovalent complex with VWF and has a biological half-life of 8 to 12 h. In the complete absence of VWF, such as occurs with type III von Willebrand disease, the half-life of factor VIII is less than 1 h. When activated factor VIII is released from VWF, it binds to the surface of activated platelets where it interacts with factor IXa.

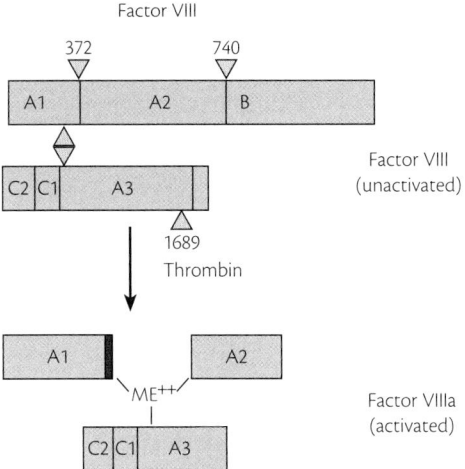

Fig. 22.6.1.8 Schematic representation of factor VIII. Activation by thrombin (or factor Xa) results in a heterotrimer non-covalently linked by metal ions (Me). Like factor Va, factor VIIIa is inactivated by activated Protein C.

VWF

VWF is synthesized by endothelial cells and stored in Weibel–Palade bodies. It also circulates in plasma although larger than normal molecular weight multimers of VWF are found in Weibel Palade bodies. It binds to glycoprotein Ib on platelets and is required for normal platelet adhesion to components of the vessel wall such as collagen. A schematic diagram of VWF is shown in Fig. 22.6.1.9. Although synthesized as a prepolypeptide with A, B, C, and D domains, it is secreted into the plasma in multimeric form with molecular mass ranging from 1000 kDa to 15 000 to 20 000 kDa. Higher molecular mass forms of VWF are secreted to the abluminal surface of the endothelial cell as one component of the extracellular matrix. The higher molecular mass VWF multimers are very effective in promoting platelet adhesion. VWF is also important in platelet aggregation. A major function of VWF is to act as a carrier protein for factor VIII. Factor VIII is associated with VWF multimers of all sizes.

HK

HK circulates in plasma, and part is bound to factor XI and prekallikrein. HK is a cofactor for both of these zymogens. Deficiency of HK is not associated with a bleeding tendency, although the partial thromboplastin times of affected subjects are prolonged.

TF

Unlike other cofactors, TF is associated with cell surfaces. Soluble TF circulating in plasma has been described but does not appear to be functional. TF may also be found in microparticles but again its functional significance has not been well established. It is composed of 263 amino acids and with a 219-amino acid extracellular domain, a 23-amino acid transmembrane domain, and a 21-amino acid intracytoplasmic domain. The characteristics of TF are shown in Table 22.6.1.7. It has a molecular mass of about 46 kDa and is constitutively expressed on several extravascular tissues such as fibroblasts and smooth muscle cells. It is not constitutively expressed on cells exposed to the circulating blood, but can be induced in endothelial cells by certain inflammatory cytokines and certain bacterial products such as endotoxin. It can also be induced in blood leucocytes. TF functions as a receptor for factor VII. When factor VII binds to TF, it is rapidly converted to factor VIIa, although the precise mechanism for its activation is not clear. The VIIa–TF complex is now thought to be the main physiological initiator of blood coagulation by activating both factor IX and factor X, each of which plays a distinct role in subsequent coagulation reactions as described below. On some cells TF exists in a 'latent' form, sometimes referred to as 'encrypted TF', as suggested by the fact that TF antigen levels on cells may be higher than TF functional activity. De-encryption can be accomplished by exposure of cells to agents such as calcium ionophores and various cytokines, but the physiologic mechanism by which this process takes place is not known.

Thrombomodulin

Thrombomodulin (TM) is a transmembrane protein synthesized by and localized to endothelial cells although it has also been found on mesothelial cells, monocytes, and squamous epithelial cells. It has a molecular mass of about 78 kDa. A chondroitin sulphate moiety is attached to TM via a serine residue. The major characteristics of TM are depicted in Table 22.6.1.7. It serves as a receptor on endothelial cells for thrombin. Thrombin bound to thrombomodulin undergoes a structural transformation such that it no longer activates platelets or clots fibrinogen, but rather activates protein C. The principal function of the TM–thrombin complex is to prevent the extension of the haemostatic clot past the site of a break or leak in the vessel wall and as such represents an important control mechanism to restrict the haemostatic plug precisely to the point of injury. Thus, under normal conditions, clot formation does not occur on the endothelial cell surfaces.

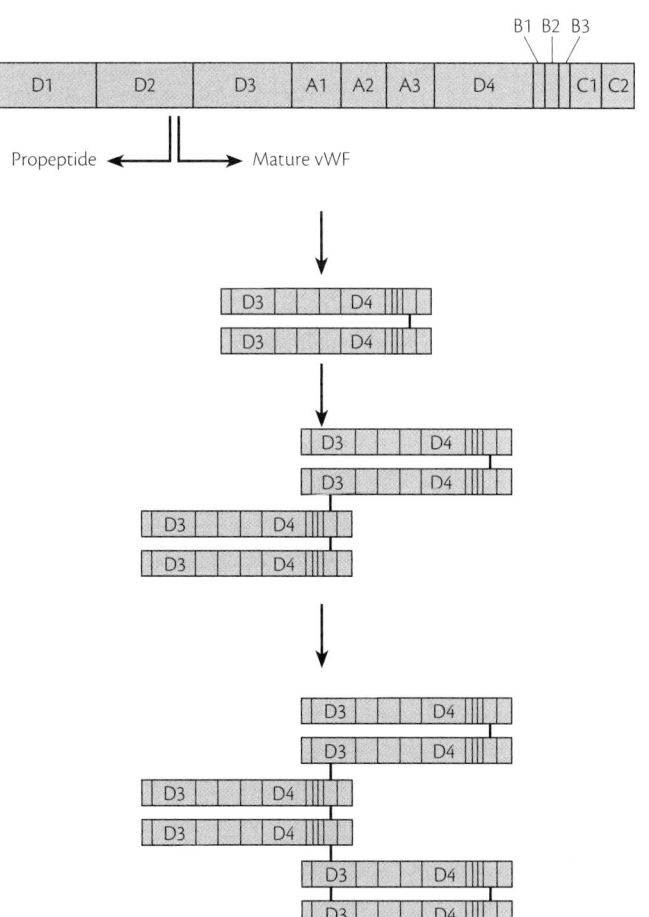

Fig. 22.6.1.9 Schematic diagram of von Willebrand factor (vWF). The formation of multimeric forms of vWF occurs through links of dimeric vWF via D³ domains.

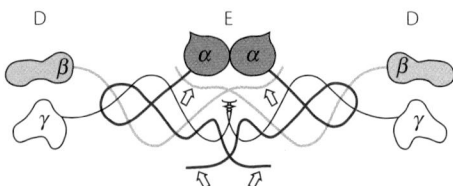

Fig. 22.6.1.10 Diagram of the structure of fibrinogen. The three chains, α, β, γ, are shown. The E domain occurs at the N-termini while the D domains are found at the C-termini. Arrows represent cleavage sites for fibrinopeptide A from the α chain and fibrinopeptide B from the β chain.

Fibrinogen

Fibrinogen is synthesized in the liver and has a molecular mass of 340 kDa. It is a dimeric glycoprotein consisting of two sets of identical chains, the α, β, and γ chains. The synthesis of each fibrinogen chain is governed by a separate gene, as depicted in Table 22.6.1.7. The normal plasma half-life of fibrinogen is about 3 to 5 days. It is also found in the α granules of platelets as a result of endocytosis. Fibrinogen is the soluble plasma precursor of the solid fibrin clot that is so necessary for haemostasis and normal wound healing. A schematic diagram of fibrinogen is shown in Fig. 22.6.1.10. It is a trinodular structure with a central E domain that includes the disulphide-linked N-termini of all six polypeptide chains. The E domain is linked to the C-terminal domains referred to as the D domains. Fibrinogen conversion to fibrin is accomplished by thrombin cleavage of two fibrinopeptides (fibrinopeptide A and fibrinopeptide B) from each of the two α and β chains, respectively, leading to the formation of the fibrin monomer. The molecular mass of each fibrinopeptide A and B is about 2500 Da. The soluble fibrin monomer then undergoes spontaneous polymerization by forming side-to-side and end-to-end interactions, resulting in protofibrils that aggregate into a visible fibrin clot composed of thicker, branched fibres. During fibrin clot formation, other proteins are occluded in the clot, including plasminogen, fibronectin, thrombospondin, and VWF. The fibrin polymerization is enhanced by calcium ions, but the polymerization process alone does not lead to a stable and impermeable fibrin clot since the fibres are held together weakly by hydrogen bonds and electrostatic forces. A stable fibrin clot requires cross-linking of the α and γ chains of fibrin by the action of activated factor XIII.

Inhibitors of the coagulation reactions

TFPI (Table 22.6.1.7)

TFPI is synthesized by endothelial cells. It has a molecular mass of about 34 to 40 kDa and serves to inhibit the initiation of coagulation. TFPI can inhibit factor Xa in a slow reaction and also inhibits the VIIa–TF–Xa complex. TFPI exists in two forms, TPFIα and TFPIβ. The latter is directly anchored to cell surfaces via glycosylphosphatidyl-inositol links. It exists in the circulation in at least three pools. One is bound to plasma lipoproteins; one pool is bound to proteoglycans on the vessel wall; and one exists in platelets. The TFPI bound to proteoglycans can be released by heparin. TFPI is a Kunitz-type inhibitor that is essential for control of coagulation at the initiation phase.

Antithrombin

The characteristics of antithrombin (AT) are also depicted in Table 22.6.1.7. Antithrombin belongs to a family of protease inhibitors

known as serpins that inhibit many proteases with a serine-active site. It is synthesized in the liver and has a plasma half-life of approximately 65 h. Its major function is to inhibit thrombin and factor Xa, although it will also inhibit the other coagulation serine proteases less well. The inhibitory action of AT is greatly enhanced by heparin, which accelerates the rate of inhibition of the serine proteases.

Protein Z-dependent protease inhibitor

This inhibitor inhibits factor Xa in the presence of calcium, phospholipids, and protein Z. It has a molecular mass of about 72 kDa. Like AT, it is also a member of the serpin family of serine protease inhibitors.

Other inhibitors of clotting factors

The major inhibitor of factor XIa is thought to be α_1-antitrypsin since it has the highest affinity for the enzyme. However, other inhibitors, namely C-1 esterase inhibitor, will also inhibit factor XIa. The other inhibitors that are of some importance in coagulation are also listed in Table 22.6.1.7.

Coagulation pathways

The coagulation reactions have been viewed as a sequential series of steps in which a enzymatic precursor (zymogen) clotting factor is converted to an active enzyme which, in turn activates another precursor, finally ending in the rapid conversion of prothrombin to thrombin. Early models of the coagulation reactions are shown in Fig. 22.6.1.11. As can be seen, when viewed in this manner, the clotting reactions appear as a waterfall or cascade, hence the terms waterfall or cascade hypotheses. Since TF was extrinsic to the blood stream, the activation of factor X by the VIIa–TF complex was termed the extrinsic system. The intrinsic system consisted entirely of clotting factors within the circulation and, upon conversion of factor IX to IXa by factor XIa, the factor IXa–VIIIa complex could also convert factor X to Xa in the presence of phospholipids.

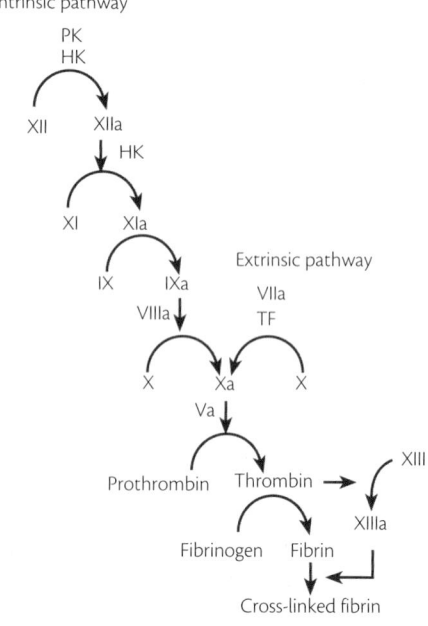

Fig. 22.6.1.11 An earlier model of blood coagulation reactions: the cascade or waterfall hypothesis of coagulation.

Although this concept of coagulation was essentially correct, it did not explain why patients with factor XII deficiency had no bleeding tendency nor why factor XI-deficient patients had only a mild bleeding tendency. It was also pointed out that defects in the intrinsic system could lead to haemorrhage in affected patients even though the extrinsic system was intact and vice versa. The demonstration that the VIIa–TF complex could activate both factor IX and factor X led several groups to conclude that the clotting reactions were, in fact, initiated by factor VIIa–TF and that the intrinsic and extrinsic systems did not exist *in vivo*. Further work demonstrated that the clotting reactions leading to a haemostatic plug were controlled in large part by cell surfaces which modulated the reactions.

Role of the TF cell

When a blood vessel is injured or ruptured, flowing blood is exposed to TF, which is bound through a transmembrane and cytoplasmic tail to cells exposed as the result of injury, e.g. pericytes, fibroblasts, and other connective tissue cells. Factor VII binds to the TF-bearing cell and is activated. In fact, it appears that the TF found in pericytes surrounding small vessels is already saturated with factor VII. As a result, the VIIa–TF complex on the TF cell activates both factor IX and factor X as shown in Fig. 22.6.1.12A. The factor Xa and IXa formed in the milieu of the TF cell play very different and distinct roles in subsequent reactions.

The role of factor Xa in the milieu of the TF cell

Factor Xa, in concert with its cofactor Va (which is found in the vicinity of TF cells) then converts prothrombin to very small amounts of thrombin, as shown in Fig. 22.6.1.12B. This amount of thrombin, though insufficient to clot fibrinogen, can, however, act as a 'primer' of subsequent coagulation reactions to accomplish the following: activate platelets; activate more factor V; dissociate factor VIII from VWF and activate factor VIII; and activate factor XI as shown in Fig. 22.6.1.12B. Factor Xa alone and in complex with VIIa–TF is then inhibited by TFPI. The activated co-factors resulting from the priming amount of thrombin in the milieu of the TF cell then occupy binding sites on the activated platelet as shown in Fig. 22.6.1.12B. Thus the main function of factor Xa formed as the result of the VIIa–TF complex is to furnish a priming amount of thrombin sufficient to initiate further subsequent reactions which take place on the activated platelet surface.

Role of factor IXa activated by the fVIIa–TF complex

Factor IXa formed by the VIIa–TF on the TF-bearing cell diffuses away from the TF cell and occupies a site on the activated platelet adjacent to its co-factor VIIIa (Fig. 22.6.1.12C). This factor IXa then plays a primary role in the subsequent burst of thrombin generation on platelet surfaces as noted below.

Role of the activated platelet

The activated platelet mass is the primary site of thrombin generation, which is highly dependent upon the amount of factor IXa formed both by the VIIa–TF cell and factor XIa, which also occupies sites on the platelet. Factor IXa in the presence of its cofactor VIIIa then recruits more factor X from solution and activates it on the activated platelet surface. This factor Xa in the presence of its cofactor Va then converts large amounts of prothrombin to thrombin sufficient to clot fibrinogen. All of these reactions are summarized in Fig. 22.6.1.13. The mass of aggregated platelets

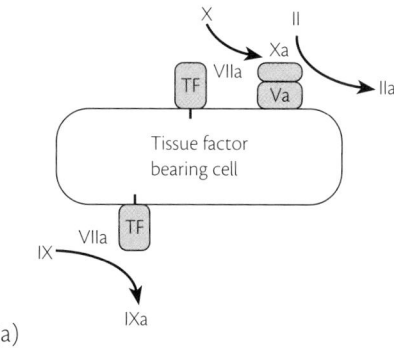

(a)

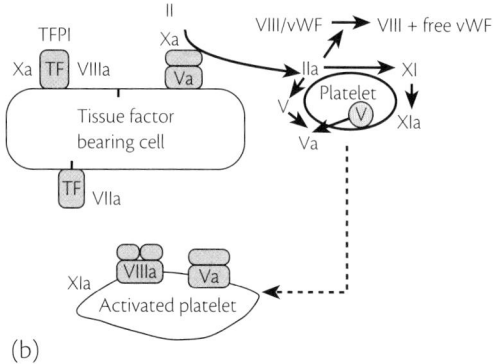

(b)

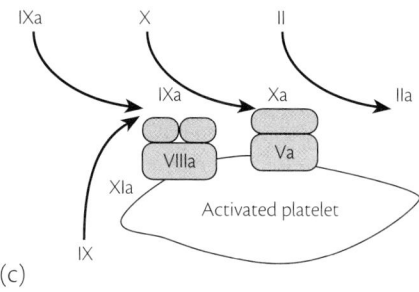

(c)

Fig. 22.6.1.12 (a) Tissue factor (TF), a transmembrane protein expressed on TF-bearing cells, acts as a receptor for factor VII, which is rapidly converted to factor VIIa. The TF–VIIa complex then accomplishes two major functions: (1) activation of factor X to Xa and (2) activation of factor IX to IXa. Factor Xa activates factor V on the TF-bearing cell and the resulting Xa–Va complex converts small amounts of prothrombin to thrombin. (b) This small amount of thrombin formed in the vicinity of the TF cell acts as a 'primer' for coagulation by: (1) activating platelets; (2) dissociating factor VIII from vWF and activating factor VIII; (3) activating factor V; and (4) activating factor XI. The activated platelets then adhere to the site of vascular injury and bind the cofactors, factors VIIIa and Va. Factor XIa also binds to platelets. The TF–VIIa–Xa complex is then inhibited by TFPI. (c) Factor IXa formed by the TF–VIIa complex associates with VIIIa on the platelet surface and recruits additional factor X from plasma to form factor Xa. The factor Xa then associates with its cofactor, factor Va, on the platelet surface to rapidly convert prothrombin to large amounts of thrombin sufficient to clot fibrinogen.

upon which these reactions take place is localized to the damaged area of the vessel wall.

Role of the endothelial cells, vessel wall, and inhibitors

The mass of platelets interspersed with fibrin forms a plug at the site of a leak in the vessel wall where the endothelial cell monolayer

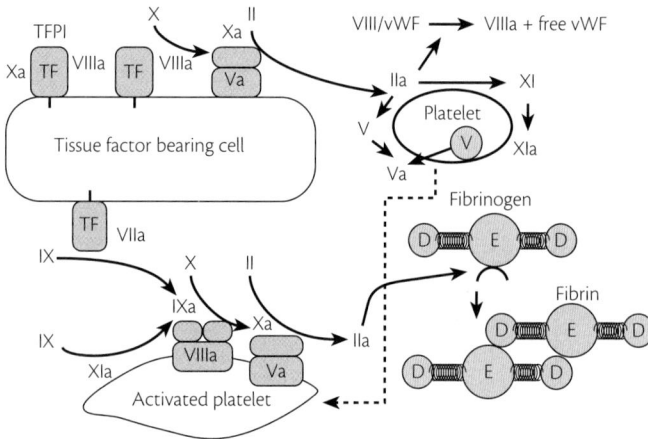

Fig. 22.6.1.13 The clotting reactions summarized. After thrombin formation, fibrinogen is converted to fibrin.

is disrupted. The question arises as how the haemostatic plug is confined to the damaged area of the vessel wall. A schematic diagram of these events is shown in Fig. 22.6.1.14. The endothelial cells express, which traps thrombin to form a TM–T complex that controls the procoagulant stimulus by activating the protein C system, resulting in inactivation of both factors Va and VIIIa on the endothelial cell surface. This series of events is enhanced by activated protein C on the EPCR. In addition, endothelial cells contain glycosoaminoglycans (GAG), some of which inhibit thrombin. AT also circulates in solution to inhibit any thrombin that escapes from the haemostatic plug. In this way the fibrin clot sealing a leak in a blood vessel wall is confined precisely to that site such that extension of the clot does not occur under normal circumstances.

Ongoing coagulation *in vivo*

It is well known that products of the coagulation reactions are found in the circulation under normal (basal) conditions. Small but definite levels of fibrinopeptides A and B can be measured. Fragment 1 + 2 derived from the N-terminal portion of prothrombin after thrombin is formed can also be detected. Activation peptides from several of the coagulation factors as well as complexes of activated factors with their inhibitors can also be found in the circulation. These observations strongly suggest that small leaks in blood vessels that occur during the stress and strain of everyday living are repaired by the ongoing formation of haemostatic

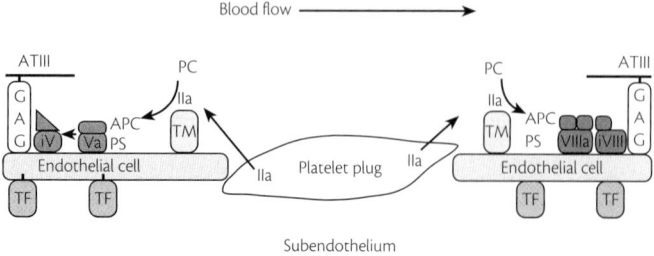

Fig. 22.6.1.14 Diagram of the haemostatic plug and the control mechanisms that restrict this plug to the site of injury and prevent extension of the clot to normal endothelium. TM, thrombomodulin; IIa, thrombin; GAG, glycosoaminoglycans; PC, protein C; APC, activated protein C; PS, protein S; TF, tissue factor; platelet plug = haemostatic plug iVIIIa, inactivated VIIIa; iVa, inactivated Va.

fibrin clots. This has been termed 'basal' coagulation, a process that allows the blood to remain fluid within the vascular tree and at the same time permits small, exquisitely controlled and confined fibrin clots to plug small leaks in the vasculature without dissemination. The fibrin plug is then removed by the fibrinolytic system following the formation of new tissue.

Role of TF in microparticles

It has been shown that microparticles shed from leucocytes and other cells possess procoagulant activity at least *in vitro* and perhaps *in vivo*. These particles have also been shown to possess TF but the physiological role of this TF *in vivo* has not been definitively demonstrated. Platelets contain pre-mRNA for TF and under certain circumstances may express TF activity but again, the physiological significance of these interesting observations has not been clearly delineated.

Fibrinolytic system

The fibrinolytic system is shown schematically in Fig. 22.6.1.15. The components of the system and their characteristics are depicted in Table 22.6.1.8. The active enzyme in the fibrinolytic system is plasmin, which is derived from its precursor, plasminogen. Plasminogen is activated to plasmin by activators. The physiologic activator is single-chain tissue plasminogen activator (tPA), which cleaves plasminogen into two-chain plasmin. Another activator of plasminogen *in vivo* is single-chain urokinase, but this appears to be more important for degradation of matrix proteins. The physiological inhibitor of plasmin is α_2-antiplasmin.

Plasminogen and tPA associate in the circulation with fibrinogen. Thus, when fibrinogen is converted to fibrin, the clot is rich in both of these proteins, which are protected from the inhibitory action of antiplasmin. Thus, clots can be lysed without interference from inhibitors, yet free plasmin in the circulation will be rapidly inhibited by its inhibitor.

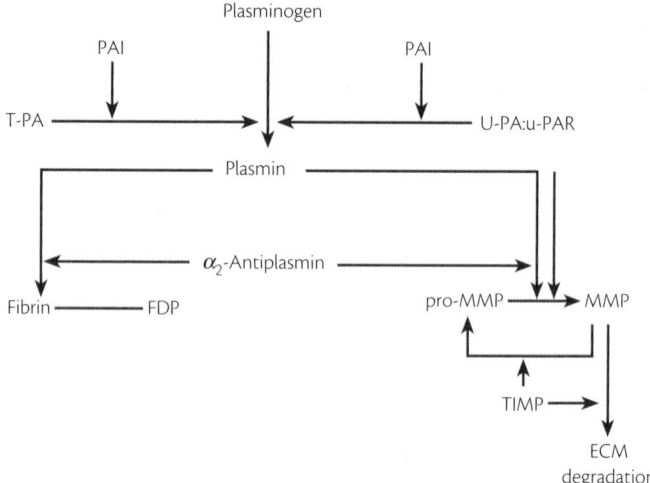

Fig. 22.6.1.15 The fibrinolytic system. Plasminogen is converted to plasmin by activators, including plasminogen activators (tPA) and urokinase (U-PA). The activators are inhibited mainly by plasminogen activator inhibitor-1 (PAI-1). Plasmin degrades fibrin and activates matrix metalloproteinases (MMP), which degrades extracellular matrix (ECM). Plasmin is inhibited by antiplasmin. FDP, fibrin degradation product; TIMP, tissue inhibitors of metalloproteinases; U-PAR, urokinase protease-activated receptor.

Table 22.6.1.8 Characteristics of the fibrinolytic system

	Plasma Mr (kDa)	Concentration (mg/l)	Chromosomal location
Plasminogen	92	20	6
Plasmin	85	–	
t-PA	68	0.005	8
u-PA	54	0.008	10
α2-antiplasmin	70	200	18
PAI-1	52	70	7
PAI-2	47, 60	0.0518	18
u-PAR	50, 60		

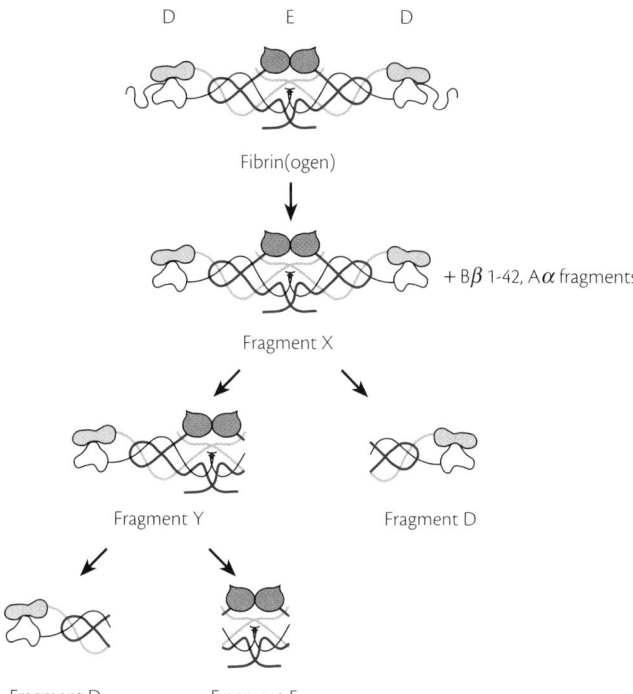

Fig. 22.6.1.16 Plasmin digestion of fibrin(ogen) results in fibrin degradation products: X, Y, D, and E. The final protolytic fragments resulting from plasmin degradation of fibrin are two molecules of fragment D and one of E.

Plasminogen

Plasminogen is synthesized in the liver and has a molecular mass of about 92 kDa. It is composed of a single chain and exists in two forms in the circulation: Glu-plasminogen and Lys-plasminogen. Glu-plasminogen has an N-terminal glutamic acid and is larger than Lys-plasminogen, which is formed in the circulation by plasmin cleavage of an arginyl bond at position 78 of the Glu form, leaving lysine as the N-terminal residue. Lys-plasminogen rapidly binds to fibrin via lysine binding sites. Thus, Lys-plasminogen is in close proximity to fibrin and protected from the action of antiplasmin. When activated, plasminogen is converted to active two-chain plasmin with a serine-active site on the heavy chain that is connected to the light chain by disulphide bonds.

The proteolytic action of plasmin is usually characterized by the proteolysis of fibrinogen and fibrin, but it can also degrade several other proteins including factor VIII, factor V, VWF, and others. The cleavage of fibrinogen and fibrin leads to the formation of fibrin(ogen) degradation products (FDP). Fibrino(gen) fragments resulting from plasmin cleavage are shown in Fig. 22.6.1.16. Fragment X is the first and largest fragment of plasmin digestion of fibrinogen. It is still clottable by thrombin, although much slower than native fibrinogen. Fragment X gives rise to fragments Y and D, and fragment Y is further proteolysed to give rise to a second fragment D plus fragment E. These fragments can be detected in a simple laboratory test using antifibrinogen antibodies coated to latex particles. However, the test is nonspecific and does not distinguish between the fibrinogen or fibrin degradation products which are quite similar, since the only difference between fibrin and fibrinogen is the absence of the small fibrinopeptides A and B in fibrin. A better test for detection of fibrin fragments is the so-called D-dimer test, which detects D-dimers resulting from the cross-linking of fibrin by factor XIIIa.

tPA

tPA is considered to be the physiological activator of plasminogen. It is synthesized in endothelial cells and has a molecular mass of about 68 kDa. It has high affinity for plasminogen. tPA circulates for the most part in complex with its inhibitor, plasminogen activator inhibitor-1 (PAI-1). The tPA–PAI-1 complex can be dissociated during the process of coagulation, and free tPA associates with fibrin, which enhances tPA activity. Single-chain tPA has catalytic activity, but when activated to the two-chain form by plasmin, the activity is increased by threefold.

Plasminogen activator inhibitor-1 (PAI-1)

PAI-1 is the physiological inhibitor of tPA. It belongs to the serpin family of inhibitors. It is synthesized in endothelial cells and has a molecular mass of 52 kDa. Elevated levels of this inhibitor have been associated with arterial and venous thromboses. PAI-2, found in the placenta, also inhibits tPA, but not as efficiently as PAI-1. PAI-3 is also known as the protein C inhibitor and inhibits plasminogen activators less efficiently than PAI-1.

Urokinase plasminogen activator

Urokinase plasminogen activator (U-PA) exists as a single-chain zymogen and is found in the kidney, the urine, and fibroblast-like cells. It activates plasminogen by proteolysis of an arginyl residue at position 561. Its main function is in wound healing and vasculogenesis, and it is active in proteolysis of the extracellular matrix. U-PA associates with the urokinase plasminogen-activator receptor (U-PAR).

Antiplasmin

Antiplasmin is the physiological inhibitor of plasmin. It has a molecular mass of about 58 kDa and is synthesized in the liver. As an inhibitor, it has three major functions: to inhibit plasminogen binding to fibrin; to inhibit the proteolytic activity of plasmin; and to bind to fibrin in a covalent manner by the action of factor XIIIa. By binding to fibrin, antiplasmin competitively inhibits the binding of plasminogen to fibrin. However, when plasminogen within the fibrin clot is converted to plasmin, the latter is protected from inhibition by antiplasmin. On the other hand, free plasmin formed in the circulation is rapidly inhibited.

TAFI

TAFI is also known as plasma procarboxypeptidase B, and it is activated to carboxypeptidase B by large amounts of thrombin in a reaction dependent upon thrombomodulin. TAFI down-regulates fibrinolysis after clot formation and serves as an important regulatory mechanism for the fibrinolytic system. TAFI acts primarily by reducing the number of high-affinity plasminogen binding sites on fibrin, the end result of which is decreased fibrinolysis.

The fibrinolytic and coagulation systems are closely interrelated. Under normal conditions, fibrin clot formation is always accompanied by fibrinolysis. The formation of the fibrin clot which contains both tPA and plasminogen, results in formation of plasmin within the clot so that clot lysis eventually ensues. It also appears that activated factor XI and factor XII enhance fibrinolytic activity. The action of the protein C system to decrease thrombin formation down-regulates the TAFI which would favour increased fibrinolysis. Although much is still unknown, it is generally accepted that both the coagulation and fibrinolytic systems are related to the general process of inflammation involving several other host defence mechanisms.

Further reading

Cines DB, *et al.* (1998). Endothelial cells in physiology and in the pathophysiology of vascular diseases. *Blood*, **91**, 3527–61.

Collen D (1999). The plasminogen (fibrolytic) system. *Thromb Haemost*, **82**, 259–70.

Coughlin SR (2005). Protease-activated receptors in haemostasis, thrombosis and vascular biology. *J Thromb Haemost*, **3**, 1800–14.

Crawley JT, *et al.* (2007). The central role of thrombin in haemostasis. *J Thromb Haemost*, **5** Suppl 1, 95–101.

Degen JL, Bugge TH, Goguen JD (2007). Fibrin and fibrinolysis in infection and host defense. *J Thromb Haemost*, **5** Suppl 1, 24–31.

Gailani D, Renne T (2007). The intrinsic pathway of coagulation: a target for treating thromboembolic disease? *J Thromb Haemost*, **5**, 1106–12.

Griffin JH, *et al.* (2007). Activated protein C. *J Thromb Haemost*, **5** Suppl 1, 73–80.

Lundblad RL, White GC 2nd (2005). The interaction of thrombin with blood platelets. *Platelets*, **16**, 373–85.

Ma YQ, Qin J, Plow EF (2007). Platelet integrin alpha(IIb)beta(3): activation mechanisms. *J Thromb Haemost*, **5**, 1345–52.

Monroe DM, Key NS (2007). The tissue factor-factor VIIa complex: procoagulant activity, regulation, and multitasking. *J Thromb Haemost*, **5**, 1097–105.

Mosesson MW (2005). Fibrinogen and fibrin structure and functions. *J Thromb Haemost*, **3**, 1894–904.

Nemerson Y (2007). My life with tissue factor. *J Thromb Haemost*, **5**, 221–3.

Nurden AT (2005). Qualitative disorders of platelets and megakaryocytes. *J Thromb Haemost*, **3**, 1773–82.

Peake I, Goodeve A (2007). Type 1 von Willebrand disease. *J Thromb Haemost*, **5** Suppl 1, 7–11.

Pober JS, Sessa WC (2007). Evolving functions of endothelial cells in inflammation. *Nat Rev Immunol*, **7**, 803–15.

Roberts HR, Hoffman M, Monroe DM (2006). A cell-based model of thrombin generation. *Semin Thromb Haemost*, **32** Suppl 1, 32–8.

Roberts HR, Monroe DM, Hoffman M (2006). Molecular biology and biochemistry of the coagulation factors and pathways of haemostasis.

In: Lichtman MA *et al.* (eds) *Williams hematology*, 7th edition, pp. 1665–93. McGraw-Hill, New York.

White GC II, Rompietti R (2007). Platelet secretion: indiscriminately spewed forth or highly orchestrated? *J Thromb Haemost*, **5**, 2006–8.

22.6.2 Evaluation of the patient with a bleeding tendency

Trevor Baglin

Essentials

Clinical assessment

An apparent bleeding tendency is a common clinical problem, with presentation varying from acute unexpected bleeding during or immediately after surgery, to spontaneous unusual or excessive bruising, purpura, epistaxis, or a chronic haemorrhagic tendency. The following are important aspects of the assessment of the patient.

Is haemostatic capacity reduced, or is there a nonhaematological cause for bleeding?—recurrent bleeding from a single site suggests a structural vascular abnormality, whereas bleeding at many different sites suggests a systemic haemostatic defect. Other elements of history or examination that suggest reduced haemostatic capacity include (1) after dental extraction—bleeding that lasted more than an hour, rebleeding, or late bleeding requiring suturing on more than one occasion; (2) after surgery—unusual or prolonged bleeding; (3) bleeding in unusual sites, e.g. into joints; (4) very extensive bruising, particularly over soft areas that are not likely to be traumatized, and bruises more than 5 cm in diameter in the absence of trauma. Ecchymoses suggest coagulation factor deficiencies (e.g. classical haemophilia, liver disease) and petechiae suggest thrombocytopenia or a vessel wall defect, but these distinctions are not invariable.

If haemostatic capacity is reduced, is it due to a heritable defect with late clinical presentation, or is it the result of a newly acquired defect?—long-standing bleeding symptoms suggest a lifelong condition, whereas recent-onset bleeding suggests an acquired disorder. If a bleeding disorder has been diagnosed and characterized in another family member, then the cause of bleeding may be easily identified, but the absence of a family history does not exclude a heritable disorder.

If the bleeding disorder is newly acquired, is it due to an anticoagulant drug?—the commonest cause of an acquired bleeding disorder is antithrombotic therapy.

Clinical investigation

The routine evaluation of many patients includes the full blood count (including platelet count), prothrombin time (PT) and activated partial thromboplastin time (APTT), but (1) the platelet count gives no indication of platelet function; (2) the PT and APTT are insensitive; hence (3) comprehensive laboratory assessment of haemostatic capacity is indicated if these are normal but the history is suggestive of an underlying bleeding disorder.

Investigations include (1) full blood count and film—severe bleeding rarely occurs in the absence of trauma with a platelet count of more than 20 to 30×10^9/litre; automated machines may not count platelets reliably in some conditions, hence a blood film must be examined; (2) PT—the time taken in seconds for a fibrin clot to form after recalcification and addition of thromboplastin; (3) APTT—the time taken in seconds for a fibrin clot to form after recalcification and exposure to a contact factor activator; (4) fibrinogen level; (5) thrombin time—the time taken in seconds for a fibrin clot to form after addition of thrombin; (6) reptilase time—prolonged by low fibrinogen levels, but not by heparin, hence useful for determining if a prolonged APTT is due to heparin; (7) individual factor assays—useful in patients with a bleeding history and guided by PT and APTT results; (8) mixing studies—can indicate if prolongation of PT or APTT is likely due to a factor deficiency or an inhibitor; (9) platelet function analysis; (10) bleeding time—now rarely used.

Treatment of bleeding

Aside from general supportive care, specific therapy can be given when a defined haemostatic abnormality is identified. Drugs that cause bleeding should be stopped. Vitamin K should be given to critically ill patients and patients with liver disease. Early and sufficient blood product support should be given to those with massive blood loss and/or dilutional coagulopathy. Judicious use of fresh frozen plasma and platelets should be given to patients with severe coagulopathy such as disseminated intravascular coagulation while the underlying condition is being treated. Patients with overt haematological disorders will require specialist care.

Introduction

An apparent bleeding tendency is a common clinical problem. In all cases a comprehensive history is needed to assess the nature and extent of the bleeding, to guide clinical examination and logically to select informative investigations. Nongenetic acquired bleeding disorders are much more frequent than heritable defects; the most common cause of an acquired bleeding disorder is antithrombotic therapy—in many instances this is due to oral anticoagulant therapy with a vitamin K antagonist such as warfarin. Some patients who bleed excessively during or after surgery have a mild underlying heritable haemostatic defect and so an important aspect of assessment is to determine if there is an heritable defect with delayed clinical presentation. Effective treatment depends on identifying the underlying cause of bleeding recognizing its clinical importance so that appropriate measures can be introduced at times of risk to prevent excess bleeding.

Clinical assessment

Presentation of a bleeding disorder varies from acute unexpected bleeding during or immediately after surgery to spontaneous unusual or excessive bruising, purpura, epistaxis or chronic haemorrhagic tendencies evolving over a more prolonged period.

With increasing use of thromboprophylaxis in medical and surgical inpatients and increasing indications for long-term antithrombotic therapy, it is imperative to consider drug-induced bleeding. In all cases a comprehensive history is needed. Most heritable disorders of haemostasis are mild, e.g. von Willebrand's disease, and abnormal bleeding may not become manifest until there is a haemostatic challenge, such as surgery or menstruation. Therefore, an important aspect of the assessment of a patient with an apparent acquired bleeding disorder is to determine if it is genuinely of recent onset. The main issues to be determined are:

* Is haemostatic capacity reduced or is there a nonhaematological cause for bleeding?

* If haemostatic capacity is reduced, is it due to a heritable defect with late clinical presentation or is it the result of a newly acquired defect?

* If newly acquired, is it due to an anticoagulant drug?

* If not due to reduced haemostatic capacity, then what are the likely circumstances responsible for abnormal bleeding?

Taking a systematic history
Assessing haemostatic capacity
The main purpose of the history is to establish whether haemostatic capacity is normal and if there is a likely explanation for a bleeding tendency. Individual features in the history, such as bruising, epistaxis, or menorrhagia, have low positive and negative predictive value in isolation and unless a systematic history is taken with consideration of the 'overall picture', one can easily be misled. Rarely is it possible to absolutely exclude a disorder or make a positive diagnosis exclusively on the basis of the clinical history. However, the history is critical: there are patients who bleed after surgery and yet the mechanism of their bleeding disorder cannot be characterized by laboratory investigations. Nevertheless, such patients should be considered to have a bleeding disorder and empirical treatment to reduce bleeding before surgical procedures should be planned. In contrast, patients with borderline abnormal laboratory tests but with no clinical bleeding tendency at times of haemostatic challenge should not be categorized as having a bleeding disorder. Such issues occur frequently when interpreting von Willebrand factor (VWF) and factor XI results because there is a poor correlation between factor levels and bleeding tendency in individuals with a familial bleeding tendency. Recurrent bleeding from a single site suggests a structural abnormality of the vascular system, while bleeding at many different sites suggests a systemic haemostatic defect.

Severity and pattern of bleeding
The circumstances of the bleeding episode should be carefully assessed. Was bleeding spontaneous or provoked, e.g. by trauma or surgery? Was the degree of bleeding excessive or the pattern of bleeding unusual? Did bleeding result in anaemia, requiring transfusion? Was the site of bleeding unusual, e.g. a joint bleed in an adult with no previous history of abnormal bleeding? Was there bleeding with previous haemostatic challenges such as surgery, trauma, dental extraction, or menstruation? Bleeding symptoms over a long time period suggest a lifelong bleeding condition, whereas recent-onset bleeding suggests an acquired disorder; however it is important to realize that a mild lifelong condition can be unmasked at times of stress such as surgery.

Purpura

Purpura describes bleeding into the skin. The extent of bleeding may be small (petechiae) or larger (bruising, also called ecchymoses). Bruising is common in patients with reduced haemostatic capacity but is also very common in patients who have no apparent defect of haemostasis. Very extensive bruising particularly over soft areas that are not likely to be traumatized and very large bruises in the absence of trauma (>5 cm diameter) are more likely in patients with reduced haemostatic capacity. Bruising over bony areas does not necessarily indicate an abnormality, and many normal children frequently have several bruises over their knees and shins. When bruising is the result of a bleeding disorder the pattern of bleeding may be suggestive of the type of underlying disorder, e.g. ecchymoses suggesting coagulation factor deficiencies such as classical haemophilia or liver disease and petechiae suggesting thrombocytopenia or a vessel wall defect. However, these distinctions are not absolute, e.g. thrombocytopenia may present with large bruises rather than petechiae. Thrombocytopenia causes petechiae, typically when the platelet count is less than 20×10^9/litre. Petechiae may occur when there is platelet dysfunction or with vascular purpuras, either of which can be congenital or acquired. Petechiae are unusual with low VWF levels but may occur in some individuals with low levels when antiplatelet drugs are prescribed or when there is an increase in hydrostatic pressure, e.g. in the arm after application of a blood-pressure cuff—the Rumpel–Leede sign.

Epistaxis

Nosebleeds are common in children in the absence of a bleeding disorder. They also occur in some adults with allergic rhinitis. Repeated bleeding from the same nostril suggests a local cause. Lifelong recurrent epistaxis can occur in von Willebrand's disease, haemophilias and hereditary haemorrhagic telangiectasia (Osler–Weber–Rendu syndrome). Recent-onset epistaxis in adults may be due to an acquired disorder such as thrombocytopenia but is surprisingly uncommon in adults with lifelong bleeding disorders such as the haemophilias and von Willebrand's disease.

Gingival bleeding

Gum bleeding in the absence of any other abnormal bleeding is usually due to gingivitis requiring improved dental hygiene. Rarely is isolated gingival bleeding due to an underlying disorder.

Menorrhagia

Menorrhagia is a common problem and not specific for a bleeding disorder. Recent-onset menorrhagia in older women is likely to be due to a gynaecological cause. The main problem in assessing menorrhagia is subjectivity, e.g. many women with von Willebrand's disease do not complain of heavy periods because they consider their own experience as 'normal'. It is important to determine the pattern: bleeding for several days with clots, the need for internal and external absorbent pads, and particularly bleeding that interrupts normal lifestyle, e.g. absence from school or work, is more likely to be abnormal and caused by an underlying haemostatic defect. Very prolonged menorrhagia, rather than heavy bleeding, is more likely to be caused by an underlying haemostatic defect.

Dental extraction

Bleeding after dental extraction is very variable in the normal population. Bleeding lasting more than an hour, rebleeding, or late bleeding requiring suturing on more than one occasion suggests a bleeding disorder. Bleeding after extraction requiring blood transfusion even on one occasion suggests a bleeding disorder. Prolonged bleeding typically occurs in patients with low VWF levels; rebleeding is typical of haemophilia.

Surgery

It is important to ask specifically about all operations, including circumcision and tonsillectomy. Abnormal bleeding during surgery or in the postoperative period may be due to antithrombotic therapy, such as warfarin or aspirin that was not stopped. Abnormal surgical bleeding may be the first presentation of a mild or moderate heritable bleeding defect if there has been no previous haemostatic challenge, e.g. a male having his first operation. It is useful to determine if the bleeding was simply local, which might be due to a local anatomical reason such as a failed suture, or if there was evidence of more generalized bleeding such as oozing from the wound or bruising at venepuncture or sites of venous cannulation. Low-dose heparin (including low-molecular-weight heparin, LMWH) is used frequently to prevent venous thrombosis and in a minority of patients this can unmask a mild bleeding tendency, such as that associated with low VWF concentrations. In most patients, low-dose heparin does not appreciably increase surgical bleeding. However, it is important to review the drug charts from the time of the operation to ensure that the correct dose of heparin was given and that no other drugs that might cause bleeding were administered.

Bleeding in unusual sites

Bleeding in an unusual site may on occasion indicate a specific diagnosis. Joint bleeding rarely occurs in the presence of normal haemostatic capacity. It usually indicates severe coagulation factor deficiency, such as severe congenital factor VIII or IX deficiency or overdose with an oral vitamin K antagonist with an INR in excess of 8.0. Umbilical stump bleeding in the neonate is typical of severe congenital factor XIII deficiency, although the condition is very rare (1 per 1 000 000 of the population). Intracerebral bleeding in an otherwise healthy neonate necessitates exclusion of severe congenital factor VIII or IX deficiency, factor XIII deficiency and severe thrombocytopenia such as occurs in neonatal alloimmune thrombocytopenia (NAIT).

Family history of bleeding

If a bleeding disorder has been diagnosed and characterized in another family member then the cause of bleeding may be easily identified. The absence of a family history does not exclude a heritable disorder. The penetrance of von Willebrand's disease is incomplete and new mutations account for one-third of new patients with haemophilia A.

Drug history

The most common cause of an acquired bleeding disorder is antithrombotic therapy. Increasingly, low-dose heparin for inpatient thromboprophylaxis and oral vitamin K antagonists, such as warfarin, and aspirin in both inpatients and outpatients are responsible for bleeding. Other causes include drug-induced thrombocytopenia and impaired platelet function due to nonsteroidal anti-inflammatory drugs.

Clinical examination

Skin

The skin should be inspected in its entirety for evidence of bleeding, noting the distribution (bony or soft areas), pattern (random or suggestive of nonaccidental injury) and size (petechiae or ecchymoses). Senile purpura occurs predominantly on the extensor surfaces of the hands and arms and the face. The lesions tend to persist for several weeks, becoming increasingly darker. Senile purpura is due to skin atrophy and resultant blood vessel fragility; it is not associated with an underlying systemic bleeding disorder. Purpura occurs with amyloid which may cause bleeding due to capillary fragility, as a result of amyloid infiltration, or rarely an acquired deficiency of factor X. Vessels are extremely fragile and bleed with very minor trauma. Amyloid may also cause proteinuria, and excess bleeding may complicate renal biopsy in these patients. Some of these patients also have myeloma causing thrombocytopenia. Petechiae with a perifollicular distribution occur in scurvy, which may also present with more widespread bleeding into joints, gastrointestinal and intracerebral bleeding. Other features include xerostomia, keratoconjunctivitis sicca, and hyperkeratosis. Dental decay is common in patients with scurvy. Treatment with vitamin C results in improvement within hours. Scurvy may be the cause of bleeding in elderly patients with a very poor diet. Purpura occurs with infections including meningococcal septicaemia and diphtheria, chickenpox, measles, and the haemorrhagic fevers of Ebola virus and Lassa fever. Purpura fulminans describes necrotic skin lesions which occur with overwhelming infection and the development of disseminated intravascular coagulation (DIC).

Allergic purpura may follow exposure to chemicals and toxins. Henoch–Schönlein purpura is the most common allergic purpura and involves principally skin, joints, gastrointestinal tract, and kidneys. It typically occurs in children after an upper respiratory tract infection due to streptococcus. The rash consists of purpuric papules over the shins, thighs, buttocks, sometimes with small ulcers, and the rash is associated with arthritis, nephritis and abdominal pain. IgA-containing immune complexes are deposited in the vessel walls. Mixed cryoglobulinaemia in patients with hepatitis C infection can produce extensive purpura in association with arthropathy and glomerulonephritis.

Psychogenic purpura refers to unexplained bruising with preceding pain in association with anxiety. It has also been referred to as 'autoerythrocyte sensitization', following reports that subcutaneous injection of the patient's own red cells can induce the lesions. However, it is uncertain if this is a genuine clinical sign, particularly as subcutaenous injection of red cells would be expected to appear as a 'bruise'.

Telangiectasia may occur in the skin and the mucous membranes. In patients with hereditary haemorrhagic telangiectasia they occur predominantly in the skin of the hands and fingertips. The lesions blanch on pressure in contrast to purpura. Telangiectasia also occur in pregnancy and liver disease, usually on the face and chest. Rarely, large cavernous haemangiomas can cause local consumption of coagulation factors and platelets resulting in a systemic bleeding disorder. Skin elasticity, scars, papules and plaques may indicate a collagen vascular disorder. Ehlers–Danlos syndrome, Marfan's syndrome, pseudoxanthoma elasticum, and osteogenesis imperfecta are associated with a bleeding tendency due to abnormal platelet–vessel wall collagen interaction. Unusual scars may be due to a dysfibrinogenaemia, Ehlers–Danlos syndrome or pseudoxanthoma elasticum. Long-term steroid therapy and Cushing's disease cause skin atrophy and bruising typically on the extensor surfaces of the hands and arms and on the thighs.

Mucosa

Telangiectasia are dilated small vessels that may be found in skin and the mucous membranes of the respiratory and gastrointestinal, urinary tracts, vagina, eye, liver, and brain in patients with hereditary haemorrhagic telangiectasia (Osler–Weber–Rendu syndrome). Recurrent epistaxis and gastrointestinal bleeding cause iron deficiency.

Musculoskeletal system

Severe haemophilia A (factor VIII deficiency) and B (factor IX deficiency) are characterized by repeated spontaneous bleeds into joints, muscles, and soft tissue. The most common joints that bleed are the ankles, knees, hips, and elbows. Acute haemarthrosis presents as an acutely swollen painful joint resulting in joint immobilization. Repeated bleeds into a joint (target joint) produces chronic haemophilic arthropathy with features of both osteoarthritis (mechanical pain on movement) and rheumatoid (inflammatory pain at rest). Muscle haematomas occur in the iliopsoas, gluteal, calf, and forearm muscles and are more insidious than joint bleeds. Compartment syndrome can complicate large bleeds and fibrosis and contractures produce dysfunction and deformity. Large haematomas can cause pseudotumours, particularly when there is chronic rebleeding. These large expanding soft tissue cysts produce mass effects including neuropathy, bone erosion and may produce chronic fistulas.

Splenomegaly

Splenomegaly can cause hypersplenism with thrombocytopenia. Patients with myeloproliferative disorders may have impaired platelet function. Essential thrombocythaemia is a myeloproliferative disorder which is particularly associated with impaired platelet function but both bleeding and thrombosis occur. In patients with very high platelet counts there can be increased consumption of VWF causing an acquired von Willebrand's syndrome. Patients with polycythaemia are particularly prone to chronic gastrointestinal bleeding. Splenomegaly may be due to portal hypertension in patients with liver disease. In these patients bleeding may be due to a systemic disorder with thrombocytopenia, platelet dysfunction, coagulation factor deficiency and production of dysfunctional factors. In addition there may be local bleeding sites such as oesophageal varices.

General aspects of examination

In addition to identifying signs that may indicate likelihood and type of a bleeding disorder, it is important to consider broader aspects. For example, is a patient anaemic due to iron deficiency as a consequence of chronic gastrointestinal blood loss? Patients with severe bleeding disorders who have been treated with human-derived blood products, in particular pooled products that have not been virally inactivated, may have chronic infections including hepatitis C and HIV. Chronic liver disease, opportunistic infections, and other complications may be evident. Bleeding as a result of liver, renal failure, or paraproteinaemia should be considered. In children the possibility of nonaccidental injury should be considered, particularly with multiple bruises around the head and neck, or a pattern of bruising in keeping with gripping or shaking. The retina should be examined for haemorrhages. In a drowsy patient or a patient with raised intracranial pressure or an acute focal neurological deficit there is the possibility of an intracranial bleed.

Investigations

Laboratory tests

These include:

- prothrombin time (PT)
- activated partial thromboplastin time (APTT)
- fibrinogen level (Fgn)
- thrombin time (TT)
- reptilase time (RT)
- factor assays
- mixing studies
- platelet function analysis

Coagulation tests are typically performed on plasma that has been separated from a venous blood sample by centrifugation. Thrombin generation takes place on phospholipid surfaces (provided by platelets normally) and so an artificial lipid preparation is added as the platelets are removed by the centrifugation. Most routine clotting tests use the time taken for a clot to appear as the endpoint of the assay. Blood is usually taken into tubes containing citrate, which chelates calcium and thereby prevents clotting. After centrifugation the plasma is removed and recalcified during the clotting assay. Clotting tests are indicated in patients with a personal or family history of bleeding. They are not generally indicated as routine preoperative screening tests as they have very low sensitivity and specificity for surgical bleeding in unselected patients. Preoperative assessment of bleeding risk is better determined by identification of a personal or family bleeding history, which should then be investigated accordingly with specific tests including coagulation factor assays, VWF level and function and platelet count and function.

Assessment of haemostasis

The history is of primary importance in determining if haemostatic capacity is genuinely reduced. Standard laboratory tests such as PT and APTT are insensitive to mild and moderate reductions of levels of coagulation factors which may be clinically significant and cause bleeding. These tests are not influenced at all by levels of VWF. Therefore, it is on the basis of the history that a decision is made on the extent of laboratory testing. The blood count and film, PT, APTT and platelet count should be measured. If these are normal but the history is suggestive of an underlying bleeding disorder, a more comprehensive laboratory assessment of haemostatic capacity is indicated. Measurement of the platelet count gives no indication of platelet function.

Blood count and film examination

Bleeding tendency increases with thrombocytopenia with a platelet count of less than 80×10^9/litre but severe bleeding rarely occurs in the absence of trauma with a platelet count greater than 20 to 30×10^9/litre. Film examination is mandatory when a bleeding disorder is suspected. Pseudothrombocytopenia due to platelet clumping can lead to an erroneous diagnosis of true thrombocytopenia if the film is not examined for clumps. Conversely, a normal platelet count may be occasionally reported in patients with true thrombocytopenia, the normal count being an artefact, e.g. due to the presence of a cryoglobulin. In these patients the thrombocytopenia is readily apparent from examination of the blood film. Abnormal platelet morphology may suggest an underlying heritable platelet defect such as Bernard–Soulier syndrome, May–Hegglin abnormality, or a grey platelet syndrome. Alternatively, a leukaemia or an acquired myeloproliferative disorder or myelodysplastic syndrome may be apparent from the blood count and film examination.

Prothrombin time (PT)

The prothrombin time is the time taken in seconds for a fibrin clot to form after recalcification and addition of thromboplastin (a preparation of tissue factor which is the protein that activates factor VII). The normal PT is about 11 to 14 s, depending on the type of thromboplastin used.

The PT is prolonged by:

- oral anticoagulant therapy (typically warfarin)
- vitamin K deficiency
- liver disease
- DIC
- dilutional coagulopathy (massive blood transfusion)
- and very rarely by congenital factor VII deficiency

Anticoagulant therapy with oral vitamin K antagonists is monitored by the INR, which is derived from the PT ratio and is a standardized method of reporting which permits comparability between laboratories. It is inappropriate to use the INR for any purpose other than measuring the intensity of oral anticoagulant therapy. For all other purposes the PT or PT ratio should be used.

Activated partial thromboplastin time (APTT)

The APTT is the time taken in seconds for a fibrin clot to form after recalcification and exposure to a contact factor activator, such as kaolin. The normal APTT is about 32 to 38 s, depending on the type of contact factor activator used.

The APTT is prolonged by:

- unfractionated heparin (LMWH has minimal effect at therapeutic levels)
- oral anticoagulant therapy (mildly; the PT is much more sensitive)
- vitamin K deficiency (mildly; the PT is more sensitive)
- liver disease (mildly; the PT is more sensitive)
- DIC
- dilutional coagulopathy (massive blood transfusion)
- severe and moderate deficiencies of clotting factors VIII, IX, or XI
- antiphospholipid antibodies (known as lupus anticoagulant activity)
- contact factor deficiency (including factor XII and prekallikrein, none of which cause bleeding)

A low factor XII level produces a marked prolongation of the APTT but deficiency is not associated with any bleeding tendency. This reflects the fact that the APTT is a nonphysiological test that, although useful for screening for deficiency of clotting factors, does not actually reflect physiological haemostasis.

Fibrinogen level

Fibrinogen levels are low in:

◆ DIC

◆ dilutional coagulopathy (massive blood transfusion)

◆ advanced liver disease

◆ following thrombolytic therapy

◆ congenital hypofibrinogenaemia (very rare)

Thrombin time (TT)

The TT is the time taken in seconds for a fibrin clot to form after addition of thrombin.

The TT is prolonged by:

◆ unfractionated heparin

◆ hypofibrinogenaemia (see above for low fibrinogen levels)

◆ fibrin degradation products (high levels may occur in DIC and after thrombolysis)

Reptilase time (RT)

This test is based on snake venom. It is prolonged by low fibrinogen levels but not by heparin and so comparison of the TT and RT is useful for determining if a prolonged APTT is due to heparin; a long TT with normal RT indicates heparin. Heparin contamination is common on samples from hospitalized patients, even though use of heparin flushes and sampling from catheters is often denied by clinical staff. Weak heparin flushes significantly prolong the APPT on samples taken from indwelling catheters. In many cases it is necessary to obtain a venous sample from a fresh venepuncture.

Factor assays

Individual factor assays are useful in patients with a bleeding history and are guided by PT and APTT results. The cascade model of coagulation is no longer considered to represent the physiological process involved in coagulation. The cascade model was derived from observation of results using the PT and APTT assays but these are not 'physiological' tests. Although the cascade model may not be 'physiologically true' it is still a useful framework for interpreting PT and APTT results. For example, in a patient with a bleeding history with a normal PT and a long APTT (not due to heparin or a lupus anticoagulant) there may be deficiency of factor VIII, IX, or XI (see Fig. 22.6.2.1). Table 22.6.2.1 summarizes the interpretation of laboratory investigations.

Mixing studies

If the PT or APTT is prolonged then mixing with normal plasma and repeating the test will indicate if the prolongation is likely due to a factor deficiency (the mix corrects the abnormality) or an inhibitor, such as heparin or a specific factor inhibitor (the mix does not correct the abnormality).

Platelet function analysis

Platelet function can be assessed at high and low shear. The Platelet Function Analyser (PFA-100) is an automated technique that measures the ability of platelets to occlude an aperture under conditions of high shear. The test is performed on a citrated blood sample within 4 h of sample collection and is abnormal in the presence of low VWF activity or platelet function defects. Thrombocytopenia causes prolonged closure and so the test requires a normal platelet count in order to assess platelet function. Platelet function at low shear rate is assessed by platelet aggregation. Aggregation studies are performed typically on platelet rich plasma prepared by slow centrifugation of citrated blood within 4 h of sample collection. There is a poor correlation with bleeding tendency except in specific congenital disorders characterized by severe platelet dysfunction, e.g. Glanzmann's thrombasthenia (GT) and Bernard–Soulier syndrome (BSS).

◆ Agonists used for aggregation studies include ADP, collagen, arachidonic acid, and adrenaline (epinephrine).

◆ Response to ristocetin is an agglutination response dependent on induced conformational change of platelet membrane proteins, e.g. glycoprotein Ib-IX-V, promoting interaction with VWF.

◆ Ristocetin induced platelet agglutination (RIPA) is carried out at high (1.2 mg/ml) and low ristocetin concentrations (0.5 mg/dl). Positive RIPA at 0.5 mg/dl is an abnormal result and is observed in type 2B von Willebrand's disease and with high VWF levels, e.g. pregnancy.

Platelet storage pool disorders (SPD) are characterized by absent platelet α or δ granules. α-Granule proteins include β-thromboglobulin (β-TG) and platelet factor 4 (PF4) which can be measured by enzyme-linked immunosorbent assay (ELISA)—these are deficient in α-granule storage pool defects. Nucleotides (ADP/ATP) can be measured by a variety of techniques including high pressure liquid chromatography and are deficient in δ-storage pool disorders. These analyses are beyond the scope of most haematology laboratories.

Bleeding time

The bleeding time is used much less frequently now that platelet function analysis at high shear is readily available. The bleeding time does not predict surgical bleeding.

Other investigations

Global tests of haemostasis

Further tests of haemostasis which assess the dynamic interaction of the individual components of haemostasis rather than the amount or function of specific components in isolation are available in some specialized laboratories. These techniques include, thromboelastography, thrombin generation, and tests of fibrinolysis.

Anatomical imaging

Specific bleeding points may be due to structural abnormalities and imaging directly by endoscopy or by CT, MRI, or angiography will be indicated in some patients.

Specific issues

Drug-induced bleeding

The most common cause of an acquired bleeding disorder is anticoagulant therapy. Platelets are integral to thrombin generation and antiplatelet drugs can be considered as anticoagulants, hence their ability to prevent thrombosis. Bleeding risk is in part determined by the potency of antiplatelet activity, e.g. the bleeding risk associated with a fibrinogen receptor antagonist (IIbIIIa inhibitor) is far greater than with aspirin or an ADP receptor antagonist such as clopidogrel. The individual response to antiplatelet therapy is extremely variable and even aspirin or clopidogrel will produce

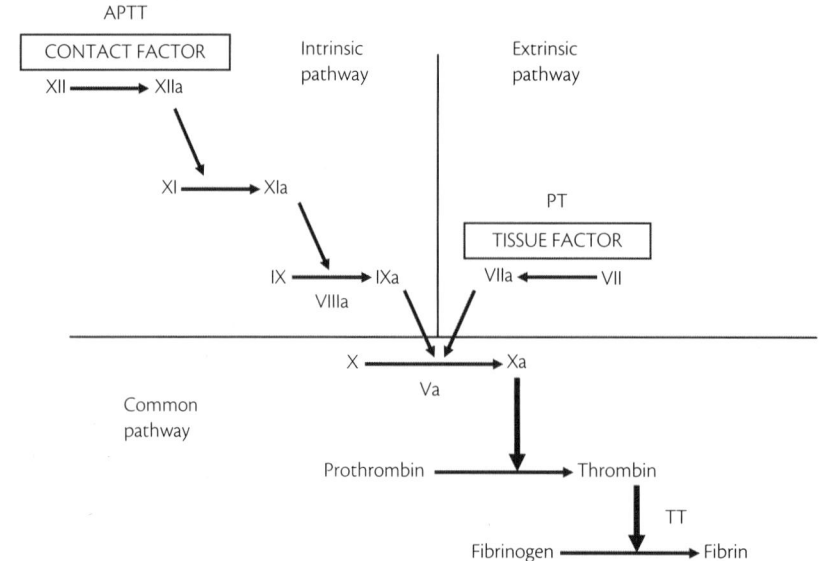

Fig. 22.6.2.1 Cascade model of coagulation. APTT, activated partial thromboplastin time; PT, prothrombin time; TT, thrombin time.

Table 22.6.2.1 Interpretation of laboratory investigations

Coagulopathy	PT	APTT	Fibrinogen	TT	Platelets	PFA
Heritable						
VWF—mild	N	N	N	N	N	Abnormal
VWF—moderate	N	N or ↑	N	N	N	Abnormal
VWD—severe	N	↑	N	N	N	Abnormal
VWD—type 2B (rare)	N	N	N	N	↓	Abnormal
VIII	N	↑	N	N	N	N
IX	N	↑	N	N	N	N
XI	N	↑	N	N	N	N
VII	↑	N	N	N	N	N
X, V, or II	↑	↑	N	N	N	N
Fibrinogen	N/↑	N/↑	↓	↑	N	N or abnormal
XIII	N	N	N	N	N	N
Thrombocytopenia	N	N	N	N	↓	Abnormal
Glanzmann's disease	N	N	N	N	N	Abnormal
Bernard–Soulier syndrome	N	N	N	N	↓	Abnormal
Acquired						
Heparin	N or ↑	↑	N	↑*	N	N
Warfarin	↑	N or ↑	N	N	N	N
Aspirin/clopidogrel	N	N	N	N	N	Abnormal
Dilutional coagulopathy	↑	↑	N or ↓	N or ↑	↓	abnormal
Renal disease	N	N	N	N	N or ↓	Abnormal
Liver disease	↑	↑	N or ↓	N or ↑	N or ↓	N or abnormal
DIC	↑	↑	N or ↓+	N or ↑	↓	abnormal
Acquired VWS	N	N or ↑	N	N	N	Abnormal
Hyperfibrinolysis	N or ↑	N or ↑	N or ↓	N or ↑	N	N or abnormal
Surgical bleeding	N	N	N	N	N	N

APTT, activated partial thromboplastin time; DIC, disseminated intravascular coagulation; PFA, platelet function analysis; PT, prothrombin time; TT, thrombin time; vWD, von Willebrand's disease, VWF, von Willebrand factor, VWS, von Willebrand's syndrome. PFA (Platelet function Analysis on the PFA-100) only performed in selected cases. In cases of complex coagulopathy PFA is abnormal primarily due to thrombocytopenia.

* With heparin the TT is prolonged but the reptilase time (RT) is normal.

+ With DIC the level of fibrin degradation products (such as D-dimer) is very high and this interferes with fibrin polymerisation which contributes with low fibrinogen levels to the prolonged thrombin time.

a significant bleeding tendency in some patients. Approximately 1 in 100 of the United Kingdom population are now receiving long-term oral anticoagulant therapy and overanticoagulation as indicated by a high INR, often due to intercurrent illness and antibiotic use, is probably responsible for the majority of life-threatening bleeds attributable to antithrombotic therapy. The INR is particularly influenced by the factor VII level, which is not the main determinant of bleeding risk. When overanticoagulation due to an oral vitamin K antagonist is reversed by intravenous vitamin K the INR may correct over several hours, but a significant bleeding tendency remains as the factor VII level rises more quickly than the other vitamin K-dependent factors. Therefore, in patients with significant bleeding reversal requires a combination of factor replacement (for immediate and effective reversal of bleeding) and vitamin K (for a sustained reversal when the response to factor replacement has decayed).

Surgical bleeding

Postoperative bleeding is a common clinical problem. It is essential to examine the drug and infusion charts and check that the dose of any drug that may affect haemostasis is not excessive. It is also imperative to determine if the site of surgery is the only site of bleeding. If this is the case, e.g. there is no bleeding from venepuncture sites or an endotracheal tube and there is no history of previous abnormal bleeding, then depending on the results of coagulation tests it is important to keep the possibility of anatomical surgical bleeding as a likely possibility. In some cases of severe bleeding the patient may have to return to theatre to look for a bleeding point. Severe surgical bleeding may result in a dilutional coagulopathy due to fluid volume replacement or DIC due to hypotensive shock with a severe exacerbation of bleeding and a complex secondary coagulopathy.

Critically ill patients

There are many potential acquired disorders of haemostasis in critically ill patients. A coagulopathy due to vitamin K deficiency occurs within a few days in critically ill patients with no oral intake. Parenteral vitamin K supplementation should be used routinely to prevent bleeding. Many critically ill patients develop DIC.

Massive transfusion and dilutional coagulopathy

A dilutional coagulopathy resulting in deficiency of clotting factors and platelets will cause abnormal bleeding in patients receiving large amounts of plasma expanders and red blood cells even in the absence of DIC. It is important to give replacement therapy with fresh frozen plasma (FFP) and platelet concentrates guided by repeated measurement of the PT, APTT, and platelet count.

Disseminated intravascular coagulation (DIC)

The major manifestations of DIC are end-organ damage due to microvascular thrombosis but the most readily apparent clinical manifestation is often bleeding due to the consumptive coagulopathy. DIC is a clinical diagnosis supported by the results of laboratory investigations with a prolonged PT and APTT, a low fibrinogen and platelet count, and elevated fibrin degradation products (such as D-dimer). Persistent oozing from venepuncture sites in patients with sepsis or in obstetric patient suggests DIC. A fibrinogen level less than 1 g/litre suggests DIC in a patient with an acquired severe bleeding disorder. The most important aspect of treatment is that of the underlying cause, e.g. sepsis, although FFP and platelet concentrates are used to treat bleeding or prevent haemorrhage associated with planned invasive procedures. A chronic form of DIC occurs in patients with malignancy.

ABO blood group-associated low VWF levels and von Willebrand's disease

The most common heritable bleeding tendency is due to a low VWF level. This may be due to genetic mutation of the VWF gene (often designated von Willebrand's disease), or more commonly the effect of epigenetic factors such as blood group O (designated blood group O-associated low VWF level). Regardless, the level of VWF appears to be an important continuous variable influencing the coagulation phenotype. The first apparent manifestation of this may be excessive surgical bleeding and as a result the patient is considered to have an acquired bleeding disorder. The history may be informative, such as a detailed menstrual history in women. It can be difficult to establish a diagnosis of a mild reduction in VWF in the immediate postoperative period as levels rise due to the stress response. Consequently, it is prudent to re-evaluate patients several weeks after an episode of abnormal surgical bleeding. VWF levels should be interpreted in relation to blood group and the clinical circumstances at the time a blood sample was taken.

Thrombocytopenia

Many drugs result in a reversible idiosyncratic thrombocytopenia. In most cases drug-induced thrombocytopenia is mild and does not cause bleeding. Notable exceptions are quinine and gold-induced thrombocytopenia, which are severe. An evaluation of drug history and cessation of possibly implicated drugs is essential in patients with acquired bleeding who are found to be thrombocytopenic. Other commonly used drugs for which there is good evidence for drug-induced thrombocytopenia include amiodarone, atorvastatin, carbamazepine, cimetidine, diclofenac, digoxin, ranitidine, co-trimoxazole, and vancomycin. Cytotoxic drugs produce a dose-dependent suppression of bone marrow platelet production and thrombocytopenic bleeding is common in oncology practice. Bone marrow suppression and bone marrow failure syndromes, such as aplastic anaemia and myelodysplasia, often result in production of dysfunctional platelets and the bleeding tendency is significantly greater than in patients with thrombocytopenia and an uncompromised marrow, such as occurs in idiopathic thrombocytopenic purpura (ITP) in which the bleeding risk is relatively low. Thrombocytopenia is common in HIV infection. Gestational thrombocytopenia occurs in 5% of pregnancies but the platelet count is rarely less than 80×10^9/litre and it is not associated with an increased bleeding tendency.

Renal disease

Bleeding risk increases with the degree of renal impairment and is due to a defect of platelet–vessel wall interaction. In most patients laboratory tests of haemostasis are normal. The bleeding time (if performed) is prolonged and platelet function tests may give variable results that do not correlate with bleeding risk. The cause of the bleeding is an accumulation of dialysable uraemic toxins including urea and phenols which inhibit platelet function and possibly VWF activity. Anaemia contributes to the bleeding tendency due to reduced coaxial streaming of platelets and a reduction in platelet–vessel wall contact. Bleeding is most commonly into the skin and mucous membranes, and gastrointestinal haemorrhage is common. Haemodialysis and peritoneal dialysis reduce the bleeding tendency without any necessarily appreciable effect on tests of platelet function. Desamino-D-arginine vasopressin (Desmopressin DDAVP) improves haemostasis. Correction of anaemia by transfusion or erythropoietin therapy to maintain the haemoglobin above 10 g/dl is beneficial. Infusion of cryoprecipitate can be considered in patients who continue to bleed despite dialysis and correction of anaemia as reports of reduced bleeding have been reported for reasons that are not completely understood. Administration of conjugated oestrogens has also been reported to reduce the bleeding tendency.

Liver disease

The PT and APTT are frequently abnormal in patients with advanced liver disease but correction of abnormalities with FFP is indicated only if there is active bleeding or in anticipation of an invasive procedure. Otherwise intravenous vitamin K can be administered. The liver is the site of synthesis of most of the proteins involved in haemostasis. In cirrhosis there is deficient production of coagulation factors compounded by production of dysfunctional factors (due to defective post-translational carboxylation) with thrombocytopenia due to portal hypertension with hypersplenism and in some case defective marrow platelet production. Platelet function is defective. In obstructive jaundice there is production of dysfunctional factors which responds initially to intravenous vitamin K. In acute hepatitis there is predominantly a consumptive coagulopathy due to DIC. In advanced liver disease and hepatoma there may be additional dysfibrinogenaemia. Hypofibrinogenaemia with a fibrinogen less than 1 g/litre occurs with fulminant hepatic failure. Reduced clearance of tissue plasminogen activator causes hyperfibrinolysis which contributes to bleeding. A variable degree of DIC may be present in patients with chronic liver disease. Acute DIC may be precipitated by infection. Transfusion of platelets, FFP and cryoprecipitate (as a source of fibrinogen) will depend on individual circumstances. Parenteral vitamin K should always be considered and frequently a trial of therapy is required, e.g. 10 mg daily for 3 days.

Acquired haemophilia and acquired von Willebrand's syndrome

Acquired inhibitors are rare and most often autoantibodies. Platelet autoantibodies result in shortened platelet survival and ITP. The bleeding manifestations of ITP are variable and often mild, as compared with thrombocytopenia associated with inadequate platelet production (see above). Rarely, an autoantibody to a specific clotting factor, such as factor VIII, produces a severe acquired bleeding disorder. An acquired von Willebrand's syndrome may be due to either an autoantibody (often an IgG paraprotein and occasionally IgM) or consumption of VWF in patients with uncontrolled essential thrombocythaemia.

Hyperfibrinolysis

Heritable defects of fibrinolysis are exceptionally rare. The fibrinolytic system may have a primary role in clot lysis as part of wound healing rather than in the immediate haemostatic response to injury. Nevertheless, pharmacological doses of fibrinolytic activators, such as recombinant tissue plasminogen activator, have an immediate lytic effect and hence clinical utility as a 'clot-busting drugs'.

Bleeding in the neonate

Bleeding in the neonate may be due to a rare heritable defect or an acquired abnormality occurring *in utero* or soon after delivery. Thrombocytopenia is present in 30 to 40% of neonates in special care baby units. Thrombocytopenia presenting in the first 72 h is most often due to chronic fetal hypoxia, often with intrauterine growth retardation, but rarely due to transplacental passage of an alloantibody to a platelet antigen (NAIT, neonatal alloimmune thrombocytopenia). Thrombocytopenia presenting after 72 h is most often in association with sepsis or necrotizing enterocolitis and is often associated with DIC. Bleeding form the umbilical stump or intracranial haemorrhage not explained by DIC or severe thrombocytopenia may be due to severe deficiency of factor VIII, IX, XIII, or afibrinogenaemia.

Treatment of bleeding

Acute bleeding

Effective treatment depends on a critical assessment of the extent and nature of bleeding and the likely cause. When a defined haemostatic abnormality is identified specific therapy can be given. Drugs that cause bleeding should be stopped. Nonhaematological causes of bleeding should be managed appropriately, e.g. dialysis and red cell transfusion in patients with renal failure. Vitamin K should be given to critically ill patients and patients with liver disease. Early and sufficient blood product support should be given to patients with massive blood loss and to those with dilutional coagulopathy. Supportive care with judicious use of FFP and platelets should be given to patients with severe coagulopathy such as DIC whilst the underlying condition is being treated. Patients with overt haematological disorders such as myelodysplasia, ITP, or factor VIII inhibitors will require specialist care. Pharmacological agents can be used to increase haemostatic capacity but should be used by clinicians with appropriate experience. Such drugs include DDAVP, tranexamic acid, and off-licence use of drugs such as recombinant factor VIIa. Aprotonin was used extensively in the past but is now used with caution because of thrombotic complications, including death, and renal impairment.

Nonacute bleeding

It is important to identify the circumstances that contribute to abnormal bleeding and to determine the likelihood of an underlying persistent bleeding tendency as this will influence future management, e.g. at times of surgery or decisions regarding antithrombotic therapy. A comprehensive drug history should identify drugs that may have to be stopped. Some individuals are particularly sensitive to the usually mild anticoagulant effect of aspirin or clopidogrel. A single episode of abnormal surgical bleeding may not be readily explained but this should be taken into consideration at times of future surgery so that mechanical rather than pharmacological thromboprophylaxis is used and any antiplatelet or anticoagulant therapy stopped with certainty.

Further reading

Baglin TP, *et al.* (2006). Guidelines on oral anticoagulation (warfarin): third edition—2005 update. *Br J Haematol*, **132**, 277–85.
Harrison P (2005). Platelet function analysis. *Blood Rev*, **19**, 111–23.

Laffan M, *et al.* (2004). The diagnosis of von Willebrand disease: a guideline from the UK Haemophilia Centre Doctors' Organization. *Haemophilia*, **10**, 199–217.

Levi M (2004). Current understanding of disseminated intravascular coagulation. *Br J Haematol*, **124**, 567–76.

Monroe DM, Hoffman M (2006). What does it take to make the perfect clot? *Arterioscl Thromb Vasc Biol*, **26**, 41–8.

Sadler JE (2003). von Willebrand disease type 1: a diagnosis in search of a disease. *Blood*, **101**, 2089–93.

22.6.3 Disorders of platelet number and function

Kathryn E. Webert and John G. Kelton

Essentials

Platelets are released from megakaryocytes in the bone marrow and circulate for 5 to 10 days before being cleared by the cells of the reticuloendothelial system. They play a critical role in haemostasis, with key features being (1) adhesion—when the wall of a blood vessel is damaged, platelets adhere to exposed collagen and other components of the subendothelium via the glycoprotein Ib receptor and other adhesive receptors; followed by (2) activation—release of thrombin, adenosine diphosphate, and arachidonic acid, which is converted by a cascade of enzymes into platelet activating agents including thromboxane A_2; and (3) aggregation—glycoprotein IIb/IIIa undergoes conformational changes, making it able to bind fibrinogen and resulting in the formation of the haemostatic plug

Thrombocytopenia

Thrombocytopenia is defined as a reduction in the number of circulating platelets to less than 150×10^9/litre. Bleeding is uncommon unless the platelet count falls below 10 to 20×10^9/litre, or unless there is abnormal platelet function.

Increased platelet destruction: autoimmune thrombocytopenia—mediated by antibodies that bind to individual platelet glycoproteins, most frequently glycoprotein IIb/IIIa. May be (1) Primary (idiopathic thrombocytopenic purpura, ITP)—a disorder of children and (typically) young or middle-aged women. May present in adults with incidentally discovered thrombocytopenia, a long history of easy bruising, or acute onset of petechiae, purpura, and bleeding. Many patients will not require specific treatment, but those with severe thrombocytopenia (platelets $<10 \times 10^9$/litre) and/or significant haemostatic impairment are treated with corticosteroids, typically oral prednisone (1 mg/kg). Second-line treatments include high-dose intravenous immunoglobulin, splenectomy, and danazol. (2) Secondary—conditions that can cause immune thrombocytopenia include systemic lupus erythematosus, drug induced (most commonly heparin, quinidine, sulfonamides, valproic acid, and gold), chronic lymphocytic leukaemia, post-transfusion purpura, and infections (e.g. HIV, varicella, Epstein–Barr virus).

Increased platelet destruction: nonimmune thrombocytopenia—disorders associated with both thrombocytopenia and fragmentation haemolysis include (1) Thrombotic thrombocytopenic purpura—manifestations include thrombocytopenia, microangiopathic haemolytic anaemia, renal impairment, fever, and ischaemic neurological findings; may be related to a deficiency of ADAMTS13 (a disintegrin and metalloprotease with thrombospondin-1-like domains); treatment is with plasmapheresis. (2) Haemolytic uraemic syndrome—presents as renal failure, microangiopathic haemolytic anaemia, and thrombocytopenia. May be epidemic in association with a diarrhoeal illness caused by enterohaemorrhagic or verotoxigenic *Escherichia coli* serotype O157:H7 or *Shigella dysenteriae* serotype I; can also be hereditary or sporadic, sometimes in association with noninfectious conditions. Aside from supportive care, treatment is usually with plasmapheresis. (3) Disseminated intravascular coagulation—patients are usually very unwell and present with fulminant bleeding and organ dysfunction, most often in the context of sepsis; characterized by large amounts of thrombin that overwhelm the physiological inhibitors of coagulation; replacement therapy with fresh frozen plasma, cryoprecipitate, and platelets should be considered.

Decreased platelet production—may rarely be congenital, but most cases are acquired, with common or important causes being (1) toxins—drugs (e.g. chemotherapeutic agents, chloramphenicol, nonsteroidal anti-inflammatory drugs, antiepileptic medications, gold), alcohol; (2) nutritional deficiencies—folate or vitamin B12; (3) bone marrow infiltration; (4) myelodysplastic syndrome.

Disorders of platelet distribution and platelet sequestration—these include (1) splenomegaly and hypersplenism; (2) haemodilution—in patients who have received large volumes of crystalloid solutions or blood products; (3) extracorporeal circulation; (4) hypothermia.

Thrombocytosis

Thrombocytosis is defined as an increase in the number of circulating platelets to more than 600×10^9/litre.

Primary thrombocytosis (thrombocythaemia)—a chronic myeloproliferative disorder often caused by mutation in the JAK2 tyrosine kinase. Presentation may be with thrombosis or bleeding. Young, asymptomatic patients do not require treatment. Low-dose aspirin can prevent thrombosis and may relieve symptoms such as headache and erythromelalgia, but it may unmask bleeding tendencies and hence should be avoided in patients with a history of bleeding. Hydroxyurea will lower the platelet count and usually reduces thrombohaemorrhagic complications.

Secondary thrombocytosis—causes include infections, malignancy, chronic inflammatory bowel disease, rheumatoid arthritis, iron deficiency, and hyposplenism.

Disorders of platelet function

Congenital disorders—these can affect platelet (1) adhesion and aggregation—e.g. Bernard–Soulier syndrome, caused by a deficiency or abnormality of platelet glycoprotein Ib/IX; (2) secretion; and (3) procoagulant activity.

Acquired disorders—most common causes of platelet dysfunction are (1) medications and toxins—e.g. aspirin, nonsteroidal anti-inflammatory agents, ticlopidine, clopidrogel, glycoprotein IIb/IIIa inhibitors; (2) systemic disorders—e.g. chronic renal failure; and (3) haematological diseases—e.g. chronic myeloproliferative disorders, myelodysplastic syndromes, dysproteinaemias.

Introduction

Platelets are the smallest of the circulating blood cells and their numbers in healthy individuals range from 150×10^9/litre to 450×10^9/litre. Platelets are released from the megakaryocytes in the bone marrow and circulate for 5 to 10 days before being cleared by the cells of the reticuloendothelial system. Disorders of platelet number and function are frequently encountered.

Platelets are discoid cells that average $4\,\mu m$ in diameter. The external membrane is a glycocalyx surface covering a phospholipid bilayer. Penetrating the membrane and traversing the platelet is a tubular system termed the open canalicular system. This system is continuous with the surface membrane and acts as a conduit for the release and uptake of nutrients and biologically active compounds. The platelet cytoskeleton is composed of three filamentous systems consisting of microtubules, microfilaments, and intermediate filaments. These tubules maintain the platelet's shape and participate in shape change, a complex process that occurs following platelet activation.

Platelets contain several organelles including α-granules, dense granules, lysosomes, peroxisomes, and mitochondria. The α-granules are the most numerous platelet granules (c.50 granules/platelet) and contain proteins synthesized by megakaryocytes, including β-thromboglobulin, platelet factor 4, thrombospondin, and von Willebrand factor (VWF). The α-granules also contain plasma-absorbed proteins such as fibrinogen, albumin, IgG, and certain coagulation factors, particularly factor V. On the α-granule membrane are a variety of proteins including P-selectin and glycoprotein IIb/IIIa. Dense granules are far fewer in number than α-granules (4–8/platelet) and are smaller. These electron-dense granules are important for platelet activation and contain ATP, serotonin, calcium, magnesium, pyrophosphate, and granulophysin. Their membranes also contain a number of platelet proteins including P-selectin, glycoprotein Ib, and glycoprotein IIb/IIIa. Lysosomal granules contain proteolytic enzymes.

Platelet surface structures

Penetrating the platelet membrane are platelet glycoproteins. Most of these glycoproteins can be classified as one of five supergene families: integrins, leucine-rich glycoproteins, immunoglobulin domain molecules, selectins, and quadraspanins. The integrin family is the most common with glycoprotein IIb/IIIa being the most abundant integrin. Glycoprotein IIb/IIIa, also known as $\alpha_{IIb}\beta_3$, is present in high numbers (40 000–50 000 surface copies per platelet) and is the key binding site for platelet aggregation. Glycoprotein Ib/IX complex is the second most abundant platelet glycoprotein with an average of 20 000 surface copies per platelet. Glycoprotein Ib is a binding site for VWF. A variety of other platelet glycoproteins are present in lower numbers such as glycoprotein Ia/IIa, the receptor for collagen. Finally, platelets carry 400 to 4000 copies of an IgG Fc receptor, which is important in heparin-induced thrombocytopenia.

Thrombopoiesis

Pluripotent stem cells produce precursors of the red and white cells and the platelets. The platelet precursor is the megakaryocyte. Megakaryocytes undergo repeated nuclear replication without cytoplasmic division. This produces very large cells with 4 to 12 times the nuclear material of other cells of the body. Platelets bud off the cytoplasm of the megakaryocytes and are released into the circulation. The mean platelet volume can be measured using a cell counter and is roughly correlated with the number of nuclei in the megakaryocyte. Thrombocytopenia usually leads to proliferation of megakaryocytes and the resultant platelets are large.

The primary regulator of megakaryopoiesis and platelet production is thrombopoietin. Thrombopoietin, an erythropoietin-like hormone, is primarily produced in the liver, with secondary sites including the kidney, bone marrow, brain, smooth muscle cells, and testes. The receptor for thrombopoietin, c-Mpl, is present on stem cells, megakaryocytes, and platelets. Binding of thrombopoietin to c-Mpl activates a variety of pathways resulting in the proliferation of megakaryocyte progenitors, an increased rate of megakaryocyte maturation, an increase in megakaryocyte nuclear mass and ploidy, and increased platelet release. Thrombopoietin is constitutively secreted and the circulating level of thrombopoietin is primarily determined by the platelet mass. Platelets bind the thrombopoietin, internalize it, and degrade it. Consequently, less is available to stimulate platelet production by megakaryocytes. When the platelet count falls, less thrombopoietin is bound to platelets resulting in increased circulating levels of thrombopoietin and increased platelet production. Platelet production is also regulated, to a lessor degree, by a number of other cytokines including interleukins 6 and 11.

The role of platelets in haemostasis

Platelets play a critical role in haemostasis. When the wall of the blood vessel is damaged, platelets adhere to exposed collagen and other components of the subendothelium. The key receptor is glycoprotein Ib linked to the vessel wall through VWF. Other adhesive receptors include glycoprotein Ia/IIa, which binds collagen. Adhesion to the vessel wall asctivates platelets and agonists such as thrombin or adenosine diphosphate are released from their granules. The prostaglandin pathway is also activated; arachidonic acid is released from the platelet membrane and converted by a cascade of enzymes into platelet activating agents including thromboxane A_2. A rate-limiting step in this pathway is catalysed by the cyclooxygenase enzyme. Aspirin, an antiplatelet agent, irreversibly inactivates this enzyme. After platelet activation, glycoprotein IIb/IIIa undergoes conformational changes making it able to bind fibrinogen. This process is termed platelet aggregation and results in the formation of the haemostatic plug. Activated platelets also contribute to the clotting cascade by providing the phospholipid membrane surface needed for many reactions leading to thrombin generation, especially the activation of factor X by a complex of factors IXa and VIIIa ('tenase' complex) and the activation of prothrombin by a complex of factors Xa and Va (prothrombinase complex).

Disorders of platelet number

Thrombocytopenia

Thrombocytopenia is defined as a reduction in the number of circulating platelets to less than the laboratory's normal reference range (typically $<150 \times 10^9$/litre). Bleeding is uncommon unless the platelet count falls below 10 to 20×10^9/litre or unless there is abnormal platelet function.

Classification of thrombocytopenia

It is convenient to classify disorders of thrombocytopenia into problems of underproduction, increased destruction, and sequestration

(Table 22.6.3.1). Since megakaryocytes originate from stem cells, it is rare to see a deficit in platelet production without abnormalities also occurring in other cell lines. Although isolated underproduction of platelets can occur, isolated thrombocytopenia usually suggests increased platelet destruction or platelet sequestration. Platelet sequestration is usually due to splenomegaly and can cause isolated thrombocytopenia, but often also causes mild leucopenia or anaemia.

History and physical examination of the thrombocytopenic patient

The physician must explore the risk of the thrombocytopenia as well as determine the underlying cause. It is important to elicit the duration of the haemostatic impairment to determine if the patient has recently ingested an antiplatelet agent such as aspirin or alcohol, which interferes with platelet function and can trigger bleeding (see Chapter 22.6.2).

The history should be guided by the potential mechanism of thrombocytopenia. For example, if increased destruction is considered, then the patient should be questioned about drugs including prescription drugs, over-the-counter medications, herbal remedies, and illicit drugs. Secondary associations of thrombocytopenia, which include systemic lupus erythematosus (SLE), HIV infection, and lymphoproliferative disorders (Box 22.6.3.1), will lead to other questions. Finally, one should obtain information about any family members with a history of thrombocytopenia or bleeding disorders.

Physical evaluation focuses on evidence of haemostatic impairment and signs of an underlying cause of the thrombocytopenia. Many patients with thrombocytopenia are asymptomatic. Only at low platelet counts will one see petechiae, which are tiny, red collections of red cells found on dependent parts of the body and sites of trauma. Petechiae are relatively specific for thrombocytopenia. Large bruises or purpura can be observed on the limbs and trunk and have a lower specificity. The risk of bleeding increases progressively from asymptomatic patients, to patients with petechiae and purpura, to patients who have mucous membrane bleeding, which is typically manifest by blood blisters in the mouth. Blood blisters usually occur on the bite margins of the oral mucosa and on the tongue. They indicate that the patient is at significant risk for bleeding and treatment is urgently required. The physical examination should focus on the examination of the joints, lymph nodes, spleen, and liver since abnormalities indicate a secondary cause of the thrombocytopenia.

Laboratory evaluation of the thrombocytopenic patient

One of the most important tasks is first to review the peripheral blood film to exclude pseudothrombocytopenia. Pseudothrombocytopenia is a laboratory artefact that causes spontaneous platelet agglutination which can be identified by the presence of platelet clumps in the peripheral blood film. Automated determination of the platelet count will be inaccurate, as the machine will not recognize the larger platelet aggregates as platelets. Pseudothrombocytopenia commonly occurs because of agglutination of the patient's platelets in ethylenediaminetetra acetic acid (EDTA). This effect occurs in 0.1% of blood samples and is caused by a clinically insignificant autoantibody which agglutinates platelets at low calcium concentrations. Often the artefact can be avoided by using an anticoagulant other than EDTA in which to collect the blood sample.

The haemoglobin concentration and white blood cell count should be determined. Cytopenias involving other cell lineages

Table 22.6.3.1 Classification of thrombocytopenia by aetiology

Aetiology of thrombocytopenia	Relative frequency
Decreased platelet production	
Acquired	
Marrow infiltration: metastatic cancer, haematological malignancies (leukaemia, lymphoma, myeloma), myelofibrosis, storage disorders (Gaucher's disease etc.), granulomatous disorders (sarcoidosis)	+++
Marrow aplasia—aplastic anaemia, postchemotherapy or radiation	+++
Amegakaryocytic thrombocytopenia	++
Ineffective thrombopoiesis—myelodysplasia, secondary to toxins (alcohol), folate and vitamin B_{12} deficiency, paroxysmal nocturnal haemoglobinuria	+
Congenital	+
Wiskott–Aldrich syndrome and variants	
Bernard–Soulier syndrome	R
May–Hegglin anomaly	R
Alport syndrome and variants	R
Other	R
Increased platelet destruction	
Immune mechanisms	
Autoimmune	
ITP	+++++
Evan's syndrome	++
Secondary to other disorders—lymphoproliferative disorders, systemic lupus erythematous, HIV infection, thyroid dysfunction, hypogammaglobulinemia, antiphospholipid antibody syndrome	+++
Alloimmune	
Neonatal alloimmune thrombocytopenia	++
Post-transfusion purpura	+
Refractoriness to platelet transfusions	+++
Immune complex mediated	R
Drug-induced	++
Nonimmune mechanisms	
DIC	++
TTP	++
HUS	++
Sepsis	++++
Malignant hypertension	++
Hypertensive disorders of pregnancy	+++
Hypersplenism	+++
Abnormal vascular surfaces	++

(Continued)

Table 22.6.3.1 *(Cont'd)* Classification of thrombocytopenia by aetiology

Decreased numbers of circulating platelets (sequestration)	
Splenomegaly	++++
Extracorporeal circulation	++++
Dilutional disorders	++
Hypothermia	++

DIC, disseminated intravascular coagulation; HUS, haemolytic uraemic syndrome; TTP, thrombotic thrombocytopenic purpura.
+ to +++++ indicates the relative frequency. R indicates it is rare.

are suggestive of disorders involving the bone marrow such as myeloproliferative or myelodysplastic diseases. The platelet count helps to determine the patient's risk of bleeding. Patients with mild thrombocytopenia (platelet count $>50 \times 10^9$/litre) have a low risk of bleeding. Patients with severe thrombocytopenia (platelet count $<20 \times 10^9$/litre) have a higher risk of bleeding and can experience spontaneous bleeding. The peripheral blood film may lead to the diagnosis of the condition causing the thrombocytopenia. Fragmented red cells or schistocytes may be seen in thrombotic thrombocytopenic purpura (TTP), haemolytic uraemic syndrome (HUS), disseminated intravascular coagulation (DIC), and renal graft rejection. Leukoerythroblastic changes in the peripheral smear, such as teardrop-shaped red blood cells, nucleated red blood cells, and immature white cells suggest infiltration of the bone marrow. The presence of abnormal circulating cells such as lymphoblasts or myeloblasts suggests a malignant process. Typical changes on the peripheral smear such as megaloblastic red blood cells and hypersegmented neutrophils suggest vitamin B_{12} or folate deficiency. The finding of atypical lymphocytes should cause one to consider the diagnosis of a viral infection. Finally, the finding of giant platelets

---

Box 22.6.3.1 Secondary associations of immune thrombocytopenia

- Infections
  - HIV
  - Varicella
  - Epstein–Barr virus
- Collagen vascular disease
  - SLE
  - Rheumatoid arthritis
- Lymphoproliferative disorders
- Chronic lymphocytic leukaemia
  - Hodgkin's disease
  - Non-Hodgkin's lymphoma
- Other
  - Antiphospholipid antibody syndrome
  - Autoimmune thyroid dysfunction
  - Sarcoidosis
  - Post bone marrow transplantation

---

on the peripheral smear suggests the diagnosis of certain congenital thrombocytopenias. Examination of the bone marrow should be considered if the aetiology of the thrombocytopenia is uncertain after the initial evaluation. Additionally, a bone marrow examination is required when abnormalities are seen on the peripheral blood smear or when multiple blood cell lineages are affected. The finding of normal or increased numbers of megakaryocytes in the marrow supports the diagnosis of peripheral destruction or sequestration of the platelets. Other laboratory investigations that may be indicated include antinuclear antibody, rheumatoid factor, thyroid stimulating hormone, and testing for HIV infection.

Disorders of increased platelet destruction

Disorders of increased platelet destruction can be subdivided into two principal categories: immune and nonimmune. Nonimmune causes include DIC, and a variety of schistocytic or haemolytic anaemias such as TTP. For most thrombocytopenic disorders caused by nonimmune mechanisms, the underlying cause is apparent and the patient's clinical presentation indicates the correct diagnosis (i.e. fever and clinical septicaemia suggest infectious causes of thrombocytopenia, fragmentation haemolysis suggests TTP or HUS).

Immune-mediated platelet disorders

Immune-mediated disorders can be caused by autoantibodies, e.g. idiopathic thrombocytopenic purpura (ITP); alloantibodies, exemplified by post-transfusion purpura; and immune complexes, as demonstrated in heparin-induced thrombocytopenia. Most immune mediated platelet disorders are caused by IgG antibodies that bind to the platelet membrane.

Autoimmune thrombocytopenia

Autoimmune thrombocytopenia is mediated by antibodies that bind to individual platelet glycoproteins, most frequently glycoprotein IIb/IIIa. The autoimmune thrombocytopenia is classified as primary if there are no underlying conditions and secondary if it is associated with a systemic disease.

Primary autoimmune thrombocytopenia (ITP) Idiopathic thrombocytopenic purpura (ITP) is one of the most common autoimmune disorders. It is a disorder of both children and adults. In young children, frequently under the age of 5, the disease presents abruptly with dramatic evidence of a bleeding tendency. At least 80% of children will have a spontaneous remission of their disease. Girls and boys are affected equally. In contrast, 80% of adults who present with ITP will have a long-standing disease. The disorder is typically seen in young and middle-aged adult women. The natural history of ITP in adults in children is different; however, the risk of bleeding and general approach to therapy is similar.

Adults with ITP can present in one of three ways. Many will be asymptomatic and will have thrombocytopenia discovered incidentally. Others will give a history of easy bruising that may have occurred for many years and, frequently, worsened with ingestion of a substance which interferes with platelet function, such as aspirin or alcohol. Finally, patients may have an acute onset of petechiae, purpura, and bleeding. From mucous membranes as commonly occurs in affected children.

Treatment of adults with idiopathic thrombocytopenic purpura The most important decision is whether the patient requires any treatment. If the patient has mild or moderate thrombocytopenia (platelet count >30–50×10^9/litre) and no history of haemostatic impairment, we would monitor this patient with periodic platelet counts every few weeks. These patients usually maintain a consistent platelet count that tends to drop only if the patient has an immune stimulus such as an infection. The decision is more difficult in patients with more severe thrombocytopenia (platelet count 20–30×10^9/litre) and who have modest signs of haemostatic impairment such as occasional bruising. We often do not treat these patients, but would alert the patient that the platelets should be raised before a haemostatic challenge such as a tooth extraction or surgery. Patients with severe thrombocytopenia (platelets $<10 \times 10^9$/litre) usually require treatment, especially if they have clinical signs of haemostatic impairment. The first line of treatment is corticosteroids, typically oral prednisone (1 mg/kg). Corticosteroids are effective in two-thirds of patients, but have predictable side-effects (Cushing's syndrome, hypertension, diabetes mellitus, osteoporosis, and mental changes). Corticosteroids should be given for as short an interval as possible, tapering the dose once the platelet count has reached haemostatically safe levels ($>100 \times 10^9$/litre). Patients who have a relapse of their thrombocytopenia may require consideration of more definitive treatment such as splenectomy.

Reticuloendothelial blockade through high-dose intravenous immunoglobulins (1 g/kg delivered over 6 h on two consecutive days) or anti-D in a rhesus positive individual (75 µg/kg) usually results in a more rapid rise in the platelet count than corticosteroids and are indicated when platelets must be urgently raised. The principal disadvantage of these treatments is that they are more expensive than corticosteroids; however, they may have fewer side effects. There is a strong correlation between the response of a patient to high-dose intravenous immunoglobulins and response to a subsequent splenectomy. About 80% of patients will respond to reticuloendothelial blockade with the peak platelet count occurring within 7 days and lasting for 4 to 8 weeks.

Splenectomy Splenectomy should be considered for patients who require ongoing medical management. Patients needing splenectomy should be vaccinated 2 weeks prior to the procedure with pneumococcal, meningococcal, and *Haemophilus influenzae* type B vaccines. The platelet count should be raised to safe levels prior to the procedure. Because of its reduced morbidity and significantly shortened hospital stay, laparoscopic splenectomy is the preferred approach. Splenectomy will result in a long-term remission or cure in about two-thirds of patients.

Second-line therapies As many as one-third of patients will not respond to splenectomy and will require an alternative therapy. Danazol, an attenuated anabolic steroid, will induce a dose-dependent rise in platelet count in some refractory patients. The typical dose ranges from 200 to 1200 mg/day. Unfortunately, it has adverse effects including dose-dependent liver enzyme abnormalities and virilization. Vincristine or vinblastine have been used in refractory patients. However, if a rise in platelet count does occur, it is generally transient. Hence, the drug needs to be given repeatedly, which invariably causes dose-dependent neurotoxicity. Patients with refractory ITP who require ongoing therapy may need aggressive immunosuppression that includes oral chemotherapy such as azathioprine, intermittent high-dose intravenous immunoglobulins, or intermittent corticosteroids.

Emergency treatment of ITP Patients with ITP who have severe bleeding require aggressive therapy including platelet transfusions, high-dose intravenous immunoglobulins, and high-dose corticosteroids, in addition to standard resuscitation including blood replacement if required.

Experimental therapies of ITP Experimental therapies for ITP include romiplostim, eltrombopag, and rituximab. Eltrombopag and romiplostim are novel thrombopoietin-stimulating proteins. Clinical studies have demonstrated increased platelet counts in patients with ITP treated with these agents. Case reports and small clinical trials of rituximab, a chimeric monoclonal anti-CD20 antibody that targets B cells, have suggested a beneficial response in patients with ITP. Larger clinical trials are ongoing investigating the effectiveness of these medications.

ITP during pregnancy ITP occurs in young women and frequently these young women will become pregnant. Most of these patients can successfully carry a child without excessive morbidity or mortality. Typically, the platelet count falls across the pregnancy and the mother may require treatment. We use high-dose intravenous immunoglobulins since corticosteroids may be associated with an increased risk of hypertensive disorders in pregnancy. About 10% of the infants born to these mothers will be thrombocytopenic, with the platelet nadir occurring several days after delivery. Very severe thrombocytopenia is uncommon (*c.*1%) and should suggest an alternative diagnosis such as alloimmune neonatal thrombocytopenia. Infant thrombocytopenia cannot be predicted by any maternal factor or serological test with the possible exception of a history of a previously affected infant. We manage these mothers with routine vaginal delivery unless there is an obstetrical indication for caesarean section.

Secondary immune thrombocytopenias A variety of medical disorders cause secondary immune thrombocytopenia (Box 22.6.3.1). The treatment for secondary immune thrombocytopenia is similar to that of ITP.

Thrombocytopenia complicating SLE Thrombocytopenia can occur in up to 25% of patients with SLE. The thrombocytopenia is usually caused by autoantibodies. Some patients will have concomitant platelet dysfunction characterized by increased bleeding and bruising. The treatment is similar to that for ITP.

A subset of patients with SLE or lupus-like disorders have antibodies which interfere with phospholipid-dependent coagulation reactions, commonly detected by an unexplained prolongation of the patient's partial thromboplastin time. These antibodies are immunoglobulins with specificity for negatively charged phospholipids and are also called lupus anticoagulant antibodies. They tend to be heterogenous in their epitope specificity with most binding phospholipid protein complexes including β_2-glycoprotein I. Another class of antibodies, the anticardiolipin antibodies, is detected by an enzyme-linked immunosorbent assay using cardiolipin as the antigen. Cardiolipin is the same antigen that is detected in the VDRL test for syphilis, which explains the false-positive VDRL test in these patients. The two classes of antibodies are distinct, but have overlapping specificities. Most anticardiolipin antibodies recognize an epitope on β_2-glycoprotein I. The term 'antiphospholipid antibodies' applies to both sets of antibodies.

Antiphospholipid antibodies are associated with venous and arterial thrombosis. The antiphospholipid antibody syndrome includes any combination of arterial and venous thrombosis, recurrent fetal losses and thrombocytopenia plus a repeatedly positive test for these antibodies. Some of these patients also have a vascular rash termed livedo reticularis. Patients can have haematological abnormalities including mild thrombocytopenia, platelet dysfunction, autoimmune haemolytic anaemia, and leucopenia. As the thrombocytopenia is usually mild, treatment is rarely necessary. The thrombotic complications dominate this syndrome. Many patients require long-term anticoagulation therapy to prevent recurrent thrombotic events.

Thrombocytopenia secondary to lymphoproliferative disorders
Immune thrombocytopenia commonly complicates chronic lymphocytic leukaemia. This should be differentiated from thrombocytopenia of underproduction, which is seen in the late stage of chronic lymphocytic leukaemia. Immune thrombocytopenia is often seen in patients with Hodgkin's disease and can predate or postdate the illness and is not a marker of disease activity.

Alloimmune thrombocytopenia

Alloimmune thrombocytopenia is caused by alloantibodies against platelet glycoproteins. There are two typical alloimmune thrombocytopenic disorders, alloimmune neonatal thrombocytopenia, and post-transfusional purpura.

Alloimmune neonatal thrombocytopenia Alloimmune neonatal thrombocytopenia is mediated by alloantibodies in maternal plasma directed against fetal platelet glycoproteins inherited from the father. This disorder can cause severe and life-threatening fetal thrombocytopenia that can occur *in utero*. The most common alloantibody responsible for this disorder is targeted against a platelet glycoprotein called PLA1 (HPA-1a) located on platelet glycoprotein IIIa.

Post-transfusion purpura In cases of post-transfusion purpura the patient, usually a woman, develops severe thrombocytopenia 5 to 12 days after receiving a transfusion of a blood product containing platelets. The thrombocytopenia is often very severe (platelet count $<10 \times 10^9$/litre). Post-transfusion purpura occurs when a patient produces an alloantibody to a specific platelet antigen that she lacks, usually PLA1. The syndrome most commonly occurs in multiparous women because previous pregnancies lead to their sensitization. Patients, including men, who have previously been transfused are also at risk.

The diagnosis of post-transfusion purpura is made by the identification of a platelet-specific antibody in a patient with acute onset of thrombocytopenia 5 to 12 days after receiving a transfusion of a blood product. Although post-transfusion purpura is most commonly seen after transfusion of packed red blood cells, all blood products, including plasma, can cause the reaction. Post-transfusion purpura is self-limited with recovery occurring within 1 to 3 weeks. However, because the condition can be lethal, treatment with plasmapheresis or intravenous immunoglobulins should be considered. Platelet transfusions should be avoided except in cases of life-threatening haemorrhage. For uncertain reasons, the frequency of post-transfusion purpura is declining.

Drug-induced thrombocytopenia

Many drugs can cause thrombocytopenia. These medications most commonly implicated include heparin, quinidine, sulfonamides, valproic acid, and gold. However, virtually every medication has been associated with thrombocytopenia.

Patients with drug-induced thrombocytopenia typically have moderate to severe thrombocytopenia. Thrombocytopenia is usually seen 1 to 2 weeks after beginning a medication, but it may occur in patients who have been taking the medication for several years. The platelet destruction is usually IgG-mediated. The thrombocytopenia usually resolves within days of stopping the causative drug. In cases of severe thrombocytopenia, the drug should be discontinued and the patient treated with reticuloendothelial blockade using either intravenous immunoglobulins or intravenous anti-D immune globulin. Treatment with corticosteroids is less effective. In cases of life-threatening haemorrhage, platelet transfusions may be required. Patients should not take the drug causing the thrombocytopenia again as it will cause thrombocytopenia with subsequent exposure.

Heparin-induced thrombocytopenia Heparin-induced thrombocytopenia develops between 5 and 12 days after the initiation of heparin therapy but if the patient has been exposed to heparin within the last 3 months, it can occur earlier. Patients develop moderate thrombocytopenia (platelet counts $40–80 \times 10^9$/litre). Patients with heparin-induced thrombocytopenia frequently develop thrombotic complications, especially deep venous thrombosis and pulmonary embolism. Other clinical associations include arterial thrombosis, skin lesions, and uncommon thrombotic events such as adrenal gland thrombosis and haemorrhage.

Heparin-induced thrombocytopenia is caused by an IgG antibody, which recognizes a complex of heparin and platelet factor 4 (PF4). The PF4–heparin–IgG immune complexes bind to platelet crystallizable fragment receptors, causing platelet activation and microparticle formation resulting in activation of coagulation.

The risk of thrombocytopenia is to be related to the type, dose, and duration of heparin administration. For example, unfractionated heparin is more immunogenic than low-molecular-weight heparin. Also, different patient populations have different risks of forming the heparin-induced thrombocytopenia IgG. For example, the risk of heparin-induced thrombocytopenia IgG is higher in orthopaedic patients than in medical patients.

The diagnosis of heparin-induced thrombocytopenia should be considered in all patients receiving heparin therapy who develop thrombocytopenia or thrombotic complications. Serological tests can be used to confirm the diagnosis of heparin-induced thrombocytopenia. Enzyme assays measure the binding of platelet antibodies to a complex of heparin and PF4. The gold standard tests are biological assays, such as the serotonin release assay.

Treatment of heparin-induced thrombocytopenia involves discontinuation of heparin. The patient should be treated with an agent that inhibits thrombin generation, such as hirudin or argatroban. Warfarin should not be used to treat acute heparin-induced thrombocytopenia because it can induce limb gangrene.

Gold-induced thrombocytopenia Gold-induced thrombocytopenia occurs in as many as 3% of patients who receive therapeutic preparations of gold salts. There appears to be a genetic predisposition to the syndrome, with HLA DR3 occurring in up to 80% of affected patients. The thrombocytopenia usually occurs within the first several months of therapy and can range from mild to severe. Treatment involves stopping the gold agent drug and supportive treatment. The thrombocytopenia can persist for many months after the discontinuation of gold. This is probably due to gold-independent autoantibodies, but may be due to the prolonged release of gold from tissue stores. Rapid correction of the thrombocytopenia may be achieved with intravenous immunoglobulins; however, a relapse of the thrombocytopenia may occur in 2 to 4 weeks.

Patients also respond to corticosteroids. Some patients with persistent thrombocytopenia may respond to splenectomy. There is less experience using a gold-chelating agent such as dimercaprol (BAL).

Nonimmune platelet disorders
Destructive thrombocytopenia and schistocytic haemolysis
Certain disorders are associated with both thrombocytopenia and schistocytic or fragmentation haemolysis. These disorders include TTP, HUS, and DIC.

TTP This is a syndrome consisting of thrombocytopenia, microangiopathic haemolytic anaemia, renal impairment, fever, and ischaemic neurological findings. TTP is an uncommon disorder, but its recognition is important because it is usually fatal if not treated.

Most cases of TTP are likely related to a deficiency of ADAMTS13 (a disintegrin and metalloprotease with thrombospondin-1-like domains) that cleaves the large VWF multimers released by endothelial cells. This deficiency may be due to reduced blood levels or due to the presence of circulating inhibitory antibodies. Patients with the familial form of TTP–HUS have decreased ADAMTS13 activity caused by genetic abnormalities. The patients also have been found to have unusually large VWF multimers which have a greater ability to react with platelets.

Most patients who develop TTP are young to middle-aged, with slightly more women affected than men. The presentation of illness may be insidious or acute. Typically, the patient has a several day history of generalized malaise, fatigue, or focal ischaemic problems. The focal ischaemic events usually involve the central nervous system and can include sudden weakness, paraesthesiae, and confusion. Approximately 50% of patients will have a neurological event.

Most adult patients with TTP do not have an associated underlying condition. Nonetheless, the initial evaluation of a patient with TTP should exclude diseases associated with TTP (Box 22.6.3.2). TTP can develop spontaneously, but is often triggered by an infection, pregnancy, or an immune challenge.

All patients with TTP have destructive thrombocytopenia. The thrombocytopenia is the best indicator of disease activity. Additional laboratory investigations demonstrate abnormalities of microangiopathic haemolytic anaemia, such as anaemia, fragmented red blood cells, and increased reticulocyte count. Serum lactate dehydrogenase and bilirubin levels are elevated. Other abnormalities include elevated serum creatinine, proteinuria, and abnormal liver function tests. Investigators have identified the presence of abnormal VWF multimers in patients with TTP.

TTP is treated with plasmapheresis. This treatment has reduced the mortality from 80% to 20%. Plasma exchange of at least one to two volumes of plasma should be performed daily. Plasma should be replaced with cryosupernatant plasma or fresh frozen plasma. Some physicians believe that cryosupernatant plasma is more beneficial because it is depleted of VWF. Plasmapheresis should be continued until the platelet count and serum lactate dehydrogenase have normalized. This generally occurs after 3 to 10 exchanges. Plasma exchange is better than plasma infusion alone. However, when plasmapheresis is not immediately available, patients should be treated initially with plasma infusion. If the initial response to plasma exchange is poor, other therapies such as glucocorticoids may be added. Additionally, the volume of plasma exchange may

---

Box 22.6.3.2 Classification of TTP

- Primary (no associated disease)
- Primary but triggered by a disorder or condition
  - Vaccination
  - Viral infection
- Secondary
  - Pregnancy
  - ITP
  - HIV infection
  - Collagen vascular disease
  - Carcinoma (typically adenocarcinoma)
  - Drug associated:
    - Allergic—quinidine, ticlopidine
    - Dose-related toxicity—mitomycin C, ciclosporin, pentostatin, gemcitabine
  - Bone marrow transplantation (allogeneic)

---

be increased. Studies involving agents such as rituximab are ongoing and appear promising. Other treatments, such as antiplatelet agents, are of uncertain benefit. With discontinuation of plasma exchange, exacerbation of disease occurs in about a third of patients. This risk of relapse can be reduced by splenectomy.

HUS This syndrome includes renal failure, microangiopathic haemolytic anaemia, and thrombocytopenia. Different types of HUS have been identified, including classic epidemic, sporadic, hereditary and sporadic in association with noninfectious conditions. Epidemic HUS is seen primarily in children and occurs in association with a diarrhoeal illness caused by enterohaemorrhagic or verotoxigenic *Escherichia coli* serotype O157:H7 or *Shigella dysenteriae* serotype I. HUS may be also associated with other bacterial, viral, and rickettsial infections. Patients have been reported to develop HUS after receiving immunizations.

Laboratory investigations demonstrate severe anaemia and thrombocytopenia. Examination of the peripheral smear shows fragmented red blood cells, burr cells, and spherocytes. Haemoglobinaemia and haemoglobinuria may be severe. Serum lactate dehydrogenase levels and other markers of red blood cell destruction are elevated. The serum creatinine is usually increased.

In children, the treatment of HUS focuses on providing supportive care with careful attention paid to fluid status and electrolyte levels. Plasma exchange should be considered in children with severe HUS. In adults, treatment of HUS generally includes plasmapheresis. Other therapies including antiplatelet agents, fibrinolytic therapy, and heparin therapy have not been shown to be beneficial, and are not recommended.

DIC DIC is a disorder in which clotting occurs within the circulation. It is characterized by large amounts of thrombin that overwhelm the physiological inhibitors of coagulation. The thrombin causes platelet aggregation resulting in thrombocytopenia and fibrinogen cleavage into fibrin, which forms the microthrombi.

The most common cause of DIC is sepsis, but DIC is associated with a large number of disorders including trauma and obstetric conditions (Box 22.6.3.3). The clinical presentation is variable, but patients with DIC are usually very unwell presenting with fulminant bleeding and organ dysfunction. Some patients have thrombotic events. Occasionally, DIC can be subclinical and detected only with laboratory tests. The diagnosis of DIC is supported by the laboratory finding of thrombocytopenia in association with fragmented red blood cells, decreased fibrinogen level, and elevated fibrinogen and fibrin degradation products such as D-dimers. Coagulation studies often show a prolonged international normalized ratio, partial thromboplastin time, and thrombin time. DIC is best managed by identifying and treating its cause. If the patient is bleeding, replacement therapy with fresh frozen plasma, cryoprecipitate, and platelets should be considered. Heparin therapy may be of benefit in patients with clinical evidence of ongoing microvascular thrombosis.

Sepsis and infection

Transient thrombocytopenia occurs with systemic infections. Thrombocytopenia occurs in 50 to 75% of patients with bacteraemia

---

Box 22.6.3.3 Causes of DIC

- Infections
  - Bacterial (Gram-negative bacilli, staphylococci, streptococci, pneumococci, meningococci, others)
  - Viral (herpes, rubella, varicella, hepatitis, variola, arboviruses, others)
  - Parasitic (malaria, kala-azar, others)
  - Rickettsial (Rocky Mountain spotted fever, others)
  - Fungal (histoplasmosis, aspergillosis, others)
- Neoplasms
  - Adenocarcinomas (prostate, breast, pancreas, lung, ovary, others)
  - Metastatic carcinoid, rhabdomyosarcoma, neuroblastoma, others
- Obstetric complications
  - placental abruption, retained dead fetus, second-trimester abortion, amniotic fluid embolism, others
- Haematological disorders
  - Acute promyelocytic leukaemia, intravascular haemolysis, histiocytic medullary reticulosis
- Vascular disorders
  - Kasabach–Merritt syndrome (giant haemangioma), aortic aneurysm
- Tissue injury
  - Crush injuries, burns, hypothermia, head injury
- Miscellaneous
  - Fat embolism, acute glomerulonephritis, snake bite, extracorporeal circulation, allograft rejection, anaphylaxis, graft versus host disease, many others

---

or fungal infections. It also occurs in association with viral infections, including HIV. The thrombocytopenia is generally mild to moderate and is not usually associated with symptoms of bleeding. The mechanism leading to the lowered platelet count is multifactorial including activation of platelets by bacterial products or mediators of inflammation; destruction due to immune mechanisms; or destruction due to chemokine-induced macrophage ingestion of platelets. Additionally, severe viral infections may lead to suppression of platelet production. Resolution of the platelet count occurs with eradication of the infection.

Thrombocytopenia associated with HIV is common, occurring in at least 20% of patients with symptomatic disease. Various mechanisms contribute to the thrombocytopenia. Some patients have immune-mediated destruction of platelets. Patients also have a defect in platelet production due to direct infection of megakaryocytes and the suppressive effects of medications. The platelet count can improve with antiretroviral therapy. Patients with severe thrombocytopenia should be treated similarly to patients with ITP including the performance of a splenectomy.

Haemophagocytic syndrome

This rare syndrome is caused by phagocytosis of haematological cells by macrophages. Adult patients can present with an acute illness consisting of fever, weight loss, hepatosplenomegaly, pancytopenia, and increased liver enzymes. Bone marrow aspiration is diagnostic and shows morphological evidence of phagocytosis of platelets, red blood cells, and granulocytes by macrophages. The haemophagocytic syndrome may be associated with infections, particularly with the Epstein–Barr virus, T-cell lymphoma, histiocytosis, or immune disorders such as SLE and Still's disease. Treatment is directed at the underlying disorder.

Decreased platelet production

Platelet production is impaired by conditions affecting megakaryocyte progenitor cells, megakaryocytes, or the bone marrow stroma. It is rare to see a deficit in platelet production without abnormalities in the production of other cell lines as well. Decreased platelet production can occur when the bone marrow is aplastic, dysplastic, or infiltrated with other cells. Diagnosis of a defect in platelet production is usually made by evaluation of the bone marrow. Disorders causing decreased platelet production may be classified as congenital or acquired.

Congenital disorders causing decreased platelet production

Thrombocytopenia in infancy is usually due to increased platelet destruction and is only rarely due to decreased production. However, various congenital disorders may result in decreased platelet production. These disorders include congenital amegakaryocytic thrombocytopenia, thrombocytopenia with absent radii syndrome, Wiskott–Aldrich syndrome, May–Hegglin anomaly, Epstein's syndrome, Fechtner's syndrome, and Sebastian platelet syndrome. Bernard–Soulier syndrome is also associated with moderate thrombocytopenia.

Acquired disorders causing decreased platelet production

Toxins Numerous drugs and toxins may cause bone marrow suppression and subsequent thrombocytopenia. Chemotherapy and irradiation cause direct destruction of megakaryocytes and other cells of the marrow. Other medications causing marrow aplasia are numerous and include chloramphenicol, nonsteroidal anti-inflammatory drugs, antiepileptic medications, and gold.

Alcohol thrombocytopenia This is the most common haematological abnormality associated with alcohol abuse. The thrombocytopenia can be due to hypersplenism (described subsequently) or alcohol suppression of the marrow. Alcohol-induced marrow suppression can cause very severe thrombocytopenia requiring treatment by platelet transfusions. Elimination of alcohol intake will induce an increase of the platelet count within days to weeks. Associated haematological abnormalities include megaloblastic anaemia and ringed sideroblasts.

Nutritional deficiencies Thrombocytopenia may occur with folate or vitamin B_{12} deficiency. The degree of thrombocytopenia is variable and may be severe. Associated haematological abnormalities include megaloblastic anaemia and hypersegmented neutrophils. Replacement of the deficient vitamin will result in recovery of the platelet count. Iron deficiency has also been associated with thrombocytopenia, although more frequently with thrombocytosis. Replacement of iron generally corrects the platelet count.

Infiltration of the bone marrow The bone marrow may become infiltrated with nonhaematopoietic or nonstromal cells. Conditions that may lead to marrow infiltration include metastatic cancer, haematological malignancies (leukaemia, lymphoma, myeloma), myelofibrosis, storage disorders, and granulomatous disorders (sarcoidosis, tuberculosis).

Acquired amegakaryocytic thrombocytopenic purpura Bone marrow aplasia is characterized by hypocellularity of the marrow. Aplasia involving more than one lineage of haematopoietic cells is called aplastic anaemia. When isolated decreased platelet production occurs, it is called amegakaryocytic thrombocytopenic purpura. This rare condition frequently progresses to aplastic anaemia. Bone marrow examination reveals absent or severely decreased numbers of megakaryocytes. The disorder may be secondary to various aetiologies including drugs, toxins, and infections, but most frequently it is idiopathic. Treatment varies with the suspected aetiology and typically is supportive, but can include intravenous IgG, corticosteroids, and immunosuppressive therapies.

Myelodysplastic syndromes Myelodysplastic syndrome can present with isolated thrombocytopenia. Examination of the bone marrow usually demonstrates abnormal megakaryocyte morphology and cytogenetic analysis reveals chromosomal abnormalities.

Disorders of platelet distribution and platelet sequestration
Splenomegaly and hypersplenism
Decreased numbers of circulating platelets may be seen in patients with splenomegaly. Normally, one-third of the circulating platelets are pooled in the spleen. With splenomegaly the size of the pool of platelets sequestered in the spleen increases, decreasing the number of circulating platelets. Increased destruction of the platelets may also occur. The thrombocytopenia is usually moderate (platelets $>40 \times 10^9$/litre). Bone marrow examination reveals normal numbers of megakaryocytes. Other laboratory abnormalities include leucocytosis with a normal differential and mild anaemia. Splenomegaly may be demonstrated by ultrasound or a liver–spleen scan. The diagnosis of hypersplenism can be confirmed by performing an autologous platelet survival test. This test will show a reduced recovery of transfused platelets (usually <30%) with a normal platelet survival. The thrombocytopenia is rarely severe enough to require treatment; however, splenectomy is curative.

Haemodilutional disorders
A low number of circulating platelets may also be seen in patients who have received large volumes of crystalloid solutions or blood products. This type of thrombocytopenia is commonly seen immediately after surgery and is generally transient. If treatment is required, the patient should receive platelet transfusions.

Extracorporeal circulation
Patients undergoing cardiopulmonary bypass commonly develop mild thrombocytopenia. The cause of the decreased platelet count is multifactorial; adherence of platelets to synthetic surfaces causes activation and damage to the platelets, haemodilution, and blood loss. The thrombocytopenia is usually mild. Generally, the platelet count recovers within 3 to 4 days to levels greater than the count preoperatively.

Hypothermia
Hypothermia is associated with transient thrombocytopenia. Decreased body temperature results in pooling of platelets in the peripheral circulation. Hypothermia may be seen in cases of environmental exposure, after prolonged surgery, and after transfusions of massive amounts of inadequately warmed blood products.

Thrombocytosis
Thrombocytosis is defined as a platelet count greater than 600×10^9/litre. An elevated platelet count may be primary (essential) or secondary to other disorders.

Thrombocythaemia
Primary thrombocytosis also known as thrombocythaemia is a chronic myeloproliferative disorder. Other chronic myeloproliferative disorders such as polycythaemia vera, myeloid metaplasia, and chronic myelogenous leukaemia can also cause an increase in platelet count.

Incidence and epidemiology
The incidence of thrombocythaemia is approximately two per 100 000 population per year. The average age at diagnosis is 60 to 80 years with men and women equally affected. Young women in their thirties may present with thrombocythaemia.

Aetiology and pathogenesis
Thrombocythaemia is probably a clonal process originating at the stem cell level leading to sustained proliferation of megakaryocytes with increased numbers of circulating platelets. A mutation in the JAK2 tyrosine kinase (JAK2V617F) is present in approximately 50% of patients with essential thrombocytosis. This mutation results in a constitutively active tyrosine kinase that is able to activate tyrosine kinase signalling when expressed with receptors including the erythropoietin receptor, the thrombopoietin receptor and the granulocyte colony-stimulating receptor. Thrombopoietin may also play a role in the pathogenesis of the disorder. Studies have shown reduction of c-Mpl protein and messenger RNA expression. This may reflect an intrinsic defect of c-Mpl transcription or decreased receptor expression that results in ineffective clearance of thrombopoietin.

Clinical findings
Two-thirds of patients have symptoms at the time of diagnosis, usually thrombosis or bleeding; however, thrombocythemia can occur in patients, typically young women, who are otherwise well. Thrombotic events are common, occurring in 20 to 30% of

patients, particularly older people. The thrombosis involves the microvasculature and patients present with headache, transient ischaemic attacks or strokes, paraesthesiae of extremities, distal extremity gangrene, and erythromelagia (burning pain and redness of the toes or fingertips). Patients with essential thrombocythaemia have an increased risk of angina pectoris and myocardial infarction. Patients at greatest risk for thrombotic events are older and have a history of thrombosis. Major bleeding complications are rare, but bruising is common.

Laboratory findings

Patients have an unexplained elevation of their platelet count, typically above 800×10^9/litre. Examination of the peripheral smear can reveal megathrombocytes and leucocytosis with immature myeloid precursor cells. Mild eosinophilia and basophilia can occur. Bone marrow evaluation shows increased cellularity, marked megakaryocytic hyperplasia, and clustering of megakaryocytes. In addition the megakaryocytes often are morphologically bizarre with nuclear pleomorphism. Bone marrow karyotypes are usually normal. The Polycythaemia Vera Study Group has suggested criteria for the diagnosis of essential thrombocythaemia (Box 22.6.3.4). The JAK2V617F mutation is found in approximately 50% of patients.

Management

Untreated, asymptomatic patients with thrombocythaemia can have a near normal life expectancy. Furthermore, the thrombotic risk in asymptomatic patients younger than 60 years of age with no history of thrombosis is not increased. Young, asymptomatic patients therefore do not require treatment, although aspirin may be given. Possible indications for treatment to lower platelet count include patients with a history of thrombotic events, patients with cardiovascular risk factors, elderly patients, and patients in whom platelet counts remain very high ($>1000 \times 10^9$/litre).

Low-dose aspirin can be used to prevent thrombosis and it may relieve symptoms such as headache and erythromelagia. However, aspirin may unmask bleeding tendencies so it should be avoided in patients with a history of bleeding. Hydroxyurea will lower the platelet count and usually reduces thrombohaemorrhagic complications. Adverse affects include myelosuppression and possibly an increased risk of leukaemic transformation. Anagrelide can effectively lower the platelet count, but its efficacy at reducing complications has not been established. A randomized clinical trial comparing hydroxyurea plus low-dose aspirin with anagrelide plus low-dose aspirin found that both regimens gave equivalent long-term control of the platelet count; however, anagrelide was associated with an increased risk of arterial thrombosis, serious haemorrhage and transformation to myelofibrosis. Interferon-α may also be used to lower platelet counts. Unfortunately, side effects including influenza-like symptoms, anorexia, and neuropsychiatric symptoms are severe enough to cause discontinuation of therapy in up to 25% of patients. Therefore, the standard of therapy for patients with essential thrombocytosis who are at high risk for thrombosis is generally considered to be hydroxyurea and low-dose aspirin.

Prognosis

The life expectancy of many patients with thrombocythaemia is near normal. However, there is a high rate of thrombotic events and 3 to 4% of patients develop leukaemia. This occurs predominantly in patients who have been treated with alkylating agents.

Box 22.6.3.4 Criteria for diagnosis of essential thrombocytosis

All of the following:

- Platelet count $>600 \times 10^9$/litre on two different occasions, separated by a 1-month interval
- Absence of identifiable cause of thrombocytosis, such as infections, inflammatory disorders, or nonhaematological malignant disorders
- Normal red cell mass (males <36 ml/kg; females < 32 ml/kg)
- Absence of significant fibrosis of the marrow
- Absence of the Philadelphia chromosome and the fusion *BCR/ABL* gene

Plus three of the following:

- Splenomegaly
- Bone marrow hypercellularity seen on biopsy (megakaryocytic hyperplasia present with aggregates of megakaryocytes)
- Absence of iron deficiency, as documented by the presence of stainable marrow iron and/or normal serum ferritin
- Females: demonstration of clonal haematopoiesis using restriction fragment length polymorphism analysis of genes present on the X chromosome
- Presence of abnormal bone marrow haematopoietic progenitor cells, as determined by the formation of endogenous erythroid and/or megakaryocytic colonies
- Abnormal platelet aggregation studies in response to epinephrine and adenosine diphosphate when the patient is not taking any drug that might impair platelet function

From: Murphy S *et al.* (1997). Experience of the Polycythemia Vera Study Group with essential thrombocythemia: a final report on diagnostic criteria, survival, and leukemic transition by treatment. *Semin Hematol*, **34**, 29–39.

Secondary thrombocytosis

Essential thrombocythaemia must be differentiated from reactive or secondary thrombocytosis. Causes of secondary thrombocytosis include infections, malignancy, chronic inflammatory bowel disease, rheumatoid arthritis, iron deficiency, and hyposplenism. Reactive thrombocytosis is not associated with symptoms related to the elevated platelet count; it is usually not harmful and does not require treatment, although the underlying cause should be determined.

Disorders of platelet function

Congenital disorders of platelet function

Patients with congenital disorders of platelet function often present with a history of easy bruising, epistaxis, menorrhagia, and prolonged bleeding after surgery or dental procedures. Some of these patients may have family members with similar problems. The various platelet abnormalities may be classified functionally into disorders of platelet adhesion, aggregation, secretion, and procoagulant activity.

Disorders of platelet adhesion and aggregation

Platelet function disorders include Bernard–Soulier syndrome which is caused by a deficiency or abnormality of platelet glycoprotein Ib/IX, and Glanzmann's thrombasthenia, caused by a deficiency of glycoprotein IIb/IIIa. Both are inherited in an autosomal recessive fashion and are very rare. The most common cause of abnormal platelet aggregation is likely a heterogeneous group of disorders characterized by abnormal platelet release of granule contents generally due to various disorders of signal transduction and internal metabolic pathways.

Disorders of platelet secretion

Disorders of platelet secretion occur when there are abnormalities of the platelet secretory pathways or if there is a deficiency of platelet granules. Grey platelet syndrome occurs when the α-granules are decreased or absent. Dense granule deficiency or platelet storage pool deficiency is due to a deficiency of dense granules. In alpha delta storage pool deficiency, both the α and dense granules are deficient.

Disorders of platelet procoagulant activity

Platelets play an important role in haemostasis by providing a phospholipid membrane on which various coagulation reactions occur. In disorders such as Scott syndrome, abnormalities of the platelet membrane impair its procoagulant activity.

Treatment

There are no definitive therapies for any of the congenital disorders of platelet function. Administration of deamino-D-arginine vasopressin (DDAVP) induces the release of VWF from endothelial cells and may improve bleeding time and haemostasis. An effect is seen within 1 to 2 h and lasts for up to 12 h. Antifibrinolytic agents, such as aminocaproic acid, may improve haemostasis. Menorrhagia may be controlled by oral contraceptive medications and perhaps by antifibrinolytic medications. In cases of life-threatening bleeding, platelet transfusions may be necessary. However, platelet transfusions can cause immunization against the platelet receptors and should be avoided.

Acquired disorders of platelet function

The most common acquired causes of platelet dysfunction are medications and toxins, systemic disorders, and haematological diseases.

Drugs

There are numerous drugs that have been shown to affect platelet function (Box 22.6.3.5). Aspirin has been demonstrated to cause a significant increase in bleeding. Aspirin acts by irreversibly inhibiting platelet cyclooxygenase resulting in decreased formation of thromboxane A_2, an agonist for platelet aggregation. Nonsteroidal anti-inflammatory agents also affect platelet function by reversibly inhibiting cyclooxygenase. Ticlopidine and clopidrogel inhibit platelet function by inhibiting the action of platelet ADP. Glycoprotein IIb/IIIa inhibitors block platelet aggregation by directly inhibiting the platelet receptor for fibrinogen, glycoprotein IIb/IIIa. β-lactam antibiotics may bind to and modify the platelet membrane resulting in abnormal platelet aggregation with ADP, adrenaline (epinephrine), and collagen. Nitrates inhibit platelet aggregation. Calcium channel blockers and β-blockers affect platelet aggregation by unknown mechanisms. Other drugs that may

---

Box 22.6.3.5 Medications affecting platelet function

- Aspirin
- Anaesthetics
  - Halothane, local anaesthetics
- Antibiotics

β-lactam antibiotics (penicillins, cephalosporins), nitrofurantoin

- Antidepressant medications
  - Serotonin reuptake inhibitors, Tricyclic antidepressants
- Antiepileptic medications
- Psychotropic drugs
- Antihistamines
- Cardiovascular medications
  - β-Blockers, calcium channel blockers, nitrates
- Chemotherapeutic drugs
  - Mithramycin, daunorubicin, BCNU (carmustine)
- Clofibrate
- Dipyridamole
- Glycoprotein IIb/IIIa inhibitors
- Nonsteroidal anti-inflammatory medications
  - Phenthiazines
- Plasma expanders
  - Dextrans, pentastarch
- Ticlopidine and clopidogrel

---

adversely affect platelet function include antiepileptic medications, tricyclic antidepressants, and phenothiazines.

Chronic renal failure

Patients with chronic renal failure or uraemia have platelet dysfunction including defects in adhesion, aggregation, secretion, and procoagulant activity. The bleeding time may be prolonged. The pathogenesis of the platelet dysfunction is unknown, but is probably secondary to toxins present in the uraemic plasma. Treatment of a bleeding uraemic patient includes prompt dialysis. DDAVP may improve haemostasis. Maintenance of a normal haematocrit may also decrease the bleeding tendency.

Cardiopulmonary bypass surgery

Excessive bleeding occurs in approximately 5 to 20% of patients undergoing cardiopulmonary bypass surgery. Studies have demonstrated decreased platelet aggregation, altered platelet surface membrane proteins, selective depletion of platelet α-granules, and evidence of *in vivo* platelet activation. An extrinsic platelet defect may occur resulting from thrombin inhibition by high doses of heparin. The aetiology of these abnormalities could be related to the hypothermia of the procedure and damage to the platelets as they pass through the pump system. The haemostatic abnormalities usually improve within hours after surgery.

Chronic myeloproliferative disorders and myelodysplastic syndromes

Disorders such as chronic myelogenous leukaemia, essential thrombocythaemia, polycythaemia vera, and myeloid metaplasia may be associated with abnormalities of platelet number and function. Abnormalities of platelet function include impaired aggregation with epinephrine, abnormal arachidonic acid metabolism, and storage pool defects. The bleeding tendency responds to treatment of the underlying disorder and correction of the associated thrombocytosis.

Dysproteinaemias

Patients with a paraproteinaemia, such as multiple myeloma or Waldenström's macroglobulinaemia, can have abnormalities in both platelet number and function. Nonspecific binding of the paraproteins to the platelet membrane may interfere with membrane surface receptors. Treatment of the disorder causing the paraproteinaemia will usually correct the bleeding problem. Plasma exchange may be necessary in the acute phase of this condition.

Further reading

Arnold DM, *et al*. (2007). Systematic review: efficacy and safety of rituximab for adults with idiopathic thrombocytopenic purpura. *Ann Intern Med*, **146**, 25–33.

Arnold DM *et al*. (2010). Combination immunosuppressant therapy for patients with chronic refractory immune thrombocytopenic purpura. *Blood*, **115**, 29–31.

George JN (2006). Management of patients with refractory immune thrombocytopenic purpura. *J Thromb Haemost*, **4**, 1664–72.

George JN (2006). Thrombotic thrombocytopenic purpura. *N Engl J Med*, **354**, 1927–35.

Gill KK, Kelton JG (2000). Management of idiopathic thrombocytopenic purpura in pregnancy. *Semin Hematol*, **37**, 275–89.

Lankford KV, Hillyer CD (2000). Thrombotic thrombocytopenic purpura: new insights in disease pathogenesis and therapy. *Transfus Med Rev*, **14**, 244–57.

Li X, *et al*. (2007). Drug-induced thrombocytopenia: an updated systematic review. *Drug Safety*, **30**, 185–6.

Nurden AT (1999). Inherited abnormalities of platelets. *Thromb Haemost*, **82**, 468–80.

Provan D. (2010). International consensus report on the investigation and management of primary immune thrombocytopenia. *Blood*, **115**,168–185.

Warkentin TE (2007). Drug-induced immune-mediated thrombocytopenia—from purpura to thrombosis. *N Engl J Med*, **356**, 891–3.

22.6.4 Genetic disorders of coagulation

Eleanor S. Pollak and Katherine A. High

Essentials

Much of what is understood about specific coagulation proteins has emerged from the careful study of hereditary disorders of blood coagulation.

Haemophilia

Haemophilia is a familial X-linked disorder due to deficiency of either factor VIII (haemophilia A) or factor IX (haemophilia B), which are components of the intrinsic enzymatic complex that activates factor X. The severity of the disease correlates with predicted concentrations of active protein, and those with activity levels below 1% are defined as having severe disease.

Clinical features and diagnosis—the main manifestations are bleeding into joints and soft tissues, with haemophilic arthropathy and joint deformity being inevitable complications in untreated patients. Other features include pseudotumours, bleeding into the urinary system, and bleeding following clinical procedures (e.g. dental extractions). Laboratory diagnosis is based on a modification of the classic activated partial thromboplastin time (aPTT) assay, with inhibitor screening used to exclude other causes of prolonged aPTT (e.g. lupus anticoagulant).

Treatment—this involves the administration of the deficient factor VIII or factor IX, most commonly 'on demand' in response to bleeding, with prophylactic treatment given before surgery. The use of recombinant factors is preferable to preparations derived from pooled human plasma samples, which have led to numerous infectious complications (hepatitis B and C, HIV). The development of inhibitory antibodies is a significant problem, particularly in patients with haemophilia A. Trials of gene therapy are being performed.

von Willebrand's disease

von Willebrand's disease is a common autosomal (dominant or recessive) disorder of platelet function caused by a functional deficiency of von Willebrand factor (VWF), which is normally synthesized by megakaryocytes, preventing degradation of factor VIII, and also by endothelial cells, enhancing platelet activation and recruitment at sites of tissue damage. It may be due to quantitative deficiency of VWF (types 1 and 3), or to defects of its platelet binding affinity (type 2).

Clinical features and diagnosis—typical presentation is with nosebleeds, menorrhagia, and easy bruising. Laboratory diagnosis involves both an antigenic test and an activity test (ristocetin cofactor), in which formalin-fixed platelet aggregation is induced due to ristocetin-enhanced VWF binding to glycoprotein complex Ib–IX.

Treatment—mild von Willebrand's disease is treated with desmopressin 1-desamino-8-D-arginine vasopressin (DDAVP), which releases factor VIII and VWF from endothelial cells. Other treatments include ε-aminocaproic acid (for patients who require dental surgery, and women with menorrhagia), oestrogens. and factor VIII concentrates.

Other hereditary disorders of coagulation

These include (1) hereditary deficiency of the plasma metalloproteinase ADAMTS13, which predisposes to thrombotic thrombocytopenic purpura; (2) combined deficiency of coagulation factors V and VIII, caused by single-gene defects in the coordinated machinery for protein trafficking and secretion; (3) factor XI deficiency—an autosomal recessive diathesis of variable severity frequently occurring in Ashkenazi Jews; (4) inherited deficiencies of factors II, V, VII, and X—these cause bleeding tendencies of varying severity and are inherited as recessive disorders; (5) deficiency of the contact activating factors, factor XIII, and fibrinogen.

Hypercoagulable diseases due to deficiencies of anticoagulant or propensity to thrombosis

Typical presentation is with deep venous thrombosis and/or pulmonary embolism, and hypercoagulable states should be considered particularly when there is 'unusual' thrombosis, e.g. superficial thrombophlebitis, mesenteric vein thrombosis, and cerebral vein thrombosis.

Antithrombin III deficiency—diagnosis is particularly difficult in the post-thrombotic period when patients frequently have lower levels of antithrombin III due either to consumption of antithrombin III during clot formation or to the decreased function seen with heparin administration. Treatment is typically with therapeutic or prophylactic low molecular weight heparin or warfarin; antithrombin III concentrate may be given during an acute event or as a prophylactic treatment to prevent further disease.

Deficiencies of protein C and protein S—in addition to thrombotic manifestations, protein C deficiency can also manifest as warfarin-induced skin necrosis and dangerously life-threatening purpura fulminans in the homozygous or compound heterozygous protein C deficient neonate.

Factor V Leiden—a single mutation in the factor Va protein, found in about 5% of people of European ancestry, leads to resistance to activated protein C and a prolonged activity. This may lead to thrombotic disease.

Prothrombin 20210 mutation—this frequent allelic variant in populations of European ancestry increases the concentration of prothrombin, thus biasing haemostatic balance towards excess formation of thrombin.

Introduction

Haemostasis, the physiological process of blood clot formation, involves a coordinated interaction between the wall of the blood vessel, platelets, and blood coagulation proteins. The haemostatic mechanism maintains a state of readiness to respond to a multitude of haemostatic stressors to prevent haemorrhage while also preventing inappropriate clot formation. Although acquired diseases of the coagulation system frequently occur with liver disease and other pathological disease states, this chapter focuses specifically on genetic disorders resulting from abnormalities and/or deficiencies of the blood coagulation proteins. More specifically, this chapter covers haemophilia, von Willebrand's disease, and deficiencies/abnormalities of fibrinogen and factors II, V, VII, X, XI, XII, and XIII. The role of an inherited increased risk for excess clotting will also be addressed. These conditions may result from either the loss of function of anticoagulant proteins (antithrombin III, protein C, and protein S) or a gain of function of procoagulant proteins (factor V Leiden and prothrombin 20210G to A).

Additionally, we briefly describe recently discovered haemostasis-related genes: *LMAN1* (previously *ERGIC-53*) and *MCFD2* linked to combined factor V/factor VIII deficiency, *ADAMTS13*, associated with thrombotic thrombocytopenic purpura (TTP), and the

gene for vitamin K epoxide reductase (*VKORC1*), the enzyme responsible for recycling vitamin K 2,3-epoxide to the enzymatically activated form.

The coagulation cascade as a haemostatic mechanism

The human blood coagulation system involves a coordinated array of reactions which generates a stable fibrin clot when needed and prevents unnecessary clot formation. The system involves numerous proteins which interact, principally on phospholipid surfaces, to create a meshwork of fibrin fragments entrapping haematopoietic cells (Fig. 22.6.4.1). The majority of coagulation enzymatic complexes involve protease enzymes. Many of these enzymes are serine proteases, and a subset of these have the distinguishing feature that their functional synthesis requires vitamin K to enable post-translational modification of glutamic acid residues in the N-terminal region; this property provides the basis of the therapeutic mechanism by which the drug warfarin prevents proper synthesis of functional factors. The principal enzyme balancing the pro- and anticoagulant forces is prothrombin, thought to be the evolutionary forerunner of the mammalian coagulation proteins. In addition to its procoagulant functions, prothrombin, once activated, provides anticoagulant and cellular mobility functions as well.

In 1905, Morawitz first described the importance of thrombin, thromboplastin, and calcium in cleaving fibrinogen to create a fibrin clot. In the early 1930s and 1940s laboratory tests were developed that relied on *in vitro* fibrin clot formation to analyse the adequacy of a patient's clotting system. The waterfall cascade of sequential activation steps resulting in a fibrin clot was elegantly

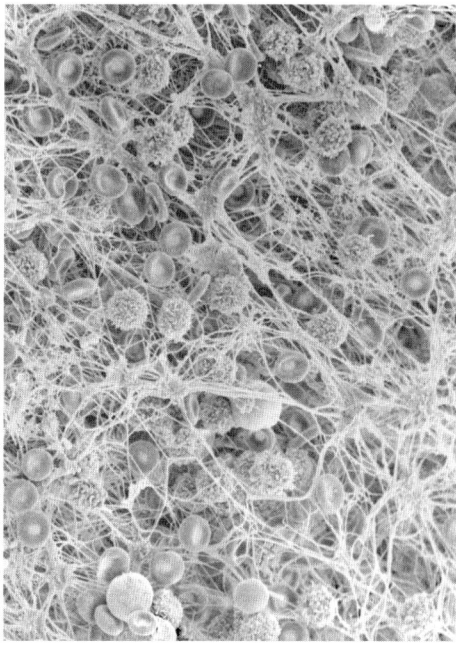

Fig. 22.6.4.1 Scanning electron micrograph of a whole blood clot. There is a meshwork of fibrin fibres emanating from platelet aggregates in which erythrocytes, lymphocytes, and other cells are trapped.
(Courtesy of John W Weisel and Chandrasekaran Nagaswami, Department of Cell and Developmental Biology, University of Pennsylvania School of Medicine, Philadelphia, PA.)

described in the early 1960s, delineating separate pathways to account for the prothrombin time and the partial thromboplastin time which the earlier laboratory tests measure. However, the set of activation steps is now better described as an interwoven, reinforcing set of reactions (Fig. 22.6.4.2). The unique specificities of the coagulation enzymes summarized in the classical coagulation cascade have been found to be more versatile in activating diverse proteins under varied conditions. However, the separate pathways, now termed the tissue factor (extrinsic) and the intrinsic pathways, help define the steps involved in the principal tests used in clinical medicine for evaluation of haemostatic proteins. For the series of reactions and specific factors involved, the time to clot formation defines the principal parameter used in clinical evaluation of the health of a patient's coagulation system. The assays (the prothrombin time (PT), the activated partial thromboplastin time (APTT), and activity levels of specific individual clotting factors) compare the time needed for clot formation in a patient's plasma with that in a control pool of plasma from normal donors.

Endothelial injury and tissue damage first trigger clot formation. The response of the platelets forms the primary phase of healing by temporarily patching the site of vascular injury. Subsequent to this initial platelet phospholipid patch, a fibrin clot provides a more solid framework for the necessary but slower cellular repair. Secondary haemostasis begins with injury-induced exposure of the integral membrane protein tissue factor to plasma proteins, enabling formation of the active enzymatic complex tissue factor–factor VIIa. The generation of tissue factor–factor VIIa then catalyses clotting by activating both factor X to factor Xa and factor IX to factor IXa. This activation primarily involves the cleavage of an arginine–isoleucine bond in a secreted plasma protein zymogen to form a two-chain active protein. Thus, once tissue injury has signalled the need for fibrin clot formation and tissue factor–factor VIIa has initiated coagulation, the haemostatic process amplifies through

the generation of factor IXa from factor IX, which is 10 times more abundant than factor VII and consequently leads precipitously to thrombin generation. Among thrombin's numerous roles is the activation of the essential procoagulant cofactors factors V and VIII. This process then further amplifies clotting by generating more thrombin through the active cofactors Va and VIIIa which then form the tenase (factor IXa/factor VIIIa) and prothrombinase (factor Xa/factor Va) complexes (see Fig. 22.6.4.1). Thrombin also activates the cross-linking enzyme (factor XIIIa) and the fibrinolytic inhibitor (TAFIa), and triggers platelet recruitment. Importantly, thrombin generation simultaneously counterbalances its procoagulation activities by inciting lysis of the clot via the release by endothelial cells of tissue plasminogen activator converting plasminogen to plasmin, the enzyme responsible for lysis of fibrin clots. Thrombin also dampens the clotting process by activating protein C that actively breaks down the critical procoagulant cofactors factors Va and VIIIa.

The basis for initiating clot formation in the PT and aPPT tests is titration of calcium into an anticoagulated plasma specimen along with a source of phospholipid. In addition, in the prothrombin time test, the source of phospholipid is a thromboplastin reagent that provides tissue factor to enable the tissue factor–factorVIIa complex to catalyse clot formation. The variation in prothrombin times, due to differences in the source of reagent tissue factor, has led to development of the international sensitivity index which creates an international normalized ratio (INR) for clinical management and the desire to synthesize a thromboplastin with an International Sensitivity Index (ISI) approaching 1.0. In the APTT test the phospholipid reagent lacks tissue factor and thus prevents formation of the tissue factor–factor VIIa complex. An activator, such as silica particles, also greatly decreases the time required for clot formation through activation of factor XII via the contact activation system.

Deficiencies of specific clotting proteins

Haemophilia

Deficiency of either factor VIII (haemophilia A) or factor IX (haemophilia B), which together make up the factor VIIIa/factor IXa intrinsic tenase enzymatic complex, results in the clinical phenotype commonly known as haemophilia. A sex-linked bleeding diathesis, now thought to be haemophilia, was described in Talmudic writings as a cause of fatal haemorrhage at circumcision. In the modern era, the disease may cause bleeding at circumcision, but haemophilia principally presents with haematoma formation, easy bruising, and bleeding at the site of venepuncture during the toddler period. The disease exists in severe, moderate, and mild forms classified as such on the basis of a clinical laboratory blood coagulation test performed to assess the level of functional coagulant protein (per cent activity of factor VIII or factor IX). The pathological problem in both haemophilia A (factor VIII deficiency) and haemophilia B (factor IX deficiency; also called Christmas disease), is the inability to form a functional tenase complex to activate factor X to factor Xa. Although factor X can still be activated to factor Xa by tissue factor–factor VIIa, the available quantities of factor VII (400 ng/ml) do not allow sufficient activation of factor X to enable clotting to occur in a physiologically timely fashion. Although patients with haemophilia may have some difficulties with immediate haemorrhage subsequent to a cutaneous or superficial injury, they characteristically have joint and deep tissue

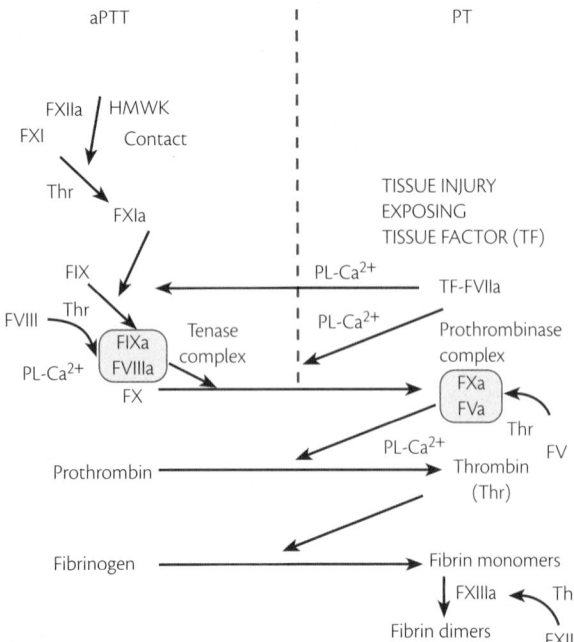

Fig. 22.6.4.2 Schematic representation of the enzymatic reactions involved in blood clot formation. APTT, activated partial thromboplastin time; PL-Ca^{2+}, phospholipids/calcium; PT, prothrombin time; Thr, thrombin.

bleeding problems as discussed below. The severity of disease is very well predicted by an *in vitro* assay for evaluation of the deficient protein level such that patients with severe disease have levels of factor activity of less than 1%, patients with moderate disease have activity levels of 1 to 5%, and patients with mild disease have activity levels of 6 to 30%. Normal factor VIII and IX levels are 50 to 200% and 75 to 125% respectively.

Numerous genetic mutations have been described accounting for the factor deficiencies causing haemophilia. In part because of the considerable difference in size between the factor VIII gene (186 kbp), and the factor IX gene (34 kbp), the ratio of the frequency of factor VIII to factor IX deficiency is between 4 and 5 to 1 (*c*.186/34 kbp). Thus, the frequency of haemophilia A is approximately 1 in 5000 to 6000 and that of haemophilia B is approximately one-fifth of that. Among affected cases, approximately 1 in 3 to 1 in 4 patients presents spontaneously without a familial inheritance pattern. One of the only differences between factor VIII and IX deficiencies is the frequency of severe disease, which occurs more commonly in factor VIII deficiency (60% of cases as compared with 45% in haemophilia B). This difference is largely attributed to the frequency of mutation due to a factor VIII gene inversion in intron 22 of the 26-exon factor VIII gene. At this locus of the factor VIII gene, a region of homology to sequences telomeric to the factor VIII gene, a recombination event results in the inability to synthesize any functional factor VIII, thus leading to severe disease (<1% functional protein activity). A less common inversion in intron 1 has also been described in 2 to 3% of severe haemophilia A patients. In both factor VIII and factor IX deficiency, milder disease is commonly due to missense mutations.

The clinical features of haemophilia predominantly include bleeding into joints and soft tissues. The incidence of central nervous system bleeding has dramatically decreased with concentrate therapy. The life expectancy of people with severe haemophilia has increased from 11 years at the beginning of the 20th century to approximately 70 years at the beginning of the 21st century. However, there was a marked decrease to 60 years in the 1980s, when the devastating effects of blood-borne viral disease again shortened average life expectancy.

In the untreated patient with severe disease, haemophilic arthropathy and joint deformity are inevitable complications. In decreasing order of involvement, the most commonly affected joints include the knee, elbow, ankle, shoulder, wrist, and hip. Recurrent bleeding episodes create a hypertrophic synovial lining with chronic inflammation; however, the pathophysiology responsible for recurrent joint bleeding remains unknown. Arthropathies commonly necessitate replacement of affected joints for pain control and improvement of mobility. Soft-tissue haemorrhages frequently complicate haemophilia; further complications due to these haemorrhages include compartment syndrome, neurological damage, and extensive blood loss from retroperitoneal bleeds. Haematoma formation, a frequent complication of haemophilia, may arise spontaneously or with trauma and require extensive factor replacement and fasciotomy, the necessity for which can be assessed by mean arterial pressure in a compartment. Intracranial haemorrhage, occurring in approximately 5% of patients, warrants immediate evaluation and treatment within the first 6 to 8 h of presentation; however, the majority of children presenting to an Emergency Department with central nervous system symptoms have not suffered from intracranial haemorrhage.

A pseudotumour, an encapsulated collection of blood most commonly originating in bone or soft tissues, is a rare but extremely serious consequence of haemophilia occurring in approximately 2% of patients. This complication is difficult to manage but may sometimes be treated with surgery at specialized haemophilia centres.

Frequently, patients with haemophilia have haematuria, the severity of which may range from self-limited episodes to gross haematuria with significant blood loss. Protease inhibitors for HIV therapy may lead to haematuria with flank pain or renal stones. Physicians should be aware of the possibility of nephrotic syndrome in patients with severe disease and high titres of antibody inhibitors receiving high-dose intravenous replacement therapy and other agents to induce tolerance.

Dental procedures warrant involvement of a haemophilia specialist. Factor replacement levels of 25 to 100% are suggested depending on the complexity of the dental procedure. Antifibrinolytics such as ε-aminocaproic acid (6-aminohexanoic acid) or tranexemic acid and fibrin sealants may be a helpful adjuvant to replacement therapy.

On account of the sex-linked inheritance pattern, haemophilia is rarely found in women unless extensive lyonization takes place in the normal gene, or the woman is born to a haemophilic father and a carrier mother. Normal vaginal delivery is considered to be relatively safe in the case of a haemophilic infant; however, vacuum extraction, midcavity forceps deliveries, and invasive fetal monitoring should be avoided because of the increased risk of formation of subgaleal and cephalic haematomas.

The laboratory diagnosis of haemophilia is based on a modification of the classic APTT assay used as a standard test for the haemostatic system. Normally patients are evaluated due to bleeding symptomatology or because of a prolonged APTT result. The APTT is a very sensitive but poorly specific screening test for haemophilia. All patients, even those with mild disease, will normally have a prolonged APTT unless there is a problem with specimen acquisition or the insensitivity of the APTT reagent. Once suspected, haemophilia can be evaluated by an inhibitor screen which involves performing a 50:50 mix of patient and normal plasma to evaluate whether the prolongation is due to a deficiency of a clotting protein or alternatively to the presence of an inhibitor. There are many causes of a prolonged APTT other than haemophilia (see Table 22.6.4.1). Classically, a phospholipid inhibitory antibody, called a lupus anticoagulant, will cause a prolongation of the APTT of the 50:50 mix due to the effect of the phospholipid inhibitory antibody on the normal pooled plasma. A lupus anticoagulant which causes a prolonged APTT may also result in a low factor VIII or factor IX level. In such cases, further testing for a lupus anticoagulant is necessary to rule out a low factor VIII due to a lupus anticoagulant as opposed to a deficiency.

Management of haemophilia predominantly involves administering the deficient protein (factor VIII or factor IX) to a patient. Factor replacement therapy is most commonly administered in a so-called 'on-demand' regimen, when a patient's symptomatology necessitates treatment. However, prophylaxis is indicated during surgery or at times of expected injury. Prophylactic therapies during early childhood are now recommended when feasible after the first major bleeding episode as a means of preventing arthropathies in patients with severe disease. Prophylactic administration during the first few years of life requires special consideration due to the

Table 22.6.4.1 Coagulation laboratory testing, plasma concentrations, and chromosomal location of coagulation proteins

Clotting factor	PT	aPTT	Half-life of protein	Plasma concentration	Inheritance (chromosome)
Fibrinogen	Increased	Increased	2–4 days	200–400 mg/dl	Autosomal (1)
Prothrombin (factor II)	Increased	Increased	3 days	100 μg/ml	Autosomal (11)
Factor V	Increased	Increased	36 h	10 μg/ml	Autosomal (1)
Factor VII	Increased	Normal	2–6 h	0.5 μg/ml	Autosomal (13)
Factor VIII	Normal	Increased	8–12 h	0.1 μg/ml	X-linked (X)
von Willebrand factor	Normal	Mildly increased in approximately 50% of cases	Several hours	10 μg/ml	Autosomal (12)
Factor IX	Normal	Increased	24 h	5 μg/ml	X-linked (X)
Factor X	Increased	Increased	40 h	10 μg/ml	Autosomal (13)
Factor XI	Normal	Increased	60–80 h	5 μg/ml	Autosomal (4)
Factor XII	Normal	Increased	50 h	30 μg/ml	Autosomal (5)
Factor XIII	Normal	Normal	9–19 days	10 μg/ml	Autosomal (6, α chain, and 1, β chain)
Protein C	Normal	Normal	6 h	5 μg/ml	Autosomal (2)
Protein S	Normal	Normal	30 h	25 μg/ml	Autosomal (3)
Antithrombin III	Normal	Normal	48 h	150 μg/ml	Autosomal (1)

Abbreviations: PT, prothrombin time; aPTT, activated partial thromboplastin time.

need for repeated intravenous access generally requiring an indwelling line. These have been associated with high rates of sepsis, particularly in children under the age of 3. Before the development of stringent purification and viricidal procedures, the transmission of viral disease was almost inevitable as each vial of plasma-derived concentrate was pooled from approximately 60 000 to as many as 400 000 donors, although the number has recently been reduced to 15 000. Tragically, most patients with severe disease treated before 1985 developed HIV. Rates of development of hepatitis B and C are also extremely high. Although drastically reduced, the potential for transmission of infectious disease has not been totally eliminated. Many recombinant preparations are prepared with human serum albumin, thus leaving a possible source of transfusion of a blood-borne disease.

Treatment
Acute bleeding episodes
Safe and effective treatment options continue to improve for the management of acute bleeding episodes for patients with haemophilia A and B. Blood products available include fresh frozen plasma (FFP) which contains both factors VIII and IX, prothrombin complex concentrates containing factors II, VII, IX, and X, activated prothrombin complex concentrates (factors IIa, VIIa, IXa, Xa), monoclonal-antibody purified factor VIII and factor IX, and recombinant factor VIII and factor IX. Recombinant factor VIIa is now approved for use in patients with inhibitors during acute bleeds. Currently trials using gene therapy approaches are under way and may provide a method for continuous prophylaxis against bleeding (see below). Recombinant or highly purified products are the optimal therapy because of the great benefit/risk ratio. Availability, ease of administration, cost, viral safety, and thrombotic risk, particularly in patients undergoing high-dose therapy or procedures with a high risk of thrombotic complications, dictate the choice of product. Cryoprecipitate, made from the precipitate of thawed frozen plasma, contains factor VIII but does not

contain factor IX. Cryoprecipitate and FFP should only be used in the haemophilia patient in an emergency setting where concentrates are not available. Inhibitor formation, the development of antibodies to the deficient protein, arises subsequent to transfusion of a blood product or factor replacement and is the major complication of treatment. An inhibitor presents an extremely difficult situation for patient management (see 'Complications of therapy' below).

Several immunoaffinity purified plasma-derived factor VIII and factor IX products are available in the United States of America and Europe and currently have excellent records of viral safety, efficacy, and lack of thrombogenicity. When concentrate is unavailable, FFP is readily available in most emergency settings. Viricidal methods using solvent detergent treatment may now be applied in production of FFP; furthermore, each unit is from a single screened donor, thus the risk of transfusion-transmitted disease is low.

Recombinant factor VIII and factor IX have been licensed for over a decade. These proteins are produced in cultured mammalian cells and purified from conditioned medium. Recombinant factor IX is devoid of human plasma whereas the recombinant factor VIII concentrates utilize human plasma-derived albumin for stabilization. Because *in vivo* coagulant activity of recombinant factor IX is only 80% of *in vitro* estimates used for labelling of product in IU/mg, it is recommended that the calculated factor IX dosage be multiplied by a factor of 1.2 for dose calculation when using recombinant factor IX. A plausible explanation for this discrepancy is a difference in post-translational modifications compared with plasma-derived factor IX.

During severe and critical bleeds it is optimal to achieve 50 to 100% factor activity levels for 7 to 10 days (e.g. for pharyngeal, retropharyngeal, retroperitoneal, and central nervous system bleeds). More modest levels of 20 to 50% for 2 to 7 days are generally adequate for dental extractions, haematuria, intramuscular or soft-tissue bleeds with dissection, or bleeds into mucous membranes. Levels of 20 to 30% for 1 to 2 days are recommended for uncomplicated haemarthroses, superficial muscle, or soft-tissue bleeds. The frequency of dosing is every 12 to 24 h for factor IX concentrates and every 8 to 12 h for factor VIII concentrates. At 24 h for factor IX and 12 h for factor VIII, the calculated amount to infuse would be one-half the initial amount of factor IX, as the half-life of factor IX is approximately 18 to 24 h.

The timing of factor level determination should be 15 to 30 min after the loading dose and immediately prior to subsequent doses for appropriate dose adjustments. When factor concentrates are used for patients with inhibitors, higher doses will most likely be required. Additionally, some authors have also reported good success and reduced cost with constant infusion regimens.

Calculation of the optimal factor concentration for administration

The number of international units (IU) of factor required is equal to:

$$\text{body weight (kg)} \times \text{desired \% increase in factor VIII or IX level} \times C$$

where C is a constant depending on the product and the source of the product. The value of C is 0.5 for administration of plasma-purified and recombinant factor VIII, 1 for administration of plasma-purified factor IX, and 1.2 for administration of recombinant factor IX.

Surgery in patients with haemophilia

When possible, treatment should be instituted by caregivers aware of major and minor adverse reactions and complications occurring in the haemophiliac population. Care should also be given in association with an experienced reference laboratory able to provide timely evaluation of a patient's response to treatment. Therapeutic factor levels should be obtained before surgery. Depending on the type of surgery, the factor level should reach levels of 50 to 100% of normal and should be maintained 2 to 7 days postprocedure. In addition to factor concentrates, fibrin glue has been recommended with circumcision, antifibrinolytics with dental procedures, aprotinin with caution in cardiac procedures, and recombinant factor VIIa and/or apheresis in patients with high-titre inhibitors. The use of aprotinin has been proposed to increase the risk of thrombogenicity. A factor level approaching 100% is recommended for brain or prostate surgery, because of a higher risk of bleeding. In patients with milder haemophilia A administration of the synthetic octapeptide desmopressin (deamino-D-arginine vasopressin, DDAVP) may be helpful in increasing factor levels. However, this is not the case for haemophilia B.

Complications of therapy

The main adverse outcomes related to treatment with concentrates include transmission of viruses when using plasma-derived products and development of inhibitory antibodies seen with both recombinant and plasma-derived products. Thrombosis has also been a complication of early complex concentrates used for patients with inhibitors.

The development of purification schemes that inactivate viruses, and the development of recombinant products, has dramatically decreased the incidence of transmission of viral disease. Early preparations of prothrombin complex concentrates presented a significant risk of thrombotic complications, but this risk has now been markedly reduced.

Inhibitor formation—the development of antibodies that inhibit clotting activity—occurs subsequent to transfusion of a blood product or factor replacement. Development of inhibitors presents difficult challenges for the management of haemophilia. Therapeutic strategies largely rely on the ability to bypass the factor VIIIa–factor IXa tenase complex. Inhibitor formation almost exclusively arises in severely affected patients and occurs in approximately 7 to 52% of patients with haemophilia A but in only about 1 to 3% of patients with haemophilia B. This difference in inhibitor formation is not completely understood, but possible explanations include the higher incidence of severe disease in haemophilia A, prenatal exposure to maternal factor IX but not factor VIII antigens due to the former's ability to pass the placenta membrane, the structural similarity between factor IX and other vitamin K-dependent proteins, the higher plasma levels of factor IX, and the greater inherent immunogenicity of factor VIII due to its larger size. One very rare but severe complication that may occur with the development of a factor IX inhibitor is the development of a potentially life-threatening anaphylactic complication following first treatment.

Therapeutic strategies for treatment of patients with inhibitors need to address the acute management of the bleeding episode as well as a longer-term treatment directed toward suppression of antibody production. Quantification of the titre of factor inhibitor involves mixing the patient's plasma with test plasma containing a known amount of factor, normally from a pool of healthy donors. After incubation, factor activity levels present in the patient's incubation mixture are compared with that in a control mixture so that the amount of inhibitory antibody can be calculated. The Bethesda unit (BU), the standard unit used to report a titre of factor inhibitor, represents the amount of inhibitor that inactivates 50% of factor activity. Acute management of bleeding in a patient with an inhibitor relies first on quantifying the BU of the inhibitor. With low-titre inhibitors (<5 BU), it may be possible to overwhelm the inhibitor with aggressive concentrate therapy. With high-titre inhibitors, it is usually necessary to bypass the inhibitor using either prothrombin complex concentrates, activated prothrombin complex concentrates, porcine factor VIII, or recombinant factor VIIa. These bypassing agents, with the exception of porcine factor VIII, largely work by directly activating factor X to factor Xa, thus bypassing the need for the intrinsic tenase complex. With porcine factor VIII, it is wise to first perform testing to ensure that the patient's inhibitor does not cross-react with the porcine factor VIII. Because of the life-threatening bleeding complications in patients with inhibitor, immune tolerance regimens have been designed with the aim of eradicating the inhibitor in the long term. Therapeutic regimens involve infusion of high-dose factor concentrates enabling a tolerance to the deficient factor. This protocol is highly effective in approximately 80% of patients.

Viral diseases

Severely affected patients treated with plasma-derived concentrates before 1985 had an extremely high rate of viral disease. Over the course of a 70-year lifespan, a patient with severe haemophilia may be exposed to donations from 70 million individuals as a result of the pooling of thousands of donor units for concentrate production. Specific laboratory tests to screen for HIV, hepatitis C, and hepatitis B, in addition to much improved donor screening procedures, have dramatically limited the number of contaminations from individuals carrying viral diseases. Solvent detergent treatment procedures, which inactivate enveloped viruses (HIV and hepatitis viruses B, C, D, and G), and heat treatment procedures used to eliminate nonenveloped viruses (hepatitis A and E viruses and parvovirus B19) have radically decreased the risk of viral infection from plasma-derived products. The viral inactivation procedures in current use include pasteurization, vapour heating, high-dry heating, and nanofiltration. Recently, β-propiolactone ultraviolet inactivation has been discontinued because of ineffective viricidal technique.

HIV In the late 1970s and early 1980s, HIV appeared in the blood supply before routine laboratory testing was developed to detect its presence. The leading cause of death in American haemophilia patients in 1982 was haemorrhage; however, contaminated blood products during the period between 1979 and 1983 led to a sharp rise in viral disease shortly thereafter. A large proportion of patients with haemophilia became infected with HIV and have subsequently died from AIDS. Risk factors for infection included the severity of the disease (severely affected patients were much more commonly affected than those with moderate or mild disease), the type of concentrate used (factor VIII vs factor IX concentrate), the viral inactivation procedures used in product preparation, and the geographical location of the patient with regard to percentage of blood products contaminated.

The incidence of HIV infection in American patients who received plasma-derived concentrates between 1979 and 1984 was lower in patients receiving factor IX complex concentrates (55%) than in those receiving factor VIII concentrates (approximately 90%). Despite the devastating consequences of HIV for affected individuals and families, the projected impact on births of patients with haemophilia over the next two centuries is small (1.79% reduction).

Hepatitides Contaminated plasma-derived products also led to significant morbidity and mortality due to hepatitis viruses. Effective viricidal techniques have greatly reduced the incidence of hepatitic viral disease in this population. In the United States of America in the late 1980s, 87% of the 345 HIV-negative and more than 99% of the HIV-positive patients showed evidence of prior infection with hepatitis B, hepatitis C, or hepatitis D viruses. Infection due to hepatitis A virus has rarely been reported in patients with haemophilia in the United States. Solvent/detergent inactivation of concentrates has been associated with a high prevalence of antibodies to hepatitis A virus.

Hepatitis B was commonly seen in patients with haemophilia until routine screening of liver enzymes and the subsequent availability of hepatitis-specific antibody and antigen tests in the 1980s. Most patients are now vaccinated against hepatitis B so that it is difficult to estimate hepatitis B infection from concentrate administration. The hepatitis delta virus, dependent on coinfection with hepatitis B virus, has also been a significant cause of illness in patients with haemophilia; its prevalence is largely attributed to the administration of prothrombin complex concentrates.

Routine testing for hepatitis C, instituted in the early 1990s, has reduced but not eliminated hepatitis C contamination in the donor pool. A variable susceptibility and morbidity is seen in response to hepatitis infection; cirrhosis was estimated at approximately 20% and liver failure at 10 to 20% 20 years after infection. Concurrent infection with HIV can accelerate complications of hepatitis C virus. There is also an increased likelihood of hepatocellular carcinoma with long-term infection with viral hepatitis.

Other infectious agents The great majority of patients with haemophilia have antibodies to parvovirus B19. This is a small, non-lipid-enveloped, highly heat-resistant virus found to contaminate plasma-derived products. Methods that inactivate other non-enveloped viruses in products have not proved to be routinely effective against this virus. Although parvovirus B19 infection is often mild and self-limited, infection with parvovirus B19 has the potential to severely compromise the health of an infected immunodeficient patient.

There is experimental evidence in animal models that cellular blood components, plasma, and plasma components have a potential, though minimal, risk of transmitting the prion disease Creutzfeldt–Jacob disease (CJD). To date, no definitive direct infection of a recipient of a blood product or blood product concentrate has been documented, although transmission has been reported from corneal and dura mater grafts and cadaveric pituitary hormones. The American Red Cross currently administers a questionnaire to screen donors for risk of prion disease. There is now concern that transmission of new variant Creutzfeldt–Jacob disease (vCJD) may differ from classical CJD and could potentially be transmitted through plasma-derived concentrates. This new variant has been associated with outbreaks of bovine spongiform encephalopathy, potentially from dietary exposure. Experimental evidence shows that bovine spongiform encephalopathy and vCJD are caused by the same infectious agent, and prion-related protein has been found in lymphoid tissue of patients with vCJD. In Europe, particular large amounts of concentrate have been removed from the market as a result of the development of vCJD in product donors.

Treatment of patients infected with hepatitis virus and/or HIV

Vaccination against hepatitis A and B is highly recommended for patients who receive concentrates and lack viral antibodies indicative of past infection. Treatment of hepatitis C with interferon-γ is associated with significant improvement in approximately one-half of patients in many but not all studies. Liver transplantation has been successful in many cases for patients with liver failure who are unresponsive to treatment. The liver transplant fortuitously corrects the deficiency of clotting protein due to synthesis of clotting factors by the orthotopic liver. However, the possibility of reinfection with viral disease is significant and must be included in management decisions.

Drug-related hepatitis in haemophilia patients has been reported subsequent to treatment of HIV, particularly in response to indinavir. Additionally, complications in HIV-positive haemophilia patients taking protease inhibitors include haematuria, intracranial bleeds, and excessive bleeding often requiring hospitalization and administration of higher than expected doses of factor concentrate to correct the bleeding. Protease inhibitor therapy should not be withheld from HIV-positive individuals with haemophilia. A 6-month prospective study of 20 haemophilia patients receiving protease inhibitors revealed only one unusual bleed, which was corrected by factor infusion.

Future directions: gene transfer as a method of treating haemophilia

The development of clotting factor concentrates resulted in a dramatic improvement in life expectancy for individuals with haemophilia. Nonetheless, this treatment strategy has a number of disadvantages. The protein must be infused intravenously, and has a relatively short half-life in the circulation. This makes chronic prophylaxis difficult, especially in small children where venous access may present a problem. In addition, the product is so expensive that only about one-quarter of the world's haemophiliacs (those in the developed world) have access to it. Although current viral inactivation techniques have largely eliminated the risk of HIV and hepatitis in plasma-derived products, there are ongoing concerns about the risk of other bloodborne diseases (CJD, transfusion-transmitted viruses) that are not easily eradicated using current techniques. These factors have fuelled interest in the development of a gene transfer approach to the treatment of haemophilia. Such an approach, if successful, would result in continuous production of a level of clotting factor adequate to prevent bleeds rather than treating bleeds after they have occurred. The level of clotting factor required for this goal can be predicted based on a generation of experience with clotting factor concentrates. Thus, in Swedish prophylaxis studies, it has been shown that maintenance of trough factor levels in the range of 1 to 3% are adequate to prevent all the life-threatening bleeds and most of the joint bleeds in boys with severe haemophilia. The validity of a target of 1 to 3% is further confirmed by the natural history of the disease; individuals with factor levels of less than 1% are severely affected, whereas those with levels of 1 to 5% have a moderately severe phenotype with a considerably lower incidence of spontaneous bleeding episodes.

Successful gene transfer approaches require three elements: a therapeutic transgene, a means of delivering it (i.e. a vector), and an appropriate target cell type in which gene transfer and expression will exert a therapeutic effect. Of the inherited diseases for which gene transfer approaches have been attempted, haemophilia has a number of advantages. First, tissue-specific expression is not required. Although clotting factors are normally synthesized in the liver, biologically active material can be synthesized in a variety of tissues, including fibroblasts, muscle cells, and endothelial cells. This allows latitude in the choice of target cell. Second, the therapeutic window is wide, since even small increases in circulating levels of factor are likely to result in some improvement in symptoms, and increases to 100% would still leave the patient within normal limits. Excellent small and large animal models of the diseases exist (murine and canine), and determination of therapeutic efficacy is in the case of haemophilia relatively straightforward, since levels of circulating factor correlate well with symptoms of the disease.

A number of different strategies for gene therapy for haemophilia have been investigated in preclinical studies, and five of these have been evaluated in early phase clinical trials conducted in the United States of America beginning in 1999. The plethora of approaches suggests that there will eventually be more than one successful combination of vector and target tissue that is safe and effective for haemophilia; this is an advantage, since the haemophilia population is a heterogeneous one, and approaches that work well in some instances, e.g. delivery of a viral vector to the liver, may be impossible for individuals with severe liver disease due to prior hepatitis C infection. Previous studies have included (1) an *ex vivo* approach in which fibroblasts from a patient are isolated from a skin biopsy, cells are expanded in culture, transfected with a plasmid expressing factor VIII, and then reimplanted on to the patient's omentum. This study showed safety in the first six patients treated, with evidence of gene transfer and expression in three out of six. (2) In a second trial, a retroviral vector expressing

B-domain deleted factor VIII was infused intravenously. This trial enrolled 13 adults with severe haemophilia A, and demonstrated that the approach was safe, but since retroviruses require a dividing target cell to achieve transduction, long-lasting expression was not achieved. Subsequent preclinical studies showed that this approach can be successful in large animals if the vector is infused into neonates, where hepatocytes are rapidly proliferating. (3) A third trial explored use of a gutted adenoviral vector to express factor VIII, but enrolled only a single subject because of short-term, reversible toxicities associated with vector infusion. (4) Intramuscular injection of a recombinant adenoassociated (AAV) viral vector expressing factor IX was also demonstrated to be safe in eight subjects with severe haemophilia B; muscle biopsies showed evidence for long-term persistence and expression of the donated gene, but circulating levels of factor IX did not reach a therapeutic range (>1%). Subsequent studies in the canine model of haemophilia have shown that delivery of the AAV vector to skeletal muscle via an intravascular infusion technique (originally developed for gene transfer in muscular dystrophy models) results in much higher levels of factor IX expression. This has not yet been tested in humans. (5) Hepatic artery infusion of an AAV vector expressing factor IX was carried out in seven subjects. Infusion of vector at the highest dose tested resulted in expression of therapeutic levels of factor IX (>10%) for a period of 4 weeks in the first subject injected with this dose. Factor IX levels gradually decreased over the ensuing 6 weeks, returning to the baseline of <1% at 10 weeks after infusion. This was subsequently demonstrated to be due to an immune response to the AAV capsid, which had not been predicted by animal models. The trial was revised to include a short course of immunosuppression at the time of vector administration, to block the T cell response to capsid until it is degraded and cleared from the cell. Short-term immunosuppression as an adjunct to vector infusion is currently being tested in multiple gene transfer studies. Currently, a second trial of AAV gene transfer to liver, utilizing an alternate AAV serotype which can be infused intravenously and still target the liver, is in the late planning stages. This will avoid the need for an interventional radiographic procedure to cannulate the hepatic artery for vector administration. The trials to date underscore the iterative nature of advances in gene transfer, with problems encountered in early phase testing in humans requiring additional studies in the laboratory or in preclinical animal models to inform the next generation of clinical studies.

Von Willebrand's disease

In 1926 Erik von Willebrand first described what we now know as von Willebrand's disease upon finding an autosomally inherited bleeding diathesis in a large kindred on the Åland islands in the Gulf of Bothnia between Sweden and Finland. Although the bleeding disorder in this family resulted in haemorrhagic death in multiple family members, the bleeding diathesis in patients with von Willebrand's disease is usually much milder. Most commonly, patients with von Willebrand's disease manifest mucosal platelet-type bleeding tendencies of varying severity. Nose bleeds, menorrhagia, and easy bruising are the most common manifestations.

The pathophysiology of von Willebrand's disease involves a functional deficiency of von Willebrand factor (VWF), a 270-kDa monomer that forms a large multimeric plasma glycoprotein of several subunits up to 100 subunits. Synthesized in the megakaryocyte and endothelial cell and stored in subcellular granules, VWF enables proper two-chain factor VIII formation and serves as a carrier, thus preventing degradation of factor VIII and lengthening the half-life of the labile factor VIII protein to around 8 h. VWF secreted by endothelial cells also binds to heparin glycosaminoglycan and to the platelet glycoprotein complex Ib–IX enhancing platelet activation and further platelet recruitment at sites of tissue damage. The interaction between platelets and VWF is thought to provide the explanation for the mucosal bleeding phenotype occurring in patients with von Willebrand's disease. These patients frequently have reduced levels of factor VIII. However, the remaining factor VIII is normally sufficient to prevent the haemophilia-type symptomatology of arthropathy and deep tissue bleeding.

The 180-kbp gene for VWF is located on chromosome 12 and consists of 52 exons. There are three types of von Willebrand's disease: types 1, 2, and 3. Types 1 and 3 are quantitative deficiencies of the VWF, but type 2 is a qualitative deficiency due to binding defects of the VWF. The inheritance of types 1 and 3 are autosomal dominant and autosomal recessive, respectively. However, rare reports of an autosomal dominant inheritance pattern for type 3 have been published. There are four principal subtypes of type 2 classified as follows: 2A, absence of high-molecular-weight VWF species causing decreased platelet-dependent function; 2B, increased affinity of VWF for platelet glycoprotein Ib–IX; 2M, platelet functional defect not caused by the absence of high molecular weight multimers; and 2N, a factor VIII binding abnormality.

Laboratory diagnosis of von Willebrand's disease involves assaying the plasma for VWF. The two principal tests are an antigenic test (VWF antigen) and an activity test (VWF ristocetin cofactor) in which formalin-fixed platelet aggregation is induced due to the ristocetin-enhanced VWF binding to glycoprotein complex Ib–IX. Comparison of the tests helps identify the enhanced ristocetin-induced aggregation seen in type 2B von Willebrand's disease where VWF ristocetin cofactor is typically much lower than VWF antigen. Other tests performed in the evaluation of von Willebrand's disease include the level of factor VIII, which is often decreased, and the APTT, which is elevated in approximately half of cases of von Willebrand's disease due to the low activity of factor VIII. Nonreducing gel immunoelectrophoresis is employed to assay the distribution of multimeric subunits of VWF with a gel containing antibody to VWF antigen. This assay is particularly relevant for visualization of the presence of low, intermediate, and high molecular weight VWF subunits. The intermediate and high molecular weight species are markedly decreased in subtypes of type 2 disease. A decreased normal pattern is seen in type 1 disease, although the decreased visual intensity may be difficult to quantify. Type 3 disease shows near absence of all subunit molecular weights. The lower limit of the normal range of VWF varies with blood type (A, B, O, AB). Thus, symptomatology must be evaluated based on normal ranges for each blood type. The bleeding time in a patient with von Willebrand's disease is most often prolonged; however, the test is no longer routinely necessary because of the non-specific nature of a positive result and the higher specificity of other testing.

The specific treatment for von Willebrand's disease varies with a patient's symptoms, the circumstances of the need for treatment, the subtype of von Willebrand's disease, laboratory results indicating the potential success of increased VWF with non-protein-based treatment, and the clinical experience with a particular patient and their biological family members. When possible, treatment based on nonblood products is preferred. The mainstay of treatment for mild disease is treatment with the synthetic octapeptide desmopressin, DDAVP. This causes release of factor VIII and VWF from endothelial cells raising the plasma VWF by approximately two- to tenfold. Thus treatment with DDAVP relies on a partial quantitative deficiency of VWF. Intravenous and nasal preparations are available. The nasal preparation allows a patient to self-administer medication at either regular intervals or on an as-needed basis. The phenomenon of tachyphylaxis, the decreased effectiveness of repeated doses of the compound, does occur, and there is usually little response after three consecutive doses. In the past, DDAVP was considered contraindicated in type 2B von Willebrand's disease because of the thrombocytopenia sometimes observed with DDAVP infusion. However, this recommendation is controversial and should be assessed on a case-by-case basis. Patients with type 3 von Willebrand's disease may lack sufficient intracellular reserves for effective therapy; thus alternative measures for such patients are usually necessary.

A trial of effectiveness of DDAVP is often indicated, particularly prior to prophylactic surgical use of the compound. The trial is normally performed after subtyping the VWF disease to ensure that DDAVP is not contraindicated, as in type 2B. Optimally, the test should not be given within 24 h of the last DDAVP infusion nor at a time of environmental stress in order to minimize problems associated with tachyphylaxis or depletion of intracellular reserves. A therapeutic trial entails measurement of VWF antigen before and 1 h after DDAVP infusion of 0.3 µg/kg. The patient should be watched carefully during this period because of possible flushing, mild anaphylactoid reactions, and possible hyponatraemia.

ε-Aminocaproic acid is frequently administered in the setting of dental surgery to inhibit fibrinolysis. However, care must be taken in administration to patients with a predisposition to thrombosis because of the potential deleterious effects of ε-aminocaproic acid in this setting. Other compounds which may be administered include oestrogens in women because of the natural positive regulation of synthesis of VWF with oestrogen compounds. This may ameliorate menorrhagia in such patients. Components in cryoprecipitate include factor VIII, fibrinogen, and factor XIII, in addition to VWF. Cryoprecipitate had been the mainstay of plasma-based therapy until the recent availability of factor VIII concentrates with preserved VWF protein such as Alphanate and Humate P. The use of cryoprecipitate, which does not undergo viral inactivation, has thus fallen out of favour.

Treatment of von Willebrand's disease with DDAVP is the method of choice in patients who respond to this therapy. DDAVP for intravenous or subcutaneous use is supplied as either a 4-µg/ml 10-ml vial or a 15-µg/ml 1- or 2-ml vial preparation. The recommended dose is 0.3 µg/kg, mixed in 30 ml normal saline, infused slowly over 30 min or 0.4 µg/kg subcutaneously. This dose may be repeated after 12 to 24 h. A DDAVP nasal spray is available in a metered dose pump which delivers 0.1 ml (150 µg) per actuation. The bottle is at a concentration of 1.5 mg/ml and contains 2.5 ml with a nasal spray pump which can deliver 25 150-µg or 12 300-µg doses. For administration, patients who weigh less than 50 kg should deliver one 150-µg spray in one nostril. For those weighing over 50 kg, one spray should be delivered in each nostril for a total dose of 300 µg. Administration may be repeated after 24 h. Precautions to take with the medication include administration no more than every 24 h or for three consecutive days unless under the supervision of personnel from a haemophilia treatment centre.

The medication should not be used in pregnant women or in children under 2 years of age. The medication should be used with caution in the elderly and in individuals with a history of cardiovascular disease.

ADAMTS13 deficiency—thrombotic thrombocytopenic purpura

The gene encoding the novel metalloproteinase ADAMTS13 (a disintegrin-like and metalloproteinase with thrombospondin type-1 motifs) was discovered in 2001. *ADAMTS13*, located on chromosome 9q34, cleaves the peptide bond at Tyr1605 to Met1606 in the A2 domain of VWF. Normally, ADAMTS13 rapidly degrades 'unusually large' VWF multimers into smaller multimers. Lack of ADAMTS13 due to familial absence or acquired inhibition may result in thrombotic thrombocytopenic purpura (TTP) with an increase of the ultralarge multimers and formation of platelet clumps and microthrombi.

Combined deficiency of coagulation cofactors factor V and factor VIII

Combined deficiency of coagulation cofactors factor V and factor VIII (F5F8D) is a rare autosomal recessive disorder due to genetic mutations in the coordinated system of protein trafficking. The disorder results from mutations in the genes for the transmembrane lectin LMAN-1 (ERGIC-53) on chromosome 18 (18q21.3-q22) or its protein complex partner MCFD2 (multiple coagulation factor deficiency 2) located on chromosome 2 (2p21). MCFD2 recruits glycoproteins factors V and VIII for endoplasmic reticulum–Golgi transport by the molecular chaperone ERGIC-53. *LMAN1* or *MCFD2* mutations that cause this rare disorder in patients result in indistinguishable clinical manifestations with mild to moderate bleeding symptomatology. Plasma antigen and activity levels of both factors V and VIII measure between 5 and 30 U/dL.

Factor XI deficiency

Factor XI deficiency is an autosomal recessive bleeding diathesis of variable severity. It was first described in 1953 as a third type of haemophilia and is thus sometimes referred to as haemophilia C or Rosenthal syndrome. The deficiency predominantly occurs in eastern European Ashkenazi Jews, accounting for more than 50% of cases. In Ashkenazi Jews the disorder is reported to occur in 5 to 11% of individuals in the heterozygous state and 0.1 to 0.3% in the homozygous state. Genetically, the mutations are grouped into three types: type I, abnormalities in the intron–exon splice boundaries; type II, mutations that result in a premature stop in translation; and type III, mutations resulting from a missense mutation.

The protein itself is an 80-kDa protein that circulates in the plasma as a zymogen in a noncovalent association with high-molecular-weight kininogen. It contains four apple domains in its protein structure, and although factor XIa is a cleaving protease, its structure differs from the serine protease coagulation proteins. Factor XI is principally activated by factor XIIa in the presence of a negatively charged surface (contact activation). The lack of any bleeding diathesis related to a severe deficiency of factor XII suggests the importance of thrombin as an alternative mechanism of *in vivo* factor XI activation.

The *in vitro* factor XI activity level does not correlate well with clinical phenotype. Family history of the bleeding complications

and the specific mutated sites are more predictive. Bleeding manifestations are rare in heterozygotes and occur in approximately 50% of homozygous patients.

Factor XI activity levels are assayed in an APTT-based test. Bleeding problems include easy bruising, epistaxis, haematuria, postpartum haemorrhage, haematomas, and menorrhagia. Haemophilia symptoms, including haemarthroses and intramuscular bleeding, are rare. Bleeding most frequently occurs after trauma or surgery. Damage to tissues rich in fibrinolytic activity, such as oral mucosa and the prostate, are more commonly associated with bleeding problems.

Therapy for patients with factor XI deficiency is indicated for symptomatic bleeding and prophylactically for surgery in patients with markedly reduced levels (i.e. below 20%), unless there is no personal or family history of any bleeding complication. FFP should be readily available at surgery for infusion in case of a bleeding emergency. Factor XI has a half-life of 60 to 80 h; 10 ml plasma/kg per day is usually adequate for maintaining haemostasis. Prophylactic therapy for most surgery includes replacement of factor XI with plasma at a loading dose of 15 ml/kg followed by 3 to 6 ml/kg every 24 h. The protective level for surgical prophylaxis is suggested as 45% for major surgery and 30% for minor surgery.

Antifibrinolytic therapy with ε-aminocaproic may be a helpful adjunct to plasma therapy; however, antifibrinolytics should be avoided in patients with haematuria or bleeding in the bladder because of possible obstruction by clots.

Deficiencies of proteins in the tissue factor and common pathways

The autosomally inherited deficiencies of factors II, V, VII, and X result in bleeding diatheses of varying severity. Such deficiencies of coagulation factor correlate poorly with tests of *in vitro* factor activity; these are thus quite different disorders from haemophilia, in which *in vitro* assessment predicts the clinical phenotype very well. These factor deficiencies can best be assessed by an initial screen using the prothrombin time as a measurement of the tissue factor pathway. Although the APTT may be prolonged with deficiencies of factors II, V, and X, but not VII, the PT is most often much more sensitive.

Factors II, VII, and X, are structurally homologous containing a signal peptide, a propeptide region necessary for recognition by the post-translational modifying enzyme γ-glutamyl carboxylase, an intermolecular binding region (two epidermal growth factor (EGF) domains in factors VII, IX, and X and two kringle domains in the prothrombin molecule), and a catalytic domain in the C-terminal of the molecule.

Deficiency of prothrombin (factor II) results from a lack of prothrombin or a malfunctional prothrombin protein. Deficiencies result in haemorrhagic manifestations. All reported patients with a prothrombin deficiency retain some prothrombin, suggesting that complete prothrombin deficiency is incompatible with life. This is consistent with the knockout mouse model which results in embryonic lethality at 9.5 to 11.5 days postcoitum in over 50% of fetuses; however, for some unknown reason, some murine fetuses are able to survive to birth but promptly die within 2 days due to haemorrhage. Patients with heterozygous prothrombin deficiency most commonly D̲e̲r̲b̲y̲ ̲H̲o̲s̲p̲i̲t̲a̲l̲s̲ ̲N̲H̲S̲ ̲F̲o̲u̲n̲d̲a̲t̲i̲o̲n̲ ing. Bleeding manifestations include easy bruising, soft-tissue haemorrhage, excessive postoperative bleeding, epistaxis, and menorrhagia in women. Haemarthroses are uncommon.

Congenital disease is characterized by a lifelong and a family bleeding history. Levels of 20 to 30% prothrombin normally prevent symptomatic bleeding. When necessary, administration of plasma is recommended at doses of 15 to 20 ml/kg followed by 3 ml/kg every 12 to 24 h. Prothrombin complex concentrates can be administered for serious bleeds and as a prophylactic before surgery. Transmission of viral disease and thromboembolic phenomena are risks of the administration of prothrombin complex concentrates.

Factor V deficiency occurs in fewer than one in a million individuals. Approximately 20% of the body's factor V reserve resides in the platelets. Thus, it is not surprising that patients with factor V deficiency tend to have mucosal bleeding manifestations including epistaxis, gastrointestinal bleeds, and menorrhagia in women. Haemarthroses, although a possible complaint, are much less common than in haemophilia. Mild to moderate bleeding may be treated by raising the factor V activity to about 20% of normal with a plasma dose of approximately 15 to 20 ml/kg followed by 3 to 6 ml/kg every 24 h. Because of the large amount of factor V stored in α granules, platelet transfusions may be an appropriate therapy. However, patients should be monitored for the possibility of generation of antiplatelet antibodies.

Factor VII deficiency presents as a variable bleeding disorder ranging from mild to severe, with a possibility of fatal intracranial haemorrhage. Patients with homozygous or compound heterozygous mutations manifest symptoms similar to those of a patient with haemophilia. However, unlike the correlation between activity levels and severity of disease in haemophilia, the *in vitro* factor VII activity clotting test provides only a relative indication of possible disease manifestations. Manifestations include haemarthrosis, arthropathies, haematoma formation, and retroperitoneal bleeding. Fatal intracranial haemorrhage is estimated to occur in approximately 16% of patients with severe disease. Levels below 10% activity most often result in bleeding manifestations. Therapy includes replacement of factor VII levels to 10 to 25% for patients undergoing most types of surgery. Treatment options include plasma at 5 to 10 ml/kg for 6 to 12 h for 1 to 2 days for minor episodes. For surgery, the recommended dose is administration of 15 to 20 ml/kg followed by maintenance doses of 3 to 6 ml/kg every 12 h.

Prothrombin complex concentrates may frequently be used to supply the factor VII along with the other vitamin K-dependent proteins. Although thrombogenicity has not been a recent problem, this does remain a potential complication.

In July 2005, recombinant coagulation factor VIIa (NovoSeven) was officially approved in the United States of America for treating patients with factor VII deficiency. Intravenous doses of 15–30 µg/kg are therapeutically effective in this setting for acute bleeds, a significantly lower dose than that used for treatment of haemophilia patients with inhibitors. However, the possible development of a factor VII inhibitor must be considered, as this has been reported. The product is administered every 2 h for prophylaxis during surgery for the first 24 h, then reduced to every 3 h 24 to 48 h postoperatively, and then further reduced according to patient symptomatology and necessity, depending on the risk of bleeding into the surgical site.

Factor X deficiency may present with symptomatology similar to that of a patient with severe haemophilia. Haemarthroses, soft tissue haemorrhages, retroperitoneal bleed, central nervous system haemorrhages, pseudotumours, and menorrhagia may occur.

Therapy with FFP includes a loading dose of 10 to 15 ml/kg followed by approximately 50% of that at 24 h.

Deficiency of the contact activating factors, factor XIII, and fibrinogen

Although the APTT is grossly prolonged (often >150 s) with deficiencies of the contact activating factors—factor XII, high-molecular-weight kininogen, and prekallikrein—these deficiencies are not associated with bleeding manifestations and will not be covered further here.

Factor XIII deficiency often presents shortly after birth with bleeding of the umbilical cord. Patients with clinical manifestations typically have factor levels of less than 1%. Factor XIII is a transglutaminase that cross-links fibrin monomers, thus stabilizing a forming fibrin clot. Patients with deficiency of factor XIII therefore have delayed wound healing and often suffer from soft tissue haemorrhages, haemarthroses, haematomas, and excessive bleeding from poorly healed wounds. Up to 25% of individuals deficient in factor XIII may experience intracranial bleeding. For unknown reasons, affected men may have oligospermia and affected women may suffer from repeated spontaneous abortions. Since routine clotting tests are normal in factor XIII deficiency, a physician must specifically request a test for factor XIII deficiency which entails a clot solubility test using 2% chloroacetic acid on a formed clot. Treatment of factor XIII deficiency involves administration of small amounts of factor XIII required to minimize bleeding complications. Prophylaxis includes using 2 to 3 ml/kg of FFP every 4 to 6 weeks or one bag of cryoprecipitate per 10 to 20 kg every 3 to 4 weeks. To prevent spontaneous abortions, products containing factor XIII can be administered every 14 to 21 days.

Afibrinogenaemia may cause dangerous haemorrhagic episodes. However, it is somewhat surprising that the mutation does not lead to embryonic death in light of the fact that the blood is incoagulable *in vitro*. The lack of necessity for fibrinogen during fetal development is supported by the viable fibrinogen knockout mouse model. Prolonged bleeding from the umbilical cord often permits early recognition of an affected child. The leading cause of death in afibrinogaemia is intracranial haemorrhage. Haemorrhages from mucous membranes occur frequently, and haemarthroses occur in approximately 20% of patients. Pregnancy-related problems include first-trimester abortion, placental abruption, and postpartum bleeding complications and may be markedly reduced by administration of fibrinogen. However, fibrinogen replacement may cause thromboembolic phenomena. The target fibrinogen level for replacement therapy is approximately 50 to 100 mg/dl. One bag of cryoprecipitate contains approximately 250 mg of fibrinogen; thus dosing of cryoprecipitate usually necessitates 5 to 10 bags per 70-kg person. Therapeutic complications include allergic reactions and the development of antifibrinogen antibodies. Thromboembolic phenomena may occur in conjunction with fibrinolytic inhibitors or oral contraceptives.

Dysfibrinogaemia results from a functional deficiency of fibrinogen associated with a malfunctional molecule, although some degree of antigen remains present. Approximately 55% of patients with dysfibrinogaemia remain asymptomatic, 25% have a bleeding tendency, and 20% may experience thrombotic episodes ranging from mild to fatal events.

Numerous combined deficiencies have been described; the underlying mutation for several of these combined deficiencies has been determined. Combined deficiency of the two structurally similar proteins factor V and factor VIII is an autosomal recessively inherited disorder of variable bleeding severity. The mechanism responsible for the disorder results from mutations in either LMAN1 (ERGIC-53), or MCFD2; these two proteins together form a Ca^{2+} dependent cargo receptor. LMAN1 is a 53-kDa transmembrane component of the endoplasmic reticulum-Golgi intermediate compartment, while MCFD2 is a soluble protein that interacts with 1:1 stoichiometry in complex with LMAN1. Mutations at this site are associated with factor levels of 4 to 30% of normal factor V and factor VIII activity and generally show mucocutaneous and postsurgical bleeding of a severity similar to that seen in individuals with a single protein deficiency at the same level. Other combined deficiencies for which a genetic mechanism has been described include deficiency of factors II, VII, IX, and X caused by a mutation in the γ-glutamyl carboxylase gene, required for a critical post-translational modification in vitamin K-dependent factors.

Hypercoagulable disease due to deficiencies of anticoagulant

Pathological diseases resulting from inappropriate clot formation in either the arterial or venous circulation are a major cause of morbidity in developed countries. The genetic contribution to this pathophysiology, particularly to thrombosis in the arterial circulation, is not well understood. Clearly cardiovascular disease represents a complex multifactorial process. The contribution of genetic causes to venous thrombotic disease is better understood; it may be associated with either an isolated deficiency of an anticoagulant protein, a malfunctional procoagulant protein, or a combination of these processes. The functional deficiencies become particularly relevant during times of increased environmental stress such as in the puerperium or in postsurgical, traumatic, or immobilized states. In addition to deficiency states, several common mutations involving a gain of function have also been described which can disrupt the delicate balance of coagulation by shifting the balance toward greater procoagulant function.

Procoagulant and anticoagulant plasma proteins interact with platelets and cellular phospholipids to promote physiological coagulation. Regulation of the formation of thrombin is the key step in the proper balance between pro- and anticoagulant functions. Anticoagulant proteins are particularly important in areas where there may be prolonged exposure of procoagulant factors and platelet phospholipids to the vessel wall, predisposing an individual to thrombotic disease. Deficiencies of anticoagulant proteins thus place a patient at an increased risk for thrombosis in the slowly flowing venous circulation. In the rapidly flowing arterial circulation, laminar flow largely prevents prolonged interaction between platelets and vessel walls.

The principal anticoagulant proteins that keep the procoagulant proteins in check include thrombomodulin, tissue factor pathway inhibitor, antithrombin III, protein C, and protein S. Thrombomodulin, an integral membrane protein expressed by endothelial cells, plays a key role in tempering the action of thrombin. Despite attempts to discover mutations in the thrombomodulin gene, only rare reports have implicated thrombomodulin in the pathophysiology of disease, although some recent studies suggest the existence of polymorphic regulation variants in the promoter region. Recently, a mutation in the small but critical protein known as tissue factor pathway inhibitor, which inhibits procoagulant function by binding to factor Xa either alone or in association with tissue factor–factor VIIa, has been suggested to be associated with a ninefold increased risk of venous thrombosis.

Deficiencies leading to a hypercoagulable state are most frequently caused by deficiencies of antithrombin III, protein C, and protein S. These anticoagulant deficiencies result from either a quantitative deficiency (type I) or a qualitative deficiency (type II). Deficiencies of any of these factors may cause life-threatening deep venous thromboses and pulmonary emboli, or may be asymptomatic. Clinical presentation relates to physical sequelae in the affected organ. In addition to deep venous thromboses and pulmonary emboli, symptomatology may include superficial thrombophlebitis, mesenteric vein thrombosis, and cerebral vein thrombosis.

Antithrombin III deficiency

A deficiency of antithrombin III was the first anticoagulant protein deficiency described which was associated with an increased risk of thrombosis. Antithrombin III is a 60-kDa glycoprotein found at high concentrations in the plasma—150 μg/ml: approximately 15- to 30-fold higher than that of many other pro- and anticoagulant proteins. Antithrombin III primarily inhibits thrombin but also inhibits factors IXa, Xa, XIa, XIIa, kallikrein, and plasmin. The ability to inhibit thrombin requires interaction with heparin, which increases the inhibitory activity several thousandfold. Historically, the risk of thrombosis in individuals deficient in antithrombin III has been thought to be higher than that seen with deficiencies of protein S or protein C, or than that seen with increased functionality of the procoagulant proteins factor V and prothrombin. Clearly the influences of gene–gene and gene–environment interactions contribute to this risk. A normal activity range for most procoagulant/anticoagulant proteins may be as low as 50%. However, the critical requirement for antithrombin III can be surmised from the 80% lower limit of a normal antithrombin III level, significantly higher than that for other coagulation proteins. This makes the diagnosis of antithrombin III deficiency particularly difficult in the post-thrombotic period when patients frequently have lower levels of antithrombin III due either to consumption of antithrombin III during clot formation or to the decreased function seen with heparin administration. Additionally, the presence of homozygous disease of antithrombin III deficiency has only been reported with rare type II deficiencies resulting from impaired heparin binding mutations. No homozygous type I deficiencies have been reported, probably because of their incompatibility with life.

The frequency of antithrombin III deficiency in patients with thrombophilia varies widely between studies. The cause of these differing frequencies has recently been carefully addressed by van Boven and colleagues. Their study clearly shows the strong influence of acquired and genetic factors which modulate the baseline risk due to one specific genetic mutation, highlighting the role of additional factors when combined with genetics. In thrombophilic family studies, the risk of thrombosis is 20 times greater than in control populations. The most frequent presentation is deep venous thrombosis with a pulmonary embolism, particularly after an inciting environmental influence such as surgery or immobilization in men or the start of oral contraceptives or pregnancy/postpartum in women. The average age of first onset is 33 years. In patients deficient in antithrombin III without a known acquired risk, the rate of incidence of thrombosis is less than 1% per year.

Therapy for antithrombin III deficiency includes prophylactic treatment with warfarin, low molecular weight heparin, and treatment of an acute event with heparin or another anticoagulant therapy, for example administration of a fibrinolytic agent in the patient presenting early enough during an acute episode. Antithrombin III concentrate may be administered for therapy of deficiency during an acute event or as a prophylactic treatment to prevent further disease.

Deficiencies of proteins C and S

Deficiencies of proteins C and S present with thrombotic manifestations similar to those seen with antithrombin III deficiency. However, in protein C deficiency an additional condition includes warfarin-induced skin necrosis and dangerously life-threatening purpura fulminans in the homozygous or compound heterozygous protein C deficient neonate. A diagnosis of protein C deficiency is found in approximately 33% of individuals with warfarin-induced skin necrosis, a condition which may lead to skin necrosis several days after initiation of warfarin therapy. The proposed mechanism for this condition is due to the earlier decrease in protein C compared with decreases in procoagulant proteins following initiation of warfarin therapy (due to the short half-life of protein C, c.6 h). It is thus 'normal' clinical practice to begin warfarin only after a patient has first been anticoagulated with heparin or another immediately-acting anticoagulant therapy.

Protein C acts in concert with its cofactor protein S to inactivate the active forms of the procoagulant cofactors, factors Va and VIIIa. Protein C is a vitamin K-dependent serine protease structurally similar to factors VII, IX, and X. Protein S is also vitamin K-dependent because of conserved N-terminus but lacks enzymatic function because of the existence of a sex-hormone binding globulin domain instead of a catalytic domain at the C-terminus. Thrombin activates protein C to activated protein C when bound to thrombomodulin, a protein which acts like an endothelial cell receptor for thrombin. Symptomatic manifestations of protein C or protein S deficiencies are similar to that of antithrombin III deficiency. Deep venous thrombosis with or without pulmonary embolism occurs in 50% of patients by the age of 30 to 45, depending on the study population. Environmental and gene–gene interactions are particularly important. As with antithrombin III deficiency, superficial thrombophlebitis, cerebral vein thrombosis, and mesenteric vein thrombosis are all possible complications. Postphlebitic syndrome presents as a complication after deep venous thrombosis in up to 50% of patients.

Factor V Leiden and the prothrombin 20210 mutation

Since 1994, two additional common mutations have been described leading to an increased risk of thrombosis. These mutations, unlike the anticoagulant protein deficiencies, are due to gain of function mutations causing either an increased resistance to inactivation in factor V (factor V Leiden) or increased levels of a procoagulant protein (prothrombin) which results in higher levels of thrombin formation.

Activated protein C (APC) resistance was first described by Dahlback in a 42-year-old man with a history of recurrent thromboses. Dahlback noted an absence of prolongation of the APTT, found after addition of APC, which is normally prolonged due to inactivation of factors Va and VIIIa. Soon thereafter, Poort and colleagues identified a single mutation as the principal cause of APC resistance in the vast majority (over 90%) of patients. The mutation leads to a decreased ability of APC to inactivate the cofactor Va due to an amino acid substitution (arginine for glutamine) at a critical hydrolysis point in the factor Va protein normally enabling inactivation.

Other non-factor-V Leiden causes of APC resistance include a haplotype in the factor V molecule, the H2 haplotype.

Factor V Leiden leads to thrombotic disease as described for hypercoagulable states due to deficiencies of anticoagulant protein. Because of the extremely high incidence of factor V Leiden in the white population (c.5%), gene–gene interactions play a particularly important role in manifestation of disease. It should be noted that the frequency of factor V Leiden in most nonwhite populations is low.

The prothrombin 20210 mutation reported in 1996 results in an increased concentration of prothrombin, also tipping the balance towards excess thrombin formation. The cause of this increase is associated with a guanine to adenine mutation at the last base of the 3′ untranslated region in the factor V gene. The mechanism by which this influences prothrombin levels is thought to be posttranscriptional.

Vitamin K epoxide reductase complex, subunit 1

The gene encoding vitamin K epoxide reductase (VKOR), the enzyme that completes the vitamin K cycle, was identified in 2004. VKOR converts vitamin K 2,3-epoxide to the enzymatically activated form. The gene was identified by two distinct techniques, a traditional positional cloning approach and a novel siRNA-aided functional screen of the predicted locus on chromosome 16. VKOR is a multisubunit complex; VKOR complex, subunit 1, (VKORC1) is a 163-amino-acid integral membrane protein (18 kDa) highly expressed in the liver. The oral anticoagulant warfarin, used in the prophylaxis of acute and chronic thromboembolic conditions, inhibits the action of vitamin-K dependent proteins. Pharmacogenetics-based dosing algorithms based on VKORC1 genotyping have been developed to account for inter-individual variation in patient response to warfarin. Additionally, differences in warfarin metabolism, largely based on variant cytochrome P450 complex alleles, are under evaluation for initiation of warfarin dosing.

Further reading

General articles about coagulation

Bin Zhang et al. (2008). Genotype-phenotype correlation in combined deficiency of factor V and factor VIII. Blood, 111, 5592–600.

Colman RW, et al. (2006). Overview of hemostasis. In: Colman RW, et al. (eds) Thrombosis and hemorrhage. J B Lippincott, Philadelphia.

Davie EW, Ratnoff OD (1964). Waterfall sequence for intrinsic blood clotting. Science, 145, 1310–12.

Gage BF, Lesko LJ (2008). Pharmacogenetics of warfarin: regulatory, scientific, and clinical issues. J Thromb Thrombolysis, 25, 45–51.

Li T, et al. (2004). Identification of the gene for vitamin K epoxide reductase. Nature, 427, 493–4.

Nichols WC, et al. (1998). Mutations in the ER-Golgi intermediate compartment protein ERGIC-53 cause combined deficiency of coagulation factors V and VIII. Cell, 93, 61–70.

Levy GG, et al. (2001). Mutations in a member of the ADAMTS gene family cause thrombotic thrombocytopenic purpura. Nature, 413, 488–94.

MacFarlane RG (1964). An enzyme cascade in the blood clotting mechanism and its function as a biochemical amplifier. Nature, 202, 498–9.

Roberts HR, Lozier JN (1992). New perspectives on the coagulation cascade. Hosp Pract, 27, 97–105, 109–12.

Haemophilia and von Willebrand's disease

Berntorp E, et al. (2006). Inhibitor treatment in haemophilias A and B: summary statement for the 2006 international consensus conference. Haemophilia, 12 Suppl 6, 1–7.

Bolton-Maggs PH (2006). Optimal haemophilia care versus the reality. *Br J Haematol*, **132**, 671–82.

Bolton-Maggs PH, *et al.* (2004). Evidence-based treatment of haemophilia. *Haemophilia*, **10** Suppl 4, 20–4.

Ota S, *et al.* (2007). Definitions for haemophilia prophylaxis and its outcomes: the Canadian consensus study. *Haemophilia*, **13**, 12–20.

Plug I, *et al.* (2006). Mortality and causes of death in patients with hemophilia, 1992–2001: a prospective cohort study. *J Thromb Haemost*, **4**, 510–16.

Ragni MV (2006). The hemophilias: factor VIII and factor IX deficiencies. In: Young N, Gerson S, High K (eds) *Clinical hematology*, Chapter 63, p. 814. Elsevier, Philadelphia.

Sadler JE, *et al.* (2006). Update on the pathophysiology and classification of von Willebrand disease: a report of the Subcommittee on von Willebrand Factor. *J Thromb Haemost*, **4**, 2103–14.

Administration of factor concentrates

Ewenstein BM, *et al.* (2004). Consensus recommendations for use of central venous access devices in haemophilia. *Haemophilia*, **10**, 629–48.

Federici AB, Mannucci PM (2007). Management of inherited von Willebrand disease in 2007. *Ann Med*, **39**, 346–58.

Manco-Johnson MJ, *et al.* (2007). Prophylaxis versus episodic treatment to prevent joint disease in boys with severe hemophilia. *N Engl J Med*, **357**, 535–44.

Yasunaga, H (2007). Risk of authoritarianism: fibrinogen-transmitted hepatitis C in Japan. *Lancet*, **370**, 2063–7.

Infectious diseases associated with haemophilia therapy

Ponte ML (2006). Insights into the management of emerging infections: regulating variant Creutzfeldt-Jakob disease transfusion risk in the UK and the US. *PLoS Med*, **3**, e34.

Posthouwer D, *et al.* (2006). Treatment of chronic hepatitis C in patients with haemophilia: a review of the literature. *Haemophilia*, **12**, 473–8.

Rumi MG, *et al.* (2004). Hepatitis C in haemophilia: lights and shadows. *Haemophilia*, **10** Suppl 4, 211–15.

Gene therapy in haemophilia

High KA (2005). Gene transfer for hemophilia: can therapeutic efficacy in large animals be safely translated to patients? *J Thromb Haemost, State of the Art 2005*, **3**, 1682.

Manno CS, *et al.* (2006). Successful transduction of liver in hemophilia by AAV-Factor IX and limitations imposed by the host immune response. *Nat Med*, **12**, 342.

Murphy SL, High KA (2008). Gene therapy for haemophilia. *Br J Haematol*, **140**, 479–87.

Nathwani AC, *et al.* (2006). Self-complementary adeno-associated virus vectors containing a novel liver-specific human factor IX expression cassette enable highly efficient transduction of murine and nonhuman primate liver. *Blood*, **107**, 2653.

Thrombotic disease

Bucciarelli P, Rosendaal FR, Tripodi A (1999). Risk of venous thromboembolism and clinical manifestations in carriers of antithrombin, protein C, protein S deficiency, or activated protein C resistance: a multicenter collaborative family study. *Arterioscl, Thromb, Vasc Biol*, **19**, 1026–33.

Mannucci, PM (2005). Laboratory detection of inherited thrombophilia: a historical perspective. *Semin Thromb Hemost*, **31**, 5–10.

Moake JL (2004). Thrombotic thrombocytopenic purpura: survival by 'giving a dam'. *Trans Am Clin Climatol Assoc*, **115**, 201–19.

Nicolaes GA, Dahlbäck B (2003). Congenital and acquired activated protein C resistance. *Semin Vasc Med*, **3**, 33–46.

Genetic databases:

Ensembl. http://www.ensembl.org [A collaborative effort between the Wellcome Trust Sanger Institute and EMBL's European Bioinformatics Institute.]

National Center for Biotechnology Information (NCBI). http://www.ncbi.nlm.nih.gov/

UCSC Genome Browser. http://genome.ucsc.edu [Developed by an academic research group at the University of California Santa Cruz, United States of America.]

22.6.5 Acquired coagulation disorders

T.E. Warkentin

Essentials

Acquired disorders of coagulation may be the consequence of many underlying conditions, and although they may share abnormality of a coagulation test, e.g. a prolonged prothrombin time, their clinical effects are diverse and often opposing.

General clinical approach

Diagnosis—most acquired disorders of coagulation can be identified by screening haemostasis tests, including (1) prothrombin time (PT); (2) activated partial prothromboplastin time (aPTT); (3) thrombin clotting time (TCT); (4) fibrinogen degradation products (FDPs); (5) the cross-linked fibrin assay (D-dimer); (6) protamine sulphate paracoagulation assay; (7) bleeding time—now rarely required or performed; and (8) complete blood count with examination of a blood film. Few bleeding disorders give normal results in all these tests, but disorders predisposed to thrombosis as a result of deficiency of natural anticoagulants (e.g. antithrombin III, protein C, protein S) must be specifically sought.

Treatment—patients with coagulopathies who are bleeding or who require surgery are usually treated with blood products such as platelets and fresh frozen plasma. Other treatments used in particular circumstances include (1) vitamin K—required for the post-translational modification of factors II, VII, IX, and X as well as the anticoagulant factors, protein C and protein S; (2) cryoprecipitate—used principally for the treatment of hypofibrinogenaemia; (3) concentrates of specific factors—used in isolated deficiencies, e.g. of factors VIII, IX, or VIIa; (4) protein C—available as an activated recombinant protein and approved for use in severe septicaemia; (5) antifibrinolytic agents—e.g. ε-aminocaproic acid and tranexamic acid; (6) desmopressin (1-desamino-8-D-arginine vasopressin, or DDAVP)—increases factor VIII and von Willebrand factor.

Prohaemorrhagic coagulation disorders

Vitamin K deficiency—most haemostatic factors are produced exclusively by the liver, including the vitamin K dependent factors II, VII, IX, and X, deficiency of which can be caused by (1) malabsorption of fat-soluble vitamins; (2) coumarin overanticoagulation—minor bleeding episodes occur in about 6 to 10% of patients per year and major bleeding episodes in 1 to 3%; (3) liver disease. Diagnosed by finding a disproportionately prolonged PT in an appropriate clinical setting.

Disseminated intravascular coagulation (DIC)—clinical manifestations range from generalized haemorrhage to widespread microvascular thrombosis, predisposing to multisystem organ dysfunction and limb necrosis. Initiated by numerous triggers, e.g. the extrinsic coagulation pathway or interleukin-6 in the context of systemic inflammation. May be caused by a wide variety of conditions, including trauma and shock, infection, obstetric complications, acute haemolysis, immunological disorders, and vascular anomalies. The presence of DIC is often indicated by abnormal coagulation tests associated with thrombocytopenia and red cell abnormalities on examination of the blood film: FDPs and D-dimers are significantly increased, and the protamine sulphate paracoagulation assay usually indicates abnormalities of clinical significance.

Immunoglobulin-mediated factor deficiency—(1) Acquired factor VIII deficiency—this is suggested by the occurrence of bleeding, either spontaneously or after minor trauma, in association with a prolonged aPTT and a normal PT, with mixing experiments with normal pooled plasma indicating the presence of an inhibitory antibody. The condition is of unknown cause in 50% of cases, with the remainder associated with other autoimmune disorders (e.g. systemic lupus erythematosus), lymphoid and other malignancies, penicillin treatment, or the postpartum state. Aside from treatment with DDAVP (mild bleeding) or purified human factor VIII (or VIIa) concentrates (severe bleeding), patients with high antibody titres may require immunosuppressive therapy, e.g. high dose intravenous immunoglobulin, rituximab. (2) Other acquired coagulation-factor deficiencies caused by antibodies.

Other acquired coagulation-factor deficiencies—these include (1) haemodilution and massive transfusion; (2) heparin and acquired heparin-like anticoagulants; (3) coagulopathies secondary to plasma-cell dyscrasias; (4) hyperfibrinolysis—which may be a result of thrombolytic therapy, malignancy, cardiopulmonary bypass procedures, or liver disease, and (5) heterogeneous coagulopathies induced by venoms (snake bites).

Prothrombotic coagulation disorders

Heparin-induced thrombocytopenia—caused by IgG antibodies which recognize complexes of platelet factor 4 and heparin, typically leading to a fall in platelet count 5 to 10 days after starting the drug (but more abruptly in patients who have recently been exposed to it). Thrombosis is caused by several factors, including activation of platelets and stimulation of tissue factor expression on endothelium and monocytes. Clinical manifestations include (1) venous thrombosis—e.g. deep vein thrombosis, pulmonary embolism; (2) arterial thrombosis—e.g. major limb artery thrombosis, stroke, myocardial infarction. Treatment includes stopping heparin and instituting alternative nonheparin anticoagulation, e.g. danaparoid, lepirudin, argatroban, fondaparinux. Coumarin therapy should be postponed until the platelet count has recovered, and heparin should usually be avoided in the future (exception: heparin use for cardiac surgery once antibodies are gone).

Adenocarcinoma-associated chronic disseminated intravascular coagulation—metastatic adenocarcinoma and other tumours may be associated with a prothrombotic state and large vessel thromboses. Tissue factor and prothrombotic cysteine proteases have been found in tumour extracts. Heparin is the preferred treatment.

Antiphospholipid antibody syndrome—caused by antibodies that are usually directed against protein cofactors such as β_2-glycoprotein I and prothrombin. Clinical manifestations include intermittent thromboses and (rarely, but most dramatically) sudden life-threatening arterial occlusions. Lupus anticoagulant activity is shown by demonstrating inhibition of phospholipid-dependent coagulation assays (most commonly by prolongation of the APTT), with antiphospholipid antibodies also detected by enzyme-immunoassay using purified phospholipids as the target antigen, e.g. anticardiolipin antibody assay. Most patients require long-term anticoagulation.

Other conditions associated with microvascular thrombosis—these include (1) thrombotic microangiopathy—e.g. thrombotic thrombocytopenic purpura; (2) coumarin-induced skin necrosis; (3) coumarin-induced venous limb gangrene; (4) purpura fulminans.

Introduction

A coagulopathy is a disorder associated with an abnormal coagulation assay result, such as a prolonged prothrombin time (PT) (often expressed as the international normalized ratio, or INR), activated partial thromboplastin time (APTT), or thrombin clotting time. Coagulopathies can be associated with either bleeding or thrombosis, and have many causes (Table 22.6.5.1). The importance of the clinical context is illustrated by two contrasting patient scenarios that have in common a prolonged INR (6.0; usual therapeutic range, 2.0–3.0) during oral anticoagulant therapy: one patient has a life-threatening intracranial *haemorrhage* complicating warfarin therapy given for a prosthetic heart valve; in contrast, another patient, who was treated for deep-vein thrombosis (DVT) complicating heparin-induced thrombocytopenia has the limb-threatening complication of warfarin-induced venous limb gangrene, caused by microvascular *thrombosis*.

Table 22.6.5.2 lists common screening tests for coagulopathy. Only a few bleeding disorders give normal results in all these tests (e.g. α_2-antiplasmin deficiency, factor XIII deficiency, type 2a von Willebrand's syndrome associated with aortic stenosis). A drawback of these assays is that only procoagulant haemostatic pathways are assessed. Thus, deficiency of a natural anticoagulant such as antithrombin or protein C must be determined by specific testing.

Agents for treating acquired disorders of coagulation

Blood products are usually indicated for the treatment of patients with coagulopathies who are bleeding or who require a major invasive procedure.

Fresh-frozen plasma (FFP)

FFP contains all the haemostatic factors at concentrations between 0.7 and 1.0 U/ml, is appropriate for liver disease, haemodilution from massive transfusion, disseminated intravascular coagulation (DIC), reversal of coumarin anticoagulation, and replacement of

Table 22.6.5.1 Coagulopathies that cause bleeding or thrombosis

Acquired coagulopathies	Comment
Prohaemorrhagic disorders	
Vitamin K deficiency or pharmacologic antagonism by coumarin	Reduced levels of vitamin K-dependent procoagulant factors (II (prothrombin), VII, IX, X)
Liver disease	Multiple factor deficiencies (although factor VIII levels are usually normal/elevated); low fibrinogen can indicate hyperfibrinolysis
Severe haemodilution/ massive transfusion	Multiple factor deficiencies; concomitant DIC in some patients
Acute DIC	Certain forms of DIC, e.g. acute head trauma, placental abruption, can lead to bleeding secondary to generalized coagulopathy, especially with fibrinogen depletion
Acquired coagulation factor inhibitor	Anti-VIII autoantibodies are most common
Heparins and related drugs	Marked APTT prolongation with heparin overdose (extreme overdose also prolongs INR); low-molecular-weight heparin overdose only minimally prolongs APTT
Heparin-like anticoagulants	Rare; associated with plasma cell disorders; minimal or no prolongation in APTT
Paraprotein-induced coagulopathies	See text and Box 22.6.5.2
Hyperfibrinolysis	Associated with prostate adenocarcinoma, advanced liver disease, post-thrombolytic therapy, post-cardiac surgery, or with aortic aneurysm
Snake envenomation	See text and Table 22.6.5.7
Prothrombotic disorders	
Heparin-induced thrombocytopenia	Strong association with venous and arterial thrombosis; about 10% to 20% of patients have decompensated DIC (elevated INR, low fibrinogen, and/or microangiopathic blood film)
Chronic DIC secondary to adenocarcinoma	Strong association with venous and arterial thrombosis; improves with (LMW) heparin; predisposes to coumarin-induced necrosis (see below)
Antiphospholipid syndrome	Prolonged APTT due to 'lupus anticoagulant' ('nonspecific inhibitor'); associated with venous and arterial thrombosis, spontaneous abortions, thrombocytopenia
Thrombotic microangiopathy	Thrombocytopenia and microangiopathic haemolysis (red cell fragmentation), platelet-vWf microthrombi within arterioles; elevated INR and APTT are occasionally seen
Coumarin-induced necrosis	Central skin or acral limb necrosis resulting from microvascular thrombosis; pathogenesis includes depletion of vitamin K-dependent natural anticoagulant, protein C
Purpura fulminans (symmetric peripheral gangrene)	Generalized areas of (sub)dermal necrosis associated with coagulopathy (neonatal, idiopathic, postvaricella, associated with septicaemia/DIC); symmetric peripheral gangrene refers to more localized syndrome affecting acral regions

Table 22.6.5.2 Screening haemostasis tests

Assay	Comment
Prothrombin time (PT), often expressed as international normalized ratio (INR)	Screen for deficiency of factors VII, X, V, II, and/ or fibrinogen (e.g. vitamin K deficiency/coumarin therapy, liver disease)
Activated partial thromboplastin time (APTT)	Screen for deficiency of factors VIII, IX, X, V, II, contact factors, and/or fibrinogen; monitor certain anticoagulants, e.g. heparin, lepirudin, argatroban
Thrombin clotting time (TT or TCT)	Screen for hypofibrinogenaemia and/or presence of heparin; some TCT assays are also sensitive to FDPs
Serum fibrin(ogen) degradation products (FDPs)	Requirement to clot blood sample can lead to false-positive results due to incomplete blood clotting (e.g. residual heparin)
Cross-linked fibrin assay (D-dimer)	Detects fibrin degradation products generated after thrombin, factor XIII, and plasmin have acted upon fibrinogen (marker for DIC and/or thrombosis)
Paracoagulation assay (e.g. protamine sulphate test)	Positive paracoagulation assay often means DIC is clinically significant and may require blood products or anticoagulant therapy
Bleeding time	Assesses primary haemostasis, i.e. vWF- mediated platelet adhesion to endothelium with secondary aggregation of platelets within haemostatic plug
Complete blood count; blood film examination	Platelet enumeration, and assessment of causes for thrombocytopenia, e.g. red cell fragments indicating microangiopathy

isolated factor deficiency (when specific factor replacement is unavailable). For a 70-kg adult with a 3-litre plasma volume, 1 litre of FFP will increase the coagulation factors by about 0.25 U/ml. In most patients, this should lead to levels greater than the minimum required for adequate haemostasis (>0.30 U/ml for most factors). Repeat FFP transfusion (e.g. 500 ml every 6 h) may be necessary if the haemostasis defect is ongoing. FFP is being supplanted by cryosupernatant as a replacement fluid for thrombotic thrombocytopenic purpura (TTP). Solvent-detergent-treated plasma, in which most blood-borne pathogens are inactivated (but not nonenveloped viruses such as hepatitis A, parvovirus B19, or the agent that causes Creutzfeldt–Jakob disease, a potential blood-borne pathogen), has become available recently, but is limited by its high cost.

Cryoprecipitate

This contains fibrinogen (0.10–0.25 g/unit), factors VIII and XIII, von Willebrand factor (VWF), and fibronectin. Its principal indication is the treatment of hypofibrinogenaemia, where it increases fibrinogen levels using just one-quarter of the volume of blood product compared with FFP. Cryoprecipitate is appropriate for patients with significant hypofibrinogenaemia, e.g. DIC, primary fibrinolysis, congenital hypofibrinogenaemia. For a bleeding patient whose fibrinogen level is about 0.5 g/l, 10 U of cryoprecipitate would probably increase the fibrinogen to above 1.0 g/l, although a lower than expected increment could occur if the patient had a higher volume of distribution (e.g. a cirrhotic patient with ascites).

Specific factor concentrates

These are available for use in patients with an isolated deficiency in certain factors, such as VIII or IX. Prothrombin complex concentrates contain the vitamin K-dependent factors, and are appropriate for the rapid reversal of severe coagulopathy related to coumarin use, or coagulopathy secondary to massive transfusion. Activated PCC (e.g. factor VIII inhibitor bypassing activity) and factor VIIa are other specialized concentrates with specific uses, for instance to manage a bleeding patient with an acquired factor VIII inhibitor. Certain other isolated factor deficiencies can be managed by specific factor concentrates, e.g. recombinant factor VIIa, factor XI, factor XIII, and fibrinogen. Protein C concentrates are available in some jurisdictions for treatment of congenital protein C deficiency, whereas recombinant activated protein C is approved for use in severe septicemia.

Pharmacological therapies

These include the antifibrinolytic agents ε-aminocaproic acid and tranexamic acid. ε-Aminocaproic acid and tranexamic acid bind to the lysine-binding sites of plasminogen; paradoxically, although increasing the susceptibility of plasminogen to proteolysis by plasminogen activator, these lysine analogues also prevent plasminogen from binding to fibrin, thus impeding fibrinolysis. Oral dosing for ε-aminocaproic acid is about 7 g (100 mg/kg) initially, followed by 3.5 g (50 mg/kg) every 4 h; similar doses are used for intravenous administration. For tranexamic acid, 1.0 to 1.5 g is given every 8 h by mouth; the dose is reduced to between 0.5 and 1.0 g every 8 h if given intravenously. Both drugs are available in 500-mg capsules. These drugs are appropriate for the treatment of hyperfibrinolysis, for instance bleeding following thrombolytic therapy or associated with cardiac or hepatic surgery. These drugs are generally contraindicated in patients with DIC, however, as blocking secondary fibrinolysis could lead to microvascular thrombosis.

Desmopressin

Desmopressin or 1-desamino-8-D-arginine vasopressin (DDAVP), a synthetic vasopressin analogue, leads to an increase in factor VIII and vWf levels that peak between 45 and 90 min after intravenous infusion (0.3 µg/kg in 50 ml normal saline over 20–30 min; maximum dose, 20 µg). Although repeat DDAVP can be given at 12- to 24-h intervals, the drug becomes less effective over time (tachyphylaxis) as endothelial stores of vWf are depleted, limiting the usual number of injections to no more than three with any treatment course. Flushing, tachycardia, mild hypotension, free-water retention (leading to dilutional hyponatraemia), and angina are occasional side effects.

Prohaemorrhagic acquired coagulation disorders

Vitamin K deficiency disorders

Vitamin K-dependent coagulation factors

Vitamin K is required for the post-translational modification of six haemostatic factors, four with procoagulant activity (factors II, VII, IX, and X), and two with anticoagulant activity (protein C, protein S). The physiological relevance of a seventh factor, factor Z, remains unclear. The enzyme vitamin K-dependent γ-glutamylcarboxylase adds a carboxyl group to each member of a cluster of glutamyl residues, thereby forming the γ-carboxyglutamyl residues crucial for enabling these six haemostatic factors to interact with phospholipid membranes in a calcium-dependent fashion. During this γ-carboxylation reaction, the reduced form of vitamin K is oxidized to vitamin K epoxide; oral anticoagulants inhibit the enzyme complex (vitamin K epoxide reductase complex) that regenerates the reduced form of vitamin K.

Diet and absorption of vitamin K

Vitamin K_1 (phylloquinone) is exclusively derived from plants; vitamin K_2 (menaquinone) is synthesized by bacteria. Green, leafy vegetables, such as broccoli, lettuce, cabbage, and spinach, are very good dietary sources of vitamin K (100–500 µg/100 mg). Vitamin K is fat-soluble, and absorption occurs primarily in the small bowel. Serum vitamin K concentrations are only between 150 and 800 pg/ml and, as hepatic storage is limited (half-life is just a few days), a regular daily intake of about 0.1 to 0.5 µg/kg is required. Although bacterial synthesis is not a major source of vitamin K in humans, antibiotic treatment nevertheless predisposes to vitamin K deficiency.

Vitamin K deficiency

Malabsorption of fat-soluble vitamins caused by biliary tract disease, or primary bowel disorders such as coeliac or inflammatory bowel disease, can cause vitamin K deficiency. An inadequate diet, particularly when combined with antibiotic therapy, is another cause. Indeed, coagulopathy can arise during a brief period of decreased intake, e.g. 1 week postoperatively.

A disproportionately prolonged PT/INR in the appropriate clinical setting suggests vitamin K deficiency (Table 22.6.5.3). The diagnosis is usually confirmed by assessing the response to vitamin K administration. Compared with the treatment of a coumarin overdose, small amounts of vitamin K are effective, e.g. 1 mg vitamin K_1 given orally or by slow intravenous infusion (over at least 30 min to minimize risk of an anaphylactoid reaction). For serious bleeding, FFP or especially prothrombin complex concentrates provides a more rapid (but transient) correction of the coagulopathy.

Coumarin overanticoagulation

Oral anticoagulants (e.g. coumarins such as warfarin and phenprocoumon) are widely used to prevent and treat thrombosis via their vitamin K antagonism. An INR target range between 2.0 and 3.0 is appropriate for most clinical indications, although a higher therapeutic range (INR 2.5–3.5) is appropriate for patients at very high risk for thrombosis (e.g. with mechanical prosthetic heart valves).

Bleeding is the major complication of coumarin, with minor and major bleeding episodes occurring in about 6 to 10% and 1 to 3% of patients per year respectively; the intracranial haemorrhage rate is between 0.25 and 1% per year. Changes in diet or alcohol consumption, poor patient compliance, and the introduction of new drugs (Table 22.6.5.4) can cause bleeding by producing coumarin overanticoagulation. In contrast, recurrent gastrointestinal or urinary tract bleeding at therapeutic levels of anticoagulation often indicates an occult gastrointestinal or renal lesion, respectively.

The treatment of nontherapeutic (elevated) INRs depends on the clinical setting (Table 22.6.5.5). Oral vitamin K_1 use is appropriate in many nonurgent conditions as it avoids the risk of anaphylactoid reactions to intravenous use, and has more predictable effects than subcutaneous injection. Much larger and prolonged vitamin K dosing (100–150 mg/day) is required to treat accidental

Table 22.6.5.3 Results of screening haemostasis assays in various clinical settings

	PT/INR	APTT	Fibrinogen	TCT	FDPs	Platelets
Vitamin K deficiency or antagonism (coumarin)	↑↑	↑	N	N	N	N
Liver disease	↑, ↑↑	N, ↑	↓, N, ↑	N, ↑	N, ↑, ↑↑	N, ↓, ↓↓
Heparin	N, sl↑	↑↑	N	↑↑	N	N, ↓
LMWH, danaparoid	N	N, sl↑	N	N, sl↑	N	N
Thrombin inhibitors	N, ↑	↑, ↑↑	N	↑↑	N	N
Thrombolytic	sl↑	N	↓, ↓↓	↑, ↑↑	↑	N, ↓
Renal disease	N	N	N	N	N	N, sl↓
Acute DIC	↑, ↑↑	↑, ↑↑	N, ↓, ↓↓	N, ↑, ↑↑	↑, ↑↑a	↓, ↓↓
Chronic DIC	N, ↑	N, sl↑	N, ↓	N, ↑	↑, ↑↑a	N, ↓, ↓↓
Primary fibrinolysis	N, sl↑	N, sl↑	↓, ↓↓	↑, ↑↑a	↑, ↑↑a	↓, N
Lupus anticoagulant	N, ↑	N, ↑, ↑↑	N	N	N	N, ↓
Factor VIII inhibitor	N	↑, ↑↑	N	N	N	N
Haemodilution	↑	↑, ↑↑	↓, ↓↓	↑, ↑↑	N	↓

a Cross-linked fibrin degradation products (D-dimer) are greater in patients with DIC, compared with primary fibrinolysis.

or deliberate overdoses of long-acting second-generation rodenticides ('superwarfarins'), such as brodifacoum.

Liver disease

Most haemostatic factors are produced exclusively by the liver. Exceptions include factor VIII (hepatic and extrahepatic synthesis), vWf (endothelium, megakaryocytes), and several factors produced by endothelium (e.g. plasminogen activator, plasminogen activator inhibitor type I (PAI-1)). Box 22.6.5.1 lists the multiple effects on haemostasis caused by liver disease. Often, bleeding is primarily related to anatomical factors, such as oesophageal varices or gastric/duodenal ulcers, though reduced hepatic synthesis of coagulation factors can be a contributing factor. Increased susceptibility to DIC via superadded illness (e.g. bacterial peritonitis), impaired clearance of activated coagulation factors, and hyperfibrinolysis are other factors.

A prolonged PT/INR is the most frequent laboratory abnormality (Table 22.6.5.3). The fibrinogen level is usually normal or increased; when hypofibrinogenaemia occurs, it generally indicates severe liver disease or hyperfibrinolysis. Fibrin(ogen)-degradation product (FDP) and D-dimer levels are often increased; thus, the laboratory picture can resemble that of DIC even in a patient who is otherwise clinically stable.

Management of hepatic coagulopathy should include a trial of vitamin K_1 (e.g. 10 mg once daily for 3 days), although this will not benefit most patients. FFP should be given to bleeding patients with a prolonged INR, or who require major invasive procedures. Retrospective studies suggest that minor invasive procedures (e.g. paracentesis, pleurocentesis) can usually be performed safely with an INR as high as 1.8. For patients suspected to have significant fibrinolysis, antifibrinolytic therapy can be tried. Prothrombin complex concentrates should only be used in emergencies, given their prothrombotic potential in this group of patients. Platelet transfusions usually provide minimal increase in the platelet count in patients with platelet sequestration caused by hypersplenism. DDAVP improves haemostasis in patients with prolonged bleeding time secondary to hepatic platelet dysfunction.

Haemodilution and massive transfusion

Coagulopathies occur in most patients who receive crystalloids, colloids, or red cell concentrates following trauma, surgery, or fluid resuscitation for other major illnesses. In many patients, no bleeding results despite moderate abnormalities in the INR, APTT, thrombin clotting time, and platelet count. The reason is that all the individual coagulation factors remain at haemostatically effective levels, even though the laboratory assays are abnormal when all the factor levels are uniformly reduced.

Massive transfusion is defined as the transfusion of blood products equivalent to the patient's total blood volume within 24 h. Red cell concentrates do not provide significant amounts of platelets or coagulation factors. Thus infusions of platelets, FFP, and, sometimes, cryoprecipitate are often needed as well. Although 'formulas' to guide transfusion therapy have been devised, individualized assessment that takes into account clinically evident bleeding, risk factors for haemorrhage, supervening DIC or fibrinolysis, acute liver insult, and laboratory test results, is preferable.

Disseminated intravascular coagulation (DIC)

DIC is a group of clinicopathological syndromes characterized by widespread activation of coagulation; there results intravascular generation of thrombin, formation of fibrin, and reactive fibrinolysis. Clinical consequences range from coagulation factor and platelet depletion, resulting in generalized haemorrhage, to widespread microvascular thrombosis, predisposing to multisystem organ dysfunction or limb necrosis. 'Acute' DIC, caused by septicaemia, trauma, and obstetrical complications, is most frequent; 'chronic' DIC, typically caused by malignancy, is often associated with a dramatic hypercoagulable state (Table 22.6.5.6). Although DIC is usually a systemic process, sometimes a localized abnormality (such as a vascular malformation or aortic aneurysm) leads to the regional activation of coagulation and resulting in the depletion of haemostatic factors.

DIC is usually triggered by the extrinsic coagulation pathway: tissue factor and factor VIIa (Fig. 22.6.5.1). The proinflammatory cytokine interleukin-6 (IL-6) is a principal mediator of DIC

Table 22.6.5.4 Drugs, food, and dietary supplement interactions with warfarin by level of supporting evidence and direction of interaction

Potentiation of warfarin's anticoagulant effect	Inhibition of warfarin's anticoagulant effect
Antimicrobials: amoxicillin/clavulanate[a], azithromycin[a], ciprofloxacin[a], clarithromycin[a], cotrimoxazole[a], erythromycin[b], fluconazole[b], isoniazid[b], itraconazole[a], levofloxacin[a], metronidazole[b], miconazole[b], tetracycline[a], voriconazole[b]	*Antimicrobials*: dicloxacillin[a], griseofulvin[b], nafcillin[b], ribavirin[b], rifampin[b]
Cardiovascular: amiodarone[b], aspirin[a], clofibrate[b], diltiazem[b], fenofibrate[b], fluvastatin[a], propafenone[b], propranolol[b], quinidine[a], ropinirole[a], simvastatin[a], sulfinpyrazone (biphasic with later inhibition)[b]	*Cardiovascular*: bosentan[a], cholestyramine[b]
Analgesics/anti-inflammatory: acetaminophen[a], aspirin[a], celecoxib[a], dextropropoxyphene[a], interferon[a], phenylbutazone[b], piroxicam[b], tramadol[a]	*Analgesics/anti-inflammatory*: azathioprine[a], mesalamine[b]
CNS drugs: alcohol (if concomitant liver disease)[b], chloral hydrate[a], citalopram[b], disulfiram[a], entacapone[b], fluvoxamine[a], phenytoin (biphasic with later inhibition)[a], sertraline[b]	*CNS drugs*: barbiturates[b], carbamazepine[b], chlordiazepoxide[a]
Food and herbal supplements: boldo-funugreek[b], danshen[a], don quai[a], fish oil[b], grapefruit[a], lyceum barbarum L[a], mango[b], PC-SPES[a], quilinggao[b]	*Food and herbal supplements*: avocado[b], ginseng[a], high vitamin K content foods and enteral feeds[b], multivitamin supplement[a], soy milk[a]
Miscellaneous: anabolic steroids[b], cimetidine[b], fluorouracil[a], gemcitabine[a], levamisole/fluorouracil[a], omeprazole[b], paclitaxel[a], tamoxifen[a], tolterodine[a], zileuton[b]	*Miscellaneous*: chelation therapy[a], influenza vaccine[a], mercaptopurine[b], raloxifene[a], sucralfate[a]

CNS, central nervous system

Level of causation: [a] probable, [b] highly probable. See Ansell *et al.* (2008) for other drugs for which level of causation is listed as 'possible' and 'highly improbable'.

Modified from Ansell J, *et al.* (2008). The pharmacology and management of the vitamin K antagonists. The Eighth ACCP Conference on Antithrombotic and Thrombolytic Therapy. *Chest*, **133** (Suppl), 160–98S.

Table 22.6.5.5 Management of non-therapeutic INRs or bleeding in patients receiving vitamin K antagonists

Clinical situation*	Guidelines[a]
INR above the therapeutic range but <5.0, no significant bleeding	Lower dose or omit dose [of vitamin K antagonist, e.g. warfarin]; monitor more frequently and resume at lower dose when INR therapeutic; if only minimally above therapeutic range, no dose reduction may be required.
INR >5.0 but <9.0, no significant bleeding	Omit next one or two doses, monitor more frequently, and resume at an appropriately adjusted dose when INR in therapeutic range.
	Alternatively, omit dose and give vitamin K (1–2.5 mg po), particularly if at increased risk of bleeding.
	If more rapid reversal is required because the patient requires urgent surgery, vitamin K (≤5 mg po) can be given with the expectation that a reduction of the INR will occur in 24 h. If the INR is still high, additional vitamin K (1–2 mg po) can be given.
INR >9.0, no clinically significant bleeding	Hold warfarin therapy and give higher dose of vitamin K (2.5–5 mg po) with the expectation that the INR will be reduced substantially in 24–48 h. Monitor more frequently and use additional vitamin K if necessary. Resume therapy at an appropriately adjusted dose when INR is therapeutic.
Serious bleeding at any elevation of INR	Hold warfarin therapy and given vitamin K (10 mg by slow IV infusion), supplemented with FFP, PCC, or rVIIa, depending on the urgency of the situation; vitamin K can be repeated q12h.
Life-threatening bleeding	Hold warfarin therapy and give FFP, PCC, or rVIIa supplemented with vitamin K (10 mg by slow IV infusion). Repeat, if necessary, depending on INR.
Administration of vitamin K	In patients with mild to moderately elevated INRs without major bleeding, given vitamin K orally rather than subcutaneously.

* If continuing warfarin therapy is indicated after high doses of vitamin K$_1$ then heparin or LMWH can be given until the effects of vitamin K have been reversed, and the patient becomes responsive to warfarin therapy. It should be noted that INR values >4.5 are less reliable than values in or near the therapeutic range. Thus, these guidelines represent an approximate guide for high INRs.

[a] Guidelines as given by the Eight American College of Physicians Conference on Antithrombotic Therapy (2008).

IV, intravenous , FFP, fresh frozen plasma; PCC, prothrombin complex concentrate; rVIIa, recombinant factor VIIa.

in septicaemia and other systemic inflammatory responses, and impairs natural anticoagulant and fibrinolytic pathways. For example, a sustained increase in PAI-1 impairs plasmin formation despite intravascular fibrin generation.

Diagnostic and treatment approach to DIC

One or more prolonged clotting times and thrombocytopenia in a patient with one of the disorders listed in Table 22.6.5.6 suggests DIC. However, similar test results are seen in patients following major surgery, emphasizing the need to interpret the laboratory data in the appropriate clinical context. Typically, cross-linked fibrin degradation products (D-dimers) are significantly increased in DIC. The protamine sulphate 'paracoagulation' test, based on visual detection of gelling of patient plasma after the addition of protamine sulphate, is a rapid test for fibrin monomers; the lower sensitivity of the test is helpful, as a positive result usually indicates clinically significant DIC associated with bleeding or thrombosis. Sometimes, specialized haemostasis assays are useful, e.g. protein C activity levels in purpura fulminans.

The cornerstone of management is treating its underlying cause and providing supportive measures. For bleeding patients, replacement of depleted haemostatic factors with FFP, cryoprecipitate, and platelet transfusions may be needed. Drotrecogin alfa (recombinant activated protein C) reduces mortality in some patients with severe septicaemia. Heparin can benefit patients with large-vessel thrombosis or acral ischaemia. The routine use of vitamin K and folate will avoid coagulation and platelet count disturbances in some patients.

Trauma and shock

Tissue injury due to trauma, burns, or hypoperfusion can cause DIC, especially when organs rich in tissue thromboplastin (e.g. the brain) are injured.

Box 22.6.5.1 Causes of bleeding and thrombosis in liver disease

Predispose to bleeding

♦ Effects of portal hypertension:

  • Oesophageal varices (bleeding site)

  • Splenomegaly (thrombocytopenia)

♦ Decreased thrombopoietin production (thrombocytopenia)

♦ Decreased procoagulant factor synthesis

♦ Abnormal coagulation factor synthesis:

  • Dysfibrinogenaemia (increased sialic acid content)

  • Descarboxylated vitamin K-dependent factors

♦ Decreased clearance of plasmin, plasminogen activators, and fibrin(ogen) degradation products

♦ Vitamin K malabsorption

♦ Platelet dysfunction

♦ Increased susceptibility to adverse hepatic effects of alcohol or other drugs

♦ Decreased α_2-antiplasmin synthesis (predisposes to hyperfibrinolysis)

Predispose to thrombosis

♦ Decreased natural anticoagulant synthesis (e.g. protein C, antithrombin)

♦ Decreased clearance of activated coagulation factors

♦ Physician reluctance to prescribe antithrombotic therapy

Table 22.6.5.6 Main causes of DIC

Acute DIC
Trauma, burns, shock
Infection
Obstetrical complications:
placental abruption
amniotic fluid embolism
pre-eclampsia/eclampsia
puerperal sepsis
saline-induced abortion
Malignancy, promyelocytic leukaemia
Allergic reactions
Severe heparin-induced thrombocytopenia
Severe haemolysis
Chronic DIC
Malignancy, especially adenocarcinoma
Obstetrical complications:
dead fetus syndrome
Chronic liver disease
Vascular anomalies:
giant haemangioma (Kasabach–Merritt syndrome)
aortic aneurysm

Infection

Gram-negative and Gram-positive bacteria can cause DIC, either from procoagulant bacterial components (e.g. endotoxin, *Staphylococcus aureus* toxin) or via the host response to infection (e.g. IL-6). The clinical spectrum ranges from prominent thrombocytopenia with minimal activation of coagulation, to marked coagulation factor and natural anticoagulant depletion. Certain infections, such as meningococcaemia, *Capnocytophaga canimorsus* (from dog bites), sometimes produce severe acquired consumptive protein C and/or antithrombin deficiency, which leads to widespread ischaemic necrosis of the extremities (symmetric peripheral gangrene) and elsewhere (purpura fulminans). Postvaricella purpura fulminans can be caused by acquired antiphospholipid antibodies that interfere with protein S.

Obstetrical complications

Acute DIC can be caused by thromboplastin-like materials released during placental abruption or amniotic fluid embolism. Pre-eclampsia too can be accompanied by DIC, although there can be clinical and laboratory overlap with other life-threatening complications of pregnancy (e.g. fatty liver of pregnancy; HELLP syndrome (haemolysis, elevated liver enzymes, low platelets). Bleeding due to hypofibrinogenaemia is often prominent in pregnancy-associated DIC. Chronic DIC can be caused by fetal death.

Acute haemolysis

Haemolysis caused by incompatible blood transfusions, certain infections (e.g. *Clostridium perfringens* septicaemia), or microangiopathic disorders such as TTP and HELLP, can sometimes be associated with DIC.

Immunological disorders

Severe allergic reactions (e.g. anaphylaxis), transplant rejection, glomerulonephritis, and other vasculitic disorders are sometimes associated with DIC. Severe heparin-induced thrombocytopenia can also be associated with overt DIC.

Vascular anomalies

Giant haemangiomas cause overt DIC in about 25% of those affected (Kasabach–Merritt syndrome). Although activation of coagulation and fibrinolysis is localized to the vascular anomaly, depletion of haemostatic factors produces a clinical and laboratory profile indistinguishable from DIC. Eradication of haemangioma by radiation, embolization, or surgery is curative. Medical therapies have included heparin, antifibrinolytic drugs (combined with cryoprecipitate to thrombose the vascular tumour), glucocorticoids, and interferon.

Disseminated intravascular coagulation also occurs in about 0.5 to 1% of patients with abdominal aortic aneurysms, which usually contain adherent thrombi.

Immunoglobulin-mediated factor deficiency

Coagulation factor inhibitors are usually IgG antibodies that bind to specific coagulation factors, and either neutralize their activity (most coagulation factor inhibitors) or result in accelerated

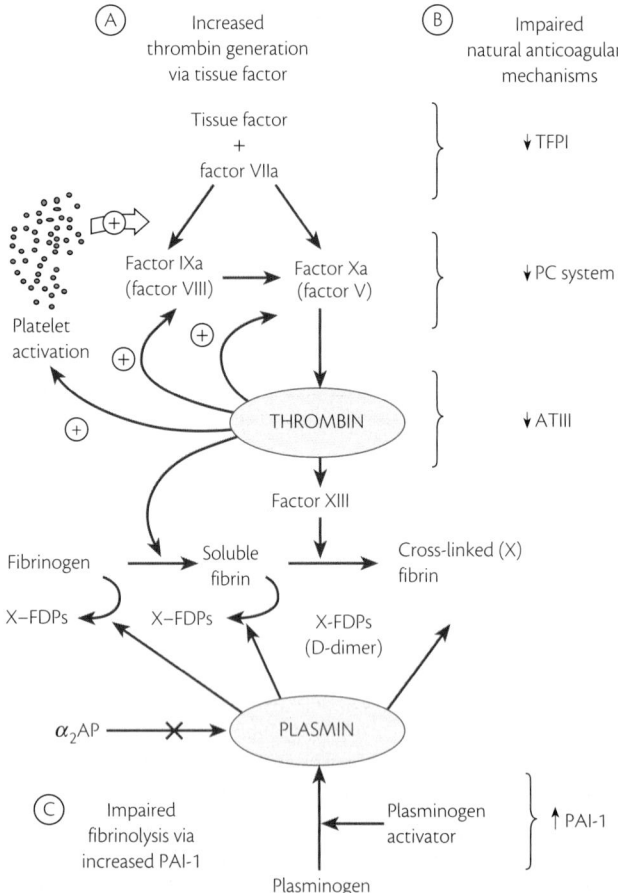

Fig. 22.6.5.1 Pathogenesis of thrombosis in DIC. (A) DIC is usually triggered by tissue factor, which activates coagulation by complexing with factor VIIa, ultimately resulting in the generation of thrombin. (B) Impaired natural anticoagulant mechanisms (e.g. excessive consumption of natural anticoagulants, or cytokine-mediated downregulation of natural anticoagulant pathways) predispose to microvascular thrombosis. (C) Impaired fibrinolysis via increased PAI-1 leads to greater microvascular thrombosis. Sometimes, hyperfibrinolysis is caused by increased plasminogen activator release, or low levels of α_2-antiplasmin. Abbreviations: α_2AP, α_2-antiplasmin; ATIII, antithrombin III; fDPs, fibrinogen degradation products; FDPs, fibrin degradation products; PAI-1, plasminogen activator inhibitor type 1; PC, protein C; TFPI, tissue-factor pathway inhibitor.

clearance (e.g. antiprothrombin antibodies associated with the antiphospholipid antibody syndrome). Acquired inhibitors against coagulation factors are rare in otherwise normal (nonhaemophiliac) individuals. Even the most common autoimmune coagulation factor deficiency (factor VIII) has an estimated incidence of only 1 per 1 000 000 per year.

Acquired factor VIII inhibitor

Acquired factor VIII deficiency should be suspected in a patient with spontaneous bleeding, or bleeding following minor trauma, that occurs in association with a prolonged APTT and a normal PT/INR (Table 22.6.5.3). Most commonly, muscle or cutaneous haematomas occur, but life-threatening retroperitoneal or intracranial haemorrhages are described; haemarthrosis is uncommon (cf. congenital haemophilia). The disorder occurs most commonly in older people (median age 60 years), affects men and women equally, and is idiopathic in 50% of cases. Other autoimmune disorders (e.g. systemic lupus erythematosus), lymphoid and other malignancies, penicillin treatment, or the postpartum state, have

been observed in some patients. About 20% of patients die of bleeding, often from their initial bleeding episode.

A rapid screening test for a coagulation factor inhibitor is performed by repeating the APTT after mixing patient plasma 50:50 with normal pooled plasma. An inhibitor is suggested by a prolongation time more than 4-s over the control, although some inhibitors require a 2-h incubation at 37°C to show inhibition. Confirmation is obtained by a specific factor assay showing reduced levels of factor VIII; inhibitor quantitation is most often performed by Bethesda assay, in which various dilutions of patient plasma are mixed with normal plasma and incubated for 2h at 37°C: a Bethesda unit is defined as the reciprocal of the plasma dilution that yields a 50% reduction in residual factor VIII activity in the test system. Unfortunately, the Bethesda assay tends to underestimate the amount of inhibitor in nonhaemophiliac patients with acquired factor VIII inhibitors.

Therapy of bleeding depends upon its severity and the amount of inhibitor present, if known. For patients with minor bleeding, detectable factor VIII levels, and low inhibitor levels (<5 Bethesda units), desmopressin (DDAVP) can be tried. Peak factor VIII levels occur between 45 and 90 min post-DDAVP, and repeat levels should be measured to assess efficacy. In other patients with low inhibitor levels but with more severe bleeding, purified human factor VIII concentrates are usually effective. One approach is to give an initial intravenous bolus of 100 U/kg, followed by a continuous infusion of factor VIII at 10 U/kg per h, with factor VIII levels measured again 4 to 6h later. Careful clinical and laboratory assessment for response is needed, since inhibitor levels may have been underestimated, or higher inhibitor levels stimulated by factor VIII use. Either prothrombin complex concentrates or recombinant factor VIIa can be given for patients refractory to human factor VIII. Activated prothrombin complex concentrates (e.g. FEIBA or Autoplex) are more effective than nonactivated prothrombin complex concentrates, but concomitant antifibrinolytic therapy should be avoided to reduce risk of thromboembolic complications. Recombinant factor VIIa may be preferable for perioperative management, since the risk for inducing postoperative thrombosis is probably lower. In desperate situations, extracorporeal immunoadsorption using staphylococcal protein A may be helpful in removing the antibodies.

Spontaneous disappearance of the inhibitor occurs in about 10 to 30% of patients, most commonly in the patient who developed her inhibitor postpartum. Nevertheless, the unpredictable clinical course, and the potential for life-threatening bleeding, means that immunosuppressive therapy should be given to most patients. The most widely adopted treatment is with corticosteroids (prednisolone, 1 mg/kg daily) in combination with cyclophosphamide (1–2 mg/kg daily), which eradicates the inhibitor in about 70% of cases. A more recent alternative is the anti-CD20 monoclonal antibody rituximab, which has been used successfully in many autoimmune conditions; the regimen consists of four separate intravenous infusions (375 mg/m² each), given at weekly intervals. Other options include combination chemotherapy (prednisone, cyclophosphamide, vincristine); ciclosporin; or high-dose intravenous IgG (1 g/kg for 2 days, or 0.4 g/kg for 5 days). Even partial remission can help reduce bleeding. Women with postpartum factor VIII inhibitors usually develop remission within 30 months, and only rarely develop recurrent factor VIII inhibitors with later pregnancies. They also may be less likely to respond to corticosteroids or other immunosuppressive therapy.

Other acquired coagulation factor deficiencies

Hypoprothrombinaemia

This should be suspected in patients with the antiphospholipid antibody syndrome, particularly if bleeding occurs or the PT/INR is prolonged. Typically, these pathogenic anti-factor II antibodies are non-neutralizing, and therefore mixing patient plasma 50:50 with normal pooled plasma can produce correction of the APTT, in contrast to other coagulation factor inhibitors.

Thrombin inhibitors

These are rare, but may cause severe bleeding. More often, patients have antibodies that react preferentially against bovine thrombin: these are formed following the use of 'fibrin glue', which contains various bovine clotting factors. Patients have prolonged PT/INR, APTT, and TCT (especially using bovine thrombin). However, it is more likely that any bleeding is the result of clinically significant anti-bovine factor V antibodies.

Factor V inhibitors

Rarely, IgG antibodies against factor V arise spontaneously or following treatment with topical bovine thrombin used at surgery. FFP usually does not provide enough factor V to treat bleeding; however, platelet transfusions are usually effective, as platelet activation causes factor V to be released into haemostatic plugs.

Factor XIII inhibitors

These inhibitors, which sometimes occur in association with isoniazid therapy, cause bleeding via impaired factor XIII-mediated cross-linking of fibrin. Factor XIII should be measured in a patient with unexplained bleeding and normal results of screening coagulation assays.

Factor X inhibitors

Factor X inhibitors are a rare cause of bleeding in patients with prolonged PT/INR and APTT. The differential diagnosis also includes amyloidosis of the AL (amyloid light chain) variety, caused by adsorption of factor X to amyloid fibrils.

Factor IX inhibitors

In nonhaemophiliac patients, factor IX inhibitors are rare and usually associated with autoimmune disease. Treatment includes PCCs or purified factor IX, and immunosuppression. The differential diagnosis of acquired, isolated, factor IX deficiency includes the nephrotic syndrome (urinary loss of factor IX).

Factor XI inhibitors

These rare inhibitors are most often observed in association with systemic lupus erythematosus, and usually do not cause bleeding or require specific treatment.

Factor VII inhibitors

Factor VII inhibitors are extremely rare, and usually do not cause bleeding or require treatment. The diagnosis is suggested by an isolated prolonged PT/INR in the absence of coumarin or vitamin K deficiency.

Acquired von Willebrand's syndrome

Rarely, bleeding is caused by a severe acquired deficiency of VWF, most often in the setting of a monoclonal gammopathy, benign or malignant. Typically, there is disproportional deficiency of the largest VWF multimers due to antibody-mediated clearance (acquired type 2a von Willebrand's syndrome). Aortic stenosis and obstructive cardiomyopathies are other causes of type 2a von Willebrand's syndrome: this explains why aortic valve replacement can cure recurrent gastrointestinal haemorrhage in patients with colonic angiodysplasia.

Heparin and acquired heparin-like anticoagulants

Bleeding is a complication of heparin treatment, particularly when the APTT is above the therapeutic range. In patients with massive accidental or deliberate heparin overdose, intravenous protamine should be given to treat bleeding complications.

Rarely, patients with spontaneous bleeding and prolonged APTT and thrombin time measurements have circulating heparin-like anticoagulants. Usually associated with multiple myeloma and other plasma-cell dyscrasias, the coagulopathy does not necessarily respond even to large-dose protamine infusion, and fatal haemorrhage can ensue. Circulating dermatan sulphate glycosaminoglycan appeared to explain the bleeding in a patient with renal failure.

Coagulopathies secondary to plasma-cell dyscrasias

Multiple myeloma, macroglobulinaemia, and other plasma-cell dyscrasias such as primary amyloidosis can cause various coagulopathies (Table 22.6.5.7). Usually, the TCT is prolonged, most often because of paraprotein-induced interference with fibrin polymerization. A long bleeding time suggests inhibition of platelet function by paraprotein; rarely, acquired von Willebrand's syndrome is the cause. Apheresis can improve haemostasis by quickly reducing paraprotein levels, as antineoplastic chemotherapy is initiated.

Hyperfibrinolysis

Activation of fibrinolysis occurs normally when fibrin clots are formed during physiological or pathological haemostasis. However, primary fibrinolysis (Table 22.6.5.3) is sometimes the major cause for bleeding, and requires specific treatment.

Thrombolytic therapy

About 0.5 to 0.7% of patients with myocardial infarction who receive thrombolysis with either streptokinase or tissue plasminogen activator (tPA) develop an intracranial haemorrhage. The thrombolytic agent should be stopped immediately in any such patient, and they should receive cryoprecipitate and an antifibrinolytic drug (e.g. tranexamic acid); platelets and FFP can help to increase factor V and VIII levels that may have been reduced by plasmin generated by thrombolysis. It can take between 24 and 36 h for fibrinogen levels to recover after stopping thrombolytic therapy.

Malignancy

Cancer-associated DIC usually causes a hypercoagulable state. However, promyelocytic leukaemia (PML) and prostatic adenocarcinoma are two malignancies commonly associated with prominent hyperfibrinolysis. Laboratory abnormalities include prolonged PT/INR, APTT, and TCT, and hypofibrinogenaemia. The use of all-*trans*-retinoic acid during induction chemotherapy of PML has reduced the frequency of life-threatening bleeding. Antifibrinolytic therapy can control bleeding in cancer-associated fibrinolysis, but there is a risk of thrombosis if tissue

Table 22.6.5.7 Venom-induced coagulopathies (selected examples)

Animal source of venom	Main biological effects (trivial name of venom component in bold)	Comments	Main distribution
Venomous snakes			
Family Viperidae SUBFAMILY CROTALINAE (PIT VIPERS*)			
Crotalus adamanteus (Eastern diamondback rattlesnake)	**Crotalase**: cleaves FPA, but not FPB, from fibrinogen (decreased fibrinogen, plasminogen; increased FDPs)	'Thrombin-like' based upon fibrinopeptide A cleavage, but does not activate platelets or factor XIII; despite 'defibrination syndrome', bleeding is uncommon	USA (coastal plain from Florida to Mississippi)
Crotalus atrox (Western diamondback rattlesnake)	**Catroxobin**: cleaves FPA from fibrinogen; other fibrinogenase activities	Also causes defibrination syndrome, usually without bleeding; venom also contains catrocollastatin-C (platelet inhibitor)	USA (California to Arkansas); Mexico
Calloselasma [Agkistrodon] rhodostoma (Malayan pit viper)	**Ancrod**: cleaves FPA from fibrinogen	Purified ancrod previously used as an antithrombotic agent	Southeast Asia
SUBFAMILY VIPERINAE (TRUE VIPERS*)			
Echis carinatus (saw-scaled viper)	**Ecarin**: activates prothrombin and platelets	Causes DIC, often with bleeding; most common cause of snake-bite mortality in the African savannah	India, Africa, Asia
Daboia russelli (Russell's viper, formerly, *Vipera russelli*)	**Russell's viper venom**: activates factor X	Causes DIC, often with bleeding; venom also causes direct nephrotoxicity	Far East
Bothrops jararacussu (jararacucu, lance-headed pit viper)	**Botrocetin**: platelet agglutination via vWF; **Jararhagin**: haemorrhagin	Venom also contains thrombin-like and factor Xa-activating enzymes, and can cause severe bleeding	Brazil
Family Elapidae** *Notechis scutatus* (tiger snake)	**Notecarin**: activates prothrombin	Fatal haemorrhage has been reported	Australia
Family Colubridae***			
Non-snake envenomations that cause coagulopathy			
Lonomia achelous (caterpillar)	Proteolysis of factor XIII; reduced fibrinogen, factor V, plasminogen, and increased FDPs also observed	Severe bleeding in humans (wound site, mucous membranes, and internal haemorrhage)	Venezuela, Brazil
Loxosceles reclusa (brown recluse spider)	Activation of endothelium, with resulting dysfunction of interactions with PMNs	Potential for severe skin lesions; systemic effects (DIC, haemolytic anaemia) occur in small minority of patients	Midwest USA

Two other families of venomous snakes (Hydrophiidae and Atractaspididae) do not cause coagulopathies.

*Pit vipers are New World snakes named for the heat-sensitive pit located between the eye and the nostril that enables the snake to detect warm-blooded prey even in darkness: the three genera of the Crotalidae family that inhabit the US are *Crotalus* (rattlesnakes), *Agkistrodon* (moccasins, including the copperheads and cottonmouths), and *Sistrurus* (massasaugas and pigmy rattlesnakes).

**With the exception of several Australian species, such as taipan, tiger snakes, brown snakes, and black snakes, elapid snake bites usually cause neurotoxicity, and only occasionally result in haemostatic abnormalities.

***The colubrid family includes: boomslang, vine snake, keel backs, and the South American 'green snake,' which can also cause bleeding.

Abbreviations: DIC, disseminated intravascular coagulation; FDP(s), fibrin(ogen) degradation product(s); FPA, fibrinopeptide A; PMNs, polymorphonuclear leucocytes; vWF, von Willebrand factor.

factor-induced DIC, rather than the release of plasminogen activator by the tumour, is primarily responsible for the coagulopathy.

Cardiopulmonary bypass surgery

Excess bleeding, defined as more than 1 litre per procedure, is a common problem following heart surgery utilizing cardiopulmonary bypass (extracorporeal circulation). About 20% of all red cell concentrates in the United States of America are given for cardiac surgical bleeding. About 5% of patients require urgent resternotomy for critical rates of blood loss (defined as >500 ml in the first 1 h; >400 ml/h in the first 2 h; >300 ml/h in the first 3 h; or >1 litre in 4 h). Re-exploration reveals bleeding vessels in two-thirds of patients; the remainder have diffuse oozing.

Thrombocytopenia, transient platelet dysfunction, and hyperfibrinolysis are the principal haemostatic defects. Typically, the platelet count falls by between 30 and 60% mainly from haemodilution, although platelet losses from bleeding and within the extracorporeal perfusion device also occur. The thrombocytopenia persists for 3 to 4 days, followed by recovery of the platelet count to values exceeding the preoperative baseline. Marked prolongation of the bleeding time (>30 min) quickly improves to under 15 min shortly after surgery, and to normal several hours later. Some platelet function defects are 'extrinsic' and reversible (e.g. hypothermia, heparin), whereas others indicate longer-lasting 'intrinsic' changes (surface glycoprotein deficiency, acquired granule depletion). Preoperative treatment with aspirin or clopidogrel also increases bleeding.

The importance of hyperfibrinolysis in postcardiac surgical bleeding is highlighted by meta-analysis of studies of high-dose aprotinin, a plasmin inhibitor derived from bovine lung: a two-thirds reduction in blood transfusion, and 50% reduction in resternotomy. However, aprotinin has been withdrawn because of concerns regarding its adverse effect profile. Other antifibrinolytic drugs that reduce bleeding include the lysine analogues, tranexamic acid (e.g. 10 mg/kg bolus before cardiopulmonary bypass; then 1 mg/kg per h, although dosing regimens vary widely) and ε-aminocaproic acid (total dose up to 20 g). Although these therapies are usually given before cardiopulmonary bypass, they may also provide benefit when used postoperatively for bleeding patients.

Management of postcardiac surgical bleeding also includes blood transfusions, especially platelets and FFP, although their benefit is unproven. Residual heparin, including heparin 'rebound', can respond to additional protamine. Desmopressin probably is ineffective. No universally accepted algorithm for management exists.

Liver disease
Hyperfibrinolysis complicating liver disease is discussed elsewhere.

Venom-induced coagulopathies (snake bites) (see also Chapter 9.2)
Envenomations can harm or kill humans generally through systemic effects, e.g. profound hypotension. Sometimes, however, life-threatening coagulopathies result.

Snake bites
In the United States of America, about 8000 bites from venomous snakes occur each year, resulting in 10 to 20 deaths. This relatively low mortality reflects the less lethal character of New World snakes, as well as the victim's usual close proximity to medical facilities and antivenin therapy. Pit vipers (rattlesnakes, copperheads, cottonmouths, massasaugas) account for 99% of snakebite poisonings in the United States. Worldwide, annually over 100,000 people are estimated to die from snakebite, many in India. Although death usually results from multiple mechanisms (such as circulatory shock, rhabdomyolysis, renal failure, pulmonary failure, neurotoxicity), bleeding is sometimes the major factor.

Venoms contain multiple digestive enzymes with a broad spectrum of activity that can include effects on human haemostasis (Box 22.6.5.2). Within a species, haemostatic effects of envenomation vary with snake age, diet, and other factors. North American rattlesnakes typically cause the 'defibrination syndrome'; despite even profound hypofibrinogenaemia, bleeding is uncommon. In contrast, venom from Old World vipers frequently cause generalized activation of the coagulation system (DIC), with a greater chance for bleeding or microvascular thrombosis. Bleeding can also result from platelet inhibitors present within venom; e.g. the platelet fibrinogen receptor antagonist echistatin (from *Echis carinatus*), or 'haemorrhagins' such as jararhagin (from *Bothrops jararacussu*) that damage endothelium.

Immediate treatment of a snake bite includes efforts to limit the venom spread (immobilizing and placing a constriction band proximal to the bite site). Rapid transport to medical facilities is crucial since antivenin therapy is the mainstay of treatment. Antivenin treatment is indicated for patients with significant pain or swelling, as well as suspected or proven haemostasis abnormalities, as these indicate envenomation rather than a 'dry bite'. Hypersensitivity testing to the antivenin should be performed to rule out pre-existing

Box 22.6.5.2 Haemostatic abnormalities associated with dysproteinaemias

- Interference with fibrinogen polymerization
- Isolated factor deficiency:
  - Factor X, fibrinogen, or α_2-antiplasmin deficiency (amyloidosis)
  - Acquired von Willebrand's disease (benign monoclonal gammopathy)
- Hyperviscosity (comprising vascular integrity)
- Circulating glycosaminoglycans (heparin-like inhibitor)
- Thrombocytopenia secondary to marrow:
  - Marrow failure (disease- or treatment-related)
  - Autoimmune thrombocytopenia
- Platelet dysfunction

hypersensitivity to horse serum. The treatment of snake bite is discussed in Chapter 9.2.

Coagulation studies should include: complete blood count (including platelets), PT/INR, APTT, TCT, fibrinogen, and FDPs. Abnormal results indicate envenomation, and are an indication for antivenin therapy. The bedside assessment of defibrination involves placing a few millilitres of blood in a clean, dry test tube at room temperature for 20 min; incoagulable blood indicates defibrination. Usually, blood products should only be given to patients with bleeding. A small clinical trial found that heparin was ineffective in patients with DIC caused by a Russell's viper bite.

Laboratory and therapeutic uses of snake venoms
Snake-venom fractions are useful for certain laboratory assays. For example, the thrombin-like enzyme batroxobin (Reptilase, *Bothrops atrox moojeni*), cleaves fibrinopeptide A from fibrinogen even in the presence of heparin. Thus, a prolonged Reptilase time indicates hypofibrinogenaemia even in heparin-containing plasma.

Ecarin activates prothrombin irrespective of its γ-carboxylation status; thus, it can be used to detect proteins induced by vitamin K antagonists to document vitamin K deficiency or dysprothrombinaemia. An ecarin clotting time is superior to the APTT for monitoring therapy with hirudin, particularly the high doses used for heart surgery. Differences in phospholipid dependency of venom prothrombin activators has led to the use of a Textarin/ecarin ratio to detect lupus anticoagulants; a ratio over 1.3 is a sensitive and relatively specific test for lupus anticoagulants.

Russell's viper venom contains a potent activator of factor X (RVV-X); the dilute Russell's viper venom time (dRVVT), performed by adding RVV-X and diluted rabbit brain phospholipid to test plasma prior to recalcification, measures the rate of formation and activity of the phospholipid-dependent prothrombinase complex in producing thrombin. The dRVVT is thereby prolonged in the presence of a lupus anticoagulant.

A commercially available protein C activator (Protac) from *Agkistrodon contortrix contortrix* (the southern copperhead) has greatly simplified assays for protein C activity, as well as in screening for defects in the protein C anticoagulant pathway.

The defibrinogenating snake venom ancrod (Arvin, derived from the Malayan pit viper *Calloselasma [Agkistrodon] rhodostoma*), which proteolyses fibrinopeptide A, was formerly used for management of heparin-induced thrombocytopenia, acute stroke, thrombotic nephropathy, and priapism. The inability to control thrombin generation is a potential drawback of this therapy. Batroxobin (Defibrase) is another defibrinogenating venom that has seen limited clinical applications.

Prothrombotic acquired coagulation disorders

Some acquired coagulation disorders are characterized by an increased risk for thrombosis, rather than bleeding. Accordingly, the appropriate treatment usually involves anticoagulant therapy, even if there are abnormal coagulation or platelet count values.

Macrovascular thrombosis

Some acquired coagulation disorders typically cause thrombosis in large veins and arteries, although small-vessel thrombi can also result.

Heparin-induced thrombocytopenia

Heparin-induced thrombocytopenia is caused by IgG antibodies that recognize multimolecular complexes of platelet factor 4 (PF4) and heparin. Thrombosis results from IgG-induced platelet activation (via platelet Fc receptors), resulting in the generation of procoagulant, platelet-derived microparticles, tissue-factor expression by endothelium and monocytes, and inactivation of heparin by PF4 released from platelets. Increased thrombin–antithrombin complex levels indicate DIC in almost all patients with this condition, although a prolonged INR and/or low fibrinogen level occurs in 10 to 20% of cases.

Typically, the fall in platelet count begins 5 to 10 days after starting heparin; however, in patients who received heparin within the past 100 days, the platelet count can fall abruptly upon resuming heparin therapy, because of residual circulating antibodies. Heparin-induced thrombocytopenia occurs in as many as 5% of certain high-risk populations: e.g. postoperative orthopaedic patients receiving unfractionated heparin for over 1 week. Heparin-induced thrombocytopenia is less frequent in patients initially treated with low-molecular-weight heparin or fondaparinux. Interestingly, heparin-induced thrombocytopenia does not usually recur with future heparin exposure, although deliberate reexposure is usually restricted to special situations (e.g. cardiac surgery), and only if platelet-activating antibodies are no longer detectable.

Most patients with heparin-induced thrombocytopenia develop venous or arterial thrombosis (Fig. 22.6.5.2), most commonly a DVT, pulmonary embolism, major limb artery thrombosis, stroke, or myocardial infarction. Acute or chronic adrenal failure from bilateral adrenal haemorrhagic necrosis (manifestation of adrenal vein thrombosis) has been described. The thrombocytopenia is typically moderate in severity (median platelet count nadir 60 × 10^9/litre), and in only 10% of patients does the platelet count fall to less than 20 × 10^9/litre. In at least 10% of patients, the platelet count never drops below 150 × 10^9/litre. This degree of thrombocytopenia in heparin-induced thrombocytopenia is much less marked than observed in classic immune-mediated drug-induced thrombocytopenia (Fig. 22.6.5.2).

Laboratory testing for HIT antibodies includes activation and antigen assays. The former assays detect antibodies via their platelet-activating properties. Commercially available antigen assays detect antibodies that bind to surface-immobilized PF4 complexed to heparin or polyvinylsulphonate. Antigen assays are more likely to detect clinically-insignificant antibodies, with the potential for a false-positive diagnosis of heparin-induced thrombocytopenia.

Treatment includes stopping heparin and instituting alternative nonheparin anticoagulation. Coumarin should not be given to patients during the acute (thrombocytopenic) phase of HIT;

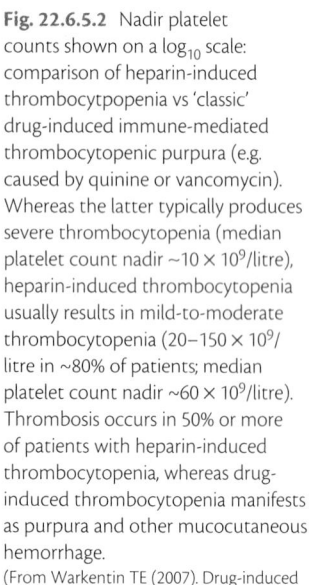

Fig. 22.6.5.2 Nadir platelet counts shown on a log₁₀ scale: comparison of heparin-induced thrombocytpopenia vs 'classic' drug-induced immune-mediated thrombocytopenic purpura (e.g. caused by quinine or vancomycin). Whereas the latter typically produces severe thrombocytopenia (median platelet count nadir ~10 × 10⁹/litre), heparin-induced thrombocytopenia usually results in mild-to-moderate thrombocytopenia (20–150 × 10⁹/litre in ~80% of patients; median platelet count nadir ~60 × 10⁹/litre). Thrombosis occurs in 50% or more of patients with heparin-induced thrombocytopenia, whereas drug-induced thrombocytopenia manifests as purpura and other mucocutaneous hemorrhage.
(From Warkentin TE (2007). Drug-induced immune-mediated thrombocytopenia—from purpura to thrombosis. *N Engl J Med*, **356**, 891–3, with permission.)

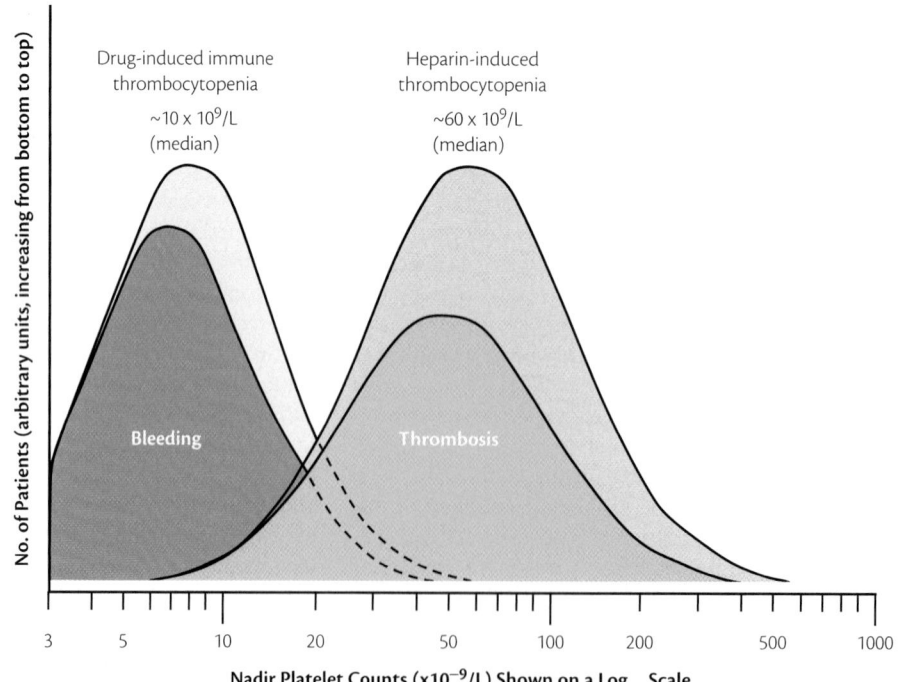

particularly in those with associated DVT, there is substantial risk of limb loss due to microvascular thrombosis (coumarin-induced venous limb gangrene). Thus, coumarin therapy should be postponed until the platelet count has recovered to at least 150×10^9/litre, and only then cautiously overlapped (over at least 5 days) with an agent that inhibits thrombin (or its generation). Suitable anticoagulants include danaparoid (a low-molecular-weight mixture of glycosaminoglycans with predominant anti-factor Xa activity), lepirudin (a recombinant hirudin with potent antithrombin activity derived from leech salivary glands), and argatroban (a synthetic small-molecule direct thrombin inhibitor); fondaparinux (synthetic factor Xa-inhibiting pentasaccharide) shows considerable promise as a treatment option. Among patients with heparin-induced thrombocytopenia, low-molecular-weight heparin (LMWH) treatment has a high risk for clinical cross-reactivity, and should be considered a contraindicated treatment for acute HIT. Some patients benefit from selected adjunctive treatments, e.g. surgical thromboembolectomy for acute arterial thrombosis of a limb. The dramatic natural history of HIT, with a risk for subsequent thrombosis of about 50% even after stopping heparin, means that an alternative anticoagulant, together with DVT surveillance, should be considered for all patients strongly suspected to have HIT.

Adenocarcinoma-associated chronic DIC
Metastatic adenocarcinoma sometimes presents as venous or arterial thrombosis accompanied by DIC. The diagnosis is suggested by an unexpected rise in the platelet count during heparin treatment, followed by an abrupt platelet count fall, together with new or progressive thrombosis, when heparin is stopped, despite therapeutic anticoagulation with warfarin. The clinical situation can mimic heparin-induced thrombocytopenia ('pseudo-HIT'), but the appropriate antibodies are absent, and the platelet count recovers during resumption of heparin (Fig. 22.6.5.3). Oral anticoagulants

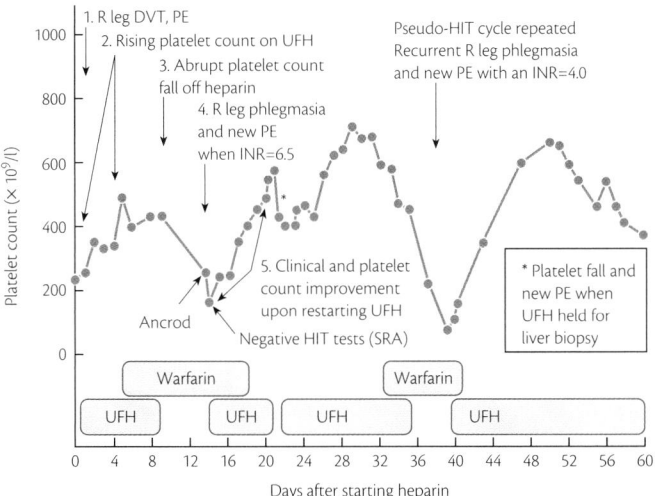

Fig. 22.6.5.3 Pseudo-HIT. Adenocarcinoma with thrombocytopenia and phlegmasia cerulea dolens after stopping unfractionated heparin. The timing of thrombocytopenia onset suggested heparin-induced thrombocytopenia prompting the use of an alternative anticoagulant (ancrod). Heparin was restarted when PF4/heparin antibodies were not detected by activation assay (serotonin-release assay [SRA]). Subsequently, heparin discontinuation led to the recurrence of thrombocytopenia and warfarin-associated phlegmasia cerulea dolens (repeat of pseudo-heparin-induced thrombocytopenia cycle). DVT, deep venous thrombosis; INR, international normalized ratio; PE, pulmonary embolism.

are ineffective, and may even cause venous limb gangrene (discussed subsequently). Heparin, especially LMWH, is the preferred treatment. Tissue factor-containing tumour vesicles, and factor Xa-activating enzymes found in tumour extracts, are two possible explanations for these procoagulant effects of adenocarcinoma.

Antiphospholipid antibody syndrome ('lupus anticoagulant')
This clinicopathological syndrome is characterized by large-vessel venous and/or arterial thrombosis, recurrent miscarriages, and thrombocytopenia. An associated 'lupus anticoagulant' (or 'non-specific inhibitor') is a prolonged APTT that results from the interference by antibodies against phospholipid-dependent coagulation reactions; these antiphospholipid antibodies are usually directed against protein cofactors such as β_2-glycoprotein I (β_2GPI) and prothrombin. Sometimes a prolonged PT/INR is caused by non-neutralizing antiprothrombin antibodies that cause hypoprothrombinaemia by increased prothrombin clearance.

Despite these laboratory abnormalities, bleeding is unusual, since severe thrombocytopenia or hypoprothrombinaemia is uncommon. More often, antiphospholipid antibodies are associated with intermittent thrombosis; rarely, the abrupt onset of life-threatening multiple vascular occlusions occurs ('catastrophic antiphospholipid antibody syndrome'). The explanation for the paradoxical association with thrombosis remains elusive, but it could be caused by antibody interactions with other protein cofactors described (e.g. activated protein C, protein S, thrombomodulin). Many patients have a thrombocytopenia that is typically mild and intermittent. Other less common complications include cardiac valvulitis and microvascular thrombosis, which can manifest as acrocyanosis, digital ulceration/gangrene, and livedo reticularis.

Antiphospholipid antibodies are detected by enzyme-immunoassay using purified phospholipids as the target antigen, e.g. the anti-cardiolipin antibody assay. Lupus anticoagulant activity is shown by demonstrating inhibition of phospholipid-dependent coagulation assays. Several assays should be performed, as anti-β_2GPI antibodies especially interfere with the conversion of prothrombin to thrombin (i.e. best detectable by the dilute Rusell's viper venom time), whereas antiprothrombin antibodies interfere most with global coagulation assays (e.g. kaolin clotting time). The coagulation times remain prolonged following mixing with normal plasma; confirmation involves adding excess phospholipid to neutralize the effects of the antiphospholipid antibodies. Not all APTT reagents are sensitive to antiphospholipid antibodies, and so these phospholipid-dependent coagulation assays should be performed in the appropriate clinical situation, even if the APTT is normal.

The term 'lupus anticoagulant' refers to the frequent occurrence of these antibodies in patients with systemic lupus erythematosus; nevertheless, most patients with the antiphospholipid antibody syndrome do not have systemic lupus erythematosus. Some patients have other autoimmune disorders, malignancy, infections, or procainamide treatment, but usually no associated condition is identified (primary antiphospholipid antibody syndrome). Many patients require long-term anticoagulation. Corticosteroids can benefit patients with bleeding caused by hypoprothrombinaemia.

Microvascular thrombosis
Some disorders of haemostasis are characterized by small-vessel thrombi, affecting either arterioles (e.g. TTP) or small venules (e.g. coumarin-induced necrosis).

Thrombotic microangiopathy

Thrombotic microangiopathy is a clinicopathological syndrome of microangiopathic haemolysis and thrombocytopenia carrying a risk for arteriolar occlusion by microaggregates of platelets and VWF, particularly affecting the kidneys and central nervous system. Microangiopathic red cell changes are characteristic, e.g. 'helmet cells' (schistocytes) and small, triangular red-cell fragments. The prototypic illness is thrombotic thrombocytopenic purpura (TTP), which typically affects adults and is idiopathic. However, familial and secondary forms of TTP also exist. The haemolytic-uraemic syndrome is a nephrotropic variant of TTP with a distinct pathogenesis, including its association with verocytotoxin-producing *Escherichia coli* acquired from eating undercooked meat (hamburger disease).

The pathogenesis of TTP involves the formation of platelet–VWF microaggregates in high shear situations (arterioles). Platelet-bound VWF levels are increased during TTP. Patients with familial TTP have ultralarge multimers of VWF during remission; these very large multimers disappear during active disease. A constitutional deficiency of a VWF-cleaving metalloproteinase (ADAMTS13) has been identified in patients with familial TTP. In many patients with nonfamilial TTP, an IgG autoantibody, which inhibits the VWF-cleaving metalloproteinase, has been identified.

The mainstays of treatment for acute TTP are corticosteroids and FFP given by infusion or apheresis. Corticosteroids, often given as prednisone 200 mg/day, may treat the autoimmune component of TTP. Provision of either FFP, or the cryoprecipitate-depleted fraction of plasma (cryosupernatant), has greatly reduced mortality in TTP, likely through several mechanisms, e.g., apheresis helps clear the pathogenic autoantibody and large VWF multimers. The monoclonal antibody rituximab, which recognizes CD20 (surface antigen on B-cell precursors), appears to be effective in many patients with refractory or relapsing TTP.

Coumarin-induced skin necrosis

Coumarin-induced skin necrosis (CISN) is characterized by necrosis of the skin and underlying subcutaneous tissues that typically begins 3 to 6 days after commencing warfarin or coumarin anticoagulants. CISN results from failure of the protein C natural anticoagulant system to downregulate thrombin generation in the microvasculature. The relatively short half-life of protein C, compared with prothrombin, explains the temporal profile of coumarin-induced skin necrosis—that is to say, a transient period of disproportionately reduced protein C activity soon after starting coumarin (Table 22.6.5.8). Furthermore, a relatively high proportion of affected patients have a hereditary abnormality of the protein C anticoagulant pathway, especially protein C deficiency. Other disorders associated with CISN include congenital deficiency in protein S or antithrombin, factor V Leiden, and HIT. The pathology is a predominantly noninflammatory, small-vessel thrombosis affecting the subcutaneous postcapillary venules and small veins.

CISN characteristically affects central (nonacral) sites with substantial underlying fatty tissues, such as the breast, buttocks, hips, and thighs (Fig. 22.6.5.4). Less common areas include the anterior abdomen, flank, back, penis, legs, arms, and face. About 75% of patients are women; one-third have multiple lesions that can be symmetrical. The earliest features are localized pain, induration, and erythema; over the next few hours, the skin lesions progress

Table 22.6.5.8 Half-lives of vitamin K-dependent procoagulant and anticoagulant factors

Procoagulant factors	Half-life (h)	Anticoagulant factors	Half-life (h)
Factor II (prothrombin)	60	Protein C	9
Factor X	40	Protein S	40–60
Factor IX	24		
Factor VII	4–6		

The longer half-life of the major procoagulant vitamin K-dependent zymogen (factor II, or prothrombin), compared with the major natural anticoagulant factor (protein C), is relevant to the pathogenesis of CISN (see text).

to central purplish or black discoloration, with blistering, subsequently demarcating to full-thickness skin necrosis. CISN is rare (1/10 000 patients treated with warfarin).

Prompt reversal of anticoagulation with vitamin K may prevent incipient coumarin-induced skin necrosis if recognized early. However, the diagnosis is usually not made until necrosis is established; at this point, it is unknown whether vitamin K, FFP, or protein C concentrates alter its natural history. In patients without HIT, warfarin is usually replaced by heparin. Many patients require surgical treatment, such as skin grafting or tissue amputation. Following recovery, it is usually safe to reintroduce warfarin provided certain precautions are taken, e.g. the gradual initiation of oral anticoagulation.

Coumarin-induced venous limb gangrene

Venous limb gangrene involves the acral (peripheral) regions of the body—most often the toes, feet, and legs, but sometimes also the fingers, hands, and arms—usually in association with DVT.

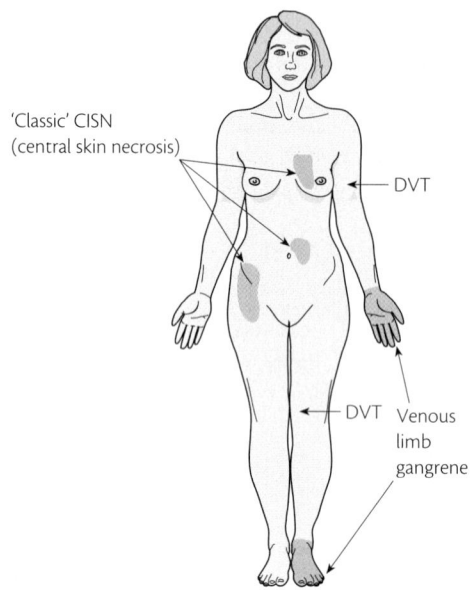

Fig. 22.6.5.4 Coumarin-induced skin necrosis: 'classic' syndrome (usually affecting central tissue sites) and coumarin-induced venous limb gangrene. Typically, an active DVT subtends the distal extremity affected by venous limb gangrene. (From Warkentin TE (1996). Heparin-induced thrombocytopenia IgG-mediated platelet activation, platelet microparticle generation, and altered procoagulant/anticoagulant balance in the pathogenesis of thrombosis and venous limb gangrene complicating heparin-induced thrombocytopenia. *Transfus Med Rev*, **10**, 249–58, with permission.)

The severity ranges from an initial stage of phlegmasia caerulea dolens ('swollen, blue, painful' limb) to extensive venous limb gangrene requiring limb amputation. Two disorders predispose to coumarin-induced venous limb gangrene: Heparin-induced thrombocytopenia and cancer-associated DIC. Recent data suggest that the supratherapeutic INR (typically >3.5) that characterizes venous limb gangrene is caused by a severe reduction in factor VII, which parallels a severe reduction in protein C activity that explains the microvascular thrombosis underlying this syndrome. Essentially, coumarin interferes with the protein C anticoagulant pathway, while at the same time it is unable to control the increased thrombin generation characteristic of heparin-induced thrombocytopenia or cancer-associated DIC.

Purpura fulminans

Purpura fulminans is a rare syndrome of DIC and microvascular thrombosis that results in multicentric ischaemic necrosis of the skin and subcutaneous tissues, predominantly affecting the extremities. The most common cause is overwhelming septicaemia, especially with meningococcus. A severe, acquired reduction in protein C activity complicating DIC is the most likely cause for the microvascular thrombosis, and some experts recommend treatment with protein C concentrates, if available. Autoantibodies against protein S have been implicated in patients with postvaricella purpura fulminans. In other patients with apparent 'idiopathic' purpura fulminans, autoantibodies that interfere with the protein C anticoagulant system have been described. Peripheral symmetric gangrene is a term sometimes used when acral regions of two or more limbs are affected.

Septicaemia and other systemic inflammatory response syndromes

Multiple organ failure often complicates septicaemia and other systemic inflammatory disease syndromes, including adult respiratory distress syndrome, fat embolism, and acute pancreatitis. Thrombocytopenia and coagulopathy are common, and some patients have DIC that could contribute to organ dysfunction via microvascular thrombosis. However, a prothrombotic basis for organ failure is usually speculative, as microthrombosis is rarely documented pathologically, and nonthrombotic microvascular disturbances that impair tissue oxygen delivery also occur.

Haemostasis in the newborn

Neonatal vitamin K deficiency

Haemorrhagic disease of the newborn caused by vitamin K deficiency was once a relatively common cause of bleeding during the first week of life, particularly in breastfed infants. Low vitamin K levels in mother's milk, and insufficient colonization of the newborn bowel by bacteria producing vitamin K, predispose to the inability to meet the infant's vitamin K requirements (1 µg/kg per day). The routine administration of vitamin K, either 1 mg given intramuscularly immediately after birth, or three oral doses of vitamin K, has led to the near disappearance of this problem in developed countries. Bleeding within 24 h of birth can occur in certain high-risk settings, e.g. mothers receiving anticonvulsants or warfarin; in these cases, the mother should receive vitamin K, 10 mg by mouth, each day for 2 weeks prior to delivery. Vitamin K deficiency occurring later in infancy despite appropriate neonatal vitamin K prophylaxis can indicate hepatobiliary or bowel disease.

Neonatal DIC

In neonates DIC commonly complicates infection, asphyxia, respiratory distress syndrome, aspiration of meconium or amniotic fluid, maternal hypertensive syndrome, hypothermia, and brain injury. This condition poses a significant risk of bleeding or thrombosis, as the immature liver has an impaired capacity to synthesize coagulation factors, and the reticuloendothelial system has a limited ability to clear activated coagulation factors. Treatment is aimed at the underlying cause of the DIC, with blood product given for the bleeding.

Neonatal purpura fulminans

Purpura fulminans can begin within hours or days following birth, often first affecting the heels or venepuncture sites. The underlying cause is usually a congenital abnormality affecting the protein C anticoagulant system (homozygous deficiency of protein C or protein S. FFP or protein C concentrates given every few days prevents a recurrence in some patients.

Further reading

Ansell J, et al. (2008). The pharmacology and management of the vitamin K antagonists. The Eighth ACCP Conference on Antithrombotic and Thrombolytic Therapy. *Chest*, **133** (Supp l), 160–98S. [Discusses the management of non-therapeutic (elevated) INRs in patients receiving oral anticoagulants; recommendations of the Eighth American College of Chest Physicians Consensus Conference on Antithrombotic Therapy.]

Asherson RA, et al. (1998). Catastrophic antiphospholipid syndrome. Clinical and laboratory features of 50 patients. *Medicine (Baltimore)*, **77**, 195–207. [Describes clinical presentations of multiorgan failure in patients with antiphospholipid antibodies.]

Bevan DH (1999). Cardiac bypass haemostasis: putting blood through the mill. *Br J Haematol*, **104**, 208–19. [Excellent review of cardiopulmonary bypass surgery and approaches to bleeding.]

Cole MS, Minifee PK, Wolma FJ (1988). Coumarin necrosis—a review of the literature. *Surgery*, **103**, 271–7. [Comprehensive review of coumarin-induced skin necrosis.]

Franchini M (2006). Acquired hemophilia A. *Hematology*, **11**, 119–25.

George JN (2006). Clinical practice. Thrombotic thrombocytopenic purpura. *N Engl J Med*, **354**, 1927–35. [Authoritative review.]

Kitchens CS (1992). Hemostatic aspects of envenomation by North American snakes. *Hematol Oncol Cl North Am*, **6**, 1189–95. [The focus is on envenomation by North American snakes, resulting in defibrination rather than true DIC syndromes.]

Levi M, Ten Cate H (1999). Disseminated intravascular coagulation. *N Engl J Med*, **341**, 586–92. [Authoritative review.]

Levine JS, Branch DW, Rauch J (2002). The antiphospholipid syndrome. *N Engl J Med*, **346**, 752–63. [Authoritative review.]

Manco-Johnson MJ, et al. (1996). Lupus anticoagulant and protein S deficiency in children with postvaricella purpura fulminans or thrombosis. *J Pediatr*, **128**, 319–23. [Provides evidence that purpura fulminans following varicella infection is usually caused by autoantibodies to protein S.]

Marsh NA (1998). Use of snake venom fractions in the coagulation laboratory. *Blood Coagul Fibrinolysis*, **9**, 395–404. [Discusses many laboratory uses of snake venom fractions.]

Oldenburg J, Watzka M, Rost S, Müller CR (2007). VKORC1: molecular target of coumarins. *J Thromb Haemost*, **5**, 1–6. [Describes the discovery and characterization of the enzyme complex inhibited by coumarins.]

Ortel TL, et al. (1994). Topical thrombin and acquired coagulation factor inhibitors: clinical spectrum and laboratory diagnosis. *Am J Hematol*, **45**, 128–35. [Summarizes acquired coagulation inhibitors that occur following treatment with topical bovine thrombin preparations ('fibrin glue').]

Sane DC, *et al.* (1989). Bleeding during thrombolytic therapy for acute myocardial infarction: mechanisms and management. *Ann Intern Med*, **111**, 1010–22. [Describes the management of post-thrombolytic hemorrhage.]

Warkentin TE, *et al.* (1997). The pathogenesis of venous limb gangrene associated with heparin-induced thrombocytopenia. *Ann Intern Med*, **127**, 804–12. [Indicates that an oral anticoagulant (warfarin) can cause deep-vein thrombosis to progress to venous limb gangrene in patients with heparin-induced thrombocytopenia.]

Warkentin TE, *et al.* (1995). Heparin-induced thrombocytopenia in patients treated with low-molecular-weight heparin or unfractionated heparin. *N Engl J Med*, **332**, 1330–5. [Provides evidence that HIT is a prothrombotic state associated with venous and arterial thrombosis that occurs less frequently with low-molecular-weight heparin.]

Warkentin TE (1996). Heparin-induced thrombocytopenia IgG-mediated platelet activation, platelet microparticle generation, and altered procoagulant/anticoagulant balance in the pathogenesis of thrombosis and venous limb gangrene complicating heparin-induced thrombocytopenia. *Transfus Med Rev*, **10**, 249–58. [Compares and contrasts the pathogenesis and clinical profile of coumarin-induced skin necrosis and coumarin-induced venous limb gangrene.]

Warkentin TE (2001). Venous limb gangrene during warfarin treatment of cancer-associated deep venous thrombosis. *Ann Intern Med*, **135**, 589–93. [Implicates warfarin in the pathogenesis of venous limb gangrene complicating cancer-associated DIC.]

Warkentin TE (2007). Drug-induced immune-mediated thrombocytopenia—from purpura to thrombosis. *N Engl J Med*, **356**, 891–3 [Compares and contrasts immune HIT with other drug-induced immune-mediated thrombocytopenia.]

Warkentin TE, Greinacher A (2007). *Heparin-induced thrombocytopenia*, 4th edition. Informa Healthcare USA, New York.

The blood in systemic disease

D.J. Weatherall

Essentials

Few diseases do not produce some alteration in the blood, and changes in the blood may give the first indication of many nonhaematological disorders.

Malignant disease

Malignant disease can cause protean haematological manifestations, including (1) leucoerythroblastic anaemia—the appearance of immature myeloid cells and nucleated red cells is a common phenomenon in disseminated malignancy, and occasionally there is a leukaemoid reaction; (2) anaemia of chronic disorders—see Chapter 22.5.5; (3) increase of the erythrocyte sedimentation rate; (4) thrombocytosis—of unknown cause, but often the first manifestation of cancer; (5) thrombocytopenia—may be due to widespread infiltration of the bone marrow, but more frequent in association with autoimmune effects of lymphomas and other tumours; (6) activation of blood coagulation pathways—this may cause thromboses as well as disseminated intravascular coagulation; adenocarcinomas that release tissue factor are characteristically responsible.

Specific tumours can cause particular haematological manifestations, most commonly iron deficiency anaemia attributable to gastrointestinal malignancy as a result of chronic haemorrhage, and much less commonly (1) microangiopathic haemolytic anaemia—may be caused by mucin-secreting adenocarcinomas; (2) autoimmune haemolytic anaemia—may occur with a wide variety of tumours; (3) pure red-cell aplasia—seen in thymoma; (4) secondary polycythaemia—caused by erythropoietin-secreting tumours, e.g. of cerebellum and kidney.

Other associations between malignancy and haematological disorders include (1) pernicious anaemia—associated with gastric cancer; (2) the effects of treatments for cancer—chemotherapy frequently causes various cytopenias and other toxic effects, including haemolysis.

Infection

Acute bacterial infections—these cause neutrophilia, but occasionally in severely ill patients there is an inadequate response or frank neutropenia, which is characteristic of salmonellosis, brucellosis, rickettsial infections, disseminated tuberculosis, or histoplasmosis.

Chronic bacterial infections—these characteristically induce the anaemia of chronic disorders, but tuberculosis may also cause leukaemoid reactions, pancytopenia, and myelofibrosis, and should be considered in any patient with an unexplained and atypical myeloproliferative disorder.

Virus infections—these generally cause mild neutropenia with lymphocytosis. Conditions of particular note include (1) Epstein–Barr virus—often associated with atypical lymphocytes, which are also found in other viral infections (e.g. cytomegalovirus). (2) Rubella and measles—often cause thrombocytopenia, and occasionally there is bleeding due to disseminated intravascular coagulation. (3) HIV/AIDS—may cause marked anaemia related to the chronic disorder, but examination of the bone marrow frequently shows dyserythropoiesis, which may be related to poor nutrition, drug toxicity and opportunistic infection. Progressive immunodeficiency is associated with lymphoma. (4) Aplastic anaemia—may occur in parvovirus B19 infection and (rarely) hepatitis B infection.

Protozoal and helminthic infections—these include (1) Malaria—can cause a range of manifestations including (a) severe anaemia of complex aetiology—typically in children; (b) thrombocytopenia—a common finding; (c) neutropenia—a common finding; (d) intravascular haemolysis—may be associated with glucose-6-phosphate dehydrogenase deficiency; (e) disseminated intravascular coagulation—probably uncommon; (f) tropical splenomegaly syndrome—can cause pancytopenia due to hypersplenism. (2) Other conditions—these include (a) Leishmaniasis—causes pancytopenia with prominent neutropenia in the early phase of infection; anaemia is due to an inappropriate marrow response and hypersplenism. (b) Hookworm infestation—one of the commonest causes of iron deficiency anaemia in the world. (c) Eosinophilia—characteristic of helminth infestation, particularly during the systemic phase.

Rheumatic and autoimmune disorders

Rheumatoid arthritis—haematological manifestations include (1) anaemia—largely attributable to the response to chronic disease, but iron deficiency due to medication-related blood loss is common; (2) Felty's syndrome—hypersplenism and immune destruction of neutrophils causes pancytopenia and marked neutropenia.

Other disorders—these include (1) systemic lupus erythematosus—anaemia is common and may be related to chronic illness, gastrointestinal blood loss attributable to medication, renal impairment, and autoimmune haemolysis; mild thrombocytopenia occurs in 10 to 25%; lupus anticoagulants and associated anticardiolipin antibodies may be associated with venous thromboembolism, arterial thromboembolism, an increased fate of fetal loss, or thrombocytopenia. (2) Polymyalgia rheumatica and temporal arteritis—may present with severe anaemia of chronic disorders and marked elevation of the erythrocyte sedimentation rate.

Other conditions

These include (1) Renal disease—complications include anaemia, mainly due to erythropoietin deficiency, and also defective haemostasis with bleeding tendency due to abnormal platelet function. (2) Gastrointestinal disease—haematological manifestations include iron deficiency due to bleeding, also malabsorption of iron, folate, and/or vitamin B_{12}. (3) Liver failure—associated with macrocytic anaemia, also with microcytic anaemia due to blood loss from peptic ulceration or bleeding varices; bleeding and haemostatic failure are common, attributable to both thrombocytopenia due to hypersplenism and failure of hepatic formation of coagulation factors V, VIII, IX, X, XI, prothrombin, and fibrinogen. (3) Alcohol—has numerous adverse effects on the blood: macrocytosis and thrombocytopenia are frequent; nutritional deficiencies of iron and folate may complicate the picture; may have direct toxic effects on megakaryocytes and impairs neutrophil function.

Numerous specific abnormalities of the blood occur in other systemic diseases, e.g. in pulmonary eosinophilia, mast-cell and neurological syndromes due to neuroacanthocytosis, and abetalipoproteinaemia.

Introduction

There are few diseases that do not produce some alteration in the blood. In this chapter some of the haematological changes associated with general systemic diseases are summarized. Many of these topics are discussed elsewhere but they are brought together to emphasize how blood changes may give the first indication of non-haematological disorders. It should be remembered that the haematological consequences of systemic disease vary considerably depending on the age of the patient. References to specific aspects of this topic in children and older people are provided in the list of further reading.

Malignant disease

The most common haematological finding in malignant disease (Table 22.7.1) is the anaemia of chronic disorders, which was described in Chapter 22.5.3. It may occur together with localized or widespread malignancy and is sometimes associated with an elevated erythrocyte sedimentation rate (ESR). It is found in patients with practically every type of carcinoma or reticulosis and is refractory to iron, but may respond to erythropoietin.

The anaemia of patients with carcinoma, particularly of the gastrointestinal tract, may be complicated by chronic blood loss and superimposed iron deficiency. Chronic bleeding of this type is often associated with a mild thrombocytosis. The chronic anorexia and general debilitation associated with advanced malignant disease may be associated with a variety of nutritional anaemias, particularly iron or folate deficiency.

Disseminated malignancy

The most common haematological change with disseminated malignancy is a leucoerythroblastic picture characterized by the presence in the blood of immature myeloid cells together with some nucleated red cells, and, sometimes, a mild reticulocytosis. The red cells often show a moderate degree of anisocytosis and poikilocytosis. This finding is very commonly accompanied by the presence of tumour cells in the bone marrow. Clinically, it can cause confusion with the diagnosis of primary myelosclerosis but splenomegaly is unusual in patients with disseminated carcinoma.

Occasionally, widespread carcinoma leads to a leukaemoid reaction with white-cell counts in the range seen in chronic myeloid leukaemia. The differentiation between these two conditions was described earlier.

The microangiopathic haemolytic anaemia of disseminated malignancy is most frequently found in association with a mucin-secreting adenocarcinoma, particularly of the stomach, breast, and lung.

Less common forms of anaemia associated with cancer

Autoimmune haemolytic anaemia is sometimes found in patients with an underlying lymphoma. It is much less common in other forms of malignancy except for the association with tumours of the ovary. However, there have been reports of autoimmune haemolysis occurring with a wide variety of tumours, including lung, stomach, breast, kidney, colon, and testis.

Pure red-cell aplasia may occasionally be the presenting feature in a patient with a tumour of the thymus. There have been occasional reports of this type of anaemia occurring in patients with carcinoma of the bronchus or lymphomas.

Finally, it should be remembered that there is an association between pernicious anaemia and carcinoma of the stomach. A patient may present with a megaloblastic anaemia associated with a malignancy of this type. In the early literature on sideroblastic anaemia, an association with carcinoma was suggested. Since acquired sideroblastic anaemia has been classified as part of the myelodysplastic syndrome there seem to have been no further reports of this association and its significance remains uncertain.

Polycythaemia

The relation between secondary polycythaemia and an underlying neoplasm is discussed in Chapter 22.3.8. It has been found in patients with renal tumours, hepatomas, hamartomas of the liver, uterine fibroids, vascular tumours and cystic adenomas of the cerebellum, and carcinoma of the lung.

Changes in the platelets and blood coagulation

An otherwise unexplained thrombocytosis may be the first indication of an underlying malignancy. It is important to remember

Table 22.7.1 Principal haematological changes in malignant disorders

Haematological change	Malignancy
Erythrocytes	
Anaemia of chronic disorders	All forms
Iron-deficiency anaemia	Gastrointestinal; cervix, uterus
Leucoerythroblastic anaemia	Stomach, breast, thyroid, prostate, bronchus, kidney
Microangiopathic haemolytic anaemia	Mucin-secreting tumours; stomach, bronchus, breast
Secondary myelosclerosis	As for leucoerythroblastic; also reticuloses
Selective red-cell aplasia	Thymus, lymphoma, bronchus
Immune haemolytic anaemia	Ovary; lymphoma; other carcinomas
Megaloblastic anaemia	Stomach; rarely others
Sideroblastic anaemia	Myelodysplastic syndrome
Polycythaemia	Kidney, liver, posterior fossa, uterus
Leucocytes	
Leucocytosis	
Leukaemoid reactions	As for leucoerythroblastic anaemia
Eosinophilia	Miscellaneous carcinomas and reticuloses
Monocytosis	All forms
Basophilia	Myeloproliferative disease; mastocytosis
Lymphopenia	Carcinoma, reticuloses
Platelets	
Thrombocytosis	Gastrointestinal with bleeding; bronchus and others without bleeding
Thrombocytopenia	As for the microangiopathies
Acquired thrombocytopathy	Macroglobulinaemia; other paraproteinaemias
Coagulation	
DIC	Prostate, many others
Primary activation of fibrinolysis	Prostate
Selective impairment of coagulation (see Table 22.7.2)	
Thrombophlebitis	All forms
Miscellaneous	
Abnormal proteins—cryofibrinogens	Prostate, others
Fetal proteins	AFP —liver and others
	CEA—gastrointestinal neoplasms
	Fetal haemoglobin—leukaemia, other tumours
Circulating tumour cells	All forms
Effects of cytotoxic drugs	All forms

AFP, α-fetoprotein; CEA, carcinoembryonic antigen; DIC, disseminated intravascular coagulation.

that this is not always associated with chronic blood loss; bronchial carcinoma may present in this way. Thrombocytopenia may sometimes occur with bone marrow infiltration by tumour cells, but is seen most frequently as a side-effect of chemotherapy. Autoimmune thrombocytopenia has been observed most commonly in association with lymphoid malignancies, but it can also occur in association with tumours of the lung, breast, and testes.

Generalized haemostatic failure (Figs. 22.7.1 and 22.7.2) associated with disseminated carcinoma is considered in detail elsewhere.

Some bleeding disorders associated with cancer seem to be due to selective impairment of coagulation. This may result from pathological inhibitors of different parts of the coagulation system or from isolated factor deficiencies. The mechanism is unknown. If the bleeding disorder is not characterized by consumption of clotting factors or fibrinolysis, a detailed analysis of the activities of the intrinsic and extrinsic pathways must be made in case a correctable lesion is present (Table 22.7.2).

Patients with cancer have an increased tendency to thrombosis. Apart from debilitation and periods of prolonged bed rest there is undoubtedly a hypercoaculable state associated with many tumours. This seems to involve a variety of procoagulants including fibrinogen and factors V, VII, VIII, IX, and XI. Low-grade disseminated intravascular coagulation (DIC) can consume anticogulants such as antithombin III, protein C, and protein S. Cancer cells can initiate clotting by releasing a tissue factor, a phenomenon which is described in patients with lung, kidney, colon, and breast cancers. The syndrome of nonbacterial thrombotic endocarditis, characterized by cerebral embolic strokes and extensive fibrin/

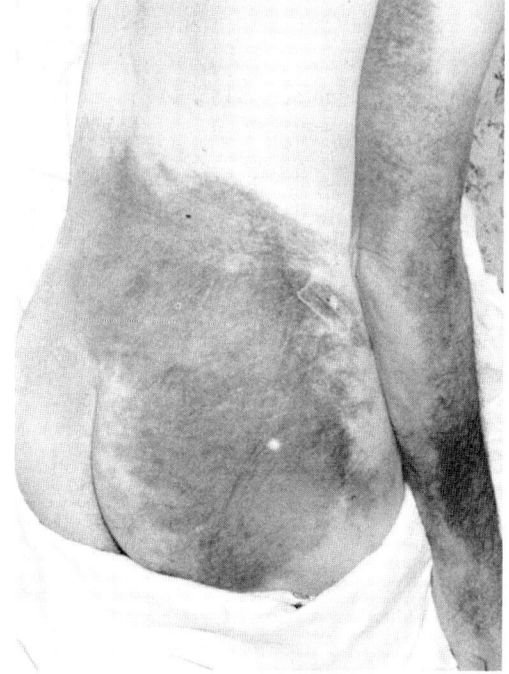

Fig. 22.7.1 Disseminated intravascular coagulation (DIC) in association with carcinoma of the prostate. The patient started to bleed extensively from the iliac-crest marrow biopsy site and from venesection sites. Marrow biopsy showed widespread tumour metastases.
(From Hardisty RM, Weatherall DJ (ed.) (1982). *Blood and its disorders*, 2nd edition. Blackwell Scientific, Oxford, with permission.)

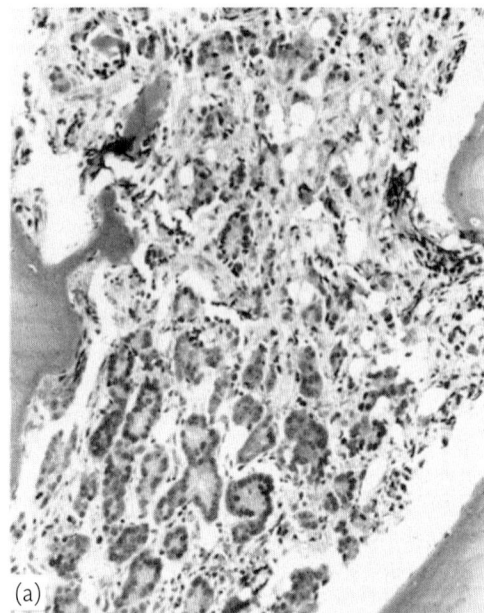

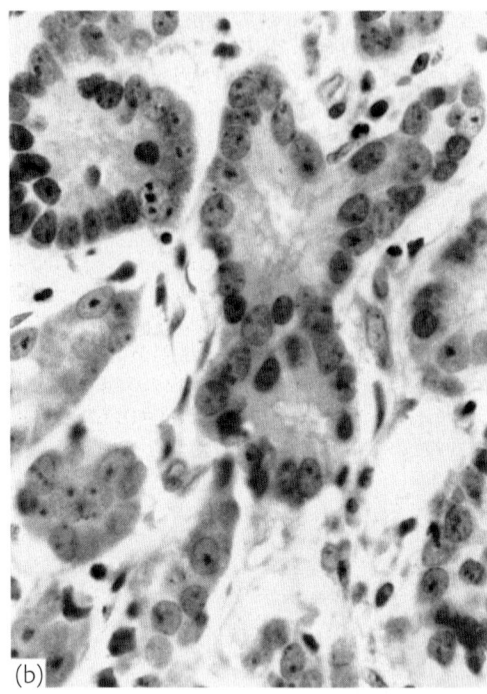

Fig. 22.7.2 Section prepared from Gardner needle biopsies from bone marrow infiltrated with neoplastic cells; the primary tumour was in the prostate. (a) haematoxylin and eosin stain, ×230; (b) haematoxylin and eosin stainstain ×920. (From Hardisty RM, Weatherall DJ (ed.) (1982). *Blood and its disorders*, 2nd edition. Blackwell Scientific, Oxford, with permission.)

platelet vegetations on the mitral and aortic valves, is most commonly associated with cancers of the lung, prostate, and pancreas.

White-cell abnormalities

In addition to the leukaemoid reaction, there are several white-cell changes that should make the clinician think about an underlying malignancy. For example, a persistent monocytosis or eosinophilia may be associated with Hodgkin's disease or with bronchial carcinoma. Persistent lymphopenia may occur in patients with Hodgkin's disease.

Haematological changes due to cancer chemotherapy

Many agents used in cancer chemotherapy depress the bone marrow, causing varying periods of neutropenia and thrombocytopenia associated with a variable anaemia. The bone marrow may also show marked myelodysplastic features. Haemolytic reactions have been associated with a number of drugs, including mitomycin C and bleomycin–cisplatin. In some cases these drugs are associated with a syndrome of microangiopathic haemolytic anaemia resembling the haemolytic uraemic syndrome. Circulating immune complexes have been observed in some cases and there have been reports of response to plasma exchange and immunosuppression. Some chemotherapeutic agents appear to cause a warm antibody type of haemolytic anaemia. In patients who are deficient in glucose-6-phosphate dehydrogenase, the administration of doxorubicin can produce a haemolytic reaction.

Haemophagocytic syndrome

This disorder, which is described later in its association with viral illness (see 'Viral infections', below), has now been reported in patients with cancer, lymphoma, and acute leukaemia. It is characterized by pancytopenia, fever, and splenomegaly; the bone marrow resembles histiocytosis with intense haemophagocytosis by macrophages.

Infection

Most of the important haematological changes in association with infection are considered in Section 7. Just a few points of particular haematological relevance are summarized below.

Acute bacterial infection

Most acute bacterial infections are associated with a neutrophil leucocytosis. This may be so marked, and associated with a 'shift

Table 22.7.2 Selective impairment of coagulation in cancer

Coagulation impairment	Disorder
Inhibitors	
Paraproteins	Plasma-cell disorders
Lupus-like	Hodgkin's disease, lymphoma, myelofibrosis, carcinoma
Factor IX inhibitor	Cancer of colon or prostate
Factor VII inhibitor	Bronchogenic carcinoma
Heparin-like	Bronchogenic carcinoma, myeloma
Isolated factor deficiencies	
Factor XIII	Acute leukaemia, chronic myeloid leukaemia
Factor XII	Chronic myeloid leukaemia
Factor XI	Melanoma
Factor X	Myeloma with amyloid
Factor VIII	Macroglobulinaemia, chronic lymphatic leukaemia, Wilms' tumour
Factor V	Chronic myeloid leukaemia, polycythaemia vera

Modified from Goldsmith GH Jr (1984). Hemostatic disorders associated with neoplasia. In: Ratnoff AD, Forbes CD (eds) *Disorders of hemostasis*, pp. 351–66. Grune & Stratton, Orlando, FA.

to the left' with production of myelocytes in the blood, that the condition may present a leukaemoid type of reaction. Occasionally, in patients who are severely ill with acute bacterial infection, the neutrophil response seems inadequate. Some may be frankly neutropenic. A number of these individuals will prove to have an underlying haematological disorder or a debilitating condition such as alcoholism, but many who recover from their infection show no such underlying abnormality. A marrow examination usually reveals a paucity of mature granulocytes. This clinical picture is particularly common in newborn infants, especially those born prematurely. Some infections seem to be particularly prone to association with a reduced white-cell count. They include salmonellosis, brucellosis, pertussis, rickettsial infections, disseminated tuberculosis (in some cases), and disseminated histoplasmosis.

Other leucocyte changes are less common in acute infection. Monocytosis has been reported in patients with typhoid fever and sometimes in brucellosis or subacute bacterial endocarditis. In endocarditis a monocytosis may be associated with the presence of undifferentiated reticuloendothelial cells in the blood that show erythrophagocytosis.

Some degree of anaemia is found almost invariably in patients with bacterial infection. It usually presents a picture of the anaemia of chronic disorders. Haemolytic anaemia may occur in severe septicaemias and is usually associated with disseminated intravascular coagulation. Some organisms, e.g. *Clostridium welchii*, produce an α-toxin that acts as a lecithinase and causes fulminating intravascular haemolysis. There is a variety of forms of the immune haemolysis associated with infection, including cold agglutinin disease in mycoplasma or Epstein–Barr virus infections; paroxysmal cold haemoglobinuria associated with syphilis; measles or measles vaccination; and others.

DIC is a common accompaniment of severe bacterial infection. Many mechanisms have been suggested, including vascular injury with activation of factor XII or the generation of procoagulants from white cells by the action of endotoxin. Thrombocytopenia is also common in patients with septicaemia. Although this may sometimes reflect DIC, the mechanism is probably more complicated. There may be quite dramatic thrombocytopenia without any other evidence of a consumption coagulopathy. Several mechanisms are involved, including suppression of platelet production by the bone marrow, damage to circulating platelets by immune complexes, endothelial damage, and direct interaction of the platelets with bacteria; phagocytosis of bacteria by platelets may provoke the rapid disappearance of platelets from the circulation.

Chronic bacterial infection

Chronic bacterial infection is usually associated with the anaemia of chronic disorders. Unusual haematological changes are sometimes ascribed to tuberculosis (Table 22.7.3). The most common change is a mild, normochromic, normocytic anaemia with a raised ESR, but more spectacular blood changes have been reported, particularly in association with disseminated tuberculosis. These clinical pictures include leukaemoid reactions, pancytopenia, myelofibrosis, and even polycythaemia. The main problem in assessing these associations is whether the reported patients had infections due to atypical mycobacteria superimposed on an underlying blood disease, or whether disseminated tuberculosis can occasionally produce a clinical picture similar to leukaemia or a myeloproliferative disease. In practice, any patient who presents with an

Table 22.7.3 Haematological changes in tuberculosis

Type of tuberculosis or therapy	Haematological changes
Type of tuberculosis	
Pulmonary	Anaemia of chronic disorders; iron-deficiency anaemia; anaemia due to therapy; high ESR
Ileocaecal	Anaemia of chronic disorders; megaloblastic anaemia due to vitamin B12 or folate deficiency; high ESR
Cryptic, miliary (aregenerative)	Leukaemoid reaction; myelosclerosis;[a] pancytopenia; polycythaemia,[a] anaemia of chronic disorders
Antituberculous drugs	
PAS or streptomycin allergy	Fever, lymphadenopathy, eosinophilia
INAH, cycloserine	Sideroblastic anaemia
Rifampicin	Thrombocytopenic purpura

[a] These reports may well represent cases of disseminated tuberculosis in patients with underlying haematological disorders (see text).

atypical myeloproliferative disorder, and who is going downhill for no apparent cause, should be investigated for tuberculosis. Attempts should be made to grow the organism from bone marrow cultures.

Viral infections

Haematological changes occur quite commonly in association with many virus illnesses. Changes associated with specific viral infections such as infectious mononucleosis are considered in Section 7.

Many viral infections are associated with a modest neutropenia and often with a relative or absolute lymphocytosis. Atypical lymphocytes are characteristic of patients with infectious mononucleosis but they may also be found in association with many other virus infections.

Rubella, acquired in childhood or adult life, is often associated with a leucocytosis and an atypical lymphocytosis. A small proportion of patients develop an acute fulminating thrombocytopenic purpura approximately 4 days after the appearance of the rash. It is usually self-limiting but fatalities have been reported. Thrombocytopenia is also common in infants with congenital rubella. This condition is also characterized by a nonimmune haemolytic episode shortly after birth. Thrombocytopenia has also been reported in association with measles. In particularly severe forms of rubella and morbilli, severe haemorrhagic states due to DIC have been seen. Similar changes occur occasionally in patients with varicella infections.

Haematological changes very similar to those seen in infectious mononucleosis can occur in patients with cytomegalovirus (CMV) infection. Infants may exhibit hepatosplenomegaly with purpura and anaemia. The anaemia is characterized by a haemolytic picture with many normoblasts in the peripheral blood. This form of anaemia may last for several weeks and may be associated with severe thrombocytopenia. There are well-documented cases of an infectious mononucleosis-like disorder occurring after transfusion with fresh blood or after perfusion for open heart surgery. This self-limiting syndrome usually occurs 1 to 3 months after blood transfusion and resolves within a few weeks. It is characterized by a moderate rise in temperature, with hepatosplenomegaly, lymphadenopathy, and transient maculopapular rashes, and a lymphocytosis indistinguishable from that of infectious mononucleosis.

The protean haematological changes that are associated with HIV/AIDS infection are outlined in Chapter 7.5.23. The virus can infect haemopoietic precursors as well as bone-marrow macrophages and stromal fibroblasts. Hence it is not surprising that the often severe anaemia associated with HIV infection produces a diverse haematological picture. The commonest finding is a variable degree of anaemia with a low reticulocyte count and mild microcytosis and hypochromia of the red cells, reflecting the anaemia of chronic disorders. However, the bone marrow often shows quite marked dyserythropoiesis, a finding which may be complicated by opportunistic infection, malnutrition and drug toxicity. Neutropenia and thrombocytopaenia are common and the condition is frequently complicated by a microangiopathic haemolytic anaemia as part of thrombotic thrombocytopenic purpura (TTP). Lupus-like inhibitors of coagulation are also observed. Finally, advancing immunodeficiency, as well as leading to a severe propensity for secondary infection, is also associated with a high frequency of lymphoma. Antiviral therapy may be associated with bone marrow depression.

Haematological complications of infectious hepatitis are rare but can be extremely severe. Coombs' positive haemolytic anaemia has been reported. There is also considerable literature on the occurrence of aplastic anaemia. This disorder seems predominantly to affect young males; the onset of aplasia is usually about 9 weeks after the onset of hepatitis. The condition is associated with a mortality in excess of 90%. In those patients who recover, the period to complete haematological normality ranges between 3 and 20 months.

Many viruses are capable of provoking severe bleeding due to intravascular coagulation. Why viruses can fire off the coagulation cascade is far from clear. Activation of factor XII due to vascular injury or damage to platelets with the release of coagulants have been suggested as possible mechanisms.

The human parvovirus has a particular affinity for red-cell progenitors. It probably causes transient red-cell aplasia quite commonly, but this only gives rise to a symptomatic anaemia in patients who have a markedly shortened red-cell survival. Thus parvovirus infection appears to be responsible for the aplastic crises in patients with sickle-cell anaemia, pyruvate kinase deficiency, or other congenital haemolytic anaemias. Viruses can cause acute damage to the bone marrow in immunesuppressed patients as part of the virus haemophagocytic syndrome.

The haematological changes associated with the viral haemorrhagic fevers are described in detail in Section 7.

Parasitic disease

The major haematological accompaniments of the parasitic diseases are described in Section 7. Those that produce important haematological changes will be briefly summarized here.

Toxoplasmosis

Congenital toxoplasmosis can produce a condition identical to erythroblastosis fetalis. The clinical picture is of a pale, hydropic infant with a large spleen and liver associated with severe anaemia, thrombocytopenia, and a leucocytosis, often with a marked eosinophilia.

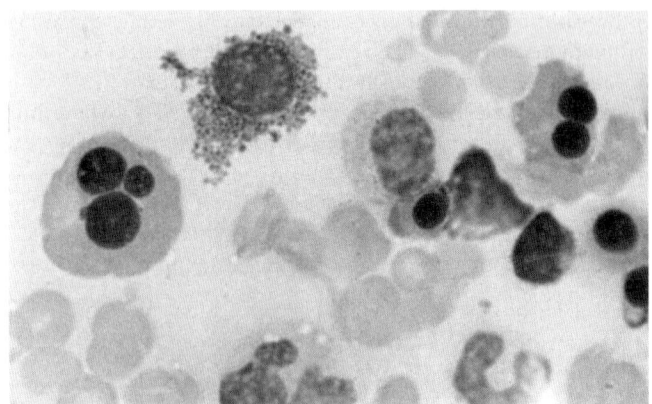

Fig. 22.7.3 Bone marrow appearances in *P. falciparum* malaria. There is marked dyserythropoiesis with several multinucleate red-cell precursors (Giemsa stain, ×800).

In adult life the acquired forms of toxoplasmosis produce a clinical disorder resembling infectious mononucleosis.

Malaria

Malaria produces a wide variety of haematological changes, the most severe of which occur during *Plasmodium falciparum* infections (Fig. 22.7.3). Severe malarial anaemia (SMA), defined by the World Health Organization as a haemoglobin value of less than 5 g/dl, has a very high mortality in babies in regions of high transmission. In older children and adults, profound anaemia is less common, at which time cerebral malaria and other complications become the major problem. Chronic, recurrent attacks of malaria are also a major cause of anaemia in many tropical countries and chronic infection with *P. vivax* is also associated with persistent anaemia.

The pathophysiology of the anaemia of malaria is extremely complex. During acute attacks there may be a massive destruction of parasitized red cells and there is strong evidence that the survival of nonparasitized cells is also shortened. There may be an added immune mechanism particularly in children, although this remains controversial. Aggregation of parasitized red cells and rosette formation may be an added factor in the shortened survival of the red cells. The haemolytic component is complicated by a poor lack of bone marrow response. There is marked dyserythropoiesis with major morphological changes of the red cell precursors. These changes are associated with a poor reticulocyte response. Recent evidence does not suggest that there is a lack of erythropoietin response to anaemia but rather that the dyserythropoiesis reflects the action of cytokines, particularly tumour necrosis factor (TNF) and also the action of haemozoin, a by-product of haemoglobin degradation, on red cell proliferation and survival.

In some patients with severe *P. falciparum* infections, there may be marked intravascular haemolysis and haemoglobinuria. The mechanism is not certain. Some of these patients may be glucose-6-phosphate dehydrogenase deficient but this is by no means the whole story. It has been suggested that some patients with fulminating malaria have DIC. This is probably uncommon and plays very little part in the pathophysiology of either the anaemia or haemorrhagic phenomena that occur. Thrombocytopenia is extremely common but is only rarely associated with evidence of consumption of blood clotting factors. In most forms of malarial infection there is a neutropenia. Monocytosis has also been described.

Several interesting haematological manifestations are associated with unusual forms of malaria. In the tropical splenomegaly syndrome, there may be anaemia, thrombocytopenia, and neutropenia, all secondary to hypersplenism. Congenital malaria infection is contracted in intrauterine life from the mother; newborn babies have a febrile illness associated with profound anaemia that appears to result from the combination of haemolysis and bone marrow suppression.

Leishmaniasis

Visceral leishmaniasis, or kala azar, is associated with hepatosplenomegaly, lymphadenopathy, and pancytopenia, particularly in young children. Early in the course of the disease there is often marked neutropenia. The marrow may be grossly infiltrated with parasitized macrophages. The anaemia is due mainly to a short red-cell survival; there is also an inappropriate marrow response and a variable degree of hypersplenism.

Hookworm

The haematological changes of hookworm infestation are described in Chapter 7.9.4. It is one of the most common causes of iron-deficiency anaemia in the world population. During the systemic phase of the illness, when the larvae invade the lungs, there may be a marked eosinophilia. During this phase the bone marrow shows a remarkable increase in the percentage of eosinophilic myelocytes, which may be out of proportion to the eosinophilia observed in the peripheral blood.

Visceral larva migrans

This condition is characterized by striking haematological changes including anaemia, a marked leucocytosis with eosinophilia, and changes in the titre of anti-A and anti-B blood-group antibodies.

Schistosomiasis

In the chronic phase of *Schistosoma mansoni* and *S. japonicum* infections there may be severe portal hypertension, splenomegaly, and the typical picture of hypersplenism.

Other trematode infestations, including clonorchiasis and paragonamiasis, are associated with eosinophilia and anaemia. Antibodies to the P_1 blood-group antigen may be found in grossly elevated titres in the blood of many patients with acute fascioliasis.

Rheumatoid arthritis and related disorders

In patients with rheumatoid arthritis, anaemia is extremely common. It usually follows the general pattern of anaemia of chronic disorders. It is occasionally complicated by genuine iron deficiency, which may result from a variety of causes including poor diet and chronic blood loss due to the effects of treatment, particularly ingestion of salicylates and nonsteroidal anti-inflammatory agents (NSAIDs) or corticosteroids. Furthermore, significant bleeding into actively inflamed joints can occur. It has been estimated that if only two knee joints were affected, the annual blood loss through this mechanism could amount to as much as 2500 ml. It is not certain how much of the iron derived from this blood is available for reutilization for haemoglobin synthesis. The diagnosis of iron deficiency complicating rheumatoid arthritis may not be straightforward; levels of serum iron and iron-binding capacity may be difficult to interpret because of coexisting inflammation. Determination of marrow stores and estimation of serum ferritin may be more helpful. Although the last two are

elevated in inflammatory conditions, a low level suggests genuine iron deficiency.

There are no particular changes in the neutrophil response in uncomplicated rheumatoid arthritis; a marked leucocytosis may reflect a response to corticosteroid therapy or a superadded infection such as a septic arthritis. The platelet count is elevated in between 20 and 50% of patients with rheumatoid arthritis. The degree of thrombocytosis parallels the degree of activity of the illness and cannot be accounted for on the grounds of associated intestinal blood loss due to drug therapy.

The haematological changes of Felty's syndrome are summarized in Chapter 24.4.1. There is anaemia, thrombocytopenia, and marked neutropenia. Although many of these changes are features of hypersplenism, recent studies on the neutropenia in this disorder indicate that it has a complex basis. Immune destruction of neutrophils may play a major part.

A variety of haematological changes are due to drug therapy for rheumatoid arthritis and related disorders. Salicylates may produce chronic blood loss, while drugs containing phenacetin produce methaemoglobinaemia and Heinz-body haemolytic anaemia that may sometimes be preceded by a marked eosinophilia. Phenylbutazone produces pancytopenia, which may be severe and irreversible; this drug has now been discontinued in the United Kingdom. Oxyphenylbutazone and penicillamine may also cause severe marrow depression. The administration of gold occasionally causes marked thrombocytopenia or pancytopenia.

The management of the haematological manifestations of rheumatoid arthritis and Felty's syndrome is unsatisfactory. The anaemia generally reflects the activity of the disease. If there is genuine iron deficiency, iron replacement therapy is indicated. The vexed question of whether intramuscular iron administration has some nonspecific effect on the anaemia of rheumatoid arthritis, even in the absence of reduced body iron stores, remains unresolved. Similarly, there is controversy about the best way to manage Felty's syndrome. After splenectomy there is sometimes a dramatic rise in the neutrophil and total leucocyte counts, but this is not always associated with a decreased incidence of infection. Some patients show no change in the white-cell count after surgery. It is difficult to advise about the best approach to the management of this condition; only if there are recurrent, life-threatening infections should splenectomy be done. Patients require extremely careful surveillance after the operation. There may be some place for the use of prophylactic antibiotics in those whose neutrophil counts do not respond.

The anaemia of rheumatoid arthritis, and related inflammatory states, may respond to erythropoietin given in the higher therapeutic dose range. This treatment is extremely expensive and its use should be reserved for those patients who have severe anaemia which is refractory to treatment of the underlying inflammatory disorder by any other means. The commonest cause of lack of response is associated iron deficiency.

Systemic lupus erythematosus and other collagen disorders

It is quite common for systemic lupus erythematosus (SLE) to present with a haematological disorder. This is not the case in the other collagen–vascular disorders.

The most common blood change in SLE is anaemia, which occurs in nearly all patients at some stage of the illness. It is usually a mild anaemia of chronic disorders, which may be complicated by blood loss from analgesics or anti-inflammatory medication, renal impairment, or haemolysis. Acquired autoimmune haemolytic anaemia may be the sole presenting feature in SLE and may antedate the appearance of other typical features by many years. The incidence of this complication varies in reported series but occurs overall in approximately 5% of cases. The Coombs' test is invariably positive with anticomplementary reagents and is positive with anti-IgG during episodes of acute haemolysis. Other forms of anaemia in SLE include those associated with hypersplenism due to splenomegaly, and the occasional occurrence of a hypocellular bone marrow, probably due to involvement of small vessels by the disease process.

The most consistent finding in the white-cell count in SLE is leukopenia, which occurs in up to half the patients at some time during the illness. This is often a combined neutropenia and lymphopenia. Mild eosinophilia occurs occasionally, particularly in association with skin involvement.

A mild thrombocytopenia occurs in 10 to 25% of all cases of SLE. More severe thrombocytopenia, producing a picture almost indistinguishable from idiopathic thrombocytopenic purpura, occurs in a small proportion of patients and may be the sole presenting feature in some. Although early reports indicated that splenectomy might be associated with a flare-up of the systemic symptoms of SLE in patients with thrombocytopenia, this has now been shown to be incorrect.

Lupus anticoagulant

This is an antibody that prolongs phospholipid-dependent coagulation tests *in vitro*. Although it received its name because it was found in patients with SLE, it occurs more frequently in patients without this disease and is associated with thrombosis rather than with bleeding. It is particularly common in patients with lupus-like autoimmune disorders without the associated criteria for the diagnosis of SLE. Originally it was thought to occur in approximately 10% of patients but using more sensitive assays it is now clear that it occurs in about 50%.

Both lupus anticoagulants and associated anticardiolipin antibodies are immunoglobulins which react with phospholipid and other molecules (platelet factor IV). They may be associated with venous thromboembolism, arterial thromboembolism, an increased fate of fetal loss, or thrombocytopenia. They are discussed in detail in Section 19.

Other collagen disorders

The haematological changes in the other collagen–vascular diseases are much less impressive. They are all associated with the anaemia of chronic disorders. Polyarteritis nodosa may be characterized by an eosinophilia.

The interesting syndrome of polymyalgia rheumatica and temporal arteritis may present to the haematologist (Chapter 19.11.4). Haematological changes are characterized by a severe anaemia of chronic disorders with a marked elevation of the ESR. The leucocyte count is usually normal, although there may occasionally be a mild eosinophilia. There is a marked increase in the α_2- and γ-globulins, although this is polyclonal in type. This blood picture can very closely resemble that of multiple myeloma or disseminated malignancy.

Renal disease

Almost all forms of renal disease are associated with haematological changes. However, by far the most important is the severe refractory anaemia that accompanies chronic renal failure.

Anaemia

Anaemia is an important and intractable complication of chronic renal failure. The correlation between the blood urea nitrogen and the haemoglobin level is inconsistent. Although erythropoietin deficiency is an important component, the anaemia has an extremely complex aetiology, which is only partly understood. The red cells of patients with chronic renal disease have a shortened survival, although they survive normally when injected into healthy recipients. Similarly, normal red cells have a shortened survival in uraemic recipients. The nature of the intracorpuscular defect has not been determined. Most red-cell enzymes are present at normal levels and the intracellular level of ATP is elevated. However, changes in membrane function have been demonstrated, in particular decreased activity of the Na^+–K^+ pumps; the toxic substances that cause these changes have not been identified.

There is also impaired red-cell production in the anaemia of chronic renal failure. The fact that the anaemia of chronic renal failure can be corrected by the administration of recombinant erythropoietin suggests that the ineffective production of this hormone due to renal damage is the major aetiological factor in the anaemia of renal failure. However, it has been found that the serum from patients on haemodialysis also inhibits the proliferation of erythroid progenitors. The suppressive activity is found in serum fractions containing material of molecular weights ranging from 47 000 to above 150 000. Interestingly, patients on continuous ambulatory peritoneal dialysis (CAPD) have higher haemoglobin levels than those on haemodialysis. It is possible this reflects the more effective removal of medium-sized molecules of this type by CAPD. Patients on haemodialysis with low haemoglobin concentrations are more likely to have fibrous replacement of their bone marrow. This has been correlated with secondary hyperparathyroidism, suggesting a role for parathyroid hormone in the bone marrow unresponsiveness and fibrosis (see Chapter 13.6).

The anaemia of chronic renal failure may be exacerbated by deficiency of iron resulting from blood loss due to excessive blood sampling, incorrect haemodialysis procedures, or bleeding due to defective platelet function (see below). A small proportion of patients with chronic renal failure develop splenomegaly and hypersplenism. Folate deficiency is found occasionally in patients on haemodialysis. There have been a few reports of nephrosis leading to severe urinary loss of transferrin and hence to a low plasma iron-binding capacity. Some patients with renal disease have chronic inflammatory lesions, which may lead to a superadded anaemia of chronic disorders.

The type of renal lesion is also an important factor in determining the severity of anaemia. For example, the renal failure of polycystic disease of the kidneys is associated with a relatively higher haemoglobin level than other forms of renal failure. It is noteworthy that the shrunken kidneys of some patients on long-term dialysis programmes develop cysts and this phenomenon is also associated with a rise in haemoglobin level. It seems likely that both these conditions are associated with a relative increase in the output of erythropoietin.

The anaemia of chronic renal failure is normochromic and normocytic unless there is associated iron deficiency. The red cells show characteristic deformities with multiple tiny spicules and contracted poikilocytes. The capacity of the red cells for oxygen transport does not seem to be impaired. There is often an increased intracellular concentration of 2,3-diphosphoglycerate (2,3-DPG) in response to anaemia and hyperphosphataemia, and the oxygen affinity of haemoglobin is decreased. This right shift in the oxygen dissociation curve may be augmented by uraemic acidosis. However, part of the advantage of the acidosis is cancelled out by the direct effect of low pH on glycolysis and 2,3-DPG production. Intensive dialysis may cause a reduction in the concentration of intracellular phosphate, which has the effect of increasing the oxygen affinity of haemoglobin. This effect may play a part in the so-called dialysis disequilibrium syndrome.

In patients with chronic renal failure who have associated iron deficiency, the red-cell indices are typical of this condition; the reduced mean corpuscle haemoglobin and volume are corrected by iron therapy.

The bone marrow in chronic renal failure shows normoblastic erythropoiesis but the degree of erythroid hyperplasia is not compatible with the degree of anaemia, indicating suppression of erythropoiesis.

The management of the anaemia of chronic renal failure is described in Chapter 21.6.

White cells

The total and differential white-cell count is usually normal in patients with chronic renal failure. However, the phagocytic activity of granulocytes may be reduced and complement activation by haemodialysis membranes may cause stasis of white cells in the pulmonary circulation with temporary granulocytopenia. Cell-mediated immunity is also depressed.

Platelets and coagulation

There is a variety of haemostatic defects in different forms of renal disease. Most forms are associated with a bleeding tendency, which is seen in its most florid form in acute renal failure. The main features are purpura, and mucosal and gastrointestinal bleeding associated with abnormal platelet function and a prolonged bleeding time; these changes are reversible by dialysis. Various mechanisms have been proposed. These include a direct action of metabolites on platelet function and a disturbance of prostaglandin balance because of a deficiency of a renal factor that modifies vascular production of prostacyclin and/or platelet endoperoxide and thromboxane synthesis. These changes result in an abnormality of the control of platelet cAMP, causing the platelets to become refractory to aggregation agents. Many conditions that lead to renal failure are also associated with thrombocytopenia. For example the circulating immune complexes found in patients with acute glomerulonephritis, polyarteritis nodosa, or lupus nephritis may be responsible for platelet activation and the release of aggregating agents. Thrombocytopenia may also be aggravated by heparin therapy or the use of immunosuppressant drugs in patients who have received kidney grafts. Mild thrombocytopenia is well recognized in patients with functioning renal allografts. This has also been found to be associated with an inability to clear the immune complexes. Graft rejection is associated with enhanced platelet aggregation and thrombocytopenia.

The nephrotic syndrome is characterized by a marked tendency to thrombosis. This also has a complex pathogenesis. Both platelet aggregation and release reactions have been shown to be enhanced in this condition. Protein loss in the urine may also play a part. It has been found that an increased loss of antithrombin III is related to thrombotic episodes. Conversely, coagulation factors IX and XIII are also lost in the urine of patients with a nephrotic syndrome; the deficiency of factor IX may be sufficient to induce bleeding.

The haematological changes associated with the haemolytic uraemic syndrome and thrombotic thrombocytopenic purpura were considered earlier in this section.

Polycythaemia

The polycythaemias associated with renal lesions and following renal transplantation are discussed in Chapter 21.7.3.

Treatment of the haematological complications of renal disease

The management of the anaemia of chronic renal failure, which has been revolutionized by the availability of recombinant erythropoietin, is considered in Chapter 21.6. The management of bleeding in patients with acute renal failure is based on correction of uraemia by dialysis and appropriate replacement therapy. Peritoneal dialysis is probably more effective in reversing abnormalities of platelet function, although there is no definite evidence that one form of dialysis is superior to another. If there is severe thrombocytopenia, platelet transfusions should be given.

Gastrointestinal and liver disease

Many of the haematological changes that occur in gastrointestinal and liver disease are described in Section 15. Here we will simply summarize the haematological manifestations of those disorders that present frequently with anaemia or defective haemostasis.

Gastrointestinal blood loss

Blood loss in excess of 20 ml/day will always result in a negative iron balance and ultimately in iron-deficiency anaemia, the time taken depending on the body stores of iron when the bleeding started.

The haematological picture shows the typical changes of iron-deficiency anaemia, with hypochromic, microcytic red-cell morphology. Occasionally, there are some clues that this blood picture is associated with chronic blood loss. Quite frequently there is a mild to moderate thrombocytosis, and if iron is being taken there may be a dimorphic blood picture (Fig. 22.7.4), red-cell polychromasia, and a low-grade reticulocytosis. It is always worth examining the peripheral blood film very carefully as it may give some clue as to the site of the blood loss. For example the presence of target cells may indicate liver disease, whereas the presence of distorted cells and Howell–Jolly bodies suggests malabsorption due to adult coeliac disease complicated by hyposplenism.

The diagnosis of the site of acute upper intestinal bleeding is considered in Chapter 15.14.2. The investigation of chronic gastrointestinal blood loss may be difficult. First, it is essential to determine whether iron-deficiency anaemia is due to a defective intake or due to excessive loss of iron. If gastrointestinal blood loss is suspected the first step is to confirm that this is occurring, by examination of several stool specimens for occult blood.

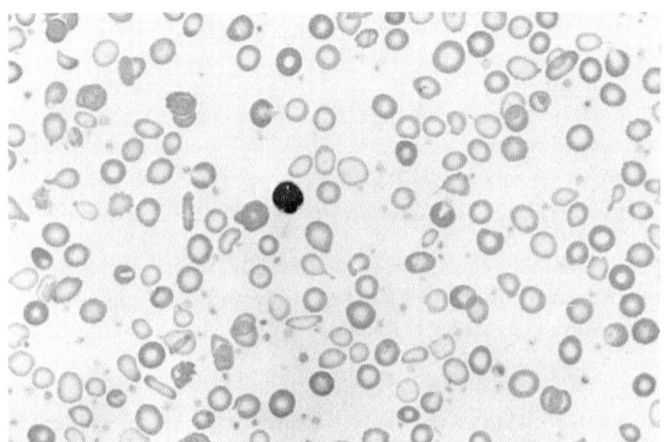

Fig. 22.7.4 Peripheral blood picture associated with gastrointestinal bleeding. The red cells show a dimorphic picture with hypochromic and normochromic forms. The platelet count is elevated, a typical finding in bleeding. (Giemsa stain, ×600).

Currently, the most commonly used method is the Haemoccult card which contains a filter paper impregnated with guaiac, or a similar commercial kit. The peroxidase activity of red blood cells releases a free oxygen radical from hydrogen peroxide (the developer) which then reacts with the guaiac to produce a blue colour. This test is simple, easy to perform following a rectal examination, and quick. Nevertheless, it is relatively insensitive, since blood loss must exceed 20 ml daily for 80 to 90% of tests to be positive (the normal loss in a healthy individual is 0.5–1.2 ml daily as measured by ^{51}Cr-labelled red cells). False-positive results may result from peroxidase or nonspecific oxidants in the diet. Thus in many screening programmes, subjects are requested to omit red meat, fresh fruit, cauliflower, swede, turnip, tomatoes, horseradish, and vitamin C supplements from their diet during the 3 days before testing. NSAIDs and aspirin may also give positive results but, since the increased blood loss is in the upper gastrointestinal tract, the haemoglobin is metabolized in the small intestine and is therefore not detected in stools by Haemoccult unless blood loss is considerable. Iron therapy does not affect guaiac-based tests. Many newer tests, which are said to be even more sensitive, are being developed but their role in clinical practice is not yet established.

Once having established that there is gastrointestinal blood loss, the next step is to determine the site. This requires a detailed history and clinical examination as outlined in the introduction to this section. The next step is a careful endoscopy, followed by sigmoidoscopy and colonoscopy. If these investigations do not provide a diagnosis, and there is persistent bleeding, the duodenum and small bowel should be studied radiologically. Occasionally it is necessary to resort to coeliac or superior mesenteric angiography, which may be useful for showing duodenal or ileal varices, bleeding from Meckel's diverticulum or nonspecific ulcers of the ileum, small bowel tumours, and vascular lesions. However, small lesions can only be visualized if there is active bleeding at the time of the examination, probably at a rate of at least 0.5 ml/min.

Inflammatory diseases of the bowel

A mild anaemia of chronic disorders is a common accompaniment of inflammatory disease of the ileum, caecum, and colon. It is observed frequently in patients with Crohn's disease, ileocaecal tuberculosis, ulcerative colitis, and other forms of proctocolitis. In many of these conditions the anaemia of chronic disorders is complicated by intermittent blood loss or dietetic iron deficiency. In some cases of extensive Crohn's disease there may be an added factor of malabsorption. Anaemia occurs in about one-third of these patients and it may be complicated by reduced vitamin B$_{12}$ or folic acid absorption. In one large survey of patients with Crohn's disease, anaemia was present in 79% of the men and 54% of women. Out of a total of 63 patients, 46 had bone marrow biopsies, and of these 39% were megaloblastic. Of this group, 11 were folate deficient, 6 were vitamin B$_{12}$ deficient, and 1 had both deficiencies. On the other hand, macrocytic anaemia is unusual in patients with ulcerative colitis and the anaemia is usually hypochromic due to blood loss. Interestingly, there have been occasional reports of autoimmune haemolytic anaemia occurring in association with ulcerative colitis; in several cases the autoantibodies showed rhesus specificity.

The anaemia of intestinal inflammatory disease may be made worse by drugs used in its management. Patients who receive salazopyrine for colitis occasionally develop an acute haemolytic anaemia associated with Heinz body formation. Bone marrow depression may occur in patients receiving immunosuppressive treatment for colitis or Crohn's disease. Ileocaecal tuberculosis may be associated with any of the bizarre haematological manifestations of tuberculosis described above, and it may be complicated by the side effects of antituberculous drug therapy.

Whipple's disease may produce a clinical picture and blood changes that can mimic several primary haematological disorders. The typical clinical triad of diarrhoea, arthropathy, and enlarged lymph nodes is usually associated with a mild normochromic, normocytic anaemia, a raised ESR, and a polymorphonuclear leucocytosis. Quite often there is associated lymphopenia or eosinophilia. Some cases present less typically. When the spleen is enlarged the condition may closely mimic a primary reticulosis. Malabsorption of vitamin B$_{12}$ or folic acid may occasionally be encountered in this disorder (see Chapter 15.10.6).

Structural disease of the stomach, and small and large bowel

The structural changes and resulting abnormalities of absorption associated with gastritis are described in detail in Chapter 15.10.1. Similarly, the various anatomical abnormalities of the small gut and malabsorption syndromes that lead to vitamin B$_{12}$ and folate deficiency are reviewed earlier in this section. The relation between gastric surgery and iron and vitamin B$_{12}$ metabolism is discussed in Chapter 22.5.4.

Most anatomical lesions of the small bowel present to the haematologist as a macrocytic anaemia with a megaloblastic bone marrow due to vitamin B$_{12}$ or folate deficiency or as a refractory iron-deficiency anaemia. Several abnormalities of the small gut are associated with the production of a relatively profuse bacterial flora that utilize vitamin B$_{12}$. These conditions include surgically produced blind loops, strictures, anastomoses between loops of small bowel, fistulas between various sections of the bowel, diverticula of the small bowel, malfunctioning gastroenterostomies, interference of gut motility in conditions such as scleroderma, Whipple's disease, postvagotomy, and after extensive gut resection, where the disorder may also produce malabsorption. All these conditions are associated with defective vitamin B$_{12}$ absorption, which can be partly corrected by the administration of broad-spectrum antibiotics but not by intrinsic factor.

Megaloblastic anaemia due to intestinal malabsorption is fully reviewed in Chapter 22.5.6. It should be remembered, however, that the malabsorption syndromes may present to the haematologist in other ways. For example, there is a very high incidence of iron-deficiency anaemia in this group and, particularly in childhood, this is the much the more common form of presentation than a megaloblastic anaemia. The peripheral blood changes of hyposplenism are quite frequently associated with an underlying malabsorption syndrome, which itself may also present with a bleeding disorder due to defective absorption of vitamin K. Patients with malabsorption syndrome frequently have biochemical evidence of vitamin E deficiency; although this may produce a slightly shortened red-cell survival, there is no evidence that vitamin E deficiency alone produces a significant degree of anaemia.

Liver disease

There is usually a moderate degree of anaemia in patients with chronic liver failure (Box 22.7.1). The red cells are normochromic or slightly macrocytic with mean corpuscle volume values ranging from 100 to 115 fl. Target cells and a variable degree of polychromasia with a slightly elevated reticulocyte count are often found. The degree of macrocytosis and target-cell formation corresponds reasonably well with the degree of liver failure. The bone marrow tends to be hypercellular with erythroid hyperplasia and macronormoblastic changes.

The actual mechanism of the anaemia of liver failure is uncertain. However, there may be many complicating factors that cause a worsening of the anaemia in this condition. Nutritional folate deficiency is very common in patients with liver disease, particularly the alcoholic form. Secondary iron deficiency is also common and usually results from chronic intestinal blood loss associated with a poor dietetic intake. Interestingly, in patients with severe portal hypertension and cirrhosis, or in those who have undergone portacaval shunt surgery, there may be some increase in iron absorption with marked haemosiderosis of the liver.

A variety of different forms of haemolytic anaemia occur in patients with liver disease. In Zieve's syndrome there is jaundice, hyperlipidaemia, and haemolytic anaemia that follows an excessive alcohol intake. Other forms of haemolytic anaemia may occur. Acute haemolysis has been well documented in patients with viral hepatitis, particularly those who are glucose-6-phosphate dehydrogenase deficient. An acquired haemolytic anaemia with a positive Coombs' test may occur occasionally in patients with chronic active hepatitis. Another form of haemolytic anaemia in liver disease, usually alcoholic cirrhosis, has been observed in which there are marked red-cell abnormalities with burr and spur-shaped forms predominating.

Bleeding and haemostatic failure are extremely common accompaniments of liver failure. They have a complex aetiology including diminished hepatic synthesis of coagulation factors V, VII, IX, X, and XI, prothrombin, and fibrinogen. In some forms of liver disease there may be malabsorption of vitamin K with reduction in the K-deficient clotting factors, and reproduction of a dysfunctional form of fibrinogen has been reported in some patients with cirrhosis and hepatocellular carcinoma. In some forms of liver failure there is enhanced fibrinolysis, due to decrease synthesis of α_2-plasmin inhibitor. In severe liver failure disseminated intravascular

---

Box 22.7.1 Haematological changes in liver disease

- Virus hepatitis
  - Haemolytic anaemia, hypoplastic anaemia
- Chronic active hepatitis
  - Immune haemolytic anaemia, hyperglobulinaemia
- Chronic liver failure
- Chronic anaemia is often complicated by:
  - Blood loss and iron deficiency
  - Alcohol, direct effect on marrow
  - Folate deficiency
  - Portal hypertension and hypersplenism
  - Acute haemolytic episodes (e.g. Zieve's syndrome, spur-cell syndrome)
- Thrombocytopenia, leucopenia, haemorrhagic diathesis due to:
  - Deficiency of vitamin K-dependent factors
  - Portal hypertension and hypersplenism
  - Increased fibrinolysis
  - Thrombocytopenia
- Portal hypertension
  - Anaemia, leucopenia, thrombocytopenia, bleeding from varices
- Obstructive jaundice
  - Mild anaemia, target-cell formation, masking of hereditary spherocytosis
- Tumours
  - Polycythaemia, leukaemoid reactions, α-fetoprotein production
- Liver transplantation
  - Haemorrhagic and hypercoagulable states

---

configuration may occur. Thrombocytopenia is extremely common in liver disease, sometimes due to hypersplenism but in other cases its pathogenesis is not clear.

The management of bleeding in liver diseases is considered in Section 15.

Haematological effects of alcohol

Because excessive consumption of alcohol is so common, it is important for clinicians to appreciate the remarkably diverse haematological manifestations that it causes. Anaemia is particularly common in chronic alcoholics. It has an extremely complex aetiology including a deficient diet, chronic blood loss, hepatic dysfunction, and the direct toxic effects of alcohol on the bone marrow.

Macrocytosis is also particularly common in chronic alcoholics. An unexplained macrocytic blood picture should always raise the possibility of alcoholism, although its absence does not rule out the diagnosis. It may be associated with normoblastic or megaloblastic erythropoiesis. In moderately severe alcoholics who are maintaining a reasonable diet, it probably reflects the direct toxic action of alcohol on the bone marrow. The normoblasts may show vacuolation, or there may be no specific changes on light microscopy. Megaloblastic anaemia is usually seen in severe alcoholics who are poorly nourished, and is due to folate deficiency. Although a folate-poor diet is the major factor, there is some evidence that alcohol plays a more direct part in interfering with folate metabolism by an unknown mechanism. It should be remembered that macrocytosis can also occur in alcoholics during a reticulocytosis in response to bleeding or alcohol withdrawal. It may also reflect coexistent liver disease. The occurrence of sideroblastic anaemia in severe alcoholics was mentioned in an earlier chapter. It is often associated with a macrocytosis or a dimorphic blood picture and occurs in severe alcoholics. The sideroblastic changes revert to normal after stopping alcohol.

Simple iron deficiency is also found commonly in alcoholics and probably reflects both a poor diet and chronic blood loss due to gastritis or bleeding varices. It may be associated with folate deficiency; the blood film is then dimorphic with macrocytes, microcytes, and hypersegmented neutrophils. Alcoholics with chronic pancreatitis may develop iron loading due to increased absorption. These changes, which are specific for alcohol, may be accompanied by any of the haematological manifestations of liver disease.

Alcohol has deleterious effects on the white cells. Severe alcoholics are prone to infection. The neutropenia of alcoholism may reflect both the toxic effect of alcohol on the marrow and folate deficiency. There is also some evidence that alcohol can interfere with neutrophil locomotion and with their ability to ingest foreign material including microorganisms.

Thrombocytopenia is commonly seen in chronic alcoholics and may occur without accompanying folate deficiency or splenomegaly. Megakaryocytes may be normal or diminished in number. Following withdrawal of alcohol the platelet count usually returns to normal, although it may become markedly elevated for a few days.

Chest disease

(See also carcinoma and tuberculosis, above, and secondary polycythaemia, Chapter 22.3.8).

Pneumonia

Most bacterial pneumonias are associated with a neutrophil leucocytosis. Two relatively common forms of pneumonia are associated with more specific haematological changes. In mycoplasma pneumonia, cold agglutinins can usually be detected in increased amounts towards the end of the first week in up to 80% of cases. The cold antibodies are polyclonal IgM to the red-cell I antigen. Although a positive Coombs' test and an increased reticulocyte count have been described in these cases, serious haemolysis is rare. Occasionally, the condition is complicated by DIC.

There is increasing evidence that in patients with pneumonia caused by *Legionella pneumophila* (Legionnaires' disease) there may be severe thrombocytopenia and, sometimes, lymphopenia. Several cases have been reported to be complicated by DIC.

Pulmonary eosinophilia (see also Section 18)

This term refers to a group of disorders that have in common a raised eosinophil count in the peripheral blood in association with pulmonary infiltrates on the chest radiograph. The exact nature of many of the disorders that constitute this syndrome is uncertain. In its simplest form there may be a brief period of respiratory distress in association with eosinophilia. This condition is sometimes called Löffler's syndrome. At the other end of the spectrum there is a severe illness associated with widespread pulmonary infiltrates and eosinophilia, which may culminate with the features of polyarteritis nodosa.

The transient disorder described by Löffler probably represents a heterogeneous group of conditions, which in many cases are associated with parasitic infection. Many parasitic disorders can cause this type of illness, including ascariasis, ankylostomiasis, trichiuriasis, taeniasis, and fascioliasis. A similar condition has been well documented as part of a hypersensitivity reaction to drugs. The most common is *p*-aminosalicylic acid but similar reactions have been observed in patients receiving penicillin, sulphonamides, and nitrofurantoin. A similar clinical picture is associated with the syndrome of allergic alveolitis, including farmer's lung, bird fancier's lung, and a variety of other occupational disorders. Another condition characterized by a marked eosinophilia with pulmonary infiltrates goes under the general term 'tropical eosinophilia'. There is considerable evidence that this disorder is due to occult filarial infection. Pulmonary eosinophilia may also be due to hypersensitivity to fungi, particularly *Aspergillus fumigatus*.

Idiopathic pulmonary haemosiderosis and Goodpasture's syndrome

These disorders occasionally present as a refractory anaemia that has the characteristics of the anaemia of chronic disorders, although it may become markedly hypochromic and microcytic due to chronic blood loss.

Skin diseases

Megaloblastic anaemia and the skin

The whole relation between skin disease and megaloblastic anaemia is extremely complex and much of the work in this field is still controversial. The subject is discussed elsewhere (see Section 23).

A proportion of patients with various dermatoses show evidence of folate depletion, at least biochemically, and in some cases, haematologically. This has been reported in patients with erythroderma, psoriasis, or extensive eczema. There is a well-documented association between malabsorption and dermatitis herpetiformis. Although megaloblastic anaemia is not found frequently in association with disorders of the skin, some patients with these conditions do have mild megaloblastic changes. Earlier reports suggested that a significant proportion of them had abnormalities of small-intestinal function and structure, leading to the descriptive term 'dermatogenic enteropathy'. This concept has been questioned and it is now agreed that a completely flat small-bowel mucosa is rarely seen in these conditions. The relation between dermatitis herpetiformis and malabsorption of the coeliac type seems to be a special case. Several series have shown a high incidence of small-bowel changes of coeliac disease in patients with this condition. Furthermore, there appears to be a high incidence of splenic hypoplasia with typical haematological changes of defective function of the spleen (see Chapter 22.4.4).

Other dermatological disorders

Several dermatological diseases have a major haematological component. Of particular importance are the systemic mast-cell syndromes, Sezary syndrome and cutaneous T-cell lymphomas, hereditary telangiectasia, and some of the inherited disorders of collagen.

Endocrine disease

Pituitary deficiency

A mild, normochromic, normocytic anaemia is very common in patients with anterior pituitary deficiency. The mechanism is not absolutely clear, although the anaemia has many features in common with that of hypothyroidism and is fully responsive to appropriate replacement therapy.

Thyroid disease

Hypothyroidism is associated with a variety of haematological changes. Anaemia is common and may be normocytic, microcytic, or macrocytic.

Severe microcytic anaemia in hypothyroidism is most commonly seen in women who have menorrhagia, which is a frequent complication of this condition. Severe macrocytosis in hypothyroidism usually indicates an associated vitamin B_{12} deficiency; there seems to be a genuine association between pernicious anaemia and myxoedema. It has been suggested that mild macrocytosis may occur in hypothyroidism in the absence of vitamin B_{12} or folate deficiency, although published series of studies have shown a remarkable variability in the incidence of this phenomenon. Some patients with severe hypothyroidism have a small proportion of misshapen red cells on their peripheral blood films.

The anaemia of uncomplicated myxoedema is normochromic and normocytic. The mechanism is still uncertain. Recent studies have shown that thyroid hormones (T_3, T_4, and reverse T_3) can potentiate the effect of erythropoietin on the formation of erythroid colonies *in vitro*. This effect appears to be mediated by receptors with β_2-adrenergic properties. It appears that the thyroid hormones have a direct effect in altering the erythropoietin responsiveness of erythroid progenitors. It has also been suggested that part of the normochromic anaemia of hypothyroidism may be a physiological adaptation to reduced oxygen requirements by the tissues.

Curiously, patients with hyperthyroidism do not have elevated haemoglobin levels. There is some recent evidence that there may be a mild increase in the red-cell mass in hyperthyroidism, but that this is compensated for by an increase in plasma volume. In some patients with severe hyperthyroidism, there is a mild anaemia associated with abnormal iron utilization.

Adrenal disease

A mild, normochromic, normocytic anaemia together with neutropenia, eosinophilia, and lymphocytosis is observed in some patients with Addison's disease. There is a variety of haematological changes following the administration of corticosteroids or endogenous overproduction of these agents. These include granulocytosis, reduced lymphocyte count, involution of lymphatic tissues, and a decrease in the eosinophil and monocyte count.

Parathyroid disease

Primary hyperparathyroidism is occasionally associated with anaemia, which responds to removal of the parathyroid glands. The relation between parathyroid disease and marrow fibrosis is discussed in Chapter 13.6.

Diabetes mellitus

The structural changes that occur in the haemoglobin of diabetic patients are discussed in Chapter 13.11.1. There have been recent reports that there may be an increase in the red-cell volume of patients with severe diabetes. The mechanism and significance of this observation remains to be clarified. Severe diabetic acidosis is associated with a marked leucocytosis, even when there is no underlying infection. Hyperosmolarity impairs neutrophil function; reduced neutrophil migration has been observed in patients with diabetic ketoacidosis or poorly controlled hyperglycaemia. Because of the high incidence of atheroma in patients with diabetes, both platelet function and vessel-wall metabolism have been studied in considerable detail in this condition. Synthesis of prostaglandin I_2 in biopsy specimens of forearm veins is reduced. A variety of changes in platelet reactivity and survival have been observed. The relation of these changes to the vascular disease of diabetes requires further clarification.

Neuropsychiatric disease

Anorexia nervosa

About one-third of patients with severe anorexia nervosa have a mild, normochromic, normocytic anaemia. In patients who are severely malnourished there may be mild neutropenia. There have been reports of the finding of irregularly shaped red blood cells in this condition. The platelet count is usually normal but there may be mild thrombocytopenia and in one study there was a marked increase in the rate of platelet aggregation.

Trauma

The brain is rich in thromboplastin activity. Acute DIC occurs quite commonly after severe head or brain injury.

Myasthenia gravis

The association between myasthenia gravis and pure red-cell aplasia is described in Chapter 24.23. An immune neutropenia has also been described as part of the myasthenia–thymoma syndrome.

Lesch–Nyhan syndrome

This X-linked recessive disorder is described in detail in Chapter 12.4. There have been occasional reports of the development of severe megaloblastic anaemia, presumably resulting from defective nucleic acid synthesis; the condition has been reversed by the administration of large doses of adenine.

Abetalipoproteinaemia

This condition is characterized by an ataxic neurological disease, retinitis pigmentosa, fat malabsorption, and the absence of chylomicrons and low-density lipoproteins. It is caused by the failure to synthesize or secrete lipoprotein-containing products of the apolipoprotein B gene. It is characterized by the presence of from 50 to 90% of acanthocytes in the peripheral blood. These are abnormal, spiky red cells, which have a moderately shortened survival. Despite these changes there is only a mild haemolytic anaemia.

Acanthocytosis with neurological disease and normal lipoproteins (amyotrophic chorea–acanthocytosis)

This syndrome is characterized by marked acanthocytosis associated with a progressive neurological disease, beginning in adolescence or adult life, which includes orofacial dyskinesia, lip and tongue biting, choreaiform movements, sensorimotor polyneuropathy, distal muscle wasting, and hypotonia. Because it has been found to follow both dominant and recessive forms of inheritance it is likely that this is a heterogeneous disorder. The cause is unknown.

Cardiac disease

There are several important haematological manifestations of cardiac disease, all of which are dealt with in more detail in Section 16. The severe haemolytic anaemia that occasionally follows the insertion of prosthetic valves, particularly the aorta, is described in Chapter 16.5.2.

A variety of abnormalities of coagulation are found in patients with cyanotic congenital heart disease. These include thrombocytopenia, low plasma fibrinogen levels, defective clot retraction, a deficiency of factors V and VII, and increased levels of fibrin degradation products. Overall, the severity of these abnormalities correlates with the degree of secondary polycythaemia. The exact mechanism is not known. In addition to the quantitative changes in blood platelets, there may also be qualitative abnormalities of platelet function. These include defects in both aggregation and release. They may be associated with a prolonged bleeding time. Again, the mechanism is not understood.

The striking haematological changes that may accompany bacterial endocarditis were mentioned earlier in this chapter. Dressler's syndrome may be associated with the anaemia of chronic disorders, atypical lymphocytes in the peripheral blood, and, certainly in the earlier descriptions of the disease, an eosinophilia of varying degree. Similar changes have been observed in the postpericardiotomy syndrome.

Haematological changes in ageing

The haematological manifestations of systemic disease, and of primary haematological disorders, are having to be assessed in increasingly aged populations. Commonly, therefore, clinicians are presented with the question as to whether changes in a patient's blood picture reflect underlying disease or whether they are the normal accompaniments of an ageing process. Although this field has been rather neglected, and from what is known it seems unlikely that ageing has a major effect on haematological parameters, a few findings are of some clinical importance.

There is a steady decrease in the volume of haematopoietic progenitors in the marrow with age and a variety of cellular, cytogenetic, and molecular alterations have been observed including chromosome shortening. The clinical significance of these findings is not yet clear although at least some of them may dispose to neoplastic transformation.

Although the results of studies of the haemoglobin or packed cell volume values of ageing populations have been conflicting, there appears to be a statistically significant fall in mean haemoglobin levels during the sixth through the eighth decades, although probably less than 1.0 g/dl and of lower magnitude in women than in men. Serum erythropoietin levels, however, do not seem to differ significantly with ageing. There are no consistent changes in the white cell count and although a variety of abnormalities of the adaptive immune system have been reported their clinical significance is still not clear. The platelet count does not change with age, and although several studies have emphasized changes in the level of coagulation factors and both procoagulant and fibrinolytic activities in older subjects the clinical significance is not clear. Some older patients show an exaggerated anticoagulant response to warfarin.

The erythrocyte sedimentation rate increases significantly with age and hence is of limited value in detecting disease in elderly patients. The C-reactive protein content of serum is also mildly elevated in older people.

Several haematological diseases, notably pernicious anaemia, increase in frequency with age and there is an unequivocal increase in the frequency of neoplastic disease of the bone marrow notably myeloma, lymphoma and leukaemia.

Although these haematological changes associated with ageing are not, in themselves, particularly striking, it should be emphasised that many old people who live in isolation may present with nutritional anaemia, particularly iron and folate deficiency, and that it is still not uncommon to observe such patients with mild or even severe haemorrhagic disorders associated with vitamin C deficiency. Indeed, there is scope for a great deal more work in defining the haematological changes consequent on ageing.

Further reading

Boxer H, *et al.* (1977). Anemia in primary hyperparathyroidism. *Arch Intern Med*, **137**, 588–90.

Hamblin TJ (ed.) (1987). Haematological problems in the elderly. *Baillière's Clin Haematol*, **1**, 271–596.

Henry DH, Hoxie JA (2006). Hematologic manifestations of AIDS. In: Hoffman R, *et al.* (eds) *Hematology: basic principles and practice*, 4th edition, pp. 2585–612. Churchill Livingstone, Philadelphia.

Herbert V (ed.) (1980). Hematologic complications of anemia in alcoholic patients. *Semin Hematol*, **17**, vols 1 and 2.

Marks PW, Rosenthal DJ (2006). Hematologic manifestation of systemic disease: infection, chronic inflammation and cancer. In: Hoffman R, *et al.* (eds) *Hematology: basic principles and practice*. 4th edition, pp. 2573–84. Churchill Livingstone, Philadelphia.

Rosovsky R, Marks PW. (2006). Hematologic manifestations of systemic disease: liver and renal disease. In: H In: Hoffman R, *et al.* (eds) *Hematology: basic principles and practice*. 4th edition, pp. 2564–71. Churchill Livingstone, Philadelphia.

Shayne M, Lichtman MA (2006). Hematology in older persons. In: Lichtman MA *et al.* (eds) *Williams hematology*, 7th edition, pp. 111–21. McGraw-Hill, New York.

St John DJB, Young GP, *et al.* (1993). Evaluation of new occult blood tests for detection of colorectal neoplasia. *Gastroenterology*, **104**, 1661–8.

Weatherall DJ, Kwiatkowski D, Roberts D (2007). Hematologic manifestations of systemic diseases in children of the developing world. In: Nathan DG, Oski FA, (eds) *Hematology of infancy and childhood*, 6th edn, pp. 1810–34. W B Saunders, Philadelphia.

Zaroulis CG, Kourides JA, Valeri CR (1978). Red cell 2,3-diphosphoglycerate and oxygen affinity of hemoglobin in patients with thyroid disorders. *Blood*, **52**, 181–5.

Blood replacement

Contents

22.8.1 Blood transfusion

P.L. Perrotta, Y. Han, and E.L. Snyder

Essentials

Transfusion of blood components is a life-saving treatment for patients with severe haemorrhage: it can also be used to replace coagulation factors and to ameliorate the effects of severe anaemia, thrombocytopenia, and impaired platelet function. However, blood transfusion has many hazards, hence its use should always be considered carefully and restricted to those who will gain benefit that outweighs the risks.

General considerations

Safe administration of blood components requires secure processes from vein to vein to prevent the wrong blood product from being given to the wrong patient. Reduction in transfusion risks is also achieved by (1) robust arrangements for the collection, storage, and delivery of appropriate supplies of blood products to their point of need; (2) better understanding of the antigenic structures on blood cells and the widespread introduction of advanced blood-group typing methods, screening for antibodies, and testing for compatibility before transfusion; (3) identification and screening for agents present in donors, as well as the use of sterile disposable materials.

Blood group systems—these include (1) ABO system—the codominantly expressed *A* and *B* genes code for glycosyl transferases that add either N-acetyl-D-galactosamine (*A* gene) or D-galactose (*B* gene) to the common precursor H antigen. Anti-A and Anti-B antibodies are 'naturally occurring' and responsible for most haemolytic transfusion reactions. (2) Rhesus system—the most clinically important Rh antigen is D because it is strongly immunogenic; anti-D is responsible for immune reactions including haemolytic disease of the newborn and immune-mediated transfusion reactions. (3) Other blood group antigens—these include Kell (K), Duffy (Fy), Kidd (Jk) and the MNS systems; multiple antibodies can develop when the range of red-cell antigens in the donor population differ from that of patients who require repeated transfusion.

Clinical use of blood components

Cellular components—these include (1) red blood cells—symptomatic anaemia; (2) leucocyte-reduced components (red blood cells and platelets)—symptomatic anaemia, reduce febrile reactions from leucocyte antibodies, alternative to cytomegalovirus-negative components, prevent HLA alloimmunization; (3) washed components (red blood cells and platelets)—remove harmful plasma antibodies; (4) platelet components—thrombocytopenia with bleeding, prophylactic transfusion, platelet function abnormalities; (5) granulocytes (obtained by apheresis)—for neutropenic patients with infection unresponsive to antibiotics (rarely used, given increased use of haemopoietic growth factors in haematological practice); donor lymphocyte infusions can induce remission of disease and improve survival by exerting a graft-vs-leukaemia effect in some bone marrow transplant recipients.

Plasma, cryoprecipitate, and plasma derivatives—these include (1) fresh frozen plasma—replacement of plasma coagulation factors for which specific factor concentrates are not available, liver disease, disseminated intravascular coagulation, hypofibrinogenaemia, thrombotic thrombocytopenic purpura; (2) cryoprecipitate—fibrinogen and factor XIII replacement, factor VIII and von Willebrand factor replacement when recombinant and virus-inactivated concentrates are not available; (3) albumin—used principally in specialized surgical practice and in the treatment of liver disease; (4) intravenous immunoglobulin—used principally for immunodeficiency syndromes, autoimmune rheumatic/vasculitic diseases, Guillain–Barré syndrome and autoimmune haemolytic anaemias; specific Rh (D) immunoglobulin is used to prevent alloimmunization in D-negative mothers; specific immunoglobulin preparations are used as antivenoms and to treat viral infections e.g. hepatitis A and B.

Complications of transfusion therapy

Immune complications—these include (1) acute intravascular haemolytic reactions—usually caused by transfusions of ABO-incompatible blood resulting from patient identification or clerical errors; manifest with sudden onset of back pain, hypotension, tachycardia, fever, chills, diaphoresis, and dyspnoea; treatment consists of immediately stopping the transfusion and providing supportive care, but can be fatal despite best management; (2) delayed haemolytic reactions—usually caused by an antibody that is initially of a titre below the limits of detection on routine screening; (3) febrile nonhaemolytic reactions—usually attributed to the development of antibodies in the recipient directed against HLA and/or leucocyte-specific antigens on donor white blood cells and platelets; (4) allergic reactions—IgE mediated; IgA-deficient patients are particularly prone to anaphylactic reactions; (5) transfusion-related acute lung injury; (6) transfusion-associated graft-vs-host disease.

Nonimmune complications—these include (1) infection—organisms commonly implicated in septic reactions include Gram-positive (staphylococci) and Gram-negative (enterobacter, yersinia, pseudomonas) bacteria. Other infections that may be transmitted from the donor include malaria, babesiosis, syphilis, leishmania, toxoplasmosis, and viral infections such as hepatitis B and C, HIV1, HIV2, and West Nile virus. Immunocompromised recipients are also at risk from human cytomegalovirus and parvovirus B19. A few patients have been shown to have acquired variant Creutzfeld–Jacob disease, probably as a result of transfusion from latently affected donors. (2) Other complications—acute problems can include circulatory overload, dilutional coagulopathy, hypocalcaemia, and hypothermia; complications of multiple blood transfusions include iron overload.

Prevention of complications—risks of alloimmunization from donor leucocytes and transmission of viruses can be avoided or reduced by (1) autologous blood salvage during surgery or acute normovolaemic haemodilution immediately before surgery; (2) improved methods for leucocyte reduction and inactivation of infectious agents. Despite much research the introduction of blood substitutes has yet to be realized in clinical practice. Use of purified recombinant haematopoietic growth factors (e.g. erythropoietin, granulocyte colony stimulating factor) has reduced the need for transfusion of blood products in many patients.

Introduction

Blood transfusion is used to treat patients with severe anaemia, haemorrhage, thrombocytopenia, and coagulation disorders. Greater understanding of red cell, platelet, and leucocyte antigen structure have greatly improved transfusion therapy. Routine blood bank procedures, including ABO typing, antibody screening, and compatibility testing, identify most patients at risk for haemolytic transfusion reactions. One of the most important technological improvements in transfusion therapy was the development of sterile, disposable, and flexible plastic containers that allow separation of whole blood into cellular (e.g. red cells, platelets) and noncellular (e.g. plasma, cryoprecipitate) components. Anticoagulants and additives currently used to collect blood allow storage of liquid suspensions of concentrated red cells for 35 to 42 days. These advances have essentially eliminated the use of whole blood.

Although the hazards of blood replacement are relatively small, the expected benefit of a transfusion must outweigh the risk to the patient. Therefore, a thorough understanding of the indications of blood transfusion is required to minimize unnecessary blood replacement and to prevent wastage of limited blood resources. Clinicians who prescribe blood transfusion must also be familiar with the risks and be able to recognize and treat transfusion reactions.

Blood group systems

ABO system

Over 250 distinct antigens have been identified on the surface of red blood cells. The most clinically important belong to the ABO system. The codominantly expressed *A* and *B* genes, located on chromosome 9, code for glycosyl transferases that add either *N*-acetyl-D-galactosamine (*A* gene) or D-galactose (*B* gene) to the common precursor H antigen (Table 22.8.1.1). The *O* gene is structurally similar to the *A* gene except for a single base deletion that eliminates production of a functional enzyme. The AB antigens are of critical importance because individuals who lack the A and/or B antigens form IgM and IgG antibodies directed against the missing antigen(s). Circulating A and B antibodies can fix complement and cause intravascular haemolysis. Anti-A and Anti-B antibodies are 'naturally occurring', i.e. they are formed without prior clinical antigenic stimulation. Presumably, individuals become immunized following exposure to carbohydrate ABO antigenic determinants commonly found in the bacterial environment. Accordingly, group A individuals produce anti-B, group B produce anti-A, and group O produce both anti-A and anti-B. Circulating A and B antibodies are of critical importance in blood therapy because they are responsible for most major haemolytic transfusion reactions.

Rh system

The Rh blood group system is composed of at least 44 distinct antigens. The five major antigens in the Rh system (D, C, c, E, and e) are responsible for most Rh-related transfusion incompatibility. It is now known that the D polypeptide is encoded at the *RHD* locus, whereas the CcEe polypeptide is coded by alleles at the *RHCE* locus. Based on the D gene frequency in North America and Europe, approximately 15% of individuals will not produce D antigen and are 'Rh negative'. Very rare individuals who lack all Rh antigens are termed 'Rh-null'. Rh-null red cells are morphologically abnormal and typically have shortened survival, resulting in a mild haemolytic anaemia.

The most clinically important Rh antigen is D because it is strongly immunogenic; the likelihood of a D-negative person developing anti-D following exposure to as little as 0.1 ml of D-positive red cells is extremely high. Anti-D is responsible for immune reactions including haemolytic disease of the newborn and immune-mediated transfusion reactions. Despite widespread use of Rh immune globulin, anti-D remains a most common cause of serious haemolytic disease of the newborn. Rh-negative women most commonly produce anti-D after exposure to D-positive red cells during pregnancy, a miscarriage, or abortion. The anti-D formed is of the IgG class and therefore can cross the placenta where it may cause potentially fatal intrauterine haemolysis in an Rh-positive fetus.

Table 22.8.1.1 ABO blood group system

ABO type	Gene(s)	Enzyme coded by gene	Resulting antigen	Antibody present in plasma	Frequency (white population)
O	*H*	L-fucosyl transferase	H	Anti-A and Anti-B	0.43
A	*A*	N-acetyl-D-galactosamine transferase	A	Anti-B	0.45
B	*B*	D-Galactosyl transferase	B	Anti-A	0.09
AB	*A* and *B*	N-acetyl-D-galactosamine and D-galactosyl transferase	AB	None	0.04

Other blood groups

Other well-characterized, clinically significant blood groups include Kell (K), Duffy (Fy), Kidd (Jk), and MNS systems. Antibodies to these blood group antigens may form following exposure to the corresponding antigens during transfusion or pregnancy and are associated with immune-mediated red cell destruction of transfused cells and HDN (Table 22.8.1.2). In most cases, compatible blood can be found for patients with red cell alloantibodies. Based on the high incidence of some red cell antigens among specific donor populations, however, some patients may be difficult to transfuse if they have developed multiple antibodies. This is particularly true in patients with sickle cell disease and other red cell disorders who require frequent transfusions. Table 22.8.1.2 lists the antigen frequencies of the most clinically relevant blood groups.

Certain blood groups are known to have particular disease associations. The Kell system is linked to chronic granulomatous disease (CGD), a congenital disease in which a decreased oxidative capacity

Table 22.8.1.2 Clinically significant blood groups

Red cell antigen	Antigen frequency[a]	Risk of haemolysis (immediate or delayed)	Risk of HDN
A, B	Variable	High (immediate)	Moderate (anti-A)
			Low (anti-B)
Rh	Variable	High (immediate and delayed)	Variable
			High to low
K	0.09	High (immediate and delayed)	High
Fy^a	White 0.66	High (delayed)	Low
	Black 0.10		
Fy^b	White 0.83	Low (delayed)	None
	Black 0.23		
Jka	0.77	Moderate (immediate and delayed)	Rare
Jkb	0.73	Moderate (immediate and delayed)	None
M	0.78	Low	Rare
N	0.72	None	None
S	0.55	Moderate (immediate and delayed)	Rare
s	0.89	Low (delayed)	Rare

[a] Antigen frequency in white population unless otherwise specified.

of neutrophils leads to recurrent, severe bacterial infections. The genetic defect seen in CGD is located on the X chromosome near the Kx Kell locus. Abnormalities described in this disease include acanthocytic red cells that are prone to mild haemolysis, cardiomyopathy, areflexia, and skeletal myopathies. The Duffy antigens, which occur at a much lower incidence among African populations, have an interesting association with malaria. Specifically, Fy(a–b–) negative red cells are resistant to *Plasmodium vivax* and *P. knowlesi* infection. Red cells from most West African blacks are Fy(a–b–) and therefore resistant to these forms of malaria.

The antibodies to the Kidd antigens are unusual in that once formed, they often fall below the level of detection and may not be detected in an already immunized patient. In this situation, transfusion of additional Kidd-positive red cells may cause a rapid, secondary immunological response, leading to formation of high-titre anti-Kidd with subsequent haemolysis and delayed transfusion reactions.

Detection of blood group antibodies

Antibody screening and antibody identification

To prepare blood for transfusion, both donor and recipient red cells are typed for ABO and Rh status using commercially available reagents. During 'front typing', red cells are reacted with antibodies directed against the A, B, and D antigens. Blood grouping is confirmed during 'back typing' in which serum/plasma is tested for the presence of expected anti-A and anti-B antibodies. Following blood grouping, serum/plasma is screened for red cell antibodies. Antibody screening is typically performed by incubating serum/plasma with two to four group O red cells that, in sum, contain all the common and clinically significant red cell antigens. If an antibody is present in the serum/plasma, it will react with the screening cell(s) and cause red cell agglutination. Antibody screening is commonly performed at room temperature (immediate phase), after incubating serum/plasma and test red cells at 37°C, and after incubation with antihuman globulin serum (Coombs phase). Some blood banks screen samples after adding various antigen–antibody enhancing substances such as polyethylene glycol and low-ionic strength saline. Most blood banks still perform 'tube testing' in which red cell agglutinates are identified in standard test tubes. A number of newer systems are being used to detect antigen–antibody reactions. These include gel systems based on the differential mobility of red cell agglutinates through gel columns and capture systems in which test red cells are immobilized on microtitre plates. Newer automated and semiautomated systems will rapidly replace tube testing for the majority of ABO grouping, Rh typing, antibody screening, and crossmatching.

If a patient's serum reacts with one or more screening cells, additional tests are performed to identify the antibody(ies). In most cases, the serum is tested against a larger commercial 'panel' of group O red cells of known antigen profile. Based on the reactivity pattern, the antibody can usually be identified. In some cases, a patient's serum may react with all panel cells. These 'panagglutinins' can be caused by (1) a single antibody directed against a high incidence antigen present on all panel test red cells; (2) multiple antibodies that in total react with all test cells; or (3) an autoantibody, in which case the patient's serum will also react with his or her own red cells (see 'Autoantibodies', below).

Compatibility testing

Routine compatibility testing is performed on red cell units before being transfused to a patient. Specifically, donor red cells are reacted with patient serum, and if no reaction is observed, the unit is considered 'crossmatch compatible'. In emergency situations, there may be insufficient time to perform compatibility testing. Many hospitals will supply group O Rh-negative red cells until a patient sample is obtained and tested. If a patient's ABO Rh status is known with certainty, then type-specific uncrossmatched blood can be provided. In either case, compatibility testing is performed on these transfused units as soon as possible. It is important to realize that supplies of O-negative blood are often limited. 'Computer crossmatches' have been instituted at many hospitals in North America. Patients with known ABO and Rh type, and who have a negative antibody screen, are provided ABO-compatible blood while omitting the crossmatch step described above. Although a true serological crossmatch is not performed, the computer crossmatch is safe in the vast majority of transfusions.

Autoantibodies

Autoantibodies consist of immunoglobulins that react with a wide range of self-antigens including membrane and intracellular components, adsorbed plasma proteins, and nuclear antigens. Patients with warm autoimmune haemolytic anaemia often require transfusion. In this case, the blood bank may have difficulty finding a 'compatible' unit of red cells because the patient's serum not only reacts with their own red cells, but also those of all donor red cells. Additional time may be required by the blood bank to exclude the presence of a significant underlying alloantibody that is obscured by the autoantibody. Upwards of 25% of previously transfused patients with warm autoimmune haemolytic anaemia may have an underlying alloantibody which can cause red cell haemolysis. Autoimmune antibodies often appear to have specificity for Rh antigens (e.g. anti-e), but the transfusion of antigen negative red cells (e.g. e-negative) is not indicated, as *in vivo* red cell survival of antigen-negative cells is usually no better than antigen-positive cells.

Clinical use of blood components

Blood component therapy refers to transfusing only the specific component that is required by a patient. Individual components are stored under optimal conditions. Plasma separated from whole blood can be further fractionated into coagulation factor concentrates, albumin, or gamma globulin. Cell separators capable of collecting platelets, plasma, granulocytes, peripheral blood stem cells, and, more recently, red blood cells, are also in widespread use across the United States of America and Europe.

Red blood cells

Red blood cells account for approximately 75% of the annual cost of transfusion therapy in the United Kingdom. Red cell units, prepared from whole blood by removing most of the plasma, are indicated for patients with acute haemorrhage or chronic anaemias (Table 22.8.1.3). Earlier preservative solutions composed of citrate, dextrose, and phosphate buffers allowed storage of red cells from 21 to 35 days. It was later observed that adenine improved cell viability by increasing intracellular ATP levels. The haematocrit of red blood cell units varies from 55% to 70% depending on the specific anticoagulant/preservative solution is used. Citrate contained in blood preservatives binds calcium to inhibit clotting and may cause hypocalcaemia and alkalosis in neonates and massively transfused patients.

Units of red cells stored refrigerated at 1 to 6°C have a shelf-life of 35 to 42 days depending on the ingredients of the preservative. During storage, the following changes are observed in red cell units: (1) a fall in pH; (2) decreases in red cell ATP and 2,3-diphosphoglycerate; (3) increased supernatant potassium; and (4) decreased supernatant glucose. Red blood cells with uncommon antigen profiles can be frozen within 6 days of collection and stored for up to 10 years. They are frozen with glycerol to avoid cell dehydration and damage during the freezing process.

The patient's overall clinical status and laboratory parameters should be considered as a whole when deciding to transfuse a patient. A decision should not be based on the haematocrit alone.

Table 22.8.1.3 Uses of blood transfusion components

Component	Indication for use
Red blood cells	Symptomatic acute and chronic anaemias
Red blood cells frozen and deglycerolized	Symptomatic anaemia, storage of red cells of rare antigen composition for up to 10 years
Leucocyte-reduced components (red blood cells and platelets)	Symptomatic anaemia, reduce febrile reactions from leucocyte antibodies, alternative to CMV-seronegative components, prevent HLA alloimmunization
Washed components (red blood cells and platelets)	Remove harmful plasma antibodies
Platelet components (pooled platelets and pheresis platelets)	Thrombocytopenia with bleeding, prophylactic transfusion, platelet function abnormalities
HLA matched/selected platelets and crossmatch-compatible platelets	HLA-alloimmunized thrombocytopenic patients with decreased platelet survival
Fresh frozen plasma	Replacement of plasma coagulation factors for which specific factor concentrates are not available, liver disease, DIC, hypofibrinogenaemia, TTP
Cryoprecipitate	Fibrinogen and factor XIII replacement, factor VIII and vWF replacement when recombinant and virus-inactivated concentrates are not available
Granulocytes by apheresis	Neutropenic patient with infection unresponsive to antibiotics

DIC, disseminated intravascular coagulation; TTP, thrombocytopenic purpura, vWF, von Willebrand factor.

Younger patients will usually tolerate a given degree of hypoxaemia and hypotension better than older patients who may have underlying coronary or myocardial disease. Evidence of symptomatic anaemia include excessive fatigue, malaise, headache, tachycardia, hypotension, and end-organ damage. Hypovolaemic shock typically ensues with acute loss (<24 h) of more than 30% of total blood volume. Initially, the haematocrit will be falsely elevated in acute haemorrhage, but will then fall with fluid resuscitation. Slowly developing, chronic anaemias are usually better tolerated than rapid onset anaemias due to the ability of the body's fluid compensatory mechanisms. Transfusion is rarely indicated when the haemoglobin (Hb) is greater than 10 g/dl, and is often not considered until the Hb is less than 7 g/dl. A patient's cardiac and pulmonary status must be considered when determining transfusion thresholds. Patients with unstable angina or acute myocardial infarction may require transfusion when the Hb is less than 10 g/dl. In the absence of active red cell destruction, transfusing a single unit will typically increase the Hb by 1 g/dl (haematocrit by 3%).

Platelets

The transfusion of platelets is in most cases a by-product of red cell separation. In the United States of America, platelets are prepared by the platelet-rich plasma method, whereas the buffy coat method is used in Europe. Each unit of 'random donor' platelets prepared by differential centrifugation of a single whole blood collection typically contains at least 5.5×10^{10} platelets suspended in 50 ml of plasma. Platelets stored under agitation at 20 to 24°C in plastic containers that allow oxygen diffusion have a shelf-life of 5 days. The risk of bacterial growth and development of platelet function abnormalities (platelet storage defect) has precluded longer storage. However, in the United States, all platelets are now tested for bacterial contamination using culture or surrogate methods (see section on septic reactions, below). 'Random donor' whole blood-derived platelets are usually administered in pools of 4 to 6 units. In the absence of conditions associated with decreased platelet survival, each unit can be expected to raise the recipient's platelet count by 5000 to 10 000/μl. Single donor platelets prepared by apheresis contain more than 3×10^{11} platelets suspended in about 200 ml plasma, equivalent to 4 to 6 average random donor platelet units. Pooled and stored, leukoreduced, whole blood-derived platelets are available in the United States. Licensed by the FDA in 2006, these products are usually manufactured in pools of 5 units and offer the benefit of allowing the use of culture techniques to detect bacterial contamination.

Platelets are not normally crossmatched with the recipient's serum. ABO type-specific platelets should be provided whenever possible because transfusing out-of-type platelets may result in poor platelet survival in the patient's circulation. Rh antigens present on the small number of contaminating red cells found in platelet concentrates are capable of immunizing an Rh-negative recipient. If Rh-negative platelet concentrates are not available for an Rh-negative patient, Rh-positive platelets can be transfused followed by administration of Rh immune globulin within 72 h of transfusion.

Platelets are provided to thrombocytopenic patients who are bleeding or to severely thrombocytopenic patients as a prophylactic measure. Spontaneous bleeding is rare when a patient's platelet count is above 20 000/μl, and studies suggest that patients who receive chemotherapy can tolerate platelet counts as low as 5000 to 10 000/μl. Postsurgical patients may require platelet transfusions to control or prevent postoperative bleeding when the platelet count is over 50 000/μl. Overall coagulation status should also be considered because patients with plasma coagulation factor disorders are more likely to bleed at marginal platelet counts. Actively bleeding patients receiving treatment with aspirin, an irreversible inhibitor of platelet function, may require transfusions at higher platelet counts, although transfused platelets will also be affected if the patient remains on aspirin.

Platelet refractoriness is a major issue for patients who are dependent on platelet transfusions. Immune and nonimmune factors may be responsible for platelet refractoriness. Common causes of diminished platelet survival post transfusion include splenomegaly, disseminated intravascular coagulation, and sepsis. Patients may become refractory to platelet transfusions through either HLA or platelet alloimmunization. Once platelet alloimmunization is documented, crossmatch-compatible platelets or HLA-matched platelets should be considered. However, these special products are not readily available in most blood banks. Increasing the dose of standard platelet concentrates can be considered until compatible platelets are identified. Leucocyte reduced blood products should be provided to patients who will require many platelet transfusions to decrease the risk of HLA alloimmunization.

Plasma, cryoprecipitate, and plasma derivatives

Plasma therapy started in the late 1940s when fractionation techniques were developed to separate plasma proteins from large pools of human plasma. Fresh frozen plasma (FFP) is prepared by separating plasma from whole blood by centrifugation and then freezing the plasma within 8 h of collection. This process maintains the activity of labile coagulation factors, particularly factors V and VIII. Many blood suppliers also prepare plasma that is frozen within 24 h of collection; this product is considered an effective alternative to FFP in most instances when plasma transfusion is necessary. Plasma should not be transfused for volume expansion because of the risk of transfusion-transmitted disease and the availability of other, safer nonplasma substitutes. The primary indications for plasma transfusion include deficiency of multiple coagulation factors as seen in liver disease and disseminated intravascular coagulation. It is often used to reverse warfarin anticoagulation urgently. Plasma is not particularly effective in replacing individual clotting factors because of the large volumes that would be required to obtain adequate factor levels. The patient's fluid and cardiovascular status may preclude the use of large amounts of plasma.

FFP is no longer the treatment of choice for coagulopathies where virally inactivated or recombinant blood products exist, such as for deficiencies of factor VIII (haemophilia A) or factor IX (haemophilia B). Fears of transmitting infectious disease with plasma transfusion remain of concern, particularly for pooled products. In addition to donor screening and testing, other strategies to decrease infectious risk that have been studied include photoinactivation and solvent detergent treatment. Furthermore, in order to decrease the risk of transfusion-related acute lung injury, in the United Kingdom, only male donor plasma has been used as a source of FFP since 2003. A similar trend has started in the United States of America.

Cryoprecipitate is prepared by thawing FFP between 1 and 6°C. Each 10- to 20-ml unit contains 100 to 350 mg fibrinogen/unit, at least 80 IU/unit factor VIII, and some von Willebrand factor.

Use of cryoprecipitate is generally reserved for patients with severe hypofibrinogenaemia (<100 mg/dl). Cryoprecipitate is not used to treat haemophilia or von Willebrand's disease in developed countries because safer alternatives are available that avoid the risk of viral transmission. Cryoprecipitate and thrombin have been combined to make 'fibrin glue'. This biological sealant works well but exposes the recipient to the risks of transfusion-transmitted disease because of the use of cryoprecipitate. Safer sealants have been developed that do not expose patients to cryoprecipitate.

Albumin is available as a 5% or 25% solution and is used to treat hypovolaemia and hypoalbuminaemia, primarily in surgical settings. Albumin is virally inactivated by heat treatment plus other viral inactivation steps, and is tested for hepatitis C virus RNA. Properly processed albumin is not considered to transmit viral disease. Readily available nonplasma colloidal solutions have replaced albumin in many situations requiring volume expansion. Intravenous immunoglobulin is used to treat patients with immune thrombocytopenia, Guillain–Barré syndrome, and autoimmune haemolytic anaemias. Prompt and adequate doses of Rh (D) immunoglobulin available in intramuscular and intravenous preparations, are used to prevent alloimmunization in D-negative patients who are exposed to D-positive red cells through transfusion or pregnancy. Rapid advances in molecular techniques led to the cloning and purification of recombinant clotting factors. Recombinant factors VIII, IX, and VIIa are available.

Granulocytes

Granulocytes are transfused primarily to neutropenic oncology patients with an absolute neutrophil count less than 500/µl and a reasonable chance of marrow recovery, who develop bacterial or fungal sepsis unresponsive to antimicrobial therapy. Granulocytes collected from nonstimulated healthy donors by apheresis contain at least 1×10^{10} neutrophils/unit and can be stored for only 24h at 20 to 24°C. Higher numbers of granulocytes can be collected when donors are stimulated by steroids and/or growth factors. The product contains a large number of red cells (20–50 ml) and must be crossmatched with the recipient's serum. Granulocytes should be irradiated because of the large number of lymphocytes present in the product. Because of their short half-life, granulocytes are usually provided daily until the patient can maintain an absolute neutrophil count above 500/µl without transfusion or until the infection resolves. Infusion of larger numbers of granulocytes allows measurable increases in recipient neutrophil counts, but the optimal dose and frequency remain undefined. Febrile reactions to granulocytes are common, the reactions being more severe when amphotericin is administered near the time of granulocyte infusion. Overall, the additional benefit of granulocyte transfusion for neutropenic patients compared to antibiotic treatment alone remains unclear.

Complications and management of transfusion therapy (Tables 22.8.1.4 and 22.8.1.5)

Acute intravascular haemolytic reactions

Acute intravascular haemolytic transfusion reactions are one of the most serious transfusion complications. ABO incompatibility remains the most common cause of immediate intravascular haemolytic reactions. Donor erythrocytes carrying either A and/or B red cell antigens bind to the recipient's anti-A and/or anti-B antibodies, resulting in complement fixation, formation of the C5b-9 membrane attack complex, and subsequent haemolysis. Biological response modifiers, such as proinflammatory cytokines

Table 22.8.1.4 Major risks of blood transfusion therapy

Immune complications	Nonimmune complications
Acute haemolytic transfusion reactions	Transfusion-associated bacterial sepsis
Delayed extravascular haemolytic reaction	Circulatory overload, cardiac failure
Febrile transfusion reaction	Viral transmission (hepatitis A, B, C, CMV, parvovirus)
Allergic transfusion reaction (urticaria and anaphylaxis)	Iron overload
Transfusion-associated sepsis	Hypocalcaemia
Alloimmunization	Hypothermia
Transfusion-associated graft-vs-host disease	Dilutional coagulopathy due to factor depletion, thrombocytopenia
Transfusion-associated acute lung injury	

Table 22.8.1.5 Symptoms, signs, and management of transfusion reactions

Reaction	Symptoms and signs	Management/treatment
Acute intravascular haemolytic reaction	Back pain, fever, hypotension, shock, dyspnoea, haemoglobinuria, haemoglobinaemia, positive direct Coombs	Stop transfusion, IV fluids, vasopressor support, maintain diuresis, corticosteroids, dialysis if indicated
Delayed extravascular haemolytic reaction	Anaemia, jaundice, fever, positive direct Coombs	Stop transfusion, fluid support, follow lab results (Hct, LDH, bilirubin)
Febrile reaction	Fever, chills, rigors, mild dyspnoea	Stop transfusion, antipyretics, consider leucoreduced product for subsequent transfusions
Allergic (mild)	Pruritis, urticaria	Antihistamines, may continue transfusion if symptoms improve in <30 min, otherwise stop transfusion
Allergic (anaphylactic)	Urticaria, bronchospasm, dyspnoea, nausea, hypotension	Stop transfusion, antihistamines, vasopressor support, corticosteroids, consider premedication or washed RBCs for subsequent transfusions
Septic reaction	Rapid onset of chills, fever, hypotension	Stop transfusion, culture sample from product and patient, vasopressor support, IV fluids, broad spectrum antibiotics
TRALI	Dyspnoea, tachypnoea, cyanosis, fever, hypotension	Respiratory support

(interleukin (IL)-1, tumour necrosis factor α (TNFα)), chemokines (IL-8), and complement fragments (C3a, C5a), also play a role in the pathophysiology of acute transfusion reactions. The sudden onset of back pain, hypotension, tachycardia, fever, chills, diaphoresis, and dyspnea are clinical characteristics of acute intravascular transfusion reactions. The symptoms usually begin soon after the transfusion is started. Laboratory studies reveal an increase in unconjugated bilirubin (typically to 2–3 mg/dl) and a marked elevation of lactate dehydrogenase. Other evidence of intravascular haemolysis include haemoglobinuria and haemoglobinaemia. The direct antiglobulin test (direct Coombs) becomes reactive due to the coating of donor red cells with the recipient's antibodies.

Acute intravascular haemolytic transfusion reactions are usually caused by transfusions of ABO-incompatible blood resulting from patient identification or clerical errors, but they can also be caused by incompatibility within other blood group (e.g. Duffy, Kidd) systems. Proper labelling of samples used by the blood bank for compatibility testing and careful identification of patients are the best ways to prevent these potentially fatal reactions. Acute haemolytic immune transfusion reactions are medical emergencies and treatment consists of immediately stopping the transfusion, close monitoring of vital signs, cardiac and airway support, and maintenance of urine output with saline diuresis with or without a loop diuretic. Dialysis should be considered in patients with renal failure.

Delayed extravascular haemolytic reactions

Delayed haemolytic transfusion reactions occur in patients who have a negative antibody screen on pretransfusion testing, but who then experience accelerated destruction of transfused red cells 3 to 14 days after transfusion. In most cases, red cell destruction is caused by an antibody that is initially of a titre below the limits of detection on routine screening. The antibody then rapidly forms on re-exposure to the offending antigen. The antibodies typically fix complement to C3 and stop, thus resulting in extravascular haemolysis. Antibodies most commonly implicated in delayed transfusion reactions are directed against Rh (E, c), Kell, Duffy, and Kidd blood group antigens. Delayed extravascular haemolytic transfusion reactions can be diagnosed by an unexpected post-transfusional fall in haematocrit, development of unconjugated hyperbilirubinaemia, and appearance of a positive direct antiglobulin test. A delay of 3 days to 2 weeks is usually seen between transfusion and the onset of extravascular haemolysis. Only rarely do delayed reactions result in intravascular haemolysis.

Febrile nonhaemolytic reactions

Febrile nonhaemolytic transfusion reactions to red blood cell and platelet transfusion are very common. They are classically attributed to the development of antibodies in the recipient directed against HLA and/or leucocyte-specific antigens on donor white blood cells and platelets. Reactions between leucoagglutinins present in the transfused product and recipient leucocyte antigens can also occur. Subsequent formation of leucocyte antigen–antibody complexes results in complement binding and release of endogenous pyrogens such as IL-1, IL-6, and TNFα. Cytokines generated by leucocytes during platelet and red cell storage may also contribute to these febrile reactions to transfusion. Symptoms may occur during or several hours after the transfusion and typically include fevers (>1°C rise) accompanied by shaking chills. Rarely, vomiting, dyspnoea, hypotension, and decreased oxygen saturation may develop. The severity of symptoms is often directly related to the number of leucocytes in the product or the rate or volume of transfusion. Leucoreduction of blood components decreases the frequency of febrile transfusion reactions. Premedication with an antipyretic can ameliorate mild febrile transfusion reactions. Corticosteroids can also minimize febrile transfusion reactions if they are administered several hours before the transfusion. Intramuscular or subcutaneous meperidine will usually resolve severe rigors within minutes. If symptoms do not resolve in less than 4 h or are especially severe, other complications such as sepsis due to contaminated blood products or a haemolytic reaction should be considered.

Allergic reactions

Allergic reactions to plasma, platelets, and red blood cells are relatively common. They present as pruritus and/or urticaria in the absence of fever. Allergic reactions are IgE mediated and most symptoms are attributed to histamine release. It may be difficult to distinguish allergic and febrile transfusion reactions when urticarial symptoms are accompanied by low-grade fever. Common symptoms and signs include erythema, papular rashes, weals, and pruritus. As in other allergic responses, symptoms are not dose-related and severe manifestations can occur following small exposures. Treatment of mild allergic reactions consists of stopping the transfusion and administering antihistamines. In a mild allergic reaction with only pruritus and hives, it is acceptable to continue transfusing the same unit, provided the symptoms promptly resolve and no accompanying fever or vasomotor instability is noted.

Severe allergic reactions with bronchospasm and cardiovascular collapse are rare and should be treated like any other anaphylactic reaction with steroids, vasopressors, and airway support. Anaphylactic transfusion reactions occur in IgA-deficient patients who have already developed anti-IgA antibodies, and then receive plasma-containing blood products. While IgA deficiency is common in the general population (1 in 700 individuals), only a subset of IgA-deficient individuals are at risk since not all of them develop the antibody. Patients with IgA deficiency who have had an anaphylactic reaction or who have demonstrated anti-IgA should receive cellular products that have been saline-washed and plasma from only IgA-deficient donors. Washed red blood cells may also benefit patients without IgA deficiency, but who have experienced repeated moderate to severe allergic transfusion reactions.

Septic reactions

Blood products can become contaminated by bacteria if a donor is bacteraemic at the time of collection or if the donor's arm is improperly cleansed before venepuncture. Transfusing blood products contaminated by bacteria is particularly dangerous and can result in profound hypotension and shock. The risk of septic transfusion reactions is higher for platelet transfusions than other blood components because platelets are stored at room temperature. As noted above, in an attempt to reduce the risk of transfusion-associated bacterial sepsis, blood collection facilities in the United States of America have implemented several strategies to detect bacterial contamination of platelet units. These include culture of the product as well as surrogate methods. The latter comprise

(1) visual inspection for loss of swirling that occurs with a change in platelet shape associated with the fall in pH; (2) direct visualization of microorganisms using the Gram stain, Wright stain, or acridine orange; and (3) the use of dipsticks for pH and glucose readings. These surrogate methods are more rapid and less costly, but also much less sensitive than culture and are being phased out. The sensitivity of culture in detecting bacterial contamination of blood products is affected by several factors, however, such as growth characteristics of the organism, timing of specimen collection, specimen volume, and the degree of initial bacterial contamination.

Organisms commonly implicated in septic transfusion reactions include Gram-positive (staphylococcus) and Gram-negative (enterobacter, yersinia, pseudomonas) bacteria. Blood cultures should be obtained from patients who develop high fevers following or during transfusion, especially if they become hypotensive. A Gram stain of the suspected contaminated product may be helpful but is often negative, and the product should be cultured if possible. Other symptoms attributed to preformed endotoxin and cytokines include skin flushing, severe rigors, and rapid-onset cardiovascular collapse. The symptoms may occur during or a minute to hours after the transfusion is completed. Treatment includes fluids, cardiorespiratory support, and broad-spectrum antibiotics.

Transfusion-related acute lung injury

Transfusion-related acute lung injury is a serious complication of blood transfusion that presents as noncardiogenic pulmonary oedema. It typically occurs within 6 h of transfusion and is clinically similar to the acute respiratory distress syndrome (ARDS). The most common clinical findings are rapid-onset dyspnoea, tachypnoea, cyanosis, fever, and hypotension. Lung auscultation reveals diffuse crackles and decreased breath sounds. Invasive cardiac monitoring demonstrates normal cardiac pressures and function with hypoxaemia and decreased pulmonary compliance. Radiographic findings include diffuse, fluffy infiltrates typical of pulmonary oedema.

In most cases, the aetiology is believed to involve an immune-mediated reaction between passively transferred donor antileucocyte antibodies present in a plasma-containing blood product with the recipient's white cells, resulting in leucocyte activation. Much less frequently, the antibodies present in the recipient may react with white cells in the transfused products. Granulocytes are first activated by HLA or other antigen–antibody complexes and then migrate to the lungs. The activated neutrophils bind to the pulmonary capillary bed via cell adhesion molecules where they release proteolytic enzymes that destroy tissue, resulting in a capillary leak syndrome and pulmonary oedema. More recently, reactive lipid products released from donor cell membranes have been associated with the development of transfusion-related lung injury.

Transfusion-related acute lung injury is a clinical diagnosis and should be suspected in patients with severe, rapid-onset respiratory distress during or soon after transfusion therapy. Definitive diagnosis requires identification of HLA and/or granulocyte antibodies in either the donor's or recipient's serum, as well as the corresponding antigens on the recipient's or donor's leucocytes. This testing is performed in only a few specialized laboratories. Most patients with this syndrome will survive with supportive care, including aggressive respiratory support with supplemental oxygen, and if necessary, mechanical ventilation. Often, the hypoxia that develops during or after transfusion is attributed to fluid overload, and diuretics are empirically administered. Although not absolutely contraindicated, diuretics may be harmful and should be used with extreme caution. Corticosteroids have no proven role in the management of transfusion-related acute lung injury. As discussed above, in order to reduce its incidence, plasma from female donors is no longer used as a source of FFP in the United Kingdom, with the United States of America beginning to follow this course as of 2007.

Transfusion-associated graft-vs-host disease

Acute graft-vs-host disease (GVHD) is a rare complication of blood transfusion, but is fatal in approximately 90% of patients. Transfusion-associated graft-vs-host disease (TA-GVHD) occurs when donor immunocompetent T and NK cells attack immunoincompetent recipient cells because these recipient cells appear foreign due to differences in major or minor histocompatibility antigens. The risk of TA-GVHD is related to the number of viable T lymphocytes transfused, the recipient's immune status, and the HLA disparity between donor and host. Therefore, multiply transfused patients who receive cells from donors who share HLA haplotypes with the recipient (i.e. blood relatives) are at greatest risk. Clinically, transfusion-associated GVHD is characterized by the acute onset of rash, abdominal pain, diarrhoea, liver abnormalities (elevated liver enzymes, hyperbilirubinaemia), and bone marrow suppression 2 to 30 days following transfusion. The maculopapular rash seen is similar to that observed in acute GVHD following bone marrow transplant, and biopsy of the skin may help confirm the diagnosis. Pancytopenia may be severe and is attributed to destruction of recipient marrow stem cells by donor lymphocytes. Immunosuppressive therapy with prednisone and ciclosporin has had little effect on TA-GVHD. Fortunately, the development of this condition can be prevented by irradiating cellular blood products before transfusion.

Transfusion-transmitted disease

Despite major improvements in blood safety during the past two decades, a small risk of transfusion-transmitted disease still remains. The use of volunteer donors and predonation screening questionnaires were the first steps taken to reduce the risk of transfusion-related hepatitis and HIV. These risks continue to drive mandated pretransfusion testing requirements in developed countries. The advent of enzyme immunoassays in the 1970s and more recently, nucleic acid amplification testing, have further decreased the risk of transfusion-transmitted disease (Table 22.8.1.6). Transfusion-transmitted disease is a persistent problem in parts of the world that do not have access to screening tests.

At present, pretransfusion testing in the United States of America and Europe includes screening for hepatitis B (HBsAg, anti-HBc, nucleic acid amplification), hepatitis C (anti-HCV, nucleic acid amplification), HIV (anti-HIV-1/2, nucleic acid amplification), human T-cell lymphotropic virus (anti-HTLV-I/II), and syphilis (RPR). Additionally, in the United States, donated blood is screened for West Nile virus (nucleic acid amplification). Serum alanine aminotransferase is measured in most European countries as a nonspecific surrogate marker of hepatitis. When positive, these tests are confirmed by supplemental or confirmatory testing.

Table 22.8.1.6 Organisms potentially transmitted by blood transfusion

Agent/organism	Estimated risk per unit transfused[a]	Pretransfusion testing
Hepatitis B virus	1:65 000	HBsAg, anti-HBc, ALT, NAT
Hepatitis C virus	1:1.9 million	anti-HCV, NAT
HIV-1/2	1:2.1 million	anti-HIV-1/2, NAT
HTLV-I/II virus	1:650 000	anti-HTLV-I/II
West Nile virus	Unknown	NAT
CMV	1:10–1:20 (see text)	Some units tested for anti-CMV antibodies
Parvovirus B19	Unknown	None
Bacterial contamination	1:1500	None
Treponema pallidum	Rare	RPR
Parasites (plasmodium, ehrlichia, *Babesia microti*)	Rare	None
vCJD	Unknown	Deferral based on history

CMV, cytomegalovirus; vCJD, variant Creutzfeldt–Jakob disease;
[a] USA figures.

Nucleic acid amplification testing for HCV and HIV is typically performed on small pools of samples.

The current estimate of the risk of transfusion-related HIV is approximately one in two million units transfused. With the introduction of screening by amplification of nucleic acid templates, the 'window period', in which the virus could be transmitted by an HIV-infected but seronegative donor, has decreased to approximately 10 days. Genomic testing for HCV RNA has also been implemented in the United States and Europe to detect seronegative yet infectious units. Nucleic acid amplification testing screening has decreased the transfusion-related hepatitis C risk by decreasing the window period to 10 to 20 days.

The first cases of transfusion-transmitted West Nile virus infection were documented in the United States in 2002; the following year, national blood donation screening for West Nile virus was initiated using nucleic acid amplification testing technology. The risk of transfusion-related transmission of this virus since instituting this screening test has not been established.

Several techniques have been developed to inactivate viruses in platelets and plasma, including solvent detergent treatment and photochemical inactivation using psoralens and long-wavelength ultraviolet light. Methods to inactivate infectious pathogens in red cells are currently under development. Due to the low risk of viral infection by transfusion and the fact that most patients who receive plasma also receive cellular blood components, the cost-effectiveness of virally inactivated plasma is unclear. Albumin, immune globulin, factor concentrates, and other plasma derivatives are treated using protocols that essentially eliminate the risk of viral transmission.

Cytomegalovirus (CMV) and parvovirus B19 are common in the general donor population, and may pose a serious threat to immunocompromised patients. Approximately 40 to 60% of blood donors have been exposed to CMV during their lifetime and subsequently are CMV seropositive. However, only about 2% of CMV-seropositive donors are actively infected and transfusing their blood to an immunocompromised recipient could cause acute CMV infection. The actual risk of post-transfusion seroconversion of a CMV-negative recipient who receives CMV-untested blood depends on the prevalence of CMV seropositivity in the donor population. As for parvovirus B19, only a few cases of transmission by blood components have been reported in immunocompetent recipients. Thus, blood donor screening tests for parvovirus have not been recommended.

Since its initial description in the United Kingdom in 1996, variant Creutzfeldt-Jakob disease (vCJD) has raised additional transfusion safety concerns. The observations from the study conducted in the United Kingdom, the Transfusion Medicine Epidemiology Review, have provided evidence that vCJD can be transmitted through blood transfusion. As of 2006, of the 66 British patients identified as having received blood from donors who went on to develop vCJD, three or four probable cases of transfusion-transmitted vCJD have been documented. These numbers may, however, be an underestimate of the overall risk of transfusion transmission of this disease. Given the long incubation period of vCJD, some surviving recipients of blood products derived from 'vCJD donors' may still develop the disease. Moreover, a significant number of deceased blood recipients may not have survived long enough to manifest clinical disease even if infected. The introduction of universal leucocyte depletion of the United Kingdom blood supply in 1999 may have reduced the risk to blood recipients.

A number of parasitic diseases are known or suspected to be transmitted by blood transfusion. These include malaria, Chagas' disease, babesiosis, leishmaniasis, and toxoplasmosis. Transmission of Lyme disease (*Borrelia burgdorferi*) by transfusion has not been documented. Infection with babesia, if untreated, can be dangerous in at-risk populations such as asplenic patients. A screening test for babesiosis is available in the United States.

Use of special blood products

Leucoreduction

Leucocytes contained in blood components can provoke febrile nonhaemolytic reactions, induce HLA alloimmunization, and transmit CMV to at-risk recipients. Leucocytes are effectively removed from red cell and platelet concentrates by leucocyte reduction filters. American standards require that units labelled 'leucoreduced' contain less than 5×10^6 white blood cells, whereas the European standard is less than 1×10^6 white blood cells per unit. Red cells are most commonly leucoreduced shortly after blood collection (prestorage leucodepletion). Filters are similarly used to leucoreduce platelet concentrates. Apheresis devices have been designed to collect leucoreduced platelets directly (process leucoreduction).

Leucoreduction has been shown to decrease the prevalence and severity of febrile transfusion reactions and the risk of HLA alloimmunization. Other generally accepted benefits of white blood cell reduction include reducing platelet refractoriness and decreasing the risk of transmitting white blood cell-related infectious agents including CMV and HTLV-I/II. Prestorage leucoreduced products are preferable because they contain less cytokines and other biological response modifiers produced by white blood cells. With the dramatic decrease in the risk of viral transmission, investigators are focusing on the immunomodulatory effects of blood transfusion. These effects specifically deal with associations between allogeneic transfusion and bacterial infection, tumour progression, and tumour recurrence. Universal leucoreduction of both red blood cells and platelets has been required and/or is being implemented in a number of European countries and in North America.

Irradiation

Blood components are irradiated to prevent potentially lethal TA-GVHD by interfering with the ability of lymphocytes to proliferate. Irradiation of blood components is indicated in bone marrow or peripheral blood stem cell transplant recipients, patients with congenital immunodeficiency states, neonates, premature infants, and during intrauterine exchange transfusion. Patients with AIDS commonly receive irradiated components, although no clear increased risk of TA-GVHD exists in this population. Standard guidelines recommend irradiating red blood cells, platelets, and granulocytes with a minimum dose of 2500 cGy. Platelets are not adversely affected by this exposure. Red cells have a maximum shelf life of only 28 days. It is not necessary to irradiate FFP or cryoprecipitate because they do not contain viable leucocytes. Bone marrow or peripheral blood stem cells must never be irradiated prior to transplant.

Cytomegalovirus-safe

CMV infection is a leading cause of morbidity and mortality in marrow and solid organ transplant patients. Most serious CMV infections that develop in these populations are a result of latent reactivation of recipient CMV, but CMV can also be transmitted by blood transfusion. Therefore, blood banks supply products that have a low potential of transmitting CMV. The available products include CMV-seronegative units prepared from donors who are CMV IgG antibody negative, and leucodepleted components. The latter refers to blood components leucoreduced in a blood centre or laboratory using 'good manufacturing practice' techniques. Studies suggest that CMV-seronegative and leucodepleted filtered products are equivalent in preventing CMV transmission. Many transfusion specialists consider leucodepleted units produced under conditions of good manufacturing practice as CMV 'safe' in that they are unlikely to transmit CMV disease. In addition to CMV-seronegative marrow and solid organ transplant recipients, CMV-seronegative or safe components are generally indicated for premature infants, during intrauterine transfusions, for patients with congenital immunodeficiencies, CMV seronegative pregnant women, and seronegative patients with HIV. The British Committee for Standards in Haematology has concluded that leucoreduced components are an 'effective alternative' to seronegative products for preventing CMV transmission by transfusion.

Alternatives to blood component therapy

Autologous transfusion

Commonly used forms of autologous transfusion include preoperative blood donation, acute normovolaemic haemodilution, and autologous blood salvage. Many blood centres provide autologous preoperative blood donation services in which a patient's blood is drawn and stored for later use, usually during a surgical procedure. The criteria for autologous donations are less stringent than those

for allogeneic donors. Preoperative blood donation can be utilized in elderly patients, although there is a higher risk of anaemia and more serious cardiovascular complications associated with the donation. Although the use of autologous blood decreases the risk of viral infection, the risk of bacterial contamination remains. Acute normovolaemic haemodilution is performed by removing blood from a patient immediately before surgery and replacing the blood volume with crystalloid or colloid solutions to maintain haemodynamic stability. The withdrawn blood is then later reinfused. Autologous blood salvage is performed by collecting and then returning blood lost during or shortly following operative procedures using intraoperative salvage devices. This technique is primarily employed in cardiac and orthopaedic surgery.

Growth factors

Haematopoietic growth factors used in transfusion therapy are designed to limit the exposure of patients to allogeneic blood. The isolation, characterization, and subsequent synthesis of erythropoietin by recombinant technology were important advances in decreasing red cell transfusions. The use of recombinant human erythropoietin has reduced the transfusion needs of some patients with renal failure and various anaemias. In the United States of America, use of recombinant human erythropoietin is being restricted due to reported adverse vascular and other events. Granulocyte colony stimulating factor (G-CSF) has been shown to decrease infection rates in neutropenic patients undergoing chemotherapy, replacing marginally effective granulocyte transfusions. Thrombopoietic growth factors, such as recombinant thrombopoietin, as well as small molecules with thrombomimetic activity, are currently being evaluated and some formulations are licensed in the United States of America.

Blood substitutes

For over a century, ongoing research has sought to develop haemoglobin-based oxygen-carrying compounds that can serve as an alternative to allogeneic red cell transfusion. The earliest products consisted of stroma-free haemoglobin, which was abandoned because of its renal toxicity, and polymerized haemoglobin. Most of these agents are not used clinically because of vasoactivity and other untoward effects; other formulations are in various phases of clinical trials. No formulation is currently licensed in the United States of America.

Further reading

Arslan O (2006). Electronic crossmatching. *Transfus Med Rev*, **20**, 75–9.
BCSH Blood Transfusion Task Force (1996). Guidelines on gamma irradiation of blood components for the prevention of transfusion-associated graft-versus-host disease. *Transfus Med*, **6**, 261–71.
Blajchman MA, Vamvakas EC (2007). The continuing risk of transfusion-transmitted infections. *N Engl J Med*, **28**, 1303–5.
Bowden RA, et al. (1995). A comparison of filtered leukocyte-reduced and cytomegalovirus (CMV) seronegative blood products for the prevention of transfusion-associated CMV infection after marrow transplant. *Blood*, **86**, 3598–603.
Brecher M (2005). *Technical manual*, 15th ed. American Association of Blood Banks, Bethesda.
Cohn E, et al. (1950). A system for separation of components of human blood. *J Am Chem Soc*, **72**, 465–74.
Contreras M (1998). The appropriate use of platelets: an update from the Edinburgh Consensus Conference. *Br J Haematol*, **101** (Suppl 1), 10–12.

Corash L (2003). Pathogen reduction technology: methods, status of clinical trials, and future prospects. *Curr Hematol Rep*, **2**, 495–502.

Daniels G, *et al.* (1996). Blood group terminology: from the ISBT Working Party. *Vox Sanguinis*, **71**, 246.

Dike AE, *et al.* (1998). Hepatitis C in blood transfusion recipients identified at the Oxford Blood Centre in the national HCV look-back programme. *Transfus Med*, **8**, 87–95.

Dobroszycki J, *et al.* (1999). A cluster of transfusion-associated babesiosis cases traced to a single asymptomatic donor. *JAMA*, **281**, 927–30.

Fisk JM, *et al.* (2007). Platelets and related products. In: Hillyer CD, *et al.* (eds.) *Blood banking and transfusion medicine*, 2nd edition, pp. 308–41. Churchill Livingstone, Philadelphia.

Friedberg RC, Donnelly SF, Mintz PD (1994). Independent roles for platelet crossmatching and HLA in the selection of platelets for alloimmunized patients. *Transfusion*, **34**, 215–20.

Goodnough LT, *et al.* (1999). Transfusion medicine. Second of two parts–blood conservation. *N Engl J Med*, **340**, 525–33.

Hebert PC, *et al.* (1999). A multicenter, randomized, controlled clinical trial of transfusion requirements in critical care. Transfusion Requirements in Critical Care Investigators, Canadian Critical Care Trials Group. *N Eng J Med*, **340**, 409–17.

Heddle N, Webert KE (2007). Febrile, allergic, and other noninfectious transfusion reactions. In: Hillyer CD, *et al.* (eds.) *Blood banking and transfusion medicine*, 2nd edition, pp. 677–90. Churchill Livingstone, Philadelphia.

Hewitt P (2007). vCJD and blood transfusion in the United Kingdom. *Transfus Clin Biol*, doi 10.1016/j.

Issitt PD, Anstee DJ, eds (1998). *Applied blood group serology*, 4th edition. Montgomery Scientific, Durham.

Klein HG, Strauss RG, Schiffer CA (1996). Granulocyte transfusion therapy. *Semin Hematol*, **33**, 359–68.

Klein HG (2005). Pathogen inactivation technology: cleansing the blood supply. *J Intern Med*, **257**, 224–37.

Kuter DJ, Begley CG (2002). Recombinant human thrombopoietin: basic biology and evaluation of clinical studies. *Blood*, **100**, 3457–69.

Liles WC, *et al.* (1997). A comparative trial of granulocyte-colony-stimulating factor and dexamethasone, separately and in combination, for the mobilization of neutrophils in the peripheral blood of normal volunteers. *Transfusion*, **37**, 182–7.

Lo YM, *et al.* (1998). Prenatal diagnosis of fetal RhD status by molecular analysis of maternal plasma. *N Engl J Med*, **339**, 1734–8.

Looney MR, Gropper MA, Matthay MA (2004). Transfusion-related acute lung injury. *Chest*, **126**, 249–58.

Luban NLC (2005). Transfusion safety: where are we today? *Anna N Y Acad Sci*, **1054**, 325–41.

Lundberg G (1994). Practice parameter for the use of fresh-frozen plasma, cryoprecipitate, and platelets. Fresh-Frozen Plasma, Cryoprecipitate, and Platelets Administration Practice Guidelines Development Task Force of the College of American Pathologists. *JAMA*, **271**, 777–81.

Marcus DM (1969). The ABO and Lewis blood-group system. Immunochemistry, genetics and relation to human disease. *N Engl J Med*, **280**, 994–1006.

Montgomery SP, *et al.* (2006). Transfusion-associated transmission of West Nile virus, United States 2003 through 2005. *Transfusion*, **46**, 2038–46.

Murphy MF (1999). New variant Creutzfeldt-Jakob disease (nvCJD): the risk of transmission by blood transfusion and the potential benefit of leukocyte-reduction of blood components. *Transfus Med Rev*, **13**, 75–83.

Novotny VM (1999). Prevention and management of platelet transfusion refractoriness. *Vox Sang*, **76**, 1–13.

Paglino JC, *et al.* (2004). Reduction of febrile but not allergic reactions to RBCs and platelets after conversion to universal prestorage leukoreduction. *Transfusion*, **44**, 16–24.

Popovsky MA, Moore SB (1985). Diagnostic and pathogenetic considerations in transfusion-related acute lung injury. *Transfusion*, **25**, 573–7.

Race R (1944). An 'incomplete' antibody in human serum. *Nature*, **153**, 771.

Reid ME, Yazdanbakhsh K (1998). Molecular insights into blood groups and implications for blood transfusion. *Curr Opin Hematol*, **5**, 93–102.

Silliman C (1999). Transfusion-related acute lung injury. *Transfus Med Rev*, **13**, 177–86.

Snyder EL (1995). The role of cytokines and adhesive molecules in febrile non-hemolytic transfusion reactions. *Immunol Invest*, **24**, 333–9.

Vogelsang GB, Hess AD (1994). Graft-versus-host disease: new directions for a persistent problem. *Blood*, **84**, 2061–7.

Wandt H, *et al.* (1998). Safety and cost effectiveness of a 10×10^9/L trigger for prophylactic platelet transfusions compared with the traditional 20×10^9/L trigger: a prospective comparative trial in 105 patients with acute myeloid leukemia. *Blood*, **91**, 3601–6.

Wiener A (1943). Genetic theory of the Rh blood types. *Proc Soc Exp Biol Med*, **54**, 316.

Winslow RM (2007). Red cell substitutes. *Semin Hematol*, **44**, 51–9.

Wroe SJ, *et al.* (2006). Clinical presentation and pre-mortem diagnosis of variant Creutzfeldt-Jakob disease associated with blood transfusion: a case report. *Lancet*, **368**, 2061–7.

Yamamoto F, *et al.* (1990). Molecular genetic basis of the histo-blood group ABO system. *Nature*, **345**, 229.

22.8.2 Haemopoietic stem cell transplantation

E.C. Gordon-Smith and Emma Morris

Essentials

Haemopoietic stem cells give rise to the blood cell lineages and the cells of the immune system, and their transplantation may be an appropriate part of the management of conditions including (1) malignant disorders—(a) haematological, e.g. leukaemia, lymphoma, myeloma; (b) nonhaematological—e.g. malignant teratoma; (2) bone marrow failure syndromes—e.g. aplastic anaemia; (3) congenital disorders—(a) haematological—e.g. Fanconi's anaemia; (b) immunological—severe combined immunodeficiency; (c) metabolic—e.g. lysosomal diseases.

Successful engraftment of haemopoietic stem cells from a healthy donor into a patient depends upon (1) overcoming immune rejection by the recipient, and (2) preventing or suppressing graft-vs-host disease, in which donor cells mount an immune attack against recipient tissues.

Identification and sources of haemopoietic stem cells

Haemopoietic stem cells are principally identified by expression of the surface antigen CD34. Sources include (1) bone marrow; (2) peripheral blood—following stimulation by infusion into the donor of certain cytokines, e.g. granulocyte colony-stimulating factor (G-CSF); (3) umbilical cord blood.

Selection of donors

Minor disparity between the HLA types of donor and recipient are allowable, but the greater the disparity the higher the frequency of complications. HLA-matched sibling donors are only available for about 1 in 3 recipients. For those without such a donor, possible sources are (1) volunteer donor banks—can provide HLA-suitable matches for about 80% of recipients with the same genetic disequilibrium as the donor pool; (2) umbilical cord blood banks.

Conditioning regimen

These include measures to induce immunosuppression (required for all transplants, excepting those from identical twin donors) and, when appropriate, eradicate diseased bone marrow. They may be (1) myeloablative—cyclophosphamide with (a) total body irradiation (TBI), or (b) busulphan, or (c) antilymphocyte globulin (ALG); (2) nonmyeloablative—fludarabine with varying combinations of (a) ALG or alemtuzumab (anti-CD52), (b) low-dose cyclophosphamide or melphalan, (c) low-dose TBI. After transplantation, donor lymphocyte infusions may be given to patients with malignant disorders for graft-vs-leukaemia or graft-vs-tumour effect.

Graft-vs-host disease (GVHD)

Acute GVHD—this major cause of transplant-related morbidity and mortality may develop at any time within the first 6 weeks after transplantation, with manifestations involving (1) skin—maculopapular rash, generalized erythroderma, desquamation and bullae; (2) liver—severity graded according to level of serum bilirubin; (3) gut—diarrhoea, persistent nausea, pain/ileus.

Chronic GVHD—may follow acute GVHD or emerge de novo several months after transplantation. Mainly affects the skin, but almost any organ may be affected, e.g. lung (broncheolitis oblterans), gut, liver, eyes (sicca syndrome), buccal mucosa, and musculoskeletal system.

Treatment—this presents a major challenge. Standard management is with ciclosporin, with or without methotrexate; alternatives include tacrolimus, sirolimus, rituximab (anti CD20), alemtuzumab, high-dose steroids, thalidomide.

Other complications and prognosis

Conditioning regimen are extremely toxic. (1) Acute—the patient is particularly vulnerable to infectious complications in a period of intense neutropenia, usually lasting 2 to 4 weeks after transplantation. Patients are managed in isolation facilities, with (as appropriate) prophylactic measures against fungal infection (fluconazole), herpes simplex (aciclovir), Gram-negative infection (ciprofloxacin), pneumocystis (co-trimoxazole). Broad-spectrum intravenous antimicrobial therapy is used to treat fevers empirically. Ganciclovir is given if routine monitoring shows evidence of cytomegalovirus reactivation. (2) Chronic—common manifestations include retardation of growth, endocrine impairment, infertility, intellectual impairment (following brain irradiation).

Prognosis—once the graft is fully established and tolerance is reconstituted, immunosuppression may be stopped. The procedure offers hope to many patients with life-threatening marrow failure or malignant disease for which no other treatment is available, but in the long term recipients have a reduced life expectancy due to relapse of the underlying disease, infection, and chronic graft-vs-host disease. There is an increased risk of solid tumours.

Introduction

The idea that haemopoietic stem cells (HSC) from the bone marrow could be transferred from a normal individual to a patient to replace defective bone marrow has a long history. With the exception of rare instances where marrow was obtained from an identical twin, such attempts in humans universally failed until an understanding of the immune processes involved in tolerance and rejection became available. Much of the pioneering work in making possible human bone marrow transplantation was carried out by E. Donnall Thomas and colleagues in the United States of America, work for which Thomas received the Nobel Prize jointly in 1990. Experiments on inbred mice had shown that lethally irradiated animals could be rescued by intravenous transfusion of bone marrow from unirradiated mice and that this protection was the result of engraftment of the normal marrow in the recipient. Successful engraftment depended upon the donor marrow being genetically acceptable by the recipient mouse or the recipient mouse being sufficiently immunosuppressed. Engraftment when there was immunological disparity between the donor and recipient was followed after a period of 2 weeks or so by a 'secondary' disease in which the recipient mouse failed to thrive and developed gastrointestinal disorders, liver failure and skin disease, leading to poor further development and eventual death from infection. This so-called 'runt disease' is the murine equivalent of graft-vs-host disease (GVHD) in humans, in which immunocompetent cells from the immunologically disparate donor mount an attack against recipient tissues. From these and other experiments in outbred animals it was recognized that transplantation of bone marrow would carry the special risk of GVHD and that histocompatibility would be a critical requirement for successful transplantation. Furthermore, considerable immunosuppression would be required to achieve engraftment in all transplants except those from syngeneic (identical twin) donors. However, it was also recognized that not only the haemopoietic but also the immune system would be replaced following myeloablation and reconstitution and that the need for immunosuppression would cease, except for the management of GVHD, once the donor immune reconstitution was complete.

Transplants in dogs demonstrated that total body irradiation and cyclophosphamide were sufficiently immunosuppressive to permit engraftment, and that GVHD could be controlled to some extent, where there was not great disparity between the histocompatibility antigens of donor and recipient, with methotrexate. The elucidation of the major histocompatibility complex (MHC) on chromosome 6 in humans, with the identification of the histocompatibility antigens at the A, B, or C (class I) and DR (class II) loci of the HLA system, finally allowed the identification of appropriate donors for human transplantation. The paramount importance of histocompatibility in haemopoietic stem cell transplantation (HSCT) has been confirmed subsequently by extensive clinical practice. The first successful transplant from a nonidentical, but HLA compatible, sibling was carried out in 1968 for a patient with severe combined immune deficiency where the underlying disease prevented rejection. Successful allogeneic transplantation from sibling donors using conditioning with total body irradiation and cyclophosphamide carried out in 1969 in Seattle by the group led by Thomas. Many thousands of such transplants have been carried out subsequently, though the indications and stage of disease for

Table 22.8.2.1 Main disorders for which haematopoietic stem cell transplantation may be appropriate[a]

Malignant disorders	
Haematological malignancies	Acute leukaemias
	Chronic myeloid leukaemia
	Non-Hodgkin's lymphoma
	Hodgkin's lymphoma
	Myeloma and other plasma cell dyscrasias
	Chronic lymphocytic leukaemia
Solid tumours	Malignant teratoma
	Ewing's sarcoma
	Renal cell carcinoma
Bone marrow failure syndromes	Myelodysplasias
	Myeloproliferative disease
	Aplastic anaemia
	Paroxysmal nocturnal haemoglobinuria
Congenital disorders	
Haematological	Fanconi anaemia
	Diamond–Blackfan anaemia
	Kostmann's syndrome
Immunological	Severe combined immune deficiency
	Chronic granulomatous disease
Metabolic	Malignant osteopetrosis
	Lysosomal storage diseases

[a] Stem cell transplantation may be considered an option according to availability of a suitable donor, the stage or severity of the disease, and the availability and effectiveness of other forms of management.

transplantation, particularly in malignant disease, are not always as clear as they might be (Table 22.8.2.1) and the problems of GVHD, graft failure, and infection remain hazards which contribute to transplant-related mortality (TRM). HSCT must always be compared with best available alternative therapies. On the other hand, better support with blood products and antibiotics, improved tissue typing techniques, and the introduction of less toxic ways of delivering conditioning to control rejection and GVHD, as well as better selection of recipients, have improved outcomes steadily over the last 40 years.

Histocompatibility complex and haemopoietic stem cell transplantation

The organization of the major histocompatibility complex (MHC) on chromosome 6, and its importance in transplantation, is described in detail in Chapter 5.5. The closeness of the relevant genes in the complex means that within families there is little crossing-over in germ-line cells and inheritance more or less follows the autosomal pattern, so that the chances of a sibling having the same HLA type as a patient is about 1 in 4. This is genotypic identity in which not only the HLA types but also many unidentified

sequences in the MHC are identical. At each HLA locus there are large numbers of possible alleles in humans leading to a potential of many millions of different histocompatibility profiles. However, within populations, certain HLA alleles tend to be associated and segregate together, 'genetic disequilibrium', so that it is theoretically and practically possible to find phenotypically identical pairs within an unrelated population.

The identification of phenotypes was originally based upon serological testing for A, B, and DR antigens. The introduction of molecular techniques for identifying DNA sequences directly has shown that there may be a large number of HLA gene products whose cognate protein molecules are assigned to the same phenotype by serological methods. HLA typing of individuals within populations has made possible the creation of large volunteer donor panels of individuals prepared to supply HSC. However, matching the MHC between unrelated pairs even by molecular techniques gives at best phenotypic identity and there are likely to be many fine genetic differences. Selection of donors by improved typing techniques has reduced the risks associated with unrelated transplants but restricted the range of appropriate donors. It has also become clear that there are very wide variations in the linkage disequilibria at MHC loci between different populations of the world so that a donor panel of one ethnic type may have a much reduced chance of providing stem cells for another.

Where there is an HLA disparity between donor and recipient, HSCT is possible, but the incidence of complications rises steadily as the degree of disparity increases. It is also apparent that the major antigens of the MHC (HLA class I and II antigens) are not the only ones important in determining the incidence and severity of GVHD. GVHD is mediated by CD4+ helper and CD8+ cytotoxic T lymphocytes. These T cells recognize allogeneic MHC molecules and minor histocompatibility antigens (self proteins where a polymorphism exists between donor and recipient) expressed on normal recipient tissues. The role of specific major and minor antigens in determining the attack, and the part played by recipient antigens in susceptibility to the disease, have not been worked out in detail. As discussed later, the cell-mediated immune attack on normal tissues causing GVHD seems to be linked to an ability to attack abnormal, particularly malignant cells, producing a graft-vs-leukaemia/lymphoma (GVL) effect. Much effort has gone into trying to identify the donor cells, which mediate the GVL effect and the antigen-presenting cells of the recipient which facilitate it, to separate GVL from GVHD, so far with inconclusive results. It appears that many target antigens of GVL and GVHD are shared. The problems and benefits of immunological disparity obviously only apply in the allogeneic transplantation setting and are absent when autologous stem cells are used to restore haemopoiesis after intensive chemotherapy.

Haemopoietic stem cells

Stem cells are defined by their ability to proliferate and differentiate into one or more specific cell lineages and also to maintain the stem cell pool by self-renewal. Haemopoietic stem cells (HSC) give rise to the blood cell lineages—red cells, granulocytes, and platelets as well as the cells of the immune system. It seems probable that a single stem cell can repopulate the blood and immune systems of an entire animal. HSC can be identified by immunophenotyping and their ability to repopulate marrow. The best *in vitro* techniques have suggested that the human HSC is closely related to precursors that carry an antigen designated CD34, lack other haemopoietic markers including CD33, and have no lineage-specific markers. Whether such cells are truly the most primitive cells that are capable of giving rise to both haemopoietic and immunological precursors is not of practical importance since successful haemopoietic reconstitution, both in allogeneic and autologous transplants, is closely related to the number of such cells present in the donation. The CD34+, CD33– cells represent some 1×10^{-3} to 10^{-4} of the cells of normal human haemopoietic marrow.

Sources of haemopoietic stem cells

HSC develop in specific sites within the bone marrow, designated niches, which include specialized cells of the bone marrow stroma. The stem cell is not fixed in its environment but may leave the marrow, enter the circulation and home once again to the marrow or to other sites depending on chemokine and cytokine signals it receives (see Chapter 4.3). Small numbers of CD34+ HSC circulate in normal blood, and this number is greatly increased during the marrow recovery after cytotoxic chemotherapy. Administration of certain cytokines, particularly granulocyte colony-stimulating factor (G-CSF), granulocyte–macrophage colony-stimulating factor (GM-CSF), and stem cell factor increases the number of circulating CD34+ cells enormously, such that for a period of a few days following treatment there are adequate numbers in the circulation to use as a source of cells for transplantation. Homing and mobilization of HSC seems to be a continuous, dynamic process—even under normal conditions.

In the early development of the fetus, haemopoiesis takes place in the liver. Fetal liver cells have been used as a source of HSC, mainly for the treatment of inherited severe combined immune deficiency. The logistics of such transplants, which require 11-week-old fetal livers, make this an impractical approach. However, research on embryonic stem cells suggests that there may be other important sources of stem cells, not only for haemopoiesis but for other types of tissue replacement. Of more immediate practical importance was the finding that umbilical cord blood (UCB) contained large numbers of cells with high proliferative potential and characteristics of stem cells. UCB has become a third practical source of donor cells. Each of these sources—bone marrow, peripheral blood, and cord blood—has advantages and disadvantages that impinge on clinical management. A critical requirement for successful transplantation is that there should be a sufficient number of stem cells. The ability to expand stem cells *ex vivo* would solve this and other requirements, but so far this has not proved to be useful clinically.

HSC from bone marrow

Until about 1993 most transplants were conducted using bone marrow stem cells, but peripheral blood mobilized HSC have steadily become the preferred option in more recent years. Much of the data concerning the success and problems of stem cell transplantation are derived from the use of bone marrow. Bone marrow is harvested with the patient under general anaesthetic by aspiration from the posterior and superior iliac crests, and if necessary the sternum. Experience has shown that some 3×10^8 nucleated cells/kg recipient body weight are required for successful engraftment and this usually involves collecting 1 to 1.5 litres of bone marrow (mixed, of course, with blood). Donors may have a

unit of blood collected before harvesting, which is returned at the end of the procedure to ameliorate the anaemia. The procedure takes 1 to 2 h and the donor usually requires brief admission to hospital to recover. Serious complications are very rare and are those associated with the general anaesthetic or local complications such as osteomyelitis or abscess formation. The advantage of this source of stem cells from the donors' viewpoint is that collection is rapid, with a maximum of 48 h involvement. The disadvantage is the need to be admitted to hospital for an anaesthetic and the pain or discomfort and anaemia that follow the procedure.

HSC from peripheral blood

HSC may be mobilized into the peripheral blood following exposure to G-CSF. For allogeneic transplantation, donors receive G-CSF (filgrastim or lenograstim) at a dose of 10 μg/kg subcutaneously daily for 5 days. The peripheral granulocyte count rises to 30 $\times 10^9$/litre or higher and CD34+ cells appear in the peripheral blood reaching a maximum 5 to 6 days after the start of treatment. Leucocytes are collected by cytopheresis with the objective of reaching more than 2×10^6 CD34+ cells/kg body weight of the recipient. Sufficient cells can usually be collected in one procedure. Attempts to increase the circulating stem cell concentration still further using additional cytokines, such as stem cell factor, have not proved to be sufficiently safe for general use. The main disadvantages for donors of this type of stem cell collection is that of bone pain or ache following the injections of G-CSF and the procedure of cytopheresis. Rare instances of splenic rupture have been recorded. There has been some concern about the theoretical potential of G-CSF to cause cytogenetic abnormalities that could lead to leukaemia; although no such effect has yet been found in normal donors given the cytokine, long-term follow-up is advisable. The main advantages are the avoidance of admission to hospital and a general anaesthetic. When autologous collection of stem cells is required, the concentration of CD34+ cells may be increased further by giving cyclophosphamide (or some other chemotherapeutic agents, such as etoposide) before starting the G-CSF. Autologous HSCT is used mainly for patients with malignant disease, for marrow rescue following further intensive chemotherapy.

The use of peripheral blood for harvesting stem cells for allogeneic transplants provides high numbers of CD34+ cells and more rapid engraftment than with bone-marrow-derived stem cells. On the other hand, peripheral blood contains more T cells and, although original concerns that acute GVHD would be unacceptably severe unless T cells were removed have proved unfounded, chronic GVHD, especially extensive disease, is, more prevalent than in bone marrow and UCB transplants and is the main non-relapse cause of mortality after peripheral blood stem cell transplants. Nevertheless, the ease of collection and advantages of rapid engraftment have meant that most autologous transplants (where GVHD is not a problem), and a majority of allogeneic transplants, are currently sourced from the peripheral blood.

HSC from umbilical cord blood

Sourcing HSC from umbilical cord blood has several theoretical and practical advantages. UCB is widely available with no risk to mother or infant donor, there is low viral contamination, the immaturity of the immune cells may theoretically reduce the risk of GVHD, and the cells may readily be stored frozen and made available rapidly for transplantation. Furthermore, a balance of umbilical cord blood stem cells from different ethnic groups to take advantage of genetic disequilibrium can be achieved and specific HLA types can be targeted. A disadvantage is the relatively small volume of UCB and hence low total numbers of HSC. UCB donations have mostly been used for children. Recently the use of double or multiple UCB donations has been introduced for adult transplants; further follow-up is needed to assess the results, though there is early evidence that the risk of chronic GVHD is less than with bone marrow or peripheral blood donations. The storage and administrative costs of UCB are high compared with sourcing at the time of transplant. A further difficulty is the lack of any back-up source of cells should the graft fail or relapse occur. For adults with impaired thymic function the lack of memory T lymphocytes for common latent viruses such as cytomegalovirus (CMV) in the donation may result in repeated reactivation episodes. There is also the theoretical risk that the UCB carries some latent infective or genetic defect which might appear years after the transplant. Nevertheless, UCB transplants are likely to increase as the practical source of HSC in the future.

Plasticity of stem cells

It has become apparent that there are present in the bone marrow, and in other tissues, cells that are totipotent in their capacity to develop into differentiated cells depending upon the molecular and cellular microenvironment to which they are exposed. Thus bone-marrow-derived cells may differentiate to cardiac muscle cells, nerve cells, striated muscle fibres, and many other tissues, whether they be ectodermal, mesodermal, or endodermal in origin. This potential is also present in embryonic stem cells. HSC have been used in phase I/II studies examining the effect on cardiac function post myocardial function and other insults. Although it is possible to identify HSC in the myocardium after such procedures, practical benefits have not yet been clearly revealed. A second class of bone marrow cells which have stem cell properties *iv vitro* and may be stem cells *in vivo* are the mesenchymal stromal (stem) cells (MSC). *In vitro* they can differentiate into a variety of mesodermal tissues. Their potential interest for HSC transplants lies in their immunomodulatory effects. Early clinical trials suggest they may be able to modify acute GVHD.

Donors for allogeneic stem cell transplantation

Problems of transplant-related morbidity and mortality, graft rejection, GVHD, and infection increase with increasing donor disparity. HLA-matched sibling donors are not only phenotypically matched for the MHC, but have genotypic identity throughout most of the MHC. This does not eliminate transplant-related morbidity and mortality, but reduces the incidence and severity of the problems compared with unrelated volunteer donors matched only phenotypically for the MHC and mismatched at minor histocompatibilty antigens. HLA-matched sibling donors are only available for about 1 in 3 recipients in populations with an average of two or three children per family. To overcome this shortfall, volunteer donor banks have been established, now including more than 10 million typed donors worldwide. These panels can provide HLA-suitable matches for about 80% of recipients with the same genetic disequilibrium as the donor pool, though finding the right match may take several weeks. Extensive immunosuppression of the

recipient is required pretransplant to prevent graft rejection and post-transplant to control GVHD. New methods of immunosuppression which allow the stepwise engraftment of donor marrow may produce a greater degree of tolerance and permit successful transplantation of HSC with some degree of HLA disparity. UCB banks have been established in many countries. Their use is likely to increase if double or multiple donations prove effective for adults.

Management of transplant recipients

Conditioning regimen

The treatment of recipients pretransplant includes measures to induce immunosuppression and eradicate diseased bone marrow. For HSC transplantation for malignant disease, most protocols contained cyclophosphamide combined either with total body irradiation (TBI), single dose or fractionated, or with alkylating agents such as busulphan. For nonmalignant conditions irradiation should be avoided. For acquired aplastic anaemia cyclophosphamide, either alone or combined with anti thymocyteglobulin (ATG), has been the major conditioning regimen. Some of the more widely used regimens are indicated in Table 22.8.2.2. The incidence and severity of GVHD was reduced by giving methotrexate in a short protocol post-transplant; the introduction of ciclosporin further improved results. Such conditioning regimens, particularly for malignant and genetic disorders, carry delayed as well as acute toxicity, particularly for children. Where radiation is used and to a lesser extent busulphan, infertility is usual, growth is retarded, and other endocrine functions may be impaired. Where transplantation is used for patients who have already received

Table 22.8.2.2 Outline of examples of conditioning regimens for allogeneic haematopoietic stem cell transplantation

Conditioning Regimen	Indications
Myeloablative	
Cyclophosphamide at 120 mg/kg + TBI of 750–1400 cGy	Acute leukaemia
	Chronic myeloid leukaemia
	Relapsed lymphoma
Cyclophosphamide at 120 mg/k + busulphan at 16 mg/kg	As above
	Thalassaemia major
	Other congenital bone marrow disorders
Cyclophosphamide at 200 mg/kg ± ALG	Acquired aplastic anaemia
Cyclophosphamide at 25 to 100 mg/kg + TBI of 200 cGy	Fanconi's anaemia
Nonmyeloablative	
Fludarabine at 30 mg/m²	Fanconi's anaemia
± ALG or alemtuzumab	Congenital disorders of haemopoiesis or immune system
+ low-dose cyclophosphamide or melphalan	
± low-dose TBI (200cGy)	Acquired aplastic anaemia
With DLIa	Malignant disorders

ALG, antilymphocyte globulin; DLI, donor lymphocyte infusions; TBI, total body irradiation. Lower doses given in single fraction, higher doses fractionated.
a Given 6 weeks or longer postinfusion to provide GVL or GVT effect.

irradiation or chemotherapy to the central nervous system, e.g. patients with a relapsed acute lymphoblastic leukaemia, intellectual impairment as well as the above problems are common.

Success of stem cell transplantation in certain malignant conditions is related to the cellular immune response to recipient cells and tissue (GVL), provided by donor lymphocytes, rather than the direct cytotoxic effect of conditioning. Repopulation of marrow by donor HSC does not require the immediate abolition of recipient marrow. Full donor chimerism may be achieved over time rather than in one step, and in some instances mixed stable chimerism of both donor and recipient cells may occur. Conditioning regimens have been introduced which do not rely on cytotoxic measures to obliterate recipient marrow and immune system, but which have increased immunosuppressive action. Such regimens include fludarabine, a highly immunosuppressive drug that is not very cytotoxic, often combined with ATG, monoclonal antibodies (e.g. alemtuzumab, anti-CD52) and/or low dose TBI. Removal of T lymphocytes from the donor preparation (T cell depletion, TCD), to reduce acute GVHD with subsequent later add-back of donor lymphocytes to reduce the chances of relapse, is also employed (Table 22.8.2.2). Results using this approach have been encouraging and reduced-intensity transplant regimens are widely used for lymphomas and leukaemias, though long-term follow-up is required. The reduced toxicity has allowed the use of HSC transplants for patients up to 60 years of age or even older.

Graft-vs-host disease (GVHD)

Acute GVHD (Fig. 22.8.2.1)

This may develop at any time within the first 6 weeks after transplant. Some acute GVHD occurs in the majority of HSCT recipients and grades II–IV in 25 to 40%. The typical features and classification of severity are summarized in Table 22.8.2.3. Grades III and IV of GVHD are a major cause of transplant-related morbidity and mortality. GVHD itself has an immunosuppressive effect which may lead to reactivation of latent viruses, particularly CMV, as well as death from fungal or bacterial infections. Liver failure, catastrophic diarrhoea, and gastrointestinal haemorrhage are other direct causes of death from GVHD.

Chronic GVHD

This mainly affects the skin, but almost any organ may be affected. Frequent sites are the lung (broncheolitis oblterans), gut, liver, eyes (sicca syndrome), buccal mucosa, and musculoskeletal syndromes. It may follow acute GVHD or arise *de novo* beyond 100 days post-transplant. The rash may vary from a mild dryness of the skin in localized areas to a major extensive scleroderma-like illness (Fig. 22.8.3.1). Chronic GVHD clearly results from histoincompatibility between donor and recipient, but the cells involved and the pathophysiology are poorly characterized and management is difficult.

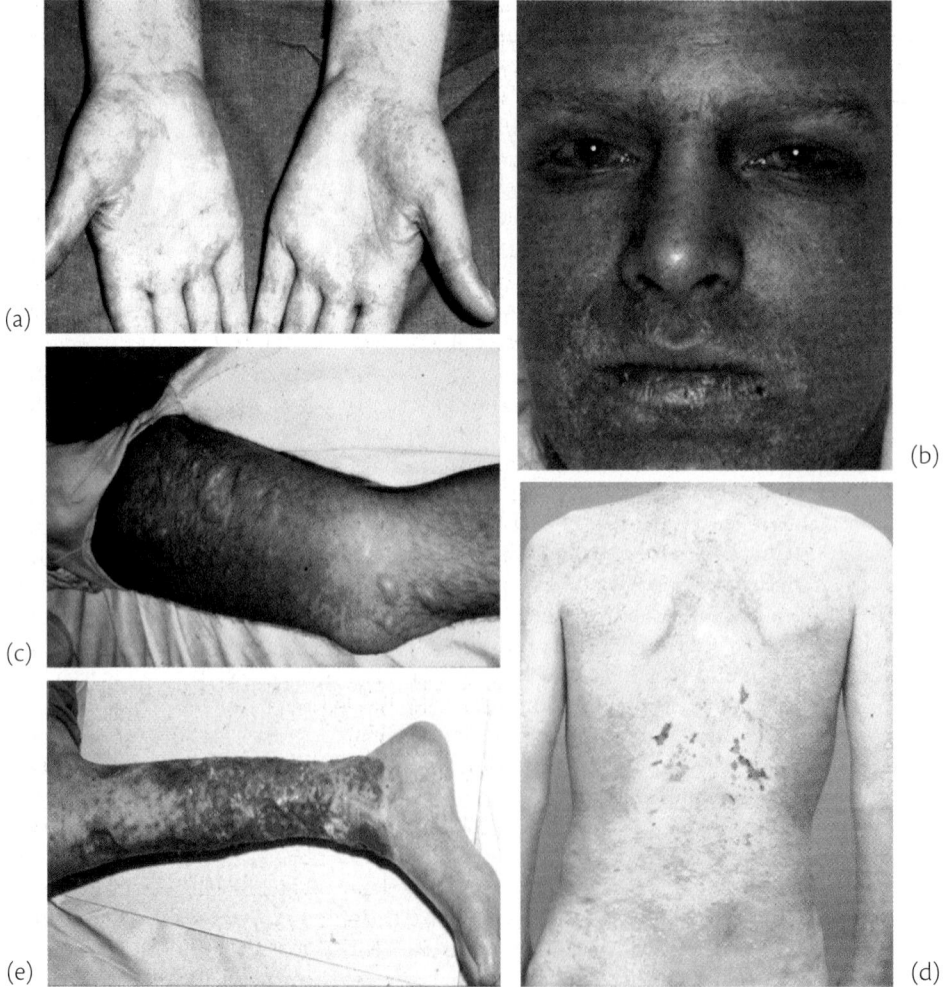

Fig. 22.8.2.1 Skin manifestations of acute and chronic GVHD. Acute GVHD: (a) grade I, skin +, showing typical palmer maculopapular rash (recovered); (b) grade IV, skin 4+, generalized erythroderma with early exfoliation; liver 3+, bilirubin >250 µmol/litre (fatal); (c) grade III, skin 4+, bullous desquamation (recovered). Chronic GVHD: (a) scleroderma-like plaques on hands; (b) sclerotic scarring on back; (c) severe ulceration and contracting scleroderma-like skin involvement.

Table 22.8.2.3 Clinical analysis of acute GVHD

Clinical stage	Organ involvement[a]		
	Skin	**Liver**	**Gut**
+	Maculopapular rash <25% of body surface	Bilirubin 30–50 μmol/litre (2–3 mg/dl)	Diarrhoea 0.5–1 litre/day and/or persistent nausea
++	Maculopapular rash 25–50% of body surface	Bilirubin 50–100 μmol/litre (3–6 mg/dl)	Diarrhoea 1–1.5 litre/day
+++	Generalized erythroderma	Bilirubin 100–250 μmol/litre (6–15 mg/dl)	Diarrhoea >1.5 litre/day
++++	Desquamation and bullas	Bilirubin > 250 μmol/litre (>15 mg/dl)	Pain ± ileus

Clinical grade	Stage			
	Skin	**Liver**	**Gut**	**Functional impairment**
0 (none)	0	0	0	0
I (mild)	+ to 2+	0	0	0
II (moderate)	+ to 3+	+	+	+
III (severe)	2+ to 3+	2+ to 3+	2+ to 3+	2+
IV (life threatening)	2+ to 4+	2+ to 4+	2+ to 4+	3+

[a] Confirmation may require biopsy.

Prevention and treatment of GVHD

Amelioration of acute GVHD with ciclosporin plus or minus methotrexate has already been discussed and the role of T-cell depletion mentioned. Methotrexate is usually given in a short course while ciclosporin is continued for 100 days or so for malignant regimens, longer in transplants for aplastic anaemia. The introduction of new immunosuppressive agents (e.g. tacrolimus, sirolimus, mycophenolate mofetil, rituximab, alemtuzumab), has led to trials of these agents in combination with ciclosporin for both prophylaxis and treatment of acute GVHD. Corticosteroids are the primary treatment option for acute GVHD; about 40% respond to high doses alone. Non- or partial responders receive a combination of the newer immunosuppressive agents. Management

of chronic GVHD is difficult. High-dose steroids together with specific anti-T cell or cytokine receptor monoclonal antibodies may be effective. Many 'novel' agents, including thalidomide, are being tested.

Immune reconstitution and infections in HSC transplantation

The immunosuppression of the conditioning, the cytotoxicity of the agents used and above all the severe depression of the immune response caused by GVHD, both acute and chronic, all contribute to the prolonged deficiency of cellular and humoral immunity and hence high risk of infection in the post-transplant period (Fig. 22.8.2.2). The duration may be exacerbated by prior chemotherapy,

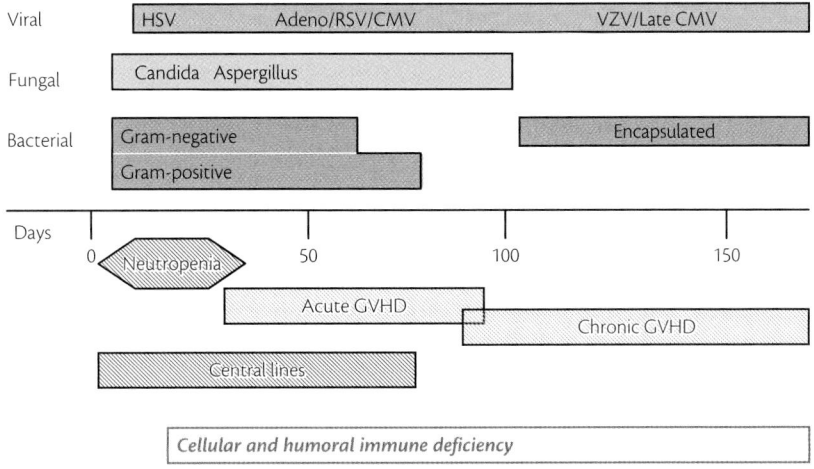

Fig. 22.8.2.2 Risk factors and timing of high-risk infections following HSCT.

TCD, and subsequent immunosuppressive treatment of GVHD. Agranulocytosis develops as soon as the conditioning regimen is started and continues until the graft is established and neutrophils return, usually after 2 to 4 weeks. During this phase bacterial and fungal infections are common. Patients are managed in isolation facilities, preferably with laminar airflow to remove environmental pathogens, particularly aspergillus. Prophylactic antibiotics including antifungals (eg fluconazole 100–400 mg/day), aciclovir 200 to 400 mg four times a day to prevent herpes simplex reactivation, and some antibacterial measures to prevent Gram-negative infection (e.g. ciprofloxacin 500 mg twice a day) are used to cover the neutropenic phase. The use of ciprofloxacin and other broad-spectrum antibiotics increases the risk of *Clostridium difficile* infection and pseudomembranous colitis. Gram positive infection, particularly by *Staphylococcus epidermidis*, is common because of the use of indwelling catheters. *Pneumocystis carinii* is a major hazard, especially when steroid treatment is given for GVHD. Co-trimoxazole 480 mg three times a week should be given until the risk of chronic GVHD has passed. CMV pneumonitis following CMV reactivation was a major cause of transplant-related mortality before the introduction of effective antiviral agents such as ganciclovir. Ganciclovir is myelosuppressive so its use following early evidence of reactivation rather than automatic prophylaxis is preferred when detection of CMV by PCR or CMV antigenaemia are available. Newer antiviral agents continue to reduce the risk of CMV disease after reactivation, together with novel cellular therapies including the adoptive transfer of CMV-specific T cells. Patients with chronic GVHD have immune deficiency similar to splenectomized patients and should receive penicillin V 250 mg twice a day (or erythromycin if allergic to penicillin) for lifelong prophylaxis against encapsulated organisms, *Streptococcus pneumoniae*, *Haemophilus influenzae*, and *Neisseria meningitides*. A revaccination programme should be instituted once cellular and humoral immunity are reconstituted, usually 1 to 2 years after the transplant.

Blood transfusions

The intense immunosuppression of conditioning produces a risk of engraftment by stem cells present in transfusion products. Where transfusion is necessary the products must be irradiated to prevent proliferation of cells.

Long-term follow-up

Life expectancy of recipients alive 2 years after transplant is reduced compared to matched controls, main causes of late death being relapse, chronic GVHD, infection, and increased risk of solid tumours. Immune suppression may be stopped once the graft is fully established and tolerance complete (usually 6 months to 2 years after transplant) but lifelong follow-up is still required.

Management of relapse

Patients transplanted for leukaemia, particularly chronic myeloid leukaemia (CML), who develop acute and/or chronic GVHD have less relapse, though not better survival, than patients without GVHD. Relapse may be effectively managed by giving donor lymphocyte infusions though this increases the risk of chronic GVHD. There is a hierarchy of GVL effect: CML being the most clear-cut, some effect in acute myeloid leukaemia (AML), less in acute lymphocytic leukaemia (ALL), and variable in lymphomas and myeloma.

Donor lymphocyte infusions now form part of the management plan post-transplant for relapse in reduced-intensity transplants when T-cell depletion is used.

Indications for haemopoietic stem cell transplantation

The main indications are shown in Table 22.8.2.1. They fall broadly into two groups. In the first, donor stem cells are used for replacement therapy— a rather crude form of gene therapy—for inherited disorders. In the second group, donor stem cells are used in malignant disease as an adjunct to chemotherapy, both through additional cytotoxicity and through the GVL effect. It is in this group that uncertainties remain as to the most appropriate timing as well as effectiveness of allogeneic transplantation. Randomized controlled trials have proved difficult to mount and much of the evidence is based on registry data or historical controls. At the same time that the results of HSC transplantations have improved, the results of chemotherapy have also become better. Nevertheless, particularly in children and younger adults, allogeneic transplantation is widely used with some success, particularly for relapsed conditions. There is a very marked inverse relationship between success of transplantation and age, children having much less transplant-related morbidity and mortality due to reduction in infection and GVHD. Children also tolerate a higher degree of HLA mismatching than adults. The upper age limit for allogeneic transplant has continued to rise as results improve and in some conditions where transplantation is the only hope of cure, e.g. CML, patients aged more than 60 years have been successfully transplanted. However, the transplant-related morbidity and mortality at this age is very marked. As would be expected, results of allogeneic transplantation are best in low-risk groups, in first complete remission or with chemosensitive disease, and are worst in relapsed and resistant disease. However, it was in this last group that the potential benefits of allogeneic transplantation were first clearly demonstrated by Thomas and his group in Seattle. In most protocols for the management of leukaemias the inclusion of allogeneic transplantation, where a suitable sibling donor is available, is considered either up-front or as a form of rescue in younger patients. The results of unrelated donor transplants consistently lag behind those of matched sibling donors and although HLA antigen-mismatched stem cells are used in desperate situations, success rates decline as transplant-related morbidity and mortality increases.

Indications for autologous transplantation

The use of autologous HSC for treatment of malignant disease can only be considered a form of rescue from increased chemotherapy since there is no GVL effect. Where there may be tumour antigens that are amenable to immune therapy, attempts have been made to induce specific immunotoxicity, so far without clear-cut benefit. On the other hand, autologous stem cell rescue does allow greatly increased intensity chemotherapy regimens for lymphoma, myeloma, and a variety of solid tumours with shortening of hospital stay— indeed, in some cases treatment can be managed in an outpatient setting—and a prolonged course of therapy with repeated rescue from stored cells. Autologous stem cells will also provide the vehicle for gene therapy once techniques for gene insertion and long-term expression become practical.

Future directions for haemopoietic stem cell transplantation

◆ Better understanding and treatment of GVHD, particularly chronic GVHD

◆ Wider use of UCB donations

◆ Further clinical trials to establish best practice, conditioning regimen and indications

◆ Harnessing the GVL effect

◆ Development of cellular therapies post transplant

Further reading

Brunstein CG, Setubal DC, Wagner JE (2007). Expanding the role of umbilical cord blood transplantation. *Br J Haematol*, **137**, 20–35.

Craddock C, Chakreverty R (2005). Stem cell transplantation. In: Hoffbrand AV, Catovsky D, Tuddenham EGD (eds) *Postgraduate haematology*, pp. 419–35. Blackwell Publishing, Oxford.

Deeg HJ (2007). How I treat refractory GVHD. *Blood*, **109**, 4119–26.

Giralt S, *et al*. (1997). Engraftment of allogeneic hematopoietic progenitor cells with purine analog-containing chemotherapy: harnessing graft-versus-leukemia without myeloablative therapy. *Blood*, **89**, 4531–6.

Kennedy-Nasser AA, Bollard CM. (2007). T cell therapies following haematopoietic stem cell transplantation: surely there must be a better way than DLI? *Bone Marrow Transplant*, **40**, 93–104.

Kolb H, *et al*. (1995). Graft-versus-leukemia effect of donor lymphocyte transfusions in marrow grafted patients. European Group for Blood and Marrow Transplantation Working Party for Chronic Myeloid Leukemia. *Blood*, **86**, 2041–50.

Körbling M, Anderlini P (2001). Peripheral blood stem cell versus bone marrow allotransplantation: does the source of hematopoietic stem cells matter? *Blood*, **98**, 2900–8.

Lee SJ (2007). New approaches for preventing and treating chronic graft-versus-host disease. *Blood*, **105**, 4200–6.

Nauta AJ, Fibbe WE (2007). Immunomodulatory properties of mesenchymal stem cells. *Blood*, **110**, 3499–506.

Peggs KS, *et al*. (2005). Clinical evidence of a graft-versus-Hodgkin's-lymphoma effect after reduced-intensity allogeneic transplantation.*Lancet*, **365**(9475), 1934–41.

Rizzo JD, *et al*. (2006). Recommended screening and preventive practices for long-term survivors after hematopoietic cell transplantation: joint recommendations of the European Group for Blood and Marrow Transplantation, Center for International Blood and Marrow Transplant Research, and the American Society for Blood and Marrow Transplantation (EBMT/CIBMTR/ASBMT). *Bone Marrow Transplant*, **37**, 249–61.

Rocha V, *et al*. (2004). Transplants of umbilical-cord blood or bone marrow from unrelated donors in adults with acute leukaemia. *N Engl J Med*, **351**, 2276–85.

Slavin S, *et al*.(1998). Nonmyeloablative stem cell transplantation and cell therapy as an alternative to conventional bone marrow transplantation with lethal cytoreduction for the treatment of malignant and nonmalignant hematologic diseases. *Blood*, **97**, 56–63.

Socié G, *et al*. (1999). Long term survival and late deaths after allogeneic marrow transplantation. Late effects working committee of the International Bone Marrow Transplant Registry. *N Engl J Med*, **341**, 14–21.

Socié G, *et al*. (2003). Non-malignant late effects after allogeneic stem cell transplantation. *Blood*, **101**, 3373–85.

Thomas ED (2005). Bone marrow transplantation from the personal viewpoint. *Int J Hematol*, **81**, 89–93.

Thomson KJ, Potter M, Mackinnon S (2005). Non-myeloablative transplantation. In: Hoffbrand AV, Catovsky D, Tuddenham EGD (eds) *Postgraduate haematology*, pp. 436–448. Blackwell Publishing, Oxford.

Thomson KJ, *et al*. (2009). Favorable long-term survival after reduced-intensity allogeneic transplantation for multiple-relapse aggressive non-Hodgkin's lymphoma. *J Clin Oncol*, **27**, 426–32.

SECTION 23

Disorders of the skin

Editor: Graham S. Ogg

23.1

Structure and function of skin

John A. McGrath

Essentials

Skin provides a mechanical barrier against the external environment, but has further roles in thermoregulation, metabolism, and the regulation of fluid balance, as well as being socially important in contributing to physical and chemical attraction between individuals.

There are more than 1000 different skin diseases, although relatively few are commonly encountered in general medical practice. However,

several skin conditions can reflect a general medical problem such as a systemic infection, or a cutaneous manifestation of internal disease (e.g. patients with underlying malignancy, endocrine disorders or chronic inflammatory diseases). An understanding of skin structure and function is also important in dealing with the common clinical scenario of 'skin failure' resulting from adverse drug reactions, burns, or extensive trauma.

Introduction

The skin is the body's largest organ. In a 70-kg individual the skin weighs over 5 kg and covers a surface area approaching 2 m^2. Structurally, skin consists of a stratified cellular epidermis (made of keratinocytes) and an underlying dermis of connective tissue (fibroblasts, collagens, elastic tissue, and ground substance) (Fig. 23.1.1). Below the dermis is a layer of subcutaneous fat, which is separated from the rest of the body by a vestigial layer of striated muscle. The skin also contains hair follicles, sweat glands, blood vessels, autonomic and sensory nerves, as well as pigment cells (melanocytes), antigen-presenting cells (e.g. Langerhans' cells), neuroendocrine (Merkel's) cells, and some resident inflammatory cells (lymphocytes and mast cells).

Origin of the skin

The skin arises by the juxtaposition of two major embryological elements: the prospective epidermis, which originates from a surface area of the early gastrula, and the prospective mesoderm, which comes into contact with the inner surface of the epidermis during gastrulation. The mesoderm not only provides the dermis, but is essential for inducing differentiation of the epidermal structures, such as the hair follicle. The melanocytes are derived from the neural crest. While the skin develops *in utero* it is covered by a special layer, the periderm, which is unique to mammals. The periderm provides some protection to the newly forming skin, as well as having a role in the uptake of carbohydrate from the amniotic fluid.

The embryonic dermis is at first very cellular, and at 6 to 14 weeks three types of cell are present: stellate cells, phagocytic macrophages,

and cells with secretory granules (either melanoblasts or mast cells). From weeks 14 to 21 fibroblasts are numerous and active, and perineural cells, pericytes, melanoblasts, Merkel's cells, and mast cells can be individually identified. The various components of the skin that can be recognized postnatally start to appear at different embryonic time-points, e.g. hair follicles and nails (9 weeks), sweat glands (9 weeks for the palms and soles, 15 weeks for other sites), and sebaceous glands (15 weeks). Touch pads become recognizable on the hands and fingers, and on the feet and toes, by 6 weeks, and reach their greatest development at 15 weeks. After this, they flatten and become indistinct. It is these areas that determine the pattern of the dermatoglyphs (fingerprints) that take their place.

Structure of the skin

Epidermis

The normal epidermis is a terminally differentiated, stratified squamous epithelium composed of keratinocytes, which progressively move from attachment to the epidermal basement membrane towards the skin surface. This process normally takes about 40 days, but is accelerated in diseases such as psoriasis. The brick-like shape of keratinocytes is provided by a cytoskeleton made of keratin intermediate filaments. As the epidermis differentiates, the keratinocytes become flattened as a result of the action of filaggrin, a protein component of keratohyalin granules, on the keratin filaments. Indeed, keratin and filaggrin comprise 80 to 90% of the mass of the epidermis.

The outermost layer of the epidermis is the stratum corneum, where the cells (now called corneocytes) have lost their nuclei

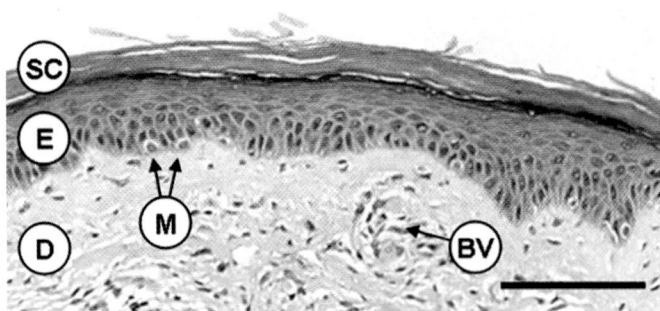

Fig. 23.1.1 Histopathological appearance of normal human skin. This light microscopic image illustrates the structural features of the outer skin layers. BV, blood vessel; D, dermis; E, epidermis; M, melanocyte; SC, stratum corneum. Haematoxylin and eosin; scale bar = 0.1 mm.

and cytoplasmic organelles. The corneocyte has a highly insoluble cornified envelope within the plasma membrane, formed by the cross-linking of soluble protein precursors including involucrin and loricrin. The latter contributes 70 to 85% of the mass of the cornified cell envelope, which also contains several lipids (fatty acids, sterols, and ceramides) released from lamellar bodies within the upper, living epidermis.

Melanocytes are located within the basal layer of the epidermis (closest to the dermis). These are dendritic cells that distribute packages of the pigment melanin (melanosomes) to surrounding keratinocytes, the process that gives skin its physical colour. The number of melanocytes does not differ much between white and black skin. Rather it is the nature of the melanin and the size of the melanosomes that account for the different appearance.

Another dendritic cell population within the epidermis is the Langerhans' cell, which is of mesenchymal origin, and originates from bone marrow. Langerhans' cells are antigen-presenting cells that process antigens encountered by the skin to local lymph nodes, and thus have a key role in adaptive immune responses in the skin.

Dermis

Collagen is the major extracellular matrix protein, comprising 80 to 85% of the dry weight of the dermis. Twenty-seven different collagens have been identified in vertebrate tissue (distinguished by roman numerals in the order of their discovery, from I to XXVII), of which at least 12 are expressed in skin. The main interstitial dermal collagens are types I and III, whereas the principal basement membrane collagen (at the junction between the dermis and the epidermis, and around dermal blood vessels, nerves, and glands) is type IV. Triple-helical collagen monomers polymerize into fibrils and fibres, which then become stabilized by the formation of complex intra- and intermolecular cross-links. Collagen fibres are extremely tough and provide skin with its tensile strength.

Elastic fibres account for no more than 2 to 4% of the extracellular matrix in the dermis, and consist of two components, elastin and microfibrils, which together give skin its elasticity and resilience. Elastic microfibrils are composed of several proteins, including fibrillin, that surround the elastin and can extend throughout the dermis in a web-like configuration to the junction between the dermis and the epidermis.

The dermis also contains a number of noncollagenous glycoproteins, including fibronectins, fibulins, and integrins, which are important components of the extracellular matrix, facilitating cell adhesion and cell motility. Between the dermal collagen and elastic tissue is the ground substance, made up of glycosaminoglycan/proteoglycan macromolecules. These contribute only 0.1 to 0.3% of the total dry weight of the dermis, but play a vital role in providing hydration, mostly via the high water-binding capacity of hyaluronic acid. Indeed, about 60% of the total weight of the dermis is composed of water.

Regional variations in skin anatomy

The thickness of the living epidermis in normal human skin shows some variation with body site, and usually measures about 0.05 to 0.1 mm, although it may be thicker in regions such as the palm and sole, where the stratum corneum can be up to 10 times thicker than in nonacral sites (Fig. 23.1.2). Likewise, the thickness of the dermis may differ considerably, from less than 0.5 mm on the eyelid to more than 5 mm on the back.

There are two main types of human skin. Glabrous (nonhairy) skin is found on the palms and soles. It has a grooved surface with alternating ridges and sulci, giving rise to the fingerprints. Glabrous skin has a compact stratum corneum, encapsulated sense organs within the dermis, and a lack of hair follicles and sebaceous glands. By contrast, hair-bearing skin has both hair follicles and sebaceous glands, but lacks encapsulated sense organs. There is also wide variation between body sites. For example, the scalp has large hair follicles that may extend into the subcutaneous fat, whereas the forehead has only small vellus hair-producing follicles, although the sebaceous glands are large. The axilla is notable because it has apocrine glands in addition to the eccrine sweat glands that are found throughout the body.

Skin renewal

The epidermis can regenerate from keratinocyte stem cells that are located in small clusters in the basal interfollicular epidermis and, in particular, in the bulge region of hair follicles. Although morphologically similar to other keratinocytes, stem cells are associated with a particular molecular profile that includes increased β_1-integrin production, as well as high levels of Notch ligand Delta 1. Other markers with altered expression in epidermal stem cells include the transferrin receptor, the nuclear export protein 14-3-3σ, and keratins 15 and 19. Not all dividing basal keratinocytes are stem cells; some cells, known as transient amplifying cells, can proliferate and divide a small number of times before undergoing terminal differentiation. Stem cells in the bulge region have the capacity to migrate (e.g. to the base of the hair follicle in follicular regeneration), as well as to differentiate into diverse lineages (e.g. hair, sebaceous glands, or interfollicular epidermis). Mesenchymal stem cells may also reside within the dermis, although the precise function of such cells in skin homeostasis or during wound healing has not been well established. Likewise, the renewal of skin cells, including keratinocytes, may be possible by cellular differentiation from other stem-cell sources such as bone marrow.

Functions of the skin

Skin provides a barrier against the external environment (Fig. 23.1.3). The cornified cell envelope and the stratum corneum restrict water loss from the skin, while keratinocyte-derived endogenous antibiotics (defensins and cathelicidins) provide an

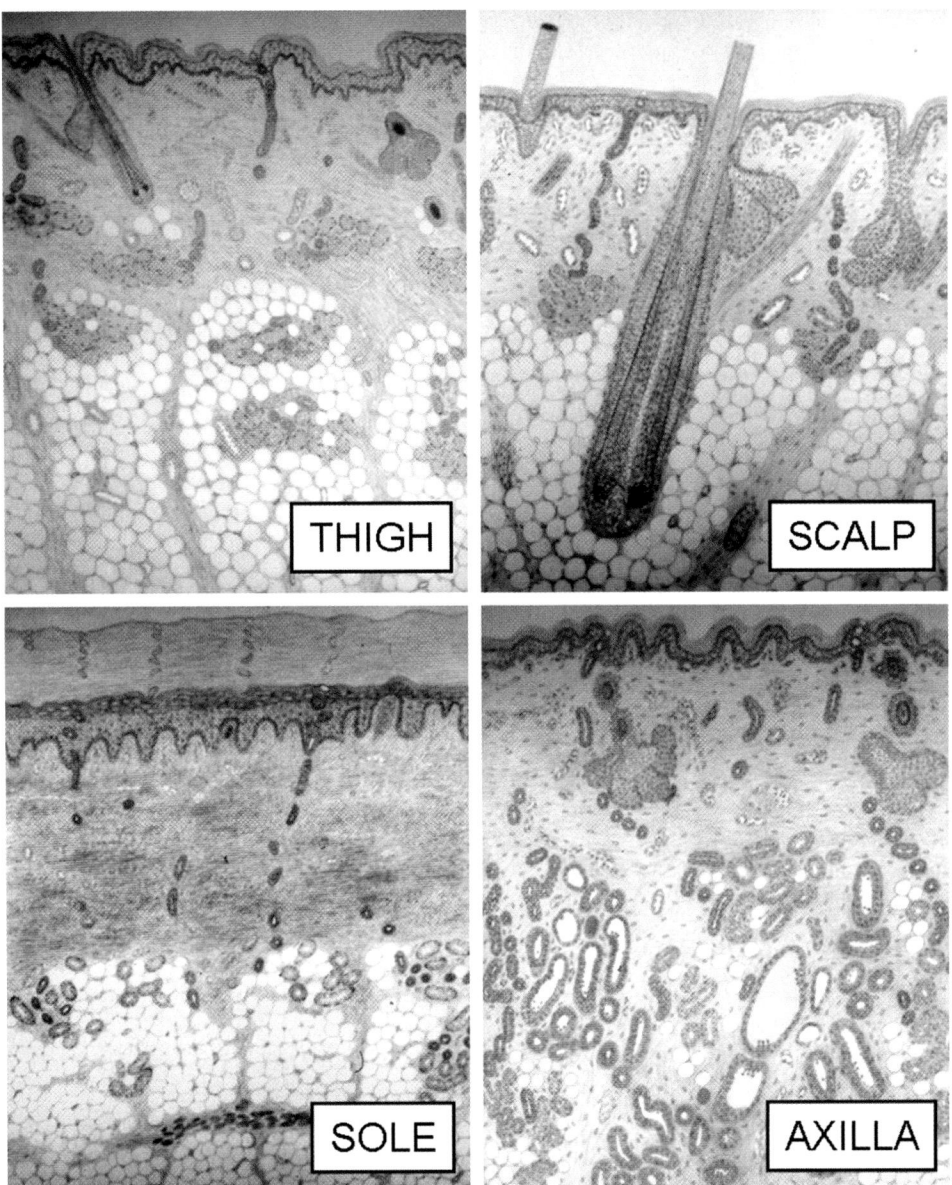

Fig. 23.1.2 Regional differences in skin anatomy. The physical differences in the structural composition of human skin at four different body sites (thigh, scalp, sole, and axilla) are depicted. Compared with thigh skin, the scalp has much larger hair follicles that extend deep into the subcutaneous fat, the sole has a thick stratum corneum, and the axilla has numerous eccrine and apocrine sweat glands.

innate immune defence against bacteria, viruses, and fungi. The epidermis also contains a network of about 2×10^9 Langerhans' cells, which serve as sentinel cells whose prime function is to survey the epidermal environment and initiate an immune response against microbial threats, although they may also contribute to immune tolerance in the skin. Melanin in keratinocytes also provides some protection against DNA damage from ultraviolet radiation.

An important function of skin is thermoregulation, and there is both a superficial and a deep vascular plexus; vasodilatation and vasoconstriction of these blood vessels helps regulate heat loss. Eccrine sweat glands, present in densities of 100 to 600/cm^2, also play a role in heat control, and may produce approximately 1 litre of sweat per hour during moderate exercise. Secretions from apocrine sweat glands, which are mainly found in the axillae, contribute to body odour (pheromones). Skin lubrication and waterproofing is provided by sebum secreted from sebaceous glands—outpouchings of hair follicles.

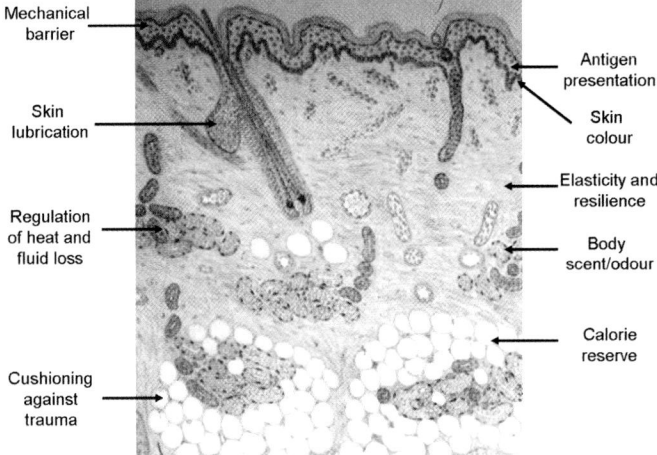

Fig. 23.1.3 Function of human normal skin. The skin has several key biological roles, from the formation of a mechanical barrier, the stratum corneum, against the external environment, to providing a calorie reserve in the subcutaneous fat.

Subcutaneous fat has an important role in cushioning trauma, as well as in providing insulation and a calorie reserve. Nails provide protection to the ends of the fingers and toes, and are important in pinching and prizing objects. Skin also has a key function in synthesizing various metabolic products, such as vitamin D.

Skin also contains motor and sensory nerves. The motor innervation of the skin is autonomic, and includes a cholinergic component to the eccrine sweat glands, and adrenergic components to both the eccrine and apocrine glands, to the smooth muscle and the arterioles, and to the arrector pili muscle (attached to hair follicles). The sensory nerve endings are of several kinds; some are free, some terminate in hair follicles, and others have expanded tips.

Failure of the skin

Epidermis

Loss of a functional epidermis has profound biological and clinical consequences involving the loss of water and electrolytes, cutaneous and systemic infection, and impaired thermoregulation. The clinical importance of an intact skin barrier has recently been highlighted by the discovery that a large number of people with atopic dermatitis (and atopic dermatitis associated with asthma) have loss-of-function mutations in filaggrin (see OMIM 135 940), an important component of the cornified cell envelope. Loss of filaggrin leads to a defective skin barrier with increased transepidermal water loss (leading to skin dryness and itching) and an increased susceptibility to allergic sensitization and infection.

As far as acquired epidermal failure is concerned, burns, trauma, and adverse drug reactions such as Stevens–Johnson syndrome and toxic epidermal necrolysis (TEN, Lyell's syndrome) can all lead to significant skin detachment and major metabolic imbalances. Stevens–Johnson syndrome can be considered a minor form of TEN, and involves less than 10% of body surface area skin detachment, with an average reported mortality of 1 to 5%, whereas TEN is characterized by more than 30% skin detachment, and an average reported mortality of 25 to 35%. Both conditions are characterized histologically by a rapid onset of keratinocyte cell death by apoptosis, a process that results in the separation of the epidermis from the dermis. Recent evidence supports a role for inflammatory cytokines and the death receptor Fas (TNF receptor superfamily, member 6) and its ligand in the pathogenesis of keratinocyte apoptosis during TEN. Fas-mediated keratinocyte apoptosis can be inhibited *in vitro* by antagonistic monoclonal antibodies to Fas, and by intravenous immunoglobulins, which have been shown to contain natural anti-Fas antibodies. Some studies in patients with TEN have indicated a benefit (reduced mortality) from intravenous immunoglobulins when used at doses greater than 2 g/kg, but this has not been clearly established. Early recognition of TEN leading to skin failure is, however, vital for optimal patient management.

Dermis

In normal skin ageing, and in photoageing (skin changes resulting from chronic sun exposure), there is reduced synthesis of interstitial collagens (type I and III), and increased synthesis of enzymes (matrix metalloproteinases) that break down dermal fibres. Paradoxically, there is an increase in elastin synthesis, although this functions poorly and contributes to the wrinkled, sagging appearance of aged skin.

More specific insight into the consequences of the failure of particular dermal components, however, has recently been determined from the molecular characterization of genetic disorders such as Ehlers–Danlos syndrome (EDS) and cutis laxa. EDS represents a collection of six diseases associated with varying degrees of hyperextensible fragile skin and loose joints. Some subtypes may also be associated with catastrophic rupture of arterial blood vessels, the bowel, or the uterus. Although the cause of the major forms of EDS is unknown, in some forms of EDS abnormalities have been detected in type V collagen (OMIM 120 190) and tenascin X (a molecular organizer of connective tissue; OMIM 600 985), and in the vascular type of EDS, in type III collagen (OMIM 120 180). Further pathology has also been demonstrated in type I procollagen (OMIM 120 160) and in two enzymes, lysyl hydroxylase (EC 1.14.11.4; OMIM 153 454) and procollagen N-endopeptidase (EC 3.4.24.14; OMIM 604 539), involved in the formation of collagen fibres.

Cutis laxa is clinically characterized by loose, sagging skin and, in some subtypes, by extracutaneous abnormalities such as emphysema, and inguinal or umbilical hernias. Mutations in the gene encoding fibulin 5 (OMIM 604 580), a protein involved in elastin fibrillogenesis, have been shown to underlie some, but not all cases of this disease. Collectively, these rare genetic diseases highlight the significant clinical consequences of the failure of specific components of the dermis, and provide evidence for their important roles in the maintenance of normal, healthy skin.

Further reading

Bergstresser PR, Costner MI (2008). Anatomy and physiology. In: *Dermatology* (eds, Bolognia J, Jorizzo J, Rapini R). Mosby Elsevier, Oxford, pp. 25–35.

Lai-Cheong JE, McGrath JA (2009). Structure and function of skin, hair and nails. *Medicine*, **37**, 223–26.

McGrath JA, Eady RAJ, Pope FM (2004). Anatomy and organization of human skin. In: *Rook's textbook of dermatology* (eds Burns T, *et al.*), Blackwell Publishing Ltd, Oxford, pp. 3.1–3.84.

Clinical approach to the diagnosis of skin disease

Vanessa Venning

Essentials

As in most medical specialities, the diagnosis of skin disease relies on careful history taking, and a thorough examination, supported in some cases by appropriate investigation. Astute physicians will also be aware that management outcomes are improved by taking account of the impact of skin disease on patients' lives, whether through discomfort, disfigurement, or disability. This section, however, is chiefly concerned with aspects of history taking and examination that inform the diagnostic process.

History taking

There are certain key points in the history of skin disease that should be specifically elicited, and these are summarized in Box 23.2.1. These should include a description of the events surrounding the onset of skin lesions: when and where the eruption started and how it progressed. Neoplasms are likely to be relatively asymptomatic and persistent, whereas inflammatory disorders may itch, scale, or ooze, and frequently fluctuate. The rapidity of fluctuation is helpful; urticaria and eczema are both intensely itchy, but are distinguished by the fluctuation of the individual lesions of urticaria over hours, rather than days or weeks as in eczemas or psoriasis. The site of onset may also give a clue to the diagnosis and cause of a rash.

The history should include an enquiry into general health, both past and present, and of skin disease, including specific enquiry about the personal and family history of psoriasis and the atopic disorders eczema, asthma, and hay fever. If more than one household member is affected this may indicate heredity or contagion. Occupation, travel or residence abroad, leisure activities, and hobbies may indicate exposure to the sun, irritant or sensitizing chemicals, or infections. Many patients will already have tried topical treatment before presentation, either self medicated or physician prescribed, and the response to these, whether beneficial or adverse, may be helpful in diagnosis. Drug-induced skin disease is important, and a full history of drugs taken for other disorders is essential.

Examination

Dermatology differs from other specialties because the disease is visible to the naked eye, and the lesions can also be touched and palpated. However, it is necessary to know what to look for and to understand what is seen and felt. To examine the skin properly the patient should ideally be undressed, and examined in a good light, preferably daylight.

Distribution

Before concentrating on the appearance of the individual lesions, much can be deduced from their distribution. The distribution of lesions in many common dermatoses is so characteristic that it frequently aids diagnosis. In some diseases the pattern may reflect regional variations in skin structure, e.g. acne vulgaris favours areas rich in pilosebaceous units, such as the face and upper torso. Other disorders are distributed according to exposure to external causative agents (e.g. points of contact with irritants/allergens or sun exposure) (Fig. 23.2.1). Gravity and stasis underpin the distribution of varicose eczema on the lower legs. The sluggish blood flow of stasis also favours immune-complex deposition, and explains the frequency of vasculitis lesions on the lower legs (Fig. 23.2.2). In other instances the factors affecting distribution are not necessarily fully understood, but nonetheless, observation of the distribution may be crucial to diagnosis. Is the skin disease localized or generalized? Is it symmetrical? What specific sites are involved? It is important to examine not only the skin itself, but also the hair and nails, and the mucous membranes (particularly inside the mouth).

Symmetry

Although the basis for the body symmetry of rashes is not fully understood, the presence or absence of symmetry serves as a useful pointer in diagnosis. Rashes showing bilateral symmetry are frequently suggestive of endogenous skin disease. The most common inflammatory dermatoses—atopic eczema and psoriasis, having a strong hereditary component in their pathogenesis, are regarded as endogenous or constitutional diseases, and both show striking

Box 23.2.1 Outline of dermatological history

- History of present skin condition
  - Duration
  - Site of onset
  - Details of spread or enlargement
  - Does it fluctuate or persist?
  - Provoking or aggravating factors
  - Symptoms, e.g. itch, burning, soreness, pain, bleeding, weeping, oozing, blisters, odour
  - Impact on quality of life
- Past history of skin disorders
- Past and present general medical history
  - Ask specifically about asthma and hay fever
- Family history
  - Ask specifically about eczema, asthma, and hay fever (the atopic disorders), and psoriasis
- Social history
  - Occupation, travel, and leisure activities
  - Particularly enquire about sun exposure and burning episodes
- Medication used to treat present skin condition
  - Topical or systemic
  - Physician prescribed or over the counter
- Drugs taken for other disorders
  - Allergies to medication, or contact allergens

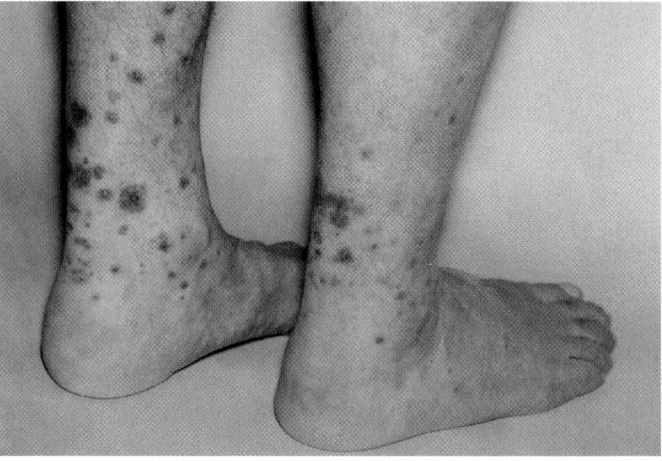

Fig. 23.2.2 These purpuric lesions are palpable rather than flat, indicating vasculitis. The distribution on the lower legs is common.

most drug eruptions, viral exanthema, erythema multiforme provoked by a cold sore or other trigger, and dermatitis herpetiformis (the rash of gluten sensitivity).

By contrast, rashes and lesions caused by exogenous factors such as the random behaviour of a biting insect, contact with allergenic or irritant substances, or with infections like bacterial impetigo are commonly, but not necessarily, asymmetric. A foot dermatitis that affects only one foot should prompt investigation for fungal infection.

Site

Certain conditions have a predilection for characteristic sites, and knowledge of the favoured sites is diagnostically important. Psoriasis favours the extensor surfaces of elbows and knees, and also affects the scalp, nails, and gluteal cleft. By contrast, atopic eczema favours the flexures (Fig. 23.2.3b), e.g. antecubital and popliteal fossae, and other sites. This distinguishes it from seborrhoeic eczema, which prefers the scalp and ears, central face (eyebrows, nasolabial folds), mid chest, and groins.

Lesions provoked by sunlight predominate on exposed skin (e.g. skin cancers, idiopathic or drug-induced photosensitive rashes, lupus erythematosus). In some sun-induced rashes there may be a sharp cut-off under clothing, or sparing of shielded sites, e.g. under the chin and behind the ears. Contact dermatitis to airborne pollens, such as those of the Compositae family (Fig. 23.2.1), or volatile allergens such as epoxy resin glues, will not spare these shielded sites, but may show a similar cut-off at the collar. The distribution of some important diseases is shown in Fig. 23.2.4.

Morphology

Many skin diseases have characteristic lesion morphology, although scratch marks, ulceration, and secondary infection may modify the appearance. A good light is essential, and a hand lens is helpful. Touch and palpation give important information about the thickness, depth, consistency, and tenderness of lesions, and whether the surface is rough or smooth. Ideally, a primary lesion should be sought for deciding lesion type, one that has not been damaged by picking, scratching, or prior application of creams or anything else likely to eradicate important clues. To aid the clear and unambiguous description of lesions, certain terms are used, the most important of which are listed in Table 23.2.1.

symmetry in the distribution of their lesions (Fig. 23.2.3). Symmetry is not confined to the major heritable skin diseases; several skin diseases are regarded as reactions to underlying triggers. Although these may not have a genetic basis, they behave like intrinsic disorders, and as such frequently show symmetry. Examples of these are

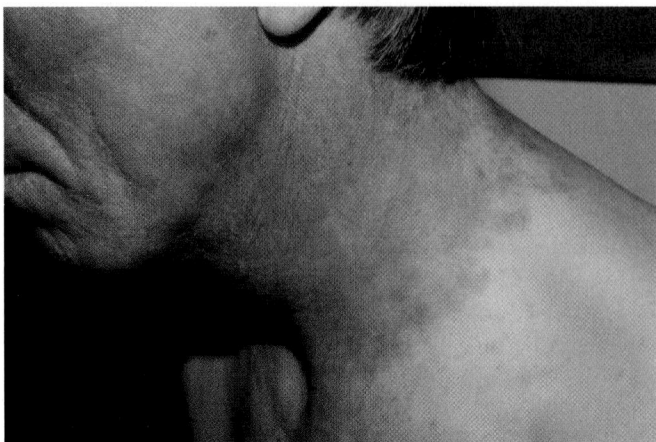

Fig. 23.2.1 Eczema confined to exposed skin. In this case resulting from contact dermatitis to an airborne allergen (Compositae pollen), but a similar cut-off under clothing can occur with photosensitivity.

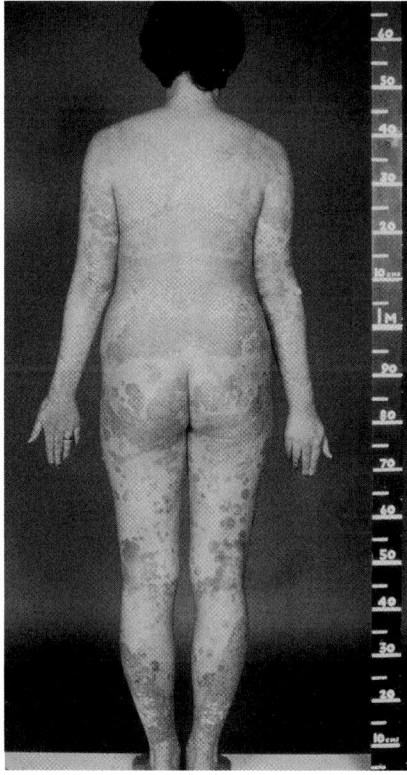

(a)

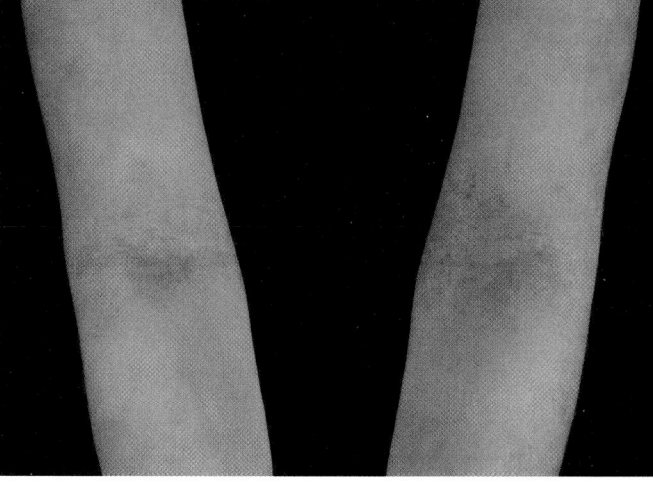

(b)

Fig. 23.2.3 Both atopic eczema and psoriasis show classical epidermal signs (scaliness), but have different distributions. Symmetry is characteristic of many endogenous skin diseases: (a) Extensive psoriasis. The symmetry of psoriatic lesions may be dramatic and striking. (b) Itchy, scaly, inflamed skin in a symmetrical flexural pattern. This is typical of atopic eczema.

The lesion type, colour, and surface characteristics should be recorded, the aim being to try to glean as much information as possible about the underlying pathology. Redness (erythema) resulting from vasodilatation of the upper dermal vasculature will blanch on pressure, and indicates inflammation. If purpuric lesions are present, attention should be paid to whether they are entirely flat (macular) or are palpable, the latter indicating a more profound degree of vascular pathology than mere leakage, and signifies the presence of vasculitis (Fig. 23.2.2).

The presence and nature of scale is a physical sign of great importance. Keratin is the principle polypeptide product of the epidermis, and constitutes up to 90% of the stratum corneum. Any disease, whether inflammatory, infective, or neoplastic, that affects the epidermis will disrupt keratin production, resulting in scaliness. The importance given to scale is indicated by the large number of synonyms used by dermatologists to describe it (scaly, keratotic, hyperkeratotic, keratinized, warty, verrucous). Scale can be particularly thick and loosely adherent in psoriasis, making it appear light in colour (silvery scale), or is sometimes dense and compacted.

Very acute inflammation of the epidermis will also result in vesiculation and oozing, as in the case of acute eczemas and superficial bacterial infections, or may result in an influx of neutrophils leading to pustule development in bacterial and candidal infections, and in some forms of psoriasis. The presence of epidermal signs (scale, vesicles, ooze, pustules) indicates that the pathology is chiefly or solely superficial, and differentiates these diseases from those that are chiefly dermal. Deep-seated dermal or subcutaneous inflammatory or neoplastic infiltrates are more likely to form lumps or swellings, which may distort the epidermis from below, but may not actually disrupt it, so that the surface is more likely to be smooth with skin markings preserved. This distinction between epidermal and dermal diseases is not of course absolute, and many disorders affect both, but this artificial separation helps to focus the examiner on the question: Where is the pathology?

The appearance of some lesions may be so characteristic that occasionally they permit an immediate confident diagnosis, an example being lichen planus when present in its most typical form, with shiny, flat-topped, mauve-coloured papules with surface white streaks (Wickham's striae). Other lesion types may not permit immediate diagnosis, but are still sufficiently distinctive as to be a useful starting point for a differential diagnosis, an example being vesicles and bullae (blisters). Common causes of blisters include burns, acute eczemas, viral infections such as Herpes spp., and infection with *Staphylococcus aureus* (bullous impetigo). Rarer causes of blisters include erythema multiforme, immunobullous diseases (e.g. pemphigoid, pemphigus), and some porphyrias.

Lesion shape and grouping

Additional diagnostic clues are afforded by the lesion shape and the way they are grouped. Distinctive lesion shapes are annular, target-shaped and linear.

Annular lesions imply inflammation spreading out centrifugally from a central focus, with clearance in the centre. This pattern is characteristic of dermatophyte fungus infection of skin (tinea corporis or ringworm; Fig. 23.2.5), which, being a superficial infection, is accompanied by subtle scaling, particularly at the margin. Granulomas in the dermis form a characteristic ring in granuloma annulare. These lesions are palpable, but the overlying epidermis is smooth. Reactive erythemas frequently assume an annular shape (also known as annular or toxic erythema; Fig. 23.2.6). The margin is red, slightly elevated, and may be very slightly scaly. Annular erythemas evolve at a variable rate; the slow enlargement of erythema chronicum migrans (the eruption of early Lyme disease) occurs at a rate of a few centimetres per day, rather than over hours, and eventually fades within a few weeks. Reactivation of inflammation at the centre of annular erythema produces target lesions characteristic of, but not exclusive to, erythema multiforme.

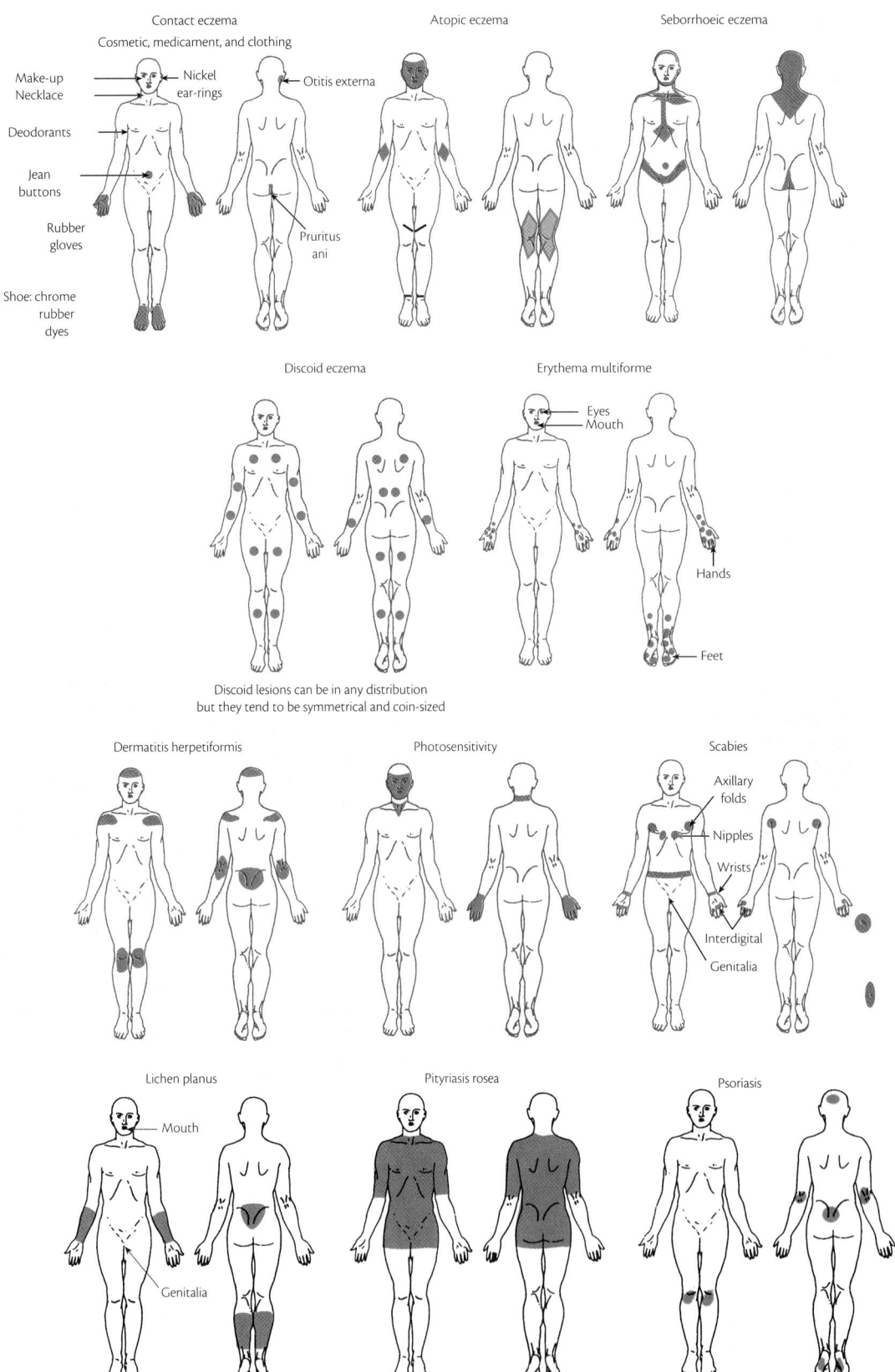

Fig. 23.2.4 Distribution of common skin diseases.

Table 23.2.1 Terminology of skin lesions

Lesion	Definition	Description
Macules	Flat (nonpalpable) lesion	Minimal changes in surface markings or texture; may merely be areas of redness, purpura, or melanin
Papules and plaques	Papules are small, circumscribed, palpable raised lesions. Plaques are larger diameter palpable lesions, often resulting from the confluence of papules	Palpable lesions may arise either from thickening of the epidermis, or from infiltration/oedema of the upper dermis, or a combination
Nodules	Circumscribed palpable masses, usually >1 cm	Usually consist of infiltrating cells (inflammatory or neoplastic) filling the dermis and/or subcutaneous tissue
Cysts	Circumscribed palpable lesions containing fluid or semisolid material	Clinically resemble nodules, but are fluid filled rather than solid (unlike vesicles and blisters, which are superficial, unlined, and contain visible fluid)
Vesicles and bullae (blisters)	Visible accumulations of fluid	Vesicles are small, bullae are >1 cm; they frequently coexist
Urticaria or wheal Angio-oedema	Urticaria is dermal oedema (can be any size). Angio-oedema is deep-seated dermal oedema extending into subcutaneous tissue	
Petechiae and purpura	Leakage of blood in the skin, which does not blanch on pressure	Petechiae(pinhead size) Purpura (a few mm diameter) Ecchymosis (larger haemorrhagic areas

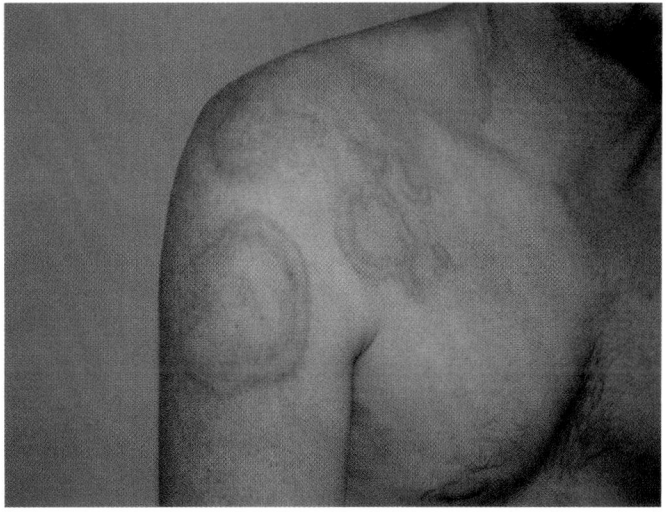

Fig. 23.2.6 Annular erythema (reactive or toxic erythema). The annular shape may suggest a fungal infection, but the overlying epidermis is smooth or only slightly scaly, indicating that the pathology lies chiefly in the dermis. The margins of these rings are elevated by dermal infiltration with inflammatory cells and oedema.

The close clustering of individual lesions into groups is sometimes distinctive. The grouping of vesicles in herpes simplex (Fig. 23.2.7) is so characteristic that other diseases that show similar lesion grouping are referred to as herpetiform, e.g. dermatitis herpetiformis. The grouping of lesions within a dermatomal distribution is seen in shingles, and reflects reactivation of the varicella–zoster virus from dorsal root ganglia.

In some conditions, a scratch or other injury localizes lesions in a linear fashion because the lesions have a predilection for damaged skin. This is known as the Koebner phenomenon, and is seen in psoriasis, lichen planus, and warts. Other lesions are roughly linear because they follow linear anatomical structures, e.g. superficial thombophlebitis and ascending lymphangitis. The shape of many congenital hamartomas may be determined by the migration of skin cells during embryogenesis, or from genetic mosaicism. Lesions may be roughly linear in shape, or assume bizarre patterns of lines and whorls (Blaschko's lines, named after the dermatologist who described the patterns in epidermal naevi). Brushing against the foliage of phototoxin-containing plants in sunlight

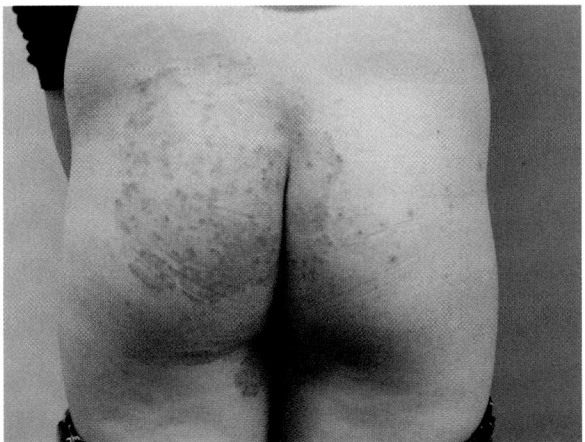

Fig. 23.2.5 Fungal infection (tinea corporis). By contrast with the endogenous diseases, this eruption is asymmetrical. The annular shape is typical. Dermatophyte fungus infections are usually very superficial, so the epidermal sign of scaliness is marked.

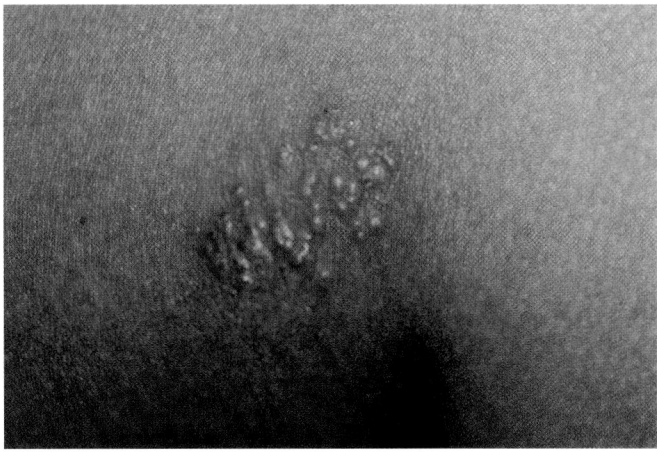

Fig. 23.2.7 Grouping of vesicles typifies herpes simplex virus infection.

produces painful linear lesions with blisters (phytophotodermatitis) and long-lasting streaks of pigmentation. Very straight-edged lines and rectilinear shapes may raise the suspicion of artefactually induced lesions (dermatitis artefacta).

Special investigations

Although it is frequently possible to diagnose a rash or lesion from its appearance, in some cases additional investigations are required.

Skin scrapings for fungal mycelia

Scales removed by gentle scraping with a scalpel blade are treated with potassium hydroxide to clear keratin and other obscuring debris, and examined by light microscopy for fungal hyphae. Culture on a suitable medium identifies the fungal species.

Biopsy

Biopsy is indicated in the evaluation of skin tumours, in the case of rashes in which there is clinical uncertainty, or when it is essential to document the diagnosis before treatment, e.g. lymphomas. The lesion or area of rash chosen for biopsy should be reasonably representative, and not be modified by scratching, picking, secondary infection, or treatment. The standard procedure is to remove a small ellipse of skin, including some underlying fat, under local anaesthesia. A punch biopsy of 4 mm diameter is frequently sufficient and convenient in a clinic setting, but is less suitable for evaluating deep pathology such as panniculitis. Small lesions (e.g. papules, small nodules, and blisters) can be entirely excised within a small ellipse. Complete excision is preferable to an incisional biopsy for the evaluation of tumours. If a blister is to be biopsied, this should be a recent one (no more than 24 h old), so that the blister depth can be judged before epithelial regeneration takes place. For standard histopathology the skin is placed in formalin.

Immunofluorescence tests

Immunofluorescence tests using fluorescein-labelled antibodies can detect skin-bound immunoglobulins or complement, and are used in the diagnosis of the immunobullous diseases such as pemphigus, pemphigoid, and dermatitis herpetiformis (see Chapter 23.4). The direct immunofluorescence test requires a skin biopsy frozen immediately in liquid nitrogen, and detects immunoreactants already bound to antigenic components of the patient's skin. The indirect test is performed using patient serum or blister fluid incubated with a substrate of normal skin or other epithelia before the application of a fluorescein-tagged antiglobulin. The indirect test is used to detect circulating antibodies directed against skin antigenic components.

Woods light examination

Examination of the skin with an ultraviolet A lamp (360 nm, Wood's light) may help to accentuate pale areas, e.g. the symmetrical irregular areas of depigmentation in vitiligo (see Chapter 23.8) or the hypopigmented ash-leaf macule of tuberous sclerosis (see Chapter 24.17). It can also demonstrate green fluorescence in some fungal infections of hair (e.g. *Microsporum canis*), or pink fluorescence in teeth and urine indicating porphyrin accumulation.

Further reading

Coulson IH, Cox NH (2010). The Diagnosis of Skin Disease.
In: *Rook's Textbook of Dermatology* (eds Burns, T. *et al.*) Blackwell.

23.3

Inherited skin disease

Irene M. Leigh and David P. Kelsell

Essentials

Most patients referred from primary care to the dermatology clinic will be seeking advice and treatment for a few common skin disorders, including psoriasis, eczema, and acne. The genetic basis of these complex conditions is being unravelled. For example, susceptibility variants have been identified in the gene for filaggrin (*FLG*), and in *SPINK5*, which link with atopic eczema.

A number of genes have been identified that predispose to malignancies of the skin, including p16 (*CDKN2A*) and *CDK4* in

melanoma, and the Patched (*PTCH1*) gene involved in Gorlin's syndrome, in which mutation carriers have an elevated risk of basal cell carcinomas. There are a myriad monogenic epidermal disorders and syndromes including blistering diseases, ichthyoses, palmoplantar keratodermas, and the ectodermal dysplasias. The genetic basis of many of these disorders have been elucidated.

Structure of the epidermis

To understand inherited skin diseases it is first necessary to understand the basic biology of the epidermis and associated basement membrane zone. The basic structure of the epidermis is illustrated in Fig. 23.3.1. The epidermis is a stratified squamous epithelium consisting predominantly of keratinocytes. The remaining small percentage of intraepidermal cells includes resident melanocytes, Langerhans' cells, and migratory leucocytes. The keratinocyte undergoes a process of terminal differentiation resulting in the stratum corneum, the critical component for the barrier function of the epidermis. The highly insoluble stratum corneum consists of a cornified envelope enclosing keratin microfibres separated by a highly lipid-rich intercellular layer. This lamellated lipid is the predominant component of the barrier, and is secreted into the extracellular space from membrane-coating granules synthesized in the stratum granulosum. The epidermis is separated from the underlying dermis by a complex basement membrane zone.

The basement membrane zone

When studied ultrastructurally, the basement membrane zone of the epidermis contains four distinct layers:

♦ the basal cell membrane of the basal keratinocyte, which contains electron-dense adhesion plaques called hemidesmosomes

♦ the electron-lucent lamina lucida, which is traversed by anchoring fibrils

♦ the electron-dense lamina densa

♦ within the sublamina densa region, the lamina fibroreticularis contains distinct anchoring structures called anchoring fibrils,

which insert into the lamina densa and loop around bundles of connective tissue collagens

The hemidesmosome

Although the morphology of this organ ultrastructurally resembles that of the desmosome (see below), there are clear differences in biochemical composition. Two major hemidesmosomal proteins were initially identified by the characterization of autoantibodies arising in bullous pemphigoid, an autoimmune mechanobullous disease of late adult life. The proteins are known as bullous pemphigoid antigen 1 (dystonin (DST); 230 kDa) and bullous pemphigoid antigen 2 (COL17A1; 180 kDa). Bullous pemphigoid antigen 2 has been identified as a unique transmembrane collagen, type XVII, which has an extracellular domain containing the immunodominant epitope of bullous pemphigoid. Bullous pemphigoid antigen 1, like plectin, a further component of hemidesmosomes, is a member of the plakin family of proteins.

Plakins have been thought to contribute to plaque structures within the hemidesmosome; other members of the plakin family include desmoplakin, envoplakin, and periplakin, and are found associated with the desmosome. Plectin and bullous pemphigoid antigen appear to interact with keratin intermediate filaments as they course towards the hemidesmosome, and bind them into the hemidesmosome structure, acting as a protein clamp. This appears to provide a stable link between the intermediate filament cytoskeleton and the basement membrane zone. Basal keratinocytes also express a number of integrins, which are members of a superfamily of receptors for extracellular matrix proteins. The major hemidesmosomal integrin is $\alpha6\beta4$ integrin, although other aspects of the basal cell membrane express $\alpha6\beta1$, $\alpha5\beta1$, $\alpha3\beta1$, $\alpha\nu\delta$, and $\alpha2\beta1$ integrins.

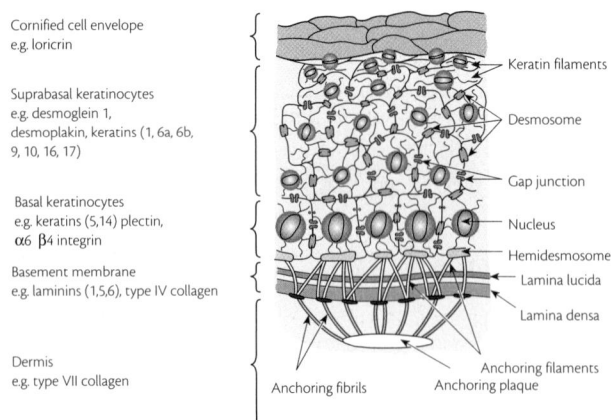

Fig. 23.3.1 A schematic representation of the epidermis indicating its organization, important structures, and site of expression of a number of skin-disease associated proteins.

The lamina lucida appears to contain a complex of laminin molecules, particularly laminins 5 and 6. It is thought that laminin 5 is the major component of the anchoring filament. The lamina densa is constructed of a meshwork of interacting type VII collagen, from which arises the anchoring fibrils of the basement membrane complex, which are made of aggregates of antiparallel dimers of type VII collagen.

Keratins

The cytoskeleton of all epithelial cells contains a number of filamentous systems, including actin, microfilaments, microtubules, and intermediate filaments. The protein that is characteristic of the intermediate filaments of all epithelial cells is the keratin family. Keratin polypeptides are segregated by two-dimensional gel electrophoresis into acidic and basic polypeptides. Fifty-four keratin genes have been identified expressed in epithelial cells and/or the hair follicle: 28 belong to the type I group and 26 to the type II group. The type II keratin gene family encodes the basic keratin polypeptides, and the type I family the acidic keratin polypeptides. Each keratin gene is expressed in a body-site and cell-type specific manner, e.g. *KRT9* is only expressed in the suprabasal layer of the palmoplantar epidermis. The keratin genes are clustered in two chromosomal regions of the human genome: the type I keratins mapping to 17q12-q21, and the type II keratins to 12q11-q13.

A keratin intermediate filament consists of both type I and type II keratin. The fundamental building block of a keratin filament is a heterodimer of a type I and type II keratin comprising four helical regions separated by nonhelical linking regions, with nonhelical head and tail domains. These heterodimers aggregate in a complex antiparallel fashion to form the intermediate filaments, which associate with both hemidesmosomes and desmosomes to provide stability to the cell and ensure its integrity. In addition to keratin mutations associated with human disease, *in vitro* and transgenic models of keratin genes harbouring mutations have shown that there are critical regions for filament assembly, particularly the helix initiation and termination motifs. The function of the head and tail domains is not entirely clear.

Desmosomes

Desmosomal proteins form a complex structure at the interface between adjacent epithelial cells. The desmosomal plaques of electron-dense material run along the cytoplasm parallel to a junctional region in which three ultrastructural bands can be seen. The plaques contain plakoglobin (which is also found in adherens junctions and is also thought to be important in cell signalling), desmoplakin, and plakophilin 1. In addition, the desmosomal cores are enriched with calcium-binding glycoproteins called desmogleins and desmocollins. These are the adhesive proteins of the desmosome, and are similar to the classical cadherins in their general structure, with five extracellular repeats that contain Ca^{2+}-binding sites, a single transmembrane region, and a cytoplasmic domain.

To date, seven human desmosomal cadherins have been identified clustered in the chromosomal region 18q11-q12. The cytoplasmic domain has binding sites for plakoglobin, plakophilin 1, and desmoplakin, linking them to the intermediate filaments. Desmoglein 1 has been identified as the dominant target antigen for the autoimmune bullous disease pemphigus foliaceus, and desmoglein 3 is the target antigen for pemphigus vulgaris.

Gap junctions

Gap junctions provide a mechanism for synchronized cellular responses to a variety of intercellular signals by regulating the diffusion of small molecules (<1 kDa) such as metabolites and ions between the cytoplasm of adjacent cells. Connexins are the major proteins of gap junctions and are encoded by a large gene family. All connexins have four transmembrane domains and two extracellular loops, with the N- and C-termini located in the cytoplasm. Connexins assemble into hexameric hemichannels (termed connexons) in the endoplasmic reticulum, and are then transported into the lipid bilayer of the plasma membrane. A connexon then docks with a connexon of an adjacent cell to form a dodecameric aqueous channel, the gap junction. These cluster together in macromolecular complexes of several hundred channels. Connexons can form either homotypic or heterotypic channels, with various channel types having distinct molecular permeabilities. Most connexins have wide tissue distribution. Those expressed in the skin include connexin 26, 31, and 43.

Disease associations with the above structural proteins have provided a molecular classification of disease to complement the classical morphological description of hereditary blistering diseases and disorders of keratinization, some of which are described below.

Epidermolysis bullosa

Genetic analysis of the heterogeneous group of mechanobullous disorders has facilitated enormous progress in understanding the function of proteins involved in the basement membrane at the dermoepidermal junction, and the role of keratins in the cytoskeleton (Table 23.3.1). The clinical phenotypes of epidermolysis bullosa correspond to different levels of skin separation within the basement membrane zone or basal keratinocyte, identified via electron microscopic examination. All cases of epidermolysis bullosa are atrophic skin disorders characterized by the blistering of mucocutaneous sites following minor trauma, and are classified according to a combination of laboratory and clinical criteria.

Epidermolysis bullosa simplex

In epidermolysis bullosa simplex, skin tissue separates at the level of the basal keratinocyte, with or without the aggregation of keratin intermediate filaments. This is the most common form of epidermolysis bullosa, and is usually inherited in an autosomal dominant fashion. Blister formation occurs in the basal keratinocytes, which

Table 23.3.1 Genetics of epidermolysis bullosa

Type of epidermolysis bullosa: site of blistering	Genetic defect (chromosome)	Associated disorder
Simplex: basal cells	Keratin 5 (12q11–q13) Keratin 14 (17q12–q21)	
Hemidesmo-somal: basal cells/ lamina lucida	Plectin (8q24) Integrin α6 (2q24–q31) Integrin β4 (17q24) Type XVII collagen (10q24)	Muscular dystrophy Pyloric atresia
Junctional: lamina lucida	Laminin α3 (18q11) Laminin β3 (1q32) Laminin γ2 (1q25–q31)	
Dystrophic: sublamina densa	Type VII collagen (3p21)	

may show aggregates of keratin filaments. Mutations in the genes encoding the basal cell-specific keratins 5 (*KRT5*; OMIM 148040) and 14 (*KRT14*; OMIM 148066) have been found to underlie epidermolysis bullosa simplex, probably leading to the cytoskeletal weakness that results in the tendency for cells to rupture on pressure. Three types of the disease are described below, and clinical pictures are shown in Fig. 23.3.2.

Epidermolysis bullosa simplex Weber–Cockayne

The soles and palms are mainly affected, but other sites may also be involved, although rarely. The blistering occurs from infancy (with walking), and is exacerbated by heat and ameliorated by cold. The blisters heal without scarring.

Epidermolysis bullosa simplex Koebner

The blisters are widespread on the scalp, trunk, arms, and legs, in addition to the palmoplantar areas. These cases may represent autosomal recessive inheritance. Nail dystrophy, oral blisters, and dental caries are common.

Epidermolysis bullosa simplex Dowling–Meara (herpetiform epidermolysis bullosa simplex)

The blistering may be very severe, and is potentially fatal in infancy. The blisters occur in groups on an erythematous bed, which heals without scarring, but hyperpigmentation and milia formation may occur. Patchy keratoderma develops in later life.

Junctional epidermolysis bullosa

In junctional epidermolysis bullosa the epidermis separates from the dermis at the lamina lucida of the basement membrane zone. Most mutations lie within genes encoding the three polypeptide subunits of laminin 5 (*LAMA3*, OMIM 600805; *LAMB3*, OMIM 15010; *LAMC2*, OMIM 150292). Clinically, the disease has been subdivided into two main categories: Herlitz (lethal) and non-Herlitz (nonlethal) forms.

Herlitz junctional epidermolysis bullosa

Blistering and erosions are present at birth, and become widespread as the skin is so fragile that it peels away on contact. The resulting lesions are slow to heal and tend to persist, becoming infected. The oropharyngeal mucosa is involved, often making feeding difficult. If the infant survives for a few months, typical crusted lesions will be seen on the nose, mouth, and jaw, and across the rest of the skin in patches. The teeth have abnormal enamel and

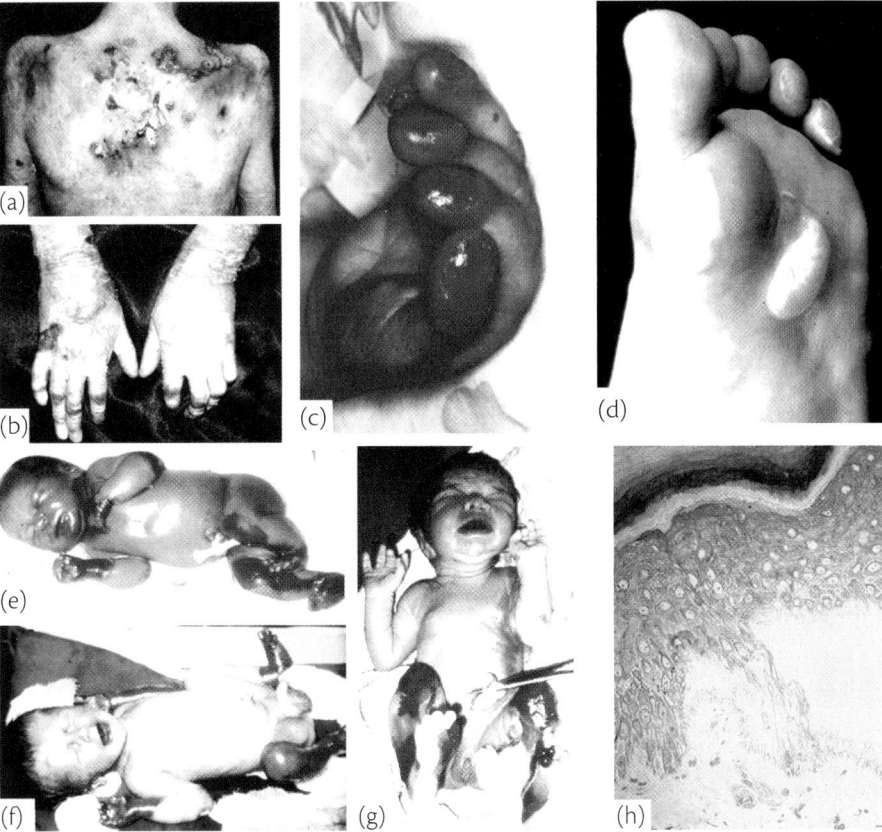

Fig. 23.3.2 Clinical photographs of the different forms of epidermolysis bullosa. (a) and (b) a patient with Hallopean–Siemans dystrophic epidermolysis bullosa; (c) the hand of an infant with Herlitz junctional epidermolysis bullosa; (d) blister on the foot of a patient with epidermolysis bullosa simplex?; (e) baby with epidermolysis bullosa simplex Dowling–Meara; (f) baby with Herlitz junctional epidermolysis bullosa; (g) baby with Hallopean–Siemans dystrophic epidermolysis bullosa; (h) intraepidermal blister from a Weber Cockayne epidermolysis bullosa simplex patient. Skin section stained with Richardson's stain.

are lost easily, as are the nails. Infants usually die from overwhelming infection.

Non-Herlitz junctional epidermolysis bullosa

Patients show generalized skin fragility and blistering, but the mucosae are less severely affected. The lesions heal leaving atrophic scars (generalized atrophic benign epidermolysis bullosa). Poor hair and tooth development is seen, and the nails are dystrophic. Large hyperpigmented patches are seen.

Dystrophic epidermolysis bullosa

In both the recessive and dominant forms of dystrophic epidermolysis bullosa, skin separation occurs below the dermoepidermal region at the level of the anchoring fibrils, and a large number of mutations have been discovered in the type VII collagen gene (COL7A1; OMIM 120120) that encodes the constituent protein of the anchoring fibrils. Scarring and dystrophy are prominent features in addition to skin fragility and blistering.

Severe generalized recessive dystrophic epidermolysis bullosa

This is the most severe form of dystrophic epidermolysis bullosa, and is very disabling in view of the deformities produced by scarring. Blisters are present at birth and recur readily at sites of trauma, especially the hands, feet, neck, shoulders, and sacrum. They heal slowly, with scarring and milia formation producing a mitten-like deformity of the hands, and clubbed feet. The severe oral lesions lead to microstomata, and the inability to protrude the tongue or open the mouth. Poor dentition leads to feeding problems. Scalp blistering and scarring gives permanent hair loss, eye involvement gives corneal erosions and opacities, and general physical development is retarded. Oesophageal and perianal strictures lead to difficulty in swallowing, and constipation. Although children often survive into adult life, multiple squamous cell carcinomas may develop in the chronically scarred skin and progress rapidly.

Dominant dystrophic epidermolysis bullosa

The skin is less fragile than in recessive dystrophic epidermolysis bullosa, and blistering is much more difficult to provoke, so that it tends to be localized to bony prominences—knees, elbows, hands, and feet. Localized scarring with milia may replace the nails. Other areas, such as the oral and anal regions, are much less affected.

Hemidesmosomal epidermolysis bullosa

Rarer forms of epidermolysis bullosa result from inherited defects in three hemidesmosomal components: plectin mutations in epidermolysis bullosa simplex with muscular dystrophy (PLEC1; OMIM 601282), type XVII collagen mutations in generalized atrophic benign epidermolysis bullosa (COL17A1; OMIM 113811), and α6β4 integrin mutations in epidermolysis bullosa with pyloric atresia (ITGB4; OMIM 147557).

Diagnosis and management of blistering in childhood

Early diagnosis is key to the management of the disease and the prognosis. The diagnosis of a baby born with blisters is often difficult on clinical grounds, so diagnosis will rest on electron microscopy of a shave skin biopsy. Immunohistochemistry is likely to be indicative in recessive cases of gene knockout, the diagnostic reagents being LH7.2 antibody to type VII collagen, and GB3 antibody to laminin 5. There is no specific treatment for any form of epidermolysis bullosa, so management centres on wound care, the

avoidance of physical trauma, and general physical and psychological support. Specialist nurses can advise on nursing babies with silk-covered dressing pads, and the use of Vaseline gauze dressings. Oral hygiene and dental care needs to be lifelong. A high-calorie and -fibre diet is essential to improve growth. Gastrostomy feeding can also help maintain body weight in children unable to eat. Finger and hand contractures require splinting at night and regular surgical release by an expert surgeon. Now that the genetic basis of epidermolysis bullosa has been identified, prenatal diagnosis by DNA-based techniques, and gene therapy by *ex vivo* techniques are actively being explored.

Hailey–Hailey disease and Darier's disease

The genetic bases of these rare autosomal dominant intraepidermal blistering diseases are mutations in the genes for calcium pumps: ATP2C1 (OMIM 604384) in Hailey–Hailey disease, and ATP2A2 (OMIM 108740) in Darier's disease. Darier's disease typically presents in the mid teenage years, with small pink and brown papules with greasy scale, and may distribute in a seborrhoeic pattern. However, the pattern and severity of the disease can be highly variable. Histology shows characteristic clefts in the epidermis, and dyskeratotic cells.

Ichthyoses

Ichthyoses manifest as dry, rough skin, with persistent scaling over most of the body, which may resemble fish scales (ichthys, Greek: fish). Congenital ichthyosis may be bullous, or associated with other abnormalities (ichthyosiform syndromes). Ichthyosis can be acquired in later life as a result of drugs such as hypocholesterolaemic agents, chronic hepatic disease, lymphoma and other malignancies, thyroid disease, chronic renal or hepatic failure, and malabsorption. When an individual's ichthyosis has improved in adult life and then worsened in late adult life it is sometimes difficult to be absolutely sure whether a patient has a congenital or an acquired ichthyosis. Progress in the understanding of the molecular and cellular biology of the ichthyoses will aid in establishing their classification and potential treatment.

Autosomal dominant ichthyosis vulgaris

This, the most common form of ichthyosis, is associated with atopic eczema in up to 50% of individuals. The condition improves in teenagers and young adults, and often worsens again with age. The clinical features present with dryness and scaling in the neonatal period, and become progressively more obvious in childhood. Scales are small, flaky, or brown, and are most pronounced on the extensor aspects of the arms and lower legs. Facial involvement is often minimal, although patients may have dandruff and increased markings on the palms and soles. Hyperlinearity of palm creases may be seen.

It is usually very well tolerated symptomatically, with only the dryness and roughness being a problem. Treatments have therefore been aimed at removing the keratotic retained stratum corneum with keratolytic agents such as salicylic acid or 1 to 5% lactic acid, other hydroxy acids, or buffered urea creams. Histopathology shows hyperkeratosis, with a diminished or absent granular cell layer, but otherwise very little abnormality at both the light and ultrastructural levels. This disease appears to be inherited in an autosomal dominant manner; however, there is variable penetrance, and difficulties in ascertainment. Loss-of-function mutations in

FLG, the gene encoding filaggrin (filament aggregating protein), underlie ichthyosis vulgaris (OMIM 135940). Filaggrin plays a role in the differentiation of the epidermis and the formation of the skin barrier.

X-linked recessive ichthyosis

This disorder is much less common than the autosomal dominant form, and predominantly affects the male children of female carriers. The scaling is usually absent for the first week of life, but progressively increases; it tends to be prominent on the arms, thighs, and lower legs, and very large adherent brown scales may involve the flexures and the face. On ultrastructural examination the granular cell layer and keratohyalin granules appear normal.

The molecular basis of this form of ichthyosis was determined from observations of low urinary oestriol secretion in the third trimester of pregnancy, and reduced steroid sulfatase activity. Subsequently, the steroid sulfatase gene was mapped to the X chromosome (*STS*; OMIM 300747), and disease-associated mutations in this gene have been identified in the vast majority of patients. Steroid sulfatase mutations lead to the abnormal breakdown of cholesterol sulfate in the stratum corneum lipids, resulting in an increase in stratum corneum thickening.

A small proportion of patients will have the additional manifestations of Kallman's syndrome, with hypogonatropic, hypogonadal, and neurological abnormalities. These result from contiguous gene defects, usually a large deletion on the short arm of the X chromosome encompassing the steroid sulfatase locus.

Bullous ichthyosiform erythroderma (epidermolytic hyperkeratosis)

This is a rare autosomal dominant ichthyosis. There is mild erythroderma at birth, and blisters and peeling may occur at sites of minor trauma. Large areas of denuded skin are often apparent after a difficult birth. In infancy, a yellow-brown hyperkeratosis develops, particularly at the sites of joint flexure, with cobble-stone keratoses present on the hands, feet, and trunk. Ridged scale may accumulate in skin creases, which are highly susceptible to bacterial and/or fungal infection, leading to a pungent body odour.

Histologically, there is lysis and clumping of the keratin filaments in the granular layer of the epidermis. Intercellular spaces are often apparent because of the rupture of suprabasal keratinocytes. Immunohistochemical studies have revealed the specific aggregation of the suprabasal keratins of the epidermis, keratins 1 and 10. Subsequently, mutations in either *KRT1* (OMIM 139350) or *KRT10* (OMIM 149080) have been shown to underlie the disease in many patients.

Ichthyosis bullosa of Siemens

This is a more rare form of bullous ichthyosis. Neonatal disease is much milder, with episodic superficial blistering occurring throughout childhood, sometimes into adulthood. The blisters occur mainly on the flexures, lower limbs, and abdomen. At these sites, a rippled grey hyperkeratosis may occur. Plate-like scaling and focal peeling (mauserung phenomenon) are usually found. There is an absence of palmoplantar keratoderma and erythroderma. Mutations in the gene encoding another suprabasal keratin, *KRT2* (OMIM 600194), have been identified as the basis of this condition. This type II keratin is expressed in many of the higher suprabasal keratinocytes.

Lamellar ichthyosis

Lamellar ichthyosis is a severe form of autosomal recessive congenital ichthyosis characterized by severe hyperkeratosis and the formation of large, often brownish-coloured plate-like scales over the whole body surface, including the face, with some flexural accentuation. The scales are present at birth, and may appear as a carapace-like sheet over the body of the newborn (collodion babies), which then sheds. Bathing-suit ichthyosis is a rare variant of lamellar ichthyosis in South African black patients, where the scale is centrally distributed on the trunk, upper limbs, scalp, and neck. Mutations in the genes encoding transglutaminase 1 (*TGM1*; OMIM 190195), a lipid transporter (*ABCA12*; OMIM 607800), ichthyin (*ICHYN*; OMIM 609383), and arachidonate lipoxygenase 3 (*ALOXE3*; OMIM 607206) and 12 (*ALOX12B*; OMIM 603741) underlie both lamellar ichthyosis and nonbullous ichthyosiform erythroderma (see below).

Nonbullous ichthyosiform erythroderma

Although these patients have a severe generalized autosomal recessive ichthyosis, and present as collodion babies, this condition differs from lamellar ichthyosis by the presence of generalized erythroderma, which contributes to the characteristic facies and ectropion. This also produces problems with temperature and fluid control. The scaling is often finer and more brawny than in lamellar ichthyosis, and inflammation and parakeratosis are additionally found on histopathology.

Netherton's syndrome

Netherton's syndrome is a severe autosomal recessive disorder often resulting in infant mortality, and is characterized by ichthyosis with erythroderma and trichorrhexis invaginata (hair-shaft abnormalities often termed bamboo hair). Scanning electron microscopy of patients' hair often also reveals torsion nodules, pili torti, and trichorrhexis nodosa. Light microscopy can show invagination of the hair cuticle into the cortex. Mutations in the gene *SPINK5* encoding LEKTI, a serine protease inhibitor, underlie Netherton's syndrome.

Sjögren–Larsson syndrome

Sjögren–Larsson syndrome is inherited as an autosomal recessive trait, and is particularly prevalent in northwestern Sweden (1 in 10 000), occurring less frequently elsewhere. The syndrome characteristically includes ichthyosis, spastic diplegia, and mild-to-moderate developmental delay. The skin disease presents as mild erythroderma at birth, with scaling developing in the first few months, which persists particularly on the face and limbs. In the flexures, neck, and periumbilical folds, an orange/brown lichenification overlaid with hyperkeratosis is a characteristic feature. In early life, neurological defects including upper motor neurone defects of the limbs, learning difficulties, and often ocular abnormalities (spots on the retina) are observed. Histologically, the affected skin displays orthohyperkeratosis, acanthosis, and papillomatosis. The genetic defect has been shown to be in the fatty aldehyde dehydrogenase gene (*FALDH*; OMIM 609523), which affects essential fatty acid metabolism.

Ichthyosis prematurity syndrome

This recessive ichthyosis has a higher prevalence in Norway and Sweden (OMIM 608649). It manifests with complications at midtrimester leading to premature birth. The babies are born with thick desquamating skin and atopic features. Mutations in the *FATP4* gene underlie this condition and is associated with defective very long chain fatty acid metabolism.

Harlequin ichthyosis

Harlequin ichthyosis is the most severe and often lethal form of recessive congenital ichthyosis. Infants born with this condition have hard, thick skin covering most of their bodies. The skin forms large diamond-shaped plates separated by deep fissures that restrict movement. These skin abnormalities also affect the shape of the eyelids, nose, lips, and ears. The impaired barrier function of the skin leads the neonates to struggle to control water loss and temperature, and they are more susceptible to infection. In addition, the tightened skin can cause breathing difficulties leading to respiratory failure. Mutations in the *ABCA12* gene encoding an ATP-binding cassette (ABC) transporter (OMIM 607800) are found in almost all harlequin ichthyosis cases.

Keratodermas

The inherited keratodermas are characterized by the presence of thickened skin on the palms and soles. Palmoplantar skin is specialized for high levels of weight bearing and friction, so the stratum corneum is much thicker (hyperkeratotic) than the rest of the epidermis. The keratodermas can be classified clinically according to the pattern of thickening on the palm and sole skin. Three distinct clinical patterns have been observed:

- diffuse—the hyperkeratotic thickening is evenly and symmetrically distributed over the palm and sole, usually manifesting at birth
- focal—hyperkeratotic plaques develop particularly at sites of weight bearing and friction; these are usually plaque-like callosites or linear thickening (striate keratoderma)
- punctate—multiple bead-like keratoses that pepper the palmoplantar skin

The keratodermas can have autosomal recessive or dominant inheritance, and may occur in syndromes. They can be further subgrouped into:

- simple—palmoplantar involvement only
- complex—associated with lesions of nonvolar skin, hair, teeth, nails, and sweat glands (including ectodermal dysplasias)
- syndromic—associated with abnormalities in other organs, including deafness, cancer, cardiomyopathy, and adrenal insufficiency.

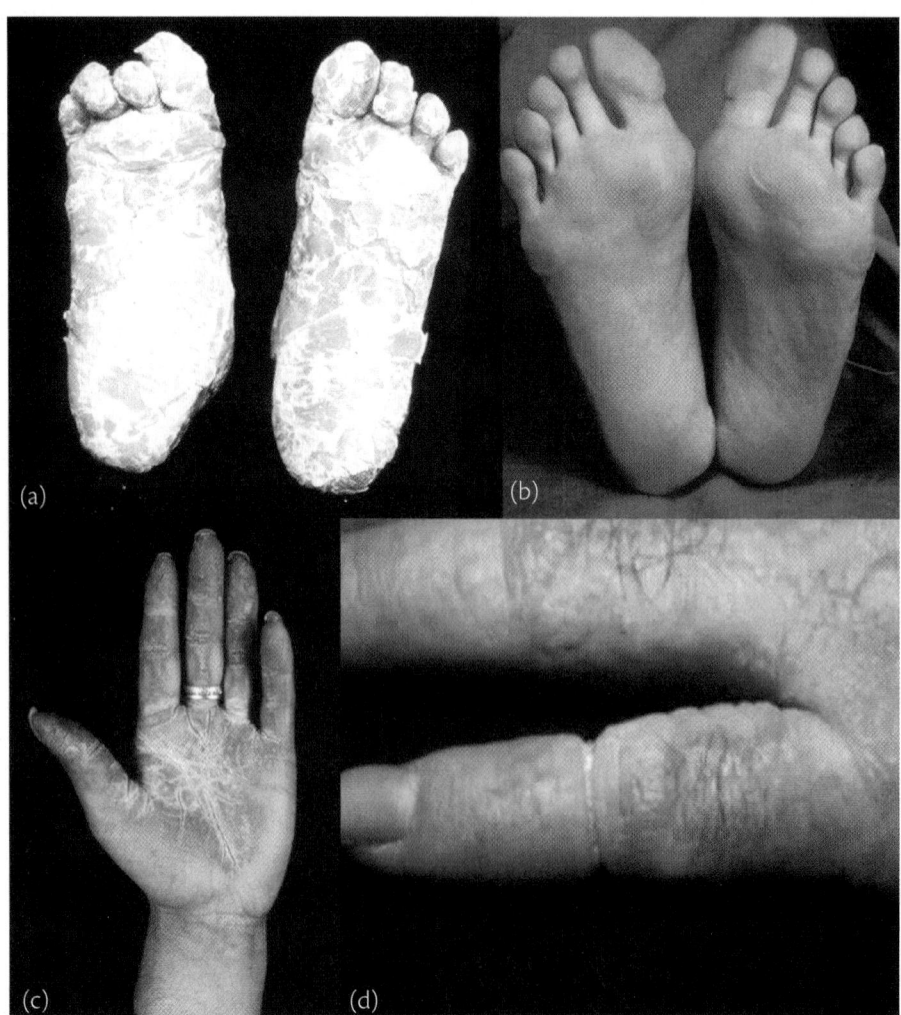

Fig. 23.3.3 Clinical photographs of: (a) bullous ichthyosiform erythroderma (BIE) and three types of keratoderma: (b) focal palmoplantar keratoderma (PPK) associated with a keratin 16 mutation; (c) striate palmoplantar keratoderma associated with a desmoglein 1 mutation; and (d) constriction around the digit from an individual with Vohwinkel's syndrome associated with a Cx26 mutation.

Table 23.3.2 Genetics of diffuse palmoplantar keratoderma (PPK)

Type of diffuse PPK	Associated disorder	Genetic defect (map location)
EPPK (epider-molytic PPK)		Keratin 9 (17q12–q21)
NEPPK (non-epidermolytic PPK)	Umbilical hyperkeratosis	Keratin 1 (12q11–q13)
NEPPK		Not known (12q11–q13)
Syndromic NEPPK (Naxos disease)	Woolly hair and cardiomyopathy	Plakoglobin (17q12–q13)
		Desmoplakin (6p23–p24)
Vohwinkel's syndrome	Sensorineural deafness	Connexin 26 (13q12)
	Ichthyosis	Loricrin (1q21)
Erythrokerato-derma variables	Generalized erythroderma	Connexin 31 (1p34–p36)
Clouston's syndrome	Alopecia, nail dystrophy, sensorineural deafness	Connexin 30 and connexin 30.3 (13q11–q12)
Hypohidrotic ectodermal dysplasia	Erythroderma, impaired sweating, hair and nail abnormalities	Plakophilin (1q32–q34)
Mal de Meleda	Hyperhidrosis and perioral erythema	SLURP-1 (8q24)

They can also be classified biologically by their underlying genetic defects (see Fig. 23.3.3 and Tables 23.3.2 and 23.3.3). This branch of the genodermatoses is genetically heterogeneous, with mutations in genes encoding keratins, desmosomal proteins, connexins, and a protease.

Diffuse palmoplantar keratodermas (PPK)

Simple—diffuse epidermolytic palmoplantar keratoderma

This condition is characterized by epidermolytic hyperkeratosis with keratin filament clumping in suprabasal keratins. This autosomal dominant disease presents with symmetrical thickening

Table 23.3.3 Genetics of focal palmoplantar keratoderma (PPK)

Type of focal PPK	Associated disorder	Genetic defect (map location)
Focal NEPPK	Follicular and orogenital hyperkeratosis	Keratin 16 (17q12–q21)
Focal NEPPK (tylosis)	Oesophageal cancer, oral and follicular hyperkeratosis	Not known (17q24q25)
Pachyonychia congenita type 1	Nail dystrophy and oral lesions	Keratin 6a (12q11–q13) Keratin 16 (17q12–q21)
Pachyonychia congenita type 2	Epidermal cysts, nail dystrophy, and oral lesions	Keratin 6b (12q11–q13) Keratin 17 (17q12–q21)
Striate PPK		Desmoglein 1 (18q12) Desmoplakin (6p21) Keratin 1 (12q11–q13)
Papillon–Lefevre		Cathepsin C (11q14)
Oculocutaneous tyrosinaemia	Photophobia, corneal ulceration, and mental retardation	Tyrosine aminotransferase (16q22)

giving a cracked, crocodile skin-like surface resulting from the underlying epidermolysis, which starts in early infancy. Most epidermolytic PPK pedigrees are linked to the type I keratin cluster on chromosome 17q12-q21, and disease is because of mutations in the palmoplantar-specfic keratin 9 (*KRT9*; OMIM 607606), the majority clustering in the helix initiation domain of the protein. However, epidermolytic PPK can also be associated with mutations in the type II keratin 1 (*KRT1*; OMIM 139350).

Simple—diffuse nonepidermolytic palmoplantar keratoderma (NEPPK)

Nonepidermolytic PPK is also inherited as an autosomal dominant trait, and is often difficult to distinguish from epidermolytic PPK because of the inconsistent finding of epidermolysis by electron microscopy in epidermolytic PPK. There is a uniform waxy yellow thickening over the palms and soles, which may spread onto the dorsum of the hands and wrists, with a sharp cut-off. It is commonly aggravated by secondary fungal infection, which may require intermittent oral antifungal agents. These often improve the keratoderma. A number of families have disease linked to 12q11-q13. A single family has a mutation in the variable head domain of keratin 1; however, in most nonepidermolyic PPK families, fine mapping of the 12q11-q13 locus has excluded abnormalities of the type II keratin genes.

Complex—erythrokeratoderma variabilis

Erythrokeratoderma variabilis is a rare autosomal dominant skin disease characterized by diffuse PPK and transient figurate red patches at various sites of varying severity. Germline mutations in connexin 31 (*GJB3*; OMIM 603324) have been identified in the affected members of some erythrokeratoderma variabilis families.

Focal keratoderma

Most focal PPKs are characterized by the presence of discoid lesions, and the majority can be regarded as complex PPKs as they are often associated with abnormalities of hair, nails, teeth, and glands.

Simple—striate PPK

This focal PPK is characterized by the presence of distinctive linear streaks on the palms and soles, and over the ventral aspects of the fingers extending onto the palms. The lesions are often more extreme on the feet. Variable nail and hair involvement with fragility or splitting is seen. Mutations in the genes for two desmosomal proteins: desmoglein 1 (*DSG1*; OMIM 125670; 18q11-12) or desmoplakin 1(*DSP*; OMIM 125647; 6p21) have been described, which result in a hemizygous gene knockout leading to haploinsufficiency of the gene product. Keratin 1 mutations have also been reported.

Complex—pachyonychia congenita type 1/focal PPK with oral mucosal hyperkeratosis

This clinical overlap syndrome presents in childhood with nail changes (pachyonychia). Typically, a subungual hyperkeratosis produces a trumpet-shaped nail, especially on the thumb, first finger, and toes. The sole lesions consist of painful callosities over weight-bearing areas; less prominent callosities occur on the palms. The gingival mucosa shows milky hyperkeratosis. Nutmeg-grater-like follicular keratoses also occur. Variable fragility and blistering can be associated with severe pain on walking. Milder nail involvement may present as splinter haemorrhages. The pathological finding of epidermolytic hyperkeratosis with keratin filament clumping suggests that keratin gene mutations underlie this disorder; this was confirmed by the identification of mutations in genes encoding keratin 6A (KRT6A; OMIM 148041) and keratin 16 (KRT16; OMIM 148067) in affected individuals from multiple families.

Complex—pachyonychia congenita type 2/steatocystoma multiplex

The palmoplantar keratoderma may be very limited, although pachyonychia nail changes present early. Multiple epidermal cysts and steatocysts are seen. Woolly scalp hair, fuzzy eyebrows, and natal teeth are also common features. The finding of keratin clumps in skin bearing keratin 17, particularly the hair follicle deep outer root sheath, suggested KRT17 (OMIM 148069) as the candidate gene, and autosomal dominant mutations have been extensively described. Mutations in KRT6B (OMIM 148042) have also been identified. The resulting pathology varies from keratin cysts, vellus hair cysts, and oil-filled cysts.

Complex—Papillon–Lefevre syndrome

This focal PPK is inherited in an autosomal recessive manner, and is marked by associated severe periodontitis and secondary ulceration, with opalescent oral mucosae. The inflammatory lesions often result in pocket formation seen pathologically. Mutations in cathepsin C, a lysosomal protease, have been shown to underlie this disorder. It is postulated that cathepsin C may be important in the processing of key structural proteins, such as keratins, in the epidermis.

Simple—punctate PPK

The palms and soles are covered by uniform bead-like hyperkeratosis with secondary broader areas of hyperkeratosis in weight-bearing areas. They may appear clinically similar to acquired punctate keratoses, but are more uniform, appear earlier in life, and have a positive family history. Rarer porokeratotic forms exist.

Syndromic keratodermas (multiple phenotypic)

PPK and deafness

A number of families with PPK and sensorineural deafness have been described. This may be due to a mutation in a single gene expressed in all affected tissues, or cosegregation of two distinct gene mutations. One such disorder is Vohwinkel's syndrome; a mutating PPK with constrictions developing around the fingers, leading to autoamputation. Autosomal dominant mutations in the genes encoding the gap junction protein connexin 26 (GJB2; OMIM 121011) have been described in families with Vohwinkel's syndrome, and other forms of PPK and sensorineural deafness. There is a genotype–phenotype correlation between the site of the GJB2 mutation and the severity of the keratoderma and extent of the hearing impairment. Mutations in the gene for loricrin (LOR; OMIM 152445), a cornified cell-envelope component of the stratum corneum, have also been identified in individuals affected with a variant form of Vohwinkel's syndrome that is associated with ichthyosis. In addition, PPK and deafness have also been associated with mutations in mitochondrial DNA.

PPK and cancer

Focal nonepidermolytic PPK and oesophageal cancer

Three pedigrees from the United Kingdom, the United States of America, and Germany have been studied in which a focal nonepidermolytic PPK with oral hyperkeratosis segregates with a high lifetime risk of squamous cell carcinoma of the oesophagus (40–91% by age 70 years). In all three families, the disease gene has been localized to a very small region within the chromosomal interval 17q24-q25. However, identification of the specific gene mutation remains elusive.

Huriez disease (sclerotylosis)

This is an autosomal dominant disease characterized by PPK, nail changes, and scleroatrophy of the distal extremities. Around 15% of individuals develop aggressive squamous cell carcinomas in their thirties and forties. It is proposed that the scarring resulting from skin fragility predisposes to the carcinomas. The Huriez disease gene has been mapped to chromosome 4q23.

PPK, woolly hair, and cardiomyopathy

Diffuse nonepidermolytic PPK with arrhythmogenic ventricular cardiomyopathy (which leads to heart failure and arrhythmias) can result from recessive mutations in the gene for either desmoplakin (DSP; OMIM 125647) or plakoglobin (JUP; OMIM 173325), two major proteins of the desmosome. Dominant desmoplakin mutations have also recently been identified, and have alerted dermatologists to the possible cardiac problems that may occur in patients with PPK and woolly hair.

Triple A syndrome

In triple A or Allgrove's syndrome, individuals have ACTH-resistant adrenal insufficiency, achalasia, and alacrima with PPK. This disease has been mapped to 12q13, and mutations in a novel gene, AAAS (OMIM 605378), have been identified. The predicted protein is a WD repeat-containing protein that may play a role in signalling, and RNA processing and transcription.

Ectodermal dysplasias

There are a very large number of ectodermal dysplasias, in which abnormalities of the skin, hair, teeth, nails, and/or sweating are seen. The clinical classification is unsatisfactory, but may become more transparent when the genetic basis of a significant number of these complexes has been classified. Two major subgroups include hidrotic and nonhidrotic ectodermal dysplasia. The concept of dysplasia in these diseases is developmental rather than premalignant.

Hidrotic ectodermal dysplasia (Clouston's syndrome)

Hidrotic ectodermal dysplasia is characterized by nail dystrophy with thick, slow-growing, discoloured, short nails. Diffuse PPK is variable, but may be severe and spread to knuckles and finger joints. Scalp hair is sparse, fine, pale, and brittle, with thin eyebrows and sparse body hair. The disease is inherited as an autosomal dominant. Mutations in connexin 30 encoded by GJB6 (OMIM 604418) underlie this condition.

Keratosis, ichthyosis, deafness syndrome

In this condition, a severe extensive and progressive erythrokeratoderma is associated with sensorineural hearing loss and vascularizing keratitis. Fatal cases have been reported. Missense germline mutations in the genes encoding connexin 26 (GJB2; OMIM 121011) and 30 (GJB6; OMIM 604418) have been found.

Ectodermal dysplasia/skin fragility syndrome

This very rare inherited disorder presents with erythema at birth and skin blistering resulting from fragility, and is associated with nail dystrophy, plantar keratoderma, and hair loss. It was initially confused with epidermolysis bullosa. It was found to be histologically associated with increased intercellular spaces and desmosomal abnormalities, which led to the discovery of plakophilin 1 mutations (*PKP1*; OMIM 601975) in sporadic cases.

Hypohidrotic ectodermal dysplasia

This X-linked recessively inherited disease is characterized by a loss of sweat glands, causing absent or reduced sweating (hypohidrosis), and total or partial loss of teeth. Patients may be very uncomfortable on exertion and are heat intolerant. The teeth are characteristically conical and the mouth dry. In severe forms the facial appearance is altered, with saddle nose, sunken cheeks, and sparse, dry, fine, short hair with absent eyebrows. The disease maps to Xq12-13.1 and is caused by mutations in the gene for ectodysplasin anhidrotic protein (*EDA*; OMIM 300451). An autosomal recessive form results from mutations in the ectodysplasin receptor (*EDAR*; OMIM 604095).

Recent advances and possible future developments

This chapter has focused on the rarer types of genetic skin diseases rather than the more common, genetically complex disorders such as eczema, psoriasis, and acne. This is largely because it is only recently that genetic studies have been performed on these latter diseases, leading to the identification of a few potential disease-associated genetic variants. By contrast, great advances have been made in understanding the molecular basis of the rarer blistering diseases, ichthyoses, and the keratodermas, with the identification of a number of important proteins involved in epidermal and also nonepidermal biology. In addition, these studies have revealed genetic heterogeneity, with mutations in different proteins causing similar clinical manifestations, e.g. Vohwinkel's syndrome can result from mutations in either connexin 26 or loricrin. With the technological ability to sequence entire human genomes and the capability for high-throughput genotyping, it is likely that the genetic basis of the more common epidermal disorders will be elucidated in the near future.

Further reading

Akiyama M, *et al.* (2005). Mutations in lipid transporter *ABCA12* in harlequin ichthyosis and functional recovery by corrective gene transfer. *J Clin Invest*, **115**, 1777–84.

Akiyama M (2006). Harlequin ichthyosis and other autosomal recessive congenital ichthyoses: the underlying genetic defects and pathomechanisms. *J Dermatol Sci*, **42**, 83–9.

De Laurenzi V, *et al.* (1996). Sjogren–Larsson syndrome is caused by mutations in the fatty aldehyde dehydrogenase gene. *Nat Genet*, **12**, 52–7.

Hu Z, *et al.* (2000). Mutations in ATP2C1, encoding a calcium pump, cause Hailey–Hailey disease. *Nat Genet*, **24**, 61–5.

Irvine AD (2005). Inherited defects in keratins. *Clin Dermatol*, **23**, 6–14.

Kelsell DP, *et al.* (2005). Mutations in ABCA12 underlie the severe congenital skin disease harlequin ichthyosis. *Am J Hum Genet*, **76**, 794–803.

Kere J, *et al.* (1996). X-linked anhidrotic (hypohidrotic) ectodermal dysplasia is caused by mutation in a novel transmembrane protein. *Nat Genet*, **13**, 409–16.

Kottke MD, Delva E, Kowalczyk AP (2006). The desmosome: cell science lessons from human diseases. *J Cell Sci*, **119**, 797–806.

Laird DW (2006). Life cycle of connexins in health and disease. *Biochem J*, **394**, 527–43.

Lefevre C, *et al.* (2003). Mutations in the transporter ABCA12 are associated with lamellar ichthyosis type 2. *Hum Mol Genet*, **12**, 2369–78.

Lefevre C, *et al.* (2004). Mutations in ichthyin a new gene on chromosome 5q33 in a new form of autosomal recessive congenital ichthyosis. *Hum Mol Genet*, **13**, 2473–82.

McGrath JA (2005). Inherited disorders of desmosomes. *Australas J Dermatol*, **46**, 221–9.

McGrath JA, Mellerio JE (2006). Epidermolysis bullosa. *Br J Hosp Med (Lond)*, **67**, 188–91.

Mikkola ML (2007). p63 in skin appendage development. *Cell Cycle*, **6**, 285–90.

Oji V, *et al.* (2006). Bathing suit ichthyosis is caused by transglutaminase-1 deficiency: evidence for a temperature-sensitive phenotype. *Hum Mol Genet*, **15**, 3083–97.

Oji V, Traupe H (2006). Ichthyoses: differential diagnosis and molecular genetics. *Eur J Dermatol*, **16**, 349–59.

Rugg EL, Leigh IM (2004). The keratins and their disorders. *Am J Med Genet C Semin Med Genet*, **131C**, 4–11.

Sakuntabhai A, *et al.* (1999). Mutations in *ATP2A2*, encoding a Ca²⁺ pump, cause Darier disease. *Nat Genet*, **21**, 271–7. Comment in: Nat Genet, **21**, 252–3.

Segre JA (2006). Epidermal differentiation complex yields a secret: mutations in the cornification protein filaggrin underlie ichthyosis vulgaris. *J Invest Dermatol*, **126**, 1202–4.

Smith FJ, *et al.* (2006). Loss-of-function mutations in the gene encoding filaggrin cause ichthyosis vulgaris. *Nat Genet*, **38**, 337–42.

Toomes C, *et al.* (1999). Loss-of-function mutations in the cathepsin C gene result in periodontal disease and palmoplantar keratosis. *Nat Genet*, **23**, 421–4.

Uitto J, Richard G (2004). Progress in epidermolysis bullosa: genetic classification and clinical implications. *Am J Med Genet C Semin Med Genet*, **131C**, 61–74.

23.4

Vesiculobullous disease

Fenella Wojnarowska

Essentials

The autoimmune blistering diseases have a dramatic clinical presentation, and are significant diseases with substantial morbidity and mortality.

The diseases can be split broadly pathologically into intraepidermal (pemphigus) and subepidermal (pemphigoid, dermatitis herpetiformis and others) groups, the former being characterized by pathogenic autoantibodies to desmosome components, and the latter by pathogenic antibodies to proteins of the basement membrane zone adhesion complex that link the epithelium/epidermis to the underlying mesenchyme/dermis (or genetic mutations of the same proteins). There are concomitant differences in clinical presentation, e.g. blistering lesions present in the subepidermal bullous diseases tend to be less easily ruptured than those observed in intraepidermal bullous diseases.

Treatment is often difficult, e.g. pemphigus vulgaris requires potent topical steroids and often systemic corticosteroids (e.g. prednisolone 45–60 mg/day), bullous pemphigoid requires topical steroids and often anti-inflammatory antibiotics or systemic corticosteroids, with both needing immunosuppressive or immunomodulatory treatments in difficult cases.

Introduction

The autoimmune vesiculobullous diseases are frequently caused by autoantibodies directed against the structural components of the skin (Tables 23.4.1 and 23.4.2, Figs. 23.4.1 and 23.4.2). The intraepidermal diseases are characterized by autoantibodies to desmosome components, the subepidermal blistering diseases by antibodies to proteins of the basement membrane zone adhesion complex that link the epithelium/epidermis to the underlying mesenchyme/dermis. Genetic counterparts for these diseases exist in which the same structural protein is mutated, also resulting in blistering (see Chapter 23.3). There is evidence for most of the autoimmune blistering diseases that the antibodies are pathogenic.

Historical perspective

Blisters are referred to in early Greek and Arabic medical texts because of their striking clinical appearance. Differentiation of the diseases was difficult until the 1960s, when immunofluorescence enabled the detection of circulating and bound skin antibodies. This lead to the identification of their target antigens (Table 23.4.1), driven by interested clinician scientists who made the clinicopathological correlations that have illuminated the molecular biology of blistering diseases.

The individual diseases (Tables 23.4.1, 23.4.2, and 23.4.3) are described in detail below.

Intraepidermal diseases: the pemphigus group

The intraepidermal diseases: pemphigus vulgaris, pemphigus foliaceus, and paraneoplastic pemphigus are characterized by autoantibodies to desmosome components, resulting in separation of the cells within the epithelium, so the blister roofs are thin and easily ruptured, forming erosions.

Pemphigus vulgaris

Aetiology, genetics, pathogenesis, and pathology

Pemphigus vulgaris is mediated by autoantibodies to desmoglein 3, the major adhesion molecule in the mucosa, neonatal epidermis, and basal layers of the epidermis (Fig. 23.4.1). These antibodies result in mucosal blistering, particularly prominent in the mouth, and in the skin of the neonate as a result of transplacental transmission of maternal antibodies. In addition, most patients also develop antibodies to desmoglein 1, which is the major adhesion molecule in the upper layers of the epidermis. The antibodies to desmoglein 1 and 3 result in the loss of cohesion in the epidermis, and splitting of the epidermis at the basal layer. Their pathogenicity has been demonstrated by transplacental transmission and animal models. Pemphigus vulgaris is associated with HLA class II antigens and with polymorphisms of desmoglein 3 in several racial groups.

Table 23.4.1 Major vesiculobullous dermatoses

Dermatosis	Frequency	Target structure	Target antigen
Intraepidermal			
Pemphigus vulgaris	Uncommon in western Europe	Desmosome	Desmoglein 1 and 3
Pemphigus foliaceus	Uncommon in western Europe	Desmosome	Desmoglein 1
Paraneoplastic pemphigus	Very rare	Desmosome	Plakins
Subepidermal			
Bullous pemphigoid	Most common in Western Europe	Hemidesmosome	BP230 (BPAg1); BP180 (BPAg2)
Mucous membrane pemphigoid	Uncommon	Hemidesmosome anchoring filament	$\alpha6\beta4$ integrins; BP180; laminin 5
Pemphigoid gestationis	1:50 000 pregnancies	Hemidesmosome	BP180
Linear IgA disease	Uncommon	Hemidesmosome	BP180 and its shed ectodomain
Epidermolysis bullosa acquisita	Rare	Anchoring fibril	Collagen VII
Dermatitis herpetiformis	Uncommon	Microfibrils	Unknown

The disease occurs worldwide, but is most common in the Middle East (Arabs, Iranians, Jews), Southeast Asia, and China. This susceptibility persists when these populations move to the West. It is rarer in northwestern Europe than in southern and eastern Europe.

Clinical features

The disease usually presents with mouth ulceration. The palate, gums, tongue, and buccal mucosa manifest painful erosions (Fig. 23.4.3). Eating is a problem and patients lose weight. The genitals may have similar erosions. The skin lesions are particularly common on the face, scalp, and upper torso, and are coin-sized thin-walled blisters that rapidly rupture to form erosions with a red base (Fig. 23.4.4), although in the healing phase they may become more scaly and heaped. In severe uncontrolled disease the patients lose fluid and may die from uncontrolled sepsis.

The diagnosis is made by the histological examination of an early blister or erosion, showing splitting of the epidermis above the basal layer with individual rounded cells (acantholysis). The gold standard is direct immunofluorescence testing (see Chapter 23.2) of perilesional skin or mucosa, and indirect immunofluorescence testing of serum on normal human skin or monkey oesophagus, demonstrating binding to the surface of the epidermal cells (Fig. 23.4.5), and in some centres, enzyme-linked immunosorbent assays (ELISA).

Treatment

Treatment is according to British Association of Dermatologists guidelines (see 'Further reading'). Initial treatment is with potent topical steroids, and if necessary systemic steroids, e.g. prednisolone 45 to 60 mg per day. Adjuvant treatment with azathioprine, mycophenolate mofetil, cyclophosphamide, and tetracyclines is used, and in recalcitrant cases rituximab and intravenous immunoglobulins (IVIG). Remission occurs in 75% of patients, but may take 10 years or more.

Pemphigus foliaceus

Aetiology, genetics, pathogenesis, and pathology

Pemphigus foliaceus is mediated by autoantibodies to desmoglein 1, which is the major adhesion molecule in the upper layers of the epidermis (Fig. 23.4.1), but not in mucous membranes. The antibodies to desmoglein 1 result in loss of cohesion in the epidermis, and superficial splitting. Their pathogenicity has been demonstrated in animal models. In staphylococcal scalded skin syndrome (Chapters 7.6.4 and 23.10), a bacterial protease digests desmoglein 1, explaining the clinical similarity. Pemphigus foliaceus associations with HLA class II antigens have been found.

Table 23.4.2 Clinical features of vesiculobullous dermatoses

Dermatosis	Clinical features	Immunofluorescence	First-line therapy
Intraepidermal			
Pemphigus vulgaris	Oral and other mucosal erosions; superficial blisters and erosions	Intercellular IgG in epithelium and oral mucosa	Steroids
Pemphigus foliaceus	Superficial erosions	Intercellular IgG in epithelium	Steroids
Paraneoplastic pemphigus	Severe mucosal lesions; blistering of skin	Intercellular and basement membrane zone IgG in epithelium and rat bladder	Unresponsive
Subepidermal			
Bullous pemphigoid	Tense blisters	Basement membrane zone IgG	Steroids
Mucous membrane pemphigoid	Mucosal blisters and erosions	Basement membrane zone IgG and IgA	Steroids; dapsone; cyclophosphamide
Pemphigoid gestationis	Tense blisters	Basement membrane zone IgG	Steroids
Linear IgA disease	Tense blisters; some mucosal lesions	Basement membrane zone IgA	Dapsone
Epidermolysis bullosa acquisita	Tense blisters; scarring	Basement membrane zone IgG	Steroids
Dermatitis herpetiformis	Uncommon	IgA granules in dermal papillae	Dapsone; gluten-free diet

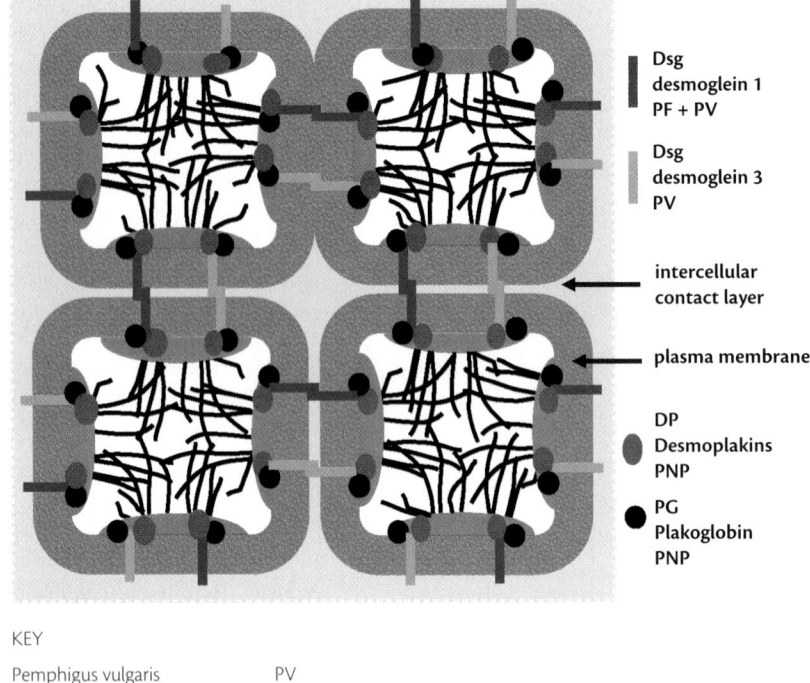

Fig. 23.4.1 The desmosome and its target antigens.

KEY

Pemphigus vulgaris	PV
Pemphigus foliaceus	PF
Paraneoplastic pemphigus	PNP

The disease is common in North Africa, the Middle East, Southeast Asia, and China. There is an endemic form in Brazil, which has a characteristic distribution along rivers in rural areas, altering with development. Many members of a household may be affected, suggesting that a bloodsucking insect is the vector for the disease (Chapter 7.12). In North Africa there is an unexplained female predominance. Drug triggers include penicillamine and other drugs with sulfhydryl groups.

Clinical features

This disease only affects the skin; the mucosae are spared. The face and upper trunk are commonly affected (Chapter 7.12, Fig. 1). The superficial layers of the skin split, giving coin-sized red scaly lesions. The diagnosis is made by histology showing superficial splitting of the epidermis. Direct and indirect immun-ofluorescence show binding to the surface of the epidermal cells (Fig. 23.4.5), and ELISA can also demonstrate antibodies to desmoglein 1.

Treatment

Initial treatment is with very potent topical steroids, and in all but the mildest cases systemic steroids (prednisolone 20–60 mg). In severe cases immunosuppressants may be required. The disease runs a prolonged course, but most patients eventually remit. It is likely that the presence of endemic foci will lead to the identification of an environmental trigger for this autoimmune disease.

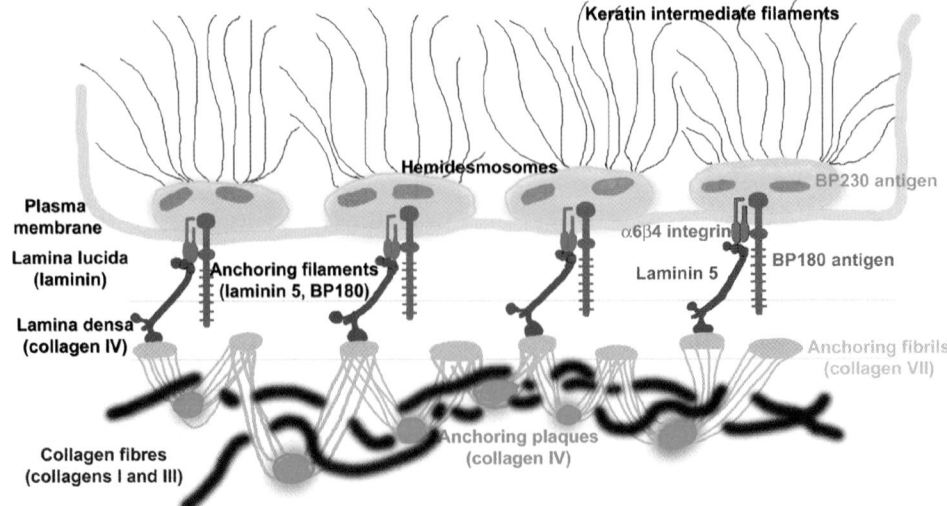

Fig. 23.4.2 The basement membrane zone of the skin and mucosa.

Table 23.4.3 Differential diagnosis of vesiculobullous dermatoses

Diagnosis	Frequency	Typical patient/circumstances
Intraepidermal		
Impetigo	Common	Children >adults
Staphylococcal scalded skin syndrome	Rare	Child <10 years
Toxic epidermal necrolysis	Rare	Usually drug induced
Subepidermal		
Viral infections		
Herpes simplex	Common	Children >adults
Varicella–zoster virus	Common	Chickenpox: children >adults Shingles: adults >children
Trauma	Common	
Burns	Common	
Insect bites	Common	
Eczema	Common	
Erythema multiforme	Common	Infections, e.g. herpes simplex Drugs
Oedema blisters	Common	Oedematous legs
Drugs		
Fixed drug eruption	Rare	e.g. paracetamol
Bullous reactions	Rare	e.g. furosemide, clindamycin
Pseudoporphyria cutanea tarda	Very rare	Drugs
Porphyria cutanea tarda	Rare	Liver damage, e.g. alcohol

Paraneoplastic pemphigus

This rare condition was not recognized until the 1980s, previous cases having been misdiagnosed as severe drug reactions or pemphigus.

Aetiology, genetics, pathogenesis, and pathology

The condition occurs in the setting of myeloproliferative disorders, in some cases linked to treatment with fludarabine, other malignancies, or Castleman's syndrome. There are autoantibodies to

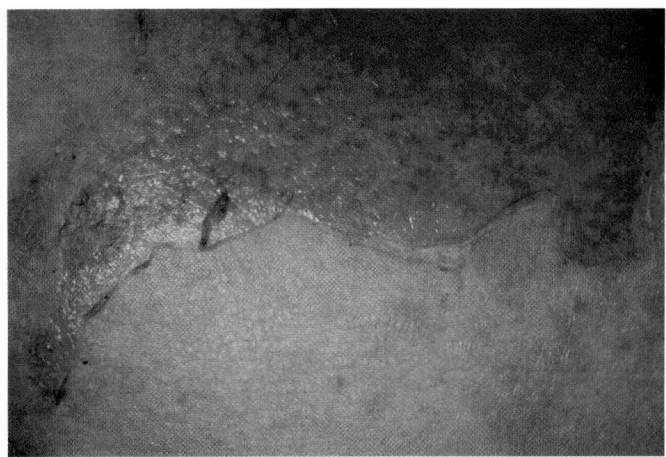

Fig. 23.4.4 Characteristic skin erosions in pemphigus vulgaris.

plakins, which are components of the desmosomes (Fig. 23.4.1), in the skin, transitional epithelium, and other epithelia.

Clinical features

The patients present with severe mucosal disease with erosions and ulceration of the oropharynx, and often also the eyes and genitalia. Skin involvement with tense blisters on the palms and soles, and around the nails, is characteristic. There may be generalized involvement, with denuding of large areas, or occasionally a lichenoid type of eruption. There may be involvement of multiple organs, and respiratory disease may be a late cause of death. Often the patient is known to have lymphoproliferative disease or other malignancy.

Histology shows splitting low in the epidermis. Immunofluorescence shows antibodies binding to epidermal cells and the basement membrane zone of skin and the transitional epithelium of rat bladder. The patient will require investigation for underlying lymphoma, other malignancy, or Castleman's disease.

Treatment

Treatment is directed at the underlying condition, combined with immunosuppression to reduce the skin and mucosal disease. The prognosis is poor, and most patients die.

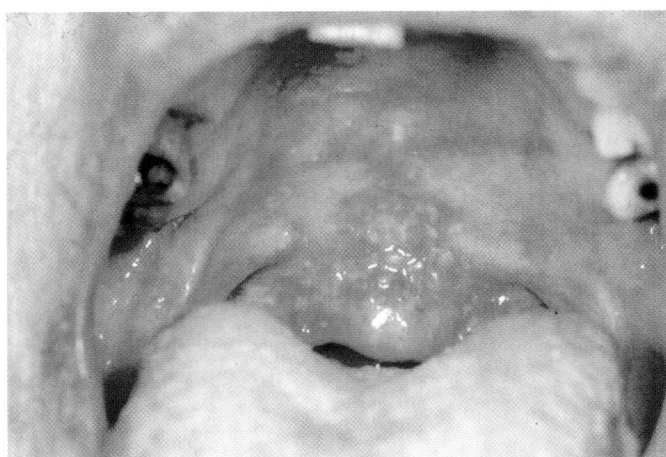

Fig. 23.4.3 Erosions on the palate in pemphigus vulgaris.

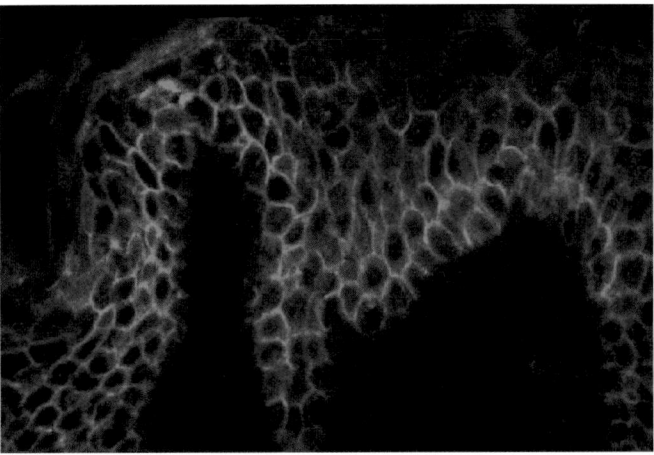

Fig. 23.4.5 Immunofluorescence demonstrating antibody binding in the epidermis in pemphigus.

Subepidermal diseases: the pemphigoid group and others

The subepidermal blistering diseases are the pemphigoid group: bullous pemphigoid, pemphigoid gestationis (see Chapter 14.13), mucous membrane pemphigoid, linear IgA disease and also, epidermolysis bullosa acquisita, and dermatitis herpetiformis. This group is characterized by the presence of autoantibodies to structural components of the basement membrane zone (Fig. 23.4.2 and Tables 23.4.1 and 23.4.2) that result in separation of the epidermis/epithelium from the dermis/mesenchyme, so that the blister roofs are thick, and intact blisters are seen. Dermatitis herpetiformis is the exception, and involves antibodies to epidermal transglutaminases.

Bullous pemphigoid

This is the most common blistering disease in the West.

Aetiology, genetics, pathogenesis, and pathology

The trigger for bullous pemphigoid is unknown, although in a few patients drugs or local trauma to the skin, e.g. an operation or radiotherapy, may initiate the disease. The disease is mediated by IgG autoantibodies to BP230 (bullous pemphigoid antigen 1; dystonin) and BP180 (bullous pemphigoid antigen 2; collagen XVII), components of the hemidesmosome (Fig. 23.4.2). Animal models have shown the antibodies to be pathogenic, and in the closely related condition pemphigoid gestationis (see Chapter 14.13), the transplacental transmission of the disease to the neonate has confirmed pathogenicity in humans. The combination of the autoantibody with the target antigen triggers an inflammatory cascade, the binding of complement, and separation of the epidermis from the dermis, visible as a blister.

Bullous pemphigoid occurs at a rate of 7 to 30 per million. It is a disease of older people, and there is an association with neurological disease, particularly multiple sclerosis in younger patients, and dementia, cardiovascular disease and Parkinson's disease in older patients.

Clinical features

The first symptom is itching. There may be a long prodromal period of weeks to years, with itching, transient urticarial lesions, or eczematous patches. When the blisters appear the diagnosis is obvious. Tense clear blisters, which may be several centimetres in size, arise from normal skin or large raised red areas (Fig. 23.4.6). The eruption is symmetrical and typically flexural, often around the groins and inner thighs, and may be attributed to a catheter rash. The mouth may have asymptomatic blisters and erosions.

The diagnosis is made clinically, and confirmed by histopathology performed on a small fresh blister, ideally taken within a 4 mm punch biopsy. This shows a subepidermal blister with intact epidermis overlying it. Direct immunofluorescence testing of perilesional skin, and indirect immunofluorescence testing of serum or blister fluid (useful in patients with mental incapacity) demonstrates the binding of IgG antibodies and complement C3 to the basement membrane (Fig. 23.4.7), with binding to the epidermal side of salt-split skin. An ELISA to detect BP180 antibodies is available in some centres.

Treatment

In the United Kingdom there are national guidelines for treatment (see 'Further reading'). Topical steroids are the standard treatment,

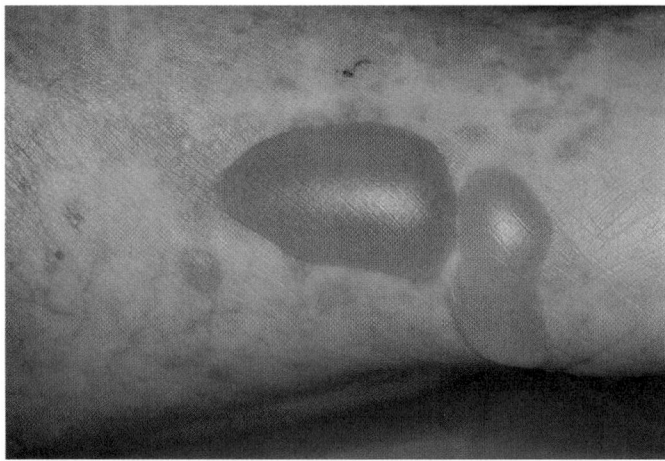

Fig. 23.4.6 Large blisters, vesicles, and red plaques in bullous pemphigoid.

combined if necessary with anti-inflammatory antibiotics (tetracyclines or erythromycin) or systemic steroids (prednisolone 20–60 mg). Immunosuppressants are added if control is difficult, azathioprine or mycophenolate mofetil most commonly, and rarely immune therapy such as IVIG, plasmapheresis, or rituximab. The aim of treatment is to suppress the disease so the patient is comfortable, the occasional blister indicating that the patient is not being over treated. The treatment is slowly tapered once the disease has been controlled. The disease usually remits within 3 to 5 years, but may be more prolonged. Mortality and morbidity are significant, and are related to steroid and immunosuppressive therapy.

With the ageing population, bullous pemphigoid will become a greater problem, and rapid safer treatments would be a great advantage. It is likely that future biological therapies will revolutionize treatment.

Mucous membrane pemphigoid (previously cicatricial pemphigoid)

This is a rare blistering disease. The patients present to multiple specialities: dermatology, oral medicine, ophthalmology, otolaryngology, and gynaecology. An international consensus in 2002 defined the disease.

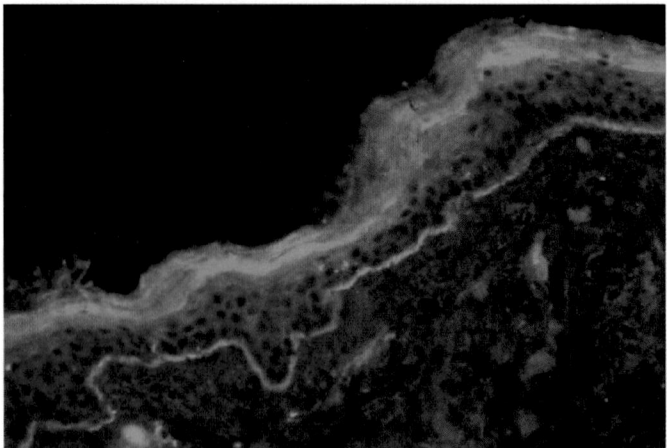

Fig. 23.4.7 IgG autoantibodies binding to the basement membrane zone in bullous and mucous membrane pemphigoid.

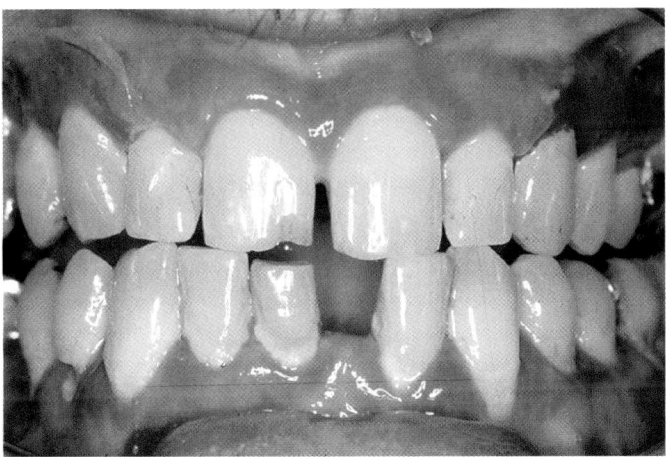

Fig. 23.4.8 Desquamative gingivitis of the gums.

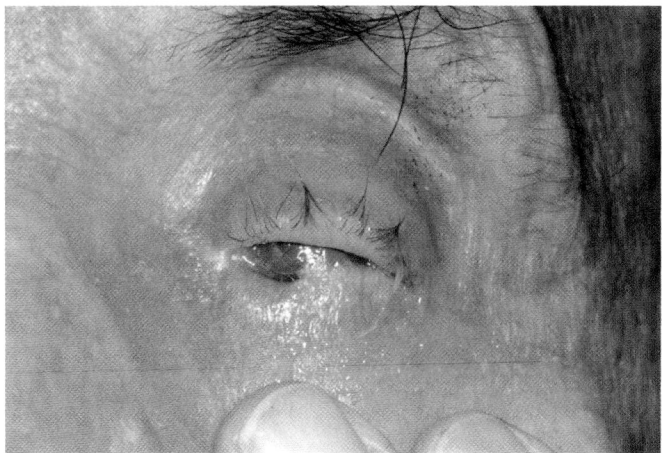

Fig. 23.4.9 End stage ocular disease, showing scarring and symblepharon.

Aetiology, genetics, pathogenesis, and pathology

The disease is mediated by IgG and IgA autoantibodies to BP180, BP230, or α6β4 integrin subunits in the hemidesmosome, or to laminin 5 or collagen VII in the adhesion complex (Table 23.4.1, Fig. 23.4.2). A dual IgG and IgA response is associated with a poorer prognosis. Experimental models have confirmed the pathogenicity of the antibodies. The combination of the antibody with antigen triggers an inflammatory cascade that results in separation of the epidermis/epithelium from the dermis/mesenchyme, and scarring.

Mucous membrane pemphigoid occurs at a rate of 1 per million, in middle aged and older people, although cases have been described in children and teenagers. There is an association with autoimmune disease, and laminin 5 mucous membrane pemphigoid has been associated with malignancy.

Clinical features

The disease predominately affects the mucosal surfaces, usually several sites, and there may additionally be skin involvement. The oral mucosa is often the first affected, with desquamative gingivitis (Fig. 23.4.8), shedding of the epithelium of the gums, giving a bright red appearance, and blisters and erosions on the buccal mucosa and the palate. This makes eating painful, and patients may lose weight. There may be hoarseness, choking, and coughing because of involvement of the oropharynx and larynx; involvement of the trachea can lead to stridor, and because of the risk of asphyxiation a tracheostomy may be necessary. Eye involvement presents with conjunctivitis and scarring, leading to symblepharon and blindness (Fig. 23.4.9), which can be rapid. Blistering and scarring of the genitals can interfere with sexual function and micturition. Skin involvement is often localized, and repeated blistering at the same site causes scarring.

The diagnosis is made clinically, and is difficult to confirm. Histology should be performed on a fresh blister. Perilesional mucosa or skin shows basement membrane antibodies on direct immunofluorescence, and serum for indirect immunofluorescence demonstrates low titre antibodies. On salt-split skin the antibodies bind to the epidermal side of the split (BP180, BP230, α6β4 integrin subunits) or to the dermal side (laminin 5, collagen VII). An ELISA is available to detect BP180 antibodies.

Treatment

A Cochrane review revealed that the evidence base for treatment was small. The international consensus discussed treatment, which is often disappointing. Topical steroids are helpful for symptom relief; systemic therapy is usually needed. Systemic steroids, anti-inflammatory antimicrobials (dapsone, sulfonamides, tetracyclines, or erythromycin), immunosuppressants, and azathioprine are most commonly used, but the best evidence is for cyclophosphamide, immunomodulators, IVIG, plasmapheresis, and rituximab. The aim of treatment is to suppress the disease to make the patient comfortable and prevent catastrophic scarring.

The disease runs a very prolonged course over decades, although it may burn out in some patients. Morbidity from mucosal scarring is significant, and is difficult to prevent even with aggressive treatment.

Linear IgA disease (linear IgA bullous dermatosis, chronic bullous disease of childhood)

This is an uncommon blistering disease in the West, and is unusual in being mediated by IgA antibodies.

Aetiology, genetics, pathogenesis, and pathology

The trigger in a few patients is drugs (e.g. vancomycin, diclofenac) or infections. The disease is mediated by IgA autoantibodies to BP180 and its physiologically shed ectodomain, BP230, and LAD285, components of the hemidesmosome (Fig. 23.4.2). It is strongly associated with the autoimmune haplotype HLA B8, DR3.

Linear IgA disease occurs at a rate of 0.5 per million. It is a disease of young children, often preschool, and there is a second peak in older people. There are large series of children from northern Africa, South Africa, and Sri Lanka.

Clinical features

Usually the onset is abrupt, with either blisters or red lesions; in adults there may be scattered groups of small papulovesicles. The lesions are typically annular, with blistering at the edges (Fig. 23.4.10). The symptoms are burning and itching. Involvement of the genitals is common in young children, and the trunk is usually affected. The mouth may have blisters and erosions.

The diagnosis is usually made clinically, confirmed by histopathology performed on a small fresh blister. Normal skin tested by direct immunofluorescence, and serum tested by indirect immunofluorescence demonstrate the binding of IgA antibodies to the basement membrane.

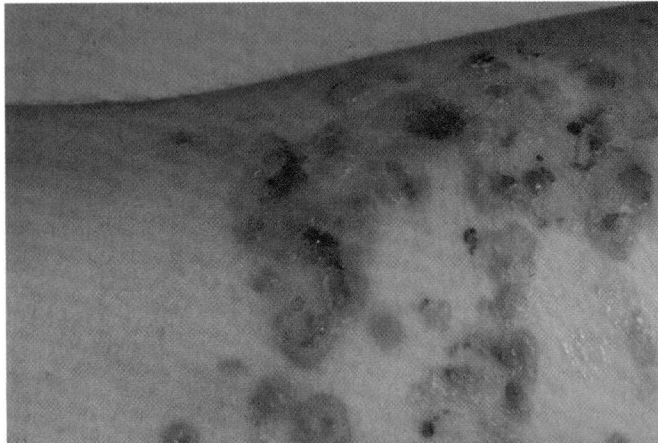

Fig. 23.4.10 Annular blistering lesions in linear IgA disease.

Treatment

Antimicrobials are the mainstay of treatment (dapsone or the sulfonamides sulfamethoxypyridazine and sulfapyridine), but some patients respond to anti-inflammatory antibiotics (tetracyclines or erythromycin). Rarely, systemic steroids or immunosuppressants are required. The disease usually remits within 3 to 5 years, but may be more prolonged.

Epidermolysis bullosa acquisita

This is one of the rarest blistering diseases.

Aetiology, genetics, pathogenesis, and pathology

Epidermolysis bullosa acquisita is sometimes associated with inflammatory bowel disease. The disease is mediated by IgG autoantibodies to collagen VII, the anchoring fibril (Fig. 23.4.6), which are pathogenic in animal models. Epidermolysis bullosa acquisita occurs at a rate of less than 0.25 per million in Western Europe. It may be more common in other regions.

Clinical features

Usually the onset is abrupt, with typically mechanobullous blisters (i.e. induced by trauma) on the hands, feet, knees and elbows. The tense blisters heal with scarring and milia (small keratin inclusion bodies) (Fig. 23.4.11). The nails may be scarred and destroyed. Mucosal involvement may be prominent, and some patients have a mucous membrane pemphigoid phenotype.

The diagnosis is made clinically and confirmed by histopathology. Direct immunofluorescence and indirect immunofluorescence testing demonstrate the binding of IgG antibodies to the basement membrane and the dermal side of split skin (Fig. 23.4.12). The demonstration of antibodies to collagen VII is essential for diagnosis.

Treatment

Treatment is difficult, and a Cochrane review found almost no reports. Dapsone or sulfonamides (sulfamethoxypyridazine or sulfapyridine) with systemic steroids can be effective, but immunosuppressants or IVIG are usually required. The disease is severe and prolonged in most cases, with scarring impairing function.

Dermatitis herpetiformis

This is a manifestation of coeliac disease, although the connection was unrecognized until the 1960s.

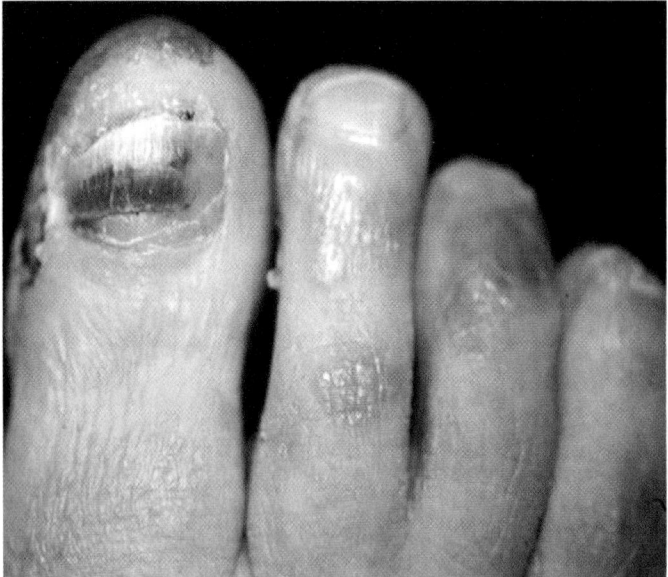

Fig. 23.4.11 Blisters, scarring, milia, and nail damage.

Aetiology, genetics, pathogenesis, and pathology

Dermatitis herpetiformis is gluten dependent (see Chapter 15.10.3). However, the mechanism by which gluten causes the skin to blister is unclear. The only autoantibodies that distinguish it from coeliac disease are IgA epidermal transglutaminases, and it may be an immune complex-mediated disease. There is a strong association with HLA DQ2 or 7, and 10% of patients have a family history of dermatitis herpetiformis or coeliac disease. The frequency of this condition is highest in western Ireland, Scandinavia, and Hungary. It is rare in non-European populations. Methods to reduce the incidence of coeliac disease would be predicted to reduce the incidence of dermatitis herpetiformis.

Clinical features

The onset is usually sudden in young adults, although childhood cases are common in Italy and Hungary, and older people can present with it. Small, intensely itchy papules and vesicles develop on the extensor surfaces of the knees, elbows, buttocks, and trunk.

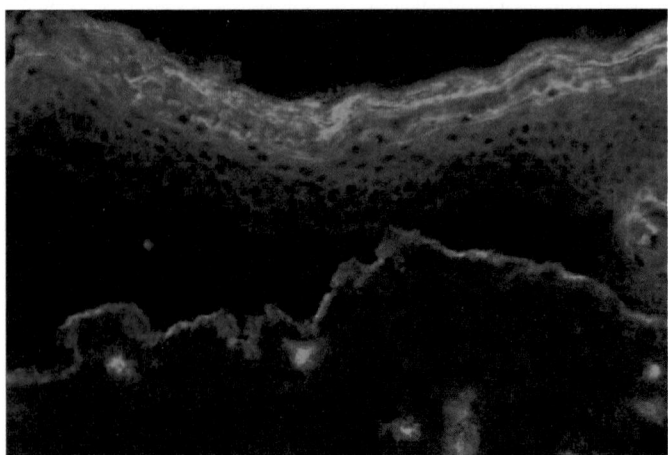

Fig. 23.4.12 IgG antibodies binding to the dermal side of the basement membrane zone of split skin.

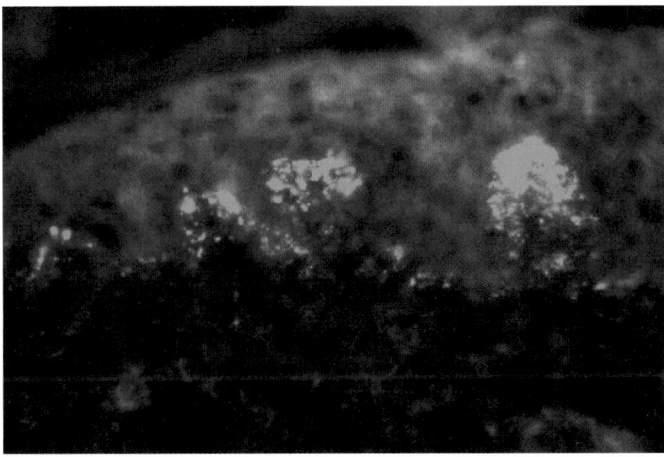

Fig. 23.4.13 Characteristic granular IgA deposits in the papillary dermis.

In partially controlled disease the lesions are often found on the scalp and chin. The lesions are so intensely itchy that it is rare to see an intact blister. There may be other autoimmune diseases present.

Histology of a fresh lesion shows papillary microabscesses filled with neutrophils. Direct immunofluorescence testing demonstrates granular deposits of IgA in the papillary dermis (Fig. 23.4.13), which are essential for diagnosis. As in coeliac disease, antiendomysial and antitransglutaminase antibodies should be sought, and the patient investigated for malabsorption and other autoimmune diseases.

Treatment

The treatment of choice is a gluten-free diet (see Chapter 15.10.3) although the malabsorption improves within weeks, the skin will not usually clear until after 2 years of strict gluten avoidance. The ingestion of gluten causes recurrence of the itching and lesions. Dapsone or sulfonamides (sulfamethoxypyridazine or sulfapyridine) will switch off the disease in 24 to 48 h, and may be slowly reduced as the gluten-free diet takes effect. Remission is dependent on strict gluten avoidance, and those electing not to have gluten-free diet will need lifelong treatment. There is an increased susceptibility to lymphoma.

Further reading

Anhalt GJ, *et al.* (1990). Paraneoplastic pemphigus. An autoimmune mucocutaneous disease associated with neoplasia. *N Engl J Med*, **20**, 1729–35.

Aoki V, *et al.* (2004). Environmental risk factors in endemic pemphigus foliaceus (fogo selvagem). *J Investig Dermatol Symp Proc*, **9**, 34–40.

Chan LS, *et al.* (2002). The first international consensus on mucous membrane pemphigoid: definition, diagnostic criteria, pathogenic factors, medical treatment, and prognostic indicators. *Arch Dermatol*, **138**, 370–9.

Collin P, Reunala T (2003). Recognition and management of the cutaneous manifestations of celiac disease: a guide for dermatologists. *Am J Clin Dermatol*, **4**, 13–20.

Fry L, *et al.* (1968). Effect of gluten-free diet on dermatological, intestinal, and haematological manifestations of dermatitis herpetiformis. *Lancet*, **16**, 557–61.

Giudice GJ, *et al.* (1993). Bullous pemphigoid and herpes gestationis autoantibodies recognize a common non-collagenous site on the BP180 ectodomain. *J Immunol*, **151**, 5742–50.

Harman KE, Albert S, Black MM (2003). Guidelines for the management of pemphigus vulgaris. *Br J Dermatol*, **149**, 926–37.

Khumalo N, *et al.* (2005). Interventions for bullous pemphigoid. *Cochrane Database Syst Rev*, **3**, CD002292.

Kirtschig G, *et al.* (2003). Interventions for mucous membrane pemphigoid and epidermolysis bullosa acquisita. *Cochrane Database Syst Rev*, **1**, CD004056.

Liu Z, *et al.* (1993). A passive transfer model of the organ-specific autoimmune disease, bullous pemphigoid, using antibodies generated against the hemidesmosomal antigen, BP180. *J Clin Invest*, **92**, 2480–8.

Stanley JR, Amagai M (2006). Pemphigus, bullous impetigo, and the staphylococcal scalded-skin syndrome. *N Engl J Med*, **26**, 1800–10.

Takahashi Y, *et al.* (1985). Experimentally induced pemphigus vulgaris in neonatal BALB/c mice: a time-course study of clinical, immunologic, ultrastructural, and cytochemical changes. *J Invest Dermatol*, **84**, 41–6.

Wojnarowska F, *et al.* (1988). Chronic bullous disease of childhood, childhood cicatricial pemphigoid, and linear IgA disease of adults. A comparative study demonstrating clinical and immunopathologic overlap. *J Am Acad Dermatol*, **19**, 792–805.

Wojnarowska F, *et al.* (2002). British Association of Dermatologists guidelines for the management of bullous pemphigoid. *Br J Dermatol*, **147**, 214–21.

23.5

Papulosquamous disease

Christopher Griffiths

Essentials

Papulosquamous diseases are typically characterized by well-demarcated areas of papules and scale, typically on an erythematous background. The differential diagnosis includes psoriasis, lichen planus, mycosis fungoides, discoid lupus erythematosus, eczema/dermatitis, drug eruptions, tinea, pityriasis versicolor, secondary syphilis, and pityriasis rosea.

The presence of significant pruritus is a useful marker to help with the differential diagnosis: lichen planus and discoid eczema are typically pruritic, whereas others, such as psoriasis, are less so. The distribution is also key to making the diagnosis, with psoriasis often showing characteristic symmetrical involvement of the extensor surfaces, scalp, and nails. Histology can be essential to reach a diagnosis and plan an appropriate approach to management.

The most common form of psoriasis is chronic plaque psoriasis, which often first affects the scalp. The nails are affected in about 50% of cases. There is no cure. Topical corticosteroids are the most commonly used treatment worldwide, but they should not be used continuously for more than 2 weeks. Dithranol has been one of the main topical treatments for many years, but is now largely superseded by vitamin D_3 analogues, e.g. calcipotriol. Phototherapy and photochemotherapy can be effective. Systemic treatments are only required in the most refractory cases.

Lichen planus is characterized by purple (violaceous) flat-topped polygonal papules that vary in size, most commonly on the flexor aspects of the wrists, the lower back, and the ankles. About 50% of patients have involvement of the mucous membranes. The skin disease is usually self limiting.

Psoriasis

Psoriasis is one of the most common and easily identifiable inflammatory skin diseases. In Western Europe the prevalence of psoriasis is estimated at 2%, but is higher in parts of Scandinavia, e.g. the Faroe Islands, where it reaches 5%. Worldwide, the disease is rare in Inuit, native American, Japanese, and Afro–Caribbean people, and has been estimated to affect just 0.3% of the general population in China. There is no evidence that the incidence of the disease is changing, by contrast with the year-on-year increase in atopic dermatitis. Overall, the sex incidence is equal, and the mean age of onset is 33 years, but 75% of cases occur before the age of 40 years. Disease starts earlier in females than males, indicating hormonal influences. Late-onset disease (type II), occurring after the age of 40 years, reaches a peak at onset between the ages of 55 and 65 years. There appears to be no association with either social class or diet.

Early-onset type I psoriasis is familial; one-third of patients have a first-degree relative with the disease. It is apparent that this form of psoriasis is genetically predetermined and polygenic. At least nine chromosomal psoriasis susceptibility loci have been identified. The most robust association is with chromosome 6p, probably involving MHC class I allele HLA Cw6, which contributes up to 50% of the risk in patients with psoriasis. No gene or gene product has thus far been definitively associated with psoriasis, but corneodesmosin, expressed solely in the upper layers of the epidermis, is a strong candidate. Type II psoriasis is not associated with HLA Cw6, and may be a separate disease.

Twin studies underscore the importance of an interaction between environment and genotype for the expression of psoriasis, and concordance is 72% in monozygotes. Environmental triggers in genetically susceptible individuals include: β-haemolytic streptococcal tonsillitis/pharyngitis; physical and psychological stress; HIV infection; drugs including β-blockers, nonsteroidal anti-inflammatories, lithium, and antimalarials; and alcohol.

Clinical features

The most common form of psoriasis, chronic plaque psoriasis or psoriasis vulgaris, accounts for 90% of cases. The characteristic features are well-circumscribed red plaques covered with silvery-white scales. These occur most commonly on the extensor aspects of the knees and elbows, the lower back, and the scalp (Figs. 23.5.1, 23.5.2), although any skin surface may be affected. Plaques are frequently strikingly symmetrical, varying in diameter from less than 1 cm to more than 10 cm. Individual plaques are dynamic, such that in active disease a plaque may clear from the centre to leave an annular or gyrate configuration that to the uninitiated could be misdiagnosed as tinea corporis. Various phenotypes of psoriasis exist:

Guttate psoriasis

Named from the Latin *guttata*, meaning a droplet. This form classically occurs 2 to 3 weeks after streptococcal pharyngitis or tonsillitis, and is the most common presentation in childhood (Fig. 23.5.3). Onset is acute, with a predominantly centripetal distribution of small (<1 cm diameter) papules. This form of psoriasis is frequently self limiting.

Erythroderma

Total skin involvement by psoriasis is known as erythroderma, although this term is also used for any inflammatory skin disease affecting more than 90% of the skin's surface area. Other diseases producing erythroderma include atopic dermatitis, lichen planus, drug eruptions, and cutaneous T-cell lymphoma. Erythroderma, particularly in older people, can lead to fluid loss, hypocalcaemia, impaired thermoregulation (both hypo- and hyperthermia), and high-output cardiac failure.

Generalized pustular psoriasis

Generalized pustular psoriasis, known also as Von Zumbusch's disease, is described as an acute onset of painful red plaques of psoriasis studded with small sterile pustules. This form of psoriasis is usually indicative of unstable disease, particularly that precipitated by infection or acute withdrawal of either systemic glucocorticosteroids or, on occasion, high-potency topical corticosteroids, leading to a rebound pustular flare. The patient is systemically unwell, with pyrexia and influenza-like symptoms.

Flexural psoriasis

Flexural psoriasis (psoriasis inversa) pertains to a form that involves the groins, axillae, and inframammary regions. Psoriasis at these sites loses many of the characteristic clinical features, in that it is shiny, nonscaly, and bright red, but retains the characteristic clear demarcation between involved and uninvolved skin.

Sebopsoriasis

This form of psoriasis occurs in the seborrhoeic sites of the nasolabial folds, eyebrows, scalp, postauricular region, and presternum. At times it may be difficult to distinguish it from seborrhoeic dermatitis.

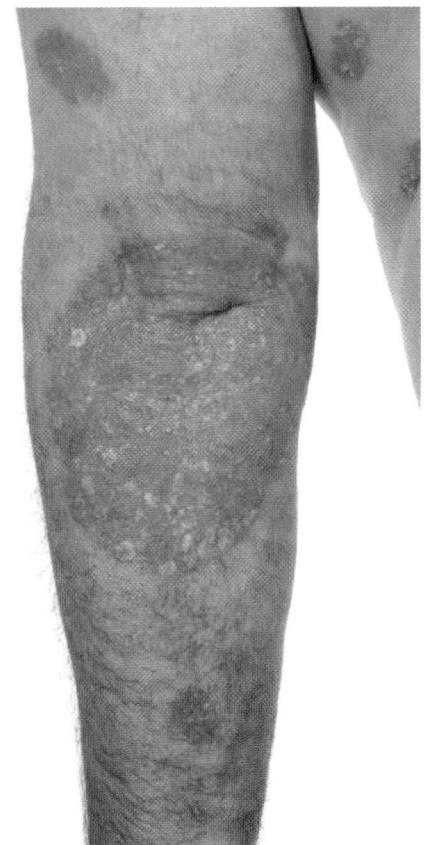

Fig. 23.5.1 Plaques of psoriasis.

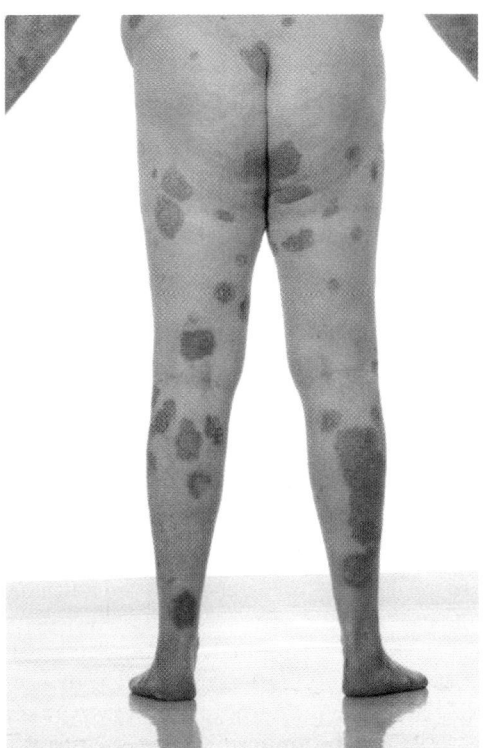

Fig. 23.5.2 Widespread chronic plaque psoriasis.

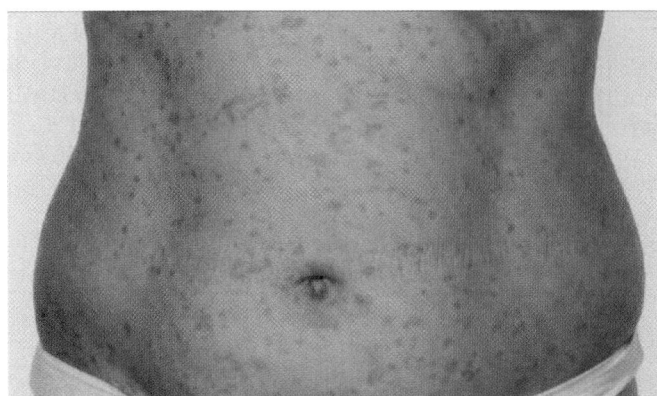

Fig. 23.5.3 Guttate psoriasis.

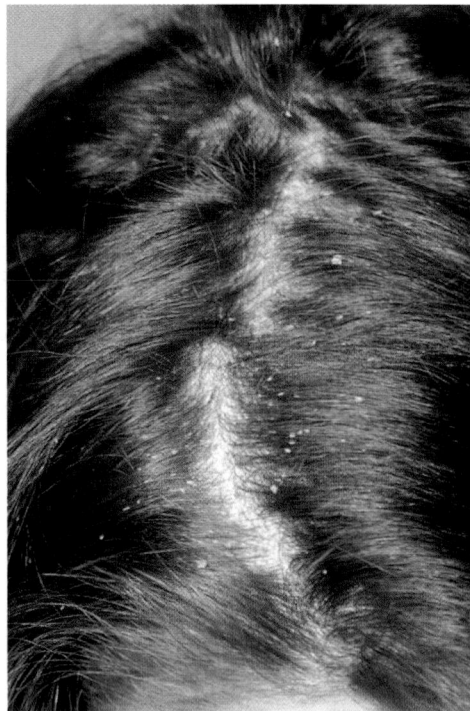

Fig. 23.5.4 Scalp involvement by psoriasis, showing tinea amiantacea.

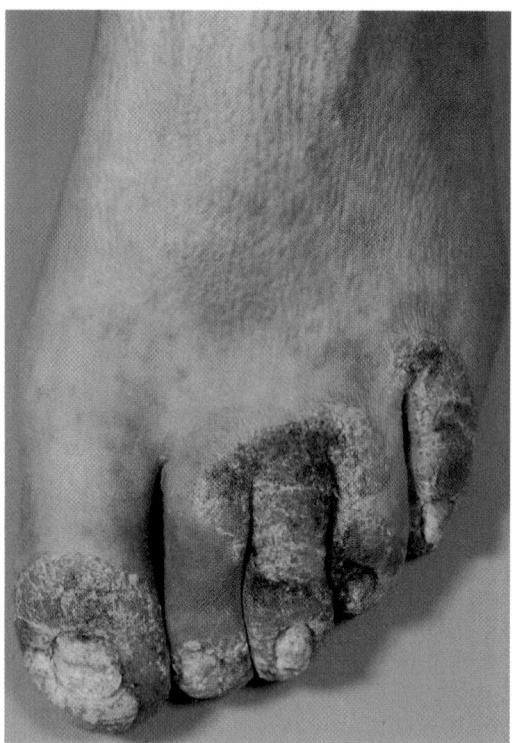

Fig. 23.5.5 Psoriatic nail dystrophy.

Scalp

The scalp is often the first and sometimes the only site to be affected by psoriasis. Paradoxically, it may be the most difficult form of psoriasis to treat. The lesions vary from typical plaques to involvement of the entire scalp, with the encroachment of scales along the hair shafts, a process known as tinea amiantacea (Fig. 23.5.4). Rarely do the lesions extend beyond the hairline. Alopecia may at times be a consequence.

Koebner phenomenon

The appearance of psoriasis at sites of recent trauma or pressure to the skin, such as under a tight waistband, is known as the isomorphic or Koebner phenomenon. Although not unique to psoriasis (it occurs also in lichen planus, viral warts, and vitiligo) it is a clinical marker of active, progressive psoriasis.

Nails

Approximately 50% of patients with psoriasis have characteristic clinical involvement of any one or up to all the finger and toe nails. The involvement of the skin of the fingers by psoriasis, and the presence of psoriatic arthritis, predispose to nail disease. The clinical features range from thimble-like pitting of the nail plate, to onycholysis (separation of the nail from the nail bed), oil spots (orange discolouration of the nail bed), and disabling nail dystrophy (Fig. 23.5.5). Patients are frequently concerned about nail disease, and may request treatment for this aspect of psoriasis alone.

Comorbid diseases

Chronic plaque psoriasis is associated with several comorbid conditions, which include:

Inflammatory bowel disease

Ten per cent of patients with inflammatory bowel disease, particularly Crohn's disease, have concomitant psoriasis.

Palmoplantar pustulosis

Now believed to be a condition separate from psoriasis, palmoplantar pustulosis has been reclassified as a comorbid condition. Yellow sterile painful pustules occur on the palms and soles, fading to brown scaled lesions. Up to 25% of patients have coexistent chronic plaque psoriasis. This is a disease of middle-aged women (female: male ratio 9:1), and more than 95% are current or previous smokers. There is an association with thyroid disease.

Psoriatic arthritis

This seronegative inflammatory arthritis occurs in more than 25% of patients with psoriasis. Most cases present either concomitantly with or after the first signs of skin disease, but on occasion (<10%) the arthritis predates psoriasis. Five clinical phenotypes of psoriatic arthritis exist: asymmetrical distal interphalangeal arthritis (most commonly and classically), oligoarthritis, polyarthritis, spondylitis, and arthritis mutilans (Fig. 23.5.6). A characteristic, perhaps pathognomonic, radiological feature is the presence of enthesitis—inflammation of a tendon sheath, particularly the Achilles. The immunogenetics of psoriatic arthritis are different from those of psoriasis, implying that the underlying pathogenic mechanisms are separate.

Metabolic syndrome

Emerging evidence suggests that patients with severe psoriasis have an increased incidence of the metabolic syndrome, particularly the components of diabetes mellitus, central obesity, hypertension, hyperlipidaemia, and coronary artery disease. There is also a three-fold increased risk of myocardial infarction in young patients with severe disease. It is unknown whether these signs are a consequence of psoriasis *per se* or of chronic inflammation, as is the case with arthritis.

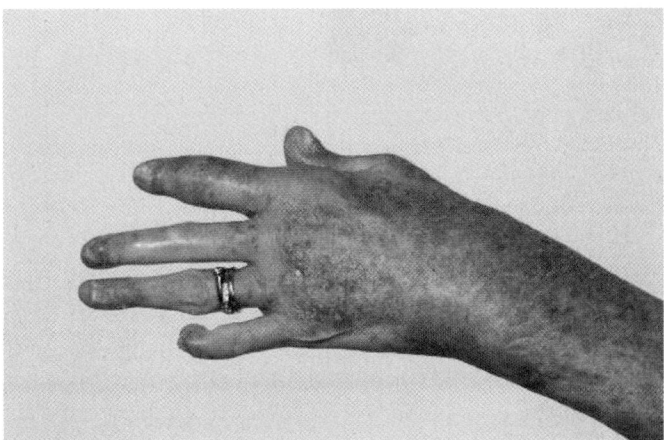

Fig. 23.5.6 Psoriasis with psoriatic arthritis.

Psychosocial aspects

Psoriasis is associated with significant impairment of quality of life. Studies have shown that this is equivalent to or worse than for other chronic diseases, including chronic obstructive airways disease, diabetes mellitus, and ischaemic heart disease. There is a significant association with clinical anxiety, depression, and suicidal ideation. Worry about the chronicity of psoriasis produces resistance to therapy.

Histology

The classical histology of psoriasis comprises epidermal keratinocyte hyperproliferation and loss of markers of differentiation, e.g. keratins 1 and 10, loss of the granular cell layer, and parakeratosis of the stratum corneum. The epidermis also contains microabscesses (of Munro) and collections of neutrophils (micropustules of Kogoj (Fig. 23.5.7)). There is, at times, a significant inflammatory infiltrate comprising predominantly T lymphocytes, with localization of CD8+ T cells in the epidermis and CD4+ T cells in the dermis. Dilated blood vessels are prominent in the dermis.

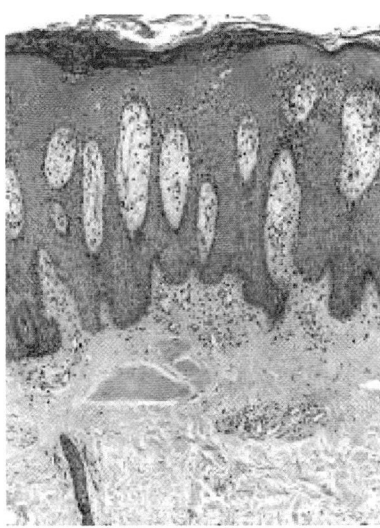

Fig. 23.5.7 Histological section of psoriasis showing epidermal acanthosis, elongation of rete ridges, and inflammation.

Pathogenesis

For many years it was believed that psoriasis was a disease primarily of keratinocytes, and that the inflammatory infiltrate was a secondary phenomenon. Current understanding of psoriasis is that it is an immune-mediated dermatosis, probably autoimmune in origin, although no autoantigen has been identified to date.

Components of the innate and adaptive immune responses play important roles in pathogenesis. CD8+ T cells within plaques are clonal, and most T cells are positive for cutaneous lymphocyte-associated antigen. It is believed that in the case of streptococcal pharyngitis there is stimulation and subsequent expansion of T cells, which cross-react with components of keratin in the epidermis. The central importance of T cells to the psoriatic process has been confirmed by the efficacy of T-cell targeted drugs including ciclosporin, an interleukin 2 (IL-2) diphtheria fusion toxin that is cytolytic for activated T cells, and biological therapies including efalizumab, a monoclonal antibody to CD11a. Natural killer and natural killer T cells also participate in the psoriatic process.

Plaques of psoriasis contain a predominance of Th1 cytokines, including interferon-γ, IL-2, and IL-12/23. By contrast, atopic dermatitis is primarily a Th2-cytokine-driven disease. This is confirmed by observations that atopic dermatitis is relatively rare in patients with psoriasis. Cytokines and chemokines of the innate immune response, including tumour necrosis factor-α (TNFα), are also present in plaques of psoriasis, and the demonstrated efficacy of biological agents targeted to TNFα has underscored the key role of this cytokine in the pathogenesis of psoriasis.

Keratinocytes are again the focus of researchers, in that the disruption of signalling in keratinocytes, either by abrogating activated protein 1 (AP-1) pathways such as jun-A, or up-regulating signal transducer and activator of transcription 3 (*STAT3*), will lead to cutaneous psoriasiform changes in the skin of transgenic mice. Angiogenesis is an underinvestigated area in psoriasis, but there is compelling evidence for significant vascular proliferation and angiogenesis in the dermis, and that this is associated with the overexpression of vascular endothelial growth factor produced by epidermal keratinocytes.

Research on the pathogenesis of psoriasis is hindered by the absence of an animal model for the disease—psoriasis occurs in no other animal but humans. The most reliable model for psoriasis is xenotransplantation, which involves transplantation of biopsies of uninvolved, clinically symptomless skin from patients with psoriasis onto the flanks of immunodeficient mice.

Management
General principles

The management of psoriasis, as with any other chronic skin disease, involves a biopsychosocial approach and an understanding of the individual patient's expectations of therapy. At present there is no cure. In the United Kingdom, 80% of patients with psoriasis can, with the use of topical agents, be treated adequately in primary care. Patients should be educated about psoriasis, e.g. it is not caused by diet, and is neither contagious nor neoplastic. An understanding of how psoriasis interferes with a patient's daily activities, and the psychosocial disability associated with anxiety and depression, are key aspects of the consultation. Indeed, cognitive behavioural therapy is often a useful adjunctive management tool. Environmental triggers of psoriasis should be ascertained, such as underlying infection, including streptococcal pharyngitis/tonsillitis, and drug triggers. Up to 50% of patients with psoriasis may enter spontaneous remission for varying periods of time, but in most cases it is a persistent and lifelong disease.

In all cases the liberal use of emollients is important. Topical therapies are aimed at directly reducing the epidermal keratinocyte proliferation or the inflammatory mediators that drive the epidermal changes.

Topical therapies
Vitamin D₃ analogues

A major advance in the topical treatment of psoriasis in the past 20 years has been the introduction of vitamin D_3 analogues. These include calcipotriol, calcitriol, and tacalcitol. All vitamin D_3 analogues directly inhibit keratinocyte proliferation, but also switch intraplaque cytokines from a Th1 to a Th2 profile. Calcipotriol and calcitriol are applied twice daily, whereas tacalcitol is used once daily. Local side effects include the irritation of uninvolved skin, and if used over an extensive body surface area, a risk of hypercalcaemia. A recent innovation has been the combination of calcipotriol with betamethasone valerate in a once-daily preparation. This enhances efficacy and reduces irritation.

Topical corticosteroids

Worldwide, topical corticosteroids are still the predominant therapy for localized chronic plaque psoriasis. If used appropriately, they can be a valuable component of the armamentarium. Medium- and high-potency topical corticosteroids in ointment formulation are the most effective, but should be used for no more than 2 weeks on a continuous basis, and not on the face or in the flexures. Higher potency steroids carry an increased risk of rebound flare on withdrawal. To minimize complications various innovative regimens are employed, such as weekends-only usage, combination with nonsteroidal drugs such as calcipotriol (see above), and tapering to less potent topical steroids.

Tazarotene

Tazarotene is the only topical vitamin A derivative available for the treatment of psoriasis. This is used once daily at night, the main limitation being a high incidence of local irritation. It is best used for recalcitrant plaques of psoriasis, particularly on the palms and soles.

Calcineurin inhibitors

The calcineurin inhibitor tacrolimus, although only approved for the treatment of atopic dermatitis, has an advantage over topical corticosteroids in that it does not produce skin atrophy. It is effective for the treatment of facial and flexural psoriasis.

Dithranol

Dithranol (formerly anthralin) has been one of the main topical treatments for psoriasis for many years. The mechanism of action is via an inhibitory effect on mitochondria. Dithranol is applied once daily, usually in a short-contact (30–60 min) outpatient regimen. Significant skin irritation, and staining of involved and uninvolved skin, clothing, and furniture nowadays limits dithranol to inpatient and day-treatment centre usage. The Ingram regimen is the combination of dithranol with ultraviolet B (UVB) phototherapy. With the advent of vitamin D_3 analogues the use of dithranol has declined significantly over the past 20 years.

Coal tar

Coal tar has been a standby of treatment for psoriasis for over 100 years; the classical psoriasis treatment, the Goeckerman regimen, involves a combination of crude coal tar with UVB phototherapy. Dissatisfaction with the cosmetic aspects of crude coal tar, in addition to skin irritation and folliculitis, has reduced its use as a routine outpatient therapy, and it is mostly limited to day-treatment centre or inpatient management of psoriasis.

Phototherapy
Broadband and narrowband UVB

Natural sunlight has been used for centuries for the treatment of psoriasis. The Dead Sea, because of its salinity and the abundant UV radiation, is a popular destination for psoriasis patients. The most effective wavelength of UV radiation for psoriasis is in the narrowband (311–313 nm) range. Narrowband UVB phototherapy is an effective treatment for psoriasis, and is superior to traditional broadband UVB phototherapy. UVB phototherapy is performed as an outpatient procedure following determination of the minimal erythema dose, based on an individual patient's skin phototype. Twenty-five year follow-up studies have not demonstrated significant increases in melanoma or nonmelanoma skin cancers in patients receiving narrowband UVB phototherapy.

Photochemotherapy

Psoralen UVA (PUVA) photochemotherapy is a combination of an ingested psoralen photosensitizer (8-methoxypsoralen or 5-methoxypsoralen), followed by exposure to UVA. This is one of the most effective treatments available for psoriasis. Apart from immediate side effects, which include nausea, headache, sunburn, and photosensitivity, there is a significant risk of premature skin ageing (photodamage) and nonmelanoma skin cancer, particularly in those who have received a cumulative dose of $1\,000\,mJ/m^2$ or 250 treatments. Side effects are reduced to some extent by bath PUVA, which involves immersion in a dilute aqueous solution of psoralen for 30 min before UVA exposure. PUVA patients should wear spectacles with plastic lenses, and avoid natural sun exposure on the day of treatment. Because of the complexities of treatment and significant skin cancer risk, the use of PUVA is declining.

Systemic therapies

Only a minority of psoriasis patients require therapy with systemic agents; most can be managed with topical therapies. However, some patients have disease that is too extensive, unstable, inflammatory, or recalcitrant for topical therapies, and thus phototherapy or systemic therapy is indicated.

Methotrexate

Methotrexate is a folic acid antagonist that inhibits DNA synthesis and thus cell replication; it also has T-cell suppressive activities. Methotrexate is the gold standard systemic therapy. Very few trials of the efficacy of methotrexate have been performed. Approximately 60% of patients achieve at least a 75% improvement in clinical severity as measured by the psoriasis area severity index (PASI).

Methotrexate is prescribed orally (occasionally intramuscularly or subcutaneously) in a once-weekly dose following a 2.5 mg test dose. Dosages range from 7.5 to 22.25 mg per week, dependent on clinical response. Folic acid 1 to 5 mg daily is added to prevent stomatitis and anaemia, and to reduce gastrointestinal side effects. Psoriasis patients receiving methotrexate require careful monitoring; they appear to have an increased risk of hepatotoxicity compared with rheumatoid arthritis patients. Traditionally, hepatotoxicity from methotrexate was assessed by liver biopsy; however, serum assay of the amino propeptide of collagen III has been shown to be a reliable measure of hepatic fibrosis, thereby obviating the need for liver biopsy in most patients. The use of pharmacogenetics may optimize the use of methotrexate by identifying individuals susceptible to hepatotoxicity and bone marrow suppression, and those likely to achieve a clinical response.

Retinoids

Oral retinoids (vitamin A derivatives) have been used in the treatment of psoriasis for over 30 years. The original third-generation retinoid used for psoriasis, etretinate, has been superseded by its natural metabolite acitretin. Monotherapy with acitretin is normally commenced at a dose of 10 to 25 mg daily. Systemic retinoids are particularly effective for the treatment of the erythrodermic and pustular variants of psoriasis. As they are not immunosuppressive, retinoids have a role in the treatment of those psoriasis patients who are HIV infected or have cancer, particularly non-melanoma skin cancer following PUVA.

Caution must be exercised when considering acitretin in women of childbearing potential, because of significant teratogenicity. Women should avoid pregnancy for up to 2 years (United Kingdom) or 3 years (United States of America) after completing acitretin treatment. Adverse psychiatric events, such as mood swings, depression, and suicidal ideation, have been reported as possible idiosyncratic reactions to the related retinoid isotretinoin. Retinoid toxicities are similar to those occurring with hypervitaminosis A, and can include mucocutaneous side effects including sticky skin, alopecia, and cheilitis. Osteoporosis, hyperlipidaemia, diffuse idiopathic skeletal hyperostosis syndrome, and pseudotumor cerebri may occur.

Combining acitretin with PUVA (Re-PUVA) significantly enhances the response to PUVA.

Ciclosporin

Ciclosporin is a highly effective, short-term therapy for moderate to severe psoriasis. It inhibits the activation of T cells as a consequence of blockade of cytoplasmic calcineurin phosphatase. Ciclosporin therapy is used for psoriasis at doses between 2.5 and 5 mg/kg per day, usually for no more than 12 weeks. Intermittent short-course therapies are recommended because of the association of long-term continuous ciclosporin therapy with nephrotoxicity and hypertension.

Unlike methotrexate or acitretin, ciclosporin is not teratogenic, thus it is the only systemic therapy that can be used in pregnancy. In those patients who have received significant PUVA there is an increased risk of nonmelanoma skin cancer. Patients may have other side effects, including hypertrichosis, gum hyperplasia, and paraesthesia. Long-term continuous therapy with ciclosporin is used on occasion at a daily dosage of 3 to 4 mg/kg, but regular monitoring of glomerular filtration rate is required. Ciclosporin has been used in combination with acitretin, low-dose methotrexate, and the newer biological agents.

Fumaric acid esters

A commercially available mixture of four fumaric acid esters (fumarates) has been used to treat psoriasis in Europe for around 50 years. They are hindered by a number of subjective side effects,

mainly gastrointestinal in nature, including abdominal cramps, diarrhoea, nausea, and flushing.

Other systemic therapies

Less frequently used second-tier systemic agents include hydroxy-carbamide, mycophenolate mofetil, sulfasalazine, azathioprine, and leflunomide. Few randomized controlled trials are available to confirm their effectiveness.

Biological agents

A major advance in the management of patients with moderate to severe psoriasis has been the introduction of biological agents. These are defined as recombinant molecules designed from the genetic sequence of existing living organisms, and are often similar or identical to proteins produced by humans. They include fusion proteins, recombinant proteins, and monoclonal antibodies, and have been in common use for diseases such as rheumatoid arthritis and Crohn's disease. There are a number of biological agents used in the management of psoriasis; these can be divided into those that target T cells and those that block cytokines, TNFα and IL-12/IL-23.

T-cell targeted agents

Alefacept Alefacept was the first biological agent specifically designed and approved for the treatment of psoriasis. It is a human leucocyte function-associated antigen 3 (LFA3)/IgG fusion protein that binds to CD2 on T cells, thereby inhibiting activation. Alefacept also produces apoptosis of memory effector CD45RO+ T cells. Delivered as a 12-week cycle of once-weekly intramuscular injections, approximately 20% of patients achieve a 75% reduction in PASI (PASI 75). Side effects are few, and monitoring involves the analysis of subsets of CD4+ and CD8+ T cells in peripheral blood. Some patients may go into long-term remission following a single cycle of therapy.

Cytokine-blocking agents

Etanercept Etanercept is a human recombinant p75 TNF receptor/Fc fusion protein that binds TNF and is self-administered subcutaneously at doses from 25 to 50 mg twice weekly. At the lower dose 34% of patients achieve PASI 75 at 12 weeks, and at the higher dose 49% of patients achieve this level of improvement. In addition to its beneficial effects on psoriasis, etanercept, in common with other TNF antagonists, is an effective treatment for psoriatic arthritis.

Infliximab Infliximab, a chimaeric monoclonal antibody, binds to and neutralizes the activity of TNFα. It is given as a 5 mg/kg intravenous infusion, with three loading infusions at 0, 2, and 6 weeks, and then subsequently at 8-week intervals. Infliximab is a highly effective, rapid-acting biological therapy in that more than 80% of patients achieve PASI 75 by 10 weeks. It can be used long term, and at 1 year 61% of patients maintain PASI 75 with a regular 8-week infusion. Infliximab is also effective for psoriatic arthritis.

Adalimumab Adalimumab, a fully human anti-TNFα monoclonal antibody, is self administered subcutaneously at a dose of 40 mg on alternate weeks. Twenty-four weeks of treatment with adalimumab significantly improves psoriasis, 54% of patients achieving PASI 75; psoriatic arthritis is improved also.

TNFα antagonist monitoring Because of the role of TNFα in granuloma formation, infections such as tuberculosis, histoplasmosis, and deep fungal infections require careful monitoring with appropriate tuberculosis screening before starting therapy. Other reported serious adverse effects with TNF antagonists include demyelination, exacerbation of pre-existing cardiac failure, development of lupus, enhanced risk of soft-tissue infections, and the potential development of nonmelanoma skin cancer in patients who have received significant PUVA. Prospective pharmacovigilance under the auspices of national registries is of importance for ascertaining the true risk of biological therapies.

Ustekinumab Ustekinumab, a fully human monoclonal antibody directed to the shared p40 subunit of IL-12 and IL-23 is self-administered subcutaneously at 0 and 4 weeks and 12 weekly thereafter at a dose of 45 mg or 90 mg. Twelve weeks of treatment significantly improves psoriasis, 70% of patients achieving PAS175, response is maintained with continuous therapy to 18 months.

Lichen planus

Lichen planus is a relatively common benign skin disease, estimated to account for 1.2% of new patients presenting to dermatology departments. It is slightly more common in women, and although occurring at all ages most commonly presents between the ages of 40 and 50 years. The familial incidence has been quoted as 11%, implying genetic susceptibility. The underlying aetiology is unknown; however, a number of drugs (gold, methyldopa) can produce a lichenoid reaction that is at times almost indistinguishable from lichen planus. In parts of Europe, including Italy and Spain, hepatitis C infection is associated with lichen planus, but this has not been noted in patients from northern Europe, the United Kingdom, and the United States of America. There is no consistent MHC association, although HLA A3 and HLA A5 have been linked.

The clinical features are highly characteristic in that lichen planus is characterized by purple (violaceous) flat-topped polygonal papules that vary in size (Fig. 23.5.8). The surface of the papules has a fine tracery of white lines known as Wickham's striae. Lichen planus can occur at sites of excoriation or scars—the Koebner phenomenon (Fig. 23.5.9). Annular lesions are seen, particularly on the penis. Although lichen planus can affect any skin surface it most commonly occurs on the flexor aspects of the wrists, the lower back, and the ankles. Hypertrophic lesions occur most commonly on the anterior shins, and involvement of the hair follicles of the scalp (lichen planopilaris) can produce significant scarring alopecia. Resolution of lesions can lead to significant postinflammatory hyperpigmentation, particularly in black and Asian skin.

Approximately 50% of patients have involvement of mucous membranes, most commonly the buccal mucosa, where the appearance is of a lacework of white streaks. Oral involvement can be significant, with painful erosions. In the absence of cutaneous manifestations oral lichen planus may present solely to dentists. The skin lesions are classically highly pruritic, but can be variable in pattern and morphology, including hypertrophic, atrophic, follicular, annular, and linear forms. Involvement of the nails occurs in approximately 10% of cases, and when present can be pathognomonic. The most common changes are longitudinal ridges caused by thinning of the nail plate, but adhesion between the dorsal nailfold, causing destruction of the lateral aspect of the nail (pterygium), is characteristic (Fig. 23.5.10). Chronic oral ulceration as a consequence of lichen planus can lead to the development of squamous cell carcinoma.

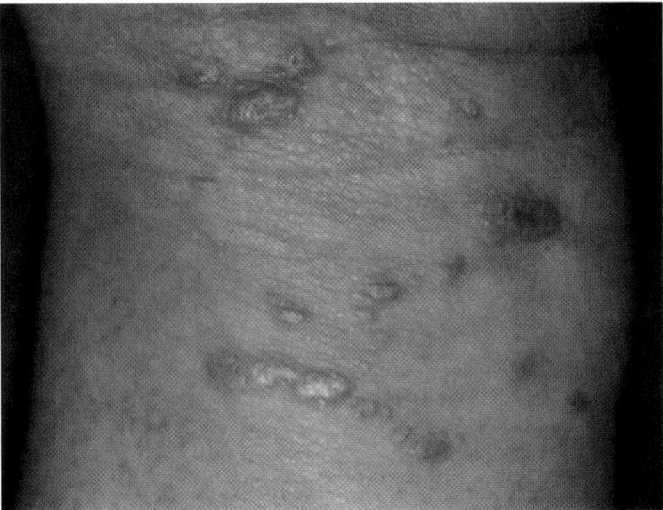

Fig. 23.5.8 Typical flat-topped polygonal papules of lichen planus.

Lichen planus and lichenoid drug eruptions are characterized histologically by thickening of the epidermis (acanthosis) and hypokeratosis, in which the basal layer of the epidermis is damaged, producing colloid bodies that may be clumped. Rete ridges of the epidermis are irregular and flattened, giving a saw-tooth appearance, and a band-like infiltrate of lymphocytes hugging the dermal–epidermal junction is a characteristic feature. Hyperpigmentation is due to pigmentary incontinence. At times, complete separation of the epidermis from the dermis may result in blister formation.

Treatment

The cutaneous disease is usually self limiting, with 85% of cases clearing spontaneously within 2 years. Oral lichen planus and scarring alopecia are difficult to treat, but local skin lesions can be treated with high-potency topical corticosteroids, e.g. clobetasol propionate 0.5%. Sometimes, systemic corticosteroids such as prednisolone, or other immunosuppressant agents such as ciclosporin, are required. Phototherapy, either PUVA or narrow-band UVB, and a variety of immunosuppressant therapies including methotrexate, azathioprine, and thalidomide, have also been used. Oral mucous membrane disease can be treated with topical corticosteroids such as triamcinolone in a carmellose and gelatine

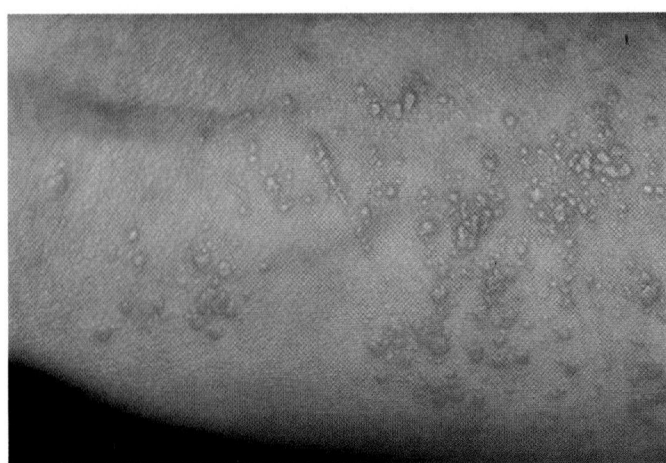

Fig. 23.5.9 Lichen planus with linear Koebner response.

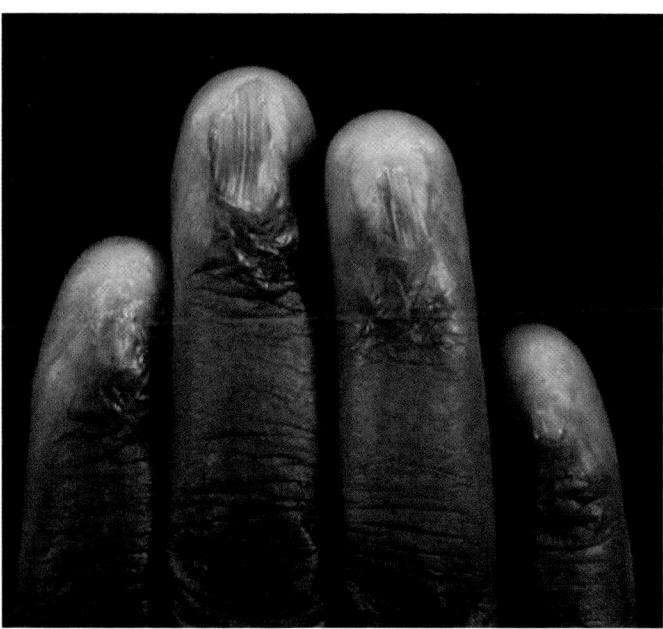

Fig. 23.5.10 Nail dystrophy from lichen planus, with pterygium.

paste that adheres to mucous surfaces, clobetasol propionate ointment, or fluticasone propionate asthma inhaler spray directed to the lesions. Ciclosporin oral rinse has also been used effectively for the treatment of oral lichen planus.

Other papulosquamous diseases

Numerous other disorders can present with a papulosquamous phenotype, including mycosis fungoides (see Chapter 23.10), discoid lupus erythematosus (see Chapter 23.7), eczema/dermatitis (see Chapter 23.6), drug eruptions (see Chapter 23.16, tinea (Chapter 23.10), pityriasis versicolor (Chapter 23.10), secondary syphilis (Chapter 7.6.6), and pityriasis rosea.

Pityriasis rosea

Most cases of pityriasis rosea occur between the ages 10 and 35 years, and onset is often seasonal. In many cases it is likely to be viral in aetiology, and various herpes viruses have been implicated. In addition, a prolonged pityriasis rosea-like rash can occur in association with various drugs, e.g. angiotensin-converting enzyme

inhibitors and hydroxychloroquine. Histology may show epidermal hyperplasia, spongiosis, and focal parakeratosis, with a superficial dermal infiltrate of lymphocytes, histiocytes, and occasional eosinophils.

Most patients with pityriasis rosea present initially with one plaque (herald patch), and then after several days many smaller plaques appear on the trunk, neck, and extremities, and sometimes other sites. In Africans, the lesions tend to be more papular. The plaques themselves are pink, with a fine peripheral scale and a well-defined and sometimes elevated margin. The scaling usually forms a ring (collarette) at the outer edge of the lesion, with its free edge inwards. Lesions are arranged with the long axes running in parallel to the ribs, resulting in a characteristic 'Christmas tree' distribution pattern. Lesions typically evolve over a few weeks, with subsequent spontaneous resolution. As secondary syphilis can mimic pityriasis rosea so closely, testing for syphilis is usually wise. The classical disease is self limiting, and no treatment is usually required.

Further reading

Breathnach SM, Black MM (2004). Lichen planus and lichenoid disorders. In: Burns DA, *et al.* (eds) *Rook's textbook of dermatology*, 7th edition. Blackwell, Oxford.

Eisen D (2003). The clinical manifestations and treatment of oral lichen planus. *Dermatol Clin*, **21**, 79–89.

Gelfand JM, *et al.* (2006). Risk of myocardial infarction in patients with psoriasis. *JAMA*, **296**, 1735–41.

Griffiths CEM, Camp RDR, Barker JNWN (2005). Psoriasis. In: Burns DA, *et al.* (eds) *Rook's textbook of dermatology*, 7th edition, pp. 35.1–35.69. Blackwell, Oxford.

Griffiths CEM, Barker JNWN (2007). Pathogenesis and clinical features of psoriasis. *Lancet*, **370**, 263–71.

Helliwell PS, Taylor WJ (2005). Classification and diagnostic criteria for psoriatic arthritis. *Ann Rheum Dis*, **64** Suppl 2, ii3–8.

Krueger JG, Bowcock A (2005). Psoriasis pathophysiology: current concepts of pathogenesis. *Ann Rheum Dis*, **64** Suppl 2, ii30–36.

Menter A, Griffiths CEM (2007). Current and future management of psoriasis. *Lancet*, **370**, 272–84.

Trembath RC, *et al.* (1997). Identification of a major susceptibility gene locus on chromosome 6p and evidence for further disease loci revealed by a two stage genome-wide search in psoriasis. *Hum Mol Genet*, **6**, 813–20.

Valdimarsson H, *et al.* (1995). Psoriasis: a T-cell-mediated autoimmune disease induced by streptococcal superantigens? *Immunol Today*, **16**, 145–9.

Dermatitis/eczema

Peter S. Friedmann

Essentials

Eczema is a characteristic pattern of skin inflammation that has many subtypes, with some induced by external factors such as irritants or skin sensitizers. Atopic eczema is due partly to a genetic susceptibility, which programmes altered immune responses and skin physiology, together with reactions to exogenous allergens and microbes, but a number of eczema patterns do not appear to have external causes.

The key points in the recognition of eczema are that the skin is reddened, may be thickened as a result of the inflammatory infiltrate and oedema, and the affected areas have ill-defined margins that break up into tiny red papules. Acute or severe eczema bubbles, blisters, and weeps. The distribution of the rash may be diagnostic, both of the type of eczema and the key causal factors.

Management requires identification and avoidance of provoking factors. The inflammation is treated with topical steroids of different potencies, supplemented with moisturizers. Newer therapies include topical calcineurin antagonists, with a range of systemic therapies being used to control the most severe types of disease.

Introduction

The term eczema is used to describe a pattern of skin inflammation characterized clinically by ill-defined areas of redness (erythema) made up of tiny individual papules (bumps). At the edges of eczema lesions the individual papules often become visible, which accounts for the lack of sharp definition (Fig. 23.6.1). Eczemas are characteristically very itchy. Microscopically, eczematous inflammation shows infiltration of T lymphocytes in both the dermis and epidermis, and the generation of oedema in the dermis, but also particularly in the epidermis. The oedema separates the epidermal cells from each other like the air spaces in a sponge (called spongiosis), but the oedema may coalesce into blisters, giving the appearance of a bubbly surface; these may leak or rupture producing serous oozing and crusting. There are many different types of eczema, some with known causation and others remaining cryptic.

Classification

There is no completely accepted classification of eczema, but it can be helpful to group eczemas in relation to what is known of their aetiology: those with mainly exogenous causation, often called dermatitis rather than eczema, and those with no known external causes (endogenous eczemas) (Box 23.6.1). The exogenous eczemas are nevertheless the consequence of interactions between external factors and host susceptibility, which may be largely genetically determined.

Contact dermatitis/eczema

This form of dermatitis/eczema is induced by external agents of different physicochemical types: substances with irritant properties that are not immunogens, those that induce T-cell-mediated allergic contact sensitivity, and ultraviolet light.

Irritant contact dermatitis

Aetiology/pathogenesis

Irritants are substances that inflict toxic damage on the epidermis. There are many types of irritant, but from a practical point of view they can be classified as surfactants (soaps/detergents), solvents (petrol, paraffin, oils), caustics (acids, alkalis, chemicals such as phenol), and miscellaneous chemicals that include nonanoic acid and dithranol (used in the treatment of psoriasis). Irritants vary greatly in their potency and hence the level of exposure required to induce an inflammatory response in skin. Individuals also vary greatly in their intrinsic resistance or susceptibility to the effects of irritants. A single exposure to mild irritants such as soaps and detergents is often insufficient to cause a clinically apparent irritant effect, which usually requires multiple exposures having a cumulative effect.

The general effect of irritants is a perturbation of the epidermal microenvironment, which is detected as a danger signal. This results in the activation of essential components of the innate immune response. Keratinocytes produce a wide range of cytokines, including

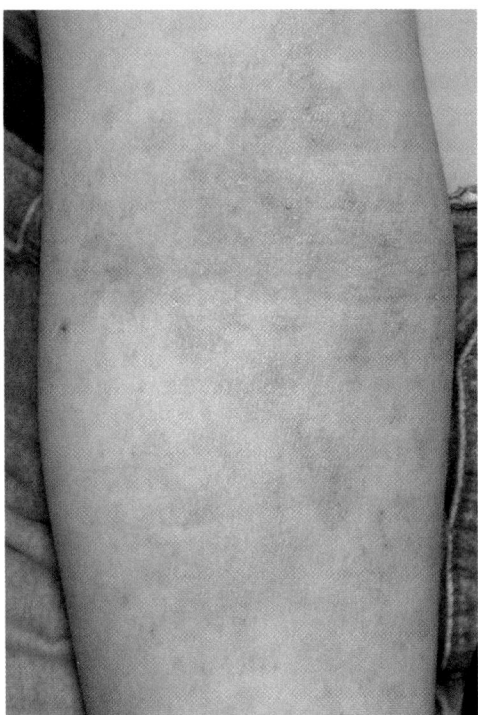

Fig. 23.6.1 Poorly defined margins of eczema.

interleukin (IL)-8, IL-18, and tumour necrosis factor-α; epidermal Langerhans' cells become activated and up to 30% may migrate into the dermis; the dermal microvasculature expresses increased levels of the adhesion molecules ICAM1, E-selectin (ELAM1), and VCAM1; and there is infiltration of lymphocytes and often neutrophil leucocytes. Repeated exposure may augment the microscopic response until it becomes clinically apparent inflammation. Most of the changes resulting from cumulative irritant insult are indistinguishable from those that follow the specific immunologically mediated process of allergic contact dermatitis.

Epidemiology

Irritant dermatitis is a major occupational skin disease. A survey in Sweden indicated that of 16 600 people who responded to a questionnaire about hand eczema, 11% had experienced eczema in the last year. Thirty five per cent of cases were irritant hand eczema, 19% allergic contact dermatitis, and 22% atopic hand eczema. In northern Germany, a large study from 1990 to 1999 examined compensation claims for occupational skin disease. The annual incidence of occupational irritant dermatitis was 4.5 cases per 10 000, compared with 4.1 cases per 10 000 of allergic contact dermatitis.

Clinical manifestations of irritant dermatitis

Under most circumstances the hands are the body site most likely to come into contact with irritants. One notable exception is the napkin area of infants, which may be in prolonged contact with alkaline (ammoniacal) urine or faecal material, and can develop irritant napkin dermatitis as a result.

The rash is erythematous with poorly defined margins, accompanied by scaling or fissures, and if more severe or acute, by eczematous blisters. The dorsa of the hands are usually more severely affected than the palmar surfaces, which probably reflects the thicker stratum corneum permeability barrier of the palms (Fig. 23.6.2). Once an irritant dermatitis has been initiated it seems to require very little and only occasional exposure to irritants to maintain a chronic dermatitis. Many patients who try to protect themselves by wearing rubber gloves find that when the hands become sweaty inside the gloves, this actually irritates and aggravates the dermatitis.

Those with a past or present history of atopic eczema are significantly more susceptible to developing irritant dermatitis from surfactants and solvents. This may reflect an impaired stratum corneum barrier and/or summation/synergism of the irritant effects and low-level subclinical inflammation of atopic eczema.

Treatment

The most important principle is avoiding further contact with irritants. The medical treatment is as for other eczemas, as outlined in 'Treatment of atopic eczema' below.

Box 23.6.1 Classification of eczema

Exogenous

Contact dermatitis

 ◆ Irritant

 ◆ Allergic

 ◆ Photoinduced

Atopic eczema

Seborrhoeic eczema/dermatitis

Photodermatitis

Endogenous

Asteatotic eczema

Dyshidrotic eczema

Varicose eczema

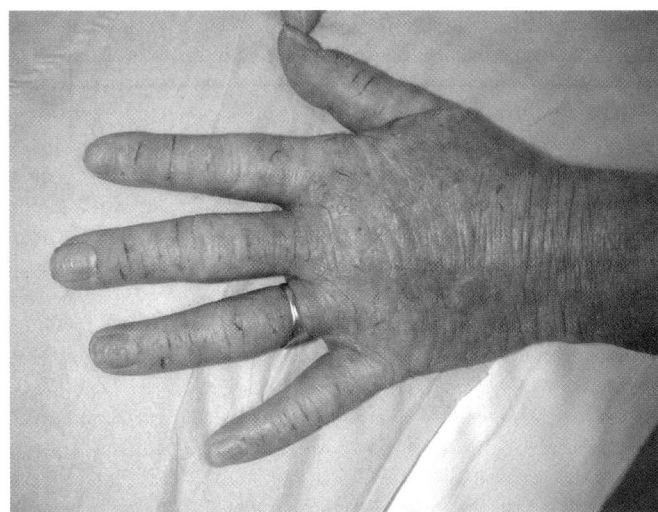

Fig. 23.6.2 Dorsal hand involvement in dermatitis.

Allergic contact dermatitis

Aetiology

Contact hypersensitivity is an acquired immune response in which T lymphocytes recognize and react to the causative molecules. Contact allergens are mostly small xenobiotic molecules, although under some circumstances proteins can act as contact sensitizers. Several factors are involved in determining whether an individual will develop contact sensitivity to a given molecule. These include the intrinsic immunogenicity of the chemical, the dose to which the individual is exposed, and the individual's susceptibility to sensitization.

Sensitizing potency of chemicals

Of the thousands of chemicals in the environment, some are clearly highly potent immunogens capable of sensitizing everyone, while others may be defined as moderate, weak, or even nonsensitizers. For small molecules to become recognizable by the T-cell receptor, they have first to act as haptens, which become bound to protein carriers. The hapten–carrier complex will be processed by dendritic antigen-presenting cells such as epidermal Langerhans' cells. Processing involves loading haptenated peptides into the major histocompatibility molecules (mainly MHC class II, but in some instances also Class I) on the surface of the antigen-presenting cell.

The sensitizing potency of chemicals is generally proportional to their protein-binding reactivity. Some compounds (haptens) are intrinsically protein reactive, others (prohaptens) are converted to protein-reactive metabolites through the actions of phase I xeno-biotic metabolizing enzymes such as the cytochrome P450 family. The overall phenotype of xenobiotic detoxification systems, including P450 and other antioxidant systems, may be an important contributor to an individual's susceptibility to sensitization. They may either detoxify reactive compounds and prevent immunogenicity, analogous to high acetylator status and resistance to drug allergy, or possibly through the failure of normal detoxification, may generate protein-reactive immunogenic intermediates.

Lessons from experimental work

The use of 2,4-dinitrochlorobenzene (DNCB) as an experimental contact sensitizer in healthy human volunteers has revealed that the human immune system obeys very reproducible dose-response relationships. Groups of individuals received different sensitizing doses of DNCB (62.5–1000 μg) on a 3 cm diameter circle of forearm skin. In proportion to the log of the sensitizing dose, there was a classical sigmoid dose-response curve for the proportion of individuals showing clinical sensitization, as detected by positive elicitation challenges applied 4 weeks later, with 100% being sensitized by 500 μg or more. Furthermore, as the sensitizing dose increased there was a log-linear increase in the strength of the response to the elicitation challenge; in other words, as the sensitizing dose increases on a log scale, so proportionately more people are sensitized, and to a greater extent.

For a chemical to induce allergic contact sensitization it must penetrate the stratum corneum. Most sensitizers are lipophilic and hence penetrate readily, but metals such as nickel, cobalt, and chromate are water soluble. Hence a major factor in augmenting sensitization by metals is mechanical penetration of the stratum corneum, as in body piercing.

The induction of contact sensitization involves the activation of hapten-specific T cells, which undergo clonal expansion resulting in the establishment of immunological memory. The next time the sensitizer is in contact with the skin it will be recognized by the memory T cells, which respond by releasing interferon-γ and other proinflammatory cytokines. This recruits other T cells to the site in a non-antigen-specific fashion. The combination of cells and cytokines generates the oedema and swelling accompanied by itch that is characteristic of allergic contact dermatitis.

Individual susceptibility

Very little is known of how individual susceptibility is controlled. There are clearly individuals who develop contact sensitivity to environmental substances more easily than others. Thus individuals who developed contact sensitivity to three or more unrelated chemicals could be sensitized experimentally by DNCB to a much greater degree than individuals with no pre-existing contact allergy. Individuals with only one contact sensitivity were intermediate in reactivity. These differences are not qualitative, but reflect the high-responder end of the normal distribution of responsiveness. The corollary of this is that there is a low-responder end of the normal distribution—individuals who appear resistant to the spontaneous development of contact sensitivities, and who give the lowest responses to any given sensitizing dose of DNCB.

There do not appear to be any major HLA associations with increased susceptibility to contact sensitization. As indicated above, one level at which susceptibility may be determined is that of intermediate metabolism, which can either detoxify or generate reactive intermediates. A second level, which has been shown at least with regard to nickel sensitivity, is the fundamental control of immunological tolerance, mediated by regulatory T lymphocytes.

Prevalence

Allergic contact sensitization and dermatitis are common; about 10% of women are sensitized to nickel. The total prevalence of contact dermatitis among the population of many countries is estimated at between 6 and 11%. The incidence of occupational contact dermatitis has been estimated to be around 0.5 to 1.9 cases per 1000 full-time workers per year (Chapter 9.4.1).

Clinical features of allergic contact dermatitis

Allergic contact dermatitis can vary from a low-grade minor nuisance—the pierced earlobes that become mildly inflamed and itchy if the earrings are left in for too long—to catastrophic and disabling acute blistering and weeping with severe oedema of the sites to which the sensitizer was applied. The key points in diagnosis are the recognition that the inflammatory process is eczematous in nature, and that the distribution on the body raises the suspicion that there is an exogenous source. Thus contact dermatitis from nickel in the metal studs and buttons of denim jeans has a characteristic distribution around the lower abdomen and hips (Fig. 23.6.3). However, in strongly sensitized individuals nickel in most metal objects, such as money, keys, cutlery, and door handles, can transfer from the fingers to other places, resulting in ill-defined eczematous areas on the face and abdomen. The relationship of these distant areas to contact sensitivity may be much less obvious.

Common sensitizers in everyday products include metals; dyes (paraphenylenediamine and other azo dyes) used for hair and clothing; preservatives (often formaldehyde releasers) found in many personal products; rubber accelerators found in rubber gloves and glue/cement used in shoe manufacture; colophony, extracted from pine resin and used to facilitate adhesion, as in

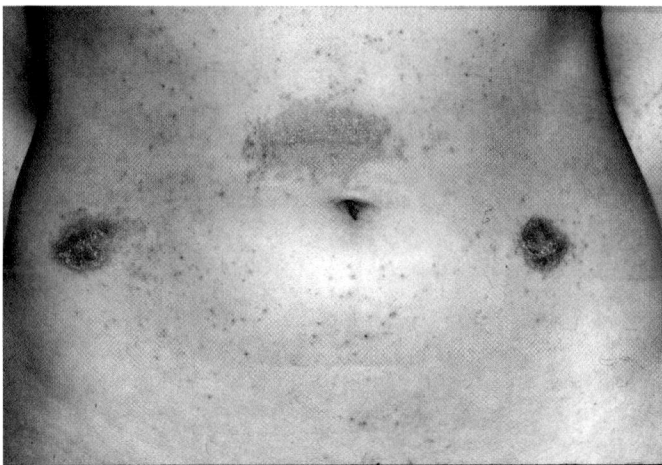

Fig. 23.6.3 Allergic contact dermatitis to nickel.

the rubbery adhesive of sticking plasters, but also in mascara and felt-tipped pens; and fragrances used in personal and domestic products.

Confirmation of causality

Contact allergens are applied to the skin of the back in patch tests. Patients are normally screened by an initial application of 40 substances (some individual, others as mixtures of a class) referred to as the European standard battery. These compounds have been selected by the International Contact Dermatitis Research Group and the European Environmental and Contact Dermatitis Research Group because they represent the groups of the most frequent sensitizers. The patch tests are applied on aluminium disc chambers held in place with hypoallergenic adhesive tape for 48 h, after which the chambers are removed and the skin assessed. Each compound or mixture is used at the highest concentration that does not normally induce a nonspecific irritant reaction. Many centres read the patch tests a second time at 72 or 96 h after application; this is said to reduce the number of false-positive tests that may result from irritant effects, and may detect responses that are slower to evolve.

The final interpretation of causality depends not only on the presence of a positive patch test, but also on the demonstration of relevance in terms of the person actually being exposed to the culprit, and it making contact with them in the areas where there is clinical dermatitis. The use of patch tests in elucidating the presence of contact allergy in patients with hand dermatitis is of great importance, as there may be major implications for the person in terms of their occupation.

Treatment

The general approach is first to identify the causal agent(s) through careful history taking, examination, and patch tests, and then avoid it. The treatment of the eczematous inflammation is summarised in 'Treatment of atopic eczema' below.

Atopic dermatitis/eczema

Definitions

The atopic state is defined when an individual's immune system responds to certain antigens by producing antibodies of the IgE class rather than the IgG class. There is considerable disagreement among dermatologists, paediatricians, and allergists over how best to define atopic eczema/dermatitis. Dermatologists define it as a diffuse symmetrical eczematous eruption that is characterized by onset in early life (infancy or childhood), and typically affects flexural sites such as the antecubital and popliteal fossae, and the hands and face. There is characteristically a personal and/or family history of allergic syndromes of asthma or rhinitis.

The main point of controversy is whether it is found only in individuals who are atopic. Among European dermatologists, atopic dermatitis is classified as extrinsic: associated with IgE-mediated allergies of mucosal systems, or intrinsic: usually of onset in adult life and not associated with the formation of allergen-specific IgE or clinical mucosal allergies. The extrinsic type accounts for around 80 to 95%, and the intrinsic type for 5 to 15% of cases of atopic eczema.

Incidence, prevalence, and natural history of atopic eczema/dermatitis

Over the last 40 years there has been a steady increase in the frequency of the atopic state and all the associated allergic syndromes of eczema, asthma, and rhinitis. While assessments for different national groups vary somewhat, it is now estimated that one-third of the population of the Western World is atopic. In the United Kingdom up to 15% of children will develop atopic eczema by the age of 12 years. The maximum incidence is during the first 2 years of life. Atopic eczema is usually the first of the atopic syndromes to develop, whereas asthma comes later, and rhinitis last—a sequence that has been called the atopic march. There are a number of patterns to the natural history, the most common being early onset and spontaneous remission during childhood. Atopic eczema affects up to 0.5% of the adult population. In some of these, the eczema has been present from early childhood, in others it recurs after a period of remission.

Clinical features

The distribution of atopic eczema varies with age. In precrawling infants it is often a diffuse symmetrical erythema with dryness affecting the head and neck, torso, and even the limbs. Once the baby starts crawling the eczema is usually distributed on the extensor surfaces of the arms, knees, and ankles, all of which are in physical and frictional contact with the floor surface on which the child is crawling. As the child becomes ambulatory the eczema tends to be distributed in the flexural areas, particularly the antecubital and popliteal fossae (Fig. 23.6.1).

In some adults, the eczema may be localized predominantly or exclusively to the head, neck, and upper chest, a pattern possibly related to the distribution of the saprophytic skin microbe *Malassezia furfur* (previously called *Pityrosporum orbiculare*).

In addition to the flexural pattern, there is a pattern comprising circular or discoid patches of eczema, sometimes called nummular (coin-shaped), scattered on the torso and limbs. This pattern is not well associated with allergic sensitization (Fig. 23.6.4).

The extent of skin involvement is one of the indicators of the overall severity, others being the degree of redness, the presence of weeping/oozing and crusting, as well as the presence of excoriation. The main symptom of eczema is itch, which can be very intense; a child can work itself into a complete frenzy of scratching, which

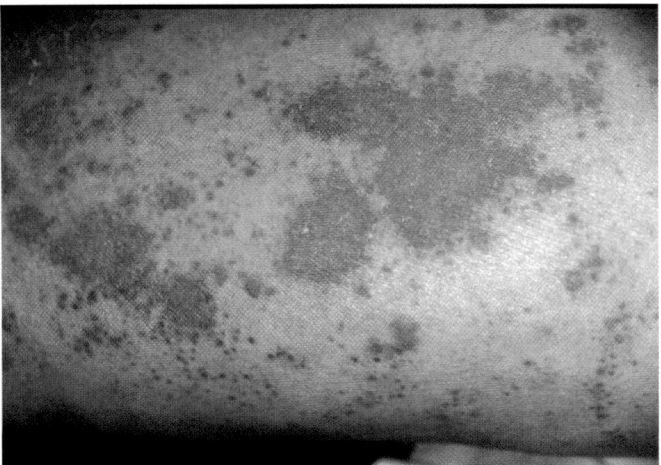

Fig. 23.6.4 Discoid eczema.

can be almost as distressing for the parents/carers because of the difficulty of relieving the symptom.

Pathogenesis of atopic eczema

The pathogenesis of atopic eczema is still remarkably obscure. There is clearly genetic programming of susceptibility, with the atopic state being determined in a polygenic manner. Twin studies show that in monozygotic twins there is a 75% concordance rate, while it is only 21% in dizygotic twins. However, what causes the susceptibility to become manifest as disease is unknown. Many observations have been made of abnormalities in the physiological functions of the skin and the immune system, but it is not clear how they fit together.

The dominant hypothesis is that the atopic state is primarily a dysregulation of the immune system, in which characteristics of the fetal immune system aimed at avoiding immune rejection between the mother and fetus somehow fail to mature into the adult immune responses designed to give protection against the extrauterine world. Thus in the fetus, T-helper cells differentiate towards the Th2 phenotype (Chapter 5.1.3 and 5.3). Following delivery, as the postnatal infant is colonized by microbes and exposed to endotoxin-producing pathogens, there is a change in the drivers of T-cell differentiation, resulting in the redirection of T-helper cells towards the Th1 phenotype. Lack of exposure to endotoxins from enteral pathogens is regarded as a major factor in the increase in the incidence of the atopic phenotype; the so-called hygiene hypothesis. So in early postnatal life the immune response of atopic individuals is directed via the Th2-derived cytokines IL-4, -5 and -13 to generate IgE, causing the activation of mast cells and eosinophils. This pattern of immune response correlates with the development of clinical atopic allergies, but it is not clear what causes the orientation to either the skin or mucosae.

Additional factors that may contribute to the altered immune response include constitutive overproduction of prostaglandin E2 and IL-10 by monocyte-macrophages, which favours Th2 differentiation. There is also evidence of constitutive overactivity of the cAMP-degrading enzyme phosphodiesterase 4. This results in the attenuation of intracellular signalling mediated via cAMP, but the consequences of this on the immune system or skin are not yet known.

Two main alterations have been detected in the skin itself. The first suggests an impaired contribution to innate immune responses. Thus, atopic eczematous skin produces decreased quantities of the antimicrobial peptides β-defensins, which have homologies with chemokines such as IL-8. This appears crucial in the increased susceptibility of atopic eczematous skin to infection by a range of microbes (see 'Microbes' below). The second alteration is the observation of a strong genetic association with mutations in the filaggrin gene. Filaggrin is a crucial component involved in the formation of the stratum corneum permeability barrier. This finding has not been confirmed in all populations studied, but it raises the important concept that altered permeability of the epidermis may be a primary factor in the development of atopic eczema.

The current working hypothesis is that atopic eczema, like other forms of eczematous inflammation, is a T-cell-mediated inflammation. However, the range of cells and mediators contributing to the pathogenesis is more complex than for other types of eczema. Thus, at the microscopic level atopic eczema is characterized by the infiltration of CD4+ T cells, and eosinophils. In acute lesions, degranulated mast cells can be seen. A factor thought to be of importance is the presence of IgE on the epidermal Langerhans' cells. Antigen-specific cell-bound IgE is thought to facilitate the presentation of very low levels of antigen to T cells, so-called antigen focusing. Atopic eczema is regarded as multifactorial; some of the recognized triggering or aggravating factors include airborne and dietary allergens, microbial colonization and infection, emotional factors, and climatic factors (temperature and humidity). There are probably other as yet unrecognized factors.

Role of allergy

There are two sides to allergy in atopic eczema: the demonstration of allergic sensitization by skin tests, and the ascertainment of the clinical significance of allergy in the provocation of an individual's eczema. There is clear evidence that immunological sensitization, reflected by the presence of specific IgE, occurs not only early in life, but even *in utero*. The pattern of allergen-specific IgE changes during the first 2 years of life from predominantly food-directed to airborne allergen-directed IgE.

Allergy to environmental airborne and/or food allergens is an important triggering factor in some, but not all individuals. There are major difficulties in determining which patients have clinically significant allergies contributing to driving the eczema. Different types of allergic response can be demonstrated with skin tests. Thus immediate, Type I, weal and flare responses can be elicited by prick tests in 80 to 95% of people with eczema. If allergens are administered by intradermal challenge, up to 30% will exhibit both immediate and late phase (6–12 h) responses. If allergens are administered by application as patch tests, depending on whether or not the stratum corneum permeability barrier is breached by prior stripping with cellophane tape, eczematous responses that replicate the clinical and histological features of eczema can be generated in up to 80% of patients. Also, if the patch-test challenge sites are inspected at the appropriate time, immediate (15 min) weal and flare responses are seen, and sometimes late phase (6 h) responses.

The practical difficulty is in determining whether these positive skin tests correlate with clinically significant allergic provocation. Most patients have current or previous mucosal allergies of asthma or rhinitis, and immediate reactions in prick tests generally correlate well with the allergic provocation of those symptoms rather than the eczema. However, very strongly positive prick-test responses to a given allergen often indicate that the allergen will aggravate the eczema. Positive patch tests with atopic allergens are reported to occur only in individuals with current or past eczema, and not in people with mucosal allergies and no eczema. Again, a strong patch-test response to a given allergen often indicates that the allergen has a significant role in provoking the eczema. Historical enquiry into which agents clearly exacerbate the eczema is usually unrewarding. One approach to establishing clinical relevance is allergen avoidance.

Allergen avoidance

This is only seriously practicable for house-dust mites, and foods. There is controversy in the literature as to the value of allergen avoidance measures. Tan *et al.* showed highly significant beneficial effects, whereas two other studies failed to show any benefit. The difference between the studies was the rigour of the dust-mite exclusion measures. Tan encased all the bedding components (duvet, pillows, and mattress) in sealed encasements, treated the carpets with a spray combining acaricidal and allergen-denaturing activity, and used a high-power high-filtration vacuum cleaner. Gutgesell used bedding encasements and a vacuum cleaner, and Oosting *et al.* only used bedding encasements. In fact in Tan's study, the combination of allergen-denaturing spray and vacuum cleaning resulted in a great reduction in the allergen load in the carpets, but the overall effect was not significantly better than that from the simple vacuum cleaner alone. So it is hard to explain why there are such differences in the results of the three studies. Dietary allergen exclusion has been explored in many studies, with the best effects being reported for infants and small children.

Microbes

Atopic eczema is highly susceptible to colonization and infection by coagulase-positive staphylococci. This was thought to result from the high relative humidity at the skin surface; even though the skin is dry to the touch the permeability barrier is defective, and there is a high transepidermal water loss. It is now known that an additional factor in the poor resistance to staphylococci is deficient production of the antimicrobial peptides β-defensins. Colonization by staphylococci that produce superantigens may lead to a general exacerbation of the eczematous inflammation. Infection by staphylococci results in folliculitis and/or acute exacerbations of eczema with weeping and crusting. Also, the development of fissures of the eyelids and/or ear lobes is usually a sign of staphylococcal infection.

Eczema is also susceptible to infection with herpes viruses, either herpes simplex or varicella–zoster. Eczema herpeticum is a potentially very serious condition that may lead to ocular damage, herpes encephalitis, or pneumonitis.

The head and neck pattern of eczema is thought to be provoked by the ubiquitous skin-surface yeast *Malassezia furfur*. Evidence is circumstantial, but is derived from the therapeutic response following treatment with imidazole antifungal agents.

Treatment of atopic eczema

The general approach is to: (1), avoid any provoking factors, i.e. irritants, contact sensitizers, or atopic allergens; (2), suppress inflammation with topical steroids (Box 23.6.2); and (3), give supporting symptomatic treatment.

Box 23.6.2 Treatment of eczema

Moisturizers/emollients
- Liquid oils or creams
- Greasy ointments

Topical steroids
- See Box 23.6.3

Topical calcineurin antagonists
- Tacrolimus
- Pimecrolimus

Systemic drugs
- Azathioprine
- Ciclosporin

Additional treatments
- Antibiotics if infected
- If wet/oozing, potassium permanganate soaks (1/10 000)

Allergen avoidance

If clear allergic provoking factors can be identified then avoidance measures can make a significant contribution to the control of atopic eczema. Dust-mite avoidance must be done properly; ideally, all three elements of the bedding (mattress, top covers, and pillows) should be encased in bags of the appropriate dust-proof material. However, these are often hot and intolerable, and replacing duvet/quilts with cotton cellular blankets that can be washed frequently is an alternative. Similarly, acrylic pillows and duvets can be subjected to hot washing and tumble drying every 3 months.

The avoidance of dietary provocations is often practised, particularly in babies and children, on an empirical basis. This should only be continued if good evidence that it is contributing can be obtained by provocation challenge.

Infection

Staphylococcal infection requires antibiotics; it is better to use systemic antibiotics for 7 to 10 days than topical forms, to reduce bacterial resistance. In patients with recurrent skin infection the use of moisturizers containing antiseptic agents in the bath or applied directly to the skin is helpful.

Itch

The mediators of itch in atopic eczema are not known, but the contribution of histamine is minimal. Although antihistamines are often given, it is more likely that the sedating effects of older antihistamines such as chlorpheniramine or trimeprazine make them better at symptom relief than nonsedating modern forms.

Skin inflammation

A crucial part of topical therapy is the use of emollient moisturizers (Box 23.6.2). These are available as liquid oils, thin creams, and thick ointments, with varying degrees of water miscibility. The application of moisturizers that the patient finds agreeable can have excellent anti-itch and soothing effects, thus reducing scratching and hence contributing to controlling the eczema. The technique of wet wrapping can be very helpful, particularly in babies and small children. This involves the initial application of a moisturizer to the limbs and torso, followed by the application of a double layer of tubular bandages, the inner layer being wetted with tepid water.

Topical steroids are the mainstay of treatment of the skin inflammation (see Box 23.6.3). In many patients, the chronic use of topical steroids may be ineffective or can result in steroid-induced side effects of striae, skin atrophy, and telangiectasia. In this case the topical calcineurin antagonists tacrolimus or pimecrolimus are indicated. If these are ineffective, a range of systemic drugs may be used. These include azathioprine, ciclosporin, methotrexate, and mycophenolate mofetil. Systemic steroids are reserved for acute rescue therapy of acute flares, but should not be used for long-term therapy.

Other forms of dermatitis/eczema

Seborrhoeic eczema

Seborrhoeic eczema is a response to the ubiquitous saprophytic skin yeast *Malassezia furfur*. The rash comprises erythematous dry areas, most classically affecting the nasolabial folds, scalp, and ears. The most minimal form of seborrhoeic eczema is dandruff; if it is more active the scalp becomes itchy and finally inflamed, with red scaly areas most typically around the hair margin. There may be circular coalescing areas on the central chest and/or upper back. Seborrhoeic eczema can mimic psoriasis, and indeed there is an entity termed sebopsoriasis, which behaves like psoriasis, but is in the distribution of seborrhoeic eczema. Most people experience minimal seborrhoeic eczema at some time. It is not known what causes the relationship with the fungus to change so that it induces an inflammatory reaction. People infected with HIV are prone to developing florid seborrhoeic eczema.

Treatment

The main treatment is with antifungal agents such as imidazoles in shampoo and topical forms; for severe cases systemic agents such as fluconazole may be used. For very symptomatic cases, low-potency topical steroids in combination with antifungal agents can be used to gain control, after which imidazole antifungals are usually sufficient for long-term control.

Dyshidrotic (pompholyx) eczema

This is an intensely itchy eruption affecting the palms and/or soles. It is characterized by tiny vesicles and blisters (pompholyx), which initially appear as small grey dots. The affected areas then become reddened, with hyperkeratotic scale that can fissure leading to painful splits. This is often a very chronic eczematous condition. It is thought that there is an associated disturbance of the structure or function of the sweat glands in the affected areas, hence the term dyshidrotic.

Differential diagnosis

It is important to exclude the presence of allergic contact dermatitis by careful history taking and diagnostic patch tests. It is also important to avoid irritants such as soaps; greasy moisturizers should be used as substitutes. Potent topical steroids are normally required, but often the condition is only poorly controlled. Systemic agents such as azathioprine may be required for the long-term control of severe cases.

Asteatotic eczema

Asteatosis indicates lack of oil/grease, a condition that develops gradually with increasing age, and that preferentially affects the lower legs. The epidermal surface becomes dry, and cracks develop in the scale. These cracks can become red and itchy, a characteristic appearance called eczema craquelé, one pattern of asteatotic eczema (Fig. 23.6.5). The other main pattern is a more typical eczematous inflammation, usually distributed on the lower legs in association with a generalized dryness and hyperkeratosis.

Treatment

The main component of treatment is replacement of the epidermal oils by the application of greasy moisturizers. In the acute phase, moderate-potency topical steroids in ointment base may be required to bring the symptoms under control.

Varicose eczema

Following deep venous thrombosis in the leg veins, the valves in the veins are damaged, causing a rise in the venous pressure gradient down the legs. Any cause of venous hypertension may reverse the direction of flow, channelling returning blood into the superficial veins. The raised pressure transmitted to the small veins and postcapillary venules results in plasma transudation, deposition of fibrin (which produces sclerosis and skin tethering), and leakage of erythrocytes, generating haemosiderin. The haemodynamic

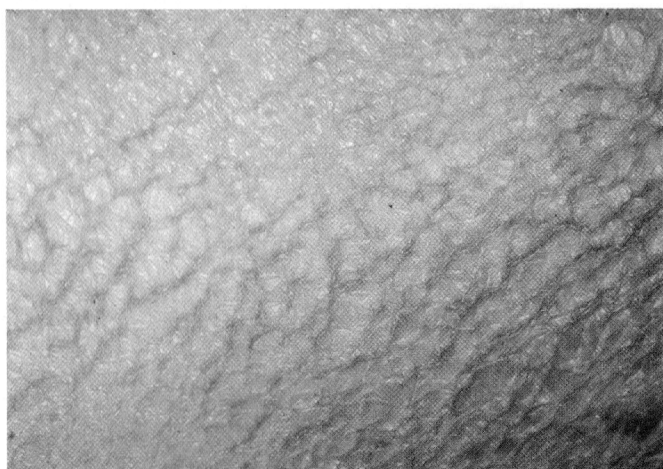

Fig. 23.6.5 Asteatotic eczema.

changes alter the nutritional provision to the skin. As part of this, perhaps by analogy with the processes underlying asteatotic eczema, there may develop a rather diffuse eczematous process. If the skin's nutritive blood supply is sufficiently compromised the tissue may break down, resulting in venous ulcer disease (Chapter 23.12.3).

Differential diagnosis

It is common for allergic contact dermatitis to develop on the lower legs affected by venous ulcers. The contact allergy is in response to ingredients of the many medicaments and impregnated bandages that are applied as part of the treatment.

Treatment

The most important component of therapy is external compression with stockings or bandages. This can improve the haemodynamics and restore the direction of venous return, with associated improvement in nutritive skin blood flow. The eczema is treated with moisturizers and a range of topical corticosteroids.

Ultraviolet-induced eczema or photodermatitis

Some people develop eczema in areas exposed to sunlight, mainly the face, neck, and dorsa of hands. There are two types of this photodermatitis; an apparently spontaneous reactivity to light, and chemically sensitized photoallergy. Many drugs can act as photoallergens, becoming converted to allergens by the combined effect of ultraviolet (UV) radiation and as yet undefined metabolic factors in the individual. Well-known examples are thiazide diuretics and quinine. The causal role is demonstrated by photopatch tests, in which the suspect chemical is applied to the back in duplicate; one test site is irradiated with long-wavelength ultraviolet (UVA), and the other is simply occluded. The role of photoallergy is shown by a positive response only at the UV-irradiated test site.

Even in people who develop apparently spontaneous photodermatitis, there is often the suspicion that plant-derived substances such as sesquiterpene lactones from the chrysanthemum family may be involved.

Treatment

This involves minimizing exposure to sunlight by wearing thick clothing and hats. Sunblock creams are only helpful if they are very thick and opaque. Potent topical steroids and even systemic agents such as azathioprine may be required.

Further reading

Calnan CD, Fregert S, Magnusson B (1976). The International Contact Dermatitis Research Group. *Cutis*, **18**, 708–10.

Cavani A, *et al.* (2003). Human CD25+ regulatory T cells maintain immune tolerance to nickel in healthy, nonallergic individuals. *J Immunol*, **171**, 5760–8.

Coenraads PJ, Smit J (1995). Epidemiology. In: Rycroft RJG, *et al.* (eds) *Textbook of contact dermatitis*, 3rd edition, pp. 133–50. Springer-Verlag, Berlin.

David TJ, *et al.* (2000). Dietary factors in established atopic dermatitis. In: Williams HC (ed) *Atopic dermatitis: The epidemiology, causes and prevention of atopic dermatitis*, pp. 193–201. Cambridge University Press, Cambridge.

de Jongh GJ, *et al.* (2005). High expression levels of keratinocyte antimicrobial proteins in psoriasis compared with atopic dermatitis. *J Invest Dermatol*, **125**, 1163–73.

Dickel H, *et al.* (2002). Importance of irritant contact dermatitis in occupational skin disease. *Am J Clin Dermatol*, **3**, 283–9.

Diepgen T (2000). Is the prevalence of atopic dermatitis increasing? In: Williams HC (ed) *Atopic dermatitis: The epidemiology, causes and prevention of atopic dermatitis*, pp. 96–109. Cambridge University Press, Cambridge.

Diepgen TL, Coenraads PJ (1999). The epidemiology of occupational contact dermatitis. *Int Arch Occup Environ Health*, **72**, 496–506.

Friedmann PS (1991). Graded continuity, or all or none—studies of the human immune response. *Clin Exp Dermatol*, **16**, 79–84.

Friedmann PS (2006). Contact sensitisation and allergic contact dermatitis: immunobiological mechanisms. *Toxicol Lett*, **162**, 49–54.

Friedmann PS, *et al.* (1993). Early time course of recruitment of immune surveillance in human skin after chemical provocation. *Clin Exp Immunol*, **91**, 351–6.

Gerberick GF, *et al.* (2000). Local lymph node assay: validation assessment for regulatory purposes. *Am J Contact Dermatitis*, **11**, 3–18.

Gutgesell C, *et al.* (2001). Double-blind placebo-controlled house dust mite control measures in adult patients with atopic dermatitis. *Br J Dermatol*, **145**, 70–4.

Kusel MM, *et al.* (2005). Support for 2 variants of eczema. *J Allergy Clin Immunol*, **116**, 1067–72.

Lachapelle JM (1995). Histopathological and immunohistopathological features of irritant and allergic contact dermatitis. In: Rycroft RJG, Menne T, Frosch PJ (eds) *Textbook of contact dermatitis*, 3rd edition, pp. 91–102. Springer-Verlag, Berlin.

Lintu P, *et al.* (2001). Systemic ketoconazole is an effective treatment of atopic dermatitis with IgE-mediated hypersensitivity to yeasts. *Allergy*, **56**, 512–17.

Meding B (1990). Epidemiology of hand eczema in an industrial city. *Acta Derm Venereol Suppl (Stockh)*, **153**, 1–43.

Miles EA, *et al.* (1996). Peripheral blood mononuclear cell proliferative responses in the first year of life in babies born to allergic parents. *Clin Exp Allergy*, **26**, 780–8.

Mudde GC, Bheekha R, Bruijnzeel-Koomen CA (1995). Consequences of IgE/CD23-mediated antigen presentation in allergy. *Immunol Today*, **16**, 380–3.

Ohmen JD, *et al.* (1995). Overexpression of IL-l0 in atopic dermatitis. Contrasting cytokine patterns with delayed-type hypersensitivity reactions. *J Immunol*, **154**, 1956–63.

Oosting AJ, *et al.* (2002). Effect of mattress encasings on atopic dermatitis outcome measures in a double-blind, placebo-controlled study: the Dutch mite avoidance study. *J Allergy Clin Immunol*, **110**, 500–6.

Palmer CN, *et al.* (2006). Common loss-of-function variants of the epidermal barrier protein filaggrin are a major predisposing factor for atopic dermatitis. *Nat Genet*, **38**, 441–6.

Patrick E, Maibach HI (1995). Predictive assays: animal and man, and *in vitro* and *in vivo*. In: Rycroft RJG, Menne T, Frosch P (eds) *Textbook of contact dermatitis*, 3rd edition, pp. 705–747. Springer-Verlag, Berlin.

Raghupathy R (2001). Pregnancy: success and failure within the Th1/Th2/Th3 paradigm. *Semin Immunol*, **13**, 219–27.

Schultz Larsen FV (1993). The epidemiology of atopic dermatitis. *Monogr Allergy*, **31**, 9–28.

Strachan DP (1989). Hay fever, hygiene, and household size. *BMJ*, **299**, 1259–60.

Tan BB, *et al.* (1996). Double-blind controlled trial of effect of housedust-mite allergen avoidance on atopic dermatitis. *Lancet*, **347**, 15–18.

Warner JA, *et al.* (1996). Prenatal sensitisation. *Pediatr Allergy Immunol*, **7**, 98–101.

Willis CM, Stephens CJM, Wilkinson JD (1993). Differential patterns of epidermal leukocyte infiltration in patch test reactions to structurally unrelated chemical irritants. *J Invest Dermatol*, **101**, 364–70.

23.7

Cutaneous vasculitis, connective tissue diseases, and urticaria

Susan Burge and Graham S. Ogg

Essentials

Vasculitis (angiitis) denotes necrotizing inflammation of the blood vessels; occlusive vasculopathy implies vascular occlusion without significant vascular inflammation. A small-vessel cutaneous vasculitis is the most common vasculitis affecting the skin, and may be the first sign of a systemic vasculitis, but 50% of patients have no systemic disease. The clinical findings must be integrated with the results of serological, pathological, and imaging studies to reach a diagnosis.

Systemic lupus erythematosus (SLE) is diagnosed if four or more of the American College of Rheumatology revised criteria for the classification of SLE are present, either sequentially or simultaneously (Chapter 19.11.2). These include four mucocutaneous signs: malar rash, discoid rash, photosensitivity, and oral ulcers. Skin lesions are the first manifestation of SLE in 23 to 28% of patients; about 73% of patients report photosensitivity, and up to 91% develop cutaneous symptoms at some stage in the evolution of their disease.

Dermatomyositis is an uncommon multisystem autoimmune disease in which inflammatory skin changes are associated with polymyositis of skeletal muscle. The clinical spectrum ranges from pure cutaneous disease, through coexisting patterns of cutaneous/ systemic disease, to isolated inflammatory polymyositis. Cutaneous involvement may precede the onset of myositis by several years, but some patients never have muscle involvement (amyotrophic dermatomyositis).

Scleroderma means thickened, fibrotic, bound-down skin. It may develop in association with a systemic connective tissue disease (systemic sclerosis) or present as a localized cutaneous problem. Localized scleroderma, unlike systemic sclerosis, is a self-limiting condition confined to the skin and subcutaneous tissue; it does not transform into systemic sclerosis. Dermatologists tend to use the term 'morphoea' for localized disease, while paediatricians and rheumatologists refer to the same condition as 'scleroderma'.

Panniculitis is inflammation of the subcutaneous fat, sometimes associated with vasculitis. It presents with erythematous subcutaneous nodules, most often on the lower leg.

Cutaneous vasculitis and occlusive vasculopathy

Historical perspective

Although some types of cutaneous vasculitis (angiitis) target vessels of a given size, the vascular lesions are patchy, and patients with the same disease may have different patterns of organ involvement, so clinical presentations are hugely variable. The most commonly used classifications of the vasculitides are those of the American College of Rheumatology in 1990, and the 1992 Chapel Hill Consensus Conference. The American College of Rheumatology classification is based on clinical, historical, and histological data, whereas the names and definitions in the Chapel Hill Consensus Conference criteria are based on histopathological findings. Unfortunately, neither system provides clinicians with robust diagnostic criteria (the American College of Rheumatology criteria had a positive predictive value of 17–29% in diagnosing vasculitic syndromes), and the systems conflict in a number of respects.

Pathogenesis

Vasculitis may be primary (idiopathic), or a secondary event in diseases associated with circulating immune complexes, such as rheumatoid arthritis, systemic lupus erythematosus, inflammatory bowel disease, infections, or malignancy. Inflammation and necrosis of blood vessel walls leads to extravasation of red blood cells, vascular obstruction, and tissue ischaemia or infarction. The clinical features depend on the size of the affected vessels, the sites involved (frequently the earliest signs are in the skin), and the intensity of the inflammation. Genetic background also influences disease expression and outcome.

Many vasculitic syndromes are caused by an immune reaction to an unidentified external or constituent antigen, although bacteria, rickettsiae, and fungi can also induce vasculitis directly, by invading vessel walls. The pattern of disease is probably influenced by the size of the immune complexes and local factors such as haemodynamics (turbulence may favour deposition of immune complexes), temperature, and hydrostatic pressure. Activated neutrophils release proteolytic enzymes, along with oxygen free radicals, that damage the vessel walls and the surrounding tissues. Tissue specificity may be determined by the expression of adhesion molecules that mediate interactions between lymphocytes and endothelial cells, as well as interactions between chemokines and chemokine receptors that direct lymphocyte traffic.

Vasculitic reaction patterns may be classified broadly into allergic angiitis (type I reaction), antibody-associated vasculitis (type II reaction), immune-complex vasculitis (type III reaction), and vasculitis associated with T-cell-mediated hypersensitivity (type IV reaction) (Box 23.7.2). The features of vasculitic syndromes overlap, and more than one type of immune reaction may be involved during the course of a single disease. The relative dominance of mechanisms also varies among patients with the same disease.

Urticarial vasculitis is the prototype of an allergic vasculitis (type I reaction). Activated Th2 lymphocytes release cytokines (interleukin (IL)-4, IL-5, and IL-13) that mediate the accumulation of mast cells, basophils, and eosinophils.

Type II immune reactions seem to predominate in Wegener's granulomatosis and microscopic polyangiitis, two vasculitides closely associated with the generation of antineutrophil cytoplasmic antibodies (ANCA). In Wegener's granulomatosis, ANCA react with proteinase 3 to produce diffuse immunofluorescent cytoplasmic staining. In microscopic polyangiitis, antibodies to cytoplasmic myeloperoxidase produce a perinuclear immunofluorescent staining pattern. Some studies suggest a direct pathogenic link between ANCA and the development of glomerulonephritis and vasculitis. ANCA might mediate vessel-wall injury and aggravate inflammation by activating neutrophils, promoting the adherence of neutrophils to vessel walls, triggering the release of tumour necrosis factor (TNF) from macrophages, and interfering with apoptosis and the clearance of neutrophils. The factors responsible for the generation and perpetuation of these autoantibodies are not clear, but in some circumstances infections may trigger the ANCA response. Type II mechanisms may also be relevant in conditions such as systemic lupus erythematosus, rheumatoid arthritis, and systemic sclerosis, when antibodies binding to endothelial cell antigens may generate a thrombogenic vasculopathy.

Henoch–Schönlein purpura, cryoglobulinaemic vasculitis, and other forms of small-vessel cutaneous vasculitis are associated with an immune complex-mediated reaction (type III reaction). Complement is activated, and Th2-type cytokines (IL-10, IL-6) may perpetuate inflammation. Most patients have polyclonal hypergammaglobulinaemia or autoantibodies. Immunoglobulins and complement can be detected in blood vessel walls.

Type IV immune reactions may underlie the granulomatous vasculitis seen in large-vessel vasculitides such as temporal arteritis and Takayasu's arteritis. Lymphocytes and monocytes invade blood vessel walls, but the infiltrate is dominated by CD4+ Th1-type cells that produce interferon-γ.

Small-vessel cutaneous vasculitis

This is also known as leukocytoclastic angiitis/vasculitis, cutaneous/small-vessel necrotizing vasculitis, allergic vasculitis, and hypersensitivity angiitis.

Aetiology and pathology

The aetiology of small-vessel cutaneous vasculitis is uncertain (idiopathic) in at least 50% of patients, but has been ascribed to infections in 15 to 20% of patients, inflammatory diseases such as connective tissue diseases in 15 to 20% of patients, drugs in 10 to 15% of patients (usually 7–21 days after commencing the drug), and malignancies, especially lymphoproliferative disorders, in 5% of patients. Prolonged exercise (long-distance walks, marathons) may trigger a cutaneous vasculitis of the leg (exercise-induced purpura).

Small-vessel cutaneous vasculitis involves dermal small vessels, predominantly postcapillary venules. The histological findings include perivascular neutrophilic inflammation extending into vessel walls, with swelling and injury of endothelial cells; necrosis of vessel walls; fibrinoid deposition around vessels (fibrinoid necrosis); and extravasation of red blood cells. The presence of nuclear dust is indicative of leukocytoclasis (fragmentation of the nuclei of neutrophils).

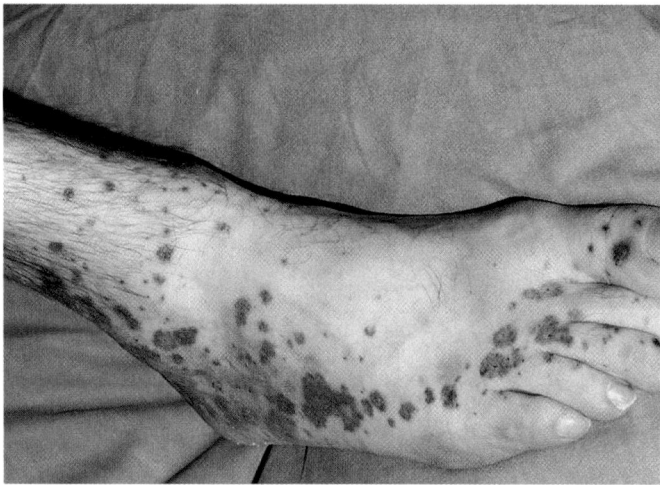

Fig. 23.7.1 Palpable purpura is the hallmark of small-vessel cutaneous vasculitis. Small oval or round purpuric papules are found in areas of stasis (below the knee), at pressure sites (elbows, sacrum, waist band), or at sites of cooling.

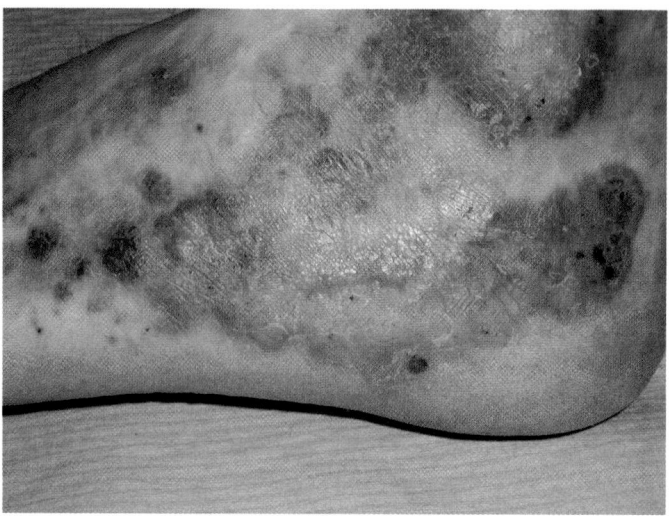

Fig. 23.7.2 Vasculitic papules have coalesced into plaques in this patient (also shown in Fig. 23.7.1) with chronic vasculitis. Stasis localizes disease and aggravates the clinical findings.

Clinical features

Palpable purpura, usually on the lower leg, is the hallmark of small-vessel cutaneous vasculitis (Fig. 23.7.1). The purpuric lesions are palpable because the purpura is accompanied by inflammation and increased vascular permeability. This contrasts with the flat petechiae and purpura seen in noninflammatory conditions such as thrombocytopenic purpura. Radial diffusion of red blood cells that have leaked from small vessels in the upper dermis produces small oval or round purpuric papules. Thrombosis with infarction is unusual in a small-vessel cutaneous vasculitis, but irregularly outlined indurated areas of haemorrhagic infarct are produced when deeper dermal or subcutaneous vessels become thrombosed in other conditions.

Early in the course of systemic vasculitis, patients may complain of rather nonspecific flu-like symptoms such as myalgia, migratory arthralgia, or synovitis. Patients present with a symmetrical purpuric rash in dependent areas such as the leg, at sites of trauma (Koebner phenomenon), pressure sites (elbows, sacrum, waist band), or sites of cooling. Oval or circular erythematous lesions rapidly become raised (palpable) and purpuric, sometimes coalescing into larger polycyclic lesions (Figs. 23.7.2, 23.7.3). Some patients develop annular purpuric lesions with haemorrhagic or vesicular centres, or superficial ulceration. Intense inflammation produces haemorrhagic bullae or pustules. Lesions fade gradually over 3 or 4 weeks leaving macular pigmentation (haemosiderin) (Fig. 23.7.3) or atrophic scars.

Differential diagnosis

Purpura does not blanch with light pressure, unlike erythema. Purpuric lesions may be divided into those that are associated with inflammatory pathology (vasculitis) and are palpable, and those that are noninflammatory and flat, i.e. macular. Scattered flat purpuric spots may be a nonspecific finding on the legs in association with inflammatory dermatoses such as psoriasis or stasis eczema. The frail sun-damaged skin on the forearms of older patients, or skin that has been thinned after prolonged exposure to corticosteroids, is prone to developing large flat bruises (ecchymoses) after minor trauma. Scurvy causes perifollicular purpura with corkscrew

hairs in the centre of the spots. Disorders associated with thrombocytopenia produce flat purpuric lesions and petechiae. Cholesterol emboli may produce asymmetrical acral petechiae and subcutaneous nodules, often in association with livedo reticularis (see 'Thrombo-occlusive vasculopathies' below). Livedo reticularis is also associated with a necrotizing vasculitis affecting deeper cutaneous vessels. Disseminated intravascular coagulation (see 'Septic vasculitis' below) produces extensive irregularly outlined haemorrhagic areas.

The vasculitic lesions in idiopathic small-vessel cutaneous vasculitis are clinically and histologically identical to the cutaneous lesions in small-vessel cutaneous vasculitis occurring as a component of a systemic disease. The clinician must rule out systemic disease and also search for other cutaneous signs of vasculitis, such as livedo reticularis or nodules.

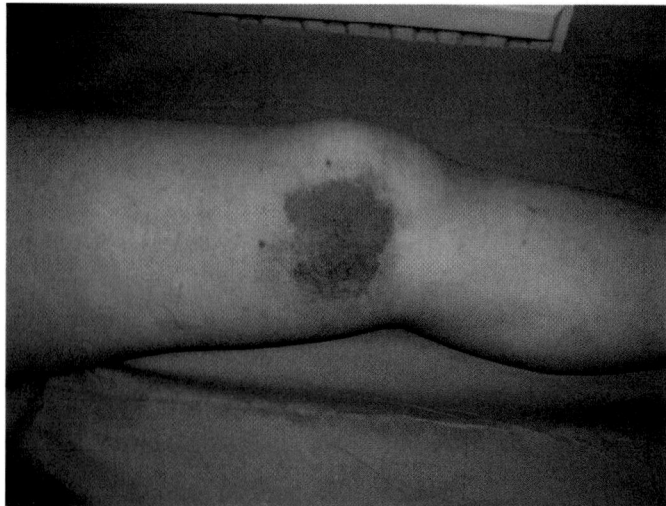

Fig. 23.7.3 This young woman has an unexplained small-vessel cutaneous vasculitis without systemic involvement, which is characterized by the sudden onset of painful purpuric plaques that resolve leaving bruising.

Clinical investigation

The history, physical examination, and investigations must determine the extent of any systemic disease and identify causative agents: drugs; infections including hepatitis B or C; or conditions associated with circulating immune complexes, such as connective tissue diseases, inflammatory bowel disease, lymphoma, multiple myeloma, leukaemia, and solid tumours.

Preliminary laboratory screening should include full blood-cell count, inflammatory markers (erythrocyte sedimentation rate, C-reactive protein), urinalysis, renal function tests, liver function tests, hepatitis B and C serology, complement levels (C3, C4), immunoglobulins, rheumatoid factor, and antinuclear antibody. Cryoglobulins should be measured if C4 is low. ANCA should only be checked if there is evidence of systemic disease. If these laboratory studies are normal, further testing to rule out a systemic vasculitis is probably not warranted unless the history and physical examination are not consistent with limited cutaneous disease. A streptococcal sore throat is a common precursor of vasculitis in children, and otitis media, dental caries, cystitis, and sinusitis occasionally play a role. In many countries tuberculosis or leprosy is the most common cause; bacterial endocarditis and meningococcal septicaemia are often missed. Other treatable infections occasionally causing vasculitis are syphilis and those caused by neisseria, rickettsiae, and mycoplasma. Although viruses cannot usually be eliminated, any history of a recent flu-like illness or vaccination may be relevant.

A skin biopsy to confirm a small-vessel cutaneous vasculitis should be taken from a palpable purpuric lesion about 12 to 24 h old. A biopsy taken too late may not show the initial injury. However, the histology is unlikely to reveal the cause of the vasculitis, exclude systemic disease, or distinguish one form of systemic vasculitis from another.

In patients with evidence of deep necrotizing vasculitis (livedo reticularis and ulcerated nodules), an incisional biopsy down to fat is necessary to detect pathology in arterioles or small arteries, but if a large-vessel vasculitis is suspected, a biopsy from involved tissue in muscle, nerve, or lung will be more informative than a skin biopsy. The investigation of the systemic vasculitides is discussed in more detail in Sections 18 and 20 in particular.

Treatment

Precipitating agents (drugs or infection) must be identified and removed, but it may still take several weeks for vasculitis to settle. Local factors that might exacerbate or localize vasculitis (cooling, stasis, trauma) should be minimized by simple measures such as warmth, leg elevation, support stockings, and exercise.

Dapsone (50–200 mg/day) is effective in controlling limited cutaneous vasculitis. Colchicine (0.6 mg twice daily) and low-dose methotrexate (10–25 mg/week) have also been recommended. Most patients with small-vessel vasculitis limited to the skin do not require systemic corticosteroids or more aggressive treatment with immunosuppressive agents.

Prognosis

Idiopathic small-vessel vasculitis confined to the skin resolves within a few weeks or months. Most patients have a single episode, but about 10% have recurrent disease that may last months or years. Exercise-induced vasculitis fades in a few days.

Increased understanding of the pathogenesis of vasculitis may lead to the development of targeted immunotherapy with monoclonal antibodies to cell adhesion molecules or cytokines that will control the autoimmune response and reduce inflammation.

Small-vessel cutaneous vasculitis associated with systemic disease

Henoch–Schönlein purpura

Pathogenesis

Henoch–Schönlein purpura is triggered by infection, often in the upper respiratory tract, and is associated with IgA immune complexes in the circulation and vessel walls. It is the most common small-vessel systemic vasculitis in children, but it may also affect adults.

Clinical features

The cutaneous signs are similar to those of other cutaneous small-vessel vasculitides, but in children the urticarial component may be more prominent than in adults. A symmetrical macular erythema develops on the extensor surfaces of the limbs, and the buttocks and back. Lesions become raised and purpuric, but regress over 10 to 14 days. In addition, children may have any combination of arthritis, gastrointestinal tract involvement, and nephritis. Infantile acute haemorrhagic oedema of the skin is a benign condition that is probably a variant of Henoch–Schönlein purpura in which the oedematous component is particularly marked.

Treatment

In the absence of severe systemic disease, treatment is supportive. Corticosteroids or dapsone may be prescribed in severe disease, although it is not known if these drugs affect the duration of illness or the frequency of relapse. Rapidly progressive renal failure is rare, and the prognosis is excellent. Relapses are usually mild and do not require treatment.

Erythema elevatum diutinum

Clinical features

This indolent cutaneous vasculitis involves the extensor surfaces of joints, and the buttocks. The purpuric red-brown papules, nodules, and plaques may persist for years, remit and relapse, or disappear. Erythema elevatum diutinum has been described in association with systemic diseases such as myeloma, myelodysplasia, acute myelogenous leukaemia, inflammatory bowel disease, relapsing polychondritis, and rheumatoid arthritis.

Cryoglobulinaemic vasculitis and occlusive vasculopathy

Aetiology, pathogenesis, and pathology

Cryoglobulins are immunoglobulins that precipitate at low temperatures and are classified according to their immunochemical composition. Type I cryoglobulins (monoclonal immunoglobulins) are present in 25% of cases; type II mixed cryoglobulins (a mixture of monoclonal and polyclonal immunoglobulins) are present in 25% of cases; and type III mixed cryoglobulins (polyclonal immunoglobulins only) are present in 50% of cases. Most patients are women aged 30 to 50 years.

Type I cryoglobulinaemia is always associated with a malignant haematological disorder such as chronic lymphatic leukaemia, multiple myeloma, or Waldenström's macroglobulinemia. The cryoglobulins obstruct the vessels rather than trigger an inflammatory vasculitis, and are associated with cold sensitivity. A skin biopsy, particularly from the edge of an ulcer, reveals an occlusive vascular disease (vasculopathy). The small cutaneous blood vessels are plugged by homogenous eosinophilic material, and there is red blood cell extravasation with a perivascular mononuclear cell infiltrate, but no vasculitis.

In most patients, hepatitis C virus (HCV) infection underlies type II mixed cryoglobulinaemia. HCV infection triggers B-cell clonal expansions, primarily in the liver. These expansions are associated with high serum levels of polyclonal rheumatoid factor and cryoglobulins, as well as monoclonal gammopathy of undetermined significance and, rarely, non-Hodgkin's B-cell lymphoma. The pathogenesis of malignant B-cell transformation is uncertain. HCV particles and nonenveloped nucleocapsid protein participate in the formation of the immune complexes that are precipitated in the vessel walls of many organs. The complexes then activate the complement cascade, producing a small-vessel vasculitis affecting venules, capillaries, and arterioles. Mixed cryoglobulinaemia may also be associated with connective tissue diseases such as rheumatoid arthritis or systemic lupus erythematosus, as well as other infections.

Clinical features

Patients with type I cryoglobulinaemia complain of Raynaud's phenomenon, mottling of the skin, or blotchy cyanosis on exposure to cold. Acrocyanosis affects the helices of the ears as well as the fingers and toes (Fig. 23.7.4). Cold-induced lesions may be urticarial and then become purpuric. Cold triggers the formation of large haemorrhagic bullae that break down to produce ulcers.

More than 90% of patients with mixed cryoglobulinaemia develop palpable purpura, and in most this is the first sign of the disease. Fifteen per cent of patients have chronic leg ulcers, usually above the malleoli. These are surrounded by purpura, but patients have no other evidence of stasis (Fig. 23.7.5). Patients may also have Raynaud's phenomenon (30%), cold urticaria (10%), arthralgia (70%), renal involvement (20–30%), and/or sensorimotor neuropathy (60%).

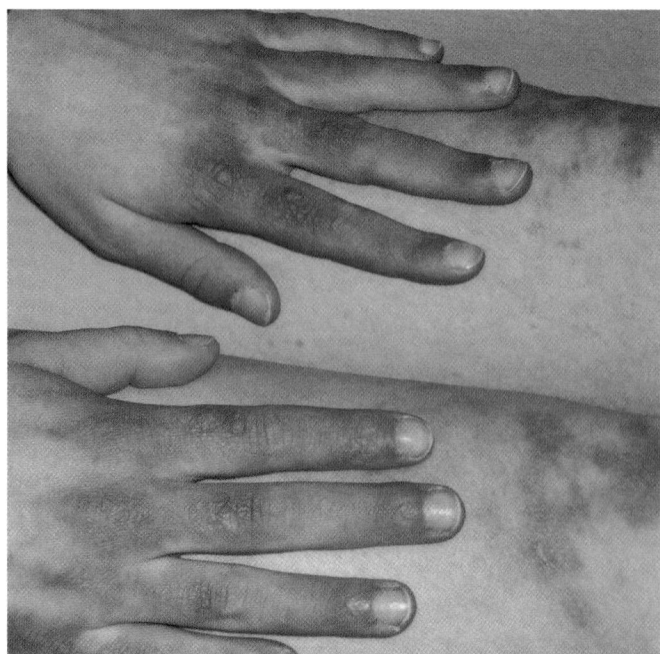

Fig. 23.7.4 Acrocyanosis of the fingers in a young girl with an urticarial vasculitis, but no systemic disease. She also had chilblain-like lesions on the ears and nose. Although cold appeared to trigger cutaneous disease, no cryoglobulins were found.

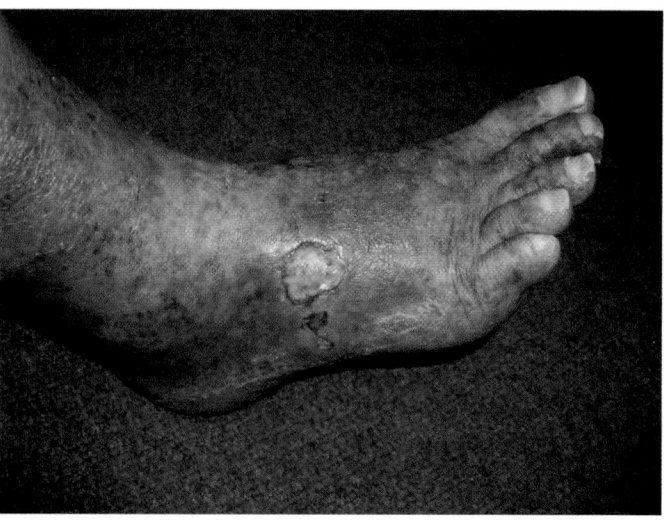

Fig. 23.7.5 Ulceration surrounded by palpable purpura in a patient with mixed cryoglobulinaemic vasculitis.

Clinical investigation

Measuring complement C4 is a useful screening test because C4 is very low in mixed cryoglobulinaemia. Cryoglobulins are present in serum, but the blood specimen taken for cryoglobulins must be kept warm (37°C) and it may be easier to send the patient than the sample to the immunology laboratory. Rheumatoid factor can sometimes be detected. Skin biopsy may show obstructive vasculopathy (Type I cryoglobulinaemia) or vasculitis (mixed cryoglobulinaemia).

Treatment

Underlying lymphoproliferative disorders or connective tissue diseases should be treated, and patients should keep warm. Compression bandaging may reduce venous stasis and improve leg ulceration. In HCV infection, interferon-α reduces viral load and cryoglobulinaemia, but about 80% of responders relapse within 6 months. Few data are available on the response of neuropathy, renal disease, or cutaneous ulceration to this treatment. The treatment for patients without HCV infection, or those with progressive disease, may involve corticosteroids in combination with cytotoxic agents. Plasmapheresis has been used to treat rapidly progressive cryoglobulinaemic vasculitis.

Urticarial vasculitis

Pathogenesis and pathology

Urticarial vasculitis occurs in association with connective tissue diseases, serum sickness (approximately 10 days after the administration of drugs or vaccines), infection (including HCV), IgM or IgG gammopathy, and haematological malignancies. Skin biopsy shows prominent dermal oedema with evidence of a leukocytoclastic vasculitis, but changes of vasculitis may be quite subtle.

Clinical features

Urticaria is characterized by the presence of a recurring itchy rash consisting of smooth erythematous papules (weals) that fade in about 24 h to leave normal skin. By contrast, the weals of urticarial vasculitis are tender or they burn, they last up to 72 h, and may resolve leaving bruising (Fig. 23.7.6). Urticarial vasculitis is associated with low complement levels in 18% of patients. This subtype is more likely to be associated with systemic disease, and patients

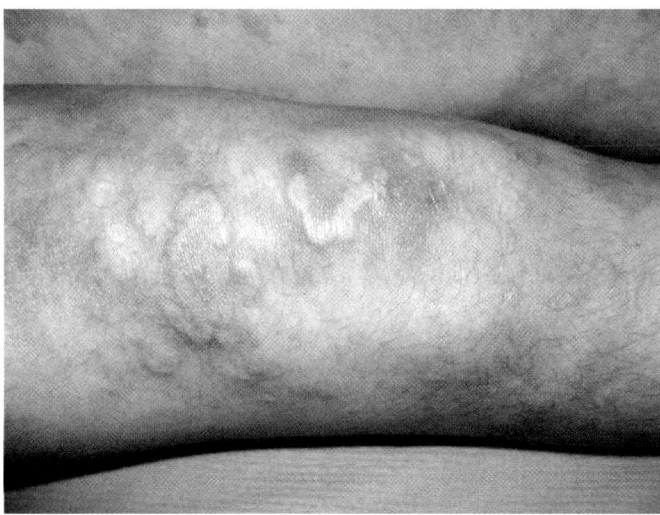

Fig. 23.7.6 Urticarial vasculitis: tender urticated papules and plaques that are associated with purpura and resolve with bruising

have a higher incidence of arthritis, asthma, and gastrointestinal symptoms than those with normal complement levels. Some patients with low complement levels have anti-C1q antibodies and overlapping features with systemic lupus erythematosus, including pleuritis, glomerulonephritis, eye symptoms, and positive anti-nuclear antibodies.

Treatment

Antihistamines or nonsteroidal anti-inflammatory drugs (NSAIDs) may be effective. Prednisolone is helpful, but alternatives such as dapsone, colchicine, or hydroxychloroquine should be considered to avoid the side effects of prolonged treatment with systemic corticosteroids.

Cutaneous vasculitis and malignancy

Small-vessel cutaneous vasculitis, erythema elevatum diutinum, and urticarial vasculitis have been described in association with lymphoproliferative disorders, e.g. Hodgkin's disease, mycosis fungoides, lymphosarcoma, adult T-cell leukaemia, multiple myeloma, and less often with solid tumours, e.g. cancer of the colon, kidney, prostate, head and neck, or breast. Vasculitis may present 2 to 4 years before the manifestation of the tumour.

Cutaneous vasculitis of medium and small vessels

Vasculitis associated with connective tissue disease

Patients with diseases such as systemic sclerosis, rheumatoid arthritis, or systemic lupus erythematosus may develop signs of small-vessel cutaneous vasculitis, including palpable purpuric lesions on the legs, palms, or digits, haemorrhagic bullae, papulonecrotic purpuric lesions, urticarial vasculitis, or punched-out necrotic ulcers. Vasculitis may also involve larger vessels, particularly in rheumatoid arthritis (Chapter 19.5) and systemic lupus erythematosus, with livedo reticularis (see 'Thrombo-occlusive vasculopathies' below), ulcers, nodules, digital gangrene, or pyoderma gangrenosum-like lesions.

ANCA-associated vasculitis

ANCA-associated vasculitis affects people of all ages, but is most common in adults in their 50s and 60s, and is the most common primary systemic vasculitis affecting adults. The three major subtypes have overlapping features:

1 Wegener's granulomatosis (granulomatous inflammation of the upper and lower airways, necrotizing small-vessel vasculitis, and necrotizing glomerulonephritis)

2 Microscopic polyangiitis (necrotizing glomerulonephritis, pulmonary capillaritis without asthma, necrotizing small-vessel vasculitis)

3 Churg–Strauss syndrome (allergic rhinitis and asthma, eosinophilia, necrotizing small-vessel vasculitis, and eosinophil-rich or granulomatous inflammation involving the respiratory tract)

Clinical features

Cutaneous lesions have been described during the course of disease in around 70% of patients, but signs of a cutaneous vasculitis are present at disease onset in more than 40% of patients with microscopic polyangiitis and 8 to 10% of those with Wegener's granulomatosis. The vasculitic phase does not develop until about 3 years after the onset of asthma in Churg–Strauss syndrome.

The cutaneous findings vary, but the most common (and least specific) finding in all three conditions is a palpable purpuric rash on the lower extremities. Progressive ulceration in Wegener's granulomatosis may resemble pyoderma gangrenosum, and can affect unusual sites such as the face, neck, or perianal skin. Livedo reticularis is found in some patients. Patients with Wegener's granulomatosis or Churg–Strauss syndrome may develop lesions associated with a large-vessel vasculitis, such as cutaneous ulcers or subcutaneous nodules. In both Wegener's granulomatosis and Churg–Strauss syndrome, ulcerated papules (papulonecrotic lesions) resembling rheumatoid nodules are found on the limbs, particularly the elbows, but can occur on the face and scalp. These diseases are discussed in further detail in other organ-specific chapters (in particular Sections 15, 18, 19, and 21).

Septic vasculitis
Pathogenesis

Organisms can damage blood vessels by direct invasion, by the release of endotoxins that provoke a thrombotic response (disseminated intravascular coagulation), or by inducing an immune-mediated vasculitis. Purpuric lesions are most often seen in infective endocarditis, meningococcaemia, gonococcaemia, Gram-negative septicaemia, and certain rickettsial infections. A septic vasculitis can follow any intravascular procedure.

Clinical features

The cutaneous signs in infective endocarditis include mucosal petechiae, Osler's nodes (tender erythematous spots on the pulps of the fingers and toes), and Janeway's lesions (nontender red or haemorrhagic macules or nodules on the palms and soles). In sub-acute disease, circulating immune complexes probably trigger a leukocytoclastic vasculitis in small vessels that is responsible for mucocutaneous lesions, but septic emboli may play a direct role in the pathogenesis of vasculitic lesions in acute disease. Unilateral emboli following a percutaneous arterial puncture may indicate a septic endarteritis. Disseminated intravascular coagulation (DIC) is a devastating disease characterized by extensive purpura, haematomas, haemorrhagic infarcts, and gangrene. Persistent cyanosis of the extremities is an early sign. DIC is not a vasculitis, but an occlusive vasculopathy in which fibrin thrombi occlude capillaries, venules, and vessels in the deeper dermis and subcutis, leading to ischaemia and infarction. DIC is discussed in detail in other organ-specific chapters, in Section 22.

The purpuric lesions of acute meningococcaemia are present on the limbs or trunk in 80 to 90% of patients within 12 to 36 h of disease onset, but may be small and few in number (Chapter 7.6.5). These lesions are followed by DIC, with large irregular indurated ecchymoses with central necrosis that may progress to extensive gangrene. Septic emboli in Gram-negative septicaemia caused by *Escherichia coli*, pseudomonas, or klebsiella produce vasculitic lesions that present as erythematous weals and papules that become irregularly purpuric and necrotic.

The immune complex-mediated febrile illnesses in patients with chronic meningococcaemia or chronic disseminated gono-coccaemia are associated with arthralgia, arthritis, and cutaneous vasculitis. Scattered purpuric papules and vesicopustules appear on the trunk and extremities in chronic meningococcaemia, but have a predilection for the palms, fingers, and soles in disseminated gonococcaemia. The histology is a leukocytoclastic vasculitis with thrombosis in small vessels.

The maculopapular rash of Rocky Mountain spotted fever is initially erythematous, but becomes petechial and purpuric within 24 to 48 h. *Rickettsia rickettsii* invades the walls of small cutaneous vessels, inducing a focal lymphocytic vasculitis with extravasation of red blood cells, and occasional thrombosis. Infections are dealt with in detail in Section 7.

Cutaneous involvement in medium- and large-vessel vasculitis

Polyarteritis nodosa

Polyarteritis nodosa is a life-threatening necrotizing segmental vasculitis that involves vessels ranging in size from arterioles to medium-sized arteries. The panarteritis results in aneurysms that may be demonstrated by arteriography of renal or mesenteric arteries. It may be associated with hepatitis B infection. Systemic complications include renal disease, hypertension, and peripheral neuropathy. Cutaneous manifestations are infrequent, but palpable purpura, indicative of a small-vessel cutaneous vasculitis, is the most common cutaneous sign (see 'Small-vessel cutaneous vasculitis' above). Signs of large-vessel disease include livedo reticularis, cutaneous nodules, ulcers, and peripheral gangrene.

Kawasaki disease

Kawasaki disease (mucocutaneous lymph node syndrome) is a multisystem vasculitis of infants and small children. The disease follows an acute course over 4 to 6 weeks, with fever, erythema of the palms and soles and/or oedema of the hands and feet, an erythematous rash, bilateral conjunctival injection, dry red lips, and cervical lymphadenopathy. Vasculitis affects large, medium, and small arteries, both external to organs and within many organs including the heart. Coronary aneurysms develop in about 20% of patients, and ischaemic heart disease causes myocardial infarction and sudden death. Intravenous gammaglobulin plus aspirin controls fever and reduces the formation of aneurysms (Chapter 18.10.8).

Cutaneous polyarteritis nodosa
Pathogenesis and pathology

A benign cutaneous form of polyarteritis nodosa has been described, but the relationship of this condition to the systemic disease is uncertain, and the cause is unknown. A necrotizing vasculitis affects small and medium-sized muscular-walled arteries in the deep dermis and subcutis.

Clinical features

Painful cutaneous nodules, purpura, ulceration, and livedo reticularis (see 'Thrombo-occlusive vasculopathies' below) occur on the lower limbs (Fig. 23.7.7). Cutaneous polyarteritis nodosa may be associated with fever, malaise, arthralgia, myalgia, and peripheral neuropathy, but major organs are not involved. The disease is chronic and recurrent.

Investigation

Patients should be screened for systemic involvement, but laboratory findings are generally unremarkable, except for leukocytosis and an elevated erythrocyte sedimentation rate. Deep incisional biopsies are necessary to demonstrate the primary vascular pathology.

Treatment

Treatment is unsatisfactory. NSAIDs may control pain, but some patients require morphine. Compression bandaging may promote healing, but may not be tolerated because of pain. Pentoxifylline and low-dose methotrexate have been recommended, but controlled trials are lacking.

Nodular vasculitis

See 'Panniculitis' below.

Large-vessel vasculitis

Temporal arteritis (giant-cell arteritis)

This is a granulomatous panarteritis with multinucleated giant cells, which affects the larger and medium-sized arteries, particularly

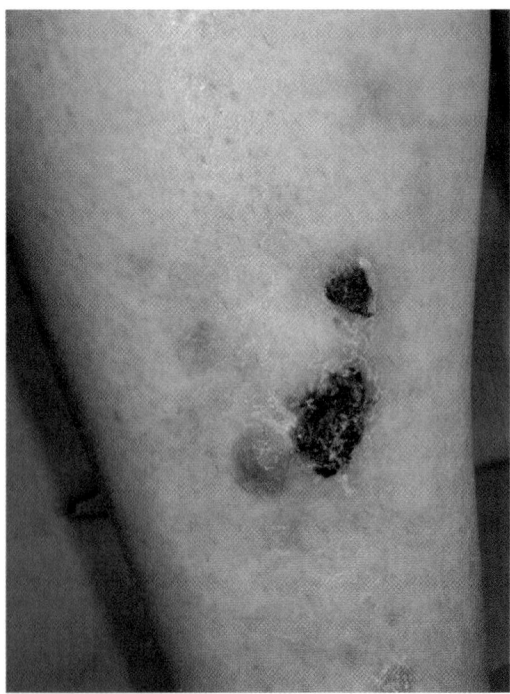

Fig. 23.7.7 Painful necrotic ulceration and livedo reticularis in a woman who also developed a sensory neuropathy in the foot. Ulceration was preceded by tender cutaneous nodules. She had no systemic disease. Ulcers healed slowly with conservative management, and neurological signs resolved. The findings were consistent with the benign cutaneous form of polyarteritis nodosa.

those of the head and neck. Patients, usually women aged over 50 years, have fever, headache, anaemia, and an elevated erythrocyte sedimentation rate. Many have polymyalgia rheumatica. The typical cutaneous lesion is a tender scalp nodule that may ulcerate. An ulcerated nodule may be misdiagnosed as a basal cell skin cancer (see Chapter 18.10.4).

Takayasu's disease

This is a chronic systemic arteritis affecting the aorta and its main branches, which occurs in patients younger than 50 years. The granulomatous arteritis is followed by fibrosis and stenosis (Chapter 16.14.4). The cutaneous manifestations include palpable purpura and ulcerated lesions resembling pyoderma gangrenosum.

Thrombo-occlusive vasculopathies

Livedo reticularis (livedo racemosa)
Clinical features
Livedo reticularis is seen most often on the legs. The skin develops a mottled reddish-purple reticulated discoloration that reflects sluggish vascular flow in the superficial dermis (Fig. 23.7.8). Some venous stasis is common. A continuous livedo network is likely to be physiological, and disappears when the skin is warmed. A broken (discontinuous) persistent livedo reticularis, sometimes with painful cutaneous ulceration and nodules (evidence of necrotizing vasculitis) (Fig. 23.7.9), occurs with hyperviscosity states (polycythaemia rubra vera, antiphospholipid antibodies, cryoglobulinaemia), large-vessel vasculitis (connective tissue diseases, polyarteritis nodosa, and Wegener's granulomatosis), and emboli, including cholesterol emboli.

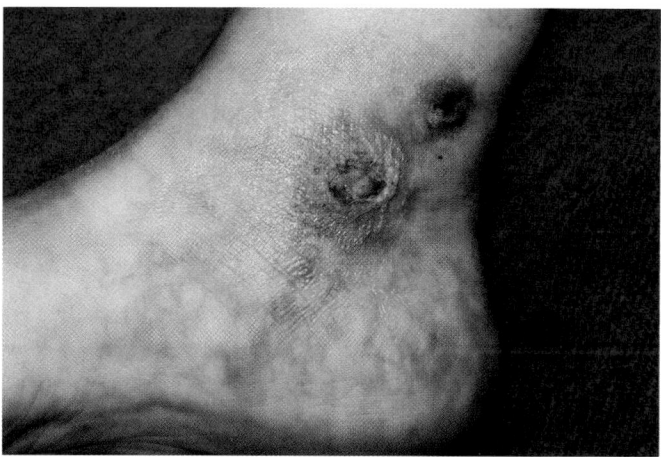

Fig. 23.7.9 Painful cutaneous ulceration, necrotizing vasculitis, and livedo reticularis in a patient with antiphospholipid antibodies.

Differential diagnosis and investigation
Erythema ab igne is a reticulated hyperpigmented staining that can develop on any skin surface after chronic exposure to heat from a radiator, open fire, or hot-water bottle. Deep biopsies from subcutaneous nodules are required to demonstrate diagnostic pathology such as cholesterol emboli.

Livedoid vasculopathy
This is also known as segmental hyalinizing vasculitis, livedo reticularis with summer/winter ulceration, livedoid vasculitis.

Pathogenesis and pathology
This idiopathic disorder affects young to middle-aged women. The condition is primarily an occlusive vasculopathy rather than a necrotizing vasculitis. Hyaline thrombi occlude small vessels in the upper and mid dermis. Occlusion may be associated with endothelial swelling, extravasation of red blood cells, fibrinoid material in vessel walls, infarction of the superficial dermis, and scattered perivascular lymphocytes. Endothelial, platelet, or lymphocyte activation with the release of proinflammatory cytokines may play some part in the pathogenesis of hypercoagulation.

Clinical features
Focal purpuric lesions on the leg break down to form small excruciatingly painful ulcers that are surrounded by a purpuric rim (Fig. 23.7.10). Ulcers heal slowly, leaving atrophie blanche (porcelain-white stellate scars with a rim of telangiectasia) and net-like hyperpigmentation. The condition pursues a chronic course, sometimes with seasonal exacerbations.

Investigation and treatment
Antiphospholipid antibodies or protein C deficiency have been detected in a few patients, but in general, investigations reveal no evidence of abnormalities in fibrinolytic or coagulation systems. Pain must be controlled. Antiplatelet therapy, antithrombotic regimens, fibrinolytic agents, and intravenous immunoglobulin have all been recommended, but there is no consensus over management, and treatment is difficult. Treatment for vasculitis with drugs such as systemic corticosteroids is ineffective.

Hypertensive ulcer (Martorell's ulcer)
Hypertensive ulcer was described in 1945. The pathogenesis may be linked to a thrombo-occlusive vasculopathy of cutaneous arterioles

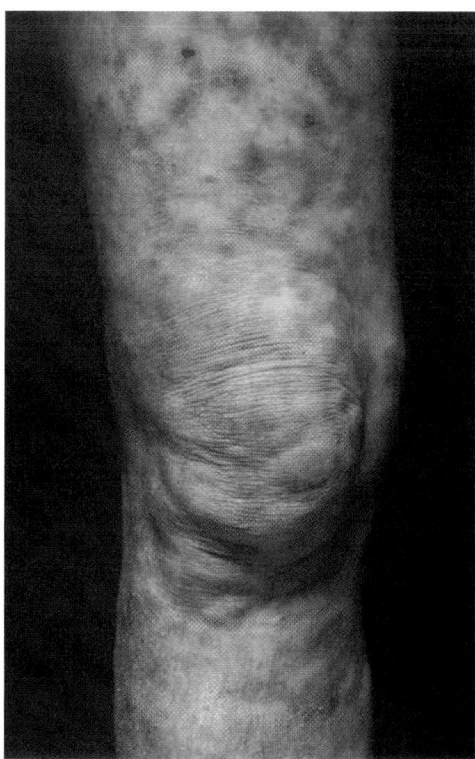

Fig. 23.7.8 Extensive livedo reticularis.

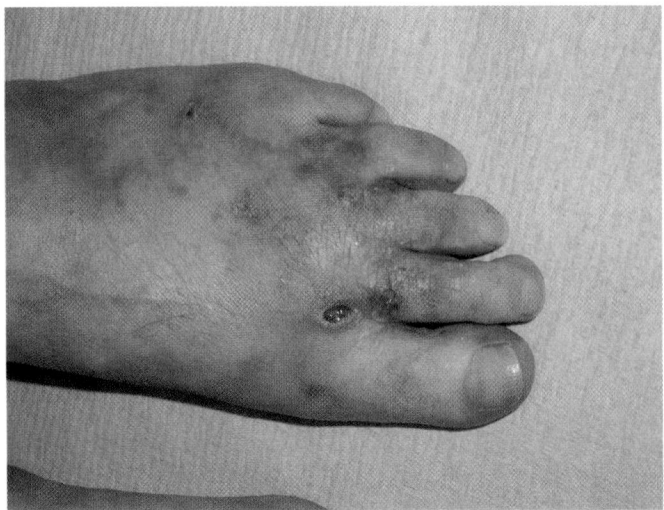

Fig. 23.7.10 Livedoid vasculopathy with small painful ulcers that eventually healed to leave porcelain-white stellate scars (atrophie blanche). This patient has no evidence of systemic disease or abnormalities in coagulation. Biopsy revealed an occlusive vasculopathy without vasculitis.

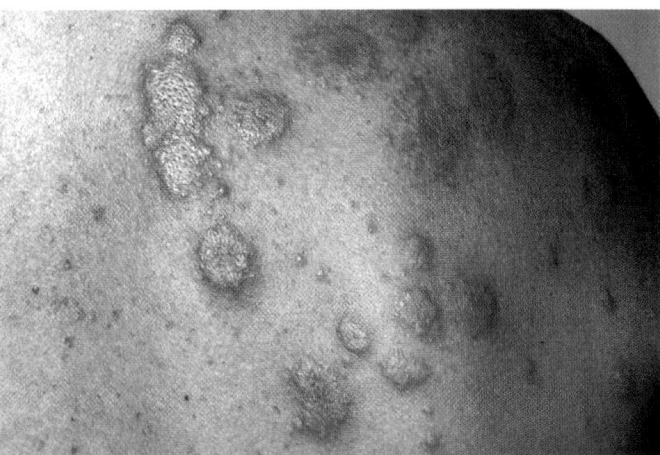

Fig. 23.7.11 Sweet's syndrome: oedematous nodules in a woman with myeloid leukaemia.

in long-standing hypertension, but the existence of this entity is controversial.

A purpuric lesion appears on the anterolateral aspect of the shin between the mid and lower third of the leg. It becomes necrotic and forms a superficial ulcer with an erythematous or purpuric rim. Patients have no signs of venous or arterial insufficiency. The ulcers, which may be bilateral, are extremely painful. Management involves the control of hypertension, pain relief, and compression bandaging.

Neutrophilic dermatoses (pustular vasculitis)

This heterogeneous group is linked by the histopathological finding of a heavy dermal infiltrate of neutrophils with leukocytoclasis, but limited evidence of vasculitis.

Sweet's syndrome (acute febrile neutrophilic dermatosis)

Sweet's syndrome was described in 1964. The condition usually affects women in their sixth decade.

Pathogenesis and pathology The cause is unknown and 50 to 70% of cases are idiopathic, but in up to 50% of cases Sweet's syndrome may be associated with malignancy (haematological or solid tumours) or immunological disease (rheumatoid arthritis, dermatomyositis, relapsing polychondritis, inflammatory bowel disease). Less frequently, a variety of infections or certain drugs such as granulocyte colony stimulating factor appear to have precipitated the disease. A skin biopsy shows a dense neutrophilic infiltrate in the upper dermis, with leukocytoclasis and nuclear dust. The dermis is oedematous. Vessels show endothelial swelling without a true vasculitis.

Clinical features The syndrome is characterized by the sudden onset of fever, neutrophilia, and tender erythematous nodules and plaques, most frequently on the face and upper trunk (Fig. 23.7.11). The plaques appear oedematous, but blisters are unusual; occasionally they may be pustular. Other features include conjunctivitis or episcleritis, oral ulcers, arthralgia, and arthritis.

Investigations and treatment Infection should be excluded by blood culture. The erythrocyte sedimentation rate is elevated, and patients have a marked neutrophilia. Underlying malignancy should be excluded by the history, physical examination, and appropriate investigations. A skin biopsy is essential to confirm the diagnosis. Most patients respond rapidly to systemic corticosteroids (0.5–1.0 mg/kg) used in association with potent topical corticosteroids, but the disease may relapse as corticosteroids are reduced. A minority of patients have chronic relapsing disease.

Bowel-associated dermatosis–arthritis syndrome

Pathogenesis This syndrome is seen in 10 to 20% of patients who have had bowel bypass surgery to treat morbid obesity, or after extensive resection of the small bowel. It occurs less frequently in patients with an abnormal segment of bowel in other diseases, such as diverticulitis or inflammatory bowel disease. The overgrowth of bacteria in a blind loop, with the deposition of immune complexes, is thought to trigger disease. The histopathological changes resemble those of Sweet's syndrome.

Clinical features The syndrome is characterized by purpuric papules and small vesicopustular lesions on the trunk and extremities. These may be associated with polyarthritis, malaise, and fever. Some patients have cryoglobulinaemia. Management should be directed at correcting the underlying cause.

Cutaneous lupus erythematosus

Aetiology and pathogenesis

Lupus erythematosus-specific skin disease (cutaneous LE) is distinct from lesions such as cutaneous vasculitis, which may occur in association with a number of connective tissue diseases. The pathogenesis of cutaneous LE is uncertain, but in genetically predisposed individuals ultraviolet (UV) light may play some part in triggering and perpetuating disease through apoptosis and the release of proinflammatory cytokines. Certain genes (e.g. the HLA 8.1 ancestral haplotype, a TNF-α gene promoter) increase susceptibility to subacute cutaneous LE (SCLE). Deficiencies in complement C2, C4, and C1q are also associated with SCLE. The role of specific autoantibodies in the pathogenesis is unproven, although it has been hypothesized that autoantigens on the surface of apoptotic cells might stimulate the immune system. Drugs that cause photosensitive SCLE skin lesions also trigger the production of Ro (SS-A) autoantibodies. The defective clearance of apoptotic debris may lead to the secondary necrosis of keratinocytes, inflammation, and further tissue damage.

Pathology

Skin biopsy shows a lichenoid (interface) dermatitis with apoptotic basal keratinocytes, a T-cell inflammatory infiltrate at the dermo–epidermal junction, periadnexal inflammation, and perivascular inflammation without vasculitis. Inflammation and basal cell damage are most marked in chronic cutaneous lesions.

The prevalence of cutaneous lupus ranges from 14.6 to 68 per 100 000 people. All races are affected. Most forms of cutaneous LE affect women more than men.

Classification

Cutaneous LE is classified into acute, subacute, and chronic subtypes (Box 23.7.3), but patients often have more than one type of lesion. The terms discoid LE (DLE) and subacute cutaneous LE (SCLE) are used in two ways: either to describe a subtype of lupus skin lesion, or to refer to subsets of patients who share certain clinical and laboratory features.

Chronic cutaneous LE

DLE is the most common form of chronic cutaneous LE (Box 23.7.3). Most discoid lesions are localized to the head and neck, but disease may be widespread (Figs. 23.7.12–23.7.17). Lupus panniculitis (lupus profundus) is a lobular panniculitis that occurs in 1 to 3% of patients with cutaneous LE (Fig. 23.7.18). Atrophy (fat loss) is disfiguring. Cold-induced chilblain lupus is characterized by purple plaques on the fingers or toes (Fig. 23.7.19); chronic lesions develop a warty surface (Fig. 23.7.20). The histology is not specific, but this pattern of disease may be associated with systemic lupus erythematosus (SLE). Lupus erythematosus tumidus is an uncommon variant that does not scar, but is associated with photosensitivity. Smooth, erythematous, urticated nodules appear on sun-exposed skin, and may persist for weeks. The diagnosis is clinical, as most patients do not have lupus antibodies, and the histology may not be diagnostic.

Subacute cutaneous LE

Subacute cutaneous LE (SCLE) was first recognized in 1979 as a distinct subtype of LE with a low risk of severe SLE. This pattern of disease is associated with photosensitivity and anti-Ro (SS-A) antibodies. SCLE may be induced by a wide range of drugs, including hydrochlorothiazide, calcium-channel blockers, angiotensin-converting enzyme inhibitors, and terbinafine.

The nonscarring scaly erythematous lesions develop in a photosensitive distribution (Figs. 23.7.21 and 23.7.22), and may be annular (Fig. 23.7.23) or, less frequently, papulosquamous (resembling psoriasis).

Women with SCLE may have infants affected by neonatal LE, because anti-Ro antibodies cross the placenta. These infants present with photosensitive cutaneous disease (usually SCLE) or congenital heart block, but rarely both. Infants may also develop transient haemolytic anaemia, thrombocytopenia, leukopenia, and elevated liver function tests. Skin signs resolve over 4 to 6 months, but heart block is permanent. Rarely, infants affected by neonatal LE develop a connective tissue disease later in life.

Box 23.7.3 Subtypes of cutaneous lupus erythematosus (LE)

Chronic cutaneous LE

Discoid LE (DLE)

◆ Most common form of chronic cutaneous LE

◆ Frequently occurs without evidence of systemic lupus erythematosus (SLE)

◆ Usually localized to the head and neck, but may be widespread

◆ Erythematous telangiectatic plaques or hyperkeratotic plaques with adherent keratotic scale

◆ Plaques on the face tend to spare the nasolabial fold

◆ Acne-like plugged lesions involve the concha of the ears

◆ Plaques may involve the vermillion border of the lips or eyelids

◆ Lichen planus-like lesions develop on the buccal mucosa

◆ Chronic plaques cause scarring and deformity

◆ Perifollicular inflammation leads to irreversible hair loss (scarring alopecia)

◆ Dyspigmentation (increased or decreased) is common in dark skins

Lupus panniculitis (lupus profundus)

◆ Subcutaneous nodules

◆ Tends to involve the shoulders, upper arms, face, and buttocks

◆ Overlying skin may be affected by DLE

◆ Fat loss is a disfiguring complication

◆ Subcutaneous nodules may calcify and ulcerate

Less common forms of CCLE

◆ Chilblain lupus

◆ Lupus erythematosus tumidus

Subacute cutaneous LE (SCLE)

◆ May have SLE, but low risk of severe disease

◆ Photosensitive

◆ Anti-Ro antibodies

◆ Superficial scaly annular lesions (common) involve the V-area of the neck, the upper trunk, upper limbs, and hands (sparing the knuckles)

◆ Papulosquamous lesions (less common) may resemble psoriasis

◆ Face is affected less often than in other forms of cutaneous LE

◆ Nonscarring, but postinflammatory hypopigmentation is common

◆ Affected mothers may have infants with neonatal LE

Acute cutaneous LE

◆ Occurs in active SLE

◆ Photosensitive

◆ Oedematous malar erythema

◆ Erythema may be generalized

◆ Evanescent and nonscarring

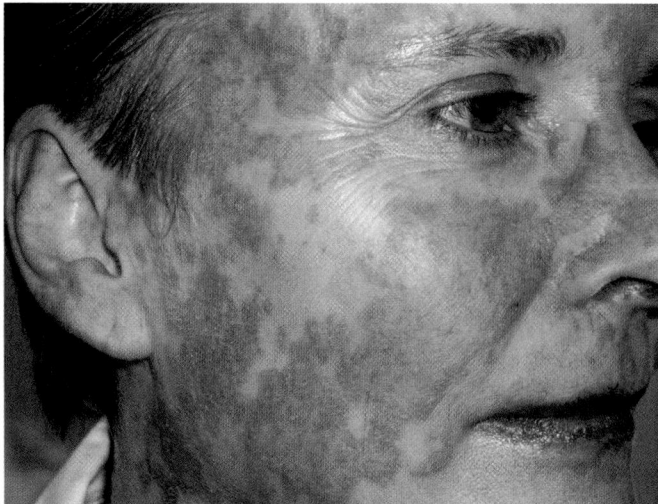

Fig. 23.7.12 Chronic erythematous telangiectatic plaques in a photosensitive distribution on the face of a woman who has systemic lupus erythematosus.

Acute cutaneous LE

The oedematous malar erythema of acute cutaneous LE develops in photosensitive patients with active SLE. The rash disappears rapidly without scarring once the patient is protected from UV light. Subepidermal bullae are an uncommon manifestation associated with antibodies to basement membrane-zone antigens, including type VII collagen.

Nonspecific cutaneous signs in SLE

Forty to seventy per cent of patients with SLE develop nonscarring alopecia. Causes include lupus hairs (hairs break off at the front of the scalp), telogen effluvium (shedding after severe illness), and alopecia areata.

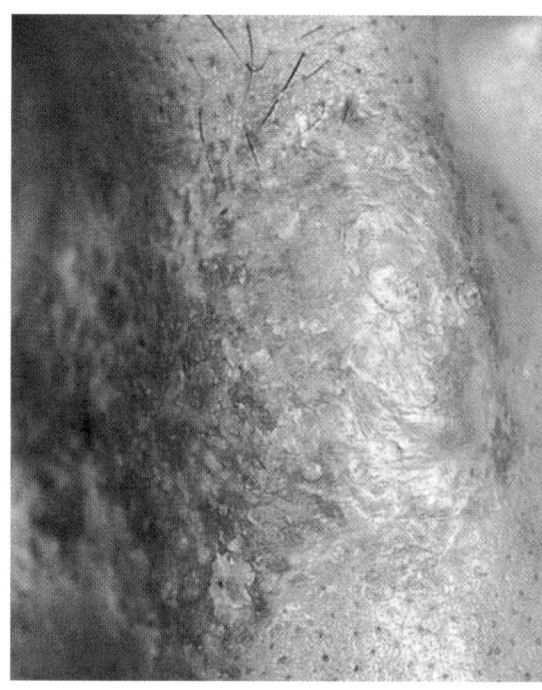

Fig. 23.7.14 Chronic discoid lupus erythematosus causes scarring and deformity, seen here on the bridge of the nose.

Patients with SLE may have periungual erythema and discrete papular telangiectasia on the palms or finger tips. Some have Raynaud's phenomenon. About 10 to 20% of patients with SLE have some form of vasculitis. Linear telangiectasia is present on the posterior nail fold (a sign of a connective tissue disease also found in dermatomyositis, systemic sclerosis, and 5% of cases of rheumatoid arthritis). Thrombosed vessels may be carried forward into a ragged cuticle. Painless red-black lesions of the nail fold or finger

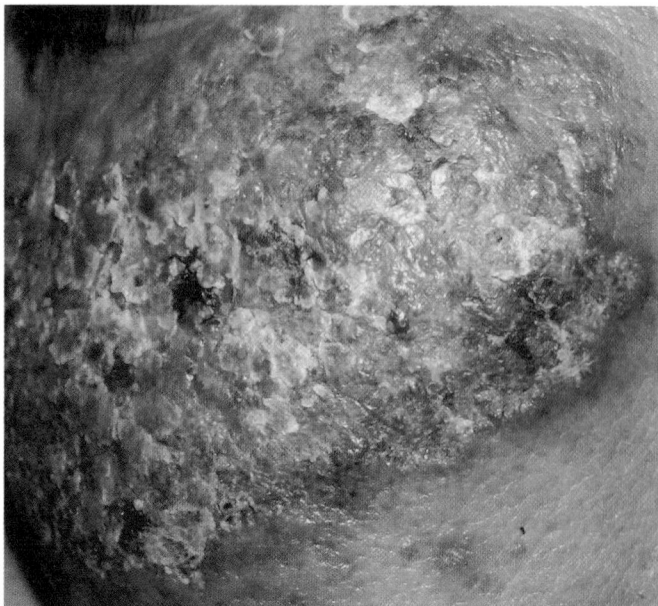

Fig. 23.7.13 This well-defined untreated plaque on the cheek is characteristic of discoid lupus erythematosus. Hyperkeratotic scale extends down dilated follicular orifices (visible as 'carpet tacks' on the underside of the scale). This woman has no other evidence of lupus erythematosus.

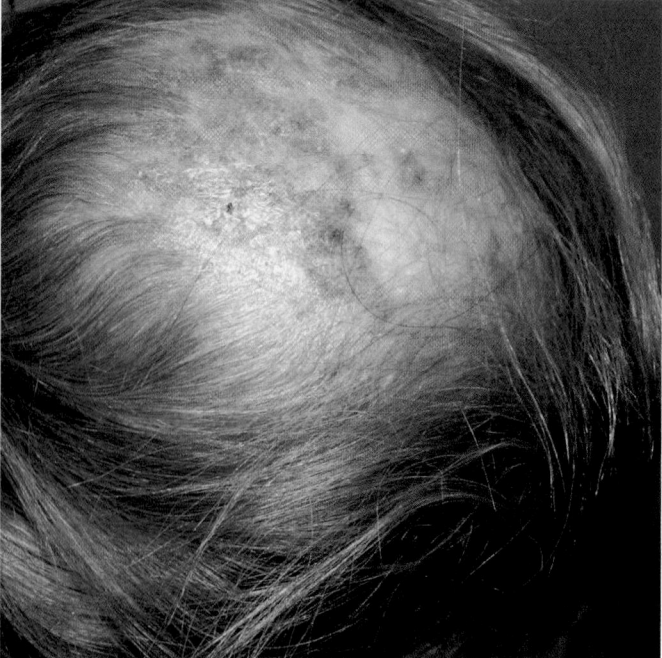

Fig. 23.7.15 Discoid lupus erythematosus in the scalp causes a scarring alopecia that may be extensive and disfiguring.

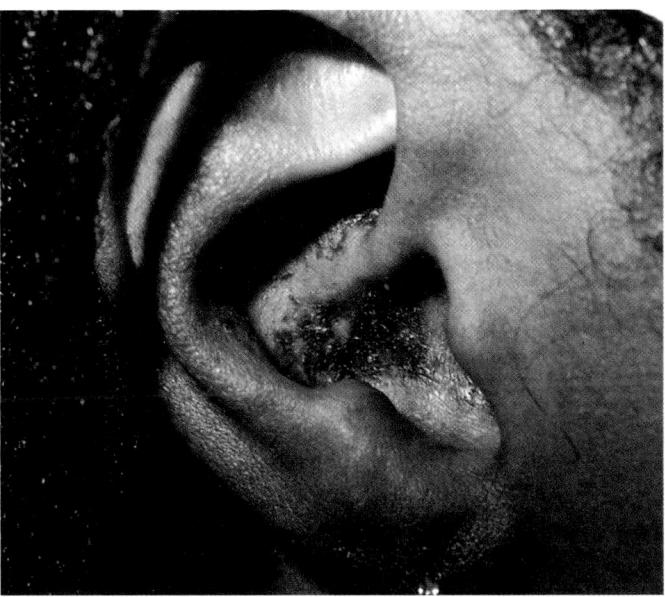

Fig. 23.7.16 The plugged lesions of discoid lupus erythematosus in the concha of the ears were misdiagnosed as acne, and in this patient with dark skin have caused hyperpigmentation.

pulp (Bywater's lesions) reflect microinfarcts of superficial dermal vessels, and are most common in rheumatoid arthritis, but may be seen in SLE (Fig. 23.7.24).

Urticaria is common in SLE, but long-lasting tender urticarial lesions that fade to leave bruises are a sign of urticarial vasculitis, sometimes an indication of an underlying complement deficiency. A small-vessel cutaneous vasculitis (palpable purpura) may be associated with cryoglobulinaemia (see 'Small-vessel cutaneous vasculitis' above).

Fixed livedo reticularis in a broken rather than a continuous physiological pattern may be linked to the antiphospholipid syndrome, recurrent thromboses, and neurological complications. Atrophie blanche, a sign of vasculitis or obstructive vasculopathy, may be present on the plantar surface of the toes (Fig. 23.7.25) or fingers.

Differential diagnosis

Red faces are common, but the distribution and morphology of the rash will provide important clues to the underlying diagnosis. Patients with a malar (butterfly) rash that spares the sun-protected

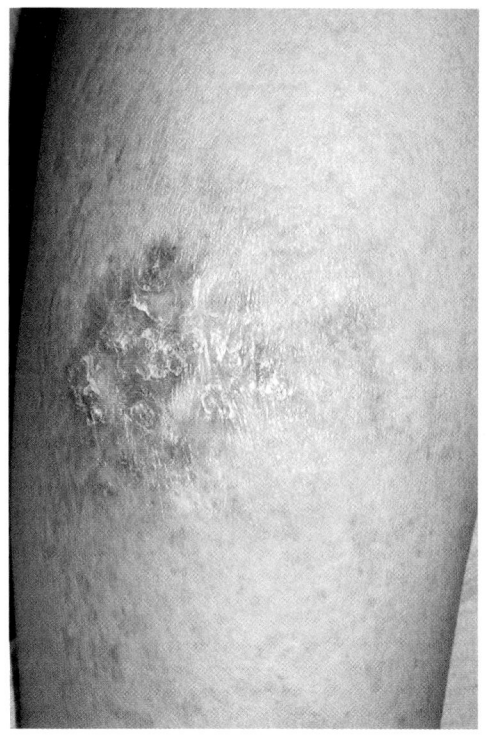

Fig. 23.7.18 Lupus panniculitis on the upper arm presented as a deep tender nodule. The overlying skin is affected by discoid lupus erythematosus. Chronic ulceration is a troublesome complication that may be precipitated by a biopsy.

skin on the eyelids, behind the ears, and under the chin may be photosensitive, but drugs cause photosensitivity more often than LE.

Pustules are not found in cutaneous LE; instead consider rosacea or steroid-induced acne (a complication in patients treating 'cutaneous LE' with potent topical steroids). Seborrhoeic dermatitis produces a superficial scaly facial erythema involving the nasolabial folds (unlike LE), mid forehead, and scalp (dandruff). Seborrhoeic dermatitis is not photosensitive, does not scar, and is not usually associated with hair loss (Chapter 23.6).

The cutaneous signs in dermatomyositis (see 'Cutaneous features of dermatomyositis' below) are similar to those of LE; however, the intense itching that plagues patients with cutaneous dermatomyositis is not a feature of cutaneous LE. Both conditions

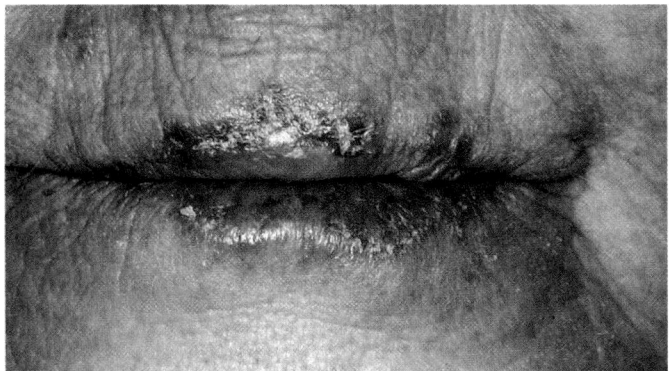

Fig. 23.7.17 Discoid plaques on the vermillion border of the lips are triggered by ultraviolet light.

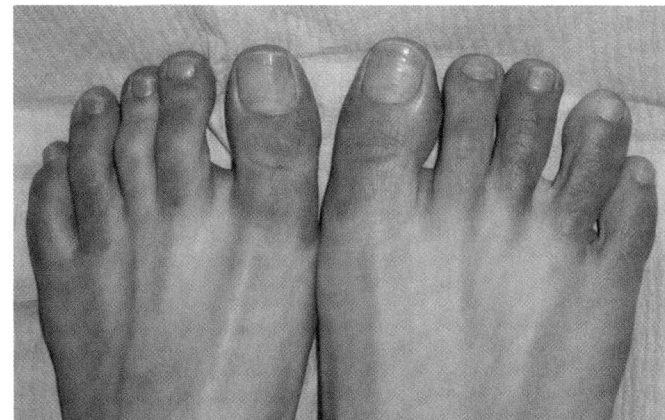

Fig. 23.7.19 Purple plaques on the toes or fingers are characteristic of chilblain-like cutaneous lupus erythematosus.

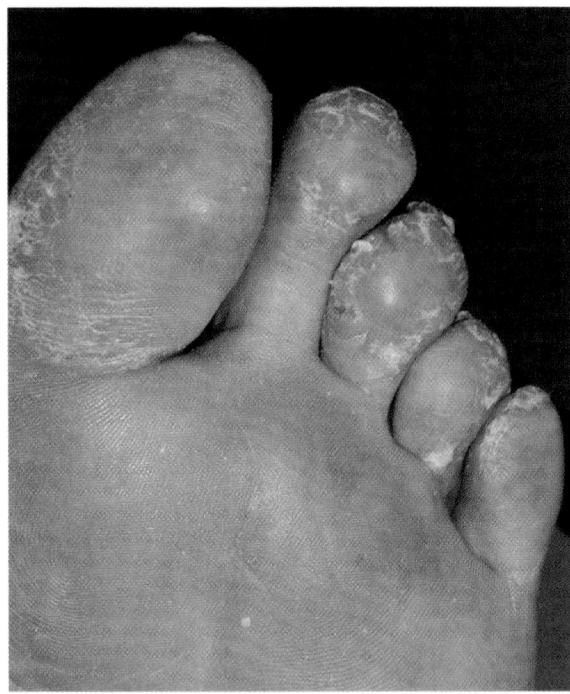

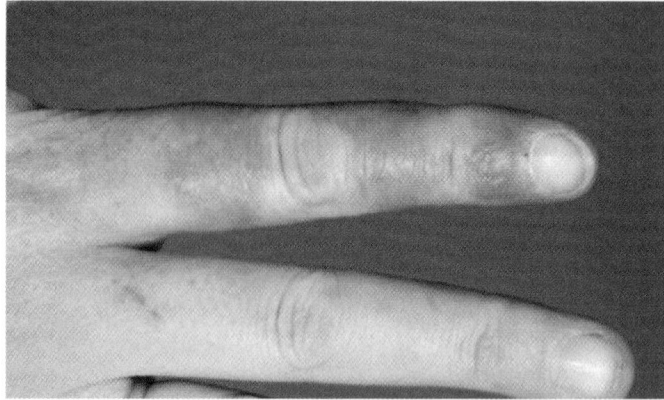

Fig. 23.7.22 Cutaneous lupus erythematosus involves the skin between the knuckles, by contrast with the scaly papules of dermatomyositis (Gottron's papules), which occur over the knuckles.

by the antimalarials used to treat cutaneous LE; check for psoriatic nail pitting or onycholysis. Hypertrophic DLE may simulate a squamous cell skin cancer.

Clinical investigation

Systemic disease should be excluded by the history, physical examination, and laboratory studies including examination of the urine, a full blood count, routine biochemistry, and immunology (antinuclear antibodies, extractable nuclear antigen, complement levels). The diagnosis should be confirmed by the histological examination of a skin biopsy. Immunofluorescence testing is not required unless the lesions are bullous. In annular SCLE,

Fig. 23.7.20 Chronic hyperkeratotic chilblain lesions may fissure.

are photosensitive, but the facial rash in dermatomyositis is more oedematous than in cutaneous LE, and tends to involve the nasolabial folds, unlike cutaneous LE. The rash of dermatomyositis targets the skin over the joints on the hands, whereas cutaneous LE tends to involve the skin between the joints (Fig. 23.7.22).

In patients with SCLE, a drug-induced aetiology must be considered. The annular lesions may be mistaken for dermatophyte infection (ringworm), but the trailing edge of scale is on the inner edge of the ring and follows the erythema (Fig. 23.7.23), whereas in dermatophyte infection, scale on the outer edge of the expanding ring is followed by erythema. SCLE must also be differentiated from erythema multiforme (Chapter 23.16) and psoriasis (Chapter 23.5). Psoriasis may coexist with cutaneous LE, and can be exacerbated

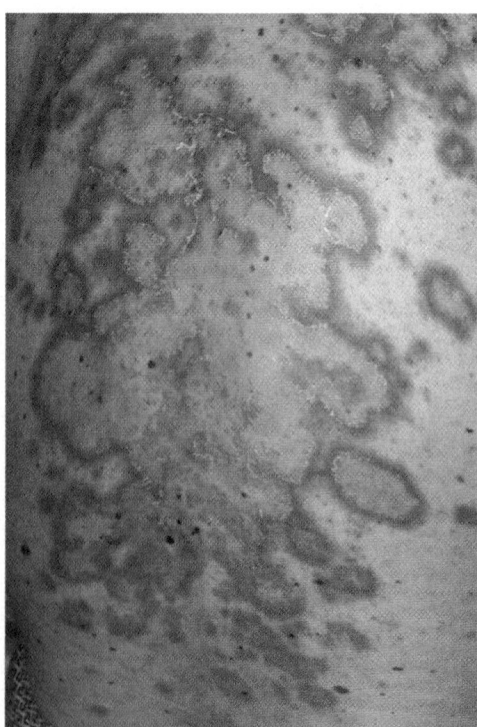

Fig. 23.7.23 Subacute cutaneous lupus erythematosus (SCLE) may adopt a striking annular configuration, when it can be confused with tinea corporis (ringworm), but typically the scale of SCLE is on the inner border of the rings, and the rash is in a photosensitive distribution.

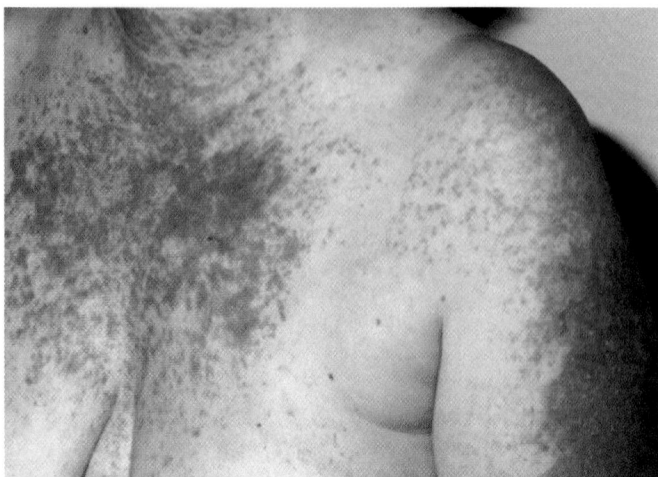

Fig. 23.7.21 Subacute cutaneous lupus erythematosus: nonscarring scaly erythematous papules are distributed in a photosensitive distribution on the chest and arms.

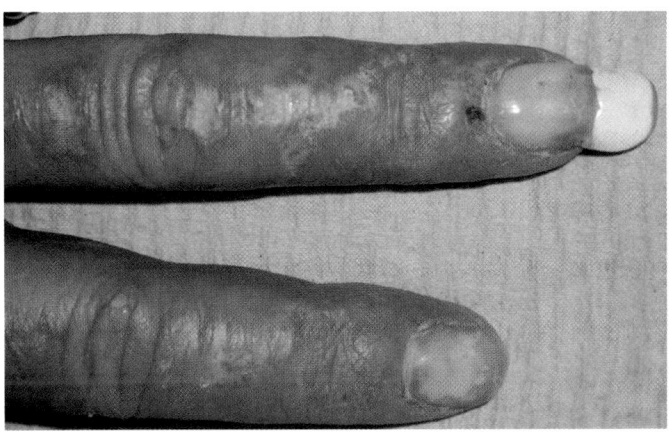

Fig. 23.7.24 Vascular involvement in systemic lupus erythematosus may present with infarcts of the nail fold (Bywater's lesions). This patient also has extensive atrophie blanche (hypopigmented atrophic skin with telangiectasia) on the dorsa of the fingers, indicative of vascular damage.

dermatophyte infection should be excluded by mycological culture of a skin scrape.

Treatment

Treatment aims to minimize scarring and pigment change by controlling cutaneous disease. Patients should be advised to stop smoking (smokers have disease that is more severe and less responsive to treatment than nonsmokers).

Photoprotection is essential (Box 23.7.4). Some patients are sensitive to both UVA (penetrates glass) and UVB, while others are sensitive to UVA alone or UVB alone. Occasionally, visible light triggers disease. Adequate sun protection will reduce the need for topical corticosteroids or systemic treatment.

Very potent topical corticosteroids are required to control inflammation and prevent scarring. Initially, the very potent topical corticosteroid clobetasol propionate should be thinly applied twice daily to all lesions, including those on the face.

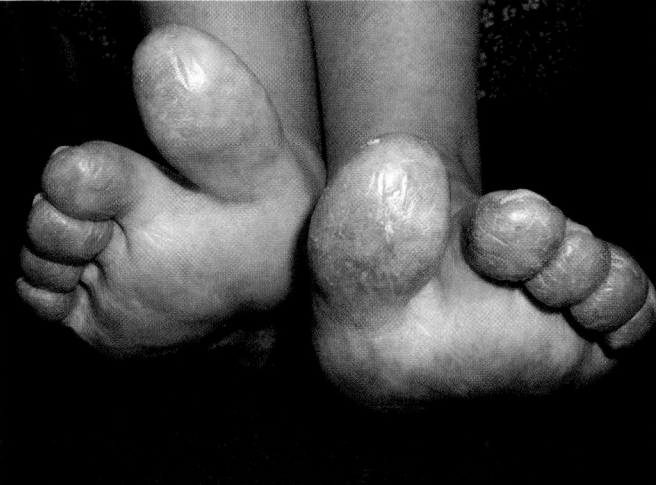

Fig. 23.7.25 This woman with systemic lupus erythematosus had no signs of active disease apart from atrophie blanche on the plantar surface of her toes. Atrophie blanche indicates either obstructive vasculopathy or vasculitis. The skin may ulcerate after minor trauma or in cold weather. It is important to examine the toes of any patient with a connective tissue disease.

Box 23.7.4 Strategies for photoprotection

- Limit sun exposure, particularly between 11.00 a.m. and 2.00 p.m.
- Wear clothing with a tight weave
- Wear wide-brimmed hats
- Use high-factor broad-spectrum sunscreens containing the physical blocker titanium dioxide to block the entire UV and visible light spectrum.
- Apply sunscreen liberally in the morning to all exposed sites
- Reapply sunscreen four hourly during the hours of sunlight

Clobetasol propionate scalp application may be used for discoid lesions in the scalp. It may take several weeks of treatment before the inflammation settles, particularly in thick discoid lesions. Atrophy is unlikely if treatment is supervised, but the strength of corticosteroid should be reduced gradually to less potent preparations such as mometasone furoate (potent) or clobetasone butyrate (moderate) as soon as the inflammation is controlled and the lesions have flattened. Sunscreens must be continued.

Patients should be shown how to apply the treatment (steroid phobia causes under treatment), and advised that treatment aims to control inflammation and further damage, but will not alter scars or pigmentation. Patients with disfiguring scars or pigment change may be referred to Red Cross camouflage clinics for advice on the use of cosmetic camouflage creams.

The calcineurin inhibitor tacrolimus ointment may be effective in cutaneous LE on the face, reducing the need for potent topical corticosteroids.

Patients with widespread cutaneous LE or localized disease that does not respond to topical treatment need systemic treatment with an antimalarial in addition to topical treatment. Hydroxychloroquine 200 mg twice daily (<6.5 mg/kg per day) is effective after about 8 to 12 weeks in most patients, and is well tolerated, but is less effective in smokers. Ocular toxicity has been reported with the related drug chloroquine, but hydroxychloroquine may be safer, provided the maximum dose is not exceeded. Visual acuity should be checked, and patients should see an optician annually. Mepacrine (quinacrine) may used in combination with hydroxychloroquine. Other options include dapsone, thalidomide, and gold.

Prognosis

SLE is most frequent in patients with acute cutaneous LE or LE-nonspecific skin lesions. One-half of patients with SCLE fulfil the criteria for SLE, but only 10 to 15% of patients presenting with SCLE develop severe manifestations of SLE. Drug-induced SCLE does not always reverse on withdrawal of the triggering drug.

DLE eventually remits in 50% of those with localized disease (confined to the head and neck). Most patients with localized chronic cutaneous disease, including lupus panniculitis and lupus erythematosus tumidus, do not develop significant systemic disease. DLE occurs with SLE in 5 to 10% of patients, but those with widespread DLE are most at risk. The course is benign and renal disease, if it occurs, is mild.

Cutaneous features of dermatomyositis

Aetiology, genetics, pathogenesis, and pathology

T lymphocytes, predominantly of the CD4+ phenotype, appear to play a pathogenetic role in mediating microvascular injury and the apoptosis of basal keratinocytes. Cytokines and chemokines released by activated T cells and keratinocytes may induce and perpetuate inflammation. UV-induced apoptosis may also play a part in the pathogenesis of skin lesions.

The cutaneous histological features include an interface dermatitis (vacuolar degeneration of basal keratinocytes and apoptosis), mild perivascular inflammation, oedema, and deposition of dermal mucin. The histological features are usually similar to those of cutaneous lupus erythematosus, but the acute vesiculobullous variant may resemble graft-versus-host disease.

Dermatomyositis affects adults and children of all races. Females are affected more often than males.

Clinical features

Skin and muscle involvement usually present within a short time of each other, but the extent of skin involvement does not correlate with severity of muscle disease. Skin and muscle problems present concurrently in 60% of patients, whereas in 10% muscle involvement precedes inflammatory cutaneous disease, and in 30% the skin involvement presents weeks or a few months before the onset of myositis. Interstitial lung disease and internal malignancy may be fatal. The term amyopathic dermatomyositis (dermatomyositis *sine* myositis) describes a subset of patients, usually female, in whom muscle involvement does not develop until up to 20 years after the onset of cutaneous dermatomyositis. These patients are still at risk of interstitial lung disease or internal malignancy.

Cutaneous dermatomyositis, unlike cutaneous lupus erythematosus, causes pruritus, burning, and pain. UV light exacerbates or triggers the rash in up to 50% of patients, but patients may not realize that the rash is photosensitive. A symmetrical violaceous or heliotrope (violet-red) erythema of the eyelids or periorbital skin is associated with fine scale and periorbital oedema or facial swelling (Figs. 23.7.26 and 23.7.27). Intense oedema may lead to blisters. Erythema also affects the cheeks, the V-area of the upper chest and neck, the posterior neck, upper back, and shoulders (shawl sign); the extensor aspects of the shoulders, arms, forearms, and fingers; and bony prominences of the elbows, knees, knuckles, and greater trochanter of the hip (holster sign). Scalp involvement may be associated with diffuse alopecia (Fig. 23.7.28).

The hands should be examined using magnification (an ophthalmoscope or dermatoscope) to assess the nail fold. Signs in the hands or nails may be diagnostic, and are listed in Box 23.7.5 (Figs. 23.7.29 to 23.7.31). Chronic inflammation results in poikiloderma (hypo- and hyperpigmentation, atrophy, and telangiectasia). Vasculopathy, with necrosis and ulceration, and cutaneous calcinosis are less common in adults than children (Fig. 23.7.32).

Dermatomyositis is associated with internal malignancy in 20 to 25% of adult patients. The increased risk may persist for 5 years after diagnosis, but is greatest in the first year, and in women. Signs linked to malignancy include corticosteroid resistance, an intense erythematous flush on the shoulders, neck, face, and scalp (malignant suffusion), and cutaneous ulceration.

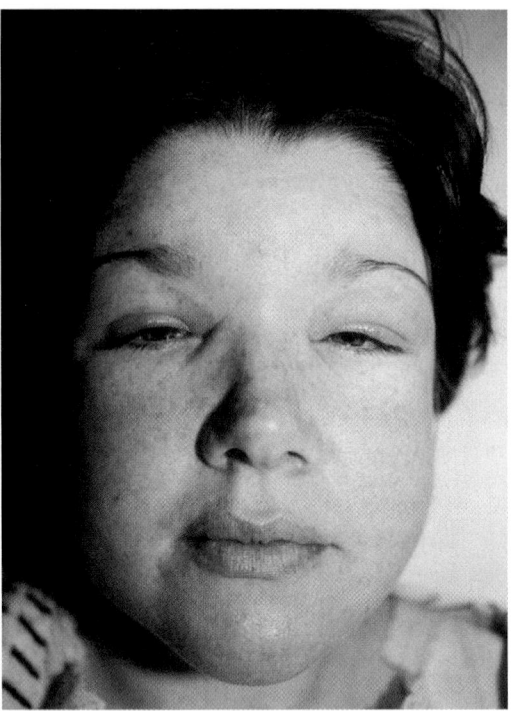

Fig. 23.7.26 Periorbital oedema and facial swelling was misdiagnosed as angio-oedema in this woman with dermatomyositis.

Differential diagnosis

Cutaneous lupus erythematosus may resemble dermatomyositis clinically and histologically, but intense pruritus is not a feature of lupus erythematosus. When cutaneous lupus erythematosus involves the hands, the rash tends to spare the joints, whereas Gottron's papules occur over the joints. Lesions tend to be oedematous in dermatomyositis, but hyperkeratotic in lupus erythematosus.

Scalp erythema and scale may be confused with seborrhoeic dermatitis, but the purplish colour, periorbital oedema, and predilection of lesions for light-exposed skin suggest dermatomyositis. Alopecia is not a feature of dermatitis. Mechanic's hands may be misdiagnosed as contact dermatitis. Facial oedema may be

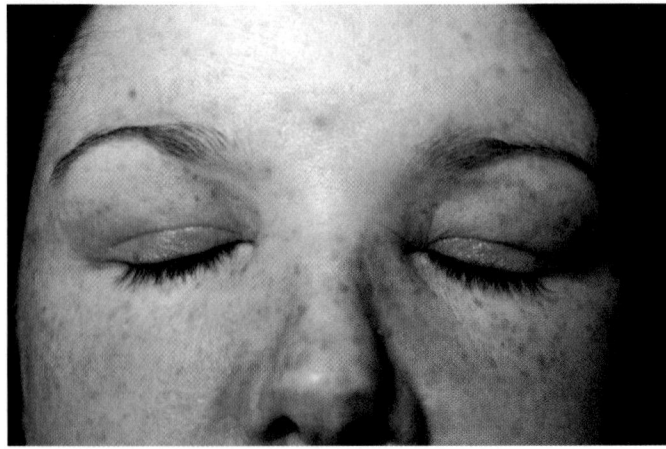

Fig. 23.7.27 The characteristic heliotrope (violet-red) erythema of the eyelids is revealed more clearly when the patient closes her eyes.
(From Harris A, *et al.* (1995). Dermatomyositis presenting in pregnancy. *Br J Dermatol*, **133**, 783–5, with permission.)

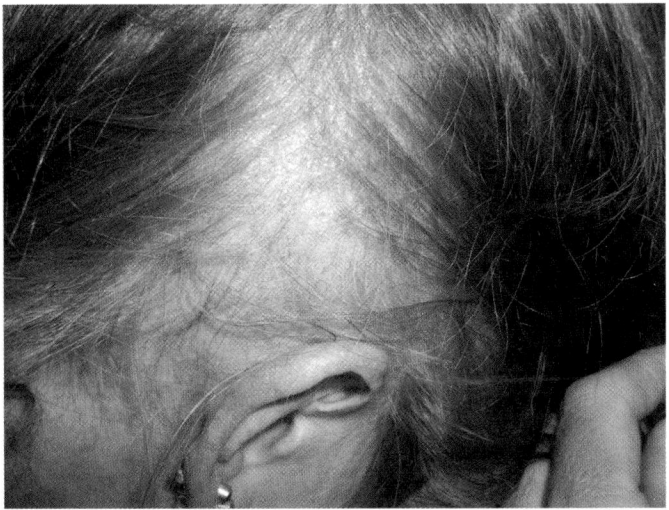

Fig. 23.7.28 Scalp erythema with hair loss may be difficult to manage in dermatomyositis, and simulates the scarring alopecia in chronic cutaneous lupus erythematosus.

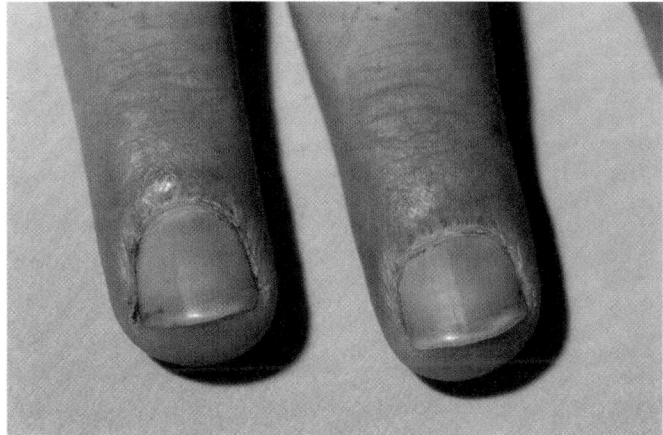

Fig. 23.7.29 Periungual erythema, tortuous nail-fold capillaries, capillary dropout (avascular areas), and/or thickened irregular cuticles with capillary haemorrhage are more common in dermatomyositis than in lupus erythematosus.

misdiagnosed as angio-oedema. Dermatomyositis may also simulate psoriasis. Dermatomyositis or a dermatomyositis-like rash has been induced by a number of drugs.

Clinical investigation

Biopsy of involved skin is helpful, but will not distinguish dermatomyositis from cutaneous lupus erythematosus. The antinuclear autoantibodies found in dermatomyositis include myositis-specific antibodies such as anti-Jo-1 (a marker for interstitial lung disease), anti-Mi-2, and anti-SRP. Myositis-associated antibodies include anti-Ro/SS-A, anti-La/SS-B, and anti-PM/Scl (marker of the systemic sclerosis/dermatomyositis overlap syndrome).

Muscle involvement should be investigated with serum muscle enzymes, electromyography, and muscle biopsy or muscle MRI (Chapter 19.11.07). Patients with pulmonary symptoms should have chest radiography as well as tests of pulmonary function.

The history taking and physical examination should be directed towards detecting underlying disease. Investigations should include chest radiography and CT of the abdomen and pelvis. Women should be offered mammography and bimanual examination of the pelvis, with cervical smear, CA125 blood levels, and transvaginal ultrasonography. Reinvestigation for internal malignancy should be considered 6-monthly for at least 2 years following the diagnosis of dermatomyositis.

Criteria for diagnosis

The diagnosis of cutaneous dermatomyositis is based on the presence of the typical cutaneous signs, with or without muscle involvement, combined with the cutaneous histology of interface dermatitis.

Box 23.7.5 Dermatomyositis: signs in the hands

♦ Periungual erythema

♦ Tortuous nail-fold capillaries and capillary dropout (avascular areas)

♦ Thickened irregular cuticles with capillary haemorrhage

♦ Gottron's papules (flat-topped violaceous scaly papules over the dorsal interphalangeal joints) are present in about one-third of patients, and are pathognomonic of dermatomyositis. Gottron's papules evolve into hypopigmented atrophic areas with irregular telangiectasia.

♦ Linear streaks of erythema over the extensor tendons of the fingers.

♦ Mechanic's hands: hyperkeratosis, scaling, and fissuring on the lateral aspects of the thumb and fingers simulates contact dermatitis

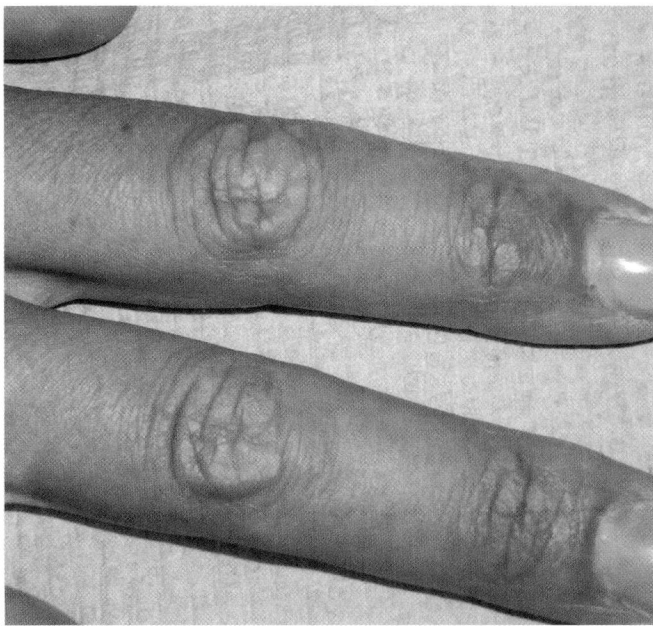

Fig. 23.7.30 Flat-topped violaceous scaly papules over the dorsal interphalangeal joints (Gottron's papules) are pathognomonic of dermatomyositis. Chronic papules develop depressed porcelain-white centers, with prominent telangiectasia.

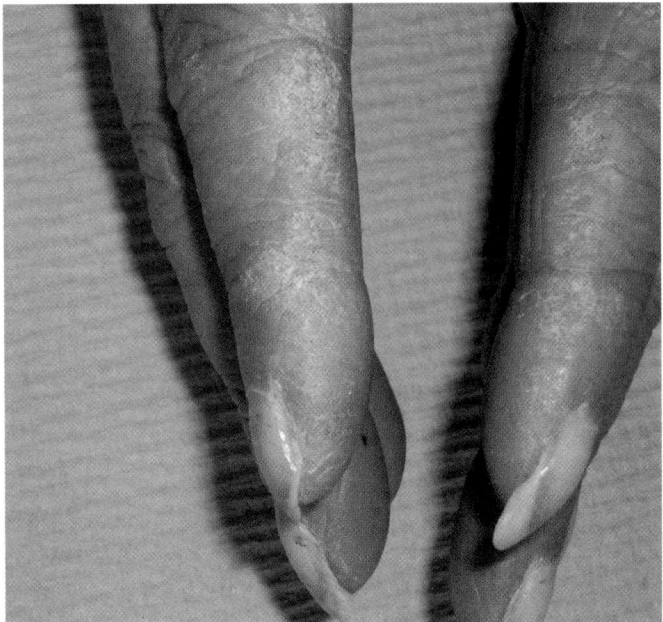

Fig. 23.7.31 Hyperkeratosis, scaling, and fissuring on the lateral aspects of the fingers (mechanic's hands) simulates contact dermatitis.

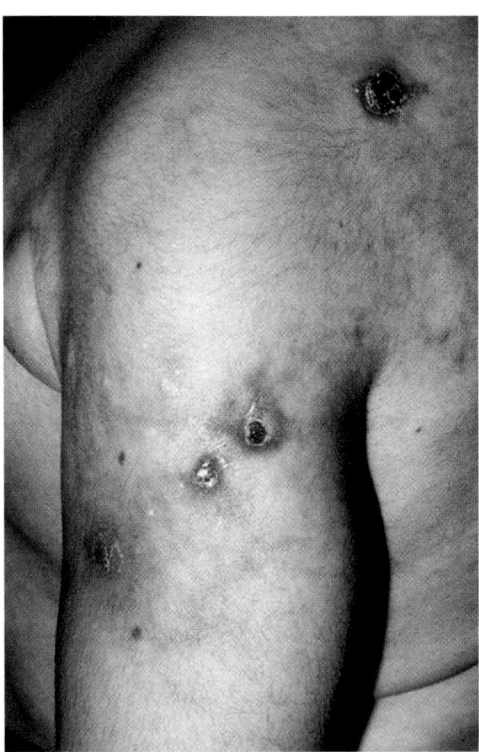

Fig. 23.7.32 Cutaneous calcinosis, necrosis, and ulceration in a 12-year-old child with chronic dermatomyositis.

Treatment

Pruritus, skin pain, and burning are difficult to manage, but may be helped by sedating antihistamines such as hydroxyzine, cooling baths, aqueous cream with 1% menthol, and moisturizers or soap substitutes to prevent dry skin (common in older people).

Cutaneous dermatomyositis is less responsive to treatment than cutaneous lupus erythematosus, but the approach is similar. Optimal topical therapy will minimize the dose of systemic immunosuppressive drugs. Protective clothing, wide-brimmed hats, and high-factor sun blocks are essential. Potent or highly potent topical corticosteroid ointments applied twice daily may control limited cutaneous disease, as may 0.1% tacrolimus ointment. Steroid lotions may relieve scalp irritation. Cosmetic camouflage can reduce disfigurement, particularly in patients with long-standing disease, and poikiloderma.

Most patients require oral therapy, but randomized controlled trials are required to evaluate treatments. Hydroxychloroquine (<6.5 mg/kg/day) can be beneficial, but takes 8 to 12 weeks to have an effect, and up to 6 months for maximal benefit. Hydroxychloroquine is less effective in cutaneous dermatomyositis than in cutaneous lupus erythematosus. Ocular toxicity has been reported with the related drug chloroquine, but hydroxychloroquine may be safer provided the maximum dose is not exceeded. Visual acuity should be checked, and patients should see an optician annually. Oral prednisolone (0.5–1 mg/kg per day) in reducing doses over 2 to 3 months may control symptomatic cutaneous disease while hydroxychloroquine is taking effect. Dapsone may be helpful (50–300 mg/day). Immunosuppressives such as methotrexate, azathioprine, ciclosporin, mycophenolate mofetil, and chlorambucil have been used with varying success in refractory skin disease. One small trial of intravenous immunoglobulin suggests that it might be helpful.

Prognosis

The prognosis is variable and unpredictable. Some patients have acute and fulminant disease, whereas in others it runs a chronic course punctuated by remissions and relapses. Skin and muscle disease tend to respond in parallel with treatment, but as immunosuppressants are gradually withdrawn, cutaneous disease may relapse without recurrence of muscle weakness.

Mechanic's hands were considered to be a cutaneous marker for the antisynthetase syndrome (idiopathic inflammatory myositis, antisynthetase antibodies such as anti-Jo-1, arthritis, Raynaud's phenomenon, high risk of interstitial lung disease), but this association has not been substantiated.

TNF-α may play a part in the pathogenesis of dermatomyositis. The efficacy of biological agents that inhibit TNF-α, such as etanercept and infliximab, has been investigated in clinical trials. Advances in biological therapies may improve treatment.

Scleroderma

Systemic sclerosis

Systemic sclerosis is reviewed in detail in Chapter 19.11.3, but the cutaneous features are discussed below.

Aetiology, genetics, pathogenesis, and pathology

Systemic sclerosis is a connective tissue disease that is characterized by collagen accumulation (fibrosis) associated with vascular injury and autoantibodies. The small arteries and microvasular beds of target organs appear to be damaged before the onset of fibrosis. Mesenchymal cells (fibroblasts, smooth muscle cells, and endothelial cells), activated by unknown stimuli, produce increased amounts of collagen, proteoglycan, and fibronectin, while lymphocyte activation produces autoantibodies and cytokines. The generation of autoantibodies is influenced by hereditary factors, including the presence of certain major histocompatibility complex

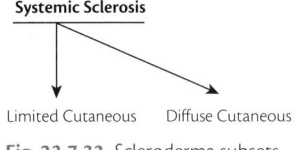

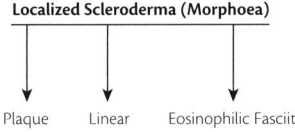

Fig. 23.7.33 Scleroderma subsets.

genes. It has been suggested that autoantibodies to basement membrane antigens might be involved in vascular injury, and that chronic activation of B cells, with release of cytokines, might play some part in the stimulation of fibroblasts and the development of skin fibrosis, but it is still not clear if autoantibodies have a direct role in the pathogenesis.

Skin biopsy shows a thickened dermis, with broad collagen bundles extending into subcutaneous fat. The walls of small vessels are thickened, with intimal fibrosis and thrombosis.

Epidemiology

The distribution of clinical subtypes and antibody prevalence varies among populations and geographic regions. The prevalence

---

Box 23.7.6 Clinical features of systemic sclerosis

Limited cutaneous systemic sclerosis

- Raynaud's phenomenon for years or decades

- Dilated nail-fold capillary loops, usually without capillary destruction

- Skin sclerosis limited to the hands, face, neck, feet, and forearms, or absent

- May have cutaneous calcinosis, telangiectasia, or oesophageal hypomotility

- Late incidence of pulmonary hypertension, with or without interstitial lung disease

- Anticentromere antibodies in 70–80%

Diffuse cutaneous systemic sclerosis

- Onset of Raynaud's phenomenon within 1 year of onset of skin changes

- Nail-fold capillary dilatation and capillary destruction (also seen in dermatomyositis and overlap syndromes)

- Skin sclerosis (tightness, thickening, nonpitting induration) affecting the arms, chest, abdomen, back, or thighs, in addition to acral sclerosis (face, feet, hands)

- Sclerodactyly (fingers and/or toes), digital pitting scars, or loss of substance of the digital finger pads (pulp loss)

- Tendon friction rubs

- Early interstitial lung disease (bibasilar pulmonary fibrosis), oliguric renal failure, diffuse gastrointestinal disease, and myocardial involvement

- Anti-DNA topoisomerase I (anti-Scl-70) antibodies in 30%

- Absence of anticentromere antibodies

---

of systemic sclerosis is reported to be between 13 and 105 to 140 per million, and it has an annual incidence of between 2.6 and 20 to 28 per million. Genetic, ethnic, and environmental factors may explain these variations. Systemic sclerosis is more common in women, and black women are most at risk. The average age of onset is between 40 and 50 years, with limited cutaneous systemic sclerosis occurring in older women more than often diffuse cutaneous disease. Raynaud's phenomenon occurs in 3 to 15% of the population.

Clinical features

Systemic sclerosis is divided into two major subtypes, depending primarily on the extent of cutaneous involvement (Fig. 23.7.33). The clinical features are given in Box 23.7.6.

Limited cutaneous systemic sclerosis

This is also known as CREST; C: calcinosis cutis, R: Raynaud's phenomenon, E:oesophageal distal hypomotility: S: sclerodactyly, T: telangiectasia.

Raynaud's phenomenon is the first sign of disease, and may precede other features by 10 to 15 years. Symmetrical thickening and tightening of the skin distal to the metacarpophalangeal joints (sclerodactyly) restricts opposition of the palms when the wrists are extended. This prayer sign indicates joint or skin pathology, or shortening of the finger flexor muscles. Well-defined telangiectatic macules (mats) appear on the hands, tongue, lips, and face (Fig. 23.7.34). Raynaud's phenomenon is associated with linear periungual nail-fold telangiectasia (usually without capillary dropout) (Figs. 23.7.35 and 23.7.36), atrophy of the finger pulps with breaking of the finger nails, resorption of bone in the terminal phalanges,

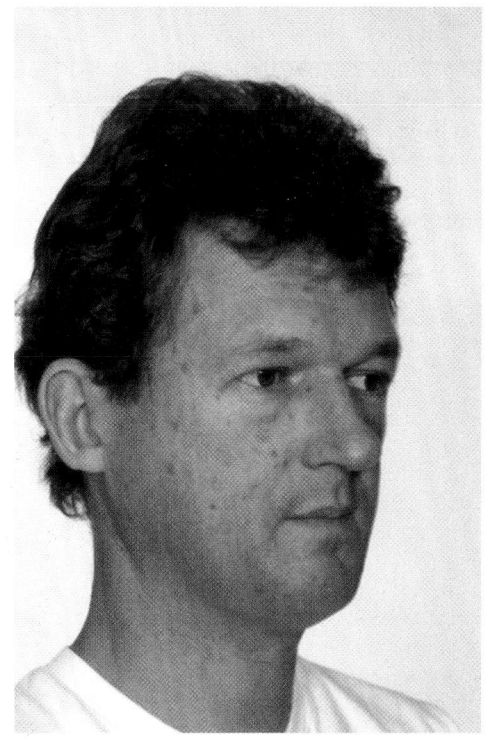

Fig. 23.7.34 Well-defined telangiectatic macules (mats) on the face of a man with long-standing limited cutaneous systemic sclerosis. This patient also has cutaneous calcinosis, Raynaud's phenomenon, oesophageal hypomotility, and anticentromere antibodies.

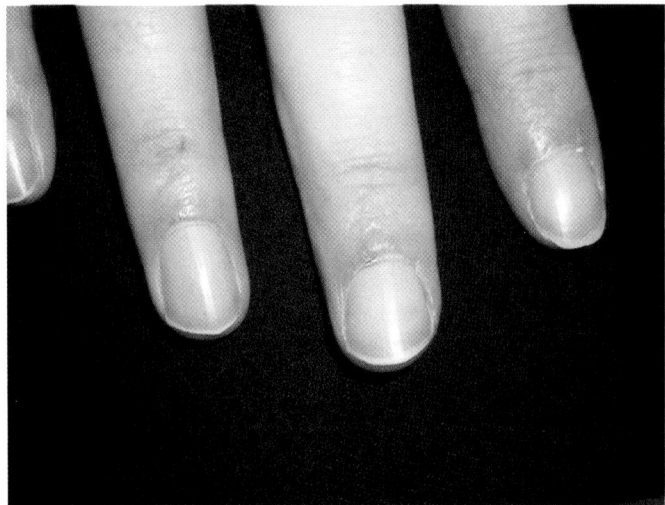

Fig. 23.7.35 Linear periungual nail-fold telangiectasia in a young female patient with limited cutaneous systemic sclerosis and Raynaud's phenomenon.

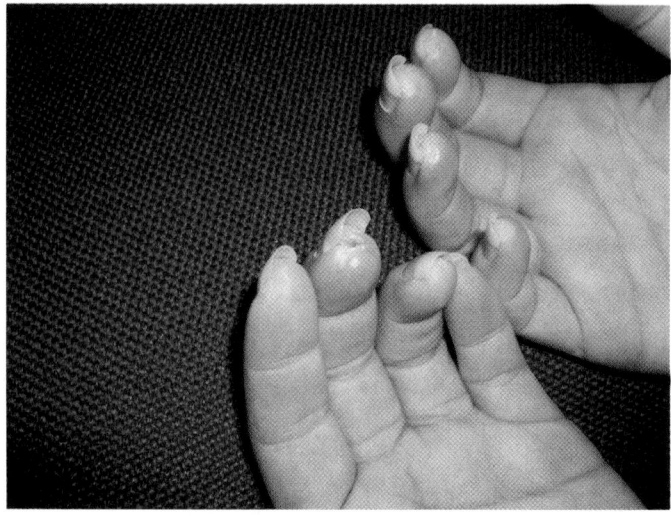

Fig. 23.7.37 Raynaud's phenomenon, atrophy of finger pulps with breaking of fingernails, calcinosis, and painful ulceration heals leaving pitted scarring of the finger tips in limited cutaneous systemic sclerosis.

and painful ischaemic ulceration that heals leaving pitted scarring of the finger tips (Fig. 23.7.37). Nodules of cutaneous calcinosis may become inflamed and ulcerate, discharging chalky material (Fig. 23.7.38). Cellulitis may complicate ulceration.

Systemic problems, such as oesophageal dysmotility causing dysphagia, interstitial lung disease with pulmonary hypertension, or biliary cirrhosis, may not develop for decades, if at all.

Diffuse cutaneous systemic sclerosis

The disease starts abruptly with the sudden onset of nonpitting oedema of the hands, feet, and face, often associated with constitutional symptoms and a rheumatoid-like arthritis. Raynaud's phenomenon usually develops within 1 year of the skin changes. Patients may complain of pruritus.

The nail-fold capillaries are distorted and irregular; fingers and toes become dusky and cyanotic. Sclerodactyly and flexion contractures produce a claw-like deformity with painful ulcerations

of the finger tips and knuckles (rat-bite necroses). Sclerosis spreads to the proximal extremities, chest, face, scalp, and trunk over 3 to 12 months, or may be present at disease onset. Facial sclerosis gives the face a mask-like stiffness with a reduced mouth aperture (Fig. 23.7.39), radial furrowing around the lips, and a pinched nose. The skin of the neck is ridged and tightened when the head is extended. This neck sign is positive in more than 90% of patients. Pigment change is common, with either generalized hyperpigmentation or focal hypo- or hyperpigmentation in areas of sclerosis.

Signs of systemic involvement include hypertension and abnormalities in gastrointestinal, pulmonary, renal, or cardiac function (Chapter 19.11.3).

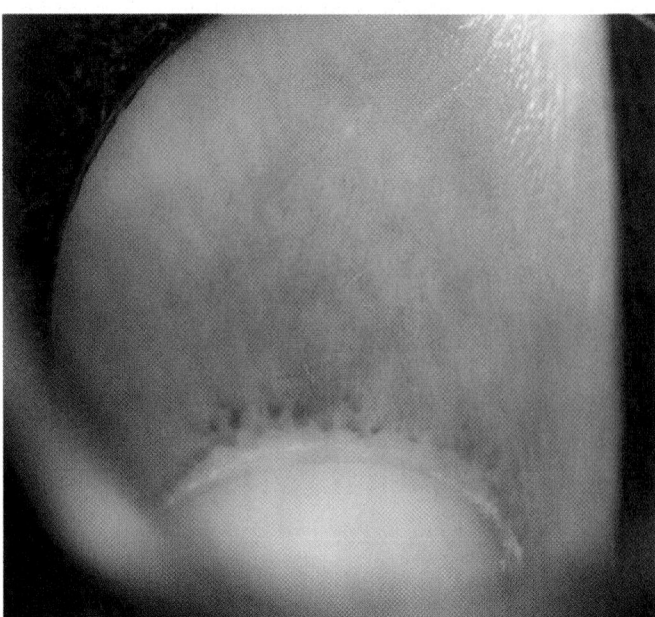

Fig. 23.7.36 Linear periungual telangiectasia in the nail fold of the patient illustrated in Fig. 23.7.35, viewed through a dermatoscope.

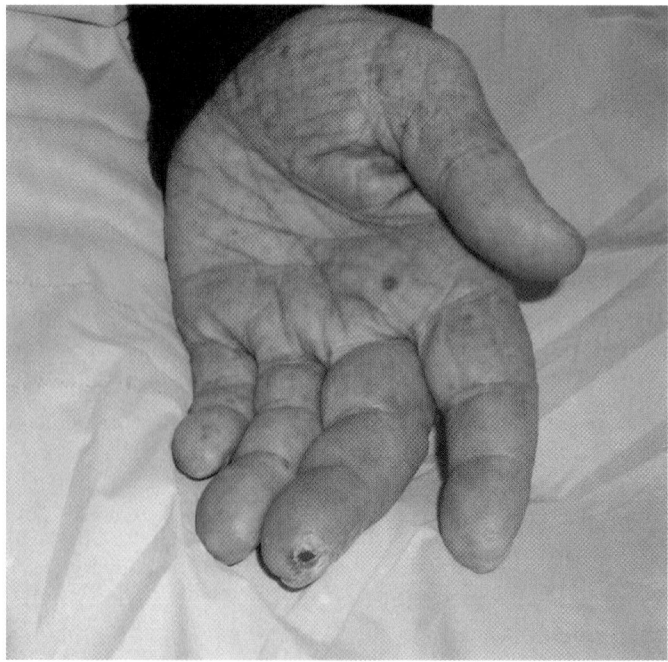

Fig. 23.7.38 Nodules of cutaneous calcinosis may become inflamed and ulcerate, discharging chalky material. Telangiectatic mats are visible on the palm and finger pulps.

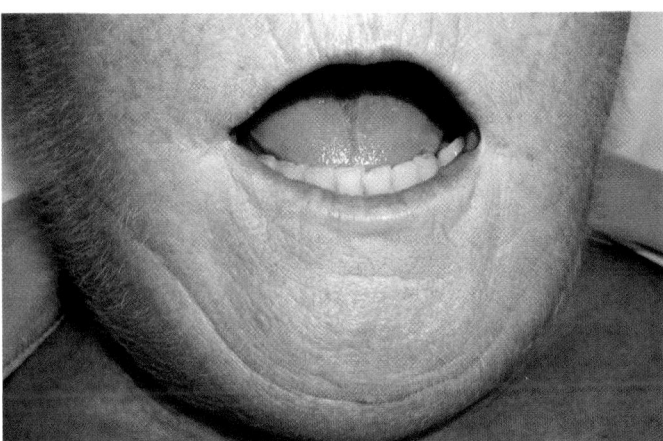

Fig. 23.7.39 Reduced mouth aperture in a patient with diffuse cutaneous systemic sclerosis.

Table 23.7.1 Autoantibodies in systemic sclerosis

Antibody	Type of sclerosis	Clinical associations
Anticentromere antibodies	Limited cutaneous sclerosis	High risk: calcinosis, ischaemic digital loss, pulmonary hypertension Low risk: pulmonary fibrosis Low mortality
Anti-Scl-70 antibodies	Diffuse cutaneous sclerosis	Pulmonary fibrosis High mortality from ventricular failure secondary to pulmonary disease
Anti-Th/To antibodies	Mild skin involvement	Severe pulmonary fibrosis Poor prognosis
Anti-RNA polymerase family antibodies	Diffuse cutaneous sclerosis	Systemic sclerosis-related renal crisis High mortality
Antifibrillarin antibodies/anti-U3 RNP antibodies	Diffuse cutaneous sclerosis	Some populations: myositis, pulmonary hypertension, renal disease

Differential diagnosis

Raynaud's phenomenon with normal nail-fold capillaries and no autoantibodies may be idiopathic or linked to problems such as β-blocker therapy, hyperviscosity syndromes, emboli, or atherosclerosis. Systemic sclerosis must be distinguished from localized forms of scleroderma (see 'Localized scleroderma' below), but these patients do not have Raynaud's phenomenon, and the nail-fold capillaries are normal. Some features of systemic sclerosis, including Raynaud's phenomenon, may be present in patients with rheumatoid arthritis, SLE, dermatomyositis/polymyositis, and Sjögren's syndrome.

Environmental agents and some drugs may induce a scleroderma-like disease (Box 23.7.7). Cutaneous thickening and induration is seen in conditions such as lipodermatosclerosis (the lower leg in venous stasis), sclerodema adultorum (triggered by infection—firm nonpitting oedema of the face, neck, trunk; increased dermal acid mucopolysaccharides), scleromyxoedema (increased dermal acid mucopolysaccharides), chronic graft-versus-host disease, and porphyria cutanea tarda (sun-exposed skin, blistering, skin fragility).

Clinical investigation

Evaluation should include the assessment of systemic involvement (lung, heart, kidney, gastrointestinal tract), functional impairment, and impact on quality of life (Chapter 19.11.3). Skin thickening is assessed by palpating and pinching the skin. Generally, a skin biopsy is not required.

Autoantibodies specific for different subtypes of systemic sclerosis, or for overlap syndromes with other connective tissue diseases, are present in 95% of patients, usually at the onset of disease

(Table 23.7.1). These persist throughout the course of the disease. Less than 1% of patients have more than one systemic sclerosis-specific antibody.

Criteria for diagnosis

Raynaud's phenomenon is defined as episodic bilateral di- or triphasic vascular reactions (pallor, cyanosis, and erythema) of the fingers, toes, ears, or nose that are provoked by cold or emotion. The diagnostic criteria for systemic sclerosis are discussed in Chapter 19.11.3.

Treatment

Moisturizers and sedating antihistamines may reduce pruritus. Patients should avoid nicotine, and keep peripheries warm (Box 23.7.8). Fingertip ulceration in Raynaud's phenomenon may be complicated by secondary infection. Moisturizers (ointments) relieve dryness and cracking of the fingers. Topical antibiotics or antibiotic–steroid combinations may be helpful in superficial ulcers. Hydrocolloid dressings may relieve pain and promote healing.

Systemic treatments to improve peripheral circulation, prevent the synthesis and release of harmful cytokines, and inhibit

---

Box 23.7.7 Agents that cause a scleroderma-like disease

- Chemicals (polyvinyl chloride, solvents, pesticides)
- Drugs (bleomycin, pentazocine, ethosuximide, penicillamine)
- Paraffin
- Contaminated rapeseed oil (toxic oil syndrome)
- L-tryptophan

Box 23.7.8 Improving peripheral circulation

- Avoid nicotine and β-blockers
- Thermal underwear to raise core temperature
- Thermal gloves and/or socks
- Thick-soled padded footwear
- Warm hands for 5 min every 4 h in warm water
- Warm hands in warm water before going outdoors
- Heat pads (purchased in outdoor activity shops)
- Hand or foot warmers (battery powered)
- Glyceryl trinitrate (nitroglycerin) patches
- Oral nifedipine

or reduce fibrosis are discussed in Chapter 19.11.3, but placebo-controlled trials are needed to evaluate these treatments.

Prognosis

Patients with systemic sclerosis have a fourfold risk of death compared with the general population, but the risk of death varies between subgroups. Renal, pulmonary, and cardiac involvement are independent adverse predictors, but as the severity of the cardiovascular, pulmonary, and renal disease correlates with the extent of cutaneous involvement, the extent of skin sclerosis is a useful marker of severity and prognosis. Ten-year survival in patients with limited cutaneous systemic sclerosis is 65 to 88%, whereas that in patients with diffuse cutaneous disease ranges from 61 to 75%. An erythrocyte sedimentation rate greater than 15 to 25 mm/h, or a haemoglobin level lower than 12.5 to 11 g/dl, is associated with a 2.5 to 3-fold increase in mortality. Specific autoantibodies provide additional prognostic information (Table 23.7.1).

Localized scleroderma

Localized scleroderma (morphoea) refers to a group of conditions in which increased collagen deposition causes skin thickening (Fig. 23.7.40). Some patients have more than one type of lesion.

Aetiology, genetics, pathogenesis, and pathology

The pathogenesis of localized scleroderma is unknown, but autoantibodies may play a role. The activation of T lymphocytes and cytokine release may stimulate dermal fibroblast proliferation and collagen production. Endothelial cells also appear to be activated. Infection with agents such as *Borrelia burgdorferi* has been implicated in the pathogenesis of some cases of morphoea, but these findings have not been substantiated.

The histological features are similar to those in the involved skin in systemic sclerosis. The histological features of eosinophilic fasciitis, a deep variant, include marked inflammation and fibrous thickening of the deep fascia and subcutis.

Epidemiology

The prevalence of localized scleroderma has been estimated to be 27 cases per million. Females are affected more often than males.

Linear scleroderma is more common in children, whereas plaque-type morphoea (the most common form of localized scleroderma) is more common in adults.

Clinical features

Plaque morphoea

Patients have one or more lesions, usually on the trunk. These start as erythematous patches that progress to indurated smooth shiny white or yellow plaques with violet borders (the lilac ring) (Fig. 23.7.40). This form of morphoea is self limiting. Inactive lesions hyperpigment (Fig. 23.7.41). Generalized morphoea is a rare variant, usually seen in adults, in which much of the skin becomes sclerotic. Internal organs are not involved, but involvement of the chest wall causes disabling restrictive lung defects.

Linear scleroderma

A unilateral sclerotic band extends along a limb. Deep atrophy may affect underlying subcutaneous tissues, including muscle and bone, so that the limb becomes shortened and wasted. The face is affected in the rare en coup de sabre linear variant in children (Fig. 23.7.42). Disfiguring hemifacial atrophy may be the end result if deeper tissues are affected. These children may also develop neurological complications (seizures, headache, and hemiparesis), eye problems, and misalignment of the jaws.

Eosinophilic fasciitis (Shulman's syndrome)

This scleroderma-like disorder involves the deep fascia, and may be triggered by vigorous exercise. Patients develop symmetrical induration of the skin and subcutaneous tissues, usually of the limbs. The reddish-brown subcutaneous plaques are initially oedematous, but become indurated and brawny. Peripheral eosinophilia is common.

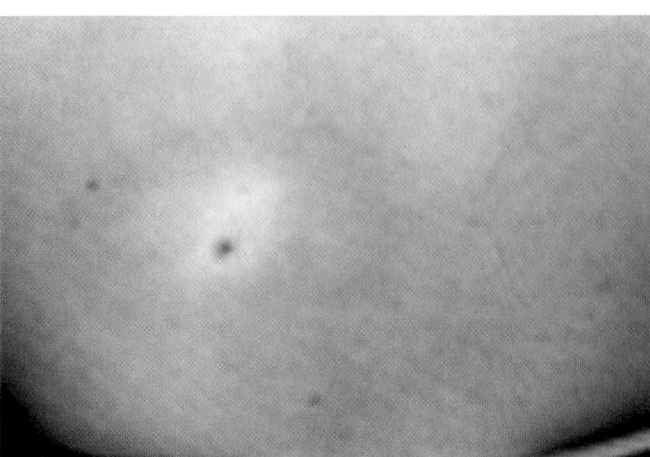

Fig. 23.7.40 Plaque morphoea is the most common form of localized scleroderma. The violet border of the indurated shiny plaque is indicative of inflammation. Plaque morphoea is self limiting, but inactive lesions may become hyperpigmented (a biopsy has been taken from the centre of the plaque).

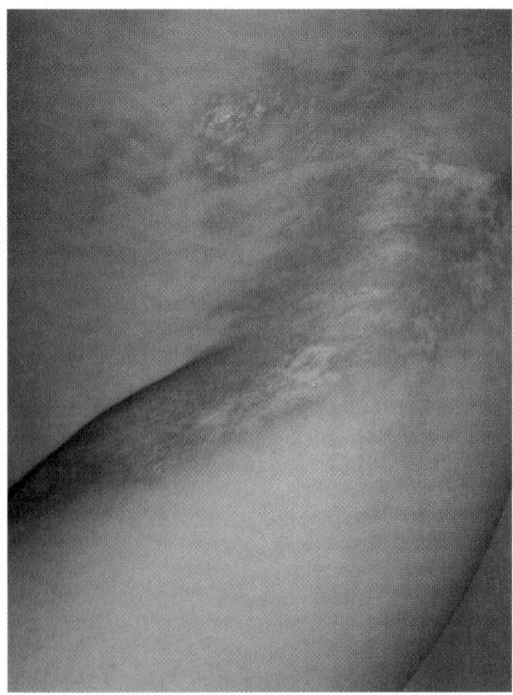

Fig. 23.7.41 The sclerotic plaque on the hip of this child is pigmenting as it softens.

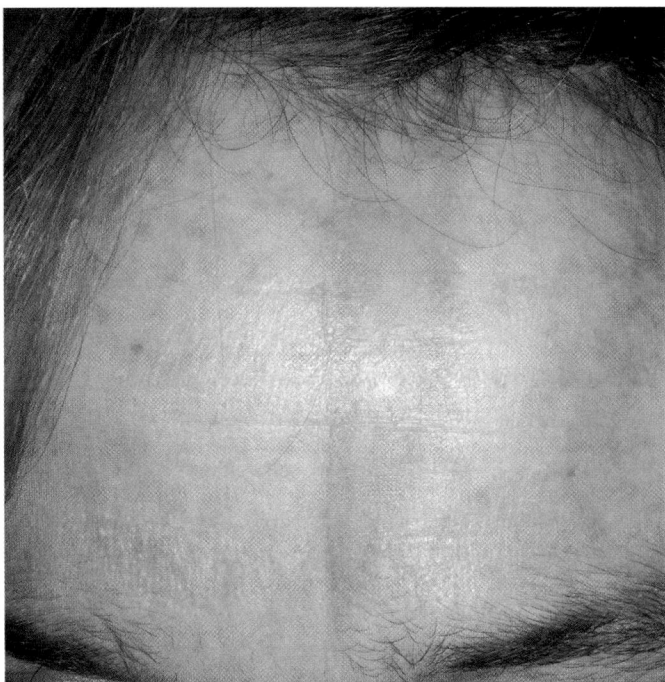

Fig. 23.7.42 En coup de sabre morphoea, now inactive, has left a linear groove on the forehead of this young woman.

Differential diagnosis

Early plaque morphoea can simulate both granuloma annulare and erythema chronicum migrans (see 'Annular erythemas' below). Extragenital lichen sclerosus resembles plaque morphoea, but in lichen sclerosus the surface is slightly hyperkeratotic with follicular plugs. Patients may also have genital lichen sclerosus. Some patients have both lichen sclerosus and morphoea.

Eosinophilic fasciitis must be differentiated from conditions such as cellulitis, deep venous thrombosis, postirradiation injury, toxic oil syndromes, and L-tryptophan-induced eosinophilia–myalgia syndrome.

Clinical investigation

A deep elliptical skin biopsy that extends from normal into abnormal skin may be helpful in diagnosing plaque morphoea, but sometimes the changes are subtle. A full-thickness biopsy that includes fascia and muscle is required in deep variants such as eosinophilic fasciitis.

Patients may have autoantibodies, including antinuclear antibodies, anti-Scl-70, anticentromere antibody, antidouble-stranded DNA, anticardiolipin antibody, and rheumatoid factor, but their significance is unclear.

Bone and joints should be evaluated in patients with linear scleroderma, and limb length discrepancy should be excluded. In linear scleroderma affecting the face, a periodic eye examination should be performed, and MRI considered to detect central nervous system involvement.

Treatment

Treatments have not been evaluated in controlled trials. Plaque morphoea remits spontaneously, and no treatment is required, but a potent topical corticosteroid ointment can be used until the inflammatory ring has settled. Psoralen UVA bath phototherapy

and low-dose UVA1 (340–400 nm) have been reported to be effective in widespread morphoea and linear scleroderma.

Linear scleroderma is difficult to manage, and a multidisciplinary approach is essential. Complications such as joint contractures or malocclusion should be addressed. Monthly intralesional triamcinolone may halt the progression of disease affecting the scalp and forehead. Intravenous methylprednisolone, oral prednisolone, and/or methotrexate have been recommended for progressive linear disease. Once the disease is inactive, reconstructive surgery can reduce deformity. Eosinophilic fasciitis eventually remits spontaneously in many patients, but oral corticosteroids, methotrexate, and azathioprine have been prescribed.

Prognosis

Plaque morphoea is a self-limiting disease that slowly resolves over 3 to 5 years. Eosinophilic fasciitis also remits spontaneously in about one-third of patients.

Rheumatoid arthritis

Rheumatoid arthritis is a chronic inflammatory arthritis in which extra-articular manifestations are common. It is discussed in detail in Chapter 19.5, but the cutaneous manifestations are outlined below.

Cutaneous features

The common cutaneous features of rheumatoid arthritis are listed in Box 23.7.9; these signs are most obvious in the hands.

Rheumatoid nodules are found in 20 to 30% of patients. Nodules are linked to both seropositivity for rheumatoid factor, and severe systemic manifestations. The firm skin-coloured nontender subcutaneous nodules are most common in areas exposed to mild trauma and pressure, e.g. the olecranon, knuckles, knees, and occiput. Rarely, nodules may ulcerate or become infected. The nodules are composed of fibrin-like material surrounded by palisading histiocytes with an outer zone of chronic inflammatory cells. Similar nodules may be found in 5 to 7% of patients with SLE.

Rheumatoid vasculitis is most common in seropositive patients with long-standing nodular disease. Vasculitis involving medium-sized cutaneous vessels presents with livedo reticularis, nodules, and painful punched-out ulcers along the lateral malleoli or pretibial region. Twenty per cent of patients with severe vasculitis have digital gangrene. Peripheral neuropathies are another common manifestation of systemic vasculitis. Small-vessel cutaneous

---

Box 23.7.9 Cutaneous features of rheumatoid arthritis

- Pale, shiny, and atrophic skin in long-standing disease
- Skin fragility and easy bruising
- Palmar erythema
- Bluish discoloration of the finger tips
- Periungual erythema
- Nails ridged longitudinally, with red lunulae
- Rheumatoid vasculitis (small and/or medium cutaneous vessels)
- Leg ulcers (multifactorial)

vasculitis manifests as palpable purpura, papulonecrotic lesions, or urticarial vasculitis (see above). Vasculitic lesions are common on the fingers, even in patients without systemic vasculitis. They include splinter haemorrhages, linear telangiectasia in the nail fold, and petechiae and brownish purpuric lesions of the nail fold or finger pulp (Bywater's lesions) that may infarct and heal leaving small scars.

Ten per cent of patients with rheumatoid arthritis have leg ulcers, but the pathogenesis is multifactorial (Fig. 23.7.43). Trauma, skin fragility, and immobility with venous stasis cause leg ulcers more often than vasculitis. Painful rapidly enlarging ulcers with undermined bluish-red borders can be caused by pyoderma gangrenosum (Fig. 23.7.44) (Chapter 23.15). Patients with Felty's syndrome (rheumatoid arthritis, leukopenia, and splenomegaly) may develop chronic leg ulcers that are refractory to treatment.

Interstitial granulomatous dermatitis with arthritis is an uncommon condition of unknown cause that may be associated with severe rheumatoid arthritis and other systemic autoimmune diseases. Tender linear indurated bands arise symmetrically on the axilla, trunk, and inner portions of the thighs. Rheumatoid neutrophilic dermatitis, another condition of unknown cause, is associated with severe rheumatoid arthritis, and is characterized by papules, plaques, nodules, and urticarial weals. Blistering diseases, including mucous membrane pemphigoid, pemphigus, epidermolysis bullosa acquisita, and subcorneal pustular dermatoses, have been reported in association with rheumatoid arthritis (Chapter 23.4).

Panniculitis

Aetiology, genetics, pathogenesis, and pathology

The panniculitides are classified histologically into predominantly septal or predominantly lobular patterns of inflammation, and some types are associated with vasculitis. Panniculitis may commence in subcutaneous fat, or be caused by dermal inflammation extending into subcutaneous fat. The common subtypes of panniculitis are listed in Box 23.7.10. Some of the panniculitides likely to be encountered by the general physician are considered below, but many are covered elsewhere in organ-specific chapters.

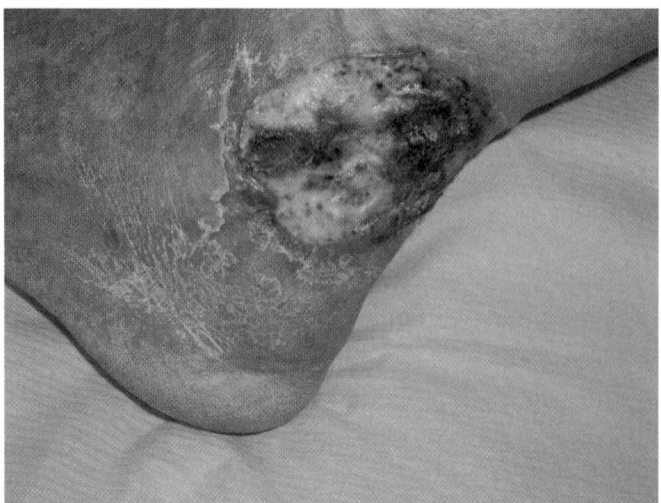

Fig. 23.7.43 Leg ulcers are common in rheumatoid arthritis, and difficult to manage. Biopsy may not be diagnostic. Stasis, trauma, and vasculitis have contributed to ulceration in this man with long-standing rheumatoid arthritis.

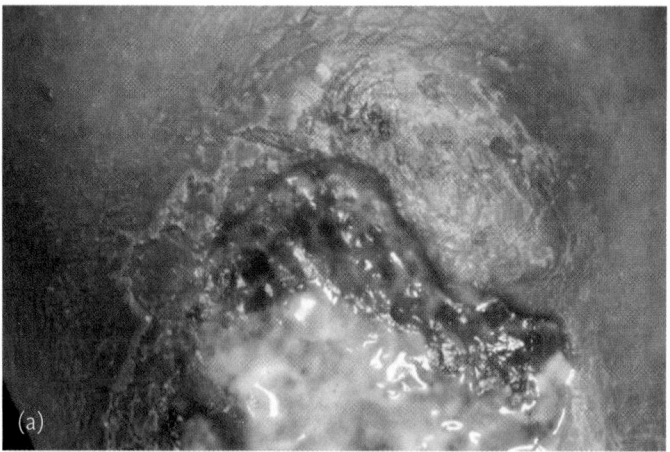

(a)

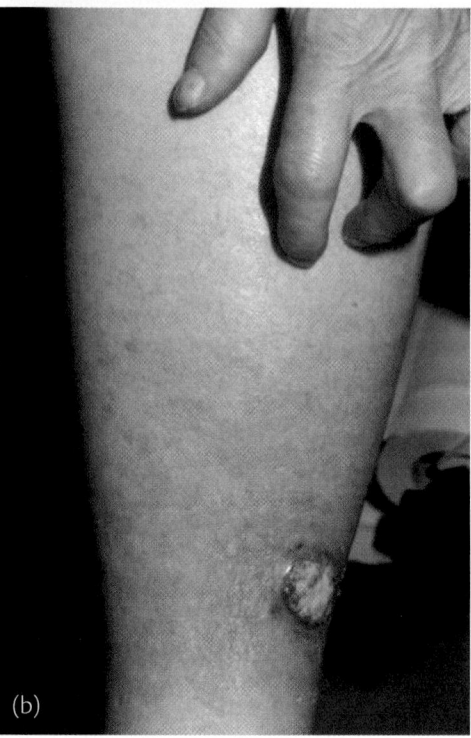

(b)

Fig. 23.7.44 Pyoderma gangrenosum presents as painful rapidly enlarging ulcers with undermined bluish-red borders. In the early stages this may respond to topical treatment with a very potent corticosteroid or tacrolimus.

Septal panniculitis

Erythema nodosum

Aetiology

The pathogenesis is unknown, but erythema nodosum may be a hypersensitivity response to an infection or an underlying inflammatory disease. Inflammation may be triggered by immune complexes deposited in the venules of the septa in subcutaneous fat. A type IV delayed hypersensitivity reaction may be involved.

Erythema nodosum is frequently linked to streptococcal infections in children. The most common associations in adults include infections (bacterial, viral, fungal), drugs, sarcoidosis (erythema nodosum and bilateral hilar adenopathy), and inflammatory bowel disease, as well as miscellaneous conditions ranging from Sweet's syndrome to pregnancy. In about one-third of cases no precipitating factor is identified.

Box 23.7.10 Subtypes of panniculitis

Septal panniculitis

With large-vessel vasculitis

- Superficial thrombophlebitis (see Chapter 23.13)
- Cutaneous polyarteritis nodosa (see above)

Without vasculitis

- Erythema nodosum
- Rheumatoid nodule (see above)
- Necrobiosis lipoidica (see Chapter 23.15)
- Scleroderma and eosinophilic fasciitis (see above)

Lobular panniculitis

With large-vessel vasculitis

- Nodular vasculitis

Without vasculitis

- α_1-Antitrypsin deficiency
- Cold panniculitis
- Sclerosing panniculitis (lipodermatosclerosis) (Fig. 23.7.45)
- Calciphylaxis
- Lupus panniculitis (lupus profundus)
- Pancreatic panniculitis
- Infective panniculitis (infection of subcutaneous fat in immunosuppressed patients)
- Traumatic or factitial panniculitis
- Cytophagic histiocytic panniculitis and subcutaneous T-cell lymphoma

(Weber–Christian disease is no longer considered to be a distinct entity)

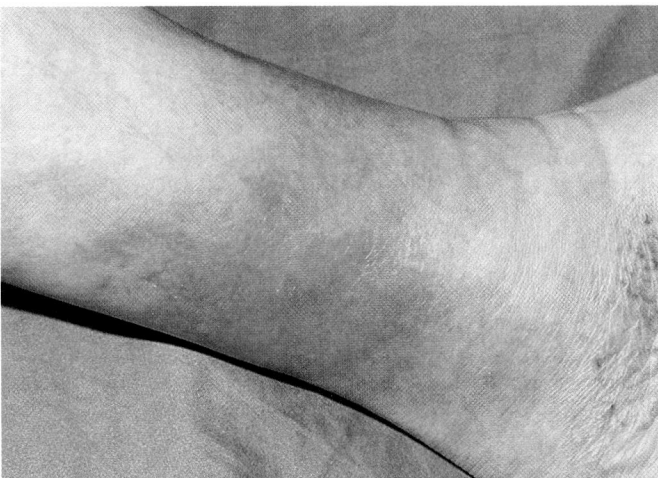

Fig. 23.7.45 Sclerosing panniculitis (lipodermatosclerosis) is a lobular panniculitis found in association with venous stasis.

Erythema nodosum is a septal panniculitis. Septa are inflamed and thickened, neutrophils are present in early lesions, a perivascular lymphocytic infiltrate is present in the overlying dermis, and variable numbers of giant cells and histiocytes form granulomas. Vasculitis is not a feature of typical erythema nodosum, but the erythema nodosum-like lesions that develop in Behçet's disease have a vasculitic histology.

Epidemiology

Erythema nodosum is the most common type of panniculitis. Most cases appear between the second and fourth decades, with a peak incidence between the ages of 20 and 30 years. It occurs more frequently in women.

Both the incidence and prevalence of associated aetiological factors vary geographically. Most cases occur in the first half of the year, possibly linked to an increase in streptococcal infections; one of the most common causes in the United Kingdom is a streptococcal sore throat. Sarcoidosis and tuberculosis are common causes where the incidence of these diseases is high. Ulcerative colitis and Crohn's disease are common associations seen in secondary care in the United Kingdom. Worldwide, erythema nodosum is commonly caused by lepromatous leprosy. This is a widespread and often very persistent reaction to local antigen, and is not typical of erythema nodosum in general. It may become pustular and necrotic.

Other associations of erythema nodosum include blastomycosis, coccidioidomycosis, *Trichophyton verrucosum*, lymphogranuloma venereum, cat-scratch disease, ornithosis, leukaemia, Epstein–Barr virus, Hodgkin's disease, tularaemia, histoplasmosis, yersinia, pregnancy, and drugs such as the contraceptive pill and sulphonamides.

Clinical features

Tender, erythematous, warm nodules measuring 1 to 5 cm or more in diameter are distributed symmetrically on the shins, ankles, and knees (Fig. 23.7.46). Less often, nodules appear on the arms or trunk. The nodules fade over 2 to 6 weeks (more quickly in children), taking on the appearance of a deep bruise. They do not ulcerate, and resolve without loss of fat or scarring. Erythema nodosum may be associated with fever, malaise, arthralgia, and headache, or problems such as abdominal pain, vomiting, or diarrhoea. A chronic migratory variant (subacute nodular migratory panniculitis; erythema nodosum migrans) is less common (Fig. 23.7.47).

Differential diagnosis

Lesions are subcutaneous and erythematous rather than purpuric. The symmetrical distribution suggests an endogenous reaction rather than an exogenous cause such as trauma, cellulitis, or insect bite. Erythema nodosum can be differentiated clinically from nodular vasculitis (erythema induratum of Bazin; see 'Nodular vasculitis' below) by the distribution of the lesions (shins rather than calves) and the absence of ulceration, atrophy, or scarring. The cord-like lesions of superficial thrombophlebitis are usually on the sides of the leg.

Investigation

Underlying causes must be excluded by history taking and examination. Investigations should be guided by the local prevalence of aetiological factors such as bacterial, viral, fungal, or protozoal infections. Preliminary investigations might include full blood count, erythrocyte sedimentation rate, urinalysis, and chest radiography. Skin biopsy is seldom required.

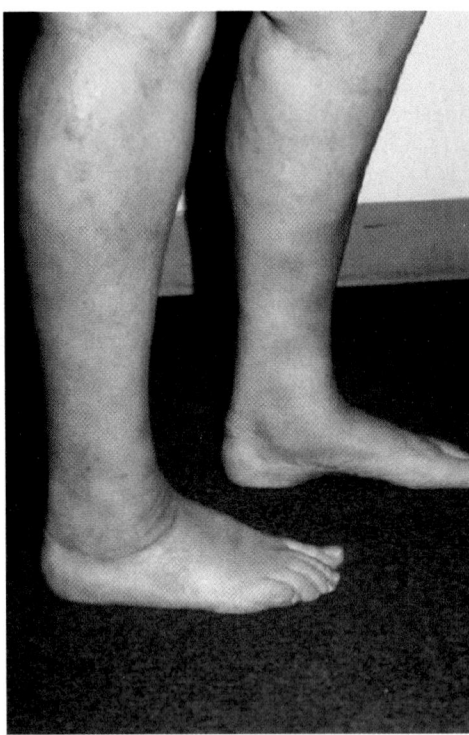

Fig. 23.7.46 Erythema nodosum presenting with tender erythematous nodules on the shins in a patient with sarcoidosis.

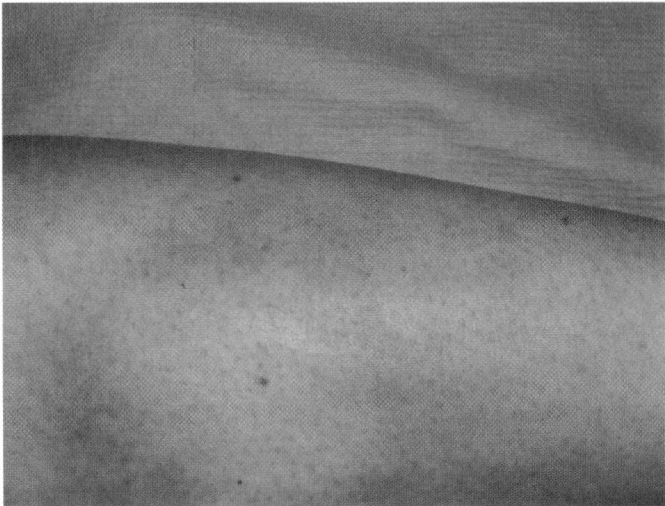

Fig. 23.7.47 The chronic migratory form of erythema nodosum presented as a tender expanding indurated lesion on the leg that persisted for several months. Panniculitis was demonstrated on biopsy. No trigger was identified.

Treatment

Underlying causes should be identified and treated. Pain relief with NSAIDs is generally all that is required. Elevation or bed rest may be helpful in acutely painful disease, and patients may benefit from support stockings to control swelling. Potassium iodide has been recommended in persistent disease. Rarely, oral corticosteroids are needed, but infection must be excluded first.

The prognosis will depend on that of the underlying disease. Idiopathic erythema nodosum is a self-limiting condition with an excellent prognosis. Relapses are uncommon.

Lobular panniculitis

Nodular vasculitis (erythema induratum of Bazin)
Aetiology
Nodular vasculitis is the most common form of lobular panniculitis with vasculitis. It is considered to be a reactive disorder. Bazin described this form of vasculitis in 1861, and a link with tuberculosis was recognized in the early 1900s. *Mycobacterium tuberculosis* DNA has been demonstrated in cutaneous biopsy specimens; however, in many patients no underlying factor is identified. Stasis and cooling play some part in the localization of disease. The pathology is a lobular panniculitis with fat necrosis and vasculitis, primarily affecting the venules and veins of the fibrous septa. This disease affects obese middle-aged women.

Clinical features
Tender indurated erythematous nodules and plaques develop slowly on the calves of fat legs, where the skin is cyanotic and cold. The subcutaneous nodules may ulcerate and heal slowly leaving atrophic scars. Recurrences are frequent. Patients tend to have evidence of venous insufficiency of the lower legs, but are otherwise healthy. Nodular vasculitis runs a protracted course over many years.

Tuberculosis should be excluded by chest radiography and the Mantoux test. A deep incisional biopsy is required to demonstrate the pathology. The indolent presentation, distribution of lesions, ulceration, and scarring differentiate nodular vasculitis from erythema nodosum.

Treatment
Tuberculosis must be treated. Venous stasis should be controlled by weight loss, compression bandages, elevation, and exercise. NSAIDs may relieve pain.

α₁-Antitrypsin deficiency
Lung and liver disease associated with deficiency in α_1-antitrypsin are discussed elsewhere (Chapter 12.13; Sections 15 and 18).

Pathogenesis, genetics, and pathology
α_1-Antitrypsin (AAT) is a circulating inhibitor of serine protease. Subnormal levels of AAT can result in panniculitis, as well as pulmonary or liver disease. The genetic variants are classified into four primary categories (Z,S,M,F). The 90 or more allelic variants of the AAT gene can be divided into three major categories of mutation, which result in enzyme deficiency, null mutations, or altered enzyme function. Enzyme function may be significantly impaired, despite normal serum levels of AAT, but most cases associated with panniculitis have the ZZ phenotype, with AAT levels below normal. The most common histological findings are an acute lobular panniculitis accompanied by neutrophils, fat necrosis, and foamy macrophages.

AAT allele studies have estimated a frequency of 116 million carriers globally, and 3.4 million individuals with the known deficiency allele combinations. Approximately 70 000 to 100 000 individuals in the United States of America and Europe have AAT deficiency. The sexes are affected equally. Adults are affected by panniculitis more often than children.

Clinical features
Recurrent erythematous plaques and nodules develop on the hips, thighs, and buttocks. Nodules may suppurate, with the release of oily material. Panniculitis is characteristically induced or exacerbated by trauma. AAT deficiency is also associated with emphysema, hepatitis, cirrhosis, vasculitis, and angio-oedema.

The proximal distribution combined with nodules that ulcerate and suppurate, helps distinguish this from other panniculitides.

Investigation and treatment

A deep biopsy of a fresh nodule will reveal a suppurative panniculitis. The serum level of AAT and the AAT phenotype are only useful if the clinical and histological findings are compatible with panniculitis associated with AAT deficiency.

This panniculitis may respond to drugs that inhibit neutrophil function, such as dapsone or colchicine. Tetracycline antibiotics may have a direct effect on serine proteases released from neutrophils, and can be helpful in some patients. NSAIDs and hydroxychloroquine have also been recommended.

Cold panniculitis

This form of panniculitis is seen most often in the winter in plump young female horse riders wearing tight clothing that provides insufficient insulation and restricts the blood supply to the subcutaneous fat. The rider develops chilblains affecting the thighs (Chiltern chaps) (Fig. 23.7.48) and buttocks (Berkshire buttocks). The ill-defined mottled bluish-red plaques resolve without scarring. Riders should be advised to wear loose-fitting warm clothing.

Weber–Christian disease

More than 70 years ago Weber used this term to describe a nodular relapsing panniculitis with fever and lipoatrophy. Many cases considered to be examples of Weber–Christian disease have subsequently been given more specific clinicopathological diagnoses, and most authors no longer consider it to be a distinct entity.

Annular erythemas

This group of disorders, also known as gyrate or figurate erythemas, is characterized by lesions that begin as red papules or macules and spread centrifugally to produce rings or arcuate shapes.

Erythema annulare centrifugum

Erythema annulare centrifugum is thought to be a hypersensitivity reaction, and has been linked to a variety of aetiological factors ranging from infection to drugs, but in most cases the cause is unknown. Lymphocytes cluster tightly around the small blood vessels in the superficial and mid dermis. Epidermal changes (spongiosis, parakeratosis) may be present in superficial lesions. It is more common in adults than children.

Clinical

Patients have one or more lesions, most often on the trunk or proximal limbs (Fig. 23.7.49). The lesions start as erythematous papules or macules, and slowly expand by 2 to 3 mm/day into well-defined annular or arcuate shapes (maximum 10 cm diameter) with central clearing, and then fade over days to weeks to leave normal skin. The trailing inner edge of the erythematous ring may be finely scaly in superficial lesions. Sometimes lesions are oedematous and vesicular; they may be itchy.

Most cases pursue a chronic course over several years, but eventually regress spontaneously.

Differential diagnosis

The scale of tinea corporis (ringworm) is more pronounced, and typically is on the outer margin of the ring. Granuloma annulare tends be less erythematous, the ring is composed of coalescing papules that give the lesion a beaded edge if the skin is stretched, lesions are smooth not scaly, and the evolution is less rapid than erythema annulare centrifugum. The cutaneous lesions of subacute cutaneous lupus erythematosus are widespread and are linked to photosensitivity. Neonatal cutaneous lupus should be considered in infants. Smooth annular lesions may also be a manifestation of urticaria, but these fade over 24 h. Erythema annulare centrifugum should also be differentiated from the other annular erythemas—erythema migrans and gyrate erythema (see below).

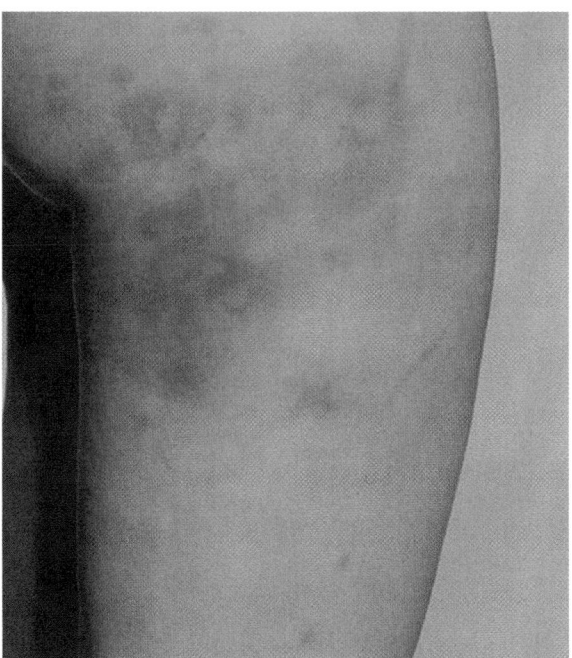

Fig. 23.7.48 Cold panniculitis causes mottled bluish-red chilblains on the thigh of a young female horse rider, so-called 'Chiltern chaps'.

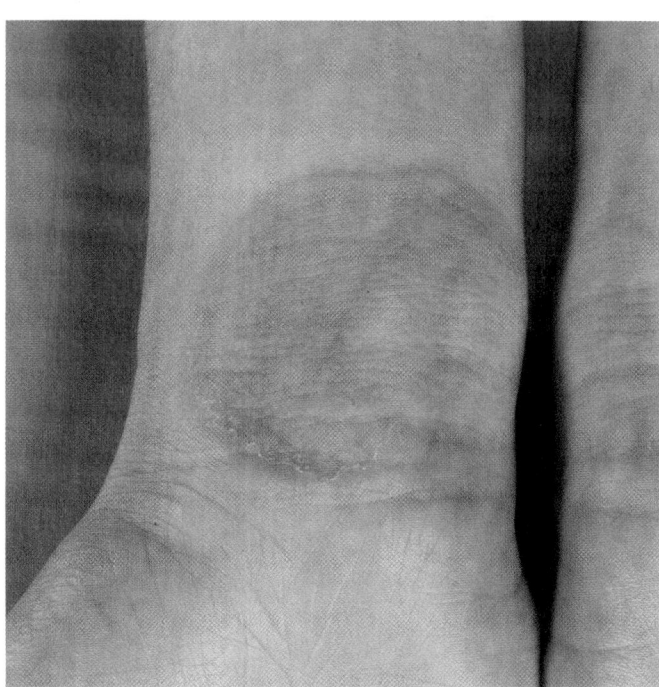

Fig. 23.7.49 Erythema annulare centrifugum is the most common of the annular erythemas. Scale is visible on the inner edge of the erythematous ring.

Investigation and treatment

Fungal infection should be excluded by taking a skin scrape for mycological culture. Topical corticosteroids may relieve irritation, but have no effect on the course of the disease.

Erythema gyratum repens

Waves of rapidly expanding (1 cm/day) erythematous concentric bands give the skin the appearance of wood grain. This is a rare manifestation of internal malignancy.

Erythema migrans

Pathogenesis

Erythema migrans is the first sign of Lyme borreliosis, an infection caused by spirochaetes of the group *Borrelia burgdorferi* sensu lato, which is transmitted by the bite of *Ixodes scapularis* and related ticks (see Chapter 7.6.32). *B. burgdorferi* sensu stricto transmits the disease in the United States of America, whereas *Borrelia garinii* and *Borrelia afzelii* cause most of the illness in Europe. Skin is infiltrated by T lymphocytes, with a predominance of CD4+ helper/inducer cells, as well as numerous plasma cells and CD68+ macrophages. Epidermal Langerhans' cells are invaded by *B. burgdorferi* in early Lyme borreliosis.

Epidemiology

Lyme borreliosis occurs with similar frequency in men and women, and affects people of all ages. The disease is found in forested areas throughout most of Europe, but particularly in Germany (Black Forest), Austria, Slovenia, and Sweden. It has been reported in Russia, Mexico, Asia, Australia, and South Africa. Lyme disease also occurs in the coastal areas of the north-east United States of America, the upper Midwest and the west coast. Birds, mice, deer, voles, and lizards are the major reservoirs of borrelia.

Clinical features

The disease is divided into three stages: early localized disease, early disseminated disease, and persisting late disease.

Erythema migrans occurs around 7 to 10 days after the tick bite in patients with early localized disease. A small erythematous macule or papule appears at the site of the bite, usually the knee, groin, or axilla. As spirochaetes spread through the skin, the erythema extends over days to weeks to produce either an annular lesion with central clearing, or a roundish erythematous patch (Fig. 23.7.50). Lesions range in size from 10 cm to more than 50 cm diameter. A papule with a punctum may be visible in the centre of the primary lesion. Erythema migrans is not scaly and the signs may be subtle, but are more obvious if the skin is warmed. The lesion may be slightly pruritic. Flu-like symptoms are common in the early localized stage.

The haematogenous spread of spirochaetes may induce additional lesions. The rash clears spontaneously, usually in 3 days to 8 weeks, but persistence for more than 1 year has been recorded.

Late cutaneous manifestations are seen more frequently in Europe than in the United States of America. Acrodermatitis chronica atrophicans is a chronic progressive skin condition characterized by bluish-red discoloration of the skin on acral surfaces (dorsa of hands and feet, lower leg). Initially the skin is swollen, but this is followed by atrophy, when the skin appears thin and wrinkled. These changes may be associated with arthritis or polyneuropathy. Lymphadenosis benigna cutis is another chronic

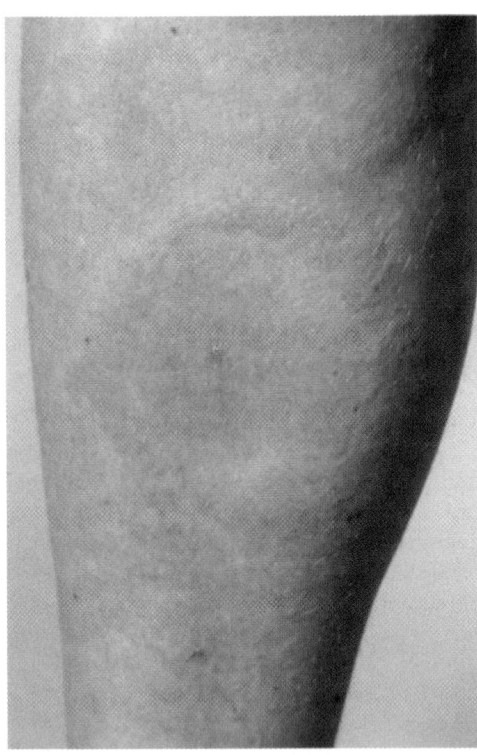

Fig. 23.7.50 Erythema migrans occurs around 7 to 10 days after the tick bite, and continues for days to weeks. Doxycycline is the treatment of choice.

manifestation of borrelia infection, in which painless erythematous nodules develop on the ear lobe, nipple, or scrotum.

Systemic manifestations (cardiac, rheumatological, ophthalmological, neurological) are discussed elsewhere (Chapters 16.7.1, 19.12, 24.11.1, Section 25).

Treatment

If the tick is attached for less than 48 h, infection is unlikely. A single 200 mg dose of doxycycline prevents Lyme borreliosis when given within 72 h of a tick bite. A 14 to 21-day course of doxycycline is recommended for early localized or disseminated infection.

The prognosis is excellent in patients with erythema migrans treated for Lyme borreliosis; persistent infection and relapses are rare. The natural course of disease in European borreliosis is not as well defined as in the United States of America, and the effect of antibiotic treatment on the long-term manifestations is uncertain.

Urticaria and angio-oedema

Introduction

Urticaria is a transient eruption of erythematous or oedematous swellings of the dermis, which are usually pruritic. Angio-oedema consists of transient swellings of deep dermal, subcutaneous, and submucosal tissues, and may coexist with urticaria. Anaphylactic/anaphylactoid episodes involve multiple organ systems and can also be associated with urticaria and angio-oedema. The latter are discussed in detail in Chapters 5.3 and 17.2. Chronic urticaria or angio-oedema is defined as disease on most days for longer than 6 weeks.

Aetiology and pathology

The principal underlying disease mechanism is mast cell degranulation, releasing both preformed mediators, e.g. histamine, and also membrane-derived mediators such as prostaglandins and leukotrienes. Together these lead to vasodilatation, increased vascular permeability, and smooth muscle contraction, among other effects. Histologically, the appearance is variable, but there may be evidence of dermal oedema and an infiltrate possibly including CD4+ T cells, monocytes, neutrophils, basophils, and eosinophils. In the setting of urticarial vasculitis there are likely to be other histological features such as leukocytoclastic vasculitis, as described earlier in the chapter.

Although IgE-mediated allergy is a frequently considered explanation for urticaria, it comprises only one mechanism through which mast cell degranulation can occur. Such degranulation can be induced through a number of mechanisms, and this has led to a reclassification of urticaria and angio-oedema based on aetiology (Table 23.7.2). It has relatively recently been recognized that up to 40 to 60% of adults with chronic urticaria have IgG antibodies specific to the alpha subunit of the high-affinity IgE receptor on mast cells, or IgG antibodies specific to IgE, suggesting an autoimmune diathesis in these patients. Indeed, 27% have antithyroglobulin antibody and/or antimicrosomal antibody. The incidence of angiotensin-converting enzyme (ACE) inhibitor-associated angio-oedema is 0.1 to 0.2%, and may result from the increased availability of bradykinin.

Hereditary C1 esterase inhibitor deficiency is an autosomal dominant disorder, but with a spontaneous mutation rate of 25% and a prevalence of 1 in 50 000. In type I disease, there is a relative deficiency of C1 esterase inhibitor, and in type II disease there are functional defects rather than loss of inhibitor levels. There may be a very rare third type with normal levels and function of C1 esterase inhibitor. Acquired C1 inhibitor deficiency may account for approximately 10% as many cases as the hereditary form of the deficiency, and can be associated with systemic disease, including lymphoproliferative and autoimmune disease. In the presence of C1 esterase inhibitor deficiency, the classical complement pathway can be excessively or inappropriately activated.

Clinical features

Urticaria is characterized by transient red raised itchy weals, varying from a few millimetres to large areas covering many centimetres. The lesions typically last less than 24 h, with no residual changes; however, the presence of more prolonged lesions, particularly when painful or associated with residual bruising, should raise the possibility of an underlying vasculitic aetiology. Angio-oedema consists of transient deeper swellings of subcutaneous or submucosal tissue, which are typically slightly more prolonged than urticarial lesions and may persist for several days. ACE inhibitor-associated angio-oedema may start many years after starting the drug, and may take months to settle after stopping. Persisting disease after termination of ACE inhibitor therapy should prompt the possibility of ACE inhibitor-exacerbated idiopathic angio-oedema.

As the typical lesions are frequently not present at examination, a detailed history is a cornerstone of diagnosis and should include the nature of the lesions, their frequency, timing, and any putative triggers, as well as other symptoms, drug history, and family history. Although delayed reactions are well described, potential allergic food triggers are typically only relevant in the 60 min before the onset of the episode. The clinical features of allergic disease are discussed in Chapters 5.3 and 16.5. It can be helpful to test for dermographism by gentle rubbing of the skin and examining for an urticarial response within a few minutes.

Table 23.7.2 Classification and investigation of urticaria/angio-oedema

Aetiology	Mechanism	Investigations
Autoimmune	IgG specific to FceRI and/or IgE	Thyroid antibodies, thyroid function, ANA Specialist centres may undertake a basophil histamine release test and an autologous serum skin test
Physical stimuli	Physical induction of mast cell degranulation	Challenge testing with appropriate stimuli, e.g. dermographism, ice cube, exercise, pressure Cryoglobulins (cold urticaria)
Allergic (IgE-mediated)	IgE specific to food, airborne allergens, drugs, e.g. penicillin, latex	Skin prick testing or specific IgE to allergen
Drug induced	Increased availability of bradykinin (ACE inhibitors), NSAIDS, opiates	Response to avoidance
C1 esterase inhibitor deficiency	Genetic or acquired	C4 and/or C1 esterase inhibitor level/function, autoimmune screen, lymphoproliferative screen
Vasculitis	Vessel wall inflammation Possible immune complex involvement	FBC, ESR, urinalysis, renal, liver, ASOT, hepatitis B/C, Ig electrophoresis, autoimmune screen, ANCA, C3, skin biopsy
Lymphoproliferative	Paraproteinaemia	Paraprotein in blood and urine
Food constituent (non-IgE), e.g. salicylates (rare)	Unknown	Response to exclusion
Infection	Parasites, viral exanthems, EBV, hepatitis B and C	Relevant serology, stool microscopy
Idiopathic	Unknown	Typically negative

ACE, angiotensin-converting enzyme; ANA, antinuclear antibody; ANCA, antineutrophil cytoplasmic antibody; ASOT, antistreptolysin O titre; EBV, Epstein–Barr virus; ESR, erythrocyte sedimentation rate; FBC, full blood count; NSAID, nonsteroidal anti-inflammatory drug.

A diagnosis of C1 esterase inhibitor deficiency is suggested by a history of recurrent episodes of angio-oedema and abdominal pain. The swellings are not typically pruritic. Although urticaria is not associated, there can be a prodromal erythema in up to 25%. Classically, the oedema develops over 12 to 36 h and takes 2 to 5 days to subside. Episodes can arise spontaneously or following minor trauma, such as dental work. Other triggers include oestrogens, ACE inhibitors, or infection.

Clinical investigation and treatment

Table 23.7.2 shows a possible investigation strategy based on the known aetiologies. The approach to the investigation of allergic disease is discussed in Chapters 5.3 and 17.2. In practice, it is not uncommon for all investigations to be normal in chronic urticaria/angio-oedema, which are then, rather unsatisfactorily, currently grouped as idiopathic. C4 is a useful screening test for untreated C1 esterase inhibitor deficiency, and if low, then C1 esterase inhibitor and/or function can be measured.

In the management of chronic idiopathic urticaria it is common practice to start with a regular long-acting nonsedating antihistamine, unless the episode frequency is low, in which case the antihistamine can be taken as required. It may be necessary to increase the dose of the antihistamine or add a different histamine to gain satisfactory control, as long as the benefits outweigh the risks. If these measures fail it may be required to consider using other approaches, such as the use of a sedating antihistamine, leukotriene-receptor antagonist, or other agent such as ciclosporin for very severe disease. It is advisable to avoid ACE inhibitors. Tranexamic acid can be a helpful adjunct to the therapy of angio-oedema. The carrying of adrenaline autoinjectors should be considered if there is a history of angio-oedema affecting the upper airway, or if there are other anaphylactoid features, subject to the absence of contraindications. Clearly, if there is an allergic cause for the urticaria/angio-oedema, or if there is a defined trigger, then the patient should be counselled on avoidance (see Chapters 5.3 and 16.5).

Acute treatment for a severe episode associated with hereditary C1 esterase inhibitor deficiency can be with C1 inhibitor concentrate or fresh frozen plasma. Prophylactic treatment of hereditary angio-oedema is often by attenuated androgens and/or tranexamic acid; there are a number of new developments in the pipeline, including genetically engineered C1 esterase inhibitor, kallikrein inhibitor, and bradykinin B2 receptor antagonist.

Prognosis

Up to 20% of patients with chronic urticaria attending hospital departments will be symptomatic 10 years after first presentation. More prolonged duration associates with more severe disease, the presence of angio-oedema, and positive antithyroid antibodies.

Further reading

Cutaneous vasculitis

Fiorentino DF (2003). Cutaneous vasculitis. *J Am Acad Dermatol*, **48**, 311–40.

Ghersetich I, *et al.* (1999). Proposal for a working classification of cutaneous vasculitis. *Clin Dermatol*, **17**, 499–503.

Jennette JC, *et al.* (1997). Small-vessel vasculitis. *N Engl J Med*, **337**, 1512–23.

Jorizzo JL (1998). Livedoid vasculopathy: what is it? *Arch Dermatol*, **134**, 491–3.

Lotti T, *et al.* (1998). Cutaneous small-vessel vasculitis. *J Am Acad Dermatol*, **39**, 667–87; quiz 88–90.

Sansonno D, *et al.* (2005). Hepatitis C virus, cryoglobulinaemia, and vasculitis: immune complex relations. *Lancet Infect Dis*, **5**, 227–36.

Cutaneous lupus erythematosus

Albrecht J, *et al.* (2004). Dermatology position paper on the revision of the 1982 ACR criteria for systemic lupus erythematosus. *Lupus*, **13**, 839–49.

Callen JP (2004). Update on the management of cutaneous lupus erythematosus. *Br J Dermatol*, **151**, 731–6.

Orteu CH, *et al.* (2001). The pathophysiology of photosensitivity in lupus erythematosus. *Photodermatol Photoimmunol Photomed*, **17**, 95–113.

Sontheimer RD (2004). Skin manifestations of systemic autoimmune connective tissue disease: diagnostics and therapeutics. *Best Pract Res Clin Rheumatol*, **18**, 429–62.

Sontheimer RD (2005). Subacute cutaneous lupus erythematosus: 25-year evolution of a prototypic subset (subphenotype) of lupus erythematosus defined by characteristic cutaneous, pathological, immunological, and genetic findings. *Autoimmun Rev*, **4**, 253–63.

Cutaneous features of dermatomyositis

Choy EH, *et al.* (2005). Immunosuppressant and immunomodulatory treatment for dermatomyositis and polymyositis. *Cochrane Database Syst Rev*, **3**, CD003643.

Gerami P, *et al.* (2006). A systematic review of adult-onset clinically amyopathic dermatomyositis (dermatomyositis sine myositis): a missing link within the spectrum of the idiopathic inflammatory myopathies. *J Am Acad Dermatol*, **54**, 597–613.

Santmyire-Rosenberger B, *et al.* (2003). Skin involvement in dermatomyositis. *Curr Opin Rheumatol*, **15**, 714–22.

Sontheimer RD (1999). Cutaneous features of classic dermatomyositis and amyopathic dermatomyositis. *Curr Opin Rheumatol*, **11**, 475–82.

Sontheimer RD (2004). The management of dermatomyositis: current treatment options. *Expert Opin Pharmacother*, **5**, 1083–99.

Scleroderma

Cepeda EJ, *et al.* (2004). Autoantibodies in systemic sclerosis and fibrosing syndromes: clinical indications and relevance. *Curr Opin Rheumatol*, **16**, 723–32.

Ioannidis JP, *et al.* (2005). Mortality in systemic sclerosis: an international meta-analysis of individual patient data. *Am J Med*, **118**, 2–10.

LeRoy EC, *et al.* (1988). Scleroderma (systemic sclerosis): classification, subsets and pathogenesis. *J Rheumatol*, **15**, 202–5.

LeRoy EC, *et al.* (2001). Criteria for the classification of early systemic sclerosis. *J Rheumatol*, **28**, 1573–6.

Meyer O (2006). Prognostic markers for systemic sclerosis. *Joint Bone Spine*, **73**, 490–4.

Nadashkevich O, Davis P, Fritzler MJ (2004). A proposal of criteria for the classification of systemic sclerosis. *Med Sci Monit*, **10**, CR615–21.

Naschitz JE, *et al.* (1996). The fasciitis-panniculitis syndromes. Clinical and pathologic features. *Medicine (Baltimore)*, **75**, 6–16.

Sapadin AN, *et al.* (2002). Treatment of scleroderma. *Arch Dermatol*, **138**, 99–105.

Zulian F, *et al.* (2005). Localised scleroderma in childhood is not just a skin disease. *Arthritis Rheum*, **52**, 2873–81.

Zulian F, *et al.* (2006). Juvenile localised scleroderma: clinical and epidemiological features in 750 children. An international study. *Rheumatology (Oxford)*, **45**, 614–20.

Rheumatoid arthritis

Jorizzo JL, *et al.* (1983). Dermatologic conditions reported in patients with rheumatoid arthritis. *J Am Acad Dermatol*, **8**, 439–57.

Sayah A, *et al.* (2005). Rheumatoid arthritis: a review of the cutaneous manifestations. *J Am Acad Dermatol*, **53**, 191–209; quiz 10–2.

Panniculitis

Requena L, *et al.* (2001). Panniculitis. Part I. Mostly septal panniculitis. *J Am Acad Dermatol*, **45**, 163–83; quiz 84–6.

Requena L, *et al.* (2001). Panniculitis. Part II. Mostly lobular panniculitis. *J Am Acad Dermatol*, **45**, 325–61; quiz 62–4.

White JW Jr, *et al.* (1998). Weber–Christian panniculitis: a review of 30 cases with this diagnosis. *J Am Acad Dermatol*, **39**, 56–62.

Annular erythemas

Dinser R, *et al.* (2005). Antibiotic treatment of Lyme borreliosis: what is the evidence? *Ann Rheum Dis*, **64**, 519–23.

Hengge UR, *et al.* (2003). Lyme borreliosis. *Lancet Infect Dis*, **3**, 489–500.

Mullegger RR (2004). Dermatological manifestations of Lyme borreliosis. *Eur J Dermatol*, **14**, 296–309.

Urticaria and angio-oedema

Gompels MM, *et al.* (2005). C1 inhibitor deficiency: consensus document. *Clin Exp Allergy*, **139**, 379–94.

Grattan CEH, Humphreys F (2007). Guidelines for evaluation and management of urticaria in adults and children. *Br J Dermatol*, **157**, 1116–23.

Kaplan AP (2002). Clinical practice. Chronic urticaria and angioedema. *N Engl J Med*, **346**, 175–9.

Powell RJ, *et al.* (2007). BSACI guidelines for the management of chronic urticaria and angio-oedema. *Clin Exp Allergy*, **37**, 631–50.

Disorders of pigmentation

Eugene Healy

Essentials

Normal human skin colour results from the reflection of light from haemoglobin in blood, and carotenoids and melanin pigmentation in skin. The melanin pigmentation is the major component determining differences in skin colour between races.

Increases and decreases in skin pigmentation (hyperpigmentation and hypopigmentation, respectively) may be localized or generalized, can result from a wide variety of physiological or pathological processes, including both genetic and acquired factors, and may reflect underlying systemic disease.

Addison's disease (primary adrenocortical hypofunction) can result in diffuse hyperpigmentation, more pronounced in sun-exposed areas, sites exposed to trauma, such as the elbows and knees, the creases of the palms and soles, surgical scars, the buccal and gingival mucosa, as well as the nipples and genital region. Numerous drugs can cause changes in pigmentation, e.g. amiodarone can cause a blue-grey discolouration of the skin whereas bleomycin can cause a flagellate pattern of hyperpigmentation.

Vitiligo is characterized by white patches of variable size, but in some darker-skinned people the margin or entire patch may be an intermediate colour of light brown (trichrome vitiligo). Patches may be generalized or segmental in distribution, and the borders are irregular. In the generalized form lesions are usually symmetrical, and the more frequently involved sites are around the orifices (eyes, nose, mouth), flexures (axillae, groins, genitals), and extensor surfaces (elbows, knees, digits). The isomorphic or Koebner phenomenon can occur, in which trauma to the skin can produce lesions at that site. The skin is usually normal otherwise, with no evidence of scaling or atrophy.

Microbial diseases such as pityriasis versicolor, leprosy, and syphilis are important infectious causes of hypopigmentation. Irrespective of cause and associations with underlying systemic disease, disorders of pigmentation can cause considerable distress to sufferers due to the visible nature of this condition.

Introduction

Melanin is synthesized in intracellular organelles called melanosomes by the melanocyte, a dendritic cell situated in the basal layer of the epidermis and in the hair follicle. There are two types of melanin, brown-black eumelanin and red-yellow phaeomelanin, and the combination of these in different proportions results in a wide variety of skin and hair colours worldwide. The biochemical pathways responsible for the synthesis of the two melanin types involve the sequential manufacture of several melanin intermediates from the precursor amino acid tyrosine, and require certain melanogenic enzymes, including tyrosinase, tyrosinase-related protein 1, and dopachrome tautomerase (tyrosinase-related protein 2) (Fig. 23.8.1).

Melanin-laden melanosomes are passed along the dendrites of the melanocyte, and into adjacent keratinocytes; approximately 40 keratinocytes receive melanin from a single melanocyte, thus forming the epidermal melanin unit. In keratinocytes, especially in the basal layer of the epidermis, the melanin becomes packaged over the nucleus to protect the DNA against incident ultraviolet (UV) radiation. Although the exact role of phaeomelanin is unclear, it is accepted that eumelanin is photoprotective, with greater quantities of eumelanin in darker-skinned races.

Some variation in pigmentation exists within and between different skin sites in most individuals, e.g. the freckling (ephelides) of fair Celtic skin, and the lighter pigmentation on the palms and soles of black skin. Increases and decreases in skin pigmentation (hyperpigmentation and hypopigmentation, respectively) can result from a wide variety of physiological and pathological processes. The degree to which alterations in pigmentation are obvious to an independent observer, and the amount of concern that they cause affected individuals, is often influenced by the patient's natural (constitutive) skin colour and the extent to which the altered pigmentation contrasts with this. However, even minor alterations in pigment can cause significant distress to patients, possibly related to the fact that mild pigmentary changes can often be detected relatively easily by individuals from the same racial group as the affected person.

Normal skin pigmentation

Skin and hair colour varies within and across populations, with variations in hair colour greater in light-skinned than more

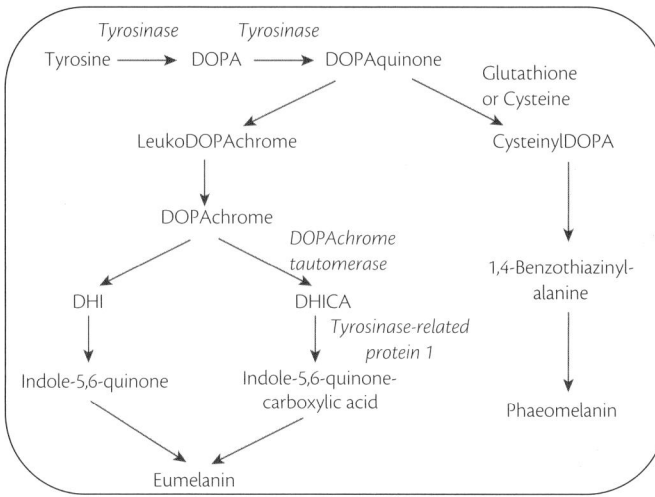

Fig. 23.8.1 Melanin synthesis pathways in the melanosome. DHI, 5,6-dihydroxyindole; DHICA, 5,6-dihydroxyindole-2-carboxylic acid; DOPA, 3,4-dihydroxyphenylalanine.

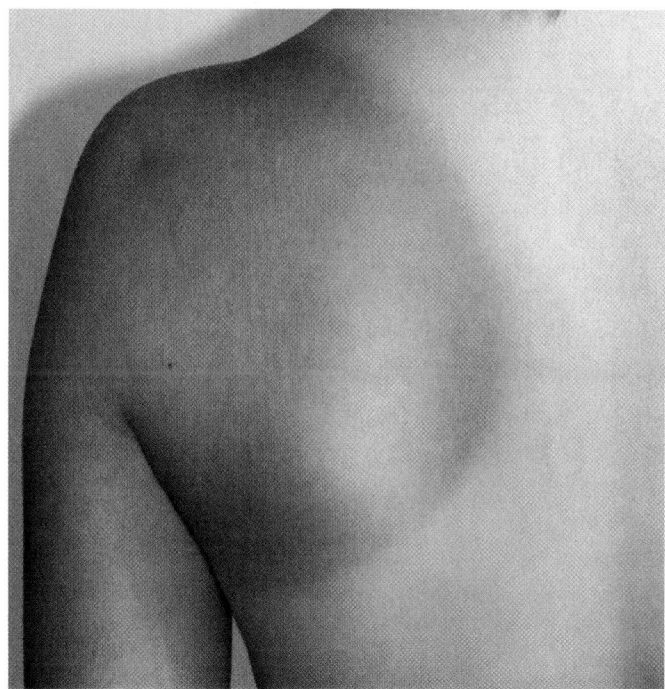

Fig. 23.8.2 Ultraviolet radiation-induced tanning in a white individual.

pigmented races. Despite the large differences in constitutive skin colour between races, similar numbers of melanocytes are present in the skin of whites, Asians, and blacks, but the melanosomes are significantly larger in black skin.

It has been estimated that variation in four to six genes accounts for most of the variation in normal human skin colour. Recent evidence suggests that a single evolutionary alteration in the *SLC24A5* gene (OMIM 609802) (substitution of threonine for alanine at codon 111) is responsible for white skin being less pigmented. In addition, certain heterozygous variants of the melanocortin 1 receptor (*MC1R*) gene cause fair skin type in whites, whereas compound heterozygous and homozygous *MC1R* variants lead to red hair. Other genes that seem relevant to variation in skin and hair pigmentation within and across populations include the *P* (OCA2) gene (OMIM 611409) and the agouti signalling protein (*ASIP*)(OMIM 600201) gene as well as the tyrosinase (TYR) (OMIM 606933), tyrosinase-related protein 1 (*TYRP1*) (OMIM 115501), *SLC45A2* (*MATP*) (OMIM 606202), *KITLG* (OMIM 184745), *SLC24A4* (OMIM 609840) and *IRF4* (601900) genes.

In general, cutaneous melanocytes are restricted to the hair follicles in nonhuman mammals and primates, and it is thought that the development of melanocytes in human skin evolved in Africa as a means of photoprotection, possibly to prevent the photodegradation of folate and/or to avoid blistering sunburn leading to infection and death in childhood and early adulthood. As human populations moved out of Africa, the subsequent lightening of skin secondary to genetic changes may either have occurred to enable the UVB-induced synthesis of vitamin D in skin, or resulted from the loss of selective pressure from UV radiation (i.e. the lack of a requirement for high-level photoprotection in places with lower UV radiation exposure).

UV radiation-induced pigmentation/ tanning

UV radiation is a frequent cause of increased skin pigmentation, with UVB and UVA both able to stimulate tanning (Fig. 23.8.2). In general, the history of sun exposure is obvious, and there is a sharp cut-off in pigmentation between exposed and unexposed sites. The speed of development, colour, and intensity of the tan differs between individuals, with people having a Celtic skin phenotype less likely to tan, or more likely to tan poorly following UV radiation exposure.

Several molecular mechanisms have been proposed to underlie the tanning response, and signalling via the melanocortin 1 receptor secondary to increased α-melanocyte stimulating hormone (αMSH) is thought to be one important mechanism. Although repeated exposure to UV radiation causes melanin synthesis and an increase in the total amount of melanin in skin, the initial changes in skin colour during tanning may result from a redistribution of some melanin to a higher level in the epidermis. In a single individual, the degree of melanin synthesis and thus the degree of tanning is dependent on the dose of UV radiation (including UV radiation intensity and duration of exposure). Whereas the increased amount of melanin in tanned skin is considered to offer greater protection against UV radiation, photoprotection by other mechanisms (e.g. thickening of the stratum corneum) is also physiologically important. It should be noted that there are some indications that tanning may be a response to DNA damage, raising questions about whether there is such a thing as a 'healthy' tan.

Hyperpigmentation

The causes of hyperpigmentation are given in Table 23.8.1.

Endocrine causes of hyperpigmentation

Several hormones can stimulate melanin synthesis in melanocytes. These include proopiomelanocortin (POMC), a peptide synthesized in the pituitary (a precursor of ACTH), αMSH (the first 13 amino acids of ACTH), and β-melanocyte stimulating hormone (βMSH). In Addison's disease (primary adrenocortical hypofunction) the lowered serum cortisol level means that there is a lack of

Table 23.8.1 Causes of skin hyperpigmentation

Type	Cause
Localized	
Lentigo type	Lentigo simplex, lentigo senilis, lentigo maligna, Peutz–Jeghers syndrome, xeroderma pigmentosum, LEOPARD syndrome, Carney complex, PUVA lentigines
Café-au-lait type	Normal skin (fewer than six), neurofibromatosis* type 1 (von Recklinghausen's disease), McCune–Albright syndrome, Fanconi's anaemia
Naevoid type	Junctional naevus, Becker's naevus, naevus spilus, naevus of Ota, naevus of Ito, Mongolian blue spot, seborrhoeic keratosis (early stage)
Drugs	Fixed drug eruption (caused by various drugs, e.g. nonsteroidal anti-inflammatories), minocycline, bleomycin-induced flagellate dermatosis
Melasma	Pregnancy, oral contraceptives, idiopathic
Infections	Erythrasma, tinea (pityriasis) versicolor
Inflammatory/postinflammatory	Lichen planus, psoriasis, eczema, trauma (e.g. burns), acne vulgaris
Miscellaneous	Incontinentia pigmenti, urticaria pigmentosa, acanthosis nigricans, morphoea, erythema ab igne, poikiloderma, tattoo ink, primary localized cutaneous amyloidosis (macular amyloidosis, lichen amyloidosis)
Generalized	
Endocrine	Addison's disease, Cushing's disease, Nelson's syndrome, ACTH- and αMSH-secreting tumours, thyrotoxicosis
Drugs	Phenothiazines/chlorpromazine, antimalarials (chloroquine, hydroxychloroquine, quinine), anticancer drugs (busulfan, cyclophosphamide, dactinomycin, doxorubicin, fluorouracil, hydroxycarbamide, methotrexate), miscellaneous (amiodarone, minocycline, phenytoin)
Ultraviolet radiation	Natural sunshine, artificial sources (broadband UVB, narrowband UVB, UVA, PUVA)
Postinflammatory	Lichen planus, psoriasis, eczema, etc.
Nutritional deficiency	Malabsorption, malnutrition
Miscellaneous	Haemochromatosis, scleroderma, porphyria cutanea tarda, liver disease, dyskeratosis congenita, Fanconi's anaemia, confluent and reticulated papillomatosis

Note that the distinction between localized and generalized is not absolute, and that generalized pigmentation may be diffuse (e.g. on the trunk) or consist of localized pigmentation on several body sites. αMSH, α-melanocyte stimulating hormone; PUVA, psoralen and UVA; UV, ultraviolet.
* Neurofibromatosis is described in Chapter 24.17

negative feedback on the pituitary synthesis of ACTH and related POMC peptides. This results in diffuse hyperpigmentation that is more pronounced in sun-exposed sites, and is similar to that observed following the exogenous administration of ACTH, αMSH, and βMSH. Pigmentation is also more evident at sites exposed to trauma, such as the elbows and knees, the creases of the palms and soles, surgical scars, and the buccal and gingival mucosa, as well as the nipples and genital region; however, the absence of hyperpigmentation does not exclude the diagnosis of Addison's disease (see Chapter 13.7.1).

Hyperpigmentation in an addisonian pattern can occur in Cushing's syndrome (raised serum cortisol), where it arises from excess ACTH

secretion from a pituitary adenoma (termed Cushing's disease), or ectopic ACTH secretion from a malignancy (e.g. bronchial small cell carcinoma, pulmonary carcinoid tumours). Similarly, diffuse marked hyperpigmentation is seen in Nelson's syndrome following bilateral adrenalectomy for pre-existing Cushing's disease, where high circulating ACTH levels from a pituitary adenoma are increased further as a result of the absence of negative feedback by cortisol from the adrenals. Generalized pigmentation of the skin can also be observed in patients with thyrotoxicosis caused by Graves' disease.

Hyperpigmentation is also common in pregnancy, with darkening of the linea alba to form the linea nigra, and pigmentation of the nipples, genital skin, and face; the hypermelanosis of the cheeks, chin, and forehead is termed melasma (see below) and is also seen in women taking oral contraceptives.

Melasma

Melasma, also known as chloasma, is a hyperpigmentary disorder affecting the face. It generally develops symmetrically as darker brown areas on the cheeks, upper lip, forehead, and chin, and is seen more frequently in women, but also affects men. It is more common in darker-skinned whites, Asians, Hispanics, and people from India and the Middle East, and is more apparent following sun exposure, sometimes fading during the winter months and relapsing during the summer.

In some cases histology shows increased melanin in the epidermis, whereas in others the melanin is in dermal melanophages. The exact pathogenesis of melasma is unclear, but several factors seem important in aggravating the condition, e.g. pregnancy, oral contraceptives, and exposure to UV radiation. Theories that have been postulated to explain its aetiology include the pigmentary effects of some unknown endocrine factor or locally produced αMSH. Some authors have suggested that the disorder is a result of a photosensitivity reaction to some allergen in cosmetic products. In addition, certain drugs (e.g. phenytoin) can induce a melasma-like condition.

Melasma may resolve after parturition or when contraceptives are discontinued, but in a proportion of cases it may last for several years. Adherence to adequate sun protection measures is imperative as part of any treatment strategy. Topical bleaching agents, such as those containing hydroquinone, can be helpful, but it is important that the concentration of hydroquinone is not greater than 2 to 4%, as higher concentrations seem more likely to cause hyperpigmentation (ochronosis), or in some cases be toxic to melanocytes and cause permanent depigmentation. Hydroquinone may also be combined with topical corticosteroids to reduce the occurrence of contact dermatitis and post-inflammatory hyperpigmentation. Other therapeutic agents include tretinoin, azelaic acid, and 4% N-acetyl-4-S-cysteaminylphenol.

Chemical and drug-induced hyperpigmentation

Increased skin pigmentation at localized skin sites can occur following contact with certain chemicals in plants and perfumes when combined with UV radiation exposure. Phytophotodermatitis is an inflammatory and hyperpigmentary reaction at a skin site that has been in contact with a plant containing furocoumarins or psoralens, and subsequently been exposed to UV radiation. The inflammation (consisting of erythema and sometimes blistering) and later pigmentation is often streaked, because of the accidental nature of the contact between the plant juices and the skin. Although less frequent, berloque dermatitis is a similar entity in which the offending agent is bergapten (5-methoxypsoralen), found in bergamot oil, which is present in some perfumes. The hands can be affected by phytophotodematitis after squeezing or slicing fruit, as this allows exposure to psoralens present in the peel. Topical treatment with nitrogen mustards can cause localized hyperpigmentation through an unknown mechanism.

Another cause of linear streaks of pigmentation secondary to exogenous agents is that following systemic therapy with the anticancer drug bleomycin, which induces a flagellate dermatosis. The exact site of the reaction and the streaky nature of the initial inflammation and later pigmentation may be caused by scratching of the skin by the patient during the bleomycin therapy.

Generalized pigmentation or more localized pigmentation of the mucosae and/or nails can be seen during treatment with a wide variety of drugs and therapeutic agents. In some situations the cause is generally obvious to the patient, e.g. during photochemotherapy for psoriasis with psoralen and UVA (PUVA). In cases of generalized pigmentation secondary to systemic medications the discolouration of the skin can vary from brown to slate grey, depending on the causative drug (Fig. 23.8.3). Medications responsible for this type of pigmentation are listed in Table 23.8.1. For example, amiodarone can cause a generalized blue-grey discolouration of the skin.

Fixed drug eruptions are localized inflammatory reactions in skin, caused by various agents including antimicrobials, analgesics/nonsteroidal anti-inflammatories, sedatives, metals, and halides. The inflammatory reaction recurs at the same skin site on each occasion the offending agent is ingested, and seems to result from specific immunological characteristics of the skin at the affected location. Multiple lesions can occur, but in most cases solitary lesions are observed. Upon resolution of the inflammation there remains in many cases a brownish discolouration caused by pigmentary incontinence resulting from damage to the basal layer of the epidermis; deposition of the melanin in dermal

macrophages causes persistence of the pigmentation for weeks to months. The skin site often becomes progressively darker as more melanin accumulates with each subsequent exposure to the drug. Discontinuation of the offending agent and its future avoidance is the treatment of choice.

Urticaria pigmentosa

Urticaria pigmentosa is the most common manifestation of a group of cutaneous mastocytosis disorders in which excess mast cells are present in the skin (Fig. 23.8.4). In the adult-onset disease, which is usually lifelong, lesions often first appear in the 20 to 40 year age group, and affect internal organs (e.g. bone marrow, liver) as well as the skin. By contrast, childhood-onset disease typically arises in the first year of life, but can appear at any time in the first decade, and tends to clear spontaneously.

The skin exhibits multiple brown or red-brown macules and papules on the trunk and limbs, which urticate on rubbing (Darier's sign), causing oedema and redness typical of a weal and flare response. In one variant of the adult disease, known as telangiectasia macularis eruptiva perstans, the disorder is characterized by multiple telangiectatic lesions on the skin. The lesions may be pruritic, and generalized flushing can occur as a result of mast cell degranulation. The cause of urticaria pigmentosa is unclear in most cases, but mutations in the *KIT* gene (OMIM 164920) have been identified in some affected individuals.

Despite the lifelong aspect of the adult disease, the prognosis is generally good, and the mainstay of treatment is to avoid substances that trigger mast cell degranulation, and to suppress the itch with antihistamines. Phototherapy (narrowband UVB or PUVA) can temporarily clear or improve the skin, but long-term phototherapy

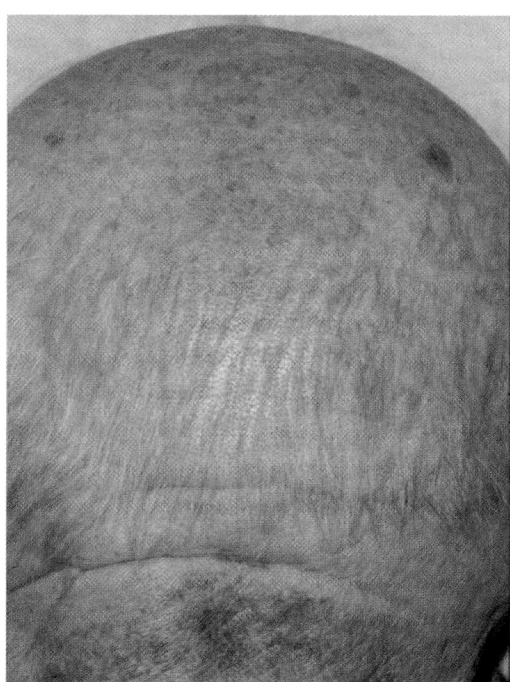

Fig. 23.8.3 Slate-grey pigmentation, diffuse on the scalp and more pronounced at the nape of the neck, secondary to oral minocycline treatment for rosacea.

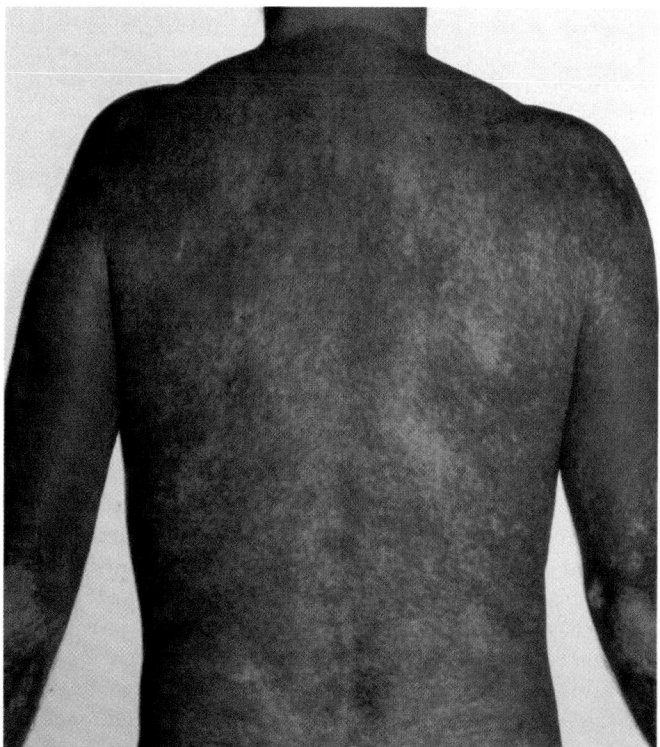

Fig. 23.8.4 Multiple pigmented macules and papules on the trunk and upper limbs in a patient with urticaria pigmentosa.

can lead to skin cancer, and the skin lesions of urticaria pigmentosa relapse when phototherapy is discontinued. Potent topical steroids can also clear the skin lesions, but the risk of steroid atrophy and systemic adrenocortical suppression limits their use.

Incontinentia pigmenti

Incontinentia pigmenti is a disorder with four recognized stages (vesiculobullous, verrucous, pigmented, and atrophic), although the lesions from the first three phases may overlap. The lesions, which are linear or grouped, tend to arise on the extremities (often on the flexor surface) and on the lateral parts of the trunk. The blistering phase, with erythematous areas and vesicles/bullae, is seen at birth or usually within the first couple of months of life; it is thought that the disease can also begin and progress in utero. The warty lesions develop between 2 and 6 weeks of life, often on an erythematous base, in whorls or patches. Later, streaks and whorls of pigmentation with an appearance suggestive of marble cake appear, and usually last for years. The pigmentation, which can appear reticulate and range from blue-grey to brown, slowly resolves leaving atrophic hypopigmented reticulate areas, especially on the calves. Abnormalities of the teeth, hair, eyes, and central nervous system can also occur.

The X-linked condition mainly affects females (more than 95% of cases), generally being prenatally lethal in males, although some cases have been reported in boys. The genetic alterations responsible for the disorder reside in the *IKBKG* (also known as NF-κB essential modulator; NEMO) gene (OMIM 300248) on chromosome Xq28; most cases are accounted for by genomic rearrangement resulting in deletion of part of the *IKBKG* gene, rather than a single base mutation at this locus.

IKBKG plays a role in the activation of NF-κB, which functions as a transcription factor controlling inflammation, immunity, and apoptosis. In affected females, due to the random inactivation of an X chromosome (lyonization), cells expressing the abnormal *IKBKG* allele undergo apoptosis, and are replaced by cells with the active *IKBKG* on the normal X chromosome. In affected males, this replacement by cells with a normal *IKBKG* gene is not possible, resulting in intrauterine mortality, or death from infection during childhood. In females, treatment for the skin lesions is usually not required, and treatment for other related problems is usually symptomatic.

McCune–Albright syndrome

Also known as Albright's syndrome, this condition consists of hyperpigmented (café-au-lait) patches, fibrous dysplasia of bones, and in females, precocious puberty (Fig. 23.8.5). The hyperpigmented patches vary in size, but are usually large with jagged borders, and develop either at birth or more commonly during the first 2 years of life. The bone lesions, which often affect the long bones, tend to develop during the first decade of life and manifest as bone pains and fractures, and sometimes deformities. Cystic spaces are seen in the cortex of affected bones on radiography. Overgrowth of the skull can lead to problems with vision and hearing. Puberty begins before 10 years of age in most females, and in the first 5 years of life in about half of all cases. Other endocrine problems are also encountered, including hyperthyroidism, hyperparathyroidism, and Cushing's syndrome.

McCune–Albright syndrome is caused by activating mutations in the stimulatory G protein gene (*GNAS*; OMIM 139320), with

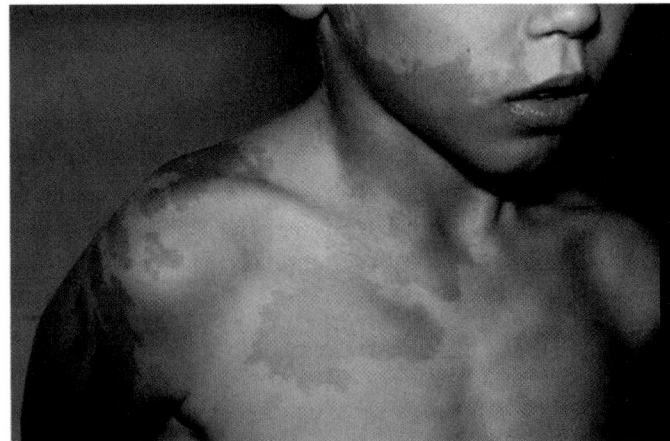

Fig. 23.8.5 Café-au-lait patches with jagged borders in a child with McCune–Albright syndrome.

the mutation frequently observed at codon 211, which normally codes for arginine in the wild-type protein. Lifespan is usually normal, and therapies are directed towards the treatment of complications. Fractures generally heal without sequelae.

Localized pigmentation caused by dermal melanocytosis

Localized dark pigmentation of the skin can arise from the formation of collections of melanocytes in the dermis during embryonic development, as a result of impaired migration of melanoblasts from the neural crest. The lesions are seen more frequently in oriental races, and have a blue or slate-brown colour.

The hyperpigmentation in naevus of Ota affects the skin on one side of the face in an area innervated by the ophthalmic and maxillary division of the trigeminal nerve, and may involve the eye (sclera, iris, retina). In naevus of Ito, the skin over the shoulder (innervated by the posterior supraclavicular and lateral brachial cutaneous nerves) is affected. The Mongolian blue spot, frequent on the lower back, occurs in most East Asian babies and is also common in black children. It usually fades during childhood; however, it may persist throughout life, whereas naevus of Ota and naevus of Ito are generally lifelong.

Post-inflammatory hyperpigmentation/ hypopigmentation

Inflammation resulting from a wide variety of causes can frequently lead to the development of dyspigmentation at that site. The condition is more common and more problematic in darker-skinned subjects. The degree of dyspigmentation varies, and can follow inflammation from exogenous stimuli (trauma, burns) as well as from inflammatory skin disorders (e.g. acne vulgaris, atopic eczema, lichen planus, lupus erythematosus, morphoea/systemic sclerosis, macular amyloid) (Fig. 23.8.6).

In cases where the hyperpigmentation arises secondarily to damage to the epidermal basal cell layer, e.g. lichen planus and lupus erythematosus, there is pigmentary incontinence by the basal epidermal cells, and subsequent phagocytosis of the melanin by macrophages (in this situation also known as melanophages) in the dermis. The tendency is for these melanophages to remain in the dermis for a long period, thus the hyperpigmentation can take many months to resolve.

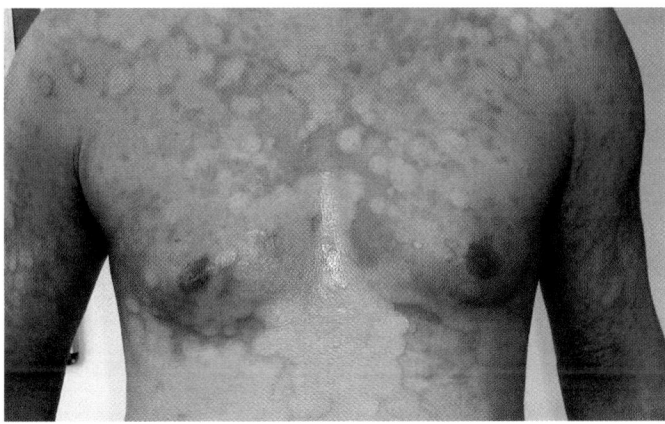

Fig. 23.8.6 Post-inflammatory hyperpigmentation on the trunk and upper limbs in a patient with psoriasis; the psoriasis has cleared in some areas (as a result of systemic antipsoriatic therapy) leaving the post-inflammatory hyperpigmentation.

Hyperpigmentation resulting from excess melanin in the epidermis can also occur as a result of inflammation, although hypopigmentation from reduced melanin transfer and increased keratinocyte mitosis is more frequent. Hypopigmentation frequently follows psoriasis, atopic eczema, discoid lupus erythematosus, systemic lupus erythematosus and pityriasis versicolor.

Hypopigmentation

The causes are hypopigmentation are given in Table 23.8.2.

Vitiligo

Vitiligo is a disorder with reduced pigmentation resulting from the death of melanocytes in the epidermis, with or without the concomitant death of melanocytes in the hair bulb. There are several

Table 23.8.2 Causes of skin hypopigmentation

Type	Cause
Localized	
Vitiligo	Includes vitiligo vulgaris, vitiligo in patients with melanoma, and in Vogt–Koyanagi–Harada syndrome
Naevus-related	Halo naevus, naevus depigmentosus, depigmentation within/around a melanoma
Postinflammatory	Eczema (pityriasis alba), psoriasis (frequently post-UV therapy), etc.
Chemical/drugs	Hydroquinones, topical corticosteroids
Congenital	Piebaldism, Waardenburg's syndrome, tuberous sclerosis*
Infective	Tinea (pityriasis) versicolor, leprosy, onchocerciasis, syphilis, yaws, pinta
Scarring	Trauma, surgical, discoid lupus erythematosus
Miscellaneous	Morphoea, lichen sclerosus, idiopathic guttate hypomelanosis, hypomelanosis of Ito
Generalized	
Congenital	Oculocutaneous albinism type I, oculocutaneous albinism type II, Prader–Willi syndrome, Angelman syndrome, Chédiak–Higashi syndrome, Hermansky–Pudlak syndrome, Griscelli syndrome
Endocrine	Hypopituitarism, hypogonadism (males)
Vitiligo	

*Tuberous sclerosis is described in Chapter 24.17.

theories as to the mechanism of melanocyte death, including loss of survival signals (e.g. reduced *KIT* expression), damage to the cell from a variety of factors (e.g. reactive oxygen species), and/or activation of the immune system (antibody and cell mediated) to recognize melanocyte-specific antigens.

The prevalence of vitiligo varies from about 0.38 to 1.78% in different populations, and the disease can begin at any age, with approximately 50% of cases affected before the age of 20 years. The condition is usually more problematic in darker-skinned individuals, who may view it as a social stigma because of the combination of significant cosmetic impairment and the incorrect suspicion by others that the hypopigmentation may be a manifestation of leprosy. Males and females are equally affected. A family history is noted in up to one-third of cases, and genetic factors are thought to be important in its susceptibility/pathogenesis, although there is some conflicting evidence from linkage and candidate gene studies over the relevant loci. In general there is no obvious cause for most patients presenting with vitiligo, but certain chemicals (hydroquinone derivatives, monobenzone, *para-tert*-butylcatechol) are toxic to melanocytes, and can cause vitiligo-like depigmentation.

The areas of hypopigmentation manifest as white patches of variable size (Fig. 23.8.7), but in some darker-skinned individuals the margin or entire patch may be an intermediate colour of light brown (trichrome vitiligo). Patches may be generalized or segmental in distribution, and the borders are irregular, similar to those of countries on a map. In the generalized form lesions are usually symmetrical, and the more frequently involved sites are around the orifices (eyes, nose, mouth), flexures (axillae, groins, genitals), and extensor surfaces (elbows, knees, digits). The isomorphic or Koebner phenomenon can occur, in which trauma to the skin can produce lesions at that site. The skin is usually normal otherwise, with no evidence of scaling or atrophy, but occasionally the lesions may undergo an initial inflammatory stage with raised erythematous (and sometimes hyperpigmented) borders.

Although usually distinct clinically, microbial diseases such as pityriasis versicolor (Chapter 23.10), leprosy (Chapter 7.6.27), and syphilis (Chapter 7.6.36) are important infectious causes of hypopigmentation. For example, in leprosy, hypomelanosis is a feature of the tuberculoid and borderline tuberculoid types; in tuberculoid

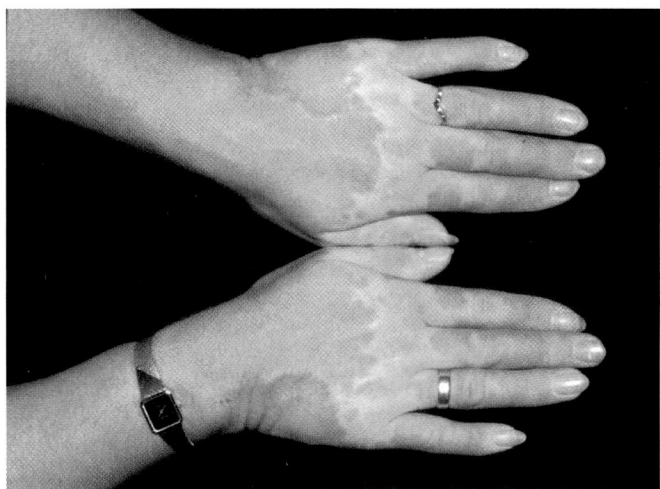

Fig. 23.8.7 Loss of skin pigmentation on the dorsa of the hands in a subject with vitiligo.

leprosy, light touch and, later, pinprick sensations are also impaired in the hypopigmented patch, there is often a lack of sweating, there may be loss of hair and an adjacent enlarged peripheral nerve may be palpable, which may be mistaken for an enlarged lymph node.

There is an association between vitiligo and several autoimmune diseases, including hyperthyroidism and hypothyroidism, pernicious anaemia, diabetes mellitus, and adrenal insufficiency (Addison's disease). Vitiligo has also been reported in patients with a number of other disorders (psoriasis, alopecia areata, lichen planus, myasthenia gravis, rheumatoid arthritis, and morphoea/scleroderma), but the relevance of these diseases in a condition that is relatively common is unclear. Halo naevi may occur in patients with vitiligo, presumably as a result of an immunogical response to melanocytes crossreacting with the melanocytic naevus cells. Similarly, vitiligo can occur in individuals with melanoma, secondary to the antitumour immune response reacting against melanocytes at other skin sites. Although squamous cell carcinoma of the skin has been reported occasionally in people with vitiligo, it is thought that the risk is not significantly increased; this may be because the skin site is generally covered by clothing, the total body surface area affected by vitiligo is limited in many cases, or because other factors protect the skin in the absence of pigment. Vitiligo *per se* does not increase the risk of melanoma because the melanocytes necessary to give rise to melanoma are missing from the epidermis at the affected skin site. Nevertheless, patients are advised to use good sun protection measures (see Chapter 23.9).

Vitiligo may last for many years, or it may repigment spontaneously. When it does repigment, the pigment initially appears around hair follicles, and is thought to represent proliferation and migration of new melanocytes from precursors in the bulge region of the follicle. In general, therapies for vitiligo are limited, and the choice of treatment often depends on the constitutive skin colour of the patient. In people with lighter skin colour, advice on the use of sunscreens may be sufficient. Potent topical steroids and/or UV radiation can be employed with varying success, but UV radiation, if unsuccessful, can exaggerate the difference in colour between normal and vitiliginous skin in darker-skinned patients. Some authors advocate the use of pseudocatalase in combination with UV radiation, whereas others have seen good cosmetic results with minigrafting of pigmented skin onto the affected sites. Cosmetic camouflage can be helpful in those cases that do not repigment spontaneously, or those failing to respond to therapy. In addition, counselling is important for those distressed by the condition.

Endocrine causes of hypopigmentation

Lighter pigmentation of skin can occur in endocrine disorders. Hypopituitarism often leads to a generalized skin pallor that is thought to result from a lack of POMC peptides, including αMSH and ACTH. Similarly, men who have hypogonadism, e.g. as a result of castration, have been reported to exhibit generalized skin pallor. The tanning response is impaired in these men, as it is in people with hypopituitarism. The administration of testosterone re-establishes UV radiation-induced tanning in hypogonadic men, whereas the administration of αMSH does likewise in cases of hypopituitarism.

Depigmentation/greying of hair

The reduction and loss of pigment in hair, resulting in its greying (canities), is a normal ageing response in adults. The initial greying seems to result from a dilution of the pigment, secondary to a progressive decline in the number and activity of melanocytes in some hairs, with the overall grey effect being the consequence of a mixture of hypopigmented/white and normal-coloured (blond, brown, etc.) hairs. Eventually the hair may appear white, as a result of most of the hairs lacking melanocytes. Canities affects most individuals, frequently beginning in the fourth and fifth decades of life (senile canities), but may occur earlier in some people (premature canities).

Rapid greying or whitening of the hair has been observed in some people as a result of diffuse alopecia areata causing generalized hair thinning on the scalp, with loss of pigmented hairs and retention of grey/white depigmented hairs. In circumscribed alopecia areata the hair loss may similarly be confined to pigmented hairs, with depigmented hairs surviving, or alternatively, during hair regrowth there may be earlier or selective regrowth of white hairs in the affected area. The presence of a localized patch of white hair, termed poliosis, can arise from a congenital or acquired defect; examples of the former include piebaldism and Waardenburg's syndrome, whereas examples of the latter include alopecia areata and vitiligo.

Piebaldism

In this autosomal dominant condition, nonpigmented patches of skin are seen on the central forehead (often in a diamond or triangular shape and in association with a white forelock) as well as on the chest, abdomen, arms, and legs. The hypopigmented areas are present at birth, and do not vary throughout life, being caused by an absence of melanocytes in the affected skin. Islands of normally pigmented skin are often seen in the hypomelanotic areas, and the hands, feet, and back are usually pigmented normally. Mutations in the *KIT* proto-oncogene (OMIM 164920), and deletions within this locus on chromosome 4q are responsible. The consequently reduced ability of the KIT ligand (stem cell factor) to signal via the KIT receptor on developing melanoblasts results in reduced survival of these cells during embryogenesis, thus causing the lack of melanocytes in affected skin sites. Treatment for piebaldism is, in general, restricted to cosmetic camouflage, photoprotection with clothing and sunscreens, and in some cases skin grafting.

Waardenburg's syndrome

Waardenburg's syndrome, the severity of which varies widely, features the following abnormalities from birth: a white forelock, white eyebrows, premature greying of the hair, heterochromatic irides, and hypomelanotic macules on the skin, in combination with lateral displacement of the inner canthi/dystopia canthorum, hypertrophy of the nasal bridge, and congenital neurosensory deafness in a proportion of cases.

There are four subgroups, types I to IV, with type II differing from type I by the absence of the lateral displacement of the inner canthi/dystopia canthorum; type III (Klein–Waardenburg syndrome) being similar to type I, but with limb abnormalities; and type IV (Waardenburg–Shah syndrome) being a combination of Waardenburg's syndrome and aganglionic megacolon (Hirschsprung's disease).

Types I and III result from defects in the *PAX3* gene (OMIM 606597), type II is caused by mutations in the microphthalmia-associated transcription factor (*MITF*; OMIM 156845) and SLUG (*SNAI2*; OMIM 602150) genes, whereas type IV is caused by alterations in the endothelin-B receptor (*EDNRB*; OMIM 131244), endothelin 3 (*EDB3*; OMIM 131242), and *SOX10* (OMIM 602229) genes. In general, the pigmentation defects seem to occur as a result of effects on MITF signalling (caused by mutations in *MITF* or in genes that control *MITF* activity), which is important for neural crest and melanocyte development. However, in cases of Waardenburg's syndrome type IV caused by *EDNRB* and *EDB3* alterations, the megacolon and pigmentation abnormalities are caused by defective EDB3/EDNRB signalling, which is necessary for the migration of neuron precursor cells to the gastrointestinal tract, and melanoblasts into skin. Similar to piebaldism, there is no simple effective treatment for the pigmentary defects in Waardenburg's syndrome.

Oculocutaneous albinism type I

In this type of albinism (OCA1) there is a lifelong absence of melanin pigment in the skin, hair, and eyes such that, irrespective of race, the skin is pink, the hair white, the irides light-coloured, and the red-eye reflex prominent. There is an absence of pigmented naevi and freckling. Photophobia, visual impairment, and nystagmus are common.

The condition is autosomal recessive, and the genetic defect responsible for the condition lies in the tyrosinase (*TYR*; OMIM 606933) gene. The tyrosinase enzyme is essential for normal melanogenesis, catalysing the production of dihydroxyphenylalanine (DOPA) and DOPAquinone in the melanin synthetic pathway (Fig. 23.8.1). Although mutations in the coding region of the *TYR* gene can inhibit the enzymatic activity of tyrosinase, there is evidence that mutant tyrosinase may fail to traffic adequately to the melanosome, where it is required for melanin synthesis. There is no specific treatment for the lack of skin pigmentation in OCA1 (or OCA2 below), but advice at an early age on appropriate photoprotective clothing and sunscreens, and limiting sun exposure, are important to reduce the risk of skin cancer development in later life.

Oculocutaneous albinism type II

Oculocutaneous albinism type II (tyrosinase-positive albinism; OCA2) is more common in black populations, whereas OCA1 is more frequent in whites. In OCA2 in whites there is absence of pigment in the skin, hair, and eyes, but pigmented naevi may be seen. In darker populations, the presence of some melanin pigmentation is seen, and blacks with this type of albinism tend to have yellow hair and pigmented freckles on their skin. Affected individuals may also have nystagmus and photophobia.

The condition is autosomal recessive, and results from mutations in the *P* gene (*OCA2*; OMIM 611409) and/or deletions of this locus on chromosome 15q. The exact function of the protein encoded by the *P* gene has been debated, but it is thought that OCA2 results from a failure of the P protein to control melanosomal pH, thus reducing tyrosinase activity. The fact that people with OCA2 in darker populations have yellow hair suggests that the net effect is an absence of eumelanin production, whereas some phaeomelanin can still be synthesized. In hotter climates, appropriate sun protection is necessary to limit the development of skin cancers, and regular monitoring of affected individuals is recommended to identify skin cancers at an early stage.

Praeder–Willi and Angelman syndromes

Both these syndromes exhibit lighter pigmentation of the skin, hair, and retina, in association with developmental delay and behavioural abnormalities. In Prader–Willi syndrome there is concomitant obesity, hypotonia, hypogonadism, and short stature. In Angelman syndrome there is hypotonia, ataxia, motor retardation, epilepsy, absence of speech, and a characteristic facies.

Cytogenetic and molecular investigations of Prader–Willi syndrome have demonstrated deletions in the paternal copy of chromosome 15q (or maternal uniparental disomy, which gives rise to two copies of chromosome 15q, both of which are maternal in origin), whereas deletions of the maternal copy of this region are observed in Angelman syndrome, suggesting that both disorders are caused by loss of function of imprinted genes on chromosome 15q. Alterations in the gene for the E6-associated protein ubiquitin-protein ligase (*UBE3A*; OMIM 601623) have been detected in Angelman syndrome, whereas the deletions in Prader–Willi syndrome affect the *SNRPN* (OMIM 182279) and *NDN* (OMIM 602117) genes.

Depigmentation in Prader–Willi syndrome seems confined to those cases with 15q deletions, and is not seen in patients with maternal uniparental disomy. Similarly, hypopigmentation is not seen in cases of Angelman syndrome with very small deletions, indicating that the affected gene in cases with hypopigmentation is located further along the same chromosome. These observations, coupled with the fact that the human *P* gene, mutations of which cause OCA2, is also located on chromosome 15q has led to the hypothesis that reduced expression of the *P* gene through haploinsufficiency is responsible for the hypopigmentation phenotype in Prader–Willi and Angelman syndromes.

Hermansky–Pudlak syndrome

The features of this rare autosomal recessive syndrome are oculocutaneous albinism, which can vary in the degree of hypopigmentation, in association with a bleeding diathesis caused by a platelet abnormality, and deposits of pigment in cells of the reticuloendothelial system. Pulmonary fibrosis and granulomatous colitis can also occur. It is more common in Puerto Ricans, but has been reported worldwide.

The underlying problem is a defect in lysosomal ceroid-lipofuscin storage affecting a number of organelles within cells, including melanosomes, lysosomes, and platelet dense granules, resulting in abnormal synthesis/development of these organelles; platelet numbers are normal, and the diagnosis is confirmed by a lack of platelet dense bodies on electron microscopy. Based on genetic heterogeneity there are eight subtypes of Hermansky–Pudlak syndrome (HPS1, HPS2, etc), which are caused by mutations in different genes; *HPS1* on chromosome 10q (OMIM 604982), *AP3B1* on 5q (causing HPS2; OMIM 603401), *HPS3* on 3q (OMIM 606118), *HPS4* on 22q (OMIM 606682), *HPS5* on 11p (OMIM 607521), *HPS6* on 10q (OMIM 607522), *DTNBP1* on 6p (resulting in HPS7; OMIM 607145), and *BLOC1S3* on 19q (causing HPS8; OMIM 609762).

Platelet transfusion is the suggested treatment of choice for bleeding episodes. Treatment with 1-desamino-8-D-arginine vasopressin (dDAVP) has been suggested to reduce the bleeding tendency in some cases, but was not shown to reduce the bleeding time in most cases in an open-label trial.

Chédiak–Higashi syndrome

This uncommon disorder consists of reduced pigmentation of the skin, hair, and eyes, with atypical inclusions in several cell types, including leucocytes, bone marrow, spleen, liver, kidney, some endocrine glands, and the mucosa of the gastrointestinal tract. Decreased retinal pigmentation, photophobia, and nystagmus may also occur. Abnormally large melanosomes are present in melanocytes, and are retained in the melanocyte rather than being transported to the associated keratinocytes in the skin, accounting for the reduced pigmentation. The giant granules in leucocytes similarly affect their function, and markedly increase susceptibility to bacterial (staphylococcal and streptococcal) and viral infections, often resulting in death during the first decade of life. In those who survive for longer, lymphadenopathy and hepatosplenomegaly develop (called the accelerated phase), with the patient ultimately dying from lymphoma. Some of these patients may develop neurological problems.

The disorder is autosomal recessive, resulting from mutations in the lysosomal trafficking regulator gene on chromosome 1q (*LYST*; OMIM 606897). It is thought that the genetic abnormality causes fusion of the secretory lysosomes in neutrophils and natural killer cells, inhibiting the secretion of proteases by these cells. This is also thought to be the case with melanosomes, where a failure to fuse to the plasma membrane of the dendrites inhibits melanosome transfer to surrounding keratinocytes. In addition, some of the clinical problems in Chédiak–Higashi syndrome may be caused by an inability to repair lesions in the plasma membrane (which seem to occur in all eukaryotic cells), because of the reduced ability of lysosomes to fuse with and therefore repair the cell membrane. There is no effective therapy for the underlying problem, and treatment is based on the complications that arise, e.g. antibiotics for infections.

Further reading

Gianfrancesco F, *et al.* (2000). Genomic rearrangement in NEMO impairs NF-kappaB activation and is a cause of incontinentia pigmenti. The International Incontinentia Pigmenti (IP) Consortium. *Nature*, **405**, 466–72.

Giebel LB, Spritz RA (1991). Mutation of the KIT (mast/stem cell growth factor receptor) protooncogene in human piebaldism. *Proc Natl Acad Sci USA*, **88**, 8696–9.

Halaban R, *et al.* (2000). Endoplasmic reticulum retention is a common defect associated with tyrosinase-negative albinism. *Proc Natl Acad Sci USA*, **97**, 5889–94.

Healy E, *et al.* (2000). Melanocortin-1-receptor gene and sun sensitivity in individuals without red hair. *Lancet*, **355**, 1072–3.

Hermansky F, Pudlak P (1959). Albinism associated with hemorrhagic diathesis and unusual pigmented reticular cells in the bone marrow: report of two cases with histochemical studies. *Blood*, **14**, 162–9.

Huynh C, *et al.* (2004). Defective lysosomal exocytosis and plasma membrane repair in Chediak-Higashi/beige cells. *Proc Natl Acad Sci USA*, **101**, 16795–800.

Kemp EH, *et al.* (2002). The melanin-concentrating hormone receptor 1, a novel target of autoantibody responses in vitiligo. *J Clin Invest*, **109**, 923–30.

Lamason RL, *et al.* (2005). SLC24A5, a putative cation exchanger, affects pigmentation in zebrafish and humans. *Science*, **310**, 1782–6.

Lee HO, Levorse JM, Shin MK (2003). The endothelin receptor-B is required for the migration of neural crest-derived melanocyte and enteric neuron precursors. *Dev Biol*, **259**, 162–75.

Lerner AB, McGuire JS (1961). Effects of alpha- and beta-melanocyte stimulating hormones on the skin colour of man. *Nature*, **189**, 176–9.

Longley BJ, *et al.* (1996). Somatic c-*KIT* activating mutation in urticaria pigmentosa and aggressive mastocytosis: establishment of clonality in a human mast cell neoplasm. *Nat Genet*, **12**, 312–14.

Miller R, Ashkar FS, Jacobi J (1970). Hyperpigmentation in thyrotoxicosis. *J Am Med Assoc*, **213**, 299.

Nelson DH, Meakin JW, Thorn GW (1960). ACTH-producing pituitary tumors following adrenalectomy for Cushing's syndrome. *Ann Intern Med*, **52**, 560–9.

Nicholls RD, Knepper JL (2001). Genome organization, function, and imprinting in Prader-Willi and Angelman syndromes. *Annu Rev Genomics Hum Genet*, **2**, 153–75.

Nishimura EK, *et al.* (2002). Dominant role of the niche in melanocyte stem-cell fate determination. *Nature*, **416**, 854–60.

Norris A, *et al.* (1996). The expression of the c-kit receptor by epidermal melanocytes may be reduced in vitiligo. *Br J Dermatol*, **134**, 299–306.

Ogg GS, *et al.* (1998). High frequency of skin-homing melanocyte-specific cytotoxic T lymphocytes in autoimmune vitiligo. *J Exp Med*, **188**, 1203–8.

Read AP, Newton VE (1997). Waardenburg syndrome. *J Med Genet*, **34**, 656–65.

Rinchik EM, *et al.* (1993). A gene for the mouse pink-eyed dilution locus and for human type II oculocutaneous albinism. *Nature*, **361**, 72–6.

Schallreuter KU, Wood JM, Berger J (1991). Low catalase levels in the epidermis of patients with vitiligo. *J Invest Dermatol*, **97**, 1081–5.

Smahi A, *et al.* (1991). Activating mutations of the stimulatory G protein in the McCune–Albright syndrome. *N Engl J Med*, **325**, 1688–95.

Spritz RA, *et al.* (2004). Novel vitiligo susceptibility loci on chromosomes 7 (*AIS2*) and 8 (*AIS3*), confirmation of *SLEV1* on chromosome 17, and their roles in an autoimmune diathesis. *Am J Hum Genet*, **74**, 188–91.

Stinchcombe JC, Page LJ, Griffiths GM (2000). Secretory lysosome biogenesis in cytotoxic T lymphocytes from normal and Chediak Higashi syndrome patients. *Traffic*, **1**, 435–44.

Sulem P, *et al.* (2007). Genetic determinants of hair, eye and skin pigmentation in Europeans. *Nat Genet*, **40**, 835–7.

Sulem P, *et al.* (2008). Two newly identified genetic determinants of pigmentation in Europeans. *Nat Genet*, **40**, 835–7.

Szabo G, *et al.* (1969). Racial differences in the fate of melanosomes in human epidermis. *Nature*, **222**, 1081–2.

Tadokoro T, *et al.* (2005). Mechanisms of skin tanning in different racial/ethnic groups in response to ultraviolet radiation. *J Invest Dermatol*, **124**, 1326–32.

Tomita, Y, *et al.* (1989). Human oculocutaneous albinism caused by single base insertion in the tyrosinase gene. *Biochem Biophys Res Commun*, **164**, 990–6.

Valverde P, *et al.* (1995). Variants of the melanocyte-stimulating hormone receptor gene are associated with red hair and fair skin in humans. *Nat Genet*, **11**, 328–30.

Wei ML (2006). Hermansky-Pudlak syndrome: a disease of protein trafficking and organelle function. *Pigment Cell Res*, **19**, 19–42.

23.9

Photosensitivity

Jane McGregor

Essentials

Normal human skin is photosensitive in that it reddens following acute sunlight exposure and tans and thickens following chronic sunlight exposure. Skin cancer, particularly nonmelanoma skin cancer, is also a consequence of high cumulative sun exposure in genetically predisposed normal individuals (predominantly those with fair skin).

Outside the range of normal photosensitivity, there are a number of conditions in which patients exhibit diverse abnormal cutaneous reactions to sunlight. These are broadly described together as the photosensivity disorders, but in fact they comprise a very heterogeneous group of skin conditions.

Abnormal cutaneous photosensitive responses range from easy sunburn (as in drug phototoxicity and the DNA repair-deficient photodermatoses) and pain (erythropoietic protoporphyria), through to complex inflammatory responses such as urticaria, eczema, or epidermal necrosis induced by specific wavelengths of sunlight, the so-called idiopathic photodermatoses. The action spectra for the induction of most of these conditions are not established.

Introduction

Sunlight is essential for life on earth. It comprises electromagnetic energy emitted from the sun of wavelengths from 10^{-7} nm (cosmic rays) to 10^7 nm (radio waves). Terrestrial solar radiation (wavelengths more than 290 nm) includes that part of the ultraviolet (UV) spectrum (290–400 nm) which is responsible for vitamin D synthesis in the skin, visible radiation (400–800 nm), required for photosynthesis, and infrared (800–17 000 nm) which provides warmth. Apart from vitamin D synthesis, it is broadly held that exposure of the skin to ultraviolet radiation is otherwise deleterious, causing sunburn and skin cancer. The so-called 'photosensitivity disorders' are in fact a very heterogeneous group of skin conditions (Table 23.9.1).

The acute effects of sunlight on normal skin

Acute effects of ultraviolet radiation (UVR) on normal human skin include erythema (redness), pigmentation (tanning), and immunosuppression, as well as diverse cellular and histological changes and are not further detailed here. Sensitivity of the skin to sunlight is genetically determined and used to define the Fitzpatrick skin type classification for white skinned individuals ranging from Celtic to Mediterranean:

- Skin type I/II—burns, tans with difficulty

- Skin type III/IV—sometimes burns, usually tans

Erythema

Maximal reddening of the skin in normal individuals following irradiation with ultraviolet B (UVB) is wavelength dependent: it occurs 7 h postirradiation at 313 nm and 12 h at 254 nm. The standard photobiological measure of photosensitivity is the minimal erythema dose (MED), which is generally defined as that dose of UV required to produce 'just perceptible erythema at 12 h following skin irradiation'.

The pharmacological changes that induce erythema have not been fully established, but histamine and prostaglandins are thought to have a role in the initiation of the response, with interleukins 1 and 6 (IL-1, IL-6) involved with the continuation of the response and also with the systemic effects, e.g. tiredness and nausea, which accompany sunburn.

Pigmentation

Pigmentation of the skin following UVR occurs in two distinct phases: immediate pigmentation and delayed tanning. Immediate pigmentation occurs during irradiation with ultraviolet A (UVA), and is maximal immediately afterwards, lasting only a few hours and probably resulting from oxidative changes and redistribution of melanin within the epidermis. Delayed tanning occurs predominantly with UVB and is maximal 72 h after irradiation. It is associated with increased numbers of melanocytes as well as increased dendritic branching, tyrosinase activity, and transfer of melanosomes to keratinocytes.

Table 23.9.1 Clinical features of the photosensitivity disorders

Nomenclature	Clinical manifestation of photosensitivity
Idiopathic photodermatoses	
Polymorphic light eruption	Acute papulovesicular rash
Actinic prurigo	Excoriations and scars
Chronic actinic dermatitis	Eczema
Solar urticaria	Urticaria
Hydroa vacciniforme	Varioliform scars
Cutaneous porphyrias	
Porphyria cutanea tarda	Skin fragility and scarring
Variegate porphyria	
Congenital erythropoietic porphyria	
Hereditary coproporphyria	
Erythropoietic protoporphyria	Pain
Drug and chemical photosensitivity	
Oral ingestion	Easy sunburn (phototoxicity)
Topical sensitization	Blistering/pigmentation (phytophotodermatitis)
DNA repair-deficient photodermatoses	
Xeroderma pigmentosum	Sunburn, premature ageing, skin cancer
Cockayne's syndrome	Sunburn
Trichothiodystrophy	Sunburn
Bloom's syndrome	Sunburn and skin cancer
Photoaggravated skin conditions	
Systemic lupus erythematosus	Induction or worsening of pre-existing condition
Dermatomyositis	
Darier's disease	
Psoriasis	
Atopic/seborrhoeic dermatitis	
Actinic lichen planus	
Bullous pemphigoid and pemphigus	
Cutaneous T-cell lymphoma	

Immune suppression

There is evidence in both animals and humans of local and systemic immunosuppression following acute and chronic exposure of the skin to UV. Experimentally this can be demonstrated by reduction in both the sensitization and elicitation phase of contact hypersensitivity following prior skin irradiation of the site of application. Clinically, it is evidenced by the reactivation of herpes simplex infection on acutely sun exposed sites.

Chronic effects of UV on the skin (photoageing and photocarcinogenesis)

Clinical manifestations of photoageing are skin type dependent to some extent. They are superimposed on changes in the skin that occur as a result of chronological ageing. The action spectrum for photoageing has not been possible to determine in humans and the relative contribution of UVB vs UVA in this process is not established. In animal models, the action spectrum for photocarcinogenesis implicates UVB.

People with skin types I/II are sun sensitive and tend to burn easily. The skin develops atrophic changes over time, with fine wrinkling, telangiectasis, and lentigines. In darker skinned individuals, chronic sun exposure causes skin thickening and coarse wrinkling, often referred to as solar elastosis. Epidemiological evidence indicates two patterns of risk for malignant change; acute intense sunburn (for basal cell carcinoma and melanoma) and chronic exposure (for actinic keratoses, squamous cell and basal cell carcinoma). Both melanoma and nonmelanoma skin cancers are more common in sun sensitive skin types I/II (see Chapter 23.14).

Cutaneous porphyrias

A detailed discussion of all aspects of porphyrias is presented in Chapter 12.5. Here we focus on the cutaneous manifestations. The cutaneous porphyrias are a group of inherited disorders of haem biosynthesis and include sporadic and familial porphyria cutanea tarda (PCT), hereditary erythropoietic porphyria (HEP), variegate porphyria, and erythropoietic protoporphyria (EPP) (Table 23.9.2). Identical skin signs may be seen where there is an acquired alteration of porphyrins, e.g. associated with porphyrin-producing hepatic tumours or in patients with sideroblastic or myeloproliferative anaemia. Photosensitivity, which includes pain, skin fragility, blistering, (Fig. 23.9.1) and scarring, derives from the interaction of porphyrins at various levels within the skin and penetrating wavelengths of UV and visible light at around 400 nm. Excess hair growth and pigmentation are also seen.

The genes for all the enzymes in the human haem biosynthetic pathway have now been characterized, affording a better understanding of the genetic basis of the porphyrias. Decreased enzyme activity is compensated by an increase in substrate in an attempt to maintain haem synthesis. Such accumulation of substrate

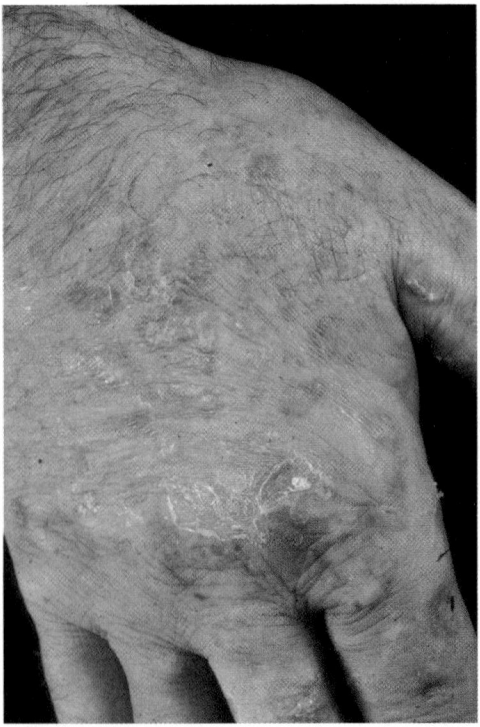

Fig. 23.9.1 Skin fragility and blistering, sometimes with milia (not visible here) is characteristic of the cutaneous porphyrias.

Table 23.9.2 Characterization and clinical features of the cutaneous porphyrias

Defective enzyme	Gene	Disorder	Photosensitivity	Other features
Uroporphyrinogen III synthase	UROS	CEP (Gunther's disease)	Blistering and skin fragility, with mutilating scarring of eyelids, earlobes, and scalp. Keratoconjunctivitis may lead to blindness.	Rare condition of variable severity. Many present in infancy with red staining of nappy due to urinary porphyrins Haemolytic anaemia and splenomegaly Erythrodontia, pathological fractures
Uroporphyrinogen decarboxylase	UROD	PCT (familial and sporadic)	Blistering, skin fragility, and milia. Skin tthickening, hyperpigmentation, and hypertrichosis.	Usually presents in adulthood. Investigate for underlying liver pathology, hepatitis, and HIV where indicated. Increased risk of hepatocellular carcinoma
Uroporphyrinogen decarboxylase	UROD	HEP	Blistering and skin fragility of variable severity.	Rare. Homo- or hetero-allelic for URO-D gene defects with variable effect on catalytic activity and clinical features from severe (CEP-like) to mild (PCT-like) phenotype
Protoporphyrinogen oxidase	PPOX	VP	Skin fragility, blistering, and scarring with milia as for PCT.	May be associated with acute abdominal pain, confusion, and convulsions, often with hyponatraemia. Increased risk of hepatocellular carcinoma
Ferrochelatase (protoporphyria)	FECH	EPP	Painful skin and oedema following sun exposure	Hepatic necrosis and liver failure reported

CEP, congenital erythropoietic porphyria; EPP, erythropoietic protoporphyria; HEP, hepatoerythropoietic porphyria; PCT, porphyria cutanea tarda; VP, variegate porphyria.

characterizes each of the porphyrias, but the clinical presentation, even within families, is very variable.

Diagnosis is by analysis of urine, blood, and faeces for porphyrins. Associated pathologies should be sought, including iron overload, haemochromatosis, liver pathology (hepatitis, cirrhosis, and hepatoma), and HIV in selected patients.

Treatment, where possible, includes sun avoidance (particularly for EPP where pain following sun exposure may be excruciating), venesection (to reduce iron load), and low dose chloroquine (both for PCT, but with monitoring for ocular toxicity), and bone marrow transplantation in selected cases (for CEP).

Drug induced photosensitivity

Many drugs can cause photosensitization in predisposed individuals, meaning that the presence of the drug in the skin of some patients alters their cutaneous response to sunlight. Here we document important and common drug photosensitivity reactions. Other exogenous photosensitizers include topical agents, such as sunscreens and plants, which contain psoralens.

The most common mechanism of photosensitivity caused by drugs is phototoxicity. Clinically this may present in a variety of ways, including urticaria or pain (see Table 23.9.3), but more usually it presents as an increased tendency to sunburn. A small number of phototoxic drugs cause pseudoporphyria (Table 23.9.3) in which the photosensitizing effect is of skin fragility and blistering.

Evidence suggests that some phototoxic drugs may also be photocarcinogenic, although this work has been done *in vitro* and with animal models and may not be clinically relevant to humans. Azathioprine and the fluoroquinolone antibiotics are two examples.

Photoallergy is an uncommon cutaneous reaction to sunlight in which, often following an acute phototoxic (erythemal) response, dermatitis occurs on the sun exposed skin some days or weeks later. This has been reported with the use of phenothiazines and also with musk ambrette, once widely used in fragrances, but which has now been withdrawn in most countries. Para-aminobenzoic acid (PABA) and benzophenones (both used in sunscreens) have also been reported as causing photoallergy, although the incidence of this reaction is low.

The DNA repair-deficient photodermatoses

Cellular organisms have evolved a complex set of DNA damage repair enzymes many of which, as a consequence of life on earth and chronic sun exposure, are directed towards the repair of UV-induced DNA damage. The best characterized of these are the seven nucleotide excision repair (NER) enzymes, one of which is defective in each of the complementation groups A–G of the rare autosomal recessive disorder known as xeroderma pigmentosum (XP), associated with easy sunburn and early onset of skin cancer. There is also a variant form of XP, with a milder phenotype, in which there is defective postreplicative translesional DNA synthesis as a result of a mutation in the human polymerase *eta* gene. The genetics of inherited cancers are further discussed in Chapter 6.3.

Other related DNA repair-defective disorders include Cockayne's syndrome, trichothiodystrophy, and Bloom's syndrome which

Table 23.9.3 Common photosensitizing drug reactions

Skin reactions following exposure to sunlight	Exogenous photosensitizers
Easy sunburn (phototoxicity)	Fluoroquinolone antibiotics, tetracyclines, chlorpromazine, thiazide diuretics, quinine, amiodarone
Pain or burning sensation (phototoxicity)	Benoxaprofen,[a] amiodarone, chlorpromazine, coal tar
Solar urticaria (phototoxicity)	Tetracyclines
Skin fragility and blistering (pseudoporphyria)	Nalidixic acid, tetracycline, naproxen, amiodarone, furosemide
Dermatitis (photoallergy)	Chlorpromazine, PABA, benzophenones
Photocarcinogenic (not established in humans)	Fluoroquinolone antibiotics, azathioprine
Redness, blistering, and hyperpigmentation	Psoralens, phytophotodermatitis (plant psoralens, e.g. in cow parsley)

PABA, *para*-aminobenzoic acid.
[a] Now withdrawn.

Table 23.9.4 DNA repair-deficient photodermatoses

Photosensitivity disorder	Molecular defect	Diagnostic test	Clinical features	Comment
XP	NER enzymes (XP complementation groups A–G)	Reduction in post-UV UDS of patients fibroblasts *in vitro*	Premature ageing, skin cancers, CNS tumours, neurological disease (variable)	Rigorous sun avoidance to prevent skin cancer. No effective treatment for neurological disorder
XP variant	Mutation in human polymerase eta — involved in translesional DNA repair	Defective post-UV daughter-strand gap repair in patients' fibroblasts	As above, but milder phenotype—may not present until adulthood with skin cancer. No neurological component	As for XP
Cockayne's syndrome (CS)	*CSA* and *CSB*—also XP genes *ERCC3B*, *ERCC2D*, and *ERCC5G*—encode transcription coupled repair proteins	Defective post-UV recovery of RNA synthesis in patients' fibroblasts	Variable penetrance. Presents in childhood—easy sunburn and facial dermatitis. Skin cancer is not a feature. Progressive neurological disability	No specific treatment available
Trichothiodystrophy (TTD)	*GTF2H5* TTD gene—also XP genes *BERCC3* and *DERCC2* (together comprise subunits of transcription factor (TF)IIH)	Amino acid hair analysis shows reduction in cysteine concentration. Reduction in post-UV UDS in patients' fibroblasts	Variable penetrance. Brittle hair, ichthyosis, and neurological abnormalities. Easy sunburn in approx 50%. Skin cancer is not a feature	No specific treatment available
Bloom's syndrome	*BS* gene—a DNA helicase	High frequency sister chromatid exchange and spontaneous mutation rate in cultured cells	Easy sunburn. Internal malignancies prevail at young age, e.g. gastro-intestinal and breast. Increased risk of skin cancer	No specific treatment available

NER, nucleotide excision repair; UDS, unscheduled DNA synthesis; UV, ultraviolet; XP, xeroderma pigmentosum.

exhibit a variable degree of acute photosensitivity to UV, but skin cancer is not a feature (Table 23.9.4).

Clinical features

Xeroderma pigmentosum patients usually present in childhood, often with a history of easy sunburn on minimal exposure. This is not an invariable feature, however, and in young children and babies, distinguishing the sunburn of XP from that of a fair skinned child without XP is not straightforward.

Later signs are more consistent, and are those associated with chronic sun exposure, but in XP patients this becomes apparent at a very early age, depending on the degree of exposure, the skin type of the child, and the severity of the disorder. This is determined to some extent by the complementation group, e.g. E and F being less severe. Skin signs include lentigines (freckles), variable pigmentation on sun exposed sites, dryness, telangiectasis, and scarring. Nonmelanoma and melanoma skin cancers occur at approximately 1000 times the frequency, and approximately 50 years earlier, than in the general population. In one large study, 50% of XP patients in the 10 to 14 year age group had skin cancer.

Ocular abnormalities are also common in XP, including keratitis, ectropion, and malignancies. Approximately 20% of XP patients develop neurological disorders of variable severity, according to their complementation group (group A XP is associated with severe progressive neurological disease in many cases).

XP patients have an increased risk of central nervous system tumours, including medulloblastoma, astrocytoma, and sarcoma. There is also a less well documented increased risk of diverse internal malignancies and, at least in the past, of premature death, the median age being approximately 40 years.

Diagnosis

Phototesting is rarely used for diagnosis since it yields variable results. Where abnormal acute photosensitivity is demonstrable,

reduced and delayed MED to UVB is seen, sometimes with a papular or vesicular reaction.

Instead, confirmation is routinely done by measuring unscheduled DNA synthesis (UDS) by the incorporation of tritiated thymidine into fibroblasts following irradiation; a significant reduction in UDS indicates the XP defect. The variant form of XP is not demonstrable by this means, however, and if suspected, requires measurement of daughter-strand gap repair—a more complicated and costly procedure.

Treatment

Once the diagnosis has been made, lifelong rigorous sun avoidance is crucial to prevent skin cancer in these patients. A topical liposomal endonuclease has recently been reported to decrease the incidence of squamous cell cancers in XP and may be a useful adjunct treatment. There is no prevention for the onset of the neurological component of XP.

The idiopathic photodermatoses

The so-called idiopathic photosensitivity disorders comprise a heterogeneous group of skin conditions in which patients exhibit abnormal immunological responses to UV. They include polymorphic light eruption, actinic prurigo, hydroa vacciniforme, solar urticaria, and chronic actinic dermatitis. Diagnosis relies on an accurate history, particularly of the onset and offset time of the eruption in relation to sun exposure, as well as a description of the eruption, since the transient nature of the acute photodermatoses means there may be nothing to see on the skin at the time of consultation.

Routine investigations include lupus serology (antinuclear antibody (ANA) and extractable nuclear antigen (ENA)), porphyrin analysis where relevant, HLA class II typing (if a diagnosis of actinic prurigo is considered), and biochemistry and haematinics

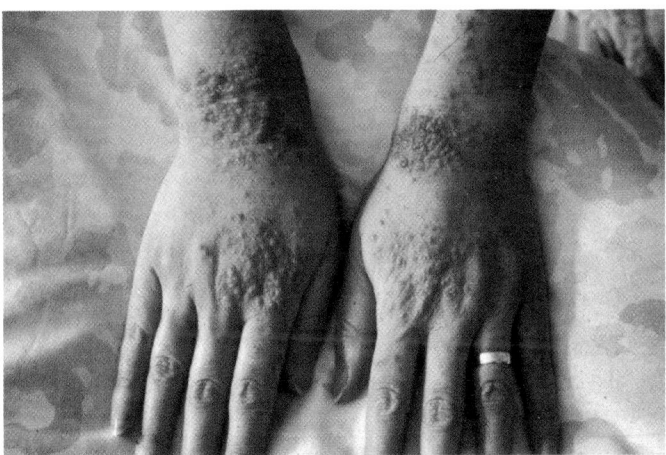

Fig. 23.9.2 Polymorphic light eruption.

if systemic medication is to be employed. Skin biopsy is not routinely undertaken but may help in selected cases where the diagnosis is in doubt, or if lupus needs to be excluded.

Monochromatic phototesting is useful in some instances to confirm a diagnosis of photosensivity and to define the provocation spectrum, particularly for solar urticaria and chronic actinic dermatitis.

Polymorphic light eruption (PMLE)

This is the most common of the photosensitivity disorders, occurring in approximately one in ten women in the United Kingdom and one in 20 to 30 men. The typical age of presentation is early adulthood, although it can occur for the first time in both younger and older patients. It occurs in all skin types.

Evidence suggests a genetic basis for PMLE, but the pathogenesis of this condition is not otherwise established. PMLE typically presents during the summer months as an itchy, papular eruption on sun exposed skin (although often sparing the face) (Fig. 23.9.2). It occurs within hours of UV exposure and usually clears within days without scarring, although occasionally a more persistent form may last a few weeks, even without re-exposure.

For milder cases, sun avoidance around midday and judicious use of sunblock is all that is required to suppress the condition, but for others oral prednisolone and/or prophylactic phototherapy

are used. PMLE recurs every year during the summer months in susceptible individuals, although it may lessen in severity with time.

Actinic prurigo (AP)

This is a rare condition which typically presents for the first time in childhood (3–10 years), with a female bias, often improving with age. It has some characteristics of PMLE, and there may be a shared genetic basis for this, but it is a much more persistent condition.

A diagnosis of AP is made on clinical grounds, supported by HLA-DR4 Class II typing which is found in 90% of individuals (compared with 30% of the general population). The subtype DRB1*0407 is frequently present.

The relationship between the onset of photosensitivity and sun exposure is much less clear for AP than for PMLE, so the diagnosis is less obvious. Often children with AP have been diagnosed as having atopic eczema, perhaps with a history of worsening during the summer months. A PMLE-like rash may occur in some patients on sun exposure, but unlike PMLE it persists, often for many months, as an excoriated, papular, and eczematized eruption on the arms, face, and legs (Fig. 23.9.3). Unusually, it may also occur on the buttocks and at this site the eruption often persists through the winter months. AP may leave hypopigmented and atrophic scars on affected sites.

Treatment includes sun avoidance and sunblock. For milder cases phototherapy, given as for PMLE, can help reduce the severity of the eruption during the summer, but for most individuals systemic therapy is required. Oral prednisolone will clear the acute eruption but is not an option for maintenance. Thalidomide is routinely used for AP and is highly effective at doses between 25 and 100 mg daily.

Hydroa vacciniforme (HV)

This is a very rare condition which presents in childhood as a papulovesicular eruption on sun exposed sites, and which classically resolves over several weeks to leave varioliform scarring, hence the name (Fig. 23.9.4). It appears that the severity of the condition lessens with time in many cases. Unlike other acute photodermatoses, there are distinct histological changes in HV, notably intraepidermal vesicle formation and focal epidermal keratinocyte necrosis which, in the appropriate clinical setting, are diagnostic.

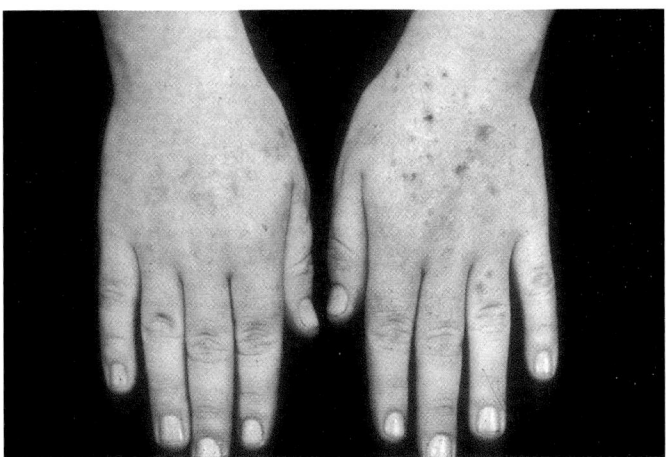

Fig 23.9.3 Actinic prurigo.

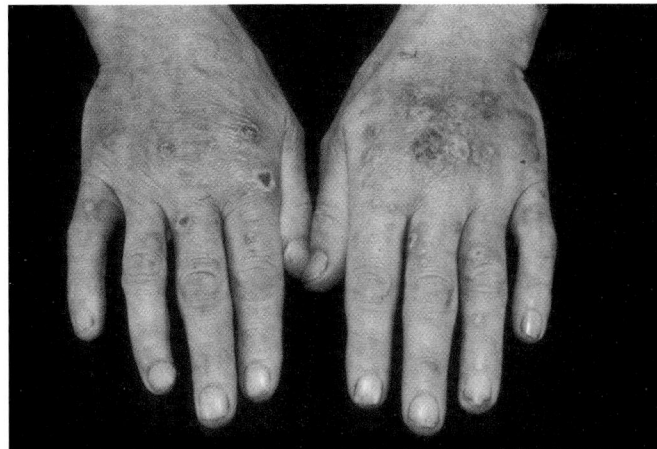

Fig 23.9.4 Hydroa vacciniforme.

The pathogenesis of the condition is not established but, like AP, the acute eruption may resemble PMLE and it is likely that it shares some genetic component of this condition. For mild cases, phototherapy is given, as for PMLE, but for others vigilant sun avoidance is the only option. There is no systemic treatment that is of proven value.

Solar urticaria

This is a rare and sometimes disabling condition in which urticaria occurs on exposed sites often following just a few minutes of sunlight. The wealing characteristically resolves within hours, although solar urticarial vasculitis has been described in which lesions persist for more than 24 h, with bruising. It can occur at any age, but is unusual in children. Like other physical urticarias, it appears to be a transient problem occurring over a number of years and then spontaneously resolving. There are no studies describing the demographics of this condition.

Monochromatic phototesting shows that urtication can occur in susceptible individuals across a wide range of wavelengths, including UV and visible light. Porphyrins should be checked since PCT and EPP can, albeit rarely, both present with solar urticaria.

Treatment involves general measures of sun avoidance and antihistamines, and may be all that is required for milder cases. Phototherapy can be helpful in selected patients, but is not suitable

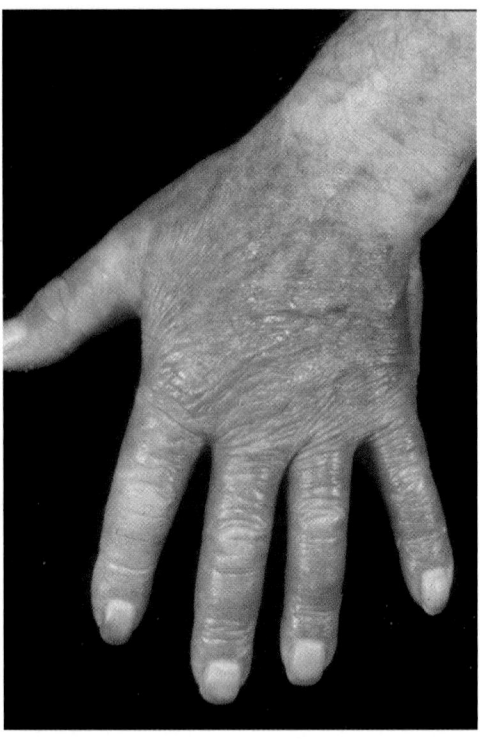

Fig. 23.9.5 Chronic actinic dermatitis.

Table 23.9.5 Photoaggravated conditions

Skin condition	Frequency affected by sun exposure	Characteristic features of photosensitivity	Phototesting	Comment
Lupus erythematosuis (LE)	Characteristically worsened	Lesions appear on sun-exposed sites, either acutely, e.g. in subacute cutaneous LE, or chronically as in discoid LE	Reduced MEDs in some cases. Simulated solar radiation may produce a polymorphic light eruption (PMLE)-like rash	Sun exposure may worsen systemic symptoms in SLE
Dermatomyositis	Unknown—probably in the order of 30% of cases	Malar rash	Variable. Reduced MEDs and PMLE-like rash	Photo-sensitivity common in those with lupus overlap
Pemphigus and Pemphigoid	Unknown, but many reports in literature	Onset of disease more common in summer months	Induction of acantholysis has been described on phototesting	
Erythema multiforme	Uncommon	Where reported, lesions occurred on sun-exposed sites	Induction of lesions on phototesting in two2 reported cases	Has been described secondary to phenylbutazone ingestion.
Darier's disease	Frequently worsened	Localized and widespread worsening of Darier's reported		Mechanism unknown
Actinic lichen planus	Characteristically induced by sun exposure	Nonpruritic grey macules appear on face, neck, and dorsum of hands	Reduced MEDs and induction of lichenoid lesions on phototesting	May be a lichenoid variant of chronic actinic dermatitis
Photoaggravated eczema/seborrhoeic dermatitis	Uncommon	Usually worsened on the face only, sparing the hands	No consistent abnormality on photo-testing which distinguishes condition from CAD	UV may act as an irritant
Viral exanthems	Commonly seen in reactivation of herpes simplex	Eruption of herpes simplex on lips	No abnormality on phototesting	Probably a result of UV-induced immunosuppression
Cutaneous T-cell lymphoma/mycosis fungoides	Uncommon but well documented	Worsening of condition on sun-exposed sites	Not consistently reported	May be difficult to distinguish from CAD
Psoriasis	Uncommon but well documented	Worsening of the condition on sun exposure	None consistently reported	Mechanisim unknown

CAD, chronic actinic dermatitis; MED, minimum erythema dose; SLE, systemic lupus erythematosus.

when the condition is severe. Ciclosporin and plasmapheresis are reported to be helpful in such instances.

Chronic actinic dermatitis (CAD)

This is a relatively common condition in the context of the photosensitivity disorders. It occurs almost exclusively in older patients (usually more than 60 years) with a male predominance. Patients are typically chronically sun exposed and many are keen gardeners. A variant of CAD has been described in younger patients with human immunodeficiency virus (HIV) disease and also, very rarely, in young atopics.

CAD presents as a chronic eczema on sun exposed sites, notably on the face and dorsum of the hands and neck (Fig. 23.9.5). Although it may worsen over the summer months, it persists throughout the year and patients may not have noticed its relationship to sun exposure. Patch testing often reveals multiple contact allergens, many to airborne antigens, such as colophony and compositae oleoresins (sesquiterpene lactone). Contact allergy to sunscreens is also common in this population.

Confirmation of the diagnosis is by monochromatic phototesting, which typically demonstrates extreme photosensitivity (markedly reduced MED responses) to UVB in particular, sometimes extending into the UVA range. Skin biopsy may occasionally be required to distinguish CAD from photosensitive mycosis fungoides or Sézary's syndrome (cutaneous lymphoma), which it may mimic.

Treatment includes general sun avoidance measures, topical steroids, and sunblock, but systemic therapy is usually also required to control the symptoms. Azathioprine, prednisolone, ciclosporin, and mycophenolate mofetil have all been used.

Photoaggravated conditions

These comprise a heterogeneous group of skin disorders which are aggravated by exposure to sunlight, although the mechanism by which this occurs is not known (Table 23.9.5). Those conditions characteristically worsened by sun exposure include lupus, dermatomyositis, bullous pemphigoid, bullous pemphigus, and Darier's disease. For others, exacerbation occurs in only a few patients, e.g. in UV-exacerbated psoriasis which is uncommon but well documented.

Further reading

Beattie PE, et al. (2003). Characteristics and prognosis of idiopathic solar urticaria: a cohort of 87 cases. *Arch Dermatol*, **139**, 1149–54.

Cleaver JE (2005). Cancer in xeroderma pigmentosum and related disorders of DNA repair. *Nat Rev Cancer*, **5**, 564–73.

Cleaver JE (2005). Splitting hairs –discovery of a new DNA repair and transcription factor for the human disease trichothiodystrophy. *DNA Repair (Amst)*, **4**, 285–7.

Clydesdale GJ, Dandie GW, Muller HK (2001). Ultraviolet light induced injury: immunological and inflammatory effects. *Immunol Cell Biol*, **79**, 547–68.

De Silva BD, McClaren K, Kavanagh GM (2000). Photosensitive mycosis fungoides or actinic reticuloid? *Br J Dermatol*, **142**, 1221–7.

Grabczynska SA, et al. (1999). Actinic prurigo and polymorphic light eruption: common pathogenesis and the importance of HLA-DR4/DRB1*0407. *Br J Dermatol*, **140**, 232–6.

Gupta G, Man I, Kemmett D (2000). Hydroa vacciniforme: a clinical and follow-up study of 17 cases. *J Acad Dermatol*, **42** part 2, 208–13.

Hawk JLM (ed) (1999). *Photodermatology*. Arnold, London.

Hickson ID (2003). RecQ helicases: caretakers of the genome. *Nat Rev Cancer*, **3**, 169–78.

Hönigsmann H (2002). Erythema and pigmentation. *Photodermatol Photoimmunol Photomed*, **18**, 75–81.

Jenkins G (2002). Molecular mechanisms of skin ageing. *Mech Ageing Dev*, **123**, 801–10.

Johnson BE, Ferguson J (1990). Drug and chemical photosensitivity. *Semin Dermatol*, **9**, 39–46.

Kerker BJ, Morison WL (1990). The photoaggravated dermatoses. *Semin Dermatol*, **9**, 70–7.

Liu G, Chen X (2006). DNA polymerase eta, the product of the xeroderma pigmentosum variant gene and a target of p53, modulates the DNA damage checkpoint and p53 activation. *Mol Cell Biol*, **26**, 1398–413.

Loveday KS (1996). Interrelationship of photocarcinogenicity, photomutagenicity and phototoxicity. *Photochemc Photobiol*, **63**, 369–72.

Menagé H, et al. (1995). Contact and photocontact sensitization in chronic actinic dermatitis: sesquiterpene lactone mix is an important allergen. *Br JDermatol*, **132**, 543–7.

Norgauer J, et al. (2003). Xeroderma pigmentosum. *Eur J Dermatol*, **13**, 4–9.

O'Donovan P, et al. (2005). Azathioprine and UVA Light Generate mutagenic oxidative DNA damage. *Science*, **309**, 1871–74.

Peters TJ, Sarkany R (2005). Porphyria for the general physician. *Clin Med*, **5**, 275–81.

Schwarz T (2205). Mechanisms of UV-induced immunesuppression. *Keio J Med*, **54**, 165–71.

Yarosh D, et al. (2001). Effect of topically applied T4 endonuclease V in liposomes on skin cancer in xeroderma pigmentosum: a randomised study. Xeroderma Pigmentosum Study Group. *Lancet*, **357**, 926–9.

23.10

Infections and the skin

Roderick J. Hay

Essentials

A huge variety of different organisms exist on healthy skin. Under certain circumstances, microbes can actively infect the skin as a primary or secondary event in cutaneous or systemic disease.

The most common causes of bacterial infection of the skin are *Staphylococcus aureus* or β-haemolytic streptococci. There are increasing reports of both hospital- and community-acquired infection by methicillin-resistant *S. aureus*. Superficial infection that spreads laterally in the upper dermis or along the subcutaneous fascia is known as cellulitis. Complications of cellulitis include septicaemia or involvement of nearby structures, hence it requires immediate antibiotic therapy.

Mycobacterium tuberculosis remains a common skin infection in many tropical areas, and syphilis, leprosy, and leishmaniasis are important skin infections in some parts of the world (see Section 7).

Dermatophytosis or ringworm is caused by mould fungi that can digest keratin (keratinophilic). The diagnosis can be confirmed in the laboratory by examining scrapings or clippings of skin, hair, or nails mounted in potassium hydroxide. Pityriasis versicolor is mainly caused by *Malassezia globosa*: it is a chronic scaly condition in which the skin becomes either hyper or hypopigmented in the affected area; macules and scales join and may become confluent over the back and chest, less commonly elsewhere.

Herpes simplex (HS) infections cause both acute as well as recurrent infections such as cold sores. Occasionally, in the immunocompromised patient these and other herpesvirus infections may disseminate, both to other parts of the skin as well as internally.

Introduction

The structure of the epidermis and its appendages such as hair and nails has been described elsewhere (see Chapters 23.1, and 23.13). The outer epidermis and the openings of the pilosebaceous units play host to a large variety of microorganisms, the majority of which are bacteria such as micrococci, coryneform bacteria, and staphylococci such as *Staphylococcus epidermidis* and *Staphylococcus saprophyticus*. These can achieve very high densities in excess of $4\log/cm^2$. However, in occluded areas and other parts of the body, anaerobic bacteria such as brevibacteria or microaerophilic organisms including *Propionibacterium acnes* are also present. Generally, these do not cause disease unless their local environment is disturbed, e.g. by occlusion or blockage of the sebaceous follicle or if they find entrance to the bloodstream through an internal appliance such as a cannula; also, these may cause disease in the presence of immunosuppression. *S. epidermidis*, for instance, is a common pathogen in neutropenic patients. Other factors that play a role in determining surface populations include ultraviolet light exposure and the presence of skin disease. Fungi, apart from members of a single genus of lipophilic (fat metabolizing) yeasts called the Malassezia species, are not commonly carried on the skin surface. These are mainly found in the openings of sebaceous follicles. A mite species, *Demodex folliculorum*, is also sometimes found on the skin surface within hair follicles. Again these organisms are normally in balance with the host and unless other conditions prevail, they do not cause disease.

In addition to these microbes that are members of the resident microflora of the skin, some bacteria may be temporarily carried as transient colonists of the skin. Examples include *Staphylococcus aureus* which colonizes the anterior nares, the axillae, or perineum in about 3 to 35% of normal healthy individuals, depending on site. In addition, these bacteria or fungi can also colonize abnormal skin surfaces; e.g. patients with psoriasis or atopic dermatitis often carry *S. aureus* on their skin lesions. Similarly, fungal species such as *Candida albicans* are occasionally carried on the skin surface, e.g. on the hands. The skin is therefore an ecological niche for a variety of microorganisms that, in turn, affect local environmental factors such as pH.

The skin may also be the focus for infections which are usually, but not invariably, caused by external pathogens. These are discussed under the heading of bacterial, fungal, viral, and ectoparasitic infections. The skin may also be affected by infections originating from other internal sites and carried via the bloodstream. Detailed accounts of diseases associated with particular organisms are also presented elsewhere, e.g. for *Mycobacterium leprae* see Chapter 7.6.27 and for *Treponema pallidum* see Chapter 7.6.35).

Cutaneous bacterial infections

Bacteria commonly cause infection of the skin either as a primary event or secondary to some pre-existing skin condition. The term 'pyoderma' is used to describe purulent infection of the skin caused by bacteria. The most common of these infections is the epidermal infection impetigo, but small abscesses such as boils or furunculosis can also result. The most common causes of pyoderma are *S. aureus* or β-haemolytic streptococci. Uncommonly, but increasingly, both hospital- and community-acquired infection by methicillin-resistant *S. aureus* (MRSA) are being reported. Infections with community-acquired methicillin-resistant staphylococci are more virulent; e.g. they are more likely to require surgical intervention and many of these strains carry the Panton–Valentine leukocidin gene which enhances virulence. Other forms of bacterial infection affecting deeper planes of the skin, e.g. dermis or subcutaneous tissue, leading to cellulitis, are also seen regularly in clinical practice. Examples of secondary bacterial infection include secondary infection of atopic dermatitis, Darier's disease, or psoriasis.

Impetigo

This is a superficial infection confined to the epidermis caused by *S. aureus* (see Chapter 7.6.4) or β-haemolytic streptococci (see Chapter 7.6.2), the cause depending, to some extent, on geography and climate. In temperate zones, the normal cause is *S. aureus* but in the tropics β-haemolytic streptococci are more common, although in about 20% of cases these organisms can both be isolated from lesions, indicating a mixed infection. In most cases this is a primary infection but it may also be secondary to other skin conditions such as eczema or scabies. Impetigo is common in primary care in temperate climates, its incidence accounting for about 20 per 1000 person years in the under 18 population, and there is some evidence to suggest that this incidence is increasing. However, it can also be found in other groups where close contact is likely, e.g. military recruits. It is more common in summer than winter. Pyoderma is more common in the tropics where it is often secondary to another skin disease such as scabies (see below).

In most European countries and the United States of America, where *S. aureus* predominates, some cases present with blistering lesions (bullous impetigo—see below). *S. aureus* produces exfoliotoxins that cleave the human cell adhesion molecule desmoglein 1(Dsg1). This results in the formation of an epidermal bulla similar to the blister formation in pemphigus foliaceus where Dsg1 is the target of an autoantibody. Very extensive blistering occurs in the childhood infection staphylococcal scalded skin syndrome (SSSS). Production of exfoliotoxin A is more associated with bullous impetigo and exfoliotoxin B with SSSS.

Impetigo usually presents with itching or discomfort in the affected area, which becomes red and the surface glazed and with a golden-coloured serous ooze. As stated previously, *S. aureus* infections may also result in bullous lesions (bullous impetigo) (Chapter 7.6.4, Fig.7.6.4.2). Impetigo is most common in children and often develops on the face or trunk, but lesions can be found elsewhere. Infected lesions may also develop from localized wounds, or insect bites, or around areas where the carriage rate is high, e.g. near eczematous plaques, or close to the nose. Patients are generally well and usually show no internal signs of infection such as fever.

Treatment consists of flucloxacillin or erythromycin, although, if the lesion is very localized, a topical antibiotic such as fusidic acid or mupirocin can be used (short-term). Impetigo is contagious particularly among children at school or in families and therefore close contacts should be screened for infection. There is little evidence to support the use of antiseptics in primary treatment, however logical. Hand washing, though, has been shown to reduce the risk of impetigo.

If the lesions penetrate deeper into the dermis they appear as well defined but localized ulcers know as ecthyma. These occur, particularly, in hot climates or where the site of infection is occluded by tight clothing. Ecthyma may also complicate other skin conditions, e.g. chickenpox. It is treated with systemic antibiotics.

Folliculitis and furunculosis

S. aureus is the usual cause of a boil or furuncle which develops around an infected hair follicle. If the infection is restricted to the superficial part of a follicle the lesion is called folliculitis, whereas if it is deeper a cutaneous abscess, the boil or furuncle, develops. Folliculitis commonly presents in hair bearing areas such as in the beard area. Lesions are small, multiple, and pustular; with the earliest symptom often being itching. Folliculitis-like lesions may also be caused by inflammatory tinea corporis and may also accompany ingrowth of curling hairs in the beard area (pseudofolliculitis) that traps skin commensal bacteria to cause a papular or pustular response.

A furuncle or boil usually starts as a solitary, tender, and inflamed nodule which, as it develops, points to form a pustular head. The patient may be febrile. Treatment is by incision to release pus followed by antibiotics (flucloxacillin or erythromycin). The most common sites for the formation of boils are the axillae or trunk areas or even the face.

Boils can develop at any age but there may a cluster of cases within the same household over a number of months suggesting transmission within the family. Although it is frequently stated that recurrent boils are indicative of underlying disease such as diabetes or immunosuppression, this is, in reality, unusual; it is more common that the individual is a bacterial carrier. Carriage of *S. aureus* is common in atopics and history of atopy is therefore quite frequent in those with recurrent furunculosis.

Lesions that resemble furuncles may appear in the axillae or groin associated with entrapment of commensals. This condition, known as hidradenitis suppurativa, is not associated with *S. aureus*, a useful clue to the diagnosis. Secondary scarring and recurrent attacks are common. There is little effective treatment for this condition (see Chapter 23.11). If several boils amalgamate the large pustular mass is called a carbuncle. Sites of predilection include the neck.

Cellulitis

Superficial infection that spreads laterally in the upper dermis or along the subcutaneous fascia is known as cellulitis. The main cause is infection with β-haemolytic streptococci (also see Chapter 7.6.2), but other common causes include *S. aureus*. Cellulitis starts as a zone of spreading erythema and tenderness with other signs of inflammation such as increased surface temperature. With streptococcal infections the patient is often systemically unwell with fever and chills. The main sites for infection are the face or the lower legs. Cellulitic infections affecting the dermis and upper subcutaneous tissue are sometimes known as erysipelas. Non-group A streptococci are also sometimes responsible.

Complications include the development of septicaemia or encroachment on adjacent structures such as the orbital cavernous sinus leading to thrombosis. Rare causes of the same syndrome include zygomycete fungi. Cellulitis requires immediate antibiotic therapy with an oral penicillin such as flucloxacillin or a macrolide antibiotic, and in systemically unwell patients with an intravenous regime. Recurrent attacks are also seen, particularly on the limbs and are often associated with lymphoedema. Management is difficult as local antisepsis and improved drainage by themselves do not appear to prevent recurrences and long-term oral penicillin V (phenoxymethylpenicillin) is often necessary for recurrent disease. However, in lower limb cellulitis there is an association with skin lesions such as the cracks caused by athlete's foot and treatment aimed to heal local skin defects, e.g. antifungals, is indicated.

In the early phases, these infections are easily confused with early necrotizing fasciitis (see Chapter 7.6.2) where the surrounding erythema spreads slowly but the patient remains unwell and the overlying skin becomes hypoaesthetic. Necrotizing fasciitis can be caused by group A streptococci but also by mixed bacterial infections after surgery or a compound fracture. The spreading erythema, dull ache, systemic reaction, and the reduction in overlying sensation should alert the physician. Surgical exploration is warranted, which then reveals necrotic and oedematous reaction in the underlying dermis and deeper fascial planes. Treatment is by early surgical debridement, which is an essential part of management in addition to systemic antibiotics.

Other bacterial skin infections

Gram-negative bacteria, such as a *Pseudomonas* species, may cause skin lesions. Most commonly these present as interdigital infections of the feet. It occurs often in those whose occupations involve wearing heavy footwear or wet working conditions. The skin becomes eroded and cracked; the toe web is also painful. If pseudomonas is present, the edge of the lesions appears greenish. Often, Gram-negative interdigital infection follows fungal infection (tinea pedis). Treatment with topical povidone-iodine or 1 to 2% acetic acid is useful, but sometimes the lesion flares up after treatment and this heralds the return of a dermatophyte infection.

Gram-negative folliculitis is a painful form of folliculitis presenting with fiery pustules on the trunk and limbs, sometimes associated with fever. It is associated with bathing in whirlpool bathtubs contaminated with Gram-negative bacteria. Ecthyma gangrenosum is a necrotic ulcerative condition which is a manifestation of disseminated *Pseudomonas* infection in patients with Gram-negative septicaemia. The lesions develop as nodules that evolve into raised plaques with a necrotic centre.

Tuberculosis of the skin and other mycobacterial infections

Mycobacterium tuberculosis is a rare cause of skin infection in most industrialized societies although it remains a regular infection seen in many tropical areas (see Chapter 7.6.25). With the increase in HIV and drug resistant tuberculosis, there have been increasing numbers of cases seen in recent years. Once common, cutaneous

tuberculosis presents with a number of different clinical forms, all of which reflect the state of the host's immunity and the route of infection to reach the skin—either through haematogenous spread, by direct spread from an underlying infected structure, e.g. lymph node or bone, or by direct inoculation into the skin. In immune individuals there are usually few organisms, which is described as paucibacillary. In other forms of infection, particularly in those who are immunocompromised, there are many organisms, which is described as multibacillary disease. The term tuberculid is used to describe skin lesions that do not contain viable organisms but that are associated with tuberculosis elsewhere. Usually, but not always, the pathogenesis is through an antigen-mediated reaction, e.g. vasculitis. Examples include erythema nodosum and erythema induratum (Bazin's disease) (see Chapter 23.7), both of which are forms of vasculitis, and which can in some countries be caused by tuberculosis among other causes. In papulonecrotic tuberculid the rash is a reaction to disseminated and particulate antigen and therefore, in some cases, if viable agents are present, this progresses to infective forms of tuberculosis such as lupus vulgaris.

The main cutaneous forms of infection seen are tuberculosis verrucosa cutis, scrofuloderma, lupus vulgaris, and papulonecrotic tuberculid. The clinical and immunological features are seen in Table 23.10.1. Cutaneous tuberculosis, e.g. miliary tuberculosis, is seen more frequently now with the spread of HIV/AIDS, although not in patients on antiretrovirals.

Nontuberculous mycobacteria may also infect the skin. These include *Mycobacterium chelonei* and *Mycobacterium fortuitum* which may cause cold abscesses, often as a result of local skin injury including needlestick injury. *Mycobacterium ulcerans* is the cause of rapidly spreading skin ulceration or Buruli ulcer (Chapter 7.6.28) seen in tropical and semitropical areas ranging from West Africa to northern Australia. It is associated with exposure to fresh water and a potential link with aquatic insects has been proposed. It is difficult to arrest the process with antibiotics and the most successful form of management is surgical excision. *Mycobacterium marinum* is an infection usually contracted from tropical fish kept

Table 23.10.1 Cutaneous forms of tuberculosis

Form	Immune status/ organisms	Clinical features	Evidence of TB elsewhere
Tuberculosis verrucosa cutis	TB +ve No organisms	Warty lesions on peripheries Slow spread	No
Scrofuloderma	TB +ve or −ve Organisms	Purplish plaques over lymph node, often in neck	Lymphadenopathy
Lupus vulgaris	TB +ve No organisms	Plaques on face or trunk Heals with central scarring Risk of squamous cell carcinoma	Uncommon
Papulonecrotic tuberculid	Usually TB −ve. Seen in healthy and HIV +ve patients. Organisms	Multiple papules, with central area of necrosis, limbs more than trunk	Often other sites, e.g. lungs

TB, tuberculosis.

Table 23.10.2 Clinical patterns and common types of human papillomavirus

Skin or mucosal infection	HPV type[a]
Common, plantar, mosaic warts	1, 2, 4
Plane warts	3, 10
Butcher's warts	7
Bowen's disease (some cases)	16
Epidermodysplasia verruciformis	3, 5, 8, 12, 36–38, and others
Condyloma acuminata (genital warts)	6, 11
Intraepithelial neoplasia, e.g. cervical dysplasia, bowenoid papulosis	16

HPV, human papillomavirus.
[a] Only commonly associated forms are shown.

in a fish tank—fish tank granuloma; however, naturally acquired infections are seen in the tropics, e.g. in association with commercial fish-farming (Chapter 7.6.26). It presents with an area of localized pustular swelling, and granulomatous infiltration or ulceration, usually on a peripheral site such as a finger. In some cases there is local lymphadenitis (sporotrichoid spread). The main differential diagnosis is sporotrichosis or leishmaniasis. Treatment with a range of different antibiotics from minocycline to rifampicin has been used.

Cutaneous fungal infections

With the exception of infections due to malassezia species, most fungal infections of the skin are extrinsic. The most common of these, dermatophytosis, is seen in all countries, whereas malassezia infections are more common in the tropics. Candida infections of the skin are less common but are seen regularly as secondary skin infections. The infections are discussed in detail in Chapter 7.7.1.

Cutaneous viral infections

Certain viruses are capable of establishing infections of the epidermis and dermis, but, strictly speaking, there are no viral commensals of the skin. The main infections are the human papillomavirus (HPV) infections (warts) and herpes zoster and simplex. These infections are discussed in detail in Section 7.5. Table 23.10.2 outlines common HPV types and associated clinical patterns.

Ectoparasitic infestations

Demodex folliculorum, an acarid mite, is a commensal on normal skin, but there are also infestations due to ectoparasites—scabies and pediculosis (lice). These are described in detail in Chapter 7.12.

Further reading

Beyt BE Jr, *et al.* (1981). Cutaneous mycobacteriosis: analysis of 34 cases with a new classification of the disease. *Medicine (Baltimore)*, **60**, 95–109.

Daikos GL, *et al.* (1998). Disseminated miliary tuberculosis of the skin in patients with AIDS: report of four cases. *Clin Infect Dis*, **27**, 205–08.

Del Giudice P, *et al.* (2006). Emergence of two populations of methicillin-resistant Staphylococcus aureus with distinct epidemiological, clinical and biological features, isolated from patients with community-acquired skin infections. *Br J Dermatol*, **154**, 118–24.

Espinal MA, *et al.* (2001). Global trends in resistance to antituberculosis drugs. World Health Organization-International Union against Tuberculosis and Lung Disease Working Group on Anti-Tuberculosis Drug Resistance Surveillance. *N Eng J Med*, **344**, 1294–303.

Koning S, *et al.* (2004). Interventions for impetigo. *Cochrane Database Syst Rev*, **2**, CD003261.

Schachner LA (2005). Treatment of uncomplicated skin and skin infections in the pediatric and adolescent patient populations. *J Drugs Dermatol*, **4** Suppl 6, S30–3.

Seal DV, Hay RJ, Middleton K (2000). *Skin and wound infection: investigation and treatment in practice.* Martin Dunitz Ltd, London.

Stanley JR, Amagai M (2006). Pemphigus, bullous impetigo, and the staphylococcal scalded-skin syndrome. *N Engl J Med*, **355**, 1800–10.

Sebaceous and sweat gland disorders

Alison Layton

Essentials

Cutaneous glands in humans include holocrine or sebaceous glands and merocrine or sweat glands. Merocrine glands are subdivided into apocrine, eccrine, and apoeccrine glands. Disorders of each of these cutaneous glands have been associated with disease.

Apocrine glands in adults are found predominantly in the axillae and anogenital regions, with a few located in the ear canal (ceruminous glands) and eyelids (Moll's glands). Associated disorders include hidradenitis suppurativa, Fox–Fordyce disease, bromhidrosis, trimethylaminuria, and chromhidrosis.

Eccrine glands are the sweat-producing glands of the skin. Many drugs and systemic diseases can influence the degree of sweating, such as thyroid disease, infection, carcinoid and cholinergic drugs. The concentration of sodium chloride in sweat is increased in cystic fibrosis.

Sebaceous glands form part of the pilosebaceous unit and are found over the entire body surface, with the exception of palms and soles. They are under the influence of androgenic hormones, especially dehydrotestosterone (DHT). Acne is a common inflammatory skin disease often associated with significant psychosocial morbidity. Early effective intervention reduces emotional and physical scarring. An understanding of pathophysiology allows topical and systemic therapies to be combined logically to target therapy.

Disorders of apocrine glands

Apocrine glands are compound sweat glands with a secretory coil that extends deep through the dermis into subcutaneous tissue and drains via a long, straight secretory duct, into a hair follicle. Their function in man is not altogether clear, but in other mammals they are responsible for sexual attraction and scent production. This is responsible for axillary and inguinal odour. The glands become larger and functionally active at puberty. The secretion is opalescent and malodorous. The glands are innervated by adrenergic fibres of the sympathetic nervous system.

Hidradenitis suppurativa (HS)

This is a chronic, inflammatory, suppurative disease affecting apocrine-gland bearing skin sites, including the axillae, groins, perineum and/or submammary area (in women). Occlusion of the follicular infundibula is the initial event in pathogenesis. This is followed by inflammation of the apocrine glands and rupture of the follicles. Painful, inflamed nodules and sterile abscesses result in sinus tract formation, fistulae, and scarring. Distinction from septic furunculosis may be difficult in the early stages. The aetiology of HS is unclear; it is more common in women than men and the incidence in England is 1:600. Patients of African descent have a higher incidence than Europeans. A familial form of HS with autosomal dominance has been described. Specific bacteria, e.g. anaerobic streptococci like *Streptococcus milleri* have been reported in HS and although cultures are frequently sterile, microbiological assessment allows treatment to be based on documented sensitivities. However, treatment is notoriously difficult. Reducing friction and moist hot environments, together with weight reduction and cotton clothing will help some patients. Localized inflammatory lesions benefit from intralesional injections using triamcinolone (5 mg/ml). Small studies have shown a combination of oral clindamycin (300 mg twice daily) and rimfampicin (600 mg daily) is also beneficial. Systemic antibiotics, including erythromycin 500 mg twice each day or minocycline 100 mg daily, are frequently used but topical clindamycin lotion is the only antibiotic that has been shown to be beneficial in a double-blind, placebo-controlled trial. Systemic steroids frequently produce dramatic improvement but recurrence is usual on withdrawal. Antiandrogen therapy alone as cyproterone acetate or in combination with ethinylestradiol has been used successfully in women. Isotretinoin produces minimal benefit and the longer acting retinoid acitretin 25 mg daily has shown more promise. Ciclosporin A and the tumour necrosis factor-α (TNFα) inhibitor infliximab have demonstrated improvement in refractory disease. Good results have been reported following radical surgical excision of involved areas with laying open of sinus tracts.

Fox–Fordyce disease

This problem relates to inflammation of the apocrine ducts and occurs most commonly in women postpuberty. Light brown or flesh coloured papules appear in areas of apocrine glands around the breasts, vulva and axillae. The lesions are frequently itchy and inflamed. If symptomatic, electrodessication of the irritable lesions will help. Other treatments advocated include topical clindamycin lotion, ultraviolet radiation, topical retinoids, oral contraceptives, and systemic retinoids.

Bromhidrosis (abnormal sweat odour)

Apocrine secretion is odourless when it is first excreted onto the surface of the skin but certain food substances, e.g. garlic, and bacterial decomposition which liberates fatty acids will influence apocrine odour. Odour is associated with bacteria, especially corynebacteria. Increased axillary pH may facilitate overgrowth of bacteria; hence deodorants that lower the pH will reduce the bacterial growth. Treatment of axillary bromhidrosis includes avoidance of relevant food substances, frequent washing, and local antibacterial substances. Surgical ablation of eccrine and apocrine glands can be beneficial in patients not helped with conservative approaches.

Trimethylaminuria (fish odour syndrome)

This unpleasant disorder occurs from excessive tertiary amine trimethylamine (TMA), appearing in eccrine and apocrine secretions as well as breath and urine. The odour is likened to rotting fish. Sufferers are unable to oxidize TMA and are homozygous for an allele which determines this impaired reaction. In the general population, 1% are heterozygous carriers of this allele. The odour is often worse after eating fish, at times of stress, or around menstruation. The condition can be diagnosed by direct estimation of TMA in the urine. A diet low in carnitine and choline may help. Short courses of neomycin or metronidazole may reduce the bacteria that degrade carnitine and choline in the gut.

Chromhidrosis

Rarely apocrine sweat can be blue/black, yellow, or green resulting from the secretion of lipofuscins. The more oxidized lipofuscins appear deeper in colour and the lighter coloured lipofuscins may fluoresce. The onset of coloured sweat starts in puberty and resolves in old age as apocrine function regresses. The axillae are most frequently affected, although areolar and facial chromhidrosis have been reported. Topical capsaicin may be beneficial.

Disorders of eccrine glands

Eccrine glands represent small tubular structures draining directly onto the skin surface. Up to four million sweat glands are present in all sites of the skin excluding mucous membranes, palms, soles, axillae, and forehead, the latter having the highest density. Sweat is formed by active secretion involving the sodium pump. After tubular resorption of electrolytes and water the sweat becomes isotonic. Sweat contains sodium, potassium chloride, lactate, urea, and ammonia. The concentration of sodium chloride in sweat is increased in cystic fibrosis. Sweat glands exhibit thermoregulatory control, the skin surface being cooled by evaporation. Eccrine glands are innervated by cholinergic fibres of the sympathetic nervous system and sweating may therefore be induced by cholinergic drugs and blocked by anticholinergic therapies. The preoptic hypothalamic sweat centre controls sweating centrally.

Hyperhidrosis or excessive sweating

This is acutely embarrassing and can manifest itself as generalized or localized disease. Underlying organic conditions should be considered as outlined in Box 23.11.1. Localized hyperhidrosis most commonly affects the palms, soles, and/or axillae.

Treatment of hyperhidrosis is not always successful. Practical advice on appropriate cotton clothing, heat avoidance, and weight reduction along with relaxation techniques and anxiolytics in selected cases may all prove helpful.

Topical anticholinergic drugs can produce local benefits without causing systemic adverse effects. Topical 0.5% glycopyrrolate

---

Box 23.11.1 Causes of generalized hyperhidrosis

- Thermoregulatory triggers
  - Hot weather/environment
  - Exercise
- Infection
  - Fever/nausea
  - Tuberculosis/malaria/brucellosis/endocarditis, etc.
- Metabolic/hormonal
  - Thyrotoxicosis, acromegaly, diabetes, Cushing's syndrome
  - Hypoglycaemia, alcohol intoxication, hyperpituitarism
  - Phaeochromocytoma
  - Menopause
- Neoplastic
  - Lymphoma
  - Carcinoid
  - Carcinoma
- Gustatory
  - Spicy/hot foods or drinks
- Neurological
  - Lesions of the sympathetic nervous system, cortex, basal ganglia, or spinal cord
  - Peripheral neuropathies
  - Familial dysautonomia (Riley–Day)
  - Congenital autonomic dysfunction with universal pain loss
  - Cold-induced profuse sweating
- Drugs
  - Cholinergic drugs
  - Fluoxetine
  - Opiate withdrawal
- Psychological
  - Anxiety
  - Fear

cream has been used with some success in gustatory hyperhidrosis associated with diabetes.

Eccrine blocking agents work by impeding the delivery of sweat to the skin surface. Soaks using 3% formalin and 10% glutaraldehyde solution help pedal hyperhidrosis but they are irritant to other sites. Aluminium chloride is the most frequently used preparation for axillae and hands but is also irritant and damages clothes.

Botulinum A injections produce blockade of neuronal acetylcholine release at the neuromuscular junction and in cholinergic autonomic neurons. Intradermal injections can reduce sweating within 48 h and have lasting effects (8 months in the axillae and 6 months in palms). Injections can be safely repeated with good effect.

Iontophoresis using tap water or anticholinergic drugs such as glycopyrronium bromide is very helpful for palmoplantar hyperhidrosis. A small, battery operated unit can be purchased for home maintenance.

While atropine-like drugs are effective for hyperhidrosis, adverse effects including dryness of the mouth, constipation, visual disturbances, and rarely glaucoma, hyperthermia, and convulsions may outweigh their benefits. Propantheline is the most frequently used preparation at 15 mg three times daily increasing as tolerated to 150 mg daily. Calcium channel blockers such as diltiazem have helped some cases. Anxiolytic agents may be beneficial where there is psychological overlay. Clonazepam and amitriptyline have both been reported to help unusual localized hyperhidrosis.

Surgical sympathectomy will result in anhidrosis. This is generally performed endoscopically and is very successful in treating palmar, axillary, and craniofacial hyperhidrosis. Postoperative compensatory hyperhidrosis frequently ensues, particularly in warmer climates and, although usually mild, it can prove disabling. Axillary hyperhidrosis may be greatly helped by surgical excision of axillary glands.

Hypohidrosis/anhidrosis

These rare problems may occur under the following conditions:

- Abnormalities of the sweat glands:

  - Prematurity—in neonates/premature babies the sweat glands function poorly.

  - Ectodermal dysplasia—this is a rare, inherited, X-linked recessive disorder in which sweat glands are either absent or decreased. Boys have characteristic facies with abnormal teeth and hair and experience heat intolerance. See Chapter 23.3.

  - Heat stroke—this is due to sweat gland exhaustion and represents a medical emergency. It is seen most often in older people exposed to a hot climate. It may occur in the young during or after prolonged exercise. Patients present with headache, cramps, fatigue, confusion, and hyperthermia. This progresses to vomiting, hypotension, oliguria, metabolic acidosis, and hyperkalaemia. Morbidity is high if they are not cooled down immediately and given fluid and electrolyte replacement.

- Abnormalities of the nervous system—any abnormality in the sympathetic tract from the hypothalamus to peripheral nerves may result in anhidrosis. The symptoms of anhidrosis include heat intolerance, nausea, dizziness, tachycardia, and hyperthermia in hot environments.

- Skin disease—anhidrosis has been reported in a number of skin diseases including, ichthyosis, psoriasis, lupus erythematosus, and morphoea and may be associated with Sjögren's syndrome. A localized loss of sweating ability may be due to tuberculoid leprosy, syringomyelia, or diabetes mellitus.

Miliaria

This results from occlusion of the eccrine ducts leading to sweat retention. Typically, it occurs in hot, humid climates, and in all ages, particularly when excessive clothing is worn and excessive sweating occurs. It may also be seen in association with high fever. Depending on the level of ductal occlusion the clinical picture can vary.

- Miliaria crystallina results from ductal plugs in the stratum corneum and presents with vesicles of 1 to 2 mm. The lesions are usually nonsymptomatic, and as they rupture desquamation of the skin occurs.

- Miliaria rubra (prickly heat) reflects intraepidermal ductal obstruction and occurs in 1:3 people exposed to hot climates. Itchy red papules typically occur at points of friction and flexures. Relief is usually gained quickly by cooling the skin.

- Miliaria profunda relates to dermal ductal occlusion and presents with pale firm papules 1 to 3 mm diameter. It is rare outside the tropics.

Disorders of sebaceous glands and the pilosebaceous unit

Sebaceous glands are an integral part of the pilosebaceous unit and are found over the entire body surface with the exception of palms and soles. The glands are multilobed and contain lipid filled cells. The lobules empty sebum into the upper hair follicle via a short duct. The sebum lubricates and waterproofs the skin and has some bactericidal and fungistatic activity. Free sebaceous glands are found in the eyelid (meibomian glands), mucous membranes (Fordyce's spots), areolar, perianal, and genital skin. The hair follicle, the hair, the sebaceous gland, arrectores pilorum muscle, and (in certain regions) the apocrine glands make up the pilosebaceous unit.

Sebaceous glands are under the influence of androgenic hormones especially dehydrotestosterone (DHT). Human sebaceous glands contain 5α-reductase, 3β-, and 17β-hydroxysteroid dehydrogenase which convert androgens to DHT. A surge of androgens at puberty is associated with the onset of acne in adolescence.

Acne

This is a polymorphic inflammatory disease of the pilosebaceous follicles, predominantly affecting the skin of the face and trunk. It is one of the most common skin diseases encountered by community physicians and dermatologists. Acne can present at any age, from neonates to mature adults, but is most prevalent and most severe during adolescence with 30% of teenagers requiring medical treatment.

The pathogenesis of acne relates to an increase in androgen-mediated sebum production, follicular hyperkeratosis, proliferation of *Propionibacterium acnes*, and inflammation. There appear to be three phases in the development of acne, an innate immune response mediated by IL-1α, followed by microcomedo formation, and then visible inflammation associated with a specific delayed-type hypersensitivity response.

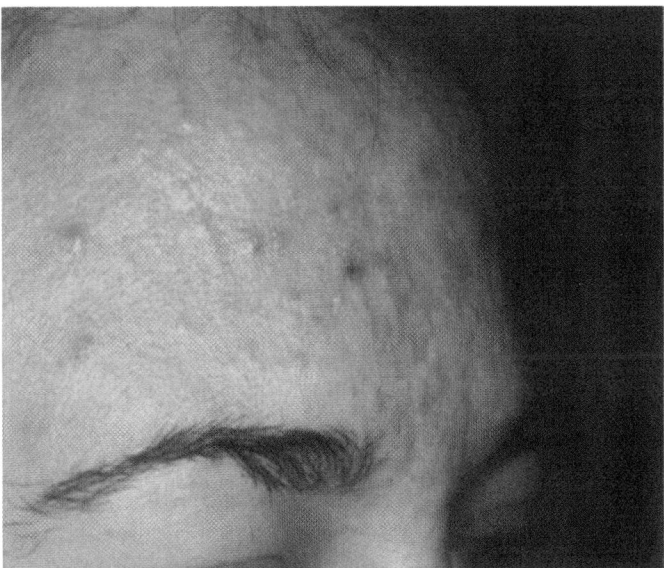

Fig. 23.11.1 Inflammatory papular acne interspersed with closed, non inflammatory lesions of the forehead.

Hyperkeratinization of the sebaceous duct is mediated by IL-1α and tumour necrosis factor-α (TNF-α) from keratinocytes and T lymphocytes. The result is hyperproliferation of keratinocytes, reduced apoptosis, and consequent hypergranulosis. The sebaceous follicle becomes blocked with dense keratin and so evolves the microcomedo, considered to be the precursor to both the non-inflammatory (blackheads/whiteheads; Fig. 23.11.1) and inflammatory lesions seen in acne. *P. acnes* colonize the skin surface and pilosebaceous ducts and bind to the Toll-like receptor 2 (TLR-2) on monocytes and neutrophils, leading to the induction of macrophage or keratinocyte secretion of IL-12. This results in the differentiation of T cells, leading to the activation of Th 1 cells when they encounter their antigen in the dermis.

The resulting inflammatory lesions embrace papules and pustules in most cases, but deeper inflamed lesions may present as acne nodules (Fig. 23.11.2). When examining acne it is useful to adopt a grading system so that improvements can be quantified.

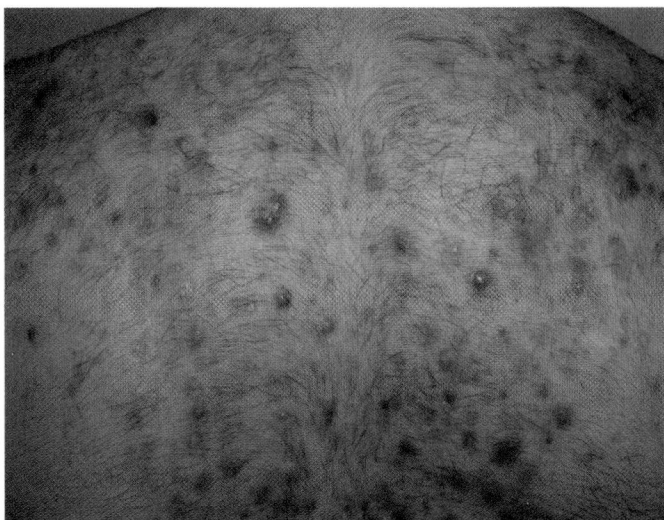

Fig. 23.11.2 Inflammatory nodular acne of the back with associated scarring.

Scars frequently occur in acne and are not necessarily related to the severity of the inflamed acne lesions.

Management

Assessment of the acne should include a thorough history, including details of family history, duration of acne, previous therapies, and response to treatments, along with careful physical examination. The majority of patients do not have an endocrine problem relating to their acne, however, polycystic ovary syndrome should be considered in women who have persistent/late-onset disease particularly if this coexists with other signs of hyperandrogenism such as hirsutism, irregular menses, or infertility. Cushingoid features, androgenic alopecia, acanthosis nigricans, and deepening of the voice may also reflect hyperandrogenism. These patients frequently have insulin resistance and are at increased risk of developing type 2 diabetes and possibly cardiovascular disease. Late-onset adrenal hyperplasia can also trigger late-onset acne in both sexes. Table 23.11.1 summarizes the investigations used to confirm or refute these diagnoses.

Response to treatment can be slow and patients must be encouraged to adhere to the chosen treatment regimen. Acne and scarring can result in significant psychological and social disability in predisposed individuals, e.g. anxiety, depression, social isolation, and interpersonal difficulties.

Topical therapies form the mainstay of treatment for mild to moderate acne. The choice of preparation will depend on the type of acne present (Table 23.11.2). Topical retinoids treat noninflammatory and inflammatory acne. They reverse hypercornification and induce proliferation of the follicular epithelium, thus helping to 'unplug' the follicle. The less anaerobic conditions that result lead to a reduction in *P. acnes*. Given the central role of the microcomedo in the early development of both noninflammatory and inflammatory lesions, most patients require a topical retinoid as part of their treatment regime. Retinoids are also now being considered for maintenance therapy. Skin irritation is a common side effect but is less problematic with the newer retinoids (topical isotretinoin and adapalene). Irritation is minimized by using

Table 23.11.1 Investigating the underlying endocrine abnormalities implicated in acne

Cause	Investigations
Polycystic ovary syndrome	Day 1–5 of menstrual cycle:
	Total and free testosterone
	LH/FSH
	SHBG
	Ultrasonography of ovaries (not mandatory but may help to support the clinical impression)
Congenital adrenal hyperplasia	17-Hydroxyprogesterone
	DHEAS
	Cortisol levels
Cushing's syndrome	Dexamethasone suppression test
Gonadal or adrenal tumours	Total and free testosterone
	DHEAS

DHEAS, dehydroepiandrosterone sulphate; LH/FSH, luteinizing/follicle-stimulating hormone ratio; SHBG, sex-hormone binding globulin.

Table 23.11.2 Topical therapies for acne: impact on aetiology

	Inflammation	Comedogenesis	Reduction in *Propionibacterium acnes*
BPO	+++	+	+++
Retinoids			
Tretinoin	+	+++	−
Isotretinoin	+	++	−
Adapalene	++	++	−
Antibiotics			
Erythromycin	+++	±	+++
Tetracycline	+++	±	+++
Clindamycin	+++	±	+++
Combination therapies			
Zinc/erythromycin	+++	+	+++
BPO/erythromycin	+++	+	+++
Isotretinoin/ erythromycin	++	+	+++
BPO/clindamycin	+++	+	+++

BPO, benzoyl peroxide.

Table 23.11.3 Systemic antibiotics for acne—dosage and adverse effects

Drug	Dosage	Adverse effects
Oxytetracycline	500 mg twice a day	Rare onycholysis, photosensitivity, benign intracranial hypertension
Erythromycin	500 mg twice a day	Gastrointestinal upset, nausea, diarrhoea all fairly common
Minocycline	100–200 mg daily	Headaches (dose dependent), pigmentary changes, autoimmune hepatitis/lupus erythematosus-like syndrome[a]
Doxycycline	100–200 mg daily	Photosensitivity (dose dependent)
Lymecycline	300–600 mg daily	Less than minocycline
Trimethoprim	200–300 mg twice a day	Rare hepatic/renal toxicity agranulocytosis

ANA, antinuclear antibody; LFT, liver function test; p-ANCA, perinuclear antineutrophilic cytoplasmic antibody.

[a] Advise, monitor LFTs, ANA, and p-ANCA in 'at risk' patients or when treatment is prolonged (>6 months). Cyclines are contraindicated in pregnancy and in children below 12 years.

lower concentrations for shorter durations. Topical retinoids are contraindicated in pregnancy.

Benzoyl peroxide (BPO) is a powerful antimicrobial agent. It decomposes to release free oxygen radicals in the sebaceous follicles, which have bactericidal and anti-inflammatory effects. BPO is active against fully sensitive and resistant strains of *P. acnes*. One high quality, randomized controlled trial demonstrated that BPO was as effective as oral oxytetracline and minocycline in mild/mild to moderate acne. BPO is available alone in concentrations of 2.5 to 10% and in combination with agents including hydroxyquinoline, erythromycin, and clindamycin. Lower concentrations are as effective as 10% and less irritant. Infrequently an allergic contact dermatitis occurs. BPO can bleach clothes and hair, so patients should be informed.

Topical antibiotics both reduce *P. acnes* and are anti-inflammatory through suppressing leucocyte chemotaxis and decreasing a proportion of proinflammatory free fatty acids and surface lipids. Topical erythromycin and clindamycin have been shown to be as effective as BPO in mild acne and are seemingly equally effective in treating moderate facial acne. As topical antibiotics drive bacterial resistance, they should be avoided as monotherapy over prolonged periods.

Evidence supports a direct correlation between *P. acnes* resistance and failure to respond to oral antibiotic treatment. Resistance to erythromycin can be reduced by using a combination of erythromycin and zinc or erythromycin and BPO peroxide.

Azelaic acid has some effect on inflamed acne lesions as it can reduce the number of *P. acnes*. It may be irritant and, rarely, photosensitivity can occur. Nicotinamide gel represents an alternative topical anti-inflammatory therapy; it has been shown to be as effective as 1% clindamycin gel and has the advantage of not promoting bacterial resistance.

Topical treatments can work synergistically when used in combination. Topical antibiotics and BPO are more effective than BPO as a single therapy. When combined with zinc, topical erythromycin has increased therapeutic efficacy. When retinoids are used in combination with antimicrobial agents, the combination produces faster results and significantly greater reductions in acne lesions. Compliance may be enhanced by using combinations products.

Systemic therapy is used for moderate to severe acne, or mild to moderate acne associated with scarring or significant psychosocial disability and/or failure to respond to topical treatment when it may be given in combination with topical therapy. Systemic antibiotic therapy (Table 23.11.3) reduces the number of *P. acnes* and *S. epidermidis* and proinflammatory mediators in the microcomedo. It also modulates the host response to these stimuli. Patients with marked seborrhoea and truncal acne respond less well to antibiotics. If oral antibiotics are to be incorporated into a regimen containing oral contraceptives, patients should still be warned about the possible decreased efficacy of the oral contraceptive, although, with the exception of rifampicin, there is currently no evidence to support the fact that commonly prescribed antibiotics either reduce blood levels and/or the effectiveness of oral contraceptives. Based on efficacy, safety, and bacterial resistance, cyclines should be used in preference to other classes of antibiotics. Oxytetracycline needs to be taken 30 min pre-food and not with milk to ensure adequate absorption. Second generation cyclines such as lymecycline (300–600 mg/day) and doxycycline (100–200 mg/day) may ensure better compliance and both have a better side effect profile than minocycline. Cyclines are contraindicated in children below 12 years of age and in pregnancy as they can affect dentition and result in inhibition of skeletal growth in the fetus.

The increasing incidence of *P. acnes* resistance to erythromycin and the link between erythromycin resistant *P. acnes* and reduced therapeutic response has resulted in the recommendation that erythromycin should be restricted. Erythromycin 1 g daily is the antibiotic of choice in pregnancy. Trimethoprim 200 to 300 mg daily is a third-line option for patients who have failed to respond to alternative antibiotics.

Combining topical and systemic treatment aids more rapid efficacy and potentially reduces the length of exposure to antibiotics, so reducing the likelihood of emerging antibiotic resistance. Antibiotic resistant *P. acnes* were first detected in the United States of America in the late 1970s. The worldwide incidence of antibiotic resistant *P. acnes* has increased significantly over the last decade. Carriage of resistant *P. acnes* can result in reduced therapeutic response to antibiotics. This is true for both erythromycin and tetracycline.

To reduce emerging resistance, oral antibiotics should only be used for 6 to 12 weeks in the first instance and only for as long as there is further clinical improvement. If the patient relapses after discontinuing the antibiotics, the same antibiotic should be restarted where possible. The addition of topical BPO can be used to try and eliminate resistant organisms.

Hormonal therapies can help females with acne whether or not their serum androgen levels are normal. They aim to reduce circulating androgen levels and/or block androgen receptors. Possible options are oestrogens, androgen receptor blockers, or agents designed to decrease the endogenous production of androgens by the ovary or adrenal gland. The oestrogen component of oral contraceptives increases sex hormone binding globulin, thus decreasing free testosterone in healthy women. Oestrogens also decrease production of ovarian androgens by suppressing secretion of pituitary gonadotropins. The progestin component of oral contraceptives minimizes the risk of endometrial cancer. However, progestins like norethisterone have intrinsic androgenic activity so may aggravate acne. Drospirenone 3 mg combined with ethinylestradiol 30 µg has been shown to have a superior effect to a third generation combined pill. However, it is not licensed in the United Kingdom as a treatment for acne.

Cyproterone acetate (CPA) has been shown to reduce sebum production and comedogenesis. CPA (2 mg) in combination with 35 mg ethinylestradiol has a licence for the treatment of severe acne in the United Kingdom and achieves significant improvement in 75 to 90% of female patients. Treatment is frequently required for 6 months before a response is seen. The relative thromboembolic risk with co-cyprindiol is slightly higher than that linked to non-antiandrogenic combined oral contraceptives but no higher than those containing third generation progestins.

Spironolactone acts as an androgen receptor blocker and inhibits 5α-reductase. In doses of 50 to 100 mg twice daily it reduces sebum production and improves acne. Side effects are dose-related and include potential hyperkalaemia, irregular menstrual periods, breast tenderness, headache, and fatigue. Although tumours have been reported in rodent models treated with spironolactone, this drug has not been directly linked with cancer in humans. There is a risk of feminization of a male fetus and thus pregnancy should be avoided.

Isotretinoin is a synthetic form of vitamin A and is effective in severe inflammatory acne that has failed to respond to other treatments. Oral isotretinoin is the only agent that impacts on the four main aetiological factors driving acne. It is a lipid soluble drug, hence its absorption is enhanced when administered with food. Oral isotretinoin should not be combined with tetracyclines as both can lead to benign intracranial hypertension. Mucocutaneous problems are the most common side effect of oral isotretinoin, including cheilitis, irritant dermatitis, and blepharoconjunctivitis. These side effects are dose dependent. Oral isotretinoin is a potent teratogen and women of childbearing age should not start therapy until a negative pregnancy test has been obtained, ideally 2 to 3 days prior to menstruation. Adequate contraception is essential for fertile, sexually active females before, during, and up to 5 weeks post-therapy. A recent European directive recommends mandatory pregnancy testing prior to the start of treatment and 5 weeks post-therapy and advocates monthly pregnancy testing throughout the treatment period. Baseline blood tests including fasting lipids and liver function should be done pretherapy and are recommended at 1 month, then 3-monthly throughout the treatment course. Adverse psychiatric events such as mood swings, depression, and suicidal ideation have been reported as possible idiosyncratic reactions to isotretinoin and must be highlighted. Epidemiological studies have not demonstrated a definite causal relationship between psychological effects and isotretinoin, but the association of depression with isotretinoin has not been satisfactorily investigated.

A number of small studies have trialled lasers, photodynamic therapy, and phototherapy with either clear blue or mixed blue-red light/radiation in inflammatory acne. Whereas some success has been reported, optimum regimes are still being assessed.

Unusual acne variants

Acne excoriée

This occurs frequently in adolescent girls and young women. Patients pick their skin leading to inflammatory lesions. Treatment can be difficult, psychological problems should be investigated, and underlying acne lesions managed with standard acne treatment. Successful treatment with habit reversal has been reported.

Dysmorphophobia

This occurs in a small number of acne patients. The patient's perception of their acne is disproportionate to their physical signs. There is often associated depression and/or obsessional neurosis. The acne should be treated in the standard fashion and psychiatric collaboration is important.

Drug-induced acne

This is well recognized. Corticosteroids are the most common offenders. Steroid acne has a monomorphic appearance and consists of noninflammatory and inflammatory lesions. Other drugs implicated include anticonvulsants, lithium, and the novel epidermal growth factor receptor (EGFR) inhibitors currently used for solid tumours.

Cosmetic acne

Various cosmetic ingredients induce comedones, in particular lanolins, petrolatum, and certain vegetable oils. Hair pomades can produce a monomorphic, low-grade acne.

Infantile acne

This is rare but may result in scarring if left untreated. Patients develop inflammatory lesions, particularly on the cheeks, usually after 3 months of age. These can evolve into deep-seated nodules and sinus tracts. Treatment is similar to adult acne, but tetracyclines should be avoided due to the risk of discoloured teeth. Topical therapies and/or oral erythromycin (125 mg twice daily) or trimethoprim (100 mg twice daily) can be used safely.

Gram-negative folliculitis

This occurs as a complication of any long-term topical or oral antibiotic therapy. It is characterized by sudden onset of multiple pustules, often localized periorally and perinasally. This results from overgrowth of Gram-negative organisms including *Escherichia coli*, proteus, pseudomonas, and klebsiella. The offending antibiotic should be stopped and changed to oral trimethoprim or ampicillin.

Oral isotretinoin generally produces a more rapid and permanent response.

Acne conglobata

This is an uncommon severe form of acne characterized by acne nodules, interconnecting sinuses, grouped comedones, and extensive scarring. Treatment is difficult and the problem usually runs a chronic course. Isotretinoin is usually the preferred therapy. Concomitant short courses of antibiotics and oral steroids may be required to control acute exacerbations.

Acne fulminans

This is rare, most frequently affecting adolescent boys. Acute erosive inflammatory lesions occur predominantly on the trunk. Associated systemic symptoms including fever, weight loss, arthralgia, and myalgia are evident. The aetiology is uncertain, but the presence of microscopic haematuria, erythema nodosum, increased response to *P. acnes* antigen on skin tests, and depressed response to intradermal purified protein derivatives are in favour of an abnormal immunological response. Oral prednisolone is the treatment of choice followed by the cautious introduction of systemic isotretinoin. A number of cases of acne fulminans have been triggered by anabolic steroids and testosterone.

Pyoderma faciale

This disorder is more common in adult women and often occurs in the context of emotional stress. These patients are not systemically unwell but the appearance of the disorder often adds considerably to the stress. Treatment with prednisolone reducing over 4 to 6 weeks and the daily application of moderate to potent topical steroid for 1 week will help. Isotretinoin should be introduced after 1 week, and, if tolerated, can be gradually increased.

SAPHO

This is the acronym for synovitis, acne, pustulosis, hyperostosis, and osteitis in which a group of overlapping joint diseases occur in conjunction with palmoplantar pustulosis and, less frequently, with psoriasis, acne, and inflammatory bowel disease.

Conclusions and the future

Acne is a common inflammatory skin disease often associated with significant psychosocial morbidity. Early effective intervention prevents emotional and physical scarring. Understanding of pathophysiology allows topical and systemic therapies to be combined logically to target the individual aetiological factors.

Research into the pathogenesis has defined acne as a T-cell mediated dermatosis. The possibilities for using immunomodulatory therapies and specific anti-inflammatory treatments are open to further developmental research studies and controlled trials. In theory, a TLR-2 antagonist, IL-1α antagonist, and cytokine therapy could be possible candidates for future acne treatment. Other possibilities include insulin sensitizing agents, 5α-reductase type 1 inhibitors, and possibly new anti-inflammatory agents such as lipoxygenase inhibitors.

Further reading

Archer JS, Archer DF (2002). Oral contraceptive efficacy and antibiotic interaction: a myth debunked. *J Am Acad Dermatol*, **46**, 917–23.

Coulson IH (2004). Disorders of sweat glands. In: Burns T, *et al.* (eds) *Rook's textbook of dermatology*, 7th Edition, pp. 45.1–45.23. Blackwell Science, Oxford.

Cunliffe WJ, Gollnick H (2001). *Acne: diagnosis and management*. Martin Dunitz Ltd, London.

Dréno B, *et al.* (2004). European recommendations on the use of oral antibiotics for acne. *Eur J Dermatol*, **14**, 391–9.

Eady EA, Gloor M, Leyden JJ (2003). Propionibacterium acnes resistance: a worldwide problem. *Dermatology*, **206**, 54–6.

European Agency for the Evaluation of Medicinal Products (2003). Committee for Proprietary Medicinal Products (CPMP). *Summary information on a referral opinion following an arbitration pursuant to article 30 of directive 2001/83/EC for roaccutane and associated names (see Annex 1). International non-proprietary name (INN): isotretinoin*. http://www.emea.europa.eu/pdfs/human/referral/roaccutane/284603en1.pdf

Garner SE, *et al.* (2003). Minocycline for acne vulgaris: efficacy and safety. *Cochrane Database Syst Rev*, **1**, CD002086.

Gollnick MD, *et al.* (2003). Management of acne: a report from a global alliance to improve outcomes in acne. *J Am Acad Dermatol*, **49** Suppl 1, S1–37.

Marqueling AL, Zane LT (2005). Depression and suicidal behaviour in acne patients treated with isotretinoin: a systematic review. *Semin Cutan Med Surg*, **24**, 92–102.

Ozolins M, *et al.* (2004). Comparison of five antimicrobial regimens for treatment of mild to moderate inflammatory facial acne vulgaris in the community: randomised controlled trial. *Lancet*, **364**, 2188–95.

Plewig G, Kligman AM (2000). *Acne and rosacea*. 3rd edition. Springer, New York.

Purdy S, de Berker D (2006). Acne. *BMJ*, **333**, 949–53.

Simpson NB, Cunliffe WJ (2004). Disorders of sebaceous glands. In: Burns T, *et al.* (eds) *Rook's textbook of dermatology*, 7th Edition, pp. 43.1–43.75. Blackwell Science, Oxford.

Thiboutot D (2004). Acne: hormonal concepts and therapy. *Clin Dermatol*, **22**, 419–28.

Blood and lymphatic vessel disorders

Peter S. Mortimer

Essentials

Bleeding into the skin may occur for local reasons or as part of a systemic disorder. The distribution of lesions is important: widespread lesions suggest a systemic problem, whereas regional lesions suggest that local factors predominate.

Widespread flat purpura without erythema should prompt a search for underlying haematological abnormalities such as platelet disorders. Larger (>1 cm) areas of purpura or bruising usually result from coagulation dysfunction. Palpable purpuric lesions, or those with a blanching component, suggest an associated inflammation as can be seen with vasculitis.

In patients with acute peripheral ischaemia it is important to exclude embolism. A pressure ulcer (decubitus ulcer, bedsore, pressure sore) is due to localized injury to the skin and/or underlying tissue as a result of pressure alone, or in combination with shear and/or friction. The presence of moisture, particularly relevant in an incontinent patient, leads to a macerated (and therefore more vulnerable) skin. Faecal soiling results in chemical damage to the skin.

Acute deep venous thrombosis (DVT, Chapter 16.16.1) may be silent but usually results in skin erythema and limb oedema. Consequences of post thrombotic vein damage include further DVT, superficial thrombophlebitis, oedema, skin changes, and eventually ulceration. Approximately 70% of leg ulcers are venous in origin; the other 30% resulting from coexistent arterial disease, diabetes, and other skin disease. Most ulcers occur in the gaiter region at or above the level of the malleoli, where the persistently elevated ambulatory venous pressure has an adverse effect on the upstream capillary microcirculation. Nearly half of all venous ulcers are associated with deep vein valvular incompetence, usually secondary to previous DVT, while the remainder result from incompetence of the superficial or communicating veins (primary varicose veins).

Introduction

Vasculogenesis represents the formation of new blood and lymphatic vessels from endothelial precursors which share an origin with haemopoietic precursors. This process is not confined to the embryo. Adult bone marrow-derived haemopoietic cells extravasate around nascent vessels and stimulate growth of resident vessels by releasing angiogenic factors. These cells can also function as haemangioblasts, producing both haemopoietic and endothelial progenitors that give rise to new blood vessels (probably not lymphatic vessels).

Angiogenesis is the growth of blood vessels through a process of sprouting and remodelling from existing vessels. The lymphatic system develops differently as most lymphatics differentiate from veins. Both blood and lymphatic vessels are crucial for organ growth in the embryo, as witnessed by mutations in some of the key genes in programming for cardiovascular and lymphatic development. For example, deletion of *FLT4* (*VEGFR3*, vascular endothelial growth factor receptor 3, the gene most responsible for lymphangiogenesis) leads to defects in blood vessel remodelling and embryonic death at mid-gestation, indicating an early blood vascular function. The formation of blood and lymphatic vessels is a complex process controlled by numerous genes and molecular players. For example, members of the *Notch* family drive the arterial gene programme; the orphan receptor COUP-TF11 regulates venous specification; and PROX1 commits venous endothelial cells to lymphatic lineage. The VEGF family of proteins seem most important for vascular and lymphatic endothelial cell sprouting, whereas platelet-derived growth factor (PDGF) and the angiopoietins are responsible for subsequent remodelling, maturation, and stability of the newly formed vessels. Close links exist between vessels and nerves; e.g. axon-guidance signals such as ephrins and semaphorins allow vessels to navigate to their targets.

Skin has been one of the most investigated tissues for understanding mechanisms of (lymph) angiogenesis, largely because it is so accessible. Angiogenesis is reactivated physiologically during wound healing and repair. In some circumstances, e.g. malignancy, the (lymph) angiogenesis activation becomes excessive and harmful so promoting the tumour growth and facilitating metastatic spread. Conversely, in arterial ischaemia the angiogenic switch is insufficient, preventing revascularization and healing of skin ulcers. In recent years, angiogenesis promoters and inhibitors have served as therapeutic targets. For example, the anti-VEGF antibody bevacizumab conveys survival benefit in the treatment of metastatic colorectal, breast, and lung cancer when combined with conventional chemotherapy but not as a monotherapy. One side effect is poorer wound healing.

Cutaneous manifestation of blood vessel disorders

As the main organ interacting with the environment, the skin vasculature has to be adaptive. The blood supply has a generous reserve to meet the requirements of wounding and repair as well as thermoregulation.

Skin disorders invariably involve the vasculature, if only because inflammation drives an increase in blood (and lymph) flow. A rash is red (erythema) because of an increase in blood flow. Surface pressure, by emptying the compressible venules and veins and reducing capillary inflow, will blanch the skin. Purpura represents extravasation of red cells from microvessels into the dermis and cannot be blanched. Simple purpura is not raised, but if it is associated with inflammatory changes of the blood vessels (vasculitis), the mass of cells and oedema makes the purpura palpable. More extensive release of red cells into the skin and subcutis (haemorrhage) will result in a bruise (ecchymosis). Differences between purpura and bruising are simply a matter of degree or depth of haemorrhage. The cause may be due to: thrombophilia; excessive intravascular pressure; weakness of the blood vessel wall or surrounding stroma (as seen with steroid therapy). Petechiae are pin point lesions of purpura (<2 mm diameter). Gravitational forces, by increasing venous and consequently capillary pressure, are likely to make purpura more evident in the lower limbs.

Telangiectases (named from Greek words meaning 'end', 'vessel', and 'extension or dilatation') are chronically widened capillaries or small vessels. They appear on the skin and mucous membranes as small, dull red, linear, stellate or punctate markings. Telangiectases (telangiectasias) represent expansion of pre-existing vessels without any obvious new vessel growth (angiogenesis). Unfortunately, clinical appearance may vary greatly according to the site, depth, and type of blood vessel involved. For example, the macular (flat) telangiectases seen in scleroderma, generalized essential telangiectasia, and port-wine stain are produced by dilatation of the postcapillary venules of the uppermost vascular plexus in the dermis. The common raised cherry angioma (Campbell de Morgan spot) is produced by spherical and tubular dilatations of capillary loops in the dermal papillae. Telangiectases are discussed in more detail below.

Angiokeratomas (as seen in Fabry's disease and the more common, harmless scrotal angiokeratoma) have the ultrastructure of collecting venules that contain valves and are dark red to black in colour. A spider angioma (spider naevus) represents high flow filling of surface capillaries by a single feeding dilated arteriole which, if blanched, will obliterate the whole spider naevus. The cutaneous lesions of hereditary haemorrhagic telangiectasia represent small arteriovenous anastomoses.

Mottling (marbling) of the skin is a physiological response to cold. Vasoconstriction to the skin results in desaturation of the slow flowing blood, leading to bluish (cyanotic) discoloration overlying the polygonal plexus of superficial venules and veins; warming restores normal flow and colour. If a similar reduction in

---

Box 23.12.1 Causes of simple purpura/ecchymoses

- ◆ Platelet disorders
  - · Thrombocytopenia (in isolation or with myeloproliferative disorders)
  - · Abnormal platelet function/anti platelet drugs (aspirin, chemotherapy)
  - · Thrombocytosis
- ◆ Coagulation disorders
  - · Haemophilia and other clotting factor deficiencies
  - · Drugs (anticoagulants)
  - · Thrombophilia (protein C and S deficiency)
  - · Disseminated intravascular coagulation and purpura fulminans
  - · Liver disease (decreased clotting factor synthesis)
- ◆ Microvascular occlusion
  - · Dysproteinaemias, e.g. hypergammaglobulinaemic purpura
  - · Cryoproteinaemias
  - · Emboli (cholesterol, oxalate, fat, myoma, septic)
  - · Sickle cell disease
- ◆ Mechanical
  - · Chronic sun damage ('senile' purpura)
  - · Corticosteroids
  - · Scurvy
  - · Amyloid
  - · Inherited collagen disorders (Ehlers–Danlos, pseudoxanthoma elasticum)
  - · Easy bruising syndrome/pinch purpura/'bite'/exercise purpura
- ◆ Raised intravascular pressure
  - · Coughing, vomiting, Valsalva manoeuvre
  - · Tourniquet
  - · 'Stasis' from chronic venous disease (varicose veins, post-thrombotic syndrome) and dependency syndrome

---

flow occurs for pathological reasons, e.g. intravascular thrombosis in antiphospholipid syndrome or vasculitis in polyarteritis nodosa, the mottling is fixed and broken up in pattern (livedo reticularis). Necrosis of the skin occurs following vascular occlusion due to intravascular coagulation, vasculitis, emboli, hyperviscosity syndromes, or vessel wall thickening.

Purpura (Box 23.12.1)

Simple macular purpura/petechiae

Bleeding into the skin may occur for local reasons or as part of a systemic disorder. Widespread flat (macular) purpura without erythema (no associated inflammation) should prompt a search for underlying haematological abnormalities such as platelet disorders. Larger (>1 cm) areas of purpura with or without ecchymoses

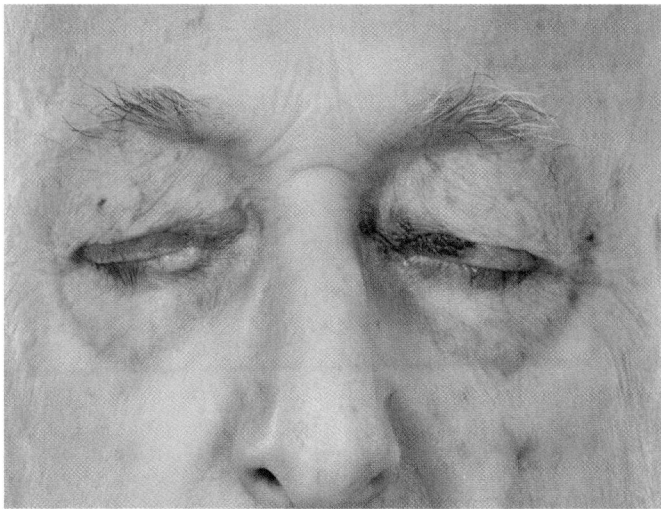

Fig. 23.12.1 Amyloid (panda sign).

usually result from coagulation dysfunction. The distribution of lesions is important: widespread lesions suggest a systemic problem whereas regional lesions suggest that local factors predominate. For example, purpura confined to the lower limbs would suggest venous hypertension (acute following a deep venous thrombosis (DVT) or chronic from long standing varicose veins); purpura in chronically sun damaged skin such as the backs of hands and forearms in older people result from weakness in the supporting collagen of the dermis, particularly in those on steroids; eyelid purpura occurs acutely with raised intravascular pressure from coughing/vomiting or chronically with systemic amyloidosis (panda sign, Fig. 23.12.1).

Palpable purpura

Palpable purpuric lesions, or those with a blanching component, suggest an associated inflammation. Care should be taken to evaluate new purpura as old lesions may show secondary inflammatory changes. Palpable purpura suggests vasculitis or some degree of vessel damage. In dysproteinaemic purpura, hypergammaglobulinaemic purpura, and cryoproteinaemia, a range of purpura may develop from macular purpura to larger necrotic lesions depending upon the size and type of blood vessel involved.

Distribution may be widespread or limited to colder or more dependent peripheries (lower legs). Larger vessel involvement may produce cutaneous necrosis or livedo reticularis.

Vasculitis (Box 23.12.2)

Vasculitis refers to inflammation and necrosis of any blood vessel (also see Chapter 21.10.2). Minor inflammation of a capillary (capillaritis) may simply increase permeability, resulting in only purpura, whereas involvement of arteries and veins will affect tissue perfusion. Vasculitis may be local or systemic, primary or secondary. Many systemic vasculitides have a cutaneous component. That cutaneous component will usually be a palpable purpura with multiple lesions distributed symmetrically and usually worse in the lower limbs. More severe inflammation from neutrophil infiltration will often manifest with pustule formation on top of the purpura. Necrosis of the lesion will produce a small black eschar after a few days. More extensive necrosis and punched out ulceration will ensue.

> **Box 23.12.2** Working classification of systemic vasculitis
>
> **Small vessel vasculitis**
> - Henoch–Schönlein purpura
> - Essential mixed cryoglobulinaemia
> - Waldenström's hypergammaglobulinaemia
> - Vasculitis associated with SLE and other connective tissue disorders and antiphospholipid syndrome
> - Urticarial vasculitis
> - Septic vasculitis
> - Eosinophilic vasculitis
> - Drug-induced
> - Reactive leprosy
> - Bowel-associated dermatosis–arthritis syndrome (BADAS)
> - Fungal infection of vessels (immunocompromised)
> - Behçet's disease
>
> **Larger vessel vasculitis**
> - Polyarteritis nodosa
>   - Systemic (including microscopic polyarteritis)
>   - Cutaneous limited
> - Granulomatous vasculitis
>   - Wegener's granulomatosis
>   - Churg–Strauss allergic granulomatosis
> - Giant cell arteritis
>   - Temporal
>   - Takayasu's
>
> SLE, systemic lupus erythematosus.

'Vasculitic' is a term inappropriately used to describe focal necrotic skin lesions that result from small infarcts due to microvascular occlusion. To understand the cause and guide treatment, a skin biopsy is essential in order to distinguish an inflammatory vasculitis responsive to systemic steroids from a vasculitis with marked fibrinoid wall changes where steroids are unlikely to be helpful. Other investigations that should be performed include measurement of complement (C4), antiphospholipid antibodies (which cause microvascular thrombosis and a secondary vasculitis), antiendothelial cell antibodies (AECA), and antineutrophilic cytoplasmic antibodies (ANCA), as well as serological tests for connective tissue disorders and screening for distant infection.

Microvascular occlusion/cutaneous necrosis

Microvascular occlusion may occur for a number of reasons (Box 23.12.3). While purpura may be the only clinical manifestation, the usual consequences are focal areas of necrosis secondary to failed perfusion, such as the digital finger tip infarcts seen in scleroderma.

Box 23.12.3 Disorders of microvascular occlusion

Intravascular

- Platelet plugging (myeloproliferative disorders)
- Cryoprecipitates (cryoglobulinaemia, cryofibrinogenaemia, cold agglutins)
- Emboli (cholesterol, crystals, septic)
- Sickle cell disease

Vessel wall

- Raynaud's disease
- Scleroderma, rheumatoid arthritis, dermatomyositis
- Fibrinoid vasculopathy/atrophie blanche

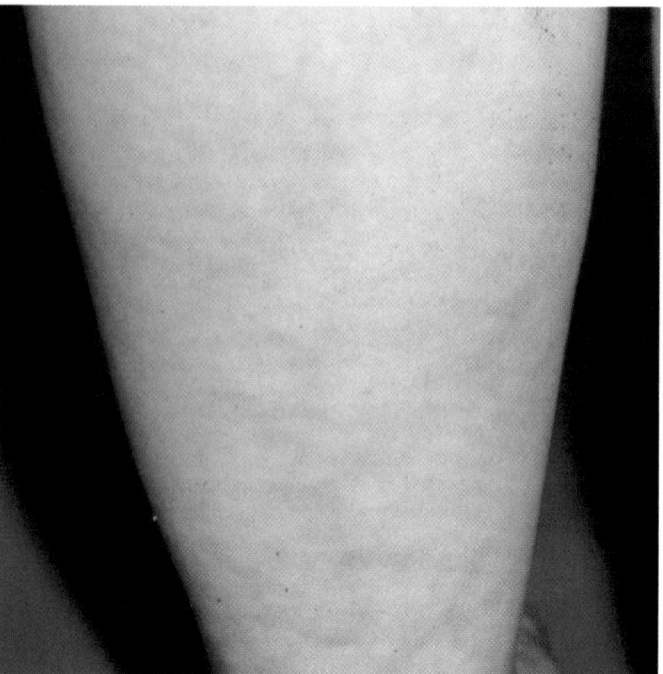

Fig. 23.12.2 Livedo reticularis.

Disturbances in blood rheology may arise from aggregation of blood contents. Alternatively, the fault may lie with the endothelial wall or lack of blood vessel conformation.

If vascular occlusion is extensive or involves larger vessels, then well demarcated areas of skin are infarcted and a black eschar forms. Terminal vessel involvement will cause peripheral gangrene. Purpura fulminans results from extensive vascular occlusion, the most important cause of which is meningococcaemia.

Livedo reticularis (Box 23.12.4)

Livedo (Fig. 23.12.2) describes a reticulate network of slow blood flow in the deep skin vascular plexus. When fixed and broken up in its pattern it is always pathological, usually representing thrombosis or vasculitis. In areas of livedo where perfusion is most compromised, purpura and necrosis will occur.

Erythema ab igne is a hyperpigmented fixed mottling resulting from prolonged application of heat to the skin. It occurs from sitting too close to a fire or from the use of heat pads applied for pain relief.

Arterial and peripheral ischaemic disorders

Arterial disease will generally compromise skin perfusion only in its advanced stages. Nevertheless, it may present with a dusky red to blue discoloration of skin in the peripheries (hand or foot)

Box 23.12.4 Livedo reticularis

- Vasculitis (large vessel)
  - Polyarteritis nodosa
  - Mixed cryoglobulinaemia
- Antiphospholipid syndrome
- Sneddon's syndrome (livedo with cerebrovascular accident)
- Calciphylaxis
- Disseminated intravascular coagulation + thrombophilia

or frank ulceration. If the ischaemia is marked, limb elevation above heart level causes skin pallor while dependency results in delayed but exaggerated hyperaemia. In such circumstances, a history of cardiovascular risk factors, intermittent claudication, and rest pain should be sought. A gross general rule is that arterial disease will cause foot ulceration particularly at sites of pressure including between the toes, whereas venous disease will cause leg ulceration (see below). If peripheral pulses cannot be palpated, simple assessment of peripheral arterial pressure can be undertaken by measuring the ankle brachial pressure index or toe pressures. Arterial pressure in the foot or ankle vessels should be the same or slightly greater than in the arm. If lower limb pressure is less than 80% of the arm, then arterial disease should be considered. Measurements can be unreliable in diabetes where calcification of the arterial wall prevents occlusion by the sphygmomanometer cuff and a false high reading may be obtained. Toe pressures are more reliable in such circumstances.

Significant arterial disease demanding investigation is uncommon when the foot pulses are easily palpable. Covert arterial disease may manifest with a reduction in oxygen delivery from anaemia, cardiac dysrhythmias, or any circumstances where cardiac output is reduced.

In patients with acute peripheral ischaemia it is important to exclude embolism. Thromboangiitis obliterans (Buerger's disease) may be difficult to distinguish from atherosclerosis. Rarer causes of ischaemia include external arterial compression (popliteal entrapment or a cervical rib), dissecting or thrombosed aneurysms, ergot poisoning, intra-arterial injections, coagulation disorders, and vasculitis.

Management of atherosclerosis includes correction of underlying cardiovascular risk factors where possible. The vast majority of patients with arterial disease die from medical comorbidities, such as myocardial infarction.

Small vessel calcification (calciphylaxis)

Calcification of arteries is common, but when it affects small arterioles as occasionally happens with hyperparathyroidism, particularly in chronic renal failure, it results in complete vascular occlusion of dermal arterioles (Fig. 23.12.3). Surrounding an area of skin infarction there is extensive livedo reticularis as well as subcutaneous induration from fat necrosis. The pathogenesis is unexplained. Uraemia and hyperphosphataemia are often more obvious than hypercalcaemia. Women are more often affected. An X-ray will reveal extensive vessel calcification and a skin biopsy will demonstrate calcium replacing dermal vessels. The prognosis is poor and treatment unsatisfactory. The management of any renal failure and normalization of the calcium phosphate product are essential. Parathyroidectomy is only indicated if hyperparathyroidism is proven.

Thromboangiitis obliterans (Buerger's disease)

This appears a distinct condition usually in young men who are heavy smokers. The aetiology is unknown but antiendothelial cell antibodies (AECA) can be present in high titre in active disease. Pathological examination shows that the arterial walls are invaded by inflammatory cells with changes being segmental or focal and resulting in thrombosis. Nerves and veins may be involved and fibrosis occurs in the later stages. Pain is usually the presenting feature because of muscle or nerve ischaemia or thrombophlebitis. Claudication of the foot is especially characteristic. Ulceration or gangrene develops early, especially around the sides of the nails or tips of digits. Recurrent superficial or deep venous thrombosis (DVT) is common. The proximal pulses, e.g. brachial or popliteal, are usually present while the distal pulses are absent. The erythrocyte sedimentation rate (ESR) and C-reactive protein (CRP) levels are usually raised, AECA are often present, and arteriography is usually diagnostic (normal proximal vessels but multiple stenoses and occlusions in distal vessels with collateralization). The differential diagnosis is early-onset atherosclerosis, embolism, diabetic vasculopathy, and connective tissue disorders.

Strict abstinence from smoking is essential. Infusion of a prostacyclin analogue has been shown to be effective, but medical treatment is otherwise unhelpful and referral to a vascular surgeon is recommended.

Sickle cell disease

Perimalleolar, painful leg ulcers develop in association with sickle cell anaemia. While the ulceration may be attributed to sickling of erythrocytes causing microvascular occlusion and skin infarction, similar ulcers have been reported in other forms of chronic haemolytic anaemia. Low, steady state levels of haemoglobin, intensity of haemolysis, and sickle cell anaemia with thalassaemia genotypes appear associated with ulceration.

Leucocyte adhesion may initiate occlusion episodes in a manner similar to venous ulceration (in the same site), indeed gravitational factors or venous disease may contribute to nonhealing of sickle cell ulcers. Secondary infection may also discourage healing, particularly in tropical climates. Treatment is unsatisfactory. Spontaneous healing may occur after some weeks irrespective of intervention; otherwise, bed rest and local compression may be necessary.

Raynaud's phenomenon/syndrome

Raynaud's phenomenon is defined as episodic digital ischaemia occurring in response to cold, emotional stimuli, or vibration. It is characterized by sequential colour changes: white—blue—red. Pallor is essential for the diagnosis but may be short-lived and be succeeded by prolonged cyanosis making distinction from acrocyanosis difficult. Raynaud's phenomenon may be primary (idiopathic), when it is referred to as Raynaud's disease, or secondary to a range of diseases, most notably connective tissue disorders.

Perniosis/acrocyanosis (cold injury)

Chilblains (perniosis) are localized, tender, red, and often itchy lesions which may blister or ulcerate. They occur as an abnormal response to cold. Perniosis of fingers and toes can be associated with cryoglobulinaemia, myelodysplastic disorders, lupus erythematosus ('chilblain' lupus), and anorexia or malnutrition. In contrast to peripheral (acral) chilblains, perniosis can occur overlying extensive subcutaneous fat, e.g. thighs, because the skin is more vulnerable to cold as a result of insulation by the fat.

Acrocyanosis is a persistent bluish mottled discoloration of the skin, usually over hands and feet. Unlike Raynaud's phenomenon where digital artery vasoconstriction occurs, it arises due to dilatation of small venules resulting in extremely slow venous flow following physiological vasoconstriction of arteriolar inflow in response to cold. The backs of the hands and fingers look blue and puffy (from oedema). While connective tissue disorders, antiphospholipid syndrome, neuropathies, and cryoglobulinaemia should be considered, the vast majority of cases are constitutional.

Frostbite is the result of acute freezing of tissues including the blood vessels. Hands, feet, ears, nose, and cheeks are most often affected. After the initial pain the affected part becomes pain free and the skin becomes shiny and white. Reperfusion injury occurs on warming with necrosis of tissue. Long-term scarring and abnormal autonomic nerve responses may occur.

Trench or (cold) immersion feet are similar, but the tissues do not freeze. Vascular occlusion results in tissue necrosis and neuropathic changes. The syndrome is not uncommon in the homeless population living in the United Kingdom.

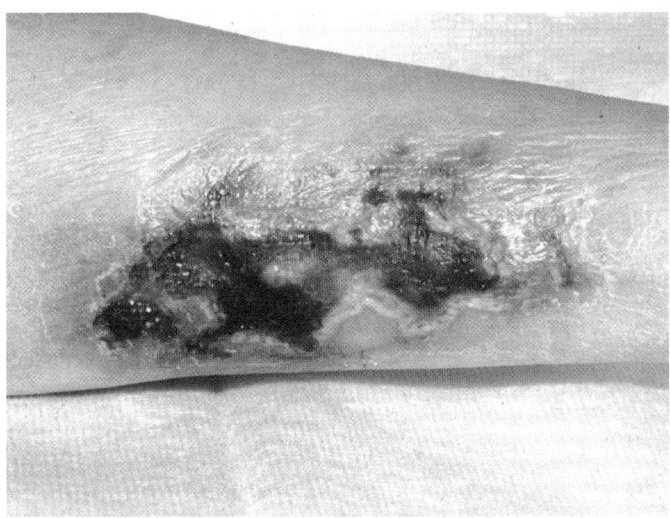

Fig. 23.12.3 Calciphylaxis.

Erythromelalgia (erythermalgia)

This is a condition of painful red extremities in which the sensation of burning is induced by warmth. Patients will complain of intolerable burning relieved only by dunking their feet in cold water or wrapping in towels kept in the freezer. There is consequently a danger of cold immersion injury. The term erythermalgia was introduced to separate primary cases (erythermalgia) from those (erythromelalgia) secondary to underlying disorders such as thrombocythaemia and other myeloproliferative disorders. The fundamental cause is now known to be a fault in sodium channels discovered by identifying mutations in the gene *SCN9A* which encodes the voltage-gated sodium channel $Na_V1.7$. Mutations alter channel gating behaviour in a manner that increases nociceptive neuron excitability. Cooling reduces the threshold of activation of the abnormal sodium channels. Although fundamentally a neuropathy, involvement of skin blood vessels results in persistent vasodilatation. Treatment with carbamazepine and similar drugs acting on sodium channels can help.

Complex regional pain syndrome—CRPS (reflex sympathetic dystrophy, causalgia, Sudeck's atrophy)

This is a syndrome of chronic pain with altered or heightened sensation, hyperhidrosis, and swelling. Allodynia is characteristic. The increased blood flow combined with a reluctance to use the limb (movement triggers pain) results in deep redness of the skin and swelling. Increased blood flow is an important diagnostic feature of early CRPS and can often be demonstrated on a three phase bone scan. Treatments include graded physical therapy and neuropathic pain relief.

Arteriovenous fistulae

Persistent arteriovenous shunts cause local venous hypertension and skin changes as a result. Arteriovenous fistulae consist of direct connections between large arteries and veins and are always pathological. Congenital forms result from a failure of embryological differentiation. Acquired forms are almost always traumatic and, if large, can cause significant cardiovascular effects. Increased warmth of the skin together with signs of increased venous pressure result, e.g. varicose veins. A palpable thrill and murmur on auscultation may be detected. Duplex ultrasonography is the investigation of choice. Embolization may be the best therapeutic option.

Pressure ulcers

A pressure ulcer (decubitus ulcer, bedsore, pressure sore) is due to localized injury to the skin and/or underlying tissue as a result of pressure alone or in combination with shear and/or friction. The presence of moisture, particularly relevant in an incontinent patient, leads to a macerated, and therefore more vulnerable, skin. Faecal soiling results in chemical damage to the skin.

Sustained pressure occurs most commonly when an individual is debilitated or paralysed and therefore cannot move to relieve pressure. Neurological deficit predisposes to a lack of movement or a lack of sensory feedback to pain as well as impaired autonomic control. Observations on patients with amyotrophic lateral sclerosis, a condition in which pressure sores are rarer, suggest a role for ciliary neutrophic factor. Defective collagen synthesis may be promoted in anaesthetic skin as well as by certain drugs such as corticosteroids. Other factors contributing to the development of pressure ulcers include arterial ischaemia, hypotension, dehydration, malnutrition, cachexia of cancer, prolonged pyrexia, hypermetabolic states, and hypoalbuminaemia. Patients undergoing extracorporeal circulation are particularly at risk.

Different classifications exist, but that of the National Pressure Ulcer Advisory Panel is simple to use. Stage I is nonblanchable erythema over a bony prominence; Stage II partial thickness loss of dermis; Stage III is ulceration into subcutaneous fat; Stage IV is exposure of muscle, bone, or joint. Deep sores will often result in more necrosis of fat or muscle than skin, so a cavity wound with undermined edges occurs.

Prevention should involve recognition of the at risk patient. A number of risk scales exist with the Norton scale being the best known. All at risk patients should have a pressure-relieving mattress in addition to frequent repositioning. Static support systems mould around the patient so distributing pressure over a greater area, while dynamic support systems vary the pressure distribution by, e.g. the use of air-fluidized and low air loss beds. The lateral position must be avoided and nursing in the prone position is advised. Any medical conditions should be controlled and the nutritional status assessed; spasticity should be relieved where possible. When pressure is relieved, necrotic tissue will separate naturally but eschar is best removed surgically. In principle, wounds heal best when moist and clear of infection and when exudate is absorbed away from wound surfaces. The choice of dressing depends upon the stage and state of the wound. Surgical debridement is necessary for removal of necrotic tissue and radical excision with reconstruction may be needed for extensive cavity wounds.

Venous disorders

Chronic venous disease

Veins are responsible for venous return. Muscles in the calf and foot compress and empty veins thereby lowering venous pressure. Valves prevent the reflux of blood. Valve failure results in minimal respite from high venous pressures during exercise. Venous pressure at the ankle is normally 70 to 100 mm Hg dropping to 0 to 30 mm Hg on exercise and remaining at approximately 55 mm Hg while sitting. Long periods spent sitting with legs dependent, reduced exercise levels, and obesity encourage venous hypertension with sustained pressures of 50 to 100 mg Hg. Venous reflux due to valve failure will result from inherent vein or valve weakness in primary varicose veins, or damage to veins usually from deep venous thrombosis. Persistently elevated venous pressure affects capillary pressure and endothelial function that results in a complex train of events which adversely affects skin viability in the gaiter region. The clinical consequences are varicose veins, oedema, haemosiderin skin pigmentation, varicose eczema, lipodermatosclerosis, and ulceration signs that are used for the CEAP Classification (class, aetiology, anatomy, pathophysiology) of chronic venous disease (CVD).

Deep venous thrombosis (DVT), post-thrombotic syndrome and venous obstruction

Acute deep venous thrombosis (DVT) may be silent but usually results in skin erythema and limb oedema. Iliac vein thrombosis may be easily missed on compression ultrasonography but should be suspected if whole limb swelling is associated with a mottled erythema. Post-thrombotic (postphlebitic) syndrome complicates

50 to 75% of DVTs. The more proximal the DVT the greater the risk. Consequences of post-thrombotic vein, and particularly valve, damage include further DVT, superficial thrombophlebitis, oedema, skin changes, and eventually ulceration.

Lipodermatosclerosis and prominent perforating veins are characteristic skin changes. Lipodermatosclerosis refers to a combination of skin and subcutaneous changes seen with chronic congestion, due to venous or lymphatic hypertension. Fat inflammation (panniculitis) combined with phlebitis and dermatitis results, over time, in fat atrophy and fibrosis which manifests as hardening and retraction of the skin, leading to the appearance of an inverse champagne-bottle shape to the gaiter region.

The most common cause of deep vein obstruction is DVT but nonthrombotic causes include iliac vein compression from pelvic tumours or aneurysms, tumours or aneurysms compressing the deep femoral vein, and a Baker's cyst may compress the popliteal vein. Abdominal obesity interferes with venous drainage, particularly in the sitting position. Retroperitoneal fibrosis can obstruct the iliac veins.

Superficial thrombophlebitis

Thrombosis in a superficial vein usually develops because of slow flow within a varicose vein. Pain, heat, and tenderness over a palpable nodule or cord is characteristic. Cellulitis may extend for some distance, making distinction from infection sometimes difficult. In the absence of any varicose veins, superficial thrombophlebitis usually occurs from trauma due to an intravenous cannula with or without extravasation of an irritating substance, e.g. chemotherapeutic agent. When recurrent or widespread, consideration should be given to the possibility of a thrombophilic state such as protein C or S deficiency, antiphospholipid syndrome, Behçet's syndrome, or underlying cancer (thrombophlebitis migrans).

Mondor's disease is diagnosed when palpable tender cords develop around the axilla, breast, or chest wall. Such cords, which may represent thrombosed veins or lymphatics, may 'bowstring' across the axilla (axillary web syndrome) and extend down the arm creating a 'guttering' effect with the limb outstretched.

Leg ulcers

Approximately 70% of leg ulcers are venous in origin; the other 30% result from coexistent arterial disease, diabetes, and rarer skin disorders (Box 23.12.5). Most ulcers occur in the gaiter region, at or above the level of the malleoli, where the persistently elevated ambulatory venous pressure has an adverse effect on the upstream capillary microcirculation. The consequent changes to the microvasculature and interstitium result in a failure of wound healing after trauma. Nearly half of all venous ulcers are associated with deep vein valvular incompetence, usually secondary to previous DVT, while the remainder results from incompetence of the superficial or communicating veins (primary varicose veins). Community surveys suggest an overall prevalence of 0.2% of the population with the highest rates in older women. Once treated, up to 72% can recur.

Capillary congestion conveys a bluish erythema to the skin often with purpura and oedema. Over time, the purpura turns to a brown 'rust' discoloration due to haemosiderin deposition. Scratching (due to 'varicose' eczema) or other trauma will lead to skin breakdown. Once ulceration has occurred, wound exudation will further

damage surrounding skin, promoting more skin inflammation (eczema/dermatitis) and necrosis. Underlying oedema will further fuel the exudation process. Indeed, leg oedema is an invariable association of a venous ulcer and always a sign of inadequate treatment. The 'congestion' resulting from the venous hypertension and oedema can cause a persistent redness to the skin resembling cellulitis from which clinical distinction can be difficult.

Box 23.12.5 Cutaneous necrosis

- Venous disease
  - Stasis, congenital, post-thrombotic
- Coagulation defects
  - Disseminated intravascular coagulopathy
  - Purpura fulminans
  - Protein C and S deficiency, antithrombin III deficiency
- Infection
  - Viral, gas gangrene, Buruli ulcer, tuberculosis, leprosy, swimming pool granuloma, Meleney's anaerobic ulcer, synergistic gangrene, streptococcal, superficial or deep fungus, syphilis, yaws, leishmaniasis
- Blood disorders
  - Hyperviscosity, dysglobulinaemia, sickle cell anaemia, spherocytosis, polycythaemia,
- Vasculitis
- Pyoderma gangrenosum
- Vasculopathy
  - Arterial disease, Buerger's disease
  - Antiphospholipid syndrome
  - Raynaud's disease
  - Calciphylaxis
- Emboli
- Metabolic
  - Hyperhomocysteinaemia
- Venoms (snake and spider bites)
- Neuropathic
  - Leprosy, diabetes
- Drugs
  - Anticoagulants
  - Ergot
  - Chemotherapy infusions
  - Illicit drugs
- Malignancy (or paraneoplastic)
  - Melanoma, squamous cell carcinoma, Kaposi's sarcoma, leukaemia, secondary deposits
- Physical damage from contact

The diagnosis of a venous ulcer is essentially clinical. Venous duplex Doppler ultrasound examination can be normal in obese patients who spend long periods in a chair, whereupon 'functional venous hypertension' occurs. Nevertheless, venous duplex Doppler is essential for identifying ulcers due to surgically correctable superficial venous incompetence. Arterial ischaemia can be excluded by measuring the ankle brachial pressure index, although it is unreliable in diabetes and other circumstances where compression by a sphygmomanometer cuff is not possible due to arterial wall calcification. Falsely high readings may be obtained and arterial duplex Doppler may be needed. Sensory testing is always important in diabetic patients, not just because impaired sensation can lead to ulceration but also because compression therapy applied unwittingly may contribute to ulceration. Any ulcer with a raised border or one that does not respond to therapy should undergo biopsy to exclude malignancy.

First-line therapy for venous ulceration is compression therapy and exercise. The concept is to reduce venous pressure, particularly during walking, by improving calf muscle pump function and by opposing gravitational venous reflux. Exercise and movement are to be encouraged and preferred to rest. Long periods spent sitting and standing are discouraged, but when resting the leg(s) should be elevated, ideally with the ulcer just above heart level, to ensure the maximum reduction in venous pressure. Falling asleep in a chair with the legs elevated on a stool is of no use. Obesity should be tackled effectively. Heart failure must be controlled as right sided failure further elevates leg venous pressures. Severe anaemia should be corrected, although chronic leg ulcers will result in a degree of chronic anaemia.

Graduated, multilayer, high compression bandage regimens capable of sustaining compression for a week at a time should be the first line of treatment. In general, it is treatment of the leg rather than the wound that is important. Nevertheless, eczema and exudation must be controlled. Antibiotics, topical or oral, are of no value unless there is clear evidence of clinical infection or if streptococci are colonizing the ulcer. Beneath the compression, a simple low adherent wound dressing is advisable.

Foot ulcers

It is unusual to see ulcers of purely venous origin below the line of the edge of the shoes, although atrophie blanche/livedoid vasculopathy (Fig. 23.12.4) can occur on the foot. Vasoconstriction operates more powerfully in the feet than the legs and it is here that the earliest effects of arterial insufficiency or neuroischaemia manifest. Pressure or friction points suffer first. In populations who do not wear protective shoes the foot is prone to infection. It was previously thought that microangiopathic arteriolar occlusion disease was responsible for the tissue necrosis in the diabetic foot. Tissue necrosis and ulceration are now believed to result from narrowing and occlusion of the main arteries of the leg below the knee, complicated by septic occlusive vasculitis of the terminal arteries. Consequently, correction of the occlusive artery disease by angioplasty and the infection by aggressive antibiotic treatment and debridement are recommended.

Telangiectasis

Telangiectases (Box 23.12.6) are chronically expanded capillaries or small venules. They usually appear in the skin as spidery red

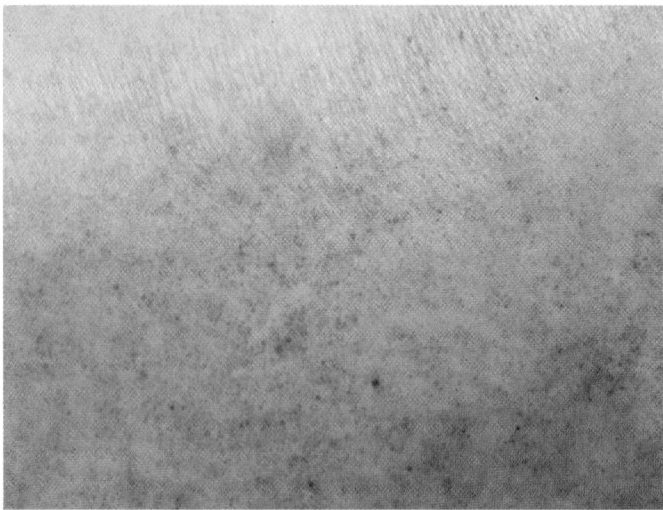

Fig. 23.12.4 Atrophie blanche represented by red dots (enlarged tortuous capillaries) between which are areas of white scarring.

lines, as on the facial cheeks, but can be punctate, as in hereditary haemorrhagic telangiectasis (HHT), or be flat red macules as seen in the mat telangiectasis of scleroderma. Telangiectases represent enlargement of pre-existing vessels without any apparent angiogenesis (conversely angiomas imply a vascular malformation due to an anomaly of embryological development or alternatively a form of tumour).

Secondary telangiectases

Telangiectases commonly represent the effect of wear and tear on the skin and are particularly frequent on ageing, light exposed skin. Atrophy of the skin and the resulting lack of dermal support to the microvasculature will result in telangiectases, as may follow

---

Box 23.12.6 Telangiectasia

Secondary

- Prolonged vasodilatation, e.g. rosacea, varicose veins
- Photoageing (sun damage, smoking)
- Spider naevi
- Radiotherapy
- Topical steroids
- Connective tissue disorders (scleroderma, lupus erythematosus, dermatomyositis)
- Mastocytosis
- Cutaneous lymphoma

Primary

- Vascular birthmarks, e.g. port-wine stain
- Hereditary haemorrhagic telangiectasia
- Ataxia—telangiectasia
- Generalized essential telangiectasia

smoking and ultra violet radiation. Prolonged vasodilatation may be followed by permanent telangiectases as in rosacea. Varicose veins are frequently the cause of telangiectases of the leg where an arborizing pattern may result. The colour of the telangiectases depends on the calibre of the dilated venule. Large dilatations (<1 mm) are dark blue and palpable. The smallest (0.1 mm), most superficial telangiectases are red and barely empty when the leg is raised. Telangiectases around the lower border of the ribs are virtually physiological in older age groups. There are increasing reports of telangiectases associated with calcium channel blocking drugs.

Connective tissue disorders

The presence of telangiectases is an important diagnostic sign in lupus erythematosus, dermatomyositis, scleroderma, and overlap syndromes. Nail-fold telangiectases can usually be seen with the naked eye, but an ophthalmoscope will reveal fewer but larger, tortuous capillaries often with haemorrhage. Scleroderma results in mat telangiectases which can mimic the telangiectases of HHT both in appearance and distribution (face and hands), but in HHT they are more obvious on mucous membranes. Telangiectases can occur with cutaneous mastocytosis and angiotropic (intravascular) lymphoma.

Spider naevi (arterial spider, spider angioma)

Spider telangiectases occur in up to 15% of a normal population and are even more common in children and pregnant women. They are characteristically found in liver disease of which they may be a presenting sign. A relationship to high oestrogen levels has been suggested.

The main vessel of the spider is an arteriole. The high blood flow fills the capillaries radiating from the vessel. Occlusion of the arteriole with a pin head blanches the whole lesion; refilling occurs first from the arteriole and is pulsatile. Spider naevi are only seen above heart level, e.g. upper body.

Cherry angiomas (Campbell de Morgan spots)

These are common in middle age, but disappear in extreme old age. They can be confused with petechiae when small and flat because they do not blanch. Larger angiomas are raised and dome-shaped. They have no known medical associations.

Venous lakes (phlebectasia)

Greatly dilated, thin-walled venules occur on the face, lips, and ears of older patients. Because they contain desaturated blood, venous lakes are dark blue to black and can be confused with melanoma until compressed and emptied.

Rosacea and flushing

Rosacea is a diagnostic term applied to a spectrum of abnormalities in the skin and eyes. Cutaneous features include persistent redness of exposed skin (usually the face) with telangiectases, flushing, oedema, erupting small inflammatory papules (pimples) and pustules, and, in chronic cases, hypertrophy of the sebaceous glands with fibrosis (rhinophyma). Ocular changes occur in more than 50% of patients and range from the common blepharitis and conjunctivitis to the rare, sight-threatening keratitis. The onset is usually between 30 and 50 years old and more common in women and in patients with fair skin. Ambient heat, alcohol, sunlight, hot

drinks, spicy food, and stress appear to exacerbate the condition. The use of topical fluorinated steroids and tacrolimus can trigger a rosacea-like eruption.

Persistent central facial erythema is the most common feature. Telangiectases are prominent and, together with inflammation, cause the red complexion. Appearances may mimic the 'butterfly' rush of lupus erythematosus, but a skin biopsy will confirm the presence of ectatic capillaries (and lymphatics) in the dermis. Inflammation may be minimal but, if present, is usually follicular (folliculitis). Photo (sun) damage and oedema frequently coexist.

Flushing is usually provoked by ambient temperature, alcohol, hot or spicy food, menopause, or anxiety. Prolonged episodes of severe flushing accompanied by sweating, flushing, sweating not limited to the face, and associated systemic symptoms such as diarrhoea, wheezing, headache, or palpitations should prompt investigation for carcinoid syndrome, phaeochromocytoma, or mastocytosis.

Treatment of the erythema and flushing component of rosacea is difficult. A therapeutic 6-week trial of antiacne-type antibiotics, e.g. oxytetracycline 500 mg twice daily or metronidazole 200 mg twice daily is worthwhile to resolve any underlying inflammation contributing to symptoms. Such first-line treatment usually works well for any papules or pustules. If telangiectases are prominent, laser therapy can be helpful. Because relapse of rosacea is common, avoidance of exacerbating factors, such as alcohol, is advised and topical metronidazole cream has proved effective.

Perioral dermatitis is a persistent erythematous eruption consisting of tiny papules and pustules primarily distributed around the mouth. It occurs predominantly in younger women and is associated with the use of topical steroids. Indeed, the steroid potency associates with risk of disease and it is important to stop steroid usage. Response to treatment with 4 weeks of oral tetracycline is usually excellent. Topical tetracycline and topical metronidazole can also be effective.

Primary telangiectases

Hereditary haemorrhagic telangiectasia (Osler–Rendu–Weber disease)

HHT is an autosomal dominant disorder characterized by epistaxis, cutaneous telangiectases, and visceral arteriovenous malformations (AVMs).

Mutations in at least two genes are responsible. *Endoglin* (*ENG*) on chromosome 9 is the gene for HHT1, where there is a higher prevalence of cerebral and pulmonary AVMs, while activin receptor-like kinase 1 (*ACVRL1* or *ALK1*) on chromosome 12 causes HHT2 which has a milder, later onset phenotype with an increased number of hepatic AVMs. *ENG* and *ALK* both encode a homodimeric integral membrane glycoprotein which is the surface receptor for TGF-β.

Recurrent epistaxis is usually the presenting symptom at, or just after, puberty but onset may begin in childhood. Telangiectases are punctate, or sometimes papular, and most commonly seen on the lips, mucous membranes, and fingers. They represent microvascular arteriovenous anastomoses causing the visible dilatation of postcapillary venules. Lesions occur on the nasal septum, nasopharynx, and throughout the gastrointestinal tract where they may be demonstrated by endoscopy or MR angiography but not by barium studies. Pulmonary AVMs cause dyspnoea, cyanosis, and clubbing and are seen on chest X-ray. Liver enlargement and cirrhosis can occur (HHT2). An association with juvenile polyposis has been described. The diagnosis is based on family history and clinical phenotype. Molecular genetic testing detects mutations in 60 to 80% of individuals. Prenatal testing is available.

In mild cases, no treatment is usually needed except the control of any anaemia, possibly including iron replacement. Tranexamic acid, by regulating the *ALK1/endoglin* pathway, may be beneficial in some patients. Symptomatic skin or mucous membrane lesions can be destroyed by cautery or laser. Recurrent nasal bleeding and pulmonary AVMs may demand more extensive surgery or embolism approaches. Antibiotic prophylaxis is recommended for dental and invasive procedures.

Ataxia-telangiectasia (Louis-Bar syndrome)

Ataxia-telangiectasia syndrome is a rare recessive disease with pleiotropic involvement of nervous and lymphoid systems caused by mutations in the ataxia telangiectasia mutated (*ATM*) gene.

Defective excision repair of DNA damaged by ultraviolet (UV) light, gamma or X-rays is responsible. The syndrome presents with telangiectases, progressive cerebellar ataxia, combined immunodeficiency, and a marked susceptibility to cancer. A diminished level, or absent, IgA is characteristic.

Telangiectases may be present as early as the second year and first appear on the bulbar conjunctiva and subsequently on the ears, eyelids, and the butterfly area of the cheeks. Bleeding is uncommon. Recurrent sinus and pulmonary infections are frequent and may dominate the clinical picture. X-ray investigation should be restricted. The laboratory diagnosis relies on increased serum α-fetoprotein levels and cellular sensitivity to ionizing radiation. Molecular, genetic, and prenatal testing for the presence of the abnormal *ATM* gene is available.

No proven treatment exists. Antioxidants such as vitamin E and α-lipoic acid are recommended. Intravenous immunoglobulin appears to reduce the number of infections.

Vascular birthmarks

Vascular birthmarks usually develop during childhood and are therefore naevoid in origin (naevus is Latin for 'maternal impression' or 'birthmark'). Many, possibly all, birthmarks represent clones of genetically altered cells arising from mosaicism during somatic mutation. It is important to distinguish between haemangiomas and vascular malformations, although it may prove difficult on clinical grounds.

Haemangiomas are proliferative blood vessel tumours, whereas vascular malformations represent structural defects arising from vascular development.

Vascular malformations can be high flow (arterial or arteriovenous fistulas) or low flow (capillary, venous, lymphatic, or mixed) types. In general, vascular malformations possess no endothelial proliferation, are present at birth, and do not involute.

Port-wine stain (naevus flammeus)

These are characterized clinically by persistent macular erythema from birth, and pathologically by ectasia of superficial dermal capillaries. Port-wine stains have a greatly diminished density of perivascular nerves. Associated eye and brain abnormalities occur in 8 to 15% of port-wine stains on the head and neck. The most significant ocular problem is glaucoma, particularly if the eyelids are involved. The Sturge–Weber syndrome represents involvement of the leptomeningeal vasculature giving rise to epilepsy and neurological deficit.

Klippel–Trénaunay syndrome

The association of a port-wine stain with tissue overgrowth and vein abnormalities usually affecting one hindquarter is termed the Klippel–Trénaunay syndrome. The port-wine stain is present from birth with excessive longitudinal bone growth occurring during childhood. Increased limb girth suggests soft tissue overgrowth. Vein abnormalities, particularly aberrant veins such as the lateral thigh vein (embryological remnant), progress from puberty. Lymphatic abnormalities (lymphoedema and lymphangioma) are not uncommon. Sometimes the whole of one side of the body is affected with hemihypertrophy. There is a high rate of thrombosis involving both superficial and deep veins. Venous ulceration may occur.

The differential diagnosis includes the Parkes Weber syndrome in which limb hypertrophy is associated with multiple arteriovenous anastomoses. The Proteus syndrome is highly variable (protean) in its clinical presentation. Mandatory general criteria include mosaic distribution of lesions, a progressive course, and a sporadic occurrence. Connective tissue naevi are pathognomonic and epidermal naevi, tissue overgrowth, lipodystrophy, and vascular malformations (including lymphatic) may occur. Mutations in *PTEN* may be present. The Proteus-like syndrome is undefined and refers to the presence of significant clinical features falling short of diagnostic criteria. The Servelle–Martorell syndrome encompasses vascular malformations associated with limb hypoplasia (shortening).

Cutis marmorata (reticulate vascular naevus)

This is a combined capillary and venous birthmark form of livedo reticularis. Appearances are very similar in that a fixed mottled or marbled look to the skin results from an uneven perfusion and slow flow in the venous component. Atrophy of skin and subcutaneous tissue makes the reticulate pattern even more livid. Limbs are most commonly involved, in which case hypoplasia of underlying bones may occur. A range of other abnormalities can occur including glaucoma, macrocephaly, and cardiac abnormalities. Because of natural improvement with time, treatment is rarely needed.

Blue rubber bleb naevus syndrome

The most typical lesions are small, compressible, blue to purple rubbery nodules occurring anywhere on the body surface as well as on lips, mouth, and penis and within the gastrointestinal tract where they frequently bleed. The resulting anaemia may be profound. Other organs including the lung and the central nervous system may be involved. Nodular blue lesions under the tongue are characteristic. Onset is usually during childhood but may be in adult life. Once developed, lesions persist for life. Treatment is directed at controlling bleeding and anaemia.

Maffucci's syndrome (dyschondroplasia with haemangiomas)

Despite the name, the soft, bluish cutaneous protrusions are not haemangiomas but small venous malformations. They persist and may grow into large lesions resembling a bunch of red grapes.

Hard nodules arising from the bones, especially on the hands and feet, represent enchondromas which are radiologically translucent. Bone growths are delayed and pathological fractures occur with slow recovery. Deformity of hands and feet may be gross. Malignancy is common, particularly chondrosarcoma but also angiosarcoma and ovarian cancer. Dyschondroplasia can occur without the vascular malformations (Ollier's disease). Patients require careful follow up with imaging or biopsy of any lesions that enlarge or cause symptoms.

Angiokeratoma corporis diffusum (Fabry's disease)

Angiokeratomas are characterized clinically by the presence of dark red to black, flat to slightly raised, vascular lesions which are most commonly seen on the scrotum where they are harmless. Histology reveals superficial vascular ectasia (expanded capillaries) with an overlying increase in surface keratin and so they represent capillary malformations rather than haemangiomas. Anderson–Fabry disease should be considered when lesions are clustered as small telangiectatic spots between the umbilicus and the knees. This is an X-linked disorder (MIM 301 500) in which deficiency of lysosomal hydrolase and galactosidase leads to deposition of globotriaosylceramide in cells throughout the body.

It causes severe, painful neuropathy with progressive renal, cardiovascular, and cerebrovascular dysfunction and early death. The surface angiokeratomas affect both skin and mucous membranes and usually appear shortly before puberty. Lesions can be up to 4 mm across but do not blanch on pressure due to the presence of red cells trapped within the ectatic capillaries. Their persistence distinguishes the lesions from purpura. Skin biopsy will confirm an angiokeratoma. The finding of albuminuria or haematuria and, more specifically, 'mulberry-like' cells in the urinary sediment suggests a diagnosis of Fabry's disease, but the finding of decreased X-galactosidase A in plasma or isolated leucocytes is diagnostic. Disease causing mutations in the *GLA* gene can be found in all affected individuals and in most carriers.

Vascular tumours

Infantile haemangioma

Usually appearing in the first year of life, these common haemangiomas characteristically have an initial proliferative and then a later involutional phase. Although previously known as a 'strawberry' naevus or haemangiomas, the terms strawberry, capillary, and cavernous have been abandoned for the preferred superficial, deep, and mixed haemangiomas. Over 60% will develop on the head and neck. The principal features distinguishing infantile haemangiomas from vascular malformations are that they are not present at birth and that they undergo spontaneous resolution. Few associations exist, but posterior fossa brain abnormalities may occur as in the PHACE(S) syndrome (posterior fossa malformations, haemangiomas, arterial anomalies, coarctation of the aorta and other cardiac defects, eye abnormalities, and sternal abnormalities). Lumbosacral haemangiomas can be a marker of spinal dysraphism.

Glomus tumour (glomangioma)

Glomus cells are modified smooth muscle cells found in glomus bodies which are believed to function as temperature receptors. Solitary glomus tumours are characteristically found in finger tips and in nail beds and are exquisitely tender. Multiple glomangiomas can be familial.

Pyogenic granuloma (lobular capillary haemangioma)

Pyogenic granuloma is a misnomer. Neither pyogenic nor granulomatous, the lobular capillary haemangiomas are benign vascular tumours that represent excessive production of granulation tissue usually in response to injury. Bleeding can be profuse and persistent. They can be indistinguishable clinically from amelanotic melanomas and should be treated by excision biopsy, although curettage will suffice if confident of the diagnosis.

Kaposi's sarcoma

Kaposi's sarcoma (KS) is a multifocal tumour characterized by dysregulated angiogenesis, a proliferation of spindle cells, and extravasation of inflammatory cells and erythrocytes. Human herpesvirus 8 appears causal.

KS is the most common cancer in HIV-infected individuals and in sub-Saharan Africa. There are four clinically distinct subsets of KS: (1) classic forms, as described originally by Kaposi, are found mainly in older men. Red to purple lesions appear on the feet and spread proximally. Usually flat patches (like purpura or purple stain) or slightly raised lesions can progress to plaques or nodules. Limb oedema (lymphoedema) frequently coexists. The characteristic colour, slow development, and multifocal distribution should suggest the diagnosis. (2) Endemic KS is found in equatorial Africa. Crops of cutaneous vascular lesions develop, usually on the lower limbs, associated with gross oedema, lymphadenopathy, and sometimes visceral involvement. (3) Iatrogenic forms result from immunosuppression in transplant patients and after cytotoxic chemotherapy. Both systemic and cutaneous involvement occurs. (4) HIV associated KS occurs most commonly in homosexual men where dark red to purple stains may appear rapidly and occur anywhere on the skin surface or mucous membranes, particularly in the soft palate.

Skin biopsy is characteristic, demonstrating a proliferation of jagged, irregular lymphatic-like vascular channels lined by a single layer of bland endothelial cells. An inflammatory infiltrate is associated with red cell extravasation and haemosiderin deposition (explaining the purple to brown skin discoloration on blanching). A network of bland spindle cells develops. Staining for HHV-8 should be positive in all tumour cells. HIV testing should be undertaken. The differential diagnosis would include causes of purpura, venous disease (lower limb only), and angiosarcoma.

No treatment may be required in asymptomatic indolent classical forms. Superficial radiotherapy is rapid and effective for localized diseases. Cases related to AIDS may regress with HAART (highly active antiretroviral therapy). Doxorubicin, bleomycin, and vincristine chemotherapy is widely regarded as first-line treatment, although liposomal anthracyclines have also proved effective in advanced disease. A reduction of immunosuppressant therapy will often resolve lesions in transplant patients, but this is not always possible without jeopardizing the transplant. Sirolimus inhibits the progression of dermal Kaposi's sarcoma in kidney transplant recipients while providing effective immunosuppression.

Angiosarcoma (lymphangiosarcoma)

This is a malignant vascular tumour arising from both vascular (and lymphatic) endothelium which occurs in three settings: (1) as a primary event on the face, scalp, or neck usually in older people; (2) associated with lymphoedema (although best described following mastectomy (Stewart–Treves syndrome)) lymphangiosarcoma can occur in any long-standing lymphoedema); and (3) postirradiation. In all types of (lymph) angiosarcoma, the first sign may be a bruise. Dark red to black plaques and nodules appear, spreading rapidly. Oedema and haemorrhage are common. The diagnosis is through skin biopsy. Defining the limits of the tumour is difficult and imaging is unhelpful. Consequently, wide excision, if possible, is the only treatment and the prognosis is poor.

Lymphatic disorders

The lymphatic system has long been a neglected area of medicine largely because, lymphoma excepting, it has not produced any life-threatening diseases nor has the technology been available to indicate the contribution of lymphatics to pathology. See Section 15 for further descriptions of lymphatic disease.

The recent discovery of specific genes and proteins, however, has catapulted lymphatic biology onto the research agenda of cancer spread, infection and inflammation, asthma, organ transplant rejection, and lymphoedema.

The lymphatic system is essentially a drain returning to the blood circulation protein and fluid unwanted by the tissues. This completes the extravascular circulation of fluid and protein and maintains tissue volume homeostasis. Lymph drainage is also an essential part of the body's immune defence. Cells such as extravasated leucocytes and activated antigen-presenting cells enter the initial lymphatics and are transported to lymph nodes where specific immune responses to foreign materials are generated.

Lymphatic capillaries are thin-walled vessels but capacious and potentially larger than nearby blood capillaries. Lymphatic capillaries absorb protein and fluid from the interstitial space and initiate lymph drainage and hence are referred to as 'initial lymphatics'. They drain into downstream 'collecting lymphatics' which, unlike initial lymphatics, possess a smooth muscle layer and valves. Intermittent changes in tissue pressures, external to initial lymphatics, are mainly responsible for lymph absorption and transport. Lymph within collecting lymphatics, however, is propelled forward by mural smooth muscle contraction with valves preventing backflow.

Lymphangiogenesis

Lymphatic vessels were discovered before the blood circulation but the first growth factors and molecular markers specific for lymphatics were discovered only 15 years ago. The gene *PROX1* commits endothelial cells from a venous to a lymphatic phenotype. Vascular endothelial growth factor (VEGF) C and D and their receptor VEGFR3 are mainly responsible for lymphatic vessel sprouting and growth. Subsequently, a signal transduction system is responsible for lymphatic endothelial cell growth, migration, maturation, and survival.

Lymph sacs appear at 6 to 7 weeks in embryos with lymphatic endothelial cells sprouting from embryonic veins in the jugular and perimesonephric areas under the influence of VEGFC. From here they migrate to form primary lymph sacs and the primary lymphatic plexus. Antibodies to cell surface markers LYVE1, VEGFR3, podoplanin (D2-40), and PROX1 enable distinction between blood and lymphatic endothelial cells.

Lymphoedema

A failure of lymph drainage causes a build-up of protein and fluid within the tissues (lymphoedema). When this occurs in the skin and subcutis the tissues become swollen and undergo characteristic changes. An increase of intralymphatic pressure (lymphatic hypertension) results in enlargement of the dermal initial lymphatics. If compliance permits, distended lymphatics bulge like blisters on the skin surface (lymphangiectasia), leading to leakage of lymph fluid (lymphorrhoea). If disruption to lymph drainage involves the lymphatics draining the intestinal lacteals, then rerouting/backflow of chylous lymph can result in leaking of milky chyle from the skin surface, particularly after a fatty meal.

Chronic distension of dermal lymphatics and accumulation of protein-rich fluid within the skin results in a cobble stone appearance to the skin (papillomatosis) and a build up of surface keratin (hyperkeratosis). This combination of features is referred to as elephantiasis (Fig. 23.12.5) because of its resemblance to elephant skin. In tropical medicine and parasitology the term elephantiasis is synonymous with lymphoedema resulting from filarial infection, but elephantiasis skin changes can occur with any form of lymphoedema irrespective of cause. If left untreated, elephantiasis progresses to marked fibrosis with little evidence of pitting oedema.

Most swelling with lymphoedema occurs in the more compliant subcutis. Fat and fibrous tissue accumulates as much as protein-rich fluid. Indeed, the pathology of lymphoedema is complex involving proliferation of inflammatory cells, adipocytes, fibroblasts, and blood vessels (angiogenesis). Lymphoedema is also discussed in Chapter 16.18.

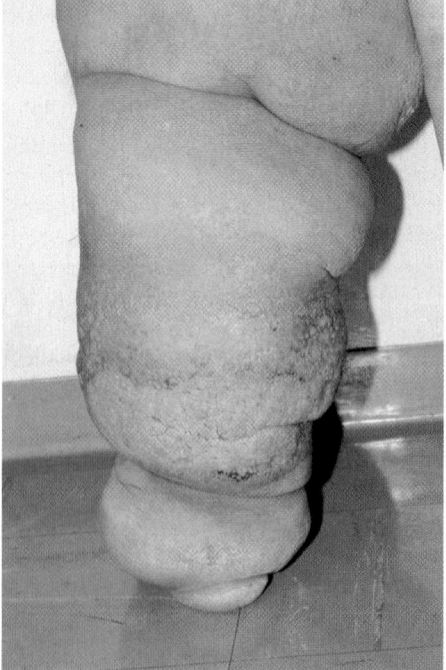

Fig. 23.12.5 Elephantiasis resulting from underlying lymphoedema. Elephantiasis refers to the thickened skin with papillomatosis and hyperkeratosis.

Infection and lymphatic failure

Recurrent infection (e.g. tinea pedis, cellulitis) is a common event in lymphoedema. It is likely that disturbances to the trafficking of immunologically active cells, such as lymphocytes and dendritic cells, compromise tissue immunosurveillance, but the exact mechanism is not known. Lymphatic vessels participate in the regulation of an inflammatory response through their role in transport of lymphocytes to and from lymph nodes. Migration of dendritic cells is mediated in part by the chemokine receptor CCR7, with lymphatic vessels expressing the ligand CCL21.

Lymphangitis

The lymphatic system has evolved in humans as a host defence mechanism. Noxious agents and predators such as bacteria, if not dealt with at the point of entry to the host, access the lymphatic system. Lymphatic vessels, together with adjoining lymph nodes, effectively act as a second line of defence preventing further onward spread and limiting systemic involvement, e.g. septicaemia.

Lymphangitis represents inflammation of the lymphatic collectors and is clinically seen as tender red streaks spreading up the limb corresponding to the inflamed vessels. Inflammation of downstream lymph nodes, known as lymphadenitis, manifests with painful, tender, swollen glands. Lymphangitis is not easily seen in the presence of oedema and a more diffuse erythema is observed making distinction from cellulitis impossible.

Cellulitis (erysipelas, acute inflammatory episodes, dermatolymphangioadenitis)

Cellulitis can result from the impaired local host defence mechanism associated with lymphatic insufficiency but, conversely, can damage lymph drainage routes and cause lymphoedema. A vicious cycle of recurrent cellulitis and worsening swelling can arise. In one epidemiological study, 64 (29%) of 218 patients identified with lymphoedema had suffered at least one attack of cellulitis within the previous 12 months with 16 (8%) experiencing more than three episodes. Any patient with recurrent attacks of cellulitis in the same leg almost certainly has compromised lymph drainage in that leg. Unlike conventional cellulitis (in an immunocompetent site), the first sign of illness is usually constitutional upset with flu-like symptoms, fever, rigors, or vomiting. Only some hours later may a blotchy rash, pain, and increased swelling appear with the diagnosis becoming clear. The typical advancing border of a spreading cellulitis is not seen with lymphoedema. Streptococcal infection is considered the likely culprit, but it is unusual to be able to isolate an organism.

A consensus document on the management of cellulitis in lymphoedema emphasizes the need to correct risk factors, e.g. skin wounds, dermatitis, tinea pedis, and the need for longer courses of antibiotics as insufficient treatment will often result in early relapse of cellulitis. When attacks occur more than twice a year, prophylactic antibiotics are indicated, e.g. penicillin V (phenoxymethylpenicillin) 500 mg daily. Prophylaxis for 2 years is recommended, although it is not unusual for cellulitis to recur as soon as antibiotics are discontinued suggesting relapse rather than the development of a new infection. In such circumstances, life-long prophylaxis is suggested.

Filarial lymphoedema

Adenitis and lymphangitis are major acute manifestations of lymphatic filariasis. Two events may present in a similar manner.

'True' filarial adenolymphangitis is caused by the death of the adult worm, whereas acute dermatolymphangioadenitis (ADLA) is equivalent to cellulitis/lymphangitis secondary to bacterial infection (usually streptococcal). Recurrent ADLA/cellulitis is a major risk factor for progression to elephantiasis. Treatment with diethylcarbamazine (DEC) has no effect on the outcome of ADLA, but scrupulous attention to skin hygiene and/or prophylactic penicillin significantly reduces the number of attacks.

Tumour metastasis

Lymphatic spread is the preferential route of metastasis for most human cancers, with sentinel lymph node assessment as the most important prognostic indicator in, e.g. melanoma, vulval and penile cancers, where growth factor stimulation of lymphatic vessels enhances lymphatic metastasis. Melanoma cells expressing VEGFC induce local lymphangiogenesis at the tumour margin. Some evidence exists to suggest that lymphatic endothelium actively attracts certain cells, by secreting chemokines such as CCL21 whose receptor CCR7 is expressed on some tumour cells. Lymph containing VEGFC stimulates downstream lymphatics to dilate and facilitate spread of clumps of tumour cells.

Carcinoma erysipeloides (carcinoma telangiectatica)

Carcinoma erysipeloides (Fig. 23.12.6) manifests clinically with a fixed erythematous patch or plaque resembling cellulitis/erysipelas but without fever. The inflamed area may show a distinct raised component due to palpable infiltrated lymphatics and oedema.

Congenital lymphatic malformations

Lymphangioma

Simple sustained dilatation of otherwise normal lymphatic vessels is termed lymphangiectasia, but when lymphatics are distended due to structural abnormalities of a tumour-like nature the term lymphangioma is best used. The most important feature of all congenital lymphangiomas is that they are not part of the normal lymph conducting system. Lymphangioma circumscriptum, as the name implies, is localized to an area of skin, subcutaneous tissue, and sometimes muscle. It consists of lymph (and sometimes blood) filled vesicles which bulge on the skin surface (Fig. 23.12.7).

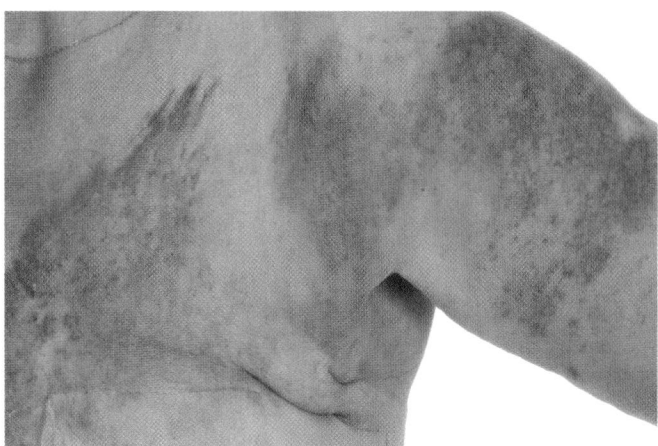

Fig. 23.12.6 Carcinoma erysipeloides indicating infiltration of breast carcinoma within dermal lymphatics. Usually associated with local oedema because of lymphatic obstruction.

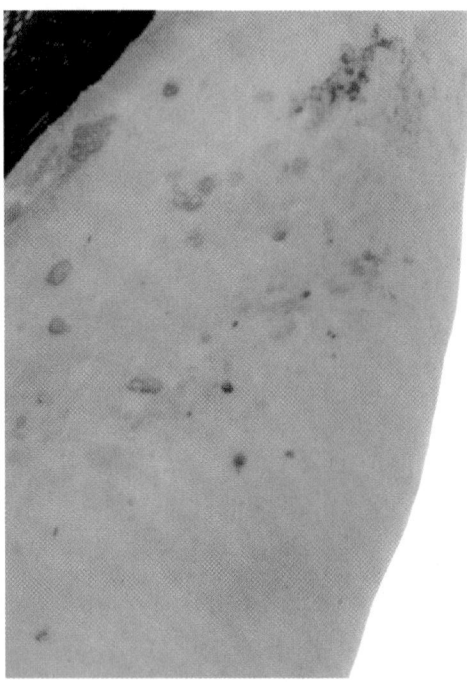

Fig. 23.12.7 Cutaneous lymphangioma as demonstrated by lymph blisters on skin surface.

The lymphangiomas may resemble blisters or may take on a more warty appearance and be mistaken for viral warts except they can leak lymph fluid. There may or may not be swelling depending upon extension into deeper tissues, but pitting oedema is absent. The term 'circumscriptum' may be misleading because deeper components may be extensive making surgical excision difficult. Although lymphangioma circumscriptum is usually evident at or soon after birth, it may present later. Radical surgery offers the only chance of cure, but a conservative approach with simple electrocautery to correct the weeping (lymphorrhoea) is advised.

Diffuse lymphangioma indicates a more extensive malformation which may involve an entire hindquarter. Limb swelling may be due either to lymphoedema or to gross dilatation of abnormal lymphatic channels, skin surface lymphangiomas may coexist with blood vascular malformations. Diffuse lymphangiomas may form part of the Klippel-Trénaunay syndrome with limb and tissue overgrowth. If the lymphangioma involves underlying bone, osteoid tissue may resorb leading to pathological fractures (Gorham's disease).

Maffucci's syndrome consists of diffuse, multiple haemolymphangiomas accompanied by severe deformities of bone and cartilage.

Cystic hygroma (cystic lymphangioma)

Cystic hygromas are large lymph cysts considered remnants of primitive lymph sacs, which is why they are found most often in the neck, groin, or retroperitoneum. Although usually present at birth, some present in adulthood after a local disturbance stimulates lymph absorption. The size of a cystic hygroma may interfere with breathing or swallowing. Episodes of infection occur in 25% of both cystic hygromas and lymphangiomas. Cystic hygromas are strikingly translucent. Repeated aspiration, sclerotherapy, or excision are treatment options.

Acquired lymphatic abnormalities

Acquired lymphangiectases (acquired lymphangioma)

Acquired or secondary lymphangiectases arise following damage to previously normal deep lymphatic vessels. Obstruction to drainage leads to back pressure and dermal backflow with subsequent dilatation of upper dermal lymphatics. They develop most often in genital skin where they are easily mistaken for warts but weeping of lymph distinguishes one from the other. Persistent leakage of lymph can be mistaken for urinary incontinence. They occur following cancer treatment (lymphadenectomy or radiotherapy) and scarring processes.

Traumatic lymph cysts (lymphoceles) and fistulae

Lymphatics severed by accidental trauma or surgery normally collapse and block with fibrin. If lymph continues to leak, it collects in the tissues forming a large pseudocyst or lymphocele (often wrongly called a 'seroma'). Should the lymphocele burst through the overlying wound, then a fistula with continuous lymph leakage can occur. The majority of lymphoceles resolve spontaneously with or without repeat aspiration.

Chylous reflux/intestinal lymphangiectasia

Chyle is lymph-rich in chylomicrons. The word chylous means juice and the milky whiteness comes from fat absorbed from intestinal lacteals. It is important to recognize that fluid in the lacteals is only white after a meal containing free fat; patients on a low or nonfat diet have clear fluid in their lacteals. Chyle, like lymph, can escape into peritoneal (chylous ascites), pleural, or pericardial cavities, joints, vagina (chylous colporrhoea), or external genitalia as well as refluxing into a lower limb with chyle leaking from the skin. Where chyle refluxes is entirely dependent on the position of incompetent lymphatics or the site and degree of any obstruction to normal lymph flow.

Primary chylous reflux arises from congenitally incompetent megalymphatics (lymphangiectasia with valve incompetence) or lymphatic hypoplasia when lymph/chyle is forced to reroute. Secondary (acquired) reflux is almost always caused by thoracic duct obstruction caused by filariasis, malignant disease, or trauma (accidental or surgery). Treatment involves reducing chyle production by following a strict, no fat diet supplemented with medium chain triglycerides and extra vitamins.

When chyle cannot pass through the lacteals, cisterna chyli, and thoracic duct as usual, it refluxes back into the villi and diffuses back through the intestinal mucosa into the lumen of the bowel. The distended intestinal lacteals are termed intestinal lymphangiectasia. A steady loss of protein, fat, and fat-soluble vitamins causes weight loss, steatorrhoea, diarrhoea, and a hypoproteinaemic oedema (protein-losing enteropathy). Intestinal lymphangiectasia usually occurs from a failure of lymphatic development in genetic forms of lymphoedema, but can rarely be acquired following radiotherapy.

Lymphatic tumours

The understanding of benign and malignant lymphatic tumours has been limited owing to a lack of specific lymphatic markers.

Lymphangiosarcoma

Lymphangiosarcoma is the only known malignant disease of lymphatics. Although well known for its association with postmastectomy lymphoedema (Stewart–Treves syndrome), it is a rare but serious complication of any chronic lymphoedema irrespective of cause. Red-brown or purple discoloration, like a bruise, appears in the skin. Nodules or raised plaques may appear later and oedema deteriorates. Limits are poorly defined and progression is rapid. Radical surgery, if performed early, may offer cure.

Kaposi's sarcoma

The phenotype of the endothelial cells of Kaposi's sarcoma (KS) may be as much lymphatic as blood vascular, but its origins may lie with a primitive cell capable of either differentiation. KS can arise in long-standing lymphoedema or indeed cause lymphoedema (see above).

Further reading

Angiogenesis/lymphangiogenesis

Alitalo K, Tammela T, Petrova TV (2005). Lymphangiogenesis in development and human disease. *Nature*, **438**, 946–53.
Carmeliet P (2005). Angiogenesis in life, disease and medicine. *Nature*, **438**, 932–6.

Calciphylaxis

Weeniq RH, *et al.* (2007). Calciphylaxis: natural history, risk factor analysis and outcome. *J Am Acad Dermatol*, **56**, 569–79.

Buerger's disease

Olin JW, Shih A (2006). Thrombangiitis obliterans (Buerger's Disease). *Curr Opin Rheumatol*, **18**, 18–24.

Sickle cell disease

Clare A, *et al.* (2002). Chronic leg ulceration in homozygous sickle cell disease; the role of venous incompetence. *Br J Haematol*, **119**, 567–71.

Erythromelalgia

Waxman SG, Dib-Hajj S (2005). Erythermalgia: molecular bases for an inherited pain syndrome. *Trends Mol Med*, **11**, 555–62.

Pressure ulcers

National Pressure Ulcer Advisory Panel. Updated staging system. http://www.npuap.org/pr2.htm

Venous disorders

Eklöf B, *et al.* (2004). Revision of the CEAP classification for chronic venous disorders: consensus statement. *J Vasc Surg*, **40**, 1248–52.
Palfreyman SJ, *et al.* (2006). Dressings for healing venous leg ulcers. *Cochrane Database Syst Rev*, **3**, CD001103.

Foot ulcers

Prompers L, *et al.* (2007). High prevalence of ischaemia, infection and serious comorbidity in patients with diabetic foot disease in Europe. Baseline results from the Eurodiale Study. *Diabetologia*, **50**, 18–25.

Rosacea

Powell FC (2005). Clinical practice. Rosacea. *N Engl J Med*, **352**, 793–803.

Vascular birthmarks

Garzon MC, *et al.* (2007). Vascular malformations: Part I. *J Am Acad Dermatol*, **56**, 353–70.
Garzon MC, *et al.* (2007). Vascular malformations. Part II: associated syndromes. *J Am Acad Dermatol*, **56**, 541–64.
Berry SA, *et al.* (1998). Klippel–Trénaunay Syndrome. *Am J Med Genet*, **79**, 319–26.
Biesecker LG, *et al.* (1999). Proteus syndrome: diagnostic criteria, differential diagnosis, and patient evaluation. *Am J Med Genet*, **84**, 389–95.

Vascular tumours

Stallone G, *et al.* (2005). Sirolimus for Kaposi's sarcoma in renal-transplant recipients. *N Eng J Med*, **352**, 1317–23.

Lymphatic disorders

Browse NL, Burnand KG, Mortimer PS (2003). *Diseases of the lymphatics*. Arnold, London.
Moffat CJ, *et al.* (2003). Lymphoedema: an underestimated health problem. *QJM*, **96**, 731–8.

Website

NCBI. *GeneTests*. http://www.ncbi.nlm.nih.gov/sites/GeneTests/ [The former genetests.org site is now hosted by NCBI. Gene reviews are available e.g. for ataxia-telangiectasia, Fabry's disease, and haemorrhagic hereditary telangiectasia].

Hair and nail disorders

David de Berker

Essentials

Nails grow continuously throughout life, except after exceptional physiological or traumatic events when they are shed. All other less disruptive influences result in changes in the colour, thickness, texture, and growth of nails and may also affect the periungual tissues. The most common local diseases affecting the nail are psoriasis, fungal nail infections, periungual eczema, and viral warts. Looking at the nails is an important part of the general examination, since changes such as clubbing or splinter haemorrhages can indicate systemic disease.

Hair growth in a healthy person is determined by body site, gender, and age. Within these parameters there are accepted norms. Disease may affect hair growth by direct action on the follicle or by indirect effects sustained through generalized physiological disturbance.

Clinicians may be called to assess specific diseases of the scalp with implications for hair growth, or specifically to address pathological patterns of hair growth where there may be underlying systemic disease.

Common diseases of the scalp include psoriasis, eczema, fungal infection, alopecia areata, and the scarring alopecias. Telogen effluvium is the most common hair problem related to general medical or surgical upset, characterized by massive shedding of hair about 6 to 10 weeks after a period of significant physiological disturbance. Where scalp hair loss presents in association with increased hair on the body or at sites associated with masculinity (hirsutism), a pathological source of androgen should be sought.

Disorders of the nails

The nail grows from the matrix and is supported by the nail bed until it reaches the free edge. At the proximal and lateral margins, it is embedded in the nail folds. Local and systemic diseases can alter the appearance and function of all four structures (Fig. 23.13.1). The most common local diseases affecting the nail are psoriasis, fungal nail infections, periungual eczema, and viral warts. Tumours other than viral warts are rare. They include squamous cell carcinoma and malignant melanoma. Systemic diseases manifested in the nail include cardiovascular, respiratory, and gastrointestinal diseases leading to clubbing; vascular phenomena (e.g. splinter haemorrhages, cyanosis) and changes in nail growth as a result of general metabolic factors influencing nail matrix function.

Psoriasis

Psoriasis affects 1.5 to 3% of the population, and nail involvement is found in up to 90% of patients at some time.

Clinical features

The most common manifestations are pitting, onycholysis, 'oily spots', transverse ridging of the dorsal surface, splinter haemorrhages, and subungual hyperkeratosis. Pits represent surface defects in the nail due to foci of psoriatic epithelium (Fig. 23.13.2). Onycholysis is separation of the nail from the nail bed arising because psoriasis of the nail bed reduces adherence of the nail. Subungual hyperkeratosis is thickening of the skin of the nail bed with psoriatic scale that cannot be lost because of the overlying nail. An oily spot is psoriasis in the nail bed. It is termed 'onycholysis' if it extends to the free edge. These signs may allow diagnosis of psoriasis at other sites. Even in the presence of obvious psoriasis elsewhere, fungal infection should be sought if the nail features are not typical, because treatable infection may be superimposed and may warrant active therapy.

Treatment

Local therapy—pitting can be concealed with lacquers, or may respond to a potent topical corticosteroid applied over 2 to 3 months to the proximal nail fold. Severe pitting and other changes may occasionally justify a trial of injection of triamcinolone acetonide, 0.1 ml of 2.5 to 5 mg/ml, into the proximal nail fold, with preliminary local anaesthetic. Onycholysis is difficult to cure and is made worse by trauma and picking. Patients should avoid leverage at the free edge by keeping the nails short and by wearing gloves during wet or dirty work. Debris caught beneath the nail should be removed with a soft nail brush. Excavation with a pointed tool (a common cleaning technique) makes the condition worse. Topical calcipotriol or potent corticosteroid ointment can be helpful. Clipping the nail back to the point of separation from the nail bed

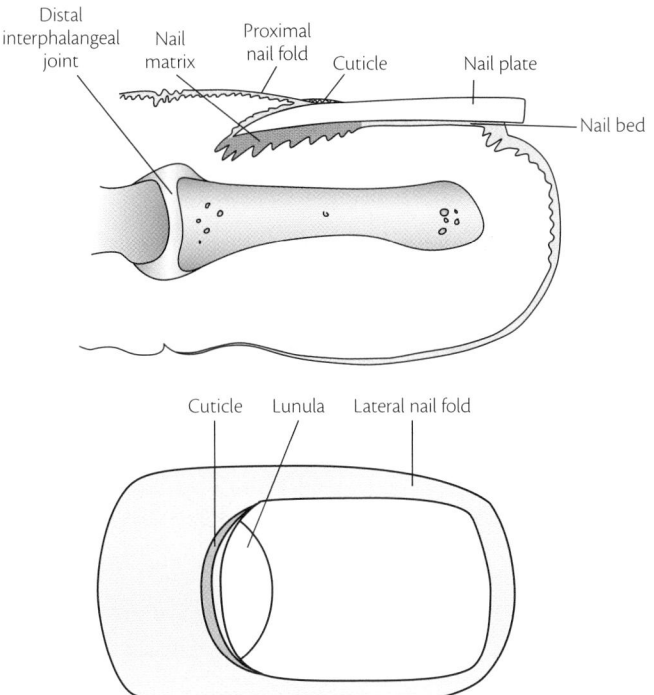

Distal interphalangeal joint — Nail matrix — Proximal nail fold — Cuticle — Nail plate — Nail bed

Cuticle — Lunula — Lateral nail fold

Fig. 23.13.1 Anatomy of the normal nail.

can facilitate treatment of nail bed psoriasis with topical therapy. Occlusion of the nail with tape is also advocated.

Systemic therapy (e.g. methotrexate, ciclosporin, acitretin or biologics) and psoralen plus ultraviolet A (UVA) can help.

Fungal nail infection

The prevalence of fungal nail disease is up to 13% in urban areas in developed countries, but less than 1% in rural Democratic Republic of Congo (formerly Zaire); enclosed footwear raising humidity probably explains the difference. The principal pathogens are dermatophyte fungi, which infect skin and nail; *Trichophyton rubrum* and *Trichophyton interdigitale* are the most common (see Chapters 7.7.1 and 23.10). The nondermatophyte fungi (e.g. *fusarium sp.*, *Scopulariopsis brevicaulis*) and yeasts (e.g. candida spp.) are uncommon pathogens. Onychomycosis is more common in damaged nails. Tinea pedis often coexists between the 4th and 5th web space or as a moccasin infection (a diffuse, scaling fungal infection affecting the sole of the foot).

Clinical features

Onychomycosis presents in one of four patterns (Fig. 23.13.3). Classic onychomycosis is where the nail thickens, becomes yellow, and is undermined by subungual hyperkeratosis. It may involve just the distal and lateral margins of the nail or be throughout, being named distal, lateral, subungual, or total dystrophic onychomycosis respectively. Superficial white onychomycosis is relatively more common in children and is the variant best treated with topical therapy. Proximal white subungual onychomycosis may present with a white proximal nail plate and no destruction in the early stages of the disease; this pattern is more common in patients who are immunosuppressed (e.g. organ transplant recipients, those with HIV infection). Candida spp. is most commonly found colonizing the damp undersurface of an onycholytic fingernail, where warmth

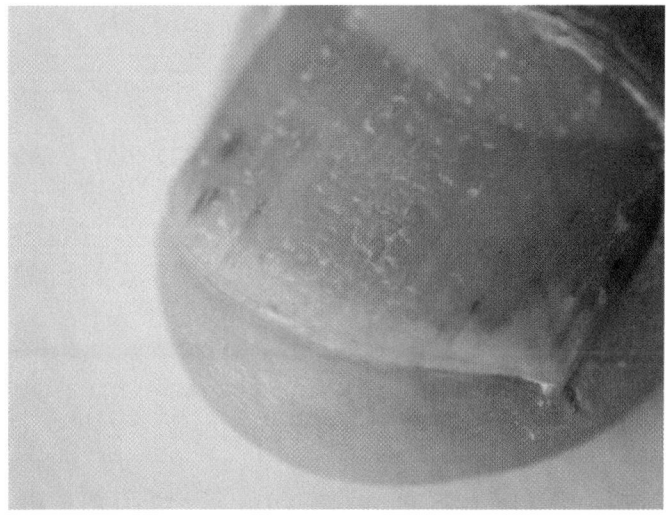

(a)

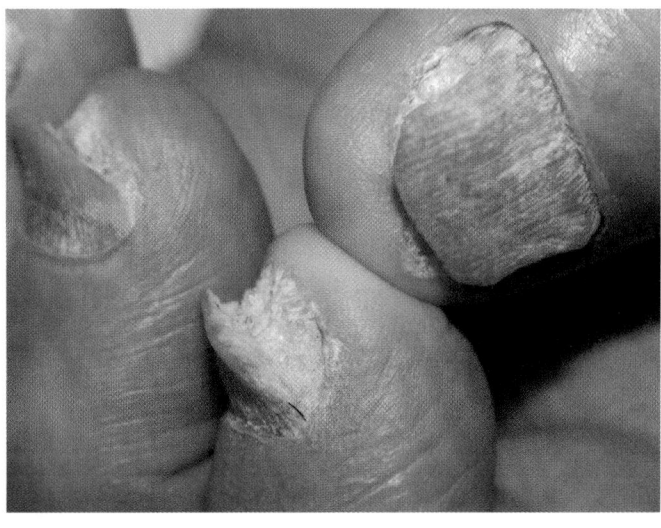

(b)

Fig. 23.13.2 (a) Psoriasis with pitting of the nail and splinter haemorrhages in the nail bed. (b) Psoriasis with marked subungual hyperkeratosis.

and humidity are common in affected individuals (e.g. caterers). There may also be factors influencing local or systemic immunity (e.g. peripheral ischaemia, Raynaud's, and diabetes mellitus).

Diagnosis

Mycological confirmation should normally be obtained before starting systemic antifungal therapy. A large sample of discoloured nail plate, with underlying soft debris, is required for a reliable result; this is best taken using heavy-duty nail clippers. The importance of making a clear diagnosis before treatment is greatest where systemic therapy is advocated. Both of the main agents have been reported as causing severe reactions such as Stevens–Johnson syndrome. Drug interactions are a particular risk with itraconazole.

Treatment

Terbinafine and itraconazole are systemic therapies for dermatophyte onychomycosis. Terbinafine is slightly more effective than itraconazole in dermatophyte infections, but possibly less effective against candida spp. Topical therapy is usually less effective than

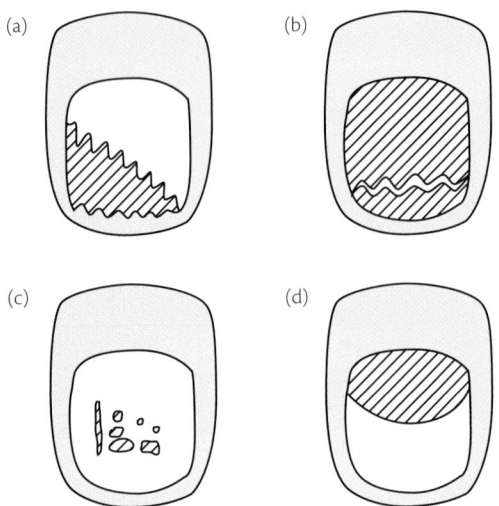

Fig. 23.13.3 Four most common variants of onychomycosis: (a) distal lateral onychomycosis; (b) total dystrophic onychomycosis; (c) superficial white onychomycosis; (d) proximal white subungual onychomycosis.

systemic therapy, being of most use in superficial or mild distal infections. Avulsion is usually warranted only in nondermatophyte infections or when systemic therapy is ineffective or contraindicated. Relapse may be diminished by vigorous treatment of local tinea pedis and avoidance of trauma through correction of orthopaedic abnormalities and the wearing of broad-fitting footwear.

Nails in systemic disease

Clubbing

This is a classic sign of various disorders (Box 23.13.1), but is seen in some healthy people. It is usually more obvious on the fingers than the toes; increased longitudinal curvature and loss of the angle between the nail at its proximal margin and the nail fold is seen. This margin is 'boggy' or fluctuant. There may be associated cyanosis if clubbing is caused by cyanotic heart disease or certain

---

Box 23.13.1 Systemic causes of clubbing

- Idiopathic/congenital
- Cardiovascular
  - Congenital cyanotic heart disease
  - Infective endocarditis
- Respiratory
  - Bronchiectasis
  - Bronchial carcinoma
  - Empyema
  - Fibrosing alveolitis
- Gastrointestinal
  - Liver disease
  - Inflammatory bowel disease
  - Malabsorption

---

pulmonary diseases. Classic changes of geometry entail the angle (Lovibond's angle) at the junction of the proximal nail fold and nail plate. Normally, this is less than 160°, but in clubbing it increases to become more than 180°. Clinically, this corresponds to the loss of a window visible between the dorsal aspects of corresponding contralateral fingers when held against each other (Schamroth's sign). Prominent clubbing may be part of hypertrophic pulmonary osteoarthropathy (HPOA) where hypertrophy of the upper and lower extremities resembles that seen in acromegaly, with additional pseudoinflammatory painful changes of the large limb joints with associated radiological and neurovascular changes. HPOA is typically associated with lung carcinoma, mesotheliomas of the pleura, and, less commonly, bronchiectasis. The diagnostic features of clubbing are shown in Fig. 23.13.4.

Splinter haemorrhages

These represent blood escaping from the longitudinal capillaries in the nail bed beneath the nail (Fig. 23.13.2a). They may have a local or systemic cause. The most common causes are trauma (e.g. manual labour) and nail psoriasis, in which nail bed vessels are more numerous and fragile. Significant systemic causes are uncommon; they include infarction of the vessels (e.g. microemboli in endocarditis) and vessel damage related to other causes of vasculitis. The likelihood of a systemic disorder is greater when there are associated nail fold infarcts than when nail bed changes are found in isolation.

Nail fold vessels

They may become prominent with dilatation, tortuosity, and haemorrhage. This can be associated with increased length and a ragged appearance of the cuticle. These changes are seen in connective tissue diseases and in particular systemic sclerosis, dermatomyositis, and systemic lupus (see Chapter 23.7).

Beau's lines

Any severe illness may lead to a transverse linear depression on each nail. Because the average rate of fingernail growth is 2 to 4 mm per month, the position of the line indicates the approximate date of onset of the original illness. A milder event may produce just a pale transverse line in the nail (see Mee's lines below).

Thyroid disease

Localized separation of the nail from the nail bed (onycholysis) is sometimes seen in thyrotoxicosis. In hypothyroidism, nail thickening is more common. A form of clubbing termed 'thyroid acropachy' occurs in Graves' disease.

Koilonychia (spooning of the nails)

This is occasionally seen in iron deficiency anaemia. It is common in the big toes of normal babies, and has been reported in mechanics performing oily work. Rickshaw pullers tend to develop traumatic toenail koilonychia.

Acquired colour changes (Table 23.13.1)

None of the classic variants of white transverse bands or zones represent firm clinical signs. The three main signs reflect vascular changes within the nail bed, unlike the fourth which represents abnormal nail production.

Terry's nail

A white nail bed obscures the lunula and extends to the distal 2 to 3 mm of the nail bed, where there is a red-brown appearance.

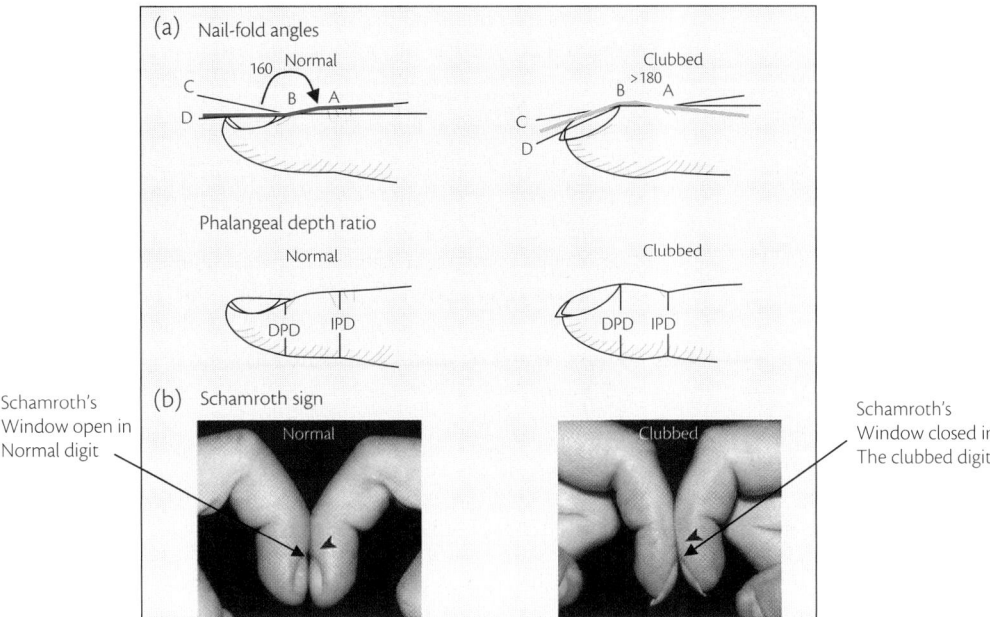

Fig. 23.13.4 Diagnostic features of clubbing. (a) The normal angle between the nail plate and the proximal nail fold is less than 160°, increasing to greater than 180° in clubbing. If the depth of the finger is measured at the interphalangeal joint (interphalangeal finger depth, IPD), it is greater than the depth as measured at the edge of the proximal nail fold (distal interphalangeal finger depth, DPD) in a normal finger. In clubbing it is the reverse. (b) When two contralateral fingers are apposed on their dorsal surfaces, a diamond-shaped window is revealed in normal fingers, bordered by the proximal nail fold and proximal nail (Schamroth's window). This is lost in clubbing.

This is sometimes associated with cirrhosis, in which setting it was originally described; it is also seen in normal ageing.

Uraemic half and half nail
This is similar to Terry's nail, but only 50% of proximal nail bed is involved and associated with uraemia in some instances.

Muehrcke's bands
These are thin, transverse white bands seen usually within the proximal part of the nail bed, but which move distally to some degree. They appear sensitive to blood albumin levels and can be dramatically reversible if it is normalized. But this association does not hold completely and they have been reported in patients postchemotherapy.

Mee's lines
These are transverse bands resembling Muehrcke's bands but the white change appears within the nail plate rather than the nail bed. This reflects a period of abnormal nail production that usually corresponds to some form of poisoning. The most common is therapeutic poisoning in the form of chemotherapy, but criminal poisoning with arsenic has been detected by this sign. Associations between acquired nail colour changes, drugs, and systemic disease are listed in Table 23.13.1.

Table 23.13.1 Systemic causes of nail discoloration

Nail colour	Location	Causes
Yellow	Nail plate	Yellow nail syndrome
White	Nail bed	Hypoalbuminaemia
Brown	Nail bed	Chronic renal disease
Blue	Nail bed	Mepacrine
	Lunula	Wilson's disease
Red	Lunula	Congestive cardiac failure, rheumatoid arthritis

Disorders of the hair

Hair arises from follicles distributed almost universally over the body surface, within the skin. In some areas it becomes dark and relatively thick in diameter such as in the axillae, groin, and beard. On the scalp it is variably pigmented and of moderate bore. On the rest of the body it is generally pale, fine, and termed vellus hair. Vellus hair is short. Length is determined by the period of growth of any single hair before the hair follicle transforms out of the growth phase (anagen) and into the resting phase (telogen), during which the hair is shed and the follicle gradually returns to the growing phase. Follicles that have an anagen phase of 1000 days or more will grow hair far longer than those where it is limited to 60 days and this reflects the situation for the scalp and eyebrow respectively. If scalp hair follicles were grafted to the eyebrow, they would retain their scalp identity and the person would grow extremely long eyebrows!

Scalp psoriasis

Scalp psoriasis may present in isolation. Equally, where signs elsewhere are equivocal, scalp changes should be sought to explore and clarify the diagnosis. Typically, there are zones of redness with moderate demarcation and variable amounts of scale. Scale can be either light and yellow or composed of dense, adherent white material that exposes pin point bleeding of the scalp when picked off. There is a predilection for the margins of the scalp, the creases behind the ears, and within the external auditory canal. There is rarely marked hair loss, but when inflammation is intense there may be shedding and, if associated with prolonged periods of dense scale, scarring can occur. Diagnosis can be confirmed by scalp biopsy where the main differential is with eczema or discoid lupus erythematosus. The main local scalp diseases, including psoriasis, as well as systemic diseases and treatments affecting hair growth are shown in Box 23.13.2.

Treatment

Patients mainly complain of itch, scale that drops onto clothing, and the appearance within the hair line. Itch can be relieved short

Box 23.13.2

The main local scalp diseases affecting hair growth are:

◆ Psoriasis

◆ Eczema

◆ Fungus

◆ Alopecia areata

◆ Scarring alopecia: lichen planopilaris and discoid lupus erythematosus

Systemic diseases/treatments affecting hair growth are:

◆ Telogen effluvium

◆ Endocrine: androgen secreting pathologies, hypopituitarism, hypo/hyperthyroidism, hypoparathyroidism, acromegaly, hyperprolactinaemia, Cushing's syndrome

◆ Iron deficiency

◆ Malnutrition

◆ Severe chronic illness

◆ Genetic syndromes

◆ Drugs, e.g. antimitotic, anticoagulants, oral contraceptives

term by washing with tar-based shampoos, but this does little more than wash away the surface scale and only provides a weak antipruritic dose of tar coupled with the detrimental irritant effects of shampoo. It does not address the underlying inflammatory process. Alcohol-based steroid preparations delivered through a nozzle are popular because they leave no residue on the hair and are easy to apply. However, the alcohol can sting in the cracked inflamed skin and the barrier function of the diseased skin is further compromised by the solvent properties of the alcohol. The best treatments entail making a mess of the hair in order to treat the scalp as for psoriasis elsewhere. This can include thick emollient based products containing tar, salicylic acid, and coconut oil massaged carefully into the scalp and left overnight before washing out. Vitamin D based products, topical steroid, and dithranol can all be used on the scalp. Systemic therapies used for widespread psoriasis also help the scalp, while phototherapy provides less benefit as the scalp is photoprotected by hair.

Eczema

Scalp eczema

This is usually part of atopic eczema and will be found with a typical history and appearance of the disease elsewhere (see Chapter 23.6). The treatments are as for the skin, with an emphasis on avoidance of irritants (use conditioner in place of shampoo and avoid alcohol-based topical products), the use of some emollient (ideal with short hair, but otherwise use steroids in lotion or cream base), and some steroid creams, gels, or foams.

Allergic contact scalp dermatitis

This can present acutely, typically in connection with paraphenylenediamine (PPD) in hair dyes. Less aggressive presentations are with allergy to ingredients in other hair cosmetics. PPD allergy may be sufficiently florid as to appear as an acute cellulitis of the scalp, descending onto the forehead. There may be significant

reversible hair shedding in the aftermath of such an episode. The allergen is determined by patch testing (see Chapter 23.6).

Irritant scalp dermatitis

This presents with gradual widespread scalp itch, dryness, and light scale with only slight inflammation. It is usually due to excess use of shampoo in someone who has a low threshold for skin irritancy—which can be part of atopy or acquired with age and loss of sebum.

Seborrhoeic dermatitis of the scalp

This is also termed pityriasis capitis. It barely itches, but presents as scaling or as 'heavy dandruff'. Redness and scale affect the nasolabial folds, eyebrows, sternum, and sometimes interscapular skin. In the scalp it may be difficult to distinguish from psoriasis, with light, yellow, slightly greasy scale. Overgrowth of normal skin pityrosporum yeasts plays a part in the disease and management can be directed at reducing the concentration of this yeast on the skin and scalp with antifungal shampoos containing azoles or selenium sulphide. Topical hydrocortisone can reduce the inflammatory component.

Fungal scalp disease (Chapter 7.7.1)

Fungus can primarily affect the hair shaft, or the scalp, or both. Where the scalp is heavily involved, it can respond either mainly with scaling or with inflammation, with some common ground between both presentations. An intense inflammatory response may produce a raised, oedematous boggy mass known as a kerion. This is usually found in a child in contact with farm animals or pets where the zoophilic fungi *Trichophyton verrucosum* or *Microsporum canis* are encountered. Transmission between humans is of anthropophilic fungi where the inflammatory response may be less. Patterns include discoid areas of hair loss, diffuse scale, diffuse pustules, kerion formation or a scalp with little scale and inflammation, and hairs that snap at the scalp surface revealing a 'black dot' of residual hair shaft. Changing urban patterns of fungal scalp disease means that this variant due to *Trichophyton tonsurans* is now the most common in western medicine. Diagnosis is by scalp scraping and hair pluck for mycology. A differential diagnosis can be sought by scalp biopsy, but this is seldom necessary in a child. Treatment is with systemic griseofulvin, itraconazole, or terbinafine. All are effective, but griseofulvin requires longer treatment and has more side effects. However, in many countries it is the only systemic agent licensed in children who are the most common sufferers. Contact tracing within the extended family is important to try to prevent relapse through reinfection. Infectivity in the early phases of treatment may be reduced with use of antifungal shampoos. A kerion may give rise to scarring hair loss long term due to the intensity of the inflammation.

Alopecia areata

The classic pattern of alopecia areata is with small discoid areas ('areata') of hair being shed in a scattered distribution on the scalp or body. The beard area in men, eyebrows, and lashes are also commonly affected. Hair loss may progress through a phase where there are residual white hairs (being lost last) followed by a smooth scalp with retained normal hair follicle openings and no apparent inflammation (Fig. 23.13.5). Scalp biopsy reveals that there is a lymphocytic inflammatory process engulfing the dermal papilla of the hair follicle. This is interpreted as an autoimmune attack on the follicle which switches off anagen, leading to shedding of hair. This attack is not always overwhelming and some follicles may

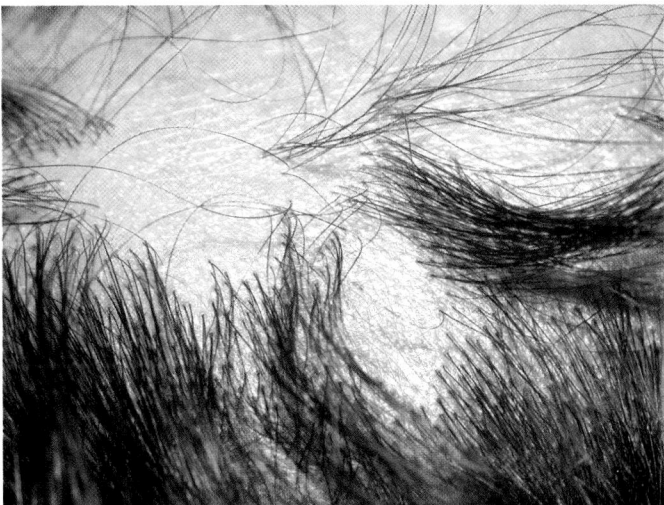

Fig. 23.13.5 Alopecia areata with smooth, unscarred scalp.

continue to produce small, short-lived, slightly dystrophic hairs with partial pigmentation. These are known clinically as 'exclamation mark' hairs because they are distally thicker and more pigmented than they are proximally.

Where all the hair on the scalp is lost, the clinical pattern is referred to as alopecia totalis, which can extend to all hair throughout the body, known as alopecia universalis. The likelihood of spontaneous regrowth of hair is between 60 and 80% for small 'areata', but substantially less for more extensive patterns and the longer the abnormal pattern persists. There is a statistical association with autoimmune thyroid disease.

Treatment

This does little to alter the natural pattern of the disease, but may suppress the immune attack on the follicle for as long as therapy is maintained. Topical, locally injected, and systemic steroid can all be used, with greater efficacy in proportion to penetration and concentration of steroid. However, the side effects of systemic steroid mean that it is not a long-term treatment option. Topical immunotherapy is the term applied to the other main treatment option where the patient is sensitized to either diphencyprone or dimethylbutyl squaric ester. These chemicals are then applied to the affected scalp at regular intervals to provoke an allergic contact dermatitis. Hair may grow in response to this in 20 to 50% of patients. These chemicals have no licence for medical use and there are problems with sensitization of medical staff and contamination of work areas, which means that these treatments are not universally accepted. Wigs and hair pieces can be very helpful and are not to be underestimated.

Scarring alopecia

Lichen planopilaris (LPP) and discoid lupus erythematosus (DLE)

These are two of the more common forms of scarring alopecia. LPP is characterized by perifollicular purplish discoloration and scale. The interfollicular skin may be normal. DLE has a more coarse pattern of scale and is more likely to affect the scalp between follicles. Where hairs have been lost, the follicles may be plugged with scale. Both conditions may leave scarring which appears as multiple hairs aggregated within one follicular opening and loss of normal follicle openings in adjacent scalp. With time, these areas may become smooth, white, or patchily pigmented. Both conditions may have signs elsewhere to help confirm the clinical diagnosis (see Chapters 23.7, 23.5, and 19.11.2). Confirmation of the diagnosis is by scalp biopsy with part sent for immunofluorescence. False positive immunofluorescence can be a problem on the scalp. Serological tests are done to exclude systemic lupus erythematosus or by way of preparation for systemic medication.

Treatment

Both conditions can be progressive and irreversible and hence brief early treatment with systemic steroid can be justified as a means of containing active disease before establishing a less toxic regimen for maintenance. Systemic hydroxychloroquine and acitretin are common options in this order for DLE and ciclosporin is an option for LPP. Doses can be minimized by coincident, locally injected, or topical potent steroid. Sun avoidance can be important for some DLE patients where photoexacerbation is noted.

Systemic diseases and hair changes

Telogen effluvium (TE) is the most common hair problem related to general medical or surgical upset. It is characterized by massive shedding of hair about 6 to 10 weeks after a period of significant physiological disturbance such as major blood loss, high fevers, or a period of active inflammatory bowel disease. The patient may not make the association with recent illness and such clues need to be actively sought when someone presents with hair loss. Anagen effluvium describes a more acute pattern where a toxic event immediately switches off the hair follicle. The typical example of this is cancer chemotherapy, where treatment is often directed at proliferative cells, inadvertently including those of the dermal papilla of the hair follicle. Other drugs such as retinoids, some anticonvulsants, and progestogens may contribute to hair loss. The list is much longer, but the data to support commonly cited drugs, such as statins, hormone replacement therapy, and atenolol is less clear.

Treatment

This entails looking for any active contributing inflammatory or other systemic precipitating factor and correcting it. The serum iron or ferritin may have some independent relevance and should be maintained within the normal range. Usually, the hair will return to normal. The exception is when the individual is of an age where normal patterns of balding are evolving. In this instance, they may find that the hair pattern returns one or two grades down the line of age-related patterned balding.

Where scalp hair loss presents in association with increased hair on the body or at sites associated with masculinity (hirsutism), a pathological source of androgen should be sought. The history is extremely important in terms of establishing the time course of change and whether the problem is part of a familial pattern. Disturbed menses will increase the index of suspicion. In someone with recent alteration of menses and evolving male-type hair changes, the concern is of an androgen secreting tumour. Where there is a family history and problems have been established over the years, often since puberty, the diagnosis is more likely to be polycystic ovary disease. Both can be screened by checking the free testosterone levels. Where it is elevated, further endocrinological, and possibly gynaecological assessment is warranted. The rash of secondary syphilis can cause a patchy pattern of hair loss scattered over the scalp like numerous 'glades in a wood'. Loss of eyebrows is a feature of lepromatous leprosy.

Further reading

Disorders of the nails

Baran R, *et al.* (eds) (2001). Baran & Dawber's diseases of the nails and their management, 3rd edition. Wiley-Blackwell.

Bergman R, *et al.* (2003). The handheld dermatoscope as a nail-fold capillaroscopic instrument. *Arch Dermatol*, **139**, 1027–30.

Daniel CR 3rd, Zaias N (1988). Pigmentary abnormalities of the nails with emphasis on systemic diseases. *Dermatol Clin*, **6**, 305–13.

de Berker D (2009). Management of psoriatic nail disease. *Semin Cutan Med Surg*, **28**, 39–43.

de Berker D (2009). Clinical practice. Fungal nail disease. *N Engl J Med*, **360** (20), 2108–16.

Epstein E (1998). How often does oral treatment of toenail onychomycosis produce a disease-free nail? *Arch Dermatol*, **134**, 1551–4.

Evans EG, Sigurgeirsson B (1999). Double blind, randomised study of continuous terbinafine compared with intermittent itraconazole in treatment of toenail onychomycosis. The LION Study Group. *BMJ*, **318**, 1031–5.

Hershko A, *et al.* (1997). Yellow nail syndrome. *Postgrad Med J*, **73**, 466–8.

Kavanaugh AF, Ritchlin CT, GRAPPA Treatment Guideline Committee (2006). Systematic review of treatments for psoriatic arthritis: an evidence based approach and basis for treatment guidelines. *J Rheumatol*, **33**, 1417–21.

Myers KA, Farquhar DR (2001). The rational clinical examination. Does this patient have clubbing? *JAMA*, **286**, 341–7.

Tosti A, Piraccini BM, Lorenzi S (2000). Onychomycosis caused by nondermatophytic molds: clinical features and response to treatment of 59 cases. *J Am Acad Dermatol*, **42**, 217–24.

Disorders of the hair

Azziz R (2003). The evaluation and management of hirsutism. *Obstet Gynecol*, **101**, 995–1007.

Friedlander SF, *et al.* (2002). Terbinafine in the treatment of Trichophyton tinea capitis: a randomized, double-blind, parallel-group, duration-finding study. *Pediatrics*, **109**, 602–7.

Fuller LC, *et al.* (2003). Diagnosis and management of scalp ringworm. *BMJ*, **326**, 539–41.

van de Kerkhof PC, Franssen ME (2001). Psoriasis of the scalp. Diagnosis and management. *Am J Clin Dermatol*, **2**, 159–65.

Harrison S, Sinclair R (2002). Telogen effluvium. *Clin Exp Dermatol*, **27**, 389–5.

MacDonald Hull SP, *et al.* (2003). Guidelines for the management of alopecia areata. *Br J Dermatol*, **149**, 692–9.

Price VH (2006). The medical treatment of cicatricial alopecia. *Semin Cutan Med Surg*, **25**, 56–9.

Rosenfield RL (2005). Clinical practice. Hirsutism. *N Engl J Med*, **353**, 2578–88.

Schwartz RA, Janusz CA, Janniger CK (2006). Seborrheic dermatitis: an overview. *Am Fam Physician*, **74**, 125–30.

Sperling LC, Solomon AR, Whiting DA (2000). A new look at scarring alopecia. *Arch Dermatol*, **136**, 235–42.

Tumours of the skin

Edel O'Toole

Essentials

A wide range of tumours, both benign and malignant, are found in skin. Benign skin lesions such as seborrhoeic keratoses and skin tags are often just a cosmetic nuisance, but some benign skin lesions can be a component of diseases with serious medical consequences, e.g. neurofibromatosis or LEOPARD syndrome.

Exposure to ultraviolet light (UVL) is a major factor leading to the development of both benign lesions, e.g. melanocytic naevi, and most skin cancers. Changes in dress style, increased travel abroad, use of sun tanning salons (sunbeds), and the depletion of the ozone layer have all contributed to increased exposure to UVL.

Skin cancer is the most common human cancer and its incidence continues to increase. It most commonly affects older, fair-skinned individuals who have had either acute intermittent exposure to UVL or chronic UVL exposure. Organ transplant recipients have a 200-fold increased risk of squamous cell carcinoma. About 2% of patients who develop skin cancer have a genetic predisposition, e.g. Gorlin's syndrome in basal cell carcinoma (BCC) and familial melanoma syndromes in malignant melanoma. Mutations in the *PTCH* gene cause Gorlin's syndrome, and loss of heterozygosity at that locus is also present in most sporadic BCC.

Nonmelanoma skin cancer is rarely fatal, but can cause a lot of morbidity. Malignant melanoma is a deadly skin cancer which is the 2nd most common cancer (excluding nonmelanoma skin cancer) in young women. Over the last 20 years, its incidence has been increasing faster than any other cancer, with an approximate doubling of rates every 10 years in countries with largely white populations. Early detection and excision of melanoma is the best way to reduce mortality, as there is no curative treatment for metastatic malignant melanoma.

Benign skin tumours

Benign nonmelanocytic tumours

Seborrhoeic keratosis

Seborrhoeic keratoses are probably the most common benign skin tumour. These lesions are usually found on the trunk in older individuals.

Clinical features

The classic seborrhoeic keratosis is a dry, brown, warty plaque with a 'stuck-on' appearance (Fig. 23.14.1). There is large variation in colour, including pale and darker lesions which may even simulate malignant melanoma. The sudden appearance of multiple seborrhoeic keratoses accompanied by the development of a malignancy is known as Leser–Trélat sign.

Treatment

If the lesion is definitely a seborrhoeic wart the patient can be reassured. As the lesions are a cosmetic nuisance, patients may request treatment which can include cryotherapy or curettage.

Sebaceous hyperplasia

Sebaceous hyperplasia is a common benign tumour of the sebaceous glands usually occurring in middle age. The lesions are usually 2 to 3 mm, skin-coloured or yellow papules with central umbilication from which a small amount of sebum can be expressed. Treatment is usually not needed, but if requested for cosmetic reasons, curettage or gentle cautery are appropriate.

Sebaceous adenoma

Sebaceous adenomas are also derived from the sebaceous glands. Tumours present as a yellow, smooth papule or nodule usually on the face or neck and are associated with Muir–Torre syndrome. This is an autosomal dominant disorder, caused by mutations in the mismatch repair genes, *MLH1* or *MSH2*, with an increased tendency to visceral cancers, particularly colorectal carcinoma.

Skin tags

Skin tags are extremely common, flesh-coloured, pedunculated skin lesions that usually occur in the flexures, particularly the neck and axillae. There is some correlation with obesity. Treatment can include cryotherapy or snip excision.

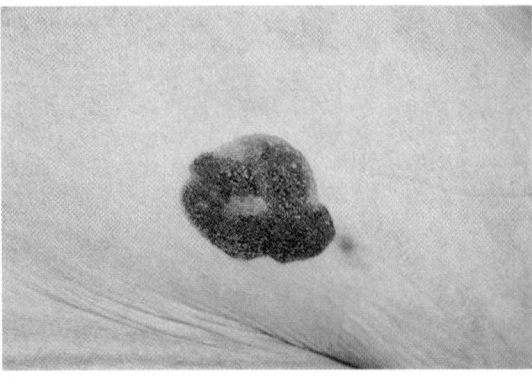

(a)

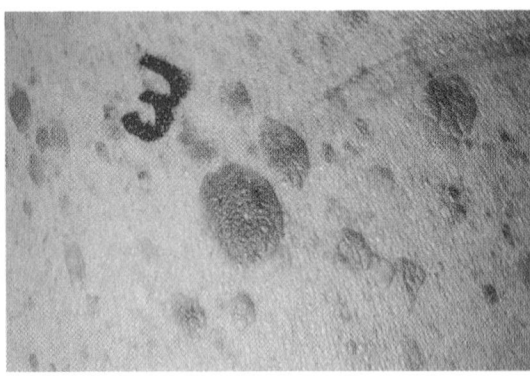

(b)

Fig. 23.14.1 Seborrhoeic warts are often multiple and may be deeply pigmented (a) or light brown (b).

Epidermoid cyst

An epidermoid cyst consists of a sphere of stratified squamous epithelium buried within the dermis. These cysts occur mainly on the face, neck and chest and have a predilection for the genitalia, where they frequently calcify. A common presentation is a dermal nodule with a small pore (punctum) on the surface. The cyst wall may rupture into the dermis, causing an intense inflammatory response followed by suppuration which may require incision and drainage. If the lesion is bothersome to the patient, it may be surgically excised.

Milia

Milia present as 1 to 2 mm white papules, most commonly on the thin skin of the periorbital region in an adult female. Histologically, the lesions are small epidermoid inclusion cysts. A 20 gauge needle may be used to extract milia.

Pilar cyst

Pilar (trichilemmal) cysts occur on the scalp, where they present as smooth, firm, mobile nodules with overlying hair. A punctum is not usually present and inflammation rarely occurs. Histologically, these cysts differ from epidermoid cysts in having the squamous epithelial lining without the granular layer. Surgical excision can be performed if required.

Dermatofibroma

The dermatofibroma is a common dermal tumour usually occurring on the limbs. There is sometimes a history of an insect bite or other trauma. The lesions are firm, pink-brown papules that may involute with time.

Xanthogranuloma

This is a benign tumour of histiocytic cells which occurs predominantly in infancy and early childhood and typically regresses spontaneously. The characteristic clinical appearance is of reddish yellow papule(s) which enlarge up to 1 cm diameter and evolve into yellow-brown plaques and macules. Resolution occurs over months or years to leave small atrophic scars. Visceral involvement may occur in the lung, liver, spleen, testes, pericardium, gastrointestinal tract, and kidney, as well as in the eye. Histologically, the lesions show a mixed dermal infiltrate with histiocytes, lymphocytes, eosinophils, and other cells. A typical feature is the presence of giant cells with a wreath-like arrangement of nuclei, the Touton giant cell.

Benign melanocytic tumours

Freckles

Freckles (ephelides) are brown macules that occur on sun-exposed areas, particularly the nose and the arms, in fair-skinned individuals. The lesions often fade in winter.

Solar lentigo

The solar lentigo is a brown patch occurring on sun-exposed skin that results from UV exposure. Multiple symmetric, hyperpigmented patches on the face, arms, and dorsa of the hands are typical.

Lentigines-associated syndromes

Extensive lentigines at a young age may indicate underlying genetic disorders such as xeroderma pigmentosum (see Chapter 23.9), Carney's (atrial cutaneous myxomas, lentigines, blue naevi, endocrine disorders, and testicular tumours) or LEOPARD (lentigines, electrocardiographic conduction defects, ocular hypertelorism, pulmonary stenosis, genital abnormalities, retardation of growth, and deafness) syndromes.

Acquired melanocytic naevi (moles)

Melanocytic naevi are benign tumours of melanocytes, and are also known as moles.

Aetiology, genetics, and pathogenesis

Acquired naevi tend to first appear and increase in number during childhood, reaching their maximum in early adulthood. There is some evidence that the number of acquired naevi may be related to UV exposure. Fair-skinned individuals and white people who live close to the equator have more acquired naevi than nonwhite populations. Naevi commonly darken or enlarge during pregnancy suggesting a degree of sex hormone responsiveness. Correlation in sex and age-adjusted naevus density in adolescence is higher in monozygotic twins than dizygotic twins suggesting a definite additional genetic effect. About 2% of the population have the atypical mole syndrome, which is associated with an increased risk of melanoma. Mutations in the *BRAF* gene, a serine/threonine kinase involved in the mitogen-activated kinase pathway, are present in about 80% of melanocytic naevi and may contribute to melanocytic hyperproliferation.

Clinical

Acquired melanocytic naevi appear and change in the childhood, teenage, and early adult years. As a rule, new melanocytic naevi do not appear after the age of 40 years. Junctional naevi are usually flat, uniformly pigmented macules that appear in childhood.

Histologically, nests of naevus cells appear at the dermoepidermal junction. Compound naevi are, usually, slightly elevated pigmented papules. They may have a smooth or papillomatous surface (Fig. 23.14.2a). Compound naevi usually increase in size during adolescence. Nests of naevus cells are found both at the dermoepidermal junction and in the dermis. Intradermal naevi are seen mainly after adolescence. These are skin-coloured, dome-shaped papules that most frequently occur on the face. A halo naevus is a clinical variant with a ring of depigmentation around an otherwise normal mole (Fig. 23.14.2b). A blue naevus usually occurs on the limbs. It appears blue-grey because the pigmentation is deep in the dermis. A Spitz naevus usually presents as a vascular-looking papule on the face in children. Atypical (dysplastic naevi) are usually more than 5 mm in diameter, have a macular component, and an indistinct margin, sometimes with background erythema. Recognition of atypical naevi is important as individuals with two or more atypical naevi, naevi in unusual locations (scalp, buttocks, dorsum of feet, and iris) and 100 or more naevi more than 2 mm in diameter (atypical mole syndrome) are at increased risk of developing malignant melanoma.

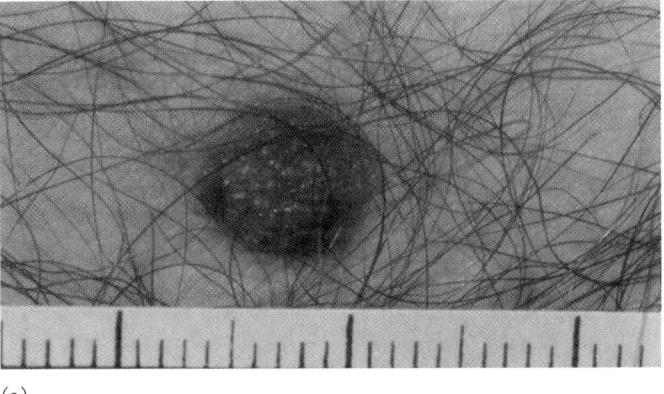

(a)

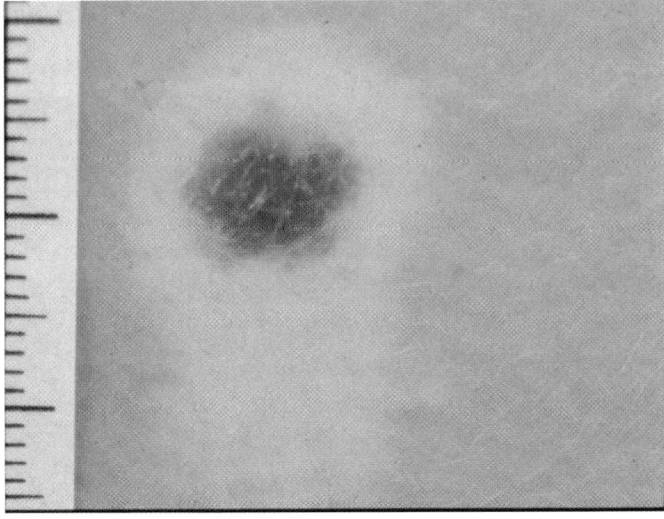

(b)

Fig. 23.14.2 (a) Benign compound naevus with papillomatous surface. (b) Halo naevus showing an area of depigmention around a benign mole. The mole may well eventually regress completely leaving a depigmented patch, which will eventually repigment.

Treatment

The malignant potential of individual naevi is low, therefore prophylactic excision of acquired melanocytic naevi to prevent transformation into melanoma is not advised. Excision of naevi is advocated where it is not possible to clinically exclude a diagnosis of melanoma. Complete excision and histological examination is advocated even when moles are removed for purely cosmetic reasons. Although the clinical differentiation of atypical naevi from melanoma is difficult, it may be facilitated by regular surveillance, automated digital imaging systems, and dermoscopy. Removal of an atypical mole is only necessary if melanoma is suspected.

Congenital melanocytic naevi
Clinical

Congenital melanocytic naevi (CMN) are proliferations of nested melanocytes that are present at birth. The term is also used to describe histologically and clinically identical lesions that appear in diameter in infancy. Small CMN (<1.5 cm in diameter) are seen in 1 to 2% of neonates, intermediate-sized lesions (1.5–20 cm) in 0.6%, and large CMN (>20 cm) in about 0.02%. Large CMN are also known as 'bathing suit naevi' because of their distribution. The lesions are tan, brown to dark brown patches or plaques at birth. They may have a smooth, nodular, or verrucous surface which may be hair-bearing. Patients with large CMN are at increased risk of developing melanoma within the CMN, in the central nervous system, and elsewhere.

Treatment

Most small and intermediate CMN may be managed by routine surveillance. The lifetime risk of malignant melanoma in a patient with a large CMN is about 7%. Parents should be instructed on proper sun avoidance and sun protection techniques including use of sunscreen and use of high-weave, sun-protective clothing. Many specialists recommend partial or complete excision of large CMN. This may require multiple surgical procedures, tissue expansion, and/or grafting. Other surgical options include curettage, dermabrasion, or laser surgery to remove the superficial naevus cells.

Premalignant lesions

Solar keratosis

Solar keratoses (also known as actinic keratoses) are erythematous scaling lesions between 2 and 10 mm in diameter, seen in fair-skinned individuals on areas of maximal sun exposure such as the face, ears, dorsum of the hands, forearms, and lower legs. Histologically, these lesions show dysplasia of the basal keratinocytes. The estimated risk of transformation into squamous cell carcinoma (SCC) is very low, approximately 1% per annum. Some small lesions resolve spontaneously, particularly with photoprotection. Treatment options include cryotherapy, topical diclofenac, 5-fluorouracil, or imiquimod, a topical immune modifier.

Bowen's disease

Bowen's disease (squamous cell carcinoma (SCC) *in situ*) presents as an asymptomatic, enlarging, erythematous, scaly plaque. Approximately 5% progress to invasive SCC. Bowen's disease affecting the glans penis is called erythroplasia of Queyrat. Bowen's disease may be misdiagnosed as tinea, psoriasis, or discoid eczema. Biopsy of a typical lesion shows full-thickness dysplasia of the epidermis.

Treatment can include cryotherapy, topical 5-fluorouracil, or photodynamic therapy.

Malignant skin tumours

Nonmelanocytic

Basal cell carcinoma

Introduction

Basal cell carcinoma (BCC) is the most common cancer in humans, which typically occurs in areas of chronic sun exposure. Basal cell carcinomas are usually slow growing and rarely metastasize.

Aetiology, genetics, pathogenesis, and pathology

The most common factor involved in the pathogenesis of BCC is exposure to ultraviolet light (UV). Fair-skinned individuals who burn easily and tan poorly are at greatest risk of developing BCC. Both cumulative lifetime UV exposure and intermittent intense sun exposure are risk factors. Other sources of UV include sunbeds and psoralen ultraviolet A (PUVA) for psoriasis. Other environmental factors leading to the development of BCC include ionizing radiation given for benign conditions (e.g. acne, tinea capitis) and arsenic ingestion. Organ transplant recipients have a 10-fold increased risk of BCC.

A number of genetic syndromes of increased susceptibility to BCC have been described. The most significant is Gorlin's syndrome (naevoid basal cell carcinoma syndrome) which is characterized by the appearance of BCCs before the age of 20, an autosomal dominant family history, palmar/plantar pits, odontogenic keratocysts, and bilamellar calcification of the falx cerebri. Mutations are present in the human *PTCH* gene, the human homologue of the drosophila patched gene *Ptch1*. Ninety per cent of sporadic nodular BCCs have loss of heterozygosity at chromosome 9q21-q31, where the *PTCH* gene is located and 70% of nodular BCCs have detectable *PTCH* gene mutations. This gene negatively regulates the hedgehog signalling pathway, which is important in epithelial cell growth during hair follicle development, and an inactivating mutation allows uncontrolled hedgehog signalling. Activating mutations in the *SMO* gene (smoothened) similarly allow for unregulated hedgehog signalling in BCC. About 40% of BCC have UV-induced transition mutations in *p53*. Polymorphisms in genes activated by exposure to UV, such as reactive oxygen species (GST, CYP450) or DNA repair (xeroderma pigmentosum), are also significantly associated with risk of BCC development.

The major histological patterns of BCC are nodular, micronodular, superficial, and morphoeic BCC. The nodular type is characterized by well-defined islands of basaloid cells with well-defined peripheral palisading. The superficial type has foci of tumour extending from the epidermis into the papillary dermis. The morphoeic subtype has tumour islands of varying size with surrounding fibrosis.

Epidemiology

Basal cell carcinoma most commonly occurs in white, fair-skinned individuals and rarely occurs in darker skin types. Although BCC more commonly occurs in men, the incidence of BCC continues to rise in women because of increased UV exposure due to changes in dress and lifestyle, including 'sun holidays' and use of sunbeds.

Prevention

The most important risk factor is cumulative lifetime UV exposure. Avoidance of exposure to UV radiation is encouraged.

Helpful preventive measures include avoidance of midday/afternoon sun, wearing a broad-brimmed hat during outdoor activities, and using sunscreens with sun protection factor (SPF) of 15 or greater (see Chapter 23.7). Patient education about the appearance of new lesions to maximize early detection should be encouraged.

Clinical features

Approximately 50% of BCCs occur on the head and neck, 30% on the upper trunk, and the remainder elsewhere. The clinical variants of BCC include nodular/nodulocystic, morphoeic, superficial, and pigmented BCCs. The nodular subtype represents about 60% of BCCs and presents as a small, pink nodule, with a translucent, pearly appearance with telangiectasia (Fig. 23.14.3a). As the lesion enlarges, central ulceration may occur ('rodent ulcer'). Although slow-growing, if neglected, these tumours may enlarge and extend deeply causing significant damage to eyelids, nose, or ears. Superficial BCC accounts for about 20% of BCCs and is more commonly found on the trunk and extremities. Typically, the lesion is a slightly scaly, pink plaque with a threadlike, translucent, raised border. Multiple lesions may be present. Melanin pigmentation may occur in both superficial and nodular BCCs, giving a pigmented variant which is more common in individuals with dark skin (Fig. 23.14.3b). Morphoeic (infiltrative) BCCs present as an indurated, ivory plaque, often resembling a scar. The name is derived from its resemblance to a plaque of localized scleroderma (morphoea). This variant of BCC is notable for its tendency to extend beyond the apparent clinical borders and a high local recurrence rate after treatment.

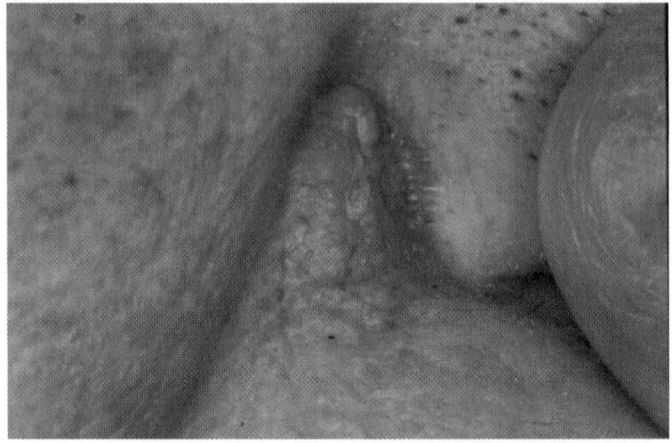

(a)

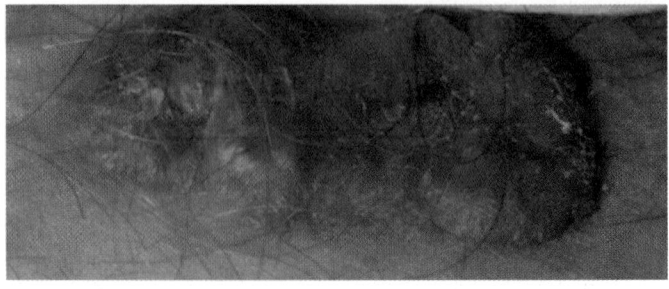

(b)

Fig. 23.14.3 (a)Basal cell carcinoma in a common location, nasal aspect of the nasolabial fold. Note the surface crusting and telangiectasia. (b) Pigmented basal cell carcinoma.

Differential diagnoses of nodulocystic BCC to consider include intradermal naevi and rarer tumours derived from appendageal structures.

Clinical investigation

A small shave or punch biopsy is usually sufficient to confirm the diagnosis and histological subtype of BCC. In some centres, scrapings for cytology can be performed to confirm the diagnosis.

Treatment

Treatments are influenced both by tumour factors (the size, site, margin, and subtype of the BCC) and patient factors (such as age, coexisting illnesses (bleeding diathesis, anticoagulant therapy, or susceptibility to bacterial endocarditis), access to specific treatments locally, and patient preference. Options for superficial BCC include topical 5-fluorouracil, cryotherapy, or more recently, imiquimod. Nodular BCC can be treated by curettage and cautery or simple excision. Morphoeic BCCs or nodular BCCs in high-risk sites ideally should be treated with Mohs' micrographic surgery, which is performed in stages with examination of the histological margins, but wide excision can be performed if this is not available. Photodynamic therapy may be useful for thin BCCs at cosmetically difficult sites. Radiotherapy can be useful in older patients where surgery is not feasible.

With appropriate patient selection, the treatments described above will give cure rates exceeding 95%. Patients who have had one BCC have a 20% risk of developing a further BCC over the following 5 years.

It is likely that over the next 5 to 10 years, further BCC tumour suppressor genes will be identified. The use of imiquimod for superficial BCC will also become more widespread. Small-molecule inhibitors of the hedgehog signalling pathway currently in clinical trials, such as cyclopamine, may well be used routinely as topical therapy in the future.

Squamous cell carcinoma

Squamous cell carcinoma (SCC) is the second most common form of skin cancer and usually occurs on sun-exposed areas in older individuals.

Aetiology, genetics, pathogenesis, and pathology

SCC is a malignant tumour of epidermal keratinocytes. The development of SCC is multifactorial, involving both genetic predisposition and environmental factors. The majority of SCCs occur on sun-exposed areas (head and neck, dorsum of hands). Individuals with type I and II skin types (who burn easily) are at greatest risk. Africans with oculocutaneous albinism, who have lost their protective melanin, also have an increased risk of SCC.

The amount of chronic cumulative sun exposure is a major risk factor for SCC. The highest incidence of SCC worldwide is in Australia, a country with a large white population and year-round sunshine. Absorption of UVB by DNA in skin keratinocytes induces unique mutations at the site of pyrimidine dimers. Ultraviolet B (UVB) irradiation also leads to the activation of cell cycle checkpoint controls and apoptotic pathways. The repair and/or elimination of such apoptotic and mutated cells from the epidermis by 'gatekeeper genes' such as p53 is important, as clonal proliferation of mutated cells may eventually lead to cancer development. Mutations in p53 are found in up to 90% of SCCs. Mutations in p16INK4a and p14ARF, as well as hypermethylation without mutation, have also been documented in SCC. Finally, mutations in

HRAS and KRAS have also been demonstrated in SCC. UVA also plays a role in SCC carcinogenesis through DNA damage, modulation of protein kinase C, and immunosuppression.

There is evidence that human papillomavirus (HPV) may play a causal role in SCC (Chapter 7.5.19). Epidermodysplasia verruciformis, a rare inherited disorder with a high risk of SCC is associated with susceptibility to infection with specific HPV types, called 'EV types', including the oncogenic HPV-5. Organ transplant recipients are highly susceptible to HPV infection, particularly warts, and have a c.200-fold risk of SCC compared to the immunocompetent population. Up to 80% of transplant SCCs have detectable EV-type HPV DNA. HPV E6 protein inhibits UV-induced apoptosis by abrogation of the proapoptotic protein, Bak, enhancing tumour survival. HPV E6 and E7 proteins also functionally inactivate p53. Azathioprine and UVA radiation have recently been shown to generate oxidative DNA damage which may be a further risk factor in organ transplant recipients.

Other documented risk factors include arsenic ingestion and exposure to chemical carcinogens such as polycyclic aromatic hydrocarbons found in soot and tar (a historical example of this is SCC of the scrotum in chimney sweeps). Other conditions predisposing to SCC include chronic ulcers (known as Marjolin's ulcer), recessive dystrophic epidermolysis bullosa (an inherited blistering disease which heals with extensive scarring), skin damage from ionizing radiation, thermal injury, and lymphoedema. Chronic infection and chronic inflammation, such as discoid lupus erythematosus, erosive lichen planus, and lichen sclerosus et atrophicus, also increase the predisposition to SCC. Mutations in nucleotide excision repair genes in xeroderma pigmentosum causing defective DNA repair result in a 1000-fold increased risk of skin cancers (both nonmelanoma and melanoma).

Epidemiology

The incidence of SCC has doubled over the last 40 years. The British Association of Dermatology estimates that there are 25 000 new cases of SCC in the United Kingdom annually, representing about one-quarter of nonmelanoma skin cancers. Men are affected 2 to 3 times more than women probably because of outdoor occupations, less protective clothing, and a greater lifetime cumulative UV radiation exposure. The success of organ transplantation and immunosuppression has also contributed to the increased incidence of SCC.

Prevention

Recommendations include photoprotection against UVA and UVB, patient education about warning signs, regular skin examination, and treatment of actinic keratoses. Systemic chemoprevention with oral retinoids may be an option for high-risk patients, e.g. organ transplant recipients with multiple SCCs.

Clinical features

The classical SCC is a pink, keratotic papule or nodule (Fig. 23.14.4) appearing on the head and neck regions on sun-damaged skin. Surface changes may include ulceration, crusting, scaling, or the presence of a cutaneous horn. As the lesion progresses, it will become nodular and/or ulcerated. These lesions are frequently tender to compression. SCC of the lip generally occurs on the vermilion border of the lip in men with a background of actinic cheilitis (the lower lips are scaly, irregularly pigmented, and atrophic). SCC of the anogenital region may present with pruritus, a palpable lump, or erosion. A full skin examination and palpation of regional lymph nodes is important.

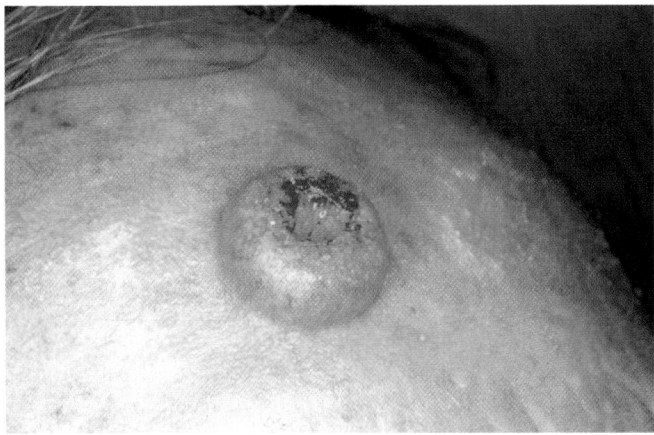

Fig. 23.14.4 Squamous cell carcinoma presenting as a nodule with central keratinization on the forehead.

The common differential diagnoses of SCC include keratoacanthoma, hypertrophic actinic keratosis, verruca vulgaris, and basal cell carcinoma.

Clinical investigation
In most patients, the clinical diagnosis of SCC is confirmed by excision and histopathology. Where there is diagnostic doubt, a small biopsy will confirm the diagnosis.

Treatment
Simple excision with a 4 mm margin of normal surrounding skin is adequate treatment for most low-risk SCC. High-risk tumours (>2 cm in diameter, depth more than 4 mm, located on ears, lip, nose, or scalp, poorly differentiated, perineural, or subcutaneous invasion and recurrent tumours) should be removed with a margin of 6 mm or ideally using Mohs' micrographic surgery. Selected small, low-risk SCCs can be treated with curettage and cautery or cryotherapy after a confirmatory biopsy. Radiotherapy can be used for nonresectable tumours.

Prognosis
The 5-year cure rate after simple excision of SCC is 92%. The overall risk of metastasis from SCC is in the range of 2 to 5%. High-risk SCCs have the greatest risk of metastasis. Chronically immunosuppressed patients also have an increased rate of metastasis. The overall 5-year survival after regional metastasis is just 25%. In addition, patients are at risk of developing a second primary skin cancer. Within 5 years, 12% cent of patients will have developed a new SCC, 43% a new BCC, and 2% a malignant melanoma.

It is likely that over the next 5 to 10 years, the use of genomic and proteomic technology will identify new therapeutic targets in cutaneous and metastatic SCC. Cyclo-oxygenase-2 inhibitors and antioxidants, e.g. green and black tea compounds, may be potentially useful as chemopreventative agents in patients with multiple actinic keratoses. There will be more aggressive management of patients with high-risk SCC, including sentinel lymph node mapping. If a role for HPV in SCC development is validated, there may be randomized clinic trials of vaccination against EV-type HPV in high-risk groups such as organ transplant recipients. The use of sirolimus, an mTOR inhibitor, instead of azathioprine in transplant immunosuppression regimes may reduce the incidence of post-transplantation cancer.

Keratoacanthoma
Keratoacanthoma is a clinically and genetically distinct subtype of SCC. A nodule with a central keratin crater develops rapidly over several weeks, stabilizes in size, and then spontaneously resolves over several months. Histologically and clinically (apart from the history), it is difficult to distinguish from a well-differentiated SCC. There are minimal mitoses or cellular atypia. Ferguson Smith syndrome is an autosomal dominant disorder presenting with multiple keratoacanthomas at a young age. Hundreds of eruptive keratoacanthomas occur in the Grzybowski variant. Keratoacanthomas are also found in Muir–Torre syndrome.

Melanocytic tumours

Malignant melanoma
Malignant melanoma (MM) is a melanocyte-derived tumour located predominantly in the skin, but also found in the eyes, leptomeninges, and oral, genital, and rectal mucous membranes. Melanoma accounts for only 4% of all skin cancers, but causes about 80% of skin cancer-related deaths worldwide.

Aetiology, genetics, pathogenesis and pathology
The development of MM is multifactorial. Risk factors include fair skin phenotype (blonde/red hair, freckles easily, blue eyes), blistering sunburn in childhood or adolescence, history of excessive UV exposure, greater than 100 melanocytic naevi, greater than 5 atypical/dysplastic naevi, personal or family history of MM, and changing moles. The presence of the atypical mole syndrome (also known as familial atypical mole melanoma syndrome) or xeroderma pigmentosum increases the risk by 500 to 1000-fold. More than 60% of melanomas arise *de novo* (no pre-existing lesion). The genetics of inherited cancers are further discussed in Chapter 6.3.

BRAF mutations occur in 70% of melanomas arising in intermittently sun-exposed sites. The receptor tyrosine kinase gene, *KIT*, is mutated in 20% of acral and mucosal melanomas. Melanocortin 1 receptor variants that cause red hair and freckling are associated with a small increase in melanoma risk (two–threefold) and an increased risk of melanoma with *BRAF* mutations. There are probably at least three other genes which underlie predisposition to familial melanoma. The most common is a gene on chromosome 9, *CDKN2A*, which codes for p16INK4a, an inhibitor of the cyclin-dependent kinases 4 and 6. In the United Kingdom, 50% of families with three or more melanoma cases have *CDKN2A* mutations, but only 12% of families with two or fewer cases. The second is the *CDK4* gene. A rare, dominant activating mutation in this gene renders it insensitive to p16 inhibition. The third is *p14ARF*, a second product of the *CDKN2A* locus. Very rare deletions of this gene have been shown to underlie susceptibility to melanoma and neural tumours. Melanoma may also occur as a second tumour in familial retinoblastoma and in the Li–Fraumeni syndrome (associated with sarcomas, brain, and breast tumours).

Histologically, a MM is an asymmetric lesion consisting of single or nested melanocytes in the epidermis (pagetoid spread), appendageal structures, and dermis. The tumour melanocytes do not mature as they descend into the dermis. The distribution of melanin is irregular and the melanocytes display atypia and mitoses. An initial radial growth phase (melanocytes proliferating in the epidermis and papillary dermis) is followed by a more aggressive vertical growth phase with more extensive spread deep into the dermis.

Epidemiology

Malignant melanoma is the most serious type of skin cancer and is primarily a disease of white individuals. It rarely occurs in black and Asian individuals. There are about 8000 new cases of MM in the United Kingdom annually and about 1800 melanoma related deaths (Cancer Research UK statistics). In the age group 20 to 39, melanoma is the second most common cancer (excluding BCC and SCC). The incidence of melanoma increases with age with a peak in the 5th decade.

Prevention

The general public should be encouraged to avoid sunburn and other excessive UV exposure. At risk individuals should use sunblock and wear protective clothing (see Chapter 23.7). Health care professionals and patients should be educated about the features of early MM as early detection of thin melanoma is the best method of reducing mortality.

Clinical features

The major clinical characteristic of melanoma is a changing mole. The seven-point checklist is useful. Major features are change in size, irregular colour, and irregular shape, while minor features are inflammation, oozing, change in sensation, and diameter 7 mm or less. Lesions with any of the major features or three of the minor features are suspicious of melanoma. The mnemonic ABCDE is also used which stands for asymmetry, border irregularity, colour variegation, diameter more than 6 mm, and evolving (changing).

Four major clinicopathological variants of MM have been identified. Superficial spreading melanoma represents about 70% of melanomas and occurs most commonly on the legs in women and on the trunk in men (Fig. 23.14.5a). It presents as a flat, pigmented lesion with variegation in colour and an irregular border. Nodular melanoma accounts for about 15 to 20% of melanomas and presents as a papule or nodule on the trunk (usually in men) or limbs. There is frequently a history of rapid growth. This variant is more likely to be amelanotic (no pigmentation) and there may be a delay in diagnosis (Fig. 23.14.5b). Lentigo maligna, also known as Hutchinson's melanotic freckle, occurs on the head and neck of older people who have been heavily exposed to sunlight. These are slow-growing *in situ* melanomas (Fig. 23.14.5c) with the potential to progress to invasive melanoma (lentigo maligna melanoma) and metastasize. Acral lentiginous melanoma occurs on palmoplantar skin (Fig. 23.14.5d) or the nail bed. It occurs in all races and therefore does not appear to be caused by exposure to the sun. A tendency to delayed diagnosis gives this variant a poor prognosis.

At presentation, 10% of cutaneous melanomas will have metastasized. The primary lesion may regress, leaving a hypopigmented patch, or the primary can be noncutaneous. Although systemic metastasis is predominantly to the lung, liver, brain, and

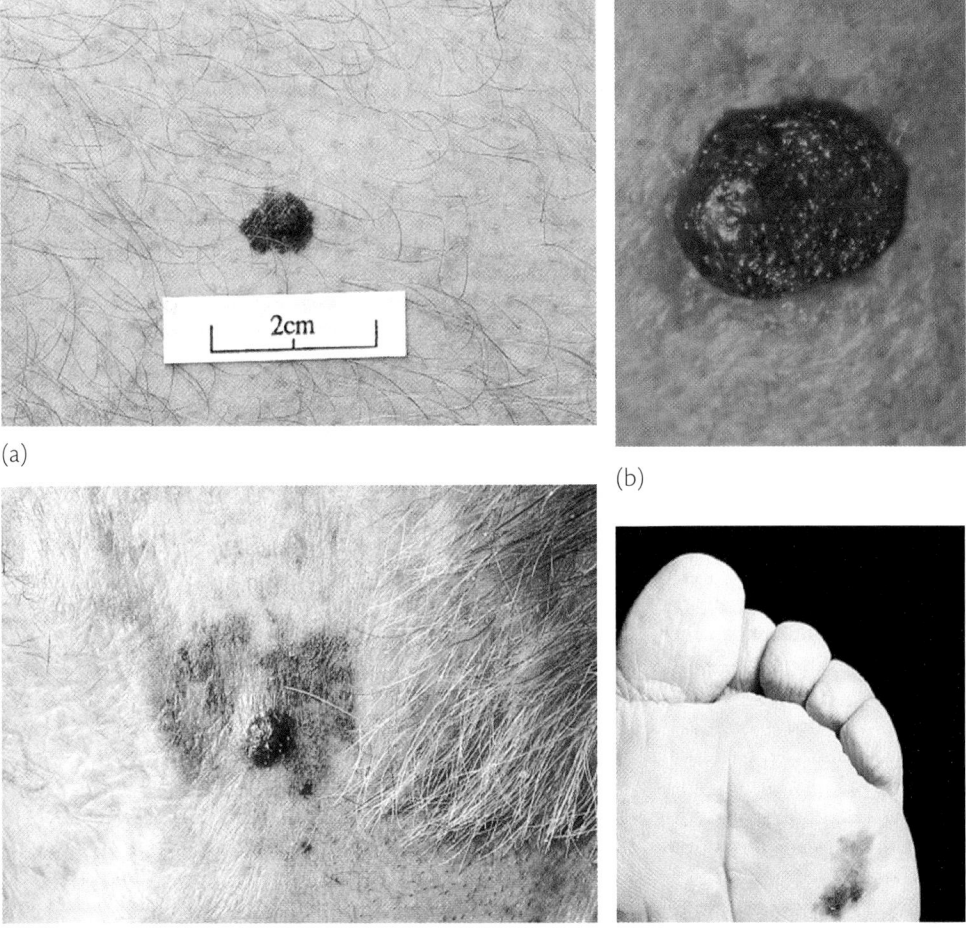

(a)

(b)

(c)

(d)

Fig. 23.14.5 Malignant melanoma: (a) superficial spreading melanoma with variegation in colour and irregular margin, (b) amelanotic (no pigment) nodular melanoma, (c) invasive nodular melanoma arising in a lentigo maligna; and (d) acral lentiginous melanoma on the sole.

bone, lesions can arise anywhere including bowel, kidney, and muscle. Localized skin metastasis is also common.

Differential diagnosis

Atypical naevi, deeply pigmented seborrhoeic warts, and pigmented BCC may all simulate melanoma. Dermoscopy may be helpful in discriminating between melanocytic and nonmelanocytic lesions. Features of MM include a broadened pigment network, multiple colours, a blue-white veil, pseudopods, and peripheral black dots and globules.

Clinical investigation

The diagnosis should always be based on a full thickness excisional biopsy down to fat with a margin of 2 mm of normal skin around the lesion. Patients with Stage IIB melanoma or higher (Breslow's thickness 2.01–4 mm without ulceration, or >4 mm or any Breslow's thickness with metastases) will require further investigation including full blood count, liver function tests, chest X-ray, lactate dehydrogenase, and CT of chest/abdomen/pelvis.

Treatment

The definitive treatment of localized disease is wide excision of the tumour with a normal skin margin of 0.5 cm for *in situ* melanoma (confined to the epidermis), 1 cm for tumours with a Breslow's thickness of 1 to 2 mm and 2 to 3 cm for thicker lesions. Sentinel node (initial draining lymph node) biopsy with selective complete clearance of regional nodes is now performed in many centres for lesions with a Breslow's thickness of more than 1 mm but remains an area of controversy.

Adjuvant therapy should be considered for those with positive lymph nodes or thick primary tumours who should be entered into available clinical trials. Multiple approaches have been tried including immunotherapy, vaccine therapy, and chemotherapy. High-dose interferon prolongs relapse-free survival, but no clear benefit in overall survival and carries significant systemic side effects.

Limited metastatic disease can be managed with excision or carbon dioxide laser ablation. Extensive recurrent disease in a limb can be treated with isolated limb perfusion with melphalan. About 15 to 20% of patients with visceral metastatic disease will have a temporary response to interleukin 2 (IL-2) or dacarbazine.

Prognosis

Breslow's thickness is the distance from the granular layer to the deepest level of the tumour and is the most important prognostic factor in MM. Patients with lesions confined to the epidermis (melanoma *in situ*) have an approximate 5-year survival rate of 100%; those less than 1 mm, 95 to 100%; between 1 and 2 mm, 80 to 96%; between 2.1 and 4 mm, 60 to 75%; and lesions of more than 4 mm in depth, 50%. If a single lymph node is involved the 5-year survival is 45 per cent, if two lymph nodes are involved, the survival rate is 28%, but this rate drops to 9% if more than four lymph nodes are involved. The median survival time following metastasis is between 5 and 16 months.

It is likely that over the next 5 to 10 years, immunotherapy may provide hope for those patients with metastatic disease. In a recent study using autologous T cells transduced with high-affinity tumour antigen (MART-1), specific T-cell receptors produced dramatic remission in metastases in 2 out of 15 patients with metastatic melanoma. Clinical trials of targeted inhibitors, e.g. Raf and Kit inhibitors, in combination with chemotherapy will continue. Advances in genomic technology should provide new targets for investigation.

Other cutaneous malignancies

Cutaneous lymphoma

Cutaneous lymphomas are rare lymphoproliferative disorders of the skin, mainly of T or B-cell origin. The most common cutaneous lymphoma is mycosis fungoides (MF), a T-cell lymphoma.

Aetiology, genetics, pathogenesis, and pathology

Clonal lymphocyte proliferation has been ascribed to viral infection, chromosomal alterations, overexpression of oncogenes, or environmental toxins. Chromosomal aberrations associated with cutaneous T-cell lymphoma include losses on chromosomes 1p (38%) and 17p (21%) and gains on chromosomes 4/4p, 18, and 17q/17. These loci contain two well-known tumour suppressor genes, *p53*(17p) and *PTEN*(10q).

Biopsy of a patch or plaque lesion in MF shows prominent atypical lymphocyte invasion of the epidermis (epidermotropism), formation of intraepidermal collections called Pautrier's microabscesses, and a band-like infiltrate in the papillary dermis. The clonal nature of the lymphocyte infiltration can be confirmed by demonstration of rearrangement of the *TCRB* gene by polymerase chain reaction. However, clonal T-cell populations are also found in inflammatory dermatoses. Immunohistochemistry shows that the lymphocytic infiltrate expresses T-cell antigens (CD2, CD3, CD4, CD5) with loss of CD7 and CD26.

Mycosis fungoides most commonly occurs in the fourth to fifth decade and is approximately twice as common in black individuals as it is in white individuals.

Clinical features

Mycosis fungoides—the typical clinical presentation of MF is with brownish-red patches and plaques. Some lesions may have an annular or serpiginous configuration and poikiloderma (telangiectasia, pigmentation and atrophy), particularly on the breasts and buttocks. Some patients will progress to develop thicker plaques and tumours. Widespread erythroderma with ulcerated tumours is the final stage of the disease. Other clinical variants that may have the immunophenotypic features of MF include granulomatous slack skin disease, follicular mucinosis and large plaque parapsoriasis.

Sézary's syndrome—this is part of the spectrum of MF and is characterized by generalized erythroderma ('red man') with scaling and pruritus, lymphadenopathy, and circulating atypical lymphoid cells (Sézary cells) which have cerebriform nuclei (usually >1000 atypical lymphocytes/mm^3).

Adult T-cell leukaemia/lymphoma—this is a high-grade CD4-positive lymphoproliferative disorder associated with infection with human T-lymphotropic virus 1 (HTLV-1). It is most common in Japan and in the Caribbean and in immigrants from these regions. The cutaneous manifestations include patches, plaques, and tumours. Atypical lymphocytes (clover leaf cells) are commonly seen in the peripheral blood. Extracutaneous manifestations include lymphadenopathy, hypercalcaemia, splenomegaly, pulmonary infiltrates, and opportunistic infections.

B-cell lymphoma—cutaneous B-cell lymphoma usually presents as grouped dermal nodules, sometimes in an annular configuration. These generally progress slowly and remain confined to the skin.

Other inflammatory skin disorders may simulate MF including psoriasis, eczema, and parapsoriasis.

Clinical investigation

A clinical diagnosis of MF is confirmed by a skin biopsy. Initial histology may be subtle and several biopsies may be required to see the histological features of MF. Initial clinical investigation of a newly diagnosed patient with MF should include a thorough history (looking for systemic symptoms such as fever, weight loss, night sweats) and examination (looking for lymphadenopathy or hepatosplenomegaly). Routine investigations should include full blood count/blood film, liver function tests, lactate dehydrogenase (an indicator of tumour load), and HTLV-1 antibodies. If lymph node enlargement is present, a lymph node aspirate/biopsy should be performed. Patients with an elevated lactate dehydrogenase (LDH), abnormal full blood count, or rapidly progressive disease should have a staging CT of chest, abdomen, and pelvis and bone marrow biopsy.

Treatment

Potent topical corticosteroids are usually the initial treatment for limited patch or plaque stage cutaneous T-cell lymphoma (CTCL). Topical nitrogen mustard is also effective in adults with patch or plaque stage disease but application is time-consuming. Superficial (patch stage) disease also responds well to narrowband UVB, but psoralen ultraviolet A (PUVA) is better for plaque stage disease. Combined treatment with α-interferon improves the duration of response. Total skin electron beam therapy is a further option. Bexarotene, a synthetic retinoid-X receptor agonist, is a promising new therapy for CTCL with response rates of up to 70%, even in tumour stage disease. Bexarotene-related toxicity includes marked hypertriglyceridaemia and hypercholesterolaemia. Photopheresis and denileukin diftitox are other options for more advanced disease. Patients with resistant early stage disease or advanced disease should be offered entry into clinical trials where available.

Prognosis

Patients with early stage disease have a similar life expectancy to their peers. Patients presenting with tumours or erythroderma have a 10-year survival of approximately 40% (tumour-node-metastasis (TMN) Stage III or higher). Poor prognostic factors include presentation with extensive thick plaques, tumours, or erythroderma, a late age of onset, or folliculotropic histology.

There are many newer agents in development/trials directed at receptors, tumour-specific genes, or signalling pathways. These include alemtuzumab, a humanized anti-CD52 antibody that targets a cell surface antigen expressed on normal and malignant T-cells, individualized dendritic cell-based vaccines, depsipeptide, a histone deacetylase inhibitor molecule (in Phase I-II clinical trials), topical tazarotene, and allogenic haematopoietic stem cell transplant.

Leukaemic infiltrates

Leukaemic infiltrates of skin are known as leukaemia cutis. Leukaemia cutis is most commonly associated with myeloid subtypes of leukaemia, particularly acute monocytic or myelomonocytic leukaemias, but may also herald the transformation of myelodysplastic syndrome to leukaemia. It is less commonly associated with lymphatic leukaemia. The most characteristic lesions of leukaemia cutis are red-brown to violaceous papules, nodules, and plaques which may be purpuric from thrombocytopenia. The lesions may localize to sites of skin trauma or surgical scars. A granulocytic sarcoma (or chloroma) presents as a rapidly growing, firm nodule that at times has a green hue. This tumour is usually

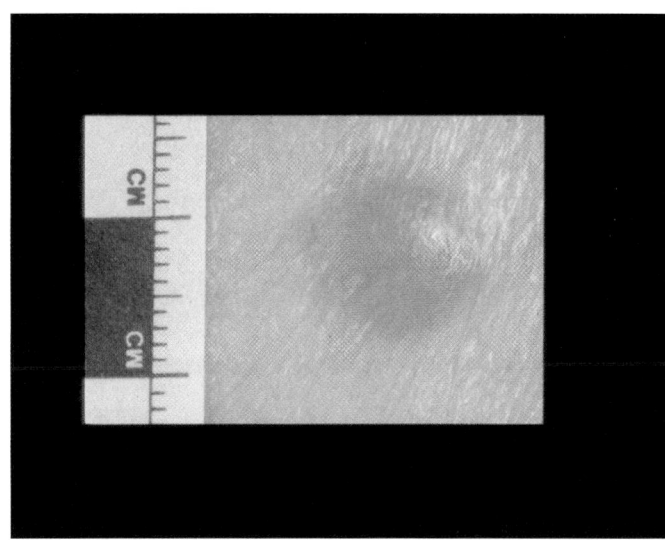

Fig. 23.14.6 Erythematous nodule on abdomen. This was a cutaneous metastasis from breast carcinoma.

associated with acute myeloid leukaemia, and the greenish colour is related to myeloperoxidase in the granulocytes. Leukaemia cutis is usually an indicator of advanced disease. If there is diagnostic doubt, immunophenotyping of a skin biopsy may be helpful.

Cutaneous metastases

Skin metastases usually occur at a late stage of disease and indicate a poor prognosis. The most common skin tumour to metastasize to the skin is malignant melanoma. Frequent visceral primary sites that metastasize to skin include breast, stomach, lung, uterus, colon, kidney, prostate gland, and ovary. Metastases from other organs are transferred via lymphatic or haematogenous spread and this occurs in about 3% of cancer cases. The presenting lesions are often rather inflammatory in appearance (Fig. 23.14.6). The most common presentation is isolated or multiple nodules. Intra-abdominal metastasis may produce an umbilical nodule, known as Sister Mary Joseph's nodule. The primary cancer is often ovarian or gastric and this may be the presenting sign. Metastases from renal cell carcinoma are often very vascular. In breast carcinoma, metastases may present as inflammatory plaques resembling erysipelas (carcinoma erysipeloides). Breast cancer may also cause dermal oedema which resembles orange peel (peau d'orange). Rarely, infiltrative breast cancer metastases can cause scarring alopecia. The presenting lesion is usually excised to confirm the diagnosis. Immunohistochemistry can be performed with tumour-specific markers to confirm the primary source.

Paget's disease (Chapter 13.8.3)

Paget's disease of the nipple is the presenting feature of about 2% of breast cancers, usually intraductal carcinoma. It occurs most frequently in the 5th or 6th decade. Early changes may be very minimal, e.g. only a very small amount of nipple discharge. An erythematous plaque subsequently develops over the nipple and areola which may simulate eczema. The main differential diagnosis is nipple eczema which is almost always bilateral. A biopsy will confirm the diagnosis.

Langerhans cell histiocytosis

Langerhans cell histiocytosis is a rare disease of unknown aetiology, but characterized histologically by a proliferation of Langerhans cells expressing CD1a and CD207, and with the presence of Birbeck granules on electron microscopy. The clinical presentation varies with the nature of organ involvement and whether it is single system or multi system disease. Skin, bone, and lymph node are the most common sites of involvement, but other systems include liver, lung, gastrointestinal, endocrine, nervous system, and haematological. The characteristic skin presentation is the presence of greasy scales on the scalp, reminiscent of seborrhoeic dermatitis. On the trunk, the lesions are discrete, yellow-brown, scaly papules, often with areas of purpura. Ulceration in the flexures and groin is a common presentation in adults. The disease is discussed in detail in Chapter 22.4.7.

Further reading

Agar NS, *et al.* (2004). The basal layer in human squamous tumors harbors more UVA than UVB fingerprint mutations: a role for UVA in human skin carcinogenesis. *Proc Natl Acad Sci U S A*, **101**, 4954–9. [Paper showing that UVA fingerprint mutations are more commonly found in the basal layer of skin, associated with the stem cell compartment.]

Ananthaswamy HN, *et al.* (1997). Sunlight and skin cancer: inhibition of p53 mutations in UV-irradiated mouse skin by sunscreens. *Nat Med*, **3**, 510–14. [Landmark paper showing that p53 mutation is an early event in IV-induced skin carcinogenesis which can be inhibited by sunscreen.]

Bishop JN, *et al.* (2007). The prevention, diagnosis, referral and management of melanoma of the skin: concise guidelines. *Clin Med*, **27**, 283–90. [Review of clinical aspects of malignant melanoma.]

Dajee M, *et al.* (2003). NF-κB blockade and oncogenic Ras trigger invasive human epidermal neoplasia. *Nature*, **421**, 639–43. [Paper showing an important role for oncogenic Ras in SCC formation.]

Euvrard S, Kanitakis J, Claudy A (2003). Skin cancers after organ transplantation. *N Engl J Med*, **348**, 1681–91. [Overview of the cutaneous malignancies occurring in organ transplant recipients.]

Fan H, *et al.* (1997). Induction of basal cell carcinoma features in transgenic human skin expressing Sonic Hedgehog. *Nature Med*, **3**, 788–92. [Paper showing that keratinocytes overexpressing Sonic Hedgehog transplanted on to mice form BCC.]

Gudbjartsson DF, *et al.* (2008). ASIP and TYR pigmentation variants associate with cutaneous melanoma and basal cell carcinoma. *Nat Genet*, **40**, 886–91. [Association of genetic variants controlling skin pigmentation with malignant melanoma and BCC.]

Hussussian CJ, *et al.* (1994). Germline p16 mutations in familial melanoma. *Nat Genet*, **8**, 15–21. [Paper showing p16 mutations in 13 out of 18 kindreds with familial melanoma.]

Landi MT, *et al.* (2006). MC1R germline variants confer risk for BRAF mutant melanoma. *Science*, **313**, 521–2. [People with MC1R polymorphisms have an increased risk of developing melanomas with BRAF mutations.]

Morgan RA, *et al.* (2006). Cancer regression in patients after transfer of genetically engineered lymphocytes. *Science*, **314**, 126–9. [Landmark paper showing sustained regression of metastatic melanoma by genetically engineering patient lymphocytes to recognize and attack melanoma cells.]

Morton DL, *et al.* (2006). Sentinel-node biopsy or nodal observation in melanoma. *N Engl J Med*, **355**, 1307–17. [This study shows that sentinel node biopsy provides important prognostic information in patients with intermediate-thickness melanoma and identifies patients with lymph node metastases whose survival can be prolonged by immediate lymphadenectomy.]

Motley R, *et al.* (2002). Multiprofessional guidelines for the management of the patient with primary cutaneous squamous cell carcinoma. *Br J Dermatol*, **146**, 18–25. [United Kingdom evidence-based guidelines on management of SCC.]

O'Donovan P, *et al.* (2005). Azathioprine and UVA light generate mutagenic oxidative DNA damage. *Science*, **309**, 1871–4. [This paper provides a scientific rationale behind the increased incidence of skin cancer in organ transplant recipients on azathioprine].

Pho L, Grossman D, Leachman SA (2006). Melanoma genetics: a review of genetic factors and clinical phenotypes in familial melanoma. *Curr Opin Oncol*, **18**, 173–9. [Review of genetics of familial melanoma.]

Prickett TD, *et al.* (2009). Analysis of the tyrosine kinome in melanoma reveals recurrent mutations in ERBB4. *Nat Genet.* **41**, 1127–32. [Mutation analysis of protein tyrosine kinase genes in melanoma identified kinase-activating ERBB4 mutations in 19% of tumours]

Stacey SN, *et al.* (2009). New common variants affecting susceptibility to basal cell carcinoma. *Nat Genet*, **41**, 909–14. [Follow-up to genome-wide association study showing new genetic variants predisposing to BCC.]

Stern RS, *et al.* (1984). Cutaneous squamous-cell carcinoma in patients treated with PUVA. *N Engl J Med*, **310**, 1156–61. [Landmark paper showing that PUVA treatment for psoriasis causes a dose-dependent increase in SCC.]

Teh MT, *et al.* (2005). Genomewide single nucleotide polymorphism microarray mapping in basal cell carcinomas unveils uniparental disomy as a key somatic event. *Cancer Res*, **65**, 8597–603. [Paper showing that more than 90% of BCCs have loss of heterozygosity on chromosome 9.]

Telfer NR, Colver GB, Morton CA (2008). British Association of Dermatologists. Guidelines for the management of basal cell carcinoma. *Br J Dermatology*, **159**, 35–48. [UK evidence-based guidelines on management of BCC.]

Thompson JF, Scolyer RA, Kefford RF (2009). Cutaneous melanoma in the era of molecular profiling. Lancet, 374, 362–65. [Brief review of melanoma genetics and treatment of advanced disease.]

Skin and systemic diseases

Clive B. Archer

Essentials

Dermatology is most interesting where it overlaps with general internal medicine. Skin lesions may be part of a systemic disease (e.g. in sarcoidosis or systemic lupus erythematosus), or they may be a manifestation of an underlying disease or process as in the case of acanthosis nigricans, which can be associated with either an underlying adenocarcinoma in older patients, or with insulin resistance and sometimes overt diabetes mellitus in younger obese patients.

Sarcoid can affect the skin in numerous ways, including erythema nodosum, nodular sarcoid lesions, multiple papules, and larger plaques, particularly on the nose, a site at which the skin changes are frequently perniotic in appearance (lupus pernio, scar sarcoidosis, and rarely angiolupoid sarcoid).

Diabetes mellitus can also affect the skin in a myriad of ways, with more common forms including granuloma annulare, necrobiosis lipoidica, diabetic dermopathy, cutaneous infections, and the consequences of neuropathy.

Liver disease may affect the skin by causing pruritus, pigmentation (grey or jaundice), vascular changes (spider naevi), porphyria cutanea tarda, dryness, and hair/nail alterations. Renal disease may affect the skin by causing pruritus, pigmentary changes, dryness, and calciphylaxis, and use of immunosuppression can lead to an increase in malignancy in some cases.

Common associations of pyoderma gangrenosum include inflammatory bowel diseases (ulcerative colitis and Crohn's disease), rheumatoid arthritis and other rheumatological disease, haematological malignancies, and monoclonal gammopathies.

The noninfectious granulomatous disorders of the skin include sarcoidosis, granuloma annulare, and necrobiosis lipoidica. Granulomatous diseases caused by bacterial infections (e.g. tuberculosis and leprosy) and fungal infections are discussed in Chapter 23.9 and Section 7.

Sarcoidosis and the skin (Chapter 18.12)

Sarcoidosis has been defined as 'a disease characterized by the formation in all or several affected organs or tissues of epithelial cell tubercles, without caseation, although fibrinoid necrosis may be present at the centre of a few, proceeding either to resolution or to the conversion of the epithelial cell tubercles into hyaline fibrous tissue'. Other changes present to a varying degree include partial or complete suppression of tuberculin and other intradermal cell-mediated immune responses, and an elevated serum calcium level. The Kveim test, which was positive in most active cases, is no longer available.

Aetiology

Many infectious agents have been put forward as the potential cause of sarcoidosis, but cultures have been negative and responses to anti-infective treatments have been disappointing. A polymerase chain reaction (PCR) study revealed the presence of various subtypes of mycobacterial DNA in 16 of 20 cases of cutaneous sarcoidosis, but the significance of these and other findings are unclear. Genetic factors may be important, HLA type, for example, seeming to influence the pattern of the disease rather than determining its occurrence.

The prevalence of sarcoidosis in developed countries is greater than 10 per 100 000 population, but an apparent increased incidence in the last 50 years is probably due to improved methods of detection.

Clinical features

Skin lesions occur in about 30% of patients with systemic sarcoidosis, but cutaneous sarcoidosis can occur without systemic disease.

The photographs have been published previously in Dr Clive Archer's books: Archer CB and Robertson SJ, *Black and White Skin Diseases—an Atlas and Text*, Blackwell Science (1995) and Archer CB, *Ethnic Dermatology—Clinical Problems and Skin Pigmentation*, Informa Healthcare (2008). We are most grateful to Stuart Robertson of the Department of Education at the St John's Institute of Dermatology, London for access to the collection of photographs at the St John's Institute of Dermatology.

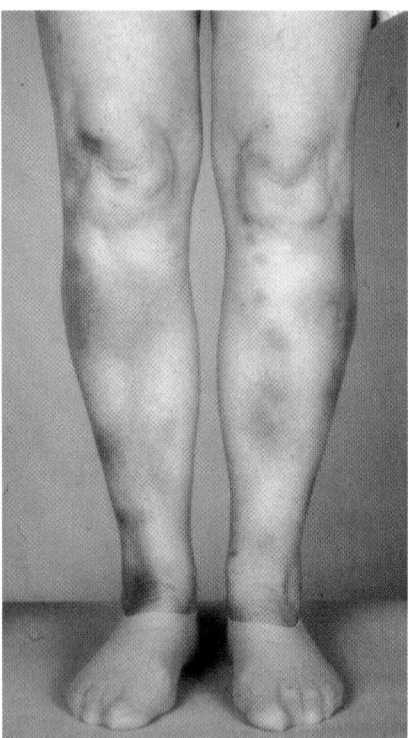

Fig. 23.15.1 Erythema nodosum, with painful bruise-like lesions on the shins.

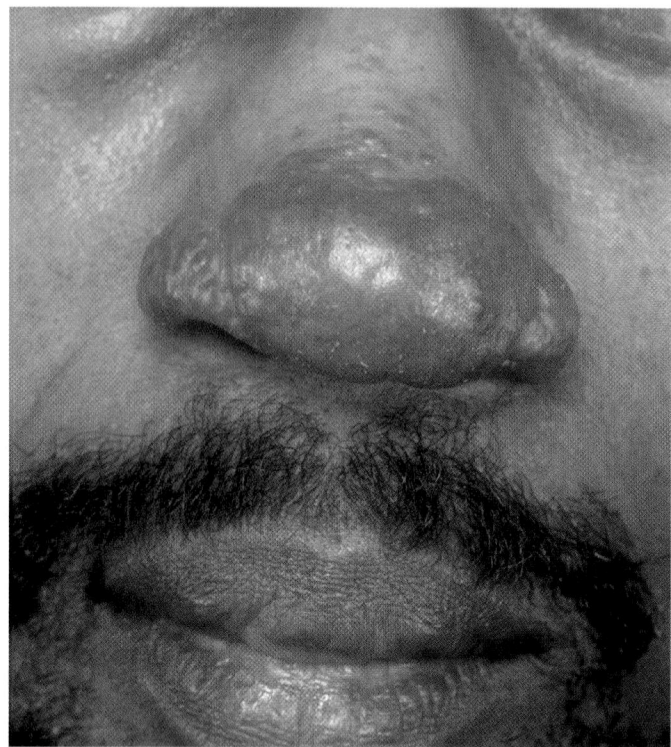

Fig. 23.15.3 Sarcoidosis on the nose of a man of Afro-Caribbean origin.

Significant pulmonary disease may be asymptomatic and the extent of skin involvement does not correlate with the extent of systemic disease.

The specific skin lesions of sarcoidosis arise from a dense accumulation of epithelioid granulomas in the dermis or subcutis and can be of variable morphology. Erythema nodosum (Fig. 23.15.1) is a nonspecific clinical feature of early or acute sarcoidosis without the characteristic sarcoidal granulomas (see Chapter 23.7). Nodular sarcoid lesions are often annular and reddish-brown or violaceous in colour. There may be multiple papules and larger plaques, particularly on the nose, a site at which the skin changes are frequently perniotic in appearance (lupus pernio) (Fig. 23.15.2). Skin lesions can affect pre-existing scars (the Koebner or isomorphic phenomenon), sometimes referred to as scar sarcoidosis. A rare but characteristic telangiectatic form of sarcoidosis, angiolupoid sarcoid, affects women, almost always on the sides of the nasal bridge, on the adjacent cheek or below the eyebrows. Sometimes the nodular lesions are solely subcutaneous, and erythrodermic and lichenoid sarcoidosis are unusual morphological forms.

Sarcoidosis is more common in black skin and in African-Americans; typical lesions include annular lesions on the nose (Fig. 23.15.3), hypopigmented macules and papules, keloid-like lesions, ulcerative, verrucous, and large nodular forms. Erythema nodosum is uncommon in black skin. In white skin the colour of the lesions ranges from yellowish to the livid violaceous colour which is most marked in lupus pernio. The epidermis is rarely affected and scarring is unusual except in the papular and annular forms.

Differential diagnosis

The differential diagnosis includes lupus vulgaris, a cutaneous form of tuberculosis, syphilis, and tuberculoid leprosy (see Chapters 23.10, 7.6.25, 7.5.27, and 7.6.36). These can usually be distinguished on histology. Other common disorders with granulomatous histology include granuloma annulare, rosacea, and Crohn's disease. Sarcoid-like reactions in a scar should be distinguished from a foreign body reaction. A granulomatous sarcoidal

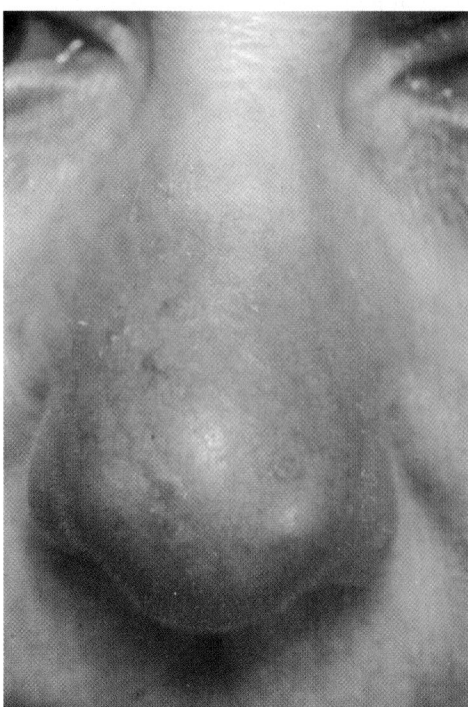

Fig. 23.15.2 Sarcoidosis, showing the violaceous lesions of lupus pernio on the nose.

reaction to any pigment of a tattoo may occur, either alone or accompanied by other signs of sarcoidosis.

Clinical investigation

A skin biopsy is usually required to show the characteristic granulomatous histology. However, a patient with erythema nodosum and bilateral hilar lymphadenopathy may not require histological confirmation of the erythema nodosum (a form of panniculitis) for the diagnosis of acute sarcoidosis to be acceptable.

A chest X-ray (radiograph) should be performed in all cases. Angiotensin-converting enzyme (ACE) is produced by sarcoidal granulomas and serum ACE is raised in about 60% of patients with systemic sarcoidosis. However, serum ACE may be elevated in diabetes mellitus and alcoholic liver disease, and is often normal in localized sarcoidosis of the skin. Serum calcium should be checked, as an increased level may lead to renal failure. Less specifically, the erythrocyte sedimentation rate (ESR) is usually raised, with a slight anaemia, neutropenia or lymphopenia, and hypergammaglobulinaemia in over 50% of patients. An ECG is required to exclude cardiac involvement.

Pulmonary function tests may be indicated and computed tomography of the chest is helpful to define lung involvement. Hand radiographs may show cystic changes in chronic disease, usually when there are clinical abnormalities in the fingers.

The most specific investigation was the Kveim test, in which sarcoidal tissue from the spleen of an affected individual was injected intradermally to produce an epithelioid cell granulomatous reaction. A positive response was the development of a reddish papule at 2 to 3 weeks. Excision at 6 weeks showed the confirmatory histology. However, this test is no longer used because of the infective risk of injecting human tissue. See Chapter 18.12 for further details of investigation of the patient with suspected sarcoidosis.

Treatment

Limited cutaneous sarcoidosis can resolve spontaneously, so a conservative approach to treatment is often adopted. Papular and subcutaneous skin lesions may settle spontaneously but lupus pernio tends to persist.

Superpotent topical corticosteroids are usually tried and can be helpful. Intralesional triamcinolone is often effective, care being taken to inject deeply to avoid atrophy of the skin. In some types of cutaneous sarcoid, e.g. lupus pernio, cosmetic camouflage advice is useful.

Other local therapies reported to be beneficial have included cryotherapy, radiotherapy, PUVA (psoralen ultraviolet A) in hypopigmented and erythrodermic sarcoidosis, pulsed dye laser in lupus pernio, and topical tacrolimus.

Commonly used systemic therapies include oral corticosteroids, pulsed intravenous corticosteroids, methotrexate, and azathioprine. The most frequent indications for systemic treatment include symptomatic pulmonary disease, ocular disease not responding to local corticosteroids, disfiguring skin disease or lymphadenopathy, hypercalcaemia, liver disease with significant dysfunction or hepatomegaly, other organ involvement such as myocardial disease, nervous system disease or renal disease, myopathy or myositis, and thrombocytopenia. See Chapter 18.12 for further details of treatment of the patient with sarcoidosis.

Prednisolone is usually prescribed at 30 to 40 mg mane and reduced over about 2 months to a maintenance dose of prednisolone 15 mg on alternate mornings. Treatment may be necessary for about 6 months, and azathioprine is often introduced for its immunosuppressive and steroid-sparing effects. Intravenous pulsed methylprednisolone, e.g. 1 g/week for 2 months, has been effective in patients with severe systemic disease.

Methotrexate is often an effective systemic agent, usually prescribed as a weekly oral dose (e.g. 7.5–25 mg weekly), with careful monitoring. The response of sarcoidosis to other drugs has been variable, including ciclosporin, chlorambucil, allopurinol, isotretinoin, thalidomide, and minocycline.

Diabetes mellitus and the skin (Chapter 13.11.1)

Skin disorders in individuals with diabetes mellitus include diabetic dermopathy, the most common skin disorder associated with diabetes, cutaneous infections, the consequences of diabetic neuropathy, acanthosis nigricans (related to insulin resistance), and, as discussed above, necrobiosis lipoidica and probably generalized granuloma annulare. Anogenital pruritus in diabetes mellitus may be caused by candidiasis or streptococcal infection, but diabetes is not a proven cause of generalized pruritus. See Chapter 13.11.1 for further discussion of diabetes.

Diabetic dermopathy (diabetic shin spots)

This occurs in about half of the patients with diabetes, men being more commonly affected than women. Diabetic dermopathy is thought to be due to microangiopathy and possible neuropathy. Reddish oval macules and slightly scaly plaques are seen on the shins, forearms, thighs, and over bony prominences, later evolving into brownish atrophic scars, the brown pigment being due to haemosiderin deposition. The presence of these lesions has been suggested to correlate with other internal complications of diabetes including retinopathy, nephropathy, and neuropathy.

Granuloma annulare

Granuloma annulare (GA) is a reaction pattern in the skin with a well-established morphology and natural history, although the aetiology and pathogenesis are unclear. A number of potential antigenic trigger factors have been suggested. There is an association between GA and diabetes mellitus but this is seen uncommonly. Granuloma annulare can occur at any age but most patients are under 30 years old, women being affected more frequently than men.

Localized GA is the most common form and presents as reddish collections of papules which form annular lesions, with palpable edges, often over the knuckles (Fig. 23.15.4) and on the elbows. Other areas of the skin may be involved and a diffuse or generalized pattern occurs uncommonly. In the generalized pattern, there are numerous skin-coloured or erythematous, slightly palpable coalescing papules, arranged symmetrically on the trunk and limbs. Annular lesions may be violaceous in colour and itching is often a feature of the generalized form. Perforating (referring to extrusion of material through the epidermis) and subcutaneous GA are uncommon patterns, the latter sometimes being difficult to distinguish from rheumatoid nodules.

It is reasonable to exclude diabetes mellitus in patients with GA, but this probably occurs in only about 5% cases of localized GA, rising to about 20% in the generalized form. The association

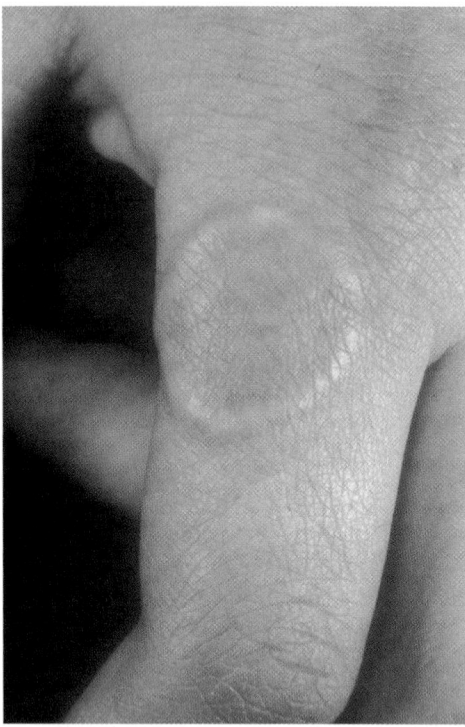

Fig. 23.15.4 Granuloma annulare, showing an annular dermal lesion on the dorsum of the hand.

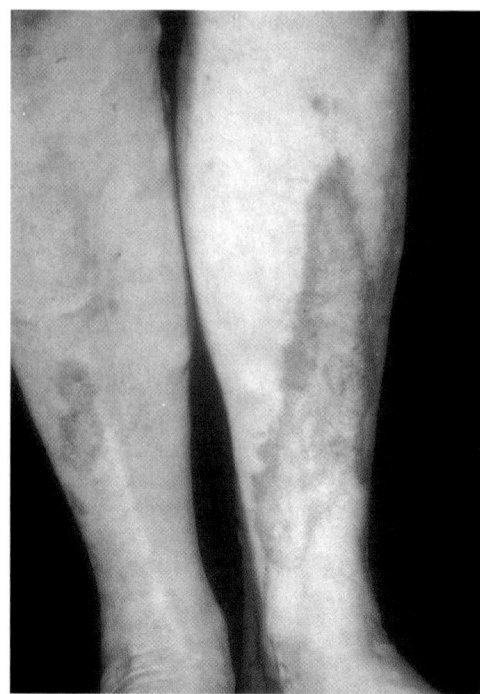

Fig. 23.15.5 Necrobiosis lipoidica, showing reddish-yellow atrophic plaques on the shins.

of GA with diabetes mellitus is debatable, however, and some relatively small studies have not shown a definite association. The distinction from necrobiosis lipoidica, more strongly associated with diabetes mellitus, is usually made histologically but GA and necrobiosis lipoidica can occur in the same patient.

The sporadic occurrence of GA and its tendency to remit spontaneously makes it difficult to assess the efficacy of treatment and in many cases no treatment is needed. Spontaneous remission would occur in about 50% of patients within 2 years but recurrence, usually at the same sites, occurs in 40%.

Potent topical corticosteroids may hasten resolution of localized GA and intralesional triamcinolone can be effective if treatment is required. Cryotherapy has also been used. PUVA seems to be effective for generalized GA. Other treatments reported to be of benefit include retinoids, ciclosporin, local injections of low-dose recombinant interferon-γ, and topical imiquimod or tacrolimus. However, better clinical studies are required in what is a sporadic disorder. In one clinical trial of generalized GA treated with oral potassium iodide, the active drug had no advantage over placebo.

Necrobiosis lipoidica

The precise pathogenesis of necrobiosis lipoidica is unknown, but impaired vascularity of the microcirculation is considered to play a role. The occurrence of diabetes mellitus in up to 60% patients who have necrobiosis lipoidica was probably overestimated previously in tertiary referral populations. Necrobiosis lipoidica may precede the development of diabetes in about one in 10 individuals. However, it does not occur exclusively in diabetes, and the term necrobiosis lipoidica diabeticorum is no longer used. It can occur at any age but usually develops in young adults and in early middle age. There is a female to male ratio of 3:1. Only about 0.3% patients with diabetes mellitus will have necrobiosis lipoidica.

Necrobiosis lipoidica occurs as reddish-yellow shiny plaques on the shins, with atrophy and telangiectasia (Fig. 23.15.5), but early lesions are less obvious. Lesions may ulcerate and a chronic course is usual. In most cases, lesions are bilateral, and they are similar in appearance whether occurring in diabetic or nondiabetic patients.

The differential diagnosis includes granuloma annulare, in which there is less necrobiosis on histology. The yellowish appearance may resemble xanthomatous lesions but this will be distinguished on histology. Necrobiotic xanthogranuloma is a rare disease in which red-orange or yellowish indurated plaques occur on the trunk and periorbital regions, associated with systemic lesions and a monoclonal gammopathy.

Treatment with a superpotent topical corticosteroid under polythene occlusion is effective in settling the active inflammatory process of necrobiosis lipoidica, but the chronic atrophic changes are not reversible and the lesions persist. Early treatment is therefore recommended. Intralesional triamcinolone has been used with good effect, and some dermatologists use perilesional triamcinolone to prevent extension of the process centrifugally. Short courses of prednisolone have been reported to arrest the process but are usually not required.

Psoralen and ultraviolet A (PUVA) using a topical psoralen has been beneficial, as has excision and grafting in severe cases. Other treatments which have been tried in the past with limited success include nicotinamide, clofazimine, pentoxifylline, ciclosporin, mycophenolate mofetil and, more recently, infliximab.

Cutaneous infections in diabetes mellitus

Skin infections due to *Staphylococcus aureus* and group A *Streptococcus haemolyticus* are common in diabetes mellitus. Infections with boils (furuncles), carbuncles (with multiple sinuses), and styes were more common before insulin and antibiotics became available, and good skin care, especially of the feet and lower legs, is essential to help prevent cellulitis. Uncommonly, diabetics are prone to soft tissue infections with a mixture of organisms, sometimes referred to as nonclostridial gas gangrene or bacterial synergistic cellulitis/gangrene, probably a form of necrotizing fasciitis. Well demarcated red areas on the legs and feet of older diabetics do not necessarily indicate cellulitis or erysipelas, and this is sometimes referred to as erysipelas-like erythema.

Candida albicans infections of the mouth, nail folds, genitals, and intertriginous zones (skinfolds) are common in diabetes. A high glucose level in the saliva seems to be related to the increased prevalence of oral candidiasis. Recurring candidal infection is thought to be the cause of an increased prevalence of phimosis in diabetic men.

Diabetic neuropathy

Older patients with diabetes mellitus are at risk of developing a peripheral neuropathy with mixed sensory and motor nerve involvement. Good foot care is essential to prevent the formation of indolent painless perforating ulcers, particularly at pressure points (e.g. from footwear or the bed). The ulcer is usually punched out and often occurs on the sole of the foot in the middle of a callosity. Diabetic ulcers are usually due to a combination of factors including microangiopathy, neuropathy, and an increased tendency to infection.

Acanthosis nigricans and insulin resistance

Acanthosis nigricans, in which there is hyperpigmentation and hyperkeratosis of the flexures (e.g. a velvety appearance in the axillae), exists in two forms. In the absence of obesity, acanthosis nigricans (Fig. 23.15.6) may be an important clinical sign of an underlying adenocarcinoma, e.g. carcinoma of the stomach. The changes of acanthosis nigricans in younger obese patients, in which

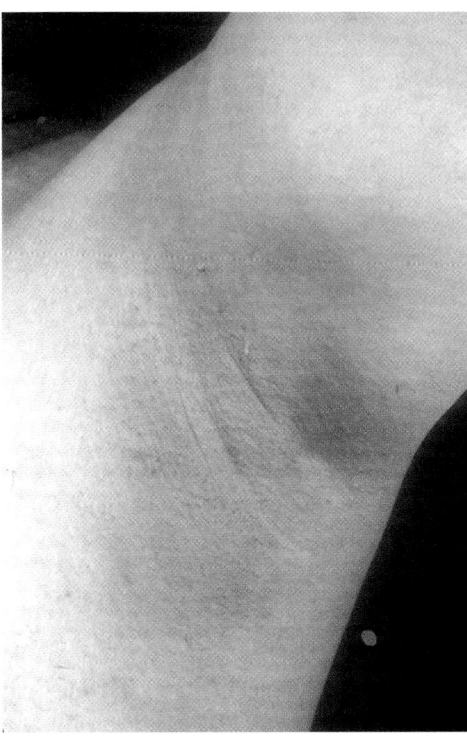

Fig. 23.15.6 Acanthosis nigricans, showing hyperpigmentation and hyperkeratosis of the axillary skin.

the nape of the neck and antecubital fossae are often involved, are associated with insulin resistance (hyperinsulinaemia) and sometimes overt diabetes mellitus. There are considered to be two syndromes of insulin resistance, type A occurring in hyperandrogenic women due to a genetic defect affecting insulin receptor function, and type B in older women with signs of immunological dysfunction.

Other skin disorders associated with diabetes mellitus
Diabetic bullae
Various forms of diabetic blisters occur, presenting as apparently spontaneous lesions mostly on the feet and hands. A typical subepidermal blister occurs on a noninflamed base and heals without scarring in a few weeks.

Skin reactions to insulin
Insulin may cause immediate or, more commonly, delayed reactions in the skin. A delayed reaction usually begins after 2 weeks as an itchy nodule at the site of the injection. It lasts for days before healing, with hyperpigmentation and sometimes scarring.

Insulin lipodystrophy is rare. Atrophic lesions at the sites of insulin injections reflect localized fat atrophy which usually persists.

Vitiligo
Vitiligo occurs more frequently in patients with diabetes mellitus, a prevalence of about 5% being reported in late-onset diabetes.

Wet gangrene of the foot
This is a late manifestation of diabetic microangiopathy, nondiabetic atherosclerotic patients tending to develop a dry form of gangrene due to large vessel disease.

Liver disease and the skin (Section 14)

Numerous systemic diseases may affect the liver and some of these will have cutaneous features (e.g. as occurs in sarcoidosis). The predominant dermatological features and dermatoses associated with liver diseases are discussed here. For a full discussion of liver disease, see Section 14.

Pruritus in liver disease
Generalized pruritus is the most common symptom associated with liver disease. It may precede the onset of jaundice and may be a feature of hepatitis. Itching is most prominent in primary biliary cirrhosis, sclerosing cholangitis, and other forms of biliary tract obstruction, being less of a problem in alcoholic cirrhosis, autoimmune chronic active hepatitis, and haemochromatosis. Improvement in hepatic itching by drugs which block the action of opiates suggests that endogenous opiates may be important in the mechanism of itching.

Treatment is directed at the underlying cause, e.g. drug withdrawal in drug-induced cholestasis, surgery for mechanical biliary obstruction. Antihistamines are usually ineffective. Other approaches have included colestyramine, rifampicin, and various forms of phototherapy.

Pigmentary changes in liver disease
Jaundice is first seen in the sclerae before it becomes generalized. Carotenaemia and drugs, including mepacrine, can also cause yellowing of the skin.

A grey hyperpigmentation may occur in chronic liver disease of any cause. There may be a yellowish tinge due to associated jaundice. The pigmentation is usually more prominent on sun-exposed sites, including the face with perioral and periorbital accentuation. Pigmentation sometimes localizes to the palmar creases, and men sometimes have increased pigmentation of the areola in association with gynaecomastia.

Vascular changes in liver disease

Some of the recognized vascular changes in liver disease are non-specific, including spider naevi (spider telangiectases/spider angiomas) and palmar erythema. Finger clubbing, thought to be due to increased digital pulp blood flow and dilation of arteriovenous anastomoses, occurs in about 15% of patients with cirrhosis.

Hair, nail, and collagen changes in liver disease

The body hair is often thinned and men tend to develop a female pubic hair pattern, due to increased production and decreased metabolism of oestrogens, associated with decreased production and increased metabolism of testosterone. Extensive loss of scalp hair may be due to zinc deficiency.

Nail colour changes include diffuse white colour, proximal white colour, and distal reddish-pink colour, and white bands. Nail plate changes include clubbing (see above), and flattened nails or koilonychia, associated with poor nutrition or altered iron metabolism. Striae occur in both sexes, especially on the lower abdomen, thighs, and buttocks.

Porphyria cutanea tarda

Porphyria cutanea tarda (PCT) is associated with chronic liver disease. In this form of porphyria, there is photosensitivity with blisters, scarring, milia (small epidermal cysts), and hyperpigmentation on sun-exposed areas (e.g. dorsa of hands and forearms) with hypertrichosis of the face (e.g. the temples). See Chapters 11.5 and 23.9.

Lichen planus

The cause of most cases of lichen planus is unknown but lichen planus has been reported in primary biliary cirrhosis, usually following treatment with penicillamine, and in chronic active hepatitis. Hepatitis C virus has also been associated with lichen planus. See Chapter 23.5.

Uncommon skin disorders

Capillaritis of the skin has also been reported in chronic active hepatitis and primary biliary cirrhosis. Other skin disorders include pityriasis lichenoides, pyoderma gangrenosum, the Gianotti–Crosti syndrome, and the signs of zinc deficiency.

Renal disease and the skin

The skin and renal system may be affected by the same disease process. This occurs in various forms of collagen diseases and vasculitis (see Chapter 23.7), in hereditary syndromes such as Fabry's disease (angioma corporis diffusum) and nail-patella syndrome, and in metabolic diseases, including calcific arteriolopathy (calciphylaxis) and primary systemic amyloidosis. Here we concentrate on the cutaneous signs of chronic renal failure, with discussion of recent findings in calcific arteriolopathy and nephrogenic fibrosing dermopathy.

Uraemic pruritus

Generalized severe pruritus occurs in about one-third of patients with renal failure, with many more patients experiencing less troublesome pruritus. In one study, up to 85% of patients on haemodialysis suffered from pruritus, the haemodialysis seeming to provoke the itching in two-thirds of them. There seems to be a correlation between pruritus and predialysis plasma urea levels, but a less obvious relationship between itching and dry skin (xerosis) and secondary hyperparathyroidism. The mechanism of pruritus is complicated, since a reduction in uraemia often does not improve the itching, and pruritus is unusual in acute renal failure. Uraemic neuropathy affects about 60% of patients with renal failure or on long-term haemodialysis and may play a role in uraemic pruritus.

The incidence of uraemic pruritus has been reported to be decreasing, which in part may be due to the use of more sophisticated techniques and equipment for dialysis. In dialysis, lowering the magnesium concentration of the dialysate has been reported to be helpful. In intractable itching, emollients and ultraviolet B (UVB) radiation are reported to be the most effective therapy. Other treatments have included UVA (without psoralen), colestyramine, activated charcoal, and erythropoietin therapy.

Pigmentary changes in chronic renal failure

Anaemia presenting as pallor is an early and common sign of chronic renal failure, resulting from reduced haemopoiesis and increased haemolysis. A greyish-brown discolouration develops in many cases, due to deposition of melanin. Increased nail pigmentation, usually confined to the distal nail, occurs in a proportion of patients. This distal brown or reddish colour, combined with a proximal white appearance gives rise to the term 'half and half' nails, a distinctive pattern seen in about 10% of patients with renal failure.

Purpura due to mild thrombocytopenia or more marked platelet dysfunction is common and may be partly corrected by dialysis. Urea frosting, in which crystalline urea is deposited on the skin, is now exceedingly rare.

Renal transplantation and the incidence of skin cancer

The incidence of skin cancers in patients who have received a renal transplant is above that of the general population, and patients often have numerous viral and dysplastic lesions on their skin, some of which will become malignant. The incidence of basal cell carcinomas (BCCs) rises in a linear fashion from the date of transplantation, but the increase in the incidence of squamous carcinomas (SCCs) rises in an exponential fashion. Sun exposure does play a major aetiological role in these immunosuppressed patients, as in the nontransplanted population. There is a high incidence in Australia with a mean nonmelanoma skin cancer (NMSC) incidence of 28.1%, with a maximum incidence of 47.1% in patients immunosuppressed for more than 20 years. The same group from Queensland noted that white patients at highest risk for developing NMSC have blue or hazel eyes, have spent a longer time living in a hot climate, and are more likely to have a pretreatment SCC. See Chapter 23.14.

Sun avoidance advice is important in all potential renal transplant patients and should be encouraged among the general population.

Calcific arteriolopathy (calciphylaxis)

Calcific arteriolopathy (calciphylaxis, calcific uraemic arteriolopathy, CUA)) is a disorder in which patients, usually with renal failure, develop large painful areas of ulceration. These can be distal involving the limbs, or can be proximal causing large areas of ulceration on the breasts, abdomen, and buttocks.

Recent studies have shown that the calcification is not the same as that seen in patients with skin necrosis, and the term calciphylaxis is considered inaccurate. CUA indicates the site of the calcification and the usual clinical state of the patients. However, CUA has been reported in patients with minimal or no renal failure, hence the author's preferred use of the term calcific arteriolopathy.

In addition to renal failure, the other major risk factors include female gender, white race, diabetes mellitus, obesity, and warfarin and the clotting disorders such as protein C and protein S deficiency. It has also been shown that the use of calcium salts and vitamin D in chronic renal failure is a risk factor. A direct role of hyperparathyroidism in the development of calcific arteriolopathy is not proven, the disease having been described in the presence of a normal parathormone level.

The usual presentation of calcific arteriolopathy is of areas of ulceration on the legs, buttocks, abdomen, or breasts which are painful and may be extensive. Livedo reticularis around the ulcers may be present. Acral ulceration can also occur, causing autoamputation. The differential diagnosis is any cause of ulceration, especially vasculitis, in which livedo reticularis may also be present. Increasing awareness of the condition is allowing the diagnosis of calcific arteriolopathy at an earlier nonulcerative stage, before the subcutaneous indurated plaques develop into ulcers.

The diagnosis of calcific arteriolopathy is usually by biopsy, the histology showing calcification of the media of small arterioles in the skin. This is associated with a brisk intimal proliferation, sometimes with fibrin thrombi visible in the lumen. Other types of vascular calcification are seen in chronic renal failure. The calcification seen in calcific arteriolopathy is no longer thought to be a passive process. The calcium deposited is hydroxyapatite, which is the same as seen in bone. This is different from the compounds found in other types of calcification.

If calcific arteriolopathy is diagnosed at the nonulcerative stage there is some evidence for the use of oral prednisolone at a dose of 30 to 50 mg mane for up to 8 weeks. If ulceration is already present, debridement of the necrotic tissue is sometimes recommended and use of antibiotics to prevent overwhelming sepsis is important. Adequate pain control is another important management measure.

The outcome is poor, with a mortality of about 60% for proximal disease and about 20% for distal disease, usually from overwhelming sepsis. Since there is such a high mortality, the approach should be to aim for prevention. The control of the hyperphosphataemia is thought to be fundamental to this. Phosphate binders are used, with some evidence showing that the non-calcium-containing binders are better. Parathyroidectomy has been found to be useful in the control of calcific arteriolopathy in some series but not in others.

Nephrogenic fibrosing dermopathy

Nephrogenic fibrosing dermopathy (NFD) is a recently reported fibrotic disease occurring in patients with renal disease. NFD was initially reported in patients with established renal failure, either on dialysis or having had a transplant, but it has since been reported in patients with chronic renal insufficiency not requiring renal replacement therapy. An association with the intravenous injection of gadolinium-based radiocontrast media has been suggested.

The clinical presentation of this rare disorder is of plaques of indurated skin on the extensor surfaces of the limbs, and scleral involvement has been described. The limbs are affected in a symmetrical manner with skin-coloured papules coalescing to form brawny plaques with a 'peau d'orange' appearance, occasionally with swelling of the hands and feet. Patients may complain of pain, pruritus, and causalgia. Most patients do not have systemic involvement, but when this is present the disease may be rapidly fatal.

The histology shows an increase in dermal collagen with a paucity of inflammatory cells. There is mucin deposition with abundant eosinophilic spindle cells in the upper dermis that stain for CD34. The disease that NFD is most similar to is scleromyxedema, but the relative sparing of the face in NFD and the lack of a paraprotein allows the diseases to be separated on clinical grounds.

The mainstay of treatment is improvement of the renal function but transplantation is not guaranteed to cure the disease. Treatments such as plasmapheresis, topical calcipotriol under occlusion, PUVA, and oral steroids have been tried, but the results are difficult to assess, since an improvement in renal function is itself an effective form of therapy.

Other systemic diseases and the skin

Pyoderma gangrenosum

Pyoderma gangrenosum (PG) is an uncommon, noninfectious neutrophilic dermatosis commonly associated with underlying systemic disease. Several clinical variants of PG have been described, including ulcerative, pustular, bullous, and vegetative forms.

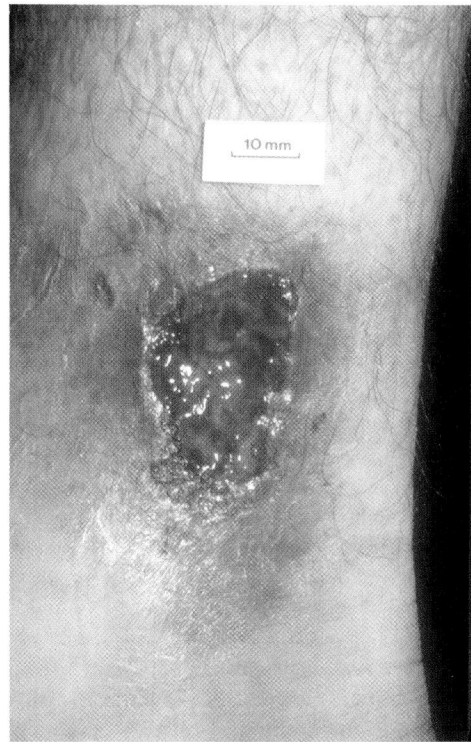

Fig. 23.15.7 Pyoderma gangrenosum, showing ulceration with a characteristically undermined edge on the lower leg.

An immune-mediated process is thought to play an important pathogenetic role, with about 50% of patients having an associated systemic disease. Common associations include inflammatory bowel diseases (ulcerative colitis and Crohn's disease), rheumatoid arthritis and other rheumatological disease, haematological malignancies, and monoclonal gammopathies.

A characteristic presentation of PG begins with small tender papules or pustules that evolve into painful ulceration with typical undermined violaceous edges (Fig. 23.15.7). Lesions may be solitary or multiple. Healing usually occurs with an atrophic cribriform scar (i.e. having a number of small holes within it). Associated symptoms include fever, malaise, myalgia, and arthralgia. Bullous PG is often associated with myeloproliferative disorders. Vegetative or superficial granulomatous PG may have superficial and deep components and is not usually associated with any systemic disease.

The diagnosis of PG is made by recognizing the characteristic clinical features and by excluding other causes of ulceration. A biopsy across the edge of a lesion, depending on the type of PG, will show a neutrophilic infiltrate, but at best the histology is 'consistent with' as opposed to 'diagnostic of' PG.

Many effective treatments for PG have been reported, the precise choice depending on disease severity as well as on the presence of an underlying systemic disease. For early or mild PG, topical therapy with a superpotent corticosteroid or tacrolimus, along with good wound care, may be sufficient. Intralesional triamcinolone may also be effective.

For more severe cases or PG resistant to topical therapy, oral prednisolone has been the mainstay of treatment. Other treatments include pulsed intravenous corticosteroids, minocycline, dapsone, and immunosuppressants such as azathioprine or ciclosporin. Ciclosporin is usually effective at a dose of less than 5 mg/kg per day. Methotrexate has been used for patients with underlying inflammatory bowel disease and, more recently, infliximab and other biological agents have been effective. Less commonly used treatments include plasmapheresis, intravenous immunoglobulin, and thalidomide.

Behçet's disease (Chapter 19.11.5)

Behçet's disease is a multisytem disease that is defined by the presence of oral aphthosis with at least two of the following: genital aphthae, synovitis, posterior uveitis, cutaneous pustular vasculitis, or meningoencephalitis, in the absence of inflammatory bowel disease or autoimmune diseases. It typically affects young adults and is uncommon in northern Europe and the United States of America, but common in Middle Eastern and Japanese populations. Here we focus on cutaneous manifestations, but see Chapter 19.11.5 for a full discussion of Behçet's disease.

Behçet's disease was named after the Turkish dermatologist who described the multisystem disease. The pathogenesis is unclear, but there may be a genetically determined response to an infectious agent. Biopsies of early aphthae or of lesions of pustular vasculitis show a leukocytoclastic vasculitis, although late lesions are lymphocytic.

The clinical course of Behçet's disease is variable, although patients typically have oral aphthae with any combination of genital aphthae, cutaneous pustular vasculitis, ocular lesions, or arthritis. Only pustular vasculitis and erythema nodosum-like nodules should be used to satisfy diagnostic criteria, although a wide range of skin findings (e.g. pyoderma gangrenosum-like lesions) may be present in patients with Behçet's disease. Posterior uveitis is the only ocular criterion for the diagnosis of Behçet's disease, but there are other ophthalmological manifestations. The posterior uveitis in Behçet's disease is due retinal vasculitis and may result in blindness. The musculoskeletal involvement in Behçet's disease is an asymmetrical, migratory, nonerosive oligoarthritis, mimicking rheumatoid arthritis. Many neurological manifestations may occur, but only meningoencephalitis is considered to be a diagnostic criterion. Vascular involvement in Behçet's disease may affect arteries and veins, leading to aneurysms or occlusions that are sometimes fatal.

The diagnosis of Behçet's disease should be suspected in any patient with recurrent and extensive oral aphthosis. Other causes of aphthosis such as inflammatory bowel disease, as well as lesions that mimic aphthae such as herpes simplex virus infection, must be excluded. The diagnosis should also be considered in young patients with deep venous thrombosis, particularly in the absence of other risk factors or thrombophilia.

A positive pathergy provocation test, read at 24 to 48 h, may further support the diagnosis.

Aphthae may be treated with topical or intralesional corticosteroids, topical tacrolimus, or with viscous lidocaine (lignocaine). Oral colchicine may also be used to treat mucocutaneous manifestations, although this option might be limited by gastrointestinal intolerance and requires monitoring for neutropenia. Dapsone in combination with colchicine has also been used successfully. Thalidomide may be effective in this situation but is becoming increasingly difficult to prescribe for women because of the risks to the foetus.

Behçet's disease with manifestations other than mucocutaneous involvement may be treated with systemic corticosteroids, although this may not control severe ocular, neurological, or nonvasculitic vascular disease. Immunosuppressive agents such as ciclosporin, azathioprine, and methotrexate have been used for patients with severe Behçet's disease.

Xanthomas

There are different forms of xanthoma. Eruptive xanthomas of the skin, often on the buttocks and limbs, may develop in patients with hyperlipoproteinaemia in association with diabetes mellitus. Control of the hyperlipoproteinaemia and diabetes usually leads to resolution of the yellowish papules. See Chapter 11.6 for more detailed discussion.

Crohn's disease and the skin

Periorificial granulomatous lesions sometimes occur in Crohn's disease. Perianal abscesses and multiple fissures with fistulae occur in about a quarter of patients. Anal tags which are oedematous or have granulomatous histology are common. Oral Crohn's disease presents as a thickened corrugated appearance of the oral mucosa and lips. Granulomatous cheilitis may precede other features of Crohn's disease.

Cutaneous Crohn's disease may also affect sites not in continuity with the bowel, and reactive dermatoses associated with Crohn's disease include oral aphthae, erythema nodosum (see Chapter 23.7), and pyoderma gangrenosum (see below), a neutrophilic dermatosis. Other skin diseases are rarely associated with Crohn's disease, and it can be difficult to distinguish perianal Crohn's disease from hidradenitis suppurativa.

Thyroid disease and the skin

Thyroid disease is discussed in detail in Chapter 13.4. However, there are a number of cutaneous manifestations of both hypothyroidism and hyperthyroidism. Skin features associated with hypothyroidism include pale and cold extremities, absence of sweating, puffy oedema of hands and face, eczema craquele and pruritus, xanthomatosis (secondary to hyperlipidaemia), coarse sparse hair, brittle/striated nails, purpura/ecchymoses, punctuate telangiectasia on arms and fingertips, and delayed wound healing. Features associated with hyperthyroidism include soft and dry skin, palmar erythema, flushing, increased sweating, fast nail growth, pruritus and urticaria, pretibial myxoedema, acropachy, and diffuse addisonian hyperpigmentation.

Pruritus without a rash

Pruritus associated with systemic disease has been dealt with elsewhere within this chapter, but individuals presenting with itch in the absence of skin disease, should be carefully assessed. It can sometimes be difficult to distinguish secondary changes associated with excoriation from primary skin disease. However, detailed history (including drug history) and thorough systemic examination are crucial. Routine initial investigations might include renal function, full blood count with differential and haematinics, thyroid function, and liver function, with consideration of other investigations dependent on the clinical findings, such as chest radiograph, HIV testing, and screening for malignancy.

Further reading

Archer CB, Robertson SJ (1995). Dermatological aspects of internal medicine. In: Archer CB, Robertson SJ *Black and white skin diseases: an atlas and text*, pp. 155–75. Blackwell Science, Oxford.

Archer CB (2008). Dermatological aspects of internal medicine. In: Archer CB. *Ethnic Dermatology—Clinical Problems and Skin Pigmentation*, pp. 110–25, Informa Healthcare, London.

Barham KL, *et al.* (2004). Vasculitis and neutrophilic vascular reactions. In: Burns T, *et al.* (eds) *Rook's textbook of dermatology*, 7th edition, pp. 49.1–49.46. Blackwell Science, Oxford.

Carroll R, *et al.* (2003). Incidence and prediction of non-melanomatous skin cancer post-renal transplantation: a prospective study in Queensland, Australia. *Am J Kidney Dis*, **41**, 676–83.

Euvrard S, Kanitakis J, Claudy A (2003). Skin cancers after organ transplantation. *N Engl J Med*, **348**, 1681–91.

Finucane KA, Archer CB (2005). Dermatological aspects of medicine: recent advances in nephrology. *Clin Exp Dermatol*, **30**, 98–102.

Gawkrodger DJ (2004). Sarcoidosis. In: Burns T, *et al.* (eds) *Rook's textbook of dermatology*, 7th edition, pp. 58.1–58.24. Blackwell Science, Oxford.

Graham RM, Cox NH (2004). Systemic disease and the skin. In: Burns T, *et al.* (eds) *Rook's textbook of dermatology*, 7th edition, pp. 59.1–59.75. Blackwell Science, Oxford.

Johns CJ, Scott PP, Schonfled SA (1989). Sarcoidosis. *Annu Rev Med*, **40**, 353–71.

Jorizzo JL (1986). Behçet's disease: an update based on the 1985 international conference in London. *Arch Dermatol*, **122**, 556–8.

Li N, *et al.* (1999). Identification of mycobacterial DNA in cutaneous lesions of sarcoidosis. *J Cutan Pathol*, **26**, 271–8.

Sarkany RPE, *et al.* (2004). Metabolic and nutritional disorders. In: Burns T, *et al.* (eds) *Rook's textbook of dermatology*, 7th edition, pp. 57.1–57.124. Blackwell Science, Oxford.

Scadding JG, Mitchell DN (eds) (1985). *Sarcoidosis*, 2nd edition, pp. 1–12. Chapman & Hall, London.

Sterling JC (2004). Virus infections. In: Burns T, *et al.* (eds) *Rook's textbook of dermatology*, 7th edition, pp. 25.1–25.83. Blackwell Science Ltd, Oxford.

Wells RS, Smith MA (1963). The natural history of granuloma annulare. *Br J Dermatol*, **75**, 199–205.

Young AW Jr, *et al.* (1973). Dermatologic evaluation of pruritus in patients on haemodialysis. *N Y State J Med*, **73**, 2670–4.

23.16

Cutaneous reactions to drugs

Peter S. Friedmann and Eugene Healy

Essentials

Adverse drug reactions (ADR) are responsible for about 5% of all hospital admissions, and 10 to 20% of hospital inpatients develop ADRs, many of which involve the skin. ADRs are classified into five groups: (1) type A (augumented)—the most common form of drug reaction, and predictable from the normal pharmacological effects of the drug or its metablite; (2) type B (bizarre)—are not predictable and reflect patient individuality; most cutaneous drug reactions, including hypersensitivity reactions, are of this type; (3) type C (chemical)—can often be predicted from the structure of the drug or its metabolites; some cutaneous reactions are of this type; (4) type D (delayed)—e.g. teratogenicity; (5) type E (end of dose)—withdrawal reactions.

Drugs can induce a very wide variety of skin lesions, ranging from maculopapular eruption/toxic erythma (the most common drug-induced rash, often due to antibiotics) through to the spectrum of erythema multiforme (characterized by target lesions), Stevens–Johnson syndrome (when mucosal surfaces are affected), and toxic epidermal necrolysis (when the blisters become confluent and affect >30% of the skin).

The key to identifying which drug may be responsible for a suspected drug reaction is a thorough clinical assessment in the form of a careful drug history and precise description of the clinical features. Immune mediated reactions require previous exposure or at least a week of ongoing exposure to induce allergic sensitization. *In vivo* or *in vitro* tests are of limited use because, for most drugs, the antigenic molecule, hapten or metabolite is not known or available.

Classification of adverse drug reactions

Adverse drug reactions may be classified as follows:

- Type A (augmented) are the most common type: predictable from the pharmacology of the drug itself or of known metabolites and dose-related—hence dose reduction may resolve the problem.

- Type B (bizarre or idiosyncratic): not predictable from the known pharmacology of the drug. The term reflects patient individuality rather than known drug mechanism of action. There is a dose relationship which is less obvious because it seems to apply at lower doses of drug than those used therapeutically. Most cutaneous drug reactions are of this type, which includes hypersensitivity.

- Type C (chemical): can often be predicted from the structure of the drug or its metabolites. Examples include paracetamol which is bioactivated in the liver to a toxic quinone imine that is hepatotoxic; and azathioprine, metabolized to 6-mercaptopurine which is myelotoxic and must be further converted by the enzyme thiopurine methyltransferase (TPMT). Some cutaneous drug reactions are of this type.

- Type D (delayed): late effects of drugs including teratogenicity and carcinogenicity.

- Type E (end of dose): withdrawal reactions that follow discontinuation of the drug; e.g. seizures after the discontinuation of benzodiazepines.

Interpretation of the clinical patterns of immune-mediated drug hypersensitivities is facilitated by reference to the classification of immune hypersensitivity mechanisms defined by Gell and Coombs (Table 23.16.1).

Factors determining susceptibility to type B reactions

Many type B reactions involve an 'allergic' response in which the immune system recognizes the drug as foreign. Most drugs are chemical entities of low molecular weight (<1000 Da). In order for small molecules to be recognized by the T-cell receptor, they must act as so-called haptens by binding to proteins which act as carriers. The hapten-conjugated protein is then cleaved to peptides which can become complexed with major histocompatibility complex (MHC) molecules. The whole structure of MHC/peptide/

Table 23.16.1 Types of hypersensitivity reaction and the underlying immune effector mechanisms

Type of hypersensitivity	Effector mechanisms
Type I **Immediate or** **anaphylactic**	IgE bound to surface of mast cells or basophils. Antigen binding causes mast cell degranulation, release of histamine and other mediators
Type II **Cytotoxic**	Antigenic determinants on cell surfaces are the target of antibodies—may be IgG or IgM. The antibodies damage cells/tissues by activating complement, or by binding to cytotoxic cells through Fcγ receptors
Type III **Immune complex**	Circulating immune complexes are deposited in vascular beds or on tissue surfaces. Complement is activated, neutrophils attracted, and their products damage tissues
Type IV **Delayed**	Effector T lymphocytes are activated after recognition of specific 'antigen'. The antigen is 'presented' associated with peptide(s) in the groove of MHC molecules. CD4+ T cells are activated via MHC class 2, CD8+ T cells are activated via MHC class 1. The cytokines released generate inflammation

IgE, immunoglobulin E; IgM, immunoglobulin M; MHC, major histocompatbility complex.
(Modified from Coombs RRA, Gell PGH (1968). Classification of allergic reactions responsible for clinical hypersensitivity and disease. In: Gell PGH, Coombs RRA (eds) *Clinical aspects of immunology*, pp. 576–96. Blackwell Scientific, Oxford.)

hapten is thought to be what the T-cell receptor recognizes. Many drug molecules are not intrinsically able to react with proteins but protein-reactive intermediate metabolites can be generated during metabolic detoxication of the drug. Normal detoxication of xenobiotics (foreign chemical substances) generally comprises two phases: phase 1 enzymes of the cytochrome P450 (CYP450) superfamily perform oxygen addition reactions. The intermediates produced may be highly toxic or reactive and so must be rapidly detoxified by phase 2 metabolism (Fig. 23.16.1). Phase 2 enzymes

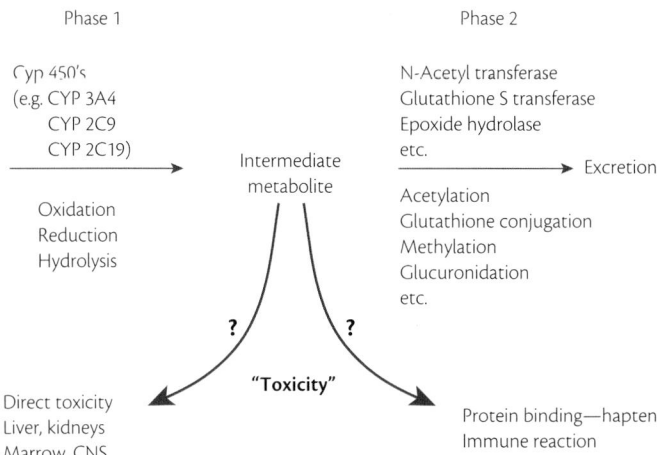

Fig. 23.16.1 Normal metabolic detoxication of drug molecules involves two phases. If there is a defect in phase 2 metabolism, reactive intermediate metabolites may persist. These can either be directly toxic to cells and tissues, or act as haptens, binding to proteins and hence initating immune reactions.

may 'neutralize' reactive epoxides by hydrolysis (epoxide hydrolase) or they attach groups such as acetate (acetyltransferases), or glutathione (glutathione S-transferase), rendering the target water-soluble and capable of excretion. One of the main hypotheses to explain what is different about the individuals who develop ADRs (at least of types B and C) suggests that phase 2 detoxication processes are deficient or fail, allowing persistence of higher levels of toxic or immunogenic intermediate metabolites. For example, individuals with slow capacity to acetylate reactive drug intermediates are generally more susceptible to adverse drug reactions, while fast acetylators are relatively resistant to such reactions. Also, HIV infection results in a general depletion of intracellular glutathione levels and it is well recognized that HIV infection predisposes to a much higher frequence of drug hypersensitivity. However, so far, this general hypothesis has not been clearly supported by identification of specific failure of detoxication.

An alternative hypothesis that is now arising is that differences in the control of the immune system exist such that individuals who develop immune hypersensitivity to a drug somehow fail to generate immunological tolerance—perhaps mediated by suppressive 'regulatory T cells'. The role of genetic factors such as HLA type being determinants of susceptibility to B reactions is suggested by the familial incidence of such reactions, but no definite associations have yet been established.

Clinical patterns of cutaneous adverse drug reactions

Any organ as well as the skin can be involved by these individual-specific reactions. There are three general classes of mechanism; nonimmunological, pseudoallergic, and true allergic.

Nonimmunological are essentially chemical toxicities (called type C in the formal classification). In susceptible individuals, chemical toxicity such as dapsone-induced neuropathy or azathioprine-induced marrow suppression occur with no involvement of immune effector mechanisms.

Pseudoallergic reactions look clinically indistinguishable from type I (immediate) hypersensitivities (see below) with full-blown anaphylaxis, asthma, urticaria, or intestinal cramps and diarrhoea. These reactions are a chemically-induced release of mediators with mast cell degranulation. Examples are intolerances to salicylates, opiates, and muscle relaxants.

Allergic/immune-mediated hypersensitivity. From Table 23.16.1 it will be seen that a range of antibody and cell-mediated effector mechanisms may be activated. The skin is commonly involved in type B reactions and is often the earliest indicator of such reactions. The pattern of reaction in the skin is an excellent indicator of the type of underlying immune effector mechanisms. When the immune system reacts to an immunogen, there is initial activation of T lymphocytes which recognize the 'antigen' when it is presented, associated with the major histocompatibility complex (MHC), by professional dendritic antigen-presenting cells. T cells of CD4+ type see antigen in the context of MHC class II, while CD8+ T cells see it in association with MHC class I. Once T helper (Th) cells are activated by this interaction through the specific T-cell receptors, they will proliferate to generate memory T cells and also, they may help B lymphocytes to make antibodies of different classes: IgM, IgG, IgA, or IgE. This takes a mimimum of 7 days and often longer. It then requires further exposure to the immunogen to elicit the immune effector mechanisms. This may be a second course of the same drug at a later date, or the availability of the drug from a continuous/ongoing exposure. Therefore, the time at which a reaction develops after exposure to a drug can give important clues when it comes to identifying the culprit drug or to ascertaining the mechanism (see below).

Type I hypersensitivity (IgE-mediated) reactions

The reaction patterns which may involve skin, range from urticaria (Fig. 23.16.2a) and angioedema to systemic anaphylaxis. Reactions after drug exposure may occur in about 15 min (immediate phase) or 6 to 24 h later (late phase). It is presumed that interaction of a drug or its immunogenic metabolite with specific IgE bound to the surface of mast cells and possibly basophils triggers the release of vasoactive mediators such as histamine, prostaglandin D_2, leukotriene C4, eosinophil and neutrophil chemotactic factors, platelet activating factor, and bradykinin.

The most common causes of IgE-mediated, drug-induced hypersensitivity are antibiotics (especially the penicillins) and anaesthetic-related drugs, particularly muscle relaxants. Anaphylaxis occurs in 1 per 10 000 courses of penicillin and leads to death in 1 to 5 per 100 000 intramuscular courses. Two surveys of over 2000 patients suffering perioperative anaphylaxis showed that only 52% were due to immune mechanisms, the others were due to pseudoallergic intolerance. Less than 50% of reactions to muscle relaxants are IgE-mediated. This is supported by the observation that the majority of patients (85%) who reacted to muscle relaxants had not had prior exposure to them.

Type II hypersensitivity reactions: cytotoxic/cytolytic mechanisms

In the skin, drug-induced type II immune hypersensitivity may manifest as pemphigus (Fig. 23.16.2b), bullous pemphigoid, or linear IgA disease. Drug-induced pemphigus can be divided into two main groups:

- Drug-dependent pemphigus—where exogenous factors such as thiol (-SH) containing drugs (e.g. D-penicillamine, captopril) cause pemphigus. Once the drug is discontinued the pemphigus usually regresses. Thiol-containing drugs induce mainly pemphigus foliaceus and erythematosus—the pemphigus usually develops within the first 12 to 24 months of commencing the drug.

- True pemphigus (drug-triggered) where the patient has the genetic predisposition (e.g. DRB1*0402, DRB1*1402, and DRB1*0701) for pemphigus, but exogenous factors such as nonthiol drugs are required to trigger the disease. Non-thiol drugs (e.g. penicillins, cephalosporins, piroxicam) trigger pemphigus vulgaris, which explains the increased mucous membrane involvement seen in these patients compared to those with penicillamine induced pemphigus. The onset of drug-triggered pemphigus is about 120 days after commencing the triggering drug and the disease does not regress after withdrawal of the causal drug, but follows the normal natural history of the disease.

Type III hypersensitivity: immune complex mediated vasculitis

Hypersensitivity vasculitis occurs when circulating immune complexes form between IgG or IgM antibodies and antigens from exogenous sources such as bacteria (streptococci), viruses, or drugs. These immune complexes deposit within the postcapillary venules causing vessel wall damage via activation of the complement cascade, with subsequent neutrophil accumulation and release of vasoactive mediators and proteases. Drug-induced vasculitis develops in the skin (Fig. 23.16.2c) and other organs approximately 8 to 10 days after exposure to the causative drug. Presumably, the immune response is directed at the combination of a drug-derived metabolite (hapten) conjugated to a self-protein. Vasculitis is a reaction pattern that may develop after exposure to a wide range of drugs including antibiotics, nonsteroidal anti-inflammatory drugs (NSAID), and cytotoxic drugs, to name but a few. There are so far no real clues as to how the drug or its metabolites are involved in the immune complexes. 'Drug' or therapeutic agents that are macromolecules—such as heparin or streptokinase—can cause vasculitis. Presumably, the substance is handled as a complete antigen in the same way as microbe-derived proteins which evoke 'allergic or hypersensitivity' vasculitis. The quality of the antibody response in terms of binding affinity determines whether immune complexes are of the type easily cleared by the reticuloendothelial system or are soluble and persist in the circulation. Thus, antibodies of intermediate to low affinity favour formation of small soluble complexes that remain in the circulation.

Type IV hypersensitivity: T lymphocyte-mediated reactions

There are two main types of T lymphocyte-mediated reaction: those from topical contact and those from systemic exposure:

- Contact allergic drug hypersensitivity due to topical drug preparations such as antibiotics, antiseptics, local anaesthetics, and corticosteroids. The clinical and immunological features of allergic contact hypersensitivity are dealt with in Chapter 23.6.

- Systemic, T cell-mediated drug hypersensitivity underlies a variety of cutaneous drug reactions such as maculopapular eruptions ('ampicillin rash'), toxic erythemas, erythema multiforme, toxic epidermal necrolysis (TEN), eczematous, lichenoid, and toxic pustuloderma reactions. Many of the published studies have mixed findings from more than one type of reaction, but individual exanthemas have been discussed by Pichler and colleagues.

Maculopapular eruption/toxic erythema

This is the most common pattern of drug-induced skin eruption and can be induced by a very wide range of drugs. Some of the main drugs causing maculopapular eruptions include antibiotics (sulphonamides, β-lactams, and trimethoprim), anticonvulsants including carbamazepine and phenytoin, allopurinol, and NSAIDs. The clinical picture can be diverse, with the rash ranging from tiny erythematous macules and papules to urticaria-like weals. This rash is differentiated from urticaria in that individual weals last days, whereas true urticarial weals only last 2 to 24 h. There is good evidence for maculopapular reactions being a T lymphocyte-mediated

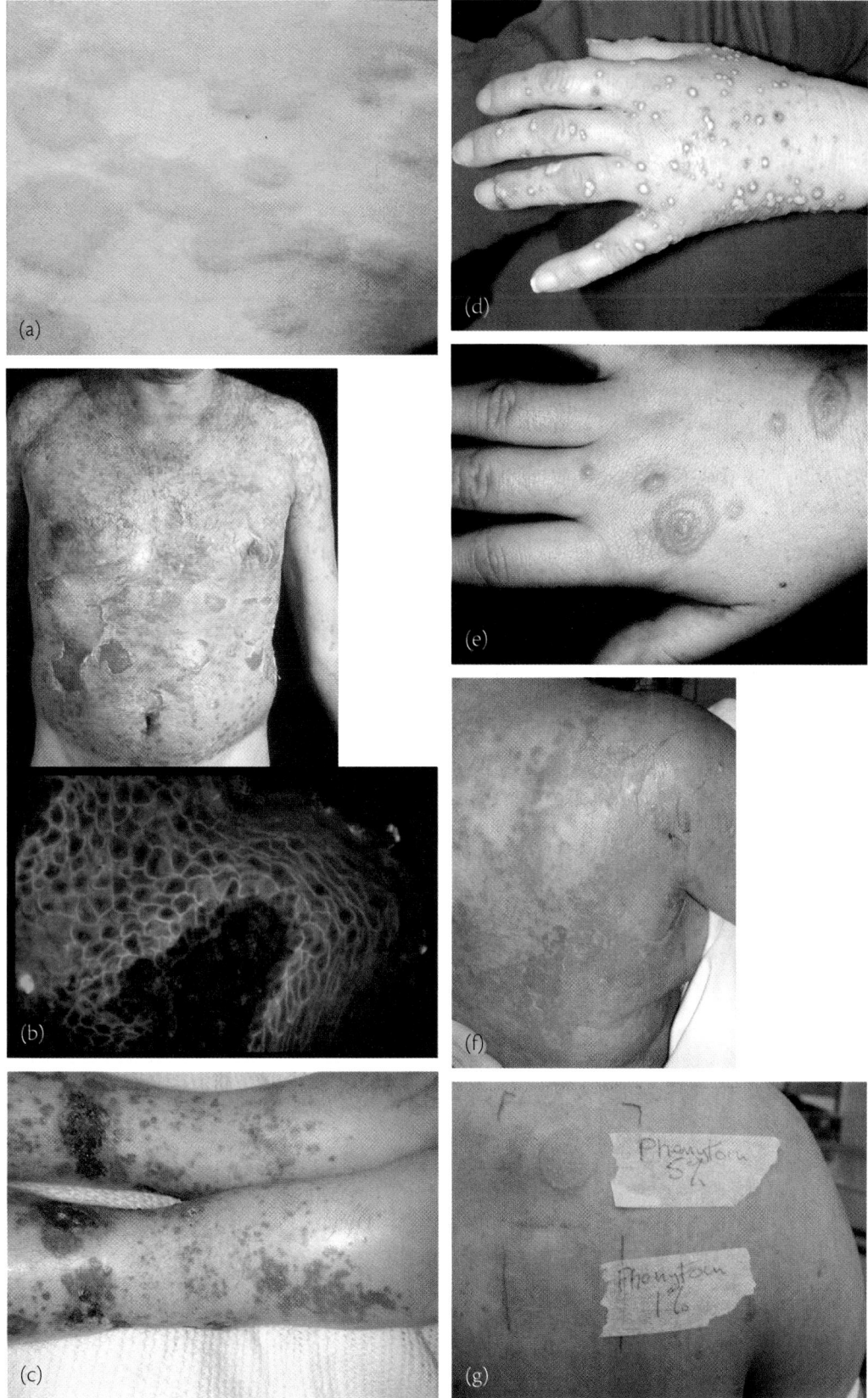

Fig. 23.16.2 Clinical patterns of cutaneous drug hypersensitivity reflecting the allergic hypersensitivity mechanisms. a) Type 1: Urticaria, b) Type 2: Pemphigus foliaceous with immunofluorescence staining of anti-desmoglein antibodies in the epidermis—so-called "chicken wire" pattern, c) Type 3: Hypersensitivity vasculitis, d) Type 4: Acute generalised exanthematous pustulosis (AGEP), e) Type 4: Erythema multiforme, f) Type 4: Toxic epidermal necrolysis (TEN), g) Positive patch tests with phenytoin in a patient who had suffered TEN.

process in that T cells are present in the lesions—predominantly CD4+ cells in the dermal infiltrate, but CD8+ cells in the epidermis and antigen-specific CD8+ T cells have been cultured from lesional skin. Positive 48-h patch tests can be elicited with the culprit drug in a proportion of cases.

Eczematous reaction

Drug-induced eczematous reactions are often a widespread eczema with a distribution that could not be explained by contact with external factors. There are often mixed features of eczema together with either urticated lesions or lichen planus-like lesions that can confuse the diagnostic picture. Eczematous reactions are mediated by CD4+ T cells.

Lichenoid reactions

Lichenoid reactions are so-called because they consist of small, flat-topped papules which may be of a dusky or mauve colour similar to spontaneously occurring lichen planus. Drug-induced lichenoid reactions usually do not involve the buccal mucosa, which helps raise the suspicion that the eruption is drug-induced. Lichenoid reactions often come on months or even years after commencing the causal drug and can take many months to resolve after withdrawal of the drug. The pathogenetic mechanisms have not yet been elucidated but it is likely to be a T cell-mediated process.

Toxic pustuloderma (Fig. 23.16.2d)

These rare reactions are characterized by widely distributed pustules often arising on an erythematous base. They can occur on the palms and soles as well as the torso and limbs. Interestingly, although the inflammatory response generates polymorph neutrophil accumulation as pus, this is due to drug-activated T lymphocytes producing large amounts of interleukin 8 which is chemotactic for neutrophils.

Erythema multiforme, Stevens–Johnson syndrome, and toxic epidermal necrolysis

The classical skin lesion of erythema multiforme (EM) is the so-called target lesion—circular, usually slightly raised, and comprising a set of concentric rings of different colours (Fig. 23.16.2e). The centres are often a dusky/cyanotic hue, while the more peripheral rings are different shades of erythematous pink or white. When the process is more aggressive the lesions blister, when 10 to 30% of body surface is affected it is called EM major, when mucosal surfaces (buccal cavity, eyes, genital mucosae) are involved it is called the Stevens–Johnson syndrome. If the blisters become confluent and more than 30% of the skin is affected, it is referred to as toxic epidermal necrolysis (TEN). In the most severe cases it may be difficult to make out the morphology of individual lesions as the involved area is a confluent mass of detaching skin. The prognosis for full-blown TEN is poor with up to 35% mortality. A scoring system (SCORTEN) awards a point for age (>40), extent of skin involvement, tachycardia more than 120 beats per minute, plasma urea more than 10 mmol/litre, glucose more than 14 mmol/litre, bicarbonate level less than 20 mmol/litre, and presence of malignancy (Table 23.16.2). Scores of 5 or worse predict 90% mortality, while a score of 2 is associated with 12.1% fatality (Table 23.16.3).

Table 23.16.2 The SCORTEN system for assessment of prognostic factors in toxic epidermal necrolysis

Independent prognostic factors	Weight
Age >40 years	1
Cancer/haematological malignancy	1
Body surface area involved at day 1 >10%	1
Serum bicarbonate level <20 mmol/litre	1
Serum glucose level >14 mmol/litre	1
Serum urea level >10 mmol/litre	1
Heart rate >120 beats/min	1

These values were derived from multivariate analysis of 23 variables in 165 patients with toxic epidermal necrolysis (TEN). Each positive criterion is given a score of 1; the correlation between SCORTEN and mortality is shown in Table 23.16.3.
Reprinted by permission from Macmillan Publishers Ltd: Journal of Investigatory Dermatology, SCORTEN: A Severity-of-Illness Score for Toxic Epidermal Necrolysis, S. Bastuji-Garin *et al*, **115**, 149–53, copyright 2000.

The immune effector mechanisms underlying EM involve both CD4+ and CD8+ T cells; T cells from the bullous lesions of TEN have been shown to be CD8+, CD56+, and have NK-like features; there may also be monocyte/macrophages within the epidermis. The epidermal necrolysis is a mass apoptosis of keratinocytes induced by increased production of Fas ligand which interacts with its receptor Fas (CD95), a member of the 'death receptor' family. See Box 23.16.1 for causes of EM.

EM may respond to treatment with systemic corticosteroids, but the epidermal necrolysis cannot be stopped with conventional anti-inflammatory or immunosuppressive agents. There is controversy as to whether high dosage intravenous immunoglobulin (IVIG) can be effective. Some studies showed good effects of IVIG, with significant reductions in expected mortality. Therapeutic success may be related to the presence of naturally occurring antibodies that neutralise Fas ligand. However, there are reports that conflict and suggest IVIG is of no value.

These reaction patterns often involve other organ systems in addition to skin, as reflected by altered liver function tests or haematological indices. The drug hypersensitivity syndrome is characterized by rash, fever, lymphadenopathy, hepatitis, and eosinophilia. The eosinophilia reflects production of large quantities of interleukin 5 by the T cells which are of the Th 2 type.

Table 23.16.3 Mortality rates and relative risks as predicted by SCORTEN

SCORTEN	Mortality rate	Odds ratio
0–1	3.2	1
2	12.1	4.1
3	35.3	14.6
4	58.3	42
>5	90	270

Reprinted by permission from Macmillan Publishers Ltd: Journal of Investigatory Dermatology, SCORTEN: A Severity-of-Illness Score for Toxic Epidermal Necrolysis, S. Bastuji-Garin *et al*, **115**, 149–53, copyright 2000.

Box 23.16.1 Some causes of erythema multiforme

- Drugs, e.g. sulphonamides, anticonvulsants, nonsteroidal anti-inflammatory drugs, and others
- Bacterial infections
- Viral infections, e.g. herpes simplex, orf, infectious mononucleosis, and others
- Histoplasmosis
- Connective tissue diseases
- Malignancy
- Hormonal, e.g. pregnancy
- Sarcoidosis

Assessment of causality

The key to identifying which drug may be responsible for a suspected drug reaction is a thorough clinical assessment in the form of a careful drug history and precise description of the clinical features. Drawing a flow diagram of the times and doses of drug administration in relation to the onset of the reaction (Fig. 23.16.3) can be very helpful. The morphology of the rash will help indicate the type of immune mechanism involved, which is relevant to possible treatment and diagnostic tests. It must be remembered that urticarial rashes, suggestive of type I (IgE/mast cell) mechanisms, are characterized by individual weals of short duration—lasting less than 24 h. Lesions that can look like urticarial weals but which last for days may indicate 'toxic erythema' or even erythema multiforme, which are mediated by T cells. Urticaria can be 'pseudoallergic', reflecting drug intolerance, in which case previous exposure may not have occurred. However, immune mediated reactions require previous exposure or at least a week of ongoing exposure to induce allergic sensitization.

Diagnostic tests

In vivo or *in vitro* tests may be carried out, but these are usually confined to research centres with an interest in drug allergy. The robustness and range of such tests is, at present, limited mainly because, for the majority of drugs, the correct antigenic molecule, hapten or metabolite is not known or available. The choice of test is important and depends on the suspected immune mechanism underlying the drug reaction. Skin testing, i.e. prick, intradermal, or patch testing is usually performed 6 weeks to 6 months after resolution of the reaction. It may, however, lead to relapse of symptoms and for this reason, low concentrations of the suspected agent are used initially. In general no tests are available for type II or III hypersensitivities.

For immediate (type I) hypersensitivities, skin prick tests can be performed with some drugs—particularly the penicillin family and some drugs available for parenteral administration such as muscle relaxants and anaesthetic induction agents. Positive reactions develop within 15 min of the challenge. The challenges should be performed in a setting with full cardiopulmonary resuscitation facilities. Quantitation of specific IgE antibodies are available for a limited range of drugs, including the penicillin family. Some centres can perform basophil degranulation tests which indicate the presence of specific IgE on the surface of basophils.

For lymphocyte-mediated reactions, patch tests with the drugs made up to 1, 5, and 10% in white soft paraffin can often produce positive responses. The drug challenge is applied on the back in special patch test chambers which are left in place for 48 h. Positive tests are erythematous areas, often raised and sometimes, in patients who have had EM/TEN, they may blister (Fig. 23.16.2g). Some centres are able to perform *in vitro* lymphocyte stimulation

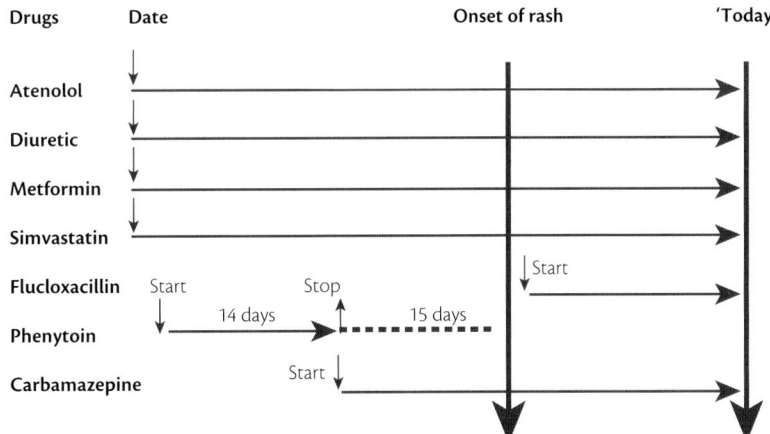

Fig. 23.16.3 A patient undergoing neurosurgery for a meningioma develops fever and rash—severe EM/TEN on the date 'Onset of Rash'. 'Today', 3 days later, dermatologists are consulted. Atenolol, the diuretic, metformin, and simvastatin had been started long before. Flucloxacillin was started after the rash erupted (so cannot be the cause). Phenytoin was started immediately postoperatively for 14 days but was discontinued because of failure to control seizures. Carbamazepine was started and has continued until 'Today'. Although the upper four drugs must be considered, they have all been administered long term and none is notorious for this type of reaction. The most likely culprits are the anticonvulsants. Carbamazepine would be the most probable as it was started 15 days before the onset of the EM/TEN. However, phenytoin was also administered for 14 days—enough time to evoke the reaction and it is probable that if it were the responsible culprit, the eruption would have commenced sooner. Sometimes hypersensitivity reactions can commence after withdrawal of a drug, but they usually start subsiding within a few days; if the culprit is still being administered the process will be likely to be exacerbating.

tests which give positive responses indicating the presence of drug-reactive T cells. Oral challenges should never be performed in patients with type I hypersensitivity where there is a question of anaphylaxis or in patients who have had Stevens–Johnson syndrome or TEN. See Chapter 23.17 for further details of management of severe reactions.

Further reading

Abuaf N, *et al.* (1999). Validation of a flow cytometric assay detecting in vitro basophil activation for the diagnosis of muscle relaxant allergy. *J Allergy Clin Immunol*, **104**, 411–18. [Describes an in vitro method for diagnosing type 1 hypersensitivity.]

Barbaud A, *et al.* (2001). Guidelines for performing skin tests with drugs in the investigation of cutaneous adverse drug reactions. *Contact Dermatitis*, **45**, 321–28. [Gives a good overview of the approach to skin testing in the diagnosis of drug allergy.]

Bastuji-Garin S, *et al.* (2000). SCORTEN: a severity-of-illness score for toxic epidermal necrolysis. *J Invest Dermatol*, **115**, 149–53. [Defines the SCORTEN system for prognosis in TEN.]

Britschgi M, *et al.* (2001). T-cell involvement in drug-induced acute generalized exanthematous pustulosis. *J Clin Invest*, **107**, 1433–41. [Demonstrates that these pustular reactions are indeed the result of T cell-derived cytokines.]

Brown KM, *et al.* (2004). Toxic epidermal necrolysis: does immunoglobulin make a difference? *J Burn Care Rehabil*, **25**, 81–8. [Showed no benefit from treatment of TEN with IVIG.]

Campione E, *et al.* (2003). High-dose intravenous immunoglobulin for severe drug reactions: efficacy in toxic epidermal necrolysis. *Acta Derm Venereol*, **83**, 430–32. [Showed a clear benefit from using IVIG in treatment of TEN.]

Cavani A, *et al.* (2003). Immunoregulation of hapten and drug induced immune reactions. *Curr Opin Allergy Clin Immunol*, **3**, 243–47. [Seminal work showing that tolerance to drugs and contact sensitizers is maintained by regulatory T cells.]

Chan HL, *et al.* (1990). The incidence of erythema multiforme, Stevens–Johnson syndrome, and toxic epidermal necrolysis. A population-based study with particular reference to reactions caused by drugs among outpatients. *Arch Dermatol*, **126**, 43–7. [A large epidemiological survey of the frequency of severe drug hypersensitivity reactions.]

Coombs RRA, Gell PGH (1968). Classification of allergic reactions responsible for clinical hypersensitivity and disease. In: Gell PGH, Coombs RRA (eds) *Clinical aspects of immunology*, pp. 576–96. Blackwell Scientific, Oxford. [The original classification of immune mechanisms involved in different patterns of allergic hypersensitivity.]

Hertl M, Merk HF (1995). Lymphocyte activation in cutaneous drug reactions. *J Invest Dermatol*, **105**, 95S–98S. [Demonstration that maculopapular drug reaction lesions contain drug-specific T lymphocytes.]

Laxenaire MC (1993). Drugs and other agents involved in anaphylactic shock occurring during anaesthesia. A French multicenter epidemiological inquiry. *Ann Fr Anesth Reanim*, **12**, 91–6. [Demonstration of the occurrence of pseudoallergic (intolerance) mechanisms in about 50% of cases of anaphylaxis induced by perianaesthetic drugs.]

Matzner Y, *et al.* (1995). Identical HLA class II alleles predispose to drug-triggered and idiopathic pemphigus vulgaris. *Acta Derm Venereol*, **75**, 12–14. [Demonstration that drug triggered pemphigus occurs in people with the identical HLA-haplotype as in patients who develop spontaneous pemphigus vulgaris.]

Park BK, Pirmohamed M, Kitteringham NR (1992). Idiosyncratic drug reactions: a mechanistic evaluation of risk factors. *Br J Clin Pharmacol*, **34**, 377–95. [Review of pharmacological and immune mechanisms involved in susceptibility to drug hypersensitivity.]

Park BK, Pirmohamed M, Kitteringham NR (1998). Role of drug disposition in drug hypersensitivity: a chemical, molecular, and clinical perspective. *Chem Res Toxicol*, **11**, 969–88. [Review in which the possibility that failure to detoxify reactive drug metabolites could be crucial to formation of allergic responses to the drug is discussed.]

Pichler W, *et al.* (2002). Pathogenesis of drug-induced exanthems. *Allergy*, **57**, 884–93. [Review of the immune mechanisms involved in the different types of drug rashes.]

Pirmohamed M, *et al.* (2004). Adverse drug reactions as cause of admission to hospital: prospective analysis of 18 820 patients. *BMJ*, **329**, 15–19. [Recent epidemiological survey that quantifies the problem of adverse drug reactions as a cause of admission to hospitals.]

Roujeau JC (1994). The spectrum of Stevens–Johnson syndrome and toxic epidermal necrolysis: a clinical classification. *J Invest Dermatol*, **102**, 28S–30S. [The account defining the clinical features required to make the diagnosis of these conditions.]

Trent JT, *et al.* (2003). Analysis of intravenous immunoglobulin for the treatment of toxic epidermal necrolysis using SCORTEN: The University of Miami Experience. *Arch Dermatol*, **139**, 39–43. [Clear evidence of a protective effect of IVIG in TEN.]

Viard I, *et al.* (1998). Inhibition of toxic epidermal necrolysis by blockade of CD95 with human intravenous immunoglobulin. *Science*, **282**, 490–93. [The first work to show the major protective effect of IVIG in TEN with analysis of mechanisms by which it acts.]

Management of skin disease

Rod Sinclair

Essentials

Topical therapy employs a vehicle (ointments, creams, lotions, gels) to deliver an active ingredient to the skin, to provide a protective barrier, or to hydrate and moisturize the skin. There are many types of topical treatments, including (1) antipruritics, e.g. calamine, are used to relieve itching; (2) keratolytics, e.g. salicylic acid, urea, are used to remove hyperkeratotic skin; (3) tars act by reducing the thickness of the epidermis; (4) corticosteroids have anti-inflammatory and immunosuppressive effects that are useful in treating many skin disorders; (5) calcipotriol (an analogue of 1,25-dihydroxycholecalciferol) reduces epidermal proliferation and is used in local treatment of plaque psoriasis; (6) retinoids influence immune function and have some anti-inflammatory activity and are used in acne; (7) antiseptics, e.g. benzoyl peroxide, chlorhexidine; (8) antifungal agents; (9) sunscreens; (10) anaesthetics/analgesics.

Other dermatological treatments include phototherapy (e.g. for psoriasis), photodynamic therapy (e.g. for actinic keratosis), and cryotherapy (e.g. for viral warts). Systemic therapies include oral retinoids, cytotoxics, and immunosuppressants.

There have been many recent advances in the topical and systemic treatments available for skin diseases and it is likely that these developments will continue. Examples include the use of calcineurin inhibitors for eczema and other diseases, immunomodulatory drugs such as imiquimod for some human papillomavirus infections, superficial basal cell carcinomas, and other diseases, and the emergence of the biological therapies as effective interventions for psoriasis and many other disorders.

General principles of therapy

Topical therapy employs a vehicle to deliver an active ingredient to the skin, to provide a protective barrier, or to hydrate and moisturize the skin.

Compliance and adherence

Noncompliance to the clinician's instructions is an important consideration in the treatment of dermatological disease where patients may be asked to apply sticky and unpleasant preparations. The incidence has been estimated at around 30%.

Helping patients to understand their disease encourages them to follow instructions from their medical attendant. Patient involvement in the decision making process can be helpful in building rapport when dealing with a chronic problem like psoriasis or atopic dermatitis.

Compliance is affected by the cost of medication so a clear indication of the likely duration, cost, and quantities needed for adequate treatment should be given, especially if the patient is financially disadvantaged.

When prescribing topical preparations, it is important to provide patients with sufficient quantities. Full body coverage requires 40 g of a cream and slightly less if applying an ointment.

Dermatological vehicles

Dermatological vehicles are composed of one or more of the following ingredients: powders, e.g. zinc oxide, starch, calamine, or talc; liquids, e.g. water, alcohol, glycerol, or propylene glycol; oils, greases, or waxes, e.g. peanut oil, castor oil, liquid paraffin, white and yellow soft paraffin, wool fat, hard paraffin, beeswax, or polyethylene glycols (macrogols). These ingredients are combined to produce ointments, creams, gels, powders, lotions, paints, tinctures, and pastes.

Ointments

Ointments consist of oils, greases, or waxes and have little or no water. They are generally greasy, but can be rendered water miscible if an emulsifying agent is included. They have emollient, protective, and occlusive properties. Greasy ointments can be sticky and difficult to remove, and are often not well received by patients. Nongreasy ointments such as macrogol ointment consist of polyethylene glycols and are water-soluble. They spread well on the skin and wash off with water. Ointments are not prone to mould or bacterial growth and therefore do not require the addition of preservatives.

Creams

Creams contain ointment and water, stabilized by an emulsifying agent. The stability and the drug-carrying ability of these finely balanced emulsions are dependent on the pH of the creams, the type and amount of emulsifying agents used, and the chemical properties of the active ingredients.

Lotions

Lotions are liquid preparations. They may be aqueous or alcoholic solutions, suspensions, or emulsions. They are easily spread, have a cooling effect, and a low risk of irritation to the skin. They are often used to deliver a thin layer of powder to the affected surface over a large or hairy area. Shake lotions such as calamine lotion tend to evaporate quickly, providing a cooling effect, but leaving a layer of powder on the skin.

Gels

Gels are water-miscible, viscous preparations which contain no oil. They contain a gelling agent such as tragacanth, gelatin, or hydroxypropyl cellulose, together with a solvent such as glycerol, propylene glycol, or alcohol, and a preservative. Gels form a durable film which stays on the skin surface longer than a water-miscible cream. They are suitable for the delivery of water-soluble drugs.

Additives

Preservatives

Preservatives are added to products with high water content, e.g. creams, lotions, and shampoos, to inhibit the growth of moulds or bacteria and prevent spoilage. All preservatives are capable of producing irritant or allergic contact dermatitis.

Absorption enhancers

A number of chemical agents can be added to the vehicle base to enhance percutaneous absorption of certain drugs. These agents include propylene glycol, dimethyl sulfoxide (DMSO), cetrimide, and sodium lauryl sulfate.

Antioxidants

Antioxidants are sometimes added to topical preparations to increase the stability of formulations that are susceptible to oxidation. These agents act either by reacting with free radicals and blocking oxidation by competing for oxidation (reducing agents), or by enhancing the action of other antioxidants.

Emulsifiers

Emulsifiers are added to stabilize complex ingredients, vehicles, and additives. For water-based preparations, the issue of ion compatibility must be considered when emulsifiers are selected.

Vehicle choice

The vehicle is a critical factor in the effectiveness of all topical therapies. Some vehicle-related key factors which may influence therapeutic outcome in topical therapy are water/lipid miscibility, occlusive properties, and durability. The following guide can be used in the selection of an appropriate vehicle or base for a particular use.

Creams and ointments are the most commonly used bases and the selection usually depends on the degree of hydration of the skin, as well as cosmetic factors. Creams are generally used on normal or moist skin. They are cosmetically acceptable for use on the face, and are suitable for use in the flexures and for application to large areas. However, some creams can be drying if the skin is already very dry. The preservatives in creams can also cause contact dermatitis in some patients.

Ointments are generally used when the skin is dry, when enhanced absorption is required (ointments are generally more effective than creams), and when avoidance of preservatives is desirable.

Lotions are generally used on wet surfaces, e.g. wet rashes (soaks or wet dressings) and oral mucosa (mouthwashes), or on hairy areas, e.g. scalp, axillae, and pubic area.

Gels are used as alternatives to lotions in hairy areas and where a drying effect is beneficial; and this applies especially to gels with an alcoholic base such as use in the treatment of acne. Gels or lotions containing alcohol should not be applied to excoriated or abraded skin, as they will sting.

Pastes are used for occlusion and protection, and where substantive effects are required, allowing the drug to stay in contact with the skin for prolonged periods. They are also used in the application of an irritant drug to a limited area of skin, e.g. dithranol or a high concentration of salicylic acid.

Moisturizers

Moisturizers can be categorized into emollient, humectant, and occlusive (see Table 23.17.1). Excessive soaking in water damages the waterproof seal on the skin, allowing a net water loss and dehydration. The best time to apply a moisturizer is immediately after a handwash or a bath.

Emollients are preparations of emulsified oils and fatty acids, which replace the natural oils in the stratum corneum. These molecules are incorporated into the epidermal structure, repairing the epidermis and providing a humidifying barrier to loss of water from between the cells of the keratin layer, which is the main source of loss, as well as from the skin surface, thereby increasing the water holding capacity of the skin.

Humectants contain chemicals that attract and retain water due to their hygroscopic or osmotic properties. They act by causing a migration of water from the epidermis to the skin surface as well as trapping water on its way out.

Occlusive preparations provide an external physical barrier over the skin surface to prevent transepidermal water loss, at the same time replacing the natural oils in the stratum corneum. They are very effective but are greasy and often not cosmetically acceptable to patients.

Topical antipruritics

Calamine

Calamine is zinc carbonate or zinc oxide powder mixed with a small amount of ferric oxide, which gives it its pink colour. It is a mild astringent and antipruritic, and is used as a soothing and protective application in dusting powders, creams, lotions, and ointments.

Table 23.17.1 Types of moisturizers

Emollient	Humectant	Occlusive
Aqueous cream	Urea 10% cream	White soft paraffin 50% in liquid paraffin
Sorbolene cream	Glycerol 10% cream	White/yellow soft paraffin
Peanut oil 5% cream		
Olive oil 10% cream		

Camphor

This is a white, crystalline ketone, which acts as a mild topical analgesic and a counterirritant. It is readily absorbed from all surfaces and systemic adverse effects such as nausea, dizziness, headache, and breathing difficulties may occur.

Menthol

Menthol is a crystalline substance obtained from mint oils or prepared synthetically. When applied topically, it will dilate blood vessels and cause a cooling and analgesic effect. It is used in creams and ointments to relieve itching in pruritus. However, it has the potential to cause allergic reactions and contact dermatitis, and may sting if applied to broken skin.

Keratolytics

Keratolytics are used to remove hyperkeratotic skin in conditions such as dermatitis, seborrhoeic dermatitis, ichthyosis, psoriasis, palmoplantar keratoderma, warts, and acne.

Salicylic acid and benzoic acid

Salicylic acid and benzoic acid are keratolytic agents with mild bacteriostatic and antifungal properties. They are both mild irritants and can themselves cause dermatitis.

Salicylic acid has been used topically as a 2 to 10% cream or ointment for hyperkeratotic dermatitis, although concentrations as high as 50% have been used in palmoplantar keratoderma. A 2% alcoholic lotion is used in acne to unblock comedones. It can be combined with liquor picis carbonis (LPC) in the treatment of psoriasis and dermatitis or with sulphur in the treatment of ichthyosis. Salicylic acid 30% in mineral oil is used to remove scale from the scalp. For warts, a 10 to 15% paint or a 20 to 72% paste can be used. Benzoic acid 6% can be used with 3% salicylic acid (Whitfield's ointment) for treating fungal infection of the skin, but specific targeted antifungal treatments are more effective (see Chapter 23.10).

Urea

Urea is a mild bactericidal keratolytic agent and promotes hydration of the skin by increasing the ability of the epidermis to absorb water. It is used as a 10% cream for moisturizing, or a 20 to 60% soak solution for the treatment of hyperkeratotic dermatitis.

Propylene glycol

Propylene glycol is a keratolytic agent with some bactericidal and fungicidal properties. A 40 to 60% solution applied under occlusion can be used to clear scaling skin in hyperkeratotic eczema.

Tars

Introduction

Tars act by reducing the thickness of the epidermis and are used for the treatment of psoriasis, dermatitis, seborrhoeic dermatitis, and dandruff. Their efficacy is enhanced when ultraviolet B (UVB) therapy is given after application of the tar. Controversies exist in relation to the potential carcinogenic and teratogenic effects, and to the increased risk of carcinogenicity with concurrent use of tar application and ultraviolet (UV) therapy. Long-term treatment with high concentration tar preparations is not encouraged.

Coal tar

Coal tar is obtained from bituminous coals at high temperature. It has anti-inflammatory, antipruritic, and mild antiseptic properties.

Crude coal tar 0.5 to 5% is included in creams, ointments, pastes, shampoos, and soaps, often in combination with salicylic acid. Coal tar solution (liquor picis carbonis or LPC), which is a 20% solution of coal tar in alcohol, is used in concentrations of 3 to 12%. Coal tar may cause skin irritation and photosensitivity, but hypersensitivity reactions are uncommon. Preparations stain clothing and skin and have a mild odour, which may affect compliance.

Pine tar

Pine tar is obtained from the destructive distillation of the wood of trees belonging to the Pinaceae family. It has antipruritic properties, but does not have the anti-inflammatory properties or photosensitizing potential of coal tar. It is included in a variety of proprietary preparations as solutions, cleansing bars, gels, and bath oils.

Ichthammol

Ichthammol is a black, viscous liquid with a strong odour, consisting of a destructive distillation product of bituminous schist or shale together with ammonium sulphate. It has a mild antibacterial effect and is used in chronic dermatitis. It is a mild skin irritant. It is included in proprietary preparations for the treatment of dermatitis, psoriasis, and acne. Ichthammol 2% in glycerol lotion has been used for the treatment of ear psoriasis.

Dithranol

Dithranol is a yellow to orange powder of synthetic trihydroxyanthracene. When used in topical preparations, its strength starts at 0.05 or 0.1% and gradually increases to 3% as required. Strengths as high as 6% have been used in severe cases. It has anti-inflammatory properties. It stains skin and many fabrics and surfaces. Liquid paraffin may be used to remove dithranol products from the skin.

Dithranol reduces proliferation of the epidermis by inhibiting enzyme metabolism and reducing mitotic turnover. As it is irritant to mucosal surfaces, inflamed skins, and other delicate skin areas, it should not be used on the face, groin, and perilesional skin. Patients with fair skin are more sensitive. Concomitant use of coal tar may reduce its irritating effect. Dithranol can be localized to the plaques by application in Lassar's paste. Application of white soft paraffin to the perilesional areas may provide further protection.

Dithranol is better absorbed through plaques of psoriasis than normal skin. There are two methods of dithranol treatment: low-strength, long-contact therapy and high-strength, short-contact therapy. It is also used in the treatment of alopecia areata. While its mode of action is unknown, it is not effective unless skin irritation is produced.

Dithranol preparations have many problems with stability, which decreases with the strength of the preparations. Addition of salicylic acid, ascorbic acid, or oxalic acid as an antioxidant stabilizes dithranol products and prevents discolouration and inactivation. White soft paraffin appears to be the most stable base, while cream bases are least stable. Dithranol must be protected from light and should be supplied in appropriate light-occlusive containers.

Topical corticosteroids

The naturally occurring hydrocortisone has anti-inflammatory and immunosuppressive effects, which are useful in treating many skin disorders. Modifications of the hydrocortisone molecule have produced a large number of agents with varying anti-inflammatory potency, which may be used systemically or topically.

Table 23.17.2 Classification of potencies of topical corticosteroids

Class I—mild	
Hydrocortisone	0.5–1%
Hydrocortisone acetate	0.5–1%
Class II—moderate	
Alclometasone dipropionate	0.05%
Betamethasone valerate	0.02, 0.05%
Triamcinolone acetonide	0.02, 0.05%
Class III—potent	
Betamethasone dipropionate	0.05%
Betamethasone valerate	0.1%
Methylprednisolone aceponate	0.1%
Mometasone furoate	0.1%
Triamcinolone acetonide	0.1%
Class IV—very potent	
Clobetasol	0.05%

The potency of topically applied corticosteroids is ranked according to clinical effectiveness and potential for adverse effects (see Table 23.17.2). Adverse effects consist of loss of dermal collagen (leading to skin atrophy, striae, fragility, and easy bruising), telangiectasia, and perioral dermatitis.

Penetration of corticosteroid to the dermis is greater on the face, the scrotum, and where conditions mimic application under occlusion, i.e. flexures and intertriginous areas. The use of the more potent corticosteroids on these sites therefore carries greater risk of local damage and should be avoided. With greater potency, there is increased risk of rebound on withdrawal and of tachyphylaxis.

Absorption of more potent agents applied to large areas may cause suppression of the hypothalamic-pituitary axis and other usual complications associated with systemic corticosteroid administration.

Topical corticosteroids should not be used on a patient where the diagnosis is uncertain. For example, patients may use topical corticosteroids for years on a groin rash where the diagnosis is tinea cruris, which is curable with correct treatment.

It is common for patients to express reluctance to use topical corticosteroids because of misconceptions about the risks of their use.

Suggested potencies and preparations for intermittent use of topical corticosteroids for chronic dermatoses are:

◆ face and flexures (hydrocortisone 1%)

◆ trunk (betamethasone valerate 0.02%, triamcinolone acetonide 0.02%)

◆ elbows/knees and palms/soles (betamethasone dipropionate 0.05%, mometasone 0.1%, methylprednisolone aceponate 0.1%)

Potent corticosteroids should be avoided on the face. However, more potent corticosteroids may be used intermittently for up to 2 weeks. The greater the potency the greater the risk of local adverse effects, particularly perioral dermatitis.

Calcipotriol

Calcipotriol is an analogue of 1,25-dihydroxycholecalciferol, the active form of vitamin D. It shares with the vitamin affinity for an intracellular receptor, combination with which reduces epidermal proliferation and inhibits interleukin 1 (IL-1) and T-cell function. It is used topically as an ointment or cream in local treatment of plaque psoriasis. Adverse effects include erythema and irritation. The theoretical possibility of hypercalcaemia, renal calculi, and ectopic calcification due to absorption is not a practical problem unless it is applied to large areas of inflamed skin. It should not be used on the face or flexures.

Retinoids

The term vitamin A refers to a group of compounds that are necessary for cellular differentiation, organ development, and production of the visual pigment in the retina. These compounds also influence immune function and have some anti-inflammatory activity.

Tretinoin creams in concentrations ranging from 0.025 to 0.1% can be used for acne and sun damage. Acne sufferers can experience some erythema, dryness, and irritation, which can be managed by decreasing the frequency of application or discontinuing the preparation.

Patients with sun-damaged skin react more vigorously to topical tretinoin, and its use should be titrated for the individual patient, starting with a daily application for 10 min before washing off. The duration of application can be increased until the preparation is eventually left on overnight.

The best results in the treatment of sun damage are not seen until the preparation has been used for 6 months but include improvement in texture, reduction of pigmentation, removal of superficial solar keratoses, and effacement of small wrinkles. Topical isotretinoin and adapalene are used in acne and may also cause drying, erythema, burning, and photosensitivity, but generally these symptoms would be less than with tretinoin.

Antiseptics

Benzoyl peroxide

Benzoyl peroxide has mild keratolytic, antiseptic, and bleaching properties. It is used in the treatment of acne as a 2.5 to 10% gel. Its antiseptic properties are probably the result of its oxidizing effect. Bleaching of clothing may occur where it is in contact with the agent. As irritation is common, caution is needed when applying it near the eyes and other mucosal surfaces. The irritation usually resolves on continued use.

Chlorhexidine

Chlorhexidine is a bisbiguanide antiseptic that is commonly used in topical preparations with or without cetrimide. It is used as the acetate, gluconate, or hydrochloride in sprays, creams, gels, solutions, dressings, and powders in concentrations ranging from 0.02 to 5%.

Chlorhexidine salts may cause skin reactions, irritate mucosal surfaces, and interrupt wound healing. Discolouration of the teeth, tongue, and the buccal cavity associated with chlorhexidine mouthwash or oral gel has been reported.

Cetrimide

Cetrimide is a quaternary ammonium antiseptic with surfactant properties. It has been used alone or with chlorhexidine in topical preparations in concentrations ranging from 0.1 to 3%. Skin sensitivity may occur, particularly with repeated and prolonged applications. Application to mucosal surfaces should be avoided.

Povidone-iodine

Povidone-iodine is an iodine complex which has antibacterial, antifungal, and antiviral properties. It is used in mouthwash/gargles, skin cleansers and antiseptic creams, ointments, solutions, and paints, in concentrations ranging from 5 to 14%. It is also used in some antiseptic swabs and wound dressings. It can cause skin irritation and is absorbed via damaged skin. Application over a large, broken skin surface is not recommended.

Triclosan

Triclosan is a bisphenol antiseptic agent commonly used in medicated soaps and topical preparations in concentrations of up to 2%. It is a mild irritant and allergic contact dermatitis has been reported.

Antifungal agents

Topical application of antifungal agents is effective for superficial cutaneous infections but is not for those involving hair or nails.

There is a large number of agents used in this way. Imidazole derivatives bifonazole, clotrimazole, econazole, miconazole, and ketoconazole have a broad spectrum of antifungal activity achieved by inhibition of ergosterol synthesis and consequent disruption of the fungal membrane. After topical application they efficiently reach keratinocytes but there is no appreciable systemic absorption. Topical imidazole preparations can be irritating but local sensitization is uncommon.

Tolnaftate is a thiocarbamate active against dermatophytes but not Candida species. Its mode of action is unknown. Terbinafine is an allylamine, which inhibits ergosterol synthesis at an earlier stage than the azoles. It is fungicidal for dermatophytes, and is also active against pityrosporum species, but less clearly useful against Candida species. Nystatin and amphotericin are polyenes active against Candida species but not dermatophytes. Various other compounds such as undecenoic acid and the keratolytics benzoic acid and salicylic acid are used to treat tinea. Amorolfine is a morpholine with a broad spectrum, which inhibits ergosterol synthesis at different sites to other antifungals. It is used as a lacquer painted onto abraded nails once or twice weekly for 6 to 12 months to treat onychomycosis.

Sunscreens

Sunscreen active agents work by either absorbing or reflecting UV radiation. Absorbent sunscreen chemicals act mainly in the UV range, whereas reflectants provide a barrier against UV, visible light, and infrared radiation. A list of the commonly used sunscreen agents is included in Table 23.17.3.

The majority of sunscreen products combine agents that absorb in the ultraviolet B (UVB) range (wavelengths 290–320 nm) with agents that absorb in the UVA range (wavelengths 320–360 nm) to provide broad-spectrum coverage. Many products also include a reflectant, such as titanium dioxide, which increases the protection but can give the skin a white appearance. Zinc oxide is used as a physical sun barrier for the protection of the ears and nose, which often receive high sun exposure.

Primary prevention is an important part of the public approach to management of skin cancer. Reduction of sunlight exposure in childhood is critical, but protection during adulthood is also important. It has been suggested that the entire spectrum of ultraviolet radiation (UVR), i.e. 290 to 400 nm, contributes to risk of skin cancer, so protection should be broad-spectrum in the UVR range. The primary approach is natural protection, involving the use of good quality clothing and hats while outdoors, seeking shade where possible, and avoiding the sun around the middle of the day. Reflected radiation may result in people receiving a high dose of UVR even when they are in the shade, and this needs to be accounted for when a canopy is being designed to reduce UVR exposure. Sunscreens are an adjunct to natural protection, not a substitute for it.

Sun protection factor (SPF) is a laboratory-derived figure classifying the relative potency of the different products. Because of the many variables determining the actual dose of UVR received, e.g. time of day, time of year, cloud cover, reflection, adequacy of application, it is not a figure which can be translated easily into the degree of protection afforded when used under normal conditions outdoors.

The SPF number applies to the ability of a sunscreen product to reduce predominantly the UVB range of the solar spectrum. There is relatively little increase in protection for large increases in SPF number after SPF15 (Table 23.17.4).

Other topical therapies

Antihistamines

Topical antihistamines are poorly absorbed and not effective in the treatment of most skin conditions. Systemic H_1 receptor antagonists should be considered when indicated.

Table 23.17.3 Commonly used sunscreen chemicals

Physical blockers (reflectants)	Zinc oxide, titanium dioxide, talc, red petrolatum
Chemical absorbers	
UVB absorbers	Salicylates—octyl salicylate, homosalate
	Cinnamates—octyl and isoamyl p-methoxycinnamate
	Camphor derivatives—4-methylbenzylidene camphor
	Aminobenzoates—p-aminobenzoic acid (PABA), padimate-O (octyl dimethyl PABA), methyl anthranilate
UVA absorbers	Benzophenones[a]—benzophenone-6, oxybenzone
	Dibenzoylmethanes—dibenzoylmethane, avobenzone (butylmethoxydibenzoylmethane)

[a] Benzophenones absorb in the UVB, UVA, and UVC ranges.

Table 23.17.4 Erythemal UVB reduction by SPF number

SPF number	% Reduction	% Penetration
2	50	50
4	75	25
8	87.5	12.5
16	93.75	6.25
32	96.88	3.13
64	98.44	1.56

Emulsifying ointment

Emulsifying ointment is a mixture of paraffin and emulsifying wax. It can act as a detergent or soap substitute and is particularly useful for patients with contact dermatitis in which the offending chemical is not known.

Lanolin

Lanolin (wool fat) is a purified anhydrous waxy substance obtained from the wool of sheep. It is used in creams and ointments to provide skin penetration properties. Lanolin is capable of absorbing about 30% of water, and hydrous lanolin is used as an ointment base. It is known to cause skin sensitivities. However, most lanolin-related sensitivities are found to be caused by residues of pesticide and detergent used on sheep. Removal of these impurities reduces the incidence of sensitization markedly.

Podophyllum

Podophyllum has an antimitotic action and is used in the treatment of warts. A combination of podophyllum resin and salicylic acid as a paint or ointment is used in the treatment of plantar warts. Podophyllotoxin 0.5% paint is used for anogenital warts. Podophyllum should not be used during pregnancy or in children.

Topical anaesthetics and analgesics

Most local anaesthetic agents are well absorbed through mucous membranes and damaged skin but absorption through intact skin is poor. However, a eutectic mixture of lidocaine and prilocaine can produce effective surface analgesia of intact skin prior to minor medical or surgical procedures, and this effect is enhanced by occlusion. Lidocaine is used in a number of products for use on oral and other mucosal surfaces and ulcers. Choline salicylate is used as a local analgesic for oral lesions.

Zinc oxide

Zinc oxide is a mild astringent used as a soothing and protective application in dusting powders, pastes, ointments, creams, and lotions, often combined with ingredients such as coal tar, ichthammol, salicylic acid, calamine, or castor oil.

Common topical preparations containing zinc oxide include calamine cream and lotion, zinc cream, ointment, and paste, Burow's emulsion, and zinc and castor oil ointment. Zinc oxide reflects UV radiation and is used in sunscreen preparations.

Fluorouracil

Fluorouracil cream is used to remove superficial solar keratoses. It is used for a period of 3 weeks on the face and on the arms and legs for 4–6 weeks, although times may vary. It causes severe chemical irritation with erythema and crusting, but heroic patients who complete a course reap significant benefits. Some irritation is needed for the preparation to be effective. It may cause some photosensitivity. If added potency is required, tretinoin can be applied along with the fluorouracil, as the two act synergistically.

Imiquimod

Imiquimod (1-(2-methylpropyl)-1H-imidazo[4,5-c]quinolin-4-amine) is an immune response modifier that binds to the toll-like receptors 7 and 8. The drug has many actions including modulation of antigen presenting cell function and consequent enhancement of effector T-cell activity. It is used topically in the treatment of external genital warts, but has no direct antiviral activity. It is also used in the treatment of actinic keratosis and superficial basal cell carcinoma (BCC). Inflammatory reactions can be a problem.

Complementary medicines in topical therapy

Aloe vera

Extract from aloe vera has been used in a variety of creams, ointments, gels, lotions, and shampoos. It has been suggested that aloe vera gel is useful for the treatment of mild burns and to promote wound healing as a result of antiseptic, anaesthetic, anti-inflammatory, antipruritic, and moisturizing properties.

While recent clinical studies have provided mixed findings about its effectiveness in the treatment of frostbite, wound healing, and cuts, its topical use appears to be nontoxic.

Tea tree (melaleuca) oil

Oil from the leaves of the tea tree *Melaleuca alternifolia* has traditionally been used for cuts, burns, and insect bites. It contains various terpene oils and sesquiterpenes. It may also contain cineole, which is known to be a skin irritant.

The antiseptic effect of tea tree oil is largely due to the presence of terpinen-4-ol. This is added to various commercial preparations. There are many *in vitro* studies demonstrating the antibacterial and antifungal effects of melaleuca oil. However, its antimicrobial activity is concentration dependent and clinical studies have not adequately demonstrated its effectiveness in the treatment of acne and skin infections such as tinea.

Phototherapy

Phototherapy involves treating patients with ultraviolet (UV) light of three types. These are shown below.

Narrowband UVB (311 nm)

The adverse effects of this treatment seem to be few. Carcinogenesis has not so far been demonstrated; however, lag times for the development of skin cancer are prolonged. Remission seems to be shorter than seen with psoralen ultraviolet A (PUVA) therapy, but the lack of long-term problems indicates that it should be the first-line form of phototherapy in most patients.

Broadband UVB (290–320 nm)

This is a tried and tested therapy, having been used for more than 80 years. It has not been shown to be carcinogenic. It is often combined with tar therapy for added efficacy.

Psoralen and ultraviolet A (PUVA) (320–400 nm)

Ultraviolet A light source is administered following pretreatment with a psoralen drug, usually methoxypsoralen 0.6 mg/kg orally, 2 h before UVA. Adverse effects include nausea and photosensitivity. Long-term use causes skin atrophy, lentigines and, after cumulative high dose, the incidence of squamous cell carcinoma is greatly increased. Long-term studies are still in progress, but it appears to also cause a small but definite increase in the incidence of melanoma.

In the management of psoriasis, both PUVA and narrowband UVB are made more efficacious by pretreatment with acitretin.

Continuation of acitretin during a course of phototherapy reduces the cumulative dose needed for clearing the psoriasis and lengthens the duration of post-treatment remissions.

Patients taking psoralens to photosensitize themselves take the drug 2 h before phototherapy. They remain photosensitive to a decreasing extent for 24 h, so while on these drugs they must protect themselves generally from natural UV light, including the wearing of suitable eye protection. A typical course of phototherapy, either PUVA or narrowband UVB, for plaque psoriasis may involve three treatments a week for 6 to 8 weeks. Patients need to stand unaided in the phototherapy apparatus for periods of up to 10 min. Claustrophobia is a relative contraindication for phototherapy.

Photodynamic therapy

Photodynamic therapy (PDT) is used to treat actinic keratosis, Bowen's disease, and superficial BCC. It involves the application of a photosensitizing cream to the target lesion followed after a few hours application of intense red light to the skin. During this time the drug is selectively modified and concentrated in diseased cells while largely clearing from normal tissue. The drug remains inactive until exposed to light. When applied, the light energy, delivered to the cancer site, chemically activates the active metabolite and creates a toxic form of oxygen which destroys the cancerous and precancerous cells with minimal damage to healthy cells. Most PDT treatment can be performed on an outpatient basis.

Principal side effects of PDT include a skin sensitivity to light for a few hours following treatment. Inflammation can occur after treatment. The reaction can be painful while the light is on (5–10 min) and local anaesthetic may be required in some cases.

Cryotherapy

Cryotherapy is very useful in the treatment of solar keratoses, superficial BCC, viral warts, small seborrhoeic keratoses, and small skin tags (acrochordons). A firm diagnosis is needed prior to consideration of cryotherapy.

Liquid nitrogen is the preferred cryogen. The method of application of the nitrogen is somewhat immaterial as the damage to the tissue is determined by the depth of the resultant ice ball and the thaw time. Nitrogen is usually applied with a cotton-tipped applicator or sprayed on with a cryotherapy gun. After cryotherapy, patients may be alarmed at the blistering reaction. If they are forewarned they are less likely to be anxious.

Systemic therapy

Oral retinoids

Isotretinoin (13-*cis*-retinoic acid) is a stereoisomer of all-*trans*-retinoic acid, which probably acts by conversion to it but has less toxicity. It is given orally in the treatment of cystic acne. Like all vitamin A analogues it is teratogenic, but in contrast to acitretin relatively rapid elimination permits the safe initiation of pregnancy from 1 to 2 months after stopping the drug. Adverse psychiatric events such as mood swings, depression, and suicidal ideation have been reported as possible idiosyncratic reactions to isotretinoin.

Acitretin has been used orally in the treatment of psoriasis and disorders of keratinization such as severe ichthyosis. It is necessary to avoid pregnancy for 2 years (3 years in the United States of America) after stopping acitretin.

More recent potent synthetic analogues known as arotinoids (adapalene and tazarotine) differ more markedly in structure from retinoic acid. They bind to retinoic acid receptors with different affinities for the different subtypes. Future developments may produce agents with selective activity and consequent reduced toxicity.

All systemic retinoids have substantial toxicity potentially manifested as:

- cheilitis
- dryness of nose, eyes, and face
- scaling of palms and soles and softening of nails
- loss of hair
- joint and muscle pain and headache
- hypertriglyceridaemia
- hypercholesterolaemia and reduced high-density lipoprotein cholesterol
- photosensitivity

Most significantly, they are teratogenic and must not be used in women who may conceive. Because of prolonged retention of etretinate in the body, pregnancy should be prevented for 2 years after the drug is ceased (3 years in the United States of America). A similar caution applies to acitretin since it is in part metabolized to etretinate. Comprehensible, practical advice on the need and means for fertility control is essential.

Cytotoxics and immunosuppressants

Corticosteroids

Oral corticosteroids have an important role in management of many skin conditions. They are the mainstay of therapy in autoimmune blistering disease and most life threatening dermatoses. While effective in atopic dermatitis, most cases can be managed with topical therapy. While also effective in psoriasis, their use in this condition is contraindicated due to the potential for severe rebound on dose reduction. Chronic stable plaque psoriasis may be converted in to generalized pustular psoriasis following discontinuation of oral steroid.

Azathioprine

Azathioprine is converted in the body to 6-mercaptopurine, an inhibitor of purine synthesis and an immunosuppressant. It also has potent anti-inflammatory properties. It is used alone or in combination with other agents, usually corticosteroids. Toxicity is mainly due to bone marrow suppression, although this is less than with agents such as cyclophosphamide. Estimation of serum levels of thiopurine methyltransferase (TPMT) help predict the risk of myelotoxicity. Gastrointestinal upset is common and may necessitate discontinuation of therapy.

Cyclophosphamide

Cyclophosphamide is a nitrogen mustard analogue which is converted to the active metabolite in the body where it exerts its immunosuppressant effects by interfering with DNA synthesis and function in B and T cells. It may be a more effective immunosuppressant than azathioprine, but this is associated with greater toxicity.

Ciclosporin

Ciclosporin is a potent inhibitor of T-cell activation and proliferation. It is variably absorbed after oral administration and extensively metabolized predominantly by CYP3A4, an isoform of the hepatic cytochrome P450 enzymes. Standard doses for psoriasis are in the range of 3 to 5 mg/kg. Use of high doses should be guided by monitoring of blood levels. The main toxicity is partially reversible renal impairment and hypertension. Its place in dermatology is in the treatment of a wide variety of inflammatory conditions such as psoriasis, atopic dermatitis, lichen planus, and bullous pemphigoid, but the difficulties in its use and the reversibility of benefit on ceasing administration markedly limit the circumstances warranting its use.

Methotrexate

Methotrexate is an inhibitor of dihydrofolate reductase. It is well absorbed after oral dosing of up to 25 mg/m². It is not metabolized to any extent and elimination depends on renal excretion, so caution and perhaps dosage adjustment is needed in the presence of renal impairment. Toxicity due to bone marrow depression and mucositis is less likely in dermatological applications than when higher doses are used, but regular monitoring with blood counts is necessary. Prolonged intake leads to hepatic fibrosis and this requires liver function to be included in the monitoring. Liver biopsy is necessary for early detection and characterization of this complication, but whether this is justified and how often it should be performed is controversial. Methotrexate is valuable in treatment of severe unresponsive psoriasis.

Hydroxyurea

Hydroxyurea blocks pyrimidine synthesis. It causes much more short-term bone marrow depression than methotrexate, necessitating frequent blood counts.

Thalidomide

Thalidomide is not generally available but is an inhibitor of tumour necrosis factor and has found a use in a number of inflammatory conditions despite its significant risks.

Bleomycin

Bleomycin has antitumour, antibacterial, and antiviral activity. It binds to DNA, causing strand scission and elimination of pyridine and purine bases. Intralesional injections are used in the treatment of unresponsive warts, although it can be extremely painful. The mechanism of action is not known.

Biological treatments

See Chapter 23.5 for an account of the currently used biological agents in the management of psoriasis. Many other potential uses have emerged and it seems likely that this will continue to develop. Anti-CD20 antibody is currently approved for the management of various forms of B-cell lymphoma, but reports are also appearing of their use in pemphigus vulgaris, paraneoplastic pemphigus, epidermolysis bullosa acquisita, dermatomyositis, and graft-versus-host disease, as well as other disorders. Off label reported uses of the tumour necrosis factor-α (TNFα) antagonists have included the treatment of hidradenitis suppurativa, pyoderma granulosum, cutaneous sarcoidoisis, cutaneous Crohn's disease, Wegener's vasculitis, autoimmune blistering diseases, Behçet's disease, graft-versus-host disease, and others, although there appears to be differences in activity between the specific TNFα antagonists. An antibody directed to the CD11a subunit of leucocyte function associated antigen 1 (LFA-1) is approved for the management of psoriasis. However, there are number of reports describing the use of anti-LFA-1 in the treatment of other skin diseases including atopic dermatitis, discoid lupus erythematosus, and others. IL-12/IL-23 pathway inhibition is increasingly being recognized as a potentially useful therapy for psoriasis. There are many other emerging biological therapies, resulting in a rapidly progressing and exciting area of therapeutics.

Antimicrobial agents

Topical administration favours development of resistance in skin flora (particularly if given long term) and is prone to cause hypersensitivity in the patient. It can be an extremely valuable approach, but should thus be cautiously employed with these caveats in mind.

Mupirocin

Mupirocin is a valuable topical antibiotic which is not used systemically. It is active mainly against Gram-positive aerobes, including most strains of staphylococci and streptococci. However, the emergence of high level mupirocin resistance in methicillin-resistant *Staphylococcus aureus* (MRSA) has been reported.

Topical mupirocin is used in the treatment of bacterial skin infections such as impetigo and infected dermatitis. Nonmacrogol based formulations are used intranasally to eradicate staphylococcal carriage.

Tetracyclines

Tetracycline itself has a very broad spectrum, but acquired resistance is common in many species of organisms.

Modifications of the basic molecule has produced many drugs, including doxycycline and minocycline, which have longer half-lives and greater potency on a weight basis but do not differ appreciably in spectrum and exhibit cross-resistance.

All tetracyclines cause some gastrointestinal symptoms and may lead to photosensitivity. They damage enamel of unerupted teeth and should not be given to children under 12 years. They should be avoided in pregnancy for the same reason but also because of the rare occurrence of hepatic necrosis in pregnant women. Except for doxycycline and minocycline they are excreted renally, and may accumulate in renal failure and further aggravate renal impairment. Minocycline is particularly prone to cause dizziness and ataxia but such symptoms can occur with others of the group and they can rarely cause benign intracranial hypertension. Minocycline in particular can cause abnormal pigmentation of mucosae and of tissues, including scars. As with all broad-spectrum antibiotics, overgrowth of resistant organisms occurs, particularly fungi in the case of Tetracyclines.

Tetracyclines are frequently used in the treatment of acne where, like other antibiotics, they probably act by suppressing proliferation of *Propionibacterium acnes*. The rationale for use in rosacea is uncertain. Tetracyclines also have anti-inflammatory effects, mediated by inhibition of neutrophil chemotaxis and phagocytosis and suppression of granuloma formation, and possibly a direct effect on vascular endothelium, which may be beneficial in a variety of skin conditions.

Erythromycin

Erythromycin is a macrolide active against Gram-positive organisms and some anaerobes. It is used both topically (as a 2% gel or solution) and systemically in the treatment of acne and rosacea. This antibiotic is suitable for use in pregnancy.

Clindamycin

Clindamycin is active against *P. acnes*. It is used topically as a lotion or gel in acne and rosacea. Oral administration carries a risk of producing pseudomembranous colitis.

Metronidazole

Metronidazole is active against anaerobes but not *P. acnes*. It is administered topically in rosacea but the mode of its action is unknown, although there is some evidence that metronidazole is effective against the demodex mite.

Dapsone and sulfapyridine

Dapsone, a sulphone used for the treatment of leprosy, and sulfapyridine, a sulfonamide, are used in dermatology for anti-inflammatory effects in a variety of inflammatory skin conditions. Dapsone is of specific value in dermatitis herpetiformis and is used in such noninfective inflammatory conditions as pyoderma gangrenosum, pemphigus, and bullous pemphigoid. Dapsone, in the doses employed, causes a considerable incidence of haemolysis (especially in patients with glucose-6-phosphate dehydrogenase (G6PD) deficiency), methaemoglobinaemia, and rash. Rarer adverse consequences are blood dyscrasias, severe skin reactions, hepatitis, fever, and malaise, which may occur alone or as part of a generalized hypersensitivity reaction.

Antifungal agents

Systemic administration of antifungals is employed to treat deep-seated infections and those involving nail and hair. The imidazole, ketoconazole was the first orally active azole but has been largely superseded by the triazoles (itraconazole and fluconazole) due to the rare occurrence of liver damage, inhibition of androgen synthesis, and interactions with many drugs due to inhibition of the cytochrome P450 3A4 pathway. The triazoles are absorbed after oral administration. Both are effective against Candida species but itraconazole is more active against filamentous fungi.

Terbinafine, an allylamine, is well absorbed when given by mouth and concentrates in the stratum corneum, including the nail bed. Gastrointestinal disturbance occurs in approximately 5% of patients and rare adverse effects include hepatitis, toxic epidermal necrolysis, blood disorders, and a reversible loss of taste.

Griseofulvin was the first orally effective agent against dermatophytes. It is less effective than the azoles and allylamines but is much cheaper. It is poorly soluble and absorption is assisted by preparations with very small particle size or by ingestion with a fatty meal. It is taken up by keratinocytes and exerts a fungistatic action in the stratum corneum which continues in hair and nails. It must be given for sufficient time for the quiescent but viable spores in the keratin to be shed. It is inactive against Candida species.

Antimalarial agents

Chloroquine and hydroxychloroquine are used as immunomodulating agents in lupus erythematosus and other connective tissue disorders. Their mode of action in these diseases is unknown. The most alarming adverse effect is a dose-related permanent retinopathy, and regular monitoring by an optometrist or ophthalmologist is necessary. They are category D drugs and their use should be avoided in pregnancy.

Antiviral agents

Aciclovir is an analogue of guanosine that is phosphorylated preferentially by herpes simplex viral thymidine kinase to then inhibit the DNA polymerase. It may be administered topically or systemically by oral or intravenous routes. When taken orally, it is poorly and variably absorbed. Its prodrug, valaciclovir, is its L-valyl ester which is much better absorbed after hydrolysis, resulting in higher and more reliable blood levels of aciclovir and permitting less frequent dosing. Famciclovir is a prodrug of penciclovir, which has the same mode of action as aciclovir. Penciclovir is also administered topically. They are all generally well tolerated.

Antiandrogens

These have a role in hirsutism, androgenic alopecia, and in acne. They should all be avoided in pregnancy.

Spironolactone

Spironolactone is a potassium-sparing diuretic which, independent of that property, is a weak antagonist of androgen receptor binding and an inhibitor of androgen biosynthesis.

Spironolactone should not be administered to patients with renal failure due to the potential for potassium retention. The patient's potassium status should be checked prior to commencing therapy and on an annual basis thereafter.

Cyproterone acetate

Cyproterone acetate is a synthetic corticosteroid with progestational and antiandrogen actions. The latter is due to competition at the dehydrotestosterone receptor and, at high doses, to inhibition of androgen synthesis. It may be used in the treatment of hirsutism and paradoxically of alopecia of the androgenetic type.

Finasteride

Finasteride inhibits the conversion of testosterone to dehydrotestosterone by the type 2 5α-reductase enzyme, which is present on hair follicle cells, thus reducing the influence of androgens. Consequently, it has a role in androgenetic alopecia in men since it does not alter the effect of androgen on the testes and hypothalamic-pituitary function.

Minoxidil

Minoxidil is a potent vasodilator. Its systemic use to treat hypertension is limited by tachycardia, fluid retention, and the undesired stimulation of hair growth. Minoxidil is used as a local application to the scalp where it acts as a nonspecific hair growth stimulant, probably by prolonging the anagen phase. This persists only while treatment is continued.

Management of skin failure

Erythema multiforme, Stevens–Johnson syndrome, toxic epidermal necrolysis

These disorders represent a spectrum ranging in severity from relatively benign erythema multiforme to life-threatening toxic

Box 23.17.1 Drug-induced rashes

Drugs that commonly cause serious reactions

- Allopurinol
- Anticonvulsants
- NSAIDs
- Sulfa drugs
- Bumetanide
- Captopril
- Furosemide
- Penicillamine
- Piroxicam
- Thiazide diuretics

Drugs less likely to cause skin reactions

- Digoxin
- Diphenhydramine hydrochloride
- Aspirin
- Aminophylline
- Prochlorperazine
- Ferrous sulphate
- Prednisone
- Codeine
- Tetracycline
- Morphine
- Regular insulin
- Warfarin
- SSRIs

NSAID, nonsteroidal anti-inflammatory drugs; SSRIs, selective serotonin reuptake inhibitors.

epidermal necrolysis. Erythema multiforme is usually secondary to infection (mainly herpes simplex) and presents with target lesions particularly on the hands and feet. It can be more generalized, with mucosal involvement. Stevens–Johnson syndrome and toxic epidermal necrolysis are both, in most cases, caused by drugs (Box 23.17.1). They are considered to be a continuum, with clinical features ranging from atypical targetoid lesions with blisters and severe mucosal involvement in Stevens–Johnson syndrome to widespread detachment of full-thickness epidermis, confluent erythema, and skin tenderness in toxic epidermal necrolysis. See also Chapter 23.16.

There is a mortality rate of up to 20% even with appropriate management in toxic epidermal necrolysis, but this was much higher several years ago. Most fatalities in patients with toxic epidermal necrolysis are the result of sepsis. If Stevens–Johnson syndrome or toxic epidermal necrolysis is suspected then hospital admission is essential. Patients with toxic epidermal necrolysis should be admitted to a burns unit. All drugs should be stopped.

Treatment consists of fluid and electrolyte replacement; maintenance of body temperature; adequate pain relief; early treatment of infection; debridement where needed; and treatment of mucosal surfaces, especially the eye, where there is a 30% long-term morbidity. The role of oral corticosteroids is controversial, but if they are to be given they need to be started early, in high doses, and should be given for short periods of time. Ciclosporin and other approaches have been reported in some recent articles to be effective. Some studies have suggested that intravenous immunoglobulin (IVIG) may be of benefit, but others have disputed this.

Staphylococcal scalded skin syndrome

Children and neonates are most susceptible. They present with irritability and raised temperature, along with skin tenderness and a scarlatiniform eruption, leading to superficial crusting initially in the flexures and around body orifices and then becoming generalized. Treatment is with supportive measures and di/flucloxacillin 2 g (children: 25–50 mg/kg up to 2 g) orally, 6-hourly. Corticosteroids are contraindicated.

Meningococcal septicaemia (Chapter 7.6.5)

A preceding, viral-like illness is followed by petechial lesions plus transient urticarial, macular, or papular lesions. The petechiae have a 'smudged' appearance and are raised with pale greyish centres. There is associated fever and there may be signs of meningitis. For further information on management, see Chapter 7.6.5.

Exfoliative dermatitis (erythroderma)

These terms are applied to any inflammatory skin disease that affects more than 90% of the body surface. The cause is not found in 10% of patients. The most common causes are dermatitis, psoriasis, drugs, lymphoma, pityriasis rubra pilaris, and Norwegian (crusted) scabies. There are profound metabolic disturbances which mean that rapid diagnosis and inpatient management are needed. These disturbances include hypothermia, fluid loss, protein and electrolyte imbalance, and haemodynamic changes. Any suspected drug should be withdrawn. Treatment is directed at the underlying cause but oral corticosteroids are effective for cases due to dermatitis or drugs.

Further reading

Dermatology Expert Group (2009). *Therapeutic guidelines: dermatology Version 3*, 3rd edition. Therapeutic Guidelines Limited, Melbourne.
Lebwohl MG, *et al.* (eds) (2006). *Treatment of skin disease. Comprehensive therapeutic strategies*, 2nd edition. Mosby Elsevier, Philadelphia.
Price CJ, Sinclair RD (2008). *Fast facts: minor surgery*. 2nd edition. Health Press, Oxford.
Rakel RE, Bope ET (2009). *Conn's current therapy*. Elsevier Science, Philadelphia.
Williams HC, *et al.* (eds) (2008). *Evidence-based dermatology*, 2nd edition. BMJ Books, London.

SECTION 24

Neurological disorders

Introduction and approach to the patient with neurological disease

Alastair Compston

Essentials

Clinical neurology uses conversation, detailed questioning and discussion, observation, structured examination, and selective investigation to formulate problems into an anatomical and pathological framework. The competent neurologist senses and probes relevant components of the history, reliably elicits the physical signs, knows which investigations are necessary and relevant, appreciates the most likely underlying diagnosis and mechanism of disease, and communicates relevant information to the patient accurately, intelligibly, and sensitively. This system has evolved over several centuries, during which much knowledge has accumulated on structure and function in health and disease, the reliability of physical signs and laboratory investigations, and the nosology of disease.

The neurological history

Although patients usually start with an account of what troubles them most, the neurologist prefers a history of the components in the order in which they occurred. It may take some time to establish this chronology. The first task is to assess the core symptoms and how they cluster. The neurologist asks enough questions to settle whether, for example: a reported episode of difficulty with speech refers to a disturbance of language (aphasia) or articulation (dysarthria); there are motor or sensory deficits in a 'heavy' limb; alterations of sensation are positive (tingling and paraesthesiae) or negative (numbness) symptoms; a disturbance of bladder function suggests neurological or urological disease; and double vision actually refers to diplopia or altered acuity. Some questions reflect the peculiarities of neurological anatomy; it may surprise the patient complaining of impaired vision on the right that the symptom is in fact unaltered by sequential closure of either eye—because it is hemianopic—or that awareness of temperature and the appreciation of pain may be disturbed in the 'good' leg in some forms of spinal cord disease (the Brown–Séquard syndrome).

Once the individual symptoms have been accurately defined, they can be grouped; from this follows an interpretation of their anatomical basis, suggesting the involvement of one or more sites. Recognition of these patterns is fundamental to interpretation of the neurological history and this synthesis directs attention to specific components of the subsequent examination. It is easy to conclude that the patient with cognitive impairment has disease of the cerebral cortex, but a more detailed history will, in addition, indicate whether this is diffuse or focal and reflects involvement of the dominant or nondominant hemispheres and the frontal, temporal, or parietal cortices. Incoordination of more than one motor skill (eye movement, speech, the limbs, and balance) necessarily indicates involvement of brainstem–cerebellar connections. The process causing a hemianopic field defect lies above and that resulting in lower cranial nerve palsies below the tentorium. The combination of motor and sensory symptoms in limbs with altered sphincter function indicates spinal cord disease; for the male patient with an unreliable bladder, the significance of linking urgency and frequency to impotence and constipation may seem strange. In turn, the coexistence of diffuse distal symmetrical motor and sensory symptoms, shoulder and pelvic girdle weakness, or ocular, bulbar, respiratory, and upper limb weakness steers the thinking towards peripheral nerve, primary muscle, and neuromuscular junction disease respectively.

As a generalization, abrupt events are vascular or electrical in origin, subacute symptoms are demyelinating or inflammatory, and symptoms that develop slowly suggest structural deficits or degeneration. The subsequent course also reveals the underlying process: self-limiting events are often vascular; paroxysmal symptoms tend to be electrical or demyelinating, depending on their duration; and progressive syndromes are compressive or degenerative.

The circumstances may be suggestive of a particular pathophysiology: trauma, preceding infection, drug exposure, or pregnancy alerts the observer to structural, demyelinating, toxic, and venous thrombotic mechanisms, respectively. Dangerous for the beginner, but nevertheless important to recognize, are the inconsistencies of exaggeration, mismatch between the severity of symptoms and altered function, and the anatomical impossibilities that usually feature in nonorganic neurological disease. Together, these pattern recognitions are the stuff of neurological diagnosis.

The neurological examination

Examination of the patient with neurological disease needs to be structured and organized without exhausting the patient and examiner through obsessive attention to irrelevant detail. Much can be learned by astute observation without formal assessment. Gross defects of cognition do not need to be confirmed by reciting telephone numbers in reverse or assembling lists of former prime ministers, defects of speech will usually be evident in conversation, many neurological diagnoses are immediately apparent from the patient's gait, and movement disorders can be observed while taking the history. That said, it is best routinely to adopt a basic core examination and do things in order because the detection of one abnormality will determine the interpretation of another. It takes only a few minutes for the experienced and adequately equipped examiner to confirm that corrected visual acuity is normal in each eye, there is no gross field defect, and the optic fundi are normal.

Although more detailed assessment will sometimes be necessary, a full range of smooth following (pursuit) eye movements in the horizontal and vertical planes can rapidly be established: this will detect obvious ophthalmoplegia and can be supplemented by cover testing of each eye during fixation on the examiner's nose, and rapid gaze from right to left—very few significant defects of eye movement will escape this rapid screen. Movement of the lower face during forced eye closure, voluntary elevation of the palate, and rapid protrusion or side-to-side movement of the tongue take a few seconds to observe and effectively cover all the lower cranial nerves. It is rarely necessary to test the sense of smell or hearing and a tuning fork is most useful for establishing that deafness is conductive and therefore probably not relevant. Before moving to the limbs, it is worth testing neck flexion in patients where the history suggests muscular or neuromuscular disease.

A sufficient routine examination of the arms would start with posture (outstretched with the eyes open and then closed): a quick look for selective muscle wasting; tone in flexion–extension and supination–pronation at the elbow and wrist respectively; strength in flexion and extension at the elbow and wrist, spreading the fingers and abduction of the thumb; coordination during movement between the patient's nose and examiner's finger (or both hands if there is gross incoordination to avoid accidental ocular injury); and the tendon reflexes. This will take the experienced examiner less than a minute. It may be necessary to establish specific patterns of muscle weakness: global loss affecting the hand in cortical disease; selective involvement of extensor groups in upper motor neuron disease; the patterns of C5 to T1 nerve root lesions; diffuse distal weakness of both extremities in peripheral neuropathy; and the subtle distinctions between radial, median, and ulnar neuropathies and C7, C8, and T1 root lesions respectively. Detailed sensory examination of the arms rarely achieves more

than can be learned from establishing that crude protective sense (recognition of a sharp pin) or discrimination (position sense and the ability to distinguish two points or perform a simple task such as manipulating a button) is intact.

Although this may involve some rearrangement of clothing, it otherwise takes almost no time to swipe the abdominal reflexes in passing, before examining the legs. Here, the structured motor examination is as for the arms, although increased tone is more easily detected by lifting the relaxed leg from the couch at the thigh, and testing internal and external rotation at the hip. Characteristic patterns of weakness are the involvement of flexors at all joints and eversion at the ankle in upper motor neuron lesions, the usual diffuse symmetrical distal involvement in peripheral neuropathy at a time when the hands may be normal, and difficulty in distinguishing injury of the lateral popliteal nerve from an L5 to S1 root lesion (in which the ankle jerk is lost) in the context of unilateral foot-drop. Proximal weakness is best detected by watching the patient walk, and the calf muscles are normally so strong as to be untestable except with the patient standing. As in the arm, coordination can be assessed only once the degree of weakness has been established. Tendon reflexes in the legs may be brisk in isolation and often spread, so that, in an upper motor neuron lesion, when one is tapped several may respond—and in either leg. Even non-neurologists rarely forget to elicit the plantar responses.

Sensory examination of the legs tends to be more reliable for protective than for discriminative sensation. In mapping a sensory level it is best to move from the relatively anaesthetic to the normal zone, noting the band of hypersensitivity that usually exists at the boundary. It is a matter of fact that many patients confuse the examination by exaggeration or elaboration of physical signs; this most commonly affects power, with the usual clues being a mismatch between the ability to walk and findings on formal assessment of muscle strength (or vice versa), and simultaneous contraction of agonist and antagonist muscles. Sensory testing is subjective and so necessarily vulnerable to inaccurate reporting, but confirming that a sensory level is present both on the abdomen and back, and on the same side on each, with a slightly higher level on the trunk, is a simple manoeuvre that may yield surprising discrepancies in the patient with nonorganic deficits.

The overall purpose of the history and examination is to assess where and through what mechanism structure and function have been affected. Detection of these patterns becomes routine for the experienced neurologist but the process represents more than just a ritual of clinical neurology. From anatomical localization follows a formulation of likely mechanisms and pathological conditions underlying the patient's symptoms and signs.

Investigation of neurological disease

The investigation of patients with neurological disease was revolutionized in the early 1970s with the introduction of CT. Before then, only the most primitive structural details of the central nervous system (CNS) could be detected by demonstrating indirectly the shape and placement of the ventricles and blood vessels, and usually at some discomfort to the patient. Function in the CNS and peripheral nervous system (PNS) was measured using neurophysiological techniques. Disruption of the blood–brain barrier and immunological activity in the CNS were assessed through analysis of the cerebrospinal fluid (CSF).

Investigation still does not replace clinical assessment but, as the chapters that follow make clear, it is now possible: to detect structural changes in most parts of the brain and spinal cord at high resolution; to distinguish many pathological appearances at these sites on the basis of differences in the MR signals; to map function within regions of interest using changes in blood flow and the use of metabolic substrates; to show variations in efferent and afferent electrical activity in the CNS and PNS; and to detect an increasing range of soluble mediators of normal and pathological function in the CSF. Taken together, these laboratory investigations still do no more than supplement clinical assessments and, in one sense, the high expectations of diagnosis make for additional difficulties in interpreting neurological illness when the images are normal, compared with the era when authoritative statements from neurologists could never be validated and necessarily went unchallenged.

The value of many routine investigations lies in confirming normality and endorsing abnormalities already strongly suspected on clinical grounds. Given the increasing sensitivity of techniques for brain imaging, altered appearances that are not necessarily of pathological significance and genuine lesions that are not relevant in the particular clinical context need to be interpreted with common sense. Overall, the trend has been for the pendulum to swing from diagnosis without adequate laboratory evidence to diagnosis made in defiance of clinical intuition. Even when an imaging abnormality has been identified, its nature may require clinical discussion in order to resolve the most likely pathological substrate—the distinction between ischaemic and inflammatory tissue often proving difficult and not all neoplastic tissue being easily identified as such.

The management of neurological disease

The first issue that confronts the doctor looking after a person with neurological disease is when to discuss and name the diagnosis. Most wait until there is sufficient clinical or laboratory evidence to rule out misdiagnosis; telling people that they have a condition when they do not is bound to cause distress and has landed some specialists in the law courts. However, overcaution and avoidance of discussion can be equally damaging, and there are many more patients who harbour bitterness over delay in learning the true nature of their illness than those who wish that they had not been told so soon, or at all. Most individuals cope extremely well even with the prospect of conditions that are known to be life threatening or have a poor prognosis for disability. Advice may be needed on alterations in lifestyle resulting from neurological disease, e.g. driving in epilepsy, and the use of drugs in pregnancy. There is a basic human need to know why a thing has happened and most patients enquire about causation but, naturally, the uppermost question is whether symptoms can be treated or the natural history of disease usefully modified.

The chapters that follow document specific treatments for particular conditions but judgement is often required in deciding whether to deploy these remedies, depending on age, significance of the symptoms for the individual, level of disability, security of the diagnosis, adverse effects, and the patient's own views. Drug treatment may be used, on an intermittent or regular basis, to suppress symptoms, e.g. intravenous methylprednisolone to reduce inflammation, anticonvulsants to suppress epilepsy, γ-aminobutyric acid agonists to deal with spasticity, or anticholinesterases to enhance transmission at the neuromuscular junction. Pharmacological options also exist for interfering with the mechanism of disease, again on an intermittent or routine basis, e.g. the use of triptans to relieve migraine or the replacement of dopamine in Parkinson's disease. In other situations, the rationale of treatment is to modify the underlying disease process, e.g. by suppressing inflammatory processes in acute postinfectious polyneuritis using intravenous gammaglobulin, treating patients with multiple sclerosis using β-interferon, and using immunosuppressants such as methotrexate and cycophosphamide in polymyositis and vasculitis respectively. Many other illustrations could be given, confirming that the age-old witticism concerning the therapeutic nihilism of clinical neurology is at best now only of historical interest and was always generally rather ill-informed. Beyond the present pharmacological achievements in drug treatment lie many opportunities for improving handicap and disability through the use of rehabilitation, which increasingly assumes centre stage in the management of neurological disease through attention to the person with impairments in a particular social and cultural setting rather than focusing on the pathophysiology of disease in an individual void. For the future, there is the prospect of enhanced regeneration in the context of diseases affecting the CNS and PNS, restoring structure and function and thereby both limiting and repairing the damage.

Mind and brain: building bridges linking neurology, psychiatry, and psychology

A. Zeman

'The great regions of the mind correspond to the great regions of the brain.'

Paul Broca

'… the master unsolved problem of biology: how the hundred million nerve cells of the brain work together to create consciousness …'

E.O. Wilson, *Consilience*, 1998

Essentials

Here is one view of the relationship between medicine and psychiatry. Physicians study, diagnose, and treat disorders of the body; psychiatrists (by contrast) study, diagnose, and treat disorders of the mind. Medicine has to do mainly with processes in objects, such as the circulation of blood to the kidneys; psychiatrists concern themselves mainly with the experiences of subjects, such as auditory hallucinations. Medical disorders are 'organic'; psychiatric disorders are 'functional'. Medicine is mainly a science; psychiatry mainly an art. The brain, on this view, occupies an ambiguous position, poised between body and mind: it is an ambiguous intermediary, a skilful interpreter between the languages of mind and body. Nevertheless, disorders of body and mind can and should be rigorously distinguished.

This chapter examines and questions these assumptions, which are not universally held but are widespread and tenacious, and have some practical importance. They influence the way that doctors approach patients and train students, and they underpin a deep theoretical problem in biology, the puzzling relationship between body and mind. A century of research on the biological basis of cognition, mood, personality and behaviour, and much recent writing in philosophy, points to the need to rethink these time-honoured beliefs.

What is the mind?

'Mind' is not a scientific term and has no strict technical definition. We use it to refer, broadly, to the capacities that enable our cognition, mood, motivation, personality, and behaviour. 'Cognition', in turn, a word derived from the Latin *cognoscere*, to know, refers to our intellectual capacities: very broadly these allow us to gain and store knowledge of the world, including each other, and to use it to guide our actions. Cognition is currently subclassified into attention, memory, executive function (the ability to organize thought and behaviour), language, perception, and praxis (our capacity for skilled action). Cognition is closely related to—but not identical with—the other aspects of mind: mood and motivation are self-explanatory; personality refers to the more or less enduring traits that characterize our conduct of our lives and our approach to other people; and behaviour is included among the elements of mind to allow for instances—such as temper tantrums—in which the outward manifestations of mental processes are their most striking feature.

It is worth noting, in passing, that because the term 'mind' is colloquial rather than technical, and because its workings are of great interest and importance to most of us, we tend to have preconceptions about its nature. These are strongly influenced by our religious and cultural backgrounds. There is, for example, a powerful human tendency, apparent across cultures and historical time, to believe that the mind can be prised apart from the body and survive its death. Whatever our own attitudes to these beliefs, they continue to exert a widespread influence.

What is consciousness?

Another complex capacity, consciousness, closely linked to mind, has attracted enormous interest over the past 20 years. The term 'consciousness' can be used to refer both to a state of arousal—wakefulness, for example, as opposed to sleep or coma—and to the contents of our awareness, e.g. 'what it is like' to be sitting and reading these words. Recent advances have allowed neuroscientists to investigate the physical basis of experiences such as these, taking due account of both the rich texture of our awareness and the immense subtlety of the related processes occurring in the brain. The advances that have made this possible include the development of functional brain imaging techniques, which are constantly revealing exquisite correlations between features of experience and events in the brain, and discoveries in psychology showing that only a part of what happens in the brain ever reaches awareness, underwriting the concept of unconscious processes. But the fundamental explanation for the current, widespread, fascination with consciousness is that its science holds out the promise of healing the ancient rift between brain and mind.

The biology of conscious and unconscious mind

Mechanism

The maintenance of wakefulness depends upon the integrity of a complex activating system located in the upper brainstem, thalamus, and basal forebrain which projects widely throughout the cerebral hemispheres to regulate conscious states. These are reflected in the rhythms of the brain's electrical activity recorded from the scalp—the electroencephalograph (EEG). The contents of awareness, by contrast, depend upon the transient activation of widespread 'neuronal assemblies', interconnected groups of neurons distributed among cortical and subcortical regions.

At any given moment, much of the potentially conscious activity in the brain occurs unconsciously; you were probably not aware, before reading this, of the tension in your left elbow. What distinguishes the neural activity of which we are aware? There are several candidates with some empirical support for each: the quantity of neural activity, related to its amplitude and duration; its quality, e.g. the degree of synchronization among participating neurons; its location in the brain, e.g. whether it is predominantly cortical or subcortical; and its connectivity, e.g. whether activity in early sensory areas does or does not propagate to cortical areas downstream. The leading current theory of awareness, the global workspace model, emphasizes the last of these four parameters, proposing that the distinctive feature of the neural activity 'in consciousness' is that it is communicated widely throughout the brain, gaining access, in particular, to the neural resources that control action and allow report.

Phylogeny: evolution of the mind

The elements of the nervous system—the neuron, its ion channels, and its chemical transmitters—date back to the origins of multicellular life. In almost every complex organism, these common elements have been exploited to create a signalling system that enables animals to respond to events around them with appropriate actions, the earliest embodiment of mind. Some animals have invested heavily in this system, allowing a progressively richer range of perceptual distinctions and a more flexible repertoire of response. This process of 'encephalization' has been particularly striking in parts of the vertebrate lineage, including our own primate line. The rapid growth of the brain, out of proportion to change in body size, has been the most striking feature of the past 5 million years of hominid evolution. It occurred in parallel with—probably both drove and was driven by—the emergence of technology, language, and culture, with the implication that the most distinctive features of the human mind are integral to our biology.

Ontogeny: individual development of mind

'Follow a child from its birth, and observe the alterations that time makes, and you shall find, as the mind by the senses comes to be more and more furnished with ideas, it comes to be more and more awake', wrote the philosopher John Locke 300 years ago. Our capacity to learn, the prerequisite for the process that Locke describes, is now thought to depend upon the plasticity of synapses: these are shaped by experience, which strengthens some and weakens others, creating neural assemblies that represent regularities in the world around us and in our behaviour. There is no shortage of material for this process: the human brain contains of the order of 10^{11} neurons, each receiving up to several thousand synapses.

The development of a human mind has another crucial dimension. The acquisition of a 'theory of mind' between the ages of around 2 and 5—the realization that we ourselves and those around us gain knowledge of the world from a fallible, limited perspective, and are therefore liable to false belief—may be the most distinctively human intellectual achievement.

Function

What is the biological purpose of the mind? Simple nervous systems are networks of communication and control, designed to ensure that the organism responds to events in the environment with appropriate actions. Complex nervous systems elaborate these processes, but the tailoring of behaviour to circumstance remains the fundamental function of the mind.

The mind–brain problem

How then are mind and brain related? The relationship is clearly intimate, but also puzzling. Traditionally, physicalism claims that what passes through our mind is identical with what happens in our brains; behaviourism asserts that statements about mental events can be reduced to statements about behaviour; functionalism suggests that mental processes can be understood in terms of transformations of sensory inputs into motor outputs. The puzzle that troubles some thinkers about mind and brain is that, seemingly, one could know everything about an organism's neural processes, behaviour, and functional design, and yet be ignorant about what it is like to be that creature. This inspires alternative 'dualistic' accounts of mind and brain, which posit an essential difference between mental and physical, or subjective and objective, entities or properties. But these dualistic theories, in turn, get into difficulty when they try to explain the undoubted interactions between mind and brain. This ancient dilemma remains unresolved: it seems likely that the solution will involve some changes in our understanding of the nature of both matter and mind.

SECTION 24 NEUROLOGICAL DISORDERS

A practical solution: a biopsychosocial approach

The mind–brain problem impinges on clinical practice. As every practising doctor knows, interactions of mind, brain, and body are constantly on view. Here are some examples:

◆ Medical problems usually come to light by way of a complex set of intervening psychological processes that occur when someone notices, ponders, and decides to present with a physical symptom.

◆ Psychological upset can manifest itself in physical symptoms, as, for example, in a panic attack or a somatoform disorder.

◆ Physical diseases commonly cause secondary psychological reactions, such as anxiety and depression

◆ Physical disease affecting the brain often gives rise directly to psychological manifestations, e.g. memory loss.

Given that the physical and mental are both constantly on show in the everyday practice of medicine, there is much to recommend taking a 'biopsychosocial' approach to every patient. This acknowledges that people cannot be divided into 'organic' and 'functional' groups: we are all compounded of body and mind. In every clinical encounter—whether in general practice, cardiology, neurology, or psychiatry—we should aim to define its biological, psychological, and social dimensions.

A theoretical solution: matter, life, and mind

In the 19th century many thinkers believed that 'life' was an irreducible phenomenon, the manifestation of an 'élan vital'. The biochemical discoveries of the 20th century revealed that life simply is the set of processes that allow organisms to utilize energy from their surroundings to reproduce themselves—and thereby made it clear how matter could give rise to life. It seems natural to ask whether mind might be explained in terms of the intelligent activities of living things, just as life has been explained in terms of the workings of organized matter. Is this a plausible ambition?

As we have seen, attempts to 'conjure' mind from brain can be met with puzzlement: there seems to be no possibility of understanding how the 'water of the brain' gives rise to the 'wine of experience'. But arguably the problem we run into here results from narrowing the frame of explanation too severely. Mind is not a mysterious emanation from the brain; it is always the activity of a human being: an activity rooted in a brain and body; the product of a long, largely forgotten history of development; embedded in the context of a human culture; and usually engaged in interaction with its physical surroundings. The brain is not a magic lamp from which we conjure the genie of mind; it is instead a great enabler, a subtle instrument enabling us to apprehend, and engage with, the rich complexities of our social and physical environment.

Conclusion

Given what science and philosophy reveal about the nature of the mind, here is an alternative view of the relationship between medicine and psychiatry: physicians and psychiatrists study, diagnose, and treat illnesses. These are physical processes linked to human experiences, the outcome of disorders of structure or function occurring in organisms. Some, medical disorders, are more easily identified or understood at the level of bodily process, others, psychiatric disorders, at the level of subjective experience, but this distinction is extremely fluid, especially so in clinical neurology. Medicine must always draw on science, to understand the physical basis of disorders, and art, and to appreciate the individual human complexities of the resulting predicaments. All our disorders affect our bodies and our minds.

Further reading

Butler C, Zeman A (2005). Neurological syndromes which can be mistaken for psychiatric conditions. *J Neurol Neurosurg Psychiatry*, **76** Suppl I, 31–8. [This paper reviews a range of symptoms and syndromes in the borderland between neurology and psychiatry.]

Clark A (2001). Where brain, body and world collide. In: Edelman G, Changeux J-P (eds) *The brain*, pp. 257–80. Transaction Publishing, London. [An introduction to the idea that to understand the mind we need to understand more than, simply, the brain.]

Cummings JL, Mega MS (2003). *Neuropsychiatry and behavioural neuroscience*. Oxford University Press, Oxford. [An up-to-date review of neuropsychiatry.]

Gazzaniga MS *et al.* (2002). *Cognitive neuroscience: the biology of the mind*. W.W. Norton & Co., New York. [A lively introduction to the neurological basis of cognitive processes.]

Laureys S (ed.) (2005). *The boundaries of consciousness. Progress in brain research*, vol 150. Elsevier, Amsterdam. [A comprehensive collection of papers on contemporary consciousness science.]

Lishman WA (1997). *Organic psychiatry: the psychological consequences of cerebral disorder*. Blackwell Science, Oxford. [A classic: an extensive, historically informed, study of the psychological and psychiatric associations of medical and neurological disorders.]

Lishman's Organic Psychiatry. Fourth edition. Edited by Anthony David, Simon Fleminger, Michael Kopelman, Simon Lovestone, John Mellers. Wiley Blackwell, Chichester, 2009.

Zeman A (2002). *Consciousness: a user's guide*. Yale University Press, New Haven, CT. [An introduction to the science and philosophy of consciousness.]

24.3

Clinical investigation of neurological disease

Contents

24.3.1 Lumbar puncture

Roger A. Barker, Wendy Phillips, and R. Rhys Davies

Essentials

Lumbar puncture provides the means to sample cerebrospinal fluid for diagnostic purposes and to remove it for some therapeutic purposes. The procedure allows measurement of the pressure of cerebrospinal fluid, its cytological composition, biochemical content, and microbial as well as serological characteristics.

Indications—the commonest diagnostic indications are clinical suspicion of central nervous system infection (meningitis, encephalitis), subarachnoid haemorrhage, and demyelinating diseases (central and peripheral); the commonest therapeutic indications are idiopathic intracranial hypertension and for intrathecal administration of drugs.

Contraindications—these include infection in the skin overlyingthe spine, evidence of intracranial hypertension, and bleeding disorders.

Acknowledgement: This chapter has been adapted from the one contributed to the 4th edition of the *Oxford Textbook of Medicine* by R A Fishman.

Indications

Lumbar puncture (LP) should be carried out only after clinical evaluation of the patient, with consideration of the potential value and hazards of the procedure. Cerebrospinal fluid (CSF) findings are important in the differential diagnosis of a range of central nervous system (CNS) infections (meningitis, and encephalitis), subarachnoid haemorrhage, confusional states, acute stroke, status epilepticus, meningeal malignancies, demyelinating diseases (central and peripheral), vasculitis, cerebral venous thrombosis, idiopathic intracranial hypertension, and normal pressure hydrocephalus.

Examination of CSF is usually necessary in patients with suspected intracranial bleeding when initial CT/MRI has not been diagnostic. LP is also helpful in patients with symptoms of raised intracranial pressure and papilloedema with normal imaging. Measurement of the opening pressure and examination of the CSF cellular constituents may distinguish idiopathic intracranial hypertension (IIH), venous sinus thrombosis, and diffuse meningitic processes such as neoplastic or inflammatory/infective meningitis.

LP is necessary in patients with suspected infection. The cellular constituents, as well as the glucose and protein concentrations, may suggest a type of organism. This may be confirmed by culture, or by using specific stains or polymerase chain reaction (PCR) for known CNS pathogens. Finally, CSF analysis is useful in the diagnosis of inflammatory disorders. Again, cellular constituents of the CSF may help to define the condition: raised protein in the absence of cells occurs with inflammatory polyneuropathies, and the detection of intrathecal immunoglobulin synthesis (i.e. oligoclonal bands on electrophoresis) may also be helpful.

LP has therapeutic as well as diagnostic uses. Drugs may be administered intrathecally in meningeal malignancies, fungal meningitis, spastic paraparesis, or spinal anaesthesia. Repeated LP (or placement of a lumbar drain) may also be used to reduce intracranial pressure in IIH, normal pressure hydrocephalus (NPH), or venous sinus thrombosis, or after surgical procedures (e.g. after acoustic neuroma excision).

Contraindications

LP is contraindicated in the presence of infection in the skin overlying the spine. A serious complication of LP is aggravation of preexisting, unrecognized, brain herniation syndrome (e.g. uncal, cerebellar, or cingulate herniation) associated with intracranial hypertension. This hazard is the basis for considering papilloedema as a relative contraindication to LP. The availability of CT/MRI has simplified the management of patients with papilloedema. If CT reveals no evidence of a mass lesion, LP is usually needed in the presence of papilloedema to establish the diagnosis of IIH and to exclude meningeal inflammation or malignancy. In most acute hospital settings, CT is obtained before LP in the presence of new neurological signs or any features of raised intracranial pressure (including drowsiness).

Thrombocytopenia and other bleeding diatheses (including therapeutic anticoagulation) predispose patients to needle-induced subarachnoid, subdural, and epidural haemorrhage. LP should be undertaken only if urgently needed when the platelet count is depressed to about 50 000/μl or below. Platelet transfusion just before the puncture is recommended if the count is below 20 000/μl or dropping rapidly. The administration of protamine to patients on heparin, and vitamin K or fresh frozen plasma to those receiving warfarin, is recommended before LP to minimize the hazard of the procedure. In patients receiving subcutaneous low-molecular-weight heparin, standard practice is to delay puncture for at least 24 h after an injection.

Complications

Complications of LP include worsening of brain herniation and spinal cord compression, subarachnoid bleeding, diplopia, radicular symptoms, backache, and headache. Infection after an LP is rare. The introduction of dermal tissue into the subarachnoid would be a theoretical risk if an unstyletted needle were used.

Headache after LP is the most common complication, occurring in about 25% of patients and usually lasting 2 to 8 days. It results from low CSF pressure due to persistent fluid leakage through the dural hole. Characteristically, pain is present in the upright position and is promptly relieved by a supine position. Aching of the neck and low back is common. The headaches are aggravated by cough or strain and may be associated with nausea, vomiting, or tinnitus. They are less likely after first-pass LP with a small needle, and if the needle stylet is reinserted before removal. The management of headache after LP depends on strict bedrest in the horizontal position for at least 12 h, adequate hydration, and simple analgesics. Caffeine may help. If conservative measures fail, the use of a 'blood patch' is indicated. The technique consists of injecting autologous blood epidurally, close to the site of the dural puncture, forming a thrombotic tamponade that seals the dural hole. Blood patches are often undertaken by anaesthetists in their obstetric practice.

Cerebrospinal fluid

Opening pressure

The CSF pressure should be measured routinely. The pressure level within the right atrium is the reference level with the patient horizontal in the lateral decubitus position. The normal lumbar CSF pressure ranges between 50 and 200 mmH$_2$O (and as high as 250 mmH$_2$O in very obese individuals). Low pressures are seen in dehydration, spinal subarachnoid block, or CSF leak (e.g. from previous LP), or may be technical in origin because of faulty needle placement. Increased pressures occur with intracranial mass lesions (when an LP should not routinely be performed), infections, acute stroke, cerebral venous occlusions, congestive heart failure, pulmonary insufficiency, and IIH.

Leucocytes and cytology

Normal CSF contains no more than five lymphocytes or mononuclear cells per microlitre. A higher white cell count indicates disease in the CNS or meninges. A stained smear of the sediment is needed for an accurate differential cell count. A variety of centrifugal and sedimentation techniques has been used. A pleocytosis occurs in a range of neoplastic, infective, and inflammatory disorders, and the changes characteristic of the various meningitides are listed in Table 24.3.1. Other disorders associated with a pleocytosis include stroke, subarachnoid haemorrhage, cerebral vasculitis, acute demyelination, and brain tumours. CSF pleocytosis may occur in inflammatory polyneuropathies but is not characteristic, and should prompt a search for an underlying cause, e.g. HIV. Eosinophilia most often accompanies parasitic infections, such as cysticercosis. Cytological studies for malignant cells are rewarding in some CNS neoplasms although this may require repeated LPs (typically three) and the involvement of specialist haematology service for flow cytometry analysis to define immunophenotype. If malignancy is suspected, it is important to obtain a large volume (e.g. 10 ml) of fresh CSF for analysis.

Bloody CSF due to needle trauma contains increased numbers of white cells contributed by the blood. A useful approximation to a true white cell count can be obtained by the following correction for the presence of the added blood: if the patient has a normal full blood count, subtract from the total white cell count (WBC per μl) one white cell for each 1000 red blood cells (RBCs) present. Thus, if bloody fluid contains 10 000 red cells and 100 white cells/μl, 10 white cells would be accounted for by the added blood and the corrected leucocyte count would be 90/μl. If the patient's full blood count reveals significant anaemia or leucocytosis, the following formula may be used to determine more accurately the number of white cells (*W*) in the spinal fluid before the blood was added:

$$w = \frac{\text{blood WBC} \times \text{cerebrospinal fluid RBC}}{\text{blood RBC}} \times 100$$

$$W = \left[(\text{blood WBC} \times \text{CSF RBC})/\text{blood RBC}\right] \times 100$$

The presence of blood in the subarachnoid space produces a secondary inflammatory response, which leads to a disproportionate increase in the number of white cells. Following an acute subarachnoid haemorrhage, this elevation in the WBC is most marked about 48 h after onset, when meningeal signs are most striking.

To correct CSF protein values for the presence of added blood due to needle trauma, subtract 0.01 g for every 1000 RBCs. Thus, if the red cell count is 10 000/μl and the total protein is 1.1 g/litre the corrected protein level would be about 1 g/litre. The corrections are reliable only if the cell count and total protein are both made on the same tube of fluid.

Blood

To differentiate between a traumatic spinal puncture and pre-existing subarachnoid haemorrhage (or subarachnoid extension of a parenchymal bleed), the fluid can be collected in a series of three tubes. In traumatic punctures, the fluid generally clears between the first and the third collections. This is detectable with the naked

Table 24.3.1 Cerebrospinal fluid findings in meningitis

Meningitis	Pressure (mmH₂O)	Leucocytes/µl	Protein (g/l)	Glucose (mmol/l)
Acute bacterial	Usually elevated	Several hundred to more than 60 000; usually a few thousand but occasionally less than 100 (especially meningococcal or early in disease). Polymorphonuclears predominate	Usually 1 to 5, occasionally more than 10	0.2 to 2.2 in most cases (in the absence of hyperglycaemia)
Tuberculous	Usually elevated; may be low with dynamic block in advanced stages	Usually 25 to 100; rarely more than 500. Lymphocytes predominate except in early stages when polymorphonuclears may account for 80 per cent of cells	Nearly always elevated, usually 1 to 2; may be much higher if dynamic block	Usually reduced; less than 2.5 in three-quarters of cases
Cryptococcal	Usually elevated	0 to 800; average 50. Lymphocytes predominate	Usually 0.2 to 5; average 1	Reduced in most cases; average 1.7 (in absence of hyperglycaemia)
Viral	Normal to moderately elevated	5 to a few hundred; but may be more than 1000, particularly with lymphocytic choriomeningitis. Lymphocytes predominate but there may be more than 80 per cent polymorphonuclears in the first few days	Frequently normal or slightly elevated; less than 1; may show greater elevation in severe cases	Normal (reduced in one-quarter of cases of mumps and herpes simplex)
Syphilitic (acute)	Usually elevated	Average 500. Usually lymphocytes; rarely polymorphonuclear	Average 1	Normal (rarely reduced)
Cysticercosis	Often increased; low with dynamic block	Increased mononuclears and polymorphonuclears with 2 to 7 per cent eosinophilia in about half of cases	Usually 0.5 to 2	Reduced in a fifth of cases
Sarcoid	Normal to considerably elevated	0 to fewer than 100 mononuclear cells	Slight to moderate elevation	Reduced in half of cases
Tumour	Normal or elevated	0 to several hundred mononuclears plus malignant cells	Elevated often to high levels	Normal or greatly reduced (low in three-quarters of carcinomatous meningitis cases)

Cerebrospinal fluid immunoglobulins are commonly increased in all of the above (including carcinomatous meningitis) as well as in multiple sclerosis and central nervous system vasculitis. Cerebrospinal fluid immunoglobulins are assessed by the IgG index: (IgG (cerebrospinal fluid) × albumin (serum))/ (IgG serum × albumin(cerebrospinal fluid)). The normal index is less than 0.65.

Oligoclonal bands (with gel electrophoresis) present in cerebrospinal fluid but absent in serum are also a measure of abnormally increased cerebrospinal fluid immunoglobulins synthesized within the CNS).

eye and may be confirmed by cell count. In subarachnoid bleeding, the blood is generally evenly admixed in the three tubes. A sample of the bloody fluid should be centrifuged and the supernatant fluid compared with tap water to exclude the presence of pigment. The supernatant fluid should be crystal clear if the red cell count is less than 100 000 cells/µl but, with more severe bloody contamination, the plasma proteins may be sufficient to cause minimal xanthochromia.

Following subarachnoid haemorrhage, the supernatant fluid usually remains clear for 2 to 4 h, or even longer, after the onset of subarachnoid bleeding. Between 12 h and 12 days after symptom onset, however, the absence of xanthochromia effectively excludes the diagnosis. After an especially traumatic puncture, some blood and xanthochromia may be present for as long as 2 to 5 days after the initial puncture. CSF protein of greater than 1.5 g/litre, irrespective of cause, may be associated with faint xanthochromia. When the protein is elevated to much higher levels, as in spinal block, inflammatory demyelinating polyneuropathies, or meningitis, the xanthochromia may be marked. Xanthochromic fluid when the protein level is less than 1.5 g/litre generally indicates recent subarachnoid haemorrhage.

Rarely, xanthochromia is due to severe jaundice, carotenaemia, or rifampicin therapy.

If there is any doubt as to whether the CSF reflects a subarachnoid haemorrhage as opposed to a bloody tap, further imaging of the vasculature is required.

Pigments

Two major pigments derived from red cells, the basis of xanthochromia after haemorrhage, may be seen in CSF—oxyhaemoglobin and bilirubin. Methaemoglobin is detected only by spectrophotometry. Oxyhaemoglobin, released with lysis of red cells, may be detected in the supernatant fluid within 2 h of a subarachnoid haemorrhage. It reaches a maximum in about the first 36 h and gradually disappears over the next 7 to 10 days. Bilirubin is produced *in vivo* by leptomeningeal cells after red cell haemolysis, and is first detected about 10 h after the onset of subarachnoid bleeding. It reaches a maximum at 48 h and may persist for 2 to 4 weeks after extensive bleeding. The severity of the meningeal signs associated with subarachnoid bleeding correlates with the inflammatory response, i.e. the leucocytic pleocytosis.

Protein

Total protein

The total protein level of CSF ranges between 0.15 and 0.5 g/litre. although an elevated protein level lacks specificity, it is an index of neurological disease reflecting a pathological increase in the permeability of endothelial cells. Greatly increased protein levels, 5 g/litre and above, are seen in meningitis, bloody fluids, or cord tumour with spinal block. Guillain–Barré syndrome or chronic inflammatory demyelinating polyneuropathies (CIDPs), diabetic radiculoneuropathy, and myxoedema may also increase the level to 1 to 3 g/litre. Low protein levels, below 0.15 g/litre, occur most often with CSF leaks due to a previous LP or traumatic dural fistula.

Immunoglobulins

A vast number of proteins may be measured in CSF but only increases in immunoglobulins are of major diagnostic importance. Such increases are indicative of an inflammatory response in the CNS and occur with immunological disorders, and bacterial, viral, spirochaetal, and fungal diseases. Immunoglobulin assays are most useful in the diagnosis of multiple sclerosis (MS), other demyelinating diseases, and CNS vasculitis. The CSF level is corrected for the entry of immunoglobulins from the serum by calculating the IgG index (see Table 24.3.1). More than one electrophoretic band in CSF ('oligoclonal bands') is also abnormal. This pattern is found in 90% of MS cases and may occur with other inflammatory processes (e.g. vasculitis and paraneoplasia). It is important to stress that, whenever a LP is performed and CSF sent, a serum sample is sent at the same time so that the necessary comparisons can be made to determine whether the inflammation is confined to the CNS (e.g. MS) or part of a multisystem disorder (e.g. systemic lupus erythematosus).

Other proteins

The 14-3-3 proteins are ubiquitous regulator proteins, and can be found in the CSF of patients with Creutzfeldt–Jakob disease. The astrocytic protein, S100β, and neuron-specific enolase may also be raised in the CSF of such patients. The sensitivity and specificity are limited. Angiotensin-converting enzyme levels are increased in neurosarcoidosis but variation between individuals undermines the value of this in diagnosis.

Glucose

The concentration of glucose in CSF is dependent on the blood concentration. The normal range of glucose concentration in CSF is between 2.5 and 4.5 mmol/litre in patients with a blood glucose between 4 and 7 mmol/litre, i.e. 60 to 80% of the normal blood level. CSF glucose values between 2.2 and 2.5 mmol/litre are usually abnormal, and values below 2.2 mmol/litre invariably so. Hyperglycaemia during the 4 h before LP results in a parallel increase in CSF glucose. The latter approaches a maximum and the CSF:blood ratio may be as low as 0.35 in the presence of a greatly elevated blood glucose level and the absence of any neurological disease. Increased CSF glucose has no further diagnostic significance. The CSF glucose level is abnormally low (hypoglycorrhachia) in several diseases of the nervous system. It is characteristic of acute purulent meningitis, and is a usual finding in tuberculous and fungal meningitis, as well as neoplastic meningitis. It is usually normal in viral meningitis, although it can be reduced in patients with mumps, herpes simplex, and zoster meningoencephalitis. CSF glucose may be reduced in other inflammatory meningitides including cysticercosis, amoebic meningitis (*Nagleria* spp.), acute syphilitic meningitis, sarcoidosis, granulomatous arteritis, and other vasculitides. Glucose levels may also be depressed in the context of subarachnoid haemorrhage (usually 4 to 8 days after the bleed) or in chemical meningitis after intrathecal injection.

The major factor responsible for reduced glucose levels is increased anaerobic glycolysis in adjacent neural tissues and, to a lesser degree, in cells that may be detected in the CSF itself. As such, the decrease in the CSF glucose level is accompanied by an inverse increase in the CSF lactate level.

Lactate

Detection of elevated CSF lactate may be useful when inborn errors of metabolism and mitochondrial disease are suspected. Although CSF lactate is more reliable than plasma lactate, it is not definitive and muscle biopsy, DNA analysis, etc. should also be performed. High CSF lactate is also seen in systemic lactic acidosis and nonspecifically when other CSF abnormalities are present. Some advocate the use of CSF lactate as a marker for bacterial versus viral meningitis, but this is not widely accepted.

Microbiological and serological reactions

The use of appropriate stains, cultures, and PCR to specific pathogens is essential in cases of suspected infection. Typically CSF is examined using standard stains (e.g. Gram stain) before culturing and PCR tests are undertaken. The involvement of an infectious disease specialist is often helpful in defining the true validity and significance of positive microbiological/serological tests. In all cases, if there is a clinical suspicion of a CNS infection, treatment should be commenced before any definite microbiological results from the CSF can be obtained.

Further reading

Fishman RA (1992). *CSF in diseases of the nervous system*, 2nd edition. W B Saunders, Philadelphia, PA.

24.3.2 Electrophysiology of the central and peripheral nervous systems

Christian Krarup

Essentials

Electrophysiological studies of the central nervous system and peripheral nervous system—the core investigations in clinical neurophysiology—include electroencephalography, evoked potentials,

Acknowledgement: I am indebted to Dr H. Høgenhaven MD for comments on the manuscript.

electromyography, and nerve conduction studies. These provide information from anatomical regions which may not be accessible to direct pathological examination, and are good for tracking changes over time. However, they do not provide direct information about pathological changes in the nervous system, hence it is often necessary to supplement electrophysiological findings by imaging or other laboratory studies, and it is mandatory to view all results in their clinical context.

Electroencephalography (EEG)

EEG is mainly used to identify and diagnose epileptic discharges in connection with paroxysmal events. The procedure is valuable for the evaluation and prognosis of disturbances of consciousness at diffuse disorders of the brain, including infectious, metabolic, and ischaemic disorders, when serial recordings are often used. EEG is of value to diagnose epilepsy caused by focal or diffuse brain diseases, but it is of limited value for detecting focal lesions, since those that affect subcortical regions cannot be detected by scalp electrodes.

Evoked potentials

Evoked potentials in the brain are obtained following sensory stimulation and used to determine the integrity of afferent and efferent pathways, principally threatened by disease in myelinated tracts or the synaptic connections by which sensory impulses are relayed. (1) Somatosensory and motor evoked potentials—these are useful for monitoring surgical procedures in the vertebral column or carried out for spinal lesions. (2) Visual evoked potentials—these are used to assess diseases of the optic nerve in for example multiple sclerosis; electroretinography recorded with contact lenses is used to assess retinal disease, and dark adapted studies may assist diagnosis of retinal degeneration. (3) Brainstem auditory evoked potentials—elicited by clicks, are complex multiphase responses determined by conduction within the cochlear nerve and the different relay steps in the lateral lemniscus; they assist in evaluating the integrity of the brainstem in diverse types of brain injury, and are also useful in localizing cochlear nerve lesions, lesions of the cochlear nucleus and brainstem tracts.

Electromyography (EMG) and nerve conduction studies

EMG is useful for determining whether weakness is caused by muscle disease or by loss of alpha-motor fibre innervation, for which nerve conduction studies—to search for loss of sensory or motor axons or disease of myelinated fibres—are usually required. Disturbances of neuromuscular transmission (e.g. myasthenia gravis and the Lambert–Eaton syndrome) require special examination of compound muscle responses evoked by repetitive motor stimulation. Single-fibre recordings of action potentials induced during voluntary activity or after repetitive stimulation allow the stability of neuromuscular transmission to be assessed.

Other electrophysiological techniques

Additional methods—e.g. cardiovascular reflexes in the study of the autonomic nervous system, respiratory movements and oxygen saturation in polysomnographic studies of sleep disturbances, and recording of force in the study of voluntary muscle—are becoming increasingly important.

Studies of the central nervous system

Electroencephalography

At electroencephalography the spontaneous ongoing activity from the cerebral cortex is recorded through electrodes placed over the scalp. In most routine studies, recordings are carried out over 30 to 60 min. In addition specialized studies may be performed to diagnose patients with particular types of epilepsy, during carotid artery endarterectomy or brain death. In patients with poorly described epileptic fits, the clinical features may require that both visual information and electroencephalographic (EEG) evidence are obtained simultaneously (video-EEG). This may, in patients who are candidates for surgical treatment of medically intractable epilepsy, be carried out over many days. In some patients additional information may be obtained with intracranial subdural, or intracerebral depth electrodes. During epilepsy surgery, an EEG is recorded directly from the cortex, so-called electrocorticography.

Indications

The main indications to obtain an EEG include paroxysmal events, convulsions, disturbed levels of consciousness, and neuroinfections. The EEG is not well suited as a screening procedure in patients with suspected focal cerebral lesions, because deep-seated lesions do not show abnormalities at EEG, if the cortex itself or its afferent projections are not affected. However, when the clinical picture in patients with the focal brain lesions is complicated by periodic changes in consciousness, convulsions, or unexplained changes in focal weakness, the EEG is necessary to establish the presence of secondary paroxysmal events. Furthermore, the EEG is often indicated in patients with encephalopathy in order to ascertain whether the clinical features are complicated by additional ictal discharges.

Serial EEGs are often necessary to assess the prognosis in patients with diffuse brain lesions. When abnormalities obtained early during a cerebral disorder (e.g. cardiac arrest associated with cerebral ischaemia) are followed by further deterioration of the EEG pattern, this indicates a poor prognosis.

Method

The recording takes place with the patient in a comfortable position in a quiet room, and is carried out by a technician who places surface or needle electrodes over the scalp according to an international, standardized system (the 10–20 system, Fig. 24.3.2.1). After placement of the electrodes, the technician ensures that the impedance of the electrodes is less than $5\,k\Omega$. The age, clinical state, and medication of the patient are indicated on the record, in particular whether the level of consciousness is normal. The session includes recording while the patient is awake, during activation procedures, and if possible during drowsiness and sleep. During the recording the technician makes notes about the patient's awareness and state of consciousness, and if events occur during the recording they should be fully described. During the recording, activity is evaluated at different electrode montages including both bipolar and unipolar recordings. Bipolar recordings are of value to localize abnormalities in focal brain areas whereas the unipolar recordings are necessary to examine more widespread and generalized disturbances.

During recording the awake patient is asked to relax with closed eyes to assess the background activity. The EEG waveforms are described in terms of their frequencies. The frequency contents of the EEG are classified into activity with frequencies of 8 to 13 Hz

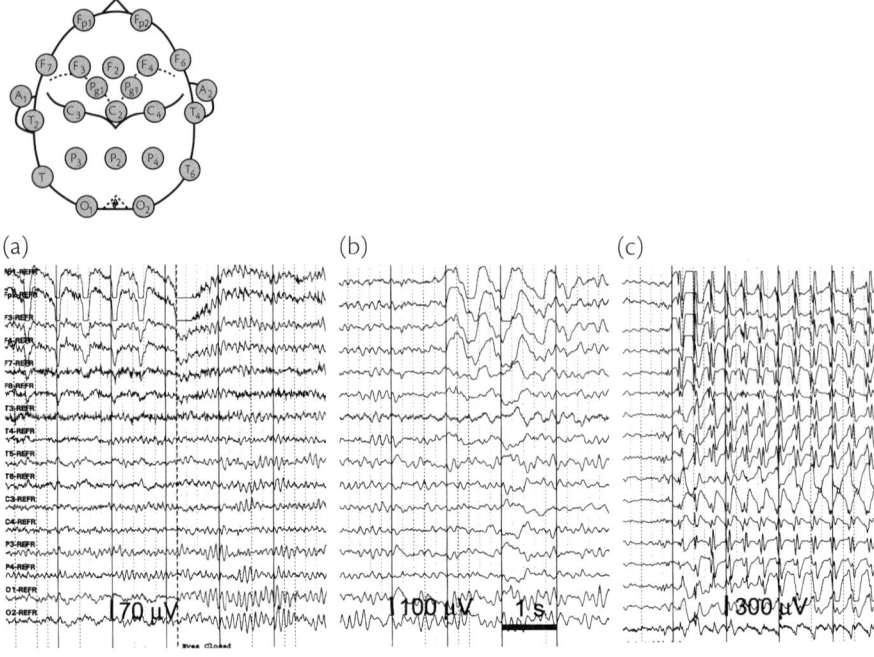

Fig. 24.3.2.1 Examples of EEG curves recorded using a common reference recording montage. Above left is shown the electrode placement using the 10–20 international system. (a) EEG from a 20-year-old normal man (aviation candidate). Eye blinking was carried out to the left of the stippled line. At the stippled line the eyes were closed and the 10-Hz background activity became prominent mainly over the posterior regions. (b) A 72-year-old woman with progressive gait abnormalities, dementia, and urine incontinence. The CT scan showed cerebral atrophy and hydrocephalus. The EEG showed high amplitude δ waves over the frontal regions. The background activity was slowed to 7 Hz. (c) An 8-year-old boy with absences. The EEG showed generalized 3-Hz spike-and-wave paroxysms.

(α activity), 3.5 to 7.5 Hz (θ activity), equal to or less than 3 Hz (δ activity), and activity above 13 Hz (β activity). The interpretation of the EEG should include a description of the background activity, and the presence of abnormal waveforms ('transients') during rest and activation procedures, and it should be indicated if changes in the background or the occurrence of abnormal waveforms occur diffusely, synchronously, or in a focal pattern (Fig. 24.3.2.2 and see Fig. 24.3.2.1b,c). Advanced algorithms to localize the distribution of waveforms (brain mapping) are now used in the diagnosis and research on epileptic and nonepileptic syndromes, and they are of particular relevance in the temporal and spatial development of transient abnormalities.

Activation procedures include hyperventilation, where the patient breathes deeply at a rate of 20/min for 2 to 4 min and followed up to 2 min after hyperventilation. In children and young adults this may elicit θ and δ activity whereas this is considered abnormal in older individuals aged over 30 years, and patients with absences may develop spike-and-(sharp)-wave patterns during hyperventilation (see Fig. 24.3.2.1c). The possible epileptogenic effect of photic stimulation is evaluated by stimulating with variable frequencies with the eyes opened and closed. In susceptible individuals spike activity limited to the occipital regions is not associated with epilepsy, but spikes or sharp waves in a more widespread distribution are indicators of a lowered epileptogenic threshold.

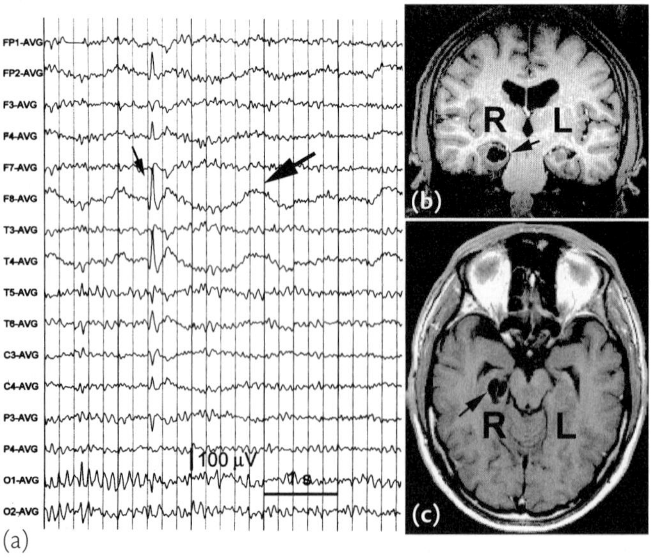

The normal EEG

The frequency content in the normal individual is highly dependent on age, the level of awareness, and medication. In the normal awake adult with closed eyes the EEG is dominated by α activity most pronounced over posterior parts of the head (see Fig. 24.3.2.1a), and is subject to modulations by changes in vigilance, e.g. it disappears when the individual opens the eyes.

In the newborn, the EEG is characterized by low-frequency activity and variable amplitudes. In premature babies, the EEG may be dominated by burst-suppression activity, which does not occur in the normal full-term baby. During maturation the background frequencies move into the α range by the early teens. Even in normal young adults, intermittent posterior slowing may be seen over the occipital regions, and become enhanced and spread to other regions during hyperventilation. This slow activity during hyperventilation is augmented by low glucose levels in the blood, and glucose should be given by mouth to individuals with excessive amounts of slow activity during hyperventilation.

Fig. 24.3.2.2 A 31-year-old man with a history of complex partial seizures. (a) The EEG showed a spike focus over the right pre- and midtemporal regions (small arrow). In addition there was a slow wave (1–2 Hz) focus over the same regions (large arrow), highly suspicious of a focal brain lesion. An average reference electrode montage was used. (b) Coronal T_1-weighted MRI after contrast injection. (c) Transverse reconstructed section. Arrows indicate the site of a cystic ring-enhancing lesion in the right hippocampal region. MRI by courtesy of the Danish Research Centre for Magnetic Resonance, Hvidovre Hospital.

During drowsiness the α activity is diminished and disappears first intermittently and subsequently completely, and is replaced by θ activity (stage 1 sleep). During stage 2 sleep (light sleep), sleep spindles (bursts of 12- to 14-Hz activity), sharp waves over the vertex, and K complexes (high-amplitude slow-wave activity) are recorded in addition to θ activity. At deeper levels of sleep (stages 3 and 4), increasing amounts of high-amplitude δ activity are recorded (often designated 'delta sleep'). If drowsiness is not recognized during the recording session, the EEG may be badly misinterpreted, and it is therefore important that the technician closely controls the level of awareness at all times.

The abnormal EEG

The abnormal EEG may be characterized by changes in the background activity, the presence of low-frequency waveforms, or epileptiform activity, or by periodic phenomena. The EEG is evaluated for the presence of abnormal frequencies or waveforms either intermittently or continuously, whether these are localized diffusely or focally, and whether they occur in a synchronous or an asynchronous distribution.

Abnormal frequencies

Slowing of the normal background activity occurs in patients with encephalopathy (e.g. ischaemic or metabolic brain disease) or degenerative brain disease (e.g. Alzheimer's disease). Focal slowing (see Fig. 24.3.2.2) and attenuation of background activity are highly suggestive of focal brain disease (e.g. stroke, tumour, or subdural haematoma). In comatose patients with pontine lesions, the EEG may be dominated by α-like activity; however, in these cases, the activity is not modulated by stimulation.

Generalized, diffuse, and focal abnormalities

Generalized abnormalities occur synchronously throughout the brain, although the amplitudes and waveforms may vary at different recording sites (see Fig. 24.3.2.1c). Diffuse abnormalities are also present over large brain areas, but the low-frequency activity or spikes/sharp waves may occur independently. It should be considered if the generalized changes occur in recordings with a single reference electrode, because this may erroneously give rise to the impression of generalization.

Generalized abnormalities are considered to have a central origin if generalization occurs from the onset, but may also be due to a focal cortical lesion if generalization occurs as a secondary phenomenon. So-called intermittent rhythmic δ activity (IRDA, see Fig. 24.3.2.1b) may occur over widespread areas of the brain, due to raised intracranial pressure, and have little localizing value. Diffuse low-frequency abnormalities, often associated with triphasic waves, indicate widespread cortical abnormalities in metabolic encephalopathies.

Spikes, sharp waves, and periodic complexes

The central role of the EEG in the diagnosis and follow-up of patients with epilepsy justifies the attention that is paid to the identification and localization of epileptic discharges. The features characteristic of epileptiform events consist of waves of various forms, usually spikes (potential duration equal or less than 70 ms) or sharp waves (potential duration of 70 to 200 ms) in a rhythmic pattern, which are of high voltage compared with the background activity and reflect hypersynchronization of neuronal discharges (see Fig. 24.3.2.1c). Spikes may be followed by a negative wave, the so-called spike–wave complex. It is unusual for an epileptic seizure to coincide with the EEG, and the diagnosis therefore relies on the presence of epileptiform discharges during interictal recordings, and the examination at the first EEG may be negative in up to 50% of patients. Repeat studies or prolonged recordings (often under video control) are frequently indicated, and proper activation procedures such as hyperventilation, photic stimulation, and possibly sleep deprivation, or the use of sedatives to ensure sleep during the study, may be needed. The diagnostic yield of repeated EEG studies has accordingly been found to show abnormalities in more than 90% of patients with a clinically established diagnosis of epilepsy.

Paroxysmal discharges may be focal or generalized in distribution according to the underlying aetiology. Recently developed focal epileptic symptoms (see Fig. 24.3.2.2) may be evidence of a brain tumour and should be thoroughly investigated with appropriate imaging studies. Epileptic activity may develop abruptly in primary generalized seizures (see Fig. 24.3.2.1c). It is, however, important to evaluate this development closely to distinguish primary from secondary seizures that develop focally and then spread to adjacent cerebral regions, and possibly with generalization to the whole brain. Detection of focal epileptic activity may require specialized electrode montages. For example, an epileptic focus in the temporal lobe may require recording through electrodes placed over the zygomatic arch or through a needle sphenoidal electrode placed at the foramen ovale. Such focal epileptic activity may, moreover, not become apparent until the patient becomes drowsy or goes to sleep.

The electrophysiological activity is usually not unambiguous for subgroups of epileptic seizures, although the particular combination of clinical characteristics, the EEG changes during seizures, and the interictal activity may be distinctive for epileptic syndromes, and the term 'electroclinical diagnosis' has been coined. Generalized 3/s spike–wave complexes are considered pathognomonic for generalized absence seizures (see Fig. 24.3.2.1c), and hypsarrhythmia (high-voltage irregular slow waves interspersed with spikes) occur almost exclusively in infantile spasms. Periodic lateralised epileptiform discharges (PLEDs) are continuous focal spike activity with a frequency of 0.5 to 3/s seen in connection with acute severe brain disease. Periodic generalized complexes of sharp waves are characteristically seen in patients with Creutzfeldt–Jakob disease, herpes simplex encephalitis, and subacute sclerosing panencephalitis, and may be present in patients with severe brain anoxia.

Evoked potentials

Evoked potentials (EPs) are CNS potentials obtained by stimulation of particular sensory receptors or fibre tracts and are carried out to examine the integrity of afferent and efferent pathways. The sensory pathways examined routinely include the visual system (visual-evoked potentials, VEPs), fibre tracts in the brainstem (brainstem auditory-evoked potentials, BAEPs), and somatosensory pathways in the dorsal columns (somatosensory-evoked potentials, SSEPs). Motor-evoked potentials (MEPs) are elicited by transcortical magnetic stimulation (TMS) of the motor cortex to study the corticospinal tracts. In the following is given a description of the main methodological questions and pathophysiological findings, whereas detailed description methods are considered beyond the scope of this chapter, and the reader is referred to the suggested literature.

Near-field and far-field responses

The responses discussed in this chapter are the modality-specific components of the EPs that reflect the propagation of action potentials in fibre tracts and cortical areas. The so-called 'event-related' potentials, although time locked to a stimulus, are not modality specific and reflect activity in neuronal networks involved in cognitive processing (e.g. P300), and are not described further.

The electrical responses recorded close to the source are the so-called near-field potentials and may arise from axons or be of postsynaptic origin. These include action potentials recorded from peripheral nerve, the spinal cord, or cortical areas. However, the activity recorded from scalp electrodes with a noncephalic reference also reflects activity in deeply located structures, far-field potentials. The origin of a number of these EP components is incompletely known, and in routine practice the latencies and amplitudes of only some of these are of clinical relevance.

Indications

The main purpose of EP studies is to ascertain the presence of pathological processes localized to myelinated fibre tracts or to the synaptic connections through which messages are relayed. The conduction velocity of the fibres is gauged by the latencies of the responses, and these are particularly susceptible to abnormalities of the myelin sheath (e.g. multiple sclerosis). However, conduction abnormalities are not specific for a particular disease, and delayed conduction may be seen in a variety of disorders including hereditary diseases, compression of nervous tissue (such as spondylotic myelopathy), and infectious diseases (such as AIDS). Thus, the constellation of EP abnormalities, the clinical setting, and other paraclinical or laboratory findings are important when the findings are interpreted in a diagnostic setting.

The amplitudes of responses are influenced by the number of conducting fibres and, in disorders characterized by fibre loss without involvement of myelin, abnormalities may be confined to a reduction in amplitude. However, the amplitude of the EP is a poor indicator of the degree of fibre loss due to the amplification that occurs at synaptic relays. Thus, a cortical response may still be recordable at SSEPs in patients with a severe neuropathy and absent peripheral nerve response. Finally, the conduction may be delayed in disorders characterized by axonal loss, possibly related to delays at synaptic transmission. Thus, in patients with amyotrophic lateral sclerosis, the MEP often shows delayed central conduction time even though the disorder is characterized by fibre loss rather than demyelination.

The use of SSEPs and MEPs has proved valuable for intraoperative monitoring during surgery on the vertebral column for scoliosis and on the spinal cord for tumours or vascular malformations. Both a reduction in amplitudes and prolongation of latencies have proved to be reliable indicators of impending damage to the spinal cord and hence the need to take measures to avoid permanent damage. In addition, the use of electromyograph (EMG) recordings from relevant muscles is helpful during scoliosis operations, by warning the surgeon that a root may be in danger by screws or other hardware.

Visual-evoked potentials

Method

The VEP is evoked by either a diffuse stroboscopic flash (flash VEP), which stimulates the whole retina, or by pattern reversal stimulation (pattern VEP), where a black-and-white chequerboard

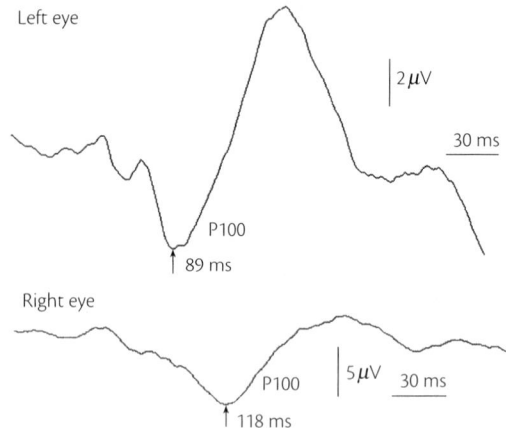

Fig. 24.3.2.3 Pattern-reversal visual-evoked potentials (VEPs; chequerboard stimulation) from a 64-year-old man showed a normal pattern VEP with a P100 latency of 89 ms from the left eye and an abnormal pattern VEP from the right eye with a latency of 118 ms (27% prolonged, upper normal limit 103 ms). The findings indicated the presence of a right-sided optic nerve lesion.

reverses position at a frequency of 2/s. The patient is seated at a distance of 1 m and gazes at the centre of the chequerboard projected on either a screen or a TV monitor. The pattern VEP is sensitive to the cooperation of the patient whereas the flash VEP can be used to ascertain whether functional connections exist between the retina and the occipital lobes. The size of each square is either 9 mm or 18 mm depending on the visual acuity. The pattern VEP is generated mainly by the central 10° of vision. The responses are recorded over the occipital lobes. At least 100, and preferably 200, sweeps are averaged to yield responses of adequate resolution.

Each eye is stimulated in turn, and in routine studies the whole visual field is stimulated; in some conditions, it is more revealing to stimulate part of the visual field. In these instances, usually the half-field is stimulated. Half-field stimulation is particularly useful in conditions with lesions localized in the visual projections behind the chiasma but require considerable expertise for interpretation.

Measurements

The pattern VEP has three main components of which the positive phase at a latency of about 100 ms is the most constant (Fig. 24.3.2.3). In clinical practice, the latency of this phase and the amplitude of the response are measured. In flash VEP, the latencies of the N70, P90 and N120 phases are measured.

Clinical correlations

Flash VEP is reduced in retinal disease and is useful in retinitis pigmentosa and patients who cannot cooperate to carry out pattern VEP, in particular children.

Monocular full-field pattern VEPs with prolonged latency to the P100 component in one eye indicates that the lesion is localized anterior to the optic chiasma (Fig. 24.3.2.3). This is most frequently due to demyelination of the optic nerve but may be due to retinal degeneration, optic nerve compression, or glaucoma. In some patients with mild optic neuritis, the latencies show only an abnormal interocular difference. The interpretation is more uncertain if bilateral prolonged latencies are found, because this may be due to lesions anywhere along the visual pathways. Interocular differences in patients with bilateral retrochiasmal lesions (e.g. spinocerebellar syndromes) are within normal range. Marked latency differences in patients with bilateral abnormalities suggest bilateral optic nerve lesions. Retrochiasmal lesions may be further examined by partial-field (half-field) studies of the individual eye.

Electroretinography

The electroretinogram (ERG) is the electrical response evoked in the retina by a flash and is due to depolarization of the interstitial Müller cells and pigmented epithelium. The ERG is recorded by a contact lens electrode or with an infraorbital surface electrode. The state of light and dark adaptation can be used to separate the function of rods and cones. The ERG is usually carried out when the VEP is missing and it is uncertain whether this may be due to a retinal problem. In such cases, the ERG may be evoked by a routine flash. Dark-adapted ERGs are carried out in the differential diagnosis of retinal degenerations and are a specialist task usually carried out in collaboration with a neuro-ophthalmologist.

Brainstem auditory-evoked potentials

Method

The auditory brainstem response is elicited by passing short-lasting clicks at an intensity of 75 to 100 dB through earphones to each ear separately. The responses of interest include the time-locked far-field responses with latencies of less than 10 ms. The brainstem-derived response consists of several phases that indicate conduction along peripheral pathways in the cochlear nerve and different relay stations of the lateral lemniscus pathways within the brainstem.

Measurements

The waves of interest are positive peaks numbered as PI to PVI, where PI, PIII, and PV are usually recorded, whereas the remaining waves may be missing even in normal individuals. PI is generated in the cochlear nerve, PII in the cochlear nucleus, PIII in the pons, and PV at the midbrain level. For clinical purposes the latency of PI is measured to ascertain peripheral conduction and the PI to PIII, PI to PV, and PIII to PV to ascertain the central conduction time within the brainstem.

Clinical correlations

The BAEP is of help in investigating the integrity of the brainstem and is used to confirm brain death in some laboratories. Its main usefulness lies in the localization of lesions at the cochlear nerve, at the entry into the brainstem (cochlear nucleus), and at different sites within the brainstem. Central abnormalities are found in 50% of patients with MS.

Somatosensory-evoked potentials

Method

The responses are evoked by repetitive stimulation (2 to 5/s) of the median nerves at the wrists and the tibial nerves behind the medial malleolus (Fig. 24.3.2.4), using a stimulus duration of 0.2 ms at a strength just sufficient to elicit a motor response. Differentiation between peripheral and central disease is obtained after stimulation of the median nerve by recording peripheral nerve responses through surface or subcutaneous needle electrodes at the supraclavicular fossa (Erb's point, designated the N9 response), from the spinal cord at C6 (designated the N13), and over the contralateral hemisphere (designated N20). At stimulation of the tibial nerves, recordings are carried out from the peripheral nerve at the popliteal fossa (or at the gluteal fold), at Th12 (designated the N23), and over the brain (onset response and P40 response). Up to 1000 responses are averaged, depending on the level of noise and the size of the response. The average is carried out in two bins to ensure reproducibility.

Measurements

The latencies to the onsets of the peripheral nerve responses are measured to calculate the peripheral conduction velocities (Fig. 24.3.2.4), to the negative peak of the spinal response, to the first negative response at the cortex after the median nerve, and to the onset and the P40 responses after tibial nerve stimulation.

The central conduction time is calculated as the differences in latencies between the spinal responses at C6 and the peak of the N20 response after median nerve stimulation, and between the spinal responses at Th12 and the onset latency (or the P40 latency) after tibial nerve stimulation. The values are compared with height-matched controls.

Clinical correlations

The SSEPs from median and tibial nerves are helpful when very proximal nerve disorders or CNS disorders are suspected. A prolonged latency of the spinal responses indicates the presence of

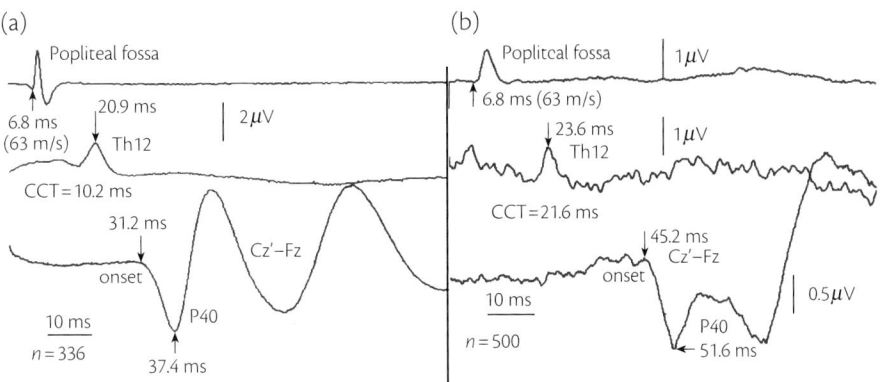

Fig. 24.3.2.4 Somatosensory-evoked potentials from (a) the right leg of a 25-year-old normal woman and (b) the left leg of a 55-year-old man with signs of myelopathy. The tibial nerve was stimulated at the medial malleolus and responses were recorded from the peripheral nerve at the popliteal fossa, the spine (T12), and the scalp. In both, the peripheral conduction velocities and spinal latencies were normal. The latencies of the cortical responses to both the 'onset' and the P40 were normal in (a) and 31% and 25% prolonged, respectively, in (b). The central conduction time was calculated as the difference between the spinal latency and the onset latency. The central conduction time was normal in (a), whereas it was 98% prolonged consistent with myelopathy in (b).

proximal plexus or root lesions, and may be differentiated from a peripheral neuropathy by a normal peripheral nerve response. SSEP studies may be extended by dermatomal stimulation in the legs and the arms to diagnose monoradicular lesions. The SSEPs are, however, particularly useful to identify spinal cord disease, and the central conduction time obtained from the upper and lower limbs separately may be used to determine the likely localization of myelopathic lesions (Fig. 24.3.2.4b). In patients with multiple sclerosis, the central conduction time often shows marked prolongation.

Motor-evoked potentials

Method

MEPs are obtained by activating focal motor cortical areas by a short-lasting strong magnetic pulse of up to 2 tesla (T) which induces a current within the excitable tissue of the cortex. In some laboratories electrical stimulation rather than magnetic stimulation is employed. However, electrical stimulation is painful; moreover, the electrical stimulus activates fibres deeper within the cerebrum than the magnetic stimulus. The two methods therefore yield results that cannot be directly compared. The descending waves from the cortex consist of D waves from cortical neurons followed by I waves that arise trans-synaptically. In addition, stimulation is performed at cervical and lumbar spinal levels. At magnetic stimulation, excitation occurs at the proximal spinal nerves rather than at the spinal cord.

The motor responses are recorded from muscles of the upper and lower limbs (including proximal and distal muscles), using surface electrodes to evaluate the compound muscle action potential (CMAP). In order to obtain 'maximal' motor responses facilitation of cortical neurons by slight voluntary contraction is necessary.

Measurements

The amplitudes and latencies of the CMAPs are measured at both cortical and spinal stimulation (Fig. 24.3.2.5). The central conduction time is obtained by calculating the differences of these latencies; however, as excitation at spinal stimulation occurs at the proximal peripheral nerve, central conduction time includes conduction along the roots. The central conduction time has therefore also been calculated by using the F-wave latency to obtain a measure of the peripheral conduction time. In central lesions the central conduction time is prolonged compared with height- and age-matched controls (Fig. 24.3.2.5b). In addition, the CMAP amplitudes of the cortical response may show reduction, indicating central axonal loss, conduction failure, or increased temporal dispersion along corticospinal fibres. The shape of the CMAP in patients with MS is often polyphasic, indicating dispersion along demyelinated central pathways.

Due to central dispersion, the amplitudes of the CMAPs are often unreliable indicators of loss of corticospinal fibres. This limitation of the methodology has been improved by the introduction of so-called triple-stimulation TMS, which through a collision technique synchronizes the corticospinal response and has been shown to be a sensitive indicator of corticospinal involvement in disease processes.

Clinical correlations

The central motor conduction time is prolonged in demyelinating disorders and the investigation is of particular value in patients suspected of MS (Fig. 24.3.2.5). However, slowing of central conduction is a nonspecific abnormality that may also be seen in patients with other causes of CNS motor disorders. In amyotrophic lateral sclerosis, for example, the central conduction time is often abnormal in an irregular pattern, although the prolongation is usually only slight. The MEPs should therefore be supplemented with other evoked potentials (pattern VEPs and SSEPs), MRI, and spinal fluid examination.

In some patients with peripheral nerve disorders, in particular acute inflammatory demyelinating (poly)neuropathy (AIDP) or CIDP, the MEP may show abnormalities indicating CNS as well as peripheral nervous system involvement. Due to the stimulation of peripheral nerves distal to the intervertebral foramen, the conduction along the spinal roots is included in the central conduction time, and slowing at this segment may therefore erroneously be localized to the CNS.

Studies of the peripheral neuromuscular system

Indications

An EMG is used to establish whether weakness is due to primary disease of muscle fibres (myopathy) or to loss of α-motor fibres (neurogenic disorders). Nerve conduction studies are carried out to ascertain loss of motor or sensory axons or disturbed function of myelinated fibres. Both types of studies are usually needed in the differential diagnosis and, as the findings are rarely specific for particular disorders, the interpretation relies on inferences from several criteria of abnormality. The degree to which the findings should be supplemented and confirmed by light or electron microscopy of nerve or muscle and other laboratory studies depends on the clinical situation. Even though subclinical involvement has

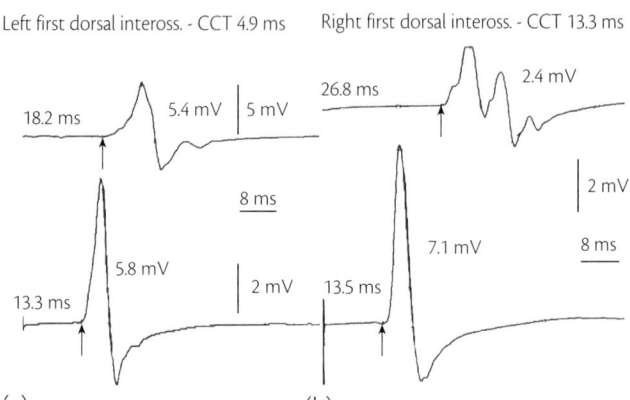

Fig. 24.3.2.5 Motor-evoked potentials obtained by magnetic stimulation from the (a) left and (b) right first dorsal interosseous muscles in a 60-year-old woman suspected of having multiple sclerosis (the pattern visual-evoked potentials (VEP) and the somatosensory-evoked potentials (SSEPs) were also abnormal). Lower traces: compound muscle action potentials (CMAPs) evoked by stimulation of the cervical spine. Upper traces: CMAPs evoked by cortical stimulation. The latencies of the responses (shown above the traces) at spinal stimulation were normal on both sides, whereas cortical latency was normal in (a) and 36% prolonged in (b). The central motor conduction time (indicated above traces) was calculated as the difference between the cortical and peripheral latencies. The central conduction time in the left arm was normal (a), whereas it was 86% prolonged in (b), consistent with a central lesion.

important implications in the diagnostic interpretation in several conditions (e.g. neurogenic changes in nonweak muscles in amyotrophic lateral sclerosis), the use of these studies to 'rule out' neuromuscular involvement in diffuse or focal pain problems should be discouraged.

Disturbance of neuromuscular transmission requires specialized studies that include recording of compound muscle responses evoked by repetitive stimulation of motor nerve fibres. In a single-fibre EMG the action potentials from individual muscle fibres are recorded during voluntary activity or repetitive stimulation to measure the stability of neuromuscular transmission.

Electromyography

Method

An EMG is carried out using needle electrodes. In routine studies most laboratories use concentric needle electrodes, with a core recording lead that has a surface area of $0.07\,mm^2$ referenced to the cannula, or insulated monopolar needles with a surface recording area of $0.17\,mm^2$ referenced to a surface electrode. The results obtained with these electrodes differ in regard to the amplitude of the motor unit potential (MUP), whereas its duration differs only slightly. The baseline is somewhat more unstable when recorded with a monopolar electrode than using a concentric needle. The signals should be recorded via a high-impedance amplifier with a frequency range of 2 Hz to 10 kHz.

Measurements

Recordings are carried out at rest, during weak voluntary activity and maximal voluntary activity (Table 24.3.2.1).

During rest the presence and type of spontaneous activity are characterized. During weak voluntary effort, individual MUPs are recorded without disturbance by other MUPs. The duration and amplitude of the MUP are measured. The duration of the MUP reflects the activity of muscle fibres of the motor unit at a distance from the recording electrode. In contrast, the very few muscle fibres placed at the tip of the concentric electrode determine the

Table 24.3.2.2 EMG criteria of neuromuscular disease

	Specific criteria	Non-specific criteria
Myopathy		
MUP during weak effort	Reduction in duration (>20% shortened)	Increased incidence of polyphasic potentials (>12%).Reduced amplitude
Recruitment pattern	Full recruitment in a weak and wasted muscle. Reduced amplitude of full recruitment pattern	Reduced recruitment pattern
Activity at rest		Fibrillation activity and positive sharp waves
Peripheral nerve and root disease		
MUP during weak effort	Increase in duration (>20% prolonged). Increase in amplitude	Increased incidence of polyphasic potentials (>12%)
Recruitment pattern	Discrete activity. Increased amplitude	Reduced recruitment pattern
Activity at rest		Fibrillation activity and positive sharp waves (4–10 sites)
Anterior horn cell disease		
MUP during weak effort	Increase in amplitude (>500% increased)	Increase in amplitude of individual MUPs (200%)
Recruitment pattern	Increased amplitude (>8 mV)	
Activity at rest	Fasciculations (malignant, intervals of >3 s)	Fasciculations (benign, intervals <1 s)

With permission from Journal of Neurology.

Table 24.3.2.1 EMG limits in normal muscle

	Normal limit
Spontaneous activity recorded at rest	
Number of sites outside endplate region with fibrillation potentials or positive sharp waves	2 sites
Voluntary activity	
1. Weak effort	
Duration of the motor-unit potential (%)	± 20[a]
Amplitude of motor-unit potential (%)	< −50, > +100[a]
Incidence of polyphasic potentials (%)	12[b]
2. Full effort	
Pattern	Full recruitment
Amplitude of envelope curves (mV)	>2 mV, <4 mV

[a] Mean of 20–25 or more MUPs compared to age-matched controls.
[b] In the deltoid and facial muscles, 25%; in the anterior tibial and lateral vastus muscles, 20%.

amplitude of the MUP. The mean amplitudes and durations of at least 20 different MUPs recorded from 10 different sites at 3 different insertions are obtained in quantitative studies. The shapes of individual MUPs are evaluated and designated as simple (fewer than five phases) or polyphasic (five or more phases). The findings are compared with age-matched control values from the investigated muscle, and the percentage deviation is calculated to ascertain whether the findings are normal or consistent with myopathy of chronic partial denervation (Tables 24.3.2.1 and 24.3.2.2).

During a maximal voluntary contraction, all motor units in the muscle are activated. The MUPs from individual motor units cannot therefore be distinguished but form an interference pattern, which according to the degree of overlap is measured semiquantitatively as a 'full', 'reduced', or 'discrete' recruitment pattern. A full recruitment pattern occurs in normal muscle but requires the patient to cooperate fully. It should therefore be noted whether the activity is recorded during maximal or submaximal effort. In addition to the degree of overlap the envelope amplitude of the main activity is measured to distinguish myopathy and neurogenic involvement.

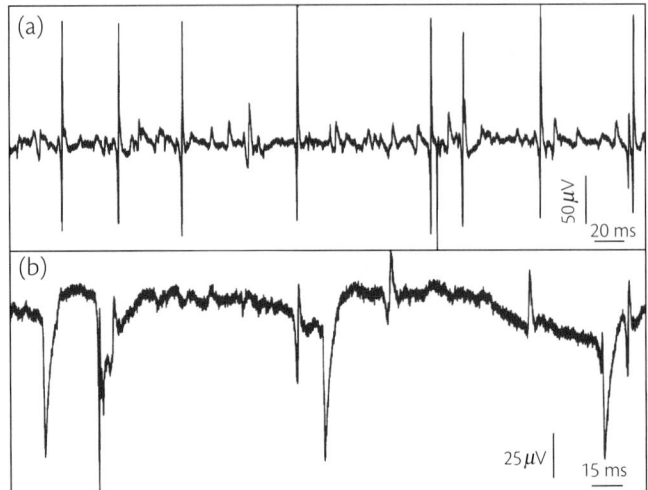

Fig. 24.3.2.6 Fibrillation potentials (a) and (b) and positive sharp waves (b) recorded from a muscle with profuse denervation activity. Fibrillation potentials arise from single muscle fibres and have a triphasic shape, duration of less than 5 ms, and variable amplitudes depending on the distance to the recording electrode. Positive sharp waves are thought to arise from damaged muscle fibres with conduction block at the recording electrode.

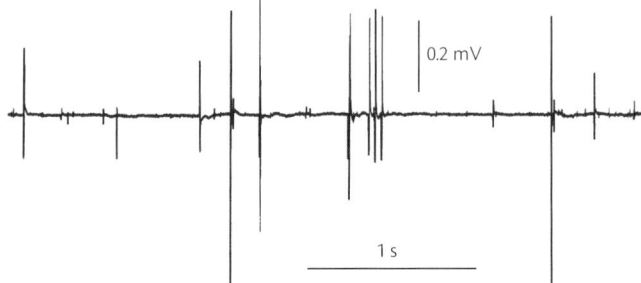

Fig. 24.3.2.7 Fasciculations recorded from the extensor digitorum communis muscle of a patient with multifocal motor neuropathy. The discharges arise from groups of muscle fibres or whole motor units and occur with irregular intervals.

Clinical correlations

Recordings at rest

The sarcolemma of the denervated muscle fibre undergoes changes, including gradual spread of acetylcholine receptors, and the resting membrane potential is reduced. Spontaneous discharges of denervated fibres occur in a cyclical pattern, and they appear as fibrillation potentials or positive sharp waves (Fig. 24.3.2.6). Fibrillation potentials have a triphasic shape, a duration of at most 5 ms, and the discharge pattern may be regular or irregular (Fig. 24.3.2.6). The positive sharp waves are considered to arise from damage to the cell membrane and indicate block of propagation at the needle-recording electrode (Fig. 24.3.2.6b). No particular pathological significance is assigned to whether the denervation activity consists of fibrillation potentials or positive sharp waves.

Continuous, nonpropagated, miniature endplate potentials (MEPPs), and in addition irregular, spontaneous, endplate potentials (EPPs) with negative onset, are recorded from the resting normal muscle within the endplate region. When recorded outside the endplate region such single-fibre potentials cannot be distinguished from fibrillation potentials. Therefore, in normal muscle spontaneous single-fibre activity may be recorded at up to 2 of 10 recording sites (see Table 24.3.2.1).

Denervation activity arises with a delay after the nerve lesion, and the lag is dependent on the length of the distal nerve stump, i.e. at very distal lesions it occurs within 5 to 10 days. Similarly, after a nerve root lesion, denervation arises after a few days in paraspinal muscles and after 2 to 3 weeks in distal extremity muscles. The presence of denervation activity indicates that the denervation is ongoing but may continue for years after the lesion if reinnervation does not take place. However, denervation activity also occurs in muscular dystrophy, inflammatory myopathy (polymyositis, dermatomyositis, and inclusion body myositis), and some metabolic myopathies (e.g. acid maltase deficiency), whereas it is rare or absent in mitochondrial myopathy. In myopathy denervation is due to segmental muscle fibre necrosis, leaving a segment of the muscle fibre denervated. Denervation activity is a nonspecific sign of neuromuscular disease (see Table 24.3.2.2).

Whereas denervation activity arises from single muscle fibres, other types of spontaneous activity are due to discharges in groups of muscle fibres, possibly the whole motor unit. These include fasciculations (defined as irregular discharges with short or long intervals of less or more than 3 s (Fig. 24.3.2.7), myotonic discharges (defined as burst of activity with gradually waxing and waning frequencies, often elicited by percussion, needle movement, or voluntary activity, and with a decreasing incidence after repeated contractions), complex repetitive discharges (defined as bursts of activity of variable duration with sudden occurrence and dropout of discharge components that may arise from single fibres), and myokymia (defined as fasciculations, doublets, or triplets occurring with variable, sometimes high frequencies). Neuromyotonia belongs in the last category of activity.

Recording at weak effort

The smallest functional unit in the muscle is the motor unit, which differs quantitatively by several orders of magnitude in different muscles; in lower extremity muscles the motor units have 1000 to 2000 muscle fibres whereas they have 5 to 10 in extraocular muscles. The motor units also differ according to the biochemical characteristics of the muscle fibres in fast contracting motor units (type II fibres) and in slowly contracting motor units (type I fibres). The diagnostic power of the EMG depends mainly on the assessment of the structural changes of the motor units as evidenced by evaluation of the MUP. The reliance on the EMG has varied considerably over the years: (1) quantitative measurements of MUPs may be utilized to gauge the overall size of the motor units, and therefore as a diagnostic indicator of whether weakness is due to neurogenic abnormalities or myopathy, as opposed to (2) qualitative evaluation, which can give only an impression of the MUP changes. The use of quantitative measurements is now more widespread and accepted because the introduction of computerized measurement devices has enabled adequate numbers of MUPs to be sampled. This may increase the use of the MUP to differentiate between neurogenic and myogenic abnormalities.

The MUP parameters include the duration, amplitude, and shape of the MUPs (Fig. 24.3.2.8). The motor units in myopathic muscle are reduced in size due to functional loss or degeneration of individual muscle fibres, and this is reflected in reduced durations and amplitudes of the MUPs (Figs. 24.3.2.9 and 24.3.2.10). In contrast

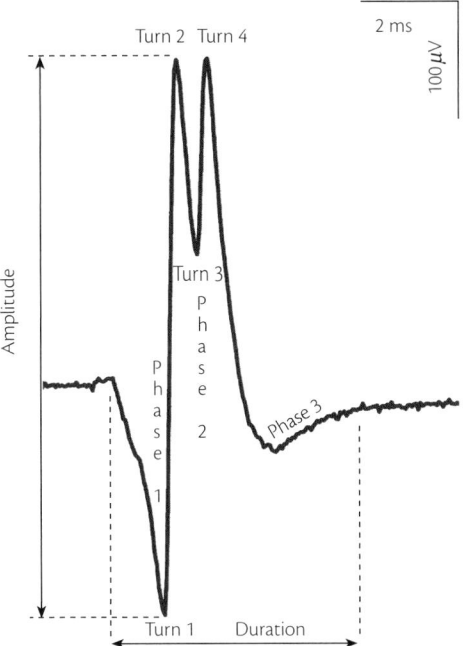

Fig. 24.3.2.8 Motor unit potential (MUP) to illustrate measurements. The duration is measured from the first deflection from the baseline to the return to the baseline. The amplitude (negative sign upwards) is measured peak to peak. The MUP has three phases and four turns (potential reversals of >100 μV). This potential is simple in shape (fewer than five phases).
From Simonetti S, Nikolic M, Krarup C (1999). Electrophysiology of the motor unit. In: Younger DS (ed.) *Textbook of motor disorders*, pp. 45–60. Lippincott Williams & Wilkins, Philadelphia, PA, with permission of the publishers.

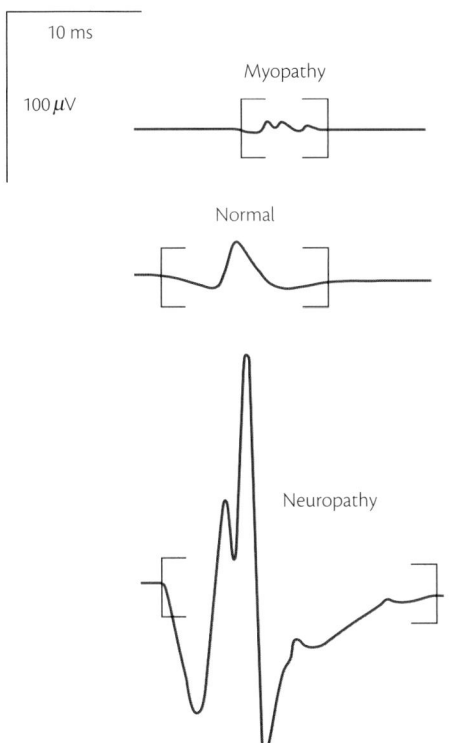

Fig. 24.3.2.9 Examples of motor unit potentials (MUPs) from patient with myopathy (top), normal individual (middle), and neuropathy (bottom).

the motor units in neurogenic lesions are enlarged due to collateral reinnervation of muscle fibres, and the mean duration of the MUPs is prolonged and the amplitude increased (Figs. 24.3.2.9 and 24.3.2.10). These changes, which indicate the presence of chronic partial denervation, tend to be more pronounced in very chronic conditions. However, in motor neuron disease, MUPs may be gigantic even in muscles without clinical weakness.

Whereas the changes in duration and amplitude are specific for either a myopathy or a neurogenic lesion, an increased incidence of polyphasic MUPs occurs both in myopathy and in neurogenic lesions, and is therefore a nonspecific sign of neuromuscular involvement (see Table 24.3.2.2). It is claimed that long-duration polyphasic MUPs are characteristic of neurogenic lesions whereas short polyphasic MUPs are seen in myopathy. However, polyphasic MUPs in myopathy have two mechanisms: (1) loss of muscle fibres in the motor unit which results in short-duration MUPs, and (2) degeneration of muscle fibres followed by regeneration and subsequent reinnervation, resulting in long-duration MUPs. The long-duration MUPs in myopathy may obscure the interpretation of the EMG, and it is therefore necessary to calculate the mean duration of simple MUPs (fewer than five phases) to avoid error.

The EMG examination should include a number of muscles according to the likely clinical diagnosis, because involvement of different muscles may vary in different disorders. In myopathy, proximal muscles in the upper and lower extremities should be examined. Some muscles show clear abnormalities characteristic of the disorder whereas others show only nonspecific changes (e.g. fibrillation potentials and increased incidence of polyphasic potentials), and several criteria should therefore be collected. In neurogenic lesions, on the other hand, distal muscles are most severely affected and may show abnormalities at an earlier stage than proximal muscles. In patients suspected of having amyotrophic lateral sclerosis, both clinically weak and nonaffected muscles should be studied and both often show neurogenic changes (see Table 24.3.2.2). As amyotrophic lateral sclerosis frequently has a focal distribution at presentation, it is important to exclude spinal root compression or peripheral nerve lesions from being the cause of the neurogenic involvement, and it is therefore customary to study several muscles in different extremities to ensure that changes are widespread.

Maximal voluntary contraction

In myopathy the number of motor units is normal, and therefore the loss of muscle fibres is associated with a full recruitment pattern with reduced amplitude (see Table 24.3.2.2). In neurogenic involvement, the loss of motor units results in a reduced recruitment pattern, often with increased amplitude due to collateral reinnervation. In advanced denervation, the number of motor units is so depleted that the recruitment pattern becomes discrete (Fig. 24.3.2.11c). In motor neuron involvement, the reduced or discrete pattern has a markedly increased amplitude, often more than 8 mV, considered typical of motor neuron disease (see Table 24.3.2.2 and Fig. 24.3.2.11c).

Specialized recordings

As indicated earlier, the amplitudes of the MUPs, in particular when recorded with a concentric needle, are markedly variable and dependent on the distance between the recording area and the closest two to three muscle fibres of the motor unit. An increased or decreased amplitude is therefore a relatively insensitive indicator of motor unit abnormalities. In order to record

54-year-old male
Muscle: vastus medialis

Number of potentials = 74
Number of polyphasic potentials = 3
Mean duration of all potentials = 11.2 ms
Mean duration of simple potentials = 11.1 ms
Mean amplitude of all potentials = 369 μV

65-year-old male
Muscle: vastus medialis

Number of potentials = 69
Number of polyphasic potentials = 9
Mean duration of all potentials = 18.7 ms
Mean duration of simple potentials = 18.6 ms
Mean amplitude of all potentials = 1212 μV

41-year-old female
Muscle: deltoideus

Number of potentials = 71
Number of polyphasic potentials = 22
Mean duration of all potentials = 8.0 ms
Mean duration of simple potentials = 6.7 ms
Mean amplitude of all potentials = 245 μV

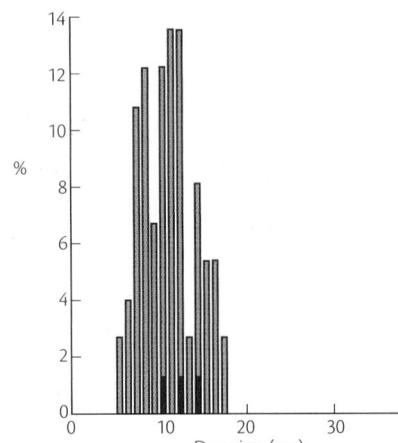 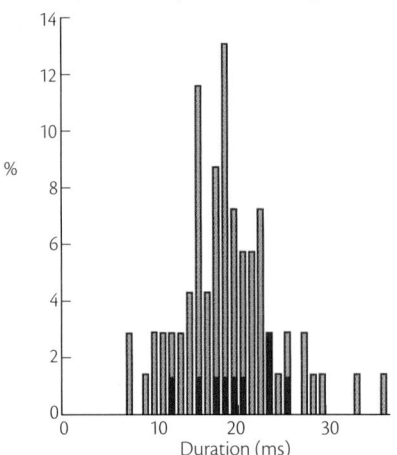 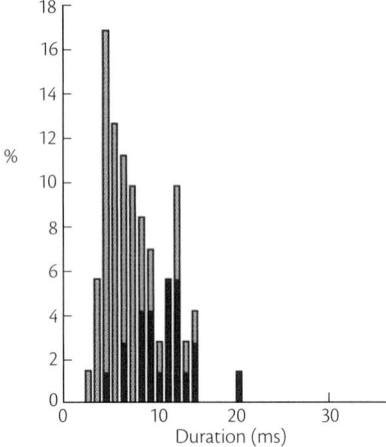

Fig. 24.3.2.10 Quantitative measurements of motor unit potentials (MUPs) from a normal individual (left), a patient with neuropathy (middle), and one with myopathy (right). The total number of MUPs analysed, the number of polyphasic MUPs, the mean duration of all MUPs, the mean duration of simple MUPs, and the mean amplitude of all MUPs are indicated above the histograms. The histograms show the distribution of the durations of simple MUPs (open bars) and polyphasic MUPs (filled bars). The amplitude and duration were markedly increased (duration: +51%; amplitude: +427%) in the patient with neuropathy. The duration was 29% diminished and the amplitude was normal in the patient with myopathy. The incidence of polyphasic MUPs was slightly increased (13% and 25%) in the patients with neuropathy and myopathy, respectively.

From Simonetti S, Nikolic M, Krarup C (1999). Electrophysiology of the motor unit. In: Younger DS (ed.) *Textbook of motor disorders*, pp. 45–60. Lippincott Williams & Wilkins, Philadelphia, PA, with permission of the publishers.

more evenly from the whole motor unit, and hence get a more reliable measure of the MUP amplitude, the macroelectrode, which consists of 15 mm of the noninsulated cannula of the needle electrode to increase the recording surface area, has been introduced. This has been useful in serial studies to follow the disintegration of the motor unit in patients with postpolio syndrome.

In contrast to the macroelectrode, the single-fibre electrode has a small recording area of 25 μm (0.005 mm²), which allows recording of the action potential from individual muscle fibres in the motor unit. The main use of the single-fibre electrode has been in the recognition of disorders of neuromuscular transmission. The timing of the discharges of two (or more) muscle fibres in the motor unit is followed during repetitive activity. Whereas the discharges are quite stable in normal muscle, they become unstable in myasthenia gravis or Lambert–Eaton syndrome. The larger variance of the discharges is termed 'increased jitter' and, in more severely affected neuromuscular transmission disturbances, some of the discharges may fall out altogether—so-called blocking. Increased jitter is also encountered in myopathy. In neurogenic lesions, where the activity of several muscle fibres may be recorded simultaneously, groups of discharges may become unstable, indicating that conduction along immature terminal sprouts may have a diminished safety factor.

The quantitation of the MUP relies on the ability to distinguish the individual MUP from the activity in other motor units. This may introduce a bias regarding the type of motor unit on which a diagnosis is based. Thus small, fatigue-resistant motor units are recruited during weak effort, whereas large motor units are activated at higher levels of activity. Methods have therefore been developed that quantitate the electrical activity during higher levels of activity. These methods have been used to investigate patients with myopathy and neurogenic involvement. They have been found to supplement the findings obtained using quantitative evaluation of the MUPs.

Nerve conduction studies

Motor and sensory nerve conduction studies of peripheral nerves are performed by recording the propagated responses evoked by supramaximal electrical stimulation of the nerve. The responses reflect summation of action potentials from individual sensory nerve fibres (the compound sensory nerve action potential—SNAP) or motor units (the CMAP), and their amplitudes represent a semiquantitative measure of the number of activated myelinated fibres. The SNAP amplitude is an expression of activity in large nerve fibres, and the CMAP amplitude is a reflection of the number of α-motor neurons. A reduction of the SNAP or the CMAP amplitudes is an indicator of fibre loss. However, the CMAP amplitude is also influenced by the size of the motor unit response. During chronic axonal loss, collateral sprouting causes an increase in the MUP, which may partially or completely compensate for the fibre loss. As reinnervation does not have the same effect on sensory nerves, the SNAP is more sensitive to determine the degree of fibre loss in chronic lesions than the amplitude of the CMAP. In order to make certain that motor fibres are affected by the pathological process, conduction studies are supplemented with an EMG.

(a)   Extensor dig. comm. - full recruitment, maximal effort

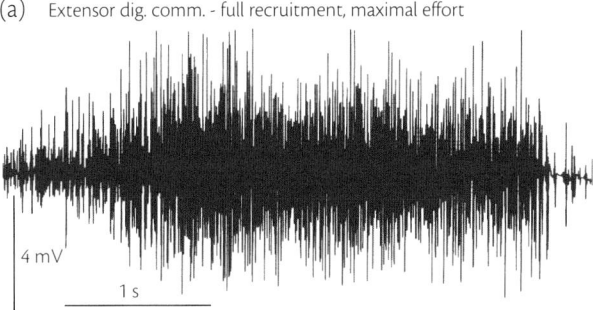

4 mV

1 s

(b)   Anterior tibial - reduced recruitment, submaximal effort

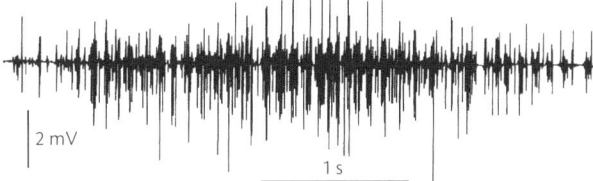

2 mV

1 s

(c)   Medial vastus - discrete pattern, maximal effort

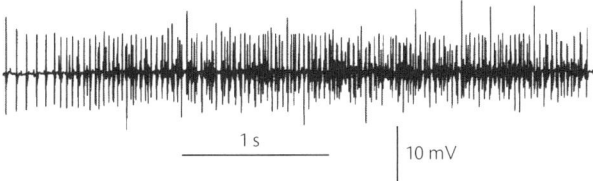

1 s   10 mV

Fig. 24.3.2.11 Electrical activity recorded during voluntary effort. In (a) the recruitment pattern was full and had a normal amplitude of 3.5 to 4 mV. In (b) the recruitment pattern was reduced. This was due to incomplete cooperation by the patient (submaximal effort), as shown by the uneven discharges that occurred in bursts. In (c) the recruitment pattern was discrete due to loss of motor units, and the amplitude was markedly increased to 8 to 10 mV as a result of collateral reinnervation (46-year-old man with motor neuron disease).

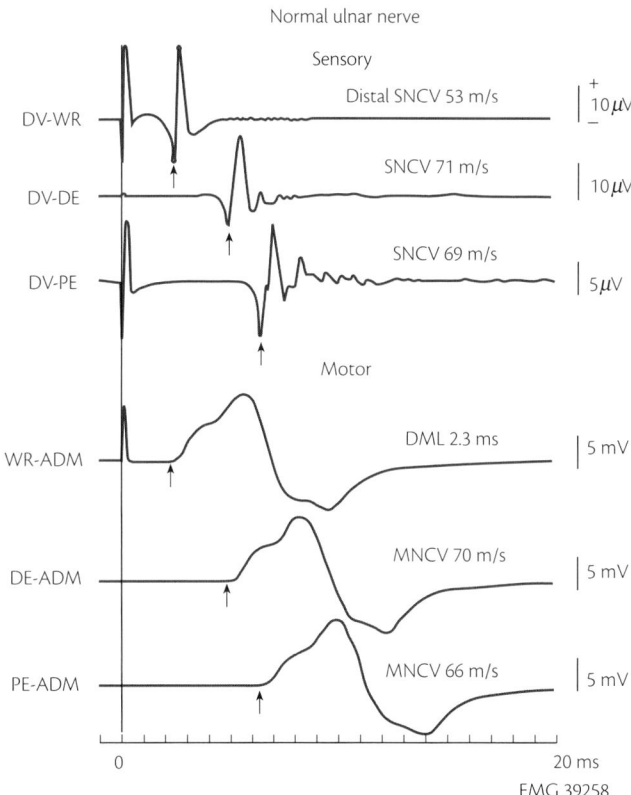

Fig. 24.3.2.12 Motor and sensory conduction studies of a normal ulnar nerve from a patient with diffuse complaints about the arm. Above: compound sensory action potentials, evoked by electrical stimulation at digit V (DV), were recorded via needle electrodes at the wrist (WR), below the elbow (DE), and above the elbow (PE). The latencies were measured to the first positive peak (arrows) and the conduction velocities (SNCVs), indicated above the traces, were calculated as indicated in the text. Below: compound muscle action potentials, evoked by stimulation at the wrist (WR), below the elbow (DE), and above the elbow (PE), were recorded via a surface electrode over the abductor digiti minimi muscle (ADM). The latencies were measured to the first deflection from the baseline (arrows). DML (distal motor latency) and MNCV (motor nerve conduction velocity) indicated above traces were obtained as described in the text.

Method

Investigations of motor and sensory fibres are carried out separately.

Motor conduction studies

The nerve is stimulated by a 0.1- to 0.2-ms duration electrical pulse applied to the nerve at well-defined sites, with the cathode (depolarizing electrode) being placed over the nerve distal to the anode. It is essential that the stimulation pulse is supramaximal to ensure that all fibres in the nerve remain activated, even though the stimulation electrode may move slightly and is defined as being 10 to 20% above the stimulus strength that elicits a maximal CMAP. The CMAP is recorded from the muscle, preferably using surface electrodes to ensure that activity from all the muscle fibres in the muscle can be 'seen' by the recording electrode. Usually a belly-tendon montage is used with the reference electrode being placed over a remote site. The response is amplified at a frequency band of 10 (or 20) Hz to 10 kHz.

Measurements The parameters include latencies, conduction velocities, amplitudes, areas, durations, and shapes of the CMAPs (Fig. 24.3.2.12). The latency is measured to the first deflection from the baseline, which is negative when the CMAP is recorded from the endplate zone. Motor conduction velocities (MNCVs) between two sites of stimulation are calculated by dividing the distance between stimulation sites by the difference in latencies (Fig. 24.3.2.12):

$$\frac{\text{Distance between stimulation sites (mm)}}{\text{Difference between distal and proximal latencies (ms)}}$$
$$= \text{MNCV (m/s)}$$

An MNCV is not calculated for the most distal site of stimulation because the latency includes conduction along terminal motor axon branches and the neuromuscular transmission delay. In this instance the delay is designated the distal motor latency (DML) (Fig. 24.3.2.12).

The CMAP amplitude (in millivolts) is measured either at the negative phase or peak to peak. The area and duration of the negative phase are useful in the evaluation of temporal dispersion or conduction block.

Sensory conduction studies

In contrast to the CMAP, the SNAP (in microvolts) is recorded directly from active nerve fibres, and it is therefore only about

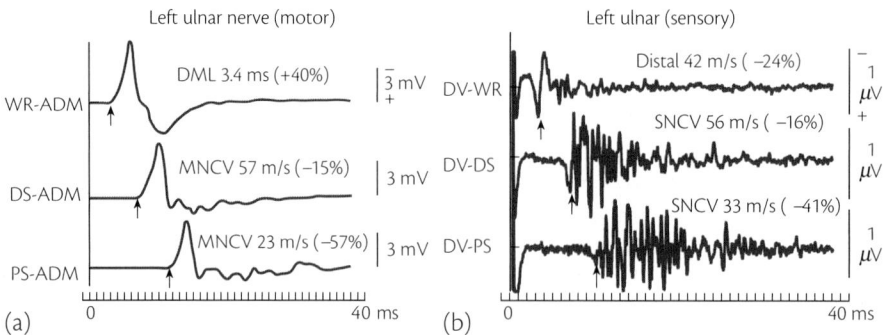

Fig. 24.3.2.13 Conduction studies in a patient with clinical signs of ulnar nerve affection. Both (a) motor and (b) sensory conduction showed a marked reduction of conduction velocities across the elbow (57% and 41% reduced between distal to the ulnar sulcus (DS) and proximal to the sulcus (PS), respectively). In addition there was motor and sensory axonal loss as indicated by the reduction in amplitudes of the compound muscle action potentials (CMAPs) and the sensory nerve action potentials (SNAPs). The mild-to-moderate slowing of conduction distal to the elbow was probably due to the loss of large fibres.

1/500th to 1/1000th of the CMAP amplitude. The response may be recorded through surface electrodes placed on the skin above the nerve or through needle electrodes placed close to the nerve. Surface electrodes are easy to apply but have a lower sensitivity than needle electrodes. In some normal, older people a SNAP from the lower limbs may, therefore, not be recorded through surface electrodes that have a resolution of about 1 μV, whereas near-nerve needle electrodes allow recording of responses with amplitudes as low as 0.1 μV. In addition the use of needle electrodes allows simultaneous recordings from several sites along the nerve, which are usually not possible using surface electrodes (see Fig. 24.3.2.12).

Sensory responses may be recorded antidromically (proximal stimulation, distal recording) or orthodromically (distal stimulation, proximal recording). The recording and reference electrodes may be placed longitudinally in relation to the nerve (bipolar recording) or the reference electrode may be placed transversely at a remote site (unipolar recording). The recording arrangements have advantages and disadvantages, the main advantage of bipolar recording being a smaller stimulus artefact and the main disadvantage that the potential recorded by the reference electrode influences the SNAP shape and amplitude. Due to the low amplitude of the SNAP, electronic averaging is usually required to obtain a clear response suitably free of noise.

Measurements The parameters include latencies, conduction velocities, amplitudes, and shapes of the compound sensory action potentials (SNAP). The latency is measured to the first positive phase of the SNAP. This indicates conduction along the largest fibres in the nerve. As the conduction path between the sites of stimulation and recording does not include synaptic transmission, a distal sensory conduction velocity (SNCV) may be calculated (see Fig. 24.3.2.12):

$$\frac{\text{Distance between stimulation and recording sites (mm)}}{\text{Latency (ms)}}$$

$$= \text{Distal SNCV (m/s)}$$

When the orthodromically conducted SNAPs are recorded at several sites along the nerve, the SNCV is calculated using a similar procedure to that used to calculate the MNCV:

$$\frac{\text{Distance between proximal and distal recording sites (mm)}}{\text{Difference between proximal and distal latencies (ms)}}$$

$$= \text{SNCV (m/s)}$$

In some laboratories, the latency of the SNAP is measured to the first negative phase. This is discouraged because this part of the response is a summation of both large and small fibres. A change in summation due to temporal dispersion therefore precludes measurements to the same group of fibres.

The amplitude of the SNAP is measured peak to peak. The shape is usually bi- or triphasic. In both axonal and demyelinating

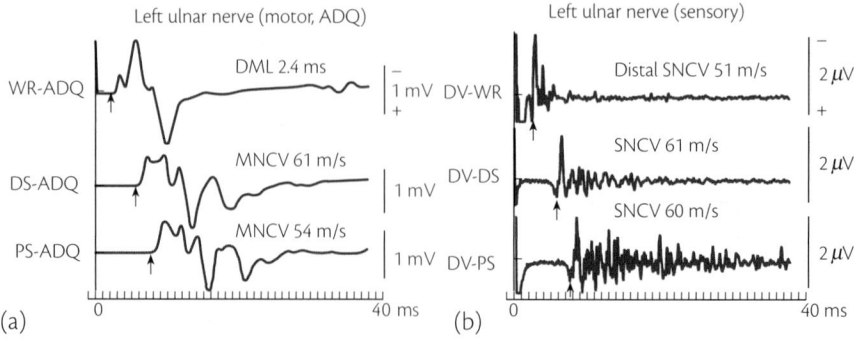

Fig. 24.3.2.14 Conduction studies in a patient with clinical signs of ulnar nerve affection, which clinically was localized at the brachial plexus or the spinal roots, as indicated by the extent of sensory complaints along the medial forearm and upper arm. Both (a) motor and (b) sensory conduction showed normal conduction velocities distal to and across the elbow. However, the amplitudes of the compound muscle action potentials (CMAPs) and the sensory nerve action potentials (SNAPs) were markedly decreased, indicating diffuse axonal loss. The loss of sensory fibres was inconsistent with a root lesion and suggested entrapment at the brachial plexus.

neuropathies the shape may become dispersed. The conduction distance has a marked influence on the shape of the SNAP due to temporal dispersion.

Clinical correlations

The motor and sensory conduction velocities (MNCVs, SNCVs) are measures of conduction of the largest motor and sensory fibres in the nerve. These limitations should be considered when the results of the studies are interpreted because, for example, a small fibre neuropathy may escape detection. Similarly, if just a single large motor fibre is preserved, the MNCV may remain normal, indicating that the conduction velocity cannot be used in isolation to establish the presence of a neuropathy.

Focal nerve lesions

The number of patients referred to the clinical neurophysiology laboratory with a question of focal nerve lesions due to compression or entrapment at root level or along the course of the nerve far outweighs other neuromuscular disorders. In entrapment and focal compression neuropathy, the main pathological abnormalities comprise demyelination at the site of the lesion and this is complicated by axonal loss in advanced lesions. Accordingly, the electrophysiological findings display disproportionate slowing of conduction at the site of the compression and, in some cases, also loss of fibres as demonstrated by reduced amplitudes of the CMAP and the SNAP. This is illustrated in Fig. 24.3.2.13 from a patient with ulnar nerve entrapment at the elbow; the MNCVs and SNCVs across the elbow were markedly reduced compared with the conduction velocities distal to the elbow, consistent with a focal demyelinating lesion. The SNAP amplitudes were in addition markedly diminished indicating axonal loss (Fig. 24.3.2.13b), and the slight reduction in SNCVs distal to the elbow is commensurate with loss of large fast-conducting fibres. The apparent sparing of the CMAP amplitude is due to collateral reinnervation masking the motor fibre loss revealed by EMG examination (see above). The slight MNCV reduction distal to the elbow is due to the fibre loss (Fig. 24.3.2.13a).

In patients with carpal tunnel syndrome, the distal motor latency of the CMAP to abductor pollicis brevis (APB), evoked by stimulation at the wrist, is prolonged, indicating slowing of conduction beneath the flexor retinaculum. However, it is difficult to stimulate motor fibres distal to the entrapment, and differential attenuation of the MNCV is therefore not assessed. To ensure that the median nerve is selectively affected, the latency to the nonaffected ulnar nerve should be normal. The SNCV, by contrast, may be tested both distal to and across the carpal tunnel, and is disproportionately reduced along this segment of the nerve compared with that distal to it. Variations on the study paradigm have been devised to increase the sensitivity of the electrophysiological studies.

On the other hand, it is usually not possible to study conduction across the compressed nerve segment directly in patients with very proximal lesions located at spinal roots or the brachial plexus across a cervical rib or band. In these situations, the anatomical distribution of EMG signs of chronic partial denervation is important in the differential diagnosis, e.g. the EMG findings in patients with apparent involvement of the ulnar nerve, due to a C8 lesion or a thoracic outlet syndrome, include abnormalities in nonulnar nerve-innervated muscles (e.g. APB and extensor digitorum communis). This distribution of motor axon loss, and the absence of focal MNCV changes at the elbow (Fig. 24.3.2.14a) show that a

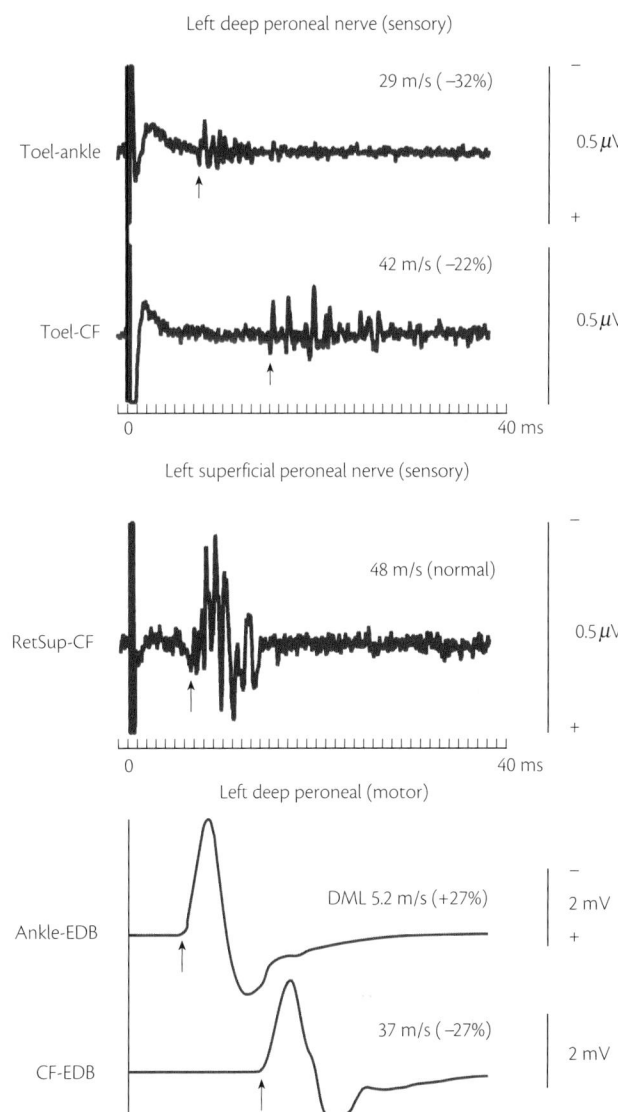

Fig. 24.3.2.15 Motor and sensory conduction studies of the peroneal nerve in a patient with diabetic neuropathy. The findings in this patient were consistent with axonal loss, primarily present in the very distal segment of the nerve. Top panel: orthodromic compound sensory nerve action potentials (SNAPs), evoked at the deep peroneal nerve in the first dorsal interstice (Toel), were recorded at the ankle (ankle) and the fibular head (CF). The amplitudes were more than 95% diminished. The sensory nerve conduction velocities (SNCVs) were moderately diminished due to large fibre loss. Middle panel: compound sensory action potential (SNAP) of the superficial peroneal nerve evoked at the superior retinaculum (RetSup) at the ankle and recorded at the CF. The amplitude was slightly diminished and the SNCV was normal. Lower panel: compound muscle action potentials (CMAPs) of the deep peroneal nerve, evoked at the ankle and the CF, were recorded at the extensor digitorum brevis muscle (EDB). The distal motor latency (DML) was prolonged and the MNCV (motor nerve conduction velocity) was reduced due to fibre loss.

nerve lesion located at the elbow is not the cause of the clinical deficit, but does not distinguish between a radicular and a brachial plexus lesion. By contrast, sensory conduction studies in root lesions usually remain normal, provided that the lesion is located proximal to the dorsal root ganglion, whereas the SNAP from the fifth digit in thoracic outlet syndrome is diminished due to sensory fibre loss at the level of the brachial plexus (Fig. 24.3.2.14b).

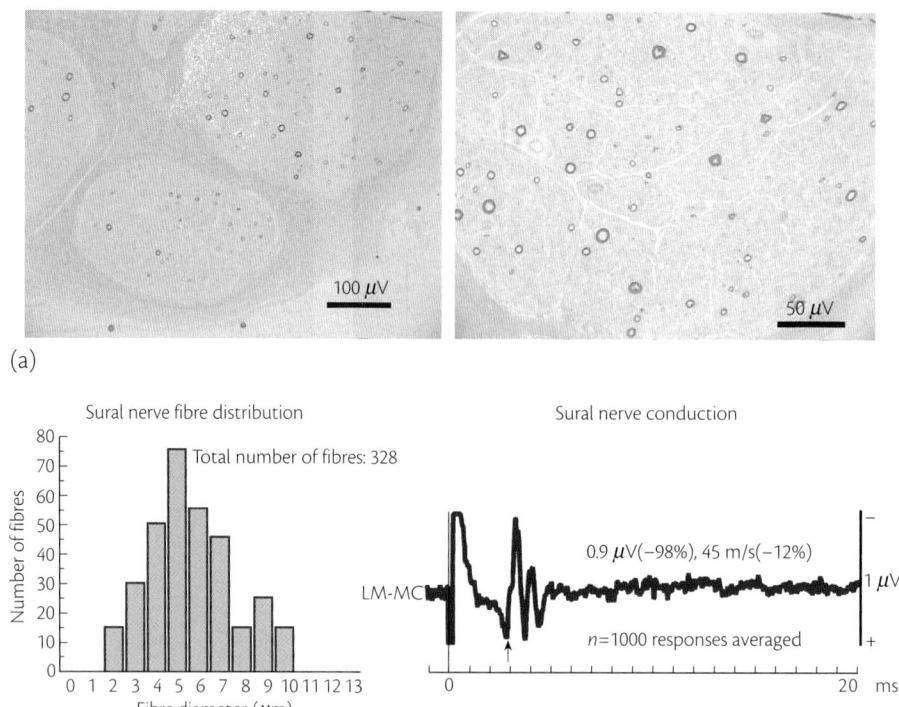

Fig. 24.3.2.16 Morphometric and electrophysiological studies of the sural nerve in a 47-year-old woman with sensory neuronopathy. (a) Transverse semithin sections of the sural nerve showed generalized severe fibre loss without evidence of degeneration or regeneration. (b) A total of 328 myelinated fibres were counted in the whole nerve. The fibre diameter distribution showed loss of both small and large fibres with a maximal diameter of 10 to 11 μm. (c) Conduction studies in the sural nerve showed pronounced reduction of the compound sensory action potential (SNAP) amplitude and dispersed shape. The sensory nerve conduction velocity (SNCV) was at the lower normal limit, consistent with the diameters of the largest fibres at morphometry.
(Histological studies by courtesy of H Schmalbruch, University of Copenhagen.)

Generalized nerve lesions (peripheral neuropathy)

The electrophysiological study in patients suspected of polyneuropathy should document the wide distribution of pathological abnormalities. It is therefore a prerequisite that several motor and sensory nerves in the upper and lower limbs are investigated. However, the study should be individually tailored to delineate the distribution of changes, and the strategy should reflect the symptoms and clinical findings, and hence the differential diagnostic questions. For example, it may be necessary to investigate some nerves bilaterally if the symptoms are asymmetrical. This would allow the investigation to show whether the patient has a mononeuropathy, a multiple mononeuropathy, or a polyneuropathy with asymmetrical features.

Axonal polyneuropathy The underlying pathology in most patients with peripheral neuropathy is axonal loss in a symmetrical distribution, primarily located at distal nerve segments and more pronounced in the legs than in the arms. The electrophysiological characteristics in these patients are due to loss of nerve fibres, which are associated with EMG signs of chronic partial denervation and conduction studies that show diminished amplitudes of evoked CMAPs and SNAPs. The remaining fibres in the nerve may conduct normally, and the MNCV and SNCV in these patients may therefore be normal or show a reduction consistent with large fibre loss (Fig. 24.3.2.15). In some patients, the pathological changes may be present primarily at the distal nerve segments, also requiring studies of these segments (Fig. 24.3.2.15).

In rarer types of neuropathy, only motor or sensory fibres are involved, and demonstration of such a distribution may have important implications in the differential diagnosis. A sensory neuropathy is illustrated in a 47-year-old woman (Fig. 24.3.2.16) with profound sensory ataxia. The motor nerve conduction studies and the EMG were normal whereas the sensory conduction studies were

profoundly abnormal, and the sural nerve biopsy showed loss of 95% of myelinated fibres (Fig. 24.3.2.16a,b). The SNCV was at the lower normal range consistent with the diameter of the largest remaining fibres being slightly diminished at about 10 μm (Fig. 24.3.2.16b,c). These findings were consistent with a sensory autoimmune neuronopathy.

Demyelinating neuropathy

Primary demyelination usually has a hereditary, inflammatory, or autoimmune basis. Although demyelinating neuropathy is rare compared with axonal neuropathy, it has become increasingly important to be able to diagnose acquired demyelinating neuropathy with a high degree of certainty because AIDP or CIDP may respond to immunomodulatory therapy. The primary electrophysiological sign of demyelination is a markedly reduced conduction velocity that is beyond the diminution caused by large fibre loss. In hereditary motor and sensory neuropathy, types I and III, the MNCVs and the SNCVs are markedly diminished to less than 50% of the lower limit of normal in all nerves, consistent with primary demyelination. In these conditions the amplitudes of the CMAPs and the SNAPs are, however, also markedly reduced and nerve biopsy confirms marked loss of myelinated nerve fibres. Pure demyelination without axonal loss does not occur in these hereditary conditions and is extremely rare in acquired demyelinating neuropathy. The distinguishing features in acquired demyelinating neuropathy include widespread demyelination, often in a multifocal pattern, as indicated by focal temporal dispersion or conduction block, or both, of CMAPs and SNAPs. Criteria have been established to assist in the diagnosis of these demyelinating neuropathies (Table 24.3.2.3).

Weakness or sensory loss does not result solely from diminished conduction velocity but is a consequence of nerve fibre loss or block of conduction between the CNS and the target muscle. Conduction block is a partial or complete inability of fibres to propagate action

Table 24.3.2.3 Criteria for the classification of acquired demyelinating polyneuropathies

Nerve conduction parameter	Albers and Kelly, 1989	Ho *et al.*, 1997	Copenhagen values	
			Upper limbs	Lower limbs
Distal motor latency	>115% of UNL (amp. nl.)	>110% of UNL (amp. nl.)	4.5 ms	6.4 ms
	>125% of UNL (amp. <nl.)	>120% of UNL (amp. <nl.)	5.4 ms	7.7 ms
Motor conduction velocity	<90% of LNL (amp. nl.)	<95% of LNL (amp. >50% of LNL)	45 m/s	35 m/s
	<80% of LNL (amp. <nl.)	<85% of LNL (amp. <50% of LNL)	38 m/s	30 m/s
Focal conduction changes	Temporal dispersion (>10–15% increased duration). Proximal/ distal amplitude ratio, <0.7	Temporal dispersion		
F-wave latency	>125% of UNL	>120% of UNL		

LNL, lower normal 95 per cent confidence limit; UNL, upper normal 96 per cent confidence limit; amp., amplitude of CMAP; nl., normal.

potentials along a segment of the nerve, and it is demonstrated by recording a larger motor or sensory response distal rather than proximal to the site of block (Fig. 24.3.2.17a). This reduction in amplitude should be greater than that which is associated with temporal dispersion of the conducting fibres, and to demonstrate block of motor fibres the CMAP should therefore show a reduction of at least 50% (Fig. 24.3.2.17a). Conduction block may occur in acquired AIDP or CIDP, and in some cases of gammopathy. It does not occur in hereditary demyelinating neuropathy and probably not in gammopathy with IgM anti-MAG antibodies. However, demyelination as a result of compression may also cause conduction block, and in demyelinating neuropathy conduction block must therefore be demonstrated outside the usual sites of entrapment or compression. The pathophysiological changes in inflammatory demyelinating diseases usually show a multifocal pattern, with some nerves showing pronounced changes whereas other nerves or nerve segments have normal conduction.

Apparent conduction block may be found in acute neuropathies due to vasculitis. However, conduction along the nerve segment

distal to a focal lesion may continue for several days before wällerian degeneration takes place, and repeat studies should therefore be carried out to exclude this possibility.

Motor disorders (motor neuron disease and motor neuropathy)
Conduction studies in motor neuron disease are normal at early stages of the disease, but at late stages the CMAP amplitudes are reduced. The DLMs of weak and wasted muscles are often prolonged and the MNCVs slightly to moderately reduced due to loss of large α-motor axons. In amyotrophic lateral sclerosis the sensory conduction studies are usually normal, although the SNAP amplitudes may be slightly diminished. Conduction studies in the diagnosis of amyotrophic lateral sclerosis are therefore mainly useful if they are normal in the face of widespread neurogenic changes on an EMG. However, patients with X-linked bulbospinal muscular atrophy (Kennedy's syndrome) are characterized by reduction of the SNAP amplitudes while the EMG examination shows abnormalities characteristic of motor neuron disease (fasciculations, widespread denervation, markedly enlarged and

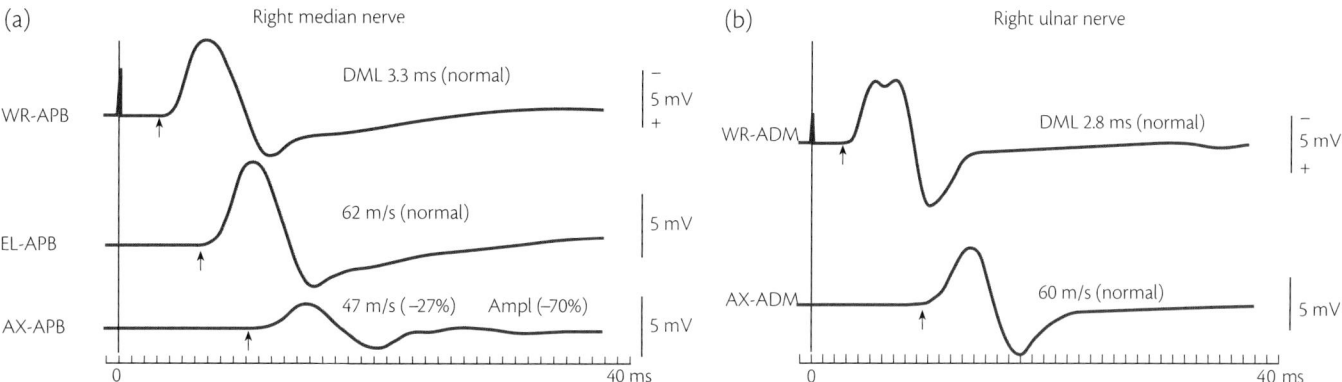

Fig. 24.3.2.17 Motor conduction studies of the median and ulnar nerves of a 29-year-old woman with electrophysiological signs of demyelinating neuropathy and clinical signs of relapsing chronic inflammatory demyelinating neuropathy. Clinical examination showed marked weakness of thenar and forearm median innervated muscles. The force in ulnar-innervated muscles was normal. (a) Compound muscle action potential (CMAP) recorded from the abductor pollicis brevis muscle (APB). Stimulation at the wrist (WR) and elbow (EL) elicited normal CMAPs, and the distal motor latency (DML) and motor nerve conduction velocity (MNCV) along the forearm were normal. On stimulation at the axilla (AX), a markedly reduced CMAP amplitude and a reduced MNCV between elbow and axilla occurred, consistent with partial conduction block. (b) Stimulation of the ulnar nerve at the wrist and axilla evoked CMAPs at abductor digiti minimi (ADM) of normal amplitudes, DML, and MNCV, indicating that motor fibres were not affected.

4768 SECTION 24 NEUROLOGICAL DISORDERS

prolonged MUPs, and discrete high-amplitude recruitment at maximal effort).

Asymmetrical or focal weakness, atrophy, fasciculations (see Fig. 24.3.2.7), without or with only slight sensory symptoms, due to multifocal motor neuropathy may be mistaken for early stages of spinal forms of motor neuron disease. The course is, however, prolonged over several years, and there is no involvement of bulbar muscles and no signs of corticospinal involvement. The electrophysiological features of these patients are distinct with conduction block of motor fibres indicating focal demyelination. Usually there is also EMG evidence of chronic partial denervation indicating fibre loss. The sensory conduction studies through affected nerve segments are normal. These patients frequently have high titres of anti-GM1 antibodies, and the patients often respond clinically and electrophysiologically to treatment with intravenous infusions of immunoglobulin. Patients with CIDP may have mainly motor symptoms with only minimal sensory deficits. Motor conduction studies in CIDP show signs of mixed demyelination, including conduction block and fibre loss, and the sensory conduction studies are abnormal with small SNAP amplitudes and often reduced SNCVs. This is an important distinction because patients with CIDP may respond to treatment with corticosteroids and other immune-modulating strategies that have no effect on multifocal motor neuropathy.

Neuromuscular transmission disorders

Myasthenia gravis and Lambert–Eaton myasthenic syndrome (LEMS) are diagnosed by single-fibre EMG (see above) or repetitive stimulation of motor nerve. The studies are carried out preferentially in proximal nerves such as the accessory nerve or the musculocutaneous nerve. Care is mandatory to reduce the effect of movement artefacts. At single stimulation the CMAP amplitudes are usually normal in myasthenia gravis but reduced in LEMS. At slow rates of stimulation of 2 to 5 Hz, decrements of the CMAP occur in both disorders. At high rates of stimulation of 20 to 50 Hz or after a maximal voluntary contraction, the CMAP is greatly increased (facilitation) in LEMS.

Further reading

Albers JW, Kelly JJ (1989). Acquired inflammatory demyelinating polyneuropathies: clinical and electrodiagnostic features. *Muscle Nerve*, 12, 435–51.

Binnie CD *et al.* (1995). EMG, nerve conduction and evoked potentials. In: Osselton JW ed. *Clinical neurophysiology*, pp. 43–321. Butterworth-Heinemann Ltd, Oxford.

Bouche P *et al.* (1999). Electrophysiological diagnosis of motor neuron disease and pure motor neuropathy. *J Neurol*, 246, 520–25.

Brown WF, Bolton CF (eds) (1993). *Clinical electromyography I*, 2nd edition. Butterworth-Heinemann, Boston, MA.

Buchthal F (1957). *An introduction to electromyography*. Scandinavian University Books, Copenhagen.

Buchthal F (1985). Electromyography in the evaluation of muscle disease. Symposium in electrodiagnosis. *Neurol Clinics*, 3, 573–98.

Buchthal F, Kamieniecka Z (1982). The diagnostic yield of quantified electromyography and quantified muscle biopsy in neuromuscular disorders. *Muscle Nerve*, 5, 265–80.

Chiappa KH (ed.) (1997). *Evoked potentials in clinical medicine*, 2nd edition. Lippincott-Raven, Philadelphia, PA.

Fuglsang-Frederiksen A (1981). *Electrical activity and force during voluntary contraction of normal and diseased muscle*. Munksgaard, Copenhagen.

Fuglsang-Frederiksen A (2000). The utility of interference pattern analysis. *Muscle Nerve*, 23, 18–36.

Ho TW *et al.* (1997). Patterns of recovery in the Guillain–Barré syndromes. *Neurology*, 48, 695–700.

Kimura J (1989). *Electrodiagnosis in diseases of nerve and muscle. Principles and practice*, 2nd edition. FA Davis Co., Philadelphia, PA.

Krarup C (1999). Pitfalls in electrodiagnosis. *J Neurol*, 246, 1115–26.

Magistris MR, *et al.* (1998). Transcranial stimulation excites virtually all motor neurons supplying the target muscle. A demonstration and a method improving the study of motor evoked potentials. *Brain*, 121, 437–50.

Mauguière F (1995). Evoked potentials. In: Osselton JW (ed.) *Clinical Neurophysiology*, pp. 325–572. Butterworth-Heinemann, Oxford.

Niedermeyer E, Lopes da Silva F (eds) (1993). *Electroencephalography. Basic principles, clinical applications, and related fields*, 3rd edition. Williams & Wilkins, Baltimore, MA.

Nuwer MR (1999). Spinal cord monitoring. *Muscle Nerve*, 22, 1620–30.

Sandberg A, Hansson B, Stålberg E (1999). Comparison between concentric needle EMG and macro EMG in patients with a history of polio. *Clin Neurophysiol*, 110, 1900–8.

Simonetti S, Nikolic M, Krarup C (1999). Electrophysiology of the motor unit. In: Younger DS (ed.) *Textbook of motor disorders*, pp. 45–60. Lippincott Williams & Wilkins, Philadelphia, PA.

Stålberg E, Trontelj JV. (1979). *Single fibre electromyography*. Mirvalle Press, Old Woking, Surrey.

24.3.3 Imaging in neurological diseases

Andrew J. Molyneux, Shelley Renowden, and Marcus Bradley

Essentials

Computed tomography (CT) and magnetic resonance imaging (MRI) are the most important imaging techniques in the diagnosis of neurological disease.

CT

During exposure to an X-ray beam, a detector array spins around the patient and measures the absorption coefficients of tissues within the beam, with the different coefficients providing image contrast. Helical and multidetector CT now allow analysis of up to 256 slices at a time (and with the prospect of more), with the patient moving continuously through the machine. This enables very rapid scanning and the ability to acquire angiographic (CT angiography and venography) and functional information (CT perfusion). A series of cross-sectional images are produced, usually in the axial plane. Iodinated contrast agents, as employed in general vascular imaging, are commonly used for image enhancement.

MRI

When the body is placed in a magnetic field, a small number of the tissue protons align themselves with the main magnetic field. They are subsequently displaced from their alignment by application of a radiofrequency gradient, and when this radiofrequency pulse terminates, the protons realign themselves with the main magnetic field, releasing a small pulse of energy as a radio signal that is detected, localized and processed by a computer to produce a cross-sectional anatomic image.

Many different and complex radio-pulse sequences are used in MRI, each of which is designed and used to answer particular clinical questions. They detect different aspects of tissue properties known as the 'relaxation times' of the protons; times that will vary according to the proton-containing tissue and the relative mobility of the protons. Gadolinium-labelled compounds, which shorten the T_1 relaxation time, are commonly used for image enhancement.

Choice of imaging modality

The choice between CT or MRI depends on a number of factors. CT is usually more readily available, is quicker to do, and is used in most acute situations, particularly in stroke and subarachnoid haemorrhage, intracranial infection, trauma, and suspected intracranial masses. MRI is now increasingly available and is the imaging modality of choice in suspected spinal pathology and also in the detailed investigation of cranial neurological diseases, particularly those affecting the white matter, epilepsy, stroke, tumours, and congenital anomalies.

Introduction

The modern imaging techniques of CT and MRI for the demonstration of structural neurological disease have developed rapidly since their first introduction in the 1970s and 1980s respectively. They have undergone further technological evolution, particularly in the last 5 years. A variety of both CT- and MRI-based techniques can provide anatomical, angiographic, and functional information. In addition, biochemical data may be obtained using MR spectroscopy (MRS).

Historical perspective

CT

CT was developed by the British scientist and engineer Godfrey Hounsfield during the early 1970s and was the first technique to provide noninvasive and cross-sectional images of the brain. It was introduced into clinical practice at the Atkinson Morley Hospital in Wimbledon, London in 1972, and the first results were published in 1973. Before this, invasive techniques such as angiography and air encephalography were required to diagnose neurological disease. CT was the beginning of a complete revolution in radiological imaging, for which Hounsfield received the Nobel Prize for medicine in 1979.

CT rapidly became the imaging modality of choice in the diagnosis of structural brain disease until the advent of MRI, developed by British scientists in Nottingham and Aberdeen, and at a similar time in California during the early 1980s. It was introduced into widespread clinical use during the late 1980s and early 1990s. However, CT still remains an essential tool, particularly in the acute situation, when MRI is contraindicated and in countries and regions where the availability cost of MRI systems is prohibitively expensive.

CT produces a series of cross-sectional images, usually in the axial plane. During exposure to an X-ray beam, a detector array spins around the patient and measures the absorption coefficients of tissues within the beam. It is the different coefficients that provide image contrast. Early machines measured a single slice at a

time but the development of helical and multidetector CT now routinely produce 64 slices, with the prospect of 256 slices at a time with the patient moving continuously through the machine. This has enabled very rapid scanning with subsecond scan times and time-resolved data, and the ability to acquire angiographic (CT angiography and venography data) and functional information (CT perfusion).

MRI

MRI is fundamentally very different from CT. No ionizing radiation is involved. It is based on the ability of a small number of protons within the body to absorb and emit radiowave energy when the body is placed within a strong magnetic field. Different tissues absorb and release radiowave energy at different rates.

When the body is placed in a magnetic field, a small number of the tissue protons (hydrogen ions) align themselves with the main magnetic field. They are subsequently displaced from their alignment by application of a radiofrequency gradient. When this radiofrequency pulse terminates, the protons realign themselves with the main magnetic field, releasing a small pulse of energy as a radio signal that is detected, localized, and processed by a computer to produce a cross-sectional anatomical image.

Many different and complex radiopulse sequences are used in MRI and are determined by the way the radiofrequency pulses are timed. They are designed and used to answer certain clinical questions in a variety of neurological circumstances. They detect different aspects of tissue properties known as 'the relaxation times of the protons'—times that will vary according to the proton-containing tissue and the relative mobility of the protons. The most basic and most commonly used sequences are termed 'T_1-weighted' and 'T_2-weighted' sequences. The appearance of these scans is quite different, e.g. fluid structures such as cerebrospinal fluid are white (high signal) on T_2-weighted and dark (low signal) on T_1-weighted images (Fig. 24.3.3.1b,c).

Some tissues such as fat (unless suppressed by a specific sequence) and some blood breakdown products (e.g. methaemoglobin) will appear bright on T_1- and T_2-weighted images. Flowing blood is usually markedly hypointense (black) on both sequences ('a signal void'), as are cortical bone and air.

Specific MR sequences have also been designed to produce noninvasive angiographic information and usually do not require an injection of a contrast agent (MR angiography and MR venography). Perfusion-weighted MRI (PWI) can assess cerebral perfusion and diffusion-weighted MRI (DWI), by assessing brownian motion of mobile protons, is useful in diagnosis of hyperacute and acute ischaemic stroke and may be also used to differentiate malignant tumour from an abscess (see later). MRS may provide useful biochemical information and may be used to grade brain tumours, differentiate malignant tumour from radiation necrosis, and malignant tumour from abscess. Functional MRI (fMRI) may localize specific brain functions, e.g. motor function, sensory function, and language, and can be useful for surgical planning where mass lesions are close to or involve eloquent cortex. White matter pathways themselves can be outlined using tractography and their infiltration or distortion by pathology demonstrated.

The resolution of modern MR scanners is submillimetre, most are 1.5 T (15 000 G and increasingly 3-T scanners are being introduced. This higher field strength (measured in tesla (T): 1 tesla = 10^4 gauss (G)) allows faster scanning and higher resolution.

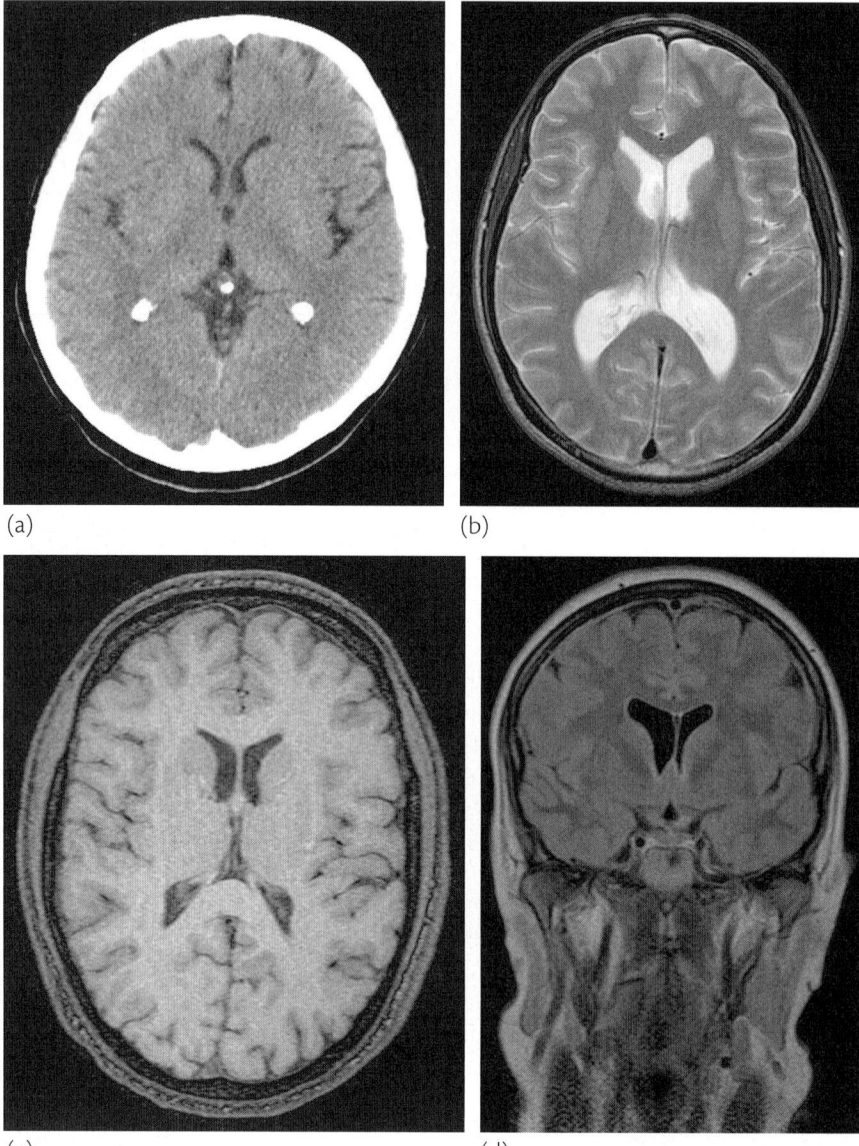

Fig. 24.3.3.1 Normal CT and MR scans of the brain at the level of the ventricles. (a) Normal CT image at the level of the lateral ventricles. (b) Normal axial T_2-weighted image of a brain at the level of the ventricular system. Note that the cerebrospinal fluid (CSF) is white, the white matter is dark, and the grey matter is lighter than the white matter. This is the most commonly used MRI sequence and it is usually the most sensitive in the detection of pathological processes. (c) Axial, T_1-weighted, unenhanced MR image, showing the cerebrospinal fluid to be dark (low signal) and the white matter lighter than the grey matter. (d) Coronal FLAIR (fluid-attenuated inversion recovery) MRI: these are T_2-weighted images but normal cerebrospinal fluid is dark on this sequence. This improves the visibility of lesions in the brain, especially adjacent to the ventricles. The mild asymmetry of the bodies of the lateral ventricles seen on this scan is within the normal range.

The sensitivity of MR for the detection of intracranial anatomy and pathology is extremely high and its multiplanar capacity is an additional advantage.

MRI may be contraindicated in patients with certain metallic implants especially cardiac pacemakers, some heart valves, older aneurysm clips, and metallic foreign bodies in the orbit. It is also optimally avoided if possible in the first trimester of pregnancy.

Contrast enhancement in brain imaging

Intravenous contrast in brain imaging is frequently used to enhance conspicuity of pathology, to determine the vascularity of structures, and to improve the demonstration of the blood vessels. In practice, it usually adds little to the specific diagnosis. It will show the extent and pattern of enhancement in tumours, abscesses, and inflammatory lesions. For CT, the same iodinated contrast agents employed in general vascular imaging are used. In MRI, gadolinium-labelled compounds, which shorten the T_1 relaxation time, are utilized and show the same patterns of enhancement as iodinated contrast media used in CT. The sensitivity of MRI contrast agents is significantly greater in the detection of metastatic lesions and the extent of tumour spread. Gadolinium enhancement is particularly useful in the assessment of meningeal disease.

Cerebral angiography

In the last 5 years CT angiography (CTA) and MR angiography (MRA) have largely replaced diagnostic, transfemoral, intra-arterial, digital subtraction angiography (DSA) for demonstration of the intra- and extracerebral vessels. Transfemoral angiography involves the selective catheterization of the carotid and/or vertebral arteries via the femoral artery and direct injection of iodinated contrast media into these arteries. It is used primarily for investigation of intracranial haemorrhage (ICH), where CTA has not demonstrated the cause, and in the investigation and assessment of complex neurovascular disorders, e.g. arteriovenous malformations. The basic techniques of DSA are used for endovascular therapy in the treatment of cerebral aneurysms, arteriovenous malformations, and fistulas.

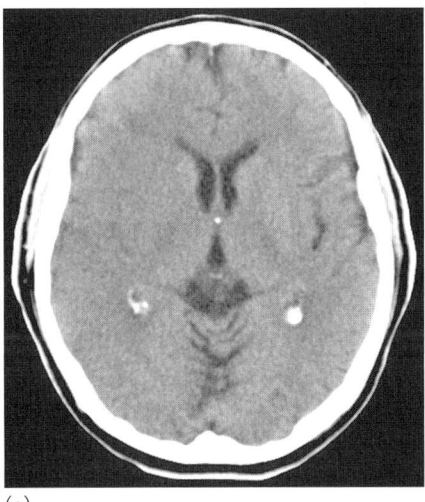

(a)

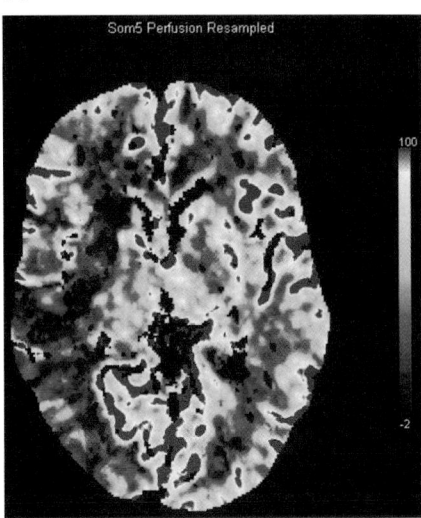

(b)

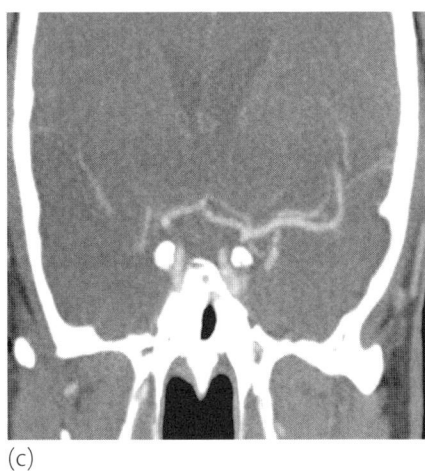

(c)

Fig. 24.3.3.2 (a) CT scan showing an acute right middle cerebral territory infarction within a few hours of onset of the neurological deficit with a left hemiplegia. Note the subtle loss of differentiation between the grey and white matter on the right side, the slight but definite reduction in attenuation, and the effacement of the sylvian fissure and cortical sulci. (b) CT perfusion image obtained with a 64-slice multidetector CT scanner showing widespread reduced perfusion and area of penumbra (blue) on the right side. (c) CT angiogram showing acute thrombus at right middle cerebral artery bifurcation.

In the investigation of a transient ischaemic attack (TIA) and minor stroke caused by suspected extracranial carotid or vertebral stenosis, Doppler ultrasonography of the neck vessels is usually the main screening test. CTA or MRA is an alternative technique and useful where carotid intervention to relieve stenosis (usually carotid endarterectomy) is planned. This has been shown to be of substantial benefit in patients with critical stenoses to prevent recurrent stroke.

Myelography

This has largely been superseded by spinal MRI. It involves a lumbar puncture and injection of water-soluble contrast into the lumbar subarachnoid space, followed by radiography to demonstrate the lumbar and cervical nerve roots and the spinal cord in patients with radiculopathy, suspected cauda equina compression, and myelopathy, when MRI cannot be performed.

Imaging of common neurological diseases

Cerebrovascular disease and stroke

The most frequent neurological presentation is acute stroke. Patients presenting with sudden onset of neurological deficit should be deemed to have suffered a vascular event until proved otherwise. In practice the clinical diagnosis of stroke is very accurate, provided that an adequate history is available. However, clinical differentiation of haemorrhage from infarction is not possible. The primary role of imaging is to identify whether the acute stroke is ischaemic or haemorrhagic and, when there is diagnostic doubt, whether a stroke has occurred. CT is the most reliable way of excluding primary intracerebral haemorrhage as a cause of acute stroke, provided that it is performed within about a week of onset. In ischaemic stroke, depending on the extent and location of infarct and timing of the examination relative to the onset of neurological deficit, it will only variably detect acute infarction.

Within hours of the ictus, CT may show a vague area of low density, loss of grey/white differentiation, or slight swelling and effacement of the sulci in the area of infarction, or it may be normal (Fig. 24.3.3.2a). In the latter especially, in hyperacute ischaemic stroke, when thrombolysis or clot extraction is contemplated, CT perfusion (CTP) (Fig. 24.3.3.2b) and CTA (Fig. 24.3.3.2c) are useful additional techniques and can be performed very quickly in a multislice CT scanner to provide information about the site and extent of arterial occlusion, and extent and location of the infarcted brain but, most important, the extent of ischaemic but potentially viable brain.

Standard MRI may also be normal within the first 6 h (except the occluded vessel may show absence of flow void) but DWI can demonstrate decreased diffusion in the ischaemic/infarcted brain within minutes of the ictus. PWI will also provide information to discriminate between ischaemic and viable brain from infarcted brain. MRA will demonstrate the site of vascular occlusion. CT techniques are of more practical value in the evaluation of hyperacute ischaemic stroke, in the United Kingdom at least.

Over the next 24 h or so, there is progressive development of a low-density area on CT involving the cortex and white matter, in a vascular distribution and with mild mass effect. Swelling increases from day 3 to day 7, and the area of infarction is progressively better defined. Loss of volume in the damaged area occurs over time from about 4 weeks (Fig. 24.3.3.3).

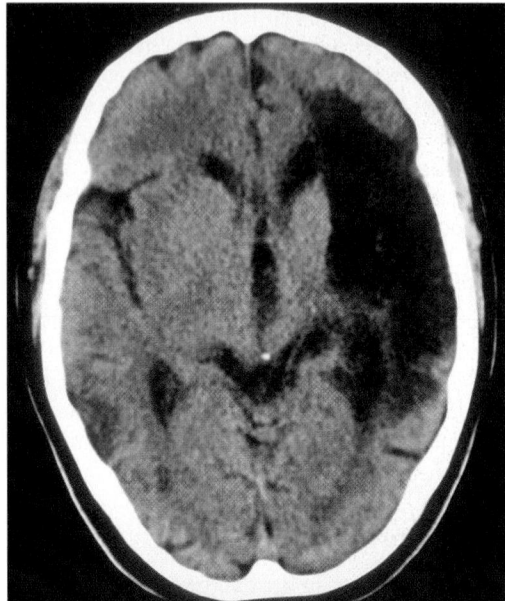

Fig. 24.3.3.3 CT showing mature left middle cerebral infarction. Note the large area of very low attenuation, with loss of volume on that side.

On MRI, an area of high T_2 signal is demonstrated, in the area of infarction, involving cortex and white matter (Fig. 24.3.3.4).

In the acute phase, there may also be some swelling around the area, representing oedema with effacement of sulci and ventricles but, with time, volume loss occurs.

Transient ischaemic attacks and minor stroke

During the 1990s it was shown in the in two large randomized trials, the North American Carotid Surgery Trial (NASCET) and the European Carotid Surgery Trial, that carotid endarterectomy significantly reduced the risk of disabling stroke or death in patients with severe carotid stenosis who had suffered a minor stroke or TIA. Recent work has shown that the risk of recurrent major stroke after a TIA or minor stroke is very high in the early period (4 weeks). Recent guidance from the National Institute for Health and Clinical Excellence (NICE) in the United Kingdom recommends that patients with these symptoms need urgent specialist assessment, including brain and carotid imaging to detect those with significant carotid stenosis. The goal is to identify patients with treatable stenosis and urgently treat other risk factors. Noninvasive imaging using Doppler ultrasonography, MRI and MRA, and CT and CTA are all used to identify these patients. MRI with DWI has the advantage of identifying with much greater sensitivity areas of acute ischaemia or small infarcts that will not be detected on CT and or on standard MRI sequences (Fig. 24.3.3.5a,b).

Intracranial haemorrhage

Acute primary intracranial bleeding (ICH) into the brain parenchyma is easily detected on CT. Fresh blood appears as an area of high density (Fig. 24.3.3.6a).

Blood generally remains hyperdense for 2 weeks but, as the clot gets broken down, it becomes the same density as brain tissue at 2 to 4 weeks, and then is of lower density than brain after 4 weeks. The speed of resolution depends on the size of the clot.

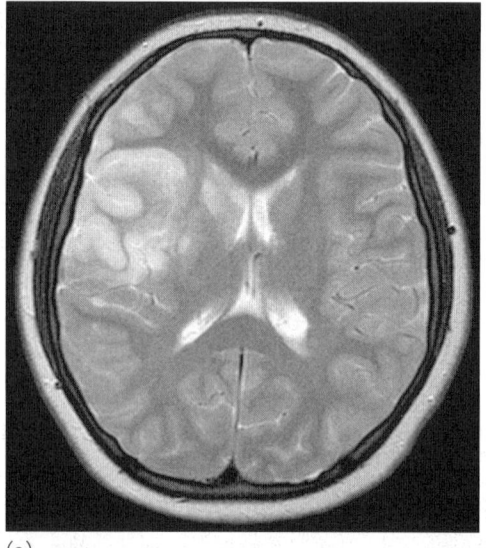

(a)

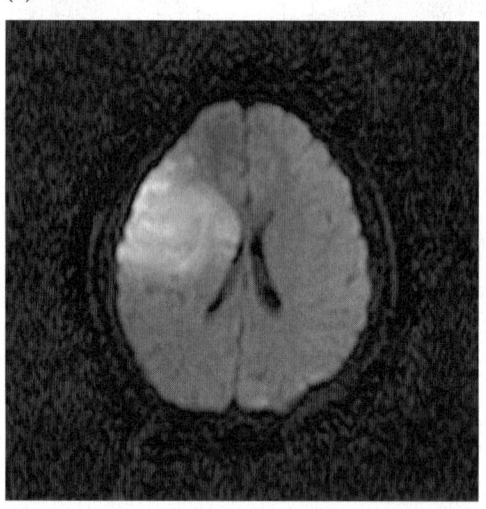

(b)

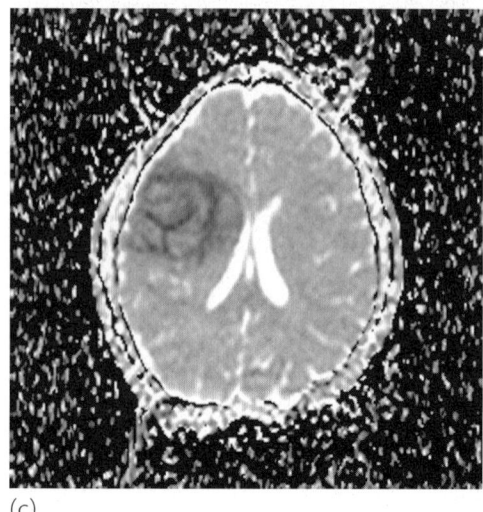

(c)

Fig. 24.3.3.4 (a) T_2-weighted MRI showing an acute middle cerebral territory infarct affecting the right temporal region. (b) MRI showing acute infarct (bright) on diffusion-weighted MR image. (c) Diffusion-weighted MRI showing the apparent diffusion coefficient (ADC map) and restricted diffusion (dark).

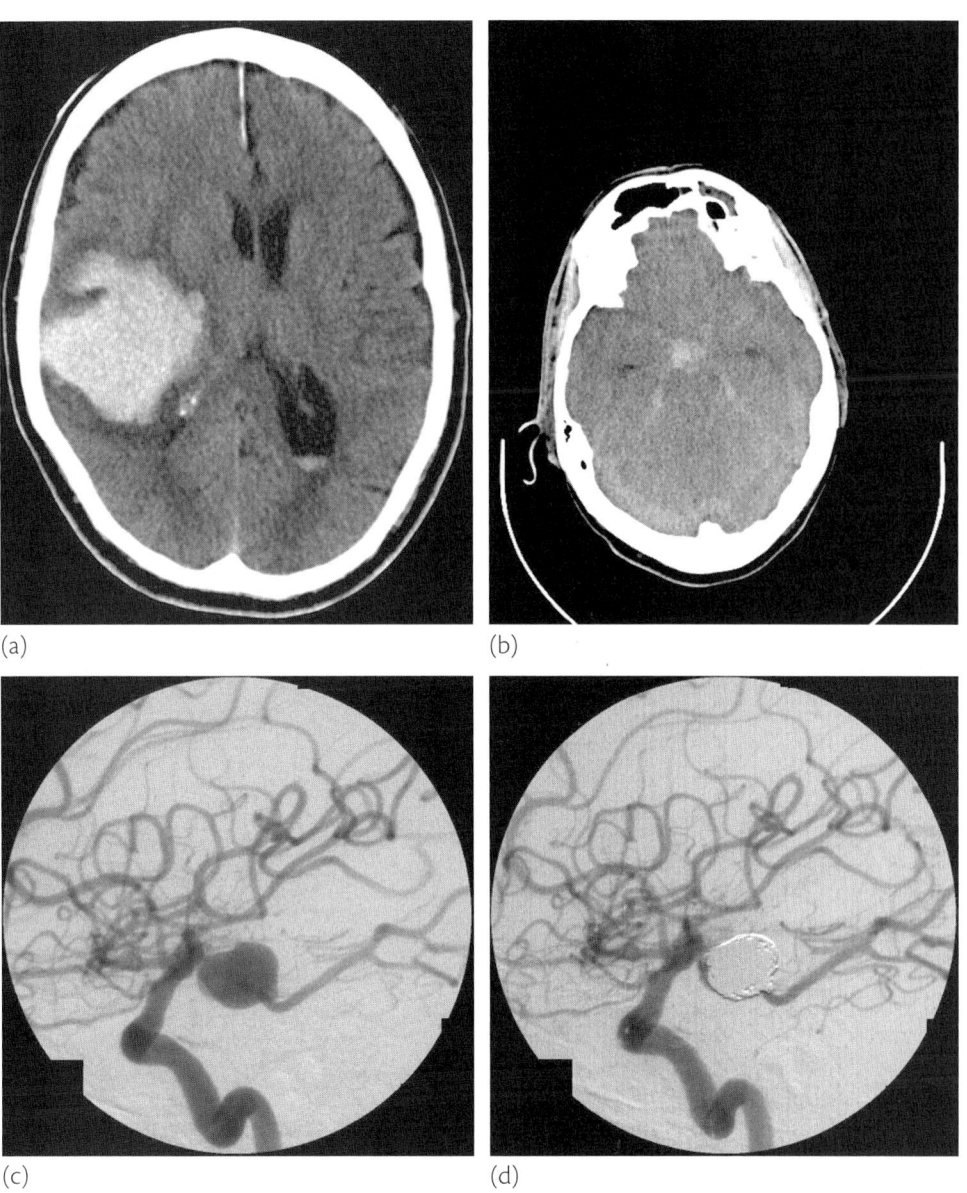

(a)

(b)

(c)

(d)

Fig. 24.3.3.5 (a) CT scan of a patient with a primary intracerebral haemorrhage in the right parietal lobe. High-attenuation area represents the acute clot. (b) CT scan of a patient with an acute subarachnoid haemorrhage from a ruptured basilar termination aneurysm, with clot in the pre-pontine cistern and around the brainstem, showing a white (as opposed to dark) cerebrospinal fluid. (c) Angiogram showing large internal carotid aneurysm at the origin of the posterior communicating artery. (d) Angiogram after placement of detachable platinum coils to occlude the aneurysm.

After an ICH, a decision must be made whether to investigate patients in more detail for the presence of an underlying lesion responsible for the haemorrhage, such as an intracranial aneurysm, vascular malformation, or occasionally a tumour. If the distribution of ICH suggests that the cause may be aneurysmal, then prompt angiographic evaluation is necessary. Otherwise, selection of which patients should undergo cerebral angiography is sometimes difficult and largely depends on the intention to treat if an underlying lesion is found. This will depend on patient's age, clinical state, location of haematoma, and patient's comorbidities.

Where there is a decision to investigate and treat, cranial MRI may also be useful. It will diagnose haemorrhage related to tumour, anatomically localize an arteriovenous malformation, and is necessary to exclude cavernous angiomas, a rare cause of haemorrhage that are angiographically occult.

Blood in the subarachnoid space after a haemorrhage (SAH) may be visible around the base of the brain as a white layer, in contrast to the normal dark outline of cerebrospinal fluid in the basal cisterns. Cranial CT performed within 24 h of a SAH is about 90% sensitive (see Fig. 24.3.3.5b). Its sensitivity diminishes thereafter depending on the extent of haemorrhage. With a large SAH, the scan will remain positive for 3 to 4 days (see Fig. 24.3.3.5b). Lack of visible blood on CT does not exclude the diagnosis of SAH, and lumbar puncture is essential if this diagnosis is suspected clinically and CT scan is negative or equivocal. It is very important not to miss a very small SAH, undetectable on CT, which may have resulted from rupture of an intracranial aneurysm. Aneurysmal SAH is potentially life threatening because re-rupture of the aneurysm is common.

All patients who survive an SAH and are in good clinical condition should undergo urgent imaging of the cerebral vessels by either CTA or DSA to detect the presence of a berry aneurysm that may be responsible for the haemorrhage. If CTA is negative, formal intra-arterial DSA is performed. Recently ruptured aneurysms

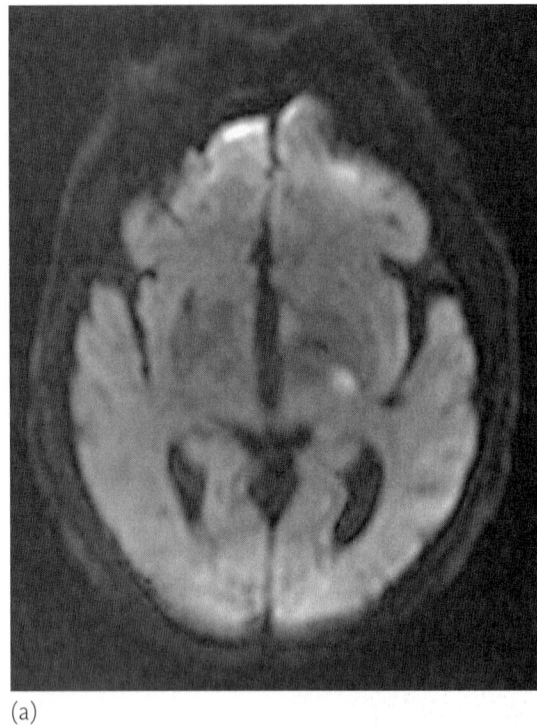

(a)

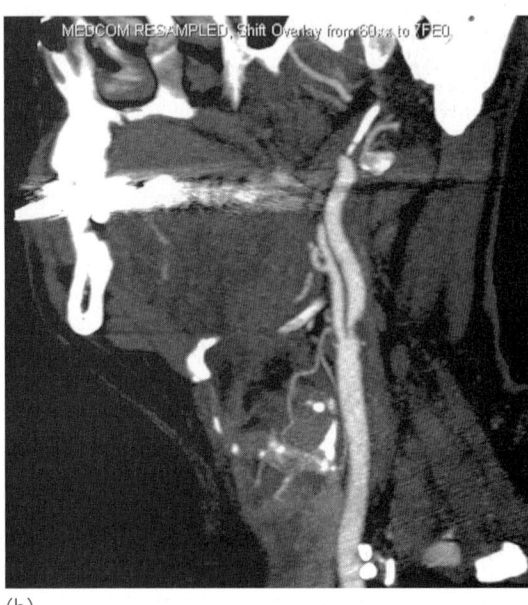

(b)

Fig. 24.3.3.6 (a) Diffusion-weighted MRI showing restricted diffusion, in a patient with a recent transient ischaemic attack (TIA), as a bright area in the left basal ganglia. (b) CT angiogram obtained on 64-slice multidetector CT (MDCT), with workstation reconstructions showing tight stenosis at the origin of the internal carotid artery.

have a high likelihood of rebleeding, as high as 30% in the first 4 weeks after the haemorrhage. Without treatment there is a 50% mortality rate at 6 months. Aneurysms should be detected and treated as soon as possible, either by endovascular techniques using detachable platinum coils (see Fig. 24.3.3.5c,d) or by neurosurgical clipping. A recent large multicentre randomized trial, the International Subarachnoid Aneurysm Trial (ISAT), has reported improved clinical outcomes at 1 year after coil embolization compared with surgical clipping.

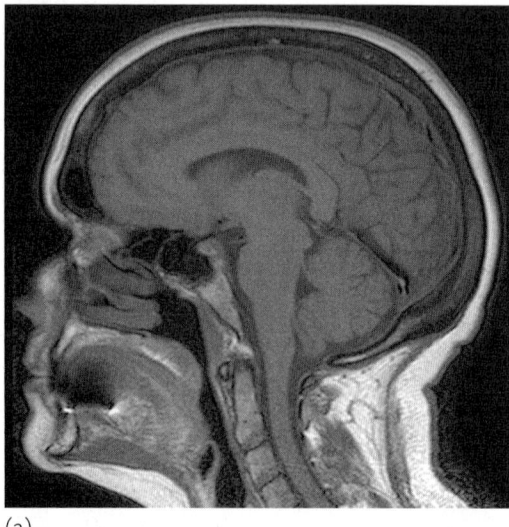

(a)

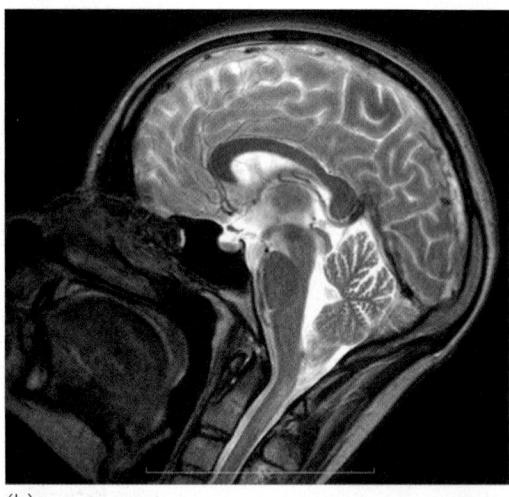

(b)

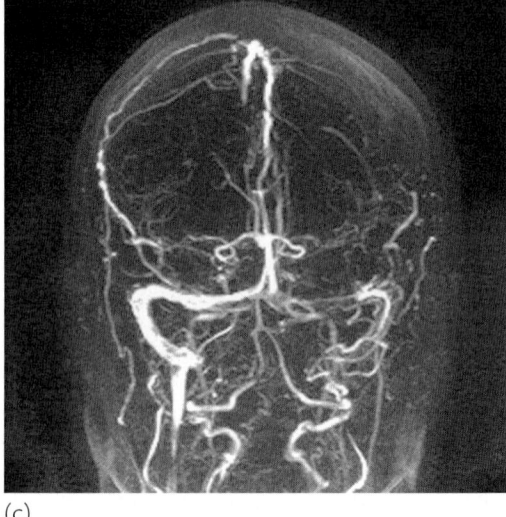

(c)

Fig. 24.3.3.7 (a) Sagittal MRI showing extensive sagittal sinus thrombus; there is intermediate signal in the sagittal sinus, but normally there would be a black flow void in this T_1-weighted sequence. (b) Sagittal T_2-weighted sequence showing clot in the superior sagittal sinus. (c) Coronal MR venogram showing lack of filling in the sagittal sinus and the left transverse sinus.

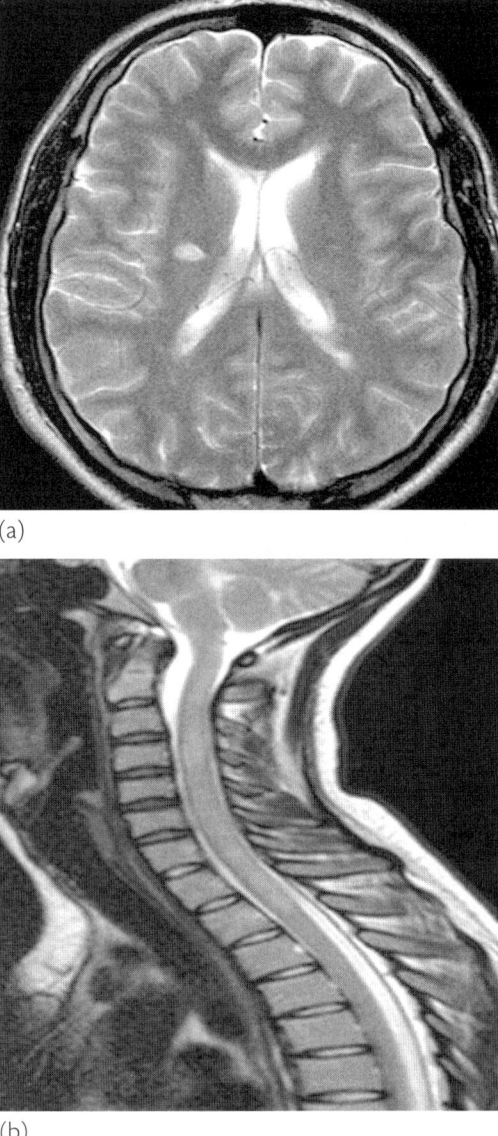

(a)

(b)

Fig. 24.3.3.8 (a) Typical ovoid-shaped white matter plaque in the deep white matter of the right hemisphere. (b) Cervical spine MRI showing a demyelinating (multiple sclerosis) plaque in the cord with swollen cervical cord and diffuse high signal. The differential is between an inflammatory process and a spinal cord tumour.

Other cerebrovascular diseases

Cerebral venous sinus thrombosis

This uncommon, potentially fatal, condition presents nonspecifically with headache, confusion, variable neurological deficits including coma, and sometimes seizures. Cranial CT may be normal or may demonstrate generalized or local cerebral swelling and/or haemorrhagic venous infarction. Dense thrombus may be seen in the occluded sinuses and veins.

The diagnosis is usually made by MRI when it is suspected, where lack of flow void is seen on some sequences (T_2 weighted) and high-signal methaemoglobin on T_1-weighted sequences are seen in thrombosed dural sinuses. Flow-sensitive MRI sequences (MR venography) demonstrate the obstructed sinus well and are sometimes useful because the signal returned by clot varies according to age of clot, and the particular sequence and field strength of the scanner (Fig. 24.3.3.7). CT venography on multislice scanners is an excellent alternative technique, readily demonstrating the extent of thrombosis.

Anticoagulation is urgently required because progression of the thrombosis can lead to ICH and fatal venous infarction. Local pharmacomechanical thrombolysis is probably successful in re-establishing flow by catheterization of the venous sinuses from the transvenous route, if the patient's clinical condition deteriorates despite anticoagulation.

Inflammatory diseases of the nervous system

Multiple sclerosis

One of the most common neurological diseases after stroke in western countries is multiple sclerosis (MS). Imaging plays a crucial role in the diagnosis but it is important to understand the MR appearances are not pathognomonic. Clinical presentation, history, and neurological examination are crucial. The typical MS plaque is a well-defined, ovoid, periventricular, white matter lesion with a long axis perpendicular to the ventricle and long axis of the brain, reflecting the perivenular inflammatory process (Fig. 24.3.3.8a).

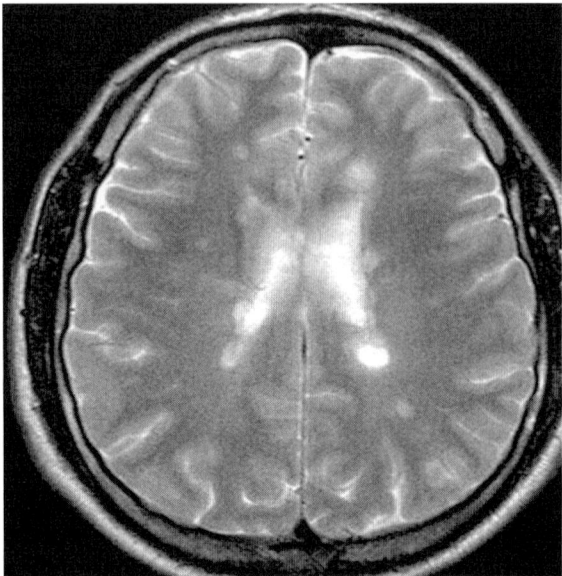

Fig. 24.3.3.9 Axial MRI T_2-weighted image showing typical lesions adjacent to the ventricles and in the white matter.

Sometimes, they enhance, may cavitate, and may be associated with oedema, and can be confused with tumours.

When patients present with symptoms of spinal cord disease (myelopathy), MRI of both the spine and brain is indicated. The entire spinal cord is imaged to exclude spinal cord compression. An inflammatory plaque may be seen in the spinal cord, often in the cervical cord (Fig. 24.3.3.8b), although failure to identify such a lesion does not mean that one is not present. If MS-type lesions are also demonstrated in the brain the chance of that patient developing clinical MS within the next 10 years is high, around 80%. The difficulty comes in older patients aged over 45 years, where, increasingly, incidental small white matter lesions may be seen normally in the brain presumably due to age-related vascular pathology.

Neoplasms

Primary intracranial tumours

The neuroimaging appearances of individual brain tumours are rarely specific. The imaging tumour differential diagnosis takes not only tumour location into account but also patient age.

Primary intracranial tumours may be broadly divided into those arising outside the brain (extrinsic, extra-axial, parasellar, pineal region, cerebellopontine angle, etc.) and those arising in the cerebral substance (intrinsic, intra-axial). The range of pathology of the locations is fundamentally different, as often is the prognosis. Differentiation between intrinsic and extrinsic lesions is usually easier on MRI than on CT because of the multiplanar capability of MRI (Fig. 24.3.3.9).

Extrinsic intracranial tumours

The most common tumours arising from structures outside the brain are meningiomas and vestibular schwannomas (often called 'acoustics') arising from nerve VIII. Both are usually benign and present with symptoms of local pressure: cranial nerve VIII tumours can produce sensorineural deafness and/or sometimes dizziness, whereas meningiomas may be incidental, and may cause seizures and/or a wide variety of deficits according to location.

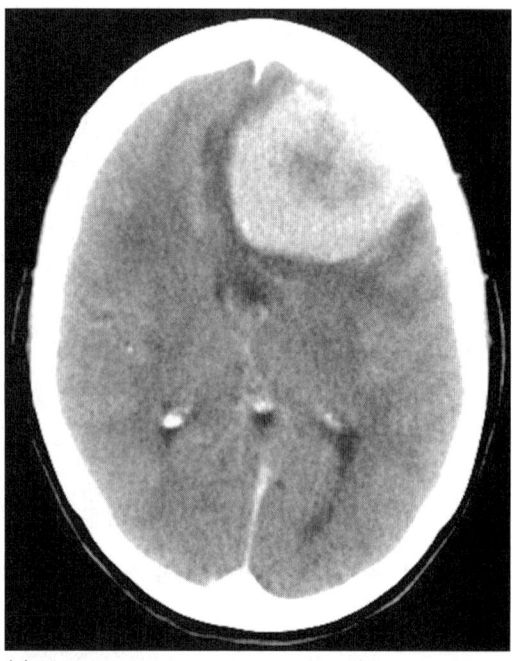

(a)

(b)

Fig. 24.3.3.10 (a) Enhanced CT scan showing left frontal convexity meningioma. (b) Coronal MRI after intravenous contrast: convexity meningioma showing broad dural origin (different patient).

The imaging characteristics of meningiomas and vestibular schwannomas are similar. CT scans usually show a slightly hyperdense mass causing local displacement of cerebral tissue. They generally enhance uniformly after the administration of intravenous contrast, although they may occasionally contain areas of low density representing necrosis or occasionally cyst formation within the tumour (Fig. 24.3.3.10a). On MRI, these lesions return a uniform intermediate signal on T_1- and T_2-weighted sequences and both show intense gadolinium enhancement (Fig. 24.3.3.10b).

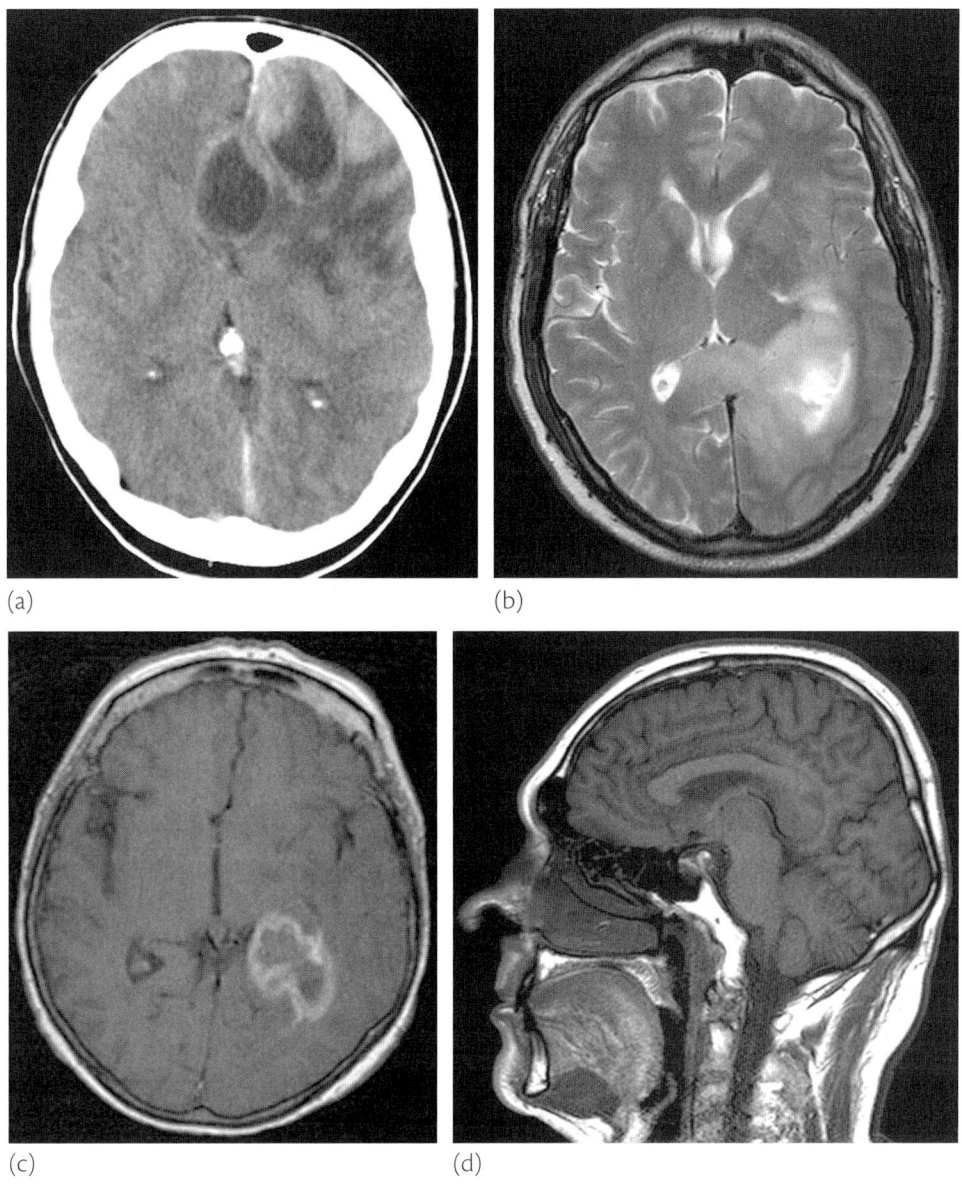

(a)   (b)

(c)   (d)

Fig. 24.3.3.11 (a) Contrast-enhanced CT scan showing a large, deeply situated mass in the left hemisphere, with considerable enhancement, and appearances typical of a glioblastoma multiforme. (b) T_2-weighted axial MRI showing diffuse infiltrating glioblastoma deeply situated in the left hemisphere and extending into the splenium of the corpus callosum; this a typical pattern of spread in this type of tumour. (c) Contrast-enhanced, axial T_1-weighted MR image of glioblastoma, showing marked irregular contrast enhancement of the margins of the tumour, with lack of central enhancement, reflecting the extensive necrosis that is often a feature of these tumours. (d) Sagittal T1-weighted image without contrast, showing the marked enlargement of the splenium of the corpus callosum depicted in the same patient.

Intrinsic cerebral tumours

Most intrinsic tumours arise from glial cells and are classified as gliomas. There are various types, e.g. astrocytoma, oligodendroglioma, oligoastrocytoma, ependymoma, and they may be benign or malignant. They are all mass lesions and most are seen as areas of low density on CT, low signal on T_1-weighted MRI, and high signal on T_2-weighted MRI, with distortion of normal structures. They may show abnormal enhancement following intravenous contrast. The presence or absence of haemorrhagic changes, necrosis, calcification, and extent of contrast enhancement will vary among tumours of different but also similar histological type. However, in general, malignant tumours are more likely to be heterogeneous with foci of necrosis, areas of haemorrhage, heterogeneous contrast enhancement, and

oedema (Fig. 24.3.3.11a). Benign tumours are more likely to be homogeneous and without haemorrhage or oedema.

MRS may enable demonstration of characteristic biochemical patterns in some cerebral tumours, enabling the distinction of malignant glioma (glioblastoma multiforme) and potentially differentiating these tumours from abscesses. DWI may also help differentiate malignant glioma from abscess and differentiate malignant glioma from lymphoma.

The current role of imaging is really primarily not to provide a precise histological diagnosis (that is the role of the neuropathologist) but rather to make the correct diagnosis of a 'brain tumour' and differentiate it from other mass lesions—acute or subacute infarcts, focal cortical dysplasias (congenital), abscesses, and inflammatory

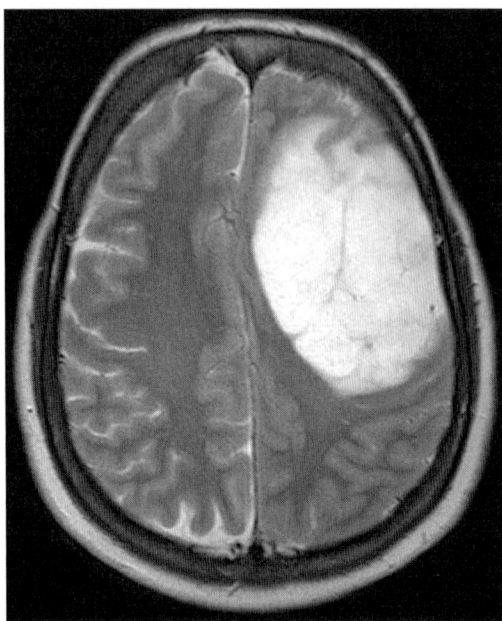

Fig. 24.3.3.12 Axial T_2-weighted MRI showing a diffuse high-signal lesion in the frontal lobe with a diffuse mass effect and sulcal effacement. These appearances are typical for a low-grade glioma.

lesions such as acute MS plaques. This is not always straightforward. Imaging is also important for precise tumour localization and determination of the relationship to eloquent cortex, and therefore is necessary for surgical planning and follow-up for assessment of surgical resection, radiotherapy, and chemotherapy treatment.

Oligodendroglioma

These tumours are the most benign of the intrinsic cerebral tumours. They often present with seizures rather than neurological deficit. Their radiological hallmark is calcification, best detected on CT. Calcification may be invisible on MRI. The time course of these tumours may be very long, often evolving over 10 to 20 years. Oligodendrogliomas may remain static for long periods (Fig. 24.3.3.12).

Posterior fossa tumours

Intrinsic posterior fossa tumours are the most common intracranial tumours in children. The most common lesion is a medulloblastoma, which usually arises in the roof of the fourth ventricle and accounts for about 30% of posterior fossa tumours in children. Other tumours commonly encountered are ependymomas, and fibrillary and pilocytic astrocytomas, both of which have a better prognosis than medulloblastomas. Medulloblastomas and ependymomas commonly metastasize down the spinal canal, producing what are known as 'drop metastases' to the lumbar or sacral region.

Other intracranial tumours

Colloid cyst

This is a very characteristic benign lesion that arises at the foramen of Munro, between the lateral and third ventricles, and presents with obstructive hydrocephalus. Colloid cysts are usually readily detectable on CT and MRI, although density and signal characteristics can vary quite widely, the location is absolutely characteristic. (Fig. 24.3.3.13).

Pituitary region tumours

MRI is the investigation of choice for suspected pituitary/parasellar lesions.

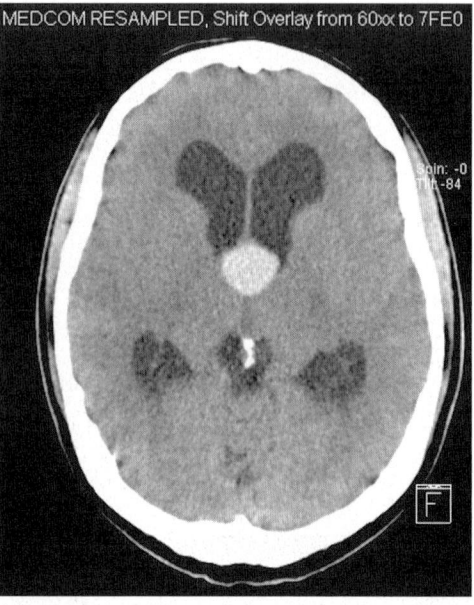

(a)

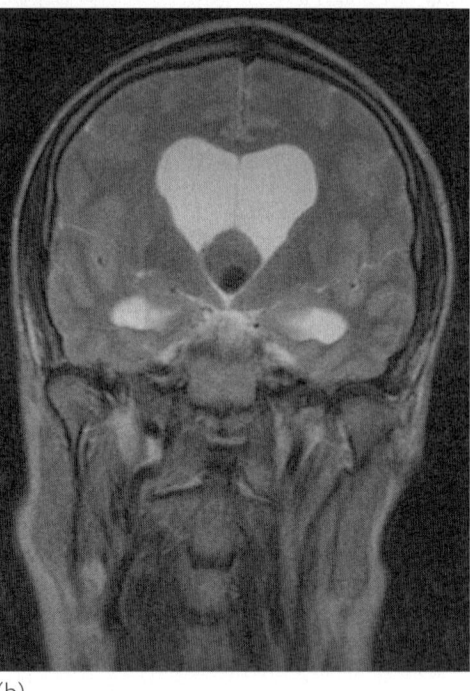

(b)

Fig. 24.3.3.13 (a) CT scan showing typical appearance of a colloid cyst (bright) on CT, but can be of any density. The location of this lesion at the foramen of Munro is absolutely characteristic and there is not really a differential diagnosis. (b) Coronal MRI showing colloid cyst in characteristic location at the foramen of Munro at the junction of the lateral and third ventricles.

Parasellar tumours, which arise outside the brain itself, are associated with a characteristic range of pathology. The most common lesion is a nonfunctioning pituitary adenoma, followed by hormonally active tumours (diagnosed initially not by MRI but by biochemical assay techniques), namely ACTH-producing tumours (Cushing's disease), prolactinomas, and growth-hormone-secreting tumours (acromegaly). All these have similar imaging characteristics, but their size varies widely: ACTH-secreting adenomas are usually very small and may not be detectable even on high-quality MRI.

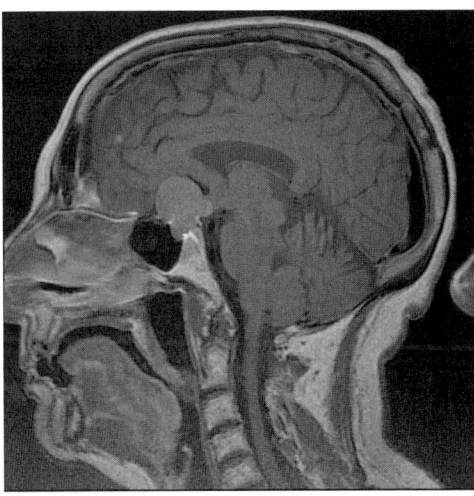

(a)

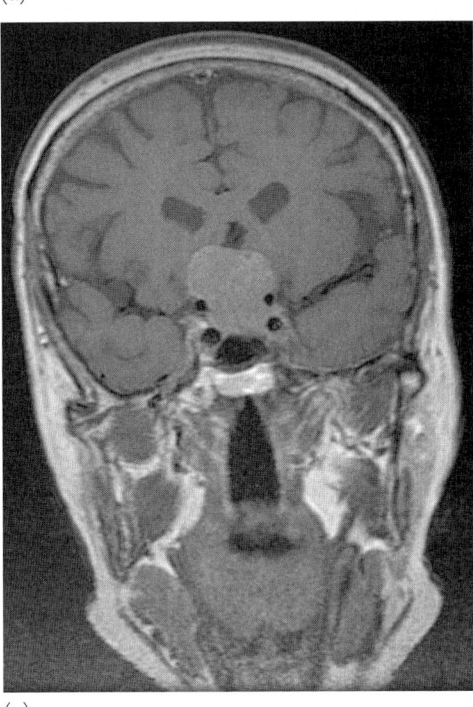

(c)

Fig. 24.3.3.14 (a) Sagittal MRI of pituitary adenoma with considerable suprasellar extension. (b) Coronal MRI of pituitary adenoma.

Nonfunctioning macroadenomas tend to present late, often with visual loss and/or pituitary failure due to the large size and optic chiasmal compression (Fig. 24.3.3.14). Lesions invading the cavernous sinus may result in ophthalmoplegia.

Meningiomas may also occur in the parasellar region and appear very similar.

Craniopharyngioma

This benign tumour arises in the hypothalamic region from remnants of Rathke's cleft, usually in young patients, and presents with visual loss and/or pituitary failure. The characteristic finding on CT is calcification. There is often a cystic as well as a solid component to the lesion.

Brainstem gliomas

These relatively uncommon tumours occur at a relatively young age. However, because of their location there is no prospect of any

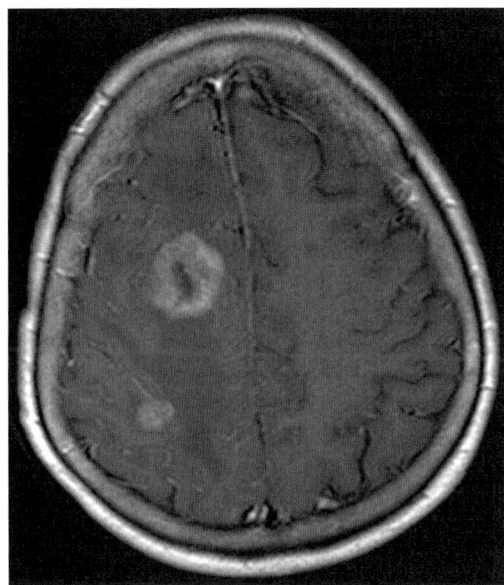

Fig. 24.3.3.15 T_1-weighted enhanced MRI showing two secondary deposits in the upper part of the right hemisphere.

surgical approach and, if any treatment is appropriate, it is usually radiotherapy. Brainstem gliomas may vary widely in their aggressiveness, from rapidly progressive lesions to indolent lesions that may remain static for many years.

Secondary cerebral tumours

These are among the most common intracranial tumours in adults and may be the presenting feature in some patients. Lung, breast, renal, and gastrointestinal tumours as well as melanomas metastasize especially to the brain.

Secondary tumours may be solitary or multiple and are fairly characteristic on the imaging, with intracranial masses (solid or cystic) surrounded by oedema and frequently with enhancement after intravenous contrast (Figs. 24.3.3.15 and 24.3.3.16). The differential

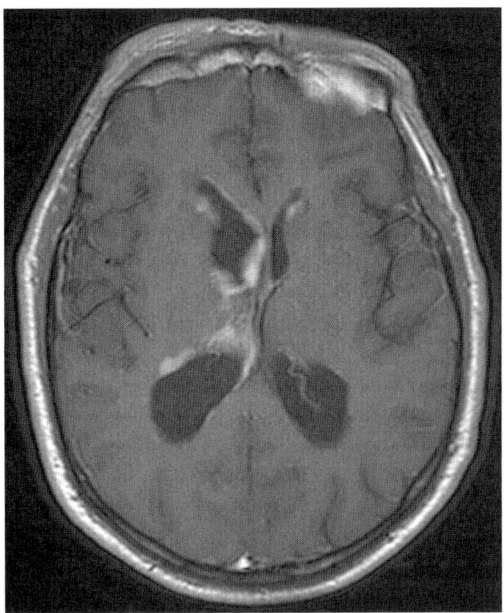

Fig. 24.3.3.16 T_1-weighted enhanced MRI showing metastases in the ventricular wall reflecting spread of disease in the subarachnoid space.

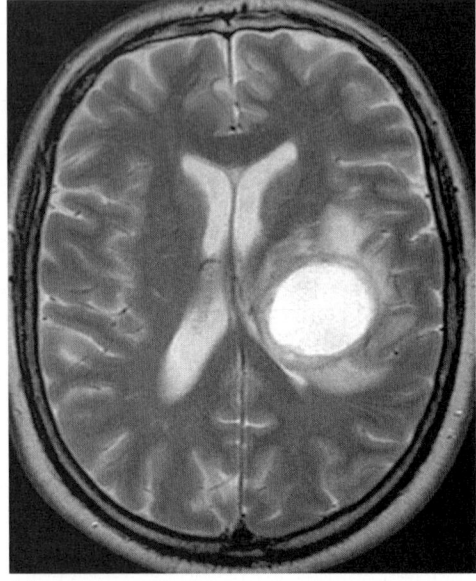

(a)

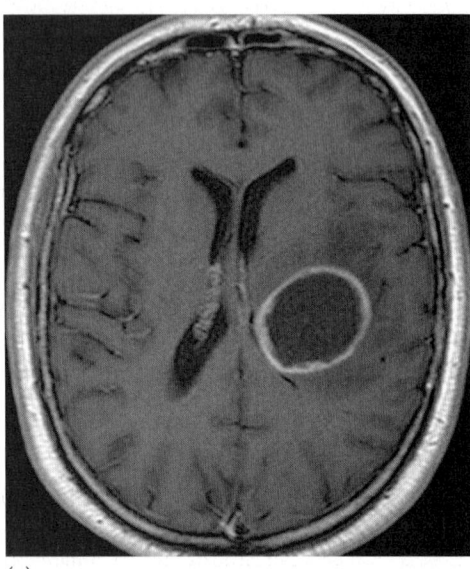

(c)

Fig. 24.3.3.17 (a) T_2-weighted MRI showing large brain abscess near the left lateral ventricle. (b) T_1-weighted MRI with contrast showing typical regular enhancement of the capsule of the abscess with surrounding oedema.

diagnosis of multiple ring-enhancing lesions in the brain is between cerebral metastases and abscesses. DWI may help to differentiate the latter which show decreased diffusion.

Malignant meningeal deposits of CNS or systemic tumours are relatively uncommon, but they do occur and may be difficult to detect on noncontrast-enhanced imaging. MRI with gadolinium enhancement is the most sensitive detection method and is more sensitive than cerebrospinal fluid cytology.

Intracranial infections

Although intracranial infections are less common in western countries than tumours, it is vital that they are detected as urgent, and definitive diagnosis and treatment are essential to their effective management.

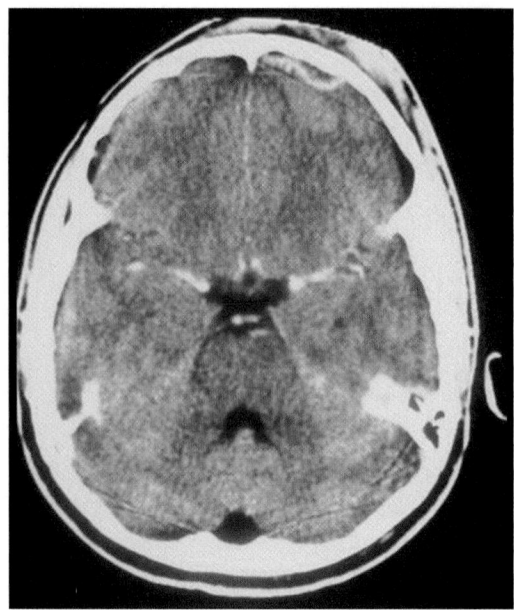

Fig. 24.3.3.18 Left frontal subdural empyema CT scan showing a collection of fluid in the left frontal subdural or extradural space in a patient with a large subdural empyema. Note that there is considerable soft-tissue swelling over the frontal region. The paranasal sinuses are often the source and show opacification (not visible on this image).

Bacterial infections

Bacterial meningitis is the most common bacterial intracranial infection. Cranial CT is usually normal in uncomplicated cases but may show meningeal enhancement and/or mild hydrocephalus. A patient who is neurologically intact and has a Glasgow Coma Scale (GCS) score of 15 does not require cranial CT before lumbar puncture. Note that mild communicating hydrocephalus is not a contraindication to lumbar puncture (see below). If a patient with suspected meningitis has a reduced GCS score or a focal deficit, cranial CT is important but antibiotics must not be delayed by imaging.

Cranial CT is often useful in diagnosing some of the complications associated with bacterial meningitis, e.g. hydrocephalus, ventriculitis, cerebral oedema, cerebral abscess, subdural empyema, cerebral infarction, and venous sinus thrombosis.

Cerebral abscess

Pyogenic brain abscesses are usually single but may be multiple. In the early stage they may not be particularly well defined and begin as an area of cerebritis, which then evolves into an abscess—a characteristic ring-enhancing mass surrounded by oedema (Fig. 24.3.3.17). MRI is particularly useful in the specific diagnosis of an abscess and its differentiation from a malignant tumour. Abscesses show decreased diffusion on DWI and have characteristic MR spectra.

If a pyogenic abscess is suspected then burr-hole aspiration is mandatory to establish the diagnosis and drain the abscess. Abscesses may be seen at various stages of evolution if associated with a septicaemic illness. The source is either blood spread or direct spread from the infection in the paranasal sinuses or the mastoid.

Subdural empyema

This is a rare, but important, intracranial infection often caused by spread from a paranasal sinus infection. Pus accumulates in the subdural space, causing a spreading cortical thrombophlebitis.

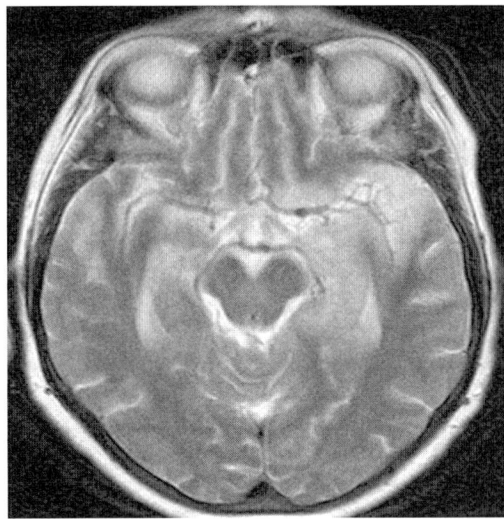

(a)

(c)

Fig. 24.3.3.19 (a) Axial T_2-weighted MRI of patient with herpes simplex encephalitis (HSE) shows bilateral hippocampal involvement with high T_2 signal, much worse on the left, and extending into the anterior part of the temporal lobe. (b) Axial T_2-weighted MRI of patient with HSE showing high T_2 signal in the left insular cortex of the temporal lobe.

Empyema is usually due to the anaerobic bacterium *Streptococcus milleri*. Such abscesses are rapidly fatal if they are not treated aggressively with antibiotics and neurosurgical drainage. CT findings are subtle. The most obvious sign may be that of sulcal effacement due to cortical swelling and contrast enhancement may emphasise the thin subdural collection of fluid, which spreads over the brain surface, often alongside the falx. MRI is more sensitive in the detection of the small subdural collections, but it is unnecessary if the diagnosis is clear on CT scans (Fig. 24.3.3.18).

The underlying brain appears swollen and tight with the sulci obliterated; it will show moderate meningeal enhancement after intravenous contrast.

Tuberculosis

This most often manifests as tuberculous meningitis, a basal meningitis, and less often as either abscesses or granulomas in the brain.

If the meninges are involved there is almost invariably a degree of hydrocephalus.

Viral encephalitis and HIV

The most common cerebral viral infection is herpes simplex encephalitis (HSE). The imaging findings are often fairly typical, although CT scan changes may be very subtle during the early phase. Cranial CT shows a mild swelling with diffuse low density in the anterior and medial temporal lobes and insular cortex, often bilateral. MRI is much more sensitive and can be fairly specific (Fig. 24.3.3.19). Later, similar changes are seen in the cingulate gyri. Classically, there is sparing of the basal ganglia.

A detailed description of HIV-related cerebral imaging findings is beyond the scope of this textbook. The incidence of HIV encephalitis and the other more commonly associated opportunistic infections has decreased since HAART (highly active retroviral therapy) became available in 1996, with the exception of progressive multifocal leucencephalopathy (PML). HAART has increased the survival of those infected with the JC virus that causes PML.

In HIV encephalitis, the white matter is damaged and MR demonstrates high signal in the deep white matter bilaterally. There is also volume loss. The white matter changes are optimally demonstrated on MRI and are not well appreciated on CT.

Toxoplasmosis produces multiple enhancing solid or cavitating nodules with oedema not distinguishable from other bacterial or fungal infections.

Cryptococcal infection causes meningitis and imaging may be normal or enlargement of the perivascular spaces may be seen because this fungus produces a mucoid material. Choroid plexitis sometimes occurs.

PML invades oligodendrocytes and causes demyelination, classically in the parieto-occipital white matter. MRI detects the disease more accurately and earlier, and is the investigation of choice.

Hydrocephalus

An understanding of hydrocephalus and its two main types is important, knowing whether it is 'safe to carry out a lumbar puncture' in a patient or not.

'Obstructive or noncommunicating hydrocephalus' is the term given to enlargement of the ventricles caused by an obstruction, usually a mass lesion in the cerebrospinal fluid pathways within the brain (i.e. between where the cerebrospinal fluid is produced from the choroid plexus in the lateral ventricles and the outflow from the fourth ventricle). It is usually caused by a tumour pressing on the ventricles or aqueduct. (Fig. 24.3.3.13a shows a colloid cyst causing obstructive hydrocephalus.)

Communicating hydrocephalus

If cerebrospinal fluid escapes from the fourth ventricle, but there is disturbance of flow around the basal cisterns or over the cortex, or there is a failure of absorption of cerebrospinal fluid, this is termed 'communicating hydrocephalus' or 'cerebrospinal fluid absorption failure hydrocephalus'. Communicating hydrocephalus occurs most commonly after an SAH or meningitis. It may require temporary ventricular or lumbar drainage. However, because cerebrospinal fluid escapes from the fourth ventricle and circulates round the spinal cerebrospinal fluid spaces, it means that it is safe to perform a lumbar puncture to measure and, if appropriate, lower cerebrospinal fluid pressure.

Congenital anomalies and paediatric imaging

Any detailed discussion of this subject is beyond the scope of this chapter, and the reader is directed to specialist texts (see also Chapter 24.17).

Where available, MRI is the investigation of choice in infants and children presenting with suspected congenital anomalies of the brain. It provides the most information and avoids exposure of young patients to ionizing radiation. The main drawback in this age group is the need for sedation or general anaesthesia. The most common indication for imaging in such patients is developmental delay or seizure disorders. It also plays a vital role in the imaging of a suspected, neonatal, hypoxic ischaemic insult and in elucidating the cause of cerebral palsy. CT is a reasonable alternative, but cannot be relied on to detect all relevant pathology, particularly in hypoxic ischaemic injury.

A wide variety of congenital anomalies is possible, ranging from minor abnormalities of neuronal migration, or localized areas of dysplastic cortex, to major anomalies of the whole brain and encephaloceles, in which there is an associated defect of the skull or spine such as a spina bifida. The most frequent is the Chiari 1 malformation of the posterior fossa associated with cerebellar ectopia. The cerebellar tonsils, classically peg-shaped, extend below the foramen magnum a distance of at least 5 mm. There may be associated syringomyelia.

Summary and possible future developments

Modern imaging techniques have revolutionized the diagnosis of neurological disease in the last 30 years. The techniques are likely to become even more sophisticated and accurate with further extension into functional imaging and spectroscopic techniques, both with MR and nuclear medicine's single-photon emission CT (SPECT) and positron emission tomography (PET).

The contribution of these techniques to the efficient and effective diagnosis of intracranial and spinal pathology, together with the ability to effectively exclude structural disease, has had a huge impact on neurological and neurosurgical clinical practice. In addition, the development of endovascular interventional neuroradiological techniques for the treatment of vascular diseases of the brain represent a major revolution in the management of patients with aneurysmal SAH and other complex neurovascular conditions.

Further reading

Atlas S (2008). *Magnetic resonance imaging of the brain and spine*, 4th edition. Lippincott Williams & Wilkins, Philadelphia.

Barkovich AJ (2005). *Paediatric neuroimaging*, 4th edition. Lipponcott Williams & Wilkins, Philadelphia.

Osborn AG, Salzman K, Barkovich AJ (2009). *Diagnostic imaging: brain*. Amirsys, Salt Lake City, UT.

24.3.4 Investigation of central motor pathways: magnetic brain stimulation

K.R. Mills

Essentials

The ability to percutaneously stimulate the central nervous system of awake humans without causing pain has opened up new areas for neurophysiological investigation in the early diagnosis of neurological disease, also furthered the understanding of normal and abnormal motor control. Magnetic stimulators are now available that can excite both upper and lower limb areas of the motor cortex, as well as cranial nerves, motor roots, and deeply sited peripheral nerves.

Clinical applications—these include: (1) measurement of central motor conduction time—this is prolonged in most cases of multiple sclerosis, the threshold is usually raised in motor neuron disease, and the technique may be useful in cerebellar ataxia, including Friedrich's ataxia; (2) assessment of completeness of spinal cord injury; and possibly (3) evaluation of neurodevelopmental delay in children with neurodegenerative and other related diseases. The technique can be used serially to monitor progress of disease or after neurological injury or to examine the effects of drugs, and it can be used safely in neonates and children.

Magnetic stimulators

The magnetic stimulator is an essentially simple device: a brief pulse of electric current is passed through a coil which then generates an intense magnetic field permeating unattenuated into the surrounding media. Any electrical conductor, such as the brain, in the vicinity of the coil will have currents induced within it; these induced currents are capable of exciting cerebral neurons. Coils are placed on the scalp and may be plane circular, figure of eight, or double cone in geometry, the last being especially effective in exciting leg areas of the motor cortex. Some magnetic stimulators produce a predominantly monophasic field pulse, others multiphasic pulses; with the former, the side of the coil next to the scalp determines which hemisphere is predominantly excited, whereas with the latter both hemispheres are about equally excited.

Physiology

If a single anodal shock is applied to the exposed cortex of a monkey and recordings are made from the pyramidal tract, it is seen that, if stimulus intensity is sufficient, an initial wave produced by direct activation of pyramidal tract neurons (the D wave) is followed by a variable number of other waves produced by indirect trans-synaptic activation (I waves) of the same pyramidal neurons. In humans a single weak stimulus to the scalp probably excites pyramidal tract cells trans-synaptically; stronger stimuli may excite the cells directly. The effect of a single stimulus is to cause a high frequency (500–1000 Hz) burst of impulses to descend in the fastest fibres of the pyramidal tract; the spinal motoneurons are engaged by these impulses and, if their excitability is high enough and there is sufficient temporal and spatial summation, the motoneurons fire, causing a muscle contraction. There is considerable convergence and divergence of pyramidal tract fibres within motoneuron pools: single spinal motoneurons receive many corticospinal inputs and, conversely, single pyramidal tract fibres branch to supply many spinal motoneurons. Intrinsic hand muscles are the most easily excited by brain stimulation but all voluntary muscles appear to be accessible via cortical stimulation.

The amplitude of response of a muscle depends on the intensity of the stimulus, to a lesser extent on coil placement on the scalp, but most potently on the degree of voluntary preactivation of the muscle. Thus the amplitude of response of an intrinsic hand muscle may be 20 to 30 times greater if the individual performs a gentle (5 to 10% maximum) voluntary contraction of the muscle. This facilitation is probably due to both cortical and spinal cord mechanisms, voluntary action increasing the effectiveness of the stimulus at the cortex, at the same time as the excitability of spinal motoneurons is increased by other pathways. The latter mechanism predominates in intrinsic hand muscles. Clearly, many factors, including mental set, affect the size of muscle response to the stimulus, and it should be emphasized that this phenomenon of response variability contrasts with the identical and reproducible responses obtained from maximal electrical peripheral nerve shocks; central motor conduction studies should not be regarded simply as an extension of nerve conduction measurements.

Single scalp shocks also bring into play inhibitory mechanisms: if an individual maintains a steady voluntary muscle contraction, the initial excitation caused by the stimulus is followed by a silent period, due to the inhibition of voluntary action. Experiments with paired cortical stimuli have established short interval intracortical inhibition where a subthreshold conditioning stimulus reduces the effects of a subsequent test stimulus if the interstimulus interval is 1 to 5 ms, and long interval intracortical inhibition, probably corresponding to the silent period (above) where the response to the second of a pair of equally intense stimuli is less if the interval between them in 50 to 150 ms.

Safety of magnetic stimulation

A number of studies have looked at the acute effects of magnetic stimuli on animals. It has been shown that magnetic stimuli have little detectable effect on the heart rate, arterial blood pressure, or cerebral blood flow in cats. Magnetic brain stimulation has no acute effects on the human electroencephalogram or on the performance of simple cognitive tests. There have currently been no reports of adverse effects in healthy humans, but, clearly, workers in the field should remain vigilant, especially for long-term effects.

It has been calculated that the total amount of power dissipated in the brain during magnetic stimulation is $1.8 \mu J/cm^3$ per stimulus and, at the maximal rate of stimulation of 0.3 Hz, the average power dissipation is $53 \mu W$, some five orders of magnitude below the basal metabolic rate of the brain.

It was considered prudent for early users of magnetic stimulation to exclude patients who had a history of epilepsy from their studies. Since then, magnetic stimulation has actually been used to attempt to localize epileptic foci in patients with intractable seizures.

Despite magnetic stimulation devices being used on many thousands of patients, many of whom must have had a predilection for epilepsy, there have been only a few reports of a fit being related to single-pulse brain stimulation.

Measurement of central motor conduction time

The latency of muscle response has a central and a peripheral component and a delay due to synaptic transmission in the spinal cord. There is good evidence that, at least with limb muscle, the connection from the pyramidal tract to spinal motoneuron is monosynaptic. The central component of conduction—central motor conduction time (CMCT)—can be estimated by subtracting from the cortex to muscle latency an estimate of the peripheral conduction time obtained either from F-wave measurement (see Chapter 24.3.2) or from responses evoked by root stimulation. In healthy individuals, the mean latency (± standard deviation) of responses in intrinsic hand muscle is 19.7 ± 1.2 ms and the CMCT is 6.1 ± 0.9 ms. The amplitude of responses from brain stimulation is usually compared with that obtained from maximal peripheral nerve stimulation; again there is great variability, but in healthy individuals the response from cortical stimuli is usually at least 15% of that from nerve stimulation. As many factors can influence these values, each laboratory should develop its own normative database.

Motor roots may be excited by both electrical and magnetic stimulators. The former method is preferable because it is not possible to obtain maximal responses in all healthy individuals with magnetic coils, even with optimal coil geometry, coil orientation, and coil position. Both devices activate motor roots at or just outside the intervertebral foramina, and so peripheral conduction time estimated by this method omits conduction in the small segment of motor root within the spinal canal, and CMCT is slightly overestimated. The method must be used, however, if F waves are unobtainable.

Compound responses from muscle may be recorded with surface electrodes, or single motor unit responses may be recorded with needle electrodes; the former method is used clinically, the latter is useful in research. A number of parameters of the surface-recorded response are useful: the maximum amplitude, the onset latency with the muscle relaxed or contracted, the threshold for evoking a response, and the variability in latency or amplitude in a series of responses.

Prolongation of CMCT has been reported in many conditions and is not specific. Delay can be produced by a variety of pathological processes: demyelination of central fibres can lead to slowing of impulse propagation in the central motor pathway; desynchronization of descending impulses can lead to loss of temporal summation at the motoneuron and delay in its firing; and loss of corticospinal axons can lead to impairment of spatial summation at motoneurons and can again delay firing.

Multiple sclerosis

In multiple sclerosis (MS), CMCT is prolonged in about 70% of cases when there are clear clinical signs of a pyramidal lesion in the particular limb being studied. The delay in some cases is very considerable: CMCT may be up to five times longer than in controls. It is likely that, in these cases, demyelination of central fibres is the

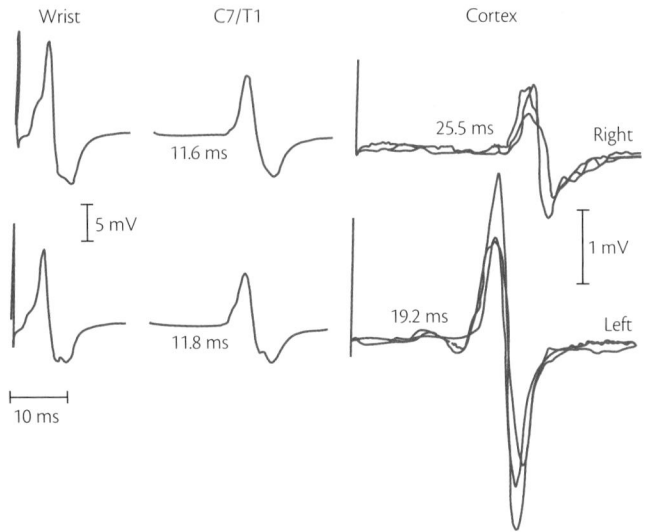

Fig. 24.3.4.1 Slowing of central motor conduction in multiple sclerosis. Compound muscle action potentials are recorded with surface electrodes over the left and right abductor digiti minimi muscles. Stimuli are given to the ulnar nerve at the wrist (left), the C7 to T1 motor roots (middle), and the motor cortex (right). Onset latencies are shown and the variability of responses from cortical stimulation can be seen. On the left central motor conduction time (CMCT) is 7.4 ms, but on the right is prolonged at 13.9 ms.

mechanism leading to delay. In other cases, delay is more modest, only a few milliseconds, and the mechanism is less certain. Abnormal central motor conduction appears to correlate most closely with exaggerated reflexes and spasticity rather than with weakness or cerebellar signs in the limb. Abnormal CMCT from leg areas of motor cortex also correlates with the finding of extensor plantar responses.

Central motor conduction can, however, be abnormal even in the absence of clinical signs. In a large series, it was found that central conduction was abnormal in 20% of cases of MS with no motor signs in the particular limb. The technique can thus be used as a screening test for MS, although it compares unfavourably with visual-evoked potentials, which have a higher rate of abnormality in the absence of clinical signs. This may merely reflect the greater accuracy with which the motor system can be examined clinically. Central motor studies may also be helpful in deciding on the importance of equivocal motor signs, such as mild impairment of fine finger movements.

Motor neuron disease

In motor neuron disease, the most common abnormality is a raised threshold for excitation of the motor cortex, although in early cases the threshold may be reduced. In many cases responses cannot be obtained even with the strongest stimuli applied in optimal conditions. CMCT may be prolonged, but usually only modestly, and responses are often reduced in amplitude in comparison with responses evoked by maximal nerve stimulation. The more muscles that are examined, the greater is the likelihood of detecting an abnormality. The test can be used to confirm an upper motor neuron component to weakness when lower motor neuron signs predominate or for detecting an upper motor neuron lesion in a limb without clinical signs.

Cerebrovascular disease

In stroke, responses in an affected limb may be normal, delayed, or absent, with abnormality grossly paralleling the clinical abnormality. Central motor conduction studies have been used to predict outcome of stroke; if performed within the first 48 h after the ictus, a poor outcome at 6 months is predicted by absent responses and a favourable outcome by normal responses. Whether the prediction is superior to that made purely on clinical grounds is uncertain, but at least the method is quantitative and can be used serially to follow recovery.

Movement disorders

Most studies have shown central motor conduction to be normal in Parkinson's disease, multiple system atrophy, Wilson's disease, Huntington's disease (including at-risk relatives), dystonia, and progressive supranuclear palsy. In some cases of Wilson's disease, central conduction delays have been found. In all these conditions, however, there may be subtle changes in motor cortex excitability detectable as a change in threshold or an abnormal inhibitory response to appropriately timed pairs of cortical stimuli.

Degenerative neurological diseases

A number of rarer degenerative diseases have been investigated with the technique: Friedreich's ataxia often shows delayed and dispersed responses, as does early onset cerebellar ataxia with retained reflexes, the severity of the abnormalities reflecting disease duration. In late-onset cerebellar degeneration, on the other hand, the responses are normal in 62% of cases. In hereditary spastic paraparesis and tropical spastic paraparesis, responses from upper limb muscles are usually normal, whereas those from the lower limbs are delayed or absent. Abnormalities of central motor conduction have also been described in some cases of hereditary motor and sensory neuropathy types I and II, the abnormalities being found especially in those patients with additional upper motor neuron signs. Central motor conduction abnormalities have also been described in a family with hereditary motor and sensory neuropathy with pyramidal signs (HMSN type V).

Spinal cord lesions

Magnetic brain stimulation has been used to assess the completeness of spinal cord injury. A variety of facilitating techniques must be used; the modulation of flexion reflexes by brain stimuli has been shown to be useful in establishing whether injury is complete; in 4 of 26 patients evidence of incomplete lesions was found in patients with clinically complete spinal cord injuries. In compressive myelopathy, by recording from a variety of upper limb muscles, CMCT can be used to localize more accurately the compressed cord segment. This can prove useful to the neurosurgeon when there are multiple levels of compression on imaging.

Paediatric applications

The central conduction time in a group of 457 normal individuals between the ages of 32 weeks and 55 years has been determined. It was found that central conduction time decreases rapidly over the first 2 years of life and then remains constant at the adult value.

In contrast, peripheral conduction increases in proportion to arm length after the age of 5 years. It is suggested that this constant central delay could be useful during the acquisition of motor skills. Central motor conduction has been studied in a range of neurological diseases in children. For example, in 13 of 20 children with an upper motor neuron syndrome of varied aetiology, the central conduction time was abnormal, but MRI and/or CT showed focal abnormalities in only 7. In 15 children with extrapyramidal syndromes, the central conduction time was normal.

Use of brain stimulation for neurosurgical monitoring

Although somatosensory motoring has been shown to be of use during neurosurgical procedures to alert the surgeon to the possibility of cord damage, the use of motor monitoring is far more relevant because paraplegia is one of the most feared, although rare, outcomes of surgery near the cord. Electrical brain stimulation and recording from the cord by epidural electrodes have been achieved; responses consist of a series of waves analogous to the D and I waves recordable in primates. Magnetic stimulation appears to produce I waves but the responses are very sensitive to anaesthetic agents and the depth of anaesthesia produced, especially nitrous oxide. If the aim of monitoring is merely to stimulate the motor cortex, there seems little to be gained by using magnetic stimuli in favour of the electrical method because the pain of the procedure is not a factor.

Further reading

Chen R, *et al.* (2008). The clinical diagnostic utility of transcranial magnetic stimulation: Report of an IFCN Committee. *Clin Neurophysiol*, **119**, 504–32.

Mills KR (1999). *Magnetic stimulation of the human nervous system*. Oxford University Press, Oxford.

Rothwell JC, *et al.* (1991). Stimulation of the human motor cortex through the scalp. *Exp Physiol*, **76**, 159–200.

Higher cerebral function

Contents

24.4.1 Disturbances of higher cerebral function

Peter J. Nestor and John R. Hodges

Essentials

Clinico-pathological and imaging studies indicate strong associations between particular disorders of cognition and focal disease in the brain, but not all focal lesions induce specific loss of higher functions. Neuropsychological research has deepened our understanding by suggesting organizational frameworks for human cognitive faculties.

Neurological basis for cognition

The neocortex around the primary sensory and motor cortices is made up of unimodal association areas, which link to heteromodal association areas, with the linkage of topographical region to specific functional attribute becoming progressively less tightly defined. Other areas of the brain that interact with these association areas in a critical way for cognition include (1) limbic system—particularly in the domains of memory and emotion; (2) basal forebrain nuclei—important to the successful encoding of memory; (3) basal ganglia—relating to attention and speed of cognitive processing; (4) brainstem reticular formation—determining the level of arousal.

Clinical testing of cognition

Regardless of the suspected disorder, the clinician should always proceed in the following way: (1) ensure adequate attention to undergo further testing—if the patient has a profound attention deficit, then their cognition cannot be properly assessed; (2) assess language comprehension—almost all tests are going to be presented with verbal instruction; (3) leave tests of executive function and praxis to the end of the examination—they often require adequate levels of function in all other cognitive domains; and (4) always ask, 'can this apparent disorder be explained in terms of a more elemental deficit?'

Particular tests of cognitive function can aid clinical diagnosis of cerebral disease and monitor treatment. It may also be possible to define the specific needs and deficiencies for which supportive aids may assist the patient.

Specific cognitive domains

Disorders of the higher functions of the brain can be described in terms of the following specific domains:

Attention—the ability to attend to a specific sensory stimulus and to maintain attention is an obligatory first step to any further cognitive processing. Breakdown in attentional processing is the central deficit in delirium or acute confusional states.

Language and related disorders—numerous terms are used to describe aphasic syndromes, but the best approach is to consider language fluency and paraphasias in spontaneous conversation, comprehension, naming, and repetition. Particular types of language and related disorders may be associated with particular anatomical lesions.

Visuospatial and perceptual disorders—a dorsal occipitoparietal pathway is concerned with spatial information and preparation for reaching ('where?' and 'how?'); a ventral occipitotemporal pathway is concerned with identifying visual stimuli ('what?'). Striking neuropsychological syndromes are seen following selective damage to one pathway.

Memory—(1) Implicit memory—unconscious memory systems, such as that responsible for conditioning as well as memory for motor tasks. (2) Explicit memory—the consciously appreciated memory, which is the category most relevant to clinical disease; divided into (a) episodic memory, referring to autobiographical recollection of personal events; typically impaired in Alzheimer's disease and lesions of the limbic system; and (b) semantic memory, referring to factual knowledge and the store of objects and meanings; lesions of the temporal lobes cause loss of this memory, with a severe incapacity to name objects and recall the meaning of words.

Apraxia—a loss of ability to carry out skilled motor tasks that cannot be explained in terms of an elementary disorder of motor control (weakness or ataxia), primary sensory disturbance, or a global impairment of cognition. Usually the result of damage to the left (dominant) hemisphere, particularly the superior parietal lobule and the premotor area of the frontal lobe.

Personality and behavioural change—alterations in complex behaviour, personality and social comportment cannot be simply defined, but are broadly associated with frontal or anterior temporal lobe pathology.

Introduction

Modern scientific study of higher cerebral function began in the late nineteenth century with the case studies of Broca and Wernicke. Their observations of language disorders associated with damage to the left hemisphere gave rise to the notion that specific mental faculties could be dissociated from each other and localized to specific regions within the cerebral hemisphere. Since that time clinicopathological and, more recently, imaging studies have established associations between specific cognitive disorders and focal brain lesions; these studies also show that some lesions do not give rise to highly specific deficits. The field of neuropsychology has offered complementary insights into this area by providing concepts of how cognitive faculties are organized.

The border between psychiatry and neurology has become less distinct; many patients with brain diseases have psychiatric symptoms, cognitive complaints are prominent in depression and schizophrenia, and a biological basis for many 'functional' psychiatric disorders is now well accepted.

Another critical area has been the study of anatomy: the finding that neocortical histology varies by region led to the development of cytoarchitectonic maps such as that of Brodmann. Brodmann's map has become a shorthand way of discussing regional specialization across the cortex. Meanwhile, anatomical studies of neural tracts have provided insights into how topographically distinct regions may interact.

Handedness and hemispheric dominance

The finding of asymmetrical functions in the human cerebral cortex led to the introduction of the term 'hemispheric dominance'. Neuroscientists often refer to cognitive processes being a function of the 'dominant' or 'nondominant' hemisphere; when such terminology is used, the 'dominant' hemisphere is synonymous with that which underpins language function. In right-handed individuals, over 95% have left hemisphere dominance; only rarely does aphasia arise from right hemisphere damage, in which circumstance it is referred to as 'crossed aphasia'. In left-handed individuals, dominance is more complex and language skills are more often shared between the hemispheres, although the left hemisphere is relatively dominant in about 70% of individuals. While the left hemisphere usually specializes in language, the nondominant hemisphere plays

an important role in spatial cognition (with damage to the frontoparietal regions resulting in spatial neglect) and particularly in face processing (with damage to the right occipitotemporal junction producing prosopagnosia).

Primary sensory input and motor output

Motor

The primary motor area lies in the precentral gyrus, immediately rostral to the central sulcus. The body is represented 'somatotopically' along the precentral gyrus: the lower limb at the superomedial and the face at the inferolateral extremity, with the upper limb in between. This is of clinical importance because the vascular supply of the superomedial region is from the anterior cerebral artery whereas the rest of the motor cortex is from the middle cerebral artery. Thus, middle cerebral artery territory infarction will affect face and upper limb with relative sparing of the lower limb, and the converse will be the case with anterior cerebral territory occlusions.

Vision

After passing from the retina, via optic nerves and tracts to the lateral geniculate body of the thalamus, visual information passes to the striate cortex of the occipital lobes (primary visual cortex) through the optic radiations (see Chapter 24.6.1). As images presented to the right visual field are represented on the left retina and conveyed to the left occipital lobe, a lesion of the latter will cause a right homonymous hemianopia (and vice versa for right occipital lesions). Fibres in each optic radiation separate such that input from the superior half of the retina (inferior visual field) runs from lateral geniculate to the striate cortex via parietal white matter whereas that from the inferior retina (superior visual field) loops down into the temporal lobe. Consequently, a lesion of the parietal lobe can cause a contralesional inferior quadrantanopic field defect whereas a temporal lobe lesion can cause a contralesional superior quadrantanopia. Large temporoparietal lesions (e.g. due to middle cerebral artery occlusion) may also cause homonymous hemianopia, which can be distinguished from that resulting from an occipital lesion by preservation of optocokinetic nystagmus in the latter but not the former.

Bilateral lesions to the primary visual cortex lead to 'cortical blindness' in which vision is lost, but, unlike blindness secondary to retinal or optic nerve diseases, pupillary reflexes are preserved. Some cortically blind individuals deny that they have any visual disorder at all (namely visual anosagnosia)—a condition known as Anton's syndrome. These cases tend to have more extensive lesions involving both striate and adjacent visual association cortices.

Somatosensory

The primary somatosensory cortex occupies the postcentral gyrus of the parietal lobe with a somatotopic representation of the body analogous to that of the primary motor area. Sensory deficits due to lesions of the thalamus, or lower components of the sensory system, cause gross abnormalities in the appreciation of touch, pinprick, temperature, and other sensations, and must be excluded before comment can be made on higher sensory function. Parietal lesions cause specific impairment of 'discriminative' sensation, including joint position sense and two-point discrimination. Parietal drift (the patient is asked, with eyes closed, to maintain the upper limbs outstretched in front of the trunk at 90°) is a sign of impairment of the former ability. It is considered specific for a contralateral parietal lesion when the drift is upward, because a downward drift may also be a consequence of subtle motor weakness. The normal separation distance at which one can discriminate one point from two varies according to body region: fingertips 3 mm, palm 1 cm, and body surface 4 to 7 cm.

Other signs of parietal sensory impairment are an inability to name numbers traced on the palm of the hand (agraphaesthesia), and an inability to name small objects (such as keys and coins) placed in the patient's hand (asterognosis). Obviously there is potential to confuse true astereognosis with a more general deficit of object naming such as that caused by loss of semantic knowledge or aphasia (see below). However, ambiguous results on parietal sensory testing can largely be avoided if the examiner adopts a methodical approach of: (1) excluding a lesion below the parietal lobe by establishing that the patient can appreciate, for instance, a pinprick or light touch; and (2) examining from the suspected normal to abnormal side to exclude a more general impairment of cognitive faculties.

Auditory

Auditory information coming from the cochlear nuclei via the inferior colliculus and the medial geniculate nucleus of the thalamus travels to the primary auditory cortex (Heschl's gyrus) in the posterosuperior temporal lobe. Clinically apparent cortical hearing impairment is uncommon due to the bilateral representation of auditory material from each ear by the cerebral cortex. Bilateral lesions of this area (as a result of strokes, prolonged hypotension, or carbon monoxide poisoning) will cause 'cortical deafness', a rare disorder manifest by inability to understand spoken language or recognize sounds although presence or absence of noise can be determined. Unlike Wernicke's aphasia (see below), individuals can understand written text and their language output is normal.

Cognitive domains

Beyond the primary sensory and motor cortices, the neocortex is made up of unimodal and heteromodal association areas. Unimodal association cortices lie adjacent to their respective primary modality whereas heteromodal association cortex is found in the prefrontal and temporoparietal regions. Moving from primary through unimodal to heteromodal association cortex, the linkage of topographical region to a specific functional attribute becomes progressively less tightly defined. Heteromodal association cortices, as the name implies, receive inputs from multiple unimodal areas, but also from non-neocortical areas. Anatomically, as the neocortex approaches the diencephalon, upon which the cerebral hemispheres sit, it transforms into a histologically distinct area: the limbic system. These areas also have critical roles in cognition, particularly in the domains of memory and emotion, and have reciprocal projections with heteromodal association cortices.

Other brain regions that have important modulatory roles on cognition include: (1) the basal forebrain nuclei, which contain cholinergic neurons that project extensively to limbic and neocortical regions and are known to be important to the successful encoding of memory; (2) the basal ganglia, which have reciprocal links to frontal association cortices and have important modulatory roles relating particularly to attention and speed of cognitive processing; and (3) brainstem reticular formation nuclei which project into the hemispheres via the thalami, the most clearly defined role for these projections being at the level of arousal.

Although the remainder of this chapter discusses various disorders of higher mental function individually, one should not view these specific deficits as a random and independent collection of phenomena. It cannot be overemphasized that one should always follow a logical sequence in assessing cognitive function so as to avoid false-positive diagnoses due to sequential effects. For example, tests of executive function that utilize analysis of complex verbal material would be beyond the grasp of a patient with Wernicke's aphasia due to the fundamental disorder of language comprehension without needing to implicate frontal lobe damage. Likewise, a patient with an acute delirium may be unable to perform even the most basic memory tasks as a consequence of the attention deficit and therefore ought not to be labelled amnesic. Therefore, regardless of the suspected disorder, one should always bear the following sequence in mind: (1) ensure adequate attention to undergo further testing; (2) as almost all tests are going to be presented with verbal instruction, assess language comprehension; and (3) as tests of executive function and praxis often require adequate levels of function in all other cognitive domains, these should be left to last. In summary, always ask: 'Can this apparent disorder be explained in terms of a more elemental deficit?'

Attention

The ability to attend to a specific sensory stimulus, such as a human voice or passage of text, and to maintain attention is an obligatory first step to any further cognitive processing. Humans are continuously bombarded with sensory stimuli from both within and between individual sensory input modalities; loss of ability to focus and sustain attention (or, alternatively, block out irrelevant 'noise') renders the individual incapable of following a specific sensory stimulus (such as a conversation) and at the same time vulnerable to random irrelevant environmental stimuli. Although disorders of the frontal lobes, basal ganglia, and ascending reticular formation are associated with poor attention, it is overly simplistic to consider attention as a localizable brain function. The most common causes of acute attention failure are diffuse brain insults such as a metabolic encephalopathy or closed head injury; breakdown in attentional processing is the central deficit in delirium or acute confusional states, the main features of which are summarized in Table 24.4.1.1.

Digit span is one of the most simple methods of assessing attention, especially in the backward condition; normal individuals have a forward span of at least six digits and a reverse span one or two digits less. The digits must be presented as individual items (read the string to be repeated at a rate of one digit per second). A common pitfall is to cluster digits as one does when reciting telephone numbers. This inflates span as each cluster becomes an individual item: compare repeating '6953–8127' with '6…9…5…3…8…1…2…7'. Ability to persevere at a given task is another way of considering attention, and can be tested by asking the patient to recite the months of the year in reverse order.

Orientation is heavily dependent on attention and is assessed by questions of time and place. Testing personal orientation adds little, because only profoundly aphasic or hysterical patients are unable to relate their own name. A recent onset of profound disorientation and attention deficit is typical of a delirium. It should be noted that many patients with episodic memory problems (such as early Alzheimer's disease) remain well oriented.

Table 24.4.1.1 The features of delirium

Onset	Usually acute/subacute
Course	Fluctuating, nocturnal exacerbations
Conscious state	May be impaired, derangement of normal sleep–wake cycle
Cognitive profile	Disoriented in time and place
	Severe impairment of attention (with knock-on effects to other cognitive domains, i.e. due to poor registration)
Psychiatric features	Incoherent and perseverative
	Mood disorders: agitation, apathy
	Visual illusions and hallucinations
	Paranoid ideas common
Physical signs	Asterixis
	May be evidence of general medical illness (pyrexia, signs of hepatic failure, etc.)

Hodges JR (ed.) (2001). *Early onset dementia: a multidisciplinary approach.* Oxford University Press, Oxford.

Language and related disorders

Numerous terms are in use to describe aphasic syndromes, although some serve more to confuse than enlighten. The terms 'expressive' and 'receptive' particularly seem to mislead: on the one hand, all patients with aphasia have some form of difficulty 'expressing' themselves and, on the other, 'receptive' aphasia is often, erroneously, taken to mean that patients have difficulty only with incoming language, but can produce their own language perfectly well. Less ambiguous terms for the two principal divisions of aphasia are 'nonfluent' and 'fluent', which correspond in classic aphasia nomenclature to Broca's and Wernicke's aphasias. The classic aphasia syndromes are, however, rarely seen in the acute stages after stroke and do not characterize the language deficits found in the dementias. A better approach is therefore to consider language fluency and paraphasias in spontaneous conversation, comprehension, naming, and repetition.

Examining patients with aphasia

Fluency and paraphasic errors

Speech can be described as fluent if the patient is able to produce some well-formed sentences or phrases even if empty or anomic (such as 'Oh, you know, the thing you put the stuff in when you're going somewhere and...). Nonfluent language, in contrast, is a consequence of breakdown of the language production and syntactic (grammatical) aspects of language, and is the hallmark of damage to Broca's area and the insula. Output is laboured or 'telegraphic', with often as few as two or three words per minute; in spite of this patients can convey meaning fairly successfully, e.g. 'I...go...hospital'.

Paraphasic errors are substitutions of a correct word for one related in sound or meaning. The former, known as phonological or phonemic paraphasias, involve the substitution of related sound fragments ('phonemes') such as 'dobble' for 'bottle'. Semantic paraphasic errors involve substitution of words of related meaning; the substituted word is typically a higher-frequency example of the same semantic category (such as 'dog' for 'fox') or else of a superordinate category (such as 'animal' for 'fox'). In more extreme circumstances, paraphasic substitutions may not be words at all ('neologisms'); fluent output with virtually continuous neologisms is an utterly incomprehensible state sometimes referred to as 'jargon aphasia'. Patients with lesions to Wernicke's area invariably make a mixture of phonemic and semantic errors. Semantic errors are also very common in Alzheimer's disease and semantic dementia. In Broca's aphasia, phonological errors predominate.

Comprehension

Some degree of impairment of language comprehension can be detected in both fluent and nonfluent aphasia. Patients with fluent aphasia have more overtly impaired comprehension of word meaning (e.g. ordinary nouns). In mild cases this can be demonstrated with semantically complex language tasks (e.g. 'Can you point to a source of artificial illumination?') or by defining uncommon words (e.g. 'What is an aubergine, accordion', etc.). Comprehension of single nouns is preserved in patients with nonfluent aphasia, but comprehension—in addition to production—of complex grammar is impaired. This can be tested with reversible passive sentences (e.g. 'The lion was eaten by the tiger; who survived?') or by asking the patient to obey syntactically complex commands (e.g. 'Touch the keys after touching the book').

Anomia

Naming is a complex task that requires the integrity of three basic processes: visual analysis, semantic knowledge (see 'Memory' below), and word production (phonology). Virtually all patients with aphasia are anomic when tested using items of low familiarity and late age of acquisition. The type of naming error and the ability to circumvent the deficit varies, however, according to the locus of damage. Patients with visuoperceptive deficits that produce visual errors (a 'head' for a 'mushroom', etc.) have retained tactile naming and can give correct responses when asked to put a name to a description ('What do we call the large grey African animal with a trunk?').

A breakdown in the central semantic process causes impairment in naming from all modalities, whereas phonological deficits produce phonological errors regardless of the mode of input.

Repetition

Lesions involving any of the perisylvian language structures are almost always associated with impaired repetition, although this may not be apparent unless multisyllabic words ('caterpillar', 'fundamental', etc.) and phrases ('no ifs, ands, or buts') are tested. Certain aphasic syndromes (see below) show either disproportionate impairment or preservation of repetition.

Aphasic syndromes

Broca's aphasia

This classic form of nonfluent aphasia is characterized by grossly distorted speech output with impaired production and comprehension of syntax. Phonological paraphasias are common and there is impaired repetition of phrases. It is associated with lesions to the left ventrolateral frontal lobe (Broca's area); owing to its close proximity to the motor cortex, when focal lesions (such as stroke or tumour) cause Broca's aphasia, it is typically associated with a right hemiparesis. The distortion of language output, often described as speech apraxia, is thought to relate to concurrent damage to structures within the insula, which is almost always affected.

Wernicke's aphasia

In Wernicke's aphasia there is fluent, although vacuous, output with a mixture of semantic and phonological paraphasic errors and often neologisms. There is also impaired comprehension of word meanings and impaired repetition. In contrast to the fundamental loss of word meaning seen in patients with semantic dementia and destruction of the left inferior temporal lobe after herpes simplex encephalitis, patients with Wernicke's aphasia have breakdown in the mapping between speech and meaning systems. Lesions localize to the posterior portion of the left superior temporal gyrus—known as Wernicke's area. As this area overlies the optic radiation, the most common neighbourhood sign is a right homonymous hemianopia.

Conduction aphasia

This form of aphasia, as the name implies, is due to a disconnection of the two principal language areas. Comprehension is relatively preserved and output is fluent, although phonemic paraphasias occur. The striking abnormality is an impairment of repetition even for single syllable words such that attempts at repeating are laboured and contain phonemic errors. Likewise, naming produces phonemic errors even for high-frequency items (such as for 'cup': 'cah...cahb...cub', etc.). Lesions producing conduction aphasia occur in the region of the supramarginal gyrus and, particularly, the underlying arcuate fasciculus, the tract linking the anterior and posterior language areas.

Global aphasia

In this devastating form of aphasia there is derangement of all aspects of language; patients with global aphasia are nonfluent and have impaired word comprehension, repetition, and naming. Language output is restricted to infrequent unintelligible noises or, at best, a single word or clichéd phrase. As the blood supply to both language areas is from the middle cerebral artery, global aphasia is not uncommon secondary to proximal occlusion of this vessel. Consequently these patients are usually also hemiplegic and hemianopic.

Atypical aphasias and the dementias

The term 'transcortical aphasia' is a legacy of an abandoned neural explanation for a distinct category of aphasia. Although the term is meaningless in its originally coined anatomical sense, it is still sometimes used to describe a distinct syndrome in which a patient with aphasia shows preservation of repetition. Patients with so-called transcortical sensory aphasia are fluent and show profound impairment in word comprehension with preserved repetition; this syndrome is also referred to as amnesic aphasia reflecting the loss of word meaning. It is seen in semantic dementia (the temporal lobe variant of frontotemporal dementia or Pick's disease) and advanced Alzheimer's disease. Earlier in Alzheimer's disease impaired naming with intact fluency and word comprehension (sometimes called anomic aphasia) is commonly seen. Impairment in language output with preserved repetition, transcortical motor aphasia, is most often associated with dorsomedial frontal lesions that involve the supplementary motor area.

Dyslexia

Patients with aphasia show dyslexic difficulties in keeping with their type of aphasia, so those with fluent aphasia will struggle to understand the meaning of words in printed form, whereas those with nonfluent aphasia have trouble with grammatical aspects of reading (particularly word endings: -ed, -ing, etc.). Within acquired dyslexia, however, dissociations have been defined for reading single words; these syndromes are known as deep and surface dyslexia.

Deep dyslexia and surface dyslexia

There may be a dissociation between ability to read orthographically regular (pronounced as they are spelt) words such as 'mint', 'flint', and 'hat', and irregular words such as 'pint', 'cellist', and 'island'. Difficulty reading the latter type is known as surface dyslexia and is one of the hallmarks of semantic dementia; for an irregular word such as 'pint' or 'yacht' to be read correctly, the reader must access knowledge of the word meaning because the graphical representation of the word alone (i.e. its 'surface' structure) will not lead to correct pronunciation. If the semantic knowledge base (located in the dominant temporal lobe) breaks down, the word can be pronounced only according to the rules of graphical-to-phonological translation and thus 'pint' will be pronounced like 'mint' (known as a 'regularization' error)—in other words, analogous to how a normal person would pronounce a nonword, such as 'rint'.

A complementary syndrome is that of deep dyslexia in which patients produce semantic paralexias when reading (reading 'prison' for 'gaol' or 'beer' for 'pint'), are unable to read nonwords, and have greater difficulty with abstract than with concrete words. This, simplistically, is thought to represent a loss of the grapheme-to-phoneme route with intact semantic knowledge (i.e. its 'deep' meaning). Deep dyslexia is typically seen in patients with extensive left hemisphere lesions and global aphasia.

Alexia without agraphia

This syndrome represents a classic disconnection syndrome of visual input from language areas due to a lesion in the left occipital lobe and adjacent splenium (disrupting input from the right occipital lobe); as such, although the right occipital cortex is capable of registering text, the information cannot be decoded by the language hemisphere. Patients are not aphasic and can write normally; they cannot read but can say words spelt out loud to them. Visual field testing shows a right homonymous hemianopia. Patients rapidly relearn how to read by identifying individual letters and reconstructing words by a laborious and slow letter-by-letter reading strategy.

Agraphia

Various acquired disorders of writing occur as homologues of other cognitive deficits, for example patients with aphasia make writing errors consistent with their aphasic syndrome (e.g. patients with Broca's aphasia will make errors in writing syntax), deep and surface dysgraphias give rise to similar errors as deep and surface dyslexia, and ideomotor apraxia (see below) will cause a disorder in motor execution such that writing will be of poor quality.

Visuospatial and perceptual disorders

The regions of the brain concerned with the higher-order analysis of visual information can be divided into a dorsal (occipitoparietal) pathway concerned with spatial information and preparation for reaching, and a ventral (occipitotemporal) pathway concerned with identifying visual stimuli. In other words, the dorsal stream is involved in 'where?' and 'how?' and the ventral with 'what?' information for a given visual stimulus. Some of the most striking neuropsychological syndromes are seen following selective damage to one stream.

The dorsal stream and Balint's syndrome

Constructional apraxia, an inability to draw or copy line drawings such as wire cubes and clock faces, is a common finding in parietal pathology, particularly with right-sided lesions. More severe breakdown in spatial cognition, causing individuals to misreach for visually guided targets, trip on steps, or collide with furniture when walking, is seen with bilateral parietal diseases (such as watershed infarction, the biparietal variant of Alzheimer's disease, and venous sinus thrombosis) and results clinically in Balint's syndrome, the features of which are simultanagnosia, optic ataxia, and ocular apraxia. Simultanagnosia is the inability to integrate and make sense of an overall visual scene in spite of preservation in the ability to identify individual elements. Such patients are relatively better at identifying small objects; this can also be demonstrated by an inability to read vertically printed words although they can be read when printed normally. Ocular apraxia describes the inability to direct gaze to a novel visual stimulus, whereas optic ataxia is the inability to reach accurately for a visually guided target.

Spatial neglect

Although considered under the visuospatial heading, spatial neglect is really a cross-modality disorder that typically involves the neglect of all sensory information (visual, tactile, auditory) from the side contralateral to the lesion. Chronic neglect virtually only occurs in the context of right parietal lobe damage. Right hemispatial neglect after an acute left parietal lesion can occur, but is usually less severe and tends to resolve within days. In addition to being a cross-modality disorder, it is not correct to define a 'hemispatial field' in purely retinotopic terms, e.g. if a patient who exhibits neglect on visual field testing has the body turned to face the neglected extrapersonal hemispace (with head and eyes fixed in the original position), the neglected space is reduced.

Visual neglect is best tested by cancellation (crossing off 'A's on a sheet of paper containing randomly arranged letters), drawing (clock, house, flower), or line bisection tasks. Patients with severe visual neglect may even appear to be hemianopic. A milder form of neglect can be elicited by 'sensory extinction' of the neglected side during bilateral sensory stimulation (visual and somatosensory at the bedside, although auditory neglect can be demonstrated experimentally). Patients often have associated hemiparesis, although as part of their neglect syndrome they may deny this impairment—a phenomenon known as anosagnosia. When presented with the hemiparetic limb they may even deny that it is their own.

The ventral stream

Lesions to the occipitotemporal pathway give rise to difficulty recognizing visual stimuli which is not a consequence of being unable to appreciate where an object is in space, as is the case in simultanagnosia. This deficit is known as visual object agnosia and has been divided further into aperceptual and associative varieties. In aperceptual agnosia, basic aspects of vision (acuity, fields, and contrast sensitivity) are intact, but patients cannot identify, or match, identical objects and have grave difficulty copying line drawings,

although knowledge of these objects is intact if tested using other inputs such as describing from name. In contrast, associative agnosia describes a state where loss of object knowledge occurs such that, although patients can copy line drawings well and match perceptually identical pictures, they cannot match nonperceptually identical images such as different angles of the same face or, for example, tell that two different types of clock are both clocks. Associative agnosia is a cross-modality disorder such that knowledge of objects is impaired in nonvisual modalities—in other words one component of generalized failure of semantic knowledge (see below). Differentiation of these agnosias requires the use of test material found only in neuropsychology laboratories. One component of object knowledge is colour, loss of which (achromatopsia) usually accompanies occipitotemporal lesions and is more accessible to bedside evaluation.

A restricted form of impaired object recognition relates to faces. Known as prosopagnosia, the person can no longer recognize previously familiar faces but can recognize their voices and have access to knowledge from their names. Usually bilateral lesions of the inferior occipitotemporal junction are responsible, although cases with lesions restricted to just the right side have been described.

Memory

Memory is divided by researchers into implicit and explicit subtypes (also known as nondeclarative and declarative, respectively). Implicit memory refers to unconscious memory systems such as that responsible for conditioning as well as memory for motor tasks such as hitting a golf ball or playing a piece of music 'by heart'. Explicit memory, in contrast, refers to consciously apprehended memory and is further divided into episodic and semantic memory. In clinical terms, when one refers to memory, it is only the explicit type of memory that is considered. When assessing memory complaints it is useful to apply a theoretically motivated approach to analysing symptoms according to the subcomponent of memory involved. In broad terms, memory subtypes can be considered under the following headings.

Working memory

Working memory refers to the amount of information that can be held by the brain 'online' (such as reading a phone number then holding it as the object of one's attention until the number can be dialled, or solving mathematical problems in the head); in the absence of rehearsal, when the focus of one's attention has moved to a novel topic for more than a few seconds, such items are lost. Working memory is also referred to as 'short-term' memory by psychologists, although this latter term is often used by patients and their doctors to describe recently acquired episodic memory (see below); it also involves aspects of attention (see above) so, to avoid confusion, the term 'working memory' is preferable. Slips of working memory are often erroneously seen by patients as the harbinger of dementia and thus these individuals are commonly referred to memory clinics: these lapses of attention (such as forgetting why you opened the refrigerator door or went into the study, or immediately forgetting a new telephone number) are common everyday symptoms which are increased with anxiety and depression, and also occur more commonly with advancing age. Complaints of this type are also common after head injury and in basal ganglia disorders.

Semantic memory

Semantic memory refers to the brain's knowledge store of, for example, objects and word meanings; it is also the term applied to knowledge of facts, such as that Paris is the capital of France, canaries are small yellow birds kept as pets, or Ronald Reagan was a president of the United States of America. Evidence from the study of semantic dementia suggests that the ventral and polar regions of the temporal lobes are particularly critical to supporting semantic knowledge. The extent to which hemispheric specialization for different types of semantic knowledge (words, objects, etc.) exists remains a subject for debate; loss of word knowledge appears to relate preferentially to left temporal damage whereas some reports suggest that face knowledge may be more dependent on the right temporal lobe.

Loss of memory for words is the usual complaint in patients with a primary disorder of semantic memory such as semantic dementia (also known as progressive fluent aphasia) and after herpes simplex virus encephalitis. However, it is important to distinguish between the occasional word-finding lapse, usually for proper nouns, which occurs normally (especially in later life), and the relentlessly progressive loss of vocabulary, which occurs in association with left temporal lobe pathology. Low-frequency words are the most vulnerable and patients with semantic dementia often have some insight into this problem in the early stages, e.g. a carpenter may complain that he can no longer remember the names of tools. People with Alzheimer's disease show a similar phenomenon, although it is usually overshadowed by their profound episodic memory deficit.

Breakdown in semantic memory manifests as an inability to name objects or drawings with the production of broad superordinate responses (such as 'animal' for 'elephant') and the inability to define the meaning of words. Category fluency (the ability to generate exemplars from a given semantic category such as types of animals, kitchen utensils, or birds) is another sensitive measure of semantic memory. Knowledge of famous people can be tested by identifying photographs and names, or asking the patient to list prime ministers in chronological order.

Episodic memory

Episodic memory refers to the event-based memories unique to each individual, in other words our recollection of personally experienced episodes (indeed, it is sometimes termed 'autobiographical' memory). Difficulty with the acquisition of new event-based memories (such as inability to recall details of a television programme or conversation with a friend despite good attention at the time) is the hallmark of early Alzheimer's disease and other causes of the amnesic syndrome (Table 24.4.1.2). Lesions that give rise to amnesia involve the limbic system of the brain (especially the hippocampi and their connections—Fig. 24.4.1.1). Although bilateral involvement is usually required to cause a full-blown amnesic syndrome, neuropsychological testing can often reveal a selective deficit in verbal or nonverbal memory in cases of left- or right-sided damage, respectively. Retrograde memory (established before the amnesic insult) is typically better than anterograde memory (established any time after) in amnesic syndromes and, within retrograde memory, very remote memory is classically (although not universally) better preserved than recent memory.

On examination, patients with amnesia have a striking inability to relate anecdotes from their recent life, although in cases of basal forebrain amnesia they may offer confabulations. Amnesia can be assessed in the clinic by asking the patient to learn some information such as a new name and address; patients with amnesic syndromes (including early Alzheimer's disease) typically repeat a name and address perfectly after two to three trials, but show very rapid forgetting and recall little or nothing after a delay of a few minutes of a distracting task.

Amnesia may occur as a temporary state as is seen with transient global amnesia (TGA), in which there is a sudden onset of severe

Table 24.4.1.2 Causes of the amnesic syndrome

Type	Common aetiologies
Transient	Transient global amnesia
	Transient epileptic amnesia
	Closed head injury (may be permanent)
	After electroconvulsive therapy
	Drugs (especially ethanol)
Anatomically defined	
Hippocampus (and adjacent mesial temporal structures)	Alzheimer's disease
	Herpes simplex encephalitis
	Limbic encephalitis (paraneoplastic; autoimmune with voltage-gated potassium antibodies)
	Watershed infarction: cardiac arrest, CO poisoning, etc.
	Complicating epilepsy surgery
Diencephalon (dorsomedial and anterior thalamus; mamillary bodies)	Korsakoff's psychosis
	Infarction (watershed, deep perforator occlusion, 'top of the basilar' syndrome)
Basal forebrain	Ruptured anterior communicating artery
	Aneurysm
Fornix	Complicating colloid cyst removal from third ventricle
Retrosplenial/posterior cingulate	Various: tumour, haemorrhage, etc. Alzheimer's disease?
Psychogenic (nonorganic)	

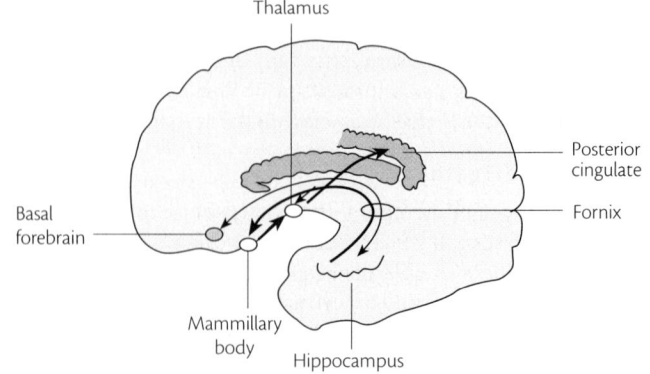

Fig. 24.4.1.1 Principal connections of structures critical to sustaining human memory.

amnesia that lasts several hours before resolution; afterwards the patient, characteristically elderly, is left with an islet of amnesia for the hours of the episode. TGA typically occurs as a solitary episode; recurrent attacks of self-limiting amnesia occasionally occur as a consequence of epileptic activity, hence the term 'transient epileptic amnesia' (TEA). Attacks of TEA are typically briefer than TGA (<1 h for TEA versus several hours for TGA) and frequently occur on waking.

Apraxia

Apraxia is defined as a loss of ability to carry out skilled motor tasks that cannot be explained in terms of an elementary disorder of motor control (weakness or ataxia), primary sensory disturbance, or a global impairment of cognition. In the early 20th century Leipmann distinguished three types of apraxia—limb–kinetic, ideomotor, and ideational—and, although these terms have suffered from a lack of universally accepted definition, they are still widely used today. In an attempt to clear up ambiguity, the terms 'production' and 'conceptual' apraxia are also now used to indicate ideomotor and ideational apraxia according to the definitions below.

Limb–kinetic apraxia refers to the loss of fine motor dexterity that can be seen, for instance, with mild pyramidal lesions (such as after recovery from stroke). In spite of apparently good strength and coordination, the person cannot manage tasks requiring fine motor control such as tying a shoelace or buttoning a shirt. As such, according to the above definition, this is not a 'true' apraxia but rather an artefact of the insensitivity of bedside tests of the motor system: in other words a primary motor deficit is unmasked only by tasks more demanding than routine tests of power and coordination.

Ideomotor (production) apraxia refers to the inability to execute the motor programme for a given task (the temporal and spatial organization of movement) in spite of adequate comprehension, as demonstrated, for instance, by the ability to describe the correct execution of the task (such as sharpening a pencil: 'You put the pointed end of the pencil into the hole then turn it') or to identify correctly a task when done by someone else. Patients with ideomotor apraxia also have problems performing meaningless (nonsymbolic) gestures.

Ideational (conceptual) apraxia, in contrast, is a loss of knowledge of actions: there is an inability to either perform or recognize a given motor task. There is also an inability to match tools correctly to their actions, so a person may select a screwdriver to hammer a nail. Unlike patients with ideomotor apraxia, they do not show disorders of the spatial and temporal aspects of action and thus their tool use, although incorrect, is fluent.

To screen for apraxia, patients should be asked to perform skilled motor tasks to verbal instruction or to imitation including both meaningful and meaningless gestures. If deficits are uncovered, tests such as correctly identifying mimes performed by the examiner and matching tools to functions should be given. Subtle disorders of praxis may be evident only with low-frequency tasks (such as using a vegetable peeler or a pencil sharpener as opposed to a knife or a hairbrush). When asked to mime an action (such as hair combing or brushing teeth), 'body part as tool' errors are often cited as evidence for apraxia: the patient uses his or her hand as the tool (e.g. rubbing an extended index finger over the teeth as a toothbrush). It is, however, not uncommon for normal individuals

to make these 'body part as tool' errors when asked to perform such tasks, hence it is essential when this type of error is committed to draw it to the person's attention and reinstruct accordingly. Normal individuals are able to correct these errors, whereas those with apraxia cannot.

In terms of the neural substrate for production (ideomotor) apraxia, the overwhelming majority of cases follow damage to the left (dominant) hemisphere. More specifically, there is evidence that a motor system incorporating the superior parietal lobule (Brodmann's areas 5 and 7) and the premotor area of the left frontal lobe are particularly critical to the temporal and spatial organization of motor programmes. Conceptual apraxia is also indicative of left hemisphere dysfunction in most cases, although whether a more specific site can be identified is contentious. It is also important where a conceptual apraxia is suspected to ensure that it is not just one manifestation of a more generalized breakdown of semantic knowledge (see Memory above)

Buccofacial apraxia represents a specific form of apraxia in which patients are unable to perform tasks such as licking the lips or blowing out matches to command. It is particularly associated with nonfluent aphasia, presumably as the motor programming of articulation and nonlinguistic buccofacial movements share a common pathway.

Personality and behavioural change

So far, disorders of higher mental function have been considered in quite discrete terms, in the sense of both the cognitive deficit and the cerebral location. Alterations in complex behaviour, personality, and social comportment cannot, however, be so simply defined, but are broadly associated with frontal or anterior temporal lobe pathology. The key to identifying such disorders is the presence of a sustained change from a previous state (thus differing from a life-long eccentric personality), which cannot be explained by a primary psychiatric diagnosis. The only reliable way to confirm such changes is by taking a separate history from a partner or other close personal acquaintance with knowledge of the patient's premorbid personality.

Prefrontal syndromes

The prefrontal cortex comprises that part of the frontal lobe rostral to the premotor area; it is classified as heteromodal association cortex and receives extensive inputs from unimodal association areas posterior to the central sulcus. The frontal lobes also have loop projections running to the basal ganglia, then the thalamus, and back to the frontal lobes. Thus, lesions along this loop (as seen in conditions such as Huntington's disease or progressive supranuclear palsy) may also share deficits in common with primary frontal lobe disorders. Anatomically, the prefrontal cortex can be divided into dorsolateral, orbital, and medial surfaces; although in many cases damage will not be restricted to just one of these regions, they provide a useful framework for considering prefrontal functions. Broadly, lesions to the dorsolateral surface are responsible for the frontal 'dysexecutive' syndrome, to the orbital surface for the classic frontal behavioural syndrome, and to the medial surface (anterior cingulate) for a profound amotivational state.

The dysexecutive syndrome

The term 'executive' refers to aspects of higher-order brain function, such as problem-solving, reasoning, and mental abstraction, which rely on the dorsolateral prefrontal lobes. It is also associated with impulsivity, susceptibility to distraction, and failure to persevere with the task at hand. Various methods are available to measure these phenomena although no single test offers foolproof sensitivity in this domain, so one should apply as many as possible if the index of suspicion is high.

The combination of letter- and category-based verbal fluency provides much useful information. In letter fluency, the patient is asked to generate as many words as they can think of beginning with a given letter in 1 min. They are instructed not to use proper nouns and not to just change the endings to create new exemplars ('go, goes, going', etc.). Neuropsychologists typically use the letters F, A, and S for this test, so it is best to choose another letter if it is likely that patients are also going to have a formal neuropsychological assessment. In category fluency, patients are asked to produce as many exemplars as possible from a given category in 1 min. Normal individuals usually generate 15 or more words on letter fluency and do slightly better on the 'animal' category. Patients with executive deficits secondary to frontal (or the subcortical loop) pathology show an exaggeration of this relationship, doing poorly on category fluency but even worse on letter fluency (patients with semantic impairments related to temporal lobe diseases such as semantic dementia and Alzheimer's disease typically show the reverse pattern of relatively worse performance on category fluency).

The 'go–no go' test offers a way of assessing impulsivity: the patient is asked to tap the desk once if the examiner does so, but, if the examiner taps twice, he should not tap at all. Patients with frontal pathology are often unable to stop themselves from tapping in both conditions. Failure to abstract meaning from proverbs ('What does "too many cooks spoil the broth" mean?') is a common test but is influenced by background intellectual ability and is culture bound. The so-called 'cognitive estimates' test can be useful ('What is the distance from London to Paris?' or 'How fast does a racehorse gallop?'), as are 'differences and similarities' ('What's the difference between a child and a dwarf?' or 'In what way are a sculpture and a piece of music similar?'). Finally, the susceptibility to irrelevant stimuli mean that the tests of attention discussed above may also be impaired.

It is important to note, however, that unlike cognitive neuropsychological tests of, for instance, memory or language, executive function—indeed cognitive functions ascribed to the frontal lobes in general—is much more inconsistently related to pathology at an individual patient level. Abilities such as problem-solving, mental flexibility, and abstraction overlap considerably with general intelligence, e.g. a patient who responds that a racehorse gallops at 100 miles/h, or, that London is 1000 miles from Paris, may simply have a poor knowledge of velocity and geography rather than being 'dysexecutive'. On the other hand, patients with unequivocal frontal lobe pathology may sometimes be hard to fault on tests of executive function, in spite of problems in day-to-day life. This stands in contrast to patients with, for example, Korsakoff's psychosis who will display evidence of amnesia regardless of how one chooses to test memory.

Orbitofrontal syndrome

The striking changes in behaviour seen in patients with prefrontal lesions relate particularly to orbital (or ventral) surface damage. An important caveat to this locationist account is that most studies derive observations from either static lesions or frontotemporal dementia, in which damage usually extends beyond the orbital frontal cortex. Although devastating in their effects on social function, such lesions are notoriously difficult to detect using standard psychometric tests. Patients lack empathy and emotional warmth, e.g. if confronted with something as serious as the admission to hospital of their partner, their primary concern may be that their mealtime routine will be disturbed. They are disinhibited and oblivious to social mores such that they may be overly familiar with strangers, disregard personal space, and make inappropriate comments or gestures (often of a sexual nature). They often make rash and irresponsible decisions such as spending money above their means. They may develop stereotyped and ritualistic behaviours such as insisting on always taking a particular route when shopping or repetitively closing doors in the home: these behaviours can be so severe as to constitute a secondary obsessive–compulsive disorder syndrome.

A useful clue is often the presence of a change in eating behaviour. Patients may become fixated on one dish; often they develop a preference for sweet foods. A lack of normal satiety means that they may overeat, often with secondary weight gain.

Imitation and utilization behaviour are dramatic phenomena related to orbital frontal lobe damage. The patient with imitation behaviour unconsciously mimics the examiner's posture and mannerisms regardless of how absurd they are: raising an arm in the air, placing a leg on the desk, or sitting on the floor. Utilization behaviour is even more striking: patients will use any object placed in their grasp. The classic example is the patient offered multiple pairs of spectacles who attempts to wear them all, one on top of another.

Amotivational states

Medial frontal lesions are particularly associated with apathy. Patients lack spontaneity, they will not initiate conversation although they can reply to specific questions. In keeping with this observation, performance on tests such as the letter fluency task, described above, is severely impoverished. If left to their own devices, they may not spontaneously move, preferring to sit in a chair staring blankly into space. This apathy has also been termed 'abulia' in the past; in its most extreme form where the individual lies motionless with no speech, the term 'akinetic mutism' has also been applied. The catatonic phenomenon of maintaining postures when the limbs are moved by the examiner may also be seen. Patients with depression also show marked apathy, although it is accompanied by both the biological features of depression (anorexia, diurnal variation, etc.) and internal symptoms of mood disturbance (pessimism, suicidal thoughts, anhedonia, etc.).

Temporal lobe syndromes

In addition to the cognitive deficits that can occur with temporal lobe lesions such as amnesia and loss of semantic knowledge, behavioural disturbances can also occur. The most severe, secondary to bilateral anterior temporal damage (including the amygdala), is the Klüver–Bucy syndrome, which comprises three characteristic features: placidity, even in threatening situations; indiscriminant hypersexuality; and oral exploration of objects. Other behaviours have been described in temporal lobe dysfunction, particularly, although not exclusively, in association with interictal temporal lobe epilepsy. These include preoccupation with religious or philosophical issues and a tendency to excessive writing.

Further reading

Baddeley AD (1999). *Essentials of human memory*. Psychology Press, Hove.

Berrios GE, Hodges JR (2000). *Memory disorders in psychiatric practice*. Cambridge University Press, Cambridge.

Driver J, Mattingley JB (1998). Parietal neglect and visual awareness. *Nat Neurosci*, **1**, 17–22.

Goodale MA, Westwood DA (2004). An evolving view of duplex vision: separate but interacting cortical pathways for perception and action. *Curr Opin Neurobiol*, **14**, 203–11.

Hodges JR (2007). *Cognitive assessment for clinicians*, 2nd edition. Oxford University Press, Oxford.

Hodges JR, Spatt J, Patterson K (1999). 'What' and 'how': evidence for the dissociation of object knowledge and mechanical problem-solving skills in the human brain. *Proc Natl Acad Sci USA*, **96**, 9444–8.

McCarthy RA, Warrington EK (1990). *Cognitive neuropsychology: a clinical introduction*. Academic Press, San Diego.

Mesulam MM (1998). From sensation to cognition. *Brain*, **121**, 1013–52.

Patterson K, Lambon-Ralph MA (1999). Selective disorders of reading? *Current Opin Neurobiol*, **9**, 235–9.

Patterson K, Nestor PJ, Rogers TT (2007). Where do you know what you know? The representation of semantic knowledge in the human brain. *Nat Rev Neurosci*, **8**, 976-87.

Rothi LJG, Heilman KM (eds) (1997). *Apraxia: the neuropsychology of action*. Psychology Press, Hove.

Stuss DT, Alexander MP (2007). Is there a dysexecutive syndrome? *Philos Trans R Soc B*, **362**, 901–15.

Tulving E, Craik FM (eds) (2000). *The Oxford handbook of memory*. Oxford University Press, New York.

Walsh K, Darby D (1999). *Neuropsychology: a clinical approach*. Churchill Livingstone, Edinburgh.

24.4.2 Alzheimer's disease and other dementias

John R. Hodges

Essentials

Dementia is defined as a syndrome consisting of progressive impairment in memory and at least one other cognitive deficit (aphasia, apraxia, agnosia, or disturbance in executive function) in the absence of another explanatory central nervous system disorder, depression or delirium.

Epidemiology and classification

Prevalence—dementia is common, affecting about 8% of all people over 65 years, rising to around 20% of those over 85 years. It is estimated that the 18 million people with dementia worldwide will increase to 34 million by the year 2025, with this increase being most marked in the developing countries.

Classification—dementia may be classified in terms of (1) its cause—these are many diseases, some of which are remediable and thus justify investigation (e.g. vitamin B_{12} deficiency, thyroid hormone deficiency), but most cases result from Alzheimer's disease, vascular disorders, or subcortical diseases of the brain; or (2) according to the pattern of cognitive loss—this alternative perspective may contribute usefully to diagnosis, to the level of care required, and allow refinement of prognosis.

Particular causes of dementia

Alzheimer's disease—the most common cause of dementia, probably caused by cerebral accumulation of the Aβ fragment of the amyloid precursor protein. The initial cognitive deficit is impairment of episodic memory (see Chapter 24.4.1), which is thought to reflect the earliest site of pathology in the medial temporal lobe structures. Progression of disease is marked by failing memory, increasing disability in managing complex day-to-day activities, mental inflexibility, and poor concentration, eventually leading on to language and visuospatial impairments, apraxia, and failure of semantic memory. Neuropsychiatric symptoms are common and behavioural problems can be prominent. Agitation, restlessness, wandering, and disinhibition cause considerable carer burden. Terminal stages are characterized by reduced speech, ambulatory difficulties, dependence, and incontinence. The mainstay of treatment is social support and increasing assistance with day-to-day activities. Cholinesterase inhibitors generally achieve modest improvements in cognition in around 25 to 50% of patients.

Frontotemporal dementia—increasingly recognized as a common cause of dementia, particularly in younger patients. Usually associated with tau or ubiquitin-positive interneuronal inclusions. Clinical presentation is with progressive changes in personality and behaviour, or (less commonly) with progressive aphasia. There is no specific treatment.

Dementia with Lewy bodies—a common cause of dementia in the elderly. Typical presentation is with progressive cognitive decline, paralleling that seen in Alzheimer's disease, but with (1) marked spontaneous fluctuations in cognitive abilities; (2) visual hallucinations; (3) spontaneous parkinsonism; and (4) exquisite sensitivity to neuroleptic medication. May respond to treatment with cholinesterase inhibitors, but neuroleptic drugs should be avoided whenever possible.

Vascular dementias—a wide variety of vascular diseases can affect the brain, with the most important vascular syndromes being (1) large infarcts, (2) lacunar infarcts, (3) small-vessel disease (Binswanger's disease), (4) cerebral amyloid angiopathy, and (5) cerebral autosomal dominant arteriopathy with subcortical infarcts and leucoencephalopathy (CADASIL).

Subcortical dementias—these include (1) Huntington's disease, (2) progressive supranuclear palsy, (3) Parkinson's disease, and (4) corticobasal degeneration.

Treatable causes of dementia—these include (1) normal-pressure hydrocephalus—the classic triad of presenting features comprises cognitive impairment, gait disturbance and incontinence; (2) chronic subdural haematomas; (3) benign tumours; (4) metabolic and endocrine disorders—including hypothyroidism, Addison's disease, and hypopituitarism; (5) deficiency states—including vitamin B_{12} deficiency; and (6) infections—including neurosyphilis and HIV infection.

Introduction

The definition of dementia has evolved from one of progressive global intellectual deterioration to a syndrome consisting of progressive impairment in memory and at least one other cognitive deficit (aphasia, apraxia, agnosia, or disturbance in executive function) in the absence of another explanatory central nervous system disorder, depression, or delirium (according to the *Diagnostic and Statistical Manual of Mental Disorders*, 4th edition (DSM-IV)). Even this recent syndrome concept is becoming inadequate, as researchers and clinicians become more aware of the specific early cognitive profiles associated with different dementia syndromes. For instance, in early Alzheimer's disease there may be isolated memory impairment many years before more widespread deficits develop.

Although the incidence of dementia is difficult to establish, community prevalence studies suggest that about 8 per cent of all people over 65 years of age suffer from dementia; this shows a marked increase with advancing age. The prevalence below 65 years is about 1:1000, this rises to 1:50 to the age of 70 and 1:20 from 70 to 80. Over 80 years of age the prevalence is 1:5.

Since dementia is predominantly a disorder of later life, it represents an increasing problem for individuals and society with the projected increase in the elderly population. It is estimated that the 18 million people with dementia worldwide will increase to 34 million by the year 2025. This increase is most marked in the developing countries, where the 11 million people with dementia in the year 2000 will reach 24 million by 2025. In the developed world, the equivalent figures are 7 million in 2000 and 11 million in 2025. In Europe alone, more than 5 million people will be affected by the year 2025.

Dementia may result from many diseases and as a consequence be remediable (e.g. metabolic disorders such as vitamin B_{12} deficiency, thyroid hormone deficiency), thus justifying extensive investigation, most cases result from Alzheimer's disease, vascular disorders or result from sub-cortical diseases of the brain. Classification of dementias according to the pattern of cognitive loss provides an alternative perspective which may contribute usefully to diagnosis, to the level of care required—and allow prognosis to be refined. At the same time, progress in the study of neurogenetics has greatly enhanced our knowledge of the pathways which lead to neuronal injury in the brain and promises greater understanding of the disease with a more unified view of molecular causation.

Dementia has numerous causes that can be classified in many ways (Table 24.4.2.1 shows a classification by aetiology). Although medical and neurological conditions cause a dementia syndrome, most of these are rare and have other neurological features that suggest the diagnosis, e.g. multiple sclerosis, the AIDS–dementia complex, and the vasculitides. Routine investigation focuses on some of these rarer causes because, although rare, they often result in a reversible dementia. An alternative classification, based on the patterns of cognitive impairment, is that of subcortical and cortical dementias as illustrated in Table 24.4.2.2. This classification shows that disease of diverse cerebral structures can result in dementia but that the resultant patterns of cognitive deficit can be very different. Alzheimer's disease is the prototypical cortical dementia. Subcortical dementias are discussed further below.

The most common causes of dementia before and after the age of 65 years are shown in Fig. 24.4.2.1. The relative frequencies of causes of dementia differ depending on age, but it is notable that

Table 24.4.2.1 Causes of dementia

Degenerative disorders

Alzheimer's disease

Frontotemporal dementia

Dementia with Lewy bodies

Parkinson's disease

Huntington's disease

Progressive supranuclear palsy

Corticobasal degeneration

Multisystem atrophy

Progressive myoclonic epilepsies

Vascular diseases

Multi-infarct disease (large vessel and lacunar infarcts)

Binswanger's disease

Primary cerebral amyloid angiopathy

Hypertensive encephalopathy

Vasculitides:

−systemic lupus erythematosus

−polyarteritis nodosa

−Behçet's disease

−giant-cell arteritis

−primary CNS angitis

CADASIL

Anoxia postcardiac arrest

Sickle-cell disease

Infections

Prion dementias:

−sporadic and familial Creutzfeldt–Jakob disease

−Gerstmann–Straussler–Scheinker syndrome

−familial fatal insomnia

AIDS dementia complex

Progressive multifocal encephalopathy

Cerebral toxoplasmosis*

Cryptococcal meningitis*

Neurosyphilis

Subacute sclerosing panencephalitis

Progressive rubella encephalitis

Viral encephalitis

Viral, bacterial, and fungal meningitides

Whipple's disease

Neoplastic causes

Primary intracerebral tumours:

−frontal gliomas crossing the corpus callosum

(butterfly glioma)

−posterior corpus callosal or midline tumours (thalamic, pineal, third ventricle)

−cerebral lymphoma

Table 24.4.2.1 (*Cont'd*) Causes of dementia

Neoplastic causes (Cont'd)
Extracerebral tumours:
–frontal meningiomas
–posterior fossa tumours (acoustic neuromas)
causing hydrocephalus
Multiple cerebral metastases
Malignant meningitis
Paraneoplastic (limbic) encephalitis
Toxic causes
Alcoholic dementia
Heavy metals:
–lead, mercury, manganese
Carbon monoxide poisoning
Drugs:
–lithium, anticholinergics, barbiturates, digitalis, neuroleptics, cimetidine, propranolol
Acquired metabolic disorders and deficiency states
Chronic renal failure
Dialysis dementia
Portosystemic encephalopathy
Hypothyroidism
Cushing's disease
Addison's disease
Panhypopituitarism
Hypoglycaemia (chronic or recurrent)
Hypoparathyroidism
Vitamin B_{12}, B_1, and folate deficiency
Malabsorption syndromes
Inherited metabolic disorders (that may present in adulthood)
Wilson's disease
Porphyria
Leucodystrophies:
–adrenoleucodystrophy
–metachromatic leucodystrophy
–globoid-cell leucodystrophy
Gangliosidoses
Niemann–Pick disease
Cerebrotendinous xanthomatosis
Adult-onset neuronal ceroid-lipofuscinosis (Kuf's disease)
Mitochondrial cytopathies
Subacute necrotizing encephalopathy (Leigh's disease)
Trauma
Major head injury
Subdural haematoma
Dementia pugilistica

Table 24.4.2.1 (*Cont'd*) Causes of dementia

Hydrostatic causes
Hydrocephalus:
–communicating (including normal pressure) and obstructive
Inflammatory
Multiple sclerosis
Sarcoidosis
Acute disseminated encephalomyelitis

* Associated with immunocompromisation.
CADASIL, cerebral autosomal dominant subcortical infarcts and leucoencephalopathy.

Alzheimer's disease is the most common cause in both groups. The genetic forms of Alzheimer's disease and other rarer causes are more common in the younger age group. Before considering the common and treatable causes of dementia, we discuss the main differential diagnoses to be considered as alternatives to dementia.

Differential diagnosis

Pseudodementia

This term has been used to describe two disorders, namely depressive pseudodementia and hysterical pseudodementia. Cognitive symptoms are common in depression, particularly in the older population. The main complaints are of poor recent memory and concentration with distractibility. There is often a lack of subjective feelings of depression, thereby making the diagnosis difficult. The telltale signs are the so-called biological features of depression, such as sleep disturbance and a loss of appetite and libido. Other common symptoms are low energy and a lack of interest in hobbies and activities. There may be a past personal or familial history of depression. The cognitive picture is of impaired attention and subsequent patchy performance on memory and frontal tasks. There may be some inconsistency in test performance and patients easily give up on a task. Language output may be sparse but paraphasic errors are not present. Even after detailed testing, it may be difficult

Table 24.4.2.2 Cortical and subcortical dementias

Feature Examples	Cortical Alzheimer's disease	Subcortical Parkinson's and Huntington's diseases
Speed of mental processing	Normal	Slowed up
Memory	Severely impaired Recognition and recall affected	Forgetfulness Recognition better
Language	Aphasia common	Normal
Frontal 'executive' abilities	Preserved in early stages	Disproportionately impaired early in disease
Visuospatial and perceptual abilities	Impaired early	Impaired late
Personality	Unconcerned	Apathetic and inert
Mood	Usually normal	Depression common

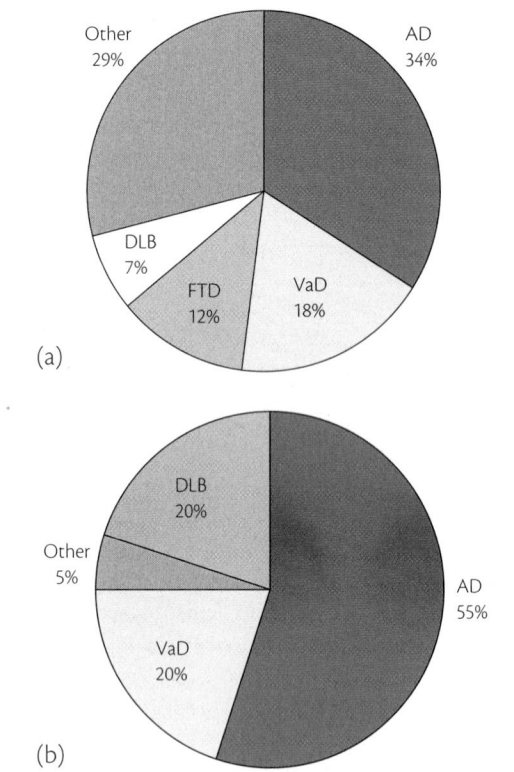

(a)

(b)

Fig. 24.4.2.1 (a) Relative frequencies of different dementia diagnoses in people under 65 years old. (b) Relative frequencies of different dementia diagnoses in people over 65 years old. AD, Alzheimer's disease; DLB, dementia with Lewy bodies; FTD, frontotemporal dementia; VaD, vascular dementia.

to distinguish depression from dementia; indeed there may also be some overlap between the syndromes in older people. For this reason, ideal practice would be for all newly presenting patients with dementia to undergo psychiatric assessment, and if any doubt remains a therapeutic trial of antidepressants may be warranted.

Hysterical pseudodementia commonly presents with a rapid onset of memory and/or intellectual impairment. There is loss of personal identity and salient personal and life events, which is unlike organic disorders of memory. There may be an obvious precipitant (such as marital problems, financial problems, or trouble with the law) and a past psychiatric history is common. 'Ganser's syndrome' is a name for the condition where the patient gives bizarrely wrong answers to questions, e.g. when asked 'How many legs does a horse have?', they reply three or five. Even with such functional states, the examiner has to be aware of the potential concomitant organic disorder exaggerating the condition, as in other conversion disorders.

Delirium

This clinical syndrome is either caused by a diffuse brain pathology (e.g. intracranial infections, head trauma, epilepsy (postictal states and nonconvulsive status), raised intracranial pressure, subarachnoid haemorrhage) or secondary to a large number of systemic illnesses or insults, including infections, metabolic derangements, hypoxia, and drugs.

The clinical features include the acute onset of attentional abnormalities and disturbance of consciousness (from clouding to coma), perceptual distortions, illusions and hallucinations,

psychomotor disturbance (hypo- or hyperactivity and rapid shifts between the two), disturbance of the sleep–wake cycle, emotional lability, and marked fluctuations in performance and behaviour. The most consistent abnormality is in attention, with a reduced ability to maintain attention to external stimuli leading to distractibility and difficulty answering questions, and to appropriately shift attention to new stimuli, leading to perseverations. The investigation and treatment need to be focused in each case on the likely precipitants (although in about 5 to 20% of older people no cause is found). Although the course and prognosis depend on the underlying diagnosis, if there is resolution of the precipitant there should be cognitive improvement to the baseline state.

Alzheimer's disease

Definition

Alzheimer's disease is the most common cause of dementia. Of the 5 to 10% of the population aged over 65 years who have some kind of cognitive decline, over 50% of cases will be due to Alzheimer's disease and, although accounting for a smaller percentage of presenile cases, Alzheimer's disease is still the single largest cause. The initial disease description by Alzheimer in 1907 was of a woman in her 50s with a progressive dementia and behavioural disturbance, who was found to have neurofibrillary tangles and amyloid plaques throughout her cerebral cortex. The term 'Alzheimer's disease' was then applied to similar cases with a presenile dementia, before it was realized that identical pathological changes were seen in most elderly demented patients. As plaques and tangles are found in a very high proportion of nondemented older individuals, debate continues about whether Alzheimer's disease represents a continuum or a distinct disease process that increases in frequency with age. With recognition of a number of causative gene mutations (see below), Alzheimer's disease is now generally believed to be a multifactorial disease with familial and sporadic forms.

Histological diagnosis remains the 'gold standard', but current research criteria, such as the widely used NINCDS-ADRDA (Table 24.4.2.3), are accurate in up to 90% of cases. Rather than merely being a diagnosis of exclusion, Alzheimer's disease is now recognized as a clinicopathological entity amenable to positive diagnosis. Much recent research has focused on methods of early and accurate diagnosis, which is particularly important in view of the advent of potential disease-modifying treatments.

Epidemiology and risk factors

Age is the most important overall risk factor for Alzheimer's disease. A positive family history is also a risk factor, although autosomal dominant presentations account for less than 5% of cases. To date, three major causative gene mutations have been established: mutations in the presenilin genes I and II on chromosome 14 and 1, respectively, and involving the amyloid precursor protein (APP) gene on chromosome 21. In these families the onset is invariably at an early age (35 to 55 years), with remarkable consistency within families and, as with Huntington's disease, penetrance is complete. Dementia is rapidly progressive and seizures and myoclonus are common. Individuals with Down's syndrome (trisomy 21) develop Alzheimer's disease during their third and fourth decades. This is thought to be due to the extra copy of the amyloid precursor gene on chromosome 21.

Table 24.4.2.3 The NINCDS-ADRDA criteria for Alzheimer's disease

Probable Alzheimer's disease
Dementia established by clinical examination, documented by the Mini-Mental State Examination (MMSE) or similar and confirmed by neuropyschological tests
Decline in memory and at least one non-memory intellectual function
Decline from previous level and continuing progression
Onset between 40 and 90 years of age
No disturbance in consciousness
Absence of systemic disorders or other brain diseases that in and of themselves could account for the progressive deficits in memory and cognition
Definite Alzheimer's disease
Clinical criteria of probable AD
Histopathological evidence of AD at postmortem or biopsy
Possible Alzheimer's disease
Patient has dementia syndrome with no other cause but clinical variation from typical for AD
Patient has second disorder that is sufficient to produce dementia but not considered the cause of the dementia
Single gradually progressive cognitive deficit in absence of other cause

NINCDS–ADRDA, National Institute of Neurological and Communicative Disorders and Stroke–Alzheimer's Disease and Related Disorders Association.

Apolipoprotein E (ApoE) is a risk factor rather than a causative gene for Alzheimer's disease in both early and late-onset cases, which at present is thought to be the single most common genetic determinant of a susceptibility to late-onset Alzheimer's disease. ApoE is a component of several classes of plasma and cerebrospinal fluid (CSF) lipoproteins. The brain is the most important site of ApoE production outside the liver, and ApoE is thought to be important in lipid homoeostasis in the brain. There are three common alleles for the *ApoE* gene: ε*2*, ε*3*, and ε*4*. One or two ε*4* alleles confer an increased risk of Alzheimer's disease and lower the age of onset in a 'dose-dependent' fashion.

Many meticulous epidemiological studies have established that women are at an increased risk for Alzheimer's disease, even after adjusting for confounding factors such as the increased longevity of women and their over-representation in the elderly population, and the increased vascular disease in men. Possible explanations include hormonal effects and the postmenopausal loss of the potentially protective effects of oestrogen. Significant head trauma in earlier life is also a risk factor that may summate with ApoE status, and there appears to be an unexplained protective effect of nonsteroidal anti-inflammatory drugs.

Pathology

Pathologically, the macroscopic features of Alzheimer's disease are cortical atrophy, particularly involving the medial temporal lobe and parietotemporal association areas, with relative sparing of the primary sensory motor and visual cortices. The pathological process is thought to start in the entorhinal cortex, hippocampus, and other medial temporal lobe structures before spreading to the temporoparietal neocortex and basal frontal cortex, and then to the

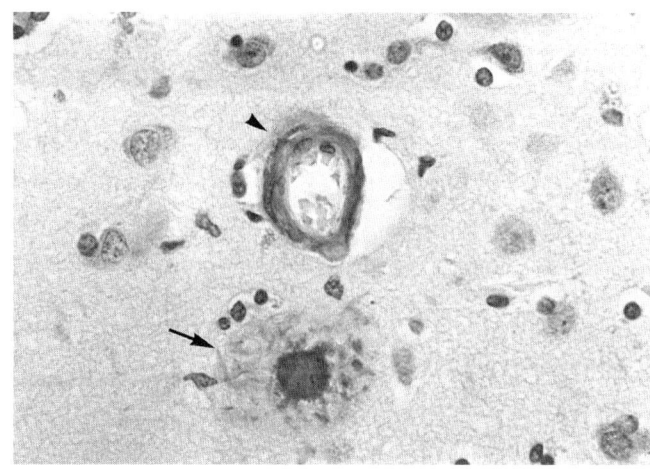

Fig. 24.4.2.2 Amyloid plaque.

other association areas. The histological hallmarks are the senile plaques and neurofibrillary tangles (Figs. 24.4.2.2 and 24.4.2.3). Neither lesion is specific for Alzheimer's disease, as both are found to a lesser extent in the ageing brain; neurofibrillary tangles are also seen in a range of diseases, including progressive supranuclear palsy, encephalitis lethargica, postencephalitic parkinsonism, cerebral trauma, and dementia pugilistica.

Neurofibrillary tangles are formed from bundles of paired helical filaments that replace the normal neuronal cytoskeleton. The central core of the paired helical filaments is the microtubule-associated protein tau. The abnormal phosphorylation of the tau protein causes the microtubular abnormalities and the subsequent collapse of the cytoskeleton. The neurofibrillary tangles are seen as intensely staining intraneuronal inclusions with silver stains or specific anti-tau immunochemistry.

The senile or neuritic plaque is the other major lesion found in Alzheimer's disease. Plaques range in size from 50 nm to 200 nm and consist of an amyloid core with a corona of argyrophilic axonal and dendritic processes, amyloid fibrils, and microglia. The amyloid core is composed of 5- to 10-nm filaments made up of a 40 to 43 amino acid peptide referred to as Aβ peptide because of its secondary structure of β-pleated sheets. The use of antibodies against Aβ reveals more widespread deposition of amyloid

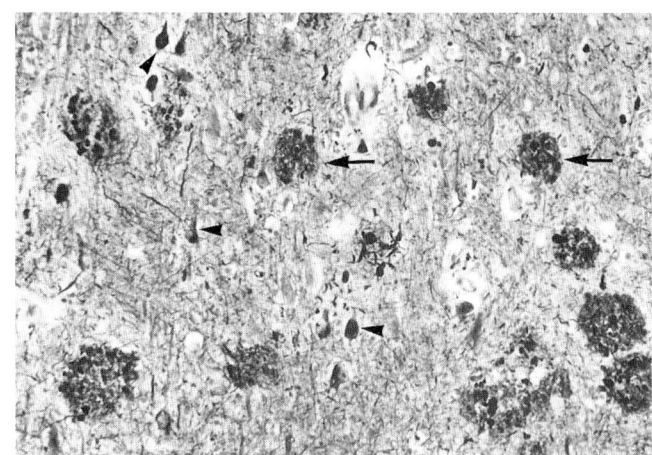

Fig. 24.4.2.3 Neurofibrillary tangle.

throughout the neocortex, especially in layers II, III, and V. The role of microvascular pathology in Alzheimer's disease remains controversial. Cerebral congophilic angiopathy can be seen in a high proportion of cases and almost certainly contributes to the hyperintense lesions commonly seen on T_2-weighted MRI.

Besides a reduction in synaptic loss from neurons, which may explain some cognitive sequelae of the pathology, there is a major loss of neurotransmitters— especially of acetylcholine. The 'cholinergic hypothesis' of neurotransmitter loss causing attentional and mnemonic dysfunction has been much investigated. There is certainly evidence of severe neuronal loss in the nucleus basalis of Meynert in the basal forebrain, the major site of cholinergic neurons, and the current therapies are aimed at improving cognitive function through inhibition of anticholinesterases. There is also disruption to other neurotransmitters including the serotonin system.

Pathophysiology

Over the past decade a great deal has been learnt about the molecular basis of Alzheimer's disease. The dominant hypothesis to explain the mechanisms leading to Alzheimer's disease is the amyloid cascade model, which states that the Aβ fragment of the APP plays an essential role in the pathogenesis (Fig. 24.4.2.4). Aβ is produced proteolytically from APP by so-called β- and γ-secretases. It is believed that the accumulation of Aβ (in particular the Aβ 42 peptide) in the brain initiates a cascade of events that ultimately leads to neuronal dysfunction, the accumulation of hyperphosphorylated tau, and cell death. The strongest argument supporting a causal role for β amyloid comes from the identification of mutations of the APP gene and the genes for presenilin 1 and 2 responsible for the early onset forms of familiar Alzheimer's disease. These mutations modify the generation of Aβ peptides in such a way that the relative proportion of the highly amyloidogenic Aβ 42 form is increased. Recent evidence suggests that, rather than the highly aggregated Aβ species, soluble oligomeric forms of Aβ may represent the neurotoxic entity that causes synaptic dysfunction. Transgenic mice expressing APP mutations have been developed. These animal models, which develop typical plaques, help to understand the role of amyloid and are ideal test beds for the development and trial usage of novel drug compounds.

Clinical features

The earliest cognitive deficit is impairment of so-called episodic memory (memories for events or episodes, including day-to-day

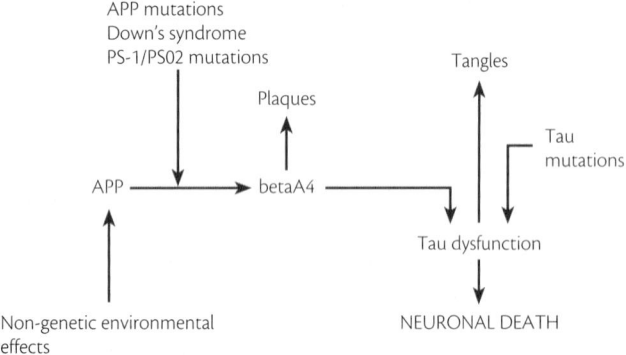

Fig. 24.4.2.4 Proposed pathogenesis of Alzheimer's disease.

memory and new learning), which is thought to reflect the earliest site of pathology in the medial temporal lobe structures. 'Mild cognitive impairment' (MCI) is a term increasingly used for people who are impaired on episodic memory tasks but who do not otherwise fit the criteria for a diagnosis of dementia. It is becoming clear that many, if not all, such people are in the predementia or early stage of Alzheimer's disease, but progression to a full-blown dementia syndrome can take several years. Recent studies indicate a conversion rate to dementia of around 10 to 20% per annum. The main clinical features at this stage are severe forgetfulness, often with repetitive questioning and impairments in social function or job performance, particularly concerning the retention of new information. As the disease progresses to mild Alzheimer's disease, memory function worsens, particularly affecting recall (e.g. forgetting recent visits or family events), increasing disability in managing complex day-to-day activities such as finances and shopping, mental inflexibility, and poor concentration, which reflects involvement of attentional and executive function.

Insight is variably affected; often patients retain a partial awareness into their difficulties but underestimate the extent of the problem. Remote memory is relatively well preserved with a temporally graded pattern (i.e. sparing of most distant memories). As the disease continues to progress patients often develop impairments in language, most typically word-finding difficulties, a shrinking vocabulary, and poor understanding of complex words and concepts. Visuospatial impairments and apraxia, which may develop at this stage, are particularly disabling, causing difficulty in dressing, cooking, and performing other daily activities. In a small subgroup of patients, language or visuospatial difficulties can be the first or most prominent presenting feature. As the cognitive deficits progress there is worsening of language function and semantic memory, and behavioural problems can be prominent.

Neuropsychiatric symptoms are also common in the earliest stages of Alzheimer's disease, particularly apathy, anxiety, and mood disturbance. Delusions and hallucinations occur in up to 50 and 30% of patients, respectively, in the later stages. Agitation, restlessness, wandering, and disinhibition also cause a considerable burden for carers. The final stages of the disease are characterized by reduced speech output (or mutism), ambulatory difficulties, dependence, and incontinence. Seizures and myoclonus are common late features. There is considerable variation in the time to this stage, but the average time from diagnosis to death is around 10 years.

Neurological examination is unremarkable in the early stages, although increased tone (often frontal resistant, or *gegenhalten*, in type) and mild extrapyramidal features can occur as the disease progresses. Reflex changes such as extensor plantar responses (Babinski's reflex) and—in contrast to frontotemporal dementia—pout, snout, and grasp reflexes occur late. In the final stages, there can be greatly increased rigidity and joint contractures.

Investigations

The aims of neuropsychological, imaging, and laboratory investigations in Alzheimer's disease are twofold: first to exclude other potentially reversible causes of dementia, and second to confirm the diagnosis of probable Alzheimer's disease. The extent and nature of investigation obviously need to be tailored to the individual, but all patients should undergo brain imaging and have a neuropsychological assessment to confirm the diagnosis of dementia.

The neuropsychological profile can also be informative in the differential diagnosis of dementia (see Table 24.4.2.2). Particularly characteristic is early impairment in delayed verbal recall of new material, followed by reduced category fluency (in which individuals are asked to generate exemplars from a given category, e.g. 'animals'), impaired naming of low-frequency words, and difficulty with complex visuospatial tasks such as copying complex figures or block design from the revised Wechsler Adult Intelligence Scale (WAIS-R).

The basic laboratory investigations required in all patients, particularly to exclude treatable causes of dementia, and some of the other investigations that may be indicated in certain cases depending on the patient's age, family history, or specific medical history are shown in Table 24.4.2.4. Research into biological markers of Alzheimer's disease has yet to yield a consistent biological or surrogate marker. Screening for specific gene mutations in young-onset familial cases is available only in specialist centres.

MRI of patients with Alzheimer's disease in the earliest stages (including MCI) show evidence of atrophy of the hippocampus and entorhinal cortex (parahippocampal gyrus) reflecting the pathology (Fig. 24.4.2.5). Unfortunately, the variability in size of these structures in normal older people means that, at present, these imaging abnormalities are not specific enough to be of predictive value. The coregistration of serial MR scans appears

Table 24.4.2.4 Recommended investigations in dementia

Routine
Full blood count and ESR
Biochemical profile:
–urea or creatinine, electrolytes, calcium, liver function
Serum vitamin B12 and RBC folate levels
Thyroid function
Serological tests for syphilis
Chest radiography
CT or MRI scan of brain
Other tests which may be indicated in certain cases
EEG (e.g. Creutzfeldt–Jakob disease and subacute sclerosing panencephalitis)
SPECT
Neuropsychological examination (confirm dementia and pattern of disease)
CSF examination
Immunological tests for vasculitides
Screening for cardiac sources of emboli
Slit-lamp examination for Kayser–Fleischer rings and caeruloplasmin estimation (Wilson's disease)
Specific blood and/or urine tests for inherited metabolic disorders
Screening for HIV infection
Genetic screening for HD mutation/ specific AD mutations if familial dementia Cerebral biopsy

ESR, erythrocyte sedimentation rate; RBC, red blood cells; CT, computed tomography; EEG, electroencephalogram; MRI, magnetic resonance imaging; SPECT, single-photon emission computed tomography; CSF, cerebrospinal fluid; HD, Huntington's disease; AD, Alzheimer's disease.

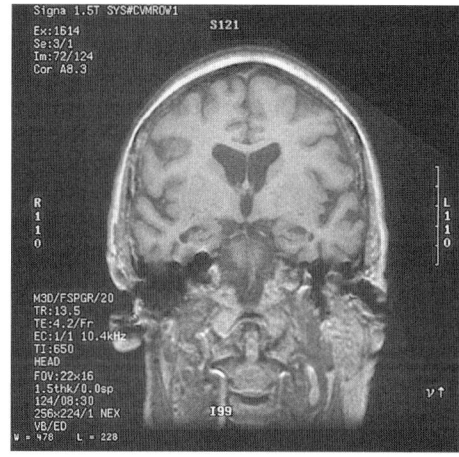
(a)

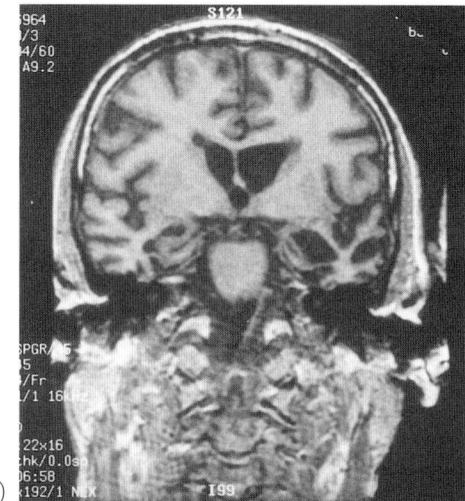
(b)

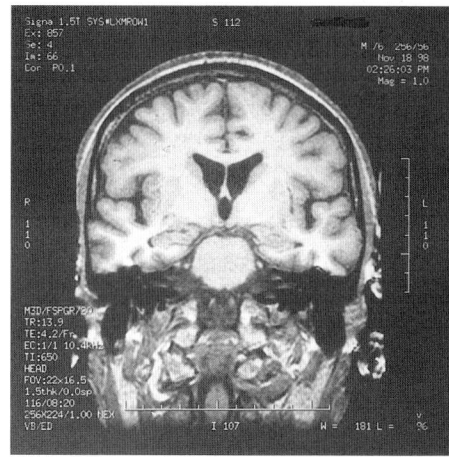
(c)

Fig. 24.4.2.5 (a) Coronal T_1-weighted MRI of a patient with early Alzheimer's disease showing bilateral early hippocampal atrophy. (b) Coronal T_1-weighted MRI of a patient with frontotemporal dementia (FTD) showing left temporal atrophy. (c) Coronal T_1-weighted MRI of a normal person.

capable of detecting abnormal rates of brain atrophy, even before the onset of clear-cut cognitive symptoms in at-risk familial cases, but it remains a research instrument. T_2-weighted MRI often reveals periventricular high-signal changes, even in 'pure' early onset cases. Single-photon emission computed tomography (SPECT) scans similarly demonstrate typical abnormalities in the parietotemporal regions but the specificity is relatively low in individual cases.

Newer technological developments, such as diffusion tensor MRI, MR spectroscopy (MRS), and position emission tomography (PET) may enhance diagnostic accuracy but are expensive and not yet suitable for routine clinical use. Very recently it has become possible to image amyloid deposition *in vivo* using a PET ligand that binds to amyloid.

Management and prognosis

The management of a patient with dementia involves many sensitive issues. It is crucial to provide medical and psychological support to patients as well as to their families and carers. During the progression of the disease there will be different treatment goals at different stages, ranging from aiding failing memory in the setting of independent living to managing behavioural problems and aggression, and eventually full supportive nursing care. There is great variation in the rate of progression, young-onset cases and those with prominent aphasia appearing to deteriorate most rapidly. On average, patients spend several years in the mild or minimal stages (although it can be as long as 5–10 years), between 4 and 5 years in the moderate disease stages, and, depending on the quality of care in the dependent stages, a year or more requiring full nursing care.

Nonpharmacological treatment

The mainstay of treatment is social support and increasing assistance with day-to-day activities. Issues such as driving and planning for future financial affairs are important and should be discussed early in the course of the disease. Throughout the course of the illness there will be different requirements for the support services listed below:

- information and education
- carer support groups
- community dementia team, including home nursing and personal care
- community services such as meals-on-wheels, community transport services, home maintenance assistance
- sitter service
- day centre
- respite care
- residential/nursing home
- diet, exercise, mental activity.

Pharmacological treatment

Pharmacological treatments can be divided into symptom- and disease-oriented approaches. Symptom modification relates to the treatment of depression, agitation, and psychotic phenomena, and requires the input from a specialist psychiatrist. The cholinesterase inhibitors donepezil, galantamine, and rivastigmine are licensed for use in the United Kingdom as is the *N*-methyl-D-aspartate (NMDA) receptor antagonist memantine. The importance of acetylcholine depletion in Alzheimer's disease is established; these cholinesterase inhibitors generally achieve modest improvements in cognition in around 25 to 50% of the patients studied. The disease-modifying effects of these drugs remain controversial. Antioxidants (such as vitamin E), ginkgo biloba, and monoamine oxidase B (MAO-B) inhibitors have shown minor benefits in some

clinical trials, although again their long-term benefit has yet to be established. Pilot trials and experimental studies are being conducted at present in this area. Ideally, the goal is to prevent patients developing further cognitive deficits and to prevent those with MCI from progressing to dementia. The epidemiological findings of protection from cognitive decline in women using hormone replacement therapy (HRT) are of interest in developing preventive strategies. Trials to look at the effect of HRT in preventing or delaying the onset of dementia have been disappointing. A number of disease-modifying drug and other therapeutic approaches have been developed based on the amyloid cascade hypothesis, ranging from inhibitors of β- and γ-secretase, anti-Aβ immunization, and tau kinase, to aggregation inhibitors.

Frontotemporal dementia

Definition

Frontotemporal dementia (FTD) is now preferred to the older term 'Pick's disease', to describe patients with focal frontal and/or temporal focal atrophy, because the underlying pathology of these syndromes is heterogeneous. Arnold Pick (1851 to 1924) first described patients with both progressive aphasia and associated severe left temporal cortical atrophy *post mortem*, and patients with behavioural disturbances associated with frontal lobe atrophy. In 1910, Alzheimer described the histological changes in patients with focal lobar degeneration as distinct from the syndrome that bears his name. Alzheimer described both argyrophilic intracytoplasmic inclusions (Pick bodies) and diffusely staining ballooned neurons (Pick cells). More recently it has become clear that the spectrum of pathology that accompanies the clinical syndromes of frontal and temporal dementias is much broader, with a range of distinct inclusions as described below. There is also considerable overlap between FTD and two categories of motor disorders: motor neuron disease (MND, also referred to as amyotrophic lateral sclerosis) and corticobasal degeneration, in terms of both clinical features and pathology.

Epidemiology

FTD is increasingly recognized as a common cause of dementia, particularly in the younger age groups (see Fig. 24.4.2.1a)— the peak incidence of onset being 45 to 65 years of age. In hospital series, the ratio FTD:Alzheimer's disease has been found to vary from 1:5 to 1:20, with men and women being equally affected. Many cases are familial, with up to 40% having an affected family member.

Pathology and genetics

The gross pathological appearance of FTD is that of profoundly atrophied frontotemporal regions which may be so severe as to produce the so-called knife-edged gyri and deep widened sulci. The histopathological hallmarks are widespread cortical and subcortical gliosis, loss of large cortical nerve cells, and microvacuolation. Immunohistochemical staining reveals two major patterns based on the presence of interneuronal inclusions. The first pattern is a build-up of either tau in the form of classic Pick bodies, diffuse neuronal and glial, and pathology typically seen in patients with mutations of the tau gene, or corticobasal degeneration. The second major pattern consists of ubiquitin-positive but tau-negative pathology, first identified in patients with MND without dementia, but then later found in those with MND-associated FTD, and more recently in patients with progranulin gene mutations. A small proportion of patients have neither tau- nor ubiquitin-positive inclusions.

About 20 to 30% of patients with FTD have a positive family history, although in some cases this may be coincidental. Two major causative gene mutations occur on chromosome 17. The first mutation, found in the late 1990s, involves the microtubule-associated protein tau gene (*MAPT*). In 2006, the second major locus close to *MAPT* was discovered, the progranulin gene. Familial MND with FTD has been linked to chromosome 9 although no gene has yet been identified.

Clinical features

The presentation of FTD mirrors the distribution of neuropathological changes; in the early stages two major presentations can be distinguished.

Frontal or behavioural presentations

Patients present with insidiously progressive changes in personality and behaviour that reflect the early locus of pathology in orbital and medial parts of the frontal lobes. There is often impaired judgement, an indifference to domestic and professional responsibilities, and a lack of initiation and apathy. Social skills deteriorate and there can be socially inappropriate behaviour, fatuousness, jocularity, abnormal sexual behaviour with disinhibition, or theft. Many patients are restless with an obsessive–compulsive and ritualized pattern of behaviour, such as pacing or hoarding. Emotional lability and mood swings are seen, but other psychiatric phenomena such as delusions and hallucinations are rare. Patients become rigid and stereotyped in their daily routines and food choices. A change in food preference towards sweet foods is very characteristic. Of importance is the fact that simple bedside cognitive screening tests such as the Mini-Mental State Examination (MMSE) are insensitive at detecting frontal abnormalities. More detailed neuropsychological tests of frontal function (such as the Wisconsin Card Sorting Test or the Stroop Test) usually show abnormalities. Speech output can be reduced with a tendency to echolalia (repeating the examiner's last phrase). Memory is relatively spared in the early stages, although it does deteriorate as the disease advances. Visuospatial function remains remarkably unaffected. Primary motor and sensory functions remain normal. Primitive reflexes such as snout, pout, and grasp develop during the disease process. Muscle fasciculations or wasting, particularly affecting the bulbar musculature, can develop in the FTD subtype associated with MND.

Language presentations

Less common than the behavioural variant is a presentation with progressive aphasia which can be of a fluent or nonfluent type. In progressive fluent aphasia, also known as semantic dementia, there is a profound loss in conceptual knowledge (or semantic memory), causing anomia and impaired comprehension of words, objects, or faces. The patient typically complains of 'loss of memory for words' and has fluent, empty speech with substitutions such as 'thing' and 'one of those', but the grammatical aspects are preserved. Naming is impaired with semantically based errors (such as 'animal' or 'horse' for zebra). Patients are unable to understand less frequent words and fail on a range of semantically based tasks such as matching words to pictures and matching pictures according to their meaning. Repetition of words and phrases is normal even though patients are unaware of their meaning. Unlike patients with Alzheimer's disease, day-to-day memory (episodic memory) with good visuospatial skills and nonverbal problem-solving ability is relatively preserved, at least in the early stages. As the disease progresses behavioural changes often emerge.

In progressive nonfluent aphasia, by contrast, there is a gradual loss of expressive language abilities with impairments in the phonological (sound based) and grammatical aspects of language production. This leads to nonfluent, agrammatical, and poorly articulated speech with phonological errors (e.g. sitter for sister or fencil for pencil). Repetition of multisyllabic words and phrases is impaired but, in contrast to semantic dementia, word comprehension and object recognition are well preserved. Orobuccal apraxia is common and some patients develop parkinsonism and limb apraxia.

Diagnosis

The diagnosis of FTD is based on the clinical, neuropsychological, and imaging assessments. The consensus broad clinical criteria are shown in Table 24.4.2.5. The differences between the various syndromes described above are obvious early in the disease, but there is increasing overlap between the temporal and frontal syndromes as the disease progresses. MRI demonstrates a characteristic pattern of frontal and/or temporal lobe atrophy: in contrast to Alzheimer's disease, the changes involve the polar and lateral temporal structures and are asymmetrical, commonly involving the left side to a greater extent (see Fig. 24.4.2.5). The functional imaging (SPECT or PET) findings mirror the structural imaging results, with reduced frontotemporal perfusion and hypometabolism.

Management and prognosis

There is no curative treatment at present, so the general management of the person with dementia and their family, as discussed above, is of prime importance. Patients with a family history of dementia should be screened for tau or progranulin mutations after appropriate genetic counselling. The prognosis can be variable with different rates of progression between individuals. The disease is progressive and the average duration from diagnosis is around 5 to 10 years.

Dementia with Lewy bodies

Definition

Since the discovery in the 1960s that patients with Lewy bodies (ubiquitin-positive inclusions) in the cortex have a distinctive pattern of dementia with features of both Parkinson's and Alzheimer's diseases, it has been increasingly recognized as an important cause of dementia. The terminology has been confusing, with multiple designations including: Lewy body dementia, dementia of Lewy body type, diffuse Lewy body disease, and cortical Lewy body disease. The consensus clinical criteria for 'dementia with Lewy bodies' (DLB), the term now preferred, are shown in Table 24.4.2.6.

Epidemiology

Dementia with Lewy bodies is a common cause of dementia in the elderly population, although the true prevalence remains unclear. As many as 12 to 36% of patients with a clinical diagnosis of Alzheimer's disease reach the pathological criteria for a diagnosis of dementia with Lewy bodies.

Table 24.4.2.5 The clinical diagnostic features of frontotemporal dementia (FTD)

Frontal syndrome

I Core features

A Insidious onset and gradual progression

B Early decline in social contact

C Early impairment in personal conduct

D Early emotional blunting

E Early loss of insight

II Supportive features

A Behavioural

    i. Decline in personal hygiene and grooming

    ii. Mental rigidity and inflexibility

    iii. Distractibility and impersistence

    iv. Hyperorality and dietary changes

    v. Perseverative and stereotyped behaviour

    vi. Utilization behaviour

B Speech and language

    i. Altered speech output:

        –aspontaneity and economy of speech

        –pressure of speech

    ii. Stereotypic speech

    iii. Echolalia

    iv. Perseveration

    v. Mutism

C Physical signs

    i. Primitive reflexes

    ii. Incontinence

    iii. Akinesia, rigidity, and tremor

    iv. Low and labile blood pressure

D Investigations

    i. Neuropsychology: significant impairment on frontal lobe tests in the absence of severe amnesia, aphasia or perceptuospatial disorder

    ii. Electroencephalography: normal on conventional EEG despite dementia

    iii. Brain imaging (structural and or functional): predominant frontal and/or anterior temporal abnormality

Semantic dementia

I Core features

A Insidious onset and gradual progression

B Language disorder characterized by:

    i. Progressive, fluent, empty spontaneous speech

    ii. Loss of word meaning, manifest by impaired naming and comprehension

    iii. Semantic paraphasias

and/or

Table 24.4.2.5 (*Cont'd*) The clinical diagnostic features of frontotemporal dementia (FTD)

C Perceptual disorder characterized by:

    i. Prosopagnosia: impaired recognition of identity of familiar faces; *and/or*

    ii. Associative agnosia: impaired recognition of object identity

D Preserved perceptual matching and drawing reproduction

E Preserved single word repetition

F Preserved ability to read aloud and write to dictation orthographically regular words

II Supportive diagnostic features

A Speech and language

    i. Pressure of speech

    ii. Idiosyncratic word use

    iii. Absence of phonemic paraphasias

    iv. Surface dyslexia and dysgraphia

    v. Preserved calculation

B Behaviour

    i. Loss of sympathy and empathy

    ii. Narrowed preoccupations

    iii. Parsimony

C Physical signs

    i. Absent or late primitive reflexes

    ii. Akinesia, rigidity, and tremor

D Investigations

E Neuropsychology

    i. Profound semantic loss, manifest in failure of word comprehension and naming, and/or face and object recognition

    ii. Preserved phonology and syntax, and elementary perceptual processing, spatial skills, and day-to-day memory

F Electroencephalography normal

G Brain imaging (structural and/or functional):

    –predominant anterior temporal abnormality (symmetrical or asymmetrical)

Progressive non-fluent aphasia

I Core diagnostic features

A Insidious onset and gradual progression

B Non-fluent spontaneous speech with at least one of the following:

    –agrammatism, phonemic paraphrasias, anomia

II Supportive diagnostic features

A Speech and language

    i. Stuttering or oral apraxia

    ii. Impaired repetition

    iii. Alexia, agraphia

    iv. Early preservation of word meaning

    v. Late mutism

Table 24.4.2.5 (*Cont'd*) The clinical diagnostic features of frontotemporal dementia (FTD)

B	Behaviour	
	i.	Early preservation of social skills
	ii.	Late behavioural changes similar to FTD
C	Physical signs:	
		–late contralateral primitive reflexes, akinesia, rigidity, and tremor
D	Investigations	
	i.	Neuropsychology: non-fluent aphasia in the absence of severe amnesia or perceptuospatial disorder
	ii.	Electroencephalopathy: normal or minor asymmetrical slowing
	iii.	Brain imaging (structural and/or functional): asymmetrical abnormality predominantly affecting dominant (usually left) hemisphere

(Adapted with permission from Neary *et al.* (1998). Frontotemporal lobar degeneration: a consensus on clinical diagnostic criteria. *Neurology* **51**, 1546–54.)

Pathology

Pathological criteria require the presence of cortical and subcortical Lewy bodies. Confusingly, there is considerable overlap with the histological features of both Parkinson's and Alzheimer's diseases, although the distribution of pathology is the key to distinguishing these conditions. Lewy bodies are intracytoplasmic eosinophilic neural inclusions formed from altered cytoskeleton components that can be seen on haematoxylin and eosin staining, but are more prominently shown using anti-ubiquitin immunohistochemistry. The major component of the Lewy body is α-synuclein and anti-synuclein immunohistochemistry in the method of choice for detecting these lesions. Cortical Lewy bodies are found in the temporal lobe, insular cortex, and cingulate gyrus, and are always accompanied by typical 'core-and-halo' Lewy bodies in the substantia nigra (the pathological hallmark of Parkinson's disease). Dystrophic ubiquitin-positive neurites are also seen in the hippocampus, amygdala, nucleus basalis of Meynert, and other brainstem nuclei.

Changes of Alzheimer disease—neurofibrillary tangles and amyloid plaques—are seen in up to 50% of cases, raising nosological issues with Alzheimer's disease. The distribution of changes is of importance in distinguishing the conditions, e.g. neurofibrillary tangles in DLB commonly spare the hippocampus, which is severely affected in Alzheimer's disease.

The neurotransmitter changes in DLB reflect the areas of pathology, with severe dopamine depletion in the basal ganglia and marked reduction in acetylcholine throughout the cortex.

Clinical features

Patients typically present with a progressive cognitive decline paralleling that seen in those with Alzheimer's disease. There are, however, a number of characteristic and distinguishing features. First, there is a tendency to marked spontaneous fluctuations in cognitive abilities, particularly alertness and attention, producing a delirious state lasting days or even weeks. Second, visual hallucinations, illusions, and fleeting misidentification phenomena occur in 50 to 80% of those with the condition even at an early stage and without drug provocation. The hallucinations are commonly well-formed images of people or animals. The marked cholinergic deficit is postulated to be the cause of their tendency to visual hallucinations. Third is the occurrence of spontaneous parkinsonism, which is usually mild in the early stages. Rigidity, gait disturbance, and bradykinesia are all common, although in contrast to patients with Parkinson's disease the tremor is usually mild, atypical (with postural and action components), and symmetrical. Repeated falls also occur. In the later stages the akinetic rigid syndrome can cause severe disabilities in mobility and swallowing, and an increase in the number of falls. Fourth, there is often an exquisite sensitivity to neuroleptic medication, producing the malignant neuroleptic syndrome (delirium, hyperpyrexia, muscle rigidity, massive elevation of creatine phosphokinase, and renal failure).

Diagnosis

Neuropsychologically there is a mixture of subcortical and cortical features, with prominent cognitive slowing plus impairment of executive (planning and organizational) abilities and visuoperceptual abilities. Compared with patients with Alzheimer's disease, those with DLB tend to have greater deficits in attention and visuospatial processing. Memory loss may be less prominent than in Alzheimer's disease. There is no diagnostic test for this condition and the diagnosis *in vivo* relies on the clinical features described above and in Table 24.4.2.6. MRI shows similar changes to Alzheimer's disease, although there is a suggestion that medial temporal lobe atrophy is less pronounced. SPECT shows occipitoparietal hypoperfusion.

Table 24.4.2.6 Clinical features of dementia with Lewy bodies

Dementia in association with:
Fluctuations in cognition (especially attention and alertness)
Visual hallucinations (typically well formed)
Mild spontaneous parkinsonism
Supportive features:
Repeated or unexplained falls, syncope, or transient loss of consciousness
Neuroleptic sensitivity syndrome
Hallucinations in other modalities
Systematized delusions

(Adapted with permission from McKeith *et al.* (1996). Consensus guidelines for the clinical and pathologic diagnosis of dementia with Lewy bodies (DLB): report of the consortium on DLB International Workshop. *Neurology* **47**, 1113–24.)

Management

The symptomatic management of this disorder is complicated by the presence of both hallucinations and an akinetic rigid syndrome. Patients are notoriously sensitive to the side effects of dopamine-enhancing medications used for the treatment of the akinetic rigid syndrome. However, although dramatic motor improvements are not to be expected, a cautious medication trial is worth attempting. Even though neuroleptic drugs should be avoided whenever possible, neuropsychiatric features, if severe, can be ameliorated with the newer atypical neuroleptics such as clozapine and olanzapine, without exacerbation of the parkinsonism. Thus, the main aim is to maintain a balance between the patient being mobile and the patient being lucid.

Marked improvement in attentional cognitive deficits in response to treatment with cholinesterase inhibitors, such as donepezil and rivastigmine, has been reported Although there have been few controlled trial reports patients with DLB may respond better than those with Alzheimer's disease to this drug therapy.

Vascular dementia

Definition and epidemiology

Vascular dementia can be defined as a dementia resulting from a cerebrovascular disorder. This is obviously a broad categorization and many different aetiologies may be included in this rubric, e.g. multiple infarcts from cardiac emboli, vasculitides including systemic lupus erythematosus, primary cerebral amyloid angiopathy, and cerebral autosomal dominant arteriopathy with subcortical infarcts and leucoencephalopathy (CADASIL). The term 'multi-infarct dementia' was introduced in the 1970s to emphasize the contribution of multiple cerebral infarcts to clinical dementia syndromes, and to replace the older label of 'atherosclerotic dementia', although it is now apparent that diffuse small-vessel disease contributes significantly in the absence of clinically overt strokes. Traditionally regarded as the second most common cause of dementia, it is increasingly difficult to estimate the true contribution of vascular disease. Postmortem studies of patients with multi-infarct dementia show that Alzheimer's disease changes commonly coexist. Conversely, the advent of sensitive instruments for detecting cerebral vascular lesions *in vivo* (MRI) has revealed that presumed vascular changes are common in patients with the clinical diagnosis of Alzheimer's disease, even in young patients with known gene mutations, and that the presence of vascular lesions may be contributing to the severity of Alzheimer's disease. Finally, it is increasingly apparent that traditional risk factors for vascular dementia—including hypertension, diabetes, and hypercholesterolaemia—are also factors that increase the likelihood of developing both vascular dementia and Alzheimer's disease.

Clinicopathological vascular syndromes

The varieties of vascular diseases that affect the brain are legion, and the resultant clinical features and underlying pathology widely different (see Table 24.4.2.1). The most important vascular syndromes are considered below.

Large infarcts

Recurrent cerebral infarcts involving multiple main arterial territories (e.g. posterior or middle cerebral artery territories), resulting from thrombosis or embolism, can cause dementia with a stepwise cognitive decline. There is commonly a history of atherosclerotic risk factors (e.g. hypertension, smoking, and hypercholesterolaemia), other evidence of atherosclerotic cardiac or peripheral vascular disease, and neurological signs on examination (e.g. spasticity, hyperreflexia, extensor plantar responses, and a pseudobulbar palsy). There are often asymmetries on the neurological examination, and gait apraxia and/or bladder dysfunction can be early features. The cognitive picture is characterized by cortical features and is dependent on the sites of the lesions. There is often severe language impairment, visuospatial disturbance, amnesia, and dyspraxia, related to lesions in the middle and posterior cerebral artery distributions. Specific syndromes can result from discrete lesions, e.g. lesions of the left angular gyrus result in a fluent aphasia, agraphia, acalculia, right–left disorientation, and finger agnosia known as Gerstmann's syndrome.

Lacunar infarcts

The small multiple lacunar lesions are caused by occlusion in the deep penetrating arterial branches. The underlying pathogenic mechanism is a distinct small-vessel arteriopathy with replacement of the muscle and elastin in the arterial wall by collagen, leading to tortuous vessel and microaneurysm formation as a result of long-standing hypertension. The basal ganglia, thalamus, and deep white matter are common sites for lesions, due to the nature of the arterial supply. These lacunes may coexist with the larger infarcts (described above), thereby contributing to a mixed picture. However, the typical presentation of the lacunar state is with a more subcortical syndrome causing impaired attention and frontal executive malfunction, forgetfulness, apathy, and emotional lability. Thalamic lacunes can result in a speech disorder and, if bilateral, in amnesia. Examination features are similar to those seen with larger infarcts, with rigidity, gait disturbance, and extrapyramidal and pyramidal signs.

Small-vessel disease (Binswanger's disease)

'Binswanger's disease' (or 'diffuse leucoaryosis') is the term applied to the radiologically defined syndrome of confluent subcortical and corpus callosal demyelination and loss of the cerebral white matter, which again typically complicates severe or accelerated hypertension. The clinical features are similar to those of the lacunar state described above. On CT there is symmetrical, diffuse, low-density periventricular hypodensity, which can be accompanied by ventricular dilatation. This is visualized with great sensitivity on T_2-weighted MRI as a diffuse white matter of high intensity. Pathologically, there is demyelination, axonal loss, and gliosis, thought to be due to diffuse ischaemia in the territory of the long perforating arteries.

Cerebral amyloid angiopathy

Amyloid is deposited in the cerebral vessels both with increasing age and in a proportion of cases with ordinary Alzheimer's disease. However, there is also a rare and sometimes familial form of cerebral amyloidosis that produces recurrent cerebral haemorrhages and an Alzheimer's disease-type dementia. Amyloid deposition in the vessel walls causes structural weakness leading to intracerebral haemorrhages and narrowing of the vessel to produce ischaemia. The haemorrhages tend to be lobar and can be recurrent.

Cerebral autosomal dominant arteriopathy with subcortical infarcts and leucoencephalopathy (CADASIL)

This recently established disorder may be a more common cause of vascular dementia than previously realized. Patients present in their early 20s with migraine-like headaches and subsequently develop stroke-like episodes, which are sometimes ascribed to migraine or may mimic the attacks of acute demyelination. A subcortical dementia syndrome develops during their fifth and sixth decades. MRI shows multiple subcortical infarcts and diffuse white-matter disease. Other clues to the diagnosis are the absence of risk factors for atherosclerotic disease and the strong family history. Pathologically there is a distinctive, nonamyloid, nonatherosclerotic angiopathy of the leptomeningeal and perforating arteries of the brain, with eosinophilic granular substance replacing smooth muscle. The diagnosis can also be confirmed with the finding of the same pathological changes in the cutaneous blood vessels in a skin biopsy. Mutations in the *notch3* gene on chromosome 19 have been reported in patients with CADASIL.

Treatment of vascular dementia

The treatment should be directed to the amelioration of any underlying cause of the vascular disorder, such as reducing cardiac embolism and treating vasculitides and hypertension. The potential for altering the progression of the disease is alluring. Nevertheless, efforts directed at altering atherosclerotic risk factors tend to produce disappointing results. The course of vascular dementia can be as severe as or even more rapid than that of Alzheimer's disease.

Subcortical dementias

Despite shortcomings, the differentiation between cortical and subcortical dementias continues to be useful in clinical practice. This classification highlights the fact that, although disease of diverse cerebral structures can result in dementia, the resultant patterns of cognitive deficits are very different. Alzheimer's disease is the prototypical cortical dementia; vascular syndromes can present with a spectrum of features from cortical to subcortical, as can dementia with Lewy bodies. Purer forms of subcortical dementia result from pathology of the basal ganglia and white matter, the prototypical examples being Huntington's disease and progressive supranuclear palsy (Steele–Richardson–Olszewski syndrome). The typical cognitive pattern is that of attentional and executive dysfunction with marked cognitive slowing (bradyphrenia), causing problems with mentation and information retrieval. Memory is moderately impaired due to reduced attention and poor registration, but is not as severely impaired as in Alzheimer's disease. There is often an associated personality change and mood disturbance with prominent apathy. Spontaneous speech is impoverished and slow.

Huntington's disease

Huntington's disease is an autosomal dominant inherited disorder with an incidence of about 4 per 100 000. The mutation is an expansion of the trinucleotide repeat (CAG) in the IT-15 gene on chromosome 4, which encodes the polyglutamine protein, huntingtin, essential for nervous system development. There is a clear dose–response relationship between the length of the CAG repeat and the age of onset of the disorder. Psychiatric symptoms, such as depression, irritability, and personality changes, often precede the motor disorder, which is typically choreiform. The other cognitive changes that develop over the next 10 to 20 years are of a subcortical pattern, with deficits in attention and concentration, executive function, and retrieval from memory.

Progressive supranuclear palsy

Progressive supranuclear palsy (PSP) is a rare, but increasingly recognized, disorder with an incidence of 1 to 2 per 100 000. The subcortical dementia is accompanied by an atypical parkinsonian syndrome. The motor deficits are symmetrical in onset, with severe rigidity in the axial muscle groups and bulbar symptoms. A supranuclear gaze palsy invariably develops, but in the early stages the only feature may be slowing of fast downward movement (saccadic slowing). Another early feature is a marked tendency to falls. The pathological features are neurofibrillary tangles, neuropil threads, and neuronal loss and gliosis in the subthalamic nucleus, red nucleus, substantia nigra, and dentate nucleus. The main neurotransmitter deficit is in dopamine. Unlike Parkinson's disease, PSP does not respond well to levodopa. The disease progresses rapidly with an average time course of around 5 years.

Parkinson's disease

Subcortical dementia occurs in about one-third to one-half of patients with Parkinson's disease, which develops at a late stage in the motor disorder in contrast to dementia with Lewy bodies.

Corticobasal degeneration

Corticobasal degeneration is a rare cause of a dementia and motor signs. Patients present with an asymmetrical akinetic rigid syndrome, together with limb apraxia, and the almost pathognomonic feature of alien limb phenomenon in which the hand(s) acts as if 'with a will of its own'. Myoclonus and dystonia also occur. Dementia is common in the later stages and there is considerable overlap with frontotemporal dementia. The pathology is focused in the frontal and parietal cortices as well as the substantia nigra, basal ganglia, and thalamus.

Treatable causes of dementia

Normal-pressure hydrocephalus

Normal-pressure hydrocephalus has a classic triad of presenting features: cognitive impairment, gait disturbance, and incontinence. The cognitive features are typically those of a subcortical dementia with frontal features and psychomotor slowing. The gait disorder is a dyspraxia and may show the pathognomonic feature of 'being stuck to the floor', although there is an absence of signs when the patient is examined in the supine position. The condition may be secondary to a prior disturbance of CSF flow (resulting from, for example, a head injury, meningitis, or a subarachnoid haemorrhage), but often no cause is found in older people. Neuroimaging shows ventricular enlargement disproportionate to the degree of cortical atrophy. The presence of periventricular lesions can make the distinction from vascular dementia difficult. The investigation and management of these patients should be undertaken by neurosurgeons, the definitive treatment being ventricular shunting. If treated early the prognosis is good.

Chronic subdural haematomas

This treatable cause of dementia is caused by head trauma. It is common in individuals at risk of recurrent head injuries, such as older people, those with alcohol problems, and people with epilepsy. Risk is also increased by coagulation disorders, either pathological or iatrogenic. The clinical features are of a subacute dementia with symptoms of raised intracranial pressure, fluctuating cognitive performance, and focal neurological signs. Diagnosis is confirmed by neuroimaging, the peripheral mass lesions may be of varying signal density on CT, depending on the age of the lesion. If the lesions are isodense with the brain tissue, the diagnosis can be easily overlooked. Treatment is by neurosurgical evacuation, except in clinically insignificant collections. Although the outcome is good, about 10 to 40% of patients have a recurrence that may require further drainage.

Benign tumours

Subfrontal meningiomas are the classic tumours that present with features of a frontal dementia. The onset is usually insidious with personality changes and other frontal features. Besides the neuropsychological abnormalities there may be anosmia or unilateral visual failure and optic atrophy. Other relatively benign midline tumours occasionally present with hydrocephalus and cognitive impairment secondary to this (e.g. colloid cysts of the third ventricle and nonsecretory pituitary tumours).

Metabolic and endocrine disorders

Metabolic derangements can give rise to acute-onset cognitive impairments, but the features are invariably those of a delirium rather than a dementia. Chronic hypocalcaemia and recurrent hypoglycaemia can result in a dementia often accompanied by ataxia and involuntary movements. Endocrine disorders can more frequently present with a dementia syndrome, with or without psychiatric features (e.g. hypothyroidism, Addison's disease, and hypopituitarism). The prominent complaints common to most disorders are mental slowing, apathy, and poor memory. Cushing's disease can present with psychiatric features, although a dementia syndrome is rarer. Although not strictly an endocrine disorder, Hashimoto's encephalopathy is a recently recognized cause of chronic delirium or dementia, often accompanied by seizures and fluctuating focal neurological signs. The diagnosis is made by finding extremely high levels of antithyroid antibodies despite a euthyroid state. Patients respond well to high-dose steroid therapy.

Deficiency states

Vitamin B_{12} deficiency can cause the classic picture of subacute combined degeneration of the spinal cord and a dementia. The dementia can be variable in severity and it is unusual to present without some features of peripheral neurological disease, at least diminished vibration sense in the lower limbs and/or sensory ataxia. Reflexes can be increased, decreased, or mixed. Although most patients have a macrocytic anaemia, neurological manifestations can occasionally occur in the absence of haematological features. Severe thiamine (vitamin B_1) deficiency results in the Wernicke–Korsakoff syndrome, with delirium, ataxia, and ophthalmoplegia. The most common causes are alcoholism and recurrent prolonged vomiting, such as hyperemesis gravidarum. If not promptly treated a chronic amnesic syndrome can occur.

Infections

Neurosyphilis, once a common cause of dementia, is now rare. The associated neurological features include pupillary abnormalities, optic atrophy, ataxia, and pyramidal signs. The diagnosis is confirmed with serology and examination of CSF. Treatment with penicillin can result in some improvement. Those at increased risk are people inadequately treated for syphilis and those infected with the human immunodeficiency virus (HIV). HIV infection is an increasingly common cause of dementia in some parts of the world. The encephalopathy (AIDS–dementia complex) is characterized by psychomotor slowing, personality change, and other features of a subcortical dementia. Examination of the CSF can show a pleocytosis and increased protein and oligoclonal bands. White-matter changes are visible on neuroimaging. Cognitive changes in patients with HIV may also be due to opportunistic infections such as cerebral toxoplasmosis and cryptococcal meningitis, and progressive multifocal leucoencephalopathy, which all require specific treatment.

Further reading

American Psychiatric Association (1994). *Diagnostic and statistical manual of mental disorders*, 4th edition (DSM-IV). American Psychiatric Association, Washington DC.

Bak TH, Hodges JR (1998). The neuropsychology of progressive supranuclear palsy. *Neurocase*, **4**, 89–94.

Berrios GE, Markova IS, Girala N (2000). Functional memory complaints: hypochondria and disorganisation. In: Berrios GE, Hodges JR (eds) *Memory disorders in psychiatric practice*, pp. 384–99. Cambridge University Press, Cambridge.

Braak H, Braak E (1991). Neuropathological staging of Alzheimer-related changes. *Acta Neuropathol (Berlin)*, **82**, 239–59.

Goedert M, Spillantini MG, Davies SW (1998). Filamentous nerve cell inclusions in neurodegenerative diseases. *Curr Opin Neurobiol*, **8**, 619–32.

Greene JDW, Hodges JR (2000). The dementias. In: Berrios GE, Hodges JR (eds) *Memory disorders in psychiatric practice*, pp. 122–63. Cambridge University Press, Cambridge.

Gregory CA, Hodges JR (1996). Frontotemporal dementia: use of consensus criteria and prevalence of psychiatric features. *Neuropsychiatry Neuropsychol Behav Neurol*, **9**, 145–53.

Harvey J et al. (1998). Genetic dissection of Alzheimer's disease and related dementias: amyloid and its relationship to tau. *Nat Neurosci*, **1**, 355–8.

Harvey RJ (2001). Epidemiology of pre-senile dementia. In: Hodges JR (ed.) *Early onset dementia*, pp. 1–23. Cambridge University Press, Cambridge.

Hodges JR, Patterson K (1995). Is semantic memory consistently impaired early in the course of Alzheimer's disease? Neuroanatomical and diagnostic implications. *Neuropsychologia*, **33**, 441–59.

Hodges JR et al. (1992). Semantic dementia: progressive fluent aphasia with temporal lobe atrophy. *Brain*, **115**, 1783–806.

Hodges JR et al. (1999). The differentiation of semantic dementia and frontal lobe dementia (temporal and frontal variants of frontotemporal dementia) from early Alzheimer's disease: a comparative neuropsychological study. *Neuropsychology*, **13**, 31–40.

Hodges JR (2007). *Frontotemporal dementia syndromes*. Cambridge University Press, Cambridge.

Jellinger K et al. (1990). Clinicopathological analysis of dementia disorders in the elderly. *J Neurol Sci*, **95**, 239–58.

Kalaria RN, Ballard C (1999). Overlap between pathology of Alzheimer's disease and vascular dementia. *Alzheimer's Disease and Associated Disorders*, **13**, S115–23.

Kalfki HW et al. (2006). Therapeutic approaches to Alzheimer's disease. *Brain*, **129**, 2840–55.

Klunk WE et al. (2004). Imaging brain amyloid in Alzheimer's disease with Pittsburgh Compound-B. *Ann Neurol*, **55**, 303–5.

Linn RT et al. (1995). The 'preclinical phase' of probable Alzheimer's disease. *Arch Neurol*, **52**, 485–90.

McKeith IG et al. (1996). Consensus guidelines for the clinical and pathologic diagnosis of dementia with Lewy bodies (DLB): report of the consortium on DLB International Workshop. *Neurology*, **47**, 1113–24.

McKeith IG. (2006). Consensus guidelines for the clinical and pathologic diagnosis of dementia with Lewy bodies (DLB): report of the Consortium on DLB International Workshop. *J Alzheimer's Dis*, 9 Suppl 3, 417–23.

McKhann G et al. (1984). Clinical diagnosis of Alzheimer's disease: report of the NINDS-ADRDA Work Group under the auspices of the Department of Health and Human Services Task Force on Alzheimer's disease. *Neurology*, **34**, 939–44.

Mackenzie IR (2007). The neuropathology and clinical phenotype of FTD with progranulin mutations. *Acta Neuropathol*, **114**, 49–54.

Masters CL, Beyreuther K (2006). Alzheimer's centennial legacy: prospects for rational therapeutic intervention targeting the Abeta amyloid pathway. *Brain*, 129(Pt 11), 2823–39.

Mesulam MM (1982). Slowly progressive aphasia without generalized dementia. *Ann Neurol*, **24**, 17–22.

Neary D *et al.* (1998). Frontotemporal lobar degeneration: a consensus on clinical diagnostic criteria. *Neurology*, **51**, 1546–54.

Rahman S *et al.* (1999). Specific cognitive deficits in early frontal variant frontotemporal dementia. *Brain*, **122**, 1469–93.

Reisberg B *et al.* (1997). Diagnosis of Alzheimer's disease. Report of an International Psychogeriatric Association Special Meeting Work Group Under the Cosponsorship of Alzheimer's Disease International, the European Federation of Neurological Societies, the World Health Organization, and the World Psychiatric Association. *Int Psychogeriatr*, **9**, S11–38.

Rockwood K *et al.* (1999). Subtypes of vascular dementia. *Alzheimer's Disease and Associated Disorders*, **13**, S59–65.

Roman GC *et al.* (1993). Vascular dementia: diagnostic criteria for research studies. Report of the NINDS-AIREN International Workshop. *Neurology*, **43**, 250–60.

Snowden JS, Neary D, Mann DMA (1996). *Fronto-temporal lobar degeneration: fronto-temporal dementia, progressive aphasia, semantic dementia*. Churchill Livingstone, Hong Kong.

van Swieten J, Spillantini MG (2007). Hereditary frontotemporal dementia caused by Tau gene mutations. *Brain Pathol*, **17**(1), 63–73.

24.5

Epilepsy and disorders of consciousness

Contents

24.5.1 Epilepsy in later childhood and adulthood

G.D. Perkin

Essentials

Epilepsy is defined as recurrent (two or more) epileptic seizures, unprovoked by any immediate identifiable cause, and is common, with a lifetime prevalence of 1.5 to 5%.

Pathophysiology

Epileptic seizures are thought to arise at cortical sites. Partial seizures begin focally; generalized seizures infer widespread, bilateral cortical involvement from the beginning. Underlying mechanisms have been best defined for absence seizures, where a thalamocortical circuit is responsible for generating synchronous burst-firing of neurones. In different types of epilepsy, roles for specific ion channels (e.g. voltage-dependent calcium channel, (T-channel)), receptors (e.g. $GABA_A$ receptors), and neurotransmitters (e.g. serotonergic) have been suggested.

Clinical features—partial seizures

These include (1) simple partial motor seizures—any part of the body can be affected, and sometimes the seizure 'marches' along the cortex, producing successive jerking of contiguous body parts; consciousness is lost with secondary generalization; (2) simple partial sensory seizures—produce paraesthesias or numbness; can march in an analogous fashion to motor seizures; (3) occipital lobe seizures—visual symptoms predominate; (4) frontal lobe seizures—commonly nocturnal; frequently associated with turning to a prone position and vocalization; (5) simple and complex partial (temporal lobe) seizures—associated with olfactory, gustatory and vertiginous sensations, and with psychic symptoms; distinguished by absence (simple) or presence (complex) of altered consciousness; various automatic activity or movement may occur (of which the patient is unaware) when consciousness is disturbed.

Clinical features—generalized seizures

These include (1) tonic-clonic seizures (grand mal epilepsy)—the tonic phase is associated with contraction of axial and then limb muscles; clonic movements appear and slowly increase in amplitude; finally all movements cease and the patient is flaccid. Injury is common; urinary and/or faecal incontinence may occur. Confusion and disorientation are usual when the patient wakes. (2) Absence seizures (petit mal)—activity suddenly ceases for 10 to 20 s, but without loss of posture. (3) Myoclonic seizures—brief, shock-like contractions of muscle, occurring either in a generalized or focal distribution. (4) Atonic seizures—result in sudden loss of muscle tone.

Status epilepticus—defined as a single seizure lasting more than 30 min or successional seizures without recovery of consciousness between.

Investigation

This may (1) provide valuable support for the diagnosis; (2) give an indication as to which part of the brain has initiated the seizure;

and (3) allow a statement as to the underlying structural process (if any). After exclusion of common metabolic precipitants, most particularly hypoglycaemia, key investigations are often electroencephalography (EEG) and structural imaging (usually MRI).

Treatment

Does the patient require anticonvulsants?—80% of patients presenting with an epileptic fit will have another one if they are untreated. The decision as to whether or not to start anticonvulsant treatment is often determined by how soon the patient wishes to start driving.

Choice of anticonvulsant—(1) Generalized seizures (tonic–clonic, absence, or myoclonic)—sodium valproate is probably the drug of choice. (2) Partial seizures, with or without generalization—carbamazepine, phenytoin and valproate are probably the drugs of choice. (3) Status epilepticus—lorazepam is probably the drug of choice.

Newer anticonvulsants and problems with anticonvulsants—eight new antiepileptic drugs have been introduced over the last 20 years: each has an individual role and profile of unwanted effects. Drug therapy induces enzymes, may require biochemical monitoring, and poses specific problems in relation to pregnancy, breast feeding, drug withdrawal and driving.

Definitions

Using guidelines developed by the International League Against Epilepsy (ILEA), epilepsy is defined as recurrent (two or more) epileptic seizures, unprovoked by any immediately identifiable cause. Excluded are febrile seizures and neonatal seizures (the latter are defined as those occurring in the first 4 weeks of life). Multiple seizures occurring within a 24-h period are considered to represent a single event. The epileptic seizure itself is defined as the clinical manifestation of an abnormal and excessive discharge of a set of brain neurons. The manifestation is a sudden transient phenomenon which may include alteration of consciousness, or motor, sensory, autonomic, or psychic events that are perceived by either the individual or an observer. Problems arise, when using the term 'epilepsy', with those individuals who may have had only two or three attacks in a lifetime. To take account of this, the terms 'active epilepsy' and 'inactive epilepsy' are used, the former referring to patients with at least one seizure in the previous 5 years, the latter to patients who have been seizure free over the same period. The definitions are further qualified, for inactive cases, according to whether the individual is taking drug therapy.

The idiopathic epilepsies are defined as those epileptic disorders (partial or generalized) that have characteristic clinical and electroencephalogram (EEG) features coupled with a genetic predisposition. Cryptogenic epilepsy defines cases of partial or generalized epilepsy in which no aetiological factor has been identified. Symptomatic seizures are those occurring in association with a known risk factor. Epileptic syndromes have been defined by the ILEA on the basis of clinical characteristics, age of onset, and EEG findings.

Epidemiology

Incidence

Most reported incidence rates lie between 40 and 70/100 000. Figures for developing countries usually exceed 100/100 000. Age-specific rates show a bimodal distribution, with the highest peak in the first decade, falling thereafter until a second peak in later life. In industrialized countries, there has been a decrease in incidence in children and an increase in older people over the last three decades.

Prevalence

Prevalence figures are more widely available. For adults, rates usually lie between 4 and 10/1000 with higher rates in resource-poor countries. Cumulative incidence (or lifetime prevalence) rates, excluding febrile seizures, are higher, producing a figure between 1.5 and 5% with up to twice that figure in resource-poor countries.

Sex

Males have slightly higher prevalence rates than females.

Socioeconomic status

Higher prevalence rates have been reported in the lower socioeconomic groups, in both developed and developing countries.

Pathophysiology

Inherent in any discussion of epilepsy mechanisms is the need to define a homogeneous population of patients in whom epilepsy occurs. Generalized tonic–clonic seizures, for example, can occur with many different epileptic syndromes. Epileptic seizures are thought to arise at cortical sites: partial seizures begin focally in the cortex and generalized seizures infer widespread, bilateral, cortical involvement from the start. An interictal discharge occurs when a group of pyramidal neurons is synchronously activated. During the discharge, the cells develop a large and prolonged depolarization, which is terminated by a hyperpolarizing potential. It is conceived that the generation of synchronized neuronal activity results from an imbalance between inhibitory (γ-aminobutyric acid (GABA)-mediated) and excitatory (glutamate-mediated) neurotransmission, the latter prevailing.

The underlying mechanisms behind epileptic discharges have been best defined for absence seizures where a thalamocortical circuit is responsible for generating synchronous burst firing of neurons. The circuit involves neocortical pyramidal neurons, thalamic relay neurons, and neurons of the nucleus reticularis thalami. The last are exclusively GABA in type. A voltage-dependent calcium channel (T channel) appears critical in allowing burst firing of neurons. After activation, the T channels acquire repolarization via GABA$_B$-receptors present on thalamic relay neurons. GABA$_A$-receptors also play an important regulatory role in synchronized thalamocortical burst firing.

Less information is available on the pathophysiological mechanisms of generalized convulsive seizures. Roles for GABA$_A$-receptors and altered serotoninergic neurotransmission have been suggested.

Classification

The ILEA classification scheme, as revised in 1989, is now widely used for epidemiological, management, and research purposes.

The scheme divides seizures into focal, generalized, and unclassifiable forms (Table 24.5.1.1).

Although it is widely used, the classification has disadvantages. The ability to determine whether consciousness is preserved, in order to make the distinction between simple and complex partial seizures, is often limited. Some individuals, although appearing alert, can be shown to have impaired awareness when carefully tested.

An elaboration of the classification consists of a list of epileptic syndromes into which, theoretically, all generalized and partial epileptic seizures can be fitted. The idiopathic generalized seizures are classified according to age of onset and seizure type. The partial seizures, attributed to dysfunction of restricted cortical areas, are predominantly classified according to their clinical features, supplemented by EEG findings. Much criticism has been made of this syndromic classification. In routine clinical practice many cases (probably the majority) are left in nonspecific categories. Moreover, the classification fails to incorporate data derived from CT or MRI.

Clinical features

Partial seizures

Simple partial motor seizures

Any part of the body can be affected by a focal motor seizure, according to the site of origin of the discharge. Sometimes the seizure remains localized to the same area (e.g. the hand) and sometimes it 'marches' along the motor cortex, producing successional jerking of contiguous body parts (Jacksonian seizures). During the focal stage, consciousness is preserved. With secondary generalization (i.e. diffuse bilateral spread) consciousness is lost. The parts of the body most commonly affected by this type of seizure correlate with their area of representation in the motor cortex. Other focal motor disturbances reflecting epileptic discharges include rotation of the head and eyes contralaterally (from the dorsolateral prefrontal cortex), tonic foot movements ipsilaterally (the paracentral lobule), and head turning with arm extension on the same side (supplementary motor cortex). After such seizures there may be paralysis of the affected part lasting for minutes or hours (Todd's paresis).

Simple partial sensory seizures

Seizures emanating from the sensory cortex produce paraesthesias or numbness. The seizure can march in an analogous fashion to a motor seizure and, similarly, can then become generalized. Where the tongue or face is involved, the symptoms are sometimes felt bilaterally. More complex sensory phenomena may be experienced and, with discharges in the second sensory area, the limb sensations can be ipsilateral, contralateral, or bilateral.

Occipital lobe seizures

Visual symptoms predominate, usually as simple rather than complex phenomena. The latter phenomena, producing alteration of size, shape, or depth of objects, are associated with seizures arising at the occipitoparietotemporal interface. In addition there may be ocular deviation, jerking, or forced closure of the eyelids. Visual hallucinations may occur.

Frontal lobe seizures

Frontal lobe seizures are commonly nocturnal and frequently associated with turning to a prone position. Vocalization is common and tends to consist of a continuous monotone with moaning or grunting. An aura before the attack is unusual. Other recognized features include pelvic thrusting, rocking of the body, and head movements. Rapid postictal recovery is common.

Simple partial (temporal lobe) seizures

The distinction between simple and complex partial seizures is difficult, based as it is on evidence of altered consciousness with the latter (Fig. 24.5.1.1). Olfactory, gustatory, and vertiginous sensations occur. The taste and smell sensations are sometimes pleasurable but often disagreeable. A metallic taste is common. Abdominal sensations also occur, which are typically ill-defined, and may ascend to the chest and throat. Psychic symptoms are more often associated with complex partial seizures. There may be intense pleasure or fear ushering in the attack. The patient can

Table 24.5.1.1 Classification of epilepsy

I. *Partial (focal, local) seizures*
A. Simple partial seizures (consciousness not impaired)
1. With motor symptoms
2. With somatosensory or special sensory symptoms
3. With autonomic symptoms
4. With psychic symptoms
B. Complex partial seizures (with impairment of consciousness)
1. Beginning as simple partial seizures and progressing to impairment of consciousness
(a) With no other features
(b) With features as in simple partial seizures
(c) with automatisms
2. With impairment of consciousness at onset
(a) With no other features
(b) With features as in simple partial seizures
(c) With automatisms
C. Partial seizures evolving to secondarily generalized seizures
1. Simple partial seizures evolving to generalized seizures
2. Complex partial seizures evolving to generalized seizures
3. Simple partial seizures evolving to complex partial seizures to generalized seizures
II. *Generalized seizures (convulsive or non-convulsive)*
A. 1. Absence seizures
2. Atypical absence seizures
B. Myoclonic seizures
C. Clonic seizures
D. Tonic seizures
E. Tonic–clonic seizures
F. Atonic seizures (astatic seizures)
III. *Unclassified epileptic seizures*

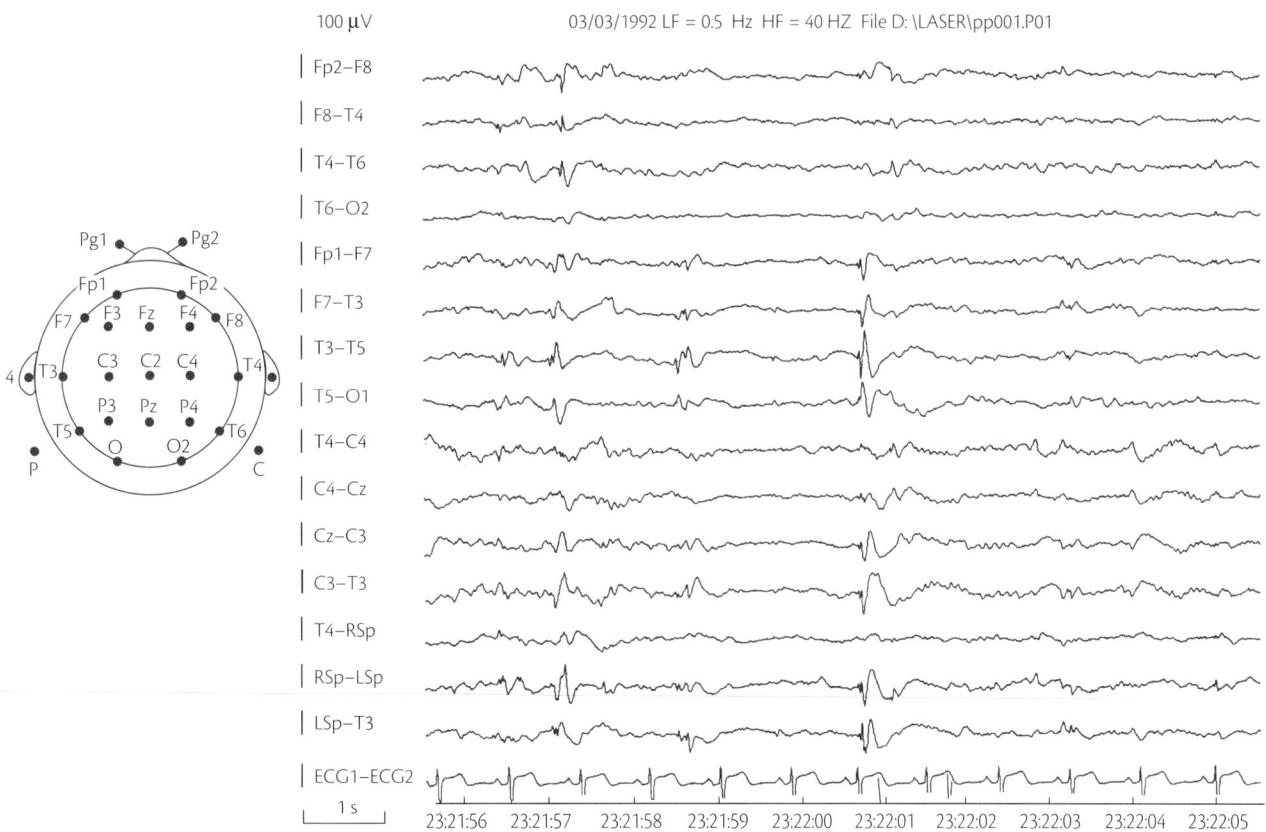

Fig. 24.5.1.1 Ictal spike and slow-wave complex in a patient with complex partial seizures. The discharges are particularly apparent over the left temporal lobe (T3 to T5), but there are some independent discharges over the right temporal lobe (T4 to T6).
(Record kindly provided by Dr David Fish.)

experience a sense of loss of personal or environmental reality (depersonalization and derealization, respectively). There may be a sense of intense familiarity (*déjà vu*) or unfamiliarity (*jamais vu*). Epileptic anger is unprovoked and rapidly subsides. Illusions are encountered, in the form of disordered visual perceptions, and visual or auditory hallucinations, sometimes of considerable complexity.

Where consciousness is disturbed, various automatic activities or movements that the patient is unaware of (automatisms) may occur. These may take the form of eating (chewing or swallowing), speaking, gesture, or more elaborate skilled activities. Some of these automatic movements are also seen with absence seizures. When elaborate, the patient may partly undress, or move about from one room to another. The symptomatology of mesial and lateral temporal lobe discharges has been distinguished, the latter having somatosensory, visual, or auditory manifestations in addition to the other features mentioned above.

Other, rarer focal seizure types are confined to childhood. In benign childhood epilepsy with centrotemporal spikes, consciousness is preserved. The sensory phenomena are usually confined to the mouth where motor activity may also occur. Speech arrest occurs if the dominant hemisphere is affected.

Any of the focal epilepsies can lead to secondary generalization. Consciousness is lost, and a tonic–clonic seizure is the usual outcome. Prolonged focal seizures (epilepsia partialis continua) lead to a repetitive or continuous focal motor activity that may last

for weeks or months and is most often the consequence of a focal cortical insult.

Generalized seizures

Tonic–clonic seizures (grand mal epilepsy)

Some patients report a premonition for hours or even days before the attack. The symptoms are usually a vague sense of loss of well-being and do not imply a focal origin for the attack. An aura lasting a few seconds before the onset, on the other hand, implies a focal origin for the attack, demanding classification as a focal seizure with secondary generalization. The tonic phase is associated with contraction of axial and then limb muscles. If upright, the patient falls heavily. Injury is common. Contraction of the jaw can lead to tongue injury. Forcible contraction of the diaphragm results in a sudden gasp or epileptic cry. Cyanosis results from a loss of respiratory activity. Subsequently clonic movements appear and slowly increase in amplitude. Gradually, periods of relaxation intervene between the clonic contractions until finally all movements cease. The patient is then flaccid. Urinary or faecal incontinence or both may occur at this stage. Subsequently the patient is liable to sleep, often heavily. If the patient wakes, initial confusion and disorientation are usual. Headache and muscle pains are common. Incomplete forms occur in which the clonic or tonic phase predominates.

In addition to injuries incurred in falling, and those resulting from biting of the cheeks or tongue (typically the lateral margin is affected), the seizures may be of such violence that vertebral compression fractures occur. Sudden death occurring soon after a tonic–clonic seizure is a recognized, although rare, complication. Its incidence lies between 1/500 and 1/1000 deaths per person-year.

Absence seizures (petit mal)

Patients are totally unaware of their absence seizures. Activity suddenly ceases but without loss of posture. Adventitious movements occur, e.g. slight contractions of the eyes or some lip movement. The head may drop slightly. More typically, the patient simply stares blankly and is unresponsive. Attacks last around 10 to 20 s (Fig. 24.5.1.2). In some cases more overt limb movement occurs.

Atypical absences are defined as attacks that begin less abruptly, last longer, and frequently lead to loss of postural tone. They usually coincide with other seizure types. Absence seizures begin in childhood and usually cease in adult life, although some 50% of patients will later develop tonic–clonic seizures.

Myoclonic seizures

Myoclonus consists of brief, shock-like contractions of muscle, occurring in either a generalized or a focal distribution. Many forms of myoclonus are nonepileptic. Those associated with epilepsy are accompanied by an ictal EEG discharge. In primary generalized epileptic myoclonus, the myoclonus is accompanied by diffuse cortical epileptic discharges.

Atonic seizures

Atonic seizures result in sudden loss of muscle tone. If the hypotonus is generalized, falls occur, often with substantial injury. The attacks begin in infancy or childhood. The episodes are brief and recovery rapid unless injury has occurred.

Status epilepticus

Status epilepticus is defined as a single seizure lasting more than 30 min or successional seizures without recovery of consciousness between. The seizures are usually tonic–clonic. Both complex partial seizures and absence seizures can occur in the form of status epilepticus. In such cases, alteration of the conscious level is likely to be the major clinical feature with little motor activity, particularly with absence seizures.

Epilepsy syndromes

The need to define epileptic syndromes arises from the fact that individual seizure types may be a manifestation of a number of differing conditions, all with individual characteristics and prognosis. The epileptic syndrome is based on a combination of seizure type, presumed localization (according to clinical features and EEG characteristics in the case of the partial seizures), and age of onset. In routine, as opposed to heavily specialized, practice only a third of patients with newly diagnosed epilepsy can be fitted into such a classification system.

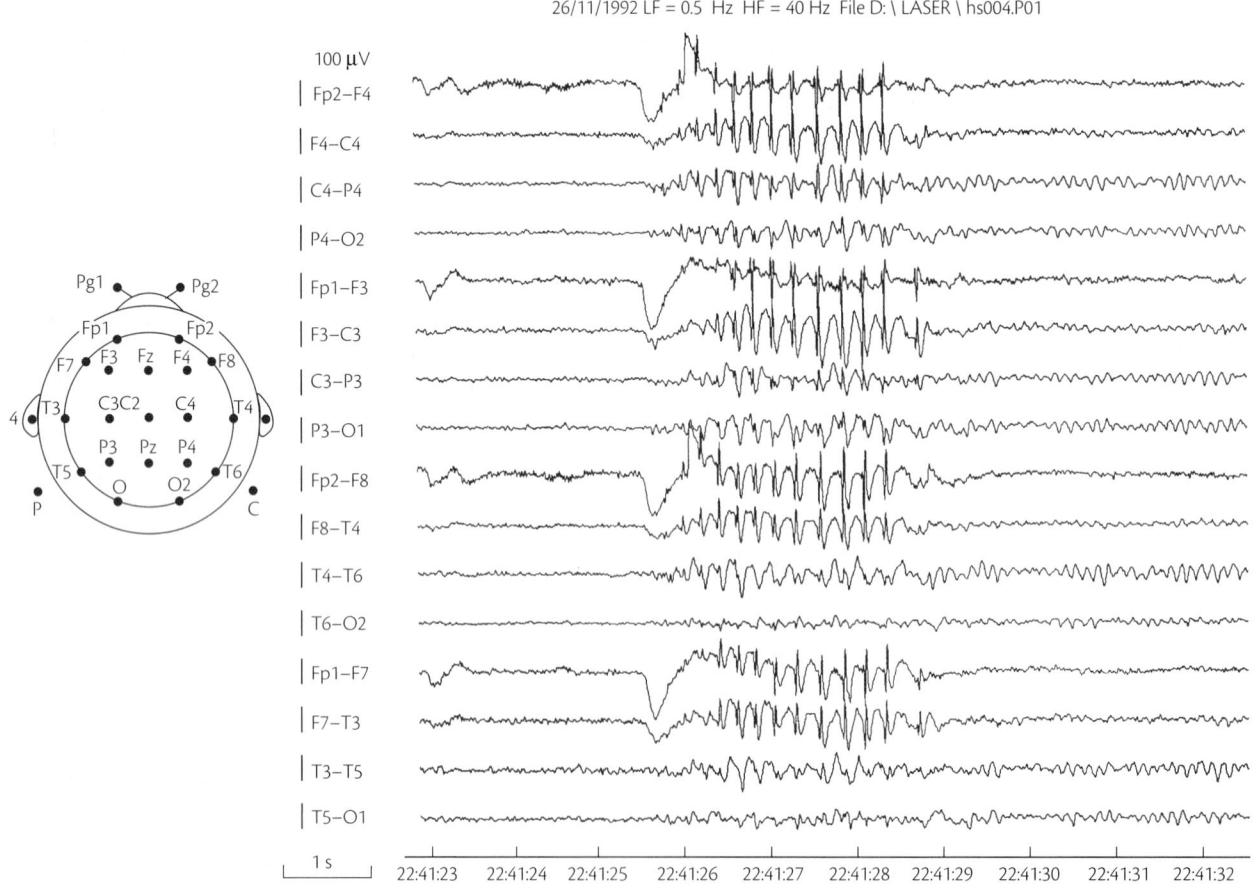

Fig. 24.5.1.2 Electroencephalogram (EEG) of a typical absence seizure. The first 2.5 s of the record are entirely normal. The event begins with a large downward deflection which records eye closure, immediately followed in all channels by a spike-and-wave discharge at a frequency of 3 cycles/s. The seizure terminates as abruptly as it began. (Record kindly provided by Dr David Fish.)

Causes of epilepsy

In most surveys, only about a quarter to a third of epilepsy cases has been attributable to a specific cause. With modern imaging methods, this proportion is likely to rise significantly.

Genetically determined

In some genetically determined disorders, epilepsy is only one feature of the condition. Many such disorders have features other than epilepsy and typically produce significant neurological disability. Examples include the forms of progressive myoclonic epilepsy associated with Lafora body disease and Unverricht–Lundborg disease. More relevant, in clinical terms, are those genetically determined conditions in which epilepsy is the sole or major manifestation.

Idiopathic generalized epilepsies

The idiopathic generalized epilepsies account for about 20 to 30% of the epilepsies and have a significant genetic influence. Childhood and juvenile absence epilepsy, juvenile myoclonic epilepsy, and generalized tonic–clonic seizures in isolation have been associated with several susceptibility loci.

Most of the idiopathic epilepsies for which the molecular basis is known are channelopathies, where mutations disrupt normal electrical transmissions between neurons. Childhood absence epilepsy is linked to a mutation in the $GABA_A$-receptor, γ_2 subunit. Autosomal dominant juvenile myoclonic epilepsy has been shown to be a channelopathy associated with a $GABA_A$-receptor, α_1-subunit mutation. A gene encoding the CLC-2 voltage-gated chloride channel (*CLCN2* gene), located on chromosome 3q26, has been found in families with idiopathic generalized epilepsy. Through association studies, it has been suggested that the α_{1A} subunit of the voltage-gated calcium channel gene (*CACNAIA*) may affect susceptibility to idiopathic generalized epilepsy. Recently, non-ion channel genes have emerged as causes of specific epilepsy syndromes.

Where ion channel or nonion channel defects have been identified, they generally account for only a minority of familial or sporadic cases of the relevant epilepsy syndrome. It has been suggested that the genetic predisposition for idiopathic epilepsy represents a continuum, in which only a small fraction follow monogenic inheritance, while the majority display oligogenic or polygenic traits.

Idiopathic focal epilepsies

Several forms of familial focal epilepsy have now been identified. Benign familial neonatal seizures are caused by mutations in the potassium channel genes, *KCNQ2* and *KCNQ3*. Benign familial infantile convulsions, which present between 4 and 8 months of life, are associated with three loci mapped to chromosomes 19, 16, and 2. Benign familial neonatal infantile seizures, an intermediate clinical variant of the previous two, are associated with mutations of the sodium channel, α_2 subunit.

Autosomal dominant, nocturnal, frontal lobe epilepsy is a childhood-onset epilepsy characterized by the clustering of nocturnal frontal lobe seizures. The syndrome has been associated with mutations in genes coding for the α_4 subunit and β_2 subunit of the neuronal nicotinic acetylcholine receptor (*CHRNA4* and *CHRNB2*).

Autosomal dominant, lateral temporal lobe epilepsy is characterized by focal seizures with auditory, visual, psychic, or dysphasic symptoms. In some families the condition is linked to mutations in the leucin-rich glioma-inactivated 1 (*LGI1*) gene—epitempin.

Febrile seizures are the most common seizure type in children, with an incidence of 2 to 5%. The inheritance is complex and the clinical pattern heterogeneous. Loci have been reported on chromosomes 6q22, 8q13–q21, 19p, 2q23–q24, and 5q14–q15. Typically, febrile seizures occur between the ages of 6 months and 3 years. Simple febrile seizures are generalized and last less than 15 min. Complex febrile seizures have focal features, are longer lasting, or recur within a 24-h period. About two-thirds of children with febrile seizures do not have a recurrence. A proportion of children with febrile seizures develop epilepsy at a later age.

Malformations of cortical development

Malformations of cortical development (MCD) are structural brain defects that are acquired during cortical development. They are a common cause of drug-refractory epilepsy in adults. The defect may be global (agyria), hemispheric (hemimegalencephaly), or focal—focal cortical dysplasia (FCD), and periventricular and subcortical nodular heterotopia (PNH and SNH).

The associated epilepsy tends to arise during childhood and adolescence. The seizure may be generalized or focal, and the type of seizure does not necessarily follow the distribution of the malformation.

EEG frequently reveals continuous epileptiform discharges in patients with FCD. MRI can detect particular signal changes in FCD, although often specialized sequencing is required.

Trauma

Approximately 70% of those individuals who eventually develop post-traumatic epilepsy will have their first seizure within 2 years of the original injury. Risk factors that predict post-traumatic epilepsy include early seizures (those occurring in the first week), a depressed skull fracture, or evidence of intracranial haemorrhage. There is no justification for the use of prophylactic anticonvulsants in the hope of preventing the development of post-traumatic seizures.

Tumour

Although adult-onset epilepsy is often equated with the presence of tumour, the cause of symptomatic epilepsy in later life is more likely to be cerebrovascular or Alzheimer's disease. The likelihood of a tumour producing seizures increases as the tumour is sited more anteriorly in the hemisphere, so that over 50% of patients with frontal lobe tumours have epilepsy. Adult-onset status, in someone without a history of epilepsy, is particularly suggestive of frontal lobe tumour. Epilepsy is more common with slow-growing tumours and may be generalized or focal in nature.

Cerebrovascular disease

The prevalence of epilepsy after stroke has been reported to lie between 6 and 15%, and appears as likely with cerebral infarction as with cerebral haemorrhage.

Infection

In large-scale surveys, infection has been considered the cause of epilepsy in 3 to 5% of cases. Differences in rate between countries are often attributed to the variable prevalence of certain aetiologies, e.g. cysticercosis. Other tropical infections that have been considered potential contributors to epilepsy prevalence include malaria, schistosomiasis, and trypanosomiasis. Epilepsy is a recognized feature of bacterial, tuberculous, and fungal meningitis, and of viral encephalitis. Epilepsy is often the first symptom of a tuberculoma.

Dementia

Patients with Alzheimer's disease of mild-to-moderate severity have a cumulative incidence of unprovoked seizures of around 8% over a 7-year period.

Multiple sclerosis

The prevalence of epilepsy in multiple sclerosis (MS) is probably of the order of 2%. Both generalized and focal seizures have been attributed to MS. Rarely, status epilepticus and epilepsia partialis continua have been recorded.

Alcohol

Alcohol lowers seizure threshold. Seizures may occur during binge drinking or during a period of withdrawal after alcohol excess.

Metabolic disorders

Seizures may occur in association with hypocalcaemia, hypercalcaemia, hypomagnesaemia, hypoglycaemia, hyponatraemia, and hypernatraemia. Severe renal and hepatic failure can both precipitate seizures.

Certain drugs are considered to lower the seizure threshold and are relatively contraindicated in patients with epilepsy. The drugs in question include the tricyclic antidepressants, the phenothiazines, and isoniazid. Rapid withdrawal of barbiturates or benzodiazepines can trigger seizures in those without a history of epilepsy.

Precipitants of epilepsy

Recognized precipitants of epilepsy include inadequate sleep, alcohol abuse, and ingestion of certain drugs. In catamenial epilepsy the attacks are confined to the menstrual period. Seizures confined to sleep are well recognized and indeed sleep EEG recordings are characteristically more likely to register abnormal discharges than recordings made in the alert individual. In reflex epilepsy, attacks are virtually inevitably triggered by a particular stimulus. Precipitants include photic stimulation, startle, noise, and movement. Rarer forms of reflex epilepsy have been linked to musical passages, eating, and performance of certain mental tasks.

Differential diagnosis

Syncope

Most individuals who faint experience a characteristic set of symptoms before loss of consciousness. These include mental slowing, fading of vision, altered hearing, malaise, and sweating. The process is the result, in varying combination, of bradycardia and profound arterial vasodilatation in skeletal muscle. Unless the individual lies down, loss of consciousness occurs and the patient falls to the ground. Characteristically the fall is gentle, and self-injury relatively uncommon. In falls associated with tonic–clonic or atonic seizures, the fall is precipitate and injury much more likely. Rarely, in complicated faints, there may be brief clonic jerks of the limbs. More commonly, multifocal myoclonus is observed, lasting a few seconds and following the loss of posture. The eyes tend to remain open. Lateral head turns, repetitive movements (such as lip licking), and hallucinations are all recognized features. After the episode there may be brief confusion and feelings of weakness, but these rapidly resolve. If, on the other hand, the upright posture is maintained (typically the individual is a soldier on parade) then stiffness of the limbs or repetitive generalized shaking occurs which is virtually indistinguishable from the movements occurring with epilepsy. Usually, however, a true tonic–clonic sequence does not occur in these circumstances.

Micturition syncope

Micturition syncope occurs predominantly in males, but of any age group. The attacks are almost always nocturnal, typically after an evening of alcohol consumption. Onset is usually during or shortly after micturition. The warning symptoms are often brief. The attacks seldom occur frequently; if they do, then the individual, if male, is advised to micturate in the sitting position.

Cough syncope

Patients with cough syncope effectively perform Valsalva's manoeuvre during a bout of prolonged coughing. Treatment is directed at the underlying chest condition.

Cardiac syncope

Various cardiac abnormalities, all having in common the endresult of failing output and reduced cerebral perfusion, are associated with syncopal attacks. Mechanisms include complete heart block, paroxysmal ventricular tachycardia or fibrillation, and supraventricular tachycardia or bradyarrhythmia. In addition to disorders of rhythm, abnormalities of ventricular contractility or obstruction of outflow can have a similar outcome, usually when increased output is required during a period of exertion. Rarely, pedunculated masses within the heart, e.g. an atrial myxoma, cause outflow obstruction when the patient assumes certain postures. Features suggesting that a cardiac lesion may be responsible for a syncopal attack include a history of cardiac disease, palpitations, or chest pain in association with the attack, and the finding of cardiac abnormalities on clinical examination.

Separate from these mechanisms are cases of syncope associated with postural hypotension. Autonomic failure resulting in postural hypotension is a feature of multisystem atrophy, certain neuropathies with autonomic fibre involvement, such as diabetes and drug therapy, e.g. with phenothiazines and tricyclic antidepressants. The correct diagnosis is usually readily established from the history.

Carotid sinus syncope

Patients with this condition usually present with either vertigo or syncopal attacks. The syncopal attacks are sometimes followed by flushing and may be triggered by pressure over the neck, e.g. during neck rotation. In most patients, the syncope is related to atrioventricular block or asystole. Occasionally, a pure vasodilator reaction occurs, with peripheral pooling of blood.

Transient ischaemic attacks

These attacks should seldom be confused with epilepsy. In some patients with carotid occlusion (or severe stenosis), attacks of limb shaking occur in which involuntary limb movements described as shaking, trembling, or twitching occur, usually for seconds. The movements, which are coarse and irregular, predominate distally. Sometimes the attacks coincide with limb weakness or speech difficulty. The attacks are not influenced by anticonvulsants but can be relieved by endarterectomy where there is an underlying carotid stenosis.

Migraine

Loss of consciousness is a recognized feature of basilar migraine. The condition presents in children or adolescents. The headache is occipital. Visual disturbances are common, along with altered sensations (typically bilateral), ataxia, and dysarthria. Typically the patient, if unconscious, can be roused. Rarely, tonic–clonic seizures are seen with the attacks.

Hyperventilation

Most patients with the hyperventilation syndrome do not develop carpopedal spasm or tetany. Rather, they have a constellation of symptoms that are liable to be confused with other conditions such as epilepsy. Those symptoms include dizziness or vertigo, weakness, paraesthesias, chest pain, and altered consciousness. Probably some 5 to 15% of patients lose consciousness during hyperventilation, but never with a tonic–clonic progression that would cause real diagnostic difficulty.

Narcolepsy and cataplexy

Narcolepsy is defined as excessive daytime sleepiness, often occurring under unusual circumstances. The onset of sleep is usually preceded by a feeling of tension, tiredness, or a noise in the head. In some patients, onset occurs without warning. At times, patients have periods of semiautomatic behaviour for which they may subsequently be amnesic.

Cataplexy is typically triggered by sudden arousal. Attacks are brief, and may lead to such loss of muscle control that the patient falls. During the attack, the patient is flaccid, the eyes may roll or diverge, and the facial muscles flicker. Despite this, the patient usually remains fully alert.

Drop attacks

Drop attacks are almost confined to women in the last third of life. Typically, while walking, the patient drops to her knees without warning. The patient is aware of the fall, and is usually able to get up quickly, provided that there is no injury. The attacks occur in otherwise fit individuals, are not due to vertebrobasilar ischaemia, and eventually remit completely. They are untreatable.

The parasomnias

Parasomnias are largely confined to children. They consist of either abnormal motor activity or excessive autonomic activity. Motor activity includes sleep starts, sleep myoclonus, bruxism, and head banging. Sleep myoclonus produces repetitive leg contraction, typically dorsiflexion of the feet. It increases with age and is usually idiopathic. Head banging, which may coincide with body rocking, is usually only seen in children or infants. The movements, which typically occur in clusters, are often accompanied by various forms of vocalization. In most cases, the child is normal. Sleep terrors usually happen within the first hour or two of sleep, occur in children, and result in a sudden cry followed by anxiety, tachycardia, sweating, and hyperkinesis. The child is not completely aware of the episodes, which sometimes necessitate short-term treatment with benzodiazepines.

Psychogenic nonepileptic seizures

Psychogenic nonepileptic seizures sometimes occur in isolation, but sometimes in those with true epilepsy. They account for 20% of the patients referred to specialist epilepsy units, usually with a diagnosis of intractable epilepsy. The prevalence is around 33/100 000 or 4% of that of epilepsy. The vast majority of people who have it are women. They are more likely to have a family history of psychiatric disorders, a past personal history of psychiatric disorder, a history of suicide attempt(s), evidence of sexual maladjustment, and current depressive symptoms. Indeed there is a substantial overlap, in terms of clinical characteristics, between psychogenic nonepileptic seizures and multiple personality disorder. In addition to the features noted above, up to 90% of patients give a history of sustained trauma, including childhood abuse, which may have been physical or sexual.

Certain features from the history should alert the physician. The attacks usually take place with witnesses present. They develop gradually rather than suddenly, and the movements displayed are often unpredictable and bizarre. Attempts to constrain the patient are resisted. Vocalization is common; incontinence is uncommon and tongue biting particularly so, but self-injury is a recognized feature. Typically the seizures are difficult to control. Serum prolactin levels taken 20 min after the event are normal, in contrast to tonic–clonic seizures where they are commonly, although not inevitably, elevated. Videotelemetry has proved of considerable value in differentiating epileptic from nonepileptic seizures. Seizures can be provoked by injections of saline, saline patches, hypnosis, hyperventilation, or photic stimulation. Management is extremely difficult, but earlier diagnosis is associated with a better outcome. Drug withdrawal is resisted by the patient, who often resents suggestions of psychiatric referral and exploration of psychological morbidity.

Investigations

Investigation of a patient with suspected epilepsy (or a single seizure) is performed for three main reasons: the investigation may provide valuable support for the diagnosis, it may give an indication as to which part of the brain has initiated the seizure, and, finally, imaging may allow a statement as to the underlying structural process, where such exists.

Routine haematological and biochemical tests should be undertaken in all patients with suspected epilepsy although they seldom point to a metabolic disturbance that has not already been recognized.

Electroencephalography

Certain facts about the EEG must be understood before interpretation is attempted. Epileptiform discharges are encountered in between 0.5 and 4% of individuals who have never had a seizure and who do not do so during a period of follow-up. Furthermore, a routine EEG in adults with established epilepsy shows epileptiform abnormalities in only some 40 to 50% of cases. With repeat recording, with or without sleep records, the figure rises to 70 or 80%. In other words, some patients with unequivocal epilepsy will have persistently normal or, at least, nonepileptic EEGs. Serial EEG recording is sometimes helpful in an attempt to define the origin of the seizure and to delineate the seizure type better. If photosensitivity is suspected (10% of individuals with seizures occurring between 1 and 7 years are photosensitive), serial recordings are appropriate, as they are in any individual with atypical status or in whom cognitive impairment might be due to subclinical epileptic activity. Where surgical intervention is being planned for the epilepsy, routine and sleep recordings are followed by videotelemetry in order to record individual attacks. For some patients, depth electrodes will be needed to establish the seizure source. Magnetoencephalography (MEG) localizes focal epileptic discharges by measuring the changes in the extracranial magnetic fields that these discharges generate. The system costs some 25 times as much as a conventional EEG system. Although in most patients spikes can be detected on both MEG and EEG, in certain patients spikes are seen with only one or other technique. It may be that MEG has a particular role in identifying focal cortical dysplasia. Depth electrodes are positioned stereotactically at sites determined by clinical and surface EEG criteria. Depth recordings are more accurate and sensitive in detecting focal discharges than either nasopharyngeal or sphenoidal electrodes, but are increasingly less used.

The EEG has also been used to attempt prediction of seizure recurrence in individuals after a single seizure of unknown cause. Epileptic discharges, in one series, predicted a seizure recurrence over 2 years of 83%, compared with a 12% rate in individuals with a normal recording. The EEG has also been used to predict seizure recurrence during or after drug withdrawal in someone whose epilepsy has gone into remission on medication. The predictive value of EEG abnormalities in such cases has varied widely from series to series.

CT

Neuroimaging is carried out in order to define whether a structural abnormality underlies the patient's epilepsy and, if so, whether some additional treatment, other than anticonvulsants, might be required. CT scanning was originally the most frequently used imaging process, before the more widespread availability of MRI. Some authors advocate MRI in all patients with epilepsy, other than for those epilepsies that are clearly idiopathic (e.g. absence seizures, juvenile myoclonic epilepsy, and benign rolandic epilepsy). In practice, this is probably unreasonable, e.g. a patient with the onset of epilepsy in the 70s or 80s, who has a normal CT (at least, with no evidence of focal pathology), hardly merits MRI if the epilepsy is well controlled.

MRI

MRI is undoubtedly both more sensitive and more specific than CT in detecting small brain lesions and abnormalities of the cerebral cortex thought to be relevant in the genesis of epilepsy (Fig. 24.5.1.3). Protocols setting out to achieve high sensitivity and specificity require T_1-weighted, thin-slice volumetric sequences, T_2 FLAIR (fluid-attenuated inversion recovery), and high-resolution T_2 spin echo. All coronal sequences need to be oriented orthogonal to the long axis of the hippocampus. The most common abnormalities detected are hippocampal sclerosis, malformations of cortical development, vascular malformations, tumours, and acquired cortical damage. MRI is particularly indicated for partial seizures, onset of generalized or unclassified seizures in adult life, patients with fixed focal clinical or neuropsychological deficit, and for those patients with poor seizure control. Quantitative measures of the hippocampi improve the diagnostic sensitivity of MRI for hippocampal sclerosis. MRI is much more sensitive than CT for detecting malformations of cortical development. MR spectroscopy (MRS), examining nuclei ^{31}P and ^{1}H, has been used for assessment

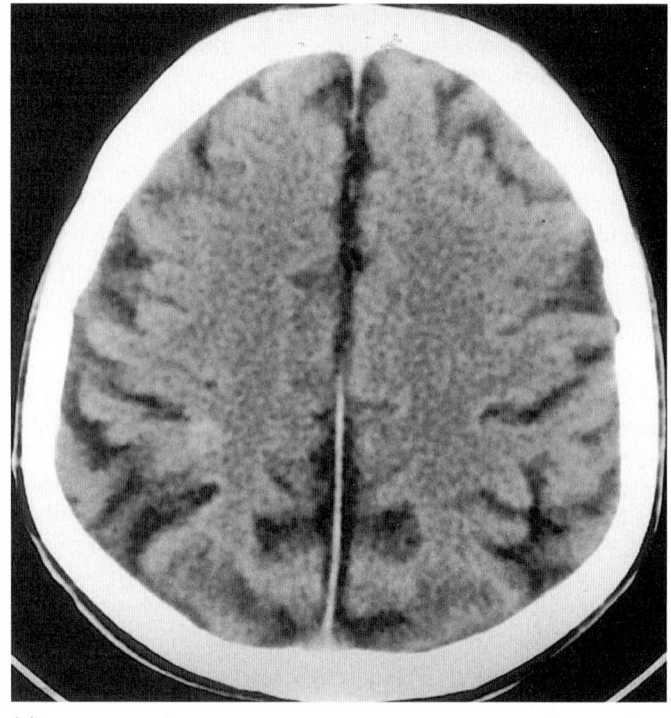

(a)

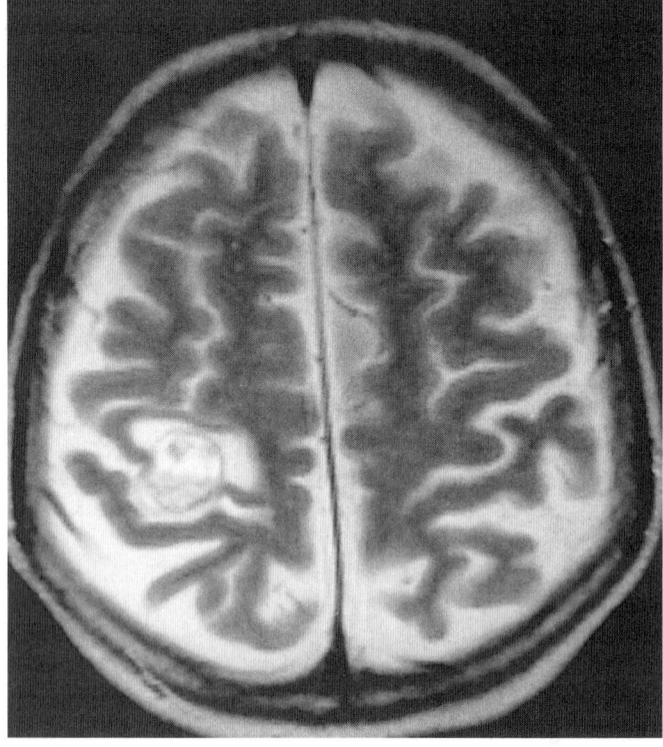

(b)

Fig. 24.5.1.3 (a) CT and (b) MRI: the readily visible cavernome on MRI is only just visible on CT.

of patients with complex partial seizures for possible surgery. Transient MRI abnormalities are a recognized occurrence in patients with epilepsy. Functional MRI is commonly used to localize the motor cortex before resection of adjacent neocortex and to lateralize language function. It is being developed to predict the consequences of temporal lobe resection on memory.

Single-photon emission computed tomography

As a result of its poor time resolution, ictal perfusion SPECT usually displays both the ictal onset zone and the seizure propagation pathways. Although it has been assumed that the region with the most intense hyperperfusion is the ictal onset zone, this is not necessarily the case. The earlier the injection is given after seizure onset, the more likely it is that the most intense focus represents the ictal onset zone. Analysis of ictal SPECT is usually done in comparison with an interictal SPECT image, using a variety of techniques.

Positron emission tomography

Interictal fluorodeoxyglucose positron emission tomography (FDG-PET) has proved a valuable tool in the presurgical evaluation of patients with refractory partial epilepsy.

FDG-PET appears to be superior to standard MRI in the detection of neuronal migration disorders. Sequential scans indicate a correlation between the extent of cortical glucose hypometabolism on PET and the quality of epilepsy control. Besides measurement of cerebral blood flow and regional cerebral glucose metabolism, PET can be used to assess the distribution of specific receptors—such as the benzodiazepine–GABA$_A$-receptor complex, using [^{11}C]fluamzenil (FMZVD) (Fig. 24.5.1.4). It appears that abnormalities in FMZVD are also linked to the pattern of recent seizure activity.

^{15}O-labelled water PET is at least as reliable as the intracarotid amytal (Wada) test for language lateralization, but this role is being rapidly supplanted by functional MRI.

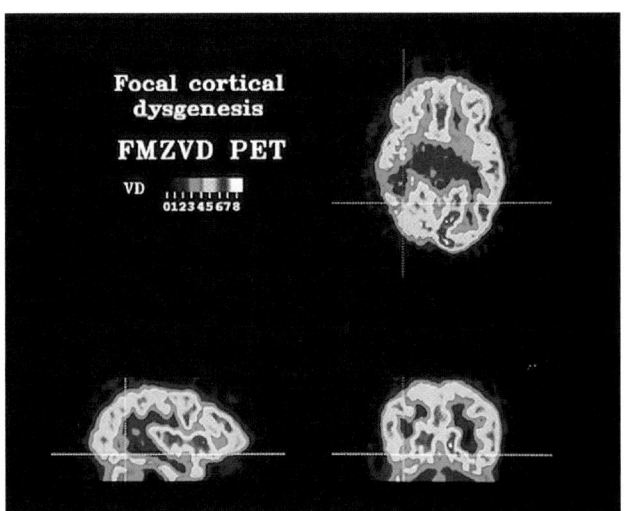

Fig. 24.5.1.4 Positron emission tomography (PET) scan showing a region of probable cortical dysplasia in the right temporal lobe. The [^{11}C]fluamzenil volume of distribution (FMZVD) is an index of γ-aminobutyric acid A (GABA$_A$)-receptor density.

It has been suggested that high uptake of α-[^{11}C]methyl-L-tryptophan (AMT) on PET occurs in a subset of epileptogenic tubers in patients with tuberous sclerosis, consistent with the location of the seizure focus.

Treatment: drug therapy

Choice of drug therapy

A number of principles can be stated in relation to drug therapy.

Does the patient require anticonvulsants?

The issue of whether isolated seizures should be treated remains unresolved. Seizure recurrence rate after a single seizure reaches 80% in untreated individuals, the vast majority recurring within 2 years of onset. Many patients prefer to defer treatment after a single seizure, a decision substantially influenced by how soon they wish to start driving. For a patient who has very infrequent seizures, say 5 or more years apart, it may seem logical to withhold medication.

Choice of anticonvulsant

An algorithm can provide some guidelines regarding drug treatment (Fig. 24.5.1.5). For generalized seizures (tonic–clonic, absence, or myoclonic) sodium valproate is the drug of choice. Further choices are determined by seizure type. There are no controlled trial data indicating the most appropriate add-on drug or combination of drugs. Myoclonus can be exacerbated by

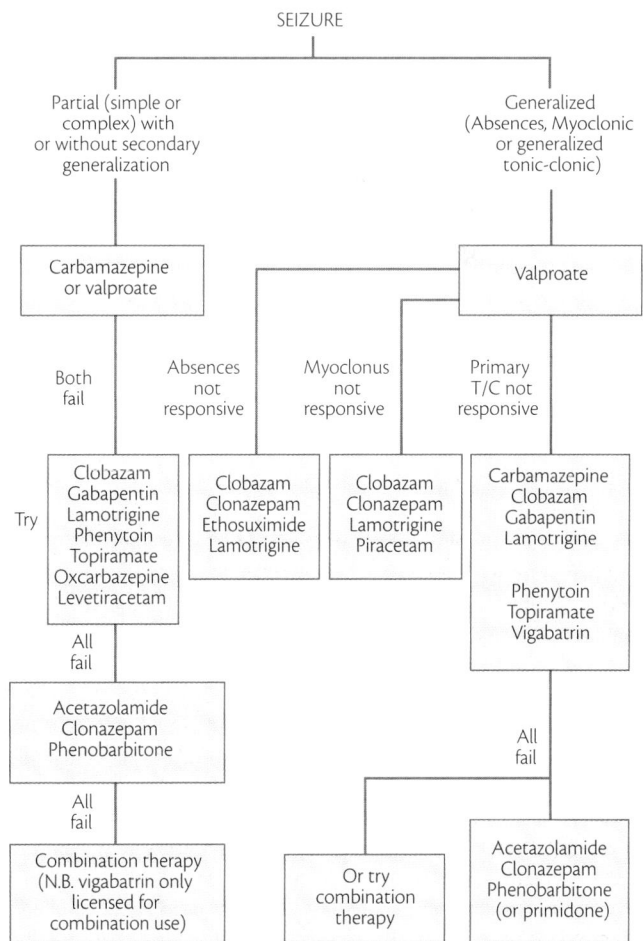

Fig. 24.5.1.5 Choice of anticonvulsant.

carbamazepine, gabapentin, and lamotrigine and absences by carbamazepine and gabapentin. For partial seizures, with or without generalization, carbamazepine, phenytoin, and valproate are probably the drugs of choice.

In addition, choice of drug will be influenced by the patient's age, sex (regarding the use of oral contraceptives and likelihood of pregnancy), and reliability of adherence to a particular drug regimen. The patient should always be started on a single drug.

Dosage

Although standard dose regimens tend to be quoted, many anticonvulsants are sometimes effective in relatively low doses. Accordingly the drug is introduced in low dosage, which is then gradually increased according to need and tolerance. Sometimes only dosages that lead to toxic serum levels appear effective. Some patients tolerate such toxic levels without difficulty.

Failure of first drug

When this occurs, a second drug should be gradually introduced without withdrawing the first. If the patient responds, the drug used originally can be slowly withdrawn.

Drug combinations

If drugs given individually have failed then drug combinations should be considered, remembering that they may interact with each other.

Generic prescribing

The bioavailability of the anticonvulsant drugs should be unaffected by whether they are prescribed generically, or as a specific branded product. Patients sometimes do not believe this assumption and prefer branded products. If they are given generic prescriptions, they should be warned that the appearance of their medication may change from prescription to prescription.

The problem of noncompliance

Noncompliance is a significant problem with anticonvulsants and is a potent cause of poor control. A full explanation of each drug's side-effect profile and its potential interactions is essential and appears conducive to improved compliance. Drugs that are given once or twice a day are preferred to ones needing more frequent prescriptions. Slow-release preparations allow drug regimens to be simplified.

Mechanisms of action (Fig. 24.5.1.6)

The prime role of GABA-mediated inhibition in the epileptic process implies that drugs that enhance $GABA_A$-receptor-mediated inhibition will have anticonvulsant activity. The $GABA_A$-receptor complex comprises at least three subunits—α, β, and δ—which appear to combine as a five-membered structure forming an anion-permeable channel. Both barbiturates and benzodiazepines act by potentiating $GABA_A$-mediated inhibition. The barbiturates bind to the β subunit to potentiate action of endogenous agonist GABA and prolong the opening time of the chloride ion channel. Benzodiazepines bind to the α subunit to potentiate the action of GABA and increase the frequency of opening of the chloride ion channel. GABA is metabolized by GABA transaminase. Vigabatrin irreversibly binds to GABA transaminase to inhibit degradation of GABA and thereby elevates brain GABA levels. GABA-mediated inhibition can also be enhanced by blocking GABA uptake into glia and neurons after its release into the synaptic cleft during synaptic transmission.

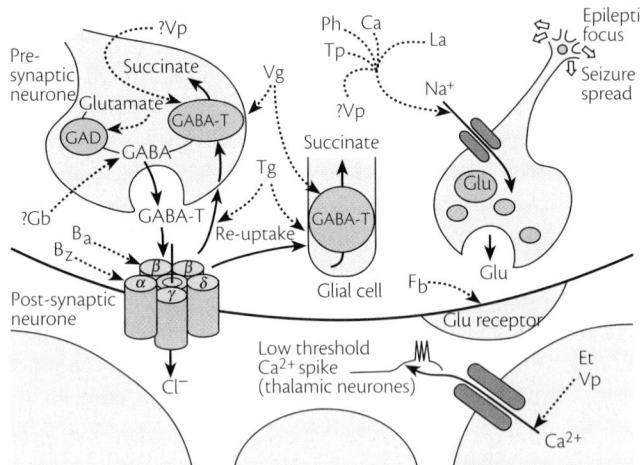

Fig. 24.5.1.6 Mechanism of action of some of the anticonvulsants. Ba, barbiturate; Bz, benzodiazepine; Ca, carbamazepine; Et, ethosuximide; Fb, felbamate; Gb, gabapentin; La, lamotrigine; Ph, phenytoin; Tg, tiagabine; Tp, topiramate; Vg, vigabatrin; Vp, valproate.

Tiagabine blocks uptake of synaptically released GABA into both presynaptic neurons and glial cells, allowing GABA to remain at its site of action for longer periods. Gabapentin acts presynaptically to promote GABA synthesis or release.

The second major neurotransmitter system involved in the genesis of epileptic activity is excitatory utilizing glutamate and, perhaps as aspartate as neurotransmitters. They act on several different receptors including α-amino-3-hydroxy-5-methylisoxazole-proprionic acid (AMPA) and N-methyl-D-aspartate (NMDA). The NMDA receptor is activated by glutamate or aspartate together with glycine. Blockade of the NMDA receptor results in antiepileptic effects.

Voltage-dependent calcium ion currents are thought to be of importance in the genesis of epileptic events. Ethosuximide acts by inhibition of one class of voltage-dependent calcium ion currents (T currents). Valproate may have a similar role. Pregabalin binds to the $\alpha_2\delta$ subunit of the voltage-dependent calcium channel.

Regulation of sodium channels also appears of relevance in the modification of the epileptic process. Phenytoin, carbamazepine, and possibly valproate reduce the rate of recovery from inactivation of depolarized voltage-dependent sodium channels, thereby blocking sustained repetitive firing of action potentials in depolarized neurons. Lamotrigine inhibits glutamate and aspartate release, suggesting that it may act at voltage-dependent sodium channels to decrease the presynaptic release of glutamate. Lamotrigine may have additional effects on calcium channels. Oxcarbazepine may act by reducing glutamate release via a blocking action on presynaptic calcium channels. Topiramate influences sodium channel activity, suggesting that its anticonvulsant properties are similar to those of phenytoin. Felbamate probably acts primarily through its effects on the NMDA receptor.

Selected drugs

Carbamazepine

Carbamazepine is a first-line drug for both partial seizures and generalized tonic–clonic seizures. In its standard form, it needs to be given three times a day, but a slow-release preparation allows twice-daily prescribing. Dosage ranges from 300 mg/day to

1600 mg/day. Sedation is common and the drug should be introduced slowly. A drug rash occurs in perhaps 3% of patients and demands immediate drug withdrawal. Signs of intoxication include drowsiness, blurred vision, and dizziness. Leucopenia occurs and can lead to a frank aplastic anaemia. Hyponatraemia and oedema are recognized features, associated with a mild degree of inappropriate antidiuretic hormone production. The drug influences atrioventricular conduction and should not be given to patients with atrioventricular conduction abnormalities unless they are already paced. The relationship between dosage and plasma concentrations is linear. Carbamazepine is a liver enzyme inducer and is teratogenic (see below).

Sodium valproate

Sodium valproate is considered, at least by some doctors, to be the drug of choice for all epilepsy types. It is not enzyme inducing, and therefore does not influence the metabolism of the oral contraceptive. Liver toxicity is a recognized, although rare, hazard. Elevated serum liver enzyme activities are more common, but usually return to normal without the need for drug withdrawal. Thrombocytopenia occurs rarely. Gastrointestinal effects are fairly common. Nausea and weight loss are seen, but appetite stimulation with weight gain is more common. Tremor occurs as a dose-related effect and hair loss, of a mild degree, is not uncommon; after a few months, hair regrowth occurs, often more curly than before. Sedation is less troublesome than with other anticonvulsants. Disturbances of menstruation are recognized. It has been suggested that the drug can trigger polycystic ovarian disease, although this may not necessarily translate to a clinically relevant condition. The dose ranges from 600 mg/day to 2500 mg/day and it is given two or three times a day. A slow-release preparation can be given once daily. Plasma levels are not a useful guide to efficacy.

Other drugs

Phenytoin

Experience with phenytoin is vast and, despite its side-effect profile and complex pharmacokinetics, large quantities of the drug continue to be prescribed. A 100-mg tablet, in the United Kingdom, costs approximately one-thirtieth of the price of a comparable dose of lamotrigine. The drug is effective in both generalized tonic–clonic seizures and the partial seizures. It has a long half-life, and can be given once daily, conveniently at bedtime. Sedation is common. Toxic effects, generally dose related, include drowsiness, ataxia, confusion, blurred vision, and dizziness. Most patients who are intoxicated with the drug have nystagmus. Permanent cerebellar ataxia and peripheral neuropathy are recorded. Other side effects or toxic effects include rashes, gum hypertrophy, thickening of the facial features, chorea, and sleep disturbance. The drug is a potent enzyme inducer and is teratogenic. The relationship between dosage and plasma concentrations is nonlinear. Once the dose exceeds 300 mg/day, increments should be pegged to 50 mg or even 25 mg at a time.

Lamotrigine

Lamotrigine is licensed for both generalized and partial seizures. Occasionally it exacerbates myoclonus. Doses seldom exceed 400 mg/day. A drug rash occurs in about 3% of patients. It interacts with enzyme-inducing anticonvulsants, which lower its plasma level. Valproate enhances lamotrigine levels. The drug can be given once daily. Originally said to be nonteratogenic, recent studies suggest that this is not the case.

Phenobarbital

Phenobarbital is a very effective anticonvulsant but often badly tolerated. Children may become hyperactive on the drug and adults (particularly older people) heavily sedated. Doses of up to 180 mg/day are used. It has a long half-life and can be given once daily. Rapid withdrawal of phenobarbital in patients who do not have epilepsy can trigger seizures. Over-rapid withdrawal in someone with epilepsy can trigger status epilepticus. Methyl phenobarbital is largely converted to phenobarbital by the liver and phenobarbital is the main metabolite of primidone, although primidone's other metabolite, phenylethylmalonamide, probably possesses anticonvulsant activity.

Vigabatrin

Vigabatrin is probably a more potent anticonvulsant than many of the other recently introduced drugs. Increasingly, it has been recognized to cause retinal damage. Up to a third of patients develop concentric constriction of the visual fields, more marked nasally than temporally. The defect is often asymptomatic and probably irreversible. It is now recommended that vigabatrin should be used only as add-on therapy where other combinations have been unsuccessful. Dosage should not exceed 3 g/day. Regular visual field analysis is mandatory.

Gabapentin

Gabapentin is used as add-on therapy for partial seizures with or without secondary generalization. Up to 4.8 g is given in three divided doses. The drug is generally well tolerated and does not interact with other anticonvulsants. Its anticonvulsant effect appears to be relatively weak.

Ethosuximide

Ethosuximide is seldom used in adults as its role is confined to the treatment of absence seizures. Gastrointestinal disturbances are common along with drowsiness, dizziness, and ataxia. Agranulocytosis or aplastic anaemia has rarely been encountered. The dose range is usually 1 to 1.5 g daily.

Clonazepam

Clonazepam is effective for tonic–clonic seizures but is particularly valuable in the treatment of myoclonic epilepsy. Sedation is a major problem, and the drug must be introduced cautiously. The maximum tolerated dose is about 8 mg/day.

Clobazam

Tolerance to clobazam tends to develop fairly readily. It is sedative. Adult dosage ranges from 30 mg daily to 60 mg daily. Used intermittently it can be very effective for the treatment of catamenial epilepsy.

Acetazolamide

Use of this drug is largely confined to childhood epilepsies.

Topiramate

This drug is licensed both for primary generalized tonic–clonic seizures and as adjunct therapy for partial seizures. It is sedative and must be introduced slowly. The total daily dose (given as a twice-daily regimen) seldom exceeds 400 mg. Nausea, anorexia, and weight loss are encountered. Behavioural disturbances are reported, including emotional lability, mood change, and aggression. There is an increased incidence of renal stones in those taking the drug.

Tiagabine

Tiagabine is a GABA uptake inhibitor, resulting in increased synaptic GABA levels. The initial dose in adults is 4 to 5 mg twice daily. Most studies have used 32 to 56 mg/day, in three divided doses. The drug is licensed as add-on therapy in refractory epilepsy. Side effects include dizziness, tiredness, tremor, and altered mood.

Oxcarbazepine

This drug is closely related to carbamazepine but is a less potent hepatic enzyme inducer. It is licensed as monotherapy or adjunctive therapy in partial seizures with or without secondary generalization. Its side-effect profile is similar to that of carbamazepine. Patients who are hypersensitive to carbamazepine should not receive oxcarbazepine. The dosage range lies between 600 and 2400 mg daily, in adults.

Levetiracetam

The mode of action of levetiracetam is not understood. It is not metabolized in the liver nor does it inhibit or induce hepatic enzymes. There are no known interactions with other anticonvulsants. Two-thirds of an oral dose are excreted unchanged in the urine. A quarter is metabolized to an inactive metabolite, also excreted in the urine.

Levetiracetam was originally licensed as adjunctive therapy in the treatment of partial seizures with or without secondary generalization and was licensed for use in idiopathic generalized epilepsy in 2006. The daily dose in adults ranges from 1000 mg to 3000 mg. The dose needs to be adjusted in the presence of renal impairment. It is not advised for use in pregnancy.

Side effects include asthenia, somnolence, headache, gastrointestinal disturbances, mood changes, and skin rash. Behavioural and neuropsychiatric side effects have been noted.

Pregabalin

Similar to gabapentin, pregabalin binds to the $\alpha_2\delta$ subunit of the voltage-dependent calcium channel in the CNS. It is used as adjunctive therapy in partial seizures with or without secondary generalization. Adverse effects include dizziness, drowsiness, blurred vision, and ataxia. There are no interactions with other anticonvulsants.

Zonisamide

Zonisamide is unrelated to other antiseizure agents. Its effect appears to come through action at sodium and calcium channels. It is licensed as adjunctive therapy in patients with partial seizures with or without secondary generalization. Somnolence is a common side effect. The drug is a sulphonamide and various toxic effects have been described including the Stevens–Johnson syndrome. It is teratogenic.

Felbamate

Felbamate is licensed for use in partial seizures. The drug has serious side effects, including liver failure and aplastic anaemia, and is used only as last-line therapy.

Particular issues

Enzyme induction

Drugs that induce liver enzymes (phenytoin, phenobarbital, carbamazepine, topiramate, and possibly lamotrigine) will alter the pharmacokinetics of other agents or drugs that undergo hepatic metabolism. Women taking an oral contraceptive pill need to take a preparation containing at least 50 µg ethinylestradiol. If breakthrough bleeding still occurs, the dose of oestrogen can be increased to a maximum of 100 µg daily. Alternatively, an injectable long-term contraceptive can be used. The interactions between anticonvulsants are complex, another reason for avoiding drug combinations where possible.

All the enzyme-inducing anticonvulsants have the potential for accelerating vitamin D metabolism. Those individuals at risk for developing vitamin D deficiency (e.g. due to poor nutrition) are at risk of developing osteomalacia or rickets when taking certain anticonvulsants.

Drug monitoring

Anticonvulsant levels are measured far too frequently. There are specific circumstances where their measurement is of value:

- to ascertain compliance
- to monitor dosage adjustment with phenytoin
- to ascertain the unpredictable effect of combining anticonvulsant preparations.

Phenytoin undergoes saturatable hepatic metabolism. Regular monitoring of the serum level is advisable, particularly after dose adjustment. Occasionally, measurement of the levels of carbamazepine, phenobarbital, and ethosuximide aids management, particularly where epilepsy control has been poor. Carbamazepine epoxide, a metabolite of carbamazepine, can sometimes be the cause of carbamazepine toxicity even when carbamazepine levels are in the therapeutic range. There is no value in the routine monitoring of levels of valproate, vigabatrin, lamotrigine, gabapentin, topiramate, clonazepam, or clobazam.

When measuring levels, the same time after the last dose should be used, wherever possible. Examples of therapeutic serum levels are given in Table 24.5.1.2. The therapeutic ranges of the anticonvulsants should be interpreted with caution. Some patients respond to a drug despite subtherapeutic levels. Others need toxic levels to achieve seizure control and can often tolerate such levels without overt difficulty.

Pregnancy

There is an increased risk of congenital malformations in women who have taken anticonvulsants during pregnancy (approximately 4 to 8% overall risk). Most evidence has accumulated for phenytoin, phenobarbital, valproate, and carbamazepine. There are very few data on the newer anticonvulsants. The critical period for development of the major malformations is from 3 weeks' gestation to 8 weeks' gestation.

Phenytoin and phenobarbital

Both these drugs are associated with cardiovascular malformations (2% risk) and cleft lip/palate syndromes (1.8% risk).

Valproate

Valproate is associated with an increased incidence of neural tube defects along with other midline abnormalities such as hypospadias, partial agenesis of the corpus callosum, and ventricular septal defects. The risk approaches 10% and is probably dose related. There is some evidence that exposure in utero leads to subsequent neurodevelopmental delay.

Table 24.5.1.2 Anticonvulsants, dosage range, and serum levels (where appropriate)

Anticonvulsant	Typical adult dose levels range (mg/24 h)	Therapeutic serum (μmol/l)
Sodium valproate	800–2500	
Phenytoin	150–350	40–80
Carbamazepine	600–1600	17–42
Phenobarbital	60–180	65–170
Lamotrigine	200–400	
Gabapentin	900–3600	
Vigabatrin	1000–3000	
Topiramate	200–400	
Tiagabine	30–45	
Ethosuximide	1000–1500	285–700
Clonazepam	2–8	
Clobazam	30–60	
Oxcarbazepine	600–2400	
Levetiracetam	1000–3000	

Carbamazepine

Carbamazepine is associated with spina bifida (1% risk) and hypospadias.

A folic acid supplement of 5 mg daily should be given to women with epilepsy who are taking valproate or carbamazepine and who are contemplating pregnancy. Doses of valproate should be less than 1000 mg/day if possible and slow-release forms of the drug prescribed. For women on other anticonvulsants, a dose of 0.4 mg/day of folic acid suffices.

Seizure frequency increases in pregnancy in about a third of patients with epilepsy. Tonic–clonic seizures are associated with an increased risk of miscarriage. Vitamin K at 20 mg/day should be given in the last month of pregnancy in women on enzyme-inducing drugs to reduce the risk of haemorrhagic disease of the newborn baby.

The epilepsy risk in the offspring of an affected patient is around 2 to 4% but higher where the epilepsy of the parent has a strong genetic basis.

Breastfeeding

All the commonly used anticonvulsants are present in low concentrations in breast milk. If the mother is on a barbiturate or a benzodiazepine, significant sedation of the baby is possible. If breastfeeding then ceases abruptly, a withdrawal reaction can occur in the infant with tremor and agitation.

Drug withdrawal

Generally medication is continued until at least a 2- to 3-year period free of seizures has been established. Approximately two-thirds of patients remain fit free after drug withdrawal. Factors known to predispose to recurrence include neurological abnormalities on examination, an underlying structural basis for the epilepsy, the need for multiple drug therapy, and a history of difficulty in establishing initial control. The EEG is of limited value in predicting outcome

although rather better in children than in adults. Any drug withdrawal should be gradual, say over 3 to 6 months. Absence seizures usually remit spontaneously in late adolescence, but juvenile myoclonic epilepsy tends to recur after drug withdrawal.

Driving

In the United Kingdom, driving must cease for 6 months after any type of seizure, providing that the patient has been assessed by an appropriate specialist and no relevant abnormalities found on investigation. If a nocturnal pattern of seizures has been established for 3 years, driving can then continue even if nocturnal seizures are still occurring. The Driver and Vehicle Licensing Agency (DVLA) prefers patients not to drive during a period of drug withdrawal, and for 6 months after the withdrawal has been completed. For drivers of large goods vehicles, a 5-year period of freedom must be established, and the criteria defined above again met. Furthermore, a continuing liability to epilepsy has to be excluded.

Status epilepticus

Status epilepticus has already been defined. The most common type is tonic–clonic status. The most common precipitants are sudden anticonvulsant withdrawal, poor compliance in a patient with known epilepsy, and alcohol abuse. The mortality figures for status epilepticus have varied substantially from series to series. In one recently published, prospective, population-based study, the overall incidence was estimated at 41 to 61/100 000 person-years with a mortality rate of 22%. Incidence rises in older people, as does mortality. From other series, overall mortality rates lie between 8 and 37%. At least half the cases occur in the absence of previous epilepsy. Although noncompliance and subtherapeutic drug levels are often quoted as causes of status, several studies have established that most individuals with epilepsy who present in status have therapeutic drug levels at or around the time of presentation. Status in the absence of previous epilepsy is followed by unprovoked seizures in about half the cases.

The diagnosis is by no means straightforward. In one study, half the patients transferred to a specialist centre for management of their status were either in pseudostatus or in drug-induced coma. The diagnosis of pseudostatus should be considered if the attacks are atypical or if the status does not respond to initial therapy. Subtle forms of status can be difficult to recognize, often presenting as coma.

Analysis of immediate management of patients in status suggests that many are given inadequate loading and maintenance doses of anticonvulsants. The patient should be moved away from possible hazard, such as broken glass, an airway established, and oxygen administered. Lorazepam is probably the drug of choice. It is given in a dose of 0.1 mg/kg intravenously at the rate of 2 mg/min. Alternatives included diazepam (Diazemuls) given intravenously in a dose of 10 to 20 mg at a rate of 5 mg/min or clonazepam given in a dose of 1 mg by slow intravenous injection.

Using the intravenous route, 50% glucose should be administered to a total volume of 50 ml after blood has been taken to establish the glucose concentration. Thiamine (Pabrinex I/V High Potency) in a dose of 250 mg should be given by slow intravenous injection over 10 min if there is suspicion of alcohol withdrawal, but remember that the infusion can produce an anaphylactic response. In addition to plasma glucose measurement, blood should be taken for urea, electrolytes (including calcium and magnesium), acid–base balance, liver function tests, and full blood count. A serum sample should be stored in case anticonvulsant or alcohol levels are required subsequently. Blood cultures should be performed if the patient is febrile.

If immediate therapy is successful and the patient is receiving phenytoin or valproate, those drugs can be given intravenously before reverting to oral therapy. If the patient is not on anticonvulsants, a phenytoin infusion at 20 mg/kg in 0.9% sodium chloride should be given at a maximum rate of 50 mg/min. An alternative is fosphenytoin, a water-soluble drug, which is metabolized to phenytoin with a half-life of 8 to 15 min. It is given intravenously in the same dose at 150 mg/min in order to achieve a comparable effect. The drug is more expensive than phenytoin but causes less phlebitis and less hypotension, and is better tolerated.

Midazolam has been developed for intranasal use and may prove of value where immediate intravenous access is difficult, e.g. in young children.

If phenytoin infusion is unsuccessful, valproate infusions can be used, with 25 mg/kg as a loading dose delivered at 3 to 6 mg/kg per min. If seizures continue phenobarbital can be considered, given at 20 mg/kg intravenously at 50 to 75 mg/min. Intramuscular or rectal paraldehyde is now seldom used, most experts suggesting a move instead to thiopental, propofol, or midazolam.

Propofol or midazolam is rapidly metabolized and has fewer hypotensive effects than the barbiturates. The suggested dose of propofol is 3 to 5 mg/kg followed by a continuous infusion of 5 to 10 mg/kg per h. Midazolam is given in an intravenous bolus of 0.2 mg/kg followed by 0.1 to 0.4 mg/kg per h.

It has been suggested that a more aggressive approach aimed at EEG burst suppression, rather than simply seizure suppression, reduces the risk of seizure recurrence after initial control.

For all the therapies used in patients with refractory status, intensive care placement is essential with the patient intubated and haemodynamic monitoring in place.

Sudden death

Patients with epilepsy have an increased risk of death compared with age- and sex-matched controls. Sudden unexpected death in epilepsy predominates in younger age groups and in those with more severe epilepsy. The median incidence in patients with refractory epilepsy has been estimated at 3.6/1000. It is likely that most of the deaths are the result of unwitnessed seizures producing respiratory complications, cardiac arrhythmias, or both.

Surgery

Despite optimal treatment, some 30% of patients with new-onset seizures continue to have attacks. A prerequisite in patient selection for surgery is accurate localization of the epileptic discharge and understanding of circumstances where a resection might prove detrimental in terms of functional deficit.

Assessment for epilepsy surgery demands localization techniques incorporating seizure characteristics, electrophysiological recording, and imaging. Equally important is the recognition by the physician that certain epilepsy syndromes are likely to be resistant to medical therapy and that early rather than delayed referral for surgical opinion is beneficial. Mesial temporal lobe epilepsy, secondary to hippocampal sclerosis, is the most common cause of medically refractory partial seizures. In most such patients, a unilateral structural abnormality can be confidently established, resection of which leads to a 70% chance of remission.

Disabling neurological complications after surgery, such as hemianopia, hemiparesis, or dysphasia, occur in about 2% of patients. Depression and psychosis are recognized complications of temporal lobectomy.

MRI characteristics of mesial temporal sclerosis include atrophy or increased signal on T_2-weighted images. The presence of atrophy is the best predictor for a good surgical outcome. Besides visual inspection, measurement of hippocampal volume and techniques for measuring the T_2 signal change are used to improve sensitivity.

SPECT and PET measure the changes in cerebral blood flow and cerebral glucose metabolism, respectively, that accompany the epileptic process. Both have relatively high sensitivity and moderate specificity for the diagnosis of temporal lobe seizures, but lower sensitivity for epilepsy arising at other sites. Interictal PET and ictal SPECT produce very similar results in predicting outcome after temporal lobectomy.

Proton MRS can contribute to recognition of the lateralization of the epileptic focus and to the identification of those patients with bilateral changes who are less likely to respond to surgery.

Continuous surface EEG monitoring is usually undertaken as part of the work-up for patients being considered for surgical intervention. The technique, however, has limitations. It often fails to detect seizure activity arising in areas distant from surface electrodes, such as the orbitofrontal cortex, and may falsely lateralize foci, particularly in the presence of large lesions. For improving EEG localization, some form of intracranial recording is necessary. Depth electrodes are used to sample deeper structures such as the hippocampus. Electrocorticography is performed at the time of surgery. Subdural electrodes, sometimes with depth electrodes, measure directly from the surface of the exposed brain.

Other less commonly performed surgical procedures include neocortical resections, lesionectomies, hemispherectomies, multilobar resections, and corpus callostomy. Hemispherectomy is performed when a diffuse epileptogenic region has been localized within one hemisphere, the other hemisphere being normal. As an alternative hemispherotomy has been devised, attempting a complete deafferentation of hemispheric neural connections with maximal preservation of cerebral tissue. Division of the corpus callosum is performed in patients with severe secondary generalized epilepsy who have disabling drop attacks. Cortical dysplasia is increasingly recognized as a cause of intractable epilepsy. MRI criteria have been developed to allow recognition of areas of focal cortical dysplasia and assist in planning the extent of cortical resection. Multiple subpial transection disconnects horizontally coursing cortical fibres over 5 mm apart while preserving vertically oriented projection fibres. Although the procedure is designed to reduce postoperative neurological deficit, it is probably less effective in seizure control compared with cortical resection.

Vagal nerve stimulation

Vagal nerve stimulation is achieved through the implantation of a small stimulator on the left vagus. The exact mechanism of action remains uncertain. The nucleus of the tractus solitarius, the main terminus for vagal afferents, has projections to the locus ceruleus, raphe nuclei, reticular formation, and other brainstem nuclei, which have been shown to influence cerebral seizure susceptibility. In patients with chronic refractory partial seizures, there is a reduction in the number of seizures, rather than their elimination. There is a suggestion that effectiveness increases with the passage of time.

The long-term role of this procedure is not yet determined, nor its role in the management of generalized seizures.

Psychiatric aspects of epilepsy

A substantial proportion of patients with poorly controlled epilepsy are likely to have psychiatric symptoms. Those symptoms may partly reflect the underlying structural process in the brain, the effects of repeated seizures, the effects of any social stigma attached to the diagnosis, and as a reaction to the patient's anticonvulsants. Psychiatric symptoms occurring around the time of the seizures tend to be affective or cognitive if before or with the seizure, but psychotic afterwards. Additional psychiatric morbidity is encountered as an interictal phenomenon. It correlates with multiple drug use, the serum concentrations of those drugs, and certain of the anticonvulsants including the newer agents, such as lamotrigine, vigabatrin, and topiramate. In addition, an adverse psychiatric outcome may follow epilepsy surgery and vagal nerve stimulation.

Patients with poorly controlled epilepsy may require referral to a clinical psychologist, partly with a view to helping in the psychological adjustment to the condition, and partly to identify specific areas of cognitive impairment that might require attention.

The role of specialist nurses and the general practitioner

Patients almost inevitably indicate some dissatisfaction with the level of information and support that they receive for their epilepsy. Studies suggest that improvement in these areas can occur using a specialist nurse, working either in general practice or in association with a hospital clinic. Where joint care is to be achieved between general practice and hospital, it is vital that good quality communication and record keeping are achieved. Giving the patient files that document vital information, including their drug regimen, is valuable. Patients prefer the continuity of care achievable through seeing the same doctor at each consultation and are more likely to adhere to medical advice under those circumstances.

Prognosis

Prognosis for patients with epilepsy followed in the community is considerably better than for a hospital-based population. Fig. 24.5.1.7 records the percentage of patients in remission (defined as being seizure free for 5 years). Factors that influence outcome adversely include a combination of complex partial and tonic–clonic seizures, clustering of seizures, abnormal physical signs, and the presence of learning difficulties. The influence of antiepileptic drugs on the natural history remains unknown and it has been suggested that a proportion of patients with epilepsy enter permanent remission regardless of treatment.

Overall care

For many patients, shared care among hospital, a specialist nurse, and general practice is ideal. Such an arrangement necessitates a reasonable level of epilepsy experience from the GP, allowing many issues to be resolved without recourse to hospital consultation. The complexities of epilepsy care in terms of new drug developments, issues relating to pregnancy, the question of nonepileptic seizures,

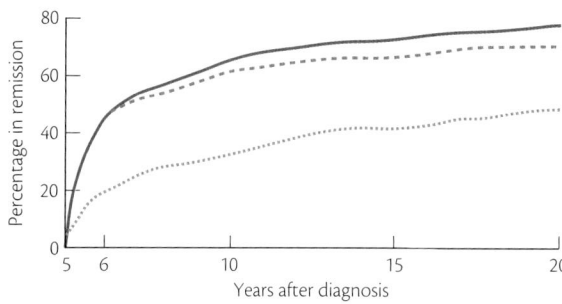

Fig. 24.5.1.7 Probability of seizure recurrence after a first epileptic seizure. The top curve indicates the percentage of patients achieving a 5-year period of remission at any time during the 20-year period of follow-up. The middle curve refers to those patients in remission for at least the last 5 years at the time of sampling. The difference between the top and middle curves represents those patients who have relapsed after achieving a 5-year remission. The bottom curve indicates the probability of being in remission while not taking anticonvulsants. The curves flatten off, indicating that remission becomes less likely the longer the seizures persist.

(Data from the National General Practice Study of Epilepsy, reproduced by kind permission.)

and the potential for surgery for many patients with poorly controlled epilepsy make the case for epilepsy clinics staffed by doctors with a particular interest in epilepsy.

Further reading

Arruda F, *et al.* (1996). Mesial atrophy and outcome after amygdalohippocampectomy or temporal lobe removal. *Ann Neurol*, **40**, 446–50.

Berg AT, Shinnar S (1994). Relapse following discontinuation of anti-epileptic drugs: a meta-analysis. *Neurology*, **44**, 601–8.

Binnie CD, Stefan H (1999). Modern electroencephalography: its role in epilepsy management. *Clin Neurophysiol*, **110**, 1671–97.

Crawford P, *et al.* (1999). Best practice guidelines for the management of women with epilepsy. *Seizure*, **8**, 201–17.

Dichter MA (1994). Emerging insights into mechanisms of epilepsy: implications for new antiepileptic drug development. *Epilepsia*, **35** Suppl 4, S51–7.

Duncan JS (1997). Imaging and epilepsy. *Brain*, **120**, 339–77. [An excellent review article, covering all aspects of imaging, including MRI, MRS, SPECT, and PET.]

Goldstein LH (1990). Behavioural and cognitive–behavioural treatment for epilepsy: a progress review. *Br J Clin Psychol*, **29**, 257–69.

Kotsopoulos IA, *et al.* (2002). Systematic review and meta-analysis of incidence studies of epilepsy and unprovoked seizures. *Epilepsia*, **43**, 1402–9.

Krishnamoorthy ES, Brown RJ, Trimble M (2001). Personality and psychopathology in non epileptic attack disorder: a prospective study. *Epilepsy Behav*, **2**, 418–22.

Lempert T, Bauer M, Schmidt D (1994). Syncope: a videometric analysis of 56 episodes of transient cerebral hypoxia. *Ann Neurol*, **36**, 233–7.

Manford M, *et al.* (1992). The national general practice study of epilepsy applied to epilepsy in a general population. *Arch Neurol*, **49**, 801–8.

Mattson RH, *et al.* (1985). Comparison of carbamazepine, phenobarbital, phenytoin, and primidone in partial and secondarily generalized tonic–clonic seizures. *NJEM*, **313**, 145–51.

Polkey CE (2004). Clinical outcome of epilepsy surgery. *Curr Opin Neurol*, **17**, 173–8.

Raymond AA, *et al.* (1995). Abnormalities of gyration, heterotopias, tuberous sclerosis, focal cortical dysplasia, microdysgenesis, dysembryoplastic neuroepithelial tumour and dysgenesis of the

---

archicortex in epilepsy. Clinical, EEG and neuro-imaging features in 100 adults patients. *Brain*, **118**, 629–60.
Ridsdale L, *et al.* (1997). The effects of nurse-run clinics for patients with epilepsy in general practice. *BMJ*, **314**, 120–2.
Saygi S, *et al.* (1992). Frontal lobe partial seizures and psychogenic seizures: comparison of clinical and ictal characteristics. *Neurology*, **42**, 1274–7.
Schmidt D (2001). Vagus nerve stimulation for the treatment of epilepsy. *Epilepsy Behav*, **2**(Pt 2), S1–5.
Tan NC, Mulley JC, Berkovic SF (2004). Genetic association studies in epilepsy: 'the truth is out there'. *Epilepsia*, **45**, 1429–42.
Tellez-Zenteno JF, Ronquillo LH, Wiebe S (2005). Sudden unexpected death in epilepsy: evidence-based analysis of incidence and risk factors. *Epilepsy Res*, **65**, 101–15.
Treiman DM (2001). Therapy of status epilepticus in adults and children. *Curr Opin Neurol*, **14**, 203–10.
Wallace H, *et al.* (1997). *Adults with poorly controlled epilepsy*. Royal College of Physicians of London, London. [An excellent short monograph with a deceptive title. Many issues are covered, including the role of electroencephalography, neuroimaging, and the issues relating to contraception and pregnancy.]

24.5.2 Narcolepsy

David Parkes

Essentials

Narcolepsy is the specific syndrome of daytime sleepiness with cataplexy, where there is a sudden loss of muscle tone—often provoked by the anticipation of emotions—leading to a tendency to fall, mouth opening, dysarthria or mutism, and facial muscle jerking. It is associated with loss of hypocretin (orexin) neurons in the hypothalamus, hypocretin-1 concentrations in the cerebrospinal fluid below 100 ng/litre, and the HLA genotype DQ B1*0602. Once established, narcolepsy is lifelong; spontaneous recovery does not occur. Treatment—which is essential to restore school performance, work, driving ability and quality of life—is with stimulant (e.g. amphetamine) and anticataplectic (e.g. clomipramine) drugs, supported by a 15-min nap once or twice a day.

Clinical features

The prevalence of narcolepsy in western Europe is about 4 per 10 000. Reported rates worldwide vary 100-fold, in part due to difficulties in case ascertainment and inexact definitions of 'narcolepsy'. Narcolepsy is as common in men as it is in women. It usually starts in adolescence, with a second peak at age 30 to 40 years. However, the age at presentation extends from under 1 to over 70. The initial symptom is usually sleepiness, followed by cataplexy within 2 years. Very occasionally this order is reversed or the gap prolonged to several decades.

Cataplexy is provoked by the anticipation of emotions such as laughter, startle, excitement, or anger, but not by fear. There is a sudden loss of muscle tone with a tendency to fall, mouth opening, dysarthria, or mutism, and facial muscle jerking. Most attacks are mild and last a few seconds but self-injury can occur. Attack frequency is markedly variable between individuals. Cataplexy is comparable to the atonia of rapid eye movement (REM) sleep but (usually) without loss of awareness. As cataplexy is seldom witnessed by the doctor, an unequivocal history using clear language is essential for diagnosis.

Sleep attacks are usually short, increased by monotony, and have a 2- to 4-h cyclicity. Automatic behaviour and failure of self-monitoring also reduce wakefulness. Sleepiness is more disabling than cataplexy and causes chronic school and work failure, broken relationships, frustration, embarrassment, poor self-image, and depression.

Insomnia, sleep paralysis, REM sleep behavioural disorder, leg restlessness, and vivid dream intrusion at the wake–sleep boundaries (hypnagogic and hypnopompic hallucinations) are common, but not specific to narcolepsy. Despite daytime sleepiness, the total sleep period over 24 h is normal due to multiple nocturnal arousals. The old concept of four symptoms—sleepiness, cataplexy, sleep paralysis, and hypnagogic hallucinations—needs revision.

Narcolepsy is often considered by the public as a 'psychiatric', 'odd', or 'amusing' condition, overused by neurologists for case demonstration and considered by primary care doctors as an excuse for laziness or to obtain amphetamines. However, early diagnosis, school and work appraisal, driving assessment, and adequate treatment are essential. Diagnosis is supported by a sleep–wake diary with simple sleepiness and cataplexy rating scales (Box 24.5.2.1).

HLA association

Ninety-five per cent of white people with narcolepsy have the HLA D-related (DR) serotype DR2 and genotype *DQ-B1*0602*. The DR association is slightly different in other ethnic groups. The HLA type is not specific to narcolepsy, being present in 25 to 30% of white people, only 1 in 500 of whom has narcolepsy. There is no present evidence of an immune defect in narcolepsy, or of definite involvement of HLA systems in normal sleep mechanisms.

One to dour per cent of all people with narcolepsy report a fully affected first-degree relative, although other relatives may have daytime sleepiness without cataplexy. In the few reported studies of monozygotic twins, there is disease discordance in up to 70% of pairs—and, in one case, cerebrospinal fluid (CSF) hypocretin-1 discordance.

Narcolepsy appears to be caused by an environmental agent in a genetically susceptible individual. The nature of this is unknown.

Hypocretin

Hypocretin-1 and -2 are neuropeptides made in dorsal and lateral hypothalamic neurons that project to the cortex, thalamus, brainstem areas, and spinal cord. They are implicated in the regulation of feeding and energy as well as the sleep–wake cycle.

In narcolepsy hypocretin neurons are lost or damaged. In normal individuals and those with non-narcoleptic sleep and neurological disorders, with the exception of rare cases of the Guillain–Barré syndrome and after head injury, CSF hypocretin-1 levels are above 200 ng/l. In around 95% of patients with narcolepsy–cataplexy hypocretin is undetectable or below 100 ng/l. The few exceptions are usually in individuals with familial or HLA-negative narcolepsy, who in any case may not have clear-cut cataplexy.

No CSF or serum antibodies to hypocretin are present. A hypocretin receptor gene mutation has been shown in dogs with narcolepsy, but not in humans with typical narcolepsy–cataplexy.

Box 24.5.2.1 Clinical features of narcoleptic syndrome

Cataplexy
- Laughter-triggered sudden antigravity and facial muscle atonia

Daytime sleepiness
- Irresistible short sleep periods at 2- to 4-h intervals, subalertness, and automatic behaviour, foremost with monotony

Night-sleep
- Latency short—seconds or minutes
- Interrupted, with frequent arousals and complaint of insomnia

Parasomnias
- Sleep paralysis, nightmares, motor restlessness, rapid eye movement (REM) behavioural disorder, minor sleep apnoea all common

Dreams
- Hallucinatory recall at unusual times: when awake, at sleep onset as well as on waking

---

Pathophysiology of narcolepsy

In narcolepsy sleep consolidation across 24 h is poor and the normal sleep cycle sequence of slow-wave sleep–REM sleep is reversed, accounting for the intrusion of dream mentation at sleep onset as well as of sleep paralysis on waking. Adult sleep patterns are not established until adolescence, and the precipitants of cataplexy in young children may be atypical.

Polysomnography in narcolepsy will detect additional pathology such as sleep apnoea, although this is usually asymptomatic and also reflects the high tendency to fall asleep in the daytime and the reversed normal sleep-phase pattern (Box 24.5.2.2). However, findings are much less specific and sensitive for diagnosis than a definite history of cataplexy, and in cases with an indefinite history may confuse rather than clarify. HLA tests will not confirm narcolepsy, although the diagnosis is unlikely if the DR2 antigen is absent.

Symptomatic narcolepsy

Typical narcolepsy–cataplexy has been associated with a wide range of other disorders. These are mostly uncommon and rarely if ever cause problems in differential diagnosis. In most cases there is an

---

Box 24.5.2.2 Investigations in the narcoleptic syndrome

- HLA—*DQ-B1*0602* allele present in 90–95%
- Hypocretin-1—lumbar daytime CSF hypocretin-1 undetectable or <110 ng/l (radioimmunoassay) in over 95% (normal level >200 ng/l)
- Polysomnography—short sleep latency by day in multiple sleep latency test (<15 min in 40% of cases); REM (rapid eye movement) activity at sleep onset (day and night: inconstant); detect sleep apnoea.

---

obvious hypothalamic, pontine, or midbrain lesion. The occasional association of narcolepsy with multiple sclerosis may result not from a brainstem lesion but from a common genetic predisposition with an over-representation of the same HLA DR antigen in both conditions.

Differential diagnosis

Sleep apnoea accompanied by sleepiness is much more common than the narcoleptic syndrome, present in up to 4% of men and 2% of women. It does not cause cataplexy.

In a small minority of cases of narcolepsy, cataplexy has not been established at presentation or the history is uncertain. Here CSF hypocretin measurement is the best guide to diagnosis and, if levels are normal, a diagnosis of non-narcoleptic hypersomnolence should be made and, if possible, the cause determined. An accurate history will avoid confusing cataplexy with epilepsy or drop attack, or misinterpretation of hypnagogic hallucinations as a symptom of schizophrenia.

In true narcolepsy failure to diagnose is more common than incorrect diagnosis. Daytime sleepiness is never normal and is rarely psychological in origin. It is sometimes wrongly attributed to insomnia although most people with insomnia have a low, not high, daytime sleep tendency. Box 24.5.2.3 shows the sleep associations.

Hypersomnolence without cataplexy

The complaint of sleepiness is common. Sleepiness must be clearly distinguished from fatigue, and a 24-h history is vital. In general, sleepiness cannot be attributed to previous minor head injury, mild depression, or viral infection other than with Epstein–Barr virus, but is not uncommon in heart failure, in ergot drug-treated Parkinson's disease, and with sedative drug overuse. Continuous positive airway pressure rarely completely reverses the symptoms in sleep apnoea. A diagnosis of idiopathic hypersomnia based on the idea of abnormal pressure for non-REM sleep, with prolonged dream-free deep sleep by night and day, sometimes with a familial or genetic basis, may occasionally be valid. In other cases, despite investigation, a cause for sleepiness cannot be determined.

Box 24.5.2.3 Sleepiness associations

Sleepiness and cataplexy
Narcoleptic syndrome
- 'Symptomatic' narcolepsy: brainstem glioma, angioma, lymphoma, encephalitis
- 'Syndromic' narcolepsy: narcoleptic syndrome-like symptoms in children with Möbius, Prader–Willi, or Niemann–Pick syndromes, or Norrie's disease

Sleepiness without cataplexy
- Narcoleptic syndrome before clinical development of cataplexy
- Family members of individuals with narcoleptic syndrome
- Other forms of daytime hypersomnolence, e.g. sleep apnoea (100 times as common as narcolepsy); 'idiopathic' hypersomnolence, many drugs, major head injury

---

Box 24.5.2.4 Treatment of narcoleptic syndrome

Daytime sleepiness, subalertness

- Dexamfetamine 5–60 mg/24h; tolerance an occasional problem, but no evidence of addiction, dependence, or abuse. Preferred treatment by most patients

- Methylphenidate 10–80 mg/24h; as for dexamfetamine

- Mazindol 2–8 mg/24h; nonamphetamine compound, less potent than above but preferred by some patients

- Modafinil 200–400 mg/24h; less potent than amphetamine, different behavioural effects

Cataplexy

- Clomipramine 10–150 mg/24h; most potent anticataplectic drug known but long-term weight gain is a major problem in treatment

- Fluoxetine 20 mg/24h; less potent alternative to clomipramine but limited side effects

Insomnia

- Avoid regular nightly treatment. Twice weekly zopiclone 7.5 mg may be appropriate

- Most 5-hydroxytryptamine (serotonin) reuptake inhibitors will reduce cataplexy and possibly sleep paralysis

- Notes:

  · Control treatment with patient sleep- and cataplexy-rating scale diary

  · Give stimulant drugs on as-needed basis (e.g. 4- to 8-h timing) with variable rather than fixed-dose schedule dependent on activity, day of week

  · Stimulants should not be given after 16.00.

  · Give sedative anticataplectic, e.g. clomipramine as single evening dose; stimulant anticataplectic, e.g. fluoxetine, as single morning dose

---

Treatment (Box 24.5.2.4)

Treatment of narcolepsy is a problem for both the doctor and the patient. The prescriber may refuse stimulant drugs because of a fear of abuse, restrict dosage to prevent tolerance, and dislike any nonfixed dose regimen. Patients may require such a regimen for good control, demand large doses, and complete freedom to overdose, not recognizing their own irritability and euphoria.

The drug of first choice for daytime sleepiness is an amphetamine. Effects are strongly dose related. Comparison of amphetamines with alternatives, including methylphenidate, mazindol, and modafinil, has not been made, although the different drugs have different subjective and objective effects on sleep, mood, and wakefulness.

Amphetamines and methylphenidate, but not modafinil, have a partial anticataplectic as well as an alerting effect. However, if cataplexy remains frequent or severe, the minimum effective dose of clomipramine or other anticataplectic should be added. These drugs may also partially control sleep paralysis. Unlike the stimulants, a single evening dose may give 24-h control.

Stimulant and anticataplectic drug treatment should be supported by a 15-min nap once or twice a day. Adequate treatment is essential to restore school performance, work, driving ability, and quality of life. This is best achieved with an as-needed, variable dose regimen dependent on factors such as day of the week, activity, and response level, and controlled by a patient-kept diary. Drug response is immediate, although sudden withdrawal may be followed by a severe rebound of sleepiness, cataplexy, or both, lasting several days.

Sweating and irritability with the stronger stimulants, mild headache with modafinil, and increased appetite, weight gain, and delayed ejaculation with clomipramine sometimes limit treatment. Acute amphetamine psychosis is not a problem in people with narcolepsy and there is no evidence that a lifetime of treatment with this causes vascular toxicity, although with cardiovascular disease low- rather than high-dose treatment is indicated. Management problems include pregnancy, with the need for the safety of mother and baby to be balanced against potential drug teratogenicity and secretion in breast milk, and prostatism with the potential for retention. A poor drug response should lead to re-evaluation of diagnosis and treatment compliance. Conventional treatment is unsatisfactory in about a fifth of people with narcolepsy. Here carefully monitored morning venlafaxine, 37.5 mg with slow increase to 275 mg/24h, may control both sleepiness and cataplexy.

Tolerance to stimulant and anticataplectic drugs develops in a third of patients. Dose revision or change to an alternative may be necessary, despite the risk of severe withdrawal effects. Psychological addiction to stimulants does not occur and there is no evidence of abuse in people with narcolepsy who have a normal personality. Very occasionally a recreational drug user will feign a history of narcolepsy to obtain stimulants and a urinary drug screen may be appropriate.

Further reading

Dauvilliers Y, Arnulf I, Mignot E (2007). Narcolepsy with cataplexy. *Lancet*, **369**, 499–511.

Johns MW (1991). A new method for measuring daytime sleepiness: the Epworth sleepiness scale. *Sleep*, **14**, 540–5.

Parkes JD, *et al.* (1998). The clinical diagnosis of the narcoleptic syndrome. *J Sleep Res*, **7**, 41–52.

24.5.3 **Sleep disorders**

Paul J. Reading

Essentials

Dysfunctional sleep is an important cause of morbidity. Sleep problems can loosely be divided into insomnias, disorders causing excessive daytime sleepiness, and parasomnias, with some conditions having elements of all three categories.

Insomnia

Chronic insomnia usually has a behavioural or psychological basis and responds best to cognitive or relaxation therapies, although secondary causes of insomnia such as restless legs syndrome may have specific therapies. Circadian rhythm disorders may also present as insomnia, and a number of neurological syndromes such as Parkinson's disease are also associated with poor quality and fragmented sleep.

Excessive daytime sleepiness

This usually has a specific identifiable cause, with sleep fragmentation or disruption due to sleep disordered breathing being the commonest reason for severe cases (see Chapter 18.5.2). However, at least 2% of excessively sleepy subjects will have a primary sleep disorder such as narcolepsy.

Narcolepsy—a primary disorder of sleep–wake regulation: inability to stay awake for more than a few hours is the most obvious symptom, which may be associated with cataplexy, sleep paralysis and hallucinations (see Chapter 24.5.3)

Parasomnias

Non-REM parasomnias—these are very common in children and rarely require investigation or treatment. Sleepwalking, confusional arousals, and night terrors occurring within 90 min of sleep form a spectrum of conditions reflecting abnormal arousals from the deepest stages of sleep. In a few cases the phenomenon persists into adulthood and may require short courses of hypnotic agents or sedative antidepressant therapy to suppress the nocturnal disturbances.

Parasomnias arising from REM sleep—these are most common in middle-aged men and may be a harbinger of a neurodegenerative syndrome such as Parkinson's disease. REM sleep behaviour disorder occurs when the mechanism to paralyse voluntary muscles during dreams in REM sleep fails, with the subsequent dream enactment sometimes causing significant physical injury. Most patients respond to clonazepam.

Circadian rhythm disorders

Circadian rhythm disorders—these are increasingly recognized. Most arise from jet lag or shift work; a few reflect abnormalities of the intrinsic clock mechanisms, of which delayed sleep phase syndrome is commonest, especially in adolescents, usually presenting with severe difficulties arising from bed for morning activities. Treatments are partially effective and include melatonin taken mid-evening and phototherapy given in the early morning.

Introduction

The need to sleep is imperative, reflecting the fact that sleepiness, similar to hunger and thirst, is a true drive state. Although its function remains largely elusive, disordered sleep can be associated with profound adverse effects on cognition, mental health, and physical well-being. Moreover, sleep-related symptoms are very common, with 25% of people reporting problems that significantly and regularly impact on daily activities.

Advances in our understanding of the neurobiology of sleep have challenged the traditional view that sleep is a passive or necessarily restful process. By contrast, rather than simply reflecting the absence of wakefulness, sleep is actively orchestrated, with a

highly reproducible and complex internal architecture. A typical pattern seen in a healthy adult is shown in Fig. 24.5.3.1. Episodes of rapid eye movement (REM) and non-REM sleep recur through the night in four or five discrete cycles. It should be recognized that occasional arousals from nocturnal sleep are normal and that seemingly random body movements or shifts in position occur regularly throughout the night. In REM sleep episodes, however, despite high levels of cerebral metabolic activity that loosely correspond to dream mentation, general motor activity is profoundly suppressed and any observable movements are confined to occasional minor jerks.

Defining disordered sleep can be difficult: most classifications are now symptom based. The recently revised *International Classification of Sleep Disorders* (ICSD-2—see 'Further reading') recognizes eight categories:

1 Insomnias
2 Sleep-related breathing disorders
3 Hypersomnias of central origin
4 Circadian rhythm sleep disorders
5 Parasomnias
6 Sleep-related movement disorders
7 Isolated symptoms, normal variants, and unresolved issues
8 Other sleep disorders.

Insomnia

Chronic insomnia is loosely defined as the perception of inadequate sleep for a period of more than 4 weeks. Such inability to fall asleep or maintain continuous sleep is a common symptom and has a number of extrinsic or secondary causes (Table 24.5.3.1). It is rare for organic cerebral pathology to underlie primary insomnia, and persistently maladaptive attitudes or behaviours are usually responsible. An index event or illness can often be identified. The common forms of primary insomnia are probably best treated by

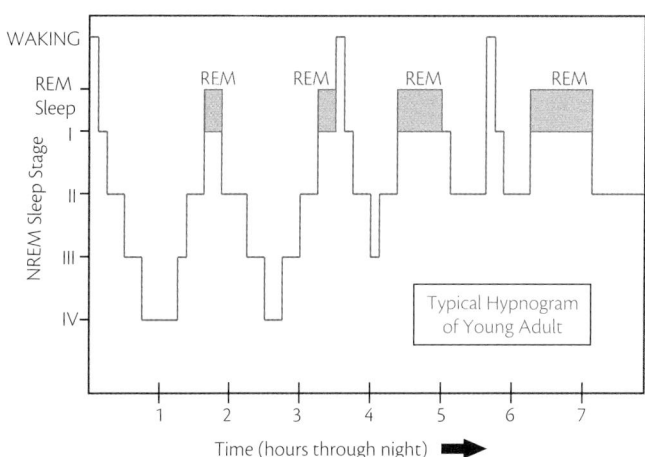

Fig. 24.5.3.1 A typical hypnogram of a young adult showing four cycles of non-rapid eye movement (non-REM) and REM sleep. Two brief awakenings are shown that can be considered normal. The proportion of deep non-REM sleep (stages III and IV) is highest in the first few hours of sleep whereas REM sleep predominates towards the end of the sleep period.

Table 24.5.3.1 Some causes of primary and secondary insomnia

Causes	Comments
Primary insomnia	
Intrinsic sleep disorders	
Psychophysiological insomnia	
Paradoxical insomnia	Sometimes called 'conditioned insomnia', formerly called 'sleep–wake misperception'
Idiopathic insomnia	History dates back to childhood
Extrinsic sleep disorders	
Poor sleep hygiene	
Environmental sleep disorder	Examples include sleep-disordered bed partners or pets interfering with sleep; usually results in daytime sleepiness
Altitude insomnia	Mild hypoxaemia produces poor sleep because of unstable respiratory control overnight
Drug-dependent insomnia	Hypnotics, stimulants, or alcohol may be responsible
Secondary insomnia	
Neurological conditions	
Restless legs syndrome	An important and treatable cause of insomnia
Parkinson's disease	Sleep fragmentation can be an integral part of the condition
Morvan's syndrome	A rare paraneoplastic or autoimmune syndrome with neuromuscular hyperexcitability and severe insomnia as cardinal features
Fatal familial insomnia	A very rare familial prion disease with significant thalamic pathology as the presumed substrate for severe insomnia
Medical disorders	
Asthma	
Gastro-oesophageal reflux	An important and often overlooked diagnosis
Chronic pain syndromes including fibromyalgia	A high percentage of light non-REM sleep is often seen
Psychiatric causes	
Secondary to medication	
Mood disorders including anxiety, depression, and mania	

REM, rapid eye movement.

behavioural modification, including a combination of cognitive–behavioural therapy and relaxation techniques. The intermittent use of short-acting hypnotics may be helpful, although long-term drug treatment is rarely beneficial.

If symptoms of inadequate sleep date back to childhood, the term 'idiopathic insomnia' is sometimes used. Although its neurobiology remains obscure, at some level this disorder probably reflects a constitutionally impaired sleep drive such that the normal homoeostatic pressure to sleep is inadequate.

The interplay between psychological distress and chronic insomnia is complex, with each element potentially fuelling the other. Psychiatric input to treat any significant mood disorder can therefore be helpful in attempting to resolve sleep-related symptoms.

Hypersomnia

Significant excessive daytime sleepiness is reported by 5% of the population and is most often due to poor quality or diminished overnight sleep (Table 24.5.3.2). It is important to distinguish true sleepiness or drowsiness from fatigue and lethargy, which often have different causes. Within the abnormally sleepy population, approximately 2% have a primary sleep disorder in which the most striking complaint is an inability to stay awake appropriately despite the desire to do so.

Narcolepsy

Introduction and clinical features
Narcolepsy is not a rare disorder, with an estimated prevalence of 1 per 2000 in white populations. However, differences in case ascertainment and the availability of sleep services have led to considerable variance in reported rates worldwide. Moreover, there is undoubtedly a spectrum of severity and many mildly affected individuals are either undiagnosed or diagnosed only after many years of symptoms. It most often starts in adolescence, with a second minor peak in early middle age. Symptoms are generally life-long, although most people with the condition develop coping strategies to minimize the impact of the syndrome.

Narcolepsy is important, not least because it is usually disabling, influencing every aspect of daily living. Many people with narcolepsy feel a sense of underachievement, partly because treatment is frequently either delayed or only partially effective. A perceived lack of medical interest in the disease, together with the adverse

Table 24.5.3.2 Some extrinsic and intrinsic causes of excessive daytime sleepiness

Intrinsic causes	Extrinsic causes
Primary causes	Sleep deprivation or insufficient sleep
Narcolepsy	Drug-related hypersomnia
Idiopathic hypersomnia	Environmental sleep disorder
Kleine–Levin syndrome (intermittent sleepiness)	Shift-work sleep disorder
Causes secondary to a chronic disorder	Jet lag
Sleep-disordered breathing	
Restless legs syndrome and periodic limb movement disorder	
Parkinson's disease	
Multiple sclerosis	
Head injuries	
Encephalitis	

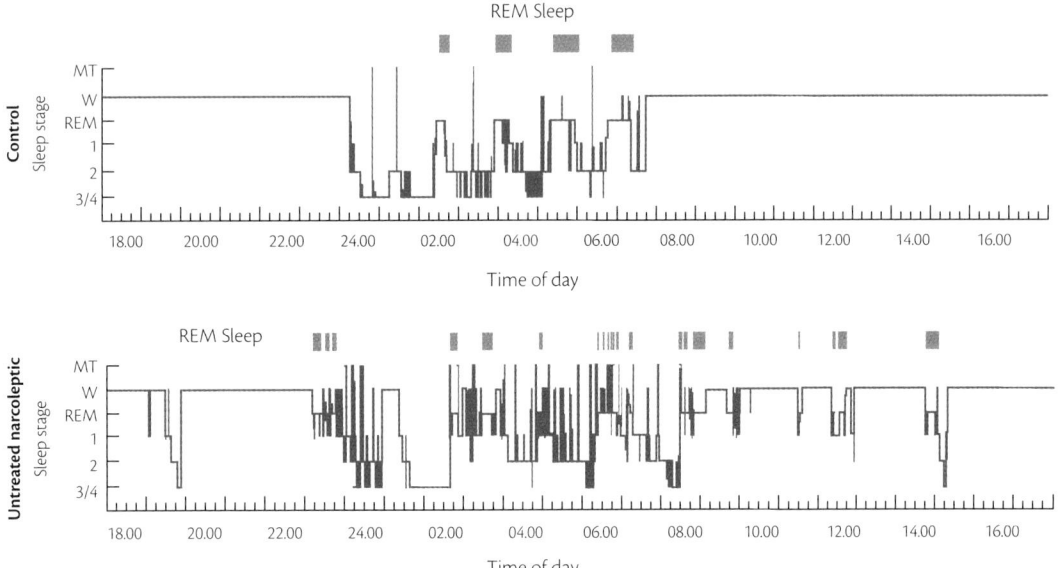

Fig. 24.5.3.2 Comparisons of typical hypnograms over 24 h in a control person and someone with untreated narcolepsy. In the narcoleptic trace, there is severe disruption of the usual pattern with numerous daytime naps containing rapid eye movement (REM) sleep. Overnight, the usual sleep architecture is disorganized in the person with narcolepsy with several awakenings and associated movement. MT, significant movements; W, wake.

effects on schooling, careers, and relationships, understandably produces frustration. Secondary mood disorders are seen in many patients.

Rather than reflecting true hypersomnolence over a 24-hour period, narcolepsy is best viewed as a primary disorder of sleep–wake regulation (Fig. 24.5.3.2), with an inability to stay awake for more than a few hours as the most obvious symptom. Indeed, excessive daytime sleepiness not explained by another disorder remains an essential diagnostic criterion. Many patients describe sudden and irresistible urges to sleep, often in public or inappropriate situations, invariably worse if they are unoccupied or bored. In contrast to most other sleep disorders, short naps lasting minutes can often be restorative. A few people with the condition are relatively unaffected by excessive daytime sleepiness and other features of the syndrome predominate.

Cataplexy

Cataplexy is a curious phenomenon, highly specific to narcolepsy and present to varying degrees in two-thirds of patients. It is particularly important to identify typical cataplexy because its presence in a person with excessive daytime sleepiness is diagnostic of narcolepsy. Full-blown episodes reflect an intrusion of profound muscle paralysis that descends over a few seconds from head to the lower limbs, often causing collapse to the floor. Identifiable triggers usually have an emotional content. Laughter or other positive emotions such as a pleasant surprise are the most common precipitants, although frustration and anger can also reliably provoke episodes. In some individuals the mere thought or anticipation of an emotional event can cause collapse. Reassuringly, attacks are rare in dangerous situations and most patients report cataplexy only when relatively relaxed in familiar environments with friends. It is therefore very uncommon for doctors to witness episodes, making a reliable history crucial for confident diagnosis. Importantly, partial or focal attacks are common and can be subtle, perhaps confined to the jaw or neck. Occasionally, an inability to tell the punchline of a joke due to a stuttering dysarthria may be the only manifestation. Facial twitching or head bobbing is very common as an episode starts and can lead to diagnostic confusion. Crucially, awareness is preserved in cataplexy, although in rare instances, when attacks last more than a minute or so, dream-like intrusions and altered consciousness may intercede. Severely affected individuals may have over 20 attacks a day, often reporting that the amusement or frustration induced by the cataplectic episodes themselves can prolong the period of weakness.

It is widely thought that cataplexy occurs because REM sleep paralysis intrudes inappropriately into the wakeful state. Indeed, as in REM sleep, a person is rendered temporarily areflexic during an episode as a result of descending inhibitory neural impulses from lower brainstem centres directly on to motor neurons. Some evidence suggests that this phenomenon may occur to a minor degree during emotion in control individuals, adding credibility to the adage 'going weak with laughter'.

Sleep paralysis and hallucinations

Sleep paralysis and hallucinations around sleep–wake transition are the other two components of the narcoleptic 'tetrad' first described in 1957. However, only 25% of patients have all four elements, and the presence of these other symptoms, particularly sleep paralysis, is not specific to narcolepsy. Sleep paralysis is usually frightening, primarily because of an inability to take deep breaths voluntarily. Most episodes occur at the point of waking, although people with narcolepsy may also report episodes at sleep onset. Accompanying sensations of being crushed, with or without vivid visual hallucinations, may add to the distress of the episodes. Similar to cataplexy, this phenomenon reflects the intrusion of REM sleep elements into the wakeful or drowsy state.

Hallucinations occurring at sleep onset (hypnagogic) or as the person wakes (hypnopompic) are usually visual and can be both vivid and disturbing, especially in children. They represent fragments of dream mentation intruding into the conscious state, reinforcing the notion that people with narcolepsy cannot adequately maintain a consistent and stable state of wakefulness or sleep.

When questioned, most people with narcolepsy have fragmented nocturnal sleep. Although this may be due to the intrusion of a parasomnia or obstructed breathing, both of which are more common in people with narcolepsy, the primary problem is one of sleep regulation and maintenance. The notion that people with narcolepsy have problems sleeping at night is counterintuitive to some but is an important addition to the original descriptions of the syndrome.

Other symptoms

In addition to obvious naps, most people with narcolepsy will experience numerous 'micro-sleeps' through the day, in which awareness during activities is compromised for a few seconds. The resulting lapses lead to automatic and inappropriate behaviours, with worrying consequences for complex and potentially dangerous tasks such as driving. Although difficult to characterize, many people with narcolepsy also report significant problems with memory and concentration as a result of their sleep–wake difficulties. Furthermore, increasing evidence suggests abnormalities of appetite, particularly at night, with cravings for sweet foods. Moderate obesity is more common in narcolepsy and may have a metabolic explanation because there is no link with excessive food intake. Indeed, some evidence suggests that overweight people with narcolepsy eat less than average.

Pathogenesis and diagnosis

Since the discovery in 1984 that Japanese people with narcolepsy were extremely likely to carry the human leucocyte antigen (HLA) haplotype DR2, an autoimmune basis for the syndrome has been thought likely. The predisposing antigen has since been established to be DQ-B1*0602, which is present in over 90% of people with narcolepsy and cataplexy and around 50% of those without cataplexy, compared with a frequency of 20% in control populations. Of interest, homozygosity for DQ-B1*0602 appears to confer an even greater risk for the syndrome. However, there remains no direct evidence for autoimmunity, in the form of either serum markers or CSF abnormalities.

A major breakthrough in understanding the neurobiology of narcolepsy occurred in 1999 when two groups independently demonstrated abnormalities of a recently described neuropeptide, hypocretin (also called orexin), in separate animal models. The well-established autosomal recessive Doberman model was shown to have dysfunctional hypocretin receptors, whereas a mouse hypocretin knockout model developed convincing clinical features of narcolepsy with cataplexy. Subsequently, it has been demonstrated that CSF hypocretin is virtually absent both in sporadic canine models and in people with narcolepsy and cataplexy. Indeed, a CSF hypocretin level of less than 110 pg/ml is now considered diagnostic. Postmortem evidence has confirmed that pathology in narcoleptic brains is confined specifically to hypocretin neurons. Confusingly, however, in rare familial narcolepsy and in sporadic cases without typical cataplexy, hypocretin levels can be preserved, implying that there is more than one pathogenic mechanism for certain forms of the syndrome.

Following the unexpected involvement of the hypocretin system in human narcolepsy, it has been intensely studied in intact animals. Around 30 000 neurons containing the peptide are confined to the lateral hypothalamus but innervate all the arousal systems in the brain. Levels of hypocretin rise towards the end of the waking day, especially in the presence of peptide hunger signals or if the person is expecting food. Activity of hypocretin neurons therefore appears to stabilize a state of wakefulness when the organism needs to be alert. In narcolepsy their absence leads to inappropriate switches between sleep and wakefulness. Moreover, transitions between behavioural states may be incomplete, explaining the intrusion of REM sleep phenomena such as paralysis into wakefulness. The mechanism by which emotional stimuli (in particular) trigger cataplexy remains elusive.

If typical cataplexy is absent and CSF hypocretin levels cannot easily be measured, a positive diagnosis of narcolepsy can be made following a multiple sleep latency test. This test measures the propensity for a person to fall asleep by recording the average length of time to reach light sleep in a conducive environment over four or five nap opportunities between 9.00 am and 3.00 pm. If the mean sleep latency is less than 8 min and REM sleep is achieved within 15 min on at least two occasions, the criteria for narcolepsy are fulfilled. Reliable results depend on ensuring a reasonable night's sleep preceding the investigation, and the test also requires a strict protocol to avoid false-negative results.

Secondary narcolepsy

Narcoleptic symptoms including cataplexy have been reported in other neurological conditions. Given the recent advances in the understanding the neurobiology of the primary syndrome, it is not surprising that pathology in the region of the hypothalamus such as tumours around the third ventricle can lead to secondary narcolepsy, presumably by depletion of hypocretin-containing neurons. However, the mechanism of severe sleepiness or sleep–wake dysregulation after head injury or as components of other conditions such as multiple sclerosis and Parkinson's disease can be difficult to explain.

The various subtypes of narcolepsy are shown in Table 24.5.3.3.

Treatment

Advice on lifestyle helps some people with narcolepsy. Planned naps, especially after meals, may improve wakefulness. Furthermore, the avoidance of large meals rich in refined carbohydrates is reportedly beneficial to some. Most people with narcolepsy, however, benefit from medication to improve daytime wakefulness (Table 24.5.3.4), although few are normalized. Modafinil is the most widely used wake-promoting agent and has partly replaced traditional psychostimulants. Its mechanism of action remains obscure, but a direct effect on arousal centres in the hypothalamus is postulated. It has no definite positive effect on cataplexy. Side effects are rare and include headache or gastrointestinal upset. Interactions with the oral contraceptive pill and uncertainty over safety in pregnancy may limit its use in young women.

In severe sleepiness or if modafinil is unsuccessful, central stimulants with a predominantly dopaminergic action, such as dexamfetamine, are helpful, especially if used flexibly. Despite prescriber concerns, it is rare for psychological addiction to occur in narcolepsy, although tolerance may require increasing doses with time. Cardiovascular side effects such as hypertension are relatively rare but necessitate caution in older people. Given the different mechanisms of action, a combination of modafinil and a psychostimulant is appropriate. Additional use of caffeine and setting aside time for planned naps may reduce the need for medication.

About a half of people with narcolepsy also require specific treatment for cataplexy. Although the evidence base is small, most antidepressants will suppress cataplexy by increasing cerebral monoaminergic activity and inhibiting the tendency to enter

Table 24.5.3.3 Subtypes of narcolepsy and associated features

	Narcolepsy with cataplexy (sporadic) (%)	Narcolepsy without cataplexy (sporadic) (%)	Familial narcolepsy (%)	Secondary (symptomatic) narcolepsy (%)
REM sleep reached within 15 min on two or more occasions in MSLT	85	100% (by definition)	Uncertain	75
HLA DQ-B1*0602 positivity	85–93	35–56	65–79	Uncertain
Presence of low or undetectable CSF Hcrt-1 levels	>90	14	38	VariableReported instances of very low levels in individual cases
Proposed or presumed pathogenesis	Autoimmune destruction of Hcrt-synthesizing neurons	Partial Hcrt deficiency	Multiple genotypes	Damage to Hcrt-containing neurons in the lateral hypothalamus
		Unknown mechanism in many	Hcrt system very rarely involved directly	

CSF, cerebrospinal fluid; HLA, human leucocyte antigen; Hcrt-1, hypocretin-1; MSLT, multiple sleep latency test; REM, rapid eye movement.

REM sleep, although the side-effect profile of most antidepressant drugs, particularly the tricyclics, may limit their usefulness. A new approach for troublesome cataplexy is to use sodium oxybate, and trial evidence suggests that this drug helps daytime sleepiness as well. It is a liquid preparation taken before bed and—due to its short half-life—once during the night if the person is awake. The effects on cataplexy are striking after several weeks of therapy, with almost 90% of attacks abolished. Inadvertent daytime naps, and objective and subjective measures of daytime sleepiness also improve. The agent appears to work, in part, by inducing deep restorative sleep early in the night, such that the sleep drive is effectively dissipated by the following morning. The drug should be used with extreme caution in any patient living alone or with young children in case confusional episodes from deep sleep are provoked. However, if disturbed nocturnal sleep is a major symptom, it appears a logical treatment given that standard benzodiazepine hypnotic agents rarely induce refreshing sleep in narcolepsy.

Following the recent findings that most people with narcolepsy are deficient in the neuropeptide hypocretin, an obvious therapeutic goal will be to develop replacement therapy. There appear to be clinical effects if hypocretin levels are increased in animal models by intracerebral infusion, hence the development of an oral analogue that penetrates the blood–brain barrier is a current pharmacological goal for treatment in humans.

Idiopathic hypersomnia

Idiopathic hypersomnia is a diagnosis of exclusion most often made when excessively sleepy patients do not fulfil the criteria for narcolepsy. Depending on precise definitions, it is probably 10 times less common than narcolepsy. Classic cases report difficulty waking in the morning followed by prolonged unrefreshing daytime naps despite long and deep nocturnal sleep. Low mood and frequent automatic behaviours are commonly reported. However, no specific narcoleptic features such as cataplexy are present, and CSF hypocretin levels are generally normal. Sleep investigations should confirm a shortened daytime sleep latency of less than 8 min, preceded by normal but prolonged nocturnal sleep. A new category of idiopathic hypersomnia without prolonged overnight sleep has been proposed, but this is controversial and distinction from atypical or monosymptomatic narcolepsy can be difficult.

As in narcolepsy, although usually with less satisfactory results, the treatment of idiopathic hypersomnia consists of modafinil alone or in combination with traditional psychostimulants.

Kleine–Levin syndrome

Kleine–Levin syndrome is a rare and poorly characterized sleep disorder most commonly seen in adolescents. The primary feature is periodic hypersomnia lasting days to weeks, recurring at intervals of weeks to months. During symptomatic periods the person is generally drowsy and usually displays abnormal behaviours. These include simple irritability, hallucinations, hypersexuality, and

Table 24.5.3.4 Commonly used drug treatments for the narcoleptic syndrome

Drug	Total 24-h dose range (mg)	Comments
Excessive daytime sleepiness		
Modafinil	200–600	Different mechanism of action to traditional psychostimulants
Dexamfetamine	5–60	Tolerance can develop but dependence rare
Methylphenidate	10–80	Similar to amphetamine but possibly smoother action; long-acting preparation available
Sodium oxybate	4.5–9 g	Taken through the night; may act synergistically with daytime stimulants
Cataplexy		
Venlafaxine	75–225	Possibly the antidepressant with most anticataplectic properties
Clomipramine	10–150	Potent but side effects often limit use
Fluoxetine	20–40	Appropriate for mild cataplexy; few side effects
Sodium oxybate	4.5–9 g	Taken at night; up to 90% of attacks may be abolished after 4 weeks of treatment
Disturbed nocturnal sleep		
Clonazepam	0.5–2	Sleep continuity improved but sleep quality not usually refreshing; intermittent rather than continuous use advisable
Sodium oxybate	4.5–9 g	Deep non-REM sleep increased; overall sleep quality improved

REM, rapid eye movement.

abnormal appetite, producing hyperphagia. Investigations are generally unhelpful, although an excess of REM sleep is occasionally seen during episodes. Intermittent hypothalamic dysfunction is a speculative but plausible mechanism to explain the symptom complex. Secondary causes are very rare and reportedly include a wide variety of neurological conditions such as multiple sclerosis and Prader–Willi syndrome.

Treatments are empirical and usually ineffective, although the syndrome tends to resolve spontaneously after several years. An amphetamine may help during episodes and lithium may be used as a prophylactic agent.

Parasomnias and sleep-related movement disorders

Parasomnias are loosely defined as intermittent undesirable events arising from sleep that are not epileptic in nature. The spectrum is large, ranging from visual imagery at sleep onset to complex motor behaviours, occasionally with violent components. Family members and bed partners are usually more concerned than the individuals themselves, who often remain oblivious to any nocturnal disturbance. Parasomnias are generally classified according to the sleep stage from which they arise, although some are not 'state dependent'.

A simple yet valid scheme to explain most parasomnias is shown in Fig. 24.5.3.3. The brain can function in three distinct and mutually exclusive states, namely wakefulness, non-REM sleep, and REM sleep. The brain normally switches seamlessly and relatively quickly between these states through the sleep–wake cycle. Most parasomnias result from abnormal state transitions such that elements of one state intrude into another: a person can be considered 'caught' for a variable period of time in a separate abnormal state somewhere between wake and sleep.

With the exception of certain REM sleep disorders, the neuroanatomical basis of parasomnias remains obscure. The high prevalence of familial aggregation suggests genetic factors and predominance in childhood implies a maturational component, particularly in non-REM parasomnias.

Parasomnias at the sleep–wake transition

It is an almost universal experience to have occasional unpleasant sensations of falling through space at the point of sleep onset, with resulting brief muscular contractions. In some individuals these hypnic jerks can regularly interfere with sleep onset and recur through the night. In others there are accompanying explosive sensory phenomena, sometimes with severe head pain as a component. Treatments with short-acting benzodiazepines may be justified in severe cases.

More complex and prolonged phenomena comprising a variety of rhythmical movements also tend to occur during extreme drowsiness just before sleep. Head banging is the most common manifestation in children. The problem tends to resolve with time, although can persist into adulthood and disturb bed partners. Various patterns of movement are seen, with the head, neck, and trunk most commonly involved. The view that the movements are semivoluntary, as part of a sleep-inducing habit, does not concord with the observation that the phenomenon arises only from deep or even REM sleep in a few individuals.

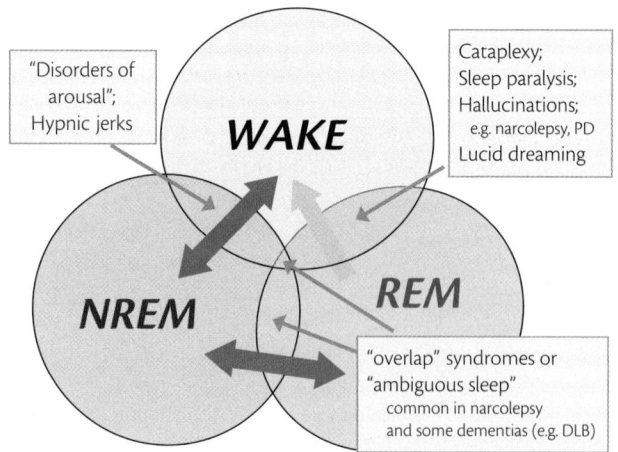

Fig. 24.5.3.3 A graphical demonstration depicting the normal transitions of the mutually exclusive states of wakefulness, non-rapid eye movement (non-REM), and REM sleep. The switch from REM sleep to wakefulness can occur directly and would normally lead to a dream experience. Most parasomnias occur because of abnormal or inefficient state transitions. Sleep-walking and related phenomena occur when a person arouses incompletely from deep non-REM sleep. Hypnic jerks may occur when the brain fails to fall asleep in its entirety. The narcoleptic symptoms of sleep paralysis, cataplexy, and hallucinations at sleep–wake transition occur when elements of REM sleep intrude into wakefulness. Parkinsonian hallucinations probably represent REM sleep imagery occurring in the drowsy wakeful state. Some individuals report the ability to control their dreams (lucid dreaming) which can be considered as wakeful consciousness intruding into the REM sleep state. In some people with narcolepsy or severe dementia, it can be very difficult to stage sleep accurately and 'overlap' syndromes producing ambiguous sleep can occur. DLB, dementia with Lewy bodies; PD, Parkinson's disease.

Parasomnias arising from deep non-REM sleep

Non-REM parasomnias are characterized by sudden but partial arousals from deep sleep, usually stage 4, resulting in behaviours for which the person usually has no subsequent clear recollection. Based on clinical features, sleep-walking, confusional arousals, and night terrors are recognized as three separate phenomena all due to abnormal arousal from deep sleep. Within this notional spectrum, however, there may be considerable overlap and the type of episodes may change with age.

In sleep-walking the person will typically leave the bedroom and may well engage in complex behaviours such as cooking and eating. Communication is possible at a basic level, but it is usually clear to observers that the person is not fully alert or responsive. Concerns often arise when there are attempts to leave the house or if there are any violent elements to the episodes.

Confusional arousals refer to brief episodes of disorientation in which the person may sit up in bed and survey the environment before returning to sleep.

Night terrors are dramatic episodes, often lasting for several minutes, in which the person suddenly arouses from sleep, typically with a loud scream and extreme agitation. Motor and autonomic indications of extreme fear are usually alarming to parents and observers.

All these arousal disorders tend to occur within an hour of sleep, when non-REM sleep is at its deepest. It is rare for events to recur through the night. If there is any recall, it is usually vague and related to a nonspecific fear or urge to leave the bedroom in the case of night terrors. Particularly deep sleep after a period of deprivation or induced by drugs (including alcohol) may increase the likelihood of events. General stress, changes in schedule, and sleeping in a new environment are further recognized precipitants.

Non-REM parasomnias are common in the first decade of life, affecting at least 6% of children on a regular basis. Persistence into adulthood occurs in around 15% of these. A confident distinction between nocturnal epilepsy and parasomnias can usually be made from clinical features alone, although investigations and video analysis may be required in some cases. Particularly in adults, overnight investigations may reveal an additional sleep disorder such as sleep apnoea or periodic leg movements that may partially arouse the person and help to trigger a parasomnia.

It is rarely appropriate to treat non-REM parasomnias with medication, especially in children. However, if disturbances are frequent or likely to cause danger, short courses of benzodiazepines such as low-dose clonazepam before bed are usually helpful. In the absence of any substantial evidence, antidepressants such as paroxetine are also used to good effect, presumably by effects on sleep architecture.

REM sleep parasomnias

REM parasomnias include nightmares, REM sleep paralysis, and REM sleep behaviour disorder. Given the propensity for REM sleep to occur late in the night, these parasomnias are typically reported between 3.00 am and 6.00 am, in contrast to the earlier occurrences of arousal disorders from non-REM sleep.

Nightmares represent arousals from unpleasant dreams and are universal experiences. However, up to 4% of adults have frequent or intrusive nightmares, often in the context of psychological stress or substance abuse. Nightmares with recurring themes are a hallmark of post-traumatic stress disorder. Some drugs, e.g. β blockers, can trigger nightmares, as may the sudden withdrawal of antidepressant agents that normally suppress REM sleep.

Symptoms of sleep paralysis seen in around 40% of people with narcolepsy can also occur as an isolated phenomenon, occasionally with a familial pattern. As in narcolepsy, the profound paralysis is usually disturbing. Typically, prolonged episodes can be aborted by a tactile stimulus from a bed partner. If treatment is thought necessary, tricyclic antidepressants are usually helpful.

An increasingly recognized REM parasomnia occurs when abnormal motor activity intrudes into REM sleep, reflecting a fault in the normal mechanisms that render dreaming individuals completely atonic. So-called REM sleep behaviour disorder is predominantly an affliction of middle-aged or elderly men and has an intimate relationship to several neurodegenerative diseases, particularly parkinsonism. Over 70% of people free of any movement disorder during wakefulness at the onset of symptoms will develop Parkinson's disease within 10 years of follow-up. The nocturnal episodes are brief and generally explosive, usually involving the arms. There is often an apparently aggressive intent, but injuries to bed partners are incidental and violence is rarely directed. In mild cases, episodes are confined to vocalization or swearing with little observable movement. If awoken during an event, dream recall is the norm, although most remain oblivious to their behaviours if their sleep remains continuous. Intriguingly, pleasant dreams or those with a sexual content are very rare, whereas reports of being chased by aggressors or attacked by animals are typical themes.

It is often appropriate to treat this parasomnia on a long-term basis to prevent injury either to the person with the condition or to the bed partner. Clonazepam in a dose range 0.25 to 2 mg is usually effective, with melatonin used as a second-line agent. If there are suspicions of an additional breathing-related sleep disorder, overnight investigations are warranted because, for example, clonazepam may worsen obstructive sleep apnoea.

Periodic leg movements of sleep

Periodic leg movements of sleep are characterized by stereotyped leg movements occurring in clusters every 30 s throughout sleep, especially in the light non-REM stages. The movements themselves tend to be fairly slow, evolving over 1 to 5 s and typically involving both legs, although one or the other may predominate. An episode tends to start with great toe extension and spreads to include ankle dorsiflexion, followed by knee and hip flexion in severe cases. It is relatively rare for individuals to be aware of the leg movements, but bed partners may complain. The phenomenon increases dramatically with age and is strongly associated with restless legs syndrome.

If periodic leg movements of sleep are demonstrated after overnight investigation, it can be difficult to gauge their clinical significance, especially if there are no associated EEG arousals. Further complications may arise if there are other reasons for fragmented sleep such as obstructive sleep apnoea, in which case leg movements may be triggered as a secondary epiphenomenon.

Treatments for restless legs syndrome also ameliorate periodic leg movements of sleep. Dopamine agonists are usually effective, although it is difficult to predict in advance whether any response will be clinically meaningful.

Circadian rhythm disorders

If both quality and quantity of sleep are normal over 24 hours but a person is unable to sleep or stay awake at the desired or expected time, a circadian rhythm disorder may be diagnosed. Most commonly this problem has a clear extrinsic cause such as shift work or long-haul jet travel, but in some situations there is almost certainly dysfunction of the internal clock mechanism. Behavioural or motivational factors may contribute to the generation of highly irregular sleep–wake especially in younger individuals.

In mammals the primary biological clock is sited in an area of the hypothalamus called the suprachiasmatic nucleus. The mechanism of the clock at a subcellular level has been extensively researched and appears very similar across all animal species, including humans. In strict isolation with no external cues, the periodicity of the human clock is around 24.3 h. In real life this rhythm is entrained precisely to 24 h primarily by light cues acting on retinal cells that contain a newly discovered retinal pigment, melanopsin. A retinal tract to the hypothalamus allows this information to influence the clock mechanism. People who are blind from birth frequently report difficulty in adapting to a conventional sleep–wake cycle because their internal clocks run a little 'slower' than average without light entrainment. Very rarely, sighted individuals also have a similar non-24-h sleep–wake disorder, the precise mechanism of which remains obscure.

Delayed sleep phase syndrome

People diagnosed with delayed sleep phase syndrome can be considered as extreme 'night owls' such that they are simply unable to sleep before 2.00 am or later. The main concern is usually the subsequent inability to wake effectively for school or work. It is important to exclude significant mood disorder as a driver for the abnormal cycle. Similarly, delayed sleep phase syndrome would not be diagnosed in those who simply prefer the solitude of night and avoid daytime interactions. Sleep diaries and wrist actigraphy can help confirm the diagnosis, which mostly affects adolescents with a prevalence estimated at 1%. Those with the condition and their families are very commonly frustrated by this sleep disorder and the relative lack of its recognition.

Treatment is difficult and starts with a strict schedule and general sleep hygiene measures. Melatonin taken around 2 h before desired sleep-onset time may help with sleep onset, but long-term use of hypnotics is usually unsuccessful. Phototherapy from a light box on waking may also help 'reset' the internal clock.

Advanced sleep phase syndrome

This is an extremely rare disorder but of interest because a familial form has been identified and the relevant gene analysed. The point mutation occurs in a period gene (*hPer2*) such that the circadian sleep–wake period is 23.3 h. This results in individuals sleeping and waking at least 4 h earlier than expected. Other indications of disturbed circadian rhythm include melatonin secretion and core temperature.

Humans also generally show 'phase advance' with increasing age. Common experience suggests that many older people will fall asleep in the evening and wake early in the day, especially in institutions where this may be encouraged as part of a convenient regimen.

Shift-work sleep disorder

An increasing number of people are employed in jobs requiring shift work in a variety of patterns. Rotating shifts, in particular, do not allow circadian rhythms to adapt and frequently lead to difficulties, either in staying awake for employment or in sleeping effectively during daylight hours. Of potential concern are the secondary effects of sleep deprivation on cognitive performance in tasks demanding sustained attention or decision-making, especially in occupations involving heavy industry or transportation. Most shift workers find it increasingly difficult to adapt their sleep–wake cycle as they age. Moreover, additional sleep problems such as obstructive sleep apnoea may worsen the situation.

If shift work is causing significant symptoms and cannot be avoided, treatment is a challenging area if simple sleep hygiene advice fails to help. Planned naps may be beneficial, and shift patterns that rotate by delaying work time rather than advancing it are generally easier to cope with. Regular medication is controversial with concerns over dependency, especially with regard to hypnotic agents. Regular caffeine may be used, and wake-promoting drugs such as modafinil have been licensed in severe shift-work sleep disorder, although the concept of shift-work sleep disorder as a problem requiring drug treatment lies uncomfortably with many doctors.

The assessment of sleep symptoms

In assessing a patient with a sleep disorder, the importance of a detailed history from the person and ideally a bed partner or close family member cannot be overemphasized. Together with a sleep diary, when appropriate, most diagnoses can be made with moderate confidence on history alone. With important exceptions, such as sleep apnoea, where quantification of the problem is important, it is relatively rare for investigations to add useful diagnostic information, but they can be invaluable if a reliable history is not available, e.g. in the case of a person who sleeps alone. The availability of facilities for studying sleep varies dramatically throughout the world, often dependent on how the tests are financed. The following section is based on a British perspective, where sleep medicine is relatively under-resourced.

Insomnia

Overnight tests are rarely useful when insomnia is an isolated symptom. In people who complain of extremely reduced overnight sleep, surrogate monitoring of sleep using wrist actigraphy may be useful in demonstrating paradoxical insomnia, in which there is a misperception of the amount of sleep obtained.

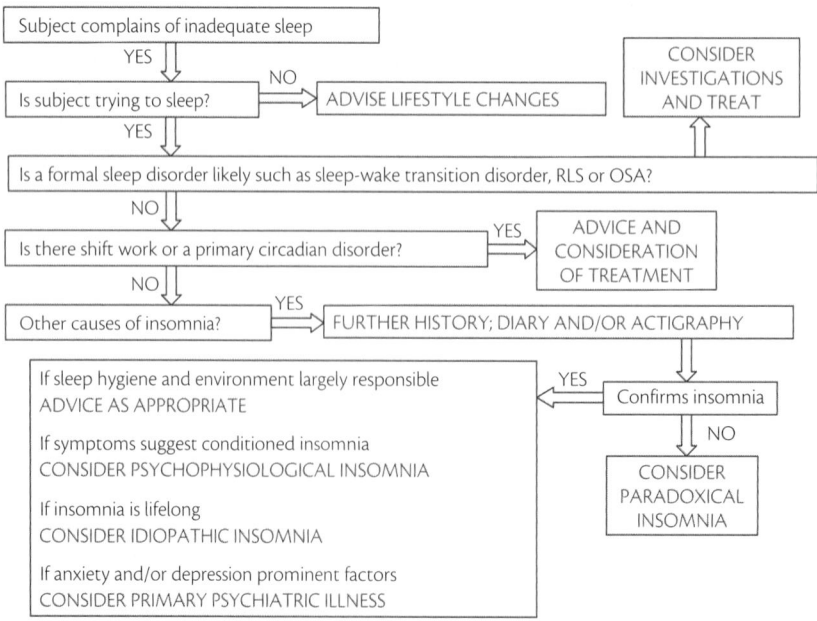

Fig. 24.5.3.4 Algorithm for the assessment of a person with insomnia. OSA, obstructive sleep apnoea; RLS, restless legs syndrome.

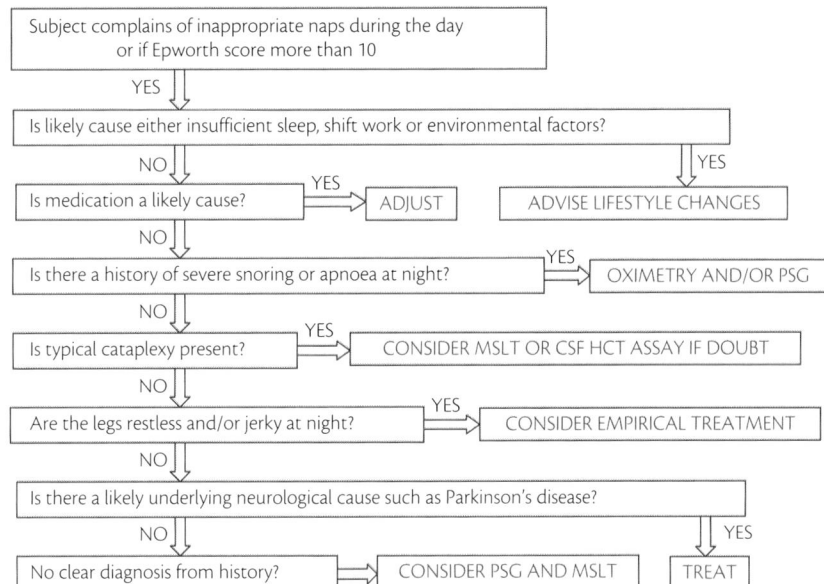

Fig. 24.5.3.5 Algorithm for the assessment of excessive daytime sleepiness. Most authorities regard a score of 10 or over on the subjective Epworth sleep scale as significant. Oximetry can usually be performed overnight in the patient's home with a finger monitor. CSF, cerebrospinal fluid; HCT, hypocretin (also called orexin); MSLT, multiple sleep latency test; PSG, polysomnography.

An algorithm for assessing chronic insomnia is shown in Fig. 24.5.3.4. Chronic insomnia associated with daytime sleepiness and frequent naps is likely to have a secondary identifiable cause.

Excessive daytime sleepiness

If excessive daytime sleepiness is the primary complaint, it is normally possible to identify an underlying cause, even if the answer is simply insufficient overnight sleep. Care should be taken in establishing that sleepiness itself is the symptom of concern and not lethargy or fatigue, which are more likely to have psychological or motivational substrates.

An algorithm for assessing a sleepy person is shown in Fig. 24.5.3.5.

Parasomnias

Non-REM parasomnias are difficult to investigate and rely on a good history to allow confident diagnosis. Capturing an event on overnight recording is rare and investigations on asymptomatic nights are usually unremarkable. Particularly in adults, an additional sleep disorder may sometimes be precipitating a parasomnia. If so, it is appropriate to perform overnight investigations to detect arousals secondary, for example, to apnoeas or leg movements. Differentiating non-REM parasomnias from nocturnal epilepsy can be difficult and video analysis—ideally of several episodes—can be crucial for diagnosis. The provision of video recorders to patients' families in order to capture events at home may be more productive and cost-effective than formal overnight recording in a hospital setting.

Further reading

American Academy of Sleep Medicine. (2005). *The International Classification of Sleep Disorders*, 2nd edition. AASM, Westchester, NY.
Arnulf I, *et al.* (2005). Kleine–Levin syndrome: a systematic review of 186 cases in the literature. *Brain*, **128**, 2763–76.
Bassetti C, Aldrich MS (1997). Idiopathic hypersomnia. A series of 42 patients. *Brain*, **120**, 1423–35.
Chemelli RM, *et al.* (1999). Narcolepsy in orexin knockout mice: molecular genetics of sleep regulation. *Cell*, **98**, 437–51.
Dauvilliers Y, Arnulf I, Mignot E (2007). Narcolepsy with cataplexy. *Lancet*, **369**, 499–511.
Frank MG (2006). The mystery of sleep function: current perspectives and future directions. *Rev Neurosci*, **17**, 375–92.
Harris CD (2005). Neurophysiology of sleep and wakefulness. *Respir Care Clin*, **11**, 567–86.
Hattar S, *et al.* (2003). Melanopsin and rod-cone photoreceptive systems account for all major accessory visual functions in mice. *Nature*, **424**, 75–81.
Lin L, *et al.* (1999). The sleep disorder canine narcolepsy is caused by a mutation in the hypocretin (orexin) receptor 2 gene. *Cell*, **98**, 365–76.
Lu BS, Zee PC (2006). Circadian rhythm sleep disorders. *Chest*, **130**, 1915–23.
Lu J, *et al.* (2006). A putative flip-flop switch for control of REM sleep. *Nature*, **441**, 589–94.
Mason TBA, Pack AI (2007). Paediatric parasomnias. *Sleep*, **30**, 141–51.
Mignot E, Nishino S (2005). Emerging therapies in narcolepsy–cataplexy. *Sleep*, **28**, 754–63.
Morin C, *et al.* (1999). Nonpharmacologic treatment of chronic insomnia. An American Academy of Sleep Medicine review. *Sleep*, **22**, 1134–56.
Nishino S, Kanbayashi T (2005). Symptomatic narcolepsy, cataplexy and hypersomnia, and their implications in the hypothalamic hypocretin/orexin system. *Sleep Med Rev*, **9**, 269–310.
Olson, EJ, Boeve BF, Silber MH (2000). Rapid eye movement sleep behaviour disorder: demographic, clinical and laboratory findings in 93 cases. *Brain*, **123**, 331–9.
Saper CB (2006). Staying awake for dinner: hypothalamic integration of sleep, feeding and circadian rhythms. *Prog Brain Res*, **153**, 243–52.
Saper CB, Chou TC, Scammell TE (2001). The sleep switch: hypothalamic control of sleep and wakefulness. *Trends Neurosci*, **24**, 726–31.
Silber MH (2001). Controversies in sleep medicine: periodic limb movements. *Sleep, Med*, **2**, 367–9.
Thannickal TC, *et al.* (2000). Reduced number of hypocretin neurons in human narcolepsy. *Neuron*, **27**, 469–74.
Turek FW (2004). Circadian rhythms: from the bench to the bedside and falling asleep. *Sleep*, **27**, 1600–2.

24.5.4 Syncope

A.J. Larner

Essentials

Syncope is the commonest identified cause of transient loss of consciousness, being ten times more frequent than epilepsy. It is a consequence of cerebral underperfusion due to reduced cardiac output, often related to reduced venous return due to decreased peripheral vascular resistance, with pooling of blood volume in dependent body parts.

Causes

These include (1) neurally mediated—vasovagal; carotid sinus; situational, e.g. cough syncope; (2) orthostatic (postural) hypotension—autonomic failure; drug-induced; volume depletion; (3) cardiac arrhythmia; (4) cardiac/vascular structural disease—e.g. aortic stenosis.

Diagnosis, prognosis, investigations, and treatment

Diagnosis is clinical, based on history of the circumstances of the event obtained from the patient and reliable eyewitnesses; there is no other diagnostic test. In most patients, particularly those under 45 years of age, the condition is benign and self-limiting, with an excellent prognosis, requiring little investigation beyond physical examination and ECG to exclude heart disease. Cardiac causes of syncope may require specific treatment.

Introduction

Syncope may be defined as a transient loss of consciousness associated with loss of postural tone consequent upon acute reduction of cerebral blood flow. Presyncope is the term sometimes used for symptomatic episodes of cerebral underperfusion that do not progress to loss of consciousness. Syncope and presyncope are among the most common problems seen in general neurology practice, although the condition overlaps with cardiology. Syncope is thus a syndrome with various causes, ranging from benign self-limiting episodes with excellent prognosis to recurrent and possibly life-threatening attacks, the latter often associated with an underlying cardiac disorder. Correct diagnosis is therefore vital, because management will depend on cause. Differential diagnosis, most particularly from epilepsy, is often required.

Pathogenesis

The pathophysiology of syncope relates to cerebral underperfusion, perhaps most particularly affecting the hindbrain. This may follow reduced cardiac venous return, consequent upon reduced peripheral vascular resistance with peripheral blood pooling, leading to reduced stroke volume and cardiac output, or to a primary cardiac disorder impairing cardiac output. Factors predisposing to and precipitating the pathophysiological changes causing syncope may be identifiable, but often the pathogenesis is multifactorial, particularly in older patients.

Distinction may be made between vasovagal, reflex, neurally mediated, or neurocardiogenic syncope, and cardiac or cardiogenic syncope; this forms the basis of classification systems for syncope (Table 24.5.4.1). In the former, reduced peripheral vascular resistance allows pooling of blood in dependent body areas, most usually the lower limbs, hence the reduced venous return and cardiac output, and cerebral underperfusion. This may be precipitated ('triggered') by activities such as standing from the sitting or lying posture, or prolonged standing. There may be a paradoxical bradycardia; standing normally induces a reflex increase in heart rate. It was this observation that led investigators to infer an increase in vagal tone and Sir Thomas Lewis to coin the term 'vasovagal'. However, the pathophysiology may, at least in some cases, relate to sympathetic withdrawal, secondary to a centrally mediated surge in the neurotransmitter serotonin. Despite hypotension and hypovolaemia, a paradoxical cerebrovascular arteriolar vasoconstriction has been observed experimentally, sometimes without cardiovascular changes ('cerebral syncope').

Carotid sinus syncope, related to carotid sinus hypersensitivity, may be precipitated by pressure on the neck or head turning, although sensitivity, as judged by carotid sinus massage, may also be found in patients without these particular triggers. Situational syncopes, such as cough or post-tussive syncope, micturition syncope, swallow syncope, and defecation syncope, may all be subsumed under the category of neurally mediated or reflex syncopes. Pathophysiologically they share similar mechanisms related to reduced venous return, sometimes associated with performance of Valsalva's manoeuvre. The latter may also be relevant in syncope associated with activities such as weight-lifting and trumpet playing.

Orthostatic (postural) hypotension of any cause, such as use of certain drugs or autonomic failure, pregnancy, or in association with anaemia or reduced circulating blood volume, may predispose

Table 24.5.4.1 Causes of syncope

Neurally mediated syncope	Vasovagal syncope
	Carotid sinus syncope
	Situational syncope—cough, sneeze, swallow, defecation, postexercise, postprandial
Orthostatic (postural) hypotension	Autonomic failure: primary, secondary
	Drug induced
	Volume depletion
Cardiac arrhythmias	Sinus node disease (e.g. sick sinus syndrome)
	Atrioventricular conduction disorders
	Paroxysmal supraventricular and ventricular tachycardias
	Inherited disorders: Brugada's syndrome; prolonged QT syndromes (Romano–Ward syndrome, Jervell–Lange–Nielsen syndrome)
Cardiac/vascular structural disease	Cardiac valvular disease (e.g. aortic stenosis)
	Acute myocardial infarction, ischaemia
	Hypertrophic obstructive cardiomyopathy
	Atrial myxoma
	Pericardial disease
	Subclavian steal syndrome

to syncope by impairing peripheral vascular resistance; likewise postprandial hypotension resulting after eating a large meal may be associated.

Cardiac syncope results from a fall in cardiac output which may be associated with arrhythmias, both brady- and tachyarrhythmias, perhaps related to ischaemic heart disease or specific disorders such as Brugada's syndrome, or with structural cardiac disease such as hypertrophic cardiomyopathy (subaortic stenosis) or valvular disease such as aortic stenosis. Vascular steal syndromes such as subclavian steal may also be associated with syncope due to diversion of blood away from hindbrain structures.

Categories of idiopathic syncope ('syncope of unknown origin') and psychogenic syncope (or, more correctly, pseudosyncope) are also described, but these are both diagnoses of exclusion. The former is a useful diagnostic category because it is associated with a better prognosis than cardiac syncope. Psychogenic pseudosyncope (pretended unconsciousness) may be associated with various psychiatric diagnoses including panic attack, somatization, factitious disorder, and frank malingering.

Epidemiology

No age group is immune from syncope, although the cause does vary with age. In neurological practice, the diagnosis is most commonly made in adolescents or young adults who typically have neurally mediated syncope, with a marked predominance of females, and in older people where the possibility of a cardiac cause or multiple factors is higher. Community-based epidemiological surveys suggest that many individuals who have a single or few syncopal episodes do not seek medical advice.

Clinical features

The clinical history is of paramount importance in making the diagnosis of syncope, far outweighing the value of any investigations. In this context, as patients are almost invariably seen after the event, the opportunity to question a reliable eyewitness, if need be by telephone, may be the most important investigation. Equally, however, the clinician should guard against too great a readiness to accept witness statements that what they saw was a 'seizure' or 'convulsion'. Symptoms before, during, and after the ictus should be ascertained. It is recognized that in older people with a higher risk of cardiac syncope the achievement of a diagnosis from the medical history is lower.

The circumstances preceding the event must be enquired about, questioning that aims to ascertain any provoking factors. Emotional or physical trauma, pain (including period pain), and fatigue may increase the risk of syncope, as may sleep deprivation, either situational or in the context of sleep-related disorders such as obstructive sleep apnoea–hypopnoea syndrome. The stuffy atmosphere of hot and crowded environments may also predispose. Attacks while in the dentist's chair, during venesection, or at the sight of blood are classic. Likewise, attacks immediately on rising from a recumbent position, after prolonged standing, or up to 90 min after a large meal are suggestive of neurally mediated syncope. Cardiac syncope may be triggered by exercise.

Patients may be able to recall some premonitory, presyncopal symptoms, sometimes prompting their own comment that they have had a 'faint' or a 'blackout'. These may include a sensation of light-headedness, as though they were going to pass out. Sometimes this is described by patients as 'dizziness', which must be distinguished from the 'spinning dizziness' encountered in vestibular disorders. Patients may recall commenting on not feeling well, or being asked by witnesses if they were feeling all right. There may be a report that sounds such as voices were audible and intelligible but increasingly distant, or there may have been tinnitus. Vision may shrink or become black, leaving just 'tunnel vision', sometimes described as a feeling of distance. Patients may feel weakness or tingling (paraesthesia), or that they 'need air', and indeed may take action to leave the room or go outside before collapsing. Evasive action such as sitting or lying may be possible if presyncopal symptoms last 1 to 2 min, as may occur in neurally mediated syncope. Nausea, sweating (diaphoresis), and feeling both hot and cold may also be remarked upon, suggesting autonomic activation; the skin may be clammy (cold and sweaty) to the touch. An enquiry about premonitory palpitations, during or independent of attacks of loss of consciousness, should also be made. However, not all syncopal episodes have premonitory symptoms, which increases the likelihood of the attack being of cardiac origin. Moreover, older people may have amnesia for the attacks, and present simply with falls of undetermined cause.

For the events during the syncopal episode, the clinician depends on eye witness accounts. These may note that the patient gradually slumps to the ground and lies still. The duration of loss of consciousness is usually brief, around 20 s, although on occasion it can be as long as minutes. Facial pallor, loss of colour, or 'greyness' may be remarked upon. There may be some twitching jerky movements of the limbs, ascribed to tonic brainstem motor activity, but not the sustained alternating tonic–clonic movements typical of a generalized epileptic seizure (unless there is a secondary anoxic seizure). Nevertheless an untrained observer may mistake myoclonic jerks for a 'convulsion' or 'seizure'. Incontinence of urine may occur even in the absence of an epileptic seizure, and some studies have not found incontinence to be a useful discriminator between seizure and syncope. A slow pulse may be detected, should any bystander be both sufficiently quickwitted and knowledgeable to assess this.

Patients should be questioned about the next thing that they remember after the blackout. As the period of loss of consciousness is brief, patients may recollect coming round in the same location where they were at onset of prodromal symptoms. Orientation to surroundings should be enquired about: generally patients are 'with it' and recognize their surroundings fairly promptly, within a minute or two of coming round, and may ask what is going on. They may recall crowds of people around them. Eyewitnesses may also attest to a rapid recovery, without a prolonged period of postictal confusion. Disorientation after a blackout increases the likelihood that it was due to a seizure, as does increasing age. Facial pallor may persist after recovery from syncope, as may skin clamminess, and nausea and vomiting. Events may recur when the patient attempts to stand again.

Historical features may also be helpful in differentiating neurally mediated from cardiac syncope with high sensitivity and specificity (Table 24.5.4.2). Presyncopal features may last longer in neurally mediated attacks, and indeed may be entirely absent in some forms of cardiac syncope. Syncope with onset during exercise or in the supine position should always prompt consideration of a cardiac cause.

Table 24.5.4.2 Clinical clues to the differentiation of neurally mediated from cardiac syncope

Neurally mediated syncope	Cardiac syncope
Onset often subacute, with prodromal symptoms: faintness, weakness, paraesthesia, nausea, sweating	Onset often sudden: palpitations, chest pain, dyspnoea may be present
Precipitating and predisposing factors: emotional upset, trauma, pain, fatigue, assumption of upright posture, prolonged standing, postexercise, postprandial, hot enclosed environments, pregnancy	Onset often spontaneous; may occur during exercise; may be history of cardiac disorder
Often standing or sitting at onset	Onset may occur standing, sitting, or supine (last should increase suspicion of cardiac syncope)
Appearance: facial pallor; usually lie still but irregular myoclonic twitches may occur; urinary incontinence may occur. May feel clammy (cold and sweaty) to touch. Bradycardia may be detected	Similar, but urinary incontinence uncommon. Heart rhythm abnormality may be detected
Postictus: rapid recovery of orientation. Further episodes of syncope may occur with standing	Similar, unless prolonged hypoxia

Table 24.5.4.3 Clinical clues to the differentiation of syncope from seizure

Syncope	Seizure
Subacute onset with prodromal features	Sudden onset, sometimes preceded by symptoms of aura (e.g. olfactory hallucinations)
Precipitating and predisposing factors often identifiable from history	Onset often spontaneous; may be predisposing factors such as sleep deprivation, missing meals, or precipitating factors such as flashing lights
Onset most often when standing or sitting	Onset may occur standing, sitting, or supine
Appearance: facial pallor; usually lie still but irregular myoclonic twitches may occur, and also urinary incontinence	May be cyanosed, or flushed. Stertorous breathing. Stereotypic tonic–clonic movements in generalized seizures. Urinary and faecal incontinence may occur. Tongue biting (sides more than tip). Injury as a consequence of fall
Recovery usually rapid, with prompt orientation to surroundings	Recovery often delayed many minutes, and no recall of event. Residual neurological signs may be present (Todd's paresis, aphasia)

Differential diagnosis

The most important differential diagnosis of syncope is epileptic seizure. Other conditions to consider may also include drop attacks, transient ischaemic attack (TIA), cataplexy, and hyperekplexia.

Patients with syncope are not infrequently reported to have had a fit or a seizure by bystanders, comments prompted perhaps by observation of the myoclonic jerks that may occur. Various historical and clinical features may argue for syncope and against epilepsy (Table 24.5.4.3), although it should be remembered that secondary anoxic epileptic seizures may complicate otherwise benign syncopal attacks, e.g. if a patient is supported by bystanders and not allowed to fall to the floor. Hence, the diagnoses of syncope and seizure are not mutually exclusive. Atonic seizures may present a particular diagnostic problem, although these most often occur in combination with other types of epileptic seizure. Features that should raise the clinical index of suspicion for seizure include lack of obvious provoking factors, amnesia for the attack, a prolonged period of loss of consciousness, an eyewitness account of typical tonic–clonic movements, attacks developing during sleep, prolonged postictal confusion, and the presence of physical injury sustained during the event (although injuries such as bony fractures and subdural haematoma may be sustained during syncope). Indeed a simple point score of historical features may distinguish syncope from seizures with sensitivity and specificity of more than 90%.

Drop attacks, unexplained falls forward onto the knees, particularly in older people, are not associated with loss of consciousness, but as patients may have little recall of these events this clinical scenario should prompt consideration of syncope. Carotid TIAs are not associated with loss of consciousness and vertebral TIAs seldom so, and the latter are invariably accompanied by other focal neurological signs (diplopia, vertigo). Cataplexy, loss of muscular tone leading to a brief fall in response to emotion such as laughter, may be a feature of the narcoleptic syndrome or occur in isolation, but is not associated with loss of consciousness, and similarly there

is no association in hyperekplexia, the pathological exaggeration of the startle response that may provoke a fall.

Clinical investigations

Clinical examination at the scene of the event is seldom possible, and delayed examination in a clinical setting may well be unremarkable. Signs of cardiac disease, arrhythmic or structural, should be sought. Checking the blood pressure in the lying and standing positions to look for orthostatic hypotension may be undertaken, but prolonged standing (minutes) may be necessary to observe a drop in blood pressure. Carotid sinus massage to look for cardioinhibitory (asystole, 'malignant syncope') and vasodepressor (hypotension) responses is best restricted to situations in which continuous ECG and blood pressure monitoring can be undertaken and resuscitation equipment is to hand (e.g. during tilt-table testing).

Of investigations, an ECG is indicated to exclude arrhythmias such as short P–R interval, prolonged corrected Q–T interval, and Brugada's syndrome (right bundle-branch block with ST-segment elevation in leads V1–V3). If a standard ECG is normal, no other investigations may be required, particularly in young and otherwise healthy individuals. Ambulatory ECG may be indicated if the clinical index of suspicion for arrhythmia is high (e.g. history of palpitations, older patient, recurrent events) but is subject to limited specificity unless rhythm disturbances correlate with clinical symptoms.

Further investigation, if required, generally falls outwith the experience and expertise of neurologists. Monitoring of cardiac rhythm with loop recorders (external, implantable) may be considered. Echocardiography may be performed when there is clinical suspicion of a valvular (e.g. aortic stenosis) or other cardiac structural abnormality (e.g. hypertrophic obstructive cardiomyopathy, atrial myxoma), or if there is a positive cardiac history or abnormal ECG, but it has no place in otherwise unexplained syncope. Head-upright tilt-table testing, a continuous passive orthostatic stress, may be used to reproduce syncope in individuals with recurrent events and no evidence of cardiac cause.

Blood tests to exclude anaemia and hyponatraemia may be appropriate. Structural brain imaging (CT, MRI) and EEG may be indicated if seizure seems more likely than syncope as the cause of loss of consciousness.

Treatment and prognosis

Treatment should be individualized according to cause. Explanation and reassurance may be the only intervention required in young individuals without heart disease and with a normal ECG as prognosis is excellent. Advice about avoiding recognized predisposing and precipitating factors of neurally mediated syncope may be appropriate, as may increasing fluid and salt intake.

Prognosis is worse for cardiac than for neurally mediated syncope, and the presence of structural heart disease is a predictor of mortality in patients with syncope. Specific treatment of cardiac arrhythmia, and valvular and other structural disorders may be required. Cardiac pacing may be indicated for certain arrhythmias, and a last resort in patients with recurrent neurally mediated syncope. Orthostatic hypotension induced by drugs (e.g. vasodilators, diuretics, phenothiazines, tricyclic antidepressants, monoamine oxidase inhibitors) may be improved by drug cessation or substitution. Autonomic failure, either primary or secondary, may be ameliorated by various strategies (e.g. volume expansion, fludrocortisone, graduated compression stockings, midodrine), and these options may also be explored as prophylaxis for recurrent syncope of noncardiac origin. Selective serotonin reuptake inhibitors such as fluoxetine, sertraline, and nefazodone have been found helpful in some circumstances.

A common issue after transient loss of consciousness due to syncope relates to driving motor vehicles and directing other forms of transport. Different jurisdictions have different rules with respect to fitness to drive, which may relate to both driver age and vehicle type (cars, motor cycles as opposed to lorries, buses). Doctors should consult these standards before advising patients on driving.

In the United Kingdom, the Driver and Vehicle Licensing Agency (DVLA) places no restrictions on patients who have a simple faint, defined as episodes with definite provocative factors, with associated prodromal symptoms, and that are unlikely to occur while sitting or lying. Even recurrent events evoke no sanction provided that the '3 Ps' (provocation, prodrome, posture) apply on each occasion. However, if loss of consciousness is likely to be unexplained syncope, patients are debarred from driving for a variable period (4 weeks to 6 months) dependent on whether the risk of recurrence is deemed to be high or low, and the type of licence applied for. A licence is revoked or refused for 1 year for lorry/bus drivers with unexplained syncope with high risk of recurrence. There are, in addition, particular standards for cough syncope (driving to cease until liability to attacks successfully controlled) and for individuals with pacemakers (for further information, see http://www.dvla.gov.uk/media/pdf/medical/aagv1.pdf).

Further reading

Arthur W, Kaye GC (2001). Current investigations used to assess syncope. *Postgrad Med J*, **77**, 20–3.
Benditt DG, *et al.* (1996). Tilt table testing for assessing syncope. American College of Cardiology. *J Am Coll Cardiol*, **28**, 263–75.
European Heart Rhythm Association (EHRA), *et al.* (2009). Guidelines for the diagnosis and management of syncope (version 2009): the Task Force for the Diagnosis and Management of Syncope of the European Society of Cardiology (ESC). *Eur Heart J*, **30**, 2631–71.

Grubb BP, Karas B (1999). Neurally mediated syncope. In: Mathias. CJ, Bannister R, eds. *Autonomic failure. A textbook of clinical disorders of the autonomic nervous system*, 4th edition, pp. 437–47. Oxford University Press, Oxford.
Hainsworth R (1999). Syncope and fainting: classification and pathophysiological basis. In: Mathias CJ, Bannister R (eds) *Autonomic failure. A textbook of clinical disorders of the autonomic nervous system*, 4th edition, pp. 428–36. Oxford University Press, Oxford.
Hartikainen JEK, Camm AJ (1999). Cardiac causes of syncope. In: Mathias CJ, Bannister R (eds) *Autonomic failure. A textbook of clinical disorders of the autonomic nervous system*, 4th edition, pp. 448–60. Oxford University Press, Oxford.
Hoefnagels WAJ, *et al.* (1991). Transient loss of consciousness: the value of the history for distinguishing seizure from syncope. *J Neurol*, **238**, 39–43.
Kapoor WN (2000). Syncope. *NEJM*, **343**, 1856–62.
Kenny RA, *et al.* (1989). Head up tilt: a useful test for investigating unexplained syncope. *Lancet*, **i**, 1352–5.
Lempert T, Bauer M, Schmidt D (1994). Syncope: a videometric analysis of 56 episodes of transient cerebral hypoxia. *Ann Neurol*, **36**, 233–7.
Lewis T (1932). A lecture on vasovagal syncope and the carotid sinus mechanism: with comments on Gower's and Nothnagel's syndrome. *BMJ*, **1**, 873–6.
Sharpey-Schafer EP (1956). Syncope. *BMJ*, **i**, 506–9.
Sheldon R, *et al.* (2006). Diagnostic criteria for vasovagal syncope based on a quantitative history. *Eur Heart J*, **27**, 344–50.
Sheldon R, *et al.* (2002). Historical criteria that distinguish syncope from seizures. *J Am Coll Cardiol*, **40**, 142–8.
Soteriades ES, *et al.* (2002). Incidence and prognosis of syncope. *NEJM*, **347**, 878–85.
Task Force on Syncope, European Society of Cardiology (2004). Guidelines on management (diagnosis and treatment) of syncope—update 2004. *Europace*, **6**, 467–537.

24.5.5 The unconscious patient

David Bates

Essentials

Prolonged loss of consciousness (coma, defined as a Glasgow Coma Score of 8 or less) is seen commonly: (1) following head injury, (2) after an overdose of sedating drugs, and (3) in the situation of 'nontraumatic coma', where there are many possible diagnoses, but the most common are postanoxic, postischaemic, systemic infection, and metabolic derangement, e.g. hypoglycaemia.

Clinical approach

Urgent assessment is required to identify and, where possible, correct the pathological cause, and protect the brain from the development of irreversible damage. Key issues are to (1) ensure adequate protection of the airway and adequate ventilation; (2) immediately exclude (and treat) rapidly reversible causes, in particular hypoglycaemia and opioid toxicity; and then (3) consider a wide range of differential diagnoses—even in 'nontraumatic coma' the patient may be harbouring delayed effects of head injury such as subdural haematomas, or meningitis arising from a basal skull fracture.

Investigations

After performing resuscitation, obtaining a history (from a witness if necessary), physical examination and bedside tests (e.g. fingerprick blood glucose), further investigation depends on the clinical context: (1) coma with focal signs or evidence of head injury—urgent brain imaging by CT or MRI; (2) coma with meningeal irritation but without focal signs—urgent brain imaging and/or lumbar puncture is required; treat before investigation if clinical suspicion of e.g. meningitis is high; (3) coma without focal lateralizing neurological signs and without meningismus—the probability of finding a focal abnormality is low; haematological/biochemical tests or a toxin screen are most likely to provide the diagnosis.

Prognosis

Brainstem reflexes are the most important clinical signs in defining prognosis: in the absence of sedative drugs, the absence for 24 h of corneal or pupillary reflexes, or of oculovestibular responses, is almost incompatible with recovery to independence, whatever the cause of coma.

Treatment

Specific treatment (if any) will depend upon the particular cause of coma, but—whatever the cause—long-term attention is required to the patient's respiration, skin, circulation, and bladder and bowel function, seizures must be controlled, and the level of consciousness should be regularly assessed and monitored. In patients in whom the prognosis is hopeless, the institution and continuation of resuscitative measures is inappropriate and will serve only to prolong the anguish of relatives and carers (see Chapter 17.8).

Definition

Normal consciousness

Consciousness is the state of awareness of the self and the environment when provided with adequate stimuli; normal consciousness is exhibited by those patients who are fully responsive to stimuli and show appropriate behaviour and speech. Patients who are asleep can be roused and then perform normally. Normal consciousness depends on the integration of activity in the ascending reticular activating substance of the brainstem and the neuronal connections between areas of the cerebral cortex. The ascending reticular activating substance determines arousal, which is shown by awakening with eye opening, motor responses, and verbal communication. The content of consciousness, which is the combination of psychological responses to feeling, emotions, and mental activity, is mediated by the cerebral cortex (Fig. 24.5.5.1).

Coma

Coma is a state of unrousable unconsciousness without any psychologically understandable response to external stimuli or inner need. The patient may appear to be asleep but is incapable of responding normally to external stimuli other than by showing eye opening to pain, flexion or extension of the muscles in the limbs to pain, and occasionally grunting or groaning in response to painful stimuli. It occurs when there is damage to the ascending reticular activating substance or bilateral damage to areas of the cerebral hemispheres, or both (Figs. 24.5.5.2–24.5.5.5).

Confusion

Patients are usually disoriented with lowered attention, an inability to express thoughts, drowsiness, and defects in memory. There is clouding of consciousness characterized by an impaired capacity to think, understand, respond to, and remember stimuli. It is important to differentiate acute confusion from dysphasia, amnesia, acute psychosis, severe depression, or dementia. Confusion is most commonly seen as the result of toxic or metabolic disturbances, particularly in older people.

Delirium

There is motor restlessness, hallucination, disorientation, and delusion. The patient is often frightened and irritable and the state can be regarded as profound confusion; both states should alert the doctor to impending coma. Delirium is most commonly seen in patients with toxic or metabolic disorders, but can be mimicked by degenerative brain disease, acute psychosis, and hypomania.

Stupor

The patient appears to be asleep and will show little or no spontaneous activity, respond only to vigorous stimulation, and then lapse back into somnolence. It may be difficult to differentiate stupor from catatonic schizophrenia or severe retarded depression, but in stupor due to organic disease the electroencephalogram (EEG) will always be abnormal.

The vegetative state

The patient breathes spontaneously, has a stable circulation, and shows cycles of eye opening and eye closure that may simulate sleep and waking, but he or she is unaware of self and environment. It can be seen transiently in the recovery from coma or it may persist to death. This state is usually seen in patients with diffuse bilateral cerebral hemisphere disturbance with an intact brainstem, although it can occur with bilateral damage to the most rostral part of the brainstem. It is most commonly seen after head injury or as the result of hypoxic–ischaemic damage after cardiac arrest. The patient appears to be awake but is unaware—a condition that frequently causes distress to carers and relatives (Fig. 24.5.5.6).

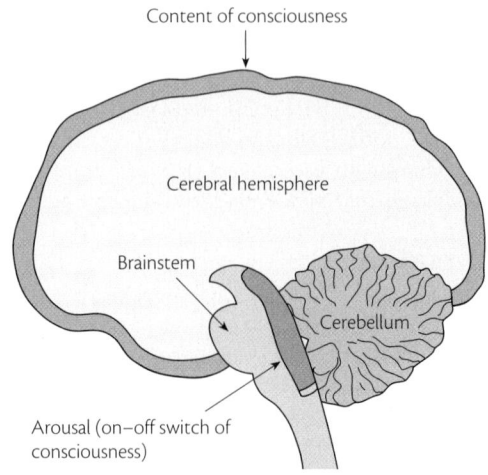

Fig. 24.5.5.1 Normal consciousness.

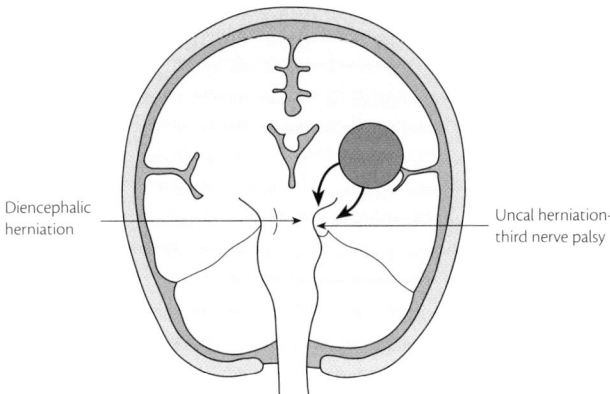

Fig. 24.5.5.2 Supratentorial mass.

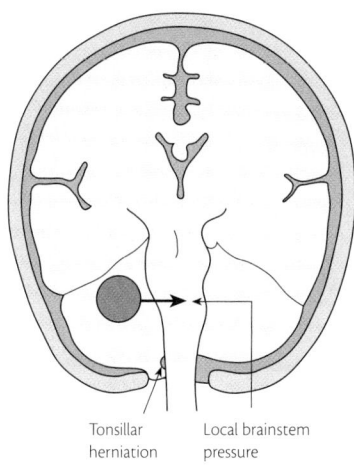

Fig. 24.5.5.4 Brainstem lesion—local pressure.

The locked-in syndrome

Damage to the ventral portion of the pons below the level of the third nerve nuclei causes total paralysis of the limbs and lower cranial nerves, but with intact consciousness (Fig. 24.5.5.7). The patient can open, elevate, and depress the eyes but cannot move the eyes horizontally, and there is no voluntary movement or speech. The diagnosis is made when the doctor recognizes that the patient is able to open the eyes voluntarily and allow them to close in response to command, and can therefore respond to verbal and sensory stimuli by blinking. The most common cause is infarction of the ventral pons, usually in a patient with hypertension, although it can also be seen with pontine tumours and multiple sclerosis, in central pontine myelinolysis after profound hyponatraemia, and after head injury. The prognosis is poor, although some patients recover, usually with residual spasticity. An EEG may help by showing an alert state, reactive to external stimuli, and neurophysiology can be used to exclude similar incapacities occurring in myasthenia gravis or the Guillain–Barré syndrome.

Psychogenic unresponsiveness

The term 'pseudo coma' or psychogenic unresponsiveness is used for patients who appear to be unconscious and in a coma but who are not. The simplest way to identify this condition is to undertake oculovestibular testing (see below), which will reveal the presence of nystagmus and indicate that the patient has an intact brainstem and cortex.

The management of the patient in a coma

History

Once the patient is stable it is important to obtain as much information as possible from those who accompanied the patient to hospital or who observed the onset of the coma. The circumstances in which consciousness was lost are of vital importance in helping to identify the diagnosis. Generally, coma is likely to present in one of three ways: the predictable progression of an underlying illness; an unpredictable event in a patient with a previously known disease; or a totally unexpected event. In the first category are patients who deteriorate after focal brainstem infarction or those with known intracranial mass lesions who show similar deterioration. In the second category are patients with recognized cardiac arrhythmia or the known risk factor of sepsis from an intravenous cannula. In the final category, it is important to distinguish whether there has been a previous history of seizures, trauma, febrile illness, or focal neurological disturbances. The history of a sudden collapse in the midst of a busy street or office indicates the need for different investigations from those required when the patient has been discovered at home in bed surrounded by empty bottles that previously contained sedative tablets. Where there is uncertainty, a telephone call to relatives and medical attendants may be useful.

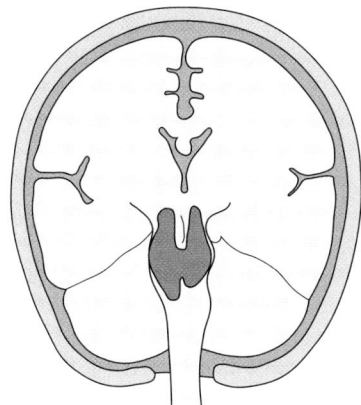

Fig. 24.5.5.3 Brainstem lesion—intrinsic.

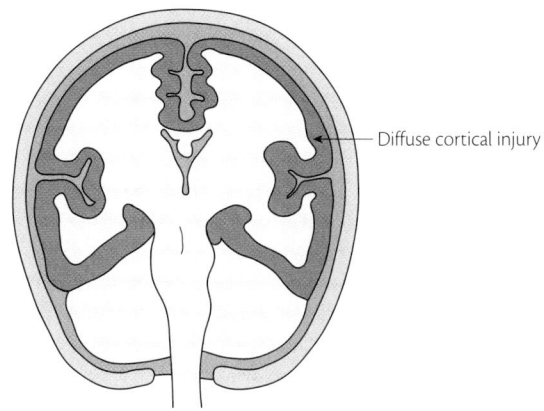

Fig. 24.5.5.5 Bihemispheric damage.

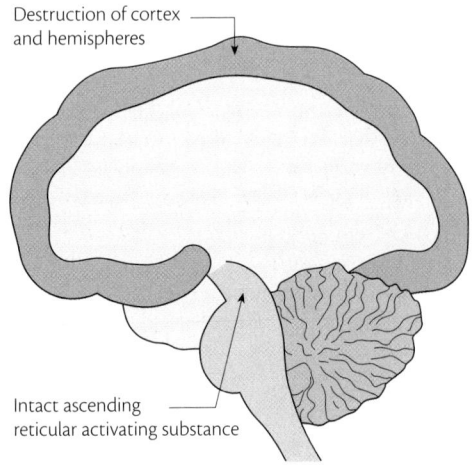

Fig. 24.5.5.6 Vegetative state.

Clinical assessment and examination

Estimation of the temperature, pulse, blood pressure, and respiratory rate, and examination of the skin, cardiovascular system, chest, and abdomen may often yield important clues in establishing the cause of a loss of consciousness. Fever, although not diagnostic, will usually indicate the presence of a systemic infection, meningitis, encephalitis, or abscess; seizures increase the likelihood of the last two diagnoses. Hypothermia is most commonly seen after exposure to low environmental temperatures, intoxication with alcohol or barbiturates, the presence of peripheral circulatory failure, or profound myxoedema. Tachy- or bradyarrhythmias, evidence for valvular heart disease, or peripheral emboli raise the possibility of a cardiogenic cause, bruits over the carotid vessels suggest cerebrovascular disease, and splinter haemorrhages suggest endocarditis or collagen vascular disease. Hypotension raises the possibility of shock, myocardial infarction, or septicaemia, and Addison's disease should be considered. Hypertension is less helpful as a clinical sign because it may be seen both as the result of cerebral insult or as an indicator of hypertensive encephalopathy.

The odour of the breath of an unconscious patient may indicate the presence of alcohol, a ketotic fetor raises the possibility of diabetes, and the fetor of hepatic or renal failure provides important clues. Clubbing of the fingernails suggests the possibility of a

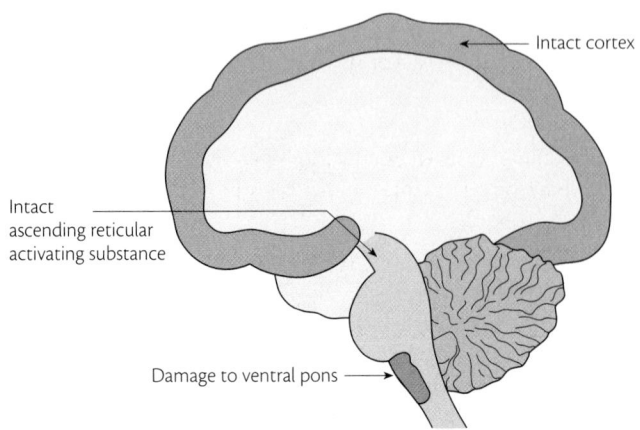

Fig. 24.5.5.7 Locked-in syndrome.

respiratory or gastrointestinal abnormality, and evidence of tracheal deviation, fluid in the chest, or collapse of the lung suggests the possibility of a respiratory cause. In the abdomen the finding of enlargement of an organ might indicate portal hypertension, polycystic kidneys, and an associated subarachnoid haemorrhage, or abnormality in the blood-forming organs. The general colour of the skin and mucous membranes might reveal anaemia, jaundice, cyanosis, or the pink discoloration of carbon monoxide poisoning. Purpura suggests a bleeding diathesis and bruising around the head indicates the possibility of trauma or a base-of-skull fracture. A rash may indicate an infective or inflammatory disease and hyperpigmentation raises the possibility of Addison's disease. The presence of puncture wounds might identify an individual who is diabetic or a recreational drug user.

Neurological examination

This requires observation and an assessment of reflex responses. The position, posture, and spontaneous movements of the patient should be noted; the skull and spine should be examined with testing for neck stiffness and Kernig's sign to identify meningeal irritation. Ophthalmoscopy will identify papilloedema, fundal haemorrhages, emboli, and subhyaloid haemorrhages; it must be remembered that the absence of papilloedema does not exclude raised intracranial pressure. The ears and fauces should be examined.

Level of consciousness

The level of consciousness must be documented by the initial observer and can then be monitored by medical and nursing staff to determine the progress of the patient and identify the need for further investigation, therapy, and decision. The most useful hierarchical grading scale to assess the level of consciousness is the Glasgow Coma Scale (GCS) in which the patient's response to graded stimuli of eye opening, motor response, and verbal response are recorded (Table 24.5.5.1); all four limbs are observed for responses to pain and the best response is recorded, although asymmetry should be noted and may identify lateralization. The scale measures consciousness and it is possible to score gradations from the fully conscious patient (eye opening, 4; motor response, 6; verbal response, 5) to the totally unresponsive patient (eye opening, 1; motor response, 1; verbal response, 1). If the level of consciousness can be shown to be improving, then urgent decisions may be delayed, but if deterioration occurs it is imperative that a decision be made about management.

Brainstem function

The brainstem reflexes identify those lesions that affect the reticular activating substance and determine the viability of the patient. Most of the reflexes involve the eyes and the pattern of respiration, although the latter may be compromised by requirements of ventilation.

Pupillary reactions

Unilateral dilatation of a pupil with lack of a light response suggests uncal herniation of the temporal lobe over the tentorium cerebrum entrapping the third nerve or due to distortion of the brainstem; it may also be seen with a posterior communicating artery aneurysm or other third nerve damage. Midbrain lesions typically cause loss of the light reflex with pupils in the midposition, lesions in the pons cause small pupils with retained light responses, and fixed dilatation of the pupils suggests significant brainstem damage but must be differentiated from the fixed dilatation caused by

Table 24.5.5.1 Neurological observation and assessment

Glasgow coma scale	Score
Eye opening	
Spontaneous	4
To speech	3
To pain	2
Nil	1
Verbal response	
Orientated	5
Confused conversation	4
Inappropriate words	3
Incomprehensible sounds	2
Nil	1
Best motor response	
Obeys	6
Localizes	5
Withdraws	4
Abnormal flexion	3
Extension response	2
Nil	1
Brainstem function	
Pupillary reactions	
Corneal responses	
Spontaneous eye movements	
Oculocephalic responses	
Oculovestribular responses	
Respiratory pattern	
Motor function	
Motor response	
Muscle tone	
Tendon reflexes	
Seizures	

atropine-like agents instilled by earlier observers. Horner's syndrome may be seen with lesions in the hypothalamus or brainstem, but can also be seen with damage to the wall of the carotid artery. Small pupils that react briskly to light raise the possibility of metabolic causes of coma such as hepatic or renal failure; drug intoxications tend not to affect the pupillary light responses.

Corneal responses

The corneal reflex is usually retained until a very deep coma occurs; if absent in a patient who appears to be otherwise in a light coma, there is a distinct possibility that the cause may be drug intoxication. The loss of the corneal reflex in the absence of drug overdose is a poor prognostic indicator.

Spontaneous eye movements

Conjugate deviation of the eyes suggests a focal hemispheric or brainstem lesion, depression of the eyes is seen with damage to the midbrain at the level of the tectum, and skew deviation of the eyes suggests a lesion at the pontomedullary junction. Incoordinate eyes suggest damage to the ocular motor or abducent nerve in the brainstem or pathways, but a minor degree of divergence of the eyes is normal in the unconscious patient. Patients in a light coma will often have normal roving eye movements, similar to those of sleep, which may be conjugate or dysconjugate. They cannot be mimicked and, when present, exclude the possibility of psychogenic unresponsiveness, when eye movements are likely to be more jerky.

Reflex eye movements are important in assessing brainstem activity. The oculocephalic response obtained by rotating the patient's head from side to side and observing the position of the eyes is likely to show doll's eye movements when the brainstem is intact, but the eyes will remain in the midposition of the head when the brainstem is depressed. Oculovestibular testing is undertaken by the installation of 50 to 200 ml of ice-cold water into an external auditory meatus. The conscious patient, and those in psychogenic coma, will develop nystagmus with the quick phase away from the side of the stimulation, indicating an active pons and intact corticopontine connections. A tonic response with conjugate movement of the eyes towards the stimulated side indicates an intact pons and suggests a supratentorial cause for the coma, whereas a dysconjugate response or no response at all implies a lesion within the brainstem.

Respiration

The techniques of ventilation limit the value of observation of respiration in patients with coma, but, if testing is possible before respiration is controlled, then deep breathing suggests acidosis, regular shallow breathing is consistent with drug overdose, long-cycle Cheyne–Stokes respiration suggests damage at the level of the diencephalon, and short-cycle Cheyne–Stokes respiration damage at the level of the medulla. Central neurogenic hyperventilation occurs with lesions in the low midbrain and upper pons, and reflex responses such as yawning, vomiting, and hiccoughing may occur with brainstem disturbances.

Motor function

Motor function is assessed as part of the level of consciousness in the GCS, but lateralizing abnormalities are important and indicate the likelihood of a focal cause, although they may occasionally be seen in the context of hepatic encephalopathy or hypoglycaemia. The presence of generalized or focal seizures implies hemispheric damage and may help in lateralization; multifocal myoclonus suggests a metabolic or anoxic cause with diffuse cortical irritation.

Investigation

After performing the resuscitation, history, examination, and assessment, the doctor should identify one of the three following states (Table 24.5.5.2).

Coma with focal signs or evidence of head injury

In such patients, whether the focal signs indicate a brainstem or supratentorial problem, a CT scan or MRI should be undertaken. A normal scan may be seen in patients with hypoglycaemia or hepatic coma and the presence of structural pathology will be identified, allowing a decision to be made about the indications for surgery or other therapy.

Table 24.5.5.2 Investigations to identify the coma state

Diagnostic category	Investigations	Causes
Coma with focal signs		
± Papilloedema	CT scan or MRI	Haematoma (extradural, subdural, parenchymal)
Hemiparesis	Chest radiograph	Infarction
Brainstem signs		Tumour
Focal seizures		Abscess
		Rarely metabolic
Coma with meningismus		
± Fever	± Imaging	Meningitis
± Fundal changes	Lumbar puncture	Encephalitis
	Blood tests	Subarachnoid haemorrhage
		Diffuse head injury
		Cerebral malaria
		Hypertensive encephalopathy
Coma alone		
History	Blood tests	Drug overdose
Systemic signs	± Lumbar puncture	Hypoxic ischaemia
	Electroencephalogram	Metabolic (diabetes, hepatatic, renal, etc.)
		Toxic (alcohol, carbon monoxide)
		Epilepsy

Coma with meningeal irritation but without focal signs

Such patients most commonly have subarachnoid haemorrhage, acute meningitis, or meningoencephalitis as the cause of their coma. Brain imaging is the ideal investigation to identify the presence of subarachnoid blood and exclude the possibility of focal collections. Depending on the results of the scan a lumbar puncture may be performed and provide diagnostic information. If the suspicion of meningitis is high, then treatment with antibiotics should be started and, in the absence of focal signs or papilloedema, lumbar puncture may precede imaging.

Coma without focal lateralizing neurological signs and without meningismus

Most patients will have suffered diffuse anoxic–ischaemic disease, metabolic derangement, or drug insult. It may be necessary to undertake imaging techniques but the probability of finding a focal abnormality is low, and it is more likely that haematological or biochemical tests or a search for toxins in the blood will provide the diagnosis, or help identify an episode of ischaemia or hypoxia in the past. There may occasionally be an indication to undertake a lumbar puncture in such patients to exclude an inflammatory or infective cause. Patients who are in a coma as the result of a drug overdose will usually be identified from the history and the circumstances of discovery, but the possibility of drug-induced coma should always be considered in patients without focal signs and without meningismus. The discrepancy in marked depression of brainstem responses in a patient who appears to be in a relatively light coma suggests a drug-induced coma, the importance of which is that such patients have a good prognosis provided that they are given adequate respiratory and circulatory support during the coma.

Prognosis

The prognosis of individual patients depends on the aetiology, depth of coma, duration of coma, and certain clinical signs.

Aetiology

Following a head injury, prognosis depends on the presence of intracranial haematoma, the age of the patient, and the severity of the systemic injury and its effects. Patients in a coma after a drug overdose have, in general, a good prognosis provided that they are adequately resuscitated and protected. Patients who are in a coma as a result of causes other than head injury or drug overdose for a period of more than 6 h have only a 10% chance of making a good recovery. Those who have had a subarachnoid haemorrhage or stroke have a less than 5% chance of making such a recovery, and those with hypoxic or ischaemic injury, typically after cardiac arrest, about 10% chance. Those with metabolic or infective causes have almost a 30% chance of making a good recovery. A vegetative state is most likely to occur after head injury or hypoxic–ischaemic damage.

Depth of coma

Patients with no response to eye opening, no focal response to pain, and a poor response to pain have a poorer outcome than those who respond with eye opening, grunting, and flexion of the limbs.

Duration of the coma

When patients have been in a coma for 6 h about 12% may make a good recovery, those who remain in a coma for 24 h have only a 10% chance of recovery, and at the end of a week only 3% of patients can be expected to make a good recovery. In general, patients who remain in a coma for more than 7 to 14 days either die or enter a continuing vegetative state.

Clinical signs

Brainstem reflexes are the most important clinical signs in defining prognosis; the absence of corneal or pupillary reflexes or of oculovestibular responses for 24 h, in the absence of sedative drugs, is almost incompatible with recovery to independence whatever the cause of the coma. Most brainstem reflexes are useful indicators of a poor prognosis but some, such as the development of nystagmus and oculovestibular testing or vocalization of any recognizable word within 48 h, identify patients with a good chance of recovery.

The value of investigations

Although the bedside tests of eye opening, motor response, and brainstem reflexes proposed by Plum *et al.* and formulated by Levy (see Further reading) have been the mainstay of assessment of the patient in coma in the accident and emergency department and intensive care unit (ICU) for two decades, there is increasing evidence that biochemical values and neurophysiological tests have a role to play. The value of the N20 wave in somatosensory-evoked potential recording (N20 SSEP) and measurement of neuron-specific enolase (NSE) in peripheral blood at varying time intervals in coma have been shown to be prognostic in the PROPAC study in centres in the Netherlands. It is suggested that the bilateral absence of N20 SSEP, or the finding of NSE serum levels greater than 33 μg/l, have a higher positive likelihood ratio and a lower false-positive rate than the clinical signs of absence of pupillary and corneal reflexes in predicting a poor outcome.

There are reservations in accepting the conclusions reached from this study, because only patients who remained unconscious at 24 h were included and 'poor outcome' was defined as death or remaining unconscious at 1 month and it was assumed that the chance of recovery of consciousness in patients remaining unconscious for 1 month was virtually nil. Nevertheless, there is logic in looking for biological parameters to identify prognosis in coma and, despite the difficulty in obtaining standardized measures of NSE and complex evoked potentials in the circumstances of most ICUs, there is the suggestion that the bilateral absence of N20 SSEP or the presence of serum NSE greater than 33 μg/l might be used to define futility of the continuance of care. At present using such criteria would result in litigation. It is, nevertheless, evident that a reproducible and validated biological marker would improve decision-making in the early management of the patient in a coma and avoid prolonging an insentient life. Further validation of such measures in large studies is warranted.

Continuation of care

The long-term care of patients in a coma may be undertaken in an ICU, on a specialist ward, in a rehabilitation unit, or in a long-stay hospital. It is important that those in whom prognosis is hopeless should not be permanently exposed to the rigors of intensive care medicine but should continue to receive basic care within routine hospital wards or a more long-stay environment. So long as patients are considered to have a potential for recovery they should be looked after in an ICU or a specialist ward. Their respiration, skin, circulation, and bladder and bowel function need attention, seizures must be controlled, and the level of consciousness should be regularly assessed and monitored. It is important that the mobility of joints and circulation to pressure areas are maintained during the long-term care of the patient, and the possibility of aspiration pneumonia, peptic ulceration, and other complications of long-term intensive care needs to be avoided. Techniques such as mechanical ventilation and steroid therapy should not be used routinely in the management of comatose patients; they do not improve prognosis and may compromise recovery. Investigations are of little help in identifying long-term prognosis because various types of EEG pattern have been recorded from patients in prolonged coma and CT scans simply show cortical atrophy with ventricular dilatation. Some somatosensory-evoked responses have been reported to show loss of the cortical component in long-term unconsciousness and positron emission tomography (PET) is reported to show metabolic underactivity, but, at present, neither test can provide decisive information as to prognosis.

A number of studies have demonstrated an important role for functional neuroimaging in the identification of residual cognitive function in the persistent vegetative state. These studies may be useful where there is concern about the accuracy of the diagnosis and the possibility that residual cognitive function is undetected, but the tests are extremely complex and subject to methodological and theoretical difficulties. Standardization of such techniques, including those assessing residual auditory function with a combination of PET and functional MRI, remains a research tool and is unlikely to have a clinical role in the near future.

Further reading

Bates D (1991). Defining prognosis in medical coma. *J Neurol Neurosurg Psychiatry*, **54**, 569–71.

Bates D (1993). The management of medical coma. *J Neurol Neurosurg Psychiatry*, **56**, 589–98.

Levy DE (1985). Predicting outcome from hypoxic–ischaemic coma. *JAMA*, **253** 1420–6.

Fisher CM (1969). The neurological examination of the comatose patient. *Acta Neurol Scand Suppl*, **45**(46), 1–56.

Pickard JD (2005). Functional imaging, electrophysiology and mechanical intervention. *Neuropsychol Rehabil*, **15**, 272–306.

Plum F, *et al.* (2007). *Diagnosis of stupor and coma*. Oxford University Press, Oxford.

Teasdale G, Jennett WB (1974). Assessment of coma and impaired consciousness: a practical scale. *Lancet*, **ii**, 81–4.

Zanbergen EJG, *et al.* (2006). Prediction of poor outcome within the first three days of post-anoxic coma. *Neurology*, **66**, 62–8.

24.5.6 Brain death and the vegetative state

P.J. Hutchinson and J.D. Pickard

Essentials

Death can be defined as the irreversible loss of the capacity for consciousness and brain stem function, combined with irreversible loss of the capacity to breathe. The irreversible cessation of brainstem function, whether caused by a primary intracranial catastrophe (e.g. trauma, haemorrhage) or the result of extracranial cranial events (e.g hypoxia), will result in the same clinical state, hence brain stem death is the same as death of the patient.

Brain death and death of the brainstem

The distinction between these is of key importance: (1) 'brain death' implies death of the entire nervous system, but focal electrical activity is often discoverable under such circumstances; (2) 'brainstem death' is an alternative term, representing irreversible loss of brainstem function. Criteria for these diagnoses have been promulgated and require formal tests (see also Chapter 17.9).

Vegetative state

This describes patients who are awake but not aware as a result of loss of cortical function, but with a functioning brain stem. The diagnosis of this condition requires documentation by skilled clinicians carried out over periods of time—care is needed to exclude the minimally conscious state or brainstem injury causing widespread paralysis, but with preserved cortical function. Recovery from the vegetative state is possible, but most patients remain severely disabled and dependent.

Declaration of permanence of the vegetative state may allow withdrawal of artificial nutrition and hydration within a legal framework in many countries; in the United Kingdom, it is a legal requirement to seek approval from a court before taking such action.

Brain death

Despite advances in prehospital, accident and emergency, and intensive care management of neurological conditions, including cerebral trauma, haemorrhage, hypoxia, and infarction, there remain many who succumb. The mechanism of death from these conditions may be sudden with cardiorespiratory decompensation and arrest, or the heart may continue to beat with respiration maintained by artificial ventilation but in the context of irreversible loss of brain function—the state of 'brain death'. The loss of brainstem function results in failure of neural transmission caudally to maintain respiration and cranially to maintain activation of the cerebrum by the reticular activating system. It is important to distinguish between the definitions of brain death and brainstem death. The original term 'brain death' (US Harvard criteria 1968) implied complete death of the whole nervous system (flat electroencephalogram or EEG) but islands of electrical activity may persist in the cortex and/or spinal reflexes may persist. This state is, however, consistent with irreversibility. In the United Kingdom, therefore, the term 'brainstem death' (death following irreversible cessation of brainstem function) is preferred. Of patients who are determined as brainstem dead, approximately half are due to trauma, a third due to spontaneous intracranial haemorrhage, and the remainder due to a number of other causes including hypoxia secondary to cardiac arrest.

Criteria for diagnosis

The current criteria in the United Kingdom for diagnosis have been defined by a working group convened in 1998 by the Royal College of Physicians on behalf of the UK conference of Medical Royal Colleges and their Faculties. The working party included doctors, nurses, lawyers, Community Health Council representatives, a member of the Patients' Association, and others representing transplant coordinators and carers. The group produced a document *A code of practice for the diagnosis of brainstem death* (see 'Further reading').

Brainstem death testing

Confirmation of brainstem death is made by formal brainstem death testing. This follows strict protocols comprising a number of stages.

Clinical prerequisites

- There should be no doubt that the patient's condition is due to irremediable brain damage of known aetiology. This may be obvious with CT confirmation of a severe head injury or spontaneous haemorrhage, but may be much more difficult to establish, e.g. after cardiac arrest with an indefinite period of hypoxia. Continued observation and investigation may be required.

- The patient is deeply unconscious. Reversible causes such as depressant drugs (e.g. narcotics, hypnotics, tranquillizers), primary hypothermia, and potentially reversible circulatory, metabolic, and endocrine causes must be excluded.

- The patient is maintained on a ventilator because spontaneous respiration has ceased. The effects of neuromuscular blocking drugs and other respiratory depressants must be excluded. Confirmation with a nerve stimulator is advisable.

Logistics

- In the United Kingdom, the diagnosis of brainstem death should be made by at least two medically qualified practitioners who fulfil the following criteria:

  - both must have been registered for more than 5 years and be competent in the conduct and interpretation of brainstem testing

  - at least one should be a consultant

  - neither should be members of the transplant team.

- Two sets of tests should always be performed. The tests may be carried out by the two practitioners separately or together. The interval between tests is at the discretion of the clinicians.

- In the United Kingdom, radiological or neurophysiological studies do not form part of the criteria unless clinical tests alone cannot be relied on, e.g. multiple facial and orbital fractures.

Tests

The following criteria must be satisfied in order to diagnose brainstem death:

- The pupils are fixed and do not respond to sharp changes in the intensity of incident light. A strong light, e.g. ophthalmoscope with ambient light dimmed, is recommended.

- The corneal absent is absent. This is tested using a wisp of cotton-wool, taking care not to damage the cornea.

- The oculovestibular reflexes are absent. After clear visualization of the tympanic membrane with an auroscope, and with the head flexed to 30° provided that no cervical injury is present, at least 50 ml of ice-cold water are injected into each external auditory meatus in turn over the course of 1 min.

- No motor response within the cranial nerve distribution can be elicited by adequate stimulation of any somatic area. In practice, there is no limb response to supraorbital pressure.

- There is no gag reflex to stimulation of the posterior pharynx with a spatula or cough reflex response to bronchial stimulation elicited by placing a suction catheter down the trachea.

- Apnoea test: no respiratory responses occur when the patient is disconnected from the ventilator. This is the last test to be performed if all the preceding tests confirm the absence of brainstem reflexes. The patient should be preoxygenated with 100% oxygen for 10 min. The patient should then be disconnected from the ventilator and observed for respiratory effort for 10 min. Oxygenation is continued by administering oxygen at a rate of 6 l/min via a fine-bore catheter down the endotracheal tube. A blood gas must be taken to ensure that the arterial pressure of carbon dioxide has reached 6.65 kPa. The patient is reconnected to the ventilator. A more detailed protocol will be included in the Code of Practice of the Diagnosis and Confirmation of Death that is under revision by the Royal Colleges and Department of Health Working Party.

Special considerations

Children

Brainstem death testing in children has been the subject of a report of a working party of the British Paediatric Association in 1991 (see

'Further reading'). In children over the age of 2 months, the brainstem death criteria should be the same as those for adults. Between 37 weeks of gestation and 2 months of age, it is rarely possible confidently to diagnose brainstem death and below 37 weeks of gestation the criteria for brainstem death cannot be applied.

Pre-existing chronic respiratory disease

Patients with pre-existing chronic respiratory disease with supranormal levels of carbon dioxide, and who depend on hypoxic drive, are special cases. Expert respiratory advice is recommended for these patients.

Action following brainstem death testing

The legal time of death is the time of completion of the first set of tests. Following conformation of brainstem death, mechanical ventilation and life support should be withdrawn. Before this it is essential to explain to relatives that brainstem death is an irretrievable state—when the brain is dead the person is dead, even though the heart may still be beating. Where appropriate, transplantation should be considered: the opportunity is offered for the relatives to discuss this with the transplant coordinator. Transplantation should be considered when there are no systemic contraindications, e.g. malignancy, and when the organs are still functioning despite the patient's final illness.

It is important that after completion of the second set of tests either the patient is taken for organ transplantation as soon as is practically possible or the patient is disconnected from the ventilator to allow a dignified death. Expeditious retrieval of organs maintains their function, so it is important, when it is a recognized that a patient is a potential organ donor, that the transplant coordinator is contacted as soon as possible and the stage that proceedings have reached is made clear. Personal experience has shown that the transplant coordinator can provide strong and essential support to the relatives, irrespective of the decision of whether or not to donate.

The vegetative state and the minimally conscious state

The term 'vegetative state' was introduced in 1972 by Jennett and Plum to describe the clinical condition resulting from loss of function in the cerebral cortex with a functioning brainstem (patients who are awake but not aware). Vegetative patients breathe spontaneously and are not ventilator dependent; another difference from brain death is that they can survive for many years if adequately fed and nursed. The most common cause of vegetative survival after acute brain damage is severe head injury, the mechanism being severe diffuse axonal injury severing the subcortical connections over a wide area. Secondary hypoxic brain damage is a contributing factor in some traumatic cases. Most nontraumatic cases result from severe hypoxia–ischaemia of the brain after a cardiac arrest, near drowning, or strangulation, while a few result from severe hypoglycaemia in people with diabetes. Other causes are acute intracranial haemorrhage or infection. In adults the vegetative state can evolve gradually during the late stages of chronic dementing conditions, and in children can result from severe congenital malformations of the brain or from progressive metabolic or chromosomal diseases affecting the brain.

At postmortem examination after acute hypoxic insults, there is commonly a widespread loss of cortical neurons. After acute traumatic and nontraumatic damage leading to vegetative survival, there is almost always severe bilateral thalamic damage, although the cortex may be relatively spared. There is also progressive degeneration over many months of neurons, nerve fibres, and their myelin sheaths remote from the site of initial damage, which is reflected during life in progressive enlargement of the ventricles as visualized by CT or MRI. Findings on the EEG are variable, but there is often loss of evoked cortical responses to somatic stimuli. Positron emission tomography in hypoxic cases shows severe depression of glucose metabolism in cortical grey matter, to levels found only in experimental deep barbiturate narcosis.

Diagnosis

In practice the diagnosis depends on characteristic clinical features recorded by skilled observers over a period of time. The patient has long periods of spontaneous eye opening (hence the inappropriateness of calling this condition irreversible or prolonged coma). The eyes or head does not track a moving object. There may be a startle reaction to a sudden noise. All four limbs are paralysed and usually spastic, with only reflex posturing and withdrawal from a painful stimulus, and often there is a grasp reflex. The face may grimace and groans may be heard but never words. There is no psychologically meaningful response to external stimuli or any learned behaviour—no evidence of a working mind. There may be emotional behaviours such as smiling, crying, or laughing but these are not related to appropriate external stimuli. It is concluded that, although awake, these patients are not aware and do not have any distress or pain. Misdiagnosis by non-experts is common, and care is needed to exclude the minimally conscious state in which there are very limited responses to indicate some return of cognitive activity. It must also be ascertained that the patient does not have the locked-in syndrome, caused by brainstem damage which results in full awareness but widespread paralysis, leaving the patient able to communicate only by a yes/no code using the sole remaining motor power—blinking the eyelids or moving the eyes. Prolonged observation in a specialized unit is required to make a secure diagnosis of the vegetative state. Recent functional brain imaging studies have revealed that a very few vegetative state patients can hear and understand before responses suggestive of minimally conscious state appear clinically.

Prognosis

Patients in a vegetative state for some time can still make some recovery. Of patients in the vegetative state 1 month after an acute insult, about half of head-injured individuals will regain some consciousness, but only a few of the nontraumatic cases do. Most who recover consciousness remain very severely disabled and dependent, particularly if they have been vegetative for several months. After head injury permanence cannot be declared until 12 months, but after nontraumatic insults it can after 6 months according to United Kingdom criteria and after 3 months in the United States of America. There is a high mortality in the first year after becoming vegetative but, once this period has been survived, patients can live for many years, if tube feeding and good nursing care are maintained and infective complications actively treated.

Action after permanence declared

There is now a consensus in many countries that survival for years in a permanent vegetative state is of no benefit to the patient, and that it is therefore appropriate to withdraw life-sustaining treatment once permanence is declared. Many courts in the United States of America and the United Kingdom have agreed that artificial nutrition and hydration is medical treatment that can be withdrawn if judged to be no longer of benefit to the patient. Once this is done a peaceful death occurs in 8 to 12 days, and the cause of death is regarded as the original brain damage. In the United Kingdom it is a legal requirement to seek court approval before withdrawing such treatment.

Further reading

Brain death

Academy of medical royal colleges. A code of practice for the diagnosis and confirmation of death. October 2008. [Most recent United Kingdom update.]

British Paediatric Association (1991). *Diagnosis of brain stem death in infants and children*. British Paediatric Association, London. [Paediatric perspective of brainstem death.]

Health Departments of Great Britain and Northern Ireland (1998). *A code of practice for the diagnosis of brain stem death*. Department of Health, London. Available at: http://www.dh.gov.uk/en/Publicationsandstatistics/Publications/PublicationsPolicyAndGuidance/DH_4009696.

Medical Royal Colleges and their Faculties in the United Kingdom (1976). Diagnosis of brain death. Conference. *BMJ*, **ii**, 1187–8.

Medical Royal Colleges and their Faculties in the United Kingdom (1979). Diagnosis of death. Conference. *BMJ*, **i**, 322. [Original descriptions of United Kingdom criteria for brainstem death.]

NHS Direct Brain Death. Available at: http://www.nhsdirect.nhs.uk/articles/article.aspx?articleId=60. [Lay description.]

Quality Standards Sub-committee of the American Academy of Neurology (1995). Practice parameters for determining brain death in adults. *Neurology* **45**, 1012–14. [Widely accepted United States criteria; available at: http://www.aan.com/professionals/practice/pdfs/pdf_1995_thru_1998/1995.45.1012.pdf.]

Youngner SJ, Arnold RM, Shapiro R (eds) (1999). *The definition of death*. Johns Hopkins University Press, Baltimore, MA. [Review of controversies, clinical, ethical, legal, and social—primarily from an American viewpoint.]

Vegetative state and minimally conscious state

Adams JH, Graham DI, Jennett B (2000). The neuropathology of the vegetative state after an acute brain insult. *Brain*, **123**, 1327–38. [Detailed pathology of 35 traumatic and 14 nontraumatic cases.]

Jennett B (2002). *The vegetative state: medical facts, ethical and legal dilemmas*. Cambridge University Press, Cambridge. [Review of medical facts, ethical issues and details of legal cases in several countries.]

Laureys S, Owen AM, Schiff ND (2004). Brain function in coma, vegetative state, and related disorders. *Lancet Neurol*, **3**, 537–46. [Recent United Kingdom review.]

Monti MM, *et al.* (2010).Willful modulation of brain activity in disorders of unconsciousness, *N Eng J Med*. [E pub ahead of print] [Original paper showing that 5154 patients in a vegetative or minimally conscious state have brain activation reflecting some brain activation reflecting some awareness and cognition.]

Multi-Society Task Force on PVS (1994). Medical aspects of the persistent vegetative state. *N Engl J Med*, **330**, 1499–507, 1572–9. [Review of world literature and prognostic data from an American perspective.]

Quality Standard Sub-Committee of the American Academy of Neurology (1995). Practice parameters: assessment and management of patients in PVS. *Neurology*, **45**, 1015–18. [Most recent American criteria.]

Wade DT, Johnston C (1999). The permanent vegetative state: practical guidance on diagnosis and management. *BMJ*, **319**, 841–4 (see also Editorial by B Jennett on pp. 796–7). [Recent United Kingdom review.]

Disorders of the special senses

Contents

24.6.1 Visual pathways

Christopher Kennard

Essentials

Visual disturbances may be caused by diseases of the optic disc, optic nerve, optic chiasm, optic tract, lateral geniculate nucleus, optic radiations, and occipital lobe of the brain, as well as other brain areas involved in complex visual processing.

Diagnosis of disturbances of the visual pathways requires both knowledge of their anatomy and physiology, and the ability to carry out a thorough neuro-ophthalmological examination which should enable (1) documentation of the character and extent of the visual disturbance, and (2) topographic localization of the lesion, so that the relevant investigative techniques, such as radiological imaging, can be appropriately requested.

Visual disturbances typically produced by particular lesions

(1) Retina—peripheral field constriction as in retinitis pigmentosa and a central field defect as in senile macular degeneration. (2) Optic nerve—'relative afferent pupillary defect'; defect of colour vision; central scotoma or arcuate defect (lesions just prior to the chiasm produce a junctional scotoma). (3) Optic chiasm—bitemporal hemianopia. (4) Optic tract—incongruous hemianopic defects. (5) Lateral geniculate nucleus—wedge-shaped homonymous field defects. (6) Optic radiations—homonymous quadrantinopia or hemianopia depending on the extent and location of the lesion (upper quadrant, temporal lobe; lower quadrant, parietal lobe). (7) Occipital lobe of the brain—(a) striate cortex—homonymous hemianopia, sometimes with macular sparing, particularly with vascular disturbances; (b) superior or inferior bank of the striate cortex—inferior or superior altitudinal defects (respectively). (8) Extrastriate areas involved in higher visual processing—can produce a wide variety of defects, including specific loss of a visual modality such as colour (achromatopsia) or movement (akinetopsia), or visual agnosia.

Clinical evaluation of visual function

Examination of visual function initially requires an accurate assessment of the visual acuity. Acuity should be tested separately in each eye using the Snellen or some other optotype chart, which contains rows of letters of diminishing size. If an impairment (>6/6) is noted, the patient should be allowed to wear spectacles or alternatively to view the chart through a pinhole, which eliminates any significant refractive error or optic media distortion. If the acuity does not improve, it is necessary to try to distinguish media opacities and retinal abnormalities from optic nerve dysfunction using the swinging flashlight test. In a darkened room each eye is alternately stimulated with a bright light, which is moved rhythmically from one eye to the other. When the light is swung from the good eye on to the defective eye, dilatation of the pupil is termed a 'relative afferent pupillary defect' (RAPD), and signifies optic nerve dysfunction. Another good indicator of an optic nerve disturbance is a defect of colour vision, which may be tested using one of several available booklets of colour plates such as the Ishihara pseudo-isochromatic plates.

The photostress test is a useful test to distinguish a maculopathy from optic nerve dysfunction. The retina of the 'normal' eye is bleached by shining a bright light at the pupil for 10 s, and measuring the time for normal acuity to be re-established. The test is repeated in the 'abnormal' eye and, if the difference in recovery time between the two eyes is greater than 60 s, the test is considered abnormal, indicating that the impairment is retinal and not due to an optic nerve disturbance.

Careful fundoscopic examination of the eye is essential to identify abnormalities of the optic media, retina, and optic nerve head.

Finally, examination of the visual fields is essential for topographic localization because, as a result of the invariate ordering of nerve fibres along the visual pathway, lesions at specific sites produce field defects of specific shapes (Fig. 24.6.1.1). Simple confrontation tests provide a qualitative method of investigating the visual fields. The examiner sits opposite the patient, maintaining a constant distance, and each eye is tested separately. With the patient fixating on the examiner's nose, he or she is asked to count stationary fingers presented on either side of the vertical meridian in each quadrant in turn. If the patient cannot identify the fingers in a particular area, they are gently wiggled and the hand moved towards fixation until they are visible to the patient, so mapping out the field defect. To examine the central field a red 5- to 10-mm hatpin is moved away from or towards the central point of fixation. The patient is asked to describe any changes in the perception of colour or brightness, and whether or not the object disappears at any point. Perimetry provides a quantitative technique for measuring the fields, but a full description is beyond the scope of this chapter.

Abnormalities of the optic disc

Optic disc anomalies

Optic nerve hypoplasia

Hypoplasia of the optic nerve can be mild or severe, unilateral or bilateral, and may be associated with normal or impaired visual function. It can occur in isolation, or be associated with central nervous system anomalies, such as the absence of the septum pellucidum in De Morsier's syndrome (septo-optic dysplasia).

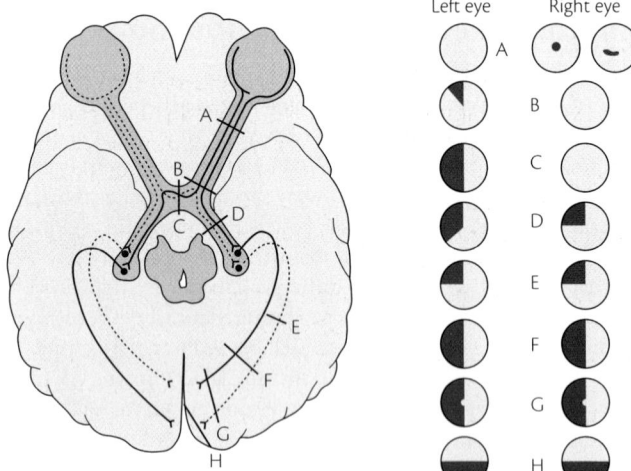

Fig. 24.6.1.1 Patterns of visual field loss due to lesions at different locations along the visual pathway: A, optic nerve lesions result in a central scotoma or arcuate defect; B, optic nerve lesions just before the chiasma produce a junctional scotoma due to ipsilateral optic nerve involvement with the inferior contralateral crossing fibres (dashed lines); C, chiasmal lesions produce bitemporal hemianopia; D, optic tract lesions result in incongruous hemianopic defects; E, F lesions of the optic radiation result in either homonymous quadrantanopia or hemianopia depending on the extent and location of the lesion (upper quadrant, temporal lobe; lower quadrant, parietal lobe); G, lesions of the striate cortex produce a homonymous hemianopia, sometimes with macular sparing, particularly with vascular disturbances; H, lesions of the superior or inferior bank of the striate cortex result in inferior or superior altitudinal defects, respectively.

Optic nerve dysplasia

Optic nerve dysplasia presents with a spectrum of abnormalities, including optic nerve colobomas, optic pits, and the morning glory syndrome, all considered to be associated with abnormal closure of the embryonic optic stalk and cup fissure. They are sometimes associated with basal encephaloceles and other forebrain anomalies.

Optic disc colobomas

These are deeply evacuated nerve head anomalies with blood vessels exiting from the margins, which are associated with defects in the retinal nerve fibre layer, leading to an appropriate visual field loss.

Optic pits

Optic pits are crater-like depressions in the optic disc with a dark-grey hue, usually situated in the temporal disc margin with an accompanying nerve fibre layer defect.

The morning glory syndrome

In this condition, an enlarged dysplastic disc is associated with an elevated, centrally retained mass of glial, embryonic glial, and vascular material, which radiates outwards in a sunburst pattern.

Tilted discs

An asymmetrically shaped, tilted disc is produced when the optic nerve leaves the globe at an extremely oblique angle. It is often associated with a crescentic zone of exposed sclera along one edge which results in elevation of the superior disc. The disc may appear hypoplastic and patients with this condition often have moderately high myopia and oblique astigmatism.

Optic nerve drusen

Drusen of the optic disc can give rise to an elevation of the optic nerve head. Drusen are intrapapillary, prelaminar, refractile concretions that arise from degenerating nerve fibres. Anomalous discs due to drusen are usually smaller than normal, have an absent central optic disc cup, and exhibit an aberrant branching pattern of the central retinal vessels. Initially the drusen are buried with simple elevation of the disc, but become more apparent in later years when they seem to give rise to a typical lumpy disc, with a scalloped margin.

Myelinated nerve fibres

In slightly less than 1% of the population some portions of retinal nerve fibres are myelinated, although normally optic nerve myelination stops at the lamina cribrosa. It appears on fundoscopy as a white area, usually adjacent to the disc, which has a centrifugal feathered edge.

Optic disc swelling

Although the terms 'optic disc swelling' and 'papilloedema' have in the past been used synonymously, it is now usual to refer only to papilloedema as optic disc swelling when it is associated with raised intracranial pressure. Other cases of optic disc swelling are due to either local abnormalities in the optic nerve or orbit, or congenital anomalies as described above.

Local causes of optic disc swelling are usually associated with impaired visual acuity and colour vision, central arcuate or altitudinal field defects, and often an afferent pupillary defect. This contrasts with papilloedema when the acuity remains normal, except in the final stages, and is usually bilateral.

Papilloedema

The evolution of the disc changes in papilloedema caused by raised intracranial pressure are usually classified into four stages: early, fully developed, chronic, and atrophic.

In early papilloedema there is disc hyperaemia, mild disc swelling with blurring of the striations of the fine peripapillary nerve fibre layer, dilatation of retinal veins with loss of spontaneous venous pulsations, and occasionally fine splinter haemorrhages at the disc margin.

In fully developed papilloedema, disc elevation is moderate to marked, and there is increased venous distension and tortuosity, an increasing number of peripapillary haemorrhages, cotton-wool spots, and dilated capillaries on the disc surface. The retinal blood vessels and disc margin become increasingly indistinct.

In chronic papilloedema, there is resolution of the haemorrhages and exudates leaving a dome-shaped ('champagne cork') disc swelling, which often contains hard exudates. White refractile bodies may appear on the disc surface, known as corpora amylacea. As time goes on there is increasing nerve fibre attrition, leading to progressive visual field loss.

Finally, there is post-papilloedema (consecutive) atrophy, in which the disc acquires a milky opalescence and the retinal vessels are sheathed.

Clinical features

Usually papilloedema is bilateral and there is an absence of visual symptoms. However, unilateral or bilateral transient visual obscurations may occur, which last a few seconds and are often associated with postural changes. Although it has been suggested that such obscurations herald permanent visual loss, there is no evidence to support this view. The longer the papilloedema persists, the more likely there is to be progressive visual field loss, which usually starts as a peripheral field constriction. Occasionally, sudden visual loss occurs in a patient with papilloedema due to ischaemic optic neuropathy.

Pathogenesis

Papilloedema is due to impairment of axonal transport in the retinal nerve fibres, leading to axonal distension, which is seen as disc swelling at the level of the prelaminar optic nerve.

Aetiology

There is a vast array of different causes leading to increased intracranial pressure, in particular space-occupying lesions such as tumours (Table 24.6.1.1).

Management

Treatment primarily depends on the underlying cause of the raised intracranial pressure. If it is due to a mass lesion that cannot be completely removed, or a nonsurgically remediable cause, a shunting procedure or medical measures, e.g. osmotic agents or diuretics such as acetazolamide, may be used. Increasingly, optic nerve sheath fenestration is being used for patients with intractable papilloedema who are developing early visual loss. This is mainly in the context of deteriorating vision in benign intracranial hypertension.

Ischaemic optic neuropathy

Ischaemic optic neuropathy is the result of infarction of the optic nerve head, and can either be arteritic, as part of giant cell arteritis, or nonarteritic (idiopathic ischaemic neuropathy,

Table 24.6.1.1 Causes of papilloedema

Mass lesions: tumours, aneurysms, granulomas, parasitic cysts
Intracranial haemorrhage: subdural haematoma, epidural haematoma, subarachnoid haemorrhage
Arteriovenous malformations
Intracranial infections: brain abscess, meningitis, encephalitis
Obstructed cranial venous outflow: dural venous sinus thrombosis, dural venous sinus infiltration, jugular vein compression, dural venous sinus arteriovenous malformation
Obstructive hydrocephalus
Brain oedema following trauma
Spinal cord tumours
Benign intracranial hypertension
(i) idiopathic   (ii) secondary to metabolic and endocrine disorders: Addison's disease, diabetic ketoacidosis, thyrotoxicosis, hypoparathyroidism, chronic uraemia (iii) secondary to toxic causes: tetracycline, nalidixic acid, steroid therapy, lithium, hypervitaminosis A
Guillain–Barré syndrome
Craniostenoses
Mucopolysaccharoidoses
Systemic illness: Behçet's syndrome, status epilepticus, Reye's syndrome, Whipple's disease, systemic lupus erythematosis, systemic hypertension, chronic respiratory insufficiency

anterior ischaemic optic neuropathy), which is the more common form of the condition.

Nonarteritic ischaemic optic neuropathy

This tends to occur in patients aged between 45 and 80 years, and is characterized by abrupt, painless, and generally nonprogressive visual loss, associated with an arcuate or altitudinal visual field loss. In almost all cases, there is optic disc oedema, often associated with one or more splinter haemorrhages at the disc margin. Although previously considered irreversible, as many as 40% of patients may show some improvement.

There is a 40% chance of involvement of the fellow eye within 5 years. Optic atrophy rapidly ensues after the ischaemic event. The cause of nonarteritic ischaemic optic neuropathy remains obscure, although it is often present on awakening in the morning, which has suggested that nocturnal hypotension, sometimes related to medication for hypertension, may be a risk factor. There is no treatment of proven benefit. The most important aspect of management is to exclude the possibility of the arteritic form, because in such cases the fellow eye is particularly vulnerable to similar involvement.

Arteritic ischaemic optic neuropathy

The arteritic form of ischaemic optic neuropathy usually occurs in giant cell (cranial, temporal) arteritis, but also occurs rarely in lupus and polyarteritis nodosa. Anyone with nonarteritic ischaemic optic neuropathy over the age of 50 should be suspected of having giant cell arteritis. This often occurs in the context of headache, malaise, weight loss, anorexia, anaemia, proximal muscle ache or stiffness, temporal artery tenderness, jaw claudication, and fever. These symptoms and signs usually precede the visual loss. The disc infarction is similar to that seen in nonarteritic ischaemic optic neuropathy.

A high index of suspicion is required for giant cell arteritis and, if suspected, an urgent erythrocyte sedimentation rate (ESR) and temporal artery biopsy should be arranged. At the same time as blood is taken for the ESR, the patient should be started on systemic steroids (prednisolone at 80 mg daily plus 200 mg intravenous hydrocortisone). In most patients the ESR is markedly elevated, as is the C-reactive protein (CRP). Occasionally the ESR may be normal. A biopsy of the superficial temporal artery should be obtained as soon as possible after the diagnosis has been considered. The biopsy will not be affected by the use of corticosteroids for at least 48 h. A positive temporal artery biopsy confirms the diagnosis of giant cell arteritis, but in 25% of patients skip areas are found in biopsy specimens, and therefore a negative biopsy may sometimes be obtained.

Steroid treatment should not be tapered or withdrawn too early, because a relapse of symptoms is common. The dose of prednisolone can be gradually tapered after 2 to 3 weeks to maintain a normal ESR and the patient asymptomatic. Treatment should be continued for at least 6 to 12 months.

Optic atrophy

Optic atrophy is the final result of a variety of disturbances to the optic nerve or retina. The disc appears pale, and there is an absence of disc vasculature and retinal nerve fibres (see Fig. 24.6.1.1).

Optic atrophy occurs after any disease process that results in death of the retinal ganglion cells with a dying back of their nerve fibres. This can, therefore, be due to diseases that directly involve the ganglion cells themselves or from damage to the axons in the pregeniculate visual pathway, resulting in retrograde atrophy. The development of optic atrophy is usually slow, dependent on its cause. In most instances the optic atrophy is bilateral, the disc appearing chalky-white in colour with clearly defined margins. The differential diagnosis of optic atrophy is considered in Table 24.6.1.2.

Optic neuritis

'Optic neuritis' is a term used to describe an idiopathic optic neuropathy or one resulting from an inflammatory, infectious, or demyelinating aetiology. In most cases the optic disc is normal on ophthalmoscopy and the term 'retrobulbar neuritis' is used. In those cases in which the optic disc is swollen, the terms 'papillitis' and 'anterior optic neuritis' are used.

Clinical features

It is important to distinguish between those features of typical optic neuritis of idiopathic or demyelinating causation and those of atypical optic neuritis. In typical optic neuritis there is usually acute unilateral loss of visual acuity and visual field, which may progress over hours or a few days, reaching its maximal effect within 1 week. Ninety per cent of patients complain of ocular pain, which is noted especially with eye movement, and which may precede the visual impairment by a few days. The visual loss may range from contrast defects with maintained acuity to no light perception. The patient is usually aged under 40 years, although optic neuritis may occur at

Table 24.6.1.2 Causes of optic disc atrophy

Deficiency states
Thiamine ('tobacco–alcohol amblyopia')
B$_{12}$(pernicious anaemia, 'tobacco amblyopia'?)
Drugs/toxins
Ethambutol
Chloromycetin
Streptomycin
Isoniazid
Chlorpropamide
Digitalis
Chloroquine
Placidyl
Antabuse
Heavy metals
Hereditary optic atrophies
Dominant (juvenile)
Leber's
Associated heredodegenerative neurological syndromes
Recessive, associated with juvenile diabetes
Demyelination
Graves' disease
Atypical glaucoma
Macular dystrophies

any age, and improvement takes place in most patients (90%) to normal or near normal visual acuity over several weeks. There may be persistent subtle residual defects of colour vision, depth perception, and contrast sensitivity, which may continue for several months. Subsequent disc pallor may occur but does not correlate closely with the level of visual recovery. An afferent pupillary defect is present in over 90% of patients with acute optic neuritis. Although optic neuritis is generally associated with a central scotoma, a wide variety of field defects may be found, ranging from a central scotoma to altitudinal and nerve fibre layer defects.

Atypical optic neuritis may involve unilateral or bilateral simultaneous onset of optic neuritis in an adult patient. There is often lack of pain and there may be other ocular findings suggestive of an inflammatory process, such as an anterior uveitis. Other features include a worsening of visual function beyond 14 days of onset, in a patient outside the 20- to 50-year age span. They may also have evidence of other systemic conditions, particularly inflammatory or infectious diseases (Table 24.6.1.3).

The evaluation of patients with optic neuritis rather depends on whether or not it is a typical or an atypical case. Typical optic neuritis probably does not necessitate any additional laboratory investigations, although an abnormal MRI of the brain significantly increases the likelihood of developing multiple sclerosis.

Those patients with atypical optic neuritis should have a chest radiograph, laboratory tests, including a blood count, biochemistry, tests for collagen and vascular disease, and for syphilis serology. Examination of the cerebrospinal fluid is probably justified in this group of patients.

Table 24.6.1.3 Causes of optic neuritis

Unknown aetiology
Multiple sclerosis
Viral infections of childhood (measles, mumps, chicken pox) with or without encephalitis
Viral encephalitides
Postviral, paraviral infections
Infectious mononucleosis
Herpes zoster
Contiguous inflammation of meninges, orbit, sinuses
Granulomatous inflammations (syphilis, tuberculosis, cryptococcosis, sarcoidosis)
Intraocular inflammations

Management

Although intravenous methylprednisolone leads to a more rapid visual recovery, at the end of 6 months the visual acuity is no better than with no treatment. Therefore, steroid treatment of patients with typical optic neuritis is unnecessary, unless there is severe ocular pain that cannot be managed with analgesics, or if there is already poor vision in the fellow eye due to some other disease process.

Heredofamilial optic neuropathies

The hereditary optic neuropathies can either be those that are autosomal dominant or recessive or those that are due to point mutations in mitochondrial DNA. The autosomal conditions usually present in childhood with impaired vision and pale optic discs.

Leber's hereditary optic neuropathy

This mitochondrial disorder develops primarily in men (approximately 14% in women) in the second to third decades of life. It is characterized by an abrupt loss of central vision in one eye, usually followed by a loss of vision in the remaining eye; this may occur weeks, months, or sometimes years later. Occasionally visual loss may occur simultaneously in the two eyes. There is no associated pain on eye movement, in contrast to acute optic neuritis, and the visual loss is usually permanent with optic atrophy and large absolute central scotomas. However, the fundoscopic picture in the acute phase often shows swelling of the papillary nerve fibre layer, circumpapillary telangiectatic microangiopathy, and tortuosity of the retinal vessels.

There is a maternal pattern of inheritance and point mutations in mitochondrial DNA, particularly at the 11778 nucleotide, and less frequently at 3460 and 14484, have been identified. The significance of the point mutation at 14484 is that a much higher percentage (37% as opposed to 4%) of patients show some visual recovery when compared with patients who have a defect at 11778. It is therefore appropriate to carry out genetic testing in those individuals presenting with atypical optic neuritis of the appropriate sex and age, even if a positive family history is not available. There is no effective treatment for this condition.

Nutritional and toxic optic neuropathies

Bilateral, slowly progressive, central visual loss with centrocaecal scotomas, and usually normal or mild temporal atrophic optic discs, characterizes optic nerve failure due to either nutritional deficiency or a toxic cause. Once a family history of one of the hereditary familial diseases has been excluded, this condition should be considered, and is usually due to a combination of alcohol abuse, deficiencies within the B-vitamin complex, and frequently a high tobacco consumption. With treatment by abstinence of the likely toxic agents and vitamin supplementation, recovery of vision usually occurs, unless the condition is so long standing that optic atrophy has intervened. Recent epidemics of optic neuropathy in Cuba and West Africa have probably been related to multiple dietary deficiencies.

Toxic optic neuropathy has been associated with ethambutol, chloramphenicol, halogenated hydroxyquinolones, lead, isoniazid, and vincristine.

Tumours of the optic nerve

Optic nerve sheath meningiomas

Although optic nerve sheath meningiomas may arise directly from the optic nerve sheath, usually in the orbital regions of the nerve, they frequently arise from the tuberculum sellae, sphenoid wing, and olfactory groove, leading to secondary invasion or compression of the nerve. Primary optic nerve sheath meningiomas, most frequently found in middle-aged women, are usually unilateral, but if bilateral raise the possibility of central neurofibromatosis type 2 (NF-2). Although most patients will have mild (2 to 4 mm) proptosis at the time of their initial consultation, they complain of dimming of vision and decreased colour vision. Visual loss progresses over years, with optic disc swelling gradually being supplanted by optic atrophy, with or without the evolution of optociliary venous (retinochoroidal anastomoses) shunt vessels.

The CT picture in patients with these tumours is most often one of diffuse narrow enlargement of the optic nerve, with bulbous swellings of the nerve in the region of the globe and orbital apex. 'Railroad-track' calcification of the optic nerve sheath in the orbit is a characteristic feature. Use of MRI has enabled optic nerve sheath meningiomas to be distinguished from optic nerve gliomas, where the former but not the latter show that the nerve is readily distinguished from the optic nerve sheath.

Management of patients with optic nerve sheath meningiomas is controversial. Although there is general agreement that nerve sheath tumours are most aggressive in children and become progressively more indolent with advancing age, there is no consensus as to the best way to treat these lesions. Clinical resection, particularly when there is intracranial spread, is usually incomplete. These patients rarely die from the meningioma and it is probably best just to observe. In some instances radiotherapy has been shown to result in some visual improvement, but should be reserved for those patients in whom there is clear evidence of progression.

Optic nerve gliomas

Optic nerve gliomas, which may also involve the chiasma, are of two distinct types. By far the more common is the benign glioma of childhood, the other being the malignant glioblastoma in adults. Approximately a quarter of cases occur in the setting of NF-1.

Benign optic nerve gliomas usually present within the first two decades of life, with a peak incidence from 1 year to 6 years of age. The usual presenting manifestations are proptosis and visual loss, which may be so mild as to be undetectable, although a profound reduction in acuity is more common. The fundus may show either papilloedema or optic atrophy.

The clinical course of childhood optic nerve gliomas is highly variable. In some, tumour enlargement proceeds slowly for a time but then reaches a plateau, whereas in others the enlargement proceeds unabated. Postmortem examination has suggested that they are in fact hamartomas rather than true neoplasms. Optic nerve gliomas are generally managed conservatively, although some practitioners favour radiation therapy for lesions with chiasmal involvement and surgery for at least those tumours restricted to the orbit.

Optic nerve gliomas of adulthood are malignant gliomas that usually arise in men aged 40 to 60 years. These patients often present with a rapid onset of visual failure, which on some occasions may mimic acute optic neuritis. The tumour rapidly progresses and the patient usually dies within a short period.

Other optic nerve tumours

Metastatic cancer may lead to optic nerve involvement, either as a result of infiltration of the meninges, as occurs with cancer of the breast and lung, or by direct tumour infiltration, as with lympho-proliferative disorders and certain types of leukaemia and non-Hodgkin's lymphoma. Paraneoplastic optic neuropathy has also been described in patients with small cell carcinoma of the lung.

Disorders of the optic chiasma

Approximately 25% of all brain tumours occur in the chiasmal region and, as half of these cases initially present with visual loss, an appreciation of the various field abnormalities is important. Although there are a number of other causes for the chiasmal syndrome, such as trauma and demyelination, these are rare. The neuro-ophthalmological signs of a compressive optic chiasmal lesion are primarily a field defect and deterioration of visual acuity, which depend on the relationship of the chiasma to the pituitary. The classic field defect of a chiasmal lesion is a bitemporal hemianopia. This may be complete or incomplete and may or may not be symmetrical. It is unusual to have a bitemporal hemianopia with no reduction in central visual acuity in at least one eye, because the optic nerve is compromised in addition to the chiasma.

In large series of patients with pituitary tumours the most common field defect is a bitemporal hemianopia (67%); less common are junctional scotoma (29%), homonymous hemianopia (7%), and prechiasmal field loss (2%). Other signs include optic disc pallor, but its absence usually denotes a virtually complete return of visual function with successful decompression.

Other causes of chiasmal compression in addition to pituitary adenomas (50 to 55%) include craniopharyngiomas (20 to 25%), meningiomas (10%), and gliomas (7%). However, there are other, noncompressive, causes of bitemporal hemianopia, including empty sella syndrome, optochiasmal arachnoiditis, and radionecrosis.

Optic tract and lateral geniculate nucleus lesions

The optic tract is the first point in the visual pathways where the ipsilateral temporal and contralateral nasal retinal nerve fibres come together, and so the field defect is usually a partial or complete homonymous hemianopia. When partial, there is often gross incongruity between the visual field defects found in each eye, which may also be found with lesions of the lateral geniculate nucleus and more rarely the optic radiations.

The most frequently encountered lesions causing the optic tract syndrome are aneurysms, craniopharyngiomas, and pituitary tumours.

Lesions of the lateral geniculate nucleus have been found to produce incongruous wedge-shaped homonymous field defects, but when the aetiology is ischaemic the defect is usually congruous.

The optic radiations

As the geniculostriate fibres leave the lateral geniculate nucleus, the ventral fibres (subserving the superior visual field) pass anteriorly around the temporal horn of the lateral ventricle to form Meyer's loop. Lesions in this region usually result in a wedge-shaped, congruous, homonymous field defect, mainly affecting the superior quadrant. The visual acuity and pupillary responses are both normal. Lesions involving the optic radiation are due to vascular occlusion, tumours (intrinsic or metastatic), or abscesses.

Although lesions of the dorsal optic radiation in the parietal lobe may result in a homonymous hemianopia primarily affecting the lower fields, large lesions usually result in a complete homonymous hemianopia with macular splitting. Damage to the parietal or occipitoparietal cortex may result in the phenomenon in the contralateral visual field called unilateral visual inattention or visual extinction. A test object presented in this field is perceived normally, but, when an identical object is similarly presented equidistant from the fixation point in the ipsilateral visual field, the stimulus in the field contralateral to the parietal lobe lesion disappears.

Occipital lobe

On reaching the occipital lobe there is a high degree of order in the fibres of the optic radiation and lesions, which usually result from infarction, trauma, or tumour, produce homonymous congruent field defects. The only features of the field defect that help localize the lesion to the occipital lobe, rather than the anterior optic radiation, are the presence of sparing of the macula or temporal crescent areas in a homonymous hemianopia.

In macula sparing there is preservation of the visual field within a region of 1 to 2° up to 10° around the fixation point in the hemianopic field. In the more usual situation the hemianopic field is split along the vertical meridian through the fixation point (macular splitting).

Altitudinal (dorsal/ventral) field defects involving either the upper or lower occipital poles may occur as a result of trauma or vascular lesions.

Cortical blindness

Cortical blindness usually indicates selective involvement of the occipital visual cortex. The essential features are: (1) complete loss of all visual sensation, (2) loss of reflex lid closure to threat, (3) normal pupillary light reactions, and (4) normal retina and full extraocular eye movements. The most common aetiology is hypoxia of the striate cortex.

Disorders of higher visual processing

In the extrastriate cortex there is parallel processing of different aspects of visual information before an organized synthesis of the visual scene can be generated. Specific lesions in one or other of these areas might be expected to give rise to an appropriate specific loss of a visual modality such as colour (achromatopsia), movement (akinetopsia), or faces (prosopagnosia).

Acquired disorders of colour vision due to lesions of the central nervous system are of two types. In one type there is an inability to see colours (dyschromatopsia or achromatopsia). These patients have lesions in the region of the lingual and fusiform gyri, which lie in the anteroinferior region of the occipital lobe. They complain that they cannot see colours and that everything looks grey or various shades of black and white. They are unable to identify the figures on pseudo-isochromatic test plates, although they are able to name the colours of brightly coloured objects correctly. Other functions such as visual acuity, object recognition, and depth perception are all normal, but there is often an associated visual field defect, usually a bilateral superior homonymous quadrantanopia. In the other type of disorder, the colour sense is normal but the naming and recognition of colour are impaired. This can occur as part of an aphasia, such as Wernicke's or anomic aphasia, in the syndrome of alexia without agraphia, or as one feature of visual agnosia (see below).

Rare cases of patients who exhibit a selective deficit of movement perception (akinetopsia) have been reported. The patients have bilateral lesions involving the lateral occipitoparietotemporal junction.

Visual agnosia

The term 'visual agnosia' refers to a rare condition in which there is an inability to recognize, name, or demonstrate the use of an object presented visually, in the absence of a language deficit, general intellectual dysfunction, or attentional disturbances. The patient is, however, able to name the object when using other sensory modalities such as touch or sound.

One classification depends on the specific category of visual material that cannot be recognized. A disturbance of recognition of objects (object agnosia), faces (prosopagnosia), or colour (colour agnosia) may occur in isolation or in various combinations. When patients are able to copy and match to sample objects that they fail to name or recognize visually, the agnosia is termed 'associative', but, if there is an inability to perform all these tasks, the agnosia is termed 'apperceptive'.

Prosopagnosia is a specific inability to recognize familiar faces despite a normal ability to recognize everyday objects and is, therefore, different from visual agnosia. Most cases of prosopagnosia are due to infarction, head injury, or hypoxia, resulting in bilateral lesions in the ventromedial aspects of the occipitotemporal region.

Visual illusions

Visual illusions occur when the visually perceived target appears altered in size, shape, colour, position in space, and number of images. The illusory type of defects may occur in the entire field of vision, or affect only the object or the background. The term 'dysmetropsia' indicates the apparent smallness (micropsia), largeness (macropsia), or irregularity of shape (metamorphopsia) of objects. Dysmetropsia usually occurs as a result of retinal disease due to distortion of the relative distance between rods and cones.

Visual hallucinations

Visual hallucinations occur under many circumstances, such as impaired visual input as in senile macular degeneration, drug withdrawal, anoxia, migraine, infection, and schizophrenia, in addition to those related to focal neurological disease in the occipital or temporal lobes. Those in the last category may be unformed, consisting of flashes of light (coloured or white), lines, or simple shapes, or they may be complex, highly organized hallucinations of people or objects.

Palinopsia

Palinopsia is a rare disorder in which there is persistence (perseveration) or recurrence of visual images after the exciting stimulus has been removed.

Further reading

Apple DJ, Rabb MF, Walsh PM (1982). Congenital anomalies of the optic disc. *Surv Ophthalmol*, **27**, 3–41.

Beck RW, ONTT Study Group (1992). A randomized, controlled trial of corticosteroids in the treatment of acute optic neuritis. *N Engl J Med*, **326**, 581–8.

Boghen DR, Glaser JS (1975). Ischaemic optic neuropathy: the clinical profile and natural history. *Brain*, **98**, 689–708.

Chung SM, Selhorst JB (1992). Cancer associated retinopathy. *Ophthalmol Clinics North Am*, **5**, 587–96.

De Renzi E (1997). Prosopagnosia. In: Finberg TE, Farah MJ (eds) *Behavioural neurology and neuropsychology*, pp. 245–55. McGraw-Hill, New York.

Dutton JJ (1992). Optic nerve sheath meningiomas. *Surv Ophthalmol*, **37**, 167–83.

Dutton JJ (1994). Gliomas of the anterior visual pathway. *Surv Ophthalmol*, **38**, 427–52.

Horton JC, Hoyt WF (1991). The representation of the visual field in human striate cortex: a revision of the classic Holme's map. *Arch Ophthalmol*, **109**, 816–24.

Humphreys GW, Riddoch MJ (1993). Object agnosias. In: Kennard C (ed.) *Visual perceptual defects*, pp. 339–59. Baillière Tindall, London.

Kölmel HW (1993). Visual illusions and hallucinations. In: Kennard C (ed.) *Visual perceptual defects*, pp. 243–64. Baillière Tindall, London.

Liu GT, *et al.* (1994). Visual morbidity in giant cell arteritis: clinical characteristics and prognosis for vision. *Ophthalmology*, **101**, 1779–85.

Manford M, Anderman F (1998). Complex visual hallucinations: clinical and neurobiological insights. *Brain*, **121**, 1819–40.

McDonald WI, Barnes D (1992). The ocular manifestations of multiple sclerosis. I. Abnormalities of the afferent visual system. *J Neurol Neurosurg Psychiatry*, **55**, 747–52.

Neetens A, Smets RM (1989). Papilloedema. *Neuro-Ophthalmology*, **9**, 81–101.

Riddoch G (1917). Dissociation in visual perceptions due to occipital injuries, with special reference to appreciation of movement. *Brain*, **40**, 15–57.

Riordan-Eva P, *et al.* (1995). The clinical features of Leber's hereditary optic neuropathy defined by the presence of a pathogenic mitochondrial DNA mutation. *Brain*, **118**, 319–37.

Rosenberg MA, Savino PJ, Glaser JS (1979). A clinical analysis of pseudo-papilloedema: I. population, laterality, acuity, refractive error, ophthalmoscopic characteristics, and coincident disease. *Arch Ophthalmol*, **97**, 65–70.

Sadun AA, *et al.* (1994). Epidemic optic neuropathy in Cuba: eye findings. *Arch Ophthalmol*, **112**, 691–9.

Sugishita M, *et al.* (1993). The problem of macular sparing after unilateral occipital lesions. *J Neurol*, **241**, 1–9.

Thompson HS (1966). Afferent pupillary defects. *Am J Ophthalmol*, **62**, 860–73.

Zeki S (1993). *A vision of the brain*. Blackwell, Oxford.

24.6.2 Eye movements and balance

Michael Strupp and Thomas Brandt

Essentials

Eye movements

The major function of eye movements is to keep the image of the visual surrounding stable on the retina, even during eye movements or head and body movements. This is achieved by (1) conjugate eye movements (both eyeballs move in parallel)—smooth pursuit, saccades, optokinetic nystagmus, vestibulo-ocular nystagmus and gaze holding; and (2) disconjugate eye movements—convergence and divergence.

Clinical examination of eye movements should comprise tests of (1) eye position, nystagmus and gaze-holding function; (2) smooth pursuit; (3) saccades. Many abnormalities of eye movements are distinctive and often indicate the site and the side of a lesion, e.g. vertical eye movements are generated and controlled in the mesencephalon, whereas horizontal eye movements in the pons.

Dizziness and vertigo

Vertigo, dizziness, and disequilibrium are common complaints of patients of all ages, particularly older people, but it can be very difficult to diagnose their cause. The complex anatomy and the physiology accounts for much of this difficulty, hence a systematic approach is crucial.

Vertigo syndromes are commonly characterized by a combination of phenomena involving (1) vertigo itself—resulting from a disturbance of cortical spatial orientation; (2) nystagmus—caused by a direction-specific imbalance in the vestibulo-ocular reflex, which activates brainstem neuronal circuitry; (3) vestibular ataxia and postural imbalance—caused by inappropriate or abnormal activation of monosynaptic and polysynaptic vestibulospinal pathways; and (4) unpleasant autonomic responses of nausea, vomiting, and anxiety—ascending and descending vestibulo-autonomic pathways activate the medullary vomiting centre.

Clinical approach—the history is of special importance, with the patient's symptoms giving an idea of the likely underlying cause and differentiating the different forms of peripheral and central vestibular vertigo. Careful and systematic examination of the ocular motor and vestibular systems often allows an exact topographic determination of the lesion. Additional laboratory investigations most often do not contribute materially to the diagnosis.

Particular causes—more than 50% of all patients presenting with dizziness, vertigo or disequilibrium in a neurological dizziness unit will be suffering from one of the following: (1) benign paroxysmal positioning vertigo; (2) phobic postural vertigo; (3) vestibular migraine; (4) Ménière's disease; (5) vestibular neuritis.

Prognosis and treatment—many forms of vertigo have a benign cause and are characterized by spontaneous recovery of vestibular function or central compensation of a peripheral vestibular tone imbalance. Most forms of vertigo can be effectively relieved by (1) pharmacological treatment—depending on the particular cause,

e.g. vestibular suppressants, antiepileptic drugs, betahistine dihydrochloride; (2) physical therapy—liberatory manoeuvres for benign paroxysmal positioning vertigo; (3) vestibular exercises and balance training—for uni- or bilateral vestibular failure or central forms of vertigo; (4) psychotherapy—in particular cognitive behavioural therapy for phobic postural vertigo; or (very rarely) (5) surgery.

Introduction

The disorders underlying vertigo and dizziness are often combined with disturbances of eye movements; reciprocal effects occur because of the anatomical and functional overlap of the vestibular and ocular motor systems. Therefore, both systems must always be tested in patients complaining of vertigo and dizziness. It is often difficult to diagnose the different forms of vertigo, oculomotor disorders, and nystagmus. The complex anatomy and the physiology account for much of this difficulty; thus a systematic approach is crucial. The history is of special importance and one should have an idea, from the symptoms reported by the patient, what the underlying cause of the vertigo is in order to differentiate the different forms of peripheral and central vestibular vertigo. Additional laboratory examinations most often do not contribute materially to the diagnosis, but, on the other hand, a careful and systematic examination of the oculomotor and vestibular systems often allows an exact topographic determination of the lesion, in particular to differentiate between central and peripheral lesions.

Eye movements

Different types of eye movements can be distinguished, each with particular functions, physiological properties, and specific anatomical substrates: smooth pursuit, saccades, optokinetic nystagmus, vestibulo-ocular nystagmus, and gaze holding (all of these are conjugate eye movements, i.e. both eyeballs move in parallel) as well as disconjugate eye movements (convergence and divergence). The major function of eye movements is to keep the image of the visual surroundings stable on the retina, even during eye or head and body movements. Normal vision relies on eye movements in two essential ways: on the one hand, eye movements make it possible to shift the gaze and to view objects of interest and, on the other, when the head or body moves during locomotion, the eyes move in a direction opposite to that of the head and compensate for these head movements, thereby preventing involuntary shifts of the visual images projected on the retina. The retinal images are kept steady. Optimal functioning of the eye movements is ensured by cooperation between the optokinetic reflex and the vestibulo-ocular reflex.

For anatomical reasons many abnormalities of eye movements are distinctive and often indicate the site and the side of a lesion, e.g. vertical eye movements are generated and controlled in the mesencephalon, whereas horizontal eye movements are generated and controlled in the pons. This is useful for topographic diagnosis, a method that can still be superior to imaging techniques. It is therefore important that the doctor examines in detail the eye movements of patients with, for example, double or blurred vision, oscillopsia (apparent movement of the visual surroundings due to retinal slip), vertigo, dizziness, or postural imbalance because they can, by this means, often differentiate between 'peripheral' and 'central' oculomotor disorders and thereby also between peripheral and central vestibular disorders. In their excellent book *Neurology of eye movements*, Leigh and Zee correctly state that 'an understanding of the properties of each functional class of eye movements will guide the physical examination; a knowledge of the neural substrate will aid topological diagnosis'.

Here the clinical examination techniques of the oculomotor system and common pathological findings, as well as the typical features of the different forms of nystagmus, are summarized.

Eye position, nystagmus, and gaze-holding function

Clinical examination should begin with examination of the eyes in nine different positions (i.e. looking straight ahead, to the right, left, up, and down, as well as diagonally right up, right down, left up, and left down) to determine ocular alignment (e.g. a possible misalignment of the eye axes), which may be accompanied by a head tilt, fixation deficits, spontaneous or fixation nystagmus, range of movement, and disorders of gaze-holding abilities. The examination can be performed with an object for fixation or a small rod-shaped flashlight. In primary position one should look for periodic eye movements, such as nystagmus (e.g. horizontal–rotatory, suppressed by fixation as in peripheral vestibular dysfunction), vertically upward (upbeat nystagmus), downward (downbeat nystagmus syndrome), or horizontal or torsional movements with only slight suppression (or increase) of intensity during fixation, as in a central vestibular dysfunction. A (nonvestibular) congenital nystagmus beats, as a rule, horizontally at various frequencies and amplitudes, and increases during fixation. So-called square-wave jerks (small saccades—0.5 to 5°) that cause the eyes to oscillate around the primary position increasingly occur in progressive supranuclear palsy or certain cerebellar syndromes. Ocular flutter (intermittent rapid bursts of horizontal oscillations without an intersaccadic interval) or opsoclonus (combined horizontal, vertical, and torsional oscillations) occurs in various disorders such as encephalitis, tumours of the brainstem or cerebellum, paraneoplastic syndromes, or in intoxication.

The examination of the eyes with Frenzel's spectacles (Fig. 24.6.2.1) is a sensitive method for detecting spontaneous nystagmus. This can also be achieved by examining one eye with an ophthalmoscope (while the other eye is covered) and simultaneously checking for movements of the optic papilla or retinal vessels, even with low, slow-phase velocities/frequencies or square-wave jerks (often observed in progressive supranuclear palsy or certain cerebellar syndromes). As the retina is behind the axis of rotation of the eyeball, the direction of any observed vertical or horizontal movement is opposite to that of the nystagmus detected with this method, i.e. a downbeat nystagmus causes a rapid, upward movement of the optic papilla or retinal vessels. It is important to simply describe the characteristics of the nystagmus and pathological eye movements. In this way most forms of nystagmus can be diagnosed even with no additional laboratory examination, because the classification is based on purely descriptive criteria. In most forms of nystagmus the initial eye movement is a slow drift (slow phase), followed by rapid corrective saccadic eye movement (quick phase) which brings the eyes back to the 'central position'. During this quick phase, cortical mechanisms suppress oscillopsia. The leading

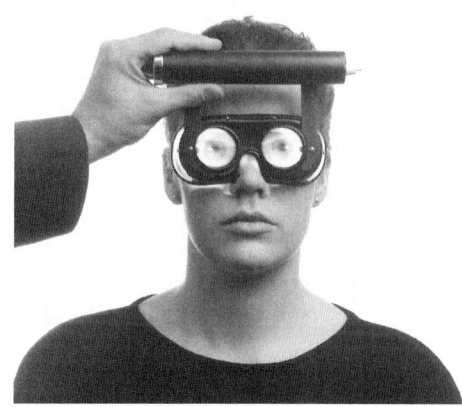

Fig. 24.6.2.1 Clinical examination with Frenzel's spectacles: the magnifying lenses (+16 D) have light inside to prevent visual fixation, which could suppress spontaneous nystagmus. Frenzel's spectacles enable the clinician to observe spontaneous eye movements better. Examination should include spontaneous and gaze-evoked nystagmus, head-shaking nystagmus (instruct the patient to rotate the head about 20 times and observe eye movements after head shaking), positioning and positional nystagmus, as well as hyperventilation-induced nystagmus.

symptoms of patients with nystagmus are blurred vision, reduced visual acuity, and oscillopsia.

After checking for possible eye movements in the primary position and misalignment of the axes of the eyes, the examiner should then establish the range of eye movements monocularly and binocularly in the eight end-positions; deficits found here can indicate, for example, extraocular muscle or nerve palsy. Gaze-holding deficits can also be determined by examining eccentric gaze position. Use of a small rod-shaped flashlight has the advantage that the corneal reflex images can be observed and thus ocular misalignments can be easily detected (note: it is important to observe the corneal reflex images from the direction of the illumination and to ensure that the patient attentively fixates the object of gaze). The flashlight also allows determination of whether the patient can fixate with one or both eyes in the end-positions. This is important for detecting a gaze-holding defect.

Gaze-evoked nystagmus can be clearly identified only when the patient fixates with both eyes. It is most often a side effect of medication (e.g. anticonvulsants, benzodiazepines) or toxins (e.g. alcohol). Horizontal gaze-evoked nystagmus can indicate a structural lesion in the area of the brainstem or cerebellum (vestibular nucleus, nucleus prepositus hypoglossi, flocculus, i.e. the neural eye velocity to position integrator). Vertical gaze-evoked nystagmus is observed in midbrain lesions involving the interstitial nucleus of Cajal. A dissociated horizontal gaze-evoked nystagmus (greater in the abducting than the adducting eye) in combination with an adduction deficit points to internuclear ophthalmoplegia due to a defect of the medial longitudinal fascicle (MLF), ipsilateral to the adduction deficit. Downbeat nystagmus usually increases in eccentric gaze position and when looking down. To examine for a so-called rebound nystagmus the patient should gaze for at least 30 s to one side and then return the eyes to the primary position; this can cause a transient nystagmus to appear with slow phases in the direction of the previous eye position. Rebound nystagmus generally indicates cerebellar dysfunction or damage to the cerebellar pathways.

Smooth pursuit

The patient is asked to visually track an object moving slowly in horizontal and vertical directions (10 to 20°/s) while keeping the head stationary. Corrective (catch-up or back-up) saccades are looked for; they indicate a smooth pursuit gain that is too low or too high (ratio of eye movement velocity to object velocity). Many anatomical structures (visual cortex, motion-sensitive areas MT, V5, frontal eye fields, dorsolateral pontine nuclei, cerebellum, and vestibular and oculomotor nuclei) are involved in smooth pursuit eye movements, which keep the image of a moving object stable on the fovea. These eye movements are influenced also by alertness, various drugs, and age. Even healthy individuals exhibit a slightly saccadic smooth pursuit during vertical downward gaze. For these reasons a saccadic smooth pursuit does not as a rule allow either an exact topographical or an aetiological classification. Marked asymmetries of smooth pursuit, however, indicate a structural lesion; strongly impaired smooth pursuit is observed in intoxication (anticonvulsants, benzodiazepines, or alcohol) as well as degenerative disorders involving the cerebellum or extrapyramidal system. A reversal of slow smooth pursuit eye movements during optokinetic stimulation is typical of congenital nystagmus (see above).

Saccades

First, it is necessary to observe spontaneous saccades triggered by visual or auditory stimuli. Then the patient is asked to glance back and forth between two horizontal or between two vertical targets. The velocity, accuracy, and the conjugacy of the saccades should be noted. Normal individuals can immediately reach the target with a fast single movement or one small corrective saccade. Slowing of saccades—often accompanied by hypometric saccades—occurs, for example, with intoxication (medication, especially anticonvulsants or benzodiazepines) or in neurodegenerative disorders. Slowing of horizontal saccades is generally observed in brainstem lesions; there is often a dysfunction of the ipsilateral paramedian pontine reticular formation (PPRF). Slowing of vertical saccades indicates a midbrain lesion in which the rostral intermedial nucleus of the medial longitudinal fascicle (riMLF) is involved, not only in ischaemic inflammatory diseases but also in neurodegenerative diseases, especially progressive supranuclear palsy.

Hypermetric saccades, which can be identified by a corrective saccade back to the object, indicate lesions of the cerebellum (especially the vermis) or the cerebellar pathways. Patients with Wallenberg's syndrome make hypermetric saccades towards the side of the lesion due to a dysfunction of the inferior cerebellar peduncle; conversely, defects of the superior cerebellar peduncle lead to contralateral hypermetric saccades. A slowing of the adducting saccade ipsilateral to a defective MLF is pathognomonic of internuclear ophthalmoplegia (INO). Delayed-onset saccades are mostly caused by supratentorial cortical disturbances.

As a general rule, it is often necessary to combine the pathological clinical findings of the different eye movement systems to differentiate between a central and a peripheral vestibular disorder, and to make an exact topographical diagnosis.

Dizziness and vertigo

Vertigo, dizziness, and disequilibrium are common complaints of patients of all ages, particularly older people. The lifetime prevalence of vertigo and dizziness is about 30%. The clinical spectrum of vertigo is broad, extending from vestibular rotatory vertigo with nausea and vomiting to presyncope light-headedness, from drug intoxication to hypoglycaemic dizziness, from visual vertigo to phobias and panic attacks, and from motion sickness to height vertigo. Appropriate preventions and treatments differ for the various types of dizziness and vertigo; they include drug therapy, physical therapy, psychotherapy, and surgery.

Vertigo usually implies a mismatch of the vestibular, visual, and somatosensory systems. These three sensory systems subserve both static and dynamic spatial orientation, locomotion, and control of posture by constantly providing reafferent cues. The sensory information is partially redundant in that two or three senses may simultaneously provide similar information about the same action. Thanks to this overlap of their functional ranges, it is possible for one sense to substitute, at least in part, for deficiencies in the others. When information from two sensory sources conflicts, the intensity of the vertigo is a function of the degree of mismatch: it is increased if information from an intact sensory system is lost as, for example, in patients with pathological vestibular vertigo who close their eyes. The distressing sensorimotor consequences of the mismatch are frequently based on our earlier experiences with orientation, balance, and locomotion, i.e. there is a mismatch between the expected and the actually perceived pattern of multisensory input.

Vertigo may thus be induced by physiological stimulation of the intact sensorimotor systems (height vertigo, motion sickness) or by pathological dysfunction of any of the stabilizing sensory systems, especially the vestibular system. The symptoms of vertigo include sensory qualities identified as arising from vestibular, visual, and somatosensory sources. As distinct from one's perception of self-motion during natural locomotion, the experience of vertigo is linked to impaired perception of a stationary environment; this perception is mediated by central nervous system (CNS) processes known as 'space constancy mechanisms'. Loss of the external stationary reference system required for orientation and postural regulation contributes to the distressing mixture of self-motion and surround motion.

Physiological and clinical vertigo syndromes are commonly characterized by a combination of phenomena involving perceptual, oculomotor, postural, and autonomic manifestations: vertigo, nystagmus, ataxia, and nausea. These four manifestations correlate with different aspects of vestibular function and emanate from different sites within the CNS:

1 The vertigo itself results from a disturbance of cortical spatial orientation.

2 Nystagmus (see above) is caused by a direction-specific imbalance in the vestibulo-ocular reflex, which activates brainstem neuronal circuitry.

3 Postural imbalance is caused by inappropriate or abnormal activation of monosynaptic and polysynaptic vestibulospinal pathways.

4 The unpleasant autonomic responses with nausea, vomiting, and anxiety travel along ascending and descending vestibuloautonomic pathways to activate the medullary vomiting centre.

More than 50% of all patients presenting with dizziness, vertigo, or disequilibrium in a neurological dizziness unit will be

Table 24.6.2.1 Relative frequency of the common syndromes of dizziness, vertigo, and disequilibrium in 10, 238 patients seen in a dizziness unit

Diagnosis	Relative frequency (%)
Benign paroxysmal positioning vertigo	18.4
Phobic postural vertigo	15.6
Central vestibular vertigo	12.7
Vestibular migraine	10.4
Menière's disease	9.3
Vestibular neuritis	7.5
Bilateral vestibulopathy	4.9
Vestibular paroxysmia	3.7
Psychogenic vertigo (without phobic postural vertigo)	3.1
Perilymph fistula (in particular superior canal dehiscence syndrome)	0.6
Unknown aetiology	3.7

Table 24.6.2.2 Pharmacological therapies for vertigo

Therapy	Type of vertigo
Vestibular suppressants	Symptomatic relief of nausea (in acute peripheral and central vestibular lesions), prevention of motion sickness
Antiepileptic drugs (carbamazepine)	Vestibular paroxysmia, vestibular epilepsy (very rare), paroxysmal dysarthria and ataxia in multiple sclerosis, other central vestibular paroxysms, superior oblique myokymia
β-Receptor blockers, antiepileptic drugs (valproic acid, topiramate)	Vestibular migraine
Betahistine dihydrochloride (high dosage (48 mg three times daily) and long term (>6–12 months)	Menière's disease
Antibiotics	Infections of the ear and temporal bone
Ototoxic antibiotics (gentamicin, transtympanically)	Menière's disease (Menière's drop attacks—'Tumarkin's otolithic crisis')
Corticosteroids	Acute vestibular neuritis, autoimmune inner ear disease, in particular Cogan's syndrome
4-Aminopyridine (5 mg three times daily) Baclofen	Downbeat or upbeat nystagmus
Acetazolamide 4-Aminopyridine	Episodic ataxia type 2
Selective serotonin reuptake inhibitors	Phobic postural vertigo

suffering from one of the five following common syndromes (Table 24.6.2.1): benign paroxysmal positioning vertigo (BPPV), phobic postural vertigo, central vertigo, vestibular migraine, Menière's disease, or vestibular neuritis.

Clinicians unfamiliar with patients complaining of dizziness can most effectively deepen their knowledge by acquainting themselves with these five most frequently met and challenging conditions of vertigo. Diagnosis and management of vertigo syndromes always require interdisciplinary thinking, and history taking is still much more important than recordings of eye movements or brain imaging techniques. Although most clinicians welcome the attempts to develop computer interview systems for use with neuro-otological

patients, and expert systems as diagnostic aids in otoneurology, their application in a clinical setting is still quite limited.

Dizziness is a vexing symptom, difficult to assess because of its purely subjective character and its variety of sensations. The sensation of spinning or rotatory vertigo is much more specific; if it persists, it undoubtedly indicates acute pathology of the labyrinth, the vestibular nerve, or the caudal brainstem, which contains the vestibular nuclei.

The patient history is the key to the diagnosis. One should focus on four aspects:

1 form of vertigo, i.e. rotatory or postural vertigo

2 duration of symptoms, which may range from attacks lasting seconds (typical for vestibular paroxysmia) to hours (typical of Menière's disease or vestibular migraine) up to ongoing symptoms for years, as in phobic postural vertigo or bilateral vestibulopathy

3 situations and circumstances when the symptoms occur (e.g. changes of head or body position typical of BPPV)

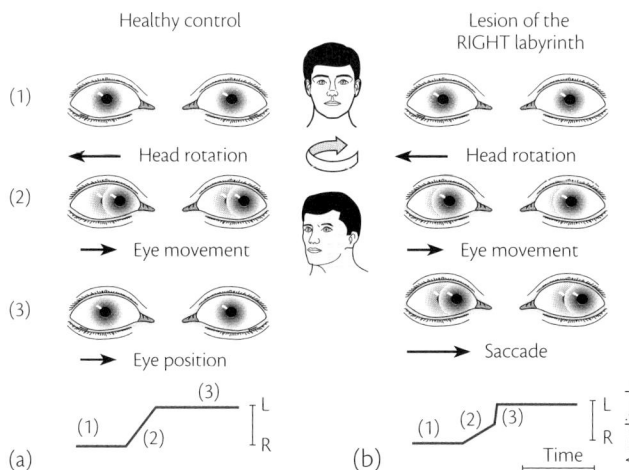

Fig. 24.6.2.2 Clinical bedside testing of the horizontal vestibulo-ocular reflex by the Halmagyi–Curthoys head-impulse test. Fast 20 to 30° rotations of the head towards the side of the lesion show the dynamic deficit of the horizontal vestibulo-ocular reflex. In contrast to the healthy control (a), the patient is not able to generate a fast controversive eye movement and has to perform a corrective (catch-up) saccade to refixate the target (b). It is important to instruct the patient to look carefully at the examiner's nose and to apply brief, high-acceleration head thrusts to detect a unilateral peripheral vestibular deficit, e.g. due to vestibular neuritis or a vestibular schwannoma.

Table 24.6.2.3 Physical therapies for vertigo

Therapy	Type of vertigo
Liberatory manoeuvres	Benign paroxysmal positioning vertigo
Vestibular exercises and balance training	Vestibular rehabilitation, central compensation of acute vestibular loss, habituation for prevention of motion sickness, improvement of balance skills (e.g. in older people)

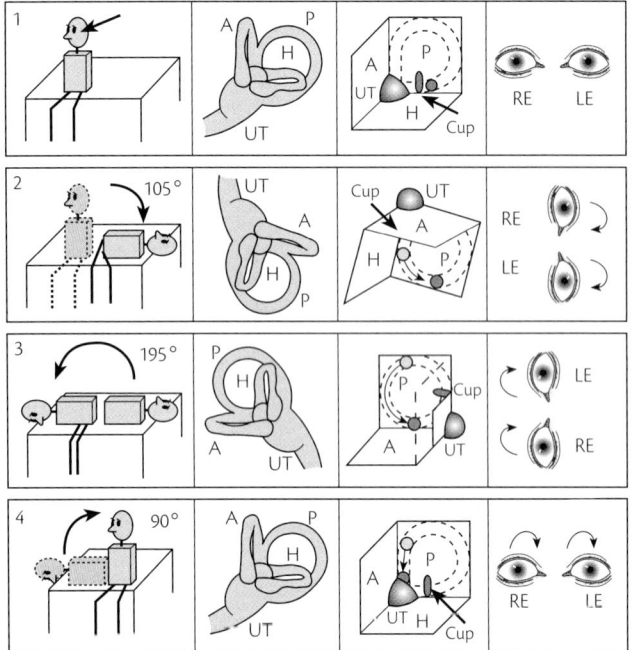

Fig. 24.6.2.3 Schematic drawing of the Semont liberatory manoeuvre in a patient with typical benign paroxysmal positioning vertigo (BPPV) of the left ear. Boxes from left to right: position of body and head, position of labyrinth in space, position and movement of the clot in the posterior canal and resulting cupula deflection, and direction of the rotatory nystagmus. The clot is depicted as an open circle within the canal; a black circle represents the final resting position of the clot. (1) In the sitting position, the head is turned horizontally 45° to the unaffected ear. The clot, which is heavier than endolymph, settles at the base of the left posterior semicircular canal. (2) The patient is tilted approximately 105° towards the left (affected) ear. The change in head position, relative to gravity, causes the clot to gravitate to the lowermost part of the canal and the cupula to deflect downwards, inducing BPPV with rotatory nystagmus beating toward the undermost ear. The patient maintains this position for 1 min. (3) The patient is turned approximately 195° with the nose down, causing the clot to move towards the exit of the canal. The endolymphatic flow again deflects the cupula such that the nystagmus beats towards the left ear, now uppermost. The patient remains in this position for 1 min. (4) The patient is slowly moved to the sitting position; this causes the clot to enter the utricular cavity. A, P, and H: anterior, posterior, and horizontal semicircular canals; Cup, cupula; UT, utricular cavity; RE, right eye; LE, left eye.
Brandt T, Steddin S, Daroff RB (1994). Therapy for benign paroxysmal positioning vertigo, revisited. *Neurology*, **44**, 796–800.

4 accompanying symptoms (e.g. hearing loss, pressure in one ear, or tinnitus typical of Menière's disease).

History taking also allows the early differentiation of vertigo and disequilibrium disorders into seven categories that serve as a practical guide for differential diagnosis:

1 dizziness and light-headedness (such as presyncopal dizziness or drug intoxication)

2 single or recurrent attacks of (rotatory) vertigo (Menière's disease, vestibular migraine)

3 sustained (rotatory) vertigo (vestibular neuritis, Wallenberg's syndrome)

4 positioning/positional vertigo (as in BPPV, central positional vertigo)

5 oscillopsia (apparent motion of the visual scene, such as in vestibular neuritis or downbeat nystagmus; it also occurs in bilateral vestibulopathy when patients walk or turn their head)

Box 24.6.2.1 Benign paroxysmal positioning vertigo (typical posterior semicircular canal type, p-BPPV)

Clinical syndrome

Brief attacks of rotational vertigo and concomitant rotatory–linear nystagmus precipitated by rapid head-trunk tilt towards the affected ear or by neck extension (when first lying down in bed, sitting up from a supine position, turning over in bed from one side to the other, extending the neck to look up):

- Latency—vertigo and nystagmus begin 1 s or more after head tilt
- Duration—attacks last less than 60 s
- Nystagmus—vertical–rotatory, with the fast phase beating upwards with a clockwise or counterclockwise rotatory component
- Reversal—when the patient returns to the seated position, vertigo and nystagmus reoccur in the opposite direction
- Fatiguability—repetition of the manoeuvres results in ever-lessening symptoms

Incidence/age/sex

Most common cause of vestibular vertigo that manifests throughout life, particularly in older people. Life-time prevalence: at least 3% with incidence peaking in the sixth and seventh decades; females exceed males by 2:1.

Pathomechanism

'Canalolithiasis' of the posterior semicircular canal; dislodged otoconia (degeneration, trauma) congeal to form a free-floating 'heavy' clot, which always gravitates to the most dependent part of the canal during changes in head position, thereby causing push or pull forces on the cupula.

Aetiology

- 'Idiopathic' forms (ageing) >95%
- Symptomatic forms due to head trauma (relatively often bilateral BPPV), After vestibular neuritis, known vestibular migraine or prolonged bed rest

Course/prognosis

Natural history is considered benign because it resolves spontaneously in 70% of the patients within days to months in most patients, persists in about 20–30% when untreated, and recurs in 30–50% after variable periods of years.

Management

- Physical liberating manoeuvres to free the canal of the 'heavy' clot (Fig. 24.6.2.3):

Semont's manoeuvre or Epley's manoeuvre (both are equally effective)
Brandt's and Daroff's manoeuvres
These are successful in almost 100% of patients within days or weeks.

Differential diagnosis

Central positional vertigo/nystagmus, vestibular migraine with positioning or positional vertigo, vestibular paroxysmia, perilymph fistula, phobic postural vertigo.

Based on Brandt T, Dieterich M, Strupp M (2010). *Vertigo and dizziness—common complaints.* 2nd edition Springer, London.

Box 24.6.2.2 Menière's disease

Clinical syndrome

◆ Recurrent attacks of vertigo, lasting longer than 20 min

◆ Fluctuating hearing loss

◆ Tinnitus

◆ Subjective fullness of the ear

◆ Rarely, vestibular drop attacks

Monosymptomatic forms possible, variable auditory and vestibular deficits in the intervals between attacks. There is no pathognomonic test to establish the diagnosis unequivocally.

Lifetime prevalence/age/sex

◆ 0.5%

◆ Affects mainly age group from 30 to 50 years

◆ Incidence in males and females roughly equal

◆ Rare in children

Pathomechanism

◆ Endolymphatic hydrops of the labyrinth due to insufficient endolymph reabsorption in the endolymphatic sac or blockage of longitudinal endolymph flow

◆ Attacks: periodic leakage or ruptures of the endolymph membrane with potassium-induced depolarization of the nerve

◆ Intervals: pressure-dependent loss of cochlear and vestibular hair cells, distortion of labyrinth structures

Aetiology

◆ Idiopathic (aetiology not known in more than 95%)

◆ Acquired, 'delayed endolymphatic hydrops' (i.e. labyrinthitis, viral autoimmunological, temporal bone trauma)

Course/prognosis

◆ Usually begins in one ear with increasing frequency of attacks and major auditory/vestibular deficit occurring during the first years

◆ After 5 years both ears are affected in 50% of the patients if not treated

Management

◆ Medical: betahistine, e.g. betahistine dihydrochloride: 48 mg three times daily for at least 6–12 months as a prophylactic treatment

◆ Destructive (in rare cases):

　• If treatment with betahistine does not prevent attacks, ototoxic antibiotics (gentamicin transtympanically in low dosages of 10 mg with long intervals of at least 4 weeks due to the delayed ototoxicity—'wait and see')

　• Vestibular nerve section (in very rare cases)

Box 24.6.2.2 (*Cont'd*) Menière's disease

Differential diagnosis

◆ Vertigo migraine

◆ Perilymph fistula

◆ Vestibular paroxysmia

◆ Vestibular neuritis

◆ Benign paroxysmal positioning vertigo

◆ Transient ischaemic attacks

◆ Cogan's syndrome

6 vertigo associated with auditory dysfunction (such as Menière's disease, Cogan's syndrome)

7 postural imbalance or to-and-fro vertigo (such as in bilateral vestibulopathy when the patient is walking).

Every patient who has vertigo or dizziness has to be examined by at least four tests: first, look for nystagmus with and without Frenzel's spectacles as described above; second, apply the head-impulse test for the vestibulo-ocular reflex. The vestibulo-ocular reflex holds images of the seen world steady on the retina during brief head rotations and locomotion. This important clinical bedside test of the horizontal vestibulo-ocular reflex is illustrated in Fig. 24.6.2.2. This test allows the doctor to find out whether there is a unilateral or bilateral peripheral vestibular deficit. Third, the Dix–Hallpike manoeuvre looks for a positioning nystagmus, i.e. BPPV. Fourth, the above detailed examination of eye movements is also important, in particular, to differentiate between peripheral and central forms of vertigo because the latter are almost always associated with central oculomotor dysfunction.

Management of the dizzy patient

The prevailing good prognosis of vertigo should be emphasized because of the following:

◆ Many forms of vertigo have a benign cause and are characterized by spontaneous recovery of vestibular function or central compensation of a peripheral vestibular tone imbalance.

◆ Most forms of vertigo can be effectively relieved by pharmacological treatment (Table 24.6.2.2), physical therapy in the form of liberating manoeuvres for BPPV (Table 24.6.2.3) or vestibular exercises and balance training for uni- or bilateral vestibular failure or central forms of vertigo, psychotherapy, in particular cognitive–behavioural therapy for phobic postural vertigo or—more and more rarely—surgery.

There is, however, no common treatment, and vestibular suppressants provide only symptomatic relief of vertigo and nausea. A specific therapeutic approach thus requires recognition of the numerous particular pathomechanisms involved. Such therapy can include causative, symptomatic, or preventive approaches.

The essential characteristics are given for benign paroxysmal positioning vertigo (Fig. 24.6.2.3, Box 24.6.2.1 and see Table 24.6.2.3), Menière's disease (Box 24.6.2.2), vestibular neuritis (Box 24.6.2.3), bilateral vestibulopathy (Box 24.6.2.4), and vestibular migraine (Box 24.6.2.5).

Box 24.6.2.3 Vestibular neuritis

Clinical syndrome

Acute onset of sustained:

◆ Rotatory vertigo

◆ Postural imbalance with falls toward the affected ear

◆ Horizontal–rotatory spontaneous nystagmus (towards the unaffected ear)

◆ Nausea and vomiting

◆ Pathological head-impulse test

◆ Unilateral hypo- or unresponsiveness in caloric testing

Incidence/age/sex

Third most common cause of peripheral vestibular vertigo that manifests throughout life (affects mainly ages 30–60 years; rare in children) without preference of sex.

Pathomechanism

Acute partial unilateral loss of labyrinthine function (horizontal and anterior semicircular canal paresis) with a vestibular tone imbalance in yaw and roll planes.

Aetiology

Most probably herpes simplex virus 1 infection of the superior division of the vestibular nerve trunk.

Course/prognosis

Spontaneous recovery within 1–6 weeks due to:

◆ Peripheral restoration of labyrinthine function (incomplete in about 50%)

◆ Central compensation of vestibular tone imbalance

◆ (Contralateral) vestibular, somatosensory, and visual substitution of the vestibular deficit

Better prognosis and higher recovery rate in children.

Management

Medical treatment

Corticosteroids (beginning, for instance, with 100 mg 6-methylprednisolone per day within 3 days after symptoms, then taper every third day by 20 mg)

Antivertiginous drugs (for instance dimenhydrinate)

Physical therapy (vestibular exercises)

Differential diagnosis

◆ Acute central brainstem lesions at the root entry zone of nerve VIII and the vestibular nucleus (multiple sclerosis plaques, small pontomedullary infarcts): 'vestibular pseudoneuritis'

◆ Midline cerebellar infarction

◆ Peripheral labyrinthine and vestibular nerve disorders, such as vascular anterior inferior cerebellar artery (AICA) infarcts or Menière's disease which may begin monosymptomatically

◆ Vestibular migraine

Box 24.6.2.4 Bilateral vestibular failure

Clinical syndrome

Symptoms

◆ Postural vertigo with unsteadiness of gait (particularly in the dark or on unlevel ground)

◆ Oscillopsia associated with head movements or when walking

◆ Episodes of vertigo early in the development of bilateral vestibular failure but not in chronic state

◆ Impaired spatial memory

Signs

◆ Bilateral pathological head-impulse test

◆ Absent or markedly reduced vestibulo-ocular reflex with bithermal caloric testing and pendular body rotation in the dark

◆ Increased postural sway with eyes closed and/or standing on foam rubber

Incidence/age/sex

◆ Often overlooked condition, in particular in older people

◆ Without preference of sex

Pathomechanism

◆ Progressive loss of bilateral labyrinthine and/or vestibular nerve function due to various aetiologies with concurrent somatosensory and visual 'compensation' (substitution) of vestibular function for spatial orientation, ocular stabilization, and postural control

◆ High-frequency deficit of the vestibulo-ocular reflex persists, however

Aetiologies

◆ Ototoxicity (ototoxic antibiotics), bilateral Menière's disease, meningitis, neurodegenerative (often associated with cerebellar degeneration and downbeat nystagmus), bilateral vestibular schwannomas in neurofibromatosis type 2, immune-mediated inner-ear disease, bilateral sequential vestibular neuritis, congenital malformations, familial vestibulopathy

◆ Aetiology remains unclear in more than 70%

Course/prognosis

Bilateral vestibular failure may develop simultaneously or sequentially, take an abrupt or slowly progressive course, and be complete or incomplete. Permanent loss of vestibular function is most frequent.

Management

◆ Prevention of bilateral vestibular failure (ototoxic drugs)

◆ Recovery from bilateral vestibular failure (immune-mediated inner-ear disease)

◆ Vestibular rehabilitation

Differential diagnosis

◆ Of the various disorders causing bilateral vestibular failure

Box 24.6.2.4 *(Cont'd)* Bilateral vestibular failure

◆ Of disorders similar in symptomatology (unsteadiness and oscillopsia):

· Cerebellar or ocular motor disorders without bilateral vestibular failure, e.g. downbeat nystagmus, which, however, is often associated with bilateral vestibulopathy

· Phobic postural vertigo

· Intoxication

· Vestibular paroxysmia

· Perilymph fistula

· Orthostatic hypotension

· Visual disorders

· Unilateral vestibular loss

Box 24.6.2.5 Vestibular migraine

Clinical features

◆ Spontaneous recurrent attacks of vertigo/dizziness (prevailing type rotational) most often lasting minutes to hours

◆ Associated with headache or other migrainous symptoms (60–70%)

◆ In most an individual history of migraine according to the HIS-II criteria

Examination findings

During the attack

◆ Pathological spontaneous or positional nystagmus (about 70%)

◆ Postural imbalance (about 90%)

During the attack-free interval

◆ Central ocular motor signs (>60%) less severe than in the attack

◆ Peripheral vestibular deficit (10–20%)

Diagnostic tests and procedures to exclude other entities

Basic tests for vestibular migraine—neuro-ophthalmological and neuro-otological examinations

Tests for Menière's disease

◆ Auditory testing

◆ Oculography with caloric irrigation

◆ Vestibular evoked myogenic potentials

Tests for transient ischemic attacks

◆ MRI

◆ Doppler ultrasonography

Tests for vestibular paroxysmia

◆ MRI (CISS sequence) of nerve VIII and treatment with carbamazepine

---

Box 24.6.2.5 *(Cont'd)* Vestibular migraine

Management

◆ Treatment of the attacks with aspirin or other NSAID and dimenhydrinate

◆ Prophylactic treatment with β-blocker, valproic acid, or topiramate if patient has more than two attacks per months

CISS sequence, constructive interference steady state gradient echo sequence; HIS-II, *The international classification of headache disorders*, 2nd edition.

Further reading

Baloh RW, Halmagyi GM (1996). *Disorders of the vestibular system*. Oxford University Press, Oxford.

Brandt T (1999). *Vertigo—its multisensory syndromes*, 2nd edition. Springer, London.

Brandt T, Dieterich M, Strupp M (2010). *Vertigo and dizziness—common complaints*. 2nd edition. Springer, London.

Brandt T, Steddin S, Daroff RB (1994). Therapy for benign paroxysmal positioning vertigo, revisited. *Neurology*, **44**, 796–800.

Bronstein A, Brandt Th, Woollacott M (1996). *Clinical disorders of balance, posture and gait*. Arnold, London.

Halmagyi GM, Curthoys IS (1988). A clinical sign of canal paresis. *Arch Neurol*, **45**, 737–9.

Herdman, SJ (2004). *Vestibular rehabilitation*, 4th edition. F A Davies, Philadelphia.

Kalla R, *et al.* (2007). 4-aminopyridine restores vertical and horizontal neural integrator function in downbeat nystagmus. *Brain*, **130**, 2441–51.

Leigh RJ, Zee DS (2006). *Neurology of eye movements*, 3rd edition. F A Davies, Philadelphia.

Strupp M, *et al.* (2004). Methylprednisolone, valacyclovir, or the combination for vestibular neuritis. *N Engl J Med*, **351**, 354–61.

Strupp M, *et al.* (2008). Long-term prophylactic treatment of attacks of vertigo in Menière's disease—comparison of a high with a low dosage of betahistine in an open trial. *Acta Otolaryngol*, **128**, 520–4.

24.6.3 Hearing

Linda M. Luxon

Essentials

Hearing loss

Hearing loss is the most common sensory impairment. The World Health Organization has estimated that at least 250 million people are affected worldwide, as are 17% of the adult population in the United Kingdom, three-quarters of these being over 60 years of age.

Clinical examination and investigation—examination includes visual inspection of the anatomy of the external ear and tympanic membrane, and tuning-fork tests to distinguish conductive from sensorineural hearing loss in some cases. Audiological investigations (1) quantify audiometric thresholds at each frequency; (2) differentiate conductive from sensorineural defects; (3) differentiate cochlear from retrocochlear abnormality; (4) identify central auditory dysfunction in the brainstem, midbrain or auditory cortex; and (5) identify a nonorganic component.

Epidemiology and causes—(1) prevalence in adults—factors include age, gender, genetic susceptibility occupational group and hazardous noise exposure. (2) Congenital hearing impairment in children—over one-half of cases are explained by factors associated with admission to a neonatal intensive-care unit genetic factors and craniofacial abnormalities. (3) Acquired hearing impairment in children—the commonest cause is a conductive hearing loss due to chronic secretory otitis media; meningitis (particularly meningococcal) is the commonest cause of acquired sensorineural hearing loss in the UK. (4) Many of the preventable causes of hearing impairment remain common in the developing world: consanguineous marriages, birth trauma, childhood infections, noise exposure, and the unlicensed sale of ototoxic drugs.

Treatment—this may involve (1) protection from noise hazards and ototoxic drugs and management of chronic secretory otitis media; (2) auditory rehabilitation—including environmental aids, instruction in communication skills, and (if accepted by the patient) hearing aids; and (sometimes) (3) surgery—restorative in some cases of conductive hearing loss; implantable devices for totally deafened adults and children.

Tinnitus

Defined as a noise in the head or ears lasting for more than 5 min, tinnitus increases in frequency with age, affecting about 20% of people >60 years, although only 4% complain of the symptom. It can be associated with many conditions, frequently in association with hearing impairment.

Management—this is primarily medical, including the following interventions: (1) psychological—explanation of the problem, and if necessary treatment of anxiety/depression; (2) prosthetic—provision of hearing aids noise generators to 'mask' tinnitus with desirable environmental noise; and (rarely) (3) pharmacological—intravenous lidocaine (lignocaine) can result in the disappearance or amelioration of tinnitus, but no oral preparation has been found to be equally effective.

Hearing impairments

Our hearing is a choice and dainty sense, and hard to mend, yet soon it may be marred. Blows, falls and noise…all these … breed tingling in the ears and hurt our hearing.
                                    Physicians of the Medical School of Salerno

Pathophysiology

For clinical purposes the ear is separated into three parts: the external, middle, and internal ear (Fig. 24.6.3.1). The external ear is important in funnelling sound to the tympanic membrane and in the localization of sound. The middle-ear ossicles connect the tympanic membrane to the oval window of the cochlea, such that sound waves cause displacement within the fluid-filled compartment of the membranous labyrinth. Within the internal ear, the mechanical activity at the oval window is transduced into neural responses by the hair cells of the organ of Corti (Fig. 24.6.3.2).

Disorders of the external and middle ear result in abnormalities of the mechanical transmission of sound from the environment to the internal ear, and give rise to a conductive hearing loss. Common examples include impacted wax, serous otitis media (glue ear), chronic otitis media, and disorders of the ossicular chain, e.g. otosclerosis, and traumatic discontinuity.

Disorders of the internal ear and cranial nerve VIII characteristically give rise to a sensorineural hearing loss, in which the perception of both bone- and air-conducted sounds is reduced and the appreciation of the intensity of sound and the frequency resolution of complex sounds are impaired. Many conditions may affect the cochlea, ranging from inherited, congenital, or iatrogenic nonsyndromal or syndromal malformations to ototoxic damage (aminoglycoside, antimalarial, loop diuretics), ischaemia including vertebrobasilar ischaemia, diabetic vasculitis, infections (mumps, rubella, syphilis, cytomegalovirus), autoimmune disorders, degenerative disorders, trauma, and idiopathic conditions such as Ménière's disease. Much doubt has been cast on so-called 'presbyacusis', which may merely reflect an accumulation of toxic/traumatic insults to the ear over many years, and recent advances in molecular biology and genetics have shown the role of genetic mutations/deletions in late-onset/progressive hearing impairments. Sudden sensorineural hearing loss, usually of cochlear origin, most commonly results from viral, vascular, or autoimmune disease. Pathology of cranial nerve VIII leading to auditory neuropathy and hearing impairment has been defined in genetic disorders, including spinocerebellar degenerations, trauma, cerebellopontine angle tumours, bony disorders such as Paget's disease, infective disorders (meningitis), and inflammatory conditions (sarcoidosis).

Central auditory disorders may be developmental or acquired in origin and present with difficulties hearing in background noise and discriminating degraded speech (e.g. over a loudspeaker), and with sound localization, often with a normal or near-normal audiogram. Unilateral neurological pathology rarely gives rise to an audiometric hearing impairment as a consequence of bilateral representation of each cochlea at every level of the central auditory

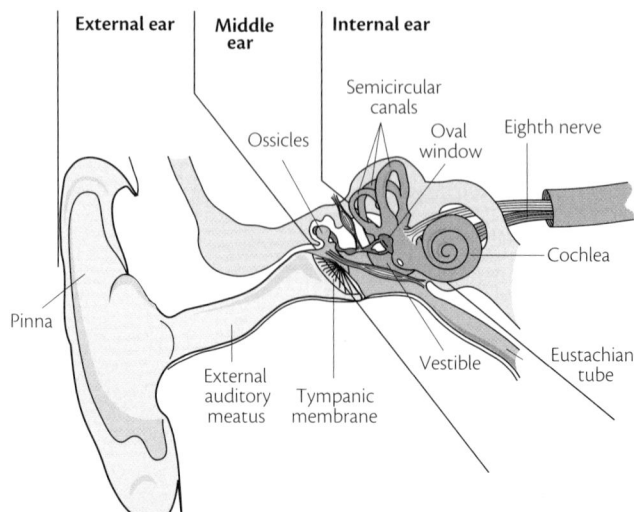

Fig. 24.6.3.1 Diagram to illustrate the anatomy of the peripheral auditory system.

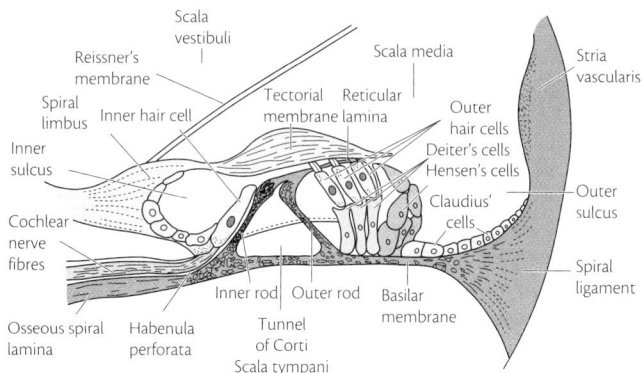

Fig. 24.6.3.2 Diagram of the organ of Corti.

pathway above the cochlear nuclei. Rarely bilateral brainstem pathology may present as a symmetrical sensorineural hearing loss, whereas bitemporal cortical pathology may give rise to cortical deafness or auditory agnosia.

Clinical examination

Clinical examination requires examination of the anatomy of the external ear to define visible signs of congenital ear disease (pits, tags, nodules, or malformations) and evidence of other craniofacial features suggestive of syndromal hearing impairment. In addition, a detailed examination of the tympanic membrane is required to define the presence of pathology within the middle ear. Wax or debris obstructing the external auditory meatus should be removed by or under the supervision of a clinician with experience in this field. Syringing should never be undertaken in the presence of an infection or if there is any possibility of a tympanic membrane perforation. Tuning-fork tests remain the most valuable clinical test of auditory function and frequently enable a clinician to distinguish a conductive from a sensorineural hearing loss (Fig. 24.6.3.3). The tests are based on two physiological facts: first, the inner ear is normally more sensitive to sound conducted by air than to that conducted by bone; second, in the presence of a purely conductive hearing loss, the affected ear is subject to less air-conducted environmental noise, making it more sensitive to bone-conducted sound. A general medical and neurological examination is mandatory to define syndromes and the plethora of general medical conditions associated with hearing impairment. A detailed vestibular assessment is also of value.

Investigations

A battery of audiological tests is required to:

◆ quantify audiometric thresholds at each frequency
◆ differentiate a conductive from a sensorineural hearing loss
◆ differentiate a cochlear from a retrocochlear abnormality
◆ identify central auditory dysfunction in the brainstem, midbrain, or auditory cortex
◆ identify a nonorganic component.

Each test can be defined as being subjective (dependent on patient cooperation) or objective (independent of patient cooperation) in terms of providing auditory data. Two pathophysiological phenomena are of importance in the differentiation of a cochlear sensorineural hearing loss from a nerve VIII or cochlear nuclei dysfunction:

◆ Loudness recruitment is defined as an abnormally rapid increase in loudness, with an increase in intensity of the stimulus, and is characteristic of disorders affecting the hair cells of the organ of Corti, but is absent in the pathology of nerve VIII.

◆ Abnormal auditory adaptation is a decline in discharge frequency with time, observed after an initial burst of neural activity in response to an adequate continuing stimulus applied to the organ of Corti. This phenomenon is characteristic of nerve VIII and brainstem auditory dysfunction.

Pure-tone audiometry is the most widely available, subjective, quantitative test of auditory thresholds. Electronically generated pure tones are delivered by earphones and the individual is required to respond to the quietest tone, at given frequencies between 125 and 8000 Hz in each ear. The sound may be delivered by air conduction (AC) or, if the tones are delivered by a bone vibrator on the mastoid process, by bone conduction (BC). In the latter test condition, as the intra-aural attenuation for a bone-conducted sound is negligible, masking of the ear not under test with narrow-band noise is mandatory. Bone-conduction thresholds significantly better than air-conduction thresholds indicate a conductive hearing loss, whereas similar bone-conduction and air-conduction thresholds are characteristic of sensorineural hearing loss (Fig. 24.6.3.4).

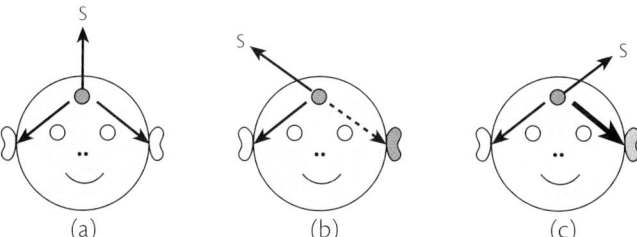

Fig. 24.6.3.3 Diagram to illustrate the Weber tuning fork test in (a) a normal individual, (b) a case of unilateral sensorineural hearing loss, and (c) a case of unilateral conductive hearing loss, in which the sound is heard more effectively in the affected ear because of the lack of masking by environmental sounds. s, sound heard; ●, tuning fork.

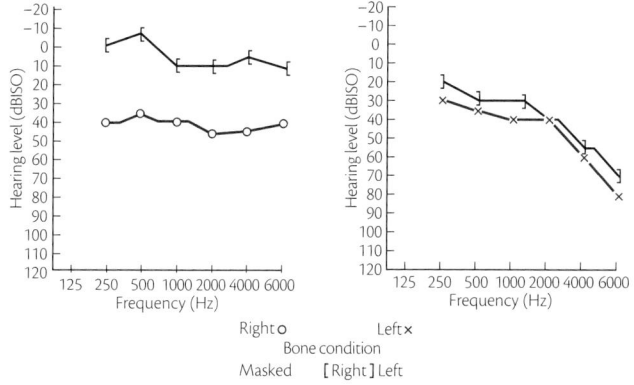

Fig. 24.6.3.4 Pure-tone audiograms showing both air- and bone-conduction thresholds and illustrating a right conductive hearing loss (a) and a left sensorineural hearing loss (b).

The stapedius muscle in the middle ear contracts bilaterally in response to loud sound directed into either ear. Using an impedance bridge, the minimum intensity of sound at a given frequency required to produce contraction of the stapedius muscle, and thus a movement of the tympanic membrane, can be measured (the acoustic reflex threshold). This objective measure enables recruitment and abnormal auditory adaptation to be measured, and allows assessment of middle-ear, cochlear, nerve VIII, and brainstem auditory function.

Otoacoustic emissions (OAEs) are weak signals that can be recorded in the ear canal and are the result of contractile properties of the outer hair cells of the cochlea. Measurement of OAEs thus provides objective information about cochlear function and has become the mainstay of universal neonatal hearing screening. Suppression of the OAEs by delivery of sound to the contralateral ear allows a measure of efferent auditory function and is of particular diagnostic value in neurological diseases affecting auditory function

Speech audiometry is a subjective test requiring the individual to repeat standard lists of words delivered at varying intensities through headphones. The responses are scored and provide an assessment of auditory discrimination. They are of particular value in assessing the efficacy of hearing-aid provision.

Electrophysiological tests provide the major objective means of assessing auditory function and siting pathology in the auditory system. Electrocochleography enables the measurement of the electrical output of the cochlea and cranial nerve VIII in response to an auditory stimulus, whereas brainstem auditory-evoked responses are of particular value in discriminating between cochlear and nerve VIII cochlear nuclei dysfunction. Recordings are obtained by averaging a series of time-locked responses generated by the major processing centres of the auditory system in response to a repetitive sound stimulus (Fig. 24.6.3.5). Analysis of the waveform must be undertaken in conjunction with knowledge of the pure-tone thresholds if appropriate, and valid conclusions about auditory function are to be obtained. Cortical- or late-evoked auditory responses are the most effective method of defining auditory threshold at each frequency in an uncooperative patient, and are essential in legal cases in which a nonorganic loss should always be excluded.

Vestibular investigations and imaging are frequently required to confirm a diagnosis, e.g. congenital inner-ear anomaly, Ménière's disease, and acoustic schwannoma, whereas cardiac, renal, gastrointestinal, endocrine, and metabolic investigations may be highly relevant in specific cases, e.g. Jervell–Lange–Neilsen syndrome, aminglycoside ototoxicity, collagen vascular disease, ulcerative colitis, Pendred's syndrome, and autoimmune disorders.

Management

Appropriate management of both acute and chronic hearing loss requires a detailed history and examination to ensure both appropriate management of related general medical and otological conditions and protection from leisure (discothèques), occupational noise hazards, and ototoxic drugs. Conductive hearing loss due to trauma, chronic middle-ear disease, or otosclerosis may be surgically remediable, whereas recent animal studies have highlighted the possible future role of antioxidants in the amelioration of sensorineural hearing loss caused by chemotherapeutic agents, aminoglycoside antibiotics, and noise. Sudden sensorineural hearing loss is deemed to be a medical emergency, but there are no randomized controlled trials confirming the efficacy of the various therapeutic interventions advocated: steroids, antiviral agents, and haemodilution techniques.

Auditory rehabilitation is a problem-solving exercise centred on each individual patient, and depends on assessing both the auditory disability of the individual and the relevance of this to other important people in the patient's life. Not only auditory impairment, but also communication skills, including lip-reading ability, the use of visual cues, and the level of speech and language, together with psychological and sociological factors, must be considered.

The remedial process may be straightforward in a highly motivated patient in whom there is an uncomplicated hearing loss. However, in the presence of a complicating factor, such as a hearing loss that is difficult to resolve with an aid or arthritis making hearing aid manipulation difficult, the particular problem must be addressed to ensure optimal use of subsequent hearing-aid provision. In patients who have a negative view of hearing aids, environmental aids and instruction in communication skills before the introduction of a hearing aid may facilitate long-term rehabilitation. In general, the provision of a hearing aid is effective only when the patient him- or herself, rather than well-meaning family members, wishes to get help.

Although hearing aids play a pivotal role in audiological rehabilitation, a detailed description of their provision and selection is outside the scope of this short review. For many patients, wearable hearing aids, which bring sound more effectively to the ear, are invaluable, but environmental aids (assisted-listening devices such as amplification systems, alerting warning devices, e.g. flashing lights connected to a doorbell or an alarm clock) may be adequate. In addition, sensory substitution systems, e.g. where visual signals are generated in response to auditory cues such as a telephone or doorbell ringing, or a baby crying, may be helpful to a hearing-impaired person.

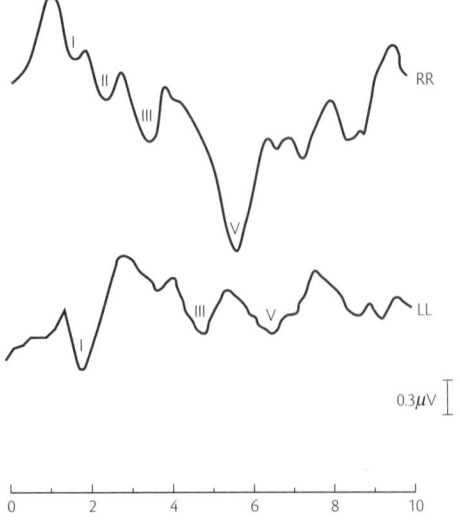

Fig. 24.6.3.5 Illustration of auditory-evoked brainstem responses showing normal waves I, II, III, and V from the right ear (RR) and delayed waves III and V from the left ear (LL), in a case of a left acoustic neurinoma.

The general principles of hearing-aid provision include the fitting of a comfortable earmould, which provides a secure mounting for the aid and a good acoustic connection between the aid and the ear canal. Hearing-aid selection involves matching the amplification required from the aid at specific frequencies with that required by the user. A particular disability experienced in most hearing-impaired people is that of hearing speech in a noisy environment and, although programmable digital processing hearing aids are of some help in this situation, conventional aids provide selective amplification of the frequencies relevant to speech, with minimal amplification at the peak frequency of background noise. Conventional aids may be divided into body-worn and head-worn aids, which can be in spectacles, behind the ear, in the ear, or in the canal in design. The major advantage of body-worn aids is the very high gain and maximum output that can be achieved, whereas the disadvantage is the unsightly nature of the device and the poor microphone placement.

Cochlear implants are electronic devices that convert sound into electrical current for the purpose of directly stimulating residual auditory nerve fibres to produce hearing sensations. The devices are implanted in the cochlea, usually with an electrode array, with an externally worn microphone and processor. Cochlear implants have been used in totally deafened adults and children with good results, and should be considered in all cases of profound acquired hearing loss and in children in whom there is good evidence of auditory nerve preservation in both congenital and acquired hearing impairment. In the bilateral absence of a functional cranial nerve VIII (e.g. neurofibromatosis) brainstem implants have been shown to be of value.

The value of counselling for the hearing-impaired person by a skilled hearing therapist must be emphasized. Such simple hearing tactics as encouraging the individual to ensure that the light is always on the speaker's face, that he or she places himself so that the better ear is towards the speaker, and sitting close to the sound source thereby minimizing background noise, can greatly improve communication ability. For profoundly hearing-impaired individuals, psychological problems associated with isolation and occupational handicaps are significant and it is therefore essential that psychological, medical, and social support are readily available.

Tinnitus

Tinnitus may be defined as a perception of sound that originates from within the head rather than from within the external world. Rarely, the sound may have an externally detectable component and is then termed 'objective tinnitus' as opposed to the more common 'subjective tinnitus'. The experience of tinnitus is universal, but the complaint of tinnitus is rare.

Many conditions are associated with tinnitus, but it is frequently, although not always, associated with hearing impairment. The proposed pathophysiological mechanisms include:

- decoupling of the stereocilia of the hair cells
- misinterpretation of auditory neural activity by higher auditory centres
- self-sustaining oscillation of the basilar membrane
- spontaneous OAEs

- an abnormality of the spontaneous resting activity of primary auditory nerve fibres, either secondary to the hypo- or hyperexcitability of damaged hair cells or as a direct consequence of the derangement of primary neurons themselves
- damage to the myelin sheath between auditory nerve fibres, allowing ephaptic transmission (cross-talk) between adjacent nerve fibres
- derangement of efferent fibres of the vestibulocochlear nerve, producing aberrant auditory behaviour.

A number of studies have demonstrated that tinnitus complaint does not correlate with psychoacoustic features of the tinnitus, but there is a significant correlation between tinnitus complaint and psychological symptoms. Importantly, the onset of tinnitus complaint may be associated with negative life events such as retirement, redundancy, bereavement, and divorce.

The assessment of tinnitus includes a detailed history, clinical examination, and audiometric investigation as outlined for hearing impairment. The most common causes of objective tinnitus include palatal myoclonus, temporomandibular joint abnormalities, vascular abnormalities such as an arteriovenous fistula, and vascular bruits. Rarely, a patulous auditory tube may give rise to tinnitus in which the patient complains of a blowing sound associated with respiration.

Bilateral subjective tinnitus with evidence of a cochlear hearing loss is associated most commonly with presbyacusis, endolymphatic hydrops, vascular labyrinthine lesions, and noise-induced hearing loss. However, it is also common with head injury, whiplash injury, ototoxicity, barotrauma, surgical intervention, and after such simple clinical practices as syringing. Unilateral subjective tinnitus, with or without an associated sensorineural hearing loss, must be fully investigated to exclude an underlying cerebellopontine angle lesion, in particular an acoustic neurinoma.

Management

The primary management of tinnitus is medical, although surgical intervention is required for the correction of arterial stenoses giving rise to bruits and for glomus jugulare tumour and arteriovenous malformations. Destructive surgery, e.g. labyrinthectomy or auditory nerve section, has no place in the management of tinnitus as there is no evidence that destruction of the peripheral cochlear elements brings about improvements in tinnitus complaint.

The medical management of tinnitus can be divided into psychological, pharmacological, and prosthetic intervention. The psychological management includes an explanation of tinnitus, reassurance that the symptom will not progressively deteriorate or indeed remain unchanged, the exclusion of sinister pathology to allay fear, and, if necessary, the appropriate formal psychiatric management of depression/anxiety. In the presence of a hearing impairment, the provision of hearing aids to 'mask' tinnitus with desirable environmental noise may be of value. In the absence of such a loss, tinnitus maskers and noise generators have been advocated to promote 'adaptation', but it must be emphasized that there is no evidence that tinnitus maskers are superior to placebo devices. Pharmacologically, intravenous lidocaine has been shown to result in the disappearance or amelioration of tinnitus, but no oral preparation has been found to be equally effective. Psychiatric drugs may be required for psychological management, although no single drug has been shown to be uniformly effective.

Tinnitus re-training therapy is a management strategy based on a neurophysiological model of tinnitus. The re-training is a combination of prosthetic and psychological intervention, which in essence provides a structured framework for the various well-established mechanisms of tinnitus management outlined above.

In conclusion, positive reassurance, appropriate psychiatric management, and prosthetic support remain the mainstays of the medical management of tinnitus.

Further reading

Gleeson M, Browning G, Luxon LM. The ear, hearing and balance. In: Browning G, Luxon LM (eds) *Scott-Brown's otorhinolaryngology, head and neck surgery*, 7th edition, Vol. 3, Part 19. Hodder Arnold, London.

Martini A, Prosser S (2003). Disorders of the inner ear in adults. In: Luxon LM, *et al.* (eds), *A textbook of audiological medicine*. Taylor & Francis, London.

Disorders of movement

Contents

24.7.1 Subcortical structures: the cerebellum, basal ganglia, and thalamus

Mark J. Edwards and Penelope Talelli

Essentials

Less is known of the function of the cerebellum, thalamus and basal ganglia than of other structures in the brain, but there is an increasing appreciation of their complex role in motor and nonmotor functions of the entire nervous system. These structures exercise functions that far exceed their previously assumed supporting parts as simple 'relay stations' between cortex and spinal cord.

The subcortical structures receive massive different inputs from the cerebral cortex and peripheral sense organs and stretch receptors. Through recurrent feedback loops this information is integrated and shaped to provide output which contributes to scaling, sequencing and timing of movement, as well as learning and automatization of motor and nonmotor behaviours.

Cerebellum

Functional neuroanatomy—the cerebellum can roughly be divided into (1) vestibulocerebellum—integration of vestibular information, (2) spinocerebellum—integration of sensory information from the body, (3) pontocerebellum—integration of information from the cortex regarding planned or on-going movement.

Function—these are proposed to be as follows: (1) a timing device for movement, (2) facilitation of motor learning, and (3) facilitation and correct scaling and harmonization of muscle activity.

Clinical features of cerebellar lesions—these include impairment of movement with dysmetria ('past-pointing'), dysdiadochokinesia, truncal and gait ataxia (in midline vermal lesions), dysarthria, and abnormal eye movements (commonly nystagmus).

Basal ganglia

Functional neuroanatomy—the basal ganglia participate in multiple parallel loops which take information from different (mainly cortical) areas and then feedback (mainly) to those same areas. Input is mainly from the striatum; output comes almost exclusively from either the globus pallidus interna or the substantia nigra pars reticulate, which send inhibitory projections to the thalamus; dopamine is the main neurotransmitter that regulates activity.

Function—four main roles are hypothesized: (1) release of desired movement from inhibitory control, (2) inhibition of undesired movement, (3) facilitation of sequential automatic movements, (4) integration of attentional, reward and emotional information into movement and learning.

Clinical features of basal ganglia lesions—these include rigidity, akinesia, and dystonia.

Thalamus

Functional neuroanatomy—the thalamus receives afferent input from the special senses, basal ganglia, cerebellum, cortex and brainstem reticular formation; efferent output is mainly directed to cortical areas and striatum.

Function—the main thalamic functions are thought to include (1) modulation of sensory information by integration of brainstem (in particular reticular activating complex) and relevant cortical information; and (2) modulation of cortical activity via cortico-thalamocortical loops.

Clinical features of thalamic lesions—these include (1) sensory abnormalities—ranging from loss to deep-seated, severe pain; (2) motor disorders—e.g. hemiplegia; and (3) movement abnormalities—e.g. myoclonus, dystonia—usually in the context of lesions also involving the basal ganglia.

Cerebellum

Gross anatomy

The cerebellum is located in the posterior fossa, bordered above by the tentorium cerebri and below by the foramen magnum. Anteriorly it borders the lower pons and medulla, separated from them by the fourth ventricle. The cerebellum is connected to the pons and medulla by the superior, middle, and inferior cerebellar peduncles. Afferents to the cerebellum enter largely through the inferior and middle peduncles, whereas most of the cerebellar efferents exit through the superior cerebellar peduncle. The cerebellum receives its blood supply from the posterior circulation via (rostrally to caudally) the superior, anteroinferior, and posteroinferior cerebellar arteries.

The anatomical divisions of the cerebellum (as is the case for the other subcortical structures discussed here, particularly the thalamus) are complicated by a number of overlapping classifications. The simplest anatomical division of the cerebellum is into the two cerebellar hemispheres and the midline structure called the vermis. A further division is into the flocculonodular lobe, comprising a nodular structure at the base of the cerebellum and an adjacent area of the hemisphere, the anterior lobe—the part of the cerebellum rostral to the primary fissure—and the posterior lobe—the part of the cerebellum caudal to the primary fissure. This division is in line with the proposed evolutionary development of the cerebellum, something that underlies an alternative classification scheme dividing the cerebellum into archicerebellum (flocculonodular lobe, receiving mainly vestibular input), paleocerebellum (anterior lobe, receiving mainly spinal cord input), and neocerebellum (posterior lobe, receiving mainly cerebral cortical input via the pons). Deep within the cerebellum are the cerebellar nuclei, which both receive input and produce output from the cerebellum. These nuclei, medially to laterally, are called the fastigial, globose, emboliform, and dentate nuclei.

Cytoarchitecture

The cellular architecture of the cerebellum is complex but remarkably uniform (Fig. 24.7.1.1). It comprises five cellular types: Purkinje cells, granule cells, basket cells, Golgi cells, and stellate cells. These are arranged in three distinct cortical layers. These are, from the outside in, the molecular layer (layer 1), the Purkinje cell layer (layer 2), and the granule cell layer (layer 3). Afferent input arrives at the cerebellum in the form of mossy fibres and climbing fibres. These are excitatory neurons arising from the input structures to the cerebellum. Only the inferior olivary complex sends mossy fibres to the cerebellum, with the rest of the input structures sending climbing fibres. These fibres may synapse on cerebellar nuclei, or ascend into the cerebellar cortex directly. The only efferents from the cerebellum are the axons of Purkinje cells.

Mossy fibres synapse with granule cells in layer 3, the axons which then ascend to layer 1, there forming parallel fibres that synapse with the dendrites of Purkinje cells directly, or synapse with basket cells and stellate cells in layer 1; these, in turn, form synaptic connections with dendrites of Purkinje cells. Climbing fibres ascend directly to layer 1 where they synapse with the dendrites of Purkinje cells. Axons of Purkinje cells give off collaterals as they descend both to adjacent Purkinje cells and to Golgi cells that lie in the outer part of layer 3.

Functional anatomy

The above brief description of cerebellar gross and cellular architecture goes some way to showing how the cerebellum is well placed to integrate a large amount of afferent information and to provide output of this integrated information to a large number of cerebral and spinal targets.

A first step to understanding the functional anatomy of the cerebellum is to consider the main input and output pathways. The cerebellum can roughly be divided into three functional areas, which receive particular inputs and produce output to particular areas either directly via the axons of Purkinje cells or via synapses of Purkinje cell axons on to cerebellar nuclei, which then connect to other structures.

Vestibulocerebellum

The main input is afferent fibres from the ipsilateral vestibular ganglion and vestibular nucleus, and the contralateral inferior olivary complex. This input either goes directly to the flocculonodular lobe or reaches there via the fastigial nucleus of the cerebellum. Output is to the vestibular nuclei either directly or via the fastigial nucleus.

Spinocerebellum

The main inputs are ipsilateral cutaneous and proprioceptive afferents from the body and face via dorsal and ventral spinocerebellar, cuneocerebellar, trigeminocerebellar, and spinoreticular tracts. Further input comes from motor and sensory areas of the cerebral cortex and vestibular nuclei via pontine reticulospinal nuclei and

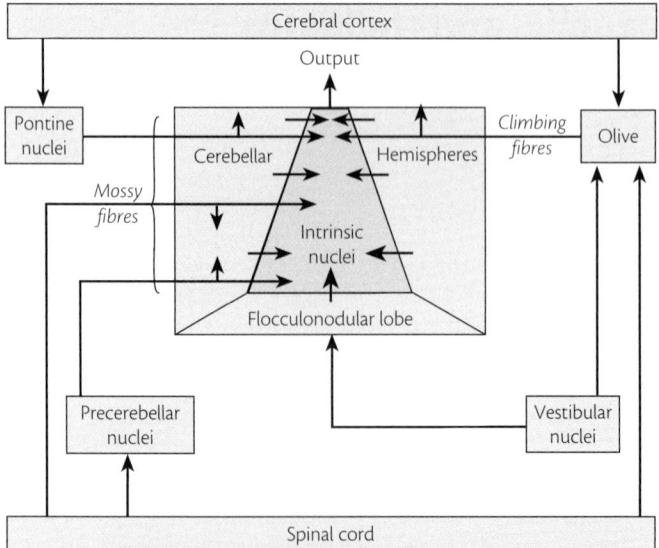

Fig. 24.7.1.1 A simplified diagram showing the principal afferents to cerebellar cortex and to intrinsic cerebellar nuclei. Both mossy (left) and climbing (right) fibre inputs project to both cortex and intrinsic nuclei.

the contralateral red nucleus, and from the contralateral inferior olivary complex. All these inputs either go directly to the anterior lobe of the cerebellum, or reach there via synapses in the globose and emboliform nuclei. Output, either direct or via these same cerebellar nuclei, goes to the pontine reticular nuclei, the contralateral red nucleus, and a major projection to the contralateral posterior division of the ventrolateral nucleus of the thalamus.

Pontocerebellum

This receives input from the contralateral pontine nuclei, which in turn receive massive input from widespread areas of cerebral cortex, in particular the frontal and parietal lobes. Input is also received from the contralateral inferior olivary complex. Input either proceeds directly to the posterior lobes of the cerebellum or reaches there via synapses in the dentate nucleus. Output (either direct or via synapses in the dentate nucleus) goes to the contralateral red nucleus and to the cortex via the contralateral posterior division of the ventrolateral nucleus of the thalamus.

Thus, in simple terms, the cerebellum has three main functional divisions: the vestibulocerebellum, concerned mainly with integrating vestibular information, the spinocerebellum, concerned mainly with integrating sensory information from the body, and the pontocerebellum, concerned mainly with integrating information from the cortex regarding planned or ongoing movement. All areas of the cerebellum also receive input from the contralateral inferior olivary complex. The inputs to the cerebellum are largely excitatory, using glutamate as a neurotransmitter. In contrast, Purkinje cells, the output cells of the cerebellum, are inhibitory, using γ-aminobutyric acid (GABA) as a neurotransmitter.

Recent advances in understanding of cerebellar functional architecture have revealed that the cerebellum appears to be divided into multiple 'modules' with similar cell structure, but receiving and giving out highly topographically organized information

(Fig. 24.7.1.2). These modules are longitudinally arranged strips of the cerebellar cortex about 1–2 mm across, each 5–6 mm in length. This modular organization has been studied in most detail in relation to receptive fields from the forelimb of the cat. This work has demonstrated that particular sensory receptive fields in the forelimb map to particular areas of the inferior olivary complex, which in turn given off projections to particular areas within cerebellar modules, called cerebellar microzones. Each area of the inferior olive may project to a variety of microzones which may be distributed widely in the cerebellar hemispheres. Crucially, however, these distributed microzones all send output to a specific area of the cerebellar output nuclei. This organizational structure (called multizonal microcomplexes) permits topographically organized input to be fed into a variety of discrete areas in the cerebellum. These discrete microzones might respond to and process a particular aspect of movement control, such as timing, direction, or scaling of movement. These various aspects of movement control could then be integrated by the common output of these areas to a particular part of the cerebellar output nuclei. Parallel fibres may in addition allow integration of information between microzones responsible for movements at a number of different muscles, but which are commonly recruited as a group or 'synergy'. This would allow for the coordination of complex multi-joint movements such as reaching and grasping.

Function and dysfunction

The main functions of the cerebellum (which are still the subject of much debate) are proposed as (1) a timing device for movement, (2) a structure that facilitates (motor) learning, and (3) a structure that allows integration of information (including information about planning of a movement and sensory feedback information on the progress of a movement) in order to facilitate correct scaling and harmonization of muscle activity.

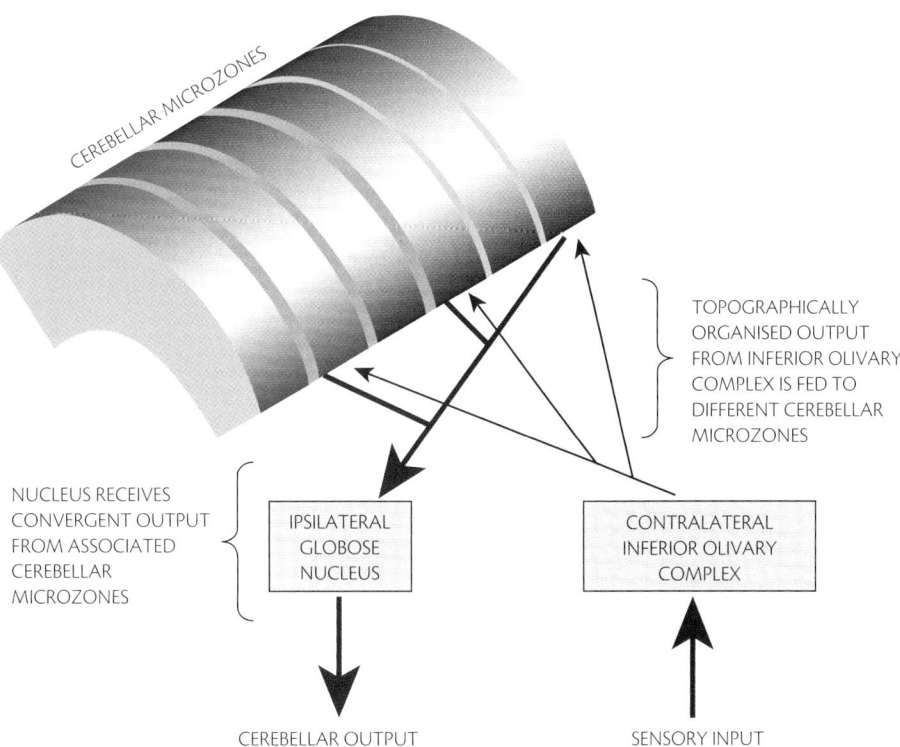

Fig. 24.7.1.2 This figure gives an example of the organisation and connections of cerebellar microzones. In this example, sensory information from the limbs (which is topographically organised) is mapped onto specific topographically arranged areas of the inferior olivary complex. Output from one of these areas is shown, which is fed to a number of different cerebellar microzones. Output from these microzones converges onto a specific area of one of the cerebellar nuclei.

In patients with cerebellar lesions a number of abnormalities can be seen in simple reaching tasks. Normal movements are usually accompanied by precisely timed agonist–antagonist–agonist bursts that allow the limb to arrive exactly at the desired target. In patients with cerebellar lesions, there is first of all a delay in movement initiation, followed by a delay in the antagonist burst so that the patient frequently overshoots the target. This is the basis for dysmetria or 'past-pointing', examined at the bedside during finger–nose or heel–shin testing. This overshoot may be a partial cause of intention tremor (worsening tremor towards the end of movement) as well as an additional effect of cerebellar lesions on the timing of activity in muscle-stretch reflex loops (via cerebellar projections to γ-motoneurons). Clinically, the timing and scaling role of the cerebellum can be assessed by looking for dysdiadochokinesia: a breakdown in force, rate, and rhythm of movement. This is often tested by asking patients to tap gently, regularly, and rapidly on a table or the examiner's hand with their fingers. This breakdown of smooth repetitive movements can even be detected by feel or by sound ('listening to the cerebellum').

Midline vermal lesions usually cause truncal and gait ataxia, often in the absence of limb ataxia. The gait is wide based and particularly precarious on turning or on heel–toe walking. Unilateral cerebellar hemispherical lesions cause deviation or falling to the ipsilateral side. Unlike a sensory ataxia, cerebellar ataxia is not made worse by shutting the eyes.

Cerebellar dysarthria may often simply manifest as slurred speech, as if intoxicated. However, in addition some patients may have either scanning or explosive speech, due to an inability to modulate its rate, rhythm, and force appropriately. Dysarthria is usually present with lesions of the vermis, whole cerebellum, or its connections, but may be absent if one lateral hemisphere alone is involved. Eye movements are frequently abnormal in disease of the cerebellum or its connections. This may relate in part to the extensive connections from vestibular areas to the cerebellum. The following eye-movement abnormalities may be seen: gaze-evoked, rebound, downbeat, or positional nystagmus, dysmetric voluntary saccades and jerky pursuit, square-wave jerks (macrosaccadic oscillations), impaired vestibulo-ocular reflex suppression, and skew deviation.

Basal ganglia

Gross anatomy

There is no complete consensus on what structures make up the basal ganglia, but most would include the caudate nucleus, putamen, globus pallidus, subthalamic nucleus, and substantia nigra (Fig. 24.7.1.3). The globus pallidus is subdivided into the globus pallidus externa and interna (GPe/GPi), and the substantia nigra is subdivided into the pars reticulata and pars compacta (SNr/SNc). As with the cerebellum and thalamus, the basal ganglia have additional nomenclature systems that are still in use. The most important term is the word 'striatum' (or sometimes neostriatum) which is used to describe the caudate nucleus and the putamen together. The globus pallidus may be called the pallidum or paleostriatum, and the globus pallidus and putamen together may be called the lentiform nucleus. The phrase 'corpus striatum' is used to refer to the caudate, putamen, and globus pallidus together.

The basal ganglia occupy a position near the base of the cerebral hemispheres. The putamen lies lateral to the thalamus, separated from it (and from most of the caudate nucleus, except anteriorly) by the internal capsule. The caudate nucleus, with its head lying anterodorsomedial to the putamen, arcs back, following, and progressively tapering with, the lateral ventricles, its tail swinging forward until its anteriorly pointing tip terminates in the amygdaloid nucleus. The pallidum lies medial to the putamen but still lateral to the internal capsule. The substantia nigra lies in the midbrain, transversely above the cerebral peduncles. Its pars reticulata, the termination of the striatonigral pathway, is below the internal segment of the globus pallidus, and its pars compacta contains the dopaminergic neurons that form the nigrostriatal pathway. Below the thalamus, medial to the internal capsule and rostral to the midbrain, is the subthalamic nucleus. Most of the caudate, putamen, and globus pallidus derive their arterial supply from the anterior circulation via the lateral lenticulostriate arteries and branches of the anterior choroidal and middle cerebral arteries. The thalamus, subthalamic region, and substantia nigra are supplied by the posterior circulation.

Functional anatomy

The basal ganglia receive a huge variety of input from the cerebral cortex, limbic system, and cerebellum. Although the role of the basal ganglia in motor control has been heavily emphasized, it is clear that the basal ganglia have a key role in many other aspects of behaviour, reflected in the diversity of input to and output from many 'nonmotor' areas of the brain.

A key concept of basal ganglia functional anatomy is their participation in several parallel loops, which take information from different (mainly cortical) areas, and then feed back, mainly to those same areas. Although the basal ganglia would seem well set

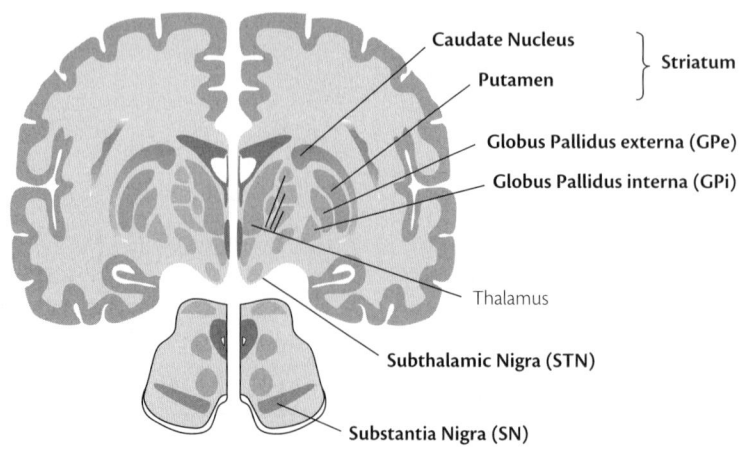

Fig. 24.7.1.3 Components of the basal ganglia seen in a coronal section of the brain.
(From Edwards *et al*. Oxford Specialist Handbook of Parkinson's Disease and Other Movement Disorders, Oxford University Press, 2008.)

Caudate Nucleus

Putamen

} Striatum

Globus Pallidus externa (GPe)

Globus Pallidus interna (GPi)

Thalamus

Subthalamic Nigra (STN)

Substantia Nigra (SN)

up to integrate information from these various loops, in fact they seem not to do so, and information is kept remarkably separate.

Five main loops are recognized: motor, oculomotor, dorsolateral prefrontal, orbitofrontal, and anterior cingulate. The motor loop has received by far the most attention, given its presumed role in movement disorders such as Parkinson's disease. The main interest has focused on how activity in this loop is modulated by the basal ganglia, and in particular how dopamine plays a role in this.

Basic basal ganglia pathways

An important first step to aid understanding of the functional organization of the basal ganglia is to consider that input to the basal ganglia, whatever its source, arrives almost exclusively at the putamen or caudate (i.e. the striatum). Therefore, the striatum is the main input structure of the basal ganglia. Output from the basal ganglia comes almost exclusively from either the GPi or the SNr. Therefore the GPi/SNr forms the main output from the basal ganglia. Crucially, these output structures send inhibitory projections to the thalamus (Fig. 24.7.1.4).

Ninety-eight per cent of the neurons in the striatum are medium spiny neurons, which mainly receive excitatory input from glutamatergic neurons of the cerebral cortex. The rest of the striatal neuronal population is made up of large nonspiny cholinergic interneurons and GABA-ergic interneurons. The medium spiny neurons are inhibitory and use GABA as their neurotransmitter. They form two main groups (bundled together in structures called 'Wilson's pencils') which have different routes to get to the output structures (GPi/SNr). One group projects directly to the GPi/SNr—the direct pathway—there colocalizing substance P and dynorphin as neurotransmitters. Activity in this pathway therefore inhibits basal ganglia output. The other group has an indirect route to the GPi/SNr, projecting first to the GPe, there colocalizing enkephalin and neurotensin as neurotransmitters. The pathway continues via an inhibitory projection from GPe to subthalamic nucleus (STN), and finally via an excitatory glutamatergic projection from STN to GPi/SNr. The net effect of activation of this indirect pathway (combining two inhibitory and one excitatory synapse) is to excite

GPi/SNr. Activity in the indirect pathway therefore facilitates basal ganglia output (see Fig. 24.7.1.4).

Output from the basal ganglia is via GABA-ergic projections from GPi and SNr to the thalamus. The projections from GPi travel in two fibre bundles through the internal capsule; the one from the outer part of GPi is called the ansa lenticularis, and the other from the inner part of GPi is called the lenticular fasciculus. After traversing the internal capsule they meet with neurons from the SNr and join to form the thalamic fasciculus, which terminates in various nuclei of the thalamus (for motor fibres this is mainly the ventrolateral medial nucleus). Additional output from GPi and SNr goes to the pedunculopontine nucleus and the superior colliculus. A crucial point is that the basal ganglia inhibits the structures to which it projects—this is vital to understand the models of basal ganglia function described below.

The most important neurotransmitter that regulates the activity of the basal ganglia is dopamine. Dopamine has different effects on the direct and indirect pathways. Dopaminergic neurons from the SNc ascend and synapse on striatal neurons (this is called the nigrostriatal pathway). Striatal neurons that will form the direct pathway express mainly dopamine D_1-receptors at the nigrostriatal synapses: these are stimulated by dopamine. In contrast, striatal neurons that will form the first projection of the indirect pathway express mainly dopamine D_2-receptors, which are inhibited by dopamine. Therefore the net effect of dopamine on the striatum is to increase direct pathway activity, decrease indirect pathway activity, and therefore reduce the inhibitory output of GPi/SNr (Fig. 24.7.1.5).

How is dopamine release controlled in the basal ganglia? The answer may lie in recent discoveries regarding the exact make-up of the striatum. It appears that, as well as the direct and indirect pathways, the striatum also sends out projections direct to the SNc which stimulate activity in dopaminergic neurons projecting to the striatal neurons that form the direct and indirect pathways. So, the striatum is not formed by a homogeneous population of medium spiny neurons, but in fact is divided into two distinct subpopulations. One population forms 'striosomes', which are more densely packed groups of medium spiny neurons that have less cholinergic input and are rich in opiate receptors. These are the neurons that send projections to the SNc (the striatonigral projection). The other

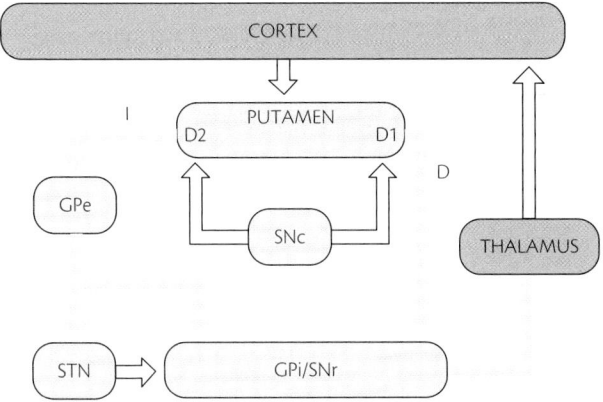

Fig. 24.7.1.4 The Direct and Indirect Pathways. Black arrows indicate inhibitory connections, white arrows indicate excitatory connections. D1=dopamine receptor type 1, D2 = dopamine receptor type 2, STN = subthalamic nucleus, GPi = globus pallidus interna, GPe = globus pallidus externa, SNc = substantia nigra pars compacta, SNr = substantia nigra pars reticulate, I = indirect pathway, D = direct pathway.
(From Edwards *et al.* Oxford Specialist Handbook of Parkinson's Disease and Other Movement Disorders, Oxford University Press, 2008.)

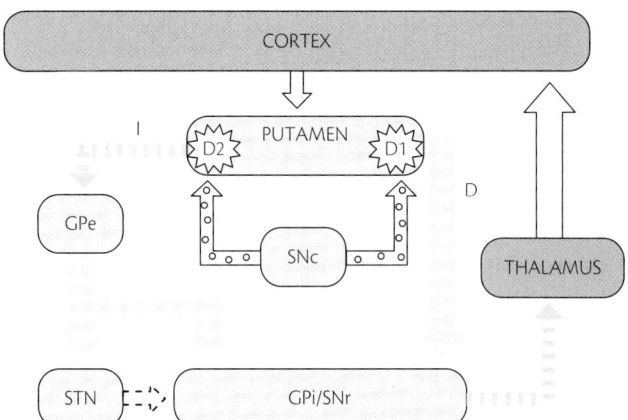

Fig. 24.7.1.5 The effect of dopamine and the direct and indirect pathways. Dopamine released from the substantia nigra pars compacta stimulates the direct pathway via its action on DI receptors and inhibits the indirect pathway via its action on D2 receptors. Abbreviations are the same as for Fig. 24.7.1.4.
(From Edwards *et al.* Oxford Specialist Handbook of Parkinson's Disease and Other Movement Disorders, Oxford University Press, 2008.)

population forms the 'matrix', which is made up of less densely packed medium spiny neurons with no output to SNc. These are the neurons that form the direct and indirect pathways. The putamen is almost all matrix, whereas the caudate has many striosomes. The striosomes receive input mainly from limbic structures, whereas the matrix receives input from a variety of cortical areas, but not limbic structures. The connections of these different striatal neurons has led to the idea of two striatal systems: the ventral striatum (striosome), which, via its connections with the limbic system, feeds emotional, reward and attentional information into the basal ganglia, and via its ability to modulate dopaminergic output from the SNr it can influence activity in the dorsal striatum (matrix).

Basic pathways and the rate model of basal ganglia function

The discussion above about the connections of the various nuclei of the basal ganglia sets the scene for the most influential model of basal ganglia function proposed by DeLong and colleagues in 1990 (against the background of work by many others). The key to understanding this model is to appreciate that:

- output from the GPi and SNr is inhibitory to the thalamus (and therefore to the cortex), and therefore, from a motor circuit point of view, an increase in rate of GPI/SNr firing is hypothesized to inhibit movement
- as the direct and indirect pathways have opposite effects on basal ganglia output, the rate model hypothesizes that they will have opposite effects on movement
- dopamine has opposing effects on the direct and indirect pathways, tending to increase direct pathway activity via D_1-receptors and decrease indirect pathway activity via D_2-receptors. The net result of dopaminergic stimulation is, therefore, to decrease GPi/SNr rate of firing, promoting movement.

This model, sometimes described as the 'rate model', is successful in explaining a number of aspects of motor dysfunction related to the basal ganglia, e.g. the pathology of Parkinson's disease leads to a dopamine-depleted state which would be predicted to decrease direct pathway activity and increase indirect pathway activity. This would tend to cause an increase in GPi/SNr (inhibitory) output to the thalamus, therefore inhibiting movement (Fig. 24.7.1.6). In contrast, hemiballism (flinging movements of the arm and leg) is known to occur frequently with damage to, or close to, the subthalamic nucleus. The rate model would predict the effect of a subthalamic nucleus lesion to be a drop in indirect pathway activity, leading to a reduction in GPi/SNr activity and a consequent increase in thalamic activity, promoting movement (Fig. 24.7.1.7). There is experimental support for this model, e.g. the finding from functional imaging studies that in Parkinson's disease there is hypermetabolism of the GPi which reverses with the administration of levodopa.

However, problems occur when considering other clinical aspects of movement disorders, e.g. a lesion of the GPi in experimental animals tends not to cause excessive movement, as the model would predict. In fact, a lesion of the GPi can be a very successful treatment for both levodopa-induced dyskinesia in Parkinson's disease and primary dystonia. In addition, the movement disorders characterized by excessive movement (the hyperkinetic movement disorders—dystonia, tremor, tics, myoclonus, chorea) are variable in their clinical features, something that is difficult to explain via a model based solely on rate of GPi/SNr firing.

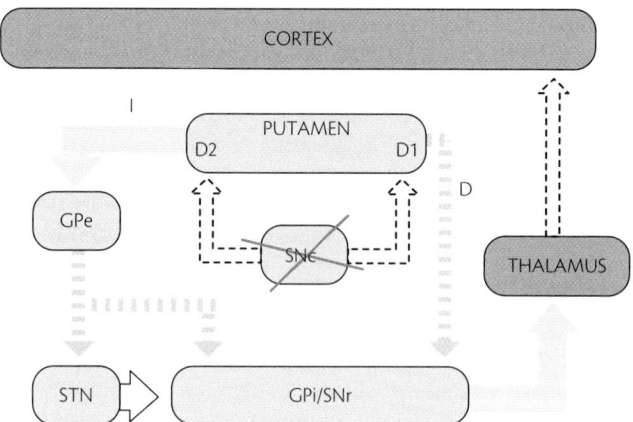

Fig. 24.7.1.6 How a lesion in the substantia nigra pars compacta can cause parkinsonism. Abbreviations are as in Fig. 24.7.1.4.
(From Edwards *et al.* Oxford Specialist Handbook of Parkinson's Disease and Other Movement Disorders, Oxford University Press, 2008.)

Beyond basic basal ganglia connections: the hyperdirect pathway and basal ganglia oscillations

The connections between the basal ganglia are considerably more complex than the rate model permits, e.g. there is a 'hyperdirect' pathway—a glutamatergic pathway that directly links the supplementary motor area (SMA) and the subthalamic nucleus. In addition, there are numerous basal ganglia–basal ganglia pathways, e.g. a direct excitatory connection from the subthalamic nucleus to GPe, and a direct inhibitory connection from GPe to GPi and SNr. These additional connections suggest the presence of two networks within the basal ganglia: an 'extrastriatal network' where the subthalamic nucleus is the main player, with links to GPe, GPi, and SNr, and a 'striatal network' that connects directly to GPi/SNr.

The development of animal models of parkinsonism, and more recent developments in human deep brain stimulation surgery for Parkinson's disease and dystonia, have permitted direct recording from the basal ganglia. These recordings have demonstrated that alterations in pattern and synchrony of basal ganglia firing may be more important than changes in rate alone. So, for

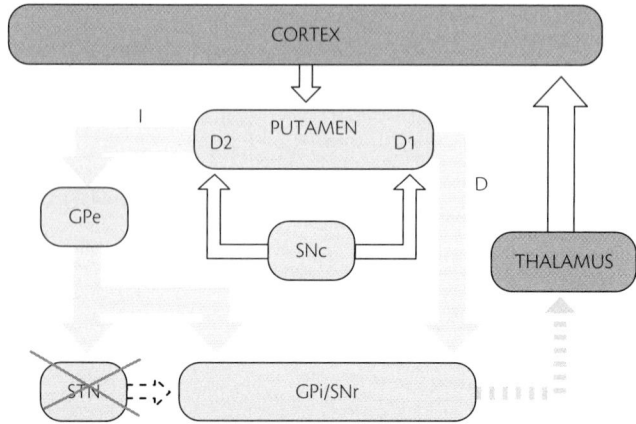

Fig. 24.7.1.7 How a lesion in the subthalamic nucleus can cause hemiballismus. Abbreviations are as in Fig. 24.7.1.4.
(From Edwards *et al.* Oxford Specialist Handbook of Parkinson's Disease and Other Movement Disorders, Oxford University Press, 2008.)

example, in patients with Parkinson's disease, direct recordings from the basal ganglia show an increase in bursting activity in the subthalamic nucleus that oscillates at a low frequency (in the beta band: 10–20 Hz) and is synchronized across the basal ganglia and motor cortex. Successful treatment with levodopa is associated with a shift to higher-frequency oscillations (into the gamma band >60 Hz).

One way to try to unify these disparate aspects of basal ganglia physiology into a functional whole is to first consider the basal ganglia as having a strong inhibitory bias. Therefore, although STN neurons fire quite consistently in response to cortical activity, fed to them via the hyperdirect pathway, this is not translated on the whole into changes in firing from basal ganglia output nuclei (GPi/SNr), due to strong inhibitory control from the striatum, and therefore the tonic inhibitory discharge of the basal ganglia output continues. However, in the presence of dopamine, this situation is reversed, and the net effect of dopamine on the direct and indirect pathways causes a shift in basal ganglia output firing, allowing the information carried in the subthalamic nucleus firing patterns to be fed through to the thalamus. This occurs in a strictly segregated way, and the topography of input is preserved.

In disease, there is a shift towards more synchronous firing within the basal ganglia with, in the case of Parkinson's disease, a shift towards low-frequency oscillations even when movement is attempted, reflecting a loss of the normal modulation of firing patterns during movement. In dystonia, a hyperkinetic disorder, the GPi shows lower firing rates compared with Parkinson's disease (as would be predicted by the rate model), but in addition there are more frequent and irregular bursts seen with long pauses of absent activity. This might link to the clinical picture of dystonia with excessive muscle activation that stops and starts with shifting coactivation of agonists and antagonists, leading to abnormal posture, writing movements, and often a jerky tremor. Synchronization of firing across the basal ganglia undermines its ability to focus and concentrate activation in a topographically discrete manner.

Function and dysfunction

The above discussion is complex, but reflects the evolving understanding of the functional role of the basal ganglia. The basal ganglia are hypothesised to have four main roles, all of which have most often been related to the motor function of the basal ganglia:

1 To release a desired movement from inhibitory control, e.g. before a desired eye movement the tonic discharge of the basal ganglia output nuclei drops, and this allows the movement to occur.

2 To inhibit undesired movement: in the motor system this would be reflected in the highly topographically organized nature of basal ganglia input and output. Therefore, as well as releasing the desired movement, the basal ganglia appear to play a key role in inhibiting other movements. This focusing role is also known as centre-surround inhibition, where the desired movement (centre) is surrounded by an area of undesired movement that is actively inhibited.

3 To facilitate sequential automatic movements: in motor learning experiments, basal ganglia activity tends to increase as learning occurs. This is thought to reflect a role for the basal ganglia in coding sequences of movements that become automated. This may explain the particular difficulty showed by patients with

Parkinson's disease in performing multi-stage automatic movements such as turning over in bed.

4 To integrate attentional, reward and emotional information into movement and learning: via the connections of the limbic system with the ventral striatum, the basal ganglia form an important location for the integration of motivational and emotional information with motor behaviour. This is particularly the case for reward-based learning. It has been suggested that the basal ganglia can be seen as integrating two aspects of reward-based learning: the 'critic'—the ventral striatum system that holds information on how motivated the organism is towards a particular goal—and the 'actor'—the dorsal striatum that holds information on the motor behaviour needed to achieve that goal.

These various functions are certainly biased towards the motor system, but it is clear, from both the discussion of basal ganglia connections above, and the symptoms displayed by patients with disorders of the basal ganglia, that nonmotor aspects of behaviour are strongly linked to the function of the basal ganglia. It may be particularly the case for motivation and reward-based learning, e.g. lesions of the caudate nucleus have been associated with the psychiatric syndrome of abulia—a syndrome of apathy and lack of motivation that is thought to reflect failure of normal reward-based motivational mechanisms.

The movement disorders are hypothesized to reflect dysfunction within the basal ganglia, although, surprisingly, it is difficult to mimic some of these disorders simply by lesions to the basal ganglia alone. Thus tics and myoclonus rarely occur in humans as a consequence solely of basal ganglia lesions. Likewise, chorea rarely occurs from lesions to the caudate nucleus alone, as one might expect given the degeneration of this nucleus in Huntington's disease. Parkinsonism, combining akinesia (slowness—bradykinesia) and progressive fatiguing of repetitive movement, rigidity (stiffness of muscles in flexion and extension), rest tremor of 5–6 Hz, and postural instability, can be seen in response to discrete lesions of the SNc. In terms of the various functions of the basal ganglia outlined above, both rigidity and akinesia could be seen as reflecting an inability to release the desired movement (akinesia) and a failure to inhibit undesired movement (rigidity). In Parkinson's disease, clear deficits in reward-related learning and performance of integrated automatic movements are seen, together with emotional and motivational problems. Dystonia can also be produced by discrete basal ganglia lesions (usually to the putamen) and, in terms of the basal ganglia functions outlined above, dystonia could reflect an inability to inhibit unwanted movement, leading to the typical clinical picture of overflow of activity into adjacent muscles and co-contraction of agonists and antagonists. The huge variety of clinical presentation of movement disorders no doubt reflects the interaction of basal ganglia dysfunction with dysfunction caused by neurological disease elsewhere in subcortical and cortical areas.

Thalamus

Gross anatomy

The two thalami sit at the head of the brainstem, their medial borders largely separated by the third ventricle, but often partially fused as the massa intermedia. They constitute the largest nuclear mass in the diencephalon (the others being the hypothalamus and subthalamus). On the lateral surface of the thalamus is the external medullary lamina, containing thalamocortical and corticothalamic fibres either entering or exiting the internal capsule. The external medullary lamina and the internal capsule are separated by a thalamic nucleus called the reticular nucleus. The internal structure of the thalamus, already complex, is further confused by the existence of different nomenclatures (the one used here being that of Wessler). Inside the thalamus the internal medullary lamina (consisting of fibres leaving or entering the various thalamic nuclei) roughly divides the thalamus into three groups of nuclei—lateral, medial, and anterior—with each subdivided into ventral and dorsal areas. There are further nuclei that are not defined by this ventral/dorsal system such as those that lie within the internal medullary lamina (the intralaminar nuclei), and others such as the lateral and medial geniculate and the pulvinar. The blood supply to the thalamus derives from the posterior circulation via the posterior cerebral arteries and perforators from the terminal part of the basilar artery.

Cytoarchitecture

Before discussing the functional anatomy of the thalamus, we briefly summarize its cellular structure. The main output cells of the thalamus are called relay cells. These form excitatory glutamatergic projections to the cortex. These cells receive multiple inputs including GABA-ergic inputs from interneurons within the thalamus, cholinergic input from the brainstem reticular formation, as well as glutamatergic input from particular cortical areas (usually those areas to which the relay cells then project back, forming corticothalamocortical loops). Relay cells have two modes of firing—a burst mode and a tonic mode—which may have different functions (see below). Relay cells are mainly contained in the dorsal thalamic nuclei (the relay nuclei), whereas nuclei in the ventral thalamus (particularly the intralaminar nuclei) project mainly to the basal ganglia via glutamatergic projections.

Functional anatomy

The thalamus is in an ideal position to modulate information flow to and from the cortex. Although previously this role had been thought of as a mainly passive relay station, it is clear that the thalamus has a much greater role in moulding the information that passes through it than previously realized.

Thalamic afferents arrive from five main sources.

1 Afferents from special senses (except olfaction): touch (from the body—ventral posterolateral nucleus; face—ventral posteromedial nucleus), taste (ventral posteromedial nucleus), vision (lateral geniculate nucleus), and hearing (medial geniculate nucleus)

2 Afferents from the output nuclei of the basal ganglia: GPi (centromedian nucleus, ventral anterior nucleus, ventral lateral nucleus oralis and medialis) and SNr (mediodorsal nucleus and ventral anterior nucleus magnocellularis)

3 Afferents from the cerebellum: ventral lateral nucleus caudalis, to the ventral posterolateral nucleus oralis

4 Cortical afferents from many cortical areas: mainly synapse on dorsal thalamic nuclei

5 Afferents from the brainstem reticular formation.

Efferents from the thalamus from three main groups:

1 Efferents from thalamic nuclei to representative areas of the cortex determined by the input to the nucleus (e.g. afferents

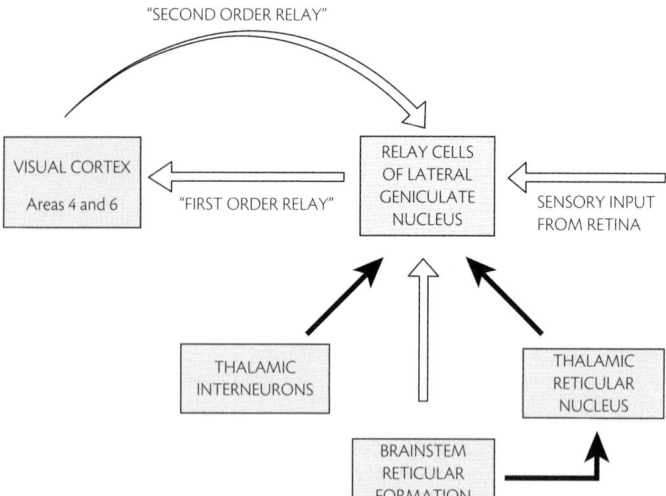

Fig. 24.7.1.8 Main connections of the Lateral Geniculate Nucleus as an example of primary and secondary relays in the thalamus. Black arrows indicate inhibitory connections, white arrows indicate excitatory connections.

from the retina project to the lateral geniculate nucleus, which then projects to the visual cortex)

2 Efferents to cortical areas that project directly to the thalamus (corticothalamocortical loops)

3 Efferents to the striatum (mainly from the intralaminar nuclei).

The functional anatomy of thalamic circuits has been most closely studied for the visual system, and this can serve as a model for other thalamic circuits (Fig. 24.7.1.8). In the visual system, the main input to be relayed to the appropriate area of cortex comes from the retina, but, interestingly, this forms only about 5% of the input to the relevant thalamic nucleus: the lateral geniculate body. The rest of the input comes from a variety of sources including inhibitory input from thalamic interneurons and the thalamic reticular nucleus, excitatory input from the brainstem reticular formation, and layer 6 of the visual cortex. Output from the lateral geniculate is then primarily to layers 4 and 6 of the visual cortex. This system therefore has a primary function: transfer of visual information from the retina to the visual cortex (sometimes called the driver function or first-order relay), but this is subject to a huge amount of modulation from other areas, both cortical and brainstem.

A secondary system, often called the higher-order relay, is distinguished from this first-order system. This system takes cortical information down to the thalamus (typically the dorsal nuclei), and then back again to the same area (corticothalamocortical loops). As for the first-order system this circuit is subject to multiple modulatory inputs at the thalamic level. Of course, the cortical areas projecting as higher-order relays may have themselves been influenced by first-order relays, leading to a complex series of loops integrating and modulating information flow to and from the cortex.

One of the most important modulating forces at work in the thalamus arises from the brainstem reticular activating complex. This is demonstrated by the massive decease in thalamic activity seen during sleep, and the potential of certain thalamic lesions to cause coma. The influence of the reticular activating complex may occur via its ability to cause the 'burst' pattern of firing in thalamic relay cells. It is hypothesized that this is a 'wake-up' signal to the cortex, causing diversion of attention to the particular input in question, following which relay cells switch to their normal regular tonic discharge.

Function and dysfunction

The above discussion clearly demonstrates the role of the thalamus as more than a neuronal rest stop on the way to and from the cortex. The main functions of the thalamus are thought to include:

◆ modulation of sensory information by integration of brainstem (in particular the reticular activating complex) and relevant cortical information

◆ modulation of cortical activity via corticothalamocortical loops.

A diverse range of clinical consequences of thalamic lesions has been described, as one would expect from a region where so many different information flows coalesce, e.g. sensory abnormalities are reported with thalamic lesions, from pure hemisensory loss to deep-seated, severe pain. Mild hemiplegia may be seen with thalamic lesions, sometimes in combination with hemisensory loss, dysaesthesia, hemiataxia, astereognosis, and hemichorea as in the thalamic syndrome of Déjèrine and Roussy. Other lesions, often spreading outside the thalamus to involve the basal ganglia, have been associated with myoclonus, dystonia, or a slow 3–4 Hz tremor of the limbs on one side of the body. Lesions of the ventral lateral nucleus caudalis (also known as the ventral intermediate nucleus) have been used as a treatment for parkinsonian and essential tremor.

Conclusions

These three subcortical structures, the cerebellum, basal ganglia, and thalamus, provide the bridge over which information passes to and from the periphery and the cerebral cortex. Through their intricate structure and interconnections they play a major role in modulating and integrating this information. The recent discovery of a hitherto unknown direct connection between the cerebellum and the basal ganglia again underlines the importance of considering these structures as part of a coordinated system rather than in isolation. The question 'What does the cerebellum/basal ganglia/thalamus do?' therefore becomes slightly nonsensical, because in fact they do nothing in isolation, and function only as part of a system. This system can certainly be affected in particular ways by dysfunction of one of its parts, but the results of discrete lesions are often hard to predict and may have wide-ranging consequences for motor and nonmotor behaviour.

Further reading

Apps R, Garwicz M (2005). Anatomical and physiological foundations of cerebellar information processing. *Nat Rev Neurosci*, **6**, 297–311. [Information about cerebellar microzones.]

Brown P (2003). Oscillatory nature of human basal ganglia activity: relationship to the pathophysiology of Parkinson's disease. *Mov Disorders*, **18**, 357–63. [Basal ganglia oscillations and disease.]

Hammond C, Bergman H, Brown P (2007). Pathological synchronization in Parkinson's disease: networks, models and treatments. *Trends Neurosci*, **30**, 357–64.

Hoshi E, *et al.* (2005). The cerebellum communicates with the basal ganglia. *Nature Neurosci*, 8: 1491–3. [Yet more complexity: this paper shows that there is a direct connection between cerebellum and basal ganglia.]

Lehericy S, *et al.* (2001). Clinical characteristics and topography of lesions in movement disorders due to thalamic lesions. *Neurology*, **57**, 1055–66.

Lera G, *et al.* (2000). A combined pattern of movement disorders resulting from posterolateral thalamic lesions of a vascular nature: a syndrome with clinico-radiologic correlation. *Mov Disorders*, **15**, 120–6.

Middleton FA, Strick PL (1994). Anatomical evidence for cerebellar and basal ganglia involvement in higher cognitive function. *Science*, **266**, 458–61. [Evidence for the importance of subcortical structures in 'higher' functions.]

Middleton FA, Strick PL (2000). Basal ganglia and cerebellar loops: motor and cognitive circuits. *Brain Res Brain Res Rev*, **31**, 236–50. [Review of cerebellar and basal ganglia anatomy and physiology.]

Nambu A (2004). A new dynamic model of the cortico-basal ganglia loop. *Prog Brain Res*, **143**, 461–6. [Model of basal ganglia function focusing on the hyperdirect pathway.]

Obeso JA, Rodriguez MC, DeLong MR (1997). Basal ganglia pathophysiology. A critical review. *Adv Neurol*, **74**, 3–18. [Difficulties with the rate model of basal ganglia function explored.]

Obeso JA, *et al.* (2000). Pathophysiologic basis of surgery for Parkinson's disease. *Neurology*, **55**, (12 Suppl 6), S7–12.

Rothwell JC (1994). *Control of human voluntary movement*, 2nd edition. Croom Helm, London. [An excellent short textbook on the physiology of human motor disorders.]

24.7.2 Parkinsonism and other extrapyramidal diseases

K. Ray Chaudhuri and Vinod K. Metta

Essentials

Parkinson's disease

Parkinson's disease affects about 0.2% of the population, including 2% of those over 80 years of age. The main pathological feature is degeneration of neuromelanin-containing neurons in the pars compacta of the substantia nigra, which leads directly and indirectly to excessive inhibition of the thalamus and consequent bradikinesia.

Clinical features—these include (1) bradykinesia—the most disabling and progressive motor symptom; (2) resting tremor (4–7 Hz)—often the presenting symptom/sign, and often unilateral; (3) rigidity—cogwheel or lead pipe; (4) postural imbalance; fixed and stooped posture; (5) gait difficulty—shuffling and small steps, with or without festination; (6) other features—hypomimia ('masked' face), freezing episodes (sudden failure of movement), seborrhoea of the scalp, mental/cognitive disturbance; (7) Hyposmia (impaired olfaction).

Investigation and treatment—there are no specific tests for Parkinson's disease and diagnosis remains clinical. However SPECT imaging with DAT Scan is a valuable adjunct to clinical suspicion of diagnosis. First-line drug treatment is with levodopa (in combination with a decarboxylase inhibitor), dopamine agonists or monoamine oxidase-B inhibitors.

Other Parkinsonian and extrapyramidal diseases

Drug-induced Parkinsonism—dopamine-blocking agents (neuroleptics) such as prochlorperazine or chlorpromazine are the most common offending agents. Vestibular sedatives (used for motion sickness) are also implicated.

Progressive supranuclear palsy—typically presents with gait disturbance and falls (backwards predominantly). Examination reveals supranuclear gaze palsy, particularly of down-gaze, with extension and rigidity of neck, a staring look due to lid retraction, and bradykinesia/akinesia.

Multiple-system atrophy—comprises a variable combination of Parkinsonism with autonomic (postural hypotension), pyramidal or cerebellar symptoms and signs. Any response to levodopa is commonly incomplete and short-lived.

Dementia with Lewy bodies—manifestations include fluctuations in cognition and attention, recurrent and persistent visual hallucinations, and Parkinsonian motor signs.

Corticobasal ganglionic degeneration—characterized by progressive gait disturbances, cortical sensory loss and stimulus-sensitive myoclonus which results in a jerky, useless hand.

Dopa-responsive dystonia—characteristically shows marked diurnal variation; may start in childhood with an odd and unusual gait; diagnosed by finding mutation in the GTP-cyclohydrolase gene; excellent and sustained response to low-dose levodopa.

Other conditions—these include Wilson's disease, neuroacanthocytosis, vascular pseudo Parkinsonism, and neuro ferritinopathy.

Other movement disorders

Dystonia—a syndrome of sustained muscle contractions, which may be focal, multifocal or generalized genetic or idiopathic. Particular causes include (1) generalized idiopathic torsion dystonia; (2) tardive dyskinesia—induced by long-term exposure to dopamine-blocking drugs; involuntary movements usually begin with the face and mouth. See Chapter 24.7.3 for further discussion.

Chorea and related disorders—chorea is an irregular, rapid, uncontrolled, involuntary, excessive movement that seems to move randomly from one part of the body to another; athetosis is a slower writhing and twisting movement. Causes include Huntington's disease and Sydenham's chorea (associated with rheumatic fever). See Chapter 24.7.3 for further discussion.

Tics—these are sudden, repetitive, stereotyped, nonrhythmic, involuntary movement (motor tic) or sound (phonic tic); when treatment is required, they generally respond to drugs that decrease dopaminergic transmission.

Introduction

The human basal ganglia is a complex functional organization, with important interconnections with the nigrostriatal pathway, which dominates the dopaminergic innervation of the striatum (caudate nucleus and the putamen). Additionally, the globus pallidus, thalamic nuclei, the subthalamic nucleus and the pedunculopontine nucleus all play important regulatory and excitatory/inhibitory roles. Neuronal loops also interconnect the basal ganglia

with the cerebellum as well as the cortex, and function is mediated by dopamine as well as a complex array of neuropeptides such as serotonin, acetylcholine, catecholamines, adenosine and gamma aminobutyric acid. See Chapter 24.7.1 for further discussion.

The principal clinical syndromes are Parkinson's disease; other syndromes with Parkinsonian features (including drug-induced Parkinsonism); progressive supranuclear palsy; multisystem atrophy; Dementia with Lewy bodies; neuroacanthosis; torsion dystonia, and chorea. Apart from the use of dopaminergic agents, several drugs have beneficial effects in the management of Parkinsonism and other extrapyramidal diseases.

Parkinson's disease was first described by the celebrated London physician James Parkinson in 1817, and later named after him by Charcot. Parkinson's disease is one of the most important disabling illnesses of later life. It is estimated to affect 1% of those aged 70 years, but is also seen in younger people, with 10% of cases occurring before the age of 50.

Epidemiology, incidence, and prevalence

The exact estimation of the incidence and prevalence of Parkinson's disease is problematic, because there is no 'in-life' marker for idiopathic Parkinson's disease; estimates of the annual incidence of Parkinson's disease are in the range of 4 to 20 per 100 000 individuals. A widely accepted figure for the prevalence of Parkinson's disease is approximately 200 per 100 000 population. In the United Kingdom, there are approximately 120 000 to 130 000 diagnosed cases, but there may be many more who remain undiagnosed. In the United States of America, it is estimated that between 750 000 and 1.5 million people have the condition.

Both the incidence and prevalence of Parkinson's disease increase with age, and the prevalence may be as high as 1 in 50 for patients over the age of 80 years. Men are 1.5 times more likely than women to develop the condition. Hospital-based studies and a limited number of epidemiological surveys in Africa have suggested that Parkinson's disease is less common in the black population, although this observation remains controversial.

Risk factors

Although Parkinson's disease was first described almost 200 years ago, it remains difficult to define exactly which individuals are at risk. The ageing process is related to the development of Parkinson's disease but is not solely responsible, because some patients develop the disease early in life. Furthermore, the type of dopamine cell loss in normal ageing differs from that in Parkinson's disease. Certain personality traits and environmental factors may increase the risk of Parkinson's disease (Box 24.7.2.1). People with a family history of Parkinson's disease, particularly first-degree relatives, are also at higher risk of developing the disease.

It has been postulated that people may be affected differently by a combination of genetic and environmental factors. A possible role of an environmental toxin was triggered by the fascinating observation that 1-methyl-4-phenyl-1,2,3,6-tetrahydropyridine (MPTP), accidentally consumed as a heroin contaminant in the United States of America in the late 1970s and early 1980s, caused an outbreak of levodopa-responsive parkinsonism. This led to the development of MPTP as an experimental agent to cause selective nigrostriatal cell loss in animal models. Recently, similar observations have been made in people in the welding trade, fuelling the hypothesis that

Box 24.7.2.1 Personality trends and environmental factors

Box 24.7.2.1 Personality trends and environmental factors

Personality trends

♦ Obsessive–compulsive disorder

Environmental factors

♦ Drinking well water

♦ Insecticide/pesticide exposure

♦ Manganese exposure (welding)

♦ N-Methyl-4-phenyl-1,2,3,6-tetrahydropyridine (MPTP)

manganese may be a causative factor. There have been conflicting reports about environmental agents that may predispose to Parkinson's disease. These are listed in Box 24.7.2.1.

Genetic factors

Individuals with a positive family history have twice the risk of developing Parkinson's disease and the risk for siblings is increased significantly if there is an affected sibling with young-onset Parkinson's disease. The risk increases further to 12 to 24% if both a sibling and a parent are affected (see Box 24.7.2.1). α-Synuclein was the first gene to be identified in a multigeneration Italian–American family (the Contursi family) as causing an aggressive parkinsonism. Since then several genes have been identified, with Parkin and *LRRK2* being the most prevalent ones (Table 24.7.2.1). *LRRK2* stands for leucine-rich repeat kinase 2 and is part of the family of Roco genes; it encodes for the protein dardarin. *LRRK2* has been associated with familial late-onset Parkinson's disease and a few cases of sporadic late-onset Parkinson's disease. However, routine genetic testing for Parkinson's disease is not available, nor is genetic counselling currently possible. The precise function of these genes is unknown, although α-synuclein is the core protein

Table 24.7.2.1 Genetics of parkinsonism

Symbol	Inheritance	Product	Location	Gene
PARK1	AD	α-Synuclein	4q21.3–q23	SNCA
PARK2	AR, juvenile onset	Parkin	6q25.2–q27	Parkin
PARK3	AD, Lewy body		2p13	–
PARK4	AD, Lewy body		4p15	–
PARK5	AD	Ubiquitin C-terminal esterase L1	4p14	UCHL1
PARK6	AR, early onset		1p35–p36	
PARK7	AR, early onset		1p36	
PARK8	AD	Dardarin	12p11.2–q13.	
PARK9	AR		1p36	–
PARK10			Unspecified	–
PARK11			2q36	

AD, autosomal dominant; AR, autosomal recessive.

in Lewy bodies whereas parkin may be active through the ubiquitin pathway.

Pathophysiology

The main pathological feature of Parkinson's disease is the degeneration of neuromelanin-containing neurons in the pars compacta of the substantia nigra (SN), which leads to deafferentation of the striatum. Normally, it has been suggested that the basal ganglia exert their motor and nonmotor effects through a complex circuitry. The two main pathways are the direct (stimulatory) and indirect (inhibitory) pathways, a balance in favour of the direct pathway being kept by regulatory control exerted by dopamine manufactured in the SN. In Parkinson's disease, dopamine cell degeneration leads to overexcitation of the direct circuit, and the resultant bradykinesia, by a complex pathway that also involves paradoxical excitation of the subthalamic nucleus and internal segment of the globus pallidus. The net result of both the direct and indirect pathways in the absence of dopamine is overexcitation of the medial globus pallidus, leading to excessive inhibition of the thalamus. Thalamic input to the motor cortex is excitatory and thus thalamocortical inhibition leads to akinesia and other symptoms of Parkinson's disease (Fig. 24.7.2.1).

Lewy bodies are intracytoplasmic eosinophilic inclusion bodies, typically found in the neurons of the SN. The pathophysiological basis of Parkinson's disease has recently been re-explored by seminal and somewhat controversial work by Heiko Braak, who has suggested that Lewy body formation, a hallmark of dopaminergic cell degeneration in Parkinson's disease, actually occurs in the brainstem, in the lower medulla and the olfactory bundle (stage 1 Parkinson's disease—Fig. 24.7.2.2a). In stage 2 more dorsal medulla and pons are involved (Fig. 24.7.2.2b) whereas it is at stage 3 that the midbrain and the SN are involved (Fig. 24.7.2.2c). According to this hypothesis, therefore, clinical Parkinson's disease is being detected only at stage 3. In support of this observation is the fact that several nonmotor features of Parkinson's disease, e.g. olfactory loss and sleep disorders such as rapid eye movement disorder (RBD), seem to occur from the brainstem and olfactory bundle involvement, and in fact precede the development of motor Parkinson's disease. A list of such nonmotor features that may actually precede the development of motor signs of Parkinson's disease and may in fact in future detect people 'at risk' of Parkinson's disease is listed in Box 24.7.2.2.

A recent twist to the pathophysiological basis of Parkinson's disease is the observation that positron emission tomography (PET) of the brain in Parkinson's disease identifies neuroinflammation in the brainstem, suggesting that the pathological process in Parkinson's disease may be initiated by an inflammatory process within the glial cells.

Symptoms and signs

Parkinsonism is a clinical syndrome and typically, when the condition appears to be idiopathic and in particular responds to levodopa therapy, it is referred to as Parkinson's disease. Often the presenting symptom is a slow resting tremor, worse at rest (4–7 Hz) and often unilateral, although up to 30% of cases do not have a tremor at onset of the disease. The presence of an obvious tremor often leads both patients and their carers to suspect Parkinson's disease and self-referral. In this context, it is important to differentiate an

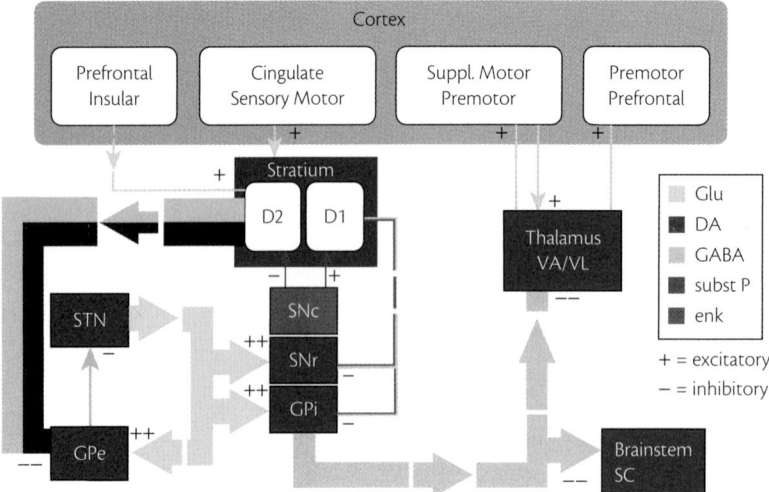

Fig. 24.7.2.1 Pathological functional anatomy of the basal ganglia in Parkinson's disease.

essential tremor from a parkinsonian tremor because the former carries a more benign prognosis and is twice as common, with a prevalence of at least 400 per 100 000 (Table 24.7.2.2).

Bradykinesia/akinesia is difficulty in initiating and slowness in executing, movement. It is the most disabling and progressive motor sign of Parkinson's disease and is a core feature for diagnosis of Parkinson's disease using the United Kingdom Parkinson's Brain Bank criteria (Box 24.7.3). It first affects fine movements such as fastening buttons, and handwriting, which becomes smaller and may progressively trail off (micrographia). Associated movements suffer and one or both arms may stop swinging when walking.

Diagnosis of parkinsonism

Gait is affected in Parkinson's disease, with difficulty starting walking, small steps, and shuffling. 'Festination' occurs when the patient appears to hurry and then stops suddenly as if rooted to the ground. The face often becomes expressionless (masked face or hypomimia) with reduced blinking. Bradykinetic laryngeal movement leads to quiet, monotonous speech that is low in volume and sometimes repetitive (palilalia).

Rigidity is usually detected on examination and patients tend to complain of muscular stiffness and pain. Parkinsonian rigidity, which can be activated by performing mirror movements in the opposite limb, presents as one of two types:

1 'lead-pipe' rigidity—a constant resistance to passive movement, in the absence of tremor

2 'cogwheel' rigidity—a superimposed clicking resistance similar to a ratchet, in the presence of tremor

Clinical assessment of Parkinson's disease is possible using several validated Parkinson's disease-specific scales and questionnaires. These include the self-rated, 30-item, nonmotor questionnaire (NMSQuest), the simple 8-item, Parkinson's disease quality-of-life questionnaire (PDQ-8), the motor scale (Unified Parkinson's disease rating scale, UPDRS), and the nonmotor scale (NMSS).

The nonmotor symptom complex

A wide range of nonmotor symptom complexes (NMSs) is also seen in Parkinson's disease from an early stage, all of which are likely to have a major effect on the health-related quality of life of patients. These symptoms include depression, dementia, sleep disorders, bowel and bladder problems, fatigue, apathy, pain, and autonomic dysfunction (see Box 24.7.2.2).

Confirmation of diagnosis

There are no specific tests for the diagnosis of Parkinson's disease, which remains clinical.

DaTSCAN

This is single photon emission computed tomography (SPECT) using the labelled cocaine derivative N-ω-fluoropropyl-2β-carboxymethoxy-3β-(4-iodophenyl)tropane (^{123}I-labelled β-CIT and ^{123}I-labelled FP-CIT (DaTSCANn, Fig. 24.7.2.3), and is recommended in guidelines from the National Institute for Health and Clinical Excellence (NICE) and widely used to support diagnosis and differentiate Parkinson's disease from essential tremor (Fig. 24.7.2.4). It labels the presynaptic dopamine transporter and this provides assessment of the presynaptic neurons, which degenerate in Parkinson's disease. Essential tremor is likely to show a normal DaTSCAN whereas in Parkinson's disease there is diminished uptake of the ligand, usually correlating with the clinically affected side, and DaTSCAN also appears to have a close correlation with the progression of Parkinson's disease. However, DaTSCAN does not differentiate between Parkinson's disease and other parkinsonian syndromes.

PET scan

Using ^{18}F-labelled dopa the PET scan has similar properties and better resolution but is currently available as a research tool only. More recently, transcranial ultrasonography has been used to reveal characteristic hyperechogenicity of the SN in patients with early Parkinson's disease, possibly suggestive of excessive iron deposition in the SN. However, this technique needs to be validated in large-scale studies before widespread use can be advocated.

CT or MRI

Scans are usually not needed for diagnosis, but a brain scan should be performed if parkinsonism is purely unilateral or otherwise

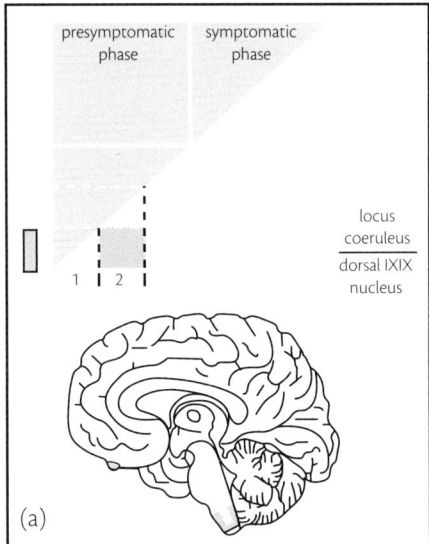

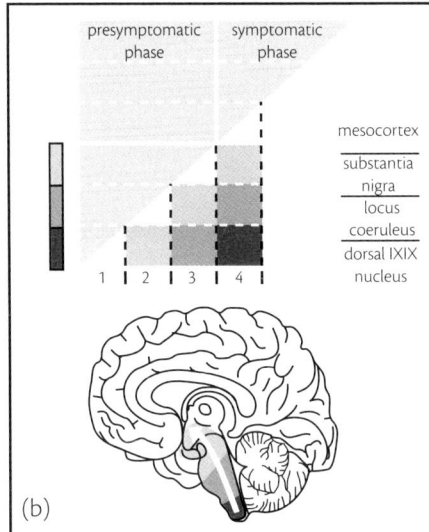

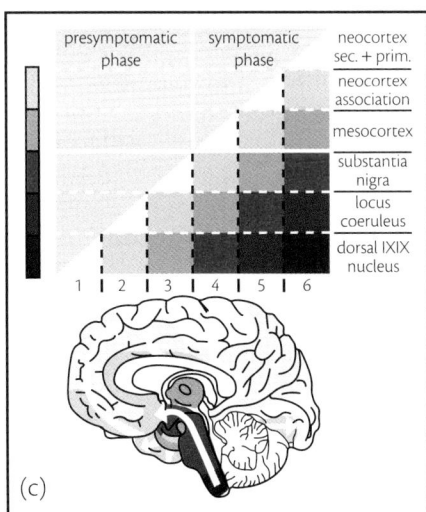

Fig. 24.7.2.2 Proposed pathophysiological basis of Parkinson's disease. (a) Stage 1 disease—Lewy body formation in the brainstem, lower medulla, and olfactory bundle. (b) Stage 2—more dorsal medulla and pons are involved. (c) Stage 3—midbrain and substantia nigra involved (Fig. 24.7.2.2c). (Colour scale relates anatomical site(s) of involvement to disease progression).

Box 24.7.2.2 The nonmotor symptom complex

Neuropsychiatric symptoms

◆ Depression, apathy, anxiety

◆ Anhedonia

◆ Attention deficit

◆ Hallucinations, illusion, delusions

◆ Dementia

◆ Obsessional behaviour (usually drug induced), repetitive behaviour

◆ Confusion

◆ Delirium (could be drug induced)

◆ Panic attacks

Sleep disorders

◆ Restless legs and periodic limb movements

◆ REM (rapid eye movement) behaviour disorder and REM loss of atonia

◆ Non-REM sleep-related movement disorders

◆ Excessive daytime somnolence

◆ Vivid dreaming

◆ Insomnia

◆ Sleep-disordered breathing

Autonomic symptoms

◆ Bladder disturbances:
  · urgency
  · nocturia
  · frequency

◆ Sweating

◆ Orthostatic hypotension (OH):
  · Falls related to OH
  · 'Coat hanger' pain

◆ Sexual dysfunction:
  · Hypersexuality (likely to be drug induced)
  · Erectile dysfunction

◆ Dry eyes (xerostomia)

Gastrointestinal symptoms

◆ Dribbling of saliva

◆ Ageusia

◆ Dysphagia/choking

◆ Reflux, vomiting

◆ Nausea

◆ Constipation

◆ Unsatisfactory voiding of bowel

◆ Faecal incontinence

(Continued)

Box 24.7.2.2 (*Cont'd*) The nonmotor symptom complex

Sensory symptoms

◆ Pain

◆ Paraesthesia

◆ Olfactory disturbance

Other symptoms

◆ Fatigue

◆ Diplopia

◆ Blurred vision

◆ Seborrhoea

◆ Weight loss

◆ Weight gain (possibly drug induced)

Box 24.7.2.3 Diagnosis of parkinsonism (Parkinson's Brain Bank criteria)

Essential features

◆ Bradykinesia and two of the following:

· Tremor (resting) and/or

· Rigidity (cogwheel or lead pipe)

· Postural imbalance, fixed, stooped posture

· Gait difficulty (shuffling, short-step gait (with or without festination)

Additional features

◆ Hypomimia ('masked' face)

◆ Freezing episodes (sudden onset failure of movement)

◆ Seborrhoea of the scalp

◆ Mental and cognitive disturbance

atypical, or if additional signs (pyramidal) are present. CT or MRI may also be used to rule out a space-occupying lesion, vascular disease, and normal-pressure hydrocephalus. MRI brain scan is preferable to a CT brain scan.

Management of Parkinson's disease

When to initiate treatment remains a key question and increasingly the modern school of thought would suggest that it may be best to start treatment at diagnosis. The decision to treat may be dictated by the following clinical issues:

◆ Involvement of the dominant hand relative to the nondominant hand and the effect on employment/occupation

◆ The particular subtype of Parkinson's disease (bradykinesia-dominant disease may require earlier treatment than tremor-dominant disease)

Table 24.7.2.2 Comparison of parkinsonian tremor and essential tremor

Feature	Parkinsonian tremor	Essential tremor
Age at onset	Usually >50 years	>10 years
Occurrence	Incidence *increases* with each decade of age	Incidence remains the *same* with each decade of age
Family history	Rare	Common
Site	Usually hands, also legs and jaw; head uncommon	Hands, head (a no–no or yes–yes motion), vocal
Characteristics	At rest; supination/pronation action reduces; mental concentration increases	Postural; flexion/extension action increases; mental concentration diminishes
Frequency (Hz)	4–7	8–12
Lead-pipe rigidity	Yes	No
Cogwheel rigidity	Yes	Rare
Alcohol	No effect	Often improves
Treatment	Dopaminergics	β-Blockers, primidone

◆ The individual sentiments of patients and carers (offer informed choice)

◆ Presence of nonmotor symptoms such as pain, depression, or sleep problems

As initiating treatment, the NICE (National Institute of Health and Clinical Excellence (UK)) guidelines recommend levodopa, dopamine agonists, or monoamine oxidase-B inhibitors. Levodopa is a precursor to dopamine, converted to dopamine by dopa decarboxylation, and restores the dopamine lost due to degeneration of striatonigral cells. The addition of a peripheral decarboxylase inhibitor that does not cross the blood–brain barrier, such as carbidopa or benserazide, inhibits dopa decarboxylase in the rest of the body and reduces side effects. The bioavailability of levodopa has been enhanced further by the emergence of drugs such as tolcapone and entacapone that inhibit catechol-*O*-methyl transferase (COMT), which also breaks down dopamine.

Evidence suggests that levodopa therapy should be started at the minimal effective dose (usually 50–100 mg/day), in combination with a decarboxylase inhibitor given three to four times daily. Doses at or above 600 mg/day may be associated with a dyskinesia rate as high as 17% at 1 year. Side effects, such as light-headedness or nausea, may be relieved by taking the medication with food or by increasing the dose of decarboxylase inhibitor or taking domperidone, which does not cross the blood–brain barrier and hence does not cause central dopamine antagonism. Controlled-release preparations of levodopa, with addition of a COMT inhibitor (entacapone) to the traditional combination of levodopa and a decarboxylase inhibitor (carbidopa), are now licensed for the treatment of later stage Parkinson's disease.

In advanced Parkinson's disease refractory to other forms of conventional therapies, intraduodenal/-jejunal infusion of levodopa (Duodopa) forms an alternative route of administration. Studies have shown that Duodopa is effective in controlling motor fluctuations in advanced Parkinson's disease and reduces dyskinesias.

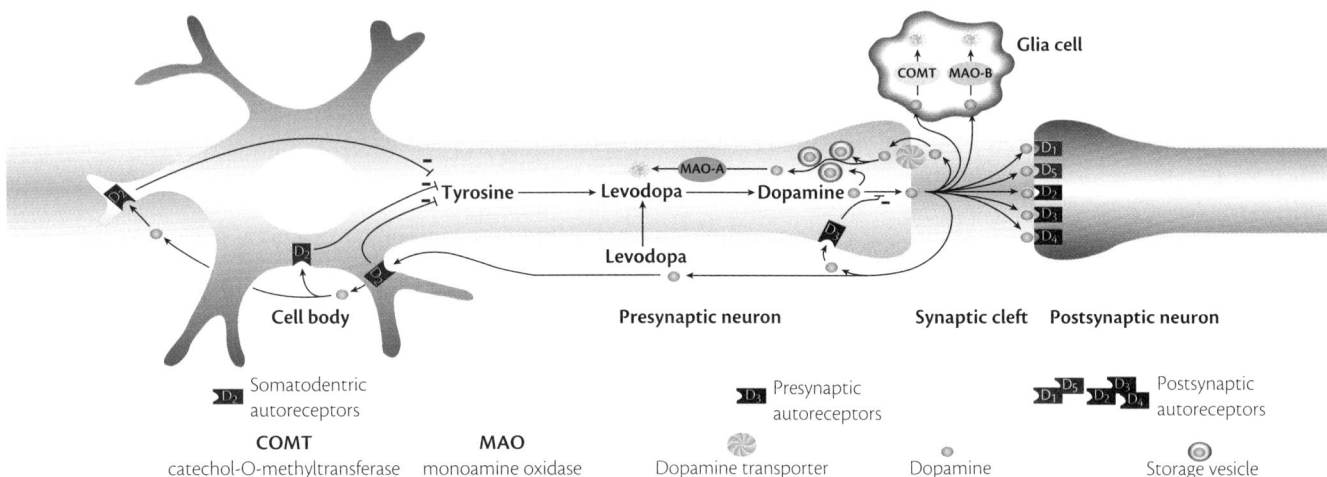

Fig. 24.7.2.3 (a) A normal DaTSCAN showing the comma appearance. (b) DaTSCAN in Parkinson's disease showing a 'dot' appearance on one side, reflecting dopaminergic loss.

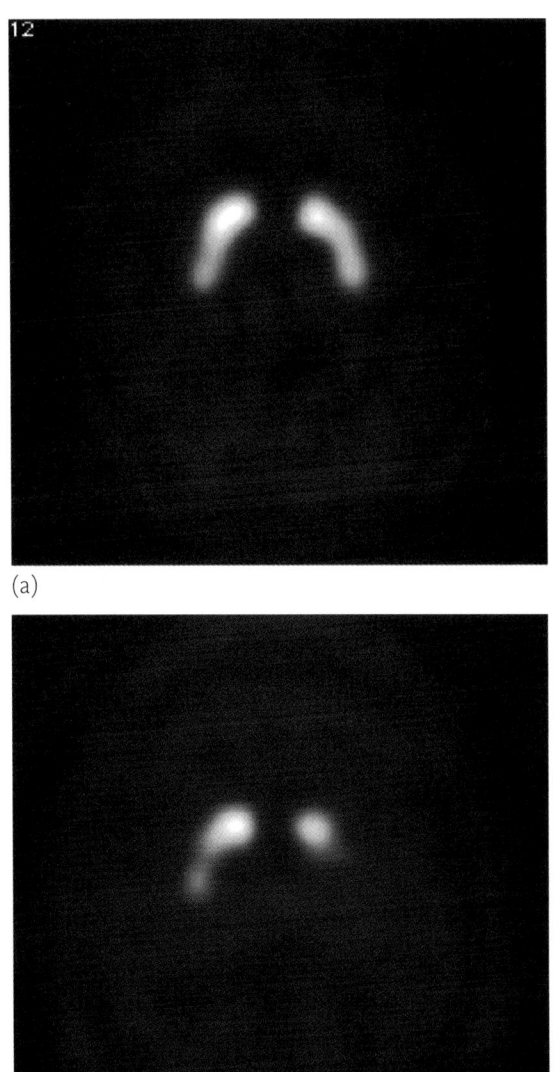

Fig. 24.7.2.4 Dopaminergic neuronal transmission.

Dopamine agonists

Dopamine agonists stimulate dopamine receptors directly and so bypass the degenerating presynaptic nigrostriatal neurons. Five types of dopamine receptors (D_1–D_5) have been identified so far; these are broadly divided into: D_1-like and D_2-like receptors. In the 1980s and 1990s ergot dopamine agonists such as bromocriptine, pergolide, and more recently cabergoline, were fashionable, whereas nonergot agonists were preferentially recommended owing to the risk of cardiac valvular fibrosis with ergot dopamine agonists. Ropinirole and pramipexole remain the two main oral nonergot dopamine agonists although recently rotigotine, a transdermal nonergot dopamine agonist patch, has been released, which is effective when given once a day and utilizes the concept of continuous dopaminergic stimulation (CDS). Both ropinorole and pramipexole are also now available as once a day therapy which leads to improved concordance with therapy in PD (Fig. 24.7.2.4). Side effects of dopamine agonists include nausea, vomiting, postural hypotension, and hallucinations/psychosis in susceptible individuals or at high doses. More specifically somnolence or sudden onset of sleep has been linked to nonergot dopamine agonists, but studies have revealed that somnolence can occur with progression of Parkinson's disease and other dopaminergic drugs as well. Patients therefore need to be warned about driving when starting on these drugs. More recently, behavioural problems such as compulsive gambling, hypersexuality, and a complex medley of impulsive behaviour has been linked to use of dopaminergic drugs, particularly dopamine agonists. The exact prevalence is unknown but can be up to 7% in susceptible individuals.

Apomorphine is a powerful nonergot dopamine agonist that is administered subcutaneously by an infusion pump in advanced cases of Parkinson's disease when oral therapy is no longer useful. Skin nodules and nausea are the main side effects. Subcutaneous apomorphine is indicated when oral or skin patch therapy is unable to control motor fluctuations.

Monoamine oxidase-B inhibitors

Selegiline 10 mg once daily or 5 mg twice daily orally (or 1.25 mg once daily by buccal administration) is a selective, irreversible blocker of intra- and extraneuronal monoamine oxidase B

(MAOB), and reduces metabolism of dopamine. Rasagiline is a new, second-generation, irreversible, selective MAOB inhibitor that is administered orally at a dosage of 0.5 to 1 mg once daily. A recent study (ADAGIO) suggest a potential disease modifying effect of rasagiline. The side effects of MAOB inhibition include hallucinations, sleep disorders, agitation, postural hypotension, and withdrawal problems.

Anticholinergics

Anticholinergics block the action of acetylcholine against dopamine within the basal ganglia. These drugs may occasionally be used as an adjunct to levodopa therapy, helping to control rest tremor and dystonia. However, they are not routinely recommended and should be used with great caution in older patients with parkinsonian syndromes because of the risk of inducing a confusional state and aggravating dementia.

Other drugs

Amantadine 100 to 400 mg daily is an antiviral agent with a moderate antiparkinsonian effect. It acts, in part, via increased dopamine synthesis and may also have an antidyskinetic action.

Patients who may require surgery

Surgery has gained popularity in selected patients when conventional pharmacological therapy has failed to control symptoms. It has a morbidity rate of approximately 2% due to strokes and infection, and a mortality rate of about 0.5%. The operation of choice is deep brain stimulation of the subthalamic nucleus (STN), which reverses the akinesia and controls dyskinesias. Patients with severe resistant unilateral tremor could have single-side thalamic stimulation of the ventral intermediate (VIM) nucleus. Other surgical approaches such as delivery of viral vectors to the striatum for gene therapy or neurotransplantation remain experimental options currently, although some such as adenosine-associated virus (AAV), a nonpathogenic virus, is being used in human trials for gene delivery.

Intrajejunal levodopa infusion

It is indicated for the treatment of advanced levodopa-responsive Parkinson's disease with severe motor fluctuations and dyskinesia . This involves giving L-dopa through jejunum via peg. It proved beneficial for nonmotor symptoms and health related quality of life in Parkinson patients.

Other parkinsonian/extrapyramidal syndromes

There are a number of degenerative diseases that have a more complex clinical picture than Parkinson's disease and a poorer response to therapy. It may be impossible to distinguish idiopathic Parkinson's disease from other parkinsonian syndromes.

Drug-induced parkinsonism

This is one of the most common causes of secondary parkinsonism, and is often misdiagnosed as Parkinson's disease because clinical features may be indistinguishable. It causes rigidity, bradykinesia, tremor, and gait disturbance, and may be asymmetrical. Although several medications are associated with secondary parkinsonism, dopamine-blocking agents (neuroleptics) such as prochlorperazine or chlorpromazine are the most common offending agents, and are often prescribed to older people for nonspecific complaints such as dizziness, and drug-induced parkinsonism may take up to 9 months to disappear. The incidence of drug-induced parkinsonism is estimated to be 15 to 40% in patients receiving neuroleptics, and its prevalence increases with age. Vestibular sedatives are also implicated .Commonly used antiemetics and anti dizziness pills needs to be monitored.

Treatment consists of withdrawal of the offending medication. If drug withdrawal is impractical, patients are given the lowest possible dose or are changed to a new atypical agent, such as clozapine or quetiapine. Occasionally emergence of parkinsonism may be permanent.

Progressive supranuclear palsy

Progressive supranuclear palsy (PSP or Steele–Richardson–Olszewski syndrome) presents with gait disturbance and falls (predominantly backwards) in over 50% of cases, and is a disease of later life. The pathological hallmark is tau protein-positive filamentous inclusions known as neurofibrillary tangles in the glia and neurons.

The clinical picture consists of supranuclear gaze palsy, particularly downgaze with extension and rigidity of the neck, a staring look due to lid retraction, and predominant truncal extensor rigidity. Varying degrees of bradykinesia, dysphagia, personality changes, and other behavioural disturbances, such as a subcortical frontal dementia, coexist. Subtype with levodopa responsiveness have been described.

Multiple-system atrophy

Multiple-system atrophy (MSA) consists of a variable combination of parkinsonism with autonomic, pyramidal, or cerebellar symptoms and signs. In the past, patients were categorized as having striatonigral type (SND) if there were dominant parkinsonian signs, olivopontocerebellar type (OPCA) if cerebellar signs predominated. These terms are no longer in use and, currently, SND and OPCA variants are called MSA-P and MSA-C, respectively. The pathological feature of MSA is the glial cytoplasmic inclusions.

The parkinsonian features of MSA include progressive bradykinesia, rigidity and postural instability, and signs that are usually bilateral. Useful clinical clues include disproportionate anterocollis, truncal dystonia (this may resemble the so-called 'Pisa syndrome'), characteristic sighing, and the presence of cold, blue hands. Autonomic failure, particularly postural hypotension, occurs early in MSA and is more severe than in idiopathic Parkinson's disease.

The response to levodopa is commonly incomplete and benefit usually declines within 1 to 2 years of treatment.

Dementia with Lewy bodies

In dementia with Lewy bodies (DLB), widespread areas of neocortex as well as the brainstem and diencephalic neurons have Lewy bodies. Parkinsonian DLB may be indistinguishable from Parkinson's disease, but these patients have early onset dementia (progressive cognitive decline interfering with normal social and occupational function) and may have hallucinations, delusions, and even psychosis in the absence of dopaminergic therapy, usually within 2 years of disease onset.

Clinical criteria for diagnosis include fluctuations in cognition and attention, recurrent and persistent visual hallucinations, and parkinsonian motor signs. Repeated early falls and neuroleptic sensitivity can be seen. Rarely, patients develop supranuclear gaze palsy; this may lead to the condition being mistaken for PSP.

Corticobasal ganglionic degeneration

Corticobasal ganglionic degeneration, also known as corticodentatonigral degeneration with neuronal achromasia, typically presents in the sixth or seventh decade with slowly progressive, unilateral development of tremor, apraxia, and rigidity in an upper limb.

The condition is characterized by progressive gait disturbances, cortical sensory loss, and stimulus-sensitive myoclonus, which results in a jerky, useless hand. A jerky, useless lower extremity is uncommon, but may occur; it is known as the alien limb phenomenon and can occur in about 50% of patients. Gait disturbance consists of a slightly wide-based, apraxic gait rather than the typical festinating gait of Parkinson's disease. Patients with corticobasal ganglionic degeneration do not benefit from levodopa, and the disease course is relentlessly progressive.

Dopa-responsive dystonia

Patients with young-onset parkinsonism manifest dystonia, which may respond to dopaminergic drugs. Those with hereditary dopa-responsive dystonia (Segawa's disease) have an excellent and sustained response to low-dose levodopa. This disorder characteristically shows marked diurnal variation, and may start in childhood with an odd and unusual gait; diagnosis can be made by checking for mutation in the GTP-cyclohydrolase gene.

Wilson's disease

Wilson's disease should be considered in every case of young-onset parkinsonism, because it is treatable and the consequences of nonrecognition can be grievous. The most common neurological manifestations include:

◆ A combination of parkinsonism and ataxia, characteristic of neurological Wilson's disease. Tremor typically involves the upper limbs and the head, and rarely the lower limbs; classically, the tremor is coarse, irregular, and present during action. Holding the arms forward and flexed horizontally may demonstrate the activity of the proximal muscles (wing-beating tremor).

◆ Kayser–Fleischer rings—rings of brownish-green pigmentation, due to copper deposition in the cornea, may be easy to recognize in patients with light-coloured irises, and are best appreciated with a careful slit-lamp examination performed by an ophthalmologist. The most useful diagnostic test results are a low serum ceruloplasmin level and a raised 24-h urinary copper excretion.

◆ Juvenile Huntington's disease, which is an autosomal dominant neurodegenerative disorder that typically presents with chorea, difficulty with gait and cognitive problems.

Neuroacanthocytosis

Neuroacanthocytosis is a rare cause of parkinsonism and typically presents with a hyperkinetic movement disorder, including chorea, tic-like features, and polyneuropathy. Acanthocytes are revealed on a fresh blood smear.

Vascular disease is a rare cause of a straightforward parkinsonian syndrome with a variety of clinical presentations. Onset is either acute or subacute, and symptoms (usually bilateral) are those seen in classic Parkinson's disease, including tremor, bradykinesia, rigidity and postural instability, and a gait disturbance with minimal upper-extremity symptoms (lower-body parkinsonism), or walking with small steps (marche à petits pas), which is characteristic of vascular disease.

Dystonia

Dystonia is a syndrome of sustained muscle contractions, which may be due to either derangement of the spinal cord or cortical mechanism or a dopaminergic dysfunction of basal ganglia. Dystonia is focal if a single area is involved, e.g. the face, oromandibular area, arm, or neck. Focal dystonias are very well treated with botulinum toxin injections.

It is multifocal if two or more noncontiguous body regions are involved, e.g. an arm and a leg with cranial muscle involvement or blepharospasm and leg dystonia. Finally, it is generalized if both legs and one other body region are involved or the whole body is involved.

Generalized idiopathic torsion dystonia

The mode of inheritance of this type of dystonia is autosomal dominant (*DYT1* gene on chromosome 9). This type of dystonia typically occurs in childhood and in early adult life. Symptoms often start in one area of the body and spread to other areas, and may present with twisted postures, turning in of the foot or arm, etc. Sometimes joints can twist; dystonia usually produces torsion—hence the term 'torsion dystonia'. Oral medications such as anticholinergic drugs, e.g. trihexyphenidyl, are often the mainstay of treatment for early onset generalized dystonia.

Tardive dyskinesia

Tardive dyskinesia is a chronic condition that is induced by long-term exposure to dopamine-blocking drugs. Major tranquillizers and antiemetics, such as metoclopramide, are the real culprits. These involuntary movements usually start with the face and mouth and cause grimacing, lip smacking, and tongue movements. They may also involve the rest of the body and produce involuntary gestures, tics, and writhing movements. Treatment for tardive dyskinesia is withdrawal of the drug responsible when possible and replacement with newer antipsychotics, e.g. quetiapine or quatrain fumarate. Clonazepam has proved to be useful. Recent studies showed that vitamins E and B_6 have a positive effect on these movement disorders.

Chorea and related disorders (see also Chapter 24.7.3)

Chorea is an irregular, rapid, uncontrolled, involuntary, excessive movement that seems to move randomly from one part of the body to another, often similar to dancing or piano playing. When chorea is severe, the movements may cause motion of the arms or legs which results in throwing. The main pathology lies in the caudate nucleus. Athetosis is a slower writhing and twisting movement. Choreoathetosis is a movement of intermediate speed, between the quick, flitting movements of chorea and the slower, writhing movements of athetosis. Chorea is closely related to ballism, which is a high-amplitude displacement of the proximal muscles.

Huntington's disease, for example, is dominantly inherited; it is caused by a mutation on chromosome 4—the Huntington gene—characterized by an expansion of CAG repeats. Huntington's disease generally starts in mid-adult life, around the age of 35 years; the Westpal variant occurs in childhood. There is no effective treatment for Huntington's disease. Tetrabenazine will reduce the involuntary movements.

Sydenham's chorea is associated with rheumatic fever, and commonly occurs in childhood with spontaneous remission usually taking place within 3 to 6 months.

Other causes of chorea are neuroacanthocytosis and systemic lupus erythematosus; it also rarely occurs in pregnancy—known as chorea gravidarum.

Tics

Tics are sudden, repetitive, stereotyped, nonrhythmic, involuntary movements (motor tics) or sounds (phonic tics). Motor tics are movement-based tics affecting discrete muscle groups.

Phonic tics are involuntary sounds produced by moving air through the nose, mouth, or throat. The characteristic feature of all tics is the patient's ability to suppress them for brief periods of 30 to 60 s.

Tics confined to a single muscle group often persist through life. When tics move around from one part of the body to another, they are termed 'chronic multiple tic', or Gilles de la Tourette's disease. The pathological basis of tics is not known, but they generally respond to drugs that decrease dopaminergic transmission. Gilles de la Tourette's syndrome can cause severe tics and noises that are socially disruptive, and in such cases a minimal but therapeutic dose of tetrabenazine, usually between 12.5 and 100 mg daily, may be helpful.

Other rare conditions

Other rare conditions to exclude are neuroacanthocytosis, neuroferrritinopathy (neuronal brain iron storage disorders), spinocerebellar atrophy.

Further reading

Albanese A, et al. (2001). Consensus statement on the role of acute dopaminergic challenge in Parkinson's disease. *Mov Disorders*, **16**, 197–201.

Albin RL, Frey KA (2003). Initial agonist treatment of Parkinson's disease: a critique. *Neurology*, **60**, 390–4.

Barbeau A, Sourkes TL, Murphy CF (1962). Les catecholamines de la maladie de Parkinson. In: Ajuriaguerra J (ed.) *Monoamines et système nerveux central*, pp. 247–62. Masson, Paris.

Birkmayer W, Hornykiewicz O (1962). Der l-Dioxyphenylalanin (=DOPA) Effekt beim Parkinson-Syndrom des Menschen: Zur Pathogenese und Behandlung der Parkinson-Akinese. *Arch Psychiatr Nervenkr*, **203**, 560–74.

Chaudhuri KR, Healy D, Schapira AHV (2006). The non-motor symptoms of Parkinson's disease. Diagnosis and management. *Lancet Neurol*, **5**, 235–45.

Chaudhuri KR, Pal S, Brefel-Courbon C (2002). Do 'sleep attacks' or 'unintended sleep episodes' occur with dopamine agonists? Is this a class effect? *Drug Safety*, **25**, 473–83.

Devos D, Defebvre L, Bordet R. (2010). Dopaminergic and non-dopaminergic pharmacological hypotheses for gait disorders in Parkinson's disease. *Fundam Clin Pharmacol*, Feb 12. [Epub ahead of print.]

Dhawan V, et al. (2006). The sleep-related problems of Parkinson's disease. *Age Ageing*, **35**, 220–8.

Fahn S, Elton R, Members of the UPDRS Development (1987). Unified Parkinson's Disease Rating Scale. In: *Recent developments in Parkinson's disease*, pp. 153–63. Macmillan Healthcare Information, Florham Park, NJ.

Fiszer U (2007). Adverse effects of dopamine agonists. *Neurol Neurochir Pol*, **41**(2 Suppl 1), S34–9.

Foltyne T, et al. (2002). The genetic basis of Parkinson's disease. *J Neurol Neurosurg Psychiatry*, **73**, 363–70.

Grossman RI, et al. (1989). Magnetic resonance imaging in Parkinson's disease and parkinsonian syndromes. *Neurology*, **39**, 1524.

Hatano T, Kubo S, Sato S, Hattori N (2009). Pathogenesis of familial Parkinson's disease: new insights based on monogenic forms of Parkinson's disease. *J Neurochem*, **111**, 1075–93.

Jankovic J (2005). Searching for a relationship between manganese and welding and Parkinson's disease. *Neurology*, **64**, 2021–8.

Kalra S, Grosset DG, Benamer HT (2010). Differentiating vascular parkinsonism from idiopathic Parkinson's disease: A systematic review. *Mov Disord*, Jan 13. [Epub ahead of print.]

Kashihara K (2007). Management of levodopa-induced dyskinesias in Parkinson's disease. *J Neurol*, **254** Suppl 5, 27–31.

Lindvall O, Kokaia Z (2010). Stem cells in human neurodegenerative disorders—time for clinical translation? *J Clin Invest*, **120**, 29–40.

Massey LA, Yousry TA (2010). Anatomy of the substantia nigra and subthalamic nucleus on MR imaging. *Neuroimaging Clin N Am*, **20**, 7–27.

Mark MH (2001). Lumping and splitting the Parkinson Plus syndromes: dementia with Lewy bodies, multiple system atrophy, progressive supranuclear palsy, and cortical-basal ganglionic degeneration. *Neurol Clinics*, **19**, 607–27, vi.

McGeer PL, McGeer EG (2008). Glial reactions in Parkinson's disease. *Mov Disorders*, **23**, 474–83.

National Institute for Health and Clinical Excellence (2006). *Clinical guidelines for management of Parkinson's disease in primary and secondary care*. Department of Health, London.

Nutt JG (2007). Continuous dopaminergic stimulation: Is it the answer to motor complications of levodopa? *Mov Disorders*, **22**, 1–9.

Nyholm D, et al. (2003). Optimising levodopa pharmacokinetics: Intestinal infusion versus oral sustained-release tablets. *Clin Neuropharmacol*, **26**, 156–63.

Olanow CW, Watts RL, Koller WC (2001). An algorithm (decision tree) for the management of Parkinson's disease (2001): treatment guidelines. *Neurology*, **56** (11 Suppl 5), S1–88.

Olanow W, Schapira AH, Rascol O (2000). Continuous dopamine-receptor stimulation in early Parkinson's disease. *Trends Neurosci*, **23**, S117–26.

Parkinson Study Group (2002). Dopamine transporter brain imaging to assess the effects of pramipexole vs levodopa on Parkinson disease progression. *JAMA*, **287**, 1653–61.

Rascol O, et al. (2000). A five year study of the incidence of dyskinesias in patients with early Parkinson's disease who were treated with ropinirole or levodopa. *N Engl J Med*, **342**, 1484–91.

Rascol O, et al. (2002). Treatment interventions for Parkinson's disease: an evidence-based assessment. *Lancet*, **359**, 1589–98.

van de Vijver RAC, et al. (2001). Estimation of incidence and prevalence of Parkinson's disease in the elderly using pharmacy records. *Pharmacoepidemiol Drug Safety*, **10**, 549–54.

Zhang Z, Roman G (1993). Worldwide occurrence of Parkinson's disease: an updated review. *Neuroepidemiology*, **12**, 195–208.

24.7.3 Movement disorders other than Parkinson's disease

Roger A. Barker and David J. Burn

Essentials

Movement disorders are considered in five main categories—dystonia, chorea, tremor, tics, and myoclonus. Each disorder may occur in several diseases, and each may be the sole manifestation of a given neurological disease, but they also may only represent a component of a more widespread disorder.

Movement disorders characteristically involve the basal ganglia and under these circumstances, neuropsychiatric manifestations—often more significant than the disturbed movement—have the greater impact on well-being.

Most treatments for movement disorders are empirical, but with greater understanding of the molecular genetics and the application of functional imaging, a more rational neurochemical basis for several disorders is emerging. Ultimately this greater understanding may lead to the development of effective therapies based on rational principles.

Particular movement disorders

Dystonias—so-called idiopathic torsion dystonia is often inherited as an autosomal dominant trait; other causes include the Dopa-responsive dystonia-Parkinsonism (Segawa's syndrome), writer's cramp and oromandibular dystonia (which responds poorly to most drugs).

Chorea—occurs in many conditions and may be a consequence of any treatment for Parkinson's disease. The most common other cause is Huntington's disease. Sydenham's chorea (St Vitus's dance), for which dopamine D_2 receptor blocking agents may be effective, and neuropsychiatric manifestations are associated with rheumatic fever and other complications of group A streptococcal infections.

Tremor—this includes 'essential' tremor, for which several candidate susceptibility gene loci have been identified.

Tics—these may be simple or complex, and arise in numerous disorders. When combined with copralalia and other sudden vocalization, Tourette's syndrome—a genetic disorder showing autosomal dominant transmission with variable penetrance—is identified. The tics may respond to neuroleptic agents, and the associated obsessive-compulsive behavioural features often benefit from clomipramine (a tricyclic agent) or fluoxetine; deep brain stimulation has been used successfully in severe cases, but is not yet established as a routine treatment.

Myoclonus—this occurs in numerous neurological diseases. It may be solitary and static, as in benign essential myoclonus, or a progressive disease with encephalopathy (progressive myoclonic encephalopathy), and it is also a feature of epilepsy. Static myoclonus after action (Lance–Adam syndrome) may develop after cerebral anoxia.

Miscellaneous movement disorders—these include (1) psychogenic conditions; (2) numerous drug-induced conditions, usually induced by anti-psychotic or anti-emetic drugs; (3) the stiff man syndrome; and (4) restless legs (Ekböm's) syndrome—a common condition.

Introduction

Movement disorders typically result from diseases of the basal ganglia and can be classified into one of five main categories: dystonia, chorea, tremor, tics, and myoclonus (see Box 24.7.3.1 for definitions). Each type of abnormal movement may occur in several diseases and many treatments are empirical. However, the study of molecular genetics and the use of functional imaging have revealed subtle neurochemical abnormalities that should facilitate the development of more rational therapies.

In this section, attention is drawn to abnormal movements that are a principal manifestation of the disease. Movement disorders have been divided into hyperkinetic and hypokinetic conditions; however, this classification may be misleading because a given disease often evolves with time. Furthermore, the disorder may be 'mixed', with different movement types present in the same patient. It is probably more useful to classify movement disorders by type, as correct identification of the phenomenology is the first step towards correct diagnosis and management.

The dystonias

Definition

Dystonias are characterized by prolonged involuntary muscle contractions, causing abnormal movements and postures. Hermann Oppenheim first used the term 'dystonia' in 1911 to describe a childhood-onset form of generalized dystonia which he called 'dystonia musculorum deformans'.

Classification

When no symptomatic cause for dystonia can be discovered, the syndrome is described as idiopathic or primary dystonia, and if generalized then the disorder is synonymous with idiopathic torsion dystonia. Secondary dystonia is due to a defined exogenous, structural, or metabolic disorder. A 'dystonia plus' syndrome constitutes dystonia in combination with other abnormalities (e.g. myoclonic dystonia) and heredodegenerative dystonia occurs when there is an underlying brain degeneration. Dystonia may affect the whole body (generalized dystonia) or adjacent parts such as an arm and neck (segmental dystonia), or may be restricted to one part (focal dystonia) as in spasmodic torticollis, dystonic writer's cramp, blepharospasm, oromandibular dystonia, and laryngeal dystonia. Age at onset may also be used to classify dystonia. Early onset disease (before the age of 26 years) usually begins in a leg or arm and less commonly in the craniocervical region. Children often develop symptoms in the legs and frequently develop segmental or generalized dystonia. Late-onset primary dystonia (onset after 26 years) commonly affects the neck and cranial musculature, and onset in a limb, particularly the leg, is much less likely. In adults the dystonia is most likely to remain confined to its site of origin as a focal dystonia.

Idiopathic dystonia is frequently inherited (see below), but the focal dystonias usually occur sporadically in middle life. However, focal dystonias may be isolated fragments of the syndrome of idiopathic torsion dystonia.

Causes of pseudodystonia (conditions that may mimic dystonia) include tonic seizures, stiff person syndrome, and other neuromuscular disorders (e.g. neuromyotonia, myotonic disorders), carpopedal spasm, head tilt resulting from posterior fossa or retropharyngeal

---

Box 24.7.3.1 Movement disorders[a]

Dystonia

Sustained spasms of muscle contraction that distort the limbs and trunk into characteristic postures—the twisted (torticollis), flexed (antecollis), or extended neck (retrocollis), the arched (lordosis) or twisted back (scoliosis), the hyperpronated arm, and plantar-flexed inverted foot. The spasms typically occur on willed action (action dystonia). Dystonic spasms may be intermittent, producing dystonic movements, which may be repetitive to give a rhythmic character or sustained to hold a fixed dystonic posture.

Athetosis

This term was originally used to describe the sinuous, writhing movements that may follow a stroke; it later became synonymous with cerebral palsy, resulting from perinatal anoxia or kernicterus. Affected infants are floppy, exhibit delayed motor milestones, and before the age of 5 years develop athetoid movements—athetoid cerebral palsy, or 'athetosis'

Tremor

A rhythmic sinusoidal movement of a body part caused by regular muscle contractions.

Chorea

A continuous flow of irregular, jerky, and explosive movements, that flit randomly from one part of the body to another. Each muscle contraction is brief, often appearing as a fragment of what might have been a normal movement, and unpredictable in timing or site (see Fig. 24.7.3.5)

Myoclonus

Rapid shock-like muscle jerks, often repetitive and sometimes rhythmic.

Tics

Similar to myoclonic jerks, but are repetitive, stereotyped movements that can be mimicked voluntarily and can be held in check by an effort of will. Simple tics are confined to a few muscles; complex tics may include quasipurposeful movements.

[a]Nearly all dyskinesias disappear in sleep, are aggravated by anxiety, and improved by relaxation. Many movement disorders merge: e.g. Huntington's disease may show chorea and dystonia, giving the appearance of 'hanging chorea'.

---

space mass lesions, and Sandifer's syndrome (gastro-oesophageal reflux in young children with associated head tilt).

Aetiology

The many metabolic and other inherited or sporadic diseases that can cause dystonia (Table 24.7.3.1 and Box 24.7.3.2) usually produce other neurological symptoms and signs. A symptomatic cause for dystonia is found in about 50% of children with the condition, but is rare in those with adult onset.

The recent identification of mutations in genes responsible for forms of dystonia gives hope for understanding its basis (Table 24.7.3.1). Abnormalities within the basal ganglia and associated cortical motor areas have been found in some patients with secondary dystonia.

Idiopathic (torsion) dystonia

Symptoms

Idiopathic (torsion) dystonia may present in childhood, when it is frequently inherited as an autosomal dominant trait, or in adult life, when a family history is unusual. In many families with early onset disease, genetic linkage studies have localized the abnormal gene mutation to the *DYT1* locus on chromosome 9q34 which codes for torsin A, a protein of unknown function expressed in the brain (including the substantia nigra). Ashkenazi Jews are particularly prone to this condition. It usually presents in children with dystonic spasms of the legs on walking, or sometimes of the arms, trunk, or neck. The condition is usually progressive when it starts in childhood; the spasms spread to all body parts, leading to severe disability within about 10 years. The intellect is preserved and there are no signs of pyramidal or sensory deficit. Speech is often spared, permitting the pursuit of intellectual employment despite severe physical disability. A spontaneous remission of symptoms occurs in about 10 to 20% of patients, usually within 5 years of onset. There is no way of predicting who will remit or when such a remission will occur. Most remissions are transitory, lasting a matter of weeks or months, but occasionally they may persist.

In adults, the condition usually presents as a focal dystonia (blepharospasm, oromandibular dystonia, spasmodic dysphonia, torticollis, axial dystonia, or dystonic writer's cramp). The legs tend to be spared, and progression is slow, with the dystonia remaining confined to its site of origin. Segmental dystonia develops in some cases.

Treatment

Dystonia is distressing and difficult to treat. Every child and young adult with dystonia should receive a trial of levodopa (e.g. Sinemet-Plus up to two tablets three times a day for 3 months), as they may have the condition of dopa-responsive dystonia–parkinsonism (see below). Occasionally, other forms of childhood-onset dystonia may also show a response, albeit incomplete, to levodopa.

The drugs that most patients find helpful, and continue to take to suppress muscle spasm, are benzodiazepines such as diazepam, often in a large dose of 20 to 50 mg daily, and an anticholinergic such as benzhexol, again in large doses (up to as much as 120 mg/day). Fifty per cent of children and 10% of adults will be helped, but adults are more sensitive to anticholinergic side effects. Dopamine-blocking drugs such as sulpiride or dopamine depletors such as tetrabenazine may help some patients, but often at the expense of drug-induced parkinsonism and unacceptable sedation. Unfortunately, dystonia is far less responsive to neuroleptics than chorea. Many other drugs have been tried in dystonia, but none has gained wide acceptance. In life-threatening dystonic crises, combination therapy may be required.

The recent interest in neurosurgery for movement disorders has extended to the treatment of dystonia, especially when the disease is advanced and disabling. Originally the thalamus was targeted for surgery but of late the target has moved to the internal part of the globus pallidum and deep brain stimulation. This therapy seems to work well in young patients with dystonia due to *DYT1* mutations.

Table 24.7.3.1 Classification of genetic dystonias[a]

Disease	Gene locus	Inheritance	Chromosome region/protein	Clinical features
Primary torsion dystonia	DYT1	Autosomal dominant	Torsin A	Late childhood. Limb, then generalized
X-linked dystonia–parkinsonian syndrome (Phillipines; Lubag's disease)	DYT3	X linked	TATA-binding protein-associated factor 1 gene (TAF1)	Onset typically 30–45 years with focal dystonia, becoming generalized, with abnormal gait, associated tremors, and parkinsonism (last may be dominant)
Dopa-responsive dystonia -parkinsonism (Segawa's syndrome)[b]	DYT5	Autosomal dominant	GTP cyclohydrolase 1 gene	Childhood. Lower limb dystonia with parkinsonism. Worse at end of day
Craniocervical dystonia parkinsonism (Mennonite/Amish)	DYT6	Autosomal dominant	8q21–22	Early adulthood. Craniocervical dystonia becoming generalized
Familial torticollis	DYT7	Autosomal dominant	18p31	Torticollis. Spasmodic dysphonia
Paroxysmal kinesiogenic or nonkinesiogenic dystonia[b]	DYT8	Autosomal dominant	Myofibrillogenesis regulator gene	Episodes of dystonia or chorea that last for seconds with movement or startle (kinesiogenic) Nonkinesiogenic episodes last for minutes to hours and are provoked by stress and certain agents
Alcohol-responsive myoclonic dystonia[b]	DYT11	Autosomal dominant	ε-Sarcoglycan gene	Myoclonic jerks compounded by dystonia. Young adults. Nonprogressive, relieved by alcohol
Rapid-onset dystonia-parkinsonism	DYT12	Autosomal dominant	Na$^+$/K$^+$ ATPase α3	
Cervical–cranial–brachial	DYT13	Autosomal dominant	1p36	Italian family with reduced penetrance
Dopa-responsive dystonia	DYT14	Autosomal dominant	14q13	Early onset lower limb dystonia, diurnal variation with later-onset parkinsonism
Myoclonus–dystonia	DYT15	Autosomal dominant	18p11	Onset in first two decades with myoclonus and dystonia, alcohol responsive; depression may be a feature

[a] Does not include DYT2 and -4 where the chromosome region has not yet been mapped.
[b] Only a proportion of cases are due to the named genetic defect.

Dopa-responsive dystonia–parkinsonism (Segawa's syndrome)

This condition is most commonly inherited as an autosomal dominant condition with incomplete penetrance and has as its defect mutations in the guanosine triphosphate cyclohydrolase 1 gene. This enzyme catalyses the production of tetrahydrobiopterin, an essential cofactor for maintaining the normal activity of tyrosine hydroxylase (TH), the rate-limiting step in the catecholamine biosynthetic pathway. The typical dopa-responsive dystonia phenotype affects the legs, which become worse as the day goes on. Rest without sleep does not help, but sleep relieves the dystonia. Many patients also have features of parkinsonism, although focal dystonia may be the presenting feature. The disease can easily be mistaken for cerebral palsy (given its lower limb predominance) or an unexplained 'spastic paraparesis' (because of brisk reflexes and variable ankle clonus). Rarer genetic causes for this condition exist, including abnormalities in the genes coding for TH itself, but in these cases there are often more widespread neurological problems such as major cognitive deficits.

This condition is characterized by a reduction in turnover of dopamine due to the abnormality in tyrosine hydroxylase activity; patients respond well to low doses of levodopa without showing any of the long-term complications encountered in Parkinson's disease.

Although very rare, the importance of this condition is that it can be easily confused with cerebral palsy and is very easy to treat.

Box 24.7.3.2 Symptomatic secondary dystonias

♦ Inherited metabolic, e.g. Wilson's disease

♦ Acquired metabolic, e.g. kernicterus

♦ Inherited possible metabolic, e.g. Hallervorden–Spatz disease or now renamed pantothenate kinase-associated neurodegeneration (PKAN)

♦ Other inherited causes, e.g. neuroacanthocytosis, Huntington's disease

♦ Miscellaneous causes, e.g. Parkinson's disease and its treatment, progressive supranuclear palsy, trauma including head trauma, cervical cord and peripheral nerve injury, anoxia/ischaemia, tumours of the basal ganglia, toxins, and drug induced

♦ Psychogenic

Spasmodic torticollis

Symptoms

Spasmodic torticollis may be the presenting feature of dystonia in childhood, but isolated spasmodic torticollis usually occurs in middle-aged or older people. The onset is usually insidious, often with initial pain, and sometimes appears to be precipitated by trauma. The dystonic spasms affect sternomastoid, splenius, and other neck muscles to cause the head to turn to one side (torticollis) (Fig. 24.7.3.1), or occasionally to extend (retrocollis) or to flex (antecollis) the neck. The spasms may be repetitive, causing a 'no–no' titubation, tremulous torticollis, or sustained hold of the posture. The trunk commonly shows a compensatory lordosis.

The condition is usually lifelong, but remissions of a year or more occur in about one-fifth of cases. Most patients are otherwise normal apart from their torticollis, although some may exhibit a postural tremor similar to that of essential tremor, and a minority may develop dystonia elsewhere. As with all types of dystonia, the frequency and intensity of the muscle spasms vary considerably, being particularly worse in conditions of mental or emotional stress. A feature characteristic of spasmodic torticollis is the 'geste antagoniste', a sensory trick in which the patient discovers some particular manual act that controls the deviation of the head. A light touch of the forefinger to the jaw may suffice, but other more complex and bizarre actions are common.

Treatment

Spasmodic torticollis, similar to other types of adult-onset focal dystonia, does not usually benefit from conventional drug therapy. The best treatment is injection of botulinum toxin A into the most affected muscles. Botulinum toxin prevents the release of acetylcholine and causes functional denervation with localized muscle weakness. Identification of the overactive muscles is a prerequisite

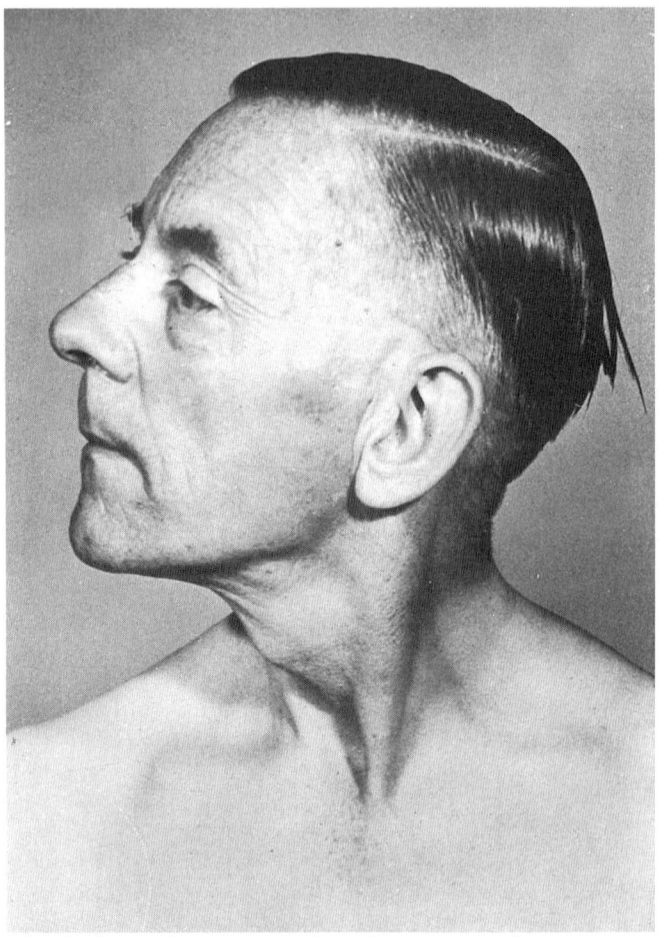

Fig. 24.7.3.1 Spasmodic torticollis in a 57-year-old man. The hypertrophy of the sternomastoid muscle is evident.

to the administration of localized injections of botulinum toxin, which, in the case of torticollis, typically involves injections into the sternomastoid and splenius muscles. These injections usually have an effect within a week although the maximum benefit is not apparent until several weeks later. Repeat injections are required approximately every 3 months as relapse, by terminal sprouting, occurs. In about 10 to 20% of patients, antibodies eventually develop to the botulinum toxin A, making it less effective with time. In these cases a switch to a botulinum toxin type F or B may be desirable; the long-term efficacy of this treatment is under investigation.

Surgery is sometimes practised and local denervation procedures are still considered in patients with otherwise intractable cervical dystonias, although the outcome from such interventions is very variable.

Dystonic writer's cramp

Symptoms

Inability to write (or to type, play a musical instrument, or use any manual instrument) has many causes but in most patients no objective neurological deficit is found other than abnormal posturing of the hand and arm on writing. Typically, the pen is gripped with great force and driven into the paper (Fig. 24.7.3.2). However, in some patients the arm adopts a typical dystonic posture and, in such cases of dystonic writer's cramp, other manual acts such as wielding a knife or a screwdriver are similarly affected. Such dystonic writer's cramp may be the initial symptom of generalized torsion dystonia, but in adults it often remains as an isolated disability. The same considerations apply to other occupational cramps, such as pianist's cramp, all of which may have their origin in abnormal plasticity and mapping of the affected limb part in the sensorimotor cortex.

Treatment

Writer's cramp, and related conditions, is usually a permanent disability. Advice to use a broad-based pen or a keyboard, or to learn to write with the opposite hand allows most to cope with everyday events, but approximately one patient in 20 will then develop dystonia in the nondominant hand. Drugs (such as benzhexol and diazepam) are rarely of benefit but botulinum toxin injections into the muscles of the affected forearm may help some patients. Electromyography may be used to guide the injections more precisely to the overactive muscles, although the functional benefits of this technique over conventional administration has yet to be clearly demonstrated. Recently some investigators have advocated restraint therapy in the affected limb with the hope that this will lead to a remapping of the sensorimotor cortex back to normal with relief of the focal task-induced dystonia. This therapy remains controversial.

Blepharospasm and oromandibular dystonia (cranial dystonia)

Symptoms

Blepharospasm refers to recurrent spasms of eye closure. Orbicularis oculi forcibly contracts for seconds or minutes, often repetitively and sometimes so frequently as to render the patient functionally blind (Fig. 24.7.3.3). Spasms of eye closure commonly occur while reading or watching television, or in bright light; they often decrease or disappear when the person is alerted or under scrutiny. Oromandibular dystonia refers to recurrent spasms of muscle contraction affecting the mouth, tongue, jaw, larynx, and

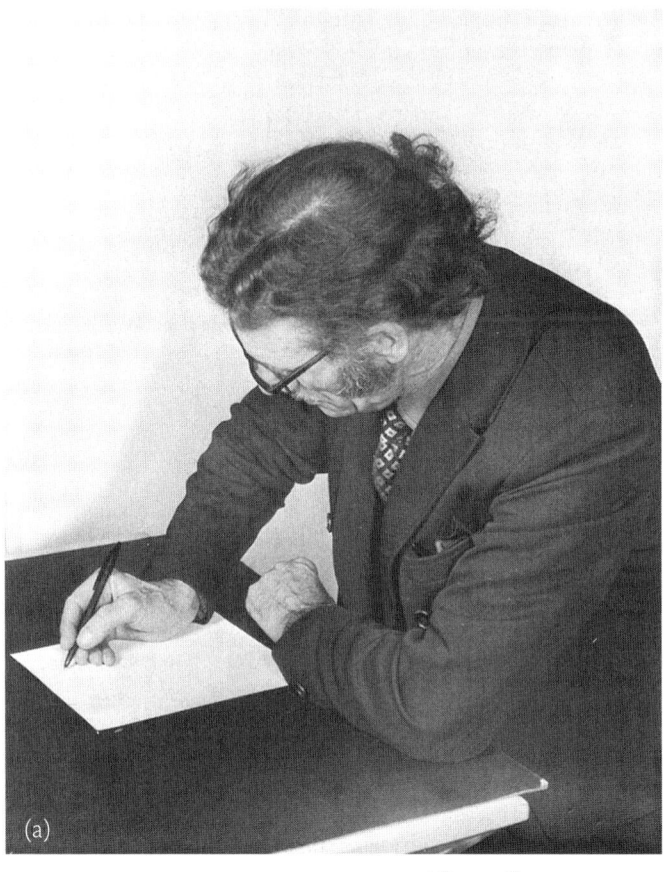

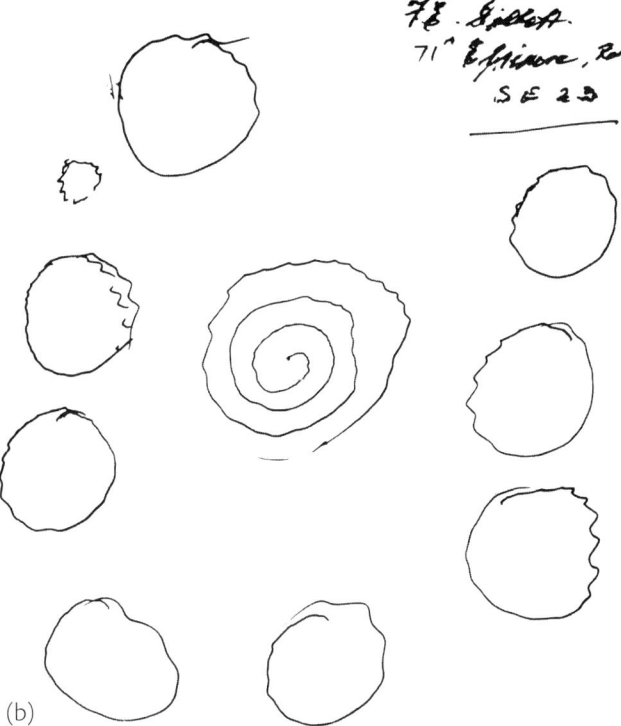

Fig. 24.7.3.2 (a) Dystonic writer's cramp in a 52-year-old man, whose right elbow rises and whose fingers grip the pen so tightly that they slide off. (b) Example of writing and drawing in this patient, showing difficulty in executing the task and thus legibility of script and ability to copy simple figures.

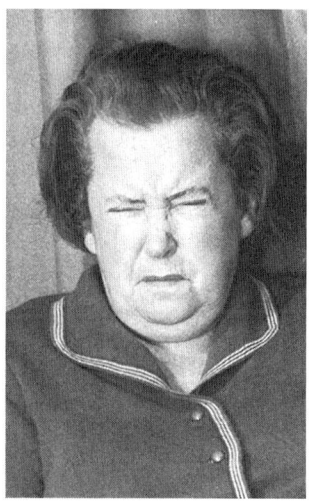

Fig. 24.7.3.3 Blepharospasm in a 57-year-old woman. Her jaw is also forcibly clamped shut, biting her gums, and some spasm of orbicularis oris is evident, in addition to the obvious spasm of orbicularis oculi.

pharynx, causing spasms of lip protrusion or retraction, jaw closure or opening (Fig. 24.7.3.4), and difficulty in speech and swallowing. Such patients may lacerate their lips and tongue or even dislocate their jaw, and are usually unable to cope with dentures. Speech may take on a characteristic, forced, strained quality, and chewing and swallowing may be impaired.

These two conditions are closely related, because the patient with blepharospasm may develop oromandibular dystonia and vice versa. The term 'Brueghel's syndrome' is often used when the dominant (or only) feature is a dystonically opened jaw, whereas Meige's syndrome has blepharospasm as its central feature. Both conditions may occur in generalized torsion dystonia, or result from drugs (often as a tardive dystonia); they also appear in isolation in late life without evident cause.

Treatment

Unfortunately, both blepharospasm and oromandibular dystonia are notoriously difficult to control with drugs (e.g. benzhexol, diazepam, and/or a neuroleptic). Surgery cannot improve oromandibular

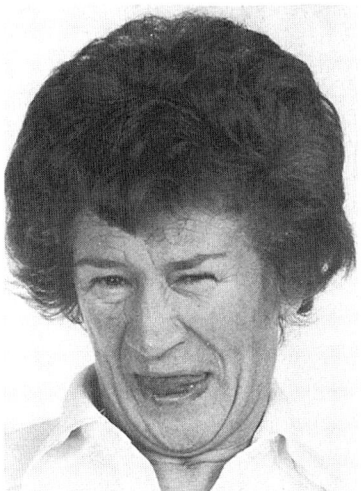

Fig. 24.7.3.4 Oromandibular dystonia in a 42-year-old woman. The spasm of forced jaw opening with tongue protrusion is evident.

dystonia but can relieve blepharospasm. The best treatment for blepharospasm is to inject botulinum toxin into orbicularis oculi, which gives relief in about 70 to 80% of cases, thereby restoring normal vision for about 3 months. The injections can be repeated as necessary. Botulinum toxin injections can be used to control some jaw spasms, although care is needed not to induce dysphagia.

Spasmodic dysphonia

Dystonic spasms of the muscles controlling the vocal folds cause spasmodic dysphonia, which impairs speech and singing, and may be severe enough to prevent communication. The most common type involves the adductor muscles, leading to a 'strangled' speech quality with pitch breaks and stops. Less common is abductor dysphonia which produces a breathy, low-volume voice. Abductor dysphonia, in particular, is often misdiagnosed as a psychogenic disorder. The diagnosis can be established by direct noninvasive visualization of the vocal folds during talking. Spasmodic dysphonia may occur in association with cranial or generalized dystonia, or appear as an isolated focal dystonia in adult life. Speech can be restored by injection of botulinum toxin into the overactive vocal muscles, identified by electromyography in specialist centres.

Paroxysmal dystonia

Focal dystonias often commence with the appearance of a dystonic posture or spasm on only one motor act (action dystonia), but there are rare, usually familial, disorders in which dramatic dystonia occurs intermittently in attacks, the patient being normal in between. These conditions are thought to be caused by mutations in genes encoding ion channels. Several families with paroxysmal dystonic choreoathetosis have now been shown to have mutations in the myofibrillogenesis regulator gene (*MR1*).

Chorea

Chorea is seen in many disorders (Table 24.7.3.2 and Fig. 24.7.3.5), but the most common cause other than the treatment of Parkinson's disease is Huntington's disease. There are also several noninherited conditions in which chorea can occur and in which treatment is beneficial.

Huntington's disease

Aetiology

Huntington's disease is an autosomal dominantly inherited condition first described in 1872 by George Huntington. It affects about 1 in 10 000 of the population and occurs in all ethnic groups worldwide; it typically presents in middle life. The genetic defect is a trinucleotide repeat disorder with an abnormal CAG expansion in exon 1 of the gene encoding huntingtin on chromosome 4. This pathological triplet (or trinucleotide) repeat codes for an expanded polyglutamine repeat in the huntingtin gene. As is common to all disorders of this type the longer repeats tend to occur in the offspring of affected men, with longer repeats occurring in the subsequent generations. This results in an earlier onset and more severe form of the disorder in subsequent generations—a phenomenon known as genetic anticipation as longer repeat sequences are associated with younger-onset, more severe forms of the disease.

The abnormal expansion of the CAG repeat in Huntington's disease to more than 36 causes a new gain of function in the mutant huntingtin with possible effects on the delivery of the growth

Table 24.7.3.2 Chorea

Hereditary	
Autosomal dominant	Huntington's disease
	Spinocerebellar ataxias
Autosomal recessive	Neuroacanthocytosis
	Wilson's disease
Other	Leigh's syndrome
Drug induced	Neuroleptics
	Anticonvulsants
	Anti-Parkinson's disease medication
	Oral contraceptive (often with a history of previous Sydenham's chorea)
Toxins	Carbon monoxide poisoning
Metabolic	Hyperthyroidism
	Pregnancy
Infection	Sydenham's chorea
Immunological	Systemic lupus erythematosus
Vascular	Infarction
	Polycythaemia
Tumours	
Trauma	Cerebral palsy
	Acquired
Age related	Senile chorea
Paroxysmal	
Psychogenic	

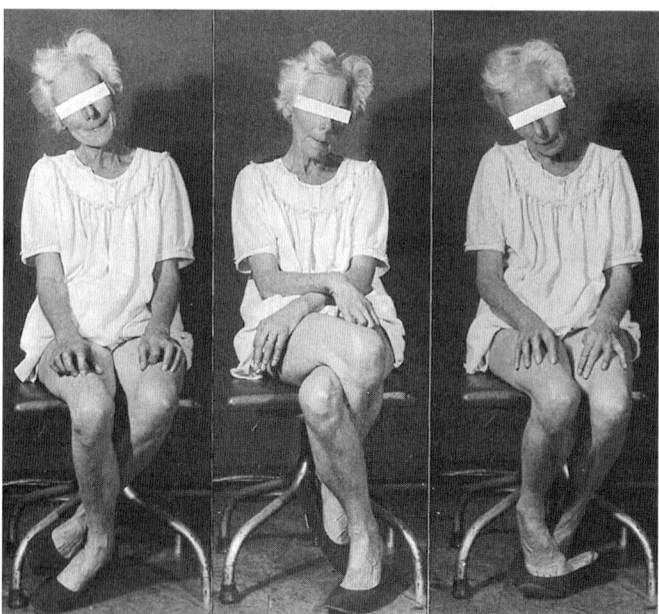

Fig. 24.7.3.5 Chorea due to polycythaemia rubra vera in a 57-year-old woman. The characteristic fleeting choreic movements are captured in these three sequential frames.

factor BDNF (brain-derived neurotropic factor) as well pathological actions through a range of intracellular protein–protein interactions. Inclusion bodies resulting from the polymerization of polyglutamine sheets in the mutant huntingtin protein develop in neurons and early on there is neuronal dysfunction ahead of cell death and loss. This loss is most marked in the striatum but cortical atrophy is also evident early on in the disease process.

Symptoms

The onset is typically insidious, usually between the ages of 30 and 50 years, and can be with motor, cognitive, and/or psychiatric symptoms and signs. The initial symptoms are frequently those of a change in personality and behaviour with a degree of irritability and impulsiveness, often with chorea that may be subtle and noticed only by a relative. Affective disorders may also occur either as part of the disease process or as a reaction to developing the disease, and thus suicide is a risk. Erratic behaviour may lead to psychiatric referral, or rarely a frank schizophrenic-like psychosis may develop. As the disease progresses, weight loss is commonly seen, cognitive deficits become more pronounced and chorea more severe, with walking, speech, and dexterity all impaired. In the later stages of the disease, many patients lose their chorea and develop increasing rigidity and akinesia, with dementia. Finally the patient becomes bedridden and death occurs about 15 to 20 years from the onset.

Huntington's disease presenting under the age of 21 (so-called juvenile Huntington's disease) often manifests with an akinetic–rigid parkinsonian syndrome without chorea (the Westphal variant), and with major behavioural problems.

Diagnosis

Despite the diverse clinical manifestations of Huntington's disease, with genetic testing the diagnosis is now straightforward although careful thought needs to be given to conducting such a test, given the widespread implications to the family and patient. However, in some cases the characteristics of the disease are not obvious and a family history is not available, which can mean that the diagnosis is overlooked (see Table 24.7.3.2).

Treatment

There is currently no cure for Huntington's disease. Drugs that modify the dopaminergic system are helpful in treating the chorea and include tetrabenazine, sulpiride, and some of the newer atypical neuroleptic drugs, such as olanzapine. Other drugs may be required for psychiatric symptoms including selective serotonin reuptake inhibitors (SSRIs) for depression, atypical neuroleptics for psychotic symptoms, and carbamazepine and sodium valproate as mood stabilizers.

A recent intervention in Huntington's disease has involved the use of neurotropic factors, such as ciliary neurotropic factor, as well as neuroprotective therapies (e.g. coenzyme Q); the benefits of these measures are uncertain. Surgical treatment for chorea is poorly documented but there has been increasing interest in the possibility of neural transplantation and deep brain stimulation in Huntington's disease.

Sooner or later respite care is required for patients with Huntington's disease. A multidisciplinary approach, including physiotherapy and dietary advice (including gastrostomy for feeding), is important, together with expert help with issues such as living wills.

Genetic testing

Predictive testing programmes are now available for individuals at risk, provided by multidisciplinary teams specializing in this condition and often directed by an experienced neurogeneticist. A nationally agreed testing protocol ensures consistency of approach.

Sydenham's chorea

Aetiology

Chorea (St Vitus's dance) associated with psychological disturbance due to rheumatic fever (rheumatic chorea) in childhood and adolescence was first described by Thomas Sydenham in 1686. Sydenham's chorea was associated with many streptococcal infections, but it is now most frequently associated with acute rheumatic fever, and as a result is rare in most parts of the world. The mechanism is thought to be antibody mediated, against epitopes within structures of the basal ganglia, which would help explain the characteristic radiological lesions seen within the basal ganglia of some affected patients. Antineural antibodies have been isolated in cases of Sydenham's chorea as well as a range of related paediatric neuropsychiatric conditions (paediatric autoimmune neuropsychiatric disorders associated with streptococci—PANDAS) and may result from cross-reactivity with elements of group A streptococcal membranes, although the pathogenic nature of these antibodies has not been demonstrated unequivocally. The nosology of PANDAS remains a contentious issue.

Symptoms

About three-quarters of cases occur between the ages of 7 and 12 years. The onset is usually gradual, but may be abrupt. The initial symptoms are often psychological, with irritability, agitation, disobedience, and inattentiveness with a frank organic confusional state occurring in about 10% of patients. Generalized chorea then appears and may worsen for a few weeks; speech is impaired in about a third of patients. The chorea is predominantly unilateral in about 20% of patients, and in severe cases is accompanied by flaccidity and subjective weakness (chorea mollis). Although cardiac disease may be found, the child usually has no fever or other manifestations of rheumatic fever.

The chorea and psychological disturbance recover over 1 to 3 months, rarely up to 6 months, but recurrences occur in about a quarter of patients over the next 2 years. Approximately a third of patients will show evidence of rheumatic cardiac involvement at the time of the illness, and about the same proportion later develop chronic rheumatic heart disease. Women who have suffered one or more attacks of Sydenham's chorea are at particular risk of developing chorea in adult life during pregnancy (chorea gravidarum), or when exposed to drugs including oral contraceptives, digoxin, or phenytoin. Although usually self-limiting, more persistent neurological deficits occasionally occur in Sydenham's chorea.

Treatment

Treatment as for rheumatic fever is necessary. The chorea may be controlled with dopamine D_2-receptor blocking agents such as sulpiride or haloperidol, or dopamine depletors such as tetrabenazine. A course of penicillin should be given, and prophylactic oral penicillin should be continued until about the age of 20 years to prevent further streptococcal infection.

Hemiballism (hemichorea)

Hemiballism refers to wild flinging or throwing movements of the arms and legs. These movements, similar to those of chorea, are irregular in timing and force, but involve the large proximal muscles of the shoulder and pelvic girdles. The occasional child or adolescent with Sydenham's chorea may present with hemiballism, but the syndrome usually occurs in older hypertensive and/or diabetic patients as the result of a stroke. The vascular lesion is classically said to involve the subthalamic nucleus, although more often than not lesions at other anatomical sites are found (e.g. Forel fields). It may appear as the hemiplegic weakness improves, when it is often accompanied by thalamic pain, although in other patients the hemiballism appears abruptly without weakness or sensory deficit. The intensity of the movements varies from mild to a severity that causes injury and requires urgent treatment.

Hemiballism due to stroke usually remits over 3 to 6 months often via a choreic phase, as the severity of the movements lessens. Treatment with haloperidol or tetrabenazine may control the hemiballism until recovery occurs, but interventional neurosurgery is occasionally required and may be beneficial.

Tremor

Three types are generally recognized—static, postural, and action tremors (Box 24.7.3.3).

1 Static tremor occurs when a relaxed limb is fully supported at rest.

2 Postural tremor appears when a part of the body is maintained in a fixed position and may also persist during movement.

3 Kinetic or action tremor occurs specifically during active voluntary movement of a body part. If the amplitude of such an action tremor increases as goal-directed movement approaches its target, this is an intention tremor.

Psychogenic tremors are generally rare. They are often of sudden onset with a variable but rarely remitting clinical course and typically affect the trunk or limb with standing and/or using the limb respectively. Psychogenic tremors are often distractible and can be entrained (i.e. the psychogenic tremor assumes the same frequency as a voluntary contralateral movement).

Psychogenic tremors

Physiological tremor has a frequency in the 7- to 11-Hz band and is typically symptomatic in states of increased sympathetic nervous activity and increased by stimulation of peripheral β_2-adrenergic receptors in muscle. The fine postural tremors associated with stress and anxiety states along with thyrotoxicosis fall into this category and usually respond to β-adrenergic-blocking drugs. Symptomatic postural tremors occur in association with many neurological disorders and can be shown to differ from physiological tremor by frequency analysis.

Essential (familial) tremor

Aetiology

This condition, which is characterized by postural tremor of the arms and head, can present at any age, although it is usually in early adult life. It is slowly progressive, generally causes mild disability, and is not associated with dystonia or parkinsonism. Its cause is

---

> **Box 24.7.3.3** Classification and types of tremor
>
> **Static or rest tremor**
> - Parkinson's disease
> - Parkinsonism (including drug induced, postencephalitic)
> - Other extrapyramidal diseases
> - Multiple sclerosis
>
> **Postural tremor**
> - Physiological tremor
> - Exaggerated physiological tremor, as in:
>   - Thyrotoxicosis
>   - Anxiety states
>   - Alcohol
>   - Drugs (e.g. sympathomimetics, antidepressants, sodium valproate, lithium)
>   - Heavy metal poisoning (i.e. mercury—the 'hatter's shakes')
> - Structural neurological disease, as in:
>   - Severe cerebellar lesions ('Holmes tremor')
>   - Wilson's disease
>   - Neurosyphilis
>   - Peripheral neuropathies (usually demyelinating)
> - Essential (familial) tremor
> - Task-specific tremors (e.g. primary writing tremor)
>
> **Kinetic or action (including intention) tremor**
> - Brainstem or cerebellar disease, as in:
>   - Multiple sclerosis
>   - Spinocerebellar degenerations
>   - Vascular disease
>   - Tumours

unknown although a positive family history is obtained in over half of such patients with a pattern of inheritance that indicates an autosomal dominant trait. Specific genes for essential tremor have not been identified yet, but susceptibility loci have been located to chromosomes 2p22 and 3q13.

No pathological or biochemical abnormality has been identified in essential tremor, although few patients have come to postmortem examination. Recent findings suggest pathological heterogeneity, with fusiform Purkinje axonal swellings in some patients' brains and extranigral Lewy bodies in other cases. Essential tremor is usually of a frequency of 5 to 8 Hz (Fig. 24.7.3.6) and has its origins in circuits of abnormal activation involving the cerebellum, red nucleus, and thalamus.

Symptoms

Tremor is present in one or both hands on maintaining a posture, as when holding a cup or glass. Handwriting becomes untidy and tremulous (Fig. 24.7.3.7). There is no tremor at rest, but a rhythmic

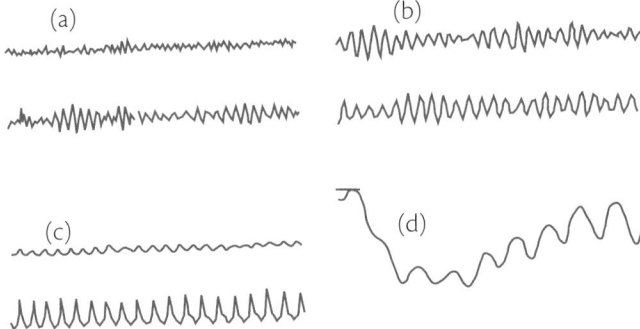

Fig. 24.7.3.6 Recordings of tremor with accelerometers placed on the right arm (above) and the left arm (below) in (a) a patient with enhanced physiological tremor of the outstretched arms (frequency 9–10 Hz), (b) a patient with benign essential tremor with the arms outstretched (frequency 7 Hz), (c) a patient with left-sided Parkinson's disease at rest (frequency 5 Hz), and (d) a patient with severe cerebellar disease and marked intention tremor when attempting to touch his nose with the right hand (frequency 2–3 Hz). All recordings are of 4 s duration. (Courtesy of Dr M Gresty.)

oscillation develops when the patient holds the arms outstretched. On movement, as in finger–nose testing, the tremor continues but does not get strikingly worse, as is the case with cerebellar intention tremor. Tremor of the head (titubation) and jaw is present in about 50% of cases, and tremor of the legs occurs in about a third. Despite the tremor, tests of coordination are usually normal, walking is unaffected, and there are no other neurological abnormalities. In some longstanding cases of essential tremor, however, mild gait ataxia and cognitive impairments have been reported.

In many patients with essential tremor small or moderate doses of alcohol may suppress the tremor, although this is highly variable and is not pathognomonic for the condition. The illness is static or only slowly progressive in most patients, causing predominantly a social disability. Individuals dependent on a manual skill may be disabled.

Other variants of the syndrome are occasionally encountered. Thus isolated, inherited head tremor may occur, with either 'yes–yes' or 'no–no' movements, and tremulous 'writer's cramp' (primary writing tremor) is recognized. Tremor of the legs on

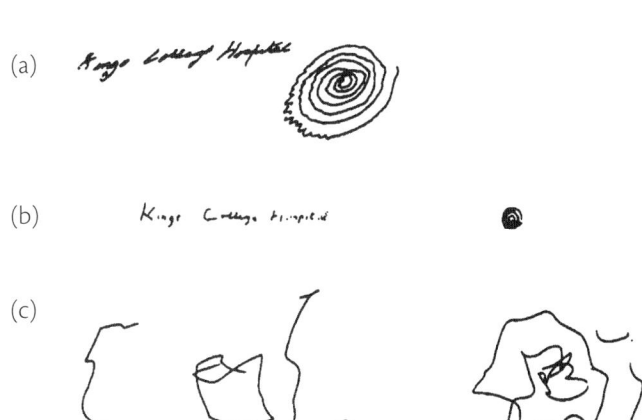

Fig. 24.7.3.7 Samples of handwriting and spiral drawings from (a) a 50-year-old woman with benign essential tremor, (b) a 38-year-old man with Parkinson's disease, and (c) a 20-year-old man with torsion dystonia (who attempts to write COLLEGE).

standing (orthostatic tremor) may occur as an isolated syndrome (primary orthostatic tremor of Heilman, high frequency 13–18 Hz) or in the context of essential tremor (5–8 Hz).

Treatment
Although alcohol may suppress the tremor effectively, and can be of value if used wisely, there is a risk of patients developing alcohol problems. Up to 50% of patients respond satisfactorily to a β-adrenergic receptor antagonist such as propranolol (up to a dose of 240 mg/day). Primidone, in standard anticonvulsant dosages, also helps some individuals but is associated with major sedative side effects and nausea at initiation. Benzodiazepines, such as clonazepam, may give some relief but are associated with tachyphylaxis. More recently gabapentin and topiramate have been shown to be of benefit in some cases. Stereotaxic thalamotomy or deep brain stimulation of the thalamus may be required in the very small number of patients whose tremor is severe.

Tics

Tics occur in several disorders (Table 24.7.3.3) and are defined as simple or complex. A simple tic is a sudden, rapid, twitch-like movement always of the same nature and at the same site, and occurs in about a quarter of all children, disappearing within a year or so (transient tic of childhood). Sometimes these persist into adult life, but are rarely considered as abnormal (chronic simple tic) such that only a minority seek assistance. Tics that are more widespread and severe, and take the form of complicated stereotyped patterns of motor action, are termed 'complex tics'.

Characteristically, complex and simple tics can be suppressed voluntarily although this causes mounting inner tension, which can be relieved only by expression of the tics. Complex multiple tics accompanied by vocal utterances, particularly swear words (coprolalia), and compulsive thoughts constitute Gilles de la Tourette's syndrome, which is an organic cerebral disease of unknown aetiology.

Gilles de la Tourette's syndrome
Aetiology
George Gilles de la Tourette described the syndrome of chronic multiple tics with vocalizations in 1885. It has been speculated that Mozart and Samuel Johnson may have been afflicted by Gilles de la Tourette's syndrome. The condition appears to be inherited as an autosomal dominant trait, with variable penetrance and so in affected families the genetic abnormality may be expressed as the full syndrome, as chronic multiple tics alone, or as an obsessive–compulsive neurosis (see below). Although the cause of this condition is unknown, the basal ganglia are believed to be involved because abnormalities within the striatum have been detected

Table 24.7.3.3 Tics

Simple tics	Transient tic of childhood
	Chronic simple tic
Multiple tics	Chronic multiple tics
	Gilles de la Tourette's syndrome
Symptomatic tics	Encephalitis lethargica
	Drug-induced tics
	Neuroacanthocytosis

using functional imaging with some subtle abnormalities within the caudate and pallidum being reported post mortem in a few cases. Furthermore, drugs acting on the basal ganglia, such as sulpiride, may control the symptoms.

Symptoms

The illness usually begins between the ages of 5 and 15 years, with multiple involuntary repetitive muscular tics that vary in site, number, frequency, and severity with time. It is more common in boys, by a factor of approximately three to one. Tics particularly affect the upper part of the body, especially the face, neck, and shoulders, more than the limbs and trunk. Typical initial symptoms are eye blinking, head nodding, sniffing, or stuttering. With time other more complex tics affecting other parts of the body appear. The motor tics are often preceded by a sensory urge (sometimes called a sensory tic), and they can be controlled, albeit temporarily, by an effort of will. Eventually, however, the patient has to 'let the tics go'.

Sooner or later, most patients with multiple tics make involuntary noises, such as grunting, squealing, yelping, sniffing, or barking. Indeed, the coexistence of such noises with multiple tics is an essential feature of Gilles de la Tourette's syndrome. In about 60% of cases the noises become transformed into swear words (coprolalia). About a third of patients also exhibit echolalia—an involuntary tendency to repeat words or sentences just spoken to them. A smaller proportion of patients also exhibit copropraxia (involuntary obscene gesturing) and echopraxia (involuntary imitation of the movements of others), as well as palilalia (involuntary repetition of their own words or sounds).

Many patients with Gilles de la Tourette's syndrome also exhibit features of an obsessive–compulsive disorder. These psychiatric manifestations of the condition may be even more disabling than the tics. A hyperactive attentional disorder is common in children.

Once established, Gilles de la Tourette's syndrome is usually lifelong, although its severity waxes and wanes. A small proportion of cases, probably fewer than 1 in 20, experience spontaneous remission of symptoms after adolescence, but in most the multiple tics and the vocalizations persist, although they usually become less prominent in adults. No other neurological abnormality develops; intellect and motor coordination are retained.

Tics secondary to other illnesses need to be excluded. As there is no imaging or genetic test yet available, the diagnosis of Gilles de la Tourette's syndrome relies on the recognition of the clinical phenotype.

Treatment

The multiple tics and the vocalizations of coprolalia cause considerable distress, social isolation, and psychological harm. Neuroleptic drugs such as sulpiride or pimozide may satisfactorily control tics, noises, and coprolalia. Tetrabenazine may also be considered. The effective dose requires careful and gradual titration because there is risk of side effects, especially the emergence of parkinsonism, depression, and tardive dyskinesia after months or years of therapy (see below). As treatment must usually be for life, the harm must be carefully balanced against the need for any form of therapy. The obsessive–compulsive symptoms of the illness may improve with drugs such as clomipramine or fluoxetine. Previously, in extreme cases psychosurgery has been undertaken with limbic leucotomies. More recently, severe cases have been treated using deep brain stimulation, although the optimal target is not yet known.

Myoclonus

Myoclonus, characterized by its sudden 'shock-like' nature, is a feature of many neurological diseases and can be classified according to its aetiology (Box 24.7.3.4).

Generalized or multifocal myoclonus can occur in four clinical settings:

1 as the solitary feature of the illness (essential myoclonus)

2 as a dominant feature of a progressive brain disease (progressive myoclonic encephalopathy)

3 as a residual feature of some transient brain insult (static myoclonic encephalopathy)

4 as a feature of obvious epilepsy (myoclonic epilepsy).

Benign essential myoclonus

This condition is a heterogeneous disorder and at its core consists of widespread myoclonus affecting all four limbs, trunk, neck, and face, occurring at about 10 to 50/min, enhanced by action and sensory stimuli, often in the context of a positive family history.

Box 24.7.3.4 Myoclonus

- Generalized myoclonus
- Essential myoclonus
- Progressive myoclonic encephalopathies[a]
  - With demonstrable metabolic cause (e.g. Lafora's body disease, mitochondrial encephalomyopathy)
  - Hereditary myoclonus with no known metabolic cause (e.g. familial myoclonic epilepsy (Unverricht–Lundborg disease))
  - Other sporadic diseases (e.g. subacute sclerosing panencephalitis, Creutzfeldt–Jakob disease, Alzheimer's disease)
  - Metabolic myoclonus (e.g. portosystemic encephalopathy, CO_2 narcosis, etc.)
- Static myoclonic encephalopathies[b] (e.g. postanoxic action myoclonus (Lance–Adams syndrome)
- Myoclonic epilepsies[c]
- Focal myoclonus
- Spinal myoclonus (secondary to spinal cord lesion, e.g. demyelination)
- Propriospinal myoclonus
- Palatal myoclonus (lesions of dentatorubro-olivary tract)
- Ocular myoclonus
- Hemifacial spasm
- Cortical myoclonus
- Epilepsia partialis continua

[a] Obvious myoclonus (with or without seizures), clearly as part of a progressive encephalopathy.
[b] Obvious myoclonus after some acute and now static cerebral insult.
[c] Obvious epilepsy as the main problem, with myoclonus.

Onset is usually in childhood or adolescence, but disability is strikingly mild, there is no progression, intellect is normal, fits do not occur, and no other deficit appears. Some patients have dystonia with their myoclonus, so-called myoclonic dystonia, and they often report that alcohol helps their jerks. Some of these patients have genetic abnormalities in the ε-sarcoglycan gene.

Progressive myoclonic encephalopathies

Most of the diseases causing a progressive myoclonic encephalopathy are described in detail elsewhere, particularly the lysosomal storage disorders and other metabolic disorders as well as the spinocerebellar degenerations. A discussion of other associated conditions lies outside the scope of this chapter.

Static myoclonic encephalopathies: postanoxic action myoclonus (Lance–Adams syndrome)

This is a distinct entity that may appear after a period of cerebral anoxia, typically respiratory arrests in the context of an acute asthmatic attack. After recovery of consciousness, such patients exhibit muscle jerks affecting the face, trunk, and limbs, often provoked by sensory stimuli, and strikingly elicited by willed voluntary action. This can affect walking, with negative myoclonus causing them to collapse as they lose the tone in their leg muscles. The condition has been associated with abnormalities of brain 5-hydroxytryptamine, as 5-hydroxytryptophan produces a marked improvement in some patients. However, the side effects of this therapy, in particular the development of the eosinophilia myalgia syndrome, have meant that other treatments such as clonazepam, piracetam, and sodium valproate are more commonly used.

Myoclonic epilepsies

In the myoclonic epilepsies, epileptic seizures are the obvious and dominant feature of the condition. There is some confusion in separating the many conditions that may cause this syndrome, which occurs particularly in children. A convenient, if arbitrary, distinction is based on the age of onset and is discussed in more detail in the section on epilepsy.

Focal myoclonus

There are a number of conditions in which myoclonic muscle jerking may be restricted to one part of the body. Some pathological processes may cause focal myoclonus limited to those segments innervated by the part of the brainstem or spinal cord affected (segmental myoclonus). Palatal myoclonus or tremor, with rhythmic contractions of the palate and clicking sounds in the ear, can be symptomatic with a lesion found within a triangle bounded by the inferior olive, dentate nucleus of the cerebellum, and red nucleus in the midbrain (Mollaret's triangle). Sometimes this spreads to the pharynx and larynx, and speech is disturbed; the ocular muscles may be involved. Similar pathologies causing cerebral damage, particularly to the cerebral cortex, may cause rhythmic repetitive focal muscle jerking associated with electrical evidence of epileptic cortical discharge in the electroencephalogram (EEG) (epilepsia partialis continua).

Spinal myoclonus

Repetitive, often rhythmic, myoclonic jerking restricted to a limb, or even to a few muscles of an arm or leg, may occur with myelitis, spinal cord tumour or angioma, or after spinal cord trauma.

The rhythmic muscle jerking occurs spontaneously, at 20 to 180/min, is not affected by peripheral stimuli, often persists in sleep, and is not associated with any change in the EEG. Anticonvulsants may help, but such segmental myoclonus is often very difficult to control.

Epilepsia partialis continua

Encephalitis, tumour, abscess, infarct, haemorrhage, or trauma to the cerebral cortex may rarely cause repetitive, rhythmic muscle jerking once or twice a second, confined to one collection of muscles, persisting even in sleep for days, weeks, or months. Usually the damage involves not only the cerebral cortex, but also deeper structures including the thalamus. As a result of its large cortical representations, the most common site of epilepsia partialis continua is the hand. Typical jacksonian focal motor fits, and grand mal seizures may also occur in such patients. The surface EEG usually shows a spike discharge over the opposite motor cortex preceding each jerk by a short interval. Treatment is with anticonvulsants, but may be difficult.

Hemifacial spasm

Hemifacial spasm occurs at a frequency of about 1 in 100 000 people and most commonly affects middle-aged or older women, and usually appears without obvious cause. Rarely, it may be symptomatic of demonstrable facial nerve compression. The condition consists of irregular, but repetitive, clonic twitching of the muscles of one side of the face. Usually those around the eyes are first involved, producing a feeling identical to the benign myokymia of the lower eyelid, which occurs in normal people when fatigued. However, the repetitive twitching spreads slowly to involve the whole face, each spasm closing the eye and drawing up the corner of the mouth. At this stage, a mild facial weakness and contraction become evident, but a frank facial palsy never develops. Facial sensation is normal and there are no other physical signs in idiopathic hemifacial spasm. The disorder is so distinctive and unilateral that it is rarely confused with other conditions. True facial myokymia, due to brainstem tumour or demyelination, consists of a continuous rippling contraction of the facial muscles, giving the appearance of a 'bag of worms'.

Treatment with drugs is usually unrewarding. Posterior fossa exploration, with separation of blood vessels from nerve VII, gives long-lasting relief and failure, when it occurs, is normally evident within the first few months after surgery. However, injection of botulinum toxin into the facial muscles, repeated every 3 to 4 months, is a simpler and effective treatment.

Other movement disorders

Restless legs syndrome (Ekböm's syndrome)

This is a common and poorly understood condition in which patients have a desire to move their extremities often in association with paraesthesiae and dysaesthesiae. This is made worse by rest and so is often mainly present at the end of the day and at night, and is relieved by activity such as walking around. It is commonly associated with periodic limb movements during sleep. In some cases there is a family history suggestive of an autosomal dominant inheritance. The aetiology of the condition is unknown, although subtle abnormalities in the dopaminergic and opioidergic systems have been demonstrated using functional imaging, although genetic studies have shown linkage to several regions. It is thought to be due to abnormal cerebellar and thalamic activation. Secondary restless legs syndrome occurs with peripheral neuropathies, uraemia, pregnancy, iron deficiency, rheumatoid arthritis, and spinal cord lesions as well as in Parkinson's disease. It responds best to the treatment of the underlying cause or in idiopathic cases to low-dose dopamine agonists.

Stiff person syndrome

This term includes a range of rare conditions that are characterized by muscle rigidity with or without spasms. The stiff person syndrome itself is characterized by axial rigidity involving the paraspinal muscles, which leads to a hyperlordotic posture of the back and an abnormal gait often described as 'walking through treacle'. Muscle spasms in response to sensory stimuli with an exaggerated startle response are common. The patients characteristically have antiglutamic acid decarboxylase (anti-GAD) antibodies, which may account for the high incidence of diabetes mellitus and other autoimmune disorders in this condition. Treatment is usually with baclofen and diazepam, although clonazepam, sodium valproate, and vigabatrin have all been used successfully. Immunosuppressive therapy may benefit some patients, especially intravenous immunoglobulin.

It can occasionally occur as a paraneoplastic syndrome when the antibodies are often against a different epitope to GAD.

Hyperekplexia

Startle is a stereotypical, developmentally protective response that involves a complex series of movements including eye closure, facial grimacing, and a typical body posture. In certain conditions it is exaggerated, and termed 'hyperekplexia'. It can be seen in a number of disorders and with a range of central nervous system lesions as well as occurring in isolation. In some cases the condition is inherited in an autosomal dominant fashion, and in these cases mutations in the glycine receptor are commonly found. In general symptoms respond to clonazepam.

Orthostatic tremor

This condition is rare and affects the legs when standing, although leg tremor can be seen in other conditions such as Parkinson's disease and essential tremor. The characteristic feature of this type of tremor is that it occurs when standing still and is relieved by moving or sitting down. The patients describe a sense of unsteadiness when standing still (e.g. in queues) such that they feel that they are going to topple only. In some patients the tremor can be heard by listening over the thigh muscles where the 15–18 Hz oscillations produce a noise akin to the sound of distant helicopters. The condition typically is idiopathic and responses best to clonazepam, gabapentin, and dopaminergic drugs.

Psychogenic movement disorders

A whole variety of movement disorders can be generated as part of a psychogenic illness of which the most common is dystonia. This can be very difficult to diagnose and treat because there is often no clear psychopathology and patients with movement disorders quite often have associated psychiatric problems consequent on their primary neurological problem. The diagnosis of psychogenic movement disorders should therefore be undertaken with great care. Useful clues are a history of unexplained medical problems and an inconsistency and variability of the abnormal movement during the consultation, especially during tasks designed to distract the patient. In addition, if the movement disorder involves an odd combination of body parts, that may suggest that it is more likely to be psychogenic in origin. However, none of these rules is absolute and many movement disorders normally show great variability, so all patients with a movement disorder should be investigated and this diagnosis is often one of exclusion made in tertiary referral centres.

Drug-induced movement disorders

The extensive use of antipsychotic neuroleptic drugs has led to much iatrogenic extrapyramidal disease. These drugs, all of which block dopamine receptors in the basal ganglia and elsewhere, are used widely to control acute psychotic behaviour, whatever its cause, and to prevent relapse of schizophrenia. Similar classes of drugs are employed as antiemetics, and to treat vertigo. The major neurological complications of these drug therapies are summarized in Table 24.7.3.4.

Akathisia refers to an irresistible and unpleasant sensation of motor restlessness, and the inability to sit or stand still, all of which may be mistaken for a recurrence of psychotic behaviour. Akathisia remits if the offending neuroleptic is withdrawn, or if the dose can be reduced sufficiently: it does not usually respond to anticholinergic drugs, but may be helped by a benzodiazepine or propranolol.

Table 24.7.3.4 Drug-induced extrapyramidal disease

Disorder	Drugs responsible	Susceptible age group	Incidence	Onset after initiation of therapy	Effect of withdrawal of drug	Treatment
Tremor	Bronchodilators, tricyclics, lithium carbonate, caffeine, SSRIs	Any	Dose-dependent, about 35%	Rapid	Disappears	Withdraw drug
Parkinsonism	Reserpine, tetrabenazine, neuroleptics, sodium valproate	Any but increases with age	Dose dependent, about 50%	Gradual, within first months	Disappears slowly, may take a year	Anticholinergics
Acute dystonia	Neuroleptics,	Children, young adults	2–5%	Acute, within first few hours or days	Disappears	Anticholinergics, diazepam
Akathisia	Neuroleptics	Any	About 30%	Gradual, within first months	Disappears	Anticholinergics
Tardive dyskinesia	Neuroleptics	Increases with age	20–40%	Delayed, but increases	May get worse; persists in about 40%	Withdraw drug, tetrabenazine

SSRIs, selective serotonin reuptake inhibitors.

Anticholinergic drugs have long been used to treat drug-induced parkinsonism if the causative neuroleptic has to be continued for psychiatric reasons, although anticholinergics are not routinely administered to those on neuroleptics. There is no good evidence that co-administration of anticholinergic drugs is 'protective' against drug-induced parkinsonism.

Acute dystonic reactions commonly include oculogyric crises, trismus, neck retraction, or torticollis, and may be mistaken for tetanus or meningitis. Although uncommon, acute dystonic reactions pose a repeated diagnostic problem in accident and emergency departments. Such reactions rapidly disappear after intravenous injection of an anticholinergic drug such as procyclidine or a benzodiazepine.

Tardive dyskinesias are the most serious of the drug-induced movement disorders because they usually persist despite drug withdrawal, or emerge as the offending agent is stopped (tardive emergent dyskinesia). About 20% of those receiving chronic neuroleptic therapy will develop tardive dyskinesia. The characteristic syndrome is one of orofacial stereotypical movements, with lip smacking and tongue protrusion, accompanied by trunk rocking and distal chorea of the hands and feet. In younger patients the picture may be dominated by axial and cranial dystonia (tardive dystonia), a condition that is largely refractory to treatment although is less likely to occur if the offending drug is discontinued within 5 years of being instituted.

Tardive dyskinesias usually appear after at least 6 months' neuroleptic drug therapy, and their incidence increases with exposure to the drugs and also with the age of the patients. Some of the more recent 'atypical' antipsychotic drugs have less of a propensity to cause this condition, presumably through their reduced dopamine D_2-receptor blocking actions. After drug withdrawal, tardive dyskinesias disappear in about 60% or more of patients over the next 3 years, but continue unaltered in the remainder. They are difficult to treat and, although the offending agent ideally should be stopped, this is often not possible. Anticholinergic drugs tend to worsen orobuccolingual dyskinesia, but may relieve tardive dystonia. Baclofen may help some patients. Deep brain stimulation of the globus pallidus may be of benefit in severe and refractory cases.

Other drugs that cause dyskinesias include levodopa in patients with Parkinson's disease. It seems likely that most such drug-induced dyskinesias are due to pharmacological effects on dopamine mechanisms in the basal ganglia, resulting in nonphysiological stimulation of the dopaminergic receptors, in contrast to the akinetic–rigid syndrome produced by dopamine depletion or blockade.

Further reading

General

Marsden CD, Fahn S (eds) (1982). *Movement disorders*, vol. I. Butterworth, London.

Marsden CD, Fahn S (eds) (1987). *Movement disorders*, vol. II. Butterworth, London.

Marsden CD, Fahn S (eds) (1994). *Movement disorders*, vol. III. Butterworth, London.

Watts RL, Koller WC (1997). *Movement disorders. Neurologic principles and practice*. McGraw-Hill, New York.

Dystonia

Berardelli A, *et al.* (1998). The pathophysiology of primary dystonia. *Brain*, **121**, 1195–212.

Dauer WT, *et al.* (1998). Current concepts on the clinical features, aetiology and management of idiopathic cervical dystonia. *Brain*, **121**, 547–60.

Nygaard TG, Wooten GF (1998). Dopa-responsive dystonia. *Neurology*, **50**, 853–5.

Bressman S (2006). Genetics of dystonia. *J Neural Transm*, **70** Suppl, 489–95.

Chorea

Cardoso F, *et al.* (2006). Seminar on choreas. *Lancet Neurol*, **5**, 589–602.

Harper PS, Bates GP, Jones L (2001). *Huntington's disease*, 3rd edition. Oxford University Press, Oxford.

Nausieda PA, *et al.* (1980). Sydenham's chorea: an update. *Neurology*, **30**, 331–4.

Walker OF (2007). Huntington's disease. *Lancet*, **369**, 218–28.

Vidakovic A, Dragasevic N, Kostic VS (1994). Hemiballism: report of 25 cases. *J Neurol Neurosurg Psychiatry*, **57**, 945–9.

Tremor

Bain P (1993). A combined clinical and neurophysiological approach to the study of patients with tremor. *J Neurol Neurosurg Psychiatry*, **69**, 839–44.

Benito-Leon J, Louis ED (2006). Essential tremor: emerging views of a common disorder. *Nat Clin Pract Neurol*, **2**, 666–78.

Elble RJ (1986). Physiological and essential tremor. *Neurology*, **36**, 225–31.

Hubble JP, Busenbark KL, Koller WC (1989). Essential tremor. *Clin Neuropharmacol*, **12**, 453–82.

Gerschalger W, *et al.* (2004). Natural history and syndromic associations of orthostatic tremor: A review of 41 cases. *Mov Disorders*, **19**, 788–95.

Myoclonus and tics

Brown P, *et al.* (1991). The hyperekplexias and their relationship to the normal startle reflex. *Brain*, **114**, 1903–28.

Fahn S, Marsden CD, Van Woert M (1986). Myoclonus. *Adv Neurol*, **43**, 1–709.

Pranzatelli MR (1994). Serotonin and human myoclonus. Rationale for the use of serotonin receptor agonists and antagonists. *Arch Neurol*, **51**, 605–17.

Rampello L, *et al.* (2006). Tic disorders: from pathophysiology to treatment. *J Neurol*, **253**, 1–15.

Other movement disorders

Bakker MJ, *et al.* (2006). Startle syndromes. *Lancet Neurol*, **5**, 513–24.

Barker RA, *et al.* (1998). Review of 23 patients affected by the stiff man syndrome: clinical subdivision into stiff trunk (man) syndrome, stiff limb syndrome and progressive encephalomyelitis with rigidity. *J Neurol Neurosurg Psychiatry*, **65**, 633–40.

Gershanik OS (1993). Drug-induced movement disorders. *Curr Opin Neurol Neurosurg*, **6**, 369–76.

24.7.4 Ataxic disorders

Nicholas Wood

Essentials

Ataxia is a feature of disorders of the cerebellum and its connections. It may be found in a large range of neurological conditions, in some of which it is the principal or main feature, but clinical assessment is complicated by the fact that few ataxic patients have disease restricted to the cerebellum alone.

Clinical features

Symptoms—common presenting complaints are (1) gait unsteadiness—particularly with lesions of the vermis, (2) limb incoordination and tremor—particularly with lesions of the cerebellar hemisphere, (3) slurring of speech, and (4) visual and oculomotor symptoms, although these are rare in pure cerebellar disease.

Signs—these include (1) a broad-based gait with a poor turn, (2) scanning dysarthria, (3) limb ataxia—manifest as dysmetria and dysdiadochokinesis, (4) intention tremor, (5) abnormal eye movements.

Key points in differential diagnosis—(1) age of onset—early onset is before 20 to 25 years; (2) rate of onset and the nature of the progression of the illness; (3) other features of neurological involvement, which enables differentiation of the 'pure' ataxias from the 'complicated' ataxias.

Investigation and treatment—high-resolution imaging, genetic testing and other investigative tools enable a diagnosis to be made in over 50% of cases. The mainstay of management is supportive: there are no drugs that help cerebellar balance problems, but active engagement in physiotherapy can help to lessen the impact of the physical disorder.

Particular causes of ataxia

Ataxias with early onset—(1) acute and subacute ataxias with onset in childhood—should raise the possibility of infectious, parainfectious or vascular conditions; (2) chronic progressive ataxias of early onset—very often genetic in aetiology, typically autosomal recessive, with the commonest cause being Friedreich's ataxia; a clear molecular genetic diagnosis can be established in some cases (e.g. abnormality of the frataxin gene in Friedreich's ataxia).

Chronic progressive ataxia—causes include (1) genetic—with inheritance typically being autosomal dominant; (2) chronic alcohol abuse—probably the most common cause of progressive cerebellar degeneration in adults; (3) deficiency disorders—e.g. vitamin E; (4) toxic agents—drugs (e.g. phenytoin), solvents and heavy metals; (5) structural lesions in the posterior fossa; and (6) other—e.g. Wilson's disease, other metabolic disorders. No cause can be found in many cases, labelled as 'idiopathic late-onset cerebellar ataxia', with the commonest pattern recognized being that of multiple system atrophy, where there is typically ataxia complicated by autonomic failure and (in some cases) Parkinsonism.

Rapid, subacute onset ataxia—should always raise the possibility of paraneoplastic or other inflammatory conditions.

Acute ataxia—the two main causes are (1) cerebellar haemorrhage—usually associated with headache, vertigo, vomiting, altered consciousness and neck stiffness; and (2) cerebellar infarction—in which cerebellar signs are usually combined with signs of brainstem ischaemia.

Introduction

The term 'ataxia' derived from the Greek means 'irregularity' or 'disorderliness'. Unsteadiness can result from a number of causes, including poor vision, impairment of postural reflexes, or a deficiency of sensory input, i.e. sensory ataxia. This chapter is devoted to the symptoms, signs, and pathological and clinical features of the disorders of the cerebellum (and its connections). There are two basic clinical rules that can be applied: (1) lesions of the vermis generally cause ataxia of midline structure (i.e. truncal and gait ataxia); and (2) output from the cerebellar hemisphere is to the contralateral cerebral hemisphere, which provides output to the contralateral limbs, so cerebellar hemisphere lesions are ipsilateral. It should, however, be noted that clinical assessment is complicated by the fact that few patients with ataxia have disease restricted to the cerebellum alone; there is often additional pathology in the brainstem, spinal cord, or elsewhere.

Symptoms of ataxic disorders

The history is critical for eliciting the most common presenting complaints: gait unsteadiness or slurring of speech. On direct enquiry many patients all admit to receiving 'jokes' or accusations of being drunk by acquaintances. The joke tends to wear thin. Some refer to 'giddiness' or 'dizziness' when they really mean unsteadiness of gait without associated vertigo or light-headedness. A particular note in the history of the age, speed of onset, and development of other features may indicate the cause. Rate of progress and any precipitating or relieving factors should also be noted. There has been a prodigious improvement in our understanding of the genetic basis of many ataxia disorders and a detailed family history is paramount (see Chapter 24.17).

Disturbances of gait

Disturbed gait is the most frequent presenting feature in ataxic disorders. Patients may report an inability to walk in a straight line and a tendency to collide with objects that others are able to avoid. If the symptoms are exaggerated in darkness, a sensory ataxia and involvement of the proprioceptive pathways may be present. Sudden changes of direction are particularly difficult. The duration of the gait disturbance should be established and it is worth asking about early motor milestones and athletic ability at school which may bring out a much longer history than previously appreciated. Collateral history should be sought, especially if an insidious onset is suspected. A question as to diurnal variation, particularly a history of morning unsteadiness that wears off later in the day, often associated with morning headache, suggests raised intracranial pressure, even if the examination is normal.

Limb incoordination and tremor

Clumsiness of the arms is often noted later in the course of the illness. Generally a tremor that is worse on action is reported and, as this worsens, patients notice clumsiness carrying objects and deterioration in their handwriting. Marked tremor is more common in multiple sclerosis than in degenerative disease. Disturbance to the midline structures may result in titubation and, in combination with action tremor in the upper limbs and only minor gait disturbance, should raise the suspicion of Wilson's disease.

Dysarthria

Abnormal speech may first be noted by friends and relatives. Classically described as having a staccato quality, this manifestation is a useful discriminatory feature against a purely sensory ataxia.

Visual and oculomotor symptoms

Visual symptoms are relatively rare in pure cerebellar disease and if present suggest brainstem disturbance, especially when there is episodic or persistent diplopia associated with ataxia. Vertical oscillopsia suggests downbeat nystagmus and a structural foramen magnum lesion should be suspected. Acute or subacute oscillopsia, with chaotic involuntary eye movements, may emerge from the history of patients with viral cerebellitis, paraneoplastic cerebellar degeneration, and the dancing eyes syndrome (opsoclonus). There are very rare degenerative ataxias associated with gradual visual loss, due to either optic neuropathy or retinopathy.

Other symptoms

Details of any headache or vomiting should be sought; their occurrence may suggest a posterior fossa mass lesion. If the history is acute then a vascular event, in particular a cerebellar haemorrhage, should be considered; a protracted course renders a tumour more likely. Ancillary signs of infection should raise the possibility of an abscess. Intermittent symptoms could indicate the presence of an episodic ataxia (see later) or, if found in the presence of malaise and fever, raise the possibility of posterior fossa cysticercosis. A history of vertigo is more suggestive of neoplastic, inflammatory, and vascular disease, than a slow degenerative process.

Direct questioning should explore the urinary system, skeletal deformities, cardiac disease and cognitive abilities, since many ataxias are associated with disease in other systems (Table 24.7.4.1).

A detailed enquiry into drug use (for both medical and recreational purposes, including alcohol) as well as occupational exposure to toxins is also required.

Signs of cerebellar disease

It is good practice to observe patients rising from a chair and shaking hands, and listening carefully to their speech. In the patient with ataxia this sequence provides much useful information about the disorder.

Gait and posture

The patient may have a broad-based gait, with a poor turn; there is often a lurching quality to the overall sequence. More detailed assessment of mild gait ataxia may be obtained by asking the patient to tandem walk (heel–toe). Asking the patient to stand still may reveal the broad base and also permits the assessment of proprioception using Romberg's test.

Speech

It is often stated that cerebellar speech is very distinctive with an explosive quality—the so-called scanning dysarthria. Although this

Table 24.7.4.1 Differential diagnosis of ataxic disorders: associated general physical signs

General physical signs	Differential diagnosis
Short stature	Mitochondrial encephalomyopathy, ataxia telangiectasia, Sjögren–Larsson syndrome, Cockayne's syndrome
Hypogonadism	Recessive ataxia with hypogonadism, ataxia telangiectasia, Sjögren-Larsson syndrome, mitochondrial encephalomyopathy, adrenoleukomyeloneuropathy
Skeletal deformity	Friedreich's ataxia, Sjögren–Larsson syndrome, many other early onset inherited ataxias, hereditary motor and sensory neuropathy
Immunodeficiency	Ataxia telangiectasia, multiple carboxylase deficiencies
Malnutrition	Vitamin E deficiency, alcoholic cerebellar degeneration
Hair	
Brittle	Argininosuccinic aciduria
Tight curls	Giant axonal neuropathy
Loss	Thallium poisoning, hypothyroidism, adrenoleukomyeloneuropathy
Low hairline	Foramen magnum lesions
Skin	
Telangiectases, particularly conjunctiva, nose, ears, flexures Extreme light sensitivity, tumours Pellagra-type rash Tendinous swellings Dry skin Pigmentation	Ataxia telangiectasia Xeroderma pigmentosum Hartnup's disease Cholestanolosis Hypothyroidism, Refsum's disease, Cockayne's syndrome Adrenoleukomyeloneuropathy
Eyes	
Kayser–Fleischer rings	Ataxia telangiectasia
Cataract	Telangiectasia
Aniridia	Wilson's disease Retinal angiomas in von-Hippel–Lindau disease Congenital rubella, cholestanolosis, Sjögren-Larsson syndrome Gillespie's syndrome
Fever	Abscess, viral cerebellitis, cysticercosis, dominant periodic ataxia, intermittent metabolic ataxias
	Haemorrhage, infarction, demyelination, posterior fossa mass lesions, intermittent metabolic ataxias
Hepatosplenomegaly	Niemann–Pick disease type C, some childhood metabolic ataxias, Wilson's disease, alcoholic cerebellar degeneration
Heart disease	
Cardiomegaly, murmurs, arrhythmias, late heart failure, abnormal ECG Conduction defects	Friedreich's ataxia Mitochondrial encephalomyopathy

is characteristic, a combination of cerebellar and spastic features is more frequent. Additional signs such as a slow moving tongue and brisk jaw jerk may confirm the spasticity.

Muscle tone

Some authorities state firmly that cerebellar disease gives rise to hypotonia, and some even include it within the symptoms. Not only do patients never complain of hypotonia, it is also rarely detectable in symmetrical, slowly progressive, or chronic disorders. Pendular knee jerks are also difficult to detect without the eye of faith; indeed, many patients with 'cerebellar' ataxic disorders have disease of the spinal cord, peripheral nerves, or both, which complicates the clinical picture.

Limb ataxia

Limb ataxia is usually assessed by seeking evidence of dysmetria and dysdiadochokinesis. Dysmetria refers to errors in the range and force of movement resulting in an erratic, jerky movement, which may under- or overshoot the target. This is most simply assessed using finger–nose and heel–shin tests. Dysdiadochokinesis is demonstrated by asking the patient to tap one hand on the other, alternately pronating and supinating the tapping hand, or rapidly opening and closing the fist. The tapping out of simple rhythms (with the hand or foot) is also useful for assessing both the rhythmicity and the force of the tap.

Traditionally, testing of coordination is undertaken after the motor and sensory tests because the presence of weakness or sensory loss can confuse the picture. It should be remembered that there is a natural asymmetry in cerebellar function, with better performance, particularly for rapid alternating movements, in the dominant limb. About 40% of patients with lesions of the cerebellar vermis do not have limb ataxia but have prominent gait ataxia.

Tremor

Intention tremor is present if a rhythmical side-to-side oscillation is seen on finger–nose testing. A combination of gross intention tremor and a postural component is often called rubral or red nucleus tremor, although peduncular tremor is probably a more accurate label. It is most commonly seen in multiple sclerosis and occasionally in late-onset degenerative ataxias. A nodding head tremor (titubation) with a frequency of 3 to 4 Hz may be seen with midline cerebellar disease.

Eye movements

It is very uncommon to find patients with cerebellar disease with a completely normal oculomotor examination. However, one may need to search hard for the abnormal signs.

In the primary position one should seek for the presence of square-wave jerks; these are inappropriate saccades that disrupt fixation and are followed by a corrective saccade within 200 ms. Assessment of pursuit usually reveals a jerkiness with saccadic intrusions. Additional isolated or multiple lesions of the cranial nerves III, IV, and VI suggest brainstem pathology. Examination of the saccadic system permits an assessment of saccadic initiation, velocity, and accuracy; the presence of an internuclear ophthalmoplegia may be found, indicated by slowness of an adducting eye, thus suggesting a diagnosis of multiple sclerosis, but can also rarely be associated with some degenerative ataxias. The vestibulo-ocular

reflex (doll's head manoeuvre) should then be used to investigate for any supranuclear component, because inability to suppress the reflex is evidence of pathology involving the vestibulocerebellum. Acute or subacute presentation of almost any of the above eye movements, especially if associated with alcohol abuse or vomiting, raises the possibility of Wernicke's encephalopathy—this requires urgent treatment with thiamine.

Gaze-evoked nystagmus is the most common type of nystagmus associated with cerebellar disease; eccentric gaze cannot be maintained, and the slow phase of the nystagmus is toward the primary position, with rapid corrective movements. Apart from down-beat nystagmus which may indicate a foramen magnum lesion, gaze evoked nystagmus is of limited localization value in most forms of ataxia. Positional nystagmus in a patient with vertigo and unsteadiness should be attributed to benign labyrinthine disease only if it is transient, torsional, and fatigable; if it does not have these features, a posterior fossa lesion should be suspected.

Other neurological signs and general examination

As the causes of ataxia are numerous, a large variety of other neurological and general physical signs may be found on examination. The range of these and their possible diagnostic significance is shown in Table 24.7.4.1.

Disorders of the cerebellum

Numerous conditions affect cerebellar function; several such as multiple sclerosis and neoplasia are discussed elsewhere. Here a classification is based on clinical characteristics.

Developmental disorders

The cerebellum has a long developmental period and is not fully mature until about 18 months of age. It is therefore susceptible to many insults, including intrauterine infections, ischaemic damage, toxins, and genetically determined syndromes (Table 24.7.4.2).

Table 24.7.4.2 Congenital inherited ataxic disorders (see also Chapter 24.17)

Syndrome	Genetics	Additional features
Joubert's syndrome	Autosomal recessive *AHI1* gene *NPHP1* gene *CEP290* Plus others with established and distinct loci	With episodic hyperpnoea, abnormal eye movements, and intellectual disability
Gillespie's syndrome	Uncertain inheritance No gene or locus known	With intellectual disability and partial aniridia
Congenital ataxia with intellectual disability and spasticity	Autosomal recessive, autosomal dominant, and X-linked NYS1—6p NYS2—X linked And others	Includes pontoneocerebellar and granule cell hypoplasia
Disequilibrium syndrome	Autosomal recessive	
Paine's syndrome	X-linked recessive ataxia— no gene identified	With spasticity, intellectual disability, and microcephaly

Some of these developmental anomalies, such as dysgenesis or agenesis of the vermis, the cerebellar hemispheres, or parts of the brainstem, give rise to congenital ataxia. These are nonprogressive disorders, and in most cases coordination improves somewhat with age.

Cerebellar dysfunction in an infant or young child may be overlooked, as it often gives rise to nonspecific abnormalities of motor development. Later there is nystagmus, obvious incoordination on reaching for objects, and truncal ataxia when first attempting to sit; intellectual disability is common but its presence usually does not provide useful diagnostic information.

Ataxia of acute or subacute onset

Cerebellar ataxia with extremely acute onset has two main causes: cerebellar haemorrhage (usually associated with headache, vertigo, vomiting, altered consciousness, and neck stiffness) and cerebellar infarction (in which cerebellar signs are usually combined with signs of brainstem ischaemia, and the presentation may mimic that of haemorrhage). Diagnosis should be made as a matter of urgency by imaging.

Subacute, reversible ataxia may occur as a result of viral infection in children aged 2 to 10 years. There is usually pyrexia, limb and gait ataxia, and dysarthria developing over hours or days. Recovery occurs over a period of weeks and is usually complete, but improvement may still be observed over 6 months. In older patients the possibility of a postinfectious encephalomyelitis, particularly that related to varicella-zoster virus infection, should be considered. The post-infectious Miller–Fisher variant of the Guillain–Barré syndrome may present with a triad that includes subacute ataxia, areflexia, and ophthalmoplegia. Nerve conduction studies and cerebrospinal fluid examination may be helpful, but the former are often normal. Other infective agents are shown in Table 24.7.4.3. Viral titres and cerebrospinal fluid examination may be helpful although serological evidence of viral infection may be difficult to establish.

Other causes of subacute ataxia include paraneoplastic disorders (see Chapter 24.21), hydrocephalus, foramen magnum compression, posterior fossa tumour (primary or secondary), abscess, or parasitic infection in any age group. Several important toxins and drugs also need to be considered, including thallium, lead, barbiturates, phenytoin, piperazine, alcohol, solvents, and antineoplastic drugs.

Table 24.7.4.3 Infections causing cerebellar disease

Viruses	Others
Echovirus	Mycoplasma pneumoniae
Coxsackievirus groups A and B	Legionella pneumoniae
Herpes simplex virus	Lyme disease
Poliovirus	Toxoplasma gondii
Epstein–Barr virus	Typhoid fever
Varicella virus	Plasmodium falciparum
Congenital rubella virus	Tick paralysis
	Prion disease

Vascular disorders of the cerebellum

Cerebrovascular disease is dealt with in detail in Chapter 24.10.1 Transient ischaemic attacks involving the vascular supply to the cerebellum rarely produce a pure ataxic syndrome and usually there are associated symptoms of brainstem dysfunction. Cerebellar infarction (from embolus or, more commonly, vertebrobasilar occlusive disease) and haemorrhage (usually on a background of hypertension or, less commonly, secondary to a vascular malformation or tumour) are relatively rare. Imaging is often necessary for early diagnosis as the later the diagnosis the worse the prognosis. Both infarction and haemorrhage may be amenable to surgical therapy, principally to relieve pressure.

Ataxia with an episodic course

These attacks may be considered bizarre and some patients are misdiagnosed as nonorganic; however, a good history can usually distinguish between the main causes (in order of frequency): drug ingestion, multiple sclerosis, transient vertebrobasilar ischaemic attacks, foramen magnum compression, intermittent obstruction of the ventricular system due to a colloid cyst or cysticercosis, and a growing list of inherited episodic ataxias (see Chapter 24.17). Autosomal dominant episodic ataxia is characterized by childhood or adolescent onset of attacks of ataxia, dysarthria, vertigo, and nystagmus. Not all patients have affected relatives. There are at least two forms of this disorder: episodic ataxia 1 (EA1) and episodic ataxia 2 (EA2).

EA1 is typified by brief attacks (minutes and occasionally hours) and clinically and electrophysiologically myokymia may be seen. Mutations in a potassium channel (Kv1.1) have been found. These patients may benefit from acetazolamide or phenytoin; between attacks patients usually have no neurological abnormalities.

In EA2 the attacks tend to be longer lasting hours or even days; they are usually associated with vertigo and consequent nausea and vomiting. The illness is more severe in childhood with associated drowsiness, headache, and fever. Although when the disease first begins the patients are well between attacks, an interictal nystagmus can be seen. As the disease progresses a slow deterioration in the ataxia is seen. MRI may reveal cerebellar atrophy. These patients tend to respond better to acetazolamide therapy than patients with EA1. Point mutations in a calcium channel gene (*CACNA1A*) have been demonstrated in some families with this disorder. However, increasingly other varieties of episodic ataxia are being recognized although the cause remains unknown.

In children and young adults, a metabolic disorder should be suspected, particularly defects of the urea cycle, aminoacidurias, Leigh's syndrome, and mitochondrial encephalomyopathies. Screening investigations include serum ammonia, pyruvate, lactate and amino acids, and urinary amino acids.

Ataxia with a chronic progressive course

Chronic alcohol abuse is probably the most common cause of progressive cerebellar degeneration in adults. Thiamine deficiency is the main (but not the sole) explanation for the chronic progressive cerebellar syndrome found in people with alcohol problems. Patients with this syndrome are frequently malnourished. Ataxia may develop during periods of abstinence, and an identical cerebellar degeneration has been observed in nonalcoholic patients with severe malnutrition. Cerebellar ataxia is common in the

Wernicke–Korsakoff syndrome, and the pathological features of both this syndrome and a cerebellar degeneration are frequently found together. With administration of thiamine some improvement may occur in early cases of alcoholic cerebellar degeneration, but, if the patient is already chairbound, the response to treatment is limited.

There are other deficiency disorders that can give rise to a progressive ataxia. There is a rare syndrome associated with zinc deficiency which responds to oral replacement therapy. Deficiency of vitamin E, either genetic (e.g. isolated vitamin E deficiency due to mutations in α-tocopherol transfer protein, or abetalipoproteinaemia) or acquired, may produce a progressive ataxia. It is important to establish the diagnosis of vitamin E deficiency as treatment with vitamin E may prevent progression of the neurological syndrome and can in rare circumstances lead to some improvement.

There are a number of toxic agents that can produce progressive cerebellar dysfunction, including pharmaceutical products, solvents, and heavy metals. The most common cause of a cerebellar syndrome due to drug toxicity in neurological practice is that associated with anticonvulsant medication, particularly phenytoin. Transient ataxia, dysarthria, and nystagmus usually develop when serum concentrations of phenytoin, carbamazepine, or barbiturates are above the therapeutic range, and remit when they return to the therapeutic range. Chronic phenytoin toxicity may cause persistent cerebellar dysfunction, and this is associated with loss of Purkinje's cells. A persistent cerebellar deficit, with dysarthria and limb and gait ataxia, and cerebellar atrophy on imaging, has also been described as a sequel to the acute encephalopathy of lithium toxicity that is usually precipitated by fever or starvation.

Recreational or accidental exposure to a number of solvents, including carbon tetrachloride and toluene, causes cerebellar ataxia along with other neurological problems, including psychosis, cognitive impairment, and pyramidal signs in the case of toluene. The neurological deficit is potentially reversible but may persist after prolonged exposure in solvent abusers. Exposure to heavy metals including inorganic mercury, lead, and thallium can also produce cerebellar damage.

Structural lesions such as posterior fossa tumours, foramen magnum compression, or hydrocephalus must be excluded by imaging studies. Tumours that may involve the posterior fossa include: astrocytomas, ependymomas, haemangioblastomas, and cranial nerve neuromas.

Paraneoplastic cerebellar degeneration (PCD) related to carcinomas of the lung or ovary usually follows a subacute course, with patients losing the ability to walk within months of onset. A variety of antineuronal antibodies may be found in these patients and help to confirm the diagnosis. Approximately half the patients with PCD have demonstrable antibodies directed against neurons in serum and CSF. The most common antibody seen in PCD is anti-Yo which specifically stains the cytoplasm of Purkinje's cells. A search for the underlying malignancy should then be undertaken involving imaging and analysis of tumour markers. Presentation with ataxia precedes diagnosis of the malignancy in 70% of cases and is usually subacute, progressing to severe disability over several months or even weeks, and then arresting. Onset may be acute and is sometimes accompanied by vertigo, mimicking a vascular event. There is severe truncal, gait, and limb ataxia, and dysarthria. Opsoclonus may be combined with myoclonus, producing a disorder in adults similar to the dancing eyes syndrome of childhood. The latter is sometimes associated with neuroblastoma. There is currently no proof that immunosuppressant therapy, or plasma exchange, improves the outlook but there are anecdotal reports of some improvement or stabilization after removal of the primary tumour. The best method of screening for the underlying malignancy is debated but standard MRI may be complemented by whole-body positron emission tomography (PET). Searching for primary tumour markers may also be useful (see review by Rees in Further reading).

Rarely, infectious agents can cause slowly progressive ataxia (see Table 24.7.4.3); these include the chronic panencephalitis of congenital rubella infection in children and, in adults, Creutzfeldt–Jakob disease (CJD), particularly the iatrogenic form, should be considered. A specific enquiry about potential risk factor exposure should be sought, especially growth hormone replacement, although in the past decade, after the introduction of stringent controls on source material, this has become extremely rare. Ataxia with psychiatric disturbance may be the presenting features of variant CJD. Multiple sclerosis only exceptionally presents as an isolated chronic progressive cerebellar syndrome.

Some conditions that are not generally considered primarily as ataxic disorders may present with clumsiness, tremor, or definite cerebellar signs, particularly in childhood or adolescence. These include Wilson's disease and several inherited neuropathies, such as hereditary motor and sensory neuropathy (HMSN; Charcot–Marie–Tooth disease, including the so-called Roussy–Levy syndrome). Although intention and postural tremor are quite frequent in the demyelinating type of HMSN (type I), dysarthria and pyramidal signs do not occur. Other chronic demyelinating neuropathies, such as chronic inflammatory and paraproteinaemic neuropathies and Refsum's disease, may give rise to prominent tremor and ataxia; the same applies to giant axonal neuropathy.

Superficial siderosis is a rare disorder that causes slowly progressive cerebellar ataxia, mainly of gait, and sensorineural deafness, often combined with spasticity, brisk reflexes, and extensor plantar responses. The diagnosis may not be suspected clinically, but the neuroradiological abnormalities are striking, MRI showing a black rim of haemosiderin around the posterior fossa structures and spinal cord, and less often the cerebral hemispheres, on *T2*-weighted images. Superficial siderosis is most commonly secondary to chronic leaking of blood into the subarachnoid space. Treatment relies on identifying the source of bleeding; chelation therapy with iron-binding agents given systemically does not appear to be effective.

After excluding acquired causes of ataxic disorders, there remains a considerable number of patients with degenerative ataxias, not all of which are overtly genetically determined. The inherited ataxias can largely be classified according to their clinical and genetic features (see below), and in a small proportion of cases a recognizable metabolic defect can be detected. It is important to make as accurate a diagnosis as possible in these disorders for the purposes of prognosis, genetic counselling, and, occasionally, specific therapy.

Progressive metabolic ataxias

Ataxia may be a minor feature of storage and other metabolic neurodegenerative disorders developing in early childhood (see Chapters 24.19). Some enzyme deficiencies that usually give rise to diffuse neurodegenerative disorders, in which ataxia is a feature, developing in infancy or early childhood, include the sphingomyelin lipidoses, which are lysosomal diseases: metachromatic leukodystrophy, galactosylceramide lipidosis (Krabbe's disease), and the β-hexosaminidase deficiencies which give rise to GM2 gangliosidosis—Tay–Sachs disease and Sandhoff's disease. Also within this group are adrenoleukomyeloneuropathy, a peroxisomal disorder, and its phenotypical variant of adrenoleukodystrophy (see Chapter 12.9). This diagnosis is supported by an increase in very long chain fatty acids or by direct genetic analysis of the AMN gene. Although X linked about 10% of carrier females may manifest neurological abnormalities. The role of diet and dietary supplements (e.g. oleic acid and Lorenzo's oil) remains to be established. Ataxia may be prominent in Niemann–Pick disease type C (juvenile dystonic lipidosis), combined with a supranuclear gaze palsy. Sphingomyelinase activity is normal, but foamy storage cells are found in the bone marrow (see Chapter 12.6).

Cholestanolosis (also called cerebrotendinous xanthomatosis—CTX) is a rare autosomal recessive disorder caused by defective bile salt metabolism, as a result of a deficiency of mitochondrial sterol 27-hydroxylase. It gives rise to ataxia, dementia, spasticity, peripheral neuropathy, cataract, and tendon xanthomas in the second decade of life. Treatment with chenodeoxycholic acid appears to improve neurological function (reviewed by Gallus—see Further reading).

Various phenotypes that are classifiable as hereditary ataxias have been described in the mitochondrial encephalomyopathies, many of which are associated with a defect of mitochondrial DNA. These include late-onset ataxic disorders associated (e.g. the Kearns–Sayre syndrome) with such features as dementia, deafness, and peripheral neuropathy. These features overlap with the syndrome of progressive myoclonic ataxia, which may also be caused by ceroid lipofuscinosis, sialidosis, or Unverricht–Lundborg disease, or the so-called Baltic myoclonus (see Chapter 24.17).

Acquired metabolic and endocrine disorders causing cerebellar dysfunction

Acquired metabolic and endocrine disorders causing cerebellar dysfunction include hepatic encephalopathy, pontine and extrapontine myelinolysis related to hyponatraemia, and hypothyroidism. The last is only very rarely a cause of a cerebellar syndrome.

Degenerative disorders

The degenerative cerebellar and spinocerebellar disorders are a complex group of diseases, most of which are genetically determined (see Chapter 24.17). In some there is an underlying metabolic disorder, and it is important to diagnose these, because there may be important implications for treatment and genetic counselling. There has been a rapid growth in our knowledge of the genetic basis of many of the spinocerebellar degenerations. The current phase of research is focused on how these genes and the abnormal proteins that they produce cause cell-specific neuropathology. Inherited ataxic disorders can be divided according to their mode of inheritance (see Table 24.7.4.2). Most autosomal recessive disorders are of early onset (less than 20 years), and autosomal dominant disorders are usually of later onset (over 20 years).

Autosomal recessive ataxias
Friedreich's ataxia

This is the most common of the autosomal recessive ataxias (Table 24.7.4.4) and accounts for at least 50% of cases of hereditary ataxia in most large series reported from Europe and the USA. The prevalence of the disease in these regions is similar—between 1 and 2 per 100 000.

The age of onset of symptoms, generally with gait ataxia, is usually between the ages of 8 and 15 years, but onset between 20 and 30 years, although fulfilling all other diagnostic criteria, have been described. In addition to the progressive ataxia, one finds a number of variable features, including dysarthria and pyramidal tract involvement. Initially this latter feature may be mild, with just extensor plantar responses, but after 5 or more years of the disease, invariably a pyramidal pattern of weakness in the legs is seen. Eventually this can lead to paralysis. Distal wasting, particularly in the upper limbs, is seen in about 50% of patients with Friedreich's ataxia. Skeletal abnormalities are also commonly found including scoliosis (85%) and foot deformities, typically pes cavus in approximately 50% of patients. Additional clinical support for one's suspicions include optic atrophy which can be seen in 25%; however, it is rare (<5%) for Friedreich's ataxia to produce major visual impairment. Deafness is found in less than 10%, but rather more have impairment of speech discrimination. Nystagmus is seen in only about 20%, but the extraocular movements are nearly always abnormal, with broken-up pursuit, dysmetric saccades, square-wave jerks, and failure of fixation suppression of the vestibulo-ocular reflex.

Investigation of patients reveals an axonal sensory neuropathy and an abnormal ECG in 65% of patients with widespread T-wave inversion. Diabetes mellitus occurs in 10% of patients with Friedreich's ataxia, and a further 10–20% have impaired glucose tolerance.

The gene frataxin was identified in 1996. The predominant mutation is a trinucleotide repeat (GAA) in intron 1 of this gene. Expansion of both alleles is found in over 96% of patients. The remaining patients have one expansion and a point mutation in the frataxin gene. This was the first autosomal recessive condition found to be caused by a dynamic repeat and it has permitted the introduction of a specific and sensitive diagnostic test, as it is a relatively simple matter to measure the repeat size. On normal chromosomes the number of GAA repeats varies from 7 to 22 units, whereas, on disease chromosomes, the range is anything from around 100 to 2000 repeats. The length of the repeat is a determinant of the age of onset and therefore to some degree influences the severity in that early onset tends to progress more rapidly.

There is now good evidence that frataxin is located in the mitochondria and appears to be involved in iron transport. Mitochondrial dysfunction does fit with the clinical picture of ataxia and neuropathy, in association with diabetes, cardiomyopathy, deafness, and optic atrophy.

Ataxic disorders associated with defective DNA repair

There are several rare disorders that are characterized at a molecular level by a reduced capacity to repair DNA. The most well known is ataxia telangiectasia. Characteristically, motor development is often delayed and ataxia noted at the time of first walking. Growth retardation and delayed sexual development are frequent, and

Table 24.7.4.4 Autosomal recessive ataxias (see also Chapter 24.17)

Syndrome	Gene defect	Clinical notes
Friedreich's ataxia	GAA repeat (and rarely point mutations in *FRDA* gene)	Neuropathy, pyramidal signs, skeletal abnormalities, diabetes, cardiomyopathy
Ataxia telangiectasia (AT) AT-like disorder	*ATM* *hMRE11*	Oculomotor apraxia, mixed movement disorder, humoral immune difficulties, increased cancer risk
Cockayne's syndrome	CS type A—*ERCC8* gene CSA type B—*ERCC6* gene	'Cachectic dwarfism' Intellectual disability Pigmentary retinopathy
Xeroderma pigmentosum	*ERCC2* but also probably genetically complex	Skin disorder and an increased risk of skin cancer
AOA1	*Aprataxin*	Oculomotor apraxia
AOA2	*Senataxin*	Oculomotor apraxia
Hypogonadism	Not known	Hypogonadotropic hypogonadism
Marinesco–Sjögren syndrome	*SIL1* on chromosome 5q31	Cataracts and intellectual disability
Progressive myoclonic ataxia (Ramsay Hunt syndrome)	Genetically complex	Epilepsy is common
Behr's and related syndromes, e.g. 3-methylglutaconic aciduria type III (Costeff's syndrome)	No gene for Behr's syndrome yet identified *OPA3* gene	Optic atrophy, spasticity, and intellectual disability
Congenital or childhood-onset deafness	Genetically complex	Syndromic diagnosis—likely to have several causes
Autosomal recessive late-onset ataxia	Heterogeneous	Wide clinical variability

Onset usually before 20 years of age.
AOAI, ataxia associated with oculomotor apraxia.

there is mild intellectual disability in some cases. A mixed movement disorder may be seen, often with a combination of ataxia, dystonia, and chorea. The cutaneous telangiectasia of ataxia telangiectasia tends to develop on the conjunctivae between the ages of 3 and 6 years, but occasionally are inconspicuous or absent in adult life. Ataxia telangiectasia is associated with abnormalities of both humoral and cell-mediated immunity. The gene for ataxia telangiectasia has now been cloned and is called *ATM* and genetic analysis can be undertaken in appropriately selected cases. A rarer clinically similar disease due to mutations in *hMRE11* has been identified and is termed 'ataxia telangiectasia-like disorder'.

Clinically related conditions, xeroderma pigmentosum and Cockayne's syndrome (see Table 24.7.4.4), are also due to defects in DNA repair; they are much rarer and associated with additional features, most frequently skin abnormalities.

Ataxia associated with oculomotor apraxia

There are two genetically distinct but clinically similar disorders associated with the distinctive feature of oculomotor apraxia—types 1 and 2. Oculomotor apraxia represents a deficit of the voluntary saccadic system and should be suspected in the presence of head thrusts or synkinetic blinking, which are used to help initiate a voluntary saccade. Ataxia associated with oculomotor apraxia type 1 (AOA1) was shown to be due to mutations in a gene called apraxia on chromosome 9p13. It is characterized by the association of ataxia with chorea early in the disease course, oculomotor apraxia, peripheral neuropathy, and variable but mild learning difficulties. MRI reveals cerebellar atrophy and serum analysis may show hypercholesterolaemia and hypoalbuminaemia.

A second condition, AOA2, is very similar clinically and also overlaps with the ataxia telangiectasia phenotype (see above).

Mutations in senataxin have been shown to cause this syndrome. α-Fetoprotein is elevated in virtually all cases and is therefore a useful screen for this disorder. It also appears that it may be more common than either ataxia telangiectasia or AOA1, accounting for approximately 8% of autosomal recessive ataxia. The other autosomal recessive ataxias are all individually rare and are listed in Table 24.7.4.4.

Testing for ATM, apraxin, and senataxin is now possible in specialized labs.

Autosomal dominant cerebellar ataxias

The autosomal dominant cerebellar ataxias (ADCAs) are a clinically and genetically complex group of neurodegenerative disorders (Table 24.7.4.5). ADCA type I is characterized by a progressive cerebellar ataxia and is variably associated with other extracerebellar neurological features such as ophthalmoplegia, optic atrophy, peripheral neuropathy, and pyramidal and extrapyramidal signs. The presence and severity of these signs are, in part, dependent on the duration of the disease. Mild or moderate dementia may occur but it is usually not a prominent early feature. ADCA type II is clinically distinguished from ADCA type I by the presence of pigmentary macular dystrophy (Fig. 24.7.4.1), whereas ADCA type III is a relatively 'pure' cerebellar syndrome and generally starts at a later age. This clinical classification is still useful, despite the tremendous improvements in our understanding of the genetic basis (see below), because it provides a framework that can be used in the clinic and helps direct the genetic evaluation.

The genetic loci causing the dominant ataxias are given the acronym SCA (spinocerebellar ataxia). At the time of publication there are 28 SCA loci identified. However, with the discovery of the genes it becomes apparent that some of these are duplicates

Table 24.7.4.5 Autosomal dominant cerebellar ataxia (ADCA): clinicogenetic classification

ADCA type	Clinical features	Genetic loci and chromosomal location	Gene
ADCA I	Cerebellar syndrome plus: Pyramidal signs Supranuclear ophthalmoplegia Extrapyramidal signs Peripheral neuropathy Dementia	SCA	Ataxin 1 CAG
		SCA2	Ataxin 2 CAG
		SCA3	Ataxin 3 CAG
		SCA8	Kelch-like 1 CTG repeat
		SCA12	PPP2R2B CAG repeat
		SCA13	KCNC3 point mutations
		SCA14	PRKCG point mutations
		SCA15	ITPR1
		SCA17	TBP CAG
ADCA II	Cerebellar syndrome plus: Pigmentary maculopathy Other signs as ADCA I	SCA7 3p12–21.1	Ataxin 7 CAG
ADCA III	'Pure' cerebellar syndrome Mild pyramidal signs	SCA5	SPTBN2 beta-III spectrin D
		SCA6	CACNL1A[a] CAG repeat
		SCA10	Ataxin 10 ATTCT repeat
		SCA11	TTBK2
		SCA27	FGF14 point mutations
Episodic ataxias (EAs)	EA1		Kv1.1
	EA2		CACNL1A[a]
	Plus others yet to be defined		

[a] SCA6 and CACNL1A are allelic variants.
Onset usually over age of 25 years. This is a list of currently identified genes and is divided by ADCA subtype to facilitate clinical relevance. (See also Chapter 24.17 for more details.)

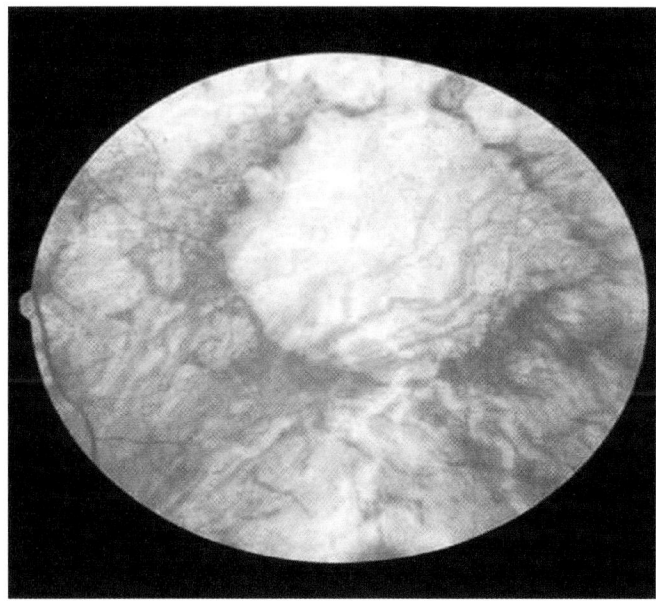

Fig. 24.7.4.1 The distinctive maculopathy in a patient with autosomal dominant cerebellar ataxia type II (see the text) associated with mutations in the human gene.

Idiopathic degenerative late-onset ataxias

About two-thirds of cases of degenerative ataxia developing in those aged over 20 years are isolated cases, and they represent a significant clinical problem; it is difficult even to know how to label them. The literature is confusing, mixing pathological terms such as olivopontocerebellar atrophy (OPCA) with clinical terms; the author prefers to use the term 'idiopathic late-onset cerebellar ataxia' (ILOCA). A proportion of patients in this group progress to develop the features of multiple-system atrophy (MSA) (see Chapter 24.7.3). These patients may have or develop facial impassivity and extrapyramidal rigidity, whereas others present with features of autonomic failure such as postural hypotension, impotence, bladder dysfunction, and a fixed cardiac rate. A cerebellar presentation occurs in about 30% of patients with MSA. The distinction of idiopathic late-onset cerebellar ataxia from MSA may therefore be difficult clinically at presentation.

Most patients with ILOCA lose the ability to walk independently between 5 and 20 years after onset, and lifespan is slightly shortened by immobility. Those who develop MSA have a particularly poor prognosis. Investigations, apart from those excluding acquired causes of cerebellar degeneration such as malignancy and hypothyroidism, tend to be unhelpful. Electrophysiological evidence of a sensory peripheral neuropathy is found in about 50%

and yet there are still more to be found. In general clinical practice five of these genes are established (*SCA1*, *-2*, *-3*, *-6*, and *-7*) (Table 24.7.4.6). Interestingly they are all caused by a similar mutational mechanism, an expansion of an exonic CAG repeat. The resultant proteins all possess an expanded polyglutamine tract and there are now at least eight conditions caused by these expansions (see Chapter 24.7.3). Other types of ADCAs are rare and mutation testing is available only for a small number of these.

Table 24.7.4.6 Clinical impact of genetics on the autosomal dominant cerebellar ataxias (ADCAs)

ADCA type	Genetic tests (widely available)	Relative contribution to each subclass (%)
I	SCA1, -2, -3	50
II	SCA7	99
III	SCA6	50

of cases, which can be a useful pointer to the presence of a degenerative multisystem disorder. CT or MRI may show cerebellar and brainstem atrophy, or pure cerebellar atrophy. The prognosis is worse in patients with clinical and radiological evidence of brainstem involvement, compared with those with a pure cerebellar syndrome and cerebellar atrophy alone on MRI.

The role of gliadin sensitivity in producing a chronic progressive ataxia, either as part of coeliac disease or as a purely neurological phenotype, is still being debated.

Recently, a newly recognized condition has been shown to be responsible for late-onset ataxia in men who develop a progressive phenotype of ataxia and tremor in association with an intermediate expansion in the fragile X gene. This has been termed FXTAS (fragile X tremor ataxia syndrome). This syndrome is being expanded as information emerges.

Further reading

Anderson NE, Rosenblum MK, Posner JB (1988). Paraneoplastic cerebellar degeneration: clinical-immunological correlations. *Ann Neurol*, **24**, 559–67.

Bomont P, *et al.* (2000). Homozygosity mapping of spinocerebellar ataxia with cerebellar atrophy and peripheral neuropathy to 9q33–34, and with hearing impairment and optic atrophy to 6p21–23. *Eur J Hum Genet*, **8**, 986–90.

Bootsma D, *et al.* (1998). Nucleotide excision repair syndromes: xeroderma pigmentosum, Cockayne syndrome and trichothiodystrophy. In: Scriver CR, Beaudet AL, Sly WS, Valle D (eds) *The metabolic basis of inherited disease*, 8th edition, pp. 245–74. McGraw Hill, New York.

Campuzano V, *et al.* (1996). Friedreich's ataxia: autosomal recessive disease caused by an intronic GAA triplet repeat expansion. *Science*, **271**, 1423–7.

Cavalier L, *et al.* (1998). Ataxia with isolated vitamin E deficiency: heterogeneity of mutations and phenotypic variability in a large number of families. *Am J Hum Genet*, **62**, 301–10.

Date H, *et al.* (2001). Early-onset ataxia with ocular motor apraxia and hypoalbuminemia is caused by mutations in a new HIT superfamily gene. *Nature Genet*, **29**, 184–8.

De Michele G, *et al.* (1989). Late onset recessive ataxia with Friedreich's disease phenotype. *J Neurol Neurosurg Psychiatry*, **52**, 1398–403.

Enevoldson PG, Sanders MD, Harding AE (1994). Autosomal dominant cerebellar ataxia with pigmentary macular dystrophy: a clinical and genetic study of eight families. *Brain*, **117**, 445–60.

Everett CM, Wood NW (2004). Trinucleotide repeats and neurodegenerative disease. *Brain*, **127**, 2385–405.

Fearnley JM, Stevens JM, Rudge P (1995). Superficial siderosis of the central nervous system. *Brain*, **118**: 1051–66.

Gallus GN, Dotti MT, Federico A (2006). Clinical and molecular diagnosis of cerebrotendinous xanthomatosis with a review of the mutations in the *CYP27A1* gene. *Neurol Sci*, **27**, 143–9.

Gilman S *et al.* (2008). Second consensus statement on the diagnosis of multiple system atrophy. *Neurology*, **71**, 670–6.

Gotoda T, *et al.* (1995). Adult-onset spinocerebellar dysfunction caused by a mutation in the gene for the α-tocopherol transfer protein. *N Engl J Med*, **333**, 1313–18.

Hadjivassiliou M, *et al.* (2003). Gluten ataxia in perspective: epidemiology, genetic susceptibility and clinical characteristics. *Brain*, **126**, 685–91.

Hanna MG, Wood NW, Kullmann D (1998). The neurological channelopathies. *J Neurol Neurosurg Psychiatry*, **65**, 427–31.

Harding AE (1981). Friedreich's ataxia: a clinical and genetic study of 90 families with an analysis of early diagnostic criteria and intrafamilial clustering of clinical features. *Brain*, **104**, 589–620.

Harding AE (1984). *The hereditary ataxias and related disorders*. Churchill Livingstone, Edinburgh.

Jacquemont S, *et al.* (2004). Penetrance of the fragile X-associated tremor/ataxia syndrome in a premutation carrier population. *JAMA*, **291**, 460–9.

Klockgether J, *et al.* (1990). Idiopathic cerebellar ataxia of late onset: natural history and MRI morphology. *J Neurol Neurosurg Psychiatry*, **53**, 297–305.

Klockgether T, *et al.* (1998). The natural history of degenerative ataxia: a retrospective study in 466 patients. *Brain*, **121**, 589–600.

Le Ber I, *et al.* (2004). Frequency and phenotypic spectrum of ataxia with oculomotor apraxia 2: a clinical and genetic study in 18 patients. *Brain*, **127**, 759–67.

Lock RJ, *et al.* (2005). Ataxia, peripheral neuropathy, and anti-gliadin antibody. Guilt by association? *J Neurol Neurosurg Psychiatry*, **76**, 1601–3.

Marsden CD, *et al.* (1990). Progressive myoclonic ataxia (the Ramsay Hunt syndrome). *Arch Neurol*, **47**, 1121–5.

Matilla-Duenas A, Goold R, Giunti P (2006). Molecular pathogenesis of spinocerebellar ataxias. Brain, 129, 1357–70.

Moreira MC, *et al.* (2004). Senataxin, the ortholog of a yeast RNA helicase, is mutant in ataxia-ocular apraxia 2. *Nature Genet*, **36**: 225–7.

Pennacchio LA, *et al.* (1996). Mutations in the gene encoding cystatin B in progressive myoclonus epilepsy (EPM1). *Science*, **271**, 1731–3.

Peterson K, *et al.* (1992). Paraneoplastic cerebellar degeneration. I. A clinical analysis of 55 anti-Yo antibody-positive patients. *Neurology*, **42**, 1931–7.

Rees J (1998). Paraneoplastic syndromes. *Curr Opin Neurol*, **11**, 633–7.

Ryan MM, Engle EC (2003). Acute ataxia in childhood. *J Child Neurol*, **18**, 309–16.

Savitsky K, *et al.* (1995). A single ataxia telangiectasia gene with a product similar to PI-3 kinase. *Science*, **268**, 1749–53.

Shams'ili S, *et al.* (2003). Paraneoplastic cerebellar degeneration associated with antineuronal antibodies: analysis of 50 patients. *Brain*, 126, 1409–18.

Stewart GE, Ironside JW (1998). New variant Creutzfeldt–Jakob disease. *Curr Opin Neurol*, **11**, 259–62.

Tranchant C, *et al.* (2003). Phenotypic variability of aprataxin gene mutations. *Neurology*, **60**, 868–70.

Watanabe H, *et al.* (2002). Progression and prognosis in multiple system atrophy: an analysis of 230 Japanese patients. *Brain*, **125**, 1070–83.

Headache

Peter J. Goadsby

Essentials

Headache is among the most common of human maladies. So much so that it is generally (and often incorrectly) assumed that it is understood, especially by doctors. The classification of headache, with formal definitions of different diagnostic entities, by the International Headache Society into (1) primary—occurring in the absence of external causes, and (2) secondary—some of which may have sinister cause, has greatly simplified the description, understanding, and management of this often challenging symptom. It also allows those headaches with serious or life-threatening consequences to be distinguished from other forms.

Pathophysiology of primary headaches

The key structures involved in producing pain appear to be the following: (1) large intracranial vessels and the dura mater, (2) trigeminal nerve, (3) higher centres in the thalamus and cortex, (4) modulatory centres in the diencephalon and brainstem.

Two of the commonest and best studied primary headaches, migraine and cluster headache, should be regarded as having a neurovascular origin. Migraine might be part of the spectrum of diseases known as channelopathies or ionopathies: the three genes currently identified as being genes responsible for familial hemiplegic migraine alter ion fluxs.

Migraine

Epidemiology and clinical features—this episodic disorder affects 12 to 15% of the population and can be highly disabling. It presents with headache, often throbbing and generally accompanied by other features such as sensitivity to light, sound, or movement, and often with nausea or (less often) vomiting, but none of the features is compulsory (the migraine aura, visual disturbances with flashing lights or zigzag lines moving across the fields or other neurological symptoms, is reported in only about 25% of patients).

Treatment—principles of management include (1) explanation—migraine is an inherited tendency to have headache and cannot therefore be 'cured'; (2) the condition can be modified and controlled by lifestyle adjustment and the use of medicines; (3) it is not life-threatening; (4) management takes time and cooperation.

Most migraine sufferers will benefit from a healthy diet, regular exercise, regular sleep patterns, avoiding excess caffeine and alcohol, and (as far as practical) modifying or minimizing changes in stress. Preventive drug treatments include pizotifen, β-blockers, some tricyclics, some anticonvulsants, flunarizine, and methysergide. Acute treatments include (often in combination with an antiemetic) nonspecific drugs such as aspirin, paracetamol and NSAIDs, and specific agents such as triptans and ergot derivatives.

Tension-type headache

Tension-type headache is common, unexplained, and completely featureless, with no nausea, no vomiting, no photophobia, no phonophobia, no osmophobia, no throbbing, and no aggravation with movement. When episodic, it is generally amenable to simple analgesics; when chronic, amitriptyline is the only proven treatment.

Trigeminal–autonomic cephalgias

Cluster headache—characterized by bouts of excruciating retro-orbital boring pain associated with ipsilateral symptoms of cranial parasympathetic activation (a red or watering eye, the nose running or blocking) or cranial sympathetic dysfunction (eyelid droop). Prevention is with agents including verapamil, lithium oral corticosteroids, and methysergide. Treatments for acute attacks include oxygen inhalation and intravenous sumatriptan.

Other conditions—these include (1) paroxysmal hemicrania, and (2) short-lasting unilateral neuralgiform headache attacks with conjunctival injection and tearing or cranial autonomic activation (SUNCT/SUNA).

Other primary headaches

Specific conditions include (1) stabbing headache, (2) cough headache, (3) exertional headache, (4) sex headache, (5) hypnic headache, (6) thunderclap headache, and (7) hemicrania continua. Many of these can present with chronic daily headaches and are often misdiagnosed as tension type headache, but they can readily be identified from the history, often leading to effective and specific treatments, an important element of which is reduction/elimination of analgesic overuse.

New daily persistent headache—this typically presents with abrupt onset of headache that then persists. Possible causes include: (1) primary—migrainous type, featureless (tension type); (2) secondary—subarachnoid haemorrhage, low cerebrospinal fluid volume headache, raised cerebrospinal fluid pressure headache, post-traumatic headache, chronic meningitis, giant cell arteritis. Effective and specific treatments are available for many of these conditions if a precise diagnosis can be made.

Secondary headache

Clinical approach—the length of the history is crucial: if this is short, the patient requires prompt attention; if this is long, then time and patience are needed rather than alacrity. Associated fever, sudden onset of pain, or the presence of neurological signs need a positive diagnosis of a benign disorder or require brain imaging with CT or MRI.

Causes and management—medically sinister headaches requiring urgent attention include subarachnoid haemorrhage, meningitis, giant cell arteritis, and raised intracranial pressure. Other important causes of secondary headache include low volume (pressure) cerebrospinal fluid, post-traumatic headache, and cerviocogenic headache. Many of these disorders require persistent diagnostic skills and investigation; but when combined with knowledge of general principles, including the anatomy and physiology of the key cranial structures, the management of headache is generally productive and beneficial for the sufferer.

General principles

To manage headache can be a source of extreme frustration or undiluted pleasure—the difference simply reflects to what extent the practitioner is familiar with the subject. A formal nosology for headache disorders is to be found in the second edition of the *International classification of headache disorders*. Although it seems obvious, the key to successful management is establishment of a clear diagnosis. The general concept is that there are primary and secondary forms of headache, following the generic medical principle that clinical syndromes may be caused by something exogenous or secondary, or may manifest anew as the primary disease process. Such a system is outlined in Table 24.8.1. Mild secondary headache, such as that seen in association with upper respiratory tract infections, is common but only rarely worrisome. The clinical dilemma remains that, although life-threatening headache is relatively uncommon in Western society, it occurs and its detection requires suitable vigilance by doctors. Primary headache, in contrast, often confers considerable disability over time and although not life threatening certainly robs patients of quality of life. Some pointers to secondary headache are listed in Box 24.8.1.

Primary headache syndromes

The primary headaches are a group of fascinating disorders in which headache and associated features are seen in the absence of any exogenous cause. The common syndromes (see Table 24.8.1) are tension-type headache, migraine, and cluster headache. Some other less well-known, indeed rarer, syndromes are mentioned because they are easily treated when diagnosed, and the most burdensome headache problems, the chronic daily headaches, are explicitly covered because concepts have altered considerably in this area in recent years.

Anatomy and physiology

The most common disabling primary headaches, migraine and cluster headache, have been studied extensively in recent times and they are now relatively well understood insofar as neurological disorders that involve the brain are concerned. In experimental animals the detailed anatomy of the connections of the pain-producing intracranial extracerebral vessels and the dura mater has built on the classic human observations of Wolff, Feindel, Penfield, McNaughton, and others. It is these structures, and not the brain itself, that are primarily involved in head pain, although it is not at all clear to what extent there is nociceptive activation as such, or simply the perception of that activation.

The key structures involved are:

- the large intracranial vessels and dura mater
- the peripheral terminals of the trigeminal nerve that innervate these structures
- the central terminals and second-order neurons of the caudal trigeminal nucleus and dorsal horns of C1 and C2: trigeminocervical complex

Table 24.8.1 Common causes of headache

Primary headache		Secondary headache	
Type	**Prevalence (%)**	**Type**	**Prevalence (%)**
Migraine	16	Systemic infection	63
Tension type	69	Head injury	4
Cluster headache	0.1	Subarachnoid haemorrhage	<1
Idiopathic stabbing	2	Vascular disorders	1
Exertional	1	Brain tumour	0.1

(After Olesen J, et al. (2005). *The headaches*. Lippincott, Williams & Wilkins, Philadelphia.)

Box 24.8.1 Warning signs in head pain

- Sudden onset of pain
- Fever
- Marked change in pain character or timing of attacks
- Neck stiffness
- Pain associated with higher centre complaints
- Pain associated with neurological disturbance, such as clumsiness or weakness
- Pain associated with local tenderness, such as of the temporal artery

◆ higher-centre processing in the thalamus, ventroposteromedial and posterior thalamus, and cortex

◆ modulatory centres in the diencephalon and brainstem, such as periaqueductal grey matter, locus ceruleus, and parts of the hypothalamus

The innervation of the large intracranial vessels and dura mater by the trigeminal nerve is known as the trigeminovascular system. Cranial parasympathetic autonomic innervation provides the basis for symptoms such as lacrimation and nasal stuffiness, which are prominent in cluster headache and paroxysmal hemicrania, although they may also be seen in migraine. It is clear from human functional imaging studies that vascular changes in migraine and cluster headache are driven by these neural vasodilator systems so that these headaches should be regarded as neurovascular. The concept of a primary vascular headache should be abandoned because it does not explain the pathogenesis of what are complex central nervous system (CNS) disorders, or necessarily predict treatment outcomes. The term 'vascular' headache has no place in modern medical practice when referring to primary headache.

Migraine is an episodic syndrome of headache with sensory sensitivity, such as to light, sound, and head movement, probably due to dysfunction of aminergic brainstem/diencephalic sensory control systems (Fig. 24.8.1). The first of the migraine genes has been identified for familial hemiplegic migraine, and includes mutations in the *CACNA1A* gene for the $Ca_V2.1$ (α_{1A}) subunit of the neuronal *P/Q* voltage-gated calcium channel, the Na^+/K^+ ATP pump α_2-subunit gene *ATP1A2*, and the voltage-gated sodium channel *SCN1A*. These findings and the clinical features of migraine suggest that it might be part of the spectrum of diseases known as channelopathies, or now ionopathies—disorders involving dysfunction of ion channel fluxes. Functional neuroimaging has suggested that brainstem regions in migraine (Fig. 24.8.2), and the posterior hypothalamic grey matter site of the human circadian pacemaker cells of the suprachiasmatic nucleus in cluster headache (Fig. 24.8.3), are good candidates for specific involvement in primary headache.

Secondary headache

It is imperative to establish in the patient presenting with any form of head pain whether there is an important secondary headache declaring itself. The headaches of subarachnoid haemorrhage, meningitis, giant cell arteritis, and raised intracranial pressure are important examples of medically sinister headaches requiring urgent attention. Perhaps the most crucial clinical feature to elicit is the length of the history. Patients with a short history require prompt attention and may require prompt investigation and management. Patients with a longer history generally require time and patience rather than alacrity. There are some important general features, including associated fever or sudden onset of pain (see Box 24.8.1); these demand attention. Patients with a history of recent-onset headache or neurological signs need a positive diagnosis of a benign disorder or require brain imaging with CT or MRI. Patients with a history of recurrent headache over a period of 1 year or more, fulfilling International Headache Society (IHS) criteria for migraine (Box 24.8.2), and with a normal physical examination, have positive brain imaging in only about 1/1000 images. In general it should be noted that a brain tumour is a rare cause

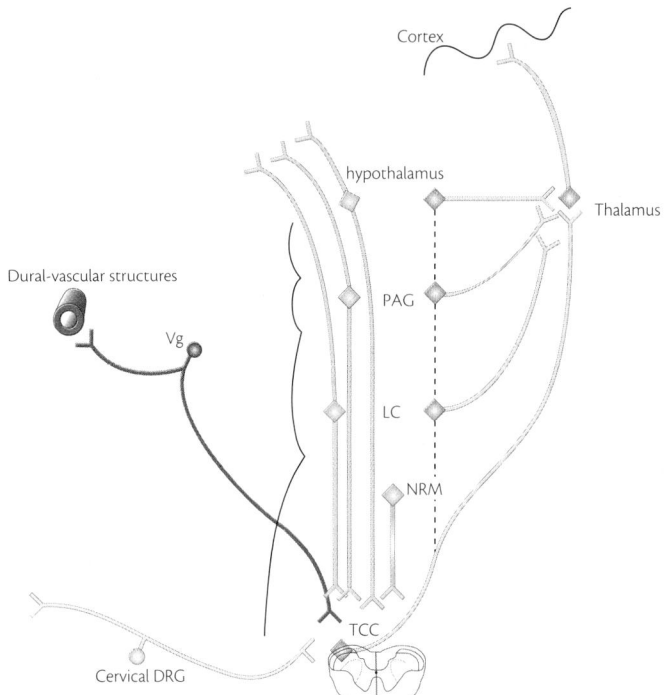

Fig. 24.8.1 Pathophysiology of migraine. Diagram of some structures involved in the transmission of trigeminovascular nociceptive input and the modulation of that input which form the basis of a model of the pathophysiology of migraine. Afferents from dural–vascular structures innervated predominantly by branches of the first (ophthalmic) division of the trigeminal nerve, with cell bodies found in the trigeminal ganglion (Vg), project to second-order neurons in the trigeminocervical complex (TCC). The TCC extends from trigeminal nucleus caudalis to the caudal portion of the dorsal horn of the C2 spinal cord. Input from cervical structures, such as joints or muscle, project through cell bodies in the upper cervical dorsal root ganglia (DRGs) to the TCC. TCC neurons project to ventrobasal thalamus (thalamus) and thence to the cortex. Sensory modulation can occur by descending influences on to the TCC that largely respect the midline (dashed line), such as those from the hypothalamus, midbrain periaqueductal grey (PAG), pontine locus ceruleus (LC), and nucleus raphe magnus (RVM). These influences are pictured as being direct but both direct and indirect projections are recognized. In addition sensory modulation can occur from at least the LC and PAG, and hypothalamic projects to thalamus nuclei as ascending systems again largely respect the midline.
(From Goadsby PJ (2005). Can we develop neurally-acting drugs for the treatment of migraine? *Nat Rev Drug Discovery*, **4**: 741–50.)

of headache, and rarely a cause of isolated long-term histories of headache. A notable exception to the general rules about secondary headache is a pituitary tumour, which can trigger underlying primary headache biology, and should always be considered, especially in the differential diagnosis of trigeminal–autonomic cephalalgias (see below).

The management of secondary headache is generally self-evident: treatment of the underlying condition, such as an infection or mass lesion. An exception is the condition of chronic posttraumatic headache in which pain persists for long periods after head injury. This is an interesting generic problem that may be seen after CNS infection, trauma, both blunt and surgical, intracranial bleeds, and other precipitants. Although the syndrome is generally self-limiting up to 3 to 5 years after the event, treatment of the headache may be required if it is disabling (see 'Chronic daily headache', below).

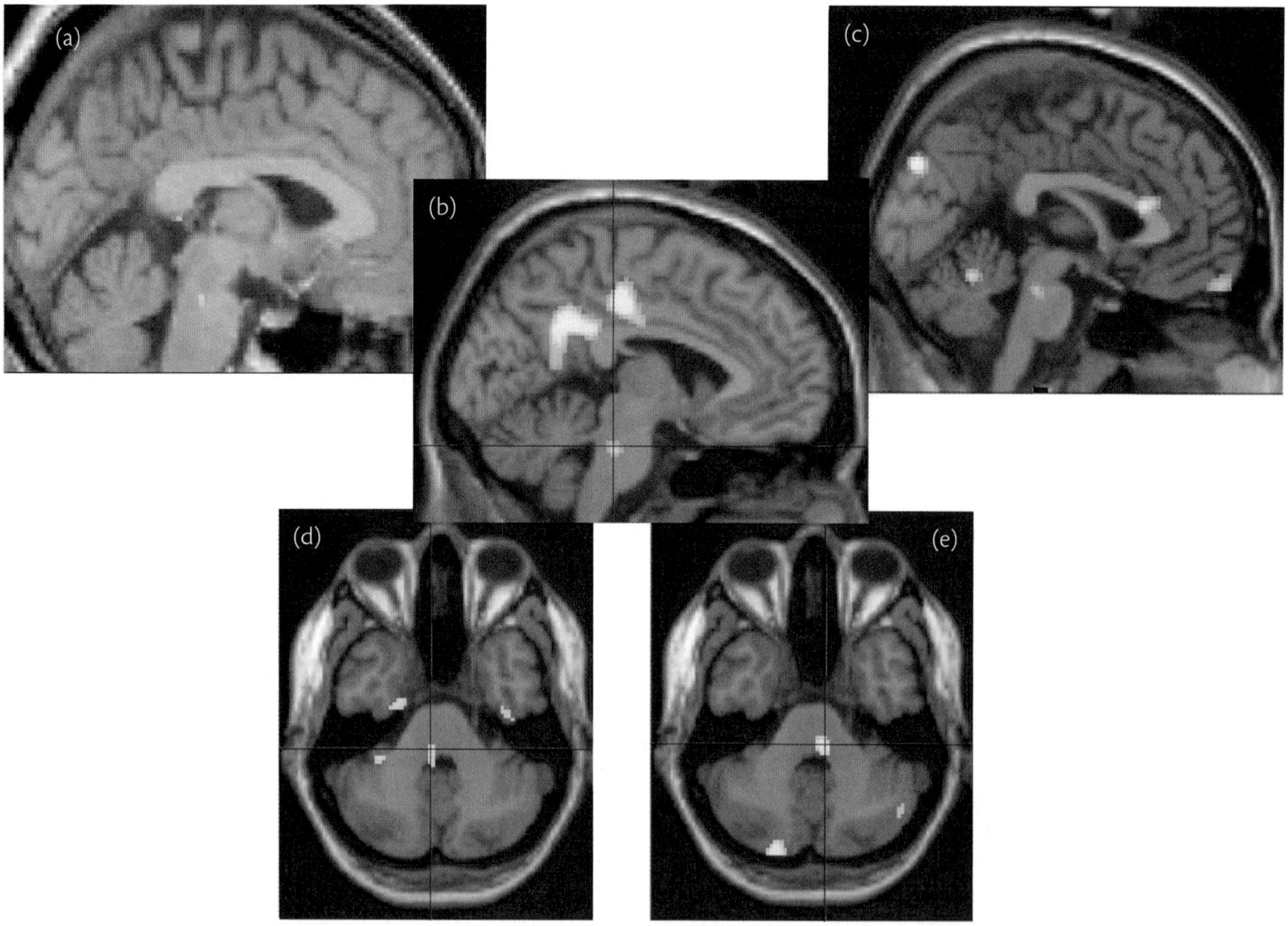

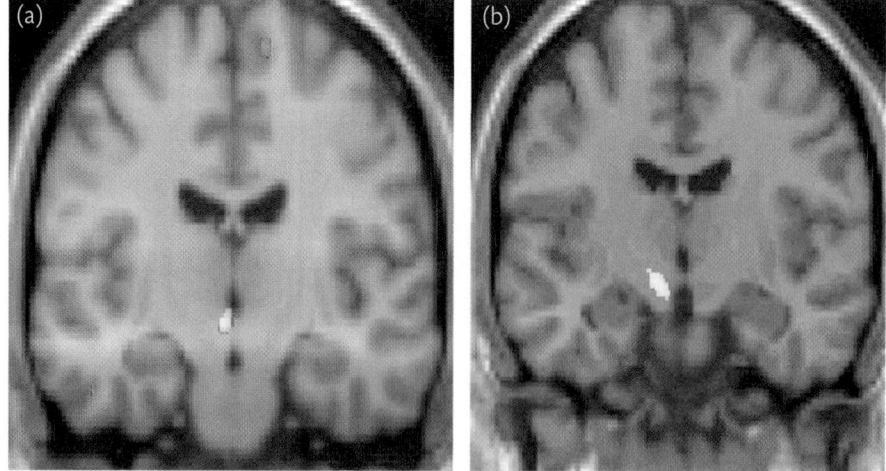

Fig. 24.8.2 Activations identified on positron emission tomography (PET) in migraine. Consistently there is dorsolateral pons activation in episodic migraine without aura, triggered by nitroglycerin (a), or spontaneously studied (b), and in chronic migraine (c). Moreover, there is lateralization to the right (d) and left (e) in this structure that parallels the unilateral presentation of the pain.
(a, from Bahra A, *et al.* (2001). Brainstem activation specific to migraine headache. *Lancet*, **357**: 1016–17; b, from Afridi S, *et al.* (2005). A PET study in spontaneous migraine. *Arch Neurol*, **62**: 1270–5; c, from Matharu MS, *et al.* (2004). Central neuromodulation in chronic migraine patients with suboccipital stimulators: a PET study. *Brain*, **127**: 220–30; d,e, from Afridi S, *et al.* (2005). A PET study exploring the laterality of brainstem activation in migraine using glyceryl trinitrate. *Brain*, **128**: 932–9.)

Fig. 24.8.3 Activations on positron emission tomography (PET) in the posterior hypothalamic grey matter in patients with acute cluster headache (a). The activation demonstrated is lateralized to the side of the pain (May *et al.*, 1998). When comparing the brains of patients with cluster headache with a control population, using an automatic anatomical technique known as voxel-based morphometry (VBM) which employs high-resolution T_1-weighted MRI, a similar region is demonstrated (b) and has increased grey matter.
a) (May *et al.*, 1998), b) (May *et al.*, 1999a).

Box 24.8.2 Simplified diagnostic criteria for migraine

Repeated attacks of headache lasting 4–72h that have these features, normal physical examination, and no other reasonable cause for the headache:

◆ At least two of:
  · Unilateral pain
  · Throbbing pain
  · Aggravation by movement
  · Moderate or severe intensity
◆ At least one of:
  · Nausea/vomiting
  · Photophobia and phonophobia

Adapted from the International Headache Society Classification (Headache Classification Committee of the International Headache Society (2004). *The international classification of headache disorders*, 2nd edn. *Cephalalgia*, **24**: 1–1604).

Migraine

Clinical features

Migraine is an episodic brain disorder that affects about 12 to 15% of the population, and can be highly disabling. It has been estimated to be the most costly neurological disorder in the European Union at more than €27 billion per year and its cost to the economy of the United States of America is a staggering US$19.6 billion per year. Migraine presents with a headache generally accompanied by features, such as sensitivity to light, sound, or movement, and often with nausea, or less often vomiting (see Box 24.8.2). None of the features is compulsory, and indeed, given that the migraine aura, visual disturbances with flashing lights or zigzag lines moving across the fields, or other neurological symptoms, are reported in only about 25% of patients, a high index of suspicion is required to diagnose migraine.

In a controlled study of patients presenting to general practitioners with a main complaint of headache over the previous 3 months, migraine was the diagnosis on more than 90% of occasions, so a high index of suspicion is well rewarded. A headache diary can often be helpful in making the diagnosis, although in reality the diary usually helps more in assessing disability or recording how often patients use acute attack treatments. Phenotyping remains an essentially clinical art, mixing experience and an understanding of the problems likely to present—good headache histories are taken, not given. In differentiating the two main primary headache syndromes seen in clinical practice, migraine at its most simple level is headache with associated features, and tension-type headache is headache that is featureless; furthermore, most disabling headache is probably migrainous in biology. By features is meant throbbing pain, or sensitivity to sensory stimuli—visual, auditory, olfactory—or to head movement itself.

Frequent migraine

If headache with associated features describes migraine attacks, then headachy describes the person who has migraines over a lifetime. It is important to realize that the word migraine can describe both the attacks using standard criteria (see Box 24.8.2) and the disorder itself, which is more than just the attack. People who have migraines (migraineurs) inherit a tendency to have headache that is amplified at various times by their interaction with their environment, the much-discussed 'triggers'. The brain of the migraineur seems more sensitive to sensory stimuli and to change; and this tendency is notably amplified in women during their menstrual cycle. People who have a migraine may have headache when they oversleep, when tired, when they skip meals, when they overexert, when stressed, or when they relax from a stressor. They are less tolerant to change, and part of successful management is to advise them to maintain regularity in their lives in the knowledge of this fluctuating biology. It is this biology that marks migraine and in clinical practice must over-ride the phenotype of individual headaches.

It has been said that migraine can never occur daily; this is simply not correct. Chronic migraine very definitely occurs and is probably the largest part of the group of headaches known collectively as chronic daily headache that presents to doctors (see below). After making a diagnosis, the second step in the clinical process is to be sure that the disease burden has been captured, how much headache patients have and, more important, what patients cannot do—what is their degree of disability? One can ask the patient

INSTRUCTIONS: Please answer the following questions about ALL your headaches you have had over the last 3 months. Write your answer in the box next to each question. Write zero if you did not do the activity in the last 3 months (Please refer to the calendar below, if necessary)

1. On how many days in the last 3 months did you miss work or school because of your headaches? .... |__|__| days

2. How many days in the last 3 months was your productivity at work or school reduced by half or more because of your headaches (*Do not include days you counted in question 1 where you missed work or school*)? .... |__|__| days

3. On how many days in the last 3 months did you **not** do household work because of your headaches? .... |__|__| days

4. How many days in the last 3 months was your productivity in household work reduced by half or more because of your headaches (*Do not include days you counted in question 3 where you did not do household work*)? .... |__|__| days

5. On how many days in the last 3 months did you miss family, social, or leisure activities because of your headaches? .... |__|__| days

    A. On how many days in the last 3 months did you have a headache? (If a headache lasted more than one day, count each day) .... |__|__| days

    B. On a scale of 0–10, on average how painful were these headaches? (*where 0 = no pain at all, and 10 = pain as bad as it can be*) .... |__|__|

Version 3.0 © Innovative Medical Research 1997

Fig. 24.8.4 Migraine Disability Assessment Score (MIDAS) questionnaire.

directly to get a flavour for this, keep a diary, or get a quick but accurate estimate using the Migraine Disability Assessment Scale (MIDAS), which is well validated and very easy to use in practice (Fig. 24.8.4).

Principles of management of migraine

After diagnosis the management of migraine begins with an explanation of some aspects of the disorder to the patient:

◆ Migraine is an inherited tendency to have headache; this is caused by the patient's genes, therefore it cannot be cured.

◆ Migraine can be modified and controlled by lifestyle adjustment and the use of medicines.

◆ Migraine is not life threatening or associated with serious illness, with the exception of women who smoke and use oestrogenic oral contraceptives, but migraine can make life a misery.

◆ Migraine management takes time and cooperation, e.g. when a headache diary has to be collected, or enquiry made about the disability.

Nonpharmacological management of migraine

This approach aims to help migrainous patients identify things making the problem worse and encourage them to modify these. Patients need to know that the brain sensitivity that is migraine varies, so that the effect of triggers will vary. Patient associations are often very helpful in supporting migraineurs to identify triggers. The knowledge that there is variability will remove considerable frustration on the patient's part, and will ring true to most as they have had the experience. The crucial lifestyle advice is to explain to the patient that migraine is a state of brain sensitivity to change. This implies that these people need to regulate their lives: healthy diet, regular exercise, regular sleep patterns, avoiding excess caffeine and alcohol, and, as far as practicable, modifying or minimizing changes in stress. The balanced life with fewer highs and lows will benefit most people who have migraines.

Preventive treatments of migraine

Patients need to understand they have an inherited, noncurable, but manageable problem. To start a preventive they need to have sufficient disability to wish to take a medicine to reduce the affects of the disease on their life. The basis of considering preventive treatment from a medical viewpoint is a combination of acute attack frequency and attack tractability that confers an unacceptable degree of disability. Patients with attacks unresponsive to abortive medications are easily considered for prevention, whereas patients with simply treated attacks may be less obvious candidates. Another important consideration is disease progress. If a patient diary shows a clear trend of an increasing frequency of attacks, it is better to initiate with prevention than wait for the problem to worsen.

A simple rule for frequency might be that for one to two headaches a month there is usually no need to start a preventive, for three to four it may be needed but not necessarily, and for five or more per month prevention should definitely be considered. Options available for treatment are covered in detail in Table 24.8.2 and vary somewhat by country. One problem with preventives is

Table 24.8.2 Preventive treatments in migraine[a]

Drug	Dose	Selected side effects
Pizotifen	0.5–2 mg daily	Weight gain Drowsiness
β-Blocker		
Propranolol	40–120 mg twice daily	Reduced energy Tiredness Postural symptoms Contraindicated in asthma
Tricyclics		
Amitriptyline Dosulepin (dothiepin) Nortriptyline	25–75 mg at night	Drowsiness *Note*: some patients are very sensitive and may only need a total dose of 10 mg, although generally 1–1.5 mg/kg body weight is required
Anticonvulsants		
Valproate	400–600 mg twice daily	Drowsiness Weight gain Tremor Hair loss Fetal abnormalities Haematological or liver abnormalities
Topiramate	50–200 mg/day	Paraesthesiae Cognitive dysfunction Weight loss Care with a family history of glaucoma Nephrolithiasis
Gabapentin	900–3600 mg daily	Dizziness Sedation
Methysergide	1–6 mg daily	Drowsiness Leg cramps Hair loss Retroperitoneal fibrosis (1 month drug holiday is required every 6 months)
Flunarizine	5–15 mg daily	Drowsiness Weight gain Depression Parkinsonism
Single studies[b]		
Lisinopril	20 mg daily	Cough
Candasartan	16 mg daily	Dizziness
Neutriceuticals[c]		Gastrointestinal upset
Riboflavin	400 mg daily	
Coenzyme Q10	100 mg three times daily	
Butterburr	75 mg twice daily	
Feverfew	6.25 mg three times daily	
No convincing controlled evidence		Verapamil
Controlled trials to demonstrate no effect		Nimodipine Clonidine SSRIs: fluoxetine

[a]Commonly used preventives are listed with reasonable doses and common side effects. The local national formulary should be consulted for detailed information.

[b] Compounds not widely considered mainstream but with a positive randomized control trial against placebo.

[c] Nonpharmaceuticals with at least one positive randomized controlled trial against placebo.

SSRI, selective serotonin reuptake inhibitor.

that they have fallen into use for migraine from other indications and often bring unwanted or intolerable side effects. It is not clear how preventives work, although it seems likely that they modify the brain sensitivity that underlies migraine. Another key clinical point is that generally each drug should be started at a low dose and gradually increased to a reasonable maximum if there is going to be a clinical effect.

Relatively little has been done in terms of systematic study of patients with more intractable forms of migraine. Neuromodulation approaches are promising, including stimulation of the occipital nerve, and functional imaging studies show that central processing of pain signals in migraine in the thalamus may be modified by such therapies. This is an exciting and developing area.

Acute attack therapies of migraine

Acute attack treatments for migraine can be usefully divided into disease-nonspecific treatments (analgesics and nonsteroidal anti-inflammatory drugs (NSAIDs)) and disease-specific treatments (ergot-related compounds and triptans). It is important to be aware that most acute attack medications seem to have a propensity to aggravate headache frequency and can induce a state of refractory daily or near-daily headache—medication overuse headache. As evidence is gathered, this seems to occur in patients with migraine: either a previous clear history or a family or personal history of headachiness. Codeine-containing compound analgesics are particularly troublesome when available in over-the-counter (OTC) preparations. Patients with migraine should be advised to avoid taking acute attack medicines on more than 2 days a week. A proportion of patients who stop taking regular analgesics will have substantial improvement in their headache with a reduction in frequency; however, for some it will not make any difference. It is crucial to emphasize to the patient that standard preventive medications often simply do not work in the presence of regular analgesic use.

Treatment strategies

Given the array of options to control an acute attack of migraine, how does one start? The simplest approach to treatment has been described as 'stepped care'. In this model all patients are treated, assuming no contraindications, with the simplest treatment, such as aspirin 900 mg or paracetamol 1000 mg with an antiemetic. Aspirin is an effective strategy, has been proven so in double-blind controlled clinical trials, and is best used in its most soluble formulations. The alternative is a strategy known as 'stratified care', by which the physician determines, or stratifies, treatment at the start, based on the likelihood of response to levels of care. An intermediate option may be described as stratified care by attack. This is what many headache authorities suggest, and what patients often do when they have the option: they use simpler options for their less severe attacks, relying on more potent options when their attacks or circumstances demand them (Table 24.8.3).

Nonspecific acute migraine attack treatments

As simple drugs, such as aspirin and paracetamol, are cheap and can be effective, dosages should be adequate and the addition of domperidone (10 mg orally) or metoclopramide (10 mg orally) can be very helpful. NSAIDs can very useful when tolerated. Their success is often limited by inappropriate dosing, and adequate doses of naproxen 500 to 1000 mg orally or rectally, with an antiemetic,

Table 24.8.3 Oral acute migraine treatments

Nonspecific treatments[a]	Specific treatments
Aspirin 900 mg	**Ergot derivatives**
Paracetamol 1000 mg	Ergotamine 1–2 mg
NSAIDs	**Triptans**
Naproxen 500–1000 mg	Sumatriptan 50 or 100 mg
Ibuprofen 400–800 mg	Naratriptan 2.5 mg
Tolfenamic acid 200 mg	Rizatriptan 10 mg
	Zolmitriptan 2.5 or 5 mg
	Eletriptan 40 or 80 mg
	Almotriptan 12.5 mg
	Frovatriptan 2.5 mg

[a] Often used with antiemetic/prokinetics, such as domperidone 10 mg or metoclopramide 10 mg.
NSIADs, nonsteroidal anti-inflammatory drugs.

ibuprofen 400 to 800 mg orally, or tolfenamic acid 200 mg orally can be extremely effective.

Specific acute migraine attack treatments

When simple analgesic measures fail or more aggressive treatment is required, the specific antimigraine treatments are required (Table 24.8.4). Although ergotamine remains a useful treatment, it can no longer be considered the treatment of choice in acute migraine. There are particular situations in which ergotamine is very helpful, but its use must be carefully controlled as ergotamine overuse produces dreadful headache in addition to a host of vascular problems. The triptans, serotonin $5HT_{1B/1D}$-receptor agonists, have revolutionized the life of many patients with migraine and are clearly the most powerful option available to stop a migraine attack. They can be rationally applied by considering their pharmacological, physicochemical, and pharmacokinetic features, as well as the formulations that are available. Recent data suggest that combining a triptan with an NSAID can improve efficacy and reduce headache recurrence.

Tension-type headache

Clinical features

As its name suggests, tension-type headache (TTH) is the least understood headache form. TTH is diagnosed often and, although the phenotype is common, much of the disabling headache that goes under the name TTH is likely to be migrainous in terms of its biology. TTH has two forms—episodic TTH, where attacks occur on fewer than 15 days a month, and chronic TTH, where attacks, on average over time, are seen on 15 days or more a month. The latter is part of the broader clinical syndrome of chronic daily headache, but these terms are not equal.

TTH has been defined by the IHS for both its episodic and chronic forms, although the admixture of symptoms allowed has consistency problems. A useful clinical approach is to diagnose TTH when the headache is completely featureless: no nausea, no vomiting, no photophobia, no phonophobia, no osmophobia, no throbbing, and no aggravation with movement. Such an approach

Table 24.8.4 Stratification of acute specific migraine treatments

Clinical situation	Treatment options
Failed analgesics/NSAIDS	*First tier*
	Sumatriptan 50 mg or 100 mg orally
	Almotriptan 12.5 mg orally
	Rizatriptan 10 mg orally
	Eletriptan 40 mg orally
	Zolmitriptan 2.5 mg orally
	Slower effect/better tolerability
	Naratriptan 2.5 mg orally
	Frovatriptan 2.5 mg orally
	Infrequent headache
	Ergotamine 1–2 mg orally
	Dihydroergotamine nasal spray 2 mg
	Dihydroergotamine 0.5 mg by inhalation
Early nausea or difficulties taking tablets	Zolmitriptan 5 mg nasal spray
	Sumatriptan 20 mg nasal spray
	Rizatriptan 10 mg MLT wafer
	Sumatriptan transdermal patch
Headache recurrence	Ergotamine 2 mg (most effective rectally/ usually with caffeine)
	Naratriptan 2.5 mg orally
	Almotriptan 12.5 mg orally
	Eletriptan 40 mg
	Dihydroergotamine 0.5 mg by inhalation
Tolerating acute treatments orally	Naratriptan 2.5 mg
	Almotriptan 12.5 mg
Early vomiting	Zolmitriptan 5 mg nasal spray
	Sumatriptan 25 mg rectally
	Sumatriptan 6 mg subcutaneously
Menstrually related headache	*Prevention*
	Ergotamine orally at night
	Oestrogen patch
	Treatment
	Triptans
	Dihydroergotamine nasal spray
Very rapidly developing symptoms	Zolmitriptan 5 mg nasal spray
	Sumatriptan 6 mg subcutaneously
	Dihydroergotamine 1 mg intramuscularly

neatly divides migraine, which has one or more of these features and is the main differential diagnosis from TTH.

Pathophysiology

The pathophysiology of TTH is very poorly understood. This results from the fact that the name implies to most that it is a product of nervous tension, for which there is no clear evidence, and the definitions employed have undoubtedly admitted patients with migraine to the studies. Moreover, the concept that TTH in some way involves muscle contraction is incorrect because the evidence is that muscle contraction is no more likely than it is in migraine. It seems likely that TTH is due to a primary disorder of CNS pain modulation alone in contrast with migraine, which is a more generalized disturbance of sensory modulation.

Management

Adopting the clinical approach to TTH outlined above results in diagnosing a headache form that is usually less disabling, more often described by patients as irritating. Its episodic form is generally amenable to simple analgesics, paracetamol, aspirin, or NSAIDs, which can be purchased over the counter. There are clear clinical studies to demonstrate that triptans in TTH alone are not helpful, although, germane to the above discussion, triptans are effective in TTH where the patient also has migraine. For chronic TTH amitriptyline is the only treatment with a clear evidence base; the other tricyclic antidepressants, selective serotonin reuptake inhibitors, or benzodiazepines have not been shown in controlled trials to be effective. Similarly, there is no controlled evidence for the use of electromyography (EMG) biofeedback, relaxation therapy, or acupuncture. Botulinum toxin has been shown reasonably clearly to be ineffective. Stress management has been shown to be an effective approach in a controlled trial.

Trigeminal–autonomic cephalalgias

Cluster headache

Cluster headache is a rare form of primary headache with a population frequency of 0.1%. It is covered in specialist books. As a clinical anchor, it is about as common as multiple sclerosis in the United Kingdom, and must be regarded as a disorder best managed by neurologists or headache specialists. It is perhaps the most painful condition of humans; in the cohort of more than 1000 patients seen at the National Hospital for Neurology and Neurosurgery in London not a single one has had a more painful experience, including childbirth, multiple fractures of the limbs, and renal stones. It is one of a group of conditions known now as trigeminal–autonomic cephalalgias (TACs), and thus needs to be differentiated from other TACs and the short-lasting headaches

Table 24.8.5 Cluster headache, other trigeminal–autonomic cephalalgias (TACs), and short-lasting headaches

TACs[a]	Other short-lasting headaches
Cluster headache	Primary stabbing headache
Paroxysmal hemicrania	Trigeminal neuralgia
SUNCT/SUNA[b] syndrome	Primary cough headache
	Primary exertional headache
	Primary sex headache
	Hypnic headache

[a] Beware of pituitary tumour-related headache in the differential diagnosis of these TACs.
[b] Short-lasting unilateral neuralgiform headache attacks with conjunctival injection and tearing/cranial autonomic features.

3.1 Diagnostic criteria:

A At least five attacks fulfilling B–D

B Severe or very severe unilateral orbital, supraorbital and/or temporal pain lasting 15–180 min if untreated

C Headache is accompanied by at least one of the following:

  (1) ipsilateral conjunctival injection and/or lacrimation

  (2) ipsilateral nasal congestion and/or rhinorrhoea

  (3) forehead and facial sweating

  (4) ipsilateral eyelid oedema

  (5) ipsilateral forehead and facial sweating

  (6) ipsilateral miosis and/or ptosis

  (7) a sense of restlessness or agitation

D Attacks have a frequency from one every other day to eight per day

E Not attributed to another disorder

3.1.1 Episodic cluster headache

Description: occurs in periods lasting 7 days to 1 year separated by pain-free periods lasting 1 month or more

Diagnostic criteria

A All fulfilling criteria A–E of 3.1

B At least two cluster periods lasting from 7 to 365 days and separated by pain-free remissions of ≥1 month

3.1.2 Chronic cluster headache

Description: attacks occur for more than 1 year without remission or with remissions lasting less than 1 month

Diagnostic criteria

A All alphabetical headings of 3.1

B Attacks recur over >1 year without remission periods or with remission periods <1 month

Headache Classification Committee of the International Headache Society, 2004.

without cranial autonomic symptoms, such as lacrimation or conjunctival injection (Table 24.8.5).

The core feature of cluster headache is periodicity, be it circadian or in terms of active and inactive bouts over weeks and months (Box 24.8.3). The typical cluster headache patient is male, with a 3:1 predominance, who has bouts of one to two attacks of relatively short duration unilateral pain every day for 8 to 10 weeks a year. They are generally perfectly well in between. Patients with cluster headache tend to move about during attacks, pacing, rocking, or even rubbing their head for relief. The pain is usually retro-orbital, boring, and very severe. It is associated with ipsilateral symptoms of cranial (parasympathetic) autonomic activation: a red or watering eye, running or blocked nose, or cranial sympathetic dysfunction—eyelid droop. Cluster headache is likely to be a disorder involving neurons in or around the central pacemaker

regions of the posterior hypothalamic grey matter (see Fig. 24.8.2). Although cluster headache patients may also experience nausea, photophobia, and phonophobia, the last two, particularly photophobia, tend to be ipsilateral to the pain only in TACs.

The TACs—cluster headache, paroxysmal hemicrania, and SUNCT syndrome—present a distinct group to be differentiated from short-lasting headaches that do not have prominent cranial autonomic syndromes, notably trigeminal neuralgia, idiopathic (primary) stabbing headache, and hypnic headache. By determining the cycling pattern, length of attack, frequency of attack, and timing of the attacks, most patients can be usefully classified. The importance of clinical classification of this group is threefold: first, the clinical phenotype determines the likely secondary causes that must be considered and appropriate investigations ordered; second, the appropriate classification gives clarity to the patient with a clear diagnosis and allows the physician to draw on available literature to comment on natural history; and third, the correct diagnosis determines therapy that can be very different in these conditions, being very good if the diagnosis is correct but largely ineffective if it is not (Table 24.8.6).

Managing cluster headache

Cluster headache is managed using acute attack treatments and preventive agents. Acute attack treatments are usually required by all cluster headache patients at some time, whereas preventives can seem almost life-saving for the patients with chronic cluster headache, and are often needed to shorten the active periods in patients with the episodic form of the disorder.

Preventive treatments

The options for preventive treatment in cluster headache depend on the bout length (Table 24.8.7). Patients with short bouts require medicines that act quickly but will not necessarily be taken for long periods, whereas those with long bouts or indeed those with chronic cluster headache require safe, effective medicines that can be taken for long periods. Verapamil is now widely considered as the first-line preventive treatment when the bout is prolonged, or in chronic cluster headache. By contrast, limited courses of oral corticosteroids or methysergide can be very useful strategies when the bout is relatively short.

Verapamil has been suggested as a useful option for the last decade and compares favourably with lithium. What has clearly emerged from clinical practice is the need to use higher doses than had initially been considered and certainly higher than those used routinely in cardiological indications. Although most patients will start on doses as low as 40 to 80 mg twice daily, doses up to 960 mg daily are often required. Side-effects, such as gingival hyperplasia, constipation, and leg swelling, are recognized, as are cardiac dysrhythmias. Verapamil can cause heart block by slowing conduction in the atrioventricular (AV) node, monitored clinically by the PR interval on the ECG. Given that the effects on the AV node take up to 10 days to manifest, 2-week intervals are recommended between dose changes on the first exposure, with ECGs before the next escalation, and routine 6-monthly ECGs after the dose has been established.

Acute attack treatment

Cluster headache attacks often peak rapidly and thus require a treatment with quick onset. Many patients with acute cluster headache respond very well to treatment with oxygen inhalation. This should be given as 100% oxygen at 10 to 12 litres/min for 15 to

Table 24.8.6 Differential diagnosis of short-lasting headaches

Feature	Cluster headache	Paroxysmal hemicrania	SUNCT/SUNA[a]	Primary stabbing headache	Trigeminal neuralgia*	Hypnic headache
Gender	M>F 3:1	F=M	M>F	F>M	F>M	M=F
Pain	Boring/ throbbing	Boring/throbbing	Stabbing/throbbing	Stabbing	Stabbing	Throbbing
Type	Very severe	Very severe	Very severe	Severe	Very severe	Moderate
Severity	Any	Any	Any	Any	V2/V3 >V1	Generalized
Cranial location						
Duration	15–180 min	2–30 min	15–600 s	Seconds–3 min	<5 s	15–30 min
Frequency	1–8/day	1–40/day	1/day–30/h	Any	Any	1–3/night
Autonomic	+	+	+	–	–	–
Alcohol	+	One-third	–	–	–	–
Cutaneous trigger to attacks	–	–	+	–	+	–
Indometacin	–	+	–	+	–	–

SUNCT, short-lasting unilateral neuralgiform headache attacks with conjunctival injection and tearing; SUNA, short-lasting unilateral neuralgiform headache attacks with cranial autonomic symptoms.

[a] SUNCT/SUNA generally has no refractory period to trigger additional attacks, although this is a very common feature of trigeminal neuralgia.

20 min. It is important to have a high flow and high oxygen content. Injectable sumatriptan 6 mg is effective, rapid in onset, and has no evidence of tachyphylaxis. Sumatriptan 20 mg and zolmitriptan 5 mg nasal sprays are effective in acute cluster headache in controlled trials, and offer a useful option. Sumatriptan is not effective when given pre-emptively as 100 mg orally three times daily, and there is no evidence that it is useful when used orally in the acute treatment of cluster headache; indeed it can be associated with medication-overuse headache problems.

Surgical treatment

The surgical treatment of cluster headache has been completely revolutionized with the introduction of neurostimulation therapies. Surgical treatment of cluster headache is reserved for the most refractory patients, typically with chronic cluster headache. Destructive procedures, such as pterygopalatinectomy or radiofrequency lesions of the trigeminal ganglion, have been used. The former, with no clear effects, and the latter being helpful, but often at significant cost, including ocular complications or anaesthesia dolorosa. Trigeminal rhizotomy has also been employed, with all the complications of radiofrequency lesions and the occasional death.

Table 24.8.7 Preventive management of cluster headache

Short-term prevention (episodic cluster headache)	Long-term prevention (episodic cluster headache and prolonged chronic cluster headache)
Prednisolone	Verapamil
Methysergide	Lithium
Verapamil	Methysergide
Greater occipital nerve injection (daily nocturnal ergotamine)	Melatonin
	?Topiramate
	?Gabapentin

? = unproven but promising.

Set against this the functional imaging work describing activations in the posterior hypothalamic region directly lead to deep brain stimulation approaches in the same region which seem to be highly effective. Occipital nerve stimulation is a further very promising and largely noninvasive approach to the management of intractable chronic cluster headache, which may become the treatment of choice in this setting over the next 5 to 10 years.

Paroxysmal hemicrania

Sjaastad and Dale (1976) first reported eight cases of a frequent unilateral severe but short-lasting headache without remission coining the term chronic paroxysmal hemicrania (CPH). The mean daily frequency of attacks varied from 7 to 22 with the pain persisting from 5 to 45 min on each occasion. The site and associated autonomic phenomena were similar to cluster headache, but the attacks of CPH were suppressed completely by indometacin.

The essential features of paroxysmal hemicrania that we have seen from a substantial cohort of patients are:

◆ unilateral, very severe pain

◆ short-lasting attacks, typically 20 min in length

◆ very frequent attacks (usually >5/day with a mean of 10)

◆ marked autonomic features ipsilateral to the pain

◆ robust, quick (<72 h), excellent response to indometacin

The pathophysiology of paroxysmal hemicrania (PH) is marked by activations on PET (positron emission tomography) in the contralateral posterior hypothalamus and contralateral ventral midbrain. The posterior hypothalamic activity is shared with cluster headache, SUNCT, and hemicrania continua, whereas the ventral midbrain activity is only seen in hemicrania continua, which remarkably is also an indometacin-sensitive primary headache.

The therapy of PH may be complicated by gastrointestinal side effects seen with indometacin, in which topiramate may be helpful. Secondary PH is more likely if the patient requires high doses (>200 mg/day) of indometacin and raised cerebrospinal fluid pressure should be suspected in apparent bilateral PH. It is worth noting that indometacin reduces cerebrospinal fluid pressure by an unknown mechanism. It is appropriate to image patients, with MRI if practical, when a diagnosis of PH is being considered.

SUNCT/SUNA

Sjaastad and colleagues (1989) reported three male patients whose brief attacks of pain in and around one eye were associated with sudden conjunctival injection and other autonomic features of cluster headache. The attacks lasted only 15 to 60 s and recurred 5 to 30 times per hour, and could be precipitated by chewing or eating certain foods, such as citrus fruits. They were not abolished by indometacin. Brain imaging has suggested that they share with cluster headache and paroxysmal hemicrania the feature on activation studies of involvement of the posterior hypothalamic region. Of the patients recognized with this problem, males dominate slightly and the paroxysms of pain may last between 5 and 300 s, although longer, duller interictal pains are recognized, as are longer attacks with a sawtooth pattern. The conjunctival injection seen with SUNCT is often the most prominent autonomic feature and tearing may be very obvious.

If one of either conjunctival injection or tearing is absent, or neither is present but another cranial autonomic symptom is seen, the term SUNA is used. The two key clinical features of SUNCT/SUNA are that the attacks can be triggered with no refractory period to triggering. The latter serves as a very useful distinction between SUNCT/SUNA and trigeminal neuralgia. SUNCT/SUNA can be treated very frequently with lamotrigine, and if that is unhelpful topiramate or gabapentin. Carbamazepine often has a useful but incomplete effect. Given what has been reported, cranial MRI with pituitary and posterior fossa views is highly recommended when SUNCT/SUNA is considered as a diagnosis.

Other primary headaches

Primary stabbing headache

Short-lived jabs of pain, defined by the Headache Classification Committee of the IHS as primary stabbing headache, are well documented in association with most types of primary headache.

The following are the essential clinical features:

◆ Pain confined to the head, although rarely is it facial

◆ Stabbing pain lasting from 1 to many seconds and occurring as a single stab or a series of stabs

◆ Recurring at irregular intervals (hours to days).

These pains have been called ice-pick pains or jabs and jolts. They generally respond to indometacin 25 to 50 mg two to three times daily. The symptoms tend to wax and wane and after a period of control on indometacin it is appropriate to withdraw treatment and observe the outcome. Most patients will not want treatment when the nature of the problem is explained and they are reassured that the attacks are not sinister in any way.

Primary cough headache

Sharp pain in the head on coughing, sneezing, straining, laughing, or stooping has long been regarded as a symptom of organic intracranial disease, commonly associated with obstruction of the cerebrospinal fluid pathways. The presence of an Arnold–Chiari malformation or any lesion causing obstruction of cerebrospinal

fluid pathways or displacing cerebral structures must be excluded before cough headache is assumed to be benign. Cerebral aneurysm, carotid stenosis, and vertebrobasilar disease may also present with cough or exertional headache as the initial symptom. The term 'benign Valsalva's manoeuvre-related headache' covers the headaches provoked by coughing, straining, or stooping but 'cough headache' is more succinct and so widely used that it is unlikely to be displaced.

The following are the essential clinical features of primary cough headache:

◆ Bilateral headache of sudden onset, lasting minutes, precipitated by coughing

◆ May be prevented by avoiding coughing

◆ Diagnosed only after structural lesions, such as posterior fossa tumour, have been excluded by neuroimaging

Indometacin is the medical treatment of choice in cough headache. Raskin followed up an observation of Sir Charles Symonds reporting that some patients with cough headache are relieved by lumbar puncture. This is a simple option when compared with prolonged use of indometacin. The mechanism of this response remains unclear.

Primary exertional headache

The relationship of this form of headache to cough headache is unclear and certainly much is shared. Indeed the relationship to migraine also requires delineation.

The following are the clinical features:

◆ Pain specifically brought on by physical exercise

◆ Bilateral and throbbing in nature at onset and may develop migrainous features in those patients susceptible to migraine

◆ Lasts from 5 min to 24 h

◆ Prevented by avoiding excessive exertion, particularly in hot weather or at high altitude.

The acute onset of headache with straining and breath-holding, as in weightlifter's headache, may be explained by acute venous distension. The development of headache after sustained exertion, particularly on a hot day, is more difficult to understand. Anginal pain may be referred to the head, probably by central connections of vagal afferents, and may present as exertional headache, so-called cardiac cephalgia. The link to exercise is the important clinical clue. Phaeochromocytoma may occasionally be responsible for exertional headache. Intracranial lesions or stenosis of the carotid arteries may have to be excluded as discussed for benign cough headache. Headache may be precipitated by any form of exercise and often has the pulsatile quality of migraine. The most obvious form of treatment is to take exercise gradually and progressively whenever possible. Indometacin at daily doses varying from 25 to 150 mg is generally very effective in benign exertional headache. Indometacin 50 mg, ergotamine tartrate 1 to 2 mg orally, dihydroergotamine by nasal spray, or methysergide 1 to 2 mg orally given 30 to 45 min before exercise are useful prophylactic measures.

Primary sex headache

Sex headache may be precipitated by masturbation or coitus and usually starts as a dull bilateral ache while sexual excitement increases, suddenly becoming intense at orgasm. The term 'orgasmic cephalgia' is not accurate because not all sex headache require orgasm. Two types of primary sex headache are recognized: a dull ache in the head and neck that intensifies as sexual excitement increases, and a sudden severe ('explosive') headache occurring at orgasm. Low cerebrospinal fluid volume headache may also be precipitated by a sexual activity and is considered as a form of new daily persistent headache (see below).

The following are the essential clinical features of a sex headache:

♦ Precipitation by sexual excitement

♦ Bilateral at onset

♦ Prevented or eased by ceasing sexual activity before orgasm

Headaches developing at the time of orgasm are not always benign, and consideration of a diagnosis of subarachnoid headache is essential. Sex headache affects men more often than women and may occur at any time during the years of sexual activity. It may develop on several occasions in succession, and then not trouble the patient again, despite no obvious change in sexual technique. In patients who stop sexual activity when the headache is first noticed it may subside within a period of 5 min to 2 h, and it is recognized that more frequent orgasm can aggravate established sex headache. About one-third of the patients with sex headache have a history of exertional headaches, but there is no excess of cough headache in patients with sex headache. In about 50% of patients, sex headache will settle in 6 months. Migraine is reported in about 25% of patients with sex headache.

Primary sex headaches are usually irregular and infrequent in occurrence, so management can often be limited to reassurance and advice about ceasing sexual activity if a milder, warning headache develops. When the condition recurs regularly or frequently, it can be prevented by the administration of propranolol; the dosage required varies from 40 mg to 200 mg daily. An alternative is the calcium channel blocking agent diltiazem 60 mg three times daily, which this author finds particularly useful in such patients. Ergotamine (1–2 mg) or indometacin (25–50 mg) taken about 30 to 45 min before sexual activity can also be helpful.

Hypnic headache

This syndrome was first described by Raskin in patients aged from 67 to 84 who had headache of a moderately severe nature which typically came on a few hours after going to sleep. These headaches last from 15 min to 30 min, are typically generalized, although may be unilateral, and can be throbbing. Patients may report falling back to sleep only to be awoken by a further attack a few hours later, with up to three repetitions of this pattern over the night. In Dodick's series of 19 patients, 16 (84%) were female and the mean age at onset was 61 ± 9 years. Headaches were bilateral in two-thirds and unilateral in one-third, and in 80% of cases mild or moderate. Three patients reported similar headaches when falling asleep during the day. None had photophobia or phonophobia and nausea is unusual.

Patients with this form of headache generally respond to a bedtime dose of lithium carbonate (200 600 mg) and in those who do not tolerate this verapamil or methysergide at bedtime may be alternative strategies. Some investigators reported that one to two cups of coffee or caffeine 60 mg orally at bedtime was helpful. This is a simple approach that is effective in about one-third of patients. An important secondary cause of hypnic headache is hypertension,

which should be carefully pursued and appropriately investigated as treatment of the blood pressure will arrest the headache problem.

Primary thunderclap headache

Sudden-onset severe headache may occur in the absence of sexual activity; the differential diagnosis includes the sentinel bleed of an intracranial aneurysm, cervicocephalic arterial dissection, and cerebral venous thrombosis. Headaches of explosive onset may also be caused by the ingestion of sympathomimetic drugs or tyramine-containing foods in a patient who is taking monoamine oxidase inhibitors, and can also be a symptom of a phaeochromocytoma. Whether thunderclap headache can be the presentation of an unruptured cerebral aneurysm is unclear. Day and Raskin (1986) reported on a woman with three episodes of sudden-onset, very severe headache who was found to have an unruptured aneurysm of the internal carotid artery, with adjacent areas of segmental vasospasm. In the absence of a CT scan or cerebrospinal fluid evidence of subarachnoid haemorrhage, studies indicate that such patients do very well, and there indeed seems to be a form of benign or primary thunderclap headache.

Wijdicks et al. (1988) followed up 71 patients whose CT scans and cerebrospinal fluid findings were negative for an average of 3.3 years: 12 patients had further such headaches and 31 (44%) later had regular episodes of migraine or TTH. Factors identified as precipitating the headache were sexual intercourse in 3 cases, coughing in 4, and exertion in 12, while the remainder had no obvious cause. A history of hypertension was found in 11 and of previous headache in 22. Markus (1991) compared the presentation of 37 patients with subarachnoid haemorrhage and 189 with a similar thunderclap headache and normal cerebrospinal fluid examination, and could not discern any characteristic to distinguish the two conditions.

Investigation of any sudden-onset severe headache, be it in the context of sexual excitement or isolated thunderclap headache, should be driven by the clinical context. The first presentation should be vigorously investigated with CT and cerebrospinal fluid examination, and where possible MRI/MR venography/MR angiography. Formal cerebral angiography should be reserved for when no primary diagnosis is forthcoming, and the clinical situation is particularly suggestive of intracranial aneurysm. Bearing in mind the entity of diffuse multifocal reversible cerebral vasospasm, which may be seen in apparent primary thunderclap headache without there being an intracranial aneurysm, caution in interpretation of the findings is crucial.

Hemicrania continua

Two patients were initially reported with this syndrome, a woman aged 63 years and a man of 53, who developed unilateral headache without obvious cause. Both patients were relieved completely by indometacin whereas other NSAIDs were of little or no benefit. Newman and colleagues (1992) reviewed the 24 previously reported cases and added 10 of their own, including some with pronounced autonomic features resembling cluster headache. They divided their case histories into remitting and unremitting forms. Of the 34 patients reviewed, 22 were women and 12 men with the age of onset ranging from 11 to 58 years. The symptoms were controlled by indometacin 75 to 150 mg daily. The following are the essential features of hemicrania continua:

♦ Unilateral pain

♦ Pain is continuous but with exacerbations that may be severe

◆ Complete resolution of pain with indometacin

◆ Exacerbations may be associated with autonomic features

Apart from analgesic overuse as an aggravating factor, and a report in an HIV-infected patient, the status of secondary hemicrania continua is unclear. Antonaci and colleagues (1998) proposed the 'Indotest' by which the intramuscular injection of indometacin 50 mg could be used as a diagnostic tool. In hemicrania continua, pain was relieved in 73 ± 66 min and the pain-free period was 13 ± 8 h. A placebo-controlled modification of this test is preferred where possible to the open-label version. Using the latter method in conjunction with PET, it has been shown that there is activation of the contralateral posterior hypothalamus and ipsilateral dorsal rostral pons in association with the headache of hemicrania continua, as well as activation of the ipsilateral ventrolateral midbrain. The alternative is a trial of oral indometacin, initially 25 mg three times daily, then 50 mg three times daily, and 75 mg three times daily. One should allow up to 2 weeks for any dose to have a useful effect. Acute treatment with sumatriptan has been employed and reported to be of no benefit. Cyclooxygenase II (COX-II) antagonists seem effective, although undesirable now, and topiramate is helpful in some patients, as is greater occipital nerve injection.

Chronic daily headache

Each of the above primary headache forms can occur very frequently. When a patient experiences headache on 15 days or more a month one can apply the broad diagnosis of chronic daily headache (CDH). CDH is not one thing but a collection of very different problems with different management strategies. Crucially not all daily headache is simply TTH (Table 24.8.8). This is the most common clinical misconception in headache, confusing the clinical phenotype with the headache biotype. Population-based

estimates of daily headache are remarkable, demonstrating that about 5% of Western populations have daily or almost daily headache. Daily headache may again be primary or secondary, and it seems clinically useful to consider the possibilities in this way when making management decisions (Table 24.8.8). It should be said that population-based studies bear out clinical practice in that a large group of refractory daily headache patients overuse various OTC preparations.

Chronic migraine

Although it is widely accepted that some of the primary headaches, TTH, cluster headache, and PH, have chronic varieties, this question seems to have become unnecessarily troublesome for migraine. Few headache authorities would argue that migraine can never ever be chronic in terms of frequency, but the issue of whether patients with frequent headache, some of which fulfils standard criteria for migraine and some for TTH, have a single migrainous biology is a very vexed one. Given that TTH describes a phenomenology that is indistinct at best, it seems unlikely that all its phenotypes will have a single biological generator.

The concept behind chronic migraine is that some patients who inherit a migrainous biology end up with CDH. The typical patient will have daily headache of a dull, nonspecific type, punctuated by more severe attacks that would often, in isolation, fulfil standard criteria for migraine. In headache speciality clinics this group is dominant, with about 90% of patients in referral headache clinics having chronic migraine, usually with medication overuse. It could be suggested that they have a biologically more difficult problem and this is the basis for their over-representation in referral centres.

If one applies the concepts outlined for TTH (see above) then the diagnosis of chronic TTH (CTTH) is made when the patient has 15 days or more a month of entirely featureless generalized dull or pressure-like pain. When any of the attacks on some days have migrainous features—nausea, photophobia, phonophobia, throbbing, or aggravation with movement—then chronic migraine is more likely to be the diagnosis. Clearly both chronic migraine and CTTH exist. Moreover, some patients must simply have coexisting CTTH and episodic migraine; however, it is simply impossible on clinical or other grounds to determine whom they are. The approach outlined probably overdiagnoses chronic migraine, taking that to be a biological entity, and underdiagnoses the coexistence of CTTH and episodic migraine. The converse would be true—if one diagnoses them all as CTTH and episodic migraine then chronic migraine is missed. In clinical practice the concept of chronic migraine is particularly helpful. Given that the lifestyle advice is identical for both TTH and migraine, and that the range of therapeutic options for preventive treatment in migraine is so much greater, the clinician loses absolutely nothing diagnosing chronic migraine, and the patient has much to gain. For research there are other imperatives.

Management

The management of CDH can be very rewarding. Most patients overusing analgesics respond very sensibly when the problem is explained.

The keys to managing daily headache are:

◆ Exclude treatable causes (see Table 24.8.8)

◆ Obtain a clear analgesic history

◆ Make a diagnosis of the primary headache type involved

Table 24.8.8 Classification of chronic daily headache

Primary		Secondary
>4 h daily	<4 h daily	
Chronic migraine[a]	Chronic cluster headache[b]	Post-traumatic
		Head injury
		Iatrogenic
		Postinfectious
Chronic tension-type headache[a]	Chronic paroxysmal hemicrania	Inflammatory, such as giant cell arteritis
		Sarcoidosis
		Behçet's syndrome
Hemicrania continua[a]	SUNCT	Chronic CNS infection
New daily persistent headache[a]	Hypnic Headache	Substance abuse headache

[a] May be complicated by analgesic overuse. In the case of substance abuse headache, the headache is completely resolved after the substance abuse is controlled (Headache Classification Committee of the International Headache Society, 2004—see 'Further reading'). Clinical experience suggests that many patients continue to have headache even after cessation of analgesic use. The residual headache probably represents the underlying headache biology.

[b] Chronic cluster headache patients may have more than 4 h/day of headache. The inclusion of the syndrome here is to emphasize that, by and large, the attacks themselves are less than 4 h duration.

CNS, central nervous system; SUNCT, short-lasting unilateral neuralgiform headache attacks with conjunctival injection and tearing.

Medication overuse

Medication overuse is defined as consuming an acute attack therapy on 10 days or more per month, expect for paracetamol where 15 days is allowed under current guidance. It is essential that analgesic overuse be reduced and eliminated if one is to see the underlying headache phenotype and start to manage the problem. Patients can reduce their use by, as an example, 10% every week or two, depending on their circumstances, or if they wish, and there is no contraindication, by immediate cessation of use. Either approach can be facilitated by first keeping a careful diary over a month or two to be sure of the size of the problem. A small dose of an NSAID, such as naproxen 500 mg twice daily if tolerated, will take the edge off the pain as analgesic use is reduced, as does a greater occipital nerve injection. It is a useful aside that NSAID overuse does not seem to be a common issue in daily headache when they are dosed once or twice daily, whereas with more frequent dosing problems may develop. When the patient has reduced analgesic use substantially a preventive should be introduced. It must be emphasized that preventive therapies most often simply do not work in the presence of analgesic overuse. Thus, the patient must reduce the analgesics or the entire attempt to use the preventive is largely wasted, although this helpful rule must have some limitations that require study. The most common cause of intractability to treatment is the use of a preventive when analgesics continue to be used regularly. For some patients this is very difficult, and often one must be blunt that some degree of pain is inevitable in the first instance if the problem is to be controlled.

Some patients with medication overuse will require admission for detoxification. Broadly this consists of two groups—those who fail outpatient withdrawal or those who have a significant complicating medical indication, such as brittle diabetes mellitus, or complicating medicines, such as opioids, where withdrawal may be problematic as an outpatient. When such patients are admitted acute medications are withdrawn completely on the first day, unless there is some contraindication. Antiemetics, such as domperidone orally or as a suppository, and fluids are administered as required, as well as clonidine for opioid withdrawal symptoms. For acute intolerable pain during the waking hours aspirin (1 g intravenously) is useful and at night chlorpromazine by injection, after ensuring adequate hydration. If the patient does not settle adequately over 3 to 5 days a course of intravenous dihydroergotamine (DHE) can be employed as Raskin described. As time goes by, one feels that DHE is indispensable in this setting. Often $5HT_3$ antagonists, such as ondansetron and granisetron, will be required with DHE because it is essential to ensure that the patient does not have significant nausea.

Preventive treatments

The tricylic antidepressants (TCAs), amitriptyline, dosulepin (dothiepin), and nortriptyline, at doses up to 1 mg/kg are very useful in patients with chronic migraine. TCAs are started in low dose (10–25 mg) daily and best given 12 h before the patient wishes to wake up to avoid excess morning sleepiness. The other very useful medications for these patients are the anticonvulsants, such as valproate, topiramate, and gabapentin. For valproate, doses up to 1500 mg daily are used, starting at 200 mg twice daily and increasing to 400 or 600 mg twice daily as tolerated over 2- to 4-week intervals. The blood count and liver enzymes should be checked at

Table 24.8.9 Differential diagnosis of New Daily Persistent Headache (NDPH)

Primary	Secondary
Migrainous type	Subarachnoid haemorrhage
Featureless (tension-type)	Low CSF volume headache
	Raised CSF pressure headache
	Post-traumatic headache[a]
	Chronic meningitis

[a] Includes postinfective forms.
CSF, cerebrospinal fluid.

baseline and the various side effects explained to patients, especially the fetal abnormalities to women. For topiramate one can start at 25 mg nightly and increase by 25 mg every 10 to 14 days to aim for 50 mg twice daily. For gabapentin the dose is 1800 to 3600 mg daily; it is very well tolerated, although probably less effective from a population viewpoint. For some patients flunarizine can be very effective, as can methysergide or phenelzine. Recently, botulinum toxin type A (onabotulinum toxin) has been shown in a randomized controlled trial to be useful in chronic migraine. One might consider its use, for example, in medically-refractory chronic migraine perhaps after three preventive classes have failed.

New daily persistent headache

New daily persistent headache (NDPH) is a clinically useful concept with a range of important possible causes because some are very treatable (Table 24.8.9). From a nosological point of view all that is mentioned here could be placed within various categories of the IHS classification, and indeed the IHS refers to primary NDPH. However, the term as employed here serves both patients and clinicians by highlighting a group of conditions, some of which are curable, and encompasses the IHS term under the primary featureless form of NDPH.

The patient with NDPH presents with a history of headache on most if not all days, starting from one day to the next. The onset of headache is abrupt, often from one moment to the next, but at least in less than a few days with three suggested as an upper limit. The typical history is for the patient to recall the exact day and circumstances, so from one moment to the next a headache develops that never leaves them. This presentation triggers certain key questions about the onset and behaviour of the pain. The pressing issues arise from considering the secondary headache possibilities. Although subarachnoid haemorrhage is listed for some logical consistency, as the headache may certainly come on from one moment to the next, it is not likely to produce diagnostic confusion in this group of patients. Suffice it to say that subarachnoid haemorrhage is so important that it must always be considered if only to be excluded, either by history or by appropriate investigation.

Primary NDPH

Initial descriptions of primary NDPH recognized that it occurs in both males and females. Migrainous features were common, with unilateral headache in about one-third and throbbing pain in about one-third. Nausea was reported in about one-half of the patients, as were photophobia and phonophobia. A number of

Box 24.8.4 Other secondary headaches

- Giant cell arteritis
- Cervicogenic headache
- Reader's paratrigeminal neuralgia
- Tolosa–Hunt syndrome
- Headache as a presentation of cervical dystonia
- Headache in temporomandibular dysfunction
- Cardiac cephalalgia
- Headache with endocrine disturbance, particularly pituitary tumour
- Neck–tongue syndrome
- Red-ear syndrome

these patients have a previous history of migraine, but not more than one might expect given the population prevalence of migraine. It is remarkable that the initial report noted that 86% of patients were headache free at 24 months. It is general experience among those interested in headache management that primary NDPH is perhaps the most intractable and least therapeutically rewarding form of headache. In general one can classify the dominant phenotype—migraine or TTH—and treat with preventives according to that subclassification.

Secondary NDPH

The secondary causes of the syndrome of NDPH are worthy of consideration, because they have distinctive clinical pictures that can guide investigation (Box 24.8.4).

Low cerebrospinal fluid volume headache

The syndrome of headache as a result of persistent low cerebrospinal fluid volume is an important diagnosis not to miss. The more immediately obvious version of this problem is encountered commonly after lumbar puncture. In that situation the headache usually settles rapidly with bed rest. In the chronic situation the patient typically presents with a history of headache from one day

to the next. The pain is generally not present on waking, worsens during the day, and is relieved by lying down. Recumbency usually improves the headache in minutes, and it takes only minutes to an hour for the pain to return when the patient is again upright. The patient may give a history of an index event: lumbar puncture or epidural injection, or a vigorous Valsalva manoeuvre, such as with lifting, straining, coughing, clearing the eustachian tubes in an aeroplane, or multiple orgasms. Patients may volunteer, or a history may be obtained, that soft drinks with caffeine provide temporary respite. Spontaneous leaks are recognized, and the clinician should not be put off the diagnosis if the headache history is typical when there is no obvious index event. As time passes from the index event the postural nature may be less obvious; certainly cases with an index event several years before the eventual diagnosis are recognized. The term 'low volume' rather than 'low pressure' is used, because there is no clear evidence at which point the pressure can be called low. Although low pressures, such as 0 to 5 are often identified, a pressure of 16 cmCSF has been recorded with a documented leak. One should be aware of the possibility of the development of subdural collections in patients with low cerebrospinal fluid volume headaches, which makes imaging before any invasive studies all the more important.

The investigation of choice is MRI with gadolinium (Fig. 24.8.5), which produces a striking pattern of diffuse pachymeningeal enhancement, although in about 10% of cases a leak can be documented without enhancement. The finding of diffuse meningeal enhancement is so typical that in the clinical context immediate treatment is appropriate. It is also common to see Chiari malformations on MRI with some degree of descent of the cerebellar tonsils. This is important because surgery in such settings simply worsens the headache problem. It seems appropriate that any patient being considered for such surgery for a headache indication should first be reviewed by a neurologist. To investigate further cerebrospinal fluid pressure may be determined, or preferably a leak sought with indium-111-labelled DPTA (diethylaminetriaminepentaacetic acid) cerebrospinal fluid studies that can demonstrate the site, early emptying of tracer into the bladder, or lack of progression of tracer over the cerebral convexities.

Treatment is bed rest in the first instance. False-positive transient improvement in persistent low cerebrospinal fluid volume

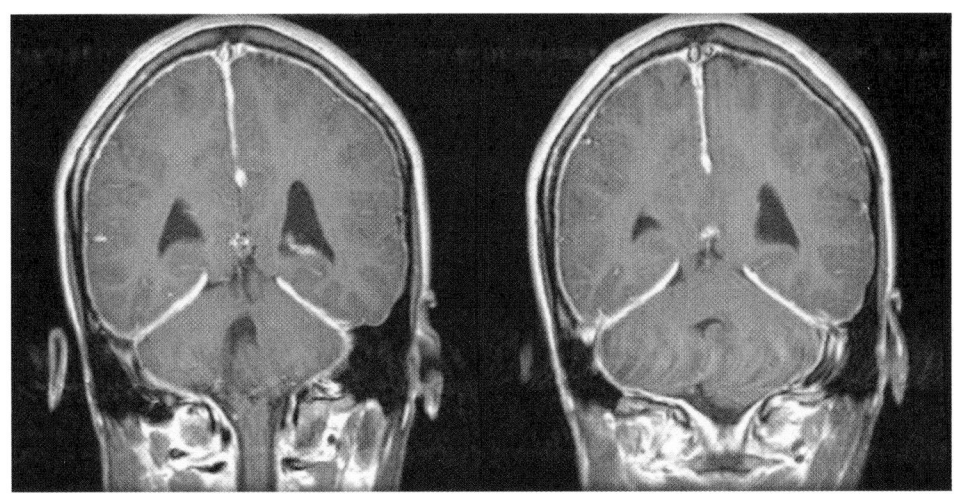

Fig. 24.8.5 MRI scan showing diffuse meningeal enhancement after gadolinium administration in a patient with low cerebrospinal fluid volume (pressure) headache.

headache with chiropractic and other similar therapies is recognized where the treatment necessitates the patient lying down for a prolonged period for the therapy. Intravenous caffeine (500 mg in 500 ml saline administered over 2 h) is a standard and often very efficacious treatment. The ECG should be checked for any arrhythmia before administration. A reasonable practice is to carry out at least two infusions separated by 4 weeks after obtaining the suggestive clinical history and MRI with enhancement. As intravenous caffeine is safe, and can be curative, by an unknown mechanism, it spares many patients the need for further tests. If that is unsuccessful, an abdominal binder may be helpful. If a leak can be identified, either by the radioisotope study or by CT myelogram, or spinal T_2-weighted MRI or more recently some radiologists using intrathecal Gd with MRI, an autologous blood patch is usually curative. In more intractable situations where as leak is not identified theophylline is a useful alternative that offers outpatient management, although its onset of action is rather slow.

Raised cerebrospinal fluid pressure headache

As is the case for low cerebrospinal fluid pressure states, raised cerebrospinal fluid pressure as a cause of headache is well recognized by neurologists. Brain imaging can often reveal the cause, such as raised pressure due to a space-occupying lesion. The particular setting in which patients enter the spectrum of NDPH are those with idiopathic intracranial hypertension who present with headache without visual problems, particularly with normal fundi. It is recognized that intractable chronic migraine can be triggered by persistently raised intracranial pressure. These patients typically give a history of generalized headache that is present on waking, and gets better as the day goes on. It is generally worse with recumbency. Visual obscurations are frequently reported. Fundal changes on raised intracranial pressure would make the diagnosis relatively straightforward, but it is in those without such changes that the history must drive the investigation. Patients often report a curious whooshing sensation in the occipital region.

Brain imaging is mandatory if raised pressure is suspected, and it is most simple in the long run to obtain an MRI scan, and include MR venography (MRV). The cerebrospinal fluid pressure should be measured by lumbar puncture, taking care to do so when the patient is symptomatic, so that both the pressure and response to removal of cerebrospinal fluid can be determined. A raised pressure and improvement in headache with removal of cerebrospinal fluid are diagnostic of the problem. The fields should be formally documented even in the absence of overt ophthalmic involvement. Initial treatment can be with acetazolamide (250–500 mg twice daily). The patient may respond in weeks with improvement in headache. If this is not effective topiramate has many actions that may be useful in this setting: carbonic anhydrase inhibition, weight loss, and neuronal membrane stabilization probably through actions on phosphorylation pathways. A small number of severely disabled patients who do not respond to medical treatment will come to intracranial pressure monitoring and even shunting. This is exceptional and not undertaken without careful work-up.

Post-traumatic headache

The issue of post-traumatic headache is vexed. The Headache Classification Committee accepts the existence of such a syndrome. Much of the scientific discussion becomes marred by the often-quoted medicolegal morass concerning delayed effects of head injury.

The term is used here to indicate trauma in a very broad way. NDPH may be seen after a blow to the head but more commonly after an infective episode, typically viral, or even malarial meningitis. A recent series identified that one-third of all patients with NDPH reported the headache starting after an influenza-like illness. The patient may note a period in which they had a significant infection: fever, neck stiffness, photophobia, and marked malaise. The headache starts during that period and never stops. Investigation reveals no current cause for the headache. It has been suggested that some patients with this syndrome have a persistent Epstein–Barr virus infection, but this syndrome is anything but clearly delineated. A complicating factor will often be that the patient had a lumbar puncture during that illness, so a persistent low cerebrospinal fluid volume headache needs to be considered first. Post-traumatic headache may be seen after carotid artery dissection, subarachnoid haemorrhage, and following intracranial surgery for a benign mass. The underlying theme seems to be that a traumatic event involving the dura mater can trigger a headache process that lasts for many years after that event.

The treatment of this form of NDPH is substantially empirical. TCAs, notably amitriptyline, and anticonvulsants, valproate, topiramate, and gabapentin, have been used with good effects. The monoamine oxidase A inhibitor phenelzine may also be useful in carefully selected patients. On the positive side, the headache seems to run a limited course of 3 to 5 years in most patients, so will eventually settle. It can certainly be very disabling in that period.

Other important forms of secondary headache (see Box 24.8.4)

Giant cell arteritis

This is an important cause of headache because delay in steroid treatment may result in blindness due to retinal artery ischaemia. It is also known as temporal arteritis or cranial arteritis. Patients are usually older with focal tenderness of the scalp, which may be provoked markedly by resting the head on the pillow. Jaw claudication provoked by chewing is a characteristic, but relatively uncommon, feature. Constitutional symptoms are common, particularly weight loss, malaise, or polymyalgia rheumatica. An elevated erythrocyte sedimentation rate (ESR) is a strong pointer to the diagnosis. The temporal artery may be tenderly inflamed, swollen, or pulseless. On suspicion of this diagnosis, steroid treatment should be started pending the result of temporal artery biopsy. Treatment is very often long term and requires careful monitoring for reactivation and the side effects of corticosteroids.

Cervicogenic headache

It is a time-honoured concept that the neck is responsible for many headaches. Unfortunately, as with much of history, the good story is often ruined by the facts. Although there is little doubt that there is a rich overlap between the innervation of intracranial pain-producing structures by the ophthalmic division of the trigeminal nerve, and the posterior fossa and high cervical innervation by branches especially of the C2 dorsal root, causality is another issue. The Headache Classification Committee recognizes that head pain can arise from the neck and labels this 'cervicogenic headache'. The term has been used by others to define a syndrome that is so poorly described as to be useless in practice. Most patients with neck discomfort and headache referred to speciality practice have migraine. They will have neck stiffness or discomfort as a premonitory symptom that can clearly persist in all stages of the attack. They may respond to local therapies, such as greater occipital nerve injection; however, this implies no more than triggering, and is to be expected. The pursuit of neck pathology and the treatment of patients with migraine by manipulative or physical means have no support in the controlled literature, and are rarely of long-lasting value.

Further reading

Afridi S, et al. (2005). A PET study in spontaneous migraine. *Arch Neurol*, **62**, 1270–5.

Afridi S, et al. (2005). A PET study exploring the laterality of brainstem activation in migraine using glyceryl trinitrate. *Brain*, **128**, 932–9.

Afridi SK, et al. (2006). Greater occipital nerve injection in primary headache syndromes—prolonged effects from a single injection. *Pain*, **122**, 126–9.

Andlin-Sobocki P, et al. (2005). Cost of disorders of the brain in Europe. *Eur J Neurol*, **12**, 1–27.

Andreou AP, Shields KG, Goadsby PJ (2010). GABA and valproate modulate trigeminovascular nociceptive transmission in the thalamus. *Neurobiology of Disease*, **37**, 314–23.

Antonaci F, Fredriksen T, Sjaastad O (2001). Cervicogenic headache: clinical presentation, diagnostic criteria, and differential diagnosis. *Current Pain Headache Rep*, **5**, 387–92.

Antonaci F, et al. (1998). Chronic paroxysmal hemicrania and hemicrania continua. Parenteral indomethacin: the 'Indotest'. *Headache*, **38**, 122–8.

Bahra A, et al. (2001). Brainstem activation specific to migraine headache. *Lancet*, **357**, 1016–17.

Bartsch T, Goadsby PJ (2005). Anatomy and physiology of pain referral in primary and cervicogenic headache disorders. *Headache Currents*, **2**, 42–8.

Bogduk N (1981). An anatomical basis for the neck–tongue syndrome. *J Neurol Neurosurg Psychiatry*, **44**, 202–8.

Brandes JL, et al. (2007). Sumatriptan–naproxen for acute treatment of migraine: a randomized trial. *JAMA*, **297**, 1443–54.

Burns B, Watkins L, Goadsby PJ (2007). Successful treatment of medically intractable cluster headache using occipital nerve stimulation (ONS). *Lancet*, **369**, 1099–106.

Cittadini E, Matharu MS, Goadsby PJ (2008). Paroxysmal hemicrania: a prospective clinical study of thirty-one cases. *Brain*, **131**, 1142–55.

Cohen AS, Goadsby PJ (2006). Functional neuroimaging of primary headache disorders. *Neurotherapeutics*, **6**, 1159–72.

Cohen AS, Matharu MS, Goadsby PJ (2006). Short-lasting unilateral neuralgiform headache attacks with conjunctival injection and tearing (SUNCT) or cranial autonomic features (SUNA). A prospective clinical study of SUNCT and SUNA. *Brain*, **129**, 2746–60.

Cohen AS, Matharu MS, Goadsby PJ (2007). Electrocardiographic abnormalities in patients with cluster headache on verapamil therapy. *Neurology*, **69**, 668–75.

Cohen AS, Burns B, Goadsby PJ(2009). High flow oxygen for treatment of cluster headache. A randomized trial. *Journal of the American Medical Association*, **302**, 2451–57.

Day JW, Raskin NH (1986). Thunderclap headache: symptom of unruptured cerebral aneurysm. *Lancet*, **2**, 1247–8.

Dodick DW, Mosek AC, Campbell JK (1998). The hypnic ('alarm clock') headache syndrome. *Cephalalgia*, **18**, 152–6.

Giffin NJ, et al. (2003). Premonitory symptoms in migraine: an electronic diary study. *Neurology*, **60**, 935–40.

Gil-Gouveia R, Goadsby PJ (2007). Secondary 'hypnic headache'. *J Neurol*, **254**, 646–54.

Goadsby PJ (2000). The pharmacology of headache. *Progress Neurobiol*, **62**, 509–25.

Goadsby PJ (2002). Pathophysiology of cluster headache: a trigeminal autonomic cephalgia. *Lancet Neurol*, **1**, 37–43.

Goadsby PJ (2002). Readers syndrome: 'Paratrigeminal' paralysis of oculo-pupillary sympathetic. *J Neurol Neurosurg Psychiatry*, **72**, 297–9.

Goadsby PJ (2004). A critical view of cervicogenic headache. In: Sjaastad O, Fredriksen TA, Bono G, Nappi G (eds) *Cervicogenic headache*, pp. 131–6. Smith-Gordon, London.

Goadsby PJ (2005). Can we develop neurally-acting drugs for the treatment of migraine? *Nat Rev Drug Discovery*, **4**, 741–50.

Goadsby PJ (2006). Is medication-overuse headache a distinct biological entity? *Nat Clin Pract Neurol*, **2**, 401.

Goadsby PJ (2007). Neurostimulation in primary headache syndromes. *Exp Rev Neurotherapeut*, **7**, 1785–9.

Goadsby PJ, Lipton RB (1997). A review of paroxysmal hemicranias, SUNCT syndrome and other short-lasting headaches with autonomic features, including new cases. *Brain*, **120**, 193–209.

Goadsby PJ, Lipton RB, Ferrari MD (2002). Migraine- current understanding and treatment. *N Engl J Med*, **346**, 257–70.

Goadsby PJ, Dodick D, Silberstein SD (2005). *Chronic daily headache for clinicians*. BC Decker Inc, Hamilton, Canada.

Headache Classification Committee of the International Headache Society (2004). *The International Classification of Headache Disorders*, 2nd edn. *Cephalalgia*, **24**, 1–160.

Hunt WE, et al. (1961). Painful ophthalmoplegia. Its relation to indolent inflammation of the cavernous sinus. *Neurology (Minneap)*, **11**, 56–62.

Irimia P, et al. (2008). Unilateral photophobia or phonophobia in migraine compared with trigeminal autonomic cephalalgias. *Cephalalgia*, **28**, 626–30.

Lance JW (1996). The red ear syndrome. *Neurology*, **47**, 617–20.

Lance JW, Goadsby PJ (2005). *Mechanism and management of headache*. Elsevier, New York.

Lance JW, Lambros J (1998). Headache associated with cardiac ischemia. *Headache*, **38**, 315–16.

Leone M, et al. (2004). Long-term follow-up of bilateral hypothalamic stimulation for intractable cluster headache. *Brain*, **127**, 2259–64.

Levy M, et al. (2005). The clinical characteristics of headache in patients with pituitary tumours. *Brain*, **128**, 1921–30.

Lipton RB, Bigal M (2006). *Migraine and other headache disorders*. Marcel Dekker, New York.

Lipton RB, et al. (2001). Prevalence and burden of migraine in the United States: data from the American Migraine Study II. *Headache*, **41**, 646–57.

Markus HS (1991). A prospective follow-up of thunderclap headache mimicking subarachnoid haemorrhage. *J Neurol Neurosurg Psychiatry*, **54**, 1117–25.

Matharu MS, et al. (2004). Central neuromodulation in chronic migraine patients with suboccipital stimulators: a PET study. *Brain*, **127**, 220–30.

Matharu MS, et al. (2004). Posterior hypothalamic and brainstem activation in hemicrania continua. *Headache*, **44**, 747–61.

Matharu MS, et al. (2006). Posterior hypothalamic activation in paroxysmal hemicrania. *Ann Neurol*, **59**, 535–45.

May A, et al. (1998). Hypothalamic activation in cluster headache attacks. *Lancet*, **352**, 275–8.

May A, et al. (1999). Correlation between structural and functional changes in brain in an idiopathic headache syndrome. *Nature Med*, **5**, 836–8.

May A, et al. (1999). Functional MRI in spontaneous attacks of SUNCT: short-lasting neuralgiform headache with conjunctival injection and tearing. *Ann Neurol*, **46**, 791–3.

Menken M, Munsat TL, Toole JF (2000). The global burden of disease study—implications for neurology. *Arch Neurol*, **57**, 418–20.

Newman LC, et al. (1992). Episodic paroxysmal hemicrania: two new cases and a literature review. *Neurology*, **42**, 964–6.

Olesen J, Goadsby PJ (1999). *Cluster headache and related conditions*, Vol. 9. Oxford University Press, Oxford.

Olesen J, et al. (2005). *The headaches*. Lippincott, Williams & Wilkins, Philadelphia.

Raskin NH (1986). Repetitive intravenous dihydroergotamine as therapy for intractable migraine. *Neurology*, **36**, 995–7.

Raskin NH (1988). The hypnic headache syndrome. *Headache*, **28**, 534–6.

Raskin NH (1995). The cough headache syndrome: treatment. *Neurology*, **45**, 1784.

Silberstein SD, Lipton RB, Goadsby PJ (2002). *Headache in clinical practice*. Martin Dunitz, London.

Sjaastad O, Dale I (1976). A new (?) clinical headache entity 'chronic paroxysmal hemicrania'. *Acta Neurol Scand*, **54**, 140–59.

Sjaastad O, et al. (1989). Shortlasting unilateral neuralgiform headache attacks with conjunctival injection, tearing, sweating, and rhinorrhea. *Cephalalgia*, **9**, 147–56.

Steiner TJ, et al. (2003). The prevalence and disability burden of adult migraine in England and their relationships to age, gender and ethnicity. *Cephalalgia*, **23**, 519–27.

Stewart WF, et al. (2003). Lost productive time and cost due to common pain conditions in the US workforce. *JAMA*, **290**, 2443–54.

Tfelt-Hansen P, et al. (2000). Ergotamine in the acute treatment of migraine- a review and European consensus. *Brain*, **123**, 9–18.

Tolosa E (1954). Periarteritic lesions of the carotid siphon with the clinical features of a carotid infraclinoidal aneurysm. *J Neurol Neurosurg Psychiatry*, **17**, 300–2.

Welch KMA, Goadsby PJ (2002). Chronic daily headache: nosology and pathophysiology. *Curr Opin Neurol*, **15**, 287–95.

Wijdicks EFM, Kerkhoff H, van Gijn J (1988). Long-term follow up of 71 patients with thunderclap headache mimicking subarachnoid haemorrhage. *Lancet*, **ii**, 68–70.

Brainstem syndromes

David Bates

Essentials

Brainstem syndromes typically cause ipsilateral cranial nerve lesions and contralateral long tract signs. They are commonly due to brainstem ischaemia, but can also be caused by neoplasia, demyelination, infective and hamartomatous lesions. Imaging, ideally with MRI rather than CT, is obligatory and only then—and possibly following other investigations to identify systemic abnormality or cerebrospinal fluid changes—can appropriate therapy be introduced.

Particular brainstem syndromes

These include: (1) Thalamic syndrome—typically presents with unpleasant dysaesthetic burning pain, often following a hemiplegic and hemianaesthetic stroke. First-line treatment is with centrally acting analgesic agents, e.g. amitriptyline. (2) Midbrain syndromes—characterized by contralateral long tract signs and ipsilateral defects of the third and fourth cranial nerves. (3) Pontine syndromes—present with ipsilateral cerebellar signs, abnormalities of ocular movements, and contralateral paralysis and impairment of sensation, with details of the deficits depending on the location of the lesion within the pons. (4) Medullary syndromes—(a) medial—causes paralysis of the tongue on the side of the lesion, with contralateral paralysis of the arm and leg, and impaired proprioception over the contralateral half of the body; (b) lateral—causes ipsilateral Horner's syndrome, vocal cord paralysis, limb ataxia and sensory loss, oscillopsia and nystagmus, and contralateral impairment of pain and thermal sensation.

Introduction

The classic presentation of brainstem syndromes, including the long tracts and deficits of cranial nerve nuclei, commonly causes crossed cranial nerve and motor or sensory long tract deficits; the cranial nerve lesions are ipsilateral to the lesion and the long tract signs are contralateral. It is important to assess the extracranial vascular supply to the posterior circulation, especially to listen for bruits over the subclavian vessels and to record the pulse and blood pressure in both upper limbs, remembering that the vertebral arteries arise from the subclavian vessels. Apart from the cranial nerve and long tract deficits, there may be ataxia, vertigo, the presence of an internuclear ophthalmoplegia and unreactive pupils, the symptoms of diplopia and oscillopsia, and the finding of nystagmus or ocular paresis.

The circulation to the brainstem is supplied by the vertebral arteries, which are the main arteries to the medulla, and then the basilar artery, which supplies the pons and midbrain. The vertebral arteries are frequently asymmetrical and commonly give rise to the large posteroinferior cerebellar arteries shortly before they join to form the basilar artery. The vertebral arteries are susceptible to trauma within the cervical spine, but the most common lesion affecting the vertebral arteries is dissection, which is probably under-recognized, and thrombosis.

The basilar artery branches are paramedian, supplying the area of the pons close to the midline, the short circumferential branches that supply the lateral two-thirds of the pons, the long circumferential branches that are the supero- and anteroinferior cerebellar arteries, and several interpeduncular branches that arise at the bifurcation of the basilar artery and supply the subthalamic and high midbrain regions.

Although most brainstem syndromes are due to vascular or inflammatory demyelinating lesions, an increasing proportion are shown on MRI to be due to cavernomas, which may or may not calcify and which were impossible to diagnose before modern imaging. The management of such cavernomas is difficult and may involve surgery or stereotactic radiotherapy. A small proportion of lesions in the brainstem are infective and inflammatory; occasionally a causative organism, commonly an adenovirus, can be identified, and may be seen as a complication of AIDS; when no identifiable infective agent is identified, the condition is termed 'Bickerstaff's encephalitis'.

The brainstem syndromes

Diencephalic syndrome

Commonly seen in children under the age of 3 years, Russell's syndrome consists of emaciation with increased appetite, euphoria, vomiting, and excessive sweating. There may also be motor hyperactivity. The differential diagnosis includes hyperthyroidism, diabetes mellitus, a tumour in the region of the fourth ventricle, such as a malformation of the great vein of Galen, and a hypothalamic tumour.

There may often be optic atrophy and rarely nystagmus. Investigation may show an elevated serum growth hormone and an MRI will show a hypothalamic mass lesion. Although contraindicated if there is a significant structural pathology, the cerebrospinal fluid may contain malignant cells or an excess of human chorionic gonadotropin in the case of germinoma.

Thalamic syndrome

Originally described by Dejerine and Roussy in 1906, thalamic pain has a particularly distressing quality. Sometimes spontaneously, but commonly after a recognized hemiplegic and hemianaesthetic stroke, the patient develops altered sensation in a hemisensory distribution together with unpleasant dysaesthetic burning pain (thalamic pain). The pain may be worsened by stimulation and is associated with hemianaesthesia, sometimes proprioceptive loss, and some evidence of hemiparesis. Anatomically the lesion is usually in the ventroposterolateral nucleus of the thalamus and is commonly caused by either a vascular event or a tumour. The investigation required is imaging and therapy is with centrally acting analgesic agents, such as amitriptyline, carbamazepine, gabapentin, and pregabalin. When pain is intractable, deep brain stimulation to the ventroposteromedial nuclei may be considered.

Tectal deafness

There is a rare syndrome associated with damage at the level of the inferior colliculi, due to either neoplasia or vascular lesions, which results in bilateral deafness with associated difficulty in coordination, weakness, and vertigo. The condition must be differentiated from bilateral conductive hearing loss, cochlear disorders, bilateral cranial nerve VIII lesions, and pure word deafness. Brain imaging will identify the lesion.

Thalamic stroke syndrome

Lesions affecting the thalamus are commonly vascular and arise from infarction within the distribution of the posterior communicating artery, the basilar, and the anterior and posterior choroidal arteries. There is usually hemiparesis with hemianopia, hemianaesthesia, and sometimes hemiataxia. There is often confusion and disorientation, and there may be language disturbance. On occasion there may be vertical gaze ophthalmoplegia, loss of pupillary reflexes, and an inability to converge the eyes. There may also be memory impairment and on occasions visual perceptual disturbances are recorded.

Midbrain syndromes

Damage to areas of the midbrain is characterized by long tract signs contralateral to the lesion with defects of cranial nerves III and IV ipsilaterally. They may occur with lesions in the brainstem or as the evolution of symptoms of rostrocaudal deterioration associated with supratentorial brain swelling (Figs. 24.9.1 and 24.9.2). They are characterized by ipsilateral cranial nerve III and IV palsies together with contralateral hemiparesis, loss of vibration, proprioception, and stereognosis, contralateral loss of pain and temperature, and an ipsilateral Horner's syndrome. Ataxia may occur and there can be eyelid ptosis, diplopia, supranuclear horizontal-gaze paresis, and an internuclear ophthalmoplegia. The association of an ipsilateral oculomotor palsy with a crossed hemiplegia due to a lesion at the base of the midbrain is called

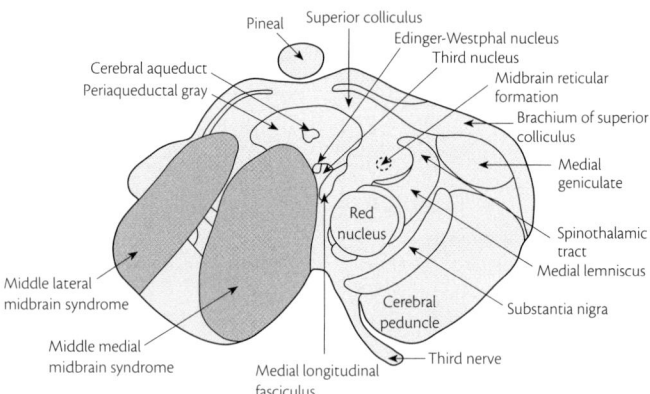

Fig. 24.9.1 Midbrain at the superior colliculus level, showing the medial and lateral territories involved with occlusive stroke in this region.

Weber's syndrome. Claude's syndrome causes an ipsilateral oculomotor palsy with contralateral cerebellar ataxia and tremor, and is due to a lesion in the tegmentum of the midbrain involving the red nucleus and nerve III nucleus. Benedikt's syndrome also involves the tegmentum of the midbrain, resulting in an oculomotor palsy with contralateral cerebellar ataxia, tremor, and corticospinal signs; it can be regarded as a combination of Claude's and Weber's syndromes. Nothnagel's syndrome occurs with unilateral or bilateral involvement of nerve III nucleus together with the superior cerebellar peduncle and causes bilateral ptosis, paralysis of gaze, and cerebellar ataxia.

Damage in the region of the dorsal midbrain results in Parinaud's syndrome in which there is paralysis of upward gaze due to damage to the supranuclear mechanisms for upward gaze, loss of accommodation, and fixed pupils. Although this may be seen with ischaemic lesions, it is more common with pineal tumours.

Pontine syndromes

Lesions in the pons and medulla are commonly identified as involving either the medial or the lateral aspect of the brainstem, depending

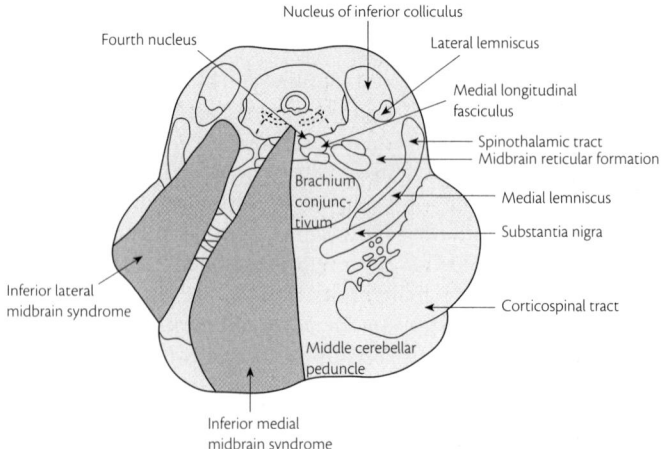

Fig. 24.9.2 Midbrain at the inferior colliculus level showing the medial and lateral territories involved with ischaemic stroke syndromes in this area.
(Reprinted with permission from DeArmond SJ, Fusco MM, Dewey MM, 1976, Structure of the human brain, 2nd edn. Oxford University Press, New York.)

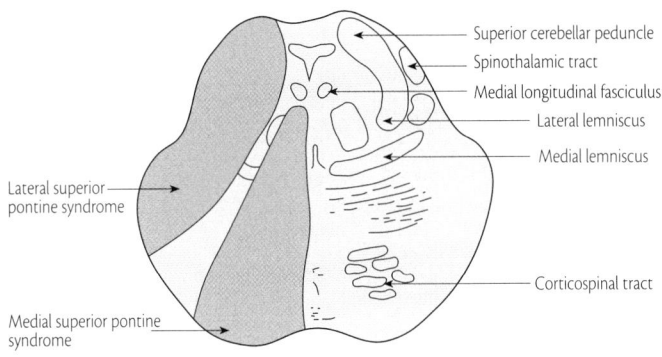

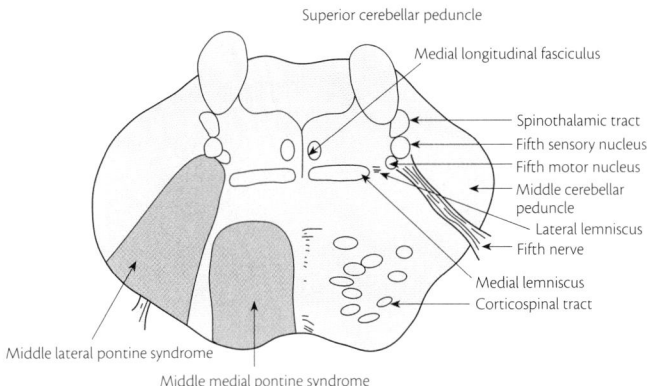

Fig. 24.9.3 Superior pontine level, showing the medial and lateral territories involved with occlusive stroke in this region.
(Reprinted with permission from Adams RD, Victor M, 1993, Principles of neurology, 5th edn. McGraw-Hill, New York.)

Fig. 24.9.4 Midpontine level, showing the medial and lateral territories involved with ischaemic stroke syndromes in this locality.
(Reprinted with permission from Adams RD, Victor M, 1993, Principles of neurology, 5th edn. McGraw-Hill, New York.)

upon whether the paramedian or short circumferential vessels from the basilar have been involved. In the pons the following three levels of damage can be identified and the basal syndrome can occur at any level.

Superior pontine syndrome

The medial superior pontine syndrome results in ipsilateral cerebellar ataxia, internuclear ophthalmoplegia, and palatal and pharyngeal myoclonus with contralateral paralysis of face, arm, and leg, and sometimes loss of sensation contralaterally. The lateral superior syndrome causes ataxia of the limbs and gait with dizziness, nausea, and vomiting; there is horizontal nystagmus, paresis of conjugate gaze towards the side of the lesion, loss of optokinetic nystagmus, and sometimes skew deviation of the eyes. There may also be an ipsilateral Horner's syndrome, and there is contralateral loss of pain and thermal sensation on the face and limbs with impaired touch, vibration, and position sense (Fig. 24.9.3).

Midpontine syndrome

The medial, midpontine syndrome causes ipsilateral ataxia of the limbs and gait with contralateral paralysis of the face, arm, and leg, deviation of the eyes away from the lesion, and variably impaired sensation contralaterally. The lateral syndrome at this level causes ataxia of the limbs on the side of the lesion together with paralysis

of the muscles of mastication and impaired sensation over the face on the same side due to damage to cranial nerve V (Figs. 24.9.4 and 24.9.5).

Inferior pontine syndrome

The medial syndrome causes paralysis of conjugate gaze to the side of the lesion, nystagmus, ataxia of limbs on the same side, and double vision on gaze to that side. Contralaterally there is paralysis of the face, arm, and leg, with impaired touch and proprioception over the opposite side of the body. The lateral syndrome involves ipsilateral, horizontal, and vertical nystagmus with vertigo and nausea, ipsilateral facial paralysis, paralysis of conjugate gaze to the side of the lesion, deafness, tinnitus, and ataxia on the side of the lesion, with impaired sensation of the face on that side. On the opposite side there is impaired sensation over half the body (Fig. 24.9.6).

Basal pontine syndrome (locked-in syndrome)

Bilateral lesions of the paramedian vessels from the basilar, commonly seen in patients with hypertension, result in infarction of the basal pontine and cause quadriplegia with loss of the ability to speak. The ascending reticular activating system is intact and

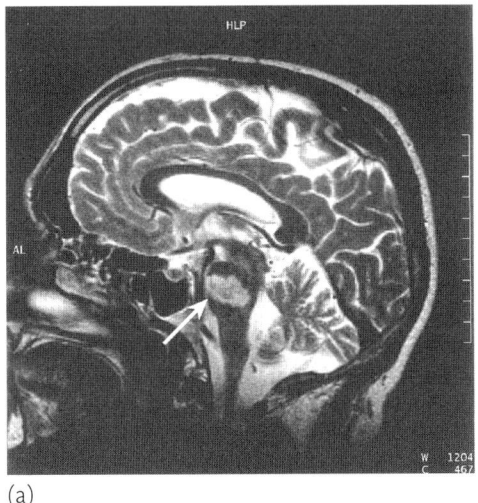

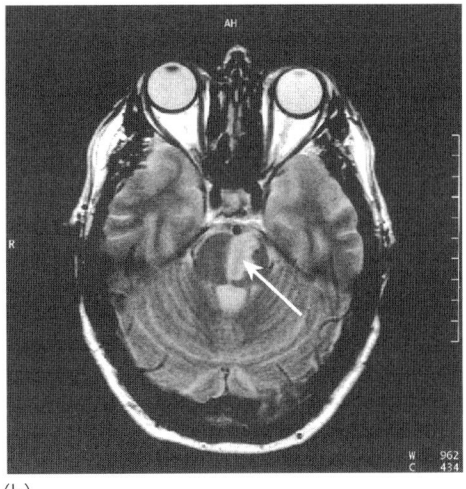

Fig. 24.9.5 MRI of a midpontine infarction.

(a)   (b)

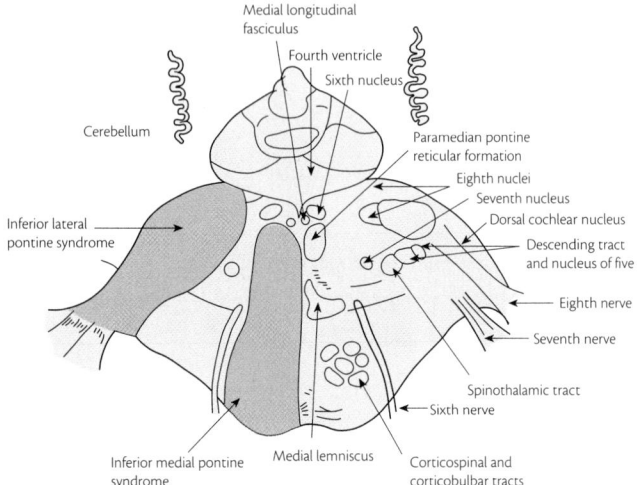

Fig. 24.9.6 Inferior pons at the level of nerve VI nucleus, showing the medial and lateral territories involved with occlusive stroke in this area.
(Reprinted with permission from Adams RD, Victor M, 1993, Principles of neurology, 5th edn. McGraw-Hill, New York.)

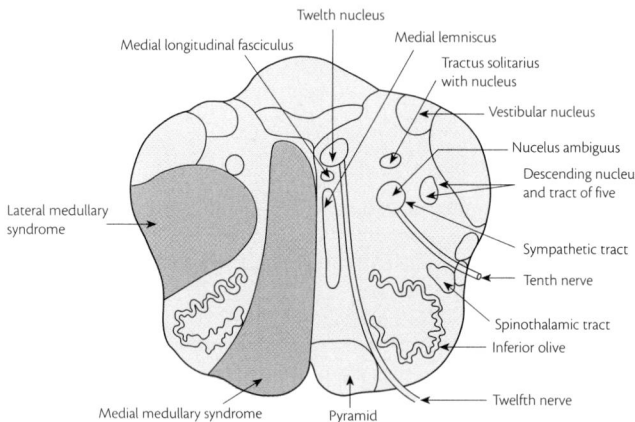

Fig. 24.9.7 Cross-section of medulla at the level of the inferior olivary complex, showing the medial and the more common lateral territory involved with ischaemic stroke in this brainstem site.
(Reprinted with permission from Adams RD, Victor M, 1993, Principles of neurology, 5th edn. McGraw-Hill, New York.)

consciousness is therefore preserved. Vertical eye movements and eye closure are all that are possible and under voluntary control in the 'locked-in syndrome'.

Pseudobulbar palsy

Bilateral lesions of the long descending tracts in the brainstem can result in pseudobulbar palsy, although this condition is more commonly seen with lesions higher in the cerebrum. The symptoms are those of spastic dysarthria, dysphagia, bilateral facial weakness with quadriparesis, and emotional lability.

Medullary syndromes

The medial medullary syndrome may occur with occlusion of the vertebral artery or a branch of the lower basilar artery; it causes paralysis and atrophy of the tongue on the side of the lesion with contralateral paralysis of the arm and leg but sparing the face and impaired tactile proprioceptive sensation over the contralateral half of the body.

The lateral medullary syndrome, eponymously called Wallenberg's syndrome, occurs most commonly with dissection or occlusion of the vertebral artery, resulting in ischaemia into the posteroinferior cerebellar artery; this causes pain, numbness, and impaired sensation of the ipsilateral half of the face with ataxia of limbs on that side, the symptoms of vertigo and nausea, double vision, and oscillopsia, and the signs of nystagmus. There is an ipsilateral Horner's syndrome, often dysphagia with paralysis of the vocal fold ipsilaterally, and loss of sensation on the arm, trunk, and leg. There is contralateral impaired pain and thermal sensation over half the body and possibly the face (Fig. 24.9.7).

A syndrome involving ipsilateral cranial nerve VII and VI palsies with a contralateral hemiplegia is called the Millard–Gubler syndrome; the involvement of cranial nerve X, causing paralysis of the soft palate and vocal fold with contralateral hemianaesthesia, is termed Avellis's syndrome and is due to a lesion in the tegmentum of the medulla.

Investigations and treatment

Once a brainstem lesion is suspected, its detection and identification will require neuroimaging, preferably by MR techniques. Other investigations, e.g. to search for systemic disease including vasculitis, immunodeficiency, or sources of emboli, may also be required. Vascular lesions within the brainstem often carry a remarkably good prognosis, but, if the syndrome appears to be evolving, the possibility of anticoagulation must be considered. In those lesions in which damage affects the medulla, it may be important to protect the airway and avoid aspiration during the early phases of the illness.

Brainstem syndromes occurring on a vascular basis are increasingly easy to diagnose because of MRI and MR angiography. Interventional angiography may be used to direct the delivery of fibrinolytic agents, attempt the rescue of an embolus, or stent a narrowed portion of the vertebral or basilar artery.

Further reading

Adams RD, Victor M (1989). *Principles of neurology*, 4th edition. McGraw-Hill, New York.
Caplan LR (1988). Vertebrobasilar system syndromes. In: Vinken PJ, Bruyn GW, Klawans HL (eds) *Handbook of clinical neurology*, pp. 390–3. Elsevier, Amsterdam.

Specific conditions affecting the central nervous system

Contents

24.10.1 Stroke: cerebrovascular disease

J. van Gijn

Essentials

Cerebrovascular diseases include many pathological conditions but the principal categories are (1) infarction—through occlusion of major arteries, small arteries or venous sinuses; and (2) haemorrhage—most often through rupture of small arteries, arterial aneurysms or capillaries.

Epidemiology

Strokes are common, with annual incidence rates for subjects aged over 55 ranging from 420 to over 1000 per 100 000. They are the most important case of disability in developed Western nations and the second most frequent cause of death after coronary heart disease. About 80% of strokes are caused by cerebral infarcts, with the remainder due to haemorrhage, with 20% of these attributable to a bleeding cerebral aneurysm. The incidence of transient ischaemic attacks (TIAs) is about 50 per 100 000.

General considerations

Strokes typically present with sudden onset of focal neurological deficit. Urgent imaging with CT or MRI allows rapid differentiation between haemorrhagic and ischaemic causes—with critical benefit for the introduction of appropriate treatment—and serial imaging may reveal the development of important complications such as rebleeding, ischaemia, or hydrocephalus that mandate specific interventions.

The consequences of stroke are often devastating: sudden loss of a large amount of brain tissue affects much more than specific, localized functions such as movement, sensation, vision, and language. Mood, initiative, sense of humour, and speed of thought are among the essential aspects of mental life that can be severely affected, but are often sadly ignored. Management of patients with stroke requires complex needs to be comprehensively addressed. The introduction of specialized clinical units for the multidisciplinary care of patients with stroke has been shown to improve clinical diagnosis and recovery, reducing the risk of death or institutionalized care by 14%.

Pathophysiology of arterial occlusive disease

Atherothrombosis is the main cause of occlusion of major arteries in the brain, typically by embolism from a source in the carotid artery, aorta, or heart. Whether occlusion of an artery supplying brain tissue actually leads to ischaemia depends on collateral pathways, which may be by (1) circle of Willis, (2) connections between extracranial and intracranial vessels, (3) leptomeningeal anastomoses.

Arterial occlusive disease—transient ischaemic attacks

These, by definition, are due to ischaemia of a part of the brain, producing symptoms/signs that last for <24 h (usually for minutes). The main presentations are with transient (1) hemiparesis, (2) dysphasia, (3) monocular visual loss, or (4) hemianopia. Without treatment (see 'Secondary prevention'), the risk of stroke after a TIA is up to 20% in the first year and 7% in subsequent years.

Arterial occlusive disease—cerebral infarction

Classification—this has been attempted on the basis of time course ('progressive', 'completed'), anatomy (which artery?), cause (e.g. large artery atherosclerosis, cardio-embolism) or functional deficit (e.g. modified Rankin scale). The Oxfordshire Community Stroke Project system provides a useful and widely accepted compromise, defining four types of cerebral infarction: (1) total anterior circulation infarcts (TACI)—with both cortical and subcortical involvement; (2) partial anterior circulation infarcts (PACI)—more restricted and predominantly cortical infarcts; (3) posterior circulation infarcts (POCI)—clearly associated with the vertebrobasilar arterial territory; (4) lacunar infarcts (LACI), confined to the territory of the deep perforating arteries.

Specific treatments—several medical interventions aim at dissolving the occluding clot, or at least preventing it from growing. Those of widest application are: (1) Thrombolysis—treatment of highly selected patients within 4.5 h of the stroke event (and the sooner the better) with intravenous recombinant tissue plasminogen activator (rt-PA) will avoid death or dependence in 55 patients per 1000 treated. (2) Antiplatelet agents—treatment with aspirin, started within 48 h of onset, will avoid death or dependence in 13 patients per 1000 treated.

Secondary prevention—aside from control of lifestyle factors (cessation of smoking, reducing overweight, daily exercise), specific measures to reduce the risk of threatened stroke include (1) Carotid endarterectomy—substantially decreases the risk of disabling or fatal stroke in patients with severe, symptomatic carotid stenosis. (2) Antiplatelet drugs—aspirin produces relative risk reduction of 13%, with addition of dipyridamole providing some further benefit; clopidogrel should be prescribed in patients who are intolerant to aspirin. (3) Anticoagulants—with embolic sources in the heart, mostly from atrial fibrillation, coumadin anticoagulants (INR 2.5–4) are the first choice in the absence of contraindications. (4) Statins—reduce the risk of stroke by about 20% per mmol/litre reduction in low-density lipoprotein (LDL) cholesterol. (5) Antihypertensive drugs—the level of blood pressure is by far the most powerful risk factor for stroke; in individuals with a history of stroke or TIA, a blood-pressure-lowering regimen reduces the risk of stroke by 25 to 50% depending on the degree of blood pressure lowering, regardless of whether or not the blood pressure at baseline was considered too high.

Venous occlusive disease

Aetiology—cerebral venous thrombosis usually occurs in the context of a combination of predisposing factors, e.g. the oral contraceptive pill, pregnancy, or postpartum, in combination with some inherited disorder of coagulation such as the factor V Leiden mutation.

Clinical features, investigation and treatment—manifestations include headache, focal deficits, seizures, and impairment of consciousness. Imaging with CT/MRI reveals 'venous' infarcts that do not correspond to a known arterial territory and evidence of the underlying sinus thrombosis. Most physicians treat with anticoagulants, but evidence for their efficacy is not strong. Mortality is 5 to 30%.

Primary intracerebral haemorrhage

Aetiology—primary intracerebral haemorrhage usually occurs in the context of a combination of (1) anatomical factors—cerebral vascular lesions or malformations, e.g. arteriovenous or cavernous malformations, ruptured perforating arteries, amyloid angiopathy; (2) haemodynamic factors—most notably blood pressure; and (3) haemostatic factors—relating to platelet function or the coagulation system, e.g. oral anticoagulants.

Clinical features, investigation and treatment—in most cases history and examination provide few clues to the cause of an intracerebral haemorrhage, but specific enquiry should always be made about use of oral anticoagulants and the possibility of malignant disease (with bleed into a metastasis), and evidence of a generalized haemostatic disorder should be sought. Brain imaging (CT or MRI) is the most important single investigation in patients with suspected intracerebral bleeding. There is no specific treatment for most patients, but therapeutic anticoagulation should be reversed, and surgical evacuation of cerebellar haematomas should be considered.

Subarachnoid haemorrhage

Aetiology—ruptured aneurysms cause 85% of nontraumatic subarachnoid haemorrhages.

Clinical features and investigation—presentation is with sudden, severe, and unusual headache, with loss of consciousness at onset in 50%. Imaging with CT is the most important investigation: scanning within 3 days reveals extravasation of blood in the basal cisterns in 95% of cases. Lumbar puncture is indicated if the history is convincing but the CT scan negative: xanthochromia of the supernatant after centrifugation of the cerebrospinal fluid sample is the diagnostic finding. CT and MR angiography are the methods of choice for demonstrating or excluding an aneurysm as the source of haemorrhage.

Treatment—aside from general nursing and supportive measures, key issues are (1) Prevention of rebleeding—without intervention, the risk of this is 30% in the month after presentation, with immediate mortality of 50%. Endovascular treatment ('coiling') is the preferred method to occlude the aneurysm and prevent rebleeding, but not all aneurysms can be treated in this way and operative clipping is still necessary for these patients. (2) Delayed cerebral ischaemia—occurs in up to 25% of patients with a ruptured aneurysm, most commonly 5 to 14 days after the initial bleed. Nimodipine reduces the frequency of cerebral ischaemia and poor outcome by about one-third.

Introduction

History

Intracerebral haemorrhage was first recorded by the Swiss physician Wepfer (1620–95) and in more detail by Morgagni (1682–1771) in Padua. Nonhaemorrhagic stroke, 'serous apoplexy', greatly puzzled the medical community until cerebral softening ('*ramollissement*') was recognized as a pathological entity in 1820 by Rostan (1790–1866), in Paris. Initially it was regarded as an inflammatory condition. The relationship of brain softening with arterial occlusion and atherosclerosis gradually dawned on the pathologists; it was firmly established by Rokitansky (1804–78) in Vienna and Virchow (1821–1902) in Berlin. The term 'infarction' was coined by Cohnheim, one of Virchow's disciples. Subarachnoid haemorrhages and their usual source, intracranial aneurysms, were first recognized at the start of the 19th century; the diagnosis could (sometimes) be made during life from the start of the 20th century. In 1931 the Edinburgh neurosurgeon Norman Dott (1897–1973) carried out the first intracranial operation for a ruptured aneurysm, by wrapping it in muscle.

Understanding cerebrovascular disease received great impetus from the advent of CT in the 1970s. Before that time, observations depended on postmortem studies and on indirect neuroradiological studies such as angiography and pneumoencephalography. CT allowed rapid and reliable distinction between haemorrhagic and ischaemic stroke during life. Subsequently, CT and the newer technique of MRI identified several subtypes of stroke, each requiring specific therapeutic measures. The rapid increase in diagnostic accuracy coincided with the emergence of the randomized clinical trial, which replaced pathophysiological reasoning as a basis for medical interventions.

Epidemiology of stroke

Worldwide, stroke is the second most common cause of death after coronary heart disease, although stroke is the most important single cause of disability in the Western world. Stroke incidence is not technically difficult to measure but requires a great deal of time and resources. The few reliable studies, mostly from industrial countries, show that age- and sex-standardized annual incidence rates for individuals aged 55 or more are between 420 and over 1000 per 100 000, depending on geographical region. More than half of strokes occur in people aged over 75 years. In western Europe the overall incidence rates are falling, despite the ageing population. The pathological type varies, even between studies with a high rate of CT, but a general estimate is that out of every five strokes four are infarcts and one a haemorrhage, and that one out the five haemorrhages is from a ruptured aneurysm (subarachnoid haemorrhage). The incidence of transient ischaemic attacks (TIAs) is about 50 per 100 000.

In terms of an average general practice of 2400 people in western Europe (1000 aged >55 years), four patients will have a stroke per annum, vs one having a TIA. Intracerebral haemorrhage will occur about twice every 3 years, and subarachnoid haemorrhage once every 8 years.

Arterial occlusive disease

The cerebral circulation and its disorders

Brain tissue is critically dependent on a constant supply of oxygen and glucose. The cerebral blood flow (c.800 ml/min) accounts for 15 to 20% of the entire cardiac output, whereas the brain (c.1350 g) accounts for only 2% of the normal adult body weight. Neurons in the brain require a constant supply of ATP to maintain concentration gradients of ions across their membranes, necessary for the generation of action potentials. The resting brain consumes energy at the same rate as a 20-W light bulb.

Whether occlusion of an artery in the brain or in the neck actually leads to ischaemia depends on collateral pathways. If an end-artery is occluded and there is no collateral circulation at all, ischaemic symptoms will occur within seconds. Neurons will start dying within minutes and within hours the entire supply area of the artery will be irreversibly damaged. In contrast, permanent occlusion of a major artery such as the internal carotid artery may be asymptomatic in the presence of adequate collateral circulation. Broadly speaking, three levels of collateral circulation can be

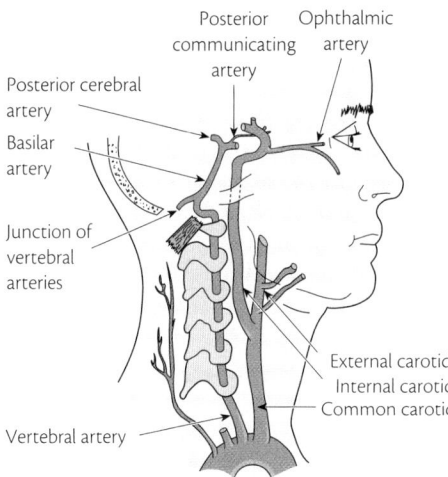

Fig. 24.10.1.1 Arterial supply of the brain. The drawing shows, on the right side, the internal carotid artery, external carotid artery, and vertebral artery. If a main artery is occluded then collateral flow may occur via the circle of Willis (see also Fig. 24.10.1.2).

distinguished (Fig. 24.10.1.1; these can be thought of as three lines of defence):

1 The circle of Willis (Fig. 24.10.1.2)—even if no blood at all is flowing to the brain from one or even both internal carotid arteries, collateral flow from the other internal carotid artery or the basilar artery, via an intact circle of Willis, may ensure an adequate blood supply in the territory of the occluded artery.

2 Connections between extracranial and intracranial vessels—if the internal carotid artery is occluded at its origin, collateral channels may develop via the external carotid artery. Branches supplying the outer orbit may connect with branches to the

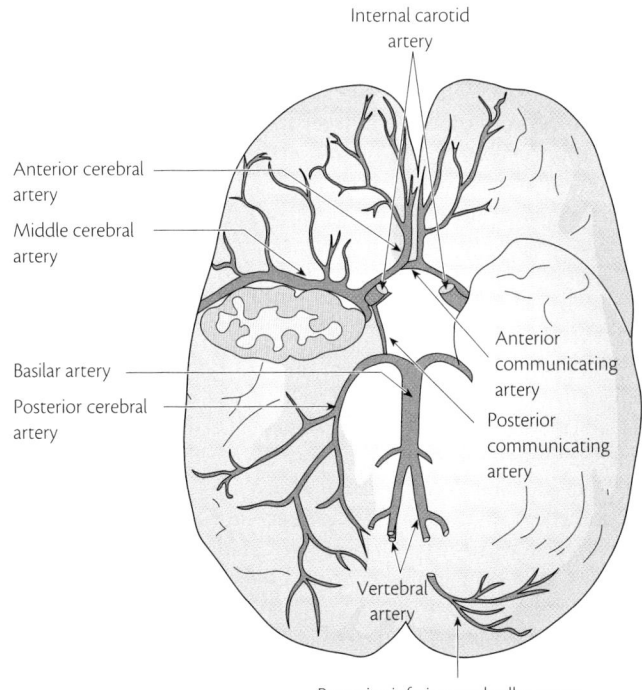

Fig. 24.10.1.2 The arterial circle of Willis, at the base of the brain.

retina, resulting in a reversed flow in the ophthalmic artery. From there, blood reaches the distal part of the internal carotid artery. Similarly, branches of the occipital arteries (normally supplying the neck muscles) may fill the basilar artery if this is occluded at its origin.

3 Leptomeningeal anastomoses—if, for example, the main stem of the middle cerebral artery is occluded, its terminal branches at the surface of the brain may anastomose with similar branches of the anterior and posterior cerebral arteries; in this way the cerebral cortex in the territory of the occluded artery is spared, partly or wholly, although the deep territory will still be ischaemic.

Atherothrombosis is the major cause of occlusion of major arteries in the brain or the neck. Two important qualifications should be made. First, atherosclerosis of intracranial arteries is relatively uncommon, at least in white people (vs black or East Asian people). This means that, in the Western world, brain infarction is usually caused by embolism, in which thrombus has been dislodged from an upstream lesion. The source can be the carotid artery, aorta, or heart. Second, atherosclerosis is not a sufficient cause in itself: not every person with severe atherosclerotic disease has an ischaemic stroke. Other relevant factors are collateral circulation, irregularity of the plaque, blood turbulence, platelet aggregation, and the balance of clotting factors.

Diagnosis of TIAs

TIAs are important to diagnose because they are potential harbingers of stroke. They precede cerebral infarction probably in only 15 to 20% (the precise proportion is uncertain because almost all such information has been retrospectively collected from patients once they have had a stroke).

The term 'transient ischaemic attack' is rather imprecise, because it tacitly implies three restrictions. To begin with, it refers only to the brain and not to angina pectoris or intermittent claudication. Also excluded is transient ischaemia of the entire brain, such as occurs in syncope or ventricular fibrillation. In medical usage, only ischaemia of a part of the brain corresponds with the term TIA. Finally, how transient is transient? Traditionally the limit for the duration of symptoms has been set at 24 h. Obviously this threshold has more to do with astronomy than with biology or disease. In fact most TIAs last minutes, not hours. The longer an attack lasts, the greater the chance that CT or MRI afterwards will show a relevant ischaemic lesion. In terms of patient management, the essential question is not whether the attack has lasted 3 minutes, 3 days, or 3 weeks, but what its cause is and how recurrences can be prevented.

What actually happens in the brain during a given period of ischaemia can often only be guessed at. The usual assumption is that an embolus, most often consisting of platelets or loosely organized thrombus, temporarily blocks an intracerebral vessel and then dissolves into smaller fragments. There is scant evidence for this phenomenon, apart from chance observations during fundoscopy, angiography, or surgery. Other explanations, applicable only to a minority, include marginal flow, secondary to severe narrowing or occlusion of arteries.

The diagnosis of a TIA is problematic. That one has to rely on the history alone is a first difficulty (it requires time, skill, and patience), but not a unique one. A greater source of error is that the term TIA is an interpretation rather than a description.

Main varieties of transient ischaemic attacks

There are four kinds of symptoms that can safely be regarded as TIAs, given that the onset is sudden (within seconds), all symptoms appear at the same time, without 'march', and there is no better explanation.

Transient weakness of one half of the body

Apart from weakness there may also have been numbness. Isolated numbness or pins and needles on one side of the body are a rare manifestation of transient cerebral ischaemia; other causes such as overbreathing are more likely. Weakness and numbness are closely related perceptions, and one should not take these or other expressions ('an arm gone dead') for granted. It is important to make sure that the problem had to do with moving the limbs or the face on one side (facial weakness on one side often manifests itself through slurred speech or drooling), and not with what it felt like when those body parts were touched or with spontaneous sensations. It is also important to verify whether the problem was in two of three body areas, and that it was not just a leg or arm gone to sleep after a nap in older people.

Transient loss of the ability to find words or to understand them

The medical term for this type of TIA is dysphasia or aphasia; in this case patients and relatives may not recognize the episode as representing a problem of language but will often describe the attack as 'confusion'. It is helpful to ask specific questions about the ability to put thoughts into words (motor dysphasia), and about having been able to understand what was said (sensory dysphasia). If a patient can write sentences but cannot speak, the cause is almost certainly psychological. A frequent problem is the distinction between dysphasia (disorder of language) and dysarthria (disorder of articulation). To ask whether pronunciation was difficult may not be very helpful. After all, in both cases the patient's thoughts are clear and the distinction between the right words and the right sounds is rather academic. A more useful question is whether the words made sense and whether they were in the right order. Dysphasia implies a lesion of the left hemisphere in right-handed people, and in 30% of strong left-handers.

Transient loss of vision in one eye

The difficulty in this case is to distinguish transient monocular blindness from loss of vision on one side in both eyes (hemianopia). Either type of attack can be interpreted by the patient as a problem in one eye. The distinction has practical implications, as monocular attacks of blindness should lead to investigation of the ipsilateral internal carotid artery in the neck with a view to angiography and surgery, whereas isolated hemianopia mostly (in 80%) reflects a disorder in the vertebrobasilar circulation, in which case treatment will often be medical. The key question to ask is whether patients have alternately covered each eye during the attack. A surprisingly large proportion of patients have done so, but they will not always offer this information without prompting. On having covered the 'good eye' in case of hemianopia, the patient should still have been able to see with the 'bad eye', although only the nasal half of the visual field. With a monocular disorder the blindness should have been complete after covering the unaffected eye.

Transient loss of vision in one hemifield

Hemianopia reflects dysfunction of the occipital lobe. It is also a common aura in migraine attacks; these auras may occur without ensuing headache, especially in older people. It is therefore important

Box 24.10.1.1 Attacks that should generally **not** be regarded as TIAs

- Any attack with loss of consciousness
- Any attack with involuntary jerking
- Any attack with positive visual phenomena (bright lights, etc.)
- Any attack with *only*:
  - numbness
  - dizziness (with or without spinning sensations)
  - double vision
  - slurred speech
  - unsteady walking

for the physician to enquire about the mode of onset: flashing lights, bright colours, zigzag lines, and a gradually expanding deficit all argue in favour of a migrainous attack rather than ischaemia in its restricted sense of a stroke warning.

Differential diagnosis of TIAs

Box 24.10.1.1 lists types of attacks that should in general not be regarded as TIAs, either because of positive phenomena such as rhythmic jerking that are incompatible with the definition of focal ischaemia, or because other causes are much more likely. In particular, the tendency to label any episode of 'dizziness' in older people as 'vertebrobasilar ischaemia' or, even worse, 'vertebrobasilar insufficiency' should be strongly resisted.

In addition, some specific disorders other than atherosclerosis may cause attacks that are more or less indistinguishable from true TIAs as defined above. They are listed in Box 24.10.1.2. These rare but important causes are reason enough to order a CT or MRI scan of the brain in patients with cerebral TIAs (not necessarily in those with transient monocular blindness). A chronic subdural haematoma should always be suspected in older people, especially if they are on anticoagulants. Hypoglycaemia should come to mind in patients with diabetes. Focal weakness may follow an epileptic seizure (Todd's paralysis) and may be misdiagnosed as a TIA if the initial jerking is missed or misinterpreted. Tumours may also cause temporary deficits without focal epilepsy. Transient global amnesia is a disorder of memory possibly caused by migrainous vasospasm or venous congestion; although technically ischaemic in nature, it is not associated with an increased risk of stroke or other vascular disease.

Box 24.10.1.2 Disorders that may mimic genuine TIAs

- Chronic subdural haematoma
- Intracranial tumour (glioma, metastasis, meningioma)
- Hypoglycaemia
- Focal deficits following a partial epileptic seizure
- Transient global amnesia
- Myasthenia gravis

Prognostic implications of TIAs

Without treatment, the risk of stroke after a TIA can be estimated at up to 20% in the first year and 7% in subsequent years, and the average risk of death, stroke, or myocardial infarction in the first 5 years at 10% per annum. Heart disease and stroke each account for about a third of all deaths. It is important to recognize that the risk of stroke is highest soon after the first episode: 8% in the first week, 12% at 1 month, and 17% at 3 months. Patients at particularly high risk can be identified by means of the ABCD score (see 'Further reading'): A for age (>60 years), B for blood pressure (>140/90 mmHg), C for clinical features (2 points for unilateral weakness, 1 point for speech disturbance without weakness), and D for duration (2 points for >60 min, 1 point for >10 min) and for diabetes (1 point). The risk of stroke within 2 days is approximately 8% in patients with a score of 6 or 7, 4% in those with a score of 4 or 5, and much less in the others.

Investigations in patients with cerebral ischaemia

There is no great difference between searching for the cause of a TIA and searching for the cause of an ischaemic stroke. Very early CT or MRI is mandatory, mainly to exclude intracerebral haemorrhage and the occasional structural lesion mimicking stroke, not so much to demonstrate infarcts. Box 24.10.1.3 lists the major and contributory causes of TIA and ischaemic stroke, with corresponding investigations. In general, first-line investigations are full blood count, erythrocyte sedimentation rate (ESR), plasma glucose, creatinine and electrolytes, plasma lipids, ECG, duplex ultrasound scanning of the arteries in the neck, and unenhanced CT or MRI of the brain.

Diagnosis of cerebral infarction
Distinction from other types of stroke

From a practical point of view, the first step is to distinguish ischaemic stroke from intracerebral haemorrhage. In the past, when a certain distinction could be made only at operation or postmortem examination, a decreased level of consciousness and headache were considered typical of intracerebral haemorrhage. After CT became available in the 1970s, it soon became clear that smaller haemorrhages are not associated with headache and drowsiness. Given that 4 out of 20 strokes are haemorrhagic, and on the assumption that half of all haemorrhages miss distinctive clinical features, a diagnosis of cerebral infarction based on clinical features alone will be wrong in approximately every tenth case. Even complex clinical scoring methods can hardly improve on this error rate.

On CT, acute parenchymal haemorrhage is of higher density than normal brain tissue (see Fig. 24.10.1.6). The hyperdensity occurs immediately—it is caused by the iron molecules in haemoglobin. Signs of infarction are more difficult to detect at an early stage. In the first decade of CT this was not possible until after 3 days, when frank tissue necrosis caused a hypodense lesion on the scan. With improved CT technology, subtle early signs of cerebral infarction have been recognized, at least when the area of infarction is large. These features include loss of normal differentiation between grey and white matter (such as the normal outline of the insular ribbon and the lentiform nucleus) (Fig. 24.10.1.3) and effacement of cortical sulci.

Box 24.10.1.3 Major and contributory 'causes' of transient ischaemic attack (TIA) or ischaemic stroke, with corresponding investigations

Investigations marked with an asterisk (*) have proven implications for management.

Arterial atheroma

- Internal carotid artery in the neck—duplex ultrasound study*
- Intracranial arteries—angiogram (with MR, CT, or catheter)

Small-vessel disease

- Aorta—transoesophageal echocardiography

Other arterial disease

- Congenital arterial anomalies—angiogram (with MR, CT, or catheter)
- Moya-moya syndrome—angiogram (with MR, CT, or catheter)
- Arterial dissection—MRI; angiogram (with MR, CT, or catheter)
- Giant cell arteritis[a]—ESR*, temporal artery biopsy*
- Systemic vasculitis—antinuclear antibodies*, tissue biopsy*
- Embolization from arterial aneurysms—MRI; angiogram (with MR, CT, or catheter)
- Cholesterol embolization syndrome—biopsy of skin, muscle, or kidney
- Meningitis, encephalitis—cerebrospinal fluid*, brain biopsy*
- Drugs of abuse—toxicological screening of urine
- Genetic conditions (MELAS, analysis of mitochondrial or nuclear DNA, CADASIL, Fabry's disease), α-galactosidase A*

- Irradiation
- Migraine

Embolism from the heart

- Atrial fibrillation—ECG*; long-term monitoring of heart rhythm*
- Recent myocardial infarction—ECG*
- Rheumatic valvular disease—echocardiogram*
- Infective endocarditis—echocardiogram*, blood cultures*
- Open foramen ovale—venography*, echocardiogram
- Atrial myxoma—echocardiogram*

Haemostatic factors

- Polycythaemia—haematocrit*
- Sickle cell disease—peripheral blood smear, sickling test
- Thrombocytosis—platelet count*
- Leukaemia—white cell count*, morphology analysis*
- Disseminated intravascular coagulation—platelet count, prothrombin, and activated partial thromboplastin times, fibrinogen, fibrinogen degradation products, D-dimers

Contributing risk factors

- Hypertension—serial measurement of blood pressure*
- Diabetes—fasting glucose*, HbA1c?
- Hypercholesterolaemia—plasma cholesterol*
- Hyperhomocysteinaemia—plasma homocysteine level

ESR, erythrocyte sedimentation rate.

[a]Only with involvement of optic nerve or occipital lobe.

Within the first few days, CT will show that the area of infarction changes into a slightly hypodense, ill-defined, and somewhat swollen lesion; towards the end of the first week it becomes more clearly demarcated and hypodense (Fig. 24.10.1.3). Occasionally there may be massive swelling with brain herniation or haemorrhagic transformation. During the second week the infarct may again gradually increase in density, because the degradation products of necrotic brain tissue more readily absorb X-rays; in the third and fourth weeks the infarcted area may even become isodense, being temporarily almost indistinguishable from normal brain, the so-called 'fogging effect'. Eventually a sharply demarcated, atrophic, hypodense (similar to cerebrospinal fluid) defect remains. It is not always possible to determine how old an infarct is, or to distinguish it from the scar of a haemorrhage that occurred weeks or years before. Intravenous injection of X-ray contrast may in the first weeks cause some enhancement of adjacent brain tissue.

The proportion of patients in whom CT shows an appropriate infarct depends not only on the time of scanning and the generation of the scanner, but also on the size of the infarct and its location; eventually more than 90% of infarcts will show up.

MRI is especially useful for demonstrating small infarcts and lesions in the posterior fossa; it is also more sensitive than CT in the early phases of brain ischaemia. Signal changes on T_2-weighted images occur after 6 to 8 h. Infarcts of any size are visible within minutes on diffusion-weighted imaging, but this technique is not yet broadly available. The distinction from intracerebral haemorrhage is less obvious than on CT, but after a few hours the paramagnetic effects of deoxyhaemoglobin can be identified.

Classification of cerebral infarction

Time course has often been the guiding principle in the classification of stroke in the era before brain imaging. From the point of view of management and prognosis, however, the distinction between 'progressive stroke' and 'completed stroke' is hardly useful, let alone that between 'permanent stroke' and 'reversible ischaemic neurological deficit' (RIND, a kind of 'extended TIA' with complete recovery within 3 or 6 weeks, depending on local convention). What counts is the eventual severity of the functional deficit and, conversely, the remaining functions that are at stake.

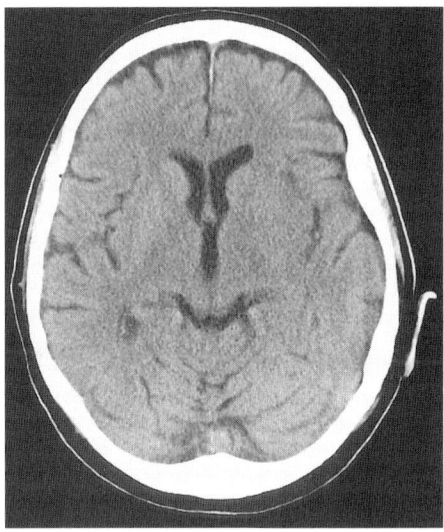

(a)

(b)

Fig. 24.10.1.3 Acute cerebral infarction in a 78-year-old man. (a) CT scan about 6 h after symptom onset. In the left brain hemisphere (on the reader's right) there are subtle changes in the region of the basal ganglia: other than on the normal side, it is difficult to distinguish the different brain nuclei and their separation by white matter. (b) CT scan 4 days after symptom onset shows marked hypodensity in the entire territory of the left middle cerebral artery.

The anatomical classification distinguishes infarcts according to the territory of major cerebral arteries: in the cerebral hemispheres infarcts can be located in the supply areas of anterior cerebral artery, middle cerebral artery, or posterior cerebral artery, or in the border zones between these three main branches; the cerebellum and brainstem are supplied by branches of the vertebral arteries and the basilar artery. The problems are that there is little if any relationship with handicap, mostly no distinction is made between partial and complete infarcts in a given territory, and the boundaries between different territories vary substantially between individuals.

Classification according to the cause of ischaemic stroke is of interest for studies aiming to describe or influence the pathophysiological background of strokes. The so-called TOAST classification, for example, distinguishes five subtypes of ischemic stroke: (1) large-artery atherosclerosis, (2) cardioembolism, (3) small-vessel occlusion, (4) stroke with other specific cause, and (5) stroke with undetermined cause. At present about 40% of patients would currently end up in the category 'unknown', even in specialized stroke services. Also the classification may change, according to the extent of ancillary investigations. Finally, and most important, the system is not suited for assessing the severity of stroke.

Rehabilitation specialists and geriatricians are more interested in the functional abilities of patients than in the niceties of neurological nosology. They mostly grade patients' disability on a scale for activities of daily life (such as the Barthel scale, which ranks 10 in-house activities in hierarchical order, from bowel continence to taking a bath), or on a scale that includes some elements of social role fulfilment ('handicap'), such as the Rankin scale (Table 24.10.1.1).

A system that strikes a useful compromise between the restrictions of lifestyle and the anatomical point of view is the classification of the Oxfordshire Community Stroke Project. Four categories are distinguished:

1 Total anterior circulation infarcts (TACIs), with both cortical and subcortical involvement, representing about one-sixth of all ischaemic strokes in the community

2 Partial anterior circulation infarcts (PACIs), with more restricted and predominantly cortical infarcts (one-third of all infarcts)

3 Posterior circulation infarcts (POCIs), clearly associated with the vertebrobasilar arterial territory (one-quarter)

4 Lacunar circulation infarcts (LACIs), confined to the territory of the deep perforating arteries (one-quarter).

Although the classes are anatomically defined, they contain important prognostic information: case fatality is highest by far in the TACI group.

Syndromes of cerebral infarction

Occlusion of the internal carotid artery may cause no symptoms at all or infarction, at its worst in the entire territory of the ipsilateral anterior and middle cerebral artery (and sometimes of the posterior cerebral artery or contralateral anterior cerebral artery as well), depending on the presence of a complete circle of Willis and

Table 24.10.1.1 Modified Rankin scale (or Oxford Handicap Scale) for measuring outcome after stroke (but suitable for other purposes as well)

Grade	Description
0	No symptoms
1	Minor symptoms that do not interfere with lifestyle
2	Symptoms that lead to some restriction of lifestyle but do not interfere with the patient's capacity to look after himself
3	Symptoms that restrict lifestyle and prevent a completely independent existence
4	Symptoms that clearly prevent independent existence though no constant attention is required
5	Totally dependent patient requiring constant attention, night and day

other collaterals. If arterial dissection is the cause of carotid occlusion, subadventitial bulging of the artery may cause Horner's syndrome and lower cranial nerve palsies, with or without infarction. Occlusion of the anterior, middle, and posterior cerebral arteries may lead to complete or partial infarction in their respective territories, depending on collaterals at the surface of the brain. Obviously, branch occlusions cause smaller infarcts. What follows is a description of syndromes associated with complete infarction in the average territory of the main cerebral arteries.

Infarcts in the area of the anterior cerebral artery cause contralateral hemiparesis, more marked in the leg than in the arm, with no or only mild sensory deficit. Other frontal lobe features include mutism, incontinence, and apathy or, conversely, disinhibition.

Middle cerebral artery infarcts, if complete, typically present with contralateral hemiplegia (most marked in the arm), sensory deficit, hemianopia, and cognitive defects such as aphasia (dominant hemisphere) or contralateral neglect (nondominant hemisphere). Massive infarction of the entire territory of the middle cerebral artery may lead to massive brain swelling followed by herniation, especially in young patients without cerebral atrophy.

Occlusion of a vertebral artery involving the origin of the posteroinferior cerebellar artery causes Wallenberg's syndrome, with ipsilateral cerebellar ataxia through infarction of the inferior part of the cerebellum, and a—for students slightly bewildering— combination of deficits from infarction of the dorsolateral medulla: decreased skin sensation in the ipsilateral half of the face and the contralateral half of the body; ipsilateral Horner's syndrome; ipsilateral weakness of the soft palate, larynx, and pharynx; and rotatory vertigo.

The full basilar artery syndrome, with infarction of most of the pons and midbrain, consists of coma, tetraparesis including facial movements, and loss of all eye movements and of pupillary and corneal reflexes. There are two characteristic partial syndromes of the basilar artery. One is the locked-in syndrome (infarction of the base of the pons), with tetraparesis including facial movements and loss of horizontal eye movements. Consciousness is preserved through sparing of the reticular formation, but patients can communicate only through vertical eye movements; these may not always be correctly interpreted or even noticed. The other is the top-of-the-basilar syndrome, with variable combinations of hemianopia or complete cortical blindness (occipital lobes), amnesia (inferior temporal lobes) and vertical gaze palsies, pupillary disturbances, and hallucinations (perforating branches to the midbrain).

The posterior cerebral artery syndrome may include hemianopia (occipital lobe), amnesia (lower temporal lobe), and oculomotor disorders or disturbances of language or visuospatial function, by involvement of perforating branches to the thalamus.

Occlusion of a single perforating artery, one of the many that originate at right angles from a large parent artery to supply a small area in the deep regions of the brain or brainstem (Fig. 24.10.1.4), may be clinically silent, or cause a so-called 'lacunar syndrome'. A necessary condition for the clinical diagnosis of a lacunar syndrome is the absence of 'cortical' deficits such as aphasia, neglect, hemianopia, or conjugate deviation of the eyes. The most common and archetypal form is pure motor stroke. In those cases the small deep infarct strategically involves corticospinal fibres (pyramidal tract) to the motor neurons of the limbs, anywhere in its course. Analogous fibres to the facial nucleus in the pons may be affected

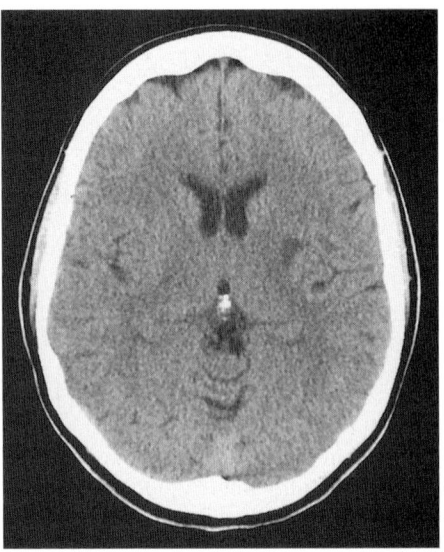

Fig. 24.10.1.4 Small, deep infarct ('lacune') in a 63-year-old woman. CT scanning shows a small area of hypodensity (distinct from sulci) in the left brain hemisphere (on the reader's right), just lateral to the internal capsule.

as well. The infarct can be located in the corona radiata, adjoining the wall of the body of the lateral ventricle, or slightly more caudally, in the posterior limb of the internal capsule, or, less commonly, in the pons or the medulla. Other 'lacunar syndromes' are sensorimotor stroke (corona radiata or internal capsule), pure sensory stroke (thalamus), and ataxic hemiparesis (usually the base of the pons). Lacunar infarcts in the brainstem may lead to an almost infinite range of syndromes, often with the name of a French 19th-century neurologist attached to it. Often such syndromes consist of an ipsilateral cranial nerve deficit and a contralateral hemiparesis.

Treatment of acute cerebral infarction

Several medical interventions aim at dissolving the occluding clot, or at least preventing it from growing: thrombolysis, antiplatelet agents, and anticoagulants. A different strategy, not yet well developed, is to protect ischaemic brain tissue. In addition, some underlying causes of stroke need urgent treatment, such as endocarditis. Before considering these specific measures, it is appropriate to consider the appropriate hospital setting in which stroke patients should be cared for.

Stroke units compared with treatment on general hospital wards

A specially organized stroke unit can be a ward or team that exclusively manages stroke patients (a dedicated stroke unit) or a ward or team that provides a generic disability service (a mixed assessment or rehabilitation unit). According to a meta-analysis of 23 randomized trials, stroke unit care reduces the risk of death or institutionalized care by 14%. The observed benefits are independent of patient age, sex, or stroke severity, and appeared to be better in stroke units based in a separate ward. No single element responsible for the benefits of organized stroke care has so far been identified, and probably there is none. The strength of stroke units lies in the integration of multidisciplinary efforts: stroke physician, nursing staff, physiotherapists, occupational therapists, speech and language therapists, rehabilitation physicians, and social workers.

Thrombolysis

Restoration of blood flow, to reperfuse the ischaemic brain as soon as possible after the cerebral artery has been occluded and, irrespective of its cause, should theoretically lead to reduction in the volume of brain damaged by ischaemia and to improvement in clinical outcome, analogous to myocardial infarction.

The main agents tested so far in stroke (18 trials in >5000 patients) are intravenous recombinant tissue plasminogen activator (rt-PA) and intravenous streptokinase, each in about one-half of the patients. Almost all were treated within 6 h of stroke onset. The evidence for efficacy is statistically significant for rt-PA, if administered within 3 h (or 4.5 h if observational studies are taken into account) and after exclusion of intracerebral haemorrhage by CT. Even within this period the adage is the sooner the better. For patients treated within 90 min the point estimates for survival with at most moderate disability improved from 54% in the placebo groups to 63% for patients in the rt-PA groups (absolute gain 9%), whereas for patients treated between 91 and 180 min after stroke onset the gain was 7% (from 57% to 64%). Taken together, a benefit of 8% means that some 12 patients have to be treated to save a single patient from death or the nursing home. These calculations have already taken into account the fact that there is a risk of secondary haemorrhage after treatment with rt-PA.

There are still many unanswered questions about thrombolysis in ischaemic stroke. The first of these is the time window. The earlier treatment is given the better, which is confirmed by subgroup analysis of patients treated within 3 h (or 4.5 h if observational studies are taken into account) but inevitably this subgroup is biased towards more severe strokes (these get to hospital quickest). Second, is one agent better than another? For rt-PA alone, the balance of risks and benefits seems more favourable than for all agents together: per 1000 patients treated, an excess of 25 fatal intracranial haemorrhages, and a net result of 55 patients avoiding death or dependence, but the difference with streptokinase is not statistically significant. Third, we can roughly identify patients in whom the risk of haemorrhage in the infarcted tissue is great (those with the most severe deficits and those with early signs of extensive infarction), but the potential benefits are also greatest in this group. More controlled studies are needed. There are many contraindications in view of the risk of cerebral haemorrhage, and only a minority of patients admitted with cerebral infarction can be treated with thrombolysis.

Antiplatelet agents

More than 99% of the evidence from randomized trials is this area relates to aspirin. The pooled results of two trials with aspirin (160–300 mg), started within 48 h of onset, concluded that 13 fewer patients are dead or dependent for every 1000 patients treated. In some 800 patients who had been inadvertently randomized after a haemorrhagic stroke there was no evidence of net hazard. Only the combination with thrombolytic treatment should be avoided, because there are indications that aspirin enhances the danger of intracerebral haemorrhage.

Anticoagulants

Anticoagulants tested in clinical trials are standard unfractionated heparin, low-molecular-weight heparins, heparinoids, oral anticoagulants, and thrombin inhibitors. There is no evidence that anticoagulant therapy reduces the odds of being dead or dependent at the end of follow-up.

Neuroprotective agents

There are many steps in the destructive cascade between vessel occlusion and irreversible cell death where pharmacological intervention might be beneficial, at least theoretically. The pharmaceutical industry has developed several compounds for clinical development and testing. There is no doubt that in animal models many neuroprotective agents, given either before or after the onset of ischaemia, reduce the area of cerebral infarction. So far, none of these agents has been proven to reduce disability in patients, despite dozens of clinical trials. Many other trials are under way, but reduction of disability by neuroprotective drugs is likely to be modest at best.

Surgical decompression of space-occupying infarcts

To prevent brain herniation and death from supratentorial infarction, a large part of the skull vault can be removed. A pooled analysis (three trials) of 93 patients randomized within 48 h of stroke onset showed not only that the case fatality rate was much lower in operated patients (22%) than in patients who were treated conservatively (71%), but also that operated patients survived significantly more often (43%) with mild or moderate disability (modified Rankin grade 3 or less, see Table 24.10.1.1), against 21% in the conservative group. This has to be weighed against an increased proportion of survivors with severe disability (modified Rankin grade 4 or 5): 35% against 7%. Also the overall benefit is less clear in subgroups of patients with aphasia, those who underwent surgery on day 2, and those over 50 years of age.

With operations for space-occupying infarcts of the cerebellum there is no controlled evidence, but less uncertainty. Without surgery swelling of a cerebellar infarct can be fatal, whereas the deficits after surgical evacuation are surprisingly mild. In some patients it is sufficient to relieve obstructive hydrocephalus by external ventricular drainage.

Secondary prevention of ischaemic stroke

In the long-term management of patients with TIAs or moderately disabling ischaemic strokes, control of lifestyle factors is a primary concern: cessation of smoking, reducing weight if overweight, and daily exercise.

Specific measures to reduce the risk of threatened stroke are mostly pharmacological. Carotid endarterectomy is the only local treatment.

Carotid endarterectomy

This operation was increasingly performed from the 1960s onwards, but not until the 1980s were two randomized trials performed, one in Europe and one in North America. In patients with severe, symptomatic, carotid stenosis (70–99% lumen diameter reduction) the risk of disabling or fatal stroke substantially decreases after endarterectomy. On average, about six patients need to undergo surgery to prevent one ipsilateral ischaemic stroke within 5 years. This basic risk difference varies with age and sex, and it levels off after 3 or more years from randomization (i.e. 3.5 years after the qualifying event). It should be kept in mind that carotid endarterectomy is indicated in only a minority (<10%) of patients with TIAs or moderately disabling ischaemic strokes: the attacks have to be in the carotid territory, the patients should be fit and willing to undergo the operation, and the angiogram should show an accessible stenosis of over 70% at the carotid bifurcation.

A possible alternative for endarterectomy is carotid stenting, with or without devices to prevent emboli being carried downstream during the procedure. Despite the less invasive nature of this procedure, it is far from certain that the balance of risks and benefits is more favourable than for endarterectomy. So far the information from clinical trials is far from definitive.

For the demonstration of severe carotid stenosis, it is no longer necessary to perform catheter angiography, at least if the results of duplex ultrasound agree with those of CT angiography or MR angiography.

Antiplatelet drugs

The preventive effect of aspirin, in different doses, has been studied in placebo-controlled randomized trials in over 8000 patients after a TIA or moderately disabling stroke. There is virtually no difference between the risk reduction for daily doses between 30 mg and 1300 mg. The overall relative risk reduction is 13% (95% confidence interval 6–19%). Side effects, mainly indigestion, nausea, heartburn, and gastrointestinal bleeding, are more common as the dose is higher. Addition of dipyridamole 200 mg twice daily to aspirin provides a further risk reduction of approximately 18%, compared with aspirin alone. Headache is a common side effect of dipyridamole; it can be avoided by starting with smaller doses.

Clopidogrel, a thienopyridine derivative, is marginally more effective than aspirin, with a relative risk reduction of 8.7% (95% confidence interval 0.3–16.5), whereas the combination of clopidogrel and aspirin has no advantage over aspirin alone; clopidogrel should be prescribed only in patients who are intolerant to aspirin.

Anticoagulants

With sources in the heart, mostly from atrial fibrillation, coumadin anticoagulants (INR 2.5–4) are the first choice in the absence of contraindications; no evidence exists for a fixed age limit. In patients with a presumed arterial cause of cerebral ischaemia, anticoagulants may prevent some ischaemic events, but this benefit is offset or even outweighed by the risk of haemorrhages, especially in the brain, depending on the intensity of anticoagulation.

Statins

The protective effect on major cardiovascular events of statins, or, with the full name of 3-hydroxy-3-methylglutaryl coenzyme A (HMG-CoA) reductase inhibitors, has been proved in clinical trials involving more than 90 000 patients with cardiovascular disease or risk factors, including cerebral ischaemia. The reduction in the 5-year incidence of major coronary events, coronary revascularization, and stroke is about 20% per mmol/litre reduction in low-density lipoprotein (LDL)-cholesterol, largely irrespective of the initial lipid profile or other presenting characteristics.

Antihypertensive drugs

Observational studies provide overwhelming evidence that the level of blood pressure is by far the most powerful risk factor for stroke. The obvious but at the same time precarious corollary that lowering the blood pressure prevents stroke has recently been confirmed by controlled evidence. In individuals with a history of stroke or TIA, a blood pressure-lowering regimen reduces the risk of stroke, regardless of whether or not the blood pressure at baseline was considered too high. The reduction of the stroke risk ranges from one-quarter to one-half, depending on the degree of blood-pressure lowering.

In conclusion, the optimal strategy for secondary prevention of stroke depends on the probable source of embolism. In patients with atrial fibrillation oral anticoagulants are the preferred treatment. Patients in sinus rhythm should be treated with a trio of drugs: an antiplatelet agent (preferably a combination of 30–300 mg aspirin once daily and dipyridamole 200 mg twice daily), a statin, and an antihypertensive agent. In most cases, baseline values for cholesterol or blood pressure should not influence the decision to administer statins and antihypertensive drugs, only the choice of the dose. In addition, patients with ischaemic events in the carotid territory should be investigated noninvasively for the presence of severe stenosis in the ipsilateral internal carotid artery, with a view to carotid endarterectomy.

Venous occlusive disease

The advent of noninvasive brain imaging methods in the last few decades has resulted in increased recognition of cerebral venous thrombosis. Before that time, physicians only rarely considered the diagnosis in patients with otherwise unexplained headache, focal deficits, seizures, impaired consciousness, or combinations of these features.

Causal factors

Unlike arterial occlusion, cerebral venous thrombosis is only rarely (in c.10%) associated with damage to the vessel wall—by infection, tumour growth, or trauma. Much more frequent causes are inherited disorders of coagulation. The most common form is factor V Leiden mutation, found in some 20% of patients without other causes. Stagnant flow (the third factor in Virchow's triad of causes of thrombosis) contributes no more than a few per cent. In 20% of patients no causal factors can be identified.

Often there is not a single cause but a combination of contributing factors, e.g. the postpartum period and protein S deficiency; pregnancy and Behçet's disease, or oral contraceptive drugs and the factor V Leiden mutation. The risk of cerebral venous thrombosis in the postpartum period increases with maternal age and with the performance of caesarean section.

In neonates, cerebral venous thrombosis is usually associated with acute systemic illness, such as shock or dehydration; in older children the most frequent underlying conditions are local infection (the leading cause before the antibiotic era), coagulopathy, and in Mediterranean countries Behçet's disease.

Diagnosis of cerebral venous thrombosis

The clinical features of cerebral venous thrombosis consist essentially of headache, focal deficits, seizures, and impairment of consciousness, in various combinations and degrees of severity. The symptoms and signs depend on which sinus is affected, and for a large part on whether the thrombotic process is limited to the dural sinus or extends to the cortical veins.

In the case of the superior sagittal sinus, which is affected in 70 to 80% of all cases, cerebral venous thrombosis alone will lead to the syndrome of intracranial hypertension, i.e. headache and papilloedema. Up to 30% of patients with so-called 'benign intracranial hypertension' (BIH) may in fact have sinus thrombosis. Papilloedema can cause transient visual obscurations and sometimes irreversible constriction of visual fields, beginning in the inferonasal quadrants. The increased pressure of the cerebrospinal fluid may also give rise to cranial nerve VI palsies, and sometimes to other cranial nerve deficits. The onset of the headache is usually gradual, but in up to 15% of patients it is sudden and may initially suggest the diagnosis of a ruptured aneurysm.

Involvement of cortical veins causes one or more areas of venous infarction, with or without haemorrhagic transformation. If the affected veins drain into the superior sagittal sinus the venous infarcts are typically located near the midline in the rolandic and parieto-occipital regions, often on both sides. In the case of the lateral sinus the venous infarct is usually located in the posterior temporal area.

Clinically the infarcts manifest themselves through epileptic seizures or focal deficits such as hemiparesis or dysphasia. If unilateral weakness develops (with thrombosis originating in the superior sagittal sinus), it tends to predominate in the leg, in keeping with the parasagittal location of most venous infarcts. Obstruction of cortical veins draining into the posterior part of the superior sagittal sinus or into the lateral sinus will commonly lead to hemianopia, dysphasia, or a confusional state. Impairment of consciousness may result from multiple lesions in the cerebral hemispheres, or from transtentorial herniation and compression of the brainstem. Either epilepsy or a focal deficit is a presenting feature in 10 to 15% of patients; in the course of the illness seizures occur in 10 to 60% of reported series, and focal deficits in 30 to 80%.

Involvement of the cortical veins alone, without sinus thrombosis and its associated signs of increased cerebrospinal fluid pressure, is an extremely rare occurrence. Thrombosis of the deep venous system, including the great vein of Galen (great cerebral vein), may lead to bilateral haemorrhagic infarction of the corpus striatum, thalamus, hypothalamus, ventral corpus callosum, medial occipital lobe, and upper part of the cerebellum. In those cases the clinical picture is often dominated by deep coma and disturbance of eye movements and pupillary reflexes.

Investigations

CT will readily show 'venous' infarcts. These do not correspond to a known arterial territory, and often show haemorrhagic transformation (Fig. 24.10.1.5); they are sometimes bilateral, in the parasagittal area, supra- as well as infratentorial, or in the deep regions of the brain. In addition, CT will often provide evidence of the underlying sinus thrombosis: the hyperdense sinus sign or, less reliable, the so-called 'empty delta sign' after injection of intravenous contrast material.

MRI has made catheter angiography redundant in the diagnosis of cerebral venous thrombosis. It is not sufficient to rely on non-visualization of a cerebral sinus on MR venography, because this may represent hypoplasia. Demonstration of the thrombus itself is essential, but this depends very much on the interval from disease onset. Three stages can be distinguished. In the acute stage (days 1–5) the thrombus appears strongly hypointense in T_2-weighted images and isointense in T_1-weighted images. In the subacute stage (up to day 15) the thrombus signal is strongly hyperintense, initially on T_1-weighted images and subsequently also on T_2-weighted images (Fig. 24.10.1.5). The third stage begins 3 or 4 weeks after symptom onset: the thrombus signal becomes isointense on T_1-weighted images but on T_2-weighted images it remains hyperintense, although often inhomogeneous. Recanalization may occur over months in up to one-third of patients, but persistent abnormalities are common and do not signify recurrent thrombosis.

Treatment and prognosis

Anticoagulant treatment is plausible, but the evidence from controlled clinical trials is sparse. In the acute phase heparin (either by intravenous route or, subcutaneously, as low-molecular-weight heparin) seems preferable to oral anticoagulants, because its intensity can be closely monitored. The evidence for heparin treatment rests on no more than 80 randomized patients; there is a nonsignificant trend towards better outcome in treated patients. At least heparin treatment seems safe, even in patients with haemorrhagic infarcts. Local thrombolysis via endovascular catheters has been performed only in uncontrolled studies.

Death rates in different series range between 5% and 30%, and probably depend more on case mix than on treatment. Residual deficits consist mostly of hemispherical deficits or visual impairment from optic atrophy.

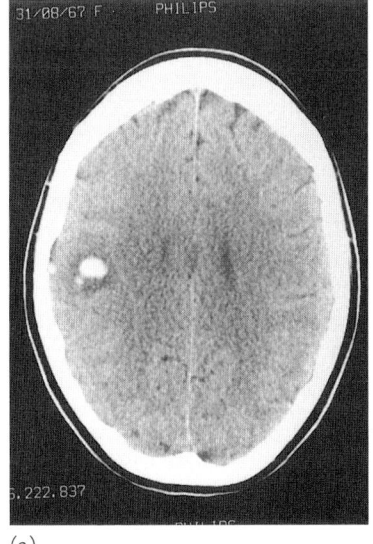

(a)

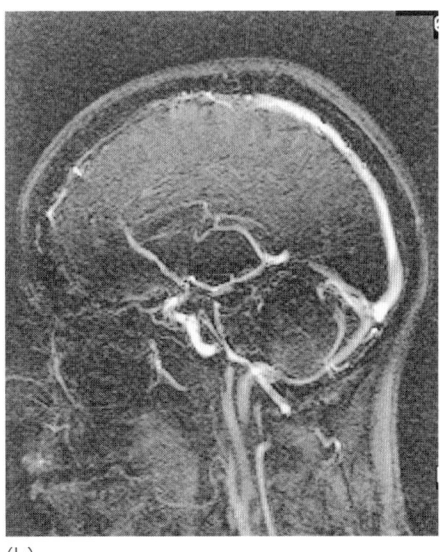

(b)

Fig. 24.10.1.5 Cerebral venous thrombosis in a 27-year-old woman. (a) This CT scan shows a small infarct with haemorrhagic transformation in the right brain hemisphere, adjacent to the top of the lateral ventricle. (b) Magnetic resonance imaging, focused on venous structures, shows non-filling of the frontal part (on the reader's left) of the superior sagittal sinus.

The risk of recurrence has seldom been systematically addressed; it is probably of the order of 10%. It seems wise to advise other means of contraception than the combined oral contraceptive 'pill' (see Chapter 8.6). In women with a peripartum episode of cerebral venous thrombosis, the available evidence does not warrant the advice to avoid a further pregnancy, although in patients with the factor V Leiden mutation the risk of a recurrent episode is probably higher than average.

Primary intracerebral haemorrhage

Causes of primary intracerebral haemorrhage

In most cases there is no single cause for primary intracerebral haemorrhage. Even in the classic example of a so-called hypertensive haemorrhage in the region of the basal ganglia, the question remains about which anatomical or other factors distinguished this patient from others, with similar degrees and duration of hypertension but without brain haemorrhage. Even a combination of recognized 'causes', such as that of hypertension and anticoagulants, does not invariably lead to intracerebral haemorrhage. In general, therefore, several causal factors combine. These can be broadly distinguished into three categories (Box 24.10.1.4): anatomical factors (lesions or malformations of brain vasculature), haemodynamic factors (blood pressure), and haemostatic factors (to do with platelet function or the coagulation system). Abnormalities of the vascular system account for the vast majority of haemorrhages. The type of underlying abnormality varies with age: below the age of 40 arteriovenous or cavernous malformations are the most common single causes, whereas between 40 and 70 the most frequent sources are ruptured perforating arteries (deep haemorrhages); in older people one also finds haemorrhages in the white matter ('lobar' haemorrhages), commonly attributed to amyloid angiopathy.

'Hypertensive' intracerebral haemorrhage

'Hypertensive' intracerebral haemorrhage results from degenerative changes in small perforating vessels, in the deep regions of the brain (basal ganglia and thalamus—Fig. 24.10.1.6), or in the cerebellum or brainstem. Risk factors other than hypertension are age, male sex and high alcohol intake. Microaneurysms occur on these vessels but are not necessarily the site of rupture. It is probable that rupture of a single small artery leads to a cascade of secondary haemorrhages from adjacent arterioles. This might explain rapid expansion of intracerebral haematomas, during a single scanning procedure or on serial scanning. A stable phase is usually reached in a matter of hours.

Deep brain haemorrhages are not always a one-time event. The recurrence rate in the first year is 7%, against 2% per year over the subsequent 6 years.

Amyloid angiopathy

This condition accounts for about 10% of intracerebral haemorrhages. Its frequency rises with age, but so does that of 'hypertensive' haemorrhage. The underlying abnormality consists of patchy deposits of amyloid in the muscle layer of small and medium-sized cortical arteries of the occipital, parietal, and frontal lobes. Amyloid can also be found in asymptomatic individuals, the proportion increasing with age. It is not found outside the brain and does not represent generalized amyloidosis. Haemorrhages associated with amyloid angiopathy typically occur at the border of the grey and white matter of the cerebral hemispheres. Recurrent haemorrhage

---

Box 24.10.1.4 Causes of primary intracerebral haemorrhage

Anatomical factors

- Lipohyalinosis (complex small vessel disease) and microaneurysms
- Cerebral amyloid angiopathy
- Saccular aneurysms
- Cerebral arteriovenous malformations
- Cavernous angiomas
- Venous angiomas
- Telangiectasias
- Dural arteriovenous fistulae
- Haemorrhagic transformation of an arterial infarct
- Intracranial venous thrombosis
- Septic arteritis and mycotic aneurysms
- Moya-moya syndrome
- Arterial dissection
- Caroticocavernous fistula

Haemodynamic factors

- Arterial hypertension
- Migraine
- Haemostatic factors
- Anticoagulants
- Antiplatelet drugs
- Thrombolytic treatment (for non-neurological indications)
- Clotting factor deficiency
- Leukaemia and thrombocytopenia

Other factors

- Intracerebral tumours
- Alcohol
- Amphetamines
- Cocaine and other drugs
- Vasculitis
- Trauma ('*Spät-Apoplexie*')

---

associated with amyloid angiopathy is much more common than with 'hypertensive' small-vessel disease. Hereditary forms of amyloid angiopathy account for only a small minority of all cases.

Possible manifestations of amyloid angiopathy other than haemorrhage are transient episodes of focal neurological deficits, and also intellectual deterioration, associated with diffuse demyelination of the subcortical white matter (leucoaraiosis).

Cerebral arteriovenous malformations

Arteriovenous malformations (AVMs) are tangles of dilated arteries and veins, without a capillary network between them. On angiography, they are recognizable by large feeding arteries and rapid

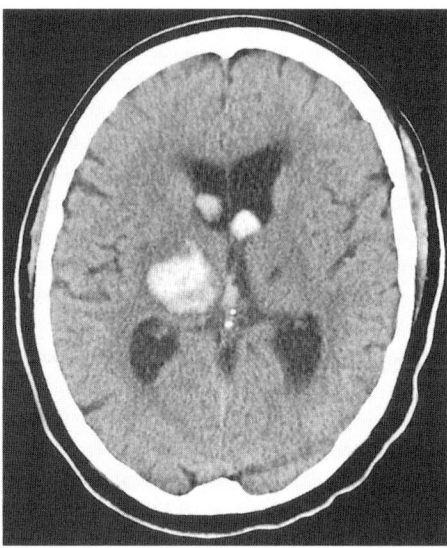

Fig. 24.10.1.6 Primary intracerebral haemorrhage in a 52-year-old man. This CT scan shows a hyperdense lesion in the right thalamus; the haemorrhage has ruptured into the ventricular system.

shunting of blood to enlarged and tortuous veins, via a central nidus of dilated vessels. Haemorrhage is the initial clinical manifestation in 50 to 60% of symptomatic AVMs. Other clinical features include epileptic seizures, headaches, and progressive neurological deficits. Demonstrable AVMs are the most common single cause of intracerebral haemorrhage in patients under 45 years (c.30%).

In 10 to 20% AVMs are associated with thin-walled saccular aneurysms. These occur on peripheral feeding arteries, not at the classic sites at the circle of Willis, and are likely sources of bleeding. In AVMs in which one or more aneurysms have formed, the annual risk of rebleeding is as high as 7%, against 2 to 3% per annum for other AVMs. If there is no associated aneurysm, the site of rupture is mostly on the venous side of the malformation.

Cavernous malformations

Cavernous malformations consist of sharply demarcated areas with widely dilated and thin-walled vascular channels, without intervening brain tissue. They are often asymptomatic and are encountered in 0.5% of routine post-mortem examinations, in the white matter or cortex of a cerebral hemisphere in about one-half of all cases, in the posterior fossa in one-third, and in the basal ganglia or thalamus in one-sixth. If a cavernous malformation is at all symptomatic, epileptic seizures are at least as common a manifestation as haemorrhage. The annual risk of haemorrhage in patients in whom the lesion presents with seizures or focal deficits is rather low, between 0.25% and 0.6%. After a first rupture, rebleeding is more frequent, around 4.5% per annum. Haemorrhages from a cavernous malformation are rarely fatal.

Familial forms of the disorder occur in several countries around the world, and should be suspected if multiple lesions are found.

Diagnosis of primary intracerebral haemorrhage

The history sometimes suggests the cause of the haemorrhage. Previous epileptic seizures should raise suspicions about the presence of an AVM, cavernous malformation, or tumour. Amyloid angiopathy should come to mind in patients over 55 years of age with a history of TIAs, intellectual deterioration, or both. A record

of long-standing hypertension indicates small vessel diseases as the most probable underlying condition in a patient with a haematoma in the basal ganglia or in the posterior fossa; on the other hand, hypertension is so common that it may coexist with other conditions. If the patient is known to have had cancer, haemorrhage into a brain metastasis is a strong possibility. The use of oral anticoagulants is a vital piece of information in patients with intracerebral haemorrhage, because their action should be neutralized as soon as possible. It is equally important to know about the use of recreational drugs, particularly cocaine and amphetamines. Finally, the circumstances preceding intracerebral haemorrhage may help to identify its cause, such as puerperium (intracranial venous thrombosis, choriocarcinoma) or neck trauma (dissection of the vertebral or carotid artery).

The physical examination will provide rather few clues to the cause of an intracerebral haemorrhage, except petechiae or bruising, which indicate a generalized haemostatic disorder, signs of malignant disease such as cutaneous melanoma, a collapsed lung or enlargement of the liver or spleen, or telangiectasias in the skin and mucous membranes. Finding a high blood pressure on admission is the rule, but only in about 50% is there evidence of long-standing hypertension. Retinal haemorrhages indicate intracranial bleeding in general, most often subarachnoid haemorrhage (SAH). Heart murmurs may be coincidental but should at least raise the possibility of infective endocarditis, as should the finding of needle marks in possible drug addicts. The neurological examination will show focal deficits corresponding to the site of the lesion, with or without a decreased level of consciousness.

Investigations should start with the usual tests of blood and serum. These will sometimes uncover a cause of intracerebral haemorrhage, such as a low platelet count or massive liver damage. Brain imaging (CT or MRI) is the single most important investigation in patients with suspected intracerebral haematomas. The location of the haematoma may to some extent indicate the underlying cause. Intraventricular extension of the haemorrhage occurs relatively often with deep, 'hypertensive' haemorrhages. A grossly irregular margin of a lobar haematoma in older patients suggests amyloid angiopathy, as do multiple or recurrent haemorrhages in the white matter. Intracranial venous thrombosis should be suspected with irregularly shaped haemorrhages in the parasagittal region. Repeat brain CT after injection of contrast may pick up underlying lesions. Sometimes these can be identified only weeks later, when the lesion is no longer obscured by mass effects.

Treatment of primary intracerebral haemorrhage

Factors predicting the chances of survival of patients with primary intracerebral haemorrhage are: level of consciousness (Glasgow Coma Scale); age; volume of haematoma (poor prognosis if supratentorial haematoma more than 50 ml), subsequent expansion of the haematoma, and intraventricular extension of haemorrhage (poor prognosis if volume >20 ml). The possible interventions outlined below of course apply only to patients who have a chance of survival.

In patients on oral anticoagulants the first step is intravenous injection of 10 to 20 mg of vitamin K, at not more than 5 mg/min, followed by infusion of a concentrate of the coagulation factors II, VII, IX, and X, or of fresh frozen plasma.

Intracranial pressure is often raised. Factors other than the local effects of the haematoma may contribute, such as fever, hypoxia, hypertension, seizures, and elevations of intrathoracic pressure. An unsolved question is the use, in comatose patients, of monitoring and, if judged appropriate, lowering intracranial pressure. There are many believers in this area but few controlled studies. Insertion of a ventricular catheter may be a definitive measure in patients with cerebellar haemorrhage and no signs of direct compression of the brainstem.

For surgical treatment of supratentorial haematoma, randomized trials have failed to show benefit, including those employing endoscopic evacuation. In patients with cerebellar haematomas there is no doubt that surgical evacuation can be life saving, often with surprisingly few neurological sequelae. Sound indications for evacuation of a cerebellar haematoma are the combination of a depressed level of consciousness with signs of progressive brainstem compression (unless all brainstem reflexes have been lost for more than a few hours, in which case a fatal outcome is unavoidable), or haematoma greater than 3 to 4 cm. If the patient has a depressed level of consciousness and hydrocephalus, without signs of brainstem compression and with a haematoma less than 3 cm, ventriculostomy can be carried out as an initial (and sometimes only) procedure.

Subarachnoid haemorrhage

Causes of subarachnoid haemorrhage

Ruptured aneurysms are by far the most common source of nontraumatic SAH, in about 85%. Around 10% are nonaneurysmal perimesencephalic haemorrhages, the remaining 5% is made up by rarities (Box 24.10.1.5).

Cerebral aneurysms are not congenital; they develop during the course of life. Therefore aneurysmal haemorrhage in a child is extremely rare. The aneurysms are saccular in shape and mostly arise at sites of arterial branching at the base of the brain, at or near the circle of Willis (Fig. 24.10.1.7). It is largely unknown why some adults develop aneurysms. There are families with two or more affected first-degree relatives, but these account for less than 5% of all SAHs. Many classic risk factors for stroke in general also apply to SAH: smoking, hypertension, heavy drinking, and oral contraceptives. Not all aneurysms rupture. Their prevalence can be estimated, from angiographic studies (for other purposes) and postmortem studies at approximately 2 to 3% in middle age, up to 5% at the end of life. On the assumption that this proportion is 1% for a standardized population across all age groups, and given that the incidence of SAH is approximately 6 per 100 000 (of the entire population), the annual risk of rupture of an aneurysm is 0.6%.

Nonaneurysmal perimesencephalic haemorrhage is a distinct and benign variety of SAH, in which the distribution of extravasated blood on the brain CT scan is different from that with aneurysms, in the cisterns around the midbrain or ventral to the pons. The angiogram is completely normal, and the long-term outcome is invariably excellent. This subtype constitutes 10% of all SAHs and two-thirds of SAHs with a normal angiogram.

Box 24.10.1.5 Causes of subarachnoid haemorrhage

- ◆ Ruptured aneurysm (85%)
- ◆ Nonaneurysmal perimesencephalic haemorrhage (of venous origin?) (10%)
- ◆ Rarities (5%)
  - Arterial dissection (transmural)
  - Cerebral arteriovenous malformation
  - Dural arteriovenous fistula
  - Pituitary apoplexy
  - Mycotic aneurysm
  - Cardiac myxoma
  - Sickle cell disease
  - Tumours
  - Spinal arteriovenous malformation or aneurysm
  - Trauma (without contusion)
  - Cocaine abuse

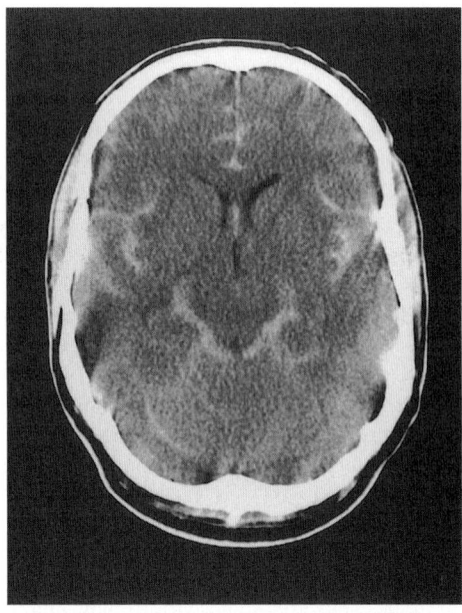

(a)

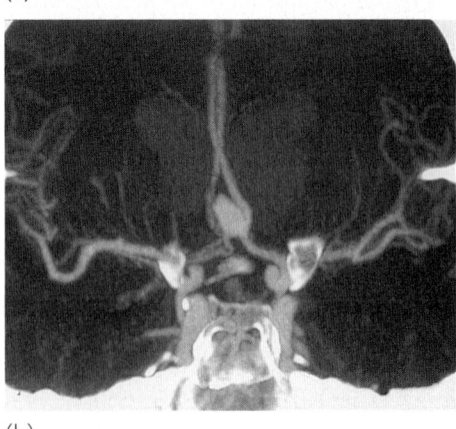

(b)

Fig. 24.10.1.7 Aneurysmal subarachnoid haemorrhage in a 31-year-old woman. (a) CT scanning shows evidence of extravasated blood throughout the basal cisterns. (b) CT angiogram, with intravenous contrast, shows an aneurysm at the anterior communicating artery.

Diagnosis of SAH

The key feature in the history is that of a sudden, severe, and unusual headache. In 50% there is loss of consciousness at onset; in them the headache may emerge only later. The diagnosis is most difficult in patients with headache as the only feature. In general practice, exceptionally sudden forms of common headaches outnumber ruptured aneurysms. The incidence of aneurysmal haemorrhage being about 6 per 100 000 population per year, the average general practitioner will, on average, see one such patient every 8 years. There are no single or combined features of the headache that distinguish reliably and at an early stage between SAH and innocuous types of sudden headache. The discomfort and cost of referring most patients for only a brief consultation in hospital are a reasonable price to pay for avoiding misdiagnosis of a ruptured aneurysm.

The physical examination is unhelpful in patients with headache alone, without loss of consciousness or focal deficits. Neck stiffness takes about 6 h to develop, so its absence soon after the onset does not exclude the diagnosis of SAH at all.

Of the investigations CT is the most important. This will show extravasation of blood in the basal cisterns of the brain in at least 95% of patients with a ruptured aneurysm, if the scan is performed within 3 days (see Fig. 24.10.1.7). After that interval the sensitivity of CT quickly decreases. In patients with a negative CT scan but a convincing history, lumbar puncture is indicated. If the cerebrospinal fluid is blood stained, it is essential to distinguish SAH reliably from a traumatic tap. For that purpose at least 6 and preferably 12 h should have elapsed from symptom onset. In case of SAH sufficient lysis of red cells will have occurred in the meantime for bilirubin and oxyhaemoglobin to have formed. These pigments give the cerebrospinal fluid a yellow tinge after centrifugation (xanthochromia); they are invariably detectable until at least 2 weeks later. The 'three tube test' (a decrease in red cells in consecutive tubes in the case of a traumatic puncture) is notoriously unreliable. If the supernatant seems crystal clear, the specimen should be stored in darkness until the absence of blood pigments is confirmed by spectrophotometry. Bilirubin can be formed only *in vivo*; its demonstration by spectrophotometry therefore proves that red blood cells cannot have been introduced during the lumbar puncture, whereas oxyhaemoglobin can be formed if a cerebrospinal fluid specimen with red blood cells is left standing before the sample is spun down. Catheter angiography is rapidly being replaced by CT and MR angiography as a method for demonstrating or excluding an aneurysm as the source of haemorrhage.

Treatment of aneurysmal SAH

Several complications may occur after a first episode of aneurysmal SAH, of which rebleeding and cerebral ischaemia are the most dreaded. Despite advances in surgical and medical management, the population-based case fatality rate is still around 50%, with half of survivors remaining more or less disabled.

As general nursing measures, continuous observation and an intravenous access are essential. A bladder catheter is necessary for monitoring fluid balance. Headache should be relieved in a stepwise approach, with paracetamol and codeine as first steps. Distressing anxiety can be alleviated with short-acting benzodiazepines. Stools should be kept soft with oral laxatives and also by an adequate intake of fluids.

Prevention of rebleeding is challenging, if only because any effective measure tends to be offset by an increased risk of ischaemia. Moreover, at least 10% of all patients with SAH suffer a further bleed within hours of the initial haemorrhage. Over the next 4 weeks the rate of rebleeding without intervention is at least 30%. The immediate case fatality of rebleeding is 50%. Endovascular treatment ('coiling') is the preferred method to occlude the aneurysm and prevent rebleeding, but not all aneurysms can be treated in this way and surgical treatment by clipping is still necessary for these patients. Antifibrinolytic drugs decrease the rate of rebleeding but do not improve overall outcome.

Delayed cerebral ischaemia occurs in up to 25% of patients with a ruptured aneurysm, mainly between day 5 and day 14 after the initial bleed. Understanding of its pathogenesis has been impeded by simplistic notions about 'vasospasm' or 'clots around vessels'. Narrowing of the arteries at the base of the brain is a factor but not a sufficient one. The total amount of subarachnoid blood is a potent risk factor, but only after rupture of an artery, and the distribution of blood in the subarachnoid space does not predict the site of ischaemia. The calcium antagonist nimodipine, in a dose of 60 mg every 4 h by mouth or nasogastric tube, reduces the frequency of cerebral ischaemia and poor outcome by about a third; its mode of action is incompletely understood. Hypertension should as a rule be left untreated; it is a compensatory reaction to maintain cerebral perfusion. The plasma volume should not be allowed to fall; hyponatraemia is caused by renal sodium depletion and not, as still often believed, by dilution as a result of inappropriate secretion of antidiuretic hormone. Fluids should therefore be replaced and not restricted. The basic intake should be at least 3 litres/day, with intravenous fluids supplementing oral intake; compensation should be made for fever or a negative fluid balance.

Further reading

Algra A, van Gijn J (1999). Cumulative meta-analysis of aspirin efficacy after cerebral ischaemia of arterial origin. *J Neurol Neurosurg Psychiatry*, **66**, 255. [Systematic review of aspirin in the secondary prevention of stroke.]

Ariesen MJ, *et al.* (2003). Risk factors for intracerebral hemorrhage in the general population: a systematic review. *Stroke*, **34**, 2060–5. [Systematic review of risk factors for intracerebral haemorrhage.]

Baigent C, *et al.* (2005). Efficacy and safety of cholesterol-lowering treatment: prospective meta-analysis of data from 90,056 participants in 14 randomised trials of statins. *Lancet*, **366**, 1267–78. [Meta-analysis of 14 randomized trials with statins in patients with cardiovascular disease or risk factors.]

Baigent C, *et al.* (2002). Collaborative meta-analysis of randomised trials of antiplatelet therapy for prevention of death, myocardial infarction, and stroke in high risk patients. *BMJ*, **324**, 71–86. [Systematic review.]

Bhatt DL, *et al.* (2006). Clopidogrel and aspirin versus aspirin alone for the prevention of atherothrombotic events. *N Engl J Med*, **354**, 1706–17. [Shows that the combination of aspirin and clopidogrel has no advantage over aspirin alone in patients at high risk of atherothrombotic events.]

Coull AJ, Lovett JK, Rothwell PM (2004). Population based study of early risk of stroke after transient ischaemic attack or minor stroke: implications for public education and organisation of services. *BMJ*, **328**, 326–8. [Shows that the risk of stroke after a transient ischaemic attack is greatest in the first week and month.]

Davis SM, *et al.* (2006). Hematoma growth is a determinant of mortality and poor outcome after intracerebral hemorrhage. *Neurology*, **66**, 1175–81. [Shows that for intracerebral haematomas not only age and initial size but also subsequent expansion are important prognostic factors.]

EAFT (European Atrial Fibrillation Trial) Study Group (1993). Secondary prevention in non-rheumatic atrial fibrillation after transient ischaemic attack or minor stroke. *Lancet*, **342**, 1255–62. [Proves effectiveness of oral anticoagulants.]

Feigin VL, *et al.* (2003). Stroke epidemiology: a review of population-based studies of incidence, prevalence, and case-fatality in the late 20th century. *Lancet Neurol*, **2**, 43–53. [Review of population-based studies of stroke incidence.]

Gent M, *et al.* (1996). A randomised, blinded, trial of clopidogrel versus aspirin in patients at risk of ischaemic events (CAPRIE). *Lancet*, **348**, 1329–39. [Shows marginal advantage of clopidogrel over aspirin.]

Gubitz G, Sandercock P, Counsell C (2004). Anticoagulants for acute ischaemic stroke. *Cochrane Database Syst Rev*, CD000024. [Systematic review.]

Hacke W, *et al.* (2004). Association of outcome with early stroke treatment: pooled analysis of ATLANTIS, ECASS, and NINDS rt-PA stroke trials. *Lancet*, **363**, 768–74. [Combined analysis of trials with rt-PA in ischaemic stroke.]

Halkes PHA, *et al.* (2006). Aspirin plus dipyridamole versus aspirin alone after cerebral ischaemia of arterial origin (ESPRIT): randomised controlled trial. *Lancet*, **367**, 1665–73. [Trial providing definitive evidence that the combination of dipyridamole and aspirin is superior to aspirin alone in the secondary prevention of stroke.]

Halkes PHA, *et al.* (2007). Medium intensity oral anticoagulants versus aspirin after cerebral ischaemia of arterial origin (ESPRIT): a randomised controlled trial. *Lancet Neurol*, **6**, 115–24. [Shows that medium intensity anticoagulation (INR 2 to 3) is ineffective in preventing major vascular events.]

Johnston SC, *et al.* (2007). Validation and refinement of scores to predict very early stroke risk after transient ischaemic attack. *Lancet*, **369**, 283–92. [Develops a simple risk score for patients with transient ischaemic attacks.]

Koudstaal PJ, *et al.* (1992). TIA, RIND, minor stroke: a continuum, or different subgroups? Dutch TIA Study Group. *J Neurol Neurosurg Psychiatry*, **55**, 95–7. [Shows how irrelevant it is to strictly distinguish ischaemic episodes of the brain according to their duration.]

MacMahon S, *et al.* (2001). Randomised trial of a perindopril-based blood-pressure-lowering regimen among 6105 individuals with previous stroke or transient ischaemic attack. *Lancet*, **358**, 1033–41. [Randomized trial of antihypertensive drugs (perindopril with or without indapamide) in more than 6000 patients with a history of transient ischaemic attack or ischaemic stroke, showing a risk reduction in normotensive as well as in hypertensive patients.]

Madden KP, *et al.* (1995). Accuracy of initial stroke subtype diagnosis in the TOAST study. *Neurology*, **45**, 1975–9. [Classification of ischaemic strokes according to cause: the initial classification is confirmed after 3 months in only two-thirds.]

Mendelow AD, *et al.* (2005). Early surgery versus initial conservative treatment in patients with spontaneous supratentorial intracerebral haematomas in the International Surgical Trial in Intracerebral Haemorrhage (STICH): a randomised trial. *Lancet*, **365**, 387–97. [Clinical trial of surgical treatment for supratentorial intracerebral haematomas, showing no overall benefit.]

Molyneux AJ, *et al.* (2005). International subarachnoid aneurysm trial (ISAT) of neurosurgical clipping versus endovascular coiling in 2143 patients with ruptured intracranial aneurysms: a randomised comparison of effects on survival, dependency, seizures, rebleeding, subgroups, and aneurysm occlusion. *Lancet*, **366**, 809–17. [Shows an advantage in survival with occlusion of ruptured aneurysms by endovascular coiling rather than clipping, maintained over several years.]

O' Collins VE, *et al.* (2006). 1,026 experimental treatments in acute stroke. *Ann Neurol*, **59**, 467–77. [Explores the question why neuroprotective drugs after cerebral ischaemia that were promising in animal studies failed to work in humans.]

Roos YBWEM, *et al.* (2003). Antifibrinolytic treatment in aneurysmal subarachnoid haemorrhage. *Cochrane Database Syst Rev*, CD001245. [Systematic review.]

Rothwell PM, *et al.* (2003). Analysis of pooled data from the randomised controlled trials of endarterectomy for symptomatic carotid stenosis. *Lancet*, **361**, 107–16. [Systematic review based on individual patient data.]

Rothwell PM, *et al.* (2004). Change in stroke incidence, mortality, case-fatality, severity, and risk factors in Oxfordshire, UK from 1981 to 2004 (Oxford Vascular Study). *Lancet*, **363**, 1925–33. [Documents a substantial decrease in the age-specific incidence of major stroke in Oxfordshire.]

Sandercock P, *et al.* (2003). Antiplatelet therapy for acute ischaemic stroke. *Cochrane Database Syst Rev*, CD000029. [Systematic review.]

Stam J (2005). Thrombosis of the cerebral veins and sinuses. *N Engl J Med*, **352**, 1791–8. [Comprehensive review article.]

Stroke Unit Trialists' Collaboration (2002). Organised inpatient (stroke unit) care for stroke. *Cochrane Database Sys Rev*, CD000197. [Systematic review showing the benefits of organized inpatient stroke care.]

Vahedi K, *et al.* (2007). Early decompressive surgery in malignant infarction of the middle cerebral artery: a pooled analysis of three randomised controlled trials. *Lancet Neurol*, **6**, 215–22. [Pooled analysis of three randomized trials.]

Van der Zwan A, *et al.* (1992). Variability of the territories of the major cerebral arteries. *J Neurosurg*, **77**, 927–40. [Shows the variability between individuals of boundaries between the territory of major cerebral arteries.]

Van Gijn J, Kerr RS, Rinkel GJE (2007). Subarachnoid haemorrhage. *Lancet*, **369**, 306–18. [Review.]

Wahlgren L, *et al.* (2008). Thrombolysis with alteplase 3–4.5 h after acute ischaemic stroke (SITS-ISTR): an observational study. *Lancet*, **372**, 1303–9. [Observational study suggesting substantial benefit of thrombolysis 3-4.5 h after stroke onset.]

Warlow CP, *et al.* (2007). *Stroke—practical management*, 3rd edition. Blackwells, Oxford. [Comprehensive monograph about cerebrovascular disease, including a chapter about the historical background.]

Zhang-Nunes SX, *et al.* (2006). The cerebral beta-amyloid angiopathies: hereditary and sporadic. *Brain Pathol*, **16**, 30–9. [Review.]

24.10.2 **Demyelinating disorders of the central nervous system**

Siddharthan Chandran and Alastair Compston

Essentials

Clinicians suspect demyelination when episodes reflecting damage to white matter tracts within the central nervous system occur in young adults. Multiple sclerosis is much the most common demyelinating disorder, but other important demyelinating diseases include postinfectious neurological disorders, metabolically mediated demyelination, and inherited leucodystrophies.

Isolated demyelinating syndromes

Acute disseminated encephalomyelitis—typically presents within days or a few weeks after an infectious illness (or more rarely following vaccination) with manifestations including headache, drowsiness, meningeal irritation, focal or generalized fits, and combinations of lesions indicating damage to the cerebrum, optic nerves, brainstem, or spinal cord. The cerebrospinal fluid contains polymorphonuclear cells and lymphocytes, with raised protein, slight reduction in glucose, and (sometimes) oligoclonal bands. MRI shows changes similar to those occurring in multiple sclerosis but the lesions are generally more extensive (and absence of lesion accrual upon serial imaging is sometimes required to exclude this diagnosis). Treatment with high-dose intravenous steroids, intravenous immunoglobulin, and/or plasmapheresis is usually given. Most patients survive, sometimes with persistent neurological deficits.

Optic neuritis—presents with pain on eye movement, followed by subacute visual loss that improves over months in 90% of patients, although defects of colour perception frequently persist. Corticosteroids accelerate recovery but do not influence long-term outcome or conversion to clinically definite multiple sclerosis (which occurs in up to 20% of patients).

Transverse myelitis—presumed to be postinfectious, this presents with pain at the site of the cord lesion, followed by weakness in the legs, sensory symptoms, and sphincter involvement. Radiological imaging may demonstrate cord swelling, and the spinal fluid shows an increased mononuclear cell count. Treatment with high-dose intravenous steroids is often given. Many patients are left with persistent disability, but there is a much lower conversion to multiple sclerosis than following optic neuritis.

Devic's disease (neuromyelitis optica)—a relapsing disorder characterized clinically by attacks of severe optic neuritis and myelitis, recovery from which is generally incomplete, leading to progressive disability, and immunologically by auto-antibodies against the water channel aquaporin-4. Treatment is with steroids, plasma exchange, and other immunosuppressants.

Multiple sclerosis

Aetiology and pathology—multiple sclerosis is widely believed to be caused by a T-cell-mediated autoimmune process. Perivascular inflammation evolves through stages of acute axonal injury, demyelination, oligodendrocyte depletion, remyelination, astrocytosis, and chronic neurodegeneration.

Epidemiology—the condition is a disease of predominantly northern European people, with a modest female predominance and an association with the class II MHC alleles *DR15* and *DQ6*.

Clinical features—these include the following: (1) Special senses—visual involvement, usually of the optic nerve, is almost invariable. (2) Motor—most patients have impaired mobility, typically as a result of spinal disease, with spasticity sometimes more problematic than weakness; incoordination due to cerebellar involvement is common. (3) Sensory—altered sensation attributable to posterior column and/or spinothalamic involvement occurs at some stage in nearly every patient. (4) Autonomic—bladder symptoms are more common in women; erectile dysfunction occurs frequently in men. (5) Eye movements—these are very commonly disturbed, the commonest sign being first-degree symmetrical horizontal jerking nystagmus. (6) Other brainstem manifestations—there can be a wide range of sustained or paroxysmal abnormalities. (7) Cognitive and affective symptoms.

Clinical course and prognosis—85% of patients have relapsing–remitting disease, with the illness typically passing through the three phases of relapse with full recovery, relapse with persistent deficits, and secondary progression. Episodes occur at random frequency, but initially average about 1.5 per year and decrease steadily thereafter. Most patients develop progressive irreversible disability within 10 to 15 years of disease onset.

Investigation—multiple sclerosis can reliably be diagnosed using clinical criteria, but investigations—electrophysiology, MRI, and cerebrospinal fluid analysis—are used to (1) demonstrate the anatomical dissemination of lesions; (2) provide evidence for intrathecal inflammation; (3) demonstrate that conduction is altered in a form consistent with demyelination; and (4) exclude conditions that mimic demyelinating disease.

Treatment—(1) Acute episodes—corticosteroids abbreviate these, but have no effect on frequency of relapse. (2) Disease-modifying treatments—agents that target the inflammatory component of disease are effective in relapsing-remitting and rapidly worsening multiple sclerosis, but there are no proven therapies for progressive disease independent of relapses. Approved therapies include β-interferons and glatiramer acetate, and use of some monoclonal antibodies (natalizumab, alemtuzumab, rituximab) shows considerable promise. (3) Symptomatic—the complex and progressive nature of disability requires a multidisciplinary approach, including attention to urinary problems, constipation, impotence, tremor, spasticity, and paroxysmal manifestations. (4) Comprehensive care—minimizing handicap by attention to social, vocational, marital, sexual, and psychological aspects of the illness remains more important to most patients than drug treatment.

Other conditions associated with demyelination

Central pontine myelinolysis—often associated with hyponatraemia, or correction of hyponatraemia (see Chapter 21.2.1), the fully evolved clinical picture is of flaccid paralysis with facial and bulbar weakness, disordered eye movements, loss of balance, and altered consciousness.

Leucodystrophies—characterized by noninflammatory demyelination, many of these conditions result from mutations affecting genes involved in myelin biology. They need to be considered in young adults with atypical syndromes combining physical and intellectual deficits, sometimes with peripheral nerve involvement, in whom imaging shows confluent lesions confined to white matter. These include (1) diffuse sclerosis (Schilder's disease), (2) Krabbe's disease, (3) adrenoleucodystrophy, (4) metachromatic leucodystrophy, (5) Pelizaeus–Merzbacher disease, and (6) adult-onset dominant leucodystrophies.

Introduction

A distinguishing feature of vertebrate development is the formation of compact glial-derived myelin ensheathing processes around axons. Myelin formation by oligodendrocytes in the central nervous system (CNS) and Schwann cells in the peripheral nervous system (PNS) has allowed the development of sophisticated and compact neural systems. Evolutionary advantage, however, is not without its drawbacks. Several diseases, inherited and acquired, loosely grouped under "demyelination" represent processes where the oligendrocyte–myelin unit appears to be the primary target, notwithstanding the intimate relationship and dependency between glia and axons.

Clinicians suspect demyelination when episodes reflecting damage to white matter tracts within the CNS occur in young adults. The paucity of specific biological markers of discrete demyelinating syndromes places an emphasis on clinical pattern—temporal and spatial—when classifying demyelining disorders. The diagnosis of multiple sclerosis, the most common demyelinating disorder, becomes probable when these symptoms and signs recur, affecting different parts of the brain and spinal cord. Other important demyelinating diseases include postinfectious neurological disorders (acute disseminated encephalomyelitis), metabolically mediated demyelination (central pontine myelinosis), and inherited leucodystrophies that may present in childhood or adulthood. Accepting differences in mechanism, presentation, and treatment, two observations can usefully be made when classifying demyelinating disorders based on presence or absence of inflammation and extent of focal versus diffuse demyelination. Multiple sclerosis is prototypic of the former and dysmylinating disorders such as leucodystrophies are representative of the latter.

Neurobiology of demyelination

Origin of oligodendrocytes

Oligodendrocytes synthesize and maintain membrane that is continuous with axonal ensheathing compact myelin. In contrast to neurons, oligodendrocytes are predominantly specified postnatally and continue to divide and migrate as oligodendrocyte precursor cells (OPCs). Identification of the *OLIG* genes has significantly advanced our understanding of the molecular regulation of developmental and adult oligodendrogenesis. In addition to its established role in specifying neurons and OPCs in the developing CNS, emerging evidence implicates Olig in self-renewal of neural stem cells and adult oligodendrogenesis in the normal and injured brain. These findings, together with accumulated insights into the proliferative, migratory and survival requirements of OPCs, have resulted in the oligodendrocyte lineage being the best characterized of all neural cells and offering potential neuroprotective therapeutic targets in the context of demyelinating disease.

Myelination

Myelination occurs when the membranous processes of mature oligodendrocytes contact and ensheathe axons. The result is compaction of myelin sheaths at two points of apposition, apparent on ultrastructural analysis as major and minor dense lines. Myelin is predominantly composed of lipids (70–80% dry weight; cholesterol, phospholipid, and galactolipids) and protein (20–30% dry weight). The major myelin-specific lipid, galactocerebroside, can be used to identify myelinating glia. The major proteins are proteolipid protein (PLP), myelin basic protein (MBP), and myelin-specific enzyme 2′,3′-cyclic nucleotide 3′-phosphohydrolase (CNP).

Myelination corresponds to the formation of segments of compact myelin around axons. Each high resistance myelin segment is separated by the unmyelinated high conductance node of Ranvier. This specialized structure, characterized by clusters of voltage-gated sodium channels, allows impulse propagation by saltatory conduction, which is more rapid, energy and space efficient than propagation along unmyelinated axons. Myelinated internodal segments contain dispersed sodium channels at a much lower density insufficient to support conduction.

Pathophysiology of demyelination

Demyelination results in predictable electrophysiological consequences including impaired saltatory conduction, decreased conduction velocity, variable degrees of conduction block, and inappropriate sensitivity to changes in temperature or mechanical displacement. Clinical manifestations of demyelination are less easily predicted. They are proportionate to the degree of redundancy in individual systems and tracts, the involvement of some being easily exposed whereas others appear able to absorb a greater degree of damage without function being impaired. As with many disorders of the nervous system, the clinical symptoms and signs may be negative (loss of function) or positive (spontaneous, involuntary and paroxysmal): either category may be equally disabling.

Partially demyelinated axons cannot transmit fast trains of impulse, which may explain symptoms that reflect physiological fatigue. Depolarization may traverse the lesion, but at reduced velocity, accounting for the characteristic delay in arrival of potentials evoked by sensory stimuli and recorded over appropriate cortical receptor zones. Partially demyelinated axons may discharge spontaneously, explaining distortions of sensation reported by many patients. Increased mechanical sensitivity manifests as movement-induced symptoms, including flashes of light on eye movement, and the electric sensation that spreads down the spine, limbs, or anterior chest wall after neck flexion—Lhermitte's symptom and sign. Increased temperature sensitivity, with a reduction in the safety factor for conduction in partially demyelinated axons, explains the temporary increase in severity of pre-existing symptoms experienced by many patients after exercise or immersion in hot water. Cold, by contrast, may improve performance. Ephaptic transmission occurs between neighbouring and partially demyelinated axons, giving rise to paroxysmal symptoms of demyelination usually manifesting as trigeminal neuralgia, ataxia, and dysarthria, or tonic brainstem seizures. These are often triggered by touch or movement.

There are several mechanisms of symptom recovery early in the course of multiple sclerosis. These include the resolution of conduction block in nerve fibres which were never demyelinated, re-establishment of conduction in persistently demyelinated axons, functional reorganization of surviving pathways, and remyelination.

Onset and recovery of conduction block and clinical impairments match the phase of acute inflammation. Transient symptoms depend on reversible conduction block caused by direct action of cytokines and inflammatory mediators (especially nitric oxide) on normal or hypomyelinated axons (Fig. 24.10.2.1). Function may be restored after demyelination by an increase in number and rearrangement of sodium channels along denuded axons, providing a variety of alternative patterns of ordered or partially disordered conduction. But channel reorganization can also be maladaptive, with the energy compromised demyelinated axon appearing vulnerable to sodium channel dependent axonal degeneration. Experimentally, remyelinated axons restore conduction of the nerve impulse and motor function. Together these observations suggest sodium channel blockade and promotion of remyelination as plausible neuroprotective strategies.

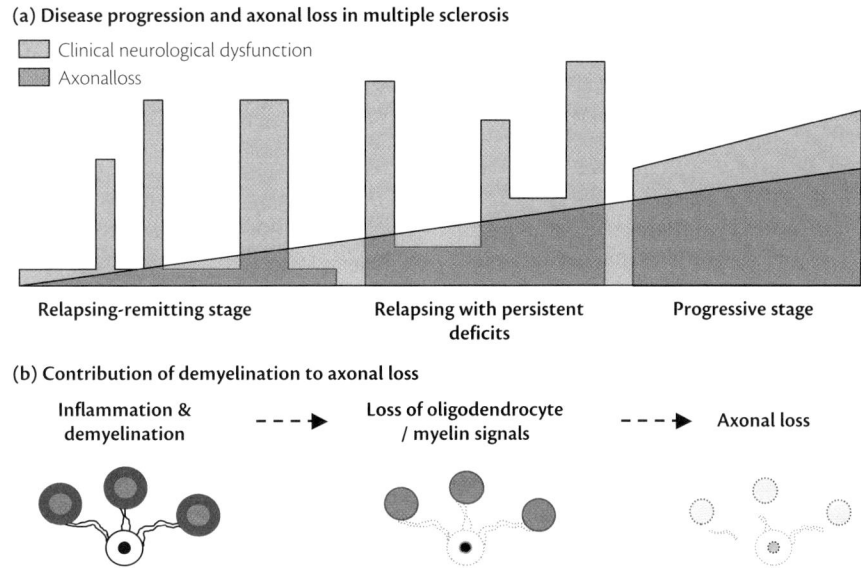

Fig. 24.10.2.1 Inflammation, demyelination, axonal loss and disease progression in multiple sclerosis. (a) The early stage of relapsing-remitting multiple sclerosis is characterized by transient neurological deficits that return to normal and pathology dominated by focal inflammation and demyelination. However, as the disease progresses neurological dysfunction becomes fixed and accumulates. The pathological correlate of the progressive phase of the disease is axonal loss. (b) The early events of demyelination and inflammation are believed to contribute to axonal loss by numerous mechanisms including loss of oligodendrocyte / myelin derived trophic and structural support. The schematic diagram shows a single oligodendrocyte (black and white) myelinating three axons (axon purple, myelin blue). Early in the course of multiple sclerosis the oligodendrocyte is damaged through inflammatory driven mechanisms resulting in demyelination of the axon. The loss of oligodendrocyte contributes and culminates in axonal loss as found in progressive multiple sclerosis.

Inflammation, neurodegeneration, and remyelination

Demyelinating disease includes conditions in which myelin fails to develop (leucodystrophies) or is lost through inflammatory (multiple sclerosis and related conditions) or metabolic (central pontine myelinolysis) mechanisms. Outstandingly the most common group is multiple sclerosis, histologically characterized by breakdown of the blood–brain barrier and multifocal inflammatory plaques. In all but the most severe forms, perivascular inflammation evolves through stages of acute axonal injury, demyelination, oligodendrocyte depletion, remyelination, astrocytosis, and chronic neurodegeneration. The order and relationship of these separate components is still debated. The resulting plaques are widely distributed, but concentrated around venous networks, the ventricles, and in the corpus callosum, the optic nerve, brainstem, and cervical cord.

Although the precise pathogenesis of inflammatory-mediated demyelination is unknown, it is widely believed to be consistent with a T-cell mediated autoimmune process. It depends on the movement of activated T cells from the periphery into the CNS. The basis of peripheral activation and the precise role and subsequent relationship between the innate and adaptive immune system in initiation and maintenance of CNS autoimmunity is unclear. Furthermore, recent experimental, clinical, and pathological insights emphasize the complex interplay between T cells (including regulatory T cells), macrophages or microglia and humoral and complement effector systems in propagating and amplifying tissue damage.

Activated T cells that encounter antigen persist within the nervous system. Recruitment of lymphocytes across the blood–brain barrier is mediated by adhesion molecules and chemokines, the latter also being important in mediating migration of inflammatory cells within the CNS. Once within the CNS, activated T cells specific for putative central antigen(s) initiate a cascade of events, including secretion of pro-inflammatory cytokines, local activation of

microglia and production of immunoglobulins that together culminate in damage to the myelin–oligodendrocyte unit. Together, these inflammatory processes lead to disruption of the myelin membrane with increased spacing, vesicular disruption, splitting, vacuolation, and fragmentation of the lamellae. This immunological formulation belies pathological heterogeneity and the complexity of evolution seen in inflammatory demyelination.

Originally, it was proposed that individual patients conform to one of four patterns: T cell infiltrates and macrophage associated tissue injury (pattern 1); antibody and complement-mediated immune reactions against cells of the oligodendrocyte lineage and myelin (pattern 2); hypoxia-like injury, resulting either from inflammation-induced vascular damage or macrophage toxins that impair mitochondrial function (pattern 3); and a genetic defect resulting in primary susceptibility of the oligodendrocytes to immune injury (pattern 4). The evidence for pathological heterogeneity—as opposed to complexity—has recently been challenged. Rather, the various pathological features are now seen as stages in the development of an ubiquitous pathological end-game in which apparent heterogeneity may disappear over time as different pathways converge on one general mechanism of demyelination—the presence of complement, antibodies, and Fc gamma receptors in phagocytic macrophages indicating that antibody—and complement-mediated myelin phagocytosis is the dominant mechanism of demyelination in established multiple sclerosis. The focus on inflammation and demyelination had until recently obscured the extent and significance of neuronal and axonal injury. Axonal injury is present at all stages of multiple sclerosis. Multiple mechanisms have been implicated, contingent on stage and pattern of disease; early axonal injury evident by axonal transection and accumulation of amyloid precursor protein tends to occur when inflammatory demyelination is prominent. Whether specific immune mediated axonal injury also occurs over and above nonspecific inflammatory collateral damage is unclear. Similarly, it is uncertain if axonal loss in normal appearing white matter merely reflects axon dropout due to time-delayed Wallerian degeneration. Chronic axonal attrition observed in the inflammatory quiescent chronic demyelinated lesion, along with other observations, implicates loss of myelin-derived signals as central to the mechanism of progressive neurodegeneration.

Recognition that neurodegeneration is the dominant pathological substrate of progressive disability raises the fundamental and as yet unanswered question of the relationship between inflammation—clinically manifest as relapse—and neurodegeneration. A widely held position, accepting that an independent axonal vulnerability may pre-exist for genetic and other reasons, is that inflammation primes and/or maintains neurodegeneration.

It has long been known that acute lesions frequently show an increase in numbers of oligodendrocyte precursors and may undergo remyelination evident as shadow plaques. Remyelination, found at all stages of disease, is histologically identified by inappropriately thin myelin lamellae, with a short internode and widened nodes of Ranvier. The finding that remyelination is associated with negligible axonal injury compared to inactive demyelinated plaques suggests remyelination is neuroprotective. The source of remyelinating cells is presumed to be the oligodendrocyte progenitor which is found in the lesions of multiple sclerosis, although recent evidence also suggests a role for adult stem cells derived from the subventricular zone.

Isolated demyelinating syndromes

The clinical expression of demyelination may be focal and monophasic. Multiple sclerosis, in contrast, is both multifocal and multiphasic. Notwithstanding that a monophasic event may occasionally appear disseminated in time, the distinction between multiple sclerosis and isolated demyelinating disorders can only be reliably made when more than one episode has occurred, affecting two or more sites, and not merely on the basis of anatomical dissemination of lesions. Longitudinal studies show that inclusion of imaging criteria increases precision in predicting likely conversion of clinically isolated syndromes to multiple sclerosis. Emerging evidence that treating high risk patients with disease modifying agents may delay conversion emphasizes the value of early accurate diagnosis.

Acute disseminated encephalomyelitis

Typically, acute disseminated encephalomyelitis, a monophasic illness, develops within days or a few weeks after an infectious illness, or more rarely following vaccination. It is usually but not invariably a disease of children and often has an explosive onset. Formerly, acute disseminated encephalomyelitis affected 1 in 1000 children with exanthematous illnesses, the risk being slightly lower following pertussis and scarlet fever than measles and rubella, but these childhood illnesses, and hence their complications, are now less prevalent. A greater variety of causative organisms has been implicated in adult-onset acute disseminated encephalomyelitis, but in both groups a presumptive diagnosis often has to be made in the absence of an identifiable preceding infection.

In the absence of biological markers, diagnosis is based on the combination of clinical, radiological, and laboratory investigations in the appropriate demographic context. However, an absence of lesion accrual upon serial imaging is sometimes required to exclude multiple sclerosis. The disorder is usually diffuse, and with a cerebral–encephalopathic flavour, but the clinical manifestations may be restricted to the brainstem, optic nerves, or spinal cord. About 50% of cases occurring after varicella infection present with a pure cerebellar syndrome. Headache, drowsiness, meningeal irritation, signs of systemic infection, focal or generalized fits, and combinations of lesions indicating damage to the cerebrum, optic nerves, brainstem, or spinal cord evolve over the course of a few days. The cerebrospinal fluid contains a mixture of polymorphonuclear cells and lymphocytes with raised protein and slight reduction in glucose; oligoclonal bands may be present. Although there is an appreciable mortality, most patients survive, sometimes with persistent neurological deficits. MRI shows changes similar to those occurring in multiple sclerosis, including gadolinium enhancement, but the lesions are more extensive, asymmetric, and frequently involve grey matter of thalamus and basal ganglia; they persist long after recovery of the clinical illness.

The hyperacute form of acute disseminated encephalomyelitis (Hurst's disease) starts with headache and progresses over hours to disorientation, confusion, drowsiness, and coma; events move quickly and the illness often proves fatal before the diagnosis has been established. The combination of pyrexia and a marked cerebrospinal fluid pleocytosis with a predominantly neutrophil response mimics pyogenic infection of the CNS, but the course is not influenced by antimicrobial treatment. Occasionally, the clinical and pathological features of acute haemorrhagic leucoencephalitis are focal and suggest a rapidly expanding tumour or herpes simplex encephalitis.

There is no evidence based standard treatment for acute disseminated encephalomyelitis. However, outcome is probably influenced by early use of high-dose intravenous steroids, but—anecdotally—there may be a more favourable response to intravenous immunoglobulin or plasmapheresis.

Some patients recovering from the initial attack subsequently relapse. In others, although the illness remains monophasic, separate sites are involved sequentially over several weeks, but the disorder does not recur. Sometimes the illness is subsequently shown to be the encephalopathic presentation of multiple sclerosis, which then follows the typical relapsing–remitting course. The nosological status of multiphasic disseminated encephalomyelitis—based on a history of episodes and atypical imaging appearances for multiple sclerosis—has not gained general acceptance.

Postvaccinial encephalomyelitis has become a rare disorder, with the definitive series collected several decades ago when vaccination against smallpox was necessary. The illness develops within 2 to 3 weeks of vaccination, with a skin rash and systemic symptoms, followed by cerebral or myelitic signs that usually recover spontaneously in due course.

Optic neuritis

Optic neuritis presents with pain on eye movement, followed by subacute visual loss which evolves over hours or days, sometimes to complete blindness; patients may be aware of selective loss of colour vision and flashes of light (phosphenes) on eye movement. Other signs of optic neuropathy at presentation include afferent pupillary defect and visual field loss. The pain disappears within a few days; vision begins to improve within 4 weeks and does so in 90% of patients over months, but defects of colour perception frequently persist.

Outside the paediatric population, optic neuritis is usually monocular; bilateral simultaneous loss, and progressive visual failure suggest alternative diagnoses. Transient visual loss, mimicking optic neuritis, also occurs in ischaemic optic neuropathy, sarcoidosis, and lupus, and a family history should be taken since the presentation of visual failure in Leber's hereditary optic neuropathy is similar to bilateral sequential optic neuritis in men.

The lesion responsible for optic neuritis can be imaged *in vivo*; inflammation within the intracanalicular portion of the nerve and long lesions are associated with delayed or incomplete recovery of vision. Correlations between imaging, symptoms, and neurophysiological changes indicate that the visual deficits in optic neuritis arise at the time of altered blood–brain barrier permeability. They are associated with conduction block and precede demyelination or axonal degeneration. In this regard, the increasing availability of optical coherence tomography is valuable as this provides a noninvasive quantitative measure of retinal nerve fibre loss, of particular interest given the association of neurodegeneration with progression.

Corticosteroids accelerate recovery but do not influence long-term outcome or alter conversion to clinically definite multiple sclerosis. Current practice tends to reserve intravenous methylprednisolone for optic neuritis in the setting of pre-existing abnormal function of the nonaffected eyes.

Acute demyelinating optic neuritis is a first manifestation of multiple sclerosis in up to 20% of patients. Brain MRI findings at presentation are invaluable in predicting conversion to clinically definite multiple sclerosis following optic neuritis. Long-term follow up of patients initially enrolled in trials to evaluate the utility of corticosteroids in optic neuritis has shown that an abnormal MRI brain scan is associated with 56% risk at 10 years compared to 22% with a normal scan. Studies that also included other isolated syndromes suggest an abnormal brain MRI predicts a conversion risk of 82% at 10 years. The presence of oligoclonal bands on cerebrospinal fluid electrophoresis during the acute phase is also a significant risk factor. An early MRI brain scan is recommended at presentation of optic neuritis in view of evidence that early treatment with β-interferons delays conversion of high risk (associated abnormal brain MRI) isolated optic neuritis to clinically definite multiple sclerosis.

Transverse myelitis

The spinal cord is vulnerable to postinfectious inflammatory damage, but as with acute disseminated encephalomyelitis in adults, the precipitating cause is often not identified. Transverse myelitis presents with pain at the site of the lesion, followed by weakness in the legs, sensory symptoms, and sphincter involvement. The weakness increases and the clinical picture is that of spinal shock—features rarely seen in acute cord lesions due to multiple sclerosis. Sphincter control is lost, but patients usually have difficulty in emptying rather than filling the bladder, unlike those with multiple sclerosis. Partial cord lesions are more typical of multiple sclerosis.

The need to exclude a structural abnormality in patients with transverse myelitis means that many patients undergo radiological investigation, which may demonstrate cord swelling. The spinal fluid shows an increased mononuclear cell count, numerically intermediate between the marked pleocytosis of acute necrotizing myelitis and the marginal abnormalities seen in multiple sclerosis; total protein is raised and oligoclonal bands may be present on electrophoresis, but the glucose is usually normal. Transverse myelitis is more common in adults than children; there is a high frequency of persistent disability, but a much lower conversion to multiple sclerosis than following optic neuritis.

Acute necrotizing myelitis causes rapidly progressive flaccid areflexic paraplegia with anaesthesia and loss of sphincter control. The intensity of inflammation results in severe pain with meningism, pyrexia, and systemic symptoms. The condition mimics cord compression, and the cerebrospinal fluid changes often resemble pyogenic or tuberculous infection of the CNS. For these reasons, treatment with high-dose intravenous steroids, which may usefully influence mortality and limit long-term disability, is often withheld. Acute necrotizing myelitis has been described in association with herpesvirus infection, and as a complication of acute lymphocytic leukaemias, lymphoma, carcinoma, and AIDS.

Devic's disease (neuromyelitis optica)

Devic's disease is an inflammatory demyelinating disorder characterized by severe optic neuritis and myelitis, occurring simultaneously or sequentially and in either order, these components usually separated by weeks or months, and one or other recurring so that the illness frequently follows a relapsing course. Cellular reaction in the cerebrospinal fluid more usually involves polymorphonuclear cells than lymphocytes, but often lacks oligoclonal bands. MRI brain findings are typically normal at onset, although asymptomatic cerebral white-matter abnormalities tend to emerge in later disease. The spinal lesion is long, extending over three or more vertebral segments, in contrast to the several short asymmetric lesions which characterize spinal MRI in multiple sclerosis. Recovery from attacks is generally incomplete and disability due to the impact of incomplete recovery from individual episodes usually emerges over time. This contrasts with multiple sclerosis where recovery from relapses is more complete but disability follows the onset of the secondary progressive phase that is typically much later in disease course and independent of relapses.

Together with these clinical and paraclinical features, the recent identification of a highly specific and sensitive auto-antibody (NMO-IgG) against the water channel aquaporin-4 antigen has clarified the relationship between neuromyelitis optica and multiple sclerosis. Demyelinating disease often follows an optico-spinal pattern in Japanese and African patients, where multiple sclerosis is otherwise rare. But, even with the use of biomarkers, the distinction from multiple sclerosis can still be confusing. Although the contribution of NMO-IgG to the pathogenesis of tissue injury is unknown, neuromyelitis optica is characterized immunohistologically by immunoglobulin and complement deposition—as in the so-called pattern II subset of pathology described in active multiple sclerosis. These insights have led to encouraging observational studies that recommend prompt use of plasma exchange and corticosteroids with subsequent maintenance immunosuppression. Similar findings have emerged from open label studies of the humanized monoclonal antibody Rituximab that selectively depletes B lymphocytes.

Isolated brainstem syndromes

The clinical symptoms and signs of isolated brainstem syndromes typically consist of disequilibrium, disturbed eye movements, facial numbness, and dysarthria, but there may be severe headache, which rightly leads to early investigation to exclude a structural lesion. Most patients progress to clinically definite multiple sclerosis. As with other isolated demyelinating syndromes, abnormal MRI outside the affected site at presentation is a risk factor for clinical conversion.

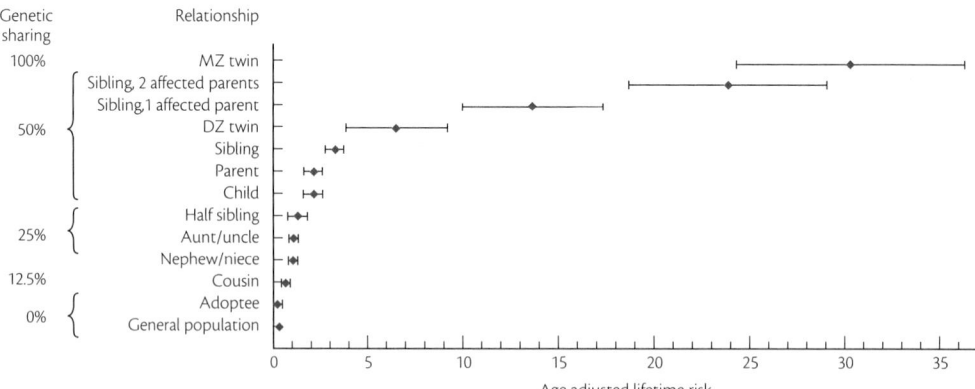

Fig. 24.10.2.2 Lifetime risk for multiple sclerosis among European people and in biological and social relatives of affected individuals. The increased risk with relatedness implicates genetic factors whereas the incomplete concordance in identical twins reflects the contribution made by environmental conditions.

Multiple sclerosis

Aetiology

The aetiology of multiple sclerosis involves an interplay between genes and the environment. It is a disease of northern European people and occurs less frequently in other racial groups with a modest female predominance. The familial recurrence rate is approximately 15%. Meta-analysis amongst relatives of probands from three population-based series shows that the age-adjusted risk is highest for siblings (3%), then parents and children (2%), with lower rates in second- and third-degree relatives. Recurrence in monozygotic twins is around 35%. Conversely, the frequency of multiple sclerosis in adoptees is similar to the population risk for Europeans. The age-adjusted risk for half-siblings is intermediate between social and biological relatives. Recurrence is higher in the children of conjugal pairs with multiple sclerosis (age-adjusted 20%) than the offspring of single affecteds (2%) (Fig. 24.10.2.2).

Population studies demonstrate an association between the linked class II MHC alleles (DR15 and DQ6) and their corresponding genotypes. Extensive searches, using association and linkage studies over many years, had—until recently—yielded very few additional candidates for susceptibility. However, large-scale genome wide association studies have begun to identify further genes that, individually, confer a modest increase in risk; these include the interleukin receptor related genes *IL2RA* and *IL7RA* and, perhaps more provisionally, HLA-C, *TYK2*, and CD58. This approach is likely to deliver further genes. The functional property of each of these newly identified genetic risk factors reinforces the idea that multiple sclerosis is an auto-immune disorder and offers a rational pathway for further studies of disease mechanisms and immunological treatments. Studies of concordance in multiplex families show that genetic factors influence the risk of progression but the responsible loci are not identified. It is assumed, but without any evidence to date, that there are also pharmacogenomic effects that determine the response to treatment. Genetic analysis may also contribute to the debate on whether multiple sclerosis is one disease. Mutations of mitochondrial DNA are responsible for a multiple sclerosis-like illness characterized by disproportionate involvement of the anterior visual pathway, although mitochondrial genes do not contribute generally to susceptibility in multiple sclerosis. A major part of future studies in the genetics of multiple sclerosis will be to resolve the question of disease heterogeneity.

The distribution of multiple sclerosis cannot be explained only on the basis of population genetics. In white South Africans and in Australia, prevalence rates are half those documented for many parts of northern Europe. There is a gradient in frequency, in both Australia and in New Zealand, that does not follow genetic clines. The risk is higher for English-speaking white people migrating into South Africa as adults than in childhood. Multiple sclerosis occurs at a low frequency in the Caribbean population, but the risk increases substantially in their first-generation descendants raised in the United Kingdom. Over and above the effect of racial predisposition, migration influences distribution of the disease. Surveys of multiple sclerosis have prompted speculation on the occurrence of post-Second World War epidemics in Iceland, the Orkneys and Shetlands, and the Faroes, but others prefer the interpretation that these merely reflect improved case recognition.

The widely accepted formulation that multiple sclerosis is the outcome of unknown environmental factors conditioned by age of exposure acting on a genetically vulnerable population has led to a largely unrewarding search for such environmental agents. The risk of developing multiple sclerosis is increased for individuals exposed to measles, mumps, rubella, and Epstein–Barr virus infection relatively late in childhood or adolescence. These studies suggest that an age-linked period of susceptibility to viral exposure exists in those wh are constitutionally at risk of developing the disease. But, noting the association with latitude, it has been suggested that the environmental effect is conferred by variable light exposure and vitamin D status rather than microbes.

Clinical symptomatology

Special senses

Visual involvement is almost invariable and most commonly affects the optic nerve (see above). The postchiasmal visual pathway is occasionally involved, resulting in hemianopic field defects. Deafness occurs in multiple sclerosis, sometimes at presentation. Feelings of unsteadiness are common. Acute brainstem demyelination causes severe positional vertigo, vomiting, ataxia, and headache. Taste may be subjectively abnormal, but ageusia is rarely described. Anosmia is reported in a high proportion of asymptomatic patients examined with more than usual thoroughness.

Motor symptoms and signs

Impaired mobility affects most patients with multiple sclerosis, usually as a result of spinal disease. Movements are slow, weakness differentially affecting extensors in the arms and flexors in the legs, and there are the expected signs of upper motor neuron lesions. Spasticity may be more problematic than weakness, and all aspects of immobility are frequently complicated by fatigue. Cerebellar involvement causes incoordination of speech, bulbar control, eye movements, the individual limbs, or balance, usually in combination with corticospinal damage. Damage to the superior cerebellar peduncle or red nucleus produces a disabling proximal wild flinging tremor, and many other movement disorders have been described. Lower motor neuron signs occur when there is extensive demyelination adjacent to the dorsal root entry zone.

Sensory symptoms and signs

Altered sensation occurs at some stage in nearly every patient with multiple sclerosis. Damage to the posterior columns in the cervical cord produces tight, burning, twisting, tearing, or pulling sensations, which are usually unpleasant. Associated loss of proprioception severely compromises function. Spinothalamic tract involvement leads to loss of thermal and pain sensation. Nonspecific tingling without accompanying signs is often described, and the commonest physical sign found in the absence of symptoms is impaired vibration sense in the legs.

Demyelination of the dorsal or lumbar segments of the spinal cord produces paraesthesias and numbness in the legs, ascending to the trunk, and sometimes associated with sacral sparing, although a characteristic sensory syndrome seen in patients with multiple sclerosis is numbness of the perineum and genitalia with disturbed sphincter function.

Autonomic involvement

Autonomic symptoms occur in most patients with multiple sclerosis. Bladder symptoms are most common in women, whereas impotence occurs frequently in males. Loss of inhibition of reflex bladder emptying, normally mediated by cholinergic neurons that contract the detrusor and relax the internal sphincter, results in urgency and frequency with incontinence when combined with immobility. With conus lesions, the problem is impaired bladder emptying. Failure to fill and empty may coexist, resulting in detrusor contractions against a closed sphincter.

Impaired control of the rectal sphincter is much less of a problem than failure of emptying. Some impotent men with multiple sclerosis retain reflex erections, in which case psychogenic factors are often invoked; but erectile failure is usually a manifestation of spinal cord disease. Mechanical difficulties, spasticity, altered sensation, skin excoriation, and indwelling catheters affect sexual performance in both sexes. Other autonomic features in multiple sclerosis occur rarely but include loss of thermoregulation leading to inappropriate sweating, fever, and hypothermia; Horner's syndrome; abnormalities of cardiac rhythm and vascular responses with acute pulmonary oedema; weight loss; and inappropriate secretion of vasopressin.

Eye movements

Abnormalities of eye movement are frequent in multiple sclerosis. They are often asymptomatic, but may manifest as double vision and oscillopsia. The commonest sign is first-degree symmetrical horizontal jerking nystagmus. Weakness of the lateral rectus is more common than isolated third and fourth nerve palsy. Internuclear ophthalmoplegia is often bilateral and may coexist with gaze paresis to produce the 'one and one half' syndrome.

Vertical up-beating nystagmus is always associated with bilateral internuclear ophthalmoplegia. Down-beating nystagmus has other important causes which can be confused with multiple sclerosis.

Ocular flutter consists of horizontal saccadic oscillations without an intersaccadic interval. Opsoclonus, in which the movements occur in all directions, is equally disabling. Ocular bobbing describes an initial rapid downward eye movement followed by slow return to the neutral position and denotes cerebellar involvement. Abrupt displacement from the primary position during central fixation (square wave jerks) occurs with severe cerebellar deficits.

Other brainstem manifestations

Facial weakness, indistinguishable from Bell's palsy, occurs in patients with multiple sclerosis, alone or in association with other signs of brainstem disease including hemifacial spasm and diffuse rippling of muscle fibres (myokymia). Exceptionally, there may be unilateral involvement of the hypoglossal and recurrent laryngeal nerves. Extensive brainstem demyelination may produce disturbances of consciousness and respiratory failure distinct from the narcolepsy syndrome, which is seen more frequently in patients with multiple sclerosis than expected by chance—an observation of immunogenetic interest in view of their shared HLA DR2 association. Occasional manifestations include the locked-in state, persistent hiccup, and the lateral medullary syndrome.

Paroxysmal symptoms are invariably brief but repetitive and usually occur in bouts lasting a few months before remitting. Symptomatic trigeminal neuralgia may begin in the first division or bilaterally, at a younger age than the idiopathic condition, and with associated signs of trigeminal involvement including motor weakness and sensory loss. It is usually associated with demyelinating lesions of the dorsal root entry zone, but may coexist with compression of the fifth cranial nerve by ectatic vessels. Other than trigeminal neuralgia, isolated involvement of the fifth nerve is rare. Paroxysmal dysarthria and ataxia with a clumsy arm, complex disturbances of sensation, and painful tetanic posturing of the limbs lasting 1 or 2 min are often triggered by movement and preceded by positive sensory symptoms on the side opposite to the muscular spasm. These are easily recognized and treated. Bursts of pain and paraesthesias, sensory distortion, itching, cough and hiccup, painful extensor spasm, akinesia, kinesogenic choreoathetosis, and complex gaze palsies—any of which may respond to anticonvulsants, especially carbamazepine—also appear to be paroxysmal manifestations of multiple sclerosis.

Cognitive and affective symptoms

Defects of visual and auditory attention occur in multiple sclerosis, sometimes at an early stage, and these are also detectable in patients with isolated demyelinating lesions. An overall impairment in IQ relates more to duration of disease, and onset of the progressive phase, affecting memory rather than language skills. Specific cognitive deficits due to hypothalamic involvement are sometimes seen, including the Korsakoff state and the syndrome of bulimia, lack of social restraint, mental inertia, and mutism. Psychotic behaviour is rare, but depression occurs more frequently than in patients with comparable neurological disability; hypomania is occasionally seen, but should not be confused with pathological laughter and crying arising from loss of central inhibition of facial and bulbar reflexes in association with extensive brainstem disease.

Rare manifestations

The list of rare clinical manifestations (some already described) includes massive cerebral lesions, aphasia, headache, fever, movement disorders, epilepsy, hypothalamic and pituitary symptoms, respiratory failure, and peripheral neuropathy. Narcolepsy, Sjögren's syndrome, ankylosing spondylitis, type I neurofibromatosis, and autoimmune thyroid disease have periodically been associated with multiple sclerosis.

Childhood multiple sclerosis

In retrospect, symptoms attributable to recurrent demyelination often affect individuals with multiple sclerosis as teenagers, but onset in the first decade also occurs; 2% of patients with multiple sclerosis present before the age of 10, and up to 10% before 16 years. Individual episodes often centred on optic neuritis and brainstem syndromes can be severe, but the long-term prognosis is surprisingly good. Fever and meningism, impaired conscious level due to cerebral oedema with swollen optic discs, and seizures are regular features and the distinction from acute disseminated encephalomyelitis can often only be made by the later occurrence of remission and relapse. A recent European study of the natural history of childhood onset disease confirms a higher female to male ratio (2.8:1), disease course that is invariably relapsing–remitting, and a delayed time by 10 years to secondary progression compared to adult onset disease. Current international guidelines recommend disease modifying treatment for childhood multiple sclerosis with active relapsing–remitting disease on lines similar to adult patients, with β-interferon being the most common first-line agent.

Clinical course and prognosis

Most patients (*c*.80%) present with relapsing–remitting disease. Typically, the illness passes through the three phases of relapse with full recovery, relapse with persistent deficits, and secondary progression (Fig. 24.10.2.1). One patient may spend several years or even a few decades in each, whereas another moves rapidly to a condition of fixed progressive disability. About 25% of patients have multiple sclerosis in a form which is not disabling, termed 'benign', and they remain ambulant. In 5%, relapses occur frequently and do not recover, leading rapidly to disability and early death from respiratory failure when the medulla is affected and from massive cerebral or spinal demyelination. Up to 15% become severely disabled within a short time. Life expectancy is at least 25 years, and a high proportion of patients die from unrelated causes.

Episodes occur at random frequency but initially average about 1.5 per year and decrease steadily thereafter. Recovery from each attack is invariably slower than onset and may be incomplete. Self-evidently, secondary progressive multiple sclerosis tends to affect whichever system has previously been involved. Progression may follow directly upon a severe relapse and be interrupted by further episodes.

In approximately 20%, multiple sclerosis is progressive from onset. The spinal cord bears the brunt of progressive multiple sclerosis, but optic nerve, cerebral, and brainstem disease may also advance slowly. Primary progressive spinal disease is the usual mode of presentation when multiple sclerosis develops beyond the fifth decade. It is characterized by an absence of acute attacks, with gradual decline from onset, and although cerebrospinal fluid analysis is similar to relapsing–remitting disease there are comparatively greater spinal and fewer brain abnormalities on MRI. Current disease modifying agents have no effect on primary progressive disease.

The prognosis is relatively good when sensory or visual symptoms dominate the illness and there is complete recovery from individual episodes; this pattern is most common in young females.

Conversely, motor involvement, especially when coordination or balance is disturbed, has a less good prognosis. The outlook is also poor in older-onset patients who are often males. Frequent, prolonged relapses with incomplete recovery and a short interval between the initial episode and first relapse carry a worse prognosis, but the main determinant of disability is onset of the progressive phase. Most patients develop progressive irreversible disability within 10–15 years of disease onset. Accumulated epidemiological evidence also argues for redundancy of the phenotypic distinction between the various forms of multiple sclerosis upon reaching the stage of fixed moderate deficit. Disability appears to be age dependent and uninfluenced by prior history of relapses. This observation in turn raises unresolved questions around the relationship between inflammation, manifesting as relapse, and neurodegeneration, the primary substrate of progression.

Prospective studies show that 9% of upper respiratory (adenovirus) and gastrointestinal infections occurring in patients with multiple sclerosis are followed by relapse and 27% of new episodes are related to infection. The emerging evidence suggests that disease activity is not increased by vaccination. Relapse rate is affected by pregnancy. There is a reduction in the prepregnancy relapse rate for each trimester, with approximately a threefold higher risk in the puerperium, and the attacks may be more severe. The clinical course is uninfluenced by breastfeeding or epidural anaesthesia. There is no evidence that trauma triggers the first or recurrent clinical manifestations of multiple sclerosis in someone who has the underlying disease process, or alters the course in individuals who have already experienced symptoms.

Laboratory investigations

Multiple sclerosis can reliably be diagnosed using clinical criteria and without laboratory support. There is no single diagnostic laboratory investigation. That said, investigations are now incorporated in revised diagnostic criteria and, under some circumstances, can supplement or replace clinical events. Taken together, laboratory investigations can be used: to demonstrate the anatomical dissemination of lesions; to provide evidence for intrathecal inflammation; to demonstrate that conduction is altered in a form consistent with demyelination; and to exclude conditions that mimic demyelinating disease.

Electrophysiology

Recent demyelination can be detected in clinically unaffected pathways using visual, auditory, somatosensory, central motor, and event-related potentials; their latencies are characteristically delayed whereas, except in acute lesions, the amplitude is unaffected. Evoked potentials add little in situations where the pathway under investigation is clinically affected. Since they provide qualitatively different information, evoked potentials remain useful as an adjunct to diagnosis despite the advent of imaging techniques.

MRI

Recent diagnostic criteria have been revised, permitting MRI-based evidence for dissemination in time and space to allow earlier diagnosis, partly to allow prompt consideration of disease-modifying treatments. The major practical application is in the investigation of individuals early in the course and, especially, those with isolated demyelinating lesions, recurrent episodes at a single site, or progressive disease affecting the spinal cord. In all these situations the first requirement is to exclude a structural lesion, especially since these can present with relapsing symptoms. Imaging any region of the nervous system, clinically affected in isolation, will reliably exclude a structural lesion that might mimic multiple sclerosis and may show changes consistent with focal demyelination, but will not distinguish the syndromes of isolated demyelination from multiple sclerosis. Once the clinically affected part has proved negative for a structural lesion, the diagnosis of multiple sclerosis also requires the demonstration of anatomically separate lesions, ideally with enhancement to identify recent lesions, or the accumulation of new imaging abnormalities over time, even if these are not expressed clinically.

Low-density lesions, corresponding to areas of demyelination, may be seen using contrast-enhanced CT or MRI, and these occasionally are mistaken for cerebral tumour or abscess. More than 95% of patients with clinically definite multiple sclerosis have periventricular lesions, and more than 90% also show discrete white matter abnormalities. Focal demyelination can also be imaged in the optic nerve, brainstem, and spinal cord.

Variations in the imaging protocol are beginning to distinguish separate components of the underlying pathological process. Imaging can distinguish inflammation (gadolinium–DTPA enhancement of T_1-weighted lesions, indicating that the lesion is of recent origin), demyelination and remyelination (magnetization transfer ratio), astrocytosis (T_2-weighted lesions, the signal arising from increased water content), and axonal damage (reduction in diffusion tensor imaging anisotrophy and N-acetylaspartate spectra with chemical shift imaging, or the presence of focal atrophy and T_1-weighted black holes). The evolving lesion starts with increased blood–brain barrier permeability that lasts for up to 4 weeks, and is revealed by demonstration of enhancement after intravenous gadolinium. These lesions may disappear, but reactivation is sometimes seen, the cycles lasting about 8 weeks. Fluid attenuated inversion recovery (FLAIR), proton-density, and T_2 sequences best demonstrate demyelination. The periventricular lesions, which characterize multiple sclerosis, correlate with areas of persistent demyelination and astrocytosis. A mixture of new, evolving, and recovering lesions may be seen in an individual patient at any one time. Lesions visible on MRI occur about 15 times more frequently than new clinical events. Eventually, there is a reduction in the frequency of new lesions as patients move from the relapsing to the progressive phases of the disease, and evidence for atrophy is then more apparent. The number or volume of lesions correlates poorly—if at all—with disease severity or course, but there is less cerebral involvement in patients who present with primary progressive disease compared with those having similar disability from secondary progression. The imaging abnormalities of multiple sclerosis are not specific and similar changes occur with inflammatory or vascular lesions and with advancing age (Fig. 24.10.2.3).

Cerebrospinal fluid

Cerebrospinal fluid analysis provides information which is complementary to imaging abnormalities and specifically useful in elderly patients suspected of having multiple sclerosis in whom MRI is less discriminating. The cell count rarely exceeds 50 lymphocytes/ml, even during periods of clinical activity, and is normal in more than 50% of patients. There is a rise in total protein (usually <1 g/litre), with a specific increase in the immunoglobulin concentration and the presence of oligoclonal bands on protein electrophoresis seen in more than 90% of cases, after correction for leakage of serum proteins through the blood–brain barrier, providing evidence for

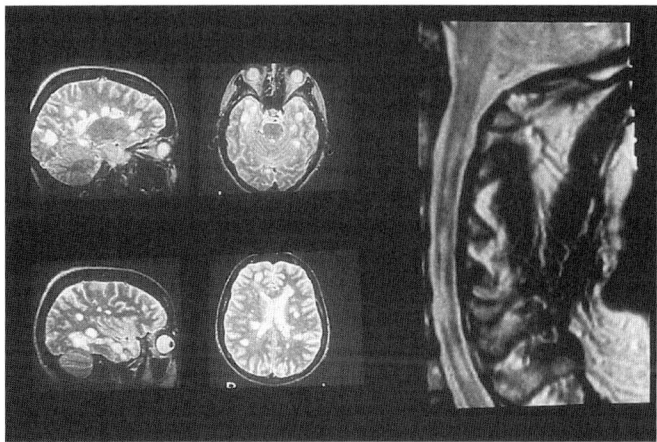

Fig. 24.10.2.3 T_2-weighted MRI abnormalities diffusely affecting the cerebrum and spinal cord in multiple sclerosis.

synthesis of immunoglobulin within the CNS. As with the imaging abnormalities, these are sensitive but not specific. Although some antibodies are directed against components of the oligodendrocyte or its myelin membranes, and others recognize extrinsic antigens including viruses, collectively these specificities only account for a minority of the bands.

Differential diagnosis

The commonest error in clinical practice is to make the diagnosis of multiple sclerosis in patients with progressive spinal disease in whom a structural lesion has not been adequately excluded. Rarely, spinal tumours present with intermittent symptoms creating difficulties for the unwary. It is not safe to assume the diagnosis of multiple sclerosis in patients with symptoms and signs restricted to a single site, whatever the clinical course without appropriate investigation. Lesions at the foramen magnum are particularly well placed to cause confusion through appearing to produce evidence for independent spinal and brainstem lesions. Errors also arise with progressive and relapsing manifestations of brainstem or spinal arteriovenous malformations.

Care must be taken in the diagnosis of multiple sclerosis when several members are affected within one family. Hereditary spastic paraplegia mimics familial multiple sclerosis, and this should also be considered in isolated cases of progressive spastic paraplegia when pyramidal manifestations occur in isolation and with disproportionate spasticity. Other familial disorders confused with multiple sclerosis include the hereditary ataxias, adult-onset leucodystrophies, and vasculopathies (CADASIL). Pedigrees with affected males and maternal inheritance may be examples of X-linked adrenoleucodystrophy, and the phenotype of multiple sclerosis occurs in families with the clinical and genetic features of Leber's hereditary optic atrophy (Harding's disease).

Clinical, immunological, and imaging abnormalities indistinguishable from multiple sclerosis occur with granulomatous and vasculitic diseases of the brain, especially the cerebral variant of systemic lupus erythematosus which often occurs in the absence of systemic manifestations or informative serology, although headache and prominent cognitive impairment are clues to vasculitic aetiology. Sarcoidosis may present with clinical involvement of the CNS, typical MRI and cerebrospinal fluid abnormalities, and without pulmonary or cutaneous manifestations; uveitis also occurs in multiple sclerosis and so is not necessarily a useful discriminator. Orogenital ulceration in a patient with the clinical manifestations of multiple sclerosis suggests the diagnosis of Behçet's disease.

Alternative diagnoses need to be considered when multiple sclerosis is diagnosed in African or Asian people in whom progressive spinal disease, sometimes with visual involvement, is more probably due to human T-lymphotropic virus type I (HTLV1) associated tropical spastic paraplegia or neuromyelitis optica (see above). Infections of the nervous system can mimic the isolated demyelinating syndromes and multiple sclerosis. These include tuberculous and other chronic meningitides, and the neurological manifestations of AIDS or Lyme disease; borreliosis can also cause a chronic or relapsing disorder of the CNS, but this is usually preceded by the characteristic painful polyradiculitis and facial palsy that epitomizes Lyme disease. Similarities between multiple sclerosis and neurosyphilis should not be forgotten in the context of opportunistic infection complicating HIV infection. The age distribution and clinical manifestations usually make it easy to distinguish subacute combined degeneration of the spinal cord from multiple sclerosis, but focal spinal lesions, accompanied by Lhermitte's sign, occur in vitamin B_{12} deficiency.

Treatment of demyelinating disease

Therapies in multiple sclerosis are aimed at managing individual symptoms, resolving acute attacks, preventing new relapses, limiting disability, and (for the future) preventing progression and repairing the damage.

Symptomatic management

The complex and progressive nature of disability requires a multidisciplinary approach to patients with multiple sclerosis. Several manifestations of the disease can be treated symptomatically. Urgency and frequency of micturition respond to drugs with anticholinergic activity (oxybutinin or propantheline). A simple means for intermittently reducing urine volume, and hence the desire to micturate, is to use intranasal desmopressin spray. When detrusor and sphincter function become uncoupled, causing impaired filling and a significant residual volume after voluntary voiding, the preferred treatment is clean self-intermittent catheterization, which is easily adopted by motivated patients retaining adequate vision and arm function; it ensures complete bladder emptying often with unimagined advantages to social activities and sleep. Other options include intravesical botox injections to reduce reflex bladder contractions or a suprapubic catheter with closure of the lower urinary tract which is preferable to an indwelling urethral catheter or, worse still, constant dribbling incontinence, which usually leads to skin excoriation. These manoeuvres have largely replaced urinary diversion through an ileal conduit, insertion of an artificial mechanical sphincter, or electrical stimulation of the spinal nerve roots in an attempt to synchronize sphincter contraction and relaxation.

Constipation in multiple sclerosis is managed by dietary alteration and the use of bulk laxatives, avoiding agents that act directly on the bowel wall. Loperamide may be useful where the predominant complaint is rectal urge incontinence. Psychological factors contribute to impotence in males with multiple sclerosis, but in most cases the complaint is a direct consequence of spinal demyelination. Trends in management have shifted from the use of mechanical devices and cavernous injection of papaverine or prostaglandin E_1 applied through the urethra, to oral treatment with sildenafil (Viagra)—a phosphodiesterase inhibitor which acts by increasing local production of nitric oxide in response to sexual stimulation.

The mainstay of pharmacological treatment for tremor is β-blockers; alternatives include anticonvulsants, isoniazid, ondansetron, and hyoscine. Physical restraint is rarely successful. Stereotactic procedures involving stimulation of the ventrolateral nucleus produce results comparable to destructive procedures, but the dividend is small. Unsteadiness arising from altered vestibular input may improve with the use of a vestibular sedative.

Fatigue as a dominant symptom in multiple sclerosis is common and frequently disabling, although its pathophysiological basis is poorly understood. It is not easy to treat noting also that separating fatigue from depression and disability is difficult. Some evidence suggests improvement with amantadine or modafinil.

Baclofen, a GABA agonist acting on spinal cord reflexes, is still the most widely used effective antispastic agent. The principal adverse effect, like most conventional anti-spasticity agents is sedation and increased weakness. Benzodiazepines also reduce spasticity by increasing presynaptic spinal inhibition. Dantrolene sodium acts by uncoupling excitation–contraction mechanisms in individual muscle fibres. It is claimed that Tizanidine, an alpha-2 agonist that modulates activity of excitatory presynaptic interneurones, reduces spasticity without increasing weakness. Patients report that spasticity and pain improve with the use of cannabis and this is still formally being evaluated. Intrathecal baclofen carries the potential advantage of selectively reducing muscle tone in affected muscles whilst leaving others intact. It is mainly appropriate for patients with advanced disease and does not seem to have any additional adverse effects compared with systemic administration. Another approach targeted at focal spasticity is loal injection of botulinum toxin. There may be a role for surgical interruption of the reflex pathways or tenotomy and peripheral nerve block with phenol or alcohol.

The paroxysmal manifestations of multiple sclerosis usually stop abruptly with the use of carbamazepine or gabapentin; this and other anticonvulsants, especially gabapentin, may also relieve trigeminal neuralgia or the more refractory forms of pain arising from spinal demyelination. Nerve block and chemical or surgical destruction of nerve fibres are sometimes an acceptable method for reducing pain in multiple sclerosis. All these sensations are coped with less well in the context of impaired mood and can respond usefully to antidepressants.

For those who develop significant disabilities and impairments, comprehensive care includes access to physical and occupational therapists, social workers, and other health-care staff with expertise in the management of chronic neurological illness. Complications are best prevented by awareness and anticipation since they usually develop quickly yet take months to resolve. Minimizing handicap by attention to social, vocational, marital, sexual, and psychological aspects of the illness is more important for many patients than drug treatment. In situations where the natural history has already led to loss of mobility, the early use of mechanical aids and home adaptations should be encouraged despite the associated stigma.

Management of the acute episode

Corticosteroids are effective in abbreviating acute demyelinating episodes in multiple sclerosis and related disorders. Although many neurologists continue to prefer the well established intravenous route, convenience and no apparent increase in adverse effects or loss of efficacy have led to increased use of high-dose oral compared to the intravenous regimen. Empirical use of plasma exchange in the treatment of fulminant steroid-resistant disease has variable efficacy but–matching its role in neuromyelitis optica—recent evidence suggests that patients with disease characterized histologically by immunoglobulin deposition and complement activation also respond to plasma exchange. However, in the absence of reliable biomarkers of pathological substrate widespread selective use of plasma exchange is not indicated. There is no evidence for reduction in relapse frequency or long-term disability using either steroids or plasma exchange.

Disease modifying treatment in multiple sclerosis

Multiple sclerosis has two distinct clinical phases, each reflecting a dominant role for inter-related pathological processes: inflammation drives activity during the relapsing – remitting (RR) stage; and neurodegeneration represents the principal substrate of progressive disability. Disease modifying agents target the inflammatory component. Efficacy has been demonstrated in the treatment of relapsing-remitting and rapidly worsening multiple sclerosis. There are no proven therapies for progressive disease independent of relapses. Development of disease modifying drugs has evolved from non-specific immunosuppressive drugs to more selective agents including humanized monoclonal antibodies targeting distinct stages in the initiation and evolution of tissue injury. Established and emerging anti-inflammatory or immune-modulatory drugs can be broadly grouped into drugs that act systemically or limit entry of inflammatory cells into the brain, and those that are thought to modify the immune environment within the brain.

β-interferons (Rebif, Avonex and Betaseron) and glatiramer acetate (Copaxone) were the first approved therapies for relapsing-remitting multiple sclerosis. The therapeutic rationale for use of the β-interferons initially was based on anti-viral properties but now rests on the catch-all hypothesis that IFN-β limits inflammation by inhibiting antigen presentation, promoting the Th-2 immune phenotype and restricting migration of cells across the blood-brain barrier. β-interferons administered subcutaneously or intramuscularly are generally well tolerated and reduce relapse frequency by around 30%. But up to 40% of patients receiving β-interferons develop neutralizing antibodies that are immunologically and biologically cross-reactive. Because of the reduction, albeit modest, in relapse frequency, initiation of treatment after a first demyelinating event will inevitably delay conversion to clinically definite multiple sclerosis. A series of trials has confirmed this prediction although it is important to understand that these results do not show that these drugs prevent the development of multiple sclerosis. The effect of β-interferon on progression is less persuasive with no convincing evidence for efficacy in the absence of on-going relapses. The focus around β-interferons has moved to timing of treatment with a plausible case being made for early initiation. The absence of reliable measures to predict disease course and separate those with benign multiple sclerosis provide counter arguments to early treatment. Glatiramer acetate has been used in multiple sclerosis on the basis that disease activity can be suppressed by mimicking the antigenic challenge initiating brain inflammation. Initial enthusiasm for the use of glatiramer acetate is conditioned by a recent Cochrane review concluding that there is little evidence for effect on relapse or progression.

In view of the modest effects of disease modifying drugs, there has been a willingness to consider more potent drugs or bone marrow transplantation in individual patients, refractory to other treatments or with above average clinical activity, using approaches that may be more effective but at the cost of increased adverse effects. Mitoxantrone, a cytotoxic agent, achieves a higher rate of conversion to disease inactivity (clinical and enhanced magnetic resonance imaging) in patients with active disease receiving monthly injections of methyl prednisolone—at least in the short term—but treatment is limited by the cumulative potential for cardiotoxicity and some cases of acute leukaemia. Accumulated experience from over 300 patients has shown that autologous haematopoietic stem cell transplantation can be effective in suppressing disease activity with evidence for stabilizing disease progression if administered at the inflammatory stage of disease. However, given the associated morbidity and mortality, treatment tends to be reserved to aggressive disease refractory to conventional treatments. A phase III study is ongoing comparing immunoablation (using combination of immune suppressant drugs) and autologous haematopoietic stem cell transplantation with Mitoxantrone in patients with severe multiple sclerosis.

The advent of humanized monoclonal antibodies allows selective treatments targeting discrete stages in the immune-pathogenesis of multiple sclerosis. Three are currently considered; natalizumab, alemtuzamab and rituximab. Natalizumab is a recombinant antibody delivered by monthly infusion that prevents activated T cells entering the brain by binding to leucocyte α4 integrin thus blocking adhesion of T cells to endothelial cells. Natalizumab offers a significant advance in efficacy over current therapies – 68% reduction in annual relapse rate and 83% reduction in gadolinium enhancing MR lesions - but six cases of progressive multifocal leucoencephalopathy (PML), two of whom had concomitant β-interferon treatment and multiple sclerosis, have qualified the indications for its use as monotherapy under a restricted prescribing programme to patients with relapsing disease who are non-responders or cannot tolerate other treatments. The relationship between natalizumab and PML may indicate impaired immune surveillance leading to reactivation or bone marrow mobilization of persistent JC virus infection. To date, no head-to-head comparisons of natalizumab against β-interferon or glatiramer acetate have been undertaken and its role in progressive disease has not been evaluated in clinical trials. Despite the salutary lesson of PML, natalizumab represents a step-change in the level of efficacy that can be achieved in relapsing-remitting multiple sclerosis. Alemtuzumab, another humanized monoclonal that targets the CD52 antigen resulting in sustained depletion of lymphocytes and monocytes, shows promising reduction in sustained accumulation of disability and annualized relapse rate in early active relapsing-remitting disease in a phase II trial against β-interferon. But, as with all other new disease modifying therapies, there are adverse effects–mild transient infusion related events and more significant secondary auto-immune disease. The experience of using alemtuzumab in secondary progressive–where despite suppression of clinical and radiological inflammatory activity disease activity continues–and relapsing-remitting multiple sclerosis provides strong evidence for the hypothesis that the contribution of inflammation wanes and becomes uncoupled from neurodegeneration as the disease matures. Rituximab, an anti-CD20 monoclonal that depletes B cells, has recently been shown in a phase II study to reduce clinical and radiological activity over 24 weeks. Its rapidity of action in suppressing radiological measures of acute activity suggests mechanisms additional to loss of pathological auto-antibodies.

Of the many other drugs undergoing clinical evaluation FTY720 (fingolimod) and cladribine are worth noting. Fingolimod is a fungal derivative that upon phosphorylation acts as a sphingosine receptor agonist and non-specifically limits lymphocyte egress from lymphoid organs. Cladribine inhibits adenosine deaminase and results in immunomodulation through selective depletion of lymphocyte subsets. Unusually both drugs are administered orally and recent clinical trials have demonstrated tolerability and efficacy against standard clinical and radiological measures of relapse and activity. Other emerging and promising oral agents include laquinimod and fumarate.

Stepping back from individual drug analyses, it is clear that a growing range of immunological therapies is becoming available: these act at different points of disease evolution and will most likely best prevent progression of disability if given early in the course before neurodegeneration is irretrievably established. This raises the dilemma of exposing individuals who may never develop disabilities from multiple sclerosis to the unpredictable hazards of prolonged immunosuppression. Apart from aiming for an ideal balance between high efficacy and low toxicity, and taking into account the preferred use of oral rather than parenteral medications and daily versus infrequent exposure, the main goal of future therapies in multiple sclerosis is to meet the unmet need of how to limit disease progression.

Neuroprotection and repair strategies

A body of evidence supports the hypothesis that chronically demyelinated axons - devoid of myelin-derived support – are vulnerable to degeneration. Spontaneously remyelinated plaques show no significant axonal injury compared to inactive demyelinated lesions. Together with the recognition that spontaneous remyelination contributes to restoration of structure and function and that neurodegeneration underlies progressive disability, this supports the idea that myelin repair will prove neuroprotective. One approach under consideration is the use of human stem cells to supplement and promote endogenous remyelination by mechanisms dependent and independent of directed differentiation.

A parallel strategy under clinical trial is the testing of putative neuroprotective agents that seek to act directly on neurons. These are hampered by incomplete understanding of the mechanisms underlying neurodegeneration, although experimental work identifies some rational candidates such as sodium channel blockade. Lamotrigine and cannabinoids are currently under randomized trial for secondary progression. Other agents that are believed to be beneficial through pleiotropic mechanisms, including statins, are also under clinical trial in the progressive phase of disease.

Central pontine myelinolysis

Central pontine myelinolysis is associated with metabolic disturbances induced by alcohol with and without Wernicke's encephalopathy, nonalcoholic cirrhosis, Wilson's disease, following hepatic transplantation, as a complication of uraemia and haemodialysis, after prolonged vomiting, and in the context of diuretic therapy. In each of these situations, affected individuals have usually been hyponatraemic before the onset of neurological symptoms. Central pontine myelinolysis seems to result from overzealous correction of a low (and occasionally also a high) serum sodium. Demyelination correlates both with the degree of hyponatraemia and rate at which this is corrected, with starting levels of less than 110 mmol/litre or rates of correction of more than 2 mmol/litre per hour substantially increasing the risk. Rapid changes in sodium are better tolerated in acute than chronic hyponatraemia. See Chapter 21.2.1 for further discussion.

The illness affects central pontine pathways and spreads centrifugally. The fully evolved clinical picture is of flaccid paralysis with facial and bulbar weakness, disordered eye movements, loss of balance, and altered consciousness. Features of severe hyponatraemia, such as epilepsy, are not usually present since pontine demyelination follows correction of the serum sodium. Extrapontine manifestations including movement disorders and other features of extrapyramidal disease may be seen. The clinical features are distinctive and present no diagnostic difficulties unless the reduction in serum sodium has been overlooked; the acute changes of central pontine myelinolysis can be imaged by MRI, with abnormalities persisting after clinical recovery. Prognosis depends on the underlying metabolic disorder. With stabilization of the serum sodium and management of bulbar failure, neurological recovery is usually complete and the condition does not recur spontaneously.

Leucodystrophies

The leucodystrophies are a heterogeneous group of conditions characterized by noninflammatory demyelination. Increasingly, these are being shown to result from mutations affecting genes which determine the synthesis, maintenance, and structure of myelin. Although rare even in paediatric practice, these need to be considered in young adults with atypical syndromes combining physical and intellectual deficits, sometimes with peripheral nerve involvement, in whom imaging shows confluent lesions confined to white matter.

Childhood-onset leucodystrophies

Diffuse sclerosis (Schilder's disease)

The term diffuse cerebral sclerosis was originally used to identify a heterogeneous group of diseases affecting cerebral white matter. Of the diseases previously classified under this heading, familial sudanophilic diffuse sclerosis, Pelizaeus–Merzbacher disease, Krabbe's diffuse sclerosis (globoid cell leucodystrophy), Canavan's diffuse sclerosis (spongy degeneration of the white matter), Alexander's disease, and metachromatic leucodystrophy are dysmyelinating leucodystrophies. Conversely, Binswager's subcortical encephalopathy is now considered a consequence of diffuse cerebral arteriosclerosis—although some cases may have been examples of CADASIL; and Balo's concentric sclerosis is now considered within the spectrum of multiple sclerosis. Many male patients previously classified as having diffuse sclerosis were probably suffering from adrenoleucodystrophy. Some of the relapsing disorders may have been examples of Leigh's disease associated with mutations of mitochondrial DNA. But even after separating these newly recognized conditions, the nosological status of diffuse sclerosis remains uncertain and some consider that, between them, acute childhood multiple sclerosis and adrenoleucodystrophy account for all the unclassified cases.

Krabbe's disease

Globoid cell leucodystrophy, an autosomal recessive condition, usually presents as an early infantile disorder. Late-onset globoid cell leucodystrophy is uncommon, almost all patients becoming symptomatic before the age of 5 years, so it is almost never confused with childhood multiple sclerosis. The clinical picture is dominated by behavioural changes with startle, progressive intellectual and motor deterioration, epilepsy, visual failure, and peripheral neuropathy leading to severe disabilities; pyrexia and other autonomic features usher in the onset of a vegetative state. Visual evoked potentials are delayed and the spinal fluid has a raised protein level but does not contain oligoclonal bands. MRI shows periventricular lesions subsequently extending into extensive white matter changes. The deficiency of α-galactocerebrosidase, best demonstrated in peripheral blood leucocytes or skin fibroblasts, leads to the accumulation of galactocerebroside in oligodendrocytes and Schwann cells, the neurotoxic molecule psychosine, and characteristic myelin-laden macrophages or globoid cells.

Adrenoleucodystrophy

This important group of disorders is characterized by deposition of saturated fatty acids in the brain and other lipid-containing tissues as a result of defective very-long-chain fatty acyl-CoA synthetase activity in peroxisomes. Mutations are present in the ABC transporter gene. The molecular defect may result from failure of the adrenoleucodystrophy gene product to anchor very-long-chain fatty acids (VLCFA) into the peroxisomal membrane or translocate these into peroxisomes. Diagnosis can be made by serum analysis of very long chain fatty acids and nerve biopsy. Evidence of adrenal insufficiency is a valuable discriminator from multiple sclerosis.

Four related syndromes share this biochemical abnormality: childhood adrenoleucodystrophy and adult-onset adrenomyeloneuropathy are X linked; neonatal adrenoleucodystrophy and Zellweger's syndrome are autosomal recessive disorders.

X-linked childhood adrenoleucodystrophy presents with behavioural disturbance, dementia, and epilepsy followed by involvement of special senses and motor systems. Although a significant proportion of children later develop adrenal insufficiency, Addison's disease may precede the neurological manifestations by several years. Treatment has been proposed with a dietary supplement containing a 4:1 mixture of glyceryl trioleate and trierucate, popularly known as Lorenzo's oil. This lowers the plasma levels of VLCFA, but does not appear to influence the phenotype in individuals with established neurological disease, although there may be a prophylactic role. Bone marrow transplantation is successful in early symptomatic cases and, in view of the inflammatory reaction, immunosuppression has also been used.

Adrenomyeloneuropathy presents in young adult men with spastic paraparesis and sensory loss in the legs; attention is drawn to an unusual cause for this otherwise common neurological problem by the associated peripheral neuropathy, but the diagnosis is frequently overlooked if adrenal insufficiency is not obvious at presentation. It may be associated with dementia later in disease course. Identification of the peroxisomal defect in easily sampled body tissues has led to the description of cases with obscure clinical manifestations; these include focal cerebral lesions, Kluver–Bucy syndrome, dementia, and spinocerebellar degeneration. Mild spastic paraparesis with sphincter involvement and peripheral neuropathy may occur in obligate heterozygote female carriers with elevated VLCFA. Carriers tend not to have adrenal insufficiency, although abnormal brain MRI and delayed evoked potentials may be present.

Autosomal recessive adrenoleucodystrophy presents in infancy with seizures, hypotonia, retardation, retinal degeneration, and hepatic involvement; females are more commonly affected than males. Although the clinical manifestations and mode of inheritance

are similar in neonatal adrenoleucodystrophy and Zellweger's syndrome, these are thought to be separate disorders.

The sensitivity and specificity of routine assays for VLCFA show that the level of hexacosanoic acid and its ratios to tetracosanoic and docosanoic acids are fully discriminating in homozygote males, irrespective of the clinical phenotype, from the day of birth if dietary supplements have not been given, providing an opportunity for mass screening; there is a false-negative rate of 15% for heterozygotes.

Metachromatic leucodystrophy

Metachromatic leucodystrophy is an autosomal recessive lysosomal storage disorder due to arylsulphatase A deficiency leading to increased urinary sulphatide excretion with a deficiency of arylsulphatase A in urine, peripheral blood leucocytes, and skin fibroblasts, or showing metachromatic material in peripheral nerve biopsies having segmental demyelination and remyelination. There is diffuse white matter involvement due to noninflammatory demyelination with loss of oligodendrocytes, axon preservation, and reactive astrocytes which, together with macrophages, contain the metachromatic material, especially in the most extensively demyelinated areas.

The clinical phenotype varies with the amount of surviving arylsulphatase A depending on heterozygosity of the mutant allele; pseudodeficiency refers to those individuals with low levels of arylsulphatase A that are sufficiently high not to display a clinical phenotype. Some affected individuals have a genetic defect of the arylsulphatase A activator and this is associated with a more complex pattern of sphingomyelin storage, biochemically and in terms of the tissue distribution.

The most common form of metachromatic leucodystrophy develops in late infancy with delayed walking due to the neuropathy, which may be painful. There are also features of brainstem involvement and the emergence of diffuse upper motor neuron signs with reduced intellectual development, optic atrophy, and death within about 5 years from presentation. In later-onset childhood cases, after several years of normal development, there are behavioural changes with poor school performance, anticipating cerebellar and upper motor neuron disability which then follows much the same course as in younger patients, although with less evidence for neuropathy. The early adult form of metachromatic leucodystrophy is rare, or perhaps seldom diagnosed, and tends to present with intellectual or emotional abnormalities. Onset with dementia and behavioural disorders is usual with ataxia, paralysis, and optic atrophy only developing at late stages; the presentation is occasionally with paraparesis or cerebellar ataxia and the condition can then more easily be mistaken for multiple sclerosis. Clinical evidence for peripheral neuropathy may be revealed by slowed nerve conduction. Treatments have included dietary manipulation with reduced vitamin A and sulphur-containing substances, and bone marrow transplantation, but the successes are limited.

Multiple sulphatase deficiency combines the features of metachromatic leucodystrophy with mucopolysaccharidosis. It also has neonatal, early childhood, and juvenile forms. The pattern of combined motor and mental regression or lack of development reflecting widespread dysmyelination with peripheral neuropathy is associated with dysmorphic features and organomegaly. The more severe phenotype also reflects extensive neuronal loss due to the combination of stored sulphatide, sulphated steroids, and mucopolysaccharides. The enzyme defects are complex involving many sulphatases including arylsulphatase A.

Pelizaeus–Merzbacher disease

The three phenotypes of X-linked Pelizaeus–Merzbacher disease usually present in childhood. The clinical features which may distinguish the otherwise ubiquitous motor and developmental delay with epilepsy are abnormal eye movements, dystonia and choreoathetosis, and laryngeal paralysis. Affected individuals often stabilize with severe disabilities and live into early adult life. Some cases do not manifest until early adult life, but here the blur with specifically different disorders becomes more apparent. MRI either fails to show myelin or depicts myelin which is immature with an atrophic brain.

The molecular defect is most frequently due to duplication of a variable length of genome containing the proteolipid protein gene. Recent evidence implicates defects in replication mechanism that leads to the complex rearrangements seen in Pelizaeus–Merzbacher disease. Proteolipid protein is normally involved in stabilizing the lamellar structure of central myelin. Gene dosage abnormalities results in oligodendrocyte loss and failure of myelination.

Adult-onset dominant leucodystrophies

Forms of dominantly inherited leucodystrophy also occur exclusively in adults and may closely resemble chronic progressive multiple sclerosis. MRI shows diffuse, nondiscrete, white-matter disease and there are no oligoclonal bands in the spinal fluid. It remains uncertain whether all the adult-onset dominant leucodystrophies are one and the same disorder, and many are difficult to distinguish from the heterogeneous group of hereditary spastic paraplegias. The various phenotypes are gradually being classified as their biochemical and genetic defects are characterized. A family with spastic paraparesis, ataxia, and mild dementia presenting in adulthood, but with onset in childhood, has been described; diffuse white matter abnormalities were present on cerebral MRI, whereas pathognomic features of the other leucodystrophies were absent. Similarly familial cases of a behavioural presentation evolving to dementia and a recent report of two unrelated families with an autosomal dominant pedigree of ataxic paraparesis associated with autonomic dysfunction hint at the range of presentations within this grouping. The relationship to a recently reported series of sporadic adult onset leucodystrophy is uncertain. Five cases with progressive cognitive and motor decline, abnormal brain MRI, and absent oligoclonal bands were described with histological features of leukodystrophy and neuroaxonal spheroids.

Further reading

Barnes D, *et al.* (1997). Randomised trial of oral and intravenous methylprednisolone in acute relapses of multiple sclerosis. *Lancet*, **349**, 902–6.

Bauer HJ, Hanefeld FA (1993). *Multiple sclerosis: its impact from childhood to old age.* W B Saunders, London.

Beck RW, *et al.* (2003). High and low risk profiles for the development of multiple sclerosis within 10 years after optic neuritis; experience of the optic neuritis treatment trial. *Arch Opthalmol*, **121**, 944–9.

Brex PA, *et al.* (2002). A longitudinal study of abnormalities on MRI and disability from multiple sclerosis. *N Engl J Med*, **346**, 158–64.

Chandran S, *et al.* (2008). Myelin repair: the role of stem and precursor cells in multiple sclerosis. *Phil Trans R Soc Lond B Biol Sci*, **363**, 171–83.

Coles AJ, *et al.* (1999). Monoclonal antibody treatment exposes three mechanisms underlying the clinical course in multiple sclerosis. *Ann Neurol*, **46**, 296–304.

Coles AJ, *et al.* (2007). Efficacy of Alemtuzumab in treatment naïve relapsing-remitting multiple sclerosis: analysis after two years of study. *Neurology*, **68** Suppl l1, A331.

Comi G, *et al.* (2001). Effect of early interferon treatment on conversion to definite multiple sclerosis: a randomised study. *Lancet*, **357**, 1576–82.

Compston DAS, *et al.* (2005). *McAlpine's multiple sclerosis.* W B Saunders, London.

Confavreux C, *et al.* (2001). Vaccinations and the risk of relapse in multiple sclerosis. Vaccines in Multiple Sclerosis Study Group. *N Engl J Med*, **344**, 319–26.

Confavreux C, *et al.* (1998). Rate of pregnancy-related relapse in multiple sclerosis. *N Engl J Med*, **339**, 285–91.

Confavreux C, Vukusic S (2006). Age at disability milestones in multiple sclerosis. *Brain*, **129**, 595–605.

Dutta R, Trapp BD (2007). Pathogenesis of axonal and neuronal damage in multiple sclerosis. *Neurology*, **68**, S22–31.

Ebers GC, *et al.* (2000). The natural history of multiple sclerosis: a geographically based study. 8: familial multiple sclerosis. *Brain*, **123**, 641–9.

Edan G, *et al.* (1997). Therapeutic effect of mitoxantrone combined with methylprednisolone in multiple sclerosis: a randomised multi-center study of active disease using MRI and clinical criteria. *J Neurol Neurosurg Psychiatry*, **62**, 112–18.

Fisniku LK, *et al.* (2008). Disability and T2 MRI lesions: a 20 year follow up of patients with relapse onset of multiple sclerosis. *Brain*, **131**, 808–17.

Hafler DA, *et al.* (2007). Risk alleles for multiple sclerosis identified by a genomewide study. *N Engl J Med*, **357**, 851–62.

IFNβ Multiple Sclerosis Study Group, University of British Columbia MS/MRI Analysis Group (1995). Interferon β-1b in the treatment of multiple sclerosis: final outcome of the randomised controlled trial. *Neurology*, **45**, 1277–85.

Jacobs LD, *et al.* (1996). Intramuscular interferon β-1a for disease progression in relapsing multiple sclerosis. *Ann Neurol*, **39**, 285–94.

Jacobs LD, *et al.* (2000). Intramuscular interferon β-1a therapy initiated during a first demyelinating event in multiple sclerosis. *N Engl J Med*, **343**, 898–904.

Jeffery ND, Blakemore WF (1997). Locomotor deficits induced by experimental spinal cord demyelination are abolished by spontaneous remyelination. *Brain*, **120**, 27–37.

Johnson K, *et al.* (1998). Extended use of glatiramer acetate (Copaxone) is well tolerated and maintains its clinical effect on multiple sclerosis relapse rate and degree of disability. *Neurology*, **50**, 701–8.

Kappos L, *et al.* (2006). Oral fingolimod for relapsing multiple sclerosis. *N Engl J Med*, **355**, 1124–40.

Kappos L, *et al.* (2007). Effect of early versus delayed interferon beta-ib treatment on disability after a first clinical event suggestive of multiple sclerosis: a 3-yr follow up analysis of the BENEFIT study. *Lancet*, **370**, 389–97.

Kieseier BC, *et al.* (2007). Treatment and treatment trials in multiple sclerosis. *Curr Opin Neurol*, **20**, 286–93.

Kremenchutzky M, *et al.* (2006). The natural history of multiple sclerosis: a geographically based study: observations on the progressive phase of the disease. *Brain*, **129**, 584–94.

Ligon KL, *et al.* (2006). Olig gene function in central nervous system development and disease. *Glia*, **54**, 1–10.

Luchinetti C, *et al.* (2000). Heterogeneity of multiple sclerosis lesions: implications for the pathogenesis of demyelination. *Ann Neurol*, **47**, 707–17.

Martenson RE, *et al.* (1992). *Myelin: biology and chemistry.* CRC Press, Boca Raton, FL.

McFarland HF, Martin R (2007). Multiple sclerosis: a complicated picture of autoimmunity. *Nat Immunol*, **8**, 913–19.

Miller HG, Stanton JB, Gibbons JL (1956). Parainfectious encephalomyelitis and related syndromes. *Q J Med*, **25**, 427–505.

Moser HW (1997). Adrenoleukodystrophy: phenotype, genetics, pathogenesis and therapy. *Brain*, **120**, 1485–508.

Noseworthy J, *et al.* (2005). Disease modifying treatments in multiple sclerosis. In: *McAlpine's multiple sclerosis*. W B Saunders, London.

Polman CH, *et al.* (2005). Diagnostic criteria for multiple sclerosis: 2005 revisions to the 'McDonald Criteria'. *Ann Neurol*, **58**, 840–6.

Polman CH, *et al.* (2006). A randomised, placebo-controlled trial of natalizumab for relapsing multiple sclerosis. *N Engl J Med*, **354**, 899–910.

Renoux R, *et al.* (2007). Natural history of multiple sclerosis with childhood onset. *N Engl J Med*, **356**, 2603–13.

Sibley WA, Bamford CR, Clark K (1985). Clinical viral infections and multiple sclerosis. *Lancet*, **i**, 1313–15.

Waxman SG (2006). Axonal conduction and injury in multiple sclerosis: the role of sodium channels. *Nat Rev Neurosci*, **7**, 932–41.

Wingerchuk DM, *et al.* (2007). The spectrum of neuromyelitis optica. *Lancet Neurol*, **6**, 805–15.

Youl BD, *et al.* (1991). The pathophysiology of acute optic neuritis: an association of gadolinium leakage with clinical and electrophysiological deficits. *Brain*, **114**, 2437–50.

24.10.3 Traumatic injuries to the head

Laurence Watkins and David G.T. Thomas

Essentials

Head injuries cause 1% of all deaths, including 15 to 20% of those in people aged 5 to 35 years, with many survivors facing long-term disability.

Pathophysiology—brain injury may be (1) primary—axonal injury and focal contusions are caused at the moment of impact; or (2) secondary—causes are (a) extracranial—e.g. hypoxia and hypotension, and (b) intracranial—e.g. haematoma, brain swelling, and infection.

Treatment

General aspects—rapid action in the 'golden hour' is often essential for success. Life-threatening extracranial injuries that affect the airway, breathing and circulation take priority, and all patients with head injuries should be assumed to have injury to the cervical spine—requiring immobilization—until this can be excluded.

Head injury—deterioration in conscious level, routinely assessed by serial recording of the Glasgow Coma Score (GCS), requires immediate action, with initial management depending on the severity of head injury. (1) Severe (GCS 3–8/15)—immediate referral to a neurosurgical unit is required; elective intubation and ventilation may be required prior to transfer; ventilation should maintain $P\text{CO}_2$ 4.0 to 4.5 kPa, and mean arterial pressure should be kept above 90 mmHg; CT scanning may be required. (2) Moderate (GCS 9–13/15)—an urgent CT scan is advisable, with urgent neurosurgical referral (and management as for severe head injury) if this reveals an intracranial abnormality. (3) Mild (GCS 14 or 15)—patients with GCS 15, no history of loss of consciousness, and none of a defined list of criteria for investigation, may be considered for discharge according to local head injury protocols. The availability of CT scanning at all times in centres receiving patients with acute head injury, together with neurological and neurointensive care facilities, is critical for the best outcomes.

Complications, prognosis, and prevention

(1) Acute subdural haematoma—rapid detection and surgical drainage is of proven value. (2) Infection—most neurosurgeons recommend early use of prophylactic antibiotics in penetrating injuries. (3) Cognitive symptoms—85% of adults with severe head injuries remain disabled at 1 year; long-term care requires multidisciplinary support in focused programmes of rehabilitation. Even 'mild' injuries can lead to significant 'postconcussional symptoms' including headache, dizziness, poor concentration, memory impairment, and personality change.

Prevention—this is a major concern for health and safety legislation, town planning and traffic laws, e.g. compulsory wearing of seat belts and crash helmets.

Epidemiology

It is estimated that each year in the United Kingdom approximately 1 million people attend hospital. Almost one-half of these are children under 16 years of age. Head injuries cause 9 deaths per 100 000 population per year in the United Kingdom. This represents 1% of all deaths, but 15 to 20% of deaths for those aged between 5 and 35 years. As mainly young people are affected, the prevalence of disability caused is very significant, with an estimated 135 000 people in the United Kingdom dependent on care after brain trauma.

In 1986, the Royal College of Surgeons of England published guidelines on the provision of surgical services for patients with head injuries. There were concerns that inappropriate treatment might lead to unnecessary death and disability. This possibility, together with increasing public expectation, led to a further working party that published updated guidelines in 1999. The availability of CT has also increased, so that now it is considered essential for all hospitals that admit patients with head injuries to have CT facilities at all times.

In 2003, the National Institute for Health and Clinical Excellence (NICE) produced comprehensive guidelines on the acute management of head injury. Most hospitals in England and Wales now use these guidelines as the basis of their head injury management protocols.

Basic concepts
Primary and secondary injury

Primary injury is the damage caused to the brain at the moment of impact. It encompasses diffuse axonal injury and focal contusions. Medicine has little to offer for primary injury; prevention, however, is a major concern for health and safety legislation, town planning, and traffic laws (such as the compulsory wearing of seat belts and crash helmets). The focus of medical intervention is the prevention of secondary damage.

The causes of secondary brain damage can be divided into extracranial (hypoxia and hypotension) and intracranial (haematoma, brain swelling, and infection).

Grading the severity of injury

Only 20% of patients are admitted to hospital and most of these are discharged in less than 48 h. About 1 in 500 of the patients attending hospital will develop intracranial haemorrhage. The doctor's task is to manage patients in such a way that the few with preventable causes of secondary injury are identified and treated effectively.

The British Society of Rehabilitation Medicine defines three broad groups depending on their Glasgow Coma Scale (GCS) score after initial resuscitation:

◆ Mild—GCS 13 to 15

◆ Moderate—GCS 9 to 12

◆ Severe—GCS 3 to 8.

This is a useful categorization for decision-making in head injury management. It should not be confused with other schemes, which are generally retrospective and used for epidemiological and statistical purposes.

The golden hour

Taking into account the practicalities of CT, interhospital transfer, and preparation for theatre, the time available for initial assessment, resuscitation, and treatment of other injuries in the hospital Emergency Department is less than 1 h. This is sometimes referred to as the 'golden hour' in which rapid action is critical to the patient's outcome.

In a typical series of patients who had surgery for acute subdural haematoma, over 70% had a functional recovery (good recovery or moderate disability) if the delay from injury to operation was less than 2 h. If the delay was between 2 and 4 h, just over 60% made a functional recovery. In contrast, for those whose operation was more than 4 h after the injury, less than 10% made a functional recovery (Fig. 24.10.3.1).

Such observations led to the Royal College of Surgeons' guideline stating that evacuation of haematoma, when required, should be done within 4 h. NICE guidelines specified that CT should be performed and assessed within 1 h of the initial request, when indicated. Despite this consensus for rapid assessment and intervention, the realities of resources and interhospital transfer still make this difficult to achieve.

Patients who 'talk and die'—the importance of deteriorating conscious level

A classic paper, by Jennett and his team, coined the phrase 'talk and die' to describe patients whose primary injury was mild, but who succumbed to secondary injury—usually an intracranial haematoma. Deterioration in conscious level is an urgent clinical sign that requires immediate action.

The GCS (Table 24.10.3.1) is now widely used in the United Kingdom and elsewhere, giving objective recording of conscious level, with a high correlation between different observers. Any deterioration is thus more likely to be noticed. When communicating about a patient with head injury, it is good practice to specify observations of each parameter, rather than to use the corresponding numerical scores, which are open to misinterpretation, e.g. a patient scoring 12 based on scores of 4 on eye opening, 3 on verbal response, and 5 on motor response should be communicated as E4, V3, M5. The overall sum should be given and should specify the denominator, to avoid confusion, e.g. 12/15. The most significant parameter

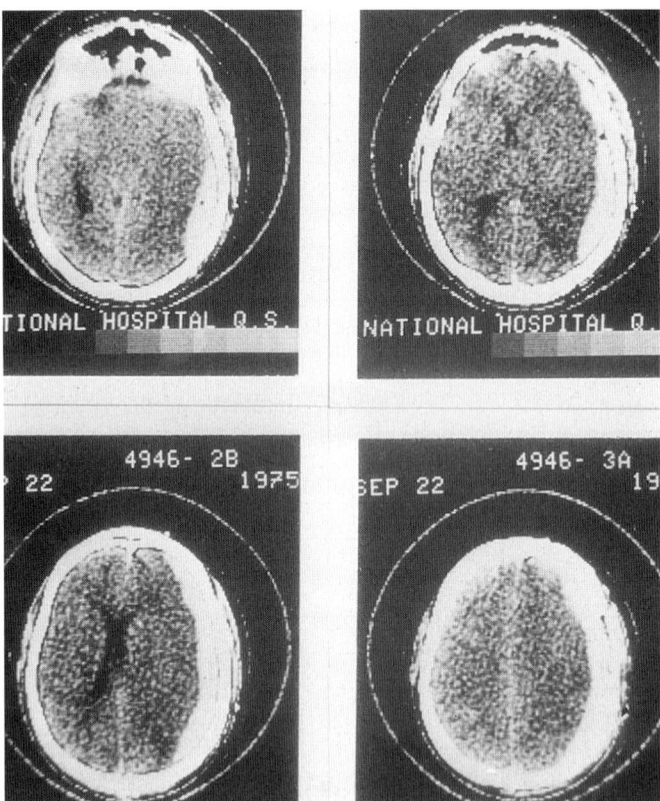

Fig. 24.10.3.1 Typical CT appearances of acute subdural haematoma. Fresh haemorrhage appears hyperdense (white). A subdural haemorrhage conforms to the surface of the brain, typically in a thin crescent. There is effacement of the lateral ventricle on the side of haematoma and midline shift away from it. An extradural haematoma, in contrast, usually appears biconvex, with well-defined edges because it is confined between the bone and dura.

in most cases is the motor score. Changes in motor score of even 1 point can reliably indicate that the patient has deteriorated.

Change in consciousness level is the most useful clinical sign in head injury assessment. Generally, a patient with primary brain injury shows a gradually improving conscious level. A patient whose consciousness level deteriorates is very likely to have a secondary brain injury and therefore requires further investigation and treatment. Consciousness level must therefore be assessed at the earliest opportunity, and then reassessed at frequent intervals.

Early management of the patient with a head injury

Extracranial injuries

Life-threatening extracranial injuries always take priority over the head injury. However severe the head trauma, the patient needs to be stabilized for safe transfer. In addition, hypotension and hypoxia are important causes of secondary brain injury. Time-consuming definitive surgery such as the internal fixation of limb fractures should, however, be postponed if possible.

Airway, breathing, and circulation are the first priorities. Management should follow the general recommendations taught in the Advanced Trauma Life Support (ATLS) courses. In particular, assessment should include consideration of respiratory problems, shock, and possible internal injuries.

Table 24.10.3.1 The Glasgow Coma Scale

Motor function	
Obeying commands	6
Localizing	5
Flexion	4
Abnormal flexion	3
Extension	2
None	1
Verbal response	
Orientated	5
Confused	4
Inappropriate words	3
Incomprehensible	2
None	1
Eye opening	
Spontaneous	4
To speech	3
To pain	2
None	1

All patients with head injury should also be assumed to have a cervical spine injury until proven otherwise. Cervical immobilization should be established, unless the patient is fully conscious, cooperative, and able to convince the examining doctor that he or she has no neck pain or tenderness, a full range of cervical movement, and no neurological deficit. There are rare exceptions to this guideline, e.g. a patient with a fixed flexion deformity due to ankylosing spondylitis might present with a cervical fracture; in that circumstance placing the neck in a 'neutral' position, in a cervical collar, might actually produce neurological injury.

Initial management of head injuries

After initial assessment, resuscitation, and stabilization of extracranial injuries, the patient is graded for the severity of the head injury. These categories then give a useful broad guide to management.

Severe

If the head injury is severe (GCS 3–8) a member of the team should immediately refer to a neurosurgical unit. If the patient's best motor response is localization or obeying, then he or she may not necessarily require ventilation, provided that oxygen saturation can be maintained at more than 95%, the $P\text{CO}_2$ at less than 6 kPa, and the $P\text{O}_2$ at more than 12 kPa on 40% inspired oxygen. If the patient's best motor response is flexion or worse, or if any of the above criteria are not met, then the patient should be electively intubated and ventilated before transfer. Ventilation should be adjusted to maintain the $P\text{CO}_2$ in the range 4.0 to 4.5 kPa. At this stage, the intracranial pressure is unknown, but should be assumed to be high; therefore a mean arterial pressure of at least 90 mmHg should be maintained.

CT scans should be performed according to the NICE guidelines. If the guidelines are followed it should be expected that a relatively high proportion of patients attending the hospital Emergency Department with a head injury will require a CT scan. In most of those cases the scan will need to be done within 1 h.

If, after discussion with the neurosurgical unit, a patient is accepted for transfer, they should be accompanied by personnel able to insert and manage an endotracheal tube and ventilation. The discussion between the two hospitals would include consideration of the risk of transfer, weighed against the benefit that is likely to be achieved. If no specialist intervention is likely, then immediate transfer may not be in the patient's best interests, especially if there is any haemodynamic instability. There may also be patients whose injuries are so severe that there is little reasonable expectation of survival.

Moderate

If the head injury were moderate (GCS 9–13), an urgent CT scan would be advisable. If the CT scan detects an intracranial abnormality, urgent neurosurgical referral is appropriate and the immediate management is similar to that for severe head injuries given above. If no abnormalities are detected on a CT, care should be taken to exclude metabolic and other causes of reduced conscious level (such as hypoglycaemia or drug overdose). If it appears that diffuse brain injury is the only cause of depressed conscious level, the care of the patient is discussed with the neurosurgical unit. In some cases transfer will be advised, whereas in others observation under the care of the Emergency Department will be appropriate. This will depend on local resources and practices. In either situation, if conscious level remains depressed at 48 h, the patient should be transferred to a neurosurgical unit for further assessment.

Mild

Most head injuries are mild (GCS 14–15). After initial assessment, the next decision is whether further investigation is required.

Patients who have a GCS of 15, no history of loss of consciousness, and none of the criteria for investigation may be considered for discharge according to the local head injury protocol. They must be under the supervision of a responsible adult and written information must be provided concerning symptoms and signs that would warrant seeking further urgent medical advice.

In this context, the criteria for CT scan include:

- GCS less than 13 at any point since the injury
- GCS less than 15 at 2 h after the injury
- Suspected open or depressed skull fracture
- Any sign of skull base fracture ('panda eye' periorbital bruising, cerebrospinal fluid flowing from nose or ear, Battle's sign, haemotympanum, subconjunctival haemorrhage with no posterior limit)
- Post-traumatic seizure
- Focal neurological deficit
- More than one episode of vomiting
- Amnesia for more than 30 min of events before the impact

If there has been any loss of consciousness or amnesia, a CT scan should also be immediately requested in patients with any of the following risk factors:

- Age 65 or older
- High-energy mechanism of injury, such as a pedestrian hit by a vehicle, an occupant ejected from a vehicle, or a fall from a height greater than 1 m (about five stairs)
- Anticoagulation or known coagulopathy
- Significant maxillofacial injuries

◆ Difficulty in assessment, whether due to extremes of age (very young or very old) or intoxication.

The validated adult rules on imaging of the head may also be safely used in children and infants, but additional criteria include:

◆ Fall from a height greater than the height of the child

◆ Tense fontanelle

◆ Any suspicion of nonaccidental injury. If nonaccidental injury is suspected in a child then a skull radiograph (as part of a skeletal survey) is also useful, together with other examination such as ophthalmology for retinal haemorrhage.

If the CT scan shows no abnormality, the patient should be admitted for observation until the consciousness level has retuned to normal. Even in those patients with a GCS of 15, they shouldbe admitted if there are other sources of concern to the clinician such as persistent vomiting, severe headache, drug or alcohol intoxication, other injuries, shock, suspected nonaccidental injury, meningism, or leak of cerebrospinal fluid. If the CT scan does show an intracranial abnormality, the care of the patient should be discussed with the neurosurgical unit. In most cases, transfer to the neurosurgical unit is advised.

Management of intracranial complications

Intracranial haematoma

In almost all cases of intracranial haematoma, urgent evacuation is indicated, bearing in mind that, the longer the delay, the greater the risk of death or disability. The above guidelines for CT scan/ transfer to neurosurgical unit are all aimed at the earliest diagnosis of the minority of patients with an intracranial haematoma.

The risk of a traumatic intracranial haematoma depends on consciousness level and whether a skull fracture is present (Table 24.10.3.2), although the decision to proceed with CT is no longer based on initial skull radiograph, but instead on the clinical features as specified in the NICE guidelines.

Even in patients with diffuse brain swelling, rather than an intracranial haematoma, neurosurgical intervention may be indicated. Intracranial pressure (ICP) monitoring can be useful in guiding therapy, such as judicious use of inotropes to maintain the cerebral perfusion pressure. In patients who have persistently raised ICP despite optimization of medical management, a decompressive craniectomy can be considered. This intervention is currently the subject of multicentre randomized trials.

Infection

Meningitis and brain abscess can develop after any head injury in which a communication has been made between the environment

Table 24.10.3.2 The risk of intracranial haematoma

Risk factor	Risk of haematoma
No skull fracture	
Oriented	1:5983
Not oriented	1:121
Skull fracture	
Oriented	1:32
Not oriented	1:4

and the intracranial contents. The most obvious example is a compound depressed fracture, where comminuted bone fragments have been forced inwards, breaching the dura. With some penetrating injuries (such as a fall on to a sharp object or assault with a pointed weapon) the visible wound may be small and appear insignificant. As the injury may have been low velocity, the patient may have a deceptively normal consciousness level. Such patients should always be referred for neurosurgical assessment.

A closed depressed fracture does not require surgery except for cosmetic reasons if it is on a visible part of the skull.

CSF rhinorrhoea or otorrhoea indicates that a skull base fracture has breached the dura. This places the patient at risk of meningitis while the cerebrospinal fluid leak continues. Ninety per cent of such cases close spontaneously within 2 weeks, and usually neurosurgical intervention is not considered until this time has elapsed. An exception is a fracture of the posterior wall of the frontal sinus, visualized on a CT scan. Such cases should be discussed with the neurosurgeon or the craniofacial team (if one exists locally) with a view to possible early anterior fossa repair.

The use of antibiotics in cerebrospinal fluid leaks is controversial, but a working party reviewing the literature concluded that the available evidence does not support the use of prophylactic antibiotics in patients with cerebrospinal fluid fistulas.

Most neurosurgeons do, however, recommend early use of prophylactic antibiotics in penetrating injuries, and there is some evidence for their use in that context.

Follow-up and late complications of head injury

Cognitive symptoms

After head injury there is a variable period before memory function returns and ongoing memories again begin to be stored. This period is referred to as post-traumatic amnesia and is a useful measure of the severity of brain damage, e.g. when questioned after recovery, a patient may not remember the accident but clearly recall being placed on a stretcher and taken into the ambulance: this would suggest a relatively short post-traumatic amnesia of a few minutes. The post-traumatic amnesia is fixed for a given injury and memories of this period do not later 'recover'.

It is also common for a patient to lose memory of events immediately before the injury. This is known as retrograde amnesia. Unlike post-traumatic amnesia, the period of retrograde amnesia often progressively reduces as the patient recovers.

Incomplete recovery after a head injury has behavioural, cognitive, emotional, social, and economic effects. For adults with severe head injuries, 85% remained disabled at 1 year following the accident. In the intermediate group, 63% remained disabled at 1 year. Even those with so-called 'minor' injuries can face considerable problems: at 3-month follow-up 79% still have headaches, 59% have symptomatic memory impairment, and 34% have not returned to work. In view of this ongoing impairment, patients who have been admitted for more than 48 h following a head injury should be referred for neuroscience involvement in their follow-up.

The most widely used measure of outcome after head injury is the Glasgow Outcome Scale (Table 24.10.3.3). These are broad categories, which miss the subtleties of impairment in many who have had mild injuries, but its wide adoption and recognition make the Glasgow Outcome Scale invaluable for statistical comparisons.

Table 24.10.3.3 The Glasgow Outcome Scale

Good recovery	Able to resume preinjury lifestyle
Moderate disability	Independent, but unable to resume full preinjury activities
Severe disability	Dependent on the care of others for the activities of daily living
Vegetative	No sign of psychologically mediated responses
Dead	

Even 'mild' injuries, with early brief loss of consciousness and an initial GCS of 14 to 15, can lead to significant symptoms that can interfere with return to previous activities. These 'postconcussional symptoms' include headache, dizziness, poor concentration, memory impairment, and personality change. The patient's relatives often report personality changes, such as 'bad temper' and lack of motivation. Such symptoms usually improve over 6 months, especially if the patient and family are warned to expect such problems and reassured that they are eventually likely to resolve.

Rehabilitation after severe head injury requires multidisciplinary input from rehabilitation neurology, physiotherapy, occupational therapy, speech and language therapy, and neuropsychology. Other specialists and therapy services are accessed as appropriate for each individual patient. At least as far as the Glasgow Outcome Scale is concerned, 60% of patients reach their final outcome category by 3 months after the injury. Ninety per cent reach their final score by the end of 6 months.

Epilepsy

Epilepsy is more common if there has been an intracranial haematoma, a depressed skull fracture, or post-traumatic amnesia of more than 24 h. A single seizure, within 1 week the injury, is of less significance than repeated seizures or those occurring after the first week. Any patient who has had a seizure, craniotomy, or depressed skull fracture should be advised not to drive or operate dangerous machinery. They should also contact the Driver and Vehicle Licensing Authority (DVLA).

Chronic subdural haematoma

The initial injury may have seemed very minor and may have occurred many weeks previously. The most common symptom is headache, progressively worsening and eventually accompanied by vomiting. There may also be a focal deficit, which can vary in severity. Increasing intracranial pressure may lead to cognitive impairment and eventually a depressed level of consciousness.

Whatever the pathophysiology, the treatment of choice is evacuation of the subdural collection and irrigation with isotonic saline at body temperature. This is a relatively small operation, which can even be performed under local anaesthetic, so even advanced age and general frailty do not contraindicate its use.

Hydrocephalus

Hydrocephalus occasionally occurs after head injury, particularly if there has been traumatic subarachnoid or intraventricular haemorrhage. It can be distinguished from post-traumatic cerebral atrophy by the appearances on the CT scan: in hydrocephalus, the sulci will be small or effaced relative to the large ventricles and there may be periventricular lucency due to interstitial oedema.

Further reading

American College of Surgeons Committee on Trauma (1997). *Advanced trauma life-support for doctors*. Student course manual, 6th edition. American College of Surgeons, Chicago.

British Society of Rehabilitation Medicine (1998). *Rehabilitation after traumatic brain injury*. British Society of Rehabilitation Medicine, London.

Commission on the Provision of Surgical Services (1986). *Report of the working party on head injuries*. Royal College of Surgeons, London.

Infection in Neurosurgery Working Party of the British Society for Antimicrobial Chemotherapy (1994). Antimicrobial prophylaxis in neurosurgery and after head injury. *Lancet*, **344**, 1547–51.

McMillan T, Greenwood R (1991). *Rehabilitation programmes for the brain injured adult: current practice and future options in the UK*. A discussion paper for the Department of Health. Department of Health, London.

Mendelow AD, Teasdale GM, Jennett B (1983). Risks of intracranial haematoma in head injured adults. *BMJ*, **287**, 1173–6.

National Institute for Clinical Excellence (2003). *Head injury. Triage, assessment, investigation and early management of head injury in infants, children and adults*. Available at: http://www.nice.org.uk/pdf/cg4niceguideline.pdf

Reilly PL, *et al.* (1975). Patients with head injury who talk and die. *Lancet*, **ii**, 375–7.

Rimel RW, *et al.* (1981). Disability caused by minor injury. *Neurosurgery*, **9**, 221–8.

Seelig JM, *et al.* (1981). Traumatic acute subdural haematoma. Major mortality reduction in comatose patients treated within 4 h. *N Engl J Med*, **304**, 1511–18.

Teasdale GM (1995). Head injury. *J Neurol Neurosurg Psychiatry*, **58**, 526–39.

Working Party on the Management of Patients with Head Injuries (1999). *Report of the Working Party on the Management of Patients with Head Injuries*. Royal College of Surgeons, London.

24.10.4 Intracranial tumours

Jeremy Rees

Essentials

Intracranial tumours represent about 2% of all cancers. There are no known risk factors apart from prior irradiation to the skull and brain and a few rare neurogenetic syndromes, e.g. neurofibromatosis, von Hippel–Lindau syndrome, Li–Fraumeni syndrome. They may be intrinsic or extrinsic, which determines potential resectability. Neuroepithelial tumours (predominantly gliomas) account for 50 to 60% of all primary tumours; 50% of secondary tumours are from the lung.

Clinical features

Typical manifestations include (1) progressive focal neurological deficit—typically subacute; present in over 50% of patients at time of diagnosis; (2) seizures—may be focal or secondarily generalized; the presenting symptom in 25 to 30% of patients with gliomas; (3) raised intracranial pressure—the classic picture of headache, vomiting, visual obscurations and papilloedema is easily recognized, but most patients present before this develops; and (4) altered mental state—cognitive and personality changes.

Diagnosis, treatment and prognosis

Diagnosis—this is made by a combination of CT/MRI scanning and pathological examination of either a biopsy or resection specimen.

Treatment—the conventional methods are (1) surgery—may be curative for extrinsic tumours, but rarely so for intrinsic tumours; (2) radiotherapy and chemotherapy—useful as adjuvant treatment; certain tumours may respond particularly well, e.g. oligodendrogliomas with chromosome 1p/19q deletion.

Prognosis—this is determined by age at presentation (young > old), performance status (high > low) and histological grade (low > high). As a general rule, survival with glioblastoma multiforme is 1 to 2 years, anaplastic gliomas 2 to 5 years, and low-grade gliomas 5 to 15 years. Tumours such as meningiomas and pituitary adenomas have over 90% 10-year survival if diagnosed before irreversible neurological damage has occurred.

Introduction

Intracranial tumours comprise primary tumours that originate from the brain, cranial nerves, pituitary gland, or meninges, and secondary tumours (metastases) that arise from organs outside the nervous system. These tumours present to many different specialists and their management is difficult because of their location and their variable clinical manifestations.

Aetiology

There are no known risk factors apart from prior irradiation to the skull and brain and a few rare neurogenetic syndromes, such as neurofibromatosis (optic nerve glioma, meningioma, vestibular schwannoma) (Fig. 24.10.4.1), von Hippel–Lindau syndrome (haemangioblastoma), and Li–Fraumeni syndrome (glioma).

Epidemiology

Intracranial tumours represent the eighth most common neoplasm in adults (c.2% of all cancers) and the second most common neoplasm in children. After stroke, intracranial tumours are the leading cause of death from neurological disease in the United Kingdom and are responsible for 7% of years of life lost from cancer before the age of 70.

The crude annual incidence for primary intracranial tumours is 7.4 per 100 000 (males 9.1/100 000, females 6.1/100 000) and for secondary tumours 14.3 per 100 000 population. There is evidence that the incidence is increasing, particularly in older patients. Different tumour types present at different ages. Supratentorial gliomas are uncommon below the age of 30 years but become increasingly prevalent thereafter. The most frequent tumours of middle life (third and fourth decades) are astrocytomas, meningiomas, pituitary adenomas, and vestibular schwannomas, whereas glioblastoma multiforme and metastases are more frequent in the fifth and six decades of life. In contrast, children tend to have infratentorial tumours: 70% of childhood primary intracranial tumours originate below the tentorium cerebelli, whereas in adults the figure is only 25%. There is a strong female preponderance of meningiomas and schwannomas, whereas gliomas are more common in men.

Pathogenesis

Gliomas are thought to arise from neoplastic transformation of glial cells. Recently, there has been increasing incidence in the role of stem cells in the origins of brain tumours—stem cells are defined as having the ability to renew themselves in perpetuity and to differentiate into mature cells. The existence of a cancer stem cell has now been proven for glioblastoma and medulloblastoma, and may explain why these tumours recur after treatment. Certain genetic lesions are associated with brain tumours. Chromosomal deletions—particularly chromosome 10, which contains multiple tumour-suppressor genes—are found in astrocytic tumours, occurring in up to 70% of glioblastomas. Mutations of a tumour-suppressor gene, *TP53*, located on chromosome 17p, have also been reported in approximately 40% of astrocytic tumours. In general the accumulation of predictable genetic alterations is associated with increasing malignant progression. Primary glioblastomas arise in older patients and are associated with amplification and overexpression of the epidermal growth factor receptor (*EGFR*) gene, whereas secondary glioblastomas occur in younger people and are associated with early loss of *TP53*.

Clinical features

With increasing sophistication of neuroimaging, tumours are being detected at an earlier stage than before. Patients typically present with one or more of four clinical syndromes:

◆ progressive neurological deficit

◆ seizures

◆ raised intracranial pressure

◆ altered mental states

The particular combination of clinical features varies depending on the location, histology, and rate of growth of the tumour, e.g. patients with low-grade gliomas present typically with a seizure disorder that may remain static for many years, whereas patients with malignant gliomas typically develop a rapidly progressive neurological deficit and raised intracranial pressure

Progressive neurological deficit

Focal neurological symptoms due to brain tumour are typically subacute and progressive, with over 50% of patients having focal signs by the time of diagnosis. Cortical tumours produce contralateral weakness, sensory loss, dysphasia, dyspraxia, and visual field loss depending on their location. Posterior fossa tumours cause ataxia and cranial nerve palsies. Vestibular schwannomas cause progressive unilateral deafness followed by ipsilateral facial sensory loss. Pituitary tumours may cause a bitemporal hemianopia if there is chiasmal compression or endocrine disturbances due to either hypopituitarism or hypersecretion of specific hormones.

Seizure disorder

Brain tumours account for about 5% of epilepsy cases although they are over-represented in cases of intractable epilepsy. Seizures are the presenting symptom in 25 to 30% of patients with gliomas and are present at some stage of the illness in 40 to 60% overall. Approximately one-half of the patients have focal seizures and the other half have secondarily generalized seizures. Low-grade gliomas are associated with seizures in over 90% of cases and these

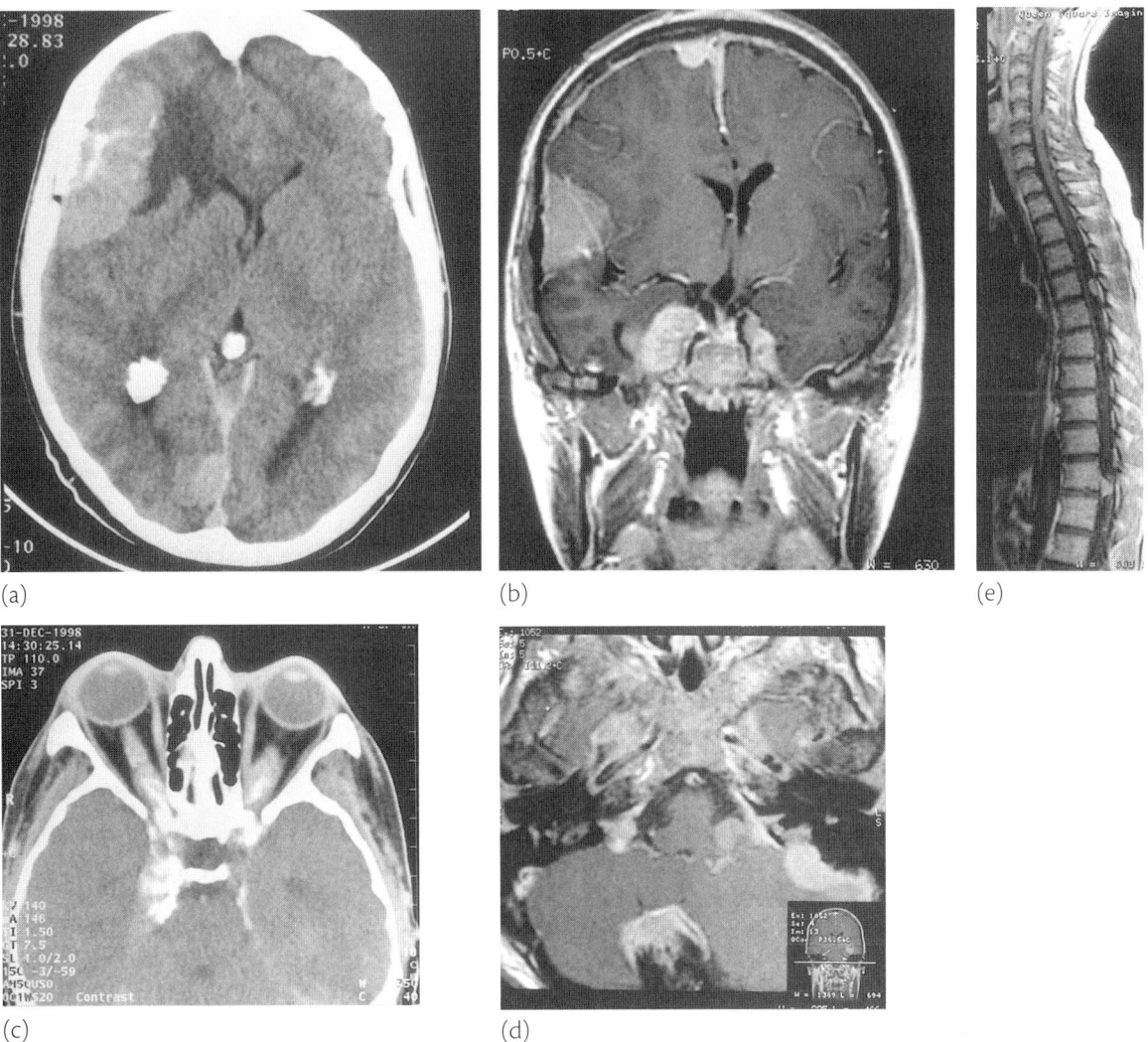

Fig. 24.10.4.1 Contrast-enhanced CT and MR scans of a patient with neurofibromatosis type 2 and multiple intracranial tumours. (a) CT of the brain with contrast enhancement showing a large right parietal convexity meningioma surrounded by vasogenic oedema exerting considerable mass effect. There is also a smaller falx meningioma in the right occipital region. (b) Coronal T_1-weighted MRI of the brain with gadolinium enhancement showing multiple meningiomas in the right temporoparietal region, right parafalcine region, and both cavernous sinuses. (c) Contrast-enhanced CT scan of the orbits showing bilateral optic nerve sheath meningiomas with intracranial extension into the right cavernous sinus, causing partial right nerve III and nerve VI palsies. (d) Axial T_1-weighted MRI of the brain with gadolinium enhancement, showing bilateral vestibular nerve schwannomas and a large fourth ventricle tumour. (e) Sagittal T_1-weighted MRI of the spinal cord with gadolinium enhancement showing three discrete meningiomas encroaching on the spinal column at midcervical, midthoracic, and upper lumbar levels.

frequently remain the only complaint for many years. Conversely, malignant gliomas have a lower frequency of seizures, presumably because of their more rapid growth and destructive characteristics. In these patients, seizures are associated with a better prognosis. Seizures are also common initial manifestations of meningiomas (40–60%) and metastases (15–20%). Supratentorial tumours and those superficially located are particularly likely to cause seizures, particularly in the frontal and temporal lobes. Todd's paresis, which may persist, is an uncommon but characteristic feature of tumour-associated epilepsy. About 10% of patients presenting anew in status epilepticus have an underlying tumour.

Raised intracranial pressure

Intracranial tumours increase intracranial pressure by a direct mass effect, provoking cerebral oedema, or producing obstructive hydrocephalus. The most common symptom of raised intracranial pressure is headache, which is the presenting symptom in 25 to 35% of patients; papilloedema is found in up to 50% of patients with headache due to tumours. The classic picture of headache, vomiting, and visual obscurations (transient fogging of vision usually on rapid changes in posture) due to raised intracranial pressure is well known and easily recognized, but most patients present before this develops. Less than 1% of patients presenting with isolated headache have a brain tumour.

Most brain tumour headaches are intermittent and nonspecific and may be indistinguishable from tension headaches. Supratentorial tumours typically produce frontal headaches, whereas posterior fossa tumours usually result in occipital headache or neck pain. Certain features of a headache are suggestive but not pathognomonic of raised intracranial pressure. These include headaches that wake the patient at night or are worse on waking and improve over the course of the day.

Mental state changes

These are an uncommon presentation of brain tumours occurring in about 20% of patients at diagnosis. Personality changes may initially be quite subtle and may show themselves as an inability to cope at work. In these cases it is essential to obtain a collateral history from relatives or colleagues at work.

Pathology

Neuroepithelial tumours (predominantly gliomas) account for approximately 50 to 60% of all primary brain tumours. The other common types are meningiomas (20%), pituitary adenomas (15%), vestibular schwannomas (5%), and primary central nervous system (CNS) lymphomas (5%). The most common sites of origin of secondary tumours are lung (50%), breast (15%), melanoma (10%), and unknown (15%).

The gliomas are a family of neoplasms that are thought to arise from astrocytes, oligodendrocytes, and ependymal cells. Astrocytomas are the most common type of glioma and are infiltrating neoplasms composed of fibrillary astrocytes. Almost all these tumours have the propensity to undergo anaplastic change to a more malignant lesion. Thus a fibrillary astrocytoma (Fig. 24.10.4.2) progresses to an anaplastic astrocytoma (Fig. 24.10.4.3) and then to the most malignant form, glioblastoma multiforme (GBM). The oligodendroglioma is characterized by the presence of uniform round nuclei with small nucleoli. This also has the propensity to undergo anaplastic change but, unlike anaplastic astrocytomas, oligodendrogliomas are frequently chemosensitive (see below).

The grading systems that have been used have attempted to describe degrees of anaplastic change and thereby correlate the histological appearances with prognosis. The most widely accepted classifications of gliomas are the World Health Organization's (WHO) three-tiered system (Table 24.10.4.1). These systems have been retrospectively applied to large series of patients and have been shown to provide reproducible and prognostically useful information. They have recently been updated to include some new diagnostic entities.

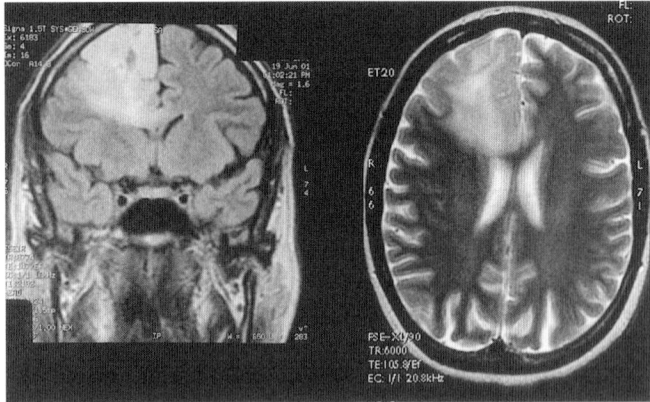

Fig. 24.10.4.2 Coronal and axial T_2-weighted MRI of the brain showing a diffuse lesion in the right frontal lobe, which returns high signal. It is seen extending from the cortex into the deep white matter and infiltrating across the corpus callosum. There is a mass effect causing compression of the frontal horn of the lateral ventricle. The tumour did not enhance with gadolinium. This patient presented with generalized seizures and has remained well after 3 years of follow-up. Biopsy revealed a fibrillary astrocytoma (WHO grade II).

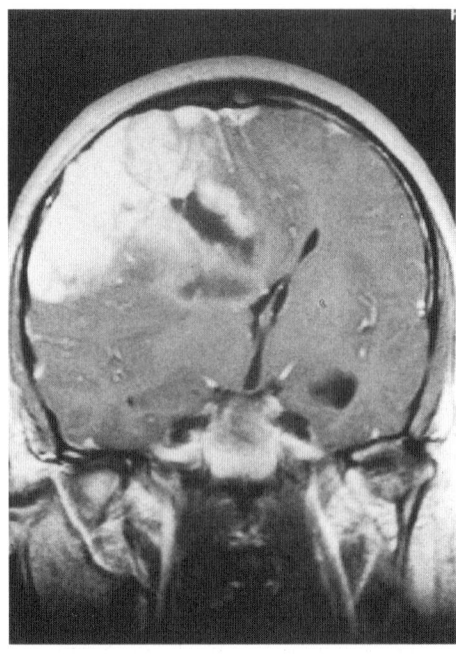

Fig. 24.10.4.3 Coronal T_1-weighted MRI of the brain with gadolinium enhancement showing a large heterogeneous enhancing tumour arising from the right frontal lobe exerting considerable mass effect in a patient presenting with a 2-month history of complex partial seizures, headaches, and papilloedema. The lesion was resected and shown to be an anaplastic astrocytoma.

Diagnosis

The diagnosis of a brain tumour is made by a combination of CT/MR scanning and pathological examination of either a biopsy or a resection specimen. Newer techniques include MR spectroscopy and metabolic imaging (single photon emission CT (SPECT) and positron emission tomography (PET)). These may permit a noninvasive method of differentiating between low-grade and high-grade gliomas and between tumour recurrence and radiation necrosis.

Treatment

The three conventional methods of treatment for brain tumours are surgery, radiotherapy, and chemotherapy. Targeted biological agents, gene therapy, and immunotherapy have still not been widely taken up because of the lack of proven benefit over and above standard therapies. In line with other areas of oncology, there is increasing use of combination therapies, particularly concomitant chemoradiation to improve survival.

Table 24.10.4.1 Pathological classification of astrocytomas

	WHO classification	St Anne–Mayo classification[a]
Pilocytic astrocytoma	I	1 (0 variables)
Diffuse/fibrillary astrocytoma	II	2 (1 variable[a])
Anaplastic astrocytoma	III	3 (2 variables[a])
Glioblastoma multiforme	IV	4 (3 or 4 variables[a])

[a] Based on presence or absence of four variables: nuclear atypia, mitoses, vascular proliferation, and necrosis. In practice, grade 2 lesions contain nuclear atypia, grade 3 mitoses, and grade 4 either or both vascular proliferation and necrosis.

Surgery

Recent advances in tumour neurosurgery include the use of computerized neuronavigation techniques, and intraoperative cortical mapping during awake craniotomy. Preoperatively, important anatomicofunctional information can be derived from functional MRI (fMRI) which allows functional localization of eloquent motor, speech, and memory cortex as well as diffusion tractography, which can delineate the anatomical relationship between tumour and important white matter tracts. These have all contributed to improving the extent of tumour resection with an attendant decrease in morbidity and mortality of neurosurgery, but an effect on overall survival has not been clearly demonstrated.

Surgery is indicated as a first-line treatment for meningiomas, nonsecreting pituitary adenomas, and vestibular schwannomas. The role of surgery in the management of primary intracranial tumours, particularly gliomas, is more controversial. Some types of glioma, e.g. pilocytic astrocytomas, can be cured by surgical resection. For most types, however, removal is not curative. Although surgery is of undoubted benefit in relieving the symptoms and signs of raised intracranial pressure or an evolving focal deficit, there are no prospective randomized data to support its use for prognostic purposes alone, particularly in patients with malignant gliomas. However, the conventional surgical wisdom in patients with low-grade gliomas is tumours that are completely or subtotally resected (leaving a residual tumour volume of <10 ml) have a better prognosis than tumours that are biopsied and treated with radiotherapy alone. Overall, about 50% of patients with medically refractory seizures derive considerable seizure reduction from surgery.

There is evidence that a combination of surgery and radiotherapy offers a survival advantage over radiotherapy alone for the treatment of solitary metastases in patients whose systemic cancer is well controlled.

Radiotherapy

Radiotherapy is the only treatment that has been proved to extend survival in patients with primary malignant brain tumours. Radiotherapy provides useful palliation in patients with low-grade gliomas. When given early, radiotherapy prolongs progression-free survival but not overall survival, compared with radiotherapy given at the time of tumour progression. Meningiomas are also partially radioresponsive and should be treated with radiotherapy where there is atypical or malignant histology or where there is recurrent tumour that is not surgically accessible.

Advances in technology have allowed greater accuracy of radiotherapy delivery and, in particular, the use of stereotactic frames that permit the focusing of radiation to a small tumour with minimal dosage to the surrounding normal tissue. This can be done either in a single high dose (stereotactic radiosurgery) or in smaller fractions (stereotactic radiotherapy) and is predominantly indicated for lesions less than 3 cm in diameter which are well circumscribed, extra-axial, and more than 5 mm away from vital structures. Intensity-modulated radiotherapy (IMRT) allows more precise 'dose painting' whereby different regions of the tumour are treated with varying doses of radiotherapy, and may be useful for the treatment of benign tumours close to vital regions, e.g. the optic nerve apparatus.

Chemotherapy

There has been increased awareness of the chemosensitivity of certain tumours, particularly anaplastic oligodendrogliomas and primary lymphomas of the nervous system in adults, and diencephalic gliomas in children. Approximately two-thirds of anaplastic oligodendrogliomas respond dramatically to a combination of treatment with procarbazine, lomustine (CCNU), and vincristine (PCV); however, recent phase III data have failed to demonstrate a survival benefit for either neoadjuvant or adjuvant PCV over and above radiotherapy in anaplastic oligodendrogliomas. The presence of combined deletions of chromosomes 1p and 19q in these tumours is a favourable prognostic factor independent of treatment modality.

Adjuvant nitrosurea chemotherapy is used in patients with malignant gliomas although it offers only a marginal survival advantage. An oral alkylating agent, temozolomide, has recently been shown to improve survival in patients with newly diagnosed glioblastoma multiforme when given together with radiotherapy and then adjuvantly. Although the improvement in median survival was modest (12.1 vs 14.6 months), the proportion of patients surviving 2 years increased from 10% to 26%. This is the first significant advance in the treatment of malignant glioma for over 30 years and has rekindled enthusiasm for chemotherapy trials in tumours previously regarded as chemoresistant. Whether this treatment can improve the survival of patients with anaplastic astrocytomas is unknown and currently being tested in clinical trials. Carmustine wafers are another recent advance that allows local delivery of carmustine (a nitrosurea) into the resection cavity of a malignant glioma, hence avoiding the systemic toxicity of these compounds. Chemotherapy does not improve survival in patients with low-grade gliomas over radiotherapy alone. There is no chemotherapy that is effective for the treatment of meningiomas. The addition of methotrexate-based chemotherapy to cranial irradiation markedly improves disease control and survival of patients with primary CNS lymphomas.

Prognosis

The three most important prognostic factors for patients with gliomas are age, performance status, and histological grade. The survival advantage for different treatments is modest in comparison. Any trial claiming a significant survival advantage for a new treatment therefore needs to show that this effect is independent of other prognostic factors. The median survival for patients with malignant gliomas varies from 6 months to 5 years dependent on the above. As a general rule, patients with GBM survive for 1 to 2 years, whereas patients with anaplastic gliomas survive for 2 to 5 years.

The outlook for patients with low-grade gliomas is considerably better, with a median survival of 5 to 15 years depending on age, preoperative performance status, histology, and tumour growth rate. Oligodendrogliomas are more chemosensitive than astrocytomas and have a more indolent course, so their prognosis is correspondingly better, with patients surviving 10 to 15 years after diagnosis.

At least 40% of primary intracranial tumours are extra-axial (not arising from within the brain substance itself) and are thus readily treatable, if not curable. Some tumours such as meningiomas and pituitary adenomas are associated with 10-year survival rate of over 90% if diagnosed before irreversible neurological damage has occurred.

Further reading

Cairncross JG, et al. (1998). Specific genetic predictors of chemotherapeutic response and survival in patients with anaplastic oligodendrogliomas. J Natl Cancer Inst, 90, 1473–9. [First study to show definitive correlation between molecular genetic analysis and chemoresponsiveness of brain tumours.]

Counsell CE, Collie DA, Grant R (1996). Incidence of intracranial tumours in the Lothian region of Scotland, 1989–90. J Neurol Neurosurg Psychiatry, 61, 143–50. [Epidemiological study in Scotland showing incidence rates more than twice those previously reported in the United Kingdom.]

Daumas-Duport C, et al. (1988). Grading of astrocytomas, a simple and reproducible method. Cancer, 62, 2152–65. [A 15-year follow-up study of a previously used grading system showing very good correlation between histological criteria and survival.]

DeAngelis LM, et al. (1992). Combined modality therapy for primary CNS lymphoma. J Clin Oncol, 10, 635–43. [Nonrandomized study showing significant improvement in disease-free survival in patients treated with chemotherapy in addition to radiotherapy.]

Forsyth P, Posner JB (1993). Headaches in patients with brain tumours, a study of 111 patients. Neurology, 43, 678–83. [Descriptive study of 111 patients with brain tumour headaches showing that the 'classic' early morning brain tumour headache is uncommon.]

Greig NH, et al. (1990). Increasing annual incidence of primary malignant brain tumours in the elderly. J Natl Cancer Inst, 82, 1621–4. [Study showing up to a 500% increase in incidence rates of malignant brain tumours in older people from the early 1970s to the mid-1980s, which may be despite more extensive uptake of imaging.]

Louis DN, et al. (2007). The 2007 WHO classification of tumours of the central nervous system. Acta Neuropathol, 114, 97–109. [Updated WHO classification system.]

Mineo JF, et al. (2007). Prognostic factors of survival time in patients with glioblastoma multiforme: a multivariate analysis of 340 patients. Acta Neurochir (Wien), 149, 245–52.

Patchell RA, et al. (1990). A randomized trial of surgery in the treatment of single metastases to the brain. N Engl J Med, 322, 494–500. [Randomized trial of surgery and radiotherapy against radiotherapy alone showing increased survival in surgical patients (median 40 compared with 15 weeks).]

Quigley MR, Maron JC (1991). The relationship between survival and extent of the resection in patients with supratentorial malignant gliomas. Neurosurgery, 29, 385–9. [Meta-analysis of over 5000 patients with malignant gliomas treated surgically showing little correlation between extent of resection and survival.]

Schomas DA, et al. (2009). Intracranial low-grade gliomas in adults: 30 years experience with long-term follow-up at Mayo Clinic. Neuro-Oncology, 11, 437–45.

Shaw EG, Scheithauer BW, O'Fallon JR (1997). Supratentorial gliomas, a comparative study by grade and histological type. J Neuro-Oncol, 31, 273–8. [Detailed analysis of survival and correlation with histology in over 500 patients with gliomas.]

Stupp R, et al. (2005). Radiotherapy plus concomitant and adjuvant temozolomide for glioblastoma. N Engl J Med, 352, 987–96. [Definitive trial showing survival benefit using chemoradiation over standard treatment of radiotherapy alone.]

Taphoorn MJB, Klein M (2004). Cognitive deficits in adult patients with brain tumours. Lancet, 3, 159–68.

van den Bent MJ, et al. (2005). Long-term efficacy of early versus delayed radiotherapy for low-grade astrocytoma and oligodendroglioma in adults: the EORTC 22845 randomised trial. Lancet, 366, 985–90. [Definitive trial examining timing of radiotherapy in adults with low-grade gliomas showing that early radiotherapy prolongs progression-free survival but not overall survival.]

Walker MD et al. (1978). Evaluation of BCNU and/or radiotherapy in the treatment of anaplastic gliomas. A cooperative clinical trial. J Neurosurg, 49, 333–43. [First randomized trial confirming survival benefit of patients with malignant gliomas treated with radiotherapy.]

24.10.5 Idiopathic intracranial hypertension

N.F. Lawton

Essentials

Idiopathic intracranial hypertension is a syndrome of raised intracranial pressure in the absence of an intracranial mass lesion, enlargement of the cerebral ventricles due to hydrocephalus, or venous thrombosis in the dural sinuses. Impaired cerebrospinal fluid absorption and raised cerebral venous pressure have both been implicated. Obese females of childbearing age are predominantly affected. Rarely, provocative factors include tetracycline, vitamin A derivatives, hypervitaminosis A, and vitamin A excess.

Clinical features

Characteristic presentation is with headache which may be typical of raised intracranial pressure but is frequently non-specific. Papilloedema is almost invariably present, but often not severe and may be unilateral; visual field defects are common. There are no focal cerebal signs, and a history of epilepsy is strongly against the diagnosis.

Diagnosis, treatment and prognosis

After brain imaging to exclude other causes of raised intracranial pressure, diagnosis depends on measurement of cerebrospinal fluid pressure higher than 200 mm. Composition of fluid is normal. Spontaneous remission and relapse is common, but treatments including the following aim to prevent symptoms and visual loss, which should be monitored by serial analysis of visual fields: (1) high-dose corticosteroids—for relief of acute crises, but not as long-term treatment; (2) drugs—the carbonic anhydrase inhibitors acetazolamide, and thiazide diuretics are used in mild cases; (3) surgery—some patients require lumboperitoneal shunts, optic nerve decompression, or other procedures; (4) intermittent lumbar puncture—particularly of use in pregnancy. Aside from visual loss, serious complications are rare.

Incidence

Idiopathic intracranial hypertension has been widely described in the literature as pseudotumour cerebri or benign intracranial hypertension. These terms can be regarded as synonyms, with the caveat that known causes of the syndrome were included under their rubric.

Idiopathic intracranial hypertension is comparatively rare in the general population with an annual incidence of approximately 1 in 100 000, but this figure rises to 19 in 100 000 in obese women of childbearing age. The disease is certainly more common in females, the preponderance over males ranging from 3:1 to 15:1. Although idiopathic intracranial hypertension is primarily a disease of young women, it may occur in childhood. Very rarely, it is familial and may occur in more than one generation.

Clinical features

It is the hallmark of idiopathic intracranial hypertension that presenting symptoms and signs are those of raised intracranial pressure alone. The diagnosis should not be entertained in the presence of neurological features that suggest a focal lesion. Furthermore, there is a remarkable preservation of consciousness and intellectual function, rarely encountered in patients with mass lesions causing raised intracranial pressure. A history of epilepsy, either generalized or focal, virtually excludes the diagnosis of idiopathic intracranial hypertension, whereas seizures may occur in patients with venous sinus thrombosis. Preservation of cerebral function also aids the distinction of idiopathic intracranial hypertension from acute viral or bacterial meningoencephalitis. Patients with idiopathic intracranial hypertension routinely present to outpatient departments and become a medical emergency when papilloedema is seen.

Headache

This is the most common symptom and is present to some degree in almost every case. The headache may be typical of raised intracranial pressure. It is then generalized, throbbing, worse on waking, and aggravated by factors that temporarily increase cerebrospinal fluid pressure such as straining, coughing, or changing posture. Not infrequently, however, headache is mild and nonspecific so that the distinction from common tension headache can be difficult. At presentation, headache has usually been present for weeks, although sometimes for months. Although up to 50% of patients complain of nausea, typical early-morning projectile vomiting is rare. Headache may be accompanied by tinnitus, which is often pulsatile in type.

Obesity

Among the medical conditions associated with idiopathic intracranial hypertension, obesity is sufficiently common to be a characteristic feature. About 90% of patients in adult series are overweight. The association with both obesity and gender is less marked in childhood.

Papilloedema

This is a virtually universal finding and the importance of fundus examination in every patient with headache cannot be overemphasized. Papilloedema is often moderate and may be unilateral. Occasionally the appearance of the optic discs may be equivocal, and fluorescein angiography is indicated to demonstrate the characteristic leakage of dye in true papilloedema.

The classic symptom of papilloedema, which is not specific to idiopathic intracranial hypertension, is a transient obscuration of vision, often described as a fleeting greyness, a halo, or a more vivid episode of 'Catherine wheels' lasting for a few seconds. Obscurations may be provoked by straining or a change in posture, but may also occur spontaneously. Persistent blurring of vision may also occur and patients may describe scotomas in the field of vision associated with optic nerve damage. Occasionally, sudden and permanent loss of vision results from infarction of the optic nerve.

Visual obscurations, persistent blurring, or scotomas are reported by 30 to 70% of patients. A history of obscurations is often elicited only by direct questioning.

Visual field defects

Together with measurement of best-corrected visual acuity, visual field analysis is an essential investigation in the examination and follow-up of patients with idiopathic intracranial hypertension. The most common defects are enlargement of the blind spots, generalized constriction of the fields, and scotomas caused by optic nerve damage. There may be a predilection for visual field loss in the inferior nasal quadrants.

Diplopia

About 30% of patients complain of horizontal diplopia due to cranial nerve VI palsy, which may be bilateral. The cause is a false localizing sign of raised intracranial pressure.

Aetiology

In most patients with idiopathic intracranial hypertension no trigger can be identified. Many clinical associations have been reported, but these may have occurred by chance. Preceding minor head injury and intercurrent infections come into this category. Furthermore, the known associations are rare with the exceptions of obesity and the predilection for females. A positive family history, vitamin deficiency, and drugs are a factor in less than 2% of cases.

Dural sinus thrombosis

Before the advent of antibiotics, benign intracranial hypertension was frequently described in chronic middle-ear disease complicated by dural sinus thrombosis. The term 'otitic hydrocephalus' was coined to describe this syndrome on the erroneous assumption that ventricular enlargement was present.

Although true 'otitic hydrocephalus' is now rare, dural sinus thrombosis remains an important differential diagnosis of idiopathic intracranial hypertension. Sinus thrombosis may complicate pregnancy, the use of oral contraceptives, head injury, venous occlusive disease due to hypercoagulability states, dehydration due to any cause, or mediastinal obstruction. Sinus thrombosis should be suspected clinically when the onset of headache is sudden and accompanied by focal signs or impaired consciousness. The clinical presentation may, however, mimic idiopathic intracranial hypertension and sinus thrombosis must be excluded radiologically.

Menstrual disorders

An association of idiopathic intracranial hypertension with pregnancy has been reported but has not been confirmed by small epidemiological studies. It is not clear whether an association with menstrual irregularity is more than would occur by chance in obese young women. An association with menarche has been reported.

In spite of the clinical associations that suggest an underlying disorder of female endocrinology, hormonal studies have not shown a consistent abnormality. The pituitary–adrenal axis is intact and occasional abnormal responses may be due to obesity rather than idiopathic intracranial hypertension. Thyroid function and prolactin secretion both appear to be normal. Vasopressin levels in cerebrospinal fluid are raised, but this is not specific and may occur in a variety of neurological diseases. Reports of a specific increase of oestrone in cerebrospinal fluid, which might link idiopathic intracranial hypertension with obesity because adipocytes are the major source of oestrone, have not been confirmed.

Deficiency states

A rare cause of intracranial hypertension in children is hypovitaminosis A due to generalized nutritional deficiency or malabsorption. In such cases the condition responds specifically to vitamin A supplements. Poisoning with vitamin A due to excessive consumption of fish or animal liver may also cause intracranial hypertension. The hypothesis that a disorder of vitamin A metabolism is an underlying cause of idiopathic intracranial hypertension continues to be debated. An increased concentration of retinol in cerebrospinal fluid has been reported.

Medication

Both tetracycline and the retinoids isotretinoin and etretinate, which are vitamin A derivatives, may cause intracranial hypertension during long-term treatment for acne. These drugs should not be used in combination. Intracranial hypertension due to tetracycline has also been reported during prophylaxis for malaria. All-*trans*-retinoic acid in treatment of acute promyelocytic leukaemia is also a cause in this category. Other drugs occasionally responsible for the syndrome include nalidixic acid, nitrofurantoin, lithium, danazol, and synthetic growth hormone. Corticosteroids may lead to intracranial hypertension during their withdrawal after chronic treatment and the syndrome may occur in Addison's disease.

Empty sella

It has been suggested that this association in about 4% of cases is caused by raised intracranial pressure in combination with incompetence of the diaphragma sellae. The theory is supported by the finding of raised pressure at lumbar puncture in some patients with empty sella, suggesting chronic idiopathic intracranial hypertension as the underlying cause. Clinical hypopituitarism does not occur, but occasionally the empty sella may harbour a prolactinoma.

Pathogenesis

The mechanism by which intracranial pressure rises is poorly understood and the contribution of various factors controversial. As the intracranial contents are housed in a rigid container, an increase in cerebrospinal fluid pressure may result from an increase in blood volume, swelling of the brain parenchyma, or an increase in the cerebrospinal fluid volume due to overproduction or malabsorption. There is little evidence to suggest that increased blood volume or cerebrospinal fluid production is an important factor. An association with thrombophilia has been reported but the significance of the finding is unclear. Recent studies have drawn attention to the possible contribution of raised cerebral venous pressure in pathogenesis.

Swelling of the brain parenchyma

Direct evidence of swelling due to cerebral oedema is slight and a single report of oedematous changes in brain biopsies has not been confirmed. However, the tendency for the ventricles to be small may indicate an increase in cerebral volume secondary to leakage from the cerebral vascular bed rather than transudation of cerebrospinal fluid from the ventricular system. Brain imaging in idiopathic intracranial hypertension does not show the periventricular leakage of cerebrospinal fluid that occurs in hydrocephalus. Although there is currently no direct evidence for vasogenic cerebral oedema, this factor cannot be ignored, because it is one mechanism for raised pressure that does not anticipate some degree of hydrocephalus. MRI studies of brain water content have been equivocal.

Decreased absorption of cerebrospinal fluid

A defect of cerebrospinal fluid absorption is widely regarded as the important factor in the pathogenesis of idiopathic intracranial hypertension. It is assumed that the defect lies in the arachnoid villi of the superior sagittal sinus where the bulk of the cerebrospinal fluid absorption takes place. The delayed clearance of radio-iodinated human serum albumin from the ventricular system after injection into the lumbar subarachnoid space is indirect evidence of reduced cerebrospinal fluid absorption. Simultaneous cannulation of the superior sagittal sinus and the subarachnoid space has shown increased resistance to cerebrospinal fluid absorption in most cases. Finally, vitamin A deficiency in rats and cows produces a rise in intracranial pressure associated with diminished absorption of cerebrospinal fluid and histological changes in the arachnoid villi, which are reversible with vitamin A supplements.

The absence of hydrocephalus in idiopathic intracranial hypertension has been cited as an objection to the theory of reduced cerebrospinal fluid absorption. It is more significant, however, that sinus thrombosis may cause intracranial hypertension by preventing cerebrospinal fluid absorption, and is similarly associated with normal or small ventricles.

Raised cerebral venous pressure

MR venography (MRV) in idiopathic intracranial hypertension may show narrowing of the lateral and sigmoid sinuses and manometry has shown consistent venous hypertension. It is not yet clear whether these findings are a primary abnormality or secondary to raised intracranial pressure. A rise in central venous pressure due to obesity has also been implicated in pathogenesis, although the significance of the finding remains unclear.

Investigations

The diagnosis of idiopathic intracranial hypertension only be confirmed can by measurement of cerebrospinal fluid pressure, but in suspected cases brain imaging is essential before proceeding to lumbar puncture.

Radiology

CT scanning may show small and slit-like cerebral ventricles that increase in volume as intracranial hypertension resolves. Sagittal sinus thrombosis may be visualized on CT scanning as the characteristic 'empty delta' sign due to clot within the sinus. MRI is far superior to CT and frequently provides graphic images of sinus thrombosis. As a result of the implications for treatment, MRV or CT venography is recommended to exclude thrombotic disease when plain imaging is normal.

Cerebrospinal fluid pressure

At lumbar puncture the opening pressure is greater than 200 mmCSF, but in simple obesity the cerebrospinal fluid pressure may be as high as 250 mm. The diagnostic significance of cerebrospinal fluid pressure must therefore be correlated with the clinical picture. It is important that cerebrospinal fluid pressure is measured in the lateral decubitus position to obtain a valid reading. In the few patients whose cerebrospinal fluid pressure is equivocal, continuous monitoring may demonstrate intermittent peaks of raised pressure.

Cerebrospinal fluid analysis

The composition of the cerebrospinal fluid in idiopathic intracranial hypertension is entirely normal and the diagnosis should not be accepted in the presence of an increase in white cells or protein concentration. The unexpected finding of a pleocytosis requires further investigation to exclude meningitic infiltration or infection, including HIV. A rare syndrome resembling idiopathic intracranial hypertension occurs in association with postinfective polyneuropathy and spinal tumours. Both conditions may lead to intracranial hypertension with papilloedema and normal-size ventricles but a marked rise in cerebrospinal fluid protein.

Management

Patients given a diagnosis of idiopathic intracranial hypertension are usually bewildered and frightened. It is important to provide a simple explanation of the nature of the condition and the rationale for treatment. Improvement has been reported with weight reduction and obese patients sholuld be offered dietary advice. In practice, however, weight loss in difficult to achieve and to maintain. With the exception of rare cases due to drug treatment, the management of idiopathic intracranial hypertension is aimed at the symptomatic reduction of intracranial pressure to protect vision and relieve headache. The methods available are difficult to evaluate because of the high spontaneous remission rate and the lack of controlled trials. Choice of treatment is further complicated by the absence of reliable risk factors for visual loss. In particular, the height of the cerebrospinal fluid pressure at diagnosis is of no prognostic significance.

In the past, repeated therapeutic lumbar puncture every 2 to 5 days has been shown to reduce cerebrospinal fluid pressure temporarily and may occasionally lead to spontaneous remission. This approach may still be useful in pregnancy, because of the risk of diuretics to the fetus. Teratogenicity of acetazolamide has been shown in animal studies.

When acute medical treatment is indicated, prednisolone 40 to 60 mg daily may be effective in relieving headache and visual obscuration due to papilloedema. However, steroids are unsatisfactory as long-term treatment because of their complications, especially in obese young females. For this reason diuretics are widely used in patients with mild symptoms. Acetazolamide, thiazide diuretics, and furosemide may relieve headache, but their efficacy in preventing slowly progressive visual loss is unproven. Acetazolamide has been favoured on the basis that carbonic anhydrase inhibition may reduce cerebrospinal fluid production, but side effects often limit its use.

As a result of the limitations of medical treatment, surgical intervention may be required, progressive visual field loss and unrelieved headache being the indications for surgery. A lumboperitoneal shunt is usually favoured, being less invasive than a ventricular approach. Unfortunately the technical failure rate of lumboperitoneal shunt is usually high and surgical revision may be required in about 50% of patients. For this reason the alternative operation,

in which the optic nerve sheath is decompressed, has recently been revived, particularly in North America. This procedure produces rapid improvement in papilloedema, occasionally in both eyes after unilateral surgery. It is not clear whether long-term improvement is due to the creation of a cerebrospinal fluid fistula in the orbit or fibrosis of the meninges preventing transmission of the high cerebrospinal fluid pressure to the optic nerve head. However, headache is often unrelieved by this procedure, and lumboperitoneal shunting may not be avoided. There is also a small risk of intraoperative visual loss as well as delayed visual loss postoperatively.

Currently it would seem reasonable to begin treatment with diuretics, reserving steroids as a temporary medical treatment in patients with severe symptoms. If surgery becomes necessary, lumboperitoneal shunting seems a logical procedure, with resort to optic nerve sheath decompression in the event of repeated shunt failure. Occasionally, subtemporal decompression may be required. Stenting of the venous sinuses in the light of MRV and manometry evidence for raised cerebral venous pressure has lead to improvement in some patients but the place of this procedure in management has yet to be established.

Prognosis

Idiopathic intracranial hypertension is a chronic condition in most patients, but spontaneous relapse and remission of symptoms are common. There is evidence that raised intracranial pressure may be found at follow-up lumbar puncture in patients whose symptoms have been in remission for several years. Serious complications of idiopathic intracranial hypertension, other than visual loss, are rare, whereas an underlying dural sinus thrombosis may lead to a fatal outcome. A degree of visual field loss persists in about 50% of patients and a loss of visual acuity, occasionally leading to blindness, in about 10%. As loss of central vision usually occurs late in the course of the disease, serial visual field analysis is the important yardstick of clinical progression.

Further reading

Ahlskog JE (1982). Pseudotumour cerebri. *Ann Intern Med*, **97**, 249–56.

Ball AK, Clarke CE (2006). Idiopathic intracranial hypertension. *Lancet Neurol*, **5**, 433–42.

Binder BK, *et al.* (2004). Idiopathic intracranial hypertension. *Neurosurgery*, **54**, 538–51.

Bruce BB, *et al.* (2009). Idiopathic intracranial hypertension in men. *Neurology*, **72**, 304–9.

McComb JG (1983). Recent research into the nature of cerebrospinal fluid formation and absorption. *J Neurosurg*, **59**, 369–83.

Rush JA (1980). Pseudotumour cerebri: clinical profile and visual outcome in 63 patients. *Mayo Clinic Proc*, **55**, 541–6.

Shah VA, *et al.* (2008). Long-term follow-up of idiopathic intracranial hypertension: the Iowa experience. *Neurology*, **70**, 634–40.

Vieira DS, *et al.* (2008). Idiopathic intracranial hypertension with and without papilloedema in a consecutive series of patients with chronic migraine. *Cephalgia*, **28**, 609–13.

Infections of the central nervous system

Contents

24.11.1   Bacterial infections

Diederik van de Beek, Jeremy Farrar, and Guy E. Thwaites

Essentials

Bacterial meningitis occurs in a number of clinical situations, including spontaneous (the most important category), post-traumatic, and device-associated (relating to cerebrospinal fluid shunts and drains). Each of these is associated with a particular pattern of infecting organisms, clinical presentation and outcome, but overall there is high morbidity and mortality.

Aetiology

(1) Adult spontaneous community-acquired meningitis—80 to 85% of cases are caused by *Neisseria meningitidis* or *Streptococcus pneumoniae* in most countries, with *Listeria monocytogenes*, aerobic Gram-negative bacilli (e.g. *Escherichia coli*), *Haemophilus influenzae* and *Staphylococcus aureus* causing most of the others. *Streptococcus suis* serotype 2 is an important cause in Asia. (2) Post-traumatic meningitis—most hospital-acquired infections are caused by aerobic Gram-negative bacilli; *S. pneumoniae* causes most community acquired disease. (3) Device-associated meningitis—most infections are nosocomial and caused by coagulase-negative staphylococci or *Staph. aureus*.

Patients with recurrent meningitis frequently have an underlying anatomical or immunological defect (particularly hypogammaglobulinaemia or complement deficiencies). In some parts of the world, HIV infection has altered the pattern of aetiological agents (and presentation and outcome of meningitis), with *Mycobacterium tuberculosis* increasingly common.

Clinical features

(1) Community-acquired meningitis—the classic triad of fever, nuchal rigidity, and altered mental status is present in just under 50% of patients. Other manifestations include rashes (particularly with meningococcal disease), seizures and focal neurological signs. Clinical tests of 'meningeal irritation' (e.g. Kernig's sign, Brudzinski's signs, and nuchal rigidity) are unreliable. Tuberculous, cryptococcal, and other fungal meningitides usually develop more slowly than pyogenic bacterial disease. (2) Post-traumatic bacterial meningitis—often indistinguishable clinically from spontaneous meningitis. (3) Device-associated meningitis—usual presentation is insidious, with features of shunt blockage such as headache, vomiting, fever, and a decreasing level of consciousness.

Investigation and treatment

Speed is of the essence—the first step in the management of acute bacterial meningitis is to obtain blood cultures and start

Acknowledgement: The authors and editors acknowledge the inclusion of material from the chapter by D A Warrell, J J Farrar, and D W M Crook in the 4th edition of the *Oxford Textbook of Medicine*.

antimicrobial therapy and (when indicated) adjunctive dexamethasone, along with providing any necessary supportive care. In the United Kingdom, family doctors are advised to give parenteral antibiotics before transferring the patient to hospital if meningococcal meningitis is suspected.

Lumbar puncture—this is the diagnostic procedure of choice if the diagnosis of bacterial meningitis cannot be ruled out, and can be safely performed without a preceding cranial CT scan to detect brain shift and evidence of herniation provided that the patient does not have any of the following: (1) signs suggesting a space-occupying lesions—papilloedema or focal neurological signs, excluding cranial nerve palsy, (2) new-onset seizure, (3) moderate-to-severe impairment of consciousness, or (4) an immunocompromised state.

The cerebrospinal fluid—the opening pressure is usually raised. Frank turbidity instantly suggests the diagnosis of pyogenic meningitis. On microscopic examination the white blood cell count is typically over 1000 cells/μl, and over 100 cells/μl in over 90% of cases, with neutrophils usually predominant, and organisms may be seen after Gram or acridine orange staining. Elevated protein and depressed glucose concentrations aid in distinction from viral meningitis. Culture of organisms has a sensitivity of about 80% in untreated cases, but this is much reduced in those who have been partially treated, when lumbar puncture results must be interpreted with particular care when attempting to differentiate viral, tuberculous, and bacterial disease. Rapid bacterial antigen tests and tests based on the polymerase chain reaction (PCR) for bacterial DNA are increasingly used.

Antimicrobial therapy—the choice of initial treatment is based on knowledge of which bacteria most commonly cause the disease, based on age and/or clinical circumstances, and on local antimicrobial susceptibility patterns. Adults with community-acquired disease would typically receive initial treatment with (1) vancomycin, with (2) ceftriaxone or cefotaxime, with (if age >50 years, alcoholism, or altered immune status) (3) ampicillin, which would then be modified based on cerebrospinal fluid culture results and in vitro susceptibility testing.

Dexamethasone—this appears to be beneficial in HIV-negative adults with confirmed bacterial meningitis, but there is no evidence for a beneficial effect in those who are HIV-positive and not on antiretroviral drugs.

Complications—these include meningoencephalitis, systemic compromise, stroke, and raised intracranial pressure. Various adjunctive therapies have been described to improve outcome in such patients, including anti-inflammatory agents, anticoagulants, and strategies to reduce intracranial pressure, but there are few randomized clinical studies with which to judge whether they are effective.

Prevention

The incidence of bacterial meningitis can be reduced by (1) vaccination—this is available against H. influenzae type b, pneumococcal and meningococcal disease; (2) chemoprophylaxis—given to close adult contacts of meningococcal disease (and children of <4 years exposed to H. influenzae type b).

Introduction

The association of headache and tinnitus with lethal inflammation of the brain was described by Hippocrates. It was not before the nineteenth century that lumbar puncture was introduced as a diagnostic procedure. Most important in the treatment of bacterial meningitis was the introduction of penicillin in 1940, which reduced the mortality rates of bacterial meningitis to an overall fatality rate of approximately 20%. Despite advances in medical care, the introduction of cranial CT and improvements in intensive care support, the mortality from bacterial meningitis remains high. The global spread of multidrug-resistant bacteria has further complicated the treatment of patients with bacterial meningitis.

Aetiology, genetics, pathogenesis, and pathology

Aetiology

Bacterial meningitis occurs in a number of clinical situations, each of which is associated with a particular pattern of infecting organisms, clinical presentation, and outcome. Spontaneous meningitis is the most important category. It can be divided into neonatal meningitis and meningitis of childhood and adulthood. Post-traumatic meningitis follows neurosurgery or fractures of the skull. Device-associated meningitis complicates the use of cerebrospinal fluid shunts and drains. Infection may also be considered as community acquired or nosocomial (hospital acquired). The bacterial species that cause meningitis vary by geographical region and according to the categories (Table 24.11.1.1). Age and local social conditions influence the attack rate and mortality of spontaneous meningitis.

Neonatal meningitis is usually caused by three species: group B streptococci (Streptococcus agalactiae), Escherichia coli, and Listeria monocytogenes. A wide range of other organisms has been reported to cause the disease. Infection mostly occurs in the postpartum period, but can occur as late as 6 weeks after birth. Prolonged rupture of membranes and low birth weight are important risk factors.

Spontaneous community-acquired meningitis in children (under 14 years of age) is usually caused by Neisseria meningitidis or Strep. pneumoniae. The national implementation of conjugated Haemophilus influenzae type b (Hib) capsular vaccine immunization programmes by many countries during the 1990s has dramatically reduced, or almost eliminated, Hib meningitis; however, meningitis caused by H. influenzae remains common in countries that have not yet implemented a national immunization programme.

In most countries, 80 to 85% of cases of spontaneous community-acquired meningitis in adults are caused by N. meningitidis and Strep. pneumoniae. L. monocytogenes, aerobic Gram-negative bacilli (such as E. coli), H. influenzae, and Staphylococcus aureus cause most of the remaining cases. Strep. suis (group R haemolytic streptococcus) serotype 2 is an important cause of meningitis (and rarely infective endocarditis and septicaemia) in Asia. Hong Kong, Thailand, China, and Vietnam all report Strep. suis as a major cause of adult meningitis.

Post-traumatic meningitis occurs in patients with skull or spinal injuries (i.e. skull fractures) or in those who have undergone head and neck or spinal surgery. It usually arises in association with a cerebrospinal fluid leak and soon after injury, but may occur

Table 24.11.1.1 Causative organisms in community-acquired adult meningitis in the Netherlands, Malawi, and Vietnam

Organism	Nationwide study, the Netherlands, 1998–2002 ($n = 696$)		Queen Elizabeth Central Hospital, Blantyre, Malawi, 1997–1999 ($n = 351$)		Centre for Tropical Diseases, Ho Chi Minh City, Vietnam, 1998–2001 ($n = 500$)	
	No.	%	No.	%	No.	%
Streptococcus pneumoniae	352	51	88	25	38	8
Strep. suis	4	1	–	–	65	13
Gram-negative bacilli	5	1	22	6	11	2
Neisseria meningitidis	257	37	64	18	9	2
Streptococcus spp.	20	3	6	2	11	2
Staphylococcus aureus	9	1	–	–	3	1
Listeria monocytogenes	30	4	–	–	–	–
Haemophilus influenzae	14	2	–	–	7	1
Mycobacterium tuberculosis culture confirmed	–	–	–	–	46	9
Probable tuberculous meningitis	–	–	44	13	210	42
Other probable bacterial meningitis	–	–	59	17	5	1
No confirmation of bacteria	–	–	68	19	90	19

many years after the trauma. The risk of developing meningitis is as high as 25% with a clinically apparent cerebrospinal fluid leak. The aetiology depends on whether the infection is acquired nosocomially or in the community. Most hospital-acquired infections are caused by aerobic Gram-negative bacilli, such as *E. coli*, *Klebsiella pneumoniae*, other Enterobacteriaceae, *Acinetobacter* spp., and *Pseudomonas* spp. Less commonly, *Strep. pneumoniae*, *H. influenzae*, *Staph. aureus*, and other normal upper respiratory tract flora cause meningitis in patients in hospital. Post-traumatic meningitis acquired in the community is caused mainly by *Strep. pneumoniae*.

Device-associated meningitis is a well-recognized entity occurring in patients with cerebrospinal fluid drains and shunts. Most infections are nosocomial and caused by coagulase-negative staphylococci (50–60%) and *Staph. aureus* (15–30%). Aerobic Gram-negative bacilli, streptococci, *Corynebacterium* spp., and *Propionibacterium acnes* are encountered. These infections usually present within a few months of inserting the device. Occasionally, *Strep. pneumoniae*, *N. meningitidis*, and *H. influenzae* are responsible.

Recurrent meningitis is an unusual (5–10% of meningitis) but well-recognized clinical category (see Chapter 24.11.2). Such cases frequently have either an underlying anatomical or an underlying immunological defect. The immune deficiencies that most often predispose to recurrent meningitis are hypogammaglobulinaemia and complement deficiencies. Consideration should be given to immunizing such patients against the most common pathogens.

Genetics

Genetic factors are major determinants of susceptibility to infectious diseases (Fig. 24.11.1.1). All individuals have single base-pair alterations (single-nucleotide polymorphisms, SNPs) in genes controlling the host response to microbes. In sepsis, identified alterations include SNPs in tumour necrosis factor (TNF) receptors, interleukin-1 (IL-1) receptors, Fcγ receptors, and Toll-like receptors (TLRs). In patients with sepsis due to *N. meningitidis*,

conflicting results on SNPs and outcome have been reported. In bacterial meningitis research on genetic factors is lacking but may provide important pathophysiological insights. Bacterial meningitis is a complex disorder in which injury is caused, in part, by the causative organism and, in part, by the host's own inflammatory response. Particular subgroups of patients with a genetic predisposition to more severe illness, potentially mediated through their innate immune response is possible, and further work in this area may help design rationale adjunct therapy.

Pathogenesis

The acquisition of infection and mode of invasion of the cerebrospinal fluid vary with the type of meningitis. However, once infection is established, the inflammatory injury and pathophysiology are similar in all types of bacterial meningitis.

The organisms that cause neonatal meningitis are acquired by the baby from the vagina and perineum during delivery or from

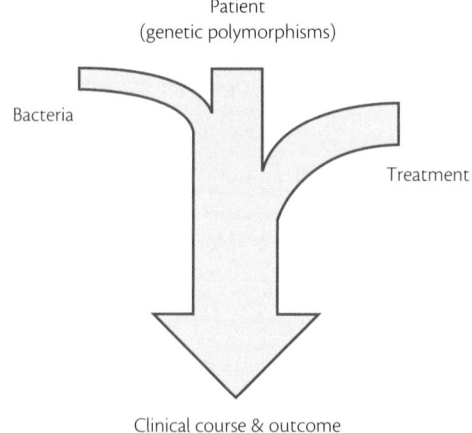

Fig. 24.11.1.1 The interaction of genotype, causative bacteria, and intervention in bacterial meningitis.

the environment soon after birth. The three main infecting species, *Strep. agalactiae* (group B streptococci), *E. coli*, and *L. monocytogenes*, invade the host and cause septicaemia and meningitis. An unusual feature of *E. coli* and many *Strep. agalactiae* strains (capsular types K1 and III, respectively) is that their capsules consist of polysialic acid. The association of this unusual type of capsule with two virulent strains suggests a role in the pathogenesis of neonatal meningitis.

Causative organisms of spontaneous meningitis, *Strep. pneumoniae* and *N. meningitidis*, are acquired by person-to-person spread (see Chapters 7.6.3 and 7.6.5). Nasopharyngeal colonization by bacteria generally leads to asymptomatic carriage. Invasion of the host is particularly likely to occur early after acquisition of the organism, before the host has developed protective immunity. Carriage is sufficient to produce immunity and resistance to disease. The greatest risk of disease, therefore, is in the first few years of life, at a time when the nonimmune host first encounters these pathogens. The precise anatomical site of invasion is not known for these pathogens. In response to the local generation of inflammatory factors, however, as seen in the presence of viral infections, the composition of surface components on target epithelial and endothelial cells changes. Binding of bacteria to up-regulated receptors (e.g. platelet-activating-factor receptors) promotes migration through the respiratory epithelium and vascular endothelium, resulting in invasive disease. Once the bacterium invades the bloodstream, the host can react with massive activation of inflammatory cascades. The main cascade pathways that are involved are the complement system, inflammatory response, and coagulation and fibrinolysis pathways. These pathways do not act independently but are able to interact. Genetic polymorphisms among components of these pathways (e.g. complement deficiencies and defects in sensing or opsonophagocytic pathways) are involved in the susceptibility to infection, as well as to severity of disease and outcome. Cytokines coordinate a wide variety of inflammatory reactions and play an important role in the initiation, maintenance, and termination of inflammatory reactions. Prominent proinflammatory cytokines include TNFα, IL-1, and IL-6. Essential parts of the inflammatory response include activation of coagulation and fibrin deposition, shifting the haemostatic balance towards thrombosis.

Pathogens can enter the central nervous system (CNS) via the bloodstream and via the blood–brain barrier, or by direct invasion through the external barrier (e.g. invade the cerebrospinal fluid directly through an anatomical defect). Shunt-associated meningitis is caused mainly by organisms that colonize the skin and contaminate the surgical wound and prosthetic material at the time of surgery. The infected shunt becomes coated with a film of adherent bacteria, commonly referred to as a 'biofilm', which is not susceptible to clinically achievable levels of antibiotic. Such infections are usually incurable unless the foreign material is removed.

The blood–brain barrier is formed by cerebral microvascular endothelial cells that restrict blood-borne pathogen invasion. Cytokines stimulate cell-surface expression of receptors, which allows binding to activated endothelial cells and invasion of bacteria into the subarachnoid space. Physiologically, concentrations of leucocytes, antibodies, and complement components in the subarachnoid space are low. This condition facilitates multiplication of bacteria, which undergo autolysis under conditions such as growth to stationary phase or exposure to antibiotics. Lysis of bacteria leads to the release of immunostimulatory and/or toxic

bacterial products. Bacterial cell-wall products (e.g. lipopolysaccharide and lipoteichoic acid), bacterial toxins (e.g. pneumolysin), and bacterial DNA induce a severe inflammatory response via binding to TLRs. TLRs play a key role in innate immunity by their capacity to recognize conserved molecular patterns shared by several microorganisms. Once engaged, TLRs transmit the activating signal into the cell and thereby initiate the induction of genes, such as costimulatory molecules and inflammatory cytokines. Thus far, 11 members of the TLR family have been identified in mammals. Whereas TLR2 is considered the key receptor for pneumococci and other Gram-positive bacteria, TLR4 seems to play an important role in meningococcal and other Gram-negative bacterial infections. TLR-mediated signalling pathways are now being elucidated. Studies in experimental pneumococcal meningitis have demonstrated that the key pathway is dependent on myeloid differentiation factor 88, which induces early phase activation of NF-κB. The inflammatory cascade induces various pathophysiological alterations, such as migration of leucocytes across the blood–brain barrier (leading to cerebrospinal fluid pleocytosis) and increased blood–brain barrier permeability. TNF-α and IL-1β stimulate the expression of chemokines and adhesion molecules, which play an important role in the influx of leucocytes from the circulation to the cerebrospinal fluid. Although Fas (CD95) and Fas ligand (FasL, CD95L) have been implicated as being involved in the acute inflammatory response by attracting neutrophils and regulating their survival, animal studies in pneumococcal meningitis have shown that they are not essential in the regulation of the acute inflammatory response during this disease. On stimulation with bacterial components, leucocytes release a broad range of potentially tissue-destructive agents that contribute to vasospasm and vasculitis, including oxidants (e.g. peroxynitrite) and proteolytic enzymes such as matrix metalloproteases. Evidence in animal studies of meningitis suggests that multiple types of programmed cell death play a central role in the complex balance among invading bacteria, the immune system, and host cells, leading to inflammation and tissue damage in infections. In addition, animal studies demonstrated that loss of ependymal cells and ciliary function expose the underlying neuronal milieu to host and bacterial cytotoxins which are likely to contribute to the neuropathology commonly observed in meningitis. The cell walls of Gram-positive bacteria and lipopolysaccharides of Gram-negative bacteria cause inflammatory change, thereby increasing vascular permeability and leading to the development of cerebral oedema.

The inflammatory reaction in meningitis is associated with a number of severe alterations in the normal physiology of the CNS (Fig. 24.11.2). (1) Permeability of the blood–brain barrier increases, which is best measured by the increased penetration of the cerebrospinal fluid by albumin. Also, antibiotic penetration of the cerebrospinal fluid is enhanced. (2) Increased intracranial pressure results from cerebral oedema secondary to an accumulation of interstitial fluid, and communicating hydrocephalus is caused by decreased cerebrospinal fluid reabsorption and cellular swelling secondary to cell injury. (3) A vasculitis may affect mainly the large vessels traversing the subarachnoid space. This vascular injury may not only disrupt the normal autoregulation of cerebral blood flow, but, in severe cases, the vessel may become obstructed with thrombus, causing a cerebral infarct. The major impact of increased intracranial pressure and vasculitis is decreased cerebral perfusion, causing general hypoxic brain injury.

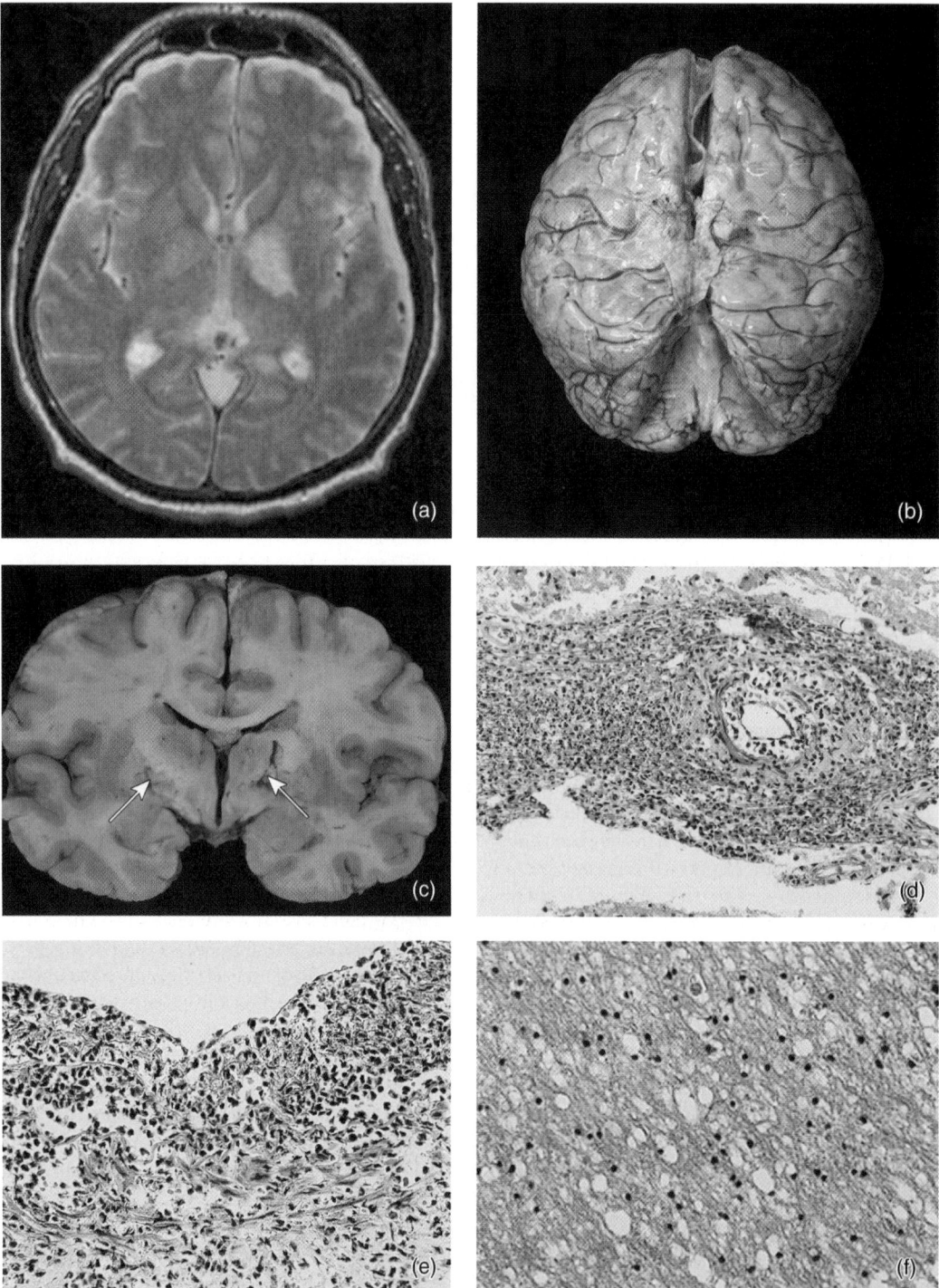

Fig. 24.11.1.2 Multiple complications in a patient with pneumococcal meningitis. (a) proton-density T_2-weighted MRI of the brain shows a transverse view of a hyperintense signal in the basal ganglia that indicates bilateral oedema. (b) A postmortem view of the brain of the same patient shows yellowish-coloured meninges as a result of extensive inflammation. (c) Confirmation of the bilateral infarction of the basal ganglia. The microscopic substrate in the same patient shows a meningeal artery with (d) lymphocytic infiltration in and around the vessel wall, (e) extensive subpial necrotizing cortical inflammation, and (f) oedema in the white matter. Published previously by van de Beek, *et al.* (2006). *Nature Clin Pract Neurol*, **2**(9), 504–16.

Pathology

There is diffuse acute inflammation of the pia arachnoid, with migration of neutrophil leucocytes and exudation of fibrin into the cerebrospinal fluid. Pus accumulates over the surface of the brain, especially around its base and the emerging cranial nerves, and around the spinal cord. The meningeal vessels are dilated and congested and may be surrounded by pus (see Fig. 24.11.1.2). Pus and fibrin are found in the ventricles and there is ventriculitis, with loss of ependymal lining and subependymal gliosis. Within the subarachnoid space and intraventricular system, infection may produce blockages of cerebrospinal fluid circulation, especially at the various foramina or in the aqueduct, causing obstructive hydrocephalus or spinal block. If reabsorption of cerebrospinal fluid across the subarachnoid granulations is prevented by a sub-arachnoid haematoma or empyema or thrombosis of the intracranial veins and venous sinuses, communicating hydrocephalus will result. In patients with meningitis, intracranial hypertension may be the result of cerebral oedema, the ventricular dilatation of hydrocephalus, or subdural or epidural collections of pus.

Cerebrovascular complications occur in 15 to 20% of patients with bacterial meningitis (see Fig. 24.11.1.2). In patients with pneumococcal meningitis, brain infarction is the cause of death in 14% of fatal episodes. Other abnormalities include subdural effusion or empyema, septic thrombosis of the cerebral venous sinuses, subarachnoid haematomas, compression of intracranial structures as a result of intracranial hypertension, and herniation of the temporal lobes or cerebellum. Gross changes, such as pressure coning, which would provide an obvious cause of death, are rarely found. In some cases death may be attributable to related septicaemia, although the familiar finding of bilateral adrenal haemorrhage (Waterhouse–Friederichsen syndrome) may well be a terminal phenomenon rather than a cause of fatal adrenal insufficiency as was once imagined. Patients with meningococcal septicaemia may develop acute pulmonary oedema. Myocarditis was a common finding in some series of patients.

Epidemiology

The attack rate of endemic meningitis caused by N. meningitidis is usually low (1–5 cases/10^5 persons per year), but occasionally the incidence of the infection may increase and even reach epidemic proportions (e.g. > 300 cases/10^5 persons per year). Crowding is thought to play a role in the epidemics occurring in military recruits, South African miners, and other groups of people crowded together in closed environments. The attack rate of N. meningitidis disease may increase secondarily to epidemics of influenza A. However, the precise origin of the major epidemics affecting regions such as sub-Saharan Africa remains unexplained. The bacterial capsule plays a role in determining the pattern of invasive disease caused by N. meningitidis. Capsulate serogroups A, B, and C occur sporadically and cause outbreaks of invasive disease, whereas serogroups Y, W, Z, W-135, and 29-E cause only occasional cases. Meningococcal virulence is related to capsule expression, expression of other surface structures, and underlying genotype.

The attack rate of Strep. pneumoniae meningitis (1–2 cases/10^5 persons per year) is remarkably constant around the world. The highest attack rate of all three bacterial species is in children under 1 year of age and falls off rapidly with increasing age. The decrease in susceptibility with increasing age results from the acquisition of protective immunity, mainly as a result of nasopharyngeal carriage. It increases in patients aged over 50 years. A high proportion of pneumococcal cases exhibit an associated infective focus. Otitis media or sinusitis is found in approximately 30% of cases and pneumonia in up to 25%. Hypogammaglobulinaemia (primary or secondary, e.g. in nephrotic syndrome and chronic lymphocytic leukaemia), sickle cell disease, splenic dysfunction or splenectomy, and previous trauma to the skull (see below) are risk factors for developing pneumococcal meningitis.

Strep. suis (group R haemolytic streptococci) serotype 2 infection is related to occupational contact with pigs or pork, but the precise epidemiology remains poorly understood. In the Netherlands the incidence of S. suis meningitis among abattoir workers and pig breeders was 3/100 000 per year. It is reported to be the most common cause of adult pyogenic meningitis in Vietnam. Possible routes of entry include skin abrasions, found in 40% of patients, and upper respiratory and gastrointestinal tracts. Splenectomized patients are particularly at risk, as with other capsulated Gram-positive organisms. Although rarely fatal Strep. suis is commonly associated with bilateral permanent deafness.

Worldwide, L. monocytogenes accounts for few cases of meningitis, with an attack rate of approximately 0.2 to 0.4 cases/10^5 persons per year or 1 to 5% of the cases of meningitis. Increased attack rates have been associated with contaminated foods such as unpasteurized soft cheeses, pâté, and poorly refrigerated precooked chicken. Meningitis due to L. monocytogenes is a disease that occurs among immunocompromised patients (e.g. attributable to immunosuppressive therapy, immunosenescence, diabetes, or malignancies) and older people. Staph. aureus causes 1 to 5% of the cases of spontaneous meningitis and usually occurs in association with infective endocarditis. Spontaneous cases of H. influenzae meningitis, both capsulate type b and non-capsulate strains, account for up to 5% of adult cases of meningitis. Aerobic Gram-negative (i.e. E. coli) meningitis occurs especially in aged, debilitated, and diabetic people. The source in these infections is usually thought to be the renal tract.

The increasing incidence of HIV infection has altered the presentation and pattern of aetiological agents causing meningitis. A large series of adult patients with meningitis who presented to the Queen Elizabeth Central Hospital in Blantyre, Malawi, was reported in 1975. At that time, meningitis comprised 2.5% of medical admissions, the most common pathogens being N. meningitidis and Strep. pneumoniae. Since then, the population of Malawi has been severely affected by the AIDS pandemic, and the HIV seroprevalence of antenatal women has climbed steadily through the 1980s to the present level of more than 30%. The changed overall pattern in this series is probably due to the influence of HIV infection; in a survey of 153 patients with invasive pneumococcal disease, HIV seroprevalence was 95%. In South Africa, HIV-infected children have more antibiotic-resistant isolates and a different clinical presentation compared with HIV-uninfected children. In adults, the HIV epidemic was found to be responsible for increasing chronic infections such as tuberculous and cryptococcal meningitides.

Another epidemiological trend is emerging of antibiotic-resistant strains of Strep. pneumoniae. Pneumococci resistance to penicillin, due to changes in its penicillin-binding proteins, was first reported in 1965. The prevalence of such resistance was limited until an epidemic of highly resistant pneumococci occurred in South Africa in 1977. Since then, resistance has developed worldwide and in some regions it occurs in a frequency up to 70%. Reports of reduced susceptibility of pneumococci to several antibiotics, including broad-spectrum cephalosporins, have also been published. In response to this epidemiological trend, recommendations for suspected and confirmed bacterial meningitis have necessarily evolved.

Prevention

Immunization

Vaccines to the three major pathogens causing community-acquired meningitis are available. H. influenzae type b capsular conjugate (Hib) vaccines are now routinely given in the developed world and there has been a dramatic reduction in the incidence of *H. influenzae* type b meningitis in these countries and invasive disease has been essentially eliminated (see Chapter 7.6.12). However, it remains an important cause of meningitis in most of the world where vaccine programmes have not been implemented.

Current pneumococcal vaccines elicit immune responses to cell-wall polysaccharides of pneumococci (Chapter 7.6.3). The current 23-valent pneumococcal polysaccharide vaccine contains capsular polysaccharides of 23 serotypes responsible for about 90% of invasive pneumococcal infections. In the United States of America, the vaccine is recommended for all people aged 65 years and older and for those aged between 2 and 64 years who are at increased risk for invasive pneumococcal disease because of underlying illnesses, such as asplenia or immunodeficiency (e.g. infection with HIV or use of immunosuppressive drugs), or renal failure. However, the vaccine is poorly immunogenic in certain groups at high risk for invasive pneumococcal infection, especially children younger than 2 years old (with relatively immature B cells), older people, and immunocompromised patients. The immune response in infants and young children can be improved by conjugation of pneumococcal polysaccharides to carrier proteins that enable activation of T cells, thereby enhancing antibody production and immunological memory.

The seven-valent pneumococcal conjugate vaccine (PCV7) consists of seven capsular polysaccharides that are among the most prevalent in children aged 6 months to 2 years, include most antibiotic-resistant types, and are highly represented in immuno-compromised and older patients. In the United States of America, the use of four doses of PCV7 is recommended for all children aged 23 months and younger and those aged 24 to 59 months with chronic illnesses, including sickle cell disease, immunocompromising conditions, and cochlear implants. In Europe, the integration of PCV7 into immunization programmes was delayed and guidelines that recommend pneumococcal immunization in children vary substantially across European countries. On the basis of current recommendations, approximately 40% of the birth cohort in Spain could be immunized, whereas this proportion in France is estimated to be 80 to 90%. The introduction of PCV7 in the United States of America has reduced the burden of invasive pneumococcal disease in children as well as in older age groups through herd immunity. As a consequence, bacterial meningitis has become a disease predominantly of adults rather than of infants and children.

Although effects on nasopharyngeal colonization are counterbalanced by strain replacement with nonvaccine strains, these immunization guidelines are expected to reduce the prevalence of antibiotic-resistant strains. Although no large increase in invasive pneumococcal disease by nonvaccine serotypes has been described, this potential side effect is an extra reason to continue active surveillance of this disease. Patients with anatomical defects leading to an increased risk of invasive pneumococcal disease (i.e. previous trauma to the skull) may be at risk of unusual pneumococcal serotypes not commonly associated with invasive disease.

Since 1905, major epidemics of meningococcal meningitis have occurred in sub-Saharan Africa every few years (see Chapter 7.6.5). For epidemic meningitis control in sub-Saharan Africa, the World Health Organization recommends a strategy of emergency immunization with meningococcal A/C polysaccharide vaccine when epidemic thresholds are exceeded. Given the relatively poor routine immunization coverage in this region, current strategies of immunization campaigns that achieve higher coverage would generally be more effective and less costly than model routine-scheduled programmes, assuming that campaigns can be rapidly implemented. In other regions of the world, invasive infections caused by *N. meningitidis* serogroup C have increased over the past 10 years, prompting the introduction of routine immunization with serogroup C meningococcal polysaccharide–protein conjugate vaccines.

Immunization should be considered in all patients with recurrent meningitis or traumatic head injury, and in splenectomized patients.

Chemoprophylaxis

The attack rate of meningitis is higher in the immediate contacts of an index case of meningococcal (up to 1000-fold) or *H. influenzae* type b meningitis (500-fold only in children under 4 years of age) than in the population at large. The administration of rifampicin or ciprofloxacin eliminates the carrier state and is assumed to eliminate the risk of secondary cases of meningitis (see Table 24.11.1.3). Close adult contacts of meningococcal disease are given either rifampicin (300 mg every 12 h for 2 days) or a single oral dose of ciprofloxacin (750 mg). Doctors, nurses, and other health care workers need not be given chemoprophylaxis unless they have given mouth-to-mouth resuscitation.

There is no evidence of benefit of antibiotics administered prophylactically to patients with skull fractures and/or cerebrospinal fluid leakage. Surgical closure of the leak is the only effective means of preventing meningitis in such cases. The prevention of device-associated meningitis relies on rigorous infection control. Ventricular and lumbar drains should be removed as soon as possible. Shunt insertion should be performed while adhering to strict aseptic techniques, and surgical antibiotic prophylaxis may also help to reduce shunt infection.

Clinical features

Community-acquired bacterial meningitis

Early diagnosis and rapid initiation of appropriate therapy are vital in the treatment of patients with bacterial meningitis. A recent study provided a systematic assessment of the sequence and development of early symptoms in children and adolescents with meningococcal disease (encompassing the spectrum of disease from sepsis to meningitis) before admission to the hospital. Classic symptoms of rash, meningismus, and impaired consciousness develop late in the pre-hospital illness, if at all. Early signs before admission in adolescents with meningococcal disease were leg pain and cold hands and feet.

Bacterial meningitis is often considered but may be difficult to recognize. The clinical presentation of a patient with bacterial meningitis may vary depending on age, underlying conditions, and severity of illness. Clinical findings of meningitis in young children are often minimal and in childhood bacterial meningitis and in older patients classic symptoms such as headache, fever, nuchal rigidity, and altered mental status may be less common than in younger and middle-aged adults. Infants may become irritable or lethargic or stop feeding, and are found to have a bulging fontanelle, separation of the cranial sutures, meningism, and opisthotonos, and they may develop convulsions. These findings are uncommon in neonates, who sometimes present with respiratory distress, diarrhoea, or jaundice.

In a prospective study on adults with bacterial meningitis, the classic triad of signs and symptoms consisting of fever, nuchal rigidity, and altered mental status was present in only 44% of the patients. Certain clinical features may predict the bacterial cause of meningitis. Predisposing conditions such as ear or sinus infections, pneumonia, immunocompromise, and dural fistulae are estimated to be present in 68 to 92% of adults with pneumococcal meningitis. Rashes occur more frequently in patients with meningococcal meningitis, with reported sensitivities of 63 to 80% and with specificities of 83 to 92%. Rash is occasionally seen in patients with echovirus type 9, leptospirosis, *Staph. aureus, Strep. pneumoniae, Strep. suis, H. influenzae, salmonella enterica* Serovar Typhi, and other infections, especially in those associated with infective endocarditis. The brownish or reddish geometrical, vasculitic rash of fulminant meningococcaemia is unmistakable and, characteristically, the toes and fingers become necrotic (Fig. 24.11.1.3).

Seizures before admission occur in 5 to 9% of all cases, and 15 to 23% of patients develop seizures during their clinical course. Cranial nerve palsy is relatively rare; most commonly affected are cranial nerves VIII (6%), III (4%), IV (3%), and VII (2%). Focal cerebral findings (aphasia, hemiparesis, and monoparesis) on admission occur in approximately 15 to 23% of patients. Papilloedema is uncommon in patients with acute bacterial meningitis (3 to 4% of patients; however, in most studies the results of fundoscopic examination were not recorded). Systemic manifestations, such as hypotension and tachycardia, occur frequently in community-acquired bacterial meningitis.

Bilateral sensorineural deafness develops early, 2 to 9 days after the start of symptoms, in most patients with *Strep. suis* type 2

meningitis. Initially associated with tinnitus this may progress to complete deafness within 24 h. Bacteria probably invade the cochlea via the cochlear aqueduct from the subarachnoid space to produce suppurative labyrinthitis and acute deafness. Associated clinical features of *Strep. suis* meningitis include nerve III palsy, septic arthritis, and purpuric skin lesions. Arthritis occurs in 7% of adults with bacterial meningitis, most commonly in meningococcal meningitis, but is also seen in 5% of patients with *Strep. suis*. Recognition of concurrent arthritis is important because prolonged antibiotic therapy is necessary.

The presence or absence of meningeal signs such as Kernig's sign, Brudzinski's signs, and nuchal rigidity are physical examination findings often documented when evaluating a patient for possible meningitis. Kernig's sign was first described in the 1880s and was originally done with the patient in the sitting position, but today is frequently done in the supine position. This test involves flexing the hip and extending the knee and a positive result is recorded when pain is elicited in the back and legs. Brudzinski's neck sign is typically done in the supine position where the head is passively flexed and is interpreted as positive when flexion at the hips to lift the legs is elicited in response. Nuchal rigidity is a clinical determination of severe neck stiffness and inability to passively flex and extend the head in a normal fashion. Local causes of neck stiffness, such as local sepsis (i.e. in the nuchal muscles or cervical lymph nodes), cervical spondylitis (particularly common in older people), temporomandibular arthritis, dental problems, and pharyngeal lesions, should be considered.

A prospective study of 297 adults evaluated Kernig's sign, Brudzinski's sign, and nuchal rigidity and their relationship to meningitis diagnosed by lumbar puncture. This study found that none of these signs accurately identified patients with meningitis. There was no correlation with moderate meningeal inflammation or with microbial evidence of infection (such as positive Gram

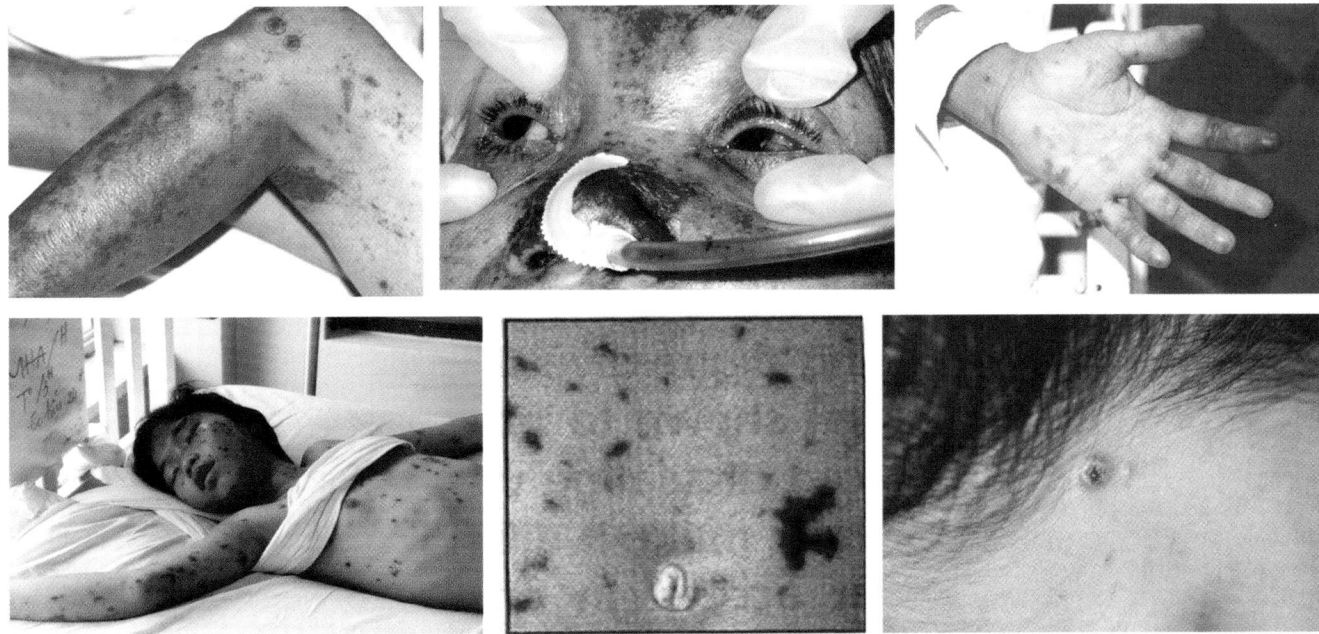

Fig. 24.11.1.3 Rashes in a patient with meningococcal meningitis.

stain or positive cultures), and Kernig's and Brudzinski's signs were found to have poor sensitivity (5%) with high specificity (95%). In this study population, 80 of 297 patients had meningitis, but only 24 had nuchal rigidity (sensitivity, 30%). Nuchal rigidity was absent in 148 of the 217 patients without meningitis (specificity, 68%). Notably, only 3 of the 297 patients had bacterial meningitis by cerebrospinal fluid culture, and nuchal rigidity failed to identify 2 of these 3 patients with bacterial meningitis.

Post-traumatic bacterial meningitis

This is often indistinguishable clinically from spontaneous meningitis. However, in obtunded or unconscious patients who have suffered a recent or previous head injury, few clinical signs may be present. A fever and deterioration in the level of consciousness or loss of vital functions may be the only signs of meningitis. Finding a cerebrospinal fluid leak adds support to the possibility of meningitis in such patients, but this is undetectable in most cases. The range of bacteria causing meningitis in these patients is broad and consideration should be given to broad-spectrum antibiotics including metronidazole for anaerobic pathogens.

Infections of cerebrospinal fluid shunts

Patients may present with clinical features typical of spontaneous meningitis, especially if virulent organisms are involved. The more usual presentation is insidious, with features of shunt blockage such as headache, vomiting, fever, and a decreasing level of consciousness. Fever is a helpful sign, but is not a constant feature and may be present in as few as 20% of cases. Shunts can be infected without causing meningitis, in which event the features of the infection will be determined by where the shunt drains. Infection of shunts draining into the venous system produces a disease similar to chronic right-sided infective endocarditis together with glomerulonephritis (shunt nephritis), whereas infection of shunts draining into the peritoneal cavity produces peritonitis.

Differential diagnosis

When a patient presents to an Emergency Department physician, primary care doctor, neurologist, or infectious disease specialist for an emergent evaluation, the patient history can help to estimate the probability of meningitis. A wide variety of patient complaints may be elicited from patients with meningitis, and a meta-analysis that included 845 patients over a 30-year period showed poor sensitivity and specificity for symptoms such as headache, nausea, and vomiting for the diagnosis of meningitis. This is not surprising since such nonspecific symptoms are found in many patients with a wide variety of clinical conditions. Viral meningitis is important in the differential diagnosis.

Meningeal irritation is seen in many acute febrile conditions, especially in children. Local infections of the nasopharynx, cervical lymph nodes, muscles, and spine may produce convincing neck stiffness. Tetanus may be easily confused with meningitis if the persisting rigidity and recurrent spasms go unnoticed. In all these conditions the cerebrospinal fluid will be normal. Subarachnoid haemorrhage can present with sudden headache, neck stiffness, and deteriorating consciousness, and a less dramatic progression of symptoms is seen in patients with some intracranial tumours.

Tuberculous and cryptococcal and other fungal meningitides usually develop more slowly than pyogenic bacterial meningitis.

They may be distinguished by examining cerebrospinal fluid. Cryptococci and free-living amoebae may be mistaken for lymphocytes in the cerebrospinal fluid unless an India-ink preparation is examined to reveal the cryptococcal capsule and the characteristic movements of amoebae. Aseptic meningitis comprises a large number of conditions, many of them caused by viruses, in which there are clinical signs of meningism and the cerebrospinal fluid is found to be abnormal (see Chapter 24.11.2). This group includes partially treated bacterial meningitis and the chemical meningitides, resulting from the introduction of irritants into the subarachnoid space (contrast media, antimicrobial agents, and contaminants of lumbar puncture and spinal anaesthesia). The cerebrospinal fluid glucose concentration may be very low. Discharge of a tuberculoma may produce a sterile tuberculin reaction, and the discharge of the contents of a craniopharyngioma or epidermoid cyst into the cerebrospinal fluid can also cause chemical meningitis.

Clinical investigations

Lumbar puncture

Once an initial patient evaluation has been completed with history and physical findings, lumbar puncture is the diagnostic procedure of choice if the diagnosis of bacterial meningitis cannot be ruled out. Characteristic findings in the cerebrospinal fluid are typically used to make the diagnosis of meningitis.

Indications for CT scan before lumbar puncture

In view of the urgent nature of this testing to make the diagnosis of meningitis, one of the issues that physicians are faced with in the hospital Emergency Department is whether neuroimaging—either CT or MRI—is required before lumbar puncture. Patients with expanding masses (e.g. subdural empyema, brain abscess, or necrotic temporal lobe in herpes simplex virus encephalitis) may present with symptoms that appear to be identical with those of bacterial meningitis. In these patients, lumbar puncture may be complicated by brain herniation. The withdrawal of cerebrospinal fluid reduces counterpressure from below, thereby adding to the effect of compression from above, increasing the brain shift that may already be present. In patients with suspected bacterial meningitis the interpretation of cranial imaging should be focused on brain shift and space around the brainstem, which may result from the pressure effects of a focal space-occupying lesion or severe diffuse brain swelling as illustrated in Fig. 24.11.1.4.

Recommendations for cranial CT and fears of herniation are based on the observed clinical deterioration of a few patients in the several to many hours after lumbar puncture and the perceived temporal relationship of lumbar puncture and herniation, but as previously mentioned proving a cause-and-effect association is very difficult based on the available data. Therefore, it is reasonable to proceed with lumbar puncture without a CT scan if the patient does not meet any of the following criteria: patients who have new-onset seizures, an immunocompromised state, signs suggestive of space-occupying lesions (papilloedema or focal neurological signs—not including cranial nerve palsy), or moderate-to-severe impairment of consciousness. Other contraindications to lumbar puncture include local skin sepsis at the site of puncture, a clinically unstable patient, and any clinical suspicion of spinal cord compression. Lumbar puncture may also be harmful in patients with coagulopathy, because of the chance of needle-induced

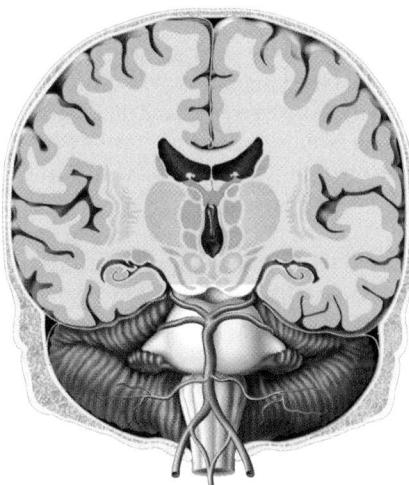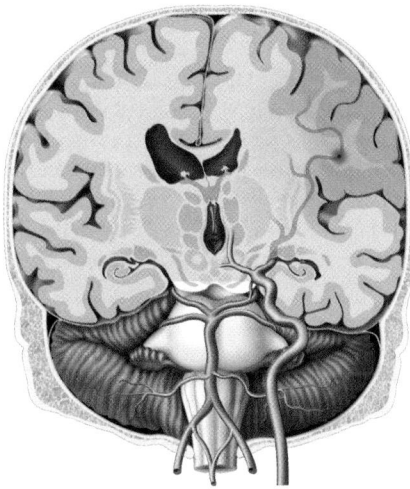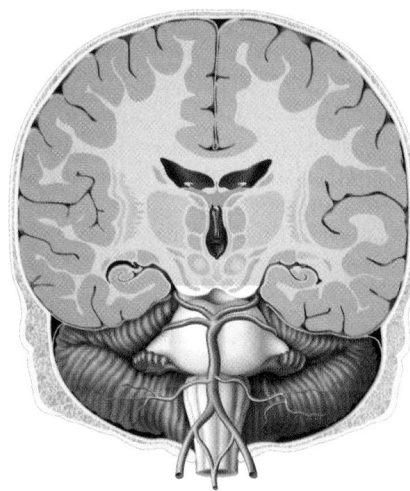

Fig. 24.11.1.4 Cranial imaging to evaluate potential contraindications for lumbar puncture should be focused on identifying signs of a focal space-occupying lesion, evidence of brain shift, and/or signs of severe diffuse brain swelling. (a) Normal brain, (b) meningitis-associated cerebral infarct causing pronounced brain shift, and (c) diffuse brain swelling associated with severe infection. Initial lumbar puncture should not be done when CT findings of significant brain shift are found, and empirical therapy for meningitis should be continued in such patients.
Published previously by Fitch and van de Beek (2007). *Lancet Infect Dis*, **7**(3), 191–200.

subarachnoid haemorrhage or of the development of spinal subdural and epidural haematomas. Contraindications for (immediate) lumbar puncture are provided in Box 24.11.1.1.

Examination of cerebrospinal fluid (see Chapter 24.3.1)

In patients with bacterial meningitis, the cerebrospinal fluid opening pressure is usually raised (>200 mmCSF), and occasionally it is markedly raised (>500 mmCSF). Frank turbidity of cerebrospinal fluid instantly suggests the diagnosis of pyogenic meningitis. Microscopic examination of cerebrospinal fluid for white cells, red cells, and organisms, the measurement of glucose and protein, and culture are important investigations in a case of possible meningitis. Classically described, the white blood cell count in bacterial meningitis is typically greater than 1000 cells/μl, although in viral meningitis it is less than 300 cells/μl—although considerable overlap exists in these categories. The neutrophil count is typically elevated in bacterial meningitis compared with viral meningitis. A raised cerebrospinal fluid white blood cell (WBC) count is present in most patients with bacterial meningitis but, rarely, the count may be normal (fewer than 6 WBC/μl, all lymphocytes) but the cerebrospinal fluid may still appear turbid because of the vast numbers of bacteria. Most cases (more than 90%) present with a count exceeding 100 WBC/μl. The measurement of protein and glucose is an important aspect of cerebrospinal fluid analysis to complement the cell counts because abnormal protein and glucose levels are typically found in bacterial disease but are relatively normal in many cases of viral meningitis. Gram or acridine orange stain of cerebrospinal fluid samples, although having reported sensitivities of only 50 to 90% can certainly help to make the diagnosis of bacterial disease with a specificity approaching 100%. Care should be taken in assessment of the cerebrospinal fluid in patients who have been partially treated with antibiotics before being seen. In this case the cerebrospinal fluid may be very difficult to interpret and the cerebrospinal fluid from partially treated pyogenic meningitis and tuberculosis (TB) meningitis can be extremely difficult. An algorithm based on readily available clinical and laboratory tests can be useful in deciding whether the patient has pyogenic meningitis or TB meningitis.

Culture of organisms has a sensitivity of approximately 80% in untreated cases, and is aided by the culture of good volumes of cerebrospinal fluid and minimizing the delay between the lumbar puncture and setting up of the culture. Organisms are recovered much less often from partially treated cases. Isolation of an organism is not only helpful in establishing the diagnosis, but allows the identification and susceptibility testing of the aetiological agent. The culture result can also be used to decide on the need for antibiotic prophylaxis, contact tracing, and other public health control measures.

A range of rapid bacterial antigen tests may be helpful in detecting the presence of bacterial capsular polysaccharide antigens of pneumococci, meningococci, *H. influenzae*, and group B streptococci. These tests may reach a sensitivity and specificity of 90% or greater for detecting specific causes of bacterial meningitis.

Box 24.11.1.1 Contraindications for immediate lumbar puncture

Neuroimaging before lumbar puncture to detect brain shift

◆ Signs of brain shift
  • Papilloedema
  • Focal neurological signs, not including cranial nerve palsy
◆ Glasgow Coma Score <10
◆ Severe immunocompromised state
◆ New-onset seizures

Other contraindications for lumbar puncture

◆ Serious skin infection at site lumbar puncture
◆ Septic shock
◆ Spinal cord compression
◆ Anticoagulant therapy or severe coagulopathy

However, in our experience these tests seldom add to the diagnostic yield of a good Gram or acridine orange stain performed on an adequate volume of cerebrospinal fluid. New molecular techniques for detecting bacteria in the cerebrospinal fluid by polymerase chain reaction (PCR) methods have emerged as powerful tools in the diagnosis of patients with negative cultures of cerebrospinal fluid; such tools have high sensitivity and specificity, although further refinements are needed before PCR can be routinely recommended.

Recurrent bacterial meningitis (see Chapter 24.11.2)

In patients with no apparent cause of recurrent meningitis or known history of head trauma, the high prevalence of remote head injury and cerebrospinal fluid leakage justifies an active search for anatomical defects and cerebrospinal fluid leakage in a patient with recurrent bacterial meningitis. Detection of β_2-transferrin in nasal discharge in cases of rhinorrhoea is a sensitive and specific method to confirm the presence of a cerebrospinal fluid leak. Optimum imaging is done by thin-slice CT of the skull base and is also the initial imaging of choice. It is important to take into account that small bone defects on CT do not prove cerebrospinal fluid leakage. T_2-weighted MRI may detect a small cerebrospinal fluid leak, but lacks fine bone detail. As cerebrospinal fluid leaks are often intermittent, the administration of intrathecal contrast will not be more accurate to prove leakage and depends on the timing of imaging. Anatomical defects and cerebrospinal fluid leakage might require consultation of a neurosurgeon or otolaryngologist to evaluate the necessity of surgical repair, which has an overall high success rate and a low mortality and morbidity.

Emergency management

Management algorithm

Although some guidelines propose an arbitrary time-based goal for antibiotic administration, others focus on disease severity and immediate antibiotic administration once the diagnosis has been considered. No prospective clinical data have determined the relationship between the timing of antimicrobial treatment and clinical outcome in patients with bacterial meningitis. However, delayed treatment is associated with a bad outcome. A retrospective study in adults with acute bacterial meningitis showed that delayed antibiotic treatment (resulting from cranial imaging or hospital transfer) contributed significantly to mortality. Another retrospective study of adults with community-acquired bacterial meningitis also identified delay in treatment with adverse outcome in patients who had deteriorated to the highest stage of prognostic severity before the first dose of antibiotics was administered. A recent prospective study of patients with pneumococcal meningitis who were admitted to the intensive care unit showed that a delay of more than 3 h between hospital admission and initiation of antimicrobial therapy was associated with an increased 3-month mortality. In patients with suspected bacterial meningitis whose lumbar puncture is postponed because of coagulopathy (e.g. disseminated intravascular coagulation), severe septic shock, or the need for cranial imaging (see Box 24.11.1.1), antimicrobial therapy should be started immediately (Fig. 24.11.1.5). In those who deteriorate clinically or who have cloudy cerebrospinal fluid (suggestive of

bacterial meningitis), antibiotic treatment should be started directly after lumbar puncture whereas in those who are clinically stable and whose cerebrospinal fluid is not cloudy treatment can be delayed until cerebrospinal fluid analysis confirms the diagnosis.

In the United Kingdom, family doctors are advised to give (parenteral) antibiotics before transferring the patient to hospital if meningococcal meningitis is suspected. However, it may be difficult to identify patients with meningococcal meningitis and to determine whether they will benefit from such pre-hospital treatment. Several retrospective studies have shown conflicting results.

Some patients with bacterial meningitis are unconscious and should be managed accordingly. Their airway should be maintained and they may need intubation to protect the airway and maintain ventilation. Monitoring in a neurological–neurosurgical intensive care unit is recommended in order to recognize changes in level of consciousness and the development of new neurological signs, monitor for subtle seizures, and effectively treat severe agitation. A urethral catheter should be inserted.

Bacterial meningitis may be associated with septic shock, which is an important predictor of outcome. Patients with meningitis and septic shock may require insertion of a Swan–Ganz catheter, to measure cardiac output, the cardiac index, systemic vascular resistance, and pulmonary wedge pressures in order to assess intravascular volume and cardiac function. Adrenocorticoid insufficiency in patients with septic shock should be treated with low doses of corticosteroids.

Care should be taken to estimate and replace imperceptible fluid loss through the skin and lungs in patients who are febrile. Patients with bacterial meningitis are at risk of acute hyponatraemia, although most cases are mild. This may result from cerebral salt wasting, the syndrome of inappropriate antidiuretic hormone secretion, or exacerbation by aggressive fluid resuscitation. Uncertainty about the mechanism creates a clinical dilemma about whether intravenous fluids should be restricted in bacterial meningitis. In children with bacterial meningitis, fluid restriction does not improve either brain oedema or outcome. It seems reasonable to maintain adult patients with meningitis in a normovolaemic state. Patients whose core temperatures exceed 40°C should be cooled using physical methods or an antipyretic to avoid brain damage and excessive fluid loss through sweating.

Antimicrobial treatment

The choice of initial antimicrobial therapy is based on which bacteria most commonly cause the disease, based on age, clinical circumstances, and prevailing antimicrobial susceptibility patterns (Table 24.11.1.2). Once the pathogen has been isolated, specific treatment based on the susceptibility of the isolate can be substituted for the empirical regimen (Table 24.11.1.3).

The pharmacokinetics and pharmacodynamics dynamics of antimicrobial agents are highly relevant. Penetration of the blood–brain barrier to reach the subarachnoid space is of paramount importance in clearing bacteria from the cerebrospinal fluid. Penetration is affected by lipophilicity, molecular weight, structure, and protein-bound fraction. Bacterial meningitis is a dynamic process and cerebrospinal fluid penetration of antimicrobials is highly dependent on the breakdown of blood–brain barrier permeability. Anti-inflammatory drugs such as dexamethasone might influence permeability and thereby interfere with cerebrospinal fluid penetration of antimicrobial agents.

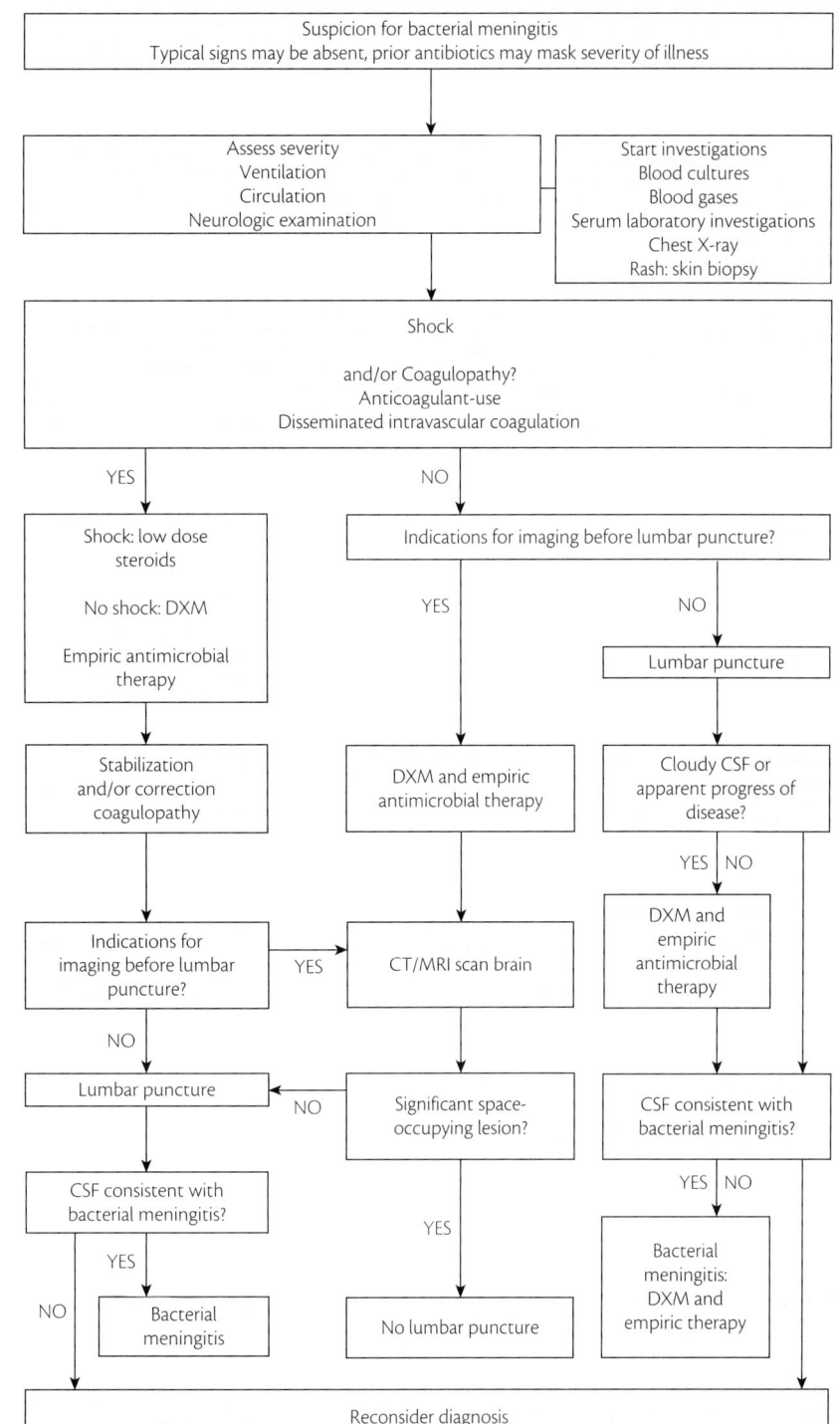

Fig. 24.11.1.5 Algorithm for the management of patients with suspected community-acquired bacterial meningitis. CSF, cerebrospinal fluid.

This material was previously published as part of an online supplementary appendix to van de Beek, *et al.* (2006). *N Engl J Med*, **354**(1), 44–53. Copyright 2006 Massachusetts Medical Society. All rights reserved.

The activity of antimicrobial drugs in infected purulent cerebrospinal fluid depends on their activity in a low pH environment, protein-bound fraction, bacterial growth rate and density, and clearance from the cerebrospinal fluid. Antibiotics target the bacterial cell wall, the bacterial cell membrane, and biosynthetic processes. Bacteriostatic antibiotics merely inhibit growth of microorganisms, whereas bactericidal agents kill the bacteria. Antibiotic-induced lysis of bacteria leads to the release of immunostimulatory cell-wall components and toxic bacterial products, which induce a severe inflammatory response through binding to TLRs.

Neonatal meningitis

This is largely caused by group B streptococci, *E. coli*, and *L. monocytogenes*. Initial treatment should, therefore, consist of penicillin or ampicillin plus a third-generation cephalosporin, preferably cefotaxime or ceftriaxone, or penicillin or ampicillin and an aminoglycoside.

Childhood meningitis

In the community, children are at risk of meningitis caused by *N. meningitidis* and *Strep. pneumoniae*, and, rarely in Hib-immunized

Table 24.11.1.2 Recommendations for empirical antimicrobial therapy in suspected community-acquired bacterial meningitis

Predisposing factor	Common bacterial pathogens	Initial intravenous antibiotic therapy
Age		
< 1 month	*Streptococcus agalactiae*, *Escherichia coli*, *Listeria monocytogenes*	Ampicillin plus cefotaxime or an aminoglycoside
1–3 months	*Strep. pneumoniae*, *Neisseria meningitidis*, *Strep. agalactiae*, *Haemophilus influenzae*, *E. coli*, *L. monocytogenes*	Ampicillin plus vancomycin plus ceftriaxone or cefotaxime[a]
3–23 months	*Strep. pneumoniae*, *N. meningitidis*, *Strep. agalactiae*, *H. influenzae*, *E. coli*	Vancomycin plus ceftriaxone or cefotaxime[a]
2–50 years	*N. meningitidis*, *Strep. pneumoniae*	Vancomycin plus ceftriaxone or cefotaxime[a]
>50 years	*N. meningitidis*, *Strep. pneumoniae*, *L. monocytogenes*, aerobic Gram-negative bacilli	Vancomycin plus ceftriaxone or cefotaxime plus ampicillin[b]
With risk factor present[c]	*Strep. pneumoniae*, *L. monocytogenes*, *H. influenzae*	Vancomycin plus ceftriaxone or cefotaxime plus ampicillin
Post-traumatic	*Strep. pneumoniae*, *H. influenzae*	Vancomycin plus ceftriaxone or cefotaxime plus ampicillin
Postneurosurgery	Coagulase-negative staphylococci, *Staph. aureus*, aerobic Gram-negative bacilli (including *Pseudomonas aeruginosa*)	Vancomycin plus ceftazidime
Cerebrospinal fluid shunt	Coagulase-negative staphylococci, *Staph. aureus*, aerobic Gram-negative bacilli (including *P. aeruginosa*), *Propionibacterium acnes*	Vancomycin plus ceftazidime

Adapted van de Beek D, *et al.* (2006). *N Engl J Med*, **354**(1), 44–53.

[a] In areas with very low penicillin-resistance rates monotherapy, penicillin may be considered.

[b] In areas with very low rates of penicillin resistance and cephalosporin resistance, combination therapy of amoxicillin and third-generation cephalosporin may be considered.

[c] Alcoholism, altered immune status.

General recommendations for intravenous empirical antibiotic treatment have included penicillin 2 MU every 4 h; amoxicillin or ampicillin 2 g every 4 h; vancomycin, 15 mg/kg every 8 h; third-generation cephalosporin: ceftriaxone 2 g every 12 h or cefotaxime 2 g every 4–6 h; ceftazidime 2 g every 8 h.

children, *H. influenzae*. Antimicrobial resistance has emerged among the three major bacterial pathogens causing meningitis. Although intermediate penicillin resistance is common in some countries, the clinical importance of penicillin resistance in the meningococcus has yet to be established.

Adult meningitis

Spontaneous meningitis in adults is usually caused by *Strep. pneumoniae* or *N. meningitidis*. Due to the worldwide emerge of multidrug-resistant strains of *Strep. pneumoniae*, some experts recommend addition of vancomycin to the initial empirical antimicrobial regimen in adult patients. Although no clinical data on the efficacy of rifampicin in patients with pneumococcal meningitis are currently available, some experts would recommend the use of this agent in combination with a third-generation cephalosporin, with or without vancomycin, in patients with pneumococcal meningitis caused by bacterial strains that, on the basis of local epidemiology, are likely to be highly resistant to penicillin or cephalosporin. *Strep. suis* remains sensitive to the β-lactams and should be treated with penicillin, cefotaxime, or ceftriaxone. Fluoroquinolones may be an alternative. In patients aged over 50 years, ampicillin should be added to the above antibiotic regimen for additional coverage of *L. monocytogenes*, which is more prevalent among this age group.

Nosocomial post-traumatic meningitis

This is caused mainly by multiresistant hospital-acquired organisms such as *K. pneumoniae*, *E. coli*, *P. aeruginosa*, and *Staph. aureus*. Depending on the pattern of susceptibility in a given hospital unit, ceftazidime (2 g intravenously, every 8 h), cefotaxime, ceftriaxone, or meropenem should be chosen. If *P. aeruginosa* infection seems likely, ceftazidime or meropenem is the preferred antibiotic.

Device- and shunt-associated meningitis

This is caused by a wide range of organisms, including meticillin-resistant staphylococci (mostly coagulase-negative staphylococci) and multiresistant aerobic bacilli. Cases with shunts and an insidious onset are probably caused by organisms of low pathogenicity, and empirical therapy is a less urgent requirement. For postoperative meningitis the first-line empirical therapy should be cefotaxime, ceftriaxone, or meropenem. If the patient has received broad-spectrum antibiotics recently or if *P. aeruginosa* is suspected, ceftazidime or meropenem should be given. Meropenem should be used if an extended-spectrum, β-lactamase organism is suspected, and flucloxacillin or vancomycin if *Staph. aureus* is likely. The infected shunt or drain will almost certainly have to be removed urgently.

Definitive antibiotic treatment

Once the aetiological agent has been isolated and its susceptibilities determined, the empirical treatment should be changed, if necessary, to an agent or agents specific for the isolate (see Table 24.11.1.3). The optimal duration of treatment has not been determined by rigorous scientific investigation; however, treatment regimens that are probably substantially in excess of the minimum necessary to achieve cure have been arrived at through wide clinical experience.

General recommendations for empirical antibiotic treatment have included ceftriaxone administered intravenously every 12 h or intravenous cefotaxime every 4 to 6 h, and/or ampicillin at 4-h intervals, or benzylpenicillin every 4 h. There are no randomized comparative clinical studies of the various dosing regimens. In general, 7 days of antimicrobial therapy are given for meningitis caused by *N. meningitidis* and *H. influenzae*, 10 to 14 days for *Strep. pneumoniae* or *Strep. suis*, and at least 21 days for *L. monocytogenes*. As these guidelines are not standardized it must be emphasized

Table 24.11.1.3 Specific antimicrobial therapy in community-acquired bacterial meningitis based on cerebrospinal fluid (cerebrospinal fluid) culture results and in vitro susceptibility testing; this material was previously published as part of an online supplementary appendix to reference

Microorganism, susceptibility	Standard therapy	Alternative therapies
Streptococcus pneumoniae		
Penicillin MIC		
< 0.1 mg/l	Benzylpenicillin or ampicillin	Cefotaxime or ceftriaxone, chloramphenicol
0.1–1.0 mg/l	Cefotaxime or ceftriaxone	Cefepime, meropenem
≥ 2.0 mg/l	Vancomycin + cefotaxime or ceftriaxone[a]	Fluoroquinolone[a]
Cefotaxime or ceftriaxone MIC		
≥ 1.0 mg/l	Vancomycin plus cefotaxime or ceftriaxone[b]	Fluoroquinolone[c]
Neisseria meningitidis		
Penicillin MIC		
< 0.1 mg/l	Benzylpenicillin or ampicillin	Cefotaxime or ceftriaxone, chloramphenicol
0.1–1.0 mg/l	Cefotaxime or ceftriaxone	Chloramphenicol, fluoroquinolone, meropenem
Listeria monocytogenes	Benzylpenicillin or ampicillin[d]	Trimethoprim–sulfamethoxazole, meropenem
Group B streptococci	Benzylpenicillin or ampicillin[d]	Cefotaxime or ceftriaxone
Escherichia coli and other Enterobacteriaceae	Cefotaxime or ceftriaxone[d]	Aztreonam,[d] fluoroquinolone, meropenem,[d] trimethoprim–sulfamethoxazole, ampicillin[d]
Pseudomonas aeruginosa	Ceftazidime[d] or cefepime[d]	Aztreonam,[d] ciprofloxacin,[d] meropenem[d]
Haemophilus influenzae		
β-Lactamase negative	Ampicillin	Cefotaxime or ceftriaxone, cefepime, chloramphenicol, fluoroquinolone
β-Lactamase positive	Cefotaxime or ceftriaxone	Cefepime, chloramphenicol, fluoroquinolone
Chemoprophylaxis[e]		
N. meningitidis	Rifampicin, ceftriaxone, ciprofloxacin, azithromycin	

Copyright 2006 Massachusetts Medical Society.

Adapted from van de Beek, *et al.* (2006). *N Engl J Med*, **354**(1), 44–53.

[a] Consider addition of rifampicin if dexamethasone is given.

[b] Consider addition of rifampicin if the MIC (minimum inhibitory concentration) of ceftriaxone is ≥2 mg/L.

[c] Gatifloxacin or moxifloxacin; no clinical data on use in patients with bacterial meningitis.

[d] Consider addition of an aminoglycoside.

[e] Prophylaxis is indicated for close contacts, who are defined as those with intimate contact, which covers those eating and sleeping in the same dwelling as well as those having close social and kissing contacts; or health-care workers who perform mouth-to-mouth resuscitation, endotracheal intubation, or endotracheal tube management. Patients with meningococcal meningitis who are treated with monotherapy of penicillin or amoxicillin (ampicillin) should also receive chemoprophylaxis, because carriage is not reliably eradicated by these drugs.

[f] General recommendations for intravenous empirical antibiotic treatment have included penicillin 2 MU every 4 h; amoxicillin or ampicillin 2 g every 4 h; vancomycin 15 mg/kg every 8 h; third-generation cephalosporin: ceftriaxone 2 g every 12 h or cefotaxime 2 g every 4–6 h; cefepime 2 g every 8 h; ceftazidime 2 g every 8 h; meropenem 2 g every 8 h; chloramphenicol 1–1.5 g every 6 h; fluoroquinolone: gatifloxacin 400 mg every 24 h or moxifloxacin 400 mg every 24 h, although no data on optimal dose needed in patients with bacterial meningitis; trimethoprim–sulfamethoxazole 5 mg/kg every 6–12 h; aztreonam 2 g every 6–8 h; ciprofloxacin 400 mg every 8–12 h; rifampicin 600 mg every 12–24 h; aminoglycoside: gentamicin 1.7 mg/kg every 8 h. The preferred dose for chemoprophylaxis: rifampicin 600 mg orally twice daily for 2 days; ceftriaxone 250 mg intramuscular; ciprofloxacin 750 mg orally; azithromycin 500 mg orally.

that the duration of therapy may need to be individualized on the basis of the patient's response

Adjunctive dexamethasone treatment

Animal models of bacterial meningitis showed that bacterial lysis, induced by antibiotic therapy, leads to inflammation in the subarachnoid space. The severity of this inflammatory response is associated with outcome and can be attenuated by treatment with steroids. On the basis of experimental meningitis studies, several clinical trials have been undertaken to determine the effects of adjunctive steroids in children and adults with bacterial meningitis.

Of several corticosteroids, the use of dexamethasone in bacterial meningitis has been investigated most extensively. Dexamethasone is a glucocorticosteroid with anti-inflammatory as well as immunosuppressive properties. It has excellent penetration into the cerebrospinal fluid. In a meta-analysis of randomized trials since 1988, adjunctive dexamethasone was shown to reduce meningitis-associated hearing loss in children with meningitis due to *H. influenzae* type b.

As the design of most available studies on adjunctive dexamethasone therapy in adults with bacterial meningitis was flawed, its value in adults was long debated. In 2002, results of a European randomized placebo-controlled trial showed that adjunctive treatment with dexamethasone, given before or with the first dose of antimicrobial therapy, improved the outcome of adult bacterial meningitis (relative risk (RR) 0.59; 95% confidence interval (CI) 0.37–0.94) and reduced its mortality (RR 0.48; 95%CI 0.24–0.96). This beneficial effect was most apparent in patients with pneumococcal meningitis, in whom the mortality rate was decreased from 34% to 14%. The benefits of adjunctive dexamethasone therapy were not undermined by an increase of severe neurological disability in patients who survived or by any corticosteroid-induced complication. In a post-hoc analysis, including only patients with pneumococcal meningitis who died within 14 days of admission, the mortality benefit of dexamethasone therapy was due entirely to reduced mortality from systemic causes such as septic shock, pneumonia, or acute respiratory distress syndrome; there was no significant reduction in mortality due to neurological causes.

Results of a subsequent quantitative review of this topic in adults, which included five clinical trials, confirmed that treatment with corticosteroids was associated with a significant reduction in mortality (RR 0.6; 95%CI 0.4–0.8) and in neurological sequelae (RR 0.6; 95%CI 0.4–1). The reduction in case fatality in patients with pneumococcal meningitis was 21% (RR 0.5; 95%CI 0.3–0.8). In meningococcal meningitis, in which the number of events was smaller, there were favourable point estimates for preventing mortality (RR 0.9; 95%CI 0.3–2.1) and neurological sequelae (RR 0.5; 95%CI 0.1–1.7), but these effects did not reach statistical significance. Adverse events were equally divided between the treatment and placebo groups. Treatment with adjunctive dexamethasone did not worsen long-term cognitive outcome in adults after bacterial meningitis. Since the publication of these results, adjunctive dexamethasone has become routine therapy in most adults with suspected bacterial meningitis.

In 2007, an updated Cochrane analysis was published on the efficacy and safety of adjunctive corticosteroids, including 20 randomized clinical trials involving 2750 people. In this analysis, adjuvant corticosteroids were associated with lower case fatality (RR 0.83; 95%CI 0.71–0.99), lower rates of severe hearing loss (RR 0.65; 95%CI 0.47 to 0.91), and long-term neurological sequelae (RR 0.67; 95%CI 0.45–1.00). Again, the effect of corticosteroids was evident in adults with bacterial meningitis. In children the beneficial effect was less convincing, although there was a trend towards a beneficial effect on hearing loss in non-H. influenzae meningitis.

In the Cochrane meta-analysis, there was a difference in efficacy of corticosteroids between high- and low-income countries. For children with bacterial meningitis admitted in high-income countries, corticosteroids showed a protective effect against severe hearing loss (RR 0.61; 95%CI 0.41–0.90), favourable point estimates for severe hearing loss associated with non-H. influenzae meningitis (RR 0.51; 95%CI 0.23–1.13), and short-term neurological sequelae (RR 0.72; 95%CI 0.39–1.33). For children in low-income countries, the use of corticosteroids was not associated with benefit. This difference was mainly caused by inclusion of the Malawian study, which included children in whom treatment began later, children who were more likely to be malnourished, and some HIV-1 positive children. There may be several reasons for the difference in efficacy of corticosteroids, such as delayed presentation, clinical severity, underlying anaemia, malnutrition, the antibiotic used and HIV-1 positivity. A recent study compared characteristics of children with culture-positive bacterial meningitis treated

in the Royal Liverpool Children's Hospital and the Children's Unit, Queen Elizabeth Central Hospital, Blantyre, Malawi; the two cohort studies were derived from time periods before the introduction of vaccines. Children in Malawi presented later and were more often comatose and malnourished, compared with children in Britain. The mortality rate from bacterial meningitis in children in Malawi was much higher than in children in Britain (41% vs 7%), even when infected with the same organisms.

Randomized studies in adults with pyogenic meningitis from Malawi and Vietnam have recently been published. In the Malawi study, dexamethasone was not associated with any significant benefit, whereas in Vietnam a significant benefit in mortality (RR 0.43; 95%CI 0.2–0.94) was seen in patients with confirmed pyogenic meningitis. These conflicting results are difficult to interpret and further large studies in developing countries may be needed.

Despite these encouraging results, the use of adjunctive dexamethasone in bacterial meningitis remains controversial. Recently a meta-analysis with individual patient data from 2029 adults and children from Malawi, Europe, Chile, and Vietnam was completed. HIV infection was confirmed or likely in approximately a third of all patients and a diagnosis of bacterial meningitis was microbiologically confirmed in 80%, most frequently with Strep. pneumoniae. Dexamethasone was not associated with a significant reduction in deaths (dexamethasone 270/1019 (27%) vs placebo 275/1010 (27%); odds ratio or OR 1.0; 95%CI 0.8–1.2), death or severe neurological sequelae or bilateral severe hearing loss (dexamethasone 43% vs placebo 44%; OR 0.9; 95%CI 0.8–1.1), death or any neurological sequelae or any hearing loss (dexamethasone 54% vs placebo 57%; OR 0.9; 95%CI 0.7–1.1), and death or severe bilateral hearing loss (dexamethasone 54% vs placebo 57%; OR 0.9; 95%CI 0.8–1.1). However, there was a suggestion that dexamethasone may reduce hearing loss among survivors (dexamethasone 24% vs placebo 30%; OR 0.8; 95%CI 0.6–1.0; $p = 0.04$). There was no effect in any prespecified subgroups including specific causative organisms, pre-dexamethasone antibiotic treatment, HIV status, or age. Pooling of mortality results with all other published trials did not change the conclusions. The use of adjunctive dexamethasone treatment was not associated with an increased risk of adverse events. Adjunctive dexamethasone in the treatment of acute bacterial meningitis does not appear to reduce deaths or neurological disability or to produce harm. There were no significant treatment effects in any of the prespecified subgroups. A post-hoc analysis showed that dexamethasone adjuvant therapy may reduce hearing loss in survivors.

By reducing permeability of the blood–brain barrier, steroids can impede penetration of antibiotics into the cerebrospinal fluid. This was shown for vancomycin in animal studies and can lead to treatment failures, especially in patients with meningitis caused by drug-resistant pneumococci in whom antibiotic regimens often include vancomycin. However, in a recent observational study, which included 14 adult patients admitted to the intensive care unit because of suspected pneumococcal meningitis, appropriate concentrations of vancomycin in the cerebrospinal fluid were obtained even when concomitant steroids were used. The dose of vancomycin used in this study was 60 mg/kg per day. Although these results suggest that dexamethasone can be used without fear of impeding vancomycin penetration into the cerebrospinal fluid of patients with pneumococcal meningitis (provided that vancomycin dosage is adequate), it is recommended that patients with bacterial meningitis due to nonsusceptible strains, treated with adjunctive dexamethasone, are carefully monitored throughout treatment.

Treatment of complications

The management of adults with bacterial meningitis can be complex and common complications are meningoencephalitis, systemic compromise, stroke, and raised intracranial pressure (ICP) (see Fig. 24.11.1.2). Various adjunctive therapies have been described to improve outcome in such patients, including anti-inflammatory agents, anticoagulant therapies, and strategies to reduce ICP. Few randomized clinical studies are available for other adjunctive therapies in adults with bacterial meningitis.

The inflammatory response in the CNS results in blood–brain barrier permeability, cerebral oedema, and increased ICP. Classically, there are two types of brain oedema: vasogenic due to blood–brain barrier disruption, resulting in extracellular water accumulation, and cytotoxic or cellular oedema due to sustained intracellular water collection. A third type, osmotic brain oedema, results from osmotic imbalances between blood and tissue.

A Dutch cohort study evaluated the effects of complications on mortality in patients with pneumococcal meningitis and compared these findings among different age groups. In older patients ($\geq$60 years), death was usually a result of systemic complications, whereas death in younger patients ($<$60 years) was predominantly due to neurological complications such as brain herniation. This observation may be explained by age-related cerebral atrophy, which allows older patients to tolerate brain swelling. These findings suggest that supportive treatments that aim to reduce ICP could be most beneficial in younger adults with pneumococcal meningitis. Methods available to reduce intracranial pressure range from simple (e.g. elevation of the head of the bed to 30°) to aggressive strategies (e.g. 'Lund concept'), although there is no evidence that ICP monitoring and treatment of increased ICP are beneficial in patients with bacterial meningitis.

The rational of hyperventilation in patients with bacterial meningitis is the interrelation of cerebral arteriolar dilatation, increased cerebral blood flow (CBF), and a subsequent rise in ICP. Hyperventilation-induced hypocapnia causes (cerebral) vasoconstriction and a reduction in CBF, resulting in lowering of the ICP. This approach has been used in patients with traumatic brain injury as well; however, the enthusiasm for hyperventilation was greatly tempered after a study on prophylactic hyperventilation in patients with severe brain injury showed a worse outcome. In bacterial meningitis, patients are often hypocapnic at the time of admission, suggesting that there is spontaneous hyperventilation. A Danish study in adults with bacterial meningitis found a decline of CBF with hyperventilation, with no change in regional CBF pattern. Therefore, experts recommend that $PaCO_2$ be maintained slightly below 'normal' during the first 24 h in patients with bacterial meningitis, i.e. 4.0 to 4.5 kPa. However, there are no published controlled trials on the effect of hyperventilation in bacterial meningitis, so recommendations in this area are based only on expert opinion.

In patients with traumatic brain injury, studies have shown that mannitol decreases blood viscosity and reduces the diameter of pial arterioles in a manner similar to the vascoconstriction produced by hyperventilation. Although osmotic tissue dehydration may still play some role, mannitol works primarily through its immediate rheological effect, by diluting the blood and increasing the deformability of erythrocytes, thereby decreasing blood viscosity and increasing CBF. This sudden increase in CBF causes autoregulatory vasoconstriction of cerebral arterioles, decreasing the intracerebral blood volume and lowering the ICP.

In bacterial meningitis, as blood–brain barrier permeability has been increased, the effect of mannitol is uncertain. There is little information from clinical and experimental studies concerning the use of mannitol in bacterial meningitis. A single dose of mannitol reduced ICP for approximately 3 h in a meningitis model. Continued intravenous infusion of mannitol attenuated the increases of regional CBF, brain water content, and ICP in a pneumococcal meningitis model.

Prognosis

In Europe and North America the overall mortality rate of patients with meningitis caused by *N. meningitidis* is about 7 to 14%, by *Strep. pneumoniae* 15 to 40%, and by group B streptococci and *L. monocytogenes* meningitis above 20%. The mortality is much higher in very young and old people, and in patients with debilitating illnesses. A study in Zaria, Nigeria demonstrated that the mortality rate of pneumococcal meningitis was 32% in patients who were fully conscious on admission, 40% in those who were confused, 54% in semiconscious patients, and 94% in those who were comatose. In Vietnam, in a prospective study of 250 cases of adult bacterial meningitis, the overall mortality rate was 13%.

Permanent neurological sequelae include intellectual impairment, deafness and other cranial nerve deficits, and hydrocephalus. The reported incidence of sensorineural deafness after meningitis ranges from 5% to 40%. A large proportion of patients recover within a few months. *N. meningitidis* and *H. influenzae* are the main causes of this complication. Permanent deafness occurs in more than 50% of patients with *Strep. suis* meningitis. It may be bilateral, complete, and associated with vestibular involvement.

Even in patients with apparently good recovery, cognitive impairment occurs frequently. In a prospective study, cognitive impairment was detected in 27% of adults who made a good recovery from pneumococcal meningitis. Results of a more recent study showed that about a third of adult survivors of bacterial meningitis experience subtle long-term cognitive impairment, which consists mainly of slight mental slowness. In this study the prevalence of cognitive impairment in patients after pneumococcal and meningococcal meningitis was similar.

Tuberculous meningitis
Epidemiology

Tuberculous meningitis (TBM) kills or disables half those who have the condition and is the most dangerous form of infection with *Mycobacterium tuberculosis*. Fortunately, it is a relatively uncommon manifestation of TB and represents around 1% of all forms of the disease. In Western countries, its incidence has fallen in parallel with TB as a whole, but for those in the less developed world TBM remains a common cause of bacterial meningitis, particularly in populations with a high prevalence of HIV infection.

Before the arrival of HIV, most cases of TBM were in young children and occurred as a complication of primary infection. Now an increased proportion of cases occur in adults with HIV coinfection.

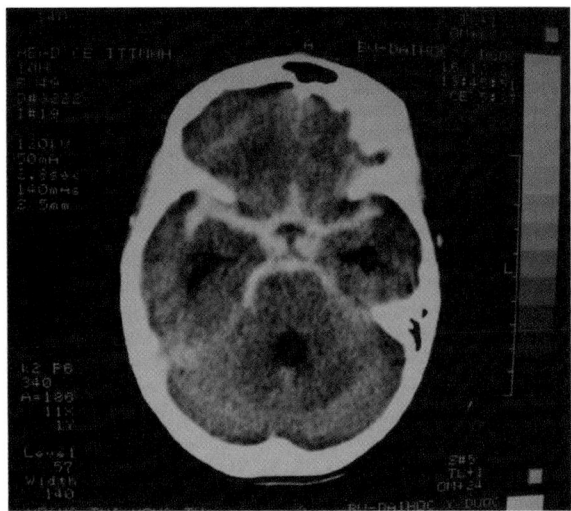

Fig. 24.11.1.6 CT of the head with contrast showing intense basal meningeal enhancement and dilated ventricles.

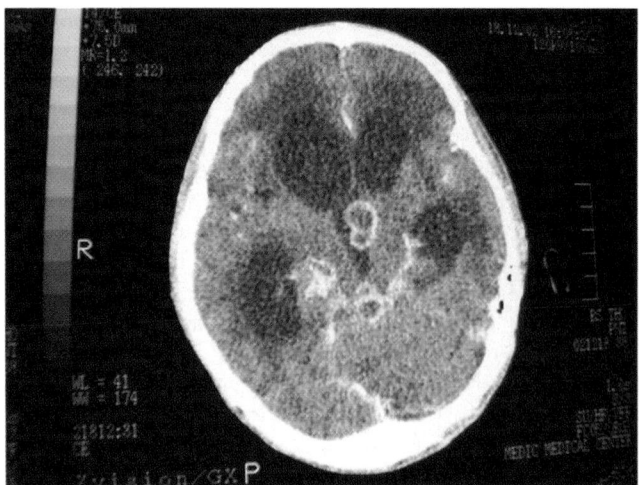

Fig. 24.11.1.7 CT of the head with contrast showing gross hydrocephalus and multiple ring-enhancing tuberculomas.

HIV infection greatly increases the risk of all forms of TB, but in particular the extrapulmonary forms such as TBM, and the risk increases as the CD4 count declines.

Pathogenesis

Understanding of the pathogenesis of TBM has progressed little since the studies of Rich and McCordock in the 1920s and 1930s. They demonstrated, through postmortem examinations of children and experiments on rabbits, that the pathogenesis of TBM requires two steps. During the first step the meninges and brain parenchyma are seeded by blood-borne bacteria with the formation of small subpial or subependymal foci of infection (or the Rich foci). In children the bacteraemia usually occurs during primary pulmonary infection and may be subclinical, whereas in adults this step may occur after new pulmonary infection or reactivation of old foci. The second step requires the rupture of a Rich focus with release of bacteria into the subarachnoid space. This heralds the onset of meningitis, which, if left untreated, will result in severe and irreversible neurological pathology. In 75% of children the onset of TBM is less than 12 months after the primary infection.

Pathology

Three processes are responsible for the neurological pathology of TBM. An adhesive exudate develops around the basal cisterns and can obstruct cerebrospinal fluid causing hydrocephalus and compromise efferent cranial nerves (Fig. 24.11.1.6). Granulomas can coalesce to form tuberculomas, or an abscess in unusual cases, causing diverse clinical consequences dependent on their anatomical location (Fig. 24.11.1.7). And an obliterative vasculitis can cause infarction and stroke syndromes, commonly involving the basal ganglia, internal capsule, and territory of the middle cerebral artery (Fig. 24.11.1.8). The severity of these complications is believed to depend on the intracerebral inflammatory response and strongly predicts outcome.

In less than 10% of cases TBM occurs with spinal involvement, usually manifest as paraplegia. Vertebral tuberculosis (Pott's disease) accounts for around a quarter of cases (Fig. 24.11.1.9) and may be associated with fusiform paravertebral abscesses (Fig. 24.11.1.10)

or a gibbus (Fig. 24.11.1.11). Extradural cord tuberculomas cause more than 60% of cases of nonosseous paraplegia, although tuberculomas can occur in any part of the cord (Fig. 24.11.1.12). Tuberculous radiculomyelitis is a rare accompaniment to TBM, characterized by a subacute paraparesis, radicular pain, and bladder dysfunction. MRI reveals loculation and obliteration of the spinal subarachnoid space with nodular intradural enhancement (Fig. 24.11.1.13).

Clinical features

If left untreated, TBM follows a slowly progressive course that leads to death in almost all cases. The first symptoms are nonspecific and unlikely to raise the suspicion of TBM. Infants may become irritable or go off their feeds, whereas older patients may complain of malaise, insomnia, lethargy, anorexia, and gradually worsening headache. These prodromal symptoms can last from 2 weeks to 8 weeks until the classic features of meningitis become more apparent. Patients commonly present to hospital at this stage, when the

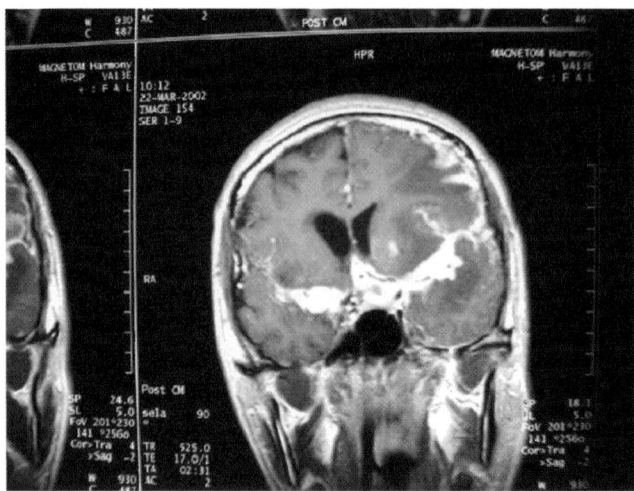

Fig. 24.11.1.8 MRI of the brain with contrast, showing intense basal enhancement with large left middle cerebral artery territory infarction and mass effect.

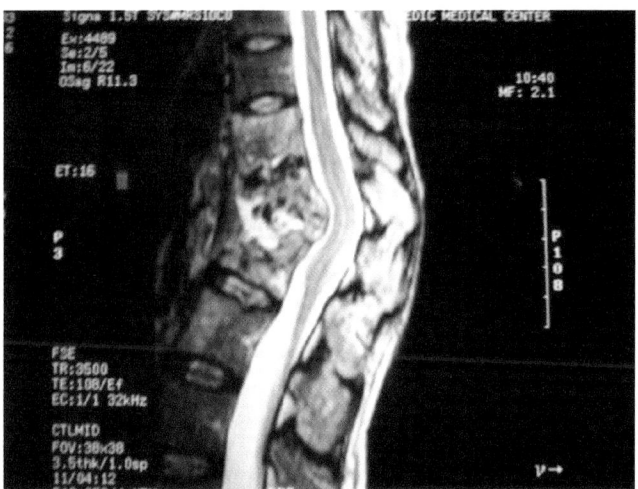

Fig. 24.11.1.9 MRI of the spine showing destruction of vertebrae and displacement of the cord.

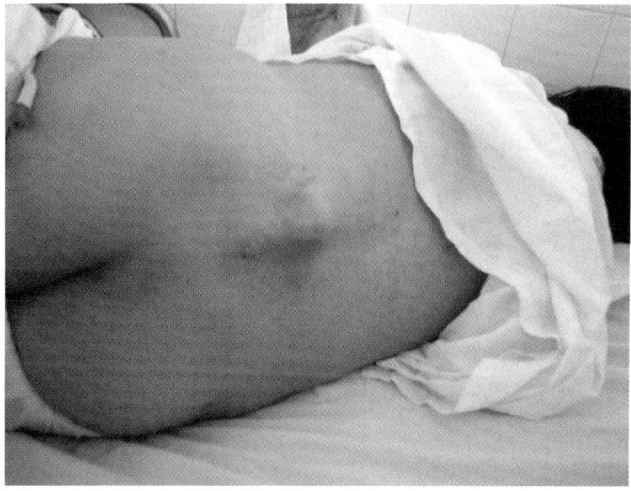

Fig. 24.11.1.11 Spinal deformity or 'gibbus' in patient with vertebral tuberculosis.

infection is well established. They will usually complain of headache and vomiting; many will present confused or comatose. Examination reveals neck stiffness in most, although it is rarely as marked as in acute pyogenic bacterial meningitis. Cranial nerve palsies are found in 25% of patients, with nerves VI, III, and VII being most commonly affected. Ten per cent of patients will present with a mono- or hemiparesis. Fundoscopy reveals papilloedema in half of patients and, occasionally, choroidal tubercles. Rarely, TBM presents as an acute meningoencephalitis that can be difficult to distinguish from pyogenic bacterial or viral meningitis. Seizures are rare in adults with TBM, but more common in children. HIV infection does not appear to alter the clinical presentation of TBM, although evidence of other extrapulmonary disease is more likely in HIV-infected patients (Fig. 24.11.1.14).

Coma occurs in advanced disease and is strongly correlated with outcome. It is usually caused by raised ICP as a result of cerebrospinal fluid obstruction and cerebral oedema. Hydrocephalus is found in 90% of children at diagnosis and 70% of adults, and is strongly associated with delayed treatment and prolonged coma. Reduced conscious level may also be caused by metabolic disturbance.

Hyponatraemia affects more than 50% of patients with TBM, although why it occurs is uncertain. Some patients have a classic syndrome of inappropriate antidiuretic hormone secretion (SIADH) but many others have reduced plasma volumes and persistent natriuresis with normal concentrations of antidiuretic hormone (ADH). Indeed, some have suggested that 'hyponatraemic natriuretic syndrome' is a better descriptive term for this common complication of TBM.

Unusual neurological manifestations of TBM are well described, particularly in the older literature. Movement disorders may follow basal ganglia infarction: tremor is the most common problem, but chorea, ballismus, and myoclonus are all reported. Tuberculomas can affect the hypothalamus and pituitary and cause disordered temperature regulation, diabetes insipidus, and panhypopituitarism on rare occasions. More controversial are cases that present with evidence of diffuse cerebral involvement but without clinical or cerebrospinal fluid signs of meningitis. 'Tuberculous encephalopathy' was first described in Indian children with disseminated TB and was characterized by coma, convulsions, involuntary movements, and pyramidal signs but with normal cerebrospinal fluid examination. It has not been reported in adults. Postmortem

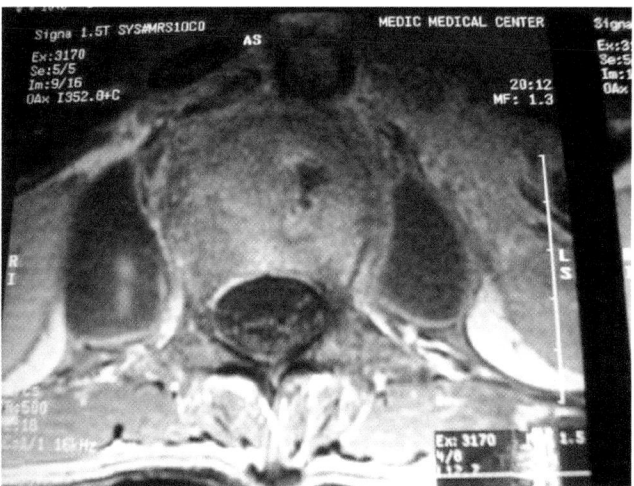

Fig. 24.11.1.10 MRI of the spine showing vertebral destruction and large, bilateral, paravertebral abscesses.

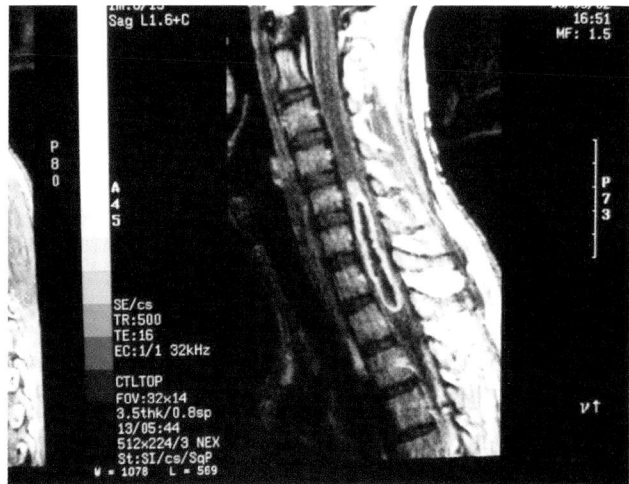

Fig. 24.11.1.12 MRI of the spine with contrast showing cavitating cervical tuberculoma.

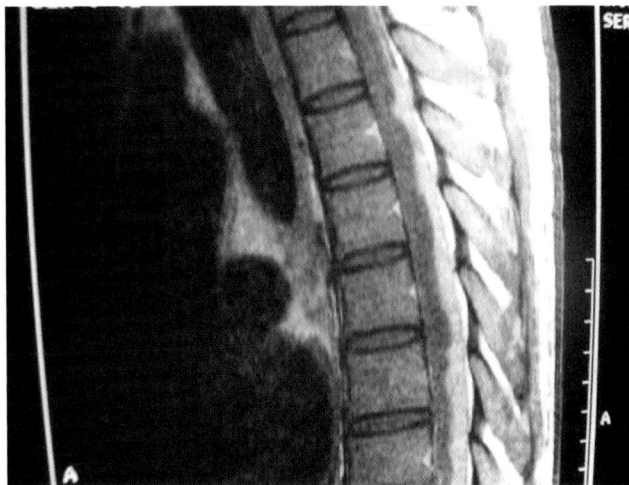

Fig. 24.11.1.13 MRI of the spine from patient with tuberculous radiculomyelitis showing meningeal thickening.

examinations revealed diffuse cerebral oedema, demyelination, and sometimes haemorrhage—features more typical of a postinfectious allergic disseminated encephalomyelitis.

Diagnosis

The diagnosis and treatment of TBM before the onset of coma are the greatest contribution that a physician can make to improve outcome. However, making the diagnosis is challenging because the clinical features of the disease are nonspecific, small numbers of bacteria in the cerebrospinal fluid reduce the sensitivity of conventional bacteriology, and alternative diagnostic methods are incompletely assessed.

The presenting clinical features of TBM are insufficiently specific to enable the diagnosis to be made on the history and examination alone. Recall of recent exposure to TB may be helpful, particularly in children, as may evidence of active extrameningeal TB on examination. Chest radiography reveals active or previous TB infection in 50%; the appearance of miliary TB is particularly useful as it strongly suggests multiorgan involvement. Skin testing with the purified protein derivative of *M. tuberculosis* is probably of limited value, except in infants.

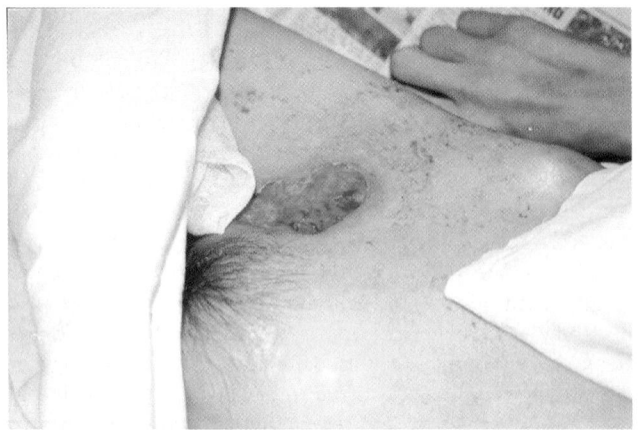

Fig. 24.11.1.14 Tuberculous, suppurating, inguinal lymphadenopathy with sinus tract formation in an HIV-infected woman with tuberculous meningitis.

Examination of the cerebrospinal fluid is an essential part of diagnosing TBM and is a safe procedure for most patients with TBM. Hydrocephalus is not a contraindication to lumbar puncture. cerebrospinal fluid pressures are usually raised (mean 30 cmH$_2$O) and the cerebrospinal fluid is typically clear and slightly xanthochromic. Much is made in the older literature of the formation of a spider's web clot in the cerebrospinal fluid from patients with TBM but the diagnostic utility of this phenomenon has never been systematically tested and is probably exaggerated. The total number of white cells in the cerebrospinal fluid varies from fewer than 5/µl to 1500/µl. Most patients will have 300 to 500 cells/µl cerebrospinal fluid but older and immunosuppressed people may have low or even normal counts. The cells are a mixture of neutrophils and lymphocytes, although lymphocytes usually form 70 to 90% of the total. Occasionally, TBM can present with a short history with 1500 to 2500 WBCs/µl in the cerebrospinal fluid, most of which are neutrophils. Cerebrospinal fluid total protein concentrations are raised in 95%, typically between 1 and 2 g/l; concentrations of more than 3 g/l suggest spinal block. The ratio cerebrospinal fluid:blood glucose concentration is less than 0.5 in 95% and is a useful way of distinguishing TBM from other lymphocytic meningitides, especially viral meningitis, in which cerebrospinal fluid:blood glucose is usually more than 0.5.

Attempts have been made to identify the clinical and cerebrospinal fluid findings predictive of TBM. In children, a history longer than 6 days, optic atrophy, focal neurological deficit, abnormal movements, and neutrophils forming less than half the total cerebrospinal fluid leucocytes were independently associated with TBM. A diagnostic rule developed in Vietnamese adults to distinguish TBM from bacterial meningitis calculated weighted scores for the variables predictive of TBM (score in brackets): age less than 36 years (0), 36 years or more (+2); peripheral blood white cell count fewer than $15\,000 \times 10^3$/ml (0), $15\,000 \times 10^3$/ml or more (+4); duration of symptoms more than 6 days (−5), 6 days or less (0); cerebrospinal fluid white cells fewer than 900/µl (0), 900/µl or more (+3); and cerebrospinal fluid neutrophils less than 75% of total cells (0), 75% or more (+4). A total score of less than 4 indicated TBM, and a score of 4 or more indicated bacterial meningitis; when applied prospectively the rule was 86% sensitive and 79% specific. However, the performance will probably differ where TB prevalence is lower and HIV prevalence higher than in Vietnam.

CT and MRI of the brain provide diagnostic information, but there are few data to indicate whether the findings can help discriminate TBM from other cerebral disorders. Basal meningeal enhancement, hydrocephalus, tuberculoma, and infarction are the cardinal neuroradiological features of TBM (see Figs. 24.11.1.1–24.11.1.3). Indeed, the presence of basal meningeal enhancement, tuberculoma, or both, was 89% sensitive and 100% specific for the diagnosis of TBM in one study. Pre-contrast hyperdensity in the basal cisterns may be a highly specific radiological sign of TBM in children. Cranial MRI is better at defining brainstem and cerebellum pathology, tuberculomas, infarcts, and the extent of inflammatory exudates, but there are no data to suggest that MRI is better than CT in discriminating TBM from other disorders. Cryptococcal meningitis, viral encephalitis, sarcoidosis, meningeal metastases, and lymphoma may all produce similar radiographic findings. The major role of neuroradiology has been in the management and follow-up of the complications of TBM requiring neurosurgery.

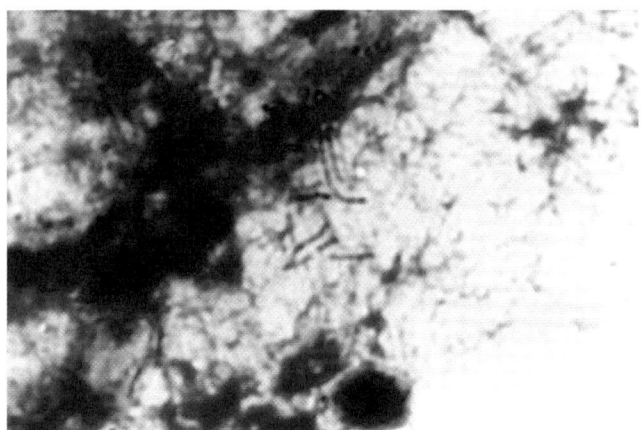

Fig. 24.11.1.15 Acid-fast bacilli of *Mycobacterium tuberculosis* stained by Ziehl–Neelsen stain in cerebrospinal fluid.

The culture of *M. tuberculosis* from the cerebrospinal fluid is the gold standard diagnostic test for TBM, but takes 2 to 6 weeks and is therefore too slow to aid clinical decision-making. Demonstrating acid-fast bacilli of *M. tuberculosis* in the cerebrospinal fluid after Zeihl–Neelsen staining is the oldest and most widely available rapid diagnostic test (Fig. 24.11.1.15), but the performance varies widely depending upon the volume of cerebrospinal fluid examined, the duration of microscopy, and the skill of the operator. Most laboratories find acid-fast bacilli in the cerebrospinal fluid of only 10 to 20% of those with TBM. Meticulous microscopy and the examination of large (>5 ml) volumes of cerebrospinal fluid can improve the sensitivity of both staining and culture to more than 60% and 80% respectively. HIV infection is also associated with better performance of bacteriology because there are higher concentrations of bacteria in the cerebrospinal fluid.

Whether molecular techniques can improve on conventional bacteriology is still unclear. In theory, nucleic acid amplification, such as that based on the PCR, should improve on bacteriology, but studies addressing their diagnostic role have failed to demonstrate an improvement because of low numbers of cases and inadequate bacteriological diagnostic comparison. A systematic review and meta-analysis calculated that commercial nucleic acid amplification assays for the diagnosis of TBM were 56% sensitive (95%CI 46–66%) and 98% specific (95%CI 97–99%). These data suggest that the sensitivity of these assays is still too low—approximately half those with a negative test will actually have the disease—and may not improve upon careful bacteriology. Studies published after the meta-analysis reinforce this conclusion and indicate that before the start of treatment careful bacteriology is as good, or better, than the currently available commercial nucleic acid amplification assays, but these methods retain their sensitivity in the face of anti-TB chemotherapy and are more useful once treatment has started. Unfortunately, there is no single test that will allow the physician to confidently rule out TBM.

Many other approaches to the diagnosis of TBM have been attempted and shown preliminary promise, but none has proved sufficiently reproducible, sensitive, specific, and practical for widespread clinical use. Commercial immunological assays based on the production of interferon-γ after stimulation with *M. tuberculosis*-specific antigens (ESAT6 and CFP10)—the T-SPOT and QuantiFERON-TB assays—have been a major advance in the diagnosis of latent TB infection, but their potential role in TBM diagnosis has not been established. Published data from small numbers of patients with TBM using an ELISPOT assay (used in the T-SPOT test) on cerebrospinal fluid suggested that it lacks sensitivity and, until further evaluation is complete, these assays cannot be recommended for the routine laboratory diagnosis of TBM.

In summary, a high index of clinical suspicion is required to diagnose TBM and, given the fatal consequences of delayed treatment, clinicians should be encouraged to initiate 'empirical' therapy in the setting of compatible clinical, epidemiological, and laboratory findings.

Differential diagnosis

TBM usually presents as a subacute lymphocytic meningitis and the differential diagnosis will depend on the age of the patient, geographical location, and immune status. In immunocompetent individuals the major differential diagnoses are partially treated pyogenic bacterial meningitis and viral meningoencephalitis. Various neoplastic infiltrations of the meninges (e.g. carcinomas, leukaemias, and lymphomas) may be more common at the extremes of age. Neurosarcoidosis can be very difficult to distinguish from TBM, as may neurosyphilis. Geographical region can suggest specific alternative diagnoses, e.g. meningitis caused by *Angiostrongylus cantonensis* or *Gnathostoma spinigerum* in south-east Asia, or by *Coccidioides* spp., *Histoplasma* spp., or cysticercosis in the Americas, can all mimic TBM. The immunosuppressed patient represents an important group often at high risk for diseases caused by mycobacteria, fungi, and herpesviruses. Cryptococcal meningitis is the major differential diagnosis of TBM in HIV-infected patients but can usually be distinguished on the basis of a cerebrospinal fluid Indian ink stain, fungal culture, or the cryptococcal antigen test. Cerebral toxoplasmosis can be difficult to differentiate from cerebral tuberculosis, especially when multiple tuberculomas are present, and cytomegalovirus (CMV) and herpes simplex virus (HSV) 1 and 2 meningoencephalitis can also cause diagnostic confusion with TBM. In most of these cases careful microbiological examination of the cerebrospinal fluid (for fungi and mycobacteria, in particular), selected use of nucleic acid amplification assays (*M. tuberculosis*, *Toxoplamsa gondii*, CMV, and HSV), and serological tests (syphilis) will allow a diagnosis to be made.

Treatment

The treatment of TBM follows the model of a short course of chemotherapy for pulmonary TB: an 'intensive phase' of treatment with four drugs, followed by a prolonged 'continuation phase' with two drugs. The first 2 months of treatment should be with isoniazid, rifampicin, pyrazinamide, and streptomycin, ethambutol, or ethionamide. The British Thoracic Society (BTS) and the Infectious Disease Society of America (IDSA) favour ethambutol as the fourth drug, although they acknowledge the lack of evidence from controlled trials. Others, particularly in South Africa, advocate ethionamide, which penetrates healthy and inflamed meninges more effectively than ethambutol or streptomycin, but can cause severe nausea and vomiting. In adults, daily single doses of 300 mg isoniazid, 600 mg rifampicin, and 2000 mg pyrazinamide provide adequate levels in the sera and cerebrospinal fluid of patients with TBM. Higher doses of these drugs are unnecessary and may result in a higher incidence of hepatotoxicity. Some advocate higher doses in children, notably in South Africa, but this approach cannot be recommended in adults. Unlike the treatment of pulmonary TB, interruptions in anti-TB chemotherapy are an independent risk factor for death from TBM.

British and American guidelines suggest between 9 and 12 months of total anti-TB treatment for TBM, although a recent systematic review concluded that 6 months might be sufficient provided that the likelihood of drug resistance is low. Isoniazid and rifampicin are considered mandatory in the continuation phase and the BTS suggests that therapy should be extended to 18 months in those unable to tolerate pyrazinamide in the intensive phase. Others recommend that pyrazinamide be given throughout treatment because of its excellent penetration across the blood–brain barrier, although there is no supporting evidence from controlled trials.

TBM caused by *M. tuberculosis* resistant to one or more first-line anti-TB drugs is an increasingly common problem. Isoniazid resistance alone does not appear to have a major impact on outcome from TBM, which is surprising given isoniazid's excellent penetration into cerebrospinal fluid and its potent early bactericidal activity. However, the combination of rifampicin and isoniazid resistance (multidrug resistance) has a major impact such that most patients will die unless second-line therapy is started early. Detecting TBM caused by multidrug-resistant organisms is difficult: patients are likely to be dead before the results of conventional susceptibility tests (which take 6–8 weeks) are available and rapid, molecular-based assays for detecting resistant organisms in cerebrospinal fluid have not been properly evaluated. In addition, the best combination, dose, and duration of second-line agents for the treatment of multidrug-resistant TBM are not known. Indeed, there are no published controlled trials addressing this issue for any form of TB. Until more data become available the treatment of multidrug-resistant TBM should follow the principles of treating drug-resistant pulmonary disease: never add a single agent to a failing regimen; use at least three previously unused drugs, one of which should be a fluoroquinolone; streptomycin resistance does not confer resistance to other aminoglycosides, therefore amikacin or kanamycin can be used; and treat for at least 18 months.

Adjunctive corticosteroids

The use of adjunctive corticosteroids has been controversial ever since they were first suggested for the management of TBM more than 50 years ago. A meta-analysis and systematic review of all controlled trials published before 2000 concluded that corticosteroids probably improved survival in children, but small trial sizes, poor treatment allocation concealment, and possible publication bias did not support clear treatment recommendations. In 2004, a controlled trial of adjunctive dexamethasone in 545 Vietnamese adults with TBM revealed that dexamethasone treatment was strongly associated with a reduced risk of death after 9 months of treatment (RR 0.69, 95%CI 0.52–0.92, $p = 0.01$), but did not prevent severe disability in the survivors. The effect of dexamethasone was consistent across all grades of disease severity, dispelling a previously held belief that corticosteroids benefited only those with more severe disease, but did not demonstrate a significant effect on death or disability in those infected with HIV. Current evidence suggests that all HIV-uninfected patients with TBM should be given dexamethasone, regardless of age or disease severity. A clear benefit of dexamethasone in HIV-infected patients has not been demonstrated,

but the trial in Vietnam suggested that it was safe and might improve survival.

There are no data from controlled trials comparing different corticosteroid regimens, so the choice of regimen should be based on those used in the published controlled trials. In adults, the following regimen was shown to improve outcome in Vietnam: those with a Glasgow Coma Scale (GCS) score of less than 15 or focal neurological deficit at the start of treatment received intravenous drug for 4 weeks (0.4 mg/kg per 24 h week 1, 0.3 mg/kg per 24 h week 2, 0.2 mg/kg per 24 h week 3, and 0.1 mg/kg per 24 h week 4) followed by 4 mg total oral drug, reducing each week by 1 mg until 0. Those without coma or neurological signs received intravenous drug for 2 weeks (0.2 mg/kg per 24 h week 1, 0.1 mg/kg per h week 2), followed by the same oral reducing course described above. In children, the South African trial demonstrated improved survival with 4 mg/kg per day of prednisolone for the first month of treatment.

Response to therapy and treatment of complications

Ninety per cent of deaths from TBM occur in the first month of treatment. The response to therapy is slow and can follow a fluctuant course. Indeed, a rapid and sustained response over a few days suggests an alternative diagnosis. Headache is often present for many weeks, even in uncomplicated cases. Fever rarely disappears within a week, and pyrexia is often observed for 6 to 8 weeks. The degree of neck rigidity at presentation varies considerably and can take 4 to 6 weeks to resolve. The cerebrospinal fluid mirrors the slow clinical response: cell counts remain elevated for 1 to 2 months, cerebrospinal fluid glucose remains low for a similar duration, and total cerebrospinal fluid protein can rise before falling slowly over many months. Transient episodes of high fever, worsening headache, and increased nuchal rigidity can occur during the first 2 months of treatment, particularly in those with more severe disease. Distinguishing self-limiting events from the onset of more serious complications is difficult. New focal neurological signs, or a fall in conscious level, rarely accompanies these transient deteriorations. Cranial imaging should be arranged urgently if new clinical signs develop during treatment. Hydrocephalus, cerebral infarction, the expansion of intracranial tuberculoma, hyponatraemia, and poor adherence to therapy are the foremost reasons for severe acute deterioration. The expansion of intracranial tuberculoma after the start of treatment is a widely reported complication and frequently labelled as a 'paradoxical' treatment reaction. Recent data suggest that 75% with TBM develop tuberculomas during therapy but only small proportions are symptomatic. Most authors suggest treatment with prolonged high-dose corticosteroids if the tuberculoma causes clinical deterioration, although there are no controlled trials to support these recommendations. There are case reports to suggest that adjunctive thalidomide may help in the management of symptomatic expanding tuberculomas. Rarely, tuberculomas coalesce to form an abscess and neurosurgical drainage may be indicated.

Hydrocephalus is a common and serious complication of TBM and can be treated with diuretics (furosemide and/or acetazolamide), serial lumbar punctures, or ventriculoperitoneal/atrial shunting. There are no data from controlled trials that determine which method of treatment is best. Some advocate early shunting in all patients with hydrocephalus, whereas others recommend shunting only for patients with noncommunicating hydrocephalus.

External ventricular drainage has been used to predict response to ventriculoperitoneal shunting but without success; others suggest that monitoring lumbar cerebrospinal fluid pressure can predict response to medical treatment. Without clear evidence physicians must balance possible benefit with the resources and experience of their surgical unit and the significant complications of shunt surgery.

Severe hyponatraemia is a common and often overlooked cause of deterioration on therapy. With the pathogenesis unclear, the best way of correcting the plasma sodium is uncertain. Sodium and fluid replacement are probably indicated in hypovolaemic hyponatraemia, whereas fluid restriction may be more appropriate in those who are euvolaemic with evidence of SIADH. There is anecdotal evidence to suggest that fludrocortisone replacement therapy and demeclocycline may be useful.

Prognosis and sequelae

TBM kills or severely disables half of the people who have the condition. Outcome is even worse in those coinfected with HIV as more than half die. Whether highly active antiretroviral therapy can improve survival is uncertain and under active investigation.

The severity of TBM has been divided into three grades, a categorization that takes its name and definitions from the 1948 British Medical Research Council (MRC) study of streptomycin in TBM treatment (Table 24.11.1.4). The grades are still used because they are good predictors of outcome: less than 10% of patients die with grade I disease, whereas 50% with grade III will not survive. A number of studies have assessed the clinical and laboratory parameters that predict outcome. Univariate analyses have suggested extremes of age, advanced stage of disease, concomitant extrameningeal TB, and evidence of raised ICP are associated with a poor outcome. Studies that have adjusted for the effect of covariables using multivariate analyses have consistently shown that treatment before the onset of coma improves outcome. A study of 434 Turkish adults revealed convulsions, coma, and delayed or interrupted treatment to be independent predictors of death. Extrameningeal TB, cranial nerve palsy, focal weakness, multiple neurological abnormalities, and drowsiness at diagnosis independently predicted later neurological disability. Permanent sequelae occur in 10 to 30% of survivors: intellectual impairment is common in infants and young children and a quarter of all patients will have cranial nerve deficits, including blindness, deafness, and squints. Ten per cent will have permanent mono-, hemi-, or paraparesis.

Prevention (see Chapter 7.6.25)

Although the efficacy of BCG immunization to prevent pulmonary TB is controversial, its ability to prevent disseminated TB (including TBM) in young children is widely accepted. Meta-analyses have

Table 24.11.1.4 The British Medical Research Council disease severity grades for tuberculous meningitis

Grade	Clinical criteria
I	Alert and oriented without focal neurological deficit
II	GCS score 14–10 with or without focal neurological deficit or GCS 15 with focal neurological deficit
III	GCS score <10 with or without focal neurological deficit

GCS, Glasgow Coma Scale.

shown that BCG immunization at birth prevents around 70% of all cases of childhood TBM and is a highly cost-effective intervention in settings with a high prevalence of TB. Whether the protection lasts into adulthood is uncertain.

TBM can also be prevented by treating the household contacts of newly diagnosed cases of pulmonary TB. The BTS recommend either 6 months of isoniazid or 3 months of isoniazid and rifampicin for Mantoux-positive contacts to prevent progression to active disease.

Possible future developments

Immunization

Despite some successes, the use of pneumococcal polysaccharide vaccines is controversial. The efficacy of the 23-valent pneumococcal polysaccharide vaccine has been extensively studied and, in a meta-analysis, its efficacy was estimated to be 38 to 53% for the prevention of invasive pneumococcal disease in adults. Although PCV7 is highly effective in children, the high costs of this vaccine limit its implementation in health care in less developed countries. In addition, duration of protection and the minimum number of doses needed for protection in conjugate vaccines are uncertain. A possible alternative or complementary approach is to develop vaccines directed against noncapsular antigens common to all pneumococcal species. Potential targets for future pneumococcal protein vaccines are neuraminidase, autolysin, pneumolysin, pneumococcal surface protein, and pneumococcal surface adhesion A.

The high variability of *N. meningitidis* emphasizes the need for a permanent global follow-up, so that public health decision-makers and vaccine manufacturers can plan the most relevant vaccine strategies and development according to the most recent epidemiological trends, while taking into account cost and logistical hurdles that are the major limitations for the less developed world. The approval of a conjugate meningococcal vaccine against serogroups A, C, Y, and W135 might lead to a further decrease in the incidence of this devastating infection. This vaccine should be included in the expanded programme of immunization.

Genetic factors

Large prospective multinational studies have to determine the role of genetic factors contributing to susceptibility and outcome in bacterial meningitis. Findings may have several implications for therapy and prevention. Existence of subgroups of patients with genetic variations or deficiencies in innate immunity that especially benefits from immunomodulatory therapy is likely. In addition, genotypes may be used to identify patients at high risk for the development of disease and those with high risk for complications. Physicians may, in the future, be able to use genetic information to dedicate immune-based therapy to modulate the response in a given patient.

Randomized clinical trials

Large trials of adjuvant dexamethasone in adults and children with acute bacterial meningitis are still needed and randomized comparative studies of various treatment regimens should be performed.

New adjunctive therapies

Experimental research has increased our knowledge about the pathophysiology of bacterial meningitis and the mechanisms involved in neuronal injury. Recent animal studies in experimental lipopolysaccharide-induced meningitis demonstrated that europium is a useful marker for quantifying blood–brain barrier permeability. Understanding and quantifying the mechanisms by which the blood–brain barrier is altered are paramount to identifying new treatment strategies. In addition, animal studies are used to study the effect of potential adjunctive therapies and the possible role of neuroprotective substances. A number of adjunctive strategies for treatment have been considered, but, thus far, all the therapies described below have been tested only in experimental bacterial meningitis models. Administration of antibodies to proinflammatory cytokines TNF-α and IL-1β decreased pleocytosis and reduced blood–brain barrier permeability in experimental bacterial meningitis. Pharmacological interference with activation of NF-κB, a transcription factor involved in the activation of many genes during bacterial meningitis, has reduced meningitis-induced CNS inflammation.

Matrix metalloproteases (MMPs) are a family of zinc-dependent matrix-degrading enzymes that can disrupt the blood–brain barrier and thereby facilitate leucocyte extravasation and brain oedema. Inhibition of MMPs reduced blood–brain barrier permeability and the extent of cortical damage in experimental meningitis. Reactive oxygen species and reactive nitrogen intermediates are involved in several aspects of the host response to bacterial infections. Antioxidants attenuate early events-associated neurological injury in bacterial meningitis and are a promising strategy in the treatment of bacterial meningitis; among these therapies, the antioxidant *N*-acetylcysteine seems to be closest to a clinical application. *N*-Acetylcysteine reduced meningeal inflammation, oxidative brain damage, cortical neuronal injury, brain oedema, ICP, cochlear injury, and hearing loss in animal models of pneumococcal meningitis. Simultaneous production of oxygen-centred and nitrogen-centred free radicals favours the production of a toxic reaction product, an oxidant called peroxynitrite. Peroxynitrite induces cytotoxicity and thereby initiates lipid peroxidation and induction of DNA single-strand breakage. Damaged DNA activates poly(ADP-ribose) polymerase (PARP) and thereby induces an energy-consuming cycle that can result in cellular energy depletion and necrotic cell death. Treatment with peroxynitrite scavengers and PARP inhibitors are other potential effective strategies in bacterial meningitis. Caspases are a family of proteases that are involved in inflammation, upstream signalling, and most forms of apoptosis. Apoptosis can be blocked pharmacologically, leading to reduced meningitis-associated intracranial complications. Potentially, the efficacy of therapeutic interventions may be enhanced by simultaneous intervention at several levels of the inflammatory cascade. Despite the benefits of these strategies in experimental models, clinical trials are needed to assess their efficacy in patients with bacterial meningitis.

Further reading

British Medical Research Council (1948). Streptomycin treatment of tuberculous meningitis. *Br Med J*, **i**, 582–97.

Dastur DK, *et al.* (1995). Pathology and pathogenetic mechanisms in neurotuberculosis. *Radiol Clin North Am*, **33**, 733–52.

Kim KS (2003). Pathogenesis of bacterial meningitis: From bacteraemia to neuronal injury. *Nature Rev Neurosci*, **4**, 376–85.

Klugman KP, *et al.* (2003). A trial of a 9-valent pneumococcal conjugate vaccine in children with and those without HIV infection. *N Engl J Med*, **349**, 1341–8.

Molyneux E, Riordan FA, Walsh A (2006). Acute bacterial meningitis in children presenting to the Royal Liverpool Children's Hospital, Liverpool, UK and the Queen Elizabeth Central Hospital in Blantyre, Malawi: a world of difference. *Ann Trop Paediatr*, **26**, 29–37.

Nguyen Thi Hoang Mai, *et al.* (2007). A randomized controlled trial of dexamethasone for Vietnamese adolescents and adults with bacterial meningitis. *N Engl J Med*, **357**, 2431–40.

Pai M, *et al.* (2003). Diagnostic accuracy of nucleic acid amplification tests for tuberculous meningitis: a systematic review and meta-analysis. *Lancet Infect Dis*, **3**, 633–43.

Rich AR, McCordock HA (1933). The pathogenesis of tuberculous meningitis. *Bull John Hopkins Hosp*, **52**, 5–37.

Scarborough M, *et al.* (2007). Corticosteroids for bacterial meningitis in adults in sub-Saharan Africa. *N Engl J Med*, **357**, 2441–50.

Schoeman JF, *et al.* (2006). Intractable intracranial tuberculous infection responsive to thalidomide: report of four cases. *J Child Neurol*, **21**, 301–8.

Stephens DS, Greenwood B, Brandtzaeg P (2007). Epidemic meningitis, meningococcaemia, and *Neisseria meningitidis*. *Lancet*, **369**, 2196–210.

Stewart SM (1953). The bacteriological diagnosis of tuberculous meningitis. *J Clin Pathol*, **6**, 241–2.

Thompson MJ, *et al.* (2006). Clinical recognition of meningococcal disease in children and adolescents. *Lancet*, **367**, 397–403.

Thwaites G, *et al.* (2002). A clinical diagnostic rule for adults with tuberculous meningitis. *Lancet*, **360**, 1287–92.

Thwaites GE, *et al.* (2005). The influence of HIV infection on clinical presentation, response to treatment, and outcome in adults with tuberculous meningitis. *J Infect Dis*, **192**, 2134–41.

Thwaites G, *et al.* (2004). A randomized, double blind, placebo controlled trial of dexamethasone for the treatment of adults with tuberculous meningitis. *N Engl J Med*, **351**, 1741–51.

van de Beek D, *et al.* (2007). Corticosteroids for acute bacterial meningitis. *Cochrane Database Syst Rev*, CD004405.

24.11.2 Viral infections

Jeremy Farrar, Bridget Wills,
Menno D. de Jong, and David A. Warrell

Essentials

Meningitis

Enteroviruses are responsible for 80 to 90% and mumps for 10 to 20% of diagnosed cases of viral meningitis, with many other viruses sometimes incriminated with considerable geographical and seasonal variation.

Clinical features and prognosis—typical presentation is with sudden onset of fever, headache, change in conscious level, and (occasionally) a stiff neck and vomiting. The specific cause may be suggested by characteristic signs outside the nervous system, e.g. swelling in the parotid region (mumps). Prognosis is excellent.

Encephalitis

Japanese encephalitis is the commonest cause of encephalitis in Asia: other causes—with considerable geographical and seasonal variation—include dengue viruses, Enteroviruses (EV71) rabies, Nipah virus, herpes simplex, West Nile virus, and mumps.

Clinical features and prognosis—most patients present with the symptoms of meningitis followed by altered consciousness, convulsions, and sometimes focal neurological signs, signs of raised intracranial pressure, or psychiatric symptoms. Some manifestations suggest particular viruses, e.g. temporal lobe features in herpes simplex encephalitis; hydrophobia in rabies; Parkinsonian and extrapyramidal features in Japanese encephalitis. Mortality and morbidity vary according to cause, but are high, e.g. mortality 10 to 40% in Japanese encephalitis, with neurological sequelae in 5 to 75% of survivors.

Myelitis

Viral 'paralytic' myelitis is classically caused by poliovirus, which has now been virtually eliminated from the Americas: other causes—with considerable geographical and seasonal variation—include Japanese encephalitis and various coxsackieviruses, echoviruses, enteroviruses and flaviviruses.

Clinical features—following a nonspecific episode of influenza-like symptoms, poliomyelitis typically presents with features of viral meningitis preceding or accompanying the development of lower motor neurone (flaccid) paralysis. Respiratory and bulbar paralysis is life-threatening. Mortality in adults is more than 20%.

Investigation

The most important investigation is lumbar puncture to allow examination of the cerebrospinal fluid (see Chapter 24.11.1 for discussion), with typical findings of (1) pleocytosis—ranging from tens to thousands of cells/µl, with lymphocytes and other mononuclear cells usually predominating; (2) modest increase in protein concentration; (3) normal glucose concentration. Some viruses can be isolated from the cerebrospinal fluid, and viruses can sometimes be cultured from distant sites, but polymerase chain reaction (PCR) technology is now used routinely for diagnosis of viral central nervous system infection.

Treatment

Aside from supportive care, aciclovir is effective in treating herpes simplex encephalitis, and hyperimmune plasma reduces mortality of Argentine haemorrhagic fever (Junin virus) and Congo Crimean haemorrhagic fever, but there is no effective specific treatment for most viral infections of the central nervous system.

Prevention

Prophylactic vaccination is available against poliomyelitis, measles, Japanese encephalitis, and rabies. Postexposure rabies vaccination is effective in preventing rabies encephalitis. Hyperimmune immunoglobulin has been used for prophylaxis of measles, herpes zoster virus, HSV-2, vaccinia, rabies, and some other infections in high-risk groups.

Other neurological disorders in which viruses play a role

These include (1) Reye's syndrome—an acute encephalopathy affecting children aged 2 to 16 years, associated with use of salicylates during the preceding viral illness. (2) Subacute sclerosing panencephalitis—caused by measles virus; typically presents with very gradual onset of altered behaviour, mild intellectual deterioration, and loss of energy and interest; periodic involuntary movements then appear; further progression is marked by intellectual deterioration, rigidity, spasticity, and increasing helplessness; there is no effective treatment; 40% of patients die within a year. (3) Progressive multifocal leucoencephalopathy—caused by opportunistic infection by papovaviruses, most commonly JC virus and the simian virus SV40; onset is usually with progressive evidence of a focal lesion of one cerebral hemisphere, before gradual development of more widespread signs; there is no effective treatment; most patients die within 6 to 12 months.

Introduction

Viruses invade and damage the central nervous system in two ways: directly, by infecting the leptomeninges, brain, and spinal cord; and, indirectly, by inducing an immunological reaction resulting in para- and postinfectious diseases. In both cases, the terms 'meningitis', 'encephalitis', and 'myelitis' are used alone or in combination. Meningitis implies inflammation of the meninges without alteration of consciousness, convulsions, or the production of focal neurological abnormalities; in encephalitis there is impairment of cerebral function, usually with an altered state of consciousness and often with convulsions and focal neurological signs; while myelitis indicates involvement of the spinal cord. Retroviral and prion diseases of the central nervous system are dealt with elsewhere (Chapters 7.5.23–25 and Chapter 24.11.5).

Virology

There is considerable geographical and seasonal variation in the kinds of viruses causing meningitis, myelitis, and encephalitis. Vulnerability varies with age and immunocompetence.

Enteroviruses are responsible for 80 to 90% of diagnosed cases of viral meningitis. Almost all the serotypes have been implicated in sporadic cases, and outbreaks have been associated with coxsackieviruses A7 and A9, EV71, all the coxsackievirus B types, and many of the echoviruses, especially 4, 6, 9, 11, 14, 16, and 30. Echovirus 13, a rare type, has caused cases in the United States of America, Australia, and Europe, and there has been an increase in echovirus 30 cases. Mumps is responsible for about 10 to 20% of cases of viral meningitis. Other causes include herpes zoster (HZV), herpes simplex virus (predominantly type 2, HSV-2), measles, adenoviruses, Epstein–Barr virus (EBV), and, in the United States of America, togaviruses, such as St Louis, eastern and western equine encephalitis, and West Nile and bunyaviruses, such as California (La Crosse) encephalitis viruses.

Poliovirus has long been considered the major cause of viral 'paralytic' myelitis throughout the world, but has now been virtually eliminated from the Americas. A confusingly similar syndrome of acute flaccid paralysis caused by Japanese encephalitis (JE) has been reported from Vietnam. Coxsackievirus A7 (AB IV) has caused occasional outbreaks, and other coxsackieviruses A and B, echoviruses, enterovirus 71, and flaviviruses (tick-borne encephalitis) have all been implicated as causes of flaccid paralysis. HZV, paralytic rabies virus, EBV, and herpesvirus simiae (B virus) can cause myelitis or ascending paralysis, and HSV-2 can cause lumbosacral myeloradiculitis.

Viruses causing encephalitis vary from country to country. JE virus is the major cause of encephalitis in Asia. There are at least 50 000 cases of JE with 15 000 deaths annually (case fatality 0.3 to 60%). The virus is transmitted by culex mosquitoes and is endemic across much of Asia and the Indian subcontinent. Dengue viruses have been implicated as a cause of encephalitis in both south-east Asia and Latin America. Rabies remains an important cause of fatal encephalomyelitis, especially in the Indian subcontinent and Africa (see Chapter 7.5.10).

In 1999 an outbreak of an encephalitic illness among pig farm and abattoir workers was reported from Singapore and Malaysia (see Chapter 7.5.7). There were 258 cases of encephalitis, with a case fatality rate of almost 40%. Subsequently, Nipah has become endemic in Bangladesh. The causative agent was a new paramyxovirus, Nipah virus, closely related to the Hendra and Manangle viruses described in Australia (see Chapter 7.5.7). Nipah virus encephalitis is a zoonosis infecting pigs and flying foxes (*Pteropus* spp.). Almost all patients infected in this outbreak had direct contact with pigs. Hendra virus has caused a few cases of equine and human encephalitis with a human fatality in Brisbane, Australia in 2008 (see Chapter 7.5.7).

In North America, herpes simplex virus is the most common cause of sporadic fatal viral encephalitis, followed by the California encephalitis group, St Louis encephalitis virus, HZV, enteroviruses, mumps, measles, and, most recently, the West Nile virus. In the United States of America, herpes simplex encephalitis has an estimated incidence of 2.3 per million population each year; HSV-1 accounts for 95% of cases; HSV-2 causes encephalitis mainly in neonates and those who are immunosuppressed, such as transplant recipients, and those with HIV infection. In 1999 there was an outbreak of West Nile infection in the eastern United States of America with a cluster of cases of encephalitis in New York and 16 human deaths. West Nile virus is a mosquito-borne flavivirus closely related to JE. It has been known to cause encephalitis in Africa, the Middle East, and southern and eastern Europe, but this was the first appearance of this virus in the New World. In endemic areas, infection with West Nile virus is usually asymptomatic or associated with a mild flu-like illness. Only occasionally does it cause encephalitis, with a case fatality rate for patients admitted to hospital in New York of 12%. The virus has now become established in migrant bird populations across the United States of America and Central America, and in 2008 there were 1370 cases with 37 fatalities in the United States of America reported by the Centers for Disease Control (CDC), Atlanta.

In the United Kingdom, mumps is the most frequently diagnosed viral encephalitis, followed by echoviruses, coxsackieviruses, measles, HSV, HZV, EBV, and adenoviruses (especially adenovirus 7). Louping ill is the only indigenous arthropod (tick)-borne encephalitis in the United Kingdom. In central and eastern Europe and Scandinavia, tick-borne encephalitis virus and Russian spring–summer encephalitis viruses are endemic. Usutu, a flavivirus, has been isolated in birds in Austria. In many developing countries rabies is an important cause of viral encephalitis. Other regional causes are Rift Valley fever virus in Africa and the Middle East, arenaviruses (Junin, Guanarito, Sabiá, Lassa, and Machupo) in Latin America and Africa, Marburg and Ebola viruses in Africa, Colorado tick fever virus in North America, and Murray Valley encephalitis virus in Australia.

Postinfectious encephalomyelitis most commonly follows measles, vaccinia, varicella, rubella, mumps, and influenza. Guillain–Barré syndrome, a sensorimotor polyneuropathy (see Chapter 24.16), has been associated with infections by EBV, cytomegalovirus (CMV), coxsackievirus B, and HZV. The decreasingly used nervous tissue vaccines for rabies may give rise to postvaccinal encephalomyelitis (see below), whereas immunization against influenza, rabies, hepatitis B, measles, and poliomyelitis has been complicated by Guillain–Barré syndrome.

Immunodeficient patients are particularly vulnerable to some viral infections. Those with depressed cell-mediated immunity (Hodgkin's disease) may develop HZV encephalitis, and CMV may cause a subacute encephalitis in patients with AIDS. In children or adults with hypogammaglobulinaemia, enteroviruses, including live-attenuated polio vaccine, may produce a progressive and fatal meningoencephalitis. Progressive multifocal leucoencephalopathy, a chronic and fatal papovavirus infection in patients with impaired cell-mediated immunity, is described below. HIV infection of the brain and meninges may be responsible for acute meningoencephalitis at the time of seroconversion and for subacute chronic encephalopathies and dementia in patients with AIDS (see Chapters 7.10.23 and 24.14.4).

Epidemiology

Many viral infections of the central nervous system (CNS) occur in seasonal peaks or as epidemics, whereas others, such as herpes simplex encephalitis, are sporadic. Epidemics of JE (see Chapter 7.5.14) occur in the summer or rainy season in northern India, Nepal, northern Thailand, Korea, Taiwan, and China. However, in southern Vietnam, Indonesia, Malaysia, southern India, and the Philippines the disease can occur all the year round, although the peak is at the start of the rainy season. This variation in the incidence of disease is an important consideration when recommending immunization. In endemic areas it is mostly a disease of children, but as the disease spreads to new regions, or nonimmune travellers visit endemic regions, nonimmune adults are also affected. The major vector is *Culex tritaeniorhynchus* mosquitoes that have been infected by first feeding on the bird (cattle egrets, herons) or mammal reservoir species. Indigenous children and nonimmune (immigrant) adults are most susceptible. Euro-Siberian tick-borne encephalitides (see Chapter 7.5.14) occur in spring and early summer when the ticks are most active but can also be acquired by drinking unpasteurized dairy products, especially goat's milk. Mumps encephalitis is most common in the late winter or early spring, whereas enterovirus infections occur most often in the summer and early autumn. Rodent-related encephalitides, such as the arenaviruses, are most common when the rodent population is at its peak, either in the fields (Machupo and Junin viruses) or in the home (lymphocytic choriomeningitis virus). Zoonotic viral infections, such as Rift Valley fever, survive periods of cold weather, during which the invertebrate–vertebrate cycle is suspended by 'overwintering' in their arthropod vectors (e.g. in the bottom of dried-up ponds) or hibernating vertebrate reservoirs. Rabies, the classic zoonosis (see Chapter 7.5.10), occurs sporadically or in microepidemics although, in Europe, historically the greatest risk of dogs becoming mad with rabies was believed to be associated with the hot weather, the 'dog days', when Sirius the dog star was in the ascendant (20 July to 15 August).

Invasion of the CNS seems to be a rare event in most viral infections. In the case of some infections, such as JE, there may be only 1 case of encephalitis for every 300 to 500 asymptomatic infections. Eastern equine encephalitis virus produces a much higher proportion of encephalitic cases than other togaviruses.

Infections by many neurotropic viruses are most frequent and severe in children and older people. Herpes simplex encephalitis affects all age groups but shows peaks of incidence in those aged between 5 and 30 years and over 50 years. When HSV-2 invades the CNS it is likely to cause a benign lymphocytic meningitis in adults, but in neonates it usually produces a severe encephalitis. Among mosquito-borne epidemic encephalitides, California encephalitis and JE are most common in children, St Louis and West Nile encephalitis in older people, whereas eastern and western equine encephalitis affect both very young and older people. Postinfectious encephalitis is most frequent in children, because it complicates the common childhood exanthematous viral infections. It is the most common demyelinating disease in the world.

Pathogenesis

Most viral infections reach the CNS from the primary site of infection and multiplication via the bloodstream, but the rabies virus enters peripheral nerves through acetylcholine and other receptors and travels to the CNS in axoplasm, employing the microtubular dynein motor system. Viruses inoculated through the skin include those transmitted by arthropods, rabies virus, herpes simplex virus, herpesvirus simiae (B virus), and lymphocytic choriomeningitis virus. Arthropod-borne viruses are presumed to replicate in local lymph nodes, the vascular endothelium, and circulating fixed macrophages, in order to sustain viraemia. Rabies virus may multiply locally in the cytoplasm of muscle cells before entering peripheral nerves. Viruses that enter through the respiratory tract (e.g. measles, mumps, varicella) or gut (enteroviruses) multiply in local lymphoid tissue before entering the bloodstream. Viraemia is a feature of most viral infections, yet invasion of the CNS is rare in most cases. The explanation for this is not known, but the CNS contains a number of intrinsic physical barriers to infectious agents such as viruses. These include the blood–brain barrier with its 'tight junctions', virus-resistant cells, and the absence of lymphatic drainage. Nonspecific mechanisms at or near the site of virus entry, such as gastric acidity and cilia in the respiratory tract, also play a protective role. In the case of rabies, HSV, and HZV, the virus enters the CNS through the peripheral nerves. Although the subarachnoid space surrounding the olfactory nerves projects through the cribriform plate and is directly beneath the nasal mucosa, this route of infection seems to be extremely rare in humans and has been proven only in a few cases of inhaled rabies virus infection and herpes simplex encephalitis. Viruses have been inoculated directly into the CNS by infected corneal transplant grafts (rabies) and prions through infected brain-surface electrodes (Creutzfeldt–Jakob disease). Herpes simplex encephalitis may complicate primary HSV infection in children and young adults, but in most cases of herpes simplex encephalitis the cause is thought to be reactivation of latent virus (HSV-1) in the trigeminal nerve, autonomic nerve roots, or brain.

Some viruses, such as the enteroviruses and mumps, usually infect the meninges rather than the parenchyma of the CNS, whereas others, such as the togaviruses, usually cause encephalitis. Different neural cells are selectively vulnerable to different neurotropic viruses. Examples are the predilection of polioviruses for motor neurons of the anterior horns of the spinal cord, and of rabies for neurons of the limbic system and cerebellar Purkinje cells. The pathological effects of viral infections on the CNS include:

- the destruction and phagocytosis of neurons (neuronophagia) as a result of either viral invasion itself or immune lysis
- demyelination
- inflammatory oedema with the compressive effects of raised intracranial pressure
- in some cases, vascular lesions

In rabies, a universally fatal encephalitis, neuronolysis is relatively mild. However, rabies virus may interfere with neurotransmission at central and peripheral synapses. It also produces severe systemic effects, following its centrifugal spread (e.g. myocarditis and cardiac arrhythmias) or its focal effects on vasomotor and respiratory centres in the brainstem and in the temporal lobes and amygdala (compare Klüver–Bucy syndrome) (see Chapter 7.5.10).

Postinfectious encephalitis and the Guillain–Barré syndrome are thought to result from sensitization to central and peripheral myelin, respectively. The animal model for the former is experimental allergic encephalomyelitis, which can be produced in a variety of animals after immunization with myelin basic protein. A similar animal model for Guillain–Barré syndrome is known as experimental allergic neuritis. It is uncertain how the preceding viral infection induces this autoimmune response. In the case of postvaccinal encephalomyelitis resulting from old-fashioned nervous tissue antirabies vaccines containing homogenized animal brain, the mechanism is still not clear. The antimyelin basic protein is not always present and is probably not the direct cause of demyelination.

The host's immune responses to viruses play a crucial role in combating infection. They may be directed against either the virus particle or the virus-infected cell, and may be humorally or cell mediated. An important local immune response at infected surfaces is provided by IgA antibody, which is present in secretions in the gut, saliva, and respiratory tract. This is important, for example, in the early stages of poliovirus infection where the antibody neutralizes the virus by combining with viral surface proteins. The systemic viral infection may also be limited by means of circulating IgG and IgM antibodies, which can neutralize the virus in a variety of different ways. Immune responses may also occur locally within the CNS, where local synthesis of immunoglobulins in response to virus infection, sometimes in an oligoclonal pattern, may be evident. Such antibody elevations may be of considerable diagnostic value (see below). Under certain conditions immune responses to viruses may themselves set in train immunopathological processes leading to disease. This may occur in a number of different ways, such as through the deposition in blood vessels of immune complexes formed between an antiviral antibody and viral antigen. In other cases, such as lymphocytic choriomeningitis virus infection, the induction of virus-specific cytotoxic T lymphocytes is itself responsible for the production of encephalitis.

Pathology

Meningitis

The basal leptomeninges, ependyma, and choroid plexus are infiltrated with mononuclear cells but the parenchyma is normal. In mumps meningitis there may be exfoliation of ependymal cells.

Poliomyelitis

Virus is distributed widely throughout the brain and spinal cord, possibly even in nonparalytic cases, but usually the only cells to suffer chromatolysis and phagocytosis are motor neurons in the anterior horns of the spinal cord, medulla, and grey matter of the precentral gyrus.

Encephalitis

Most viral encephalitides are characterized by lymphocytic infiltration of the meninges and perivascular cuffing (in the Virchow–Robin spaces) in the cortex and underlying white matter, by lymphocytes, plasma cells, histiocytes, and some neutrophils, and proliferation of microglia with the formation of glial nodules. Neuronolysis and demyelination are variable in their degree and location. Infected neurons may show characteristic inclusion bodies in their nuclei (measles, HSV, and adenoviruses) or cytoplasm (Negri's bodies in rabies). Microhaemorrhages and foci of necrosis may be found.

Herpes simplex encephalitis

Characteristic features of this condition are gross cerebral oedema and severe haemorrhagic and necrotizing encephalitis, which is often asymmetrically localized to the inferior and medial parts of the temporal lobe, the insula, and the orbital part of the frontal lobe. Histological sections show eosinophilic Cowdry type A intranuclear inclusions with margination of chromatin in neurons, oligodendrocytes, and astrocytes, inflammatory and haemorrhagic perivascular reactions, but no demyelination. Cowdry type A inclusions are also found in HZV and CMV encephalitides. The unique cerebral localization of herpes simplex encephalitis has not been satisfactorily explained, but is probably the result of viral spread along specific neural pathways rather than a differential susceptibility of particular cell populations. A popular idea is that HSV spreads along olfactory pathways to the base of the brain and temporal lobes, but it is also possible that virus may spread from the trigeminal ganglia through sensory fibres innervating the dura near these regions. This latter mechanism is consistent with the discovery of latent HSV-1 in the trigeminal, superior cervical, and vagal ganglia in a high proportion of normal individuals, irrespective of whether they have a history of mucocutaneous herpes infections ('cold sores'). Latent HSV-1 might be reactivated by a variety of stimuli, such as sunlight, fever, trauma, and stress; however, the actual mechanisms underlying its latency and reactivation in the nervous system are not yet fully understood. If herpes simplex encephalitis is caused by the reactivation of latent virus, its rarity, despite ubiquitous asymptomatic infection in humans, is hard to explain.

Japanese encephalitis

Microscopic appearances are typical of other viral encephalitides: there is oedema, congestion, and focal haemorrhages of the brain and meninges, and perivascular cuffing, neuronophagia, and glial nodules of the brain parenchyma. Neuronolysis and neuronophagia are unusually widespread in the thalamus, basal ganglia, brainstem, cerebellum (where there is marked destruction of Purkinje's cells), and the spinal cord. Viral antigen is localized to neurons, especially in the brainstem, thalamus, and basal ganglia.

Nipah virus encephalitis

Pathological studies on the brains of fatal cases demonstrated that the endothelium of small blood vessels in the CNS was particularly susceptible to infection. This led to disseminated endothelial damage and syncytium formation, vasculitis, thrombosis, ischaemia, and microinfarction. There was also evidence of neuronal infection by the virus that may have contributed to neurological dysfunction.

West Nile virus encephalitis

Pathological changes include varying degrees of neuronal necrosis in the grey matter, with infiltrates of microglia and polymorphonuclear leucocytes, perivascular cuffing, neuronal degeneration, and neuronophagia. Viral antigens were demonstrated in neurons and in areas of necrosis. No antigen was detected in other major organs, including lung, liver, spleen, and kidney. The major pathological lesions were seen in the brainstem and spinal cord.

Enterovirus 71

There is severe perivascular cuffing, parenchymal inflammation, and neuronophagia in the spinal cord, brainstem, and diencephalon, and in focal areas in the cerebellum and cerebrum. Although no viral inclusions were detected, immunohistochemistry showed viral antigen in the neuronal cytoplasm. Inflammation was often more extensive than neuronal infection, suggesting that other indirect factors may be involved in tissue damage in addition to the effects of direct viral invasion.

Tick-borne encephalitis (see Chapter 7.5.14)

A feverish illness accompanied by myalgia, headache, and fatigue develops 4 to 28 days after the tick bite. Between 1 and 33 days later, about one-third of the patients will develop meningitis, meningoencephalomyelitis, myelitis, or meningoradiculitis.

Clinical features

Meningitis

A prodromal influenza-like illness, followed by a brief remission of symptoms, is typical of lymphocytic choriomeningitis viral infection, and some outbreaks of enteroviral meningitis (e.g. echovirus 9), but in most cases of viral meningitis symptoms start suddenly. There is usually fever, headache, change in conscious level, and occasionally a stiff neck, and vomiting, especially in children. Nausea, anorexia, abdominal pain, myalgias, and sore throat are particularly common in enteroviral meningitis. Myalgia is particularly severe with coxsackievirus B infections. As in acute bacterial meningitis, infants usually present with vague irritability and a tense fontanelle, and young children with fever and irritability or lethargy. Conjunctival injection, pharyngitis, and cervical lymphadenopathy may be found. Macular or petechial exanthems or enanthemas are seen with coxsackievirus A and B and echovirus infections (especially echovirus 9). Vesicles on the hands, feet, and mouth have been reported with coxsackievirus A16 and enterovirus 71 infections. By definition, the level of consciousness is normal in simple meningitis. Neurological features include vertigo, nystagmus, cerebellar ataxia, facial spasms, and involuntary movements.

The specific cause of viral meningitis may be suggested by characteristic signs outside the nervous system, such as genital or rectal vesicles in the sexually active age group (HSV-2), HZV skin lesions, swelling in the parotid region (mumps, and occasionally coxsackie-, lymphocytic choriomeningitis, and EBV), orchitis (mumps and lymphocytic choriomeningitis virus), and arthritis (lymphocytic choriomeningitis virus). However, potentially helpful features, such as gastrointestinal symptoms associated with enteroviral infections and parotitis associated with mumps, may be completely absent in patients with meningitis.

Mollaret's meningitis (benign recurrent aseptic meningitis or benign recurrent lymphocytic meningitis)

This is a sporadic condition presenting between the ages of 5 and 60 years. The symptoms are typical of acute meningitis—malaise, fever, vomiting, neck stiffness, convulsions, and coma. There is complete spontaneous recovery, usually within a few days, and symptom-free intervals lasting from a few days to years. About half the patients develop other neurological disturbances including hallucinations, diplopia, cranial nerve lesions, and signs of an upper motor neuron lesion. Pleocytosis is usually less than 3000/µl, with a predominance of lymphocytes, monocytes, and large endothelial (Mollaret's) cells, but occasionally neutrophils are in the majority. The protein level in cerebrospinal fluid is mildly increased, with increased gammaglobulin. The cerebrospinal fluid glucose concentration may be decreased. HSV-2 and HSV-1, human herpesvirus 6, and EBV have been implicated by polymerase chain reaction (PCR) detection. However, some argue that the term 'Mollaret's meningitis' should be restricted to idiopathic recurrent aseptic meningitis.

Differential diagnosis of recurrent meningitis

An important differential diagnosis is recurrent purulent meningitis that is often attributable to a congenital or traumatic defect providing access to the subarachnoid space, such as congenital occult spina bifida or fracture of the base of the skull. A cerebrospinal fluid leak may be apparent in about 50% of the cases with post-traumatic recurrent meningitis. The head trauma may have occurred many years earlier and a connection with the subarachnoid space may be clinically inapparent. Rarely, recurrent meningitis may arise from episodes of recurrent sepsis of a parameningeal focus (e.g. sinusitis or mastoiditis) or from a complement deficiency. Deficiency in a number of the components of the complement pathway has been detected in patients with recurrent meningitis. *Neisseria meningitidis* meningitis caused consecutively by different serogroups is the usual presentation in these cases.

Other causes of recurrent meningitis include Behçet's syndrome, Vogt–Koyanagi–Harada syndrome, sarcoidosis, and systemic lupus erythematosus (see Chapter 24.20), and undiagnosed viral meningitis (e.g. that due to encephalomyocarditis virus).

Paralytic poliomyelitis

Poliomyelitis (see Chapter 7.5.8) is acquired by droplet spread from the respiratory tract or by the faecal–oral route. The 'minor illness', coinciding with viraemia, is a nonspecific episode of influenza-like symptoms—fever, headache, sore throat, malaise, and mild gastrointestinal symptoms—which resolves in a few days. Most of those infected have no further symptoms but, in a minority,

the 'major illness' follows, sometimes after a few days' remission of symptoms. The features are those of viral meningitis: muscle pain, spasms, and sensory disturbances may precede or accompany the development of lower motor neuron (flaccid) paralysis. Any combination of motor unit deficits may be seen. Respiratory and bulbar paralysis is life threatening. Encephalitis is rare. The most common causes of death are aspiration and airway obstruction, resulting from bulbar paralysis and paralysis of respiratory muscles. Disturbances of respiratory and cardiac rhythm, thought to be the result of damage to medullary vasomotor and respiratory centres, are extremely uncommon. Other complications include impaired control of body temperature and blood pressure, gastrointestinal haemorrhage, aspiration pneumonia, and paralysis of the bladder and bowel. The time course of the illness is illustrated in Fig. 24.11.2.1.

Encephalitis

Most patients with viral encephalitis present with the symptoms of meningitis (fever, headache, neck stiffness, vomiting), followed by altered consciousness, convulsions, and sometimes focal neurological signs, signs of raised intracranial pressure, or psychiatric symptoms.

Herpes simplex encephalitis

This relatively common sporadic encephalitis may occur in any age group. In neonates, it is caused by HSV-2.

As well as the usual clinical features of severe viral encephalitis, patients with herpes simplex encephalitis have symptoms related to the focal nature of the encephalitis (frontal and temporal cortex and limbic system) (Fig. 24.11.2.2). These include behavioural abnormalities, olfactory and gustatory hallucinations, anosmia,

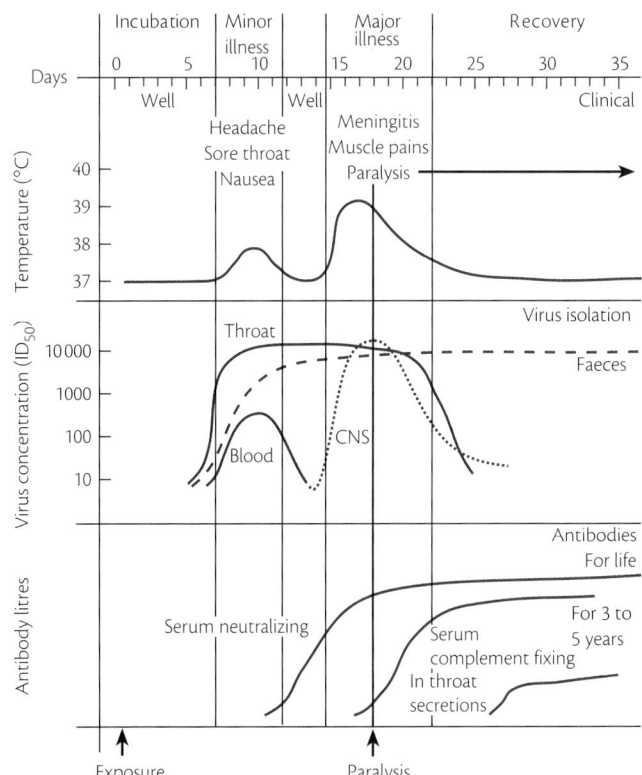

Fig. 24.11.2.1 Time course of paralytic poliomyelitis.

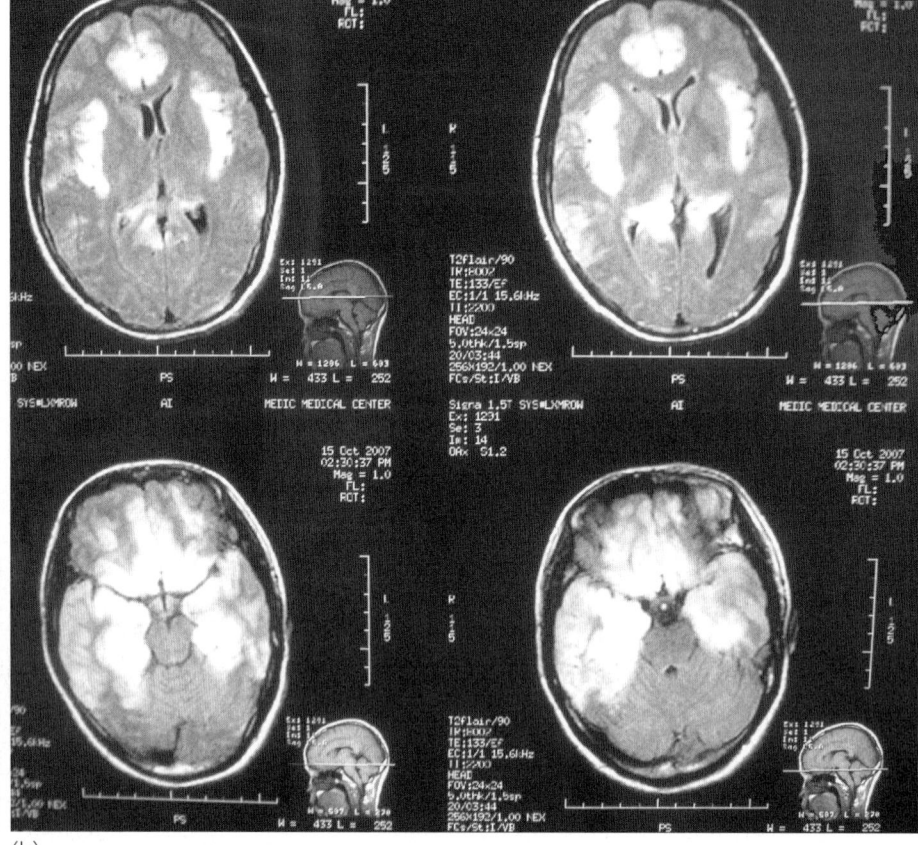

Fig. 24.11.2.2 MR scans of herpes simplex encephalitis in two Vietnamese patients showing the characteristic bilateral and extensive damage particularly to the temporal lobes but often extending to other parts of the cerebral cortex.

amnesia, expressive aphasia, and temporal lobe seizures. Herpetic skin or mucosal lesions are rarely found, except in the case of acute genital HSV-2 infection, or proctitis, and a past history of 'cold sores' does not affect the chances of the infection being due to HSV. Most deaths occur within the first 2 weeks.

Japanese encephalitis (see Chapter 7.5.14)

After an incubation period of 7 to 14 days, patients develop non-specific prodromal symptoms (fever, headache, malaise, and nausea) lasting 2 to 3 days. Neurological symptoms begin with headache, deteriorating level of consciousness, and generalized convulsions, which may result in status epilepticus. Fever persists for 6 to 7 days and, in survivors, neurological symptoms may persist for several weeks. Parkinsonian and extrapyramidal features occur frequently and choreoathetoid movement disorders or severe dystonias can last for many months (Fig. 24.11.2.3). The case fatality rate is 30% in those admitted to hospital. Most deaths occur in the first 7 to 10 days from respiratory failure, aspiration pneumonias, intracranial hypertension, and uncontrolled seizures. Up to 50% of survivors suffer from intellectual impairment, psychiatric problems, persistent epilepsy, or a vegetative state (Fig. 24.11.2.4a) with spastic quadriparesis and evidence of basal ganglia involvement (Fig. 24.11.2.5), such as dystonia of the limbs and trunk, rigidity, and tremor (Fig. 24.11.2.4b).

Nipah virus encephalitis (see Chapter 7.5.7)

The main clinical features of Nipah virus encephalitis are fever, headache, dizziness, reduced consciousness, and prominent brainstem dysfunction. Distinctive signs included myoclonus, areflexia, hypotonia, hypertension, and tachycardia, suggesting extensive brainstem and spinal cord involvement. MRI during the acute illness shows widespread focal lesions in subcortical and deep white matter and, to a lesser extent, in grey matter on $T2$-weighted sequences (Fig. 24.11.2.6). Long-term sequelae are common in Nipah encephalitis.

West Nile virus encephalitis

The most common clinical features are encephalitis, meningitis, fever, weakness, and headache following an incubation period of 3 to 15 days. Infection usually results in an acute febrile episode with no CNS involvement. In unusual cases or, as in the United States of America, when the virus is introduced into a naïve population, the incidence of encephalitis rises particularly in older people. An erythematous rash of the neck, trunk, and limbs is present in 20% of cases. Patients over 50 years of age were most at risk of developing encephalitis, but all age groups are affected in endemic areas. Muscle weakness, areflexia, and diffuse flaccid paralysis in association with an axonal polyneuropathy were also reported. MRI of the brain demonstrated enhancement of the meninges and periventricular areas. There is no specific treatment.

Enterovirus 71

As the goal of poliomyelitis eradication appears more achievable, another enterovirus is emerging as a significant cause of acute neurological disease in Asia. Enterovirus 71 (EV71) was first recognized in 1969 and is responsible for a variety of clinical manifestations,

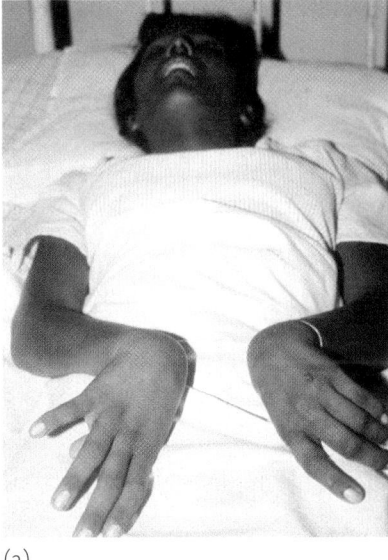

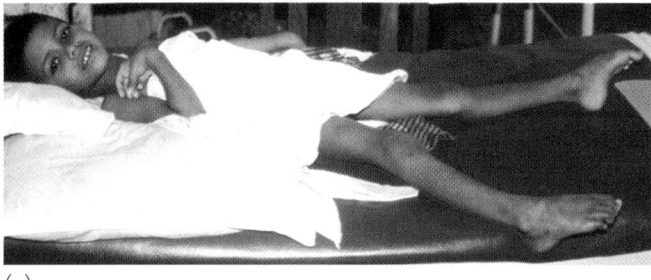

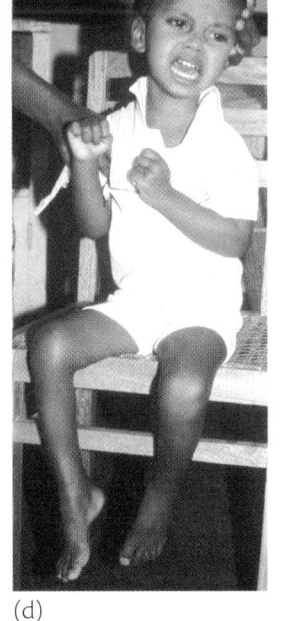

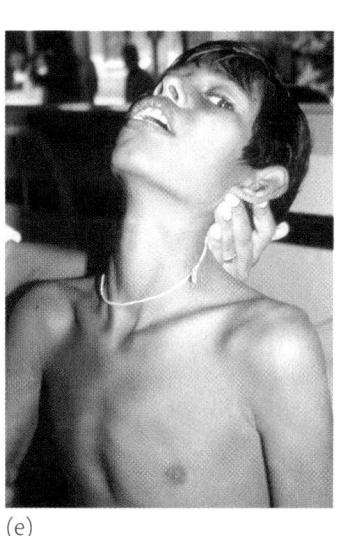

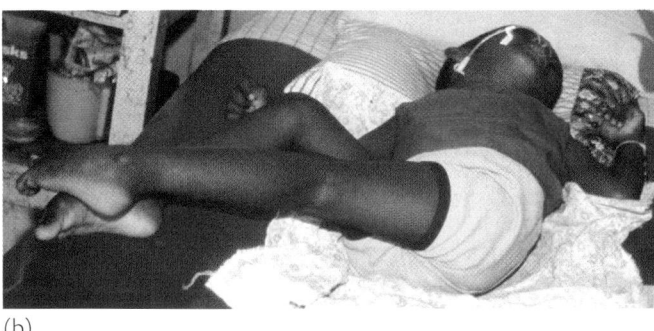

Fig. 24.11.2.3 Japanese encephalitis in Anuradhapura, Sri Lanka. (a) Comatose female patient showing symmetrical chorioathetotic movements of the upper limbs. (b) Comatose child showing dystonic movements of the upper and lower limbs. (c) Convalescent child, conscious but with residual dystonia of all four limbs. (d) Convalescent child with floppy head and involuntary movements of all four limbs. (e) Convalescent boy with residual weakness of the neck flexors. (Courtesy of Dr D T D J Abeysekera.)

including: hand, foot, and mouth disease; aseptic meningitis; meningoencephalitis; and acute flaccid paralysis. In an outbreak of hand, foot, and mouth disease in Malaysia, a number of young children developed fatal encephalomyelitis, dying within a few hours of presentation with cardiovascular instability and severe pulmonary oedema. Postmortem examination in four cases revealed major involvement of the brainstem and spinal cord, with EV71 being isolated from brain tissue in all cases; there was no apparent cardiac pathology and the virus was not isolated from the myocardium. Molecular characterization of these four viruses and others isolated concurrently suggest that at least two potentially virulent EV71 strains were circulating during the outbreak. An adenovirus was also thought to have complicated the infection in 60% of the children dying with a similar clinical picture. It is possible that coinfection with the two viruses may have resulted in severe disease.

Postinfectious encephalomyelitis

Sudden convulsions, coma, fever, or pareses appear 10 to 14 days after the start of immunization (vaccinia or nervous tissue rabies vaccine) or after infection with measles, varicella, rubella, mumps, or influenza. In the case of measles, varicella, and rubella, encephalitic

symptoms develop 2 to 12 days after the rash has appeared, and in mumps before or after parotid swelling. Involuntary movements, cranial nerve lesions (VII and III), pupillary abnormalities, nystagmus, ataxia, and upper motor neuron signs are common.

Diagnosis

Clinical and epidemiological details

The time of year, known current epidemics, the patient's age, occupation, animal contacts, and countries or states visited recently may help to narrow down the possibilities. A specific diagnosis may be suggested by distinctive clinical features of the encephalitis itself (e.g. hydrophobia in rabies, temporal lobe features in herpes simplex encephalitis) or of the associated infection (e.g. mumps parotitis, measles rash, skin and mucosal lesions of herpesviruses, and gastrointestinal symptoms associated with enteroviral infections).

Laboratory investigations

These should aim to demonstrate a specific viral agent (particularly important for the potentially treatable herpesvirus infections) or exclude potentially treatable nonviral causes of meningitis or encephalomyelitis (Table 24.11.2.1). The most important investigation is

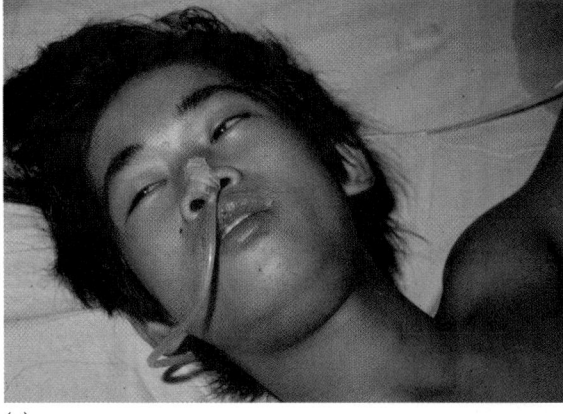

(a)

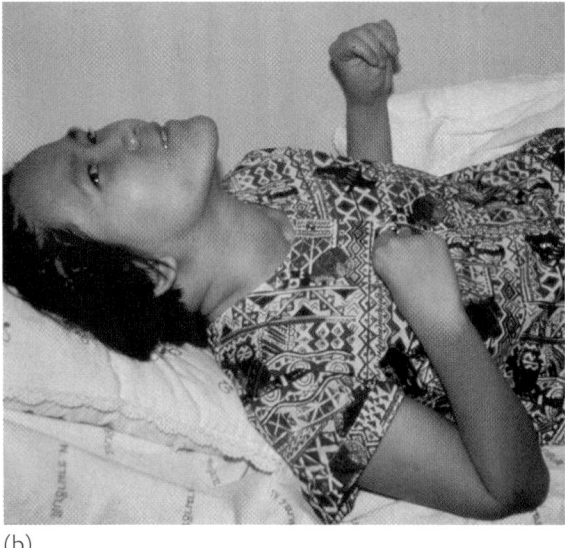

(b)

Fig. 24.11.2.4 (a) Vietnamese patient in a vegetative state after Japanese encephalitis. (b) Thai patient with severe neurological sequelae after Japanese encephalitis.
(a, copyright D A Warrell; b, courtesy of the late Professor Prida Phuapradit.)

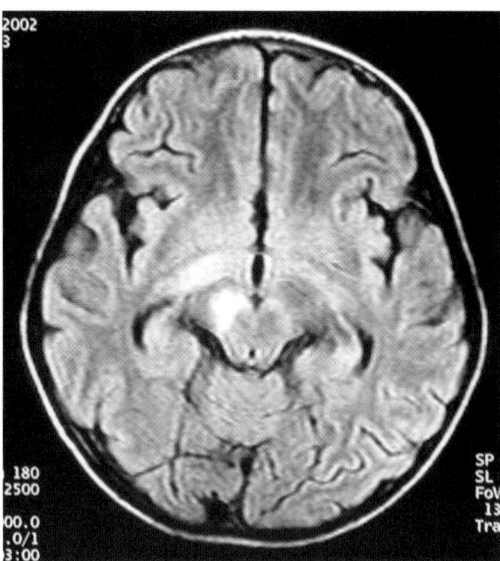

Fig. 24.11.2.5 MRI evidence of basal ganglia, cerebellar peduncles, and substantia nigra in Japanese encephalitis.

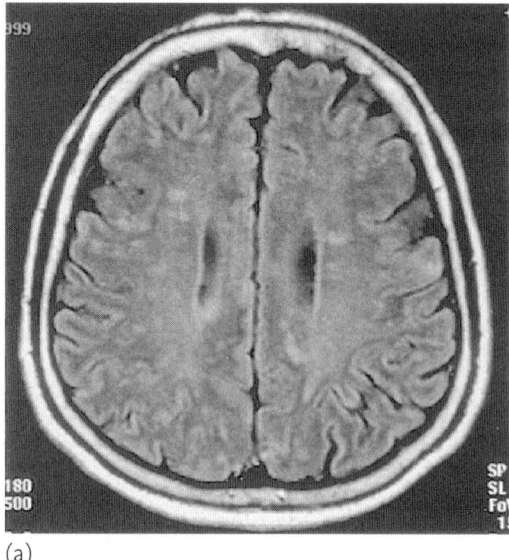

(a)

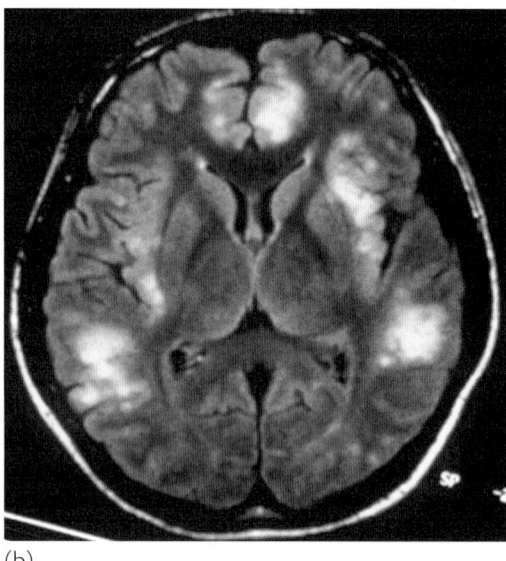

(b)

Fig. 24.11.2.6 MRI of two patients with Nipah virus encephalitis. Acute Nipah virus encephalitis in a 57-year-old pig farmer showing multiple focal lesions in the grey–white matter junction. These are areas of infarction secondary to vasculitis.
(a, courtesy of Drs B J Abdullah and Sazilah Sarj, Kuala Lumpur, Malaysia.)

examination of the cerebrospinal fluid. Contraindications to lumbar puncture are the same as for acute bacterial meningitis (see Chapters 24.3.1 and 24.11.1). If there are lateralizing neurological signs or evidence of raised intracranial pressure, a CT or MRI scan should be performed to exclude an intracranial mass lesion before contemplating a lumbar puncture. Cerebrospinal fluid pressure is especially increased in herpes simplex encephalitis, where there is intense cerebral oedema. Pleocytosis ranges from tens to thousands of cells per microlitre. Lymphocytes and other mononuclear cells predominate, except in the early stages of some infections (e.g. enteroviruses, herpes simplex encephalitis). The cerebrospinal fluid contains erythrocytes or is xanthochromic in haemorrhagic encephalitides such as herpes simplex encephalitis and acute necrotic leucoencephalitis. Protein concentration is usually increased in the range of 50 to 150 mg/dl with an increasing

Table 24.11.2.1 Causes of aseptic meningitis,[a] with or without encephalitis or myelitis, other than viruses and postinfectious/postvaccinal syndromes

Cause	Diagnostic clinical feature or investigation
Bacteria	
Acute bacterial meningitis (partially treated)	CSF antigen detection (CIE, LA), repeated CSF examination
Intracranial/spinal abscess or empyema (parameningeal infections)	Physical examination (exclude otitis media, trauma, dermoid sinus, etc.), radiographs, CT/MRI, myelogram
Brucella spp.	CSF, blood culture, serology
Cat-scratch disease bacillus	Warthin–Starry stain of skin and lymph nodes, skin test
Mycobacteria	CSF microscopy, LA, culture; Mantoux test, chest radiograph
Mycoplasma spp.	CSF and serum IgM (IFA)
Spirochaetes spp.	
Leptospira spp.	Serology
Relapsing fevers	Blood smear, mouse inoculation
Lyme disease	Serology (EIA, IFA), culture, skin biopsy, CSF IgG (EIA IFT)
Syphilis	Serology (FTA-abs test) serum and CSF
Spirillum minus	Microscopy of wound or lymph-node aspirates, mouse inoculation
Rickettsiae	
(Rocky Mountain spotted fever, murine, epidemic, scrub typhus)	Serology (Weil–Felix), skin biopsy IFT (RMSF)
Fungi	
Blastomyces spp.	CSF culture, EIA, demonstration at other sites, lung, skin, biopsy
Candida spp.	CSF culture (repeated)
Coccidioides spp.	CSF CFT, culture, microscopy
Cryptococcus spp.	CSF India ink, LA—beware false positive with surface condensate on agar
Histoplasma spp.	CSF culture (repeated), demonstration at other sites, blood smear (buffy coat) serum, urine, CSF antigen detection (RIA)
Protozoa	
Amoeba (*Acanthamoeba* spp., *Naegleria* spp., *Balamuthia* spp.)	CSF microscopy (fresh wet preparation + India ink), culture
Malaria (cerebral)	Blood smears
Toxoplasma spp.	(Immunocompromised patients—AIDS) CSF animal inoculation, serology, brain biopsy
Trypanosomiasis (African and South American)	Blood smear (buffy coat), lymph node aspirate, CSF microscopy, and IgM, serology, xenodiagnosis
Helminths	
Angiostrongylus cantonensis	CSF larvae, eosinophilia
Cysticercosis	CT/MRI, radiographs, examination for subcutaneous cysts, CSF CFT, histology

Table 24.11.2.1 (*Cont'd*) Causes of aseptic meningitis,[a] with or without encephalitis or myelitis, other than viruses and postinfectious/postvaccinal syndromes

Cause	Diagnostic clinical feature or investigation
Gnathostoma spinigerum	Cutaneous migratory swelling, CSF eosinophilia
Hydatid disease	Casoni test, serology, CT/MR scan, radiographs
Paragonimus spp.	CSF ova, eosinophils, serology, CT/MR scan or skull radiograph, histology
Schistosomiasis	Low transverse myelitis, ova in urine or stool, CT/MRI, CSF eosinophilia, myelogram, histology
Sparganosis	Histology, CT/MR scan
Strongyloides stercoralis	(Immunocompromised patients) larvae, ova in stool, duodenal fluid, etc.
Other	
Behçet's syndrome	Clinical syndrome
Carcinomas, cysts, leukaemias, lymphomas	CSF cytology, evidence of condition elsewhere
Chemical	Recent lumbar puncture, spinal anaesthesia, myelography, isotope cisternography
Drugs	Nonsteroidal anti-inflammatory agents immunomodulators, antimicrobials (e.g. trimethoprim)
Kawasaki's disease	Clinical features, echocardiography, coronary angiography, etc.
Lead encephalopathy	Blood lead, blood smear, urinary coproporphyrins
Mollaret's meningitis	Recurrence, CSF 'Mollaret's' cells (PCR for HSV)
Sarcoidosis	Histology, Kveim's test, Mantoux test, serum Ca^{2+}, ACE
Systemic lupus erythematosus and other collagen/vascular diseases	Antinuclear antibodies, DNA antibodies, lupus erythematosus cells
Vogt–Koyanagi–Harada syndrome	Clinical syndrome
Whipple's disease	Clinical features, jejunal histology

[a] Aseptic meningitis: CSF pleocytosis but no bacteria stainable by Gram's method and no growth on standard bacterial culture media.

ACE, angiotensin-converting enzyme; CFT, complement fixation test; CIE, countercurrent immunoelectrophoresis; CSF, cerebrospinal fluid; EIA, enzyme immunoassay; FTA-abs, fixed treponema antibody absorption test; HSV, herpes simplex virus; IFA, immunofluorescent antibody; LA, latex agglutination; PCR, polymerase chain reaction; RIA, radioimmunoassay; RMSF, Rocky Mountain spotted fever.

proportion of IgG as the disease progresses. Leakage of serum IgG into the cerebrospinal fluid and intrathecal IgG synthesis, indicated by a monoclonal band, are responsible. Cerebrospinal fluid glucose concentration is usually normal or increased towards the level in a blood sample taken simultaneously, but low levels are occasionally reported, especially in mumps and lymphocytic choriomeningitis virus infections. Cerebrospinal fluid examination may be misleading if it is normal: as it is at the first examination in 10 to 15% of patients with herpes simplex encephalitis; if there is a predominantly neutrophil pleocytosis; or if the glucose concentration is low.

Virology

Full laboratory resources allow a specific virus to be implicated in 70 to 75% of cases of lymphocytic meningitis and in 30 to 40% of patients with meningoencephalitis (Table 24.11.2.2). At appropriate stages of the illness, a rapid diagnosis by direct immunofluorescence may be made of HSV (skin and brain), HZV (skin lesion scrapings), rabies (skin sections and brain), measles (nasopharyngeal aspirate), and some nonviral causes such as Rocky Mountain spotted fever (skin). Electron microscopy of skin lesions will identify a herpesvirus. Some viruses can be isolated from the cerebrospinal fluid (e.g. mumps, enteroviruses, lymphocytic choriomeningitis virus, central European encephalitides, louping ill, and HIV). Virus cultured from a distant site may help with the diagnosis (e.g. polio and other enteroviruses from stool, or arthropod-borne viruses from blood culture), but they may not be related to the neurological symptoms (e.g. CMV from the pharynx or urine, HSV from skin or mucosa, or adenovirus seen in stool by electron microscopy). Specific viral IgM can be detected in serum for mumps, EBV, CMV, or measles, or using a μ-capture technique in the cerebrospinal fluid for JE virus. This method is being used increasingly to detect IgM to other viruses. The viraemia associated with JE is very brief and isolation from cerebrospinal fluid difficult. Virus can occasionally be isolated from postmortem material. A viral diagnosis is often delayed until a rising convalescent antibody titre is found by an appropriate technique. This is usually the case for mumps, coxsackieviruses, and most arthropod-borne viruses.

An important diagnostic advance has been the introduction of PCR technology for the routine diagnosis of a viral infection of the CNS. PCR greatly amplifies the amount of viral nucleic acid in the test sample, enabling the identification of HSV in the cerebrospinal fluid of suspected cases of herpes simplex encephalitis within a short time of the onset of symptoms. PCR is now the investigation of choice for the rapid diagnosis of HSV encephalitis, having

Table 24.11.2.2 Specimens for the virological diagnosis of acute meningitis or meningoencephalomyelitis

| Virus | Specimens for virus isolation/identification | | | | | | Serology | |
	Throat swab	Stool	CSF	Blood	Other specimens	PCR CSF	Acute	Convalescent
Adenovirus	++[a]	+	–	?[b]	?[b]	+		
Arenavirus								
Lymphocytic choriomeningitis	–	–	+++	+	?[b]	+	+2–3 months	
Enteroviruses								
Polioviruses	+	+++	–	–	++[c d]	+	+	
Coxsackievirus and echoviruses[f]	+	+++	+++	–		+	+	
Herpesviruses								
Cytomegalovirus	–	–	–	–	Urine[a]	+	+[a]	+
Epstein–Barr	+[a]	–	–	–		+	+[a]	+
Herpes simplex								
Type 1	+[a]	–	+	–	Brain	+++	+[a]	
Type 2	–	–	+	–	Vesicular fluid	+	+[a]	+
Herpesvirus simiae (B)	–	–	–	–	Vesicular fluid	–	+[a]	+
Herpes varicella-zoster	–	–	+	–	Vesicular fluid	+[b]	+[a]	+
Mumps	+++	–	++	–	Saliva, urine	?[b]	+	+
Rhabdoviruses								
Rabies	–	–	+	–	Skin biopsy, saliva, brain	+	+	+
Retroviruses								
HIV-1	–	–	+	+++		+++[e]	+++	–
HIV-2	–	–	+	+++		?	+++	–
HTLV-1	–	–	+	–		+	+++	–
Togaviruses	–	–	+	++		+[e]	+	+

CSF, cerebrospinal fluid; HTLV, human T-lymphotropic virus; PCR, polymerase chain reaction.

[a] Isolations or antibody responses may represent non-specific activation

[b] Too few data to indicate general usefulness in diagnosis

[c] Also serum/blood

[d] Also stool

[e] Also brain tissue

[f] Some Coxsackie A serotypes (especially A1–6) cannot be grown on cells.

a sensitivity of 95% and a specificity of 100%. The application of microchip and real-time PCR technology may further aid the rapid diagnosis of encephalitis. It is hoped that molecular techniques may aid the early diagnosis of a greater variety of CNS viral infections in the future (Table 24.11.2.2).

Brain biopsy

For the rapid diagnosis of viral encephalitides such as progressive multifocal leucoencephalopathy there is still no substitute for brain biopsy, but few would regard this inherently risky procedure as being justified. Electroencephalography (EEG), CT or MRI, angiography, or technetium scans can help to direct the surgeon towards the affected area of brain.

Imaging of the brain and spinal cord

MRI of the brain and spinal cord can be extremely useful for the diagnosis of the site, nature, and extent of mass lesions and associated oedema, sub- and epidural empyemas, meningitis, cerebritis, and ventriculitis, the presence of intracranial hypertension, hydrocephalus, cerebral and brainstem herniation, demyelination, and other anatomical abnormalities (see Chapter 24.3.3).

Some viral encephalitides do have characteristic lesions on MRI. Some 94% of patients with HSV have high-signal T_2-hyperintense lesions in the medial and inferior temporal regions, and JE is associated with characteristic lesions in the basal ganglia. More discrete high-signal intensity 2- to 7-mm lesions, particularly in the subcortical and deep white matter of the cerebral hemispheres, have been associated with Nipah virus infection. However, these classic descriptions often overlap and the general features of oedema, infarction, and high signal on the T_2-weighted images are commonly seen in a variety of viral infections of the CNS.

Differential diagnosis

Viral infections of the CNS must be distinguished from the many other conditions that produce similar clinical features and cerebrospinal fluid abnormalities (see Table 24.11.2.1). The differential diagnosis of viral meningitis includes the other causes of aseptic meningitis, such as partially treated bacterial meningitis, tuberculous meningitis, spirochaetal infections (leptospirosis, borreliosis, Lyme disease, and syphilis), and fungal, amoebic, neoplastic, granulomatous, and idiopathic meningitides. Viral myelitides must be distinguished from other causes of transverse myelitis and the Brown–Séquard syndrome. These include spinal compression by tumours, abscesses, helminths or their ova, or vertebral disease.

The differential diagnosis of paralytic poliomyelitis includes: postinfectious and other immunopathic polyneuroradiculopathies, such as Guillain–Barré syndrome and Landry's ascending paralysis; metabolic neuropathies such as acute porphyria; paralytic rabies; neoplastic polyradiculopathies; and rarities, such as tick paralysis and herpesvirus simiae (B virus) infection. The lack of objective sensory loss in poliomyelitis usually distinguishes it from these other entities.

The differential diagnosis of viral encephalitis includes other infective encephalopathies: bacterial, fungal, protozoal, and parasitic; intracranial abscesses and neoplasms; toxic and metabolic encephalopathies; and heat stroke. The diagnosis of 'viral encephalitis' should not be made too hastily, because it may condemn the patient with concealed cerebral malaria or some other curable encephalopathy to delayed treatment or even death.

Treatment

Antiviral chemotherapy

Aciclovir is effective in treating herpes simplex encephalitis. This subject is also discussed in Chapter 7.5.2. In view of this remarkable lack of serious toxicity, treatment can be started as soon as herpes simplex encephalitis is suspected clinically. Therapy with aciclovir should be started immediately on suspicion of encephalitis. Aciclovir is also the treatment for CNS associated V2V infections. There is no convincing evidence for its efficacy in CMV infections of the CNS. For CMV infections garciclovir or toscarnet should be considered. The rare, but very dangerous, encephalomyelitis caused by herpesvirus simiae B should be treated with aciclovir. Ribavirin is effective against some RNA viruses, such as those causing Lassa fever, haemorrhagic fever with renal syndrome, and possibly Argentine haemorrhagic fever, Rift Valley fever, and Congo Crimean haemorrhagic fever.

Interferons have been used by intravenous, intrathecal, or intraventricular routes in the treatment of JE, rabies, HZV, and other herpesvirus encephalitides, but have not proved effective.

Hyperimmune plasma given within 8 days of the start of symptoms has reduced the mortality rate of Argentine haemorrhagic fever (Junin virus) from between 20% and 30% to 1% and 3%. Hyperimmune human globulin has also proved effective in the treatment of Congo Crimean haemorrhagic fever. It is widely used in Asia for the treatment of enterovirus 71, although evidence from randomized controlled trials is lacking.

Supportive treatment

Corticosteroids have been used in the treatment of most of the viral encephalomyelitides, both in an attempt to combat cerebral oedema (especially in herpes simplex encephalitis) and for their other anti-inflammatory effects. Convincing evidence of benefit from controlled trials is lacking, but the immunosuppressive effects of corticosteroids have not led to obvious clinical deterioration. Corticosteroids or ACTH has also been used for postinfectious and postvaccinal encephalomyelitides, but the evidence for their efficacy is not convincing and, as they may exacerbate latent rabies in experimental animals, should be used only in life-threatening cases of rabies postvaccinal encephalomyelitis. Severe intracranial hypertension should be treated with intravenous mannitol or mechanical hyperventilation. Nursing and general care are the same as for acute bacterial meningitis and tuberculous meningitis. Seizures should be controlled with phenytoin or phenobarbital, fever lowered by cooling, respiratory failure treated by mechanical ventilation, and attention given to fluid, electrolyte, and acid–base balance. Hyponatraemia is attributable to inappropriate secretion of antidiuretic hormone in some cases.

Prognosis and sequelae

Viral meningitis has an excellent prognosis, but some patients with HSV-2 infection have recurrent attacks with spinal cord or nerve root involvement. Case fatality rates of some viral encephalomyelitides are as follows: rabies 100%; herpes simplex encephalitis (untreated) 40 to more than 75% (highest in neonates and those over 30 years old); eastern equine encephalitis 50%; JE 10 to 40%; measles 10 to 20%; varicella 10 to 30%; western equine encephalitis 8%; St Louis encephalitis 3%; California encephalitis, Venezuelan encephalitis, and mumps less than 1%. The mortality rate of paralytic poliomyelitis increases from 5% in young children to more than 20% in adults. Postinfectious and postvaccinal encephalomyelitides carry case fatality rates of 15 to 40%.

Neurological sequelae are found in 5 to 75% of survivors of JE and herpes simplex encephalitis, and are common in infants. They include intellectual impairment, loss of memory, speech abnormalities (including subtle expressive aphasias), hemiparesis, ataxia, dystonic brainstem and cranial nerve lesions, recurrent convulsions, and various behavioural and personality disturbances. Sequelae are common with postinfectious encephalomyelitis. An unusual sequel to paralytic poliomyelitis developing after an interval of many years is a condition characterized by progressive muscle weakness and wasting, attributable to depletion of anterior horn cells, which has some similarities to motor neuron disease.

Prevention

Prophylactic immunization against poliomyelitis and measles has virtually eradicated encephalitides caused by these viruses in many communities. Postexposure rabies immunization has also proved effective in preventing rabies encephalitis, and tissue-culture rabies vaccines are used increasingly for pre-exposure prophylaxis. A formalin-inactivated, adult mouse-brain vaccine is manufactured in Osaka for JE. It is effective and carries a very low risk of objective neurological complications (one in a million courses). An alternative live-attenuated vaccine, SA 14-14-2, has been developed in China, and has been shown to be both safe and effective in over 200 million Chinese and Indian children. Promising future vaccine candidates are currently being evaluated in nonhuman primate models, including a chimaeric live-attenuated JEV/yellow fever virus combination and two poxvirus-vectored recombinant JE vaccines. Travellers to endemic regions should be immunized.

Since the outbreak of West Nile infection in the United States of America, several vaccine candidates have already been identified and immune protection against infection demonstrated in several animal models: human trials have been planned. There have been no reports of such success against Nipah virus. Vaccines for use in humans have been prepared against a number of other arthropod-borne viruses (e.g. European tick-borne encephalitis).

Hyperimmune immunoglobulin has been used for prophylaxis (and in some cases attempted treatment) of measles, HZV, HSV-2, vaccinia, and rabies, and some other infections in high-risk groups. Immunocompromised patients, such as those with leukaemia, who are household contacts of a case of HZV infection, should be given prophylactic hyperimmune globulin and, if they develop skin lesions, they should be treated with aciclovir to prevent the development of severe disease.

Interferons have been used with some success to prevent herpesvirus infections, e.g. CMV in high-risk groups such as renal transplant recipients. However, the evidence does not yet justify their recommendation.

Caesarean section before rupture of the membranes in a full-term pregnant woman with genital herpes may prevent HSV-2 encephalitis in the neonate. If the herpetic lesions are discovered during or after vaginal delivery, topical aciclovir should be applied to the eyes of the neonate, as they are the most likely portal of entry.

Arthropod-borne viral encephalitides can be prevented by avoiding or controlling the arthropod vectors (e.g. by the use of mosquito nets, insect repellents, insecticides), by attempting to control the numbers of wild vertebrate reservoir species, or by immunizing domestic animals, such as horses (eastern and western equine encephalitides) and pigs (JE). To control rabies, the principal wild mammalian vectors can be immunized (e.g. wild foxes, racoons, and black-backed jackals have been immunized by distributing oral vaccine in bait). Domestic dogs and cats should be immunized. To prevent the viral encephalitides transmissible from laboratory animals (e.g. lymphocytic choriomeningitis from mice and rats, herpesvirus simiae b from monkeys) their screening, quarantine, handling, and housing should be strictly controlled.

Reye's syndrome

Reye's syndrome is an acute encephalopathy affecting children between the ages of 2 and 16 years. It is rapidly fatal in 10 to 40% of cases. The defining characteristics are sudden impairment of consciousness, increase in serum aminotransferase concentrations (or, if a biopsy is done, a fatty liver), and the exclusion of other diseases. Symptoms develop a few days after varicella or an upper respiratory tract or gastrointestinal illness. Clusters of cases (median age 11 years) have been associated with influenza B epidemics, although sporadic cases (median age 6 years) have followed varicella, coxsackievirus, dengue, and other viral infections. Studies in the United States of America have demonstrated an association between Reye's syndrome and the use of salicylates, but not of paracetamol, during the preceding viral illness. This has led the United Kingdom Committee on Safety of Medicines to recommend that aspirin should not be given to children under 12 years of age, unless specifically indicated for childhood rheumatic conditions. Aflatoxin has been implicated in Thailand. In the United States of America, the annual incidence of Reye's syndrome in those under 18 years old is 0.42 per 100 000 urban dwellers and 1.8 per 100 000 rural and suburban dwellers.

The child is nauseated and retches or vomits for 1 or 2 days before becoming confused or comatose and requiring admission to hospital. Most are afebrile and have hepatosplenomegaly but no jaundice at presentation. Fever develops later. The cerebrospinal fluid is usually normal or contains a few mononuclear cells. Irritability, extreme agitation, aggression, and delirium are succeeded by coma and death in 2 to 3 days. Decorticate and decerebrate posturing and convulsions may be partly attributable to hypoglycaemia, which occurs in most cases. There is rapid neurological deterioration with loss of pupillary and oculovestibular reflexes, evidence of increased intracranial pressure, deepening coma, and death. Neurological sequelae are common in survivors. Blood ammonia is increased in almost all cases. The characteristic histological abnormality is fatty droplets in the liver cells. Mitochondrial abnormalities, but no inflammatory changes, have also been seen in neurons and hepatocytes.

The differential diagnosis includes inborn errors of metabolism, acute hepatic encephalopathy, especially associated with poisoning, infective encephalopathies such as cerebral malaria (usually distinguishable by a positive blood smear), or bacterial, viral, and fungal meningoencephalitides (distinguished by characteristic cerebrospinal fluid abnormalities).

There is no specific treatment, but mortality can be reduced by treating hypoglycaemia, cerebral oedema, respiratory failure, fluid and electrolyte disturbances, and other complications. These measures are also considered in Chapter 24.11.1.

Other viral infections or disorders in which viruses play a role in the pathogenesis of neurological disease

Subacute sclerosing panencephalitis

This disorder (see also Chapter 7.5.6) is a form of subacute encephalitis affecting children and young adults due to persistent infection with the measles virus. The cumbersome title, usually abbreviated to SSPE, is derived from the conditions formerly known as subacute sclerosing leucoencephalitis and inclusion-body encephalitis, now known to be the same disease.

Aetiology

An infective cause was long suspected and there is now conclusive evidence to incriminate the measles virus. Measles virus antibody titres are extremely high in the blood and cerebrospinal fluid, measles antigen has been demonstrated in the brain, and the virus has sometimes been isolated, but only with difficulty. Most affected children have had measles at an unusually early age and there is a mean interval of some 6 years between infection and the onset of encephalitis. The disease can occur in children immunized with live measles virus, but the risk is much lower than that following the natural disease.

The measles virus in subacute sclerosing panencephalitis appears to be incomplete, as the matrix (M) protein required to attach the nucleocapsid to the cytoplasmic membrane before budding is deficient or absent. It is not known whether the absence of M protein from the brain is the result of an abnormality of the virus or of the host, and, if the latter, whether inborn or acquired. Current thought is that, during the long symptom-free interval between infection and appearance of disease, viral material accumulates, eventually leading to cell damage. The paradox of high antimeasles antibodies, except against M protein, and persistent virus has not been explained. The comparatively early age of clinical measles in affected children, often below the age of 2 years, suggests that the immature immune system permits entry and persistence of the virus in the brain.

Pathology

As its name implies, both grey matter and white matter show the changes of encephalitis, with perivascular cuffing and more diffuse cellular infiltration, neuronal loss, and myelin destruction, with variable glial scarring or sclerosis. Acidophilic nuclear inclusion bodies are never profuse and may not be detected. No visceral lesions are found.

Clinical features

In the great majority, the onset is in the first two decades, but young adults may also be affected. The disease is twice as common in boys as in girls. Incidence has fallen sharply in countries where measles immunization is at a high level; the annual incidence in England and Wales has fallen from 20 to around 5. Subacute sclerosing panencephalitis remains relatively common in parts of eastern Europe, Egypt, and the Lebanon. No convincing predisposing factors have been identified and, in particular, immunosuppressed children are not at special risk but they may occasionally develop acute measles inclusion-body encephalitis.

The speed of onset is extremely variable, but there is usually a prolonged period of altered behaviour, mild intellectual deterioration, and loss of energy and interest, often misinterpreted as sloth or neurosis. After some weeks or months increasing clumsiness or the appearance of focal neurological symptoms draws attention to the organic nature of the disease. Periodic involuntary movements then appear, the most common form being myoclonus, consisting of a stereotyped jerk or lapse of posture involving the limbs, often asymmetrically, occurring every 3 to 6 s. The myoclonus may result in sudden falls, which are occasionally the presenting symptom. Visual signs may be prominent, with papilloedema, retinitis, optic atrophy, or cortical blindness. Choroidoretinal scarring is present in 30% of cases. In other cases the onset is relatively abrupt with no recognizable prodromal stage. There is no fever or other evidence of systemic infection.

Further progression is marked by intellectual deterioration, rigidity and spasticity, and increasing helplessness. Some 40% of patients die within a year, but a similar proportion survive for more than 2 years. A period of apparent arrest is common and in some patients, particularly at the upper end of the age range, substantial remission and prolonged survival occur. Even in such cases there may be radiological evidence of continued cerebral damage and it is probable that the disease is always eventually fatal.

Investigation

There is no significant pleocytosis in the cerebrospinal fluid and total protein is not increased, but there is evidence of intrathecal synthesis of immunoglobulin and oligoclonal bands of IgG. Although the measles antibody titres in blood and cerebrospinal fluid are usually raised to high levels, occasionally they overlap control values. In established disease, the EEG shows highly characteristic periodic discharges, synchronous with the myoclonus, but persisting in the absence of the movements. The CT scan shows low-density, white-matter lesions and cerebral atrophy.

Treatment

There is no effective treatment for subacute sclerosing panencephalitis. Isoprinosine 100 mg/kg daily by mouth, in divided, doses possibly prolongs survival, particularly in older patients with disease of slow onset, but adequately controlled trials are naturally difficult to mount. Interferon given by intraventricular catheter has been reported to induce partial remission.

Progressive multifocal leucoencephalopathy (see Chapters 7.5.19, 7.5.23, and 24.11.4)

This disease is caused by opportunistic infection by papovaviruses, most commonly JC virus and the simian virus SV40. A high proportion of normal adults have antibodies to the former and the agent appears to be ubiquitous. The reservoir of SV40 is in monkeys and the agent was apparently transmitted in early types of poliomyelitis vaccine, without evident ill-effects. These viruses are potentially oncogenic, but are nonpathogenic for humans unless the immune system has been compromised.

Progressive multifocal leucoencephalopathy thus occurs in patients already affected by such conditions as lympho- or myeloproliferative diseases, sarcoidosis, and other chronic granulomatous diseases, or, more recently, AIDS, and also in those who are therapeutically immunosuppressed. Most patients are aged over 50 years but, with the spread of AIDS, younger people are being affected, with a male preponderance, and the disease is no longer rare.

Pathology

The virus particularly invades the nuclei of the oligodendroglia and, as a result, there is demyelination of the white matter of the cerebral hemisphere, spreading from numerous foci. The cerebellum and brainstem are less often involved and the spinal cord is spared. Abnormal giant forms of oligodendrocytes with eosinophilic inclusions are seen microscopically, and arrays of intranuclear virus particles can often be identified by electron microscopy. JC virus antigen can be identified by immunofluorescence or immunohistochemistry. DNA probing has revealed unintegrated virus in oligodendrocytes, astrocytes, endothelial cells, and extraneural organs such as kidney, liver, lung, spleen, and lymph nodes.

Clinical features

The onset is usually with progressive signs of a focal lesion of one cerebral hemisphere, limb weakness, aphasia, or visual field defects such as homonymous hemianopia. More widespread signs gradually develop, leading to personality changes, intellectual deterioration, dysarthria or fluent aphasia, and bilateral weakness. Fits are rare. There is no systemic evidence of infection. Spontaneous temporary arrest or partial remission is common but eventual progression causes death in 6 to 12 months, although far more chronic cases are on record, with survival, exceptionally, to 5 years.

Investigation

The cerebrospinal fluid is normal apart from occasionally a mild elevation of protein and slight pleocytosis, and is not under increased pressure. The EEG shows a bilateral excess of slow activity. The CT scan may at first show little abnormality, but eventually large, non-enhancing, low-density lesions appear in the cerebral white matter. MRI is more sensitive. Serum antibodies are of no diagnostic help but the response in the cerebrospinal fluid has not been fully evaluated. The diagnosis can be confirmed only by cerebral biopsy, but it is essential that white matter be included in the specimen. This may be important to distinguish lymphoma and, rarely, herpes simplex encephalitis involving white matter.

Treatment

No treatment is of proven value, but cytosine arabinoside has sometimes appeared to induce partial remission.

Progressive rubella panencephalitis

This extremely rare disorder (see Chapter 7.5.13) may follow congenital rubella or rubella in early childhood. It evolves insidiously some 10 years after the original illness and is characterized by progressive intellectual impairment with behaviour changes, fits, ataxia, spasticity, optic atrophy, and macular degeneration. Pathological changes are those of encephalitis with perivascular infiltration. The cerebrospinal fluid may show a slight rise in white cell and protein content, elevation of gammaglobulin and of antirubella antibodies to an extent greater than the rise in the serum level, suggesting local production of antibody within the CNS. The EEG may show changes similar to those seen in subacute sclerosing panencephalitis due to measles virus. The mechanism responsible for the appearance of this disorder is unknown and there is no effective treatment.

Vogt–Koyanagi–Harada syndrome

The cause of this rare syndrome is thought to be an inflammatory autoimmune reaction to an unidentified viral infection. The disorder affects tissues having a common embryological origin, the uvea and leptomeninges and the melanoblasts, ocular pigments, and auditory labyrinth pigments originating from the neural crest. The dermatological features consist of patchy whitening of eyelashes, eyebrows and scalp hair, alopecia, and vitiligo. Neurological manifestations include meningoencephalitis, raised intracranial pressure, neurosensory deafness, tinnitus, nystagmus, ataxia, ocular palsies, and focal cerebral deficits. Ocular features are those of uveitis with pain and photophobia, more generalized inflammation of the eye, retinopathy, and impaired visual acuity. The condition tends to be self-limiting but may result in serious permanent ocular and neurological deficits. Steroids and immunosuppressive drugs have been used and are said to arrest the progression of at least some features of the disorder.

Viral causes of psychiatric illness

Mental changes are common in patients with encephalitis. Influenza, infectious mononucleosis, and infectious hepatitis are sometimes followed by psychiatric sequelae, in particular a depressive reaction. Psychosis after encephalitis lethargica has been reported on occasions. Chronic fatigue syndrome (see Chapter 26.5.4) has been attributed to viral encephalitis.

Other possible virus infections in which the nervous system is involved

Acute disseminated encephalomyelitis is considered in Chapter 24.10.2 and Behçet's syndrome in Chapters 19.11.5, 23.15, and 24.20.

Further reading

Baringer JR (2008). Herpes simplex infections of the nervous system. *Neurol Clin*, **26**, 657–74, viii.

De Jong MD, *et al.* (2005). Fatal avian influenza A (H5N1) in a child presenting with diarrhea followed by coma. *N Engl J Med*, **352**, 686–91.

Ghosh D, Basu A (2009). Japanese encephalitis-a pathological and clinical perspective. *PLoS Negl Trop Dis*, **3**, e437.

Goh KJ, *et al.* (2000). Clinical features of Nipah virus encephalitis among pig farmers in Malaysia. *N Engl J Med*, **342**, 1229–35.

Gyure KA (2009). West Nile virus infections. *J Neuropathol Exp Neurol*, **68**, 1053–60.

Mansfield KL, Johnson N, Phipps LP, *et al.* (2009). Tick-borne encephalitis virus—a review of an emerging zoonosis. *J Gen Virol*, **90**, 1781–94.

Ooi MH, *et al.* (2007). Human enterovirus 71 disease in Sarawak, Malaysia: a prospective clinical, virological, and molecular epidemiological study. *Clin Infect Dis*, **44**, 646–56.

Sejvar JJ, *et al.* (2007). Long-term neurological and functional outcome in Nipah virus infection. *Ann Neurol*, **62**, 235–42.

Sonneville R, Klein I, de Broucker T, Wolff M (2009). Post-infectious encephalitis in adults: diagnosis and management. *J Infect.*, **58**, 321–8.

Tauber E, Dewasthaly S (2008). Japanese encephalitis vaccines—needs, flaws and achievements. *Biol Chem*, **389**, 547–50.

Tyler KL (2004). Herpes simplex virus infections of the central nervous system: encephalitis and meningitis, including Mollaret's. *Herpes*, **11** Suppl 2, 57A–64A.

Tyler KL (2009). Emerging viral infections of the central nervous system. *Arch Neurol.*, **66**, 939–48, 1065–74.

Weber T (2008). Progressive multifocal leucoencephalopathy. *Neurol Clin*, **26**, 833–54, x–xi.

24.11.3 Intracranial abscesses

T.P. Lawrence and R.S.C. Kerr

Essentials

The incidence of intracranial abscess is low in countries where antimicrobial treatment for infections is widespread (e.g. 2–3 per million in the United Kingdom), but they remain frequent causes of space-occupying masses in developing countries.

Aetiology—abscesses may be classified by (1) Route of transmission, including (a) direct—from a local source of infection, e.g. otitis media; (b) haematogenous—from a distant source, e.g. endocarditis, bronchiectasis, other septic lung conditions; or (c) following cranial surgery or fracture. (2) Microbiology—the commonest organisms are aerobic, anaerobic and micro-aerophilic streptococci, *Staphylococcus aureus*, and bacteroides, but up to 25% of abscesses are sterile. Immunodeficient patients are at increased risk.

Clinical features and investigation—typical presentations include headache, focal neurological symptoms/signs, seizures, meningism/meningitis, and signs of raised intracranial pressure. The investigations of choice are either CT scanning, with and without contrast, or MRI. Confirmation of diagnosis, usually by culture, follows aspiration/excision.

Treatment and prognosis—aside from supportive care and (where possible) identification and treatment of any underlying cause, treatment requires (1) abscess drainage by stereotactic surgical aspiration or excision by craniotomy, and (2) long-term antimicrobial therapy. Early intervention offers the best chance of recovery: without intervention, intracranial abscesses are fatal; appropriate treatment reduces overall mortality to about 10%, but long-term complications from neurological deficit and epilepsy remain frequent in survivors.

Introduction

Intracranial abscesses, although less common since the introduction of antibiotics and improved treatment of systemic infections, still cause significant morbidity and mortality. The incidence is approximately 2 to 3 per million population per year in the United Kingdom, but far greater in developing countries where intracranial abscesses account for up to 8% of all intracranial space-occupying lesions, compared with 2% in developed countries. The use of modern imaging techniques and a combination of antibiotics and image-guided surgery has resulted in a reduction in morbidity and mortality in these patients. Abscesses can occur at any age but there is a peak at 30 to 50 years with a male:female ratio of 1.8:1 to 4:1.

Intracranial abscesses can be categorized according to their anatomical location, occurring in the extradural space, subdural space, or intraparenchyma. Occasionally, abscesses exist in more than one tissue plane. Intracerebral and subdural abscesses may rupture into the subarachnoid space and be accompanied by meningitis. Intracerebral pus may rupture into the ventricular system and produce ventriculitis.

Aetiology

The aetiology can be divided according to the route of transmission:

- Direct—microorganisms spreading from a local source of infection such as otitis media, mastoiditis, paranasal sinusitis, or dental infection.

- Haematogenous—microorganisms spreading from a distant source such as a right-to-left shunt secondary to cyanotic congenital heart disease in children or subacute endocarditis, bronchiectasis, and lung abscesses in adults.

Abscesses can also form after intracranial surgery or cranial trauma. Immunodeficient patients are at increased risk of developing abscesses, either secondary to conditions such as AIDS or leukaemia or iatrogenic.

It is also thought that ischaemic brain tissue may encourage bacterial invasion and therefore abscesses can develop in closed head injuries and following cerebral infarcts, although this is rare.

The most common intracranial abscess is found within the intracerebral compartment, with about 60% related to middle-ear infection and 20% to frontal sinusitis. In about 10% of cases no primary source of infection can be identified. Owing to their strong connection with sinus and middle-ear disease, most intracerebral abscesses are found within the frontal or temporal lobes, or within the cerebellum. Infection disseminated through the bloodstream from more distant sites may result in multiple abscesses in any part of the brain.

Microbiology

The most common organisms associated with intracranial abscesses are aerobic, anaerobic, and microaerophilic streptococci, *Staphylococcus aureus*, and bacteroides. However, up to 25% of culture samples are sterile.

Cerebral abscesses associated with otitis media, mastoiditis, and nasal sinusitis usually show a mixed growth of anaerobic and aerobic organisms including anaerobic and microaerophilic streptococci and bacteroides, *Strep. viridans* and *Staph. aureus* are also frequently seen. Listeria tend to produce areas of focal cerebritis rather than true abscesses. Abscesses associated with frontoethmoidal sinusitis are usually due to *Strep. milleri* and *Strep. angiosus*. With trauma the organism is often *Staph. aureus* or one of the Enterobacteriaceae.

Pathology

There are four distinct histological stages in the pathogenesis of intracranial abscesses. Spread of microorganisms, either direct or haematogenous, causes parenchymal damage after occlusion of the small vessels. The initial stage is early cerebritis (days 0–3) characterized by a local inflammatory response with perivascular and parenchymal neutrophil infiltration. During late cerebritis (days 3–9) a central necrotic area forms with macrophage infiltration. A reticulin network forms around the necrotic area in the early capsular stage (up to day 14) with parenchymal oedema. This is followed by the formation of a collagen capsule with distinct zones of neovascularization during the late capsular stage (after day 14). Perilesional cerebral oedema continues and gliosis takes place. The areas of oedematous brain may exert considerable mass effect.

In the case of direct spread, infection within an accessory air sinus or the petrous bone may cause an area of localized osteitis just above the dura. This can then spread intracranially. Initially it may be entirely confined to the extradural space, but will eventually penetrate the dura and spread subdurally. If the adjacent arachnoid is stuck to the inflamed patch of dura then it may spread into the subarachnoid space to give meningitis. If the subarachnoid space has been obliterated, it may penetrate the brain to produce initially a focal cerebritis. Large intracerebral abscesses can rupture into the ventricular system, producing a ventriculitis.

Clinical features

Presentation depends upon the site, size, and number of lesions, and the involvement of neighbouring structures such as the cerebral ventricles and the venous sinuses. The signs are therefore legion, but the diagnosis should be considered in any case where there is an obvious primary source of infection associated with evidence of raised intracranial pressure, focal neurological signs, headache, epileptic seizures, or meningeal irritation.

Extradural abscess may be difficult to detect clinically, but can sometimes manifest as severe, unremitting, localized headache in association with sinusitis or mastoiditis. Patients with subdural empyema frequently appear toxic, with a swinging pyrexia, severe headache, a depressed level of consciousness, contralateral hemiparesis, papilloedema, meningeal irritation, and seizures. There is often an accompanying frontal sinusitis with tenderness of the forehead, erythema, and swelling of the eyelids.

Diagnosis

If a brain abscess is suspected, predisposing sources of infection, including possible distant sites, should be carefully sought. Intracranial abscesses derived from haematogenous spread are often more fulminating in their course than those associated with direct spread. CT scans of the skull base, including views of the mastoids and other skull sinuses, should be performed. Plain radiographs of the mastoids and sinuses may reveal infection.

The investigations of choice for all forms of suspected intracranial abscess are either CT scanning, with and without contrast, or MRI. CT will normally demonstrate both extradural and subdural empyema and show intracerebral abscesses as ring-enhancing lesions with low-attenuation centres (Fig. 24.11.3.1). The CT and MRI appearances correlate closely with the pathogenesis. During the early stages of cerebritis areas of hypodensity may be very subtle with minimal contrast enhancement. At this stage MRI may reveal oedema and some ring enhancement not evident on CT. Subdural empyema may initially be thinly spread over the cerebral cortex, producing relatively little midline shift, appearing virtually isodense with brain on CT. Under such circumstances, contrast-enhanced MRI (particularly with coronal views) is of great value. Diffusion-weighted imaging (DWI) with MRI can help differentiate a pyogenic abscess from other ring-enhancing lesions. Proton MR spectroscopy can be used to show peaks of lactate and cytosolic amino acids present in abscesses.

The principal differential diagnoses in an intracranial abscess are meningitis, subdural haematoma, and intracranial tumour. It is not always possible to differentiate between intracerebral abscess and tumour on a CT scan, particularly when there is an appearance of ring enhancement, and it is largely for this reason that the biopsy

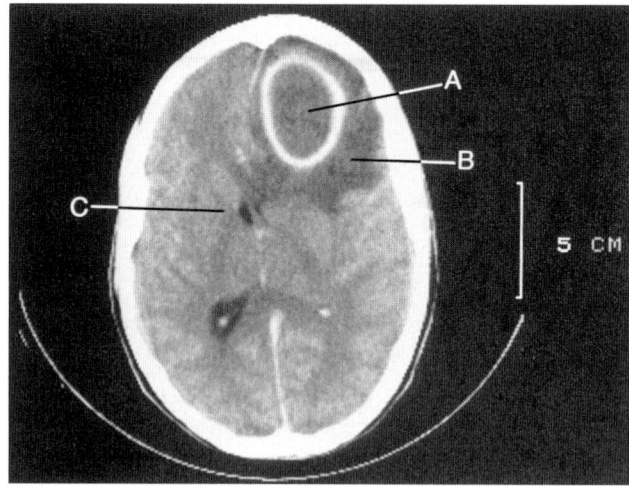

Fig. 24.11.3.1 Contrast CT scan showing large right frontal cerebral abscess (a) with surrounding oedema (b) and ventricular compression (c).

of suspected cerebral tumour is advocated in nearly all such cases. MRI, however, tends to show a low-signal capsule on T_2-weighted images and may be helpful in making this differentiation.

One obvious concern is to differentiate between bacterial meningitis and intracerebral abscess. Both may present with pyrexia, neck stiffness, and some focal signs, but if there is any evidence of raised intracranial pressure, or any other supportive evidence of cerebral abscess, a lumbar puncture should be strictly avoided until a neurosurgical opinion has been sought. Lumbar puncture in the presence of cerebral abscess can lead to tonsillar or tentorial herniation. The cerebrospinal fluid can be entirely normal in intracranial abscesses.

Management

Treatment includes identifying and treating the underlying cause and image-guided stereotactic surgical aspiration or excision of the abscess by craniotomy combined with long-term antibiotics. Selected patients can be managed without surgical intervention. This tends to be limited to those who have multiple or inaccessible abscesses and those in whom surgery is contraindicated due to poor general medical condition. However, without biopsy the diagnosis cannot be confirmed and the pathogens cannot be identified. Therefore tissue should be obtained if at all possible.

Early diagnosis and treatment are essential to good outcome. The damaging effect of abscesses results from parenchymal displacement and oedema rather than destruction of tissue, so neurological deficits may be reversible. Treatment is aimed at identifying the causative agent, obtaining antibiotic sensitivities, and reducing mass effect. Early management includes the following steps: culturing blood and any extracranial infective lesion, obtaining tissue and starting appropriate intravenous antibiotics, administration of anticonvulsant agents, and, in cases of grossly depressed level of consciousness and massive cerebral oedema seen on a CT scan, giving intravenous dexamethasone. Steroids decrease cerebral oedma but are also thought to prevent antibiotic penetration. Therefore they should only be used in patients with mass effect on CT.

Pus from the suspected primary site of infection should be collected immediately and both aerobic and anaerobic cultures obtained. The intracranial pus must be similarly cultured.

High dose intravenous empirical antibiotics should be commenced immediately without waiting for the culture report, and subsequently changed in the light of the sensitivity findings. The antimicrobial regimen should include penicillin, metronidazole, ampicillin, and either gentamicin or chloramphenicol, depending on the likely source of infection and the infective agent. Although antibiotics have good penetration into cerebrospinal fluid, the acidic environment of the abscess means that the efficacy of the antibiotic may be reduced. Intravenous antibiotics should be continued for more than 6 to 8 weeks before reverting to oral medication. Microbiologists should be involved in decisions regarding length and nature of antibiotic treatment.

Most supratentorial abscesses can be sterilized by aspiration through a burr hole. The direct administration of antibiotics through the burr hole, is sometimes employed. Aspiration is often repeated several times, but in about 30% of cases a single aspiration will suffice. Once the abscess is sterile, the capsule will shrink and finally form an irregular gliotic scar within the brain. Shrinkage of the abscess must be checked by serial CT scans. Subdural empyema should be evacuated through a craniotomy rather than burr holes, as very frequently the pus can spread widely, particularly alongside the falx cerebri. Extradural empyema is evacuated through a burr hole, or through a craniotomy for larger collections to allow complete excision of the abscess. Advances in image-guided stereotactic surgery have resulted in far more accurate and safe targeting of all intracranial lesions including abscesses and should be used to aid any surgical intervention.

Cerebellar abscesses, when diagnosed early, may be aspirated through a burr hole, but immediate total excision is often recommended because the small volume of the posterior cranial fossa leaves little latitude in terms of tonsillar herniation and death.

Prognosis

The mortality rate from intracranial abscesses has been reduced from 40 to 60% to around 10% since the introduction of CT scanners. The main problems remain those of late diagnosis and resistant bacteria. Epilepsy and permanent disability still occur in up to 50% of cases. Temporal lobe abscess, subdural empyema, and abscesses that rupture into the ventricles have a worse prognosis. Fungal abscesses can occur in transplant recipients and carry a mortality rate close to 100%.

Further reading

Kao PT, et al. (2003). Brain abscesses: Clinical analysis of 53 cases. J Microbiol Immunol Infect, 36, 129–36.
Kastrup O, Wanke I, Maschke M (2008). Neuroimaging of infections of the central nervous system. Semin Neurol, 28, 511–22.
Lorber B (1997). Listeriosis. Clin Infect Dis, 24, 1–9.
Mathisen GE, Johnson JP (1997). Brain abscess. Clin Infect Dis, 25, 763–79.
Report of the Quality Standards Subcommittee of the American Academy of Neurology (1998). Evaluation and management of intracranial mass lesions in AIDS. Neurology, 50, 21–6.
Sharma R, Mohandas K, Cooke RPD (2009). Intracranial abscesses: changes in epidemiology and management over five decades in Merseyside. Infection, 37, 39–43.

24.11.4 Neurosyphilis and neuro-AIDS

Hadi Manji

Essentials

Neurosyphilis

Invasion of the central nervous system occurs early in the course of syphilis infection. Neurosyphilis causes meningitis, myeloradiculopathy due to pachymeningitis, and gummatous cord and brain lesions; endarteritis may cause infarction.

Clinical features—these are protean: neurosyphilis should always be considered in the diagnosis of neurological disorders without a convincing explanation, including (1) stroke—especially in young patients; (2) ocular abnormalities—e.g. optic neuritis, choroidoretinitis, pupillary abnormalities; (3) unexplained cranial nerve disease, including sensorineural deafness and vertigo; (4) dementia—low-grade meningo-encephalitis is associated with generalized changes in the brain and occasionally with frontotemporal dementia; (5) tabes dorsalis—a sensory ataxia caused by disease of the dorsal roots, ganglia and posterior columns.

Diagnosis, treatment, and prognosis—diagnosis requires specific serological tests and examination of the cerebrospinal fluid (see Chapter 7.6.36). Treatment with antimicrobials is often curative in patients with meningitic or meningovascular disease, but is only partially effective in those with late forms of dementia or tabes. Follow-up after treatment should include repeat examinations of the cerebrospinal fluid until the cell count is restored to normal limits.

Neurological complications of HIV infection

The neurological sequel of HIV infection include (1) opportunistic infections—e.g. cryptococcal meningitis; toxoplasma encephalitis; tuberculous meningitis and tuberculomata; cytomegalovirus encephalitis, cauda equina syndrome; vasculitic neuropathy; progressive multifocal leucoencephalopathy (PML) and (2) neoplasms—e.g. primary CNS lymphoma.

HIV itself also affects the central and peripheral nervous systems causing HIV associated neurocognitive syndromes including dementia, vacuolar myelopathy and peripheral neuropathy.

The introduction of highly active antiretroviral therapies has greatly reduced the frequency of all such problems in patients with access to treatment. However, newer complications are now increasingly recognized—e.g. immune reconstitution inflammatory syndrome (IRIS).

Neurosyphilis

The incidence of primary and secondary syphilis in the United Kingdom (excluding Scotland) increased from 223 in 1999 to 2500 in 2008. It is more common in the United States of America, Russia, and eastern Europe, as well as in the developing world. As syphilis, similar to other ulcerating genital infections such as herpes and chancroid, is an independent risk factor for the acquisition and transmission of infection with the HIV, the disease has once again come under scrutiny. In addition, there are recent anecdotal reports of *Treponema pallidum* being more neurovirulent and with a greater risk of treatment failure in those dually infected with HIV.

Invasion of the CNS occurs early in the course of syphilis infection. *T. pallidum* has been isolated from the cerebrospinal fluid of up to 40% of neurologically asymptomatic patients with untreated primary and secondary syphilis. Despite this, cohort studies of untreated patients suggest that symptomatic late syphilis (neurosyphilis, cardiovascular syphilis, and gummas) occurs in 15 to 40% of such individuals; the Oslo study documented an incidence of clinical neurosyphilis in 9.4%. Thus, it would seem as if, at least in the immunocompetent patient, *T. pallidum* has a low virulence for the CNS.

Clinical features (Table 24.11.4.1)

Acquired syphilis is divided into an early, potentially infectious stage (primary, secondary, and early latent where less than 2 years have elapsed since infection) and a late, noninfectious stage (late latent where more than 2 years have elapsed—gummatous, cardiovascular, and neurosyphilis). Although there is a rough time course to the development of the various neurological syndromes, there is considerable overlap; these syndromes are, in reality, part of the spectrum of disease.

Neurosyphilis may include meningitis (acute and chronic), a myeloradiculopathy due to a pachymeningitis, and granulomatous lesions (gummas) that present as space-occupying lesions within the brain, spinal cord, or epidural space, causing compression. Meningovascular syphilis involves the small- and medium-sized arteries, typically causing an endarteritis (Heubner's endarteritis obliterans), resulting in infarction. The so-called late manifestations of neurosyphilis result from a low-grade meningoencephalitis. In patients with general paralysis (also called general paralysis of the insane or dementia paralytica), the focus is on the frontotemporal cortex. Therefore, during the early stages, vague symptoms may include personality and mood changes, with impaired faculties of concentration and attention being the presenting features; memory difficulties develop later.

In tabes dorsalis (taboparesis), which may coexist with general paralysis, the clinical presentation results from involvement of the dorsal roots and ganglia as well as the posterior columns within the spinal cord, with the resultant emphasis on a sensory ataxia. Diabetes may produce a similar clinical picture with a neuropathy and pupillary abnormalities (diabetic pseudotabes).

The optic nerve could be involved with or without other evidence of neurosyphilis, but must always be treated as if it were part of a systemic infection. Uveitis, chorioretinitis, optic neuritis, papillitis, and optic atrophy have all been reported at different stages of the disease. Extraocular presentations include nerve palsies involving the eye muscles and a superior orbital fissure syndrome. Although the Argyll Robertson pupil may occur in any form of the disease, it is generally encountered in tabes dorsalis. The pupils are small and irregular, being unreactive to light, but constrict normally to accommodation and convergence. Unilateral involvement is rare. The light/near dissociation is the result of gliosis in the periaqueductal grey midbrain tegmentum, which may also account for the bilateral ptosis seen in some individuals.

Diagnosis

Neurosyphilis has a myriad of neurological manifestations and therefore the diagnosis enters the differential of most neurological conditions (see Table 24.11.4.1). Treatment in the early stages of the disease (i.e. of the meningitic and meningovascular syndromes) may well result in recovery, whereas the late forms—with general paralysis and tabes dorsalis—may cease to progress with only partial recovery. These common neurological presentations include stroke, and should enter the differential diagnosis especially in younger patients, chorioretinitis, optic neuropathy of unknown cause, and single or multiple cranial neuropathies, particularly those involving cranial nerve VIII with vertigo and sensorineural deafness. Syphilis serology should be routinely performed in patients with dementia and psychiatric illnesses.

The serum reaginic tests, Venereal Diseases Research Laboratory (VDRL) test and rapid plasma reagin test (RPR), are always or almost always positive in secondary syphilis when the first neurological complications may be encountered. However, a false-negative result may occur due to the prozone phenomenon if undiluted serum is used. This occurs in 1 to 2% of cases of secondary syphilis and is due to blockage of agglutination caused by the saturation of antigenic sites by excess antibody. The specific serological tests—*T. pallidum* haemagglutination test (TPHA), *T. pallidum* particle agglutination test (TPPA), fluorescent treponemal antibody absorption test (FTA-abs), and the treponemal enzyme immunoassay (EIA)—are invariably positive.

In late syphilis (meningovascular syphilis, gummatous, general paralysis, and tabes dorsalis), the serum VDRL/RPR tests are negative in 30% of untreated cases. All the specific tests have a sensitivity approaching 100%, so that a negative treponemal antigen test has an extremely high predictive value for excluding neurosyphilis.

It is recommended that all patients with positive syphilis serology who have ocular and/or neurological symptoms and signs should undergo cerebrospinal fluid examination, as should patients with latent infection of unknown duration. In order for these tests to be correctly interpreted, it is important that the cerebrospinal fluid is not significantly (macroscopically) contaminated with blood.

In patients with neurosyphilis there is usually a lymphocytic pleocytosis (>5 cells/μl), with an elevated protein (>0.4 g/l). In the late stages, particularly in tabes, the cerebrospinal fluid may be quiescent. A reactive CSF VDRL establishes the diagnosis of active neurosyphilis, but a nonreactive test does not exclude it. The sensitivity of the CSF VDRL is 50%, with a specificity of 100%. A nonreactive CSF FTA-abs or TPHA excludes the diagnosis. However, a reactive CSF FTA-abs or TPHA does not establish the diagnosis because the presence of treponemal antibodies in the cerebrospinal fluid

Table 24.11.4.1 Clinical features of neurosyphilis

		Syphilitic meningitis	Meningovascular	General paralysis	Tabes dorsalis
Time course	Acute	Within first year; may occur during secondary syphilis	Months to years after infection, average 7 years	15–20 years	20–25 years
	Chronic	20–25 years			
Clinical features	Acute	Cranial nerve palsies (III, VI, VII, VIII), hydrocephalus	Stroke (hemiparesis, dysphasia), seizures, cranial nerve palsies, encephalitic syndrome, anterior spinal artery syndrome	Frontal–temporal dementia, psychiatric symptoms (delusions, apathy), personality change, seizures, dysarthria, tremor (tongue, face, hands), Argyll Robertson pupils, optic atrophy	Lightning pains (limbs, viscera); loss of pain and temperature (Charcot's joints), joint position (sensory ataxia, positive Romberg's sign), areflexia, sluggish pupils(early), autonomic and sphincter dysfunction
	Chronic	Myeloradiculopathy			

could result from passive transfer from the blood, or from a previous episode of treated syphilis. The sensitivity for the CSF FTA-abs is 100%, with a specificity of 30%.

The role of the polymerase chain reaction (PCR) in the diagnosis of neurosyphilis is unclear at present, because the technique cannot discriminate between viable and nonviable organisms. *T. pallidum* DNA has been detected in cerebrospinal fluid up to 3 years after intravenous treatment with penicillin.

Treatment

In patients with symptomatic neurosyphilis or ocular disease, the World Health Organization/United Nations Programme on HIV/AIDS (WHO/UNAIDS) as well as the Centers for Disease Control (CDC) recommend treatment with benzylpenicillin (2–4 MU intravenously every 4 h for 14 days). In the United Kingdom the preference is for procaine penicillin (1.8–2.4 MIU intramuscularly once daily, plus probenecid 500 mg by mouth four times daily, for 17–21 days). The alternative is intravenous benzylpenicillin (3 to 4 MU intravenously every 4 h for 17–21 days). In patients with a history of penicillin allergy one option is to perform skin testing to confirm the allergy and to then consider desensitization. The other is to treat with doxycycline 200 mg by mouth four times daily for 28 days.

After treatment of neurosyphilis, a repeat lumbar puncture should be performed at 6-monthly intervals until the cell count is normal. The cell count should have decreased by 6 months and be entirely normal by 2 years. The CSF VDRL may take years to become nonreactive.

Syphilis in the era of HIV

Since the onset of the AIDS epidemic there have been numerous reports of an accelerated course of syphilis and of treatment failures in patients who are dually infected. Compared with nonimmunosuppressed individuals there certainly does seem to be a higher than expected rate of cases of syphilitic meningitis and meninogovascular syphilis. To date, however, there are no denominator data. As cell-mediated immunity, which is necessary to eradicate *T. pallidum*, may be impaired in HIV infection, this seems plausible.

As a result of altered B-cell function there has been concern about serological tests. However, these are usually positive or may show a delayed response in the occasional case.

There is still debate as to whether or not patients with HIV and early syphilis who are neurologically asymptomatic should have a cerebrospinal fluid examination. Any cerebrospinal fluid cytochemical abnormalities could be due to either HIV or syphilis. In view of the treatment failures reported with benzathinepenicillin some authorities suggest that all HIV patients with early syphilis should be treated with neurosyphilis treatment regimens.

Neuro-AIDS (the neurological complications of HIV infection)

Soon after the onset of the AIDS epidemic in 1981, it became clear that the nervous system was frequently involved. However, opportunistic infections such as toxoplasmosis and cryptococcal meningitis, as well as neoplasms (such as primary central nervous system lymphoma, PCNSL) accounted for only 30% of the neurological problems encountered. It also became evident that, in the later stages of the AIDS illness, patients developed neurological complications due to the HIV itself. This included a progressive decline in cognitive function in association with motor abnormalities—the HIV–dementia complex or as it is now known as HIV associated neurocognitive disorder (HAND).

Neurological disorders are the AIDS-defining illness in up to 20% of cases. Over the course of the illness the prevalence of neurological complications increases up to 70%. These include other opportunistic infections and tumours, as well as the HIV-related problems of dementia, vacuolar myelopathy, and distal sensory peripheral neuropathy (DSPN).

Prior to the advent of highly active antiretroviral therapies (HAART), at postmortem examination more than 90% of the brains from patients dying of AIDS show evidence of HIV encephalitis and/or of one of the opportunistic infections such as CMV.

During the last 10 years, with the introduction of HAART, there has been a dramatic decline in the incidence of neurological opportunistic infections as well as HIV-related disorders such as HIV–dementia. The downside has been an increase in the peripheral nerve complications of some of the antiretroviral drugs. However, these are expensive drugs and are out of reach for most HIV-infected individuals worldwide.

Clinical approach

All areas of the neuraxis are vulnerable in individuals infected with HIV. Differing pathological processes occur simultaneously in various parts of the nervous system. Thus, Occam's razor—the principle of diagnostic parsimony, often used in medicine—does not always apply. Another aspect to be considered is the possibility of simultaneous infection with more than one organism, e.g. meningitis due to *Mycobacterium tuberculosis* or *Cryptococcus neoformans*. Mass lesions in the brain, with some not responding to antitoxoplasma therapy, could be due to lymphoma or another infective cause such as a tuberculoma.

The nervous system is involved early in the course of infection, as evidenced by neurological seroconversion illnesses such as an aseptic meningitis, encephalitis, and the Guillain–Barré syndrome. Furthermore, during the asymptomatic phase of the illness (i.e. when patients are well), the cerebrospinal fluid shows abnormalities in up to 60% of cases. This may be a lymphocytic pleocytosis of up to 50 cells/mm³, an elevated protein, or the presence of oligoclonal bands. The cerebrospinal fluid glucose level is usually normal. Therefore, these cytobiochemical markers are unhelpful in making a diagnosis of a meningitic or encephalitic illness. Reliance is therefore placed on specific markers such as the cryptococcal antigen or antibody tests such as the CSF VDRL or TPHA tests.

As a result of the impaired immune response, a rise in antibody titres to specific infections may not occur, especially during the later stages of HIV infection. Furthermore, the typical clinical picture—the presentation of which, at least in some infections, such as meningitis, is the result of a brisk inflammatory response such as fever—may not occur. In cryptococcal meningitis, only a third of patients exhibit the classic signs of meningism, i.e. neck stiffness, photophobia, and positive Kernig's sign.

The specific type of opportunistic complications encountered depends on a number of factors, including the degree of immunosuppression. During the early stages when individuals are relatively immunocompetent, with CD4 counts above 500/µl, autoimmune disorders such as demyelinating neuropathies may occur. With CD4 counts of between 200 and 500/µl, multidermatomal herpes zoster infections and tuberculosis (TB) may present. Once the level declines below 200/µl, patients are vulnerable to all the major opportunistic infections and the complications due to HIV itself. Symptomatic infection with CMV tends to occur at very low levels below 50/µl. With the introduction of HAART, these guidelines are less robust because, despite immunreconstitution, pathogen-specific memory T-cell clones may not have been fully restored.

Opportunistic infections

Toxoplasmosis

Toxoplasma gondii, whose definitive host includes members of the cat family with humans as the intermediate hosts, is an obligate intracellular protozoan. Human infection occurs through the ingestion of tissue cysts in undercooked meat. Variations in dietary habits therefore explain the differing seroprevalence rates worldwide—90% in French adults compared with 50% of residents in the United Kingdom. Symptomatic toxoplasmosis is usually due to a reactivation of latent infection in individuals with HIV. The risk of an HIV-infected patient who is seropositive for IgG *T. gondii* antibody developing toxoplasmosis is around 25%.

Toxoplasmosis is the most common cause of mass lesions in the brains of patients with HIV infection, including those in areas where TB is endemic. The clinical presentation is variable, but headache, confusion, seizures, and focal neurological deficits such as hemiplegia, dysphasia, and visual field defects are the most common. Other presentations described include: a variety of movement disorders (choreoathetosis, dystonia, and hemiparkinsonism); psychiatric illness such as depression; brainstem syndromes; and a rapidly progressive diffuse encephalitis. Rarely, the spinal cord may be involved with myelitis or cauda equina syndrome.

A definitive diagnosis of toxoplasma encephalitis can be made only by brain biopsy. With increasing experience and pragmatism, it is now standard practice to treat any HIV-infected individual who has a low CD4 count and multiple lesions on imaging with antitoxoplasma therapy (Fig. 24.11.4.1). A response, clinically and radiologically, confirms the diagnosis. Although a negative blood toxoplasma serology result makes the diagnosis less likely, this may occur in up to 17% of cases. This loss of seropositivity may be the result of impaired antibody synthesis with increasing immunosuppression. It is therefore useful to document an individual's toxoplasma serostatus on first diagnosis of HIV positivity. For similar reasons, the expected rise in IgM and IgG levels does not occur. A single lesion on MRI is most likely to be due to lymphoma. A single lesion on CT should, if possible, be followed by MRI, which is a more sensitive method of detecting lesions, particularly in the posterior fossa (Fig. 24.11.4.2).

The main differential diagnosis is that of primary CNS lymphoma, which presents at similar CD4 counts and has a similar presentation both clinically and on imaging studies (Box 24.11.4.1).

A response is seen in 90% of patients by the second week of treatment (Table 24.11.4.2). It is necessary to reimage 2 weeks after treatment even if there is clinical evidence of improvement, because occasionally some lesions improve but others due to, for example, *Mycobacterium tuberculosis*, continue to enlarge, which then makes it necessary to consider a biopsy. The radiological improvement generally lags behind the clinical improvement. Secondary prophylaxis is required after resolution of the acute episode.

Patients infected with HIV who are seropositive for IgG against *T. gondii* should be offered primary prophylaxis with 980 mg co-trimoxazole (trimethoprim and sulfamethoxazole) when their

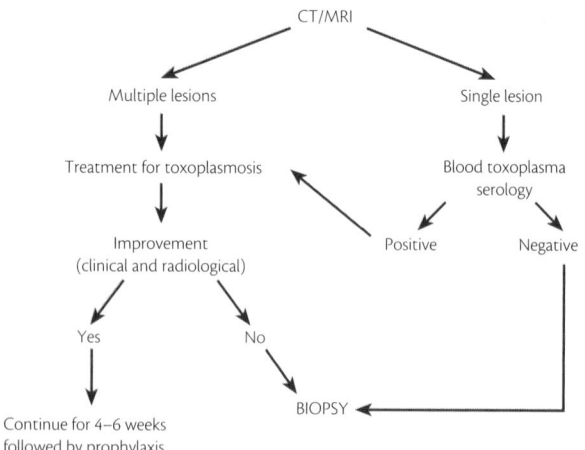

Notes: (i) MRI may detect lesions not apparent on CT; (ii) In patients with significant mass effect and danger of herniation additional treatment with a reducing course of dexamathsone is necessary.
Any deterioration subsequently on reduction of the steroids requires consideration of a biopsy.

Fig. 24.11.4.1 Management of mass lesions in AIDS.

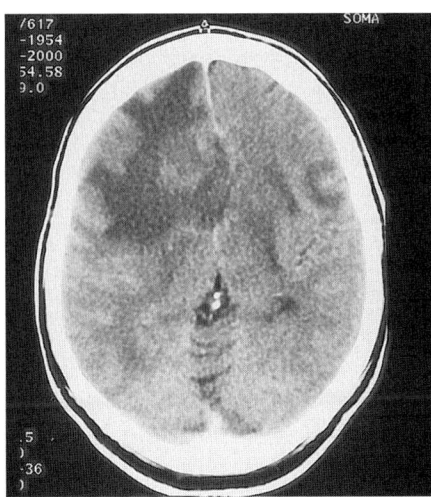

Fig. 24.11.4.2 Cranial CT: multiple lesions with mass effect and cerebral oedema due to toxoplasmosis.

CD4 count falls below 100/mm³. This will confer crossprotection against *Pneumocystis jirovecii* pneumonia. After the initiation of HAART, primary prophylaxis maybe discontinued after successful suppression of HIV viral replication and the CD4 counts exceed 200 cells/mm³ for 3 months. Maintenance therapy after an episode of toxoplasmosis may be discontinued after 6 months of successful suppression of HIV viral replication and a CD4 >200 cells/mm³.

Cryptococcus neoformans

This encapsulated yeast is a ubiquitous organism in the environment acquired by humans through inhalation. Although disseminated infection can involve the skin, bones, lungs, eyes, and prostate,

---

Box 24.11.4.1 Focal neurological syndromes

Infections

♦ *Toxoplasma gondii* (abscesses, encephalitis)*

♦ JC virus (PML)*

♦ *Mycobacterium tuberculosis* (tuberculoma)*

♦ Fungal microabscesses (*Cryptococcus neoformans*,

♦ *Histoplasma capsulatum, Candida albicans, Aspergillus fumigatus*)

♦ Cytomegalovirus

Neoplasms

♦ Primary CNS lymphoma*

♦ Metastatic tumours (non-Hodgkin's lymphoma, Kaposi's sarcoma)

Cerebrovascular

♦ Ischaemic stroke (coagulopathies)

♦ Embolic stroke (bacterial and nonbacterial endocarditis)

♦ Vasculitis (meningovascular syphilis, herpes zoster)

*Most common.

---

symptomatic infection with *C. neoformans* most often presents as meningitis.

Cryptococcal infection is the most common infectious cause of meningitis in patients with AIDS (Box 24.11.4.2). Although the presentation may be acute, it is usually subacute with symptoms of malaise, headache, fever, and vomiting. The classic signs of meningism—neck stiffness, photophobia, and Kernig's sign—are present in only one-third of patients. Other, less common symptoms include altered mental status, seizures, and focal neurological signs. The last are the result of parenchymal cryptococcal abscesses.

Brain imaging is usually normal, although the basal meningitis may result in hydrocephalus or sometimes, particularly on MRI, small abscesses—cryptococcomas—may be evident.

Cerebrospinal fluid examination is essential for the diagnosis, with culture of the fungus being the 'gold standard'. The cytochemical markers in the cerebrospinal fluid may be normal. India ink staining of the cerebrospinal fluid will reveal the fungal hyphae in 70 to 80% of cases and cryptococcal antigen is detected in over 90%. Cryptococcal antigen is also detected in the blood in over 90% of patients, and should be measured together with the cerebrospinal fluid level because in occasionally reported cases of fulminant cryptococcal meningitis the cerebrospinal fluid may be negative and the blood positive. The blood antigen measurement may be used as a screening test in patients presenting with symptoms of early infection such as headache. However, it should be appreciated that a negative result does not completely exclude the diagnosis of cryptococcal meningitis.

Treatment with amphotericin B remains the drug of choice for the treatment of severe cases of cryptococcal meningitis. The mortality rate still remains around 10%. Features that have been identified with a poor outcome include a relapse infection, abnormal mental status, cerebrospinal fluid cryptoccal antigen titre over 1:1024, cerebrospinal fluid white cell count more than 20 cells/mm³, positive India ink staining, hyponatraemia, and positive culture from an extrameningeal site. A cerebrospinal fluid opening pressure of more than 250 mmH₂O is also a marker of poor prognosis. In milder cases, where none of these features is present, oral fluconazole may be used. Although combination with 5-flucytosine has been shown to improve outcome in non-AIDS patients, this has not been confirmed in patients with AIDS. However, the combination should be considered in fulminant cases.

A specific complication that requires close monitoring is the development of raised intracranial pressure due to obstruction of the arachnoid villi and cerebral oedema. This should be managed with repeated lumbar puncture or, if necessary, by the insertion of a lumbar or ventricular drain.

Maintenance therapy is essential, with relapse rates approaching 100% if secondary prophylaxis with oral fluconazole is not adhered to. The serum cryptococcal antigen titre is not useful in predicting relapse. The timing for the initiation of HAART after an episode of meningitis is not clear cut due to the risk of precipitation of the immune reconstitution syndrome (IRIS). After 6 months of HIV viral load suppression and a CD4 count less than 200 cells/µl with HAART, it seems safe to discontinue secondary prophylaxis.

JC virus

Progressive multifocal leucoencephalopathy (PML) is caused by the reactivation of latent JC virus (JCV). This polyomavirus

Table 24.11.4.2 Treatment of neurological opportunistic infections

Infection	Drug	Dose	Duration	Side effects	Notes
Toxoplasmosis					
Acute	Pyrimethamine +	Loading dose of 200 mg, then 75 mg orally	4–6 weeks	Myelosuppression	
	Sulfadiazine	6–8 g/day orally or intravenously	4–6 weeks	Nephrotoxicity, renal calculi, crystalluria	Clindamycin 2.4 g/day oral or intravenously is an alternative to sulfadiazine. Side effect pseudomembranous colitis
	Folinic acid	15 mg/day orally	4–6 weeks		To counteract the myelosuppressive effects of pyrimethamine
Maintenance	Pyrimethamine +	25–50 mg/day orally	Indefinitely		
	Sulfadiazine +	2 g/day orally	Indefinitely		Clindamycin 1.2 g/day
	Folinic acid	15 mg/day orally	Indefinitely		
Primary prophylaxis	Trimethoprim +	80 mg/day orally		Nausea, Stevens–Johnson syndrome, thrombocytopenia	CD4 count < 200/μl and toxoplasma serology positive
	Sulfamethoxazole	400 mg/day orally			
Cryptococcal meningitis					
Acute	Amphotericin B ±	0.6–1.0 mg/kg per day intravenously	At least 2–4 weeks until symptoms resolve and CSF culture negative	Hypokalaemia, renal failure, anaemia	Via central line because of thrombophlebitis. In mild cases fluconazole 400 mg initially i.v. then continued orally
	5-Flucytosine	100 mg/kg per day	2–4 weeks	Myelosuppression	
Maintenance	Fluconazole	200–400 mg/day orally	Indefinitely	Nausea, vomiting, abnormal liver function tests	Amphotericin 1 mg/kg per week if intolerant or relapse on fluconazole

infection is acquired by most of the population during childhood as a banal upper respiratory infection. The virus is frequently found in the urine of healthy individuals. Before the AIDS epidemic, PML was a rare condition encountered in patients immunosuppressed as a result of haematological malignancies, drugs used in the treatment of post-transplant recipients, autoimmune disorders such as systemic lupus erythematosus (SLE), and granulomatous disorders such as sarcoidosis. Nowadays, underlying HIV infection accounts for 85% of cases.

Before the introduction of HAART, the incidence of PML was 4%. The clinical presentation is subacute, with progressive focal neurological deficits such as a hemiparesis, visual field defects, and a cerebellar syndrome. The disorder is not restricted to the white matter because patients may also develop dysphasia and seizures. Occasional patients may present with a progressive dementia with focal neurological signs.

MRI characteristically shows multiple areas of high signal on T_1-weighted images and a low signal on T_2-weighted ones (Fig. 24.11.4.3). There is little or no enhancement, with no mass effect or oedema around the lesions. Blood serological testing is unhelpful because 80% of the general population is seropositive. It is possible to confirm the diagnosis of PML by isolating JC viral DNA in cerebrospinal fluid by PCR techniques. This has a sensitivity of 75% with a specificity of 95%. In PCR-negative cases it may be necessary either to repeat the cerebrospinal fluid examination or to perform a brain biopsy. The typical histological features show areas of focal demyelination, bizarre enlarged astrocytes, and abnormal oligodendrocytes with inclusion bodies that stain for JC viral antigens.

There is, to date, no specific treatment for PML. Cytosine arabinoside, both intravenous and intrathecal, has been shown to be ineffective. However, improving immune function with HAART has been shown to improve survival times from a median survival of 10 weeks to 40 weeks. Cidofovir, an anti-CMV drug, in one multicentre study showed no significant additional benefit over HAART alone. Recently, there are anecdotal data suggesting that the anti-malarial drug mefloquine and the antidepressant mirtazipine may have some beneficial effecs. Adequate trial results are awaited.

Cytomegalovirus

The neurological complications from this herpesvirus results from reactivation in severely immunocompromised patients. Almost all

---

Box 24.11.4.2 Meningitis in HIV infection

Infections

- *Cryptococcus neoformans*
- *Mycobacterium tuberculosis*
- *Listeria monocytogenes*
- *Treponema pallidum*

Neoplasms

- Metastatic non-Hodgkin's lymphoma

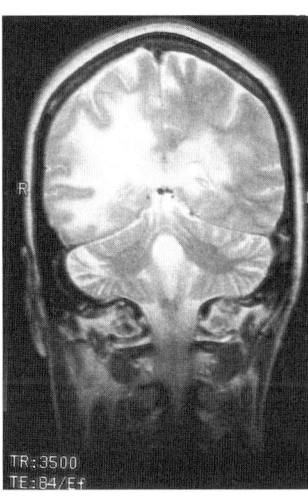

Fig. 24.11.4.3 T_2-weighted MRI in a patient with progressive multifocal leucoencephalopathy.

patients infected with HIV are seropositive for CMV. Postmortem studies of the brains of patients who died from AIDS show evidence of CMV in 25% of cases. However, clinical CMV disease, apart from CMV retinitis, is rare.

CMV retinitis is the most common manifestation of CMV disease and can affect up to 20% of patients with AIDS. The slowly progressive necrotizing retinitis results in characteristic white irregular lesions with central necrosis and haemorrhages—the cheese and tomato ketchup appearance. Retinal detachment may occur in patients with extensive retinal involvement. The retinitis presents with symptoms of reduced visual acuity, floaters, and loss of peripheral vision. As the condition may be asymptomatic in the early stages, regular ophthalmological screening is recommended for high-risk patients with CD4 counts below 50 cells/µl.

A necrotizing ventriculoencephalitis has been described, usually in patients with evidence of CMV disease elsewhere (Box 24.11.4.3). The onset is subacute over a period of days or weeks with confusion, seizures, and brainstem signs such as internuclear ophthalmoplegia, ataxia, and cranial nerve palsies. Imaging studies typically show periventricular enhancement.

CMV polyradiculopathy presents over a period of days with back pain, leg weakness, sensory impairment, and sphincter disturbance.

Box 24.11.4.3 Encephalitis in HIV

Virus

- Cytomegalovirus
- Herpes simplex
- Herpes zoster
- Human herpesvirus 6?

Protozoa

- Toxoplasmosis

The differential diagnosis includes syphilitic polyradiculopathy and infiltration with metastatic lymphoma. The cerebrospinal fluid reveals a polymorphonuclear leucocytosis which is unusual for a viral infection. Early recognition and treatment are necessary to stabilize and, in some cases, improve the neurological impairment.

Drugs licensed for the treatment of CMV disease include ganciclovir, cidofovir, and foscarnet. Oral ganciclovir is prescribed for secondary prophylaxis.

Opportunistic tumours

PCNSL is the second most common cause of mass lesions after toxoplasmosis in adults, and the most common in children with AIDS. Histologically, this is a high-grade, non-Hodgkin's, B-cell lymphoma. Recent evidence suggests that the Epstein–Barr virus is causally linked to PCNSL, with the identification of the viral DNA incorporated into that of the neoplastic cells.

The common presenting symptoms are those of headache with focal neurological deficits, altered level of consciousness, and seizures.

Brain imaging reveals enhancing mass lesions with surrounding oedema and mass effect. These are similar to those found in toxoplasmosis. PCNSL is more likely to present as a single mass lesion than toxoplasmosis and is also more likely to invade the ventricular walls. Recent studies using thallium-201 single photon emission computed tomography (SPECT) suggest that it may be possible to differentiate between an abscess and a tumour, with the former having little uptake compared with the high uptake of the mitotically active lymphoma.

There is no effective treatment for PCNSL. Whole-brain radiotherapy provides, at best, only a modest benefit, with most patients succumbing within 2 months. Current evidence suggests that HAART may improve survival in this group of patients.

HIV associated neurological disorders (HAND)

(Previously known as HIV–dementia complex)

Before the introduction of HAART (and in areas of the world where these drugs are still unavailable) approximately 15 to 20% of individuals infected with HIV developed a variably progressive dementia with associated motor deficits. HAND is now classified to three degrees – asymptomatic neurocognitive disorder (ANI), mild neurocognitive impairment (MND) with only mild functional effects and HIV dementia (HAD) where there is marked functional impairment. In children, a similar HIV-1-associated progressive encephalopathy occurs more frequently than with opportunistic infections. This usually occurs within the context of severe immunosuppression in those with a CD4 count of less than 200/mm³. In around 3% of cases, HIV–dementia is the AIDS-defining illness. Large cohort studies, using clinical, MRI, and neuropsychological methods, have largely discounted the early reports of evidence of cognitive changes in asymptomatic HIV-positive patients.

The clinical presentation in the early stages is with vague symptoms of apathy, mood changes, and difficulty with memory and concentration. These are features of a subcortical dementia with no features of cortical involvement such as language, visuospatial, or calculation difficulties. This picture may be mimicked by depression, metabolic encephalopathy, and drugs, both therapeutic and recreational. At this stage, there may be few physical signs apart from brisk reflexes, impaired fine finger movements, and unsteady gait.

Later, the memory impairments are obvious, as is the psychomotor retardation—which may progress to frank mutism and a global dementia. Some patients develop seizures. The motor signs due to the associated vacuolar myelopathy with a spastic paraparesis and sphincter disturbances are also present in a significant number of patients (Box 24.11.4.4). In addition, some patients will have the HIV-related distal sensory peripheral neuropathy. Thus, this group will have absent ankle jerks and extensor plantar responses.

The diagnosis of the HIV–dementia is made by clinical assessment—there are usually no focal signs and the tempo of the disorder is an insidious one. Investigations are performed to exclude other infection or neoplastic pathologies, and therefore necessitate imaging, preferably with MRI, and a cerebrospinal fluid examination. MRI may show evidence of cerebral atrophy with compensatory ventricular dilatation, a diffuse white-matter high signal on T_2-weighted images with no enhancement. A cerebrospinal fluid examination may be nonspecifically abnormal with a pleocytosis, elevated protein level, and oligoclonal bands. It important to exclude cryptococcal and tuberculous meningitis as well as neurosyphilis. The HIV RNA viral load in cerebrospinal fluid correlates with the severity of clinical dementia, but there is too much overlap between nondemented and demented patients for the measurement to be of use as a diagnostic aid. There is no correlation between the plasma HIV RNA viral load and dementia. Electroencephalography (EEG) may be normal in the early stages, with nonspecific diffuse slowing developing shown later.

The pathology of the HIV–dementia is a spectrum ranging from diffuse myelin pallor, microglial nodules—which are nonspecific and may be found in CMV encephalitis—to multinucleated giant cells that are indicative of productive brain infection and cortical neuronal loss. There is no clear correlation between the clinical and pathological findings.

The mechanisms of disease in the HIV–dementia are still unclear. It is, however, evident that HIV predominantly infects the microglial and astrocytic cells rather than neurons or oligodendrocytes. One hypothesis for the entry of the virus into the CNS is the 'Trojan horse' theory, with invasion occurring by infected peripheral blood monocytes penetrating a blood–brain barrier that has been disrupted by damage to the capillary endothelial cells. Neuronal damage is subsequently caused by viral toxins (e.g. Gp120) and cytokines (e.g. tumour necrosis factor α) released from activated macrophages.

After the introduction of zidovudine in 1987, there was a dramatic reduction in the incidence of HIV-associated dementia. One clinical study looking specifically at the effect of zidovudine on cognitive function confirmed its beneficial effect, albeit at dosages much higher than those currently used. With the introduction of the newer antiretroviral drugs—most of which have poor penetration into the cerebrospinal fluid and presumably the brain—there is concern that, despite the reduction of plasma HIV viral loads, the CNS may develop into a safe sanctuary for the virus from which reinfection could occur. It is clear, however, that suppressing the systemic viral load is important in the prevention and progression of HIV-associated dementia perhaps by reducing the trafficking of virus into the CNS. Recently published studies confirm that these newer therapies improve cognitive function and it seems prudent, until further data become available, to use drug combinations to which the virus is sensitive with those that best penetrate the cerebrospinal fluid to treat HIV–dementia.

HIV-associated neuropathy

The most common neurological complication encountered in patients infected with HIV is DSPN, which may occur in 30% of those with AIDS (Box 24.11.4.5). It is a significant cause of morbidity.

Typically, patients complain of numbness of the soles of the feet together with shooting pains and paraesthesiae developing over a period of months. There is little or no weakness. The hands are infrequently involved. The ankle jerks are depressed or absent. Sensory testing reveals impaired pain and temperature perception as well as vibration.

Further investigations are usually unnecessary in a patient with a CD4 count below 200 and showing the typical clinical picture, but it is always worth checking the blood sugar, vitamin B_{12} level, and syphilis serology. It is important to enquire about alcohol intake and the possibility of an excess intake of vitamin B_6.

Neurophysiological and pathological studies suggest this to be a length-dependent axonal neuropathy. Productive HIV infection has not been found in pathological specimens and the underlying mechanisms, similar to those for HIV dementia, are linked to macrophage activation products.

As antiretroviral therapy has no benefit, treatment is symptomatic with the use of tricyclic antidepressants and anticonvulsant drugs such as gabapentin.

The nucleoside analogues didanosine (ddI), zalcitabine (ddC), and stavudine (d4T) cause a dose-dependent sensory neuropathy

---

Box 24.11.4.4 Myelopathy in HIV

Infections

- HIV-associated vacuolar myelopathy*
- Herpes zoster*
- Cytomegalovirus
- HTLV-1 (coinfection)
- *Treponema pallidum*
- Toxoplasmosis
- Epidural abscess

Neoplasm

- Metastatic non-Hodgkin's lymphoma

Other causes

- Vitamin B_{12}

HTLV-1, human T-cell leukaemia/lymphoma virus-1.
*Most common.

HIV related

- Axonal neuropathy (distal sensory peripheral neuropathy)*
- Demyelinating neuropathy—acute (Guillain–Barré syndrome), chronic (chronic inflammatory demyelinating neuropathy)
- Vasculitic (mononeuritis multiplex)
- Diffuse inflammatory lymphocytic syndrome
- Lower motor neuron syndrome (resembling motor neuron disease)

Drugs

- Antiretrovirals (ddI, ddC, d4T)*
- Isoniazid
- Thalidomide
- Dapsone
- Metronidazole (high dose)
- Vincristine

CMV related

- Vasculitic (mononeuritis multiplex)
- Lumbosacral polyradiculopathy

Others

- Syphilis (polyradiculopathy)
- Metastatic non-Hodgkin's lymphoma (polyradiculopathy)
- Ganglioneuritis
- Autonomic neuropathy

*Most common.

The management in such cases is difficult but includes treatment of the appropriate organism and may warrant corticosteroids. In life-threatening situations stopping the HAART may be necessary.

Further reading

Brew B (2001). *HIV neurology.* Oxford University Press, Oxford.
Clinical Effectiveness Group (1999). National guideline for the management of early syphilis. *Sex Transm Infect,* **75** Suppl 1, S29–33.
Clinical Effectiveness Group (1999). National guideline for the management of late syphilis. *Sex Transm Infect,* **75** Suppl 1, S34–7.
French P (2007). Syphilis. Clinical review. *BMJ,* **334**, 143–7.
Gendleman H, *et al.* (eds) (2005). *The neurology of AIDS,* 2nd edition. Oxford University Press, Oxford.
Harrison MJ, McArthur JC (1995). *AIDS and neurology. Clinical Neurology and neurosurgery monographs.* Churchill Livingstone, Edinburgh.
Koralnik I (2006). Progressive Multifocal Leucoencephalopathy Revisited: Has the Disease Outgrown Its Name. *Ann Neurol,* **60**, 162–173.
Letendre S, *et al.* (2008). Validation of the CNS Penetration Effectiveness Rank for Quantifying Antiretroviral Penetration into the Central Nervous System. *Arch Neurol,* **65**(1), 65–70.
Seminars in Neurology (1999). Vol. 19. *Thieme Medical Publishers,* Amsterdam. [Whole volume devoted to HIV neurology.]
Stoll M, Schmidt RE (2003). Immune Restoration Inflammatory Syndromes: The Dark Side of Successful Antiretroviral Treatment. *Current Infectious Disease Reports,* **5**, 266–276.
Swartz MN, Healy BP, Musher DM (1999). Late syphilis. In: Holmes KK, *et al.* (eds) *Sexually transmitted diseases,* pp. 487–509. McGraw-Hill, New York.

24.11.5 Human prion diseases

R.G. Will

Essentials

Prion protein (for proteinacious infectious particle) is a membrane-associated glycoprotein present in all mammalian species. Its normal function is unknown, but in prion diseases (also known as transmissible spongiform encephalopathies) a post-translationally modified form of the protein, partially resistant to protease digestion, is deposited in the brain and associated—after long incubation periods—with neuronal dysfunction and death.

Particular prion diseases

Creutzfeldt–Jakob disease (CJD)—several forms are recognized: (1) Sporadic—a rare condition typically presenting in late middle age with a rapidly progressive dementia associated with a range of neurological signs, most commonly myoclonus of the limbs, cerebellar ataxia and rigidity. Few patients survive for more than 2 years. (2) Hereditary—dominant pattern of inheritance; age at death is typically 5 to 10 years younger than in sporadic disease. (3) Iatrogenic—exposures in or adjacent to the nervous system (e.g. neurosurgical instruments, dura mater grafts, corneal transplants) typically present in a similar manner to sporadic disease; peripheral exposure to infection (pituitary hormones) usually manifests with progressive

that may be indistinguishable from DSPN. Clues to this drug-induced neuropathy include the shorter history of weeks rather than months, and the improvement on stopping the offending drug. However, there may be a continued worsening of symptoms for a period of 4 to 8 weeks after stopping—the phenomenon of 'coasting'. The underlying mechanism appears to be the impairment of mitochondrial protein synthesis.

Neurological immune reconstitution inflammatory syndrome (IRIS)

The introduction of HAART results in the recovery of CD4 T lymphocytes including memory T-cells. This may result in the 'paradoxical deterioration of clinical or laboratory markers including imaging studies despite a favourable response in the viral load and CD4 count' due to reaction against latent antigens. Neurological immune reconstitution inflammatory syndrome has now been described with *Mycobacterium tuberculosis* causing meningitis and brain abscesses, cryptococcal meningitis, CMV with the development of vitritis, uveitis, and cystoid macular oedema, and PML with MRI showing enhancement and biopsies inflammatory infiltrates.

cerebellar ataxia. (4) Variant—bovine spongiform encephalopathy (BSE) was identified in 1986 as a prion disease in cattle, with the favoured hypothesis being that contamination of feed, probably with tissues from the central nervous system of affected animals. Variant CJD is caused by transmission of BSE to humans. Typical presentation is with psychiatric symptoms, followed after a period of months by progressive ataxia, dementia, and choreiform or dystonic involuntary movements which often evolve into myoclonus. It is likely that the maximum number of cases will be no more than a few hundred, with the mean age at death being 30 years.

Kuru—in Papua New Guinea this disease was transmitted in the course of ritual cannibalism, which ceased by 1960, hence there have been no cases in people born after 1959. Typical presentation was with headache and limb pain, progressing to a cerebellar syndrome, with eventual immobility.

Investigation, treatment, and prevention

Investigation—there is no test for the presence of the infectious agent, hence diagnosis depends on the recognition of clinical characteristics, sometimes supported by (1) electroencephalography—periodic triphasic complexes are seen in 60 to 70% of cases of sporadic CJD and in some cases of iatrogenic CJD; (2) cerebrospinal fluid analysis—elevation of 14-3-3 protein in the cerebrospinal fluid is about 90% sensitive and specific for sporadic CJD, but less useful for variant CJD; (3) MRI—with appropriate imaging protocols, localized abnormalities may be seen in the caudate nucleus and putamen in sporadic CJD, and the pulvinar region of the posterior thalamus in variant CJD; (4) tissue biopsy of brain or tonsil.

Treatment and prevention—there is nothing that influences the clinical course of human prion diseases, nor any treatment to prevent the development of neurological disease after infection.

Introduction

Prion diseases, also known as transmissible spongiform encephalopathies, are fatal disorders of the central nervous system affecting both humans and animals. The clinical features and patterns of occurrence of these diseases vary, but they are linked by a number of characteristics including experimental and natural transmissibility, shared neuropathological features, prolonged incubation periods measured in years, and the deposition of prion protein, which may be the causal agent, in the brain of the host. Prion diseases have become the subject of intense scientific and public interest because of the likelihood that they are caused by a novel disease mechanism and because of the implications for public health following the identification of a new human prion disease, variant Creutzfeldt–Jakob disease (vCJD), and the evidence that it is caused by the transmission to humans of a cattle prion disease, bovine spongiform encephalopathy (BSE).

There have been remarkable scientific advances in the understanding of prion diseases and it is hoped that this may lead to the identification of a diagnostic test in life for the presence of infection and to therapies to prevent the development of disease. Human prion diseases have attained a public notoriety disproportionate to the overall burden of disease caused by these rare conditions. However, the transmission an animal prion disease to humans has been a tragedy and the prolonged incubation periods characteristic

of this group of diseases indicate that the eventual consequences of BSE for public health both in the United Kingdom and in other countries remain unpredictable.

Historical perspective

Scrapie was first transmitted experimentally from sheep to sheep in 1936 and to laboratory mice in 1961, but laboratory transmission of human prion diseases was not achieved until 1966 (kuru) and 1968 (Creutzfeldt–Jakob disease, CJD). The seminal discovery that apparently neurodegenerative diseases were transmissible stimulated extensive research into the nature of the infectious agent and attempts to identify the source of infection in CJD. Table 24.11.5.1 sets out the principal prion diseases known to affect the brains of animal species and humans.

Aetiology, genetics, pathogenesis, and pathology

No bacterium or virus has been isolated in these diseases and there is no immunological response to infection. This is of central importance as there is, as yet, no serological test to identify the presence of infection during the incubation period of any prion disease. The transmissible agent is remarkably resistant to inactivation procedures, including those that disrupt nucleic acids. In 1982 Prusiner proposed that the protein deposited in the central nervous system (CNS) in these diseases was itself the causal agent. Purified infectious fractions of brain contain prion protein (for proteinacious infectious particle),which is a major, and perhaps the only, component of the infectious agent. This membrane-associated glycoprotein is present in all mammalian species. The normal function of prion protein is unknown. In prion diseases a post-translationally modified form of the protein, partially resistant to protease digestion, is deposited in the brain and is associated with neuronal dysfunction and death.

There is a range of experimental evidence supporting the hypothesis that the disease-associated form of prion protein is

Table 24.11.5.1 The spongiform encephalopathies

Disorder	Species
Sporadic Creutzfeldt–Jakob disease	Human
Inherited Creutzfeldt–Jakob disease (includes Gerstmann–Straussler–Scheinker and fatal familial insomnia)	Human
Iatrogenic Creutzfeldt–Jakob disease	Human
Kuru	Human
Variant Creutzfeldt–Jakob disease*	Human
Scrapie	Sheep/goat/moufflon
Transmissible mink encephalopathy	Mink
Chronic wasting disease	Deer/elk
Bovine spongiform encephalopathy*	Cattle
Feline spongiform encephalopathy*	Cat/cheetah/puma/ocelot/tiger
Spongiform encephalopathy of captive exotic ungulates*	Kudu/nyala/oryx/gemsbok/eland

* These disorders are associated with the same infectious agent (bovine spongiform encephalopathy).

the causal agent in prion diseases, most notably a series of elegant studies in transgenic rodents and the recent description of synthetic infectious prions. Cellular expression of prion protein is necessary for the development of the neuropathological changes and the disease. Hereditary forms of human prion disease are associated with, and perhaps caused by, mutations of the prion protein gene. However, the occurrence of multiple strains of the infectious agent and the stability of the transmission characteristics of the bovine spongiform encephalopathy (BSE) agent in the laboratory after cross-species transmission are not readily explained by the prion theory. The importance of prion protein as a determinant of disease expression has become increasingly clear in human prion disease. The phenotype of different clinicopathological subtypes of CJD is related to the deposition in the brain of different types of prion protein, probably reflecting distinct tertiary protein structures, despite the identical amino acid sequences of the normal and disease-associated forms of prion protein.

In experimental transmission of prion diseases there are a number of key determinants of the efficiency of transmission, as judged by the incubation periods in recipient animals and the proportion of these animals that develop disease. The route of inoculation influences these variables. The intracerebral route is the most efficient. Intravenous, intraperitoneal, and oral routes are decreasingly efficient. The incubation period is inversely related to the infective dose, while the strain of the infectious agent influences both the incubation period and whether recipient animals develop disease. In some transmission studies, e.g. transmission of BSE to hamsters or transmission of scrapie to chimpanzees, recipient animals do not develop disease even after intracerebral inoculation of high levels of infectivity. Within-species transmission is more efficient than cross-species transmission and this 'species barrier' to transmission is influenced by characteristics of both the host and the infective agent. The relative homology of amino acid sequences of prion proteins between species is not the only determinant of the species barrier. The relative efficiency of transmission between species cannot be predicted.

After oral exposure, the agent replicates in the lymphoreticular system, including the spleen and lymph nodes, before entering the thoracic spinal cord or brainstem, probably via the autonomic nervous system, and then spreading caudally to the brain. Moderate levels of infectivity plateau in the lymphoreticular system and are not associated with organ dysfunction, while in the spinal cord and brain high levels of infectivity develop, e.g. 10^{12} infectious units per gram of brain in one model of hamster scrapie, leading to neuronal death and clinical disease. In some experimental and natural prion diseases, infectivity in the lymphoreticular system can be detected at about a third of the total incubation period by inoculation of tissues of the lymphoreticular system, such as spleen, into recipient animals. The implication is that, in the absence of an *in vivo* serological test for the presence of infectivity, animals or humans incubating a prion disease may harbour significant infectivity in some organs or tissues but cannot be identified as being infected. This has important implications for the control and public health implications of prion diseases.

Human prion diseases

Human prion diseases may be classified as sporadic, inherited, or acquired (Table 24.11.5.2).

Table 24.11.5.2 Human prion diseases

Sporadic	Creutzfeldt–Jakob disease
Inherited	Familial Creutzfeldt–Jakob disease Gerstmann–Straussler–Scheinker syndrome Fatal familial insomnia
Acquired	Iatrogenic Creutzfeldt–Jakob disease Variant Creutzfeldt–Jakob disease Kuru

Sporadic CJD
Epidemiology

Sporadic CJD is a rare disease, with an annual incidence of about 1 case per million population. The disease occurs worldwide and the cause is unknown, with no convincing evidence of an environmental source of infection and in particular no proven link with the animal prion diseases. The regional clusters of cases identified in some countries are unusual and may reflect the chance aggregation of a rare phenomenon. Overall the geographical and temporal distribution of cases of sporadic CJD appear to be random and case–control studies have demonstrated no consistent risk factors for the development of disease, with no good evidence of an increased risk through occupation, dietary factors, or animal contact. The currently favoured hypothesis is that sporadic CJD is caused by a spontaneous mutation of prion protein to the abnormal form, which acts as a template for protein self-replication and eventual disease.

Clinical features

Clinically, sporadic CJD presents with a rapidly progressive dementia associated with a range of neurological signs, most commonly myoclonus of the limbs, cerebellar ataxia, and rigidity. Less common features include dysphasia, pyramidal or extrapyramidal signs, primitive reflexes, cortical blindness, and lower motor neuron signs. Despite the predominantly cortical neuropathology epilepsy is rare. The rapidity of the progression of neurological deficits and cognitive decline is distinct from most other causes of dementia and the mean survival is only about 4 months from clinical onset, although in about 10% of cases the illness is more prolonged and a small minority of patients survive for 2 years or more (Fig. 24.11.5.1). Terminally there is often a state of akinetic mutism.

Although the clinical presentation in sporadic CJD is relatively stereotyped, a minority of cases present atypically, e.g. acutely mimicking stroke, with cortical blindness, or with an initially pure cerebellar syndrome.

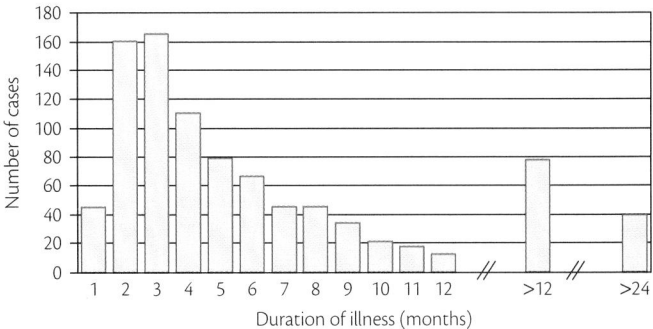

Fig. 24.11.5.1 Sporadic Creutzfeldt–Jakob disease: survival.

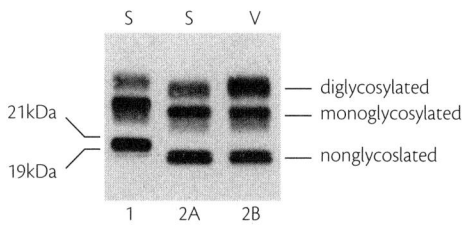

Fig. 24.11.5.2 Western blot of brain tissue showing type 1 and type 2 prion proteins. Lane 1 is sporadic Creutzfeldt–Jakob disease, lane 2A is sporadic Creutzfeldt–Jakob disease, and lane 2B is variant Creutzfeldt–Jakob disease. Type 2A and type 2B have the same mobility but are differentiated by the relative proportions of different glycoforms—in variant Creutzfeldt–Jakob disease there is an excess of the diglycosylated form.

The neuropathological characteristics of sporadic CJD include spongiform change, neuronal loss, and astrocytosis in the cerebral and cerebellar cortex, in accordance with the neurological signs seen in life. Neuropathological changes are widespread and deposition of prion protein can be detected with immunocytochemical techniques. In about 10% of cases there are cortical deposits of prion protein in the form of amyloid plaques. There is heterogeneity in the distribution and morphology of the neuropathological changes, which correlate in part with the clinical phenotype and with two isotypes of prion protein that can be distinguished on western blots of brain tissue (Fig. 24.11.5.2).

Sporadic CJD is mainly a disease of late middle age (Fig. 24.11.5.3) with a mean age at death of 67 years. In most systematic studies males and females are affected with equal frequency.

The human prion protein gene is situated on chromosome 20 and contains a polymorphic region at codon 129, which expresses either methionine or valine. Methionine homozygosity (MM) at codon 129 increases susceptibility to sporadic CJD (Table 24.11.5.3). The genotype distribution in sporadic cases is MM 70%, valine homozygous (VV) 17%, and heterozygous (MV) 13% in contrast to the genotype distribution in the normal white population. There is accumulating evidence that the disease phenotype in sporadic CJD, as well as susceptibility, is influenced by an interplay between the codon 129 genotype and the prion protein type. The classic form of sporadic CJD, representing the great majority of cases, is associated with type 1 prion protein and an MM or MV genotype, whereas alternative combinations of prion protein isotype and codon 129 genotype are often associated with atypical phenotypes.

Hereditary prion diseases

Epidemiology

Familial clusters of CJD account for about 10% of all cases and within pedigrees there is a dominant pattern of inheritance. The paradox of a transmissible disease that is also inherited was clarified by the identification of a mutation at codon 102 of the prion protein gene in two families affected by Gerstmann–Straussler–Scheinker (GSS) syndrome, a condition known to be a human prion disease on the basis of the neuropathology and laboratory transmissibility. More than 30 prion protein gene mutations, including point and insertional mutations, have now been identified in familial CJD or GSS syndrome (Table 24.11.5.4), and all cases of hereditary human prion disease to date have been found to have a mutation of the prion protein gene. Fatal familial insomnia was first identified as a prion disease following the identification of a mutation at codon 178 of the prion protein gene in affected family members, and it was only later that transmission in the laboratory confirmed the status of fatal familial insomnia as a prion disease. The current hypothesis is that mutations of the prion protein gene lead to an instability in the structure of prion protein and an increased chance of a spontaneous transformation of prion protein to the abnormal self-replicating disease-associated form. With the exception of the prion disease associated with a mutation at codon 200 of the prion protein gene, all hereditary human prion diseases are fully penetrant.

The incidence of CJD in localized areas of Slovakia and in Libyan-born Israelis was discovered many years ago to be 60 to 100 times greater than expected. Possible explanations for these clusters included excessive dietary exposure to sheep scrapie and a high coefficient of inbreeding. Following the identification of the mutations of prion protein in human disease, genetic studies have shown that in both clusters there is a high population frequency of mutations at codon 200 of the prion protein gene, and that the excess of cases of CJD is due to an excess of familial cases, with an expected background incidence of sporadic cases.

Clinical features

Overall the age at death in hereditary prion diseases is about 5 to 10 years earlier than in sporadic CJD, but the duration of clinical illness is often more prolonged and the clinical features vary with the underlying mutation. With some mutations, notably the codon 200 mutation, the clinical course is similar to sporadic CJD, but cases of hereditary prion disease may present with ataxia, e.g. GSS syndrome, or with a highly atypical phenotype such as fatal familial

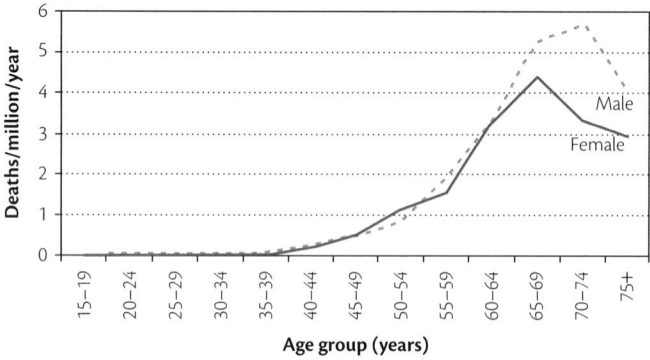

Fig. 24.11.5.3 Age- and sex-specific mortality rates from sporadic Creutzfeldt–Jakob disease in the United Kingdom, 1995 to 2007.

Table 24.11.5.3 Percentage of codon 129 genotypes in the normal population and in different forms of Creutzfeldt–Jakob disease, and in Kuru

	Genotype		
	MM	**MV**	**VV**
Normal population	39	50	11
Sporadic Creutzfeldt–Jakob disease	70	13	17
Iatrogenic Creutzfeldt–Jakob disease central	74	20	6
peripheral	48	21	32
Variant Creutzfeldt–Jakob disease	100	0	0
Kuru	30	45	25

Table 24.11.5.4 Inherited prion diseases—mutations of the prion protein gene

Creutzfeldt–Jakob disease phenotype
D178N-129V
V180I-129M
T183A-129M
E200K-129M
H208R-129M
V210I-129M
M232R-129M

Fatal familial insomnia phenotype
D178N-129M

Phenotype of GSS syndrome
P102L-129M
P102L-129M-219K
P102L-129V
P105L-129V
A117V-129V
Y145STOP-129M
F198S-129V
Q212P
Q217R-129V

Heterogeneous phenotype: insertional mutations
Ins 24 bp-129M
Ins 48 bp-129M
Ins 96 bp-129M
Ins 96 bp-129V
Ins 120 bp-129M
Ins 144 bp-129M
Ins 168 bp-129M
Ins 192 bp-129V
Ins 216 bp-129M

GSS: Gerstmann–Straussler–Scheinker.

insomnia in which the early clinical features include dysautonomia and insomnia. There may be variation in the clinical phenotype both within and between families even if these are associated with the same underlying mutation in the prion protein gene.

Neuropathologically there is great heterogeneity in hereditary prion diseases, and as with the clinical phenotype there is an overall relationship between the neuropathological features and the specific prion protein gene mutation, although there can be great variation within and between pedigrees. The neuropathology can be similar to sporadic CJD but in a significant proportion of hereditary prion diseases there is amyloid plaque formation and in fatal familial insomnia gliosis and neuronal loss may be restricted to the thalamus.

In some forms of hereditary prion disease the codon 129, genotype may influence clinical characteristics, including age at death and the neuropathology. Variation at this locus has a profound effect on the disease phenotype in association with mutations at codon 178 of the prion protein gene. Cases with a codon 178 mutation and a methionine at codon 129 of the prion protein gene develop fatal familial insomnia, whereas with valine at codon 129 the phenotype is similar to sporadic CJD.

Iatrogenic CJD

Epidemiology

CJD has been transmitted accidentally in the course of medical treatment by neurosurgical instruments, corneal grafts, cadaveric dura mater grafts, and human pituitary-derived hormones (Table 24.11.5.5). The presumption is that infection from individuals with CJD was transmitted to uninfected individuals via these procedures and there is strong circumstantial evidence that this has occurred. In the two transmissions by corneal grafts the donors died of sporadic CJD, and in the neurosurgical transmissions there was a clear temporal link between surgical procedures on CJD cases and patients operated on using the same instruments who subsequently developed CJD. It is presumed that some human dura mater grafts and human pituitary hormones came from individuals with CJD and there may have been cross-contamination in the production process, leading to dissemination of infection. Infection via human pituitary growth hormone has been demonstrated in laboratory transmission studies. All cases of iatrogenic transmission of sporadic CJD have involved surgical instruments, grafts, or hormonal products potentially contaminated by CNS tissue and, by implication, high levels of infectivity.

Clinical features

There is a distinction between the clinical features in iatrogenic CJD which depends on the route of inoculation. In exposures in or adjacent to the nervous system (neurosurgical instruments, dura mater grafts, and corneal transplants) most cases present with a progressive dementia similar to sporadic CJD. With a peripheral route of exposure to infection (pituitary hormones) there is a progressive cerebellar ataxia and cognitive impairment develops late in the clinical course, if at all.

The incubation period also varies according to the route of exposure to infection. With central exposure the mean incubation period ranges from about 18 months, similar to the incubation periods in primates after experimental intracerebral inoculation, to 6 years with dura mater grafts. With a peripheral route of exposure the mean incubation period is about 12 years, but may extend to over 30 years, which is similar to the extended incubation periods in kuru, a human prion disease also caused by a peripheral route of exposure to infection.

Table 24.11.5.5 Iatrogenic Creutzfeldt–Jakob disease worldwide

Mode	No. of cases	Mean incubation period (years)	Clinical
Neurosurgery	4	1.6	Visual/cerebellar/dementia
Depth electrodes	2	1.5	Dementia
Corneal transplant	2	15.5*	Dementia
Dura mater	114	6	Visual/cerebellar/dementia
Human growth hormone	139	12	Cerebellar
Human gonadotrophin	4	13	Cerebellar

* Range 1.5 to 26.5 years.

Homozygosity at codon 129 of the prion protein gene, either MM or VV, increases susceptibility to human growth hormone-related CJD and heterozygosity may lead to a more prolonged incubation period. In dura mater-related CJD 81% of cases have an MM genotype, similar to the proportion of sporadic cases with this genotype, but the codon 129 genotype does not influence the incubation period.

Measures to reduce the risk of iatrogenic transmission of CJD have been introduced in many countries. There are strict selection criteria for obtaining corneal grafts, recombinant growth hormone replaced human growth hormone in 1985, and human dura mater grafts have not been licensed in the United Kingdom since the early 1990s.

Variant CJD

Epidemiology

Bovine spongiform encephalopathy was identified in 1986 as a novel prion disease in cattle in the United Kingdom, and is thought to have been caused by feeding cattle material contaminated with sheep scrapie or, perhaps, a previously unrecognized endemic prion disease of cattle. Bovine-to-bovine recycling of infection through cattle feed amplified the epidemic and there have now been over 180 000 cases of BSE in the United Kingdom. Small numbers of cases of BSE have been identified in other countries, mainly in Europe.

In 1996 10 cases of a novel form of human prion disease, variant Creuzefeldt–Jakob disease (vCJD), were identified in the United Kingdom and a causal link with BSE was proposed as this was a new disease occurring only in the United Kingdom, the country with the greatest potential human exposure to BSE. Up to January 2010 there have been 167 primary cases of vCJD in the United Kingdom, 25 in France, and a limited number of cases in some other countries (Table 24.11.5.6). The mean age at death in vCJD is 30 years (range 14–75 years, Fig. 24.11.5.4) contrasting with a

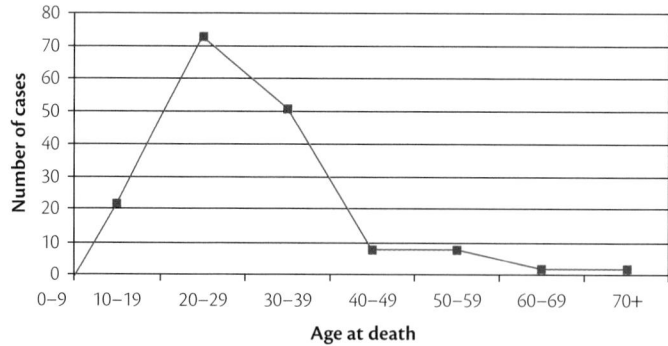

Fig. 24.11.5.4 Age distribution of cases of variant Creutzfeldt–Jakob disease in the United Kingdom (March 2008).

mean age at death in sporadic CJD of 67 years. The hypothesis that vCJD is caused by the BSE agent has been supported by the consistent disease phenotype, and in particular the neuropathology which is distinct from other human prion diseases, the failure to identify similar cases in the past either in the United Kingdom or elsewhere, and laboratory transmission studies that have shown a remarkable similarity between the transmission characteristics of BSE and vCJD in mice.

Cases of vCJD have been identified from throughout the United Kingdom, and risk factors include residence in the United Kingdom and an MM genotype at codon 129 of the prion protein gene. All the United Kingdom cases and some of the cases in other countries (see Table 24.11.5.6) had been resident in the United Kingdom during the 1980s to early 1990s, when human exposure to BSE was likely to have been maximal. However, many of the cases outside the United Kingdom had never visited the United Kingdom, implying that exposure to BSE must have occurred in the country of origin to indigenous BSE or export from the United Kingdom of cattle or food products. The favoured hypothesis is that transmission of BSE to humans was through contamination of food, probably with tissues from the CNS such as brain or spinal cord which are known to contain high levels of infectivity in cattle infected with BSE. All tested cases of vCJD to date have been MM homozygotes at codon 129 of the prion protein gene. This genotype is also present in about 70% of cases of sporadic CJD and may represent a susceptibility factor for the development of vCJD. Variation at this locus can, however, influence the incubation period and disease phenotype and it is possible that cases of human infection with BSE may yet be identified in individuals with a VV or MV genetic background.

The possible future number of cases of vCJD is unknown, but the outbreak in the United Kingdom peaked in 1999/2000 with a subsequent decrease in the annual number of deaths (Fig. 24.11.5.5). Early predictions estimated a total of 100 to over 136 000 cases of vCJD in the United Kingdom, but recent estimates are more conservative, predicting a maximum of no more than a few hundred cases There are, however, a number of uncertainties that make accurate prediction problematic, including the mean incubation period of BSE in humans, the level of the species barrier between bovines and humans, and the possibility of future cases in a non-MM genetic background. The identification of three cases of vCJD and one subclinical infection caused by transmission of the infectious agent through blood transfusion has raised concerns about the possibility of other routes of secondary transmission, e.g. through contaminated surgical instruments.

Table 24.11.5.6 Variant Creutzfeldt-Jakob disease worldwide

Country	Total number of primary cases (Number alive)	Total number of secondary cases: blood transfusion (Number alive)	Cumulative residence in UK > 6 months during period 1980–1996
UK	167 (3)	3 (0)	170
France	25 (1)	–	1
Republic of Ireland	4 (0)	–	2
Italy	2 (1)	–	0
USA	3† (0)	–	2
Canada	1 (0)	–	1
Saudi Arabia	1 (1)	–	0
Japan	1* (0)	–	0
Netherlands	3 (0)	–	0
Portugal	2 (0)	–	0
Spain	5 (0)	–	0

† The third US patient with vCJD was born and raised in Saudi Arabia and has lived permanently in the United States since 2005. According to US case-report, the patient was most likely infected as a child when living in Saudi Arabia.

* The case from Japan had resided in the UK for 24 days in the period 1980–1996.

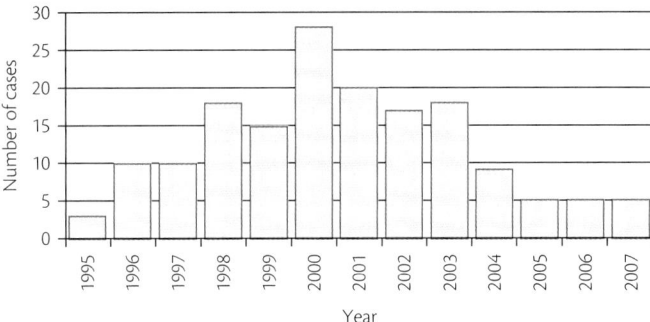

Fig. 24.11.5.5 Variant Creutzfeldt–Jakob disease: number of deaths per year in the United Kingdom (March 2008).

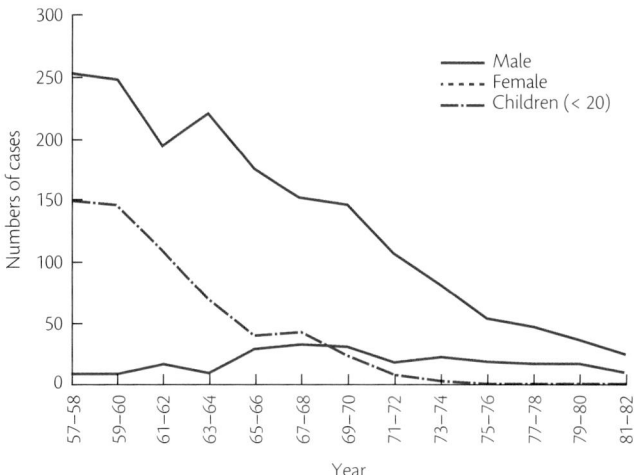

Fig. 24.11.5.6 Kuru: numbers of cases by age, sex, and time.

Clinical features

The clinical features of vCJD are relatively distinct from other forms of human prion disease, including sporadic and iatrogenic CJD. Patients present with psychiatric symptoms, including depression, withdrawal, and anxiety, followed after a period of months by progressive ataxia, dementia, and choreiform or dystonic involuntary movements, which often evolve into myoclonus. The terminal stages are similar to sporadic CJD, but the overall duration of illness, median 14 months, is significantly more prolonged. The distinctive neuropathological characteristic of vCJD is the widespread deposition of prion protein in deposits with a halo of spongiform change, so-called florid plaques, throughout the cerebral and cerebellar cortex, in addition to the spongiform change, neuronal loss, and gliosis seen in other human prion diseases.

Kuru

Epidemiology

The transmissibility of human prion diseases was first demonstrated in 1966 with the transmission of a spongiform encephalopathy to chimpanzees 18 to 21 months after intracerebral inoculation of a brain extract from a patient who had died of kuru. This seminal experiment followed years of clinical, epidemiological, and anthropological research in the Fore region of Papua New Guinea where kuru was endemic. In the early 1960s kuru caused over half of all deaths in the affected population and there have been more than 3000 deaths from kuru in the at-risk population of 30 000 people.

The epidemiological characteristics of kuru are unusual with familial aggregation of cases and a high incidence of disease in women and children in the early years of the epidemic. Since 1960 there has been a decline in the incidence, particularly in women and children (Fig. 24.11.5.6), and there have been no cases in children born after 1959. After extensive investigation into a possible genetic or toxic origin, anthropological research established that kuru was transmitted in the course of ritual cannibalism. As a mark of respect, relatives consumed affected individuals and virtually all tissues were consumed, including the brain and viscera. Although men took part in these rituals, women and children are thought to have consumed the internal organs such as the brain, which contained the highest levels of infectivity. It is also possible that there was transcutaneous transmission through rubbing of tissue on the skin. Detailed investigation of individual cannibalistic events has shown that a number of members of the same family, including those who came from different areas, developed kuru after attending a single cannibalistic rite. Ritual cannibalism ceased by 1960, explaining the subsequent decline in incidence of kuru, but there are still occasional cases with incubation periods exceeding 40 years. It is of interest that at the height of the epidemic many hundreds of women were affected by kuru during pregnancy and breastfed their children, but none of these children later developed kuru.

Clinical features

Clinically kuru presented with a cerebellar syndrome, initially truncal ataxia and titubation, followed by ataxia of gait and dysarthria. A prodromal phase of headache and limb pain was common and hypotonia was a prominent early feature. Involuntary movements such as myoclonus and rigidity of the limbs did not occur, in contrast to other forms of human prion disease. Terminally patients became immobile and communication was often impossible because of severe dysarthria. Dementia did not occur, and even in the terminal akinetic and mute state patients could obey simple commands. In children the clinical features were similar, but in the early stages there were often brainstem signs such as strabismus, nystagmus, and ptosis. The total duration of illness ranged from 12 months to 18 months in adults and 3 months to 12 months in children.

In kuru, neuropathological changes were most apparent in the cerebellum, consistent with the clinical features. Neuronal loss and intense cerebellar astrocytosis were uniform findings and about three-quarters of cases had amyloid plaque deposition, particularly in the granule cell layer of the cerebellum. The cerebral cortex showed mild spongiform change. The similarity of the neuropathology of kuru to scrapie was commented on by Hadlow in 1959, prompting the transmission studies which later demonstrated that kuru, similar to scrapie, was experimentally transmissible.

By using stored samples, analysis of the influence of the codon 129 polymorphism of the prion protein gene on susceptibility to kuru has shown that homozygosity, either MM or VV, increases susceptibility and that heterozygotes may have a more prolonged incubation period. The analysis of codon 129 genotype in kuru is complicated by the limited number of tested cases and the possible effect of the high mortality rate on the codon 129 distribution in a closed population.

The diagnosis of human prion diseases

Human prion diseases are rare, but the high public profile of CJD and vCJD has resulted in an increase in the number of cases in which the diagnosis of one of these diseases is suspected. Accurate diagnosis of any condition, including patients suffering from a human prion disease, is essential but the exclusion of a diagnosis is also important, particularly for a fatal and untreatable condition. Although symptomatic treatment, e.g. for involuntary movements, can be helpful in human prion diseases, there is currently no available treatment that influences the clinical course or any treatment to prevent the development of neurological disease after infection. An important objective is to improve diagnostic accuracy in human prion diseases and in particular to allow early diagnosis. In the absence of a test for the presence of the infectious agent, diagnosis depends on the recognition of the clinical characteristics of human prion diseases supported by a range of investigations, some of which have been developed in recent years. Diagnostic criteria for sporadic, iatrogenic, familial, and vCJD have been formulated and validated (Tables 24.11.5.7 and 24.11.5.8). In all human prion diseases a definite diagnosis can be made only by the examination of brain tissue, usually post-mortem.

In most cases of sporadic CJD the diagnosis is made in life because of the multifocal neurological deficits, the development of myoclonus, and in particular the rapidity in the progression of cognitive impairment. The clinical picture is distinct from more common forms of dementia. In forms of sporadic CJD with early focal neurological features, such as a cerebellar syndrome, the rapid evolution of other neurological deficits and dementia suggests the diagnosis of CJD. Diagnosis can be difficult in cases of sporadic CJD with atypical features such as long duration of illness, and in these cases investigations such as MRI of the brain can be helpful. There is increasing evidence that cases of sporadic CJD may be atypical if there is an underlying MV or VV codon 129 prion protein genotype.

Hereditary prion diseases are often suspected because of a family history of a similar disorder, but in a significant proportion of cases of CJD associated with a prion protein gene mutation there is a family history of another neurodegenerative disorder or

Table 24.11.5.7 Diagnostic criteria for sporadic Creutzfeldt–Jakob disease

I	Rapidly progressive dementia
IIA	Myoclonus
IIB	Visual or cerebellar problems
IIC	Pyramidal or extrapyramidal features
IID	Akinetic mutism
III	Typical electroencephalogram
Definite	Neuropathologically/immunocytochemically confirmed
Probable	I + two of II + III
	or
	Possible + positive 14-3-3
Possible	I + two of II + duration less than 2 years

Table 24.11.5.8 Diagnostic criteria for variant Creutzfeldt–Jakob disease

IA	Progressive neuropsychiatric disorder
IB	Duration of illness more than 6 months
IC	Routine investigations do not suggest an alternative diagnosis
ID	No history of potential iatrogenic exposur
IIA	Early psychiatric symptoms[*]
IIB	Persistent painful sensory symptoms[†]
IIC	Ataxia
IID	Myoclonus or chorea or dystonia
IIE	Dementia
IIIA	Electroencephalogram does not show the typical appearance of sporadic Creutzfeldt–Jakob disease (or no electroencephalogram performed)[‡]
IIIB	Bilateral pulvinar high signal on magnetic resonance scan
IVA	Positive tonsil biopsy
Definite	IA + neuropathological confirmation of variant Creutzfeldt–Jakob disease[§]
Probable	I + four out of five of II + IIIA + IIIB
Probable	I + IVA
Possible	I + four out of five of II + IIIA

[*] Depression, anxiety, apathy, withdrawal, delusions.
[†] This includes both frank pain and/or unpleasant dysaesthesia.
[‡] Generalized triphasic periodic complexes at approximately one per second.
[§] Spongiform change and extensive deposition of prion protein with florid plaques, throughout the cerebrum and cerebellum.

no relevant family history. The gradual clinical progression in many forms of hereditary human prion disease makes accurate diagnosis difficult and the diagnosis may be recognized in life only after prion protein gene analysis. Genetic testing should be carried only out with fully informed consent.

The diagnosis of iatrogenic CJD depends on the identification of a relevant risk factor, e.g. previous treatment with human growth hormone, and an assessment of the neurological presentation. Most patients with growth hormone-related CJD present with a cerebellar syndrome, whereas after central iatrogenic exposure to infection the clinical picture is usually similar to that of sporadic CJD. The utility of specialist investigation in iatrogenic CJD is uncertain because of their rarity, but positive findings on MRI of the brain and/or the 14-3-3 CSF test may support the diagnosis.

The clinical picture in the later stages of vCJD is similar to that of sporadic CJD and, although the recognition of the diagnosis in the first cases of this new disease was difficult, the clinical phenotype is now well known and the diagnosis is usually apparent after neurological signs develop, often in young patients in an age group in which dementia is very unusual. Diagnosis in the early stages is, however, difficult as there is a period of many months in which the clinical picture is dominated by psychiatric symptoms, including depression, anxiety, and withdrawal. Clues to the possibility of vCJD include cognitive impairment, subtle gait ataxia, and persistent painful sensory symptoms in combination with the psychiatric symptoms.

Table 24.11.5.9 Clinical features of sporadic and variant Creutzfeldt—Jakob disease

Feature	Sporadic CJD	Variant CJD
Mean age at death	67 years	30 years
Median illness duration	4 months	14 months
Symptoms at onset:		
Cognitive impairment	70%	10%
Psychiatric (depression, anxiety etc)	<5%	70%
Painful sensory symptoms	<1%	20%
Signs during clinical course:		
Dementia	100%	100%
Ataxia	80%	100%
Involuntary movements:		
Myoclonus	95%	70%
Chorea	<5%	50%
Dystonia	<5%	25%

The clinical features of sporadic and vCJD are compared in Table 24.11.5.9.

Investigations in human prion disease

Many of the investigations carried out in suspected cases of human prion disease do not show any specific disease-related abnormality, but help to exclude other diagnoses, some potentially treatable. The interpretation of the results of investigations depends on the clinical picture because the sensitivity and specificity of surrogate markers for prion disease, such as 14-3-3 CSF analysis (see below), depend on clearly defining the characteristics of the patients in which the test has been carried out.

Routine haematological and biochemical tests are usually normal. About a third of cases of sporadic or vCJD may have minor abnormalities in liver function tests.

The EEG shows periodic triphasic complexes at about 1/s in 60 to 70% of cases of sporadic CJD (Fig. 24.11.5.7) and in some

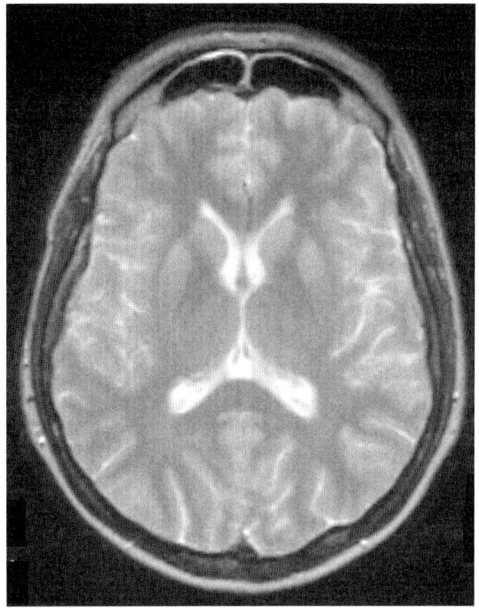

Fig. 24.11.5.8 MR image of sporadic Creutzfeldt—Jakob disease showing high-signal changes symmetrically in the caudate and putamen.

cases of iatrogenic CJD after central exposure to infection. These EEG changes are relatively specific, but similar appearances can be seen in hepatic encephalopathy, lithium or metrizamide toxicity, metabolic disturbance, and rarely in other forms of dementia such as Alzheimer's disease.

There is no CSF pleocytosis in any form of human prion disease, but CSF protein is elevated in about a third of cases. Elevation of the 14-3-3 CSF protein, a marker for neuronal damage, has a sensitivity and specificity of about 90% in the diagnosis of sporadic CJD, but is less useful in the diagnosis of vCJD.

A CT scan of the brain is usually normal, but can show nonspecific cerebral atrophy. MRI of the brain shows a high signal on

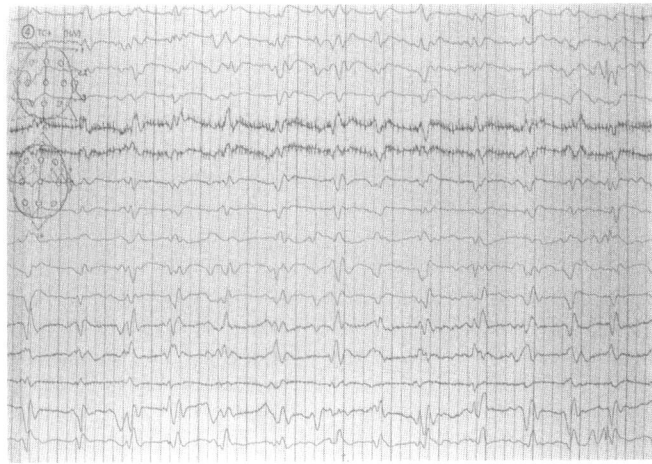

Fig. 24.11.5.7 Typical electroencephalogram in sporadic Creutzfeldt—Jakob disease.

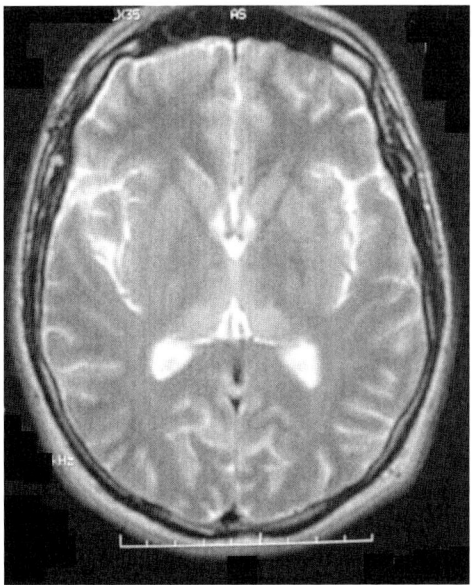

Fig. 24.11.5.9 MR image of variant Creutzfeldt—Jakob disease showing high-signal symmetrically in the posterior thalamus.

Table 24.11.5.10 Investigations in sporadic and variant Creutzfeldt—Jakob disease

Test	Result	Sporadic CJD	Variant CJD
CSF 14-3-3	Positive	90%	50%
EEG	Periodic triphasic complexes	65%	<1%
Tonsil biopsy	Positive for prion protein	0%	95%
MRI brain scan	High signal in caudate putamen	70%	15%
(DWI/FLAIR)	High signal in pulvinar	<1%	95%

diffusion-weighted imaging (DWI) or FLAIR images in the caudate nucleus and putamen in about 70% of cases of sporadic CJD (Fig. 24.11.5.8), but the sensitivity and specificity of these abnormalities have not been formally assessed. In vCJD about 95% of cases show a high signal on DWI or FLAIR images in the pulvinar region of the posterior thalamus (Fig. 24.11.5.9) and in the appropriate clinical context these abnormalities have a high sensitivity and specificity for the diagnosis of vCJD. To date all cases of vCJD classified as 'probable', a diagnosis requiring the abnormalities on MRI, that have come to postmortem examination have been confirmed as vCJD.

Brain biopsy can allow the confirmation of the diagnosis of a human prion disease in life, but this investigation has risks and is mainly carried out when there is a realistic possibility of an alternative diagnosis. Tonsil biopsy in vCJD can increase the likelihood of the diagnosis in life, but this procedure is also invasive and, although early diagnosis is important for the relatives of the patient and for clinicians, it does not benefit the patient.

The outcome of investigations in sporadic and vCJD are shown in Table 24.11.5.10.

Further reading

Bradley, et al. (2006). Variant CJD (vCJD) and bovine spongiform encephalopathy (BSE): 10 and 20 years on: Part 1. *Folia Neuropathol,* **44,** 93–101.

Brown P (2008). Transmissible spongiform encephalopathy in the 21st century. *Neurology,* **70,** 713–22.

Cali I, et al. (2006). Classification of sporadic Creutzfeldt–Jakob disease revisited. *Brain,* **129,** 2266–77.

Collee JG, et al (2006). Variant CJD (vCJD) and bovine spongiform encephalopathy (BSE): 10 and 20 years on: Part 2. *Folia Neuropathol,* **44,** 102–10.

Collinge J, et al. (2006). Kuru in the 21st century—an acquired human prion disease with very long incubation periods. *Lancet,* **367,** 2068–74.

Collins SJ, et al. (2006). Determinants of diagnostic investigation sensitivities across the clinical spectrum of sporadic Creutzfeldt–Jakob disease. *Brain,* **129,** 2278–87.

De Armond SJ, et al. (2003). Perspectives on prion biology, prion disease pathogenesis, and pharmacologic approaches to treatment. *Clin Lab Med,* **23,** 1–41.

Mead S, et al. (2009). A novel protective prion protein variant that colocalizes with kuru exposure. *N Engl J Med,* **361,** 2056–65.

Wadsworth JDF, et al. (2007). Update on human prion disease. *Biochim Biophys Acta,* **1772,** 598–609.

Disorders of cranial nerves

R.A.C. Hughes and P.K. Thomas†

Essentials

The 12 cranial nerves are peripheral nerves except for the optic nerve which is a central nervous system tract. Disorders of particular note include the following:

Olfactory (I) nerve—anosmia is most commonly encountered as a sequel to head injury.

Third, fourth, and sixth cranial nerves—complete lesions lead to the following deficits (1) third nerve—a dilated and unreactive pupil, complete ptosis, and loss of upward, downward and medial movement of the eye; (2) fourth nerve—extorsion of the eye when the patient looks outwards, with diplopia when gaze is directed downwards and medially; (3) sixth nerve—convergent strabismus, with inability to abduct the affected eye and diplopia maximal on lateral gaze to the affected side. The third, fourth, and sixth nerves may be affected singly or in combination: in older patients the commonest cause is vascular disease of the nerves themselves or their nuclei in the brainstem. Other causes of lesions include (1) false localizing signs—third or sixth nerve palsies related to displacement of the brainstem produced by supratentorial space-occupying lesions; (2) intracavernous aneurysm of the internal carotid artery—third, fourth, and sixth nerve lesions. Lesions of these nerves can be mimicked by myasthenia gravis.

Pupillary abnormalities—these include (1) constriction (miosis)—due to paralysis of the sympathetic innervation (Horner's syndrome); (2) dilatation—due to lesions of the third nerve.

Trigeminal nerve—pathology causes numbness and tingling of the side of the face and scalp back to the vertex, loss of the corneal reflex and deviation of the jaw to the affected side. May be affected by intramedullary lesions, during the intracranial part of its course, and extracranially. Trigeminal neuralgia is usually due to compression of the nerve by aberrant vessels in the posterior fossa. It is characterized by paroxysms of intense pain strictly confined to the nerve's distribution and often responsive to carbamazepine.

Facial nerve—in upper (but not lower) motor neuron lesions there is relative preservation of power in the upper facial muscles. In Bell's palsy, onset is rapid and frequently heralded or accompanied by aching pain in or around the ear: treatment with prednisolone improves the prognosis. Hemifacial spasm is characterized by irregular clonic or simultaneous twitching movements of the facial muscles, usually of insidious onset; injections of botulinum toxin may be helpful.

Glossopharyngeal nerve—rarely affected in isolation, when it is very difficult to detect any neurological deficit; usually affected in combination with the vagus nerve.

Vagus nerve—important symptoms of damage relate to pharyngeal and laryngeal innervation producing a bulbar palsy with dysphonia, dysarthria and dysphagia. Causes include brainstem stroke, motor neuron disease, and malignant infiltration anywhere along the course of the nerve and cranial polyneuropathy.

Spinal accessory nerve—may be affected by lesions, often neoplastic, in the region of the jugular foramen, but more commonly by injuries to the neck or by operations for the removal of cervical glands.

Hypoglossal nerve—may be affected by tumours in the region of the anterior condyloid foramen, or by tumours or penetrating injuries in the neck. The commonest cause of bilateral lesions is the progressive bulbar palsy variant of motor neuron disease.

The olfactory nerve

Loss of the sense of smell (anosmia) is most commonly encountered as a sequel to head injury and is probably related to severance of the central processes of the olfactory neurons as they pass through the cribriform plate to the olfactory bulb. It is usually permanent. Distortion of olfaction (parosmia) may occur and may be persistent.

The sense of smell is occasionally congenitally absent or may be acutely and permanently lost after a coryzal infection. Bilateral anosmia is frequently accompanied by impairment of taste related to reduced detection of the volatile substances that impart flavours to foods. Unilateral anosmia may occur in olfactory groove meningiomas or other subfrontal tumours. This is usually not detected by the patient.

---

† It is with regret that we report the death of Professor P K Thomas during the preparation of this edition of the textbook.

The central connections of the olfactory pathways are complex and include projections to the temporal lobes, hypothalamus, septal region, and amygdaloid nuclei. Olfactory hallucinations occur as a manifestation of temporal lobe epilepsy. Identification of odours may be impaired after bilateral medial temporal lesions and may be defective in multiple sclerosis, possibly as the result of demyelination in the olfactory tracts. Reduced sense of smell occurs in idiopathic Parkinson's disease but not other forms. Complaints of hypersensitivity of the sense of smell commonly have a psychoneurotic basis and persistent olfactory hallucinations may be reported by psychotic patients. Persistent parosmia is sometimes produced by lesions of the temporal lobe.

Third, fourth, and sixth cranial nerves

The third, or oculomotor, nerve supplies all the external ocular muscles with the exception of the superior oblique and lateral rectus. It also carries the parasympathetic innervation of the preganglionic pupilloconstrictor fibres of the iris. A complete third nerve lesion produces a dilated and unreactive pupil, complete ptosis, and loss of upward, downward, and medial movement of the eye. The eye becomes deviated laterally and slightly downwards. Diplopia is only experienced when the lid is lifted.

The fourth or trochlear nerve supplies the superior oblique muscle. Following a lesion of this nerve, there is extorsion of the eye when the patient looks outwards. When the patient looks downwards and medially, diplopia is experienced. This is particularly disturbing because looking downwards is important for walking and especially descending stairs. The patient may compensate for this by tilting the head to the opposite side.

The sixth or abducent nerve supplies the lateral rectus. A lesion of this nerve causes convergent strabismus, inability to abduct the affected eye, and diplopia which is maximal on lateral gaze to the affected side.

The third, fourth, and sixth nerves may be affected singly or in combination, and the paralysis may be complete or partial. In some instances, the lesion is within the brainstem, where it may affect either the nuclei or the intramedullary portions of the nerve fibres. In older patients, the commonest cause is vascular disease.

Extramedullary lesions of the third, fourth, and sixth nerves are more frequent and may occur at any point along their course, either intracranially or within the orbit. A third nerve palsy may develop in the region of the tentorial hiatus as a false localizing sign related to displacement of the brainstem produced by supratentorial space-occupying lesions. Unilateral or bilateral sixth nerve palsies may also arise as a consequence of raised intracranial pressure, probably caused by traction, again secondary to brainstem displacement. These nerves can be involved singly or together in conditions such as chronic basal meningitis or carcinoma of the skull base. Gradenigo's syndrome comprises a sixth nerve palsy and pain of trigeminal distribution. It is produced by a lesion at the apex of the petrous temporal bone. As this syndrome was most commonly infective in origin and related to chronic middle ear disease, it is now much less frequent.

The third, fourth, and sixth nerves traverse the cavernous sinus, as do the first and second divisions of the trigeminal nerve. In this situation, they are most commonly damaged by an intracavernous aneurysm of the internal carotid artery. The third nerve is affected more often than the fourth or sixth. The consequent internal and external ophthalmoplegia is frequently accompanied by pain, and sometimes sensory loss and paraesthesiae in the corresponding frontal region related to compression of the first division of the trigeminal nerve. Sometimes pain occurs in the cheek from damage to the maxillary division. In the superior orbital fissure syndrome, caused for example by a tumour invading the fissure, a total ophthalmoplegia may result, associated with pain and sensory loss in the distribution of the first division of the trigeminal nerve. The eye is often proptosed because of obstruction of the ophthalmic vein. The Tolosa–Hunt syndrome consists of a painful external ophthalmoplegia related to a granulomatous angiitis. Within the orbit, the third, fourth, and sixth nerves may be affected by conditions such as tumours and granulomas. They may be damaged as a result of trauma at any point along their course and may be affected singly or in combination or as part of a cranial neuropathy, of which diabetes, the Fisher syndrome, Lyme borreliosis, vasculitis, and sarcoidosis are the most important examples. Internal and external ophthalmoplegias are common and this list of nerve lesions causing the syndrome is by no means exhaustive. External ophthalmoplegia may also be caused by myasthenia or myopathy.

Pupillary abnormalities

Constriction of the pupil (miosis) occurs as a result of paralysis of the sympathetic innervation of the pupillodilator fibres of the iris and may be accompanied by the other features of Horner's syndrome, mild ptosis and vasodilatation and anhidrosis of the face on the same side. The ocular manifestations may be encountered alone if the damage is restricted to the intracranial portion of the sympathetic plexus around the carotid artery. Raeder's syndrome consists of these components of Horner's syndrome together with involvement of the first division of the trigeminal nerve. It may be caused by tumours of the skull base. Miosis may also be produced by the local action of cholinergic drugs and by morphine and related compounds.

Pupillary dilatation may be caused by lesions of the third nerve. The isolated third nerve palsies of presumed vascular origin that may occur in diabetes mellitus characteristically spare the pupil. In contradistinction, compressive lesions of the nerve, for instance by an aneurysm or transtentorial brain herniation, involve the pupil prominently and early. Anticholinergic drugs, such as atropine and related substances, and cocaine also cause pupillary dilatation.

The Argyll–Robertson pupil is small, fails to react to light, but constricts on ocular convergence, and, if bilateral, the pupils are frequently unequal in size (anisocoria). The pupil may be irregular in outline and does not dilate fully in response to mydriatics. Argyll–Robertson pupils are almost always related to neurosyphilis but somewhat similar pupils are occasionally encountered in diabetic neuropathy, in some hereditary neuropathies and following the use of atropine-like eyedrops.

In the Holmes–Adie syndrome, the pupil is tonic and reacts abnormally slowly both to light and on convergence, but particularly so for the response to illumination. A very bright light may be required to demonstrate any pupillary constriction. If the patient remains in a dark room for some minutes, the pupil slowly dilates. The condition may be unilateral or bilateral and is commoner in women than men. Tonic pupils may be associated with absence or depression of the tendon reflexes and occasionally with anhidrosis in the limbs.

Trigeminal nerve

The fifth cranial nerve is predominantly sensory in function, but also innervates the muscles of mastication. It emerges from the pons and runs forwards to the Gasserian ganglion which is situated in Meckel's cave near the apex of the petrous temporal bone. The three sensory divisions of the nerve run anteriorly from the ganglion. The first or frontal division passes through the cavernous sinus and the superior orbital fissure. Its branches supply sensation to the anterior part of the scalp, the forehead, and the eye, including the conjunctiva and cornea. The second or maxillary division leaves the skull through the foramen rotundum, traverses the infraorbital canal, and supplies the cheek. The mandibular division emerges from the skull through the foramen ovale to reach the infratemporal fossa with the motor root with which it unites to form a single trunk. It is distributed to the lower lip, chin, and the lower part of the cheek, and its auriculotemporal branch supplies the tragus of the ear and temple. It also supplies the inner aspect of the cheek and the anterior two-thirds of the tongue, and its lingual branch carries taste fibres from the anterior two-thirds of the tongue which leave it in the chorda tympani to join the facial nerve. It is important that the skin over the angle of the jaw is supplied from the second cervical nerve root, and the absence of this 'trigeminal notch' may be useful in distinguishing hysterical or feigned loss of sensation on the face which usually follows the angle of the jaw. The motor root innervates temporalis, masseter, pterygoids, mylohyoid, the anterior belly of the digastric, and also tensor tympani and tensor palati muscles. With unilateral paralysis of the masticatory muscles, the jaw is pushed towards the affected side on opening by the unopposed external pterygoid on the unaffected side.

The trigeminal nerve may be affected by intramedullary lesions. It may be damaged during the intracranial part of its course. Its branches may be compromised extracranially. A vestibular Schwannoma or other space-occupying lesion in the cerebellopontine angle may compress the nerve in the posterior fossa or the nucleus of its descending root in the brainstem. Loss of corneal sensation is usually the earliest feature. Reference has already been made to involvement of the nerve in association with damage to the sixth nerve at the apex of the petrous temporal bone (Gradenigo's syndrome), as has involvement of the first and second divisions in the cavernous sinus, or the first division in the superior orbital fissure.

Trigeminal neuralgia

Symptoms

This condition is characterized by paroxysms of intense pain strictly confined to the distribution of the trigeminal nerve. It is generally encountered in individuals over the age of 50 years. It is most commonly caused by the impingement of vascular loops on the sensory root of the trigeminal nerve in the posterior fossa. It may be due to multiple sclerosis, especially in younger patients. Rarely, compression of the nerve is responsible, for example by tumours in the cerebellopontine angle.

The salient feature of the disorder is pain, which is usually unilateral and is felt either within the territory of one division of the nerve only, or may involve two adjacent divisions or affect the whole territory of the nerve. Less commonly it is bilateral.

The pain occurs in brief searing paroxysms, each attack lasting only a matter of seconds. The pain is often described as piercing or knife-like. Its intense quality may cause the patient to screw up their face in agony, hence the use of the term 'tic douloureux' to describe the condition. The paroxysms may be spontaneous or provoked by movements of the face and jaw, by touching the skin, or by draughts of cold air on the face. Eating and speaking may become extremely difficult. 'Trigger spots' on the skin of the face may be present, the touching of which provokes the paroxysms. The attacks may be followed by less severe pain of a dull, boring character and by tenderness of the skin in the affected area. Fortunately the attacks usually cease at night.

The quality of the pain is characteristic, and when trigeminal neuralgia is present the diagnosis is not usually missed, especially if a paroxysm is witnessed. The usual mistake is to regard as trigeminal neuralgia pain that is due to some other cause, and since there are many conditions that give rise to facial pain, the opportunities for error are numerous. Pain that is of a continuous character is not trigeminal neuralgia and some other cause must be sought. Absence of provocation by eating, talking, or the touching of trigger spots also makes the diagnosis unlikely. Once the diagnosis is accepted, it is essential to exclude compressive lesions affecting the nerve.

In the early stages, remissions lasting for months or years are usual, but in older patients remissions, if they occur, are likely to be brief. In all cases the remissions tend to become shorter as time goes on, and without treatment the condition persists for the rest of the patient's life.

The distribution of the pain is usually in the first or second divisions of the nerve or both. The third division is rarely affected primarily, but pain may spread into it from the second division.

Treatment

The introduction of carbamazepine revolutionized treatment of this distressing condition. In a high proportion of cases, the paroxysms can be abolished or reduced. It is best to start with a low dose of 100 mg of a slow-release preparation twice a day and build up the dose every 2 days until control is achieved. Doses larger than 500 mg twice daily often cause ataxia and drowsiness, and some patients experience these at low doses. Allergic skin rashes occur and patients should be warned and advised to stop the drug if they do because of the danger of exfoliative dermatitis. Hyponatraemia is another common complication. Bone marrow depression may develop but is very rare.

If carbamazepine is not successful, or if the patient fails to tolerate it, oxcarbazepine, lamotrigine, or gabapentin can be tried, although they lack a solid evidence base from randomized controlled trials. If medical treatment is inadequate surgical exploration of the main sensory root or thermocoagulation of the ganglion may have to be considered. These should be undertaken only if the disorder is established so that a prolonged natural remission is unlikely to occur. Exploration of the sensory root in the posterior fossa and separation of the root from vascular loops is often curative. Despite the risks of craniotomy, this procedure is worth considering in younger patients with intolerable pain. In older patients prolonged, but not usually permanent, relief can be obtained by thermocoagulation of the trigeminal ganglion. The persistent analgesia and sometimes painful dysaesthesiae, called 'anaesthesia dolorosa', following thermocoagulation may sometimes be as or more troublesome than the original condition. When the first division is made anaesthetic, damage to the cornea leading to scarring has to be avoided. It may be possible to limit the anaesthesia to the affected area, sparing, for instance, the eye if the first division is not involved by the pain. If the cornea is anaesthetized, it must be protected by attaching a guard to the wing of the frame of eyeglasses.

Ophthalmic herpes zoster

In elderly individuals, the fifth nerve is prone to involvement in herpes zoster, the first division being most vulnerable, giving rise to the distressing condition of ophthalmic herpes. The clinical features and treatment of herpes zoster are considered elsewhere (see Chapter 7.5.2). An unfortunate sequel may be visual impairment from residual corneal scarring. Particularly in older subjects, postherpetic neuralgia may also be a sequel. This gives rise to persistent and unremitting spontaneous pain associated with cutaneous hyperaesthesia in the affected area. Treatment may be difficult. Antidepressants are the most effective drugs and there is more evidence for amitryptiline than other agents. Antiepileptic drugs, especially carbamazepine, are often used and there is evidence from randomized trials to support the use of gabapentin. There is limited evidence to support the use of topical lignocaine (lidocaine).

Isolated trigeminal neuropathy

Rarely, a slowly progressive isolated unilateral or bilateral affection of the trigeminal nerve may occur as a manifestation of Sjögren's syndrome either without other features or with undifferentiated connective tissue disease or progressive systemic sclerosis. Amyloidosis is another rare cause. Most cases are idiopathic.

Facial nerve

The seventh cranial nerve is largely motor. The nerve traverses the facial canal in the petrous temporal bone in close relationship to the middle ear and emerges at the stylomastoid foramen. Its branches pass forward through the parotid gland to be distributed to the muscles of the face and the platysma. Within the petrous bone, a branch is given to the stapedius muscle. The chorda tympani, carrying the taste fibres from the anterior two-thirds of the tongue, joins the nerve within the facial canal and a small branch supplies cutaneous sensation to the external auditory meatus. The nerve also carries preganglionic parasympathetic fibres destined for the lachrymal gland.

The distinction between upper and lower motor neuron lesions of the facial muscles is usually easy. In general, with upper motor neuron lesions there is relative preservation of power in the upper facial muscles, because these have a representation in both cerebral hemispheres. There is no loss of tone with upper motor neuron lesions, so that the sagging of the face that is an unsightly feature of lower motor neuron palsy does not occur.

In common with the trigeminal nerve, the facial nerve may be affected by tumours in the cerebellopontine angle. In the past, it was often involved in middle ear infections. It may be involved in meningeal carcinomatosis, fractures, and tumours of the skull base, in a variety of cranial neuropathies, and cephalic herpes zoster, but the most common lesion by far is Bell's palsy. More peripherally, the nerve may be compromised in tumours of the parotid gland.

Bell's palsy

This term describes idiopathic facial palsy and is usually unilateral facial paralysis of relatively rapid onset due to a lesion of the nerve within the facial canal. Taste may also be affected. It has an annual incidence of 20 to 32 per 100 000 and may develop at any age, most commonly between 20 and 50 years, and affects both sexes equally. There is some, but inconclusive, evidence that it is a manifestation of herpes simplex infection. In the acute stage, the nerve is swollen and compression within the facial canal may contribute to the damage to the nerve fibres.

The onset is rapid and is frequently heralded or accompanied by aching pain below the ear or in the mastoid region. This clears within a few days and is not present in every case. The paralysis usually reaches its maximum severity after 1 or sometimes 2 days. Complete paralysis may occur. This may cause a mild dysarthria and some difficulty in eating because of food collecting between the gums and the inner sides of the cheek and the escape of fluid when drinking. The face sags, and on smiling is drawn across to the unaffected side. Paralysis of orbicularis oculi renders voluntary eye closure impossible and, particularly in the older subject, ectropion develops. This can result in conjunctival injury from foreign bodies or conjunctivitis. If the paralysis is partial, the lower face is usually affected to a greater extent than the upper.

In the more severe cases, loss of taste over the anterior two-thirds of the tongue is often present, and paralysis of the stapedius muscle may result in a lack of tolerance for high-pitched or loud sounds, called hyperacousis.

Bell's palsy has to be distinguished from selective lesions of the facial nerve within the brainstem, in which instance taste will not be affected. Lesions in the brainstem almost always cause fifth or sixth nerves palsies and long tract symptoms or signs as well. With respect to peripheral lesions, middle ear disease requires exclusion. Facial paralysis may also be caused by herpes zoster as described below. A lesion of the facial nerve may be part of a more generalized disorder of which diabetes, Lyme borreliosis, and sarcoidosis are the most important. Bell's palsy is rarely bilateral and bilateral facial paralysis would raise the possibility of another disorder, such as sarcoidosis, Guillain–Barré syndrome, or Lyme borreliosis.

In approximately 85% of patients with Bell's palsy, especially those with mild weakness, the paralysis is the result of a local conduction block within the facial canal without axonal degeneration. The conduction block is presumably the consequence of segmental demyelination. Provided that such cases do not progress to more severe weakness, remyelination is rapid and all recover fully within a few weeks. In cases where there is total paralysis, axonal degeneration is likely to have occurred so that recovery has to take place by axonal regeneration, which is slow. Evidence of reinnervation does not appear in under 3 months and the ultimate recovery is often incomplete or may fail to occur altogether. After reinnervation the regenerated axons may form inappropriate connections, causing synkinesis and crocodile tears. In synkinesis, blinking results in a simultaneous twitch of the angle of the mouth. Crocodile tears are caused by aberrant parasympathetic reinnervation so that food elicits weeping instead of salivation.

Axons remain excitable distal to the lesion for 3 or 4 days after interruption. It is therefore not possible to be certain from electrodiagnostic tests whether axonal degeneration has taken place until later. After that stage, electrical stimulation of the facial nerve at the stylomastoid foramen will still elicit a muscle contraction if the paralysis is due to conduction block, whereas none will be obtained if axonal degeneration has taken place.

Because most patients with Bell's palsy recover completely, it was difficult to discover from observational studies whether different treatments helped. However, in a large high-quality trial the percentage of patients with complete recovery after 9 months was significantly increased from 81.6% without to 94.4% with prednisolone, 25 mg twice daily for 10 days. Another trial obtained similar results with prednisolone 60 mg daily for 5 days and then a reducing dose for the next 5 days. In the same trials oral aciclovir made no difference. There is no evidence of efficacy from antiviral agents alone although it is still possible that they might have a small effect when used in conjunction with corticosteroids. In patients with severe palsy causing ectropion, stitching the lateral parts of the eyelids, lateral tarsorrhaphy, may be performed to protect the eye. Electrical stimulation of the paralysed facial muscles has not been shown to have a significant effect on the ultimate prognosis.

In those cases in which regeneration is inadequate, cosmetic operations may be considered to counteract the facial deformity. The angle of the mouth may be elevated by a fascial sling attached to the temporalis fascia, but the result is never highly satisfactory. Restoration of facial tone may be achieved by anastomosis of the hypoglossal to the facial nerve, but at the expense of denervation of the tongue on that side. Any operation should not be contemplated before an adequate length of time has been allowed for regeneration. This should be of the order of one year.

Facial paralysis related to 'geniculate' herpes zoster (Ramsay–Hunt syndrome)

Facial paralysis of rapid onset accompanied by severe pain in and around the external auditory meatus and in the throat may accompany 'cephalic zoster'. Vesicles may be detectable in the ear and ulceration in the fauces, or anywhere on the head. Occasionally there is concomitant vertigo, tinnitus, and some deafness due to involvement of the eighth nerve ('otic herpes zoster'). Prognosis for recovery of the facial paralysis is stated to be less good than in Bell's palsy. It is not known whether antiviral agents or corticosteroids are helpful.

Hemifacial spasm

This consists of a unilateral disturbance affecting the facial muscles, producing irregular clonic or simultaneous twitching movements of the facial muscles, usually of insidious onset. It most commonly occurs in middle-aged women. There may be a mild degree of facial weakness, but not severe paralysis. Usually no underlying cause is demonstrable. The condition selectively affects the facial nerve, within the brainstem or in the posterior fossa. Hemifacial spasm is painless. If it is associated with pain, there may be a lesion in the cerebellopontine angle compressing both the trigeminal and facial nerves.

It begins with intermittent twitching of the facial muscles such as around the eye or at the angle of the mouth. These movements gradually become more frequent and extend to involve the rest of the facial muscles, often gradually advancing over the course of some years. If they become severe, the face is contorted by irregular clonic spasms which may keep the eye closed for prolonged periods. The facial distortion is often a considerable embarrassment to the patient, who finds that the spasms tend to be aggravated by emotional stress.

In severe cases, injections of botulinum toxin may be helpful, but these have to be repeated. If exaggeration by emotional factors is evident, the administration of diazepam or a similar preparation may produce a marginal improvement. Neurosurgical intervention to relieve compression of the facial nerve by aberrant vessels in the posterior fossa may be helpful in selected cases.

The condition must be distinguished from benign fasciculation of the face, which usually occurs around the eyes, related to fatigue or emotional tension, and from facial myokymia that is occasionally encountered as a manifestation of multiple sclerosis. The latter consists of a persisting irregular rippling movement of the facial muscles that usually subsides after a week or two. These conditions can be distinguished by electromyography (see Chapter 24.3.2).

Glossopharyngeal nerve

The ninth cranial nerve leaves the skull through the jugular foramen, closely related to the tenth nerve. It supplies the stylopharyngeus muscle and the constrictor muscles of the pharynx. Parasympathetic fibres are supplied to the parotid gland. Sensory fibres are carried from the posterior third of the tongue, the ear, the fauces, and the nasopharynx, and chemoreceptor and baroreceptor afferents from the carotid sinus.

The glossopharyngeal nerve is rarely affected in isolation. If it is affected alone, it is very difficult to detect the deficits expected from its anatomical distribution. Lesions usually occur in conjunction with involvement of the vagus and give rise to some dysphagia, impaired pharyngeal sensation, and loss of taste over the posterior third of the tongue. It may be affected in the jugular foramen syndrome, along with the tenth and eleventh nerves, of which glomus tumours or metastatic carcinomas are the commonest causes. The nerve may also be involved in diphtheritic neuropathy, Fisher syndrome and in cranial polyneuropathy.

Glossopharyngeal neuralgia is rare and resembles trigeminal neuralgia but with symptoms in the distribution of the glossopharyngeal nerve. As with trigeminal neuralgia, it is most often encountered in elderly subjects, and the pain may initially be confined to individual branches. Thus it may be felt deep in the ear, related to the tympanic branch, or in the throat, related to the pharyngeal branches. It usually responds to treatment with carbamazepine. If that and other antiepileptic drugs fail, surgical treatment, usually section of the nerve, may be required.

Vagus nerve

The tenth cranial nerve is structurally complex. Within the skull it is joined by the cranial division of the eleventh nerve. It leaves the skull through the jugular foramen. Cutaneous sensory fibres are carried from the external ear and visceral afferent fibres are carried from the pharynx, larynx, trachea, oesophagus, and the thoracic and abdominal viscera. Motor fibres supply the striated musculature of the palate and pharynx and, through the internal, external and recurrent laryngeal nerves, the muscles of the larynx. Parasympathetic fibres innervate the parotid gland (through the glossopharyngeal nerve), the heart, and the abdominal viscera.

The important symptoms of damage to the vagal nerve are those relating to pharyngeal and laryngeal innervation. The cells of origin in the nucleus ambiguus of the medulla may be damaged in the lateral medullary syndrome, motor neuron disease, and acute bulbar poliomyelitis, leading to dysphagia and dysphonia. Involvement along with the glossopharyngeal nerve in the jugular foramen syndrome has already been mentioned. The recurrent laryngeal nerve may be damaged during operations on the thyroid gland or by tumours within the neck, or within the thorax, usually due to carcinoma of the bronchus. The nerve on the left is vulnerable to damage by an aneurysm of the aortic arch. Isolated and unexplained lesions of the recurrent laryngeal nerve are not uncommon.

Nuclear or high vagal lesions, as well as involving the larynx, cause palatal and pharyngeal paralysis. If unilateral, there are few symptoms from palatopharyngeal paralysis. The uvula is pulled up to the opposite side on phonation and pharyngeal sensation is impaired on the affected side. With bilateral paralysis, the palate is paretic leading to nasality of the voice and nasal regurgitation of liquids on attempts at swallowing. Bilateral palatopharyngeal paralysis may be encountered in motor neuron disease, bulbar poliomyelitis, diphtheritic neuropathy, and cranial polyneuropathy.

Unilateral intrinsic laryngeal paralysis from lesions of the recurrent nerve may be asymptomatic or give rise to hoarseness of the voice. If the superior laryngeal nerve is also involved leading to paralysis of the cricothyroid muscle, the affected cord lies in a paramedian or cadaveric position. The effects of bilateral lesions of the recurrent laryngeal nerves depend upon the degree of approximation of the vocal cords. Lesions of insidious onset give rise to dysphonia and also to stridor on exertion. In partial lesions, close approximation of the cords may result from selective paralysis of the abductor muscles, giving rise to limitation of the airway and sometimes necessitating tracheostomy. With bilateral lesions involving both the recurrent and superior laryngeal nerves, both cords are paralysed and in the cadaveric position. Phonation is impossible.

Spinal accessory nerve

The spinal accessory portion of the eleventh cranial nerve arises from the upper cervical cord and the lower medulla. The nerve passes through the foramen magnum and joins the cranial portion of the nerve before emerging from the skull through the jugular foramen. The spinal accessory nerve then separates and supplies the sternomastoid and trapezius muscles, the latter also receiving an innervation from the cervical plexus.

The nerve may be affected by lesions, often neoplastic, in the region of the jugular foramen, but more commonly it is damaged by injuries to the neck or by operations for the removal of cervical glands, particularly as it crosses the posterior triangle of the neck. Isolated and unexplained lesions of the nerve are occasionally encountered.

Unilateral paralysis of the sternomastoid usually passes unnoticed by the patient. The muscle does not stand out when the head is turned to the opposite side. Paralysis of the trapezius, on the other hand, causes difficulty in lifting the arm above the horizontal, in shrugging the shoulder, and in approximating the scapula to the midline and therefore also in carrying the extended arm backwards. The shoulder droops when the arm is hanging at the side and there is moderate winging of the scapula which is accentuated when the patient attempts to elevate the arm laterally.

The hypoglossal nerve

The twelfth cranial nerve supplies all the muscles of the tongue, both intrinsic and extrinsic. It leaves the skull through the anterior condyloid foramen. A unilateral lesion of the hypoglossal nerve causes weakness and atrophy of the tongue on the affected side. When protruded, the tongue deviates to the affected side. Articulation is unaffected. The nerve may be affected by tumours in the region of the anterior condyloid foramen, or by tumours or penetrating injuries in the neck. If damage is the result of a unilateral lower brainstem lesion, it is usually combined with a contralateral hemiplegia.

Bilateral lesions give rise to generalized wasting of the tongue. Wasting of the tongue is usually accompanied by fasciculation which is best detected with the tongue at rest. Protrusion becomes impossible and articulation is disturbed. The commonest cause is the progressive bulbar palsy variant of motor neuron disease.

Further reading

Asbury AK, *et al.* (1970). Oculomotor palsy in diabetic mellitus: a clinicopathological study. *Brain*, **93**, 555–66.

Brodal A (1965). *The cranial nerves*, 2nd edition. Blackwell Scientific, Oxford.

Dyck PJ, Thomas PK (2005). *Peripheral neuropathy*, 4th edition. Elsevier Saunders, Philadelphia.

Kennard C (2007). How to examine eye movements. *Practical Neurol*, **7**, 326–30.

Leigh JR, Zee DS (2006). *The neurology of eye movements*. Oxford University Press, New York.

Lockhart P, *et al.*(2009). Antiviral treatment for Bell's palsy (idiopathic facial paralysis). *Cochrane Database of Systematic Reviews*, Issue 4. Art. No.: CD001869.

Sullivan F, *et al.* (2007). Early treatment with prednisolone or acyclovir in Bell's palsy. *N Engl J Med*, **357**, 1598–607.

Younge BR (1966). Paralysis of cranial nerves III, IV and VI: causes and prognosis of 1000 cases. *Arch Ophthalmol*, **99**, 76–89.

24.13

Disorders of the spinal cord

Contents

24.13.1 Diseases of the spinal cord

A.J. Larner

Essentials

The spinal cord is subject to numerous pathological processes that can arise within (intramedullary) and/or extrinsic to the cord (extramedullary lesions).

Clinical features

Symptoms and signs suggestive of spinal cord disease include (1) motor—weakness and alteration in tone; acute cord lesions produce flaccidity ('spinal shock') and chronic processes spasticity, with hyper-reflexia, clonus ,and upgoing plantar responses; pathological processes targeting lower motor neurons in the anterior horns typically produce early muscle wasting and fasciculation; (2) sensory—including numbness, loss of sensation, tingling, sensory ataxia; the demonstration of a sensory level and analysis of specific sensory deficit patterns are of particular importance in localizing the site, and therefore the likely cause, of any lesion; and (3) autonomic—sphincter dysfunction, most commonly affecting bladder function.

Other clinical features may give clues to the cause of spinal cord disease, e.g. multiple sclerosis, systemic lupus erythematosus (SLE), neurofibromatosis.

Investigation

Intramedullary and extramedullary pathologies may produce distinguishable symptom profiles, but the clinical distinction can only ever be probabilistic. If there is acute onset of myelopathy, and/or structural disease is suspected, imaging of the cord is mandatory, with MRI the investigation of choice. Once structural lesions are excluded, further investigation depends on suspected cause (e.g. neurogenetic testing for some hereditary spastic paraplegias and spinocerebellar ataxias), and on geographical location or travel history (e.g. schistosome ova in faeces). Examination of the cerebrospinal fluid may be required.

Particular conditions affecting the spinal cord

Many diseases can affect the spinal cord. Those of particular note include (1) spondylotic myelopathy—the most common cause of progressive myelopathy due to cord compression; (2) multiple sclerosis—may present as an isolated cord syndrome, usually partial rather than complete; (3) transverse myelitis—most commonly affects the thoracic cord; there may be a preceding history of infection, and cerebrospinal fluid analysis may disclose an infective agent; (4) subacute combined degeneration of the cord—demyelination of the posterior and lateral columns due to vitamin B_{12} deficiency; may occur in the absence of haematological abnormality; (5) genetic disorders—hereditary spastic paraplegia is usually an autosomal dominant disorder; causative mutations have been described in several genes; (6) vascular disorders—anterior spinal artery occlusion can infarct whole or part of the anterior two-thirds of the cord; (7) syringomyelia; (8) injury/trauma—see Chapter 24.13.1; (9) motor neuron disease—see Chapter 24.15.

Treatment and prognosis

Specific medical and surgical treatments are determined by the particular cause of myelopathy. These may arrest progression, but function that has been lost does not usually recover. Prognosis of acute cord compression is directly related to the time delay between symptom onset and relief of compression. Chronic disability as a consequence of spinal cord disease requires intensive neurorehabilitation.

Introduction

Disease within the substance of the spinal cord, intramedullary myelopathy, may result from a wide variety of pathological causes. Myelopathy may also result from pathology located outside the spinal cord (extramedullary) but within structures immediately adjacent to the cord, either intradural or extradural, affecting normal cord function (Table 24.13.1.1). Clinical features may sometimes give clues to both the pathological nature and anatomical location of disease (Table 24.13.1.2), but these have been greatly augmented with the development of MRI studies of the spinal cord.

Aetiology, pathogenesis

The spinal cord and its addenda may be affected by inflammatory, demyelinating, metabolic, infective, neoplastic, vascular, and iatrogenic disorders (Table 24.13.1.1). Chronic progressive myelopathy should always prompt consideration of a structural lesion such as a tumour, intrinsic or extrinsic, but cervical spondylotic change with osteophyte formation, with or without concurrent intervertebral disc degeneration and prolapse, is the most common cause of progressive cord compression. Acute cord syndromes may result from trauma or vascular pathology, and infective disorders (myelitis) may develop rapidly. Inflammatory lesions tend to evolve over hours to days, although sometimes present in a chronic progressive fashion.

Clinical features

The clinical features of spinal cord disease, the symptoms and signs and their temporal progression, may give clues to disease localization (Table 24.13.1.2) and pathogenesis. Symptoms and signs suggestive of spinal cord disease may be motor (weakness, spasticity), sensory (numbness, loss of sensation, tingling, sensory ataxia), and autonomic (sphincter dysfunction). Acute and chronic pathologies may result in differing patterns of symptoms and signs, the former sometimes evolving to the latter.

Considering motor symptoms, weakness may affect all limbs (quadriparesis) or only the legs (paraparesis). The most severe presentation, for example after cord transection, is with complete absence of power (quadriplegia, paraplegia). Exceptionally with extramedullary cervical cord lesions a triparesis may be seen, sometimes evolving in a sequential ('round the clock') pattern: arm, ipsilateral leg, contralateral leg. Alterations in tonus accompany weakness, in acute lesions flaccidity ('spinal shock') but with more chronic processes spasticity with clonus, along with pathological accentuation of myotatic (tendon, phasic) reflexes (hyperreflexia), loss of cutaneous reflexes, and upgoing plantar responses (Babinski's sign). Muscle wasting is a late sign with upper motor neuron pathology. Concurrent radiculopathy or neuropathy may however modulate the typical upper motor neuron signs, for example the absent ankle jerks with upgoing plantars sometimes seen in subacute combined degeneration of the cord in which there is concurrent neuropathy or in motor neuron disease with both upper and lower motor neuron involvement, or the segmental reflex depression in a compressive cervical myeloradiculopathy. Inversion of reflexes (i.e. movement opposite to that usually seen, such as elbow extension when eliciting the supinator reflex) may occur when pathology affects both the local reflex arc and segments higher in the cord.

High spinal cord lesions may affect segments innervating the diaphragm (C3–5) with subsequent respiratory compromise, particularly acute lesions, hence the need for respiratory monitoring in these circumstances. Because of the root values of myotatic and cutaneous reflexes, their pathological alteration may be of localizing value.

Pathological processes targeting lower motor neurons in the anterior horns of the spinal cord typically produce early muscle wasting and fasciculation. Motor neuron disease is the commonest cause of these signs, sometimes in isolation ('progressive muscular atrophy'), but they may also occur following certain viral infections (poliomyelitis, enterovirus 71, flaviviruses such as Japanese encephalitis virus). A subacute motor neuronopathy is also described in association with underlying lymphoma.

Spinal cord pathologies are often accompanied by a localizing sensory level, which may be defined clinically as the spinal segment below which sensation is altered and above which it is intact. Because pain fibres forming the spinothalamic tracts ascend in the posterior horns for two or three segments prior to decussation through the ventral commissure, contralateral loss or reduction of pain and temperature sensation may be associated with a level two or three segments above the site of pathology. The deficit associated with a sensory level may be complete, affecting all modalities, for example in cord transection ('sawn off') or complete transverse myelopathies, but more often it is partial.

Specific sensory deficit patterns have particular localizing implications. Because of the anatomical separation within the cord of the pathways subserving the sensory modalities of pain and temperature (spinothalamic) and proprioception (dorsal column), dissociated sensory loss may occur. Central cord pathologies such as syringomyelia selectively involve decussating spinothalamic pathways within the ventral commissure resulting in impaired pain and temperature sensation, often in suspended ('cape-like', cuirasse, 'bathing suit') distribution, dependent on the exact level of the syrinx. Osteoarthropathy due to loss of pain fibres (Charcot joints) may also occur in syringomyelia. Anterior spinal artery syndrome also spares the dorsal columns. Conversely, the dorsal columns are preferentially affected in disorders such as subacute combined degeneration of the cord. Focal cervical cord pathology, most typically demyelination, may be accompanied by Lhermitte's sign, tingling paraesthesia radiating like an electric shock into arms and legs on neck flexion; there may be a motor equivalent, increased limb weakness on neck flexion (McArdle's sign). Both signs reflect mechanosensitivity and impaired impulse transmission in demyelinated axons. Preservation of pain and temperature sensation in sacral dermatomes ('sacral sparing') below a sensory level may be seen with intramedullary lesions as a result of the topographical lamination of fibres in the spinothalamic tracts, ventrolateral fibres of sacral origin being most external and hence later involved with expanding intramedullary lesions.

Although ataxia is sometimes thought of as a motor symptom, it may also be a consequence of sensory dysfunction, specifically when afferent proprioceptive information is degraded or lost. Sensory ataxia, as distinct from cerebellar or optic ataxia, results in falling or markedly increased sway when standing with the eyes closed (Romberg's sign) and impaired heel–toe (tandem) walking ('dynamic Romberg's sign'). Pseudoathetosis, involuntary movements in the outstretched hands ('piano-playing fingers'), may also be seen. Dorsal column pathologies are particularly associated with

Table 24.13.1.1 Causes of myelopathy

Pathological process[a]	Intramedullary	Extramedullary
Structural—developmental	Syringomyelia related to Chiari malformation Spina bifida, spinal dysraphism, diastematomyelia	Chiari malformation Tethered cord syndrome Platybasia/basilar invagination Arteriovenous malformations Arachnoid cysts (e.g. in Marfan syndrome) Achondroplasia
Structural—acquired/trauma	Cord transection Contusion/haematoma Haematomyelia Central cord syndrome (hyperextension injury) Whiplash (hyperextension/flexion injury) Spinal cord injury without radiologic abnormality (SCIWORA)	Intervertebral disc prolapse Osteophytes Spinal stenosis Vertebral fracture (e.g. wedge fracture with vertebral metastasis) Atlanto-axial subluxation (rheumatoid arthritis) Ossification of the posterior longitudinal ligament Dural herniation of the spinal cord
Structural—neoplasia	Astrocytoma/glioma Ependymoma Medulloblastoma Metastases	Intradural: meningioma neurofibroma; lipoma (± spina bifida) Extradural: myeloma, lymphoma, sarcoma, haemangioblastoma, chordoma Metastases Leukaemic meningeal infiltration
Neuronal degeneration/hereditary	Motor neuron disease Other motor neuron diseases: spinal muscular atrophies Hereditary spastic paraplegia (HSP) Spinocerebellar ataxias (SCA) Familial Alzheimer's disease with presenilin-1 gene deletion (exon 9) Familial British dementia	N/A
Inflammation	Transverse myelitis (idiopathic > clinically isolated syndrome) Sarcoidosis Systemic lupus erythematosus Sjögren's syndrome Behçet's disease Giant cell arteritis Paraneoplastic myelitis Necrotizing myelitis (Foix–Alajouanine syndrome)	Arachnoiditis (e.g. related to radiological contrast media, ankylosing spondylitis) Discitis
Demyelination	Multiple sclerosis Acute disseminated encephalomyelitis (ADEM) Neuromyelitis otica (NMO)/Devic's disease.	N/A
Metabolic/nutritional	Vitamin B_{12} deficiency (subacute combined degeneration of the cord) Adrenomyeloneuropathy Vitamin E deficiency Copper deficiency associated myelopathy Lathyrism Konzo ?Myelopathy associated with inflammatory bowel disease Krabbe's globoid cell leukodystrophy.	Paget's disease ('osteitis deformans')
Infection	Viral: poliomyelitis, HIV, HTLV-1 (tropical spastic paraparesis), enterovirus, herpes simplex 1 and 2, herpes zoster, EBV, CMV, HHV6 Spirochaetal: neurosyphilis (tabes dorsalis) Bacterial: brucellosis Parasitic: schistosomiasis Atypicals: mycoplasma.	Spinal abscess: epidural, subdural Empyema Osteomyelitis (e.g staphylococcal) Osteitis (e.g. TB (Pott's disease), syphilis) Parasitic cysts (echinococcus)
Vascular	Cord ischaemia/infarction: anterior spinal artery syndrome Aortic aneurysm Fibrocartilaginous embolism Decompression sickness Haematomyelia/haematoma: into metastasis or vascular malformation, primary coagulation disorder.	Arteriovenous malformations: dural arteriovenous fistula, arteriovenous malformations, cavernous angioma
Iatrogenic	Surgery of aortic aneurysm: anterior spinal artery syndrome Lumbar puncture: direct trauma to cord Radiation myelopathy Vaccination-related myelopathy Drugs: anticoagulants (bleed into cord); heroin; subacute myelo-optic neuropathy (SMON) with clioquinol	Lumbar puncture: spinal subdural haematoma

CMV, cytomegalovirus; EBV, Epstein–Barr virus; HHV, human herpesvirus; HTLV-1, human T-lymphotropic virus type 1.
[a] NB: These are not necessarily mutually exclusive.

Table 24.13.1.2 Clinical clues to differentation of intramedullary from extramedullary myelopathy

Symptoms/signs	Intramedullary	Extramedullary
Sensory	Central (funicular) distribution of pain may occur. Patterns of sensory loss may be: dissociated (spinothalamic > dorsal column modalities, or vice versa) including classic Brown-Séquard syndrome; suspended (cape-like, cuirasse); sacral sparing. Vibratory sensibility more often affected than proprioception	Pain may be radicular or vertebral in distribution. Sensory signs not usually marked until the later stages and all modalities often involved. Brown-Séquard syndrome may be more common with extrinsic than intrinsic pathologies
Motor	Lower motor neuron signs at the level of the lesion(s) may be prominent and diffuse; upper motor neuron signs of spastic paraparesis below the level of the lesion tend to occur late. Combination of upper and lower motor neuron signs more likely to reflect intrinsic than extrinsic pathology	Sequential spastic paraparesis below the level of the lesion. Upper motor neuron signs occur early; lower motor neuron signs unusual and if present typically have segmental (radicular) distribution
Autonomic	Bladder involvement common, often early symptom; slow to recover	May have bladder urgency, impotence

sensory ataxia, classically the tabes dorsalis form of neurosyphilis, also sometimes known as locomotor ataxia.

Autonomic features associated with spinal cord pathology are most typically those related to sphincter, particularly bladder, function. Acute spinal cord lesions may result in urinary retention, e.g. cauda equina compression with central L1 disc prolapse, although sometimes the pathology may be many segments rostral to the clinical signs. Inflammatory and chronic lesions, for example multiple sclerosis, may be associated with urinary frequency, urgency and urge incontinence with urodynamic evidence of detrusor muscle hyperreflexia and detrusor sphincter dyssynergia. Loss of awareness of bladder fullness with urinary retention and overflow (atonic bladder) may result from chronic disease, as in tabes dorsalis. Cord damage may also result in constipation or faecal urgency or incontinence, and sexual (e.g. erectile) dysfunction. Loss of or excessive sweating may be observed in syringomyelia. Horner's syndrome may be associated with cord pathology since the sympathetic afferents originate there, for example isolated Horner's syndrome has been reported with syringomyelia.

Although the two- or three-segment mismatch between a clinically-defined pain sensory level and the location of cord pathology is easily explicable on the basis of the known anatomy of spinal cord connections, other clinical signs distant from pathology are less easy to explain. Such false localizing signs in the cord include the association of foramen magnum or upper cervical cord lesions with paraesthesia in the hands, intrinsic hand muscle wasting ('remote atrophy') and distal upper limb areflexia, a gestalt more suggestive of lower cervical myeloradiculopathy. Similarly, a midthoracic sensory level ('girdle sensation') with spastic paraparesis may occur with lower cervical or upper thoracic compressive pathology.

Intramedullary and extramedullary pathologies may produce distinguishable symptom profiles (Table 24.13.1.2) but the clinical distinction can only ever be probabilistic, and further investigation by means of spinal cord imaging, ideally with MRI, is indicated. The syndrome originally described by Brown-Séquard in the context of traumatic cord hemisection consists of ipsilateral spastic weakness with or without segmental lower motor neuron signs at the level of the lesion, with dissociated sensory loss comprising ipsilateral proprioceptive loss and contralateral pain and temperature loss below the level of the lesion. This pattern may occur with various pathologies including prolapsed disc, intra- and extramedullary tumours, and multiple sclerosis.

Other clinical features may give clues to the aetiological diagnosis of myelopathy. A history of hindbrain headache may indicate a

Chiari malformation. Likewise other clinical signs may be informative: a segmental rash may be seen acutely with varicella zoster, and clinical stigmata may point to the diagnosis of systemic lupus erythematosus (SLE), neurofibromatosis, Paget's disease, and rheumatoid arthritis.

Differential diagnosis

The particular pattern of symptoms and signs may allow differentiation of myelopathy from disorders of nerve roots (radiculopathy), although because of their close proximity to the cord simultaneous segmental involvement is not uncommon (radiculomyelopathy) particularly with cervical spinal lesions; likewise peripheral nerves (neuropathy), although certain disease processes simultaneously affect both (myeloneuropathy). Lesions of the conus may be difficult to differentiate from the cauda equina syndrome of multiple radiculopathies, although often both are present.

Clinical investigation

If there is acute onset of myelopathy, and/or structural disease is suspected, imaging of the cord is mandatory and magnetic resonance imaging (MRI) the investigation of choice, usually requiring axial and sagittal sequences with T_1- and T_2-weighting, with or without gadolinium contrast. Appearances may diagnose structural abnormalities such as spondylotic compression, disc prolapse, intrinsic or extrinsic tumours, syringomyelia, Chiari malformations, abscess, or haematoma. Arteriovenous malformations may be seen, although it remains the case that on occasion myelography will reveal vascular anomalies not seen on MRI. Further definition of these vascular lesions with selective spinal angiography or magnetic resonance (MR) angiography may be helpful in planning appropriate treatment. Neurosurgical biopsy of mass lesions may on occasion be required.

Intrinsic cord disease may have characteristic appearances on MRI. Typical demyelinating lesions of multiple sclerosis usually extend for no more than one vertebral segment and may be multiple, whereas more extensive lesions ('longitudinal myelitis') suggest infective, postinfectious, or vascular disease. These lesions may be associated with enhancement on post-contrast scans. Certain viral myelitides, such as poliomyelitis or enterovirus 71, may produce signal change confined to the anterior horns, consistent with a purely motor syndrome. MR spectroscopy of cord lesions may prove difficult because of partial volume effects in selected voxels.

Once structural lesions are excluded, further investigation of myelopathy will be dependent on suspected cause, and on geographical location or travel history. Blood tests may include haematological parameters such as full blood count and film, ESR, and vitamin B_{12} level. Biochemical analyses are seldom helpful other than for specific entities, such as angiotensin converting enzyme (ACE) for sarcoidosis, and very long chain fatty acids for adrenoleukodystrophy which may be associated with the typical electrolyte changes of Addison's disease. Raised alkaline phosphatase may alert to a possible diagnosis of Paget's disease. Serology for VDRL, autoantibodies including double-stranded DNA, antiphospholipid antibodies and gastric parietal cell antibodies may be required if specific diseases are suspected. Serology for infective agents may encompass viral (HIV, human T-lymphotropic virus type 1 (HTLV-1), enterovirus 71, Epstein–Barr virus (EBV), cytomegalovirus (CMV), varicella zoster, coxsackievirus, poliovirus), bacterial (brucella, tuberculosis), spirochaetal (syphilis) and parasitic (schistosomiasis) causes of myelopathy. In the appropriate geographical distribution or with positive travel history, a search for schistosome ova in faeces may be undertaken.

Neurogenetic testing, following appropriate genetic counselling, is available for some of the many genetic loci which have been defined for the hereditary spastic paraplegias (SPG) and spinocerebellar ataxias (SCA). Adrenoleukodystrophy has been linked to over 500 different mutations in the ATP-binding cassette *ABCD1* gene.

Examination of the cerebrospinal fluid may be required. Depending on the clinical scenario, this may require analysis for cell count, protein, glucose, xanthochromia, oligoclonal bands, serology, cytology, angiotensin converting enzyme, and polymerase chain reaction for infective agents such as viruses and tuberculosis.

Neurophysiological investigations (electromyography (EMG), nerve conduction studies) have little direct role in the diagnosis of cord syndromes, although EMG may be diagnostic for motor neuron disease, but may help to define concurrent radiculopathies or neuropathies which may focus differential diagnostic considerations. Somatosensory evoked potential studies may confirm a clinically defined spinal cord lesion, or provide evidence of a subclinical lesion, for example in multiple sclerosis, as may visual evoked potential studies. However, MRI is more sensitive in this regard. Central motor conduction times to muscles in lower (e.g. tibialis anterior) or upper limb (e.g. abductor digiti minimi) may indicate cord pathology, often being abnormal in transverse myelopathies, but this investigation is not widely available.

Criteria for diagnosis

Clinical features of some of the more common causes of myelopathy are briefly presented.

The spinal cord is one the sites of predilection for demyelinating diseases. Multiple sclerosis (MS) may present as an isolated cord syndrome, usually partial rather than complete. Clues to the diagnosis may be typical MRI features in the cord, concurrent demyelination on brain MRI, and acellular cerebrospinal fluid with oligoclonal bands. Distinct from this acute presentation is a progressive myelopathy, either following (secondary) or without prior relapsing episodes (primary progressive MS). Neuromyelitis optica (NMO), also known as Devic's syndrome, is an inflammatory demyelinating disorder of spinal cord and optic nerves, sometimes associated with antibodies to aquaporin-4.

Transverse myelitis most commonly affects the thoracic cord. If complete, there is paralysis, sensory loss, and incontinence, often with an acute flaccid paraparesis or paraplegia. There may be a preceding history of infection. MRI often reveals extensive longitudinal abnormal signal over several contiguous spinal segments, unlike the pattern typical of MS. Differential diagnosis of such 'longitudinal myelitis' includes infective (viral), postinfectious, and postvaccination myelitides, and collagen vascular diseases. Cerebrospinal fluid analysis may disclose an infective agent, including coxsackieviruses, polioviruses, enterovirus 71, flaviviruses (Japanese encephalitis, West Nile virus), some of which have a predilection for the anterior horn cells producing a largely or exclusively motor picture and MR signal change confined to the anterior horns. HTLV-1 more typically produces a chronic spastic paraparesis, also known as HTLV-1-associated myelopathy (HAM), and was probably the agent responsible for 'tropical spastic paraparesis'. The vacuolar myelopathy associated with HIV infection may be overlooked clinically because of other neurological involvement and is often defined only post-mortem. Postinfectious myelitis may be a variant of acute disseminated encephalomyelitis (ADEM). Collagen vascular diseases such as SLE, with or without antiphospholipid antibodies, may be associated, and sometimes presents, with an acute myelitis which, as in the case of postinfectious myelitis, is associated with raised cerebrospinal fluid cell count and protein but without oligoclonal bands. A depressed cerebrospinal fluid glucose level has sometimes been reported in SLE transverse myelitis.

A syndrome of acute necrotizing myelitis, sometimes known as Foix–Alajouanine syndrome, may merge with the severe end of the transverse myelitis spectrum. This condition may be associated with vascular pathologies (see below), or haematological or lung neoplasms, and hence represent a paraneoplastic syndrome, although more usually these latter manifest as an encephalomyelitis. Some episodes of transverse myelitis resist all diagnostic efforts to define their aetiology and hence by a process of exclusion may be classified as idiopathic transverse myelitis, diagnostic criteria for which have been published.

In subacute combined degeneration of the cord due to vitamin B_{12} (cobalamin) deficiency, myelopathy is due to demyelination of spinal cord white matter tracts, specifically the posterior and lateral columns. MRI of the cervical spinal cord may show evidence of posterior column high signal intensity extending over several segments, unlike the appearances of multiple sclerosis, which resolves with vitamin B_{12} repletion. Although vitamin B_{12} deficiency may occur in the context of pernicious anaemia, myelopathy may also occur in the absence of haematological abnormality. A Schilling test to examine B_{12} absorption may be required. Elevated serum levels of homocysteine and methylmalonic acid, the substrates for cobalamin-dependent enzymes, may be helpful when there is diagnostic uncertainty and vitamin B_{12} levels are borderline. A concurrent peripheral neuropathy, usually of axonal type, may be clinically and/or neurophysiologically evident. Overuse of nitrous oxide analgesia may produce a similar clinical syndrome, due to functional B_{12} deficiency, as may acquired copper deficiency, often in the context of intestinal resection. This disorder is associated with low serum copper and caeruloplasmin levels and increased signal in the dorsal columns on MRI. First described in 2001, this may be the human equivalent of swayback disease seen in ruminants with copper deficiency. Vitamin E deficiency may be acquired, in the context of intestinal fat malabsorption, including patients with cystic fibrosis, or result from an autosomal recessive genetic disorder due to mutations in the α-tocopherol gene (OMIM#277460). Ataxia is both cerebellar and spinal in these disorders and may respond to vitamin E supplements.

Other genetic disorders may present with a spinal cord syndrome. Hereditary spastic paraplegia is a heterogeneous group of motor system disorders typified by lower limb spasticity which greatly predominates over weakness. There may in addition be mild diminution of lower limb vibration and proprioception, and in complicated cases there may be additional clinical features such as seizures, cognitive impairment or frank dementia, peripheral neuropathy, amyotrophy, or extrapyramidal features. Most instances are inherited as autosomal dominant disorders although recessive and X-linked variants are described, with over 25 genetic loci (SPG) defined. Deterministic mutations have been discovered in genes encoding the proteins spastin, atlastin, parpalegin, and spartin.

Adrenoleukodystrophy is an X-linked recessive peroxisomal disorder (OMIM#300100) with variable clinical phenotype related to age. Whereas children and adolescents have a cerebral presentation with personality and intellectual changes leading to dementia, young adult males often present with a progressive spastic paraparesis with a mild distal polyneuropathy, adrenomyeloneuropathy (AMN), with delayed cerebral involvement. There may be additional adrenal insufficiency. Positive family history may alert clinicians to the diagnosis. Some female heterozygotes (carriers) may manifest an AMN-like syndrome with mild spastic paraparesis. Cord imaging in AMN may show atrophy but no signal abnormality.

Friedreich's ataxia, the most common autosomal recessive cerebellar ataxia (OMIM#229300), may present with a spastic paraparesis with extensor plantars accompanied by absent ankle jerks due to the concurrent axonal sensory polyneuropathy. The autosomal dominant cerebellar ataxias form a heterogeneous group, linked to over 25 different genetic loci, many associated with trinucleotide repeat expansions. The phenotype is of a progressive cerebellar syndrome with or without additional neurological features which may include spastic paraparesis.

Although typically an exclusively cognitive disorder, variants of Alzheimer's disease with spastic paraparesis have been described in association with mutations in the presenilin-1 gene (OMIM#104300), most particularly the exon 9 deletion. These patients also manifest a pathological phenotype, cotton wool plaques of amyloid protein, which although not totally specific are seldom seen in other cases. Familial British dementia, originally described as Worster–Drought syndrome and now characterized as one of the hereditary cerebral amyloid angiopathies, resulting from stop codon mutations in the *ITM2B* (A-Bri) gene (OMIM#176500), typically presents with presenile dementia which is later complicated by cerebellar ataxia and spastic paraparesis.

Vascular disorders of the spinal cord encompass both arterial infarction and haemorrhage or venous hypertension; venous infarction is uncommon. Cord ischaemia has been postulated to contribute to spondylotic myelopathy and delayed radiation myelopathy. Arterial infarction is most commonly due to anterior spinal artery occlusion, for example during thoraco-abdominal aneurysm repair. In this syndrome, because of the respective watersheds of anterior and posterior spinal arteries, the whole or part of the anterior two-thirds of the cord may be infarcted with loss of descending motor and ascending sensory pathway integrity but with preservation of dorsal column function. Hypoperfusion of the cord may be responsible for the myelopathies associated with fibrocartilaginous embolism, often associated with back injury, and with air embolism in decompression sickness (Caisson disease).

Haemorrhage and/or venous hypertension occur with spinal vascular malformations, which may broadly be divided into dural arteriovenous fistulas (AVF), usually acquired, and arteriovenous malformations (AVM), usually of developmental origin. Spinal dural AVFs typically present in middle age and beyond, most commonly in men, with a progressive painful myelopathy. Venous hypertension results in cord hypoxia which may progress to irreversible necrosis (Foix–Alajouanine syndrome; subacute necrotizing myelopathy). Stepwise progression may occur. In contrast, spinal AVMs tend to present at a younger age than AVFs, with a mean in the third decade but sometimes in childhood. AVMs may be at any cord level, on the surface, within the parenchyma, or both. High-flow lesions may also have arterial aneurysms on the supplying vessels. Spinal haemorrhage is the typical clinical manifestation, presenting with acute painful paraplegia, back pain, sciatica, with or without meningism and disturbance of consciousness; blood may track intracranially, simulating subarachnoid haemorrhage. Progressive neurological dysfunction is less often seen than with AVFs. The presence of a spinal bruit and/or segmentally related cutaneous malformations may give a clue to the presence of an intradural AVM. Spinal vascular malformations may occur in association with similar lesions in other organs or cutaneous angiomas, for example in neurofibromatosis, with haemangioblastomas or cerebral aneurysms, and in specific syndromes (Cobbs, Klippel–Trénaunay–Weber). Cavernous malformations may also occur in the spinal cord.

A syrinx is a fluid-filled cavity within the spinal cord (syringomyelia) or brainstem (syringobulbia) which may be connected to a dilated central canal or separate from it. Most are associated with Chiari-type hindbrain anomalies, sometimes with concurrent hydrocephalus, but there are also associations with spinal trauma, spinal tumours, arachnoiditis, and inflammatory/demyelinating disorders of the spinal cord such as MS and NMO.

Treatment and prognosis

Treatment of myelopathy is, of course, dependent on establishing aetiology. Structural lesions may require neurosurgical intervention, sometimes acutely to save or salvage cord function. With acute compressive lesions, prognosis is directly related to the time delay between symptom onset and relief of compression. Infective mass lesions may require debridement and systemic antibiotics. Foramen magnum decompression may be undertaken for syringomyelia associated with Chiari malformation. Certain spinal cord vascular malformations may be amenable to endovascular treatment, or targeted (stereotactic) radiotherapy to shrink lesion size and reduce haemorrhagic risk. Radiotherapy of vertebral metastases causing cord compression is often undertaken.

Specific treatment is sometimes available. Vitamin B_{12} myelopathy may remit with vitamin repletion, although it is well recognized that there is an inverse relationship between duration of deficiency and extent of recovery following repletion. Dysaesthesia and proprioceptive deficits often persist, although these may be related in part to concurrent peripheral nerve involvement. Likewise, with copper deficiency myelopathy neurological decline is halted but seldom reversed by copper repletion. Cord compression with Paget's disease may respond to specific treatment (bisphosphonates).

Steroids are often prescribed for inflammatory and necrotizing myelitides, sometimes with clinical improvement, although this may simply be a hastening of recovery which would have occurred anyway. Partial syndromes are said to be more likely to improve, complete syndromes less so, perhaps reflecting the fact that the former are more likely to be manifestations of MS. More specific immunosuppressive regimes may be required in SLE, and anticoagulation in the antiphospholipid antibody syndrome.

Residual or progressive deficits in sensorimotor and sphincter function resulting from myelopathy may benefit from targeted symptomatic and neurorehabilitation strategies, including physiotherapy and occupational therapy. Symptom management may include agents for spasticity (oral baclofen, tizanidine, dantrolene; focal injections of botulinum toxin; intrathecal baclofen), pain (antineuropathic pain medications such as pregabalin, gabapentin), bladder dysfunction (anticholinergic medications, clean intermittent self catheterization, suprapubic catheterization), and erectile dysfunction (sildenafil).

Further reading

Al-Deeb SM, et al. (1997). Acute transverse myelitis. A localized form of postinfectious encephalomyelitis. *Brain*, **120**, 1115–22.
Aminoff MJ (1976). *Spinal angiomas.* Blackwell Scientific, Oxford.
Critchley E, Eisen A (1992). *Diseases of the spinal cord.* Springer-Verlag, London.
Depienne C, et al. (2007). Hereditary spastic paraplegias: an update. *Curr Opin Neurol*, **20**, 674–80.
Engelhardt P, Trostdorf E (1997). Zur Differentialdiagnose des Brown-Sequard-Syndroms. *Nervenarzt*, **48**, 45–9.
Hadjipavlou AG, et al. (2001). Paget's disease of the spine and its management. *Eur Spine J*, **10**, 370–84.
Kincaid O, Lipton HL (2006), Viral myelitis: an update. *Curr Neurol Neurosci Rep*, **6**, 469–74.
Kumar N (2006). Copper deficiency myelopathy (human swayback). *Mayo Clin Proc*, **81**, 1371–84.
Larner AJ (2003). False localising signs. *J Neurol Neurosurg Psychiatry*, **74**, 415–18.
Larner AJ (2006). *A dictionary of neurological signs*, 2nd edition. Springer, New York.
Larner AJ, Muqit MMK, Glickman S (2002). Concurrent syrinx and inflammatory central nervous system disease detected by magnetic resonance imaging. An illustrative case and review of the literature. *Medicine (Baltimore)*, **81**, 41–50.
Larner AJ, et al. (1997). MRI appearances in subacute combined degeneration of the spinal cord due to vitamin B$_{12}$ deficiency. *J Neurol Neurosurg Psychiatry*, **62**, 99–100.
Miller D (2001). Spinal cord disorders. In: Donaghy M (ed.). *Brain's diseases of the nervous system*, 11th edition. Oxford University Press, Oxford, pp. 601–30.
Polman CH, et al. (2005). Diagnostic criteria for multiple sclerosis: 2005 revisions to the McDonald criteria. *Ann Neurol*, **58**, 840–6.
Scott TF, et al. (1998). Transverse myelitis. Comparison with spinal cord presentations of multiple sclerosis. *Neurology*, **50**, 429–33.
Solomon T, et al. (1998). Poliomyelitis-like illness due to Japanese encephalitis virus. *Lancet*, **351**, 1094–7.
Transverse Myelitis Consortium Working Group (2002). Proposed diagnostic criteria and nosology of acute transverse myelitis. *Neurology* **59**, 499–505.
Wingerchuk DM, et al. (2006). New NMO criteria incorporating aquaporin-4 biomarker. *Neurology*, **66**, 1485–9.
Wong SH, et al. (2008). Myelopathy but normal MRI: where next? *Pract Neurol*, **8**, 90–102.

24.13.2 Spinal cord injury and its management

M.P. Barnes

Essentials

Spinal cord injury most commonly affects young men as a consequence of road traffic accidents, violence, and sports injuries; falls are a common cause in older patients.

Early acute management

Appropriate management of the individual at the scene of an accident is vital to avoid unnecessary worsening of a spinal cord injury. Those who are unconscious should be assumed to have a cervical spine injury until proven otherwise, with (1) the head and neck held firmly (as far as possible) in a neutral position using (if available) a semi-rigid collar, and (2) transportation on a spinal board with a head immobilizer.

Investigation—spinal injury cannot be determined solely by examination. There are often very few local signs, hence radiological investigation is essential. Plain radiography will usually reveal the fracture or dislocation, but bony abnormalities are occasionally minimal or absent; MRI is now recognized to be the best imaging technique.

Treatment—injuries to the cervical spine will usually receive skeletal traction applied through skull calipers; thoracic and lumbar injuries require simple support of the patient in the correct posture. Other interventions include (1) surgery—e.g. fusion and internal fixation, anterior or posterior decompression (or some combination of these); practice varies considerably, but many spinal centres recommend surgical intervention if neurological symptoms are deteriorating; (2) steroids—high-dose methyl prednisolone, started within 8 h of injury, improves neurological outcome.

Management in the spinal cord injury centre

Spine—in the neurologically intact person, surgery allows the individual to be mobilized more quickly, but there is no convincing evidence that the endpoint of rehabilitation is delayed by conservative treatment.

Medical problems during the period of immobilization—these include (1) Respiratory—the intercostal muscles and (in high cervical lesions) diaphragm may be paralysed; regular chest physiotherapy is vital as the commonest cause of a decline in respiratory function is the retention of secretions; prophylactic anti-coagulation is advisable. (2) Pressure sores—these ought to be preventable. (3) Bladder—key matters to be considered are (a) is there impairment of renal function?; (b) is there failure of bladder emptying?—residual urine can predispose to infection or stone formation and contributes to impairment of renal function; most cases of failure of bladder emptying require mechanical drainage, preferably by intermittent clean self-catheterization; and (c) is there detrusor hyperreflexia?—anticholinergics (e.g. oxybutynin) are generally most effective. (4) Bowel care—in the initial period of spinal shock the bowel remains flaccid and should not be allowed to over-distend. (5) Autonomic dysreflexia—most commonly seen with cervical cord injuries above the sympathetic outflow and characterized by an exaggerated autonomic response to a stimulus below the level of the lesion; management consists of trying to avoid precipitating stimuli and use of antihypertensive agents. (6) Spasticity and contractures—passive stretching of the spastic muscles and regular standing regimes can be helpful; advise from a neurological physiotherapist on appropriate positioning and seating is essential; antispastic drugs should be used with care because they induce significant tiredness and weakness. (7) Pain and dysaesthesia—usually respond reasonably well to the use of carbamazepine, tricyclic antidepressants, gabapentin, or pregabalin.

Rehabilitation—a coordinated multidisciplinary team can improve functional outcome. Principles are based around the concepts of impairment, activity and participation restriction, with the aim being to work with the disabled person and their family in partnership, a key element being the setting of realistic goals that should be specific, measurable, achievable, relevant, and time limited (SMART).

Long-term issues

Spinal cord injury affects all domains of life, so a very wide range of issues may need to be addressed, including those related to discharge home, emotional problems, sexual life, fertility, leisure pursuits, driving, employment, and information. Later medical complications include pathological fractures, post-traumatic syringomyelia, and respiratory compromise (in those with high cervical cord lesions).

Prognosis

With appropriate management, initial mortality from spinal cord injury is less than 5%. Life expectancy in paraplegia is only modestly reduced, although people with tetraplegia still die prematurely. The major causes of late death are now those experienced by the general population (e.g. cancer, myocardial infarction), although excess deaths from renal failure or respiratory infection persist in those with tetraplegia.

Introduction

Remarkable improvements can be made to the survival of patients with spinal cord injury; great advances have also been made toward improving the quality of life of those so injured, principally as result of contemporary interventions used in rehabilitation medicine.

In the early part of the 20th century about 9 out of every 10 people with a spinal cord injury died within 1 year and only 1% survived in the long term. With the advent of spinal cord injury centres, these outcomes have been greatly improved. Coordinated, multidisciplinary care provided at such centres has significantly reduced mortality and improved quality of life. However, it is only the last decade or so that modern rehabilitation techniques have reduced initial mortality to less than 5%. Indeed, life expectancy has improved to the extent that the major causes of late death in spinal injury are now those experienced by the general population, such as cancer and myocardial infarction. Excess deaths from renal failure or respiratory infection persist in those with tetraplegia, and although life expectancy in those with paraplegia is only modestly

reduced, people with tetraplegia still die prematurely. A 20-year-old male would normally be expected to live for a further 65 years, but this is reduced to about 50 to 55 years in those with paraplegia. The best survival figures in tetraplegia are about 80% of normal, but figures from some centres report less than two-thirds of those injured have a normal life expectancy. Nonetheless, results continue to improve and a recent study from Australia reports an 86% overall 10 year survival.

Epidemiology

The annual incidence of spinal cord injury varies and has been reported between 10 and 50 cases per million population per year. The mean age of injury is about 33 years although the mode is 19 years. Most injuries occur in males (c.82%). The most common cause is road traffic accidents (c.40%). Regrettably, spinal cord injury from violence (either self-harm or criminal assault) is increasing, particularly in the United States of America. In the older age group falls become more common. Table 24.13.2.1 summarizes the leading causes.

The proportion of injuries from road traffic accidents has seen a modest reduction in recent years, probably due to the introduction of seat-belt legislation and improved safety features on cars. Hopefully improved safety of vehicles and improved traffic regulation, particularly speed control in urban areas, will further reduce the incidence in coming years. There is some evidence in the last decade that the incidence of spinal injury has plateaued, having been increasing in previous decades. There seems, however, to be an increase in the incidence of elderly people who sustain spinal injuries during falls mainly at home, many of whom develop tetraplegia. Regrettably the commonest result of spinal injury is tetraplegia (c.60%) and the proportion of tetraplegia compared to paraplegia is still increasing.

Management

Early acute management

The appropriate management of the individual at the scene of an accident is vital in order to avoid unnecessary worsening of a spinal cord injury. If the individual is unconscious then it should be assumed there is an injury to the cervical spine until proven otherwise. Until this diagnosis can be ruled out the head and neck should, as far as possible, be held firmly in a neutral position. This is normally achieved at the scene of an accident by immobilization in a semi-rigid collar, but if this is not available alternative improvised methods of stabilizing the head and neck should be initiated. The individual should not be placed in the coma position, as this

Table 24.13.2.1 Causes of spinal cord injury—comparison of causes in the United Kingdom and the United States of America

Cause	UK (%)	USA (%)
Road traffic accidents	35	43
Violence	7	19
Sports injuries	21	11
Falls (domestic and industrial)	36	19
Other	1	8

will rotate the cervical spine, but is best placed, if other injuries allow, in a lateral position with the head kept in line with the spine by the underlying arm. If any movement is necessary the person should be 'log rolled' to ensure that the spine is kept in a straight and neutral position at all times. Usually transportation is on a spinal board with a head immobilizer. Speed of evacuation is important, particularly if there are other life-threatening injuries. Preferably the individual should be transferred to a regional spinal injuries unit but obviously they may need resuscitation and other life-threatening injuries may need treatment at the nearest Emergency Department. It is worth recalling that the diagnosis of intra-abdominal injury can be very difficult in people with spinal cord injuries. The initial phase of spinal shock will tend to give rise to paralytic ileus and abdominal distension, which can further confuse the situation if abdominal injury is suspected.

Obviously both a general and neurological examination is vital—particularly to determine the neurological level of the lesion. Figure 24.13.2.1 illustrates the myotomes, dermatomes, and reflexes as an aide memoire. Table 24.13.2.2 summarizes likely functional outcome according to lesion level.

Spinal injury, however, cannot be determined solely by examination and often there are very few local signs. There may be some bruising, tenderness or deformity but equally there may be no clue on examination about the actual nature and extent of the underlying bone injury. Thus, radiological investigation is essential and should preferably only be undertaken in a unit familiar with the management of those with spinal injury. In a radiology department it is still important to remember that spinal movement must be minimal. Usually radiography will clearly reveal the fracture or dislocation, although occasionally bony abnormalities are minimal or absent. This is particularly true in older people with underlying cervical spondylosis when tetraplegia can result from hyperextension injury without fracture or dislocation. Radiographic examination can also be normal in children when spinal traction injury can occur without evidence of bony damage. MRI is now recognized to be probably the best investigation technique for spinal cord injury.

Initial management of people with injuries to the cervical spine usually consists of skeletal traction applied through skull calipers. Traction will help to stabilize and splint the spine and can also reduce fractures and dislocations. There are a number of different calipers available; Fig. 24.13.2.2 illustrates one type, the Cones calipers.

The amount of traction applied will vary according to the type, level and extent of injury but will be in the order of 0.5 to 2 kg for upper cervical injuries and somewhat more, around 4 kg, for lower cervical spinal injuries. Sometimes if the spine is dislocated reduction is achieved by incrementally increasing the weight of traction every few minutes under close neurological monitoring. Mobilization in a halo brace can be safely used instead of traction in people with compression fractures of the cervical spine. It is advisable, however, to await recovery from spinal shock before mobilizing a person with neurological damage.

For thoracic and lumbar injuries standard treatment is simple support of the individual in the correct posture, usually with a pillow under the lumbar spine to maintain the normal lordosis.

Surgical compared with conservative treatment

In most cases skull traction for cervical injuries and conservative postural treatment for thoracolumbar injuries is quite sufficient and operative intervention is not necessary. It has long been a

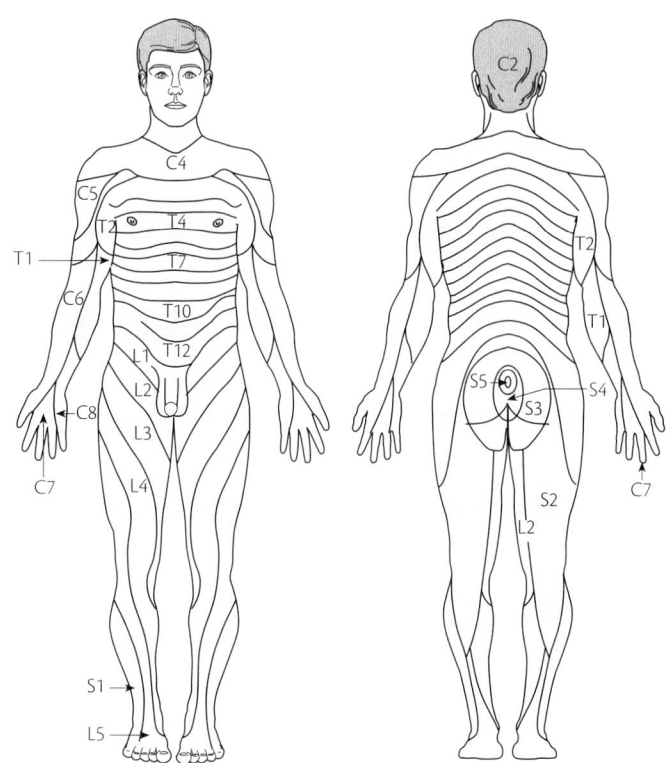

Myotomes		Reflexes
Muscle group	*Nerve supply*	
Diaphragm	C(3), 4 (5)	
Shoulder abductors	C5	
Elbow flexors	C5, 6	Biceps jerk C5, 6
Supinators/pronators	C6	Supinator jerk C6
Wrist extensors	C6	
Wrist flexors	C7	
Elbow extensors	C7	Triceps jerk C7
Finger extensors	C7	
Finger flexors	C8	
Intrinsic hand muscles	T1	Abdominal reflex T8-12
Hip flexors	L1, 2	
Hip adductors	L2, 3	
Knee extensors	L3, 4	Knee jerk L3,4
Ankle dorsiflexors	L4, 5	
Toe extensors	L5	
Knee flexors	L4, 5 S1	
Ankle plantar flexors	S1, 2	Ankle jerk S1, 2
Toe flexors	S1, 2	
Anal sphincter	S2, 3, 4	Bulbocavernosus reflex S3, 4
		Anal reflex S5
		Plantar reflex

Fig. 24.13.2.1 An aide memoire to examination—summary of the dermatomes, myotomes, and associated reflexes.

source of controversy whether operative intervention and fusion aids neurological recovery. Practice varies from country to country and indeed from centre to centre. In a broad-based survey in the United States of America, 60% of people underwent spinal surgery; most of them underwent fusion and internal fixation. Increasing numbers also undergo anterior or posterior decompression of the spinal cord with or without internal fixation and fusion. However, practice in the United States of America tends to be more orientated towards surgical intervention than practice in the United Kingdom and other parts of western Europe. In the United Kingdom surgical intervention will tend to be reserved for those

Table 24.13.2.2 Expected residual functional ability according to the level of lesion

Level of injury—complete lesions	
Lesion below C3	Dependent on others for all care
	Diaphragm paralysed, needs permanent ventilation or diaphragm pacing
	Chin-, head-, or breath-controlled electric wheelchair
Lesion below C4	Dependent on others for all care
	Can breathe independently using diaphragm
	Can shrug shoulders
	Can use electric wheelchair with chin control
	Can type/use computer with a mouth stick
	Environmental control system operated by shoulder shrug or mouthpiece
Lesion below C5	Can move shoulders and flex elbows
	Can eat with a feeding strap/universal cuff
	Can wash face, comb hair, clean teeth—using feeding strap/universal cuff
	Can write using individually designed splint and wrist support
	Can help in dressing upper half of body
	Can push manual wheelchair short distances on the flat provided that pushing gloves are used with capstan rims on the wheels
	May be able to transfer across level surfaces using sliding board and a helper
	Electric wheelchair needed for functional mobility
Lesion below C6	Can extend wrists
	Still needs strap to eat and for self-care
	Can write using individually designed splint but may not need wrist support
	Can dress upper half of body unaided
	Can help in dressing lower half of body
	Can propel wheelchair up gentle slopes
	Can be independent in bed, car, and toilet transfers
	Can drive with hand controls
Lesion below C7	Full wrist movement and some hand function, but no finger flexion or fine hand movements
	Can do all transfers, eat, and dress independently
	Can drive with hand controls
Lesion below C8	All hand muscles expect intrinsics preserved
	Wheelchair independent, but difficulty in going up and down kerbs
	Can drive with hand controls
Lesion below T1	Complete innervation of arms
	Totally independent wheelchair life
	Can drive with hand controls

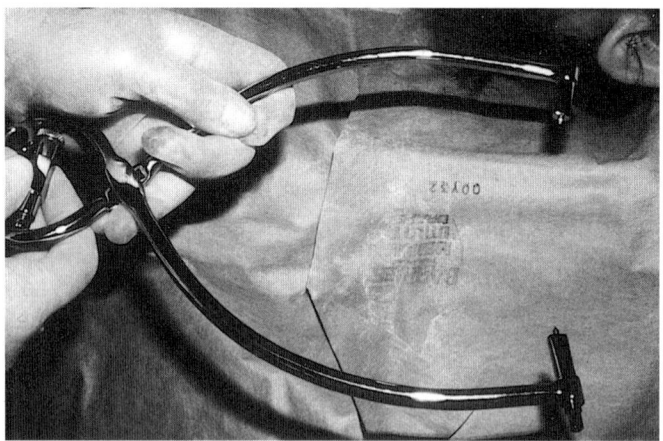

Fig. 24.13.2.2 Skull traction using Gardner–Wells calliper.

with unstable displaced fractures, and conservative management would be the normal practice for stable and/or undisplaced fractures. However, if the neurological symptoms are deteriorating then many spinal centres would now recommend surgical intervention.

Use of steroids

Another treatment intervention that can be considered in the very early stages after injury is a short course of high-dose methyl prednisolone. There is some evidence that such intervention, started within 8 h of injury, improves neurological outcome. However, this is not totally accepted and there is wide variation in practice between centres. The results of definitive trials are still awaited.

Management in the spinal cord injury centre

Initial management will consist of resuscitation, treatment of associated injuries, and containment of the biomechanical instability of the spine by either conservative or by surgical means. However, the individual should be transferred to a recognized spinal injury centre as soon as possible. There is clear evidence that outcome is maximized, both physically and psychologically, if individuals are managed in such centres as opposed to a less coordinated and less experienced approach in other hospital settings.

Problems in management

The injured person will either be managed conservatively or surgically. The advantage of surgery in the neurologically intact person is that the individual can be mobilized more quickly. If a conservative approach is adopted mobilization is delayed and active rehabilitation is obviously difficult in the first few weeks. There is, however, no convincing evidence to suggest that the endpoint of rehabilitation is delayed by conservative treatment. Cervical spine traction is normally maintained for around 6 weeks and then monitored for signs of bony union and stability. Once the fracture site is stable the individual can be gradually sat up in bed while continuing with cervical support. A profiling bed, which enables a more natural seated position, is most useful. In the early few weeks a halo brace can be used instead of skull traction. The advantage of this brace (see Fig. 24.13.2.3) is to allow early mobilization. The halo brace is kept on for 10 to 12 weeks until the site is stable.

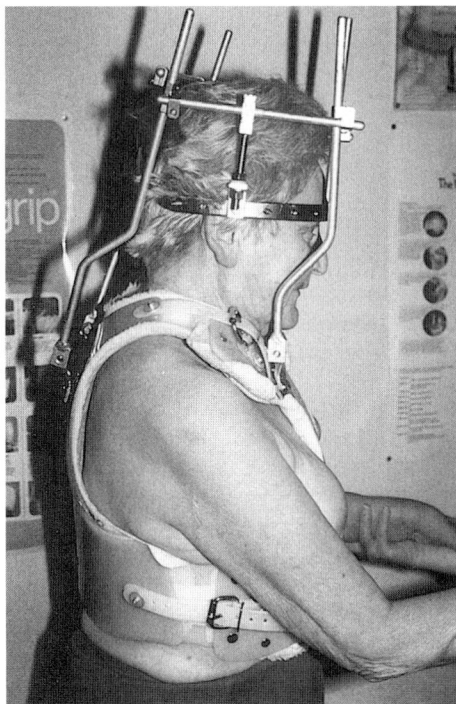

Fig. 24.13.2.3 Halo brace.

In those with thoracolumbar injuries, usually managed conservatively, the period of bed rest will usually last from 6 to 12 weeks followed by bracing and gradual mobilization, assuming that the fracture site is stable.

Over this initial period of immobilization a number of medical problems can occur.

Respiratory problems

Respiratory insufficiency can occur in people with injuries of the cervical cord. Intercostal muscles may be paralysed and in high cervical lesions the diaphragm can also be paralysed. However, even in people with lower lesions respiratory problems can still occur from associated injuries such as rib or sternal fractures. In the early hours and days respiratory function should be monitored carefully and ventilation may be required. Respiratory function can decline several hours or even days after injury and can be due to the development of spinal cord oedema. Regular chest physiotherapy is vital at this time as the commonest cause of a decline in respiratory function is the retention of secretions. Pulmonary embolism is also a risk, particularly in those who are immobilized, and prophylactic anticoagulation is advisable from an early stage prior to mobilization.

Pressure sores

Regrettably, the development of pressure sores still occurs but really ought to be preventable. Sores are commonest where there are bony prominences near the skin such as the ischial tuberosity, greater trochanter, sacrum, heel, and sometimes at the back of the head in those with skull traction. A key to prevention is awareness of the potential problem, vigilance, and regular changes of position in bed and regular lifting in the wheelchair. There are now a large range of commercial mattresses and wheelchair cushions that relieve pressure. When lifting or positioning, shear forces should be avoided as far as possible and obviously the individual should never be dragged over sheets or from the wheelchair. The skin should be kept clean and particular care should be taken to avoid any urine or faecal soiling. If a sore does occur the area must be kept clean, any dead tissue removed, and there should be complete relief of pressure from that area until it is fully healed. Occasionally surgery is indicated for larger or deeply infected sores which otherwise will take too long to heal. Education of the injured person and their family is essential. Despite awareness of the problem, around 25% of people still develop a pressure sore during their rehabilitation phase. About 15% of people will develop a pressure sore in the 1 year following discharge and this figure increases still further with time such that by year 10 about 15% of those with incomplete lesions and 28% of those with complete lesions will have developed at least one pressure sore. Septicaemia from the pressure sores is still responsible for around 10% of spinal injury deaths.

Bladder disorders

In the early part of the 20th century problems, usually infection, of the urinary system were responsible for at least half of spinal cord injury deaths. There has been very significant progress in the management of bladder and kidney disorders, but nevertheless urinary tract complications are still a residual cause of mortality and morbidity.

In the period of spinal shock the bladder is usually noncontractile and over this time catheterization may be appropriate. Once spinal shock begins to wear off the commonest problem is of detrusor hyperreflexia, which usually gives rise to frequent passage of small quantities of urine associated with urgency. However, other possibilities include detrusor sphincter dyssynergia and detrusor hyporeflexia. The latter will tend to occur when there is damage to the sacral nerves S2, 3, and 4.

The management of urinary disorders usually involves satisfactory answers to three questions: (1) Is there impairment of renal function? (2) Is there a failure of bladder emptying? (3) Is there detrusor hyperreflexia?

Is there impairment of renal function?

Screening of the upper urinary tract is important both in the short and long term. Intravenous urography should be used in the early months after injury, but long-term follow-up can often be carried out by renal ultrasound scanning or plain abdominal radiography. Late complications are possible, such as renal calculi. Cystometrography is also vital for determining the exact nature of the underlying bladder and sphincter condition.

Is there a failure of bladder emptying?

Residual urine greater than 100 ml is generally accepted as the level at which intervention is necessary. Residual urine can predispose to infection and stone formation and contributes to impairment of renal function, particularly if the failure to empty is associated with high intravesical pressure and back-pressure up to the kidney. Occasionally failure of emptying can be managed by artificial stimulation such as suprapubic tapping or perineal stimulation. However, in most cases failure of bladder emptying requires mechanical drainage. The most useful method is intermittent clean self-catheterization. This is carried out by the disabled person or sometimes by a carer four or five times every 24 h such that volumes in the bladder are kept to less than 500 ml. Intermittent self-catheterization has revolutionized the management of the bladder problems in those with spinal injury. Occasionally anticholinergic drugs such as propantheline, oxybutynin, or imipramine may help to reduce detrusor activity. Condom drainage in the male is helpful to prevent leakage between catheterization. If intermittent self-catheterization is not possible, a silastic indwelling catheter might need to be used. However, suprapubic catheterization is far better in the long term and associated with fewer problems. Regrettably there are many problems of catheterization including leakage, blockage, stone formation, and infection.

Is there detrusor hyperreflexia?

A small number of people can control minor problems with the detrusor hyperreflexia by rigid bladder drill, emptying the bladder at frequent and regular intervals. However, most people need some form of oral medication; anticholinergics are the most effective and oxybutynin the most common. Propantheline and imipramine are alternatives. Once again, protection against the embarrassment of leakage is often necessary and is more readily achieved in men with the use of condom drainage. In women a variety of absorbent pads can be worn. Advice from a specially trained nurse continence adviser can be invaluable, whatever the nature of the problem.

A whole variety of surgical techniques may be applicable in particular circumstances. An endoscopic distal sphincterotomy can be useful in those with reflex bladder emptying. The technique of bladder augmentation with an ileocystoplasty can also be helpful to allow for sufficient capacity for intermittent clean self-catheterization. Urinary diversion techniques are fortunately now needed less frequently. Recent advances include artificial urinary sphincters for treating neuropathic incontinence. Some centres also now employ sacral anterior nerve root stimulators which can be used in some people with supra sacral cord lesions. The individual has a radio linked implant to stimulate the S2, S3, and S4 anterior nerve roots and by activating the implant the bladder can be emptied. Occasionally a similar implant can also be used to assist in defecation and in obtaining penile erection.

Incontinence can be a major disability and handicap, and indeed if it is not treated properly the complications can be life threatening. Long-term follow-up is essential and proper management can make significant reductions in long-term risks and produce major improvements in the quality of life.

Bowel care

In the initial period of spinal shock the bowel remains flaccid and should not be allowed to overdistend, with the risk of constipation and overflow incontinence. Manual evacuation is usually carried out until bowel activity returns. Eventually reflex emptying can occur in those with predominant upper motor neuron lesions or the bowel can remain flaccid in those with lower motor neuron involvement. In the former, bowel evacuation can usually be triggered by glycerine suppository and/or by anal digital stimulation. In those with flaccid bowel there is a continuing need to evacuate manually or by straining using abdominal muscles. Advice on proper diet is also required. A good quality high-fibre diet together with a high fluid intake is the most helpful.

Autonomic dysreflexia

This is a potentially fatal problem most commonly seen in those with cervical cord injuries above the sympathetic outflow but can occur in those with high thoracic lesions above T6. It is characterized by an exaggerated autonomic response to a stimulus below the level of the lesion. Stimuli can include distension of the pelvic organs such as bladder, colon, and rectum. Such distension induces sympathetic activity resulting in vasoconstriction and hypertension. Other stimuli include catheterization, urinary infections, sexual intercourse, pressure sores, and even tight clothing. Surgical procedures can also induce the reflex. Symptoms will include headaches, sweating, vasodilatation, nasal obstruction, paraesthesia, and anxiety. Significant hypertension occurs. The problem occurs in around 50 to 80% of those at risk and most cases occur between 2 months and 12 months after injury. Other than awareness of the problem and avoidance of the necessary stimuli, attention is directed to reduction of the blood pressure. Sitting the person upright is usually helpful. Sublingual nifedipine can be used, or in more severe cases intravenous hydralazine. Chlorpromazine, nitroprusside and diazoxide are also possibilities. Occasionally the sympathetic reflex activity may have to be blocked by spinal epidural anaesthetic.

Spasticity and contractures

Spasticity occurs in an upper motor lesion with intact spinal reflex arcs below the level of the lesion. It is usually worse in those with incomplete lesions. Spasticity can be functionally useful and the individual can sometimes use flexor or extension spasms as an aid to dressing. However, usually spasticity produces functional problems as well as causing pain. In the long term there is a significant risk of muscle contractures. Initial management focuses on removing any unnecessary exacerbating factors such as pressure sores, tight catheter leg bags, or even urinary infections and constipation. Treatment should always involve the use of an expert neurological physiotherapist who will advise on appropriate positioning and seating. In the early stages passive stretching of the spastic muscles and regular standing regimes can be helpful and in the longer term such regimes can often be carried out by the disabled person and their carers. Antispastic drugs should always be used with care as they induce significant tiredness and weakness. However, they can provide some useful background antispastic effect. Baclofen, dantrium, and tizanidine are the commonest prescribed. Oral cannabis (or at least a 50:50 ratio of THC and cannabidiol) may also be helpful and positive trials have been undertaken, but the agent is not yet licensed (except in Canada for neuropathic pain management).

However, often spasticity is localized and focal treatment is more appropriate. Nerve blocks with phenol and alcohol can be used. However, the intramuscular use of botulinum toxin is probably the most useful agent in the management of focal spasticity. The toxin is injected directly into the muscle and will block the release of acetylcholine from the nerve endings. This produces muscle relaxation over 3 or 4 days which lasts about 3 months. Occasionally more severe spasticity will need other measures such as the use of intrathecal baclofen. If contractures have resulted then often surgical correction by tenotomy, tendon lengthening, or muscle division is the only method that will get the limb back into a functionally useful position. Aggressive early management of spasticity is important in order to maximize any neurological recovery and prevent unnecessary complications.

Heterotopic ossification

This term is used when bone develops in an abnormal anatomical position in soft tissues. The prevalence in spinal cord injury is reported to vary between 5 and 50%. It commonly occurs around the hips and knees. It will cause a decrease range of movement as well as localized swelling and joint effusion. It will normally occur in the first few months after the injury and will only rarely begin later than one year post injury. Unfortunately treatment is difficult. Etidronate disodium is probably the most useful treatment. In severe cases surgical intervention can be required but is usually unsatisfactory. Some centres now use prophylactic etidronate disodium for about a year.

Deep venous thrombosis

Deep venous thrombosis (DVT) still remains a significant complication after spinal injury, with a small risk of death from pulmonary embolism. The risk is highest in the early days and weeks. Low-molecular-weight heparin or warfarin are usually used as a prophylactic, but some centres now use external pneumatic calf compression.

Pain and dysaesthesia

Peripheral pain is quite common in the early weeks after injury. Unfortunately burning pain can also continue for some months. It usually responds reasonably well to the use of carbamazepine, tricyclic antidepressants, gabapentin, or pregabalin. Pain from other sources such as osteoarthritis can also occur. It should be remembered that people with spinal cord injury do not always appreciate pain, or it is manifested in different ways, such as autonomic dysreflexia or worsening of spasticity. Other modalities such as transcutaneous nerve stimulation, acupuncture, and psychological techniques, such as relaxation and hypnotherapy or alleviation of depressive illness, can all help. Spinal cord stimulation is occasionally used and sometimes surgical techniques, such as dorsal root entry zone radiofrequency coagulation can be used. Other causes of pain such as nerve root compression should also be borne in mind.

Rehabilitation

There is no evidence that rehabilitation can promote natural recovery, but there is ample evidence that a coordinated multidisciplinary team can improve functional outcome for the person with a spinal cord injury. The team can ensure that functional abilities are maximized and that physical and psychological complications are kept to a minimum. The coordinated team input is vital in the early weeks and months after injury, but it is equally important that the team maintains contact over the period of discharge and indeed into the longer term.

Principles of rehabilitation

There is not room in this chapter to dwell on the basic principles of rehabilitation. However, it is important to state that modern rehabilitation practice is somewhat different from other medical specialities. It is based on the principles of education, and is a process in which the disabled person and the family must be involved for it to have any meaning. Rehabilitation should go beyond the narrower confines of physical disease but should also deal with the psychological consequences of physical disability and with the social milieu in which the disabled person has to operate. Rehabilitation is based around the concepts of impairment, activity, and participation restriction as outlined by the World Health Organization (WHO) in 2001. 'Impairment' is a simply a term that describes loss or abnormality of psychological, physiological, or anatomical

structure or function. Rehabilitation must go beyond impairment and should place such impairment within a functional context. 'Participation' describes the social context of disability. Rehabilitation can be defined as an active and dynamic process by which a disabled person is helped to acquire knowledge and skills in order to maximize physical, psychological, and social function. The basic nature of rehabilitation is to work with the disabled person and their family in partnership. The professional should impart accurate information and advice, give guidance on prognosis and natural history, and help the individual establish realistic goals in an appropriate social context. A key to successful rehabilitation is goal setting. The first goal should be a long-distance strategic aim. In the context of spinal cord injury this could, for example, include enabling the person to return to their previous home fully competent in wheelchair use. The overall strategic goal can also have a number of long-term subgoals in different spheres of life such as employment, home, and leisure. Once the long-term goal has been determined, steps will need to be defined in order to achieve that goal which in turn will involve the setting of a number of short- and medium-term goals. These shorter-term aims should be clearly stated. A useful mnemonic is SMART, which implies the goals should be Specific, Measurable, Achievable, Relevant, and Time limited. The implication of goal setting is that the team and indeed the disabled person should know when the goals have been achieved. Thus, valid and reliable outcome measures are important tools. It is not possible or desirable to outline tools that should always be used in spinal cord injury. The outcome measures will depend on the goals set. However, it is often useful to employ a general disability measure such as the Functional Independence Measure or, in the short term, the more physically orientated Barthel Score. Some of the standard scales employed in spinal cord injury are frankly of little value in monitoring progress. First to be developed was the Frankel Score. This has now been modified, at least in the United States of America, by the 1992 revised American Spinal Injury Association classification (see Table 24.13.2.3). This scale is now widely quoted in the spinal cord literature, but mainly

Table 24.13.2.3 American Spinal Injury Association classification (modified Frankel classification)

Grade	Loss of function	Comments
A	Complete	No sensory or motor function preserved in sacral segments S4/5
B	Incomplete	Sensory but not motor function is preserved below the neurological level and extends through the sacral segments S4/5
C	Incomplete	Motor function is preserved below the neurological level and the majority of key muscles below the neurological level have a muscle grade less than 3
D	Incomplete	Motor function is preserved below the neurological level and the majority of key muscles below the neurological level have a muscle grade greater than or equal to 3
E	Normal	Sensory and motor function is normal

Note: the key muscles are C5 (elbow flexors), C6 (wrist extensors), C7 (elbow extensors), C8 (finger flexors), T1 (small finger adductors), L2 (hip flexors), L3 (knee extensors), ankle dorsiflexors, long toe extensors and ankle plantar flexors.

in terms of helping to determine natural history and prognosis; it is not a tool for monitoring goal attainment.

Rehabilitation team

Obviously medical input is vital to the team, particularly in the early acute stages of management. Spinal cord injury consultants are now trained rehabilitation specialists and do not necessarily have surgical qualifications, at least in the United Kingdom. However, the training is comprehensive and obviously the consultants are able to manage the day-to-day medical, surgical, and rehabilitation aspects of spinal injuries. Spinal cord injury centres will always need input from a variety of other medical and surgical consultants. Nursing staff on the ward, who will have 24-h daily contact with the patients, are also clearly vital and many nurses will now have additional spinal cord injury or other specialist qualifications such as continence advisers or expertise in the management of sexual problems. The physiotherapist comes into play in the very early stages of management to minimize chest complications, particularly in those with high cervical cord lesions. Physiotherapy advice is helpful for appropriate positioning in bed and to prevent the complication of spasticity. However, once a patient is beginning to mobilize, the physiotherapist will be the key person to advise on wheelchair choice and teaching the individual to become familiar with the wheelchair and how to control the wheelchair in different circumstances. There are a number of advanced wheelchair skills that will eventually be learnt, such as back wheel balancing to allow manoeuvrability over rough ground and up kerbs, and sideways jumping for manoeuvrability in limited space. In those with lower cord lesions the physiotherapist could be involved in limited gait training using calipers and crutches. Orthotic devices such as the reciprocating gait orthosis (RGO) and hip guidance orthosis (HGO) may be considered in some cases. Recent development of the use of supported body weight gait training also emphasizes the key role of the physiotherapist. The physiotherapist can also help in the context of social participation by encouraging and assisting with the development of sporting activities. However, this latter assistance clearly overlaps with the role of the occupational therapist. The occupational therapist is usually concerned with assisting people to reach the highest level of physical and psychological independence, particularly with regard to personal care and appropriate adaptation of the home, work, and leisure environments. For example, the occupational therapist will be involved in the design of appropriate splinting to assist those with high cord lesions, such as writing or typing splints and feeding straps. There are now a significant variety of increasingly sophisticated assistive technology devices, which will enable even those with profound disabilities to remain reasonably independent. For example, environmental control equipment enables an individual to control simple aspects of life around the house, such as a door intercom, turning lights on and off, turning the pages of a book, controlling the television and telephone, and using a computer. These devices can now be controlled even by those with high tetraplegia using mouth sticks or breath control. The occupational therapist will often be involved in such advice, particularly at the time of discharge back into the home environment. If necessary, a psychologist may be particularly useful in enabling the person to make an emotional adjustment to their new disability. The social worker is likely to be involved with the family as a whole and only a small part of the job is to advise on disability benefits. Most of the social worker's task is to ensure that the disabled person and family integrate and adapt to the new disability as smoothly as possible. Others, such as vocational advisers, specialist nurses, and dietitians will all need to be involved at some point as part of a comprehensive spinal injury team.

Long-term issues in spinal cord injury

Discharge home

A particularly difficult time for the injured person is discharge home. Often the person will have spent several weeks or months in a spinal cord centre and returning home can be a traumatic process both for them and their family. Brief trial home visits will almost certainly have been carried out beforehand. These are particularly important to ensure that the house is appropriately adapted. Obviously in some cases a new house or bungalow will need to be purchased. A number of adaptations regarding access, both internal and external, hoisting gear, adaptations to the toilet, bathroom, and kitchen may all be required before the individual can return home. Environmental control equipment may need to be prescribed and installed. Psychological support is also vital over this period, not only for the injured person but also for their family. Anxiety and depressive illness are both quite common and will need active intervention. The community services and the primary care team will need to be involved. Planned discharges are vital and should involve a case conference between the hospital and community staff in order to ensure a smooth handover. However, at this time many people with spinal cord injuries will wish to move away from the more paternalistic hospital care that was important in the first few weeks after their injury. Most will choose to live as independently as possible, albeit with the help of their family or a personal assistant. Advice on the available financial support is important. If financial compensation from a personal injury claim is ongoing then (in the United Kingdom) a solicitor can be helpful at this point in order to arrange interim payments from the Court towards home adaptations, transport, and personal care.

Emotional problems

Obviously there are profound changes in a person's life following spinal cord injury. The refocusing of life ambitions can be a frustrating, anxious or depressing time. The attitude of family and friends will have further bearing over the period of adjustment. Regrettably, clinical depression is common and at some point occurs in at least 50% of individuals. Suicide can also occur. Although such problems are not always preventable, anxiety, depression, and adjustment problems can be alleviated by appropriate intervention. The role of medication, at least in the short term, can be helpful but probably most assistance can be gained from cognitive therapy or other forms of counselling and psychological support. Contact with others in similar circumstances can often be helpful and may be facilitated through the various peer support groups.

Sexual life

Sexual ability depends on the level and completeness of the spinal lesion. Sexual readjustment is an important part of the rehabilitation process for both men and women and for both the injured person and their partner. Self-image and self-confidence can be severely affected. Individuals should be counselled about the totality of sexuality, as there is a tendency for discussions to focus on penetrative sexual intercourse. In both sexes absence of genital sensation can be compensated for by use of other erogenous zones such as the breasts, neck, and mouth. Orgasm is sometimes possible even in complete spinal cord lesions. In women problems can result from lack of vaginal lubrication. For men there are various techniques and devices to restore erectile capacity. Most people with complete upper motor neuron lesions will have reflex but not psychogenic erections, but these are often not always sustained or strong enough for intercourse. In those with parasympathetic lesions reflex erections are usually not possible. Satisfactory erection can often be achieved either by the use of intracavernosal drugs or mechanical means such as vacuum erection aids and compressive retainer rings. However, the introduction of sildenafil has reduced the need for mechanical or injected assistance.

Fertility

Fertility is not usually reduced in women, although some can go through a time of amenorrhoea. However, fertility is generally reduced in men who have low sperm counts with diminished motility. Sometimes if ejaculation is not possible during intercourse it can be induced by direct stimulation or by electroejaculation. Fertility can also be improved by some of the modern assistive conception techniques such as in vitro fertilization and intracytoplasmic sperm injection. Women with spinal cord injury who become pregnant may have some problems in labour, particularly if the lesion is complete above T10. Autonomic dysreflexia is also a risk during labour. However, spinal cord injury is not in itself an indication for caesarean section.

Later medical complications

All the complications listed above in the acute phase can of course occur later. This is why it is so important for the multidisciplinary team to keep an overview of the individual in the long term. A few other problems are more likely to occur in the long term.

- Pathological fractures—there is a higher risk of osteoporosis in paralysed limbs and thus pathological fractures may occur with minimal trauma. For example, a minor fall from a chair or even a flexor spasm secondary to spasticity can result in a fractured leg. Treatment should usually be conservative.

- Post-traumatic syringomyelia—this occurs in about 4% of people and consists of an ascending myelopathy due to secondary cavitation in the central part of the spinal cord. The problem is commonly delayed several years after injury. It usually presents with pain in the arm with a characteristic disassociated sensory loss—reduced pain and temperature sensation but preservation of proprioception. Motor loss occurs of the lower motor neuron type and occasionally sensory loss can spread up to the face (syringobulbia). Additional motor loss can occur which is of the lower motor neuron type. Surgical treatment including decompression and drainage of the cavity may be necessary.

- Respiratory management—those with high cervical cord lesions with lost diaphragmatic function obviously require long-term ventilatory support. There are modern portable ventilators that can be readily mounted on a wheelchair. Speech is entirely possible with an uncuffed tracheostomy tube, which allows air to escape to the larynx. In some people it is possible to implant a phrenic nerve stimulator to achieve diaphragmatic ventilation.

Regrettably, it is still the case that individuals with long-term ventilator dependent requirements have significantly more morbidity and mortality than those with lower lesions.

Leisure pursuits

There are now a wide variety of leisure pursuits possible for those with spinal cord injury. Integration to able-bodied clubs and pursuits is obviously to be encouraged. However, there are also a reasonable range of sports and other clubs for those with spinal injuries. Wheelchair skills can be finely tuned to develop expertise in a variety of sports. Slowly physical access is improving to leisure and social outlets. Recent legislation, such as the Disability Discrimination Act in the United Kingdom, should further improve the situation.

Driving

Access to a motor vehicle is vital in modern society. Driving should be entirely possible for people with spinal cord injury, with the probable exception of those with very high cervical cord lesions. Automatic transmission is vital and hand controls are usually essential. Hand controls enable the individual to control the accelerator and brake functions from a lever or other device near the steering wheel. A variety of infrared devices to control secondary functions such as windscreen wipers, lights, and horn are now available. Very light powered steering makes life easier for those with weak grip. Those with higher cord lesions who still retain some useful shoulder and upper arm function can still drive a car using a variety of commercial devices attached to the steering wheel. A number of techniques can be taught to stow wheelchairs safely for those with paraplegia, and for those with higher lesions there are a number of mechanical wheelchair stowage devices. It is also quite possible to adapt a suitable vehicle to enable people to drive from their wheelchair. Financial advice is often required, combined with advice on the range and type of adaptations. In the United Kingdom there are now a number of driving assessment centres, often attached to rehabilitation centres.

Employment

Overall between 25 and 35% of people with spinal cord injuries return to work, either in their original occupation or into a new job after a period of retraining. The chances of employment are higher in the younger population and in those who already had a job at the time of injury. There is also positive correlation with the number of years in education. Employment should become more prevalent as the ability to work at home becomes more readily acceptable. The individual should be encouraged to contact the disablement employment advisers (in the United Kingdom) who can provide both advice and financial help in order to return to work. In other cases careers advice or retraining to obtain new qualifications may be more appropriate.

Information

The key to independence is access to good-quality information. In most countries there are now voluntary organizations that can provide good quality information and advice. These organizations can also act as pressure groups and many have been instrumental in promoting increased awareness and improved legislation for disabled people. The internet now provides an excellent source of information and advice, and training in computer literacy should certainly be encouraged by the rehabilitation team.

Conclusion and future prospects

Spinal cord injury can cause a range of challenges to the multidisciplinary rehabilitation team. As yet we cannot repair the injured spinal cord in humans, but developments in basic neuroscience are beginning to translate into practice. Repair of spinal injury, e.g. by transplant of glial cells cultured from the adult olfactory system, may be possible in the near future. There is also progress in the use of neuroprotective agents in the acute phase. Other modalities, such as the use of anti-NOGO monoclonal antibodies to augment plasticity and regeneration may also have a role to play in the future. However, our current inability to influence natural history should certainly not inhibit active and dynamic rehabilitation in order for the spinal cord injured person to resume as normal a life as possible. Significant improvements to overall survival and quality of life have been achieved in recent years with the application of modern rehabilitation and surgical practice as well as greater social awareness and understanding.

Further reading

Baptiste DC, Fehlings MG (2007). Update on the treatment of spinal cord injury. *Prog Brain Res*, **161**, 217–33. [a very good update on future repair possibilities.]

Blackwell TL, *et al.* (2000). *Spinal cord injury desk reference: guidelines for life care planning and case management*. Demos Medical Publishing, New York. [Probably the best guide to longer-term spinal issues—American orientated.]

Ditunno JF (1999). Predicting recovery after spinal cord injury: a rehabilitation imperative. *Arch Phys Med Rehabil*, **80**, 361–363. [A source of references regarding natural history.]

Dobkin B, *et al.* (2006). Weight-supported treadmill training vs over-ground training for walking after acute incomplete SCI. *Neurology*, **66**, 484–93. [A useful summary of this important new technique for gait training.]

Phys Med Rehabil Clin North Am. May 2007 issue. [A thoroughly up-to-date review of spinal cord injury issues. the May 2006 issue of *Prog Brain Res* also covers many related topics.]

Sisto S, Druin E, Macht-Sliwinski M (2008). *Spinal cord injuries:management and rehabilitation*. Mosby, St Louis. [The most up-to-date textbook.]

Trieschmann RB (1988). *Spinal cord injuries—psychological, social and vocational rehabilitation*, 2nd edition. Demos Medical Publications, New York. [One of the few volumes to thoroughly discuss the psychological, social and vocational problems after spinal injury; despite its age, it still remains very relevant.]

Wade DT (1992). *Measurement in neurological rehabilitation*. Oxford University Press, Oxford. [An invaluable textbook outlining a number of important and useful outcome scales.]

World Health Organization (1998). *The world health report. Life in the 21st century—vision overall*. WHO, Geneva. [A useful reference for a number of world health issues and in particular includes a discussion of the new classification of impairments, activities and participation.]

Spinal Injuries Association. SIA House, 2 Trueman Place, Oldbrook, Milton Keynes, MK6 2HH, UK. Telephone 0845 678 6633; fax 0845 070 6911; freephone advice line 0800 980 0501; http://www.spinal.co.uk [The association for spinal cord injured people—a good source of further information and advice.]

Diseases of the autonomic nervous system

Christopher J. Mathias

Essentials

The autonomic nervous system innervates all organs, producing predominantly involuntary and automatic actions that are mediated by two principal efferent pathways, the sympathetic and parasympathetic, which are neurochemically and anatomically distinct. Numerous synaptic relays and neurotransmitters allow the autonomic control of organ function at local and central levels to be integrated with the requirements of the whole body.

The peripheral and central components of the autonomic nervous system are frequently affected by diseases, conditions, or toxins. Autonomic disorders are described as (1) primary—without defined cause, including multiple system atrophy and acute/subacute dysautonomias; or (2) secondary—with specific defects or as a consequence of other conditions, including diabetes mellitus, Riley–Day syndrome, amyloid neuropathy, dopamine β-hydroxylase deficiency, spinal cord injury, and many drugs.

Clinical features

Failure of the autonomic nervous system—manifestations may be (1) sympathetic—adrenergic failure causes postural hypotension and (in men) disturbed ejaculation; cholinergic disturbances interfere with sweating; (2) parasympathetic—causing a fixed heart rate, erectile failure, and disturbed emptying of the urinary bladder and large intestine.

Overactivity of the autonomic nervous system—manifestations may be (1) sympathetic—characterized by hypertension, tachycardia and excessive sweating; (2) parasympathetic—leading to bradycardia. Mixed effects, peripherally and centrally, lead to complex clinical manifestations.

Investigation

Autonomic screening tests include (1) cardiovascular—(a) physiological—e.g. head-up tilt, heart rate responses, (b) biochemical—e.g. plasma noradrenaline, adrenaline, and dopamine levels, (c) pharmacological—e.g. clonidine growth-hormone stimulation; (2) sweating—e.g. thermoregulatory response to increasing core temperature by $1\,°C$. Autonomic dysfunction may also be suggested by a wide variety of other tests, including those of gastrointestinal, urinary/renal, sexual, respiratory and eye function.

Treatment

Symptomatic—(1) Orthostatic hypotension—management requires an approach combining (a) nonpharmacological measures—e.g. avoidance of sudden standing, high salt intake; and (b) pharmacological measures—e.g. fludrocortisone, sympathomimetics (e.g. ephedrine, midodrine). (2) Other symptoms—combined pharmacological and physical interventions can improve urinary incontinence, gastrointestinal motility disorders, and sexual dysfunction. Care is required to manipulate autonomic activity in patients with parkinsonian manifestations because the autonomic aspects are frequently exacerbated by antiparkinsonian agents.

Specific—some causes of autonomic dysfunction are treatable, e.g. infusions of immunoglobulin and plasmapheresis for immune-mediated neuropathy; hepatic transplantation in familial amyloid polyneuropathy.

Introduction

The autonomic nervous system has two principal efferent pathways, sympathetic and parasympathetic, that innervate and influence every organ in the body (Fig. 24.14.1). Autonomic actions are predominantly involuntary and automatic, as indicated by the term 'autonomic' first proposed by Langley in 1898. The structure of the autonomic system, with numerous synapses centrally and peripherally, as well as multiple neurotransmitters, provides flexible control of organ function locally and in an integrated manner—as in the maintenance of systemic blood pressure and body temperature. Disease of the autonomic nervous system may cause local or systemic effects.

Basic principles

The autonomic nervous system is primarily a visceromotor system, in which each efferent pathway is influenced in a variety of ways.

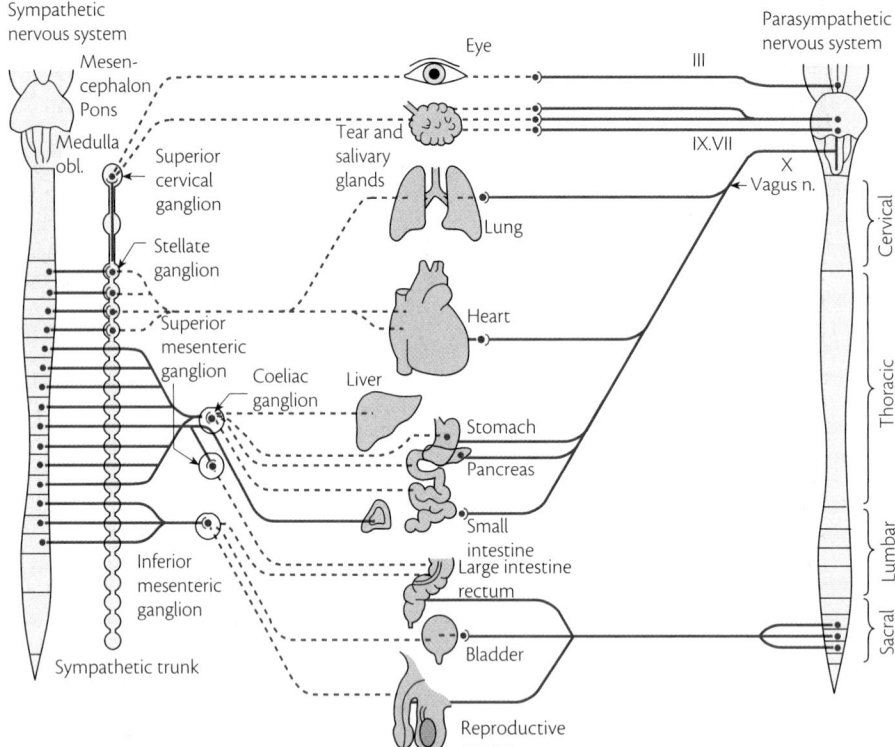

Fig. 24.14.1 Sympathetic (thoracolumbar) and parasympathetic (cranial and sacral) pathways that innervate a variety of organs. In: Schmidt RF, Lang F (eds) *Physiologie des Menschen*, 30th edition. Springer Verlag, Heidelberg.

Feedback and central integration are important and virtually every sensory pathway can influence its activity. For example, in spinal cord lesions, activation of visceral, skin, and muscle receptors below the level of the lesion influences autonomic activity and blood pressure through the spinal pathways, while heart rate responses to classic afferent baroreceptor pathways are retained. Key cerebral autonomic centres are in the hypothalamus, midbrain (Edinger–Westphal nucleus and locus ceruleus), and brain stem (nucleus tractus solitarius and vagal nuclei), and through intracerebral connections. Many other areas affect autonomic activity. Examples are the insular cortex, anterior cingulate gyrus, and amygdala, which are important in processing emotion and autonomic effects. Parasympathetic efferent pathways are craniosacral and sympathetic efferents are thoracolumbar; each has pre- and postganglionic fibres. The sympathetic ganglia are placed further from target organs than the parasympathetic ganglia.

Autonomic nerve terminals at target organs vary in complexity; they have the capacity to synthesize neurotransmitters and a host of mechanisms affects uptake and interaction with local or blood-borne chemicals (Fig. 24.14.2). There are differences between organs, especially the gastrointestinal system, in which the enteric nervous system is considered as a third autonomic division. The multiplicity of neural pathways, transmitters, and modulators results in selective control of responses in specific vascular territories and organs, making it a highly complex but precisely regulated and integrated system.

Classification

Diseases of the autonomic nervous system may result in central or peripheral damage or derangement; these may be primary with no known cause or secondary with specific abnormalities (dopamine β-hydroxylase deficiency), or strong associations with other diseases (Holmes–Adie syndrome or diabetes mellitus) (Table 24.14.1). Intermittent autonomic dysfunction may cause cardiovascular or sudomotor abnormalities (neurally mediated syncope or primary hyperhidrosis) (Box 24.14.1). Drugs are a common cause of autonomic dysfunction (Box 24.14.2).

Classification may be considered in various ways. Dysfunction may be localized (Box 24.14.3) or widespread. Diseases may result from lesions that are central (multiple system atrophy), spinal (spinal cord transection), or peripheral (pure autonomic failure), or from a highly specific biochemical deficit (dopamine β-hydroxylase deficiency). Some are age related, with presentation at birth (Riley–Day syndrome), second decade (vasovagal syncope), or adulthood (familial amyloid polyneuropathy). Autonomic failure commonly causes underactivity, but the reverse, overactivity, causes paroxysmal hypertension during autonomic dysreflexia in high spinal cord injuries. In neurally mediated syncope there is a combination of vagal overactivity and sympathetic withdrawal.

Clinical features

Sympathetic adrenergic failure causes orthostatic hypotension and ejaculatory failure in men, while sympathetic cholinergic failure causes anhidrosis. Parasympathetic failure results in a fixed heart rate, a sluggish urinary bladder and large bowel, and, in men, erectile dysfunction. With overactivity there may be hypertension, tachycardia, and hyperhidrosis, although parasympathetic overactivity causes bradycardia. In autonomic disorders there are many clinical manifestations, which may cause diagnostic difficulties, especially when the disorder is generalized.

The presenting complaints often provide clues. Palmar hyperhidrosis or gustatory sweating may indicate a localized disorder, or be a harbinger of widespread autonomic impairment, as the latter may complicate diabetes mellitus. A cardinal feature is orthostatic

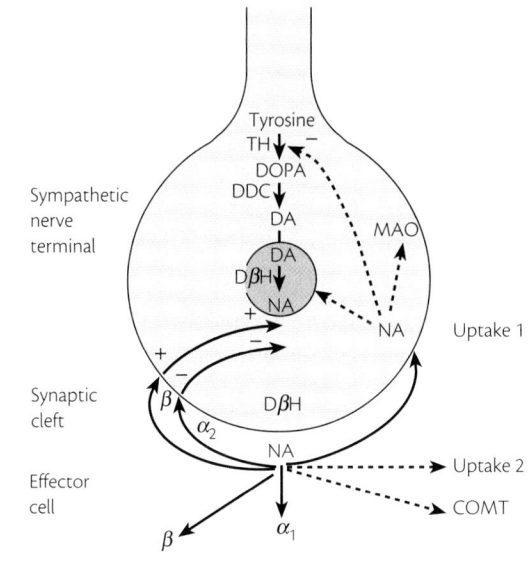

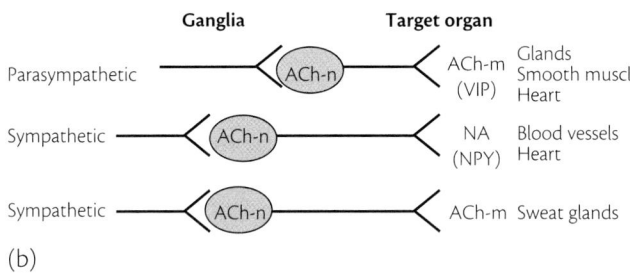

Fig. 24.14.2 Schema of some pathways in the formation, release, and metabolism of noradrenaline from sympathetic nerve terminals. Tyrosine is converted into dihydroxyphenylalanine (dopa) by tyrosine hydroxylase (TH). Dopa is converted into dopamine (DA) by dopa decarboxylase (DDC). In the vesicles, dopamine is converted into noradrenaline (NA) by dopamine β-hydroxylase. Nerve impulses release both dopamine β-hydroxylase and noradrenaline into the synaptic cleft by exocytosis. Noradrenaline acts predominantly on α_1-adrenoceptors but has actions on β-adrenoceptors on the effector cell of target organs. It also has presynaptic adrenoceptor effects. Those acting on α_2-adrenoceptors inhibit noradrenaline release and those on β-adrenoceptors stimulate noradrenaline release. Noradrenaline may be taken up by a neuronal process (uptake 1) into the cytosol, where it may inhibit further formation of dopa through the rate-limiting enzyme tyrosine hydroxylase. Noradrenaline may be taken into vesicles or metabolized by monoamine oxidase (MAO) in the mitochondria. Noradrenaline may be taken up by a higher-capacity, but lower-affinity, extraneuronal process (uptake 2) into peripheral tissues, such as vascular and cardiac muscle and certain glands. Noradrenaline is also metabolized by catechol-O-methyl transferase (COMT). Thus, noradrenaline measured in plasma is the overspill not affected by these numerous processes. (b) Outline of the major transmitters at autonomic ganglia and postganglionic sites on target organs supplied by the parasympathetic and sympathetic efferent pathways. The acetylcholine (ACh) receptor at all ganglia is of the nicotinic subtype (ACh-n). Ganglionic blockers such as hexamethonium thus prevent both parasympathetic and sympathetic activation. Atropine, however, acts only on the muscarinic (ACh-m) receptors at postganglionic parasympathetic and sympathetic cholinergic sites. The cotransmitters, along with the primary transmitters, are also indicated. NPY, neuropeptide Y; VIP, vasoactive intestinal peptide.

a) (From: Mathias CJ (2004) Disorders of the autonomic nervous system. In: Neurology in Clinical Practice. 4th edition. Eds. WG Bradley, RB Daroff, GM Fenichel, Jancovich J. Butterworth-Heinemann, Boston, USA, 2403-2240.) b) (From: Mathias CJ (1998). Autonomic disorders. In: Bogousslavsky J, Fisher M, eds. Textbook of neurology, pp 519–45. Butterworth-Heinemann, Massachusetts.)

Table 24.14.1 Classification of disorders resulting in autonomic dysfunction

Primary (aetiology unknown)	
Acute/subacute dysautonomias	Pure pandysautonomia
	Pandysautonomia with neurological features
	Pure cholinergic dysautonomia
Chronic autonomic failure syndromes	Pure autonomic failure
	Multiple system atrophy (Shy–Drager syndrome)
	Autonomic failure with Parkinson's disease
Secondary	
Congenital	Nerve growth factor deficiency
Hereditary:	
Autosomal dominant trait	Familial amyloid neuropathy
	Porphyria
Autosomal recessive trait	Familial dysautonomia (Riley–Day syndrome)
	Dopamine β-hydroxylase deficiency
	Aromatic L-amino acid decarboxylase deficiency
X-linked recessive	Fabry's disease
Metabolic diseases	Diabetes mellitus
	Chronic renal failure
	Chronic liver disease
	Vitamin B_{12} deficiency
	Alcohol induced
Inflammatory	Guillain–Barré syndrome
	Transverse myelitis
Infections:	
Bacterial	Tetanus, leprosy
Viral	HIV infection
Parasitic	Chagas' disease
Prion	Fatal familial insomnia
Neoplasia	Brain tumours—especially of the third ventricle or posterior fossa
	Paraneoplastic, to include adenocarcinomas of lung and pancreas, and Lambert–Eaton syndrome
Connective tissue disorders	Rheumatoid arthritis
	Systemic lupus erythematosus
	Mixed connective tissue disease
Surgery	Regional sympathectomy—upper limbs, splanchnic denervation
	Vagotomy and drainage procedures—'dumping syndrome'
	Organ transplantation—heart, kidney

(Continued)

Table 24.14.1 (*Cont'd*) Classification of disorders resulting in autonomic dysfunction

Primary (aetiology unknown)	
Trauma	Spinal cord transection
Miscellaneous	Subarachnoid haemorrhage
	Syringobulbia and syringomyelia
Intermittent autonomic dysfunction	See Box 24.14.1
Drugs	See Box 24.14.2

(From Mathias CJ (2003)).

(postural) hypotension (defined as a decrease in systolic blood pressure of more than 20 mmHg and in diastolic pressure of less than 10 mmHg on standing or head-up tilt—Fig. 24.14.3); this impairs perfusion of vital organs such as the brain. The symptoms vary from fainting (syncope, loss of consciousness), sometimes with ensuing injury, to fatigue and lethargy. Numerous factors in daily life enhance or reduce hypotension (Box 24.14.4). Some patients recognize these, with the self-introduction of corrective measures. Large meals, refined carbohydrate, and alcohol, which enhance postprandial hypotension, are avoided. Many sit down, lie flat, or assume curious postures, such as squatting or stooping, which now are recognized as raising blood pressure (Fig. 24.14.4). With time, symptoms of orthostatic hypotension wane, for reasons such as improved cerebrovascular autoregulation. In neurally mediated syncope, venepuncture or pain (in vasovagal syncope) or cervical movements and pressure (in carotid sinus hypersensitivity) cause hypotension and bradycardia. A history of impaired sweating and temperature intolerance, urinary disturbances, sexual dysfunction (in men), and gastrointestinal derangement (constipation), especially together with orthostatic hypotension, should suggest a generalized autonomic disorder (Table 24.14.2).

In the Riley–Day syndrome (familial dysautonomia) there is a history of consanguinity, usually in the Ashkenazi Jewish population. A family history is often elicited in vasovagal syncope and expected

Box 24.14.1 Intermittent autonomic dysfunction

- Autonomic (neurally) mediated syncope
  - Vasovagal syncope
  - Carotid sinus hypersensitivity
- Situational syncope
  - Micturition syncope
  - Swallow syncope
  - With glossopharyngeal neuralgia
  - Defecation syncope
  - Laughter-induced syncope
- Postural tachycardia syndrome
- Primary or essential hyperhidrosis

Box 24.14.2 Drugs, chemicals, poisons, and toxins causing autonomic dysfunction

Decreasing sympathetic activity

Centrally acting

- Clonidine
- Methyldopa
- Moxonodine
- Reserpine
- Barbiturates
- Anaesthetics

Peripherally acting

- Sympathetic nerve endings (guanethidine, bethanidine)
- α-Adrenoceptor blockade (phenoxybenzamine)
- β-Adrenoceptor blockade (propranolol)

Increasing sympathetic activity

- Amphetamines
- Releasing noradrenaline (tyramine)
- Uptake blockers (imipramine)
- Monoamine oxidase A inhibitors (tranylcypromine)
- β-Adrenoceptor stimulants (isoprenaline)

Decreasing parasympathetic activity

- Antidepressants (imipramine)
- Tranquillizers (phenothiazines)
- Antidysrhythmics (disopyramide)
- Anticholinergics (atropine, probanthine, benzatropine)
- Toxins (botulinum)

Increasing parasympathetic activity

- Cholinomimetics (carbachol, bethanechol, pilocarpine, mushroom poisoning)
- Anticholinesterases
- Reversible carbamate inhibitors (pyridostigmine, neostigmine)
- Organophosphorus inhibitors (parathion, sarin)

Miscellaneous

- Alcohol, thiamine (vitamin B deficiency)
- Vincristine, perhexiline maleate
- Thallium, arsenic, mercury
- Mercury poisoning ('pink' disease)
- Ciguatera toxicity
- Jellyfish and marine animal venoms
- First-dose effects of drugs (prazosin, captopril)
- Withdrawal of chronically used drugs (opiates, clonidine, alcohol)

From Mathias CJ (2003).

Box 24.14.3 Examples of localized autonomic disorders

- Holmes–Adie pupil
- Horner's syndrome
- Crocodile tears (Bogorad's syndrome)
- Gustatory sweating (Frey's syndrome)
- Reflex sympathetic dystrophy
- Idiopathic palmar/axillary hyperhidrosis
- Chagas' disease[a]

Surgical procedures[b]

- Sympathectomy—regional
- Vagotomy and gastric drainage procedures in 'dumping syndrome'
- Organ transplantation—heart, lungs

From Mathias CJ (2003).
[a]Listed here because it targets intrinsic cholinergic plexus in the heart and gut.
[b]Surgery may cause some of the disorders listed above such as Frey's syndrome after parotid surgery.

in familial amyloid polyneuropathy. A drug history, including exposure to chemicals, toxins, and poisons, is important.

A detailed clinical examination is necessary. Pupillary and associated ocular abnormalities occur in Horner's syndrome. To assess orthostatic hypotension, blood pressure should be measured with the patient lying flat, and after standing (or sitting if not possible). A fall in systolic blood pressure of less than 20 mmHg in the presence of appropriate symptoms does not exclude autonomic failure. Indeed, orthostatic hypotension may be unmasked, or enhanced, by factors such as ingestion of food and exercise. Furthermore, in the presence of vascular disease (such as carotid artery stenosis) even a small fall in blood pressure results in cerebral ischaemia. Lack of additional neurological features favours pure autonomic failure (with a good prognosis), while associated parkinsonism or cerebellar dysfunction suggests multiple system atrophy. Several disorders causing a peripheral neuropathy result in autonomic impairment. Basic bedside testing for glycosuria (in diabetes mellitus) or proteinuria (in systemic amyloidosis) provides important information.

Investigations

When an autonomic disorder is suspected, the first step is to determine if autonomic function is normal or abnormal. Autonomic screening tests (Box 24.14.5) have their value, but also their limitations. The majority are directed towards cardiovascular assessment and exclusion of autonomic underactivity. Tests of other systems are increasingly being made available. Normal screening results do not necessarily exclude an autonomic disorder, because, on the basis of the history and clinical examination, additional tests such as carotid sinus massage may be needed in patients with syncope. If autonomic tests are abnormal, further evaluation will determine the site and extent of the autonomic lesion, the functional deficit, and

whether it results from a primary or secondary disorder, because an accurate diagnosis is essential for prognosis and appropriate management. Thus, a 24-h ambulatory blood pressure profile and the effects of stimuli in daily life (such as food and exercise) help to manage orthostatic hypotension, while plasma catecholamine measurements (Fig. 24.14.5) and the clonidine growth hormone-stimulation test may separate out the different primary autonomic failure syndromes. Investigations may be needed to diagnose underlying diseases, and include neuroimaging studies (MRI or CT), serum amyloid protein (SAP) scans, sural nerve biopsy (with specific staining with monoclonal antibodies), detection of antibodies to specific receptors (such as the nicotinic acetylcholine receptor), and genetic testing. These tests should be combined with non-neurological investigations depending on the suspected diagnosis.

Management

This varies depending on the autonomic disease, the systems affected, and the functional autonomic deficit, and whether the disorder is primary or secondary. Treatment should take the underlying condition into account, e.g. in parkinsonian syndromes, where autonomic features may be worsened by antiparkinsonian therapy. In some diseases simple intervention is effective, such as unblocking a urinary catheter to resolve autonomic dysreflexia in high spinal cord lesions. In some, immunological therapy (intravenous gammaglobulin, plasma exchange) can reverse the autonomic neuropathy. Complex procedures such as liver transplantation are needed to reduce variant transthyretin levels in familial amyloid polyneuropathy. Multidisciplinary expertise may be needed, as in the Riley–Day syndrome and multiple system atrophy, to prevent complications, enhance survival, and improve quality of life. A combined approach is needed to reduce orthostatic hypotension, overcome urinary incontinence, alleviate gastrointestinal disturbances, and treat sexual dysfunction.

The management of orthostatic hypotension is outlined in Box 24.14.6 and Table 24.14.3; in individual disorders, modification is needed.

Individual autonomic disorders
Primary autonomic failure

The onset is usually slow and insidious in chronic autonomic failure, unlike the acute/subacute dysautonomias.

Chronic autonomic failure

The most common of these disorders is multiple system atrophy where there is additional neurological disease, unlike pure autonomic failure. Patients are usually middle aged at presentation although, with increasing awareness, it is being diagnosed in younger patients.

In pure autonomic failure, diagnosis is usually considered because of orthostatic hypotension. Nocturia (rather than incontinence) is frequent, presumably because fluid shifts from the peripheral to the central compartment elevate blood pressure and improve renal perfusion. Constipation often occurs. In temperate climates, hypohidrosis may not be recognized, unlike tropical areas where heat intolerance and collapse may occur. In men, impotence is common. The clinical and laboratory findings indicate widespread sympathetic failure, usually with parasympathetic deficits. Physiological and biochemical tests, along with limited neuropathological data, indicate a peripheral autonomic lesion. Management is directed predominantly towards reducing

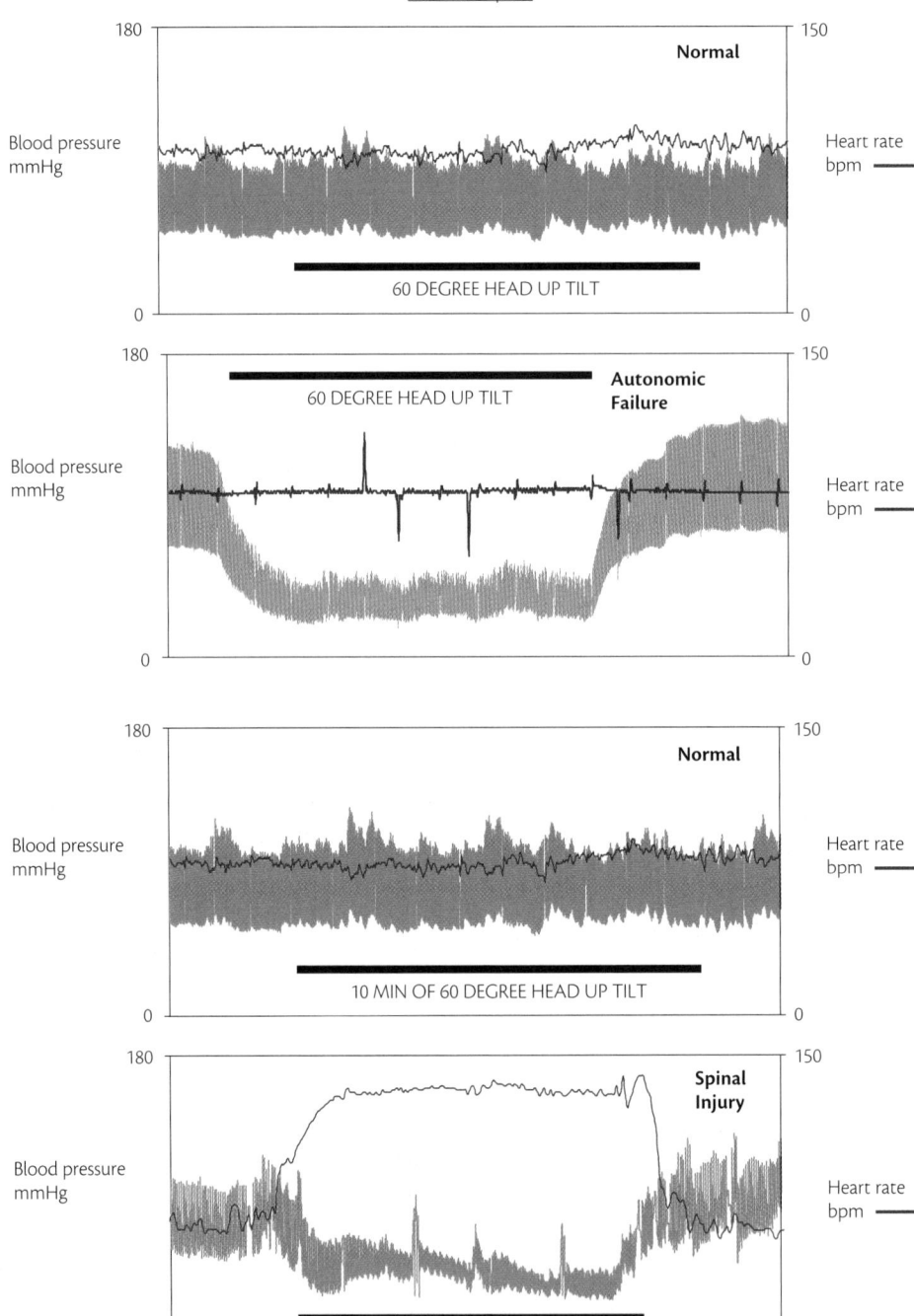

Fig. 24.14.3 (a) Blood pressure and heart rate before, during, and after head-up tilt in a normal individual (upper panel), and in a patient with autonomic failure (lower panel). In the normal individual there is no fall in blood pressure during head-up tilt, unlike a patient with autonomic failure in whom blood pressure falls promptly and remains low with a blood pressure overshoot on return to the horizontal. In this patient there is only a minimal change in heart rate despite the marked blood pressure fall. In each individual continuous blood pressure and heart rate were recorded noninvasively. (b) Blood pressure and heart rate measured continuously in a patient with a high cervical spinal cord lesion. There is a fall in blood pressure because of impairment of the sympathetic outflow disrupted in the cervical spine. Heart rate rises because of withdrawal of vagal activity in response to the rise in pressure.
(a) (Adapted from Mathias CJ. Orthostatic hypotension and orthostatic intolerance. In: Endocrinology 5th ed. Eds. De Groot, Jameson, Grossman. Elsevier, Philadelphia, PA, USA 2006, 2613–2632).
(b) (From: Mathias CJ. Orthostatic hypotension and orthostatic intolerance. In: Endocrinology. 5th ed. Eds. LJ De Groot, JL Jameson, de Kretser D, Grossman AB, Marshall JC, Melmed S, Potts JT, Weir GC. Elsevier, Philadelphia, PA, USA 2006, 2613–2632).

orthostatic hypotension. Although recovery does not occur, the overall prognosis in pure autonomic failure is good.

Multiple system atrophy is a nonfamilial and sporadic disorder with autonomic features and additional neurological (parkinsonian, cerebellar, and pyramidal) features (see Box 24.14.5) that occur at any stage and in any combination, in an unpredictable manner. Thus, patients may initially consult a range of specialists. It is randomly progressive, which adds to the difficulty of diagnosis. It is synonymous with Shy–Drager syndrome, the former name.

In multiple system atrophy the additional neurological features are predominantly parkinsonian; in a smaller number they are cerebellar and, as the disease advances, there is usually a mixture of features (Fig. 24.14.6). The neuropathological findings include striatonigral degeneration in multiple system atrophy (parkinsonian) and olivopontocerebellar degeneration in multiple system atrophy (cerebellar), with both changes often seen in either form. There is cell loss in various brain-stem nuclei (including the vagal nuclei), in the intermediolateral cell mass in the thoracic and lumbar spinal cord, and in Onuf's nucleus in the sacral spinal cord, which accounts for the various autonomic and allied abnormalities. The paravertebral ganglia and visceral (enteric) plexus are spared. A specific feature is the presence of intracytoplasmic, argyrophilic, oligodendrocyte inclusion bodies, within the brain and spinal cord. Most patients with multiple system atrophy have parkinsonian

---

Box 24.14.4 Factors influencing orthostatic hypotension

- Speed of positional change
- Time of day (worse in the morning)
- Prolonged recumbency
- Warm environment (hot weather, central heating, hot bath)
- Raising intrathoracic pressure: micturition, defecation, or coughing
- Food and alcohol ingestion
- Water ingestion[a]
- Physical exertion
- Manoeuvres and positions (bending forward, abdominal compression, leg crossing, squatting, activating calf muscle pump)[b]
- Drugs with vasoactive properties (including dopaminergic agents)

Adapted from Mathias CJ (2003).

[a]Raises supine blood pressure in chronic autonomic failure.

[b]These manoeuvres usually reduce the postural fall in blood pressure, unlike the others.

Table 24.14.2 Some of the clinical manifestations and possible presentations in primary chronic autonomic failure syndromes[a]

Cardiovascular	Orthostatic hypotension
Sudomotor	Anhidrosis, heat intolerance
Gastrointestinal	Constipation, occasionally diarrhoea, oropharyngeal dysphagia
Renal and urinary bladder	Nocturia, frequency, urgency, incontinence, retention
Sexual	Erectile and ejaculatory failure in men
Ocular	Aniscoria, Horner's syndrome
Respiratory	Stridor, involuntary inspiratory gasps, apnoeic episodes
Other neurological deficits	Parkinsonian and cerebellar/pyramidal features

[a] Certain features, such as oropharyngeal dysphagia and respiratory abnormalities (including those resulting from laryngeal fold paresis), occur in multiple system atrophy rather than in pure autonomic failure.

From Mathias CJ 1997 and 2003.

---

features and distinguishing multiple system atrophy from idiopathic Parkinson's disease, especially in the early stages, is difficult. Thus, the true prevalence and incidence of multiple system atrophy are not known. At postmortem examination up to a quarter of patients previously considered to have Parkinson's disease have the characteristic neuropathological features of multiple system atrophy.

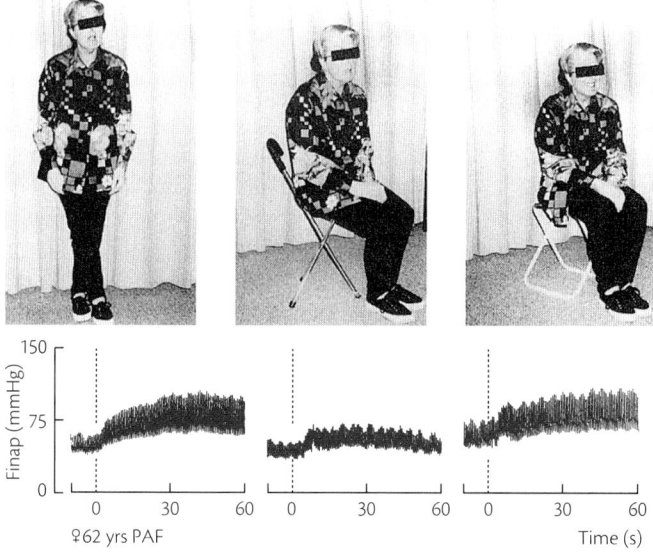

Fig. 24.14.4 The effect on finger arterial blood pressure (Finapres) of standing in the crossed-leg position, with leg muscle contraction (left), and sitting on a Derby chair (middle) or fishing chair (right), in a patient with orthostatic hypotension. Orthostatic symptoms were present initially when standing and disappeared on crossing legs and sitting on the fishing chair. Sitting on a Derby chair caused the least rise in blood pressure and did not relieve the patient's symptoms completely. (From Smith AAJ, Hardjowijono MA, Wieling W (1997). Are portable folding chairs useful to combat orthostatic hypotension? *Ann Neurol* **42**, 975–8.)

In multiple system atrophy (parkinsonian), bradykinesia and rigidity are often bilateral, with minimal or no tremor, unlike Parkinson's disease; however, this may not be a useful discriminator in an individual. Lack of a motor response to L-dopa is not indicative of multiple system atrophy, because two-thirds respond initially, although refractoriness and side effects eventually reduce the benefit. The presence of autonomic failure (especially orthostatic hypotension) and unexplained genitourinary symptoms with sphincter disturbance should alert one to the possibility of multiple system atrophy in patients with parkinsonian or cerebellar signs. Oropharyngeal dysphagia and respiratory abnormalities favour multiple system atrophy, although these often occur later. The combination of cardiovascular autonomic failure and an abnormal urethral/anal sphincter electromyogram, with characteristic clinical features, are virtually confirmatory of multiple system atrophy. Additional evaluation includes neuroimaging studies using MRI, positron emission tomography, and proton magnetic resonance spectroscopy of the basal ganglia, which are abnormal, at least in established cases. Clonidine growth hormone testing, based on α_2-adrenoceptor stimulation of the hypothalamus with release of human growth hormone-releasing factor, distinguishes central from peripheral autonomic failure and separates Parkinson's disease from multiple system atrophy (Fig. 24.14.7); whether this is the case in the early stages of parkinsonism and in patients on dopaminergic agents (which are growth hormone secretagogues) remains to be resolved.

The prognosis in multiple system atrophy is poor compared with idiopathic Parkinson's disease and pure autonomic failure. Akinesia and rigidity often worsen, with increasing refractoriness and side effects (including orthostatic hypotension) from antiparkinsonian therapy. As the disease advances there is often considerable immobility and difficulty in communication. In multiple system atrophy (cerebellar), worsening truncal ataxia causes falls and an inability to stand upright; orthostatic hypotension compounds the disabilities. Incoordination of the upper limbs, speech defects, and nystagmus result in further disabilities.

Respiratory complications include obstructive apnoea (caused by laryngeal abductor cord paresis) and central apnoea may necessitate tracheostomy. Oropharyngeal dysphagia enhances the risk of aspiration, especially when vocal fold paresis is present; a percutaneous feeding gastrostomy may be needed. Urinary bladder

Box 24.14.5 Investigations in autonomic failure

Cardiovascular

Physiological

- Head-up tilt, standing; Valsalva's manoeuvre
- Pressor stimuli: isometric exercise, cutaneous cold, mental arithmetic
- Heart rate responses: deep breathing, hyperventilation, standing, head-up tilt
- Liquid meal challenge
- Exercise testing
- Carotid sinus massage

Biochemical

- Basal plasma noradrenaline, adrenaline, and dopamine levels
- Plasma noradrenaline: supine and standing
- Urinary catecholamines

Pharmacological

- Noradrenaline—α-adrenoceptors, vascular
- Isoprenaline—β-adrenoceptors, vascular and cardiac
- Tyramine—pressor and noradrenaline response
- Edrophonium—noradrenaline response
- Clonidine—growth hormone response
- Atropine—heart rate response

Sweating

- Thermoregulatory: increase core temperature by 1 °C
- Sweat gland response to intradermal acetylcholine
- Sympathetic skin response

Gastrointestinal

- Barium studies, videocinefluoroscopy, endoscopy, gastric-emptying studies, anal sphincter electromyography

Renal function and urinary tract

- Day and night urine volumes and sodium/potassium excretion
- Urodynamic studies, intravenous urography, ultrasound examination, urethral sphincter electromyography

Sexual function

- Penile plethysmography
- Intracavernosal papaverine

Respiratory

- Laryngoscopy
- Sleep studies to assess apnoea/oxygen desaturation

Eye

- Lacrimal function: Schirmer's test
- Pupillary function: pharmacological and physiological

From Mathias and Bannister (2002).

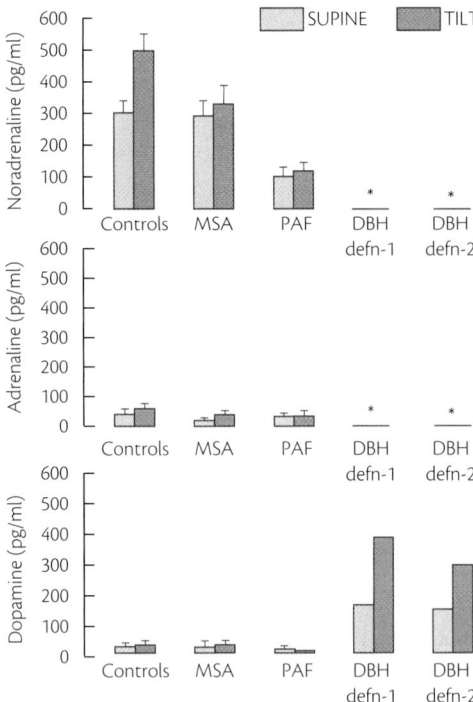

Fig. 24.14.5 Plasma noradrenaline, adrenaline, and dopamine concentrations (measured by high-performance liquid chromatography) in normal individuals (controls), patients with multiple system atrophy (MSA), patients with pure autonomic failure (PAF), and two individual patients with dopamine β-hydroxylase deficiency (DβH defn) while supine and after head-up tilt to 45° for 10 min. The asterisk indicates levels below the detection limits for the assay, which are less than 5 pg/ml for noradrenaline and adrenaline and less than 20 pg/ml for dopamine. Bars indicate ± standard error of the mean (SEM). (Adapted from Mathias CJ, Bannister R (2002). Investigation of autonomic disorders. In: Mathias CJ, Bannister R (eds) *A textbook of clinical disorders of the autonomic nervous system*, 4th edition, pp. 169–95. Oxford University Press, Oxford.)

dysfunction is distressing, and its management, together with management of constipation and, if appropriate, treatment of sexual dysfunction is important in improving quality of life. There is often a need for specialist therapists, including speech and language therapists, physiotherapists, dietitians, and occupational therapists. As the neurological decline is inexorable, supportive therapy is crucial in management of multiple system atrophy, and should incorporate the family, carers, and community along with the primary care medical practitioner and therapists.

Orthostatic hypotension and other features of autonomic failure appear more common in Parkinson's disease than previously thought. A current hypothesis places nonmotor lesions in the olfactory and brain-stem areas, including vagal nuclei, before onset of parkinsonian features. In Parkinson's disease the autonomic lesions appear peripheral and thus similar to pure autonomic failure. This is based on low basal plasma noradrenaline levels, and radionuclide and positron emission tomography studies, which indicate cardiac postganglionic sympathetic denervation. This is distinct from multiple system atrophy where the lesions are preganglionic. Orthostatic hypotension and autonomic failure may precede the motor and cognitive decline in diffuse Lewy body disease.

Acute/subacute dysautonomias

These disorders are relatively rare and consist of three main varieties: pure pandysautonomia (with features of both sympathetic and

Box 24.14.6 Outline of nonpharmacological and pharmacological measures in the management of postural hypotension due to neurogenic failure

Nonpharmacological measures

To be avoided

- Sudden head-up postural change (especially on waking)
- Prolonged recumbency
- Straining during micturition and defecation
- High environmental temperature (including hot baths)
- 'Severe' exertion
- Large meals (especially with refined carbohydrate)
- Alcohol
- Drugs with vasodepressor properties

To be introduced

- Head-up tilt during sleep
- Small, frequent meals
- High salt intake
- Judicious exercise (including swimming)
- Body positions and manoeuvres

To be considered

- Water ingestion
- Elastic stockings
- Abdominal binders

Pharmacological measures

- Starter drug—fludrocortisone
- Sympathomimetics—ephedrine or midodrine
- Specific targeting—octreotide, desmopression, or erythro-poietin

Adapted from Mathias CJ 2003b.

Table 24.14.3 Drugs used in the treatment of orthostatic hypotension

Site of action	Drugs	Predominant action
Plasma volume: expansion	Fludrocortisone	Mineralocorticoid effects—increased plasma volume
		Sensitization of α-adrenoreceptors
Kidney: reducing diuresis	Desmopressin	Vasopressin$_2$-receptors on renal tubules
Vessels: vasoconstriction (adrenoceptor mediated)	Ephedrine	Indirectly acting sympathomimetics
Resistance vessels	Midodrine,[a] phenylephrine, methylphenidate	Directly acting sympathomimetics
	Tyramine	Release of noradrenaline
	Clonidine	Postsynaptic α_2-adrenoceptor agonist
	Yohimibine	Presynaptic α_2-adrenoceptor antagonist
	L-Dopa	Prodrug resulting in formation of noradrenaline
Capacitance vessels	Dihydroergotamine	Direct action on α-adrenoceptors
Vessels: vasoconstriction (nonadrenoceptor mediated)	Triglycyl-lysine-vasopressin (glypressin)	Vasopressin$_1$-receptors on blood vessels
Vessels: prevention of vasodilatation	Propranolol	Blockade of β_2-adrenoceptors
	Indometacin	Prevents prostaglandin synthesis
	Metoclopramide	Blockade of dopamine receptors
Vessels: prevention of postprandial hypotension		
Autonomic ganglia	Caffeine	
	Pyridostigmine	Blockade of adenosine receptors
		Acetylcholine esterase inhibition
Heart: stimulation action	Pindolol, xamoterol	Intrinsic sympathomimetic
Red cell mass: increase	Erythropoietin	Stimulates red cell production

[a] Through its active metabolite.
(Adapted from Mathias CJ (2003). Autonomic diseases—management. *J Neurol Neurosurg Psychiatry* **74**, 42–7.)

parasympathetic failure); pandysautonomia with additional neurological features usually indicative of a peripheral neuropathy; and pure cholinergic dysautonomia. The prognosis in pandysautonomias is variable, with substantial recovery in some. Recovery after immunoglobulin therapy favours an immunological basis, and the possibility of a Guillain–Barré syndrome variant. In pure cholinergic dysautonomia, described mainly in children and young adults, there is widespread parasympathetic failure with blurred vision, dry eyes, xerostomia, dysphagia with middle and lower oesophagus involvement, severe constipation, and urinary retention. Clinical findings include dilated pupils, an elevated heart rate, dry and warm skin, a distended abdomen, and a palpable urinary bladder. Anhidrosis may result in hyperthermia. The term 'cholinergic' is used because both parasympathetic and cholinergic sympathetic pathways (to sweat glands) are affected. Sympathetic vasoconstrictor function is preserved and orthostatic hypotension does not occur.

Recovery is poor, but the prognosis is good if the condition is detected early. Management includes supportive therapy and adequate fluid and nutrient replacement of losses due to gastrointestinal and sudomotor failure. Barium studies should be avoided because contrast medium accumulates in the atonic colon. The differential diagnosis includes exposure to drugs, poisons, and toxins

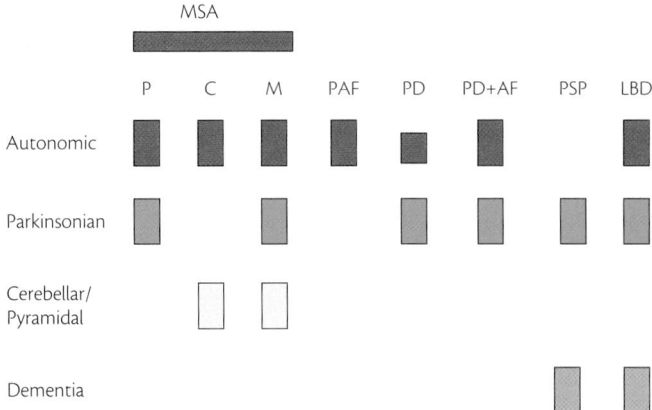

Fig. 24.14.6 The major clinical features in parkinsonian syndromes and in allied disorders with autonomic failure. These include the three major neurological forms of multiple system atrophy—the parkinsonian form (MSA-P, also called striatonigral degeneration), the cerebellar form (MSA-C, also called olivopontocerebellar atrophy), and the multiple or mixed form (MSA-M, which has features of both other forms)—pure autonomic failure (PAF), idiopathic Parkinson's disease (IPD), Parkinson's disease with autonomic failure (PD+AF), progressive supranuclear palsy (PSP), and diffuse Lewy body disease (LBD). (Adapted from Mathias CJ (1997). Autonomic disorders and their recognition. *N Engl J Med* **310**, 721–4; and Mathias CJ (2005). Cardiovascular autonomic dysfunction in Parkinson's disease and parkinsonian syndromes. In: Ebadi M, Pfeiffer RF (eds) *Parkinson's disease*, pp. 295–317. CRC Press LLC, New York.)

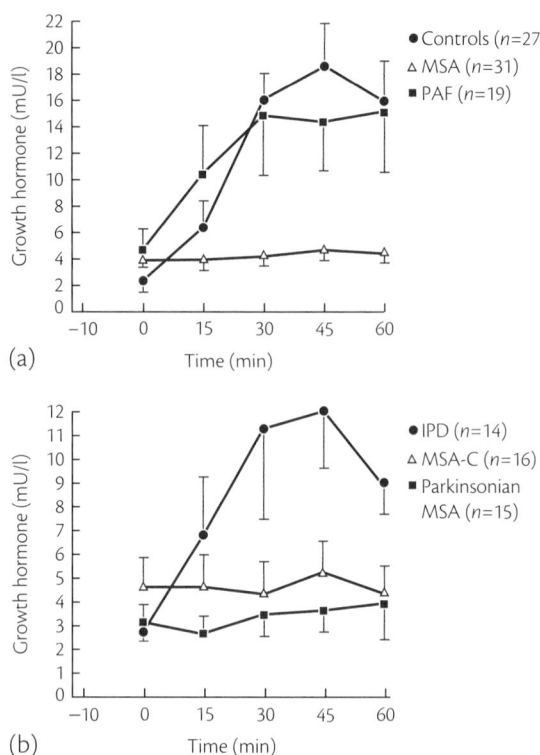

Fig. 24.14.7 (a) Serum growth hormone (GH) concentrations before (0) and at 15-min intervals for 60 min after clonidine (2 µg/kg per min) in normal individuals (controls), and in patients with pure autonomic failure (PAF) and multiple system atrophy (MSA). GH concentrations rise in controls and in patients with PAF with a peripheral lesion; there is no rise in patients with MSA with a central lesion. (b) Lack of serum GH response to clonidine in MSA (the cerebellar form and the parkinsonian forms) in contrast to patients with idiopathic Parkinson's disease with no autonomic deficit (IPD), in whom there is a significant rise in GH levels.
a) From Thomaides T *et al.* (1992). The growth hormone response to clonidine in central and peripheral primary autonomic failure. *Lancet* **340**, 263–6. b) From Kimber JR, Watson L, Mathias CJ (1997). Distinction of idiopathic Parkinson's disease from multiple system atrophy by stimulation of growth hormone release with clonidine. *Lancet* **349**, 1877–81.

with anticholinergic effects. Similar autonomic features occur in thorn apple (*Datura stramonium*) seed poisoning; the poisoning is associated with hallucinations, hyperreflexia, and clonic jerking movements, and recovery occurs in a few days. Botulism B affects cholinergic systems but spares motor systems, and substantial recovery is expected within 3 months of exposure.

Secondary disorders

Many disorders are associated with autonomic failure; a few are described here.

Riley–Day syndrome (familial dysautonomia)

This is a recessive genetic defect characterized by absent lingual fungiform papillae, lack of corneal reflexes, absence of overflow emotional tears, decreased deep tendon reflexes, and a diminished response to pain and temperature; the disease occurs typically in children of Ashkenazi Jewish extraction. An abnormal intradermal histamine skin test (absent axon flare) and pupillary hypersensitivity to cholinomimetics provide diagnostic confirmation. Prenatal diagnosis is possible with the genetic markers linked to chromosome 9 (q31). Autonomic underactivity and overactivity include lability of blood pressure (hypertension and orthostatic hypotension), intermittent hyperhidrosis, periodic vomiting, dysphagia, constipation, and diarrhoea. The neurological abnormalities include emotional and behavioural disturbances, and sensory deficits that result in injury to skin and joints. Skeletal problems (scoliosis), and respiratory (aspiration) and renal failure contribute to a poor prognosis. Anticipation of complications and adequate therapy have extended survival into adulthood.

Amyloid neuropathy

Deposition of amyloid into autonomic nerves can occur in reactive systemic (AA) amyloidosis (in chronic inflammatory disorders) or in immunoglobulin light chain (AL) amyloidosis (with lymphomas).

In familial amyloid polyneuropathy the sensory, motor, and autonomic abnormalities result from deposition in peripheral nerves of mutated variant transthyretin, produced mainly in the liver. Symptoms of a sensory and motor neuropathy often begin in adulthood in the lower limbs in Portuguese, Japanese, and Swedish forms (familial amyloid polyneuropathy I), and in the upper limbs in Indian/Swiss and German/Maryland forms (familial amyloid polyneuropathy II). These and other forms are now classified by the chemical and molecular nature of abnormal fibrillary protein, immunologically related to transthyretin. The most common is based on the first point mutations in the transthyretin gene associated with familial amyloid polyneuropathy—methionine-30 in the Portuguese form. The cardiovascular, gastrointestinal, and urinary systems are affected at variable stages, with the disease progressing relentlessly. Autonomic symptoms and signs may be dissociated, leading to underrecognition of the autonomic deficit. Liver transplantation reduces variant transthyretin levels and prevents progression of neuropathy. Its ability to reverse neuropathy is unclear, emphasizing the need for intervention before nerve damage occurs.

Dopamine β-hydroxylase deficiency

This rare disorder (with 14 patients reported, 2 of whom are siblings) was recognized in the mid-1980s. Enzymatic deficiency probably occurs at birth but presentation is often in childhood. Orthostatic hypotension has been the clue to recognition. The clinical features indicate sympathetic adrenergic failure, with sparing of sympathetic cholinergic and parasympathetic function; thus sweating is preserved and urinary bladder and bowel functions appear normal. In men, erection is possible but ejaculation difficult to achieve. Basal levels of plasma noradrenaline and adrenaline are undetectable but dopamine is abnormally elevated. Sympathetic nerve terminals, except for the enzymatic and functional defect, are otherwise intact, as demonstrated by electron microscopy, immunohistochemistry, and sympathetic microneurography.

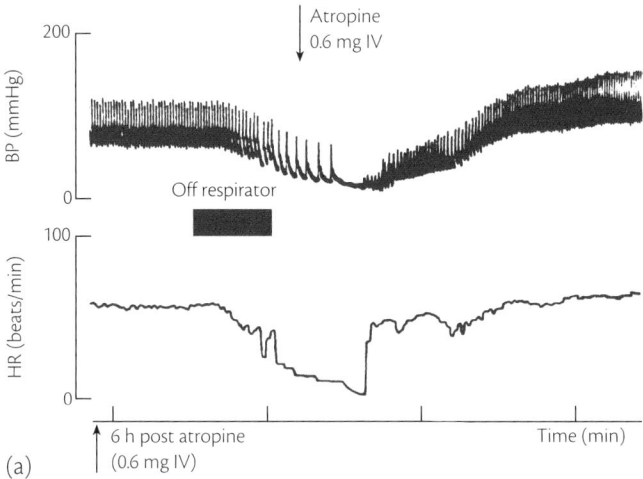

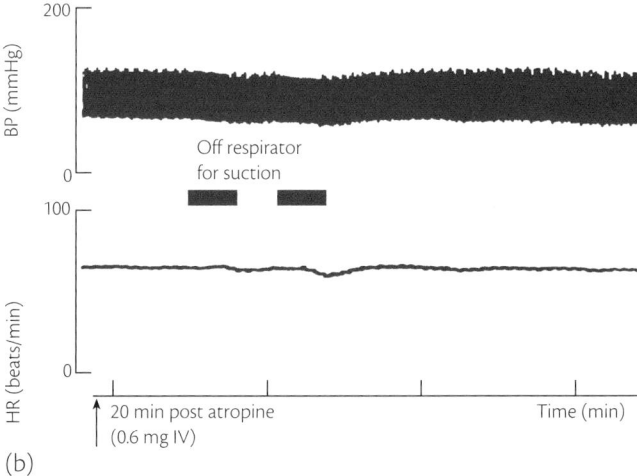

Fig. 24.14.8 (a) The effect of disconnecting the respirator (as required for aspirating the airways) on the blood pressure (BP) and heart rate (HR) of a recently injured tetraplegic patient (C4–5 lesion) in spinal shock, 6 h after the last dose of intravenous atropine. Sinus bradycardia and cardiac arrest (also observed on the ECG) were reversed by reconnection, intravenous atropine, and external cardiac massage. (b) The effect of tracheal suction 20 min after atropine. Disconnection from the respirator and tracheal suction did not lower either heart rate or blood pressure.
a) (From Frankel HL, Mathias CJ, Spalding JMK (1975). Mechanisms of reflex cardiac arrest in tetraplegic patients. Lancet ii, 1183–5.) b) (From Mathias CJ (1976). Bradycardia and cardiac arrest during tracheal suction—mechanisms in tetraplegic patients. European Journal of Intensive Care Medicine 2, 147–56.)

Effective treatment is with the prodrug L-dihydroxyphenylserine, which has a structure similar to noradrenaline and is converted by the enzyme dopa-decarboxylase (abundantly present in extraneuronal tissue such as liver and kidneys) to noradrenaline (see Fig. 24.14.2a).

Diabetes mellitus

In patients with long-standing diabetes, especially those on insulin, there is a high incidence of peripheral and autonomic neuropathy. Vagal denervation occurs earlier, impairing heart rate variability. Reduced sympathetic activity, e.g. in the feet, may increase blood flow substantially at an early stage before detection of neuropathy. Orthostatic hypotension may be enhanced by insulin. There may be sweating abnormalities (gustatory sweating), delayed stomach emptying (gastroparesis diabeticorum), impaired urinary bladder function (diabetic cystopathy), and impotence. Diarrhoea may be extremely distressing.

Spinal cord injuries

Autonomic dysfunction affecting many systems occurs in spinal injuries, depending on the lesion level and the degree of completeness. Cardiovascular dysfunction may be life threatening, especially in high lesions, in the acute phase in spinal shock, because lack of sympathetic activity with increased vagal tone may cause bradycardia and cardiac arrest (Fig. 24.14.8). After a few weeks, spinal shock passes and isolated spinal reflex activity returns; in cervical and high thoracic lesions, abnormal spinal activation results in the syndrome of autonomic dysreflexia. This is induced by cutaneous, skeletal muscle, or visceral stimuli below the level of the lesion. Thus, severe muscle spasms, an anal fissure, or a blocked urethral catheter can result in paroxysmal hypertension (due to increased spinal sympathetic nerve activity, independent of normal cerebral pathways) with associated bradycardia (because of preserved baroreceptor afferents and vagal efferent pathways—Fig. 24.14.9). Patients with lesions below T6 are spared. Patients with high lesions

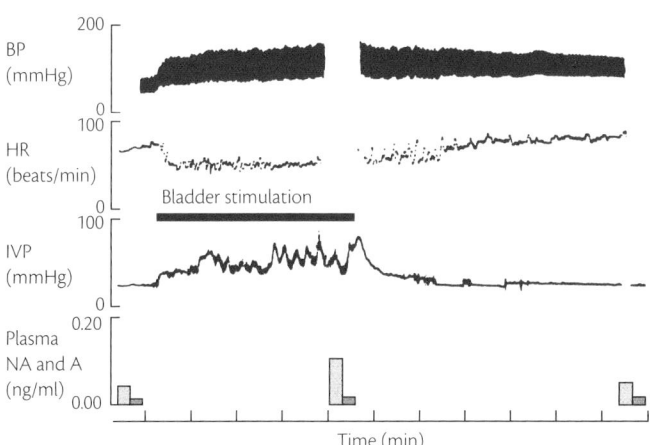

Fig. 24.14.9 Blood pressure (BP), heart rate (HR), intravesical pressure (IVP), and plasma noradrenaline (NA) and adrenaline (A) concentrations in a tetraplegic patient before, during, and after bladder stimulation induced by suprapubic percussion of the anterior abdominal wall. The rise in BP is accompanied by a fall in heart rate as a result of increased vagal activity in response to the rise in blood pressure. The level of plasma noradrenaline (open histograms), but not adrenaline (filled histograms), rises, suggesting an increase in sympathetic neural activity independent of adrenomedullary activation.
(From Mathias CJ, Frankel HL (1986). The neurological and hormonal control of blood vessels and heart in spinal man. *J Autonom Nervous Syst* Suppl, 457–64.)

are also prone to orthostatic hypotension, which compounds difficulties in management, especially shortly after injury.

Drugs

Dysfunction may result from an autonomic neuropathy (as induced by alcohol, vincristine, and perhexiline maleate) or through pharmacological effects. The latter may be expected with the sympatholytic agents, or may be a minor unexpected effect in susceptible individuals. An example is the anticholinergic bladder effects of disopyramide, which may cause urinary retention in patients with prostatic hyperplasia. A variety of toxins and poisons, including mushroom toxicity and botulism, as well as nerve gases such as sarin, affect the autonomic nervous system. The first-dose effect of angiotensin-converting enzyme (ACE) inhibitors and

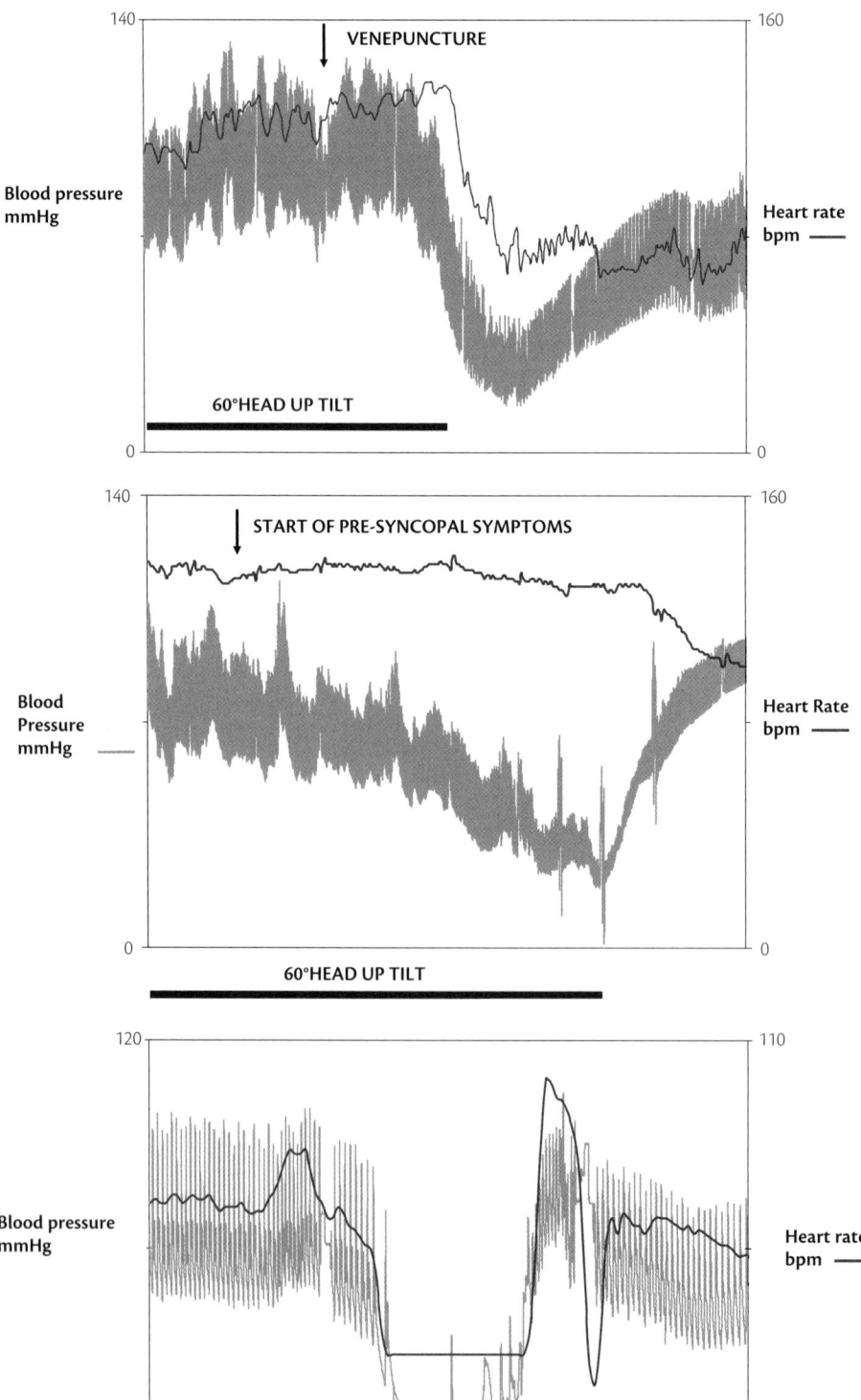

Fig. 24.14.10 (a) Blood pressure and heart rate with continuous recordings in a patient with the mixed (cardioinhibitory and vasodepressor) form of vasovagal syncope.
(b) Blood pressure and heart rate with continuous recordings in a patient with the predominantly vasodepressor form of vasovagal syncope.
(c) Blood pressure and heart rate with continuous recordings in a patient with the cardioinhibitory form of vasovagal syncope.
(In: Endocrinology. 5th ed. Eds. LJ De Groot, JL Jameson, de Kretser D, Grossman AB, Marshall JC, Melmed S, Potts JT, Weir GC. Elsevier, Philadelphia, PA, USA 2006, 2613–2632.)

prazosin may be mediated by the Jarisch–Bezold reflex. Autonomic overactivity may occur during withdrawal of clonidine, alcohol, and opiates.

Intermittent autonomic dysfunction

There is usually no damage to autonomic nerves and autonomic dysfunction is often short-lived.

Autonomic (neurally) mediated syncope

Syncope (fainting, loss of consciousness) may result from an intermittent and transient abnormality with increased cardiac parasympathetic (causing severe bradycardia, cardioinhibition) and sympathetic withdrawal (causing hypotensive vasodepression). The episodes may be cardioinhibitory, vasodepressor, or mixed (Fig. 24.14.10). There are three major groups: vasovagal syncope, carotid sinus hypersensitivity, and situational syncope. Between episodes, screening autonomic tests usually reveal no abnormalities. The most common disorder is vasovagal syncope. This is often familial and more likely in females; it may present in the early teenage years and is induced by stimuli such as the sight of blood, pain, needles, and at times even discussion of venepuncture. Hypotension is more likely in the upright position and may occur while standing still, especially in warm weather, and with salt and fluid depletion.

Testing includes head-up tilt, which sometimes may need to be prolonged for about 45 minutes, or with introduction of a provocative stimulus such as venepuncture, ideally during head-up tilt. A variety of physiological (head-up tilt plus lower body negative pressure) or pharmacological (isoprenaline infusions or glyceryl trinitrate) stimuli have been used to unmask an episode, but may result in false-positive results. Cardiac conduction disorders and other causes of syncope (neurological or metabolic) should be excluded. Treatment includes reducing or preventing exposure to precipitating causes and behavioural psychotherapy in patients with phobias. Added salt, fluid repletion, and exercise are often useful. Techniques to increase sympathetic activity and maintain or raise blood pressure (such as sustained hand grip) and to prevent pooling (calf muscle activation) are helpful, especially in patients who have a warning window of symptoms before syncope. Sitting down, or lying flat, with the legs raised should prevent most episodes. Drugs such as fludrocortisone, vasopressor agents (ephedrine and midodrine), and antidepressants such as the serotonin selective reuptake inhibitors (SSRIs) have been used. β-Adrenergic blockers provide no benefit in most cases. The long-term prognosis is favourable.

In older people, carotid sinus hypersensitivity is increasingly recognized, especially in those with falls of otherwise unknown cause(Fig. 24.14.11). A classic history of syncope induced by head movements or collar tightening may be provided, although in many the precipitating factors are unclear. Carotid sinus massage should be performed in the laboratory with the requisite precautions, ideally using continuous blood pressure and heart rate recordings, with the patient also tilted head up, because hypotension is more likely to occur when sympathetic activation is needed. Treatment, especially of the cardioinhibitory forms, includes a cardiac demand pacemaker; vasodepressor forms may require pressor agents. Surgical denervation of the carotid sinus has been used successfully, especially where unilateral hypersensitivity occurs.

A variety of other stimuli, acting through short-lived autonomic mechanisms, can also cause syncope, considered under situational syncope. This may be together with factors such as heat or drugs that cause vasodilatation or reduce intravascular volume, thus increasing the tendency to hypotension and syncope. Examples include syncope associated with glossopharyngeal neuralgia (caused by swallowing), or induced by micturition, defecation, coughing, laughing, and playing wind instruments.

Postural tachycardia syndrome

This disorder is often observed in people below the age of 50 years, mainly women, with dizziness on postural change or with modest exertion. The symptoms appear to disrupt lives almost disproportionately. There is a substantial rise in heart rate (over 30 beats/min or to 120 beats/min) without orthostatic hypotension, hence the term 'postural (orthostatic) tachycardia syndrome', or PoTS (Fig. 24.14.12). Syncope may occur. Associated disorders include a partial autonomic neuropathy, chronic fatigue syndrome, mitral valve prolapse, and hyperventilation. A noradrenaline transporter deficit, rarely genetically caused, or as a result of drugs, may be causative. A common association is the joint hypermobility syndrome (Ehlers–Danlos syndrome III). The relationship of PoTS to previously considered psychosomatic disorders, such as soldier's heart

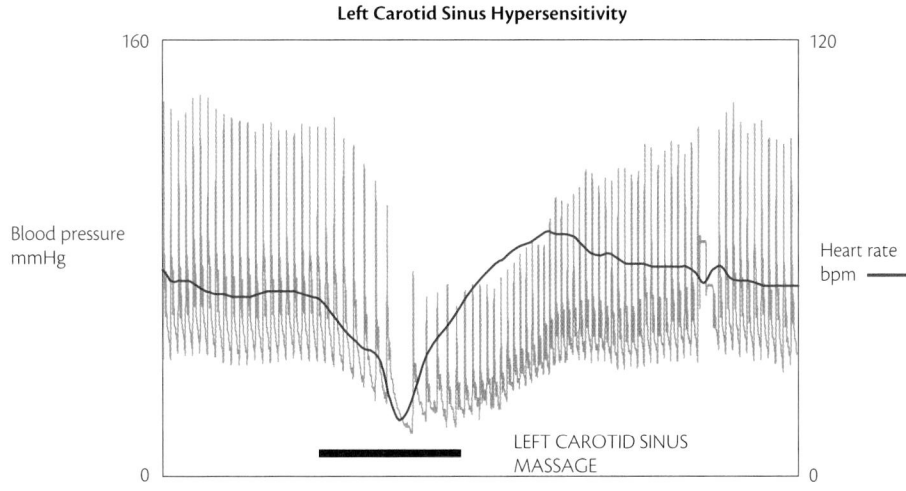

Left Carotid Sinus Hypersensitivity

Blood pressure mmHg

Heart rate bpm ——

LEFT CAROTID SINUS MASSAGE

Fig. 24.14.11 Continuous blood pressure and heart rate measured noninvasively in a patient with falls of unknown aetiology. Left carotid sinus massage caused a fall in both heart rate and blood pressure. The findings indicate the mixed (cardioinhibitory and vasodepressor) form of carotid sinus hypersensitivity.

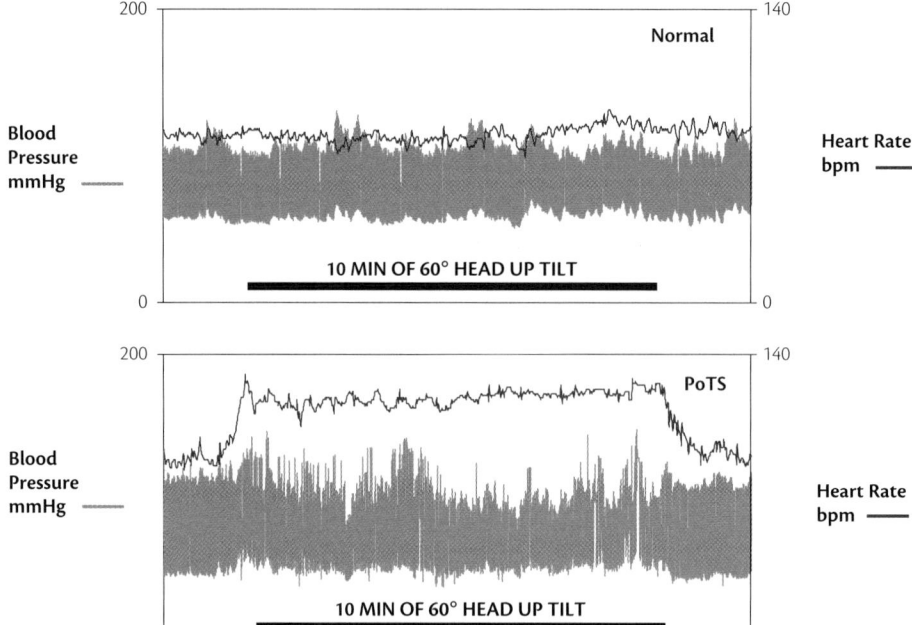

Fig. 24.14.12 Blood pressure and heart rate measured continuously before, during, and after 60° head-up tilt in a normal person (upper panel), and in a patient with the postural tachycardia syndrome (PoTS) (lower panel).
(Adapted from Mathias CJ, Bannister R (2002)).

or da Costa's syndrome, is not known. Investigation should include the causes and associated factors, which is an integral part of management. Treatment includes nonpharmacological measures as used in neurally mediated syncope, such as salt and fluid repletion and graded exercise. Similarly drugs to raise blood pressure may be used, except for excluding those that increase heart rate, such as ephedrine. Cardioselective β-adrenergic blockers have a role, but not when the tachycardia is in response to vascular pooling when upright. The selective sinus node blocker, ivabradine, may have a role in reducing tachycardia. Spontaneous recovery may occur in some.

Primary or essential hyperhidrosis

Excessive sweating without an underlying cause (such as hyperthyroidism, infection, etc.) may be familial or sporadic, and it may be localized, involving areas such as the palms, axillae, soles of the feet, or the face. In some there is widespread sweating. It can be distressing and socially destructive. Factors that provoke sweating include stress, heat, and exercise. In primary hyperhidrosis, investigation reveals no underlying pathology or autonomic deficit. Treatment options include percutaneous surgical sympathectomy for upper limb and facial sweating; in some, after surgery a complication is compensatory hyperhidrosis in the innervated areas, which some find worse than the original problem; treatment is with low doses of clonidine and anticholinergics (such as probanthine), iontophoresis for palmar and plantar sweating, and botulinum toxin injections for localized areas. Cognitive–behavioural therapy and anxiolytics, including SSRIs, have a role.

Further reading

Appenzeller O, Oribe E (eds) (1997). *The autonomic nervous system*, 5th edition. Elsevier Biomedical, Amsterdam.

Low PA (ed.) (1997). *Clinical autonomic disorders*, 2nd edition. Little Brown & Co., Boston, MA.

Mathias CJ (2003). Autonomic diseases—clinical features and laboratory evaluation. *J Neurol Neurosurg Psychiatry*, **74**, 31–41.

Mathias CJ (2003). Autonomic diseases—management. *J Neurol Neurosurg Psychiatry*, **74**, 42–7.

Mathias CJ, Bannister R (2002). *Autonomic failure: a textbook of clinical disorders of the autonomic nervous system*, 4th edition. Oxford University Press, Oxford.

Mathias CJ (2009). Autonomic Dysfunction. *In Neurology: A Queen Square Textbook*. (Eds. Clarke, C., Howard, R., Rossor, M. and Shorvon, S.D). pp 871–982. Oxford: Wiley Blackwell.

24.15

The motor neuron diseases

Michael Donaghy

Essentials

Motor neuron diseases are a family of conditions that lead to selective loss of function of the lower and/or upper motor neurons controlling the voluntary muscles of the limbs or bulbar region. Precise diagnosis is essential for prognosis, identification of those diseases with genetic implications, and for (in a very few cases) specific treatment.

Clinical features, diagnosis, and treatment

Clinical signs of lower motor neuron involvement are muscle wasting, fasciculation, and flaccid weakness; upper motor neuron involvement produces spasticity, clonus, extensor plantar responses and weakness. Sensation and cognition are generally normal on simple clinical assessment.

Accurate diagnosis depends on (1) clinical and electrophysiological classification as to whether the disease involves the upper or the lower motor neurons, or both; augmented by (2) the age of onset; (3) the rate of deterioration; and (4) whether there is familial occurrence.

Motor neuron diseases are incurable for the most part, hence treatment must aim to overcome, or minimize, the diverse disabilities.

Particular motor neuron diseases

Amyotrophic lateral sclerosis—a diffuse neurodegenerative disorder of (usually) unknown cause, with the brunt borne by motor neurons. Typically presents with (1) bulbar symptoms—dysphagia, dysphonia, and inhalation of foodstuffs; or (2) spinal symptoms—usually wasting and weakness of one limb. Upper and lower motor neuron signs in all three body regions are required for a definite diagnosis. There is no specific curative treatment: the disease progresses relentlessly, with few surviving beyond 5 years from diagnosis.

Lower motor neuron syndromes—these disorders generally follow a much more benign course than amyotrophic lateral sclerosis, and include (1) proximal childhood spinal muscular atrophy with SMN mutations, (2) other inherited spinal muscular atrophies, (3) hexosaminidase deficiency, (4) X-linked recessive bulbospinal neuronopathy (Kennedy's disease), (5) hereditary bulbar palsy of infancy and childhood, (6) monomelic, focal, and segmental motor neuronopathies, (7) postirradiation lumbosacral radiculopathy, (8) postpolio syndrome, and (9) multifocal motor neuropathy with conduction block—which may improve with high-dose intravenous human immunoglobulin therapy.

Upper motor neuron syndromes—these are the rarest forms of motor neuron disease and include (1) primary lateral sclerosis, (2) hereditary spastic paraplegia, (3) lathyrism, and (4) konzo.

Introduction

Motor neuron diseases result from selective loss of function of the lower and/or upper motor neurons controlling the voluntary muscles of the limbs or bulbar region. The term 'motor neuron disease' is best used to describe a family of diseases within which there is extensive differential diagnosis (Table 24.15.1); in the past the term has been used synonymously with amyotrophic lateral sclerosis (ALS), one of the most serious of these conditions. Precise diagnosis is essential for prognosis, for identifying those diseases with genetic implications, and appropriate use of immunosuppressant therapy for patients with certain acquired lower motor neuron disorders.

Accurate diagnosis requires clinical and electrophysiological classification as to whether the disease involves the upper or the lower motor neurons, or both. This anatomical differentiation is augmented by the age of onset, the rate of deterioration, and familial occurrence. Sensation and cognition are generally normal on simple clinical assessment, but several motor neuron disorders manifest other neurological features, such as ALS with frontotemporal dementia.

Motor neuron diseases are incurable for the most part and hence treatment must aim to overcome, or minimize, the diverse disabilities. Malnutrition due to dysphagia can be circumvented by nasogastric tube feeding or percutaneous endoscopic gastrostomy (PEG). Various forms of assisted respiration offset respiratory muscle weakness, including intermittent positive pressure ventilation (NIPPV) via a nasal mask. Limb spasticity can be reduced by baclofen, dantrolene, or diazepam. Wheelchairs and arm appliances may overcome inadequate limb function. Electronic communication devices should be supplied to those whose speech is incomprehensible. Amitriptyline may help contain the embarrassing emotional lability of pseudobulbar palsy. Housing and workplace modifications can allow patients to maintain independence despite their disability.

The motor neuron diseases, particularly ALS, are a focus of intensive neuroscience research. Therapeutic discoveries from the study of the human disease and animal models may affect the course of this disease in the foreseeable future.

Combined upper and lower motor neuron syndromes

Amyotrophic lateral sclerosis

Amyotrophic lateral sclerosis occurs worldwide, usually with an incidence of about 2 per 100 000 population and a prevalence of 6 per 100 000. It is more common in men and the incidence increases with advancing age; it is unusual before the fifth decade of life. The cause of the common sporadic form of amyotrophic lateral sclerosis is quite unknown. Its incidence is particularly high in areas of the western Pacific, particularly in Guam and the Japanese Kii Peninsula, where it tends to occur in younger adults and can be associated with dementia or parkinsonism. However, it is generally agreed now that this is a different disease, characterized by tau pathology rather than ubiquitinated inclusions.

Autosomal dominant inheritance is evident in approximately 5% of patients with adult-onset amyotrophic lateral sclerosis. Roughly 20% of familial amyotrophic lateral sclerosis is associated with more than 100 different missense mutations of the Cu/Zn superoxide dismutase (SOD1) gene on chromosome 21, which catalyses conversion of toxic superoxide anion radicals to hydrogen peroxide. The disease associated with various SOD1 mutations shows varying degrees of penetrance and a variable phenotype. It tends to begin earlier in adulthood and may involve minor sensory symptoms. SOD1 mutations are thought to damage cells by toxic gain of function, although protein misfolding may cause intracellular inclusions. Mutations of other genes associated with amyotrophic lateral sclerosis include Alsin and senataxin in juvenile forms, and a variety of other loci have been identified.

Amyotrophic lateral sclerosis is increasingly viewed as a diffuse neurodegenerative disorder with the brunt borne by motor neurons, which are particularly large neurons supporting long axons. The process of neuronal cell death may reflect a cascade process variously involving genetic factors, oxidative stress, excitotoxicity due to glutamate, mitochondrial dysfunction, perturbed axonal transport and cytoskeleton formation, intracellular protein aggregation, inflammatory cascade, apoptotic cascades, and toxic factors. Until the triggering events are understood, the question of disease subtypes and the design of pharmacological interventions will remain elusive.

Pathology

Lower motor neurons are lost from clinically affected areas of the spinal cord and brain stem. Surviving neurons may show intracytoplasmic inclusions, both the almost invariable ubiquitinated form and eosinophilic Bunina bodies, and proximal axonal accumulations of neurofilaments (spheroids). The motor cortex is depleted of Betz cells and the pyramidal tracts degenerate. There is relative sparing of Onuf's nucleus in the sacral spinal cord, and the brainstem ocular motor nuclei, which explains the preservation of micturition control and eye movements respectively. It is becoming increasingly recognized that other populations of neurons can also degenerate in motor neuron disease even though this is not usually evident clinically. These include peripheral sensory neurons and Clarke's column neurons. Up to 10% of patients develop a mild dementia, often of a frontal lobe type. These recent findings show that either amyotrophic lateral sclerosis is a generalized neurodegenerative disorder, in which the motor neurons take the vast brunt of the disease, or it sometimes overlaps with other neurodegenerations. However, for the practical purpose of clinical diagnosis early in the disease, amyotrophic lateral sclerosis should be regarded as having purely motor manifestations.

Clinical features

At presentation, patients have either bulbar or spinal symptoms, although both usually become evident as the disease progresses. The El Escorial research diagnostic criteria for amyotrophic lateral sclerosis require evidence of both upper and lower motor neuron signs in all three body regions for a definite diagnosis, with lesser involvements for probable or possible diagnosis. In everyday practice most diagnoses are made at these earlier, incomplete stages.

The bulbar form causes dysphagia, dysphonia, and inhalation of foodstuffs due to weakness of the tongue, pharynx, and larynx. The tongue is wasted, weak, and fasciculating, palatal movements are reduced, and the ability to cough explosively is lost due to vocal cord paralysis. This bulbar palsy is usually accompanied, or even preceded, by varying degrees of pseudobulbar involvement. The tongue is spastic and immobile with 'hot potato' speech and difficulty in inhibiting emotional responses such as laughing or crying. Ventilatory respiratory failure may develop due to weakness of the diaphragm and intercostal muscles. Occasionally, amyotrophic lateral sclerosis can present with dyspnoea. Diaphragm weakness can be detected clinically by noting that the upper abdomen is drawn inwards, rather than outwards, during the second half of inspiration. Furthermore, the forced vital capacity is substantially lower when the patient is lying down compared with standing, because the weight of the liver no longer assists diaphragmatic descent.

The spinal form of amyotrophic lateral sclerosis usually presents with wasting and weakness of one limb, usually as intrinsic hand muscle wasting or foot drop. Occasionally the initial weakness predominantly affects the musculature of the shoulder girdle. Asymptomatic involvement of other limbs is often evident on examination. It is diagnostically important to demonstrate combined upper and lower motor neuron signs in at least two limbs. Wasted fasciculating muscles exhibiting clonus or hyper-reflexia are also a helpful finding. With time the limbs become useless due to progressive denervation. Patients become wheelchair or bed bound, or unable to use their arms for grooming or feeding. Despite enforced recumbency, decubitus ulcers are relatively unusual because autonomic regulation of skin blood flow and secretion is unaffected. Sphincter control is not affected, although practical difficulties in excretion may result from immobility and abdominal wall weakness preventing the exertion of intra-abdominal pressure.

Table 24.15.1 Classification of the motor neuron diseases

Disease	Inheritance[a]	Age of onset[b]
Combined upper and lower motor neuron syndromes		
Amyotrophic lateral sclerosis:		
sporadic	–	A, E
familial adult onset		
familial juvenile onset	AR	C
Lower motor neuron syndromes		
Hereditary		
Proximal childhood SMA (with *SMN* mutations):		
type I Werdnig Hoffman disease	AR	I
type II intermediate form	AR	I
type III Wohlfart–Kugelberg–Welander disease	AR	C
type IV adult onset	AR	A
Acute infantile SMA (without *SMN* mutations)	Vary	C
Autosomal dominant proximal SMA	AD	A
Distal SMA:		
with respiratory distress		C
slowly progressive	AR	C, A
with upper limb predominance		C, A
with lower limb predominance	AD	C, A
with vocal fold paralysis		A
scapuloperoneal		C, A
Acquired		
Monomelic, focal and segmental SMA		A
Multifocal motor neuropathy with conduction block		A, E
Acute poliomyelitis		
Postpolio syndrome		
Postirradiation		
Bulbar		
Kennedy's disease	X	A
Brown–Vialetto–van Laere syndrome	AR	I, C, A
Fazio–Londe disease		C
Upper motor neuron syndromes		
Primary lateral sclerosis		A, E
Hereditary spastic paraplegia	AD	A, E
Lathyrism		A
Konzo		A

SMA, spinal muscular atrophy.
[a] Inheritance: AD, autosomal dominant; AR, autosomal recessive; X, X linked.
[b] Onset: I, infantile; C, childhood; A, adult (15–50 years); E, older person.

Clinical variants

Many consider progressive bulbar palsy and the pure lower and upper motor neuron variants, known as progressive muscular atrophy and primary lateral sclerosis, to be variants of amyotrophic lateral sclerosis. Segmental variants with head drop, flail arms, or progressive paraparesis seem to occur particularly in older people and often progress slowly to produce generalized muscle denervation late in the disease, if at all. The Madras form from southern India produces prominent arm and later leg involvement as part of a generalized motor neuron disease in young adults, half of whom also become deaf.

Prognosis

Amyotrophic lateral sclerosis progresses relentlessly, in both the severity and the extent of muscular involvement. Death commonly results from ventilatory respiratory failure or from inhalational pneumonia, and malnutrition often plays a part. The median survival from first symptoms in those with bulbar onset is approximately 20 months, with survival beyond 5 years being rare. The alternative diagnosis of X-linked bulbospinal neuronopathy should be considered in such long survivors. The median survival for those with spinal onset is approximately 29 months with almost 15% surviving 5 years. Although a subacute and reversible syndrome resembling spinal amyotrophic lateral sclerosis has been described, this is so extraordinarily rare that it should not influence the physician's prognosis.

Differential diagnosis and investigation

A diagnosis of amyotrophic lateral sclerosis is usually depressingly obvious on simple clinical grounds. Often only electrophysiological investigation is necessary to confirm denervation and to exclude a potentially treatable myopathy or demyelinating neuropathy. Sometimes upper motor neuron involvement is not clinically demonstrable, particularly in patients with absent Babinski's responses due to severely denervated toe extensor muscles. Unfortunately, measurement of central motor conduction after electromagnetic stimulation of the brain is less reliable for revealing upper motor neuron involvement in such cases than had been hoped. If patients present with the combination of arm denervation and upper motor neuron signs in the legs, the cervical spinal canal should be imaged with MRI to exclude a compressive lesion, most often spondylitic radiculomyelopathy.

The usual diagnostic problem lies in differentiating amyotrophic lateral sclerosis from other motor neuron diseases. A lack of upper motor neuron involvement should raise the possibility of alternative diagnoses. The postpolio syndrome causes slow deterioration in limb or bulbar function some decades after acute poliomyelitis. X-linked bulbospinal neuronopathy is much more slowly progressive than bulbar amyotrophic lateral sclerosis, grimacing usually evokes characteristic lower facial contractions; gynaecomastia, diabetes mellitus, or abnormal sensory nerve conduction is often evident, and other male family members may be affected. Multifocal motor neuropathy or neuronopathy usually develops insidiously, characteristically producing marked weakness with little wasting; it predominantly affects the arms, may be associated with paraproteinaemia or antiganglioside antibodies, and may involve motor nerve slowing or conduction block. Adult-onset proximal hereditary motor neuronopathy is very slowly progressive, with early and symmetrical involvement of the proximal muscles; it rarely involves the bulbar muscles. Benign fasciculation syndromes without evidence of denervation, usually affecting young adults, do not evolve into motor neuron disease. Myopathic disorders, particularly the bulbar presentations of inclusion body myositis and myasthenia gravis, should always be borne in mind. The possible occurrence of motor neuron disease as a paraneoplastic disorder is still in dispute.

Giving the diagnosis

Doctors or relatives are sometimes tempted on compassionate grounds not to tell patients about their diagnosis of amyotrophic lateral sclerosis. When patients eventually detect this conspiracy of secrecy it can lead to serious loss of trust at a time when death looms and trustworthy relationships are of inestimable value. When given the opportunity, patients usually indicate that they wish to know the name of the disease and the likely outcome, and they may even wish for a detailed discussion of the probable modes of death. Judgement is required to soften the blow of grim news while giving an honest appraisal of the condition. Of course, questions should be answered honestly, although sometimes it may be preferable to discuss them in stages with the partner present in order to soften the blow early on in the course of the disease. Once a patient has been told the diagnosis, the doctor must address the particular issues presented by that patient's own brand of amyotrophic lateral sclerosis before he or she becomes upset by the summary information that they may glean from lay reference books, newspapers/magazines, or the internet.

Treatment

No treatment is known to cure amyotrophic lateral sclerosis. Trials of drug therapy have concentrated on slowing the downhill progression of disability or improving survival. The antiglutamate agent riluzole, administered orally, has been licensed for treatment of amyotrophic lateral sclerosis. The 100 mg dosage improved the chance of tracheostomy-free survival at 18 months by an extra 35%, although there was no significant benefit on muscle function. Criticisms of this study have included the nature of Cox's model of statistical adjustment, and it should be noted that more of the placebo group had bulbar features at entry to the study. Riluzole is generally well tolerated by patients; nausea, gastrointestinal upset, and raised transaminase enzyme levels may occur and usually resolve with a dose reduction. Ineffective therapeutic trials have included mixtures of branched-chain amino acids, dextromorphan, total lymphoid irradiation, the free radical scavenger acetylcysteine, gabapentin, creatine, and vitamin E.

Much can be done to overcome disability and alleviate distress by the care team of speech and language therapist, physiotherapist, occupational therapist, social worker, and physician. The Motor Neuron Disease Association is often able to provide equipment promptly. Severe dysphagia is most effectively bypassed by percutaneous endoscopic gastrostomy. Preferably the patient or the carer should have good hand function and vision so that they can change nutrient bags at home. If video-swallow shows that cricopharyngeal spasm is responsible for dysphagia, cricopharyngeal myotomy may help. Speech failure can be circumvented by computer-assisted communication devices operated through a practical modality, such as pressure, blowing, head nodding, or blinking, depending on which muscles remain strong.

Decisions about the advisability of instituting assisted respiration pose complex practical and ethical dilemmas. Patients with diaphragm weakness and nocturnal dyspnoea may be helped by intermittent positive airway pressure delivered by facemask. Endotracheal intubation and ventilation are rarely to be recommended in a disease causing such ubiquitous and irreversible weakness.

Lower motor neuron syndromes

These forms of motor neuron disease generally follow a much more benign course than amyotrophic lateral sclerosis. They include syndromes previously described as spinal muscular atrophy and progressive muscular atrophy. Differential diagnosis within the lower motor neuron syndromes depends principally upon attention to the age of onset, the pattern of the weakness, and a possible family history.

Proximal childhood spinal muscular atrophy with SMN mutations

This group of lower motor neuron degenerations is associated with deletions at 5q13 of the *SMN1* survival motor neuron gene. The variable phenotype is explained by the difference in copy number of an almost identical gene, *SMN2*. The precise role of *SMN* has not been elucidated, but ribonucleoprotein or gene-splicing regulation is a likely function.

Type I: acute infantile form (Werdnig–Hoffmann disease)

This is one of the most common fatal autosomal recessive disorders of children. The disease frequency of approximately 1 in 25 000 in England results from a gene frequency of 1 in 160. Before the age of 6 months, babies become inactive, weak, and hypotonic, feed poorly, and are slow to attain motor milestones. They may be born with limb deformities and, in retrospect, fetal movements have been often absent or sparse. The tongue is weak and may fasciculate. Head control is poor and the infant's areflexic and proximally wasted limbs tend to assume a frog-like position. Respiratory movements are decreased with prominent involvement of the intercostal muscles. Half the infants die by 6 months, and almost all have succumbed by 18 months, usually to respiratory complications.

Type II: intermediate form

This produces muscle weakness before 18 months; children can sit but never walk, and usually die in adolescence.

Type III: chronic childhood form (Kugelberg–Welander disease)

This form develops at any time after the age of 18 months to the early teens. It is also autosomal recessive, may be genetically heterogeneous, and may start discordantly within families. It can resemble Werdnig–Hoffmann disease if the onset is early, but follows a comparatively benign course. More than 90% of patients are able to walk or sit unsupported at some time, although these abilities are often lost eventually. Tongue involvement occurs in only half, and significant dysphagia is unusual. Some patients develop respiratory insufficiency as a result of intercostal muscle involvement. The proximal limb weakness and wasting are only slowly progressive and may stabilize spontaneously. Those with severe early weakness often develop secondary spinal and joint deformities.

The prognosis varies, although survival into middle age is usual. It is important, although initially difficult, to differentiate those with infantile onset and no family history from types I and II infantile-onset forms.

Type IV: adult-onset form
This unusual autosomal recessive adult form starts from 15 to 60 years of age, usually in the fourth decade. Slowly progressive proximal limb weakness ensues, but significant disability for walking does not usually occur until the sixth or seventh decade. Life expectancy is only slightly reduced. Distal muscles can also be involved and the tendon reflexes are usually lost, but bulbar involvement is uncommon. The lack of either upper motor neuron signs or bulbar involvement, and the rather indolent progression, distinguish this from amyotrophic lateral sclerosis.

Other inherited spinal muscular atrophies
Autosomal dominant forms are rare, and fall into two groups with onset in childhood and early middle age respectively. Mutations of the VAPB gene (vesicle-associated membrane protein) at 20q13.3 are present in some Brazilian families. The limb weakness is predominantly proximal. Bulbar involvement does occur, although it is unusual. The childhood form may stabilize at adolescence and some patients retain walking ability into middle or old age. The adult-onset form causes more severe disability. The lack of upper motor neuron signs distinguishes these conditions from hereditary amyotrophic lateral sclerosis.

Autosomal recessive and dominant distal spinal muscular atrophies not associated with SMN mutations occur. Some resemble the type II Charcot–Marie–Tooth disease polyneuropathy. Various forms are recognized with leg or arm predominance, respiratory distress, vocal fold paralysis, and scapuloperoneal distribution. Occasional acute infantile forms are part of more complex disorders, variously involving pontocerebellar hypoplasia, arthrogryposis, bone fractures, and lethal congenital contractures.

Hexosaminidase deficiency
Autosomal recessive GM2 gangliosidosis presents a variable neurological picture, occasionally as a pure motor neuron syndrome due to lower and, rarely, upper motor neuron involvement. More usually there are also other neurological abnormalities such as cerebellar ataxia or dementia. Hexosaminidase assays should be reserved for those patients with early onset of unusual motor neuron disorders, particularly in those of Ashkenazi Jewish extraction.

X-linked recessive bulbospinal neuronopathy (Kennedy's disease)
This disorder occurs only in men, with onset in the third to fifth decades of life. It is due to a mutation causing CAG (cytosine–adenine–guanine) repeat sequences of increased length within the androgen receptor gene. Molecular genetic analysis now forms the basis of a diagnostic test. Weakness usually first affects hand or pelvic girdle muscles and the bulbar symptoms may not be evident until 20 years later, if at all. Cramps are prominent and fasciculations are usually visible in the limb, tongue, and facial muscles. Characteristically, muscle contractions around the chin are induced by pursing the lips or grimacing. The disorder is only slowly progressive. Most patients survive into their seventh or eight decade except when bulbar involvement is unusually severe. The disorder

is often misdiagnosed as amyotrophic lateral sclerosis until the unusually slow deterioration is questioned. Unlike amyotrophic lateral sclerosis, there are no upper motor neuron signs and patients commonly show gynaecomastia, diabetes mellitus, and absent sensory nerve action potentials.

Hereditary bulbar palsy of infancy and childhood
The Brown–Violetto–van Laere syndrome presents in the teens with bilateral sensorineural deafness, followed some years later by bulbar, facial, limb, and sometimes respiratory muscle weakness. Fazio–Londe disease is an autosomal recessive bulbar palsy of childhood, without deafness, and respiratory muscle involvement may lead to death within a few years.

Monomelic, focal, and segmental motor neuronopathies
These conditions are also known as chronic asymmetrical or focal spinal muscular atrophy, or monomelic motor neuron disease. Currently, the disorder is generally known as monomelic amyotrophy. Although most commonly described in Asia, especially Japan, it is seen regularly elsewhere in the world. It usually occurs sporadically and most patients are young men. It presents with distal wasting and weakness of one hand or forearm. This progresses steadily for the first 2 years before either stabilizing or settling to a slow rate of subsequent progression. Initially there may be concern that this is the first presentation of amyotrophic lateral sclerosis, but the expected upper motor neuron and bulbar involvement fails to materialize, and spread to other limbs is unusual. Nerve conduction studies are necessary to exclude focal entrapment neuropathies or multifocal motor neuropathy with conduction block. MRI of the cervical spine will detect syringomyelia or other spinal cord disease. Forms affecting a leg have been described, particularly from India.

Postirradiation lumbosacral radiculopathy
This may follow months or years of inclusion of the lower thoracic and upper lumbar spine in irradiation fields treating testicular tumours or lymphomas. It usually affects both legs, although occasionally one, and later causes mild symptoms affecting the sphincters and sensation. It is painless, and electrophysiology does not reveal the myokymic discharges or abnormal sensory nerve action potentials of irradiation plexopathy. The normal imaging of the lumbosacral plexus and cauda equina, and the absence of pain, exclude tumour recurrence.

Postpolio syndrome
After two or more decades, very slowly progressive weakness may affect muscles previously involved by acute paralytic poliomyelitis. Although this predominantly affects the limbs, approximately half the cases also have mild choking or dysphagia and weakness of the respiratory muscles, which may lead to hypercapnic respiratory failure. The sluggish deterioration, lack of upper motor neuron involvement, and previous history serve to distinguish postpolio syndrome from amyotrophic lateral sclerosis. Electromyography reveals the giant motor units typical of extensive reinnervation during recovery from previous acute poliomyelitis. At least equally commonly, late deterioration after polio is due to a secondary degenerative arthritis or fibromyalgia.

Multifocal motor neuropathy with conduction block

Patients with these conditions may present at any stage of adult life with multifocal and slowly progressive muscle weakness for as long as 20 years. The clinical picture is immensely variable. Distal limb muscles are mainly involved, often notably asymmetrical. The first symptoms and most severe weakness usually affect the arms. A third present with drop of an individual finger. Characteristically, severely weakened muscles show little or no wasting. Reflex loss is generally restricted to markedly affected muscles. The condition is neurophysiologically heterogeneous, ranging from muscle denervation to multifocal conduction block in motor nerves, and occasionally a diffusely demyelinating, pure, motor peripheral neuropathy. Early cases may show no such diagnostic electrophysiological abnormality. Serum antibodies to GM1 gangliosides are detectable in a third of cases, but are of no proven pathogenic significance. This antibody assay currently lacks specificity as positives are sometimes found in other neurological diseases.

These motor neuropathies usually progress insidiously, sometimes in a stepwise manner. Spontaneous remissions occur only occasionally, and usually in the subacute subgroup. It is important to detect the subgroup of patients with either multifocal motor conduction block or diffuse demyelinating neuropathy, because improvement may follow immunosuppressant therapy. Although cyclophosphamide is reportedly effective, its potential toxicity should limit its use to those patients with severely disabling and progressive weakness. High-dose intravenous human immunoglobulin (IvIg) therapy can produce dramatic improvement lasting 6 to 8 weeks and repeated administration is the mainstay of treatment in severely symptomatic patients. With IvIg administered sufficiently regularly to prevent end-of-dose deterioration, progressive motor axonal loss can be largely or completely prevented. Unfortunately, steroid therapy does not improve multifocal motor neuropathy, and may precipitate further deterioration.

Upper motor neuron syndromes

The pure upper motor neuron syndromes are the rarest forms of motor neuron disease. They should be considered only after MRI has excluded structural or demyelinating disease of the spinal cord, foramen magnum, or brain. Severe spasticity often overshadows weakness in these purely upper motor neuron diseases, but unfortunately antispasticity medications are often relatively ineffective. Rarely, similar upper motor neuron syndromes may be seen with syphilis and HTLV-I (human T-lymphocytic virus type I) infection. Deficiencies of vitamins B_{12} and E need to be considered along with L-dopa-responsive dystonia and adrenomyeloneuropathy.

Primary lateral sclerosis

Generally considered as a variant of amyotrophic lateral sclerosis, this rare sporadic form of motor neuron disease has an average age of onset of 50 years, and slow progression thereafter for an average of 15 years. The clinical features are all attributable to symmetrical degeneration of the upper motor neurons destined for the spinal cord and of the bulbar motor neurons. Spasticity and weakness usually start insidiously in the legs and ascend ultimately to involve the bulbar muscles. Less commonly patients present with an isolated spastic dysarthria, a symptom of pseudobulbar palsy. Pseudobulbar emotional lability may be distressing for these patients, given their normal cognition, and it often responds well to amitriptyline. Bladder function is generally preserved, at least until the later stages. Electromyography does not reveal the muscle denervation expected in predominantly upper motor neuron forms of amyotrophic lateral sclerosis, although in many patients this develops belatedly. MRI may reveal atrophy of the precentral gyrus motor cortex, reflecting loss of the Betz cells from which the pyramidal tract originates. Central motor conduction is notably delayed after electromagnetic stimulation of the motor cortex.

Hereditary spastic paraplegia

Various forms of slowly progressive, symmetrical, spastic paraparesis may be inherited, most usually on an autosomal dominant basis with onset in the fourth to sixth decades. The degree of leg spasticity often outweighs the severity of the weakness. Bulbar involvement is very rare, and arm function may be well preserved despite severe leg involvement. The condition is slowly progressive. It may remain asymptomatic in some family members, coming to light only when a familial basis for the disease is sought. Sphincter control is not impaired, but sexual impotence can develop. More than 30 genetic loci are involved, with genes identified in half. Clinically the hereditary spastic paraplegias are most conveniently divided into 'pure' and 'complicated' forms, the latter involving various features such as distal amyotrophy, intellectual impairment, dementia, pigmentary retinopathy, optic atrophy, extrapyramidal features, sensory neuropathy, ataxia, or epilepsy.

The various genetic entities produce a range of neurodevelopmental and neurodegenerative disorders. The autosomal dominant disorders are usually 'pure' and involve abnormalities of various genes for proteins involved in intra-axonal trafficking, such as spastin, atlastin, or KIF5A, while other genetic mutations involved heat shock protein 60 and seipin. The less common autosomal recessive forms often produce 'complicated' phenotypes and mutations include those for paraplegin, spartin, and maspardin. X-linked mutations are rare and generally present in childhood with 'complicated' phenotypes.

Lathyrism

Neurolathyrism is a spastic paraparesis caused by regular consumption of the chickling pea (*Lathyrus sativus*) for some months. It is endemic in parts of India and outbreaks have occurred in China, Africa, and central Europe at times of famine. Patients, usually young men, present either subacutely or chronically with a spastic paraparesis and a characteristic scissoring gait in which the balls of the feet take most of the weight. Once it has developed, neurolathyrism is usually not progressive, but little or no recovery occurs even after chickling pea consumption ceases. A plant-derived excitotoxic amino acid, BOAA, is considered pathogenic.

Konzo

Konzo is a form of tropical myelopathy which can occur in epidemics at times of famine in sub-Saharan Africa. It seems to be due to dietary cyanogen consumption, resulting from insufficient soaking of the cassava roots used to produce flour. There is an abrupt onset of symmetrical spastic paraparesis, which is nonprogressive but permanent. Blood cyanide levels are raised at the onset of disease.

Further reading

Anon (1997). Riluzole for amyotrophic lateral sclerosis. *Drug Therapeut Bull*, **35**, 11–12.

Atsuta N, *et al.* (2006). Natural history of spinal and bulbar muscular atrophy (SBMA): a study of 223 Japanese patients. *Brain*, **129**, 1446–55.

Bowen J, *et al.* (1997). The post-irradiation lower motor neuron syndrome. Neuronopathy or radiculopathy? *Brain*, **119**, 1429–39.

Lacomblez L, *et al.* (1996). Dose-ranging study of Riluzole in amyotrophic lateral sclerosis. *Lancet*, **347**, 1425–31.

La Spada AR, *et al.* (1991). Androgen receptor gene mutations in X-linked spinal and bulbar muscular atrophy. *Nature*, **352**, 77–9.

Le Forestier N, *et al.* (2001). Does primary lateral sclerosis exist? A study of 20 patients and a review of the literature. *Brain*, **124**, 89–99.

Ludolph AC, *et al.* (1987). Studies on the aetiology and pathogenesis of motor neuron diseases. I Lathyrism: clinical findings in established cases. *Brain*, **110**, 149–66.

McShane MA, *et al.* (1993). Progressive bulbar paralysis of childhood. A reappraisal of Fazio–Londe disease. *Brain*, **115**, 1889–900.

Ringholz GM, *et al.* (2005). Prevalence and patterns of cognitive impairment in sporadic ALS. *Neurology*, **65**, 586–90.

Rosen DR, *et al.* (1993). Mutations in Cu-Zn superoxide dismutase gene are associated with familial amyotrophic lateral sclerosis. *Nature*, **362**, 59–62.

Shaw PM (2009). The motor neuron disorders. In: Donaghy M (ed.) *Brain's diseases of the nervous system*, 12th edition. Oxford University Press, Oxford.

Slee M, *et al.* (2007). Multifocal motor neuropathy: the diagnostic spectrum and response to treatment. *Neurology*, **69**, 1680–7.

Trojan DA, Cashman NR (2005). Post-poliomyelitis syndrome. *Muscle Nerve*, **31**, 6–19.

Tylleskär T, *et al.* (1992). Cassava cyanogens and Konzo, an upper motor neuron disease found in Africa. *Lancet*, **339**, 208–11.

Diseases of the peripheral nerves

R.A.C. Hughes and P.K. Thomas[†]

Essentials

Disorders of peripheral nerve function can be categorized in terms of the site of the primary disturbance. (1) Neuronopathies—conditions that lead to death of the neuron cell body and axon. (2) Axonal neuropathies—conditions that affect axons which may be focal, as in local injury, or multifocal, as in vasculitis, or symmetrical and diffuse as in metabolic or toxic disorders (3) Demyelinating neuropathies in which the myelin sheaths are damaged and the axons are relatively preserved. Combinations of axonal and demyelinating pathology are common. (4) Interstitial neuropathy in which there is infiltration of the endoneurium for instance by granuloma or amyloid.

Clinical features

Peripheral neuropathy characteristically causes predominantly distal muscle weakness—with or without atrophy—sensory changes and signs of autonomic malfunction, either alone or in combination. These occur in an anatomical distribution appropriate to the nerve or nerves affected, with three broad categories recognized: (1) mononeuropathy—a lesion of an isolated peripheral nerve (2) multifocal neuropathy/mononeuropathy); and (3) polyneuropathy—diffuse and bilaterally symmetrical disturbance of function.

Investigation

The diagnosis can usually be made from the history and examination. Diagnosis of both localized and generalized neuropathies may be confirmed by nerve conduction studies of motor and sensory fibres. Simple investigations for diabetes mellitus, B_{12} deficiency and other medical causes are sufficient for the diagnosis of many cases. Cerebrospinal fluid examination, may be useful—especially in suspected inflammatory demyelinating polyradiculopathy. When the diagnosis is not revealed by simple tests an extensive range of investigations for rare causes may be needed.

Nerve biopsy is rarely be required and is principally useful for the detection of vasculitis which cannot be diagnosed in any less invasive way.

Particular peripheral neuropathies

Lesions of individual nerves—with clinical consequences determined by the normal function of that nerve (and any redundancy of innervation). Common conditions include median nerve compression due to carpal tunnel syndrome, and damage to the ulnar nerve at the elbow and the common peroneal nerve at the fibular head.

Generalized neuropathies—causes include (1) diabetes mellitus—most commonly producing a symmetrical sensory polyneuropathy; autonomic neuropathy may be debilitating; (2) alcohol—usually in association with thiamine deficiency (3) other metabolic/endocrine disorders—e.g. amyloidosis, uraemia, myxoedema, acromegaly, critical illness polyneuropathy; (4) toxic—including industrial/environmental (e.g. acrylamide, lead, thallium) and dr (e.g. cisplatin, isoniazid, vincristine, thalidomide) substances; (5) deficiencies—e.g. thiamine, vitamin B_{12}; (6) inflammatory—e.g. Guillain–Barré syndrome, chronic inflammatory demyelinating polyradiculoneuropathy, multifocal motor neuropathy, paraprotein associated neuropathy; (7) infection related—leprosy Lyme borreliosis, HIV-1 infection; (8) granulomatous—sarcoidosis; (9) vasculitic disorders; (10) neoplastic and paraneoplastic—most often with bronchial or ovarian malignancy; (11) genetic conditions—e.g. porphyria, familial amyloid polyneuropathy, Charcot–Marie–Tooth (hereditary motor and sensory neuropathy) disease, hereditary neuropathy with liability to pressure palsies, Refsum's disease; and (12) chronic idiopathic axonal polyneuropathy—the cause of about 25% of cases of late onset symmetrical polyneuropathy remains unknown despite extensive investigation.

[†] It is with regret that we report the death of Professor P K Thomas during the preparation of this edition of the textbook.

Introduction

Structure of peripheral nerves

The peripheral nerves consist of bundles (fascicles) of unmyelinated and myelinated axons that have their cell bodies in the anterior horns of the spinal cord, dorsal root ganglia, or autonomic ganglia. The fascicles are surrounded by a lamellated cellular sheath, the perineurium, which provides a diffusion barrier that separates the intrafascicular or endoneurial compartment from the extracellular tissues. Peripheral nerve trunks usually consist of several fascicles bound together by the mainly collagenous epineurial connective tissue. The nutrient vessels connect with a longitudinal anastomotic network of arterioles and venules in the epineurium. This, in turn, communicates through perforating vessels with a longitudinal, intrafascicular, capillary anastomotic network. This anastomotic system is extremely efficient: experimentally it is very difficult to produce ischaemia of nerve trunks by ligation of nutrient vessels. The occurrence of an ischaemic neuropathy therefore implies widespread vascular insufficiency. A blood–nerve barrier, comparable to the blood–brain barrier, exists in peripheral nerves (except in the sensory and autonomic ganglia and at motor nerve terminals). This, together with the diffusion barrier provided by the perineurium, regulates the composition of the endoneurial connective tissue fluid and thus the ionic environment of the nerve fibres.

Physiological aspects

All nerve fibres, whether myelinated or unmyelinated, are closely related to satellite cells, the cells of Schwann. They may provide metabolic support for the axons, which often extend for very considerable distances from their perikarya. In myelinated fibres, the myelin segments are derived by the spiralling of the surface membrane of Schwann cells around the axons. The axon is exposed at the nodes of Ranvier, which represent the gaps between adjacent myelin segments. Conduction in unmyelinated axons takes place by the spread of a continuous wave of depolarization, the action potential, which migrates along the axolemma. In myelinated fibres, because of the high electrical resistance of the lipid in the myelin lamellae, the generation of the action potential is restricted to the nodes of Ranvier. Conduction is therefore saltatory, jumping from one node to the next by local currents that traverse the axon and the extracellular tissue fluid. By this means, conduction velocity is increased from about 1 m/s in unmyelinated axons to 60 to 70 m/s in the largest myelinated fibres.

Most of the synthetic mechanisms in neurons are sited in the cell bodies. Synthesized materials are then transported down the axons to the termination of the fibres by an active transport system. This involves a fast system with a rate of about 400 mm/day, and a slow system, in which the structural proteins travel at 1 to 2 mm/day. The system is bidirectional: there is also a retrograde system transporting materials, including neurotrophic factors, back from the periphery to the cell body. The retrograde system may be involved in the regulation of protein synthesis in the cell body and probably carries the signal for chromatolysis, which follows transection.

Disorders affecting peripheral nerves

Disorders of peripheral nerve function can be categorized in terms of the site of the primary disturbance. Conditions that lead to the death of the neuron as a whole, with the loss of the cell body and the axon, are categorized as neuronopathies. Conditions that have a selective effect on axons are termed 'axonal neuropathies'. A selective effect on axonal conduction is seen in poisoning with tetrodotoxin, which blocks the sodium channels at the nodes. Focal axonal lesions occur as a result of insults such as trauma or ischaemia. Axonal interruption leads to wallerian-type degeneration below the site of injury. Recovery has to take place by axonal regeneration which is a slow process: the rate of axonal regeneration is about 1 to 2 mm/day.

Generalized axonal neuropathies often lead to a selective degeneration of the distal portion of the fibres, which then extend proximally. The axons are said to 'die back' towards the cell bodies. This pattern is seen in many toxic neuropathies and neuropathies due to nutritional deficiency. In these conditions, the axonal breakdown may result either from interference with enzymes involved in glycolysis which provide the metabolic energy for axonal transport mechanisms, or from cofactor deficiency or inactivation. As the enzymes are synthesized in the cell bodies and then transported down the axons, the further the distance from the cell body the greater the likelihood of metabolic insufficiency occurring. This probably accounts for the distal distribution of many such neuropathies, because longer axons will be more vulnerable. Again recovery has to take place by axonal regeneration. In many distal axonal neuropathies that involve the peripheral nervous system, not only does the degeneration affect the distal parts of the motor and sensory axons in the periphery, but also the terminal parts of the centrally directed axons derived from the dorsal root ganglion cells degenerate. Thus degeneration may be found in the rostral portions of the posterior columns. This process has been referred to as central–peripheral distal axonopathy. Neuropathy from iminodipropionitrile blocks the slow axonal transport system and leads to large swellings in the proximal parts of the axons that contain aggregations of neurofilaments (proximal axonopathy).

Other neuropathies primarily affect the myelin, either directly, or through interference with Schwann cell function. The consequence is a selective demyelination with relative preservation of axonal integrity. This may be restricted to the region of the nodes of Ranvier (paranodal demyelination) or involve whole internodal segments (segmental demyelination) with consequent conduction block. The selective myelin damage may occur, for example, as the result of a cell-mediated attack on myelin by sensitized mononuclear cells, which is a possible explanation for the acute inflammatory demyelinating polyradiculoneuropathy (AIDP) form of Guillain–Barré syndrome. Another instance is in diphtheritic neuropathy where the demyelination is secondary to an interference with Schwann cell protein metabolism. Local compression by a tourniquet also gives rise to selective damage to myelin through mechanical effects, although more severe pressure causes axonal interruption. In diffuse demyelinating neuropathies, the distribution of the clinical effects, as for distal axonal neuropathies, is often maximal peripherally. Presumably, this is a statistical effect: the longer the nerve fibre, the more likely it is to develop a region of demyelinating conduction block.

Recovery after paranodal or segmental demyelination occurs by remyelination. Initially, the newly formed myelin segments are short and thin, which results in an abnormally slow conduction velocity. Such reductions in conduction velocity may be focal, e.g. in relation to localized myelin damage in entrapment neuropathies, or widespread as in most inherited demyelinating neuropathies. In the latter, motor nerve conduction velocity is sometimes reduced to 10 m/s or less.

Finally, in other neuropathies the nerve fibres may be secondarily damaged by processes that primarily affect the connective tissues of nerves or of the vasa nervorum. Usually a combination of demyelination and axonal loss occurs.

Clinical categories of neuropathy: mononeuropathy, multiple mononeuropathy, and polyneuropathy

Peripheral neuropathies may be divided into two broad categories depending on the distribution of the involvement. The first category comprises lesions of isolated peripheral nerves or nerve roots termed 'mononeuropathy' or multiple isolated lesions termed multiple mononeuropathy or multifocal neuropathy. The lesions in a widespread multifocal neuropathy may summate to produce a symmetrical disturbance, but the history or a careful examination may indicate the involvement of individual nerves. Isolated or multiple isolated peripheral nerve lesions arise from conditions that produce localized damage, such as mechanical injury, nerve entrapment, thermal, electrical, or radiation injury, vascular causes, granulomatous, neoplastic, or other infiltrations, and nerve tumours.

Second, there may be a diffuse and bilaterally symmetrical disturbance of function which can be designated polyneuropathy. When such a process affects the spinal roots, or affects the roots as well as the peripheral nerve trunks, the term 'polyradiculoneuropathy' is more appropriate. In general terms, polyneuropathies result from causes that act diffusely on the peripheral nervous system, such as metabolic disturbances, toxic agents, deficiency states, and some autoimmune disorders. Isolated nerve lesions may sometimes be superimposed on a symmetrical polyneuropathy, as a consequence, for example, of pressure lesions in a patient confined to bed. In certain peripheral nerve disorders, there is an abnormal susceptibility to pressure lesions.

Symptomatology

Weakness or paralysis may be due to either conduction block in the motor nerve fibres or axonal degeneration. Conduction block is related to demyelination with preservation of axonal continuity (neurapraxia). Recovery may occur by remyelination and may be rapid and complete. This can be the situation in localized nerve lesions, e.g. 'Saturday night' palsy of the radial nerve, or in more widespread polyneuropathies, such as in the acute inflammatory demyelinating polyradiculoneuropathy form of Guillain–Barré syndrome (see below). If axonal interruption takes place, axonal degeneration occurs below the site of interruption. The muscle weakness is accompanied by atrophy and electromyographic signs of denervation. If the interruption is reversible, recovery has to take place by axonal regeneration which is often slow and incomplete. An important recovery mechanism in conditions in which muscles become partially denervated is reinnervation of denervated muscle fibres by collateral sprouting from the remaining intact axons.

In generalized symmetrical polyneuropathies, the muscle weakness and wasting are commonly peripheral in distribution and begin in the lower limbs. This results in bilateral foot drop and a 'steppage' gait in which an affected individual lifts the feet to an abnormal extent to avoid catching the toes on the ground. Involvement of the upper limbs begins with weakness and wasting of the small hand muscles, and usually weakness of the finger and wrist extensors, before the forearm flexor muscles. At times, a symmetrical involvement of the proximal limb muscles occurs in

peripheral nerve disorders, e.g. in AIDP. Fasciculation due to spontaneous contraction of isolated motor units is most often a feature of anterior horn cell disease but may be encountered in peripheral neuropathies, as may muscle cramps. Postural tremor, mainly affecting the upper limbs and resembling essential tremor, may be seen in patients with chronic demyelinating polyneuropathies with slow conduction velocity. This 'neuropathic tremor' is most often encountered in Charcot–Marie–Tooth disease type 1, chronic inflammatory demyelinating polyradiculoneuropathy (CIDP), and IgM paraprotein-associated demyelinating neuropathy. A rare manifestation of peripheral neuropathy is the occurrence of continuous repetitive discharges in motor nerve fibres, leading to generalized muscular rigidity or 'neuromyotonia' (Isaacs' syndrome, continuous motor unit activity syndrome).

Loss of the tendon reflexes is a frequent accompaniment of a peripheral neuropathy, and usually first affects the ankle jerks.

Sensory symptoms and sensory loss in symmetrical polyneuropathies are usually distal in distribution, giving rise to the 'glove-and-stocking' pattern of involvement. Only rarely is a proximal pattern encountered. The sensory loss may affect all modalities or be restricted to certain forms of sensation. If the loss is restricted, two broad patterns are discernible. In the first, the impairment predominantly affects the sensations of joint position, vibration and light touch, corresponding to a predominant loss of function in the larger myelinated nerve fibres. Loss of joint position sensation may cause sensory ataxia, which can resemble that in cerebellar disease. When very severe it may also cause 'pseudoathetosis', i.e. involuntary movements, most often of the fingers and hands: this is revealed when a patient holds the arms outstretched with the eyes closed. In the second pattern of selective sensory loss, pain and temperature sensibility are predominantly affected, often associated with loss of autonomic function, corresponding to a predominant loss of small myelinated and unmyelinated axons. 'Trophic changes' and pain may complicate such small fibre neuropathies, and include loss of the protective effect of pain sensation with the consequent development of persistent ulceration or more extensive tissue loss, most commonly in the feet, and neuropathic joint degeneration (Charcot's joints).

Paraesthesiae are a frequent feature in peripheral neuropathy. They are usually of a tingling nature ('pins and needles'), but, especially in 'small fibre' neuropathies, may involve thermal sensations, most often with a burning quality. The paraesthesiae may be aggravated by touching or stroking the skin. Stimuli that are not normally painful may acquire an unpleasant quality (allodynia). Painful stimuli may give rise to an excessive or hyperpathic response, in which a mildly painful stimulus, e.g. a pinprick, is abnormally intense. With repeated stimulation at the same site, the pain that is felt may spread widely and reach an intolerable intensity. An unusual symptom encountered most often in uraemic neuropathy is that of 'restless legs'. Affected individuals experience sensations in the feet and legs that they find difficult to describe but which are temporarily relieved by moving them. Restless legs syndrome is not uncommon in otherwise healthy individuals.

Spontaneous pains of an aching or lancinating character may complicate a number of generalized polyneuropathies. Severe paroxysms of lancinating pain occur in trigeminal neuralgia in which the lesion is at or close to the point of entry of the sensory roots into the pons. Causalgia constitutes a particularly troublesome painful syndrome, most often after injuries of the median nerve, lower trunk of the brachial plexus, or tibial nerve. It is a severe persistent pain, often with a burning quality, which may be aggravated by emotional factors. Sympathectomy relieves some cases.

Disturbances of autonomic function are occasionally the primary abnormality in a peripheral neuropathy, as in rare syndromes of primary autoimmune autonomic neuropathy and familial dysautonomia. More commonly they accompany other manifestations, either with localized peripheral nerve lesions and/or with generalized neuropathies, such as acute inflammatory demyelinating polyradiculoneuropathy or diabetic polyneuropathy.

Diagnosis and investigation

The history and physical examination frequently indicate that the disturbance has affected the peripheral nerves. If confirmation is required, this may usually be obtained by nerve conduction studies. Conduction may be examined in motor and sensory nerve fibres, and can give evidence of both localized and generalized neuropathies. Severely reduced conduction velocity may occur as a result of segmental demyelination or because of conduction in regenerating axons of small calibre after axonal degeneration.

Examination of the cerebrospinal fluid may be helpful in the diagnosis of the cause of a peripheral neuropathy. In symmetrical axonal neuropathy, the cerebrospinal fluid is usually normal. In CIDP, the protein concentration is usually increased, often to more than 1000 mg/l. The protein concentration is also usually increased in Guillain–Barré syndrome, especially after the first week, whereas the cell count remains normal or only shows a small number of lymphocytes. The cell count is usually increased in neuropathies associated with HIV infection and in Lyme disease.

Nerve biopsy is rarely required in establishing the existence of a peripheral neuropathy, but may be of diagnostic value in establishing the cause, especially in vasculitis and other multifocal inflammatory disorders and in amyloid. It is best performed in centres with special expertise in nerve biopsy because it is an invasive procedure that cannot easily be repeated. Also, special processing and staining techniques are necessary to avoid fixation artefacts and provide high-quality immunohistochemistry, morphology, and electron microscopy.

Individual nerves

Phrenic nerve (C2–4)

This nerve innervates the diaphragm. When the diaphragm is totally paralysed, the normal protrusion of the upper abdomen during inspiration is lost, or is replaced by retraction (paradoxical movement). Radiographically, paralysis may be detected by unilateral or bilateral elevation of the diaphragm in a chest radiograph and its failure to descend on inspiration. The phrenic nerve may be involved in its course through the neck or thorax by wounds or tumours such as bronchial carcinoma, and it is sometimes affected in idiopathic brachial plexus neuropathy (neuralgic amyotrophy).

Nerve to serratus anterior (C5–7)

The serratus anterior acts as a fixator of the scapula, holding the scapula against the chest wall when forward pressure is exerted by the arm. It is involved in forward movement of the shoulder, as in a rapier thrust, and in elevation of the arm, when it rotates the scapula. When serratus anterior is paralysed in isolation, the position of the scapula is almost normal at rest but, if the extended arm is pushed forward against resistance, 'winging' of the scapula becomes more evident. The vertebral border, particularly in its lower portion, stands away from the chest wall. The nerve to serratus anterior may be involved in penetrating wounds, but usually in association with damage to the brachial plexus. It may be injured by forcible depression of the shoulder. Serratus anterior weakness is a common component of idiopathic brachial plexus neuropathy (neuralgic amyotrophy) and it is not infrequently encountered as an isolated and unexplained lesion.

Brachial plexus

The brachial plexus may be affected by intrinsic lesions, neoplastic infiltration, penetrating wounds of the neck, in fractures and dislocations of the shoulder and clavicle, as a result of traction on the arm, or by pressure from an aneurysm or a cervical rib.

Neuralgic amyotrophy

This condition has been described under a variety of terms, including 'idiopathic brachial plexus neuropathy' and 'paralytic brachial neuritis'. It may follow immunizing procedures, in particular the administration of antitetanus serum or operations, or occur without a recognizable antecedent event. It can occur on a genetic basis as an autosomal dominant disorder, hereditary neuralgic amyotrophy, with variable penetrance. This is often caused by mutations in the gene encoding septin-9, a cytoskeletal filament-forming protein involved in the mitotic spindle.

The disorder develops acutely with intense pain in the shoulder region which may take some weeks to subside completely, although generally it ceases after a few days. Paralysis of the muscles of the shoulder girdle becomes evident within a day or two of the onset of the pain, sometimes also of the arms or of the diaphragm. It may be unilateral or bilateral and associated with sensory loss. More distal upper limb muscles may at times be affected, as may the phrenic nerve and, occasionally, the recurrent laryngeal nerve. The cerebrospinal fluid is consistently normal. The affected muscles show electromyographic evidence of denervation. Recovery is variable but may ultimately be satisfactory. Not all cases recover fully and recurrences may occur. A comparable disorder can affect the lumbosacral plexus (idiopathic lumbosacral plexopathy).

The pattern of muscle involvement and sensory disturbances suggests that neuralgic amyotrophy affects the brachial plexus in a patchy manner. An immune reaction is assumed but not established. The condition takes the same course whether or not it follows immunization. Corticosteroids do not appear to influence the initial pain but may improve the ultimate outcome but this needs confirmation with a randomized controlled trial which is now in progress.

Postirradiation brachial plexopathy

Brachial plexus damage may occur as a sequel to radiotherapy for breast carcinoma or tumours in the neck. The onset of symptoms is usually several years after treatment, but may be within months. It can be difficult to distinguish from tumour recurrence but is less likely to be painful. MRI, and especially positron emission tomography, may be helpful in diagnosis.

Traction lesions

Traction on the arm may result in damage to the plexus itself or may lead to avulsion of the spinal roots from the cord. If the roots are avulsed, sensory nerve action potentials from affected fingers will be preserved despite total anaesthesia, and the histamine flare response will be preserved in anaesthetized skin. This follows from the fact that the nerve fibres are interrupted proximal to the dorsal root ganglia and therefore the peripheral sensory axons do not degenerate.

In severe traction lesions, commonly encountered in current medical practice as a result of motorcycle or aircraft accidents, the whole of the plexus may be damaged. With forcible downward displacement of the shoulder, as when someone is thrown forwards and the shoulder strikes against an obstacle, only the upper part of the plexus, involving the contribution from the fifth and sixth cervical nerve roots, may be damaged. This may also be encountered as a birth injury from traction on the head, or on the trunk in a breech presentation (Erb's palsy), and rarely in anaesthetized patients during surgery or in individuals carrying heavy rucksacks. Selective injury to the lower part of the plexus involving the contributions from the eighth cervical and first thoracic nerve roots occurs as a result of traction with the arm extended, as when an individual falls from a height and tries to save himself by hanging on to a ledge. It may also occur as a birth injury following traction with the arm extended (Klumpke's paralysis), but is less common than upper plexus damage.

Selective damage to the upper portion of the plexus (C5 and C6 roots or upper trunk) results in paralysis of deltoid, biceps, brachialis, brachioradialis, and sometimes supraspinatus, infraspinatus, and subscapularis. If the roots are avulsed from the cord, the rhomboids, serratus anterior, levator scapulae, and the scalene muscles will be affected. The arm hangs at the side, internally rotated at the shoulder, with the elbow extended and the forearm pronated in the 'waiter's tip' position. Abduction at the shoulder and flexion at the elbow are not possible. The biceps and brachioradialis jerks are lost. Sensory loss affects the lateral aspect of the shoulder and upper arm and the radial border of the forearm. Selective paralysis of the lower brachial plexus (C8, T1) results in paralysis of all the intrinsic hand muscles and a consequent claw-hand deformity, weakness of the medial finger and wrist flexors, and sensory loss along the medial border of the forearm and hand and over the medial two fingers. Cervical sympathetic paralysis, giving rise to Horner's syndrome, is frequently associated.

When the spinal roots are avulsed from the cord, regeneration is impossible and intractable spontaneous pain may be a highly troublesome sequel. Where the injury is distal to the dorsal root ganglia, lesions of the upper portion of the brachial plexus recover more satisfactorily than lower plexus lesions. The value of surgical repair is still a controversial issue. In Erb's form of birth injury, weakness of abduction at the shoulder and flexion at the elbow often persist, although there may be little residual sensory loss. Full recovery takes place in about a third of cases. It is less likely to occur with lower plexus injuries or if the whole plexus is involved. Early recognition and the application of measures to reduce the risk of joint contractures are important. Surgical treatment may be considered soon after the injury in cases where the nerve roots have been avulsed.

Thoracic outlet syndromes

The contribution of the eighth cervical and first thoracic roots to the brachial plexus may be damaged by angulation over an abnormal rib or, more usually, a fibrous band arising from the seventh cervical vertebra and attached to the first rib. The subclavian artery may be affected by cervical ribs, giving rise to aneurysmal dilatation and

vascular symptoms such as Raynaud's phenomenon and embolic phenomena, but the simultaneous occurrence of both neural and vascular phenomena is rare.

Damage to the lower part of the brachial plexus leads to weakness and wasting of the small hand muscles, and of the medial forearm wrist and finger flexors. Occasionally, there is selective wasting of the thenar pad in the hand, mimicking to some extent the appearance of carpal tunnel syndrome. Numbness, pain, and paraesthesiae occur along the inner border of the forearm and hand, extending into the medial two fingers. The pain tends to be provoked by carrying heavy articles with the hand on the affected side. Horner's syndrome may be a feature. Nerve conduction studies are helpful when there are difficulties in distinguishing a cervical rib syndrome from a lesion of the ulnar or median nerves on clinical grounds. Surgical removal of the rib or fibrous band often leads to abolition of the pain and paraesthesiae, but recovery of power in the small hand muscles is usually disappointing.

Neoplastic involvement

Tumours may arise locally in the brachial plexus, such as a neurofibroma in neurofibromatosis type I (von Recklinghausen's disease) or a solitary schwannoma, or the plexus may be invaded by tumours arising in other structures. The most common is involvement of the lower part of the plexus by an apical carcinoma of the lung (Pancoast's tumour), which gives rise to wasting and weakness of the small hand muscles and of the medial forearm wrist and finger flexors, pain and sensory loss affecting the medial border of the forearm and hand, and cervical sympathetic paralysis. Other tumours that may invade the brachial plexus include carcinoma of the breast and malignant lymphomas affecting the lymph glands in the root of the neck.

Radial nerve (C5–8)

The long course of the radial nerve and its position in relation to the humerus make this nerve unusually susceptible to external compression. It is a continuation of the posterior cord of the brachial plexus. In the upper arm, it supplies triceps and anconeus, and the skin on the back of the arm, just above the elbow through the posterior cutaneous nerve of the arm. The lateral aspect of the lower part of the upper arm is supplied by the lower lateral brachial cutaneous branch and the dorsal aspect of the forearm, by the posterior cutaneous nerve of the forearm. Muscular branches of the radial nerve innervate brachioradialis and extensor carpi radialis longus and brevis. The superficial branch of the nerve is its continuation. It descends along the radial border of the forearm and supplies the skin over the dorsum of the hand and the thumb, index, and middle fingers. The deep branch forms the posterior interosseus nerve which winds around the lateral aspect of the radius, passes through supinator, which it supplies, and innervates extensor digitorum, extensor digiti minimi, extensor carpi ulnaris, and often extensor carpi radialis brevis, abductor pollicis longus, extensor pollicis longus and brevis, and extensor indicis.

The nerve may be injured in wounds of the axilla so that the paralysis includes triceps, resulting in loss of extension at the elbow. The most frequent type of injury is compression of the nerve in the middle third of the arm against the humerus. This is encountered as 'Saturday night palsy' in which an individual falls asleep when intoxicated with the upper arm over the arm of a chair. Triceps is spared, but brachioradialis, supinator, and all the forearm extensor muscles are paralysed. Sensory impairment is limited to the dorsum of the hand. Commonly the lesion consists of a localized conduction block so that muscle wasting does not occur and a muscle response can be obtained on electrical stimulation of the nerve below the level of the lesion. Recovery is complete within a matter of weeks. A cock-up wrist splint may be helpful while recovery is awaited. At times, there is some associated axonal degeneration so that electromyographic evidence of denervation is detectable and full recovery is correspondingly delayed.

Many muscles not supplied by the radial nerve work at a disadvantage when the wrist and finger extensors are paralysed. These defects must not be mistaken for signs of injury to other nerves. Owing to the flexed position of the wrist, gripping is impaired, but, if the power of the wrist and finger flexors is tested with the wrist extended, it can be shown to be normal. The action of the interossei in abducting and adducting the fingers is also feeble when the wrist is flexed, but full power is demonstrable if these muscles are tested with the hand resting flat on a table so that the fingers are maintained in extension.

A lesion of the posterior interosseus nerve gives rise to weakness confined to abduction and extension of the thumb, and extension of the fingers and extensor carpi ulnaris. Supinator is spared, together with brachioradialis and the radial wrist extensors, and there is no sensory loss. The nerve may be compressed, usually under the arcade of Frohse. This is formed by a sharp band of fibrous tissue, which binds together the superficial and deep heads of the supinator muscle as they arise from the lateral epicondyle of the humerus and lateral border of the radius. Surgical exploration and decompression should be performed if the palsy lasts more than 12 weeks.

Axillary nerve (C5, C6)

This is a branch of the posterior cord of the brachial plexus. It supplies deltoid and teres minor and the skin over deltoid through the upper lateral brachial cutaneous nerve. It may be damaged in injuries to the shoulder and the chief symptom is an almost complete inability to raise the arm at the shoulder. In the past, it was sometimes injured by pressure from a crutch ('crutch palsy').

Musculocutaneous nerve (C5, C6)

This nerve is rarely damaged alone, but may be involved in injuries to the brachial plexus. It supplies coracobrachialis, biceps, and brachialis, and the skin over the lateral aspect of the forearm through the lateral cutaneous nerve of the forearm. Flexion at the elbow is still possible by brachioradialis, but is weak, and sensation may be impaired along the radial border of the forearm.

Median nerve (C6–8, T1)

The median nerve arises from the medial and lateral cords of the brachial plexus and descends with the brachial artery through the upper arm, entering the forearm deep to the bicipital aponeurosis. It has no muscular branches above the elbow. It supplies all the muscles in the anterior aspect of the forearm except flexor carpi ulnaris and the medial half of flexor digitorum profundus. The main trunk of the nerve supplies pronator teres, flexor carpi radialis, palmaris longus, and flexor digitorum superficialis. Through the anterior interosseus branch, it also supplies the lateral aspect of flexor digitorum profundus, flexor pollicis longus, and pronator quadratus. The main trunk passes deep to the flexor retinaculum

of the wrist and its recurrent muscular branch supplies abductor pollicis brevis and opponens pollicis, and contributes to the innervation of flexor pollicis brevis. It also supplies the lateral two lumbrical muscles, the skin of the lateral aspect of the palm, and the lateral three and a half digits over their palmar aspects and terminal parts of their dorsal aspects.

Lesions in the forearm

The median nerve may be injured in the region of the elbow or compressed at the level of the pronator teres muscle. Entrapment neuropathies in the upper forearm are, however, uncommon. Occasionally the anterior interosseus branch is involved in isolation.

Complete lesions of the median nerve at the elbow give rise to paralysis of pronator teres, the radial flexor of the wrist, the long finger flexors except the ulnar half of the deep flexor, most of the muscles of the thenar eminence, and the two radial lumbricals. In brief, there is an inability to flex the index finger and the distal phalanx of the thumb, flexion of the middle finger is weak, and opposition of the thumb is defective. The appearance of the hand has been described as simian; it shows ulnar deviation, the index and middle fingers are more extended than normal, and the thumb lies in the same plane as the fingers.

In more detail, pronation is incomplete and defective. The patient attempts to overcome this by rotating the whole limb at the shoulder. Paralysis of the wrist flexors is evident when attempts are made to flex against resistance. The tendon of flexor carpi ulnaris stands out alone and the hand goes into ulnar deviation. Flexion of the fingers is good in the ulnar two fingers, although weaker than normal. The index finger cannot be flexed and the middle finger only incompletely. Flexion at the metacarpophalangeal joints is possible in all fingers, including the index, and flexion at these joints with extension at the interphalangeal joints is accomplished by interossei and the lumbricals. If the proximal phalanx of the thumb is immobilized, it will be found that flexion of the terminal phalanx is abolished because of paralysis of flexor pollicis longus. Paralysis of the thenar muscles gives rise to defective abduction and opposition of the thumb. By means of the adductor, the thumb can be drawn into the palm, but, as the radial fingers cannot be flexed or the thumb opposed, it is impossible to place the tip of the thumb on the fingers.

Sensory loss is evident over the lateral three and a half digits and the lateral aspect of the palm, although individual variations occur. There is almost complete anaesthesia over the two terminal phalanges of the index and middle fingers. This degree of sensory loss, combined with the motor deficit, renders the thumb and index fingers almost useless and makes paralysis of the median the most serious single nerve lesion in the upper limb.

Vasomotor and trophic changes often ensue. The skin in the distribution of the median nerve tends to become reddened, dry, and atrophic. The pulp of the affected fingers becomes atrophic and ulceration occasionally develops in the tip of the index finger. The nails may become white and atrophic.

After a total transection of the nerve in the region of the elbow, even with a satisfactory surgical repair, recovery is slow and rarely complete, particularly with respect to the innervation of the hand.

With partial lesions of the median nerve in the arm or forearm, causalgia may be a troublesome consequence. The pain develops at any time from a few hours to 45 days after the injury. The pain is severe and unremitting, and frequently has a burning or smarting quality. Upon this may be superimposed severe paroxysms of pain provoked by either touching or jarring the limb or emotional distress. Vasomotor and sudomotor changes may be associated. The skin usually becomes dry and scaly, but excessive sweating may be a feature. The patient adopts a protective attitude towards the limb, so that fixation of the joints of the fingers and wrist may develop, together with atrophic changes in the skin and subcutaneous tissue. About 80% of cases of true causalgia are relieved by sympathectomy. Untreated, the pain gradually subsides over months or years.

Lesions at the wrist

The superficial situation of the median nerve at the wrist renders it liable to injury as a result of lacerations sustained by falling against a window with the hand outstretched or in suicide attempts. It may also be damaged as an occupational hazard by individuals who exert repeated pressure on the butt of the hand.

Much the most common lesion at this site is the carpal tunnel syndrome, in which the median nerve is compressed as it passes deep to the flexor retinaculum. The usual presentation is with acroparaesthesiae, which consist of numbness, tingling, and burning sensations felt in the hand and fingers; the pain sometimes radiates up the forearm as far as the elbow or even as high as the shoulder or root of the neck. The paraesthesiae are sometimes restricted to the radial fingers, but may affect all the digits because some fibres from the median nerve are distributed to the fifth finger through communication with the ulnar nerve in the palm. The attacks of pain and paraesthesiae are most common at night and often wake the patient from sleep. They are then relieved by shaking the hand. The hand tends to feel numb and useless on waking in the morning but recovers after it has been used for some minutes. The symptoms may recur during the day after use, or at times if the patient sits with the hands immobile and hanging down. Such symptoms of acroparaesthesiae may persist for many years without the appearance of symptoms of median nerve damage. In some patients, weakness of the thenar muscles develops, particularly of abduction of the thumb, and is associated with atrophy of the lateral aspect of the thenar eminence (Fig. 24.16.1). Sensory loss may appear over the tips of the median innervated fingers. Occasionally patients present with symptoms of median nerve deficit in the hand without attacks of acroparaesthesiae having occurred, or motor and sensory signs may be discovered incidentally in the absence of symptoms, particularly in older individuals.

The symptoms are usually characteristic, with abnormal signs not being found except in advanced cases. At times percussion over the carpal tunnel may elicit Tinel's sign, or symptoms may be provoked by hyperextension of the wrist or sustained flexion (Phalen's sign). Neither sign is very specific or sensitive. Confirmation can usually be obtained by nerve conduction studies.

Carpal tunnel syndrome is much more common in women than men and its lifetime prevalence is 10%. It is commonly associated with excessive use of the hands. It may develop as a consequence of involvement of the wrist joint in rheumatoid arthritis or osteoarthritis, or deformity related to an old fracture. Predisposing causes are pregnancy, obesity, myxoedema, acromegaly, and infiltration of the flexor retinaculum in primary and hereditary amyloidosis. A twin study has shown a strong genetic component to the development of carpal tunnel syndrome.

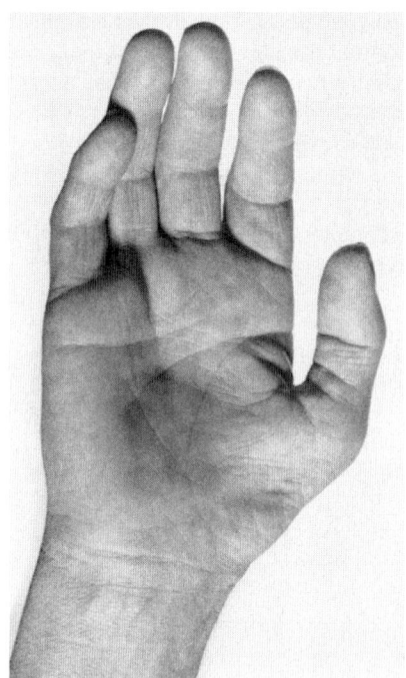

Fig. 24.16.1 Thenar wasting in a patient with a severe median nerve lesion.

Fluctuation of symptoms is common and spontaneous recovery occurs in about 20% of patients. A conservative approach to treatment is appropriate initially. Rest and weight reduction are helpful. Splinting of the wrist in a neutral position to reduce movement during the day and night may also be useful. If the symptoms persist despite these conservative measures, the choice lies between corticosteroid injection and surgical decompression by dividing the flexor retinaculum. About half the patients obtain satisfactory relief from corticosteroid injection alone. The average success rate from surgery is higher, about 75%, but it is more inconvenient and may be complicated by a painful scar. About 7% of patients report that their hands are worse after the operation than before. Patients presenting with marked signs of carpal tunnel compression, muscle weakness and wasting, or sensory loss need to undergo decompression to prevent further damage. Symptoms that were previously intermittent usually recover completely but permanent symptoms may not.

Ulnar nerve (C7, C8, T1)

The ulnar nerve arises from the medial cord of the plexus, usually with a contribution from the lateral cord. It descends in the medial side of the upper arm, passes around the elbow in the ulnar groove, and enters the forearm under an aponeurotic band between the humeral and ulnar heads of flexor carpi ulnaris. It then runs superficial to flexor digitorum profundus to the wrist and enters the hand between the pisiform bone and the hook of the hamate, superficial to flexor retinaculum. After penetrating the hypothenar muscles, its deep branch crosses the palm and ends in flexor pollicis brevis.

In the upper arm, branches arise that supply flexor carpi ulnaris and the medial part of flexor digitorum profundus. In the forearm, the dorsal branch arises, winds around the ulna and supplies the skin over the dorsal aspect of the hand and the medial one and a half fingers. In the hand, a superficial branch supplies palmaris brevis and the skin over the medial aspect of the palm and the medial one and half fingers. The deep branch, after supplying the hypothenar muscles, innervates interossei, the third and fourth lumbricals, adductor pollicis, and part of flexor pollicis brevis.

Lesions at the elbow

Total paralysis from lesions at this level, including the branches to flexor carpi ulnaris and flexor digitorum profundus, gives rise to wasting along the medial side of the forearm flexor mass. There is weakness of flexion of the fourth and fifth fingers. If the proximal portions of these fingers are held immobilized, flexion of the terminal phalanges is not possible. When the hand is flexed to the ulnar side against resistance, the tendon of flexor carpi ulnaris is not palpable. Paralysis of the hypothenar muscles abolishes abduction of the fifth finger. Paralysis of interossei and the medial two lumbricals gives rise to the 'claw-hand' deformity (Fig. 24.16.2). The action of these muscles is to flex the fingers at the metacarpophalangeal joints with the fingers extended at the interphalangeal joints. In claw hand, the posture of the fingers is opposite to this, namely extension of the metacarpophalangeal joints with flexion at the interphalangeal joints. Although all the interossei are paralysed, the defect is seen mainly in the ulnar fingers because the radial lumbricals supplied by the median nerve are still active. The long extensors of the fingers, being unopposed, overextend the proximal joints, and flexor digitorum superficialis flexes the proximal interphalangeal joints.

In the hand, there is wasting of the hypothenar muscles, interossei, and the medial part of the thenar eminence. Movements of abduction and adduction of the fingers are weak, as is adduction of the extended thumb against the palm. Sensory loss affects the dorsal and palmar aspects of the medial side of the hand and the medial one and a half fingers.

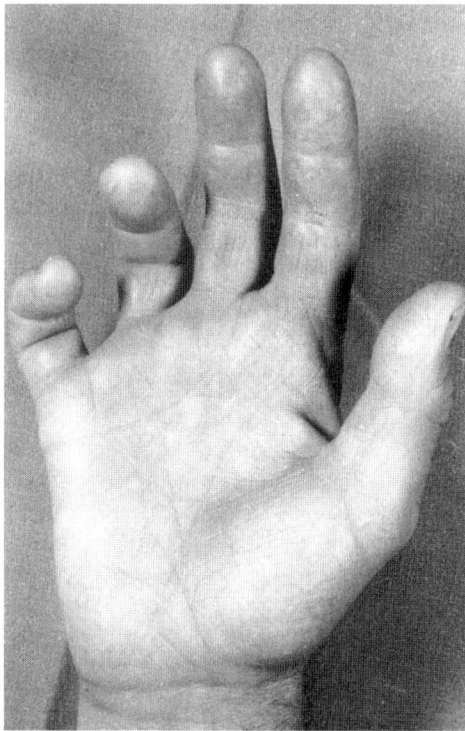

Fig. 24.16.2 'Claw-hand' deformity in a patient with an ulnar nerve lesion.

The ulnar nerve may be damaged by dislocations or fracture dislocations at the elbow and is sometimes compressed in individuals who habitually lean on their elbows. Entrapment may occur in the cubital tunnel as the nerve underlies the aponeurotic band between the two heads of flexor carpi ulnaris. This is most likely to occur in those performing heavy manual work or if there is an excessive carrying angle at the elbow, as may occur after a previous malunited supracondylar fracture of the humerus ('tardy ulnar palsy'). The medial wall of the cubital tunnel is formed by the elbow joint; osteoarthritis of the elbow can lead to osteophytic encroachment on the tunnel and compression of the ulnar nerve. In the cubital tunnel syndrome, the ulnar nerve is often palpably enlarged in the ulnar groove and for a short distance proximally. Ulnar nerve lesions are not infrequent in leprosy. Here the enlargement of the nerve tends to be maximal at a little distance above the elbow.

If the nerve is compressed in the cubital tunnel, exploration and decompression by slitting the aponeurosis may suffice. When it is suspected that the nerve has been subjected to repeated compression at the elbow, surgical transposition to the front of the medial epicondyle should be considered. Decompression of the nerve is the safer operation because transposition puts the blood supply of the nerve at risk.

Lesions at the wrist or in the hand

Damage to the nerve at the wrist will spare the dorsal branch, so that cutaneous sensation over the dorsum of the hand and fingers is spared. A lesion just proximal to the wrist will give rise to sensory impairment on the palmar aspect of the hand and fingers alone, and weakness of all the ulnar-innervated intrinsic hand muscles. A slightly more distal lesion spares the superficial branch of the nerve and therefore produces no sensory deficit. Finally, damage to the deep palmar branch spares the hypothenar muscles, but causes weakness of the other ulnar-innervated small hand muscles. Lesions at the wrist or in the hand are usually the result of compression by ganglia or by repeated occupational trauma. Damage to the deep palmar branch, for example, may be caused by firm pressure in the palm from a screwdriver or drill. If occupational pressure is the cause, recovery follows cessation of the precipitating cause. Should improvement fail to occur after an appropriate interval, surgical exploration to establish whether a ganglion is present is merited.

It is not always easy on clinical grounds to decide whether the lesion is at the elbow or the wrist. Compression of the nerve in the cubital tunnel, for example, may spare the branches to flexor carpi ulnaris and flexor digitorum profundus. In these circumstances, nerve conduction studies may be helpful, as they may in distinguishing between lesions of the ulnar nerve and damage to the eighth cervical and first thoracic spinal roots. MRI is now used to help localize the lesion site.

Lumbosacral plexus

Lesions of the lumbosacral plexus are not common. The plexus may be involved in pelvic malignancy, such as from carcinoma of the uterine cervix, bladder, prostate, or rectum, or be the site of a local neural tumour. It may be compressed by a haematoma in patients receiving anticoagulant therapy or who have haemophilia, or be involved in fractures of the pelvis. The lumbosacral cord may be compressed against the rim of the pelvis by the fetal head during parturition, with consequent weakness of the anterior tibial and peroneal muscles, and sensory impairment in the distribution of the fourth and fifth lumbar dermatomes. The superior gluteal nerve may also be affected. Recovery is initially good but may not be complete. The plexus may be affected in diabetic amyotrophy. Rare instances of idiopathic lumbosacral plexopathy are encountered, comparable to the corresponding disorder that affects the brachial plexus.

Femoral nerve (L2–4)

This nerve arises from the lumbar plexus, crosses the iliac fossa between psoas and iliacus, and enters the thigh deep to the middle of the inguinal ligament. In the iliac fossa it supplies iliacus and, in the thigh, pectineus, sartorius, and quadriceps femoris, and anterior cutaneous branches to the front of the thigh. The continuation of the femoral nerve is the saphenous nerve, which supplies the skin over the medial aspect of the lower leg as far as the medial malleolus.

Damage to the femoral nerve causes weakness of knee extension, wasting of quadriceps, loss of the knee jerk, and sensory impairment over the front of the thigh and in the distribution of the saphenous nerve. With a proximal lesion, there may also be weakness of hip flexion from paralysis of iliacus.

The femoral nerve may be injured in fractures of the pelvis or femur, in dislocations of the hip, and at times during operations on the pelvis or hip. It may be involved by psoas abscesses or tumours, or implicated in wounds of the thigh. It is commonly involved in large psoas muscle haematomas in individuals with haemophilia (see Section 22) and in diabetic amyotrophy. Owing to the rapid dispersion of the branches in the thigh, partial lesions are common from wounds at this site. The nerve to quadriceps is most often injured, and the resulting paralysis causes considerable difficulty in walking because the knee cannot be locked in extension and gives way, especially when descending stairs. The saphenous nerve is sometimes damaged in surgery for the treatment of varicose veins.

Obturator nerve (L2–4)

The nerve emerges from the lateral border of psoas, crosses the lateral wall of the pelvis, and enters the thigh through the obturator foramen where it supplies gracilis, adductor longus and brevis, adductor magnus, obturator externus, and sometimes also pectineus, and the skin over the lower medial aspect of the thigh.

Damage to the obturator nerve results in weakness of adduction and internal rotation at the hip, pain in the groin, and sensory impairment on the medial part of the thigh. The nerve may be involved in pelvic fractures, hip and pelvic surgery, and neoplastic infiltration, and can be damaged by the fetal head or forceps during parturition.

Lateral cutaneous nerve of the thigh (L2, L3)

This nerve arises from the lumbar plexus, passes obliquely across iliacus and enters the thigh under the lateral part of the inguinal ligament. It supplies the skin over the anterolateral aspect of the thigh.

Meralgia paraesthetica is an entrapment neuropathy resulting from compression of this nerve as it passes under the inguinal ligament. It is more common in men and obese individuals and may be unilateral or bilateral. The symptoms consist of numbness in the territory of the nerve, combined with tingling or burning paraesthesiae provoked by prolonged standing or after excessive walking. Weight loss may be helpful, and in many instances the condition subsides spontaneously. Decompression of the nerve is rarely necessary.

Sciatic nerve (L4, L5, S1–3)

The sciatic nerve enters the thigh through the sciatic notch. It is composed of the tibial and peroneal divisions which are usually bound together within a common sheath, the tibial division lying medially. It descends through the posterior aspect of the thigh, initially deep to gluteus maximus, and supplies semitendinosus, semimembranosus, and the long head of biceps through its peroneal division. It separates into the tibial and common peroneal nerves in the lower thigh, which supply all the muscles below the knee, and both nerves contribute to the formation of the sural nerve.

Total interruption of the sciatic nerve gives rise to foot drop. Walking is possible, but the patient cannot stand on the toes or the heel of the affected foot and the ankle is unstable. All movement below the knee is paralysed. If the injury is in the upper thigh, flexion of the knee is also weak. The skin is completely anaesthetized over the entire foot except for the medial border which is supplied by the saphenous nerve. Pressure sores may develop. The anaesthesia extends upwards on the posterolateral aspect of the calf in its lower two-thirds. The sense of joint position is abolished in the foot and toes. Beyond this area of complete anaesthesia, there is a wide zone in which sensibility may be diminished. Sweating is absent on the sole and dorsum of the foot, but is preserved on the medial side. The ankle jerk is lost but the knee jerk is retained.

The sciatic nerve may be involved in pelvic tumours and can be injured by fractures of the pelvis or femur or during hip replacement operations. After the radial and ulnar, it is implicated in gunshot wounds more frequently than any other nerve. Partial injury of the tibial division may be followed by causalgia. Incomplete lesions of the nerve may be caused by pressure of the nerve against the hard edge of a chair in individuals who fall asleep while intoxicated. Similar lesions may occur in people with diabetes, in whom the peripheral nerves are more susceptible to pressure neuropathy.

The syndrome of root pain and sciatica is considered in Chapter 19.4.

Tibial nerve (L4, L5, S1–3)

After separating from the peroneal division of the sciatic nerve in the lower thigh, this nerve passes through the popliteal fossa and enters the calf deep to gastrocnemius through the fibrous arch of soleus. It descends through the calf to the medial side of the ankle, passes beneath the flexor retinaculum, and divides into the medial and lateral plantar nerves. It supplies popliteus, all the muscles of the calf, and, through the plantar nerves, the small muscles of the sole of the foot and sensation to the sole.

When the nerve is interrupted, the patient is unable to plantarflex or invert the foot, flex the toes, or stand on the ball of the foot. Paralysis of interossei leads to a claw-like deformity of the toes. Sensation is lost over the sole. Causalgia may arise after partial lesions. Injury to the distal portion of the nerve by a penetrating injury or deep wound of the calf gives rise to paralysis of the intrinsic muscles of the foot but spares the muscles acting at the ankle. Sensation is lost on the sole of the foot and this may be accompanied by pain. If the injury is distal to the origin of the branches to flexor hallucis longus and flexor digitorum longus, the lesion may escape detection because paralysis of the small foot muscles and sensory loss over the sole may be overlooked.

The tibial nerve is very occasionally compressed under the flexor retinaculum (tarsal tunnel syndrome), usually precipitated by osteoarthritis or post-traumatic deformities at the ankle, or teno-synovitis. Burning pain and tingling paraesthesiae occur in the sole, usually after prolonged standing or walking. The condition is generally unilateral. Careful examination may demonstrate wasting of the intrinsic muscles in the medial aspect of the foot, and sensory impairment over the sole. Nerve conduction studies may be helpful diagnostically. Treatment is by surgical section of flexor retinaculum.

Morton's metatarsalgia is a syndrome of severe lancinating pain, usually in one of the web spaces at the base of the toes, especially the third web space. The pain occurs especially on walking. Removing the shoe and massaging the foot or manipulating the toes may bring relief. The condition is most common in middle-aged people, especially women. Its pathology is uncertain, although it is often held to be due to formation of a neuroma. Orthoses are often tried and decompressive operations or excision of the neuroma is commonly recommended without adequate evidence to determine which is the best treatment.

Common peroneal nerve (L4, L5, S1, S2)

After separating from the tibial division of the sciatic nerve in the lower part of the thigh, the common peroneal nerve descends through the popliteal fossa, winds around the neck of the fibula, and divides into its superficial and deep branches. The superficial peroneal nerve passes down in front of the fibula, supplies peroneus longus and brevis, and emerges in the lower leg, supplying the skin on the lateral aspect of the lower leg. It crosses the extensor retinaculum and supplies the skin on the dorsum of the foot and the second to fifth toes. The deep peroneal branch continues to wind around the fibula, pierces the anterior intermuscular septum, and descends on the anterior interosseous membrane. It innervates tibialis anterior, extensor digitorum longus, extensor hallucis longus, and peroneus tertius. It passes deep to the extensor retinaculum after which it supplies extensor digitorum brevis and the skin of the adjacent sides of the first and second toes.

Damage to the common peroneal nerve is more frequent than injury to its two branches because of its vulnerable superficial position at the neck of the fibula. It gives rise to foot drop, with paralysis both of dorsiflexion and eversion at the ankle and of toe extension. Cutaneous sensation is impaired over the lateral aspect of the lower leg and ankle, and on the dorsum of the foot.

The common peroneal nerve may be compressed at the neck of the fibula by habitually sitting with the legs crossed, prolonged squatting, pressure during sleep or while anaesthetized, and various other events. It can be damaged by traction caused by fractures of the tibia and fibula, and is sometimes damaged by ischaemia in the anterior tibial compartment syndrome. Paralysis caused by external pressure frequently gives rise to a local conduction block with satisfactory recovery within a few weeks. A foot-drop orthosis may be helpful while recovery is awaited.

Sural nerve (L5, S1–2)

This arises from the sciatic nerve and descends to the back of the calf, winds around to the lateral side of the ankle, and reaches the lateral border of the foot. It supplies the skin in this distribution. Sensory impairment occasionally results from pressure on the nerve as it lies in a superficial situation in the back of the calf. This nerve

is the one most commonly chosen on the rare occasions when a nerve biopsy is needed.

Generalized neuropathies

Neuropathies related to metabolic and endocrine disorders

Diabetes mellitus

A significant degree of peripheral neuropathy develops in about 15% of patients with diabetes, although a substantially greater number have either minor symptoms without signs or evidence of a subclinical neuropathy on clinical examination or based on abnormalities of nerve conduction. In general, the neuropathies that appear can be divided into symmetrical sensory and autonomic polyneuropathies, on the one hand, and isolated peripheral nerve lesions or multifocal neuropathies, on the other. Mixed syndromes are common.

The most common form is a symmetrical sensory polyneuropathy, giving rise to numbness and tingling paraesthesiae in the toes and feet, and less often in the fingers. Aching or lancinating pains in the feet and legs, particularly at night, may be a troublesome feature. Examination reveals loss of vibration sense in the feet, depression of the ankle jerks, and distal cutaneous sensory impairment. Neuropathic plantar ulcers, and occasionally Charcot's joints, are an important complication. Loss of the sense of pain results in perforating ulcers on the feet and neuropathic joint degeneration, particularly in the toes and tarsal joints; impaired postural sense may give rise to an ataxic gait. An acute painful diabetic neuropathy also occurs which predominantly affects the lower limbs. The onset is often associated with poor diabetic control and precipitate weight loss ('diabetic neuropathic cachexia'). Some patients have a pure small fibre neuropathy with pain, reduced temperature, and pinprick sensation, but normal reflexes and preserved vibration, and light touch and position sensation.

Autonomic neuropathy frequently accompanies the sensory neuropathy and may be the salient manifestation, and rarely occurs in isolation. Pupillary disturbances usually take the form of a reduced response to light. Gustatory facial sweating provoked by the smell and taste of food can be troublesome. Anhidrosis may occur distally in the limbs; if it is extensive and also affects the trunk, heat intolerance can result. Symptoms referable to the alimentary tract include dysphagia from oesophageal involvement, episodes of vomiting related to gastric atony (gastroparesis), and episodic nocturnal diarrhoea, often alternating with periods of constipation. Those related to the genitourinary system include erectile dysfunction, retrograde ejaculation, bladder atony with difficulty in voiding, and urinary retention with overflow. Vascular denervation sometimes results in orthostatic hypotension, and cardiac denervation may be demonstrable by an elevated resting heart rate and the absence of beat-to-beat variation with respiration. The risk and progression of diabetic polyneuropathy are reduced by strict glycaemic control.

Isolated nerve lesions tend to occur more commonly in older people with diabetes. At times they develop insidiously, but at other times they have an abrupt onset with pain. Of the cranial nerves, the nerves to the external ocular muscles, particularly the third and sixth, and also the facial nerve, are affected most often. In contradistinction to the effects of compression of the third nerve by a carotid aneurysm, pupillary innervation is often spared.

On the trunk, isolated root lesions may occur. In the limbs, the lesions tend to occur at the common sites of compression or entrapment. It seems likely that the nerves of people with diabetes exhibit an excessive vulnerability to damage from pressure.

Diabetic amyotrophy (also known as diabetic lumbosacral radiculoplexus neuropathy or proximal diabetic neuropathy) represents a particular example of a multifocal neuropathy that develops usually in older obese individuals with diabetes. It consists of an asymmetrical proximal motor syndrome that affects the anterior thigh muscles and hip flexors, and sometimes also the anterolateral muscles of the lower leg. Less commonly it is symmetrical. Its onset may be acute or insidious and is often accompanied by pain, particularly at night. There is generally little or no associated sensory loss. The knee jerks are usually depressed or absent. Inflammatory lesions including vasculitis have been demonstrated in peripheral nerves in proximal diabetic neuropathy, leading to trials of immunomodulatory therapy, which have not been conclusive.

The causation of diabetic neuropathy is uncertain. It tends to occur more often in people with poorly controlled diabetes, but the correlation is not close. In type 2 diabetes it may be the presenting symptom or occur for the first time on initiation of treatment with insulin. There is evidence to suggest that diabetic microangiopathy is important in the genesis of isolated nerve lesions. Metabolic factors are probably more important in the origin of the symmetrical polyneuropathies, but their nature is uncertain. An increased concentration of sorbitol in nerves secondary to hyperglycaemia may be involved in causing nerve fibre dysfunction. People with diabetes are more at risk of developing some other neuropathies including entrapment neuropathies and chemotherapy-induced neuropathy. Patients with impaired glucose tolerance or impaired fasting glycaemia also have an increased risk of neuropathy, even if they do not have diabetes.

Focal peripheral nerve lesions and diabetic amyotrophy, if of acute onset, may recover adequately, as does acute painful diabetic neuropathy when satisfactory glycaemic control is achieved. Symmetrical sensory and autonomic neuropathy, once established, recovers less satisfactorily, even with good diabetic control. Correcting the hyperglycaemia by continuous subcutaneous insulin infusion or transplantation of the pancreas stabilizes the neuropathy. Trials of aldose reductase inhibitors to reduce sorbitol accumulation have not given clear evidence of improvement in neuropathy.

Care of the feet is vitally important in diabetic sensory neuropathy, to prevent the development of chronic ulceration. Pain may be helped by tricyclic antidepressants, duloxetine, antiepileptic drugs, especially pregabalin, gabapentin, or carbamazepine, or tramadol. Hypotension can be improved by raising the head of the bed at night, high fluid and salt intake, and compression stockings. More severe cases may require treatment with the α-agonist midodrine and fludrocortisone. Gastroparesis may respond to metoclopramide, domperidone, or erythromycin. In extreme cases, persistent vomiting may necessitate a roux-en-Y gastroenterostomy. Diabetic diarrhoea can be helped by low-dose tetracycline or diphenoxylate, loperamide, or codeine phosphate. An atonic bladder can be managed in the earlier stages by regular voiding, lower abdominal compression, and straining. More severe cases should undergo urodynamic studies and are usually best managed by intermittent self-catheterisation. Urinary tract infections should be treated promptly. Bladder neck resection can be useful in carefully selected cases. Erectile dysfunction may be treated with one of the phosphodiesterase inhibitors, sildenafil, tadalafil, or vardenafil, and in the UK their use is funded by the NHS for diabetic neuropathy. If such treatment fails, referral to a specialist clinic should be made and intrapenile injections of alprostadil (prostaglandin E_1) may be considered.

Amyloidosis

The various forms of amyloid disease are described in Chapter 12.12.3. The peripheral nerves may be involved in primary amyloidosis due to plasma cell dyscrasia and in amyloidosis related to myeloma (light chain amyloidosis). There are also several dominantly inherited forms of amyloid neuropathy, the most important of which are the result of mutations in the gene for transthyretin (*TTR*), including the Portuguese type (see later). Isolated lesions may occur from the infiltration of amyloid into nerves or from compression of the median nerve in the carpal tunnel because of deposits in the flexor retinaculum. More strikingly, a generalized neuropathy may develop. It begins with selective loss of pain and temperature sensation in the feet, and later in the hands. Motor involvement, loss of tendon reflexes, and impairment of other sensory modalities occur later. Autonomic involvement is an early feature, causing impotence, orthostatic hypotension, bladder atony, and disturbances of alimentary function. Amyloid deposits are present in the peripheral nerve trunks, which may be enlarged, and in the dorsal root and sympathetic ganglia.

No treatment influences the progress of the neuropathy apart from liver transplantation in neuropathy due to *TTR* mutations (see Chapter 12.12.3). The use of stem cell transplantation is being explored in amyloidosis related to malignant plasma cell dyscrasias. The spontaneous pains are sometimes improved by antiepileptic (pregabalin, gabapentin, or carbamazepine) or tricyclic antidepressant drugs. Care must be taken to prevent damage to the anaesthetized feet, lower legs, and hands. Autonomic symptoms may require treatment as described for diabetic neuropathy.

Carpal tunnel syndrome is frequent in patients on long-term haemodialysis, related to deposition of amyloid in the flexor retinaculum derived from retained β_2-microglobulin.

Uraemia

Uraemic neuropathy did not become a clinical problem until the advent of treatment of end-stage renal failure by haemodialysis. It occurs in patients with severe chronic renal failure. It was most often seen in patients undergoing treatment with periodic haemodialysis but is now much less frequently a problem. The symptoms are usually predominantly sensory, with numbness and tingling paraesthesiae, and burning in the feet. Restless legs syndrome and cramps are often conspicuous (see Section 24.24). A distal motor neuropathy may be associated and occasional cases are purely motor. The condition is not necessarily improved by increased haemodialysis but does improve after kidney transplantation. Failure to clear 'middle molecules' that are toxic to axons has been proposed but not proved to be the mechanism. The nerve trunks in the arm and forearm are at risk during surgery for placing arteriovenous anastomoses for dialysis. Symptoms may be produced by surgical damage, ischaemia, sometimes partly attributable to shunting, and compression.

Myxoedema

Compression of the median nerve in the carpal tunnel in myxoedema has already been discussed. Rarely a generalized mixed motor and sensory neuropathy develops. This improves on treatment of the hypothyroidism. The slow contraction and relaxation observed in the tendon reflexes is due not to a disturbance of peripheral nerve function, but to an alteration in the contractile mechanism of the muscle fibres.

Acromegaly (see Chapter 13.2)

In addition to carpal tunnel syndrome, acromegaly may cause a sensory and motor polyneuropathy. This may occur independently of diabetes mellitus and the peripheral nerves are thickened because of an overgrowth of endoneurial and perineurial connective tissue. A similar neuropathy is occasionally observed in pituitary gigantism.

Critical illness polyneuropathy

A generalized polyneuropathy involving widespread axonal degeneration may be encountered in patients in intensive care units with sepsis and multiple-organ failure. The neuropathy is discovered when attempts are made to wean the patient from the ventilator and is difficult to distinguish from critical illness myopathy. Both may occur together. The precise cause of critical illness polyneuropathy is unknown. It is particularly likely to occur after the use of prolonged neuromuscular junction blockade and high-dose corticosteroids. Despite the development of severe wasting and weakness, satisfactory recovery may occur if the critical illness itself can be cured.

Other metabolic disorders

Symmetrical sensory and autonomic polyneuropathy probably does occur with cirrhosis but most cases are the result of the alcoholism that is its most common cause. A mild, painful, sensory neuropathy is occasionally encountered in primary biliary cirrhosis, sometimes related to xanthomatous deposits in the cutaneous nerve trunks. A motor neuropathy, especially affecting the hands, is a rare consequence of severe recurrent hypoglycaemia due to an insulinoma.

Toxic neuropathies

Industrial, environmental, and pharmaceutical substances

Acrylamide

Acrylamide monomer was formerly a cause of peripheral neuropathy because it was absorbed through the skin by workers manufacturing the nontoxic polymers used in waterproofing and other industries. It caused a distal sensory and motor neuropathy with prominent numbness and disequilibrium. Distal axonal degeneration occurred and slow improvement followed cessation of exposure. With proper safety precautions this neuropathy should not occur.

Arsenic

Arsenical poisoning is occasionally seen as a result of accidental or homicidal ingestion of insecticides containing arsenic, or from indigenous medicines in India. Gastrointestinal symptoms develop after acute ingestion, followed by a mixed sensory and motor neuropathy after 1 to 3 weeks. Desquamation of the skin of the feet and hands takes place after about 6 weeks, and white lines (Mees' lines) appear in the nails. With ingestion of smaller quantities on a chronic basis, gastrointestinal symptoms are less obtrusive and a slowly progressive neuropathy makes its appearance. The skin may become generally pigmented or show focal 'raindrop' pigmentation, and hyperkeratosis of the palms of the hands and soles of the feet may appear. Slow recovery from the neuropathy occurs with removal from exposure. Chelating agents are of value in treating the non-neurological complications, but it is uncertain whether they are effective for the neuropathy.

Lead

Lead neuropathy is now rare in the United Kingdom, although it was encountered as a consequence of the contamination of drinking water by lead pipes in old buildings. Subclinical neuropathy may be detectable in lead workers. It remains a hazard in certain parts of the world from the use of lead glazes in pottery. Lead poisoning usually causes a triad of abdominal pain with constipation, anaemia, and neuropathy. The neuropathy is predominantly motor and affects the upper much more than the lower limbs. It is frequently asymmetrical and typically produces weakness of first the finger and then the wrist extensors. The 'lead colic' that may occur is probably a manifestation of autonomic involvement. Severe chronic lead poisoning causes bluish discoloration of the gums just below the teeth, especially if they are carious. The neuropathy improves on cessation of lead intake. Chelating agents accelerate removal of lead but it is uncertain which of dimercaprol, edetate, penicillamine, and 2,3-dimercaptosuccinic acid (DMSA) is the best.

Mercury

Exposure to inorganic mercury salts and organic mercurial compounds may lead to neurological damage. There was as an outbreak of poisoning in Minamata Bay related to the consumption of fish contaminated by organic mercury. Dementia, cortical blindness, and ataxia occur, together with paraesthesiae, the last due perhaps to involvement of the dorsal root ganglia. Peripheral neuropathy was also a component of 'pink disease' in infants, consisting of anaemia, light sensitivity, skin rash, weight loss, and hypotonia. It was caused by the inorganic mercury in teething powders.

Thallium

This is present in certain pesticides and rodent poisons, and was formerly used as a depilatory agent. Accidental or homicidal poisoning is occasionally encountered. Acute ingestion causes nausea, vomiting, and diarrhoea. In severe cases coma develops rapidly. In milder cases there are central nervous symptoms including anxiety and choreoathetosis, and the development of a progressive, very painful, sensory and motor neuropathy. Alopecia develops later, after about 2 or 3 weeks, and renal damage may occur. Both Prussian blue to bind thallium in the gut and chelating agents to clear thallium from the body have been used as treatment.

Organophosphates

Organophospates, especially tri-*ortho*-cresylphosphate, have been widely used as lubricants and insecticides. The original description of organophosphate poisoning was in relation to illegal liquor distillation in the United States of America during the prohibition era (ginger jake paralysis). A large outbreak occurred in Morocco from contaminated cooking oil. Accidental or suicidal acute poisoning with high doses causes an acute muscarinic syndrome with diarrhoea, sweating, salivation, and meiosis. After 12 hours to 4 days patients develop generalized weakness, possibly due to neuromuscular blockade, confusion, and even coma. Recovery from this begins after 1 or 2 weeks. However, between 1 and 3 weeks after the acute exposure, some patients develop a subacute predominantly motor neuropathy—'organophosphate-induced delayed peripheral neuropathy'. Recovery is slow and often incomplete.

Claims that chronic, very-low-dose exposure to the organophosphates in agricultural insecticides causes peripheral neuropathy have not been proven.

Other industrial substances

Carbon disulphide, used in the manufacture of rayon, occasionally gives rise to a mild sensory neuropathy. Neuropathy may occur as a result of industrial exposure to the organic solvents *n*-hexane and methyl-*n*-butyl ketone. The former is also encountered as a consequence of solvent abuse; *n*-hexane, which has an intoxicant action, has been used as a solvent in certain glues. Other industrial agents causing neuropathy are ethylene oxide and methyl bromide. Trichlorethylene (or an impurity) has caused trigeminal neuropathy.

Iatrogenic

Bortezomib

Various different neuropathies have been described with the proteosome inhibitor bortezomib, an antineoplastic agent used for multiple myeloma. These include a painful subacute sensory axonal neuropathy and a more acute sensory and motor neuropathy that can resemble Guillain–Barré syndrome.

Isoniazid

A mixed motor and sensory neuropathy may be produced by isoniazid and is more likely to occur in individuals who acetylate the drug slowly. The neuropathy is related to interference with pyridoxine metabolism. Axonal degeneration occurs in the peripheral nerves. The neuropathy recovers slowly when the patient stops taking the drug; this may be prevented by giving pyridoxine, which does not interfere with the antituberculous action of the isoniazid.

Nitrofurantoin

Excessively high blood levels of nitofurantoin as may occur in patients with reduced renal function, can cause a rapid-onset mixed motor and sensory neuropathy, which may be confused with Guillain–Barré syndrome.

Nucleoside analogue reverse transcriptase inhibitors

The nucleoside analogue reverse transcriptase inhibitors (zalcitabine, didanosine, and stavudine) all cause a dose-dependent, subacute, painful, sensory axonal neuropathy. The neuropathy continues to progress for some weeks after the patient stops taking the drug but this eventually improves. It may be difficult to distinguish from the painful neuropathy caused by HIV itself and withdrawal of the drug is usually necessary to make the distinction.

Phenytoin

After taking phenytoin for a prolonged period, patients may report symptoms of a mild sensory neuropathy. More commonly the neuropathy is asymptomatic but detectable on clinical and especially neurophysiological examination.

Platinum

Both cisplatin and carboplatin may cause a predominantly sensory neuropathy after taking several courses. Recovery from the neuropathy is often poor. Ototoxicity is more frequent, causing high-tone deafness and tinnitus.

Pyridoxine

Pyridoxine, if taken in large doses as 'megavitamin therapy', causes a severe sensory neuropathy with numbness of the feet and an unsteady gait. It is disputed whether chronic doses as low as 100 mg daily cause neuropathy, the daily requirement being only 2 mg.

Taxanes

The taxanes, paclitaxel and docetaxel, used in the treatment of neoplasia, cause a dose-dependent, predominantly sensory axonal neuropathy. It presents with numbness and paraesthesiae in the feet and worsens with each dose. With high doses weakness develops. If the drug is stopped the neuropathy worsens for some weeks before improving, a phenomenon called 'coasting'.

Thalidomide

Thalidomide, which has found a niche in the treatment of some vasculitides and multiple myeloma, also causes a dose-dependent, predominantly sensory neuropathy. It presents with painful paraesthesiae and cramps in the legs. It may be associated with palmar erythema, brittle nails, and tremor. It improves if the drug is stopped.

Vincristine

Vincristine produces a dose-dependent axonal neuropathy, and its therapeutic use in neoplasia is limited by this side effect. Patients first develop distal paraesthesiae and lose their ankle reflexes. If the drug is continued, they gradually develop distal sensory loss and may eventually develop weakness that comes on quite rapidly. The neuropathy improves satisfactorily if the drug is withdrawn.

Other substances

Other drugs that may give rise to neuropathy are doxorubicin, amiodarone, chloroquine (with myopathy), dapsone, disulfiram, ethambutol, gold, metronidazole, misonidazole, nitrous oxide (with a myelopathy), podophyllin, suramin, and zimeldine. This list is not exhaustive and if a patient with an unexplained neuropathy is taking drugs of any sort, it is worth checking whether any of the drugs is reported to cause neuropathy.

Deficiency neuropathies

Coeliac disease

There is an association between coeliac disease and some neurological syndromes including cerebellar ataxia and peripheral neuropathy. In patients with malnutrition or vitamin deficiency, this is easily explained. Most patients with neurological manifestations experience preceding gastrointestinal symptoms before developing peripheral neuropathy. Nevertheless some patients do develop a peripheral neuropathy, usually a symmetrical, distal, sensory axonal neuropathy, in their absence. This now justifies at least screening for antibodies associated with coeliac disease in patients with otherwise unexplained axonal neuropathy. Whether the associated neuropathy is caused by subtle nutritional deficiency or an unidentified toxic factor is not known. Regardless of this, improvement after institution of a gluten-free diet has been reported.

Thiamine deficiency (see also Chapter 11.2)

Thiamine deficiency is the cause of dry beri-beri which occurs in severely malnourished communities, especially those subsisting on diets largely made up of polished rice, and medical conditions that reduce thiamine intake, most commonly chronic alcohol abuse, and after gastric surgery. Initial symptoms of fatigue, irritability, and cramps are followed by the development of painful numbness in the feet. In severe cases, involvement of the recurrent laryngeal nerves may lead to hoarseness of the voice. The neuropathy may be associated with a cardiomyopathy ('wet beri-beri'). The diagnosis may be supported by a reduced activity of erythrocyte transketolase. This enzyme requires thiamine as a cofactor. Distal axonal degeneration occurs in the peripheral nerves and slow recovery ensues with vitamin replacement.

Strachan's syndrome

Strachan's syndrome, originally described in Jamaica but also observed in other parts of the world under conditions of nutritional deprivation, is characterized by the combination of a painful sensory neuropathy, optic neuropathy, and deafness, in association with orogenital dermatitis. There may also be features of a myelopathy. It is assumed to be due to deficiency of the B vitamins, but the precise deficit has not been identified. It improves with B vitamin and folate supplementation.

Alcoholic neuropathy

This usually occurs on a background of nutritional deficiency. The dietary intake of the person with alcohol problems is high in carbohydrates and low in vitamins. Moreover, such individuals are known to have a reduced capacity to absorb thiamine. A direct toxic effect of alcohol on peripheral nerves may also be involved. The clinical features of alcoholic neuropathy are similar to those of thiamine deficiency. Other deficiency states may coexist, such as the Wernicke–Korsakoff syndrome. Improvement may take place with vitamin replacement and reduced alcohol intake, but it is beset with the usual difficulties met in treating patients with alcohol problems.

Pyridoxine deficiency

As well as high doses of pyridoxine causing neuropathy, as described above, pyridoxine deficiency may contribute to the neuropathy that occurs in nutritional deficiency states. Isoniazid neuropathy is related to an interference with pyridoxine metabolism.

Vitamin E deficiency

Vitamin E deficiency occurs in some hereditary disorders and in hepatobiliary and bowel disorders that impair its absorption. It produces a multisystem neurological disorder in which cerebellar ataxia is the most prominent problem but peripheral neuropathy also occurs. It may be diagnosed by measuring plasma concentrations of α-tocopherol, the most active form of vitamin E.

Vitamin B$_{12}$ deficiency

Vitamin B$_{12}$ deficiency, from whatever cause, may be responsible for the development of a distal sensory neuropathy, with 'glove-and-stocking' sensory loss and paraesthesiae, and areflexia, either in isolation or in association with a myelopathy or other central nervous system manifestations. Haematological changes are not always present. The peripheral neuropathy improves more satisfactorily with treatment than the central disturbances. This condition is considered in detail in Chapter 22.5.6. A peripheral neuropathy is one component of Nigerian ataxic neuropathy, in which the other features are posterior column degeneration, sensorineural deafness, and optic atrophy. It has been suggested that an interference with vitamin B$_{12}$ metabolism by cyanide derived from cassava in the diet, combined with nutritional deficiency, is responsible.

Inflammatory and postinfective neuropathies

Leprosy

Peripheral nerve involvement in leprosy is considered in Chapter 7.6.27.

Guillain–Barré syndrome

Guillain–Barré syndrome is the most common cause of acute neuromuscular paralysis in developed countries. Its annual incidence is between 1 and 2 per 100 000 throughout the world, being more common in men and older people. It consists of weakness of two or more limbs developing over a few days, with extremes of a few hours to up to 4 weeks. The tendon reflexes are lost. The illness often but not necessarily causes paraesthesiae, pain, and sensory loss. There are no signs of central nervous involvement. In two-thirds of cases there has been an infective illness between 1 and 6 weeks, most commonly 1 or 2 weeks earlier. The infection is most commonly an uncharacterized upper respiratory tract infection but alternatively gastroenteritis. About 25% of cases are due to preceding *Campylobacter jejuni* infection, but 15% result from a preceding cytomegalovirus infection, 5 to 10% from Epstein–Barr virus, and 1 to 5% from mycoplasma. Many other associated infections have been reported but not proved by large-scale epidemiological studies.

The onset is usually with the simultaneous development of weakness of the limbs, paraesthesiae, and numbness. Pain, including pain in the back, may be a prominent and confusing feature, especially in children. Weakness may be proximal, distal, or generalized in distribution, but is usually fairly symmetrical. The facial and bulbar muscles are commonly involved and sometimes the ocular muscles. About 25% of patients develop such severe respiratory muscle weakness for which they need intubation and artificial ventilation. Rarely a complete 'locked-in' state may develop. Autonomic disturbances include tachycardia, hypertension, and then later postural hypotension, bladder atony, and ileus. Papilloedema sometimes develops, possibly related to impaired resorption of cerebrospinal fluid as a result of the elevated protein content.

This same clinical picture may be caused by any of three pathological entities. In Europe and North America, AIDP is the underlying pathology in more than 90% of cases. Its pathogenesis is unclear but the hypothesis that it is due to a T-cell-mediated autoimmune response to one of several peripheral nerve myelin proteins is giving way to the idea that it is caused by a complement-fixing antibody directed against an unidentified ganglioside or combination of gangliosides. In China, Japan, and Mexico most cases are caused by acute motor axonal neuropathy. In such cases preceding *Campylobacter jejuni* infection is common and antibodies to the ganglioside GM1, GD1a, or both are usually present in the serum. Epitopes resembling the terminal sugars are present in the bacterial walls of the *Campylobacter jejuni* strains, which induce acute motor axonal neuropathy. The antibodies probably produce the neuropathy by reacting with gangliosides on the axolemma or at the motor nerve terminals, then blocking nerve conduction or inducing axonal degeneration. There is also a less common axonal motor and sensory neuropathy.

In AIDP, nerve conduction studies reveal evidence of motor nerve conduction block, slowing of motor nerve conduction, often multifocal, and reduced sensory nerve action potential amplitudes. In the axonal forms of the disease, the changes are those of an axonal neuropathy. During the first week, routine neurophysiological tests may be normal. Accurate identification of the neurophysiological type may require serial studies. The cerebrospinal fluid usually has an increased protein concentration, often markedly increased, and normal but sometimes slightly increased cell count (rarely more than 10 and by definition not more than 50/μl). The cells are lymphocytes and do not include neutrophils. There is no diagnostic test but antibodies to gangliosides, especially GM1, may be present, most commonly in the axonal forms of the disease.

Diagnosis is therefore largely clinical, supported by the neuro-physiological and cerebrospinal fluid findings. The differential diagnoses are acute muscle dysfunction (including hypo- or hyper-kalaemia), neuromuscular junction disorders, other causes of neuropathy (including drugs, toxins, porphyria, and vasculitis), and cauda equina, cord, and brain-stem causes of paralysis.

The prognosis is very variable. About a quarter have a benign course, never losing the ability to walk. About a quarter require artificial ventilation, accounting for most of the 5% who die, and 20% are left with persistent disability so severe that they need help walking. Of the remainder, most are able to walk with help by 1 month and without aid by 3 months, and return to work or their usual activities by 6 months. Some patients have persistent fatigue.

The mainstays of treatment are careful monitoring for the development of respiratory failure and cardiac arrhythmia, pro-phylactic enoxaparin for bed-bound adult patients and excellent intensive care. Plasma exchange and intravenous immunoglobulin have both been shown to improve the rate and extent of recovery if given within the first 2, and perhaps 4 weeks. Controlled trials of treatment with corticosteroids have shown no beneficial effects. Pain may be a significant problem and require nonsteroidal anti-inflammatory drugs, amitriptyline, or pregabalin, and in severe cases opiates. Careful positioning and physiotherapy are important to avoid pressure sores and contractures. Exercise programmes are probably useful for fatigue.

Fisher's syndrome

A syndrome of ophthalmoplegia, ataxia, and loss of the tendon reflexes was described by Miller Fisher in 1956 and is often called the Miller Fisher syndrome or more correctly Fisher's syndrome. Similar to Guillain–Barré syndrome, it commonly follows an infection, progresses for a few days, and then plateaus and eventually improves. As in Guillain–Barré syndrome, the cerebrospinal fluid protein concentration is usually increased. Facial and bulbar palsies also occur and are accepted as part of the syndrome, but patients with associated limb weakness are regarded as having an overlap with Guillain–Barré syndrome. In the pure cases, motor nerve conduction remains normal but sensory action potentials disappear. The prognosis is excellent even without immunotherapy. The diagnosis is usually straightforward, but confusion with botulism and diphtheritic neuropathy may arise. In most patients with Fisher's syndrome, antibodies to ganglioside GQ1b are present in the serum and are probably important in causing terminal nerve damage. Formes frustes of Fisher's syndrome, with only some of the features, are sometimes encountered.

The features of ophthalmoplegia, ataxia, and, paradoxically, loss of the tendon reflexes may occur with another relatively benign condition, Bickerstaff's brain-stem encephalitis. Signs of central nervous system involvement, including altered consciousness and extensor plantar responses, are also present. In addition there may be an increased cerebrospinal fluid cell count and abnormalities in the brain stem may be visible on MRI. Antibodies to ganglioside GQ1b may also be present in the serum of patients with Bickerstaff's encephalitis.

Chronic inflammatory demyelinating polyradiculoneuropathy

Chronic inflammatory demyelinating polyradiculoneuropathy (CIDP) is a chronic progressive or relapsing disorder with weakness and sensory changes in the limbs developing over more than 8 weeks. Patients whose symptoms develop in less than 4 weeks are regarded as having the AIDP form of Guillain–Barré syndrome, whereas those whose symptoms progress over 4 to 8 weeks are considered to have subacute inflammatory demyelinating polyra-diculoneuropathy. The three disorders probably constitute a spectrum. CIDP has emerged as an important treatable form of chronic neuropathy which has to be distinguished from the many less treatable causes of chronic axonal neuropathy. Electrophysiological tests are key to making the distinction. The hallmarks of CIDP are multifocal slowing of motor nerve conduction, often with partial conduction blocks, and prolonged duration of compound muscle action potentials. Sensory nerve action potentials are often reduced or absent. In typical cases, the clinical features are symmetrical but about 10% of patients have a multifocal disorder called the Lewis–Sumner syndrome or multifocal acquired demyelinating sensory and motor neuropathy.

Most patients with CIDP respond to treatment with corticosteroids, intravenous immunoglobulin, or plasma exchange. Prolonged treatment is necessary; it is hazardous with corticosteroids, expensive with intravenous immunoglobulin, and inconvenient with plasma exchange. Cytotoxic drugs, such as azathioprine, methotrexate, and ciclosporin, are often used and have appeared helpful in refractory cases but their efficacy has not been proved with randomized trials and controversy exists about which to choose.

Multifocal motor neuropathy

Multifocal motor neuropathy is a pure motor syndrome of weakness and wasting predominantly in the upper limbs, probably caused by antibodies to ganglioside GM1. The diagnosis depends on identifying multiple regions of motor nerve conduction block with preserved sensory nerve conduction through the same nerve segment. Most patients respond to intravenous immunoglobulin but this needs to be repeated approximately every month. Immunosuppressive drugs are often tried in severe cases but have not been proved to work in trials. Multifocal motor neuropathy may be worsened by corticosteroids.

Paraprotein-associated neuropathy

Malignant plasma cell dyscrasias may affect the peripheral nervous system. Multiple myeloma deposits may compress spinal nerve roots, causing pain and radicular symptoms as well as cord compression. Multiple myeloma is very rarely associated with an axonal neuropathy, possibly as a paraneoplastic manifestation. AL amyloidosis may cause peripheral nerve as well as other tissue infiltration and a severe neuropathy. Waldenström's macroglobulinaemia may be associated with an axonal or demyelinating neuropathy, which resembles the syndrome of IgM monoclonal gammopathy of undetermined significance (MGUS) and antibodies to myelin-associated glycoprotein described below.

The mixed cryoglobulins in essential cryoglobulinaemia, sometimes associated with hepatitis C infection, cause a multiple mononeuropathy which is thought to be due the fact that cryoglobulins are circulating immune complexes. The treatment is that of the underlying condition.

Osteosclerotic myeloma and solitary plasmacytomas may both be associated with a paraneoplastic demyelinating neuropathy the pathogenesis of which is unclear. Removal of the neoplasm is often curative. By contrast the POEMS syndrome (**p**olyneuropathy, **o**rganomegaly, **o**edema, **M** protein, and **s**kin changes) is much more difficult to treat. This multisystem disorder is associated with very high concentrations of vascular endothelial growth factor in the plasma. Polyneuropathy is a required feature for the diagnosis and is usually a mixed axonal and demyelinating neuropathy. Papilloedema, peripheral oedema, skin pigmentation, and endocrinopathy may occur. It does not respond to corticosteroids or conventional immunotherapy but, if there is a localised sclerotic myeloma, it may respond to irradiation. Otherwise good results have been reported from peripheral blood stem cell transplantation and thalidomide-like drugs.

The most common association between peripheral neuropathy and a paraprotein is the coincidence with MGUS. Both peripheral neuropathy and MGUS become more common with advancing age, so the association is not necessarily causative. This is particularly true of paraproteins and axonal neuropathy. If there is no evidence of amyloid or a malignant plasma cell dyscrasia, an association between a paraprotein and an axonal neuropathy is probably coincidental because relevant autoantibody properties of the paraprotein have very rarely been described. The association between IgG and IgA MGUS and demyelinating neuropathy may also be coincidental, because these patients, and some of those with IgM MGUS, behave in every respect like patients with CIDP who have no paraprotein. It is always essential to look for evidence of an underlying plasma cell dyscrasia, which might be a solitary myeloma or plasmacytoma and may be difficult to find.

In patients with an IgM MGUS and demyelinating neuropathy, a search should be made for antibodies to myelin-associated glycoprotein because there is a not uncommon syndrome in which these are present. The characteristic features are of a very slowly progressive sensory, then sensory and motor demyelinating neuropathy, often with a postural tremor. Nerve biopsies show widely spaced myelin lamellae, with the wide spacing and demyelination attributed to the antibody properties of the IgM paraprotein. The slow progression is fortunate because treatment is difficult. Although success has been claimed for chlorambucil and fludarabine, convincing evidence of efficacy has yet to be provided. One small trial showed modest benefit from the anti-CD20 B cell marker rituximab and a larger trial is under way.

Other rare syndromes of particular neuropathies associated with paraproteins having interesting and potentially relevant autoantibodies are gradually emerging. In the CANOMAD syndrome (**c**hronic **a**taxic **n**europathy, **o**phthalmoplegia, Ig**M** paraprotein, cold **a**gglutinins, and **d**isialosyl antibodies), antibodies are present against gangliosides with two sialic acid groups (disialosyl). The neuropathy is mixed axonal and demyelinating. The condition is so rare that it is not possible to make firm statements about treatment, but it can be very disabling and intravenous immunoglobulin can produce striking repeated short-term benefit. It is likely that other MGUS-associated neuropathies are due to as yet unidentified antibody properties of their paraproteins.

Lyme borreliosis

Lyme borreliosis is a multisystem disease caused by tick-borne spirochaetes belonging to the genus *Borrelia* (see Chapter 7.6.32). About 3 months after infection and without necessarily having had a preceding rash or arthritis, a small proportion of infected patients develop lymphocytic meningitis, facial palsy, painful radicular symptoms, and rarely a more severe generalized asymmetrical polyradiculoneuropathy. Some develop peripheral nerve lesions without ever having symptomatic meningitis. Serum antibodies to *Borrelia* are helpful in diagnosis but are common in endemic areas. In a hospital setting measurement of serum/cerebrospinal fluid antibody index is very specific but does not detect all cases. Nerve biopsies are not usually needed to make the diagnosis but do show extensive inflammatory infiltrates although the spirochaetes are not identifiable. Treatment is usually given in the form of parenteral penicillin or ceftriaxone but oral doxycycline is a possible alternative for mild cases.

HIV infection

A variety of neuropathies may be related to HIV-1 infection, particularly types tending to occur in different phases of the disease. At the time of seroconversion or soon afterwards Guillain–Barré syndrome, CIDP or multifocal vasculitic neuropathy may develop and precede other features of HIV infection. In the later AIDS phase, a distal symmetrical polyneuropathy is common. It is a slowly progressive disorder that may be painful and has to be distinguished from the toxic neuropathy produced by reverse transcriptase inhibitors mentioned earlier. In advanced cases an aggressive lumbosacral polyradiculoneuropathy from cytomegalovirus infection is encountered. HIV infection and its treatment are discussed in Chapter 7.5.23.

Sarcoid neuropathy

Facial palsy is the most common peripheral nerve manifestation of sarcoidosis (see Chapter 18.12). It may be bilateral and accompanied by uveitis and parotitis. Less commonly subacute or fluctuating multiple cranial nerve palsies occur. More rarely, almost any pattern of peripheral neuropathy has been seen, including multiple mononeuropathy and a Guillain–Barré syndrome-like picture, albeit usually more subacute. Other manifestations of sarcoidosis, such as erythema nodosum, arthritis, enlarged lymph nodes, uveitis, and abnormal chest radiographs, are not always present and the diagnosis has to be considered in a wide range of neuropathies. The cerebrospinal fluid is abnormal in about half the patients with peripheral nerve disorders due to sarcoidosis. If an accessible nerve can be biopsied, sarcoid granulomas in the nerve tissue clinch the diagnosis. Corticosteroids are the mainstay of treatment and their use is usually justified in patients with significant peripheral nerve involvement.

Diphtheritic neuropathy

Diphtheria (Chapter 7.6.1) used to be a serious, even fatal, disease of children. It was almost completely prevented in children by the advent of immunization. As immunity wanes, occasional cases are now seen in adults. It is most commonly caused by infection of the pharynx, occasionally by infection of wounds. Peripheral neuropathy is caused by the release of an exotoxin that interferes with Schwann cell function, probably by affecting protein synthesis, and produces segmental demyelination. The nerves are not invaded by the bacterium. In pharyngeal infection patients develop numbness of the tongue and face and a bulbar palsy, between 2 and 7 weeks after the infection. The bulbar palsy and respiratory involvement may be so severe as to require artificial ventilation. Paralysis of accommodation and sometimes of the external ocular muscles may occur. Weakness and sensory loss then develop in the limbs, sometimes as the bulbar palsy is beginning to improve. The disease also causes myocarditis. Nerve conduction studies show slowing of motor nerve conduction. The cerebrospinal fluid protein concentration becomes increased and the cell count may be raised. In particular in those cases with a normal cell count, there is a possibility of confusion with Guillain–Barré syndrome. Diagnosis can be made by culturing *Corynebacterium diphtheriae* from the throat, or identifying its toxin or DNA in throat swabs. Treatment is supportive because it is doubtful whether giving antitoxin will help once the peripheral neuropathy has developed.

Vasculitic neuropathy

Vasculitic neuropathy usually presents as a painful mononeuropathy or multiple mononeuropathy, but can present as a symmetrical polyneuropathy, and pain is sometimes absent. More commonly pain develops in the course of an established vasculitic disorder. Peripheral nerve involvement is characteristic and common in polyarteritis nodosa and Churg–Strauss syndrome. It also occurs in Wegener's granulomatosis, hypersensitivity vasculitis, rheumatoid arthritis, relapsing polychondritis, and systemic lupus erythematosus. In rheumatoid arthritis, carpal tunnel syndrome and ulnar nerve lesions due to joint derangement are the most common peripheral nerve manifestations, but a florid multiple mononeuropathy and sometimes a slowly distal sensory neuropathy, or one restricted to the digital nerves, also occurs. In some cases vasculitic neuropathy heralds the identification of an underlying carcinoma or lymphoma. In rare cases, vasculitis is confined to nerves not only at presentation but also during follow-up, a condition called nonsystemic vasculitic neuropathy. Vasculitic neuropathy may be diagnosed from the clinical picture, if it is typical, such as multiple mononeuropathy in Churg–Strauss syndrome, or from the clinical picture and antineutrophil cytoplasmic antibodies in polyarteritis nodosa.

Often the diagnosis has been or can be made by biopsy of another affected tissue. If the diagnosis is in doubt biopsy of an affected nerve will usually reveal evidence of vasculitis, including inflammatory cell infiltration, occlusion, and fibrinoid necrosis of the epineurial blood vessels. To achieve maximum benefit from a nerve biopsy, it needs to be removed without crushing the tissue, processed with special techniques, and interpreted by an experienced observer, so it is best performed in specialist centres. Detection of vasculitis is one of the principal reasons for performing a nerve biopsy. Treatment of vasculitic neuropathy is the same as the treatment for the underlying disorder. Corticosteroids in the form of oral prednisolone are the mainstay of treatment. In many, especially severe cases, an immunosuppressive agent is also given. A regimen of oral or intravenous cyclophosphamide for 3 months followed by azathioprine is commonly used.

Sjögren's syndrome is another cause of a vasculitic neuropathy but it also causes an ataxic sensory neuropathy related to dorsal root ganglionitis and a painful small fibre neuropathy (see below). Sometimes the trigeminal ganglion is affected in isolation.

Neoplastic and paraneoplastic neuropathy

Direct invasion of cranial nerves or spinal roots may occur in cases of malignant infiltration of the meninges and of the cervical and lumbosacral plexus from local malignancies. Malignant infiltration is usually painful. Infiltration of peripheral nerve trunks is seen most commonly from malignant lymphomas. Rarely, generalized infiltration may occur to produce a multiple mononeuropathy or even an acute neuropathy resembling Guillain–Barré syndrome.

Peripheral neuropathy may develop as a nonmetastatic, 'paraneoplastic' complication of carcinoma, most often bronchial or gastric, and very occasionally with lymphoma. The occurrence of a number of autoantibodies specific for these paraneoplastic manifestations makes it likely that it is an autoimmune condition. The underlying neoplasm often pursues an unusually indolent course, suggesting that the autoimmune process is holding the neoplasm in check. Perhaps for this reason, the neuropathy may antedate the discovery of the carcinoma by as much as 2 or 3 years. A wide variety of clinical pictures has been reported. A characteristic picture is the subacute sensory neuronopathy associated with a small cell lung carcinoma and antibodies to a nuclear protein called Hu. However, subacute sensory neuronopathy also occurs in association with many other neoplasms. Carcinoma of the bronchus is associated with other types of neuropathy, including a slowly progressive mixed sensory and motor neuropathy. Paraneoplastic neurological syndromes often occur in combinations. Gynaecological cancers are particularly associated with a cerebellar syndrome and antibodies to Purkinje cells (anti-Yo antibodies). Peripheral neuropathy may be part of this syndrome. Anti-Hu antibodies are often associated with limbic encephalitis as well as peripheral neuropathy. Paraneoplastic neuropathies may regress after removal of the underlying tumour, but may also not benefit. In a small number of cases in which treatment has been started very early, immunotherapy with corticosteroids, intravenous immunoglobulin, or plasma exchange has been followed by improvement of the neuropathy.

Genetic neuropathies

Porphyria (see also Chapter 12.5)

A predominantly motor neuropathy may complicate acute attacks in the autosomal dominant disorders of acute intermittent and variegated porphyria and hereditary coproporphyria, and in the recessively inherited δ-aminolaevulinic acid dehydratase deficiency. The neuropathy is usually preceded by colicky abdominal pain and mental disturbances including confusion, psychosis, and epilepsy. It develops acutely and resembles Guillain–Barré syndrome. It is often predominantly proximal, affects the motor more than sensory nerves and may affect the cranial nerves. The tendon reflexes are reduced in keeping with the weakness. Minor sensory symptoms including patchy paraesthesiae occur. Autonomic features include tachycardia, hypertension, pupillary dilatation, constipation, and sweating. Muscle atrophy due to axonal degeneration may be severe so that recovery is slow and often incomplete.

Attacks may be provoked by a variety of drugs, including barbiturates, sulphonamides, and the contraceptive pill, alcohol, and starvation (see Chapter 12.5). Prevention of attacks by the avoidance of precipitating factors is essential. Acute attacks should be treated with intravenous glucose and haematin to reduce the formation of porphyrin precursors.

Familial amyloid polyneuropathy

In addition to the axonal polyneuropathy that occurs in AL amyloid, a number of inherited amyloid neuropathies have been recognized. The most common are those related to point mutations in the gene for transthyretin, formerly known as prealbumin. The most common of these mutations is the Portuguese type where there is a substitution of valine for methionine in the transthyretin molecule. The neuropathy begins with the involvement of small nerve fibres, leading to a distal loss of pain and temperature sensation and autonomic failure. Spontaneous pain is often a feature and a mutilating acropathy frequently develops. The onset is commonly in the fourth or fifth decade and the disorder is slowly progressive, leading to death within about 10 years. Transthyretin is produced mainly in the liver and liver transplantation may halt progression of the disease. The same mutation occurs in Sweden, Japan, and other parts of the world, but the phenotype in these other communities varies. The neuropathy may not develop until the sixth decade or later and may sometimes have features of CIDP. Hereditary amyloid neuropathy can also be caused by mutations in the gene for other proteins and these have differing clinical features. In the Iowa form, the amyloid is derived from a mutated form of apolipoprotein A1 and causes a painful predominantly sensory neuropathy. In the Finnish form, there is a mutation in the gene for the plasma protein gelsolin, and the neuropathy affects the cranial nerves and is associated with a corneal lattice dystrophy.

Charcot–Marie–Tooth disease

Charcot–Marie–Tooth (hereditary motor and sensory neuropathy, peroneal muscular atrophy) disease usually presents during childhood or adolescence with difficulty in walking or because of foot deformity. It is genetically heterogeneous. Charcot–Marie–Tooth disease type 1 (CMT1) is caused by a demyelinating neuropathy with markedly slowed nerve conduction velocities (ulnar nerve motor conduction velocity <38 m/s). Charcot–Marie–Tooth disease type 2 (CMT2) is due to an axonal neuropathy with relatively preserved conduction velocities (ulnar nerve motor conduction velocity >38 m/s). Both CMT1 and CMT2 are themselves genetically heterogeneous. There is also a less common X-linked form, which may be demyelinating or axonal, in which the nerve conduction velocities are intermediate.

The clinical pictures of all three general forms of CMT are similar. Foot deformity is common and consists of a high arch, or pes cavus, and clawing of the toes, sometimes with an equinovarus deformity. Muscle weakness tends to affect the lower leg muscles and may give rise to bilateral foot drop with a 'steppage' gait. The muscle wasting is often restricted to below the knees, producing a 'stork' or 'inverted champagne bottle' leg appearance (Fig. 24.16.3). Weakness and wasting of the small hand muscles may appear later. The tendon reflexes become depressed or lost, and there is a variable degree of distal sensory loss. Progress of the disease is slow and cases with little disability or that are asymptomatic are common.

The most common from of CMT is CMT1a, accounting for 70% of all cases. It is caused by duplication of the gene for peripheral myelin protein 22 (*PMP22*). The onset is most frequently in the first decade. Foot deformity and scoliosis occur more often than in CMT2, sensory loss and ataxia tend to be greater, and generalized tendon areflexia is usual. Weakness in the hands appears earlier. The peripheral nerves may be thickened because of an excess of connective tissue and reduplication of the Schwann cells concentrically around axons to form the appearance in cross-section of an 'onion bulb'. Cases with ataxia and upper limb tremor are sometimes referred to as the Roussy–Lévy syndrome. Other causes of CMT1 include mutations of *PMP22* and also of the gene that codes for P0, the major peripheral nerve myelin structural glycoprotein. The most common genetic cause of CMT2 is a mutation in the gene for mitofusin 2 (*MFN2*) but this accounts for only 20% of cases. Other causes include mutations in the genes for P0 or the neurofilament light chain (NEFL). X-linked CMT is due to mutations in the gene for connexin 32; women may be asymptomatic or only mildly affected by an axonal neuropathy whereas men usually have a somewhat multifocal demyelinating neuropathy. The genetic diagnosis of CMT is in a rapid stage of development. The list of responsible genes is already much longer than the

common examples mentioned and rare autosomal recessive forms occur. The diagnosis of the common gene mutations can usually be made from the clinical picture, neurophysiological studies, and molecular genetic tests. If not it may be necessary to resort to nerve biopsy.

Affected individuals may be helped by the use of orthotic appliances and sometimes by surgical correction of foot deformity or tendon transfer. After successful treatment of mouse models for CMT1a, trials of vitamin C, an essential cofactor for Schwann cell cultures, are under way in the human disease. Preliminary results are not encouraging.

Hereditary neuropathy with liability to pressure palsies

This is an autosomal dominant disorder in which affected individuals develop recurrent focal peripheral nerve or brachial plexus lesions produced by compression or stretch injury. It has been shown to usually be caused by a deletion of the *PMP22* gene which is duplicated in CMT1a. Nerve fibres show focal regions of myelin thickening resembling little sausages, leading to the term 'tomaculous neuropathy' from the Latin 'tomacula' which means sausages.

Congenital hypomyelinating neuropathy

Rarely CMT presents in infancy or early childhood with a very severe progressive sensory and motor neuropathy and extremely slow nerve-conduction velocities. This used to be called Dejerine–Sottas disease or CMT3. Pathologically, there is hypomyelination and extensive demyelination in the peripheral nerves, with onion bulbs and a thickened peripheral nerve trunk. These cases may be due to new mutations of *PMP22*, early growth response gene 2 (*EGR2*), or other genes.

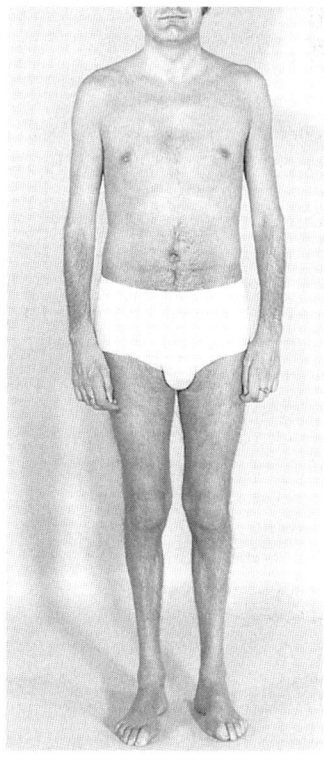

Fig. 24.16.3 Patient with Charcot–Marie–Tooth disease type 1 (CMT1) showing symmetrical distal lower limb muscle wasting.

Distal hereditary motor neuropathies

Rare hereditary pure motor neuropathies resemble CMT but lack any sensory involvement. Eleven different disorders have already been described, of which the most common are due to mutations in the heat shock protein genes *HSP27* and *HSP22*. Some have striking clinical features that help predict the diagnosis such as mutations in the *GARS* (glycyl-tRNA synthetase) gene or *BSCL2* (Beradinelli–Seip congenital lipodystrophy) gene, which both present with wasting and weakness of the small hand muscles. However, distal wasting and weakness are sometimes caused not by a neuropathy but by a myopathy, a distinction that can readily be made by electromyography, which shows a myopathic instead of a denervation pattern in the distal muscles.

Refsum's disease

Refsum's disease is a rare, autosomal recessive, multisystem disorder causing features including mixed motor and sensory polyneuropathy ataxia, pigmentary retinal degeneration, anosmia, pupillary abnormalities, deafness, cardiomyopathy, and ichthyosis. The presentation is usually with night blindness during adolescence or early adult life and the course may be steadily progressive or relapsing. The peripheral nerves become thickened and display hypertrophic changes. Nerve conduction velocity is usually severely reduced. The disorder is due to mutations in the gene *PHYH* coding for the peroxisomal enzyme, phytanoyl-CoA hydroxylase, and causing a deficiency in the ability to metabolize phytanic acid, a long-chain fatty acid that accumulates in the blood and tissues. Phytanic acid is largely of dietary origin, and clinical improvement may be achieved with diets low in phytanic acid. Plasma exchange is effective for acute episodes of deterioration. The disease is genetically heterogeneous.

Hereditary sensory and autonomic neuropathies

Hereditary sensory and autonomic neuropathies (HSANs) are much less common than CMT. As the name implies they are usually predominantly sensory and autonomic but motor involvement does occur, leading sometimes to overlap with the phenotype of CMT. In the autosomal dominant disorder HSAN-I, the predominant symptoms are usually sensory with few autonomic features, but occasional early motor involvement. The disease is due to a mutation of the serine palmitoyl transferase (*SPTLC*) gene. In the autosomal recessive HSAN-II there is severe sensory involvement with onset in the first two decades. HSAN-III is familial dysautonomia, also called the Riley–Day syndrome, an autosomal recessive disorder due to a mutation in the *IKBA* gene encountered almost entirely in Israeli Ashkenazi Jews.

Aplasia of peripheral autonomic neurons leads to a variety of symptoms, including absence of tears, unexplained pyrexia, cutaneous blotching, and episodic sweating attacks. These symptoms are present at birth and accompanied by congenital insensitivity to pain related to an associated sensory neuropathy. In early infancy, there is usually difficulty in feeding because of poor sucking, and repeated episodes of aspiration pneumonia. Later, stunted growth and often kyphoscoliosis become evident. HSAN-IV is an autosomal recessive disorder affecting mainly the unmyelinated nerve fibre; it causes severe sensory loss and intellectual impairment. HSAN-V is autosomal recessive and genetically heterogeneous. Mutations in the gene for neurotrophic tyrosine kinase receptor type 1 mainly affect small myelinated nerve fibres whereas those in the gene for nerve growth factor β mainly affect unmyelinated nerve fibres. Both cause congenital insensitivity to pain. Most cases of 'congenital insensitivity to pain' are probably examples of small fibre neuropathies. In all these diseases, the sensory loss often leads to a mutilating acropathy, with neuropathic joint degeneration and chronic cutaneous ulceration, particularly of the feet (Fig. 24.16.4).

Other hereditary neuropathies (see also **Section 12**)

Peripheral nerve involvement occurs in metachromatic and globoid cell leucodystrophy, adrenomyeloneuropathy, Fabry's disease, hereditary high-density lipoprotein deficiency (Tangier disease), hereditary abetalipoproteinaemia, and cholestanolosis. Giant axonal neuropathy is a rare, childhood-onset, autosomal recessive disorder characterized by segmental axonal enlargements containing accumulations of neurofilaments due to a mutation in the gogaxonin gene. Affected children usually have abnormally curly kinky hair and may have central nervous system abnormalities.

Chronic idiopathic axonal polyneuropathy

Despite extensive investigation, the cause of about a quarter of cases of late-onset symmetrical polyneuropathy remains unknown. Such cases are probably heterogeneous and may reflect underlying diagnoses that have not yet been discovered, such as alcohol abuse, carcinoma, or CMT2. For those in whom no cause can be found the term 'chronic idiopathic axonal polyneuropathy' is often used and some of these may have a disease of their own. It occurs in the sixth decade or later and causes a slowly progressive, predominantly sensory neuropathy. Numbness and paraesthesiae, often painful, spread from the toes up the legs and become associated with unsteadiness.

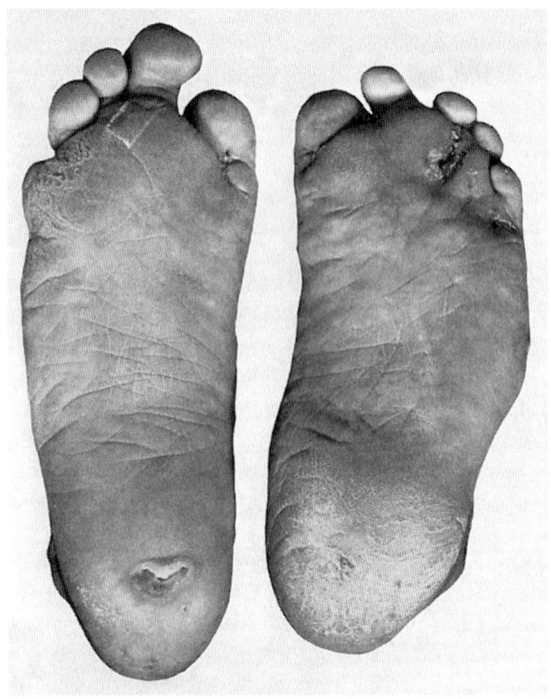

Fig. 24.16.4 Chronic foot ulceration and deformity in a case of hereditary sensory neuropathy.

It progresses very slowly over years and rarely becomes seriously disabling, although the pain may be distressing and require treatment with drugs, such as amitriptyline, pregabalin, or tramadol. In some patients, there is evidence of impaired glucose tolerance or hyperlipidaemia, and it is likely that in some the underlying cause is related to the metabolic syndrome.

Small fibre neuropathy

A particular example of chronic idiopathic axonal neuropathy is small fibre neuropathy. In this the symptoms are confined to painful paraesthesiae with paradoxical alteration of pain sensation, heightened awareness of pain (hyperpathia), and distortion of sensation so that normally nonpainful stimuli appear painful (allodynia). Pain and temperature sensation are impaired in the extremities. In these patients sensory modalities conveyed by the large-diameter nerve fibres—light touch, vibration sensation, and joint position—remain intact. Conventional clinical neurophysiological tests do not identify any abnormality because the sensory nerve action potentials derive from the large, not the small, nerve fibres. Skin biopsies show diminution of naked axons crossing the junction between the dermis and the epidermis. Quantitative sensory testing detects abnormal temperature thresholds. These investigations are used in some specialist centres to support the diagnosis which otherwise has to be made on clinical grounds. Diabetes and Sjögren's syndrome are possible causes but many cases are idiopathic. Drugs such as amitriptyline, pregabalin, and tramadol provide some relief but the condition is often distressingly resistant to treatment.

Further reading

Asbury AK, Thomas PK (1995). *Peripheral nerve disorders. A practical approach*, 2nd edition. Butterworths, London.
Birch R, Bonney C, Wynn Parry CB (1998). *Surgical disorders of the peripheral nerves*. Churchill Livingstone, Edinburgh.
Dyck PJ, Thomas PK (1999). *Diabetic neuropathy*, 2nd edition. W B Saunders, Philadelphia.
Dyck PJ, Thomas PK (2005). *Peripheral neuropathy*, 4th edition. W B Saunders, Philadelphia.
Hadden RD, *et al.* (2006). European Federation of Neurological Societies/Peripheral Nerve Society guideline on management of paraproteinaemic demyelinating neuropathies. *J Peripheral Nerv Syst*, **11**, 9–19.
Halperin JJ, *et al.* (2007). Practice parameter: treatment of nervous system Lyme disease (an evidence-based review). *Neurology*, **69**, 91–102.
Hughes R, *et al.* (2007). Peripheral nerve disorders. In: Candelise L *et al.* (eds) *Evidence-based neurology. Management of neurological disorders*, pp. 244–57. BMJ Books, London.
Hughes RAC, Cornblath DR (2005). Guillain–Barré syndrome. *Lancet*, **366**, 1653–66.
Hughes RAC, *et al.* (2005). European Federation of Neurological Societies/Peripheral Nerve Society guideline on management of chronic inflammatory demyelinating polyradiculoneuropathy. *J Peripheral Nerv Syst*, **10**, 220–8.
Hughes RAC, *et al.* (2006). Guideline on Management of multifocal motor neuropathy: Report of a joint task force. *J Peripheral Nerv Syst*, **11**, 1–8.
Hughes RAC, *et al.* (2005). Supportive care for Guillain–Barré syndrome. *Arch Neurol*, **62**, 1194–8.
Reilly MM, Shy ME (2009). Diagnosis and new treatments in genetic neuropathies. *J Neurol Neurosurg Psychiatry*, **80**, 1304–14.
Stewart JD (2000). *Focal peripheral neuropathies*, 3rd edition. Lippincott, Williams & Wilkins, Philadelphia.
van Alfen N, van Engelen BG (2006). The clinical spectrum of neuralgic amyotrophy in 246 cases. *Brain*, **129**, 438–50.

Website

National Center for Biotechnology Information. *Online Mendelian Inheritance in Man (OMIM)*. http://www.ncbi.nlm.nih.gov/sites/entrez?db=omim

Inherited neurodegenerative diseases

Edwin H. Kolodny and Swati Sathe

Essentials

Many nervous system disorders have a genetic basis, but may be difficult to diagnose because of nonspecific signs, slow progression, and lack of any family history.

Neurodegenerative disorders present an enormous challenge because of the complexity of the nervous system, the broad clinical and genetic heterogeneity characteristic of these diseases, and the progressive and generally irreversible nature of their neuropathology. A mutated gene is generally at fault, resulting in decreased production of a structural or regulatory protein important for the development or normal functioning of a special part of the nervous system.

Clinical approach

A systematic approach to the inherited neurodegenerative diseases involves analysis of (1) principal presenting signs—in most cases these will relate to one neuroanatomical region or pathology specific to that disease, e.g. the brain cortex in dementias; (2) time of onset; (3) mechanism of inheritance—the family history is obviously a key component, and specific enquiry regarding parental consanguinity must always be made; (4) extraneural clues—e.g. specific signs involving the eyes, skin, connective tissues, or visceral organs; (5) metabolic derangements—in an appropriate clinical context investigation may reveal evidence of disorders of pathways involving amino acids, organic acids, lipids, carbohydrates, purines and pyrimidines, heavy metals, porphyrins, and vitamins; (6) relevant genetic tests.

Making the diagnosis—careful correlation of presenting signs with specific components of the nervous system will demystify most neurodegenerative diseases. Judicious use of neurophysiological, neuropsychological, neuroradiological, and neuropathological testing narrows the possibilities, but ultimately the diagnosis may depend upon a biochemical test or the demonstration of a DNA abnormality within a particular gene.

Management—because of their complexity, it is recommended that patients with a neurodegenerative condition receive consultation from a multidisciplinary team involving both clinical specialists (e.g.—as required—neurologist, ophthalmologist, orthopaedic surgeon, radiologist, physiotherapist) and laboratory scientists (e.g.—as required—cytogeneticists, pathologists, biochemists, and molecular geneticists).

Particular inherited neurodegenerative diseases

Neurocutaneous syndromes (phakomatoses)—e.g. neurofibromatosis (1 and 2), tuberous sclerosis, von Hippel–Lindau disease, Sturge–Weber syndrome. These involve defects in tumor suppressor genes that lead to distinctive skin lesions in combination with tumors of brain and other organs.

Defects in DNA repair—e.g. xeroderma pigmentosum, ataxia telangiectasia, Cockayne's syndrome. Present with a wide range of abnormalities, including in many conditions a propensity to various cancers and skin abnormalities.

Dementia—this is a common feature of many neurodegenerative conditions and the result of abnormal protein aggregation within cortical neurons in Alzheimer's disease, frontotemporal dementia, dementia with Lewy bodies, and prion protein diseases.

Inherited epilepsy syndromes—these are often caused by defects in genes regulating voltage- or ligand-gated ion channels, but epilepsy is also a feature of several lysosomal storage diseases and many other inborn metabolic disorders.

Leucodystrophies—these are disorders which have a genetic basis, a progressive clinical course, primary involvement of white matter, and a demonstrable biochemical or molecular defect. The primary leukodystrophies can be classified into three subgroups: (1) classic dysmyelinative disorders—e.g. X-linked adrenoleukodystrophy, metachromatic leukodystrophy; (2) hypomyelinative with delayed or decreased myelin production—e.g. Pelizaeus–Merzbacher disease; and (3) vacuolating myelinopathies—e.g. Canavan's disease. Secondary inherited leukodystrophies include

---

The tables are a guide to the established disease genes but are not comprehensive as new discoveries in neurogenetics are occurring at a rapid pace. For further listings, the reader should consult the Human Gene Bank (http://www.hgmd.cf.ac.uk) and Gene Clinics (http://www.geneclinics.org).

(1) metabolic disorders—e.g. various mitochondrial and lysosomal storage diseases, amino and organic acidemias, some glycogen storage diseases; (2) vascular disorders—e.g. CADASIL (cerebral autosomal dominant arteriopathy with subcortical infarcts and leukoencephalopathy).

Movement disorders—basal ganglia pathology is a principal feature of these conditions, which include Wilson's disease, Huntington's disease, and Parkinson's disease. The hereditary ataxias, e.g. Friedreich's ataxia, involve primarily the cerebellum and/or spinocerebellar tracts. In the hereditary spastic paraplegias the pyramidal tracts of the spinal cord are a major site of pathology, whereas motor neuron involvement is characteristic of the spinal muscular atrophies and amyotrophic lateral sclerosis. Failure of motor function can arise due to primary diseases of muscle, as in the hereditary myopathies and muscular dystrophies.

Future prospects

The search for new therapeutic agents for rare inherited neurogenerative diseases is currently exploring a wide range of possible interventions, including small chaperone molecules that target misfolded proteins, immunization against aberrant protein aggregations, antisense oligonucleotides, interference RNA, neural stem cells that repair complex neural circuitries, and drugs with neuroprotective and anti-inflammatory effects.

Introduction

As a result of the rapid expansion of molecular genetics into clinical medicine, we are currently witnessing monumental advances in our understanding of inherited diseases of the nervous system. In assessing patients with neurodegenerative diseases, the clinician can become overwhelmed by the growing list of diagnostic possibilities and available tests. Therefore, a systematic approach is needed that will narrow the differential diagnosis, reduce the time needed to determine an exact cause, permit earlier therapeutic interventions, and remove uncertainty in counselling patients and their relatives about prognosis and risk to other family members.

The earliest clinical signs in most inherited diseases of the nervous system refer to one neuroanatomical region or pathology specific to that disease. It may be the brain cortex as in dementias, the underlying white matter as in many leucodystrophies, the pyramidal tract as in the hereditary spastic paraplegias, the extrapyramidal system affected in various movement disorders, or cerebellar–spinal pathways typical of the spinocerebellar degenerations. Primary affection of the peripheral nervous system may lead to spinal muscular atrophy, peripheral neuropathy, or a myopathy. Therefore, it behoves the clinician to take note of the earliest signs and symptoms and to extract from the examination an indication of the principal anatomical system(s) involved.

The age at which clinical signs and symptoms appear provides the second major criterion for reaching an accurate diagnosis. Admittedly, elucidation of the molecular defects in classic forms of neurogenetic disorders has permitted an expansion of the phenotypic spectrum to include both earlier onset of more severe variants as well as later, adult-onset forms of disease. Thus the practitioner experienced in geriatrics cannot ignore the possibility of a typical childhood-onset disorder first appearing in late adult life, nor can the paediatrician discount the likelihood of a classic adult-onset condition presenting in childhood.

A third guide to consider is the mode of inheritance. Family history is obviously a key component but may be lacking, especially in autosomal recessive disease. Knowledge of consanguinity can, however, be helpful in this regard. Other inheritance patterns especially common in neurological diseases include the repeat nucleotide expansion disorders and mitochondrial inheritance. The clinician interested in neurogenetics should also become familiar with other disease-causing genetic mechanisms such as the effects of genetic imprinting (parent-of-origin effect), uniparental disomy, chromosomal disorders, and the effects of spontaneously occurring major rearrangements within and between chromosomes. Modifier genes may also have a profound effect on penetrance, i.e. whether a disease-causing gene is expressed or remains silent.

Another means of classification of neurogenetic diseases utilizes extraneural clues such as the presence of specific signs involving the eyes, skin, connective tissues, or visceral organs, e.g. certain inborn errors of metabolism may present with corneal clouding or cataracts, abnormalities in skin pigmentation, or enlargement of the liver and/or spleen. Yet another method of classifying the inherited neurodegenerative diseases focuses on the metabolic derangements that occur in each (see Section 12). Thus, we refer to disorders of pathways involving amino acids, organic acids, lipids, carbohydrates, purines and pyrimidines, heavy metals, porphyrins, and vitamins. Often it is also possible to localize the abnormality to a particular subcellular element such as the mitochondria, lysosome, or peroxisome.

Although ultimately it will be helpful to obtain a specific DNA diagnosis, many tools are available to assist the clinician in obtaining the correct clinical diagnosis. These include various neuroimaging techniques, neurophysiology studies, microscopic studies of blood cells and tissue biopsies, and biochemical analyses of blood, urine, cerebrospinal fluid, and cultured skin cells. Judicious choices of confirmatory studies need thoughtful consideration of the history and clinical findings, and family history, often in consultation with a neurometabolic disease specialist.

Many inherited diseases of the nervous system present only after a prolonged presymptomatic period of several decades. This creates difficulties in attempting to reverse a pathological process that is advanced and already associated with significant cell loss, and in counselling and preventing further cases within the same family. Therefore, where there are therapies, prospects for newborn screening are being considered. In cases of severe morbidity within families of an as yet untreatable disease, prenatal diagnosis, often using preimplantation testing, may be considered. Use of this technology presupposes knowledge of a specific genetic marker for the disease in question.

Neurocutaneous syndromes (phacomatoses)

The phacomatoses are recognized by distinctive skin lesions that appear in childhood and the subsequent appearance of tumours in the brain and other organs. Several of these diseases involve defects in tumour-suppressor genes.

Neurofibromatosis 1

Neurofibromatosis 1 (NF1), also called von Recklinghausen's disease, is the most common of the phacomatoses, with a prevalence of 1 in 3000. The first feature to appear are café-au-lait macules which may be present at birth or appear during the first few months of life. There must be six or more café-au-lait spots for abnormality to be considered. Axillary freckling occurs next, usually by school age, followed by Lisch's nodules (melanotic hamartomas of the iris) gradually developing and then neurofibromas at puberty, which are made of Schwann cells, fibroblasts, and mast cells. These tumours may be cutaneous or subcutaneous, or extend into multiple nerves forming plexiform neurofibromas. About one-quarter of patients develop plexiform neurofibromas, which can in turn develop into malignant peripheral nerve sheath tumours, which have a poor overall survival rate. A small percentage of patients develop optic pathway gliomas, which do not appear to cause any ophthalmological symptoms. T_2-weighted MR images of brain reveal high-intensity, nonenhancing lesions, most often found in the brainstem, thalamus, cerebellum, and basal ganglia. These tend to disappear by late adolescence or early adulthood. Scolisis and dysplastic bone changes also occur. Among these changes are sphenoid wing dysplasia and bowing of the long bones. Phaeochromocytoma, renal artery stenosis, and precocious puberty are also encountered. Learning disabilities, intellectual impairment, seizure disorder, and psychiatric manifestations may appear in a small percentage of patients.

The neurofibromas are benign tumours derived from the nerve sheath and contain multiple cell types. Pilocytic astrocytomas also develop most commonly in the optic nerve, chiasma, and tract. The *NF1* gene maps to chromosome 17q11.2 and codes for neurofibromin, a GTPase-activating protein that silences the proto-oncogene p21-*ras*. The disease is inherited as an autosomal dominant trait, which is often inherited from a more mildly affected parent. Random somatic mutation of the one remaining functional *NF1* gene is believed to be required for tumour formation.

Most cases of NF1 require no treatment. Neurofibromas causing pressure symptoms may necessitate excision and others may merit removal for cosmetic reasons. Rapid expansion of a tumour, the development of pain, and loss of neural function suggest malignant change, and this occurs most often during adolescence or in young adults. The development of hypertension will require investigation for phaeochromocytoma, and spinal deformity may need orthopaedic attention. Follow-up annually in a multidisciplinary neurofibromatosis clinic is advisable.

Neurofibromatosis 2

Neurofibromatosis 2 (NF2) is also autosomal dominant but is much less common than NF1. Its principal manifestation is the occurrence of bilateral vestibular schwannomas. Approximately one-half of all patients also develop meningiomas and spinal ependymomas. Children with more serious disease may have other cranial and peripheral nerve tumours. Adults with NF2 usually have unilateral hearing loss, often associated with tinnitus. Cataracts are a common ocular finding.

Recommended diagnostic testing includes brain and spinal MRI to assess for tumours. Audiological work-up and brainstem auditory-evoked responses are also useful in assessing cranial nerve VIII function. In cases of bilateral hearing loss, a cochlear implant may be beneficial.

The *NF2* gene is located on the long arm of chromosome 22 and encodes merlin, a protein expressed in neurons, the lens of the eye, blood vessels, leptomeningeal cells, astrocytes, gonadal tissue, and Schwann cells. As in the case of neurofibromin, merlin mediates growth suppression and the development of NF2 requires a second hit to the remaining normal *NF2* gene. The loss of *NF2* expression is also seen in 30 to 70% of sporadic meningiomas and almost all sporadic schwannomas. Segmental neurofibromatosis affecting a restricted area of the body may be due to somatic mutations.

Tuberous sclerosis (Bourneville's disease)

The clinical features of tuberous sclerosis (TS) are intellectual impairment, infantile spasms, epilepsy, and the occurrence of retinal hamartomas and characteristic skin lesions. The disorder is dominantly inherited, but may be transmitted by individuals who are asymptomatic and show only minimal clinical evidence of the disease. Isolated cases are frequent, compromising as many as 80 or 90% of index cases. Many probably represent new mutations; others are transmitted by gene carriers with trivial manifestations. Genetic heterogeneity has now been established, with separate loci on chromosomes 9q34 (*TSC1*) and 16p13.3 (*TSC2*). The *TSC1* gene product hamartin and the *TSC2*-derived protein tuberin form a complex that interrupts mTOR (mammalian target of rapamycin) signalling which is involved in regulating cell growth. This leads to abnormally high levels of mTOR. Tuberin also binds p27, which has been implicated in regulating cell cycle progression. Mutations have been identified in 85% of patients with TS, of whom 85% are *TSC2*. Those with *TSC1* mutation have a less severe disease phenotype.

The earliest cutaneous lesions are irregular foliate areas of depigmentation over the trunk. These patches are readily identified when viewed under ultraviolet (UV) illumination using Woods' lamp. Facial angiofibromas ('adenoma sebaceum') are a second type of skin lesion that develops over the cheeks in a 'butterfly' distribution and on the forehead with multiple small warty elevations. Finally, a 'shagreen patch' may be present over the lower back. This consists of an area of elevated roughened skin with a yellowish tinge, which has been likened to shark skin. An ungual or periungual fibroma is present after puberty and in adult life.

The cerebral changes give rise to intellectual impairment, which is evident in early life and may be static or involve a slowly progressive cognitive decline, often complicated by a behavioural disorder. Infantile spasms or epilepsy with recurrent generalized or focal seizures may occur in association with intellectual impairment or in individuals of normal intelligence. The cerebral lesions, which are demonstrable by CT or MRI, are typified by nodular or tuberous masses composed of proliferated glial cells and enlarged distorted neurons. They may become calcified, and are found scattered throughout the cerebral cortex; they also extend into the ventricles to produce an appearance that was considered to resemble 'candle guttering' when seen in pneumoencephalograms. Gliomas sometimes arise in these lesions.

Retinal tumours, termed phacomas, may be present, and cardiac rhabdomyomas occasionally arise as well as hamartomas of the lungs and kidneys. Polycystic disease of the kidneys may also be associated.

Treatment consists of control of the epilepsy and management of the intellectual impairment and behavioural disorder. Facial angiofibromas have been successfully treated by laser ablation, and angiomyolipomas by embolization. Surgery is indicated if brain tumour size increases or if seizure foci are localized within abnormal brain tissue.

Von Hippel–Lindau disease

Von Hippel–Lindau disease (VHL) is characterized by central nervous system (CNS) and retinal haemangioblastomas, renal cell carcinoma, and phaeochromocytomas. Renal and pancreatic cysts, tumours of the pancreas, cyst adenomas of the epididymis and broad ligament, and endolymphatic sac tumours of the inner ear are also frequent. The incidence of this autosomal dominant tumour-suppressor syndrome is estimated at 1 in 35 000 live births.

The retinal lesions consist of angiomatous vascular malformations. The cerebellar lesion is a haemangioblastoma, often cystic, which may slowly expand and require surgical treatment. Such tumours may be associated with polycythaemia.

The VHL gene is located on chromosome 3p25–26. Inactivation of its protein product pVHL leads to up-regulation of several growth factors, including vascular endothelial growth factor and erythropoietin.

Patients with VHL require imaging of the CNS and spinal cord, monitoring of blood pressure and catecholamine metabolites, and an annual eye examination. Surgical removal is required for symptomatic tumours.

Sturge–Weber syndrome

The classic manifestations of Sturge–Weber syndrome (SWS) are a port-wine stain in the V1–V2 distribution of the trigeminal nerve, ipsilateral leptomeningeal angiomas, glaucoma, and other vascular eye abnormalities. Seizures, intellectual impairment, and focal neurological deficits are frequent. CT of the brain reveals calcifications in the involved leptomeningeal vessels. SWS is sporadic and its cause obscure.

Bannayan–Riley–Ruvalcaba syndrome

This rare autosomal dominant disorder is characterized by macrocephaly, intestinal hamartomatous polyps, lipomas, pigmented maculae of the glans penis, developmental delay, and intellectual impairment. Germline mutations in the PTEN (phosphatase tensin homologue deleted on chromosome TEN) are found in two-thirds of individuals with Bannayan–Riley–Ruvalcaba syndrome. PTEN, a tumour suppressor gene, has been mapped to chromosome 10q23.3.

Defects in DNA repair

As in the phacomatoses, the diseases involving defects in DNA repair cause skin abnormalities, neurological manifestations, and tumours although the tumours are outside the CNS.

Xeroderma pigmentosum

Xeroderma pigmentosum (XP) begins in childhood, with skin ageing and skin cancers after exposure to sunlight. Neurological manifestations occur in 20% of patients and include progressive mental deterioration, cerebral atrophy, sensorineural deafness, choreoathetosis, cerebellar ataxia, peripheral neuropathy, and growth retardation. Ocular signs include photophobia, conjunctival erythema, keratitis, and tumours.

XP is recessively inherited with an estimated incidence of 1 in 100 000 to 1 in 1 000 000. Eight different causative genes have been mapped, which are involved in either nucleotide excision repair or post-DNA replication translation synthesis. In the most severely affected form, the XP-A gene, mapped to chromosome 9q34.1, is defective. The protein product of this gene has a much higher affinity for UV-damaged DNA than undamaged DNA, indicating a role for this protein in damage recognition.

For treatment, total protection from sun exposure and UV-emitting lamps is employed along with topical retinoid derivatives.

Ataxia telangiectasia

This autosomal recessive disorder presents in early childhood with unsteady gait and truncal instability. Gaze initiation failure, choreoathetosis, and recurrent infections develop, followed by ocular telangiectasias between age 4 and 7 years. Later, cutaneous telangiectasias appear on the face, hands, and feet, the hair becomes prematurely grey, and lymph nodes are atrophic. Sexual infantilism, hepatic dysfunction, and insulin-resistant diabetes develops in older patients. Speech becomes incomprehensible, mental functioning declines, and, by the teens, the child has lost the ability to walk. Cancer develops in 38%, mainly in the form of lymphoreticular tumours and acute T-cell leukaemias. Older patients develop epithelial tumours in various organs. There is also an increase in the incidence of cancer in heterozygotes, especially breast cancer in women. Death occurs in the second decade.

Laboratory tests reveal an elevated serum α-fetoprotein, low levels of IgA and IgG2, poor responsiveness to common antigens, and an increased sensitivity of the patient's chromosomes to irradiation. ATM, the defective gene, located on chromosome 11q22–23, is a large protein kinase that serves as a regulator of the cell cycle checkpoint in response to breaks in double-stranded DNA.

On neuropathological examination there is a degeneration of the Purkinje and granule cells of the cerebellum, loss of anterior horn cells and dorsal root ganglion cells of the spinal cord, and loss of medullated fibres in peripheral nerves of some cases. General pathology studies show absence or abnormal development of the thymus and all lymphoid system elements.

Management of patients with ataxia telangiectasia involves the control of infections with antibiotics, monitoring for early signs of malignancy, the avoidance of multiple X-ray exposures, and the use of antitumour drugs rather than radiation therapy.

Cockayne's syndrome

In the classic form of this rare, autosomal recessive, multisystem, degenerative disease, symptoms start at the end of the first year or beginning of the second year. Psychomotor development is retarded; there is growth failure and progressive mental and motor deterioration. The face assumes a wizened, progeria-like appearance with sunken orbits, large beak-like nose, prominent ears, and narrow mouth and chin. The hair is sparse and the skin thin and photosensitive, but skin cancer does not occur. Eye signs include photophobia, decreased lacrimation, cataracts, retinal pigmentary degeneration, optic atrophy, strabismus, and nystagmus. Neurological signs consist of nerve deafness, dysarthria, tremor, ataxia, and peripheral neuropathy. Death occurs in the second or third decade. An earlier-onset connatal type II variant and a later-onset type III form have also been described.

CT of the brain reveals calcifications in the basal ganglia and dentate nuclei, and on MRI there are white matter changes. Histological studies disclose both central and peripheral nerve demyelination.

Nucleotide excision repair of actively transcribed genes is impaired in Cockayne's syndrome. After UV damage in Cockayne's syndrome (CS), cells, DNA replication, and RNA synthesis fail to recover rapidly as in normal cells. Two complementation groups have been demonstrated, designated CSA and CSB. The CSA gene maps to chromosome 5 and the CSB gene to chromosome 10q11. The large majority of Cockayne's syndrome patients have mutations in the CSB gene designated *ERCCG*.

Dementia syndromes

The major dementia syndromes are disorders of abnormal protein aggregation. Both genetic and sporadic forms of each illness exist and overlap has been found with parkinsonian–dementia syndromes. This section surveys the clinical genetics of dementia. See Chapter 24.4.2 for a more detailed account.

Alzheimer's disease

Alzheimer's disease accounts for about two-thirds of cases of progressive dementia. It begins with the insidious onset of loss of recent memory, increasing forgetfulness, disorientation, decreased abstraction ability, and word-finding difficulty. Behavioural problems arise including agitation, restlessness, insomnia, paranoia, and sometimes delusions or hallucinations. Depression is common. As the disease progresses the patient becomes increasingly immobile, incontinent, and mute with death occurring one to two decades after symptom onset.

Pathologically, amyloid-bearing neurotic plagues and neurofibrillary tangles are present within the cortex and subcortical nuclei. The neurotic plaques contain extracellular deposits of amyloid β-protein (Aβ) intimately associated with dystrophic neurites, activated microglia within the amyloid deposit, and reactive fibrillary astocytes surrounding the lesion. The tangles consist of masses of abnormal paired helical filaments (PHFs) and straight filaments in the perinuclear cytoplasm of selected neurons. The PHFs contain insoluble aggregates of the microtubule-associated protein tau in a hyperphosphorylated, largely insoluble form, often conjugated with ubiquitin. Fibrillar Aβ deposits are also found in the basement membranes of cerebral capillaries, arterioles, and small arteries.

Although the age of onset patients is over 60 years in most Alzheimer's disease, a small number of patients have a presenile onset. These cases are the result of genetic mutations, in the amyloid precursor protein gene (*APP*) on chromosome 21, the presenilin 1 gene on chromosome 14, or its homologous gene, presenilin 2, on chromosome 1. When mutated each of these genes cause over-production of the amyloid precursor protein. Also, the elevated dosage of the *APP* gene in Down's syndrome readily explains the early onset of Alzheimer's disease in patients with trisomy 21. Patients with the E4 allele of apolipoprotein E (apo-E4) also have increased susceptibility to Alzheimer's disease.

Positron emission tomography (PET) and single photon emission CT (SPECT) are being used as adjunctive tests for patients with probable Alzheimer's disease. For treatment, anticholinesterase inhibitors, antidepressants, and atypical antipsychotic agents are used. Current studies in transgenic Alzheimer's disease animal models offer a possible basis for immunological approaches to remove Aβ aggregates.

Frontotemporal dementia

Frontotemporal dementia (FTD) is the second most common cause of presenile dementia, accounting for 12 to 25% of the total. Originally, the concept of FTD arose with the recognition of dementia with Pick's bodies (silver-staining intraneuronal inclusions) in the presence of circumscribed atrophy of the frontotemporal regions. However, as Pick's bodies are present in a minority of cases, this finding is no longer an essential component of FTD.

Although the unifying theme in FTD is focal atrophy of the frontal lobes, temporal lobes, or both, either unilaterally or bilaterally, with greater pathology in the anterior than the posterior temporal lobe, FTD includes related disorders with substantial clinical and pathological overlap such as progressive supranuclear palsy and corticobasal degeneration.

FTD presents in the sixth decade in three subtypes. In the frontal variant, behavioural changes predominate. Patients with predominantly left hemisphere involvement experience progressive language deficits (nonfluent aphasia). In cases of left anterior lobe atrophy, there is progressive loss of the knowledge of words and objects (semantic dementia). However, patients ultimately progress to more global impairment in frontal and temporal lobe functions. Some patients will also develop parkinsonian features or motor neuron disease. SPECT shows bifrontal and bitemporal hypoperfusion.

In approximately one-half of patients with FTD, there are accumulations of insoluble hyperphosphorylated tau proteins in neurons and/or glial cells with little or no Aβ pathology. The microtubule-associated protein tau (*MAPT*) gene located on chromosome 17q21 is expressed predominantly in axons of central and peripheral nervous system neurons. Mutations in *MAPT* have been detected in familial cases, suggesting that they are pathogenic for FTD.

However, many FTD patients are negative for tau protein accumulation but are ubiquitin positive. Many of these patients, including both familial and sporadic forms, accumulate TDP-43 protein in the ubiquitin inclusions. This protein, which is encoded by a gene on chromosome 1, is involved in transcriptional repression and alternative splicing, and is also found in the motor neuron disease variant of FTD. Another FTD variant, NIFTD, is associated with abnormal neuronal aggregates of α-internexin. Tau-negative ubiquinated inclusions have also been noted in a few FTD patients with mutations in the progranulin (*PGRN*) gene on chromosome 17q21.31.

Patients with FTD are managed symptomatically. Serotonin selective reuptake inhibitors and atypical antipsychotic agents have been useful.

Dementia with Lewy bodies (see Chapter 24.4.2)

Lewy body dementia (DLB) is distinguished by the presence of intracytoplasmic aggregates of α-synuclein and other proteins within neurons, especially the CA2/3 region of the hippocampus. They are seen as well in some patients with Parkinson's disease and in others with Alzheimer's disease. The apoE4 allele frequency is increased in DLB but the association is not as strong as in Alzheimer's disease. Mutations in the α-synuclein gene and oxidative stress also favour aggregation of the protein.

Clinically, there is overlap with Alzheimer's disease. Signs include fluctuating cognition, recurrent visual hallucinations, parkinsonism, rapid eye movement (REM) sleep disorder, and depression.

Treatment with acetylcholinesterase inhibitors can be beneficial but adverse cognitive reactions have been encountered to antipsychotic agents.

Prion disorders (see Chapter 24.11.5)

Prion diseases have in common the accumulation of an abnormal isoform of the normal human protein PrP. The manner in which the conformational change from the normal form, PrP^c, into the abnormal form, PrP^{sc}, is unknown but the PrP^{sc} form then becomes infectious. Prion diseases cause a spongiform change within brains associated with astrogliosis and neuronal loss. Most cases are sporadic but 15% have a familial basis and 1% are iatrogenic, arising from transplanted tissues or pituitary extracts obtained from infected individuals or from incomplete decontamination of surgical instruments.

Creutzfeldt–Jakob disease (CJD) generally presents between ages 50 and 70 with dementia, myoclonus, and ataxia. It is rapidly progressive with death usually within less than 1 year. The EEG of many of the patients contains 1- to 2-Hz triphasic periodic sharp waves. On MRI, hyperintensity is detectable on FLAIR and DWIs (diffusion-weighted images) in the neocortex, basal ganglia, thalamus, and cerebellum.

A variant of CJD (vCJD), believed to be caused by transmission of bovine spongiform encephalopathy (BSE or 'mad cow disease') to humans, has been seen in young adults (average age 29 years). It presents with psychiatric symptoms, painful dysaesthesias, ataxia, dementia, and a movement disorder. The median survival is longer than in CJD (c.14.5 months). Diagnosis requires brain or tonsillar biopsy to demonstrate PrP^{sc}. The pathology of vCJD is distinctive with diffuse vacuolization and PrP-containing plaques surrounded by a halo of the spongiform change.

Another variant, Gerstmann–Sträussler–Scheinker syndrome (GSS), is an inherited form that occurs at an earlier age than CJD and progresses more slowly, with death resulting in 2 to 10 years. Signs include ataxia, decreased reflexes, and dementia. Amyotrophy and parkinsonian signs may also appear. EEG changes such as those in CJD are not present. Mild cerebral or cerebellar atrophy is present but there are fewer vacuolar changes than in CJD. There are extensive PrP-amyloid plaques and in some cases also neurofibrillary tangles.

In fatal familial insomnia (FFI), the insomnia is untreatable but cognitive function is spared until late in the disease. Other signs are ataxia, pyramidal and extrapyramidal dysfunction, and dysautonomia. Pathological examination reveals almost no vacuolization but neuronal loss and gliosis are found in the thalamus, inferior olives, and to a lesser degree in the cerebellum.

The PrP protein is encoded on chromosome 20. A codon 129 polymorphism with homozygosity for methionine or valine results in greater susceptibility for sporadic or iatrogenic CJD, whereas heterozygosity at this codon is protective. Methionine homozygosity at this codon results in increased susceptibility to vCJD. FFI is associated with a mutation at codon 178 plus methionine on the polymorphic codon 129. If a valine residue is present at the polymorphic codon 129, CJD results rather than FFI. Amino acid substitutions at several other codons cause GSS.

Epilepsy—genetic aspects

Seizures, i.e. the paroxysmal, spontaneous, involuntary discharge of cortical neurons, result from abnormalities in the regulation of neuronal excitability. The genetic bases for many of the idiopathic generalized epilepsies are now known. In many instances, these involve genes regulating voltage- or ligand-gated ion channels. Both clinical and genetic heterogeneity occur.

Benign familial neonatal convulsions

Apnoea and focal or generalized seizures begin in the first week of life and remit after some weeks or months. They may recur in later life in 10% of individuals. Although development is normal in most, a small proportion of patients may develop neurological sequelae. Three separate loci for benign familial neonatal convulsions (BFNCs) have been found. Each involves mutations in a voltage-gated potassium channel gene, KCNQ2 on chromosome 20q13, KCNQ3 on chromosome 8q24, and a third locus that maps to chromosome 5.

Benign familial infantile convulsions

The onset of seizures is between 3 and 8 months; the seizures consist of clusters of behavioural arrest, horizontal deviation of head and eyes, and limb jerking. They stop by 1 year of age. The interictal EEG is normal. Linkage to genes on chromosomes 16q and 2 have been suggested, including one family with a SCN2A (sodium channel) mutation.

Generalized epilepsy with febrile seizures-plus

Seizures often first occur in early childhood in association with fever but continue after the age of 6 in the absence of fever. In most children, neurological development is normal and the seizures stop in mid-adolescence. Various sodium channel genes have been implicated, including SCN1A encoded on chromosome 2q24, SCN1B located on 19q13.1, and SCN2A, also mapped to chromosome 2q24. Mutations in the γ-aminobutyric acid (GABA) receptor γ-subunit gene, GABRG2, located on chromosome 5q34 have also been found in the generalized epilepsy with febrile seizures-plus (GEFS+) phenotype.

More severe mutations in the same sodium channel genes have also been identified in children with severe myoclonic epilepsy of infancy (SMEI). The clinical course in these children similarly begins with a febrile illness but then recurs without fever and with the development of psychomotor retardation by year 2.

Generalized epilepsy with febrile seizures and absence

These individuals have clinical features similar to GEFS+ but absence seizures tend to predominate. These patients have mutations in GABA-receptor genes including GABRD, mapped to chromosome 1p36, and GABRG2, on chromosome 5q34.

Juvenile myoclonic epilepsy

Juvenile myoclonic epilepsy (JME) may comprise 5 to 10% of epilepsy patients. Such individuals present between age 8 and 20 with myoclonic jerks on awakening in the morning, possibly proceeding to generalized tonic–clonic seizures. About one-third will also have absence seizures. The EEG demonstrates bilateral symmetrical 4 to 6 Hz polyspike–wave complexes.

Both autosomal dominant and autosomal recessive modes of inheritance have been suggested. Genes implicated in JME include EFHC1 located on chromosome 6p12–p11, BRD2 mapped to chromosome 6p21.3, CACNB4, a calcium channel gene, on chromosome 2q22–23, *CLCN2*, a chloride channel gene, encoded on chromosome 3q26, and the GABA receptor gene, *GABRA1*, found on chromosome 5q34. A voltage-dependent potassium channel gene, *KCNQ3* (chromosome 8q24), a calcium-activated potassium channel gene, *KCNMB3*, and a nicotinic acetylcholine receptor gene, *CHRNA-7* (chromosome 15q14) have also been implicated in various JME family studies. Thus, JME is a complex epilepsy syndrome with significant genetic heterogeneity.

Childhood and juvenile absence epilepsy

Childhood and juvenile absence epilepsy (CAE) is estimated to occur in 13 to 17% of individuals with epilepsy. It is present in children aged 4 and 10, and is characterized by multiple daily episodes of impairment in consciousness in association with generalized 3-Hz spike-and-wave discharges. Fluttering of the eyelids, mouth movements, and myoclonic jerks of the extremities may accompany the periods of absence. Two-thirds will stop having seizures although others will go on to have JME or continued absences and generalized seizures as adults. Those with juvenile-onset absence epilepsy have less impairment in consciousness but may progress to have generalized tonic–clonic seizures as adults. Loci identified with CAE include the GABA$_A$ receptor subunit *GABRG2* (chromosome 5q34) and the voltage-gated chloride channel *CLCN2* (chromosome 3q26).

Progressive myoclonus epilepsy

The progressive myoclonic epilepsies include three lysosomal storage diseases—the neuronal ceroid lipofuscinoses, neuronopathic Gaucher's disease, and the cherry-red spot–myoclonus epilepsy syndrome—a mitochondrial disorder—myoclonus epilepsy with ragged red fibres (MERFF)—and two other entities—Lafora's body disease and Unverricht–Lundborg disease (Baltic myoclonus epilepsy syndrome). They are characterized by progressive neurological deterioration, various seizure types including polymyoclonus, which becomes unresponsive to antiepileptic medication, and dementia. Levetiracetam has been helpful in some cases.

Neuronal ceroid lipofuscinoses

This class of hereditary neurodegenerative lysosomal storage diseases is a common cause of childhood-onset seizures with an estimated incidence of 1 in 25 000. Common features are decline in cognition and motor functions, and blindness. Autofluorescent lipopigment accumulates within neurons and inclusion bodies characteristic of each variant can be seen by electron microscopy (EM).

Infantile neuronal ceroid lipofuscinosis (CLN1) is characterized by blindness before age 2, seizures, and marked cerebral atrophy. The ultrastructural appearance of the stored substance is predominantly granular, osmiophilic, dense material. Late infantile CLN2 patients present at age 2 to 3 with sleeplessness, seizures, and then visual loss. Curvilinear bodies are present on electron microscopy. The juvenile-onset patients (CLN3) develop retinal pigmentary degeneration in mid to late childhood and then seizures, and, as teens, cerebellar and extrapyramidal signs appear. On electron microscopy a pattern of fingerprint bodies predominates. Death in infantile NCL (CLN1) occurs in childhood whereas survival into adolescence or adult life is the norm for the other variants. See Chapter 12.6 for further details about the neuronal ceroid lipofuscinoses.

Neuronopathic Gaucher's disease

Gaucher's disease is characterized by lysosomal storage of the glycosphingolipid, glucocerebroside, within the reticuloendothelical system, involving principally the spleen, liver, and bone. It is due to deficiency of the hydrolytic enzyme, glucocerebroside β-glucosidase, encoded on chromosome 1; in the most common type 1 patient it rarely causes CNS complications. However, patients with the rare type 2 form fail to develop neurologically, become cachectic, with multiple brainstem signs and seizures. In the type 2 patient, death usually occurs before the age of 2 from pneumonia.

Approximately 5% of patients with Gaucher's disease worldwide have, in addition to visceromegaly, slowly progressive neurological involvement which includes gaze initiation failure, strabismus, developmental delay, and, in a few patients, cardiac symptoms. Some develop myoclonic seizures, which progress in frequency and severity and become unresponsive to anticonvulsant therapy.

Diagnosis of this autosomal recessive disease can be made by assay of blood β-glucosidase activity. Enzyme replacement therapy is effective in correcting the haematological abnormalities (anaemia, thrombocytopenia), and promotes reduction in the size of the liver and spleen but has proved ineffective in halting the progression of the myoclonic encephalopathy.

Cherry-red spot–myoclonus epilepsy syndrome (sialidosis type 1)

This autosomal recessive lysosomal storage disease begins in late childhood or early adolescence with action myoclonus. Subsequently, generalized seizures and polymyoclonus develop. A cherry-red spot may be seen in the macula early in the course of the disease, with blindness ensuing before significant cognitive decline occurs. Eventually the patient becomes bedridden and totally disabled by multiple myoclonic jerks. Vacuolated lymphocytes are present in peripheral blood and foamy histiocytes may be found in the bone marrow. Within urine, there is a marked increased in sialic acid-containing oligosaccharides. The disorder is due to a deficiency of lysosomal α-neuraminidase located on chromosome 6p21.3.

Myoclonic epilepsy with ragged red fibres

Patients with MERFF present in early adult life with short stature, myoclonus, seizures, ataxia, muscle weakness, and sensory neuropathy. Subsequently, dementia, hearing loss, and optic atrophy occur. This is a lactic acidosis and ragged red fibres are seen on a muscle biopsy with Gomori's trichrome stain. The principal neuropathological findings are degeneration of the dentate nuclei and superior cerebellar peduncles, the spinocerebellar tracts and the posterior columns of the spinal cord. The cause in most cases is a point mutation at position 8344 of the mitochondrial gene for tRNA^{Lys}.

Lafora's body disease

This autosomal recessive disease begins in late childhood or early adolescence and progresses to death within 5 years. Tonic–clonic and myoclonic seizures, polymyoclonus, and progressive mental deterioration occur. Cerebellar ataxia, optic atrophy, rigidity, and exaggerated reflexes develop later. On MRI there is moderate cerebellar atrophy and intracellular inclusion bodies composed of polyglucosan are present within neurons of the cerebral cortex, cerebellar dentate nuclei, liver, muscle, and axillary sweat glands. The last is a preferred site for a diagnostic biopsy. Most patients have a mutation in the *EPM2A* gene located on chromosome 6q23–25 coding for the protein laforin. A few patients have a mutation in *EPM2B* instead which codes for malin.

Unverricht–Lundberg disease (Baltic myoclonus)

This autosomal recessive progressive encephalopathy is particularly frequent in Finland and Estonia, hence the term 'Baltic myoclonus'. Onset is in childhood or adolescence and begins with generalized seizures. They are more frequent on awakening. Various stimuli will intensify the polymyoclonic activity. Cerebellar ataxia, dysarthria, pyramidal signs, distal muscle wasting, and over time mental deterioration become evident. Nerve cell loss occurs in the cerebellar cortex, dentate nuclei, and thalami, and sometimes also in the basal ganglia, brainstem, and anterior horn cells of the spinal cord. This disorder is caused by a sequence alteration in the cystatin B gene (*CSTB*) on chromosome 21, which involves expansion of a dodecamer (CCCCGCCCCGCG) in the 5-′flanking area of *CSTB*. A few patients with point mutations have also been described. Some patients have benefited from 5-hydroxytryptophan, piracetam, or baclofen, but the condition may be worsened by phenytoin which should be avoided.

Pyridoxine-dependent seizures

The seizures in neonatal-onset epileptic encephalopathy are resistant to antiepileptic drugs but respond immediately to the administration of pyridoxine in greater than the normal physiological requirement. Plasma and urinary levels of δ1-piperidine-6-carboxylate (P6C) and α-aminoadipic semialdehyde (α-AASA) are increased due to mutations in *ALDHTAI*, the gene encoding antiquitin, an α-AASA dehydrogenase. The accumulating P6C inactivates pyridoxal-5-phosphate, which is needed for GABA production, a central inhibitory neurotransmitter. Failure to recognize and treat this condition early can lead to permanent brain damage and lifelong intellectual impairment.

Glucose transporter 1 deficiency syndrome

Clinical manifestations of this infantile-onset disorder include severe seizures, intermittent ataxia, confusion, movement abnormalities, spasticity, sleep disturbances, and recurrent headaches. There is deceleration of head growth with acquired microcephaly, developmental delay, and cognitive impairments. Early appearance of episodic eye movements simulating opsoclonus has led to work-up for an occult neuroblastoma.

The absolute level of cerebrospinal fluid glucose is low and cerebrospinal fluid lactate concentration is also reduced. The disorder is due to new heterozygous mutations in *GLUTI*, which encodes a glucose transporter that is highly expressed in brain and red blood cells. The diagnosis may be confirmed by measuring the uptake of 3-*O*-methyl-D-glucose into erythrocytes. The seizures are refractory to conventional anticonvulsant medications and are exacerbated by phenobarbital, but respond to a ketogenic diet.

Alpers' syndrome

Progressive encephalopathy with intractable seizures, diffuse neuronal degeneration, and cortical spongiosis with and without liver disease are features of Alpers' disease. It usually affects infants and young children but rare juvenile cases are also known.

Development delay may precede the onset of seizures, which may start abruptly and consist of various types in individual patients including a marked myoclonic component. Marked motor retardation and intellectual impairment with blindness ensue. Liver dysfunction with jaundice and hepatomegaly may develop. CT and MRI show progressive cerebral atrophy. Mutations in the gene coding for the catalytic subunit of the mitochondrial DNA (mtDNA) polymerase γ (*POLGI*) have been found in a wide phenotypic spectrum of patients with this autosomal recessive disease.

Menkes' kinky hair disease

This X-linked disorder of copper transport causes profound neurological deterioration with the early onset of seizures, abnormal face and hair, hypothermia, skeletal abnormalities, and arterial degeneration. The scalp hair is sparse, stubby, and greyish in colour. Under a microscope, the hairs are seen to be twisted and display partial breaks. Seizures including myoclonic jerks are almost constant and survival is generally less than 2 years. Serum copper and ceruloplasmin levels are very low, and brain copper is reduced due to poor absorption of copper from the intestine. The disease is caused by mutations in the *ATP7A (MNK)* gene encoded on chromosome Xq13.3.

Dentatorubral-pallidoluysian atrophy

See under 'Hereditary ataxias'.

Epileptic encephalopathy due to other inborn errors of metabolism

Numerous hereditary metabolic encephalopathies other than those described above are associated with seizures. In the neonatal period and early infancy these include disorders of amino acids and organic acids, urea cycle disorders, biotinidase deficiency, peroxisomal and mitochondrial diseases, sulphite oxidase deficiency, and 3-phosphoglycerate dehydrogenase deficiency. Seizures presenting in the late infantile and early childhood period may indicate a lysosomal disorder, GABA transaminase deficiency, or creatine synthase deficiency. Disorders to consider when seizures present in later childhood or adolescence include, in addition to those listed above, acute intermittent porphyria and early onset Huntington's disease. In all cases in which the diagnosis is obscure, routine work-up should include a metabolic screen of blood and urine, plasma amino acids, total, free, and acylcarnitines, urine organic acids, brain CT or MRI, very-long-chain fatty acids for peroxisomal disease, blood lactate and pyruvate for mitochondrial disorders, and skin biopsy for electron microscopy to rule out a lysosomal disease.

Leucodystrophies

The term 'leucodystrophy' is applied to those diseases that have a genetic basis, a progressive clinical course, primary involvement of white matter, and a demonstrable biochemical or molecular defect. In contrast, the leucoencephalopathies are those disorders of white matter that lack the genetic, progressive, or other qualities of the leucodystrophies.

Primary leucodystrophies are those inherited diseases with predominately white matter involvement whereas, in secondary leucodystrophies, the involvement of brain grey matter and other structures leads to destruction of both axons and myelin by a more diffuse process.

The primary leucodystrophies can be classified into three subgroups: (1) classic dysmyelinative disorders; (2) hypomyelinative disorders with delayed or decreased myelin production; and (3) vacuolating myelinopathies. Within the category of the secondary leucodystrophies are metabolic, mitochondrial, and muscular dystrophy, and various syndromic (genetic) disorders.

Classic dysmyelinative leucodystrophies

Adrenoleucodystrophy (see also Chapter 12.9)

X-linked adrenoleucodystrophy (X-ALD), caused by a defect in the gene *ABCD1*, is the most common peroxisomal disorder with a pan-ethnic disease incidence of 1 in 20 000 males. *ABCD1*, which maps to Xq28, codes for a peroxisomal membrane protein that is a member of the ATP-binding cassette transporter superfamily. Alterations in *ABCD1* result in defective peroxisomal β oxidation and the accumulation in all tissues of saturated very-long-chain fatty acids (VLCFAs), particularly hexacosaenoic (C26:0) and tetracosaenoic (C24:0) acids. Phenotypic manifestations of X-ALD range from childhood-, adolescent-, and adult-onset, rapidly progressive cerebral forms, usually seen in affected males, to an adult-onset, slowly progressive myeloneuropathic form in males and carrier females. Varying degrees of primary adrenal insufficiency (Addison's disease) are invariably found in affected males whereas this endocrine disorder very rarely appears in females. Definitive diagnosis is established in males by demonstration of elevated levels of VLCFAs, which show abnormally high concentrations of C26:0 as well as high ratios of C24:0 and C26:0 to C22:0. As the test results for VLCFAs may be falsely negative or equivocal in 10 to 15% of heterozygous women, mutation analysis of the *ABCD1* gene is often recommended to confirm the carrier state.

The childhood cerebral form usually presents between 4 and 8 years of age with behavioural symptoms. The child becomes withdrawn and less verbal, and has difficulty with auditory and visual discrimination. Spastic paraparesis, incontinence, seizures, and feeding difficulties ensue with rapid progression to a vegetative state. MRI of the brain shows a characteristic pattern of demyelination, found in approximately 80% of cases, involving confluent T_2-weighted hyperintensity and T_1-weighted prolongation of the deep parieto-occipital white matter, which progresses in a centrifugal manner within a caudorostral direction. There is gadolinium enhancement on T_1-weighted imaging at the periphery of the involved white matter corresponding to regions of active demyelination and inflammation. A reverse pattern with frontal involvement is seen in another 15% of cases.

Adults with adrenomyeloneuropathy (AMN) present with a slowly progressive paraparesis, together with sensory and sphincter disturbances. It is associated with a noninflammatory distal axonopathy involving the dorsal column and corticospinal tract in the lower thoracic and lumbar regions, as well as more proximal segments of the corticospinal tracts in the internal capsule. In 30 to 40% of all male patients with AMN, there is inflammatory cerebral involvement detectable at the earlier stages of presentation or several years later. MRI often shows no abnormalities in the AMN phenotype, apart from infrequent spinal cord atrophy and T_2-weighted hyperintensity. Of males affected by X-ALD 70% have Addison's disease, in most instances associated with cerebral ALD or AMN; however, a smaller proportion of patients may have an 'Addison-only' phenotype of X-ALD, which is indistinguishable from Addison's disease attributable to other causes. Plasma VLCFA assay should, therefore, be performed in all patients with idiopathic Addison's disease, especially males. Pathologically, ballooning of cytoplasm with the presence of lamellar cytoplasmic inclusions is seen initially, most prominently in the zona fasciculata, followed by cytolytic cell death at a later stage. Approximately 50% of women who are heterozygous for X-ALD develop an AMN-like syndrome, typically occurring in the late 30s; progression is slower than in affected males.

Treatment includes general supportive care and symptomatic treatment for the patient. Adrenal hormone replacement therapy can be life saving, so all male patients should be adequately monitored for adrenal insufficiency. Lorenzo's oil, which is a 4:1 mixture of glyceryl trioleate and glyceryl trierucate, combined with moderate reduction of fat in the diet, normalizes or significantly lowers the levels of plasma VLCFAs, although it does not significantly alter the rate of progression in symptomatic individuals. Lorenzo's oil may provide a preventive benefit in asymptomatic boys aged between 18 months and 8 years who are at the greatest risk for the development of the cerebral form of X-ALD and for whom the brain MRI is normal. Haematopoietic stem cell transplantation (HSCT) provides the most favourable outcome in children at the early stage of the illness with 5-year survival rates of 92%, and a superior neurological and functional status compared with the group that have not received a transplant. As HSCT may accelerate the rate of progression, it is contraindicated in patients with advanced cerebral involvement. Other approaches, including phenylbutyrate, arginine butyrate, and lovastatin, as well as long-term gene replacement therapy, are under investigation. A new method for newborn screening is being developed which may alter the detection, monitoring, and treatment of X-ALD based on the measurement of C26:0 lysophosphatidylcholine applied to samples of dried blood on a filter-paper matrix. As X-ALD poses a significant burden to patients and families, professional genetic counselling is recommended. X-ALD heterozygous screening for women, together with prenatal diagnosis and preimplantation diagnosis, is available for families at risk.

Metachromatic leucodystrophy

Metachromatic leucodystrophy (MLD) is a sulphatide lipidosis caused by a deficiency of the lysosomal enzyme sulphatidase (arylsulphatase A, ASA), which catalyses the first step in the degradation of the sulphatide, 3-O-sulphogalactosyl-ceramide (cerebroside sulphate), or, in a few rare instances, a deficiency of cofactor saposin B (Sap-B). This leads to the accumulation of the substrate, cerebroside sulphate, in the white matter of the CNS and peripheral nervous system, which when stained with cresyl violet or toluidene blue reveal a brownish or reddish birefringence (metachromasia). There is another distinct clinical form of ASA deficiency, multiple sulphatase deficiency, in which at least seven different sulphatases are defective due to an abnormality in their processing and functional maturation. MLD is an autosomal recessive disorder with an estimated frequency of 1 in 121 000, ranging between 1 in 40 000 and 1 in 300 000. Diagnosis is based on demonstration of low ASA activity levels in the peripheral blood leucocytes or skin fibroblasts. About 10% of the general population has a pseudodeficiency of ASA, i.e. low activity on testing *in vitro* due to the presence of a polymorphism but with no clinical neurological disease. This needs to be excluded before a conclusive diagnosis of MLD is made. Increased excretion of urinary sulphatides is indicative of true ASA deficiency, whereas urinary sulphatides are normal in pseudodeficiency.

Most patients are equally divided between late-infantile and juvenile onset, and about 20% of patients have an onset in adolescence or later. In the late-infantile form, the clinical signs begin between 15 months and 2 years with frequent falls followed by the inability to walk, flaccid weakness, and peripheral neuropathy. The ability to sit without support is lost between 2 and 3 years of age. Speech becomes slow and indistinct, truncal titubation develops, optic atrophy becomes apparent, and deep tendon reflexes are initially diminished and then lost. Spasticity develops in the legs but the arms remain hypotonic. Spinal root and peripheral nerve involvement cause exquisite sensitivity to touch. Electrophysiological testing shows slowing of the motor and sensory nerve conduction velocities. The cerebrospinal fluid protein level is elevated. Brain MRI T_2-weighted images reveal centrifugally expanding, progressive, confluent, symmetrical white matter disease, with posteroanterior gradient. In the later stages of late-infantile MLD children are quadriplegic and spastic, with decerebrate, decorticate, or dystonic posturing, in association with loss of speech, seizures, hypertonic fits, bulbar palsy, and blindness. Death occurs 1 to 7 years after the onset of symptoms.

Juvenile MLD presents between age 4 and 12 years, with poor school performance and gait imbalance, followed by confusion and inability to follow directions. The speech becomes slurred; spasticity and inability to walk ensue. Tremor, tonic spasms, and seizures may also occur. There is visual failure. Peripheral neuropathy is common but not invariable. Most patients with juvenile MLD do not live into adulthood.

Adult MLD presents insidiously in late adolescence or early adult life with deterioration in school performance, disorganized thinking, poor memory, and a schizophrenia-like psychosis. The widespread use of MRI, which shows preferential involvement of the subcortical white matter in the frontal regions in the adult-onset form, has improved recognition of this variant in psychiatric patients. The gait is ataxic with pyramidal signs such as hypertonia and hyperreflexia. Peripheral neuropathy may or may not be associated with the adult-onset variant of MLD. Incontinence can develop relatively early. Despite the presence of optic atrophy, vision and the patient's awareness of his or her environment are preserved until the end-stage of the disease. The progression is usually slower than in the early onset disease with spastic quadriparesis, decorticate posturing, and pathological reflexes noted after 5 to 10 years, but survival for several decades is possible.

Progression of MLD may be slowed or halted when bone marrow transplantation (BMT) or umbilical cord stem cell transplantation is undertaken in presymptomatic patients or early in the course of the disease when neuropsychological signs are not advanced.

Multiple sulphatase deficiency (Austin's disease)
Mutations in *SUMF1*, which encodes a protein (the human C(α)-formylglycine-generating enzyme) involved in the processing of the catalytic site of all sulphatases, lead to a defective post-translational modification of several sulphatases and a neurovisceral disorder, multiple sulphatase deficiency (MSD), characterized by tissue accumulation of sulphatides, glycosaminoglycans (mucopolysaccharides), and cholesteryl sulphate. The clinical features of MSD overlap between the neurological findings of early infantile MLD and the dysmorphic facial features and skeletal deformities

(i.e. dysostosis multiplex) seen with mucopolysaccharidosis (MPS). Urinary excretion of sulphatides, heparan sulphate, and dermatan sulphate is high. Clinical features include ichthyosis in young infants with psychomotor retardation, hepatosplenomegaly, deafness, and peripheral neuropathy. Diagnosis of MSD is based on characteristic clinical manifestations and demonstration of deficiencies of the arylsulphatases A, B (*N*-acetylgalactosamine-4-sulphate sulphatase), and C (steroid sulphatase), and four other sulphatases involved in the degradation of specific glycosaminoglycans.

Globoid cell leucodystrophy (Krabbe's disease)
Collier and Greenfield described unusual 'globoid' cells in the white matter of patients with acute infantile diffuse 'sclerosis', a condition reported initially in two siblings by Krabbe, a Danish neurologist, in 1916. This condition, now termed Krabbe's disease, is caused by deficiency of galactocerebroside β-galactosidase (β-GALC; galactosylceramidase), which normally cleaves galactosylceramide into ceramide and galactose. Pathologically, there is rapid destruction of myelin and myelin-forming cells, i.e. oligodendrocytes and Schwann cells with reactive astrocytic gliosis and tissue infiltration by multinucleated macrophages, i.e. globoid cells filled with PAS (periodic acid–Schiff)-positive materials. Psychosine (galactosylsphingosine), a toxic metabolite that accumulates in the brain, is considered to be detrimental to the myelin-forming cells. Disease incidence in the general population is estimated at 1 in 200 000. The diagnosis of Krabbe's disease is made based on deficient β-GALC activity in peripheral leucocytes or cultured skin fibroblasts. There are at least 40 reported mutations in the β-GALC gene that cause Krabbe's disease.

Most cases present as an early infantile form, with an onset between 3 and 6 months of life. They have marked irritability, rapidly progressive generalized rigidity, and tonic spasms. Clenched fists and myoclonic jerks may be the earliest noted signs. Blindness and optic atrophy with pendular nystagmus develop later. The earliest objective findings in Krabbe's disease are abnormalities of the brainstem auditory-evoked response (ABR) as well as the visual-evoked potential (VEP). Brain MRI shows symmetrical T_2-weighted signal abnormalities in the periventricular region of the posterior cerebral hemispheres. Nerve conduction studies reveal markedly reduced nerve conduction velocities, while cerebrospinal fluid protein is elevated. Visceral organs as well as the skeletal system are unaffected. Death occurs between the ages of 1 and 2 years secondary to respiratory difficulties and/or bronchopneumonia.

About 10 to 15% of patients present with the late-infantile or juvenile form of the disease at approximately 5 years of age. They have a progressive gait disorder, spastic paraparesis, and cerebellar ataxia. Dystonia and visual failure may be associated. Behavioural changes and intellectual impairment may be the presenting features in juvenile-onset patients.

There is no definitive treatment for Krabbe's disease. Low-dose morphine may be effective in controlling the irritability. HSCT, using umbilical cord blood, is effective in modifying the clinical course and improving the neurological status of infantile Krabbe's disease; however, it is most effective if performed in the presymptomatic stages. Newborn screening has been recommended for early detection and intervention to improve outcome.

Alexander's disease
Alexander's disease, a sporadic autosomal dominant condition, first reported by WS Alexander in 1949, is an unusual form of

leucodystrophy presenting clinically and pathologically with white matter dysfunction but caused by mutations in the rod domain of the glial fibrillary acidic protein *(GFAP)* gene, resulting primarily in astrocytic dysfunction. A pathological hallmark of Alexander's disease is the presence in the astrocytes of eosinophilic, refractile, often rod-shaped, cytoplasmic inclusions termed 'Rosenthal fibres', which contain the intermediate filament protein GFAP in association with αβ-crystalline, small heat-shock proteins. These are predominantly distributed in the subependymal, subpial, and perivascular regions, in the basal ganglia and thalamus, and in the brainstem. There is widespread myelin deficiency in infantile cases associated frequently with cystic degeneration and cavitation. The arcuate fibres as well as occipital lobes and cerebellum are spared. In the juvenile-onset form the white matter degenerates whereas adult-onset disease may have only patchy zones of myelin pallor or cavitation.

The most common infantile form, with age of onset between birth and 2 years, is a relentlessly progressive lethal condition presenting as megalencephaly, seizures, hydrocephalus, and psychomotor retardation, and progressing to spastic quadriplegia. Survival varies from a few weeks to several years, but rarely beyond the early teens.

Juvenile-onset Alexander's disease between ages of 4 and 10 years presents with slowly progressive ataxia, spasticity, and bulbar signs, including speech and swallowing difficulties with relatively preserved intellect. The adult-onset presentation is heterogeneous, ranging from a presentation similar to juvenile-onset Alexander's disease and slowly progressive dementia to relapsing–remitting neurological symptoms mimicking multiple sclerosis that becomes recognizable as Alexander's disease upon neuropathological examination.

Classic brain MRI findings in the infantile presentation include extensive white matter involvement, with frontotemporal predominance, abnormalities of the basal ganglia, especially the caudate, and sometimes the thalami, and in some cases contrast enhancement associated with variable ventricular enlargement. Periventricular structures may appear swollen and cystic. Alexander's disease should be entertained in the differential diagnosis, especially in juvenile or adult cases, when brain MRI shows predominant or isolated involvement of posterior fossa structures, multifocal, tumour-like, brainstem lesions and brainstem atrophy, diffuse signal changes involving the basal ganglia, thalamus, or both, with contrast enhancement, as well as a garland-like appearance of the ventricular wall.

Hypomyelinative leucodystrophies

Pelizaeus–Merzbacher disease

Pelizaeus–Merzbacher disease (PMD), the prototypical X-linked recessive hypomyelinating disorder, is caused by alterations in the proteolipid protein (PLP) gene *(PLP)*, which in oligodentrocytes encodes two major CNS myelin proteins: PLP and its spliced isoform DM20. The phenotypic spectrum of PMD ranges from PMD type II (connatal form) >PMD type III (transitional form) >PMD type I (classic form) >spastic paraplegia type 2 (SPG2; complicated form) >SPG2 (pure form), and is closely related to the genotype. Missense mutations in the highly conserved region of the DM20-related protein family cause the most severe forms, whereas substitutions of less conserved amino acids, as well as gene alterations that do not affect the DM20 isoform such as duplications, truncations,

or deletions, cause less severe forms of PMD and SPG2. Large duplications including the entire *PLP* gene are the most frequently encountered mutations. Seitelberger delineated the neuropathological characteristics in PMD, which correlate well with the severity of the clinical presentation. The common pathological characteristics include lack or reduction of myelin sheaths in large areas of the white matter, with a patchy appearance of relatively conserved thin myelin islets, resulting in a 'tigroid' pattern. The structure of neurons and their processes including axons is well preserved.

The typical early manifestations of the more common classic form include hypotonia, nystagmus, and delayed motor development within the first year of life, followed by spasticity, cerebellar dysfunction, dystonia, and choreoathetotic movements and then disappearance of the nystagmus. Seizures may or may not be present. Patients often show slow development in the first decade of life; up to 45% of patients may be able to assume a sitting posture and some may be able to walk and acquire language capabilities. Slow deterioration begins in the second decade until death in mid-adulthood. In the connatal form there is congenital psychomotor developmental arrest with feeding problems, stridor, and spasticity, leading to progressive contracture of extremities, often accompanied by seizures. Death occurs in the first decade of life.

In patients with SPG2, which is allelic to PMD based on partial overlap of clinical manifestations with PMD and the discovery of *PLP1* mutations in SPG2, normal motor development occurs in the first year of life, but progressive weakness and spasticity of the lower limbs develop between the ages of 2 and 10. In addition some clinical features seen in PMD, such as nystagmus, optic atrophy, ataxia, dysarthria, and intellectual impairment, although less prominent, may be associated with SPG2. Later-onset spastic diplegia with no additional neurological complications (the pure form of SPG2) has also been reported. Most female carriers of PLP mutations are asymptomatic; however, in rare families, including the family described by Pelizaeus, manifestations ranging from mild spastic diplegia to progressive leucodystrophy with dementia have been reported. Female carriers for *PLP* mutations causing a mild phenotype in males tend to be symptomatic, whereas those carrying mutations causing severe phenotypes in males are usually asymptomatic in female carriers. This may be related to a skewed pattern of X inactivation in cells in which the mutated X chromosome is active or to the elimination of oligodendrocytes expressing severe mutations during early myelination, unlike those expressing milder mutations that persist.

The fact that PMD is characterized by delay in myelination and not by demyelination is reflected in T_2-weighted images on brain MRI as diffuse hyperintensity, which typically involves all the white matter, unlike many other demyelinating leucodystrophies, where abnormalities are often confined to specific regions. T_1-weighted signals from white matter in PMD are usually normal or isointense. Extensive but nonprogressive abnormalities of multimodal evoked potentials are observed in PMD. Electromyogram and nerve conduction studies are normal.

Currently, there is no definitive therapy for PMD. Symptomatic management of spasticity, feeding difficulties, and dystonia is recommended.

18q– syndrome

18q– syndrome, one of the most common chromosomal deletion syndromes, was first described by DeGrouchy in 1964. The clinical picture is distinguished by several dysmorphic features including short stature, microcephaly, midface hypoplasia, malformed ears, stenotic ear canals, flat philtrum, carp-shaped mouth, prognathism, tapered fingers, proximal thumbs, and prominent fingerprint whirls, as well as numerous neurological deficiencies such as hypotonia, hearing loss, nystagmus, and intellectual impairment. MRI studies show a high incidence of dysmyelination in about 95% of cases. The deleted 2-Mb region of 18q22–23 contains seven known genes, one of which encodes for myelin basic protein (MBP), which is a key structural protein of CNS myelin. As the deletion most often involves the distal portion of the long arm of chromosome 18 from q21 to qter, haploinsufficiency of MBP is implicated in the delayed or incomplete development of myelin seen on brain MRI; however, proton MR spectroscopy (MRS) studies suggest the possibility of active demyelination or increased myelin turnover. The characteristic pattern of dysmyelination on brain MRI T_2-weighted images, which shows low grey matter–white matter contrast, persists in individuals with 18q− beyond their first decade. The severity of dysmyelination appears to correlate with the severity of other features of the 18q syndrome, implicating the role of other deleted genes more proximal to the MBP locus in defective myelination in these patients.

Pelizaeus–Merzbacher-like disease with *GJA12* mutations

Following the first report by Uhlenberg *et al.* in 2004 several groups have reported children with Pelizaeus–Merzbacher-like disease (PMLD) with mutations in *GJA12*, which encodes connexin 47 (Cx47), and is highly expressed in oligodendrocytes. Patients with PMLD and *GJA12* mutations show the characteristic clinical symptoms such as nystagmus and impaired motor development in infancy, followed by ataxia, choreoathetotic movements, dysarthria, and progressive spasticity. Up to 70% of these patients have been reported to acquire walking capability; their intellectual functions were well preserved compared with their motor impairment. Epileptic seizures and peripheral neuropathy have been reported in a few cases. In patients with *GJA12* progression of mutations is slower, their cognition is better preserved, and there is partial myelination of pyramidal tracts compared with classic PMD. Brain MRI is similar to that of PMD with high T_2-weighted signal throughout the cerebral white matter and pyramidal tracts.

Most recently, a consanguineous Israeli Bedouin kindred with clinical and radiological findings compatible with PMLD has been identified with a homozygous missense mutation in *HSPD1*, encoding the mitochondrial heat-shock protein 60 (Hsp60).

Severe hypomyelination associated with increased *N*-acetylaspartylglutamate in the cerebrospinal fluid

A rare disorder that must be considered in the differential diagnosis of connatal forms of PMD has been reported in two unrelated girls with almost complete absence of myelin on cerebral MRI, as shown by a homogeneous high signal of white matter on T_2-weighted images and a low signal on T_1-weighted images in association with highly elevated concentrations of *N*-acetylaspartylglutamate (NAAG) in their cerebrospinal fluid. Clinical features include |rotatory nystagmus within the first 2 months, epilepsy, feeding difficulty, and acquired microcephaly. Initial pyramidal signs were followed by hypotonia and loss of reflexes secondary to peripheral neuropathy. No mutation could be found in the gene encoding the NAAG-degrading enzyme.

Hypomyelination with atrophy of the basal ganglia and cerebellum

In 2002, van der Knaap *et al.* described seven unrelated patients without parental consanguinity who had a previously unidentified leucodystrophy with an MRI picture of diffuse myelin deficiency in the central white matter and atrophy of the neostriatum (caudate and putamen) and cerebellum (vermis greater than hemispheres). The clinical picture was progressive but variable, ranging from visual failure and absent motor development to being able to walk supported or unsupported, but with frequent falls associated with learning disability without severe intellectual impairment. Later manifestations included increasing spasticity, ataxia, and extrapyramidal abnormalities. On MRI, there was diffuse myelin deficiency with high signal intensity on T_2-weighted images in the cerebral white matter including the corpus callosum, internal capsule, and pyramidal tracts in the midbrain and pons. With progression of the disease there was dilatation of the lateral ventricles and atrophy of the caudate nucleus, putamen, and cerebellum. The genetic cause and the pathogenesis of this condition have not been elucidated.

Hypomyelination and congenital cataract

Hypomyelination and congenital cataract (HCC) is an autosomal recessive hypomyelinating leucodystrophy, described by Zara *et al.* in 2006, caused by deficiency of hyccin, a membrane protein implicated in both central and peripheral myelination. In addition, there is progressive neurological impairment and congenital cataract. Most patients have cataract surgery within their first few months and intellectual impairment and developmental delay are evident by 1 year. Almost all achieve the ability to walk with support but lose this ability over time due to slowly progressive pyramidal and cerebellar dysfunction, as well as peripheral neuropathy manifesting as lower limb muscle weakness and wasting. Neurological findings include dysarthria, truncal hypotonia, brisk tendon reflexes, and bilateral extensor plantar responses along with cerebellar signs, such as truncal titubation and intention tremor. Brain MRI shows diffuse cerebral hypomyelination and progressive white matter atrophy with preservation of the cortex and deep grey matter structures. Electrophysiological studies show evidence of demyelination as well as axonal pathology in most patients.

Leucoencephalopathy with ataxia, hypodontia, and hypomyelination

Wolf *et al.* in 2005 described four patients with early onset progressive ataxia, short stature, and a distinctive pattern of hypodontia, hypomyelination, and cerebellar atrophy. Motor development was normal or slightly delayed and mental development was mildly retarded. Brain MRI T_2-weighted images show a diffusely hyperintense signal and a normal hyperintense signal on T_1-weighted images compatible with mild-to-moderate hypomyelination. Cerebellar atrophy, particularly in the vermis, was also noted. Extensive genetic as well as metabolic investigation failed to reveal the aetiology of this probable autosomal recessive disorder.

Vacuolating leucoencephalopathies

Canavan's disease

Aspartoacylase, expressed exclusively in the CNS in oligodendrocytes, normally hydrolyses NAA which is derived from neurons to aspartic acid and acetate. The acetate moiety is presumably further utilized as a building block for myelin lipids. Canavan's disease, an autosomal recessive disorder caused by deficiency of aspartoacylase, leads to a build-up of NAA in the brain, as well as to NAA acidaemia and NAA aciduria. Pathologically, intermyelinic oedema, widespread vacuolation in the lower layers of the cerebral cortex, and subcortical white matter and lack of myelin occur, along with astrocytic swelling and mitochondrial changes resulting in spongy degeneration of the brain white matter. Canavan's disease is pan-ethnic but there is a high prevalence of the carrier state, estimated at 1 in 37 to 1 in 50, in the Ashkenazi Jewish community. Two point mutations (at positions 693C and 854A in the coding sequence) are responsible for 97% of mutant alleles in Ashkenazi Jews, whereas C914A is the most common mutation among non-Jews, found in 40% of mutant alleles. Most cases present early in infancy but a few milder cases with a later onset have been encountered. Infants with Canavan's disease appear normal at birth, but developmental delay and hypotonia, including head lag, are evident between 2 and 6 months of age followed by macrocephaly and severe impairment of motor development by 1 year.

Optic atrophy, spasticity, and often seizures soon ensue with the affected children become increasingly debilitated with age, and unable to move voluntarily or to swallow. Death typically occurs before adolescence. Urine organic acid screen showing elevation of urine NAA is often the first diagnostic clue in evaluation of patients with Canavan's disease. Diffuse loss of white matter including the subcortical U-fibres, which are usually spared in most other forms of leucodystrophy, is evident on brain MRI. There is a marked increase in the NAA peak in brain white matter on MRS. The deficiency in aspartoacylase activity can be confirmed in cultured skin fibroblasts from patients but enzyme determinations in cultured amniotic fluid cells are not reliable.

Calcium acetate has been tried in Canavan's disease to replace the deficient acetate and acetazolamide has been used to slow the pace of macrocephaly. Gene therapy for Canavan's disease has thus far not been successful. Prevention strategies have included testing for carriers in Ashkenazi Jewish couples and prenatal diagnosis in at risk pregnancies using NAA quantification in amniotic fluid and molecular analyses of chorionic villous cells and amniocytes.

Megalencephalic leucoencephalopathy with subcortical cysts

Megalencephalic leucoencephalopathy with subcortical cysts (MLSC) is an autosomal recessive disorder caused by alteration in the gene mapped to chromosome 22qtel, which encodes a membrane protein that is highly expressed in brain, especially in astrocytes. Based on the pattern of localization it is speculated that the MLC1 protein is involved in astrocytic regulation and/or transport of ions or other substances. At least 50 mutations have been found thus far in *MLC1*; however, members of the Agarwal ethnic group of northern India, in whom the disease is more prevalent, share a common homozygous mutation, 320insC, suggesting a founder effect. Histopathology shows a spongiform leucoencephalopathy in the subcortical white matter without cortical involvement. The outermost lamellae of myelin sheaths contain countless vacuoles with sparing the middle or inner parts of myelin sheaths. Although most vacuoles are covered by single myelin lamellae, some vacuoles were partially covered by multi-lamellar myelin sheaths or oligodendroglial cell extensions.

MLSC is characterized clinically by macrocephaly noted within the first year or at birth, slow progressive decline in motor functions including ataxia and spastic paraparesis several years later, leading to inability to walk, and seizures in about 60% of patients. Cognitive functions are only mildly impaired with some decline in the second decade. Characteristic MRI findings that distinguish MLSC from other megalencephalic leucodystrophies include diffusely abnormal and swollen cortical cerebral white matter and bilateral cystic changes, the appearance of which resembles that of cerebrospinal fluid in all sequences, especially in the temporal lobes, occasionally in the frontoparietal regions but sparing the occipital lobes. In addition, the cerebellar white matter may exhibit mildly abnormal T_2 signal but there is no swelling. Eventually the swelling resolves and cortical atrophy develops. The number and size of the cysts progressively increase, such that they eventually occupy a significant portion of the frontoparietal cortex. The EEG shows multifocal epileptiform discharges. Supportive treatment, including treatment of seizures, is recommended.

Vanishing white-matter disease (childhood ataxia with CNS hypomyelination)

Childhood ataxia with CNS hypomyelination (CACH), a pan-ethnic autosomal recessive disease, also described as vanishing white matter disease (VWM) or myelinopathia centralis diffusa, was first identified in 1992. Astute use of molecular genetics in a population of a limited geographical region in the eastern part of the Netherlands led to the discovery that mutations in any one of the five subunits of eukaryotic translation initiation factor 2B (eIF2B) cause CACH/VWM and the recognition of a wider clinical spectrum. The eIF2B protein complex has a key regulatory role in protein synthesis through initiation of translation. Regulation of the activity of eIF2 is a protective mechanism for cells in response to stress. Mutated eIF2B could impair the ability of cells to regulate protein synthesis, resulting in increased susceptibility to various physiological stress conditions. On gross examination of the brain, the cortical grey matter is of normal consistency in marked contrast to the white matter of the centrum semiovale which is softened, atrophic, and gelatinous. There is rarefaction with moderate-to-severe vacuolation of the white matter with relative sparing of axons and subcortical U-fibres. The distinguishing feature of CACH/VWM is the presence of foamy oligodendrocytes, which on ultrastructural analysis show abnormal abundant cytoplasm containing membranous structures and numerically increased and morphologically abnormal mitochondria. Abnormally shaped coarse astrocytes and gliosis are present. In the severe forms, there is a reduction of the number of astrocytes and possibly astrocyte progenitors, but not of oligodendrocyte progenitors

Clinically, early development and head circumference are normal while some patients may present with speech and cognitive delay. The most common initial presentation is new-onset ataxia between ages 1 and 5 years. The disorder may be heralded by coma or a dysmetric tremor following mild head trauma or a febrile illness and apparently, even after an acute fright, can occur spontaneously. Subsequent deterioration is generally progressive with gait difficulty, cerebellar signs, pyramidal signs, dysarthria, and seizures. The course is often remitting–relapsing and patients may remain stable for years at any phase of the illness. Dysphagia and optic atrophy are seen late in the disease; the peripheral nervous system is usually unaffected. Death typically occurs during the first or second decade of life. There is a wide phenotypic spectrum which includes congenital forms with manifestations in organs besides the brain, a rapidly as well as a subacutely fatal infantile form, a slowly progressive form with onset after age 5 years that is often associated with ovarian insufficiency (dysgenesis), termed 'ovarioleucodystrophy syndrome', and an adult-onset disease variant. Brain MRI shows symmetrically and diffusely abnormal subcortical white matter with hypointense signal on T_1-weighted MRI and hyperintense signal intensity on T_2 images with sparing of the cortex. Cystic degeneration with a radiating stripe-like pattern or cavitation within the white matter is best seen on proton density or FLAIR sequences; there is no gadolinium enhancement of these lesions on post-contrast T_1-weighted MRI.

Supportive management such as avoidance of stress situations, use of antipyretics and antibiotics, physical therapy for motor disabilities, and carbamazepine for seizures is recommended. In families with a known mutation prenatal diagnosis can be offered.

Progressive cavitatory leucoencephalopathy

Progressive cavitatory leucoencephalopathy (PCL) was initially reported in 2005 by Naidu *et al.* as childhood-onset progressive cavitatory leucoencephalopathy associated with an increase in lactate in brain, blood, and cerebrospinal fluid. There may be subtle developmental delay followed by acute onset of irritability or neurological deficits occurring after 2 years of age, followed by steady or intermittent clinical deterioration with death between 11 months and 14 years of life. Brain MRI shows irregular asymmetrical patchy areas of white matter abnormality that evolved to multicystic degeneration. MRS shows elevated lactate in the affected structures. PCL appears to be a distinct genetic entity, possibly involving mitochondrial dysfunction, but the exact molecular basis is yet to be elucidated.

Secondary inherited leucoencephalopathies

Metabolic disorders
Mitochondrial diseases
See Chapter 24.24.5 for further description.

Lysosomal storage diseases
See Chapter 12.8 for further description.

Amino acidaemias
Neurological manifestations including leucoencephalopathy are frequently present in the amino and organic acidaemias (see Chapter 12.2). Patients with maple syrup urine disease (MSUD) were reported after a relaxed treatment protocol to have myelin abnormalities demonstrated on T_2-weighted brain MRI as increased signal in the mesencephalon and/or brainstem (cerebral peduncles and dorsal brainstem), less so in the basal ganglia–thalamus and globus pallidus, and less prominent areas of decreased signal intensity in T_1-weighted images. More severely involved patients had supratentorial changes, especially in the occipital periventricular and cerebellar white matter. The myelin abnormality may be due to chronic exposure of the brain to branched-chain amino acids or to a deficit of essential large neutral amino acids, the transport of which across the blood–brain barrier is impaired by an excess of the branched-chain amino acids.

In phenylketonuria (PKU), white matter changes on MRI are typical of the adolescent and adult with PKU. However, the distribution of MRI signal abnormality is most marked in supratentorial regions and only in more severe cases does it extend into the basal ganglia, brainstem, or cerebellum.

Organic acidaemias
Cerebral MRI has revealed bilateral white matter changes in several organic acidopathies, including L-2-hydroxyglutaric aciduria, 2-methyl-3-hydroxybutyryl-CoA dehydrogenase deficiency, and 3-hydroxy-3-methylglutaryl-CoA lyase deficiency.

Glycogen storage disease type IV/adult polyglucosan body storage disease
Glycogen storage disease type IV (GSD IV), an autosomal recessive disorder, results from deficient activity of the branching enzyme 1,4-glucan-6-glucosyltransferase mapped to chromosome 3p14. It presents in infancy with severe liver disease, causing cirrhosis, portal hypertension, and early death. A fatal neonatal neuromuscular form and a milder nonprogressive hepatic form are known.

A late-onset variant, referred to as adult polyglucosan storage disease (APBD), first described in 1971, is characterized by onset in the fifth or sixth decade of progressive upper and lower motor neuron dysfunction, sensory polyneuropathy, bladder and bowel incontinence, and, in some patients, dementia. Not all patients with APBD have deficiency of the glycogen-branching enzyme. Neurophysiological studies reveal an axonal sensorimotor peripheral neuropathy. The MRI shows extensive, nonenhancing, bilateral, symmetrical, periventricular and subcortical white matter changes with the T_2 signal abnormality extending to the cervicomedullary junction. There is progressive atrophy of the brain and spinal cord. Sural nerve biopsy, which can be diagnostic, shows frequent enlargements of myelinated fibres that stain positive with PAS. PAS-positive inclusions are also found within skeletal muscle fibres and the apocrine gland cells of the skin.

Congenital muscular dystrophy
See Chapter 24.24.2.

Sjögren–Larsson syndrome
Sjögren–Larsson syndrome (SLS) is an autosomal recessive disorder resulting from mutations in the gene for the microsomal enzyme fatty aldehyde dehydrogenase (FALDH), first described in 1957 by Sjögren and Larsson in a consanguineous cohort from the county of Vasterbotten in northern Sweden. The worldwide prevalence of this pan-ethnic disorder is probably less than 0.4 per 100 000. FALDH catalyses the oxidation of medium- and long-chain fatty aldehydes to the corresponding carboxylic acids. Deficiency in FALDH leads to elevation of free fatty alcohols in the plasma and leukotriene B_4 (LTB_4) in the urine. The accumulation of fatty alcohols or aldehyde-modified marcromolecules disrupts the integrity of multilamellar membranes in skin and myelin. Neuropathologically, there is reduction in myelinated nerve fibres in cerebral and cerebellar white matter, loss of neurons in the cortex and basal ganglia, and deposition of pigments. PAS-positive lipoid substances are found in the subpial, subependymal, and perivascular glial layers as well as in cerebral and cerebellar white matter, and there are perivascular macrophages containing lipofuscin-like pigments and spheroid bodies in the neuropili of several brainstem nuclei.

Babies with the condition may be born preterm with ichthyosis, which is generalized brownish-yellow in colour and associated with a severe pruritus. Developmental delay and spasticity are apparent by the first or second year, leading to contractures in the lower extremities and wheelchair dependency. Cognition is impaired in most patients. Pseudobulbar dysarthria, delayed speech, and seizures are common. Ophthalmological abnormalities include photophobia, macular dystrophy, and decreased visual acuity. After several years, glistening white dots surround the macular region of the retina. EEG shows symmetrical slow background activity with no epileptiform pattern. Cerebral MRI studies reveal multifocal areas of delayed myelination, hyperintense signal abnormality in the periventricular zone, and mild ventricular enlargement in the oldest patients. On MRS of the cerebral white matter and basal ganglia, there is a distinct diagnostic sharp lipid peak, believed to arise from the accumulation of long-chain fatty alcohols or aldehydes.

Treatment has been attempted with a low-fat diet supplemented with medium-chain fatty acids but was not successful. Beneficial effects have been described using the LTB_4 synthesis inhibitor Zileuton. The hypolipidaemic drug, bezafibrate, has been shown to induce residual FALDH activity in patient fibroblasts and may be a therapeutic option.

Cerebrotendinous xanthomatosis

This rare but underdiagnosed disorder should always be considered in the differential diagnosis of a leucodystrophy, because it is a treatable condition. Among Moroccan Jews the incidence of cerebrotendinous xanthomatosis (CTX) is 1 in 108 and in the general US population its prevalence is estimated to be 3 to 5 in 100 000. The 5α-dihydro-derivative of cholesterol, cholestanol, is increased 10- to 100-fold in CTX. It is present in the diet but its accumulation in the nervous system apparently results from increased endogenous production and impairment to its egress as a result of the blood–brain barrier. Mutations in the sterol 27-hydroxylase gene (*CYP27*) cause a block in bile acid synthesis, leading to absence of chenodeoxycholic acid in the bile and excretion of bile alcohols (bile acid precursors) in the bile and urine. Absence of the endproduct upregulates endogenous bile acid synthesis.

Symptoms commonly appear in childhood or during the second decade, but patients may present in the neonatal period or in middle age. There may be difficulty in school due to slowly progressive intellectual impairment, behavioural difficulties, and psychiatric symptoms. Other manifestations include cataracts, tendon and tuberous xanthomas (especially of the Achilles tendon), diarrhoea, osteoporosis, and bone fractures. Within the neonatal period, prolonged cholestatic jaundice may be observed. Eye signs in addition to cataracts include optic disc pallor, premature retinal senescence, palpebral xanthelasmas, corneal lipoid arcus, and proptosis. Neurological findings almost invariably develop and include cerebellar and pyramidal tract signs, peripheral neuropathy, and seizures.

Imaging studies disclose diffuse brain and spinal cord atrophy and brain white matter hypodensity. The cerebellar white matter is especially involved and there is hypersensitivity of the dentate nuclei bilaterally on the FLAIR sequence. A mainly spinal cord syndrome can occur with white matter abnormalities in the lateral and dorsal columns of the spinal cord.

Long-term oral therapy with chenodeoxycholic acid (750 mg/day), most effective in presymptomatic individuals, has been shown to suppress the abnormal bile acid synthesis, correct the biochemical abnormalities, and reverse the progression of CTX. Although HMG-CoA (hydroxymethylglutaryl coenzyme A) reductase inhibitors reduce serum cholesterol levels, caution is exercised because they can exacerbate the mitochondrial impairment.

Vascular disorders
CADASIL

CADASIL, cerebral autosomal dominant arteriopathy with subcortical infarcts and leucoencephalopathy, an adult-onset autosomal dominant disorder, is caused by mutations in *Notch3* encoded on chromosome 19p13. The major pathology is in small and median-sized arteries within the brain's white matter. The smooth muscle cells of the media are replaced with deposits of basophilic, granular, electron-dense material known as granular osmophilic material (GOM). There are 34 epithelial growth factor-like repeats (EGFRs) comprising the extracellular domain of the *Notch3* receptor, each containing six cysteine residues that form disulphide linkages. Almost all mutations causing CADASIL result in the gain or loss of a cysteine. Diagnosis can be confirmed by *Notch3* gene sequencing or by electron microscopic evaluation of a skin biopsy for the presence of GOM.

The clinical course is characterized by a history of migraine with or without aura in the late second or third decade (30 to 40% of patients), onset of cerebrovascular disease between 30 and 60 years of age, progressing to dementia, with MRI of the brain showing diffuse white matter lesions and subcortical infarcts. Later stages of the disease are characterized by transient ischaemic attacks (TIAs), strokes, behavioural changes, and memory loss. There is usually a family history with one parent or close relative with a similar clinical course. Vascular risk factors such as hypertension and atherosclerosis are usually absent.

Patchy white matter involvement on brain MRI may be noticed in childhood in asymptomatic patients. By the third or fourth decade, the white matter lesions have coalesced. Involvement of the anterior temporal lobes is a distinct and diagnostic feature. Infarcts may also be seen in the basal ganglia and brainstem, and the external capsules are also affected.

A young-adult onset arteriosclerotic leucoencephalopathy, termed CARASIL because of its autosomal recessive mode of inheritance, has been described in Japanese patients with many similarities to CADASIL. It is accompanied by alopecia and back pain.

Acetazolamide has been used in reducing migraine-like attacks. Antiplatelet agents and statin drugs are also prescribed for stroke prevention but there are no studies demonstrating their efficacy.

Hereditary endotheliopathy with retinopathy, nephropathy, and stroke

Hereditary endotheliopathy with retinopathy, nephropathy, and stroke (HERNS) is a rare autosomal dominant syndrome presenting, as the name implies, with retinopathy, nephropathy, and stroke. Electron microscopic studies reveal a vasculopathy consisting of multilayered basement membrane in capillary and arteriolar endothelial cells in the brain and other organs. Renal insufficiency with proteinuria and haematuria, and progressive visual loss due to macular oedema, capillary dropout and perifoveal microangiopathic telangiectases, are characteristic. Neurological symptoms appearing in the third and fourth decades include migraine-like headaches, psychiatric dysfunction, dysarthria, hemiparesis, and apraxia. Brain MRI demonstrates frontoparietal, contrast-enhancing, subcortical lesions with surrounding oedema.

Three other dominantly inherited cerebroretinal vasculopathies with leucoencephalopathy have also been described. Two, in addition to HERNS, show linkage to the same chromosome 3p21 locus. The third condition, hereditary infantile hemiparesis, retinal arteriolar tortuosity, and leucoencephalopathy, is not linked to chromosome 3p21. The leucoencephalopathy is accompanied by dilatation of perivascular spaces, microbleeds, and, in two of six symptomatic family members, silent deep cerebral infarcts.

Other leucoencephalopathies with childhood onset

Aicardi–Goutières syndrome

Aicardi–Goutières syndrome (AGS), an autosomal recessive leucoencephalopathy, is associated with developmental arrest, intracerebral calcifications, and chronic cerebrospinal fluid lymphocytosis. Mutations in the genes encoding any of the three subunits of human ribonuclease H2 enzyme (RNase H2) located on chromosomes 3p21 (*AGS1*), 13q14.3 (*AGS2*), and 11q13.2 (*AGS3*) can cause AGS. RNase H2 serves in antiviral defence by degrading DNA–RNA hybrids formed in the process of reverse transcription. By analogy with double-stranded (ds)RNA and dsDNA, which are known to stimulate interferon-α production, it is suggested that the DNA–RNA hybrids formed during retroviral reproduction will also stimulate interferon-α production. Reduced destruction of these hybrids because of mutations in RNase H2 subunits will therefore lead to overproduction of interferon-α and the phenotypic appearance of an *in utero* viral infection.

A very early encephalopathy noted in the first month, or a delayed onset by 6 to 10 months with loss of acquired skills and secondary microcephaly, spasticity, truncal hypotonia, and dystonic posturing, is the usual manifestation. The children are severely developmentally delayed, have no purposeful speech, and do not walk. Generalized seizures occur in 30% of patients. Serial CT scans demonstrate progressive periventricular, basal ganglia and subcortical calcifications, cerebral atrophy, and loss of white matter. Some patients develop swelling and acrocyanosis of the toes with peeling of the skin with no coolness of the extremities. There is a persistent synthesis of cerebrospinal fluid interferon-α as well as thrombocytopenia, hepatosplenomegaly, elevated hepatic transaminases, and intermittent fever, all of which suggest a congenital viral infection. However, TORCH studies are negative and no infectious cause has been found.

Cockayne's syndrome

See 'Defects in DNA repair', earlier in this chapter.

Other leucoencephalopathies with adult onset

Fragile-X tremor ataxia syndrome

See Chapter 24.7.5.

Autosomal dominant leucodystrophy

The locus for autosomal dominant leucodystrophy (ADLD), a condition described in 1984 in an Irish–American kindred, was mapped in a large Swedish family to chromosome 5q23, and subsequently a tandem genomic duplication in the gene encoding the nuclear membrane protein lamin B1 (*LMNB1*) was identified as the cause of ADLD. Pathology shows white matter degeneration with microscopic vacuolation, preservation of U-fibres as well as of the grey matter, and absence of an inflammatory response or gliosis. The initial clinical presentation involves abnormalities of the autonomic nervous system, including bowel and bladder dysfunction, impotence, orthostatic hypotension, and decreased sweating in the fourth or fifth decade. A slowly progressive course with loss of fine motor skills and other pyramidal tract and cerebellar signs is noted.

Survival after symptom onset is 20 years. CT scans show white matter lucencies in the frontoparietal region progressing to the parietal and occipital lobes, corresponding with brain MRI T_2-weighted signal changes in these areas as well as in the brainstem and cerebellar white matter.

Hereditary diffuse leucoencephalopathy with spheroids

Hereditary diffuse leucoenphalopathy with spheroids (HDLS), also known as leucoencephalopathy with neuroaxonal spheroids (LENAS), is an autosomal dominant, progressive, neurodegenerative disease pathologically characterized by generalized demyelination of white matter, including that of the descending tracts in the brainstem, with sparing of U-fibres. Neuroaxonal spheroids are scattered throughout the vacuolated white matter, which stain for ubiquitin. The mean age of onset in a large Swedish pedigree with 17 affected individuals was 36 years (range 8 to 60 years) and mean age at death 57 years (range 39 to 89 years). Psychiatric as well as neurological features dominate the picture with depression, anxiety, and aggressiveness, in addition to dementia, seizures, gait imbalance, and urinary incontinence. The brain MRI shows atrophy and patchy white matter changes in the frontal and frontoparietal areas, extending through the posterior limb of the internal capsule into the pyramidal tracts of the brainstem.

Movement disorders

Wilson's disease (see Chapter 12.7.2)

Wilson's disease is an autosomal recessive disorder of copper metabolism causing liver cirrhosis and neurological dysfunction in untreated individuals. It is caused by mutations in the *ATP7B* gene on chromosome 13q14.3. Copper transport is defective, leading to low serum copper and ceruloplasmin, an excess of urinary copper excretion, and copper deposition in tissues including the liver, kidney, brain, and cornea. Approximately 40% of patients first present with signs of liver disease including recurrent episodes of jaundice and portal hypertension. Neurological signs may herald the onset of the disease in 40% of cases but only after late childhood or adolescence. The first sign may be tremor in one arm or rigidity about the mouth with dysarthria and dysphagia. A masked face and characteristic grin develop and chewing and swallowing become difficult. Rigidity, tremor, dyskinesias, and speech and gait difficulties develop. Other extrapyramidal signs may appear such as choreoathetosis and in some cases cerebellar ataxia and intention myoclonus.

A psychiatric disturbance is the main presenting feature in 20% of patients with loss of emotional control, cognitive change, and intellectual decline. On MRI of the brain signal changes are noted in the caudate and lenticular nuclei and the thalami and dentate nuclei, with cerebral and cerebellar atrophy in long-standing cases. PET scans demonstrate reduction in the regional cerebral metabolic rate of glucose consumption, especially in the striatum and cerebellum.

Neuropathological studies reveal pigmentation and spongy degeneration of the putamen and to a lesser extent the dentate nuclei, substantia nigra, cerebellar cortex, and thalamic and midbrain nuclei. In addition to the loss of neurons and axonal degeneration, giant protoplasmic astrocytes (Alzheimer's cells) and Opalski's cells are found, the latter being present particularly in grey matter.

Diagnosis is aided by the measurement of serum ceruloplasmin and urinary copper. More definitive are the assay of hepatic copper (>3.9 μmol/g dry weight versus 0.2 to 0.6 μmol in normal liver) from a liver biopsy and/or screening for mutations in the *ATP7B* gene. In a mixed European population, one mutation, H1069Q, accounts for 35 to 45% of disease-causing alleles. Among Asians, 57% of the alleles contain the R778L mutation and, in Russian patients, 40 to 45% have the H714Q and delC2337 mutations. About 1% of the population are carriers.

Copper-chelating agents are used to treat Wilson's disease. Triethylene tetramine (trientine) and ammonium tetrathiomolybdate are favoured because they have no side effects compared with an earlier drug, penicillamine, which was associated with initial worsening of neurological symptoms. Zinc salts are also used to block intestinal absorption of copper. In many cases, the liver damage and neurological signs and symptoms are reversed within 1 to 2 years of initiating therapy and asymptomatic patients remain free of overt disease.

Huntington's disease

Huntington's disease is most often a disease of mid-adult life but 6 to 12% of those with the condition develop symptoms before age 20. It presents with changes in personality and behaviour as well as with involuntary motor movements. Either one can occur before the other. Memory deficits, agitation, depression, impulsiveness, delusions and hallucinations, and poor judgement may occur. Over time patients develop hand clumsiness, gait abnormalities, parkinsonism, chorea, dystonia, dysphagia, and tremor, as well as oculomotor disturbances. In juvenile patients, the clinical picture is one of bradykinesia, rigidity, seizures, and dementia. Global decline in cognition occurs with average survival of 10 years in juvenile-onset and 15 to 20 years in adult-onset patients.

Brain imaging discloses marked flattening of the head of the caudate nucleus and atrophy of the putamen. In juvenile patients there is also generalized brain atrophy with loss of cerebellar Purkinje's cells. Even before caudate atrophy appears on CT or MRI, PET may demonstrate hypometabolism in the caudate nucleus.

Huntington's disease is an autosomal dominant disorder with an incidence of 3 to 7 in 100000. It is caused in most cases by a CAG triplet repeat expansion in exon 1 of the *IT15* gene on chromosome 4q16.3, which codes for the protein huntingtin. Fewer than 26 CAG repeats at this locus is normal; over 40 repeats is characteristic of patients with Huntington's disease and more than 70 occur in the severe juvenile variant. A paternal origin of the expanded repeat is found in 80% of juvenile patients whereas small expansions or even contractions in repeat length are found in the children of women who have Huntington's disease.

Therapy for the symptoms of Huntington's disease includes neuroleptics, antiparkinsonian agents, psychotropic drugs, and a supportive stimulating environment. Family members seeking information about their risk of developing Huntington's disease should seek psychological assessment and review of their options from a genetic counselling service.

Huntington's disease-like syndromes

A small percentage of patients with Huntington's disease-like (HDL) syndrome may test negative for a CAG repeat expansion in *IT15* and could, in fact, have another genetic disorder. Four such HDL syndromes have been described: HDL1 is an autosomal dominant disorder caused by extra octapeptide repeats in the prion protein (PRNP) gene on chromosome 20p12. HDL2, especially common in the black South African population, is caused by a CTG–CAG triplet-repeat expansion in the junctophilin 3 (*JPH3*) gene on chromosome 16q24.3. An autosomal recessive variant present in Saudi Arabia has been named HDL3 and maps to chromosome 4p15.3. HDL4 is an autosomal dominant, triplet-repeat disorder caused by mutation of the TATA box-binding protein (*TBP*) gene located on chromosome 6q27. This is synonymous with spinocerebellar ataxia type 17. As only 93% of those with the classic clinical phenotype of Huntington's disease have a Huntington's disease-associated *IT15* gene mutation, these HDL syndromes should be considered as alternative diagnoses in the absence of a family history or failure to show the classic Huntington's disease molecular lesion.

Parkinson's disease

Parkinson's disease is the second most common neurodegenerative disorder after Alzheimer's disease. Incidence rates are 8 to 18/100 000 person-years with a higher prevalence among men than among women and an average age of onset of 60 years. The cardinal clinical features are tremor at rest, slowed movement (bradykinesia), rigidity, and postural instability. Secondary motor symptoms include hypomimia, dysarthria, dysphagia, sialorrhoea, decreased arm swing, shuffling gait, micrographia, positive glabellar reflex, blepharospasm, and dystonia. Motor block or freezing is particularly disabling, involving a sudden inability to move the feet. Common nonmotor manifestations are autonomic failure, cognitive decline, depression, apathy, hallucinations, and sleep disorders.

Patients with onset below age 50 have the tremor-dominant form of Parkinson's disease and slower progression of their disease than older patients who have postural instability gait difficulty with more rapid disease progression. Younger patients are also at higher risk for levodopa-induced dyskinesias than older patients.

Symptoms begin typically after 50 to 80% of dopaminergic neurons in the substantia nigra are no longer functional. The remaining intact nigral neurons may contain intracytoplasmic inclusions (Lewy bodies) composed of aggregates of α-synuclein. Neuroimaging studies with PET and SPECT are useful tools for imaging presynaptic dopaminergic neurons.

The diagnosis of Parkinson's disease is a clinical one and includes response of symptoms to levodopa. Other disorders with parkinsonian-like symptoms include multiple system atrophy, progressive supranuclear palsy, corticobasal degeneration, essential tremor, drug-induced parkinsonism, postencephalitic disorders, Lewy body dementia, and Alzheimer's disease. It is also prominent in certain genetic neurodegenerations: SCA2 and SCA3, Huntington's disease, dopa-responsive dystonia, familial prion disease, frontotemporal dementia, Wilson's disease, and X-linked dystonia–parkinsonism syndrome (Lubag). Most of these other diseases do not, however, respond to levodopa.

Disease susceptibility is increased by serious head trauma, exposure to environmental toxins (MPTP, pesticides), drinking well water, and rural living. Pathogenesis is believed to result from mitochondrial dysfunction (especially complex 1 deficiency), oxidative stress, and misfolding and impaired trafficking of α-synuclein.

Although 75 to 90% of cases are sporadic, single gene abnormalities have been identified in a subset of Parkinson's disease patients.

These include autosomal dominant, autosomal recessive, and X-linked forms. The most common known cause of familial and sporadic parkinsonism is mutations in the *LRRK2* (leucine-rich repeat kinase 2) gene. The gene is located on chromosome 12q12 and encodes the protein dardarin. The most frequent and best-studied mutation is G2019S, which accounts for 1.5% of all index cases with late-onset, classic parkinsonism. It is especially frequent among North African Arabs and Ashkenazi Jews with Parkinson's disease. The lifetime penetrance is 32% so many carriers may have no sign of disease on neurological examination. *LRRK2* is highly expressed in striatal neurons that receive dopaminergic input.

The α-synuclein (*SNCA*) gene was the first to be linked to familial parkinsonism. Besides point mutations, duplication of this gene is also observed in cases of Parkinson's disease. The phenotypic spectrum of *SNCA*, which is mapped to chromosome 4q21–q23, is broad and penetrance similar to *LRRK2*. Both *LRRK2* and *SNCA* are inherited as autosomal dominant genes.

Mutations in a third gene, *PRKN*, linked to chromosome 6q25.2–q27, are responsible for half the early onset cases of autosomal recessive Parkinson's disease. The gene product parkin is involved in proteasomal degradation of target proteins and may therefore play a role in Lewy body formation. Other known genes with autosomal recessive inheritance identified with mutations in Parkinson's disease are *PINK1* (chromosome 1 p35–p36), encoding PTEN-induced putative kinase 1, and *DJ-1* (chromosome 1p36), producing protein DJ-1.

Other much rarer neurogenic forms of parkinsonism are also described involving mutations in only a single or very small number of families. Linkage to other loci has been described but the genes responsible have not yet been identified. In addition, several susceptibility genes have been mapped in familial cases of Parkinson's disease. One of these, the glucocerebrosidase gene, is mutated more often in patients with Parkinson's disease than would be expected by chance alone. This observation has been verified in both Ashkenazi Jews who are at higher risk for Gaucher's disease, an autosomal recessive disease caused by glucocerebrosidase deficiency, and non-Jews. Whether the cause is an elevated level of glucocerebroside at the cellular level or the presence of mutated protein, either of which might promote aggregation of α-synuclein, has not been demonstrated.

Pantothenate kinase-associated neurodegeneration

This autosomal recessive neurodegenerative disorder of brain iron accumulation and pantothenate kinase deficiency represents a phenotypic spectrum of which there are three main variants. Classic pantothenate kinase-associated neurodegeneration (PKAN) manifests in childhood before age 6 years (mean 3.4 years) with gait and postural difficulties. Extrapyramidal findings are predominant with dystonia, rigidity, and choreoathetosis. Dysarthria occurs early and tremor may also be present. Corticospinal tract involvement with spasticity, hyperflexia, and Babinski's signs, as well as cognitive decline, are also common findings. About two-thirds of typical patients develop retinopathy and a few have optic atrophy. Most become nonambulatory within 15 years of disease onset.

In patients with the atypical form of PKAN, the onset is in the second to third decade, and progression of disease is slower with most patients continuing to walk for 15 or more years. The extrapyramidal signs are less severe and corticospinal tract involvement including spasticity and hyperflexia is common. Patients with the atypical variant are also more likely to have psychiatric symptoms, speech difficulties, and cognitive decline.

MRI shows bilateral areas of hyperintensity within a region of hypointensity in the medial global pallidus on T_2-weighted images, producing the 'eye of the tiger' sign. PKAN is due to mutations in the gene on chromosome 20p13–p12.3 encoding pantothenate kinase 2 (*PANK2*), which is a key regulatory enzyme in the biosynthesis of coenzyme A from pantothenate (vitamin B_5), and deficiency of which may cause oxidative stress in the iron-rich globus pallidus.

A third disorder, HARP, is allelic to PKAN. In addition to the early onset of extrapyramidal signs (dystonia, choreoathetosis, and rigidity), spasticity and dementia, retinal pigmentary degeneration, hypoprebetalipoproteinaemia, and acanthocytosis occur. Neuropathological features include bilateral degeneration of the globus pallidus and substantia nigra pars reticulata, deposition of iron in the affected regions, and neuronal axonal spheroids. These patients also have the 'eye of the tiger' sign on MRI and mutations within the *PANK2* gene.

Neurocanthocytosis

Several rare hereditary neurodegenerative diseases are associated with abnormally appearing red blood cells referred to as acanthocytes. These are contracted erythrocytes containing irregularly spaced, thorny surface projections and are best visualized under a scanning electron microscope. As described above, they are present in a small percentage of patients with PKAN. They are also present in three other movement disorders, autosomal recessive chorea–acanthosis, X-linked McLeod's syndrome, and HDL2, and in abetalipoproteinaemia. Acanthocytosis is also a predisposing factor for nonketotic, hyperglycaemia-induced hemichorea–hemiballism in patients with diabetes.

Bassen–Kornzweig syndrome

Acanthocytosis was first recognized in conjunction with Bassen–Kornzweig syndrome. This is an autosomal recessive disorder manifested by fat malabsorption, pigmentary degeneration of the retina, progressive ataxia, and neuropathy. Serum apolipoprotein B-containing lipoproteins (apoB), and very-low-density (VLDLs) and low-density lipoproteins (LDLs) are absent, causing very low serum cholesterol and triglyceride levels and deficiency of fat-soluble vitamins A, E, and K. Myelinated fibres in the posterior columns, spinocerebellar tracts, and peripheral nerves are affected. Progression of the disease can be slowed by treatment with high doses of vitamin E supplemented with vitamin A.

Chorea–acanthocytosis

Chorea–acanthocytosis is an autosomal recessive disorder manifesting clinically between ages 20 and 40 (mean 35 years), with chorea and involuntary movements in the orofacial region. However, in 42% of cases, seizures may precede other clinical manifestations by up to 15 years. The orofacial and buccal dyskinesias with tongue thrusting can cause tongue and lip biting, vocalizations, dysphagia, and dysarthria. Repetitive motor tics, dystonia, trunk spasms, and bizarre gait occur and can proceed to parkinsonism. Neuropsychiatric symptoms may precede or accompany the movement disorder. A personality change associated with obsessive–compulsive behaviour, depression, agitation, and cognitive decline is common. Autonomic disturbances include paroxysmal dyspnoea, sleep disturbance, and orthostatic hypotension.

Other manifestations are ocular motor impairments, distal muscle weakness and atrophy, peripheral neuropathy, and areflexia. Those patients with seizures may present with temporal lobe epilepsy and may require multidrug therapy. The use of carbamazepine or lamotrigine in these individuals may exacerbate the movement disorder. Patients with chorea–acanthocytosis are not candidates for epilepsy surgery. In most patients muscle creatine phosphokinase is elevated in the serum. The percentage of acanthocytes in the blood varies from 5% to 50%.

The findings on neuroimaging are similar to those in Huntington's disease. There is caudate atrophy, often more generalized, with an increased T_2-weighted signal abnormality on MRI of the caudate and putamen. PET studies show a reduction in blood flow and glucose metabolism in the caudate, putamen, and frontal cortex, and reduction in [18F]fluorodopa uptake in the posterior putamen.

Neuropathology examinations confirm atrophy of the caudate, putamen, and to a lesser extent the pallidum and ventrolateral part of the substantia nigra. On muscle biopsy there is neurogenic muscle atrophy and, in peripheral nerve biopsies, depletion of large myelinated fibres. Ultrastructural studies of peripheral nerve reveal axonal swellings filled with accumulations of neurofilaments.

Chorea–acanthocytosis is the result of mutations in the VPS13A ('vascular protein sorting') gene on chromosome 9q21. This codes for chorein, which is believed to be involved in trafficking of membrane proteins between cellular compartments. The presence of a specific deletion in French–Canadian patients and another in Japanese families suggests a founder effect in these two populations. The diagnosis of chorea–acanthocytosis may be confirmed by western blot analysis for chorein deficiency or molecular sequencing of VPS13A.

McLeod's syndrome

This rare, X-linked disorder has many of the clinical manifestations of chorea–acanthocytosis. It develops in men in the fifth decade and has a slowly progressive course. Women may show symptoms but they are generally milder. Limb chorea and facial hyperkinesia are common but lip and tongue biting are rare and parkinsonism is generally not present. As the disease progresses, many patients will manifest dystonic movements, epileptic seizures, cognitive impairment, and psychological disturbances. Other nervous system signs include muscle weakness and atrophy, and areflexia. Hepatomegaly and splenomegaly may occur and two-thirds of patients develop cardiac disease leading to severe cardiomyopathy and death.

The neuroimaging findings are similar to those in chorea–acanthocytosis and Huntington's disease with atrophy of the caudate nucleus and abnormal signals in the basal ganglia on MRI. SPECT indicates a reduction in striatal dopamine D_2-receptors. Analysis by PET discloses absent metabolism of the basal ganglia and reduced metabolism in the frontal and parietal cortex.

Muscle biopsy specimens reveal type 2 fibre atrophy and serum levels of muscle creatine kinase are elevated. Nerve biopsies confirm electrophysiological findings of axonal degeneration.

McLeod's syndrome is caused by absence of functional XK gene product. The XK gene is located on chromosome Xp21 and expresses the precursor substance for Kell antigen, the third most important blood group system after ABO and rhesus. Therefore, in McLeod's syndrome, Kell antigens are extremely reduced or absent. Kell is an endothelin-processing enzyme and, as endothelins serve as basal ganglia neurotransmitters, the deficiency of Kell could be relevant to the pathogenesis of McLeod's syndrome.

Huntington's disease-like 2

HDL2 is an autosomal dominant disorder appearing in the third or fourth decade with chorea, dystonia or parkinsonism, and progressive cognitive impairments. It is due to a CTG/CAG repeat expansion in the junctophilin 3 gene (JPH3) on chromosome 16q24.3. Age of onset is inversely proportional to the size of the repeat expansion. The gene product, junctophilin 3, seems to have a role in junctional membrane structures.

Treatment of the neuroacanthosis syndrome

As in Huntington's disease, treatment is symptomatic. To control the choreiform movements, dopaminergic function is reduced through the use of atypical antipsychotic agents or tetrabenazine. Focal dystonia interfering with eating may be treated with botulinum toxin injection into the genioglossus muscle. Anticonvulsants such as phenytoin, clonazapam, and valproate are used to treat seizures, and pharmacotherapy is also directed towards the psychiatric issues. Lesioning of the subthalamic nucleus or globus pallidus pars interna and deep brain stimulation have been used to treat chorea with mixed results. Patients with McLeod's syndrome should have periodic Holter monitoring and echocardiography for arrhythmia and cardiomyopathy. They should also have autologous blood banked to avoid potential blood transfusion reactions. Physical, occupational, and speech and language therapy are valuable adjuncts as are nutritional consultation and assistive devices.

Hereditary ataxias

Friedreich's ataxia

This disorder is an example of a spinocerebellar degeneration and is dominated by progressive ataxia with an onset in childhood or adolescence. The condition is inherited as an autosomal recessive trait and afflicts 1 in 30 000 individuals. The gene responsible has been localized to chromosome 9q13–q21 and is due to an expanded GAA repeat in a noncoding region of the gene for frataxin, a mitochondrial protein involved in iron homoeostasis. Degeneration of the larger dorsal root ganglion cells occurs, with consequent loss of the larger myelinated fibres in the peripheral nerves and degeneration in the dorsal columns. Degeneration is also evident in Clarke's column, the spinocerebellar tracts, and the corticospinal pathways. There is variable loss of Purkinje's cells in the cerebellum.

The average age of onset is 11 to 12 years, but cases of later onset may occur. The initial symptom is almost invariably ataxia of gait, although foot or spinal deformity may antedate this. At first it is noted that the child walks awkwardly with a tendency to stumble and fall readily; in cases of early onset, walking may never have been normal. As the disease progresses, the gait slowly becomes more irregular and clumsy. The patient walks on a broad base and tends to lurch from side to side. Involvement of the upper limbs develops later, at first giving rise to clumsiness of fine movements, subsequently for all movements. A coarse intention tremor becomes obvious. The trunk is also affected, leading to oscillation of the body when standing or sitting unsupported. A regular tremor of the head (titubation) occasionally appears. Nystagmus is present in about a quarter of the cases. Dysarthria of cerebellar type develops and may become severe enough to make speech almost unintelligible.

Initially weakness is not obtrusive, but this develops as the disease advances, starting in the legs and later involving the upper limbs. It results from degeneration in the corticospinal pathways and tends to vary in severity between cases. The plantar responses become extensor, but tone is not usually increased because of the accompanying disturbance of the afferent fibres from muscle spindles. There may be mild wasting of the anterior tibial and small hand muscles related to loss of anterior horn cells. Bladder and bowel function is usually unaffected.

Loss of the larger dorsal root ganglion cells leads to impairment of the sense of joint position, of vibration, and to some extent of touch–pressure sensibility, initially distally in the limbs. The impairment of proprioception superimposes a sensory element on the cerebellar ataxia. The tendon reflexes are depressed or absent.

Apart from occasional nystagmus, the ocular movements are usually intact. The pupils are unaffected. Optic atrophy is present in about a third of cases and 10% develop sensorineural deafness with particular difficulty in speech discrimination.

Associated skeletal deformities are common, in particular foot deformities (pes cavus and pes equinovarus) and kyphoscoliosis. Contractures of the knees may develop in the later stages. ECG demonstrates widespread T-wave inversion and ventricular hypertrophy in almost 70% of patients. Echocardiography may suggest the presence of hypertrophic obstructive cardiomyopathy, but these findings are not specific and the ECG is a more sensitive indicator of cardiomyopathy. The ECG changes are present early in the disease and tend not to be associated with symptoms. Cardiac failure occurs late and is usually precipitated by supraventricular arrhythmias.

Although progressive dementia is not a feature of the disease, reduced intelligence is present in some cases. There is an increased incidence of diabetes mellitus in Friedreich's ataxia (10%).

The disease is slowly progressive, the average age of death being in the latter part of the fourth decade. The foot and spinal deformities may require orthopaedic correction. Current therapeutic trials aim to counter the effects of oxidative stress using free radical scavengers such as idebenone or mitochondrial enhancers such as coenzyme Q_1, and to increase expression of frataxin with histone deacetylase inhibitors. Ultimately patients become bedridden. Death is usually from an intercurrent infection or cardiac failure.

Autosomal dominant spinocerebellar ataxias

This category of hereditary ataxias includes at least 29 clinically and genetically heterogeneous disorders. Although each is associated with extensive cerebellar atrophy involving all cellular layers and the deep cerebellar nuclei, many have involvement of the brainstem. In some, there is also involvement of the basal ganglia, cerebral cortex, spinal cord, and peripheral nerves. Other features are relatively unique such as retinal degeneration in SCA7 and epilepsy in SCA10. Action tremor is a feature of SCA12 and psychiatric manifestations, chorea, parkinsonism, and dementia occur in SCA17. The prevalence rates in different European regions range from 0.9 in 100 000 to 3.0 in 100 000.

Based on their molecular genetics, three major classes of SCAs can be delineated. The first are the polyglutamine diseases, so called because the defective gene in each contains a CAG repeat expansion that encodes an unstable polyglutamine tract. These six SCAs, namely SCA1, -2, -3, -6, -7, and -17, account for more than 50% of affected families worldwide.

The second group also involves nucleotide repeat expansions but they are in noncoding regions of the gene. In this category are SCA8, -10, and -12. The third category includes SCAs with conventional mutations in specific genes. Four are known: SCA5, -13, -14, and -27.

The repeat expansions are subject to the phenomenon of anticipation in which with each succeeding generation the expansion enlarges and, the larger the expansion, the earlier the onset and the more severe the disease. This is particularly severe in SCA7. A summary of the clinical and genetics of the SCAs is presented in Table 24.17.1.

The various symptoms are managed with conventional therapies. The extrapyramidal features in SCA3 may respond to levodopa and acetazolamide has helped patients with SCA6 due to repeat expansion in a voltage-sensitive calcium channel gene (*CACNA1A*).

Familial episodic ataxia

Severe types of episodic ataxia (EA) are known. The attacks in EA1 last a few minutes and occur several times a day. They can be precipitated by exercise or startle and are associated with facial and manual myokymia, which may persist between attacks. It is caused by mutations in the potassium channel gene *KCNA1*, which maps to chromosome 12p13.

The episodes in EA2 may last hours to days and can be precipitated by stress, exercise, or fatigue. Interictal diplopia and headache have occurred. EA2 is allelic to familial hemiplegic migraine and is caused by mutations in the calcium channel gene *CACNA1A4* on chromosome 19p13. Acetazolamide has been used to treat both EA1 and EA2 but is more effective in EA2.

At least four other hereditary forms of episodic ataxia have been described. EA5 is attributed to mutation in a gene encoding a calcium channel β subunit. The cause of EA6 is a mutation in a gene encoding a glutamate transporter.

Dentatorubral-pallidoluysian atrophy

Dentatorubral-pallidoluysian atrophy (DRPLA) is a rare autosomal dominant neurodegeneration caused by a glutamine-encoding repeat expansion in the atrophin gene on chromosome 12p13.3. Ataxia, dystonia, and dementia are characteristic.

Juvenile patients develop progressive myoclonic epilepsy whereas, in those patients with symptoms beginning after age 20, choreoathetosis and psychiatric difficulties are more prominent. The MRI and neuropathological examinations show cerebellar and brainstem atrophy, especially of the pontine tegmentum. Nerve cell loss and gliosis occur in the dentate nucleus, red nucleus, pallidum, and corpus luysi. Degenerative changes are also found in the striatum, cerebellar cortex, and corticospinal tract. The caudate nuclei are normal and the ventricles may be enlarged.

Most patients inherit the disease from their father but, if from their mother, symptoms begin earlier and are more severe even though the degree of expansion is smaller than in the case of paternal transmission. An allelic form of this disease, known as Haw River syndrome, has been described in an African–American family.

Fragile X tremor/ataxia syndrome

The fragile X syndrome is an X-linked disorder with an estimated incidence of 1 in 4000. Cardinal manifestations in the male are developmental delay, intellectual impairment, dysmorphic facial features, large testes, and autistic features. It is due to expansion of

Table 24.17.1 Classification of spinocerebellar ataxias (SCAs)

SCA type	Gene locus	Symptoms
SCA1	6p23; CAG expansion in *ATXN1* gene; polyQ disease	Ataxia with ophthalmoparesis, and pyramidal and extrapyramidal findings
SCA2	12q24; CAG expansion in ATXN2 gene; poly Q disease	Ataxia with slow saccades, peripheral neuropathy; less frequent extrapyramidal findings
Machado–Joseph disease/SCA3	14q32; CAG expansion in *ATXN3* gene; polyQ disease	Ataxia with ophthalmoparesis; pyramidal, extrapyramidal, and amyotrophic signs
SCA4	16q22	Ataxia with sensory axonal neuropathy and pyramidal signs
SCA5	11p13; mutations in *SPTBN2* gene	Relative pure cerebellar ataxia with dysarthria; includes Lincoln descendants
SCA6	19p13; CAG expansion *CACNA1a* gene; polyQ disease	Pure cerebellar ataxia with dysarthria, nystagmus; occasional mild sensory loss
SCA7	3p14; CAG expansion in *ATXN7* gene; polyQ disease	Ataxia with ophthalmoparesis, retinal degeneration, dysarthria, variable pyramidal signs
SCA8	13q21; CTG/CAG expansion in *ATXN8* gene	Gait ataxia, dysarthria, nystagmus, spasticity, and reduced vibratory sensation
SCA10	22q13; ATTCT expansion in *ATXN10* gene	Gait ataxia, dysarthria, nystagmus, frequent seizures; neuropathy
SCA11	15q14–q21.3 by linkage	Slowly progressive, relatively mild gait and limb ataxia
SCA12	5q32; noncoding CAG expansion in *PPP2R2B*	Ataxia with tremor; dysarthria, increased reflexes; occasional dystonia, late-onset dementia
SCA13	19q13.3–q14.4; mutations in *KCNC3* gene	Ataxia, varying onset including childhood; occasional delayed motor development and intellectual impairment
SCA14	19q13.4; mutations in *PRKCG* gene	Ataxia with dysarthria; facial myokymia; occasional myoclonus, dystonia; vibratory loss; late onset can be pure ataxia
SCA15	3p24.2-3pter	Slowly progressive, relatively pure cerebellar ataxia
SCA16	3p26.2-pter	Ataxia with head tremor, dysarthria
SCA17	6q27; CAG expansion in *TBP* gene; polyQ disease	Ataxia with dementia, extrapyramidal signs; widespread cerebral and cerebellar atrophy
SCA18	7q22–q32	Ataxia with sensorimotor neuropathy
SCA19	1p21–q21	Slowly progressive ataxia hyporeflexia, cognitive impairment; occasional tremor and myoclonus
SCA20	Chromosome 11	Ataxia with dysarthria; dentate calcification on CT
SCA21	7p21–p15	Ataxia with dysarthria, extrapyramidal features, cognitive defects; hyporeflexia
SCA22	1p21–q23	Pure cerebellar ataxia with dysarthria, nystagmus
SCA23	20p13–12.3	Slowly progressive ataxia with vibration loss
SCA25	2p21–p13	Ataxia with severe sensory neuropathy; gastrointestinal symptoms
SCA26	19p13.3	Pure cerebellar ataxia with dysarthria
SCA27	13q34; mutations in *FGF14* gene	Ataxia with tremor; orofacial dyskinesias; psychiatric symptoms and cognitive deficits
SCA28	18p11.22–q11.2	Ataxia with dysarthria, ophthalmoparesis, hyperreflexia
SCA29	3p26	Early onset, nonprogressive ataxia, vermian hypoplasia

Soong B-W and Paulson HL. Current Opinion in Neurology 2007; 20:438–446.

a CGG repeat (more than 230 methylated repeats) in the 5′-untranslated region of the fragile X gene, *FMRI*. Some females with the same molecular defect are affected but less severely than males.

Older males with a premutation allele (55 to 200 CGG repeats) will develop progressive gait ataxia and intention tremor, in association with neuropsychiatric abnormalities, parkinsonism, autonomic dysfunction, and peripheral neuropathy. Neuropsychological tests reveal deficits in executive functioning and memory. Anxiety, agitation, apathy, and depression are part of the neuropsychiatric profile. Penetrance of the disorder is age related, with 17% of adult premutation carriers manifesting tremor and ataxia in the 50- to 59-year age group and 75% in the cohort aged over 80 years.

MRI reveals cerebral atrophy, ventricular widening, thinning of the corpus callosum, and volume loss of the middle cerebral peduncles, cerebellar cortex, pons, and midbrain. Abnormal signal intensity in the cerebral white matter is also observed. Neuropathological studies confirm the presence of significant cerebral and cerebellar white matter disease. Eosinophilic intranuclear inclusions are found in neurons and astroglial cells of the brain and spinal cord proportionate to the CGG repeat length.

The prevalence of fragile X tremor/ataxia syndrome (FXTAS) in men aged 50 years or more is estimated to be 1 in 3000. Female premutation carriers are at risk for premature ovarian failure and early menopause, but are rarely affected with FXTAS. Men aged 50 or older with sporadic ataxia and a hyperintense signal on MRI in the middle cerebellar peduncles, as well as women with premature ovarian failure, should be offered screening for the fragile X premutation allele.

Other hereditary metabolic and degenerative ataxias

Numerous other hereditary metabolic diseases not already discussed in this chapter can cause cerebellar ataxia. These include abetalipoproteinaemia (compare Baseen–Kornzweig syndrome), ataxia with vitamin E deficiency (AVED), Leigh's syndrome (compare Chapter 24.24.5), pyruvate dehydrogenase deficiency, Refsum's disease, congenital defect of glycosylation, succinic semialdehyde deficiency, and juvenile neuroaxonal dystrophy.

Mitochondrial diseases (see Chapter 24.24.5)

Mitochondrial disorders constitute the most common neurometabolic disease of childhood with an estimated risk of 1 in 5000.

Mitochondrial genetics is complicated by the fact that mitochondria have their own DNA (mtDNA) but the vast majority of mitochondrial proteins are encoded by nuclear DNA (nDNA). Therefore, the inheritance pattern of mitochondrial diseases may be autosomal dominant or recessive, if secondary to a nuclear gene defect, or else maternally inherited or sporadic, if the mitochondrial genome is mutated. Mitochondria are ubiquitous in every tissue in the body, each cell containing many thousands of copies, all originating from the oocyte of the mother. Patients with pathogenic mtDNA mutations possess a mixture of mutated and wild-type mtDNA creating heteroplasmy. As the percentage of mutated mtDNA can vary among offspring within the same family and from organ to organ in the same individual, disease expression is highly variable. For a full description of mitochondrial diseases, see Chapter 24.24.5.

Lysosomal diseases (see Chapter 12.8)

Approximately 70 diseases are known in which failure to degrade one or more macromolecules results in their accumulation within tissues (Table 24.17.2). Together these disorders have an incidence of 1 in 5000 to 7000 births. The stored materials are byproducts of the cellular turnover of complex glycoproteins, glycolipids, glycosaminoglycans (mucopolysaccharides), and oligosaccharides.

Clinical genetics

Among Ashkenazi Jews, the frequency of the carrier state for certain of the lysosomal storage diseases (LSDs) is higher than in the general population. For this reason, screening of young adults and couples before conception or in the early stages of a pregnancy is being done to determine their carrier status for these disorders, which include Tay–Sachs disease, Niemann–Pick disease types A and B, and mucolipidosis IV. In each pregnancy of a couple in which both partners are carriers of the same recessive trait, there is a 25% risk of an affected fetus; monitoring of their pregnancies by amniocentesis or chronic villous biopsy could permit interruption at an early stage if the tests prove positive.

As, among Ashkenazi Jews, Gaucher's disease does not ordinarily cause neurodegeneration, pregnancy monitoring of carrier–carrier couples for Gaucher's disease is generally not done. Another type of prevention programme, popular among the Orthodox Jewish population, involves nonstigmatizing premarital testing permitting marriages to be arranged that avoid the possibility of two carriers for the same disease trait marrying.

Families in which an affected child has already been born can access prenatal testing of the conceptus using either information on the mutations present in the family or through testing of enzyme activity in the chorionic villous cells or the cultured amniotic fluid cells. Newborn screening is also being developed for those LSDs in which an intervention, such as umbilical cord stem cell transplantation, may be done in the early newborn period to prevent disease progression. In all cases in which a diagnosis of an LSD is made, family members should be offered genetic counselling and should be encouraged to inform relatives of their increased risk of carrying the trait for the disease.

Whereas lysosomal enzymes are ubiquitously expressed, the substrate on which they act may be confined to a single organ or system, as in Krabbe's disease, or distributed more widely causing multisystemic manifestations, as in Gaucher's disease. Signs of disease manifestations may become evident prenatally, at birth, or at any time from infancy to adulthood. Here LSDs that involve the central and/or peripheral nervous system are considered.

Sphingolipidoses

The sphingolipidoses are characterized by abnormalities in the metabolism of various glycolipid substrates that are present within membranes of nerve cells and myelin. Most of these disorders are neurodegenerative in nature.

Glycosphingolipids (GSLs) undergo degradation within lysosomes through the sequential action of specific acid hydrolases with the assistance of nonenzymatic glycoprotein cofactors, so-called sphingolipid activator proteins (or saposins [SAPs]). Ultrastructural studies of tissues from patients with GSL storage diseases typically reveal the presence of characteristic inclusions such as the membranous cytoplasmic bodies (MCBs) present in patients with G_{M1} and G_{M2} gangliosidoses.

Gangliosidoses

The gangliosides are a group of complex lipids with a ceramide backbone, to which hexoses and sialic acids are attached. They are found predominantly in brain grey matter. Disorders of ganglioside metabolism are classified according to the specific enzyme deficiency and the resultant accumulation of its substrates. The nomenclature of these substrates was assigned by Svennerholm, based on the placement of their sialic acid residues and their distinct chromatographic mobility. Each disorder is further categorized by age of onset into classic (early or late) infantile or later-onset (juvenile or adult) forms. Age of onset and degree of disease expression are influenced, in part, by the degree of residual enzyme activity. Secondary ganglioside accumulation occurs in other LSDs such as the MPSs and Niemann–Pick disease type C.

G_{M1} gangliosidosis

G_{M1} gangliosidosis, caused by deficiency of the enzyme β-galactosidase (β-Gal), is associated with the neuronal storage of the monosialoganglioside G_{M1}. Normally 20% of all gangliosides

Table 24.17.2 Lysosomal storage diseases

Stored substrate	Disease	Enzyme/protein deficiency	Gene locus
Sphingolipids			
G_{M2} gangliosides, glycolipids, globoside oligosaccharides	Tay–Sachs disease	α Subunit of β-hexoaminidase	15q23–24
	G_{M2} gangliosides (three types)	β Subunit of β-hexoaminidase	5q13
	Sandhoff's disease	G_{M2} activator	5q32–33
	G_{M2} gangliosides		
	G_{M2} gangliosides, AB variant		
G_{M1} gangliosides, oligosaccharides, keratin sulphate, glycolipids	G_{M1} gangliosides (three types)	β-Galactosidase	3p21-3pter
Sulphatides	Metachromatic leucodystrophy	Arylsulphatase A (galactose-3-sulphatase)	22q13.31-qter
G_{M1} gangliosides, sphingomyelin, glycolipids, sulphatide	Metachromatic leucodystrophy variant	Saposin B activator	10q21
Galactosylceramides	Krabbe's disease	Galactocerebrosidase	14q31
α-Galactosylsphingolipids, oligosaccharides	Fabry's disease	α-Galactosidase A	Xq22
Glucosylceramide, globosides	Gaucher's disease (three types)[a]	β-Glucosidase	1q21
Glucosylceramide, globosides	Gaucher's disease (variant)	Saposin C	10q21
Ceramide	Farber's disease (seven types)	Acid ceramidase	8p22–21.2
Sphingomyelin	Niemann–Pick disease types A and B	Sphingomyelinase	11p15.1–15.4
Mucopolysaccharides (glycosaminoglycans)			
Dermatan sulphate and heparin sulphate	MPS I, Hurler–Scheie	α-L-Iduronidase	4p16.3
	MPS II, Hunter	Iduronate-2-sulphatase	Xq27.3–28
Heparan sulphate	MPS IIIA, Sanfilippo A	Sulphamidase	17q25.3
	MPS IIIB, Sanfilippo B	α-N-Acetylglucosaminidase	17q21.1
	MPS IIIC, Sanfilippo C	Acetyl-CoA:α-glucosaminide-N-acetyltransferase	
	MPS IIID, Sanfilippo D	N-acetylglucosamine-6-sulphatase	12q14
Keratan sulphate	MPS IVA, Morquio A	Galactosamine-6-sulphatase	16q24.3
	MPS IVB, Morquio B	β-D-Galactosidase	3p21.33
Dermatan sulphate	MPS VI, Maroteaux–Lamy	N-Acetylgalactosamine-4-sulphatase	5q13–14
Dermatan sulphate and heparan sulphate	MPS VII, sly	Hyaluronidase	7q21.1–22
Hyaluronan	MPS IX	β-D-Glucuronidase	3p21.3
Glycogen			
Glycogen	Pompe's disease, glycogen storage disease type IIA	α-D-Glucosidase	17q25
Glycogen	Danon's disease	Lysosomal associated membrane protein-2 (LAMP-2)	Xq24
Oligosaccharides/glycopeptides			
α-Mannoside	α-Mannosidosis	α-Mannosidase	19p13.2–q12
β-Mannoside	β-Mannosidosis	β-Mannosidase	4q22-25
α-Fucosides, glycolipids	α-Fucosidosis	α-Fucosidase	1p34.1–36.1
α-N-Acetylgalactosaminide	Schindler–Kanzaki disease	α-N-Acetylgalactosaminidase	22q13.1–13.
Sialyloligosaccharides	Sialidosis	α-Neuraminidase	6p21.3
Aspartylglucosamine	Aspartylglucosaminuria	Aspartylglucosaminidase	4q34-35

Table 24.17.2 (*Cont'd*) Lysosomal storage diseases

Stored substrate	Disease	Enzyme/protein deficiency	Gene locus
Multiple enzyme deficiencies			
Glycolipids, oligosaccharides	Mucolipidosis II (I-cell disease); mucolipidosis III (pseudo-Hurler's polydystrophy)—three complementation groups)	N-Acetylglucosamine-1-phosphotransferase	4q21–q23
	Mucolipidosis III subtype C		γ subunit mutations on 16p
	Galactosialidosis	Protective protein/cathepsin A	20
Sulphatides, glycolipids, glycosaminoglycans	Multiple sulphatases	SUMF-1	3p26
Lipids			
Cholesterol esters	Wolman's disease, cholesteryl ester storage disease	Acid lipase	10q23.2–q23.3
Cholesterol, sphingomyelin	Niemann–Pick disease type C	NPC1; HE1	18q11–12; 14124.3
Monosaccharides/amino acid monomers			
Sialic acid, glucuronic acid	Salla's disease, infantile free sialic acid storage disease	Sialin	6q14–15
Cystine	Cystinosis	Cystinosis	17p13
Peptides			
Bone proteins	Pyknodysostosis	Cathepsin K	1q21
S-Acylated proteins			
Palmitoylated proteins	Infantile neuronal ceroid lipofuscinosis	Palmitoyl-protein thioesterase	1p32
Pepstatin-insensitive lyosomal peptidase	Late infantile neuronal ceroid lipofuscinosis	Pepstatin-insensitive lysosomal peptidase	11p15

found in the brain and 80% of gangliosides in myelin are the monosialoganglioside G_{M1}. Several other substrates of β-galactosidase, including galactose-containing glycoproteins, N-acetylgalactosamine, lactose, and keratan sulphate (a glycosaminoglycan), also accumulate and this may explain the presence of dysmorphic facial features reminiscent of the MPS disorders in the early infantile form of G_{M1} gangliosidosis. Histological examination of the brain in infantile G_{M1} gangliosidosis shows neurons and glial cells with distended cytoplasm and eccentrically placed pyknotic nuclei. Electron microscopy shows concentrically arranged inclusion bodies, which largely replace normal cytoplasmic constituents. In later-onset forms marked G_{M1} ganglioside storage is seen in the basal ganglia.

Early infantile G_{M1} gangliosidosis presents with hypotonia, feeding difficulties, and failure to thrive in the first weeks of life. A macular cherry-red spot is found in about 50% of cases, and there is a startle response similar to that seen in Tay–Sachs disease. Cherry-red spot represents the appearance of the normal ganglion cell-free region of fovea against the pale retina, where lipid-laden ganglion cells produce a white ring or halo. Dysmorphic facial features such as frontal bossing, wide depressed nasal bridge, gingival hypertrophy, or thickened alveolar ridges are prominent. Hepatosplenomegaly as well as bone deformities referred to as dysostosis multiplex, similar to those found in the MPS disorders, including hypoplasia and anterior beaking of the thoracolumbar vertebrae and widening of the diaphysis of long bone, are also noted. Cardiac complications include enlargement of the heart with thickening of the heart

valves and endocardial fibroelastosis, leading to valvular incompetence and cardiac failure. Hydrops fetalis may be the presenting feature at birth in 6% of cases.

The course is relentlessly progressive leading to spasticity, tonic spasms, and pyramidal signs with decerebrate rigidity by the second year with or without seizures. Respiratory failure and bronchopneumonia lead to death, usually by 2 years.

The late infantile form has an onset usually between 12 and 18 months, often with walking difficulty and frequent falls. Facial dysmorphism, skeletal deformities, and organomegaly are less prominent. Progression of the disease leads to seizures, spastic quadriparesis, and pseudobulbar signs such as drooling and dysphagia. Death occurs between the ages of 3 and 10 years.

The juvenile or late-onset form is a protracted illness with dysarthria, dystonia and mild-to-moderate intellectual impairment, usually developing in late childhood or adolescence, but signs and symptoms may be delayed until the third or fourth decade of life. There is vacuolation of peripheral blood lymphocytes, and the presence of galactose-containing oligosaccharides and keratan sulphate in urine, findings that help to distinguish G_{M1} gangliosidosis from mucolipidosis II (I-cell disease), because both can present with dysmorphic facial features and hepatosplenomegaly. Diagnosis is established by assay of β-Gal activity in peripheral blood leucocytes and cultured skin fibroblasts, or prenatally using cultured chorionic villous sample (CVS) or amniocytes. Only symptomatic treatment is available. A chemical chaperone therapy with N-octyl-4-epi-β-valienamine (NOEV) has been shown to be effective in mice.

G$_{M2}$ gangliosidoses

The G$_{M2}$ gangliosidoses are a group of heterogeneous clinical variants associated with the neuronal storage of the monosialoganglioside G$_{M2}$, caused by mutations in genes encoding the α (Tay–Sachs disease) or β (Sandhoff's disease) subunit of hexosaminidase A (Hex-A) or the G$_{M2}$ activator protein (in the AB variant). The Hex-A enzyme, with molecular mass of approximately 100 kDa, is a trimer consisting of one α- and two β-subunits, encoded by genes situated on different chromosomes. Mutations in the β-subunit lead to deficiency of Hex-B as well, which is a tetrameric homopolymer of β subunits. The B1 variant of G$_{M2}$ gangliosidosis, which has a high incidence in Portugal, results from altered substrate specificity of Hex-A. In this variant the mutated enzyme retains the ability to degrade the artificial substrate used in diagnostic assays, but not the natural substrate *in vivo* or the sulphated artificial substrate.

Ultrastructural examination reveals neuronal G$_{M2}$ ganglioside storage throughout the cortex and the deep grey nuclei, the spinal cord, and the autonomic ganglia. Characteristic pathological features are axonal hillock enlargement, known as meganeurite formation, and sprouting of new synapse-covered dendritic neurites at the axon hillock termed 'ectopic dendritogenesis', as well as axonal spheroid formation or neuroaxonal dystrophy. Spheroids are focal enlargements of various sizes distributed along myelinated and unmyelinated axons in the grey and white matter, consisting of multivesicular and dense bodies, mitochondria, and other organelles. This suggests that there is defective endocytic trafficking within axons. The incidence in the general population has been estimated at 1 in 112 000 live births, although the disease was highly prevalent among Ashkenazi Jews (1 in 3900 live births). Successful implementation of carrier screening programmes for at-risk couples has remedied this situation.

The 'classic' infantile form of Tay–Sachs disease (TSD), named after a British ophthalmologist, Warren Tay, and an American neurologist, Bernard Sachs, presents in infancy with psychomotor deterioration, poor head control, easy startle, axial hypotonia, bilateral pyramidal signs, and cortical blindness (pupillary responses are preserved). A characteristic hallmark of the disease is the presence of a macular cherry-red spot. In the second year of life, brain enlargement and not hydrocephalus leads to progressive megalencephaly; however, with further loss of the neurons and gliosis, the ventricles dilate. Progressive neurological deterioration leads to a spastic state and cachexia. Generalized tonic–clonic and simple motor seizures can occur in the terminal stages. Death usually occurs between 3 and 5 years of age. The AB variant, caused by deficiency of the G$_{M2}$ activator, has a phenotype that is indistinguishable from the infantile form. This diagnosis is suspected when the laboratory test results for assays of Hex-A and -B enzyme activity using artificial substrates are normal and the clinical presentation suggests gangliosidoses.

The later-onset forms of G$_{M2}$ gangliosidosis follow a protracted course and there is no ethnic predilection. Differences in the age of onset and disease progression, presumably determined by the severity of the underlying mutation, distinguish the childhood form, which has an onset between ages 3 and 6 years (chronic G$_{M2}$ gangliosidosis) from the adult-onset variant or late-onset TSD (LOTS), appearing in the teens or early adulthood. The phenotype of the B1 variant is similar to that of the childhood-onset form. Affected children develop dysarthria and gait difficulty, due to spastic paraparesis, which may be accompanied by tonic–clonic

or myoclonic seizures. Disease progression is marked by spasticity, rigidity, and dementia, ending in a vegetative state leading to death by the age of 15 years. Proximal muscle weakness, ataxia with cerebellar atrophy, and fasciculations are prominent in the later-onset forms, often leading to a wheelchair-dependent state. Psychiatric disturbances, including frank psychosis, may be the initial manifestation of disease, particularly among adult-onset patients. Late-onset G$_{M2}$ gangliosidosis should be considered in the differential diagnosis of adult patients with signs of lower motor neuron and cerebellar dysfunction. Vision and optic fundi are normal, although some cognitive decline is frequently encountered. Adult-onset patients may live into their 50s or 60s.

Sandhoff's disease (SD), a pan-ethnic disorder, is caused by mutations in the β-subunit of Hex-A and -B. Although the age of onset and clinical course are similar to TSD, organomegaly, *N*-acetylglucosamine-containing oligosaccharides in urine, and occasional cardiomyopathy are distinguishing features. Extremely rare cases of juvenile or late-onset SD have been reported.

The diagnosis is ascertained by assays of total hexosaminidase and Hex-A activity in leucocytes, and cultured skin fibroblasts complemented by analysis of the underlying Hex-A gene mutations. Prenatal diagnosis of the G$_{M2}$ gangliosidoses is available. Biochemical and/or molecular tests are preformed on cultured cells obtained by CVS or amniocentesis.

There is no definitive therapy for G$_{M2}$ gangliosidoses. However, substrate reduction therapy, based on the inhibition of glucosylceramide synthesis using the iminosugar miglustat, and gene therapy are under investigation.

Fabry's disease (see Chapter 12.6)
Gaucher's disease

Gaucher's disease, the most common lysosomal storage disorder with an estimated frequency of about 1 in 50 000, is caused by the deficiency of the lysosomal enzyme glucocerebrosidase (acid β-glucosidase), leading to the accumulation of its substrate, glucocerebroside (glucosylceramide) within cells of monocyte/macrophage lineage. The three major clinical subtypes are delineated based on the presence or absence of neurological involvement as well as the age of onset, rapidity of disease progression, and the rate and severity of neurological deterioration, when present.

Type I Gaucher's disease, a pan-ethnic disorder with high prevalence among the Ashkenazi Jewish population (carrier frequency about 1 in 20), refers to the non-neuropathic disease associated with hepatosplenomegaly, anaemia and thrombocytopenia, pulmonary involvement, and bone disease (see Chapter 12.8). Recent evidence suggests an association with Lewy body disorders, including Parkinson's disease, in a small proportion of patients and carriers of acid β-glucosidase mutations.

In type II Gaucher's disease, disease onset is before 12 months of age. In this acute neuropathic form, infants develop spasticity with head retraction (opisthotonus), dysphagia, and a rapidly fatal course; death usually occurs between 2 and 3 years of age. Laryngeal stridor, trismus, and aspiration pneumonia are frequent complications.

Type III Gaucher's disease, found in about 5% of patients with Gaucher's disease, is a chronic disorder with variable age of onset, usually before the age of 10 years. Neurological features include gaze initiation failure, tonic–clonic and myoclonic seizures, ataxia, and extrapyramidal rigidity. Severe pulmonary involvement is often present. The Norbottnian variant of type III Gaucher's disease presents with neurological problems which may be restricted to supranuclear horizontal gaze palsy despite the presence of significant extra-neurological systemic problems.

In contrast to the large amount of lipid stored in the liver and spleen, there is no significant accumulation of glucocerebroside in the brain. Severe glucocerebrosidase deficiency leads to production of glucosylsphingosine (psychosine), an alternative neurotoxic metabolic byproduct, which could play a contributory role in the primary neurological involvement seen in certain subtypes of Gaucher's disease. Neuropathological studies reveal lipid-filled cells in the perivascular Virchow–Robin spaces and neuronophagic microglial nodules in several regions of the brain (e.g. cortex, thalamus, basal ganglia, brainstem, and cerebellum) and in the spinal cord.

Enzyme replacement therapy (ERT) is now the mainstay of treatment for Gaucher's disease, although it does not alter the course of neurological deterioration in patients with type II Gaucher's disease. Recently, substrate reduction therapy (SRT) has been shown to be effective in ameliorating several clinical features of Gaucher's disease, although its role in neuropathic Gaucher's disease still has to be elucidated.

Niemann–Pick disease, including types A and B

Niemann–Pick disease (NPD) represents a group of autosomal recessive disorders causing progressive storage of sphingomyelin (phosphorylcholine) in the reticuloendothelial system. NPD subtypes A (infantile neuropathic) and B (later-onset non-neuropathic) represent the spectrum of allelic variants associated with mutations of the ASM gene, resulting in primary deficiency of sphingomyelinase. NPD subtypes C and D are also allelic disorders due to mutations of either the *NPC1* or the *NPC2* gene, which may be associated with mild secondary ASM deficiency. Mutations in NPC1 or -2 leads to disruption in the trafficking and/or metabolism of cholesterol and sphingolipid.

Early infantile NPD type A presents within the first few weeks or months with failure to thrive and hepatomegaly, followed by neurological regression and the appearance of the macular cherry-red spot, ultimately leading to liver failure with ascites and jaundice, cachexia, rigidity, and opisthotonus. Death occurs in the second or third year of life. NPD type B is associated with visceral involvement and pulmonary infiltration in late infancy or early childhood. There are vacuoles within peripheral lymphocytes and monocytes, as well as foam cells in the bone marrow. Deficient ASM activity in leucocytes or cultured skin fibroblasts confirms the diagnosis of NPD types A and B.

NPD type C has an estimated incidence of 1 in 150 000. Mutations in the gene *NPC1*, which encodes a large transmembrane glycoprotein localized primarily in the late endosomes, causes approximately 95% of cases, whereas a smaller group of patients has been shown to have a defect of the *NPC2* gene, which encodes a small soluble lysosomal protein with cholesterol-binding properties. It is a neurovisceral lipid storage disorder neuropathologically characterized by axonal spheroids, intraneuronal cytoplasmic inclusions, and neuronal loss.

About 50 to 60% of cases are considered to have the classic presentation with a benign, self-limiting jaundice in early infancy, followed by normal initial development. Between the ages of 3 and 8 years these children develop hepatosplenomegaly, clumsiness, ataxia, and supranuclear vertical gaze palsy, accompanied by blinking or head thrusting, eventually progressing to dysarthria, dysphagia, and dementia. Extrapyramidal signs, such as dystonia and choreoathetosis, in addition to cataplexy, psychosis, and seizures, are other neuropsychiatric features. A severe form of NPD type C presents at birth with ascites, jaundice, and a rapidly progressive fatal course. NPD type D was described among the French Acadians in Nova Scotia (Canada) with a disease onset usually between age 2 and 4 years. A founder mutation in *NPC1* has subsequently been described in this population.

Management of patients with NPD type C is primarily symptomatic. A trial using substrate reduction therapy with miglustat is under way for NPD type C.

Metachromatic leucodystrophy (sulphatide lipidosis)
See 'Leucodystrophies' above.

Krabbe's disease (globoid cell leucodystrophy) See 'Leucodystrophies' above.

Mucopolysaccharidoses (for individual discussion see Chapter 12.8) The MPSs are a group of heterogeneous disorders resulting from deficiency of lysosomal glycosidases and sulphatases involved in the sequential degradation of glycosaminoglycans (GAGs). Each follows an autosomal recessive inheritance pattern except MPS II, which is X linked. Their collective incidence is estimated at about 1 in 25 000 to 1 in 50 000. Incomplete hydrolysis and accumulation of GAGs leads to deposition of different types of intralysosomal inclusion bodies in tissues, the most characteristic of which are the zebra bodies. Increased urinary excretion of the substrates dermatan sulphate, heparan sulphate, keratan sulphate, and chondroitin sulphate is often used as a screening test for MPS in suspected cases; however, a definitive diagnosis of a particular MPS subtype is based on specific enzyme assays using plasma, leucocytes, or cultured skin fibroblasts.

Despite being aetiologically distinct, several non-neurological clinical features are shared by MPSs, mainly coarse facial features and dysostosis multiplex. The latter refers to the typical skeletal and radiographic findings, e.g. bullet-shaped phalanges, and flattening and anterior beaking of the vertebral bodies. Ophthalmic complications include corneal opacity, pigmentary retinal degeneration, optic atrophy, and glaucoma. Developmental regression is noted in several MPS subtypes. Hydrocephalus can result from the deposition of GAGs and histiocytic infiltration in the meninges, i.e. pachymeningitis. GAG storage at various sites may lead to nerve compression syndromes such as carpal tunnel syndrome and spinal cord compression.

MPS type I See Chapter 12.8 for further discussion.

Glycoproteinoses Deficiency of lysosomal exoglycosidases involved in the hydrolysis of the carbohydrate side chains attached to the peptide backbone of glycoproteins by the *N*-glycosidic asparagine links leads to disorders of glycoprotein degradation termed the 'glycoproteinoses'. The clinical features of glycoproteinoses are similar to the MPS disorders, such as coarsening of facial features, dysostosis multiplex, intellectual impairment, and hepatosplenomegaly. Patients with glycoproteinoses have excessive urinary excretion of oligosaccharides; however, identification of the underlying enzyme deficiency requires assays use of leucocytes or cultured skin fibroblasts.

Mannosidosis Mannosidosis results from a deficiency of either α- or β-mannosidase. Two clinical forms of α-mannosidosis are distinguished based on the age of onset. The more severe infantile form (type I) is associated with severe mental deterioration, facial dysmorphism, dysostosis multiplex, and hepatosplenomegaly, with death occurring usually between the ages of 3 and 10 years. In the relatively milder type II form intellectual impairment is evident by 2 or 3 years of age with delayed speech and poor motor performance. There are superficial corneal opacities, spoke-like posterior lens opacities, deafness, subtle facial dysmorphism, and skeletal abnormalities on radiographs. The clinical course is protracted, extending into adulthood. Late neurological complications include hydrocephalus and spastic quadriplegia. Widening of the diploic space with underdevelopment of the sinuses and prominent periventricular Virchow–Robin spaces are seen on MRI of the brain. Destructive arthropathy due to storage of oligosaccharides may be seen in children and adults. β-Mannosidosis presents with severe psychomotor retardation, hearing loss, and seizures.

Fucosidosis Deficiency of α-fucosidase leads to accumulation of fucose-containing oligosaccharides, glycopeptides, and, to a lesser extent, mucopolysaccharides and glycolipids in tissues associated with their excessive urinary excretion. There is prominent neurological dysfunction in all subtypes. The early onset form with neurological deterioration between 6 and 18 months of age rapidly progresses to a decerebrate state. The later-onset form is relatively slowly progressive; neurological regression occurs in the second or third year of life. Death usually occurs between the ages of 4 and 6 years in both subtypes. A third group of patients may show slowly progressive neurological deterioration into adolescence or adulthood. Brain MRI shows extensive and progressive changes in the signal intensity of the white matter and the internal medullary laminae of the thalami, as well as high signal intensity on T_1-weighted images and low signal intensity on T_2-weighted and FLAIR images in the globus pallidus and substantia nigra. The diagnosis is based on demonstration of decreased α-fucosidase activity in leucocytes or cultured skin fibroblasts.

Aspartylglucosaminuria

Aspartylglucosaminuria is described largely in Finland and results from a deficiency of aspartylglucosaminidase (AGA). This enzyme cleaves the bond between asparagine and *N*-acetylglucosamine of N-linked glycoproteins. Speech problems and severe behavioural abnormalities, with alternating periods of hyperactivity and apathy, are predominant in the clinical picture. Recurrent infections and diarrhoea are common in the early months and years of life. Insidious motor and mental deterioration, often with seizures, develop between the ages of 5 and 15 years. Mild coarsening of the facial features and skeletal abnormalities such as deformities of the vertebrae, periosteal thickening of the long bones, and thickening of the calvarium are evident by adolescence.

Increased aspartylglucosamine in urine and decreased AGA activity in plasma, leucocytes, or cultured skin fibroblasts confirm the diagnosis.

Sialidosis

Sialidosis types I and II are clinical variants associated with the deficiency of α-neuraminidase (sialidase) and increased urinary excretion of sialyloligosaccharides. In sialidosis type I progressive visual loss with a typical eye finding of a macular cherry-red spot, myoclonus, and seizures develop in late childhood or adolescence. Irregular myoclonic jerks are precipitated by action, sensory stimuli, emotional upset, menstruation, and smoking. The progressive

nature of the disease leads to difficulties with speech, walking, and feeding, followed by blindness, optic atrophy, and intellectual deterioration. Brain imaging shows cerebral and cerebellar atrophy.

In sialidosis type II, also known as mucolipidosis type I, there are neurological, visceral, and skeletal abnormalities including dysostosis multiplex, a Hurler-like phenotype, intellectual impairment, and hepatosplenomegaly. The diagnosis is based on deficient α-neuraminidase activity, preferably in cultured skin fibroblasts or leucocytes.

Galactosialidosis results from the combined deficiency of α-neuraminidase and β-galactosidase, due to defects in the protein cathepsin A (PPCA), which offers protection against rapid proteolytic degradation. It is clinically characterized by cerebellar ataxia, myoclonus, and visual failure in late childhood or adolescence. Additional features include the cherry-red macular spot, dysmorphic facial features, hepatomegaly, and skeletal changes.

The diagnosis of galactosialidosis is based on deficient activity of both α-neuraminidase and β-Gal in leucocytes or cultured skin fibroblasts, and/or mutations in the gene encoding the PPCA. Galactosialidosis can be distinguished from G_{M1} gangliosidosis by normal β-Gal activity in serum or plasma, unlike G_{M1} gangliosidosis.

Schindler's/Kanzaki's disease (α-N-acetylgalactosaminidase deficiency)

This rare disorder, initially described by D Schindler, is a form of neuroaxonal dystrophy, which results from deficiency of a glycosylhydrolase, α-*N*-acetylgalactosaminidase (NAGA). Progressive motor and mental deterioration, with myoclonic seizures, pyramidal signs with hyperreflexia, hypotonia, and optic atrophy were described in two brothers who were bedridden by age 4 years. Subsequently, in 1989, Kanzaki and colleagues described a group of adult Japanese patients, without overt neurological manifestations and diffuse angiokeratoma, who had NAGA deficiency and increased urinary excretion of several glycopeptides.

Mucolipidoses

The mucolipidoses feature the combined tissue storage of GAGs and sphingolipids and are a group of disorders with clinical features similar to MPSs, except for the absence of urinary excretion of GAGs.

Mucolipidosis type I or sialidosis type II

This condition is described under 'Sialidosis' above.

Mucolipidosis type II and type III

Mucolipidosis type II (I-cell disease) and type III (pseudo-Hurler's polydystrophy) are caused by abnormal transport of newly synthesized enzymes to the lysosome. I-cell disease manifests with progressive severe psychomotor retardation, dysmorphic facial features, gingival hypertrophy, and dysostosis multiplex. ML-III has a similar clinical picture; in addition stiffness of the fingers and shoulder, a 'claw-hand' deformity, short stature, and scoliosis may be noted. Mild coarsening of the face, corneal clouding, and retinopathy with progressive bone and cardiac valve involvement are also commonly seen.

The diagnosis of ML-II and -III is based on a demonstration of markedly increased lysosomal enzyme activities in the plasma while the corresponding activities in leucocytes and cultured skin fibroblasts are markedly decreased.

Mucolipidosis type IV

Mucolipidosis IV (ML-IV) is caused by mutations in the gene *MCOLN1*, mapped to chromosome 19p13.3–13.2. It encodes a protein called mucolipin, which normally functions as a calcium (Ca^{2+})-permeable cation channel but is also involved in lysosomal biogenesis and membrane trafficking. The disease has a protracted course characterized by early arrest in neurological development, corneal clouding, absent speech, intellectual impairment, and motor retardation, with no dysmorphic facial features, hepatosplenomegaly, or skeletal abnormalities. ML-IV is prevalent among the Ashkenazi Jewish population with two common mutations accounting for 95% of the alleles. Electron microscopic examination of conjunctival and skin biopsies shows characteristic lysosomal inclusions as well as enlarged lysosomes in all cell types. However, molecular genetic analysis of common mutations is often used for diagnostic purposes.

Glycogen storage disease type II (Pompe's disease)
See Chapter 12.3.1.

Sialic acid storage disorders
These autosomal recessive disorders, caused by mutations in the sialin gene, SLC17A5, encoding a protein involved in the transport of sialic acid (N-acetylneuraminic acid), include the following allelic disorders: infantile free sialic acid storage disease (ISSD) and Salla's disease (or the Finnish variant). The severe infantile form (ISSD) presents with nonimmune hydrops, hypertrophic cardiomyopathy, ascites, hepatosplenomegaly, inguinal hernias, coarse facies, and dysotosis multiple, causing death in the first 2 years of life. Clinical features of the juvenile form include developmental delay and growth retardation, seen in early childhood with mild coarsening of the facial features, hepatomegaly, and psychomotor retardation.

In Salla's disease, named after a region in north-eastern Finland, affected children manifest with mild coarsening of features, exotropia, hypotonia, ataxia, and learning disabilities during the first year of life without visceromegaly or skeletal abnormalities.

Increased amounts of free sialic acid are found in the serum and urine, as well as in cultured skin fibroblasts and several tissues, including the brain

Neuronal ceroid lipofuscinoses
The neuronal ceroid lipofuscinoses (NCLs) represent a group of childhood-onset disorders with a combined prevalence of approximately 1 in 12 500 births characterized by the intralysosomal aggregation of autofluorescent proteinaceous ageing pigments, i.e. ceroid and lipofuscin. There are eight major subtypes based on age at onset, presentation, and pathological findings. The infantile form of NCL, caused by mutations in CLN1, the gene encoding the enzyme palmitoyl protein thioesterase 1 (PPT1), presents with deceleration of head growth, muscular hypotonia, ataxia, motor clumsiness, irritability, sleep disturbance, and visual failure after a period of normal development during the first year. Rapid developmental deterioration occurs during the second year of life with loss of all motor abilities and social interest, blindness and increasing spasticity, seizures, and myoclonus. Fine motor skills are affected with purposeless, characteristic hand movements (hyperkinesias) such as those seen in Rett's syndrome.

Late infantile NCL, caused by mutations in CLN2, which encodes the enzyme tripeptidyl-peptidase 1, presents at approximately the third year of life with unexpected delay of psychomotor development or epilepsy of sudden onset. Seizures are generalized tonic–clonic or partial, frequently of a severe myoclonic type, which may soon become resistant to drug treatment.

Juvenile NCL, caused by mutations in CLN3, presents with visual failure, noticed around the age of 4 to 7 years leading to blindness usually within a few years, gradual psychomotor deterioration during early school years, and seizures at about age 10 years. Adult-onset (Kufs') disease with onset around 30 years of age is distinguished from the other subtypes by the absence of visual failure.

Intralysosomal inclusions, described as osmiophilic granular deposits, curvilinear bodies, or fingerprint deposits that are somewhat specific for each subcategory of NCL, are observed by electron microscopy of the skin. Enzyme estimation of PPT1, and tripeptidyl-peptidase 1 (TPP1), activity in peripheral blood leucocytes is diagnostic for CLN1- and CLN2-related disorders respectively. Treatment is symptomatic with aggressive control of the seizure disorder. Gene therapy for the late infantile variant is under investigation.

Motor neuron diseases
Spinal muscular atrophy
Spinal muscular atrophy (SMA) is an autosomal recessive disease characterized by degeneration of spinal cord motor neurons causing muscle weakness and atrophy. It occurs in 1 in 10 000 births and has a carrier frequency of 1 in 40 to 1 in 60. Three major clinical subtypes of childhood-onset SMA are recognized. All three subtypes are the result of deletions or mutations in the SMN1 gene located on chromosome 5q13.

Type I, also referred to as Werdnig–Hoffman disease, begins in the first 6 months of life with severe hypotonia, absent tendon reflexes, and failure to achieve independent sitting. Their weakness of intercostal muscles leads to respiratory insufficiency and early death.

Type II SMA starts in early childhood before age 18 months. The child can sit independently but cannot stand or walk unassisted. A milder type III form known as Kugelberg–Welander disease develops in childhood after independent walking is achieved but weakness progresses, leading to wheelchair dependence.

Electromyographic (EMG) studies reveal spontaneous activity including sharp waves, fasciculations, and fibrillations suggestive of degeneration. The muscle biopsy demonstrates grouped atrophy with islands of hypertrophic fibres consistent with neurogenic atrophy.

The SMN protein is ubiquitous but the neuron is particularly vulnerable to SMN deficiency because of its role in axonal transport of mRNAs in motor neurons. The severity of SMA is correlated with the extent of truncation of the SMN protein, i.e. the degree of gene deletion, e.g. type I patients are more likely to have deletions of both exon 7 and exon 8 whereas type II patients are usually missing exon 7 but retain exon 8. A homologous gene, SMN2, is retained in SMA and has been induced to produce full-length SMN protein in cell culture and animal models of SMA using inhibitors of histone deacetylase. However, clinical trials in SMA patients showed no improvement in functional motor scores.

Other rarer forms of SMA
A severe lethal form of SMA with arthrogryposis has been mapped to Xp11. Another severe infantile form, spinal muscular atrophy with respiratory distress type 1 (SMARD1), produces eventration of the diaphragm, causing respiratory failure and death.

Distal SMA is inherited as an autosomal recessive, autosomal dominant, and sporadic disease. It causes distal limb weakness and progresses slowly. At least four genetic loci have been demonstrated.

In Kennedy's disease, there is spinal and bulbar muscular atrophy and gynaecomastia. This X-linked disease is due to an expansion of a CAG trinucleotide repeat in the first exon of the androgen receptor gene (*SBMA*) on chromosome Xq13. A list of genes associated with lower motor neuron disease is shown in Table 24.17.3.

Amyotrophic lateral sclerosis (see also Chapter 24.15)

Amyotrophic lateral sclerosis (ALS) causes degeneration of motor neurons in the motor cortex, brainstem, and spinal cord. Symptoms of progressive limb weakness with involvement of bulbar and respiratory muscles begin in the fifth or sixth decade of life and in most cases result in death 3 to 5 years later. Spasticity occurs due to upper motor neuron involvement, which may precede distal limb weakness by a year or more (primary lateral sclerosis). The prevalence is 2 to 3 in 100 000 with a male:female ratio of 1.3:1.6:1.

Motor neurons exhibit immunoreactivity for neurofilament proteins and ubiquitin. The proximal segments of motor axons are often swollen and distal motor axons undergo wallerian degeneration.

Finally cell bodies shrink and dendrites become attenuated. Most cases are sporadic but approximately 10% of the total are familial. Penetrance for ALS in these familial forms is, however, incomplete.

ALS-1

Mutations in the *SOD1* gene on chromosome 21q22.11 account for 10 to 20% of autosomal dominant familial ALS cases. More than 120 mutations in this gene have been identified, of which A4V accounts for half of all North American cases. *SOD1* encodes Cu/Zn superoxide dismutase 1, an enzyme that catalyses the conversion of oxygen radicals to oxygen and hydrogen peroxide. The mutant protein is believed to cause aggregation of proteins through a toxic gain-of-function property affecting axonal transport.

ALS-2

A juvenile-onset autosomal recessive form of ALS is due to mutations in the gene *ALS2* on chromosome 2q33, encoding alsin. Symptoms begin in the first or second decade and progress slowly for 10 to 15 years. Mutations in alsin have also been observed in patients with hereditary spastic paraplegia and primary lateral sclerosis.

Table 24.17.3 Cloned genes causing lower motor neuron disease

Disease	Locus	Mode	Protein	Attribute/Function	Aggregation
CMT2A	1p36	AD	Mitofuscin	Mitochondrial GTPase	
CMT2B	3q13	AD	RAB7	GTPase	
CMT2D	7p14	AD	GARS	Aminoacyl-tRNA synthetase	
CMT2E	12q13	AD	NFL	Cytoskeletal protein	Yes
CMT2F	7q11	AD	HSPB1	Chaperone protein	Yes
CMT2L	12q24	AD	HSPB8	Chaperone protein	Yes
CMTDIB	19q12	AD	Dynamin 2	GTPase	
CMTDIC	1p34	AD	YARS	Aminoacyl-tRNA synthetase	
HMN5	11q13	AD	Seipin	ER membrane protein	Yes
HMN7	2p13	AD	Dynactin 1	Microtubular motor	Yes
CMT2A	1q21	AR/AD	Lamin A/C	Nuclear membrane	
CMT2K	8q21	AR/AD	GDAP1	Mitochondrial protein	
ALS1	21q	AD	SODI	Superoxide dismutase	Yes
ALS2	2q33	AR	Alsin	Guanine exchange factor	
ALS4	9q34	AD	Senataxin	RNA helicase	
ALS8	20q13	AD	VAPB	Endosome membrane protein	Yes
ALS-ANG	14q11	AD	Angiogenin	RNase	
BSMA	Xq12	X linked	Androgen receptor	Transcription factor	Yes
SMA	5q	AR	SMN protein	RNA-binding protein	
SMARD1	11q13	AR	IGHMPB2	Transcription factor	

AD, autosomal dominant; ALS, amyotrophic lateral sclerosis; ANG, angiogenin; AR, autosomal recessive; BSMA, bulbospinal muscular atrophy; CMT, Charcot–Marie–Tooth disease; ER, endoplasmic reticulum; GARS, glycine aminoacyl-tRNA synthetase; GDAP1, ganglioside-induced, differentiation-associated protein 1; GTPase, guanosine triphosphatase; HMN, hereditary motor neuropathy; IGHMPB2, immunoglobulin μ-binding protein 2; NFL, light neurofilament; RAB7, ras-associated protein 7; SMA, spinal muscular atrophy; SMARD1, spinal muscular atrophy with respiratory distress type 1; SMN, sensory motor neuropathy; SOD1, superoxide dismutase 1; tRNA, transfer RNA; VAPB, vesicle-associated, membrane protein-associated protein B; YARS, tyrosyl aminoacyl-tRNA synthetase.
Canete-Soler R, Schlaeper W (2007). *Ann Neurol*, **62**, 8–14, with permission.

ALS-4

ALS-4 is another juvenile-onset form of ALS. It maps to chromosome 9q34 and follows an autosomal dominant mode of inheritance. The abnormal gene, *SETX*, codes for senataxin, which is also mutated in ataxia–oculomotor apraxia type 2.

ALS-5

This locus on chromosome 15q15.1-q21 is also associated with a juvenile-onset autosomal dominant form of familial ALS.

DCTN1

A mutation in the p150 subunit of dynactin encoded by *DCTN1* has been identified with a slowly progressive autosomal form of ALS.

Other genes associated with familial ALS have been designated *ALS3* on chromosome 18q21, *ALS6* located on chromosome 16q12, and *ALS7* mapped to chromosome 20q13. Mutations in the TAR–DNA-binding protein (TDP-43) gene *TARDBP* located on chromosome 1p36.22 are yet another cause of familial and sporadic ALS. ALS has also been associated with frontotemporal dementia, leading to the identification of additional loci on chromosome 9 as well as on 17q21, where the *MAPT* gene is located. It also appears that the expression level of the *SMN* gene can confer an increased

risk for developing ALS. Cloned genes implicated in lower motor neuron disease are set out in Table 24.17.3.

Hereditary spastic paraplegia

The hereditary spastic paraplegias (HSPs) are a heterogeneous group of diseases characterized by spastic weakness in the legs, pyramidal tract signs, urinary urgency, and mild diminution in vibratory sensation in the feet. Neurological signs are bilateral and symmetrical, and confined to the lower limbs. There are pure and complicated forms of HSPs. The complicated or complex forms include added signs such as ataxia, peripheral neuropathy, cerebellar atrophy, thin corpus callosum, extrapyramidal signs, visual dysfunction, deafness, ichthyosis, learning disabilities, and seizures.

There are multiple genes and loci involved with autosomal dominant, autosomal recessive, and X-linked forms delineated (compare Tables 24.17.4 and 24.17.5). Penetrance and disease severity can vary even within the same family. The autosomal dominant (AD) forms are primarily of the pure type and comprise 70 to 80% of all HSPs. Of these the most common is SPG4, responsible for approximately 40% of the total. The SPG4 locus is on chromosome 2p22 and codes for spastin. Mean age of onset is

Table 24.17.4 Autosomal dominant and X-linked forms of hereditary spastic paraplegias (HSPs)

Locus	Chromosome region	Gene of protein	Discriminating features
Autosomal dominant			
Pure forms			
SPG3A	14q12–q21	*Atlastin*	Predominantly early onset
SPG4	2p22	*Spastin*	
SPG6	15q11.2-q12	*NIPA1*	Predominantly adult onset
SPG8	8q24	*KIAAO196*	Predominantly adult onset
SPG10	23q13	*KIF5A*	Predominantly early onset
SPG12	19q13	Unknown	Predominantly early onset
SPG13	2q24–q34	*HSP60*	Predominantly adult onset
SPG19	9q33–q34	Unknown	Predominantly adult onset
SPG31	2p12	*REEP1*	Predominantly adult onset
SPG33	10q24.2	*ZFYVE27*	
SPG37	8p21.1–q13.3	Unknown	
Complex forms			
SAX1	12p13	Unknown	Spastic ataxia
SPG9	10q23.3–q24.2	Unknown	Cataract, motor neuropathy, short stature, skeletal abnormalities, gastro-oesophageal reflux
SPG17	11q12–q14	*BSCL2/Seipin*	Silver's syndrome—severe distal wasting
SPG29	1p31–p21		Sensorineural hearing impairment, pes cavus, neonatal hyperbilirubinaemia without kernicterus, hiatal hernia
X linked			
SPG1	Xq28	*L1CAM*	Onset in infancy, corpus callosum hypoplasia, retardation adducted thumbs, spastic paraplegia, hydrocephalus
SPG2	Xq21	*PLP*	Early onset, quadriparesis, congenital nystagmus, intellectual impairment, seizures
SPG16	Xq11.2	Unknown	Onset in infancy, pure spastic paraplegia (severe)

Depienne C, *et al.* (2007). *Curr Opin Neurol*, **20**, 674–80, with permission.

Table 24.17.5 Autosomal recessive forms of hereditary spastic paraplegias (HSPs)

Gene	Protein	Locus	Age at onset (years)	Associated Signs
Pure forms				
SPG5	Unknown	8p	1–40	
SPG24	Unknown	13q	1	
SPG28	Unknown	14q	6–15	
SPG30	Unknown	2q	12–21	
Complex forms				
SPG7	Paraplegin	16q	11–42	Cerebellar signs, PNP, pes cavus, optic atrophy
SPG14	Unknown	3q	~30	Distal motor neuropathy, intellectual impairment, pes cavus, visual agnosia
SPG27	Unknown	10q	2–45	Cerebellar ataxia, PNP, intellectual impairment, microcephaly, facial and skeletal dysmorphia, blepharophimosis
SPG11 (AR-HSP-TCC)	Spatacsin	15q	1–23	Intellectual or cognitive impairment, PNP, TCC
SPG15 (Kjellin's syndrome)	Unknown	14q	13–23	Pigmented maculopathy, wasting, dysarthria, cerebellar signs, intellectual impairment
SPG20 (Troyer syndrome)	Spartin	13q	Early childhood	Intellectual impairment, cerebellar signs, developmental delay and short stature
SPG21 (Mast syndrome)	Maspardin	15q	20–40	Extrapyramidal syndrome, premature ageing, cognitive decline, dysarthria, TCC, periventricular white matter hyperintensities, cataract, dystonia, cerebellar signs, PNP, chorea, distal wasting
SPG23 (Lison syndrome)	Unknown	1q	Early childhood	Abnormalities of skin and hair pigmentation, facial and skeletal dysmorphia, postural tremor, cognitive impairment, premature ageing
SPG25	Unknown	6q	30–46	Prolapsed intervertebral discs, multiple disc herniation, bilateral cataract, congenital glaucoma
SPG26	Unknown	12cen	22–42	Intellectual impairment, distal muscle wasting, dysarthria, PNP
SPG32	Unknown	14q	6–7	Pontine dysraphia, intellectual impairment, TCC
TCC + epilepsy	Unknown	8q	1–7	Mental deterioration, epilepsy, TCC
SPOAN	Unknown	11q	Infancy	Optic atrophy, PNP
ARSACS	Sacsin	13q	Early childhood	Ataxia, dysarthria, distal wasting, nystagmus, retinal striation, PNP
ARSAL	Unknown	2q	Variable	Spastic ataxia with leucodystrophy
SAX2	Unknown	17p	Variable	Cerebellar ataxia dysarthria

AR, autosomal recessive; ARSACS, autosomal recessive spastic ataxia of Charlevoix Saguenay; ARSAL, autosomal recessive spastic ataxia with frequent leucoencephalopathy; PNP, polyneuropathy; SAX2, spastic ataxia 2; SPOAN, spastic paraplegia, optic atrophy, and neuropathy; TCC, thin corpus callosum.
Depienne C, et al. (2007). *Curr Opin Neurol*, **20**, 674–80, with permission.

30 years but an earlier age of onset occurs in the presence of a rare ser44leu spastin polymorphism.

The second most frequent AD HSP gene is *SPG3A*, coding for atlastin. It accounts for 10% of cases. It begins in childhood or adolescence but is otherwise indistinguishable from SPG4 HSP. The third most frequently gene affected is *REEP1*, causing SPG31. If SPG6 is included, these four forms account for approximately 65% of the AD HSP cases.

Of the autosomal recessive (AR) forms, 16 loci are known. Five involve a thin corpus callosum and mental impairment. The most frequent is SPG11, representing approximately half of the AR cases. It has an early onset (mean age 11.8 years) and patients become wheelchair bound in their third or fourth decade. Other features are mild-to-moderate intellectual impairment, abnormal appearance

of the white matter, and pseudobulbar dysarthria. Complex HSPs with cerebellar ataxia occur in *ARSACS*, *SAX2*, *ARSAL*, and *SAX1*. Cerebellar atrophy is observable on MRI. For further details consult Tables 24.17.4 and 24.17.5.

According to Fink, several pathogenic mechanisms may be involved in the HSPs including: (1) abnormalities in primary axonal transport; (2) Golgi abnormalities; (3) mitochondrial dysfunction; (4) myelin abnormalities; and (5) abnormal corticospinal tract development. Particularly in sporadic cases of HSP it is important to rule out other neurological diseases that may present with spastic paraplegia. These include a wide variety of conditions such as multiple sclerosis, primary lateral sclerosis, thoracic cord tumours, infections, and metabolic diseases. Examples of the last include disorders of intermediary metabolism, such as cobalamin C deficiency, arginase deficiency, biotinidase deficiency, phenylke-tonuria and nonketotic hyperglycaemia, dopamine synthesis defects, and cerebral folate deficiency, and disorders of complex molecule metabolism, including cerebrotendinous xanthomatosis, adrenom-yeloneuropathy, metachromatic leucodystrophy, Krabbe's disease, Sjögren–Larsson syndrome, and polyglucosan body disease.

Spasticity may be alleviated by oral baclofen or dantrolene, or micturition, improved by oxybutynin, with foot drop improved by ankle–foot orthoses, and general fitness and weakness addressed with physical therapy.

Hereditary neuropathies

Hereditary neuropathies affect approximately 1 in 2500 individuals and therefore are the most common inherited diseases of the nervous system. Phenotypically, demyelination and/or axonal loss leads to progressive dysfunction of motor, sensory, and/or autonomic nerves in a length-dependent manner. The first descriptions by Charcot, Marie, and Tooth more than a century ago were of a dominantly inherited progressive disorder affecting both motor and sensory axons. The term 'Charcot–Marie–Tooth disease' (CMT) continues to be used to describe a genetically heterogeneous disorder of insidious onset and slow progression affecting primarily peripheral nerves in a nonsyndromic manner.

The individual variants of inherited neuropathies may be classified according to clinical, electrophysiological, histological, and molecular genetic features. In most cases the mode of inheritance is AD but AR forms and an X-linked variant are also described. Demyelinating forms are defined by a median nerve conduction velocity (NCV) below 38 m/s, and axonal subtypes are based on median NCV above 38 m/s. A third category is now recognized with an intermediate NCV of 25 to 40 m/s. Although demyelinating disease suggests primary involvement of the Schwann cell and an axonal disorder might indicate predominately axon dysfunction, both are likely to become involved due to the interdependence of the Schwann cell and axon.

Table 24.17.6 lists the nonsyndromic inherited neuropathies and the Mutation Database of Inherited Peripheral Neuropathies (http://www.molgen.ua.ac.be/CMTMutations) may be consulted for more detail on the molecular genetics of each disorder.

Duplication of the *PMP22* (peripheral myelin protein 22) gene accounts for 70% of all patients with hereditary neuropathy. These individuals present with distal muscle weakness in the legs, diminished or absent deep tendon reflexes, and impaired sensation. As a result of weakness of the intrinsic foot muscles, patients develop foot deformities, i.e. pes cavus or hammer toe. There is atrophy of the calf muscles and a high steppage gait. Later the weakness can progress to affect the hands and forearms with weakness of intrinsic hand muscles, leading to a 'claw-hand' deformity. Onset is before the second decade, but progression is slow so that by age 40 almost all patients are still ambulatory.

Nerve biopsy shows thinly myelinated axons and reduction in myelinated axons, especially in the large fibres. Nerve conduction velocities are slow, even well before clinical onset of disease. However, motor amplitudes and number of motor units correlate with clinical disability so that axonal loss and not conduction velocity is a better measure of disease severity.

Deletion of one copy of the *PMP22* gene will cause hereditary neuropathy with liability to pressure palsies (HNPP). These patients

Table 24.17.6 Nonsyndromic inherited neuropathies

Disease	Locus	Gene
CMT1 (dominant demyelinating)		
HNPP	17p11	PMP22
CMT1A	17p11	PMP22
CMT1B	1q22–23	MPZ
CMT1C	16p13	SIMPLE
CMT1D	10q21	EGR2
CMT1X	Xq13.1	GJB1
Dominant intermediate CMT		
DI-CMTA	10q24.1–25	
DI-CMTB	19p12–13.2	DMN2
DI-CMTC	1p35	YARS
CMT2 (autosomal dominant axonal/neuronal)		
CMT2A1	1p36.2	KIF1B
CMT2A2	1p36.2	MFN2
CMT2B	3q21	RAB7
CMT2C	12q23–24	
CMT2D	7p15	GARS
CMT2E	8p21	NEFL
CMT2F	7q11.23	HSPB1
CMT2G	12q12–q13.3	
CMT2	3q13.1	
CMT2-PO	1q22	MPZ
CMT2L	12q24	HSPB8
Hereditary neuralgic amyotrophy	17q25	SEPT9
Severe (dominant or recessive) demyelinating neuropathies		
Déjérine–Sottas neuropathy/	17p11	PMP22
HMSN-III/CMT3	1p22	MPZ
	Xq13.1	GJB1
	10q21	EGR2
	19q13.1	PRX
	8p21	NEFL
Congenital hypomyelinating neuropathy	10q21	EGR2
	17p11	PMP22
	1p22	MPZ
Autosomal recessive demyelinating neuropathy (CMT4)		
CMT4A	8q13–q21.1	GDAP1
CMT4B	11q22	MTMR2
CMT4B-2	11p15	MTMR13
CMT4C	5q32	SH3TC2
CMT4D-Lom	8q24.3	NDRG1
CMT4E	10q21	EGR2
CMT4F	19q13	PRX
HMSN-R	10q23.2	
CMT4H	12p11.21–q13.11	

(Continued)

Table 24.17.6 (*Cont'd*) Nonsyndromic inherited neuropathies

Disease	Locus	Gene
Autosomal recessive demyelinating neuropathy (CMT4)		
CMT4A	8q13–q21.1	GDAP1
CMT4B-1	11q22	MTMR2
CMT4B-2	11p15	MTMR13
CMT4C	5q32	SH3TC2
CMT4D-Lom	8q24.3	NDRG1
CMT4E	10q21	EGR2
CMT4F	19q13	PRX
HMSN-R	10q23.2	
CMT4H	12p11.21–q13.11	
Autosomal recessive axonal neuropathy		
AR-CMT2A	1q21.2	LMNA
AR-CMT2B	19q13.3	MED25
Early onset/neonatal		
CMT2K	8q13–q21.1	GDAP1
Congenital	5q deletion	
Hereditary sensory and autonomic neuropathies (HSANs)		
HSAN1	9q22.1–22.3 dominant	SPTLC1
HSAN1B	3p22–24 dominant	
HSAN2	12p13.33 recessive	HSN2
HSAN3	9q31 recessive	IKBKAP
HSAN4	1q21–q22 recessive	NTRKA
HSAN5	1p163.1 recessive	NGFB
Primary erythermalgia	2q24 dominant	SCN9A
Cold-induced sweating	19p12 recessive	CRLF1
HSN with cough and gastro-oesophageal reflux	3p22–p24 dominant	
Hereditary motor neuropathies (HMNs)		
HMN I	Dominant	
HMN II	12q24 dominant	HSPB8
HMN II	7q11.23 dominant	HSPB1
HMN III and IV	11q13 recessive	
HMN V	7p15 dominant	GARS
HMN V	11q13 dominant	BSCL2
HMN VI/SMARD1	11q13.2–13.4 recessive	IGHMBP2
HMN VII	2p13 dominant	DCTN1
HMN VII	2q14 dominant	
HMN X-linked	Xq13.1–q21	
HMN/ALS4	9q34 dominant	SETX
Congenital distal SMA	12q23–q24 dominant	
HMN Jerash	9p21.1–p12 recessive	

Lippincott Williams & Wilkins, Philadelphia 2008. p. 437.

have episodic mononeuropathies due to nerve compression but may recover with little or no deficit. Some patients experience a progressive generalized sensorimotor neuropathy and a third will have absent ankle jerks. On neuropsychological testing distal motor latencies are prolonged, sensory velocities are mildly slowed, and conduction block is seen. Nerve biopsies reveal focal thickenings, sequential demyelination, and remyelination. Point mutations in *PMP22* and *MPZ* can also cause HNPP.

Other causes of autosomal dominant demyelinating CMT are mutations in the *GJB1* (gap-junction B1) gene responsible for 8 to 10% of patients with nonsyndromic inherited neuropathies, *MPZ* (myelin protein zero) mutations identified in 3% of patients, and *PMP22* mutations accounting for an additional 1.5% of patients. *GJB1* is X linked so that affected women have a later onset and milder symptoms. In this variant, known as CMT1X, sensory loss may be more prominent than in other CMT1 subtypes. Other genes with mutations contributing to the autosomal dominant demyelinating class of neuropathies are *L1TAF* (liposaccharide-induced tumour necrosis factor-α) and *EGR* (early growth response-2).

The autosomal recessive demyelinating neuropathies are classified under CMT4. These are rare and more likely in populations with a high rate of consanguinity. They manifest in childhood and their nerve biopsies show redundant loops of myelin in onion bulb formations, hence the alternative label of Déjérine–Sottas neuropathy (DSN). CMT4D due to mutations in *NDRG1* (*N-myc* downstream-regulated gene-1) is found in gypsies and is associated with hearing loss and dysmorphic features. Children with CMT4F due to mutations in *PRX* (periaxin) have marked slowing in motor NCVs and severe axonal loss.

The autosomal dominant axonal neuropathies are classified as CMT2 variants and may involve not only axonal loss but also primary nerve cell body abnormalities. A quarter of these patients have mutations in *MFN2* which encodes mitofusin-2, a protein required for mitochondrial fusion. This is an early onset neuropathy and is sometimes accompanied by optic atrophy and/or sensorineural hearing loss.

Recurrent episodes of focal neuropathy of the brachial plexus are characteristic of hereditary neuralgic amyotrophy. The episode begins with a sharp, aching, or burning pain in the arm and is followed by weakness and sensory disturbances within days. Cranial and phrenic nerve involvement also occur. Although some recovery occurs, axonal loss in the affected muscles is seen on EMG. Mutations in *SEPT9* are the cause.

Another class are the dominant intermediate CMTs (DI-CMTs) in which forearm nerve conduction velocities are between 30 and 40 m/s. The histological features are more typical of axonal loss than demyelination. Mutations in *DMN2* encoding dynamin-2 and in *YARS* encoding tyrosyl-tRNA synthase can result in DI-CMT. Some mutations in *GJB1*, *GDAP1*, *MPZ*, and *NEFL* may also fit this criterion.

The hereditary sensory and autonomic neuropathies (HSANs) spare the motor neurons or axons. The onset of HSANI is in the second or third decade. It is associated with burning pain in the feet and plantar ulcers, and is slowly progressive. Autosomal dominant inheritance of either a *SPTLC1* (long chain base subunit 1 of serine palmitoyl transferase) or *RAB7* (Ras related in brain 7) mutation is responsible.

HSANII is manifested by sensory loss of all modalities and ulcers of the fingers and feet. It is caused by autosomal recessive mutations in the *HSN2* gene.

HSANIII, also known as Riley–Day syndrome and familial dys-autonomia, is caused by a recessive mutation in *IKBKAP* (inhibitor of κ light polypeptide gene enhancer in B cells, kinase complex-associated protein). Almost all patients are of Ashkenazi Jewish ancestry. It is noted at birth with vomiting and swallowing difficulties, autonomic disturbances, and absence of fungiform papillae of the tongue. Areflexia, poor coordination, emotional lability, and kyphoscoliosis are other features. Autonomic crises are common and can lead to sudden death. There is a marked decrease in the number of unmyelinated fibres and the number of neurons in the autonomic and spinal ganglia are decreased.

HSANIV is associated with anhidrosis and congenital insensitivity to pain, leading to self-mutilation. Unmyelinated fibres are completely absent. This autosomal recessive disorder is due to mutations in *NTRKA* (neuron tyrosine kinase A).

HSANV—a rare congenital disorder—is manifested by a selective loss of pain sensation with other sensory modalities, motor strength and tendon reflexes remaining normal. Decreased sweating is also noted. Sensory nerve-evoked potentials are normal. The disease is caused by recessive mutations in the *NGFB* (nerve growth factor β) gene.

The hereditary motor neuropathies (HMNs) begin in childhood or early adulthood with distal weakness affecting the extensor muscles of the feet. Sensory responses are normal but there is reduced amplitude of the motor responses and denervation by needle EMG. Most of these disorders show autosomal dominant inheritance (see Table 24.17.6). Upper limb weakness is characteristic of HMNV and a vocal fold paralysis is a feature of HMNVII.

Inherited myopathies (see also Chapter 24.24.4)

Hereditary forms of muscle disease may be classified according to age of onset, location of muscle weakness, and pathological mechanism. Thus, separate classes of muscle disease are recognized, namely congenital myopathies, proximal and distal myopathies, dystrinopathies, myotonic dystrophies, ion channels disorders, and inclusion body myopathies. In this section we describe degenerative muscular disease of the hereditary type. The more benign and relatively nonprogressive hereditary myopathies, such as central core, nemaline, and centronuclear myopathies, are considered to be a separate category due to their nondegenerative nature. Most congenital muscular dystrophies (CMDs), some limb-girdle muscular dystrophies (LGMDs), and Duchenne and Becker muscular dystrophies are caused by pathogenic mutations of proteins involved in the dystrophin–glycoprotein complex (DGC), which provides structural support to the muscle cell membrane and participates in signalling across the cell membrane. These proteins include dystrophin, syntrophin, neuronal nitric oxide synthase (nNOS), and dystrobrevin, which are associated with the cytoplasmic surface of the cell membrane; the sarcoglycans (α, β, γ, and δ) and β-dystroglycan, which span the membrane, and α-dystroglycan, which connects to the extracellular matrix. On a pathophysiological basis, muscular dystrophies may be viewed as a mismatch between muscle breakdown and muscle repair, leading to increased susceptibility of a muscle to injury and a cascade of events that lead to cell death. These disorders are characterized by proximal muscle weakness and markedly elevated creatine kinase (CK) values during the period of maximum muscle breakdown.

Duchenne and Becker muscular dystrophies

Duchenne muscular dystrophy (DMD) is the most common X-linked recessive lethal genetic disorder in children, affecting primarily skeletal and cardiac muscle. Approximately 1 in 3500 boys born is affected with DMD; approximately a third of cases arise from a new genetic mutation. In skeletal muscle, the *DMD* gene produces a large protein molecule of 427 kDa designated dystrophin, the central component of the DGC. This complex, which includes dystroglycans and sarcoglycans, spans the muscle sarcolemma, providing a linkage between the intracellular cytoskeleton and the extracellular matrix. Dystrophin localizes to the cytoplasmic surface of skeletal muscle membrane in a subsarcolemmal location. In DMD, all components of DGC are normally synthesized but not properly assembled or integrated into the sarcolemma. Boys with DMD have a progressive and predictable deterioration of skeletal and cardiac muscle function due to lack of dystrophin, which is critical for muscle membrane stability. Without dystrophin, muscle contraction leads to membrane damage and activation of the inflammatory cascade, progressing to muscle necrosis, fibrosis, and loss of function.

Becker muscular dystrophy (BMD) is a less severe form of dystrophinopathy. The pattern of muscle wasting closely resembles that seen in DMD but BMD patients walk beyond the age of 15 years. First symptoms usually develop between age 5 and 15 years, but onset may be delayed into the third or fourth decade.

Supportive measures for DMD include physical therapy and night splints to prevent contractures, and segmental spinal stabilization in later stages when scoliosis occurs. Prednisone and deflazacort have both been shown to increase muscle strength, pulmonary function, and functional ability in double-blind randomized controlled trials, providing long-term benefits of prolonged independence. Gene therapy using adenoviral vectors raised much hope in the past, but was unsuccessful because of their tendency to immunogenicity and their large size, which limited diffusion in the muscle tissue. A phase I clinical trial of myoblast transplantation into dystrophic muscle, which will give rise to dystrophin-expressing myofibres, has been completed. Limitations of this therapy include poor survival and migration of myoblasts and also possibly an immune response to donor myoblasts. Exon skipping of dystrophin gene exons, which contain a mutation using antisense oligonucleotides to splice out selected exons from the pre-mRNA, at or next to the mutation site, is a promising potential therapy for DMD and other recessive muscular dystrophies. Skipping specific exons is expected to restore the reading frame and result in the production of internally deleted, but essentially functional, dystrophin as observed in the milder BMD, thus providing significant functional improvement of DMD.

Emery–Dreifuss muscular dystrophy

Emery–Dreifuss muscular dystrophy (EDMD) is an X-linked, autosomal dominant and, more rarely, autosomal recessive condition. The gene responsible for X-linked EDMD, *EMD*, encodes a ubiquitous transmembrane protein of the nuclear envelope inner membrane, emerin. The gene mutated in autosomal dominant and recessive forms of EDMD is *LMNA*, and located on chromosome 1, encoding two major somatic cell polypeptides, lamins A and C, which are intermediate filament proteins associated with the nuclear envelope inner membrane. Mutations in *LMNA* have been shown to cause several very different human diseases (laminopathies) other than muscular dystrophies such as partial lipodystrophy syndromes, a peripheral neuropathy, and accelerated ageing disorders such as Hutchinson–Gilford progeria syndrome. Even though these proteins are rather ubiquitously expressed, the reason for relative tissue specificity of EDMD, affecting cardiac muscle and certain skeletal muscles and tendons, is not clear.

The clinical triad of EDMD consists of: (1) slowly progressive muscle weakness and wasting in a scapulohumeroperoneal distribution; (2) early contractures of the elbows, ankles, and posterior neck; and (3) cardiac conduction defects, cardiomyopathy, or both. Contractures affecting the elbows, neck extensor muscles, and Achilles tendons are followed by slowly progressive muscle weakness and wasting in a humeroperoneal distribution (biceps, triceps, and peroneal), usually at the end of the second decade of life. Cardiac disease starting at the end of the second decade occurs in virtually all cases of EDMD and bears no direct relationship to the severity of the skeletal muscle involvement. Over time, dilated cardiomyopathy develops, complicated by ventricular tachydysrhythmias, which may cause sudden cardiac death. Timely insertion of an implantable defibrillator can be a lifesaving measure.

Fascioscapulohumeral muscular dystrophy

Fascioscapulohumeral dystrophy (FSHD) is autosomal dominant with 10 to 30% of cases being sporadic; it is the third most common form of inherited muscular dystrophy after Duchenne dystrophy and myotonic dystrophy. The FSHD locus, mapped to the subtelomeric portion of chromosome 4 (4q35), is composed mainly of a polymorphic repeat structure consisting of 3.3-kilobase repeat elements designated D4Z4. The number of repeat units varies from 11 to more than 100 in the general population, whereas in patients with FSHD there is a deletion of an integral number of these units, so that they exhibit an allele containing 10 or fewer repeat units.

Limb-girdle muscular dystrophies

Twenty-one molecularly characterized forms of limb-girdle muscular dystrophy (LGMD) have been described thus far, comprising a clinically and genetically widely heterogeneous grouping. The subclassification of the classic groups of autosomal dominant LGMD (AD-LGMD or LGMD1) and autosomal recessive LGMD (AR-LGMD or LGMD2) is based on the involved proteins and the underlying genetic defects. The dominantly inherited disorders are phenotypically milder than the recessively inherited forms. Although proximal muscle weakness is considered a clinical hallmark of LGMD, presentation with distal myopathy or myofibrillar myopathy is being increasingly recognized. Cranial, ocular, and bulbar muscles, as well as the heart and brain, are generally spared. Patients usually present in adolescence or young adulthood, but childhood-onset disorders mimicking BMD are also known. The incidence of different LGMDs is dependent on ethnicity and geographical location. Molecular diagnosis is complex because mutations have been described in a large number of genes, very few of which are recurrent mutations, with the exception of LGMD2D. Overlap in clinical presentation with allelic disorders, such as LGMD1B, and autosomal dominant forms with LGMD2B and Miyoshi's distal myopathy further complicates molecular analysis. Western blot or immunohistochemistry of muscle biopsy specimens for protein analysis is helpful in delineating the precise diagnosis. However, missense mutations may not lead to complete absence of proteins, e.g. missense mutations in myotilin (LGMD1A), and absence of a protein may be secondary to mutations in a related protein, as seen in the sarcoglycanopathies (LGMD2C-F). See Tables 24.17.7 and 24.17.8 for molecular classification and clinical features of AD and AR LGMDs respectively.

Myotonic dystrophies

Myotonic dystrophies (DMs) types I and II are, in general, late-onset autosomal dominant multisystem disorders characterized by myotonia, muscular dystrophy, posterior iridescent cataracts, endocrine, and heart involvement. DM type I (DM1) is caused by an expanded CTG repeat in the 3′-untranslated region of the dystrophia myotonica–protein kinase (*DMPK*) gene, which is mapped to 19q13. It has an incidence of about 13 in 100 000. The expansion size varies from 80 to 4000 in affected patients, while clinically normal individuals have 50 to 100 repeats. Intergenerational instability, especially with maternal transmission, may cause expansion of several thousand repeats in a single generation. Phenotypic correlation with age of onset exists with the expansion size up to 400 CTG repeats, but not for longer repeats. In DM type II (DM2), a CCTG expansion was identified in intron 1 of the zinc finger protein 9 (*ZNF9*) gene, mapped to 3q21. The incidence of DM2 is estimated at 1 in 1000. The underlying pathogenic mechanism in DM is disruption of mRNA metabolism and dominant negative effects of RNA containing the CUG and CCUG expansions, leading to accumulation of ribonuclear inclusions in the nuclei of DM cells.

DM1 may present at any age from the pre-/postnatal period to adulthood with the largest number of CTG repeats (more than 1500) identified in congenital myotonic dystrophy. Infants present with hypotonia, talipes equinovarus, other contractures, and immobility; there may be a history of hydrops fetalis or polyhydramnios with reduced fetal movements. Bilateral weakness of facial, jaw, and palatal muscles causing an open mouth, tent-formed upper lip, and a high arched palate, along with a weak cry, poor suck, and feeding difficulties, are commonly present. Tendon reflexes are absent. Mechanical ventilation may be necessary due to respiratory insufficiency. Later complications include aspiration, delayed speech and motor development, and psychomotor impairment. Unlike in myotonia congenita, clinical and electrophysiological myotonia is seldom evident. EMG analysis and clinical examination of the mother may be more informative. In the childhood-onset form, speech and learning disabilities with or without distal weakness, cardiological problems, and myotonia are the presenting features. The classic adult-onset form presents with bilateral facial weakness, mild ptosis, and weakness of neck flexors, followed by wasting of sternocleidomastoid and temporal muscles. Distal weakness includes weakness of finger flexors and ankle dorsiflexors. Grip and percussion myotonia are commonly seen. Myotonia of bulbar, tongue, and facial muscles can lead to speech, mastication, and swallowing difficulty. The spectrum of cardiac involvement varies from conduction abnormalities with arrhythmia and conduction block to sudden cardiac death. Cognitive decline as well as psychological dysfunction are often present. Posterior capsular cataracts are well described but retinal degeneration is also known. Endocrine abnormalities include hypotestosteronism with testicular atrophy as well as insulin resistance with

Table 24.17.7 Molecular classification and clinical features of autosomal dominant limb-girdle muscular dystrophy (LGMD)

Disease name	Locus name	Gene symbol	Chromosomal locus	Protein product	Onset (years) (average)	Presentation		Late findings
						Symptoms	Signs	
LGMD1A (myotilinopathy)	LGMD1A	TTID	5q31	Myotilin	18–35 (27)	Proximal weakness	Tight Achilles tendons Nasal, dysarthric speech (50%)	Distal weakness
LGMD1B	LGMD1B	LMNA	1q21.2	Lamin A/C	Birth to adulthood; about half with childhood onset	Proximal lower limb weakness		Mild contractures of elbows Arrhythmia and other cardiac complications (25–45 years) Sudden death
Caveolinopathy	LGMD1C	CAV3	3p25	Caveolin-3	About 5	Cramping Mild-to-moderate proximal weakness Rippling muscle disease	Calf hypertrophy	
LGMD1D	CMD1F	Unknown	6q23	Unknown	< 25	Dilated cardiomyopathy Cardiac conduction defect Proximal muscle weakness		All individuals remain ambulatory
LGMD1E	LGMD1E	Unknown	7q	Unknown	9–49	Proximal lower and upper limb weakness	Pelger–Huet anomaly	Contractures Dysphagia
LGMD1F	LGMD1F	Unknown	7q31.1-q32.2	Unknown	1–58	Proximal lower and upper limb weakness	Serum creatine kinase (normal to 20×normal)	Distal weakness
LGMD1G	LGMD1G	Unknown	4q21	Unknown	30–47	Proximal lower limb weakness	Progressive limitation of finger and toe flexion	Proximal upper limb weakness

http://www.ncbi.nlm.nih.gov/bookshelf/br.fcgi?book=gene&part=lgmd-overview.

diabetes. Significant disability ensues by the fifth or sixth decade compounded by diaphragmatic weakness, leading to aspiration, chest infections, and respiratory failure. A cardiac pacemaker may be lifesaving in preventing sudden cardiac death.

A congenital form of DM2 is not described. The clinical presentation of DM2 in childhood- and adult-onset forms is similar to DM1, except that patients experience exercise-induced fatigue. In DM2, weakness of the iliopsoas muscle causes difficulty rising from a chair or squatting position and difficulty climbing stairs is more prominent. In general, the phenotype is considered milder in DM2 with fewer frequent respiratory and cardiac complications.

The management of patients with myotonic dystrophies involves symptomatic therapy for motor and mental impairment, psychiatric treatment for behavioural problems, cataract surgery, cardiac evaluation, regular follow-up, pacemaker implantation, monitoring of respiratory function, prevention of aspiration, and prompt treatment of pneumonia. Appropriate attention should be given to endocrine abnormalities and physical therapy should be employed diligently. Drugs known to reduce myotonia, such as mexiletine, phenytoin, and carbamazepine, may be tried.

Congenital muscular dystrophy

The congenital muscular dystrophies (CMDs) comprise a group of autosomal recessive disorders presenting at birth or in early infancy with significant muscular weakness, hypotonia, respiratory insufficiency, bulbar dysfunction, and arthrogryposis. Muscle biopsy shows typical dystrophic changes such as variability in fibre size, endomysial and perimysial connective tissue proliferation, and fat infiltration in areas of muscle fibre loss with varying degrees of necrosis and regeneration. Immunohistochemistry is useful in delineating a particular subtype based on the absence of merosin staining (merosin negative CMD, MDC1A), or the presence of normal merosin staining and expression of β-dystroglycan but absent or reduced glycosylated α-dystroglycan, with preservation of core α-dystroglycan staining (dystroglycanopathies). CMDs are classified based on the underlying genetic defect, namely mutations in genes affecting extracellular matrix proteins, in genes affecting membrane receptors, and in the gene for an endoplasmic reticulum protein. Ultimately, all gene defects lead to an abnormal connection between the extracellular matrix and the DGC.

Table 24.17.8 Molecular classification and clinical features of autosomal recessive limb-girdle muscular dystrophy (LGMD)

Disease	Protein	Gene	Relative prevalence/founder mutations	Creatine kinase levels (IU/litre)	Age of onset (years)	Respiratory involvement	Cardiac involvement	Clinical clues
LGMD2A	Calpain3	CAPN3	One of the most common forms of AR-LGMD worldwide; founder mutations in Basques (2362_2363delinsTCATCT) and in eastern Europeans (550delA)	Normal to 50×	1st to 2nd decades (2–40 years)	–	–	Preferential involvement of posterior thigh muscles; ankle contractures; scapular winging
LGMD2B	Dysferlin	DYSF	More common in southern than northern Europe; founder mutations in several populations	10–100×	2nd to 3rd decades (10–73)	±	–	Distal weakness and wasting; muscle pain and/or swelling; good athletic performance in childhood; inflammatory cells in muscle biopsy
LGMD2C	γ-Sarcoglycan	SGCG	Present worldwide; founder mutations in North Africans (521delT) and gypsies (848G>A)	10–100×	1st decade (3–20)	+	+	Calf hypertrophy; scapular winging
LGMD2D	α-Sarcoglycan	SGCA	Present worldwide; most frequent sarcoglycan form in all populations; common mutation (229C>T), especially in northern Europe	10–100×	1st decade (3–40)	+	Rare	Calf hypertrophy; scapular winging
LGMD2E	β-Sarcoglycan	SGCB	Common in northern and southern Indiana Amish	10–100×	1st decade (3–20)	+	+	Calf hypertrophy; scapular winging
LGMD2F	δ-Sarcoglycan	SGCD	Rare all over the world; common mutation (del656C) in African–Brazilian	10–100×	1st decade (3–20)	+	+	Calf hypertrophy
LGMD2G	Telethonin	TCAP	Rarely reported outside Brazil	Normal to 30×	2nd decade (9–15)	–	±	Calf hypertrophy or hypotrophy distal leg weakness
LGMD2H	TRIM32	TRIM32	Only recently reported outside Hutterite population of Canada	Normal to 20×	2nd decade (1–44)	–	±	Possible mild facial weakness; small vacuoles in muscle fibres
LGMD2I	Fukutin-related protein	FKRP	Relatively frequent in northern Europe; founder mutation in northern Europeans (826C>A)	10–100×	1st to 2nd decade (2–40)	+	+	Calf hypertrophy; myoglobinuria; muscle pain
LGMD2J	Titin	TTN	Reported only in Finland	Normal to 25×	1st decade (5–20)	–	–	Distal weakness described; proximal–distal myopathy with associated cardiomyopathy recently described
LGMD2K	O-Mannosyl transferase-1	POMT1	Few reported LGMD cases (Turkish and English families)	10–50×	Birth–6 years	+	–	Microcephaly and cognitive impairment; muscle hypertrophy (thigh and calf)
LGMD2L[a]	Fukutin	FKTN	Few reported LGMD cases	5–100×	<1 years	?	–	Motor function deterioration during infections
LGMD2M[a]	O-Mannose β-1, 2-N-acetylglucosaminyl transferase	POMGn1	Only one reported LGMD case	20–60×	12 years	?	?	Rapidly progressive
LGMD2N[a]	O-Mannosyl transferases-2	POMT2	Few reported LGMD cases	15×	<2 years	?	–/?	Calf hypertrophy; possible cognitive impairment
LGMD?[a]	?	11p13	Reported in French Canadian families	Normal to 30×	3rd decade (11–50)	?	–	Quadriceps atrophy

[a] No international agreement has been reached for the nomenclature of this LGMD.

Limb–girdle muscular dystrophies. *Curr Opin Neurol*, Oct; **21**(5), 576–584.

Muscular weakness in CMD is static or slowly progressive. Muscle hypertrophy of tongue and calf may be seen. Clinically, CMDs may be classified based on the presence or absence of brain malformation. Most patients with the common form of CMD, MDC1A, caused by laminin α_2 or merosin deficiency, are mentally normal but T_2-weighted imaging on brain MRI consistently shows the presence of widespread cerebral white matter abnormalities, often most marked in the periventricular and frontal U-fibres after the age of 6 months. A sensorimotor peripheral neuropathy is also present. Patients with CMD with fukutin-related protein are described as having mild learning disabilities and cerebellar cysts. Patients with CMD with rigid spine disease and Ullrich's myopathy, as well as its later onset milder allelic form, Bethlem myopathy, have normal mental capacity as well as a normal brain MRI.

The unifying feature of complex CMD is a disorder of neuronal migration referred to as cobblestone cortex, which results in lissencephaly in the most severe form. Walker–Warburg syndrome (WWS), the most severe of the dystroglycanopathies, presents at birth. Patients lack spontaneous movements, and have marked hypotonia and microcephaly. Hydrocephalus secondary to aqueductal stenosis represents a serious complication. Patients are blind and several ocular abnormalities are described, including microphthalmia, cataracts, iris malformations, glaucoma, retinal dysplasia with or without retinal detachment, colobomas of the retina, and hypoplastic optic nerves. Fukuyama's congenital muscular dystrophy (FCMD) and muscle–eye–brain (MEB) disease are more common in Japan and Finland, respectively. MEB disease has a more severe phenotype with persistent bedridden state and death during the first year of life. FCMD is associated with severe intellectual impairment, cardiomyopathy, seizures, and ocular abnormalities, but not blindness. Characteristic brain malformations found include polymicrogyria, pachygyria, and agyria of the cerebrum and cerebellum (type II lissencephaly). The cerebral cortex is highly disorganized, showing no recognizable lamination and neuronal overmigration into the leptomeninges.

Further reading

Lyon G, Kolodny EH, Pastores GM (2006). Neurology of Hereditary Metabolic Diseases of Children. McGraw-Hill, New York.
Rosenberg RN, DiMauro S, Paulson HL, Ptacek L, Nestler EJ (eds.) (2008). The Molecular and Genetic Basis of Neurologic and Psychiatric Disease. 4th ed. Wolters Kluwer/Lippincott Williams & Wilkins, Philadelphia.
Tidball JG, Spencer MJ (2003). Skipping to new gene therapies for muscular dystrophy. Nat Med, 9, 997–8.
Van Haren K, et al. (2004). The life and death of oligodendrocytes in vanishing white matter disease. J Neuropathol Exp Neurol, 63, 618–30.

Websites

The tables are a guide to the established disease genes but are not comprehensive because new discoveries in neurogenetics occur at a rapid pace. For further listings, the reader should consult the websites below.

Human Genome Variation Society. Mutation database of inherited peripheral neuropathies. http://www.molgen.ua.ac.be/CMTMutations
Institute of Medical Genetics in Cardiff. Human gene mutation database. http://www.hgmd.cf.ac.uk/ac/index.php
National Center for Biotechnology Information. Gene tests. http://www.ncbi.nlm.nih.gov/sites/GeneTests/?db=GeneTests
Online Mendelian Inheritance in Man http://www.ncbi.nlm.nih.gov/omim/

Patient support and information

Alzheimer Foundation http://alzfnd.org
Charcot-Marie-Tooth Association http://www.cmtfoundation.org
Children's Tumor Foundation. http://www.ctf.org
Climb (Children living with inherited metabolic diseases http://www.climb.org.uk
Genetic Alliance http://geneticalliance.org
Muscular Dystrophy Association http://wwwmdausa.org
National Organization for Rare Disorders (NORD) http://www.rarediseases.org/info/contact.html
National Tay-Sachs and Allied Diseases Association http://www.ntsad.org
Neurofibromatosis, Inc. http://www.nfinc.org
Tuberous Sclerosis Alliance. http://www.tsalliance.org/

Developmental abnormalities of the central nervous system

C.M. Verity, C. ffrench-Constant, and H.V. Firth

Essentials

The brain and spinal cord arise from a sheet of cells that develop through a series of distinct transformations into the final complex structure. Congenital abnormalities of the central nervous system are considered in the context of this process, which may fail at distinct stages of development.

General clinical approach

A rigorous approach to the diagnosis of and counselling for developmental abnormalities of the central nervous system is required. Referral for specialist advice is recommended because of the far-reaching consequences of misdiagnosis. Many abnormalities can be identified by detailed ultrasonography, and MRI *in utero* is proving to be particularly useful for accurate investigation of the fetal brain. Prenatal diagnosis and termination is available for some conditions. In the absence of a specific diagnosis genetic advice is usually limited and empirical, but where a specific gene is implicated parental questions can often be accurately addressed. Where there are strong environmental factors, it is imperative to reduce the risk to future pregnancies by taking appropriate measures, e.g. folic acid or iodide supplementation before conception.

Neural tube defects

Clinical features and epidemiology—neural tube defects such as spina bifida and anencephaly reflect a failure of closure of the ectoderm folds that normally fuse 18 to 26 days after ovulation. Prevalence rates are very variable, but are over 8 per 1000 births in several regions. Most cases are caused by interactions between genes and environmental factors such as nutritional folic acid.

Screening—many serious (open) neural tube defects lead to an increased concentration of α-fetoprotein in maternal serum, and at-risk women with this elevated biomarker on screening—or those with a history of an affected pregnancy—are recommended to have fetal ultrasonography from 12 weeks onwards. This screening method has largely supplemented measurement of

α-fetoprotein and neuronal acetylcholinesterase in amniotic fluid obtained by amniocentesis, but this remains an alternative for prenatal diagnosis.

Prevention—the incidence of neural tube defects can be markedly reduced by avoidance of certain drugs in pregnancy (e.g. folate antagonists, anticonvulsants), as well as by preconceptual supplementation of folic acid (400 µg daily), which has been effectively introduced in some countries by fortification of foods with folic acid.

Treatment and prognosis—the major focus is on prevention, but neurosurgical procedures are employed for closure and for relief of hydrocephalus by diversion of cerebrospinal fluid through shunt procedures. The outcomes and prognosis of affected children vary greatly and surgical management remains controversial, except for those with mild abnormalities.

Other developmental abnormalities of the spinal cord—these include syringomyelia, which usually presents in later life and is associated with the Chiari malformation and hydrocephalus. Agenesis of the sacrum with abnormalities of the distal cord is associated with maternal diabetes mellitus.

Disorders of regionalization of the fully formed neural tube

Numerous genes, including those encoding signalling molecules that induce the expression of homeotic genes involved throughout evolution in regional and segmental development, are implicated in the complex process of regionalization of the neural tube. Disorders affecting these pathways often involve gene–environment interactions and give rise to abnormalities of the specification of cells in the forebrain, midbrain, hindbrain, and spinal cord, e.g. holoprosencephaly.

Holoprosencephaly—this condition may vary from severe to mild developmental abnormalities affecting the formation of the cerebral hemispheres, eyes, palate and mouth. At least nine genes

Acknowledgements: We are very grateful to Dr Nagui Antoun (Addenbrooke's Hospital, Cambridge), Dr Fred Pickworth (Norfolk and Norwich Hospital), and Mr Paul Chamberlain (John Radcliffe Hospital, Oxford) for the scans shown in this chapter and for advice on their interpretation. Many thanks to Mr Michael Cafferkey (Senior Illustrator, Medical Photography and Illustration, Addenbrooke's Hospital, Cambridge) for producing Figs. 24.18.1 and 24.18.4.

have been implicated, including *sonic hedgehog* and its signature receptor, *patched*. The different associations and variants of the condition reflect defects in one or more of the stages leading to formation of the rostral parts of the brain and associated structures. Maternal diabetes possibly increases the probability of this abnormality in the infant.

Disorders of cortical development

Numerous genetic determinants have been identified for disorders of cortical development such as microcephaly and lissencephaly, which reflect abnormalities of proliferation and cellular migration (respectively). Microcephaly may also be caused by environmental influences in pregnancy, including radiation, drugs, and maternal hyperphenylalanemia (a preventable factor of importance in the management of women with phenylketonuria).

Disorders of development of other parts of the brain

Hindbrain—development is disturbed in the Chiari II malformations and the Dandy–Walker syndrome (a kind of agenesis of the vermis, with dilatation of the fourth ventricle and enlargement of the posterior fossa; associated with trisomies 13 and 18).

Complex malformations of the brain and cord—many types are recognized, including agenesis of the corpus callosum and porencephaly. These disorders are rare, but are increased in children with other developmental abnormalities. They may be caused by mutations in as yet unknown genes, chromosomal rearrangement, and some rare metabolic syndromes.

Disorders of the developing brain caused by extrinsic factors

Hydrocephalus—this results from expansion of the ventricles secondary to a block in the normal flow pathway of cerebrospinal fluid.

It may be (1) communicating—due to failure of reabsorption of cerebrospinal fluid, e.g. following subarachnoid bleeding or (2) obstructive/noncommunicating—due to blockage at one of the ventricular levels. Mental retardation can result from both the damage associated with ventricular expansion and other abnormalities associated with the underlying cause of the problem.

Alcohol—fetal alcohol syndrome is one of the commonest causes of learning difficulty and neurobehavioural disturbance in young children. Other clinical features include microcephaly, structural anomalies of the brain such as partial or complete agenesis of the corpus callosum, cerebellar hypoplasia, and a dysmorphic appearance.

Congenital infections—e.g. toxoplasmosis, herpes simplex, cytomegalovirus, rubella, and syphilis. Primary maternal infection is implicated in most instances, hence measures to prevent these infections are important.

Maternal iodine deficiency—this leads to cretinism (spastic diplegia and deafness), which is a common, potentially preventable disorder in many regions of the world that can be addressed by screening for neonatal hypothyroidism.

Cerebral palsies

These are an important but heterogeneous group of nonprogressive disorders of the immature brain that cause defects of movement and posture that may have associated manifestations such as deafness, seizures and learning difficulties. Several clear genetic factors have been identified, and environmental exposure to toxins such as carbon monoxide, alcohol, and methyl mercury may also be responsible. Although cerebral palsy has in the past been attributed to 'asphyxia' at birth, this view is now changing; premature infants are at a greatly increased risk.

Normal development of the human central nervous system

The human central nervous system (CNS), like that of all vertebrates, develops from a two-dimensional sheet of cells into a complex three-dimensional structure. A range of abnormalities results from failures at distinct stages of development. This chapter uses the normal development of the human CNS as a framework to discuss these disorders. Only structural abnormalities of the CNS that are present at birth have been included, not the numerous metabolic and degenerative disorders that can affect the infant brain.

Malformations resulting from abnormalities in the major steps of CNS formation

Disorders of neural tube formation

The nervous system develops from a tube formed when part of the embryonic ectoderm folds and separates from the remaining ectoderm (Fig. 24.18.1). Closure of this tube starts at a level corresponding to the future hindbrain/spinal cord junction and then proceeds towards both the head (rostrally) and the tail (caudally).

This process generates the entire neural tube except for the most caudal part, which is formed by thickening of the neural plate and the subsequent formation of a cavity. A population of cells (the neural crest) then migrates out of the dorsal part of this tube to form the peripheral nervous system, while those that remain in the tube form the CNS. The neural tube usually fuses completely between 18 and 26 days after ovulation. Failure of closure leads to malformations that represent the most common congenital abnormalities in most countries and include anencephaly, encephalocele, spina bifida, and spina bifida occulta. They are malformations of the neuroectoderm, which are associated to a variable extent with abnormalities of the surrounding mesodermal structures. The term 'dysraphism' is used when there is continuity between the posterior neuroectoderm and cutaneous ectoderm.

Epidemiology

The prevalence of neural tube defects varies according to geography and race. High rates (more than 8 per 1000 births) have been reported in Northern Ireland, Egypt, India, and China. There are worldwide reports of decreasing prevalence rates. In England there was a peak in 1954 to 1955 followed by a substantial decline which started in the early 1970s, so that by 1994 the prevalence of neural

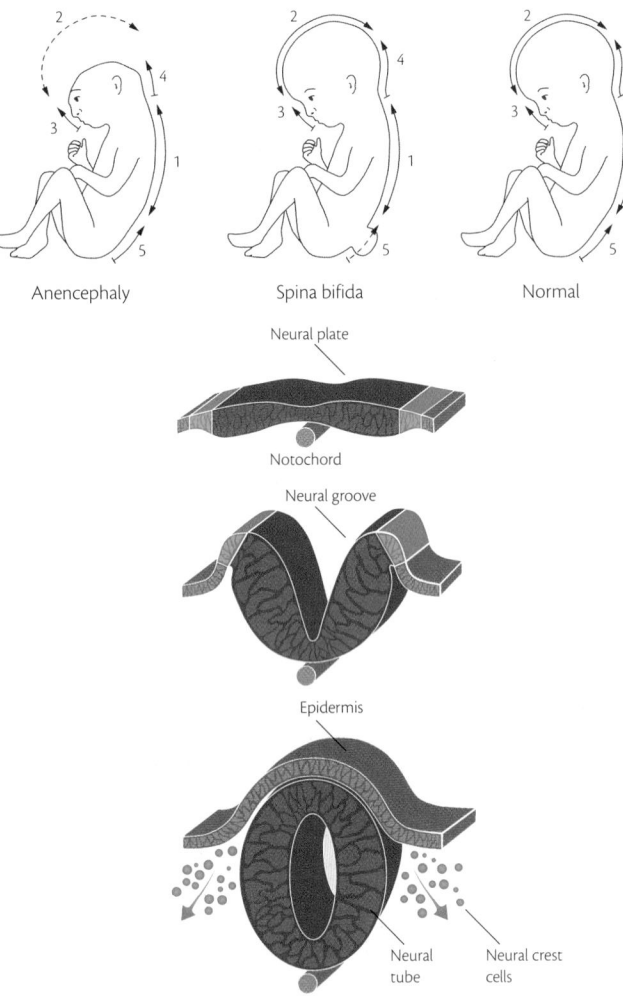

Fig. 24.18.1 The upper part of the diagram illustrates defects that arise from errors in the multisite closure of the neural tube. The coloured section shows how the embryonic ectoderm separates, folds, and closes to form the neural tube.

Anencephaly   Spina bifida   Normal

Neural plate
Notochord
Neural groove
Epidermis
Neural tube   Neural crest cells

tube defects in England and Wales was just under 0.8 per 1000 total births, with anencephaly and spina bifida of approximately equal prevalence and together making up 95% of all neural tube defects. The epidemiological evidence suggests that this decrease was not entirely due to prenatal screening, and the decline also preceded the widespread use of periconceptual vitamin supplementation, so some of the decrease remains unexplained.

Aetiology
Genetic factors
Most neural tube defects result from a complex interaction between several genes and environmental factors, but a minority occur as part of a mendelian disorder (e.g. Meckel's syndrome). All isolated (i.e. nonsyndromic) defects are aetiologically related and, if one member of a family is affected, there is an increased risk in the relatives for all types of neural tube defect. Major genes have been identified that cause neural tube defects in the mouse, but their relevance to human defects is still not clear. Some genes have been shown to alter risk, e.g. mutations in the methylene tetrahydrofolate reductase gene are associated with elevated blood homocysteine levels in pregnant women and a twofold increased risk of neural tube defects. At this time, however, genetic investigations

offer little in the management of families with one member having an isolated neural tube defect.

Environmental factors
Periconceptual multiple vitamin supplements containing folic acid have been shown to substantially reduce the incidence of neural tube defects. In England it is currently recommended that women who are planning pregnancy should take 400 μg folic acid daily before conception and during the first 12 weeks of pregnancy. To prevent recurrence of neural tube defects the dose should be 4 to 5 mg/day. In the United Kingdom, the Food Standards Agency has recommended the mandatory addition of folic acid to bread or flour. In North America fortification of certain foodstuffs with folic acid has been mandatory since 1998. Countries that have instituted folic acid fortification policies have seen reductions in neural tube defects of 27 to 50%.

Some drugs taken during pregnancy may increase the risk of neural tube defects in the fetus, including sodium valproate and folic acid antagonists such as trimethoprim, triamterene, carbamazepine, phenytoin, phenobarbitone, and primidone.

Prenatal diagnosis
α-Fetoprotein levels in maternal serum
The fetal liver is the main source of α-fetoprotein (AFP), which leaks through open neural tube defects into the amniotic fluid and then into maternal blood. The consequent abnormal increase in maternal serum AFP is best detected at 16 to 18 weeks of pregnancy. Maternal serum screening does not detect closed defects (those covered by skin).

Ultrasonography
This is recommended for all at-risk women—those with positive serum AFP screening, those who have had one or more affected child and those taking drugs associated with neural tube defects in the fetus. Anencephaly can be detected by ultrasonography from week 12 of gestation and spina bifida from 16 to 20 weeks (Fig. 24.18.2a, b), although even the best ultrasonographers may occasionally miss spina bifida, particularly in the L5–S2 region, the quality of ultrasonography has meant that direct sampling of the amniotic fluid—amniocentesis—has been largely superseded. However, when adequate ultrasound images cannot be obtained, amniocentesis with measurement of AFP and assay of neuronal acetylcholinesterase does provide an alternative method of prenatal diagnosis.

Cranial abnormalities of neural tube closure
Anencephaly
This is a lethal defect that results from failure of fusion of the rostral folds of the neural tube. The cranial vault is absent and an angiomatous membranous mass lies on the floor of the cranium. The eyes are protuberant as a result of shallow orbits and there is variable involvement of the spinal cord. Before the advent of prenatal diagnosis by ultrasonography most anencephalic babies were born in the last 3 months of gestation; now an increasing number of such pregnancies are terminated. In live-born anencephalic babies the initial neurological examination may be surprisingly normal if brainstem structures are reasonably intact. However, the infants usually die in hours or days.

Cephaloceles
A cephalocele is a herniation of the cranial contents through a skull defect. There are several subtypes: a cranial meningocele contains

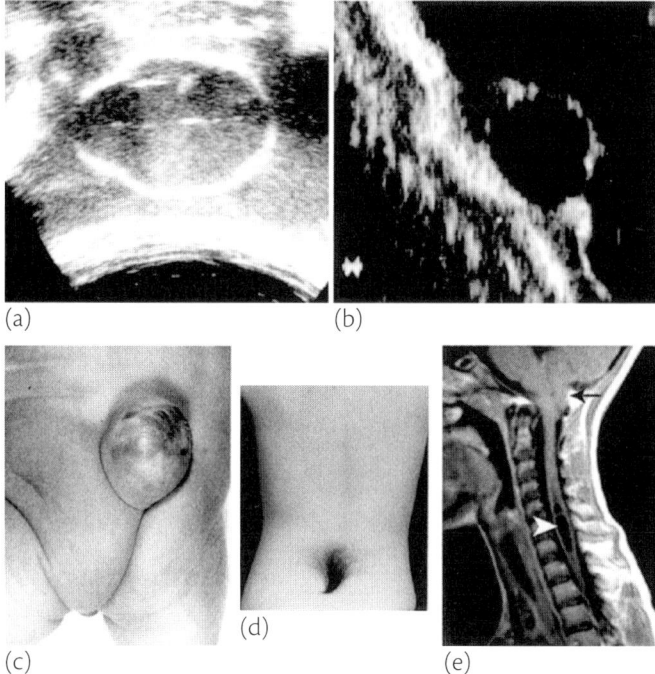

Myelomeningocele

This spinal defect represents the abnormality found in 80 to 90% of children with spina bifida cystica. It is lumbosacral in about 80% of cases and consists of a sac covered with a thin membrane that may leak cerebrospinal fluid (Fig. 24.18.2c). Neurological abnormalities depend on the level of the lesion. There is usually a mixture of upper and lower motor neuron signs, disturbance of bladder and bowel sphincters, and bladder detrusor dysfunction. The sensory level correlates with the severity of abnormalities in the urinary tract and is also related to long-term disability. Higher lesions of the cord are associated with bladder outlet obstruction, dilatation of the upper urinary tract, and chronic pyelonephritis.

Hydrocephalus complicates about 90% of cases of lumbosacral meningomyelocele. Usually it is associated with the Chiari II malformation, where there is downward displacement of the cerebellar vermis or tonsils through the foramen magnum to overlap the spinal cord. The fourth ventricle is elongated and the midbrain distorted, causing palsies from involvement of the lower cranial nerves and central apnoea (which may be misdiagnosed as epilepsy in older children). Hydrocephalus may also be due to aqueduct stenosis or have no clear structural cause. If there is evidence of progressive ventricular dilatation (often detected by ultrasonography) or signs of increasing intracranial pressure, insertion of a ventriculoperitoneal shunt is usually necessary.

Meningocele

Here there is protrusion of the meninges outside the spinal canal: the sac does not contain any neural tissue. Meningoceles account for about 5% of cases of spina bifida cystica. There is no associated hydrocephalus and the neurological examination is usually normal. They must be distinguished from meningomyeloceles because the prognosis is so different.

Spina bifida occulta

This term is often applied to a defect of the posterior arch of one or more lumbar or sacral vertebrae (usually L5 and S1). It is found incidentally by radiography in 25% of children admitted to hospital and may be a normal variant. However, if examination of the skin over the spine reveals a naevus, hairy patch (Fig. 24.18.2d), dimple, sinus, or subcutaneous mass, further evaluation including MRI of the spinal cord is indicated. A number of clinical abnormalities may be found on examination. Spinal cord malformation may cause an asymmetrical lower motor neuron weakness with wasting, deformity, and diminished reflexes in the lower limb, or progressive gait disturbance with spasticity. Either presentation may be associated with disturbed bladder control. Dorsal dermal sinuses may connect the skin surface to the dura or an intradural dermoid cyst. An open sinus tract can cause recurrent meningitis so ideally it should be explored and excised before infections occur. Lipomyelomeningoceles present as a bulge in the lumbosacral region, usually lateral to the midline. They consist of a lipoma or lipofibroma attached to a low-lying abnormal spinal cord and are often associated with a meningocele. Diastematomyelia is the presence of a sagittal cleft that divides the spinal cord into two halves, each surrounded by its own pia mater. A bony or cartilaginous spur may transfix the cord, fixing it in a low position as the child grows. The cleft is usually in the low thoracic or lumbar region, but cervical clefts have been reported.

Fig. 24.18.2 (a) Prenatal ultrasonography of a child with a neural tube defect, showing the 'lemon sign' resulting from the change in shape of the back of the skull (on the left-hand side in the image) which is associated with the Chiari II malformation described in the text. (b) Prenatal ultrasonography of a child with a neural tube defect, showing a cystic lumbar meningomyelocele in the caudal neural tube. (c) Lumbar meningomyelocele: photograph of a newborn infant. (d) Chiari I malformation and syringomyelia in an asymptomatic girl aged 11 years. Photograph of tuft of hair seen over the lumbar region at birth. The associated central nervous system malformations are shown in (e). (e) Chiari I malformation and syringomyelia. T_1-weighted sagittal MRI shows that there is herniation of the cerebellar tonsils through the foramen magnum (arrow) and a syrinx of the lower cervical spinal cord (C5–7) (arrow head). The associated tuft of lumbar hair is shown in (d).

only meninges, an encephalocele contains brain tissue, and a ventriculocele contains part of the ventricle within the herniated portion of the brain. Cephaloceles are less common than anencephaly or spina bifida, occurring in 1 to 3 per 10 000 live births. Posterior cephaloceles are the most common group in Western countries and most are occipital encephaloceles, whereas anterior cephaloceles are more common in some parts of Asia. Anterior cephaloceles are associated with other brain abnormalities such as agenesis of the corpus callosum, abnormal gyration, or, in the case of posterior defects below the tentorium, cerebellar defects. They may be part of a recognized syndrome so it is important to look for abnormalities in other parts of the body.

Spinal abnormalities of neural tube closure
Spina bifida

This can be divided into spina bifida occulta, which consists of failure of closure of the vertebral arches without an external lesion, and spina bifida cystica in which there is a cystic lesion on the back. The lesion may be either a meningocele without neural tissue or a myelomeningocele in which the spinal cord is a component of the cyst wall. The term 'rachischisis' is used for the most severe defect, which is a widely patent dorsal opening of the spine, often associated with anencephaly.

If any abnormality involving the cord or nerve roots is found there may be a good case for neurosurgical intervention. The aim is to free the spinal cord from its abnormal attachments to allow for growth and prevent further damage. Early intervention may prevent worsening motor deficits and urological complications, but the indications for intervention are controversial.

Other developmental abnormalities of the spinal cord

Syringomyelia

This is a tubular cavitation of the spinal cord that is often associated with the Chiari I malformation and hydrocephalus (Fig. 24.18.2e). It tends to be in the cervical region but may involve the whole cord. It rarely becomes symptomatic in children. Treatment is controversial. Shunting of the abnormal cavity is sometimes performed and posterior fossa exploration may be undertaken if there is a Chiari I malformation.

Sacral agenesis

This is strongly associated with maternal diabetes mellitus. Absence of the sacrum and coccyx is usually associated with abnormalities of the lumbosacral cord. There may be arthrogryposis at birth (defined as a fixed deformity of one or more joints). A flaccid neurogenic bladder causes incontinence and there are sensory and motor deficits in the legs.

Management of neural tube defects

The major emphasis is on primary prevention. It is recommended that women planning to conceive supplement their diet with folic acid, which reduces the risk of neural tube defects. Screening of maternal serum for AFP is possible and prenatal diagnosis by ultrasonography and amniocentesis is available. This is discussed above.

Treatment of infants with meningomyeloceles became possible with the development of ventriculoatrial and ventriculoperitoneal shunts. In the early 1960s it was argued that closure of the defect within 24 h of birth reduced mortality and morbidity by avoiding infection and reducing trauma to the exposed neural tissue. However, selective surgical management is not universally practised and is a controversial area. Lorber reported four adverse criteria that he thought were contraindications to treatment: a high level of paraplegia, clinically evident hydrocephalus at birth, lumbar kyphosis, and the presence of other major malformations. However, even using these criteria, the outcome was uncertain; many infants survived even though they did not have closure of the defect within 24 h, and some children with a supposedly good prognosis were left with major disabilities after surgery.

Disorders of regionalization

Once the neural tube has developed, specification of different regions and individual cells within these regions occurs. This patterning occurs in both the rostrocaudal and dorsoventral axes. The three basic regions of the CNS (forebrain, midbrain, and hindbrain) develop at the rostral end of the tube, with the spinal cord more caudally. Within the developing cord the specification of the different populations of neural precursors (neural crest, sensory neurons, interneurons, glial cells, and motor neurons) is observed in progressively more ventral locations. This process reflects the interaction between genes whose expression defines individual territories or cell types and diffusible signalling molecules secreted by adjacent areas of the embryo. Of particular importance are the extracellular signalling molecules such as sonic hedgehog required for ventral induction, and a family of genes called homoeotic genes. Most of these encode proteins containing a conserved homoeodomain motif that binds DNA sequences involved in the regulation of expression of other genes, so controlling cell differentiation.

Failure of normal development of the most rostral portion of the neural tube (the mediobasal prosencephalon) and associated structures caused by disturbances in the process of ventral induction may result in various abnormalities of the brain and face. The most severe CNS abnormality is holoprosencephaly in which there is failure of the prosencephalon to separate into two cerebral hemispheres. The mildest is olfactory aplasia with no other cerebral malformations. The severity of the associated facial abnormalities tends to parallel those in the brain. In the most severe facial abnormality there is anophthalmia and absence of the nose. However, there may be just mild hypotelorism (closely set eyes) or a single central incisor tooth, or the face may be normal.

Holoprosencephaly (prosencephaly)

This occurs with a frequency of approximately 1 in 14 000 births. There is failure of formation of the two cerebral hemispheres, resulting in abnormalities of varying severity. There are many possible causes that act within a short vulnerable period, because ventral induction probably occurs before 23 days. Environmental factors are important and it is at least 20 times more common in the infants of mothers with diabetes than in the general population. In addition, there are a number of genetic causes, with at least 12 genetic loci and 9 holoprosencephaly (*HPE*) genes identified in humans. One (*HPE3* on chromosome 7q36) is the sonic hedgehog gene, and mutations in *PTCH*, the receptor for sonic hedgehog, have also been found in some individuals with holoprosencephaly. A number of chromosomal abnormalities have been recognized in association with holoprosencephaly, including trisomy and other abnormalities of chromosome 13, partial deletion of the short arm of chromosome 18, ring chromosome 18, and partial trisomy of chromosome 7.

In alobar holoprosencephaly, the completely undivided forebrain is in the shape of a horseshoe surrounding a single cavity. The thalami are fused but the brain stem and cerebellum are well developed. The associated facial abnormalities are severe—there may be anophthalmia or cyclopia in which there is a single orbit. In holoprosencephaly with median cleft lip there is marked hypotelorism. In semilobar holoprosencephaly the brain is divided into two hemispheres posteriorly but anteriorly the two hemispheres are fused (Fig. 24.18.3). In lobar holoprosencephaly there is almost complete separation of the hemispheres and the face may be normal. The head is usually microcephalic unless there is associated hydrocephalus.

In some families in which the condition is inherited in autosomal dominant pattern the severity can be variable, with some family members having only minor features and others with holoprosencephaly. When providing genetic counselling it is therefore important to look for minor signs in both parents of an affected child.

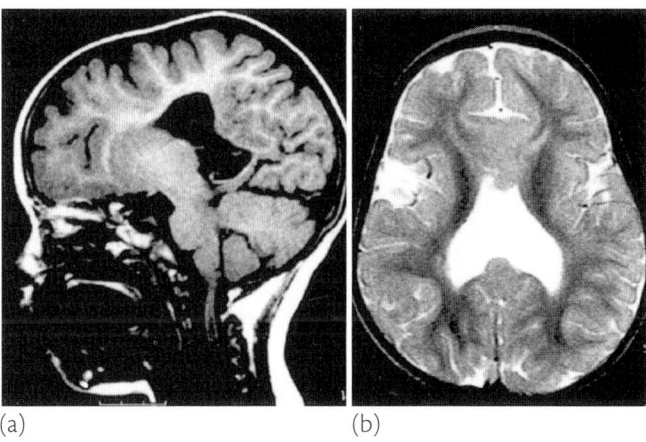

(a)   (b)

Fig. 24.18.3 (a) Semilobar holoprosencephaly in a girl aged 2 years imaged with T_1-weighted sagittal MRI. This midline view shows absence of the corpus callosum and fusion of the frontal lobes. (b) Semilobar holoprosencephaly in the same patient using T_2-weighted axial MRI. There is fusion of the frontal lobes of both cerebral hemispheres and a common central ventricle.

The signs include orbital hypotelorism, median cleft lip, flat nose with or without a single nostril, anosmia, and a single central incisor. Prenatal diagnosis can be made by ultrasonography from week 16 of pregnancy, with orbital hypotelorism an important feature for antenatal diagnosis.

The most severely affected infants die in the neonatal period. Less severely affected patients may live for months or years. The survivors often develop infantile spasms or other seizures. Some patients with significant structural abnormalities may survive to adulthood but usually there are severe learning difficulties. Associated anomalies include congenital heart disease, scalp defects, and polydactyly. Holoprosencephaly may be part of syndromes such as the Meckel syndrome and Aicardi syndrome.

Disorders of cortical development

Modern brain imaging, in particular MRI, has resulted in the identification of many previously unrecognized developmental abnormalities of the cerebral cortex. The best characterized of these arise from defects in one of two basic processes in cortical development. The first is the proliferation of the stem cell population which generates all the neurons required for the cortex. This occurs throughout fetal development in the region next to the ventricle. The second is the migration of the newly formed neurons away from this ventricular region into the overlying cortex to form appropriate connections with other neurons. Abnormalities in migration are shown schematically in Fig. 24.18.4.

Disorders of proliferation

Microcephaly

A failure of proliferation results in a reduced number of cells, causing a head that is disproportionately small (less than the 0.4th centile) in relation to the rest of the body. This microcephaly is often associated with significant additional abnormalities of the nervous system such as pyramidal tract signs and learning difficulties. Autosomal recessive primary microcephaly is the term used to describe a genetically determined form of microcephaly previously known as 'microcephaly vera', with a severe and nonprogressive reduction in head circumference (more that 4 standard deviations

below the mean for age) associated with mild-to-moderate learning disability but normal height, weight, and appearance. Eight gene loci have been identified so far, *MCPH1* to *MCPH6*. Of these, five genes have been cloned including (*MCPH1* (microcephalin), *MCPCH3* (*CDK5RAP2*), *MCPCH5* (*ASPM*—which accounts for 50% of cases), and *MCPCH6* (*CENPJ*). All encode centrosomal proteins that are crucial for cell division. The fifth gene is *MCPH7* (SCL/TAL1-interrupting locus (STIL)). In some types of genetic microcephaly the head size may not become abnormal until as late as 32 to 34 weeks of gestation or even after birth.

Nongenetic causes of microcephaly include ionizing radiation in the first two trimesters of the pregnancy, intrauterine infections, alcohol, drugs and other chemicals, circulatory disturbance, and perinatal hypoxic–ischaemic events. Poor dietary control in mothers with phenylketonuria is also an important and preventable cause of microcephaly, because the fetal brain is very sensitive to the toxic effects of phenylalanine. When there is a significant perinatal insult to the brain, the head circumference may be normal at birth, with subsequent failure of growth in the first few months of life.

Macrocephaly

The term 'macrocephaly' is used when the head circumference is above the normal range for the age, sex, and race of the child. This may result from abnormalities outside the brain parenchyma such as hydrocephalus, arachnoid cysts, congenital abnormalities of the cerebral veins, fluid collections over the surface of the brain, or abnormalities of the skull. Cranial imaging is necessary to make the diagnosis. The subsequent discussion deals only with megalencephaly, which is increased size of the brain itself. This may result from an increased number of cells but, unlike the microcephalies, we have no clear understanding of the aetiology in most cases.

Although many normal individuals have large heads, megalencephaly can be associated with significant learning difficulties, autism, neurological abnormalities, and seizures, and this combination of features can have a genetic basis. The brains may have bulky gyri and usually all parts of the cerebrum are diffusely enlarged, with normal-sized or mildly enlarged ventricles. Occasionally, particular parts of the brain such as the cerebellum are disproportionately large. No consistent microscopic alterations are reported in the cortex, but minor anomalies such as small heterotopias may be found. The abnormality may be part of a specific disorder, e.g. one of the neurocutaneous syndromes, or an overgrowth disorder such as Sotos' syndrome (OMIM 117550). Large heads can run in families ('familial megalencephaly'), in some of which there may be no abnormalities, and it is important to check the head circumference of the parents.

Hemimegalencephaly or unilateral megalencephaly may involve all parts of the brain on the same side or there may be enlargement of one hemisphere only. This can be associated with other neurological problems such as intractable seizures. It may also be associated with marked developmental delay, hemiparesis, and overgrowth of one side of the face.

Disorders of migration

Migration defects occur when neurons generated by the division of stem cells in the ventricular region fail to reach their intended destination in the cerebral cortex. The different classes of defect are illustrated schematically in Fig. 24.18.4. If neurons fail to leave the ventricular zone entirely, periventricular heterotopias result.

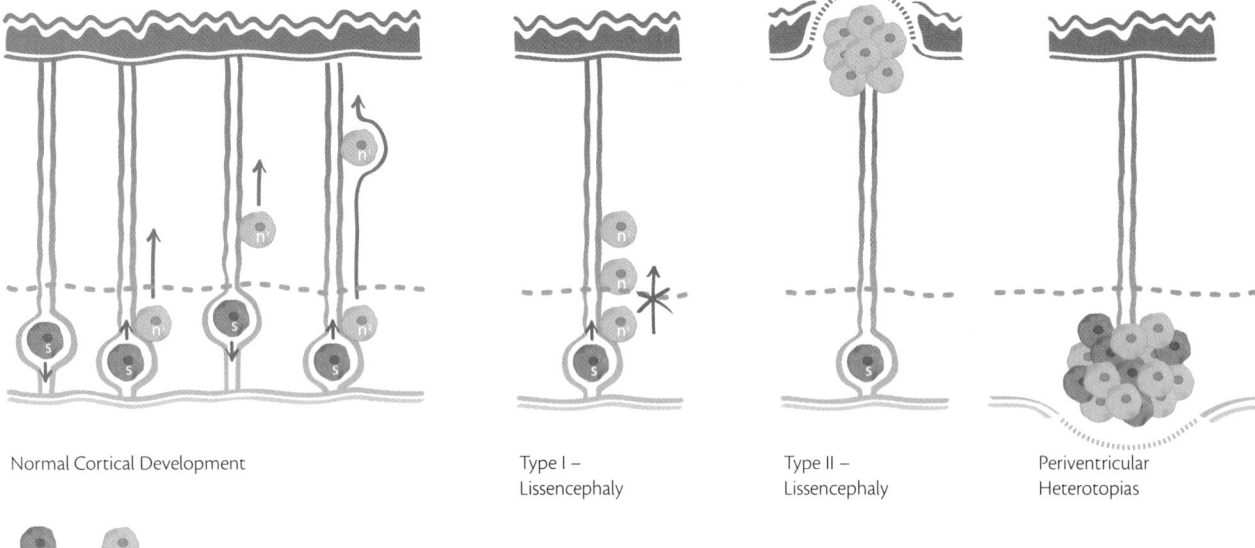

Normal Cortical Development

Type I – Lissencephaly

Type II – Lissencephaly

Periventricular Heterotopias

s — stem cell   n — neuronal precursor

Fig. 24.18.4 Diagrammatic representation of the cerebral cortex showing normal development and neuronal migration defects. In type I lissencephaly neurons fail to reach their intended destination. In type II lissencephaly there is overmigration of neuroglial precursors through a disrupted pial- to glial-limiting membrane, resulting in nodules of ectopic neurons. If neurons fail to leave the ventricular zone entirely, periventricular heterotopias result.

If neurons leave the ventricular zone but then fail to complete their migration in the cortex, this causes a group of disorders of varying severity. There may be complete absence of gyri, in which case the term 'agyria' is used. Pachygyria describes a reduced number of broadened and flat gyri with less folding of the cortex than normal. There may be varying degrees of agyria–pachygyria in the same brain. The term 'lissencephaly' (Greek: smooth brain) is commonly used to describe the spectrum of malformations from complete agyria to regional pachygyria. If, however, only a subpopulation of neurons is affected and the others complete their migration normally, this results in nodular or subcortical band heterotopias. Migration disorders are found as part of recognized genetic syndromes and there are also acquired types as a result of intrauterine infections, circulatory disturbances, and toxins (alcohol or phenytoin, for example). The classification of these disorders is evolving as a result of rapid advances in brain imaging and molecular biology.

Type I or classic lissencephaly

This is the most common type and is characterized by a smooth or almost smooth cerebral surface. The cortex is thickened (10–20 mm) usually with no other major brain malformations, although agenesis of the corpus callosum or severe cerebellar hypoplasia can be seen due, in the latter, to mutations in the *reelin* (*RELN*) gene. Infants with type I or classic lissencephaly may be divided into those who have the isolated lissencephaly sequence with no dysmorphic features (the majority) and those with the dysmorphic features of the Miller–Dieker syndrome (OMIM 247200). Currently, five genes have been identified that cause or contribute to type I lissencephaly in humans: *LIS1*, *14-3-3*, *DCX*, *RELN*, and *ARX*. *DCX* (double cortin) is on the X chromosome, explaining why inheritance of lissencephaly is in some cases X linked. While affected males in these families show the full isolated lissencephaly sequence phenotype, carrier females can show band heterotopia, in which a subset of neurons fails to complete migration and forms bilateral symmetrical ribbons of grey matter in the

centrum semiovale. This is thought to reflect X inactivation of the normal *DCX* gene in these neurons, while those that inactivate the mutation-containing X chromosome migrate normally.

In Miller–Dieker syndrome there is a severe seizure disorder with severe/profound hypotonia and developmental delay accompanied by postnatal growth deficiency and microcephaly. The dysmorphic features include a tall narrow forehead, a depressed nasal bridge, anteverted nares, midfacial hypoplasia, a prominent upper lip with a thin vermilion border, retrognathism, and hypervascularization of the retina. About 50 to 70% of cases have a deletion of chromosome 17p13.3 visible by light microscopy and almost all the remainder have a submicroscopic deletion demonstrable by either fluorescent *in situ* hybridization of chromosomes using DNA probes or microarray-based comparative genomic hybridisation. This region includes the *LIS1* gene. It has been suggested that deletions of *LIS1* cause the lissencephaly seen in the Miller–Dieker syndrome and that the facial dysmorphism is caused by loss of adjacent genes.

The diagnosis of type I lissencephaly is made by CT or MRI, which shows a thick cortical plate with no or few sulci separated from the white matter by an undulating border (Fig. 24.18.5a). Prenatal diagnosis is not possible by ultrasonography before 24 weeks because tertiary sulci do not appear before then.

Type II or 'cobblestone' lissencephaly

This is a completely different malformation from type I lissencephaly. The smooth cortex has a granular surface and the meninges are thickened due to mesenchymal proliferation. The cerebellum is small with an absent vermis and the pyramidal tracts are usually absent. Hydrocephalus is present in 75% of cases. Microscopically there is complete disorganization of the cortex which consists of neurons separated by bundles of gliomesenchymal tissue continuous with the meninges. More deeply, there is a thin layer of white matter lying above islands of heterotopic grey matter. These abnormalities are thought to result from overmigration of

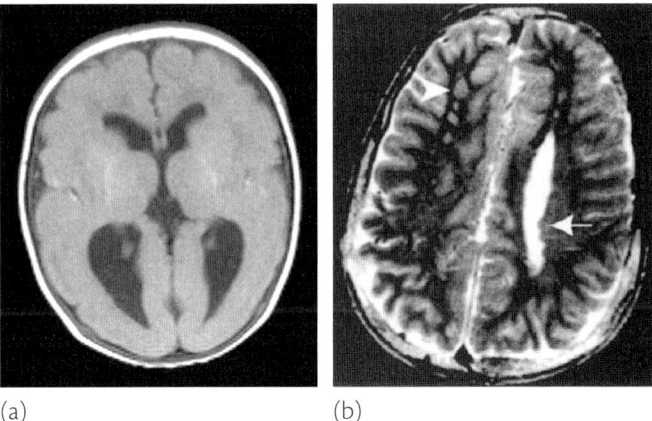

(a)   (b)

Fig. 24.18.5 (a) Lissencephaly type I in a boy with a de novo deletion in the *LIS1* gene on chromosome 17. T_2-weighted axial MRI shows agyria of the parietal and occipital lobes of the brain, with pachygyria of the frontal lobes. This anterior-to-posterior severity gradient is characteristic of *LIS1* deletions or mutations. (b) Nodular heterotopias in a boy aged 13 years. The T_2-weighted axial image shows that the nodular heterotopias are subependymal (arrow) and subcortical (arrow head).

neuroglial precursors through a disrupted pial–glial limiting membrane, resulting in the nodules of ectopic neurons that generate the granular texture of the brain. This is caused in some cases by abnormalities of adhesion molecules, such as dystroglycan—responsible for anchoring the endfeet of the glial cells that define the migratory pathway of the neurons to the overlying pial membrane. As these same adhesion molecules are required for attachment of muscle fibres and retinal cells to their overlying basement membranes, many type II lissencephaly syndromes are associated with muscle and eye abnormalities. These disorders constitute a group of autosomal recessive congenital muscular dystrophies (CMDs) associated with defects in *O*-glycosylation of α-dystroglycan, which includes Walker–Warburg syndrome, Fukuyama cerebral and muscular dystrophy, and muscle–eye–brain disease. The most severe forms of these diseases often have a fetal presentation.

Heterotopias

Periventricular heterotopias are abnormally placed groups of neurons that have failed to start or complete their migration. These often cause seizures and may be associated with intellectual impairment. Failure of migration results in the neurons remaining in the ventricular region, under the ependymal cells that line the ventricle, generating periventricular or subependymal heterotopias (see Fig. 24.18.5b). These may be the result of single gene disorders such as a mutation in the filamin A (*FLNA*) gene on the X chromosome. Filamin protein reorganizes the cytoskeleton, consistent with a role in cell migration. Families with periventricular heterotopia have been described in which females are affected whereas affected males appear to die before or soon after birth. Just as in *DCX* mutations, discussed above, it is likely that the heterotopias present in affected females result from X inactivation of the normal *FLNA* gene in those cells, whereas those cells inactivating the abnormal *FLNA* gene migrate normally. Males have only one X chromosome and so all cells will fail to migrate—a lethal phenotype. A failure to complete migration generates subcortical heterotopias, which can be divided into two groups: nodular heterotopias of grey matter are found in association with other migration disorders (see Fig. 24.18.5b) and subcortical laminar heterotopias, also known as band heterotopias, as discussed above.

Nonlissencephalic cortical dysgenesis

Polymicrogyria (microgyria) is the most important type of abnormality in this section. The surface of the cortex can be relatively smooth, resembling pachygyria, because the small gyri pile up on each other to form a thickened cortex. The histology of polymicrogyria varies, suggesting that different migration defects are responsible for the failure to form the normal six-layered cortex, but the aetiology remains poorly understood. In unlayered microgyria, there is a single cell layer between the white matter below the cortex and the molecular layer on the surface. In classic four-layered microgyria, the cortex consists of a molecular layer, an upper dense layer, a layer of low cellular density containing myelinated fibres, and a deep cellular layer. It is suggested that the developmental disturbance occurs near the fifth month of pregnancy. Case reports of polymicrogyria in the infant brain after maternal trauma or asphyxiation during the pregnancy suggest that the abnormality may sometimes be due to failure of cerebral perfusion with resulting hypoxia. The clinical manifestations of polymicrogyria depend on the location and extent of the abnormalities. Small patches may be found incidentally in the absence of symptoms, but there may be involvement of the whole cortex, resulting in developmental delay. A substantial proportion of cases have a genetic basis, so referral for a genetics opinion is recommended.

Other disorders of cortical development

Cortical microdysgenesis or dyplasia

Microscopic abnormalities of cortical structure have been described in the brains of patients with epilepsy or learning difficulties, and have also been reported in autism, schizophrenia, and fetal alcohol syndrome. These abnormalities include persistence of the subpial layer, aggregates of large neurons in the plexiform zone, a fragmented appearance of the superficial neuronal layers, excess ectopic cells in the cortex, and excess numbers of cells in the molecular layer. Their causes and the extent to which these cause global abnormalities in brain function remain unknown, as such abnormalities can be found in normal individuals. However, they do cause cortical excitability in generalized epilepsy, and localized temporal lobe cortical dysgenesis might lead to dyslexia. Focal cortical dysplasias are an important cause of early onset seizures that may be focal or generalized (Fig. 24.18.6) and patients with refractory epilepsy should therefore have the best possible neuroimaging even if they have generalized seizures.

Disorders of cortical organization

Once migration is complete, the neurons begin the complex tasks of elaborating dendrites and axons, and forming synapses to establish the connectivity required for correct functioning of the human brain. These tasks remain poorly understood, but there is increasing interest in their abnormalities because they may represent important causes of epilepsy and developmental delay. Although subtle compared with the gross anatomical defects created by the migration disorders, it is likely that this group of disorders will become increasingly well recognized as imaging and other investigative techniques improve.

Malformations of posterior fossa structures

Once regionalization has been completed, the developmental processes that generate the cerebellum and brain stem are distinct from those responsible for cortical development. Consequently, although some genetic mutations result in abnormalities in both anterior

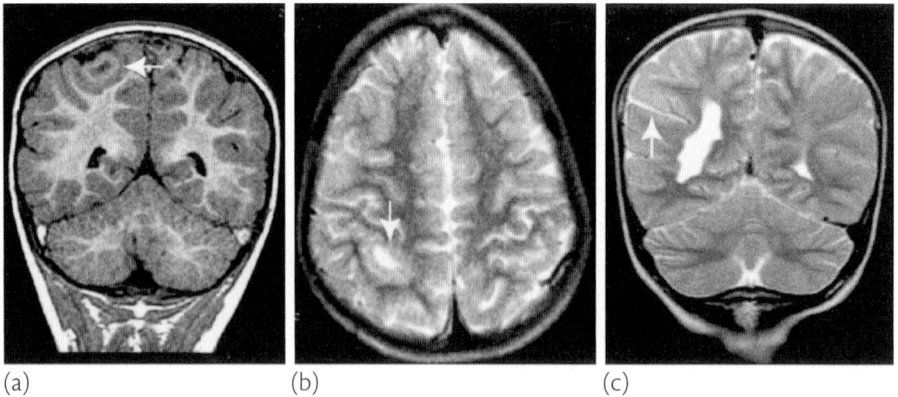

Fig. 24.18.6 (a) Cortical dysplasia in a boy aged 4 years. Focal seizures started at 1 year of age and consisted of a giggle, flexion of the left arm, and a vacant stare. T_1-weighted coronal MRI shows cortical dysplasia in the right parietal region (arrow). (b) The same patient. On T_2-weighted axial MRI, the cortical dysplasia is marked with an arrow. (c) Cortical dysplasia in a boy aged 3 years. Seizures commenced at 9 months of age and consisted of daytime absences and nocturnal generalized tonic–clonic seizures. A T_2-weighted coronal MRI shows an abnormal fissure in the cortex on the right (arrow). The right lateral ventricle is abnormal in size and shape.

and posterior fossae (e.g. *RELN* and the type II lissencephalies), there are a number of specific posterior fossa malformations. These are now identified using prenatal ultrasonography and MRI, which is superior to CT for showing posterior fossa structures. Recently, cilia-related genes have been implicated in several congenital disorders characterized by cerebellar abnormalities such as Joubert syndrome, Meckel–Gruber syndrome, Bardet–Biedl syndrome, and orofaciodigital syndrome, suggesting that cilia may play a role in cerebellar development.

Aplasia and hypoplasia of the cerebellum

This is a heterogeneous group of conditions that affect cerebellar development in various ways; total cerebellar aplasia is exceptional and unilateral hypoplasia occurs infrequently. Neocerebellar aplasia (Fig. 24.18.7a) is characterized by a small vermis and extreme smallness or absence of the cerebellar hemispheres, except for persistent flocculus. There may be associated anomalies in the brain stem such as dysplasia of the inferior olivary nucleus and other brain-stem nuclei.

Some cases are associated with genetic syndromes, many of which are poorly defined. Recent attention has been drawn to a group of disorders classified under the broad headings of pontocerebellar hypoplasia or olivopontocerebellar atrophy. Pontocerebellar hypoplasia is found in carbohydrate-deficient glycoprotein syndrome type 1 and cerebromuscular dystrophies (Walker–Warburg syndrome, Fukuyama syndrome, and muscle–eye–brain diseases—see above). There are at least two types of autosomal recessive pontocerebellar hypoplasia (types I and II). MRI demonstrates cerebellar hypoplasia together with a hypoplastic ventral pons. It has been speculated that some of these cases are due to mutations of *engrailed* genes which are essential for the development of the segmental precursors of the pons and cerebellum in the mouse brain.

The Chiari malformations

There are four types: the most common, Chiari II malformation, is usually associated with a meningomyelocele and is dealt with earlier under neural tube defects. In Chiari I malformation there is downward displacement of the lower cerebellum, including the tonsils. It rarely causes symptoms in childhood but may be associated with

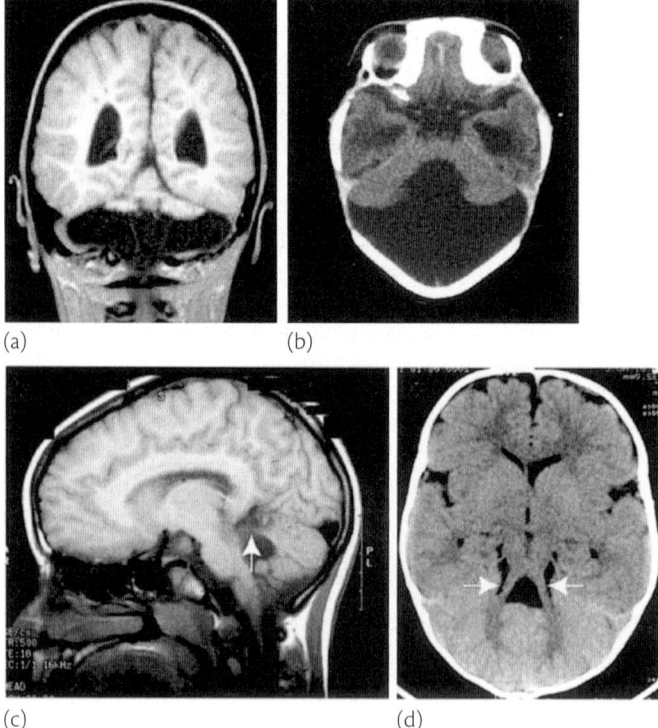

Fig. 24.18.7 (a) Cerebellar hypoplasia in a boy aged 5 years, who was born preterm at 26 weeks of gestation, with no neurological problems apart from absence seizures of unknown cause. T_1-weighted coronal MRI shows almost complete absence of the cerebellar hemispheres and hypoplasia of the cerebellar vermis. (b) Dandy–Walker malformation in a 1-year-old girl. Axial CT shows absence of the roof of the fourth ventricle. A large cyst is continuous with the fourth ventricle and fills the posterior fossa. (c) Joubert syndrome in a girl aged 10 years. T_1-weighted sagittal MRI shows that the superior cerebellar peduncles run horizontally (arrow) and the cerebellar vermis is absent. (d) Joubert syndrome in a girl aged 9 months who is hypotonic and visually unresponsive, with 'wandering' nystagmus. Axial CT shows the superior cerebellar peduncles (arrows) run horizontally and stand out because of the absence of the vermis ('molar tooth sign'). The prominent fourth ventricle has a typical shape (sometimes looking like a 'bat's wing').

hydrocephalus and syringomyelia. Chiari III malformation consists of downward displacement of the cerebellum into a posterior encephalocele and Chiari IV malformation is a form of cerebellar hypoplasia.

Abnormalities of the vermis

Dandy–Walker malformation and Dandy–Walker variant

The Dandy–Walker malformation (Fig. 24.18.7b) consists of the following triad:

- complete or partial agenesis of the vermis

- cystic dilatation of the fourth ventricle

- enlarged posterior fossa with upward displacement of lateral sinuses, tentorium, and torcula, while a variant form lacks posterior fossa enlargement

There is an association between Dandy–Walker malformations and chromosomal abnormalities including trisomies 13 and 18, and the malformation is listed as a feature of 80 syndromes in the London Dysmorphology Database. Prenatal ultrasound studies may reveal the abnormality at 18 weeks gestation, 3 weeks after the development of the inferior vermis, and show that most fetuses with the Dandy–Walker malformation have other anomalies including ventriculomegaly, holoprosencephaly, agenesis of the corpus callosum, occipital encephaloceles, abnormal migration of the inferior olive, and structural heart defects. Fetal MRI may be helpful in clarifying the nature of the brain anomaly.

The clinical features of the Dandy–Walker malformation range from severe learning disabilities and physical impairments to normal development. The abnormality is often recognized only when the infant is investigated for signs of hydrocephalus, which may not become apparent until late in the first year of life, or later in life with learning difficulties. Cerebellar signs tend not to be prominent, but cranial nerve palsies, nystagmus, and truncal ataxia have been described.

Radiological diagnosis is relatively straightforward for the complete Dandy–Walker malformation, although without sagittal MRI the variant may be difficult to distinguish from a prominent cisterna magna or a retrocerebellar arachnoid cyst.

Joubert syndrome

This rare autosomal recessive disorder is characterized by brain-stem and cerebellar malformations. It is genetically heterogeneous and several genes encoding cilial and basal-body proteins have now been implicated (e.g. *RPGRIP1L*). Features include absence or hypoplasia of the posteroinferior part of the cerebellar vermis. In some cases, enlargement of the fourth ventricle and the cisterna magna has been reported. Microscopically, heterotopias have been seen in the cerebellar hemispheres with fragmentation of the dentate nuclei. Brain-stem abnormalities include absence of pyramidal decussation, abnormal inferior olivary nuclei, and subtle dysplasias in the nuclei of the solitary and descending trigeminal tracts and of the dorsal columns.

The common clinical abnormalities are marked hypotonia (particularly in the neonatal period and infancy), poor balance (walking occurs in 50% of cases and is late—at approximately 4 years), and variable cognitive problems (some affected children are unable to talk but others develop language, read, and write). The associated abnormalities are dysmorphic facial features, episodic hyperpnoea and/or apnoea in up to 75% of patients (most marked in the neonatal period), eye abnormalities, and microcystic renal disease.

Typically CT or MRI shows the 'molar tooth' sign in the axial plane, which consists of: (1) a deeper than normal posterior interpeduncular fossa, (2) prominent or thickened superior cerebellar peduncles, and (3) vermian hypoplasia or dysplasia. MRI in the coronal and axial plane shows clefting of the vermis; in the sagittal plane it shows an abnormally shaped and rostrally placed fourth ventricle (Fig. 24.18.7c, d).

Complex malformations of the CNS

Thus far we have presented the disorders of cortical development resulting from defects in a single part of the developmental process. However, this is oversimplistic, because many of these parts occur simultaneously (and will therefore all be affected by teratogens or other extrinsic perturbations) or rely on the timely completion of a prior step for their initiation. As a result there are a number of well-recognized cortical malformations that cannot be ascribed precisely to abnormalities in one step or the major steps in development and result in more complex defects.

Agenesis of the corpus callosum

The true prevalence of this abnormality is not accurately known because it can be present without any symptoms. Estimated prevalence has varied from 0.05 per 10 000 to 70 per 10 000 in the general population, increasing to 230 per 10 000 in children with developmental disabilities. In the normal developing brain the first fibres cross the midline at 11 to 12 weeks to form the corpus callosum, which extends back in the occipital direction to assume the adult form by 18 to 20 weeks. There are two types of 'true' callosal agenesis: defects in which axons are unable to cross the midline and defects in which the commissural axons or their parent cell bodies fail to form in the cerebral cortex. The former is probably the most common type, although the latter is seen in the Walker–Warburg syndrome and other types of lissencephaly. There are also two secondary types: absence associated with major malformations of the embryonic forebrain, such as holoprosencephaly, and degeneration or atrophy, as is seen in some syndromes in which the corpus callosum is thinned but not shortened. When agenesis of the corpus callosum is the only lesion there may be no symptoms, although tests of perception and language may demonstrate disturbances of integration of hemispherical function. However, even if there is no clearly defined syndrome, some patients have learning disabilities, seizures, or cerebral palsy.

Isolated callosal agenesis may be inherited as an autosomal recessive, autosomal dominant, or X-linked recessive trait. It has also been associated with several chromosomal rearrangements, including trisomy 18, trisomy 13, many deletions and duplications, and more than 20 autosomal and many X-linked malformation syndromes, e.g. Mowat–Wilson syndrome and Pitt–Hopkins syndrome. Callosal agenesis may be seen in fetal alcohol syndrome and is often seen in metabolic disorders including glutaric aciduria type 2, peroxisomal disorders, pyruvate dehydrogenase deficiency, and nonketotic hyperglycinaemia.

Diagnosis is based on brain imaging (Fig. 24.18.8). The abnormalities that can be found are widely spaced parallel lateral ventricles, colpocephaly (enlarged posterior horns of the lateral ventricles), upward displacement of the third ventricle, absent callosal tissue or midline dorsal cyst. Prenatal ultrasonography allows diagnosis from week 20 of gestation. After birth MRI is best because it gives sagittal views of the corpus callosum. The scan should be carefully reviewed for other midline anomalies (such as

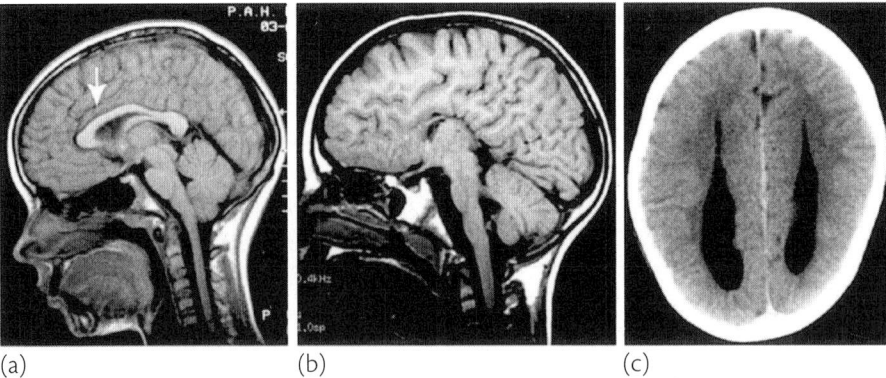

Fig. 24.18.8 (a) Normal brain in a girl aged 2 years. A T_1-weighted sagittal MRI shows normal corpus callosum and cingulate gyrus (arrow). (b) Agenesis of the corpus callosum in a girl aged 6 years who has microcephaly and moderate learning difficulties. A T_1-weighted sagittal MRI shows absence of the corpus callosum and of the cingulate gyrus, which normally runs parallel to the corpus callosum. (c) Agenesis of the corpus callosum in the same girl as in (b). Axial CT shows typical appearance of parallel lateral cerebral ventricles, with divergence of the anterior horns of the ventricles and colpocephaly (dilated posterior part of the lateral ventricles).

agenesis of the septum pellucidum) or generalized defects (such as lissencephaly). The eyes may show optic nerve hypoplasia (as seen in septo-optic dysplasia) or choroidal lacunae (as seen in Aicardi syndrome). Neonates with seizures or other significant neurological problems may have an underlying metabolic disorder, e.g. non-ketotic hyperglycinaemia (raised cerebrospinal fluid glycine) or a mitochondrial disease (raised cerebrospinal fluid lactate).

Porencephaly

The term 'porencephaly' is often used indiscriminately for all large cavities in the brains of infants, but should be reserved for circumscribed hemispherical necrosis that occurs *in utero* before the adult features of the hemisphere are fully developed (Fig. 24.18.9b). The developmental origin of such lesions is shown by their smooth walls and disturbances in the development of the adjoining cortex. These disturbances may take the form of polymicrogyria or local distortion of the gyral pattern. In contrast, areas of damage resulting from insults in the terminal phase of the pregnancy or in postnatal life have irregular shaggy walls, and do not alter the gyral environment except by atrophy or scarring.

Schizencephaly

This term is used to describe clefts that traverse the full thickness of the hemisphere, connecting the ventricle to the subarachnoid space. They are described as type I or 'fused lip' when the walls of the cleft are opposed, and type II or 'open lip' when cerebrospinal fluid separates the walls (Fig. 24.18.9d). Some authors think that the clefts are usually the result of destruction of brain tissue and the term 'porencephaly' should be used for them all. However, there is now evidence that some of them are genetic, because familial and sporadic cases have been recognized in association with mutations in the homoeobox gene *EMX2*. This is one of the vertebrate homoeobox

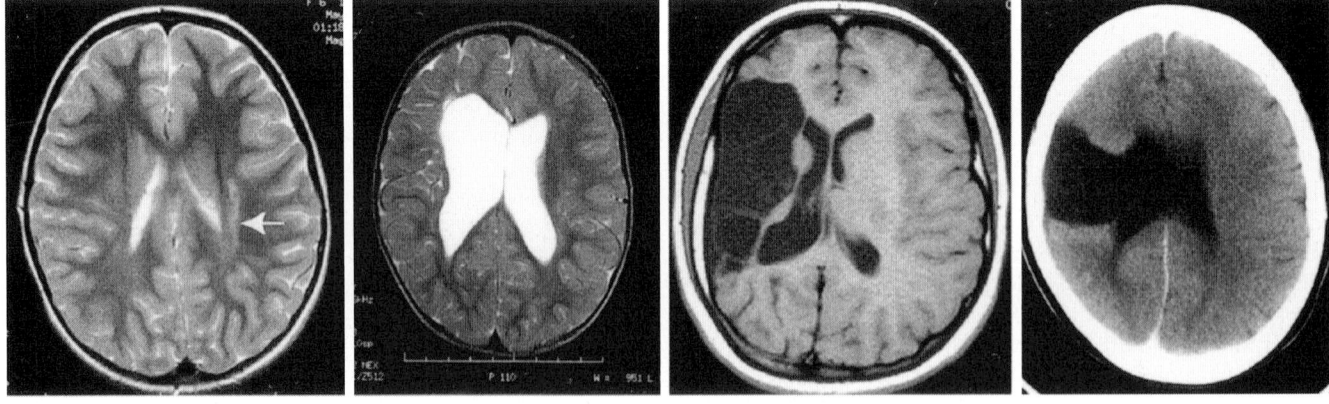

Fig. 24.18.9 (a) Cerebral palsy: spastic diplegia. Probable periventricular leucomalacia in a girl aged 6 years. There was threatened premature labour at 29 and 32 weeks, but she was born at term with no perinatal problems. She walked late with a diplegic gait. T_2-weighted axial MRI shows abnormal signal change lateral to the body of the left lateral ventricle and posterolateral to the posterior horn of the left lateral ventricle (arrow). This is a characteristic distribution of periventricular leucomalacia, but such appearances should be interpreted with caution because there are other causes of white matter abnormalities in children (e.g. the leukodystrophies). (b) Cerebral palsy: left hemiplegia. Porencephalic cyst in a boy aged 18 months. He was delivered by forceps at 38 weeks with no resuscitation, but nasogastric feeding for several days after birth. At 10 months of age he was not moving the left arm normally. T_2-weighted axial MRI shows that there is dilatation of the anterior horn of the right lateral ventricle with loss of overlying cerebral cortex and a small periventricular cyst adjacent to the anterior horn of the right lateral ventricle. These abnormalities may result from periventricular leucomalacia. Such loss of tissue due to *in utero* damage of the developing brain is called a porencephalic cyst. (c) Cerebral palsy: left hemiplegia. Tissue loss in middle cerebral artery territory in a young woman aged 17 years. There were no perinatal problems, reduced movement of the left arm from 6 months of age, nocturnal generalized tonic–clonic seizures from 4 years of age, normal intelligence, abnormal posture of the left hand, and shortening of the left leg. T_1-weighted axial MRI shows that there is a loculated cystic lesion in the distribution of the supply of the middle cerebral artery. Also *ex vacuo* enlargement of the right lateral ventricle and small ipsilateral left hemicranium. (d) Open-lip schizencephaly in a 49-year-old woman. An axial CT scan shows that there is a wide cleft joining the right lateral ventricle to the subarachnoid space.

genes thought to play a role in patterning the forebrain. The clefts are frequently bilateral and symmetrical, the most severe form being large bilateral defects. Even when unilateral, they are often combined with cortical dysplasia of the opposite hemisphere. Clinical features are variable, depending on the site and size of the lesion. Epilepsy is common and there may be hemiplegia, quadriplegia, and learning difficulties of variable degree. The diagnosis is made by MRI.

Hydranencephaly

In this condition the cerebral hemispheres are almost completely replaced by fluid-filled sacs. The defect typically corresponds to the territory of the anterior and middle cerebral arteries, although the major cranial arteries do not usually show evidence of obstruction. Preservation of the temporal lobes and the tentorial parts of the occipital lobes is common, but the extent of preservation of the basal ganglia varies. The cause of hydranencephaly is not clear in many cases. It has been described after intoxication of pregnant women with gas at about week 25 of gestation. It can result from intrauterine infections and has been described in association with a proliferative vasculopathy.

Affected infants may be born after a normal pregnancy and be surprisingly normal on neurological examination for the first few weeks of life. Gradually they become hypertonic and irritable and develop infantile spasms, which is surprising because of the almost complete lack of cerebral hemispheres. The head may enlarge because of associated hydrocephalus. The diagnosis can be made by transillumination of the skull, which lights up like a lantern in a darkened room. Similar appearances can be caused by hydrocephalus with a very thin cortical mantle, so MRI is indicated to confirm the diagnosis. Infants with hydranencephaly often die in a few months, but they may survive for several years and may need a ventriculoperitoneal cerebrospinal fluid shunt if there is progressive hydrocephalus.

Septo-optic dysplasia

This is the association of optic nerve hypoplasia with absence of the septum pellucidum. Disturbances of the hypothalamopituitary axis may occur. The most severely affected patients are blind and have severe learning difficulties. The optic discs have a characteristic double contour: the true disc at the centre is small and there is a peripheral ring about the size of a normal optic nerve head. It is important to search for evidence of endocrine disturbance when these abnormal discs are identified—deficiencies of growth hormone, corticotrophin, luteinizing hormone, and follicle-stimulating hormone have been described, together with hypoglycaemia and diabetes insipidus. Most cases are sporadic, but a homozygous mutation in the homoeobox gene *HESX1* has been identified in familial septo-optic dysplasia. Also some sporadic cases of the more common mild forms of pituitary hypoplasia are associated with heterozygous mutations of the *HESX1* gene.

Disorders of the developing brain caused by extrinsic factors

In the sections above we classified the malformations of the developing brain by their anatomical location, taking advantage of the advances in imaging that have greatly increased our ability to diagnose these conditions. However, clinical problems can arise from extrinsic factors that affect the entire CNS, and we now consider the most important of these—hydrocephalus, alcohol, and infections.

Hydrocephalus

This results from expansion of the ventricles secondary to a block in the normal flow pathway of cerebrospinal fluid. Cerebrospinal fluid is produced by the choroid plexus in the lateral ventricles, from where it flows through the foramen of Munro into the third ventricle and then the fourth ventricle via the aqueduct of Sylvius. It leaves the ventricular system via small openings in the roof of the fourth ventricle, and the foramina of Magendie and Luschka. From here the fluid flows in the subarachnoid space before being reabsorbed into the blood supply via arachnoid villi.

Two major forms of hydrocephalus are recognized: in communicating hydrocephalus the ventricular pathways are clear and a failure of reabsorption (after, for example, a bleed into the subarachnoid space) results in increased cerebrospinal fluid volume; in obstructive or noncommunicating hydrocephalus the blockage occurs at one of the ventricular levels, with expansion of the ventricular system above the block (Fig. 24.18.10). The major clinical sign that results is increasing head circumference following the ventricular enlargement, and this allows the distinction from cases in which increased ventricular size resulting from cerebral atrophy is associated with a decreased head circumference. Learning difficulties can result from both the damage associated with ventricular expansion and other abnormalities related to the underlying cause of the problem.

Sometimes hydrocephalus is genetically determined; stenosis of the aqueduct between the third and fourth ventricles can result from mutations in the cell adhesion molecule L1-CAM. Hydrocephalus then occurs in association with hypoplasia of the corpus callosum, learning difficulties, spastic paraplegia, and adducted thumbs. This X-linked syndrome has been given the unfortunate acronym CRASH syndrome and mutations in L1-CAM are found in as many as 75% of cases with a family history and 15% of apparently isolated cases. The developmental abnormalities of the cerebellum in both the Dandy–Walker syndrome and the Arnold–Chiari malformation (see above) may also be associated with obstructive hydrocephalus. Although treatment via a ventriculoperitoneal shunt can relieve the obstruction, the other problems associated with these abnormalities remain.

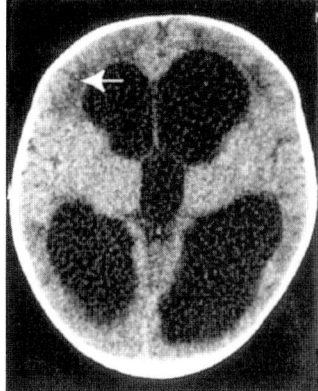

Fig. 24.18.10 Aqueduct stenosis in a boy aged 1 month with a bulging anterior fontanelle and increasing head circumference. Axial CT shows a gross dilatation of the third and lateral ventricles (the fourth ventricle is not shown, but was normal in size). Note the periventricular low density due to transependymal exudation of cerebrospinal fluid under pressure (arrow).

Alcohol

Worldwide, alcohol is one of the most common causes of learning difficulty and neurobehavioural disturbance in young children. The incidence of fetal alcohol syndrome depends on geographical location. An international survey in 1997 found that in the United States of America the incidence per 1000 live births in Seattle was 2.8 and in Cleveland it was 4.6. The combined rate of fetal alcohol syndrome and alcohol-related neurodevelopmental disorder in Seattle was estimated at almost 1% of all live births. Clinical features include microcephaly, structural anomalies of the brain such as partial or complete agenesis of the corpus callosum, cerebellar hypoplasia, and a dysmorphic appearance. These children may have impaired fine motor skills, sensorineural deafness, poor hand–eye coordination, and a poor tandem gait. An alcohol-related neurodevelopmental disorder is also recognized that includes learning difficulties, poor impulse control, problems with social perception, deficits in higher level receptive and expressive language, poor capacity for abstraction, and difficulties with memory, attention, and judgement. The causes of these clinical features remain undefined, but animal studies show that alcohol is likely to affect multiple steps in CNS development including migration and neuronal survival.

Both regular and binge drinking can cause fetal alcohol syndrome and alcohol-related neurodevelopmental disorder. Unlike many other teratogens, alcohol has harmful effects throughout pregnancy and it remains unclear whether any amount of alcohol can be considered safe. Certainly, there is a significant risk of fetal alcohol syndrome associated with high-dose exposure (estimated blood alcohol concentrations of 150 mg/dl or more, at least weekly for several weeks in the first trimester).

Congenital infections

Cytomegalovirus, herpes simplex virus, parvovirus, rubella, syphilis, toxoplasmosis, and varicella virus are all recognized as teratogens, with primary infection rather than reinfection of the mother during pregnancy being more likely to result in congenital infection. Congenital infection should always be considered in the differential diagnosis of microcephaly. Intracranial calcification identified on cranial ultrasonography or CT (calcification is not picked up well by MRI) during the investigation of developmental delay or seizures suggests congenital infection, especially cytomegalovirus or toxoplasmosis. Ophthalmological assessment may show chorioretinitis (pigmentary retinopathy) or cataract, the former being characteristic of intrauterine infection by cytomegalovirus or toxoplasmosis. Sensorineural deafness is a common sequel to congenital infection with cytomegalovirus, rubella, and toxoplasmosis.

Cytomegalovirus

Although the risk of maternal–fetal transmission with primary cytomegalovirus infection is as high as 40%, fewer than 10% of infants with intrauterine infection are symptomatic at birth. Of those, approximately 90% have one or more of microcephaly, periventricular calcification, chorioretinitis, optic atrophy, and sensorineural deafness. Of the 90% of infants who are asymptomatic at birth, approximately 15% have sequelae including sensorineural deafness and/or developmental delay.

Herpes simplex virus

Intrauterine infection with herpes simplex virus is rare and neonatal infection acquired at the time of delivery is a more common cause of neurodisability than congenital infection. Congenitally affected infants may have microcephaly, chorioretinitis, and microphthalmos. Neonatal infection may cause meningitis and encephalitis with resulting neurological damage. The risks of perinatally acquired infection may be reduced by appropriate obstetric intervention (such as delivery by caesarean section for women with active genital lesions resulting from herpes simplex virus) and by treatment of affected neonates with aciclovir.

Rubella

The classic triad of defects associated with congenital rubella syndrome is sensorineural deafness, congenital heart disease, and eye abnormalities (retinopathy, cataracts, microphthalmos, and congenital glaucoma). Microcephaly and developmental delay may also occur. The spectrum of defects in an individual child is determined by the stage of pregnancy at which intrauterine infection occurs. The risk of congenital infection is more than 90% before 10 weeks and falls to zero beyond 18 weeks.

Toxoplasmosis

The risk of intrauterine infection with toxoplasmosis increases with the stage of pregnancy at which the mother acquires her primary infection; however, the sequelae of intrauterine infection diminish with advancing gestation. Congenital toxoplasmosis syndrome includes hydrocephalus, intracranial calcification, microcephaly, seizures, and developmental delay. There may also be sensorineural deafness and chorioretinitis with visual impairment.

Varicella

Congenital varicella syndrome follows primary maternal varicella occurring at 1 to 20 weeks of gestation, but the risk of sequelae is small at around 2%. Cataracts and chorioretinitis may occur together with hypoplasia of the optic disc. Microcephaly and porencephaly have been described.

The cerebral palsies

Although the conditions above are classified by aetiology or by anatomy, one important group of disorders is conventionally classified by their clinical presentation. These are the cerebral palsies, defined as a heterogeneous collection of nonprogressive disorders of movement and posture resulting from defects or lesions of the immature brain. Although the underlying causes of the cerebral palsy syndromes are by definition not progressive, the symptoms and signs of cerebral palsy do change with age, e.g. some children who are destined to have major problems with spasticity are initially very hypotonic. In some cases it can therefore be difficult to be sure whether or not a child with suspected cerebral palsy has a progressive underlying disorder. It may be necessary to allow the passage of time and children may be 3 or 4 years old before the diagnosis of cerebral palsy can be made with confidence. Whatever the age at diagnosis, with the recent advances in imaging and genetics it is not satisfactory to label a child with neurological problems as having 'cerebral palsy' and go no further. It is important to determine the type and distribution of the abnormality of motor control and evaluate other potential neurological problems, such as learning difficulties, epilepsy, and hearing or visual loss.

Classification

Patients may be classified according to the type of motor abnormality as follows: spastic, dyskinetic (dystonic or athetoid), ataxic, or hypotonic. The clinical picture is rarely clear cut and individuals may exhibit complex mixtures of motor disability. Patients are then subclassified according to the distribution of motor abnormality—in diplegia the legs are involved more than the arms, in quadriplegia all four limbs are involved, and in hemiplegia just one side of the body is involved.

Epidemiology

Overall, cerebral palsy rates since the mid-1950s have remained remarkably constant at about 2 to 2.5 per 1000 live births, although there have been some fluctuations with time. In 1970 the rate fell to 1.5 in Sweden, Western Australia and Mersey (United Kingdom), rising again in the 1980s. In contrast, cerebral palsy rates stratified by birth weight do show marked changes with time. Most population-based registers have shown increases in rates in infants of very low birth weight (<1500 g) since the 1970s. For instance, in Mersey in the early 1970s the rate in infants of very low birth weight fluctuated around 10 per 1000 live births. In the late 1970s the rate increased sharply to about 50 per 1000 live births, presumably because more children of very low birth weight were surviving with neurological deficits. This increase was seen for all cerebral palsy types. However, to put the increasing cerebral palsy rates in survivors of very low birth weight in perspective, during this time an increasing proportion of patients were also surviving unimpaired. Although the risk of cerebral palsy is higher for preterm infants, the key observation is that most children with cerebral palsy are born at term. Overall rates are therefore determined mainly by the numbers of term infants born with cerebral palsy (and have remained fairly constant), with the much rarer very-low-birth-weight survivors with cerebral palsy having relatively little effect on overall rates.

Aetiology

Although it has been thought that cerebral palsy results primarily from 'birth asphyxia', recent studies suggest that abnormal events around the time of birth play only a limited role. Genetic causes are clearly important because families have been reported in which spastic diplegia and quadriplegia (often with associated learning difficulties) appear to be inherited in autosomal recessive, autosomal dominant, or X-linked recessive patterns. There can be a significant recurrence risk to future children, particularly in populations where consanguineous marriage is relatively common. The highest risk of recurrence is in the category of children with ataxic cerebral palsy. However, there are many conditions that cause ataxia in children, making it important to search for an underlying cause before giving genetic advice, rather than to 'lump' this group together and give an overall recurrence risk.

Other possible causes include maternal iodine deficiency in early pregnancy which may cause endemic cretinism (spastic diplegia and deafness). Abnormal thyroid function in pregnancy may play a role in developed countries. Exposure to toxins during pregnancy may cause cerebral palsy—recognized examples are methylmercury, alcohol, and carbon monoxide poisoning. Viral infections and some fetal malformation syndromes discussed above can cause cerebral palsy. Finally, postnatal causes include CNS infections, accidental and nonaccidental head injuries, cerebrovascular accidents, and hypoxia (suffocation, near drowning).

Factors shown to increase the risk of cerebral palsy

The rate of cerebral palsy among neonatal survivors born very prematurely is up to 30 times higher than among those born at term. Cerebral ultrasound scans performed in newborn babies have shown that the strongest predictor of cerebral palsy in these infants is periventricular leucomalacia. This term is used for abnormal echolucency, often associated with cystic change, which is found particularly in the white matter dorsolateral to the lateral ventricles (see Fig. 24.18.9a). Babies born small for their gestational age are also at increased risk of cerebral palsy and the risk increases with the degree of birth weight deficit. The underlying mechanism is not clear and it should be noted that most small-for-date infants do not have cerebral palsy. Finally, the prevalence of cerebral palsy is much higher in twins than in singletons, particularly in those who survive after the other twin has died *in utero* and in monochorionic twins. The risk rises with the number of fetuses carried. Causes include low birth weight, congenital anomalies, cord entanglement, and abnormal vascular connections.

The role of birth asphyxia

An important and controversial question that has significant medicolegal implications is the role of birth asphyxia in cerebral palsy. Although there may be some cases caused by intrapartum events that are preventable, these are likely to be rare. The best evidence for this comes from studies examining the impact of intensive electronic monitoring of the fetal heart rate during labour. These studies have found an increase in caesarean section rates and a reduced rate of neonatal seizures. There was, however, no impact on the rates of cerebral palsy. In addition, the proportion of cerebral palsy cases associated with intrapartum events has been estimated by several epidemiological studies to be only about 10%. Currently, then, it is likely that many cases of cerebral palsy are wrongly attributed to an acute event during labour. In 1999, a consensus statement for the International Cerebral Palsy Task Force outlined a template for defining a causal relationship between acute intrapartum events and cerebral palsy. The statement emphasized the difficulty of retrospectively identifying the antenatal causes of cerebral palsy in the individual case and the nonspecific nature of the clinical signs that lead to the suspicion of fetal hypoxia in labour.

Brain imaging in children with cerebral palsy

The most common lesion in preterm infants is periventricular leucomalacia, which is necrosis of periventricular white matter in the watershed regions dorsal and lateral to the lateral ventricle (see Fig. 24.18.9a). This is said to be characteristic of damage in the early third trimester. In term infants there are a number of different findings, said to occur only in infants born at or near term. These are infarcts in the arterial border zones in the parasagittal regions, leading to cortical and subcortical injury, bilateral lesions of the basal ganglia and the thalamus, areas of subcortical leucomalacia, and multicystic leucomalacia (replacement of the brain tissue by fluid-filled cysts). Children with hemiplegias are sometimes found to have periventricular leucomalacia, porencephalic cysts (see Fig. 24.18.9b), or cortical/subcortical lesions in the middle cerebral artery territory distribution (see Fig. 24.18.9c). The lesions tend to be unilateral, but bilateral lesions are seen. Rarely they may have schizencephaly (see Fig. 24.18.9d), focal pachygyria, or focal heterotopia.

Clinical approach to diagnosis and genetic counselling

Assessing the nervous system in children

History

General

The importance of the history cannot be overemphasized. Children may give a history themselves, but usually the parents or carers are an essential source of information, amplified by teachers, therapists, and other health professionals.

Past history

The pregnancy details are important. Significant events in the first trimester may include a threatened miscarriage, hyperemesis, or a viral infection, or the mother may have been taking medication. Later there may have been unsatisfactory fetal growth or reduced fetal movements. The perinatal history is relevant, including weeks of gestation at delivery, and details of labour, birth weight, and head circumference. In the neonatal period the infant may have required treatment for early hypoglycaemia, seizures, breathing, or feeding difficulties. A developmental history is essential—particular areas of concern in infants are lack of social response, absence of a social smile, poor fixing and following of the eyes, and lack of symmetrical organized limb movements. Later a characteristic pattern of delayed development may emerge, e.g. global delay is found in the most severe brain abnormalities or there may be mainly motor delay in the milder forms of cerebral palsy.

Family and social history

A three-generation family tree is required, with details of consanguinity, epilepsy, motor disorders, and learning disabilities. Considerable effort may be needed to obtain relevant facts—some families conceal or do not know about relatives with severe disability, perhaps because they are in institutions. Social factors are important in determining the environment in which the child grows up and they also determine the quality of care available for a child with significant disability.

Examination

Observation of spontaneous activity is essential. It may be helpful to use toys, bricks, beads for threading, paper, and crayons. The quality and symmetry of spontaneous movements should be noted and also any abnormal movements. If possible it is best to assess muscle power by watching the child run, jump, and climb stairs. Fine motor function can be assessed while the child is drawing or threading beads. The conventional examination of the nervous system may be difficult in infants or young children, e.g. examination of the cranial nerves should be made a game by using a toy to observe eye movements and by encouraging the child to smile, whistle, close the jaw tight, stick out the tongue, and so on. The examiner may need to adapt the order of events or even come back later—a useful assessment cannot be made if an infant is deeply asleep or upset and crying.

Developmental assessment may be undertaken using one of the standardized schedules, such as the Bailey Scales of Infant Development or the Denver Developmental Screening Test. Later the Wechsler Preschool and Primary Scale of Intelligence (WPPSI) and the Wechsler Intelligence Scale for Children (Revised) (WISC-R) may be used, usually by a psychologist.

Dysmorphic features are particularly relevant in the context of a suspected abnormality of the nervous system. There may be birthmarks (port-wine stain in Sturge–Weber syndrome or midline skin abnormalities such as hairy patches or dimples over the spine in neural tube defects). Other important skin abnormalities may appear in infancy or early childhood. Examples are the pale ash-leaf patches, shagreen patches, and angiofibromas of the face ('adenoma sebaceum'), which are found in tuberous sclerosis, or the café-au-lait patches and axillary freckling found in neurofibromatosis type I.

A full eye examination is essential. In babies it may be necessary to dilate the eyes and come back to perform fundoscopy while the child is feeding (and therefore preoccupied!). Indirect ophthalmoscopy by an experienced ophthalmologist is probably best. There may be abnormalities of the iris (such as colobomas in trisomy 13 and CHARGE syndrome, Lisch nodules in neurofibromatosis type I, or Kayser–Fleischer rings in Wilson's disease). Pale hypoplastic optic nerve heads are seen in septo-optic dysplasia and other congenital and acquired conditions. Significant retinal abnormalities include the chorioretinitis seen in congenital toxoplasmosis or cytomegalovirus infections and the retinal 'lacunae' seen in Aicardi syndrome.

Growth should be assessed by measuring weight, length (height), and head circumference, and plotting them on up-to-date growth charts. The head circumference should be related to the age of the child and to the other measurements. Changes with time may be significant, e.g. after a severe perinatal insult the head circumference may initially be in the normal range and then fall progressively further below the expected centile line in the first few months of life, so dating the insult to the brain.

Investigations

Cranial MRI is the cornerstone of investigations in children or adults with suspected disorders of CNS development. It is important to discuss the investigation with a neuroradiologist because special imaging sequences not normally performed may be required to visualize relevant abnormalities, e.g. subependymal nodules in tuberous sclerosis. Infants and young children may require sedation or anaesthesia for the procedure. CT does not provide the resolution of CNS structure obtained with MRI, but may be valuable if intracerebral calcification is suspected (as in tuberous sclerosis or cytomegalovirus infection).

Further investigations will depend on the specific diagnosis in question. Metabolic disorders can cause structural abnormalities in the developing CNS and routine investigations that may be appropriate include plasma and urine amino acids, together with urine organic acids. In addition, further specific investigations may be indicated, e.g. in suspected Zellweger's syndrome which is associated with pachygyria and caused by abnormalities of very-long-chain fatty acid metabolism.

Developmental anomalies of the CNS are seen in many chromosomal disorders and so a karyotype is an important investigation. The diagnostic yield of 'molecular karytyping', using array-CGH (microarray-based comparative genomic hybridization) or high-density SNP arrays is significantly higher than with routine light microscopy. Fluorescent *in situ* hybridization studies of chromosome regions using labelled probes that will bind (hybridize) to specific gene sequences may detect microdeletion syndromes such as in Miller–Dieker syndrome by revealing an absence of fluorescent labelling on one of the pair of chromosomes.

These investigations may point to a diagnosis for which one or more genes have been shown to be responsible. A detailed clinical work-up is important, because the choice of which gene, of the approximately 23 500 genes in the human genome, to interrogate is based on the clinical assessment. Sequencing genes is often an expensive and laborious investigation. However, these investigations may allow confirmation of the diagnosis and accurate assessment of risks for other family members following extended family testing.

It is important to remember that molecular genetic techniques are improving very rapidly and new tests will become available. Next generation sequencing technologies are likely to transform the diagnosis of genetically heterogeneous conditions such as cerebellar hypoplasia in the forseeable future. It is therefore valuable to take blood in order to extract and store DNA (or establish a lymphoblastoid cell line) if no precise diagnosis can be reached, especially if life expectancy is short. Immediately after death it may be appropriate to obtain a muscle or liver biopsy to help establish a diagnosis. Skin may be also obtained at this time to establish a fibroblast culture enabling further genetic and biochemical testing. Later other tissues can be frozen if a full postmortem examination is performed. The ability to perform new tests many years after the death of the index case may be extremely valuable to other family members concerned about risks to their own offspring.

Risk assessment, genetic counselling, and prenatal diagnosis

Many families request genetic advice regarding a developmental disorder of the nervous system and they usually have four questions in mind:

◆ What is it?

◆ Why did it happen?

◆ Will it happen again?

◆ What can be done to reduce the chance of it happening again, or to detect it if it does?

If it is possible to make a specific genetic diagnosis, e.g. by identifying a pathogenic mutation, these questions can often be answered very accurately. In contrast, in the absence of a specific diagnosis, genetic advice is usually limited to empirical estimates. It is important to note that providing accurate genetic advice about developmental anomalies of the nervous system is a challenging task and that errors have far-reaching consequences for the families concerned. Referral for specialist advice by geneticists is strongly recommended.

Prenatal diagnosis and termination of affected pregnancies is only one of a range of reproductive options open to parents at increased risk of having children with neurodevelopmental abnormalities, but for many couples it is the option of choice. When a specific diagnosis has been made and a chromosomal anomaly, genetic mutation, or biochemical defect has been identified, it is usually possible to offer prenatal diagnosis by chorionic villous sampling at 11 to 12 weeks' gestation in a future pregnancy. Detailed ultrasonography may be helpful in some instances such as suspected neural tube defects. Ultrasonography has the potential to detect some structural anomalies but it does not provide information about key aspects of neurodevelopment, such as cognition, behaviour, vision, or hearing, and these limitations need to be discussed with parents. Although ultrasonography remains the initial investigation of choice for evaluating the fetus *in utero*, fast MRI is increasingly being used to image the fetal brain if there is concern about the ultrasound images. MRI provides better images of CNS abnormalities and is not limited by interference from bony structures, so that posterior fossa abnormalities can be seen. *In utero* MRI is becoming increasingly valuable in antenatal counselling.

For most developmental disorders of the nervous system, preimplantation genetic diagnosis (PGD) is not yet feasible, but with the development of preimplantation genetic haplotyping, the range of genetic disorders amenable to PGD is increasing rapidly and up-to-date advice should be sought. For a condition following mendelian inheritance, the option of donor gametes could be discussed. For conditions with a strong environmental component, it is imperative that measures are taken to minimize the risk of exposure in a future pregnancy, such as periconceptual supplementation with high-dose folate, which has been shown to reduce the risk of recurrence of neural tube defects (see above).

Further reading

Aicardi J (1998). *Diseases of the nervous system in childhood*, 2nd edition. MacKeith Press, London.

Baraitser M (1997). *The genetics of neurological disorders*, 3rd edition. Oxford University Press, Oxford.

Baraitser M, Winter R (2005). *The Baraitser–Winter neurogenetics database*. London Medical Databases. RAmEx Ars Medica, Los Angeles.

Barkovitch AJ (2005). *Pediatric neuroimaging*, 4th edition. Lippincott-Raven, Philadelphia, PA.

Cox J, *et al.* (2006). What primary microcephaly can tell us about brain growth. *Trends Mol Med* **12**, 358–66.

Ferretti P, *et al.* (2006). *Embryos, genes and birth defects*, 2nd revised edition. John Wiley & Sons Ltd, Chichester.

Firth HV, Hurst JA, Hall JG (2005). *Oxford desk reference clinical genetics*. Oxford University Press, Oxford.

Friede RL (1989). *Developmental neuropathology*, 2nd (revised and expanded) edition. Springer-Verlag, Berlin.

Gleeson JG, Walsh CA (2000). Neuronal migration disorders: from genetic diseases to developmental mechanisms. *Trends Neurosci*, **23**, 352–9.

Govaert P, de Vries LS (1997). *An atlas of neonatal brain sonography*. Clinics in Developmental Medicine No. 141–2. MacKeith Press, London.

Griffiths PD, *et al.* (2006). Imaging the fetal spine using in utero MR: diagnostic accuracy and impact on management. *Pediatr Radiol*, **36**, 927–33.

Maclennan A, for the International Cerebral Palsy Task Force (1999). A template for defining a causal relationship between acute intrapartum events and cerebral palsy: international consensus statement. *BMJ*, **319**, 1054–9.

Miller G, Clark GD (1998). *The cerebral palsies. Causes, consequences, and management.* (eds) Butterworth-Heinemann, Boston, MA.

Mochida GH, Walsh CA (2004). Genetic basis of developmental malformations of the cerebral cortex (review). *Arch Neurol*, **61**, 637–40.

Stanley F, Blair E, Alberman E (2000). *Cerebral palsies: epidemiology and causal pathways.* Clinics in Developmental Medicine No. 151. MacKeith Press, London.

Thornton GK, Woods CG (2009). Primary microcephaly: do all roads lead to Rome? *Trends Genet*, Nov; **25**(11), 501–10. [Epub 2009 Oct 21.]

Wallis D, Muenke M (2000). Mutations in holoprosencephaly. *Human Mutation*, **16**, 99–108.

Websites

National Center for Biotechnology Information. *GeneReviews*. http://www.ncbi.nlm.nih.gov/sites/GeneTests/review?db=GeneTests

National Center for Biotechnology Information. *Online Mendelian Inheritance in Man (OMIM)*. http://www.ncbi.nlm.nih.gov/sites/entrez?db=OMIM

Acquired metabolic disorders and the nervous system

Neil Scolding and C.D. Marsden

Essentials

A very wide range of systemic disorders of metabolism can have neurological consequences. Conditions of particular note include the following:

Major organ diseases

Anoxic brain damage—cardiac arrest is a relatively common cause of global cerebral anoxia; other causes include suffocation, anaesthetic catastrophes, drowning, or acute carbon monoxide poisoning. The consequences depend on the duration of anoxia: (1) brief—manifests as syncope; (2) longer lasting (up to perhaps 5 min)—there is rapid loss of consciousness, generalized fits, dilated pupils, and bilateral extensor plantar responses; long-term course and prognosis are unpredictable; (3) more sustained (longer than a few minutes)—permanent or prolonged but reversible brain damage.

Other conditions—these include (1) hepatic failure—acute hepatic coma and chronic hepatic encephalopathy; (2) respiratory disease—chronic respiratory failure causing hypercarbic encephalopathy; obstructive sleep apnoea; (3) renal failure—neurological manifestations include uraemic encephalopathy, symmetrical sensorimotor polyneuropathy, myopathy, dialysis disequilibrium syndrome, dialysis dementia; (4) critical illness polyneuropathy.

Endocrine disorders

Many endocrine disorders can have neurological manifestations, including: (1) Phaeochromocytoma—anxiety, headache; complications of accelerated phase hypertension. (2) Cushing's syndrome—proximal myopathy, psychiatric disorders, direct consequences of pituitary tumour. (3) Adrenal insufficiency—adrenal crisis may manifest with depressed consciousness and/or neurological complications of hypoglycaemia or hyponatraemia. (4) Thyroid disease—thyrotoxicosis can cause myopathy, chorea and mania; hypothyroidism can present with a confusional state or coma and is often associated with a myopathy. (5) Diabetes mellitus—complications include mononeuritis, diabetic amyotrophy, peripheral neuropathy, autonomic neuropathy, and those due to hypoglycaemia.

Ionic abnormalities

(1) Hyponatraemia—nonspecific symptoms may appear when the plasma sodium drops below about 120 mmol/litre; fits and coma are usually associated with plasma sodium values below 110 mmol/litre. The condition and its treatment (see Chapter 21.2.1) can be associated with central pontine myelinolysis. (2) Hypernatraemia—may cause drowsiness or (in severe cases) coma; (3) Hypercalcaemia—muscle weakness, lassitude, and a mild encephalopathy are common; (4) Hypocalcaemia—causes neuromuscular irritability, tetany with a Chvostek's sign, and mild encephalopathy; severe hypocalcaemia may cause fits, psychosis, and coma.

Alcohol

Effects of alcohol on the nervous system, aside from those that are acute and transient, include (1) delirium tremens—an agitated confused state, with signs of sympathetic overactivity, that typically develops rapidly several days after ethanol abstinence in chronic abusers; (2) Wernicke–Korsakoff syndrome—classically manifesting with confusion, ophthalmoplegia and ataxia; treatment with thiamine should be given on suspicion; (3) peripheral neuropathy; (4) cerebellar degeneration; (5) dementia; (6) myopathy.

*Acknowledgement: Much of the late Professor C D Marsden's original chapter structure and text for the third edition has been retained.

Introduction

There are (at least) three common prejudices concerning acquired metabolic diseases and their central and peripheral nervous system complications: that they are boring, and belong only in books of lists and tables; that they are rare; and that little if anything has changed on the subject for the past half-century or so. Most neurologists are not excessively moved by a litany of the neurological complications of diabetes mellitus; and it is indeed true that the descriptions of the clinical features of Wernicke's and Korsakoff's syndromes have not really been bettered—i.e. significantly altered—since these eponymous disorders were first identified. However, the dramatic, serious, and not uncommon neurological picture of central pontine myelinolysis and its still uncertain metabolic cause(s); the emergence of new(-ish) disorders such as superficial siderosis and E-induced water intoxication; the changing face and context of other disorders—iatrogenic Cushing's syndrome, chemotherapy-induced nutritional and metabolic disruption; all these help to emphasize the importance and impact of acquired neurometabolic diseases. This chapter aims to deal with these, or to point elsewhere in this text to where the others are covered.

Metabolic complications of systemic disease

Cardiovascular disease: anoxic brain damage

Cerebral anoxia is caused by insufficient cerebral blood flow, reduced oxygen availability, reduced oxygen carriage by the blood, or metabolic interference with the utilization of oxygen, alone or in combination. Thus, cardiac arrest is a relatively common cause of global cerebral anoxia; others as diverse as suffocation, anaesthetic catastrophes, drowning, or acute carbon monoxide poisoning can produce similar results.

Brief global ischaemic anoxia causes syncope. If the episode is prolonged, myoclonic jerks or tonic–clonic seizures may occur. Still more protracted insults may precipitate a period of confusion and residual amnesia.

More lasting acute severe anoxia rapidly leads to loss of consciousness, generalized fits, dilated pupils, and bilateral extensor plantar responses. Periods of anoxia up to perhaps 5 min may cause transient coma with recovery of consciousness. Delayed postanoxic encephalopathy, characterized pathologically by demyelination in the hemispheres and in the basal ganglia, may follow within 1 to 2 weeks, often commencing with increasing irritability, apathy, and confusion. Frank dementia may emerge, or an amnesic syndrome in less severe cases, and there may also be pseudobulbar palsy and other pyramidal signs, gait ataxia, and incontinence, and/or an akinetic–rigid syndrome with or without dystonia. Some patients may be severely disabled by action myoclonus. The course and prognosis in prolonged cerebral anoxia are most unpredictable: residual deficits may be permanent; slow (months to years) but often considerable recovery may emerge; or the condition may progress occur over weeks to months.

Yet more sustained oxygen deprivation—more than a few minutes—results in permanent or prolonged but reversible brain damage. Irreversible coma may be accompanied by flaccidity, loss of all reflex function except heart beat and tendon jerks, fixed, dilated pupils and a flat electroencephalogram. (Drugs and hypothermia may also cause a flat electroencephalogram, but recovery is possible.) Such patients may be said to have suffered irreversible brain death if all signs of brainstem function are absent on repeated examination over 12 to 24 h. Other, less severely affected patients show partial recovery of brainstem reflex function, such as pupillary responses, reflex eye movements, and muscle tone, and may breath spontaneously. However, no sign of consciousness or intelligent response to the external world occurs, and they may remain in such a 'persistent vegetative state' for months or years.

Subacute or gradual anoxia may occur in severe anaemia, heart failure, pulmonary disease, or exposure to high altitude ('mountain sickness'). It produces inattentiveness, fatigue, headache, and intellectual deterioration, followed by memory difficulties and ataxia.

Cerebral anoxia is also the main cause of neurological symptoms in a number of other systemic conditions. Disseminated intravascular coagulation (DIC; see Section 22), can produce headache and difficulty in concentration, vertigo, blurred vision, and speech difficulties. Such confusion and disorientation may progress to stupor and coma with focal or generalized signs of brain disturbance. Spontaneous bleeding is common, in the form of petechiae in the skin or optic fundus, purpura, and even intracranial haemorrhage. Cerebral malaria (see Chapter 7.8.2) should always be borne in mind as a cause of unexplained coma in patients recently returning from an infective area. Most patients describe chills and fever for a few days prior to the onset of lethargy, stupor, and finally coma. The diagnosis is established by finding the parasite in fixed smears of the blood.

Fat embolism follows severe trauma, particularly to the limbs, but may also be a complication of burns and other severe system disturbance. Multiple pulmonary microemboli of fat may lead to progressive hypoxia and respiratory failure. Multiple cerebral microemboli produce confusion, lethargy, stupor, and finally coma. Symptoms often begin hours to days after the original injury, and are accompanied by fever and hyperventilation. A characteristic petechial rash usually develops over the upper half of the body on the second to third day after injury. There may also be fundal haemorrhages. The respiratory features range from the appearance of linear streaks radiating from the hilar region, or patchy opacities on the chest, to the fully developed adult respiratory distress syndrome (ARDS; see Section 18). Clotting abnormalities range from mild thrombocytopenia to acute DIC (see Section 22). Management consists of correcting hypoxia, in severe cases with positive end-expiratory pressure (PEEP) ventilation, and correction of the coagulation disorder (see Section 22). Improvements in cardiac surgical techniques have greatly reduced neurological complications, but some patients still emerge from the anaesthetic with signs of diffuse or focal brain damage. If they survive the acute episode, the prognosis usually is good.

Hepatic failure (see also Section 15)

Acute hepatic coma

This occurs with massive liver necrosis due to severe hepatitis or poisons. In other patients, who may have relatively well-preserved liver function but extensive portosystemic shunts, coma may be precipitated by a sudden intake of nitrogenous substances as (effectively) occurs with gastrointestinal bleeding, infections, or high-protein diets. Personality and cognitive changes progress if unchecked to confusion, apathy, and lack of concentration, or occasionally excitement requiring sedation, followed by stupor and coma in hours or days. Characteristic findings are asterixis ('liver flap'), in which the outstretched hands show postural lapses or negative myoclonus, and hepatic foetor. Chorea and pyramidal signs may appear as the patient lapses into coma. Decerebrate posturing is common at this stage, and focal deficits such as hemiplegia may occur. Nystagmus, conjugate deviation of the eyes, skew deviation, and even disconjugate eye movements may be evident, but reflex eye movements and pupillary responses are preserved, until the patient becomes totally unresponsive and dies. Paroxysmal and later persistent high-voltage triphasic slow waves are present in the electroencephalogram until death is imminent.

Many metabolic abnormalities may contribute to the cause of hepatic coma, including marked hyperammonaemia (>145 μmol/litre or 200mg/dl), hypoglycaemia and hyperventilation producing a respiratory alkalosis. Altered amino acids and neurotransmitters (especially γ-aminobutyric acid, GABA), formation of toxic amines such as octopamine, and short-chain fatty acids have also been incriminated. Intravascular coagulation and other coagulation defects complicate damage to the brain. Glial oedema is seen; cerebral oedema can raise intracranial pressure seriously or even fatally.

Hepatic coma carries a high mortality, but if the patient can be kept alive, liver regeneration and recovery may occur. Treatment includes correcting where possible the precipitant, sterilizing the bowel, correction of metabolic and bleeding abnormalities, the administration of lactulose, and haemoperfusion or other techniques to remove toxins (see Chapter 15.22.4). The benzodiazepine antagonist flumazenil may help. Intracranial pressure monitoring is fraught with hazards, not least the coagulopathy, but mannitol (though not dexamethasone) is of proven benefit in lowering intracranial pressure in this context. Liver transplantation is often considered if rather rarely practicable.

Chronic hepatic encephalopathy

This refers to the development of changes in intellect, cognitive function, and consciousness, often accompanied by other neurological signs (such as tremor or chorea, an akinetic–rigid syndrome, ataxia, or even spastic paraparesis) occurring in those with chronic liver failure, particularly in patients with extensive portosystemic anastomoses. (For Wilson's disease see Chapter 12.7.2.) Again, the precise nature of the substances responsible for chronic hepatic encephalopathy has not been established. Characteristically, the disorder fluctuates—with episodes of marked confusion, excitement, or frank hepatic coma. In addition, intellectual changes, parkinsonism, ataxia, or spasticity may gradually progress. Treatment consists of a low-protein diet and antibiotics to sterilize the gut, and the administration of lactulose. Shunting procedures appear increasingly promising.

A hepatic or portal-systemic myelopathy has also been documented.

Respiratory disease

Hyperventilation causes hypocarbia and alkalosis, resulting in parasthaesia, especially perioral, light-headedness and unsteadiness, visual disturbances, and occasionally carpopedal spasm; syncope may follow.

Chronic respiratory failure causes what is essentially a low-grade chronic hypoxia and hypercarbic encephalopathy, with the defining features of confusion and headache accompanied by a myoclonic or asterictic tremor and papilloedema. Mechanical devices for delivering domiciliary oxygen have transformed the management of this disorder, and the quality of life of its sufferers.

Obstructive sleep apnoea is characterized by conspicuous snoring and an often obese habitus. Early morning headache and inattentiveness or irritability with excessive daytime sleepiness occur (see Chapter 18.5.2).

Critical illness polyneuropathy

An axonal neuropathy can develop subacutely but often asymptomatically in (often anaesthetized) patients on intensive care units suffering multiorgan failure and/or sepsis, only revealing itself as they otherwise improve. Its cause is unkown. The prognosis is variable; it may slowly improve in patients whose underlying disease allows sufficient time for recovery. A myopathy is often also present; indeed the term 'critical illness neuromyopathy' may be preferable.

Renal failure

Renal failure (see Section 21) is associated with a variety of neurological complications. Uraemic encephalopathy is now uncommon but still seen. Patients become progressively drowsy, stuporose, and finally comatose. Hyperventilation, multifocal myoclonus, tremor, asterixis, tetany, and generalized fits occur. Eye movements and pupillary reactions are not affected. Uraemia, metabolic acidosis, hyperkalaemia, disorders of calcium, sodium, and water balance, and hypertensive encephalopathy all contribute to the clinical picture. Dialysis rapidly reverses the metabolic abnormalities of uraemia, but the encephalopathy may take days to clear. Other complications of chronic renal failure include myopathy due to chronic hypocalcaemia, and a symmetrical sensorimotor polyneuropathy, often subacutely progressive and disabling. It may be resistant to dialysis, but renal transplantation has been associated with a slow and sustained improvement.

Iatrogenic disease in renal failure

Some patients develop the 'dialysis disequilibrium syndrome' during correction of their uraemic abnormalities. Rapid correction of the metabolic changes, primarily through creating a significant brain–plasma osmotic gradient, leads to the emergence of asterixis, myoclonus, delirium, generalized convulsions, stupor, and even coma. Raised intracranial pressure with papilloedema may occur. Chronic dialysis—perhaps 3 to 7 years—may precipitate dialysis dementia if dialysate with a high aluminium content has been used. Such patients begin to develop speech hesitancy and arrest, then intellectual and cognitive abnormalities, convulsions, myoclonus, and sometimes focal neurological abnormalities. Death usually follows within a year.

Wernicke's encephalopathy (see below) can occur, due to chronic dialysis without thiamine supplements.

Patients with renal disease are particularly prone to develop toxic complications of drugs normally excreted in the urine—e.g. peripheral neuropathy due to nitrofurantoin, labyrinthine damage due to streptomycin, or optic atrophy due to ethambutol.

Metabolic disorders due to endocrine disease (see Section 13)

Adrenal disease

Phaeochromocytoma

Phaeochromocytoma causes paroxysms of anxiety, tremor, headache, and palpitations—combined with the serious consequences of malignant hypertension. The associations with von Hippel–Lindau disease, multiple endocrine neoplasia syndromes, ataxia telangiectasia, and Sturge–Weber syndrome should not be overlooked.

Cushing's syndrome

Endogenous Cushing's syndrome in two-thirds of cases is due to a pituitary ACTH-secreting adenoma—conventionally termed Cushing's disease. Ectopic ACTH-secreting malignant neoplasms and ACTH-independent adrenal tumours represent the other principal causes of endogenous disease; iatrogenic hyperadrenalism produces similar neurological symptoms. The systemic features are described in Chapter 13.7.1. Neurological complications include: (1) proximal myopathy, which can be severe and painful; (2) psychiatric disorders, ranging from mild mood disturbance through moderate depression (common) to severe psychosis; (3) a benign intracranial hypertension-like picture; and (4) direct consequences of a pituitary tumour, particularly optic chiasmal compression.

Adrenal insufficiency

Hypoadrenalism due to primary adrenal failure (Addison's disease) or ACTH deficiency (from pituitary disease or chronic steroid treatment) causes weakness, lassitude, nausea, and diarrhoea; and stupor or coma may be precipitated by surgical procedures or other acute illness. Hypotension (especially postural), hyponatraemia, hyperkalaemia, and often hypoglycaemia (see Chapter 13.7.1) occur: each may be symptomatic—indeed, attacks of hyperkalaemic periodic paralysis may occur. Amnesic deficits, depression, and impaired concentration progressing to confusion are relatively common. Addisonian crises may be accompanied by generalized convulsions, which are attributed to hyponatraemia and water intoxication. Benign intracranial hypertension with papilloedema and a proximal myopathy may also occur.

X-linked adrenoleukodystrophy

This is discussed in Chapter 12.9.

Thyroid disease

Thyroid disease carries one set of metabolic complications, directly related to abnormal thyroxine levels, and another sharing the same autoimmune origin (and eponyms)—Hashimoto's encephalopathy and Grave's ophthalmopathy. Here only the former will be considered.

Thyrotoxicosis

The features of hyperthyroidism include anxiety, tremor, tachycardia, and insomnia. Chorea or mania may occur. A severe proximal myopathy is not uncommon, and rarely myasthenia gravis is seen. Thyroxine-responsive hypokalaemic periodic paralysis is well reported.

Myxoedema

Hypothyroidism may present with lethargy progressing to a toxic confusional state or a subacute hypothermic, hypotensive coma. The latter (which may be provoked by infection, trauma, exposure to cold, or sedation), together with the occasionally seen psychosis or dementing illness ('myxoedema madness') responds to (judicious) thyroxine hormone replacement. Ataxia occurs in 5 to 10% of patients with hypothyroidism, and improves with thyroxine replacement.

Hypothyroid myopathy is characterized by proximal weakness with stiffness, aching, and cramps, and pseudomyotonic delayed muscle relaxation evident on tapping tendons or muscle bellies (with percussion-induced muscle ridging). Muscle hypertrophy (Hoffmann's syndrome) is rare. Carpal tunnel syndrome may occur as a a result of deposits of myxoedematous tissue around the median nerve of the wrist, and rarely this may cause a diffuse peripheral neuropathy.

Diabetes mellitus

Diabetes mellitus (Chapter 13.11.1) causes a wide variety of neurological disturbances. Centrally, stupor or coma may be produced by hyperosmolality, ketoacidosis, lactic acidosis, spontaneous (prediabetic) or iatrogenic hypoglycaemia, uraemia, or hypertensive encephalopathy. Transient ischaemic attacks and stroke due to cerebral arteriosclerosis and hypertension are common in patients with diabetes.

Peripherally, nerve damage may occur in patients with established diabetes, or may be the presenting feature of the illness; it is described in more detail in Chapters 13.11.1 and 24.16. The following syndromes are recognized:

◆ Single painful nerve lesions (mononeuritis)—isolated ocular nerve palsies, Bell's palsy, a lateral popliteal nerve palsy, or an intercostal neuropathy are common and may result from haemorrhage or infarction of the nerve

◆ Carpal tunnel syndrome, an ulnar nerve palsy, or other compression neuropathies may result from the undue susceptibility of peripheral nerves in diabetes to pressure

◆ Mononeuritis multiplex may occur, with a microvascular basis

◆ Diabetic amyotrophy refers to a proximal motor neuropathy causing the subacute weakness and wasting, often with pain, affecting quadriceps muscles, usually asymmetrically. It is probably due to ischaemia or haemorrhage in the femoral nerve or lumbosacral plexus

◆ A distal symmetrical peripheral neuropathy in diabetes may take the form of a mild asymptomatic sensory neuropathy with loss of vibration sense in the feet and absent ankle jerks. Less commonly, there is severe and progressive sensorimotor neuropathy affecting the legs before the arms

◆ Autonomic neuropathy is common, producing impotence, diarrhoea, loss of sweating, and abnormal pupils which may be irregular, and unreactive to light, mimicking Argyll Robertson pupils. Autonomic neuropathy causes orthostatic hypotension, syncope, and sometimes abrupt cardiac arrest in patients with diabetes

It should be recalled that diabetes may occur as a feature of a number of genetically determined neurological diseases, including Friedreich's ataxia, X-linked spinomuscular atrophy, mitochondrial cytopathies, myotonic dystrophy, and Wolfram's syndrome; it is also associated with the stiff man syndrome.

Hypoglycaemia

Hypoglycaemic coma can be difficult to diagnose and dangerous. In any case of coma, stupor, or confusion of unknown cause, and in newly presenting status epilepticus, blood should be drawn for glucose analysis and insulin levels, and then 25 g of glucose (with thiamine) should be administered intravenously. Such an injection can do no harm and may save life.

The commonest cause of hypoglycaemia is insulin overdose, or excessive hypoglycaemic drug intake. Hyperinsulinism due to an adenoma of the islets of Langerhans in the pancreas is uncommon, as is hypoglycaemia due to prediabetes or a retroperitoneal sarcoma. Hypoglycaemia may also occur in alcoholism and liver disease, after gastric surgery, and in a variety of rare metabolic conditions.

Hypoglycaemia presents in four ways: (1) as an organic toxic confusional state, sleepy confusion, bizarre behaviour, or mania; (2) as unexplained coma with brainstem dysfunction, including decerebrate spasms and neurogenic hyperventilation, but with preserved oculocephalic reflexes and pupillary responses; (3) as a (normally reversible) stroke-like illness with focal deficit; and (4) as epilepsy. Hyperinsulinism, very rarely, also causes predominantly motor peripheral neuropathy.

Hyperinsulinism is difficult to diagnose on occasion, but can be established by satisfying the criteria for Whipple's triad, i.e. symptoms of hypoglycaemia, associated with a low blood sugar and a disproportionately high serum insulin, and clinical response to glucose replacement. A 72-h fast, measuring morning blood sugar and insulin levels, will detect nearly all pancreatic islet cell adenomas (see Chapter 15.24.3).

Metabolic disorders due to ionic or acid–base abnormalities

Hyponatraemia or 'water intoxication'

The normal serum osmolality is 290 ± 5 mosmol/kg; serum osmolality below about 260 or above about 330 mosmol/kg is likely to produce cerebral changes. Sodium is the most abundant serum cation, so that hyponatraemia is almost always the cause of hypoosmolality. (Serum osmolality is approximately equal to double the serum sodium concentration plus 10, provided glucose and urea levels are normal.) In hyponatraemia, body water is increased relative to solute, causing water excess in the brain.

Rapid changes in serum sodium osmolality produce much greater neurological effects than chronic hyponatraemia. Hyponatraemia occurs in renal disease, as a result of excessive intravenous water infusions, due to excessive diarrhoea, vomiting, or sweating, or may result from the inappropriate secretion of antidiuretic hormone (SIADH) in bronchial carcinoma, focal hypothalamic damage due to neoplasm or infection, or diffuse acute brain disease resulting from head injury, meningitis, or encephalitis, or subarachnoid haemorrhage. (It is, however, noteworthy that in the latter acute situations, salt-wasting may also cause hyponatraemia, in which circumstances fluid restriction exacerbates the problem: hypovolaemia distinguishes salt-wasting from the eu- or hypervolaemia of vasopressin excess.) Patients with hyponatraemia become confused and restless, and develop asterixis, multifocal myoclonus, generalized convulsions, stupor, and coma. Symptoms may appear when the plasma sodium drops below about 120 mmol/litre, and fits and coma usually are associated with plasma sodium values below 110 mmol/litre. A few patients with chronic hyponatraemia may develop the syndrome of central pontine myelinolysis (see below). Treatment is by water restriction; infusions of hypertonic saline are not advised.

Central pontine myelinolysis

This was first described 50 years ago. It is often associated with hyponatraemia, and more particularly with rapid correction of serum sodium by parenteral hypertonic fluids: correction by no less than 1 to 2 mmol/litre per hour, or 8 mmol/litre per day, is allegedly safe. The disorder is also seen in alcoholics, in severe liver and renal disease, and other metabolic disturbances. The disease is characterized by a rapidly progressive flaccid or spastic quadriplegia, with involvement of bulbar muscles producing dysarthria and dysphagia. Consciousness and eye movement may remain intact. At worst the patient may be unable to speak or swallow, or to move any muscle except those of the eyes. Death is common, but remarkable recovery may occur. Extrapontine myelinolysis is also now well recognized.

Hypernatraemia

The common cause of hyperosmolality is diabetes, producing severe hyperglycaemia. Hyperosmolality due to hypernatraemia is rare, except in those who dehydrate in hot climates. Chronic uncompensated water loss in untreated diabetes insipidus may result in mild hypernatraemia, but such patients only develop severe hypernatraemia if they fail to drink. Patients with simple diabetes insipidus usually maintain thirst, but if intercurrent illness leads to excessive water loss and restricted water intake, they may become dehydrated, drowsy, stuporose, and unconscious. Simple diabetes insipidus may be due to pituitary surgery, trauma, or pituitary tumours. If pathology extends into the hypothalamic region, not only may secretion of vasopressin be deficient, but thirst regulation may also be abolished. Hypothalamic damage causing severe hypernatraemia may occur in large pituitary tumours, craniopharyngiomas, hypothalamic tumours, sarcoidosis, or Hand–Schüller–Christian disease. Loss of thirst in such patients often precipitates hypernatraemic coma with serum sodium rising above 160–170 mmol/litre. Hypernatraemia may also occur as a result of severe water depletion, particularly in children with intense diarrhoea.

Hypercalcaemia (see Chapter 13.6)

A high serum calcium may be due to primary hyperparathyroidism, immobilization, sarcoidosis, vitamin D intoxication, or multiple bony metastases. Symptoms include anorexia, nausea, vomiting, intense thirst, polyuria, and polydipsia. Muscle weakness, lassitude, and a mild encephalopathy are common. The latter may produce delusions and changes in mood so that many such patients are initially treated for a psychiatric condition. A toxic confusional state with lethargy and stupor, sometimes with generalized or focal seizures and papilloedema, also may occur. A more severe syndrome with pyramidal signs, ataxia, and an internuclear ophthalmoplegia is also described.

Hypocalcaemia (see Chapter 13.6)

Reduced serum calcium concentration may be caused by parathyroid or thyroid surgery, chronic renal failure, or chronic anticonvulsant drug treatment. It also occurs in primary idiopathic hypoparathyroidism (when the serum parathormone level is low), and in pseudohypoparathyroidism (in which the serum parathormone level is normal or high, and there is no response to parathyroid hormone; skeletal deformities and dysmorphism also are present). Pseudopseudohypoparathyroidism is a syndrome with similar skeletal and dysmorphic abnormalities but normal serum calcium and parathormone levels. Hypocalcaemia causes neuromuscular irritability, tetany with a Chvostek's sign, and mild encephalopathy. Severe hypocalcaemia produces generalized convulsions, psychosis, stupor, and coma. Raised intracranial pressure with papilloedema may occur in hypoparathyroidism. Hypocalcaemia is commonly misdiagnosed as mental retardation, dementia, or epilepsy. Skin changes and cataracts are characteristic. Calcification in basal ganglia on skull radiograph or CT may be evident. Rarely, basal ganglia calcification may be associated with extrapyramidal disorders.

Magnesium

Renal disease may impair the ability to excrete magnesium, which is cardiotoxic. Hypomagnesaemia, due to inadequate intake or excessive renal or gastrointestinal loss, causes secondary hypocalcaemia; the former rarely occurs without the latter, and the neurological complications often attributed to low magnesium are precisely those of hypocalcaemia. Hypermagnesaemia may cause an encephalopathy with decreased or absent tendon jerks; the latter may progress to a flaccid paralysis.

Potassium

Hypokalaemia, often caused by diuretics, causes myalgia and proximal myopathy; rhabdomyolysis can occur. Hyperkalaemia can precipitate areflexic flaccid paralysis, which may be fully reversible with correction of the serum potassium. The periodic paralyses are discussed in Chapter 21.2.2.

Acid–base disturbances

Systemic acidosis and alkalosis (see Chapter 12.11) occur in many diseases causing metabolic coma, but of the four acid–base balance disorders (respiratory or metabolic acidosis or alkalosis), only respiratory acidosis directly causes stupor and coma. Hypoxia associated with respiratory acidosis may be important in producing neurological abnormalities. Metabolic acidosis, by itself, usually only causes delirium or, at most, drowsiness. Even severe disorders of acid–base balance usually do not impair brain function since the central nervous system possesses a powerful acid–base homeostatic armoury, including compensatory changes in respiratory rate and cerebral blood flow, and cellular buffering in nervous tissue. Coma in metabolic acidosis due to diabetic ketosis or hyperosmolality, lactic acidosis, uraemia, alcohol poisoning, or intake of ethylene glycol, methyl alcohol, or paraldehyde is usually due to associated metabolic abnormalities or direct effects of other toxins in these conditions. Severe respiratory acidosis produces a reduction in alertness parallel to the degree of acidosis. Respiratory alkalosis, although constricting cerebral arterioles and decreasing cerebral blood flow, rarely interferes with cerebral function. A patient in coma with respiratory alkalosis due to hyperventilation has some other condition such as sepsis, hepatic disease, pulmonary infarction, or salicylate overdose. Even severe metabolic alkalosis only produces a confusional state rather than coma.

Alcohol and the nervous system

Alcohol damages the nervous system in many ways, some the result of acute or chronic poisoning, others of associated vitamin deficiency. This section mainly addresses the neurological consequences of chronic, excessive alcohol intake, not the transient acute effects of alcohol.

Delirium tremens

This develops several days after ethanol abstinence in chronic abusers. Usually rapid in onset, there is an agitated confused state, with signs of sympathetic overactivity. Circulatory collapse may contribute to the 5 to 10% mortality. It is generally distinguished from the less severe alcohol withdrawal syndrome, characterized by broadly similar symptoms that occur sooner—within hours of withdrawal—and are usually self limiting. Ethanol withdrawal seizures represent a not uncommon cause of late-onset fits. Benzodiazepines have transformed the management of delirium tremens and the alcohol withdrawal syndrome, and significantly reduced its mortality.

Wernicke–Korsakoff syndrome

Inadequate intake of thiamine, of whatever cause, may lead to foci of marked hyperaemia with multiple small haemorrhages affecting particularly the upper brainstem, hypothalamus, and thalamus adjacent to the third ventricle, and the mammillary bodies. Histologically there is a proliferation of dilated capillaries with perivascular haemorrhage. There may be associated alcohol-induced damage to the cerebral cortex, cerebellum, and peripheral nerves.

Such pathology can be produced in animals by a diet deficient in thiamine. Thiamine deficiency can be demonstrated in patients with the Wernicke–Korsakoff syndrome, and administration of thiamine can reverse many of the symptoms and signs of this syndrome. (Wernicke's and Korsakoff's syndromes probably represent the acute and chronic consequences of the same pathological process.) Thiamine and its pyrophosphate are cofactors to at least four enzymes—pyruvate decarboxylase, α-ketoglutarate dehydrogenase, the branched-chain ketoacid decarboxylase system, and transketolase. Thiamine deficiency results in reduced conversion of pyruvate to acetyl coenzyme A, causing elevated plasma and tissue pyruvate levels, with decreased flux through the Krebs cycle, reducing ATP production, and impairing energy supply.

Alcoholism combined with an inadequate diet is the commonest cause of the Wernicke–Korsakoff syndrome. Malnutrition in prisoners of war, or at times of famine, may also be responsible. Chronic vomiting, e.g. during pregnancy or due to gastrointestinal disease, systemic malignancy, prolonged intravenous feeding, and anorexia nervosa are rarer causes.

The onset may be insidious or subacute with increasing lethargy and inattentiveness, which develops into a typical confusional state with disorientation in time and place, loss of memory, and altered consciousness. Ophthalmoplegia develops with diplopia. The most common eye signs are nystagmus on lateral or vertical gaze, cranial nerve VI palsies, or defects of conjugate gaze. Retinal haemorrhages may occur. Most patients who are alcoholics will also have signs of a peripheral neuropathy, and many exhibit ataxia—the third classically described feature. Hypothermia may appear. Wernicke's encephalopathy is a medical emergency: untreated, the patient lapses into stupor and then coma, and dies—the mortality untreated is 20%.

In less acute cases, or in those recovering from the acute confusional phase, the characteristic features of the Korsakoff psychosis will appear. The patient has an often very severe gross amnesic defect for recent events, such that new information cannot be retained for more than a matter of minutes or hours. The patient is disorientated in time and place, but alert. Despite the severe defect of recent memory, the remote past is usually accurately recalled. Gaps in memory are filled by imaginary and often graphic accounts (confabulation).

The diagnosis is clinical. The cerebrospinal fluid is usually normal, although the protein may be slightly raised. Brain scanning can be normal, although patients who are alcoholic (and fall often) may have subdural haematomata, or atrophy. Demonstration of reduced red-cell transketolase activity, or of raised plasma pyruvate levels, is often invalidated by intake of food as soon as the patient comes under supervision.

The Wernicke–Korsakoff syndrome must be considered in any individual with unexplained confusion, stupor, or coma, particularly in the presence of eye signs, a peripheral neuropathy, or a history of alcoholism or excessive vomiting. Thiamine should be given to all such patients, usually in the form of two to three pairs of high-potency intravenous Pabrinex ampoules every 8 h for several days, or until oral vitamin B complex preparations can be taken. A particular problem arises commonly in the Emergency Department when patients exhibiting stupor or coma of unknown cause are admitted. All such patients should be given high-dose thiamine and glucose parenterally—if glucose is given without thiamine to a patient with Wernicke–Korsakoff syndrome, rapid deterioration and death can follow. Those who are thiamine deficient cannot handle the glucose load.

Effective treatment will restore consciousness and reverse eye signs, the latter usually within hours, but unfortunately the Korsakoff amnesic syndrome frequently does not resolve. The earlier the treatment, the better the chances of recovery, hence treatment on suspicion as a medical emergency.

Alcoholic peripheral neuropathy
(see also Chapter 24.16)

Although thiamine deficiency has long been considered responsible for the peripheral neuropathy associated with chronic alcoholism, a direct toxic effect has also been proposed. Pathologically, the picture of peripheral nerve damage is very similar to that seen in beriberi—a predominantly axonal neuropathy of the 'dying back' type, affecting somatic and sometimes autonomic nerves.

Alcoholic peripheral neuropathy predominantly involves sensory nerves, producing distal parasthesias in the feet, followed by the hands, and characteristic pain. The last may be intense and agonizing. Squeezing the calves or scratching the soles of the feet may cause severe discomfort. At a later stage, weakness and wasting of the distal limb muscles follows, with areflexia. Evidence of autonomic neuropathy may be seen in abnormal pupillary reactions and tachycardia, although postural hypotension is rare and the sphincters are usually spared.

Alcohol must be proscribed and high-potency vitamin B is given parenterally for some 10 days and then orally. The prognosis depends on how early treatment is initiated. Symptoms may take weeks to subside and in more severe cases recovery may take many months or may be incomplete.

Alcoholic cerebellar degeneration

Some patients who are alcoholic may develop a relatively pure syndrome of midline cerebellar ataxia, with a progressive unsteadiness of gait and of leg movements, and little or no involvement of the arms. Speech is not affected, and nystagmus is not present. Many such patients also have evidence of alcoholic peripheral neuropathy. Pathologically there is degeneration of the cerebellar cortex, particularly of the Purkinje cells, and also of the olivary nuclei. Changes in the cerebellum characteristically affect the anterior and superior parts of the vermis and hemispheres—often visible on MRI scans. This complication of alcoholism does not seem to be due to thiamine deficiency, though alcohol withdrawal and vitamin replacement can lead to recovery.

Alcoholic dementia (see Section 26)

In the past, there has been debate over whether alcoholism produces dementia, or whether the occasionally seen permanent cognitive deficits are rather the chronic consequences (or variants) of Wernicke–Korsakoff syndrome.

Certainly, a large proportion of those who habitually take excessive alcohol develop cognitive deficits varying from mild changes to severe diffuse global dementia, with atrophy of the cerebral cortex and enlargement of the cerebral ventricles. The dementia has the usual features of personality change, loss of memory, impairment of intellect, and emotional instability, with failure at work or in personal relationships. The gradual drift into destitution is all too familiar. Head injuries in alcoholic bouts and epilepsy may occur and contribute to the overall final picture. The fully developed case of the 'down and out' is an antisocial demented individual, with dysarthric speech, tremor, an ataxic gait, and a peripheral neuropathy, who still forlornly or aggressively clutches the bottle and a bag of residual belongings.

Treatment by withdrawal of alcohol (if possible) and vitamin replacement can lead to some improvement and occasionally to partial reversal of cerebral atrophy on scanning. However, the prognosis is generally poor, not least because of the difficulties of persuading those addicted to alcohol to stop drinking.

Marchiafava–Bignami disease

This rare disease was first described in Italian drinkers of crude red wine, but occurs in other alcohol abusers too. It presents with subacute dementia, progressing rapidly to fits, spasticity or rigidity, and paralysis, culminating in coma and death within a few months. Pathologically there is widespread demyelination and axonal damage in the corpus callosum and the central white matter of the cerebral hemispheres (all of which may be readily disclosed by MRI), also involving the optic chiasma and middle cerebellar peduncles. Abstinence stabilizes but rarely reverses the syndrome.

Alcoholic myopathy

Acute alcohol poisoning can produce a dramatic toxic myopathy. There is severe pain, muscle tenderness, oedema, and weakness, which may be associated with myoglobinuria, renal damage, and hyperkalaemia. Arrhythmias may occur. The syndrome is reversible if the necessary intensive support is available. A subacute painless myopathy resolving after withdrawal of alcohol has also been described. Chronic alcoholism is associated commonly with a painless proximal myopathy with marked muscle wasting and occasionally with coexistent cardiomyopathy; again abstinence may slowly improve the outcome.

Tobacco–alcohol amblyopia

Another uncommon complication of alcohol occurs in combination with strong tobacco. The patient develops sudden or subacute bilateral visual failure, associated with bilateral centrocaecal scotomas. The condition has been attributed to cyanide in tobacco causing a disorder of vitamin B_{12} metabolism. Visual failure and optic atrophy may occur in patients with pernicious anaemia, particularly those who smoke. A related condition is tropical amblyopia, occurring in Africa. This has been related to excessive consumption of cassava root containing cyanide. Treatment of these conditions is with hydroxycobalamine injections.

Ecstasy

'Ecstasy' (3,4-methylenedioxymethamphetamine, MDMA) has been a widely used recreational drug for two decades or more. Fatalities have been reported, but more common neurological sequelae include (1) hyperpyrexia and rhabdomyolysis with multi-organ failure; (2) hyponatraemia and its complications (largely caused by deliberate water self-intoxication, possibly intentional, to avoid (1); (3) bruxism and trismus; (4) serotonin syndrome; (5) more direct and, it is suggested, lasting, toxic effects on glia, neurons and/or cerebral endothelia.

Superficial siderosis of the CNS

Superficial siderosis is an unusual nervous system disorder recognized only recently. The four principal clinical manifestations are progressive ataxia; cranial polyneuropathy, particularly sensorineural deafness; myelopathy causing a spastic tetraparesis; and progressive dementia. Headaches occasionally feature. Cerebrospinal fluid examination reveals xanthochromia which, importantly, persists with repeated examination. MRI is diagnostic, with low signal intensity on T_2-weighted images apparent at the surface of the cerebellum, cranial nerves, brainstem, spinal cord, and more deeply on the borders of the dentate and basal ganglia. Iron deposition can be shown by high-strength MRI, corresponding to pathological descriptions of subpial siderotic deposits in the meninges. Repeated subarachnoid haemorrhage, cerebral tumours, or past surgery are recognized causes of this syndrome, but often none is historically evident; repeated subclinical haemorrhage is postulated but not proven. No treatments are of proven benefit.

Further reading

Metabolic complications of major organ disease

Lim C, *et al.* (2004). The neurological and cognitive sequelae of cardiac arrest. *Neurology*, **63**, 1774–8.

Polkey MI, *et al.* (1999). Respiratory aspects of neurological disease. *J Neurol Neurosurg Psychiatr*, **66**, 5–15.

Seidi O. (2007). Neurology and renal disorders. *Clin Med*, **7**, 165–70.

Lewis M, Howdle PD. (2003) The neurology of liver failure. *Q J Med*, **96**, 623–33.

Metabolic disorders due to endocrine disease

Shaw P (1998). Neurological complications of thyroid disease. In: Goetz CG, Aminoff MJ (eds) *Handbook of clinical neurology* **26** (70) *Systemic diseases Part II*, pp. 81–110. Elsevier Science, Amsterdam.

Watkins PJ, Thomas PK (1997). Diabetes mellitus and the nervous system. *J Neurol Neursurg Psychiatr*, **65**, 620–32.

Metabolic disorders due to ionic or acid–base abnormalities

Abrams GM, Jay C (1998). Neurological complications of mineral metabolism and parathyroid disease. In: Goetz CG, Aminoff MJ (eds) *Handbook of clinical neurology* 26 (70) *Systemic diseases Part II*, pp. 111–129. Elsevier Science, Amsterdam.

Martin RJ (2004). Central pontine and extrapontine myelinolysis: the osmotic demyelination syndromes. *J Neurol Neurosurg Psychiatr*, **75** Suppl 3, 22–8.

Alcohol and the nervous system

McIntosh C, Chick J. (2004) Alcohol and the nervous system. *J Neurol Neurosurg Psychiatr*, **75** Suppl 3, 16–21.

Harper C, Giles M, Finlay-Jones R (1986). Clinical signs in the Wernicke–Korsakoff complex: a retrospective analysis of 131 cases diagnosed at necropsy. *J Neurol Neurosurg Psychiatr*, **49**, 341–5.

Miscellaneous metabolic and deficiency disorders of the nervous system

Hall AP and Henry JA (2006) Acute toxic effects of 'Ecstasy' (MDMA) and related compounds: overview of pathophysiology and clinical management. *Br J Anaes*, **96**, 678–685.

Kumar N (2007). Superficial siderosis: associations and therapeutic implications. *Arch Neurol*, **64**, 491–496.

Young GB (1995). Neurologic complications of systemic critical illness. *Neurol Clin*, **13**, 645–58.

Neurological complications of systemic disease

Neil Scolding

Essentials

Primary neuroimmune disorders such as multiple sclerosis or the Guillain–Barré syndrome are well recognized (and described elsewhere in this section), but there are numerous diverse systemic inflammatory, infective, or immunological disorders that can affect the nervous system.

Autoimmune rheumatic and vasculitic disorders

Autoimmune rheumatic disorders—(1) Systemic lupus erythematosus—neurological manifestations include headache, acute or subacute encephalopathy, fits, myelitis, strokes and movement disorders (including chorea and other extrapyramidal disorders), ataxia and brainstem abnormalities, cranial and peripheral neuropathies, and psychiatric and cognitive disturbances. Risk of stroke is particularly associated with the lupus anticoagulant and the primary antiphospholipid syndrome. (2) Other conditions—(a) rheumatoid arthritis: mononeuritis, cervical cord compression; (b) Sjögren's syndrome: sensory neuropathy, myositis, various central nervous system complications; (c) Reiter's disease: polyneuritis, radiculitis, various central nervous system manifestations.

Vasculitides—neurological features include (1) mixed sensory and motor neuropathy—usually rapidly progressive and often painful;

(2) central nervous system disease—protean manifestations reflect focal or multifocal infarction, or diffuse ischaemia. Conditions of particular note include (1) giant cell arteritis—anterior ischaemic optic neuropathy is a feared and common complication; (2) Behçet's disease—cerebral venous sinus thrombosis is one of the more specific serious complications; (3) sarcoidosis—often manifests with optic and other cranial neuropathies.

Other autoimmune disorders

(1) Ulcerative colitis and Crohn's disease—may be associated with cerebrovascular accidents, epileptic seizures and (rarely) slowly progressive myelopathy. (2) Whipple's disease—a wide variety of neurological manifestations are recognized. (3) Coeliac disease—malabsorption may lead to neurological sequelae; progressive (spino)cerebellar degeneration is a recognized (but unexplained) complication.

Thyroid disease—hyperthyroidism and myxoedema both carry neurological complications (see Chapter 24.19), but thyroid disease may be associated with immunologically driven neurological complications including (1) dysthyroid eye disease—Graves' ophthalmoplegia; (2) Hashimoto's thyroiditis-associated encephalopathy.

Introduction

The range and breadth of diseases of the nervous system caused by immunological, infective, or inflammatory disturbances is very large. Involvement of the nervous system in a systemic inflammatory disease is no less common than idiopathic immune disorders. In this account a brief overview is provided; and the aim is not to be comprehensive. More detailed accounts of the disorders can be found in other chapters.

Systemic lupus erythematosus (SLE) (see Chapter 19.11.2)

SLE is not rare, with a prevalence of perhaps 30 in 100 000. Its incidence has more than tripled over the past 40 years. Like many autoimmune diseases, it occurs far more in women than men (probably >10 times more, and especially in the childbearing years), and those of African-Caribbean and Asian racial origin.

The neurologist should not (but usually does) omit direct enquiry and focused systemic examination to exclude fever and general malaise, skin changes—classically, the malar butterfly rash and/or photosensitivity, and large and small joint arthritis. Glomerulonephritis, pleurisy and pneumonitis, pericarditis and (so-called) Libmann–Sachs endocarditis, and haematological disorders—anaemia, thrombocytopoenia, leukocytopoenia and the generation of circulating anticoagulants—also occur. Other laboratory abnormalities include the presence of a variety of autoantibodies, including antinuclear antibodies (ANA) and anti-native

Box 24.20.1 American College of Rheumatology diagnostic criteria for SLE

'a person shall be said to have SLE if 4 or more of the 11 criteria are present, serially or simultaneously, during any interval of observation'

- Malar flush
- Discoid rash
- Photosensitivity
- Oral ulcers
- Arthritis
- Serositis (pleurisy or pericarditis)
- Renal disorder (proteinuria >0.5 g/24 h or cellular casts)
- Neurological disorder (seizures, psychosis; other causes excluded)
- Haematological disorder (haemolytic anaemia, leukopenia or lymphopenia on two or more occasions, or thrombocytopenia)
- Immunological disorder—LE cells, or anti-dsDNA or anti-Sm or persistent false-positive syphilis serology
- Antinuclear autoantibodies

DNA antibodies. The diagnosis—particularly for research and therapeutic trial purposes—is now commonly based on the widely accepted revised diagnostic criteria suggested by the American College of Rheumatology (Box 24.20.1). The presence of any four (or more) of the listed features, 'serially or simultaneously, during *any interval* of observation' [my italics] are sufficient for the diagnosis, with an estimated specificity and sensitivity of 96%.

Neurological complications

Neurological involvement in SLE is seen in perhaps 50% of cases; neurological presentation, in perhaps 3% of cases—though some suggest the true figure is higher. Central nervous system (CNS) disease is much commoner than neuromuscular involvement, and is a poor prognostic sign, reducing the overall survival figures, and representing the third commonest cause of death (after renal involvement and iatrogenic causes).

An enormous variety of CNS complications can occur, reflecting two broad pathogenetic mechanisms—thromboembolic (triggered either by changes in endothelial surfaces, or by coagulation disturbances, including lupus anticoagulant activity), and more direct autoimmune events affecting the target tissue—neurons or glia—in which soluble and cellular mediators are implicated.

Headache (including that associated with dural sinus thrombosis), acute or subacute encephalopathy, fits, myelitis, strokes and movement disorders (including chorea and other extrapyramidal disorders), ataxia and brainstem abnormalities, and cranial and peripheral neuropathies are all seen in the context of SLE. Psychiatric and cognitive disturbances have also long been associated.

Stroke, the lupus anticoagulant, and the primary phospholipid syndrome

The thrombotic tendency in patients with SLE and lupus anticoagulant (LA) manifests itself principally in the form of stroke and recurrent spontaneous abortion. Intra-abdominal and deep venous thrombosis, and peripheral arterial thrombosis are also seen. Thrombocytopoenia is a key additional feature. Importantly, Hughes also showed that a similar clinical picture was associated with the presence of anticardiolipin antibody (ACA) and/or LA in patients without serological or clinical evidence of SLE, and introduced the term 'antiphospholipid syndrome' (APS).

ACAs represent an independent risk factor for stroke. CNS thrombosis in patients with primary or secondary APS takes the form of completed arterial stroke, repeated transient ischaemic attacks (TIAs), multi-infarct dementia, and cerebral venous sinus thrombosis. Vascular visual problems, including amaurosis fugax and ischaemic retinopathy, also occur. Chorea too is associated with antiphospholipid antibodies; but the putative link with migraine may be factitious.

A severe acute ischaemic encephalopathy is also described, with confusion, obtundation, an hyperreflexic quadriparesis (usually asymmetrical), with or without systemic disturbances (dermatological and renal). Examination of the cerebrospinal fluid may show only a raised protein; a fatal outcome is common. The disorder may represent a focal variant of the recently described 'catastrophic antiphospholipid syndrome', in which there is severe multiorgan failure and a mortality of the order of 60%.

There are both clinical and pathological similarities between microangiopathic complications of lupus and the syndrome of thrombotic thrombocytopoenic purpura. In this latter uncommon disorder, multiorgan involvement is also seen, with hepatic and renal disease, and fever, together with thrombocytopoenia and an associated pupuric rash and other haemorrhagic complications. Neurologically, an encephalopathy occurs, often with fits, with or without focal deficits. Pathologically, there are widespread microangiopathic changes in the brain and systemically. Plasma exchange is commonly recommended.

Diagnosis of CNS lupus

It is clearly vital in such cases to exclude infectious complications of immune suppressants or steroids, now a major cause of death in patients with SLE. Serological tests are positive in 75 to 85% of cases, and the ESR is commonly elevated (contrasting with the CRP which usually is not)—but neither a normal ESR nor negative serology at the time of neurological episode allows a confident exclusion of neurological lupus as the underlying cause. MRI changes are common, though neither invariable nor specific. Abnormal scans are commoner in individuals with focal events, and normal scans in patients with more diffuse problems, such as headaches, meningism, memory impairment, confusion, and seizures. Examination of the cerebrospinal fluid reveals some form of abnormality (raised protein or a neutrophil or lymphocyte pleocytosis) in 40 to 50% of cases; Oligoclonal band analysis of the cerebrospinal fluid is positive in perhaps 20%—all changes which can resolve with successful immunotherapy. A skin biopsy can be extremely helpful in suspected lupus.

Management of neuropsychiatric lupus

Symptomatic therapies are important in patients with encephalopathies, epilepsy, and/or psychiatric ailments. Disease-modifying therapeutic efforts fall into two categories depending on the presumed underlying mechanisms—stroke prevention in cerebral ischaemia, particularly that associated with ACA, probably best achieved with moderate to high dose warfarin, and immuno-therapy of 'other' CNS complications. Here, intravenous methyl-prednisolone, followed by oral steroid treatment is the mainstay of treatment. Cyclophosphamide may be exhibited for severe or steroid-resistant disease, with azathioprine to maintain remission and spare steroids. Plasmapheresis synchronized with cyclophos-phamide, and intravenous immunoglobulin, may prove useful. More recent attention has focused on the promising role of the anti-B cell monoclonal antibody rituximab. Anti-tumour necrosis factor α (TNFα) therapy may actually increase disease activity.

Rheumatoid arthritis

An inflammatory peripheral neuropathy occurs in approximately 30% of seropositive rheumatoid cases. A relatively benign mono-neuritis is typical, but a more severe and aggressive axonal polyneu-ropathy or mononeuritis multiplex may be seen when rheumatoid arthritis is accompanied by a vasculitis. More common than either are entrapment neuropathies of conventional distribution, precipitated by synovial swelling. Pannus formation and cervical spine subluxation with resulting cord compression represent the commonest cause of CNS involvement. More rarely, rheumatoid vasculitis, or deposition of rheumatoid nodules, may involve the CNS; the former warrants treatment with cyclophosphamide and steroids. Recent excitement has emerged concerning the potential therapeutic role of anti-TNF and anti-B-cell therapies.

Sjögren's syndrome

Sjögren's syndrome characteristically comprises a triad of (1) kera-toconjunctivitis sicca, and (2) xerostomia, occurring in approxi-mately 50% of cases (3) in the context of another connective tissue disease, usually rheumatoid arthritis. Speckled antinuclear anti-bodies anti-Ro (SS-A) or anti-La (SS-B) are present in up to 75 to 80% of patients. Conventionally, the principal neurological mani-festations have been held to be peripheral, with descriptions both of a mainly sensory neuropathy and of myositis. Trigeminal sensory neuropathy is also classically described.

More recently, attention has been drawn to various CNS compli-cations of the disorder, with seizures, focal stroke-like or brainstem neurological deficits, and encephalopathy with or without an aseptic meningitis, often with raised cerebrospinal fluid pressure, protein level, and white cell count, together with oligoclonal immu-noglobulin bands. Psychiatric abnormalities may occur; spinal cord involvement may take the form of an acute transverse myelitis, a chronic myelopathy, or intraspinal haemorrhage. Occasionally, the features resemble those of multiple sclerosis (optic neuropathy is particularly associated), though most such patients have additional features of peripheral neuropathy or myositis.

Steroids may be insufficient for patients with CNS complications of Sjögren's syndrome; more powerful immunosuppressants are probably more useful, though, as is so often the case, their value is yet to be proven objectively.

Systemic sclerosis

Systemic sclerosis results from the excessive deposition of collagen in the skin, and other affected tissues. The cutaneous manifestation, scleroderma, may exist in isolation, but in multisystem disease, it is accompanied by Raynaud's phenomenon, calcinosis and atrophy of subcutaneous tissues, telangiectasia, and oesophageal strictures.

Neurological complications are not common. PNS disease pre-dominates, particularly painful trigeminal neuropathy; myopathy, with an elevated CPK also occurs. A myelopathy may be associated. No treatment is of proven benefit.

Mixed connective tissue disease

In this disorder, features of scleroderma, polymyositis and systemic lupus erythematosus coincide, and high levels of antibodies directed against extractable nuclear antigens—ribonucleoproteins or RNP—are found (Table 7.1). Rheumatoid factor is also often present. In common with both systemic sclerosis and Sjögren's syndrome, trigeminal neuralgia and/or sensory neuropathy are described.

Seronegative arthritides
Ankylosing spondylitis

Neurological disease in the setting of ankylosing spondylitis usually reflects advanced bony disease; a cauda equina syndrome is well reported, unexplained, and difficult to treat.

Reiter's disease

The clinical triad of seronegative arthropathy, nonspecific urethri-tis, and conjunctivitis, usually following venereal or dysenteric infection, constitute Reiter's syndrome. As many as 25% of patients are reported to have neurological features Peripherally, radiculitis and polyneuritis occur; CNS disorders include aseptic menin-goencephalitis, seizures, and psychiatric disturbances, particularly paranoid psychosis. Cranial neuropathies, pyramidal signs and myelopathy are also reported. A recent report suggests that ciclosporin may be of value in severe Reiter's disease.

Psoriasis

Psoriasis is included as the third seronegative arthropathy, but its neurology is not extensive. Cord compression from cervical psori-atic spondylosis is described, but reports of a complicating polyneuritis have not been substantiated.

Vasculitis

The clinical and histopathological picture of CNS vasculitis is seen in three contexts. (1) Primary or idiopathic isolated CNS vasculitis can occur, wherein symptoms are confined to the nervous system. (2) There are a number of primary systemic vasculitides, usually involving the lungs and/or kidneys—e.g. polyarteritis and Wegener's granulomatosis—which can also secondarily affect the nervous system. (3) Various systemic conditions can include vasculitis—occasionally with neurological involvement—among their complications. These range from rheumatological or connec-tive tissue diseases, to drugs, toxins, and infections. In both primary and secondary vasculitis of the nervous system, neurological fea-tures arise from inflammation and necrosis of the vasculature—principally through infarction.

Clinical features

The picture of peripheral nerve vasculitis is relatively straightfor-ward: a mixed sensory and motor neuropathy, usually rapidly progressive, and often painful. About 50% of patients present with mononeuritis multiplex, the remainder with a more diffuse asym-metrical polyneuropathy or a distal symmetric neuropathy.

CNS disease is infinitely more varied—focal or multifocal infarction or diffuse ischaemia affecting any part of the brain, explaining the protean manifestations, the wide variation in disease activity, course, and severity, and the absence of a pathognomic or even typical clinical picture. Thus, in primary and secondary intracranial vasculitis, headache (perhaps 50% of cases), focal and generalized seizures (10–20%), acute and subacute encephalopathies, progressive cognitive changes, behavioural disturbances, chorea, myoclonus and other movement disorders, optic and other cranial neuropathies are all seen. (Although it is included in many accounts, the conventional clinical picture of isolated large vessel stroke, so resembling atheromatous thromboembolic stroke as to cause diagnostic confusion, is profoundly uncommon.) The course is commonly acute or subacute, but monophasic, chronic progressive, and spontaneously relapsing–remitting presentations all occur.

Despite this range, three broad phenotypes of presentation may be delineated: (1) resembling atypical multiple sclerosis ('MS-plus')—with a relapsing–remitting course, and features such as optic neuropathy and brainstem episodes accompanied by other features less common in multiple sclerosis—seizures, severe and persisting headaches, encephalopathic episodes, or hemispheric stroke-like episodes; (2) acute or subacute encephalopathy, with headache with an acute confusional state, progressing to drowsiness and coma; (3) intracranial mass lesion—with headache, drowsiness, focal signs and (often) raised intracranial pressure. This grouping carries neither pathological nor therapeutic implications, but may help improve recognition of this condition. Systemic features—fever and night sweats, livedo reticulares, or oligoarthropathy—may be present (though often only revealed on direct enquiry) even in so-called isolated CNS vasculitis.

Diagnosis and management

The diagnosis of cerebral vasculitis involves the exclusion of alternative possibilities (Table 24.20.1), the confirmation of intracranial vasculitis, and pursuit of the causes of the vasculitic process.

Confirming cerebral vasculitis

No single simple investigation is universally useful in confirming cerebral vasculitis. Serological markers, including ANCA, are important. Spinal fluid examination is, like ESR testing, often abnormal, but lacks specificity, with changes in cell count and/or protein in 65 to 80% of cases; oligoclonal immunoglobulin bands may be present. Cerebrospinal fluid pressure is frequently raised, as may be the glucose level. MRI may disclose ischaemic areas, periventricular white matter lesions, haemorrhagic lesions, and parenchymal or meningeal enhancing areas, but lacks both specificity and sensitivity. Contrast angiography may show segmental (often multifocal) narrowing and areas of localized dilatation or beading, often with areas of occlusion, rarely also with aneurysms. Again, though these changes are not specific, and angiography carries a false negative rate of up to 50%, and a risk of 10% for transient neurological deficit, and of 1% for permanent deficit. MR angiography is not sufficiently sensitive for most CNS vasculitides but is valuable in imaging of large vessel disorders such as Takayasu's arteritis and classical polyarteritis nodosa (PAN). Nuclear imaging of labelled leucocytes and examination of the ocular vasculature may be useful.

Histopathological confirmation, biopsying an abnormal area of brain where possible, or by 'blind' biopsy, incorporating meninges,

Table 24.20.1 Some disorders that may mimic cerebral vasculitis

Other vasculopathies	Infections
Susac's syndrome	Lyme disease
Homocysteinuria	AIDS
Ehlers–Danlos syndrome	Endocarditis
Radiation vasculopathy	Whipple's disease
Köhlmeyer–Degos disease	Viral encephalitis
Fibromuscular dysplasia	Legionella/mycoplasma pneumonia
Fabry's disease	**Tumours and malignancy**
Moyamoya disease	Atrial myxoma
Amyloid angiopathy	Multifocal glioma
CADASIL	Cerebral lymphoma
Marfan's syndrome	Paraneoplastic disease
Pseudoxanthoma elasticum	**Other disorders**
Viral or fungal vasculitis	Multiple cholesterol emboli
Other immune/inflammatory diseases	Thrombotic thrombocytopoenic purpura
Sarcoidosis	Cerebral sinus thrombosis
Lupus and anti-phospholipid disease	Mitochondrial disease
Behçet's syndrome	
Multiple sclerosis/ADEM	
Thyroid encephalopathy	

ADEM, acute disseminated encephalomyelitis; CADASIL, cerebral autosomal dominant arteriopathy with subcortical infarcts and leukoencephalopathy.

and nondominant temporal white and grey matter, is important. Biopsy may reveal an underlying process not otherwise suspected with profound therapeutic implications, such as infective or neoplastic (principally lymphomatous) vasculopathies, but is not a trivial procedure, carrying a risk of serious morbidity estimated at 0.5 to 2%—though immune suppressant treatment may have a higher morbidity than biopsy, emphasizing the rationale behind this procedure.

A vasculitic process having been confirmed, the specific defining characteristics of the primary and secondary vasculitides must be painstakingly sought.

Neurological vasculitis complicating systemic vasculitides

Wegener's granulomatosis predominantly affects the upper and lower respiratory tracts—nose (often with destructive cartilaginous change causing saddle nose deformity), sinuses, larynx, trachea and lungs. Ocular involvement may occur; renal disease is usual. cANCA is positive, with proteinase-3 specificity, and the biopsy is characteristic, with granulomatous vasculitis. Microscopic polyangiitis is a multisystem small-vessel vasculitis which can involve almost any organ, or may rarely be confined to a single organ. Renal involvement is almost invariable. The diagnosis usually rests upon a combination of renal biopsy and ANCA serology (commonly pANCA). Classical PAN is now recognized as an unusual disorder which may have some overlap and coexist with microscopic polyangiitis, but often occurs alone. Medium-sized vessels are affected in PAN, and the kidneys are again commonly involved; renal angiography may reveal microaneurysms. pANCA testing is also often positive in Churg–Strauss syndrome, a multisystem disease characterized pathologically by a granulomatous necrotizing vasculitis, and clinically by prominent asthma with an eosinophilia. Small vessel vasculitis commonly affects postcapillary venules. The skin is most commonly involved, usually with purpura or urticaria; the common presence of an allergic precipitant has led historically to the term 'hypersensitivity vasculitis' often being used synonymously in this context; 'cutaneous leukocytoclastic vasculitis' is the currently preferred term.

In all these disorders, PNS involvement, with mononeuritis multiplex, is considerably more common than CNS disease, ranging from up to 70% of classical polyarteritis nodosa and microscopic polyangiitis cases, to around 30% of patients with Wegener's disease. CNS disease can, however, also occur. Direct effects of the granulomatous process—either by contiguous invasive spread, or from remote metastatic granulomata—represent a mode of neurological involvement unique to Wegener's disease. Middle ear disease may lead to cranial nerve VII and VIII neuropathies.

Neurological vasculitis complicating nonvasculitic systemic disorders

Although the clinical picture of cerebral vasculitis may closely be mimicked by SLE, a noninflammatory vasculopathy is far more commonly responsible—though occasional instances of vasculitis are described. In contrast, seropositive rheumatoid disease is a well-recognized precipitant of vasculitic mononeuritis multiplex and (far more rarely) of CNS vasculitis. There are rare reports of CNS vasculitis in the context of systemic sclerosis, Sjögren's syndrome, and mixed connective tissue disease. The clinical features of cryoglobulinaemia represent the combined consequences of hyperviscosity and of immune complex deposition-triggered vasculitis, particularly in mixed cryoglobulinaemia, when associated with hepatitis C infection. Skin disease, with purpura progressing to necrotic ulceration, and renal and joint involvement are common. The diagnosis, however, will only be made if blood is collected into a plain tube, immediately placed in water and kept at a temperature at 37 °C, taken to the laboratory and tested forthwith. Peripheral neuropathy occurs in a quarter of patients with essential cryoglobulinaemia; CNS involvement is rare. Peripheral nerve disease, and/or histologically and angiographically evident vasculitis of the CNS, usually in the context of granulomatous meningitis, may occur in sarcoidosis.

Drug-induced vasculitis

The issue of vasculitis and drugs is complex. The most compelling evidence of a direct association relates to amphetamines, with clinical and histological evidence of multisystem necrotizing vasculitis. The majority of strokes occurring with cocaine abuse are associated with arterial spasm, platelet aggregation, severe abrupt hypertension, or migrainous phenomena, not vasculitis, although histologically proven cerebral vasculitis does occur.

Infections

At least three mechanisms may underlie microbe-related vascular damage—direct invasion, immune complex formation and deposition, and (in part related to the second), secondary cryoglobulinaemia. Although the association of hepatitis C infection with cryoglobulinaemia and small-vessel vasculitis has been stressed above, other infections, including hepatitis B, Epstein–Barr virus (EBV), cytomegalovirus (CMV), Lyme disease, syphilis, malaria, and coccidiomycosis have all also been linked to mixed cryoglobulinaemia.

Primary invasion of the vascular wall by the infectious agent is, however, the commonest precipitant of infection-associated vasculitis. Histoplasma, coccidioides, and aspergillus are among the fungal causes of this picture, usually confined to immune-suppressed patients (including individuals with diabetes mellitus). In HIV infection, CMV and toxoplasma may precipitate vasculitis, and syphilitic cerebral vasculitis has re-emerged in the context of HIV. More general bacterial causes of meningeal or cerebral infection—mycobacteria, pneumococci, and *Haemophilus influenzae*—may also trigger intracranial vasculitis.

Herpes zoster can precipitate cerebral vasculitis in approximately 0.5% of cases, usually causing a monophasic illness, with hemiparesis contralateral to the eye disease. However, more generalized necrotizing and granulomatous vasculitis can also occur.

Malignancy, lymphomatoid granulomatosis, and malignant angioendothelioma

Leukocytoclastic vasculitis (often dermatological) may occur in association with a variety of cancers as a paraneoplastic phenomenon. CNS disease in the context of Hodgkin's disease with a pathological picture indistinguishable from conventional isolated CNS angiitis is reported. Lymphomatoid granulomatosis is a lymphomatous disorder centred on the vascular wall, with destructive change and secondary inflammatory infiltration lending the appearance of true vasculitis; the infiltrating neoplastic cell is of T-lymphocyte derivation. Cutaneous and pulmonary involvement are common, with nodular cavitating lung infiltrates, and neurological manifestations occur in 25–30% of cases; they are the presenting feature in approximately 20%. Neoplastic or malignant angioendotheliosis is also a rare, nosologically separate disorder, wherein the neoplastic process is intravascular, i.e. within the lumen, and the lymphomatous cells are B-cell derived, and characteristically do not invade the vascular wall. The neurological features of each disorder are similar, largely representing those of cerebral vasculitic disease; in malignant angioendotheliomatosis lung involvement is not the rule; characteristic skin manifestations occur.

Treatment of cerebral vasculitis

Retrospective analyses support the use of cyclophosphamide with steroids in vasculitis. In proven cerebral vasculitis a 3 to 4 month induction regime might comprise high-dose intravenous, then oral steroids, with oral or pulsed intravenous cyclophosphamide; this is followed by a maintenance regime of alternate day steroids with azathioprine. In resistant disease, methotrexate (10–25 mg once weekly; again, with steroids), or intravenous immunoglobulin may be useful. Cyclophosphamide is associated with haemorrhagic cystitis (less likely with adequate hydration and mesna cover), bladder cancer, other malignancies, infertility, cardiotoxicity, and pulmonary fibrosis. Biological agents—monoclonal antibodies and TNF receptor antagonists—have shown promise.

Two eponymous primary disorders may involve the CNS. Cogan's syndrome is an unusual disorder, mostly affecting young adults, characterized by recurrent episodes of interstitial keratitis and/or scleritis with vestibulo-auditory symptoms, which may be complicated by CNS, peripheral nervous system, or systemic vasculitis. In Eale's disease, an isolated retinal vasculitis occurs, causing visual loss; again, neurological complications are well described.

Giant cell arteritis

Giant cell arteritis, the commonest large-vessel vasculitis, rarely affects individuals less than 55 years of age. It affects women twice as commonly as men, with an overall prevalence of 1 in 1000. Generally it presents with uni- or bilateral scalp pain, often severe, with exquisite tenderness. Additional symptoms include jaw claudication, and polymyalgia rheumatica, with stiffness and aching of the shoulder girdle, worse in the mornings, and occasionally general malaise. The affected temporal artery (-ies) may be thickened and cord-like, often nonpulsatile, and tender. A raised ESR, often accompanied by a normochromic normocytic anaemia, must be followed by temporal artery biopsy—a specimen of several centimetres length is recommended to help avoid false-negative results, which may occur because of the focal or multifocal nature of the disorder.

Histopathological examination of the vessel reveals changes of vasculitis, with an inflammatory infiltrate comprising mononuclear and giant cells; the latter phagocytose the elastic laminae, causing characteristic fragmentation. Immunoglobulin and complement deposits are apparent in lesions, but activated T-cells predominate in the inflammatory infiltrate, suggesting cell-mediated immune damage. Vasculitic changes may still be apparent in biopsies taken 14 days or more after the commencement of steroids.

Neurological complications

Blindness occurs in approximately one-sixth of treated patients with temporal arteritis, as a consequence of anterior ischaemic optic neuropathy following vasculitic involvement of the posterior ciliary arteries and/or the ophthalmic artery, from which they are derived. A typical picture comprises (locally) painless loss of acuity, commonly severe, often with an altitudinal field defect. The fundal appearances may be normal, although swelling (usually mild) may be seen. Intracranial involvement is much less common; vertebral artery involvement is typical. An elevated platelet count should be considered a risk factor for permanent visual loss.

Treatment

Oral steroids should be used immediately there is serious suspicion of the disease, and in high doses (60–80 mg/day) in view of the risk of permanent blindness. The dose is generally reduced slowly (5 mg decrements weekly) after 4 to 7 days to a maintenance dose of perhaps 10 mg daily; thereafter, some would suggest continuing for 12 to 24 months before closely monitored phased withdrawal. Such a duration of steroid therapy, particularly in this elderly population, should direct attention to the treatable or preventable long-term consequences of corticosteroids, particularly osteoporosis, diabetes, cataract, and peptic ulceration.

Behçet's disease

Behçet's disease is a chronic relapsing multisystem inflammatory disorder whose clinical manifestations vary. The classical triad of recurrent uveitis with oral and genital aphthous ulceration remains clinically useful, though formal diagnostic criteria have now been proposed and generally adopted. Recurrent oral ulceration (at least three times in one 12-month period) is an absolute criterion; any

two of (1) recurrent genital ulceration, (2) uveitis (anterior or posterior) or retinal vasculitis, (3) skin lesions, including erythema nodosum, or acneiform nodules, pseudofolliculitis or papulopustular lesions, or (4) a positive pathergy test (read at 24–48 h) are also required to confirm the diagnosis.

Approximately one-third of patients develop neurological involvement, although this includes the very common occurrence of benign headache. Neurological presentation may occur in up to one-fifth of cases. Cerebral venous sinus thrombosis is one of the more specific serious complications; others include sterile meningoencephalitis, encephalopathy, brainstem syndromes, cranial neuropathies, movement disorders, and cortical sensory and motor deficits. Psychiatric and progressive cognitive manifestations are reported. Investigation may reveal an active CSF, and oligoclonal IgA and IgM bands—but apparently not IgG—may be present. Evoked potentials may be diagnostically useful. MRI abnormalities are nonspecific.

Treatment

Recent retrospective studies indicate an improved survival in patients with CNS Behçet's treated with steroids and immunosuppressants. The place of thalidomide in steroid-unresponsive Behçet's is currently under review; chlorambucil is often advocated. Anti-TNF based therapy may be valuable. Monitoring treatment is difficult—neither the ESR nor CRP levels are useful; MRI might have such a role.

Sarcoidosis

Sarcoidosis is a multisystem granulomatous disease of unknown aetiology commonly affecting the lungs and, in approximately 5% of patients, the nervous system. Optic and other cranial neuropathies (especially involving the facial nerve), often due to meningeal infiltration, and brain stem and spinal cord disease are the commoner manifestations. Cognitive and neuropsychiatric abnormalities are reported. Peripheral nerve and muscle involvement is also well described.

The diagnosis can be difficult: presentation with isolated neurological deficits may be commoner in sarcoidosis than in other systemic inflammatory or immunological conditions. Serum and CSF angiotensin converting enzyme (ACE) levels may be elevated; the CSF may reveal more general abnormalities of protein or cell count and oligoclonal bands may be present. Whole-body gallium scanning remains a useful indicator of systemic disease. Cranial MRI may show multiple white-matter lesions or meningeal enhancement. The diagnosis is confirmed where possible by biopsy, either of cerebral or meningeal tissue, or of lung or conjunctiva where appropriate.

The mainstay of medical treatment in neurosarcoidosis is corticosteroids, though response rates as low as 29% have been reported. Methotrexate, azathioprine, hydroxychloroquine, and cyclophosphamide have been used in steroid-resistant cases. TNF inhibition appears very promising.

Organ-specific autoimmune disease

Ulcerative colitis and Crohn's Disease

The neurological complications of ulcerative colitis (see Chapter 15.12) and Crohn's disease (see Chapter 15.11), seen in around 5% of patients, are similar. Three types of CNS disease have been associated: (1) cerebrovascular accidents, mostly precipitated by the hypercoagulable state, and including venous or arterial thromboembolism, cerebral sinus venous thrombosis and (more rarely and less explicably) vasculitis; (2) epileptic seizures, focal and generalized, and not always in connection with dehydration or sepsis; and, in some reports, (3) a slowly progressive myelopathy.

Peripheral neuropathy is seen in 0.5 to 1.0% of cases; an acute Guillain–Barré syndrome is the commonest phenotype. Lastly, myopathy, sometimes of metabolic origin but mostly inflammatory, is also reported.

Whipple's disease

Whipple's disease (see Chapter 15.10.6) is an uncommon multisystem disorder characterized by arthropathy, respiratory symptoms, anaemia, fever, erythema nodosum and severe wasting in addition to steatorrhoea and abdominal distension, caused by *Tropheryma whippelii*. Approximately 10% of patients have neurological involvement; 5% present in this way. A wide variety of features is seen (Box 24.20.2).

Diagnosis and management

Up to 20% of cases of cerebral Whipple's disease occur in the absence of gastrointestinal or indeed other systemic symptoms. CT and MRI scanning may be normal, although the latter can also reveal non-specific abnormalities—multiple high signal intensity areas on T_2-weighted images, or more striking enhancing mass lesions warranting biopsy. Similarly, the cerebrospinal fluid may be normal, or show an elevated protein and/or raised cell count; widely varying ratios of monocytes and polymorphonucleocytes are reported. One-third of cerebrospinal fluid samples may reveal pathognomic periodic acid–Schiff-positive bacilli; repeat spinal fluid examination increases this yield. Approximately 30% of cases have a noninformative small-bowel biopsy, though electron microscopy increases the sensitivity. Lymph node biopsy can also be useful. Polymerase chain reaction (PCR) analysis of blood, lymph node, spinal fluid, small-bowel tissue, or brain is increasingly used.

Whipple's disease usually responds to tetracyclines, penicillin, or, more commonly nowadays, co-trimoxazole. Prompt treatment is vital in patients with neurological disease, which may (if untreated) run a profoundly aggressive and not unusually rapidly fatal course.

Box 24.20.2 Neurological features of Whipple's disease (in approximate order of frequency)

- Cognitive changes, dementia, and/or psychiatric disease
- Supranuclear gaze palsy
- Pyramidal signs
- Hypothalamic features—somnolence, polydipsia, increased appetite, hypogonadism
- Myoclonus—oculo-masticatory myorythmia
- Cranial neuropathies
- Fits
- Eye disease—keratitis, uveitis, papilloedema, ptosis
- Ataxia

Successful reversal of neurological deficits, including cognitive impairment, may follow antibiotic treatment.

Coeliac disease

Coeliac disease (nontropical sprue) is an immunologically-mediated disorder resulting from intolerance to dietary gluten; it causes weight loss with steatorrhoea and/or diarrhoea, and malabsorption (see Chapter 15.10.3). In common with other enteropathies, neurological sequelae of a predictable nature may complicate coeliac disease as a direct consequence of malabsorption. CNS complications apparently unrelated to deficiency states may also occur in perhaps 10% of patients. Rarely, vasculitis is responsible, but the cause of the most commonly described and distinctive CNS association, a progressive cerebellar or spinocerebellar degeneration, with eye movement disorders, myoclonus, and occasionally epilepsy, remains unresolved.

Major psychiatric complications and dementia are well described as a significant cause of morbidity, and have been studied in detail.

Thyroid disease

Hyperthyroidism and myxoedema both carry neurological complications generally considered direct consequences of abnormal thyroxine levels—anxiety, tremor, occasionally chorea, etc., in thyrotoxicosis, and lethargy, myopathy, and dementia in hypothyroidism (see Chapter 13.4). By contrast, Grave's ophthalmoplegia and Hashimoto's encephalopathy are both thought to be immunologically driven.

In dysthyroid eye disease, the orbit and extraocular muscles are oedematous and infiltrated with inflammatory cells and glycosaminoglycans, resulting in proptosis and a restrictive ophthalmopathy. Upgaze limitation is the commonest presenting sign. Vision is occasionally threatened by a complicating infiltrative or compressive optic neuropathy. Circulating TSH receptor-stimulating antibodies cross-reactive with orbital fibroblasts are found. Steroid treatment and radiotherapy are equally effective.

Hashimoto's encephalopathy exhibits female:male ratio of up to 9:1. Most cases are clinically and biochemically euthyroid at presentation, and two modes of presentation occur. The relapsing-remitting variety causes stroke-like episodes, with or without mild cognitive impairment, focal or generalized seizures, and episodes of encephalopathy. The second group present with a more diffuse progressive disease, with dementia, psychotic features, seizures, and occasionally myoclonus, tremor and/or ataxia; focal neurological deficits are uncommon.

Imaging by CT or even MR is often normal, as is angiography, though isotope brain scanning may show patchy uptake. Spinal fluid examination may reveal a raised protein level but typically a normal cell count. Very high titres of antithyroid antibodies are found, usually antimicrosomal. Most patients respond well to steroid treatment; some have received further immunosuppressive therapy, such as cyclophosphamide or azathioprine.

Further reading

Adams M, *et al.* (1987). Whipple's disease confined to the central nervous system. *Ann Neurol*, **21**, 104–8.
Akman-Demir G, Serdaroglu P, Tasci B (1999). Clinical patterns of neurological involvement in Behcet's disease: evaluation of 200 patients. The Neuro-Behcet Study Group. *Brain*, **122**, 2171–82.

Asherson RA (2005). Multiorgan failure and antiphospholipid antibodies: the catastrophic antiphospholipid (Asherson's) syndrome. *Immunobiology*, **210**, 727–33.

Andonopoulos AP, *et al.* (1990). The spectrum of neurological involvement in Sjogren's syndrome. *Br J Rheumatol*, **29**, 21–23.

Bathon JM, Moreland LW, DiBartolomeo AG (1989). Inflammatory central nervous system involvement in rheumatoid arthritis. *Semin Arthritis Rheum*, **18**, 258–66.

Brey RL, *et al.* (2002). Neuropsychiatric syndromes in lupus: prevalence using standardized definitions. *Neurology*, **58**, 1214–20.

Caselli RJ, Hunder GG (1994). Neurologic complications of giant cell (temporal) arteritis. *Semin.Neurol*, **14**, 349–53.

Cerinic MM, *et al.* (1996). The nervous system in systemic sclerosis (scleroderma). Clinical features and pathogenetic mechanisms. *Rheum Dis Clin North Am*, **22**, 879–92.

Cooke WT, Smith WT (1966). Neurological disorders associated with adult coeliac disease. *Brain*, **89**, 683–722.

Dresner SC, Kennerdell JS (1985). Dysthyroid orbitopathy. *Neurology*, **35**, 1628–34.

Dyck PJ, *et al.* (1987). Nonsystemic vasculitic neuropathy. *Brain*, **110**, 843–854.

Elsehety A, Bertorini TE (1997). Neurologic and neuropsychiatric complications of Crohn's disease. *South Med J*, **90**, 606–10.

Furst DE, *et al.* (2005). Updated consensus statement on biological agents, specifically tumour necrosis factor α (TNFα) blocking agents and interleukin-1 receptor antagonist (IL-1ra), for the treatment of rheumatic diseases, 2005. *Ann Rheum Dis*, **64** Suppl 4, iv2–14.

Ginzler EM, Dvorkina O (2005). Newer therapeutic approaches for systemic lupus erythematosus. *Rheum Dis Clin North Am*, **31**, 315–28.

Higashida J, *et al.* (2005). Safety and efficacy of rituximab in patients with rheumatoid arthritis refractory to disease modifying antirheumatic drugs and anti-tumor necrosis factor-alpha treatment. *J Rheumatol*, **32**, 2109–15.

Hochberg MC (1997). Updating the American College of Rheumatology revised criteria for the classification of systemic lupus erythematosus. *Arthritis Rheum*, **40**, 1725.

Hughes GR (1993). The antiphospholipid syndrome: ten years on. *Lancet* **342**, 341–4.

Joseph FG, Scolding NJ (2002). Cerebral vasculitis—a practical approach. *Pract Neurol*, **2**, 80–93.

Joseph FG, Scolding NJ (2007). Neuro-Behcet's disease in Caucasians: a study of 22 patients. *Eur J Neurol*, **14**, 174–80.

Joseph FG, Lammie GA, Scolding NJ (2007). CNS lupus: a study of 41 patients. *Neurology*, **69**, 644–54.

Levine SR, Brey RL (1996). Neurological aspects of antiphospholipid antibody syndrome. *Lupus*, **5**, 347–53.

Louis ED, *et al.* (1996). Diagnostic guidelines in central nervous system Whipple's disease. *Ann Neurol*, **40**, 561–8.

Matthews WB (1968). The neurological complications of ankylosing spondylitis. *J Neurol Sci*, **6**, 561–73.

Nishino H, *et al.* (1993). Neurological involvement in Wegener's granulomatosis: an analysis of 324 consecutive patients at the Mayo Clinic. *Ann Neurol*, **33**, 4–9.

Pincelli C, *et al.* (1994). Psoriasis and the nervous system. *Acta Dermatol Venereol Suppl Stockh*, **186**, 60–1.

Scolding NJ (1999). *Immunological and Inflammatory diseases of the central nervous system*, pp. 210–58. Butterworth-Heinemann, Oxford.

Scolding NJ, Joseph FG (2002). The neuropathology and pathogenesis of systemic lupus erythematosus. *Neuropathol Appl Neurobiol*, **28**, 173–89.

Scolding NJ, *et al.* (2005). Aβ-related angiitis: primary angiitis of the central nervous system associated with cerebral amyloid angiopathy. *Brain*, **128**, 500–15.

Thatayatikom A, White AJ (2006). Rituximab: A promising therapy in systemic lupus erythematosus. *Autoimmun Rev*, **5**, 18–24.

Unger L, Kayser M, Nusslein HG (2003). Successful treatment of severe rheumatoid vasculitis by infliximab. *Ann Rheum Dis*, **62**, 587–9.

Zajicek JP (1999). Sarcoidosis and the nervous system. In: Scolding NJ (ed.) *Immunological and inflammatory diseases of the central nervous system*, pp. 193–209. Butterworth-Heinemann, Oxford.

Paraneoplastic neurological syndromes

Jeremy Rees, Jerry Posner, and Angela Vincent

Essentials

Paraneoplastic neurological syndromes are disorders caused by the presence of an underlying tumour, but not due to either direct or metastatic invasion, or to recognized metabolic or endocrine complications. They are thought to arise from an autoimmune response to onconeural tumour antigens which are also expressed by the central or peripheral nervous system.

Paraneoplastic syndromes are rare but important because (1) they often develop before the cancer has been identified, (2) serological testing for specific anti-neuronal (onconeural) antibodies may identify a neurological disorder as paraneoplastic and strongly suggests the location of the underlying tumour and/or predicts its prognosis.

Epidemiology—the most common tumours associated with paraneoplastic syndromes are lung (both small-cell lung cancer (SCLC) and non-SCLC), ovary, breast, thymus, lymph nodes (Hodgkin's disease and non-Hodgkin's lymphoma) and testis.

Treatment—a few paraneoplastic syndromes respond to immunosuppression or to treatment of the underlying cancer, particularly encephalitides with germ cell tumors, but treatment is unrewarding for most and the patients remain with stable but often severe neurological disability even if the cancer is cured.

Specific syndromes

Brain and cranial nerves—(1) cerebellar degeneration—most common with lung cancer (especially SCLC), breast and gynaecological cancer, and Hodgkin's disease; (2) opsoclonus/myoclonus; (3) limbic encephalitis (see Chapter 24.22); (4) brainstem encephalitis; (5) cancer-associated retinopathy.

Neuromuscular junction and muscle (see Chapter 24.23)

(1) Lambert–Eaton myasthenic syndrome—typically associated with SCLC; (2) myasthenia gravis—occurs in 30% of patients with thymomas; (3) polymyositis/dermatomyositis; (4) neuromyotonia; (5) peripheral neuropathies.

Spinal cord and dorsal root ganglia—(1) necrotizing myelopathy; (2) motor neuron disease (some cases); (3) myelitis; (4) sensory neuronopathy; (5) peripheral neuropathies.

Incidence

Paraneoplastic neurological syndromes (PNS) are very rare, probably affecting fewer than 1% of patients with cancers of all types. In one series of almost 1500 patients, only 3 had paraneoplastic cerebellar degeneration, and none had subacute sensory neuronopathy. The most frequent PNS is the Lambert–Eaton myasthenic syndrome (LEMS), which affects about 3% of patients with small-cell lung cancer (SCLC). In a surveillance study of all PNS from the United Kingdom, the female:male ratio was greater than 3:1, the median age of onset of PNS was 66 years and only 11% of patients were less than 50 years at presentation. The PNS preceded the diagnosis of cancer in 84% of patients.

Despite their low incidence, paraneoplastic syndromes are important for several reasons.

- They often develop before the cancer has been identified and so their presence may lead to the detection of small and potentially curable cancers.

- The presence of specific antibodies in the serum of patients with a PNS identifies the neurological disorder as paraneoplastic and may strongly suggest the location of the underlying tumour.

- The PNS is often more disabling than the cancer and, in some instances, may be the cause of death.

- A PNS or an antibody associated with a PNS (see below) may predict a less aggressive course for the cancer.

- Paraneoplastic antibodies identify proteins normally restricted to neurons that are of importance in the development and maintenance of the nervous system (see 'Further reading').

The syndromes

The clinical syndromes may be focal or diffuse involving single or multiple parts of the nervous system. The most well-characterized syndromes (termed 'classical' by Graus et al.) are those that should always arouse suspicion of an associated cancer, and are listed

Table 24.21.1 Classical paraneoplastic neurological syndromes[*]

Example(s)	Area most affected
Limbic encephalitis (dementia)	Cerebral hemisphere(s)
Cerebellar degeneration	Cerebellum
Opsoclonus–myoclonus	Brainstem
Carcinoma-associated retinopathy	Retina
Necrotizing myelopathy	Spinal cord
Stiff person syndrome[*]	Spinal cord
Sensory neuronopathy	Dorsal root ganglia
Sensory/sensorimotor neuropathy[*]	Peripheral nerve
Autonomic neuropathy[*]	Peripheral nerve
Lambert–Eaton myasthenic syndrome	Neuromuscular junction
Dermatomyositis	Muscle
Encephalomyelitis	Diffuse

[*] Syndromes that are most often non-paraneoplastic.

in Table 24.21.1. These syndromes are commonly, but not always, associated with antibodies to certain onconeural antigens which point to the most likely tumours (Table 24.21.2), and will be described in detail below.

Onconeural antibodies

These antibodies help to diagnose the syndrome as being paraneoplastic and may point to a specific underlying tumour. For example, a patient with paraneoplastic cerebellar degeneration (PCD) who has serum anti-Yo antibodies will almost always have a breast, ovarian, or other gynaecological cancer. Patients with PCD associated with nongynaecological cancers have other antibodies that react with Purkinje cells or do not have antibodies identifiable by current techniques. The main antigens (Table 24.21.2) are not described here, but most are cytoplasmic or nuclear proteins although some, e.g. voltage-gated calcium channels, are membrane proteins that are accessible to circulating antibodies.

Some autoantibodies are associated with specific tumours but widely varying paraneoplastic syndromes. For example, the anti-Hu antibody (Fig. 24.21.1) is almost always associated with SCLC (occasionally neuroblastoma or prostate cancer), but may be found in several different clinical syndromes usually encompassed by the term 'encephalomyelitis'. The clinical abnormalities include limbic encephalitis, PCD, brainstem encephalitis, sensory neuronopathy, and autonomic failure. Some or all of these clinical abnormalities may be found in the same patient.

Not all patients with a classical syndrome and associated tumour have onconeural antibodies. Thus the absence of a positive antibody should not be taken as evidence that the patient has a non-paraneoplastic form of disease. In some conditions, there are no identified antibodies. A good example is opsoclonus–myoclonus associated with neuroblastoma in children. Most observers believe that this paraneoplastic disorder is immune-mediated. The failure to find a disease- or tumour- specific antibody does not mean that one is not present, only that current techniques have not identified it. As techniques improve, new antibodies are regularly being reported; of particular interest is the recent discovery of antibodies

Table 24.21.2 Onconeural antibody associated paraneoplastic disorders

Antibody	Neuronal reactivity	Cloned genes	Tumour	Clinical syndromes
Anti-Hu	Nucleus>cytoplasm (all neuron)	HuD, HuC,Nel-N1	SCLC, neuroblastoma, sarcoma, prostate	PEM, PSN, PCD, autonomic neuropathy
Anti-Yo	Cytoplasm, Purkinje cells	CDR34, CDR62	Ovary, breast, lung	PCD
Anti-Ri	Nucleus>cytoplasm (CNS neurons)	Nova	Breast, gynaecological cancer, lung, bladder	Ataxia/opsoclonus
Anti-Tr	Cytoplasm, Purkinje cells	Not known	Hodgkin's disease	PCD
Anti-VGCC	Presynaptic neuromuscular junction	P/Q type VGCC, MysB	VGCC, SCLC	LEMS
Anti-VGKC	Presynaptic: neuromuscular junction and CNS	VGKCs and associated proteins	Thymoma, SCLC	Neuromyotonia, autonomic, limbic encephalitis or combinations of these (Morvan's syndrome)
Anti-Retinal	Photoreceptor, ganglion cells	Recoverin and others	SCLC, melanoma, gynaecological	CAR, MAR
Anti-Amphiphysin	Presynaptic	Amphiphysin	Breast, SCLC	Stiff person syndrome, PEM
Anti-CRMP5 (Anti- CV2)	Oligodendrocytes cytoplasm,	CRMP5 (POP66)	SCLC, thymoma	PEM, PCD, chorea, sensory neuropathy, autonomic neuropathy
Anti-Ma1	Neurons (subnucleus)	Ma1	Lung, others	Brainstem, PCD
Anti-Ma2	Neurons (subnucleus)	Ma2	Testis	Limbic brainstem encephalitis
Anti-NMDAR	Cytoplasmic membrane of hippocampal neurons	EFA6A	Ovarian teratoma	Limbic encephalitis with prominent neuropsychiatric features progressing to movement disorders, fall in consciousness and autonomic instability
Anti-ganglionic AChR	Ganglionic synapses	α_3-containing ganglionic AChR	SCLC, thymoma	Dysautonomia

AChR, acetylcholine receptor; SCLC, small-cell lung cancer; VGCC, voltage-gated calcium channels. For other abbreviations, see text.

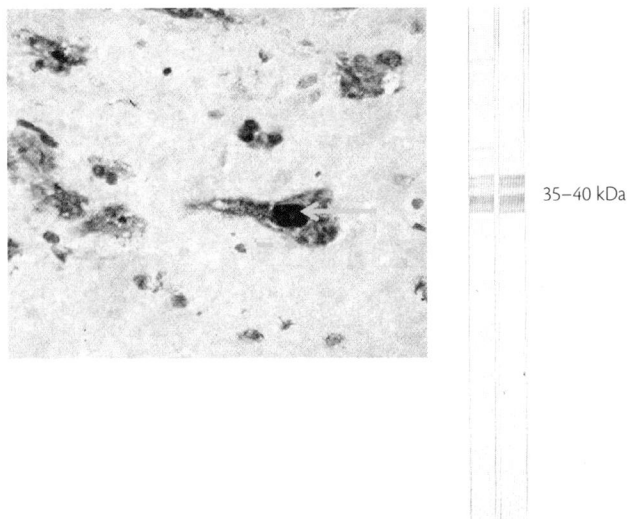

35–40 kDa

Fig. 24.21.1 Anti-Hu antibodies: serum immunoreactivity with rat brainstem counterstained showing strong nuclear staining (solid arrow) and weaker cytoplasmic staining (dashed arrow) typical of anti-Hu (anti ANNA 1) antibodies. Western blot shows a 'ladder' pattern of bands between 35 and 40 kDa. (DAB-peroxidase counterstained with haematoxylin and eosin). The patient was a woman with subacute cerebellar degeneration who was subsequently found to have lung cancer.
(Courtesy of Elizabeth Amyes, University of Oxford.)

directed against N-methyl-D-aspartate receptors (NMDAR) on hippocampal neurons in young female patients and children with a progressive encephalopathy, patients with including some associated with ovarian teratomas (see 'Further reading').

Tumours associated with PNS

The most common tumours associated with PNS are found in lung (both SCLC and non-SCLC), ovary, breast, thymus, lymph nodes (both Hodgkin's disease and non-Hodgkin's lymphoma), and testis. In a recent European survey, other tumours were also identified suggesting that whole-body scanning is appropriate in the diagnostic work-up of patients with suspected PNS.

Diagnosis

Certain clinical clues suggest that a neurological disorder may be a PNS. The onset is usually rapid; in some cases the symptoms develop overnight so that a stroke is initially suspected. Most PNS are progressive initially then stabilize after weeks to months, although more slowly progressive syndromes may occur. Recovery is rare in most of the CNS syndromes, probably because of irreversible neuronal loss and degeneration, although spontaneous resolution and improvement after oncological treatment have been reported.

The neurological disorders are usually severe. Most patients have substantial disability by the time they first consult a physician. Mild or waxing and waning neurological symptoms are rarely paraneoplastic. For example, the patient with PCD is usually unable to walk or sit unsupported, unable to write, and sometimes, because of the oscillopsia associated with nystagmus, unable to read.

The neurological findings are often characteristic. A subacutely developing pancerebellar disorder, the rapid development of opsoclonus (see below), or the development of LEMS strongly suggests

cancer as the underlying cause. However, none of these syndromes, even the most characteristic, is invariably associated with cancer. Thus, only about one-half of patients with LEMS have cancer and only about 10% of patients with myasthenia gravis have a tumour (almost always thymoma). Probably about one-half of the patients with subacute cerebellar degeneration have cancer. Limbic encephalitis was thought of as paraneoplastic but it is now clear that nonparaneoplastic forms can be identified, and are much more common (Chapter 24.22).

Imaging in suspected PNS is often not informative. Indeed, one of the clues to the presence of a PNS is the relative normality of imaging in a patient with such severe clinical symptoms and signs. Occasionally MRI may show high signal within one or both medial temporal lobes (limbic encephalitis) or brainstem (brainstem encephalitis) and very rarely diffuse oedema of the cerebellum (PCD). The cerebrospinal fluid may show pleocytosis (30–40 cells), elevated protein, increased IgG, and oligoclonal bands particularly early in the course of disease which then settles within a few weeks of onset. The immunoglobulin abnormalities usually persist. In a patient with a known cancer, the diagnosis of PNS should usually only be made after exclusion of the more common neurological complications of cancer (Box 24.21.1), unless an onconeural antibody is found in the serum.

In a patient without a known cancer, particularly when conventional imaging studies (radiography, CT, ultrasonography, and mammography) are negative, the appropriate use of whole-body fluorodeoxyglucose positron emission tomography (FDG-PET) may show a FDG-avid 'hot spot' suggestive of an occult malignancy

---

Box 24.21.1 Neurological complications of cancer

Metastases
- Brain
- Spinal cord
- Leptomeninges
- Cranial and/or peripheral nerves

Nonmetastatic effects of cancer
- Metabolic disorders:
  - Organ failure
  - Endocrinopathies
  - Nutritional deficiencies
  - Tumour secretion of ectopic substances e.g. hypercalcaemia
- Vascular disorders:
  - Haemorrhage
  - Infarction
- Infection:
- Side effects of therapy:
  - Surgery
  - Irradiation
  - Chemotherapy

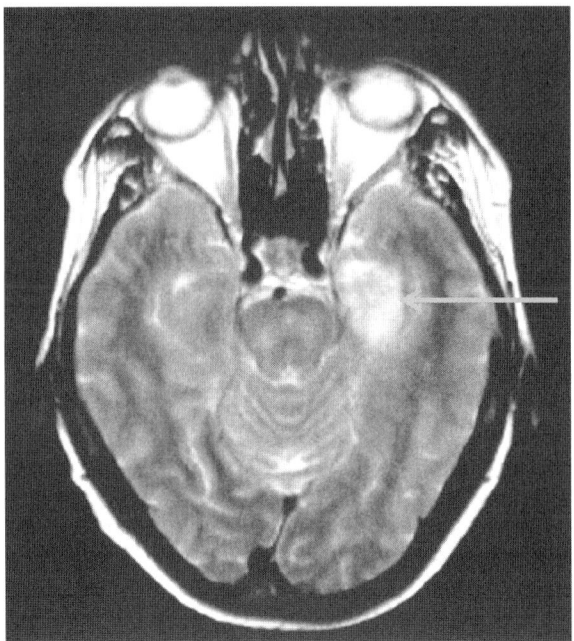

Fig. 24.21.2 Axial T2W MRI brain of patient with limbic encephalitis showing high signal in left medial temporal lobe (arrow).

(Fig. 24.21.2). Blood tumour markers are rarely helpful in this clinical context. If an onconeural antibody is present and the search for an underlying cancer is negative, the physician is obliged to follow the patient carefully, searching periodically for a cancer.

The difficulties of defining and hence diagnosing PND have been carefully considered by an international panel of neurological experts who have established guidelines for more rigorous diagnostic criteria. The aim of these guidelines has been to facilitate diagnosis, classification, and collaborative research. They rely on the definition of 'classical' paraneoplastic syndromes and 'well-characterized' onconeural autoantibodies. On this basis a condition could be diagnosed as paraneoplastic based on a descending hierarchy of factors: (1) presence or absence of 'classical' syndrome; (2) presence or absence of cancer; (3) presence or absence of 'well-characterized' antineuronal antibodies, and (4) exclusion of other possible causes of a similar neurological syndrome particularly malignant meningitis. On the basis of combinations of these criteria, the diagnosis of a PND is now either 'definite' or 'possible'. (See 'Further reading'.)

Pathogenesis

Current evidence suggests that PNS result from an autoimmune reaction to 'onconeural' antigens in the tumour. These antigens are those that are normally restricted to the nervous system (or the testis, which is also an immunologically privileged site). The immune system therefore recognizes the antigen as foreign and some patients mount an immune response. The immune response may have the beneficial effect of slowing tumour growth but it can also damage those parts of the nervous system that express the antigen. Although many PNS are associated with specific neuronal autoantibodies, there is limited evidence that those directed against cytoplasmic or nuclear antigens are pathogenic. T lymphocytes recognizing these or other onconeural antigens, and other cellular immune mechanisms, are the likely pathogenic agents in these conditions. In contrast, antibodies directed against membrane ion channels or receptors for neurotransmitters (e.g. anti-voltage gated calcium and potassium channels, glutamate receptors) are pathogenic but are also often present in nonparaneoplastic forms of the disease.

Treatment

Some PNS, such as LEMS, respond to immunosuppression or to treatment of the underlying cancer (Table 24.21.3). Some syndromes, such as opsoclonus–myoclonus, may remit spontaneously, but for most PNS treatment is unrewarding and the patients remain with severe neurological disability even if the cancer is cured. Treatments usually involve immunosuppression with plasma exchange, intravenous immunoglobulin, steroids, or cytotoxics particularly for those syndromes associated with onconeural autoantibodies. It is possible that the rapid onset of the syndromes does not allow sufficient time for accurate early diagnosis and for treatment to begin before irreversible neural damage has occurred. With earlier diagnosis, therapy may be more successful. However, as mentioned above, a number of the 'classical' paraneoplastic conditions appear to exist in nonparaneoplastic forms (e.g. limbic encephalitis with potassium channel antibodies) and may respond to immunotherapies; therefore, if onconeural antibodies are absent, and no cancer is found, a trial of immunotherapy should be considered. There has been recent interest in rituximab (anti-CD20 monoclonal Ab) which has shown modest benefit in a small open trial of patients with PNS.

Specific syndromes

Brain and cranial nerves (Box 24.21.2)

Paraneoplastic cerebellar degeneration (PCD)

PCD may complicate any malignant tumour but is most common with lung cancer (especially SCLC), breast and gynaecological cancer, and Hodgkin's disease. Males and females are both affected and the age incidence reflects the age distribution of the underlying cancer. Neurological manifestations precede detection of the associated tumour in over one-half of patients, rarely by more than five years, or PCD may develop after diagnosis of the neoplasm. In some instances, the tumour is not found until autopsy. Typically, the disorder begins as gait ataxia that progresses over a few days to weeks to severe truncal and appendicular ataxia with dysarthria and nystagmus. The nystagmus is frequently downbeating. Vertigo with or without nausea and vomiting is common and many patients complain of diplopia. The cerebellar signs are bilateral but may be asymmetrical. The cerebellar deficit usually stabilizes but, by then, the patient is often incapacitated. Spontaneous improvement sometimes occurs, particularly when associated with Hodgkin's disease. Some patients will also be found to be mildly cognitively impaired and demonstrate extensor plantar reflexes or sensory changes suggesting a more widespread encephalomyelitis.

The cerebrospinal fluid may be normal, but there is usually a pleocytosis within the first few months, and raised protein and oligoclonal bands may also be present. Cytological examination of the cerebrospinal fluid and contrast-enhanced MRI of the neuraxis rule out leptomeningeal metastases. MRI scans typically

Table 24.21.3 Treatment of paraneoplastic neurological syndromes

Syndrome	Treatment
Paraneoplastic syndromes that usually respond to treatment	
Lambert–Eaton myasthenic syndrome (LEMS)	Tumour therapy, plasma exchange, intravenous immunoglobulin, 3,4 diaminopyridine
Myasthenia gravis	Tumour therapy, plasma exchange, intravenous immunoglobulin, immunosuppressants
Dermatomyositis	Steroids, immunosuppressants, intravenous immunoglobulin
Opsoclonus–myoclonus (children)	Steroids, ACTH, tumour therapy
Limbic encephalitis or progressive syndromes with antibodies to cell surface antigens, eg. VGKC, NMDAR	Tumour therapy, plasma exchange, intravenous immunoglobulin, immunosuppressants
Neuromyotonia	Plasma exchange
Demylinating neuropathy (osteosclerotic myeloma)	Tumour therapy, radiation, bevacizumab
Paraneoplastic syndromes that may respond to treatment	
Opsoclonus–myoclonus (adults)	Steroids, tumour therapy, protein A column, clonazepam, diazepam, baclofen
Paraneoplastic cerebellar degeneration (Hodgkin's disease)	Tumour therapy
Opsoclonus/ataxia (anti-Ri)	Steroids, cyclophosphamide
Paraneoplastic syndromes that usually do not respond to treatment	
Paraneoplastic cerebellar degeneration (gynaecological cancers):	
Small-cell lung cancer (irrespective of anti-Hu)	
Anti-Yo antibodies (cancer of ovary, breast)	
Paraneoplastic encephalomyelitis/sensory neuronopathy (often anti-Hu positive):	
Limbic encephalopathy (except with anti-VGKC or anti-NMDAR antibodies)	
Cerebellar degeneration	
Brainstem encephalitis	
Necrotizing myelopathy	
Sensory neuronopathy	
Autonomic dysfunction (central or peripheral)	
Cancer-associated retinopathy	
Paraneoplastic syndromes that may improve spontaneously	
Acute motor neuronopathy and lymphoma	
Paraneoplastic cerebellar degeneration associated with Hodgkin's disease	
Acute polyradiculopathy associated with Hodgkin's disease	
Opsoclonus–myoclonus (children or adults)	

are normal early, but later show signs of progressive cerebellar atrophy with prominent cerebellar folia and a dilated fourth ventricle.

The pathological hallmark of paraneoplastic cerebellar degeneration is loss of Purkinje cells, affecting all parts of the cerebellum. Less striking changes in the cerebellar cortex may include thinning of the molecular layer with microglial proliferation and astrocytic gliosis, proliferation of Bergmann astrocytes, and slight thinning of the granular layer with decreased numbers of granule cells.

When typical, the clinical picture of PCD is almost pathognomonic. When atypical, the disorder must be distinguished from a cerebellar tumour (primary or metastatic) and from leptomeningeal metastases (by MRI and cerebrospinal fluid examination, respectively), from late-onset, nonparaneoplastic cerebellar degenerations, cerebellar haemorrhage and infarction, abscess, prion diseases, cerebellar ataxia related to 5-fluorouracil or high-dose cytarabine, and metabolic disorders, especially alcoholic cerebellar degeneration.

There have been occasional reports of a partial or near-complete remission of paraneoplastic cerebellar degeneration following treatment of the primary tumour. This is very unusual, however, and most patients do not improve even when treatment is begun early in the illness, before Purkinje cells are irreversibly damaged. Plasmapheresis, corticosteroids, immunosuppressive drugs and, more recently, intravenous immune globlulin (IVIG) and rituximab have all been tried and may lead to mild symptomatic improvement in the ataxia. PCD may occasionally be associated with LEMS, both associated with SCLC. Recognition and treatment of the peripheral symptoms can lead to overall clinical benefits.

Opsoclonus–myoclonus

Opsoclonus is a disorder of eye movements consisting of almost continuous chaotic, multidirectional, involuntary, high-amplitude conjugate saccades that are often accompanied by synchronous blinking of the lids. It is usually considered to be a paraneoplastic syndrome complicating 2% of childhood neuroblastoma (dancing eyes syndrome) or a variety of tumours in adults, particularly breast cancer and SCLC, but there are cases that appear to be non-paraneoplastic and self-limiting (see below).

Opsoclonus may be an isolated neurological sign, but is often accompanied by myoclonus of the trunk, limbs, head, diaphragm, larynx, pharynx, and palate, and ataxia, hence the term opsoclonus–myoclonus or opsoclonus–myoclonus ataxia. Neurological symptoms precede identification of the neuroblastoma in at least 50% of patients, and the tumour may be missed by abdominal examination; thus, recognition of the neurological syndrome is an important clue to the presence of a neuroblastoma. There are preliminary reports of antibodies to neuroblastoma cell lines but no specific antigen has been defined. When a neuroblastoma is associated with opsoclonus–myoclonus, there is a higher than expected incidence of intrathoracic tumours and of tumours with a benign histology. The prognosis of the neuroblastoma is better if opsoclonus–myoclonus is associated than when there is no neurological complication, an observation not explained by earlier diagnosis when neurological symptoms are present. The neurological disorder responds to ACTH and to intravenous immunoglobulin but not to prednisone. However, most patients suffer residual neurological damage, usually cognitive.

Opsoclonus–myoclonus is less common in adults, and in those cases is often nonparaneoplastic. Nevertheless, about 20% of adult patients reported with opsoclonus–myoclonus have an underlying cancer. The neurological symptoms usually precede diagnosis of the tumour and commonly progress over several weeks, although more rapid or slower progression may be observed. The cerebrospinal fluid may show a mild pleocytosis and an elevated protein. The MRI is usually normal. Neuropathological findings have been variable. In some patients there are no identifiable abnormalities. In others, the changes resembled those

of PCD with a loss of Purkinje cells, inflammatory infiltrates in the brainstem, Bergmann gliosis, and loss of cells from the granular layer of the cerebellum.

The prognosis for recovery or partial remission of the neurological disorder is better for opsoclonus–myoclonus than it is for PCD. Improvement may follow treatment of the underlying tumour, and spontaneous partial remissions occur. Differential diagnosis includes nonparaneoplastic conditions such as viral inections, postinfectious encephalitis, hydrocephalus, thalamic haemorrhage, and toxic encephalopathies from thallium or lithium, amitriptyline overdose, and diabetic hyperosmolar coma.

Limbic encephalitis

Limbic encephalitis may occur as an isolated finding or as a more extensive encephalomyelitis. The neurological symptoms often precede diagnosis of the tumour by up to 2 years; sometimes the cancer is not detected until autopsy. Symptoms usually progress over several weeks but the course may be more insidious. Anxiety and depression are common early symptoms, but the most striking feature is a severe impairment of episodic memory. Other manifestations include agitation, confusion, hallucinations, and partial or generalized seizures. The symptoms may spread to include other brain functions, e.g. the hypothalamus, with changes in appetite or sleep, e.g. hypersomnia. Progressive dementia usually occurs, but occasionally there may be a spontaneous remission; more and more of these cases are now known to be non paraneoplastic associated with antibodies to voltage-gated potassium channels (Chapter 24.22). Indeed this test should now be sent off in any patient presenting with a rapidly progressive amnesic syndrome, as it is treatable. The cerebrospinal fluid commonly shows a pleocytosis and an elevated protein concentration in PNS cases. MR scans are usually normal but medial temporal abnormalities have been reported (Fig. 24.21.3).

Inflammatory pathological changes affect the grey matter of the hippocampus, cingulate gyrus, pyriform cortex, orbital surfaces of the frontal lobes, insula, and the amygdala. No treatment has proved uniformly beneficial although spontaneous remissions have been reported and some patients have improved after treatment of the underlying tumour. If onconeural antibodies are negative and there is no evidence of a tumour, immunosuppression should be considered as recent studies have identified antibodies against novel cell-membrane antigens (nCMAg such as VGKCs, NMDARs) which are associated with a favourable prognosis.

Brainstem encephalitis

Paraneoplastic brainstem encephalitis is often associated with clinical and pathological evidence of encephalomyelitis elsewhere within the central and peripheral nervous systems, but may occur as the dominant or an isolated clinical finding. It is commonly associated with SCLC, but an identical clinicopathological syndrome may be seen in the absence of a malignancy.

The clinical features vary according to the brainstem structures involved in the pathological process. Common manifestations include vertigo, ataxia, nystagmus, vomiting, bulbar palsy, oculomotor disorders, and corticospinal tract dysfunction. Less common clinical features include deafness, myoclonus of the branchial musculature, central alveolar hypoventilation presenting with respiratory failure. Basal ganglia involvement produces movement disorders including chorea or Parkinson's syndrome, these being more commonly seen in patients with anti-CV2 antibodies.

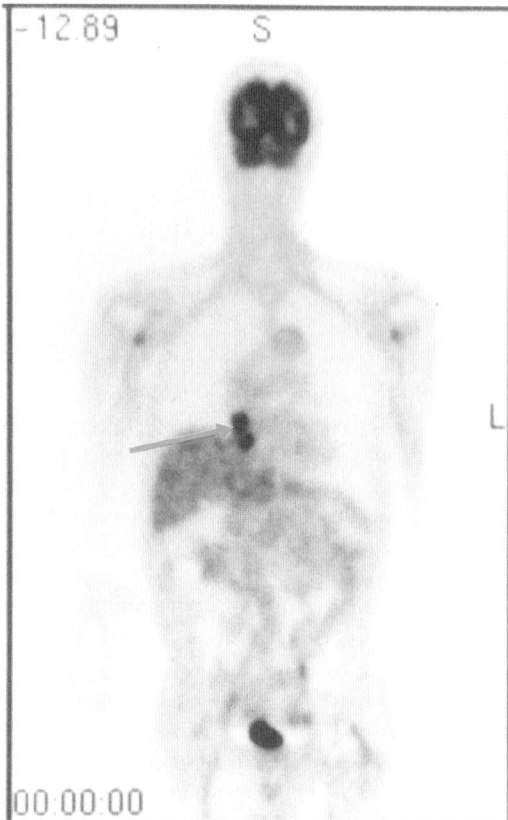

Fig. 24.21.3 Whole body FDG-PET scan showing two hot spots in right middle lobe (arrow) from patient with cerebellar degeneration and anti-Hu antibodies in whom chest radiography and CT of the thorax were both negative. Subsequent biopsy confirmed small-cell lung cancer.

Neurological symptoms may develop before or after discovery of the malignancy. The pathological changes are identical to those observed in other forms of paraneoplastic encephalomyelitis.

Visual loss
PNS can affect retinal photoreceptors, either rods or cones or both. They can cause a retinal vasculitis or optic neuropathy. Paraneoplastic retinal degeneration, also called cancer-associated retinopathy (CAR), usually occurs in association with SCLC, melanoma, and gynaecological tumours. Typically, the visual symptoms include episodic visual obscurations, night blindness, light-induced glare, photosensitivity, and impaired colour vision. Visual symptoms usually precede the diagnosis of cancer. The symptoms progress to painless visual loss. They may begin unilaterally but usually become bilateral. Visual testing demonstrates peripheral and ring scotomas and loss of acuity. Fundoscopic examination may reveal arteriolar narrowing and abnormal mottling of the retinal pigment epithelium. The electroretinogram is abnormal. Cerebrospinal fluid is typically normal, although elevated immunoglobulin levels have been reported. Inflammatory cells are sometimes seen in the vitreous by slit-lamp examination. Retinal antibodies (e.g. recoverin), although well recognized, are not routinely available in most countries.

Pathologically, CAR is associated with a loss of photoreceptors and ganglion cells with inflammatory infiltrates and macrophages. The other parts of the optic pathway are preserved, although a loss of myelin and lymphocytic infiltration of the optic nerve may occur.

Box 24.21.3 Paraneoplastic syndromes affecting spinal cord and dorsal root ganglia

- Sensory neuronopathy
- Necrotizing myelopathy
- Subacute motor neuronopathy
- Motor neuron disease (primary lateral sclerosis)
- Myelitis (as part of encephalomyelitis)

Treatment of CAR is usually unsuccessful although a recent report describes improvement in some patients with the use of intravenous immunoglobulin. The condition is not recognized very frequently, and there may be nonparaneoplastic forms that are difficult to distinguish.

Spinal cord and dorsal root ganglia (Box 24.21.3)
Necrotizing myelopathy
This is an extremely rare PNS. The initial symptoms of muscle weakness and sensory loss in the arms and legs may be asymmetrical, but eventually signs become bilateral and symmetrical. Back or radicular pain may precede other neurological signs. Cerebrospinal fluid abnormalities may include an elevated level of protein and a mild pleocytosis. Swelling of the spinal cord may be apparent on MRI. Typically, the neurological deficit progresses rapidly over days or a few weeks, ultimately leading to respiratory failure and death. There is no effective treatment.

Pathologically, there is widespread necrosis of the spinal cord, often most marked in the thoracic segments. The necrosis involves all components of the spinal cord with white matter usually more affected than grey matter.

Motor neuron disease (amyotrophic lateral sclerosis)
There is controversy as to whether motor neuron disease (MND) can be regarded as a classical PNS. It is likely to be paraneoplastic in three distinct groups of patients; the first with a rapidly progressive amyotrophic lateral sclerosis picture associated with anti-Hu antibodies; the second with primary lateral sclerosis and breast cancer; and the third with a subacute motor neuronopathy associated with lymphoma. Classical MND in a patient with a previous history of cancer is probably not paraneoplastic, merely reflecting the occurrence of two reasonably common diseases of older age in the same patient separated in time.

Myelitis
Paraneoplastic myelitis is usually a part of the encephalomyelitis syndrome with inflammatory lesions elsewhere in the brain and dorsal root ganglia as well as the spinal cord. The clinical picture is dominated by the radicular element of a myeloradiculitis and is characterized by patchy wasting and weakness of muscles, sometimes combined with fasciculations. The upper extremities are often more severely affected than the legs, reflecting predominant involvement of the cervical spinal cord. There may be striking weakness of neck and intercostal muscles, resulting in respiratory failure. Sensory symptoms and autonomic dysfunction may be present.

Sensory neuronopathy
Paraneoplastic sensory neuronopathy is most commonly associated with SCLC. Symptoms typically begin before the cancer is

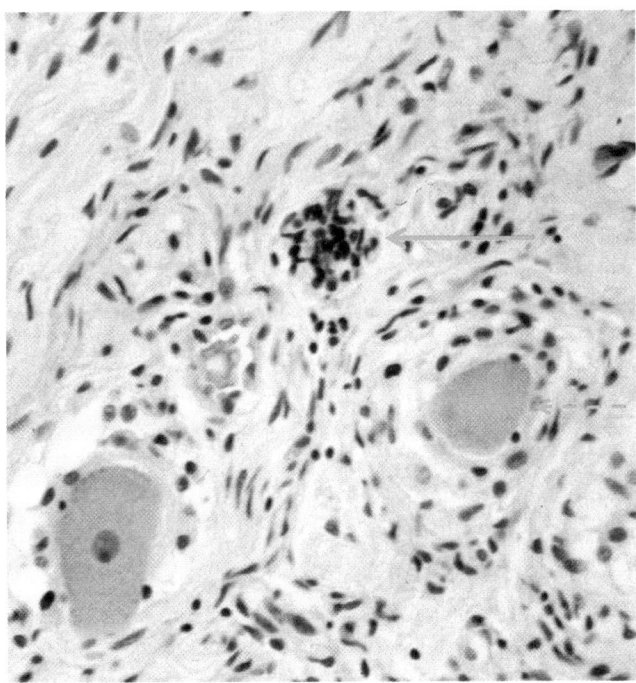

Fig. 24.21.4 Sensory ganglionitis: dorsal root ganglion with hypercellular nodules marking the site of ganglion cell degeneration. Another ganglion cell (dashed arrow) is in the process of degenerating. A healthy ganglion cell is shown in the bottom left-hand corner of the plate.

identified, with dysaesthetic pain and numbness in the legs or occasionally in the arm(s), face, or trunk. The symptoms may be asymmetrical at onset but progress over days to several weeks to involve the limbs, trunk, and sometimes the face, causing a severe sensory ataxia. All sensory modalities are affected. Deep tendon reflexes are lost but motor function is preserved. Occasional patients have a mild and indolent neuropathy. The cerebrospinal fluid is typically inflammatory.

Early pathological changes are limited mostly to the dorsal root ganglia, in which both a loss of neurons and the presence of lymphocytic inflammatory infiltrates are noted (Fig. 24.21.4). About 50% of patients with paraneoplastic sensory neuronopathy have pathological changes that may be clinically inapparent in other regions of the nervous system. As with other PND, this disorder rarely responds to treatment.

Peripheral nerves (Box 24.21.4)

Sensory and sensorimotor neuropathy
Peripheral neuropathies, particularly mild distal sensorimotor neuropathies, are common in patients with cancer and may be due to the metabolic or nutritional effects of late cancer, or associated with certain drugs, e.g. cisplatin.

Some patients not known to have cancer, and who are not evidently systemically ill, present to the neurologist with a peripheral neuropathy that may be quite severe and disabling. It is estimated that about 10% of those patients whose initial evaluations do not reveal an obvious cause (such as vitamin B12 deficiency, alcohol or diabetes), will eventually prove to have cancer as the underlying reason for the peripheral neuropathy. Paraneoplastic peripheral neuropathy may take several clinical and pathological forms. The most common is the distal, symmetrical, subacutely developing,

Box 24.21.4 Paraneoplastic syndromes affecting peripheral nerves

- Subacute or chronic sensorimotor peripheral neuropathy
- Mononeuritis multiplex and microvasculitis of peripheral nerve
- Brachial neuritis
- Autonomic neuropathy (as part of anti-Hu syndrome)
- Demyelinating peripheral neuropathy (myeloma or plasma-cytoma)

sensory neuropathy which may be either axonal or demyelinating. A relatively pure sensory neuropathy, a mononeuritis multiplex due to microvasculitis, an acute polyradiculopathy, a focal neuropathy such as brachial neuritis, or an autonomic neuropathy may also be paraneoplastic. Most of these neuropathies are not associated with autoantibodies and the diagnosis is often one of exclusion.

Neuromuscular junction and muscle (Box 24.21.5)

Paraneoplastic disorders of the neuromuscular junction include the Lambert–Eaton myasthenic syndrome, myasthenia gravis and acquired neuromyotoia. These disorders have a common pathogenetic mechanism—they are caused by antibodies against ion channels and, whether paraneoplastic or not, they respond to immunological treatment. They are described in more detail in Chapter 24.22. Finally, because of its similarity to neuromyotonia, the stiff person syndrome is also included in this section. Whereas the more common non-paraneoplastic form is associated with antbodies to glutamic acid decarboxylase, the presence of amphiphysin or other onconeural antibodies should raise the suspicion of a tumour.

Lambert–Eaton myasthenic syndrome (LEMS)
LEMS results from a reduced release of acetylcholine at presynaptic nerve terminals. The same P/Q-type voltage-gated calcium channels are found in small-cell lung cancers. Interestingly, the richest source of P/Q-type voltage-gated calcium channels is the cerebellum, perhaps explaining the occasional relationship of PCD and LEMS.

LEMS can be treated either by immune suppression or by treatment of the underlying cancer when present. Patients with SCLC associated with LEMS have a better prognosis than patients with SCLC who do not develop a paraneoplastic disorder, but this could be partly due to earlier diagnosis.

Myasthenia gravis
Myasthenia gravis occurs in 30% of patients with thymomas, and approximately 10% of patients with myasthenia gravis are found to

Box 24.21.5 Paraneoplastic syndromes affecting neuromuscular junction and muscle

- Lambert–Eaton myasthenic syndrome
- Myasthenia gravis
- Dermatomyositis, polymyositis, acute necrotizing myopathy
- Neuromyotonia

have a thymoma. Usually the two are diagnosed synchronously but rarely myasthenia may develop many years after the thymoma, sometimes in association with other autoimmune diseases, e.g. red-cell aplasia.

Polymyositis and dermatomyositis

Only a minority of patients, usually older people, with polymyositis or dermatomyositis have an underlying malignancy as the cause. Dermatomyositis with typical cutaneous changes is more likely to be paraneoplastic than polymyositis. Females and males are affected in approximately equal numbers. Symptoms of muscle weakness generally precede identification of the cancer. The tumour may be at any site, but breast, lung, ovarian, and gastric malignancies are the most common.

Corticosteroids, ciclosporin, and other immunosuppressants have been used successfully. Other reports suggest that high-dose IVIG is useful in patients unresponsive to other forms of immunosuppression.

Neuromyotonia and stiff person syndrome

Muscle cramps are a common complication of cancer, sometimes related to electrolyte imbalance or induced by chemotherapy. A much rarer but clinically significant PNS is acquired neuromyotonia. The disorder is characterized by muscle stiffness, cramps, and obviously rippling and twitching muscles, sometimes leading to sustained abnormal postures. Relaxation after voluntary contraction is delayed. Symptoms persist during sleep (and are abolished by curare). Sudden prolonged bursts of high-frequency, involuntary, repetitive muscle action potentials are seen on electromyography.

The muscle spasms and rigidity are sometimes precipitated by activity, forcing patients to become sedentary. The disorder arises from peripheral nerves and is sometimes a part of the encephalomyelitis syndrome. The disorder is usually nonparaneoplastic,

but may be associated with cancer including thymomas and SCLC. Antibodies against voltage-gated potassium channels are often positive (Chapter 24.22). Plasma exchange improves the patient's condition; but they often respond to anticonvulsants alone. Injection of IgG from affected patients into experimental animals can reproduce evidence of peripheral nerve hyperexcitability.

The stiff person syndrome may superficially resemble neuromyotonia, but has a central origin and is usually not paraneoplastic. This rare disorder is clinically characterized by stiffness and rigidity, with episodic spasms of axial muscles. A variant of the syndrome affects the limbs. Painful reflex spasms can occur in response to tactile stimuli or startle. Muscle action potentials are normal on electromyography but the activity is continuous and excessive and increased by voluntary activity. The disorder is usually autoimmune, associated with antibodies against glutamic acid dehydroxylase; since this antibody is also important in type 1 diabetes, the assay is widely available. When paraneoplastic, it can be associated with lung or breast tumours often with the appropriate onconeural antibody.

Further reading

Candler PM, *et al.* (2004). A follow up study of patients with paraneoplastic neurological disease in the United Kingdom. *J Neurol Neurosurg Psychiatry*, **75**, 1411–15.
Dalmau J, Rosenfeld MR (2008). Paraneoplastic syndromes of the CNS. *Lancet Neurol*, **7**, 327–40. Review.
Darnell RB, Posner JB (2006). Paraneoplastic syndromes affecting the nervous system. *Semin Oncol*, **33**, 270–98.
Graus F, *et al.* (2004). Recommended diagnostic criteria for paraneoplastic neurological syndromes. *J Neurol Neurosurg Psychiatry*, **75**, 1135–40.
Graus F, Saiz A, Dalmau J (2009). Antibodies and neural autoimmune disorders of the CNS. *J Neurol*, Dec 25 [Epub ahead of print.]
Vedeler CA, *et al.* (2006). Management of paraneoplastic neurological syndromes: report of an EFNS Task Force. *Eur J Neurol*, **13**, 682–90.

Autoimmune limbic encephalitis and Morvan's syndrome

Camilla Buckley and Angela Vincent

Essentials

Autoimmune limbic encephalitis—typical presentation is with acute or subacute onset of short term memory loss, seizures and disorientation. MRI characteristically shows striking abnormalities in the hippocampus. Antibodies against voltage-gated potassium channels (VGKC) are found in a high proportion and are probably pathogenic. Aside from supportive care, treatment is with immunosuppression, often comprising corticosteroids with intravenous immunoglobulin and/or plasma exchange.

Morvan's syndrome—a very rare condition presenting with varying degrees of neuromyotonia, memory loss, confusion, sleep disturbance, and autonomic features. About 50% have VGKC antibodies.

Autoimmune limbic encephalitis (LE)

Epidemiology

Since its first recognition in 2001, 100s of patients have been identified with this condition. Preliminary epidemiology suggests that it is more common in men (2:1) and that the median age at onset is 65 years. As yet, the phenotype has been recognized only in patients over the age of 18 years at onset.

Clinical features

The classic presentation is with subacute onset of short-term memory loss, seizures, disorientation, with psychological disturbance or hallucinations. Additional features that may occur are sleep disturbance, autonomic dysfunction, and neuromyotonia but these would be more typical of Morvan's syndrome (see below). The most striking feature on examination is the profound disorientation and memory loss, leading to poor performance on bedside cognitive tests such as the Mini-Mental State Examination. Neuromyotonia (see Chapter 24.21) may be evident, but often the examination is otherwise unremarkable. Recently patients have been identified who developed only one aspect of the syndrome (e.g. isolated memory loss or isolated temporal or frontal seizures), but were otherwise similar to those with the full syndrome. Some patients report an influenza-like illness 1 to 2 weeks earlier.

Investigations

Hyponatraemia is present in 80% of patients, usually accompanied by a low plasma and urine osmolarity. Other routine blood tests are normal. The cerebrospinal fluid is often normal but may show a mild pleocytosis. Voltage-gated potassium channel (VGKC) antibody titres are characteristically very high in these patients (more than 400 pmol/litre and often more than 1000 pmol/litre (normal range less than 100 pmol/litre)), and higher than the titres commonly found in patients with neuromyotonia (usually less than 400 pmol/litre) (Fig. 24.22.1b). MRI shows striking abnormalities in 70% of patients and it is often these that lead the clinician to suspect the diagnosis and request the confirmatory serological test (Fig. 24.22.1a). The most classic change is high signal restricted to the hippocampus (either unilaterally or bilaterally), best seen on T_2-weighted or FLAIR (fluid-attenuated inversion recovery) sequences, with associated swelling of the affected area. A few patients have more widespread areas of increased signal in the medial temporal lobes and amygdala. LE associated with VGKC antibodies can occasionally (<10%) be a paraneoplastic disorder and so all patients should undergo appropriate imaging to detect any underlying malignancy (e.g. thymoma or small-cell lung cancer).

Treatment

Initially patients often require fluid restriction to mange the hyponatraemia, antiepileptic drugs for their seizures, antipsychotic drugs to control paranoid ideation, and plasma exchange or intravenous immunoglobulin (IVIG) for acute immunosuppression. The choice of antiepileptics is complicated by the hyponatraemia, which can be profound. Often the seizures do not respond well to antiepileptics alone and do not start to reduce in frequency until immunosuppression has been established.

There have been no randomized controlled trials to determine the most effective immunosuppressive regimens in these patients and so currently the protocols are similar to those used to treat patients with autoimmune disorders of the neuromuscular junction

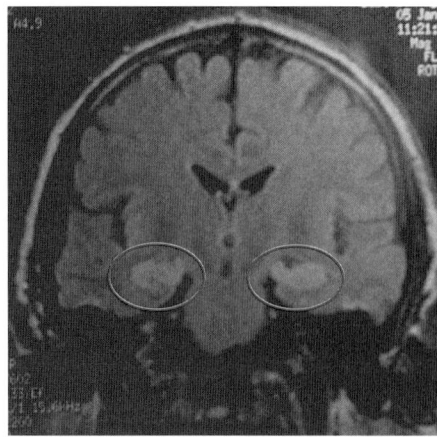
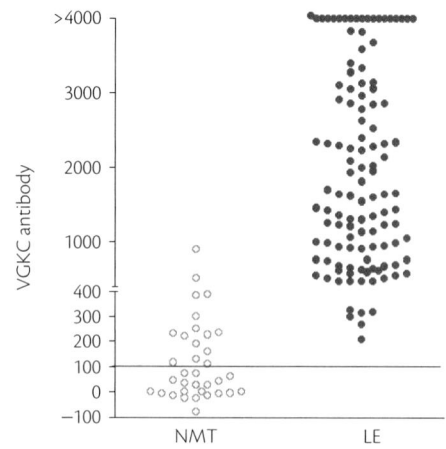

Fig. 24.22.1 (a) T_2-weighted coronal MRI of the brain with the red circles highlighting the abnormal high signal bilaterally in the hippocampi in a patient with limbic encephalitis (LE) associated with voltage-gated potassium channel (VGKC) antibodies. (b) VGKC antibody levels in patients with LE compared with those in patients with neuromyotonia (NMT). The horizontal line denotes the cut-off for healthy individuals. Only 40 to 50% of patients with NMT have positive values. Patients with LE associated with positive VGKC antibodies usually have values more than 400 pmol/litre. Morvan's syndrome patients have titres between 0 and 1000 pmol/litre (not shown).

(see Chapter 24.23). Corticosteroids appear to be a particularly important component because longer-term follow-up suggests that those treated with IVIG alone respond less well than those treated with IVIG and steroids. Although early treatment is recommended, as it appears to be associated with improved prognosis, even late introduction of steroids and other immunosuppression can be beneficial.

Differential diagnosis

Acutely the differential diagnosis lies mainly with infectious causes of LE, the most common being herpes simplex encephalitis (HSE), and most patients will have a CSF polymerase chain reaction for HSE performed on admission, particularly if they have a high fever and severe headache. Korsakoff's pyschosis can present similarly and so an accurate alcohol history and suggestive blood tests such as liver function tests and mean cell volume (MCV) should be performed.

The other main differential lies with paraneoplastic LE, so all patients need imaging to detect associated tumours and, in the right context, it may be appropriate to look for the particular antibodies seen with these disorders (see Chapter 24.21). Other forms of potentially immunotherapy-responsive LE are now being recognized some of which are associated with antibodies to other neuronal surface antigens (e.g. N-methyl-D-aspartate receptor, see Chapter 24.21) and may not be paraneoplastic. Morvan's syndrome, although very rare, can present similarly to LE and is distinguished by additional peripheral and autonomic features (see below). In addition (as with the autoimmune disorders of the neuromuscular junction), there are patients with a similar clinical phenotype who respond to immunomodulatory therapies, but in whom no antibody is detectable by current methods, although new diagnostic tests will undoubtedly emerge.

Pathogenesis

VGKC LE is probably an immune-mediated disorder given the time course of patients' clinical, serological, and radiological responses to immunosuppression. VGKC is a transmembrane protein that is densely expressed in the hippocampus. Genetic mutations in VGKC can cause seizures both in mice and in humans and, as the channel is involved in stabilizing the membrane potential, its dysfunction will result in neuronal hyperexcitability. It is likely that the antibodies have a direct role in the pathogenesis, but they may just be a very useful clinical biomarker for this treatable immune-mediated disorder. Recent evidence indicates that some of the antibodies are directed against proteins that are closely complexed with the VGKCs.

Morvan's syndrome

This is a very rare condition in which patients present with varying degrees of neuromyotonia, central nervous system symptoms such as memory loss, confusion, and sleep disturbance, and additional autonomic features such as constipation and cardiac arrhythmias. Very few cases have been described, but about 50% have VGKC antibodies, usually at levels intermediate between neuromyotonia and VGKC LE. Thymoma is more common than in VGKC LE or neuromyotonia (probably 60%), but most patients do well with thymectomy, if appropriate, and immunosuppression, and some appear to have a self-limiting disease.

Further reading

Ances BM *et al.* (2005). Treatment-responsive limbic encephalitis identified by neuropil antibodies: MRI and PET correlates. *Brain*, **128**(Pt 8), 1764–77.

Buckley C *et al.* (2001). Potassium channel antibodies in two patients with reversible limbic encephalitis. *Ann Neurol*, **50**, 73–8.

Buckley C, Vincent A (2005). Autoimmune channelopathies. *Nature Clin Pract Neurol*, **1**, 22–33.

Graus F, *et al.* (2008). Neuronal surface antigen antibodies in limbic encephalitis: clinical-immunologic associations. *Neurology*, **71**, 930–6.

Vincent A *et al.* (2004). Potassium channel antibody-associated encephalopathy: a potentially immunotherapy-responsive form of limbic encephalitis. *Brain*, **127**(Pt 3), 701–12.

Disorders of the neuromuscular junction

David Hilton-Jones and Jacqueline Palace

Essentials

Two fundamentally different pathological processes are associated with disease at the neuromuscular junction: (1) acquired disorders in which autoantibodies are directed against nerve or muscle receptor or ion channels; (2) rare inherited conditions in which the defect may be pre- or postsynaptic.

Myasthenia gravis

Aetiology and epidemiology—the fundamental disorder is loss of functional acetylcholine receptors most frequently as a result of binding of anti-acetylcholine receptor (anti-AChR) antibodies. Incidence is about 10 per million population and prevalence about 8 per 100 000, with a marked female bias in cases aged under 40 years and male preponderance in those over 50 years. Thymomas occur in about 10% of cases.

Clinical features and diagnosis—the most characteristic feature is fatiguability, meaning demonstrable weakness (without muscle pain) precipitated by repeated or sustained muscular activity. In more than 50% cases this first manifests as diplopia and ptosis. For practical purposes, a positive anti-AChR or anti-MuSK antibody test is confirmatory and no further diagnostic investigations are required; electromyography and the intravenous edrophonium test are helpful in seronegative patients. The presence of a thymoma can only be assessed by CT or MRI of the thorax.

Treatment and prognosis—thymomas require excision, but this in itself will not improve myasthenia. Anticholinesterase drugs (e.g. pyridostigmine) give symptomatic improvement in most patients, and may be sufficient in those with very mild disease. Other management is determined by the type of disease: (1) ocular myasthenia—alternate-day prednisolone with/without steroid sparing agents (e.g. azathioprine); (2) early-onset seropositive disease—some patients benefit from thymectomy, with prednisolone and azathioprine indicated for those who do not, and other immunosuppressants in those who are refractory; (3) late onset, anti-MuSK, and seronegative diseases—most respond to immunosuppression; (4) myasthenic crisis—supportive care with intubation and assisted ventilation may be required; plasma exchange and intravenous immunoglobulin may both lead to rapid improvement. Overall prognosis is good, with over 90% achieving near-normal functional recovery.

Lambert–Eaton myasthenic syndrome

A presynaptic disorder, often occurring in patients with small-cell lung cancer, associated with the presence of antibodies that reduce the number of functional presynaptic P/Q-type voltage-gated calcium channels (VGKC). The condition is characterized by limb-girdle weakness and symptoms of autonomic dysfunction. Pyridostigmine may offer some symptomatic benefit, but 3,4-diaminopyridine is more effective and the drug of choice. In cancer associated disease, removal of the tumour often leads to improvement; immunosuppression can be effective when an associated cancer is unlikely.

Other conditions

These include (1) congenital myasthenic syndromes—usually autosomal recessive; various forms include presynaptic, endplate acetylcholinesterase deficiency, and postsynaptic; (2) neuromyotonia—may be idiopathic, but recognized associations include tumour and acquired demyelinating polyneuropathies; the main clinical features are muscle stiffness, cramps, and twitching; electromyography shows highly characteristic features; most patients gain symptomatic relief from carbamazepine, phenytoin or lamotrigine.

Neuromuscular transmission

Anatomically there are three main components to the neuromuscular junction (Fig. 24.23.1). The presynaptic component is the motor nerve terminal, which contains packages (quanta) of acetylcholine, each of which contains several thousand molecules of acetylcholine. This is separated from the postsynaptic acetylcholine receptors, which sit atop the terminal expansions of the junctional folds of the muscle fibre membrane, by the synaptic space. The nerve fibre membrane contains voltage-gated sodium, potassium, and calcium channels. Voltage-gated sodium channels are also present postsynaptically, at the base of the clefts of the junctional folds.

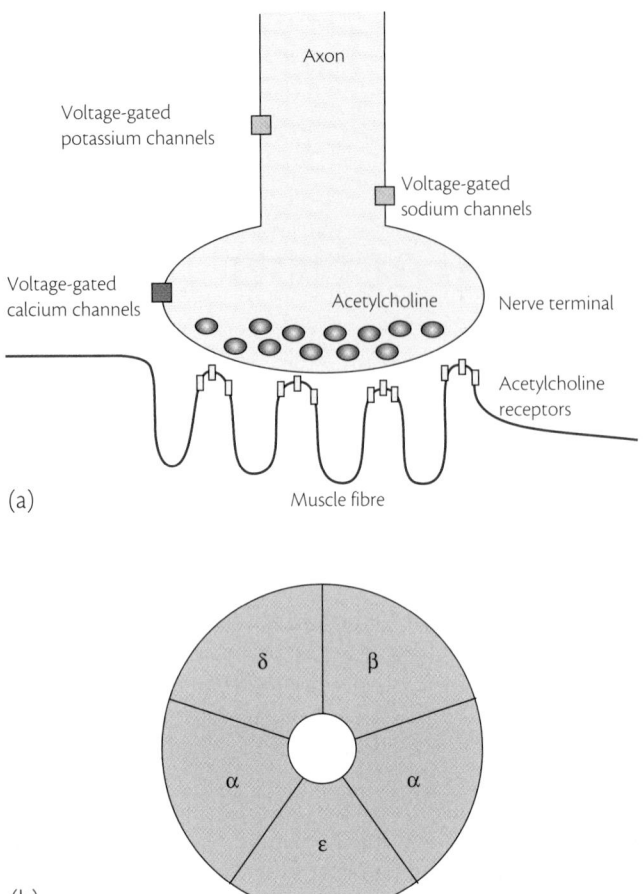

(a)

(b)

Fig. 24.23.1 Diagrammatic representation of the neuromuscular junction demonstrating the molecules that are targets for autoimmune and genetic diseases. (b) Cartoon of the organization of the subunits of the nicotinic acetylcholine receptor. These subunits form a channel in the membrane (central hole), which opens when acetylcholine (ACh) binds. The adult form differs from the fetal form by substitution of the γ subunit with an ϵ subunit. Antibodies in myasthenia bind to both forms, often to the main immunogenic region on the α subunits. Antibodies in rare cases of fetal arthrogryposis bind to the γ subunit close to the ACh-binding site.

The nicotinic acetylcholine receptor is a pentameric structure composed of four different subunits—α, β, γ, and δ in fetal muscle, and α, β, ϵ, and δ in adult muscle. It is configured to produce a central ion channel. Structurally and functionally there are similarities to voltage-gated ion channels, but the acetylcholine receptor is a ligand-gated channel, the ligand being acetylcholine.

Depolarization of the motor nerve terminal is dependent on voltage-gated sodium channels. Repolarization is the result of inactivation of these sodium channels and opening of voltage-gated potassium channels. During depolarization, voltage-gated calcium channels open—the influx of calcium ions into the nerve terminal triggers release (by exocytosis) of quanta of acetylcholine.

The acetylcholine binds to the α subunits of the acetylcholine receptors. This alters the conformation of the channel, allowing cations (mainly sodium) to enter the muscle fibre. This influx generates the endplate potential, which in turn activates voltage-gated sodium channels. These trigger the action potential that is propagated away from the neuromuscular junction, along the muscle fibre, and initiates contraction. Spontaneous release of individual

quanta of acetylcholine, as opposed to the multiple release triggered by a nerve action potential, gives rise to miniature endplate potentials, which can be recorded by a microelectrode inserted into the muscle fibre. These are of insufficient amplitude to trigger an action potential in the muscle fibre membrane.

The action of acetylcholine on acetylcholine receptors is terminated by the hydrolysis of acetylcholine by the enzyme acetylcholinesterase, which is anchored to the basal lamina by a collagen-like molecule, ColQ (see Fig. 24.23.1).

The acquired neuromuscular junction disorders are associated with antibodies directed against one of the ion channels (Table 24.23.1). The fact that there are three autoimmune disorders known to affect such a small region may be explained by the neuromuscular junction, unlike the peripheral nerve, not being contained within the blood–nerve barrier, which stops just short of the nerve terminal, and thus being potentially exposed to circulating humoral attack. The inherited disorders may affect presynaptic processes (acetylcholine resynthesis, packaging, or release), acetylcholinesterase binding, or postsynaptic function (acetylcholine receptor numbers or localization). Pathogenic mechanisms are considered in more detail when discussing individual disorders.

Myasthenia gravis

This is by far the most common of the conditions discussed in this chapter and it responds favourably to treatment. In general, over 90% of patients can be returned to normal function, although in most this represents a pharmacological remission and the patient remains dependent on treatment.

Epidemiology

All ethnic groups are affected. The annual incidence is about 10 per million population, and the prevalence about 8 per 100 000. All ages may be affected. There is a marked female bias in patients below age 40 years, who are often HLA B8-DR3, whereas over the age of 50 years men predominate, and myasthenia is increasingly recognized in very elderly people. A rather different pattern is seen in people of Asian origin; prepubertal onset is very common, the disease is often purely ocular, and there is a strong association with HLA DRw9.

Pathogenesis

The fundamental disorder in myasthenia gravis is loss of functional acetylcholine receptors as a result of binding of anti-acetylcholine receptor (anti-AChR) antibodies. High-affinity immunoglobulin IgG class antibodies can be detected, by the standard assay used for diagnostic purposes, in 85% of patients with generalized myasthenia and about half of those with purely ocular myasthenia (so-called seropositive cases). Antibodies bind to the main immunogenic region of the α subunits of the acetylcholine receptor, and

Table 24.23.1 Ion channels responsible for the different clinical disorders

Ion channel	Clinical disorder
Acetylcholine receptor	Myasthenia gravis
Voltage-gated calcium channel	Lambert–Eaton myasthenic syndrome
Voltage-gated potassium channel	Acquired neuromyotonia

also to other sites on the surface of the receptor. Patients who do not have antibodies detected by this assay are classified as seronegative. However, there is overwhelming evidence even in these patients that their disease is immune mediated: their clinical characteristics are similar to those of seropositive patients, they respond to plasma exchange and immunosuppressant therapy, their plasma can induce neuromuscular transmission dysfunction when injected into animals, and the infants of such mothers may be born with neonatal myasthenia (see below), indicating transplacental transfer of a humoral component.

Recently it has been shown that in up to half of so-called seronegative cases there is an antibody directed against muscle-specific tyrosine kinase (MuSK) which has a role in receptor clustering (see Fig. 24.23.1). The exact pathogenic mechanism in these anti-MuSK cases remains uncertain but, as noted below, such patients have a rather characteristic clinical presentation. Recent evidence suggests that low-affinity anti-AChR antibodies may be present in those patients with neither AChR nor MuSK antibodies.

Loss of functional acetylcholine receptors by antibody binding is due to complement-mediated lysis, acceleration of internalization and degradation, and blocking of acetylcholine binding. Morphological consequences include widening of the synaptic cleft and a marked reduction of the postsynaptic folds of the muscle fibre membrane.

Although the efferent limb of the immune response, described above, has been reasonably well characterized, numerous questions remain to be answered about the afferent limb. Susceptibility to myasthenia gravis is associated with particular immune response genes with correlation to different haplotypes relating to the age of onset of the disease (particularly HLA B8-DR3 in younger patients). These observations are not of immediate relevance to routine clinical practice. In contrast, knowledge about involvement of the thymus is relevant to classification and management.

The thymus has a key role in the process of inducing immune tolerance, by removal of self-antigen T-cell clones, and it is not normally a source of autoantibodies. The acetylcholine receptor is, however, expressed on thymic myoid cells and in early onset, anti-AChR antibody-positive patients there is hyperplasia of the thymic medulla, with germinal centres surrounded by a T-cell zone. In the germinal centres there is enrichment of acetylcholine receptor-specific T cells and B/plasma cells. On the basis of these observations, and the beneficial response to thymectomy, there seems little doubt that the thymus is involved in the pathogenesis of myasthenia gravis, but exactly how has yet to be elucidated. Identification of the mechanism may well be important in developing immune-specific treatment.

In late-onset cases and anti-AChR antibody-negative patients, the thymus is typically much less abnormal or atrophic (which is normal in later life), although some pathological changes have been noted and thymectomy is often performed in younger patients. Patients with anti-MuSK antibodies show very little thymic pathology and probably do not benefit from the operation.

Thymomas occur in about 10% of cases. They are locally invasive (notably affecting the pleura and pericardium) and may seed within the pleural cavity. These patients are almost invariably anti-AChR antibody positive. Surgical excision is required because of local tumour invasiveness, but, in contrast to those patients with thymic hyperplasia, this does not usually ameliorate the myasthenic symptoms.

Table 24.23.2 The four main subgroups of myasthenia gravis

	Age of onset (years)		Thymoma	Sero-negative
	<40	>40		
Thymus	Hyperplasia	Atrophy	Thymoma	?Normal/atrophy
Anti-AChR antibody titre	High	Low	Intermediate	Absent

Based on the presence or absence of antibodies detected by the routine clinical assay and the state of the thymus gland, five main subgroups of patients can be identified (Table 24.23.2)–the fifth group being MuSK positive patient. Penicillamine-induced myasthenia, which generally recovers after drug withdrawal, is clinically similar to the idiopathic disease and the patients are anti-AChR antibody positive.

Clinical features

Myasthenia gravis causes skeletal muscle weakness, but the most characteristic feature is fatigability. The term 'fatigue' causes some confusion because it may have different meanings to a clinician, physiologist, and layperson. Thus, the fatigue of chronic fatigue syndrome is quite different from that of myasthenia. Simply put, fatigue in myasthenia gravis manifests itself by increasing demonstrable weakness, without muscle pain, precipitated by repeated or sustained muscular activity. Symptoms fluctuate from day to day and week to week, which may in part explain the common delay in diagnosis and suspicions as to its genuineness. Other factors that can exacerbate the weakness include heat, emotional factors, menstruation, intercurrent infections, and drugs that interfere with neuromuscular transmission (aminoglycoside antibiotics, quinine, quinidine, β-blockers, procainamide, and neuromuscular-blocking drugs related to anaesthesia).

In over half of patients the presenting symptoms relate to extraocular muscle weakness (diplopia and ptosis); these muscles will be involved in over 90% of patients at some stage during the disease. The next most frequent presentation is with limb–girdle weakness. Typically, as the disease worsens, the weakness spreads from the extraocular muscles to the lower facial and bulbar muscles (causing dysarthria and dysphagia), to the neck, and then to the limbs. However, there are many variations on this theme. A relatively common presentation in older patients, typically men, is with selective weakness of neck extension—as they walk the head drops forwards and they arrive in the clinic holding up the head with a hand under the chin. Relatively selective weakness of finger extension and abduction is common. In patients with anti-MuSK antibodies there is a female preponderance, prevalent oculobulbar involvement sometimes with facial muscle and tongue atrophy, often very limited limb involvement, and a high frequency of ventilatory insufficiency.

On examination, weakness may or may not be evident—fatigue can be demonstrated in limb muscles, but is often most striking around the eyes and with respect to bulbar muscles. Fatigable ptosis is a striking sign (Fig. 24.23.2). As the patients give their history, the fatigue of bulbar muscles may be revealed by increasing dysarthria. A potentially misleading sign is 'pseudo-internuclear ophthalmoplegia', which may be bilateral—failure of adduction due to weakness of the medial recti. Eye movements may show striking fatigue. With increasing severity, the weakness at rest may be so marked that it is difficult to demonstrate fatigue. Respiratory muscle

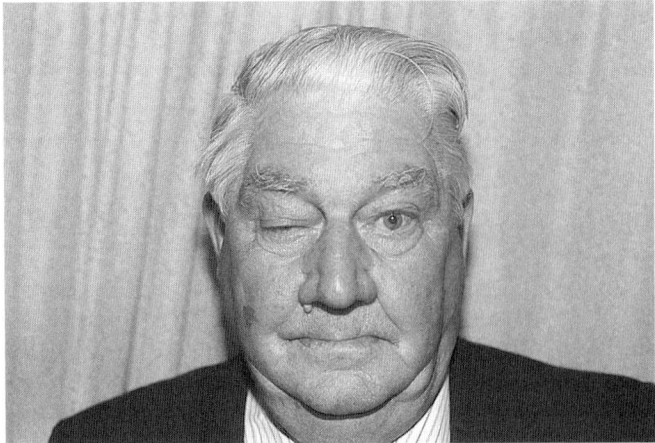

(a)

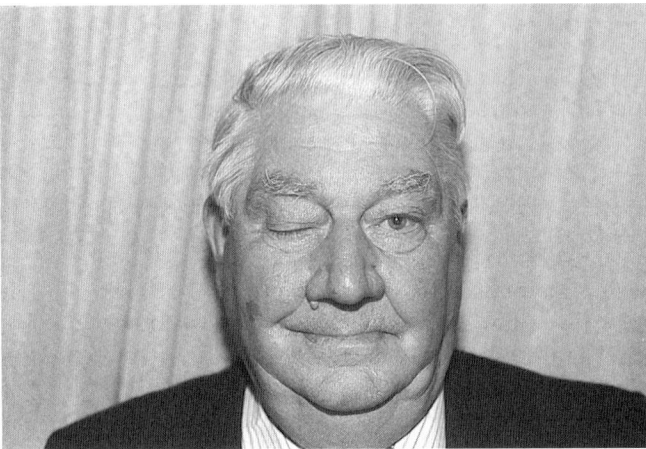

(b)

Fig. 24.23.2 Fatigable ptosis in myasthenia gravis.

weakness may be out of proportion to limb weakness; it is best assessed by measuring the vital capacity (not peak flow), and its effects by monitoring oxygen saturation. Muscle wasting is seen only in undertreated patients with long-established disease, although it is more common in patients with anti-MuSK antibodies. The tendon reflexes are normal, and indeed often rather brisk. There are no abnormal sensory signs.

There is an increased incidence of other autoimmune diseases, particularly thyroid disease (about 3% of patients) and less frequently rheumatoid arthritis, systemic lupus erythematosus, polymyositis, and acquired neuromyotonia. Coexistence of myasthenia and Lambert–Eaton myasthenic syndrome (LEMS) has been reported.

Natural course

This is very variable. In some patients the disorder remains confined to the extraocular muscles (ocular myasthenia gravis). If that is the case for more than 2 years, and particularly if the patient is seronegative, the development of generalized disease is unlikely. Older studies, before the introduction of immunosuppressive therapies, suggest that the disease reaches maximum severity within 7 years. In one study, the interval between onset and the first episode of maximal weakness ('myasthenic crisis') was less than 36 months in over 80% of patients. Permanent spontaneous remission occurs, but is

rare—of the order of 1% per annum. On the other hand, particularly early in the course of the disease, there may be protracted periods of spontaneous remission, sometimes lasting several years.

Diagnosis

This is based on the clinical picture, supported by appropriate laboratory results. For practical purposes, a positive anti-AChR or anti-MuSK antibody test is confirmatory and no further diagnostic investigations are required. In seronegative patients, electromyography (EMG) and the intravenous edrophonium (Tensilon) test are helpful. Although the edrophonium test (demonstration of improvement with a short-acting cholinesterase inhibitor) has a long pedigree and sound pharmacological basis, there are concerns about its use, particularly by doctors who are inexperienced. The patient is given 600 μg atropine intravenously; this blocks the potentially unpleasant muscarinic effects of the edrophonium and also acts as a single-blind placebo for the patient. The test dose of 2 mg edrophonium follows, which in some patients is sufficient to give a diagnostic response. If not, a further 8 mg edrophonium is given. There must be an easily assessable measure of improvement—most commonly degree of ptosis. The test is therefore likely to be of most use in patients with purely ocular symptoms and signs. Rarely, cardiorespiratory collapse may occur. False-negative and false-positive results are not uncommon.

The conventional EMG measure for diagnosing myasthenia gravis is the demonstration of a decremental response of the compound muscle action potential in response to repetitive nerve stimulation at 3 Hz. More sensitive, but not specific and only available in specialist centres, is the presence of increased jitter and blocking, as assessed by single-fibre EMG.

The presence of a thymoma can be assessed only by CT or MRI of the thorax.

Differential diagnosis

There are few difficulties in the presence of extraocular muscle involvement and readily demonstrable fatigue, although there can be confusion with LEMS and congenital myasthenic syndromes. Diagnostic difficulties can occur when, as occasionally happens, eye signs and fatigue are absent. Amyotrophic lateral sclerosis with little wasting may be suspected. Conversely, in long-established myasthenia, muscle wasting may be misleading. More difficult is seronegative, purely ocular myasthenia; the most important differential diagnosis is mitochondrial cytopathy, in which increased jitter may also occur. Other diagnoses to consider include oculopharyngeal muscular dystrophy and thyroid ophthalmopathy.

Botulism, caused by food poisoning, an infected wound, or clostridial overgrowth in the gastrointestinal tract in infants, may need to be considered. Features of autonomic malfunction are usually present.

Treatment

As noted, thymomas require excision, but this in itself will not improve the myasthenia. Management of patients with thymic tumours follows the same guidelines given here.

Anticholinesterase drugs, by reducing acetylcholine breakdown, give symptomatic improvement in most patients, and may be sufficient in those with very mild disease. Pyridostigmine is the drug of choice, given orally four or five times daily, starting at 30 mg/dose and increasing if required to 60 mg/dose with a maximum dose of

360 mg/day. Abdominal cramping is a common side effect, relating to muscarinic overstimulation, and responds to propantheline, ideally taken 30 min before each dose of pyridostigmine. If an adequate response is not obtained at this dose of pyridostigmine, further increases should not be made and other forms of therapy should be considered. The management of ocular myasthenia differs somewhat from the generalized form of the disease, the latter also depending on age of onset and antibody status.

Ocular myasthenia

If anticholinesterase drugs have given an inadequate response, alternate-day prednisolone therapy should be introduced. A suitable starting daily dose is 5 mg, increasing by 5 mg every fourth dose (or weekly) until an adequate response has been obtained (often, for an adult, a dose of around 30 mg) or a maximum acceptable dose (around 0.75 mg/kg body weight) has been reached. Once remission has been achieved, the pyridostigmine can be withdrawn, and then the prednisolone reduced slowly—initially by 5 mg/month, but when down to 20 mg by as little as 1 mg/month). Azathioprine (see below) may be added if there is an inadequate response or the minimal effective dose of prednisolone is deemed to be unacceptably high. Ocular muscle surgery can be beneficial if there is a poor or incomplete response to treatment and if the defect appears to be fixed.

Early onset, seropositive myasthenia

Many, but not all, of these patients benefit from thymectomy. Up to a third enter remission, and a further half improve if given immunosuppressive treatments. These benefits are occasionally rapid, but more typically develop over the following 1 to 2 years, possibly longer. The conventional approach is through a sternal split. There is concern that less invasive surgical procedures risk leaving behind thymic remnants which will negate the benefits of the operation. Thymectomy should be performed in centres experienced in such surgery and with the support of appropriately trained anaesthetists and neurologists.

For those patients who do not respond adequately to anticholinesterase drugs and thymectomy, immunosuppression with prednisolone and azathioprine is indicated. Introduction of prednisolone may exacerbate myasthenic weakness and should generally be done in hospital. The starting dose is 10 mg on alternate days, increasing by 10 mg/dose until the patient reaches the target dose of 1 to 1.5 mg/kg body weight per dose. When remission has been achieved the dose is slowly reduced, as for ocular myasthenia, until the minimal effective dose has been established. A controlled trial has shown the benefits of the addition of azathioprine (2.5 mg/kg body weight per day); the starting dose is 25 or 50 mg daily, increased by 25 or 50 mg daily, each week (or more rapidly as an inpatient) until the target dose is reached. During introduction, weekly tests of full blood count and liver function are required. When established, testing can be reduced gradually to 3 monthly. When available, thiopurine methyltransferase (TPMT) activity analysis may be used to identify those at risk of azathioprine toxicity, but even in low-risk patients there should be regular haematological monitoring. Azathioprine takes over 6 months to take maximal effect, after which time it may be possible to reduce prednisolone to a minimum

For those who do not respond to, or are intolerant of, prednisolone and/or azathioprine, other immunosuppressant drugs, such as ciclosporin, methotrexate, mycophenolate mofetil, and cyclophosphamide, may be used.

Late-onset myasthenia

This form of myasthenia is increasing recognized with many cases, of both sexes, presenting over the age of 70 years. Although not formally assessed, it appears that these patients do not benefit significantly from thymectomy. Most respond to the immunosuppressant regimen described above.

Anti-MuSK and seronegative myasthenia

Patients with such a myasthenia do no appear to respond to thymectomy. Seronegative myasthenia generally responds well to the immunosuppressant regimen outlined above. Patients with anti-MuSK antibodies seem to be much more resistant to anticholinesterases and immunosuppression than anti-AChR-positive patients, and other immunosuppressant drugs are often required.

Myasthenic crisis

Intubation and assisted ventilation may be required. Plasma exchange and intravenous immunoglobulin may both lead to a rapid improvement (within 1 to 2 weeks) in strength, but the beneficial effects start to wear off within about 8 weeks. However, this gives useful time in which to establish an immunosuppressant regimen, as discussed above.

Plasma exchange and intravenous immunoglobulin are also useful in preparing myasthenic patients for thymectomy and may reduce the likelihood of deterioration consequent upon the introduction of prednisolone.

Osteoporosis is an important concern in patients receiving long-term, high-dose prednisolone. A bone density determination should be carried out before starting such therapy, and repeated periodically, as appropriate. Local guidelines should be followed; these will advise on general physical measures, assess dietary calcium intake, and indicate the need to introduce calcium/vitamin D or a bisphosphonate, and the place of hormone replacement therapy for postmenopausal women.

Prognosis

The outlook for most patients with myasthenia is good, with over 90% achieving near-normal functional recovery. Death is most likely to occur during a myasthenic crisis early in the course of the disease. The response to thymectomy has been noted. Unwanted effects relating to the immunosuppressant drugs may have an important influence on the outcome.

Myasthenia in pregnancy

Pregnancy has no significant long-term effect on myasthenia, but relapse may be more common in the puerperium. Some 10% of infants born to myasthenic mothers have transient neonatal myasthenia due to transplacental passage of maternal anti-AChR antibodies. Symptoms include feeding and respiratory difficulties, generalized weakness, and, less commonly, ptosis. They resolve within a few weeks.

Immunosuppressive treatment should be maintained during pregnancy to ensure good control of the mother's myasthenia and to reduce the likelihood of neonatal weakness.

Much more rarely, the infant is born with arthrogryposis multiplex congenita, secondary to profound intrauterine weakness and lack of movement. This relates to maternal antibodies that target the fetal form of the acetylcholine receptor, which is present at the neuromuscular junction until the last weeks of pregnancy, and in some cases the mother herself has been asymptomatic.

Future research

This may provide a better understanding of the immune processes involved, and thus lead to the development of selective treatments that avoid generalized immune suppression or other unwanted effects of the currently available drugs.

Lambert–Eaton myasthenic syndrome (LEMS)

LEMS is a presynaptic disorder, characterized by limb–girdle weakness and symptoms of autonomic dysfunction, which is often associated with small-cell lung cancer. Delayed diagnosis is common. Symptomatic and immunosuppressant therapies are available.

Epidemiology

Some 60% of patients have cancer-associated LEMS, usually caused by small-cell lung cancer and much more rarely by other tumours; in these cases the peak presentation is in the fourth to sixth decades. The other 40% have non-cancer-associated LEMS and may present from childhood onwards. It is estimated that 3% of patients with small-cell lung cancer develop LEMS, but that the diagnosis is frequently not made. The weakness is often attributed to nonspecific cachectic effects and the disorder is neither suspected nor investigated. LEMS, similar to many other paraneoplastic disorders (see Chapter 24.21), may predate the appearance of the cancer by as much as 5 years.

Pathogenesis

Both forms are associated with IgG class antibodies, which reduce the number of functional presynaptic P-/Q-type voltage-gated calcium channels (VGCCs) by cross-linking adjacent channels. This causes reduced calcium influx and therefore reduced quantal release of acetylcholine. As in myasthenia, patients with LEMS have an increased incidence of other forms of autoimmune disease, including a rare association with acquired myasthenia gravis.

Small-cell lung cancers express VGCCs and it is proposed that the tumour triggers an antibody response to those channels; the antibodies then cross-react with the calcium channels at the neuromuscular junction, causing LEMS.

Clinical features

Most patients present with an abnormality of gait and complain that their legs feel heavy or weak. Symptomatic upper limb weakness tends to present later. Autonomic dysfunction is common, but infrequently volunteered, and includes dryness of the mouth and constipation. In men, impotence may predate limb weakness. Compared with myasthenia gravis, ocular symptoms are rarely severe or particularly troublesome, and bulbar weakness is rare.

On examination, mild ptosis and diplopia may be evident. The abnormality of gait is often more striking than demonstrable weakness when testing on the examination couch. This is partly because of the phenomenon of postexertional potentiation. Physiologically, with sustained effort, there is mobilization of nerve calcium stores and consequently increased quantal release of acetylcholine.

Clinically, this augmentation is apparent in two ways: first, strength increases after a few seconds of maximal effort; second, the tendon reflexes, which are reduced or absent, increase or appear following 10 to 15 s of maximal contraction of the relevant muscle. Sensory testing is normal.

Diagnosis

Single-fibre electromyography, as in myasthenia gravis, shows increased jitter and blocking, and repetitive nerve stimulation studies show decrement at certain frequencies. However, the characteristic neurophysiological finding, which reflects the clinical observations made above, is of a small-amplitude compound muscle action potential that shows potentiation, sometimes enormous, 15 s after voluntary maximal contraction. Diagnosis is confirmed by demonstrating the presence of anti-VGCC antibodies, which are detectable in up to 90% of cases.

Treatment

Pyridostigmine may offer some symptomatic benefit, but 3,4-diaminopyridine is more effective and the drug of choice. 3,4-Diaminopyridine blocks the voltage-gated potassium channels (see Fig. 24.23.1), thereby prolonging the duration of the nerve action potential, resulting in a greater influx of calcium. The maximum dose of 3,4-diaminopyridine is 100 mg daily.

When an associated cancer is unlikely (young patients, non-smokers, more than 5 years since onset, and no cancer apparent), treatment with alternate-day prednisolone (up to 1.5 mg/kg body weight per dose) and azathioprine (2.5 mg/kg body weight per day), as in myasthenia gravis, can be highly effective.

In a smoker in whom a cancer is not identified at presentation, it is prudent to repeat chest imaging (CT or MRI) yearly for 5 years.

In cancer-associated LEMS, removal of the tumour often leads to symptomatic improvement. Although there is some reluctance to use immunosuppression in patients with known cancer, alternate-day prednisolone may be used if there has been an inadequate symptomatic response to 3,4-diaminopyridine.

Plasma exchange and intravenous immunoglobulin both give short-term benefit and can be used in cancer-associated and non-cancer-associated LEMS.

Prognosis

In cancer-associated LEMS, the prognosis is largely determined by the tumour. In non-cancer-associated LEMS many patients can be rendered asymptomatic, but some prove very resistant to treatment.

Congenital myasthenic syndromes

This is a rare group of conditions with an overall prevalence of the order of 1 in 200 000 population according to our calculations in the United Kingdom. They are genetically determined (usually autosomal recessive—so a history of consanguinity is common), nonautoimmune disorders. Major clinical features include onset in infancy, fatigable weakness, a decremental response to repetitive nerve stimulation, and absence of AChR or MuSK antibodies. A significant exception to this generalization is the classic slow-channel syndrome, which may present in infancy or adult life, and is inherited as an autosomal dominant trait. The syndromes may be classified on the basis of the site of the defect of neuromuscular transmission, but this is not always certain. A revised classification is likely to evolve as the molecular basis of each is identified. Diagnosis depends on electrophysiological tests, morphological studies of the endplate region in muscle biopsy specimens, and increasingly on identification of the specific genetic defect.

Presynaptic disorders

These are the least well characterized of the myasthenic disorders. They include disorders of acetylcholine resynthesis caused by choline acetyltransferase mutations (previously known as familial infantile myasthenia, now called congenital myasthenic syndrome with episodic apnoea), and a condition with paucity of synaptic vesicles and reduced quantal release. Symptoms respond to anticholinesterase drugs.

Endplate acetylcholinesterase deficiency

Fatigable weakness is usually evident from birth. A single nerve stimulus may give rise to a repetitive compound muscle action potential response. The molecular basis is a mutation within the ColQ polypeptide gene. ColQ anchors acetylcholinesterase to the basal lamina. In the absence of the enzyme the acetylcholine receptors have a prolonged exposure to acetylcholine, leading to damage to the neuromuscular junction. Anticholinesterase drugs, not surprisingly, are ineffective. No specific treatments are available.

Postsynaptic disorders

These disorders are associated with mutations in the genes that encode the AChR subunits or associated AChR-clustering proteins. They may affect the number of receptors, the receptor-presenting area, or the kinetic properties of the central ion channel.

The most common disorder in the United Kingdom is acetylcholine receptor deficiency, which is most frequently caused by mutations in the ε-subunit gene. Presentation is at birth or within the first few years of life. There is generalized weakness, delayed motor milestones, feeding difficulties, and extraocular muscle involvement. There is a good response to anticholinesterase drugs and 3,4-diaminopyridine.

The fast-channel syndrome is phenotypically similar to acetylcholine receptor deficiency and may be associated with α-, δ-, or ε-subunit mutations. The mechanism is altered kinetics of the receptor ion channel.

The slow-channel syndrome is also a kinetic disorder, associated with mutations in different subunits and different domains within those subunits. It is an autosomal dominant disorder with variable penetrance which may not become symptomatic until adult life or may remain subclinical. It tends to be progressive and characteristically produces weakness of periscapular muscles and finger extensors. As in endplate acetylcholinesterase deficiency, electromyography may show a repetitive response to a single nerve stimulus. Anticholinesterase drugs are unhelpful, but quinidine or fluoxetine may be beneficial.

Mutations in rapsyn, an AChR-clustering protein, is associated with a common mutation (N88K), thus aiding screening. The rapsyn defect leads to reduced numbers of clustered AChRs. This condition usually presents in infancy and is characterized by squint without limitation of eye movements and mild resolving joint contractures. Such children often have unexplained and acute crises in muscle weakness, and bulbar and respiratory function,

and the diagnosis is crucial because this phenotype responds so well to anticholinesterases. Occasionally adulthood-onset cases are described with a very mild phenotype.

DOK7 mutations have been recently described in cases of CMS with a limb–girdle phenotype, and normal eye movements in most cases. Although DOK7 is a postsynaptic protein that interacts with MuSK (see Fig. 24.23.1), both the pre- and postsynaptic regions are small. This disorder generally responds poorly to anticholinesterases, but is occasionally helped by 3,4-diaminopyridine and ephedrine.

Neuromyotonia

This term describes a condition in which peripheral nerve overactivity leads to spontaneous muscle activity. It is thus quite different from classic myotonia, which relates to an abnormality of muscle fibre membrane activity. Neuromyotonia may be seen in association with a variety of inherited disorders (notably neuropathies and spinal muscular atrophy), but the most common form is acquired; this form may be idiopathic, but recognized associations include tumour (thymoma—sometimes also in association with myasthenia gravis; bronchial carcinoma) and acquired demyelinating polyneuropathies. Most acquired cases are autoimmune in origin and about 50% have antibodies directed against voltage-gated potassium channels (VGKCs) in the peripheral nerve (see Fig. 24.23.1), for which an assay is now available. As noted above, activation of these channels is an important factor in nerve repolarization—the symptoms of neuromyotonia can be understood in terms of reduced numbers of potassium channels, prolonged depolarization, and excessive release of acetylcholine.

The main clinical features are muscle stiffness, cramps, and twitching (myokymia), which may be localized or generalized. Voluntary muscle contraction may precipitate or exacerbate the abnormal activity. The myokymia persists during sleep and general anaesthesia. Additional symptoms include peripheral paraesthesias and excess sweating, and, rarely, mood change, disturbed sleep, and hallucinations. These central symptoms are part of a condition called Morvan's syndrome which is discussed elsewhere (see Chapter 24.22).

Apart from the muscle twitching (which may be confused with the fasciculation of denervation), physical examination may be normal. Mild weakness may be evident, proximally or distally. In long-standing cases, muscle hypertrophy (simply a form of work hypertrophy) may be present. Tendon reflexes may be reduced.

Electromyography shows highly characteristic, and diagnostic, doublet, triplet, or multiplet motor unit discharges, or periods of continuous motor unit discharge, with a high (up to 300 Hz) intraburst frequency. Fibrillation and fasciculation potentials may also be seen. Further confirmation of the diagnosis comes from anti-VGKC antibody assay, which is positive in about 50% of cases using the currently available assay. Chest imaging should be considered to exclude thymoma and bronchial carcinoma.

Most patients gain symptomatic relief from carbamazepine, phenytoin, or lamotrigine. If the benefit is insufficient, immunosuppression with prednisolone and azathioprine is often helpful. Intractable cases may respond to plasma exchange and intravenous immunoglobulin.

Further reading

Neurobiology of myasthenic syndromes

Vincent A (2007). Myasthenia gravis and myasthenic syndromes. In: Gilman S (ed.) *Neurobiology of disease.* Elsevier Academic Press, Burlington, MA.

Myasthenia gravis

Evoli A *et al.* (2003). Clinical correlates with anti-MuSK antibodies in generalized seronegative myasthenia gravis. *Brain,* **126,** 2304–11.

Newsom-Davis J, Besson D (2001). Myasthenia gravis and myasthenic syndromes: autoimmune and genetic disorders. In: Karpati G, Hilton-Jones D, Griggs R (eds) *Disorders of voluntary muscle.* Cambridge University Press, Cambridge.

Lambert–Eaton syndrome

Maddison P, Newsom-Davis J (2005). Treatment for Lambert–Eaton myasthenic syndrome. *Cochrane Database Syst Rev,* **2,** CD003279.

Wirtz PW *et al.* (2002). Differences in clinical features between the Lambert–Eaton myasthenic syndrome with and without cancer: an analysis of 227 published cases. *Clin Neurol Neurosurg,* **104,** 359–63.

Wirtz PW *et al.* (2005). Lambert–Eaton myasthenic syndrome has a more progressive course in patients with lung cancer. *Muscle Nerve,* **32,** 226–9.

Congenital myasthenic syndromes

Burke G *et al.* (2003). Rapsyn mutations in hereditary myasthenia: distinct early- and late-onset phenotypes. *Neurology,* **61,** 826–8.

Engel AG, Sine SM (2005). Current understanding of congenital myasthenic syndromes. *Curr Opin Pharmacol,* **5,** 308–21.

Palace J *et al.* (2007). Clinical features of the DOK7 neuromuscular junction synaptopathy. *Brain,* **130,** 1507–15.

Neuromyotonia

Hart IK *et al.* (2002). Phenotypic variants of autoimmune peripheral nerve hyperexcitability. *Brain,* **125,** 1887–95.

Maddison P (2006). Neuromyotonia. *Clin Neurophysiol,* **117,** 2118–27.

24.24

Disorders of muscle

Contents

24.24.1 Structure and function of muscle

M.G. Hanna

Essentials

The motor unit—the final common pathway for all voluntary muscle activity—is composed of an anterior horn cell, its peripheral axon, the axon terminal branches, the associated neuromuscular junctions, and the muscle fibres innervated.

Muscle cells—these are multinucleate units with unique structures adapted for response to metabolic, nervous, and autocrine signals. Their key elements being (1) sarcolemma—complex structured proteins maintain the integrity of the muscle fibre membrane, which contains specialized regions (motor endplates) by which innervating nerves interact at synapses; (2) contractile components—biochemical interactions between actin and myosin filaments are initiated by calcium ions released from the sarcoplasmic reticulum; contraction is powered by chemical energy released by the hydrolysis of ATP, in globular regions of myosin, after they form crosslinks with actin.

Different types of motor units—there are two biochemical variants (1) type 1—rich in mitochondria and specialized for oxidative metabolism of fat; (2) type 2—larger fibres with abundant glycogen that generate energy by glycosis and are critical for short-lived muscle contraction. All muscles contain populations of both fibre types, but differ in their proportions and functions.

Clinical perspective—knowledge of the underlying molecular cell biology, neurophysiology, and biochemical energetics of muscle provides a useful basis for understanding the symptoms, signs, and pathogenesis of clinical disorders affecting the muscles. Mutations in sarcolemmal proteins, such as dystrophin, cause diseases with widespread affects on skeletal muscle function, the heart, and survival.

Basic anatomy of skeletal muscle

We possess more than 150 voluntary (skeletal) muscles, most of which are attached to the skeleton at both ends through tendons. Complex voluntary movements of the body are achieved by integrated activity of different skeletal muscle groups. To the naked eye a transverse section of any skeletal muscle reveals small units known as muscle fascicles. Each skeletal muscle fascicle is composed of many basic structural units known as muscle fibres (Fig. 24.24.1.1). Muscle fibres are cylindrical structures that may be several centimetres long and 50 to 100 μm in diameter. A muscle fibre is a highly specialized cell. Similar to any other cell it has a membrane (the sarcolemma), contains cytoplasm (the sarcoplasm), and has an endoplasmic reticulum (the sarcoplasmic reticulum), as well as other subcellular organelles such as mitochondria. However, unlike cells from many other tissues, muscle cells are multinucleate. Typically the nuclei are positioned at the edges of the muscle fibre. The sarcolemma of muscle fibres possesses specialized regions known as motor endplates. These endplate regions are the points at which the axon innervating a muscle fibre forms synapses.

Release of acetylcholine from the presynaptic region transmits the axonal action potential to the muscle fibre membrane by binding to postsynaptic acetylcholine receptors located in the sarcolemma

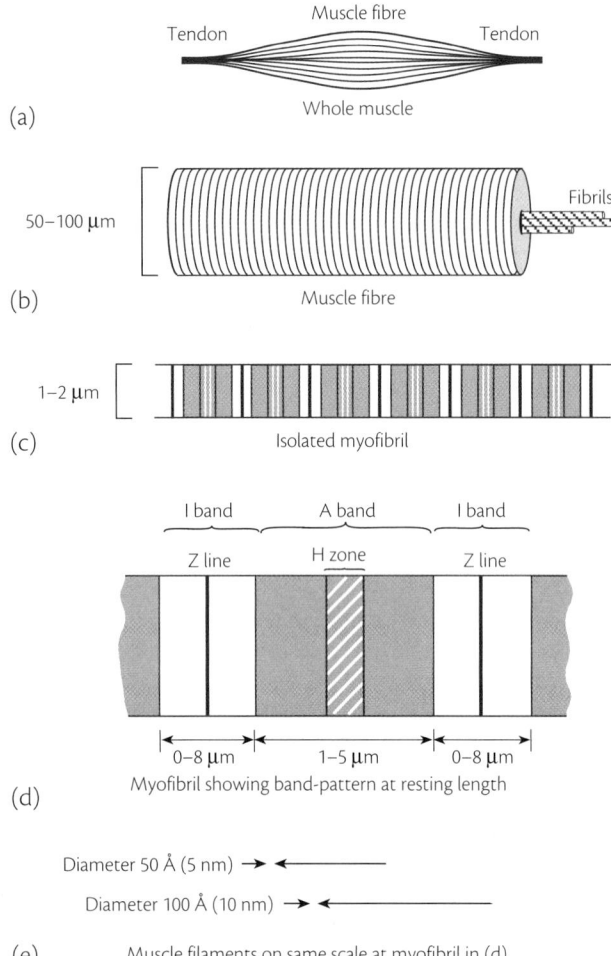

Fig. 24.24.1.1 The dimensions and arrangement of the contractile components in a muscle. The whole muscle (a) is made up of fibres (b) that contain cross-striated myofibrils (c, d). These are constructed of two types of protein filaments (e), put together as shown in Fig. 24.24.1.2.

protein filaments. In life, myofibrils are transparent on routine light microscopy, but, if viewed with a polarizing microscope, a typical pattern of cross-striations can be seen within individual myofibrils. The correct understanding of the basic microscopic anatomy of this pattern of cross-striations was critical to the discovery of the sliding filament theory of skeletal muscle contraction.

The sliding filament theory of skeletal muscle contraction

The protein filaments contained within myofibrils are of two types: the thin filaments are composed of actin, tropomyosin, and troponin, and the thick filaments of myosin (Fig. 24.24.1.2). The thick filaments are approximately twice the diameter of the thin filaments.

The thick filaments are lined up to form the A bands, whereas the array of thin filaments forms the less dense I bands. The lighter H bands in the centre of the A bands are the regions where, when the muscle is relaxed, the thin filaments do not overlap the thick filaments. The Z lines transect the myofibrils and connect to the thin filaments. If a transverse section through the A band is examined under the electron microscope, each thick filament is found to be surrounded by six thin filaments in a regular hexagonal array (see Fig. 24.24.1.2). The myosin molecules have large globular heads at their C-terminal portions (Fig. 24.24.1.3), and the heads contain an actin-binding site that hydrolyses ATP. During muscle contraction, cross-linkages occur between the heads of the myosin and the actin molecules (Fig. 24.24.1.3).

The thin filaments are composed of two chains of actin that form a long double helix. Tropomyosin molecules are long filaments located in the groove between the two chains of actin. Troponin molecules are small globular units located at intervals along the tropomyosin molecules. Troponin has three components: troponin T, responsible for binding to tropomyosin; troponin I, which inhibits the interaction of actin and myosin; and troponin C, which contains the binding sites for the Ca^{2+} ions that initiate contraction (see Fig. 24.24.1.3).

at the endplate. The sarcolemma is differentially permeable to ions. This allows different concentrations of ions to be maintained inside and outside the membrane, and is critical in maintaining the resting membrane potential. A chain of important structural proteins maintains the integrity of the sarcolemma by linking intracellular muscle fibre cytoskeletal proteins to the extracellular matrix. These structural proteins include dystrophin (located in a subsarcolemmal distribution), the dystrophin-associated glycoprotein complex (a trans-sarcolemmal protein complex), and laminin (located extracellularly). These important proteins may be dysfunctional in certain forms of genetic muscle diseases (see Chapter 24.24.2).

After staining, or if suitably illuminated, muscle fibres are seen to have regular cross-striations that extend right across the inside of the fibre, dividing it up into sarcomeres (see Fig. 24.24.1.1). The parts of the cross-striations are identified by letters: the light I band is divided by the dark Z line and the dark A band has the lighter H zone in its centre. The region between two adjacent Z lines is called a sarcomere. The cross-striations are due to the presence of the principal contractile filamentous proteins, actin and myosin, in the sarcoplasm. These filamentous proteins are arranged in rod-like structures known as myofibrils. A single myofibril contains many

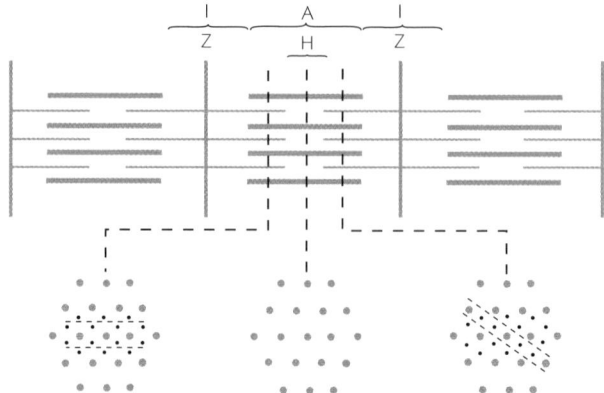

Fig. 24.24.1.2 Diagram illustrating the arrangement of the different kinds of protein filament (thick filaments: myosin; thin filaments: actin) in a myofibril. At the top are three sarcomeres drawn as they would appear in longitudinal section. Below are transverse sections through the H zone and other parts of the A band where the thick and thin filaments interdigitate. The plane of section determines whether, in electron micrographs, there seem to be one or two thin (actin) filaments between two thick (myosin) ones.
(Reproduced from Huxley and Hanson, 1960, with permission.)

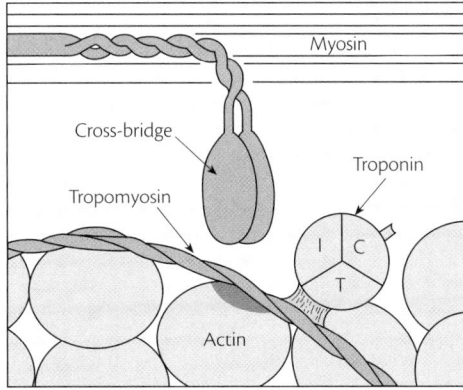

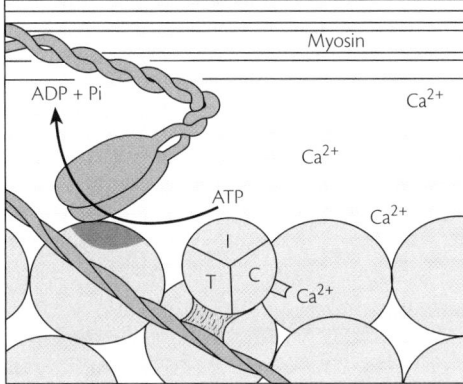

Fig. 24.24.1.3 Initiation of muscle contraction by Ca^{2+} ions. The cross-bridges (heads of myosin molecules) attach to binding sites on actin (striped areas) and swivel when tropomyosin is displaced laterally by binding of Ca^{2+} ions to troponin C. (Modified from Katz AM, 1975, Congestive heart failure. New England Journal of Medicine 293, 1184.)

The process by which shortening of the contractile elements of muscle is brought about is sliding of the thin filaments over the thick filaments. The width of the A band is constant, whereas the Z lines move closer together when the muscle contracts and further apart when it is stretched. The sliding during muscle contraction is produced by breaking and reforming the cross-linkages between actin and myosin. The immediate source of energy for contraction is hydrolysis of ATP localized to the myosin head.

Neural activation of muscle fibres—the motor unit

The motor unit is the final common pathway for all voluntary muscle activity. It is composed of an anterior horn cell (located within the spinal cord), its peripheral axon, the axon terminal branches, the associated neuromuscular junctions, and the muscle fibres innervated. The muscle fibres of a single motor unit are spatially dispersed throughout a muscle and only a few fibres innervated by the same anterior horn cell are contiguous. The number of motor units varies greatly between muscles, from approximately 1000 in leg muscles to 100 in intrinsic hand muscles. The number of muscle fibres per motor unit also varies greatly, and motor units differ in physiological and biochemical characteristics. Two main types of motor units are recognized, each composed of a single muscle fibre type. Type 1 muscle fibres contain many mitochondria and are slightly smaller than type 2 muscle fibres because they contain myofibrils, which are more slender. Type 1 fibres contain a

high concentration of oxidative enzymes and more fat; type 2 fibres are larger, contain fewer mitochondria, but have a higher concentration of glycogen and enzymes involved in anaerobic metabolism such as myophosphorylase. All skeletal muscles contain a mixture of both fibre types, typically in a chequerboard pattern when stained appropriately (with the myofibrillar ATPase reaction) and visualized under light microscopy (Fig. 24.24.1.4). Type 1 fibres are also known as slow fibres because they contract and relax slowly and are abundant in muscles concerned mainly with maintaining posture. In contrast, type 2 fibres contract and relax quickly and are also known as twitch fibres. Type 2 fibres can be further subdivided into type 2a and 2b based on their intensity of staining with myofibrillar ATPase reaction at different pH values (Table 24.24.1.1).

Normally muscle fibres do not contract in isolation; rather the muscle fibres that comprise the motor unit contract together in response to depolarization of an anterior horn cell. Such depolarization is transmitted along the axon until it invades the nerve terminal. This results in opening of voltage-gated calcium channels located in the presynaptic membrane. Calcium enters the nerve terminal down an electrochemical gradient. The resulting increase in presynaptic calcium concentration promotes fusion of acetylcholine-containing vesicles normally present in the nerve terminal with the presynaptic membrane. Quanta of acetylcholine are released into the synaptic cleft and diffuse to the postsynaptic membrane to bind to and activate acetylcholine receptors. Acetycholine binding causes opening of its receptor channel, allowing cations to enter the muscle fibre in the endplate region. This cation flux depolarizes the postsynaptic membrane, resulting in a mini-endplate potential. The summation of endplate potentials results in the excitation of the postsynaptic membrane, which is then conducted along the muscle fibre membrane. The excitation is transmitted into the muscle fibre by invaginations of the sarcolemma known as the T-tubule system. Activation of calcium channels in the T-tubule system membrane results in opening of calcium channels in the sarcoplasmic reticulum. Calcium is

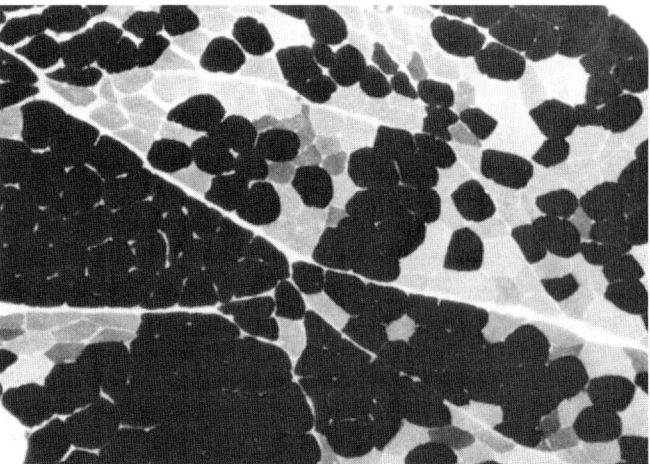

Fig. 24.24.1.4 A transverse section of human skeletal muscle obtained by biopsy from a patient with spinal muscular atrophy stained for the myofibrillar ATPase reaction after preincubation at pH 4.6. There is extensive evidence of fibre type grouping, particularly of the type 1 fibres, resulting from reinnervation. Magnification ×150.
(Kindly supplied by Dr Margaret Johnson.)

Table 24.24.1.1 Histochemical and physiological characteristics of the three major types of muscle fibre

	Fibre type		
	1	2A	2B
Enzyme reactions			
NADH–tetrazolium reductase and SDH	+++	++	+
Myofibrillar ATPase:			
pH 9.4	+	+++	+++
pH 4.6	+++	–	+++
pH 4.3	+++	–	–
Phosphorylase	+	+++	+++
Physiological properties			
Twitch speeds	Slow	Fast	Fast
Fatigue resistance	+++	++	+
Nomenclature			
Peter et al. (1972)	Slow twitch Oxidative	Fast twitch Oxidative–glycolytic	Fast twitch Glycolytic
Burle et al. (1971)	S (slow contracting)	FR (fast contracting, fatigue resistant)	FF (fast contracting, fast fatigue)

From Walton JN, Mastaglia FL (1980).

then released into the muscle fibre cytoplasm, initiating muscle contraction.

Energy production in skeletal muscle

Resting skeletal muscle requires remarkably little energy, but the need for energy production may increase dramatically in response to exercise, because energy is required for muscle contraction. ATP is the main source of energy in muscle. It is required for shortening of the contractile filaments and for the active reuptake of calcium into the sarcoplasmic reticulum after each muscle contraction. Maintenance of electrochemical gradients across the sarcolemma also requires ATP. Resynthesis of ATP from ADP is essential for normal muscle function. The two main energy-producing pathways in muscle are glycolysis in the sarcoplasm and oxidative phosphorylation in the mitochondria. Resynthesis of ATP from ADP is also aided by phosphocreatine and the creatine kinase reaction. Creatine kinase catalyses the transfer of high-energy phosphate from phosphocreatine to ADP in circumstances in which ATP demand may outstrip ATP production, e.g. at the very start of exercise before oxidative phosphorylation or glycolysis is activated. Glycolysis is the main pathway of ATP synthesis in anaerobic conditions and results in the generation of lactate. Oxidative phosphorylation is the major ATP-generating pathway in aerobic conditions. The main fuel sources in skeletal muscle are glucose, glycogen, and fatty acids. In anaerobic conditions, glycogen is the main energy source. In aerobic exercise, glycogen and glucose are utilized initially, but, after approximately 30 min, fatty acids are the main energy source. In resting aerobic muscle, fatty acids provide the principal source of fuel. Several muscle diseases are recognized in which energy metabolism is impaired; these are known as the metabolic myopathies.

Diseases of human skeletal muscle: overview

Human muscle diseases may be conveniently divided into those that are genetically determined and those that are acquired (Box 24.24.1.1).

The clinical history in muscle diseases

Although a muscle biopsy is usually needed to determine the exact type of muscle disease, the clinical history and examination are usually sufficient to determine whether a muscle disease is present or absent. As many muscle diseases are genetically determined, it is particularly important to consider the family history. A careful drug history is also essential.

Although many diseases may affect skeletal muscle (see Box 24.24.1.1), there are three main symptoms with which patients may present: muscular pain, muscular weakness, and fatigability. A further important but less common symptom is darkening of the urine (pigmenturia) due to release of myoglobin from damaged muscle, which occurs particularly in the metabolic myopathies. Unless pigmenturia has been dramatic, patients may not volunteer this symptom. Muscle pain is a common symptom, but in only about a third of patients presenting with this symptom will an underlying muscle disease be identified. In those without a definable muscle disease, many are considered to have a psychogenic cause for their muscle pain, although some may have as yet undefined disorders of muscle metabolism.

Sometimes it can be difficult for the patient and the physician to distinguish between pain originating in muscle and that originating in joints or bones. Certain rheumatological diseases may result in joint pain as well as muscle pain, e.g. systemic lupus erythematosus may cause arthritis and polymyositis. Muscle pains may take

---

Box 24.24.1.1 A simple classification of human muscle diseases

Genetically determined muscle diseases

◆ Muscular dystrophies, such as Duchenne/Becker

◆ Congenital myopathies, such as nemaline

◆ Muscle ion channel disorders, such as hyper-/hypokalaemic periodic paralysis

◆ Metabolic myopathies, such as McArdle's disease (myophosphorylase deficiency) and mitchondrial myopathies

Acquired muscle diseases

◆ Inflammatory muscle diseases, such as polymyositis/dermatomyositis

◆ Degenerative muscle diseases, such as inclusion body myositis

◆ Endocrine muscle diseases, such as hyper-/hypothyroid myopathies

◆ Toxic and drug-induced muscle diseases, due to alcohol/corticosteroids the form of cramps, which are involuntary contractions of muscle groups. Simple muscle cramps are not uncommon in older people and frequently occur at night. There is usually no underlying muscle disease but drugs such as diuretics (which induce hypokalaemia) may be implicated. In younger patients, muscle cramps may be the presenting feature of a metabolic muscle disease such as McArdle's disease. Muscle pain brought on by exertion is a particular feature of the metabolic muscle diseases. Muscle contractures may also be a source of muscle pain in patients with metabolic myopathies. Patients experience a pain similar to a cramp, but, unlike a cramp, electromyography reveals that a contracture is electrically silent.

Muscle weakness is a common feature of muscle diseases and the distribution of weakness in most of these diseases is in the proximal limb muscles. Patients may complain of difficulty performing tasks that involve lifting their arms up to or above the head, such as brushing hair. Proximal lower limb muscle weakness causes difficulties getting out of low chairs and in climbing stairs. Muscle diseases often affect the limb musculature symmetrically, although there are important exceptions to this, e.g. one of the common autosomal dominant muscular dystrophies, fascioscapulohumeral muscular dystrophy, often affects the limb muscles in an asymmetrical fashion. Some muscle diseases may affect the facial musculature as well as that of the limb. Symptoms may include difficulty in whistling, closing the eyes, or articulating. Respiratory muscle disease may cause breathlessness. It is important to determine the natural history of muscle weakness. In most genetically determined muscle diseases, weakness progresses slowly over years; occasionally patients may experience attacks of weakness separated by periods when they seem to have normal strength, as in the periodic paralyses. The muscle weakness in the inflammatory muscle diseases usually develops more rapidly.

Fatigability is defined as an increase in weakness with exercise. Patients may say that they can start a particular physical activity but the longer they continue the weaker they become. They may also complain that they become weaker as the day goes on. Myasthenia gravis, a disorder of neuromuscular transmission, is the principal cause of fatigability. In patients with myasthenia gravis, fatigability can usually be demonstrated at the bedside. Patients with metabolic muscle diseases may also experience fatigability.

The physical examination in muscle disease

The examination may be broadly divided into two aspects: first, an examination is made to establish whether there are any clues to the cause of the muscle disease. In this context, the general physical examination is very important. Particular attention is paid to eliciting signs that might indicate an underlying endocrine or rheumatological disorder, e.g. signs of hyper-/hypothyroidism, Cushing's syndrome, or rheumatological disorders such as systemic lupus erythematosus. Inspection of the skin may reveal the appearances of dermatomyositis. The second part of the examination involves examining the muscular system to determine the extent and severity of the condition; this may also give further clues to the aetiology. The muscles are inspected for any atrophy or hypertrophy (as occurs in some muscular dystrophies) or for any spontaneous activity of the muscle fibres (such as fasciculation, which might indicate an anterior horn cell disorder).

The muscles should be palpated for any tenderness or swelling, which may occur in inflammatory muscle diseases. Myotonia is a delayed relaxation of muscle after contraction, and may be observed by asking the patient to clench the fist and then open it rapidly. A patient with myotonia is unable to open the clenched fist rapidly due to an inability to relax the contracted muscles quickly. Myotonia may also be evident on percussion of muscle. The examination of muscle power is carried out systematically, starting with the cranial musculature before proceeding to the arms and legs. The degree of weakness is assessed with reference to the Medical Research Council grading scale (0 to 5). The distribution of weakness is also noted, because different muscle diseases have characteristic patterns of weakness. Bedside assessment of respiratory muscles including the diaphragm is also important, although detailed assessment of these muscles requires formal spirometry. Finally, the tendon reflexes are elicited. These are generally preserved in acquired muscle diseases, except when there is advanced weakness; however, they may be lost relatively early in the course of dystrophies.

Investigating the patient with muscle disease

Investigations are generally instituted only when the history and examination have provided clear evidence that the patient has symptoms and/or signs of muscle disease. The investigations are aimed primarily at determining the exact type of muscle disease because it is essential to establish whether the patient has a treatable muscle disease, such as an inflammatory myopathy. Many investigations of increasing complexity and invasiveness are available.

Simple blood tests allow an assessment of the endocrine and nutritional status of the patient (such as thyroid function, the consumption of excess alcohol, or the presence of vitamin D deficiency). Measurement of blood creatine kinase is important because this can be an indicator of the degree of muscle fibre damage or necrosis. Creatine kinase is generally elevated in inflammatory muscle diseases and in many of the muscular dystrophies.

Increasingly, DNA-based testing is available from simple blood samples. This can be particularly helpful and in some situations may obviate the need for further more invasive tests, such as a muscle biopsy, e.g. if analysis of the dystrophin gene on the X chromosome identifies a pathogenic mutation known to associate with Duchenne muscular dystrophy, the diagnosis is confirmed. It is likely that there will be greater availability of DNA-based tests for genetic muscle disease in the future and this will become an increasingly important aid to diagnosis.

The diagnosis of metabolic muscle diseases may be achieved by specific dynamic tests, e.g. McArdle's disease can be diagnosed using the ischaemic lactate test, and mitochondrial disease may be suspected on the basis of subanaerobic exercise tests (both these tests are described in the relevant section).

Detailed nerve conduction studies and electromyography (EMG) are useful in determining whether a patient has a neuropathy, a defect in neuromuscular junction transmission, or a myopathy. EMG is useful in characterizing any spontaneous activity of muscle, such as fasciculations or myotonia. Although EMG is generally useful in confirming the presence of a myopathy, it is less useful in determining the cause.

Muscle biopsy allows a detailed analysis of the internal architecture of muscle and is an extremely valuable and safe investigation in carefully selected patients. Using a range of histochemical stains, histochemical enzyme reactions, and immunological techniques on frozen muscle biopsy sections, much information of diagnostic use can be obtained. Different muscle diseases often reveal characteristic patterns of abnormalities, which are usually identified

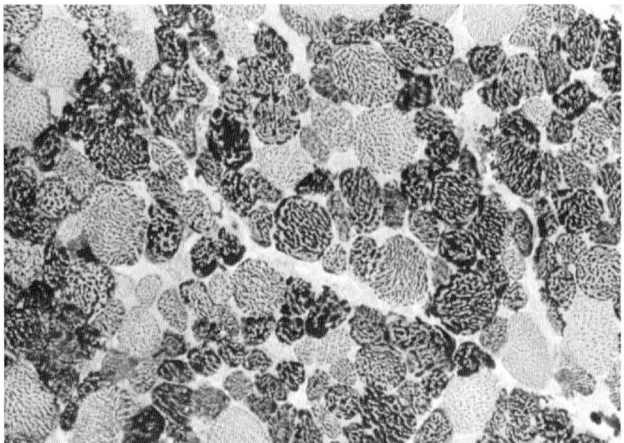

Fig. 24.24.1.5 A transverse section of human skeletal muscle obtained from a patient with carnitine deficiency and stained with Sudan black B. The massive accumulation of neutral fat, especially with the type 1 fibres, is evident. Magnification ×196.

by light microscopic techniques. Using basic histochemical stains, the features of different muscular dystrophies are generally similar, the most common features being marked variations in fibre diameter, internal nuclei, fibre splitting, fibre necrosis and regeneration, and increase in connective tissue. However, a more precise diagnosis of the type of muscular dystrophy can now be obtained by immunostaining techniques. Antibodies that are raised against specific membrane proteins allow quantitative analysis, e.g. staining using antibodies directed against dystrophin reveals no or very little dystrophin in cases of Duchenne muscular dystrophy. Prominent inflammatory infiltrates are typically seen in muscle sections from patients with inflammatory myopathies. Figs. 24.24.1.5, 24.24.1.6, and 24.24.1.7 show the muscle biopsy features of some of the metabolic myopathies. In some cases the changes seen on the biopsy clearly indicate a myopathic process, but it is not possible to be more specific in the absence of typical immunological, inflammatory, or metabolic changes.

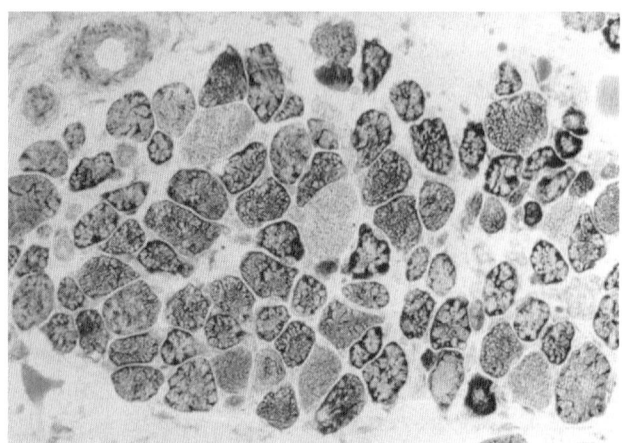

Fig. 24.24.1.6 A transverse section of skeletal muscle obtained from a patient with mitochondrial myopathy, stained for the MADH-TR reaction. The type 1 fibres are darkly stained and show the typical reticulated appearance of so-called 'ragged-red fibres' with massive mitochondria, particularly in many fibres just deep to the sarcolemma. Magnification ×384.
(Kindly supplied by Dr Margaret Johnson.)

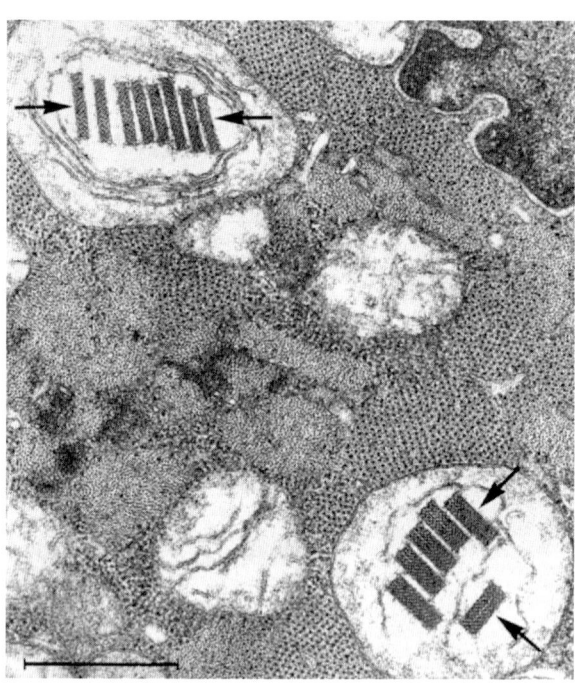

Fig. 24.24.1.7 A transverse section of a biopsy specimen obtained from one quadriceps muscle in a patient with mitochondrial myopathy, showing arrays of paracrystalline inclusions in the damaged mitochondria. Bar = 1 μm.
(Kindly supplied by Dr Michael Cullen.)

Further reading

Hughes BW, Kusner LL, Kaminski HJ (2006). Molecular architecture of the neuromuscular junction. *Muscle Nerve*, **33**, 445–61.

Huxley HE, Hanson J (1972). In: Bourne GH, ed. *The structure and function of muscle*, Vol 1. 2nd edition. Academic Press, New York.

Larsson L, Edström L, Lindegren B, *et al.* (1991). MHC composition and enzyme-histochemical and physiological properties of a novel fast-twitch motor unit type. *Am J Physiol*, **261**, 93–101.

Smerdu V, Karsch-Mizrachi I, Campione M (1994). Type IIx myosin heavy chain transcripts are expressed in type IIb fibers of human skeletal muscle. *Am J Physiol*, **267**, C1723–8.

Walton JN, Mastaglia FL (1980). The molecular basis of muscle disease. In: Thompson RHS, Davison AN (eds) *The molecular basis of neuropathology*. Edward Arnold, London.

24.24.2 **Muscular dystrophy**

K. Bushby

Essentials

Muscular dystrophies are primary, genetically determined, disorders of muscle. All cause muscle weakness, which is usually progressive. They are challenging to classify, but clinical characteristics can be combined with genetic and molecular information to obtain a useful operational nomenclature for prognosis and family counselling. In general, diagnosis is guided by the age at which clinical manifestations appear and the rate at which muscle function is lost, but unusual features such as muscle pain and rhabdomyolysis may also contribute to the identification of a particular hereditary muscle disorder.

Congenital muscular dystrophies

These are defined by their very early childhood onset. Molecularly based subclassification allows the recognition of various subgroups including those associated with mutations in/causing: (1) laminin A2, (2) abnormal glycosylation of α-dystroglycan; (3) collagen VI—Ullrich congenital muscular dystrophy, (4) selenoprotein 1 gene.

Dystrophin deficiency

Duchenne and Becker muscular dystrophy are X-linked diseases that are both caused by mutations (mostly deletions) in the *dystrophin* gene.

Clinical features—(1) Duchenne muscular dystrophy—all affected boys are symptomatic within the first 3 years of life; motor milestones and speech are frequently delayed; there is a pronounced waddling gait on attempting to run. Hypertrophy of the calf muscles is almost universal. (2) Becker muscular dystrophy—mean age at onset is 11 years; typically manifests with difficulty with high steps and climbing hills; may suffer muscle pain after exercise; frequently have hypertrophy involving the same muscle groups as seen in Duchenne muscular dystrophy.

Investigation, diagnosis and prevention—serum creatine kinase is always massively elevated, but the level does not distinguish the severity of the disease. Molecular confirmation of the diagnosis is essential to assist in defining prognosis and allow provision of appropriate genetic counselling.

Prognosis and complications—the prognosis of 'dystrophinopathies' is highly variable. Untreated patients with Duchenne muscular dystrophy lose the ability to walk by the age of 12, but corticosteroids can delay deterioration. Scoliosis, respiratory failure and cardiomyopathy develop during the teenage years. With appropriate multidisciplinary supportive care, survival into or beyond the late twenties and thirties is becoming more common.

Other muscular dystrophies

Facioscapulohumeral muscular dystrophy is an autosomal dominant disease sometimes arising as the result of a new dominant mutation, affected individuals manifest early symptoms, typically including facial weakness, shoulder girdle weakness and foot drop, by their teens or twenties. Serum creatine kinase may be normal or mildly elevated. Diagnosis can be confirmed in 95% of cases by demonstration of a deletion close to the telomere of chromosome 4q. The condition is slowly progressive; complications rarely include scoliosis and respiratory failure.

Emery–Dreifuss muscular dystrophy—caused by mutation of any one of several genes encoding components of the nuclear envelope (e.g. *emerin, lamin A/C*). May present at any age, with contractures of the ankles and elbows and rigidity of the spine often predating any clear weakness. Prognosis is determined by ability to manage life-threatening cardiac arrhythmias.

Limb girdle muscular dystrophies—these comprise a range of disorders that cause weakness of the proximal musculature. Important considerations in any case are (1) could it be a dominant disease?—e.g. limb girdle muscular dystrophy 1B (allelic with autosomal dominant Emery–Dreifuss muscular dystrophy), Bethlem myopathy; (2) age of presentation and rate of progression—these give important clues to likely diagnosis; (3) investigations—creatine kinase is greatly elevated in all forms of autosomal recessive limb girdle muscular dystrophy; EMG confirms a primary myopathic process; muscle biopsy shows dystrophic changes on standard analysis, with more specialized testing for diagnosis of e.g. sarcoglycanopathies, calpainopathy, dysferlinopathy.

Oculopharyngeal muscular dystrophy—typically presents in the sixth decade with ptosis, dysphagia to solids, and dysphonia. Associated with an expanded triplet repeat in the gene for poly(A) binding protein 2.

Introduction

Muscular dystrophy is not a single disease. Many different types of muscular dystrophy can be recognized: all are primary, genetically determined disorders of muscle and all cause muscle weakness, which is usually progressive. The various types of muscular dystrophy share several characteristic findings on muscle biopsy, most notably a variation of fibre size, evidence of muscle fibre necrosis, and usually replacement of muscle tissue by fat and fibrous tissue. These pathological findings are often, but not always, accompanied by elevation of the serum creatine kinase. Although the key clinical sign in muscular dystrophy is muscle weakness, the distribution of that weakness and the association with other features such as wasting, hypertrophy, and joint contractures are the most helpful defining features in making a clinical diagnosis, together with age at presentation and rate of progression. Unusual presenting manifestations of muscular dystrophy are muscle pain, rhabdomyolysis, myoglobinuria and cardiomyopathy.

Complications may include cardiac and respiratory failure or anaesthetic problems. These complications may be relatively specific to particular types of muscular dystrophy. Taken together with the clinical findings in any patient, precise diagnostic tests (through either DNA analysis or protein analysis of a muscle biopsy sample) are available for most of these disorders, as knowledge of the underlying mechanism of disease for each of these entities has increased. Confirmation of the type of muscular dystrophy in any individual patient is critical to the provision of appropriate management, prognostic advice, and genetic counselling. No form of muscular dystrophy is currently curable, although various experimental therapeutic procedures are under investigation.

Classification of the muscular dystrophies

Various classifications of the muscular dystrophies have been proposed, reflecting historical advances in the understanding of this group of diseases (Box 24.24.2.1). The current basis for classification combines an appreciation of the clinical features with the ability to determine the molecular basis for the disease. Therefore the eponymous names (e.g. Duchenne muscular dystrophy) still in common usage reflect the detailed clinical descriptions provided by early clinicians; other disease names reflect the recognized pattern of muscle involvement in a particular condition (e.g. facioscapulohumeral muscular dystrophy). Disease designations based on the genetic or protein defect in a particular disorder (e.g. dystrophinopathy) are becoming more widely used, reflecting the fact that some disorders previously believed to be clinically distinct actually represent different manifestations of lesions at the same locus. Genetic analysis has also revealed an unsuspected level of heterogeneity with different genetic causes for disorders that show superficial clinical similarities. This can be seen most strikingly within the 'limb–girdle' and congenital groups of muscular dystrophies.

The pathophysiology of the muscular dystrophies

Biochemical and physiological experiments failed to shed any light on the mechanisms by which muscular dystrophy could arise, and it has only been since the cloning of the dystrophin gene (*DMD*) in 1987 that progress has been made. It is now quite clear that proteins involved in several different functions within the muscle cell can, when altered or absent, cause muscle damage and account for the pathological and clinical features of a muscular dystrophy. Some of these proteins are components of the membrane of the muscle fibre that may have a structural or signalling role, others are components of the nuclear envelope or muscle-specific enzymes (Fig. 24.24.2.1).

General points on the diagnosis of muscular dystrophy

Box 24.24.2.2 summarizes some of the major considerations for arriving at the correct diagnosis of a muscular dystrophy. History taking at the time of presentation (Box 24.24.2.3) may be particularly informative. The clinical history may be pathognomonic. Detailed diagnostic information is given in the following text relating to specific diseases. The main tools for specific diagnosis in muscular dystrophy are the use of antibodies for immunolabelling of muscle biopsy sections and/or the application of specific DNA-based genetic analysis.

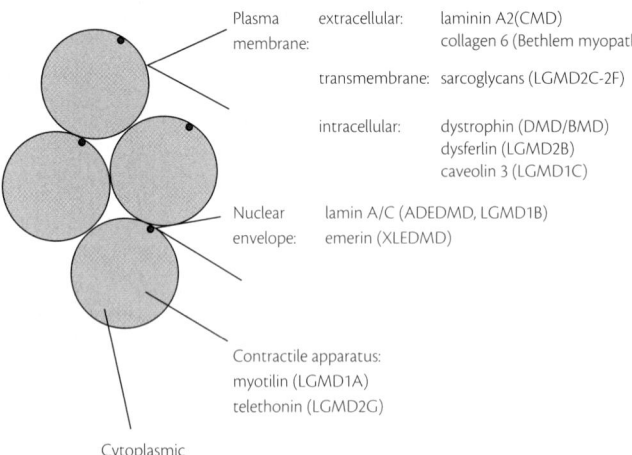

Fig. 24.24.2.1 Schematic diagram to show localization within the muscle fibre (where known) of some of the proteins involved in producing a dystrophic phenotype.

General points on the management of the muscular dystrophies

Despite the fact that no cures for muscular dystrophy have been established, there are many management issues that may be important or specific to the various types. However, as yet there is little systematic or comprehensive clinical research into management and randomized trials of management regimens are few and far between. It is nevertheless appropriate, where possible, that patients with a diagnosis or a suspected diagnosis of muscular dystrophy should be referred to a specialist clinic. The multidisciplinary approach of these clinics ensures that patients have access to the full range of diagnostic facilities, are able to obtain specialized physiotherapy advice, and can obtain accurate genetic counselling where this is required. Access to patient support organizations and their staff is also of paramount importance. The diagnosis of any kind of muscular dystrophy, in that it inevitably implies a progressive and incurable disease, possibly with implications for children or other relatives, is a considerable burden and one that needs to be recognized and supported.

The congenital muscular dystrophies

The congenital muscular dystrophies (CMDs) are defined by their very early childhood onset. They comprise a number of disorders

Box 24.24.2.3 History taking in muscle disease

- Question in detail about early motor development.

- Eliciting what actually were the first symptoms experienced by a patient may be difficult but is important in highlighting the initial pattern of muscle involvement—lower limb versus upper limb/ proximal versus distal musculature.

- Asking 'when were you at your fastest' may be informative in determining age of peak motor performance.

- Ask about performance at school sports.

- Particularly useful indicators in that respect are the ability to climb ropes (upper girdle weakness), muscle pain on running, a tendency to spend all the time in goal at football(!).

- Do not assume that difficulty climbing stairs always indicates proximal muscle weakness—it may reflect an inability to push up on the toes.

- Ask specifically about the ability to stand on tiptoe/stand on heels. The need to wear heels on shoes at all times may indicate Achilles tendon contractures.

- Patients who had early Achilles tendon contractures may have had them operated on before being referred for diagnosis. Ask about this.

with different molecular pathological bases for the diseases. For their presentation, see Box 24.24.2.4.

Differential diagnosis

In the neonatal and early childhood presentation the main clinical diagnostic confusion (after excluding central causes of hypotonia) may be with spinal muscular atrophy (check *SMN* gene for characteristic deletions), congenital myotonic dystrophy (facial weakness

Box 24.24.2.4 Presentation of congenital muscular dystrophies

Neonatal presentation

- Hypotonia, which may be prenatal

- Feeding problems (usually mild)

- Joint contractures, especially knees, hips, and ankles (Fig. 24.24.2.2)

- Joint laxity that may coexist with contractures at other joints

Early childhood presentation

- Delayed motor milestones

- Failure to thrive

- Repeated respiratory infections

Later childhood presentation (rare)

- Mainly proximal muscle symptoms

- History of delayed motor milestones

- Rigid spine, contractures of ankles, hips, and knees

is usually more pronounced and diagnosis can be excluded on genetic testing), and congenital myopathy (may be distinguished on muscle biopsy). In all of these conditions, serum creatine kinase is either normal or much lower than seen in many congenital muscular dystrophies.

With later childhood presentation the differential diagnosis is as above, plus Duchenne muscular dystrophy (though calf hypertrophy is usually more pronounced and serum creatine kinase is typically higher—biopsy will exclude the diagnosis) or childhood presentation of a limb–girdle type of muscular dystrophy.

Classification

There are several recognized forms of congenital muscular dystrophy and, as there is considerable heterogeneity in the group that remains, additional entities are ultimately likely to be distinguished at the genetic level. The diagnostic classification of this group of diseases was previously very clinically based, but is moving increasingly into a molecularly based subclassification (see Chapter 24.17). This allows the recognition of various subgroups of

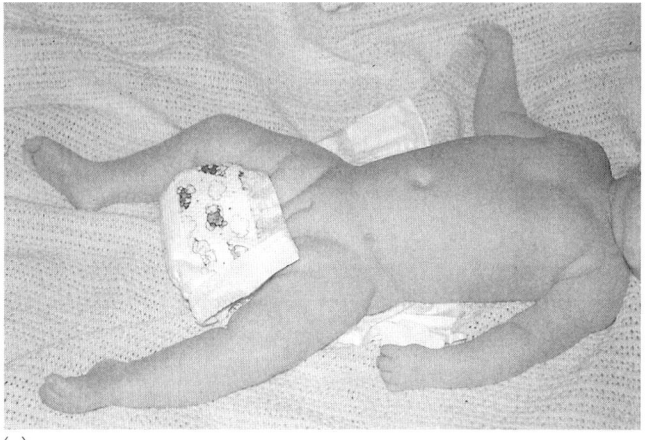

(a)

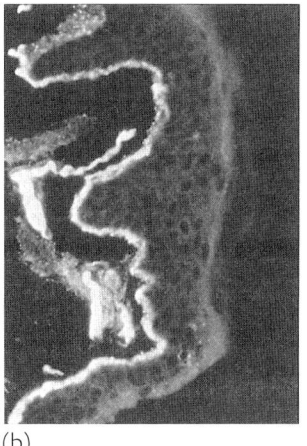
(b)

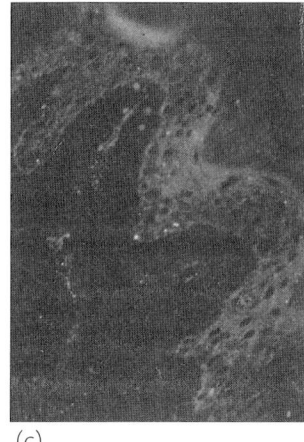
(c)

Fig. 24.24.2.2 (a) Typical clinical picture of a baby presenting with merosin-negative muscular dystrophy. Note the hypotonic posture, and mild contractures of the hips, knees, and ankles. (b, c) Immunofluorescence picture of skin biopsy labelled with an antibody to laminin A2 (merosin), showing normal and absent labelling patterns. This investigation can be carried out on a variety of tissues including skin, muscle, and placenta.

Table 24.24.2.1 The congenital muscular dystrophies

	MDC1A	CMD with abnormal glycosylation of alpha dystroglycan	Ullrich Congenital muscular dystrophy	RSMD1	Others
Molecular basis	Mutations in laminin A2 (previously known as merosin)	Mutations in fukutin, FKRP, LARGE, POMT1, POMgT and others	Mutations in collagen 6A1, 2 and 3	Mutations in selenoprotein 1	Various other causes of CMD have been described including mutations in integrin alpha 7 and lamin A/C
Diagnostic tests	Absence of laminin A2 labelling in muscle and skin, mutation testing	Abnormal labelling of alpha dystroglycans in muscle, mutation testing	Frequent absence or abnormality of collagen VI immunolabelling in muscle or cultured fibroblasts. Mutation testing.	Immunolabelling in muscle typically normal. Diagnosis established on mutation testing	Depends on causative gene which will need to be directed by protein and mutation testing
Additional features	White matter radiolucency on MRI, approx 30% have epilepsy. May have restricted eye movements	Very variable brain phenotype ranging from normal to severe lissencephaly. Eye phenotype is also variable from normal to micro-opthalmia	Characteristic pattern of joint hyperlaxity distally with proximal contractures. May be abnormal skin including keloid scarring and hyperkeratosis	Typical rigid and side sliding spine develops in first decade. Early respiratory failure while ambulation maintained	Depends on causative gene- with laminopathy typically see early rigidity of the spine and high risk of cardiac abnormalities
Notes	Progressive development of severe contractures, scoliosis, feeding and respiratory problems require close follow up	This highly variable group includes the clinical entities of Fukuyama muscular dystrophy, Walker Warburg, and Muscle eye brain disease. Other genes remain to be identified responsible for secondary loss of alpha dystroglycan. Milder allelic forms of all of these diseases exist.	Though UCMD is typically autosomal recessive, de novo dominant mutations are increasingly recognized. A milder allelic form (Bethlem myopathy) exists	Selenoprotein 1 gene mutations are also responsible for multiminicore disease	As molecular testing becomes increasingly applied, CMD phenotypes associated with mutations in various genes are likely to be identified

CMD: laminin α_2 (LAMA2) associated CMD (MDC1A), the types of CMD involving abnormal glycosylation of α-dystroglycan (where there is frequent eye and/or brain involvement as well as muscle weakness), CMD associated with collagen VI mutations (Ullrich congenital muscular dystrophy or UCMD), and rigid spine muscular dystrophy-1 (RSMD1) due to mutations in the selenoprotein-1 gene (Table 24.24.2.1). Cases of CMD due to mutations in genes also causing other types of muscular dystrophy are also increasingly recognized, for example with mutations in lamin A/C.

Establishing the diagnosis

Serum creatine kinase may, in some forms of congenital muscular dystrophy, be normal, but is typically elevated at least twofold, and up to twentyfold or more in the laminin A2-deficient group and the α-dystroglycanopathies. Muscle biopsy shows dystrophic changes and examination for LAMA2, α-dystroglycans, and collagen VI in muscle, or for LAMA2 and collagen VI; skin is also used to distinguish cases with normal and abnormal or absent protein. MRI of the brain is a useful adjunct to diagnosis because it will confirm the presence of white matter changes, which are always present after age 6 months in primary LAMA2 deficiency, and the characteristic brain malformations in the types of CMD associated with α-dystroglycanopathy (see Table 24.24.2.1).

Prognosis and management

The overall prognosis depends on the type of CMD and individual severity in the patient because there can be major variability even within the different subgroups. Children with the most severe forms are at risk of dying in early childhood. If they survive this period, with appropriate management of feeding problems, and respiratory and (in a minority) cardiac complications, survival into adult life is the norm. The muscle weakness in congenital muscular dystrophy may be relatively static, but the complications of that weakness can be severe, and vary according to the precise diagnosis. The degree of muscle weakness is quite variable. In primary laminin A2-deficient CMD, the severity of the disease correlates roughly with the abundance of laminin A2 in the muscle, with children completely lacking laminin A2 rarely achieving independent ambulation. Others may learn to walk independently but this is usually much later than usual, and these children may later lose this ability.

For all types of CMD, joint contractures and scoliosis are major complications of the disease and cause much additional disability, requiring careful management by physiotherapy, standing regimens, orthoses, and surgery where appropriate. Feeding problems may be intractable and lead to chronic malnutrition unless treated by nasogastric or gastrostomy feeding. Malnutrition may contribute to susceptibility to chest infections, which is also heightened by weakness of the respiratory muscles. These children are at risk of respiratory failure and their follow-up should include monitoring for this complication, which can be effectively managed by the provision of noninvasive home nocturnal ventilation. Cardiac failure is a relatively rare complication in CMD but has been reported in MDC1A and the α-dystroglycanopathies.

Fukuyama congenital muscular dystrophy (FCMD), muscle–eye–brain disease (MEBD), Walker–Warburg syndrome (WWS), and other diseases within the α-dystroglycanopathy spectrum may be dominated by intellectual and visual handicap. In MDC1A, brain changes on MRI are typically asymptomatic. In UCMD intellectual development is normal but respiratory failure is a major risk in the first decade. RSMD1 overall carries a generally much milder prognosis with respect to mobility, but this may mask a serious risk of respiratory failure and scoliosis, both generally necessitating intervention by the end of the first decade, often while still ambulant.

Genetic counselling

All these disorders are autosomal recessive in inheritance, although new dominant mutations in one or other of the collagen VI genes complicate genetic counselling in UCMD and the lamin A/C mutations typically seen associated with a CMD phenotype tend to be de novo. As the molecular basis for these disorders has recently become much better established, specific diagnosis should be attempted in all cases in order to allow proper direction of management as well as prenatal and carrier testing where requested.

Dystrophin deficiency

This group, including two of the most common forms of muscular dystrophy—Duchenne and Becker muscular dystrophy—involve the same gene and protein. These are X-linked diseases, caused by mutations, most of which are deletions, in the dystrophin gene (*DMD*).

Presentation

Duchenne muscular dystrophy (OMIM 300377)

- All patients are symptomatic within the first 3 years of life although the mean age at diagnosis is 4 years 10 months.

- Motor milestones are often delayed (half the cases are not walking by 18 months).

- Speech is also frequently delayed.

- Patient is unable to run: there is a pronounced waddling gait on attempting to rush.

- Patient is unable to jump with both feet together or to hop: there is no spring in the step.

- 'Climbs up legs' on rising from the floor: Gower's manoeuvre.

- Rarely presents with anaesthetic complications.

Becker muscular dystrophy (OMIM 300376)

- The mean age at onset of Becker muscular dystrophy is 11 years, although the range of age at presentation is extremely wide and the diagnosis may be made at any age, particularly if there is a family history.

- A proportion will have had delayed motor milestones (this may correlate as much with reduction in IQ as with major motor problems at that age).

- Many describe being unable to keep up with peers at school.

- There is difficulty with high steps and climbing hills.

- Muscle pains after exercise are a common complaint, especially in teenagers (rarely myoglobinuria).

Manifesting carriers of Duchenne muscular dystrophy/Becker muscular dystrophy

A highly variable group, who may occasionally be as severely affected as those with Duchenne muscular dystrophy or more or less mildly than those with Becker muscular dystrophy. Up to 10% may be at risk of cardiac complications of their carrier status.

Dystrophin-associated cardiomyopathy

There are symptoms and signs of hypertrophy progressing to dilated cardiomyopathy in the absence of major muscle symptoms. Some patients have an elevated serum creatine kinase.

Establishing the diagnosis

The clinical presentation of Duchenne muscular dystrophy (DMD) is very characteristic. Hypertrophy of the calf muscles is almost universal (Fig. 24.24.2.3a), sometimes accompanied by muscle hypertrophy elsewhere, most frequently involving deltoid, parts of the quadriceps, the tongue, and masseters. Wasting of the pectoral and scapular muscles leads to hypotonia around the shoulders, detected as the child 'slipping through the hands' on being lifted. In the lower limbs, quadriceps power is weaker than that of the hamstrings. Formal examination of a small child may be difficult, and the main clinical tool is observation of walking, attempting to run, jump, and climb stairs, and to rise from the floor. It is imperative to give the child space to attempt to run, as this will bring out the lack of spring in the step and the lack of fluidity of the attempted running.

Becker muscular dystrophy (BMD) has been described as a 'slow motion version of Duchenne muscular dystrophy', in that the pattern of muscle involvement in these two allelic disorders is essentially identical (Fig. 24.24.2.3c), but progresses at a much slower rate in BMD. Patients with BMD may be quite strong on formal muscle examination, but tend to show subtle signs of proximal muscle weakness on climbing stairs or running. They frequently have hypertrophy involving the same muscle groups as seen in DMD. Some patients have pes cavus.

Serum creatine kinase is always massively elevated, even to more than 200 times normal, but levels of serum creatine kinase do not distinguish the severity of the disease. Muscle biopsy and electromyography are nonspecifically but generally severely dystrophic. The muscle biopsy in BMD may also show some grouped fibre atrophy reminiscent of a 'neurogenic' pathology. Molecular confirmation of the diagnosis is essential to assist in defining prognosis and to provide appropriate genetic counselling. Genetic analysis readily confirms the diagnosis in the 60 to 80% of patients in whom a deletion of the dystrophin gene is present. Current standards of diagnosis include the need to establish precisely the endpoint of any deletion, and also to allow screening for duplications of the dystrophin gene. This is achievable through techniques such as multiple ligation probe amplification (MLPA). For patients in

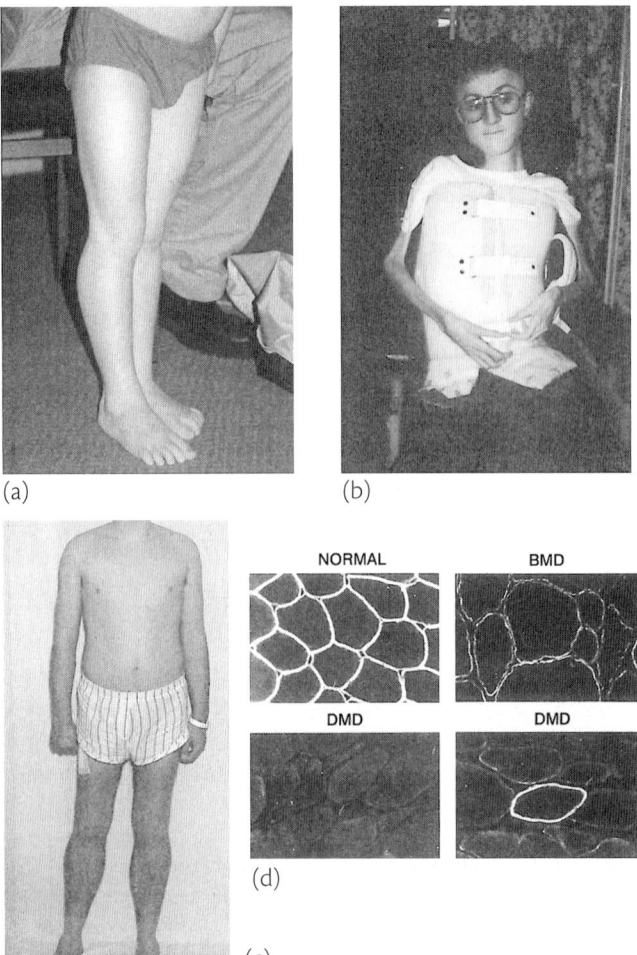

Fig. 24.24.2.3 (a) Child with Duchenne muscular dystrophy at presentation, showing the marked calf and quadriceps hypertrophy and tendency to rise onto the toes. (b) Teenage boy in the later stages of the disease, showing the complications of marked immobility, scoliosis, and muscle wasting. This young man has now been maintained on home nocturnal ventilation successfully for more than 7 years. (c) Clinical pattern at presentation in a young man with Becker muscular dystrophy. Note hypertrophic muscles in calves and quadriceps and mild wasting around the shoulder girdle. (d) Immunocytochemical analysis of dystrophin in normal muscle, Becker muscular dystrophy muscle, and Duchenne muscular dystrophy muscle. In normal muscle, dystrophin labels evenly around the periphery of the muscle fibres. This labelling is typically patchy and reduced in Becker muscular dystrophy, and is either completely or almost completely absent in Duchenne muscular dystrophy.

whom deletion and duplication analysis are negative, testing for point mutations via direct sequencing is mandatory, although, before proceeding to this still costly analysis, it is useful to consider a muscle biopsy by which, in all patients, the diagnosis can be established by not finding or finding reduced dystrophin in the muscle biopsy (Fig. 24.24.2.3d). This analysis also allows the distinction of dystrophinopathy from the much rarer (in most populations) limb–girdle types of muscular dystrophy. Precision of the exact mutation is important for offering carrier testing to the mother and other family members (important to establish the risk of any cardiac problems as well as to allow genetic advice for future pregnancies) and also to allow future access to the mutation-specific treatments that are currently under development, such as antisense oligonucleotide-mediated exon skipping and stop codon suppression.

Prognosis

Within the 'dystrophinopathy' group the prognosis is highly variable. By definition, untreated patients with DMD lose the ability to walk by the age of 12. The development of scoliosis, respiratory failure, and cardiomyopathy (Box 24.24.2.5) during the teenage years can all be managed so that survival into or beyond the late 20s and 30s is becoming more common. Patients with BMD are ambulant beyond 16 years of age, and may remain able to walk independently into their fifth decade or later. These patients are susceptible to cardiac failure at any age from the teens onward and should be monitored for this complication on a regular basis (Box 24.24.2.5). Respiratory failure is a late complication in BMD and correlates with very late-stage disease. The lifespan in BMD may be normal, or reduced in more severe disease. An 'intermediate' group is also recognized, patients losing ambulation between age 12 and 16: their overall prognosis is also intermediate between DMD and BMD. Around 8% of carriers of DMD or BMD may develop some signs of the disease: rarely this is in a full-blown form comparable to the disease in boys. In practice, there is a continuum of severity with the highest incidence in the DMD group (birth incidence 1 in 3500 male live births). As the lifespan is so much longer in the BMD group, however, the prevalence of the two conditions is roughly similar (about 24 per million population in north-east England).

Over the whole group, there is a correlation between dystrophin abundance (as measured in a muscle biopsy sample) and severity: children with completely absent dystrophin tend to be confined to a wheelchair slightly earlier than children whose biopsies contain low levels of dystrophin. Patients with BMD have much higher levels of dystrophin (see Fig. 24.24.2.3). These dystrophin levels also correlate in most cases with the type of mutation found in the dystrophin gene—in DMD most deletions are out of frame, not supporting the production of dystrophin, whereas BMD patients typically have in-frame deletions, allowing the production of a reduced amount of dystrophin of a slightly smaller size.

Although these correlations are useful in a general sense, they are not absolutely predictive of outcome in an individual case, and must always be taken in the context of the clinical features of the patient. They can be useful, however, in giving the best possible guide to prognosis, especially in those patients who present early with no clinical clues as to the severity of the disease, or who are

---

Box 24.24.2.5 Practice point: cardiac involvement in dystrophinopathy

- All patients with dystrophinopathy are at risk of developing cardiomyopathy which progresses with age. It is frequently asymptomatic, and needs to be sought through full cardiac assessment including echocardiography, as treatment with antifailure medication may improve function and prognosis.

- Cardiac transplantation has been used successfully in patients with Becker muscular dystrophy and manifesting carriers of dystrophinopathy.

- Cardiac compromise is the major determinant of operative risk in boys with Duchenne muscular dystrophy, and all should have a full cardiac assessment in advance of any surgery at any age.

identified by neonatal screening or the incidental finding of a high serum creatine kinase level.

Management

DMD is essentially a predictable disease with complications that need to be proactively sought and managed in different systems. Although, in the past, a nihilistic attitude to management in DMD was widespread, evidence of the benefits of proactive management is now available and all patients should have access to the highest possible care. The key to proper management is a team specializing in neuromuscular management who can oversee the coordination of input from physiotherapy, orthopaedic, cardiac, and respiratory specialists. Input from other specialties, including occupational therapy, educational psychology, and gastrointestinal medicine, may also be required.

Duchenne muscular dystrophy: the early stages

Proper management of a child with DMD starts with awareness of the possibility of the diagnosis in any boy who is not walking by the age of 18 months or whose mobility is poor compared with that of his peers. The current mean age at diagnosis of almost 5 years reflects a typical but unacceptable delay of at least 2 years since the onset of disease was noticed by the parents. The principal impetus to early diagnosis is currently the ability to offer parents the option of prenatal diagnosis in subsequent pregnancies. When specific treatments become available, there is likely also to be a need to implement such treatments before the disease is too advanced.

Once the diagnosis has been considered, measurement of the serum creatine kinase will confirm the suspicion and ideally a referral to a specialist unit should be made at this stage. The specialist unit should have rapid-track access to DNA diagnostic and muscle biopsy facilities to confirm the diagnosis as quickly as possible. DMD is a devastating diagnosis, and should be given to the family following guidelines for the best practice for disclosure of bad news: the parents should be seen together wherever possible in complete privacy, they should have time to sit and ask questions, and have access to experienced staff for support and further information. Access to support groups and the relevant national charity is appropriate. Supporting information should also be passed immediately to the GP, health visitor, and school who may never have looked after a child with this type of condition before.

As DMD is an X-linked condition, early access to genetic counselling is also vital shortly after diagnosis (Box 24.24.2.6).

In the early stages of the disease it is advisable for the child to be introduced to a community physiotherapist for advice on stretching, which at this stage usually concentrates on the ankles and hips, with emphasis on the maintenance of symmetry. Boys frequently develop a toe-walking gait which partially compensates for their proximal muscle weakness—walking splints or ankle–foot orthoses are therefore not appropriate at this stage and any early Achilles tendon contractures are better managed through passive stretching and night-time below-knee splints. At the point at which walking becomes impossible independently, the child can often be rehabilitated in long leg callipers or knee–ankle–foot orthoses. Lengthening of the Achilles tendon is often necessary to allow the child to do well with knee–ankle–foot orthoses. The length of time that children walk in knee–ankle–foot orthoses varies from child to child—residual muscle strength is probably the best predictor of

Box 24.24.2.6 Genetic counselling in dystrophinopathy is an essential part of the management of any family where a diagnosis of dystrophinopathy has been made because the potential implications go far beyond the index case

- These are X-linked diseases.
- The new mutation rate in the dystrophin gene is high.
- Most cases of Duchenne muscular dystrophy are born now in families with no prior history of the disease.
- None the less, even in these families, other female relatives (through the maternal line) are at risk of being carriers.
- The essential piece of information is the delineation of the dystrophin mutation in the affected child (easy to find in the 60 per cent in whom the mutation is a deletion, harder and much more specialized if it is not).
- In the presence of a known mutation, female relatives can be offered testing directly to see if they are carriers or not.
- They may choose to have prenatal diagnosis on the basis of that testing.
- Even if mothers of boys with Duchenne muscular dystrophy can be shown not to be somatic carriers of the mutation in their son, they still may have a proportion of egg cells containing the mutation (a situation known as 'germline mosaicism'). They therefore remain at a 10 to 20 per cent risk of having another affected child in a future pregnancy.
- Boys with Duchenne muscular dystrophy do not often have children, but men with Becker muscular dystrophy often do (overall fitness reduced to around 2/3). All of their daughters are obligate carriers of Becker muscular dystrophy, but none of their sons are at risk.

how long a child will use them for mobility, but motivation on the part of the child's family and school is also a key factor.

Over the past 5 years, an increasing consensus has been developing that use of corticosteroids (prednisolone at a dose of 0.75 mg/kg per day or deflazacort at a dose of 0.9 mg/kg per day, and alternative dose-limiting regimens, have also been suggested but not tested to date against the daily regimens) is the gold standard for the preservation of strength in ambulant boys with DMD. Controlled trials show a clear benefit for strength and respiratory function for up to 18 months, and uncontrolled long-term cohort studies report a significant delay in loss of ambulation, a reduction in the development of scoliosis, and a protective effect on respiratory and possibly also cardiac function. It is likely that earlier introduction of corticosteroids (at the time when the child's motor function is plateauing, before a significant loss of function) leads to a better benefit. Close monitoring for the side effects of corticosteroids is of course indicated to minimize the potentially harmful effects of the treatment. In DMD the most commonly reported side effects are weight gain (which can be addressed with careful attention to diet), reduction in height, and behavioural side effects, which may respond to a change in timing of dosage to evening instead of morning, as well as to standard psychological means to improve behaviour management. A further concern is the development of significant osteoporosis, which is a risk in any case in boys with

DMD but which may be exacerbated, particularly in the lumbar spine, by steroid usage. Current guidelines do not recommend the prophylactic use of bisphosphonates in this patient group, but intravenous bisphosphonate treatment is certainly indicated if there is a problem with symptomatic fracture, and this need not be an indication for discontinuation of steroid treatment.

Duchenne muscular dystrophy: after mobility is lost

Inevitably there comes a point in DMD where even the ability to stand supported in knee–ankle–foot orthoses is lost and the child is confined permanently to a wheelchair. The prompt provision of an electric chair with indoor and outdoor access is critical to the best possible maintenance of independence. Seating in the chair should also be carefully addressed to promote an upright and symmetrical posture. Scoliosis is seen in around 90% of patients with DMD who have not been treated with steroids, and spinal surgery in an experienced setting is a good way to restore posture and comfort, and has an additive effect on survival. The long-term cohort studies of patients treated with corticosteroids suggest that scoliosis is seen at a much lower frequency in this group. Physiotherapy priorities for all boys shift towards postural support, the prevention and containment of contractures, and respiratory maintenance. Measurements of forced vital capacity (FVC) carried out regularly provide an indication of the trend of respiratory function—FVC usually plateaus soon after confinement to a wheelchair and thereafter falls. There is some preliminary evidence that corticosteroids may be of use at this phase of the disease, as well, in improving and maintaining FVC. The timing of surgery for scoliosis therefore needs to take this variable into account, although cardiomyopathy is probably an even greater risk factor in the timing of surgery (see Box 24.24.2.5).

As FVC falls further, boys are at serious risk of chest infections and ultimately nocturnal respiratory failure. Respiratory care should begin early with prompt access to antibiotics at the first sign of any infection, support for and augmentation of coughing, and access to immunizations. Patients are at risk of hypercapnia, and oxygen should not be administered without proper monitoring of blood gases and a low threshold for initiating respiratory support. Symptoms of respiratory failure may be extremely insidious and totally missed unless explicitly sought (Box 24.24.2.7). Routine overnight pulse oximetry (which can readily be carried out at home provided that the equipment is available) can show a trend of deteriorating overnight oxygenation and, together with the monitoring of symptoms, highlight the time at which elective nocturnal respiratory support, ideally at least through noninvasive means initially, should be provided. Such respiratory support abolishes symptoms, reduces the tendency to chest infections, and undoubtedly improves lifespan with a good quality of life.

In the late stages of DMD, nutrition may be of concern. Loss of weight occurs in most boys as the disease progresses, and issues of diet and the possibility of supplemental nutrition (possibly by gastrostomy) need to be addressed.

The actual cause and timing of death in DMD is hard to predict. Some patients will die of a particularly severe chest infection. In others cardiomyopathy may be difficult to control or a cardiac arrhythmia may arise. Any medical intervention at the later stages should be carefully managed by an experienced team. Early onset of cardiomyopathy is a poor prognostic sign. Talking about death to these patients and their parents, helping them to prepare and

---

Box 24.24.2.7 Respiratory failure in neuromuscular disease is a complication which needs to be specifically sought

- It may be the result of intercostal muscle or diaphragmatic weakness or a combination of the two. The presence of a scoliosis or other spinal deformity may be an additional factor.

- Nocturnal problems tend to dominate.

- Frank symptoms of morning CO_2 retention may be seen (poor colour, morning sickness, headaches, confusion) but these are late symptoms and the problem should be detected by investigation or careful history taking before this stage.

- Increasing frequency of chest infections may indicate incipient respiratory failure.

- Subtle signs include loss of appetite and weight loss, loss of energy and enthusiasm.

- Poor sleep, increasing wakefulness at night, inability to lie flat may also be seen together with a tendency to fall asleep during the day.

- Difficulties swallowing and difficulty completing sentences may also be seen.

- In many muscle diseases, the main risk of respiratory failure is when the patient is no longer able to walk independently and weakness is pronounced (for example Duchenne muscular dystrophy, Becker muscular dystrophy, congenital muscular dystrophy, facioscapulohumeral muscular dystrophy, limb girdle muscular dystrophy, etc.).

- In other muscle diseases, respiratory failure may be an earlier feature and present while the patient is still ambulant (for example multicore and other congenital myopathies, some forms of congenital muscular dystrophy)

---

also addressing their fears and uncertainties, is another important but easily neglected aspect of management.

Education

On average, children with DMD have an IQ around 1 standard deviation below the normal mean; often a striking verbal performance deficit is observed and there is a deficit in number span. Learning problems are not progressive. Additional behavioural phenotypes may complicate the pattern of learning needs, including a tendency to behaviour in the autistic spectrum in some children. Schooling should offer the best possible environment for learning, taking into account the profile of needs of the individual child, and including full attention to information technology equipment, while supporting the very real physical needs of the child. Families and areas vary as to whether this will be best provided through mainstream or special schooling. With a good education and medical support, boys with DMD and the appropriate intellectual potential can go on to higher education, and should be encouraged to do so.

Becker muscular dystrophy

Management issues in BMD tend to cover the same broad areas as DMD, but with the deterioration in muscle function over a much longer timescale. Certain complications, such as scoliosis, are very unusual. Other complications, such as cramping muscle pains after exercise, which can be a particular problem in the teenage years, are more common. Despite the fact that BMD is much milder than DMD, it can represent a considerable and insurmountable disability for the person who has it, and problems with adjustment, poor self-esteem, and poor body image are all fairly common in this group. There are no hard data to define completely any intellectual problems in BMD, but on average it is likely that this group has a general reduction in IQ, although probably not to the extent seen in DMD. Cardiac complications may occur at any age in BMD and require proactive surveillance and management (see Box 24.24.2.5): respiratory complications tend to be a feature of the late stages of the disease.

Fascioscapulohumeral muscular dystrophy

Fascioscapulohumeral muscular dystrophy is an example of a muscular dystrophy named for the most characteristic pattern of muscle involvement observed (that of involvement of the facial, scapular, and humeral muscles predominantly). However, other muscle groups usually become involved with time and may even be involved at onset.

Presentation

◆ Age at presentation is variable. Most affected individuals manifest some symptoms by their teens or twenties. Occasionally symptoms may be very minor, even late in adult life.

◆ Symptoms may, unusually for a muscular dystrophy, be very markedly asymmetrical.

Early symptoms typically include facial weakness (inability to bury eyelashes or puff cheeks; this often goes unnoticed), shoulder–girdle weakness manifesting as problems in reaching high shelves, changing light bulbs, or climbing ropes, and foot-drop.

An infantile form of fascioscapulohumeral muscular dystrophy is recognized with early childhood onset, extremely marked facial weakness, and progressive weakness of both the shoulder and pelvic girdle musculature. Lumbar lordosis may be profound. Hearing loss and retinal telangiectasia may be seen in any patient with fascioscapulohumeral muscular dystrophy but are particularly associated with this most severe form of the disease.

Differential diagnosis

The clinical pattern of fascioscapulohumeral muscular dystrophy can be very distinctive, and the asymmetry of muscle involvement is a major clue. However, facial weakness may be very variable and, if it is absent or subtle, confusion can arise with forms of limb–girdle muscular dystrophy.

Diagnostic investigations

Serum creatine kinase may be normal or mildly elevated. Muscle biopsy and electromyography (EMG) provide supportive evidence for a muscular dystrophy; some inflammatory features are sometimes also seen in the biopsy. Most cases (if not all) of fascioscapulohumeral muscular dystrophy are linked to chromosome 4q35. Although the nature of the gene responsible for fascioscapulohumeral muscular dystrophy is not yet known, a DNA-based test is available that can confirm the diagnosis in 95% of cases. This test involves the demonstration of a DNA deletion that is consistently associated with the disease. It is likely that this deletion alters the expression of a gene or genes close to the telomere of chromosome 4q (position effect variegation).

Prognosis and management

Infantile fascioscapulohumeral muscular dystrophy is a progressive disease that leads to early confinement to a wheelchair and the development of such complications as scoliosis and respiratory failure. This condition is most frequently seen as a result of a new dominant mutation in cases with no family history, and these children often have particularly large DNA deletions on chromosome 4. The development of a lumbar lordosis, seen also in later-onset fascioscapulohumeral muscular dystrophy, together with secondary hip flexion contractures, can be very disabling. Bracing may be partially successful at controlling the lordosis, but at the expense of some loss of mobility.

More typically, fascioscapulohumeral muscular dystrophy is a slowly progressive disease. As the disease progresses it can involve the proximal as well as the distal lower limb muscles. Around 20% of patients with fascioscapulohumeral muscular dystrophy will become unable to walk independently, most when aged over 40. Involvement of the proximal lower limbs before the age of 20 years is a poor prognostic sign, indicating an increased likelihood of wheelchair use. Some patients describe progression as being stepwise in nature, with periods of faster deterioration alternating with phases of plateauing of their symptoms. Foot-drop is a common complaint, which can be helped by the provision of daytime ankle–foot orthoses. A significant proportion of patients with fascioscapulohumeral muscular dystrophy complain of painful muscles, for which no cause can be found and for which pain relief may be difficult. Some patients find swimming or a small dose of antidepressants useful for this symptom. More severely affected patients with fascioscapulohumeral muscular dystrophy may develop respiratory failure or swallowing problems, and these complications should be sought. Cardiomyopathy is rarely reported.

Genetic counselling

Fascioscapulohumeral muscular dystrophy is an autosomal dominant disease and as such an affected person has a 50% chance of transmission to his or her offspring, regardless of sex. Use of the new DNA diagnostic techniques has shown that up to 30% of cases of fascioscapulohumeral muscular dystrophy may represent new dominant mutations. Germline mosaicism is also common. Genetic analysis has also shown a higher proportion of asymptomatic gene carriers than expected, with females overrepresented in this group. The availability of a relatively straightforward genetic test in this disorder has opened up the possibility of presymptomatic and prenatal testing, which were previously impossible. However, despite an overall correlation between the size of the deletion found and the severity of the symptoms, the DNA test is not useful in predicting the severity of the disease—people in individual families with apparently the same sized deletion may have a very variable experience of the disease (Fig. 24.24.2.4).

Emery–Dreifuss muscular dystrophy (OMIM 300384)

Classic Emery–Dreifuss muscular dystrophy (EDMD) has a highly characteristic phenotype. X-linked recessive, autosomal dominant, and (very rare) autosomal recessive forms are recognized, and the

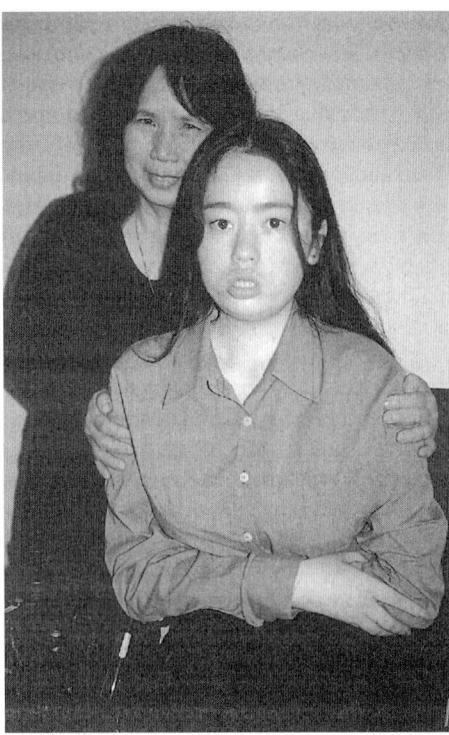

Fig. 24.24.2.4 Mother and daughter with fascioscapulohumeral muscular dystrophy. The mother is extremely mildly affected and has minimal symptoms. By contrast the daughter was affected from early childhood and has been wheelchair dependent outside from her early teens. Note the daughter's expressionless face and her posture—she is leaning forward due to a combination of her marked lumbar lordosis, a major feature of the condition, and hip flexion contractures.

genes involved in these conditions encode proteins that are components of the nuclear envelope (Fig. 24.24.2.5). The gene involved in X-linked EDMD is emerin (*EMD*), and that involved in autosomal dominant and autosomal recessive EDMD is lamin A/C (*LMNA/LMNC*). Other genes have also been implicated in patients with an emery-dreifuss phenotype including nesprin and FHL1.

Presentation

- ◆ Patients may present at any age, most typically in the early teens, although symptoms may be present much earlier than that.

- ◆ Contractures of the ankles and elbows and rigidity of the spine often predate any clear weakness.

- ◆ Consequently, these patients have frequently had Achilles tendon release before the diagnosis is suspected.

- ◆ Weakness and wasting are typically humeroperoneal in distribution.

A key part of these conditions, which may rarely be seen at presentation, is cardiac involvement, most typically arrhythmias (see below). Several alternative phenotypes (A form of congenital muscular dystrophy limb–girdle muscular dystrophy 1B and a pure cardiac disease—Box 24.24.2.8 and see Fig. 24.24.2.5) exist in combination with mutations in the same gene as autosomal dominant EDMD (lamin A/C). Lamin A/C mutations are also described in several diseases where there is no predominant muscle phenotype, including partial lipodystrophy, some forms of progeria syndromes, mandibuloacral dysplasia, and a form of peripheral neuropathy.

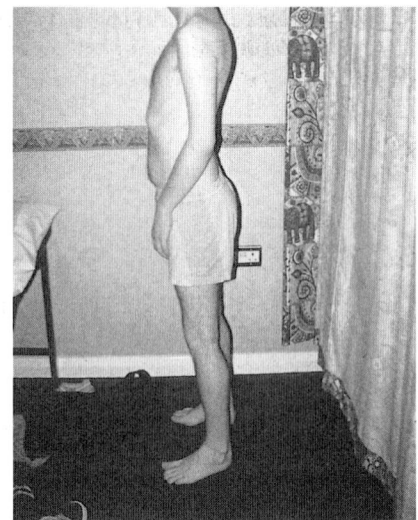

(a)

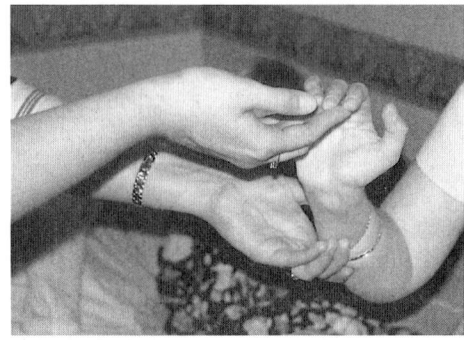

(b)

Fig. 24.24.2.5 Muscular dystrophy phenotypes characterized by prominent contractures. (a) This patient has autosomal dominant Emery-Dreifuss muscular dystrophy, with a proven mutation in his lamin A/C gene. The elbow and Achilles tendon contractures seen here, combined with his markedly rigid spine, are very similar to the pattern of contractures and weakness seen in the X-linked form of the disease. (b) Bethlem myopathy in a woman with marked contractures of the elbows, ankles, and spine. In addition she has finger flexion contractures, demonstrated here by attempting to straighten the fingers with the wrist extended.

Some patients may show overlapping features of these different syndromes. Laminopathy is much more phenotypically diverse than X-linked EDMD and a high index of suspicion of this disorder is necessary, especially due to the almost inevitable life-threatening cardiac complications.

Confirming the diagnosis

Serum creatine kinase is typically mildly elevated in EDMD. Muscle biopsy shows nonspecific histological features: in X-linked EDMD, emerin is absent in muscle and skin. Detection of mutation in the emerin gene is necessary to offer genetic counselling to female relatives at risk of being carriers.

The involvement of lamin A/C (the gene responsible for autosomal dominant EDMD) cannot be determined by antibody analysis in muscle, but requires the demonstration of a lamin A/C mutation. A secondary deficiency of laminin β-1 may be seen in muscle from some patients with autosomal dominant EDMD, but is not specific to this condition. Many lamin A/C mutations arise anew, and germline mosaicism is common. Use of specific genetic testing has shown that, in fact, in contradistinction to what had

- Forms of congenital muscular dystrophy, Emery-dreifuss muscular dystrophy and limb-girdle muscular dystrophy are all caused my mutations in lamin A/C, a component of the nuclear envelope.

- The phenotype is variable, depending on age at onset and the presence or not of contractures as a major component of the phenotype.

- Where contractures are present, these typically involve the elbows, Achilles tendons, and spine. In these patients, there is often a humeroperoneal pattern of muscle weakness as in X-linked Emery Dreifuss muscular dystrophy.

- Where contractures are less of a feature, patients typically present with proximal muscle weakness.

- In all groups, cardiac involvement is the most important complication. Arrythmias may lead to sudden death and should be sought and treated appropriately.

- A phenotype with exclusively cardiac involvement has also been described.

- New mutations and germline mosaicism is common in this group.

been previously reported, autosomal dominant EDMD is more frequent than the classically described X-linked form.

Differential diagnosis

Other muscular dystrophies may present with contractures as an important component (see Fig. 24.24.2.5). Some forms of CMD may be associated with contractures and a rigid spine. Bethlem myopathy may present congenitally (often with torticollis) or in early childhood: here finger flexion contractures, elicited especially on wrist extension, are more prominent and cardiac involvement is not associated. Bethlem myopathy is itself genetically heterogeneous, involving mutations in any of the genes for collagen VI-α1, -α2, and -α3. The condition is allelic to the much more severe CMD, UCMD. Unlike in UCMD, where examination of skin and muscle frequently shows an abnormality of collagen VI expression, in Bethlem myopathy collagen VI labelling in muscle may be normal. Immunoanalysis of cultured fibroblasts may be a useful diagnostic tool before proceeding to mutation analysis, which is time-consuming due to the large size of the three genes to be screened and the presence of many polymorphisms. Similar to autosomal dominant EDMD, some cases of Bethlem myopathy show a secondary reduction in laminin β_1 staining in muscle biopsy: the significance of this is uncertain. Patients with Bethlem myopathy may show skin abnormalities such as follicular hyperkeratosis and abnormal scarring.

In some cases, calpainopathy (limb–girdle muscular dystrophy 2A) may be associated with contractures of the ankles, elbows, fingers, and paraspinal muscles. However, the associated weakness here is predominantly proximal and of a characteristic distribution (see below). These patients typically have a higher creatine kinase, absent calpain 3 on biopsy, and *CAPN3* mutations.

Prognosis and management

The prognosis in EDMD relates almost directly to the ability to manage the life-threatening arrhythmias to which every patient with either the X-linked or dominant form is susceptible. Severe arrhythmias are inevitable by the third decade. All patients with this diagnosis should therefore be under regular cardiological review, and once a rhythm disturbance has been detected cardiac pacing may be life saving. However, in autosomal dominant EDMD evidence suggests that the risk of ventricular arrhythmias necessitates the use of an implantable defibrillator. In this condition there is also a risk of cardiomyopathy, which may be less amenable to routine treatment.

Management of the contractures in EDMD is the other main issue, and will involve close liaison with a physiotherapist. Operative treatment of contractures, especially at the Achilles tendons, is commonly performed, but, although such surgery does work in the short term, contractures often recur. With increasing age, however, contractures frequently stabilize. Muscle weakness may worsen but progression is usually very slow. Rigidity of the spine may complicate weakness of the respiratory muscles and nocturnal respiratory support may be needed. Monitoring should include regular assessment of FVC when sitting and lying, and symptom enquiry for any symptoms of respiratory impairment.

The limb–girdle muscular dystrophies

The broad definition of the term 'limb–girdle muscular dystrophy' comes from the classification of Walton and Nattrass in 1954, when the term was suggested to describe those patients with weakness of the proximal musculature who did not fulfil the criteria for either the X-linked muscular dystrophies or fascioscapulohumeral muscular dystrophy. The term has always encompassed a heterogeneous group of disorders: now that many of them can be distinguished at the gene or protein level it is no longer sufficient to use it without qualification as to the specific type of disease (Table 24.24.2.2). The type of limb–girdle muscular dystrophy may be suggested by the precise pattern of muscle involvement, with confirmation from a combination of genetic and protein analysis. The ability to provide a precise diagnosis in limb–girdle muscular dystrophy has greatly improved the prognostic and genetic information that can be given to these patients.

The approach to diagnosis in limb–girdle muscular dystrophy

Could it be dominant disease?

Autosomal dominant limb–girdle muscular dystrophy (LGMD) represents only around 10% of the total LGMD population, and LGMD1A, -1C, -1D, and -1E have been very rarely reported. In families with a dominant history the most likely diagnoses are fascioscapulohumeral muscular dystrophy (exclude fascioscapulohumeral muscular dystrophy on DNA analysis especially if there is any suspicion of facial weakness), LGMD1B (allelic with autosomal dominant EDMD—see Box 24.24.2.8), and Bethlem myopathy. New mutations are common, however, so, if the clinical features are suggestive of one of these disorders, the diagnosis should be pursued even in the absence of a family history.

Features that should raise the suspicion of dominant disease are less marked elevation of creatine kinase (typically normal to five times normal in dominant disease and much higher than this in active recessive disease), or the presence of early and prominent contractures.

Table 24.24.2.2 Recessive types of limb-girdle muscular dystrophy

	Type of muscular dystrophy (gene symbol)			
	Calpainopathy (LGMD 2A) (CAPN3)	Dysferlinopathy (LGMD 2B/MM) (DYSF)	Sarcoglycanopathies (LGMD 2C–2F) (SGCA, SGCB, SGCC, SGCD)	LGMD 2I
Distribution	Worldwide, some isolates (e.g. Reunion, Amish, Basque)	Worldwide. Founder effect in Libyan Jewish population. ?Others	Worldwide. Regional differences in different types	Worldwide
Status of diagnosis	Protein, mutations	Protein, mutations	Protein, mutations (may not be readily found in all patients)	Mutations in FKRP
Protein	Calpain 3 deficiency detectable by monoclonal antibody on blots	Dysferlin deficiency detectable on sections and blots	◆ Dystrophin may be mildly abnormal ◆ γ and α may see selective reduction ◆ β and δ mostly see depletion of all	Secondary reduction in laminin A2 or laminin β1 in some muscle biopsies
Mutations	Widely distributed, few recurrent. All types of mutation seen, large deletions rare. Changes may be non-pathogenic. Except in homozygotes, difficult to correlate mutation type with rate of progression	Widely distributed, few so far recurrent	◆ α R77C seen in 42% of chromosomes ◆ γ two predominant mutations, N. African and gypsy. Otherwise mutations very heterogeneous ◆ Missense mutations mainly in extracellular domain	Common mutation (C826A) responsible for many cases
Age at onset	Typically 8–15, may be from early childhood or adulthood	Most present around 20 (± 5 years). Onset not in first decade	α most variable—may be from childhood to adulthood. γ, β, δ tend to be more severe. Majority of all types will present in first decade	Congenital form may be very severe: ranges to very mild disease in LGMD group
Mode of presentation and selective muscle involvement	Highly selective pattern of muscle involvement wasting post. compartment of thighs, scapular winging. Sparing of hip abductors. Relative involvement of muscle groups important	Variable. May be: ◆ lower limbs first ◆ proximal alone, mixed proximal/distal alone ◆ distal presentation most commonly posterior, may be anterior	Weakness, toe walking, muscle pains/cramps are typical presentations. Main muscles—shoulder girdle involvement more prominent than DMD, scapular involvement, hamstrings more than quadriceps, lordosis, foot drop in some before loss of mobility	Proximal muscle weakness
Early development	Motor milestones normal; physical prowess in childhood may be less good than peers	Normal—good athletic prowess	Motor milestones less delayed than DMD, even if later very severe	Normal in LGMD cases
Rate of progression	May not be linear—can see rapid change with no gender effect. Otherwise gradual with time. Age at death probably typically in 60s	Usually slow—some more rapidly progressive Cases have similar age at onset	Variability main feature: ◆ poor correlation between age at onset/progression ◆ rate of progression very variable ◆ may be great intrafamilial variation, even with sibs	Variable, usually mild
Age of confinement to wheelchair	20–30+	Typically beyond 30s. Seems to be normal lifespan	Earliest 9 years. Variability in mild cases very marked. Occasional asymptomatic cases in adult life (esp. α). Typically even most severe cases live to 30s	In mild cases 40+
Atrophy	Posterior compartment of thighs, latissimus dorsi	Typically distal LL, biceps—may be very selective. Atrophy of proximal deltoid, hypertrophy of distal	Anterior and posterior thighs, shoulder girdle	Proximal
Hypertrophy	Occasionally see calf hypertrophy	Very rare—a few cases have transient calf hypertrophy at presentation which may be painful	Common in calves, also elsewhere. May be macroglossia	Common in calf muscles

Contractures	AT contractures common. Occasionally more widespread	No	AT contractures, lordosis, hip flexion contractures (may be problem in rehab). Scoliosis less common than DMD even when WCB	Not common in LGMD forms
Facial involvement	Mild facial weakness unusual. Also macroglossia very occasionally seen	No facial weakness	No facial weakness, may see macroglossia. In later stages typical transverse smile	Mild facial weakness common
Cardiac status	Normal	Normal	α usually not present (one Dutch patient). β, γ, δ may be important	Cardiomyopathy significant complication
Respiratory status	Respiratory impairment may be significant in some	Normal	Common, may be at later stage than DMD	Some cases require nocturnal ventilation
Intellectual function	Normal	Normal	Normal	Normal
Creatine kinase	10–100× normal	May be low or mildly raised in young presymptomatic cases, rising to huge elevation by early teens. Very high in active phase of disease, falling with age	10–100× normal	10–100 × normal
Biopsy	Dystrophic	Dystrophic plus inflammation, may be perivascular or more widespread	Dystrophic	Dystrophic
Other	Muscle imaging confirms highly selective pattern of muscle involvement	Muscle imaging may reveal asymptomatic proximal changes in distal onset and vice versa. Phenotypes may vary with same mutation and between sibs	Genotype–phenotype correlations: α-null tend to be more severe; β truncating very severe, huge variation with missense. Majority in γ are truncating mutations. δ mutations so far are rare	Allelic with a form of congenital muscular dystrophy
Note	Finnish anterior tibial MD homozygotes may show reduction of calpain on blots	May have been misdiagnosed as polymyositis or distal myopathy	Main differential diagnosis is with dystrophinopathy. Occasional cases may resemble calpainopathy. No clinical guidelines to distinguish subgroups, though very mild disease most likely to be α	N/K

Abbreviations: LGMD, limb girdle muscular dystrophy; DMD, Duchenne muscular dystrophy; WCB, wheelchair bound; N/K, not known; LL, lower limbs; AT, Achilles tendon.

As knowledge of the disorders within the autosomal dominant LGMD classification has grown, together with a greater understanding of the other phenotypes that have been identified in association with mutations in the same genes, a key feature of these diseases has clearly emerged as variability. So, for example, LGMD1A is due to mutations in myotilin, which is also responsible for a form of myofibrillar myopathy. Patients in this group may have mutations in a range of different genes and the phenotypes may be very variable, including both proximal and distal muscle weakness, and cardiac and respiratory complications. LGMD1B or laminopathy has already been discussed in the section on EDMD—a very high index of suspicion of this diagnosis is definitely required. Caveolin 3 mutations, responsible for LGMD1C, are also now recognized in a form of rippling muscle disease, as well as in patients presenting with myalgia or hypercalcaemia. Therefore, a broad level of knowledge about the possible diagnostic features in these different disorders is necessary when taking the family tree for these patients, as well as is in the individual clinical assessments required—rippling, for example, may be seen only if specifically elicited.

What is the age and nature of the presentation?

Variability in the age of presentation and the rate of progression is usual in the various autosomal recessive types of LGMD. However, some broad conclusions can be helpful (Fig. 24.24.2.6). Childhood presentation is most common in sarcoglycanopathy, which may superficially resemble dystrophinopathy, with frequent calf (and other muscle) hypertrophy. Adult-onset cases are less frequent and are essentially 'Becker like' in presentation. However, whatever the age at presentation, in sarcoglycanopathy, quadriceps is almost always stronger than the hamstrings. This is the reverse of the pattern seen in dystrophin deficiency. Another important differential diagnosis in a 'Becker-like' (including the presence of calf hypertrophy and cardiomyopathy) presentation is LGMD2I, which is the most common form of LGMD in northern Europe. Calpainopathy may present with early childhood symptoms, especially contractures of the Achilles tendons, but onset is most commonly between 8 and 15 years of age. Dysferlinopathy typically presents in the late teens or early twenties, and early features may include proximal weakness or distal involvement (usually manifesting as difficulty standing on tiptoe).

Which investigations should be performed?

Serum creatine kinase is greatly elevated in all forms of autosomal recessive LGMD, but may be only marginally elevated or within the normal range in autosomal dominant LGMD. EMG confirms a primary myopathic process and standard analysis of the muscle biopsy shows dystrophic changes (which, especially in dysferlinopathy, can be accompanied by evidence of inflammation). Specialized investigations are always necessary to attempt to determine the type of LGMD, and require a muscle biopsy as the starting point for immunologically based diagnosis (Fig. 24.24.2.7), together with the clinical features.

Scheme for specialized investigations

Do the clinical features or family history suggest a specific disorder (Boxes 24.24.2.9–24.24.2.11)? If so look for that first.

The sarcoglycanopathies

Dystrophin staining may be mildly abnormal in these patients, reflecting the close and interdependent relationship between the

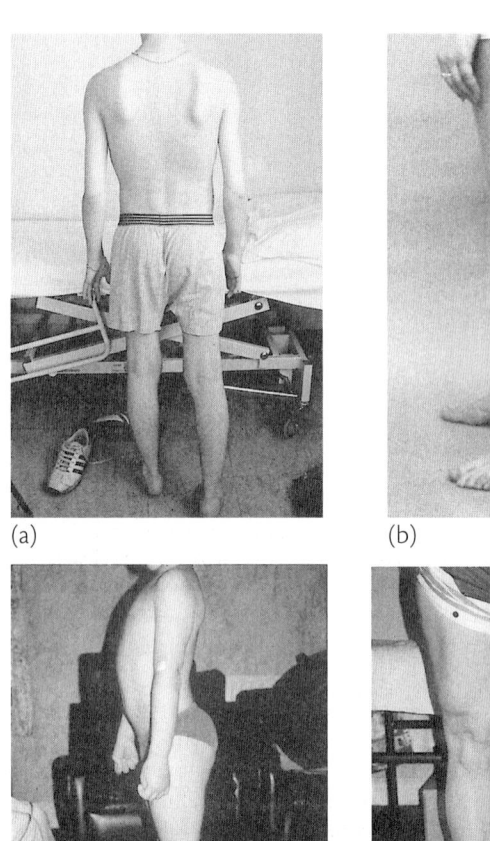
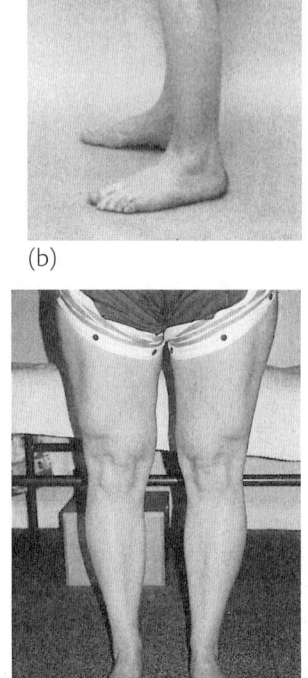

Fig. 24.24.2.6 Typical clinical pictures of patients with different types of autosomal recessive limb–girdle muscular dystrophy (LGMD). (a) Calpainopathy or LGMD2A. Note the predominantly atrophic pattern of muscle involvement and Achilles tendon contractures. The stance is often wide based due to the imbalance of the hip abductors and adductors and tight Achilles tendon. (b) Dysferlin deficiency or LGMD2B. Note the wasting of the posterior calf muscles and flat-footed stance. (c) Child with γ-sarcoglycanopathy or LGMD2C. Note the lordotic posture and scapular winging, both of which may be more marked at presentation in sarcoglycanopathy than in dystrophin deficiency. (d) Adult with γ-sarcoglycanopathy, to illustrate the variability in severity of sarcoglycan deficiencies and the muscular hypertrophy, which may be as marked or more marked than in dystrophin deficiency.

proteins of the dystrophin-associated complex; however, the predominant abnormality on immunolabelling or immunoblotting will be the absence or reduction of one or more of the sarcoglycans. The pattern of reduction of these proteins may give a clue as to the primary gene involvement. Detection of the mutation is necessary to offer prenatal diagnosis and specific genetic counselling.

Calpainopathy

Here the sarcoglycans are normal, as is dystrophin. Currently available antibodies to calpain 3 do not work on tissue sections but need to be used on immunoblotting. Detection of reduced or absent calpain on immunoblotting (see Fig. 24.24.2.7) indicates the need to search for calpain 3 mutations, which are highly variable, are

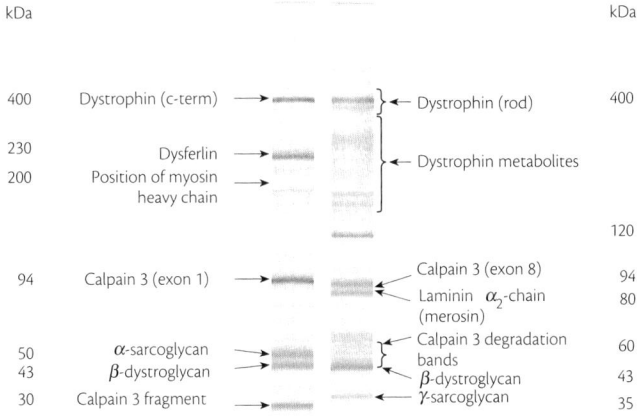

Fig. 24.24.2.7 Multiplex western blotting as an approach to diagnosis in limb–girdle muscular dystrophy. Two strips of a western blot of control human skeletal muscle protein extracts immunostained with a mixture of antibodies to the proteins indicated. Absence or reduced intensity of a particular species, compared with the other proteins labelled in the same lane, can indicate which gene and protein are implicated in that patient's disease. (Courtesy of Dr L V B Anderson, University of Newcastle upon Tyne.)

generally nonrecurrent, and may involve any part of the large (24 exons) gene. Studies consistently report a level of around 20 to 25% of nondetection of the second mutation in calpain 3, suggesting the presence of a significant number of mutations missed by current screening technologies. A secondary reduction in calpain 3 may be seen in some cases of dysferlin deficiency. The situation at the muscle biopsy level is also complicated by the fact that patients with mutations, especially in the autocatalytic domain of calpain 3, show normal protein expression on immunoblotting. A multidisciplinary approach to diagnosis in calpainopathy, including the recognition of often a very characteristic phenotype, together with protein and genetic testing, is still required.

Box 24.24.2.9 Clinical features of sarcoglycanopathies

- Most frequently present in childhood, but may present at any age. Intrafamilial variability is common.
- These conditions are most closely related clinically to dystrophinopathy which will be the major differential diagnosis and have a similar spectrum of severity.
- Typically motor milestones are less delayed than in dystrophinopathy.
- Muscle hypertrophy is common.
- Intelligence is not affected.
- Cardiomyopathy is an important complication, though not universal, and should be sought through careful surveillance.
- Respiratory failure is an important late complication.
- Scoliosis is seen in the most severely affected individuals.
- Prognosis overall is typically better than dystrophinopathy presenting at a similar age.

Box 24.24.2.10 Clinical features of calpainopathy

- This is the most common form of limb girdle muscular dystrophy in most populations.
- May present at any age but typically 8 to 15 years.
- Highly selective muscle involvement: posterior thigh weakness, and wasting; scapular winging common at onset.
- Muscle hypertrophy rare—tends to be predominantly atrophic pattern.
- Preservation of hip abductor muscles even at late stages contributes to characteristic wide-based stance.
- Most have Achilles tendon contractures: a subgroup presents with much more prominent contractures in an Emery Dreifuss muscular dystrophy-like pattern.
- Progression is variable but never as fast as Duchenne muscular dystrophy.
- Cardiac involvement is not common but respiratory impairment may be seen in late stages.
- Prognosis in all but the most severe and early onset cases is good.

Box 24.24.2.11 Dysferlinopathy: clinical features

- Presentation most commonly in late teens or early twenties.
- Patients often report good muscle prowess before onset of disease. Serum creatine kinase may not be massively elevated in presymptomatic cases.
- Occasional patients present with unilateral calf swelling which may be tender and lead to the clinical diagnosis of myositis.
- Primary muscle involvement is always in the lower limbs, with absence of upper girdle involvement at onset.
- Lower limb involvement may be of proximal muscles or distal muscles. The distal muscles involved first are typically posterior (leading to difficulty standing on tiptoe as an early feature) but may be anterior.
- Progression is typically slow and life expectancy is not reduced. This is the usually mildest type of limg girdle muscular dystrophy.
- Cardiomyopathy is not reported and respiratory involvement is usually mild and at a very late stage only.
- This phenotype is genetically heterogeneous, with another locus for Miyoshi myopathy on chromosome 10.
- The main differential diagnosis, especially in patients presenting with distal weakness, may be an alternative form of distal myopathy. Typically here the creatine kinase is not so high.

Dysferlinopathy

Here, all other proteins with the possible exception of calpain 3 are within the normal range, and deficiency of dysferlin can be demonstrated on tissue sections or immunoblotting. Decreased or absent dysferlin in muscle is an indication to proceed to mutation detection. The dysferlin gene is very large (55 exons) and, as with the other forms of LGMD, mutations are highly variable.

LGMD2I and other forms of LGMD with abnormal glycosylation of α dystroglycan

It is increasingly recognized that mutations in the same genes which can cause a congenital muscular dystrophy with abnormal glycosylation of α dystroglycan can also cause a much milder lgmd phenotype. This milder phenotype is actually the more common presentation with mutations in FKRP (LGMD2I) which is a relatively common cause of LGMD in northern Europe where there is a founder mutation. The diagnostic clue in these cases is abnormal α dystroglycan on muscle immunolabelling sometimes associated with a secondary reduction also in laminin A2 especially on immunoblotting.

Other forms of limb–girdle muscular dystrophy

Additional rare forms of LGMD have also been described. LGMD2G is mainly seen in Brazil and is due to mutations in telethonin. LGMD2H is restricted mainly to the Hutterite population of Canada and is due to mutations in TRIM32. Homozygous titin mutations in Finland (where a distal myopathy due to titin mutations is relatively common) cause LGMD2J. LGMD2L is due to mutations in TMEM16 and mutations in this gene also cause a form of Miyoshi myopathy. The existence of families with an LGMD phenotype but no detectable mutations to date suggests that novel muscular dystrophy genes remain to be identified and this process is likely to be accelerated by the application of the rapid sequencing technologies that are currently coming on line.

Management

Once the diagnosis is secure, management should include monitoring and treatment for the specific complications of the various subtypes. Attention needs to be given to the particular prevalence of cardiac or respiratory involvement and appropriate surveillance and treatment initiated. If a clear diagnosis is not possible (e.g. where appropriate samples are not available or where the diagnosis cannot be reached even after exhaustive investigation), the management should, as a minimum, include physiotherapy and regular cardiac and respiratory surveillance.

Oculopharyngeal muscular dystrophy

Oculopharyngeal muscular dystrophy is unusual in that it has an exceptionally late presentation.

Presentation

◆ Presentation is typically in the sixth decade.

◆ It commonly presents with ptosis, dysphagia to solids, and dysphonia, which may be as severe as in myotonic dystrophy.

◆ Other features include ophthalmoparesis, facial weakness, and proximal muscle weakness.

Diagnosis

The muscle biopsy in oculopharyngeal muscular dystrophy typically shows the presence of rimmed vacuoles and intranuclear inclusions. DNA analysis confirms the presence of an expanded guanine–cytosine–guanine repeat in the poly(A)-binding protein 2 gene.

Prognosis and management

Ptosis can be managed surgically, but frequently recurs. Dysphagia may respond, at least partially, to surgical intervention with myotomy of the cricopharyngeal muscle and other annular muscle fibres. Potentially life-threatening complications may include aspiration pneumonia and regurgitation. Progression of the limb muscle weakness is highly variable.

Genetic counselling

Oculopharyngeal muscular dystrophy is an autosomal dominant disorder. Genetic analysis offers the potential for presymptomatic testing if this is specifically sought.

Prospects for specific treatment in muscular dystrophy

Drug treatments have a limited place in the treatment of muscular dystrophy at present, apart from the use of corticosteroids in DMD. Treatments to modify the underlying disease are entering clinical trials. Gene transfer experiments in animal models have proved the general feasibility of this approach to these genetic diseases, at least on a small scale. Modification of mutations, either by drugs or by other means, is an area of research, as is the concept of up-regulating the production of ancillary proteins.

Supportive treatment for patients and their families remains the mainstay of treatment at present, and this is likely to be the case for the current generation of patients at least. This treatment is ideally provided through a specialized multidisciplinary team, bringing together with the 'myologist' the skills of medical and associated colleagues from physiotherapy, occupational therapy, genetics, cardiology, respiratory medicine, and orthopaedics.

Further reading

With the rate of change, over the last few years, in the information available about genetically determined diseases, the most up-to-date reviews of the subject may be found on the internet rather than in traditional textbooks. Chapter 24.17 provides a compelling genetic framework for a molecular classification of inherited dystrophy of muscle.

Bushby K, *et al.* for the DMD Care Considerations Working Group (2009). Diagnosis and management of Duchenne muscular dystrophy, parts 1 and 2. *Lancet Neurol*, Nov 27. [Epub ahead of print] [A comprehensive review of care in Duchenne muscular dystrophy, providing a framework for the multidisciplinary approach to management of muscle diseases in general.]

Engel, A (ed.) (2004). *Myology* 3rd revised edition. MacGraw Hill. [A wide ranging guide to muscle disease.]

Karpati G, Hilton-Jones D, Bushby K, Griggs RH (eds.) (2010). *Disorders of Voluntary Muscle* 8th edition. Cambridge University Press. [Another multi-author book covering wide aspects of the field.]

Websites

National Center for Biotechnology Information (NCBI). *Online Mendelian Inheritance in Man (OMIM).* http://www.ncbi.nlm.nih.gov/sites/entrez?db=omim [Provides a good starting point for up-to-date information on a range of subjects.]

Neuromuscular Disorders Online gene table http://www.musclegenetable.org/. [This updated resource contains information on the current state of knowledge about the involvement of specific genes and proteins in muscle diseases.]

Leiden University Medical Center. *Leiden Muscular Dystrophy pages.* http://www.dmd.nl [Offers specific information on the muscular dystrophies.]

24.24.3 Myotonia

David Hilton-Jones

Essentials

Myotonia is defined at an electrical level as repetitive discharge of the muscle fibre membrane after initial activation, which occurs due to dysfunction of the membrane's ion channels, most commonly the chloride channel, less commonly the sodium channel. This manifests clinically as stiffness of the muscle and delayed relaxation after voluntary contraction, e.g. difficulty relaxing the grip after clenching the fingers, and stiffness in the thigh muscles and difficulty walking on first moving after rest.

Particular myotonic disorders

Useful clinical distinction can be made between (1) myotonic dystrophies—multisystem disorders in which weakness is a significant feature, and (2) nondystrophic myotonias.

Myotonic dystrophy type 1 (Steinert's disease)—caused by expansion of an unstable trinucleotide repeat in the myotonic dystrophy protein kinase (DMPK) gene, leading to myotonia through altered splicing of the chloride channel gene. There are four main patterns of disease: (1) congenital; (2) childhood onset; (3) classic or early adult onset; (4) late onset, asymptomatic or oligosymptomatic. The classic form of the disease is the most frequent cause of myotonia and the most prevalent muscular dystrophy in adults (c.1 in 8000). In addition to myotonia and a characteristic pattern of weakness affecting the facial muscles and (unusually for a myopathic disorder) distal limbs, other features include premature male pattern balding, cataracts, central nervous system involvement (cognitive change, excessive daytime sleepiness), cardiac conduction abnormalities (which may lead to sudden death), gastroenterological involvement (dysphagia), and respiratory problems. Recurrent chest infections are common due to the combination of muscular weakness and the tendency to aspirate, and death is often secondary to pneumonia. The underlying trinucleotide repeat is unstable and increases in size during meiosis, giving rise to anticipation in which the disease has an earlier onset in the offspring of affected individuals.

Myotonic dystrophy type 2 (proximal myotonic myopathy)—caused by a quadruplet repeat expansion in the zinc finger 9 protein (ZNF9) gene that leads to disruption of normal RNA processing and altered splicing patterns of numerous genes. Clinical features are similar to type 1, but with proximal (rather than distal) weakness and less evident anticipation.

Nondystrophic myotonias—mutations affecting the skeletal muscle chloride channel (CLCN-1) gene give rise to the rare condition myotonia congenita, which can be inherited as either an autosomal dominant or recessive trait. Myotonia is striking; leg stiffness causing difficulty walking is the major feature, but persistent weakness is uncommon.

Introduction

Myotonia can be considered as a symptom, a physical sign, or a neurophysiological phenomenon, but understanding is perhaps best served by discussing these in the reverse order.

The basic neurophysiological finding is of repetitive muscle-fibre action potentials following a stimulus, which may be voluntary contraction or muscle percussion. The repetitive electrical activity causes muscle contraction, and thus myotonia is characterized by delayed muscle fibre relaxation after such a stimulus. Electromyography demonstrates the repetitive firing. Characteristically, the discharge gradually declines in amplitude and frequency, producing the so-called 'dive-bomber' sound in the monitoring loudspeaker. The term 'myotonia', and apparently related terms such as 'paramyotonia' and 'neuromyotonia', cause much confusion. Various diseases accompanied by myotonia have different molecular origins and many associated symptoms and signs

As a physical sign, myotonia is demonstrated either as delayed muscle relaxation following voluntary contraction (e.g. grip myotonia—Fig. 24.24.3.1), or as persistent muscle dimpling following percussion (percussion myotonia—Fig. 24.24.3.2).

As a symptom, complaints relating to myotonia differ between patients with myotonic dystrophy, which is by far the most common cause of myotonia, and those with myotonia congenita. In myotonic dystrophy, even when grip myotonia is readily evident on examination, the patient may offer no symptoms. They are more likely to complain of hand weakness than of myotonia. When the myotonia is symptomatic, the patient complains of difficulty releasing objects after a tight grip. This is sometimes striking. One patient first noted grip myotonia in early adult life, when he was appointed as a teacher at a school—as his future headmaster shook his hand to congratulate him, he was embarrassingly unable to release his grip. In myotonic dystrophy, bulbar symptoms relating to myotonia are quite common—patients complain of their tongue or jaw 'locking' when speaking or swallowing, and tongue myotonia on percussion may be demonstrated.

By contrast, in myotonia congenita weakness is absent and the myotonia, which is generalized, is problematic, particularly in the lower limbs. Patients complain of stiffness that is most evident on trying to initiate movement after rest. Thus, the patient who has been sitting in the waiting room rises and walks with profound leg stiffness, somewhat reminiscent of spasticity, into the consulting room. A classic presentation is the soldier on the parade ground—after

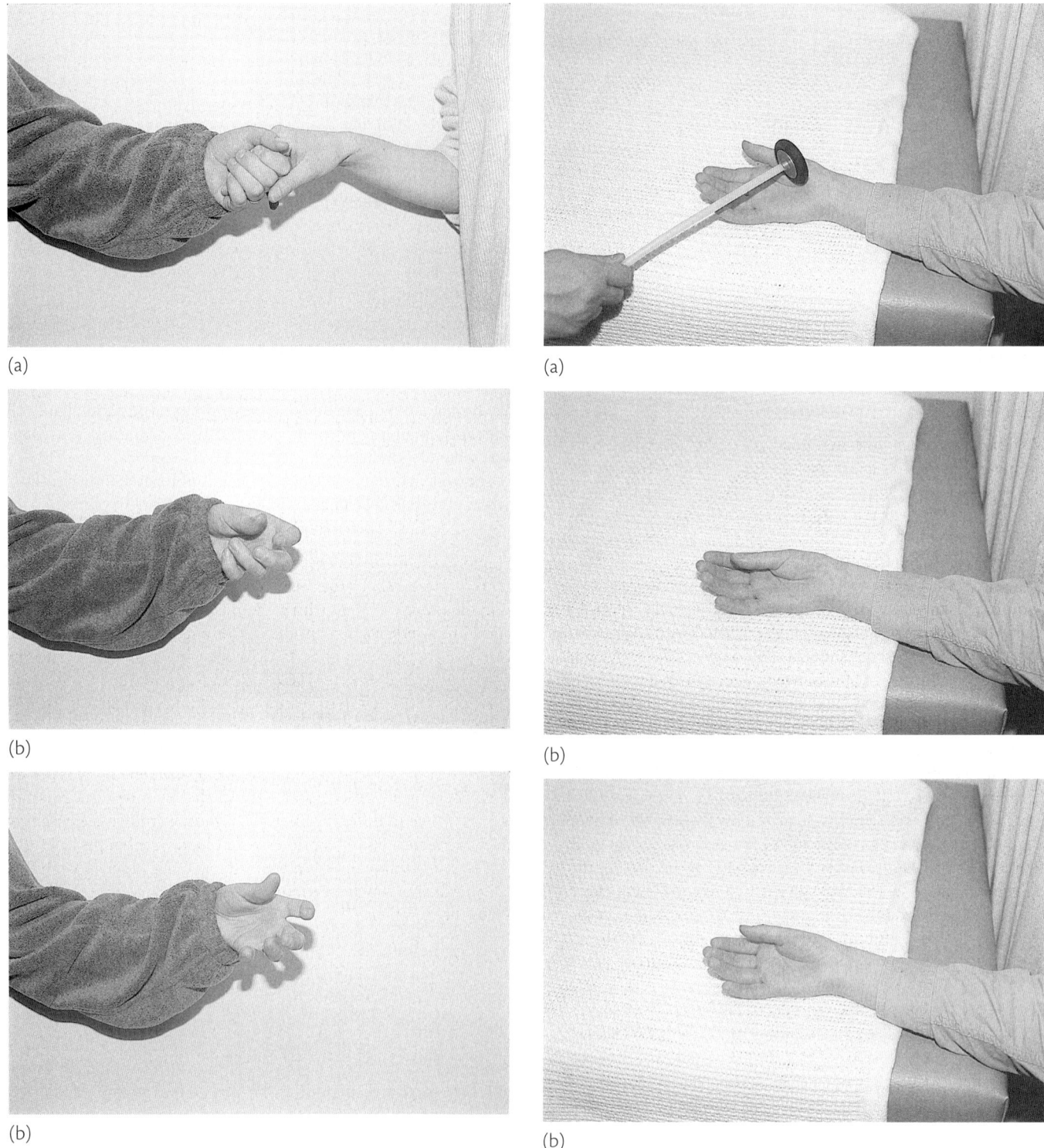

(a)

(b)

(b)

Fig. 24.24.3.1 Grip myotonia: the patient was asked to grip the examiner's fingers tightly for 3 s, and then to release the grip as rapidly as possible. The two photographs were taken at 3-s intervals.

(a)

(b)

(b)

Fig. 24.24.3.2 Percussion myotonia: following a sharp tap, the thenar eminence muscles contract and then relax slowly (photographs taken at 3-s intervals).

a prolonged period 'standing to attention', the order to march results in his falling due to leg muscle stiffness. One such patient also demonstrated marked grip myotonia—on an unfortunate occasion he alighted from a bus but, unable to release his grip from the handrail before the bus departed, was dragged along the road.

In most disorders, myotonia lessens with repeated activity of the muscle. Thus, the sign becomes less striking with repeated percussion of the thenar eminence or attempts to demonstrate grip myotonia. As a symptom, for example, the leg stiffness in myotonia congenita lessens as the patient continues to walk. In paramyotonia the reverse is seen, with myotonia increasing with activity—so-called

Table 24.24.3.1 Classification of myotonic disorders

Myotonic dystrophies (multisystem myotonic myopathies)	Nondystrophic myotonias
DM1: myotonic dystrophy type 1 (chromosome 19q)	Chloride channelopathies: myotonia congenita (chromosome 7q)
DM2: myotonic dystrophy type 2 (chromosome 3q)	Sodium channelopathies: paramyotonia congenita (chromosome 17q)
	Schwartz–Jampel syndrome: chondrodystrophic myotonia (chromosome 1p)

paradoxical myotonia. Some, but by no means all, patients complain that their myotonia is worse in the cold. This is again a particular characteristic of paramyotonia.

Classification of myotonic disorders

As with many other inherited neuromuscular disorders, nomenclature and classification are currently in a state of flux as molecular mechanisms are being unravelled. For clinical purposes a useful distinction is between those multisystem disorders in which weakness is a significant feature, and which are therefore referred to as dystrophies, and the nondystrophic myotonias (Table 24.24.3.1).

Classic myotonic dystrophy was previously called dystrophia myotonica, which gave rise to the abbreviation DM. It shows no genetic heterogeneity, all cases being associated with a trinucleotide repeat expansion in the 3′-untranslated region of a novel protein kinase gene (*DMPK*) on chromosome 19q. This locus and clinical disorder are referred to as DM1. A closely related condition, previously called proximal myotonic myopathy (PROMM), is caused by a quadruplet repeat expansion in intron 1 of the zinc finger 9 protein gene (*ZNF9*) on chromosome 3q and is referred to as DM2.

The most common nondystrophic myotonias are the autosomal dominant and recessive forms of myotonia congenita, both of which are caused by mutations of the skeletal muscle chloride channel gene (*CLCN1*). Different mutations of the skeletal muscle sodium channel gene (*SCN4A*) give rise to hyperkalaemic periodic paralysis and related disorders, including paramyotonia congenita. These chloride and sodium channelopathies, together with the calcium channel disorders causing hypokalaemic periodic paralysis, are discussed further in Chapter 24.24.5.

Schwartz–Jampel syndrome is a very rare recessive disorder of infantile onset, characterized by skeletal abnormalities (chondrodysplasia), abnormal facial appearance, and abnormal muscle electrical activity. Electromyography shows periods of continuous electrical activity, which are probably neural in origin. It is caused by mutations in the *HSPG2* gene, encoding the basement membrane protein perlecan.

Myotonic dystrophy type 1 (DM1)

DM1 is the most frequent cause of myotonia and indeed is also the most prevalent muscular dystrophy in adults. It is a multisystem disorder that has very important (but sometimes rather neglected) manifestations other than skeletal muscle dysfunction, involving cardiac conduction tissues, smooth muscle, eyes, and the central nervous system. Clinical severity ranges from death *in utero* to a condition so mild that it may be asymptomatic and with no abnormal physical signs in old age. The molecular basis is now known (an

expansion of an unstable trinucleotide repeat in a gene coding for a novel protein kinase, DMPK). There is strong evidence that the molecular mechanism in both DM1 and DM2 is disruption of normal RNA processing which causes altered splicing patterns of numerous genes, including the chloride channel gene (compare myotonia congenita)—this explains the myotonia—and the insulin receptor gene, causing insulin resistance. Myotonic dystrophy provides a dramatic example of the phenomenon of 'anticipation', by which succeeding generations may be much more severely affected than their predecessors, and this correlates with the size of the genetic expansion.

Epidemiology

The disease is seen worldwide, with a particularly high frequency in French Canadians in Quebec (originating from a single immigrant couple). Incidence and prevalence figures are unreliable, and probably mostly underestimates, because of the difficulty in identifying asymptomatic individuals. A generally accepted prevalence value is 8/100 000 population.

Pathogenesis

The molecular basis is the expansion of a trinucleotide (cytosine–thymine–guanine, CTG) repeat sequence in the 3′-untranslated region of the myotonic dystrophy protein kinase (*DMPK*) gene on chromosome 19q. In the normal population the size of the repeat is in the range CTG_{5-37}, with a trimodal distribution of 5, 11 to 17, and 19 to 37 repeats. Expansions in the range CTG_{37-49} are believed to represent premutations. Individuals with myotonic dystrophy have repeats in the range $CTG_{50-5000}$ and, as noted below, there is a correlation between the size of the repeat and clinical severity, and an inverse correlation between repeat size and age of onset.

A fundamental concept is that the expanded gene is unstable. It is mitotically unstable, and so the size of the gene increases with age. There is somatic mosaicism, so that the expansion is not the same size in different tissues. Diagnostic studies are based on measurement of the expansion size in blood lymphocyte DNA.

More important is intergenerational CTG-repeat instability, which explains why the disease tends to increase in severity in subsequent generations. The gender of the parent of origin is important. In most transmissions the allele size increases. However, there appears to be a threshold limit for sperm, and males never transmit the very large expansions associated with congenital myotonic dystrophy (see below), which occurs only when the mother is the gene carrier. There is some evidence of meiotic drive, which leads to preferred transmission of the abnormal expanded allele.

Clinical features

From the above it is apparent that there is a continuous distribution of expanded allele size, and a relationship between allele size and disease severity and between allele size and age of onset. While accepting that some patients will fall between these categories, for practical clinical purposes myotonic dystrophy can be considered to give rise to four main patterns of disease:

- congenital
- childhood onset
- classic or early adult onset
- late onset, asymptomatic, or oligosymptomatic

Table 24.24.3.2 Main clinical features of myotonic dystrophy

System	Manifestations
Neuromuscular	Weakness
	Myotonia
Ocular	Cataract
Central nervous system	Excessive daytime sleepiness
	Low IQ
	Sensorineural deafness
Cardiovascular	Heart block
	Dysrhythmias
	Sudden death
Respiratory	Recurrent infections
	Sleep apnoea
Hair	Premature balding
Gastrointestinal	Dysphagia
	Irritable bowel syndrome
	Pseudo-obstruction

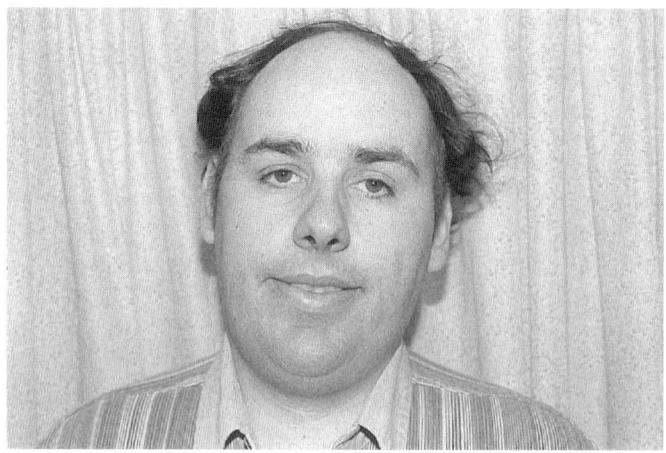

Fig. 24.24.3.3 Adult-onset myotonic dystrophy: typical facial features (see text).

As it is the best known, and illustrates the multifarious manifestations of myotonic dystrophy, the classic form is discussed first.

Classic form

Onset is in adolescence or early adult life. The principal manifestations are summarized in Table 24.24.3.2. A number of rarer or clinically less important associations are also recognized, including reduced fertility, testicular atrophy, insulin resistance (but rarely overt diabetes), retinopathy, eye movement disorder, peripheral neuropathy, disturbed tests of endocrine function, hypotension, pilomatrixomas, and reduced levels of immunoglobulins and complement.

Skeletal and smooth muscle

The features of myotonia have already been discussed. The distribution of muscle weakness is highly characteristic. Wasting and weakness of the facial muscles, combined with premature male-pattern balding, give rise to the typical facial appearance of the condition (Fig. 24.24.3.3). The temporalis muscle is atrophic, giving a sunken appearance over the temples. There is ptosis. Eye closure is weak and in severe cases the sclera may remain visible. The jaw tends to hang down. Neck flexion is weak and in some, but not all, patients there is evident atrophy of the sternomastoid muscles. In the limbs, and in marked contrast to most other myopathic disorders, the weakness is predominantly distal. In the upper limbs there is weakness and wasting of the small hand muscles and of the long wrist, and finger flexor and extensor muscles in the forearm. There is often profound weakness of grip and the patient complains of difficulty with tasks such as wringing out a cloth and removing the lid from a bottle. A simple hand-held dynamometer reveals the extent of the weakness—whereas a normal woman would easily exceed 35 kg, patients of either sex may manage only 1 or 2 kg. In the lower limbs there is weakness of ankle dorsiflexion, presenting as tripping easily and foot-drop. As the disease advances, weakness becomes evident more proximally, but the marked distal predilection remains throughout.

Bulbar muscle weakness presents with dysarthria and dysphagia. Smooth muscle involvement contributes towards the dysphagia. Symptoms akin to those of irritable bowel syndrome are frequent. Constipation is also common and pseudo-obstruction rare. There may be evidence of incoordinate uterine contraction in labour.

Ocular

Cataracts develop at an early age. The initial manifestation is multicoloured opacities in the subcapsular regions, readily seen on slit-lamp examination. Identification of cataracts used to be important in screening asymptomatic family members for the disease, but that has now been replaced by DNA testing. In practice, the cataracts are managed as any other cataracts, being operated on when vision is significantly impaired. Early onset cataracts should always raise the suspicion of myotonic dystrophy.

Central nervous system

Central nervous system (CNS) disease is expressed in two main ways. As a group, patients with myotonic dystrophy have a lower intelligence than average, but many mildly affected patients have intelligence within the normal range. They are often perceived as apathetic or lacking self-motivation. There is neuropsychological evidence of specific defects of frontal lobe functioning. The second principal feature is excessive daytime sleepiness, which affects over three-quarters of patients, some profoundly. This appears to be a central phenomenon and is only rarely attributable to obstructive sleep apnoea/nocturnal sleep disturbance.

Cardiovascular

Cardiovascular dysfunction is arguably the most important extra-muscular manifestation of myotonic dystrophy and is probably responsible for most of the not infrequently reported cases of sudden death. The most commonly recognized pattern is of progressive conduction disturbance. Thus, in very early cases the ECG is normal. Subsequently, the PR interval gradually lengthens until first-degree block is present. Later features include bundle-branch and complete heart block. Tachyarrhythmias also occur, most frequently atrial flutter or fibrillation, but also ventricular arrhythmias, which may be fatal. Symptoms include palpitation, dizzy spells, and fainting. Prolonged ECG monitoring and sometimes intracardiac electrophysiological studies are indicated if such symptoms are reported, or the standard ECG shows significant change. All patients should have an ECG annually, and be advised to report any cardiac symptoms immediately. Rhythm disturbances precipitated by anaesthesia or surgery are common, as are respiratory problems. For these reasons, patients should carry a medical alert bracelet/medallion and, for elective admissions for surgery, be reminded to inform the anaesthetist of their diagnosis. The latter is particularly important for asymptomatic individuals diagnosed on the basis of DNA studies following family screening, because they may not consider themselves to be at risk; they are. Although there is some correlation between cardiac involvement and overall severity of the myotonic dystrophy, it is not absolute and individuals with minimal muscle involvement may have significant ECG changes.

Heart muscle disease, as opposed to disordered cardiac conducting tissues, is not clinically significant and routine echocardiography is not required.

Respiratory

Recurrent chest infections are common and relate to respiratory muscle weakness and the tendency to aspirate. In advanced disease, death is often secondary to pneumonia. Respiratory insufficiency may become apparent following anaesthesia, with difficulty in weaning from the ventilator. Chronic hypoventilation and sleep fragmentation may cause excessive daytime sleepiness, but in practice are much less common than the presumed central mechanism already mentioned. However, it must be considered and excluded (e.g. by overnight oximetry and blood gas measurements) if felt to be a possibility. Particular warning features would include a history of disturbed night-time sleep, snoring, waking with headaches, and the development of secondary polycythaemia.

Congenital form

By definition, this form of myotonic dystrophy is evident at birth, but the spectrum of early onset myotonic dystrophy is much wider, as noted below. The exclusive (with only very rare exceptions) maternal transmission of congenital myotonic dystrophy has already been discussed. Many fetuses carrying large expansions are aborted spontaneously in early pregnancy and there is a high rate of fetal wastage. As a result of the unstable nature of the CTG repeat and the associated phenomenon of anticipation, it is not uncommon for the mother to be unaware of her own diagnosis at the time of birth. In that situation, the diagnosis in the infant is not always immediately apparent, because there are no entirely specific clinical features.

There is often a history of polyhydramnios and poor fetal movement in the pregnancy. The child is born hypotonic ('floppy') and talipes is present in about half. Respiratory and feeding difficulties may necessitate assisted ventilation or an oxygen tent, and feeding by nasogastric tube. Some die in the neonatal period from respiratory complications, but, somewhat surprisingly, there are few further deaths in the survivors until the late teens and early adult life. There is generalized weakness, including the face—the jaw hangs open and the mouth has a characteristic tented or carp-like (as in fish) appearance. Myotonia is not evident clinically and even electromyographically may not appear for several years.

In those who survive, hypotonia resolves and motor function improves over the following few years, but during adolescence the features of the classic adult form of the disease appear (Fig. 24.24.3.4).

Cognitive impairment is invariable and may be severe. Most require special needs schooling. Bowel involvement is common,

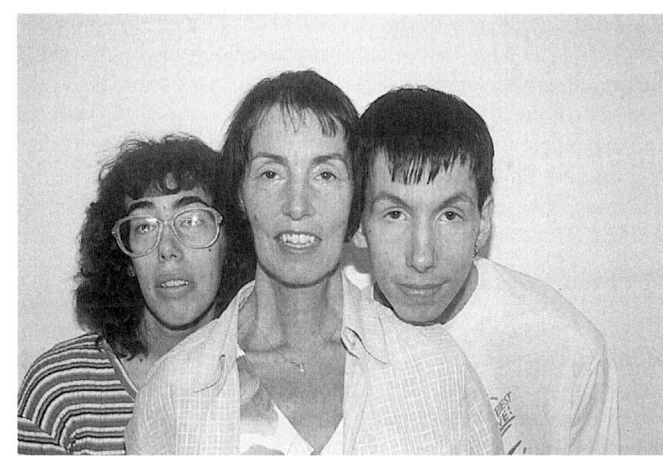

Fig. 24.24.3.4 Myotonic dystrophy: the affected mother's two children have the congenital form of the disease.

with faecal soiling and irregular bowel habit. Curiously, cataracts are relatively uncommon.

The overall prognosis is poor. Some 25% die in the first 18 months of life, most in the neonatal period. Half survive into the mid-30s, death most commonly resulting from respiratory involvement, but with a proportion of sudden deaths almost certainly due to cardiac conduction defects. Few achieve an independent adult life.

Childhood-onset form

It is only recently that the specific problems of childhood-onset disease have been recognized. By definition, such children do not have evidence of disease at birth. Motor milestones may be delayed. Problems are often first recognized around the start of schooling with evidence of cognitive delay and poor language development. Dysarthria is common. Fatigue and slowness of activities are often striking. Facial weakness is almost invariable, together with weakness of neck flexion.

Late-onset form

This form is associated with a small CTG-repeat expansion. It is typically asymptomatic or oligosymptomatic, and diagnosed during family studies or by an alert ophthalmologist when the patient presents with cataracts. Skeletal muscle disease may be absent, or confined to mild myotonia and weakness restricted to the hands. Balding may be a feature. It is not uncommon to see the parents of a patient with the classic adult form of the disease and not be able to identify the transmitting parent on clinical examination.

Importantly, even patients with such minimal symptoms may occasionally develop significant cardiac conduction problems and they should have annual electrocardiograms.

Management

The essential management issues in myotonic dystrophy are:

- genetic counselling
- annual ECG
- anaesthetic risks
- physical therapies
- cataract surgery

A particular concern relates to the genetic phenomenon of anticipation and the potential for an asymptomatic mother, ignorant of the diagnosis, to give birth to a congenitally affected child. When the diagnosis of myotonic dystrophy is established in a family member it is imperative that at-risk relatives are offered screening. Prenatal diagnosis, by chorionic villous sampling, can then be offered.

Annual ECG should be performed in all patients. They and their medical attendants must be aware of the cardiorespiratory complications associated with anaesthesia. They should be encouraged to wear an appropriate medical alert bracelet or medallion. A few patients require nocturnal positive-pressure ventilation by facemask, but most excessive daytime sleepiness is not related to respiratory insufficiency. Recurrent chest infections are common. Annual influenza immunization should be advised. Pneumococcal immunization is also given but is of uncertain value.

Physiotherapy, and occupational and speech and language therapy all have a role, as does the use of orthotic devices (e.g. for foot drop). Bowel problems in the congenital form require specific advice and counselling.

Excessive daytime sleepiness may respond, sometimes dramatically, to modafinil (but sleep-related breathing abnormalities should be excluded).

Cataract surgery is required when vision is significantly impaired.

Myotonic dystrophy type 2 (DM2)

Despite the similarity in name, and overlapping clinical features, there should generally be little difficulty distinguishing this condition from DM1. There appears to be remarkable variability in the incidence of this disorder between countries, possibly partly explained by not being able to identify it. Thus, in Germany DM2 appears to be about as prevalent as DM1; it is common in North America, but only a handful of families have been identified in the United Kingdom.

Similar to DM1, the underlying molecular basis is an unstable nucleotide repeat expansion in an untranslated part of a gene, the consequences of which seem to be mediated through disruption of RNA metabolism.

Despite the superficial similarities to myotonic dystrophy, there are also differences. Onset, or at least presentation, is usually in mid-adult life. Muscle pain and stiffness, particularly affecting the thighs, are common, and sometimes presenting, symptoms. The pattern and distribution of myotonia are similar to DM1, although, in contrast to DM1, early proximal weakness is usually evident, but hand weakness may also be prominent. Cataracts may be indistinguishable from those seen in myotonic dystrophy. Cardiac conduction problems appear to be less common. Male hypogonadism and deafness occur. A congenital form of DM2 has not been described. Cognitive involvement appears to be rare and excessive daytime sleepiness does not appear to be a major feature.

Further reading

Myotonic dystrophy type 1

Brook JD, et al. (1992). Molecular basis of myotonic dystrophy: expansion of a trinucleotide (CTG) repeat in the 3′ end of a transcript encoding a protein kinase family member. *Cell*, **68**, 799–808.
Harper P (2001). *Myotonic dystrophy*, 3rd edition. W B Saunders, London.
Harper P, et al. (2004). *Myotonic dystrophy: present management, future therapy*. Oxford University Press, Oxford.
Reardon W, et al. (1993). The natural history of congenital myotonic dystrophy: mortality and long term clinical aspects. *Arch Dis Childh*, **68**, 177–81.

Myotonic dystrophy type 2

Day JW, et al. (2003). Myotonic dystrophy type 2: molecular, diagnostic and clinical spectrum. *Neurology*, **60**, 657–64.
Ranum LPW, et al. (1998). Genetic mapping of a second myotonic dystrophy locus. *Nat Genet*, **19**, 196–8.

Molecular basis of myotonic dystrophy

Machuca-Tzili L et al. (2005). Clinical and molecular aspects of the myotonic dystrophies: A review. *Muscle Nerve*, **32**, 1–18.

24.24.4 Metabolic and endocrine disorders

David Hilton-Jones and Richard Edwards[†]

Essentials

Disturbances of the biochemical or ionic balance of muscle resulting in impaired muscle function can be caused by a disparate group of conditions, including primary inherited disorders affecting enzymes or ion channels, and secondary disorders in which metabolic or endocrine disequilibrium disturbs normal function.

Primary metabolic myopathies

The primary metabolic myopathies are mostly autosomal recessive disorders in which lack of activity of a specific enzyme impairs ATP generation. Clinical presentation is with exercised-induced symptoms, but there are fundamental differences in manifestations depending upon whether the enzyme defect affects glycogen/glucose metabolism or fatty acid metabolism, reflecting the very different contributions that these pathways make to energy production depending on the nature of the exercise.

Disorders of glycogen and glucose metabolism—these include: (1) Myophosphorylase deficiency (Mc Ardle's disease)—the commonest (but still very rare) glycogenosis; symptoms usually start in childhood, but are often not recognized at that time; cardinal features are pain, weakness, and stiffness of muscles early in exercise, relieved by rest; strenuous exercise may precipitate rhabdomyolysis and acute kidney injury. Diagnosis is established by histochemical demonstration of the absence of phosphorylase staining (or by enzyme assay) on muscle biopsy, or by genetic studies. There is no specific treatment. (2) Acid maltase deficiency—typically presents with a slowly progressive, painless, proximal myopathy; diaphragmatic involvement is common and can lead to presentation with respiratory failure; there are no exercise-induced symptoms. Enzyme replacement therapy may benefit some patients. (3) Other conditions—these include debrancher enzyme deficiency and phosphofructokinase deficiency.

[†] It is with regret that we report the death of Professor Richard Edwards during the preparation of this edition of the textbook.

Disorders of fatty acid metabolism—these include: (1) Carnitine palmitoyltransferase deficiency—symptoms are precipitated by sustained exercise (e.g. long-distance running) or prolonged fasting, and severe episodes may precipitate rhabdomyolysis and acute kidney injury; diagnosis requires enzyme assay; treatment with a high carbohydrate, low fat diet may reduce the number of attacks. (2) Other conditions—these include myoadenylate deaminase deficiency and defects of β-oxidation.

Secondary metabolic and endocrine myopathies

Endocrine myopathies—nearly all form of endocrine disturbance can be associated with weakness, typically relatively mild and involving the proximal muscles. The commonest precipitating conditions are Cushing's syndrome (including iatrogenic steroid excess), and hypo- and hyperthyroidism. Weakness resolves when the hormone imbalance is corrected.

Disorders of calcium, vitamin D, and parathyroid hormone metabolism—myopathy is a feature of osteomalacia, primary hyperparathyroidism, renal osteodystrophy, dialysis osteodystrophy and ischaemic myopathy.

Other conditions—(1) Alcohol excess—alcoholics frequently have muscle weakness, but it is often unclear whether the primary cause is myopathic or neuropathic. Alcoholic rhabdomyolysis typically follows a binge. (2) Drug-induced myopathies—the commonest cause is statins.

Skeletal muscle channelopathies

These rare inherited disorders affect muscle membrane ion channels, resulting in altered electrical characteristics: (1) period paralysis—underlying mutations affect either the sodium or calcium channels; manifest with episodic weakness; (2) myotonic dystrophies—see Chapter 24.24.3; (3) malignant hyperthermia—caused by mutations in the calcium channel associated ryanodine receptor; muscle relaxants and anaesthetic agents may trigger generalized muscle contraction with rapid rise in body temperature that can be fatal if untreated.

Introduction

This section deals with disorders of voluntary muscle that arise as the result of either a disturbance of muscle metabolism or disordered ion flux. In many cases precise mechanisms have yet to be defined.

The term 'metabolic myopathy' is applied to those disorders in which there is a primary defect, usually an enzyme deficiency, in the biochemical pathways associated with energy generation (adenosine triphosphate or ATP synthesis). This group includes the mitochondrial disorders, which are some of the most common causes of primary metabolic myopathy seen in clinical practice.

Endocrine myopathies and nutritional and toxic myopathies, including those that are drug induced, can be considered as secondary (acquired) metabolic myopathies.

Defects in genes coding for subunits of the skeletal muscle sodium and calcium channels underlie primary hyperkalaemic and hypokalaemic periodic paralysis, respectively. Both autosomal dominant and autosomal recessive myotonia congenita are caused by mutation in the skeletal muscle chloride channel. Mutations affecting two skeletal muscle calcium channels, the dihydropyridine (DHPR) and ryanodine (RYR1) receptors, are associated with malignant hyperthermia (MH). The congenital myopathy central core disease is allelic to MH and is associated with *RYR1* mutations.

The cardinal symptoms of myopathy are weakness, fatigue, and/ or pain; altered excitability may also occur. It is important that the physician appreciates several points. There are nonspecific effects, such as loss of muscle, that may be far more important as a cause of weakness than the energetic consequences of the biochemical defect. Visual inspection and circumference measurements tend to underestimate the extent of wasting, which may be better documented by quantitative scanning methods (MRI or CT).

Not all the biochemical abnormalities cause symptoms. Clinical expression of the underlying defect depends on the habitual demands on the muscle for movement and weight lifting.

A patient with a metabolic myopathy may have common, non-myopathic, musculoskeletal complaints that have no relation to the inherited or acquired defect.

Muscle symptoms may have no physiological connection with the underlying defect and may be consequences of somatization or other psychological processes.

The practical assessment of metabolic myopathy should include consideration of the World Health Organization's (WHO's) *International classification of impairments, disabilities, and handicaps* (ICIDH-2) (2000)—a classification of the functioning and disability criteria of impairment, activities, and participation (revised from the ICIDH of the WHO from 1980). In this generic consideration, the relationship between antigravity muscle strength and the body weight to be carried is crucial: performance may be improved as much or more by weight reduction as by therapeutic attempts to reverse the myopathy, provided that calorie restriction does not aggravate the metabolic defect, e.g. in the case of carnitine palmitoyltransferase deficiency, where carbohydrate starvation may exacerbate the energy supply problem of the underlying enzyme defect.

An objective assessment of a response to treatment requires the measurement of individual muscle strength and/or timing of the performance of tasks relevant to the patient's symptoms, and the everyday life demands placed on the diseased muscles.

Metabolic myopathies are unusual or rare conditions that are very variable in presentation. They are not easy to discuss in the light of current, evidence-based health-care philosophies, which are largely based on the results of randomized controlled trials (RCTs) of therapeutic interventions. The treatments of the metabolic myopathies tend to fall under the general rubric of 'orphan drugs' and 'orphan diseases', because, as with other rare diseases, a commercial return on the investment in research and development to deliver effective treatments is unlikely. Furthermore, in view of their rarity, there is little or no chance of formal treatment evaluation by RCTs. These conditions are therefore still to be evaluated by thoughtful clinical research employing the most relevant modern biochemical and physiological approaches.

The patient with a metabolic myopathy is a person, and therefore far more important and complex to understand and help than the underlying metabolic diagnosis, difficult though that may be. It is essential to the humane and effective management of such a patient to see the individual as coping in a personal and social sense despite the metabolic impairment. The aim is to determine what is likely to best improve the patient's overall quality of life. Here, as with other disabilities, the constructive analysis and recommendations

Table 24.24.4.1 Key features of disability evaluation and management in metabolic myopathy

Body	Person	Society
Impairment	**Activities (limitations)**	**Participation (restriction)**
Metabolism/function/ structure		
Severity, localization, duration	Difficulties, duration, assistance needed	Extent, facilitators, environmental demands of barriers
Harmful consequences, e.g. myoglobinuria, falls	Physical and mental adaptive responses	Positive or negative psychosocial factors
Treatment options: modification of chemistry by diet or drugs?	Counselling for exercise behaviour modification; avoidance of excessive weight gain; mechanical solutions, e.g. wheelchair/ bicycle	Better popular understanding of side effects of prescription drugs and alcohol; positive attitudes to assisting those with locomotor disability, improved access

Developed from World Health Organization (2000). *International classification of functioning and disability ICIDH-2*. Geneva, WHO. Available at: http://www3.who.int/ icf/icftemplate.

of the WHO are useful as a basis for working with the patient to determine an individual management plan (Table 24.24.4.1).

Primary metabolic myopathies

The principal energy currency of living cells is ATP. Whereas in most organs the rate of ATP utilization is fairly constant, in voluntary muscle the change from rest to strenuous activity may increase the demand on ATP generation several thousandfold. If that demand is not met, contractile failure (i.e. fatigue or weakness) will develop and may be accompanied by the destruction of muscle fibres. In many of the primary metabolic myopathies it is often assumed that exercise-induced symptoms relate to a failure of ATP generation and, although this is probably not always correct, it is a useful generalization. Although exercise-induced symptoms are often a striking feature of this type of metabolic myopathy, they are not always present. Some patients develop a chronic progressive myopathy.

The main fuels providing energy for ATP generation in skeletal muscle are glycogen, fatty acids, and glucose (Fig. 24.24.4.1). Their relative contributions depend upon the state of nutrition and, more importantly, the level and duration of exercise. A gross over-simplification of these pathways aids understanding of the clinical features of the different forms of metabolic myopathy.

At rest, the main fuel source is circulating free fatty acids, with a lesser contribution from circulating glucose. Small amounts of ATP may be generated directly from glycolysis, but the production of the energy-rich electron carriers (reduced nicotinamide adenine dinucleotide or NADH and reduced flavin adenine dinucleotide (FADH$_2$) from fatty acid β-oxidation, and the citric acid cycle) is more important. Transfer of electrons to molecular oxygen through the electron transport chain of the mitochondria releases energy for the generation of ATP (oxidative phosphorylation)

The increased demand on ATP generation during early strenuous exercise cannot be met by oxidative pathways. The resting blood flow provides an inadequate delivery of oxygen and substrate, and compression of blood vessels by the contracting muscle exacerbates the problem. ATP is therefore generated by the

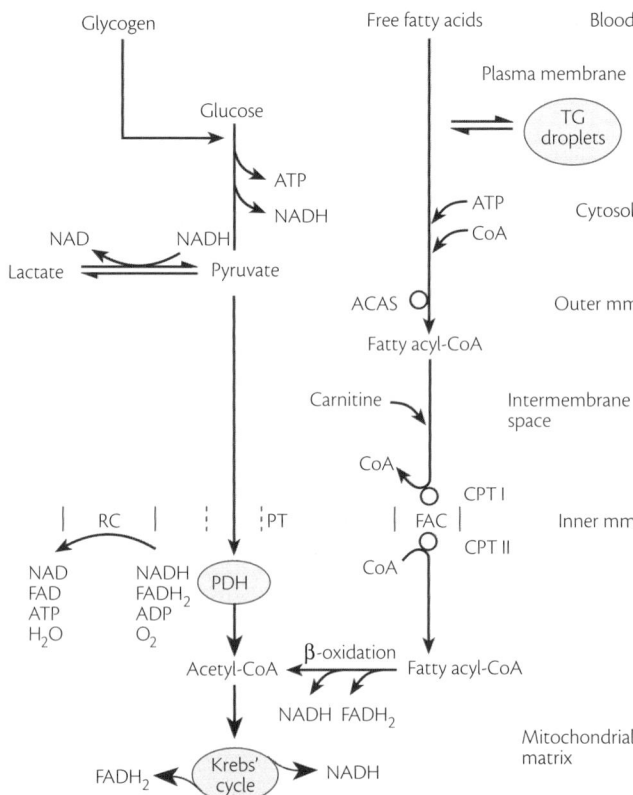

Fig. 24.24.4.1 Major pathways associated with energy production in skeletal muscle. ACAS, acyl-CoA synthetase; ADP, adenosine diphosphate; ATP, adenosine triphosphate; CoA, coenzyme A; CPT, carnitine palmitoyl transferase; FAC, fatty acylcarnitine; FAD, flavin adenine dinucleotide; FADH$_2$, reduced FAD; mm, mitochondrial membrane; NAD, nicotinamide adenine dinucleotide; NADH, reduced NAD; PDH, pyruvate dehydrogenase complex; PT, pyruvate translocase; RC, respiratory chain; TG, triglyceride.

breakdown of muscle fibre stores of glycogen (anaerobic glycolysis). The relative lack of oxygen leads to increasing levels of NADH and pyruvate. NADH accumulation would inhibit glycolysis, and thus ATP generation, and is avoided by the reduction of pyruvate to lactate, explaining the lactic acidosis seen in disorders of oxidative metabolism.

Adaptive processes occur as exercise continues; muscle blood flow increases, the respiratory rate rises, and free fatty acids are mobilized from adipose stores. Glycogen stores in muscle become depleted and circulating free fatty acids become the main energy source, with a very small contribution from circulating glucose.

Certain deductions can be made from the above that are largely borne out in clinical practice. Disorders of glycogen and glucose metabolism are typically asymptomatic at rest, but produce symptoms early in exercise when anaerobic glycolysis is important for energy supply. If low levels of exercise can be sustained, symptoms can improve as fatty acid oxidation increases ('second wind' phenomenon in McArdle's disease). Disorders of fatty acid metabolism, insufficient to cause symptoms at rest, are likely to be exposed by sustained exercise and fasting. The central role of oxidative phosphorylation explains why disorders of the respiratory chain may be symptomatic at rest. The clinical presentation will also depend upon whether the enzyme defect is restricted to skeletal muscle or is more generalized, thereby causing dysfunction of other tissues and organs. Systemic features may dominate in disorders of β oxidation and in mitochondrial disorders, but are absent in McArdle's disease because the defective enzyme is muscle specific.

Disorders of glycogen and glucose metabolism (see also Chapter 12.3)

Several of the glycogenoses show significant skeletal muscle involvement. The major pathways of metabolism, and the enzymes associated with these disorders, are shown in Fig. 24.24.4.2. They are autosomal recessive disorders, except for the X-linked recessive, phosphoglycerate kinase deficiency. In most of these disorders serum creatine kinase (CK) is elevated at rest, and massively so after exercise-induced muscle damage.

Acid maltase deficiency (type II glycogenosis)

Acid maltase is a lysosomal enzyme not directly involved in energetic pathways, and exercise-induced symptoms are absent. In the infantile form (Pompe's disease) there is widespread organomegaly as well as skeletal muscle involvement, and death occurs by the age of 2 years due to cardiac or respiratory failure. The adult form is of considerable importance and has probably been underdiagnosed. The most obvious feature is a slowly progressive, painless, proximal myopathy. Diaphragmatic involvement is an important characteristic, and some of these patients first present with respiratory failure. Nocturnal noninvasive ventilation alleviates sleep-disordered breathing and may prolong survival for many years. Muscle biopsy showing glycogen-containing vacuoles is usually suggestive, but the definitive diagnosis is established by enzyme assay in muscle, fibroblasts, or leucocytes, or by demonstrating glycogen granules by periodic acid–Schiff (PAS) staining in lymphocytes on a peripheral blood film.

Enzyme replacement therapy has been shown to be effective in the severe infantile form, substantially prolonging survival. Less evidence is available for the late-onset form (see Chapter 12.3.1).

Myophosphorylase deficiency (type V glycogenosis—McArdle's disease)

The onset of symptoms is usually during childhood, although they are often not recognized at that time, and the cardinal features are pain, weakness, and stiffness of muscles early in exercise, relieved by rest. The prevalence is estimated to be around 1 in 100 000 population but many cases are undiagnosed. Strenuous exercise, such as helping to push a car or lift heavy furniture, may induce painful, electrically silent, muscle contractures. Muscle fibre breakdown is reflected in myalgia and myoglobinuria (dark red/black urine), which, if severe, may cause renal failure. Muscle breakdown is accompanied by a large release of CK into the blood, and a failure to see such a rise in serum CK levels should cast doubt on a diagnosis of myoglobinuria. Conversely, if renal failure is present, then no myoglobinuria may be seen and the only evidence of rhabdomyolysis is the raised CK level. Exercise-induced symptoms may ease ('second wind' phenomenon) if low levels of activity are maintained, as circulating free fatty acids and glucose become available as alternative fuels.

Progressive proximal weakness frequently develops in middle age and is sometimes the mode of presentation in late-onset cases.

Failure of lactate generation (accompanied by increased blood ammonia and hypoxanthine concentrations) during forearm exercise is consistent with the diagnosis. However, this is not specific

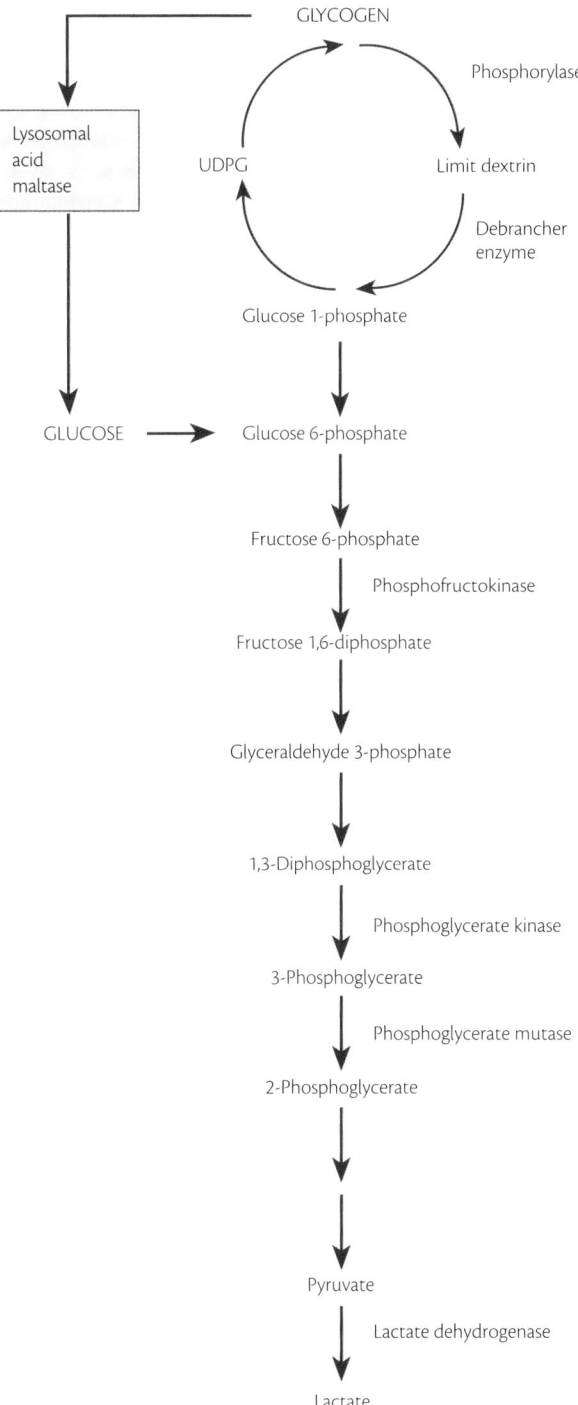

Fig. 24.24.4.2 Pathways of glycogenolysis and glycolysis. Enzymes known to be associated with particular clinical syndromes are shown.

because it also occurs in other glycogenolysis disorders, and may be seen to some extent in acquired conditions such as alcoholic myopathy or hypothyroidism. Also, the test may give a misleading ('false-negative') result if the myophosphorylase deficiency is only partial. The definitive diagnosis is established by histochemical demonstration of the absence of phosphorylase staining (or by enzyme assay) on muscle biopsy, or by genetic studies of the coding and expression of muscle phosphorylase.

Debrancher enzyme deficiency (type III glycogenosis— Cori–Forbes disease)

In infancy and childhood the main features of this disorder are hepatomegaly, hypoglycaemia, and failure to thrive. During adolescence muscle symptoms become more prominent. A small group of patients first present during adult life with muscle symptoms, but may give a history of a protuberant abdomen in childhood. Both exercise intolerance (although less striking than in McArdle's disease) and a slowly progressive proximal myopathy are present.

Some patients develop a potentially fatal cardiomyopathy.

The forearm exercise test shows impaired, but not absent, lactate generation, muscle biopsy shows glycogen accumulation, and the administration of glucagon fails to produce a hyperglycaemic response. Enzyme assay can be performed on muscle, liver, erythrocytes, and leucocytes.

Phosphofructokinase deficiency (type VII glycogenosis— Tarui's disease)

The clinical picture is very similar to that of myophosphorylase deficiency, but a phosphofructokinase (PFK) deficiency in erythrocytes leads to the additional features of haemolytic anaemia and gout. It is very much rarer than myophosphorylase deficiency. Unlike patients with myophosphorylase deficiency, ingested glucose does not improve exercise tolerance in those with PFK deficiency because of the position of PFK in the sequence of enzymes in the glycolytic pathway (see Fig. 24.24.4.2), and indeed may worsen symptoms (sometime called the 'out-of-wind' phenomenon). Diagnosis is established by enzyme assay in muscle.

Defects of distal glycolysis

Deficiencies of phosphoglycerate kinase, phosphoglycerate mutase, and lactate dehydrogenase have been found but are all extremely rare. All three are associated with exercise intolerance and myoglobinuria. It is possible that other defects of glycolysis, causing similar symptoms, remain to be discovered.

Treatment

With the exception of the recent introduction of enzyme replacement therapy for acid maltase deficiency there is, as yet, no specific treatment for any of the disorders described above. Attempts at dietary manipulation have generally proved unsuccessful. Patients must be aware of the risk to renal function from myoglobinuria, and try to avoid intense exercise. There is evidence, in patients with muscle pain due to McArdle's disease and other metabolic myopathies, that maintaining a reasonable level of aerobic fitness is beneficial, by sustaining sufficient activity of muscle mitochondria to provide energy from oxidative phosphorylation to adapt to the deficiencies in energy availability from glycogenolysis.

Disorders of lipid metabolism

Unlike glycolysis, lipid metabolism is entirely dependent on oxidative processes. Moreover, there is a close relationship between the disorders described below and defects of the mitochondrial respiratory chain, e.g. lipid accumulation in muscle is a common histological feature in respiratory chain disorders.

Free fatty acids, mainly from the blood but also from triglyceride droplets stored within muscle fibres, are a major fuel at rest and during sustained exercise (see Fig. 24.24.4.1). They are converted to fatty acyl-CoA at the outer mitochondrial membrane which, within the mitochondrial matrix, can undergo β oxidation. A transport system involving carnitine and the enzyme system carnitine palmitoyltransferase (CPT) is required to enable fatty acyl-CoA to cross the inner mitochondrial membrane. Defects involving carnitine, CPT, and β oxidation are recognized.

Carnitine deficiency

Secondary carnitine deficiency is common and seen in association with many primary metabolic disorders, including defects of fatty acid oxidation and respiratory chain disorders. Primary carnitine deficiency is very rare and is caused by a defective carnitine transporter, OCTN2. It may cause varying combinations of myopathy, hypoketotic hypoglycaemia, and hepatic encephalopathy.

Defects of β oxidation

Many enzyme deficiencies have been described, but clinical features are limited. They may present during the neonatal period with hypotonia, hypoglycaemia, cardiomyopathy, failure to thrive, and early death. Such defects may be a cause of some cases of sudden infant death syndrome. Later-onset cases develop Reye's syndrome-like crises, muscle weakness, and cardiomyopathy. Secondary carnitine deficiency is common. A high-carbohydrate and low-fat diet may help.

Carnitine palmitoyltransferase deficiency

This rare autosomal recessive disorder shows a male predominance. Symptoms are precipitated by sustained exercise (e.g. a route march) or prolonged fasting, and consist of muscle pain followed by myoglobinuria, which may cause renal failure. The diagnosis may be strongly suggested by tandem mass spectrometry, looking at the acylcarnitine profile, in a blood sample taken after an overnight fast, but confirmation requires enzyme assay, usually on cultured fibroblasts. A high-carbohydrate, low-fat diet may reduce the number of attacks.

Myoadenylate deaminase deficiency

Deficiency of myoadenylate deaminase has been suggested as a cause of exercise-induced myalgia, weakness, and cramps but its exact status remains controversial. It has been described as an incidental finding in muscle needle biopsies taken from normal volunteers to study muscle chemistry in sports science research. The enzyme catalyses the reaction adenosine monophosphate (AMP) → inosine monophosphate (IMP) + ammonia (NH_3). Theoretically, this reaction may aid ATP production by removing AMP and increasing flux through the adenylate kinase reaction 2ADP → ATP + AMP. The diagnosis is established from the absence of a rise in the plasma ammonia level during forearm exercise testing and from the histochemical demonstration of absent enzyme activity.

Endocrine myopathies

Although weakness is a common symptom in many endocrine disorders, the mechanisms are generally poorly understood. However, the myopathy responds to treatment of the underlying hormonal disorder, and extensive investigation of the myopathic component is rarely required. The most common pattern is limb-girdle weakness.

Thyroid disorders (see also Chapter 13.4)

Thyrotoxicosis

Typically, weakness develops shortly after the onset of other thyrotoxic symptoms, and 80% of patients have demonstrable weakness at presentation. The shoulder-girdle muscles tend to be involved before the pelvic musculature. Muscle atrophy is usually slight. Asymmetrical and distal weakness, myalgia, cramps, and fasciculations are rare findings.

The serum CK level is usually normal, but electromyography shows features consistent with muscle disease. The myopathy responds to treatment of the thyrotoxicosis.

Thyrotoxic periodic paralysis

Most cases have been reported in individuals from the Orient, with a strong male predominance. Clinical features closely mimic those of familial hypokalaemic periodic paralysis. The weakness is disproportionate to any muscle wasting. The onset of paralytic attacks usually follows the development of hyperthyroid symptoms but the attacks cease when the patient is rendered euthyroid. A genetic basis has not been established.

Thyroid ophthalmopathy (Graves' ophthalmoplegia)

The classic features of this condition include eyelid lag, retraction, and swelling, as well as progressive swelling of the extraocular muscles and orbital soft tissues, leading to proptosis and diplopia and, in severe cases, corneal ulceration, papilloedema, and optic atrophy. An extremely important, but often missed, variant is the patient who presents with minimal diplopia only.

In mild cases, MRI or CT is useful for detecting extraocular muscle swelling. Simple tests of thyroid function may be normal. Estimation of antithyroglobulin and antimicrosomal antibodies, and the performance of a thyrotropin-releasing hormone (TRH) stimulation test may be required. Thyroid-stimulating immunoglobulins are present in most patients.

If thyrotoxic, the patient should be rendered euthyroid. Lid retraction may respond to topical 10% guanethidine. Persisting major eye problems may require high-dose prednisolone, plasma exchange, or orbital decompression. Tarsorrhaphy protects the cornea.

Thyroid disease and myasthenia

Patients with myasthenia gravis have an increased incidence of thyroid disease, including hyperthyroidism, hypothyroidism, Hashimoto's thyroiditis, and increased antibodies to thyroglobulin or microsomal fractions. Thyroid disease may pre-date or follow the onset of myasthenia and must be considered as a cause of deterioration in an otherwise stable patient with myasthenia. Some 5% of patients with myasthenia will develop thyroid disease, but only about 0.1% of thyrotoxic patients develop myasthenia.

Hypothyroidism

Although hypothyroid myopathy may be asymptomatic, mild weakness is probably present in most patients. Muscle biopsy characteristically shows evidence of type II (fast twitch, glycolytic, high intrinsic force) muscle fibre atrophy with type I fibre dominance. Even in the absence of weakness the serum CK level is often markedly raised. Slow relaxation of the tendon jerks may be present in isolation. Muscle pain and cramps are common. In children, the combination of hypothyroidism, weakness, and muscle hypertrophy is referred to as the Kocher–Debré–Semelaigne syndrome. In adults, Hoffman's syndrome describes the combination of hypothyroidism, weakness, muscle hypertrophy, cramps, and myoedema (the formation of a localized ridge of muscle following direct percussion). They probably represent variants of the same disorder.

All hypothyroid myopathic symptoms respond to thyroxine replacement.

Pituitary–adrenal axis disorders

Clinically, the most important of these is iatrogenic steroid myopathy, discussed below under 'Glucocorticoid excess'.

Acromegaly

Proximal weakness, pelvic more than shoulder girdle, is present in about half of patients. Common complaints include tiredness, weakness, and myalgia; muscle wasting is slight. Serum CK levels are normal or slightly raised. Normalizing growth hormone levels improves the myopathy, but recovery may be incomplete.

Hypopituitarism

Growth hormone deficiency in childhood impairs muscle and skeletal development proportionately; weakness is not usually a feature. In adults, panhypopituitarism causes generalized weakness and fatigue, which usually responds to thyroxine and cortisone replacement therapy. Replacement of growth hormone in growth hormone-deficient adults has been associated with varying degrees of improvement in the strength of wasted muscles.

Glucocorticoid excess

ACTH excess, from either a functioning pituitary adenoma or ectopic production, is usually associated with high glucocorticoid levels, producing pituitary or ectopic Cushing's syndrome. Weakness is common and thought to relate to glucocorticoid excess. Weakness may occur in Nelson's syndrome, in which there is a high level of ACTH but no glucocorticoid excess.

The myopathy associated with Cushing's syndrome is probably related to glucocorticoid excess, and the clinical features are essentially the same as those of iatrogenic steroid myopathy. The 9α-fluorinated steroids, including dexamethasone, triamcinolone, and betamethasone, appear to have the greatest myopathic potential. Topical steroids can cause myopathy.

The most common picture is of a slowly progressive limb-girdle wasting and weakness, pelvic more than shoulder girdle, often accompanied by myalgia. The drug-induced form may have a more acute onset. Myopathy without other features of glucocorticoid excess is unusual. The serum CK level is usually normal and muscle biopsy shows nonspecific type II fibre atrophy.

Steroid withdrawal is followed by recovery over several months. If steroid therapy for the primary disorder has to be continued then a nonfluorinated compound such as prednisolone should be used, preferably on an alternate-day basis. Successful treatment of Cushing's syndrome leads to recovery.

Conn's syndrome

Weakness is present in about 75% of patients and is due to the associated hypokalaemia. Secondary hypokalaemic periodic paralysis may occur.

Addison's disease

Weakness, fatigue, and myalgia occur in up to half of patients. Rare myopathic presentations include progressive flexion contractures and secondary hyperkalaemic periodic paralysis.

The serum CK level is normal or slightly increased. Glucocorticoid replacement therapy is curative.

Disorders of calcium, vitamin D, and parathyroid hormone metabolism (see also Chapter 13.6)

There are complex interactions of vitamin D metabolism, calcium and phosphate homeostasis, and parathyroid hormone activity. Myopathy occurs in several clinical situations, but the precise pathophysiological mechanisms are unclear.

Osteomalacia

Weakness is the presenting symptom in a third of patients, affecting predominantly the pelvic girdle musculature. Bone pain is prominent. The serum CK level is usually normal. Muscle biopsy may show type II fibre atrophy, sometimes severe.

The pain responds fairly rapidly to vitamin D treatment, but the weakness recovers more slowly and may be incomplete.

Primary hyperparathyroidism

Myalgia, stiffness, and complaints of fatigue are common, but overt weakness is rare. Symptoms resolve when the underlying parathyroid adenoma is removed and serum calcium levels fall.

Renal osteodystrophy

End-stage renal failure is frequently accompanied by a predominantly pelvic girdle myopathy, sometimes with buttock and thigh pain. Symptoms respond to dialysis, transplantation, or vitamin D treatment.

Dialysis osteodystrophy

Some patients undergoing dialysis develop a severe myopathy with bone pain, fractures, and vitamin D resistance. It probably relates to aluminium toxicity. Fatigue and muscle weakness are common. Objective muscle testing is needed to distinguish true changes in muscle function from the nonspecific causes of fatigue and ill-health seen in patients on dialysis.

Ischaemic myopathy

Rarely, a painful ischaemic myopathy with arterial narrowing due to calcium deposition complicates renal failure. Skin ulceration and bowel infarction may also occur.

Nutritional and toxic myopathies

Although malnutrition causes muscle wasting, specific myopathic effects of nutritional deficiencies are uncommon, a notable exception being vitamin D deficiency, discussed above. Myopathies due to ingested toxins are relatively more common than the inherited metabolic myopathies and include those due to alcohol, and therapeutic drug excess or idiosyncrasy.

Alcoholic myopathies

People with chronic alcohol problems may develop subacute or slowly progressive, proximal muscle weakness with mild-to-moderate wasting and muscle biopsy evidence of type II fibre atrophy, mainly affecting the lower limbs. Occasionally the wasting is more generalized, as alcoholism may be associated with neurogenic muscle atrophy secondary to concomitant thiamine deficiency and more generalized malnutrition. It is thus still debated whether the so-called chronic alcoholic myopathy is purely myopathic, neuropathic, or both, and whether the cause is a direct toxic effect of alcohol or a secondary phenomenon, perhaps relating to malnutrition. Abstinence may lead to some degree of recovery.

Much more dramatic is acute alcoholic myopathy ('alcoholic rhabdomyolysis'), which usually occurs during or shortly after a binge. There may be widespread cramps, pain, and weakness. However, the most striking feature is the development of extremely painful muscle swelling, which may be localized or generalized. Myoglobinuria presents a threat to renal function, and hyperkalaemia may be present in severe cases. The serum CK is elevated and muscle biopsy shows acute necrosis. Recovery, which may be incomplete, occurs over several weeks.

Vitamin E deficiency

Vitamin E deficiency probably causes a myopathy, but interpretation is confused by the presence of additional neurological problems including neuropathy and ataxia.

Drug-induced myopathies

Drug-induced neuromuscular disorders are common, under-recognized, and under-reported. Numerous drugs have been implicated, several mechanisms are responsible (Table 24.24.4.2), and some drugs can affect both muscle and peripheral nerves (e.g. vincristine, D-penicillamine, and perhexiline). Arguably the most important is statin-induced myopathy, because myopathic symptoms are relatively common and their prescription is becoming ever more widespread, with over-the-counter preparations being available in some countries. A small percentage of patients develop myalgia, usually with elevation of the serum CK. The symptoms resolve on drug withdrawal. Much more rarely, statins may induce rhabdomyolysis/myoglobinuria, and deaths have been reported. There remains debate as to whether a pre-existing myopathy, symptomatic or not, increases the risk of stain-induced myopathy

Skeletal muscle channelopathies

There has been an explosion in the identification of central and peripheral nervous system and cardiac disorders caused by ion channel dysfunction. Ion channels may be ligand gated or voltage gated. In the field of muscle diseases, the most important ligand-gated channel is the skeletal muscle nicotinic acetylcholine receptor, at the neuromuscular junction. Antibody-mediated destruction underlies acquired myasthenia gravis, whereas inherited mutations of genes coding for the subunits of the receptor are the basis of several forms of congenital myasthenic syndrome. Acquired neuromyotonia and Lambert–Eaton myasthenic syndrome are caused by antibody-mediated damage to the voltage-gated potassium and calcium channels, respectively, of the terminal axon, and are discussed, together with myasthenia gravis and the myasthenic syndromes, in Chapter 24.17.

The following section is concerned with inherited disorders of skeletal muscle voltage-gated sodium, calcium, and chloride channels. In passing, it should be noted that channelopathies are not confined to muscle, and note was made above of two neuronal channelopathies. Other disorders caused by an inherited channel defect include certain forms of epilepsy (nocturnal frontal lobe epilepsy, benign neonatal convulsions), episodic ataxia, hemiplegic migraine, deafness, night blindness, cardiac long QT syndromes, and nephrolithiasis.

Periodic paralyses

Marked hypokalaemia and hyperkalaemia from whatever cause may produce weakness or paralysis (secondary periodic paralysis). The primary periodic paralyses are familial, dominantly inherited

Table 24.24.4.2 Drug-induced myopathies

Focal damage/fibrosis	Intramuscular
	Opiates
	Antibiotics
	Paraldehyde
Necrosis	Heroin
	Clofibrate
	ε-Aminocaproic acid
Myoglobinuria/ rhabdomyolysis	Heroin
	Methadone
	Amphetamines
	Barbiturates
	Diazepam
	Isoniazid
	Carbenoxolone
	Phenformin
	Amphotericin B
	Statins
Inflammatory myopathy	Procainamide
	D-Penicillamine
Hypokalaemic weakness	Diuretics
	Carbenoxolone
	Liquorice
	Purgatives
Subacute or painless proximal myopathy	Corticosteroids
	Chloroquine
	β-Blockers
Myasthenia	D-Penicillamine
	Aminoglycosides
Malignant hyperthermia	Suxamethonium
	Cyclopropane
	Halothane
	Enflurane
	Ketamine

disorders being characterized by recurrent attacks of paralysis. These have previously been subdivided into hyperkalaemic, hypokalaemic, and normokalaemic forms on the basis of changes in the serum potassium level during attacks. Recent evidence has shown that the primary abnormality in the hyperkalaemic and normokalaemic forms is a mutation affecting the adult skeletal muscle sodium channel, whereas the hypokalaemic form is caused by a mutation affecting the skeletal muscle calcium channel.

Hypokalaemic periodic paralysis

Attacks usually start during the second decade of life and then vary in frequency from daily to years between episodes. Weakness may be present on waking or develop during the day, typically in response to a heavy carbohydrate meal or during rest after strenuous exercise. The weakness involves the legs more than the arms, proximal muscles more than distal, and may be asymmetrical. Bulbar and respiratory muscle weakness is rare. Attacks last from hours to several days. The tendon reflexes may be depressed or lost during an attack. Permanent and progressive proximal weakness often develop by middle age. The serum potassium level typically falls during an attack, but not necessarily outside the normal range.

The disorder is caused by a mutation in the *CACNA1S* gene (on chromosome 1) encoding the DHPR component of the skeletal muscle calcium channel. The DHPR is located within the transverse tubular system, and acts as a voltage sensor for the RYR1 component of the calcium channel, which is located in the sarcoplasmic reticulum and is responsible for triggering calcium release and thus muscle contraction. Different mutations in the same gene, and mutations in the *RYR1* gene, are associated with malignant hyperthermia (see below).

Acetazolamide is the treatment of choice to prevent attacks. Acute attacks respond to oral potassium, given as an unsweetened aqueous solution.

Apparently identical attacks may occur in association with thyrotoxicosis and resolve when the patient is rendered euthyroid.

Hyperkalaemic periodic paralysis

Attacks tend to start at an earlier age than in the hypokalaemic form, and do not last as long. Precipitants include cold, fasting, rest after exercise, pregnancy, alcohol intake, and potassium loading. Readily utilized carbohydrate sources, such as a sweet drink, may abort an attack. A progressive proximal myopathy may also develop. Myotonia is present in some patients (see below). The serum potassium level may rise during an attack, but the change is often slight.

The underlying abnormality is a mutation within the *SCNA4* gene (on chromosome 17) encoding the α-subunit of the skeletal muscle sodium channel.

Mild attacks respond to carbohydrate ingestion. Kaliuretic diuretics usually prevent attacks.

Paramyotonia congenita

Paramyotonia congenita describes a dominantly inherited condition characterized by cold-induced weakness and muscle stiffness (paramyotonia), which is sometimes accompanied by periodic paralysis. The relationship between this disorder and primary hyperkalaemic periodic paralysis had been much debated, but recent evidence has shown that hyperkalaemic periodic paralysis, hyperkalaemic periodic paralysis with myotonia, paramyotonia congenita, and paramyotonia congenita with periodic paralysis are allelic disorders involving the *SCNA4* gene (on chromosome 17) encoding the α-subunit of the skeletal muscle sodium channel.

Myotonia congenita

Autosomal dominant (Thomsen's disease) and recessive (Becker-type) forms of this condition are recognized, with the recessive type being much more common. Onset tends to be earlier in the dominant form but both usually become apparent in childhood. There is muscle stiffness, worse after rest and exacerbated by cold, minimal or no weakness, readily demonstrable percussion myotonia, and muscle hypertrophy, which tends to be more marked in the recessive form.

Both the recessive and dominant forms are caused by mutations in the *CLCN1* gene (on chromosome 7) encoding the skeletal muscle chloride channel.

Malignant hyperthermia

The main features of this autosomal dominant disorder are a rapidly rising body temperature and generalized muscular rigidity during anaesthesia. Additional features include skin mottling, cyanosis, tachypnoea, tachycardia, cardiac dysrhythmias, and autonomic instability. Attacks in susceptible individuals may be triggered by suxamethonium and anaesthetic agents (halothane, cyclopropane, enflurane, ketamine). A similar, but probably different, disorder may be associated with heavy exercise in very hot conditions (e.g. recruits undergoing route marches on mountains during a hot summer).

Attacks are life threatening. Treatment consists of withdrawing the offending agent and providing general supportive measures and intravenous dantrolene 2 mg/kg body weight.

Disturbed calcium homeostasis underlies the attacks, with excessive Ca^{2+} influx into the sarcoplasmic reticulum. The disorder is genetically heterogeneous. In many families the underlying abnormality affects the skeletal muscle calcium channel with a mutation in either the *RYR1* gene (on chromosome 19) or the *CACNA1S* gene (on chromosome 1). *RYR1* mutations may also cause central core disease (CCD)—CCD and MH are allelic disorders and may occur together in the same individual or independently. Other *CACNA1S* gene mutations cause hypokalaemic periodic paralysis.

Screening for MH susceptibility involves muscle biopsy and *in vitro* testing for a reduced contractile threshold to halothane and caffeine. It is hoped that specific molecular biological tests will become available. A significant practical problem is the management of family members who fear that they may be at risk. As with those patients who have suffered hyperpyrexia under anaesthesia (even in those in whom repeated exposure has not led to a consistent reoccurrence), it is advisable for those individuals of proven or suspected risk to wear, at all times, some form of bracelet or locket giving details of the risk, in case they are casualties in an emergency such as a road accident.

Myoglobinuria

This important symptom and sign must be differentiated from haematuria and haemoglobinuria. Red cells are visible on microscopy in the former but not in the latter. In all three conditions, the haemoperoxidase stick test is positive.

Myoglobin is a protein that acts as an oxygen store within skeletal muscle fibres. Myoglobinuria causes a dark-brown/red discoloration of the urine, the main concern being that the protein can cause renal tubular necrosis and thus renal failure. Numerous disorders are known to be associated with myoglobinuria (Table 24.24.4.3). In the metabolic disorders, the presumed mechanism is failure of substrate utilization or supply when energy demands increase during exercise or starvation. In other disorders, there is disruption of

Table 24.24.4.3 Causes of myoglobinuria

Metabolic	Glycogenoses
	Carnitine palmitoyl transferase deficiency
	Severe electrolyte disturbance
Excessive activity/ temperature	Marathon running
	Military training
	Status epilepticus
	Malignant hyperthermia
	Neuroleptic malignant syndrome
Drugs and toxins	Several drugs (see Table 24.24.4.2)
	Venoms and animal toxins
Infection	Viral
	Toxic shock
	Clostridial infection/gangrene
Ischaemia and trauma	Crush
	Coma
	Any cause of severe ischaemia
	Compartment syndrome
	Electric shock
Inflammatory myopathies	Dermatomyositis
	Polymyositis

the plasma membrane. Apparently idiopathic cases are probably due to an unidentified metabolic defect or infection.

Rhabdomyolysis is considered further in Section 28.

Further reading

Brini M (2004). Ryanodine receptor defects in muscle genetic diseases. *Biochem Biophys Res Commun*, **322**, 1245–55.

Christopher-Stine L (2006). Statin-myopathy: an update. *Curr Opin Rheumatol*, **18**, 647–53.

Engel AG, Franzini-Armstrong C, eds (2004). *Myology*, 3rd edition. McGraw-Hill, New York.

Hanna M. (2006). Genetic neurological channelopathies. *Nature Clin Pract Neurol*, **2**, 252–63.

Karpati G, Hilton-Jones D, Griggs R (eds) (2001). *Disorders of voluntary muscle*, 7th edition. Cambridge University Press, Cambridge.

Mastaglia F (2006). Drug induced myopathies. *Pract Neurol*, **6**, 4–13.

Mastaglia F, Hilton-Jones D (2007). *Handbook of neurology—myopathies*. Elsevier, Amsterdam.

Wagenmakers AJM, Coakley JH, Edwards RHT (1988). The metabolic consequences of reduced habitual activities in patients with muscle pain and disease. *Ergonomics*, **31**, 1519–27.

World Health Organization (1980). *International classification of impairments, disabilities, and handicaps*. WHO, Geneva.

World Health Organization (2000). *International classification of functioning and disability ICIDH-2*. WHO, Geneva. http://www3.who.int/icf/icftemplate.

24.24.5 Mitochondrial encephalomyopathies

P.F. Chinnery and D.M. Turnbull

Essentials

Mitochondrial encephalomyopathies are caused by primary defects in the respiratory chain that lead to disturbed generation of ATP by aerobic metabolism, which characteristically impairs the function of high-demand tissues such as the brain, eye, cardiac and skeletal muscle, as well as endocrine organs. The numerous proteins involved in this chain are encoded by genes in mitochondrial or nuclear DNA, mutations in many of which can lead to clinical disorders.

Clinical features

The clinical presentations of mitochondrial encephalomyopathies are highly variable: the same clinical syndrome can be caused by different genetic defects, and the same genetic defect may present in a variety of different ways. Several characteristic syndromes are described, including those produced by the following:

Large-scale single deletions of mitochondrial genome—typically cause progressive ophthalmoplegia and ptosis, and limb muscles may be affected; can also cause an extended phenotype of cerebellar ataxia, pigmentary retinopathy, sensorineural deafness, diabetes mellitus and heart block (Kearns–Sayre syndrome).

Pearson's syndrome—pancreatic exocrine failure and hypoplastic bone marrow with sideroblastic anaemia in infancy; survivors may develop features of Kearns–Saye syndrome. Point mutations in the mitochondrial genome—may be present in adult life and are the major cause of visual loss in young adult males (Leber's hereditary optic neuropathy). Other syndromes include Leigh's syndrome—subacute necrotizing encephalomyopathy, with characteristic lesions in basal ganglia, cerebellum, and brainstem.

Nuclear genetic mutations with autosomal recessive inheritance—typically present in infants and children.

Investigation and treatment

Investigation—aside from general investigations to characterize the pattern and nature of organ involvement, the diagnostic strategy depends on the clinical context: (1) Inherited cases—in many patients it is possible to identify a specific clinical syndrome with a clear maternal family history suggestive of a mitochondrially inherited disorder. Under these circumstances it is appropriate (after counselling) to proceed directly to molecular genetic testing. (2) Sporadic cases—the key investigation is muscle biopsy for biochemical studies of oxidative phosphorylation, leading on to targeted molecular analysis of suitable samples of mitochondrial and nuclear DNA.

Treatment—there is no definitive treatment for patients with mitochondrial disease, except for those with deficiency of coenzyme Q_{10}. Management is aimed at minimizing disability, preventing complications, and genetic counselling. Multidisciplinary expertise is needed to provide adequate nutrition and physiotherapy, and to address endocrinological, cardiac and ophthalmic complications.

Introduction

Mitochondria are ubiquitous intracellular organelles that are involved in many different metabolic pathways. Disorders of intermediary metabolism (such as fatty acid β-oxidation or tricarboxylic acid cycle defects) involve mitochondrial enzymes, but the term 'mitochondrial encephalomyopathy' usually means a disease which is due to an abnormality of the final common pathway of energy metabolism—the mitochondrial respiratory chain, which is linked to the production of ATP by oxidative phosphorylation (OXPHOS). The respiratory chain is essential for aerobic metabolism, and respiratory chain defects characteristically affect tissues and organs that are heavily dependent upon oxidative metabolism (such as the central nervous system, the eye, skeletal muscle, myocardium, and endocrine organs).

Recent studies have demonstrated the central role of the mitochondrion in the pathophysiology of well-established diseases such as Friedreich's ataxia and Wilson's disease, and mitochondrial abnormalities have been described in common sporadic disorders including idiopathic Parkinson's disease, but these are not primarily disorders of the mitochondrial respiratory chain and are not considered further here.

Biochemistry and genetics of the respiratory chain

The intermediary metabolism of carbohydrates, amino acids, and fatty acids generates the reduced cofactors NADH, NADPH, and $FADH_2$. These cofactors transfer electrons to the mitochondrial respiratory chain. As the electrons are passed through complexes I to IV of the respiratory chain along the inner mitochondrial membrane, protons are pumped out of the mitochondrial matrix into the intermembrane space. This creates an electrochemical gradient that is harnessed by complex V (ATP synthase) to generate ATP from ADP. Each respiratory chain complex contains many polypeptide subunits, some of which are coded by genes within the nucleus and some of which are encoded by the mitochondrial genome. Although all of the polypeptides encoded in mitochondrial DNA (mtDNA) have been known for over two decades, many nuclear genes involved in mitochondrial biogenesis have yet to be characterized in detail.

The mitochondrial genome encodes seven complex I subunits (NADH-ubiquinone oxidoreductase), one of the complex III subunits (ubiquinol-cytochrome c oxidoreductase), three of the complex IV (cytochrome c oxidase) subunits, and the ATPase 6 and ATPase 8 subunits of complex V. Interspaced between the protein-encoding genes are two ribosomal RNA genes (12S and 16S rRNA), and 22 transfer RNA genes that provide the necessary RNA components for the mitochondrial translation machinery. The remaining polypeptides, including all of the complex II subunits, are synthesized from nuclear gene transcripts within the cytosol. These are subsequently imported into the mitochondria through the inner and outer membrane translocation complexes. There are many additional proteins that are essential for the normal assembly and function of the mitochondrial respiratory chain. As a result, mitochondrial respiratory chain disorders can be due to mutations affecting both nuclear and mitochondrial genes.

The classification and investigation of mitochondrial respiratory chain disorders has been revolutionized by the recent advances in our understanding of the underlying genetic defects affecting both mtDNA and nuclear DNA (Table 24.24.5.1).

Table 24.24.5.1 Genetic basis of mitochondrial encephalomyopathies

Nuclear DNA defects

Nuclear genetic disorders of the mitochondrial respiratory chain, mutations in structural subunits

	Leigh's syndrome (complex I deficiency—mutations in *NDUFS1, NDUFS4, NDUFS7, NDUFS8, NDUFV1*. Complex II deficiency, *SDHA*)
	Cardiomyopathy and encephalopathy (complex I deficiency, mutations in *NDUFS2*)
	Optic atrophy and ataxia (complex II deficiency—mutations in *SDHA*)
	Hypokalaemia and lactic acidosis (complex III, mutations in *UQCRB*)

Nuclear genetic disorders of the mitochondrial respiratory chain, mutations in assembly factors:

	Leigh's syndrome (mutations in *SURF I* and *LRPPRC*)
	Hepatopathy and ketoacidosis (mutations in *SCO1*)
	Cardiomyopathy and encephalopathy (mutations in *SCO2*)
	Leucodystrophy and renal tubulopathy (mutations in *COX10*)
	Hypertrophic cardiomyopathy (mutations in *COX15*)
	Encephalopathy, liver failure, renal tubulopathy (with complex III deficiency, mutations in *BCS1L*)
	Encephalopathy (with complex V deficiency, mutations in *ATP12*)

Nuclear genetic disorders of the mitochondrial respiratory chain, mutations in translation factors:

	Leigh's syndrome, Liver failure and lactic acidosis (mutations in *EFG1*)
	Lactic acidosis, developmental failure and dysmophism (mutations in *MRPS16*)
	Myopathy and sideroblastic anemia (mutations in *PUS1*)
	Leukodystrophy and polymicrogyria (mutations in *EFTu*)

Nuclear genetic disorders associated with multiple mtDNA deletions or mtDNA depletion:

	Autosomal progressive external ophthalmoplegia (mutations in *POLG, POLG2, PEO1* and *SLC25A4*)
	Mitochondrial neurogastrointestinal encephalomyopathy (thymidine phosphorylase deficiency—mutations in *TP*)
	Alpers-Huttenlocher syndrome (mutations in *POLG* and *MPV*)

Disorders of the lipid mileu

Co-enzyme Q$_{10}$ deficiency (mutations in *COQ2*)—new genetic defects now described from Hirano *et al.*

Barth syndrome (mutations in *TAZ*)

Mitochondrial DNA defects

Rearrangements (deletions and duplications):

	Chronic progressive external ophthalmoplegia
	Kearns–Sayre syndrome
	Diabetes and deafness

Table 24.24.5.1 *(Cont'd)* Genetic basis of mitochondrial encephalomyopathies

Point mutations:[a]

Protein-encoding genes	Leber's hereditary optic neuropathy (G11778A, T14484C, G3460A)
	Neurogenic weakness with ataxia and retinitis pigmentosa/Leigh's syndrome (T8993G/C)
tRNA genes	MELAS (A3243G, T3271C, A3251G)
	MERRF (A8344G, T8356C)
	Chronic progressive external ophthalmoplegia (A3243G, T4274C)
	Myopathy (T14709C, A12320G)
	Cardiomyopathy (A3243G, A4269G)
	Diabetes and deafness (A3243G, C12258A)
	Encephalomyopathy (G1606A, T10010C)
rRNA genes	Non-syndromic sensorineural deafness (A7445G)
	Aminoglycoside-induced non-syndromic deafness (A1555G)

*mtDNA nucleotide positions refer to the L-chain. Many different pathogenic point mutations of the mitochondrial genome have been identified with only the most common or best characterized mentioned here.

Basic mitochondrial genetics

There are two main differences between nuclear DNA and mtDNA that are important for the expression and transmission of mitochondrial genetic disease, as follows.

Heteroplasmy and the threshold effect

Each mammalian cell contains over 1000 copies of the small (16.5 kb) mitochondrial genome. Individuals with mtDNA disease often harbour a mixture of mutated and wild-type (normal) mtDNA—a situation known as heteroplasmy. Single cells only express a respiratory chain defect when the proportion of mutated mtDNA exceeds a critical threshold with low levels of wild type mtDNA. Different organs, and even adjacent cells within the same organ, may contain different amounts of mutated mtDNA. This variability, coupled with tissue-specific differences in the threshold and the varied dependence of different organs on oxidative metabolism, explains in part why certain tissues are preferentially affected in patients with mtDNA disease. In general, postmitotic (nondividing) tissues such as neurons, skeletal and cardiac muscle, and endocrine organs harbour much higher levels of mutated mtDNA and are often clinically involved. In contrast, rapidly dividing tissues such as the bone marrow are only rarely clinically affected (one example is Pearson's syndrome—see below).

Maternal inheritance and the transmission of heteroplasmy

After fertilization of the oocyte, sperm mtDNA is actively degraded. As a consequence, mtDNA is transmitted exclusively down the maternal line. This means that affected males with mtDNA disease cannot transmit the genetic defect. Deleted molecules are rarely, if ever, transmitted from clinically affected females to their offspring.

By contrast, a female harbouring a heteroplasmic mtDNA point mutation, or mtDNA duplications, may transmit a variable amount of mutated mtDNA to her children. Early during development of the female germ line, the number of mtDNA molecules within each oocyte is reduced before being subsequently amplified to reach a final number of more than 100 000 in each mature oocyte. This restriction and amplification (also called the mitochondrial 'genetic bottleneck') contributes to the variability between individual oocytes, and the different levels of mutant mtDNA seen in the offspring of a single female.

Clinical presentation of respiratory chain disorders

Mitochondrial encephalomyopathies are highly variable both clinically and at the genetic level. The same clinical syndrome can be caused by different genetic defects (which may be within nuclear or mitochondrial genes), but the same genetic defect may present in a variety of different ways. In general, adults who present with mitochondrial disease are often found to have a defect of mtDNA. Children often present with different clinical features and are more likely to have a nuclear genetic defect. It is often possible to identify well-defined clinical syndromes, but many patients present with a collection of clinical features that are highly suggestive of respiratory chain disease but do not fit into a discrete clinical category.

Defined clinical syndromes (Table 24.24.5.2)

Large-scale deletions can cause chronic progressive external ophthalmoplegia and bilateral ptosis (PEO). Some of these patients have limited limb muscle involvement. In contrast, similar deletions may also cause chronic progressive external ophthalmoplegia with bilateral sensorineural deafness, cerebellar ataxia, pigmentary retinopathy, diabetes mellitus, and cardiac conduction defects leading to complete heart block. When this begins in teenage years and is associated with a raised cerebrospinal fluid protein, it is called the Kearns–Sayre syndrome (KSS), which is a progressive neurological disorder associated with severe disability. Hypoparathyroidism and hypothyroidism are well-recognized features of KSS. The vast majority of cases of chronic PEO and KSS. These two syndromes are the extremes of a spectrum of disease and many individuals lie somewhere between the pure extraocular muscle and severe central neurological phenotypes.

Pearson's syndrome of exocrine pancreatic failure, sideroblastic anaemia, and marrow panhypoplasia is usually due to a mtDNA deletion. Pearson's syndrome also presents in infancy and a number of individuals who have survived into later childhood subsequently developed the Kearns–Sayre phenotype.

Although many patients with PEO and KSS are sporadic cases, PEO can also be inherited as either an autosomal dominant (adPEO) or recessive (arPEO) trait. A high incidence of psychiatric disease, a parkinsonian syndrome, and primary gonadal failure have also been documented in some families. Some cases have a profound peripheral neuropathy and ataxia (referred to as SANDO, sensory ataxic neuropathy with dysarthria and ophthalmoparesis), and some family members present with adult-onset ataxia without ophthalmoplegia (also called mitochondrial recessive ataxia syndrome, MIRAS) which is common in Scandinavia. Mutations in the gene encoding the mitochondrial polymerase (polγ, encoded by the nuclear gene POLG) are a major cause of adPEO and arPEO.

Table 24.24.5.2 Clinical syndromes

Disorder	Primary features	Additional features
Alpers–Huttenlocher syndrome	Encephalopathy with seizures	Developmental delay
	Liver failure	Hypotonia
Chronic progressive external ophthalmoplegia	External ophthalmoplegia and bilateral ptosis	Proximal myopathy
Kearns–Sayre syndrome	Progressive external ophthalmoplegia onset before age 20 with pigmentary retinopathy, plus one of the following: Cerebrospinal fluid protein >1 g/litre, cerebellar ataxia, or heart block	Bilateral deafness Myopathy Dysphagia Diabetes mellitus Hypoparathyroidism Dementia
Pearson's syndrome	Sideroblastic anaemia of childhood Pancytopenia Exocrine pancreatic failure	Renal tubular defects
Mitochondrial encephalomyopathy with lactic acidosis and stroke-like episodes (MELAS)	Stroke-like episodes before age 40 years Seizures and/or dementia Lactic acidosis Myopathy	Diabetes mellitus Cardiomyopathy (hypertrophic leading to dilated) Bilateral deafness Cerebellar ataxia
Mitochondrial neurogastrointestinal encephalomyopathy (MNGIE)	Gastrointestinal pseudo-obstruction Myopathy Leukoencephalopathy Peripheral neuropathy	
Myoclonic epilepsy with ragged-red fibres (MERRF)	Myoclonus Seizures Cerebellar ataxia Myopathy	Dementia Optic atrophy Bilateral deafness Peripheral neuropathy Spasticity Multiple lipomas
Leber's hereditary optic neuropathy	Subacute bilateral visual failure Males:females approximately 4:1 Median age of onset 24 years	Dystonia Cardiac pre-excitation syndromes
Leigh's syndrome	Subacute relapsing encephalopathy with cerebellar and brainstem signs	Basal ganglia lucencies
Infantile myopathy and lactic acidosis (fatal and nonfatal forms)	Hypotonia in the first year of life Feeding and respiratory difficulties	Fatal form may be associated with a cardiomyopathy and/or the Toni–Fanconi–Debre syndrome

adPEO can also be caused by mutations in PEO1 (which codes for the mtDNA helicase Twinkle), SLC25A4 (which codes for the adenine nucleotide translocase ANT1), and POLG2 (which codes for the accessory subunit of polγ).

Pathogenic point mutations of mtDNA are more common than rearrangements. This is partly because mtDNA deletions cause sporadic disease, whereas many mtDNA point mutations are transmitted down the maternal line. The m.3243A>G mutation in the leucine (UUR) tRNA gene was first described in a patient with mitochondrial encephalomyopathy with lactic acidosis and stroke-like episodes (MELAS). Different families harbouring the same genetic defect may have different phenotypes. For example, some families harbouring m.3243A>G have predominantly diabetes and deafness, some have chronic progressive external ophthalmoplegia, and some present with hypertrophic cardiomyopathy. It is currently not known why this is the case but it is likely that additional nuclear genetic factors play an important role in modifying the expression of the primary mtDNA defect. This single mutation is important since it has been estimated that between 0.5 and 1.5% of cases of diabetes mellitus in the general population are associated with the m.3243A>G mutation.

Patients may present with myoclonic epilepsy, ataxia, optic atrophy, and have ragged-red fibres in skeletal muscle (MERRF) and this may also be due to a point mutation of mtDNA (e.g. A8344G).

mtDNA mutations are the major cause of visual loss in young adult males. About one-half of all males who harbour one of three point mutations of mtDNA (m.11778G>A, m.14484T>C, m.3460G>A) develop bilateral sequential visual loss in the second or third decade—a disorder known as Leber hereditary optic neuropathy (LHON). The majority of individuals with these mutations are homoplasmic, harbouring only mutated mtDNA. It is not clear why the disease only affects approximately one-half of the males and 10% of females who inherit the primary mtDNA defect. Environmental factors, such as alcohol and tobacco, may explain the variable penetrance of this disorder; however, additional, as yet unknown, nuclear genetic factors may also be important in modulating the phenotype.

Leigh's syndrome (subacute necrotizing encephalomyopathy) is a relapsing encephalopathy with prominent cerebellar and brainstem signs that usually presents in childhood and is associated with characteristic neuroimaging abnormalities involving the basal ganglia. Leigh's syndrome can be due to an X-linked pyruvate dehydrogenase deficiency or a defect of the mitochondrial respiratory chain. Complex I deficiency or cytochrome c oxidase deficiency are common findings in Leigh's syndrome. In these patients it may be possible to identify recessive mutations in nuclear complex I genes, or genes involved in the assembly of the respiratory chain complexes (for example *SURF1*). Point mutations at position m.8993 in the ATPase 6 gene of mtDNA may cause neurogenic weakness with ataxia and retinitis pigmentosa. These particular mutations are also associated with some forms of childhood Leigh's syndrome.

Alpers–Huttenlocher syndrome is a severe autosomal recessive hepatoencephalopathy with intractable seizures and visual failure which presents in early childhood and is associated with depletion (loss) of mtDNA in affected tissues. Mutations in *POLG* are a major cause of Alpers–Huttenlocher syndrome, and mutations in *MPV* also cause liver disease. Other causes of mtDNA depletion include mutations in *TK2* (encoding thymine kinase) which presents with a progressive childhood myopathy or spinal muscular atrophy, *DGUOK* (encoding dexyguanosine kinase) which presents in childhood with a myopathy and liver failure, and *SUCLA2* (coding for ADP-forming succinyl-CoA synthase) which presents in early childhood with an encephalomyopathy.

Cytochrome c oxidase deficiency may also present in childhood with an infantile myopathy and a severe lactic acidosis, which may

also be associated with a cardiomyopathy and the Toni–Fanconi–Debre syndrome. Despite maximal supportive intervention, this is usually a fatal disorder and a severe depletion of mtDNA occurs in a proportion of these cases. It is important to recognize that isolated myopathy and lactic acidosis may be self-limiting, often with a significant improvement by 1 year of age and complete resolution by the age of 3 years.

Coenzyme Q_{10} deficiency can present in childhood with recurrent myoglobinuria, myopathy and seizures. In some families it presents with an infantile encephalomyopathy with renal tubular defects. Finally, it may also present with ataxia and variable involvement of other regions of the central nervous system, peripheral nerve, and muscle. Mutations in genes coding for enzymes involved in the biosynthesis of coenzyme Q_{10} have been found in some families.

Nonspecific clinical presentations

The foregoing diseases and numerous other syndromes may strongly suggest a mitochondrial aetiology (Fig. 24.24.5.1 and Table 24.24.5.2), many patients do not present with a characteristic phenotype. Children may present in the neonatal period with a metabolic encephalopathy and systemic lactic acidosis, often associated with hepatic and cardiac failure. This may be associated with depletion in the total amount of mtDNA within affected tissues (see above). This syndrome may be fatal, and in some the liver failure is precipitated by exposure to Sodium Valproate, but it may also be a self-limiting disorder. Childhood presentations may be even less specific, with neonatal hypotonia, feeding and respiratory difficulties, and failure to thrive. A respiratory chain defect should be considered in any patient who has a disease with multiple organ involvement, particularly if there are central neurological features (such as seizures and dementia), a myopathy, cardiomyopathy, and endocrine abnormalities such as diabetes mellitus (Fig. 24.24.5.1). Bilateral sensorineural deafness and ocular features (retinopathy, optic atrophy, ptosis, and ophthalmoparesis) are common. Renal tubular defects, gastrointestinal hypomotility, cervical lipomatosis, and psychiatric features are also well described in patients with respiratory chain disease.

Investigation of respiratory chain disease

The investigation of patients with a suspected mitochondrial encephalomyopathy involves the careful assimilation of clinical and laboratory data. In a significant proportion of cases (such as Leber's hereditary optic neuropathy), it is possible to identify a specific clinical syndrome with a clear maternal family history. Under these circumstances it is appropriate to carry out a molecular genetic test on a blood sample. In many situations, particularly in sporadic cases, this is not appropriate because the clinical features overlap with those of many other disorders. Even if the patient has a mitochondrial disorder, numerous different genetic defects may be responsible, some of which will not be detectable by analysis of blood samples.

Investigations fall into two main groups: clinical investigations used to characterize the pattern and nature of the different organs involved, and specific investigations to identify the biochemical or genetic abnormality.

General clinical investigations

It is essential to search for the more common features of respiratory chain disease, especially those which are potentially treatable. This includes cardiac assessment (ECG and echocardiography) and

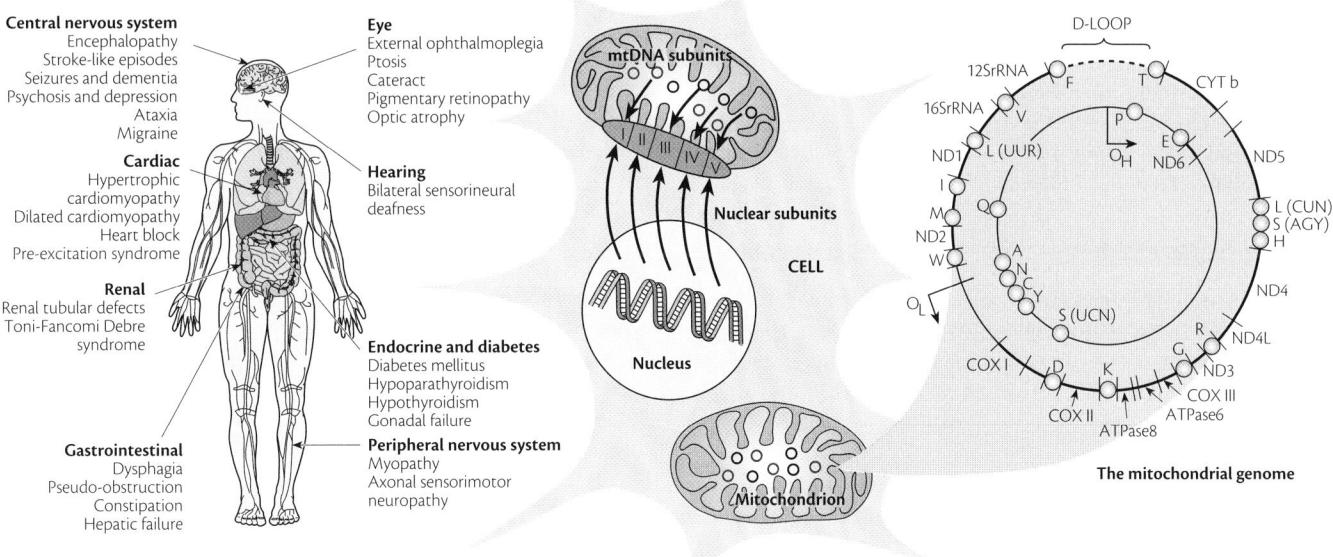

Fig. 24.24.5.1 The clinical features and biochemical and molecular genetic basis of mitochondrial encephalomyopathies.

endocrine assessment (oral glucose tolerance test, thyroid function tests, alkaline phosphatase, fasting calcium, and parathyroid hormone levels). The organic and amino acids in urine may be abnormal even in the absence of overt tubular disease. Measuring blood and cerebrospinal fluid lactate levels is more helpful in the investigation of children than adults. These measurements must be interpreted with caution because there are many causes of blood and cerebrospinal fluid lactic acidosis, including fever, sepsis, dehydration, seizures, and stroke. The cerebrospinal fluid protein may be elevated. The serum creatine kinase level may be raised but is often normal. Neurophysiological studies may identify a myopathy or neuropathy. Electroencephalography may reveal diffuse slow-wave activity consistent with a subacute encephalopathy, or evidence of seizure activity. Cerebral imaging may be abnormal, showing lesions of the basal ganglia, high signal in the white matter on MRI, or generalized cerebral atrophy.

Specific investigations

A skeletal muscle biopsy is invaluable in the investigation of respiratory chain disease. Histochemical and biochemical investigations, in conjunction with the clinical assessment, often indicate where the underlying genetic abnormality must lie.

Histochemistry and biochemistry

Histochemical analysis may reveal subsarcolemmal accumulation of mitochondria (so-called 'ragged red' fibres), or cytochrome *c* oxidase deficiency. A mosaic of cytochrome *c* oxidase-positive and cytochrome *c* oxidase-negative muscle fibres suggests an underlying primary mtDNA defect or a secondary defect of mtDNA as seen in patients with *POLG* mutations. Patients who have cytochrome *c* oxidase deficiency due to a nuclear genetic defect usually have a global deficiency of this enzyme affecting all muscle fibres. Electron microscopy may identify paracrystalline inclusions in the intermembrane space, but these are non-specific and may be seen in other nonmitochondrial disorders. Respiratory chain complex assays can be carried out on various tissues. Skeletal muscle or affected tissue is preferable, but cultured fibroblasts are useful in

the investigation of childhood mitochondrial disease. Measurement of the individual respiratory chain complexes determines whether an individual has multiple complex defects that would suggest an underlying mtDNA defect, involving either a tRNA gene or a large deletion. Isolated complex defects may be due to mutations in either mitochondrial or nuclear genes. Co-enzyme Q_{10} can be measured directly in affected tissues.

Molecular genetic investigations

Under certain circumstances, the clinical and biochemical features may point towards a specific genetic defect, and it may be possible to detect this abnormality in a blood sample. Children presenting with Leigh's syndrome and who have an isolated deficiency of one of the respiratory chain subunits may have a point mutation within the nuclear-encoded respiratory chain subunit or assembly genes. These have been identified by direct sequencing of the appropriate exons.

For some mtDNA defects (particularly mtDNA deletions) the abnormality is not detectable in a DNA sample extracted from blood, and the analysis of DNA extracted from muscle is essential to establish the diagnosis. The first stage is to look for mtDNA rearrangements or mtDNA depletion by long-range polymerase chain reaction (PCR) or real-time PCR. This is followed by PCR and restriction fragment length polymorphism (RFLP) analysis for common point mutations. Many patients with mitochondrial disease have a previously unrecognized mtDNA defect and it is necessary to sequence directly the mitochondrial genome. Interpretation of the sequence data can be extremely difficult. mtDNA is highly polymorphic and any two normal individuals may differ by up to 60 base pairs. In the strictest sense, a mutation can only be considered to be pathogenic if it has arisen independently several times in the population, it is not seen in controls, and it is associated with a potential disease mechanism. These stringent criteria depend upon a good knowledge of polymorphic sites in the background population. If a novel base change is heteroplasmic, this suggests that it is of relatively recent onset. Family, tissue segregation, and single cell studies may show that higher levels of the mutation are associated with mitochondrial dysfunction and disease, which strongly suggests that the mutation is causing the disease. Specific nuclear genes (e.g. *POLG*) are usually sequenced after initial mtDNA analysis identifies a secondary defect of mtDNA (multiple deletions or depletion). Although there may be a corresponding histochemical or biochemical defect, this may not be detectable in readily available tissues.

Management

There is currently no definitive treatment for patients with mitochondrial disease, except for patients with deficiency of coenzyme Q_{10}. Management is aimed at minimizing disability, preventing complications, and genetic counselling.

Supportive care and surveillance

Many patients with mitochondrial disorders require follow-up over many decades. An integrated approach is essential involving the primary physician, other specialist physicians (ophthalmology, diabetes, and cardiology), specialist nurses, physiotherapists, and speech therapists. Vigilant clinical monitoring over many years can prevent the development of complications, such as those secondary to cardiac and endocrine involvement. Specific procedures may be indicated at various stages of disease. These include cardiac pacing, ptosis correction, cataract surgery, and percutaneous gastrostomy.

Genetic counselling

The detailed investigation of patients with respiratory chain disease usually leads to a specific molecular genetic diagnosis, particularly in adults. This has profound implications on the counselling given to patients and their families. Most children with respiratory chain disease are compound heterozygotes with recessive nuclear gene mutations. Some adults have a recessive disorder, or adPEO. If it is possible to identify the causative mutations in both the offspring and parents, then this will allow confident genetic counselling for the whole family. If, as in many cases, it is not possible to identify the underlying gene defect, or the genetic defect in the affected child cannot be traced back to the parents, then counselling is less straightforward. The clinical penetrance of many recently identified nuclear gene defects has yet to be established, generating considerable uncertainty when counselling families

If a causative primary mtDNA defect is identified, then the implications for counselling are distinctly different. Males cannot transmit pathogenic mtDNA defects. Patients who carry mtDNA deletions rarely have a family history suggestive of mtDNA disease, and there is no significant risk that they will transmit the mtDNA defect to any offspring. There are a few rare exceptions to this rule where the propensity to develop mtDNA deletions is transmitted as an autosomal dominant or autosomal recessive trait. By contrast, women harbouring pathogenic mtDNA point mutations may transmit the genetic defect to their offspring. The mitochondrial genetic 'bottleneck' leads to a variation in the proportion of mutated mtDNA that is transmitted to any offspring (see above). It is therefore possible for a female to have mildly affected as well as severely affected children. The risk of having affected offspring varies from mutation to mutation, and although there does appear to be a relationship between the level of mutated mtDNA in the mother and the risk of affected offspring, there are insufficient data from prospective studies to allow accurate risk prediction.

Prognosis

In general the prognosis depends upon the extent of central neurological involvement. Patients with Leber's hereditary optic neuropathy rarely have significant central neurological features and have a normal lifespan. The prospect for visual recovery varies. After the initial nadir, individuals harbouring the m.11778G>A mutation are the least likely to regain functional vision, whilst those harbouring the m.14484T>C mutation are the most likely to regain their sight.

Children presenting with an encephalopathy have a poor prognosis. Although residual neurological deficits are common after repeated childhood encephalopathic episodes, the disease may enter a more stable 'chronic' phase during teenage years and adulthood. A similar course may be seen in adults presenting with a relapsing encephalopathy. In contrast, a large proportion of adults with mtDNA defects and chronic progressive external ophthalmoplegia have very mild disease that may remain limited to the extraocular muscles for many decades. For specific mtDNA mutations, there also appears to be a relationship between the proportion of mutated mtDNA in skeletal muscle and the severity of the disease. Although the proportion of mutated mtDNA in muscle may give some guide to prognosis, there is insufficient information available to allow accurate prognostic counselling based upon these determinations. A significant proportion of patients have distinct phenotypes associated with unique genetic defects and the prognosis must be guarded in these families. There is limited natural history data for nuclear genetic disorders based on retrospective notes review (e.g. for specific *POLG* mutations).

Pharmacological treatments and novel approaches under development

Standard doses of vitamin C and K, thiamine, riboflavin, and ubiquinone (coenzyme Q_{10}) may be of some benefit, particularly in patients with isolated Q_{10} deficiency. These treatments have no significant side effects and are relatively cheap, but their efficacy is largely based on anecdotal reports. Dichloracetate can be used to reduce lactic acid levels but may cause an irreversible toxic neuropathy and is therefore not favoured. Exercise is important for patients with mtDNA disease, and isometric muscle contraction may lead to an improvement in muscle strength. Finally, several centres are investigating methods for correcting the underlying mtDNA defect by gene therapy.

Further reading

Anderson S, *et al.* (1981). Sequence and organization of the human mitochondrial genome. *Nature*, **290**, 457–65.

Andrews RM, *et al.* (1999). Reanalysis and revision of the Cambridge Reference Sequence. *Nat Genet*, **23**, 147. [Benchmark reference sequences for normal human mtDNA.]

Brown DT, *et al.* (2006) Transmission of mitochondrial DNA disorders: possibilities for the future. *Lancet*, **368**, 87–9. [Discussion of the complexities of inheritance of mtDNA]

Chinnery PF, *et al.* (1998). MELAS and MERRF: the relationship between maternal mutation load and the frequency of clinically affected offspring. *Brain*, **121**, 1889–94. [First paper to show a relationship between maternal mutation load and the outcome of pregnancy.]

Harding AE, *et al.* (1995). Pedigree analysis in Leber hereditary optic neuropathy families with a pathogenic mtDNA mutation. *Am J Hum Genet*, **57**, 77–86. [Important paper summarizing the risks of blindness for the most common mutations causing Leber hereditary optic neuropathy.]

Horvath R, *et al.* (2006). Phenotypic spectrum associated with mutations of the mitochondrial polymerase gamma gene. *Brain*, **129**, 1674–84. [Description of a large cohort with mutations in the coding for the mitochondrial DNA polymerase.]

Hudson G, Chinnery PF (2006). Mitochondrial DNA polymerase-gamma and human disease. *Hum Mol Genet*, **15 Spec No 2**, R244–52. [Contemporary review of the clinical and molecular genetics of human diseases due to mutations in the gene coding for the mitochondrial DNA polymerase.]

Janssen RJ, *et al.* (2006). Mitochondrial complex I: structure, function and pathology. *J Inherit Metab Dis*, **29**, 499–515. [Review of the most common biochemical defect seen in patients with mitochondrial disease, especially children.]

Kaufmann P, *et al.* (2006) Dichloroacetate causes toxic neuropathy in MELAS: a randomized, controlled clinical trial. *Neurology*, **66**, 324–30. [Randomized controlled trial for the treatment of a mitochondrial disorder.]

Lightowlers RN, *et al.* (1997). Mammalian mitochondrial genetics: heredity, heteroplasmy and disease. *Trends Genet*, **13**, 450–5. [Discussion of the basic principles of mitochondrial genetics.]

Schapira AH (2006). Mitochondrial disease. *Lancet*, **368**, 70–82. [Review of the role of mitochondria in human disease, including the role of mitochondria in complex diseases and ageing.]

Smeitink J, van den Heuvel L (1999). Human miotochondrial complex I in health and disease. *Am J Hum Genet*, **64**, 1505–10. [Comprehensive review of nuclear complex I genes and human disease.]

Spinazzola A, *et al.* MPV17 encodes an inner mitochondrial membrane protein and is mutated in infantile hepatic mitochondrial DNA depletion. *Nat Genet*, **38**, 570–5. [State of the art approach to identifying a mtDNA depletion gene.]

Taylor RW, Turnbull DM. (2005) Mitochondrial DNA mutations in human disease. *Nat Rev Genet*, **6**, 389–402. [Review discussing the role of mtDNA mutations in disease.]

Zeviani M, Di Donato S. (2004) Mitochondrial disorders. *Brain*, **127**, 2153–72. [Comprehensive review of mitochondrial disease.]

24.24.6 Primary (tropical) pyomyositis

David A. Warrell

Essentials

Pyomyositis is a primary intramuscular abscess, not tracking from adjacent structures. Formerly a disease almost exclusively of tropical developing countries, it is now seen increasingly in patients in Western countries who have underlying diseases and immunosuppression, notably HIV infection.

Aetiology—transient bacteraemia may seed an abscess in a focal area of previously damaged muscle if there is immunocompromise. The predisposing vulnerability of apparently healthy younger people in the tropics is unexplained, but malnutrition and preceding arboviral or helminthic infections are postulated. *Staphylococcus aureus* accounts for 90% of tropical and 70% of nontropical cases.

Clinical features, investigation and treatment—pyomyositis may evolve through subacute, suppurative, and septicaemic phases over weeks or months. Early clinical evidence is local swelling and tenderness in a muscle, often with minimal systemic signs. Diagnosis is confirmed by imaging, ideally gadolinium-enhanced MRI. Treatment requires (1) drainage by open surgery or image-guided needle aspiration—whenever there is suppuration; (2) antibiotics—initial regimen must cover *S. aureus*, but should then be guided by culture findings.

Definition

The term 'pyomyositis' should be restricted to primary muscle abscesses arising within skeletal muscles. This condition must be distinguished from abscesses extending into muscle either from subcutaneous sites following infection through the skin, or from adjacent osteomyelitis, septic arthritis or suppuration originating in other tissues. Originally reported almost exclusively from tropical developing countries, hence 'tropical pyomyositis', it is now increasingly diagnosed in temperate developed countries in people with underlying medical conditions especially associated with immunosuppression.

Epidemiology

Pyomyositis has been reported from most parts of tropical Africa, Malaysia, Thailand, India, Indonesia, Oceania, Central and South America, and the Caribbean. In many of these countries it is common, accounting for 4% of admissions to a hospital in Uganda in the 1960s and for 2.2% of all surgical admissions to a hospital in eastern Ecuador in the 1990s. In temperate climates, pyomyositis has been reported increasingly since the 1970s and especially since the emergence of the HIV epidemic. It can occur at any age but is commoner in males. In the tropics, previously healthy people are infected and the peak incidence is in the second decade. In the United States of America, the mean age at diagnosis was 34 years (range 2 weeks to 92 years). Most of the patients had an underlying disease, such as diabetes mellitus, chronic liver disease, or immunosuppression.

Aetiology

Predisposition and pathogenesis

Some patients remember preceding trauma to the affected muscle. A muscle haematoma or tear from nonpenetrating trauma (even massage) or the stress of intense exertion, or an area of muscle damaged by myositis, might provide the nidus for blood-borne bacterial infection. Suggested predisposing causes for tropical pyomyositis include a viral infection (e.g. arbovirus), general debilitation/malnutrition, nematode infections such as toxocariasis, *Lagochilascaris minor*, *Oesophagostomum* spp. and filariae, and sickle cell disease. Most helminth-associated abscesses should not be termed 'pyomyositis' as they are inter- rather than intramuscular. For example, guinea worm *Dracunculus medinensis* (see Chapter 7.9.3) can cause deep intermuscular abscesses that become secondarily infected with *Staphylococcus aureus*. In Africa and South America, pyomyositis is relatively more common in indigenous peoples.

Underlying medical conditions predisposing to nontropical pyomyositis include diabetes mellitus, chronic liver disease, haematological and other malignancies under chemotherapy, rheumatic and autoimmune disorders treated with immunomodulating drugs, and intravenous drug abuse. HIV immunosuppressed patients become susceptible when their circulating CD4 count falls below $100/mm^3$. Increased carriage of *Staph. aureus*, neutropenia, defective neutrophil and cell-mediated immunity, presence of long term intravenous lines and underlying muscle damage caused by HIV or antiretroviral drugs may contribute to their risk.

Microbiology

Staph. aureus accounts for 90% of tropical and 70% of nontropical cases. In Western countries, community-acquired methicillin-resistant *S. aureus* (MRSA) is implicated. Those with Panton Valentine leukocidin genes may cause more severe disease. *Streptococcus pyogenes* (usually group A (but also groups B – *Strep. galactiae*, C and G) is responsible for a few cases, but tropical pyomyositis must be distinguished from streptococcal necrotizing myositis (also known as peracute streptococcal pyomyositis or spontaneous streptococcal gangrenous myositis) which is more fulminant and diffuse and has a very high mortality (see Chapter 7.6.2). Other isolates have included *Strep. pneumoniae*, *Haemophilus influenzae*, and mycobacteria. In Thailand, most cases of pyomyositis are caused by *Burkholderia pseudomallei*. In nontropical cases of pyomyositis, Gram-negative bacteria such as *Escherichia coli*, *Klebsiella pneumoniae*, pseudomonas, salmonella, and acinetobacter; anaerobes, such as clostridium and fusobacterium; and fungi such as candida spp. and *Blastomyces dermatiditis* may be cultured (Chapter 7.2.4).

Pathology

The abscesses may be large, are usually loculated, and are situated within skeletal muscles beneath the deep fascia. Histologically, there is focal muscle necrosis with an infiltration of mononuclear cells and inflammatory oedema.

Clinical features

Any skeletal muscle may be involved, but those of the trunk and lower limbs are the most commonly affected, especially gluteal and thigh muscles. Usually there is a single localized abscess, but multiple abscesses in distantly separated muscles can occur. Untreated pyomyositis may evolve through three phases.

1 Subacute phase—the earliest symptom is pain with ill-defined induration and tenderness of the affected muscle associated with intermittent fever and chills lasting 1 to 3 weeks.

2 Suppurative phase—after 10 to 21 days the abscess swelling enlarges and becomes tender and hot but is usually nonfluctuant and may persist for months. Usually, there is no local lymphadenopathy. Although the overlying skin is sometimes red and oedematous, it is not the source or portal of infection in strictly defined pyomyositis. Complications include compartment syndrome and spread of infection from the affected muscle to contiguous structures such as bones, joints, viscera, and serosal cavities.

3 Septicaemic phase—there is spread of infection with metastatic abscess formation in lungs, pleura, pericardium, liver, heart valves, and elsewhere and the risk of septic shock and fatal multisystem failure.

Investigations

Peripheral neutrophil leucocytosis is usual but not invariable since, in nontropical cases, neutropenia is a predisposing factor. The frequency of eosinophilia in tropical pyomyositis may reflect its prevalence in endemic populations or a specific role of helminths in abscess formation. Despite muscle destruction at the site of the abscess, serum concentrations of breakdown products such as myoglobin, creatine kinase, aldolase and aspartate aminotransferase may remain normal. Myoglobinaemia, myoglobinuria, and acute renal failure are rare. (See 'Imaging' and 'Microbiology' below).

Prognosis

Case fatality reported in large series of cases of pyomyositis ranges from less than 1 to 4%. It is less than 1.5% in tropical pyomyositis but in some groups of nontropical cases with immunosuppression it may exceed 25%.

Diagnosis

Imaging

Plain radiographs show nonspecific displacement of soft tissues, oedema, blurring of tissue planes and, in long-standing cases, adjacent periostial reaction and osteosclerosis. Ultrasound, CT, and especially gadolinium-enhanced MRI scans are the most useful investigations for confirming the diagnosis, localizing abscesses, and guiding needles for diagnostic and therapeutic aspiration. Radionuclide leucocyte scans are less useful for precise anatomical localization.

Microbiology

Repeated aerobic and anaerobic cultures may be required for specific aetiological diagnosis. Cultures for mycobacteria and fungi are indicated in immunosuppressed patients. In tropical pyomyositis, blood cultures are positive in less than 5% of cases but in nontropical cases with underlying disease seen in Western countries, yields from 30 to 50% may be expected. Pus obtained by needle aspiration and open surgery should be examined by Gram- and Ziehl-Nielsen staining and cultured.

Differential diagnosis

This includes intra- and intermuscular abscesses secondary to infection in neighbouring organs and tissues such as osteomyelitis and septic arthritis; muscle haematomas and tears; deep vein thrombosis; tumours of connective tissue or muscle such as rhabdomyosarcoma; localized myalgia as in leptospirosis; and the inflammatory and allergic swellings resulting from the migration of helminths such as *Loa loa* (Calabar swelling), *Gnathostoma*, *Paragonimus*, and sparganum. Tuberculous 'cold abcsesses' are typically more indolent and less tender. Depending on which muscle is involved, other diagnoses may be suspected such as hip or sacroiliac joint pathology (obtutator externus/internus or iliacus muscles); acute abdomen or hepatic or splenic abscesses (abdominal muscles); appendicitis (iliopsoas muscle); ischiorectal abscess (levator ani muscle); Lemierre's syndrome (cervical muscles); epidural abscess (pyriformis or paraspinal muscles); sciatica (pyriformis or gluteal muscles).

Treatment

In the early stages, antibiotic treatment alone may be effective, but once there is suppuration early drainage by needle aspiration, or by full surgical exploration with debridement, is essential. Abscesses are often loculated, making needle aspiration inadequate. Intravenous antibiotic treatment should be initiated for 1 to 2 weeks followed by oral treatment to complete a 4- to 6-week course. Since *Staph. aureus* is the commonest cause of primary pyomyositis, treatment with a β-lactamase-resistant penicillin (flucloxacillin, oxacillin, nafcillin) should be started immediately. Where MRSA is common, vancomycin may be more appropriate and in immunosuppressed patients, a combination of vancomycin with carabapenem or piperacillin-tazobactam is recommended. If group A streptococcus is cultured, benzyl penicillin and clindamycin are the drugs of choice. Clindamycin is also indicated for anaerobic infections.

Further reading

Chiu SK, *et al.* (2008). Impact of underlying diseases on the clinical characteristics and outcome of primary pyomyositis. *J Microbiol Immunol Infect*, **41**, 286–93.

Crum, NF (2004). Bacterial pyomyositis in the United States. *Am J Med*, **117**, 420–8.

Crum-Cianflone NF (2008). Bacterial, fungal, parasitic, and viral myositis. *Clin Microbiol Rev*, **21**, 473–94.

Gibson RK, Rosenthal SJ, Lukert BP (1984). Pyomyositis: increasing recognition in temperate climates. *American J Med*, **77**, 768–72.

Jacobsen KH, Fleming LC, Ribeiro PS (2010). Pyomyositis in Amazonian Ecuador. *Trans R Soc Trop Med Hyg*. Jan 30 [Epub ahead of print.]

Levin MJ, Gardner P, Waldvogel FA (1971). 'Tropical' pyomyositis. An unusual infection due to *Staphylococcus aureus*. *N Engl J Med*, **284**, 196–8.

Marcus RT, Foster WD (1968). Observations on the clinical features, aetiology and geographical distribution of pyomyositis in East Africa. *East Afr Med J*. **45**, 167–76.

Smith PG, *et al.* (1978). The epidemiology of tropical myositis in the Mengo districts of Uganda. *Trans Roy Soc Trop Med Hyg*, **72**, 46–53.

Soler R, *et al.* (2000). Magnetic resonance imaging of pyomyositis in 43 cases. *Eur J Radiol*, **35**, 59–64.

Vassilopoulos D, *et al.* (1997). Musculoskeletal infections in patients with human immuno-deficiency virus infection. *Medicine (Baltimore)* **76**, 284–94.

SECTION 25

The eye

25.1

The eye in general medicine

Peggy Frith

Essentials

All physicians should be aware of important eye symptoms, learn how to examine the eye, and in particular be proficient with the ophthalmoscope. Common presentations include (1) red eye—may be due to conjunctivitis, episcleritis, scleritis, iritis, keratitis, or acute glaucoma, some of which require urgent specialist opinion; (2) dry eye—which may have a systemic cause, particularly if accompanied by dryness of the mouth (sicca syndrome), e.g. Sjögren's syndrome; (3) loss of vision—which, when it affects one eye, is associated with a relative afferent pupillary defect and can be caused by central retinal artery occlusion, ischaemic central retinal vein occlusion, ischaemic optic neuropathy, optic neuritis, extensive retinal detachment, advanced unilateral glaucoma, and optic nerve compression.

Visual loss—the predominant causes vary according to country: conditions such as glaucoma and macular degeneration predominate in affluent populations, whereas infections and dietary deficiencies (vitamin A) cause blindness in the poor.

Diabetes mellitus—retinopathy is the most common serious eye complication and the commonest reason for blind registration of younger adults in industrialized populations. It can be classified as (1) background—microaneurysms, dot/blot haemorrhages, and hard exudates; (2) maculopathy—where hard exudates within one optic disc diameter of the fovea threaten vision; (3) ischaemic and preproliferative—with changes including multiple blot haemorrhages, dilatation, beading, looping, or tortuosity of the larger retinal veins, or multiple cotton wool spots; (4) proliferative—with tufts of new vessels on the optic nerve head itself or in the peripheral retina. Screening for retinopathy is imperative as laser treatment arrests progression of maculopathy and controls neovascularization.

Hypertension—long-standing high blood pressure and ageing produce similar changes; arterioles are narrowed, irregular or tortuous, and the wall may be thickened (sclerosis), showing an increase in reflected light described as 'copper' or 'silver' wiring. There may appear to be 'nipping' in at arteriovenous crossings where the underlying vein appears to be constricted. Most important is to identify the patient with changes of accelerated hypertension—haemorrhages, cotton wool spots, and papilloedema—which requires urgent management (see Chapter 16.17.5).

Ocular vascular occlusion—includes (1) retinal vascular occlusion—caused by embolic occlusion of the retinal artery or *in situ* retinal vein occlusion, this is a common cause of unilateral blindness, especially in older patients; (2) occlusion of vessels supplying the optic nerve—giant cell arteritis causes occlusion of ciliary branches of the ophthalmic artery, with acute ischaemia of the optic nerve and irretrievable visual loss, preventable with high-dose corticosteroid.

Systemic inflammatory disorders—many of these may affect the eye, including (1) sarcoidosis—may cause conjunctival granulomas, uveitis or optic neuropathy; (2) Behçet's syndrome—characterized by potentially blinding panuveitis and occlusive retinal vasculitis; (3) giant cell arteritis; (4) rheumatoid arthritis—causes keratoconjunctivitis sicca and sometimes ischaemic necrotizing scleritis; (5) ankylosing spondylitis—a common cause of iritis in younger people; (6) Reiter's syndrome—comprises iritis with arthritis, urethritis, or colitis; (7) juvenile chronic arthritis—associated with potentially damaging recurrent iritis; (8) Wegener's granulomatosis and other vasculitides—red eye can signify episcleritis, necrotizing scleritis, or potentially perforating keratitis; (9) systemic lupus erythematosus—also affects the coat of the eye, and can cause retinal vascular occlusions or ischaemic optic neuropathy.

Haematological disorders—retinal changes are common in haematological disorders, even if vision is normal. The eyes may be involved in (1) leukaemias—can cause retinal haemorrhages and Roth spots (focal collections of white cells), various ocular infiltrations, and the eye may be affected by infections, chemotherapy or radiotherapy; (2) lymphomas—may occur around or inside one or both eyes; (3) bleeding diatheses—may cause pronounced or repeated subconjunctival haemorrhage, hyphaema, or vitreous haemorrhage; (4) clotting tendencies—are associated with retinal vascular occlusion, especially venous; (5) sickling haemoglobinopathies—may cause retinal neovascularization with risk of haemorrhage, hence screening is recommended, with laser treatment if required.

Infectious diseases—the eye can be involved by many infections, including (1) bacterial—conjunctivitis, metastatic endophthalmitis, uveitis (tuberculosis, leprosy, syphilis); (2) chlamydial—genital serotypes cause acute conjunctivitis; trachoma is the most common cause of chronic conjunctivitis, affecting at least 600 million people worldwide, with about 6 million (preventably) blinded; (3) viral—most commonly adenoviral conjunctivitis; measles may cause a scarring corneal inflammation, an important cause of blindness in undernourished children; cytomegalovirus causes progressive retinitis with characteristic haemorrhages and patchy retinal necrosis, particularly in patients with AIDS; (4) fungal—metastatic endophthalmitis is usually caused by *Candida albicans*; infection in or around the orbit is characteristic of invasive mucormycosis; (5) protozoal—*Toxoplasma gondii* can cause congenital infection of the retina and underlying choroids; (6) helminth—onchocerciasis or 'river blindness' is still a common cause of blindness, particularly in Africa.

Thyroid disease—eye signs result either from imbalance of thyroid hormones, or from an immunological disorder of both the thyroid (Grave's disease) and retro-orbital tissues, which is the commonest cause of proptosis (exophthalmos).

Inherited disorders—the eye may be discriminant in diagnosis of many inherited disorders, including Marfan's syndrome (dislocated lenses), neurofibromatosis (Lisch nodules on the iris), and von Hippel–Lindau syndrome (retinal angiomas).

Disorders of the eye in general medicine

Because the eye may be involved in so many diseases, it is essential that clinicians are familiar with ocular manifestations. They should be aware of important eye symptoms, learn how to examine the eye, and, in particular, be proficient with the ophthalmoscope. Ocular findings may point to a particular systemic disorder and, in some cases, when an eye complication may need specific treatment, referral to an ophthalmologist is warranted. Occasionally, the need for referral is urgent.

Red eye

The pattern of redness will suggest a possible diagnosis and associated features help to confirm this, as shown in Table 25.1.1. Slit-lamp examination will show specific signs in some types of conjunctivitis, the staining pattern of corneal lesions, cells diagnostic of anterior uveitis within the chambers, and raised eye pressure of glaucoma. Iritis is described further with ankylosing spondylitis, and scleritis with rheumatoid arthritis (below).

Dry eye

Lack of tears may have a systemic cause, particularly if there is also dryness of the mouth—sicca syndrome. Sicca with an identifiable systemic association is known as Sjögren's syndrome, as with rheumatoid arthritis, systemic sclerosis, mixed connective tissue disease, graft-vs-host disease, or sarcoidosis. The eyes feel gritty and are red or sticky (see 'Rheumatoid arthritis', below). Artificial tear replacement can help, but severely dry eyes are a miserable problem that can be very difficult to manage.

Loss of vision

A clear history of the visual loss is important. 'Floaters' are characteristic of posterior uveitis. Visual acuity should be measured in each eye, using glasses or a pinhole to correct for error of focus. Major impairment of vision in one eye gives an asymmetrical pupil response to a bright light, for which there is a limited number of important causes involving the retina or the optic nerve (Box 25.1.1).

Table 25.1.1 Findings in the red eye

Finding	Features	Possible causes or associations
Conjunctivitis	Redness of conjunctiva—both eye and inside lid Discomfort, rather than pain or photophobia Sticky discharge Follicles may be visible	Bacterial or viral infection Sicca—corneal staining likely
Episcleritis	Redness of eyeball only, may be sectorial Discomfort, rather than pain Common not serious and no threat to sight	Identifiable systemic inflammatory in a minority, but may progress to scleritis if secondary
Scleritis	Redness as episcleritis—may be intense and bluish Pain—which may be intense Uncommon Serious disorder with threat to sight	Identifiable systemic inflammatory in c.50% Rheumatoid arthritis Wegener's granulomatosis Others—SLE[a], relapsing polychondritis
Iritis	Redness mostly around the cornea, may be bluish	Ankylosing spondylitis
Anterior uveitis	Pain and photophobia usual Corneal precipitates may be visible Pupil small and may festoon on dilating	Sarcoidosis Behçet's syndrome Some infections
Keratitis	Redness often sectorial and adjacent to lesion	Herpes virus infection
Corneal inflammation	Pain, photophobia, and watering usual Fluorescein staining will highlight	Vasculitis, typically Wegener's granulomatosis—occasionally Cogan's syndrome—rare
Acute glaucoma	Redness of the entire eye, often bluish Pain may be intense and vomiting common Uncommon Cornea steamy Eye feels cricket-ball hard Pupil dilated, oval, and fixed	Dilating drops—rare if using tropicamide 1% alone

[a]SLE, systemic lupus erythematosus.

Box 25.1.1 Some important causes of a relative afferent pupil defect (RAPD)

- Central retinal artery occlusion
- Ischaemic central retinal vein occlusion
- Ischaemic optic neuropathy (may be associated with giant cell arteritis)
- Optic neuritis (may be associated with multiple sclerosis)
- Extensive retinal detachment
- Advanced unilateral glaucoma
- Optic nerve compression (may be associated with thyroid ophthalmopathy or extrinsic/intrinsic tumour)

Warning!

- Test the visual acuities and pupil responses carefully before dilating the pupils to examine the retina
- The greater the discrepancy in acuities, the greater the expectation of RAPD
- It is rare for cataract or vitreous opacity to unbalance the pupil responses, and amblyopia does not affect the response
- If a retinal cause cannot be identified by careful direct ophthalmoscopy, an optic neuropathy is likely

Box 25.1.2 Some causes of retinal cotton wool spots

- Diabetes
- Accelerated hypertension
- Retinal vein occlusion (if ischaemic)
- Microemboli
- Hyperviscosity
- Severe anaemia, especially pernicious anaemia
- Giant cell arteritis
- Acute pancreatitis
- Vasculitis such as active SLE[a]
- HIV retinopathy
- Migraine attack
- Traumatic, secondary to chest compression (Purtscher's retinopathy)

[a]SLE, systemic lupus erythematosus.

Examination of the eye

The ophthalmoscope

The optic nerve head is usually visible through an undilated pupil, but it is impossible to assess the retina reliably without using a mydriatic. Short-acting drops such as tropicamide (1%) work within 15 min and the effect lasts about 2 h, with minimal risk of causing acute glaucoma. The pupils should not be dilated if the patient has had recent head injury or is in coma. The central fovea is seen if the patient looks directly into the light, and, in diabetic patients, the area temporal to the fovea should also be examined. A clouded view suggests opacity in the lens or vitreous, best seen by adjusting focus at the pupil margin to give a red reflection against which opacities stand out as black shadows, especially if the pupil is dilated. The peripheral retina, as in sickle-cell retinopathy, is best seen with the indirect ophthalmoscope.

Superficial flame-shaped haemorrhages, though not unique to hypertension, demand measurement of blood pressure. Deeper dot and blot haemorrhages temporal to the macula suggest diabetes or a haematological disorder if bilateral, or vein occlusion if unilateral or localized. Dense subhyaloid haemorrhage, confined between the retina and the vitreous which may sediment to a flat top, is typical of bleeding from diabetic new vessels or secondary to a bleeding diathesis. Most haemorrhages are asymptomatic and will resolve, but vision falls if the fovea is involved or if blood leaks into the vitreous itself, causing floaters.

Shiny, hard exudates consist of protein and lipid; if in circles—'circinate'—focal vascular leakage may suggest diabetes, whereas a star forms at the fovea as retinal oedema resolves after treatment of hypertension or papilloedema. Commonly confused with exudates are retinal drusen which are more uniform and discrete, usually scattered around the retina or congregated close to the fovea.

Cotton wool spots are fluffy, pale patches indicating swollen nerve-fibre axons at sites of microvascular closure. They are always significant (Box 25.1.2). Active focal retinal inflammation may resemble cotton wool spots, but consists of cells which spill into the vitreous. These are visible using slit-lamp magnification, as in active toxoplasmosis, cytomegalovirus retinitis, sarcoidosis, Behçet's disease, or ocular lymphoma. Discrete, punched-out scars suggest healed foci in the retina and/or underlying choroid; their morphology may be characteristic of a particular diagnosis.

Fluorescein angiography

Retinal angiography defines the type and severity of retinal vascular disorder. Fluorescein dye, injected intravenously, demonstrates patterns of perfusion both in the retina and underlying choroid, outlining abnormalities such as microaneurysms and identifying sites of closure, or leakage from damaged retinal capillaries or new vessels. Angiography is valuable diagnostically and indicates when and where laser treatment is needed. Anaphylactic reactions and even fatalities have been reported, so patients must be carefully selected.

Visual fields

The visual fields should be examined in selected patients with visual loss, as even large defects may go unnoticed. A unilateral central or altitudinal (top or bottom of field) defect suggests an anterior lesion—in the retina or optic nerve. A bitemporal defect implicates the optic chiasm, and a homonymous defect the visual path posterior to the chiasm. With bilateral occipital infarction, visual loss may be difficult to define: pupil reactions are normal. If there is unaccountably poor vision in one eye, a defect of focus or an amblyopic (lazy) eye resulting from a squint or refractive error in childhood may be responsible—the first should improve with a pinhole, but the second will not.

Eye changes in diabetes

Retinopathy, the most common serious eye complication in diabetes, is the principal reason for blind registration of younger adults in industrialized populations. Annual retinal screening is essential, as early treatment can prevent blindness and patients with sight-threatening changes are often asymptomatic.

Older diabetic patients may have cataract, glaucoma, stroke, retinal vein occlusion, and, occasionally, diabetic ischaemic optic neuropathy.

Pathological changes in the diabetic retina

It is unclear why the retina is so commonly affected by diabetes, whereas cerebral capillaries appear to be spared. In humans and experimental animals, the earliest histological change is retinal capillary basement-membrane thickening associated with increase of laminin and type IV collagen. Surrounding pericytes become sparse and are eventually lost. Endothelial cells also degenerate and may be lost, so that microaneurysms herniate through the defective capillary wall. Blood and plasma may leak into the retina, causing dot and blot haemorrhages and hard exudate. Later, small vessels may become occluded and collateral channels form at the edge of avascular areas. Abnormal capillaries here or on the optic nerve head may then begin to bud into tufts of new vessels—neovascularization—which grow forwards into the vitreous. These are fragile and may bleed spontaneously, in front of the retina or into the vitreous.

Basement-membrane thickening may be related to glycation of proteins and increase in cytokine activity. Endothelial cells are regulated by pericytes and may control local fibroblast growth factors. Retinal hyperperfusion may occur in the earlier stages, as in the kidney. The stimulus for the formation of new vessels is partly due to growth factors, such as vascular endothelial growth factor, explaining why proliferation is rare before puberty.

Incidence, progression, risk factors, and prognosis for diabetic retinopathy

Macular damage impairs detailed vision, whereas vitreous haemorrhage or retinal detachment associated with proliferative disease can cause more extensive visual loss.

In the Wisconsin study involving nearly 2500 patients, the overall prevalence of retinopathy was 50.1%, but only 2.2% had high-risk features for severe visual loss: new vessels on the optic disc or larger tufts of new vessels elsewhere in the retina which had already bled. In the 'younger' group, the prevalence of moderate visual impairment was 1.4%, and of legal blindness 3.2%. Within 4 years, 2.4% developed new proliferative retinopathy, 9.4% significant visual impairment, and 2.3% legal blindness, despite laser treatment. Before puberty, the risk was zero, rising to 24% in elderly patients with severe macular exudates and in younger patients with high-risk proliferative features.

Risk factors for the development or progression of retinopathy include age and duration of diabetes, quality of diabetic control, ethnicity (Pima Indians and Mexican Americans have a higher incidence), hypertension, smoking, pregnancy, and current severity of retinopathy.

Clinical findings in diabetic retina

Vision is usually good despite early retinopathy, though blurred vision may be a presenting symptom associated with hyperglycaemia. Foveal involvement by oedema, exudates, or ischaemia makes reading difficult, and there is a tendency to develop permanent macular damage. Vasoproliferation consequent to ischaemia may

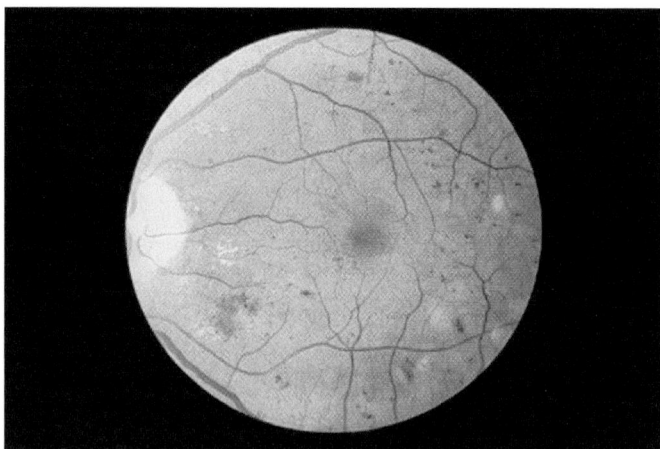

Fig. 25.1.1 Diabetic, background retinopathy. The hallmarks of background retinal changes are red dots (either microaneurysms or small haemorrhages) and blots (larger haemorrhages) together with glinting hard exudates which are no closer than one disc diameter from the central fovea and vision is normal.

cause acute haemorrhage; vitreous blood causes multiple, small floaters like a cloud of insects or a cobweb, and a massive bleed results in profound visual impairment. Most vitreous haemorrhage clears, but eventual vitreous fibrosis may distort and detach the retina, often irretrievably.

Background retinopathy

The early findings are microaneurysms—small, round, red dots—sparse, scattered haemorrhages in dot or blot pattern and hard exudates, particularly temporal to the macula (Fig. 25.1.1). Fluorescein angiography distinguishes microaneurysms from dot haemorrhages.

Maculopathy

Hard exudates form at foci of leakage from abnormally permeable capillaries, as macrophages process the fluid into lipid and protein residues, characteristically in a ring or 'circinate' pattern rarely found in nondiabetic retinopathies (Fig. 25.1.2). Exudates within

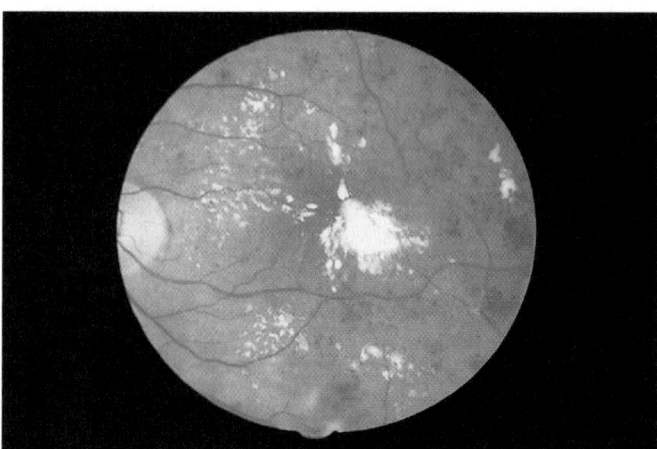

Fig. 25.1.2 Diabetic, maculopathy. Hard exudate, containing lipid and protein which has leaked from damaged retinal capillaries, has congregated at the fovea. Central vision is irretrievably impaired. Diabetes may present in this way, especially in the elderly.

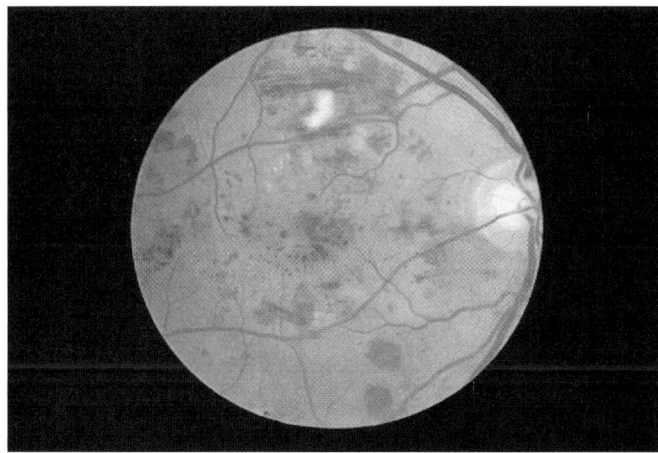

Fig. 25.1.3 Diabetic, ischaemic retinopathy. Capillary ischaemia creates multiple cotton wool spots—microinfarcts within the nerve fibre layer. Other features are dilatation of retinal veins and multiple blot haemorrhages. Frank proliferation of new vessels is almost inevitable and the retinal changes must be carefully observed.

one optic disc diameter of the fovea threaten vision. Laser burns applied focally to leaking areas usually prevent progression.

Ischaemia and preproliferation

Worse prognostic signs of ischaemic changes include multiple blot haemorrhages, dilatation, beading, looping, or tortuosity of the larger retinal veins, or multiple cotton wool spots (Fig. 25.1.3).

Proliferation of new vessels

Buds adjacent to ischaemic areas progress to tufts of new vessels on the optic nerve head itself—'disc new vessels'—or in the peripheral retina—'new vessels elsewhere' (Fig. 25.1.4). New vessels may bleed into the retina or the vitreous (Fig. 25.1.5), and after repeated haemorrhage the retina may fibrose, tear, or detach. Any patient with suspected new vessels should be referred early and assessed for urgent laser treatment. New vessels on the iris (rubeosis) visible with the slit lamp carry the risk of glaucoma.

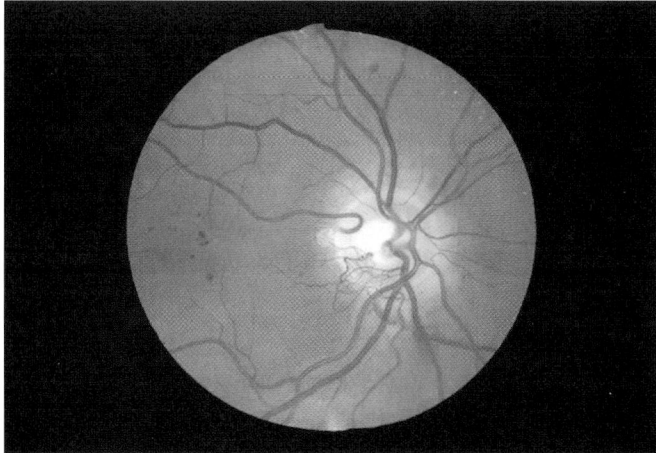

Fig. 25.1.4 Diabetic, proliferative retinopathy. New vessels have formed on the inferior part of the optic disc. They are fine, looping, and aimless. There may be others in the peripheral retina. If the vessels bleed, vision will become acutely obscured by 'floaters'.

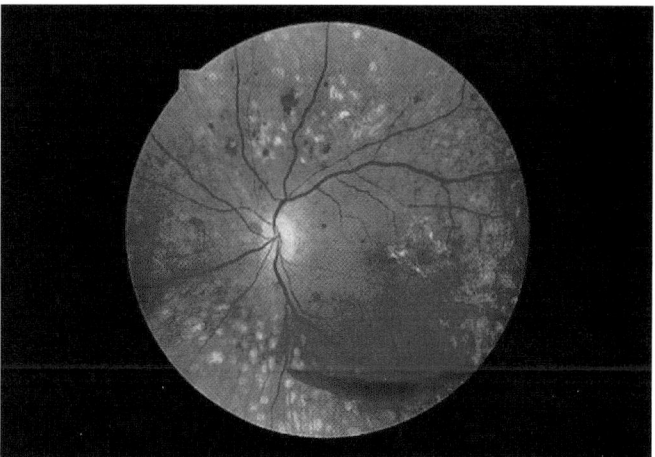

Fig. 25.1.5 Diabetic, preretinal haemorrhage and laser scars. Neovascular fronds may bleed in front of the retina or into the vitreous, obscuring vision acutely. Here blood has sedimented into a characteristic 'boat' shape and multiple laser scars have been placed outside the major vascular arcades. There are haemorrhages and hard exudate temporal to the fovea.

Management of diabetic retinopathy

Control of blood sugar and lipids, blood pressure, weight, and smoking are all important. The value of aspirin is unproven.

Screening programme

All adult diabetics should have a retinal examination at presentation and then annually. Pregnant diabetics, and those with exudation or ischaemia, should be screened every few months by a hospital specialist. Table 25.1.2 outlines a practical programme.

Laser treatment

Foveal leakage may be reduced by timely focal laser treatment. In about two-thirds of patients with macular oedema, laser treatment can arrest progression in the relatively short term. With neovascularization, early treatment can reduce the incidence of visual loss by about 60%. Proliferative retinopathy is treated by pan-retinal photocoagulative (PRP) laser destruction of the ischaemic peripheral retina. This will cause constriction of peripheral visual field and a degree of night blindness. Direct coagulation of the vessels themselves is not successful.

Surgery is a salvage measure for selected patients with opaque vitreous, retinal distortion, or detachment. Patients with irretrievably

Table 25.1.2 Practical screening programme for diabetic retinopathy

Retinopathy type	Prognosis[a] untreated	Action[b]	Appropriate treatment	Rescreening interval
None	0.3	Rescreen	Optimize risk factors	2–3 years
Background	3	Rescreen	Warn to report symptoms	1 year
Exudative	20	Refer	Focal laser	3–6 months
Ischaemic	30	Refer	Observe closely	3 months
Proliferative	50	Refer ASAP	Panretinal laser	Monthly till regress

ASAP, as soon as possible.

[a] Approximate % untreated eyes likely to be blind in 5 years.

[b] Intensify scrutiny (1) in pregnancy; (2) with rapid progression of retinopathy; (3) with intensification of diabetic control.

poor vision need specialist advice about how to live with their handicap.

Other visual complications of diabetes

Diabetes accelerates the development of cataract. Diabetic patients are suitable for lens implantation, but are more prone to operative complications.

If retinal haemorrhages appear acutely, or within a sector in one eye, retinal vein occlusion should be considered. Associated ischaemia increases the risk of secondary glaucoma and intractable rubeotic glaucoma may result from neovascularization of aqueous drainage channels.

Palsies of cranial nerves III, IV, or VI—often painful—may cause double vision, which usually improves within weeks and can be managed by a spectacle prism. Occasional patients develop an acute ischaemic optic neuropathy with a pale, swollen optic nerve head and poor vision. Stroke can cause homonymous hemianopia.

Rarely, lipaemia retinalis associated with extreme hypertriglyceridaemia in acute ketoacidosis can be a presentation, usually in a comatose patient. Major retinal vessels appear pink or white due to opalescent fat. The appearance reverses with metabolic control and vision remains normal.

The eye in hypertension

In the hypertensive patient, retinal changes will help determine if treatment is necessary, if it is adequate, or if it is needed urgently. Description of individual features is preferable to grading (Box 25.1.3). Unless the pupil is dilated, it is easy to miss or to underestimate retinal changes, and a bright halogen bulb with green ('red-free') filter helps accentuate small haemorrhages. Haemorrhages or cotton wool spots, indicating acute changes, are most likely to be seen around the optic nerve head and major vessels.

Long-standing hypertension and ageing produce similar changes. Arterioles are narrowed, irregular, or tortuous and the wall may be thickened (sclerosis), showing an increase in reflected light described as 'copper' or 'silver wiring'. There may be nipping in at arteriovenous crossings where the underlying vein appears to be

---

Box 25.1.3 Grading of hypertensive retinopathy

Perhaps the best-known grading of hypertensive retinopathy is the Keith–Wagner classification:

♦ Grade 1—mild narrowing or sclerosis of retinal arteries

♦ Grade 2—moderate to marked narrowing or sclerosis and arteriovenous crossing changes

♦ Grade 3—in addition, haemorrhages or cotton wool spots

♦ Grade 4—in addition, swelling of the optic nerve head (papilloedema)

Grades 3 and 4 indicate severe, accelerated, or 'malignant' retinopathy, though the prognosis is similar for grades 3 and 4. Blood pressure high enough to damage the renal and cerebral circulation is best recognized by inspecting retinal vessels, even in the absence of visual symptoms. Diastolic pressure likely to be associated with severe retinal changes is usually at least 110 mmHg at some time, and proteinuria is usual.

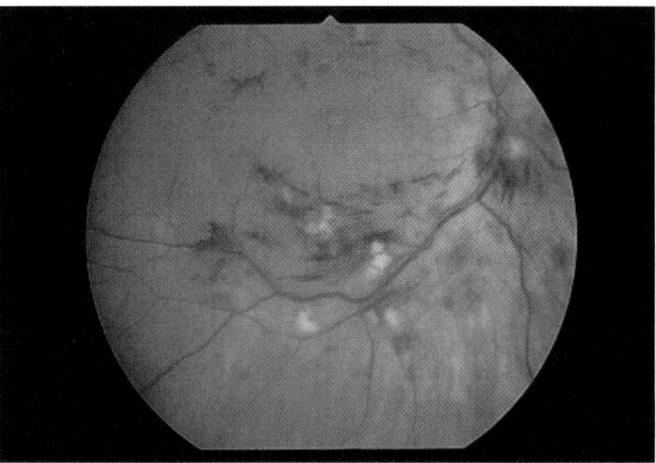

Fig. 25.1.6 Hypertension, accelerated. Multiple flame shaped haemorrhages, microinfarcts, and swelling of the optic disc margin are characteristic features of accelerated hypertension. Vision may be normal, yet the changes dictate immediate treatment to reduce blood pressure. The diastolic level is usually greater than 110 mmHg and proteinuria is to be expected.

constricted. Long-standing changes often persist despite treatment of hypertension.

Significance of retinal changes

Acute, severe retinal changes indicate either leakage or closure of smaller vessels. Flame haemorrhages are seen particularly around the vessel trunks above and below the macula (Fig. 25.1.6). These indicate leakage of blood from fine, superficial, capillary branches supplying the nerve-fibre layer. Bleeding deeper in the retina forms blot-like haemorrhages which, if widespread or in a wedge from an arteriovenous crossing, may indicate occlusion of the central, or a branch, retinal vein. Haemorrhages resolve with treatment of hypertension and vision usually recovers.

Cotton wool spots indicate closure of capillaries supplying the nerve fibres. These microinfarcts cause stasis of axoplasmic flow and intra-axonal contents accumulate, distending the fibres and producing a pale, fluffy focus. Spots gradually resolve with treatment. In the absence of hypertension, an inflammatory vasculitis such as systemic lupus erythematosus (SLE) should be considered (see Box 25.1.2).

Hypertensive damage causes disruption of retinal endothelial tight junctions so that fluid, protein, and lipid leak into the extracellular spaces within the retina. These are removed by macrophages and processed into shiny, hard exudates, which may persist for many months. Hard exudates, implying leakage for more than a matter of days, are common in resolving hypertensive retinopathy as a characteristic foveal star. In hypertension, exudate rarely forms the ring-shaped circinate pattern typical of diabetes.

Papilloedema implies hypertensive damage to the disc capillaries or cerebral oedema with raised intracranial pressure attributable to hypertension. Sudden reduction of blood pressure may cause acute, sometimes irreversible, loss of vision with a risk of stroke.

Histopathology

In the early phases of severe retinopathy, there is disruption of endothelial cells or tight junctions followed by vessel-wall damage leading to occlusion, sometimes with fibrinoid necrosis or frank thrombosis.

Nonretinal eye changes in hypertension

Occasionally, patients with severe hypertension—especially those with eclampsia or renal failure—may suffer pronounced visual loss secondary to occlusive changes in the vessels supplying the optic nerve head or in the choroid underlying the retina itself. The tissues become swollen and pale and the retina may become detached by fluid. Rarely, patients with secondary hypertension may have eye manifestations of genetic disorders such as neurofibromatosis, von Hippel–Lindau syndrome, or Sipple's syndrome (see below).

Ocular vascular occlusion

Retinal vascular occlusion is a common cause of blindness, especially in elderly patients. It can be a valuable warning of vascular disease elsewhere, particularly in the brain.

Retinal artery occlusion

Occlusion of the central retinal artery or its branches is almost always embolic—emboli arising from the carotid artery (cervical or intracranial) or in the heart. Visual loss is abrupt, with permanent loss of function once the retina has infarcted. Central artery occlusion results in profound loss of vision, whereas branch occlusion often causes a horizontal (altitudinal) defect which the patient may be able to define accurately. Prognosis for the fellow eye is good, especially if an underlying cause can be corrected (Table 25.1.3).

Clinical findings

Initially, the infarcted retina swells and becomes opaque, leaving a 'cherry-red' spot at the fovea, revealing the intact underlying choroidal circulation. The territory of an occluded branch artery may become whitened for a week or so (Fig. 25.1.7), subsiding to leave thinned retina and narrowed, often sheathed, vessels. The optic nerve head may atrophy over ensuing months as the nerve fibres die. If much of the retina is infarcted, there is a reduction in the afferent pupil response which persists when other signs have subsided. Emboli may be visible at any stage in the central or branch vessels, often at a bifurcation. Most emboli are small, glistening, white pieces of cholesterol from atheromatous plaques.

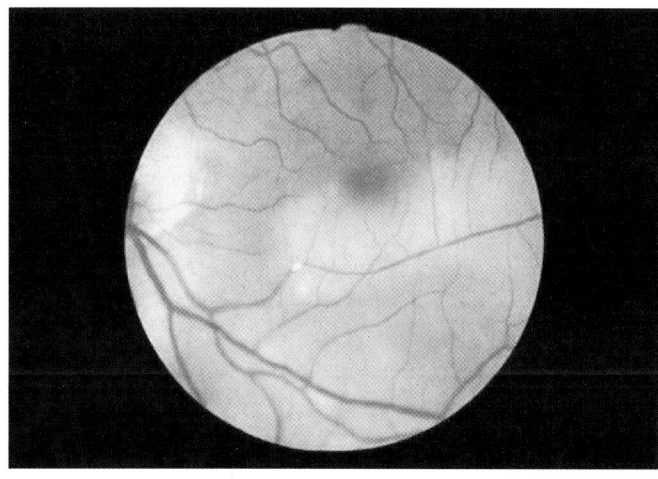

Fig. 25.1.7 Branch retinal artery occlusion. A small white embolus is lodged at the third bifurcation of the inferotemporal branch retinal artery, occluding it. The local retina is oedematous and non-functioning, producing an acute superior scotoma in the left eye. The likely origin is from the ipsilateral carotid or the heart.

Larger, round, solid, white emboli, which usually lodge proximally within or near the disc in the larger vessels, may have come from a calcified heart valve, whereas fibrin and platelet emboli from a thrombosed plaque or cardiac thrombus may look dark or grey.

Associated findings may include an ipsilateral carotid bruit, heart murmur, or dysrhythmia—particularly atrial fibrillation—absent peripheral pulses or bruits at other sites, and hypertension.

Investigation and management

No treatment is worthwhile acutely, apart from firm ocular massage, which may dislodge an unstable central embolus. Risk factors are assessed by measuring blood pressure, full blood count, blood sugar, lipids, and renal function. Even in the absence of a bruit, carotid Doppler ultrasonography is useful to detect atheromatous plaque at the bifurcation, with a view to carotid surgery.

Management involves reducing risk factors such as smoking, hypertension, obesity, or other abnormalities. Patients unsuitable for endarterectomy are offered long-term aspirin.

Amaurosis fugax

Transient retinal ischaemia causes brief episodes of blindness limited to one eye, known as amaurosis fugax. These episodes usually last for a few seconds, rarely longer than a few minutes, total or partial, and commonly affecting the upper or lower half 'like a blind moving up or down'. Recovery is usually complete, most attacks are painless, and associated symptoms are rare—there may be a history of cerebral transient ischaemic attacks on other occasions. Emboli have been seen passing through the retinal circulation during an attack, moving from central to branch arterioles as they disperse.

Retinal vein occlusion

Retinal venous occlusion usually occurs *in situ*. Risk factors include age, hypertension, diabetes, haematological disorders, and glaucoma (Box 25.1.4). Symptoms develop less abruptly than with arterial occlusion—commonly, the patient wakes with blurred vision. With a central vein occlusion, haemorrhages are scattered throughout the fundus in the characteristic 'bloodstorm' pattern (Fig. 25.1.8), often with cotton wool spots. Less complete block causes

Table 25.1.3 Associations with retinal artery occlusion

Vascular embolic	Atheroma—commonly from carotid bifurcation, carotid siphon, or aortic arch
	Paradoxical embolus (rare)
Cardiac	Thrombus from left atrium or ventricle—with AF, MI, or cardiomyopathy
	Myxoma
	Mitral valve prolapse (mechanism of occlusion not established)
	Aortic or mitral valve degeneration or prosthesis
	Endocarditis
Vasculitis	Giant cell arteritis—in a minority
	Takayasu aortitis

AF, atrial fibrillation; MI, myocardial infarct; SLE, systemic lupus erythematosus.

- Hypertension
- Diabetes
- Smoking
- Hyperlipidaemia
- Haematological—raised cell or platelet count, or hyperviscosity such as myeloma
- Glaucoma
- Clotting tendency—antiphospholipid syndrome, deficiency of protein S, C, or antithrombin III, Leiden mutation
- Vasculitis—sarcoidosis, Behçet's syndrome, associated with retinal periphlebitis
- Hormonal therapy—hormone replacement therapy or oral contraceptive

sparse, scattered haemorrhages. Branch vein occlusion, usually at an arteriovenous crossing, causes a wedge-shaped sector of haemorrhage in the area of drainage, its apex towards the optic disc. Vision may improve, depending on the state of the fovea, and the outlook for the opposite eye is good if risk factors are minimized. If the retina is ischaemic, the risk of retinal new vessel formation may be prevented by laser treatment. Acute signs of occlusion may persist for many weeks or months. Curly collateral vessels may develop at the disc or within the peripheral retina.

Investigation and management

Blood pressure, blood sugar, full blood count, and ESR should be measured. Ocular pressure is checked, as glaucoma is a treatable risk factor. Plasma protein electrophoresis, viscosity, and blood coagulation—including antiphospholipid antibodies or lupus anticoagulant in younger patients—are tested, particularly if the changes are recurrent, bilateral, or associated with thrombosis

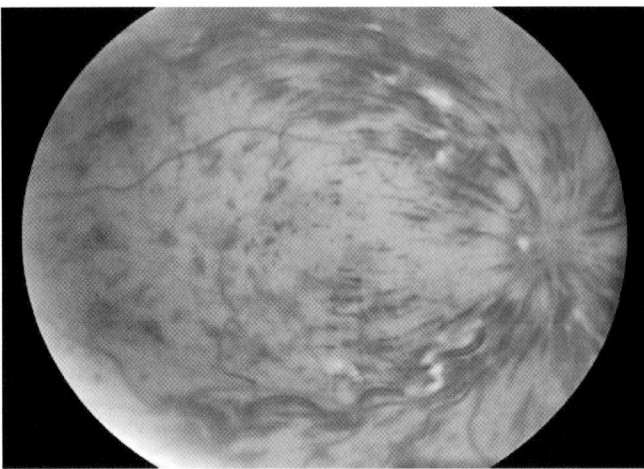

Fig. 25.1.8 Central retinal vein occlusion. Blockage of the draining central retinal vein results in a 'bloodstorm' appearance with profuse flame haemorrhages forming between the nerve fibres in all quadrants. Cotton wool spots representing microinfarcts are often also present. Vision is acutely blurred as the fovea becomes oedematous.

elsewhere. Other possibilities include sarcoidosis or Behçet's disease, particularly if the patient describes floaters or the slit-lamp examination shows inflammatory cells within the vitreous. Risk factors such as blood pressure, smoking, and obesity must be addressed, but the benefit of long-term aspirin is unproven.

Chronic ocular ischaemia

Eye ischaemia is associated with arterial disease anywhere from the aortic arch to the ophthalmic artery. The eye is often painful and red with impaired vision. Slit-lamp examination shows intraocular pressure is low and there are dilated vessels on the iris with protein flare in the anterior chamber. Cataract may obscure dilated and tortuous retinal vessels, often with scattered haemorrhages. New vessels may form. In younger patients, this syndrome may suggest congenital or acquired proximal arterial occlusion, particularly Takayasu's arteritis. In older patients, arterial surgery may save and even improve vision.

Occlusion of vessels supplying the optic nerve

Giant-cell arteritis is associated with occlusion of ciliary, rather than central retinal, branches of the ophthalmic artery, causing acute ischaemia of the optic nerve (see below). Some patients, especially smokers, have noninflammatory occlusion from atheroma. Rarely, acute optic nerve ischaemia, sometimes bilateral, is associated with catastrophic postpartum or gastrointestinal haemorrhage; prognosis for recovery of vision is poor.

The eye in systemic inflammatory disorders

Sarcoidosis

External eye

Sarcoid granulomas in the conjunctiva are multiple, small, solid, and characteristically yellowish. Visible granulomata can be easily biopsied under slit-lamp magnification using anaesthetic drops. Gritty, dry eye is common, with fluorescein staining of the cornea and reduced Schirmer's test (see 'Rheumatoid arthritis', below); lacrimal glands may be enlarged.

Uveitis

Iritis—anterior uveitis—is common in sarcoidosis and may be bilateral, recurrent, sometimes severe, and potentially damaging. The eye is red, painful, and photophobic. Large, greasy, 'mutton-fat' precipitates are seen by slit-lamp examination on the internal surface of the cornea. Granulomata may be visible in the iris—Busacca's within, and Koeppe's at the pupil margin. Repeated attacks of iritis can cause cataract or glaucoma; hypercalcaemia may be associated with corneal band keratopathy.

Posterior uveitis is associated with cells in the vitreous and floaters, which may obscure the view of the fundus and aggregate into characteristic vitreous 'snowballs'. Granulomata in the retina or choroids form pale foci, seen behind a haze of cells. Vision may be further impaired by fluid leaking from inflamed capillaries at the fovea. Inflammatory occlusive retinal phlebitis of branch veins, causing focal retinal haemorrhages and subsequent sheathing, strongly suggests sarcoidosis. Differential diagnoses are Behçet's syndrome or idiopathic retinal vasculitis. Fluorescein angiography shows a segmental pattern of retinal venous leakage.

Sarcoid can also cause optic neuropathy and sarcoid granulomata in the orbit may cause exophthalmos or involve cranial nerves.

Corticosteroids are given topically for iritis and may be injected locally for posterior uveitis. Patients with persistent posterior uveitis may need long-term systemic immunosuppression.

Behçet's syndrome

Uveitis—anterior or posterior or both (panuveitis)—is one key, defining feature of Behçet's syndrome. Recurrent attacks can progressively damage the eye. In Japan and Turkey, Behçet's syndrome is the commonest cause of blinding uveitis—the incidence in northern Japan is about 1 per 10 000 population, of whom roughly 75% have ocular inflammation at some stage. Blindness results in 50% of eyes within 5 years of the first ocular attack, if untreated. Males with the HLA B5 haplotype, particularly the BW51 subtype, are at highest risk of severe eye disease.

Ocular inflammation is usually bilateral, sometimes with a gap of many years sequentially between onset in each eye. Iritis is typically very acute, with pain, redness, and photophobia. Hypopyon is characteristic, but not unique to Behçet's syndrome (Fig. 25.1.9). Attacks may settle spontaneously, but the eye may be damaged, so short, intensive courses of corticosteroid drops with mydriatic are indicated.

Posterior uveitis, with inflammatory cells in the vitreous, is typically a retinal vasculitis. Occlusion of inflamed branch veins causes haemorrhages and cotton wool spots (Fig. 25.1.10). Acute focal retinal infiltrates of polymorphonuclear leucocytes may appear as white, fluffy patches, which are strongly suggestive of Behçet's syndrome. Leakage may cause foveal oedema with a fall in visual acuity and distortion of central vision, and vision is permanently affected if occlusion involves the fovea—fluorescein angiography defines the severity of leakage and closure. With recurrent attacks, the retina gradually dies, vessels become sheathed, and the optic nerve head atrophies. Neovascularization may cause vitreous haemorrhage.

Management is difficult. No regime of immunosuppression tolerable in the long term will prevent all inflammation. Systemic corticosteroids limit acute damage and a longer-term agent such as

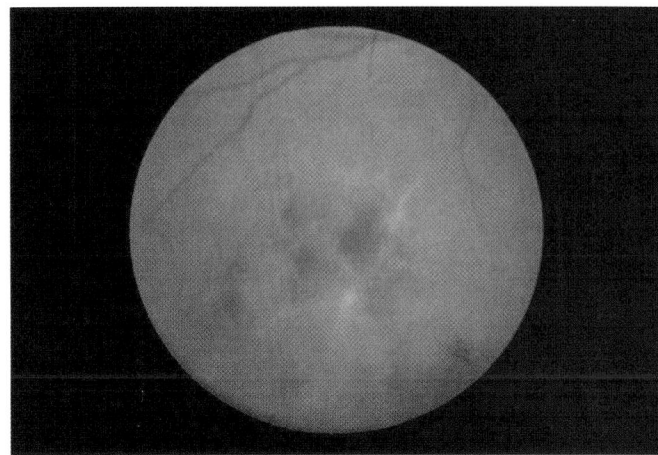

Fig. 25.1.10 Behçet's retinitis. Occlusion of blood vessels, usually venous, in the peripheral retina produces a wedge of haemorrhage with whitening of the vascular wall. The view is hazy due to inflammatory cells within the vitreous. The retina is ischaemic, function is lost, and neovascularization may occur. Repeated episodes may damage vision irretrievably.

azathiaprine may be added. Clorambucil, colchicine, or ciclosporin A may be helpful, though their impact on blindness is uncertain.

Histopathology

In a patient dying of cerebral involvement 10 years after the onset of treated eye disease, there were collections of T4 lymphocytes within and around walls of retinal vessels. Despite heavy immunosuppression, many cells were positive for interleukin 2 (IL-2), and HLA DR-positive cells were found.

Giant-cell arteritis

Irretrievable visual loss is a feared complication, which may be bilateral. Once the patient is on systemic corticosteroid treatment the risk of visual loss and blindness falls, provided initial doses are adequate. Patients presenting with visual loss are at high risk of further loss in the presenting eye or of rapid involvement of the second. They should be immediately started on high doses until symptoms, ESR, and C-reactive protein (CRP) are controlled—this usually takes days, rather than weeks. In patients presenting with bilateral involvement, intravenous methylprednisolone is justified. Temporal artery biopsy is valuable, as it may confirm the diagnosis and the need for continued treatment in patients with visual loss.

Vision may be lost overnight or during the daytime, and patients may have experienced episodes of transient visual loss in the preceding weeks or days. Initially, loss may be partial, involving either the top- or bottom-half of the visual field, but it often becomes total. The infarcted optic nerve head is characteristically pale and swollen (Fig. 25.1.11). The afferent pupillary response is usually decreased compared with the normal eye. Occlusion of the central retinal artery, producing a pale retina and cherry-red foveal spot, is uncommon.

Rheumatoid arthritis

The commonest problem is keratoconjunctivitis sicca, due to autoimmune damage to lacrimal tissue with lymphocytic infiltration and destructive fibrosis. The eyes are uncomfortable, gritty,

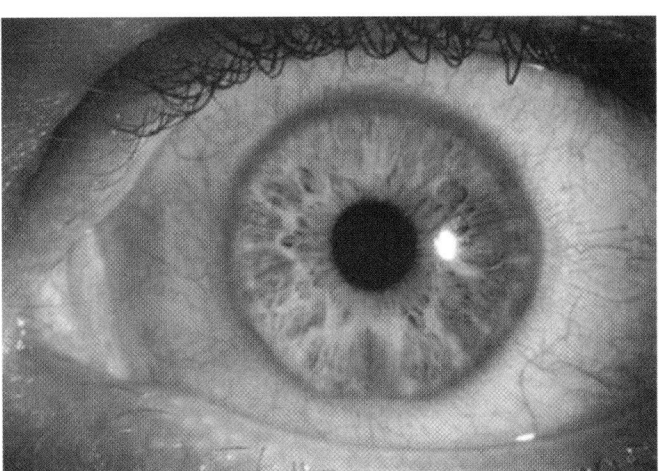

Fig. 25.1.9 Behçet's hypopyon iritis. The eye is red, painful and photophobic. White cells within the anterior chamber have sedimented into a characteristic hypopyon at the base. If bacterial endophthalmitis is excluded, Behçet's syndrome is a likely cause of this acute, intense, sterile iritis.

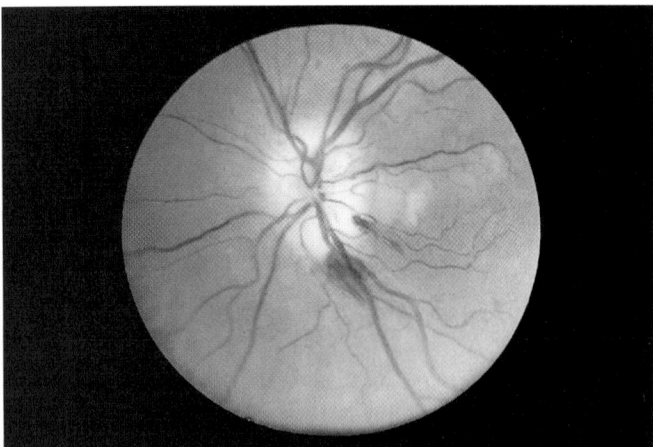

Fig. 25.1.11 Giant cell arteritis, optic disc infarction. The optic nerve head is infarcted, due to occlusion of multiple ciliary branch arterioles which supply it. The disc is pale and swollen, and juxtapapillary haemorrhage has formed. Vision is poor and will not recover. The other eye is at immediate risk unless the systemic inflammatory process is controlled.

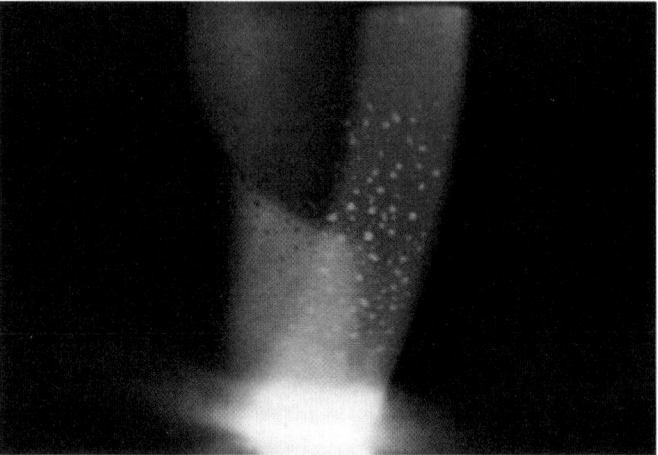

Fig. 25.1.13 Iritis in ankylosing spondylitis. The slit lamp displays cells within the anterior chamber which have sedimented on to the interior surface of the cornea as white keratic precipitates. These are the hallmarks of iritis (anterior uveitis). The eye is usually red and painful. A frequent association is with ankylosing spondylitis and HLA B27 haplotype.

and often sticky as a result of low-grade lid infection and poor flushing of the eye surface. Signs include reduced Schirmer's test and staining of the conjunctiva with fluorescein where epithelial cells are shed, particularly from the cornea exposed between the eyelids. Symptoms may respond to topical tear substitutes such as hypromellose. In some patients, filaments of adherent mucus may disperse with topical acetylcysteine treatment (e.g. Ilube). Severe dry eye is best managed by a specialist, who will watch for complications such as corneal ulceration. Other systemic conditions associated with Sjögren's syndrome include systemic sclerosis, mixed connective tissue disease, lupus erythematosus, sarcoidosis, and lymphoma.

Scleritis is usually found in patients with active vasculitis and raised plasma CRP. The eye may not be particularly painful or red, so the rheumatoid patient with eye symptoms should be referred for specialist assessment even if the eye is white. Necrotizing scleritis

is an ischaemic vasculitis and so responds best to systemic immunosuppression with corticosteroids, sometimes with a cytotoxic agent. Pulsed intravenous treatment may be needed to control the acute attack as untreated scleritis may cause scleral thinning (Fig. 25.1.13), corneal ulceration, or perforation. Patients are rarely suitable for corneal grafting.

Ankylosing spondylitis

Ankylosing spondylitis is the commonest cause of iritis in younger patients, particularly men, who should be asked about pain and stiffness of the spine or sacroiliac joints. Radiographs of lumbar spine or sacroiliac joints or HLA B27 haplotype may be positive. One-third of patients with ankylosing spondylitis will develop eye features at some stage.

The eye is painful, aching, photophobic, and red. The slit lamp shows cells diagnostic of iritis floating in the anterior chamber and sedimented on the back surface of the cornea as keratic precipitates (Fig. 25.1.14). Inflammatory cells usually clear quite rapidly within 1 to 2 weeks of treatment with topical corticosteroids. In the iris posterior synechiae may form, often with the iris constricted; mydriatic drops, which prevent these adhesions, should be continued until inflammation has settled so that the iris eventually regains mobility. Patients with ankylosing spondylitis should be warned that recurrent iritis should be treated early and effectively—there is a 50% chance of recurrence, and acute damage must be minimized on each occasion.

Reiter's syndrome

Arthritis, urethritis, cervicitis, or colitis together with red eye suggests Reiter's syndrome, especially in HLA B27-positive patients. A self-limiting, sterile conjunctivitis is common in the early stages, causing a red, sticky eye. Later, iritis may be the dominant recurrent feature. Features and management are similar to ankylosing spondylitis. Other differential diagnoses of arthritis with iritis include sarcoidosis, Behçet's syndrome, psoriasis, and gonorrhoea: with intestinal involvement, inflammatory bowel disease or Whipple's disease.

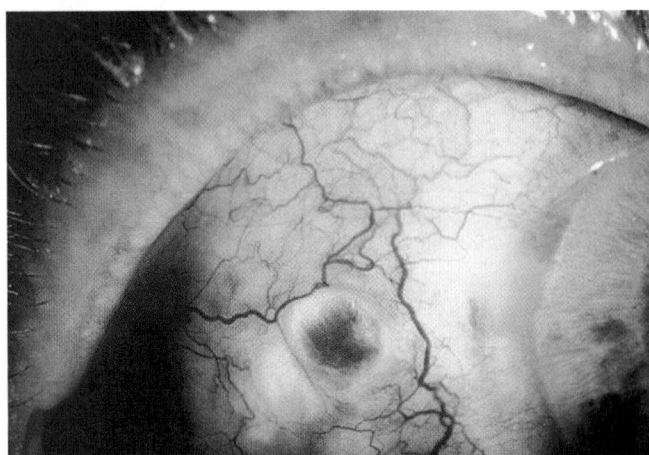

Fig. 25.1.12 Scleromalacia in rheumatoid arthritis. Vasculitis results in focal ischaemia, with translucency and thinning of the sclera: the coat of the eye may perforate. The most common associated systemic disorder is rheumatoid arthritis. The eye is usually red, and pain may be intense.

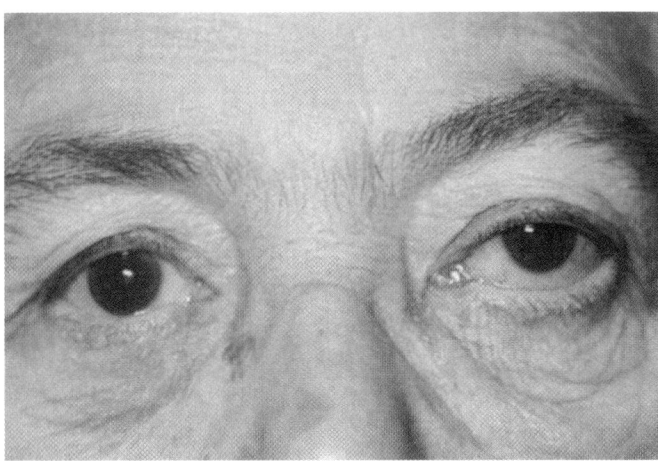

Fig. 25.1.14 Wegener's granulomatosis of the orbit. An inflammatory mass behind the left eye has displaced it forwards and upwards and the eye moves poorly due to involvement of motor nerves within the orbit. The optic nerve may also be involved. Biopsy confirmed granulomatous vasculitis and ANCA was positive. The adjacent sinuses were involved, with bone loss demonstrated on CT scan.

Juvenile chronic arthritis

Children most at risk have chronic seronegative pauciarticular arthritis, perhaps involving only one digit or ankle, especially younger antinuclear antibody (ANA)-positive girls. The picture is usually one of a low-grade, recurrent iritis over several months or years. There may be no symptoms, nor redness of the eye, in the early stages; slit-lamp examination is essential. Cells appear in the anterior chamber when inflammation is active. Untreated, inflammation can damage the cornea, lens, and aqueous drainage causing band keratopathy, cataract, glaucoma, and risk of blindness. Topical treatment may prevent secondary problems, but some patients will lose useful vision in both eyes. Other causes of iritis in children include sarcoidosis, ankylosing spondylitis, toxocariasis, and masquerade syndromes such as leukaemia or retinoblastoma.

Wegener's granulomatosis

Many patients notice that their eyes become red with episcleritis when Wegener's granulomatosis is active, and occasionally there is a more severe painful necrotizing scleritis. This typically involves the cornea; slit-lamp examination reveals infiltrates of inflammatory cells in the peripheral cornea. There is the risk of thinning and perforation of cornea or sclera. The eye is acutely red and may be intensely painful, sometimes preventing sleep. Sight-threatening sclerokeratitis responds poorly to topical treatment and requires systemic immunosuppression; a pulsed intravenous regime may be needed for initial control.

In patients with 'limited' Wegener's granulomatosis of the upper airway, the orbit may be involved, usually secondary to disease in the adjacent sinuses, but sometimes in isolation. Retro-orbital granuloma produces proptosis, usually painful, which may involve cranial nerves, including the optic nerve, with an acute threat to vision (Fig. 25.1.12). Some patients have a positive antineutrophil cytoplasmic antibody (ANCA) test though the titres may be low. Many respond to immunosuppression, but high doses may be required for local control.

Polyarteritis nodosa

Inflammation of the eye coat, similar to Wegener's granulomatosis, may produce episcleritis, scleritis, or keratitis. Complications may be severe, requiring systemic immunosuppression. The retinal vessels may be involved, with or without hypertensive changes, and branch arteriolar closure is characteristic. Uveitis is not a feature.

Relapsing polychondritis

This systemic inflammatory disorder involving cartilage is associated with inflammation of the eye coat, similar to rheumatoid arthritis. Half the patients will have eye features at some stage. Episcleritis and scleritis are most common, sometimes with severe corneal features similar to Wegener's granulomatosis. Uveitis, Sjögren's syndrome, and ischaemic optic neuropathy also occur.

Systemic lupus erythematosus

Episcleritis may occur with exacerbations in systemic lupus activity; the more serious scleritis is uncommon. Retinal vascular occlusions, particularly venous but sometimes branch arterial, may be linked with the antiphospholipid syndrome. Retinopathy with cotton wool spots is associated with active vasculitis, anaemia, and perhaps moderate hypertension. Ischaemic optic neuropathy with acute irretrievable loss of vision is unusual. Some patients, particularly those with mixed connective tissue disease, have Sjögren's syndrome. Uveitis is not a feature of SLE. Cutaneous lupus may involve the eyelids causing oedema, and the lid margins may develop scarring, inflammatory plaques.

Multiple sclerosis

Posterior uveitis can occur in multiple sclerosis. Low-grade, subtle changes are common, such as sheathing of the peripheral retinal veins with scant vitreous inflammatory cells, and fluorescein angiography reveals leakage from the retinal veins, even though the retina itself does not contain myelin. Association of ocular and neurological features also occur in sarcoidosis and Behçet's syndrome, but in these the eye inflammation is usually more pronounced.

Vogt–Koyanagi–Harada syndrome

This curious and uncommon clinical syndrome is comprised of bilateral panuveitis, deafness, and/or meningo-encephalitis with cerebrospinal fluid lymphocytosis in the acute stages. Patients are almost exclusively east Asian, and there are HLA associations. Inflammatory cells collect focally within the retinal pigment epithelium and may cause fluid detachment of the retina, associated with decreased vision. There is a response to systemic corticosteroids, with relapses if the dose is reduced. In the chronic phase of the disease, there is depigmentation of skin, hair, or eyelashes (poliosis).

Cogan's syndrome

Eye inflammation may be associated with deafness and/or vestibular dysfunction and proximal aortitis or inflammation of medium-sized arteries. Keratitis with patchy cell infiltration in the corneal stroma may lead to corneal vascularization, as in syphilitic keratitis. Some patients have anterior uveitis, scleritis, or retinitis. The disorder responds to systemic corticosteroid, which may prevent total deafness if given early enough, and may be life saving in aortitis.

Takayasu's arteritis

This inflammatory disorder involving large arteries can cause an aortic arch syndrome, with raised ESR and CRP, typically in younger patients. There may be amaurosis fugax, retinal vascular changes suggesting chronic ocular ischaemia, scleritis, or iritis.

Dermatomyositis

Purple coloration of the eyelids and oedema of the lids and conjunctiva are typical findings; retinal ischaemia with cotton wool spots is less common.

Kawasaki's disease

Bilateral conjunctivitis without discharge is a cardinal feature of Kawasaki's syndrome, characteristically found in young children. Other features are fever, rash, lymphadenopathy, and involvement of other mucosae and the nails. Slit-lamp examination may show inflammatory cells in the anterior chamber and/or cornea, but the eyes do not need specific treatment.

Inflammatory bowel disease

About 10% of patients with Crohn's disease have episcleritis, scleritis, or iritis. Corneal or retinal inflammation is uncommon. Episodes of episcleritis may be associated with exacerbation of the bowel disorder. Eye problems are less common in ulcerative colitis.

Pancreatitis

Ischaemic retinopathy and acute visual loss may occur. There is retinal oedema with cotton wool spots. Fluorescein angiography shows closure of branch retinal arterioles and capillaries, with patches of retinal nonperfusion.

Whipple's disease

This rare disorder is suggested by the association of a malabsorbing enteropathy with arthritis and ocular inflammation or particular neurological features. Retinal haemorrhages, diffuse retinal and choroidal vasculitis with cells in the vitreous, or keratitis are characteristic. Central nervous system features include cranial nerve palsies, papilloedema, and brainstem involvement. The diagnosis is confirmed by small-bowel biopsy (see Chapter 15.10.6).

Ocular features of blood disorders

Retinal changes are common in haematological disorders, even if vision is normal. Bilateral changes result from anaemia, hyperviscosity, and haemostatic abnormalities. The signs are easily missed unless the pupils are dilated.

Bilateral retinal haemorrhages suggest a blood disorder if blood pressure and blood sugar are normal—full blood count, ESR, and plasma protein electrophoresis should be checked. Hypoxia and/or hyperviscosity cause retinal vein enlargement, scattered retinal haemorrhages, and cotton wool spots. Roth spots—haemorrhages with a white centre—typical of endocarditis, also occur in leukaemia and hyperviscosity. Blood may leak in front of the retina to form a dense, rounded, often boat-shaped, subhyaloid blotch; leakage into the vitreous will cause clouding of vision with floaters.

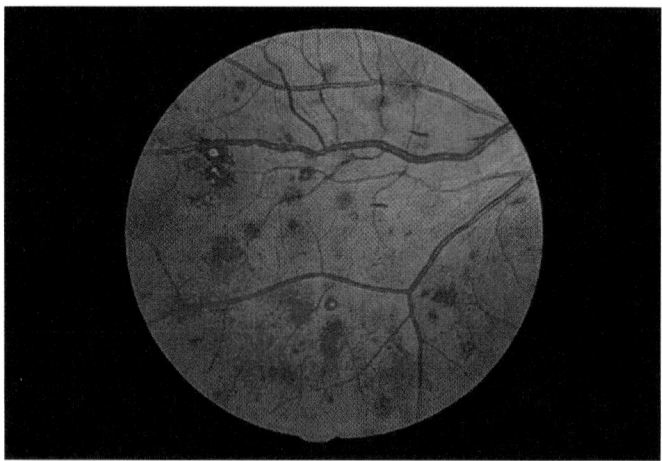

Fig. 25.1.15 Retinal haemorrhages in leukaemia. Multiple and bilateral retinal haemorrhages suggest a blood dyscrasia, if underlying diabetes and hypertension are excluded. In this case, the peripheral lymphocyte count was considerably raised, consistent with chronic lymphocytic leukaemia. Some haemorrhages have a white centre (Roth spot).

Leukaemias

Although retinopathy is common in acute and chronic leukaemias, it may be asymptomatic. Retinal haemorrhages are nonspecific, though Roth spots represent focal collections of white cells (Fig. 25.1.15). If the white cell count is very high, frank infiltration of the retina or optic nerve head causes pale, fluffy areas, and leukaemic cells may spill into the vitreous. Chronic leukaemias may cause a 'slow flow' picture from chronic retinal hypoxia. Retinopathy may improve with chemotherapy. In acute lymphoblastic leukaemia, collections of cells may form on the iris, masquerading as iritis, or a mass presenting retro-orbitally may cause proptosis. Ocular infiltrations may respond to radiotherapy. Associated infections, including orbital mucormycosis, and chemotherapy or radiotherapy may affect the eye. Bone marrow transplantation is associated with cataract, and graft-vs-host disease may cause conjunctival scarring with severe dry eye.

Lymphomas

Lymphoma may occur around or inside one or both eyes. Non-Hodgkin's, low-grade, B-cell lymphomas occur in isolation, in disseminated disease, or in relapse. Externally, they form firm swellings in the eyelid or conjunctiva, resembling smoked salmon. In the orbit, lymphomas may cause neuro-ophthalmic signs. T-cell tumours may infiltrate the internal eye, particularly the iris or choroid. The rare ocular reticulum cell sarcoma—'histiocytic' lymphoma—can masquerade as uveitis, but with a pale mass in the choroid or retina visible through a cloudy vitreous. The monoclonal cells may spread from or to the brain, typically to the frontal or temporal lobes, so repeated cranial scanning is necessary. Immunocytochemistry of cells obtained by vitreous biopsy is diagnostic. Ocular lymphomas usually respond to local radiotherapy.

Bleeding diatheses

Pronounced or repeated subconjunctival haemorrhage, hyphaema, or vitreous haemorrhage may suggest a bleeding diathesis. Bleeding may be spontaneous, or follow minor trauma or eye surgery. In haemophilia, bleeding around or inside the orbit may compress the optic or other cranial nerves.

Clotting tendencies

Thrombophilias, including factor V Leiden, protein S, protein C, or antithrombin III deficiencies, are associated with retinal vascular occlusion, especially in the veins. Closure of choroidal vessels affects vision if fluid exudes to detach the retina; this pattern suggests thrombotic thrombocytopenic purpura (TTP) or diffuse intravascular coagulation (DIC). Retinal venous or arterial occlusions occur in SLE with lupus anticoagulant or antiphospholipid antibodies. The optic nerve head may be involved, causing amaurosis fugax or ischaemic optic neuropathy. A full clotting screen is indicated in patients with retinal vein thrombosis if another site is involved, if episodes are multiple, or there is a family history of thrombosis at any site. Myeloma should also be considered.

Sickling haemoglobinopathies

Though minor eye features are common in the sickling haemoglobinopathies, major eye features occur in less than one-half of patients. They are more common with mixed heterozygosity—see below. Unilateral blindness is uncommon, even in SC patients, and so bilateral blindness is rare. As early treatment improves prognosis, screening the retina of high-risk patients is important.

Retinal neovascularization

Sickling in terminal branches of retinal arterioles produces peripheral ischaemia with the potential for neovascularization. Prevalence of new vessels is related to age, as most form between the ages of 10 and 25 years; rarely after 40. In SC patients, risk of blindness peaks between age 20 and 30. Severe retinal ischaemia with new vessel formation is twice as common in haemoglobin SC and SThal as in SS. The risk of vitreous haemorrhage, with poorer prognosis, is related to the number and size of new vessels.

Patients must be screened with fully dilated pupils using the indirect ophthalmoscope or an accessory lens at the slit lamp. The earliest sign of peripheral ischaemia is closure of arterioles in the superior temporal sector (stage I) with a paler background and narrow/white vessels. If these areas extend and become confluent, anastomotic loops form (stage II), and then tufts of new vessels (stage III). As the tufts grow forwards into the vitreous, they often look like 'coral seafans'. Fluorescein angiography reveals profusely leaking new vessels whose size can be assessed. Many new vessel tufts will autoinfarct from sickling in the feeder arteriole; these will not then bleed but others may form, so the patient must still be observed.

There are no symptoms until vitreous haemorrhage occurs (stage IV). Small haemorrhages produce a sudden shower of small floaters, like midges. Large haemorrhages cause sudden, marked cloudiness with reduced red reflex. If the retina is distorted or detached (stage V) there may be flashes of light and a visual field defect. Some patients lose central vision with macular ischaemia, foveal haemorrhage, or central retinal artery occlusion. Retinal vein occlusion is not associated with sickling.

Screening and treatment of sickle retinopathy

Annual retinal screening is recommended for patients aged between 20 and 30, especially those with SC and SThal disease. New vessels should be reassessed every few months—if they do not auto-infarct and their size increases or vitreous haemorrhage occurs, laser treatment should cause regression and reduce risk of blindness.

Other eye features

Conjunctival signs, more marked in haemoglobin SS than SC, are linear, saccular, or comma-shaped dilatations of small conjunctival vessels, more prominent in children and after topical application of phenylephrine drops.

Bleeding into the peripheral retina is usually asymptomatic and does not threaten vision. It causes a round 'salmon patch' which resolves over several weeks to leave iridescent haemosiderin spots in the superficial retina. Deeper haemorrhages damage the underlying retinal pigment layer leaving a permanent, black 'sunburst' scar.

The risk of both acute painful and chronic painless glaucoma is increased. Orbital infarction and pneumococcal endophthalmitis are both rare complications. Patients may suffer a stroke affecting the visual field.

Infectious diseases and the eye

Organisms on the surface of the eye can be identified from swabs. Treatment for superficial eye infections is by topical antimicrobial drops or ointments. Infections inside the eye are identified from their pattern of involvement; it is rarely necessary to aspirate material from inside the eye. Internal infections demand systemic therapy; the choice is partly dictated by penetration into the eye cavities. Rarely, drugs are injected directly into the vitreous to supplement systemic treatment in achieving high intraocular levels.

Bacterial infections

The commonest bacterial eye infection is conjunctivitis caused by *Staphylococcus aureus*, haemophilus, or the pneumococci. Topical chloramphenicol is effective as drops—hourly for the first 24 h then thrice daily for several days—with ointment at night. Cellulitis is usually caused by the same organisms—haemophilus is common in children—and systemic amoxicillin is the regimen of choice. Orbital spread is an ophthalmic emergency requiring hospitalization. If the patient is systemically ill or has orbital signs of proptosis, double vision, or loss of vision, a scan is indicated and intravenous treatment is warranted.

Metastatic endophthalmitis results when blood-borne bacteria seed to the internal eye (Fig. 25.1.16). The commonest sources are

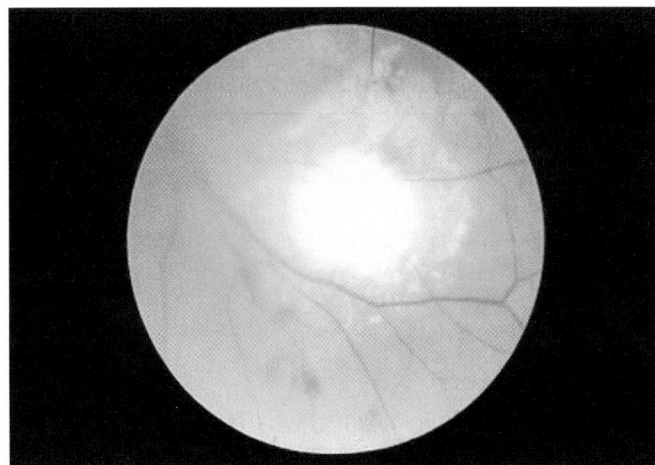

Fig. 25.1.16 Metastatic staphylococcal endophthalmitis. Blood borne organisms may settle in the eye, forming a focal abscess in the choroid, breaking through the adjacent retina into the vitreous which becomes hazy with inflammatory cells. This patient had poorly-controlled diabetes and a staphylococcal skin infection.

skin, urinary, and cardiac. The most likely organisms are staphylococci or streptococci. *Bacillus cereus* and fungi (see below) may complicate intravenous drug abuse and unusual opportunistic organisms must also be considered in immunosuppressed patients or those with poorly controlled diabetes. There is visual impairment with pain. Cells and debris within the eye chambers blur the ophthalmoscopic view, though a pale chorioretinal focus of infection may be visible. Blood, urine, and cerebrospinal fluid cultures are necessary. Tapping of the internal eye for vitreous microscopy and culture is justified in some cases. In infective endocarditis, retinal haemorrhages and microembolic infarcts are common, classically in the form of Roth spots.

Tuberculosis can cause indolent granulomatous uveitis, either of the iris or choroid. In leprosy, the eye is more frequently involved, with a risk of blindness—a specific iritis and cataracts occur in the lepromatous form and corneal scarring complicates facial palsy and/or reduced corneal sensation.

In syphilis, uveitis or neuroretinitis occur in the secondary stage and optic neuropathy or Argyll Robertson pupils in the tertiary stage. Congenital syphilis is associated with interstitial keratitis and a 'salt-and-pepper' retinopathy. *Leptospira icterohaemorrhagiae* commonly causes an early conjunctivitis with subconjuctival haemorrhages, and a late uveitis. Late Lyme disease may cause ocular inflammation.

The gonococcus causes a marked purulent conjunctivitis in the newborn or in those sexually exposed. Tularaemia is associated with a severe granulomatous conjunctivitis with local lymph node enlargement. Botulism causes paralysis of the ocular muscles, sometimes with autonomic signs, with diphtheria as a differential diagnosis. Brucellosis can cause optic neuritis or uveitis and should be considered especially in slaughterhouse or farm workers. Actinomycetes can infect the tear canaliculi. Rarely, nocardia can infect the internal eye with a focal chorioretinitis.

Chlamydial eye infection (see Chapter 7.6.44)

The genital serotypes of chlamydia cause acute conjunctivitis. The eye is red and sticky, and lymphoid follicles are found in the conjunctiva lining the eyelids. Infection is persistent, responding only partially to topical chloramphenicol. Systemic tetracycline or erythromycin, with topical tetracycline, is effective.

Trachoma is the most common cause of chronic conjunctivitis, a preventable cause of blindness worldwide. At least 600 million people are infected, and about 6 million blinded. *Chlamydia trachomatis* serotypes A to C cause chronic conjunctivitis with follicles, which look like pale grains of rice in the conjunctiva. Scarring of the lids associated with in-turning eyelashes may accelerate corneal scarring. The diagnosis is confirmed by seeing inclusions in conjunctival scrapes or by culturing the organism from swabs. The World Health Organization recommendations for control are topical tetracycline ointment twice daily for 7 days 6 times a year, or six doses of oral doxycycline 5 mg/kg given monthly.

Viral infections and the eye

Adenoviral conjunctivitis is the most common viral infection, usually caused by highly contagious, potentially epidemic types 3, 4, 7, 8, or 19. The eye is acutely red and uncomfortable with watering, but scanty discharge. Lymphoid follicles may be visible in the conjunctiva lining the eyelids and the preauricular node may be enlarged. Symptoms may continue for some weeks, but recovery is usually uneventful and treatment rarely necessary. The most important differential diagnosis is chlamydial infection, in which eye discharge is more profuse.

Measles, meningococcal, or disseminated gonococcal, infection may be implicated in systemically ill patients with fever, rash, and red eyes. In some parts of the world, relapsing fevers (borreliosis) or rickettsioses may be the underlying infection. Conjunctivitis with marked local lymphadenopathy (oculoglandular syndrome) may be attributable to adenovirus, chlamydia, mumps, or other (rarer) causes.

Primary herpes simplex can cause conjunctivitis. Secondary herpes is associated with recurrent attacks of dendritic corneal ulceration which, especially if treated with topical corticosteroid, can result in corneal scarring and poor vision. Herpes zoster can cause corneal ulceration, iritis, glaucoma, and delayed cranial nerve palsies, including optic neuropathy or Adie pupil. Patients with ophthalmic shingles should be referred for slit-lamp examination if there is red eye or visual impairment. All herpes viruses can cause retinal infection, particularly in the immunosuppressed; simplex and zoster can cause potentially blinding necrotizing retinitis, which progresses rapidly and may respond poorly to systemic antiviral therapy.

Particularly in patients with AIDS, cytomegalovirus causes progressive retinitis with characteristic haemorrhages and patchy retinal necrosis (see below). In transplant patients, cytomegalovirus infection may respond to reduction of immunosuppression.

Measles may cause a scarring corneal inflammation—an important cause of blindness in undernourished children. Inflammation of the internal eye is less common. Neuro-ophthalmic associations occur in subacute sclerosing panencephalitis (SSPE). Congenital rubella and varicella are associated with cataract and retinopathy in infancy. Iritis is characteristic of mumps. Molluscum contagiosum, cowpox, and orf can cause lid infection.

Fungal infections

Indolent fungal keratitis is associated with contact lens wear, diabetes, exposure to inoculation in the garden or field, and intravenous opiate abuse. Metastatic endophthalmitis is usually caused by *Candida albicans* in association with immunosuppression, irradiation, intravenous drug use or abuse, and poorly controlled diabetes. Small, dense, white 'snowballs' are seen in the vitreous with white foci of infection visible in the choroid and overlying retina (Fig. 25.1.17). Retinal haemorrhage is uncommon. Diagnosis can be confirmed by vitreous biopsy, which provides the opportunity to inject antifungal agent into the eye. The differential diagnosis of a white focus with a hazy vitreous full of cells includes purulent endophthalmitis, toxoplasmosis, intraocular lymphoma, sarcoid, or tuberculosis.

Infection in or around the orbit is characteristic of invasive mucormycosis in the same groups at risk of candidiasis, especially debilitated patients under treatment for haematological malignancies and in severe diabetic ketoacidosis. The infection spreads rapidly, often involving the vascular supply and producing tissue necrosis—blackening of the hard palate is pathognomonic. Medical treatment is combined with surgical debridement, but prognosis is poor.

In endemic areas such as the Mississippi basin (United States of America), *Histoplasma capsulatum* produces a multifocal, scarring chorioretinitis described as 'histospots'.

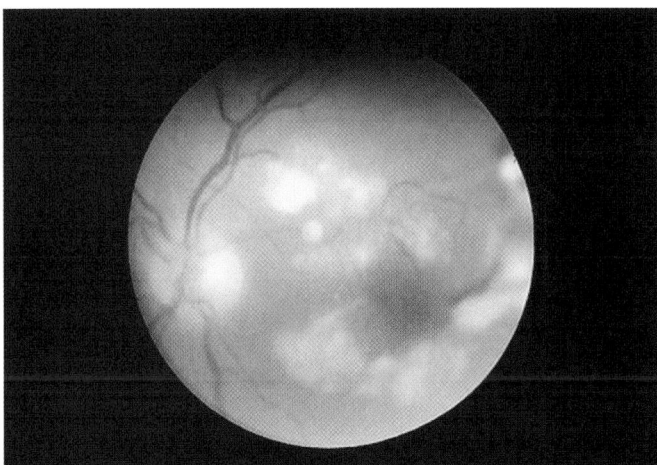

Fig. 25.1.17 Candida endophthalmitis. Fungal infection of the eye interior forms white 'snowballs' within the vitreous and retina. The organism is usually blood borne and may enter the circulation with intravenously injected agents, including heroin. Infection is indolent, with a relatively white eye and little pain. Vitrectomy and intravitreal antimicrobial treatment may be necessary.

Rickettsial infection

There are petechial haemorrhages of the bulbar conjunctiva with marked redness, and retinal haemorrhages also occur.

Protozoal infections

Toxoplasma gondii can cause congenital infection of the retina and underlying choroid if the mother acquired a primary infection in pregnancy; this is especially common in France and Brazil. The primary scar may involve the macula or optic nerve head and results in congenitally poor vision. More commonly, an asymptomatic scar reactivates later in life, releasing cells into the vitreous (Fig. 25.1.18); an inactive scar may be visible in the other eye. Patients present with visual blurring and often describe floaters. Presumptive diagnosis is based on clinical findings and positive blood serology. Acute attacks are best treated promptly, by an ophthalmologist, with several weeks of combined systemic clindamycin or co-trimoxazole together with corticosteroid. Some infants have associated cerebral toxoplasmosis.

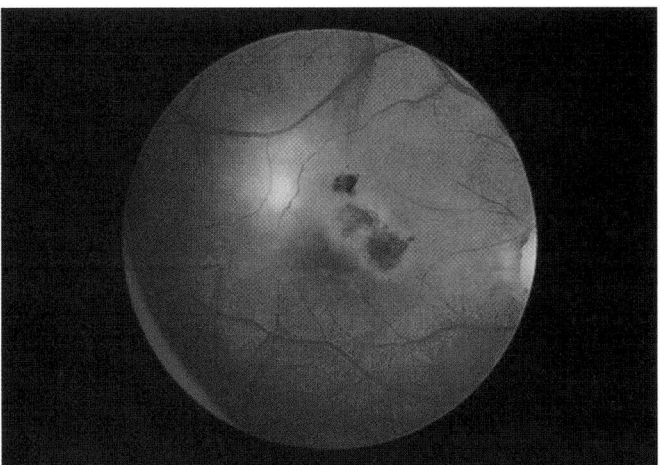

Fig. 25.1.18 Toxoplasmosis. A fluffy fresh focus of infection within the choroid and retina is found adjacent to an old pigmented scar, typical of toxoplasmosis. The organism encysts within the retina and may reactivate sporadically in this way.

Retinal haemorrhages are commonly found in patients with cerebral malaria (see Chapter 7.8.2). Retinal toxicity has not been reported with standard use of antimalarials, but has been reported with chloroquine abuse.

Ulcers and nodules of cutaneous leishmaniasis may be seen on the eyelids in endemic areas. Retinal haemorrhages are common in kala-azar, particularly when there is associated anaemia. Keratosis may occur in African trypanosomiasis. In Latin America, oedema of the eyelids, lacrimal gland, and local lymph nodes (Romaña's sign) develops in the weeks following a periocular bite by a reduviid 'kissing' bug transmitting *Trypanosoma cruzi*—the causative agent of Chaga's disease.

Acanthamoeba can cause an indolent and potentially blinding keratitis in contact lens wearers or after corneal abrasion.

Pneumocystis jiroveci choroiditis is discussed in Chapter 7.7.5.

Helminth infections

Onchocerciasis or 'river blindness' (see Chapter 7.9.1) was a common cause of blindness particularly in Africa. Microfilariae lodge particularly in the choroid causing insidiously progressive, destructive, and scarring chorio-retinitis. Targeted widespread use of ivermectin has produced tangible reduction in blindness. Lymphatic filariasis rarely affects the eye.

Nematode worms *Toxocara canis* (see Chapter 7.9.5) form a visible mass beneath the retina with uveitis and, sometimes, whitening of the pupil, of which the differential diagnosis is a tumour such as retinoblastoma.

Some adult worms invade the eye surface. Loa-loa (see Chapter 7.9.1) may be felt by the patient and is visible to an observer beneath the bulbar conjunctiva; it may be removed surgically. In Japan, the fly-transmitted 'oriental eye worm' thelazia occurs in the conjunctival sac. In South-East Asia, gnathostoma infects the eyelids or internal eye, where the larvae may be visible with slit-lamp magnification.

When undercooked pork is eaten, trichinosis (*Trichinella spiralis* infection) affects extraocular muscles, causing pain, periorbital oedema, proptosis, and defective eye movements. There may be internal eye involvement.

Sparganosis (see Chapter 7.10.4) can cause conjunctivitis, swelling, itching, proptosis, and blindness.

The larval form of cysticercosis may be visible inside the eye in either chamber, looking like a motile pearl or *toxocara*-like mass. Posterior uveitis and retinitis may occur. Orbital involvement is rare, though orbital cysts—typically calcified—may occur in patients with hydatid disease.

In schistosomiasis, an urticarial conjunctivitis is associated with egg deposition, but the interior of the eye is rarely involved.

Myiasis can involve the eye and orbit—ophthalmomyiasis externa (Chapter 7.12).

HIV and AIDS (see also Chapters 7.5.23 and 7.5.24)

Eye signs are common, particularly in the later stages of AIDS. The retina and optic nerve head are most commonly involved. In patients with coexisting central nervous system infection, eye features may provide an important clue, although definitive diagnosis in life by retinal biopsy is rarely justified. The cellular response within the eye is scantier than usual. Opportunistic pathogens tend to be facultative intracellular agents. Cytomegalovirus retinitis is the most common problem in people with AIDS in industrialized countries,

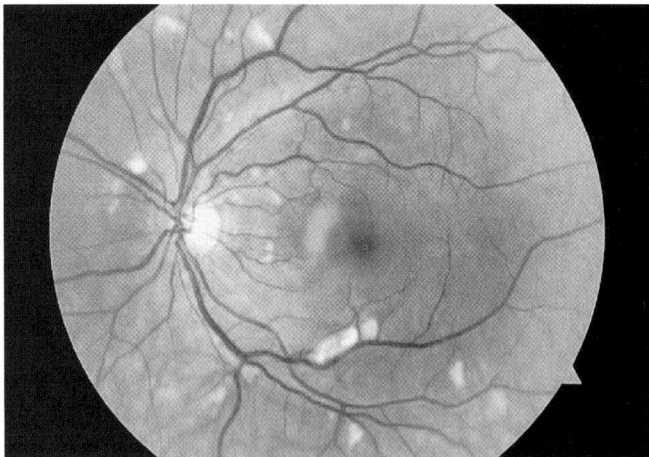

Fig. 25.1.19 Cotton wool spots. Retinal microinfarcts are due to occlusion of capillaries which supply the nerve fibre layer. These multiple 'cotton wool spots' are found associated with microemboli, as after cardiac surgery employing bypass. In patients with AIDS they may form especially at the time of pulmonary infection, for instance with *Pneumocystis carinii*.

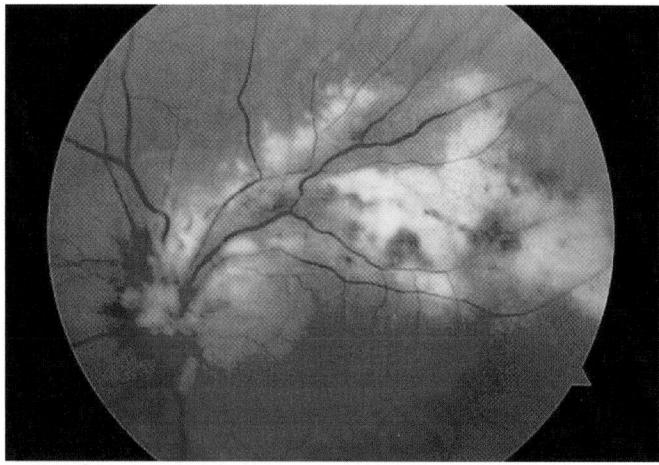

Fig. 25.1.20 CMV retinitis. The appearance of focal, fluffy, pale retinal necrosis with haemorrhages is characteristic of infection with cytomegalovirus. The area expands relentlessly, spreading along the branch vessels, unless treatment with virustatic agent is instituted or the CD4 lymphocyte count can be improved. The usual underlying disorder is AIDS.

though rarely seen in haemophiliacs. In Africa, nonspecific retinopathy and herpes zoster ophthalmicus are more common.

Retinal microvascular disease is common. Cotton wool spots (Fig. 25.1.19) are seen in relatively early HIV infection, with haemorrhages, Roth spots, and microaneurysms. There may be closure and sheathing of the peripheral retinal venous branches and occasional microvascular closure around the fovea producing visual loss. This retinal pattern is common in patients in Africa, particularly children.

Cytomegalovirus retinitis

This was the most common ocular complication in sexually acquired HIV infection in the United Kingdom and United States of America, affecting about one in three of such patients in the later stages of AIDS when the peripheral CD4 T-cell count fell below 100/µl. Since the introduction of highly active antiretroviral therapy (HAART) the incidence has fallen and the prognosis improved strikingly (see Chapter 7.5.23).

The typical appearance is of patchy areas of pale crumbled-looking retina with associated scattered haemorrhages—'pizza retinitis'—most commonly around branch vessels (Fig. 25.1.20). These are areas of cytomegalovirus replication with oedematous and necrotic retina and some cellular infiltration, mostly neutrophils and macrophages; the cell response within the eye cavity is usually scanty, though symptomatic floaters are usual. The patches spread contiguously from their borders and, untreated, enlarge week by week. Retinal death eventually results in blindness. Before the introduction of HAART, the average life expectancy of AIDS patients with cytomegalovirus retinitis was about 9 months.

Differential diagnoses of these appearances include cotton wool spots, HIV retinopathy, branch retinal vein occlusion (all with no vitreous cells), syphilis, toxoplasmosis, early acute retinal necrosis, candidiasis, cryptococcal infection, or lymphoma (all with vitreous cells). Definitive diagnosis is difficult—serology discourages a diagnosis only if repeatedly negative and polymerase chain reaction (PCR) testing of vitreous aspirate may be helpful.

An adequate dose of systemic virustatic—cidofovir, ganciclovir, or foscarnet—damps down the infection. The lesions become

atrophic with resolution of the pale and haemorrhagic features and arrest of spread. Ganciclovir treatment is initiated with 2 weeks of twice-daily intravenous doses of 5 mg/kg. The dose is reduced if there is renal impairment. The daily maintenance dose is 5 mg/kg intravenously or 3 g orally, though maintenance treatment for retinitis in patients whose CD4 count cannot be elevated is now optimally with oral valganciclovir. The most important side effect is bone marrow suppression. To avoid toxicity, ganciclovir may be given by direct injection into the eye (vitreous), but this is rarely justified as the treatment must be repeated perhaps weekly, and the infection is usually bilateral and widespread in the body.

In patients with cytomegalovirus retinitis, the low CD4 cell count must be improved with highly active antiretroviral therapy; once the count is securely above 100/µl, maintenance therapy for cytomegalovirus may usually be suspended. Spread of retinitis will occur if treatment is interrupted and if the CD4 cell count remains low, breakthrough of retinitis is common; this is treated by repeating the induction course of ganciclovir or by switching to foscarnet or cidofovir. Ophthalmic supervision is important, as it is more accurate to assess the lesions by indirect ophthalmoscopy, preferably with serial retinal photographs to document progression at the edges of lesions.

Other infections

HIV infection is a common association of herpes zoster ophthalmicus, especially in nonindustrial countries. Retinal infection with herpes zoster or simplex may also cause rapidly spreading retinal death, as acute retinal necrosis (ARN) or progressive outer retinal necrosis (PORN) with pale oedematous areas lacking the crumbled texture and haemorrhages characteristic of cytomegalovirus retinitis. There is often involvement of the optic nerve with optic neuritis, and sometimes there may be encephalitis. Vision can be lost bilaterally, within days, if untreated. Intravenous aciclovir or cidofovir may halt spread within the retina.

Syphilis in HIV infection may cause iritis or optic neuritis, often bilaterally. There may be retinitis with a vitreous cell reaction, abnormal cerebrospinal fluid, or other signs of central nervous system involvement. Nonspecific treponemal serology may be negative, so specific tests must be done. Eye complications are treated with benzathine penicillin, using a regime suitable for central nervous system infection.

Toxoplasmal choroido-retinitis in HIV-infected patients may show a fluffy, focal retinal lesion with cells in both chambers. These signs may explain accompanying optic neuritis or encephalitis. Treatment is with clindamycin; occasionally, systemic corticosteroid may be indicated.

Pneumocystis jiroveci may occasionally cause a multifocal choroidoretinitis with multiple, pale, rounded patches visible beneath the retina, and cryptococcus may present an acute optic neuropathy associated with meningitis.

Disorders of the thyroid and parathyroid

Eye signs result either from imbalance of thyroid hormones, or from an immunological disorder of both the thyroid (Graves' disease) and retro-orbital tissues. This, the most common cause of proptosis—synonymous with exophthalmos—is referred to as 'Graves' ophthalmopathy' or 'ophthalmic Graves' disease'.

Cosmetic concerns and eye discomfort are common, but a threat to vision is an acute emergency. Evolution of eye signs is often independent of current thyroid status: the patient may be euthyroid, hyperthyroid, or hypothyroid at presentation, and correction of hormonal imbalance may not affect eye features (Box 25.1.5). Commonly, orbital disease appears in patients who have become hypothyroid after treatment for hyperthyroidism.

Orbital features result from infiltration of tissues by T cells, stimulated by autoantibodies which cross-react with adipocytes. Initially, fibroblasts are stimulated to produce mucilaginous material and oedema within fat and muscle, which ultimately leads to fibrosis and atrophy.

The eyelids may be swollen, especially on waking, in both hyper- and hypothyroidism. In hyperthyroidism, upper lid retraction reveals white sclera above the cornea and there is lid lag. Raised orbital pressure causes congestion, swelling, (chemosis), and redness of the eye, particularly over the visible tendon insertions of the lateral rectus muscles (Fig. 25.1.21). Diplopia is common—it is usually vertical and worse on looking upwards, and is also worse on waking.

Proptosis causes white sclera to appear, often asymmetrically, below the lower corneal margin. This can be measured from the bony rim of the orbit using an exophthalmometer, which gives a useful assessment of progression.

Thyroid function and autoantibody tests may be normal in patients with typical eye disease. Scans, especially coronal MRI views, typically show enlargement of ocular muscles. Severe protrusion with upper lid retraction exposes the cornea to damage from

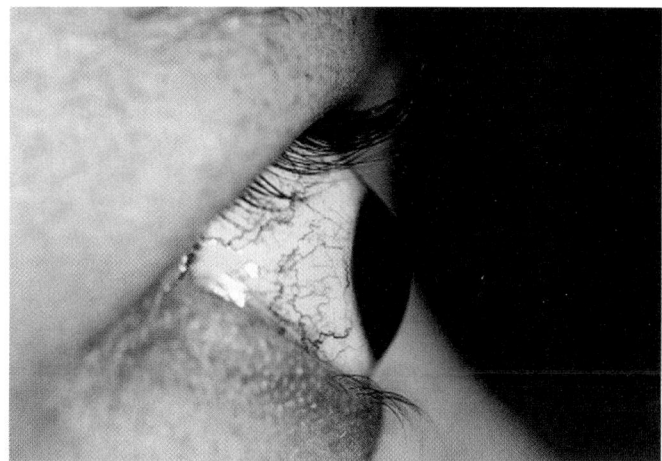

Fig. 25.1.21 Thyroid eye disease with exophthalmos. Inflammation of orbital tissues—fat and muscles—causes protrustion of the eye—exophthalmos or proptosis. The eyelids also become swollen and the conjunctiva congested. Autoimmune thyroid disease (Graves' disease) is the most common underlying disorder

corneal abrasion, and ulceration, even perforation, can develop rapidly; so patients with a protruding eye, impaired blinking, pain, or fluorescein staining of the cornea are an ophthalmic emergency.

Orbital pressure may be highest in patients without much proptosis, as protrusion has a decompressing effect. Optic nerve compression causes visual blurring, perhaps with a central scotoma, loss of colour definition, or relative afferent pupillary defect. The optic nerve head may be swollen. Scanning shows enlarged extraocular muscles. Immediate management is necessary to retrieve vision, as optic nerve compression needs urgent orbital decompression—medically, using high-dose systemic corticosteroid, or surgically, by removing bone from the orbital walls, or by orbital radiotherapy in severe cases.

Cosmetic orbital surgery is rarely justified, but upper lid surgery is sometimes worthwhile. Discomfort is difficult to treat; simple artificial tears may be tried. Immunosuppression seems justified for active orbital inflammation. Initially, diplopia is best managed with a plastic Fresnel prism stuck on to a spectacle lens. Stable diplopia may need a permanent spectacle prism, surgery, or botulinum toxin injection. Corneal exposure demands temporary taping of the lids, or single lid suture under local anaesthesia, or, if prolonged, lateral tarsorrhaphy.

Differential diagnosis

Few conditions mimic thyroid eye disease in having bilateral, if asymmetrical, signs. Upper lid signs are particularly helpful in suggesting this diagnosis. Another cause of one congested protuberant eye is an orbital mass, usually unilateral. Orbital pseudotumour or myositis is characteristically more painful and a carotico-cavernous arteriovenous fistula typically causes a frontotemporal bruit. These conditions are partly differentiated by their neuroradiological features.

Parathyroid disorders

Hyperparathyroidism producing hypercalcaemia may cause calcium deposition as band keratopathy—a lacey opacity which spreads horizontally from the corneal margins inwards. The eyes may be red, and they feel gritty.

Box 25.1.5 Werner's classification of thyroid eye disease

◆ Class 0: signs and symptoms both absent

◆ Class 1: signs without symptoms

◆ Class 2: both symptoms and signs of soft-tissue involvement

◆ Class 3: proptosis indicating orbital involvement

◆ Class 4: eye muscle involvement with double vision

◆ Class 5: secondary corneal involvement

◆ Class 6: optic nerve involvement with loss of vision

In hypoparathyroidism and pseudohypoparathyroidism, hypocalcaemia causes lens opacities—small, white, or coloured crystals beneath the lens capsule which may not impair vision. Papilloedema from intracranial hypertension is rare, and is reversed by correcting hypocalcaemia.

Multiple endocrine neoplasia (MEN) syndrome

In type IIb of this rare autosomal dominant condition, prominent corneal nerves are easily detected by slit-lamp examination. Conjunctival neuromas and thickened eyelids may occur.

The eye in diagnosis of inherited conditions (Table 25.1.4)

Marfan's syndrome (see Chapter 20.2)

Most patients have reduced vision, commonly due to myopia and astigmatism, which may be inferred from their spectacle lenses. Slit-lamp examination reveals lens dislocation upwards (Fig. 25.1.22), best assessed if the pupil is dilated. The iris may tremble with eye movement—iridodonesis—because of poor support by an abnormally mobile lens. The dislocated lenses are best retained and careful correction of focus can improve vision dramatically; in early childhood, this may prevent permanent amblyopia. Differential diagnoses of dislocated lenses are isolated ectopia lentis (without other marfanoid features) and homocystinuria (with marfanoid habitus).

Neurofibromatosis

Most patients have raised, yellowish, or brown, multiple, Lisch nodules of the iris visible by slit lamp which must be distinguished from common, simple, flat, iris freckles. Corneal, retinal, or orbital neurofibromas/schwannomas may be found. There is an increased incidence of glaucoma. Screening and management of intracranial tumours associated with neurofibromatosis type 1, including optic nerve or chiasmal gliomas, is controversial (see Chapter 24.17). Neurofibromatosis type 2 is associated with posterior subcapsular cataracts.

von Hippel–Lindau syndrome

Retinal angiomas may be the presenting, and sole, features. These are usually bilateral, multiple, and sited in the mid-peripheral retina, so indirect ophthalmoscopy is advised. The initial lesion is very small, no bigger than a microaneurysm, but it enlarges, developing dilated, tortuous feeder and draining retinal vessels and a characteristic angiographic pattern. Early, peripheral angiomas may be destroyed by laser, preferably before they enlarge, bleed, or cause retinal detachment. Juxtapapillary angiomas at the optic nerve head may affect vision early in their development and are difficult to treat (Fig. 25.1.23). Prolonged eye follow-up is necessary.

Inherited premalignant conditions

Gardner's syndrome is deep retinal pigmentation with polyposis coli. The dark retinal patches—multiple and usually bilateral—are best seen by indirect ophthalmoscopy.

Neurofibromatosis type 1 (see above) may be associated with malignant visual pathway gliomas.

Absence of the iris (aniridia) is associated with renal Wilm's tumour, especially if there is a chromosome 11p deletion.

Table 25.1.4 Eye findings in some inherited disorders

Eyelid	
Epicanthus	Turner's syndrome (XO), trisomy 18 (Edward's syndrome), Down's syndrome, deletions 13q, 18, 4p, 5p
Ptosis	Kearns–Sayre disease, myotonic dystrophy, Turner's syndrome (XO), 13q deletion
Conjunctiva	
Telangiectasia	Osler–Weber–Rendu syndrome, Louis–Bar syndrome, Sturge–Weber syndrome, Fabry's disease, fucosidosis
Pingueculae	Gaucher's disease
Cornea	
Kayser–Fleischer ring	Wilson's disease
Cornea verticillata	Fabry's disease
Corneal crystals	Cystinosis
Corneal clouding	Mucolipidoses, mucopolysaccharidoses, Lowe's syndrome, X-linked ichthyosis, tyrosinaemia, Tangier, trisomy 18
Thickened corneal nerves	Multiple endocrine neoplasia type IIb
Keratoconus	Down's syndrome
Iris	
Iris tremor (iridodonesis)	Marfan's syndrome
Lisch nodule	Neurofibromatosis type 1
Iris transillumination	Albinism
Aniridia (absent iris)	Wilm's tumour/11p deletion
Coloboma (cat eye)	Trisomy 22
Brushfield spots	Down's syndrome
Lens	
Lens dislocation	Marfan's syndrome, homocystinuria, ectopia lentis
Lenticonus	Alport's syndrome
Cataract, infantile	Galactosaemia, galactokinase deficiency, Down's syndrome, Lowe's syndrome
Cataract, childhood	Skeletal, chromosomal, and dermatological syndromes
Cataract, adult	Myotonic dystrophy, Wilson's disease, neurofibromatosis type 2, Fabry's disease, mannosidosis
Retina	
Retinal angioma	von Hippel–Lindau disease, Sturge–Weber syndrome
Retinal phakoma	Tuberous sclerosis, neurofibromatosis type 1
Angioid streaks	Pseudoxanthoma elasticum
Retinal dysplasia	Norrie's disease, incontinentia pigmenti
Macular abnormality	Batten's disease, Farber's disease, Gaucher's disease
Macular cherry-red spot	Sialidosis, Niemann–Pick disease, Tay–Sachs disease
Pigmentary retinopathy	Usher's disease, mitochondrial myopathy (some), Refsum's disease, Kearns–Sayre disease, abetalipoproteinaemia, Hurler's syndrome, Laurence–Moon–Biedl syndrome
Pigmented patches	Gardner's syndrome
Gyrate atrophy	Hyperornithinaemia
Retinoblastoma	13q deletion
Vascular anomaly	Fucosidosis
Crystals	Cystinosis, oxalosis, Alport's syndrome

Table 25.1.4 *(Cont'd)* Eye findings in some inherited disorders

Sclera	
Blue sclera	Osteogenesis imperfecta
Thinned sclera	Ehler's–Danlos syndrome
Pigmented sclera	Alkaptonuria
Glaucoma	Neurofibromatosis type 1, Sturge–Weber syndrome

Retinoblastoma, when associated with deletion of chromosome 13q, is inheritable as dominant with high penetrance, together with other tumours such as osteosarcomas.

In multiple endocrine neoplasia (MEN) syndrome type IIB, associated especially with thyroid malignancy, there are enlarged corneal nerves and other ocular abnormalities (see above).

von Hippel–Lindau syndrome is associated with malignant renal tumours.

Ocular drug toxicity

Few drugs require ophthalmic screening, but visual loss can result from acute poisoning.

Corticosteroids

Lens opacities, which are typically posterior and subcapsular and produce light scatter with glare, are visible by slit lamp or ophthalmoscope if set to catch the red reflex in focus, particularly if the pupil is dilated. Surgery may be necessary. Topical corticosteroid eye drops may cause secondary glaucoma.

Antimalarials

The risks of chloroquine are discussed in Chapter 7.8.2. Patients may develop a dose-dependant, progressive retinal toxicity of the 'bull's eye' type with permanent reduction in central vision (Fig. 25.1.24). Hydroxychloroquine carries a lower risk of retinal damage. Monitoring is recommended only in patients taking more than the standard upper dose of 400 mg daily.

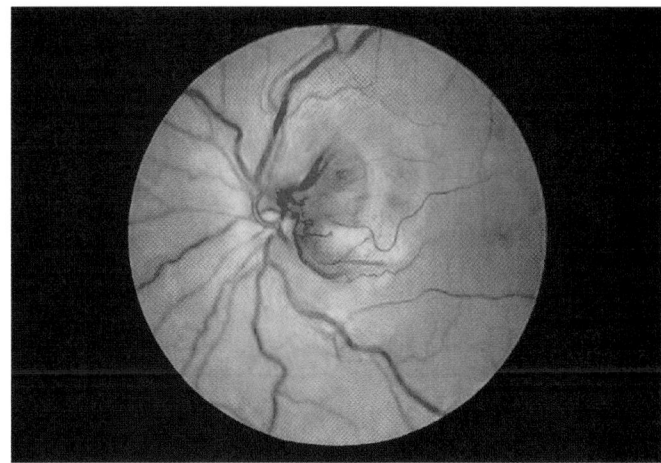

Fig. 25.1.23 Von Hippel Lindau. Angiomas of the retina are an important early feature of this dominantly inherited condition. They begin as small red lesions which expand. Here the angioma is next to the optic disc, a characteristic position which makes management difficult and visual prognosis poor.

Ethambutol (see Chapter 7.6.25)

Toxicity, rare at doses of 15 mg/kg or less, is usually related to total dose, and is, therefore, least likely in the first 6 months of treatment. However, idiosyncratic toxicity in the first few weeks has been reported. Patients should be warned to report any change in visual clarity or colour vision and, if they develop such symptoms of optic neuropathy, should stop taking the drug immediately. Visual acuity, colour vision (100 Hue test), and optic disc appearance should be monitored 3-monthly during treatment. Previous optic nerve damage increases the risk. Early changes usually recover if the drug is stopped.

Eye signs in poisonings (see Chapter 9.1)

Quinine poisoning can blind by damaging the retina and optic nerve head. Antifreeze may contain either or both ethylene glycol and methyl alcohol, both or either of which can cause irreversible blindness. Cyanide in raw cassava can blind similarly.

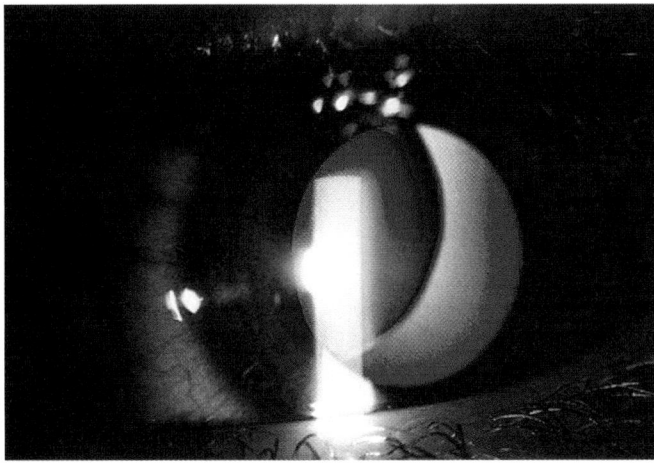

Fig. 25.1.22 Marfan's syndrome. Dislocation of the lens is sometimes easily visible, though lesser degrees may need careful examination using the slit lamp after dilatation of the pupil. The lens may also be unstable, trembling on eye movement. The most common underlying cause is Marfan's syndrome, with deficiency of fibrillin in the suspensory fibres and upward displacement.

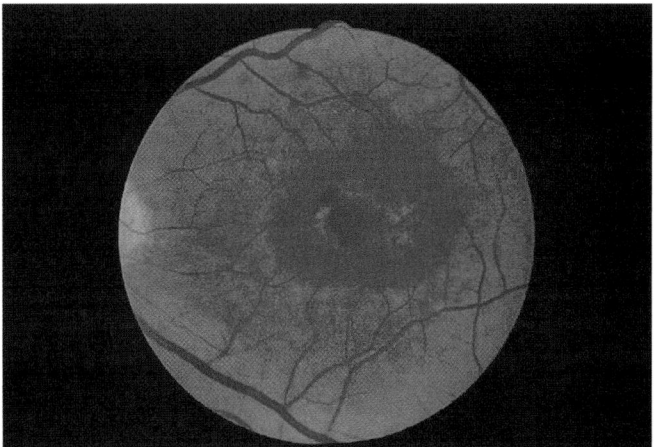

Fig. 25.1.24 Bull's eye maculopathy. Toxicity at the macula caused by chloroquine results in a concentric target-like pigmentary appearance. The features are reversible in the early, asymptomatic, stages, but once loss of central visual acuity occurs, this may progress despite stopping the drug. Hydroxychloroquine appears to carry a lesser risk.

Organophosphate pesticides and other anticholinesterases constrict the pupil by parasympathetic stimulation—vision is not affected. Opiates also constrict the pupil. Atropine-like compounds, including nightshade berries, dilate the pupils.

The external eye is vulnerable to ammonia, alkalis (including lime, cement, and plaster), acids, and some riot-control agents. Primary treatment is prolonged irrigation for up to 20 min, using tap water (or even milk, if necessary), followed by specialist referral.

Blindness worldwide

More than 45 million people are blind worldwide and perhaps two-thirds of these have visual impairment that prevents self-sufficiency. The World Health Organization defines blindness as a binocular vision of 6/60 (or 20/200, equivalent to the largest letter on the Snellen chart) or less.

Trauma

Physical or chemical eye injuries are a common cause of visual loss where prevention and treatment are poor. Emergency eye surgery and antibiotics save vision.

Cataract

There is no known method of preventing cataract, which remains the most common cause of blindness in populations with limited surgical services. As the lens ages, its protein structure changes and the lens opacifies. Malnutrition, dehydration, diabetes, and perhaps sunlight accelerate lens ageing. In some populations, primitive surgical 'couching' or dislodging of the lens within the eye makes matters worse. Implanting artificial lenses is practicable in many countries, but in others, even if surgery is successful, correction by spectacles needed afterwards is often unsatisfactory. In poorer countries, attention is focused on organizing the training and deployment of mobile surgical teams to carry out as many effective operations as possible.

Glaucoma

Nerve fibres within the rim of the optic nerve head are damaged by a sustained high intraocular pressure and impaired blood supply. The central cup of the nerve head enlarges, and visual field is irretrievably lost long before central acuity is affected, so the early stages are usually asymptomatic and painless. Even in wealthy populations, screening for early glaucoma is difficult and some patients progress to blindness despite all efforts. Those most at risk have a first-degree relative with glaucoma.

Age-related macular degeneration

The central retina around the fovea has an extraordinarily high metabolic turnover. In some patients, the efficiency of recycling metabolic products fails, abnormal material is deposited in the retina, and tissue integrity breaks down. Drusen may form around the fovea, which do not themselves impair vision but they may herald formation of aberrant new vessels which grow into the fovea from the choroid beneath. Leakage and bleeding create a scar with an irregular 'disciform' shape. This permanently damages the fovea and the patient loses detailed central vision, though peripheral vision allows independent navigation. Only a few patients at an early stage of the 'wet' type of degeneration are ever likely to benefit from laser coagulation, even with the advent of specific photodynamic therapy.

Diabetic retinopathy

This remains an important cause of blindness in diabetic patients, who predominate in blind registers of younger patients in wealthier countries. Major problems are organization of effective screening programmes and deployment of laser treatment. More than 50% of diabetic blindness is preventable if laser is given early enough—see section above.

Trachoma

Blindness occurs in populations who have poor eye hygiene and repeated fly-borne infection. Vaccination is not feasible. The only effective means of control, other then sanitary improvement, is intermittent topical or systemic tetracycline treatment. Surgery for established scarring is less effective on a mass scale.

Vitamin A deficiency (xerophthalmia)

This most commonly affects young children and may destroy the whole eye. Lack of vitamin A causes conjunctival and corneal dryness and keratinization (xerosis) with characteristic Bitot's spots. The cornea softens (keratomalacia), ulcerates, and may perforate and become infected, resulting in painful and disfiguring endophthalmitis. Vitamin A is found in many green leafy vegetables and palm oil. Measles keratitis increases the risk of corneal scarring in malnourished children.

Onchocerciasis (river blindness)

This is estimated to cause blindness in 1 million people. Recently the disease has been largely contained, thanks to vector control and widespread use of annual ivermectin.

Further reading

Inherited conditions

Traboulsi E (2006). A Compendium of Inherited Disorders and the Eye (American Academy of Ophthalmology Monograph Series). Oxford University Press, USA.

Nahum Y and Spierer A (2008). Ocular features of Marfan syndrome: diagnosis and management. *Isr Med Assoc J*, Mar; **10**(3), 179–81.

Systemic inflammatory diseases

Imrie FR and Dick AD (2007). Biologics in the treatment of Uveitis. *Curr Opin Ophthalmol*, Nov; **18**(6), 481–6.

Deuter *et al.* (2008). Behcet's disease: Ocular effects and treatment. *Progress in Retinal and Eye Research*, **27**(1), 111–136.

Pakrou *et al.* (2006). Wegener's granulomatosis: ophthalmic manifestations and management. *Semin Arthritis Rheum*, Apr; **35**(5), 284–92.

Davies JB and Rao PK (2008). Ocular manifestations of systemic lupus erythematosus. *Curr Opin Ophthalmol*, . **19**(6), 512–8.

Hall JK (2008). Giant-cell arteritis. *Curr Opin Ophthalmol*, Nov; **19**(6), 454–60.

Margolis and Lowder (2007). Sarcoidosis. *Curr Opin Ophthalmol*, Nov; **18**(6), 470–5.

Vascular occlusion

Rehak and Rehak (2008). Branch Retinal Vein Occlusion: Pathogenesis, Visual Prognosis and Treatment Modalities. *Curr Eye Res*, Feb; **33**(2): 111–131.

Hypertension

Wong and Mitchell (2007). The eye in hypertension. *Lancet*, **369**(9559), 425–35.

Diabetes

Klein BE (2007). Overview of epidemiologic studies of diabetic retinopathy. *Ophthalmic Epidemiol*, Aug; **14**(4), 179–83.

The Diabetes Control and Complications Trial/Epidemiology of Diabetes Interventions and Complications Research Group (2000). Retinopathy and nephropathy in patients with type 1 diabetes four years after a trial of intensive therapy. *N Engl J Med*, Feb 10; **342**(6), 381–9.

O'Doherty M et al. (2008). Interventions for diabetic macular oedema: a systematic review of the literature. *Br J Ophthalmol*, Dec; **92**(12), 1581–90

Scanlon PH (2008). The English national screening programme for sight-threatening diabetic retinopathy. *J Med Screen*, **15**(1), 1–4.

Mohamed et al. (2007). Management of diabetic retinopathy: a systematic review. *JAMA*, Aug; **298**(8), 902–16.

Jeganathan et al. (2008). Ocular associations of diabetes other than diabetic retinopathy. *Diabetes Care*, Sep; **31**(9), 1905–12.

Caldwell et al. (2003). Vascular endothelial growth factor and diabetic retinopathy: pathophysiological mechanisms and treatment perspectives. *Diabetes Metab Res Rev*, Dec; **19**(6), 442–55.

Infectious diseases

Bonfioli AA and Orefice F (2005). Toxoplasmosis. *Semin Ophthalmol*, Sep; **20**(3), 129–41.

Mets MB and Chhabra MS (2008). Eye manifestations of intrauterine infections and their impact on childhood blindness. *Surv Ophthalmol*, Apr; **53**(2), 95–111.

Feman et al. (2002). Endophthalmitis in patients with disseminated fungal disease. *Trans Am Ophthalmol Soc*, **100,** 67–70.

Stanek G and Strle F (2003). Lyme borreliosis. *Lancet*, Nov; **362**(9396), 1639–47.

Holland GN (2008). AIDS and ophthalmology: the first quarter century. *Am J Ophthalmol*, Mar; **145**(3), 397–408.

Blood disorders

Russo et al. (2008). Orbital and ocular manifestations of acute childhood leukemia: clinical and statistical analysis of 180 patients. *Eur J Ophthalmol*, Aug; **18**(4), 619–23.

Downes et al. (2005). Incidence and natural history of proliferative sickle cell retinopathy: observations from a cohort study. *Ophthalmology*, Nov; **112**(11), 1869–75.

Emerson GG and Lutty GA (2005). Effects of sickle cell disease on the eye: clinical features and treatment. *Hematol Oncol Clin North Am*, Oct; **19**(5), 957–73.

Thyroid

Perros et al. (2009). Thyroid Eye Disease. *BMJ*, Mar; **338,** b560.

Ocular drug toxicity

Fraunfelder FT (2008). Clinical Ocular Toxicology: Drug-Induced Ocular Side Effects. Saunders Elsevier.

World blindness

Foster A et al. (1992). Epidemiology of childhood blindness. *Eye*, **6,**173–6.

Congdon et al. (2003). Important causes of visual impairment in the world today. *JAMA*, **290**(15), 2057–60.

Rahi JS (2007). Childhood blindness: a UK epidemiological perspective. *Eye*, ct; **21**(10), 1249–53.

SECTION 26

Psychiatry and drug related problems

General introduction

Michael Sharpe

Essentials

All physicians who deal with patients experience situations where psychiatric knowledge, skills, and attitudes are relevant. This section of the book provides (1) guidance on how to take a psychiatric history and perform a mental state examination in a medical patient; (2) information about those psychiatric diagnoses most relevant to general medical practice; (3) practical advice on the management of depression and anxiety when it coexists with disease, medically unexplained somatic symptoms, deliberate self-harm, and acute behavioural problems; and (4) detailed information on the common and clinically important problems of alcohol and substance misuse.

Introduction and overview

Physicians face diagnostic and management problems every day for which knowledge of disease biology alone does not provide the answer and to which psychiatric knowledge, skills, and attitudes are relevant. Examples include the patient with whom the doctor finds it hard to form a working relationship, patients who are severely emotionally distressed, and those who present with physical symptoms that are found not to be explained by disease. It is therefore unfortunate that psychiatry and medicine have become so divorced from one another, and that psychiatry has consequently become so inaccessible to the physician. The historical separation of psychiatry from the rest of medicine still shapes our thinking and practice, and also the organization of our health services. Indeed, in recent years, trends in both medicine and psychiatry have served to widen that historical separation: modern medicine has focused increasingly on understanding the molecular biology of disease and less on the whole patient, while psychiatry has focused increasingly on the psychoses and less on the more common psychological problems that are common in medical patients.

Psychiatric knowledge that is of relevance to medical practice includes a practically useful (if imperfect) system of classifying conditions that is associated with a range of pharmacological and psychological treatments, each with a substantial evidence base for its effectiveness. Relevant psychiatric skills include the ability to manage the interview with the patient in an effective way, to assess the patient's psychological state as well as their physical state, and to find out about the patient's own understanding of their illness. The psychiatric attitude of nonjudgemental acceptance of deviance may also be helpful to the physician. It is no secret that some physicians are dismissive towards patients whom they perceive as 'psychiatric'. A doctor who is comfortable with and tolerant of patients who have medically unexplained symptoms, illogical fears, or difficult behaviour, is likely to be better able both to help these patients and to enjoy their medical practice.

Although most physicians do a great deal of what may be referred to as 'psychiatry' themselves, specialist psychiatric help is not infrequently required. Unfortunately, appropriate specialist psychiatric and psychological services are frequently hard to access because of administrative and geographical separation and an associated lack of understanding of medical problems. Fortunately, in recent years there has been a slow but steady growth in general hospital-based psychiatry and psychology services that are dedicated to the needs of medical patients. These services offer improved access and greater acceptability to patients and also are better equipped to manage the problems that are common in medical patients. These services are often referred to as liaison psychiatry (linking psychiatry and medicine), psychological medicine (specializing in psychological aspects of medicine), and in the United States of America and parts of Europe, psychosomatic medicine (medicine that links mind and body).

The sections on specific psychiatric topics that follow provide a practical and hopefully accessible summary of those aspects of the assessment and management of patients conventionally termed 'psychiatric', but which are in fact central to the practice of all of medicine. They include:

◆ Guidance on how to take a psychiatric history and perform a mental state examination in a medical patient in a way that can be readily accomplished in a medical setting

◆ Information about those psychiatric diagnoses most relevant to general medical practice, including organic mental disorders (delirium and dementia), emotional disorders (depression and anxiety), reactions to stressors, somatoform disorders (medically unexplained symptoms), and eating disorders, as well as more basic coverage of the less commonly encountered, but important, psychiatric diagnosis of bipolar disorder, schizophrenia, and obsessive–compulsive disorder

◆ Practical advice on the management of depression and anxiety when it coexists with disease, medically unexplained somatic symptoms, deliberate self-harm, and acute behavioural problems

◆ Detailed information on the highly prevalent and clinically important problem of alcohol and substance misuse

While some readers might regard this section as merely an unnecessary 'add on' to a medical textbook, of questionable relevance to the practising physician, I hope others will see it as helpful in providing a much needed, more integrated approach to medicine.

For the interested reader who wishes to find out more about psychiatry in general, and psychiatry as relevant to the practicing physician in particular, a number of standard texts are listed below.

Further reading

Gelder M, Mayou R, Cowen P (eds) (2001). *Shorter Oxford textbook of psychiatry*, 4th edition. Oxford University Press, Oxford.

Levenson JL (ed) (2005). *Textbook of psychosomatic medicine*, 1st edition. American Psychiatric Publishing Inc., Washington DC.

Mayou R, Sharpe M, Carson A (eds) (2003). *ABC of psychological medicine*. BMJ Books, London.

Royal College of Physicians and Royal College of Psychiatrists (2003). *The psychological care of medical patients: a practical guide—A report of a joint working party of the Royal College of Physicians and Royal College of Psychiatrists*, 2nd revised edition. Royal College of Physicians, London.

Sharpe M (2004). Psychiatry in relation to other areas of medicine. In: Johnstone EC, *et al.* (eds) *Companion to psychiatric studies*, 7th edition, pp. 683–700. Churchill Livingstone, Edinburgh.

Taking a psychiatric history from a medical patient

Eleanor Feldman

Essentials

It is important to screen for mental health problems: they are common in general medical patients and failure to recognize and deal with them will often interfere with the management of the physical health of the patient.

Depression can kill, and if by screening you identify depression, you should ask about hopelessness and suicidal ideation (how to do this sensitively is discussed in Chapter 26.5.2). To be ill and in discomfort is generally to be unhappy: modified diagnostic criteria for depression are required in the medically ill, emphasis being placed on a predominantly negative thinking style that is pervasive.

Heavy alcohol use can cause insomnia and mood and anxiety disorders: incorrect advice and treatment will be given if the alcohol problem is missed.

Stress, anxiety, and depression can be the main reasons for physical symptoms, a process which is termed somatization. The patient's suffering will increase if the doctor, having taken reasonable steps to exclude organic disease, fails to recognize the diagnosis and presses on with organizing more and more tests or specialist referrals, and much money will be wasted.

Introduction

This chapter covers issues that physicians and surgeons need to know about concerning psychiatric history taking in general hospital patients. It would not be appropriate for a non-psychiatrist to attempt to take a full psychiatric history, involving as it does at least a one hour's discussion covering relationships in the family of origin and a detailed biography to establish premorbid personality and aetiological factors, plus further discussion with at least one other informant. However, all patients should be screened for the most common problems: cognitive dysfunction, mood disorder, anxiety states, and alcohol and substance misuse. The assessment of cognitive dysfunction is predominantly a matter of mental state examination rather than taking a history and is covered in Chapters 26.4 and 29.2. Substance misuse is covered in some detail in Section 26.7. Chapter 26.5.2 covers how to assess a patient following attempted suicide, and the diagnostic features of patients with eating disorders are discussed in Chapter 26.5.6.

It is not necessary to screen routinely for psychotic symptoms as functional psychosis rarely presents for the first time in general hospital cases. If hallucinations and delusions do emerge during an inpatient's stay, then the most likely cause is an acute organic brain syndrome: careful testing of orientation in time and observation for fluctuations in conscious level will usually confirm delirium. If in doubt, psychiatric advice should be sought.

Screening questions in routine assessment

Depression and anxiety

Many patients seen in general hospitals will have diagnosable mental health problems (Tables 26.2.1 and 26.2.2). Frequently these will impinge on the physical health and well-being of the patient. Stress affects the immune response; depression and anxiety are often comorbid with physical illness, either preceding it, or arising largely as a result of it; depressed and anxious people frequently have increased worry about physical health and experience minor physical symptoms as severe and intolerable. Antidepressants may help.

Screening for depression and anxiety need not take much time (Box 26.2.1). However, if the patient gives positive answers, it is helpful for these to be explored in more depth when time allows and in a private interview room. Patients will be aware when you are under pressure or in a rush, and this will inhibit them from telling you important things and you from wanting to hear about them. Indicating that you think something is important and will come back to them when you can set aside more time is very helpful and reassuring to the patient.

Questions about mood disorder are best construed as part of an enquiry into general health and the 'person as a whole', and most patients are pleased to discover that their physician takes an interest in their general well-being. Starting with a nondirective enquiry about sleep before coming into hospital (most patients have sleep

Table 26.2.1 Prevalence of psychiatric disorders in 453 medical inpatients

Psychiatric disorder	Men (%)	Women (%)
Anxiety/depression	12 (4–6)[a]	16 (8–10)[a]
Alcohol problems	18	4
Dementia and delirium (patients over 70 years only)	23	38

[a] Expected figures in the general population.

disturbance in hospital) is a natural way to link physical and emotional health: difficulty sleeping is a common denominator in stress, anxiety, and depression, and a description of a disturbed sleep pattern may also assist you in distinguishing endogenous depression characterized by early morning wakening and diurnal mood variation. The reasons for any sleep disturbance, whatever they may be, are important in general health and will often reveal what troubles and worries a patient. Again ask this nondirectively: do not be tempted to offer the patient a multiple choice of explanations. By open questioning you will guide the patient into revealing what difficulties they are facing, and most will find it a relief to tell you. At this stage it is best to listen empathically and let the patient tell you their story. It may seem to you that you are doing nothing, but the patient gains great relief by being heard and understood, and you are gaining their trust and eliciting valuable information.

The rare patient who objects to a sensitive enquiry intended to be helpful will have a reason to be defensive, and a history from the family practitioner or another informant will usually explain all. If you find the patient evasive and there always seem to be reasons why there is no one else you can talk to, so that you cannot even confirm the patient's identity, be aware that this is characteristic of those with factitious disorder using a false identity.

It is also advisable to screen for a past history of mental disorder, either when screening for the patient's past medical history, or if you have already elicited current mental health problems. Use the vernacular language of the culture of that patient; e.g. in my own culture it would be: 'Have you ever had any troubles with your nerves or had to see a doctor about your nerves?'. Positive answers should then be explored nondirectively by saying something like: 'Tell me more about that'. This means that there need be only a few screening questions to lead effectively into a discussion of most mood disorders, worries, and stress. As important as the questions themselves will be, the way in which they are asked, the time available for discussion, and the physician's own willingness to listen and take note, are equally—if not more—important.

Table 26.2.2 Prevalence of anxiety/depression in medical outpatients according to final medical diagnosis

	Definite organic pathology (n = 91)	Recognized ssyndromes (e.g. irritable bowel syndrome, fibromyalgia) (n = 42)	No organic diagnosis (n = 58)
Anxiety/ depression (%)	12	43	33

Box 26.2.1 Screening and probing questions for mood and anxiety disorder

Screening for current problems

- How have you been sleeping (before you came into hospital)?

Probing: sleep, worry, and mood

If not sleeping well, ask about the pattern of, and perceived reason for, sleep disturbance:

- Is it difficulty getting off to sleep?—If Yes: how long before you fall asleep?
- Are you woken intermittently? Why? (may be due to physical symptoms)—Do you get back to sleep easily?
- Do you wake early and find you can't get back to sleep?—If Yes: how early?

If they have good nights and bad nights:

- What proportion are good or bad; is it 50:50, or better or worse than that?

If sleeping badly:

- Why do you think you are sleeping badly? (This is a natural opportunity for patients to reveal what is worrying them)
- Are you kept awake with worries going round and round your mind?

At this point you will find out what is bothering the patient—after they have confided this in you, it is then empathic to ask:

- How have you been feeling in your spirits?

If a patient reveals problems, it is appropriate now to ask about their previous mental health.

Screening for past mental health problems

Have you ever:

- Had trouble with your nerves?
- Seen a doctor about your nerves?
- Taken tablets for your nerves or to help you sleep?

Alcohol use history

Insomnia and mood and anxiety disorders may be associated with heavy alcohol use. This alone may depress mood and give rise to early morning wakening, appetite changes, and weight loss. For this reason, a diagnosis of depressive illness cannot be made until the patient has been through alcohol withdrawal and been dry for a few weeks. If the alcohol problem is missed, incorrect advice and treatment will be given. Epilepsy may have been misdiagnosed in a patient with alcohol withdrawal seizures.

Patients are often defensive when they have an alcohol problem and persistent probing is needed to elicit the precise amount. Questions need to be asked as a routine and in a nonjudgmental, friendly way. It is important to know the average intake in terms of units, rather than a vague qualitative response such as 'social drinking' or 'moderate drinking': in some countries, manufacturers are now expected to record the units of alcohol by volume on labels, but as a guide see Box 26.2.2. The CAGE (cut down, annoyed by

---

Box 26.2.2 Units of alcohol

1 unit = ½ pint ordinary strength beer/lager/cider (3.5% ABV)
       = 25 ml measure of spirit (40% ABV)
       = 125 ml glass of wine (9% ABV)

ABV, alcohol by volume.

---

criticism, guilty about drinking, eye-opener drinks) questions may also be asked as a routine in anyone who drinks excessively (Box 26.2.3).

Somatized anxiety and depression

Stress, anxiety, and depression can also be the main reasons for physical symptoms (Box 26.2.4). When patients experience the unpleasant physical symptoms that arise from their bodily reactions to emotional states, it is natural for them to complain of these to their medical attendants rather than present their primary complaint as an emotional disorder, which they will often regard as secondary to their physical symptoms, or make no connection at all. This is the common phenomenon known as somatization.

Misinterpretation by patients and their doctors of the symptoms of chronic tension, as well as sympathetic hyperarousal and hyperventilation in panic disorder, may lead to inappropriate extensive searches for organic abnormalities and provide no relief from suffering for the patient. Indeed, the patient's suffering increases as they are left with continuing uncertainty as to the cause of very distressing symptoms, and they become sensitive to the increasing scepticism and exasperation displayed by their doctors. In a study at a cardiac clinic in London, United Kingdom, 50 to 60% of patients had normal cardiac function on investigation, and many of these were experiencing the palpitations, dyspnoea, and chest discomfort of anxiety; 21% showed evidence of hyperventilation. The common physical effects of hyperarousal and hyperventilation affect most organ systems and parts of the body from head (ache) to toe (tingling) (Table 26.2.4), and so these patients find their way into every specialist clinic in the hospital.

Box 26.2.3 Screening for alcohol problems

Routine questions

On an average week, how much alcohol do you drink?
What do you like to have (spirits, wine, beer, etc.)?
How many measures/glasses/pints?
How often do you drink that much?
Did you use to drink much more than that?
If so, when and how much?

CAGE questions

Do you feel you should cut down on your drinking?
Does anyone annoy you or get on your nerves by telling you to cut down your drinking?
Do you feel bad or guilty about your drinking?
Do you have a drink first thing in the morning to steady your nerves or get rid of a hangover (eye-opener)?
A positive answer to one or more questions is indicative of problems.

Box 26.2.4 Some common physical symptoms of anxiety/depression

Common physical symptoms of anxiety

- Dry mouth
- Difficulty swallowing, lump in throat, choking
- Chest discomfort: pain or tightness
- Breathing difficulty, feeling of smothering—can't 'catch breath'
- Heart pounding, missing beats, beating faster
- Fear of dying/heart attack/collapse in an attack
- Sweating, e.g. palms of hands
- Trembling or shaking of hands or limbs/legs wobbly or 'like jelly'
- Hot or cold sweats, flushes
- Butterflies in stomach, abdominal discomfort, nausea
- Vomiting
- Diarrhoea
- Light-headedness, dizziness, feeling faint
- Tingling or numbness in hands, feet, or around mouth (secondary to hyperventilation)
- Urinary frequency
- Headache
- Any musculoskeletal pain (especially back, neck, shoulders) including tenderness
- Sleep disturbance (getting off to sleep and broken sleep and/or bad dreams)

Common physical symptoms of depression

- Symptoms of anxiety as above (depression and anxiety often coexist)
- Tiredness, can be extreme lethargy
- Physically slowed up
- Pain
- Loss of appetite
- Weight loss
- Loss of libido
- Poor sleep with early morning wakening

If you have patients with unexplained physical symptoms, then the most acceptable way of exploring the possibility of somatization is to enquire systematically about all the common symptoms listed in Table 26.2.4. Patients often have a few more symptoms that are not on the list, which they are usually not at all bothered by. Once organic causes have been excluded, the diagnosis of panic disorder can be made on the history of physical symptoms alone, and an explanation can be given to the patient in terms of the physiological effects of adrenaline plus hyperventilation. It is

> **Box 26.2.5** Endicott's criteria for depression in the medically ill
>
> Presence of five out of these nine symptoms for at least 2 weeks:
>
> 1 *Fearful or depressed appearance*
>
> 2 Social withdrawal or decreased talkativeness
>
> 3 Psychomotor retardation or agitation
>
> 4 Depressed mood, subjective or observed
>
> 5 Marked diminished interest or pleasure in most of the activities, most of the day
>
> 6 *Brooding self-pity or pessimism*
>
> 7 Feelings of worthlessness or excessive or inappropriate guilt
>
> 8 Recurrent thoughts of death or suicide
>
> 9 *Mood is nonreactive to environmental events*
>
> Symptoms in italics replace DSM-IV-TR[a] symptoms as follows:
> Weight change
> Sleep disturbance
> Fatigue or energy loss
> Diminished ability to think, concentrate; indecisiveness
>
> Diagnostic and statistical manual of mental disorder, third edition, revised (1987).

particularly important that the physician makes it clear that the symptoms are genuine, and that the tests only show that nothing is wrong because we do not use tests for the transient physiological changes accounting for the symptoms.

Treatments for panic disorder include low doses of antidepressants and cognitive behavioural therapy: these give very good results. Most patients will accept psychiatric referral if it is made clear: (1) that you do believe their symptoms are real (which they are); (2) you are not saying that they are mad, or making it up, or it is all in their minds; and (3) that there are treatments that are effective and not addictive or harmful. It helps if you know the psychiatrist and know what the patient is likely to experience. Left untreated these patients may become severely disabled and continue to undergo expensive and unnecessary medical investigation.

Recognizing depression in someone with good reasons to be unhappy

To be ill and in discomfort is generally to be unhappy, and the more serious the illness, the greater the pain, the greater the loss and the tragedy, so much more the misery. Worry about health and fears for the future are to be expected. How can a doctor tell when an ill person's unhappiness amounts to a depressive illness requiring specific intervention, and when is it an appropriate adjustment reaction to grievous circumstance? Some of the cardinal diagnostic features of depressive illness much emphasized in general psychiatric practice are of little use in these situations, so that in patients with physical reasons for poor appetite and weight loss, and sleep disturbed by pain or other physical symptoms, we must look for other indicators of mood disorder. Endicott has thus suggested modifications to the diagnostic criteria for depression (Box 26.2.5). The emphasis is placed on the predominantly negative thinking style that is pervasive. A depressed person cannot be cheered up when nice things happen, will not be interested in things they used to enjoy, will be excessively pessimistic, and have an exaggerated sense of guilt and worthlessness.

Further reading

American Psychiatric Association (2000). *Diagnostic and statistical manual of mental disorders*, 4th edition, text revision (DSM-IV-TR). American Psychiatric Publishing Inc., Washington DC.

Bass C, *et al.* (1988). Panic anxiety and hyperventilation in patients with chest pain, *Q J Med*, **69**, 949–59.

Endicott J (1984). Measurement of depression in patients with cancer. *Cancer*, **53**, 2243–8.

Feldman E, *et al.* (1987). Psychiatric disorder in medical in-patients. *Q J Med*, **63**, 405–12.

Mayfield DG, Johnstone RGM (1980). Screening techniques and prevalence estimation in alcoholism. In: Fann WE, *et al.* (eds) *Phenomenology and treatment of alcoholism*, pp. 33–44. Spectrum, New York.

van Hemert AM, *et al.* (1993). Psychiatric disorders in relation to medical illness among patients of a general medical out-patient clinic. *Psychol Med*, **23**, 167–73.

Acute behavioural emergencies

Eleanor Feldman

Essentials

Acute behavioural problems can present in any unit in a general hospital. The first priority is to discover whether or not the patient is severely physically ill and suffering from delirium, in which case—apart from managing the behavioural disturbance—treatment clearly needs to be directed towards the primary cause.

General principles of management—all patients with behavioural disturbance need to be cared for in appropriate facilities: rooms should be well-lit, with an observation window and more than one outwardly opening door; furniture and fittings should not be usable as weapons; and there should be an easily accessible panic button. Staff need to remain calm and polite.

Medication—early intervention is desirable to bring disturbed behaviour under control as soon as possible if nondrug calming measures fail. Oral medication should be offered first, e.g. lorazepam 2 mg every 1 to 2 h (with higher dosing depending on response, maximum daily dose 20–40 mg). If this is refused, then the most rapidly effective and safest major tranquillizer is haloperidol, 5 to 10 mg every 1 h (maximum daily dose about 80 mg) given by intramuscular injection. Reduced doses should be used in older people, and patients should not be left unattended in the hours following rapid tranquillization: they require frequent assessment for conscious level, vital signs, and evidence of dystonia, with an antiparkinsonian drug such as procyclidine advisable prophylactically.

Introduction

Compromised cerebral function can lead to acute behavioural problems in any unit in a general hospital, but behavioural emergencies are most frequently encountered in the Emergency Departments and on wards to which deliberate self-harm patients have been admitted. The physician needs to be able to evaluate the causes of disturbance, understand how to calm the situation before resorting to sedation, know what emergency medication may safely be used if required, and have a confident understanding of their own, and other hospital staff's, legal rights and duties under local jurisdiction. While all hospitals should have specialist help available from a psychiatrist, in many circumstances a physician will be the first doctor on the scene and may need to take immediate action to prevent harm.

Evaluating the causes of disturbance

The first priority is to discover whether or not the patient is severely physically ill with compromised cerebral function and suffering from delirium. Delirium is a term often used interchangeably with such phrases as 'toxic confusional state', 'acute confusional state', and 'acute organic brain syndrome'. It accounts for most acute behavioural disturbances arising in physically unwell patients in a general hospital who have no previous history of mental or behavioural disorder. Delirium in a young adult may signal severe life-threatening illness, but most patients will be old, many with a degree of dementia onto which the delirium is superimposed. In older people, delirium often persists for several days beyond the correction of abnormal test results, and confused older people should not be declared 'medically fit' for discharge merely because their test results have returned to normal values.

Delirium is a reversible organic mental syndrome with an acute or subacute onset, typically fluctuating in severity, and often worse at night. Patients will have disturbed attention and concentration and no clear memory of events once they recover. They may be somnolent and have decreased psychomotor activity, or have the opposite with agitation and aggression. Mood changes occur, as do delusions (usually fleeting) and hallucinations, with the latter being in any sensory modality, commonly visual. Clinical features present in delirium are listed in Table 26.3.1.

Where mood disorder, delusions, and hallucinations are prominent, the patient's history and cognitive function are particularly helpful in distinguishing delirium from acute functional psychoses such as schizophrenia, mania, or psychotic depression. The most sensitive indicator of generalized cognitive dysfunction is disorientation in time, which may be subtle (Table 26.3.1). The underlying cause of the delirium must be found and treated, but in the meantime any behavioural disturbance needs to be managed. Table 26.3.2 lists the causes of delirium.

Table 26.3.1 Clinical features of delirium

History

Onset	Acute, often at night
Course	Fluctuating, with lucid intervals; typically worse at night
Duration	Brief, from hours to weeks if untreated
Sleep–wake cycle	Always disrupted

Cognitive function

Awareness	Reduced
Alertness	Abnormally low or high
Attention	Impaired, causing distractibility; fluctuates over the course of the day
Orientation	Impairment for time is the most sensitive indicator, and may be subtle, e.g. correct day and date, but mistaking morning for afternoon. Impairment for place indicates more severe impairment. Impairment for person only is compatible with most severe generalized cognitive dysfunction
Memory	Always impaired. After recovery there is little or no memory for recent events during the period of disturbance

Other features of mental state

Speech	Incoherent, hesitant, slow, or rapid
Mood	Mood changes may be prominent and take any form; irritability is common
Thinking	Disorganized and delusional, delusions tend to fluctuate and not be fixed
Perceptions	Illusions and hallucinations, commonly visual

Table 26.3.2 Causes of delirium

Intoxication by drugs and poisons	A wide range of drugs, including tricyclic antidepressants, anticholinergics, hypnotic sedatives, antiparkinsonian agents, anticonvulsants, digoxin, etc
	Alcohol, illicit drugs, inhaled solvents
	Industrial poisons
Withdrawal syndromes	Especially of alcohol and hypnotic sedatives
Infections	Systemic or intracranial (meningitis, encephalitis)
Metabolic encephalopathies	Acid–base or electrolyte imbalance
	Hypoglycaemia
	Hypoxia, hypercapnia
	Hepatic or renal failure
	Wernicke's encephalopathy and other vitamin B deficiencies
	Endocrine disorders. e.g. Cushing's disease, Addison's disease
	Porphyria
Multifocal and diffuse brain disease	Anoxia
	Vasculitis
	Cerebrovascular disease
	Raised intracranial pressure, hydrocephalus
Head trauma	
Epilepsy, including postictal states and nonconvulsive status	
Focal brain lesions, particularly to the brainstem or right hemisphere	

It is worth noting that a patient who appears disorientated in person but shows no sign of other cognitive impairment is not delirious, but they may be in a dissociative state, or possibly be presenting with a factitious disorder.

How to calm the situation before resorting to sedation

General principles apply to the management of all patients with behavioural disturbance, whatever the cause.

Staff behaviour

Patients who are disorientated and psychotic are often in a state of nightmarish terror, while those disinhibited by drugs or alcohol are less in control of their aggressive tendencies. In all cases staff need to remain calm and polite in their dealings with patients, as anxiety and hostility on their part will only serve to escalate fear and aggression. Speech should be gentle, calm, and soft spoken, but also clear, confident, and honest. The patient should be treated with normal respect and staff should not forget to introduce themselves and explain what is happening at every point. The same few staff should have contact with a disorientated patient and, for inpatients, catering staff and cleaners should be kept away. Disorientated patients need to be reminded repeatedly where they are and what is happening. Nonverbal communication should mirror this calm and gentle approach. Touching the patient without permission or getting too close may be misinterpreted as an attack. An unpredictable patient should never be seen without support staff being present in the background and within earshot. Furthermore, the patient should not be backed into a corner of the room, and staff should remain close to the door. No attempts to control and restrain a patient should be made unless staff are trained in these techniques.

Facilities in Emergency Departments

Emergency Departments need an interview room designed for use with behaviourally disturbed patients. This should be situated within sight and hearing of Emergency Department staff, not isolated in an inaccessible part of the department, nor at the end of a corridor. It should be well-lit and in a good state of decoration, in quiet calming colours. No furniture or fittings should be usable as weapons. In the interests of safety the room should have more than one outwardly opening door and an observation window so that the occupants can be seen from outside. There should be an easily accessible 'panic button' with connection to the staff area nearby.

Facilities on an inpatient unit

Acutely disturbed inpatients are best managed in a well-lit, single-bedded room: delirious patients are more prone to visual misperceptions in the shadows of half light. The room should be sparsely furnished with no objects that can be used as weapons. The door should have an observational glass panel. If the room is not on the ground floor, the window in the room should be made safe, with reinforced glass and a means of preventing it from being fully opened. The room should be fitted with an appropriate alarm system.

What emergency medication may be safely used if required?

It may be necessary to sedate a patient when all other efforts to calm them and make the situation safe have failed. The reality is that there is usually much less capacity to contain behavioural disturbance in a general hospital than would be the case on a psychiatric unit: specialist psychiatric nurses are not usually available, ward layout is not designed for patients with disturbed behaviour, and other ill patients in the vicinity may be placed at risk. Early intervention is desirable to bring disturbed behaviour under control as soon as possible if nondrug calming measures fail. Nonetheless, the decision to restrain and sedate a patient is not to be undertaken lightly. While this experience may not be recalled by someone with delirium, it is very traumatic for a person who is fully orientated and aware, and this includes someone with psychosis. They could develop post-traumatic stress disorder, and the experience may seriously compromise their future cooperation with required medical and psychiatric treatment. The intervention must be carried out with kindness and as gently as possible. The general principles whereby medication can be used as safely as possible are summarized in Box 26.3.1.

Minor tranquillizers

The benzodiazepines are sedative drugs with low toxicity and reversibility, and hence represent the safest first line treatment in the general hospital setting. Their principal adverse effect is respiratory depression, and prolonged use results in tolerance and dependence. They raise the seizure threshold and may be used as anticonvulsants, and so are helpful in cases where there is a risk of seizures and in other conditions where major tranquillizers are contraindicated. Flumazenil allows rapid reversal of respiratory depression. Its short half-life (1 h) means repeated administration may be necessary. There have been concerns about paradoxical disinhibition and release of aggression with benzodiazepines, but these have been overstated in the past and, at less than 1%, are no greater than with placebo.

In general, intramuscular lorazepam appears as effective as a sedative as intramuscular haloperidol, even in mania, and has fewer adverse effects. In a small study in patients with mania the peak reduction in agitation occurred 60 to 120 min after oral administration, but 45 to 75 min after intramuscular and 5 to 10 min after intravenous injection. It appeared more effective than haloperidol during the first 2 h if patients were already receiving antipsychotic drugs: 10 patients who received lorazepam on one occasion and haloperidol on another spent less time in seclusion after lorazepam medication. Doses reported in studies have ranged from 2 to 10 mg every 1 to 2 h. The maximum single dose reported is 40 mg and maximum daily doses from about 20 to 40 mg. No serious adverse effects have been reported with lorazepam use over 1 to 2 weeks. Ataxia has occurred above 10 mg/day, with nausea and confusion at the highest doses. When given by intramuscular injection lorazepam should be diluted with an equal volume of water or saline for injection.

Diazepam is poorly and erratically absorbed after intramuscular injection, making it less suitable for emergency sedation than

Box 26.3.1 Using sedation in cases of behavioural emergencies: dos and don'ts

Do:

- Offer oral medication as a syrup before resorting to the parenteral route
- Use drugs that are well absorbed intramuscularly
- Use dose titration with repeated smaller doses in cases where the cause of the disturbance is unknown
- Carefully record the patient's mental state and time and dose of drugs used
- Observe patients carefully following rapid tranquillization
- Record a treatment plan in the notes for continuation of medication, and review this regularly
- Use antiparkinsonian drugs with neuroleptics to prevent dystonic reactions
- Use reduced doses for older patients

Don't:

- Sedate patients with head injuries: observation of conscious level is an indicator of clinical state
- Use major tranquillizers where seizures are a risk, e.g. known epilepsy, alcohol withdrawal
- Give drugs intravenously
- Use a depot medication for rapid tranquillization
- Use drugs with parkinsonian side effects if parkinsonism is present

lorazepam. It has a long half-life and accumulation is likely with repeated doses. Intravenous diazepam is effective in calming behavioural disturbance within 15 min, the Diazemuls preparation causing less venous inflammation.

It is often useful to combine a major tranquillizer with a benzodiazepine for the most effective safe sedation. The most studied combination has been parenteral haloperidol with lorazepam. It has been claimed that this reduces the total dose of antipsychotic required, but there are case reports where an intravenous combination of these drugs has caused cardiorespiratory arrest. In an open trial, the combination of haloperidol and lorazepam given intramuscularly was effective more rapidly than either drug alone, occurring within 30 min in most patients, compared to nearing 60 min for most receiving a single drug.

Major tranquillizers

Major tranquillizers in common usage in emergencies include chlorpromazine and haloperidol. These are generally safe and effective for rapid tranquillization. Both lower the seizure threshold and should be avoided in patients at risk of seizures, including those in alcohol withdrawal. They are also to be avoided in patients with pre-existing parkinsonism and have proved dangerous in dementia with Lewy bodies. Hypotension is the most common of the potentially serious side effects and is most frequent with chlorpromazine. Extrapyramidal side effects are also relatively frequent, making the use of an antiparkinsonian drug such as procyclidine advisable prophylactically, especially in patients with organic brain syndromes. Acute dystonic reactions may be confused with the severe neck stiffness of meningitis or a spastic posture, thereby adding to diagnostic difficulty in organic brain syndromes of unknown cause. For a patient in spinal traction, a dystonic reaction would be very dangerous. The most hazardous complication overall is cardiorespiratory arrest: the true incidence of this is unknown, but it is less of a risk with haloperidol than with chlorpromazine.

Haloperidol has been widely studied with regard to its rapidity of action: intramuscular injection brings about a quicker improvement than oral administration, with significant improvement within 30 min at minimum, although 1 to 2 h is more usual. The usual intramuscular dose is 5 to 10 mg, repeated every 60 min, to a maximum dose over 24 h of around 80 mg. Doses in older people should be much lower: Jacoby recommends a single small dose of no more than 2 mg oral haloperidol, with effect assessed after 1 h, and in general no more than 6 to 9 mg given orally over 24 h. The patient should be assessed between doses rather than given a regular regimen because individual response is unpredictable such that doses need careful titration to avoid oversedation and severe extrapyramidal effects.

Chlorpromazine is less rapidly effective than haloperidol and carries the greater risk of cardiovascular side effects, hence it need not be used when haloperidol is available. If it is all that is available, then a dose of 50 to 100 mg chlorpromazine would be appropriate for a first dose to assess the patient's response. The oral route should always be offered first, but where this fails the intramuscular route is generally preferred over the intravenous on grounds of safety and ease of access. A reasonable general assumption is about a 2:1, oral:parenteral equivalent dose.

In summary, haloperidol is the most rapidly effective major tranquillizer by the safe and convenient intramuscular route. Small doses of haloperidol should be preferred in older people.

Atypical antipsychotics

New drugs designed for the first line treatment of schizophrenia have become available in recent years, including amisulpride, aripiprazole, olanzapine, quetiapine, risperidone, and zotepine. As a group these are termed 'atypical antipsychotics' and they have the advantage of less frequent extrapyramidal side effects. They are expensive compared with the older antipsychotic drugs and offer no advantage in emergency use over the benzodiazepines if the only desired outcome is rapid sedation. However, they are the treatment of choice in initiating what is likely to be more long-term antipsychotic treatment in either acute schizophrenia or mania where their greater tolerability may enhance compliance, but this is a matter for prescribing by a psychiatrist rather than a general hospital physician.

Olanzapine and risperidone are associated with an increased risk of stroke in older patients with dementia. The increase in absolute risk has been reported to be 2%, but cohort studies in large populations of routine clinical patients have not found this. However, they should be used with caution in older people, and their potential benefit needs to be weighed against this increase in risk.

Drug interactions

Pharmaceutical formularies contain further information on drug interactions and these should be consulted for patients taking other drugs including alcohol, antiepileptic drugs, L-dopa, and lithium.

The management of different syndromes

Psychosis

A psychiatrist should be contacted as soon as possible if a nonorganic psychotic illness such as schizophrenia, mania, or psychotic depression is suspected. Where disturbance is extreme and the patient represents a risk to themselves or others, the recommended drug for urgent sedation is lorazepam 2 to 4 mg orally or intramuscularly. The benzodiazepine antagonist, flumazenil, should be available in case of respiratory depression. Evidence from the notes of a known psychiatric patient may suggest that higher doses may be required. Older people should be treated with half the normal adult doses. A psychiatrist may then choose to initiate treatment with an atypical antipsychotic as above.

Alcohol and drug states

Patients with alcohol withdrawal and disturbed behaviour should be treated acutely with diazepam 10 mg orally or lorazepam 2 mg intramuscularly. They should then be placed on an alcohol withdrawal regimen including thiamine to prevent Wernicke's encephalopathy.

Care following tranquillization

Patients should not be left unattended in the hours following rapid tranquillization. Observations should be recorded every 15 min for 1 h on a form detailing the following information:

1 Conscious level:
   a. awake and active
   b. awake and calm
   c. asleep but rousable
   d. asleep and unrousable

2 Respiratory rate, blood pressure, and oxygen saturation in patients in conscious levels 1(c) and 1(d)—arterial gases should be measured if oxygen saturation is less than 92%.

3 Blood pressure should always be measured if antipsychotic drugs have been given.

4 Reassessment at 1 h to look for evidence of dystonia.

When the acute situation has been calmed, a decision should be made as to whether parenteral or oral medication should be used to keep things under control, also regarding the need for specialist advice. There should be further consideration of the overall treatment plan and levels of nursing and medical observation. There should be a daily reassessment of mental state, and specialist advice should be sought if the patient remains disturbed after 3 days.

Legal rights and duties under local jurisdiction

Unlike clinical matters, legal issues are limited by state and national boundaries. Most states and countries will have statute laws covering the treatment of mental disorders in situations of non-consent, but these laws may not allow treatment for coexisting medical disorders where the treatment of the latter is not a recognized treatment of the mental disorder. Clinicians require an understanding of local statute law and common law covering circumstances where patients have a diminished capacity to give meaningful consent to medical intervention in their best interests. This aspect of clinicians' training has often been neglected, and the law in this area may be confusing for clinicians who must apply it in an emergency situation. While psychiatrists may have a good understanding of statute law in relation to the treatment of mental disorders, they may be less conversant with the legal issues surrounding non-consent for the treatment of physical illness. Hospital managers can assist their staff by drawing up guidance in conjunction with their legal advisors, the professions concerned, and any standing body or commission involved in the monitoring and regulation of statutory powers relevant to these circumstances.

Further reading

Gill SS, *et al.* (2005). Atypical antipsychotic drugs and risk of ischaemic stroke: population based retrospective cohort study. *BMJ*, **330**, 445.

Friedman T (2000). Medical management of acute behavioural disturbance in the general hospital. In: Peveler R, Feldman E, Friedman T (eds) *Liaison psychiatry: planning services for specialist settings*, pp. 51–60. Gaskell, London.

Hodges JR (1994). *Cognitive assessment for clinicians*. Oxford Medical Publications, Oxford.

Jacoby R (1998). Drugs causing confusion and drugs to treat confusion. *Prescr J*, **38**, 242–8.

Royal College of Physicians (2006). *The prevention, diagnosis and management of delirium in older people. National Guidelines*. Royal College of Physicians, London.

Storer D (2000). Liaison psychiatry services in the accident and emergency department. In: Peveler R, Feldman E, Friedman T (eds) *Liaison psychiatry: planning services for specialist settings*, pp. 14–26. Gaskell, London.

Neuropsychiatric disorders

Mervi L.S. Pitkanen, Tom Stevens,
and Michael D. Kopelman

Essentials

Neuropsychiatry is concerned with disorders of affect, cognition, and behaviour that arise from overt disorder in cerebral function, or from indirect effects of extracerebral disease.

The clinician needs to have a practical approach to the assessment, investigation, and management of patients manifesting cognitive and behavioural change, and to be aware of the specific cerebral and extracerebral disorders that commonly involve or are accompanied by cognitive or behavioural change.

In the assessment and classification of mental and behavioural disorders it is crucial to: (1) distinguish between acute and chronic disorders—particularly between delirium and dementia; (2) distinguish between cognitive and psychiatric disorder—misdiagnosis of depression presenting as a 'pseudodementia', or of delirium as psychosis, are errors that can have dire consequences for the patient; (3) determine whether cognitive impairment is specific or generalized—specific impairments are more likely to be due to a focal brain lesion; and (4) determine whether any underlying condition is reversible or irreversible.

Acute cognitive and behavioural disturbance

Delirium—can be caused by a very wide range of conditions and needs to be distinguished from acute psychosis, which can be difficult. Features that support the diagnosis of delirium are: (1) deficits of attention that may range from distractibility and inability to follow complicated conversations, through an almost complete inability to register information or to concentrate (manifest poor performance on serial subtraction test), progressing in the extreme case to diminished consciousness and coma; (2) attentional difficulties that tend to have a sudden onset and to fluctuate over time; (3) muddled thinking and speech showing considerable perseveration; (4) illusions and hallucinations that tend to include a strong visual component, although auditory hallucinations and misperceptions are common; and (5) delusions are usually simple, persecutory in nature, fluctuating, and transient.

Psychiatric disorders—a past history of psychiatric contact or treatment should be sought in all those with behavioural disturbance. In patients with an underlying psychiatric disorder there is usually a background of insidious behavioural disturbance or personality change. Delusions in psychotic disorders tend to be complex, bizarre, and consistently held, visual hallucinations are rare, and marked attentional and memory deficits are not typical (see Chapter 26.5.7).

Alcohol and substance misuse—about one-quarter of all male medical admissions have a current or previous alcohol problem, and such patients are vulnerable to a large number of complications that may precipitate delirium.

Clinical approach—it is necessary to consider a wide range of factors and medical conditions that can both predispose to and precipitate delirium. A history of alcohol and/or illicit substance misuse is of particular importance. Although not always easy, a thorough physical examination with particular attention to the neurological system is essential. A routine screen—including full blood count, electrolyte, and γ-glutamyl transferase (GGT) measurements, liver and thyroid function tests, glucose estimation, and C-reactive protein (CRP)/erythrocyte sedimentation rate (ESR)—is required, as this might indicate delirium where the diagnosis is in doubt. Infection is implicated in around one-third of hospital inpatients who are delirious, and a midstream urine sample (MSU) and chest radiograph are usually warranted. Relevant history and findings on physical examination determine the need for more specific investigation, e.g. brain CT, lumbar puncture, malarial blood film.

Management—delirium is a medical emergency. Management consists of treating the underlying causes and containment of any behavioural disturbance with general measures in the first instance, including nursing in a bright, simple room with minimal changes in staff and good lighting at night. Where sedation is required, then a regular oral antipsychotic such as haloperidol can be administered (see Chapter 26.3).

Chronic and subacute cognitive and behavioural disturbance

The diagnostic challenges in this group of patients are exemplified by the complex differentiation between dementia and depression or 'depressive pseudodementia'.

Dementia—this is a progressive neurodegenerative syndrome involving a pervasive impairment of higher cortical functions resulting from widespread brain pathology. Reversible causes must be excluded. A typical diagnostic screen will include a full blood count, electrolyte and metabolic screen, thyroid screen, vitamin B_{12} and folate levels, syphilis serology, urinalysis, chest radiography, electrocardiography, and CT/MRI brain imaging. In some cases, lumbar puncture, electroencephalography, and (rarely) brain biopsy will be required. Functional brain imaging is likely to assume greater importance in the future.

Focal cognitive disorders—a variety of neuropsychiatric syndromes may arise from regional cerebral impairments of diverse cause and may present in the absence of generalized cognitive impairment: frontal lobe, temporal lobe, parietal lobe, and diencephalic syndromes are recognized.

Organic comorbidity in psychiatric disorders

Missing an underlying 'organic' diagnosis remains a continuing concern for clinicians responsible for the assessment and treatment of new cases of an apparent psychiatric disorder. (1) Organic psychotic disorder—debate remains over the degree of investigation appropriate at the onset of psychosis. Patients with cognitive impairment, abnormal neurological signs, atypical illnesses not responding to treatment, or other indications from the history, certainly warrant further investigations. Where appropriate, this should include neuroimaging, electroencephalography, syphilis serology, and other investigations indicated by the clinical picture. (2) Organic mood disorder—a variety of medical conditions are associated with prominent affective disorder. (3) Organic personality disorder—insidious changes in personality may reflect frontal lobe pathology.

Introduction

Neuropsychiatry is concerned with disorders of affect, cognition, and behaviour that arise from overt disorder in cerebral function, or from indirect effects of extracerebral disease. The term has largely replaced the earlier expression 'organic psychiatry', which originated in the classification of mental disorders as either 'organic' or 'functional' on the basis of the presence or absence of pathological changes in the brain. The latter distinction has become increasingly ambiguous as a result of the development of new methods for detecting abnormal brain pathology and pathophysiology in so-called 'functional' disorders such as depression and schizophrenia. Indeed, the most recent version of the *Diagnostic and statistical manual of mental disorders*, 4th edition (DSM-IV, American Psychiatric Association) states, 'the term organic mental disorder is no longer used in DSM-IV because it incorrectly implies that 'non-organic' mental disorders do not have a biological basis'. Nevertheless, a creative conflict has always pertained between neurological and psychological theories of behaviour and, in the absence of satisfactory alternatives, these terms have retained a place in clinical practice. In part, this serves to demarcate the uneasy and shifting boundary between disorders predominantly diagnosed and managed by physicians and psychiatrists, respectively.

In this chapter, we provide a consideration of practical issues related to the assessment, investigation, and management of patients manifesting cognitive and behavioural change, and we discuss specific cerebral and extracerebral disorders that commonly involve or are accompanied by cognitive or behavioural change. Our intention is to help in the identification of possible diagnoses causing particular behavioural features, and also to alert clinicians to the likely neuropsychiatric sequelae of specific medical disorders.

Assessment and differential diagnosis of patients with cognitive and behavioural change

The assessment and classification of mental and behavioural disorders is a frequent source of misunderstanding and confusion for clinicians, the process being undermined by the absence of robust clinical and laboratory markers for these conditions. Moreover, the clinical terminology used to describe certain symptoms and signs (such as 'confusion') is often unsatisfactory and unreliable. Although the major systems of classification are broadly similar, they continue to use different terminology: e.g. the World Health Organization's *International statistical classification of diseases and health-related problems*, 10th revision (ICD-10) retains the term 'organic disorders', whereas DSM-IV uses the broad grouping 'delirium, dementia, amnesic, and other cognitive disorders'. In addition, some of the operational diagnoses may have little validity in assisting the clinician to determine the appropriate investigation and treatment, e.g. the ICD-10 'unspecified organic personality and behavioural disorders due to brain disease, damage, and dysfunction'. Kopelman and Fleminger proposed a few principles that should be considered in revising ICD-10 and DSM-IV: the existing classification should be simplified; new syndromes should be incorporated where they have pathological justification; links to other specialist diagnostic classifications should be made; a broader range of 'neuropsychiatric disorders' should be incorporated, including alcohol-related organic disorders, head injury, sleep disorders, and if possible also 'psychogenic syndromes'; progressive, degenerative disorders need to be clearly distinguished from nonprogressive syndromes, and some gradation of severity needs to be built; and finally the definitions need to be concise and accurate. Nevertheless, there is consensus on the essential clinical features of these disorders, and in this section we shall describe their assessment on the basis of a number of core features underpinning the differential diagnosis.

Acute versus chronic disorder

The differentiation of acute and chronic cognitive disorder essentially determines the boundary between delirium and dementia. This distinction should be apparent from the history and mode of presentation, although difficulties may arise where a clear history is lacking due to disturbed communication or the absence of an adequate informant. However, they can usually be distinguished on the basis that conspicuous impairment of attention is typical of an acute disorder, together with a fluctuating course and prominent perceptual disturbance, but the 'acute vs chronic' disorder—where there is a delirium superimposed on a chronic cognitive disorder— should not be overlooked. Caution is also needed in patients in hospital where protracted periods of delirium exceeding 6 months have been reported.

Cognitive versus psychiatric disorder

The distinction between a cognitive and a psychiatric disorder is not always easy. It is important to recognize that an apparent cognitive abnormality may be seen in psychiatric disorders such as schizophrenia and depression. In depression, impairment of memory and concentration together with somatic complaints may lead to a misleading impression of dementia, so-called 'pseudodementia' or 'reversible dementia'. Likewise, the distinction between acute psychotic disorders and delirium can be difficult where both conditions show behavioural disturbance and disturbed communication. The risks associated with the wrongful categorization of delirium as psychosis are high: delirium is a medical emergency with high morbidity and mortality, and it is potentially reversible. Likewise, the attribution of a psychiatric disorder as delirium or dementia bears costs in terms of performing unnecessary investigations and pursuing the wrong therapy in an inappropriate setting, thereby compounding any illness behaviour.

Specific versus generalized cognitive impairment

If cognitive impairment is identified, it needs to be determined whether this is generalized to many cognitive functions or affects a specific function such as memory, planning, perception, language, or attention. Identification of a specific impairment, such as the amnesic syndrome, offers important clues as to the aetiology and management, and is more likely to result from a focal brain lesion (as opposed to an extracerebral disorder).

Reversible versus irreversible

The range of causes for any psychiatric or cognitive impairment needs to be fully assessed. In particular, it is essential that those conditions that can be reversed or arrested should be specifically considered. Also, it is important to note that many of the psychiatric and cognitive disturbances caused by underlying organic conditions have a time window for their reversibility, which is usually only in the early phases of the disease, although recent studies suggest that true reversibility of cognitive impairment in the older patient is actually very uncommon.

Acute cognitive and behavioural disturbance

A wide range of disorders may cause acute emotional and behavioural disturbances (Box 26.4.1). One of the most problematic aspects of assessment is the distinction between an acute psychotic episode and delirium. The clinical features of delirium (also known as 'acute organic brain syndrome' or 'acute confusional state') and of the 'functional' psychoses typical of schizophrenia or affective disorder share a number of characteristics. First, both involve a pervasive disruption of thought, cognition, communication, and behaviour in the patient, hence presenting particular difficulties in assessment. Second, both conditions may involve abnormalities of perception in the form of hallucinations or illusions; abnormalities of belief, in the form of delusions or overvalued ideas; psychomotor abnormalities, including hypo or hyperactivity; disturbance of the sleep–wake cycle; and emotional disturbance encompassing the

---

> **Box 26.4.1** Causes of acute behavioural change
>
> - Delirium
> - Alcohol and substance misuse
> - Psychosis
> - Personality disorder
> - Acute stress reaction
> - Adjustment disorder
> - Depression
> - Dissociative disorder
> - Malingering

---

range from depression to irritability and euphoria. These similarities cause practical difficulties in diagnostic differentiation, and they also hint that an absolute distinction between 'functional' psychosis and 'medical' delirium is probably untenable.

Delirium

A thorough history of the antecedents and onset of any behavioural and mental disturbance, as well as details of any past medical or psychiatric disorder, will yield important clues as to the likelihood of an organic aetiology to behavioural change. A drug history should be sought, in particular regarding use of anticholinergic agents.

The uncooperative or mute patient presents a particular challenge as important historical details may not be forthcoming, such as head injury, substance misuse, foreign travel, diabetes, or other medical disorders. Furthermore, accurately eliciting a mental and cognitive state is problematic, and it is in this group that a history from an informant, ward staff, or relatives is especially important. The diagnosis of delirium should be suspected where the history of behavioural disturbance is of recent onset, fluctuating, and there is evidence of deterioration at night. Difficulty in communicating with a patient is frequently the first indication of an underlying delirium.

Older people and general hospital inpatients are particularly vulnerable to delirium and there is an expanding literature advocating prevention through early detection and assertive management of risk factors including dehydration, sensory impairment, immobility, sleep deprivation, and cognitive impairment (Box 26.4.2). A prevalence of between 10% and 20% has been identified in hospital inpatients. Any change of environment such as a recent admission to residential care or pre-existing cognitive impairment will heighten this vulnerability. Among inpatients the problem is compounded by inadequate information, impersonal environments, and confusing exposure to a myriad of different professionals. It is common for the diagnosis to be missed where there is no overt agitation or antisocial behaviour.

Behavioural changes seen with delirium include irritability, repetitive purposeless movements, and disorganization or difficulty performing routine tasks such as undressing. It is important to recognize that patients may be both overactive and noisy or inactive and slow.

The predominant clinical feature of delirium has been described as 'clouding of consciousness' or 'clouding of the sensorium'. There are no consensus definitions for these terms and they are not clear

Box 26.4.2 Risk factors predisposing to delirium

- Age
- Sensory impairment
- Male
- Cognitive impairment
- Depression
- Immobility
- Dehydration
- Alcohol and substance misuse
- Severity of physical illness
- Postoperative and intensive care

in practice, but have traditionally been used to describe a combination of orientation, attention, and memory deficits. Consequently, deficits of attention are stressed in diagnostic criteria, which in the delirious patient may range from distractibility and inability to follow complicated conversations, through an almost complete inability to register information or to concentrate, progressing in the extreme case to diminished consciousness and coma. Furthermore, such attentional difficulties tend to have a sudden onset and to fluctuate over time. Thinking tends to be muddled and speech may show considerable perseveration. The illusions and hallucinations associated with delirium tend to include a strong visual component, although auditory hallucinations and misperceptions are common. Delusions are usually simple, persecutory in nature, fluctuating, and transient.

It should be noted that if delirium and cognitive impairment are simply assessed by orientation in time, place, and person, then 'mild' or 'early' delirium may be missed, and it is therefore important to use additional tests of concentration and memory. All patients should be screened with a small battery of bedside cognitive tests that include specific tests of concentration such as serial subtractions and an assessment of memory for recent events and new information. The Mini-Mental State Examination (MMSE), is often used, but should be supplemented with a few additional memory and other tests.

Psychiatric disorder

The characteristic clinical features of psychiatric disorders are covered in Chapter 26.5.7. Here we will discuss the features of acute behavioural disturbance that are suggestive of a psychotic illness or other psychiatric disorder. This issue is especially important in the emergency medical setting where such patients may be perceived as 'time-wasting' and 'not medical', and their medical needs may be crucially neglected.

A past history of psychiatric contact or treatment should be sought in all those with behavioural disturbance, as this is an indicator of putative psychiatric causation. In those with an underlying psychiatric disorder there is usually a background of insidious behavioural disturbance or personality change, and this will often become apparent from any informant. Delusions in psychotic disorders tend to be complex, bizarre, and consistently held, but this may not be so in early cases. Visual hallucinations are rare in psychosis. Marked attentional and memory deficits are not typical

of psychosis, although more subtle attentional problems and a range of other cognitive deficits may be present. Distractibility as a consequence of internal experiences may give the impression of confusion and attentional impairment, but careful cognitive assessment will usually indicate preserved function.

Delirium in those with psychiatric disorder

The diagnosis of delirium is particularly difficult in those with a history of severe psychiatric disorder and/or learning disability. Difficulty in communicating with and examining such patients, who may have baseline cognitive impairment, means that delirium is particularly likely to be overlooked. Patients with severe mental illness will often attend for emergency consultations where the initial impression is of deterioration in their mental state, often coupled with a recent history of failing to comply with prescribed treatment or a disengagement from services provided. It should always be remembered that there is a high rate of undiagnosed physical illnesses in this population, and their risk of delirium is also raised because of serious side effects from psychotropic medication, including neuroleptic malignant syndrome and lithium toxicity that can result in a deteriorating mental state. In addition, other aspects of these patients' behaviour place them at risk of physical illness, such as coexisting substance and alcohol dependency.

Alcohol and substance misuse

About one-quarter of all male medical admissions have been found to have a current or previous alcohol problem. Such individuals commonly attend accident and emergency departments in a state of withdrawal or intoxication that engender negative attitudes from clinical staff. Often there is an expectation that the behavioural disturbance is due to intoxication or a withdrawal syndrome, without adequate assessment of any other physical pathology. Alternatively, such patients may attempt to minimize their alcohol and drug history so that the contribution of these to their complaints may not be immediately apparent.

Patients with a history of excessive alcohol consumption are vulnerable to a large number of complications that may precipitate delirium (Box 26.4.3) and care is needed to assess all of these possibilities. The onset of hallucinations may be mistakenly labelled as a consequence of delirium tremens without consideration of other 'organic' or 'functional' disorders.

Delirium tremens carries a mortality risk of about 5% and there is a danger that a withdrawal or intoxication syndrome may mask the emergence of other complications of alcohol and substance misuse. A history of recent blackouts or seizures should alert the physician to the possibility of hypoglycaemia or epilepsy. A careful assessment of the mental state is needed to differentiate 'functional' disorders, such as alcoholic hallucinosis, from schizophrenia as treatment of a mental disorder may be overlooked. Physical examination should include a careful assessment for signs of cirrhosis or acute hepatic encephalopathy, and Wernicke's encephalopathy should always be considered since it may be seen in up to 3% of all admissions for alcohol complications (see Chapter 26.7.1).

Investigation

It is necessary to consider a wide range of factors and medical conditions that can both predispose to (Box 26.4.2) and precipitate (Table 26.4.1) delirium. A history of alcohol and/or illicit substance misuse may offer important indicators of aetiology. Although not

Box 26.4.3 Causes of behavioural disturbance associated with a history of alcohol dependency

- Alcohol intoxication
- Alcohol withdrawal
- Alcoholic blackouts
- Delirium tremens
- Wernicke's encephalopathy
- Head injury
- Intracranial haemorrhage
- Pneumonia
- Tuberculosis
- Hepatic encephalopathy
- Epilepsy
- Hypoglycaemia
- Hypomagnesaemia
- Withdrawal and other alcohol-related seizures
- Alcoholic hallucinosis

always easy, a thorough physical examination, with particular attention to the neurological system, is essential in the assessment of all patients with acute disturbance. In addition, a routine screen—including full blood count, electrolyte and γ-glutamyl transferase (GGT) measurements, liver and thyroid function tests, glucose estimation, and C-reactive protein (CRP)/erythrocyte sedimentation rate (ESR)—is required, as this might indicate delirium where the diagnosis is in doubt. Infection is implicated in around one-third of hospital inpatients who are delirious, and a midstream urine sample (MSU) and chest radiograph are usually warranted in addition to routine blood testing in these patients.

Table 26.4.1 Precipitants of delirium

Infection	Pneumonia, urinary tract infection, septicaemia, any other infection, e.g. HIV, malaria, encephalitis etc.
Iatrogenic	Drug toxicity—anticonvulsants, psychotropics, anticholinergics, opiates
Vitamin deficiencies	Thiamine, nicotinic acid, and vitamin B_{12} deficiency
Epileptic	Complex partial seizures, postictal states, petit mal epilepsy
Metabolic	Hypoxia, hypercapnia, electrolyte and acid–base disturbances, liver disease, uraemia, hypothermia, hyperthermia, and porphyria
Endocrine	Hypoglycaemia, hypo- and hyperthyroidism, addisonian crisis, hypo- and hyperparathyroidism, hypopituitarism
Trauma	Head injury, acute post-traumatic psychosis
Vascular	Cerebrovascular accident, subarachnoid haemorrhage, hypertensive encephalopathy
Toxic	Alcohol and drug withdrawal and intoxication, carbon monoxide poisoning

Relevant history and findings on physical examination usually guide more specific investigation. Encephalitis and intracerebral haemorrhage sometimes present with acute disturbance and cognitive impairment with no additional abnormalities in the history or clinical examination. An urgent CT or MRI of the head is indicated where the immediate cause of acute cognitive impairment is not apparent or there are focal neurological signs. Appropriate tests for infectious diseases such as malaria, trypanosomiasis, typhoid fever, and typhus will also need to be considered when there is a history of foreign travel. An EEG with evidence of progressive cortical slowing may suggest a delirium and the need for more extensive investigations where the diagnosis is in doubt.

Management

Delirium is a medical emergency and management essentially consists of treating the underlying causes. Containment of any behavioural disturbance should involve general measures in the first instance, rather than psychotropic drug treatment, although sedation is necessary in some cases. Careful and repeated explanation of the diagnosis, investigations, and treatment to the patient and relatives is important. The patient should be nursed in a bright, simple room with minimal changes in staff and good lighting at night to reduce perceptual disturbance. Drugs, especially psychoactive and anticholinergic agents that may exacerbate confusion, should be reduced to a minimum. Where sedation is required, then a regular oral antipsychotic such as haloperidol can be administered, although the clinician should be alert to the powerful antidopaminergic side effects of these drugs (see Chapter 26.3 for further discussion of these issues).

Chronic and subacute cognitive and behavioural disturbance

In the assessment of patients with a more insidious onset of cognitive and psychiatric disturbances there can again be uncertainty as to the relative aetiological roles of organic or behavioural factors. This may lead to unnecessary investigations at both considerable expense and discomfort to the patient, with attention diverted from appropriate management. Moreover, failure to consider a treatable cerebral disorder such as a space-occupying lesion may lead to avoidable and irreversible brain damage. Box 26.4.4 outlines a list of cognitive and psychiatric disorders that may exhibit evidence of cognitive impairment.

The diagnostic challenges in this group of patients are exemplified by the complex differentiation between dementia and depression or 'depressive pseudodementia', where there are changes in behaviour, mood, intellectual functioning, and cognitive performance. Differentiation is complicated by the fact that depressed mood is a frequent prodrome for an emerging dementia such as Alzheimer's. Furthermore, depression is a common complication or consequence of Alzheimer's and other dementias. It is therefore essential in the clinical setting that the relative contributions of behavioural and pathological factors in any given case are considered, and that assessment includes a thorough physical, neurological, and psychiatric examination.

Dementia

Dementia is a progressive neurodegenerative syndrome involving a pervasive impairment of higher cortical functions resulting from

Box 26.4.4 Disorders presenting with chronic/subacute cognitive and behavioural disturbance

Cognitive

◆ Dementia

◆ Frontal lobe syndrome

◆ Amnesic disorder

Psychiatric

◆ Depression

◆ Schizophrenia

◆ Dissociative disorder

Table 26.4.3 Causes of dementia

Degenerative	Alzheimer's, cerebrovascular disease, Pick's disease, Creutzfeldt–Jakob disease, Parkinson's disease, multiple sclerosis, normal-pressure hydrocephalus
Infection	HIV, neurosyphilis, Whipple's disease
Metabolic	Renal dialysis (aluminium toxicity), liver failure, metachromatic leukodystrophy
Endocrine	Hypothyroidism
Vitamin deficiency	Vitamin B_{12} and folate deficiency, pellagra
Space-occupying	Subdural haemorrhage, tumour
Traumatic	Punch-drunk syndrome
Genetic	Wilson's disease, Huntington's chorea
Autoimmune	SLE, APS
Anoxia	Respiratory failure, cardiac arrest, CO poisoning
Toxic	Alcohol dementia, heavy metal poisoning (lead, arsenic, mercury, and thallium)

APS, antiphospholipid antibody syndrome; SLE, systemic lupus erythematosus.

widespread brain pathology, the extent of which is best determined by formal neuropsychological assessment using instruments such as the revised Wechsler Adult Intelligence Scale (WAIS-R or WAIS-III), as well as standard memory and executive tests. The aetiology and characteristic clinical features of dementia are described in detail in Chapters 24.4.2 and 29.2, summarized in Table 26.4.2, and the most important causes are shown in Table 26.4.3.

In the investigation of dementia it is essential to identify or exclude reversible causes: this should therefore include a full blood count, electrolyte and metabolic screen, thyroid screen, vitamin B_{12} and folate levels, syphilis serology, urinalysis, chest radiography, and electrocardiography. Imaging techniques are continually improving and are crucially important in the diagnosis of dementia (see section on 'Focal disorders'). In some cases, EEG and cerebrospinal fluid examination are essential. Brain biopsy can be of additional assistance when justified by the clinical setting. However, one should keep in mind that choosing the appropriate investigation is dependent on the nature of clinical presentation: e.g. any suggestion of sporadic Creutzfeldt–Jakob disease (CJD) would make an EEG essential; focal neurological signs would indicate the need for early neuroimaging to exclude a space-occupying lesion; a known history of HIV infection may warrant a lumbar puncture; evidence of extrapyramidal disturbance should alert the clinician to the possibility of Wilson's disease, necessitating serum copper and caeruloplasmin level investigation and slit lamp examination for Kayser–Fleischer rings.

Table 26.4.2 Clinical features of dementia

Behaviour	Disorganized, inappropriate, and distractible behaviour. Lack of interest and initiative. Personality change, antisocial behaviour, sleep disturbance, incontinence. Self-neglect
Mood	Anxiety, agitation, irritability, and depression. Lability of mood.
Thinking and perception	Delusions, illusions, and hallucinations
Cognition	Disorientation, recent and remote memory impairment, deficits in language; comprehension, production, recognition. Apraxia and agnosia
Insight	Impaired

The presence of a family history of early-onset cognitive impairment may raise the possibility of predictive and diagnostic genetic testing after appropriate counselling. These can be used in Huntington's disease (*huntingtin* or *HTT* gene), familial Alzheimer's disease (FAD) (three genes responsible for autosomal dominant FAD have been identified: amyloid precursor protein gene (*APP*), presenilin 1 (*PSEN1*) gene, and presenilin 2 (*PSEN2*) gene), as well as in familial frontotemporal dementia (*MAPT* gene). However, a number of risks to such testing need to be considered, including psychological effects (i.e. depression, plans of suicide), prenatal diagnosis and testing of children, impact on insurances and employment, legal aspects, possible third-party coercion, and an understanding of the test limitations (see Chapter 24.17 for further discussion of these issues).

Focal cognitive disorders

Focal degenerative disorders were described long ago by Pick and others, but little recent attention was given to the reports of focal or lobar atrophy until Mesulam reported about primary progressive aphasia in 1982. A variety of neuropsychiatric syndromes may arise from regional cerebral impairments of diverse cause and may present in the absence of generalized cognitive impairment. However, classifying these syndromes has been difficult and the terminology remains confusing. Broadly, the frontal variant and temporal lobe variants of frontotemporal dementia have been distinguished, and—within the temporal lobe variant—progressive aphasia may be 'fluent' (as in 'semantic dementia') or nonfluent. However, the underlying histopathology has been shown to be very heterogeneous even within these broad lobar variants.

Frontal lobe syndromes

Particular neuropsychiatric interest is attached to the consequences of damage to the anterior regions of the brain. These are frequently neurologically 'silent', but they can also result in remarkable alterations in behaviour and personality, with preservation of spatial skills as well as cognitive functions such as memory and intelligence. Thus, neuropsychiatric manifestations may be the only signs of frontal brain disease, and psychiatric disturbance may be an impediment to medical management. Two clinical syndromes (which frequently coexist) are recognized. The first is characterized by emotional blunting, lack of empathy, indifference, and loss of initiative and motivation with impoverished speech and communication to the extreme of mutism. The second is characterized by decline in social conduct, loss of social awareness, disinhibition, impulsivity (occasionally with aggression), poor attention and concentration span, and decline in personal hygiene and grooming: in general, such patients are excessively talkative and may confabulate spontaneously. In addition, mental rigidity, fixed ideation, and stereotyped behaviours—including mannerisms or ritualistic preoccupations—are common. Both of these syndromes have been subsumed under the term 'dysexecutive syndrome' (also known as 'strategy application disorder'), which attempts a unitary cognitive psychological perspective on the condition. Interesting parallels have been drawn between the clinical frontal lobe syndrome and features of neurological conditions such as Parkinson's disease and psychiatric disorders such as the negative syndrome in schizophrenia: in both these examples it is thought that impaired dopaminergic neurotransmission in prefrontal brain regions gives rise to the particular symptomatology.

Temporal lobe syndromes

A variety of syndromes are recognized following temporal lobe damage depending upon the particular area affected. Personality disturbance may be seen, although usually with neurological impairments. A particular variant of this is Klüver–Bucy syndrome following bilateral lesions to the medial and lateral temporal lobes: this results in placidity, hyperorality, bulimia, abnormal sexual behaviour, and visual agnosia. It is a rare neurobehavioural condition but can be seen in patients with extensive temporal lobe damage as a result of post-traumatic, postinfectious, and degenerative (dementias) disorders.

Hemisphere specific, language dominant temporal lobe lesions may produce aphasia, 'surface' dyslexia, and/or dysgraphia, frequently accompanied by neurological impairments on the contralateral side. Progressive aphasia can be fluent or nonfluent. Nondominant lesions may particularly affect facial, spatial, or autobiographical memory, or may appear to be cognitively 'silent'. There is a recognized association between temporal lobe lesions, particularly those giving rise to epileptic activity, and psychosis, which may bear striking similarities with that seen in schizophrenia or affective disorder. Severe bilateral mediotemporal lobe damage usually gives rise to a profound amnesic syndrome, with an almost complete loss of the ability to learn new material (anterograde amnesia) and a variable degree of retrograde loss of memory. Pathology in the left inferior and lateral temporal gyri can produce severe deficits in semantic memory as seen in progressive fluent aphasia.

Parietal lobe syndromes

The parietal lobes play a critical role in numerous cognitive functions such as attention, spatial representation, working memory, mental calculation, eye movements, and the guidance of actions. However, perhaps the main role of the parietal lobes is in determination of what is attended and what is ignored, in the representation of space, and in the aspects of sensorimotor conversions. Balint's syndrome, caused by bilateral parietal damage, is a particularly striking disorder characterized by gaze apraxia, optic ataxia, and simultanagnosia. It causes impairment in space representation, while visual processing of basic perceptual features (colour and form) is spared.

Damage to the inferior parietal region may result in a profound neglect, which is thought to be an attentional impairment, not a perceptual deficit, although it can be difficult to fully distinguish between the two. Theories about inferior parietal lobe involvement in attentional processing suggest that either (1) it is involved in the disengagement of attention—patients with unilateral parietal damage have difficulty disengaging spatial attention from the ipsilesional visual field, making it difficult to direct attention to contralesional stimuli—and/or (2) it participates in the detection of salient items embedded in a rapid sequence of events and in maintaining or controlling attention over time.

The posterior parietal cortex plays a critical role in multimodal spatial integration and in the fusion of different coordinates into a unified representation of space.

Hemisphere differences between right and left also appear to be important: right inferior and temporal parietal lobe lesions commonly lead to neglect, whereas damage to the homologous region in the left hemisphere can lead to an apraxic syndrome.

Diencephalic syndromes

Lesions to the deep midline structures of the thalamus, the anterior nucleus, and mamillary bodies, as well as the degeneration of key fibre tracts connecting the limbic structures, are associated with amnesic syndrome, particularly exemplified by the Wernicke–Korsakoff syndrome. The crucial pathology here is thought to involve neuronal loss, gliosis, and microhaemorrhages that produce disruption of complex mammillothalamic circuits. Pathology in the paraventricular and periaqueductal grey matter, and in the frontal lobes, is also common. Clinically the condition is characterized by profound anterograde amnesia relative to any generalized cognitive impairment, and is usually associated with disorientation in time. Typically, these patients also perseverate when faced with shifts in the task demands. An interaction between ethanol neurotoxicity and thiamine deficiency has been postulated, contributing to the development of behavioural alterations and cerebral damage. An amnesic syndrome can also be caused by herpes simplex encephalitis, carbon monoxide poisoning, cerebral anoxia, thalamic infarction, subarachnoid haemorrhage, head injury, deep midline space-occupying lesions, or tuberculous meningitis.

Investigation

Cognitive assessment

Neuropsychological tests require the patient's cooperation and may fail to discriminate reliably between a cognitive and a psychiatric disorder. However, they may furnish important indications of localized cerebral dysfunction, and they assist the clinician in monitoring the (treatment) progress of any cognitive impairment; they give valuable information about daily functioning; and they help in planning rehabilitation and intervention programmes. A wide range of tests is available to evaluate patterns of disability.

Brain imaging

Also important in investigating suspected neuropsychiatric disorders are brain imaging techniques, the technology and application of which has expanded greatly in recent years. For structural imaging, CT is able to reveal most cerebral lesions, but should nowadays be reserved for the investigation of symptoms of acute onset, where time is of essence and management decisions must be made rapidly. In more insidious, less acute contexts, the structural brain imaging of choice is MRI, which allows both a higher spatial resolution with fine anatomical detail and a choice of endogenous/exogenous tissue contrast modalities, producing greater diagnostic yield. MRI is more sensitive than CT in identifying small vascular lesions or demyelination, but less sensitive in detecting calcified lesions. Sequential estimation of cerebral atrophy and quantitative approaches can facilitate the accurate assessment of disease progression. More sophisticated techniques, such as serial volumetric imaging and voxel compression subtraction, with emphases on a quantitative approach, have been developed to reveal changes over time. However, the time consuming nature of these procedures prevents their widespread use as diagnostic tools. Diffusion tensor imaging MRI (DTI) can be used to determine the integrity of subcortical fibre tracts *in vivo*, but is generally restricted to research settings.

The past decade has also seen an enormous expansion in functional brain imaging that allows assessment of brain regional engagement during cognitive processing. Changes in regional cerebral blood flow using positron emission tomography (PET), or in regional haemoglobin oxygenation status using blood oxygenation level dependent (BOLD) functional MRI (fMRI), can be measured during cognitive performance. Magnetic resonance spectroscopy (MRS) allows noninvasive *in vivo* analysis of neurochemicals and their metabolites, and over the last two decades has been performed in patients with a range of neurological and psychiatric disorders to help understand the underlying pathological mechanisms, to monitor long-term changes with or without drug therapy, and to identify differences between diagnostic groups. More recently, changes in MRS measures have been correlated with cognitive performance in normal populations and in patients with cognitive disorders. Magnetic resonance perfusion (MRP), magnetic resonance diffusion (MRD) weighted imaging, and single photon emission computed tomography (SPECT), can help to identify subtle pathophysiological changes in the brain, before structural changes are present, thereby offering the potential for accurate and early diagnosis. Even though these functional imaging techniques are mainly used in research settings at present, they may well offer clinical value to diagnostic classification in the future (see Chapter 24.3.3 for further discussion).

Neurophysiology

The EEG is frequently employed in the investigation of neuropsychiatric disorder as it is both widely available and a sensitive, if relatively nonspecific, indicator of cerebral dysfunction. Focal abnormalities are characteristic of epilepsy that may, in turn, reflect vascular change. Diffuse slowing (i.e. a shift to lower frequency ranges) is a sensitive indicator of brain dysfunction arising from metabolic and degenerative processes that correlates with the degree of cognitive impairment, although with relatively little specificity. Characteristic EEG changes are associated with Huntington's disease (pronounced flattening of traces), sporadic Creutzfeldt–Jakob disease (repetitive and triphasic spike discharges), and in association with specific drugs. Medial temporal slowing can be suggestive of early Alzheimer's dementia (see Chapter 24.3.2 for further discussion).

Organic comorbidity in psychiatric disorders

Missing an underlying 'organic' diagnosis remains a continuing concern for clinicians responsible for the assessment and treatment of new cases of an apparent psychiatric disorder. The diagnosis of secondary psychotic/affective/personality disorder is used according to DSM-IV if the psychopathology is comparable to that of idiopathic disorder but caused by an organic brain disease. However, in many cases the causal relationship between the organic dysfunction and the psychiatric symptoms remains unclear. Therefore, instead of using the 'organic' diagnosis, the concept of comorbidity is widely used. Table 26.4.4 outlines some common brain disorders causing psychiatric disorder.

'Organic psychotic disorder'

Clinical experience and numerous case reports attest to the wide range of disorders that may emerge following the initial diagnosis of a 'functional' psychosis. One follow-up study of a sample of patients with first-episode schizophrenia found that 15 out of 268 had a neurological disorder that appeared relevant to the mental state, with 13 out of these 15 having salient features in the medical history or neurological signs that could have alerted the clinician to the underlying disorder, the two exceptions both having a diagnosis of neurosyphilis. HIV is increasingly prevalent in this population and one recent cohort identified a known diagnosis of HIV in about 6% of the patients, with many subjects not tested. An assessment of risk factors for HIV is therefore required in all the new cases of psychotic disorder. Overall, the literature suggests that the risk of missing underlying medical or neurological disorder is relatively low, provided that a thorough clinical assessment is performed.

Some debate remains over the degree of investigation appropriate at the onset of psychosis. Patients with cognitive impairment, abnormal neurological signs, atypical illnesses not responding to treatment, or other indications from the history, certainly warrant further investigations. Where appropriate this should include neuroimaging, electroencephalography, syphilis serology, and other investigations indicated by the clinical picture. Increasingly, neuroimaging provides important information relevant to the management of the particular case, although in the absence of specific indications the identification of treatable neurological disease is low.

Table 26.4.4 Neuropsychiatric causes of psychiatric disorders

Intracranial disorder	Cerebrovascular stroke, head injury, Parkinson's disease, multiple sclerosis, brain tumour, epilepsy, Huntington's disease, postencephalitic
Endocrine disorder	Hypothyroidism, hyperthyroidism, hyperparathyroidism, hypopituitarism, Addison's disease, Cushing's disease, hypoglycaemia, diabetes mellitus
Systemic disorder	Hepatic failure, renal failure, pernicious anaemia, rheumatoid arthritis, systemic lupus erythematosus, malignant neoplasia, viral infection (particularly infectious mononucleosis, influenza)
Pharmacological causes	Corticosteroids, oestrogens (e.g. hormone replacement therapy), oral contraceptives, L-DOPA, clonidine, methylphenidate, withdrawal from stimulant agents, e.g. amphetamines

'Organic mood disorder'

A variety of medical conditions are associated with prominent affective disorder, including anxiety, elation, and depressive symptoms. In many of these there appears to be a direct relationship between the presence of brain disease and depression, and the latter does not just seem to reflect the disabling social consequences of chronic disease, although the 'psychological reaction' to the disablement may well be an important contributory factor, e.g. there is accumulating evidence suggesting that depression in Parkinson's disease is secondary to the underlying neuroanatomical degeneration, rather than simply a reaction to the psychosocial stress and disability. Furthermore, the severity of depression may correlate with the 'objective' disability or the prognosis of the disorder or cognitive impairment, and in some disorders, such as multiple sclerosis, can be associated with either euphoria or depression, or mood swings between the two extremes.

'Organic personality disorder'

'Organic personality disorder' is an unhappy term employed in ICD-10 to denote acute or (more typically) insidious changes in personality, defined as a significant alteration in the habitual disposition and behaviour of a patient from their premorbid state. The syndrome is well recognized, although often in retrospect, and may often reflect frontal lobe pathology. Most prominently affected is the degree of emotional expression and levels of activity in the absence of pronounced cognitive alterations, except where 'higher level' functions such as planning complex actions or anticipation of social and emotional consequences are affected. Table 26.4.5 outlines some of the common causes.

Advances in brain imaging have led to a progressive increase in studies focusing on structural markers of human personality. These suggest a relationship between personality change and atrophy, particularly in the frontal lobes, but also in supplementary motor area grey matter, right anterior cingulate cortex, or the whole brain. Functional imaging studies have identified a number of personality traits supposedly associated with alterations in central metabolism, neurotransmitter function, or cerebral blood flow. However, these findings have not yet been closely related to neuropsychiatric symptoms.

Specific conditions giving rise to neuropsychiatric symptoms

This section attempts to address two aspects of neuropsychiatric problems associated with medical conditions: (1) to prompt the recognition and exploration of psychiatric abnormality in 'high risk'

Table 26.4.5 Causes of 'organic personality disorder'

Intracerebral insult	Cerebrovascular stroke, head injury, tumour (frequently frontal/sphenoidal meningioma), abscess, encephalitis (frequently herpes encephalitis, which has a recognized tropism for frontotemporal brain regions), subdural haematomas (chronic)
Neurodegenerative conditions	Huntington's disease, Wilson's disease (hepatolenticular degeneration), Pick's disease, Creutzfeldt–Jakob disease, subcortical dementias

conditions where such associations are well recognized; and (2) to encourage appropriate medical examination and investigation in the presence of outwardly psychiatric abnormality.

Psychological or psychiatric disorder may become manifest as an adjustment reaction to medical disability, malaise, and handicap, and this can affect not only the patient, but also family members, who often bear the practical burden of care. Psychiatric disorder may also result from a specific compromise of cerebral function, either directly or systemically mediated. For example, postoperative psychiatric disturbance is common and usually the result of infective, metabolic, or drug-induced delirium. However, the circumstances of operation may lead to the precipitation of disorientation in the presence of an insidious dementia, or a withdrawal syndrome in an alcohol-dependent individual. Furthermore, the emotional reaction in response to life-threatening and life-altering circumstances may be profound following major surgery. These factors interact, and the ultimate expression of mental disturbance depends upon a particular patient's premorbid disposition and social circumstances, as well as specific illness factors. Nevertheless, the recognition and specific ascertainment of the presence of mental disturbance in certain conditions has profound diagnostic and prognostic importance.

Neurological disorders

Cerebrovascular disorders

The psychiatric complications associated with stroke illustrate the relevance of a neuropsychiatric perspective. Early studies recognized distinct emotional reactions associated with cerebral damage. These include the catastrophic reaction (often extreme or disproportionate emotional outburst to small demands), an indifference reaction (associated with fatuous mood, indifference to failures, and unilateral neglect and anosognosia), and pathological laughter/crying reaction (also known rather pejoratively as 'emotional incontinence', where emotional displays occur seemingly spontaneously or to trivial provocation). The mood consequences of stroke are often disproportionate to the objective disability and it is important to screen for depression and anxiety in the first months after a stroke. The relationship between mood disorder and lesion location has been contentious, although there is an emerging consensus that anterior lesions are more associated with depression.

Cerebral tumours

Cerebral tumours are frequently associated with neuropsychiatric disability, ranging from understandable reactions to the diagnosis to frank syndromes resulting from impaired brain function. Minor psychological disturbance including anxiety, depression, and occasionally hysterical symptoms may be seen before the medical diagnosis is made, and specific signs of cerebral pathology need to be excluded in this group of patients. The regional syndromes outlined above are notable in cases of primary or secondary cerebral tumours, in particular when the tumour is rapidly progressive or where multiple brain regions are involved with metastases.

The most common adult-onset primary tumour is the ostensibly 'benign' meningioma, which is notoriously slow growing (estimates of growth indicate that at diagnosis it has often been present for some 10 to 15 years) and hence cerebral function is only slowly compromised. Coupled with their propensity for a frontal location, in which there may be few frank neurological signs, this can lead to tragic cases where the cause of progressive personality deterioration is missed.

More dramatic impairments of cerebral function are particularly associated with rapidly progressive tumours in which raised intracranial pressure, irritative epileptic phenomena, and an overall distortion in brain structure may combine to produce delirium and dementia.

There can be remote effects of malignant disease on cerebral function: hypercalcaemia may present with an acute confusional state or with other psychological/psychiatric manifestations, and some forms of lung carcinoma (in particular) secrete growth factor/endocrine hormones that result in neurodegenerative changes and a dementia-like picture. Furthermore, both episodic and prolonged confusional states have been reported in malignant disease in the absence of a clear metabolic disturbance or focal brain involvement, e.g. in diffuse leptomeningeal disease. Recent studies suggest that cognitive function is an important outcome measure in patients with brain tumours and is an independent prognostic factor in the survival of glioma patients. Moreover, cognitive deterioration may be the first indicator of progressive disease following treatment.

Head injury

Head injury often leads to impairment in personality, affect, and social/occupational function that is more prominent than the objective dysfunction would suggest. The wide range of neuropsychiatric sequelae recognized after head injury are outlined in Box 26.4.5. The most disabling and distressing problems for both patients and carers are often the emotional and behavioural effects and, in particular, personality change. This may reflect the vulnerability of the anterior temporal poles, frontal polar regions, and the orbitofrontal cortex to closed head injuries. After traumatic brain injury the risk of suicide increases threefold, with around 15% attempting suicide in the first 5 years after injury.

Impairment of consciousness is characteristic after all but the most mild head injuries and features of delirium are often seen after severe injuries. The period of post-traumatic amnesia represents the time that elapses between the moment of injury and the restoration of continuing memory for everyday events. This remains an important predictor of outcome, correlated with personality change as well as intellectual impairment and neurological disorder. By contrast, memory loss for the events of the trauma itself sometimes appears to protect against the development of post-traumatic stress disorder.

Cognitive impairment following head injury is usually more apparent after a post-traumatic amnesia exceeding 24 h, and testing reveals that Performance IQ is more vulnerable to the effects of trauma than Verbal IQ. Penetrating and localized injuries tend to result in more focal cognitive deficits dependent on the site of injury. Dysexecutive syndrome and anterograde memory impairment are commonly seen. In rare cases head injuries may predispose to Alzheimer's disease.

Personality change is particularly common after severe head injury and frontal lobe damage, including irritability, impatience, apathy, and lability of mood. There is also an inability to learn from experience, with poor judgement and lack of initiative. Aggression and sexual disinhibition may necessitate high levels of subsequent care and are predicted by early agitation after head injury. Delusional disorders are frequently observed in the early stages of

Box 26.4.5 Neuropsychiatric consequences of head injury

◆ Delirium

◆ Focal cognitive disorder (frontal lobe syndrome, amnestic disorder)

◆ Global cognitive disorder

◆ Subdural haematoma

◆ Post-traumatic epilepsy

◆ Delusional syndrome and hallucinosis

◆ Affective syndrome

◆ Post-traumatic disorder

◆ Anxiety disorder

◆ Personality change

◆ Conversion disorders

◆ Postconcussional syndrome

◆ Alcohol misuse

recovery and may reflect the persistence of disordered cognition; mood and anxiety disorders are also often seen. Premorbid alcohol misuse may have predisposed to the trauma and alcohol tolerance can decline markedly after severe injury. Problems with heavy drinking are common in this group, which may reflect poor insight and drinking in response to stressful circumstances. Caution is needed to exclude chronic subdural haematoma and post-traumatic epilepsy before ascribing emotional and behavioural change to a psychiatric diagnosis.

Complex rehabilitation strategies are often needed to manage this group of patients and novel pharmacological managements are being assessed.

Epilepsy

In assessing epilepsy it is important to establish the extent of underlying cerebral damage giving rise to the epileptic discharge, as well as the nature and severity of any cognitive impairment. While compatible with normal intelligence, epilepsy is more common in patients with a learning disability, and is related to its severity, presumably as both epilepsy and a learning difficulty arise from underlying cerebral dysfunction. Thus, the capacity of individuals to manage their epilepsy is highly variable and poses an important problem for management. Furthermore, there can be a relationship between emotional state and epileptic seizures, indicative of an important brain–mind correlation.

The neuropsychiatric consequences of epilepsy are best considered in terms of peri-ictal and interictal disorders, which are outlined in Table 26.4.6. This has important implications for management in which the focus should be on optimal control of seizures. Psychotropic medication can decrease the seizure threshold and possible interactions with anticonvulsants should be considered. The S2-D2 (refers to antagonism of atypical antipsychotics at the dopamine type 2 receptor and the serotonin type 2A receptor) or atypical neuroleptics are current first-line treatments for psychosis and are also used in aggression and irritability; olanzapine, risperidone, and quetiapine are particularly recommended.

Selective serotonin reuptake inhibitors (SSRI) are generally agreed to be safe treatments for depression in patients with epilepsy (see Chapter 24.5.1 for further discussion).

Subacute encephalopathies

A well recognized manifestation of acute cerebral infection or encephalitis is a dramatic behavioural disturbance that may involve violence and delirium. This is a relatively common diagnostic problem, and it is clearly of vital importance to make a correct diagnosis. Of particular note are, firstly, that the particular groups relatively predisposed to the development of encephalitis are alcohol and drug misusers, where attitudes of medical staff may exert a pejorative effect, and secondly, that the disordered behaviour may be sufficiently extreme to render medical examination and management difficult.

Herpes simplex encephalitis is particularly implicated in such presentations, perhaps as the most common encephalitis and also because of tropism of the virus to frontal and temporal regions. Damage in these areas may lead to psychosis, abnormalities in cognitive or social processing, or a syndrome resembling autism, particularly early in the course of disease. However, these presentations rarely persist in isolation and are less common than paresis or seizures. Furthermore, it is quite common that frontotemporal damage in these patients causes persistent behavioural deficits.

Other forms of encephalitis can also produce striking behavioural change, e.g. Epstein–Barr virus may lead to visual metamorphosis ('Alice in Wonderland' syndrome; an unusual syndrome characterized by visual hallucinations and bizarre perceptual distortions of form, size, movement, and colour, where objects appear larger or smaller than their actual size, associated with an abnormal sense of time or place), occasionally with persistent complications.

Intracranial infections

Neurosyphilis

Neurosyphilis can result in several different syndromes from infection of the brain, meninges or spinal cord. While its incidence is still rather low, neurosyphilis has become more common due to an increased prevalence of immunosuppression. The presentation can be subtle, atypical, often monosymptomatic, and it can present with psychiatric symptoms alone. Patients with neurosyphilis may show a normal MRI head scan, or bilateral mesiotemporal T2 hyperintensity, or meningeal thickening. A wide range of neuroimaging findings can resemble those found in herpes simplex encephalitis, mesial temporal sclerosis, leukoaraiosis, normal pressure hydrocephalus, and glioblastoma multiforme. However, neurosyphilis most commonly adopts either a meningeal form (leptomeningeal granulomas that may also occur intra-axially) or a vascular form (typically presenting with cortical and subcortical infarcts), which often occur together. CSF findings can vary from positive oligoclonal IgG bands and high IgG index to pleocytosis with or without CSF venereal disease research laboratory test (VDRL). Clinicians should be aware that dementia in young patients with temporal lobe atrophy and/or vascular damage can be caused by syphilis, and therefore these findings necessitate CSF and syphilis testing (see Chapter 24.11.4 for further discussion).

Human immunodeficiency virus

Human immunodeficiency virus (HIV) is a neurotropic virus that enters the brain within 2 weeks of initial infection. Combination antiretroviral therapies have changed the course of the illness, but many patients with HIV still show signs of associated neurocognitive dysfunction. The clinical features of HIV-associated neurocognitive impairment are thought to reflect widespread synaptodendritic problems in the fronto-striato-thalamo-cortical circuit. Patients typically have problems with executive functions (e.g. abstraction, processing speed, verbal fluency, decision making, and attention) as well as with learning new information. It has also been postulated that prospective memory is particularly affected, i.e. ability to execute a future intention. The severity of cognitive decline can increase with age and in association with high viral loads and reduced CD4$^+$ cell counts, as well as in association with age-related decline in functioning of fronto-striato-thalamo-cortical circuitry. Cognitive impairment can predict mortality, independent of clinical stage or CD4$^+$ cell counts.

There is also an overall increased susceptibility of patients with HIV to develop a major psychiatric disorder: new-onset psychosis is reported in up to 15% and can occur without encephalopathy. The putative involvement of subcortical dopaminergic systems, particularly basal ganglia structures, is supported by high rates of antipsychotic-related extrapyramidal symptoms and neuropathological studies in HIV-infected patients.

Mood disorders are common in patients with HIV and effective treatment may result in considerable health and economic benefits. Depressive disorders are reported among 20 to 40%; they are commonly unrecognized but respond to appropriate treatment interventions in 80 to 90% of cases. Mania without pre-existing bipolar disorder or family history is found in 8% of patients in the late stages of disease, typically in the context of dementia and CNS involvement; early in HIV infection, episodes of mania are more commonly related to pre-existing bipolar disorder or family history (see Chapter 24.11.4 for further discussion).

Variant Creutzfeldt–Jakob disease

Variant Creutzfeldt–Jakob disease (vCJD) appears to present in a much younger population (mean age at death is 29 years) than the sporadic variant (mean age at death is 63). Difficulties occur in

Table 26.4.6 Neuropsychiatric complications of epilepsy

Ictal and peri-ictal disorders	
Prodromal states Complex partial seizures	Tension, irritability, and depression may be seen Automatisms, distortions of perception, hallucinations, déjà vu, unusual disturbances of memory, thinking Sudden changes in affect.
Interictal disorders Nonepileptic seizures Cognitive impairment	Seen in about one-third of those attending specialist epilepsy centres. Associated with physical and sexual abuse. This usually reflects underlying brain damage, and developmental consequences of repeated seizures and treatment with anticonvulsants. Associated with duration and frequency of previous seizures
Personality	Probably only related to severe epilepsy where there is underlying brain damage.
Schizophrenia-like psychosis	Associated with temporal lobe epilepsy.
Depression	Suicide is four times more frequent in epileptics: those with adverse social factors and temporal lobe epilepsy are particularly at risk

diagnosis because the early symptoms of vCJD are often nonspecific, such as anorexia, mild insomnia, apathy, mood swings, and personality changes, and prominent neurological signs are lacking. Neurological examination in the early stages is usually normal, but subsequent neurological decline is characterized by progressive ataxia, paraesthesia in legs and face, unusual aches and pains in hands, feet, face and lumbar region, and cognitive impairment. Careful clinical assessment remains the most important element in the early detection of symptomatic disease.

The most useful noninvasive investigation in advanced cases has been MRI imaging, particularly fluid attenuated inversion recovery (FLAIR) sequence. The pulvinar sign (a symmetrical region of signal hyperintensity in the pulvinar nucleus of the thalamus) has been reported to have sensitivity of up to 95% in the appropriate clinical context. EEG generally does not show the typical appearances of sporadic CJD. Definitive diagnosis of vCJD is based on neuropathological findings, obtained by brain biopsy, and supplemented by prion protein (PrP) immunohistochemistry and molecular strain typing by Western blotting of human brain tissue. Because PrP immunoreactivity is present in the tonsils of vCJD patients, tonsil biopsy has been proposed as a less invasive alternative to brain biopsy. The WHO published diagnostic criteria for sporadic CJD in 2001, suggesting that neuropathological examination (biopsy) is not mandatory for the confirmation of the diagnosis (see Chapter 24.11.5 for further discussion).

Neurodegenerative conditions
Multiple sclerosis
Affective disorders are common in multiple sclerosis (MS) and have been divided into four categories; depressive disorder, bipolar affective disorder, euphoria, and pseudobulbar affect. Both bipolar affective disorder and depression are more common in patients with MS than in the general population, with the lifetime prevalence for the latter being 50%. Euphoria is more common in patients with advanced disease, with a median prevalence of 25%. Pseudobulbar affect is found in about 10% of MS patients.

It is important not to dismiss these symptoms as they all are associated with significant morbidity and mortality. Furthermore, a strong association between affective disorder and cognitive impairment (40–65%) is recognized in MS. Depression can exert particularly adverse effects on the executive component of working memory. Cognitive functions in progressive MS subtypes are likely to decline across time, particularly on tasks requiring concurrent multiple abilities, i.e. visuospatial ability and processing speed or working memory and processing speed. Cognitive impairment in MS may reflect several underlying defects such as lesion severity, changes in neuronal signaling caused by axonal degeneration, and demyelination. Neurotransmitter changes are also recognized, e.g. a decline in choline acetyltransferase activity, and there are a number of studies showing benefits with acetylcholine esterase inhibitors. MS can also occasionally present as a cortical variant alone, with significant psychiatric complaints prior to sensory and motor presentations.

Parkinson's disease and movement disorders
There are four particular aspects of neuropsychiatric disturbance relevant to the consideration of idiopathic and atypical parkinsonian syndromes, including multisystem atrophy:

1 A prodromal period without frank movement disorder is well recognized and may be typified by sleep disturbances, depression, as well as sensory and autonomic dysfunction, possibly reflecting the non-dopaminergic-cell dysfunction. Interestingly, these nonmotor symptoms are also prominent in advanced stages of the disorders.

2 Dopaminergic replacement therapy, whether with cholinergic antagonists, dopamine agonists, or levodopa (L-DOPA), is associated with a substantial incidence of psychosis and delirium. However, the neuronal degeneration of the pedunculopontine nucleus, locus coeruleus, and the dopaminergic raphe nuclei may also play a role.

3 There is a strong association between Parkinson's disease and depression (10–50%), with possibly a more significant biological than purely reactive basis. Depression is characterized by a feeling of guilt, lack of self-esteem, sadness, and remorse.

4 Many patients develop 'diffuse' (extranigrostriatal) Lewy body disease, characterized by a progressive dysexecutive syndrome with impairment of visuospatial abilities and memory against a background of loss of response to dopaminergic drugs.

Particular mention should be made here of the iatrogenic movement disorder attendant upon antipsychotic and antidepressant medication. The mechanisms underlying this drug-induced movement disorder are largely unclear, but drug-induced movement disorders are generally reversible once the medication is removed, suggesting that the drugs produce an interference with neuronal function (see Chapter 24.7.2 for further discussion).

Learning disability
Although beyond the immediate scope of this chapter, the diverse conditions that give rise to learning disorders have been the subject of intense recent interest. In particular, their strong associations with attention deficit-hyperactivity disorder (ADHD), fetal alcohol syndrome, and autism have underscored a probable neuropsychiatric basis. Interestingly, studies suggest a critical role of the prefrontal cortex and its connections to the parietal cortex and striatum in children with ADHD in divided attention tasks, in inhibiting distraction and prepotent responses, and in maintaining the information 'on line' in working memory. From a neurodevelopmental perspective, attention deficit in children is strongly linked to conduct disorder and may have diverse consequences in adulthood, providing a precursor for some instances of personality disorder, traditionally not viewed in neuropsychiatric terms (see Chapter 24.18 for further discussion).

Another relevant area of interest is the concept of behavioural phenotypes, where consistent behavioural abnormalities are associated with distinct genotypic abnormalities. For example, the frequently occurring chromosomal disorders of Down's syndrome, Turner's syndrome, and Klinefelter's syndrome have distinct and consistent neuropsychiatric aspects, albeit of variable degree. In Turner's syndrome, overall IQ is variable but distinct difficulties in visuospatial function give rise to large Verbal-Performance IQ deficits.

Extracerebral disorders
Endocrine disorders
Endocrine disorder has an important influence on mental function and there are characteristic associations with neuropsychiatric disorder. The use of 'routine' blood tests of endocrine function has resulted in the earlier detection of problems, such that florid states are now rarely seen. The focus of clinical interest in this area is

upon 'preclinical' endocrine dysfunction, the complications arising from the disorder, and treatment.

Diabetes mellitus

The neuropsychiatric aspects of diabetes mellitus (DM), both insulin-dependent (IDDM) and non-insulin-dependent (NIDDM) forms, may be considered in four aspects:

1 The syndrome itself and the constraints of optimal management have a considerable impact on the lives of people with the disorder. The disorder is stigmatizing, especially in the young, and is associated with significant morbidity and mortality. There is a risk of impaired psychological development, personality difficulties, and affective disorder. There is clear evidence of a relationship between 'stress', emotional disturbance, and impaired glycaemic control, although whether this is mediated directly or indirectly (through neglect of diet and treatment) is unclear.

2 Increased prevalence of psychological disturbance has been reported, particularly with IDDM. Anxiety disorder has been linked to poor glycaemic control, which in turn relates to fear of hypoglycaemia. IDDM-associated hypoglycaemic episodes can also cause frank automatisms.

3 Cognitive dysfunction in diabetic subjects has been recognized since the early 20th century. Both IDDM and NIDDM are associated with slowing of mental speed and diminished mental flexibility, and NIDDM is also associated with deficits in actual learning and memory processing. Several studies have shown that the rate of cognitive decline is accelerated in older people with NIDDM. There are several proposed pathophysiological mechanisms linking diabetes to changes in the brain and cognitive decline, including atherosclerosis (macroangiopathy, increased risk of stroke), microvascular disease (microangiopathy, small vessel disease), glucose toxicity (advanced protein glycation and oxidative stress, 'advanced aging'), and insulin mediated changes (increased secretion and decreased breakdown of the amyloid). Neuroimaging studies suggest that the appearances of the brain in patients with diabetes resemble that of normal aging, but appear to develop at a younger age than in normal population.

4 The incidence of dementia is higher in people with diabetes compared with the normal population. However, the risk factors and mechanisms underlying the association between diabetes, accelerated cognitive decline, and vascular dementia still need to be identified.

Thyroid disorder

It is rare for classical presentations of thyroid disease to be missed in clinical practice, but interesting to note that surveys reveal that more than 5% of attendees at psychiatric consultations have an abnormality in thyroid function. While not all of this group would benefit from treatment for thyroid disease, it underscores the insidious nature of thyroid dysfunction. The rule should be to exclude this whenever suspicions are aroused. In particular, hypothyroidism may commonly manifest as apathy, depression, memory impairment, and dementia with prominent cognitive slowing: the condition may be reversible if recognized and treated early, but rarely so in long-lasting cases of hypothyroidism. Neonatal hypothyroidism or 'cretinism' is now rare as a result of routine screening, but this indicates the importance of adequate thyroid function for cerebral development. Occasionally, adult hypothyroidism may be associated with psychosis (most commonly a delirium with prominent agitation), famously termed 'myxoedema madness'.

Hyperthyroidism is commonly associated with a subjective feeling of tension, irritability, and high arousal. Initially this may be confused with anxiety, but in more severe cases behaviour can be frankly disturbed, although the individual concerned generally retains insight. However, it should be noted that studies show no clear association between anxiety or depression and serum concentration of thyroid hormones. In a similar way, no strict relationship has been found between severity of symptoms of hyperthyroidism and degree of elevation in thyroid hormones concentrations. Hypomania is rare but has been reported. Thyroid 'crises' with delirium are occasionally seen following radioiodine treatment.

Both hypothyroidism and hyperthyroidism are common consequences of lithium treatment in bipolar affective disorder. This introduces the possibility of confusing a thyroid disorder with the recurrence of an affective disorder, although it should be effectively excluded by the routine monitoring of lithium treatment.

Hashimoto's encephalopathy is an uncommon condition of presumed autoimmune aetiology characterized by the presence of high titres of antithyroid microsomal/peroxidase antibodies. The condition can follow a relapsing and remitting course, with features including confusion, cognitive decline, hallucinations, stroke-like episodes, myoclonus, or seizures. Thyroid function is typically normal. Treatment with corticosteroids is almost always effective.

Cushing's syndrome

It is estimated that more than 70% of patients with Cushing's syndrome can present psychiatric problems, ranging from anxiety and agitated depression to psychosis. Some degree of psychiatric disturbance frequently persists even after treatment. Furthermore, impairment in anterograde memory and cognition is common and can persist for at least a year after treatment. These effects are associated with a reduction in apparent brain volume, particularly in the hippocampal formation, which have been shown to be only partially reversible after correction of hypercortisolaemia. Exogenous steroids have also been shown to reduce hippocampal volume and to impair declarative memory.

Phaeochromocytoma

Phaeochromocytoma can mimic endocrine, cardiovascular, and neurological, as well as psychiatric conditions. The latter include panic and anxiety disorder, depressive disorder, and substance misuse. Common symptoms include dizziness, tremulousness, palpitations, and the subjective feeling of intense fear, leading to confusion with anxiety and panic attacks. The diagnostic feature is the elevation of blood pressure during an attack, and if such attacks are reported, routine testing for adrenergic metabolites should be conducted. Attacks are occasionally of sufficient intensity to lead to confusion and delirium.

Pituitary disorder

Panhypopituitarism with consequent adrenal failure produces a characteristic neuropsychiatric picture with apathy, fatigue, weight loss, inability to attend and concentrate, and memory impairment. The disorder may be confused with chronic fatigue, depression, or even dementia, and the weight loss has been confused with anorexia nervosa, although neither appetite disturbance nor distorted body image is usually found. Acromegaly can also result in a rather characteristic apathy and lack of concern, with occasional depression and irritability, perhaps reflecting a degree of global hypopituitarism.

There are two other particular neuropsychiatric issues that arise in consideration of a pituitary disorder. First, cerebral irradiation of pituitary tumours may give rise to collateral damage to adjacent brain structures, and there are reports of memory impairment, perhaps reflecting diencephalic and/or hippocampal damage. Second, endocrine replacement therapy following pituitary ablation may be suboptimal, indeed replacement of sex steroids is occasionally omitted because of their propensity to release sexual drive, which may be inappropriate.

Gonadal dysfunction
Contrary to previous beliefs, the menopause is not necessarily associated with psychological problems in healthy women. However, the following risk factors have been associated with affective disturbance: psychiatric problems; poor social, educational, occupational, and health status; stressful life events; high body mass index (BMI); cigarette smoking; as well as negative attitudes towards menopause and ageing. Successful treatments for mood disturbance include hormone therapy and psychological interventions, particularly cognitive behavioural therapy. Furthermore, increasing evidence supports the hypothesis that oestrogen treatment can have positive effects on cognitive performance in aging. The initiation of oestrogen treatment at the time of menopause, or soon after ovariectomy, is considered to provide a window of opportunity for the protection of memory in women. Imaging studies provide evidence of the neuroprotective role of oestrogen, particularly on the hippocampal volume in aging, and that it may lose its effectiveness after a specific period of time.

While significant advances have been made in our understanding of the modulatory effects of ovarian hormones on cognition in women, relatively little attention has been directed towards understanding the role of gonadal steroids on the modulation of cognitive functions in men. However, there are some studies which suggest that low premorbid testosterone levels are associated with a higher risk for Alzheimer's disease. Furthermore, it may be that low testosterone has a selective effect on memory consolidation. Preliminary data suggest that replacement therapy can modify the deficits. However, one should note that the adverse effects the low testosterone levels have on mood, arousal, and attention may also indirectly affect higher cognitive functions.

Neuropsychiatric systemic lupus erythematosus (SLE) and antiphospholipid antibody syndrome (APS)
Neuropsychiatric SLE is becoming an increasingly prevalent manifestation of SLE, estimated to affect 14 to 75% of patients and able to cause chronic irreversible brain injury. The American College of Rheumatology has recently revised its definition of neuropsychiatric SLE, distinguishing 12 types of central neurological involvement. There is no single diagnostic test that is sensitive or specific, hence the diagnosis depends on the combination of rheumatological examination, immunoserology, and brain imaging as well as psychiatric and neuropsychological tests in the presence of lupus disease activity. Recent neuropsychological investigations suggest that patients with SLE have particularly poor performance on verbal and memory tests. Furthermore, about 10 to 40% of patients have

depression, for which risk factors are thought to include direct brain damage, concomitant neuropsychiatric disorders, steroid administration, and the patient's response to the burden of the disease.

The clinical antiphospholipid antibody syndrome (APS) is found in 30% of patients with SLE or may occur in isolation. It is characterized by venous and arterial thromboses and neurological disease in the presence of antiphospholipid antibodies.

Voltage-gated potassium channel antibody-mediated syndromes
In the last few years, the role of channelopathies has been recognized in acute or transient neuropsychiatric disorders. Evidence has accumulated that voltage-gated antibodies to potassium channels are involved in certain limbic syndromes, and in some patients with subacute onset of unexplained epilepsy. Voltage-gated potassium channel (VGKC) antibodies were initially identified in patients with Isaac's syndrome, which is an acquired syndrome of peripheral nerve hyperexcitability. Patients may present with myokymia and often have hyperhidrosis. Subsequently, two VGKC antibody syndromes have been described with CNS manifestations: limbic encephalitis and Morvan's syndrome. Limbic encephalitis is an inflammatory disorder affecting prominently the mesial temporal lobes and characterized by confusion, disorientation, amnesia, personality change, and seizures. Patients develop acute or subacute memory loss and confusion, progressing over days or weeks to temporal lobe/partial complex epileptic seizures. Cognitive impairment is typically profound, with significant retrograde and anterograde amnesia. MRI usually shows high signal in the hippocampal region(s). In Morvan's syndrome, the peripheral and the CNS manifestations of the VGKC antibody syndromes coexist, characterized by severe and persistent insomnia, autonomic instability, lability of affect, cognitive impairment, hallucinations, and peripheral hyperexcitability. Patients with limbic encephalitis or Morvan's syndrome may improve spontaneously over time, but this is unusual. Treatment usually consists of immunotherapies similar to those employed for myasthenia gravis and other autoimmune disorders.

Further reading
Alper KR, Barry JJ, Balabanov AJ (2002). Treatment of psychosis, aggression, and irritability in patients with epilepsy. *Epilepsy Behav*, **3** Suppl 1, 13–8.

Arnsten AFT (2009). ADHD and The Prefrontal Cortex. *J Pediatrics*, **154**(5) S1, 1–S43.

Basson R (2008). Women's sexual function and dysfunction: current uncertainties, future directions – REVIEW. *International Journal of Impotence Research*, **20**, 466–78.

Biessels GJ, et al. (2006). Risk of dementia in diabetes mellitus: a systematic review. *Lancet Neurol*, **5**, 64–74.

Binetti G, et al. (2006). Areas of intervention for genetic counselling of dementia: Cross-cultural comparison between Italians and Americans. *Patient Educ Couns*, **64**, 285–93.

Bourne RS, Tahir TA, Borthwick M, Sampson EL (2008). Drug treatment of delirium: Past, present and future. *J Psychoso Res*, **65**(3), 273–82.

Brinar VV, Habek M (2007). Dementia and white-matter demyelination in young patient with neurosyphilis. *Lancet*, **368**(9554), 2258.

Bunevicius R, Velickiene D, Prange AJ Jr (2005). Mood and anxiety disorders in women with treated hyperthyroidism and ophthalmopathy caused by Graves' disease. *Gen Hosp Psychiatry*, **27**, 133–9.

Burns A, Gallagley A, Byrne J (2004). Delirium. *J Neurol Neurosurg Psychiatry*, **75**, 362–367.

Cruess DG, et al. (2003). Prevalence, diagnosis, and pharmacological treatment of mood disorders in HIV disease. *Biol Psychiatry*, **54**, 307–16.

Culham JC, Kanwisher NG (2001). Neuroimaging of cognitive functions in human parietal cortex. *Curr Opin Neurobiol*, **11**, 157–63.

David *et al.* (2009). *Lishman's Organic Psychiatry*. 4th Ed. Wiley-Blackwell.

Dickerson BC, Eichenbaum H (2009). The Episodic Memory System: Neurocircuitry and Disorders. *Neuropsychopharmacology REVIEWS*, 1–19. 10.1038/npp.2009.126

d'Ydewalle G, Van Damme I (2007). Memory and the Korsakoff syndrome: Not remembering what is remembered. *Neuropsychologia*, **45**, 905–20.

Eller M, Williams DR (2009). Biological fluid biomarkers in neurodegenerative parkinsonism – Review. *Nature Reviews Neurology*, **5**, 561–70.

Ekstrand JR, *et al.* (2004). The presence of psychiatric disorders reduces the likelihood of neurologic disease among referrals to a neurology clinic. *J Psychosom Res*, **57**, 11–6.

Feinstein A (2006). Mood disorder in multiple sclerosis and the effects on cognition. *J Neurol Sci*, **245**, 63–6.

Ferguson SM, Rayport M (2006). Pathogenesis of psychosis in epilepsy. the 'seesaw' theory: myth or reality? *Int Rev Neurobiol*, **76**, 45–61.

Finberg KE (2004). Mad cow disease in the United States: an update on bovine spongiform encephalopathy and variant Creutzfeldt–Jakob disease. *Clin Microbiol Newsl*, **26**, 113–18.

Florian Holsboer (2008). How can we realize the promise of personalized antidepressant medicines? *Nature Reviews Neuroscience*, **9**, 638–46.

Folstein MF, Folstein SE, McHugh PR (1975). 'Mini mental state'. A practical method for grading the cognitive state of patients for the clinician. *J Psychiatr Res*, **12**, 189–98.

Fong TG, Tulebaev SR, Inouye SK (2009). Delirium in elderly adults: diagnosis, prevention and treatment. *Nature Reviews Neurology*, **5**, 210–20.

Frackowiak RSJ, *et al.* (eds) (1997). *Human brain function*. Academic Press Inc.

Giaconne G, Mangieri M, Capobianco R, *et al.* (2008). Tauopathy in human and experimental variant Creutzfeldt-Jakob disease. *Neurobiology of Aging*, **29**(12), 240–3.

Götz J, Ittner LM (2008). Animal models of Alzheimer's disease and frontotemporal dementia. *Nature Reviews Neuroscience*, **9**, 532–44.

Gouveia PA, *et al.* (2007). Disorders in planning and strategy application in frontal lobe lesion patients. *Brain Cogn*, **63**, 240–6.

Gupta N, de Jonghe J, Schieveld J, Leonard M, Meagher D (2008). Delirium phenomenology: What can we learn from symptoms of delirium. *J Psychosomc Res*, **65**(3), 215–22.

Harisingani R (2005). Where are the reversible dementias? *J Am Geriatr Soc*, **53**, 1066–8.

Hebb DO (1945). Man's frontal lobe: a critical review. *Arch Neurol Psychiatry*, **54**, 10–24.

Hillman CH, Erickson KI, Kramer AF (2008). Be smart, exercise your heart: exercise effects on brain and cognition. *Nature Reviews Neuroscience*, **9**, 58–65.

Huijbregts SC, *et al.* (2006). Cognitive impairment and decline in different MS subtypes. *J Neurol Sci*, **245**, 187–94.

Hunter M, Rendall M (2007). Bio-psycho-socio-cultural perspectives on menopause. *Best Pract Res Clin Obstet Gynaecol*, **21**, 261–74.

Husain M, Nachev P (2007). Space and the parietal cortex. *Trends Cogn Sci*, **11**, 30–6.

Hyman SE (2008). A glimmer of light for neuropsychiatric disorders. *Nature*, **455**, 890–93.

Janowsky JS (2006). Thinking with your gonads: testosterone and cognition. *Trends Cogn Sci*, **10**, 77–82.

Kanner AM (2003). Depression in epilepsy: a frequently neglected multifaceted disorder. *Epilepsy Behav*, **4** Suppl 4, 11–9.

Karp G, *et al.* (2009). Syphilis and HIV co-infection - Review article. *Eur J Int Med*, **20**(1), 9–13.

Kopelman MD (1994). Structured psychiatric interview: psychiatric history and assessment of the mental state. *Br J Hosp Med*, **52**, 93–8.

Kopelman MD (1995). The Korsakoff syndrome. *Br J Psychiatry*, **166**, 154–73.

Kopelman MD (2002). Disorders of memory. *Brain*, **125**, 2152–90.

Kopelman MD, Fleminger S (2002). Experience and perspectives on the classification of organic mental disorders. *Psychopathology*, **35**, 76–81.

Lee Y-S, Silva AJ (2009). The molecular and cellular biology of enhanced cognition. *Nature Reviews Neuroscience*, **10**, 126–40.

Lipkin WI, Hornig M (2004). Psychotropic viruses. *Curr Opin Microbiol*, **7**, 420–5.

Mesulam MM (1982). Slowly progressive aphasia without generalized dementia. *Ann Neurol*, **11**, 592–98.

Michaud L, *et al.* (2007). Delirium: guidelines for general hospitals. *J Psychosom Res*, **62**, 371–83.

Minden SL, *et al.* (2005). Predictors and outcomes of delirium. *Gen Hospital Psychiatry*, **27**, 209–14.

Oksenberg JR, Baranzini SE, Sawcer S, Hauser SL (2008). The genetics of multiple sclerosis: SNPs to pathways to pathogenesis -Review. *Nature Reviews Genetics*, **9**, 516–26.

Okuda DT (2009). Unanticipated demyelinating pathology of the CNS - Review. *Nature Reviews Neurology*, **5**, 591–7.

Park Y-M, Che H-J, Im C-H, *et al.* (2008). Decreased synchronization and its correlation with symptom severity in Alzheimer's disease. *Neurosci Res*, **62**(2), 112–7.

Peng F, Hu X, Zhong X, *et al.* (2008). CT and MRI findings in HIV-negative neurosyphilis. *Eur J Radiology*, **66**(1), 1–6.

Perrin RJ, Fagan AM, Holtzman DM (2009). Multimodal techniques for diagnosis and prognosis of Alzheimer's disease. *Nature Nature*, **461**, 916–22.

Pitel AL, Beaunieux H, Guillery-Girard B, *et al.* (2009). How do Korsakoff patients learn new concepts? *Neuropsychologia*, **47**(3), 879–86.

Ponholzer A, *et al.* (2009). Serum androgen levels and their association to depression and Alzheimer dementia in a cohort of 75-year-old men over 5 years: results of the VITA study - ORIGINAL ARTICLE. *International Journal of Impotence Research*, **21**, 187–91.

Postle BR (2006). Working memory as an emergent property of the mind and brain. *Neuroscience*, **139**, 23–38.

Rademakers R, Rovelet-Lecrux A (2009). Recent Insights into molecular genetics of dementia. *TINS*, **32**(8), 451–61.

Rolfson D (2002). The causes of delirium. In: Lindesay J, Rockwood K, Macdonald A (eds) *Delirium in the elderly*, pp. 101–22. Oxford University Press, Oxford.

Rumboldt Z, Thurnher MM, Gupta RK (2007). Central nervous system infections. *Sem Roentgenol*, **42**, 62–91.

Rutter M, Taylor E (eds) (2005). *Child and adolescent psychiatry*, 4th edition. Wiley-Blackwell.

Sacks O (1995). *An anthropologist on Mars*. Picador, London.

Santosa M, Kövaria E, Hofd PR, *et al.* (2009). The impact of vascular burden on late-life depression - Review. *Brain Res Reviews*, In Press.

Savage LM, Roland J, Klintsova A (2007). Selective septohippocampal—but not forebrain amygdalar—cholinergic dysfunction in diencephalic amnesia. *Brain Res*, **1139**, 210–19.

Schwartz JM, Marsh L (2000). The psychiatric perspectives of epilepsy. *Psychosomatics*, **41**, 31–8.

Silver JM, Yudofsky SC, Hales RE (eds) (1994). *Neuropsychiatry of traumatic brain injury*. American Psychiatric Press, Washington DC.

Stefanova E, *et al.* (2006). Depression predicts the pattern of cognitive impairment in early Parkinson's disease. *J Neurol Sci*, **248**, 131–7.

Stuss DT, Anderson V (2004). The frontal lobes and theory of mind: developmental concepts from adult focal lesion research. *Brain Cogn*, **55**, 69–83.

Tairyan K, Illes J (2009). Imaging genetics and the power of combined technologies: a perspective from neuroethics. *Neuroscience*, **164**(1), 7–15.

Taphoorn MJ, Klein M (2004). Cognitive deficits in adult patients with brain tumours. *Lancet Neurol*, **3**, 159–68.

Turner MS, *et al.* (2007). Qualitatively different memory impairments across frontal lobe subgroups. *Neuropsychologia*, **45**, 1540–52.

Vincent A, Lang B, Kleopa KA (2006). Autoimmune channelopathies and related neurological disorders. *Neuron*, **52**, 123–38.

von Gunten A, *et al.* (2006). Neural substrates of cognitive and behavioral deficits in atypical Alzheimer's disease. *Brain Res Rev*, **51**, 176–211.

Wichowicz HM, Cubala WJ, Slawek J (2006). Wilson's disease associated with delusional disorder. *Psychiatry Clin Neurosci*, **60**, 758–60.

Whalley LJ, Dick FD, McNeill G (2006). A life-course approach to the aetiology of late-onset dementias. *Lancet Neurol*, **5**, 87–96.

World Health Organization (1992). The ICD-10 classification of mental and behavioural disorders. World Health Organization, Geneva.

Wright CI, *et al.* (2007). Neuroanatomical correlates of personality in the elderly. *Neuroimage*, **35**, 263–72.

Yeap BB (2009). Are declining testosterone levels a major risk factor for ill-health in aging men? REVIEW. *Int J Impotence Res*, **21**, 24–36.

Zandman-Goddard G, Chapman J, Shoenfeld Y (2007). Autoantibodies involved in neuropsychiatric SLE and antiphospholipid syndrome. *Semin Arthritis Rheum*, **36**, 297–315.

Zarei M (2006). Clinical characteristics of cortical multiple sclerosis. *J Neurol Sci*, **245**, 53–8.

26.5

Psychiatric disorders as they concern the physician

Contents

26.5.1 Grief, stress, and post-traumatic stress disorder

Tim Dalgleish, Jenny Yiend, and
Ann-Marie J. Golden

Essentials

Grief—this is the constellation of psychological responses to the loss of a loved one. Normal grief arguably develops in stages and dissipates in strength and impact over time. Some people (14–34%) suffer from pathological grief, where intense emotional distress and impairment of functioning persist for 6 months or more. This is often comorbid with other psychiatric disorders. Grief—and pathological grief in particular—carry an increased risk of mortality in the bereaved person, hence treatment of pathological grief using psychological therapy is advised.

Stress—the term can refer either to an external object, event, or situation that is the source of ongoing emotional distress, or to the constellation of psychological responses, dominated by elevated physiological arousal, that comprise an individual's subjective experience in response to such stimuli. A subdiagnostic level of stress is common and is a risk factor for numerous physical health problems. Stress of this nature can frequently be ameliorated by lifestyle changes.

Pathological stress responses—these include acute stress disorder and post-traumatic stress disorder (PTSD), which occur in response to extremely stressful events. PTSD is characterized by (1) re-experiencing of the stressful event—e.g. nightmares, images, and flashbacks; (2) sustained avoidance of reminders of the event or of stimuli that might trigger re-experiencing; and (3) hyperarousal—e.g. sleep disturbance, irritability.

Management—debriefing in the early stages is not recommended as a routine intervention for all who have been exposed to traumatic events. However, PTSD is a disabling condition that is often comorbid with other psychiatric problems. Trauma-focused psychological interventions are the treatment of choice, with pharmacological interventions being a second-line treatment for those who do not wish to engage in a psychological intervention.

Grief

Introduction

Grief could be described as a natural response to an objectively significant loss, most commonly the death of a loved one, although whether the boundaries defining a 'significant loss' should be stretched further (and if so, how far) remains controversial. It involves primarily psychological reactions, although it may also lead to social and physical responses. 'Normal grief', which requires no clinical intervention, can be distinguished from 'pathological grief', also variously called 'atypical, traumatic, neurotic, morbid, complicated, or unresolved grief'.

However, it should be stated clearly at the outset that the concept of an abnormal form of grief is not represented in current official diagnostic manuals, and as such is not an established clinical condition. Indeed, the lack of consensus over terminology in the literature illustrates the urgent need for quality research to establish clear and universally accepted diagnostic criteria. Despite this confusion, many professionals now recognize some form of abnormal grief response as an appropriate target for active intervention, the key features being: (1) an excessive intensity of the grief reaction (inappropriate within the culture) which includes pathological yearning; and (2) an unusually prolonged duration. This gathering consensus has led to proposals for the establishment of complicated grief as a formal diagnosis in the forthcoming 5th edition of the Diagnostic and Statistical Manual of Mental Disorders (DSM) to be published by the American Psychiatric Association (due in May 2013).

Epidemiology

Considering the ubiquity of bereavement, the consequences of grief are of global importance. Incidence rates for pathological grief are not available; estimates of prevalence vary from 14 to 34%, based primarily on samples drawn from the United States of America and Europe. In geographical areas prone to natural disasters and places engaged in active military conflict these rates will obviously rise significantly in line with death rates, and in such cases particular attention should be paid to the concurrent trauma that will have accompanied the loss (see 'Stress', below).

Mortality

Much evidence shows that the bereaved in general (irrespective of whether a pathological response develops) are at greater risk of dying themselves than would be expected given mortality rates in the population at large. Mortality is elevated by a factor of two to three, applying not only to spousal loss, but also to parental, sibling, and child loss. These findings have proven robust across cultures and generations. The point of highest risk is the weeks and months immediately following the loss, although the data suggest it remains elevated for several years. This evidence should alert the clinician to pay particular attention to all forms of presenting grief, whether normal or pathological.

Within a bereaved population additional factors moderate this mortality risk, although it remains elevated for all subgroups. Thus, the younger bereaved are at a higher relative risk of death themselves than the older, as are widowers compared to widows (although remarriage selectively reduces the risk in widowers). The cause of bereavement is also important, mortality risk being particularly elevated for bereavements involving suicide, accidents, liver cirrhosis, and heart disease.

Hard evidence concerning the underlying reason for reduced longevity following bereavement is scarce, but factors both directly and indirectly related to the loss may be involved. For example, psychological consequences such as the loss of the will to live might directly lead to increased suicides and carelessness. Indirectly, the change in lifestyle necessitated by bereavement may lead to the adoption of health-impairing behaviours (neglect of diet, exercise, general well-being) or may create psychological stress, which in turn could have serious negative consequences for health (see 'Stress', below).

Psychiatric comorbidity

Acute bereavement is associated with an increased risk for a range of psychiatric disorders, including major depression, panic disorder, generalized anxiety disorder (GAD) and post-traumatic stress disorder (PTSD). Any of these may occur comorbidly with pathological grief, when between 17 and 31% will also meet criteria for major depression, 13% panic disorder, 39% GAD, and 9% PTSD. However, these figures should be treated with caution since the criteria for 'pathological' and the timing and consistency of assessment can greatly affect the results. But what is clear is that the rate of comorbidity following bereavement is significant, with estimates suggesting more than half of the bereaved suffer from two disorders. Hence, having diagnosed one disorder in the bereaved patient (be it psychiatric or pathological grief), the clinician should be particularly alert to the possible presence of additional, complicating disorders. It is unclear whether this comorbidity is best conceived as the presence of one disorder predisposing the patient to additional pathology, or simply the presence of two coexisting disorders whose symptoms may or may not aggravate each other. Whichever, it is essential that both domains of symptoms are separately monitored and, to the extent that it differs, treatment for both disorders is given.

Clinical features
Normal grief
The literature on normal grief reveals that we have not yet precisely characterized the process or clearly demarcated its boundaries. Many theorists propose that there are distinct 'stages' of grief, and while opinions vary about the precise number and nature of stages, it is common to consider at least three. These are:

◆ an initial period of shock, including emotional numbing and disbelief. This stage may last from hours to weeks.

◆ a subsequent phase of acute mourning, involving an acknowledgement of the death together with intense emotional states that typically engulf the individual in periodic 'waves' of feeling. Somatic discomfort, social withdrawal, and preoccupation with thoughts of the deceased may accompany this. There may also be 'identification' with the deceased, in which the individual adopts characteristic behaviours, mannerisms, or habits of the loved one, and may even experience physical symptoms associated with the cause of death ('grief facsimile symptoms'). This phase may last for several months.

◆ a period of restoration of normal function during which the characteristics of acute mourning are gradually replaced by feeling able to continue with life. A shift in focus occurs away from the deceased and towards the future. While memories and a sense of loss may remain, there is recognition of having grieved and a will to move on.

More recent theories have placed less emphasis on chronological stages, preferring instead to consider particular domains or clusters of symptoms that may fluctuate in intensity throughout the period of grieving. Table 26.5.1.1 summarizes some of these symptoms of grief.

Pathological grief
The concept of 'abnormal' grief superseding what might be construed as normal and therefore requiring medical intervention is not currently an officially acknowledged pathology. However, many

Table 26.5.1.1 Symptoms of normal grief

Psychological					Social	Physical
Emotional	**Cognitive**	**Behavioural**	**Perceptual**	**Pathological**		
Longing, yearning for deceased	Disbelief, shock	Searching, seeking out things and places associated with the deceased	Hallucinations	Despair	Social withdrawal and isolation	Sighing
Numbness	Preoccupying thoughts of the deceased	Aimlessness	Illusions	Arousal	Social inhibition	Crying
Sadness, nostalgia	Loss of interest, meaning	Avoidance	Dreams, nightmares	Anxiety, panic	Loss of compassion for others	Insomnia
Anger	Intrusive, unpleasant images	Identification behaviours (mimicking habits of the deceased)		Anorexia-like symptoms	Problems functioning at work	Fatigue, lethargy, apathy
Irritability	Mental disorganization (trouble concentrating, making decisions)	Coping strategies		Suicidal ideation		Vague somatic symptoms
Guilt	Acceptance and remembering	New commitments				
Loneliness						

Box 26.5.1.1 Proposed criteria for complicated grief

Criterion A

♦ Yearning, pining, longing for the deceased.

Yearning must be experienced at least daily over the past month or to a distressing or disruptive degree.

Criterion B

In the past month, the person must experience four of the following eight symptoms as marked or extreme.

1 Trouble accepting the death

2 Inability trusting others since the death

3 Excessive bitterness over the death

4 Feeling uneasy about moving on with one's life (e.g. difficulty forming new relationships)

5 Feeling emotionally numb or detached from others since the death

6 Feeling life is empty or meaningless without the deceased

7 Feeling the future holds no meaning or prospect for fulfilment without the deceased

8 Feeling agitated, jumpy, or on edge since the death

Criterion C

♦ Yearning and at least one criterion B item must cause marked dysfunction in social, occupational, or other important domains.

Criterion D

♦ Yearning and at least one criterion B item must last at least 6 months.

Criteria A, B, C, D must be met for a diagnosis of complicated grief.

workers are calling for a set of universally accepted diagnostic criteria to be developed, and, in the meantime, Prigerson and colleagues have proposed a preliminary set for what they have termed complicated grief that should prove helpful to the practising clinician. These represent a consensus opinion and as such incorporate a variety of perspectives on grief and its manifestations. They are formulated in the DSM style in Box 26.5.1.1.

Several features are worth noting.

♦ Diagnosis requires the actual death of a significant other, thereby excluding any other forms of loss (physical separation, loss of nonhuman objects—animals, body parts, material possessions). This remains controversial.

♦ Observable psychological distress in response to the death is essential, although it may be delayed. Thus, a total nonresponse (the absence of any observable or reported signs of grief), which may be of concern to the practising clinician, would not warrant a positive diagnosis. In such cases the best approach may be close monitoring of the patient over time, together with probing for signs of intrusive thoughts or behaviours relating to the deceased, despite emotional numbing.

♦ Criterion B represents symptoms of particular severity. They fall into four broad categories: numbing (1, 5), disorganized behaviour or experience (2, 4, 6, 7), hyperarousal (8), and bitterness (3). The recommendation is that at least four of these eight symptoms should be present for a positive diagnosis in addition to the core response of distressing yearning, longing, and preoccupation listed under criterion A.

♦ Criteria C and D are central to distinguishing normal from pathological grief. They embody the notion, described earlier and consistent throughout DSM-IV, that there must be significant impairment of functioning together with an abnormally long duration of symptoms. The latter is set at 6 months, based on previous evidence that if complicated grief is diagnosed at least 6 months after loss then this reliably identifies individuals persistently affected by grief.

The core domains for positive diagnosis can therefore be summarized as severity, duration, and functioning.

Differential diagnosis

Bereavement and comorbid psychiatric disorder

DSM-IV criteria for the diagnosis of major depression include specific guidelines for the circumstances of bereavement. This acknowledges that depressive-like symptoms will be fairly ubiquitous following bereavement and criteria are therefore more stringent. Specifically, either a 6-month (rather than a 2-week) duration of symptoms is required, or alternatively the presence of particular symptoms such as marked functional impairment, psychotic symptoms, or suicidal ideation is necessary. Although no specific guidelines for other comorbid psychiatric disorders are given, the clinician would be well advised to apply similar principles of increased severity or extended duration before making a positive diagnosis.

Pathological grief and comorbid psychiatric disorder

Pathological grief, by the working definition given above, occurs exclusively in the circumstances of the death of a significant other. While this objective criterion helpfully restricts diagnosis, it remains necessary to distinguish between this and other possible psychiatric disorders that may follow bereavement.

- Major depressive episode—is distinguished by a pervasive and general depressed mood disturbance, in contrast to the episodic pangs of grief focused around the absence of the deceased. Other characteristic symptoms of pathological grief are absent.

- Panic disorder and GAD—are distinguished primarily by the absence of characteristic symptoms of pathological grief, and in the former by the presence of acute episodes of severe anxiety or panic attacks.

- PTSD—this is perhaps the most problematic differential diagnosis. Could pathological grief be construed as a specific example of PTSD? Only further research will resolve this question. For the present we suggest that the following features be considered: pathological grief, in contrast to PTSD, does not require exposure to an objectively traumatic event (although this may occur in cases of violent death). In pathological grief, symptoms of avoidance and hyperarousal are less prominent than in PTSD, and avoidance is not among the proposed criteria for complicated grief. Symptoms of pathological grief are centred on the deceased person (pining, searching for them, sensitivity for signs of them in the environment), whereas those of PTSD centre around the traumatic event itself (re-experiencing the trauma, intrusive thoughts about the trauma, general hypervigilance). Finally, where both disorders are suspected, it is advisable to focus treatment initially on PTSD.

Treatment

Normal grief will resolve spontaneously over time. Treatment options for pathological grief fall into the categories of pharmacology, psychotherapies, cognitive/behavioural therapies, and self-help strategies. In common with other psychological disorders, maximum benefit may often be obtained by the prudent combination of drugs with psychological treatments. In practice, individual circumstances and the local availability of treatments will inevitably impose restrictions.

Pharmacology

The few studies available looking specifically at drug treatments following bereavement suggest that both tricyclic antidepressants and selective serotonin reuptake inhibitors (SSRIs) may provide effective relief of symptoms. The tricyclics appear to be more confined in their effects, influencing primarily depressive symptoms, whereas the SSRIs may have a broader action, additionally counteracting symptoms reflecting trauma, such as avoidance and emotional numbing. SSRIs have the additional advantage of more tolerable side effects, as well as being safer in overdose. Individual circumstances, side effect profiles, and any known personal or family history of response to treatment can act as a guide in the selection of therapy.

Psychotherapies

Psychodynamic forms of psychotherapy tend to be favoured over those of a psychoanalytical persuasion. The former centre around the developing relationship between therapist and client, and focus on ongoing changes in the presenting psychological processes observed in the client. Current opinion suggests that this form of psychotherapy may yield more effective results within a shorter time frame than psychoanalytical techniques, which tend to focus more on a re-evaluation of personal history as the means to personal change.

Psychotherapies that have been used specifically to treat the bereaved include crisis intervention and brief dynamic psychotherapy. One study of crisis intervention psychotherapy, given immediately after the loss, lasted for several months and involved reviewing aspects of the lost relationship within the context of the psychodynamic relationship. A significant reduction in symptoms was noted. By contrast, in a study of a psychodynamic therapy starting several months after the loss, only a marginal symptom improvement was found.

Cognitive/behavioural therapies

Cognitive behavioural therapy (CBT) is a popular form of treatment for many psychological disorders. It combines behavioural techniques, such as relaxation and exposure, with cognitive restructuring in which the patient is encouraged to identify and alter maladaptive styles of thinking that are thought to maintain ongoing psychological distress. There is promising initial data for the efficacy of CBT-based therapy for complicated grief, with two randomized controlled trials currently published.

Exclusively behavioural techniques have also been used. These involve exposure to feared or avoided stimuli in order to produce habituation, and may also incorporate relaxation techniques to aid this process. Guided mourning and trauma desensitization are two such treatments: both appear to selectively reduce somatic and avoidance symptoms, having less of an effect on depressive symptoms and preoccupations with the deceased.

Self-help

Self-help groups should not be overlooked as a possible supplement to treatment, either to aid transition following successful treatment, or in a preventive capacity. Some evidence suggests that, with appropriately trained group leaders, benefits conferred may be equivalent to some of the more formal treatments discussed above.

Finally, the reader is referred to an excellent text by Jacobs, an expert in the area, which outlines one possible practical approach to treatment endorsed by the author (see p. 81 therein), as well as a diagnosis/treatment algorithm (see p. 76 therein).

Prognosis

Pathological grief responses may be chronic and unremitting without medical intervention, and a prolonged course of 2 years or more is likely where symptoms persist beyond the first year. In the case of normal grief, most of the acute symptoms of mourning may be expected to dissipate within several months to a year, but some level of emotional involvement may persist indefinitely. Those at higher risk of a pathological grief response may include the young, women, those who suffer multiple losses, and those who have suffered childhood loss. The risk is increased following sudden, unexpected, violent, or suicidal death. An ambivalent or insecure relationship to the deceased ('attachment disturbance') also increases risk, as do personality traits such as neuroticism, dependency, and schizoid personality. Finally, transient features displayed in an individual, such as the inability to accept an imminent death, or severe distress during a terminal illness, increase that individual's risk for pathological grief.

Prevention

Primary measures fall largely in the domain of social policy, such as gun control, safe driving practice, or healthy living styles. These can directly reduce deaths due to unnatural causes. However, the clinician may also play a role by moderating the impact of death, particularly when it is sudden or unexpected. This would include allowing ample time to be spent with a dying or indeed a deceased patient in a quiet and supportive atmosphere, which can enable associated others to more effectively assimilate their loss.

Secondary prevention might include screening bereaved populations at high risk. At the level of the individual this would involve ascertaining the risk profile of a recently bereaved patient and, where this is high, maintaining contact, monitoring progress, and providing early intervention where appropriate.

Tertiary prevention, to moderate the extent of disability, can be implemented by considering appropriate medium- to long-term treatments. Patients may well present late in the course of pathological grief, prompted only by severe functional impairment or social pressure. Although early intervention is preferable, an appropriate selection from the treatment options discussed above is still likely to confer some benefit.

Areas of controversy needing further research

Perhaps the main controversy of concern to clinicians is whether the concept of 'pathological grief' warrants a distinct diagnostic category, or whether it is best subsumed under existing pathologies such as PTSD or major depression. The high comorbidities and the question marks concerning differential diagnosis support the latter view; factor analysis of symptom clusters, their differential response to drugs, and the distinct risk profiles support the former. However, the question of labelling becomes clinically unimportant to the extent that the treatment for these pathologies overlaps.

Other controversies are the model of distinct 'stages of grief', which some advocate more than others; the extent to which the absence of grief might be considered pathological; the duration of normal grief, which some argue is indefinite; the nature of the grief object, which some restrict to the death of an intimate, while others

extend far more broadly to include nondeath and nonhuman loss. The following issues also warrant investigation: cultural differences in the expression and experience of grief; the factors responsible for the relationship between bereavement and increased health and mortality risks.

Stress and post-traumatic stress disorder

Introduction

Stress and stressors

Stress often refers to an external object, event, or situation that causes physical and psychological effects on an individual as a result of increased levels of arousal. These effects are usually experienced as unpleasant and undesirable, although there is a close correspondence with the excitement that occurs when a positive, desirable interpretation is adopted, e.g. during dangerous sports. The term 'stress' is perhaps more appropriately used to refer to the subjective experience of these effects, and the agent causing them is more accurately termed 'the stressor'.

Societal and lifestyle changes in developed nations, as well as media coverage, have given prominence to the role of stressors and their adverse effects, although in practice these are prevalent universally. While a moderate degree of stress can be helpful to enhance performance, chronic stress is indeed associated with negative outcomes. Stress can be a risk factor for various physical health problems, most notably coronary heart disease, infectious diseases, immune function, and cancer. In addition 'background stress' (the presence of low-level chronic stressors) is known to potentiate an individual's negative response to acute stressors, and thus can be considered a vulnerability factor for negative outcome. Within psychiatry the effect of stressors has been extensively studied. They are known to raise the probability of relapse and, more controversially, are believed to play a part in triggering the onset of some disorders. Examples include schizophrenia, where interventions developed to reduce the levels of interpersonal stress within families ('expressed emotion') have proved effective. Similarly, in major depression much research has been conducted on the role of 'life events' (e.g. death of a spouse, loss of a job, going on holiday).

For the patient without psychiatric disorder the adverse effects of stressors can usually be addressed through lifestyle changes such as increased exercise, improved diet, relaxation techniques, reduction of working hours, and delegation of responsibilities. All these measures require an adjustment of personal priorities, which some may be unwilling to do. Where stress arises from unavoidable personal circumstances (e.g. caregiving, financial or relationship problems), the role of the clinician includes referral to appropriate support services to enable the stressors to be addressed at their source.

An additional option, provided within the DSM-IV system, is a diagnosis of adjustment disorder. This may be appropriate where a discrete, identifiable stressor exists and causes either significant impairment in functioning, or distress beyond that which would normally be expected given the nature of the stress. However, this disorder (by definition) is time-limited by and closely coupled to the external stressor itself, although it may be classed as chronic where the stressor or its consequences persist indefinitely. Specifically, symptoms must commence within 3 months of the onset of the stressor and cease within 6 months of its termination. It is also of note that bereavement is specifically excluded as a qualifying stressor. Nevertheless, where these criteria are fulfilled and other psychiatric diagnoses have been excluded, the clinician may wish to offer appropriate psychological interventions as described below.

Trauma

We will use the term 'trauma' where extreme stress occurs in response to an acute, intense episode brought about by a specific, objectively identifiable, external event. A trauma (defined under Clinical features, below) may be distinguished from a stressor primarily in terms of the objective intensity and severity of the experience or incident. It is now recognized that some people exposed to such a trauma go on to develop a clinical pathology, post-traumatic stress disorder (PTSD). PTSD, the subject of the rest of this section, was first introduced into the diagnostic nomenclature in 1980 with the publication of DSM-III, and it subsequently appeared in the World Health Organization's International Classification of Diseases (ICD) in 1992.

Epidemiology

Traumatic events are common, estimates suggesting that most Americans will experience at least 1 trauma over a lifetime. The lifetime prevalence of PTSD in the general population is between 1 and 14% according to DSM-IV, with a recent review suggesting this level is higher in women (10–12%) than men (5%). Estimates of lifetime prevalence among trauma victims vary widely according to the criteria and populations sampled, but somewhere between 3 and 58% of people who experience a trauma will go on to develop PTSD at some time in their lives, although more recent reviews put the figure as high as 60 to 80%. Clearly, geographical factors will influence these figures, leading to significant increases in areas prone to natural disasters or human conflict. In common with most psychiatric disorders there appears to be high comorbidity in PTSD, with 80% of sufferers meeting the criteria for at least one other psychiatric disorder.

Clinical features

The primary, essential feature for a positive diagnosis of PTSD is the prior experience of an objectively traumatic event. DSM-IV distinguishes two components: first, the nature of the event itself, which should involve an 'actual or perceived threat to life or physical integrity'—typical events including active combat, rape or other assault, natural disasters, and serious accidents. Witnessing such events is also included within the concept of 'experiencing'. Second, individuals should have an extreme emotional response to the event, which DSM-IV describes as intense fear, helplessness, or horror.

A pathological reaction to such a trauma is characterized by symptoms that fall into three clinically observed domains: re-experiencing, avoidance/numbing, and hyperarousal. Avoidance and numbing may be better considered separately, although DSM-IV does not do so. Typical examples of these symptoms are as follows.

◆ Re-experiencing—including nightmares, flashbacks, intrusive thoughts, and images relating to the trauma. Such symptoms have often been considered to be the hallmark of PTSD.

◆ Avoidance—typically anything that could remind the individual of or be associated with the trauma is avoided. This can include people, places, activities, and conversations.

◆ Numbing—emotional responsiveness is generally reduced. This may include an inability to experience certain feelings and feelings of detachment or other dissociative symptoms (e.g. depersonalization, dissociative amnesia, derealization).

◆ Hyperarousal—this includes insomnia, anger, irritability, hypervigilance, problems with concentration, exaggerated startle.

DSM-IV requires at least one symptom of re-experiencing, three of avoidance/numbing, and two of hyperarousal to be present for a positive diagnosis. It also currently specifies three subtypes of PTSD—acute, chronic (where symptoms have lasted under or over 3 months, respectively), and delayed onset (where 6 months or more have elapsed after the stressor before the emergence of symptoms).

DSM-IV also introduced a new, related diagnostic category—acute stress disorder (ASD)—which essentially is an acute form of PTSD. The symptoms are identical, but the diagnosis can be made as early as 2 days post-trauma, thereby encouraging earlier intervention. Persistence of symptoms beyond 1 month results in the diagnosis reverting to PTSD. For ASD, three of five dissociative/numbing symptoms are required, reflecting the belief that these are predictive of longer term psychopathology. Although the diagnosis remains controversial, it does provide the clinician with a clear indication for early intervention in some cases.

Differential diagnosis

Normal reactions to trauma

As with grief, the key features that distinguish PTSD from non-pathological reactions to trauma are intensity, duration, and effect on functioning. The intensity of the pathological reaction is captured by the nature of the symptoms themselves, with the presence of numbing symptoms thought to be the most effective distinguisher of victims with PTSD from those without. In addition, symptoms must have been present for at least 1 month and must be causing clinically significant distress or impairment in functioning.

Other psychiatric conditions

Subsets of the features of PTSD often overlap with other psychiatric conditions, but distinguishing characteristics are usually present. First, in PTSD there is an instigating traumatic event, which is not required for any of the other anxiety disorders. Second, the symptoms of nightmares and flashbacks are specific for PTSD and do not characterize other anxiety disorders. Third, emotional numbing, which occurs in the place of the normally expected emotional reactions, is strongly and uniquely characteristic to PTSD.

PTSD, considered to be an anxiety disorder, shares several anxiety-related symptoms, particularly from the hyperarousal cluster. Hypervigilance, sleep disturbance, irritability, and concentration problems are all common to GAD. Similarly, fear and avoidance are common to the phobias. Intrusive thoughts may also occur in obsessive–compulsive disorder (OCD), major depression, and GAD. Conversely, PTSD sufferers may exhibit compulsive behaviours of the type associated with OCD, such as repetitive cleansing procedures, or continual checking of locks and security devices, perhaps following rape or other kinds of assault. Although rates of comorbidity are indeed high (see above), dual diagnoses should only be made where the full criteria for both disorders are met.

Treatment

In March 2005, the National Institute for Health and Clinical Excellence (NICE) in the United Kingdom produced guidance for the screening and treatment of PTSD in children and adults. The key priorities for implementation for adults are listed in Box 26.5.1.2. The main points are that debriefing is not recommended as a routine intervention for all in the early stages, that trauma-focused psychological interventions are the treatment of choice, and that pharmacological interventions are a second-line treatment for those who do not wish to engage in a psychological intervention.

Crisis intervention

This approach, also called 'psychological debriefing', aims to treat all survivors of a trauma in the hope of reducing subsequent pathology. It takes place in a single session, within days of the incident, most forms of treatment being given individually or in small groups. Typically, there are several structured phases including

---

> ### Box 26.5.1.2 Key priorities for implementation for adults with PTSD
>
> #### Initial response to trauma
>
> ◆ For individuals who have experienced a traumatic event, the systematic provision to that individual alone of brief, single session interventions (often referred to as debriefing) that focus on the traumatic incident, should not be routine practice when delivering services.
>
> ◆ Where symptoms are mild and have been present for less than 4 weeks after the trauma, watchful waiting, as a way of managing the difficulties presented by people with post-traumatic stress disorder (PTSD), should be considered. A follow-up contact should be arranged within 1 month.
>
> #### Trauma-focused psychological treatment
>
> ◆ Trauma-focused cognitive behavioural therapy should be offered to those with severe post-traumatic symptoms or with severe PTSD in the first month after the traumatic event. These treatments should normally be provided on an individual, outpatient basis.
>
> ◆ All people with PTSD should be offered a course of trauma-focused psychological treatment, e. g. trauma-focused cognitive behavioural therapy (CBT) or eye movement desensitization and reprocessing (EMDR). These treatments should normally be provided on an individual, outpatient basis.
>
> #### Drug treatments for adults
>
> ◆ Drug treatments for PTSD should not be used as a routine, first-line treatment for adults (in general use or by specialist mental health professionals) in preference to a trauma-focused psychological therapy.
>
> ◆ Drug treatments (paroxetine or mirtazapine for general use, and amitriptyline or phenelzine for initiation only by mental health specialists) should be considered for the treatment of PTSD in adults who express a preference not to engage in trauma-focused psychological treatment.
>
> Post Traumatic Stress Disorder: The management of PTSD in adults and children in primary and secondary care, National Clinical Practice Guideline Number 26, National Collaborating Center for Mental Health. Reproduced with permission of the Royal College of Psychiatrists and the British Psychological Society, 2005.

---

each individual sharing their own general perspective ('recreating the event'), their thoughts at the time, the worst aspect of the event, and their reactions to it. There is usually also a teaching element, covering common reactions to trauma and how to deal with them.

Without doubt participants subjectively feel this type of intervention to be helpful and valuable. However, the research findings do not demonstrate efficacy a recent review revealed that there have been few randomized controlled trials, but that these show little observable benefit, some even reporting a negative outcome. Currently, the NICE guidelines are against the use of debriefing as an indiscriminate, immediate intervention. The treatment options discussed below are suitable for individuals who go on to develop PTSD following trauma.

Pharmacological treatments

The main difficulty regarding drug treatment is the dearth of clinical trials, hence what follows is based primarily on clinical experience.

Antiadrenergic agents

β-Blockers are effective in the short term in reducing symptoms of hyperarousal and re-experiencing. Patients respond quickly, although tolerance is likely to develop. They are perhaps most appropriate for those whose individual prognosis is good, or where immediate symptom relief is required, before pursuing other treatment options.

Antidepressants

Most antidepressants provide at least some symptom relief, but the benefits are generally modest for classes such as tricyclics and monoamine oxidase inhibitors (MAOIs), and issues of side effect profiles and overdose safety mean that SSRIs tend to be preferred. Recent data suggests that SSRIs may be effective in reducing symptoms from all symptom domains, and, therefore, they are currently the preferred option for the long-term drug treatment of PTSD. Two additional points are worth noting. First, uncertainty persists about the speed of action of these drugs, with estimates for the onset of beneficial effects varying between 2 weeks and 1 month. Patients should therefore be prepared for some delay. Second, some SSRI side effects, such as arousal and insomnia, although usually short-lived, will be particularly difficult for the patient with PTSD to tolerate. Paroxetine is currently the only drug with a United Kingdom product licence for PTSD.

Psychological treatments

Many different types of psychological therapy have been used to treat patients with PTSD, most appearing to impart some benefit in terms of symptom relief and improved psychological and social functioning, but longer term benefits remain unclear. Similarly, the potential for additional gains to be made by combining psychological treatments with each other or with drugs remains largely unexplored. Some of the more common therapies employed are discussed below.

Cognitive behavioural therapies

These are one of the psychological treatments of first choice for patients with PTSD recommended by NICE because most are relatively brief and have a well-established efficacy, both from clinical experience and empirical research. Treatments focus specifically on trauma-related material. Therapies may differ in the particular components included, but generally they comprise one or more of exposure treatments, anxiety management, and cognitive intervention.

Exposure treatments Exposure treatments involve repeated exposure to trauma-related material on the basis that this will reduce undesirable responses, either through simple habituation or as a result of concurrent cognitive reprocessing. Treatments vary in the type of exposure used. Imaginal techniques involve the patient reliving (describing verbally, writing down, or role playing) the trauma within the treatment room. *In vivo* exposure involves confronting, in real-life but safe situations, places or objects that provide reminders of the trauma. Other variables include the length of exposure (brief or prolonged) and the level of arousal induced (high or low). Prolonged imaginal exposure is currently the favoured technique of many therapists for the treatment of PTSD because of its relative efficacy and time efficiency.

Some forms of exposure treatment, e.g. systematic desensitization, adopt a hierarchical approach in which exposure is graded in difficulty, starting with least feared stimuli and progressing in tandem with patient improvement. Relaxation procedures may also be employed: these are known to be unnecessary for treatment efficacy, but may help to encourage patient participation in an initially unpleasant procedure.

Exposure techniques are time efficient and easy for patients to learn. Good quality, consistent data supports their efficacy. However, as noted, compliance may be a genuine problem, particularly in those with prominent avoidance symptoms.

Anxiety management Anxiety management training aims to teach patients to control and cope with their symptoms, rather than focusing on elimination or cure. Stress inoculation training is one such technique that has been commonly used for PTSD. Treatment usually involves components of both education and skills training. The latter may include deep relaxation, quick relaxation, breathing control, thought stopping, and role play. Anxiety management programmes are more complex to administer and more intellectually demanding for patients than other treatment options. However, they are likely to be particularly appropriate for PTSD patients with symptoms of chronic, general arousal. In addition, they may be indicated at later stages, e.g. where maximal benefit has been achieved from other treatment options and the patient is left with residual symptoms.

Cognitive intervention Cognitive interventions are directed at thoughts and appraisals associated with the trauma and its affective consequences. They involve challenging beliefs such as 'I will never be the same again', 'I have lost my mind', 'the world is a dangerous and unpredictable place'. Challenging involves working with the client to gather evidence to refute such cognitions and working to overcome habitual coping responses that serve to perpetuate the beliefs, e.g. becoming withdrawn from the world.

Psychotherapies Both psychodynamic and psychoanalytical techniques (see 'Grief', above) have been used to treat PTSD. Such therapies tend to vary enormously in nature, encompassing individual and group approaches and lasting anywhere from a few sessions to over a year. The available data reveals improvements following treatment, but methodological flaws preclude any clear conclusions. It may well be advisable to pursue alternatives where they exist.

Hypnotherapy Hypnosis has reportedly been used with some success, but there is a lack of sound published data to confirm this, although one controlled study suggests that it is effective and may be particularly suitable for reducing intrusive symptoms (re-experiencing cluster).

Eye movement desensitization and reprocessing (EMDR) EMDR involves focusing on a disturbing, trauma-related thought or image, while visually tracking a movement, e.g. the therapist's finger. The primary components are therefore production of saccadic eye movements and exposure. EMDR is the remaining therapy advocated by NICE for the treatment of PTSD.

Prognosis

Several treatments are effective in reducing symptoms and improving quality of life, but it seems that the magnitude of these benefits is limited. Many sufferers retain some symptoms despite having received optimal treatment. Little data exists on the efficacy of combining treatment options (e.g. drugs alongside psychological techniques), but it may be appropriate to consider this in resistant cases. It may be appropriate to shift goals towards rehabilitation and the successful management of symptoms where residual symptoms persist.

What factors influence the chance of recovery following exposure to trauma? Known risk factors for the development of PTSD and poor outcome include the following: the severity of (including proximity to) the trauma; bereavement as a result of the trauma; presence of a pre- or comorbid psychiatric disorder; certain personality traits, e.g. neuroticism; low intelligence; a prior history of trauma, and the absence of adequate social and psychological support. Recent reviews suggest that neither age nor ethnic group interacts with pathological response to trauma, though women are at greater risk, and that PTSD symptom expression is similar across age groups and cultures.

Areas of controversy needing further research

Controversial issues largely overlap with those requiring further research in this relatively newly recognized area. Particular attention should be paid to: drug treatment for PTSD; combined treatment approaches for PTSD; long-term outcomes following trauma; the diagnostic category of acute stress disorder; PTSD and psychosis; acute stress disorder and PTSD in children, especially very young children; postconcussional syndrome—a category provided for further study (Appendix B, DSM-IV: symptoms occur following a closed head injury with concussion and include cognitive (attention and memory), emotional (anxiety, depression, irritability), and physical (sleep problems, fatigue, headache) problems).

Further reading

American Psychiatric Association (1994). *Diagnostic and statistical manual of mental disorders*, 4th edition. American Psychiatric Press Inc., Washington DC.

Boelen PA, *et al.* (2007). Treatment of complicated grief: a comparison between cognitive-behavioral therapy and supportive counseling. *J Consult Clin Psychol*, **75**, 277–284.

Breslau N, *et al.* (1998). Trauma and posttraumatic stress disorder in the community: the 1996 Detroit Area Survey of Trauma. *Arch Gen Psychiatry*, **55**, 626–32.

Brewin CR, Andrews B, Valentine JD (2000). Meta-analysis of risk factors for posttraumatic stress disorder in trauma-exposed adults. *J Consult Clin Psychol*, **68**, 748–66.

Brom D, Kleber RJ, Defares PB (1989). Brief psychotherapy for posttraumatic stress disorders. *J Consult Clin Psychol*, **57**, 607–12.

Bryant RA, Harvey AG (1997). Acute stress disorder: a critical review of diagnostic issues. *Clin Psychol Rev*, **17**, 757–73.

Davis LL, *et al.* (1997). Post-traumatic stress disorder and serotonin: new directions for research and treatment. *J Psychiatry Neurosci*, **22**, 318–26.

Foa EB, Keane TM, Friedman MJ (eds) (2000). *Effective treatments of PTSD.* Guilford Press, New York.

Greenwood DC, *et al.* (1996). Coronary heart disease: a review of the role of psychosocial stress and social support. *J Public Health Med*, **18**, 221–31.

Gump BB, Matthews KA (1999). Do background stressors influence reactivity to and recovery from acute stressors?. *J Appl Soc Psychol*, **29**, 469–94.

Irwin M, Pike J (1993). Bereavement, depressive symptoms and immune function. In: Stroebe MS, Stroebe W, Hansson RO (eds) *Handbook of bereavement: theory, research, and intervention*, pp. 160–71. Cambridge University Press, Cambridge.

Jacobs S (1999). *Traumatic grief: diagnosis, treatment and prevention.* Brunner Mazel, Philadelphia.

Jacobs S, Mazure C, Prigerson H (2000). Diagnostic criteria for traumatic grief. *Death Stud*, **24**, 185–99.

Kleber RJ, Brom D (1987). Psychotherapy and pathological grief controlled outcome study. *Isr J Psychiatry Relat Sci*, **24**, 99–109.

Krysinska K, Lester D (2010). Post-traumatic stress disorder and suicide risk: a systematic review. *Arch Suicide Res*, **14**, 1–23.

Lichtenthal WG, Cruess DG, Prigerson HG (2004). A case for establishing complicated grief as a distinct mental disorder in DSM-V. *Clin Psychol Rev*, **24**, 637–62.

Maciejewski PK, *et al.* (2007). An empirical examination of the stage theory of grief. *JAMA*, **297**, 716–23.

Marmar CR, *et al.* (1988). A controlled trial of brief psychotherapy and mutual-help group treatment of conjugal bereavement. *Am J Psychiatry*, **145**, 203–9.

Marshall RD, Spitzer R, Liebowitz MR (1999). Review and critique of the new DSM-IV diagnosis of acute stress disorder. *Am J Psychiatry*, **156**, 1677–85.

Mawson D, *et al.* (1981). Guided mourning for morbid grief: a controlled study. *Br J Psychiatry*, **138**, 185–93.

National Institute for Clinical Excellence (2005). *Post-traumatic stress disorder: the management of PTSD in adults and children in primary and secondary care (Clinical Guide 26)*, National Institute for Clinical Excellence, London.

Prigerson HG, *et al.* (1995). Inventory of Complicated Grief: a scale to measure maladaptive symptoms of loss. *Psychiatry Res*, **59**, 65–79.

Raphael B (1977). Preventive intervention with the recently bereaved. *Arch Gen Psychiatry*, **34**, 1450–4.

Shapiro F (1995). *Eye movement desensitization and reprocessing: basic principles, protocols and procedures.* Guilford Press, New York.

Shear K, *et al.* (2005). Treatment of complicated grief: a randomized controlled trial. *JAMA*, **293**, 2601–08.

Simon RI (1999). Chronic posttraumatic stress disorder: a review and checklist of factors influencing prognosis. *Harv Rev Psychiatry*, **6**, 304–12.

Solomon SD (1997). Psychosocial treatment of posttraumatic stress disorder. *In Session-Psychother*, **3**, 27–41.

Solomon SD, Davidson JR (1997). Trauma: prevalence, impairment, service use, and cost. *J Clin Psychiatry*, **58** Suppl 9, 5–11.

Stroebe MS, Stroebe W, Hansson RO (eds) (1993). *Handbook of bereavement: theory, research, and intervention.* Cambridge University Press, Cambridge.

Weintraub D, Ruskin PE (1999). Posttraumatic stress disorder in the elderly: a review. *Harv Rev Psychiatry*, **7**, 144–52.

World Health Organization (1992). *The ICD-10 classification of mental and behavioural disorders: clinical descriptions and diagnostic guidelines.* World Health Organization, Geneva.

26.5.2 The patient who has attempted suicide

Keith Hawton

Essentials

Attempted suicide includes all acts of intentional self-poisoning or self-injury, with most cases seen in hospitals involving self-poisoning. It is a substantial health care problem in many countries, especially in young people, hence all large general hospitals should have dedicated services for patients who have attempted suicide.

Background—attempted suicide occurs in relation to a range of factors, including psychiatric disorders, life events and problems, and difficulties in coping. Many people (12–25%) repeat the act within a year, with 1 to 2% dying by suicide within a year, and 3 to 5% within 8 to 10 years.

Management—it is imperative that patients should not only receive adequate physical care, but that their psychiatric and psychosocial problems and needs are assessed. A brief assessment of all patients should be conducted on arrival in the emergency department to assess psychiatric status and risk. Those who refuse physical care should be assessed for capacity to do so and for possible mental illness that may allow compulsory treatment. Detailed psychosocial assessment should be conducted by a member of the psychiatric service, including assessment of suicidal intent, other motives for the act, life events and problems, psychiatric disorder, risk of repetition of the attempt and of suicide, and coping resources and supports. Aftercare may include a range of pharmacological and psychosocial treatments.

Introduction

The term 'attempted suicide' includes acts of intentional self-harm, in other words self-poisoning or self-injury. In many ways this is a misleading term because the primary motivation for and aim of deliberate self-harm is often not death but some other purpose, such as communication of distress, blotting out an unbearable state of mind, or trying to change the behaviour of other people. However, the impact of such 'nonsuicidal' intentions may be enhanced by patients claiming that the act was a suicidal one. Nevertheless, many acts involve major suicidal intent, and because of this and the popularity of the term 'attempted suicide' among physicians, this terminology will be used throughout this chapter.

Attempted suicide is a big and increasing health care problem in most developed (and some developing) countries. In the United Kingdom, there are about 200 000 general hospital presentations for self-poisoning or self-injury each year. Two-thirds of patients are under 35 years of age. Attempts occur in older children, but the behaviour becomes more common in adolescence, increasing rapidly in frequency in females from the age of 12 years, with peak rates in the late teens and early twenties. In men, rates increase more slowly with age, peaking in the mid- to late-twenties. Attempted suicide rates in men are closely related to suicide rates.

Most hospital-referred attempts involve self-poisoning. In the United Kingdom, the substances most frequently involved are nonopioid analgesics, particularly paracetamol and paracetamol-containing compounds, and psychotropic agents, especially anti-depressants and minor tranquillizers. Most self-injuries involve patients cutting themselves. In developing countries, more toxic substances, such as pesticides, are often used for self-poisoning, with consequent higher fatality rates.

Many patient characteristics and problems can lead to attempted suicide, including psychiatric disorders (especially depression, substance abuse, and anxiety disorders), personality difficulties, and poor coping resources. The more common life difficulties experienced by patients include interpersonal problems and broken relationships (especially in the young), employment difficulties, legal problems, and alcohol and drug misuse.

Attempted suicide is often repeated, with at least 12 to 25% of people repeating the act within a year. In the United Kingdom, between 1 and 2% die by suicide within a year and 3 to 5% within 8 to 10 years. In older patients the risk of suicide is higher.

This chapter focuses on the management of those who present to hospital after attempted suicide. It is imperative that patients should not only receive adequate physical care but that their psychiatric and psychosocial problems and needs are assessed.

Arrival of patients at the general hospital

In addition to the immediate assessment of the medical consequences of self-poisoning or self-injury, emergency department staff should be capable of conducting a brief assessment or triage of a patient's psychiatric status and risk. In particular, they need to determine whether a patient has a serious psychiatric disorder (e.g. psychosis or severe depression) and/or is actively suicidal such that urgent attention by the psychiatric service is required. Dangerous tablets or other potential methods of self-harm should be removed.

Staff should be aware that patients often leave hospital emergency departments before a psychiatric assessment can be conducted. Such patients tend to have a history of substance abuse and previous attempts, and may show behavioural disturbance while in the department. Many have features associated with suicide risk and tend to present to hospital with further repeat attempts more often than patients who are assessed in the emergency department. These facts highlight the need for emergency staff to have basic skills in assessment, and for them to be able to obtain urgent psychiatric assessment readily when they judge it to be necessary. Where a patient is thought to be at serious risk but wanting to leave hospital, medical staff can—in the United Kingdom at least—restrain the patient under common law until a psychiatric opinion can be obtained and, if necessary, a Mental Health Act order completed.

Giving medical care to those who have attempted suicide

Management of the medical complications of suicide attempts is dealt with in Chapter 9.1. Difficulty for physicians commonly arises when patients who have attempted suicide refuse potentially life-saving treatment for the physical consequences of their acts. This problem most often presents in those who have poisoned themselves, such as with large overdoses of paracetamol, in which early treatment can prevent the development of potentially fatal liver damage. The dilemma is whether to instigate such treatment against a patient's will.

In the United Kingdom, the issue primarily comes down to one of mental capacity. To show that patients have the capacity to refuse treatment, they:

1 must be able to understand and retain information on the treatment proposed, its indications, and its main benefits, as well as possible risks and the consequences of nontreatment

2 must be shown to believe that information

3 must be capable of weighing up the information in order to arrive at a conclusion

If a clinician instigates treatment against a patient's wishes in spite of the patient appearing to have capacity, then the clinician is at risk of being accused of assault. Where the patient is judged as lacking capacity, essential treatment can either be instigated directly by a physician, or after the patient has been placed on a Mental Health Order because of the degree of mental illness, in which case the treatment for the physical condition is given because the suicide attempt is judged to have resulted from mental illness.

In situations of dire emergency most clinicians would instigate essential treatment to save the patient's life and then try to sort out the legal issues afterwards. Such understandable action is unlikely to lead to successful litigation if the clinician acted in a way that they judged at the time to be in the patient's best interest.

Psychosocial assessment

Psychosocial assessment should not usually take place until a patient has recovered from any acute medical effects of an attempt. Clearly more urgent assessment is indicated if the patient is severely disturbed or regarded as being at acute risk. In some centres general medical and nursing staff may have to carry out these assessments, either because this is local policy or because of the inadequacy of the local psychiatric service. General hospital staff should in any case be familiar with how to conduct an assessment so that they can do this at times of emergency.

A semistructured assessment procedure is recommended. The main factors that should be covered are listed in Box 26.5.2.1. A useful way of assessing the events and the patient's problems that preceded the act, the nature of the attempt, possible motivation, and suicidal intent, is to obtain a very detailed account of the few days leading up to the act. Whenever possible the patient's account should be supplemented by enquiry of other informants such as a partner, relatives, and friends. Information should also be sought from professionals and others involved in the patient's care, including the general practitioner.

Suicidal intent and other motives

Suicidal intent (that is to say, the extent to which the patient wished to die at the time of the attempt) can usefully be assessed by examining the circumstances of the act and the explanation given by the patient and by the relatives or friends. Circumstances suggesting high suicidal intent include:

◆ act carried out in isolation

◆ act timed so that intervention unlikely

◆ precautions taken to avoid discovery

Box 26.5.2.1 Factors that should be covered in the assessment of patients having attempted suicide

- Life events that preceded the attempt
- Motives for the act, including suicidal intent and other reasons
- Problems faced by the patient
- Psychiatric disorder
- Personality traits and disorder
- Alcohol and drug misuse
- Family and personal history
- Current circumstances, such as:
  - social (e.g. extent of social relationships)
  - domestic (e.g. living alone or with others)
  - occupation (e.g. whether employed)
- Psychiatric history, including previous suicide attempts
- Risk of a further attempt
- Risk of suicide
- Coping resources and supports

- preparations made in anticipation of death (e.g. making a will, organizing insurance)
- preparations made for the act (e.g. purchasing means, saving up tablets)
- communicating intent to others beforehand
- extensive premeditation
- leaving a note
- not alerting potential helpers after the act

It is also important to take account of what the patient and others say about the purpose of the act. About one-third of patients will say that they definitely wanted to die, although in some cases the circumstances of the act will suggest otherwise. However, there is a small but important group of patients who will claim they did not wish to die when the circumstances strongly suggest high suicidal intent—such patients may be at increased risk of making a repeat attempt, which has a high chance of being fatal. Scoring

---

Box 26.5.2.2 Common motives or intentions for attempted suicide

- To die
- To escape from an unbearable situation
- To get relief from a distressed state of mind
- To change the behaviour of others
- To show desperation to others
- To get back at other people/make them feel guilty
- To get help

---

systems can assist in the assessment of suicidal intent, e.g. Beck suicide intent scale.

It is extremely important to recognize that the apparent physical danger of an overdose is a poor and potentially misleading measure of the extent to which a patient may have wanted to die. Many patients do not recognize the relative dangers of substances taken in overdose. Thus, a small overdose of a benzodiazepine hypnotic or even an antibiotic may represent a serious attempt at suicide for some patients, whereas a large overdose of a highly dangerous analgesic might be taken with low intent by others. People in the medical and allied professions represent an exception, and usually the danger of their acts is a good measure of intent. Very dangerous self-injuries are often associated with high suicidal intent, but this is not always so.

Assessment of the motives or intentions underlying deliberate self-poisoning and self-injury should be based on the precedents, circumstances of the act, the patient's account, that of other informants, and deduction by the clinician. Common motives or intentions for attempted suicide are shown in Box 26.5.2.2.

Risk of repetition of attempts and of suicide

Estimation of the risk of repetition and of suicide following attempted suicide, both short-term and long-term, is a very important part of the assessment. Factors associated with an increased risk of a repeat suicide attempt and of suicide are shown in Box 26.5.2.3, but it is essential to recognize that such predictive measures are notoriously imprecise. Patients who show risk factors for repetition have a high risk of repeating, but many repeaters—possibly more than half—do not demonstrate many risk factors. For suicide, this is also because the risk of suicide is relatively low.

Coping resources and supports

Assessment of coping resources and supports should be based on past behaviour under stress and the patient's account of whom they can turn to for support. It is particularly important to assess whether the patient has specific difficulties in problem solving as these can be an important target for psychosocial therapy. The best evidence for such difficulties will be a description of the methods used to solve problems in the past. It is always important to determine whether current problem solving is impaired by depression or other psychiatric disorders.

Care after attempted suicide

Some patients who have attempted suicide may appear ambivalent about accepting help, or even frankly dismissive of it. This may be understandable in the context of acts that often represent attempts at interpersonal communication or have other functions unconnected with help-seeking. Furthermore, many patients come from socioeconomic backgrounds in which they are unfamiliar with help-seeking for emotional problems, hence clinicians may have to work hard in some cases to explain to patients how treatment might be of benefit. These factors also mean that a brief psychological intervention, such as problem solving, is likely to be more acceptable to many patients than more lengthy therapeutic approaches.

The assessment procedure can itself be highly therapeutic. Patients may be provided with their first opportunity to discuss their difficulties with a clinician. Joint interviews with family members can help highlight issues that need addressing and assist with communication problems.

Box 26.5.2.3 Factors associated with an increased risk of a repeat suicide attempt and of suicide

Suicide attempt

- Previous attempt(s)
- Personality disorder
- Alcohol or drug abuse
- Previous psychiatric treatment
- Unemployment
- Lower social class
- Criminal record
- History of violence
- Single, divorced, or separated

Suicide

- Older age
- Male gender
- Unemployed or retired
- Separated, divorced, or widowed
- Living alone
- Poor physical health
- Psychiatric disorder (particularly depression, alcoholism, schizophrenia, and antisocial personality disorder)
- High suicidal intent in current episode
- Violent method involved in current attempt (e.g. attempted hanging, jumping)
- Leaving a suicide note
- Previous attempt(s)

Some patients thought to be at high risk of suicide refuse psychiatric treatment when this is judged to be essential. Management comes down to a judgement of whether the patient is suffering, or likely to be suffering, from a mental illness that necessitates hospital assessment and/or treatment. In most countries, if a patient thought to be at serious risk and/or mentally ill has presented to a general hospital following attempted suicide but is refusing to stay for a psychiatric assessment, emergency department staff would be judged to be acting reasonably if they restrained the patient under 'common law' until a psychiatric opinion could be obtained.

Major psychiatric disorders should receive appropriate pharmacological treatment, although care in prescribing should be exercised where there is ongoing risk of self-poisoning. There is increasing evidence for the efficacy of psychological treatments for patients who have attempted suicide in terms of the prevention of repetition of attempts and effects on depression, hopelessness, and life problems. Cognitive behavioural therapy appears to be particularly effective. Intensive and prolonged psychological therapy also appears to be helpful for women with a history of multiple acts of self-harm and borderline personality disorder. Efforts to keep in contact with patients, such as by telephoning or home visiting, may improve compliance with treatment.

Clinical services for patients who have attempted suicide

At one time, the assessment of patients who attempted suicide was regarded as primarily the responsibility of psychiatrists. Increases in the clinical responsibilities of nonmedical clinical staff and findings from research have resulted in a major change in the pattern of services in many places. In the United Kingdom, it has been demonstrated that nurses, social workers, and other clinicians can assess these patients reliably, make effective aftercare arrangements, and provide effective therapy. This has resulted in official guidelines that reflect these findings.

It is imperative that staff of whatever discipline who are involved in this work have reasonable background experience and skills in the management of patients with emotional and psychiatric disorders, and that they be properly trained in the assessment and treatment of patients who have attempted suicide. They must also have support from senior psychiatrists, especially for patients with severe psychiatric disorders and where compulsory admission to hospital may be required. They must also be highly motivated and have good support systems in place because working with such patients can be extremely demanding.

The functioning of a service for patients who have attempted suicide but do not require physical treatment in specialized settings (e.g. in an intensive care unit) can be improved if they are admitted to a short stay medical ward, rather than to a large number of wards. The attitudes of general medical and nursing staff to these patients can be negative, especially towards those whose acts they perceive as having a low suicidal intent. Clinical experience shows that attitudes are far more favourable when admission to a single ward is possible, when general medical and nursing staff acquire experience in managing these patients, and also develop closer working relationships with members of the service for attempted suicide.

The development of high quality general hospital services for patients who attempt suicide should be a major element in any national or local suicide prevention strategy.

Specific subgroups of patients

Alcohol and drug abusers

Many patients who attempt suicide have problems related to alcohol and drug abuse, and these factors—especially alcohol abuse—increase the risk of both repetition and eventual suicide. All attempters should be screened for substance abuse. Recognition of such problems in the general hospital may provide a special opportunity for treatment, which may be an important factor in preventing further suicidal behaviour as well as reducing physical and social harm.

Children and very young adolescents

These are usually admitted to a paediatric ward where this is available in the general hospital. It is advisable that all very young attempters be admitted to hospital rather than be dealt with in the emergency department since they require particularly careful and often prolonged assessment, including interviews with their families and the possible involvement of community statutory services (e.g. social services).

Elderly patients

Attempted suicide in older patients, while much less common than in younger people, very often involves high suicidal intent and a high risk of subsequent suicide. Routine admission to a medical bed is therefore also recommended for this group. Close links should be established with the local psychogeriatric service (if one exists) so that clinicians from the service can provide assessment and make arrangements for aftercare.

Further reading

Boyce P, *et al.* (2003). Summary Australian and New Zealand clinical practice guideline for the management of adult deliberate self-harm (2003). *Australas Psychiatry,* **11,** 150–55.

Cooper J, *et al.* (2005). Suicide after deliberate self-harm: a 4-year cohort study. *Am J Psychiatry,* **162,** 297–303.

Harriss L, Hawton K, Zahl D (2005). Value of measuring suicidal intent in the assessment of people attending hospital following self-poisoning or self-injury. *Br J Psychiatry,* **186,** 60–6.

Hawton K (2000). General hospital management of suicide attempters. In: Hawton K, Van Heeringen K (eds) *The international handbook of suicide and attempted suicide,* pp. 519–537. Wiley & Sons, Chichester.

Hawton K, *et al.* (1998). Deliberate self-harm: systematic review of efficacy of psychosocial and pharmacological treatments in preventing repetition. *BMJ,* **317,** 441–47.

Hawton K, Harriss L (2006). Deliberate self harm in people aged 60 years and over: characteristics and outcome of a 20 year cohort. *Int J Geriatr Psychiatry,* **21,** 572–81.

Hawton K, *et al.* (2003). Deliberate self-harm in Oxford, 1990-2000: a time of change in patient characteristics. *Psychol Med,* **33,** 987–95.

Hawton K, James A (2005). Suicide and deliberate self harm in young people. *BMJ,* **330,** 891–94.

Hawton K, Van Heeringen K (2000). *The international handbook of suicide and attempted suicide.* Wiley, Chichester.

Hawton K, Zahl D, Weatherall R (2003). Suicide following deliberate self-harm: long-term follow-up of patients who presented to a general hospital. *Br J Psychiatry,* **182,** 537–42.

National Collaborating Centre for Mental Health (2004). *Self-harm: the short-term physical and psychological management and secondary prevention of self-harm in primary and secondary care (full guideline) Clinical Guideline 16.* National Institute for Health and Clinical Excellence, London.

Royal College of Psychiatrists (1994). *The general hospital management of adult deliberate self-harm. Council report CR32.* Royal College of Psychiatrists, London.

Royal College of Psychiatrists (1998). *Managing deliberate self-harm in young people. Council report CR63.* Royal College of Psychiatrists, London.

Royal College of Psychiatrists (2004). *Assessment following self-harm in adults. Council report CR122.* Royal College of Psychiatrists, London.

Skegg K (2005). Self-harm. *Lancet,* **366,** 1471–83.

26.5.3 Medically unexplained symptoms in patients attending medical clinics

Michael Sharpe

Essentials

Patients commonly present to doctors with symptoms, and doctors seek disease to explain these symptoms. However, in about one-third of medical outpatients the symptoms remain inadequately explained by disease, even after exhaustive assessment. The size of the problem of medically unexplained symptoms, their cost to services, and public health importance are all becoming increasingly clear.

Medically unexplained symptoms may be described as due to somatization, or as somatoform or functional symptoms—common examples being pain, fatigue, and weakness. They may also be described in terms of a functional somatic syndrome diagnosis such as irritable bowel syndrome, fibromyalgia, or chronic fatigue syndrome.

Clinical approach—patients with medically unexplained symptoms may have substantial disability, distress, and a poor prognosis. Most doctors still regard such symptoms as purely mental in origin, but it has become increasingly obvious that such an approach is both scientifically inadequate and practically unhelpful. Patients regard a purely mental explanation as dismissive and stigmatizing, and physicians find it frustrating as it does not help them manage the patient. The evidence favours a more complex understanding of aetiology in which genetic vulnerability, early experience, and life stress interact to produce symptoms that are associated with reversible changes in the nervous system and associated function. Developments in neuroscience combined with increasing consumerism amongst patients require that we take a more positive approach to this neglected area of medical research and practice.

Management—to be effective, this requires more than simply the exclusion of disease: (1) the patient needs their symptoms to be taken seriously; (2) it is important to seek other symptoms of depression and anxiety that are commonly associated; (3) a positive diagnosis needs to be made (often as a functional somatic syndrome with or without associated depression or anxiety) and appropriate explanation for the symptoms (in terms or reversible changes in bodily function) given to the patient; (4) a practical management plan is required, including education about the symptoms and a gradual return to normal activity. The so-called antidepressants drugs may be effective even if the patient is not depressed; (5) some patients may require referral for specialist treatment, there being most evidence of efficacy for cognitive behavioural therapy (CBT).

Introduction

Definition and terminology

Various terms have been used to describe symptoms unexplained by identifiable disease. These include:

* Medically unexplained—A useful and simple operational term, but a negative one with the potential disadvantage of suggesting that psychophysiological explanations are not 'medical'.

* Functional—Originally meaning a disturbance of bodily function rather than of bodily structure, it is unfortunate that this term is now used pejoratively by some doctors to mean 'all in the mind', although it appears to be acceptable to patients who understand it in its original meaning.

* Somatization—A widely used term implying a psychological problem that has become expressed somatically. It should arguably be restricted to cases where the somatic symptoms are plausibly understood as an expression of emotional disorder.

Table 26.5.3.1 Functional somatic syndrome by medical specialty

Gastroenterology	Irritable bowel syndrome, nonulcer dyspepsia
Gynaecology	Premenstrual syndrome, chronic pelvic pain
Rheumatology	Fibromyalgia
Cardiology	Atypical or non-cardiac chest pain
Respiratory medicine	Hyperventilation syndrome
Infectious diseases	Chronic (postviral) fatigue syndrome
Neurology	Tension headache, nonepileptic attacks,
Dentistry	Temporomandibular joint dysfunction, atypical facial pain
Ear, nose, and throat	Globus syndrome
Allergy	Multiple chemical sensitivity

◆ Conversion—Used specifically to refer to loss of function such as weakness of a limb. Embodies the (unproven) assumption (as for somatization) that the symptoms are due to a 'conversion' of psychological problems into somatic symptoms.

◆ Somatoform—A diagnostic category in the psychiatric classifications. Intended to be atheoretical but obviously linked to the idea of somatization and implying a mental disorder in physical form.

There is no entirely satisfactory term: the best term for scientific use is probably 'medically unexplained', or perhaps better 'unexplained by identifiable disease'. However, most textbooks and computer databases use the terms 'somatoform' and 'somatization', and patients prefer 'functional'.

Symptoms

Almost any symptom can remain medically unexplained, even after exhaustive medical assessment. Common examples include pain (including back pain, chest pain, abdominal pain, and headache); fatigue and weakness; dizziness; 'fits' and funny turns.

Syndromes

Unexplained symptoms have been grouped into syndromes. Each medical specialty has at least one of these (Table 26.5.3.1): rheumatologists label prominent muscle pain and tenderness as fibromyalgia; gastroenterologists describe abdominal pain with altered bowel habit as irritable bowel syndrome; and infectious disease specialists refer to chronic fatigue and myalgia as postviral or chronic fatigue syndrome. It has been argued that these 'functional syndromes' are not really separate conditions but merely a reflection of the tendency of specialists to focus only on those symptoms that relate to their (organ based) specialty. The research literature offers support for this hypothesis by revealing substantial overlap between these syndromes in their constituent symptoms, proposed aetiological factors, and response to treatment.

The significance of medically unexplained symptoms and syndromes

Medically unexplained symptoms are a common and important, but remarkably neglected, medical problem. They account for a substantial proportion of the work of most doctors and are the reason for approximately a third of new medical outpatient consultations.

Although sometimes dismissed as merely the 'worried well', these patients often suffer more disability and distress than patients whose symptoms are explained by disease. They are also expensive to the health care system because they attend multiple specialist services where they receive extensive but unproductive investigation and treatment. Doctors working in these services not surprisingly find them 'difficult to help'. The size and importance of this clinical problem makes it all the more curious so that few doctors take any special interest in it.

Historical perspective

Throughout history patients have presented with somatic symptoms that their doctors could not explain in terms of objectively identifiable disease. Modern medical advances have improved the precision with which disease can be identified, but have not solved the problem. Many patients still present with symptoms that remain unexplained by disease even after state of the art investigation and they still present a challenge to doctors.

The explanations that have been proposed for medically unexplained symptoms have varied over time. The early ideas located their cause in a disturbance of a bodily organ, often the uterus. Attention then moved to the peripheral nervous system, later the central nervous system, and more recently the mind. These changing aetiological theories have been reflected in the terms used to describe the symptoms: the organ theory gave rise to 'hysterical' (referring to the uterus) and 'hypochondriacal' (below the ribs); the nervous system theory to 'nervous', 'functional nervous' (malfunctioning nerves), and neurasthenic (weak nerves); and the mental theory to 'psychological,' 'psychogenic', and somatization (mental problems made somatic).

The changing theories have produced changing approaches to management. Early treatments focused on the organ believed to be giving rise to the symptoms. Consequently, manipulations of, and even removal of, the female reproductive organs were carried out. When the proposed explanation shifted to the peripheral nervous system the preferred treatments became nerve tonics, electrical stimulation, and other methods that were intended to regenerate nervous energy. As interest shifted to the central nervous system, hypnosis became a favoured treatment and was used by famous physicians such as Charcot. It was only in the 20th century, following the work of Freud and the rise in popularity of psychoanalysis, that medically unexplained symptoms came to be seen as a 'mental' problem requiring psychiatric rather than medical treatment. This view persisted for most of the 20th century.

Most doctors still regard medically unexplained symptoms as purely mental in origin, but it has become increasingly obvious that such an approach is both scientifically inadequate and practically unhelpful. Developments in neuroscience have supplemented previous studies demonstrating a variety of associated physiological changes and indicate that many so called unexplained symptoms have a basis in the functioning of the nervous system. In practice, patients regard a purely mental explanation as dismissive and stigmatizing, and physicians find it frustrating as it does not help them manage the patient. A better approach is required, and one that sees such symptoms as not only psychological but also having a basis in changed nervous system functioning offers both a new research paradigm and better ways of talking to patients about their symptoms. Although offering new opportunities this idea is

Table 26.5.3.2 The aetiology of medically unexplained symptoms

	Predisposing	Precipitating	Perpetuating
Biological	Genetic	Acute illness or injury	Neuro-physiological mechanisms
			Effects of reduced activity
Psychological	Childhood abuse	Stresses	Fears and beliefs about symptoms
			Anxiety or depression
			Adoption of a disabled lifestyle
Interpersonal	Childhood experience of illness	Conflicts, e.g. at work	Iatrogenesis and lack of effective treatment
			Financial and other gain from being ill
			Behaviour of family, doctors, and others

in fact a rediscovery of the concept of functional disorders that was in common usage in the 1890s.

Aetiology and pathophysiology

The precise aetiology of many medically unexplained symptoms is unknown, but there is evidence of an aetiological role for biological, psychological, and interpersonal factors. For any given case, rather than seeking a single cause for the patient's symptoms, it is probably better to consider the relative contribution of these factors. They may be conveniently considered as having predisposing, precipitating, or perpetuating influences on the symptoms (Table 26.5.3.2). Perpetuating factors are especially important to identify as they offer targets for treatment. For example, a person may be predisposed by virtue of genetics or childhood experience to develop irritable bowel syndrome. This may have been precipitated by a combination of infection and psychological stress. The symptoms are then perpetuated by a vicious circle of changed bowel motility, fear of gastrointestinal disease, and iatrogenic overinvestigation. Effective management addresses these perpetuating factors.

Although the physiological mechanisms of symptom production are not fully understood, many putative mechanisms have been identified. These interact with psychological and interpersonal factors to perpetuate the illness. Hence, overbreathing gives rise to paraesthesiae and dizziness (by lowering plasma carbon dioxide). These symptoms may be interpreted by the patient as indicating a 'stroke' and lead to increased lead to anxiety and the seeking of medical care. Medical attention may inadvertently increase the fear about stroke and consequently the anxiety, leading to further hyperventilation, more symptoms and so on. A number of putative physiological mechanisms are listed in Table 26.5.3.3.

Epidemiology

Medically unexplained somatic symptoms are extremely common in the general population of all countries. However, only some of the people experiencing them will seek medical attention, usually because of concern about the cause or because of severe discomfort or disability.

Table 26.5.3.3 Examples of possible physiological mechanisms for medically unexplained physical symptoms that are supported by evidence

Noncardiac chest pain	Chest wall pain and paraesthesiae from over breathing
Localized chronic pain	Neuronal plasticity
Fibromyalgia	Changed overall CNS pain sensitivity
Chronic fatigue	Neuroendocrine changes
Irritable bowel	Changed neuronal control of bowel motility

- Primary care—Medically unexplained symptoms are the principal reason for a quarter to a half of all consultations in primary care, but only a few are referred to hospital clinics.

- Hospital outpatient care—At specialist outpatient clinics a third of all new patients have symptoms that remain inadequately explained by disease, even after exhaustive assessment. Some are admitted to hospital.

- Hospital inpatient care—While only a few patients with medically unexplained complaints become inpatients, these can be particularly costly to the service and are at high risk of iatrogenic harm, e.g. from unnecessary surgery.

Prevention

We do not know enough about the aetiology of medically unexplained symptoms to know which primary preventive strategies are effective. However, there is increasing evidence that while genetic factors play a part, the interpersonal and economic factors of parenting, the stigma of psychiatric illness, and the nature of our current benefit and litigation systems are relevant and reversible influences. For secondary prevention, effective early management probably reduces the risk of chronicity, whereas poor explanation, overinvestigation, and inappropriate medical treatment probably increase it. Tertiary prevention can be achieved by effective management of the patient with chronic established symptoms and by limiting iatrogenic harm.

Clinical features

Pointers to a patient having medically unexplained complaints may be apparent even before the initial consultation. The referral letter and medical notes may record frequent attendance at medical services, numerous negative (and often repeated) investigations, and a previous history of repeated unsuccessful surgery. At the consultation the presentation of multiple symptoms is strongly suggestive. However, the only way of confidently diagnosing complaints as medically unexplained is to complete the appropriate history, examination, and investigation. It should also be remembered that patients may have some symptoms that are explained by disease and others that are unexplained, for example the co-occurrence of epilepsy and nonepileptic attacks.

It is important to remember that many (but not all) unexplained medical complaints are somatic symptoms of depression or anxiety, most medically unexplained complaints reflect genuine suffering and disability, and the deliberate manufacturing of complaints is uncommon in ordinary (non-medico-legal) medical practice.

Differential diagnosis

The main medical differential diagnosis for medically unexplained symptoms is from symptoms due to disease. Diagnostic difficulties are likely to occur with unusual presentations of common diseases and with rare diseases. While missing diagnosis of serious disease is an appropriate concern, the evidence indicates that once a patient has been carefully assessed the emergence of a 'missed' disease at a later date is uncommon.

Patient assessment

When assessing the patient the main tasks are to:

◆ Make it clear that you are taking the symptoms seriously.

◆ Clarify the nature of the presenting symptoms. For example, what does the patient really mean by fatigue? Is it lack of energy (nonspecific), sleepiness (suggesting a sleep problem), or lack of motivation (suggesting depression)?

◆ Find out what other symptoms the patient has. It is worth asking for an exhaustive list: the more symptoms, the more likely it is that they will all be medically unexplained.

◆ Ask the patient what they think or fear is wrong with them. This can reveal why they have presented (e.g. 'I am worried that it could be cancer').

◆ Ask about life 'stresses'. This may be why the patient is presenting now.

◆ Seek evidence of depression and anxiety. This is often best done towards the end of the consultation so that the patient does not feel they are being dismissed as 'just psychiatric'. Stigma can be minimized by linking depression and anxiety with 'understandable' causes such as stress or the symptoms themselves.

◆ Physically examine the patient. This may reveal unsuspected signs of disease. It also helps to convince the patient that they have been taken seriously and properly assessed.

◆ Do not omit reasonable investigations. Misdiagnosis is relatively uncommon, but more likely when the patient looks 'psychiatric'. A balance must be struck between the risk of missing disease and the iatrogenic psychological harm from overinvestigation.

Management

The general principles of management are outlined in Box 26.5.3.1.

Giving reassurance, explanation, and advice

As well as being reassured that there is no evidence they have an unpleasant disease, patients require a positive diagnosis and a credible explanation for their symptoms. They also need practical advice on what to do.

Reassurance

The provision of appropriate reassurance is an important part of the medical consultation. To be effective it must be based on the patient's concerns, not just on those of the doctor. Hence it is important to ask the patient what they are worried they have, before reassuring them that they don't. Many patients report the physical examination as particularly reassuring. A detailed explanation of what any investigations show can also help. Clearly it is unwise to state categorically to any patient that they have no disease, but appropriate to explain that the probability they have the disease they fear is very low and why. Beware of the patient who repeatedly asks for reassurance about the same disease—they may have health anxiety (hypochondriasis). This is considered further below.

Giving a diagnosis and explanation

Patients benefit from a positive diagnosis, and the failure to offer one may set them off on an unhelpful search. Clearly the diagnosis must be appropriate; it may be 'functional symptoms' or a named functional syndrome (such as irritable bowel syndrome). This diagnosis should then be elaborated with an explanation of why the patient has the symptoms. While our understanding is imperfect, we do have some evidence about aetiology as described above. Explanations that include both psychological and biological factors and emphasize their reversibility helpfully set the scene for treatment (see below). Some explanations are probably unhelpful. Dismissing the symptoms as 'just psychological' or 'all in the mind' is likely to reduce the patient's confidence in the doctor and reduce the value of their reassurance. Colluding with the patient's belief that their symptoms are explained by an untreatable disease (such as myalgic encephalopathy or chronic Lyme's disease) when they are not is likely to make them less willing to accept appropriate treatment and to encourage invalidity.

Giving practical advice

After diagnosis and explanation, a positive plan of action that specifies both what the patient can change and what the doctor will do is required. The patient can be advised how to overcome the illness perpetuating factors, e.g. by becoming more active or by addressing stress. The doctor can provide accurate information about the illness, review progress, prescribe (e.g. an antidepressant drug), and if appropriate refer (e.g. to physiotherapy or psychology).

Writing to the patient as well as to the general practitioner to summarize the conclusions of the medical assessment and the proposed plan of action usefully reinforces messages that may otherwise be easily forgotten.

Box 26.5.3.1 Principles of general management of medically unexplained symptoms

◆ Exclude disease, but avoid unnecessary investigation or referral

◆ Seek specific treatable psychiatric syndromes

◆ Demonstrate to the patient that you believe their complaint(s)

◆ Take a full and sympathetic history

◆ Give the patient a diagnosis of a functional symptom or syndrome

◆ Give the patient a positive explanation, including but not overemphasizing psychological factors

◆ Encourage a return to normal functioning

◆ Consider prescribing antidepressant drugs

Prescribing antidepressant drugs

The so-called antidepressant drugs are most likely to be of benefit when the patient is depressed or anxious, but they can also reduce symptoms in patients who are not depressed or anxious. A systematic review of their use in patients with functional syndromes found them to be moderately effective. The odds ratio for improvement with antidepressant drug treatment compared with placebo was 3.4, but a high dropout rate from treatment was also noted, emphasizing the need for careful explanation and follow-up to ensure adherence.

For these drugs to be accepted by the patient, a clear explanation that minimizes stigma of why they are being prescribed is required. One of the following two approaches is suggested: the first is to explain that the term 'antidepressant' is a misnomer and that the drugs are actually broad-spectrum 'nerve tonics' of proven value for symptoms such as difficulty sleeping and pain, as well as for depression; the second is to be explicit that they are being prescribed for depression or anxiety, but to emphasize that these emotional problem are an understandable reaction to the somatic symptoms.

Referral for psychological or psychiatric management

A referral for specialized psychological treatment may be required when simple measures and antidepressant drugs are insufficient to relieve the patient's symptoms. The most widely used are behavioural or cognitive behavioural therapy (CBT), which aims to help the patient change thinking (cognitions) and ways of coping (behaviour) that are perpetuating symptoms. A systematic review of CBT for medically unexplained symptoms found that it was significantly superior to nonspecific treatment or no treatment in 70% of trials. Individual behavioural components of CBT, such as graded exercises, are less studied but also of value.

The decision to refer to specialist services will be based on the physician's assessment of the patient and on knowledge of what services are available. While ideally all medical clinics would have dedicated specialist psychiatric or psychology services, in practice this is rarely the case. Consequently, it is wise to find out before the need to refer arises which local practitioners are interested in physical symptoms and willing to accept referrals. If the options are few it may be necessary to make the case for better services.

Reasons to refer to include: to psychology for specialist CBT; to psychiatry if the patient is judged to be at risk of self-harm; to psychiatry or psychology if the patient has severe emotional distress; to a specialist service, e.g. for chronic pain or chronic fatigue syndrome (CFS). When explaining the referral to the patient, it is wise to be positive about the service you are referring to and to emphasize that the referral does not mean you regard the patient's symptoms as 'all in the mind'.

A patient is more likely to attend for a referral if you have said: 'I see you have real and troublesome symptoms. I am pleased to tell you that you do not have serious disease but I am sorry to say that I do not have a simple cure that I can prescribe. However, I can recommend and refer you to a specialist service for your problem', than if you have told them: 'There is clearly nothing wrong with you; it must all be in your mind. There is nothing to do now but to refer you to the shrinks.'

Management of the chronic complex patient

Advice for the management of patients with chronic persistent symptoms is shown in Box 26.5.3.2.

> **Box 26.5.3.2** Management of patients with chronic, persistent symptoms
>
> - Try to be proactive, not reactive; see the patient at regular, fixed intervals, not on demand
> - Aim to broaden the agenda with the patient to include non-medical problems
> - Reduce or taper unnecessary drugs
> - Minimize the contact the patient has with other specialists or practitioners
> - Try to coopt a relative as a therapeutic ally to implement your management goal
> - Aim for containment of demands, damage limitation, and avoidance of iatrogenic harm
> - Encourage the patient (and yourself) to think in terms of coping rather than curing

What happens in practice?

In practice, management of medically unexplained symptoms is frequently suboptimal, and iatrogenic psychological and physical harm from unhelpful explanations, unnecessary tests, and ineffective medical and surgical treatments is probably common. The evidence based treatments of antidepressant drugs and CBT are rarely offered and frequently refused by patients. Specific services such as psychological services for chronic pain are often not available. We surely could do better.

Prognosis

The prognosis for those patients whose symptoms are sufficiently severe and persistent to lead to referral to a specialist service is often poor. It is not uncommon for symptoms and disability to persist for years, but this reflects in part a failure to provide treatment. The prognosis is best for those patients who were well before the onset of symptoms and who have clear depressive and anxiety disorders. It is worst for those patients with long-standing multiple symptoms.

Specific syndromes

Classification

There are parallel medical and psychiatric classificatory schemes for medically unexplained symptoms, which is confusing. The former emphasizes the nature of the symptom and lists functional syndromes by organ system as in Table 26.5.3.1; the latter emphasizes the number of symptoms and associated psychological factors and is shown in Table 26.5.3.4.

The implication of these parallel, overlapping classifications is that most patients will qualify for both a medical and a psychiatric diagnosis. Both may be useful in guiding management and prognostication, hence a combined medical/psychiatric diagnosis such as 'irritable bowel syndrome/anxiety disorder' is probably more useful than either alone. An alternative multidimensional classification system that unifies the medical and psychiatric approach would be preferable: an example is shown in Box 26.5.3.3.

Table 26.5.3.4 The main psychiatric diagnostic categories of medically unexplained symptoms

Main feature	Diagnosis
Predominantly worry about disease	Hypochondriasis
Predominantly concern about symptoms	Somatization (somatic presentation of depression and anxiety)
Small number of symptoms	Simple somatoform disorders
Chronic multiple symptoms	Somatization disorder (Briquet's syndrome)
Loss of function	Conversion disorder
Dislike of body parts	Body dysmorphic disorder
Other unusual presentations	
Deliberate deception	Factitious disorder and malingering (including Münchausen's syndrome)

Common syndromes

This section addresses specific aspects of the main psychiatric diagnoses for medically unexplained symptoms listed in Box 26.5.3.3.

Predominant worry about disease: health anxiety or hypochondriasis

The central feature of hypochondriasis is a persistent preoccupation with the possibility that one has a serious or progressive medical condition. These fears persist despite the fact that repeated investigations and examinations have identified no such condition, and appropriate reassurance has been given (see Example 26.5.3.1).

Predominant concern about symptoms: somatic presentation of depression and anxiety

One of the most common causes of medically unexplained somatic symptoms is undiagnosed depressive and anxiety disorders. Because depression is (erroneously) thought of as a purely 'mental illness', it is readily forgotten that it also has prominent somatic symptoms. These include fatigue, pain (often of chronic widespread nature), and loss of weight and appetite.

Somatic symptoms of anxiety in generalized form (generalized anxiety disorder) or episodic severe form (panic disorder) include fatigue, dizziness, paraesthesias, chest pain and palpitations, and shortness of breath (especially 'getting enough breath in'). See Example 26.5.3.2.

Predominant concern about symptoms: simple somatoform disorders

This diagnosis refers to the patient with a single or small number of somatic complaints that do not appear to be expressions of depressive or anxiety disorders. It includes so-called undifferentiated

> **Box 26.5.3.3** A multidimensional classificatory scheme of medically unexplained symptoms
>
> ◆ Duration of illness
> ◆ Number of symptoms
> ◆ Degree of disability
> ◆ Severity of depression/anxiety
> ◆ Patients fears/beliefs

somatoform disorder and somatoform pain disorder. The most commonly encountered clinical problem in this category is chronic medically unexplained persistent pain, such as chronic back pain or chronic headache. The physical symptoms may have commenced after a trivial injury or accident, but the subsequent disability is out of proportion to the objective findings (see Example 26.5.3.3).

Chronic multiple symptoms: somatization disorder (Briquet's syndrome)

Somatization disorder, or Briquet's syndrome, is a term used to describe patients—mostly women—who have a lifelong history of multiple recurrent somatic complaints referable to multiple bodily systems. Such patients are relatively easy to identify as although the current presenting complaint may be of only one or two symptoms, scrutiny of the past medical notes reveals a long history of outpatient visits to different clinics with medically unexplained symptoms such as abdominal pain and bloating, diffuse muscular pains and tenderness, and chronic lassitude. A history of childhood abuse and unnecessary surgery is common (see Example 26.5.3.4).

Example 26.5.3.1

The patient is a young woman. Her urgent referral is faxed to you by her general practitioner (GP). She has attended the general practice clinic daily for the last 2 weeks with headache. The history reveals that her father died of a brain tumour 2 years ago and when he presented to the GP was told it was only a 'tension headache'. Examination is normal but she is very anxious indeed and repeatedly asks for your reassurance that she doesn't have a brain tumour. She wants a brain scan.

Management and prognosis

Assessment should aim to clarify the patient's fears. A useful question is: 'what is your worst fear?' The patient's fear makes their anxiety and behaviour understandable. For example, if the patient thinks, 'I have a brain tumour', she will be understandably anxious and keen to seek urgent medical attention. The symptom (headache) leads to thoughts ('I have a brain tumour') that in turn lead to anxiety, to certain coping behaviours (visiting doctors and requesting a scan). The more she seeks reassurance the stronger the worry she has a brain tumour becomes and so on in a vicious circle. Eliciting this sequence from the patient, and describing it to them, perhaps using a diagram, aids explanation. While is it is appropriate to reassure them that they do not have a tumour, responding to requests for repeated reassurance or investigations can paradoxically worsen the patient's worry. In this circumstance the patient can be told, 'I have already reassured you a number of times; every time I do this it makes you feel better for a short period. But we know if I keep doing this it will make your worries stronger and make you want yet more reassurance and more tests. So I am not going to reassure you again or do any more tests'.

Depressive disorder is common in such patients, in which case effective treatment of depression may resolve the problem. There is also some evidence for the effectiveness of CBT in health anxiety. While most acute cases resolve, the condition can become chronic. In a few patients the concern with disease is delusional in intensity, and these should be referred to a psychiatrist.

Example 26.5.3.2

A 40-year-old man presents to the Emergency Department with acute chest pain and breathlessness with fatigue. Examination and investigations are negative. Only after admission to hospital does a junior doctor examine the patient's mental state and find that he has symptoms of both depression and severe episodic anxiety associated with overbreathing and many other somatic symptoms. The diagnosis is depressive disorder with associated panic disorder.

Management and prognosis

Treatment is by making a positive diagnosis, providing reassurance and explanation, and treating the depression and anxiety. This can be achieved most simply by prescribing an antidepressant agent with appropriate explanation and active follow-up to ensure adherence. In some cases psychological treatment may also be required. The prognosis for recovery within 6 months is good, although there is a risk of relapse. Patients should continue to take the antidepressant drug for at least 6 months after they have recovered in order to prevent early relapse. Antidepressant drugs can initially make anxiety worse, and short-term prescription of benzodiazepines may also be required.

Loss of function: conversion disorder

Conversion disorder refers to the loss of function of a body part or to abnormal body movements. Examples are transient medically unexplained blindness, paralysis of a limb, or nonepileptic attacks. These symptoms are regarded as not being produced intentionally (in distinction to factitious disorder and malingering—see below), but rather 'subconsciously'. In practice this distinction can be difficult to make. Persistence of functional impairment even when the patient believes they are not being observed suggests that the symptoms are not deliberately feigned. Other often quoted signs of conversion disorder such as 'belle indifference' (smiling indifference to disability) are unreliable. Acute presentations may have arisen in the context of severe interpersonal stress, conflict, or physical injury. The patient may have experienced a family member with similar symptoms (see Example 26.5.3.5).

Example 26.5.3.3

A middle-aged man presents with pain in his back. He believes that his symptoms are a result of lifting heavy items at work and is engaged in litigation against his former employer. There is a history of depression some 12 months ago, but this has largely resolved. Physical examination is normal. The patient walks with a stick and seems concerned to demonstrate to you how ill he is.

Management and prognosis

As well as diagnosis explanation and symptomatic treatment (including pain management programmes), antidepressant drugs may be tried on an empirical basis. There is a role for CBT. Improvement may occur over many months. The prognosis for acute problems is fairly good, but for established symptoms with associated disability is poor. Legal proceedings complicate management and probably worsen prognosis.

Example 26.5.3.4

The patient is a middle-aged woman, referred to as a 'heart-sink' patient by the referring GP. She presents with dizziness, bloating of her stomach, and generalized weakness. She has three volumes of medical notes documenting her previous presentations with a range of symptoms including pain in various places, irritable bowel, menstrual problems, and transient loss of sight. She has had many investigations, as well as a hysterectomy and three laparotomies. She is taking a long list of prescribed medications including oral opioids, but review of her notes does not reveal any convincing evidence of disease. Examination reveals only a number of operation scars.

Management and prognosis

If possible, it is desirable to review the case notes before seeing the patient. It is also worth considering why the patient, who has a chronic condition, has been referred now. The GP may be feeling more frustrated or helpless than usual in the face of repeated complaints, the patient may have seen a different GP who was unaware of her history, or the patient's presentation may have changed, raising concern about disease. If the presentation justifies it, reasonable efforts must be made to exclude disease—but also noting what investigations have already been done. The general approach should be one of helping patient and GP to cope with a chronic illness, rather than investigation and cure. Some practical management strategies are listed in Box 26.5.3.2. Depression is common in such patients, makes symptoms worse and should be treated. Long-term but infrequent follow-up (by a hospital doctor, GP, psychiatrist, or a combination of these) is desirable to prevent iatrogenic harm. The condition is very likely to persist.

Dislike of a body part: body dysmorphic disorder

Patients who are dissatisfied with some aspect of their bodily appearance or shape may find their way into the clinics of physicians and surgeons. Some of these patients are preoccupied with a perceived defect in appearance, such as a large nose. Others have more substantial concerns, such as disliking a limb sufficiently to request its amputation. Even in the presence of a minor physical abnormality, the person's concern appears to be markedly excessive (see Example 26.5.3.6).

Other unusual presentations

Atypical eating disorders

Some patients who attend with symptoms of abdominal pain after food, vomiting, anorexia, or constipation may have a covert eating disorder. Judicious enquiry about weight loss, amenorrhoea, and laxative use may help to establish the correct diagnosis. See Chapter 26.5.6 for further discussion.

Chronic constipation that has not responded to conventional treatment

Patients may present with a history of constipation for two or three decades that has proved unresponsive to all treatment. In such cases there is often no identifiable medical cause, but they may be referred to surgeons for colectomy. All require a thorough psychiatric assessment before major decisions about treatment are implemented.

Example 26.5.3.5

A young woman is referred for sudden onset of weakness of her left side and a stroke is suspected. She reports being unable to move her left arm and leg. Enquiry reveals that she was sexually assaulted the week before her symptoms began. She herself offers no explanation for the symptoms. On examination her left arm and leg appear weak, with a 'collapsing' pattern, but there are no abnormalities of reflexes. An MRI brain scan is normal.

Management and prognosis

An acute case of conversion disorder such as this needs to be given a diagnosis, a positive explanation that describes how reversible brain malfunction causes the symptoms, and a plan of gradual return to normal function. However, there have been very few clinical trials of treatment. Physiotherapy may be useful. Depression should be sought and treated if present. The prognosis is good for cases of acute onset, but in established cases it is poor and long-term invalidism with dependence on state benefits is common, although referral to a physical rehabilitation service may be helpful.

Treatment with biofeedback may benefit some patients, but is not generally available.

Loin pain haematuria syndrome

This is a rare syndrome that is poorly understood but thought to be a somatoform disorder. Patients may abuse opioid analgesics, and some are thought to simulate their pain. It is unwise to carry out renal autotransplantation because it often fails to cure the pain, which may recur on the opposite side of the body, and puts the patient at risk of the complications of surgery.

Deliberate deception

Factitious disorder

Patients with factitious disorder deliberately feign or simulate illness in order to obtain medical attention. The term 'factitious disorder' is preferable to the eponym Munchausen's syndrome, because this stereotype is often misleading. The label of 'Munchausen's syndrome' is generally applied to wandering, untreatable, male sociopaths, whereas most patients with factitious disorders are women working in medically related occupations. They often report a large number of childhood illnesses and operations. High rates of substance abuse, mood disorder, and personality

Example 26.5.3.6

A 30-year-old woman complains about the shape of her nose and blames this for her inability to find a partner and for many other difficulties in her life. She requests plastic surgery.

Management and prognosis

In the absence of a conspicuous physical abnormality or deformity, it is usually prudent to seek a psychiatric opinion. There is some evidence for the effectiveness of CBT. Surgery may have good psychological results where there is a single clear abnormality to correct, but should only be carried out after careful assessment.

Example 26.5.3.7

A student nurse is repeatedly admitted to hospital with breakdown of an abdominal surgical wound. She is observed rubbing faeces into the wound. When confronted with this she discharges herself immediately.

Management and prognosis

A 'supportive confrontation' is generally recommended, but there have been few systematic studies of management. This means presenting the patient with the evidence that they have been manufacturing symptoms and signs, while suggesting that they have an emotional problem for which help and support is offered. Ideally, the physician and psychiatrist do this jointly. There is some evidence that psychological support following hospital discharge may be associated with an improved outcome. Patients with stable social networks have a better prognosis.

disorder have been reported. Some patients exaggerate genuine disease (usually chronic) to create dramatic medical emergencies (see Example 26.5.3.7).

Malingering

The term malingering is not a medical diagnosis. It refers to the behaviour of the deliberately simulating or exaggerating symptoms for obvious and understandable gain, e.g. monetary compensation, disabled status, avoidance of criminal prosecution, or conscription. It is differentiated from factitious disorder in which the aim of simulation is simply to get medical attention. Doctors are often reluctant to describe a patient as malingering lest it adversely affect their health care, occupation, or legal case. However, malingering does occur, especially in medico-legal contexts. It can be hard to detect reliably in a medical consultation and is often detected by covert video surveillance that reveals the patient vigorously engaging in an activity (such as playing sport) that they have reported they are unable to do. There is probably a continuum of behaviour from the minor embellishment of symptoms to frank malingering (see Example 26.5.3.8).

Areas of uncertainty and controversy

Many aspects of the nature and management of medically unexplained somatic symptoms are controversial. The core issue is whether they are best regarded as a psychiatric/psychological problem or as a medical condition. This issue has been played out particularly prominently in the debate over the chronic fatigue syndrome/myalgic encephalomyelitis (see Chapter 26.5.4). A consideration of the changing medical fashions for the explanation of such symptoms over the last few hundred years should encourage humility and suggests that current controversies may tell us more about the inadequacies of our conceptualization of illness and our health services than they do about the patients.

Likely developments over the next few years

The size of the problem of medically unexplained symptoms, its cost to services, and its public health importance is becoming increasingly clear. A likely scientific development that will come from brain imaging studies is the better understanding of the

Example 26.5.3.8

A 30-year-old man is seen in order to produce a legal report in relation to his claim for compensation. He reports severe back pain following a car accident 2 years ago and presents in a wheelchair. There are no neurological signs and no muscle wasting. He is later seen walking to his car and lifting his wheelchair into the boot.

Management and prognosis

Malingering is a behaviour, not a medical diagnosis. If management is required, it is by confrontation. Often the identification of malingering ends the behaviour (and the legal case).

neuropsychological mechanisms of symptom production, both medically unexplained and associated with disease. Better drugs for a variety of symptoms are a likely development, although psychological treatments are likely to remain important. A more consumerist attitude from symptomatic patients who will be less willing to be told that 'there is nothing wrong with them' is to be expected. These factors will drive better management and better services for symptoms in general. We can expect the development of more symptom treatment programmes that coexist with current disease oriented disease management, as exemplified by some existing pain and palliative care services.

Further reading

Barsky AJ, Borus JF (1999). Functional somatic syndromes. *Ann Intern Med*, **130**, 910–21.

Barsky AJ (1998). A comprehensive approach to the chronically somatizing patient. *J Psychosom Res*, **45**, 301–6.

Bass C, May S (2002). Chronic multiple functional somatic symptoms. *BMJ*, **325**, 323–26.

Bass C, Gill D (2000). Factitious disorders and malingering. In: Gelder M, *et al.* (eds) *New Oxford textbook of psychiatry*, pp. 1126–32. Oxford University Press, Oxford.

Drossman DA (1995). Diagnosing and treating patients with refractory functional gastrointestinal disorders. *Ann Intern Med*, **123**, 688–97.

Henningsen, P, Zipfel, S, Herzog, W. (2007), Management of functional somatic syndromes, *The Lancet*, **369**, 946–55.

Hotopf M (2004). Preventing somatization. *Psychol Med*, **34**, 195–98.

Kroenke K, Swindle R (2000). Cognitive–behavioral therapy for somatization and symptom syndromes: a critical review of controlled clinical trials. *Psychother Psychosom*, **69**, 205–15.

Mayou R, *et al.* (2005). Somatoform disorders: time for a new approach in DSM-V. *Am J Psychiatry*, **162**, 847–55.

Mayou RA, Bass C, Sharpe M (1995). *Treatment of functional somatic symptoms*. Oxford University Press, Oxford.

O'Malley PG, *et al.* (1999). Antidepressant therapy for unexplained symptoms and symptom syndromes. *J Fam Pract*, **48**, 980–90.

Royal College of Physicians, Royal College of Psychiatrists (2003). *The psychological care of medical patients: a practical guide*. Royal College of Physicians, London.

Smith RC (1991). Somatization disorder: defining its role in clinical medicine. *J Gen Intern Med*, **6**, 168–75.

Veale D (2004). Body dysmorphic disorder. *Postgrad Med J*, **80**, 67–71.

Wessely S, Nimnuan C, Sharpe M (1999). Functional somatic syndromes: one or many?. *Lancet*, **354**, 936–9.

26.5.4 Chronic fatigue syndrome (postviral fatigue syndrome, neurasthenia, and myalgic encephalomyelitis)

Michael Sharpe

Essentials

Chronic fatigue syndrome (CFS) is also known as postviral fatigue syndrome, neurasthenia, and myalgic encephalomyelitis. All describe an idiopathic syndrome characterized by disabling fatigue and other symptoms occurring chronically and exacerbated by minimal exertion.

Aetiology and pathogenesis—it is likely that multiple factors operate to predispose, precipitate, and perpetuate CFS: (1) predisposing factors—some individuals may be predisposed to develop CFS by virtue of genetics, personality, or other vulnerability; (2) precipitating factors—the condition may be precipitated by factors such as infection or psychological stresses; (3) perpetuating factors—for practical management the most important factors are those that perpetuate the illness and consequently act as barriers to recovery, including modifiable psychological, biological, behavioural, and social factors. Studies have reported a variety of biological abnormalities: few have been confirmed, but the most robust are (1) altered brain function, and (2) reduced hypothalamic-pituitary-adrenal axis responsiveness, although it is not clear if these are primary or secondary to inactivity.

Clinical context—important obstacles to recovery in many cases include (1) the psychological factors of fear and misconception about symptoms; (2) emotional distress; and (3) coping by becoming inactive or adopting a pattern of fluctuating levels of activity. The boundary with depression, anxiety, and other functional syndromes such as fibromyalgia is unclear.

Management and prognosis—this requires that the doctor excludes treatable conditions that may cause fatigue, demonstrates acceptance of the reality of the symptoms, addresses misconceptions about them, and refers for rehabilitative behavioural treatments when these are available and acceptable to the patient. There is no proven drug therapy and the prognosis without treatment is poor.

Introduction

Fatigue is an imprecise term with many meanings. In clinical medicine the symptom of fatigue implies a subjective feeling of lack of energy and endurance. While fatigue after exertion is a normal phenomenon, it is abnormal when it is disproportionate to exertion, persistent, and associated with impaired function. A variety

Acknowledgement: I am grateful to Simon Wessely, Peter White, and David Wilks for comments on this chapter.

of names have been given to this condition when it is unexplained by another diagnosis: chronic fatigue syndrome (CFS), postviral fatigue syndrome (PVFS), neurasthenia, and myalgic encephalomyelitis (ME). CFS is one of the most disputed illnesses in current medical practice, with strong differences of opinion about aetiology and treatment. Even the name is disputed and the unsatisfactory compromise term CFS/ME increasingly used.

Historical perspective

Illness characterized by chronic fatigue but without a clear pathological basis has a long history. In the 19th century it attracted a diagnosis of 'neurasthenia', but by the early 20th century this term fell into disuse. It is probable that patients continued to present to doctors with similar symptoms but received other diagnoses such as depression, brucellosis, and Epstein–Barr virus infection. As well as sporadic cases there have been occasional reports of apparent epidemics over the last 50 years, with one that occurred among staff at the Royal Free Hospital, London, United Kingdom in 1955 giving rise to the term myalgic encephalomyelitis (ME). By 1988 it had become increasingly accepted that most cases of chronic disabling fatigue were not caused by an infection or inflammation of the brain and the purely descriptive term chronic fatigue syndrome (CFS) was introduced. At the beginning of the 21st century the cause and treatment of this syndrome remain controversial.

Aetiology

There is no established pathology or cause for CFS, but a number of biological, psychological, and social factors have been identified that may play a role in the onset and perpetuation of illness. It is unlikely that all cases have the same cause.

Biological factors

A range of factors have been proposed but none established.

Genetic

Twin studies suggest that CFS is moderately heritable. Preliminary studies suggesting the involvement of specific genes require replication.

Infection

Patients presenting with CFS often give a history suggestive of acute infection at the outset, hence the term 'postviral fatigue syndrome'. A number of viruses including retroviruses have been reported as causes but to date none have an established aetiological role. Prospective studies confirm that fatigue states lasting several months can follow infections such as Epstein–Barr virus and Q fever. However, the available evidence does not support the hypothesis that chronic occult infection is commonly a cause of CFS.

Immune dysfunction

Minor immune abnormalities, most commonly mild activation, have been detected in some patients with CFS. Cytokines can cause fatigue, but no consistent immune abnormality or casual link of these with symptoms has been established. The role of immune factors in CFS remains of interest but is still unclear.

Dysfunction of the central nervous system

There is evidence for abnormalities in neuroendocrine tests of serotonergic function and in functional neuroimaging. However, abnormalities in similar domains have been found in patients with depression and anxiety disorders, hence the specificity and clinical utility of such tests remains to be established.

Endocrine dysfunction

Some of the most robust biological findings in CFS relate to the hypothalamic-pituitary-adrenal axis. The main finding has been under-responsiveness of the axis, but it remains unclear whether this is cause or consequence of CFS. Replacement therapy with low-dose hydrocortisone has been reported to produce short-term symptomatic relief. However, the balance of risks and benefits of this treatment is not yet established.

Inactivity

Some patients with chronic fatigue syndrome are profoundly inactive. This may lead to muscle wasting, changes in the cardiovascular response to exertion, and postural hypotension. The consequent intolerance of activity may perpetuate the illness by leading to symptoms that are interpreted as worsening of illness and further avoidance.

Idiopathic postural hypotension (neurally mediated hypotension)

A tendency to postural hypotension has been reported in some patients with CFS, particularly young women. The aetiological and treatment implications of this observation remain unclear.

Sleep disorder

Various sleep abnormalities have been reported as associated with CFS. They include both specific sleep disorders, such as restless legs syndrome, and nonspecific abnormalities, such as fragmentation of sleep. These may contribute to daytime fatigue in at least some cases.

Psychological and behavioural factors

There is evidence that these may perpetuate chronic fatigue syndrome.

Stress

Many patients describe major life stresses preceding illness onset, and it has therefore been suggested that at least some cases of CFS may be stress related.

Emotional disorder

Many patients seen in hospital clinics who meet criteria for CFS also meet criteria for depressive and anxiety disorders. Fatigue is a symptom of depression and anxiety. In many but not all cases CFS may be confounded with these emotional disorders, which remain the main differential diagnosis.

Fears and beliefs about symptoms

Patients often have misconceptions about the nature of their illness that may perpetuate it, including beliefs that activity that exacerbates symptoms is harmful and that CFS is an untreatable neurological disease.

Coping behaviour

A number of coping behaviours may be associated with poorer outcome. These may result from the beliefs described above and include excessive avoidance of physical activities (leading to chronic disability), the repeated seeking of (ineffective) medical care, and a failure to address psychological and social problems (such as stressful employment).

Social and iatrogenic factors

Information about CFS or ME—whether from doctors, patient groups, or the media—that leads patients to see their illness as mysterious, with a hopeless prognosis, and best treated by rest, is likely to inhibit efforts toward rehabilitation.

Epidemiology

Prevalence

One-quarter of people complain of persistent fatigue, but population studies in the United Kingdom and United States of America suggest that only about 0.5% could be regarded as having CFS, most of whom are aged between 20 and 40, with a predominance of women. The syndrome is also seen in children and adolescents, but less commonly.

Epidemics

Epidemics of a chronic fatigue-like syndrome have been described from various parts of the globe. This observation is compatible with, but does not establish, an infective cause. It remains unclear whether these were true epidemics and also whether the clinical picture reported is similar to that of cases of sporadic CFS.

Prevention

As the cause is unknown there is no specific primary prevention. Secondary prevention is important as it is likely that good early management and avoidance of iatrogenesis will reduce the risk of chronicity.

Clinical features

CFS is defined by symptoms alone.

Symptoms

The principal symptom is chronic mental and physical fatigue, tiredness, or exhaustion that is exacerbated by activity. Patients often report being able to perform activities for brief periods, but subsequently experiencing severe fatigue for hours or days thereafter. Other commonly associated symptoms include impaired memory and concentration, muscular and joint pain, unrefreshing sleep, dizziness and breathlessness, headache, tender lymph glands, and sore throat.

Patients often describe day-to-day fluctuations, irrespective of activity. Periods of almost complete recovery may be followed by relapse, often sufficiently severe to make normal daily activity impossible. Depression and anxiety are common, and some patients suffer panic attacks.

Patients and their relatives may hold strong beliefs about the nature and aetiology of their illness (see section on Aetiology), and it is important to take these into account when discussing treatment.

Physical signs

Physical examination is typically unremarkable. Complaints of fever and lymphadenopathy are not confirmed on examination. The presence of definite physical signs (such as objectively measured fever) should not be ascribed to the syndrome and alternative diagnoses should be sought.

Differential diagnosis

Almost any disease may present with fatigue. The differential diagnosis of idiopathic CFS is correspondingly large (Table 26.5.4.1). The nature of the fatigue may offer useful clues:

♦ Muscular diseases should be considered if the patient has objective weakness, no psychological symptoms, and a family history.

♦ Prominent sleepiness suggests a sleep disorder, e.g. prominent snoring and morning headaches in the obese patient raise the possibility of obstructive sleep apnoea.

♦ Depression is suggested by fatigue that is worse in the morning and accompanied by loss of motivation, interest, and pleasure. Other symptoms of depression may include sadness, loss of appetite and weight, and feelings of pessimism and failure.

♦ Anxiety is also associated with fatigue and may give rise to many of the somatic symptoms of chronic fatigue syndrome such as muscle pain, impaired concentration, and poor sleep. Severe episodic anxiety (panic) may be described as episodic severe symptoms followed by hours of fatigue.

Table 26.5.4.1 Conditions to be considered in the differential diagnosis of chronic fatigue syndrome

Nature of symptoms	Possible condition
General	Occult malignancy
	Autoimmune disease
	Endocrine disease
	Cardiac, respiratory, or renal failure
Gastroenterological	Malabsorption including coeliac disease
Neurological	Disseminated sclerosis
	Myasthenia gravis
	Parkinson's disease
	Early dementia
	Cerebrovascular disease
Infectious disease	Chronic active hepatitis (B or C)
	Lyme borreliosis
	HIV
	Tuberculosis
Respiratory disease	Nocturnal asthma
	Obstructive sleep apnoea
Chronic toxicity	Alcohol
	Solvents
	Heavy metals
	Irradiation
Psychiatric	Major depressive disorder
	Dysthymia
	Anxiety and panic disorder
	Somatization disorder

◆ Somatization disorder is suggested by a lifelong pattern of many physical symptoms referable to multiple bodily systems, with a history of unproductive investigation and unsuccessful treatments.

Clinical investigation

There are no specific diagnostic tests and no characteristic abnormalities on laboratory investigations that are conducted purely to exclude other diseases. All patients should have a full blood count, erythrocyte sedimentation rate or C-reactive protein, basic biochemistry screen, creatine kinase, random blood glucose, urine analysis, thyroid function, and (possibly) serological screening tests for autoimmune inflammatory disorders (antinuclear antibody test). Further investigation depends on the clinical findings and differential diagnoses under consideration.

Criteria for diagnosis

The current international consensus definition reported by Fukuda and colleagues is shown in Table 26.5.4.2. Guidelines on its application have been published by Reeves and colleagues in 2003.

Treatment

General management

The doctor should listen to the patient's story and ask about his or her own understanding of the illness. It is usually also worth seeing the partner or relevant family members. It is important to address misunderstandings about the nature of the illness, and especially to make clear that it is not progressive or life-threatening (see below). A positive explanation of CFS as a 'dysfunction of the central nervous system', emphasizing potential reversibility, is often helpful. The adverse physiological and psychological effects of prolonged bed rest should be explained, and the patient encouraged to avoid extremes of both inactivity and exertion. An initial hospital appointment that achieves all the above usually requires at least 45 min. An evidence-based self-help book may be recommended (such as *Chronic fatigue syndrome (CSF/ME): the facts*; see Further reading).

Drug therapy

There is no drug therapy of proven efficacy. A trial of an antidepressant drug may be considered if there is evidence of depression. It is advisable to choose a nonsedating type and to start with a low dose, which may reduce anxiety, improve the quality of sleep, and reduce pain, but it is important to give a recommended dose if there is evidence that the patient has a depressive disorder.

Rehabilitation, graded activity, and cognitive behavioural therapy (CBT)

The rehabilitative behavioural treatments of slowly graded activity or exercise programmes and CBT have been found to be more effective than conventional management in systematic reviews of randomized trials. They are currently the mainstay of management, but they are not effective in all patients and require both careful explanation and therapists skilled in their delivery to patients with CFS.

It is particularly important that patients do not interpret referral for a behavioural treatment as the doctor implying that their illness is imaginary. It can be explained that the most likely cause of fatigue in CFS is changes in brain and neuroendocrine function and that these can be reversed by these therapies. General physical rehabilitation services may be useful for patients with chronic severe disability.

Other treatments

Many other treatments have been proposed, but none has been adequately evaluated. Many unproved and often unscientific therapies are offered, some at considerable expense to the patient, hence patients should be cautioned about the potential risks of pursuing unproven treatments unless they are part of a clinical trial.

Prognosis

The prognosis for functional recovery is relatively good for patients seen in general practice. It is poorer for those severe enough to be referred to hospital clinics. A long history, multiple symptoms, and entrenched belief that the illness is irreversible predict a particularly poor prognosis. Rehabilitative treatments can improve the patient's ability to function. There is no mortality associated with CFS other than suicide, which may reflect unrecognized depressive illness and the physical consequences of severe and prolonged disability.

Other issues

CFS can be associated with severe chronic disability and occupational impairment, with severe economic implications for patient, employer, and insurer. The ambiguous status of CFS as an accepted disease makes disputes in these areas especially difficult to resolve.

Areas of controversy

Almost all aspects of chronic fatigue syndrome are controversial. Most controversy has centred on whether it is most appropriately

Table 26.5.4.2 International consensus definition of chronic fatigue syndrome

1. Complaint of fatigue
Of new onset
Not relieved by rest
Duration at least 6 months
2. At least four of the following additional symptoms
Subjective memory impairment
Sore throat
Tender lymph nodes
Muscle pain–Joint pain
Headache
Unrefreshing sleep
Post-exertional malaise lasting >24 h
3. Impairment of functioning
4. Other conditions that might explain fatigue excluded

Fukuda K *et al.* (1994). Chronic fatigue syndrome: a comprehensive approach to its definition and management. Annals of Internal Medicine 121, 953–9.

regarded as a medical or a psychiatric syndrome. This debate should be seen in the context of the stigma associated with psychiatric illness but often prevents patients receiving potentially effective treatment.

Likely future developments

Although there is likely to be increased acceptance of CFS as a 'real' illness, it is also likely that aetiologically subgroups will be identified. The most likely area for increased understanding will come from studies of altered brain function. It is possible that pharmacological agents with antifatigue action will be identified, but it is more likely that there will be increasing evidence for and provision of rehabilitative behavioural treatments.

Further reading

Campling F, Sharpe M (2008). *Chronic fatigue syndrome (CFS/ME): the facts* 2nd edition. Oxford University Press, Oxford.

Chambers D, *et al.* (2006). Interventions for the treatment, management and rehabilitation of patients with chronic fatigue syndrome/myalgic encephalomyelitis: an updated systematic review. *J R Soc Med*, **99**, 506–20.

Fukuda K, *et al.* (1994). The chronic fatigue syndrome: a comprehensive approach to its definition and management. International Chronic Fatigue Syndrome Study Group. *Ann Intern Med*, **121**, 953–9.

Henningsen P, Zipfel S, Herzog W (2007). Management of functional somatic syndromes. *Lancet*, **369**, 946–55.

Prins JB, van der Meer JW, Bleijenberg G (2006). Chronic fatigue syndrome. *Lancet*, **367**, 346–55.

National Institute for Health and Clinical Excellence. *Chronic fatigue syndrome/myalgic encephalomyelitis (or encephalopathy); diagnosis and management. Clinical guidelines CG53.* http://guidance.nice.org.uk/CG53.

Reeves WC, *et al.* (2003). Identification of ambiguities in the 1994 chronic fatigue syndrome research case definition and recommendations for resolution. *BMC Health Serv Res*, **3**, 25.

Wessely S, Nimnuan C, Sharpe M (1999). Functional somatic syndromes: one or many? *Lancet*, **354**, 936–9.

Wessely S, Sharpe M, Hotopf M (1998). *Chronic fatigue and its syndromes.* Oxford University Press, Oxford.

26.5.5 Anxiety and depression

Lydia Chwastiak and Wayne J. Katon

Essentials

Depression is common, with point prevalence in Western industrialized nations about 3% for men and 7% for women, and lifetime risk is about 10% for men and 20% for women. Depression is the leading cause of years lived with disability. Physicians fail to make an accurate diagnosis in at least half of those with depressive or anxiety disorders.

Pathophysiological hypotheses involve abnormalities in the hypothalamic–pituitary axis, levels of particular neurotransmitters (particularly noradrenaline, serotonin, and dopamine), and neuro-anatomical changes.

Clinical features

Patients with depression or anxiety initially present with physical complaints 50 to 70% of the time, and these conditions are associated with an amplification of physical symptoms, additional functional impairment, and a decreased ability to adhere to medication and important lifestyle changes (exercise and diet) in patients with chronic medical illness.

Major depressive episodes—these last at least 2 weeks and are characterized by at least one of the two primary criteria—(1) depressed mood, or (2) loss of interest or pleasure in nearly all activities—together with at least five of nine other criteria.

Panic attacks—these are characterized by the sudden onset of intense apprehension, fear or terror, and by the abrupt development (within 10 min) of at least four of a number of symptoms.

Generalized anxiety disorder—this is characterized by constant, nonepisodic anxiety that affects patients for more than 6 months and interferes with normal function.

Management

Patients should be reassured: (1) that they are not 'crazy', nor are their symptoms a manifestation of their own failure or shortcomings; (2) with proper treatment, these disorders almost always improve or remit, but relapses and recurrences can occur and so follow-up is essential; (3) a variety of treatments are available.

Psychosocial interventions—these are effective for ambulatory medical patients with psychiatric disorders, the three short-term psychotherapies used to specifically target the symptoms of major depression being cognitive behavioural therapy, interpersonal psychotherapy, and problem solving therapy.

Antidepressant therapy—the decision to prescribe should be based on the number of symptoms, the level of dysfunction, and previous episodes of depression or anxiety. The different classes of antidepressant drugs show virtually equivalent efficacy, hence the choice of medication should be made on issues such as side effects, cost, adherence, and physician familiarity and comfort with prescribing particular agents. The selective serotonin reuptake inhibitors (SSRIs) have become the first-line treatment for major depression, dysthymia, and panic disorder, primarily because their improved side effect profiles are associated with improved adherence to treatment. About 40 to 50% of patients with major depression respond to an antidepressant within 3 weeks after reaching a therapeutic plasma level, and up to 80% will respond if initial nonresponders are switched to another class of antidepressant, or with augmentation strategies using additional medication or psychotherapy. Treatment should be continued for between 6 and 9 months after a first major depressive episode. Pharmacotherapy should be discontinued slowly over a period of 7 to 21 days: if tapered too quickly, almost all antidepressants can produce withdrawal syndromes.

Electroconvulsive therapy (ECT)—this remains the most effective treatment available for depression: it can be life-saving in some cases, and in frail older patients it may be safer than antidepressants.

Prognosis and need for specialist referral

Many patients (30–40%) who respond to treatment remain at substantial risk of relapse during the subsequent 12 months, with risk factors for relapse being: (1) persistence of subthreshold depressive symptoms; (2) history of three or more previous episodes of major depression; and (3) chronic mood symptoms for more than 2 years.

Referral to a psychiatrist should be considered when: (1) the physician is confused about the primary diagnosis; (2) adequate treatment does not lead to an improvement in symptoms within 10 to 12 weeks, or several medication trials have failed; (3) there is suicidal behaviour.

Introduction

Depression and anxiety are more commonly seen in primary care than any other condition except hypertension. Over half of all patients with mental health disorders are cared for solely by a primary care provider, and many seek help from their physician because they attribute symptoms of depression and anxiety to a physical problem. Physicians fail to make an accurate diagnosis in at least 50% of those with depressive or anxiety disorders. This failure occurs because of time limitations, lack of knowledge, focus on presenting physical symptoms, both the physician and patient perceiving depression as a 'normal' response to stressors, fear of opening 'Pandora's box', and the stigma associated with psychiatric illness. Only about half of those patients who are accurately diagnosed with major depression receive the dose and duration of treatment with antidepressants that meets United States of America Agency for Health Care Policy and Research (AHCPR) guidelines. Fewer than half of patients with anxiety disorders in primary care are treated with specific medications or psychotherapy.

Early recognition of depressive and anxiety disorders is important because they can be treated effectively, often in primary care. The detection and treatment of anxiety and depression can prevent patient discomfort and unnecessary expensive diagnostic investigations, which are often ordered to investigate unexplained physical symptoms. More serious complications may also be prevented, such as the progression of psychiatric illness, loss of employment and impairment of social roles, decreased adherence to medical treatment, and suicide.

Epidemiology

Depression and anxiety are very common and frequently follow a recurrent or a chronic course. The National Comorbidity Survey (NCS) found using structured psychiatric interviews that almost 50% of community respondents in the United States had at least one lifetime DSM-III-R (Diagnostic and Statistical Manual of Mental Disorders, third edition, revised) psychiatric disorder. Major depression was the most common of these, with a lifetime prevalence of 17.3% and a 12-month prevalence rate of 10.3%. The point prevalence of depression in western industrialized nations is from 2.3 to 3.2% for men and 4.5 to 9.3% for women; lifetime risk is 7 to 12% for men and 20 to 25% women. The reasons for gender differences are poorly understood but are thought to include endocrine, biological, and sociocultural factors: women have been found to have experienced higher rates of childhood (especially sexual) abuse.

The prevalence rates of depression are higher for medical patients than for the general population: 6 to 10% of primary care patients and 10 to 14% medical inpatients meet the criteria for major depression. In patients with at least two chronic physical illnesses, the 12-month prevalence rate of major depression was 12.5%. Major depression is commonly associated with cardiovascular disease (prevalence rate of 15–23%), diabetes (prevalence rate of 11–15%), chronic obstructive pulmonary disease (prevalence rate of 10–20%), cancer (15–30%), cerebrovascular accidents (12–34%), chronic pain (33–35%), and Parkinson's disease (40%). Depression and panic disorder are also common in patients with 'medically unexplained' syndromes (Table 26.5.5.1, and Chapter 26.5.4).

About 16% of people experience an anxiety disorder sometime during their lifetime. These are more common in women, with a lifetime prevalence of panic disorder in 5%, compared to 2% in men. Only one-quarter to one-third of patients with panic disorder or post-traumatic stress disorder (PTSD, see Chapter 26.5.1) present to a mental health setting, with one-third presenting to an emergency room and over a third to their primary physician.

Most patients (80%) meeting criteria for a psychiatric disorder also have one or more comorbid psychiatric disorders: almost half the cases of depression and anxiety occur in the same patients at the same time. About 25% of patients with major depression, dysthymia, and anxiety disorders also have a history of substance abuse.

Impact

Depression is the leading cause of years lived with disability. In the United States of America, the estimated total annual cost of major depression was 83.1 billion dollars in 2000, of which 31% were direct medical costs, 7% were suicide-related mortality costs, and 62% were workplace costs. This increase in medical costs is secondary to the many medically unexplained symptoms these patients experience as well as the adverse effect of depression on self-care (adherence to diet, exercise, cessation of smoking and taking medications) in those with comorbid, chronic medical illness.

Table 26.5.5.1 Prevalence of depression and panic disorder

	Prevalence (%)	
	Panic disorder	Major depression
Community	1–3	3–5
Primary care	7	6–10
Medical inpatients	2–3	10–14
High utilizers of primary care	22	25
Chest pain and negative angiography	33–43	40
Irritable bowel syndrome	29	35
Unexplained dizziness	13	12
Headaches	5–15	9–25
Chronic fatigue	11–30	30–50
Fibromyalgia	20–30	30–60

Patients with anxiety and depression make more emergency visits, primary care visits, and more telephone calls to their physicians, have more medical tests and evaluations, take more medications, and are more likely to be admitted to hospital for a medical disorder than patients who do not have these disorders. As many as 50% of 'high utilizers' of medical care services have a current depressive or anxiety disorder. Even after controlling for age and pre-existing medical comorbidity, patients with depression receive two to four times as much nonpsychiatric medical care as patients without depression, and those with panic disorder and PTSD use two to three times as many services as other primary care patients.

Depressive and anxiety disorders are associated with an amplification of physical symptoms, additional functional impairment, and a decreased ability to adhere to medication and important lifestyle changes (exercise and diet) in patients with chronic medical illness. Depression reduces the effectiveness of rehabilitation in older patients with stroke, Parkinson's disease, heart disease, fractures, and pulmonary disease. Effective treatment of major depression reduces physical symptom burden and functional impairment in patients with chronic medical illness. In patients with depression and diabetes, effective treatment of depression was associated with savings in total medical costs.

The indirect costs of depression and anxiety include absenteeism from work, adverse effects on family roles, and shortened lifespan. In the WHO study in primary care, depression was associated with 6.1 disability days per month—as much or more than eight chronic illnesses, including coronary artery disease and arthritis. Anxiety disorders usually strike people at the beginning of their working lives and may last for many years. Some studies report that over half of those with panic disorder or PTSD are not working, with others forced to take lower-paying or part-time jobs near their homes. The lost economic productivity is easier to quantify than the other indirect costs: lost earning time of family or friends bringing patients to treatment, decreased efficiency at work, the toll on families, the future costs to society of children reared by an unemployed or housebound parent. The role functioning of patients with panic disorder and PTSD has been found to be substantially lower than that of patients with chronic medical illnesses, but higher than that of depressed patients.

Pathophysiology

Depressive and anxiety disorders are complex syndromes that are diagnosed based on clinical criteria. Pathophysiological hypotheses for these disorders involve abnormalities in the hypothalamic–pituitary axis, levels of particular neurotransmitters, and neuroanatomical changes.

Data support an underlying genetic component for major depression, panic disorder, generalized anxiety disorder, and obsessive–compulsive disorder. There are significantly higher rates of depression and panic disorder in first-degree relatives of patients with these disorders. Twin studies have shown a higher rate of concordance for monozygotic compared to dizygotic twins in patients with panic disorder and major depression.

Mood disorders are associated with dysregulation of the biogenic amines: noradrenaline (norepinephrine), serotonin, and dopamine are the three neurotransmitters most implicated. In animal models, long-term treatment with virtually all antidepressants is associated with a decrease in the sensitivity of postsynaptic β-adrenergic and serotonin-2 receptors. Anxiety disorders are associated with abnormalities of the same neurotransmitters as well as in receptors of the neurotransmitter γ-aminobutyric acid (GABA), an inhibitory neurotransmitter found mainly in the cerebral cortex.

A variety of neuroendocrine abnormalities have been reported in patients with mood disorders, but it is unclear whether these are the cause of the mood disorder, or reflect an underlying brain disorder. Among the more consistent observations in patients with major depression is dysfunction of the hypothalamic–pituitary–adrenal (HPA) axis, presenting as elevation of basal cortisol, dexamethasone-mediated negative feedback resistance, increased cerebrospinal fluid levels of corticotropin-releasing factor (CRF), and an ACTH response to challenge with exogenous CRF. These features appear to be markers of state rather than trait: they usually normalize after successful treatment.

There is evidence suggesting that panic disorder is associated with specific biological abnormalities in the central nervous system. It may result from an abnormally sensitive fear network, which includes the prefrontal cortex, insula, thalamus, amygdala, and projections to the locus coeruleus, hypothalamus, periaqueductal grey substance, and peribrachial nucleus. Selective serotonin reuptake inhibitors (SSRIs), tricyclic antidepressants, monoamine oxidase inhibitors (MAOIs), and benzodiazepines all decrease the firing rates of selected neurons in this fear network, such as those in the locus coeruleus. Studies of patients with PTSD have shown increased central noradrenaline levels, down-regulated central adrenergic receptors, and chronically decreased glucocorticoid levels.

Diagnosis and clinical manifestations

Patients with depression or anxiety initially present with physical complaints 50 to 70% of the time. They often complain of vague symptoms or report multiple somatic symptoms in a variety of anatomical locations, or experience greater dysfunction than can be attributed to their known medical disorders. Patients with panic disorder and PTSD often selectively focus on the somatic components of anxiety, such as chest pain or palpitations, attributing their increased anxiety and tension to the frightening nature of somatic symptoms.

When depression or anxiety is suspected, simple screening questions may be helpful: 'Are you feeling sad, blue, or depressed?'; 'Have you lost interest and pleasure in most things you usually enjoy?'; 'Do you have sudden episodes or attacks where your heart beats fast, your chest is tight, it feels hard to breathe and you feel shaky?' For PTSD, inquiry about persistent nightmares or flashbacks (daytime memories of trauma) after a traumatic event is an effective screen. The physician should enquire about the patient's explanatory model for his or her symptoms: 'Why do you think you get these symptoms?'

History is the single best diagnostic tool. The physician should elicit the patient's concerns and fears, current life situation, family and other support systems, and concurrent medical problems. A family history of psychiatric problems (depression, anxiety, substance use disorders) should also be obtained. In the United States of America, the Patient Health Questionnaire-9 (PHQ-9) has been the depression tool recommended to screen for depressives as well as monitor progress of depression treatment. Screening questions about a childhood or adult history of physical or sexual abuse, or of domestic violence, are important and can be woven into the usual questions about family medical history. Adverse childhood and adult traumatic experiences are associated with an increased risk of anxiety and affective disorders in adulthood. Over half of the depressed women in one primary care study reported experiencing physical abuse as adults.

The physician should explain carefully that anxiety and depression reflect a biological predisposition that is provoked during a period of life stress. Risk factors that predispose patients to anxiety or depression include a personal or family history of depression or substance abuse, serious medical illness, lack of social support, or a history of early childhood trauma or neglect. Risk factors that can precipitate an acute episode or perpetuate the disorder include poor physical health, divorce, poor interpersonal relationships, illness or death in a family member, trauma, low socioeconomic status, or a stressful work situation.

Depression and dysthymia

Major depressive episodes last at least 2 weeks and are characterized by at least five of nine criteria, including at least one of the two primary criteria of depressed mood and loss of interest or pleasure in nearly all activities (Table 26.5.5.2). There are two to three times as many people with 'minor' depressive symptoms that fall short of major depression criteria: these have a higher rate of spontaneous recovery.

Physical symptoms of depression are predictive of a good response to treatment: those with middle insomnia (awakening between 02.00 and 04.00 h) or a diurnal variation in mood are more likely to respond to antidepressant medications.

Several dimensions of depression severity should be assessed: the frequency and chronicity of depressive symptoms, the impact of depression on the patient's ability to function, the potential for suicide, and the presence of psychotic or manic symptoms. Dysthymic disorder is characterized by a chronically depressed mood that occurs most of the day, more days than not, for at least 2 years. It is associated with many features of major depression but differs in its onset, duration, persistence, and severity of symptoms. Dysthymia is associated with impaired functioning and may not remit spontaneously, and most patients with this condition have also experienced recurrent major depressive episodes.

Anxiety

Patients with anxiety have cognitive, affective, and somatic symptoms. The key feature distinguishing panic disorder from other anxiety disorders is the episodic nature of the attacks. Panic attacks are characterized by the sudden onset of intense apprehension, fear or terror, and by the abrupt development of at least four of the

Table 26.5.5.2 DSM-IV criteria for major depressive episode

Five (or more) of the following symptoms, present most of the time for the past 2 weeks; at least one of the symptoms is either depressed mood or loss of interest or pleasure:

- ◆ Depressed mood
- ◆ Loss of interest or pleasure in activities
- ◆ Weight loss or gain (change of >5% per cent of body weight in a month)
- ◆ Sleep disorder (insomnia or hypersomnia)
- ◆ Psychomotor agitation or retardation
- ◆ Fatigue or loss of energy
- ◆ Feelings of worthlessness, or excessive or inappropriate guilt
- ◆ Diminished ability to concentrate or make decisions
- ◆ Recurrent thoughts of death or suicidal ideation, plan or attempt

Diagnostic and statistical manual of mental disorder, third edition, revised (1987).

Table 26.5.5.3 DSM-IV criteria for panic disorder

Both 1 and 2:	
1. Recurrent unexpected panic attacks: discrete period of intense fear or discomfort, in which four (or more) of the following symptoms develop abruptly and reach a peak within 10 min:	
Palpitations	Dizziness
Sweating	Derealization or depersonalization
Trembling or shaking	Fear of losing control or going crazy
Shortness of breath or choking	Fear of dying
Chest pain	Chills or hot flushes
Nausea or abdominal distress	
2. At least one of the attacks has been followed by 1 month (or more) of one (or more) of the following:	
Persistent concern about having additional attacks	
Worry about the implications of the attack or its consequences	
A significant change in behaviour related to the attacks	

Diagnostic and statistical manual of mental disorder, third edition, revised (1987).

symptoms listed in Table 26.5.5.3, reaching a peak within 10 min. Panic disorder is diagnosed when attacks are recurrent, produce persistent fear, or become significantly disruptive to the patient's life. Post-traumatic stress disorder (PTSD) is associated with exposure to a traumatic event and persistent re-experiencing of the event in dreams and flashbacks, persistent avoidance of stimuli associated with the trauma and numbing of general responsiveness, and persistent symptoms of increased arousal (i.e. startling easily, sleep problems) (see Chapter 26.5.1).

Suicide

The risk of suicide should be evaluated in all patients with depressive and anxiety disorders. The risk of suicide attempts and suicidal ideation more than doubles in depressed patients with comorbid anxiety or physical illness. Other risk factors for suicide include gender (older white males are at highest risk), alcoholism, severe medical illness, psychosis, and lack of social support. The topic of suicidal ideation can be approached gradually with a nonspecific question such as, 'Do you ever feel so discouraged that life does not seem worth living?'

Asking about suicide will not increase a patient's risk. Enquiries about suicide can reassure the patient and enable the physician and patient together to make a plan to prevent suicide, including deciding together whether emergency psychiatric consultation or hospitalization is necessary. Physicians should consider using a 'no harm contract', meaning that patients are simply asked to contract with the physician in writing that they will contact the physician if they think that they are losing control of a suicidal impulse. Although data on the effectiveness of this technique are not available, it seems sensible and is standard clinical practice in many centres.

For further discussion of these issues see Chapter 26.5.2.

Investigation

An adequate diagnostic workup for anxiety or depression may include a complete blood screen, urinalysis, and routine laboratory tests of renal and liver function. Selected patients should receive an electrocardiogram or chest radiograph. Thyroid function studies are recommended in perimenopausal or postmenopausal women.

Given the sizeable differential diagnosis for a patient presenting with anxiety or depression, the extent of workup must be tailored for each case.

Treatment

While depression and anxiety are usually recurrent or chronic disorders, their clinical course can be markedly improved with timely, evidence-based treatments. Many patients can be treated successfully by primary care or general physicians.

Physicians should educate patients about the nature of depression or anxiety and how symptoms can be managed. They should explore background problems, define treatment goals, and dispel negative perceptions (e.g. that antidepressant therapy is addictive). Patients should be reassured that they are not 'crazy', nor are their symptoms a manifestation of their own failure or shortcomings.

There are several important educational points to cover. Depression and anxiety are common and are associated with important physiological changes. With proper treatment these disorders almost always improve or remit, but relapses and recurrences can occur and so follow-up is essential. Physicians should enquire about the patient's concerns regarding a diagnosis of depression or anxiety, also their worries about medical disorders. Raising the possibility of referral to a psychiatrist or other mental health professional early may make it easier to accept later.

Patients should be educated about the types of available treatments. Identifying the patient's desires and goals for treatment can provide a focus for the management of problems that can otherwise seem to be poorly defined and overwhelming. This can also increase patients' sense of participation in their care. Successful disease management programmes developed for asthma and diabetes that have emphasized educating patients to be partners in their medical care have resulted in significant improvements in adherence to treatment and in outcomes: similar approaches have been shown to be successful in managing those with depression and panic disorder.

Pharmacotherapy

The decision to prescribe antidepressant therapy should be based on the number of symptoms, the level of dysfunction, and previous episodes of depression or anxiety. Before initiating antidepressant therapy the physician should educate the patient regarding potential side effects, the need to take medication regularly, and the usual time period and course to recovery.

The different classes of antidepressant drugs show virtually equivalent efficacy in the treatment of outpatients with major depressive disorder. The consensus on the pharmacotherapy of panic disorder also described equivalent efficacy of SSRIs, tricyclic antidepressants (TCAs), serotonin noradrenaline reuptake inhibitors (SNRIs), MAOIs, and high potency benzodiazepines. For other forms of anxiety (social phobia and PTSD) there is more evidence of the efficacy of SSRIs and MAOIs compared to TCAs.

The choice of medication should therefore be made on issues other than efficacy, such as side effects (Table 26.5.5.4), cost, adherence, and physician familiarity and comfort with prescribing particular agents. Primary care providers should become familiar with one or two medications with minimal side effects from each of the major classes of antidepressants: SSRIs, TCAs, and newer atypical antidepressants. In each case, the aim is to optimize treatment benefit and lower risk. Factors to be considered include the possibility

of side effects, history of response or a failure to respond, possible drug interactions, the presence of other psychiatric or medical conditions, familial response to a specific agent, and patient age.

Randomized controlled trials have failed to show efficacy for antidepressant medication in patients with minor depression, largely because the placebo response rate is so high. Watchful waiting is appropriate for these patients, although the physician should recognize that they are at a higher risk of developing a major depressive episode.

Classes of medications

For a discussion of the pharmacology, side effects, and interactions of tricyclic antidepressants, SSRIs, MAOIs, and other agents used in the treatment of anxiety and depression, see Chapter 26.6.1.

The SSRIs have become the first-line treatment for major depression, dysthymia, and panic disorder, primarily because their improved side effect profiles are associated with improved adherence to treatment. In the primary care setting patients are significantly more likely to discontinue TCAs than SSRIs, with those started on an SSRI being 7.5 times more likely to take medication consistent in dosage and duration with treatment guideline recommendations. The initial prescription of fluoxetine results in fewer side effects, a lower rate of medication switching, and no difference in clinical outcomes, quality of life outcomes, or overall treatment costs when compared to TCAs. Given that most SSRIs are now sold as generics, the costs compared to TCAs are comparable.

Selective serotonin reuptake inhibitors (SSRIs)

The advent of the SSRIs (fluoxetine, paroxetine, sertraline, fluvoxamine, citalopram) and the newer atypical antidepressants (bupropion (previously called amfebutanone), venlafaxine, and duloxetine) has significantly increased the number of patients receiving pharmacological treatment for depression and anxiety in a primary care setting. These new agents have fewer, adverse side effects and are safer for treating older patients and those with comorbid medical illnesses. SSRIs are also much safer than the tricyclic antidepressants if taken in overdose. They do not cause postural hypotension or cardiac conduction delay.

These agents have the advantage that the starting dose may also be an effective treating dose. This is most clearly the case for fluoxetine (20 mg), but may also be true for paroxetine (20 mg), sertraline (50 mg), and citalopram (20 mg). The frail older patients and those with liver disease require smaller starting doses (generally one-half of the usual recommended starting dose). Fluoxetine has the longest half-life (24–27 h) and a long-acting active metabolite (half-life of 7 days). The other SSRIs and duloxetine have half-lives of about 24 h and have no active metabolites with longer half-lives. This allows once-daily dosing and rapid washout. Bupropion, venlafaxine, and nefazodone have shorter half-lives (14 h), so must be given at least twice a day; sustained release forms of amfebutanone and venlafaxine can be taken once daily.

Table 26.5.5.4 describes common side effects of these medications: those such as anxiety, insomnia, nausea, headache, and agitation occur in fewer than 20% of patients. When they do occur, they are usually mild and may respond to a reduction in the dose of medication. Sexual dysfunction (decreased libido and anorgasmia) occurs in up to one-third of patients treated with SSRIs and may be alleviated by the addition of bupropion (100–200 mg per day in divided doses) or buspirone (30–60 mg). Strategies for the management of other common side effects are listed in Table 26.5.5.5.

Table 26.5.5.4 Side effects of medications used to treat depression and anxiety

	Sedation, fatigue	Anticholinergic	Dizziness	Insomnia; Aagitation	Headache	Weight gain	GI	Anorgasmia
TCA								
Amitriptyline	3+	3+	3+	0	0	2+	1+	1+
Desipramine	1+	1+	1+	1+	0	2+	1+	1+
Doxepin	3+	3+	3+	0	0	2+	1+	1+
Imipramine	2+	3+	3+	1+	0	2+	1+	1+
Nortriptyline	2+	2+	1+	0	0	2+	0	1+
Protriptyline	1+	3+	1+	1+	0	2+	1+	1+
Other heterocyclic								
Trazodone	3+	0	2+	0	0	2+	0	0
SSRIs								
Fluoxetine	0	0	0	2+	1+	0	1+	2+
Sertraline	1+	0	0	1+	0	0	2+	2+
Paroxetine	1+	1+	0	1+	0	0	2+	2+
Fluvoxamine	0	0	0	1+	0	1+	2+	2+
Citalopram	1+	0	0	1+	0	0	0	1+
Atypical antidepressants								
Buproprion [a]	0	0	0	1+	0	0	0	1+
Venlafaxine	0	0	0	1+	0	0	2+	1+
Nefazodone	1+	0	0	1+	0	0	0	0
Mirtazapine	2+	0	0	0	0	1+	0	0
Duloxetine	0	1+	1+	1+	0	0	2+	0

GI, gastrointestinal; TCA, tricyclic antidepressant; SSRIs, selective serotonin-reuptake inhibitors; * buproprion
GI, gastrointestinal; SSRI, selective serotonin reuptake inhibitor; TCA, tricyclic antidepressant.
[a]Previously known as amfebutanone.

Patients with anxiety disorders are especially sensitive to the SSRI side effects of jitteriness, restlessness, agitation, and insomnia. Low doses should be prescribed initially (5–10 mg paroxetine; 12.5–25 mg of sertraline; 25 mg fluvoxamine; 5 mg fluoxetine) for approximately 1 week, then gradually increasing to full therapeutic doses. To completely alleviate panic attacks in most cases requires: 20 to 50 mg paroxetine, citalopram, or fluoxetine; 50 to 200 mg of sertraline; and 100 to 300 mg of fluvoxamine and 150 to 300 mg of venlafaxine. Similar schedules and dosages are used to treat patients with social phobia, PTSD, and generalized anxiety disorder.

Most SSRIs (but not bupropion) inhibit the cytochrome P450 system in the liver, thus potentially leading to drug interactions (see Chapter 26.6.1). Amfebutamone is an effective antidepressant that may be especially useful because it does not cause the sexual side effects common to the SSRIs, but it has been associated with a slight increase in prevalence of seizures compared to other antidepressants. The medication should not be given to individuals at risk for seizures (those with a history of seizures or head injury, or—for reasons that are unclear—bulimia), and should never be administered in a single dose greater than 200 mg. The starting dose of 75 mg twice per day should be increased every week to achieve a therapeutic dose of between 300 and 450 mg/day. The sustained-release form of bupropion may have a decreased risk of seizures due to being associated with lower peak serum levels.

Tricyclic antidepressants

The heterocyclic medications include the tricyclic antidepressants and several other agents that are similar in structure, including maprotiline, amoxapine, and trazodone. These medications are similar in their side effects and dosing strategies (see Chapter 26.6.1).

Table 26.5.5.5 Managing the side-effects of pharmacotherapy

Insomnia	Move dose to early part of the day
	Add trazodone 50–100 mg at bedtime or nortriptyline 25 mg at bedtime
	Switch to paroxetine or fluvoxamine
Nausea or diarrhoea	Take medication with food
	Reduce dose for 4–7 days, then reintroduce higher dose
	Add H$_2$ blocker
	Switch to nortriptyline
Sedation	Move dose to bedtime
	Switch to fluoxetine or sertraline
Anorgasmia	Add buproprion 100 mg once or twice per day
	Weekend drug holidays (not fluoxetine)
	Switch to buproprion

Low starting doses are required, with a gradual increase to a therapeutic level. For treating depression, panic disorder, or PTSD, physicians should begin at 10 to 25 mg of imipramine, gradually increasing the dose by 10 to 25 mg every 4 or 5 days. The ultimate dosage is variable, with some patients responding at a low dosage (50–100 mg), and others needing up to 300 mg. Plasma levels can be measured, but these function primarily as indicators of whether or not the patient is taking the medication: clinicians should treat the patient and not the blood level, since many with high or low blood levels may do very well clinically. Nortriptyline is an exception: it has a therapeutic window (50–150 ng/ml)—levels below or above this are less likely to lead to remission of depression.

Other agents

For the few patients with anxiety disorders who do not tolerate SSRIs or TCAs, high-potency benzodiazepines may be an effective second-line treatment. Alprazolam, lorazepam, and clonazepam have all been shown to be more effective than placebo for the treatment of panic disorder. Patients can be started at 0.25 mg clonazepam three times per day, gradually increasing by 0.25 mg every 2 to 3 days until the attacks stop. Symptoms of generalized anxiety disorder can be alleviated in most cases with a clonazepam dose between 0.25 and 0.5 mg twice daily and 1 mg two or three times daily, or lorazepam 0.5 to 1 mg three times daily. These agents are best used in conjunction with an SSRI or TCA at the beginning of treatment. After 6 to 8 weeks, when the antidepressant begins to have its optimal effects in treating anxiety symptoms, the benzodiazepine can usually be tapered with a 10% dose reduction per week.

Buspirone is an azapirone with affinity for 5-HT1A and dopamine receptors that has been approved for the treatment of patients with generalized anxiety disorder. It is nonsedating, and there are no withdrawal symptoms with abrupt discontinuation. There are also no synergistic effects with alcohol. Buspirone is typically effective at doses of 30 to 60 mg, divided two or three times daily. Common side effects include dizziness, nausea, headache, and nervousness. These can be reduced by using lower starting doses of 5 mg two or three times daily and advancing as tolerated.

β-Adrenergic blockers may be useful for treating performance anxiety. Propranolol is used at doses of 10 to 80 mg per day (ideally taken 2 h before the anticipated exposure). Atenolol at 25 to 100 mg may be preferred since it has fewer CNS side effects (exacerbating depression). The α-blocker prazosin has been found to be more effective than placebo in treating nightmares in patients with PTSD.

MAOIs are potentially the most effective class of medication for panic or certain types of depression. However, their regular use in primary care or by general physicians is precluded by the lack of familiarity with these agents, and the potential for hypertensive crisis that can ensue from not following a low tyramine diet or taking an over-the-counter stimulant medication (like pseudoephedrine).

Alternative treatments

Clinicians need to ask patients in a routine and nonjudgemental manner about their use of alternative treatments, and should know enough about the more common ones to assess for deleterious effects or interactions. St John's wort has been widely used in Europe. A recent meta-analysis found it to be more effective than placebo and of similar effectiveness to low dose TCAs in the short-term treatment of mild depression. However, a recent study comparing treatment with an SSRI versus St John's wort found that St John's wort was less effective in treating major depression.

Gastrointestinal effects including nausea, pain, loss of appetite, and diarrhoea occurred at a rate of 0.55% in a German study of 3250 patients taking 300 mg three times a day. It may cause a sunburn-like reaction, mucosal inflammation, pruritus, and can lead to significant depression of the blood level of ciclosporin (or tacrolimus) in organ transplant recipients, even leading to rejection.

Special issues in pregnancy

Mild post-partum 'blues' occur in 30 to 75% of women immediately after delivery. Symptoms include labile mood, tearfulness, irritability, anxiety, and sleep and appetite disturbances lasting 4 to 10 days. Patients should be evaluated for post-partum major depression if physical symptoms and depressed mood persist for 2 weeks, which occurs in about 10%. Symptoms usually begin during the third trimester. A history of depression, limited social support, marital conflict, and ambivalence about the pregnancy increase the risk of depression during pregnancy and in the post-partum period.

Pharmacotherapy for depression during pregnancy requires an assessment of the risks and benefits of treatment for both mother and fetus. The risks of not treating major depression may include suicide, poor maternal and fetal nutrition, low birth weight and preterm labour, obstetric complications, and the continuation of depression into the post-partum period, with effects on mother and child bonding. Interpersonal psychotherapy has been shown to be effective in decreasing depression and helpful in resolving interpersonal and psychosocial conflicts without exposing the mother or fetus to medications. Although psychotherapy is the first-line treatment for mild to moderate depression during pregnancy or after the birth of a child, antidepressant treatment may be warranted in severe major depression.

The use of selective serotonin reuptake inhibitors (SSRIs) and selective norepinephrine reuptake inhibitors for the treatment of depression during pregnancy should be individualized based on their respective risks and benefits. Although the majority of early reports of SSRI treatment during pregnancy did not identify an increased risk for birth defects, in 2005 the Food and Drug Administration (FDA) issued an advisory indicating that early exposure to paroxetine may increase the risk for cardiac defects. In response, two large-scale case- control studies were published, and overall, SSRI exposure was not associated with congenital heart problems in these studies, suggesting that SSRI exposure is associated with a small absolute risk for major defects. Findings on the relationship of minor physical anomalies to SSRI exposure, however, have been inconsistent. Although a higher risk for three or more minor anomalies in fluoxetine-exposed infants has been reported, no increased risk has been found in newborns exposed to sertraline or SSRIs generally, compared to unexposed newborns. Studies of SSRI use later in pregnancy have suggested significantly lower maternal weight gain and infant birth weight after exposure to fluoxetine after 25 weeks' gestation. Exposure to SSRIs late in pregnancy has been associated with short-term complications in newborns including jitteriness, mild respiratory distress, excessively rapid respiration, weak cry, poor muscle tone, and admission to the neonatal intensive care unit. There have also been several reports of less favorable Apgar scores associated with third-trimester SSRI exposure, and a specific association between late-pregnancy fluoxetine exposure and persistent pulmonary hypertension of the newborn.

Data regarding the excretion of antidepressants in breast milk are limited. The American Academy of Pediatrics Committee on

Drugs concluded: 'antidepressants are drugs whose effect on nursing infants is unknown but may be of concern'. Several studies have shown only small amounts of SSRIs in breast milk and infant serum samples. Children have been followed through their enrolment in kindergarten with no evidence of negative effects on global intelligence, language, or behaviour.

Monitoring

Regular visits are essential for patients with depression and anxiety. Brief visits every 2 weeks are usually indicated during the first 6 weeks of treatment to evaluate the dosage and side effects of medications, and any changes in the patient's condition. With appropriate counselling beforehand and a regular discussion of side effects, patients are more likely to adhere to a full medication trial, which can also be encouraged by telephone monitoring. The physician should record the main symptoms that the patient presents at the beginning of treatment, and review these at each follow-up visit. The treatment response should be evaluated after they have been on a therapeutic dose of medication for 4 weeks. Simply asking the patient to note the degree of progress on a scale of 1 to 5 can be helpful in assessing either an improvement or worsening of the target symptoms, e.g. by using empirically validated, self-rating scales, such as the PHQ-9, administered at initial diagnosis and at each follow-up. A 25% or greater reduction in baseline symptoms constitutes a reasonable basis for extending the initial treatment. If there has been no response or only a partial response in symptoms, the dose of the medication should be increased to the upper therapeutic range.

Because only 40% of patients with major depression improve over 4 to 6 months during treatment in usual primary care, researchers have developed health care models to improve quality of depression care in primary care systems. A recent meta-analysis of 37 studies reported that collaborative care models were twice as effective as usual care in achieving adherence to antidepressant medication at 6 months and were associated with improved depression outcomes for as long as 2 to 5 years. Collaborative care has two core components: (1) designation of allied health professionals or mental health professionals (called depression care managers) to support primary care providers by helping educate patients about depression, providing close patient follow-up, tracking depression outcomes, side effects and treatment adherence, and facilitating additional visits or treatments with the primary care physician for patients with persistent symptoms; and (2) consultation focusing on patients whose depression is not improving as expected by a designated psychiatrist, who provides backup and case load supervision for the depression care manager and clinical advice/decision support to primary care doctors.

About 40 to 50% of patients with major depression respond to an antidepressant within 3 weeks after reaching a therapeutic plasma level. This success rate can be as high as 80% by switching initial nonresponders to another class of antidepressant, or by augmentation strategies using additional medication or psychotherapy. However, if a patient fails to improve adequately with first-line therapy, the diagnosis and the treatment plan must be reassessed. There may be unrecognized comorbid anxiety or substance abuse, and treatment failure is commonly due to inadequate dosing or lack of adherence to medication.

Once the patient is stabilized on a medication (usually 6–12 weeks), monthly visits are important for support. If chronic prophylactic treatment is necessary, visits every 3 months are usually appropriate. Consensus statements recommend a treatment period of between 6 and 9 months after a first major depressive episode. Pharmacotherapy should be discontinued slowly over a period of 7 to 21 days. If tapered too quickly almost all antidepressants (except fluoxetine) can produce withdrawal syndromes that include sleep disturbance, mood changes, anxiety, sensory disturbance, malaise, muscle aches, vertigo, sweating, fatigue, and gastrointestinal upset.

Patients who have remitted during the acute phase of pharmacotherapy for anxiety and depressive disorders remain at substantial risk of relapse during the subsequent 12 months: 37.1% of depressed primary care patients experience further depressive symptoms during this time. There are three main risk factors associated with relapse: (1) persistence of subthreshold depressive symptoms; (2) history of three or more previous episodes of major depression; and (3) chronic mood symptoms for more than 2 years. Patients with two of these risk factors are approximately three times more likely to relapse than those without. Between 50 and 60% of patients who have had a single major depressive episode will have a second one; 70% of those who have two episodes will have a third; and 90% of those who have had three episodes will have a fourth. For patients with three or more depressive episodes or dysthymia and major depression, the AHCPR guidelines recommend treatment for 2 years or more.

The optimal duration of treatment for anxiety disorders has not been as well established by controlled studies. Treatment is recommended for 6 to 9 months after the first episode. Maintenance therapy should be considered for those with either a chronic history since adolescence, or three or more recurrences. Panic disorder and PTSD are recurrent or chronic diseases in most cases. In a review of 16 studies, most patients with panic disorder had improvement in symptoms with treatment, but few experienced complete resolution. As panic disorder progresses, attacks become more frequent and are preceded by anticipatory anxiety. Patients may begin to associate environmental events with anxiety, leading to avoidance behaviour. The disorder may culminate in agoraphobia: being afraid to leave the house because of the association with panic attacks.

Electroconvulsive therapy (ECT)

ECT remains the most effective treatment available for depression: it can be life-saving in some cases, and in the frail older patient it may be safer than antidepressants. Some reversible short-term memory loss is a common side effect, but this reverts to normal in almost all cases. Patients with recurrent depression who receive effective ECT treatment should be treated with prophylactic medication or maintenance ECT once the acute course of the treatment has finished.

Psychotherapy

Randomized controlled trials support the efficacy of psychosocial interventions provided to ambulatory medical patients with psychiatric disorders. Problem solving skills and other behavioural techniques, most of which can be provided as simple self-help materials, are part of the psychosocial support that general physicians can provide in a disease management programme for depressive or anxiety disorders. As in all chronic illnesses, lifestyle changes should be reinforced: good sleep habits, adequate exercise, and minimization of caffeine and alcohol intake.

There are three short-term psychotherapies used to specifically target the symptoms of major depression: cognitive behavioural therapy (CBT), interpersonal psychotherapy (IPT), and problem solving therapy (PST). CBT is directed at the negative and distorted thinking patterns and subsequent maladaptive behaviours that often accompany depressive episodes. IPT helps the patient learn to manage the current interpersonal relationship difficulties that are sometimes related to the development and maintenance of depressive symptoms. PST helps activate patients to break down global problems to smaller units that they can begin to attempt to solve.

Patients with major depression treated with CBT and IPT experience as much relief from symptoms by 16 weeks, and those with PST by 11 weeks, as those taking medication alone. Given these findings, physicians need not rely as heavily on drug treatments as they typically have, and should consider psychosocial interventions if the patient prefers them and they are available.

In a meta-analysis of studies on panic disorder and PTSD, psychological coping strategies involving relaxation training, cognitive restructuring, and exposure worked comparably with both antidepressant and benzodiazepine medications. The combined somatic exposure and cognitive therapy (or exposure to traumatic memories in patients with PTSD) helps patients confront and alter maladaptive cognitions (e.g. catastrophic thoughts of a heart attack or stroke when experiencing rapid heartbeat). A meta-analysis of the treatment of generalized anxiety disorder concluded that CBT is more efficacious than control treatments and at least equal in efficacy to anxiolytics.

See Chapter 26.6.2 for further discussion.

Specialty referral

Referral to a psychiatrist should be considered when the physician is confused about the primary diagnosis, as in distinguishing an anxiety disorder from depression with anxiety or substance abuse disorder. Referrals should also be made when adequate treatment does not lead to an improvement in symptoms within 10 to 12 weeks, or several medication trials have failed. Patients with suicidal behaviour also require specialty care (see Chapter 26.5.2).

Other disorders

Generalized anxiety disorder

Generalized anxiety disorder is characterized by constant, nonepisodic anxiety that affects patients for more than 6 months and interferes with normal function. Lifetime prevalence rates are 5.1% in community samples. Medical problems such as hyperthyroidism should be ruled out as the cause of the symptoms of motor tension and autonomic hyperactivity. This disorder can be treated effectively with SSRIs, TCAs, SNRIs, buspirone, and benzodiazepines; the first four classes should be tried first, given their lower potential for habituation and dependence.

Specific phobias

Specific phobias are characterized by episodic anxiety in response to a specific precipitant, with intense excessive fear making patients avoid the situation. Examples of stimuli for simple phobias are airplanes, heights, and insects, although most patients with simple phobias do not seek care for the condition. Social phobia is the fear of humiliation or failure in public situations (such as public speaking, meeting strangers, and eating in restaurants), and many with this condition also have major depression (58.3% of cases of social phobia), or other anxiety disorders (panic disorder, 27.8%; generalized

anxiety disorder, 30.6%). Since social phobia usually begins in childhood or adolescence, patients often consider marked social anxiety and avoidance as part of their personality.

Recent studies have shown that SSRIs are more effective than placebo in the treatment of social phobia; effective cognitive behavioural techniques have also been developed. Propranolol (10–80 mg) may be useful for treating nongeneralized social phobia that occurs in one situation, such as public speaking.

Obsessive–compulsive disorder

Obsessive–compulsive disorder (OCD) is characterized by regular intrusive thoughts or obsessions about aggression, sex, religion, theft, or loss—or other covering mental rituals such as counting objects or letters. Patients may also have persistent rituals or compulsions that are so frequent or complex that they interfere with normal function. They experience these obsessions and compulsions as intrusive, silly, and upsetting. Most patients with OCD have experienced major depressive episodes. Pharmacological treatment is indicated: although clomipramine has been the first-line treatment for many years, recent randomized controlled trials have shown SSRIs to be as effective. Treatment with SSRIs should continue for at least 10 weeks before it is considered ineffective. Randomized trials have shown behavioural treatments to be effective; these focus on exposure to feared activities and prevention of compulsive responses.

Further reading

Ballenger JC, et al. (1998). Consensus statement on panic disorder from the International Consensus Group on Depression and Anxiety. *J Clin Psychiatry*, **59** Suppl 8, 47–54.

Brown C, Schulberg HC (1995). The efficacy of psychosocial treatments in primary care. A review of randomized clinical trials. *Gen Hosp Psychiatry*, **17**, 414–24.

Agency for Health Care Policy and Research (1993). *Depression in primary care, vols.1 and 2. Clinical practice guidelines No. 5*. US Departments of Health and Human Services, Rockville Maryland.

Edlund MJ (1990). The economics of anxiety. *Psychiatr Med*, **8**, 15–26.

Gaynes BN, Warden D, Trivedi MH, Wisniewski SR, Fava M, Rush AJ (2009). What did STAR*D teach us? Results from a large-scale, practical, clinical trial for patients with depression. *Psychiatr Serv*, **60**(11), 1439–45.

Greenberg PE, Kessler RC, Birnbaum HG, Leong SA, Lowe SW, Berglund PA, Corey-Lisle PK (2003). The economic burden of depression in the United States: how did it change between 1990 and 2000? *J Clin Psychiatry*, **64**(12), 1465–75.

Katerndahl DA, Realini JP (1995). Where do panic attack sufferers seek care? *J Fam Pract*, **40**, 237–43.

Katon W (2006). Clinical practice. Panic disorder. *N Engl J Med*, **354**, 2360–67.

Katon W, et al. (1990). Distressed high utilizers of medical care. DSM-III diagnoses and treatment needs. *Gen Hosp Psychiatry*, **12**, 355–62.

Katon W, et al. (1992). Adequacy and duration of antidepressant treatment in primary care. *Med Care*, **30**, 67–76.

Katon W, et al. (2006). Cost-effectiveness and net benefit of enhanced treatment of depression for older adults with diabetes and depression. *Diabetes Care*, **29**, 265–70.

Kessler RC, et al. (1994). Lifetime and 12-month prevalence of DSM-III-R psychiatric disorders in the United States. Results of the National Comorbidity Survey. *Arch Gen Psychiatry*, **51**, 8–19.

Kim HL, Streltzer J, Goebert D (1999). St. John's wort for depression: a meta-analysis of well-defined clinical trials. *J Nerv Ment Dis*, **187**, 532–8.

Kulin NA, et al. (1998). Pregnancy outcome following maternal use of the new selective serotonin reuptake inhibitors: a prospective controlled multicenter study. *JAMA*, **279**, 609–10.

Lin EH, *et al.* (1998). Relapse of depression in primary care. Rate and clinical predictors. *Arch Fam Med*, **7**, 443–9.

Mynors-Wallis LM, *et al.* (1995). Randomised controlled trial comparing problem solving treatment with amitriptyline and placebo for major depression in primary care. *BMJ*, **310**, 441–5.

Ormel J, *et al.* (1994). Common mental disorders and disability across cultures. Results from the WHO Collaborative Study on Psychological Problems in General Health Care. *JAMA*, **272**, 1741–8.

Roy-Byrne P, Craske MG, Stein MB (2006). Panic disorder. *Lancet*, **368**, 1023–32.

Schulberg HC, *et al.* (1998). Treating major depression in primary care practice: an update of the Agency for Health Care Policy and Research Practice Guidelines. *Arch Gen Psychiatry*, **55**, 1121–7.

Simon GE, vonKorff M, Barlow W (1995). Health care costs of primary care patients with recognized depression. *Arch Gen Psychiatry*, **52**, 850–6.

Spitzer RL, *et al.* (1995). Health-related quality of life in primary care patients with mental disorders. Results from the PRIME-MD 1000 study. *JAMA*, **274**, 1511–17.

Stein MB, *et al.* (1999). Social phobia in the primary care medical setting. *J Fam Pract*, **48**, 514–19.

Wells KB, *et al.* (1989). The functioning and well-being of depressed patients. Results from the Medical Outcomes Study. *JAMA*, **262**, 914–19.

Wisner KL *et al.* (2009). Major Depression and Antidepressant Treatment: Impact on Pregnancy and Neonatal Outcomes. *Am J Psychiatry*, **166**, 557–66.

26.5.6 Eating disorders

Christopher G. Fairburn

Essentials

Eating disorders affect about 5% of adolescent girls and young adult women. They are much less common among men. They typically begin in adolescence and may run a chronic course, interfering with psychological, physical, and social functioning.

Three eating disorders are distinguished: (1) anorexia nervosa; (2) bulimia nervosa; and (3) a residual diagnostic category—the most common seen in routine clinical practice— termed 'eating disorder not otherwise specified' (eating disorder NOS). They all share a distinctive 'core psychopathology', the overevaluation of shape and weight, and patients frequently move between the categories, hence a case may be made for adopting a 'transdiagnostic' perspective.

The aetiology of the eating disorders is complex and ill-understood: there is a genetic predisposition, and some specific environmental risk factors have been implicated.

Clinical features and diagnosis

In anorexia nervosa the pursuit of weight loss leads patients to engage in a severe and selective restriction of food intake, with foods viewed as fattening being avoided. The same eating habits

Acknowledgement: Christopher G Fairburn is supported by a Principal Research Fellowship (046386) from the Wellcome Trust.

are seen in patients with bulimia nervosa, the main distinguishing feature being that the attempts to restrict food intake are punctuated by repeated episodes of binge eating. Three subgroups within eating disorder NOS may be recognized: (1) those that just fail to meet diagnostic criteria for anorexia nervosa or bulimia nervosa; (2) those that are mixed in character between anorexia nervosa and bulimia nervosa; and (3) binge eating disorder.

Aside from low body weight (body mass index <17.5), a wide range of physical abnormalities is present in anorexia nervosa, some of which can be life-threatening, e.g. cardiac arrhythmia. These appear to be largely secondary to the disturbed eating habits and compromised nutritional state: most are reversed by restoration of healthy eating habits and sound nutrition. The weight of most patients with bulimia nervosa is in the healthy range (body mass index 20–25) due to the effects of the undereating and overeating cancelling each other out.

The diagnosis of an eating disorder is made on positive grounds by using the history and mental state examination to detect the characteristic behavioural and attitudinal features—not by simply ruling out possible physical causes.

Management

Eating disorders are difficult to treat and impose a significant burden on health services.

Bulimia nervosa—in this condition: (1) the most effective treatment is a specific type of cognitive behaviour therapy (CBT) that focuses on modifying the specific behaviours and ways of thinking that maintain these conditions; (2) antidepressant drugs have an 'antibulimic' effect; and (3) no consistent predictors of outcome have been identified.

Anorexia nervosa—there is little evidence on which to base treatment, but it would generally be agreed that the following aspects are important: (1) patients need to be helped to see that they need change; (2) weight needs to be restored; (3) patients' overevaluation of shape and weight, their eating habits, and their general psychosocial functioning all need to be addressed, perhaps in younger patients by family-based treatment.

Eating disorder NOS—there is very little information regarding treatment, but an adaptation of the CBT for bulimia nervosa appears to be useful.

Prevention—the idea of trying to stop schoolgirls from developing eating disorders is clearly attractive, but there is a danger of magnifying concerns about shape and weight rather than reducing them, and there is potential for conflict between emphasis on the risks of undue dieting and advice directed at the prevention of obesity.

Classification and diagnosis

The classification of the eating disorders and their principal diagnostic criteria are shown in Box 26.5.6.1. There are two specified eating disorders, anorexia nervosa and bulimia nervosa, and in addition a residual category termed 'eating disorder not otherwise specified' (eating disorder NOS). This is reserved for eating disorders of clinical severity that do not meet the diagnostic criteria for anorexia nervosa or bulimia nervosa.

Box 26.5.6.1 Classification and diagnosis of eating disorders

Definition of an eating disorder

- There is a definite disturbance of eating habits or weight control behaviour.

- Either this disturbance, or associated core eating disorder features (disturbance of eating, extreme weight control behaviour, and the overevaluation of shape or weight), results in a clinically significant impairment of physical health or psychosocial functioning.

- The behavioural disturbance is not secondary to any general medical disorder or to any other psychiatric condition.

Classification of eating disorders

- Anorexia nervosa

- Bulimia nervosa

- Eating disorder not otherwise specified (eating disorder NOS):
  Binge eating disorder (a provisional new diagnosis, currently subsumed under eating disorder NOS)

Principal diagnostic criteria

Anorexia nervosa

- Overevaluation of shape and weight (i.e. judging self-worth largely, or exclusively, in terms of shape and weight)

- Active maintenance of an unduly low body weight (e.g. body mass index ≤17.5)

- Amenorrhoea (in postmenarcheal females who are not taking an oral contraceptive)—this criterion is often omitted.

Bulimia nervosa

- Overevaluation of shape and weight (i.e. judging self-worth largely, or exclusively, in terms of shape and weight)

- Recurrent binge eating (i.e. recurrent episodes of uncontrolled overeating)

- Extreme weight control behaviour (e.g. strict dietary restriction, frequent self-induced vomiting, or laxative misuse)

- Diagnostic criteria for anorexia nervosa are not met

Eating disorder NOS

- Eating disorders of clinical severity that do not conform to the diagnostic criteria for anorexia nervosa or bulimia nervosa

Binge eating disorder

- Recurrent binge eating in the absence of the extreme weight control behaviour seen in bulimia nervosa

---

The relationship between the three diagnoses is represented diagrammatically in Fig. 26.5.6.1. The two overlapping inner circles represent anorexia nervosa (the smaller circle) and bulimia nervosa (the larger circle) respectively, the area of potential overlap being that occupied by those people who would meet the diagnostic

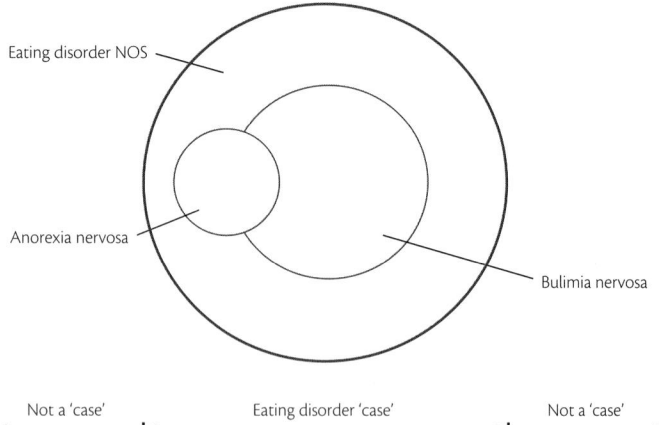

Fig. 26.5.6.1 A schematic representation of the relationship between anorexia nervosa, bulimia nervosa, and eating disorder NOS.
(Reprinted from Behaviour Research and Therapy, 43, Fairburn, C. G. & Bohn, K, Eating disorder NOS (EDNOS): an example of the troublesome' Not Otherwise Specified', 691–701, Copyright 2005, with permission from Elsevier.)

criteria for both disorders but for the rule that the diagnosis of anorexia nervosa trumps that of bulimia nervosa (see Box 26.5.6.1). Surrounding these two circles is an outer circle that defines the boundary between having an eating disorder, a state of clinical significance, and having a lesser, nonclinical, eating problem. It is this boundary that demarcates what is, and is not, an eating disorder. Within the outer circle, but outside the two inner circles, lies eating disorder NOS.

It has recently been proposed that an additional eating disorder be recognized, termed 'binge eating disorder'. This is somewhat different in nature to the other three disorders and is currently subsumed under the rubric of eating disorder NOS.

General clinical features

Anorexia nervosa, bulimia nervosa, and most cases of eating disorder NOS share a distinctive 'core psychopathology' that is essentially the same in women and men, adults and adolescents: the overevaluation of shape and weight. Whereas most people evaluate themselves on the basis of their perceived performance in a variety of domains of life (such as the quality of their relationships; their work performance; their sporting prowess; etc.), people with eating disorders judge their self-worth largely, or even exclusively, in terms of their shape and weight and their ability to control them. This psychopathology is peculiar to the eating disorders and is rare in the general population. It should be distinguished from body shape dissatisfaction, which refers to the dislike of one's appearance, and from body dysmorphic disorder where there is overconcern with the appearance of a specific body part.

The overevaluation of shape and weight results in the pursuit of weight loss and an intense fear of weight gain and fatness. Most other features of these disorders are secondary to this psychopathology and its consequences (e.g. undereating; becoming severely underweight). Thus, in anorexia nervosa there is a sustained and successful pursuit of weight loss that results in patients becoming severely underweight. This pursuit is not seen as a problem: rather, it is viewed as appropriate and, as a consequence, patients have little desire to change. Often it is other people who are responsible for these patients entering treatment. In bulimia nervosa, equivalent attempts to restrict food intake are punctuated by repeated episodes of loss of control over eating (binges). Generally these binges are aversive and a source of distress, and they result in patients seeking help. For this reason patients with bulimia nervosa are easier to engage in treatment, although because of the accompanying shame and secrecy there is typically a delay of many years before they divulge their eating problem.

The core psychopathology of anorexia nervosa and bulimia nervosa has other expressions too. Many patients mislabel adverse physical and emotional states as 'feeling fat' and equate this with actually being fat, and many repeatedly scrutinize their bodies focusing on parts that they dislike, which may contribute to them overestimating their size. Others actively avoid seeing their bodies, assuming that they look fat and disgusting. Equivalent behaviour is seen with respect to weighing, with many patients weighing themselves frequently and as a result becoming preoccupied with trivial day-to-day fluctuations, whereas others actively avoid knowing their weight while nevertheless remaining highly concerned about it.

Anorexia nervosa

In anorexia nervosa the pursuit of weight loss leads patients to engage in a severe and selective restriction of food intake, with foods viewed as fattening being avoided. Generally, there is no true 'anorexia' (in the sense of a loss of appetite). The undereating may be an expression of other motives too, including asceticism, competitiveness, and a desire to attract attention from others. In the early stages of the disorder undereating may be a goal in its own right, the patient valuing the sense of self-control that it imparts.

Some patients also engage in a type of exercising that contributes to their weight loss. This is characterized by a strong drive to exercise, a tendency to overexercise, and giving exercise precedence over other aspects of life. Self-induced vomiting and other extreme forms of weight control (such as the misuse of laxatives or diuretics) are practised by a subgroup, and an overlapping group has episodes of loss of control over eating, although the amount eaten may not be objectively large. Depressive and anxiety features, irritability, lability of mood, impaired concentration, loss of sexual appetite, and obsessional symptoms are also frequently present. Typically, these features get worse as weight is lost and improve with weight regain. Interest in the outside world diminishes as patients become underweight with the result that most are socially withdrawn and isolated: this too tends to reverse with weight regain.

Bulimia nervosa

The eating habits of patients with bulimia nervosa resemble those seen in anorexia nervosa, the main distinguishing feature being that the attempts to restrict food intake are punctuated by repeated episodes of binge eating. The frequency of these episodes ranges from once or twice a week (the diagnostic threshold) to several times a day, and the amount eaten per episode varies, but is typically between 1000 and 2000 kcals. In most cases, each binge is followed by compensatory self-induced vomiting or laxative misuse, although there is a subgroup of patients who do not 'purge'.

The weight of most patients with bulimia nervosa is in the healthy range (body mass index between 20 and 25) due to the effects of the undereating and overeating cancelling each other out. As a result these patients do not experience the secondary psychosocial and physical effects of maintaining a very low weight. Depressive and anxiety features are prominent—indeed more so than in anorexia nervosa—and there is a subgroup who engage in substance misuse or self-injury or both (also found among some anorexia nervosa patients who binge eat).

Eating disorder NOS

The psychopathology of eating disorder NOS closely resembles that seen in anorexia nervosa and bulimia nervosa, and is of comparable duration and severity. It is helpful to distinguish three subgroups within eating disorder NOS, although there is no sharp boundary between them. The first comprises cases that closely resemble anorexia nervosa or bulimia nervosa but just fail to meet their diagnostic criteria. The second and largest subgroup consists of cases in which the clinical features of anorexia nervosa and bulimia nervosa are combined in a different way to that seen in the two prototypic disorders: such states may be thought of as 'mixed' in character. Patients with binge eating disorder form the third subgroup: they report binge eating, much as in bulimia nervosa, but their eating habits outside the binges are quite different, with there being a tendency to overeat outside the binges. Indeed, the eating habits of patients with binge eating disorder resemble those of people with obesity, albeit with binges superimposed. Self-induced vomiting and laxative misuse are not present, nor is there any tendency to overexercise. Most patients with binge eating disorder are overweight or meet criteria for obesity (body mass index ≥ 30).

Development and subsequent course

Anorexia nervosa typically starts in mid teenage years with the onset of dietary restriction that becomes progressively more extreme and inflexible. In its early stages the disorder may be self-limiting and treatment-responsive, but if it persists it tends to become entrenched and needs more intensive treatment. In 10 to 20% of cases it proves intractable and unremitting. Even in patients who recover, residual features are common, particularly some degree of overconcern about shape, weight, and eating. A frequent occurrence is the development of binge eating and, in about half the cases, progression on to full bulimia nervosa.

Most prominent among the favourable prognostic factors are an early age of onset and a short history, whereas unfavourable prognostic factors include a long history, severe weight loss, and binge eating and vomiting. Anorexia nervosa is the one eating disorder to be associated with a raised mortality rate, the standardized mortality ratio over the first 10 years from presentation being about 10: most deaths are either a direct result of medical complications or due to suicide.

Bulimia nervosa has a slightly later age of onset, typically in late adolescence or early adulthood. It usually starts in much the same way as anorexia nervosa, indeed—in about a quarter of cases—the diagnostic criteria for anorexia nervosa are met for a time. Eventually, however, episodes of binge eating interrupt the dietary restriction and, as a result, body weight rises to normal or near normal levels. The disorder is highly self-perpetuating, hence patients often present with an unremitting history of eight or more years of disturbed eating, and even 5 to 10 years after presentation between a third and a half still have an eating disorder of clinical severity, although in many cases it has changed into a 'mixed' form of eating disorder NOS. No consistent predictors of outcome have been identified, but there is evidence that childhood obesity, low self-esteem, and signs of personality disturbance are associated with a worse prognosis.

Almost nothing is known about the development and course of eating disorder NOS. Most patients present in their adolescence or twenties, as in bulimia nervosa, and with a comparable length of history. Between a quarter and a third have had anorexia nervosa or bulimia nervosa in the past, their present state being simply the latest expression of an evolving eating disorder.

Binge eating disorder has a rather different age of presentation and course: most are middle-aged, and a third or more are men. This is quite unlike patients with the other forms of eating disorder, who are generally adolescents or young adults and female (about 10% are male). Binge eating disorder also differs in its course in that it tends to be phasic rather than persistent, with most patients reporting sustained periods when they were prone to binge eat and other times when they were in control of their eating. Throughout, these patients have a general tendency to overeat and gain weight. Few report a history of anorexia nervosa or bulimia nervosa. Whether binge eating disorder should be classed as an eating disorder is a matter of debate.

Epidemiology

There is limited reliable information on the distribution of eating disorders, hence the findings must be regarded as tentative and imprecise. The data come from studies of Western samples; virtually nothing is known about the distribution of eating disorders elsewhere. Within Western samples, most is known about the distribution of eating disorders among young adults; there have been few studies of children and adolescents.

Anorexia nervosa is rare. Even within adolescent girls or young adult women, the group thought to be at greatest risk, prevalence figures are low at 0% to 0.9%. Outside this age group, and in boys and men, anorexia nervosa is likely to be even less common. Figures for the incidence of anorexia nervosa are particularly suspect as most are based on cases detected medically. They suggest that anorexia nervosa became more common in the second half of the 20th century, and especially so in adolescent females, but the apparent increase could well be due to greater help-seeking, better detection, and changes in diagnostic practice rather than any true increase in the incidence of the disorder. In clinical samples anorexia nervosa is the least common of the three eating disorder diagnoses, comprising 10% to 15% of adult cases. In adolescent samples the proportion is higher. The ratio of females to males is about 10 to 1 in adults but somewhat lower in adolescents.

Unlike anorexia nervosa, epidemiological data indicate that bulimia nervosa is more a disorder of early adulthood than adolescence, with most cases being in their twenties. It is more common than anorexia nervosa, in part because the age group at risk is broader (18–40-year-old women) and in part because the point prevalence rate is higher (1–2%). There are no reliable data on the prevalence of bulimia nervosa in boys or men. Clinical experience suggests that bulimia nervosa became considerably more common in the 1970s and 1980s, and limited epidemiological data support this, although there is evidence that the rise has now ceased. The explanation for these changes is not clear. What is known is that most cases of bulimia nervosa are not in treatment and the subgroup that is receiving help is atypical in that the eating disorder is more severe and there is greater psychiatric comorbidity. Within clinical samples male cases are unusual. Bulimia nervosa comprises about 30% to 40% of adult eating disorder cases.

The most glaring gap in knowledge about the epidemiology of eating disorders is the total absence of reliable data on the prevalence and incidence of eating disorder NOS in community samples. Studies of adolescents and young adults often report detecting large numbers of people with 'partial' or 'atypical' syndromes, but the status of these cases is unclear in the absence of an agreed definition of eating disorder NOS. What is now well-established is that eating disorder NOS is the most common eating disorder diagnosis among adults who present for treatment, comprising 50% to 60% of cases, and the same is true of adolescents. As with anorexia nervosa and bulimia nervosa, it is women that are primarily affected.

Pathogenesis

Research on the pathogenesis of the eating disorders has focused almost exclusively on anorexia nervosa and bulimia nervosa. It is clear that there is a genetic predisposition and a range of environmental risk factors, and there is some information regarding the identity and relative importance of these contributions. However, virtually nothing is known about the individual causal processes involved, or how they interact and vary across the development and maintenance of the disorders.

Genetic factors

Eating disorders and some associated traits run in families. A shared familial liability is suggested by cross-transmission between anorexia nervosa, bulimia nervosa, and the atypical eating disorders. The prevalence of substance abuse is increased, especially among the relatives of bulimic probands, but there seems to be no cross-transmission. There is also a raised prevalence of depression, the pattern of familial transmission being unclear. In addition, there is evidence of familial coaggregation of anorexia nervosa and obsessional and perfectionist traits.

In the absence of adoption studies, twin designs have been used to establish the genetic contribution to the familiality of eating disorders. Clinic samples show concordance for anorexia nervosa of around 55% in monozygotic twins and 5% in dizygotic twins, with the corresponding figures for bulimia nervosa being 35% and 30% respectively. These findings suggest a significant heritability to anorexia nervosa but not to bulimia nervosa. Despite this, there is uncertainty as to the size of the genetic contribution to both disorders because of differing point estimates and wide confidence intervals. The same applies to the contributions of individual-specific and shared (common) environmental factors. A number of issues affect the interpretation of the data, e.g. there has been insufficient power to detect shared environmental effects, and established diagnostic criteria have been broadened considerably to increase the number of 'affected' twins available for analysis.

Genetic association studies have focussed in particular on polymorphisms in 5-HT (serotonin)-related genes because this neurotransmitter system is important in regulation of eating and mood, but a range of other polymorphisms have also been investigated. However, no associations with eating disorders have been clearly replicated or confirmed in a family study or by meta-analysis. There has been one multicentre, genome-wide linkage study, which found linkage peaks for anorexia nervosa and bulimia nervosa on chromosomes 1, 4, 10, and 14. A further analysis, which covaried for related behavioural traits, identified a different locus on chromosome 1, as well as loci on chromosomes 2 and 13. All these findings await replication.

Other risk factors

Many other risk factors have been implicated (Box 26.5.6.2). These differ in nature and specificity: some are adverse premorbid experiences of the type associated with many psychiatric disorders (e.g. childhood sexual abuse); others appear to predispose especially to bulimia nervosa (e.g. childhood and parental obesity, early menarche, parental alcoholism), some of which may operate by sensitizing the person to her or his shape, thereby encouraging dieting. This effect is most likely to be seen in women in Western societies in view of the social pressure on them to be slim. Yet other risk factors are character traits, the two most prominent being low

self-esteem and perfectionism, the latter being a particularly common antecedent of anorexia nervosa.

Neurobiological findings

There has been extensive research into the neurobiology of eating disorders, focusing on neuropeptide and monoamine (especially 5-HT) systems thought to be central to the physiology of eating and weight regulation. Of the various central and peripheral abnormalities reported, many are likely to be secondary to the aberrant eating and associated weight loss. However, some aspects of 5-HT function and its receptors remain abnormal after recovery, leading to speculation that there is a monoamine abnormality trait that may predispose to the development of eating disorders or to associated characteristics such as perfectionism. Furthermore, normal dieting in healthy women has been shown to alter central 5-HT function, providing a potential mechanism by which eating disorders might be precipitated in women vulnerable for other reasons.

Brain functional imaging studies have identified altered activity in the frontal, cingulate, temporal, and parietal cortical regions in both anorexia nervosa and bulimia nervosa, and there is some evidence that these alterations persist after recovery. Whether they are a consequence of the eating disorder or have somehow contributed to it is not known.

Psychological processes

Specific psychological theories have been proposed to account for the development and maintenance of eating disorders, the most influential in terms of treatment being cognitive behavioural theories. In brief, these propose that the restriction of food intake that characterises the onset of many eating disorders has two main origins, both of which may operate in tandem. The first is a need to feel 'in control' of life, which gets displaced onto controlling eating. The second is overevaluation of shape and weight in those who have been sensitized to their appearance. In both instances, the resulting dietary restriction is highly reinforcing. Subsequently, other processes begin to operate and serve to maintain the eating disorder. These include social withdrawal, the fact that extreme and rigid dietary restraint promotes binge eating in certain individuals, and the negative impact of binge eating on concerns about shape and the sense of being in control. There is increasing evidence that correcting these processes is necessary for recovery.

Medical complications

The physical abnormalities seen in anorexia nervosa are striking but appear to be largely secondary to the patients' disturbed eating habits and their compromised nutritional state: most are reversed by restoration of healthy eating habits and sound nutrition, with the possible exception of reduced bone density. The principal features are listed in Box 26.5.6.3.

The abnormalities found in bulimia nervosa are usually minor unless vomiting, or laxative, or diuretic misuse are frequent, in which case there is risk of electrolyte disturbance. Patients who vomit frequently are also at risk of dental damage. Equivalent physical abnormalities are found in cases of eating disorder NOS in which body weight is very low or there is a high frequency of purging. There are no established medical complications of binge eating disorder per se (other than those secondary to comorbid obesity).

Box 26.5.6.2 Principal risk factors for anorexia nervosa and bulimia nervosa

General factors

- Female
- Adolescence and early adulthood
- Living in a Western society

Individual-specific factors
Family history

- Eating disorder of any type
- Depression
- Substance abuse, especially alcoholism (bulimia nervosa)
- Obesity (bulimia nervosa)

Premorbid experiences

- Obstetric complications
- Adverse parenting (especially low contact, high expectations, parental discord)
- Sexual abuse
- Family dieting
- Critical comments about eating, shape, or weight from family and others
- Occupational and recreational pressure to be slim

Premorbid characteristics

- Low self-esteem
- Perfectionism (anorexia nervosa and, to a lesser extent, bulimia nervosa)
- Neuroticism
- Anxiety and anxiety disorders
- Obesity (bulimia nervosa)
- Early menarche (bulimia nervosa)
- Type 1 diabetes (bulimia nervosa)

Box 26.5.6.3 Principal physical features of anorexia nervosa

Physical symptoms

- Heightened sensitivity to cold
- Gastrointestinal symptoms (e.g. constipation, fullness after eating, bloatedness)
- Dizziness and syncope
- Amenorrhoea (in women not taking an oral contraceptive); low sexual appetite; infertility
- Poor sleep with early morning wakening

Physical signs

- Emaciation; stunted growth and failure of breast development (if prepubertal onset)
- Dry skin; hair loss; fine downy hair (lanugo) on the back, forearms, and side of the face; in patients with hypercarotenaemia, orange discolouration of the skin of the palms and soles
- Swelling of parotid and submandibular glands (especially in bulimia nervosa)
- Erosion of inner surface of front teeth (perimylolysis) in those who vomit frequently
- Cold hands and feet (acrocyanosis); hypothermia
- Bradycardia; orthostatic hypotension; cardiac arrhythmias (especially in underweight patients and those with electrolyte abnormalities)
- Dependent oedema (complicating the evaluation of body weight)
- Weak proximal muscles (elicited as difficulty rising from a squatting position)

Abnormalities on physical investigation

Endocrine

- Low LH, FSH, and oestradiol
- Low T_3, T_4 in low normal range, normal TSH ('low T_3 syndrome')
- Mild elevation of plasma cortisol

- Elevated growth hormone
- Severe hypoglycaemia (rare)

Cardiovascular

- ECG abnormalities (especially in those with electrolyte disturbance): conduction defects, especially enhanced QT/RR slope, of major concern

Gastrointestinal

- Delayed gastric emptying; delayed small bowel transit time
- Decreased colonic motility (secondary to chronic laxative misuse)
- Acute gastric dilatation (rare, secondary to binge eating or excessive refeeding)

Haematological

- Moderate normocytic, normochromic anaemia
- Mild leucopenia with relative lymphocytosis
- Thrombocytopenia

Other metabolic abnormalities

- Hypercholesterolaemia
- Increased serum carotene
- Hypophosphataemia (exaggerated during refeeding)
- Dehydration
- Electrolyte disturbance (varied in form; present in those who vomit frequently or misuse large quantities of laxatives or diuretics): vomiting—metabolic alkalosis and hypokalaemia; laxative misuse—metabolic acidosis, hyponatraemia, hypokalaemia

Other abnormalities

- Osteopenia and osteoporosis, especially of the spine (with heightened fracture risk)
- Enlarged cerebral ventricles and external cerebrospinal fluid spaces (pseudoatrophy)

FSH, follicle-stimulating hormone; LH, luteinizing hormone; T_3, triiodothyronine; T_4, thyroxine; TSH, thyroid-stimulating hormone.

The panoply of physical abnormalities seen in the eating disorders can cloud thinking about diagnosis and management. The diagnosis of an eating disorder is made on positive grounds by using the history and mental state examination to detect the characteristic behavioural and attitudinal features, not by simply ruling out possible physical causes. No laboratory tests are required to make the diagnosis of an eating disorder and, unless there are positive reasons to suspect the presence of physical disease, no tests are required to exclude other general medical disorders. The management of any physical abnormalities should focus on the correction of the eating disorder. It is, for example, wrong to treat starvation-induced hypothyroidism with

thyroxine, but life-threatening complications must be addressed and the patient's nutritional state needs to be optimized.

Osteopenia and osteoporosis deserve particular mention: these are especially common in longstanding cases of anorexia nervosa and are associated with substantially increased fracture risk. The pathophysiology is ill-understood and there is uncertainty over management. Restoration of a healthy weight and an adequate diet, and with them the resumption of spontaneous menstruation, appear to be of central importance. The benefits of calcium supplementation and oestrogen replacement are unclear, and no other treatment has been shown to be of value.

Management

Bulimia nervosa

There have been over 70 randomized controlled trials evaluating treatments for bulimia nervosa and the main findings are reasonably consistent. Although almost all the trials have been 'efficacy' rather than 'effectiveness' studies, there are good reasons to think that their findings are relevant to management in most settings.

The research has generated three robust findings. First, the most effective treatment is a specific type of cognitive behaviour therapy (CBT) that focuses on modifying the specific behaviours and ways of thinking that maintain these patients' eating disorder. It typically involves about 20 individual treatment sessions over 5 months and results in substantial improvement with (on intention to treat analyses) more than half the patients making a complete and lasting recovery. The remainder range in outcome from markedly improved to not improved at all. The second finding is that antidepressant drugs have an 'antibulimic' effect. They may produce a rapid decline in the frequency of binge eating and purging, and an improvement in mood, but the effect is not as great as that obtained with CBT and, more importantly, the limited evidence suggests it is often not sustained. The third research finding is a negative one: no consistent predictors of outcome have been identified.

Three less robust findings have also emerged. First, combining CBT with antidepressant drugs results in few consistent benefits over CBT alone. Second, findings from two trials suggest that a short-term focal psychotherapy termed 'interpersonal psychotherapy' may be as effective as CBT, but it takes considerably longer to work. Third, simple, largely behavioural, treatments (including forms of self-help) that include elements of CBT may help a subset of patients, but they are unlikely to be sufficient for most.

In summary, CBT is the clear treatment of choice for bulimia nervosa. It is not a panacea but it has the potential to benefit many patients. Having said this, clinical experience and research evidence suggest that few patients receive it. Arguably, the main role for antidepressant drugs is as a readily-delivered initial intervention (possibly provided in primary care), the second step being full CBT (delivered by a trained therapist). It is not possible to formulate evidence-based guidelines for the treatment of patients who do not respond to CBT.

Anorexia nervosa

There has been a very limited amount of research on anorexia nervosa, in part because it is uncommon and in part because its treatment is often complex and lengthy. The following comments therefore simply reflect mainstream current opinion. In principle, there are four aspects to management. The first is to help patients see that they need help and to maintain their motivation thereafter, which is crucial given their reluctance to change.

The second aspect is weight restoration. This is needed to reverse malnutrition and of itself usually leading to substantial improvement in the patient's overall state. It may be achieved on an outpatient, day patient, or inpatient basis, their relative merits being the subject of debate. Indications for hospitalization include risk of suicide, severe interpersonal problems at home, and failure of less intensive methods. Physical indications include a very low weight, rapid weight loss, and the presence of medical complications such as marked oedema, severe electrolyte disturbance, hypoglycaemia, or significant intercurrent infection. Under such circumstances admission should be to a general medical ward or a psychiatric unit with good access to general medical help. In either case it is a great advantage if staff are experienced in the management of anorexia nervosa. Hospitalization is invariably a preliminary to subsequent outpatient treatment. The third aspect of management is addressing patients' overevaluation of shape and weight, their eating habits, and their general psychosocial functioning. There is no single way to do this.

One approach that has some research support is a family-based treatment that appears to be of most value with younger patients and thus is mainly used with adolescents. CBT is a logical alternative for older patients, not least given its effectiveness in bulimia nervosa. However, its use in anorexia nervosa has not been well described and, at present, there is little evidence to support it. Both forms of treatment require training to implement them and both are best conducted on an outpatient basis.

The fourth aspect of management is only relevant to a small minority of cases. It is the use of compulsory treatment. Reconciling respect for patients' wishes and their right to receive good treatment can be difficult, and compulsory treatment, though legally permissible in many countries, should never be undertaken lightly. Drug treatment does not have an established place in the management of anorexia nervosa.

Eating disorder NOS

Binge eating disorder aside, the treatment of eating disorder NOS has barely been studied, a remarkable omission given its prevalence. The only advice that can be given is for clinicians to follow bulimia nervosa treatment guidelines in cases in which there is binge eating, and anorexia nervosa guidelines with patients whose weight is low. Alternatively, there is a new 'transdiagnostic' form of CBT that has been designed for the full range of eating disorders seen amongst adults.

There is a growing body of evidence concerning the treatment of binge eating disorder. Various treatments show promise, the greatest support being for an adaptation of the CBT for bulimia nervosa that has a marked effect on the binge eating of these patients, although it has little effect on their body weight.

Prevention

Programmes for the prevention of anorexia nervosa and bulimia nervosa have been developed, but none has been satisfactorily evaluated. The primary prevention programmes tend to focus on schoolgirls, the group most at risk. However, two specific difficulties have been encountered: first, there is a danger of magnifying concerns about shape and weight rather than reducing them; and second, there is potential for conflict between the content of these programmes, which tend to emphasize the risks of undue dieting, and those directed at the prevention of obesity.

Further reading

Fairburn CG (2008). Eating disorders and cognitive behavior therapy. Guilford Press, New York.

Grilo CM (2006). *Eating and weight disorders*. Psychology Press, Hove and New York.

Mitchell JE, Crow S (2006). Medical complications of anorexia nervosa and bulimia nervosa. *Curr Opin Psychiatry*, **19**, 438–43.

National Institute for Clinical Excellence (2004). *Eating disorders. Core interventions in the treatment and management of eating disorders in primary and secondary care.* National Institute for Clinical Excellence, London.

Palmer B (ed) (2000). *Helping people with eating disorders.* Wiley, Chichester.

26.5.7 Schizophrenia, bipolar disorder, obsessive–compulsive disorder, and personality disorder

Stephen Lawrie

Essentials

Schizophrenia—is characterized by phenomena that qualitatively differ from everyday experience. These may be 'positive symptoms', commonly auditory hallucinations and/or bizarre delusions, or 'negative symptoms', commonly including a loss of emotion (flat affect), apathy, self-neglect, and social withdrawal. Acute positive symptoms generally respond well to any antipsychotic drug, but prognosis is often poor, with most suffering chronic symptoms, numerous relapses, unemployment, and social isolation.

Bipolar disorder ('manic depression')—the key features are episodic increases or decreases in mood, thoughts, and activity. Patients who are hypomanic feel 'high', report rapid thoughts, have limitless energy, require little sleep, and are disinhibited—problems that become uncontrollable if they become manic. If depressed, mood is low. Hypomania generally responds well to antipsychotic drugs. Lithium is also effective and remains the mainstay of treatment. Carbamazepine and sodium valproate are alternative mood stabilizers. Recurrence is the norm.

Obsessive–compulsive disorder—is characterized by recurrent, unwanted ideas or images that are recognized by the patient as their own, and repeated behaviours or mental acts (rituals) to relieve tension. Patients are commonly ill for years before they come to psychiatric attention. Both drugs (the tricyclic antidepressant clomipramine, and selective serotonin reuptake inhibitors (SSRIs)) and psychotherapy are effective. A chronic waxing and waning course is typical.

Personality disorders—people with personality disorders are common, disabled, and often regarded as 'problem patients'. They are defined by having culturally abnormal experience or behaviour, with onset in early adulthood, which is pervasive and inflexible, leading to distress or impairment. Few treatments have been evaluated: cognitive therapy may reduce the frequency of deliberate self-harm; dysthymia responds to antidepressants; paranoid, schizotypal, and borderline patients may benefit from antipsychotic drugs; and those with obsessional personality disorder may respond to SSRIs.

Schizophrenia

Schizophrenia is characterized by phenomena that qualitatively differ from everyday experience: delusions, hallucinations, disorganized speech/behaviour, and negative symptoms. Onset is in early adulthood (median age 25 years). Men tend to get the illness earlier, more severely, and possibly more often than women. The incidence is only 15 in 100 000 of the population per year, but the prevalence is about 5 in 1000 due to chronicity, and the lifetime risk is 1%.

Aetiology

Recent research, using reliable diagnostic criteria based on clinical features since diagnostic laboratory tests are not available, has established that schizophrenia is multifactorial, with polygenic, neurobiological, and psychosocial components.

Genetic factors account for 80% of the liability to schizophrenia: having an affected relative increases the risk 5 to 50 times, depending on the relationship. Several plausible genes, such as neuregulin 1, have been identified in recent years. Other risk factors include obstetric complications, developmental problems, and cannabis use, but these only double the risk. Stressful life events can be precipitants, but only in those otherwise predisposed.

There are subtle abnormalities of brain structure and function (particularly of the temporal and frontal lobes) in both chronic and first episode cases. Developmental abnormalities in brain structure (e.g. hippocampal volume) and function (e.g. dopamine sensitivity), probably exacerbated by drug and/or stress related changes around onset, are thought to disrupt frontotemporal integration and bring on symptoms, but direct evidence is limited.

Clinical features

Hallucinations and delusions are 'positive symptoms', meaning that they are abnormal by their presence. Hallucinations are perceptions in the absence of stimuli. They are usually auditory voices speaking the patients' thoughts or commenting on their actions. Hallucinations in other senses can occur but suggest a neurological disorder. Delusions are unshakeable false beliefs. Persecutory ('paranoid') delusions are common but occur in all psychoses. Delusions of passivity (actions or feelings 'made' by external forces) and other bizarre beliefs are more specific. The other positive symptom is thought disorder—an illogical sequence of thoughts (as revealed in speech).

'Negative symptoms' are features that are abnormal by their absence: these commonly include a loss of emotion (flat affect), apathy, self-neglect, and social withdrawal. These may be prodromal, but are more common in chronic patients.

Differential diagnosis

Prodromal symptoms can be similar to depression. Drug intoxication can cause positive symptoms, but also disorientation. Neurological causes, e.g. temporal lobe epilepsy or brain tumours, are rare. Delusions of passivity can be confused with obsessional ideas, but the latter are recognized as one's own. Negative symptoms can be confused with depression or parkinsonism. The distinction of schizophrenia from bipolar disorder is based on whether psychotic or affective features predominate; occasionally, if both are notably present, a diagnosis of schizoaffective disorder is appropriate.

Management

Acute positive symptoms generally respond well to any antipsychotic drug (Table 26.5.7.1). These work by dopamine receptor blockade. The main adverse effects are sedation, weight gain, and extrapyramidal syndromes (acute dystonia, akathisia, parkinsonism, tardive dyskinesia), which are best avoided by minimizing dosage, but dystonias and parkinsonism respond to anticholinergics. Medication should be continued for at least 2 years after an acute episode to reduce relapse rates. See Chapter 26.6.1 for further discussion.

Patients often refuse medication, due to adverse effects or lack of insight. Some are suitable for depot medication (intramuscular injections of esterified antipsychotics, see Table 26.5.7.1). The second generation antipsychotics generally cause fewer extrapyramidal problems but more weight gain. It is claimed that they are effective in those with negative and treatment-resistant positive symptoms, but clozapine is the only proven such treatment. Clozapine is the definitive and arguably only 'atypical' antipsychotic, but carries a considerable risk of neutropenia and agranulocytosis. These treatments are not contraindicated in pregnancy, as they confer only a small increased risk of teratogenicity and an untreated psychosis is often more dangerous.

There are few effective nondrug treatments. Illness education reduces relapse rates, as does teaching social skills, but these may primarily work by improving drug compliance. Early enthusiasm for cognitive therapy, as a means to reduce symptoms and relapse rates, is waning. Vocational rehabilitation helps to get people back to work.

Table 26.5.7.1 Commonly used antipsychotic drugs

Type/name of drug	Optimal dose[a]	Main side effects
Phenothiazines		
Chlorpromazine	400–600 mg/day	Sedation
Thioridazine	400–600 mg/day	Anticholinergic
Trifluoperazine	20–30 mg/day	Extrapyramidal
Butyrophenones		
Haloperidol	8–12 mg/day	Extrapyramidal
Benzamides		
Sulpiride	800–1200 mg/day	Minimal
Pimozide	8–10 mg/day	Minimal
Depot injections		
Flupentixol decanoate	40 mg every 2 weeks	Extrapyramidal
Fluphenazine decanoate	25 mg every 2 weeks	Extrapyramidal
Haloperidol decanoate	100 mg monthly	Extrapyramidal
Second-generation drugs		
Risperidone	6 mg/day	Extrapyramidal
Olanzapine	15 mg/day	Weight gain
Quetiapine	300–600 mg/day	Sedation
Amisulpiride	800–1200 mg/day	Agitation
Atypicals		
Clozapine	300–600 mg/day	Hypersalivation

[a] This dose of chlorpromazine is established from meta-analyses. Others are calculated as chlorpromazine equivalents, but these are uncertain for depot, second generation, and atypical drugs.

Primary prevention is not a realistic prospect until better understanding of the pathogenesis of schizophrenia allows early detection. There is some evidence that earlier treatments may be associated with a slightly better prognosis, but the trials are small and rarely blind.

Prognosis

The prognosis is generally poor. About 25% of patients will only have one or two episodes, but most will suffer chronic symptoms, numerous relapses, unemployment, and social isolation. Most patients smoke heavily, and many abuse alcohol/drugs, resulting in a high premature mortality rate—especially from myocardial infarction. Suicide is all too common, leading to 5 to 10% of deaths.

Bipolar disorder (BPD)

The key features of bipolar disorder ('manic depression') are episodic increases or decreases in mood, thoughts, and activity, lasting at least 1 week. The prevalence, incidence, and lifetime risk of BPD are similar to schizophrenia (at 0.5%, 0.01%, and 1%, respectively). The sex incidence is equal in BPD, the mean age at onset is 21 years in both sexes, and bipolar II ('highs' that do not cause disability) is twice as common as bipolar I.

Aetiology

The risk factors for BPD are similar to those for schizophrenia. Genetic influences are equally strong, and some of the genes almost certainly overlap, but other associations are weaker in BPD. There may be more specific abnormalities in monoamine metabolism and neuroendocrine function, and a first 'high' may be precipitated by antidepressants, stimulants, steroids, or childbirth.

Clinical features

Patients who are 'hypomanic' feel 'high', report rapid thoughts, have limitless energy, require little sleep, and are 'disinhibited', i.e. they are overfamiliar and take risks. They speak quickly ('pressure of speech') and jump between topics ('flight of ideas'), but with logical connections between thoughts. If 'manic', these problems are uncontrollable without treatment and patients can be a risk to themselves and others. Manic patients often have delusions and hallucinations, but these are usually mood congruent—e.g. grandiose delusions of special abilities.

If depressed, mood is low, activities are not enjoyed (anhedonia), interests are diminished, energy is low, sleep is disturbed, appetite is reduced, and weight may fall. Patients typically think they are worthless, the future is hopeless, and they may be suicidal. Severe melancholic depression is accompanied by early morning wakening, diurnal mood variation (feeling worst in the morning), and psychomotor retardation (head down, expressionless face, little spontaneous activity). Any psychotic symptoms are again mood congruent, e.g. delusions of sin or voices criticizing the patient.

Occasionally there are mixed states, where patients have some features of (hypo)mania and depression simultaneously.

Differential diagnosis

Around one-third of patients will have several depressive episodes before their first 'high'. With no previous history, especially if old, (hypo)mania may rarely be attributable to thyroid disease or dementia. In established cases, the main differential is schizophrenia as individual symptoms can be similar (e.g. low mood vs flat affect, flight of ideas vs thought disorder), but the key is that BPD is an episodic disturbance of mood.

Management

The treatment of depression is discussed in Chapter 26.6.5, but antidepressants (particularly tricyclics) should be used with care in depressed patients with BPD as they can cause 'switching' into (hypo)mania—especially if patients are not on prophylactic lithium, carbamazepine, or valproate. Lamotrigine and quetiapine are alternatives, but with limited support from randomized clinical trials.

'High' patients may reject treatment, but most will later report feeling out of control and gratitude for being treated. (Hypo)mania generally responds well to antipsychotic drugs (Table 26.5.7.1). Lithium is also effective, particularly with high serum levels (c. 1.0 mmol/litre). Carbamazepine and sodium valproate are alternative mood stabilizers, with fewer adverse effects, but may be less effective. 'Rapid cycling disorder' (four or more illness episodes annually) and acute mixed episodes are probably best treated with mood stabilizers and/or antipsychotics.

Prophylaxis is required if patients have two or more episodes in 5 years. Lithium (maintained at 0.5–1.0 mmol/litre) is the treatment of choice as it reduces both (hypo)manic and depressive relapses, and reduces suicide rates. Common adverse effects are dose-related and include diarrhoea, tremor, thirst, polyuria, and weight gain. Long-term effects can include hypothyroidism and renal impairment. Lithium is excreted in competition with sodium, hence thiazide diuretics, nonsteroidal agents, and dehydration can precipitate toxicity. Sudden vomiting, coarse tremor, sedation, or dysarthria require urgent medical treatment to avoid seizures, renal failure, and death.

Lithium is contraindicated in pregnancy and breastfeeding because it increases the rate of Fallot's tetralogy 10- to 20-fold and can cause neonatal toxicity. Carbamazepine and sodium valproate are associated with spina bifida. Best practice is therefore to use antipsychotics for symptom control until after delivery. Mood stabilizers should then be reinstituted, and bottle feeding commended, as relapse is very common postnatally.

Early diagnosis and self-medication can minimize relapses in established cases, but primary prevention is not presently possible.

Prognosis

Acute episodes generally respond to treatment, but 10% of patients will be ill for a year and 50% of (hypo)manic patients immediately become depressed. Recurrence is the norm and becomes more frequent with age. Many patients have chronic symptoms between episodes, such that only about one-third of patients fully recover. Employment and social difficulties are common. The annual mortality from cardiovascular collapse or suicide before treatment was possible was 10%; but premature mortality remains unacceptably high.

Obsessive–compulsive disorder (OCD)

OCD is characterized by recurrent, unwanted ideas or images that are recognized as one's own and repeated behaviours or mental acts ('rituals') to relieve tension. It was originally viewed as a neurosis, but the *Diagnostic and statistical manual of mental disorders*, 4th edition (DSM-IV) does not use this ambiguous term and classifies OCD as an anxiety state. OCD is common, with a prevalence of 1% and lifetime risk of 2 to 3%. Onset occurs at all ages, with peaks in the first and fourth decades, and a slight excess in women.

Aetiology

OCD runs in families, but twin studies are inconclusive. Obsessional personality is a risk factor, as is Tourette's syndrome. OCD can arise after lesions of the frontal lobes and basal ganglia, which are regions also implicated by studies of brain structure and function in patients. Follow-up functional imaging has found recovery is associated with normalized activity in these areas of the brain. Effective drugs all inhibit serotonin (5-hydroxytryptamine, 5-HT) reuptake, and neurochemical evidence also suggests postsynaptic serotoninergic hypersensitivity and/or low synaptic 5-HT concentrations.

Clinical features

Patients are commonly ill for years before they come to psychiatric attention. Obsessions are recurrent, resisted, and unwanted, but regarded as one's own. There may be a fear of contamination, excessive doubt over actions, a somatic concern, a desire for precision, or an aggressive or sexual impulse. Several obsessions usually coexist. Obsessional slowness and precision are more common in men.

Compulsions are repetitive behaviours or mental acts based on obsessions: they are usually performed to reduce anxiety and are not in themselves pleasurable. Checking, cleaning, and counting are the most common acts. Most are performed in private as they are recognized as senseless.

Differential diagnosis

Rituals and superstitions are common in childhood and only pathological if they cause distress. Distinguishing OCD from depression/anxiety can be difficult, as secondary depression is frequent in OCD and there is often an obsessional quality to thoughts in depression and anxiety. Obsessions can appear to be similar to phobias, but people with OCD may actually seek out anxiety-provoking stimuli whereas phobics avoid them.

Management

Both drugs and psychotherapy are effective in OCD. The tricyclic antidepressant clomipramine and the selective serotonin reuptake inhibitors (SSRIs) work, but high doses may be required. Clomipramine is probably most effective, particularly in treating patients with comorbid depression, but has unpleasant adverse effects (sedation, weight gain, anticholinergic). Response to treatment may take months and symptoms tend to return if drugs are stopped.

The most effective psychotherapeutic techniques are cognitive and behavioural. Most therapists now combine cognitive therapy, in which faulty beliefs of impending catastrophe and exaggerated responsibility are challenged, with the standard treatment. Behavioural therapy begins with making a complete list of obsessions, compulsions, and avoidance behaviour, which is arranged in an anxiety-provoking hierarchy. Exposure to anxiety-provoking stimuli (with or without therapist 'modelling') and response prevention (avoiding rituals by persuasion, monitoring, or adopting alternative behaviours) may also involve family members. Recent trials suggest that the combination of antidepressants and exposure may be best of all.

Table 26.5.7.2 Personality disorders

Type	Prevalence[a]	Essential features	Associated disorders	Possible treatments
Eccentric				
Paranoid	2% generally 5% outpatients 20% inpatients	Suspicious; distrustful	Paranoid psychoses; depression	Antipsychotics
Schizoid	3% generally	Social detachment; emotional restriction	Brief psychotic episodes; depression	None known
Schizotypal	3% generally	Strange ideas or experiences; social discomfort	Schizophrenia; depression	Antipsychotics
Emotional				
Histrionic	2–3% generally 10–15% patients	Attention-seeking; overemotional; seductive	Somatization disorder; conversion; depression	None known
Antisocial (psychopathic)	3% generally 50% prisoners	Callous disregard for others	Substance abuse; depression	None known
Narcissistic	1% generally 10% patients	Grandiose; need for admiration; lack of empathy	Depression; anorexia; substance abuse	None known
Borderline	2% generally 10% outpatients 20% inpatients	Unstable moods and relationships; impulsive	Depression; anorexia; substance abuse	Antipsychotics; cognitive therapy
Anxious				
Obsessive–compulsive	1% generally 5% patients	Perfectionistic; controlled	Obsessive–compulsive disorder	SSRIs
Dependent	30% patients	Clinging; submissive; need for care	Depression; anxiety	None known
Avoidant	1% generally 10% outpatients	Social inhibition; fear of criticism; timid	Anxiety states	Psychotherapy

SSRI, selective serotonin reuptake inhibitor.
[a]Refers to prevalence in psychiatric settings.

Prognosis

Most patients improve with treatment but have relapses. Some cases progressively deteriorate, particularly men with an early onset. Recent studies challenge the convention that suicide is rare.

Personality disorder (PD)

PD is commonly seen as distinct from psychiatric 'illness' and untreatable, which is ironic given that many PDs were originally described because they had links to particular psychiatric disorders, and that recent research has rediscovered these and found possible treatments. It is defined as culturally abnormal experience or behaviour, with onset in early adulthood, that is pervasive and inflexible, leading to distress or impairment. Only a brief description of subtypes (Table 26.5.7.2) and specific points is possible here.

Aetiology

Paranoid and borderline traits are clearly heritable, and schizotypy is genetically and biologically linked to schizophrenia. Paranoid and antisocial PDs are more common in men; borderline, histrionic, and dependent PDs in women. Childhood adversity, such as low parental affection and/or harsh punishment, is a general risk factor, but specific effects are difficult to identify. Child sexual abuse, for example, may be linked to self-harm and substance abuse rather than any particular PD. People with antisocial PD have mild frontal lobe deficits—and similar head trauma related changes in personality have been described. Several neuroimaging studies have reported abnormalities in borderline PD and functional correlates of personality dimensions like impulsiveness, aggression, and neuroticism.

Clinical features

Many patients meet more than one set of PD criteria. Some borderline patients report auditory and visual hallucinations. Dysthymia (formerly depressive PD) and cyclothymia (also formerly a PD) are now seen as mild depression and bipolar disorder, respectively. Paranoid, schizotypal, obsessional, and avoidant PDs may be similarly reclassified in the future. About one-half of all prisoners will have antisocial PD, but most people with antisocial PD are not prisoners.

Differential diagnosis

The main differential is with the associated psychiatric disorder and other PDs. As a rule, the eccentric cluster can present similarly to schizophrenia, the emotional cluster like bipolar disorder, and the anxious cluster with anxiety states. Borderline PD can cause diagnostic difficulties with both schizophrenia and BPD, but psychotic experiences tend to be transient in the former.

Management

Clinical management has conservative aims, but pressure is being put on psychiatrists to do more. Few treatments have been evaluated for PD *per se*. Cognitive therapy may generally reduce the frequency of deliberate self-harm. Dysthymia responds to antidepressants; paranoid, schizotypal, and borderline patients may benefit from antipsychotic drugs; and obsessional PD may respond to SSRIs.

Prognosis

Recurrent deliberate self-harm and eventual suicide is common. Patients with PDs who develop other psychiatric disorders also have a poor prognosis for that disorder, although recent studies suggest that many PDs will ease and sometimes even spontaneously remit with time.

Further reading

Schizophrenia

Harrison PJ, Weinberger DR (2005). Schizophrenia genes, gene expression, and neuropathology: on the matter of their convergence. *Mol Psychiatry*, **10**, 40–68 (errata in *Mol Psychiatry*, 10, 420 and *Mol Psychiatry*, 10, 804).

Johnstone EC, *et al.* (eds) (2004). *Companion to psychiatric studies*, 6th edition. Churchill Livingstone, Edinburgh.

Lewis DA, Gonzalez-Burgos G (2006). Pathophysiologically based treatment interventions in schizophrenia. *Nat Med*, **12**, 1016–22.

Naeem Z, McIntosh A, Lawrie SM (2006). Schizophrenia. In: *Clinical evidence concise*, pp. 383–7. BMJ Publishing Group, London.

Bipolar disorder

Belmaker RH (2004). Bipolar disorder. *N Engl J Med*, **351**, 476–86.

Geddes J (2006). Bipolar disorder. In: *Clinical evidence (concise)*, pp. 344–8. BMJ Publishing Group, London.

Kupfer DJ (2005). The increasing medical burden in bipolar disorder. *JAMA*, **293**, 2528–30.

Obsessive–compulsive disordr

Heyman I, Mataix-Cols D, Fineberg NA (2006). Obsessive-compulsive disorder. *BMJ*, **333**, 424–9.

Jenike MA (2004). Clinical practice. Obsessive–compulsive disorder. *N Engl J Med*, **350**, 259–65.

Personality disorder

American Psychiatric Association (1994). *The diagnostic and statistical manual of mental disorders (DSM-IV)*, 4th edition. APA, Washington DC.

Johnson JG, *et al.* (2006). Parenting behaviors associated with risk for offspring personality disorder during adulthood. *Arch Gen Psychiatry*, **63**, 579–87.

Lieb K, *et al.* (2004). Borderline personality disorder. *Lancet*, **364**, 453–61.

Psychiatric treatments

Contents

26.6.1 Psychopharmacology in medical practice

Philip J. Cowen

Essentials

Psychotropic drugs play an indispensable role in the treatment of severe psychiatric illness such as schizophrenia and bipolar disorder. They are often used to treat other conditions, particularly depression and anxiety disorders, but for these disorders nondrug treatments are effective and—if available—are often preferred by patients.

Antidepressants—newer drugs, particularly selective serotonin reuptake inhibitors (SSRIs), have replaced traditional tricyclic antidepressants in the treatment of depression. These are somewhat better tolerated and, with the exception of venlafaxine, are safer in overdose. All patients should be monitored carefully following the introduction of antidepressant medication because the risk of suicidal behaviour appears to be higher at this time. Patients with recurrent depression often benefit from maintenance treatment with antidepressants.

Lithium—this continues to be the leading mood stabilizing agent prescribed for the treatment of bipolar disorder in the United Kingdom, but it has significant adverse effects that particularly involve the kidneys and central nervous system. It also has a narrow therapeutic index and drug interactions carry a high risk of serious toxicity. For these reasons there is growing use of anticonvulsant drugs such as sodium valproate as alternatives to lithium.

Antipsychotics—in the treatment of schizophrenia, atypical antipsychotic drugs are replacing conventional agents such as haloperidol and chlorpromazine because of their better perceived adverse effect profile, particularly with regard to extrapyramidal movement disorders. However, some atypical agents, particularly clozapine and olanzapine, cause excessive weight gain and have been linked with type 2 diabetes and disturbances in lipid metabolism. Of these agents, only clozapine has clearly superior efficacy relative to conventional agents, but it carries a risk of agranulocytosis and hence the need for weekly blood count monitoring complicates its use.

Benzodiazepines—use of these drugs for the treatment of anxiety and insomnia continues to decline because of their recognized liability to cause tolerance and dependence. They are indicated only for short-term use, preferably on an as needed basis. The same advice applies to other hypnotic agents such as the 'Z' drugs. Where psychological treatments are not effective or unavailable, antidepressants treatment—particularly with SSRIs—can be used to treat a range of anxiety disorders, including obsessive–compulsive disorder.

Introduction

Psychotropic drugs are widely used in medical practice, hence most clinicians are likely to have under their care a number of patients receiving treatment with psychoactive medication (Table 26.6.1.1). Practitioners therefore need to have an understanding of the uses and unwanted effects of psychotropic drugs, particularly of the way in which such medication can interact with drugs used to treat other medical disorders.

Most psychotropic drugs are prescribed for the treatment of depressive and anxiety disorders. This reflects the frequency of these conditions in both primary care and general hospital settings; accordingly, drug treatment for anxiety and depression will often be instituted both by general practitioners and hospital clinicians. Similarly, while the principal use of antipsychotic drugs is in the treatment of schizophrenia, such agents are also frequently used in general hospitals in the management of organic psychoses. Finally, while treatment with mood stabilizing drugs, such as lithium, will generally be initiated by psychiatrists, patients receiving long-term therapy may well require treatment for coexisting medical disorders; because of which, a knowledge of the effects of lithium on

Table 26.6.1.1 Classification of clinical psychotropic drugs

Name	Examples of classes	Indications
Antipsychotic	Phenothiazines Butyrophenones Substituted benzamides	Acute treatment of schizophrenia and mania, prophylaxis of schizophrenia
Antidepressant	Tricyclic antidepressants Monoamine oxidase inhibitors Selective serotonin reuptake Inhibitors (SSRIs)	Major depression (acute treatment and prophylaxis), anxiety disorders, obsessive–compulsive disorder (SSRIs)
Mood stabilizer	Lithium Carbamazepine Valproate	Acute treatment of mania, prophylaxis of recurrent mood disorder
Anxiolytic	Benzodiazepines Azapirones (buspirone)	Generalized anxiety disorder
Hypnotic	Benzodiazepines Cyclopyrrolones (zopiclone) Imidazopyridines (zolpidem)	Insomnia

5-HT, 5-hydroxytryptamine.

different body systems and its liability to produce adverse drug interactions will be required.

For many psychiatric conditions, particularly anxiety and depressive disorders, psychological treatments are as effective as psychotropic drugs and may have other advantages (Box 26.6.1.1). Hence, if appropriate psychological treatments are available they may be considered before the use of drug therapy.

Drug overdose

The effects of deliberate or accidental overdose of psychotropic drugs will also involve physicians (see Chapters 9.1 and 26.5.2). Related to this is the general point that when prescribing psychotropic drugs, particularly for depressed patients, the risk of overdose should always be considered. If such a risk is present, the practitioner should: (1) ensure that medication is dispensed in small amounts; (2) consider asking a close relative to supervise the medication; (3) use a relatively nontoxic drug, if possible.

Pharmacokinetic factors

Most psychotropic drugs are highly lipophilic and well absorbed from the gastrointestinal tract. They are metabolized by the liver to water-soluble derivatives that are eliminated by the kidneys. Therefore, their half-life will be prolonged in patients with hepatic

Box 26.6.1.1 Possible advantages of cognitive behavioural therapy (CBT) compared to psychotropic drugs

- Fewer adverse effects
- Better long-term efficacy
- Reduced risk of relapse
- Better for patient's self-esteem

Box 26.6.1.2 Effects of sudden discontinuation of an SSRI

- Sleep disturbance—insomnia, nightmares
- Mood symptoms—irritability, anxiety, emotional lability
- Gastrointestinal symptoms—nausea, diarrhoea
- Sensory—electric shock sensations, light-headedness, vertigo
- Somatic—headache, lethargy, sweating

or renal impairment and in older patients. Where psychotropic medication is added to another drug treatment the possibility of drug interaction must be considered. For example, some selective serotonin reuptake inhibitors (SSRIs) are potent inhibitors of hepatic cytochrome P450 enzymes and can thereby increase plasma levels of coadministered drugs such as warfarin.

Withdrawal of psychotropic medication

Psychotropic and many other classes of drugs produce neuroadaptive changes during their repeated administration. Readjustment has to occur when drug treatment is stopped, and this may appear clinically as a withdrawal or abstinence syndrome. Characteristic abstinence syndromes have been described for the antidepressants, particularly SSRIs (Box 26.6.1.2) and anxiolytics, while the sudden discontinuation of lithium can provoke a 'rebound' mania. It is therefore prudent to withdraw psychotropic drugs slowly whenever possible. It is also important to be able to distinguish withdrawal syndromes from relapse of the disorder being treated.

Compliance and concordance with treatment

Compliance is an even greater problem when prescribing psychotropic drugs than it is in general therapeutics. Psychoactive drugs frequently have unpleasant side effects and, while side effects are experienced early in treatment, several days may elapse before a therapeutic response is evident. In addition, patients may not see the need for treatment or believe that it can help them. Careful explanation accompanied by written instructions can help to ensure that necessary medication is taken.

It is increasingly recognized that the successful and safe use of medication requires a collaborative relationship between patient and doctor. The term 'concordance' may be preferred to 'compliance', which carries the implicit assumption that the patient's task is to obey instructions. It is therefore important to acquire an understanding of the patient's attitude to their illness as well as its treatment. For example, discussion that helps patients to weigh the advantages and disadvantages of drug treatment ('compliance therapy') has been shown to benefit those with schizophrenia.

Antidepressant drugs

All currently employed antidepressant drugs increase the activity of serotoninergic (5-hydroxytryptamine, 5-HT) and/or noradrenergic neurons in the CNS through one mechanism or another. The pharmacological actions of both noradrenaline (norepinephrine) and 5-HT in the synapse are terminated by specific reuptake pumps that draw these neurotransmitters back into the presynaptic nerve ending. Most antidepressants potentiate the action of 5-HT and noradrenaline by blocking this reuptake process.

Serotonin reuptake inhibitors (SSRIs)

The actions of SSRIs are confined to blockade of the reuptake of 5-HT and their use is associated with a sustained increase in brain 5-HT neurotransmission.

Principal drugs

These are citalopram, escitalopram, fluoxetine, fluvoxamine, paroxetine, and sertraline.

Indications and use

With the availability of generic forms of citalopram, sertraline and fluoxetine, SSRIs are now first-line treatment for moderate to severe depression. They are modestly better tolerated than tricyclic antidepressants, lack significant cardiotoxicity, and are relatively safe in overdose. They are generally nonsedating and can be given in a single dose once daily. There are few important therapeutic differences between them. If treatment is successful, it is usual to continue the antidepressant for 4 to 6 months (so called 'continuation therapy'). This reduces the risk of early relapse by about half. Some patients with recurrent depressive illness require long-term prophylactic treatment with antidepressant drugs. This should be considered in those who have had more than two episodes of depression in the previous 5 years, particularly if the episodes have been severe in terms of symptomatology and impact on work and social functioning.

Adverse effects

The main adverse effects of SSRIs are shown in Table 26.6.1.2. They can cause activation and agitation early in treatment and there has been controversy as to whether this might be associated with an increased risk of suicidal behaviour when therapy is initiated.

There is some evidence for an effect of this nature in young people and, with the exception of fluoxetine, SSRIs are contraindicated in the treatment of depression in patients less than 18 years of age. The evidence for a prosuicidal effect of SSRIs in adults is more equivocal and, at a population level, some studies show a decreased suicide rate correlating with SSRI prescription. However, it does seem likely that the initiation of antidepressant drug treatment of any kind is associated with an increased risk of self-harm in the first weeks of treatment. Whether this represents a specific pharmacological effect is unclear. In practical terms, however, it suggests that depressed patients should be carefully monitored in the days after starting antidepressant medication and that medication should be prescribed in limited amounts.

Drug interactions

SSRIs, with the exception of citalopram and escitalopram, slow the metabolism of numerous other drugs including warfarin, theophylline, anticonvulsants, antipsychotics, and tricyclic antidepressants. Dangerous interactions, characterized by 5-HT neurotoxicity, have been reported between SSRIs and monoamine oxidase inhibitors. This may be particularly problematic with fluoxetine, whose active metabolite norfluoxetine has a half-life of 7 to 10 days. At least 5 weeks should therefore elapse between stopping fluoxetine and prescribing a monoamine oxidase inhibitor. SSRIs may also produce 5-HT toxicity in combination with lithium. SSRIs may increase the risk of upper gastrointestinal bleeding, particularly if given in conjunction with nonsteroidal anti-inflammatory drugs (NSAIDs).

Other, newer antidepressants

Principal drugs

These can be classified as follows:

- selective noradrenaline reuptake inhibitors—reboxetine
- selective serotonin-noradrenaline reuptake inhibitors—duloxetine, venlafaxine
- monoamine receptor antagonists—mirtazapine, trazodone

Reboxetine inhibits only the reuptake of noradrenaline. Venlafaxine is a potent blocker of 5-HT reuptake and at higher doses blocks the reuptake of noradrenaline as well. Duloxetine has a similar action. Both trazodone and mirtazapine are 5-HT_2 receptor antagonists and block α_1-adrenoceptors in addition, which gives them a sedating profile. Mirtazapine also blocks inhibitory presynaptic α_2-adrenoceptors, resulting in an increased release of noradrenaline.

Indications and use

These antidepressants can be used to treat patients in whom SSRIs are poorly tolerated or ineffective. The lack of sedation associated with reboxetine, duloxetine, and venlafaxine can be beneficial in outpatients striving to carry out their usual activities. With the exception of venlafaxine these drugs lack significant cardiotoxicity and are relatively safe in overdose.

Adverse effects

The main adverse effects of the other, newer antidepressants are shown in Table 26.6.1.2. The major distinction between compounds is whether or not they are sedating. The sedating antidepressants have the advantage of improving sleep at an early stage, but they

Table 26.6.1.2 Newer antidepressants

Drug	Mechanism	Adverse effects
SSRIs	5-HT reuptake blockade	Nausea, insomnia, headache, anxiety, rash, sweating, sexual dysfunction, low sodium state, extrapyramidal movement disorders (rare), seizure (rare)
Venlafaxine, duloxetine	5-HT and noradrenaline reuptake blockade	Nausea, headache, insomnia, sweating, anxiety, hypertension, sexual dysfunction, seizure (rare), overdose toxicity (venlafaxine)
Reboxetine	Noradrenaline reuptake blockade	Dry mouth, sweating, constipation, insomnia
Trazodone	5-HT_2-receptor antagonism α_1-Aadrenoceptor blockade	Sedation, dizziness, nausea, postural hypotension, priapism (rare), cardiac arrhythmias (rare), seizure (rare)
Mirtazapine	$5\text{-HT}_2/\alpha_2$-receptor agonist	Sedation, weight gain, abnormal liver function tests, reversible agranulocytosis (rare), seizure (rare)

5-HT, 5-hydroxytryptamine; SSRI, selective serotonin reuptake inhibitor.

may impair cognitive function, while the reverse is true for duloxetine, venlafaxine, and reboxetine which may impair sleep.

Drug interactions

Duloxetine and venlafaxine, like SSRIs, potentiate 5-HT function and therefore can cause serious 5-HT neurotoxicity when combined with monoamine oxidase inhibitors (MAOIs). Toxicity can also occur in combination with lithium. Trazodone and mirtazapine may increase the sedative effects of other centrally acting drugs. Reboxetine should not be given with other agents that might potentiate noradrenaline function (such as MAOIs) or increase blood pressure (such as ergot derivatives).

Tricyclic antidepressants

Tricyclic antidepressants (TCAs) inhibit the neuronal uptake of noradrenaline and 5-HT. They have numerous other pharmacological properties, but these are thought to contribute to their adverse effect profile rather than their therapeutic activity. However, some of these adverse effects, e.g. sedation, can prove beneficial in certain circumstances.

Principal drugs

These are amitriptyline, clomipramine, desmethylimipramine, dosulepin, doxepin, imipramine, lofepramine, and nortriptyline.

Indications and use

TCAs are now prescribed somewhat less for depression than are SSRIs, but they still retain a role in patients with severe or treatment-resistant depression or in those who have shown a good previous clinical response. Many tricyclics are sedating, which can be helpful in patients with sleep disturbance and anxiety. To obtain tolerance to side effects, it is usual to begin treatment at a low dose, e.g. 25 to 50 mg of amitriptyline at night, and to increase the amount over about 2 to 3 weeks to the usual therapeutic dose, which ranges between 75 and 150 mg daily for amitriptyline and imipramine.

Adverse effects

TCAs possess antagonist properties at a variety of neurotransmitter receptors, including muscarinic cholinergic receptors, α_1-adrenoceptors, and H1 histamine receptors. These receptor antagonist effects account for much of the adverse effect profile of these agents, particularly their anticholinergic properties (Table 26.6.1.3). TCAs also possess membrane stabilizing effects; these underlie their most serious side effect of cardiotoxicity, which can be particularly problematic in tricyclic overdose, where ingestion of less than 1 g can sometimes prove fatal. Lofepramine, however, is relatively safe in overdose. TCAs should be used with caution in patients with cardiovascular disease. They also lower the seizure threshold and can thereby aggravate pre-existing epilepsy or sometimes cause seizures *de novo*.

Drug interactions

TCAs antagonize the hypotensive effects of $\alpha2$-adrenoceptor agonists such as clonidine, but can be safely combined with thiazides and angiotensin-converting enzyme (ACE) inhibitors. The ability of TCAs to block noradrenaline reuptake can lead to hypertension with systemically administered noradrenaline and adrenaline (epinephrine). TCAs should not be used in conjunction with antiarrhythmic drugs, particularly amiodarone. Plasma levels of

Table 26.6.1.3 Some adverse effects of tricyclic antidepressants

Pharmacological action	Adverse effects
Muscarinic receptor blockade (anticholinergic)	Dry mouth, tachycardia, blurred vision, glaucoma, constipation, urinary retention, sexual dysfunction, cognitive impairment
α_1-Adrenoceptor blockade	Drowsiness, postural hypotension, sexual dysfunction, cognitive impairment
Histamine H_1 receptor blockade	Drowsiness, weight gain
Membrane stabilizing properties	Cardiac conduction defects, cardiac arrhythmias, epileptic seizures, overdose toxicity
Other	Rash, oedema, leucopenia, elevated liver enzymes

TCAs can be increased by numerous other drugs including cimetidine, sodium valproate, calcium channel blockers, and selective serotonin reuptake inhibitors (SSRIs).

Monoamine oxidase inhibitors

Monoamine oxidase inhibitors (MAOIs) block the enzyme monoamine oxidase, which deaminates the neurotransmitters 5-HT, noradrenaline, and dopamine. There are two forms of monoamine oxidase, known as type A (which deaminates noradrenaline and 5-HT) and type B (which preferentially deaminates dopamine and tyramine). Conventional MAOIs irreversibly deactivate both type A and type B monoamine oxidase. This has two main consequences of importance for MAOI use: (1) there is a potential for serious food and drug interactions; and (2) the consequent drug and food restrictions need to be continued for 2 weeks after cessation of MAOI treatment so that new monoamine oxidase can be synthesized.

Moclobemide is a reversible MAOI that selectively inhibits type A monoamine oxidase only. This leads to an increase in brain noradrenaline and 5-HT levels, but other amines such as tyramine are little affected. These factors make moclobemide much less likely than the older MAOIs to produce adverse food and drug interactions, giving it a significant safety advantage. However, while moclobemide has been shown to be effective in the treatment of moderately depressed outpatients, studies have not thus far demonstrated its efficacy in the patient groups for whom conventional MAOI treatment is currently reserved (see below).

Principal drugs

These are isocarboxazid, phenelzine, tranylcypromine, and moclobemide.

Indications and use

Conventional MAOIs are now regarded as third-line antidepressant treatment and are reserved for depressed patients who have failed to respond to multiple drug and other treatments. However, MAOIs can have useful effects in such patients, which is why they have retained a therapeutic role.

Phenelzine and tranylcypromine are the two most commonly prescribed MAOIs, the usual therapeutic dose for phenelzine being between 30 and 90 mg daily. As with TCAs, patients should be informed about side effects and advised that a therapeutic response from MAOIs may not be apparent for 3 to 4 weeks. Once a response is obtained, it is usually necessary to continue treatment for several months.

Adverse effects

MAOIs may cause the following side effects:

* central nervous system—dizziness, muscular twitching, insomnia, confusion, mania

* cardiovascular—tachycardia, postural hypotension, hypertension

* other—dry mouth, blurred vision, impotence, peripheral oedema, hepatocellular damage, leucopenia

Food and drug interactions

The main hazard of conventional MAOI treatment is through interaction with indirect sympathomimetics, i.e. agents that release noradrenaline from nerve endings. The usual source of interaction is tyramine in certain foodstuffs, especially cheese and meat extracts. Tyramine is usually metabolized by monoamine oxidase in the gut wall and liver, but in patients taking MAOIs large amounts may enter the systemic circulation, resulting in hypertension and even cerebrovascular accidents. Similar adverse effects have been reported when sympathomimetic drugs, e.g. amphetamines or ephedrine, are administered to patients taking MAOIs. Ephedrine or its derivatives are frequently present in cold cures: patients must therefore be warned against self-medication without seeking advice.

Hypertensive episodes resulting from the interaction of sympathomimetic drugs and MAOIs are best treated with an $\alpha 1$-adrenoceptor antagonist. Chlorpromazine is an alternative, if a selective agent is unavailable.

MAOIs also produce important interactions with other commonly used drugs, including opioids, insulin, and oral hypoglycaemic agents. Except in special circumstances, combination with TCAs is best avoided. Combination with clomipramine, SSRIs, and venlafaxine can cause a 5-HT neurotoxicity syndrome and is contraindicated.

From the foregoing, it will be apparent that conventional MAOIs should only be prescribed to patients capable of adhering to the necessary dietary restrictions. Written instructions listing prohibited foods should be provided. No additional medication should be given until the possibility of an adverse drug interaction has been excluded.

Moclobemide

Moclobemide is well tolerated, although insomnia and nausea may occur. Unlike conventional MAOIs, it does not cause significant interaction with tyramine, and adverse drug interactions also seem to be less likely. However, caution is recommended when prescribing with opioids, and combined use with SSRIs and sympathomimetic agents should be avoided. Because of the reversible nature of moclobemide's interaction with monoamine oxidase and its short half-life (about 3 h), normal monoamine oxidase activity is restored within a day of stopping treatment.

Mood stabilizing drugs

Lithium

Lithium salts have inhibitory effects on receptor-transduction systems, particularly second messengers such as cAMP and phosphoinositol. Lithium also produces marked increases in some aspects of brain 5-HT function.

Indications and use

The main uses of lithium are:

* prophylaxis of recurrent affective disorders, especially manic depressive illness

* acute treatment of mania

* augmentation of antidepressant medication in patients with resistant depression

Lithium remains a leading pharmacological treatment for the maintenance phase of bipolar disorder. However, because of its potential toxicity and limited tolerability, anticonvulsant treatments are being used more widely for this purpose, particularly in the United States of America.

The excretion of lithium from the body is critically dependent on the kidneys. Since there is little margin between therapeutic plasma levels of lithium (0.5–0.8 mmol/litre) and those causing toxicity (>1.2 mmol/litre), the introduction of lithium therapy should be preceded by clinical and laboratory assessment of renal function. Renal function tests should include urinalysis and measurement of plasma creatinine and electrolyte levels: note should be taken if there is any suggestion of impaired renal function (reduced estimated GFR (eGFR)).

Patients should initially be treated with 200 to 400 mg daily of lithium carbonate, usually as a single dose at night. Slow-release preparations of lithium are available, but their pharmacokinetics in vivo are very similar to those of the standard preparation. Dosage should be adjusted every 5 to 7 days on the basis of plasma lithium determinations obtained approximately 12 h after the last dose. Plasma levels of 0.5 to 0.8 mmol/litre are usually satisfactory for prophylaxis of recurrent mood disorders, but some patients—particularly those with an acute manic episode—may require higher levels (0.8–1.0 mmol/litre). Most patients achieve adequate plasma levels with lithium carbonate dosages of between 600 and 1200 mg daily, and following this their lithium requirement is generally stable.

In the absence of clinical indications, it is usually sufficient to check lithium levels every 2 to 3 months and repeat renal function tests every 6 months. Lithium can also cause hypothyroidism, so thyroid function tests should be performed prior to treatment and at 6-monthly intervals thereafter. If necessary, lithium can be combined with thyroxine replacement therapy. Sudden withdrawal of lithium in bipolar patients can cause an acute rebound mania and should be avoided if at all possible.

Adverse effects

Side effects of lithium are shown in Table 26.6.1.4. The most important concern the effects of lithium on the kidneys. Some degree of thirst and polyuria is common, and a few patients develop nephrogenic diabetes insipidus, probably caused by lithium blocking the effect of ADH on the renal tubule. Most patients taking lithium have a demonstrable impairment of tubular concentrating ability, although this is rarely of clinical significance. Glomerular function is less affected by lithium, but glomerular damage and interstitial fibrosis have been reported following lithium toxicity. There are also reports that long-term lithium treatment, even at therapeutic plasma levels, can occasionally cause long-term renal impairment

Table 26.6.1.4 Some adverse effects of lithium

Central nervous system	Drowsiness, lethargy, headache, memory impairment, fine tremor
Cardiovascular system	Conduction defects (rare)
Gastrointestinal system	Nausea, vomiting, diarrhoea
Genitourinary system	Polydipsia, polyuria, nephrogenic diabetes insipidus
Endocrine system	Hypothyroidism ($T_4 \downarrow$ TSH $\uparrow$), hyperglycaemia, hyperparathyroidism
Other	Leucocytosis, skin rash, weight gain
Signs of toxicity (plasma level: >1.2 mmol/litre)	Nausea, vomiting, coarse tremor, drowsiness, dysarthria, seizures, coma, renal failure, cardiovascular collapse

T_4, thyroxine; TSH, thyroid stimulating hormone.

and renal failure. However, this risk is manageable provided the plasma concentration of lithium is kept within the therapeutic range and episodes of toxicity avoided. An increasing level of creatinine/decreasing level of eGFR (a fall of more than 5 ml/min per year, or to a value <45 ml/min) should prompt referral to a renal physician.

Up to 80% of the lithium filtered by the renal glomerulus is reabsorbed by the proximal tubule. Conditions such as diarrhoea and excessive sweating, which induce renal sodium retention, also result in increased lithium reabsorption by the kidney and elevated plasma lithium levels.

Drug interactions

As noted above, the narrow therapeutic index of lithium means that drug interactions that raise plasma lithium levels can have serious clinical consequences (see below). Important interactions can occur with:

◆ Diuretics—through their effect on sodium excretion, thiazides increase lithium reabsorption and can produce lithium toxicity unless the dose of lithium is reduced and plasma concentration carefully monitored. Loop and potassium-sparing diuretics are less likely to alter lithium clearance, but it is prudent to monitor lithium levels carefully when using these drugs.

◆ NSAIDs—plasma lithium levels may be increased by concomitant administration of NSAIDs

◆ Antihypertensives—lithium levels can be increased by ACE inhibitors and angiotensin II receptor antagonists.

◆ Other—lithium levels may be increased by metronidazole and lowered by theophylline and antacids. While the effects of lithium on cardiac conduction are usually considered benign, the effects of cardiac glycosides on conduction may be potentiated. Lithium can cause neurotoxicity (at normal plasma levels) with calcium channel blockers and carbamazepine, and may also increase the liability of antipsychotic drugs to cause extrapyramidal movement disorders.

Toxicity

Acute lithium toxicity usually appears at a plasma level above 1.2 mmol/litre. Early signs are coarse tremor, drowsiness, and dysarthria.

Higher plasma concentrations (>2.0 mmol/litre) can lead to seizures, coma, and death. Since lithium toxicity is potentially fatal, any suspicion of intoxication should lead to the immediate withdrawal of lithium treatment and close monitoring of serum lithium and plasma electrolyte and creatinine concentrations. Severely ill patients with high serum lithium levels may require dialysis.

Carbamazepine

Carbamazepine blocks neuronal sodium channels, as do certain other anticonvulsant drugs. The relationship of this effect to its therapeutic actions in affective disorder is uncertain.

Indications and use

Carbamazepine is effective in the acute treatment of mania and in the prophylaxis of bipolar affective disorder. It is used in patients who have difficulty tolerating or fail to respond to lithium therapy, when it may be given in combination with lithium.

The dose range of carbamazepine employed to treat patients with affective illness is similar to that used in the treatment of seizure disorders. Initial treatment should be with 100 mg of carbamazepine twice daily, with the dose increased according to tolerance over the next 2 to 4 weeks. The effective dose range in the treatment of bipolar disorder is generally between 600 and 1200 mg daily, although some patients require higher doses. Plasma level monitoring may be used to help avoid toxicity.

Side effects

Dizziness, drowsiness, and nausea are common early in treatment, particularly with rapid dose titration, but tolerance to these effects usually develops. Persistent ataxia and diplopia may indicate plasma carbamazepine levels in the toxic range. A moderate degree of leucopenia is often seen during carbamazepine treatment and agranulocytosis can occasionally develop, such that it is prudent to monitor the white cell count as well as the carbamazepine level during treatment. Skin rashes are also quite common. Other rarer adverse effects include hyponatraemia and liver cell damage. Circulating thyroid hormone level may be lowered by carbamazepine treatment, but thyroid-stimulating hormone (TSH) levels generally remain in the normal range and clinical hypothyroidism is unusual. Carbamazepine can impair cardiac conduction and should be used with caution in patients with cardiovascular disease.

Drug interactions

Carbamazepine increases the metabolism of a number of other drugs, including TCAs, haloperidol, oral contraceptive agents, warfarin, and other anticonvulsants. A similar mechanism may underlie the decline in the plasma carbamazepine level sometimes seen during continued treatment. The carbamazepine level may be increased by erythromycin and by some calcium channel blockers, such as diltiazem and verapamil. Neurotoxicity has been reported when carbamazepine is combined with lithium.

Sodium valproate

Valproate is a simple branched-chain fatty acid with a mode of action that is unclear, although there is some evidence that it can slow the breakdown of the inhibitory neurotransmitter γ-aminobutyric acid (GABA). This action could account for its anticonvulsant properties, but whether it also underlies the psychotropic effects is unclear.

Indications and use

Like carbamazepine, sodium valproate was first introduced as an anticonvulsant. Recent studies have shown that it is effective in the management of acute mania. In the United States of America valproate is widely used in the longer term prophylaxis of bipolar disorder, but the evidence for this indication from randomized trials is not particularly strong.

Valproate can be started at a dose of 200 to 400 mg daily, which may be increased once or twice weekly to between 1 and 2 g daily. Plasma levels of valproate do not correlate well with either its anticonvulsant or mood stabilizing effects, but it has been suggested that efficacy in the treatment of mood disorders is usually apparent when plasma levels are above 50 µg/ml.

Side effects

Common side effects of valproate include gastrointestinal disturbances, tremor, sedation, weight gain, and transient hair loss. Serious side effects are rare, but fatal hepatic toxicity has been reported, as has acute pancreatitis. Valproate may also cause thrombocytopenia and inhibit platelet aggregation, and increases in plasma ammonia have been reported.

Drug interactions

Valproate potentiates the effects of central sedatives. It has been reported to increase the side effects of other anticonvulsants (without necessarily improving anticonvulsant control). It may increase plasma levels of phenytoin and TCAs.

Other drugs

Although not licensed for this indication in the United Kingdom, the anticonvulsant drug lamotrigine is increasingly used to treat depression in patients with bipolar disorder. Atypical antipsychotic drugs such as olanzapine and quetiapine (see below) are also employed in the treatment of bipolar illness.

Antipsychotic drugs

Antipsychotic drugs, also known as major tranquillizers or neuroleptics, are a group of agents of varied structure that are used to treat schizophrenia and other psychoses. Conventional or typical antipsychotic agents have in common the ability to block dopamine receptors in the central nervous system, and it is likely that their antipsychotic effect is caused by blockade of dopamine D_2 receptors in mesolimbic regions of the brain. Blockade of D_2 receptors in striatum explains the common occurrence of various kinds of extrapyramidal movement disorders.

Atypical antipsychotic drugs have been developed more recently. These have a varied pharmacology, but a lower likelihood than conventional agents of producing extrapyramidal side effects at therapeutic doses. Some are highly selective dopamine D_2 receptor antagonists with selectivity for mesolimbic dopamine receptors, e.g. amisulpride. Others (e.g. risperidone, olanzapine, and quetiapine) have high affinities for the 5-HT$_2$ receptor that exceed their affinities for the D_2 receptor. Finally, clozapine is also a potent 5-HT$_2$ receptor antagonist but a weak D_2 receptor antagonist, which accounts for its particularly low risk of inducing extrapyramidal movement disorders.

Principal drugs

These are:

- conventional (typical) antipsychotic drugs—chlorpromazine, haloperidol, flupentixol, fluphenazine, loxapine, pimozide, thioridazine, and trifluoperazine

- atypical antipsychotic drugs—amisulpride, aripiprazole, olanzapine, quetiapine, and risperidone

Indications and use

Antipsychotic drugs are used mainly in the management of schizophrenia. They are also used to treat mania and are sometimes given to depressed patients who have psychotic symptoms or who are particularly agitated. Some atypical antipsychotic drugs (for example, olanzapine and quetiapine), are helpful in the maintenance treatment of bipolar disorder and quetiapine has useful effects in the treatment of bipolar depression. Antipsychotic drugs are also used in the management of disturbed behaviour arising from other medical causes (e.g. confusional states), but their use as nonspecific tranquillizing agents should be limited to short-term use because of potentially serious side effects. In this respect it is worth noting that some groups of demented patients (particularly those with Lewy body type dementia) may suffer severe extrapyramidal effects from comparatively low doses of antipsychotic drugs, and patients with dementia also appear to be at increased risk of adverse cardiovascular events, particularly stroke, during antipsychotic drug treatment.

The treatment of patients with schizophrenia or mania with antipsychotic drugs requires careful monitoring and persistence because the full therapeutic response may be delayed for some weeks. Furthermore, the dose of antipsychotic drug required may vary considerably from patient to patient, and also within the same patient at different stages of the illness. Lower doses of conventional antipsychotic drugs are now employed for the treatment of these disorders, since positron emission tomography (PET) imaging studies have revealed that an adequate blockade of dopamine D_2 receptors can be obtained with oral doses of 5 to 10 mg of haloperidol daily or 200 to 400 mg of chlorpromazine. Higher doses of these agents can produce sedation and behavioural calming, but at the expense of movement disorders and decreased compliance subsequently.

If a patient has responded to an antipsychotic drug, it is usual to continue the medication for a number of months into remission. It is frequently necessary to administer medication on a long-term basis to prevent relapse, in which case the use of long-acting intramuscular preparations will improve compliance. The decanoates of fluphenazine, flupentixol, and haloperidol are most commonly used, and a depot preparation of the atypical agent risperidone is also available.

Atypical antipsychotic drugs are generally used for new cases of schizophrenia and are also indicated when patients experience extrapyramidal movement disorders on modest doses of typical agents. Clozapine can be effective in up to 30% of patients with schizophrenia whose symptoms have not responded to other antipsychotic drugs (both typical and atypical). It is effective in the treatment of both positive and negative symptoms of schizophrenia; the latter often showing a poor response to other antipsychotic drugs.

Adverse effects
Movement disorders

Through their blockade of brain dopamine receptors, typical antipsychotic drugs produce a variety of extrapyramidal movement

Table 26.6.1.5 Extrapyramidal disorders and antipsychotic drugs

Disorder	Description	Treatments employed
Dystonic reaction	Involuntary muscle contraction, especially face and jaw, oculogyric crisis	1. Benzatropine (1–2 mg IM or IV) 2. Diazepam (10 mg IV)
Akathisia	Sense of subjective motor restlessness, continual pacing	1. Reduce dose of antipsychotic drug 2. Benzatropine (1–6 mg daily) 3. Propranolol (40–120 mg daily) 4. Diazepam (10–30 mg daily)
Parkinsonism	Rigidity, bradykinesia, tremor	1. Reduce dose of neuroleptic 2. Benzatropine (1–6 mg daily)
Tardive dyskinesia (late onset)	Choreoathetoid movements, especially tongue, lips, and jaw	1. Withdraw antipsychotic drug 2. Vitamin E 3. Atypical antipsychotic drug
Neuroleptic malignant syndrome (rare)	Fever, muscular rigidity, coma, death	1. Discontinue neuroleptic 2. Intensive care support 3. Bromocriptine 4. Dantrolene

IM, intramuscular; IV, intravenous.

disorders that can mimic signs of basal ganglia disease (Table 26.6.1.5). Many patients exhibit symptoms of parkinsonism very similar to those of the idiopathic disorder, although tremor is less prominent. A side effect that appears early in treatment is acute dystonia, which can present with abnormal postures or dramatic muscular spasms involving the face and limbs. Laryngeal spasm with respiratory distress can also occur. A history of recent antipsychotic drug use can help avoid misdiagnoses (e.g. it is not unusual for such reactions to be viewed as 'hysterical'). Another movement disorder that patients find very distressing is akathisia, which is a state of motor restlessness, often with agitation and dysphoria. Distinguishing this reaction from symptoms arising from the underlying psychiatric disorder may not be easy.

All these movement disorders may be treated by a reduction in dosage of the antipsychotic drug or by the introduction of anticholinergic medication such as benztropine. However, anticholinergic drugs should not be prescribed routinely with antipsychotic medication because of the risk of misuse for their euphoriant effects.

Later in treatment, tardive dyskinesia may develop. This consists of involuntary repetitive movements, usually involving the tongue and lips, though other parts of the body may be involved. The condition may be associated with a supersensitivity of postsynaptic dopamine receptors in the basal ganglia. Unfortunately, this disorder cannot be treated easily, and anticholinergic medication may make it worse. If possible, the antipsychotic drug should be stopped, but this decision is often difficult because of the risk of relapse of the psychiatric disorder.

Atypical antipsychotic drugs are less likely to cause movement disorders. Risperidone, however, is a potent D_2 receptor antagonist as well as a 5-HT$_2$ receptor antagonist and can produce some movement disorders at the upper end of its dose range (above 4–6 mg daily). Atypical antipsychotic drugs, particularly clozapine, are generally less likely to cause tardive dyskinesia.

Neuroleptic malignant syndrome

A rare, but potentially very serious, reaction to antipsychotic drugs is the neuroleptic malignant syndrome (Table 26.6.1.5). This is characterized by fever, rigidity, and altered consciousness, together with tachycardia and labile blood pressure. Laboratory investigations usually reveal a leucocytosis together with a markedly raised serum level of creatinine phosphokinase. Antipsychotic drug treatment should be withdrawn immediately if the neuroleptic malignant syndrome is suspected. Management in an intensive care facility may be needed to deal with cardiovascular, respiratory, and renal complications. Treatment with a dopamine receptor agonist such as bromocriptine and the antispasticity agent dantrolene may be beneficial.

Weight gain and diabetes

Many antipsychotic drugs can cause weight gain, but the risk is greater with certain atypical agents, particularly clozapine, olanzapine, and quetiapine. These drugs are also associated with a greater risk of type 2 diabetes than conventional agents, as well as disturbances in lipid profile. Patients taking atypical antipsychotics should therefore be monitored regularly for weight gain and disturbances in glucose and lipid metabolism.

Other side effects of antipsychotic drugs

Antipsychotic drugs such as chlorpromazine can produce a variety of side effects due to blockade of muscarinic receptors and α-adrenoceptors (Table 26.6.1.2). Other side effects include:

- endocrine—elevated prolactin levels, amenorrhoea, and galactorrhoea (not seen with atypical agents except amisulpride and risperidone)
- skin—rashes, pigmentation, and photosensitivity (especially phenothiazines)
- other—precipitation of seizures, hypothermia (especially chlorpromazine), cardiac arrhythmias (pimozide, thioridazine), weight gain, cholestatic hepatitis, leucopenia, and retinitis pigmentosa (thioridazine in doses >800 mg daily)

The most common side effects of atypical antipsychotic drugs are shown in Table 26.6.1.6.

Drug interactions

Antipsychotic drugs potentiate the effects of other central sedatives. They may delay the hepatic metabolism of TCAs and antiepileptic drugs, leading to increased plasma levels of these agents. The hypotensive properties of chlorpromazine and thioridazine may enhance the effects of antihypertensive drugs. Antipsychotic drugs, particularly pimozide and thioridazine, can increase the QT interval and should not be given with other drugs likely to potentiate this effect, such as antiarrhythmics, astemizole, terfenadine, and TCAs. There are also reports of an increased risk of cardiac arrhythmias when pimozide has been combined with clarithromycin and erythromycin. Clozapine should not be given with any agent likely to potentiate its depressant effect on the white cell count such as carbamazepine, co-trimoxazole, and penicillamine. SSRIs slow the hepatic metabolism and increase blood levels of several antipsychotic drugs, including haloperidol, risperidone, and clozapine.

Antianxiety agents

Benzodiazepines

Benzodiazepines enhance the action of the neurotransmitter γ-aminobutyric acid (GABA) in the central nervous system by

Table 26.6.1.6 Atypical antipsychotics

Drug	EPS	Prolactin	Weight gain	Adverse effects
Amisulpiride	+	↑	+	Insomnia, agitation, nausea, constipation, QT prolongation (rare)
Clozapine	0	0	+++	Agranulocytosis—white cell monitoring mandatory, myocarditis and myopathy (rare), fatigue, drowsiness, hypersalivation, sweating, tachycardia, postural hypotension, nausea, constipation, ileus, urinary retention, diabetes
Olanzapine	+/0	0	+++	Somnolence, dizziness, oedema, hypotension, dry mouth, constipation, diabetes
Quetiapine	0	0	++	Somnolence, dizziness, postural hypotension, dry mouth, abnormal liver function tests, QT prolongation (transient), diabetes
Risperidone	+	↑	+	Insomnia, agitation, anxiety, headache, impaired concentration, nausea, abdominal pain

0, not present; +, sometimes; ++, often; +++, can be excessive; EPS, extrapyramidal symptoms.

binding to a specific benzodiazepine receptor located in a complex with a GABA receptor and a chloride ion channel. The pharmacological effects of benzodiazepines are attributed to the facilitation of GABA neurotransmission.

Principal drugs

These are alprazolam, chlordiazepoxide, diazepam, flurazepam, lorazepam, lormetazepam, nitrazepam, and temazepam.

Indications and use

The prescription of benzodiazepines is decreasing following concern about their liability to produce dependence. Alternative therapies are available for most anxiety related disorders, and it is recommended that the drug treatment of anxiety and insomnia should be limited to a few weeks' duration. The main indication for the use of benzodiazepines is to help patients in a crisis, when generalized anxiety and insomnia are causing functional impairment and reducing their ability to cope. Patients should be advised that the drug treatment will be of short duration to help them manage their immediate difficulties.

All benzodiazepines have hypnotic and anxiolytic properties, the main difference between them of clinical importance being their length of action. Derivatives with short half-lives, such as temazepam, are suitable hypnotics because of their relative lack of a hangover effect. Other benzodiazepines, e.g. diazepam, have long half-lives and are metabolized to active compounds. These may be used for the treatment of anxiety, either in the form of regular dosing, or on the now preferred 'as required' basis with an agreed maximum daily dose.

Side effects and interactions

Benzodiazepines have a low acute toxicity. Their adverse effects are extensions of their clinical effects and include the following: drowsiness, psychomotor impairment, dizziness, ataxia, and paradoxical aggression (rare). Benzodiazepines potentiate the effects of other centrally acting sedatives, particularly alcohol. The effects of benzodiazepines are potentiated by cimetidine.

Patients who have taken clinical doses of a benzodiazepine for more than a few weeks may show a withdrawal syndrome when the medication is stopped. In many respects this syndrome resembles an anxiety state, but perceptual disturbances and acute dysphoria may also occur. It is thus apparent that benzodiazepines can cause physical dependence, and although the withdrawal syndrome is less severe than that seen following the cessation of barbiturates, patients frequently find it difficult to stop their medication. A gradual reduction is usually best. Generally, withdrawal from a long-acting benzodiazepine is easier than from a short-acting preparation, and if patients taking short-acting benzodiazepines have difficulty withdrawing, then a switch to a long-acting preparation may be helpful.

Other drugs that increase brain GABA function

A number of nonbenzodiazepine agents with short half-lives (the Z drugs) also increase GABA function and are licensed as hypnotics. Whether the Z drugs have advantages over short-acting benzodiazepines such as temazepam is disputed. The treatment of insomnia with either benzodiazepines or the Z drugs should be short-term to avoid dependence.

Zopiclone, zolpidem, and zaleplon (the Z drugs)

Zopiclone is a cyclopyrrolone derivative marketed for the treatment of insomnia. It binds to a site close to the benzodiazepine receptor and thereby facilitates brain GABA function. By contrast to the benzodiazepines, which reduce the amount of slow-wave (deep) sleep at night, zopiclone has little effect on sleep architecture and is relatively free from a daytime 'hangover' effect. It is claimed to be less likely than benzodiazepine hypnotics to produce tolerance and withdrawal effects, but cases have been reported. The most common adverse effects of zopiclone include bitter taste, nausea, dry mouth, irritability, and headache.

Zolpidem is an imidazopyridine derivative that also binds to a site close to the benzodiazepine receptor. It has a very short duration of action and, like zopiclone, has little effect on sleep architecture or daytime performance. Its possible adverse effects include nausea, dizziness, headaches, and diarrhoea. Zaleplon is a pyrazolopyrimidine derivative with pharmacological properties similar to zopiclone and zolpidem, but its half-life is only about an hour such that it can be used to reinduce sleep after nocturnal waking.

Clomethiazole

Clomethiazole also binds at the GABA receptor complex, but its clinical effects resemble those of barbiturates rather more than those of the benzodiazepines. It can cause serious respiratory depression in overdose, particularly in combination with alcohol. Because of its short half-life (4–5 h), clomethiazole is used as a hypnotic in older people, but again only short-term use is recommended.

Drugs altering monoamine function

Buspirone

Buspirone is a 5-HT$_{1A}$ receptor agonist structurally unrelated to benzodiazepines. It is effective in the treatment of generalized anxiety disorder (less so in patients previously exposed to benzodiazepines), but has a slow onset of action (1–3 weeks). Unlike benzodiazepines, buspirone does not cause significant sedation or cognitive impairment and appears unlikely to cause dependence. It does not have hypnotic properties. Side effects include nervousness, dizziness, and headache.

Other drugs

SSRIs and TCAs are effective in the management of patients with a range of anxiety disorders, including generalized anxiety and phobic states. They are generally preferred to benzodiazepines for the treatment of agoraphobia with and without panic attacks. SSRIs are also effective in the treatment of obsessive–compulsive disorder and social phobia, but TCAs (with the exception of clomipramine) are not.

Further reading

Anderson IM, *et al.* (2008). Evidence based guidelines for treating depressive disorders with antidepressants: A revision of the 2000 British Association for Psychopharmacology guidelines. *Journal of Psychopharmacology*, **22**, 343–396.

Baldwin DS, *et al.* (2005). Evidence-based guidelines for the pharmacological treatment of anxiety disorders: recommendations from the British Association of Psychopharmacology. *J Psychopharmacol*, **19**, 567–96.

Cowen PJ (2005). New drugs, old problems. Revisiting pharmacological management of treatment-resistant depression. *Adv Psychiatr Treat*, **11**, 19–27.

Ferrier N, Ferrie LJ, Macritchie KA (2006). Revisiting lithium therapy. *Adv Psychiatr Treat*, **12**, 256–664.

Gartside SE, Cowen PJ (2006). Pharmacology of drugs used in the treatment of mood disorders. *Psychiatry*, **5**, 162–166.

Gelder MG, Harrison PJ, Cowen PJ (2006). Drugs and other physical treatments. In:, *The shorter Oxford textbook of psychiatry, OUP*, 5th edition, pp. 518–76, Oxford University Press, Oxford.

Goodwin GM *et al.* (2009). Evidence-based guidelines for treating bipolar disorder: revised second edition—recommendations from the British Association of Psychopharmacology. http://www.bap.org.uk/pdfs/Bipolar_guidelines.pdf

National Institute for Clinical Excellence (2004). *Anxiety: Management of anxiety (panic disorder with and without agoraphobia, and generalized anxiety disorder) in adults in primary, secondary and community care. Guideline 22*, National Institute for Clinical Excellence, London. http://www.nice.org.uk

National Institute for Clinical Excellence (2009). Schizophrenia. National Clinical Practice Guideline 82. National Institute for Clinical Excellence, London. http://www.nice.org.uk

National Institute for Clinical Excellence (2009). The treatment and management of depression in adults. *National Clinical Practice Guideline* 90, National Institute for Clinical Excellence, London. http://www.nice.org.uk

National Institute for Health and Clinical Excellence (2004). *Insomnia—newer hypnotic drugs. Zaleplon, zolpidem and zopiclone for the management of insomnia. Technology Appraisal Guidance TA77*. http://guidance.nice.org.uk/TA77

National Institute for Health and Clinical Excellence (2006). *Bipolar disorder: The management of bipolar disorder in adults, children and adolescents, in primary and secondary care. Guideline CG38*. http://www.nice.org.uk/CG38 National Institute for Clinical Excellence, London. http://www.nice.org.uk.

Stahl SM (2008). *Essential psychopharmacology*, 3rd edition. Cambridge University Press, Cambridge.

Taylor D, Paton C, Kerwin D (2007). *The Maudsley prescribing guidelines*, 9th edition. Martin Dunitz, London.

26.6.2 **Psychological treatment in medical practice**

Michael Sharpe and Simon Wessely

Essentials

Patients have minds as well as bodies, and medical treatment must often address both if it is to be effective.

Psychological treatments—these may be divided into general and specialist types. All medical consultations have an important and inescapable psychological effect, hence all physicians are general psychotherapists. All medical consultations have the potential for both psychological help and for harm. Helpful consultations educate the patient, reassure them, and achieve adherence to treatment. Harmful consultations leave the patient confused or with inaccurate ideas about their health, increase anxiety, and make adherence to the physician's treatment less likely. Being able to deliver a psychologically helpful consultation is therefore a core medical skill.

Specialist psychological treatments—these also have an important role in medical practice. Referral to specialist services may be needed for patients who are distressed by their disease or its treatment, and for those who have medically unexplained symptoms (see Chapter 26.5.3). Short- and medium-term structured therapies such as cognitive behavioural therapy (CBT) are evidence-based treatments for these problems. Before the need to make a referral arises, physicians should familiarize themselves with what psychological treatments are available for their patients, how long they will have to wait to be seen, and how they will be received.

What is psychological treatment?

Psychological treatments in medicine come in two main forms: general and specific. General psychological treatments are an integral aspect of medical practice as all medical consultations have a psychological impact on the patient, whether for good or ill. In this sense, all doctors are in the business of delivering psychological treatment. Specialist psychological treatments come in a variety of types of 'psychotherapy' such as counselling or cognitive behavioural therapy (CBT).

General psychological treatment and the medical consultation

The psychotherapeutic importance of the medical encounter was perhaps better acknowledged and described at a time when physicians had less to offer in terms of biological investigations and treatments, and consequently had to place more emphasis on what they could achieve by simply talking with the patient. Despite the power of modern 21st century drug and surgical therapies, the general psychotherapeutic aspects of the consultation remain critical to the effective practice of medicine. This is especially the case when there is diagnostic uncertainty or when the patient is distressed. An important development in recent years has been training in communication skills for both medical students and for trained physicians.

Psychotherapeutic consultations (doing good)

The key ingredients of the psychotherapeutic consultation are those described by Jerome Frank as common to all psychological treatments:

♦ Establishing a good, confiding, and collaborative relationship with the patient

♦ Convincing the patient that whatever the nature of their problem they can be trusted to help

♦ Offering an acceptable and convincing explanation for what is wrong with the patient

♦ Providing a positive and credible plan of action for addressing the problem.

Although medical encounters are often suboptimal in these psychotherapeutic ingredients, they can be easily improved. The ingredients are listed in Table 26.6.2.1 and described below.

Attention must be paid to the physical arrangements for the consultation. The days when patients were first told that they have cancer on an open ward round may have gone, but many consultations still offer scant privacy and little opportunity for the patient to ask questions. Some consultations will simply take time, and while other professionals such as nurses can supplement the doctor's role in listening and explaining, it is important that time and privacy are recognized, and if necessary insisted on by the doctors, as the essential therapeutic tools that, like drugs, will only work in appropriate dose.

Taking an interest in the patient's symptoms (even those that are not of diagnostic value) and their fears about these (even if they appear illogical) is important. Unless this is done, the patient is likely to feel that they have not been listened to and will consequently ignore the doctor's advice. It is hard to give effective reassurance without taking the trouble to find out what the patient fears: time spent on such matters is not therefore a mere distraction

Table 26.6.2.1 General psychotherapeutic aspects of the medical consultation

Prepare	Ensure adequate time and privacy for the consultation, and that you have the information you need
Listen	Listen to the patient's concerns about symptoms and accept as problems in their own right and not only as pointers to disease. Ask about their worries
Explain	Explain what you understand to be wrong, including a diagnosis. Reassure about unfounded worries
Plan	Agree a plan with the patient that includes actions for both them and you. Ensure that they don't feel dismissed or helpless. Summarize in writing

from the diagnostic process, but is a critical aspect of the fundamental task of helping the patient to feel better.

A clear explantion of the problem is required. All too often patients complain that doctors told them what they didn't have, but not what they did have. This usually happens when the patient's complaints are not adequately explained by identifiable disease and they have medically unexplained symptoms (see Chapter 26.5.3).

Even when a clear explanation cannot be given, a positive plan of action usually can. There is evidence that such a positive approach has a beneficial effect on the patient's well-being. The provision of hope, a practical plan, and an expectation of improvement have long been ingredients of the doctor–patient relationship. Although the hope offered should not be false, e.g. If the patient has a terminal condition, the message can still be a positive one; the symptoms will be managed and the doctor will provide ongoing help for them. A written summary— perhaps as a copy to the letter to another doctor—is often helpful.

Psychological iatrogenesis and the consultation (doing harm)

Like all powerful treatments, the consultation has the potential to do harm as well as good. Iatrogenesis does not only result from prescribing the wrong drug or doing the wrong operation, but also from what doctors say to patients. Iatrogenic psychological harm can result from:

♦ Dismissive messages: e.g. telling a patient with medically unexplained symptoms 'there is nothing wrong with you—it's 'all in your mind' or 'you are imagining it'. This will not only damage your relationship with the patient, but may also send him or her into the arms of less scrupulous practitioners.

♦ Ill-considered or unhelpful explanation for the illness: e.g. telling the person who is depressed that it's 'probably a virus', or a person with back pain that they have a 'weak ligament'. This can send false messages about why they are unwell, what might be the outcome, and what treatment they should seek.

♦ Excessively optimistic predictions: e.g. telling a patient who has not yet been adequately assessed 'I'm sure it's nothing serious'. This may lead to the patient losing faith in the doctor who made the predictions (and to legal redress) if it turns out to be incorrect.

♦ Excessively pessimistic predictions: e.g. telling a person with possible multiple sclerosis, 'it's probably best if you just come to terms with the idea of a wheelchair now'. This is likely to lead to unnecessary distress.

♦ Poorly thought out or ill-informed advice: e.g. telling a patient with indigestion to avoid all foods that are associated with the symptoms. For some patients this can fuel excessive dietary restriction. An elegant demonstration of this type of problem was found in a study of schoolchildren whose parents were told (sometimes incorrectly) that their children had abnormal hearts and should avoid exertion: at follow-up many years later the children with normal hearts were found to be still restricting their activity as much as those who really did have heart disease.

Specialist psychological treatments

Specialist psychological treatments may be broadly divided into: (a) simple counselling type treatments; (b) more intense but brief psychotherapies such as CBT; (c) longer-term treatments such as psychodynamic psychotherapy. Specific psychotherapies have a potentially important role in the management of medical patients by providing evidence-based treatments for improving symptoms such as fatigue and pain, reducing emotional distress, and improving adherence to medical treatments. There is a strong argument that patients would benefit from better integration of these psychotherapies into general medical care.

Counselling

Counselling can help patients to express distress and talk through acute problems such as the diagnosis of cancer. Whereas the provision of reassurance and emotional support is clearly important, whether or not this qualifies as a specialist 'treatment' that needs to be given by a mental health professional is doubtful. Rather, it could be regarded as a generic skill that should ideally be possessed by all health workers.

Brief psychotherapies

Problem solving therapy (PST)

This is a brief (typically six to eight sessions) simple psychological treatment that aims to help patients feel more in control of practical problems they face. It teaches them to define the problems clearly, to tackle them one at a time, and to work out clear strategies to overcome them. It is effective for depression.

Cognitive behavioural therapy (CBT)

CBT is a more complex treatment usually given over 10 to 20 sessions. The cognitive aspects refer to helping the patient to re-evaluate and optimize their understanding of their illness. The behavioural part involves helping them to cope more effectively by reducing unhelpful behaviours such as excessive checking of symptoms and increasing normal activities. It is effective in the treatment of patients with depression, anxiety, and panic disorders and also in the treatment of medically unexplained somatic symptoms (see Chapter 26.5.3). It has been shown in randomized trials to be effective for the functional syndromes of chronic unexplained pain, chronic fatigue syndrome, irritable bowel syndrome, and noncardiac chest pain.

Longer term psychological treatments

For people with problems not amenable to brief therapy, such as ongoing difficulty in adjusting to disease and/or personality problems, there is a case for longer term psychological therapy planned to last many months or even years. However, both the availability of such therapy and the evidence for its effectiveness is limited.

Making a referral for specialist psychological treatment

The first requirement for making a referral for specialist psychological treatment is to find out what services are available and what types of referrals are accepted by them. The second is to make sure that the patient understands why they have been referred and to explain the referral in a way that ensures that they are likely to attend.

Psychological treatment services

Psychological treatment services would ideally be located in organizational and geographical proximity to the medical consultation. In reality they rarely are, hence physicians are often unfamiliar with them. It is therefore desirable for the physician to familiarize themselves with what is available, how long the patient will have to wait, and how the patient will be received before the need to make a referral arises.

Making the referral

It is often helpful to discuss the referral with the service to ensure it is appropriate before telling the patient. For example, the patient's psychological problems may appear obvious to the physician but regarded as untreatable personality disorder by the service being referred to. If medical investigation or treatment is ongoing it will help if uncertainties are made explicit in the referral letter and new findings communicated to the therapist as they arise.

Explaining the referral to the patient

The first, and perhaps most important, aspect of explaining the referral to the patient is to make is clear that you are not implying that their illness is 'imaginary' or 'all in their mind', but rather that there is a psychological aspect to their problems that deserves attention. The second is to convey a positive attitude towards psychotherapy as a sensible treatment approach with a good chance of helping. It is even better if you can explain to the patient what they can expect during the therapy. Finally, it is important, if appropriate, to make sure the patient knows that you will if required see them after the psychological treatment has finished, thereby making it clear that you do not regard referral simply as a way of disposing of them but rather as an essential and valuable supplement to their medical care.

Further reading

Andrews G (1996). Talk that works: the rise of cognitive behaviour therapy. *BMJ*, **313**, 1501–2.

Clark DM, Fairburn CG (1997). *Science and practice of cognitive behaviour therapy*. Oxford University Press, Oxford.

Fallowfield L, *et al.* (2002). Efficacy of a Cancer Research UK communication skills training model for oncologists: a randomised controlled trial. *Lancet*, **359**, 650–6.

Frank JD (1967). *Persuasion and healing. A comparative study of psychotherapy*. The Johns Hopkins University Press, Baltimore, MD.

Guthrie E (1996). Emotional disorder in chronic illness: psychotherapeutic interventions. *Br J Psychiatry*, **168**, 265–73.

Kroenke K, Swindle R (2000). Cognitive–behavioral therapy for somatization and symptom syndromes: a literature synthesis. *Psychother Psychosom*, **69**, 205–15.

Stone J, *et al.* (2002). What should we say to patients with symptoms unexplained by disease? The 'number needed to offend'. *BMJ*, **325**, 1449–50.

Thomas KB (1987). General practice consultations: is there any point in being positive? *Br Med J (Clin Res Ed)*, **294**, 1200–2.

26.7

Alcohol and drug-related problems

Contents

26.7.1 Alcohol and drug dependence

Mary E. McCaul, Gary S. Wand, and Yngvild K. Olsen

Essentials

Alcohol and drug dependence are diagnosed based on the clustering of characteristic physiological and behavioural symptoms. Since there is considerable diagnostic overlap with a variety of medical and psychiatric conditions, a careful history of a patient's substance use, associated problems, and familial patterns of substance misuse is important.

Epidemiology and aetiology—alcohol use is widespread in Europe and North America, with about 1 in 10 people meeting the criteria for alcohol dependence during their lifetime. Genetics, comorbid psychiatric illness, personality factors, and environmental/social factors all influence the likelihood of development of alcohol and drug use disorders.

Pathological effects—alcohol consumption affects virtually every major organ system, with the primary causes of excess mortality including liver disease, severe respiratory infections, cancer of the upper respiratory and digestive systems, cardiovascular disease, suicides, and violence. While drug use is also associated with increased pathology, these effects are often the result of methods of administration or lifestyle rather than direct drug toxicity. Heavy or binge alcohol use during pregnancy can result in fetal alcohol syndrome, the leading preventable cause of mental retardation in North America and Europe. Other common adverse infant outcomes from both alcohol and drug use include reduced birth weight, decreased cognitive and learning abilities, and behavioural problems.

Management—this must focus on both management of the acute withdrawal syndrome associated with discontinuation of regular alcohol or drug use and long-term maintenance of abstinence/sobriety. (1) Alcohol withdrawal management—benzodiazepines remain the mainstay, with flexible, symptom-driven dose protocols appearing to provide greater relief at lower overall medication doses compared with more traditional, fixed-dose regimens. (2) Opioid withdrawal management—buprenorphine, typically in a sublingual formulation, is used. (3) Stimulant withdrawal management, e.g. amphetamines, cocaine—symptoms are primarily psychological rather than physical; antidepressants and/or noncardioselective β-blockers are sometimes employed but there is mixed evidence of effectiveness. Psychosocial treatments including motivational interventions, cognitive behavioural therapies, and supportive therapies are the primary interventions used in the outpatient setting. There is increasing interest in pharmacotherapies to support alcohol abstinence; naltrexone (oral and depot formulations) and acamprosate are now approved for use in North America and most European countries.

Pain—this is often undertreated in drug abusing patients due to providers' concerns about medication misuse, hyperalgesia in this patient population, and tolerance to opioid drugs. Acute pain in drug-abusing patients can be successfully managed using the same protocols as with any patient, with the possible exception of the need to use higher medication doses. Chronic pain management can be more complex and requires careful assessment and monitoring by the provider.

Marijuana, nicotine, sedative, hallucinogen, and inhalant use—see Chapter 9.1.

Diagnosis

In the 1970s, Edwards and Gross first characterized the alcohol dependence syndrome. Today, this syndrome forms the basis of alcohol and other drug dependence criteria for both major diagnostic systems: the World Health Organization International Statistical Classification of Diseases and Health-related Problems, 10th revision (ICD-10) and the American Psychiatric Association Diagnostic and Statistical Manual of Mental Disorders, 4th edition (DSM-IV). For a diagnosis of dependence, both systems require a clustering of at least three symptoms during a 12-month period (Box 26.7.1.1).

In DSM-IV, dependence is subtyped by the presence/absence of physiological withdrawal and tolerance, and recovery status is characterized by duration (early vs sustained remission) and symptom status (partial vs full remission). International studies have found remarkable consistency in the dependence syndrome across diverse geographical and cultural settings, suggesting that fundamental biological processes underpin the disorder.

By contrast, cross-cultural reliability has not been established for the less severe diagnoses of harmful use (ICD-10) and substance abuse (DSM-IV), defined by the negative consequences of alcohol and drug use. This may stem from the greater subjectivity of defining 'harm' within a particular social and cultural context, compared to the more physically based dependence symptoms of withdrawal and tolerance. Similarly, specific levels of hazardous alcohol consumption have not been defined: acceptable amounts vary across cultures, time, and individuals as a function of health, pregnancy, age, and gender.

It is sometimes difficult to disentangle the signs and symptoms of substance abuse and dependence from other common psychiatric and medical conditions. Given their prevalence, alcohol and other drug use should be explored carefully with every patient; there are few socioeconomic, racial/ethnic, or educational predictors of who may experience these problems. Key issues to explore are:

- substance use vs abstention
- recent, lifetime, and heaviest use patterns
- any problems associated with use
- family history of alcohol or drug problems

Additionally, certain behaviours often suggest hazardous levels of substance use, including:

Box 26.7.1.1 Diagnostic criteria for substance dependence

1 Tolerance (i.e. increasing amounts of drug needed to achieve the desired effect)

2 Characteristic physiological withdrawal

3 Difficulties in controlling onset, termination, or amount of substance use

4 Neglect of important social, occupational, or recreational activities because of substance use

5 Increased time required to obtain, use, or recover from substance use

6 Continued use despite persistent negative physical or psychological consequences

---

- cigarette smoking
- missing work
- neglecting family responsibilities
- poor nutrition and hygiene
- high rates of injury and accidents

While not diagnostic, laboratory assessments can be useful for:

- confirming recent alcohol or drug use
- providing information about alcohol and drug sensitive physical problems
- monitoring progress of treatment

To confirm recent use, measurements are made of current alcohol or drug concentrations in blood, urine, or other body fluids. Blood alcohol levels are typically measured in milligrams of alcohol per decilitre of blood and can be readily obtained from breath or blood samples. Impairment from alcohol is common above 50 mg/dl and climbs steeply as the blood alcohol level reaches 100 mg/dl and higher. A very elevated value without significant impairment indicates high alcohol tolerance resulting from chronic, heavy drinking. Urine or blood toxicology screens are commonly effective in detecting most illicit drugs for up to 72 h following use.

A variety of biomarkers have been examined for the detection of heavy drinking; these laboratory tests include liver enzymes (aspartate aminotransferase (AST), alanine aminotransferase (ALT), γ-glutamyl transferase (GGT)), and estimation of macrocytosis by mean cell volume (MCV). Recently, carbohydrate-deficient transferrin (CDT) and phosphatidyliethanal (PEth) levels have been shown to be fairly sensitive and specific for detection of moderate and heavy alcohol consumption. Although various non-alcohol-related diseases produce similar changes in many markers to those produced by excessive alcohol use, laboratory markers in combination with a brief screening instrument can be clinically helpful in identifying those patients in need of more in-depth assessment. The usefulness of combining two or more markers for detection of heavy drinking is being investigated. Elevation in markers should prompt the provider to carefully assess alcohol and drug use and can provide an opportunity for brief counselling (see Chapter 26.7.2).

Epidemiology of alcohol and drug use, abuse, and dependence

There is considerable cultural variation in alcohol and drug use patterns and definitions of harmful or pathological levels of consumption. In North America and Europe the use of alcohol is widespread, and in a recent multinational study about one-quarter of primary health care patients reported at least one alcohol related problem in the last year. The North American and European lifetime prevalence of alcohol dependence is about 9% (range: 5.5% in the Netherlands to 14.3% in the United States of America). Alcohol is ranked as the third leading risk factor for disease in North America and Europe.

In comparison to alcohol use, the prevalence of drug use in Europe and North America is considerably lower: about one-third of people report lifetime drug use, but the prevalence of drug dependence is about 4% (range: 0.7% in Mexico to 7.5% in the United States of America). Globally, the use of substances other than alcohol is generally considered socially aberrant. In the

United States of America there was a large increase in the prevalence of cocaine use during the 1970s and 1980s, and currently about 10% of people report lifetime cocaine use, 2% report use in the past year, and 1% report current use. In the United States of America less than 1% of the population reports heroin use in the past year. Use of most illicit drugs peaks in young adults and then declines with age.

Aetiology of alcohol and drug dependence

Many people have tried alcohol or drugs, but only a subset develop dependence, with an interplay of genetic, psychological, and environmental factors increasing dependence vulnerability. A family history of alcohol or drug dependence remains one of the strongest predictors of risk, with heritability estimates for alcohol dependence ranging from 45 to 65% for men and women. Genetic factors associated with an increased risk for alcohol dependence may include inborn abnormalities in dopamine, opioid, γ-aminobutyric acid (GABA), glutamate, and serotonin neurotransmitter systems. By contrast, specific polymorphisms in the liver enzymes ADH (alcohol dehydrogenase) and ALDH (aldehyde dehydrogenase) can be protective against alcohol use disorders, these polymorphisms encoding for isoforms of ADH and ALDH that cause rapid accumulation of acetylaldehyde, a toxic by-product of alcohol metabolism that limits alcohol intake.

Drugs of abuse influence multiple brain neurotransmitter systems and many of these primary responses lead to secondary effects involving dopamine. For example, morphine and heroin first bind to opioid receptors, which then increase the activity of midbrain mesolimbic dopamine neurons that send projections to interconnected forebrain structures such as the prefrontal cortex and striatum. Drugs such as amphetamine and cocaine act directly by increasing dopamine levels at the nucleus accumbens, a key region at the base of the striatum that mediates the rewarding effects of these drugs as well as those of ethanol. Opioid antagonists block ethanol-induced release of nucleus accumbens dopamine, implicating opioidergic activity as an intermediary between ethanol consumption and dopamine release.

In addition to brain regions that mediate reward and reinforcement, neural circuitry that modulates negative emotional states generated in part through activation of circuits in the amygdala are involved in craving and relapse. For example, the negative emotional aspects of alcohol withdrawal appear to involve at least two neuropeptides expressed in the amygdala: corticotropin-releasing factor (CRF), which is associated with an increased stress response and negative affect, and neuropeptide Y (NPY), a neuropeptide with anxiolytic properties. Genetic, psychological, and environmental effects on the mesolimbic and amygdala systems may contribute to individual differences in dependence vulnerability and relapse.

Psychological factors also appear to increase a person's vulnerability for alcohol or drug dependence. There are strong associations between affective (anxiety and mood) disorders and substance use disorders. These relationships are observed internationally despite large differences in the prevalence of these disorders around the world. Anxiety disorders are very likely to predate the onset of the substance use disorders, suggesting aetiological significance. By contrast, mood disorders do not have so strong a temporal relationship. In a United States of America household survey, over three-quarters of alcohol dependent people were diagnosed with at least one additional psychiatric disorder, with anxiety disorders having the highest prevalence, particularly among women. Antisocial personality disorder also increases the risk of alcohol dependence about fourfold for men and over fivefold for women. Cross-cultural consistency in patterns of comorbidity suggests that, while cultural factors may influence the availability and type of substance exposure, the associations between psychopathology as risk factors and the sequelae of substance disorders are probably independent of particular cultural norms and standards.

Finally, environmental and social processes—including marital discord, parental hostility, poor parental monitoring, and high parental tolerance of adolescent drinking—influence a person's vulnerability for alcohol and drug dependence.

Pathology and pathogenesis
Alcohol-related pathology

Age-adjusted morbidity and mortality rates increase as a function of the amount and duration of alcohol consumption, and these rates are increased two- to threefold among chronic, heavy drinkers. Alcohol consumption affects virtually every major organ system. The primary causes of excess mortality include liver disease, severe respiratory infections, cancer of the upper respiratory and digestive systems, cardiovascular disease, suicides, and violence.

Gastrointestinal

Heavy alcohol use is associated with acute abdominal pain, nausea, and vomiting. With regular, heavy alcohol use, a variety of medical complications involving the gastrointestinal tract and related organ systems can develop. Oesophageal disorders include oesophagitis, oesophageal varices, and oesophageal mucosal tears with bleeding. Common upper gastrointestinal symptoms are gastritis, duodenitis, ulcer disease, and pancreatitis. Some of these effects result from direct mucosal irritation by alcohol.

Liver

The liver receives portal blood directly from the intestines and is the primary site of alcohol metabolism. Liver damage is one of the most common health consequences of chronic, heavy drinking. Two main types of alcohol-related liver injury are inflammation (alcoholic hepatitis) and progressive scarring (fibrosis or cirrhosis), the mechanisms of the toxic effects being shown in Box 26.7.1.2. Despite multiple pathways for alcohol-induced hepatic injury, only some chronic, heavy drinkers experience serious liver damage. Vulnerability to liver injury may result from genetic variations in the enzymes that metabolize alcohol (ADH and ALDH) and in cytochrome P4502E1 activity. Women experience higher rates of hepatic injury at lower cumulative alcohol levels than men. This has been attributed to a toxic interaction of female sex hormones and alcohol-metabolizing enzymes, and also to lower levels of gastric ADH in women compared to men, resulting in reduced first-pass metabolism in the stomach and higher blood alcohol levels following equivalent alcohol doses. Hepatic injury is also facilitated by nutritional factors, including depletion of antioxidant vitamins and glutathione; diet high in polyunsaturated fats or iron; and other medical conditions including infection with hepatitis B and C viruses. For further discussion, see Chapters 15.21 and 15.22.

Cardiovascular

In healthy individuals, moderate alcohol use reduces mortality from atherosclerotic cardiovascular disease, due in part to alcohol's

---

Box 26.7.1.2 Mechanisms for alcohol's toxic effects on the liver

- Peroxidation of liver cells, resulting from the interaction of free radicals and superoxide anions produced during the metabolism of alcohol with proteins, lipids, and DNA

- Increased hypoxia and associated damage, secondary to increased production of vasoconstrictors by Kupffer cells and endothelial cells in liver sinusoids

- Reduced production of protective eicosanoids (such as pros-taglandins) and increased production of toxic eicosanoids (such as thromboxane B$_2$)

- Accumulation of acetaldehyde (the first oxidative metabolite of alcohol) in the liver, thereby increasing the risk of free-radical production, acetaldehyde–protein adduct formation, and acetaldehyde-induced impairment of protein secretion. Acetaldehyde–protein adducts stimulate collagen production, leading to fibrosis and cirrhosis

- Increased production of cytokines, including TNFα and TGFβ, associated with Kupffer cell stimulation

TGFβ, transforming growth factor β; TNFα, tumour necrosis factor α.

---

effects of decreasing low-density lipoprotein (LDL) and increasing high-density lipoprotein (HDL) cholesterol. By contrast, heavy drinking is associated with an increased risk for cardiac arrhythmias, cardiomyopathy, sudden cardiac death, systolic and diastolic hypertension, thereby increasing stroke risk as well. In those with established arrhythmias, hypertension, or hyperlipoproteinaemia, even moderate alcohol use may aggravate symptoms.

Pulmonary

At high doses, alcohol decreases respiratory rate, airflow, and oxygen transport, hence increasing pulmonary disease symptoms in affected patients. Alcohol also reduces key pulmonary defences against infection, including mucociliary clearance; macrophage mobilization, killing, and clearance; and phospholipid metabolism. These actions directly contribute to the increased rates of pulmonary infections (e.g. pneumococcal and Gram-negative pneumonias) in chronic, heavy drinkers.

Neurological

Chronic, heavy alcohol consumption causes structural changes in the brain, particularly in the cerebellum, limbic system, diencephalon, and cerebral cortex. Enlargement of the ventricles and widening of the fissures and sulci over the cerebral hemispheres suggest cortical atrophy. Severely dependent patients may experience a significantly decreased blood flow in the frontal, cortical, and periventricular regions of the cerebral cortex.

A variety of cognitive deficits have been associated with regular, heavy alcohol use, including slowed information processing; poor attention; difficulties with abstraction, solving problems, and learning new information; and reduced visuospatial abilities. Chronic irreversible damage includes ataxia and gait disturbances, polyneuropathy, dementia, and the Wernicke–Korsakoff syndrome. These are discussed further in Chapter 24.19.

Endocrinological

Endocrine abnormalities result from the direct toxic effects of chronic, heavy alcohol use and indirect effects associated with alcohol-related liver disease and malnutrition. Chronic alcohol exposure is particularly damaging to the gonadal axis, resulting in impaired sex hormone production. Male alcoholics often develop gynaecomastia, impotence, and testicular atrophy. Alcohol dependent women often develop menstrual abnormalities. Both sexes have a higher incidence of osteoporosis resulting in part from reduced sex hormone levels.

Chronic, heavy alcohol use is also associated with activation of the hypothalamic-pituitary-adrenal axis (HPA), especially during acute alcohol withdrawal. Some alcoholics develop clinical and biochemical features of Cushing's syndrome or the 'pseudo-Cushing's syndrome'. By contrast, HPA responsiveness is temporarily dampened following alcohol withdrawal. As alcohol dependent individuals cycle through periods of intoxication and withdrawal, the HPA cycles through hyper- and hypoactivity. This alcohol-induced cyclical pattern of corticotropin-releasing factor (CRF) and cortisol secretion may induce various pathological states. For instance, episodes of sustained hypercortisolism may exacerbate osteoporosis, diabetes mellitus, and hypertension, as well as impairing growth, reproductive ability, and immune function. Furthermore, hypercortisolism accompanying alcohol withdrawal increases excitatory amino acid levels within the central nervous system (CNS), resulting in neurotoxicity and worsening withdrawal symptoms such as seizures.

Other alcohol-related endocrine abnormalities are shown in Box 26.7.1.3.

Cancer

Heavy alcohol consumption significantly increases the risk of oesophageal cancer through the local actions of alcohol-metabolizing enzymes on oesophageal cells, and by the increased production of cytochrome P4502E1 in the oesophageal mucosa. This risk is considerably increased by smoking, which has a strikingly high prevalence in heavy drinkers. Other cancers increased by chronic heavy alcohol use include breast, thyroid, skin, laryngeal, and nasopharyngeal. Compromised immune function associated with heavy drinking may contribute to these elevated cancer rates.

Injury

Accidental injuries are a major cause of increased morbidity and mortality among chronic, heavy drinkers. Alcohol use has been implicated in 15 to 63% of fall fatalities, 33 to 61% of burn fatalities, and 44% of fatal traffic accidents. In a study of emergency room patients admitted for blunt or penetrating trauma, almost half had a positive blood alcohol level (as do half of all those who die from unintentional injuries).

Stimulant-related pathology

Stimulants including amphetamines and cocaine work primarily on three CNS neurotransmitters, noradrenaline, serotonin, and dopamine. They acutely increase noradrenaline neuronal activity by increasing presynaptic synthesis and blocking reuptake from the synaptic cleft, leading to effects shown in Box 26.7.1.4. Noradrenaline levels in the brain decrease in the longer term, leading to depression, confusion, restlessness, suicidal ideation, and irritability.

Box 26.7.1.3 Other alcohol-related endocrine abnormalities

Pituitary–gonadal axis

◆ Decreased LH and FSH

◆ Decreased testosterone and oestrogen

◆ Impotence, gynaecomastia, testicular atrophy, and infertility in men

◆ Menstrual abnormalities and infertility in women

Pituitary–adrenal axis

◆ Hypercortisolism

◆ Altered glucocorticoid negative feedback—reduced cortisol response to stress during early abstinence

Bones

◆ Osteoporosis

Carbohydrate metabolism

◆ Glucose intolerance

◆ Alcoholic hypoglycaemia

◆ Alcoholic ketoacidosis

◆ Lactic acidosis

Lipid abnormalities

◆ Hypertriglyceridaemia

Electrolyte abnormalities

◆ Low calcium and magnesium

◆ Sodium retention

LH, luteinizing hormone; FSH, follicle-stimulating hormone.

Stimulants also acutely diminish CNS serotonin activity, contributing to insomnia. Effects on dopamine transmission, particularly in ventral tegmental/corticomesolimbic regions, are thought to mediate the high potential of stimulants for abuse. Acutely, dopamine transmission is increased, but chronic cocaine use depletes central dopamine levels, such that short-term euphoria, increased energy, and alertness are followed by depression and subsequent drug administration.

Box 26.7.1.4 Acute physical effects of stimulants

◆ Hypertension

◆ Tachycardia

◆ Dilated pupils

◆ Diaphoresis

◆ Vasoconstriction

◆ Tremor

Drug-related pathology often results from the method of administration and lifestyle issues (e.g. prostitution) in addition to direct drug toxicity. Chronic intranasal administration increases rhinitis, maxillary sinusitis and necrosis, and perforation of the nasal septum. Smoked cocaine increases pulmonary complications including pneumonitis, obliterative bronchiolitis, asthma, and pulmonary haemorrhage. Finally, intravenous administration increases the risk of infectious diseases, including human immunodeficiency virus (HIV) infection, endocarditis, hepatitis, and sepsis, as well as abscesses and cellulitis at the injection site.

Cocaine use is associated with a number of other serious medical problems, particularly cardiovascular complications, including cardiac arrhythmias, myocardial infarction, myocarditis, cardiomyopathy, endocarditis, and aortic dissection. Myocarditis was present in approximately 20% of regular cocaine users in one autopsy study.

A serious neurological complication of cocaine use and a leading cause of cocaine-associated deaths are seizures. The seizure threshold decreases with repeated cocaine use and associated kindling (the phenomenon whereby repeated, neural stimulation increases vulnerability for seizures to occur). Additionally, acute cocaine use increases the risk of stroke secondary to focal artery vasospasm, thrombosis, and elevated blood pressure. Chronic use can result in significant hypoperfusion in the frontal, periventricular, and temporoparietal areas, changes that have been linked to deficits in attention, concentration, learning, visual and verbal memory, and visuomotor integration.

Stimulant use can lead to significant psychiatric symptoms, both acutely and chronically. Acute symptoms include grandiosity, impulsiveness, and aggression. Common complications of chronic use include panic attacks, paranoia, depression, delirium, and hypersomnia.

Medical problems are more frequent among female than male drug abusers. Common complaints include infections, anaemia, sexually transmitted diseases (particularly gonorrhoea, trichomonas, and chlamydia), hepatitis, urinary tract infections, and gynaecological problems. Substance-abusing women are at an increased risk of developing a variety of reproductive dysfunctions compared with other women, including amenorrhoea, anovulation, luteal phase dysfunction, ovarian atrophy, spontaneous abortion, and early menopause.

Opioid-related pathology

As described above for stimulants, the pathology associated with regular heroin use often results from the method of drug administration and lifestyle issues. Approximately one-quarter of heroin dependent individuals die from homicide, suicide, accidents, and infectious disease within 10 to 20 years of initiating regular use.

Infections including abscesses, cellulitis, endocarditis, and septicaemia are common among opioid users. Many stem from intravenous drug administration, the use of unsterile injection equipment, and contaminated drugs. Infection with the hepatitis C virus, associated with an increased mortality rate, is a growing concern among intravenous drug users. In the United States of America, as many as two-thirds of patients seeking drug treatment are positive for hepatitis C; hepatitis B is also fairly common. Both contribute to the liver dysfunction frequently observed in these patients.

More than 30% of adult and 50% of paediatric AIDS (acquired immunodeficiency syndrome) cases in the United States of America are directly or indirectly associated with intravenous drug use, and in both the United States of America and Europe over one-third of drug treatment patients are infected with HIV. As a result, more aggressive harm reduction strategies are recommended by some to reduce the spread of HIV, and needle exchange programmes in which drug dependent users can exchange used for new injection equipment are increasing. Other sexually transmitted diseases including syphilis, gonorrhoea, trichomonas, and chlamydia also are common, especially among female drug users.

Tuberculosis (TB) emerged in the 1990s as a significant concern among intravenous drug users, with its rising prevalence attributed to increased susceptibility to TB infection among HIV-positive, immunocompromised drug users, and the emergence of antibiotic-resistant strains of the tubercle bacillus.

Pregnancy complications

Alcohol-related pregnancy complications

Although many women reduce unhealthy behaviours during pregnancy, including alcohol and drug use and cigarette smoking, about one in five women in the United States of America reports drinking alcohol while pregnant and 1 in 25 reports binge drinking during pregnancy. Thus, alcohol use remains high during pregnancy despite well-documented and publicized maternal and fetal risks. Because no safe alcohol limits have been established during pregnancy, women are targeted for early intervention at lower alcohol use levels during pregnancy.

At its most extreme, alcohol consumption during pregnancy can result in the fetal alcohol syndrome—characterized by facial dysmorphology, growth retardation, and CNS disorders—which is the most common preventable cause of mental retardation. The current global estimated incidence of fetal alcohol syndrome is about 1 in 1000 live births in the general obstetric population and 25 per 1000 births among alcohol dependent women. Other more common alcohol-related birth defects include reductions in weight, height, and head circumference; decreased cognitive abilities and school achievement; and an increased risk of behavioural problems such as attention deficits and impulsiveness.

Stimulant- and opiate-related pregnancy complications

Rates of illicit drug use among pregnant women range from less than 1% to about 25% depending on the sample under study. Across a variety of drug classes, drug-abusing women experience a clinically significant increase in obstetric complications compared with non-drug-using women, and the overall morbidity for drug-exposed neonates is over twice that of non-drug-exposed neonates (Table 26.7.1.1).

The most obvious neonatal complication associated with maternal drug abuse is withdrawal. Neonatal stimulant withdrawal symptoms include tremors, irritability, high-pitched and excessive crying, poor feeding, and abnormal sleep patterns.

Neonatal opiate withdrawal symptoms are very similar to those of adults, and include CNS hyperirritability, loose stools and other gastrointestinal dysfunction, nasal stuffiness, yawning, sneezing, increased lacrimation, and fever.

Drug-using women generally participate in fewer prenatal services than non-drug-using women, compromising the delivery of adequate prenatal care for these more complicated pregnancies.

Table 26.7.1.1 Obstetric complications of cocaine and heroin dependence

Cocaine	Heroin
Maternal complications	
Spontaneous abortion	Spontaneous abortion
Reduced maternal weight gain	Placental insufficiency
Placental abruption	Amnionitis/chorioamnionitis
Preterm labour	Pre-eclampsia/eclampsia
Precipitous delivery	Toxaemia
Neonatal drug withdrawal	Placental abruption
	Premature labour
	Premature rupture of membranes
	Postpartum haemorrhage
Fetal and neonatal complications	
Intrauterine growth retardation	Intrauterine growth retardation
Low birth weight	Low birth weight
Increased risk of intrauterine and perinatal infections (hepatitis, STDs, HIV)	Increased risk of intrauterine and perinatal infections (hepatitis, STDs, HIV)
Neonatal drug withdrawal	Prematurity
Anaemia	Suboptimal APGAR scores
Decreased length, head circumference	Neonatal drug withdrawal
Cardiac abnormalities	

STDs, sexually transmitted diseases.

Maternal and infant opiate-related morbidity and mortality are significantly improved among women receiving opioid replacement treatment. Maintenance has also been shown to improve the frequency of prenatal care, decrease illicit drug use, improve nutritional status, and decrease risky lifestyles. Infants of methadone-maintained mothers need to be closely monitored and (in most cases) treated for opiate withdrawal, typically using morphine sulphate or other opioid. Symptom onset is often delayed and duration may be unusually prolonged because of reduced metabolic clearance.

Treatment

Once an individual has developed alcohol or drug dependence, the course of the illness is often chronic, with intermittent episodes of recovery and relapse. The goals of treatment do not include cure but focus on minimizing withdrawal, achieving recovery quickly, and avoiding relapse to the extent possible. Inpatient settings and short-term residential programmes have traditionally been used for the early phases of treatment, particularly acute detoxification, with outpatient settings providing longer term, abstinence maintenance treatments. With growing concern over the cost-effectiveness of services, outpatient utilization has increased across all treatment phases.

Acute withdrawal management

Alcohol withdrawal

Alcohol withdrawal is potentially life-threatening. However, fewer than 10% of alcohol dependent patients are at risk for

---

Box 26.7.1.5 Symptoms of alcohol withdrawal

- Tremor
- Sweating
- Headache
- Restlessness
- Anxiety
- Nausea/vomiting
- Disorientation
- Hallucinations
- Seizures

Box 26.7.1.6 Acute opioid withdrawal symptoms

- Gastrointestinal distress—cramping, diarrhoea, nausea, vomiting
- Arthralgias or myalgias
- Increased respiratory rate
- Lacrimation
- Yawning
- Rhinorrhoea
- Piloerection
- Anxiety, restlessness, and irritability
- Tachycardia and hypertension

---

severe withdrawal symptoms, which appear within the first 24 h after drinking cessation, intensify, and then decrease over 2 to 3 days. Symptoms generally result from disinhibition of the γ-aminobutyrate (GABAergic) system and the resulting overactivation of the autonomic nervous system. Primary symptoms are shown in Box 26.7.1.5.

The level of alcohol consumption typically determines symptom severity, but comorbid medical conditions can exacerbate the problem and complicate its management.

Repeated, unmedicated withdrawal episodes may increase the risk of future alcohol withdrawal seizures (kindling), and hence withdrawal management using benzodiazepines is recommended for most patients. Symptom-driven protocols that base medication frequency and dosage on regular withdrawal severity assessments are increasingly preferred over traditional fixed-dose regimens. The Clinical Institute Withdrawal Assessment for Alcohol, revised scale (CIWA-Ar) combines patient self-report and objective withdrawal indicators and provides an easily quantified measure to guide dosing decisions. These flexible dosing protocols often decrease the total amount and duration of medication as well as the severity of withdrawal symptoms.

Recently, anticonvulsant medications have been examined for effectiveness in managing alcohol withdrawal. Generally, these medications appear to provide comparable suppression of withdrawal symptoms to the benzodiazepines. Possible advantages include reduced abuse liability and adverse events, and an improved safety profile in terms of potentiation of alcohol intoxication effects on cognitive and psychomotor performance. For most patients, alcohol withdrawal can be successfully treated on an outpatient basis.

Stimulant withdrawal

Stimulant withdrawal is characterized by primarily psychological rather than physical symptoms. The acute 'crash' following discontinuation of intense cocaine use is notable for depression, agitation, cocaine craving, and hypersomnia. Prolonged withdrawal symptoms include anhedonia, anergia, and cocaine craving.

Chronic cocaine use increases brain noradrenaline and serotonin, hence these systems have been the target for cocaine withdrawal management. Although the use of antidepressants has become popular for the treatment of dysphoric symptoms accompanying cocaine cessation, larger, well-controlled studies have provided little evidence for their effectiveness. Because the noradrenergic system is

involved in cardiovascular responses following cocaine use, adrenergic blockers such as propranolol have also been examined for management of cocaine withdrawal and relapse, and there is suggestive evidence that they may provide some benefit in cocaine dependent patients experiencing more severe withdrawal symptoms.

Opioid withdrawal

Opioids produce a very characteristic withdrawal syndrome, although the speed of onset and duration vary as a function of the half-life of the particular drug. Heroin or morphine withdrawal begins 8 to 12 h following the last dose and subsides over 5 to 7 days. Methadone withdrawal begins 12 to 16 h after the last dose, peaks in approximately 3 days, and can persist for 3 weeks or longer. Acute opioid withdrawal symptoms are shown in Box 26.7.1.6.

Multiple ancillary agents (Table 26.7.1.2) are used for symptomatic relief of opioid withdrawal, although these are typically only effective in alleviating milder symptoms, and are generally dosed on an as needed basis. Buprenorphine, a mixed agonist and antagonist drug, may offer particular advantages for opioid withdrawal management. Short-term, symptom-driven buprenorphine protocols have been successfully used for withdrawal management for opiate dependent patients.

Early intervention

Given the high prevalence of alcohol and drug disorders, all physicians treat patients with these problems. It is estimated that as many as 20% of primary care patients and 25 to 40% of inpatients are alcohol dependent or problem drinkers. Physicians should

Table 26.7.1.2 Ancillary medications for opioid withdrawal symptom relief

Medication	Suggested dose
Co-phenotrope (diphenoxylate and atropine)	10 mg or 2 tabs PO every 6 h
Dicyclomine	10 mg PO every 6 h
Methocarbamol	750 mg PO every 4–6 h
Ibuprofen	600 mg PO every 6 h
Clonidine	Variable

PO, by mouth.

routinely enquire about drinking and other drug use (prescribed and illicit), and facilitate the identification, referral and management of patients with these problems.

Most alcohol-related health consequences are experienced not by those who are alcohol dependent, but by the much larger group of heavy drinkers whose problems are at an early or relatively mild stage. Brief advice on setting safe drinking limits can have a significant and sustained impact on drinking levels in this at-risk population. These interventions begin with a focused assessment of alcohol and drug use and related problems, followed by a brief, highly directive interaction in which the health professional provides personalized feedback based on the assessment findings (e.g. elevated liver function test results or other medical problems, absenteeism or lateness at work, marital distress). Finally, the provider offers specific drinking reduction strategies, such as goal setting for 'sensible' drinking and assigning relevant reading materials. Brief interventions reduce overall alcohol use, binge drinking episodes, and hospital admissions and are easily conducted in various health care settings, including that of primary care (for further discussion see Chapter 26.7.2).

Long-term abstinence maintenance

Psychosocial treatments

Most long-term, abstinence-oriented treatments are provided in outpatient rather than inpatient facilities. Outpatient programmes typically offer assessment and diagnosis, individual and group therapy, and referral for other needed services. Outpatient services have increasingly introduced focused, empirically validated treatment interventions, such as cognitive behavioural skills training programmes, relapse prevention groups, and marital and family therapy. Family involvement in treatment and patient participation in community-based, self-help programmes such as Alcoholics Anonymous (AA) can improve long-term, post-treatment outcomes.

Retention for longer rather than shorter periods in outpatient treatment is associated with improved long-term, postdischarge outcomes across alcohol, cocaine, and opiate treatments. For drug dependent patients receiving outpatient psychosocial treatments, retention in care for 90 days or longer is associated with a reduced risk of relapse. Abstinence-focused as compared with drinking moderation treatments appear most effective for promoting long-term recovery in people with dependence disorders.

Pharmacological treatments

Alcohol pharmacotherapy

There is considerable interest in developing medications to use in conjunction with psychosocial therapies to improve treatment retention and reduce relapse. Until recently, the only pharmacotherapy for alcoholism was disulfiram, an alcohol sensitizing medication that produces flushing, nausea, vomiting, increased blood pressure, and heart rate when combined with alcohol. However, there is limited empirical support for the effectiveness of disulfiram because of poor patient acceptance and compliance.

As described above, various neurotransmitter systems contribute to alcohol reward, tolerance, and dependence; this provides an empirical basis for the development of pharmacotherapies to treat alcohol craving or reduce alcohol reward or intoxication. If persistent and intrusive thoughts about drinking (in other words, craving) and within-treatment 'slips' could be effectively treated,

this would improve patients' retention in psychosocial services and decrease their risk of more sustained relapse. Opioid receptor antagonists (such as naltrexone) decrease craving and alcohol consumption, while improving objective markers of drinking such as liver function test results. Of particular interest, naltrexone appears to reduce the risk of full blown relapse among patients who slip. A long-acting (30-day), depot formulation of naltrexone is now available to improve medication compliance. Acamprosate, an *N*-methyl-d-aspartate (NMDA) receptor antagonist, also increases abstinence and improves treatment retention; it is widely marketed in Europe and has been approved by the Food and Drug Administration (FDA) for alcoholism treatment in the United States of America. Finally, there is growing interest in medications that modulate the serotonin, GABA and glutamate systems (such as topiramate and ondansetron) for treatment of alcohol dependence.

Alcohol dependent patients with a concurrent psychiatric disorder are at increased risk of substance abuse treatment noncompliance, relapse, psychosocial and interpersonal problems, greater severity of psychiatric symptoms, and suicide attempt and completion. The psychiatric disorder often requires treatment concurrently with the substance use disorder and may not improve simply as a result of reduced alcohol and drug use (e.g. serotonergic medications may be effective in reducing drinking in alcohol dependent patients with concurrent major depression, possibly secondary to improvements in mood and overall psychosocial functioning). The nonbenzodiazepine anxiolytic, buspirone, has also been found to increase substance abuse treatment participation and duration, and improve outcomes on measures of anxiety, depression, and global psychopathology compared to placebo treatment, although not all reports are favourable.

Stimulant pharmacotherapy

There has been little progress in identifying effective pharmacological treatments for stimulant dependence and, as a result, psychosocial treatments remain the mainstay of care. Because chronic cocaine use depletes brain dopamine levels, pharmacotherapeutic research has focused predominantly on dopamine agonists. Recently, the GABA system has become a target for cocaine medication development due to the role of GABA in inhibiting dopamine activity and evidence of depleted GABA brain levels in chronic cocaine users. GABA enhancers, including topiramate, baclofen, and tiagabine, have shown some promise in reducing cocaine use in small-scale clinical trials; however, a recent multi-site study of baclofen did not. Their widespread adoption awaits further study.

Opioid pharmacotherapy

Because of the high morbidity and mortality associated with heroin use, opioid substitution therapy is the treatment of choice in the United States of America and Europe, and generally recommended for opioid dependent people who have failed in prior drug-free treatments. Opioid substitution therapy replaces the use of illicit, short-acting, injected, impure drugs with longer and orally active medications of known potency and purity. Outcomes include withdrawal symptom suppression, reduced drug craving, blockade of the euphoric effects of heroin or other opioid administration, and patient engagement with rehabilitative services.

Individual and group counselling and urine testing for illicit drugs are part of routine care in most programs. HIV/AIDS has heightened the importance of treatment approaches focused on reducing or eliminating injection drug use as opposed to achieving drug-free status. Methadone is commonly used for short- and long-term management of heroin and other opioid dependence. Buprenorphine, a mixed agonist and antagonist drug, may offer particular advantages for opioid dependent treatment.

Pain management in drug dependent patients

Drug dependence often complicates pain management. Physicians may be hesitant to use strong pain medications with these patients, worrying about exacerbation of addiction, medication diversion, and personal liability. As a result, current or past drug use is a risk factor for the undertreatment of pain. The fact that drug dependent people are actually more sensitive to pain (i.e. have lower pain thresholds in physiological studies) than nondependent individuals further complicates management. It is unclear whether this pain intolerance precedes the onset of drug use or is a neurobiological consequence of prolonged drug exposure. Hyperalgesia also may occur in patients maintained on methadone or other opioids. For patients in recovery from drug dependence, untreated or undertreated pain can be a powerful trigger for relapse.

The approach to drug dependent patients in acute pain only significantly differs from that of nondependent patients in that higher doses of pain medication may be required to achieve an equivalent level of pain control. This holds true even for patients maintained on methadone. For opioid dependent patients receiving buprenorphine treatment, this medication should be withheld in cases of acute injury where full agonist opioids are needed. Once the need for pain medications is past, buprenorphine can be reinitiated.

In substance dependent patients with chronic pain, pain management is more complex and requires attention to both concerns. The initial approach includes a thorough pain assessment (Table 26.7.1.3); identification of other psychiatric disorders; inquiry about ongoing substance use, treatment status, and frequency of treatment interactions; and discussion with the patient about realistic goals for pain management.

As complete elimination of chronic pain is unlikely, maximizing function while minimizing pain intensity should be the focus. Written agreements outlining goals, potential pharmacological and nonpharmacological objectives, expectations for substance abuse treatment, and appropriate procedures for handling medications,

Box 26.7.1.7 Indications for opioid medications in chronic pain

1 Moderate to severe persistent pain
2 Pain has significant impact on function and quality of life
3 Failure to improve function with non-opioids alone
4 Patient agreement to close monitoring of opioid medications

All four indications should exist before initiating opioids.

can clarify treatment parameters for both patient and provider. In cases where opioids are used, additional details can be added, such as methods for monitoring prescription drug use and consequences for inappropriate medication-related behaviour.

Effective pain regimens typically combine pharmacological and nonpharmacological interventions; input from multiple disciplines is often needed in implementing a comprehensive therapeutic strategy. While research supporting the efficacy of nonpharmacological interventions is limited, regimens often include physical therapy, acupuncture, or massage therapy. Pharmacological regimens typically start with nonopioid agents, either singly or in combination, chosen to target the particular type of pain. For mild to moderate pain, dosing can be on an as needed basis, while more severe pain usually requires around the clock medication. Reassessment of function and pain intensity after each medication or dosing change is crucial to determining treatment response.

There are several indications for stepping up treatment to include prescription opioids, even in patients with a history of drug dependence (Box 26.7.1.7). Long-acting opioids—either in sustained release or patch formulation—are favoured, reserving short-acting agents for breakthrough pain. Frequent follow-up should focus on assessment of function, pain intensity, side effects, and development of cravings, with medications adjusted as needed. Monitoring for prescription opioid misuse may include random urine toxicology testing, pill counts at every visit, and review of the continuum of aberrant medication-taking behaviours (Table 26.7.1.4).

If there is enough evidence to suggest misuse or abuse of medications, a frank discussion with the patient and discontinuation of opioids is warranted. It is important to emphasize that addiction treatment is a vital therapeutic component for patients with drug dependence receiving prescription opioids for chronic pain.

Likely future developments

We are gaining a better understanding of factors that contribute to the initiation and escalation of alcohol and drug use. For over three decades we have known that there are genetic influences on the development of alcohol dependence; research is now beginning to identify specific genes and proteins that may alter susceptibility. The neurotransmitter systems involved in alcohol and drug reward, dependence, and withdrawal are becoming better understood and provide exciting pathways for pharmacotherapy development: medications that interact with glutamate, GABA, cannabinoids, CRF, and neuropeptide Y are of particular interest. Knowledge of the mechanisms of alcohol- and drug-related pathologies is expanding and leading to more effective, symptom- and disease-specific interventions. A fundamental goal of much of this research

Table 26.7.1.3 Elements of initial pain assessment

Element	Validated instruments
Intensity	Visual Analogue Scale
Location	
Duration	
Aggravating and alleviating factors	
Description	
Associated symptoms	
Impact on function	McGill Pain Questionnaire
	Brief Pain Inventory
Prior laboratory and imaging tests	
Past treatments and response	

Table 26.7.1.4 Continuum of aberrant drug-taking behaviours

Less serious	→	→	More serious
Aggressively complaining about need for medication	Claiming multiple pain medicine allergies	Frequent unscheduled clinic visits for early refills	Injecting an oral formulation
Asking for specific medications by name	Visiting multiple doctors for controlled substances prescription	Refusing diagnostic workup or consultation	Forging prescriptions
Requesting to have medication dose increased	Hoarding medication	Consistent disruptive behaviour in clinic	Selling medications
Taking a few extra, unauthorized doses on occasion	Frequent calls to clinic	Obtaining controlled substances medications from family members	Use of aliases
	Using a controlled substance for nonpain relief purposes (e.g. to enhance mood, as sleep aid)	Pattern of lost or stolen prescriptions	More concern about the drug than their medical problem that persists beyond the third clinic visit
	Unwilling to sign controlled substances agreement	Anger or irritability when questioned closely about pain	Obtaining controlled medications from illicit sources
		Unwilling to consider other medications or nonpharmacological treatments	Consistently calling outside of clinic hours or when a particular physician is on call who prescribes controlled substances
		Frequent unauthorized dose escalations after being told that is inappropriate	Deterioration at home or work or reduction of social activities because of medication side effects

will be the identification of individual differences that alter susceptibility to alcohol and drug misuse, the pathological consequences of excessive use, and ultimately treatment response—all in order to more effectively target prevention and intervention approaches to the affected individual.

Further reading

Aceijas C, et al. (2004). Global overview of injecting drug use and HIV infection among injecting drug users. *AIDS*, **18**, 2295–303.

Ait-Daoud N, Malcolm RJ Jr, Johnson BA (2006). An overview of medications for the treatment of alcohol withdrawal and alcohol dependence with an emphasis on the use of older and newer anticonvulsants. *Addict Behav*, **31**, 1628–49.

American Psychiatric Association (1994). *Diagnostic and statistical manual of mental disorders (DSM-IV)*, 4th edition. American Psychiatric Association, Washington, DC.

Anton RF, Swift RM (2003). Current pharmacotherapies of alcoholism: a U.S. perspective. *Am J Addict*, **12** Suppl 1, S53–68.

Bau PF, Bau CH, Rosito GA, Manfroi WC, Fuchs FD (2007). Alcohol consumption, cardiovascular health, and endothelial function markers. *Alcohol*, **41**, 479–88.

Compton WM, et al. (2005). Developments in the epidemiology of drug use and drug use disorders. *Am J Psychiatry*, **162**, 1494–502.

Fiellin DA, Friedland GH, Gourevitch MN (2006). Opioid dependence: rationale for and efficacy of existing and new treatments. *Clin Infect Dis*, **43** Suppl 4, S173–7.

Floyd RL, et al. (2005). Recognition and prevention of fetal alcohol syndrome. *Obstet Gynecol*, **106**, 1059–64.

Gelernter J, Kranzler HR (2009). Genetics of alcohol dependence. *Hum Genet*, **126**, 91–9.

Gowing L, Ali R, White JM (2009). Buprenorphine for the management of opioid withdrawal. *Cochrane Database of Systematic Reviews*, **3**. Art. No.: CD002025.

Guerri C, Bazinet A, Riley EP (2009). Foetal Alcohol Spectrum Disorders and alterations in brain and behaviour. *Alcohol Alcohol*, **44**, 108–14.

Hannuksela ML, Liisanantti MK, Nissinen AE, Savolainen MJ (2007). Biochemical markers of alcoholism. *Clin Chem Lab Med*, **45**, 953–61.

Heilig M, Egli M (2006). Pharmacological treatment of alcohol dependence: target symptoms and target mechanisms. *Pharmacol Ther*, **111**, 855–76.

Johnson BA (2008). Update on neuropharmacological treatments for alcoholism: scientific basis and clinical findings. *Biochemical Pharmacology*, **75**, 34–56.

Kuczkowski KM (2007). The effects of drug abuse on pregnancy. *Curr Opin Obstet Gynecol*, **19**, 578–85.

Leggio L, Kenna GA, Swift RM (2008). New developments for the pharmacological treatment of alcohol withdrawal syndrome. A focus on non-benzodiazepine GABAergic medications. *Prog Neuropsychopharmacol Biol Psychiatry*, **32**, 1106–17.

Li TK (2008). Quantifying the risk for alcohol-use and alcohol-attributable health disorders: present findings and future research needs. *J Gastroenterol Hepatol*, **23**, S2–8.

Lieber CS (2004). Alcoholic fatty liver: its pathogenesis and mechanism of progression to inflammation and fibrosis. *Alcohol*, **34**, 9–19.

Mann K (2004). Pharmacotherapy of alcohol dependence: a review of the clinical data. *CNS Drugs*, **18**, 485–504.

Mathers BM, Degenhardt L, Phillips B, Wiessing L, Hickman M, Strathdee SA, Wodak A, Panda S, Tyndall M, Toufik A, Mattick RP; 2007 Reference Group to the UN on HIV and Injecting Drug Use. (2008). Global epidemiology of injecting drug use and HIV among people who inject drugs: a systematic review. *Lancet*, **372**, 1733–45.

Miller PM, Anton RF (2004). Biochemical alcohol screening in primary health care. *Addict Behav*, **29**, 1427–37.

Montoya ID, Vocci F (2008). Novel medications to treat addictive disorders. *Curr Psychiatry Rep*, **10**, 392–8.

O'Connor AD, Rusyniak DE, Bruno A (2005). Cerebrovascular and cardiovascular complications of alcohol and sympathomimetic drug abuse. *Med Clin North Am*, **89**, 1343–58.

Olsen Y, Alford DP (2006). Chronic pain management in patients with substance use disorders. *Adv Stud Med*, **6**, 537–549.

Oroszi G, Goldman D (2004). Alcoholism: genes and mechanisms. *Pharmacogenomics*, **5**, 1037–48.

Oswald LM, Wand GS (2004). Opioids and alcoholism. *Physiol Behav*, **81**, 339–58.

Puddey IB, Beilin LJ (2006). Alcohol is bad for blood pressure. *Clin Exp Pharmacol Physiol*, **33**, 847–52.

Quertemont E (2004). Genetic polymorphism in ethanol metabolism: acetaldehyde contribution to alcohol abuse and alcoholism. *Mol Psychiatry*, **9**, 570–81.

Rehm J, Taylor B, Room R (2006). Global burden of disease from alcohol, illicit drugs and tobacco. *Drug Alcohol Rev*, **25**, 503–13.

Reuben, A (2008). Alcohol and the liver. *Curr Opin Gastroenterology*, 24, 328–38.

Room R, Babor T, Rehm J (2005). Alcohol and public health. *Lancet*, **365**, 519–30.

Sofuoglu M, Kosten TR (2006). Emerging pharmacological strategies in the fight against cocaine addiction. *Expert Opin Emerg Drugs*, 11, 91–8.

Stotts AL, Dodrill CL, Kosten TR (2009). Opioid dependence treatment: options in pharmacotherapy. *Expert Opin Pharmacother*, **10**, 1727–40.

Uhart M, Wand GS (2009). Stress, alcohol and drug interaction: an update of human research. *Addict Biol*, **14**, 43–64.

Valdez GR, Koob GF (2004). Allostasis and dysregulation of corticotropin-releasing factor and neuropeptide Y systems: implications for the development of alcoholism. *Pharmacol Biochem Behav*, **79**, 671–89.

Wagner CL, et al. (1998). The impact of prenatal drug exposure on the neonate. *Obstet Gynecol Clin North Am*, **25**, 169–94.

26.7.2 Brief interventions against excessive alcohol consumption

Nick Heather and Eileen Kaner

Essentials

Treatment and prevention of alcohol-related harm includes attention to the full range of alcohol problems that occur, including hazardous and harmful drinking as well as alcohol dependence. The prevalence of these problems is high, amounting to about one in four of the adult population of the United Kingdom, which is similar to the numbers who smoke.

Definition and role—screening and brief alcohol interventions are secondary prevention activities involving early identification of alcohol-related risk or harm, followed by advice or counselling to help reduce this risk or harm. Screening and brief interventions delivered opportunistically in medical settings have a crucial role to play in improving public health.

Screening instrument—that of choice is the alcohol use disorders identification test (AUDIT), shorter versions of which are available for use in situations where time for screening is limited.

Aim and efficacy of brief interventions—the usual goal is to reduce drinking to low-risk levels, and there is very good evidence from numerous randomized controlled trials that the alcohol consumption

of hazardous and harmful drinkers can be reduced to this target, with the number needed to treat (NNT) for a successful outcome of brief alcohol intervention being about eight, which compares favourably with physicians' advice to quit smoking.

Delivery of brief intervention—there are two basic methods: (1) simple brief intervention—comprising simple, structured advice that can be delivered by someone without extensive training in 3 to 5 min; and (2) extended brief intervention—brief behavioural counselling that takes from 20 to 30 min, possibly involves repeat consultations, and needs training to deliver.

Introduction

Harm caused by excessive drinking extends far beyond 'alcoholism' or severe alcohol dependence. Alcohol-related problems can be of many different kinds—medical, interpersonal, social, psychological, financial, vocational, legal—and can be associated with varying levels and patterns of drinking. For example, problems related to acute alcohol intoxication, such as accidents, violence, and public disorder offences, need not involve high levels of alcohol dependence. When those at risk of harm are added to those who have already incurred it, the number of individuals whose lives may be adversely affected in some way by their drinking approaches one in four of the adult population (see prevalence below) and is therefore similar to the number whose health is directly affected by smoking.

Among specialists in the treatment and prevention of alcohol problems, there is now a consensus that a prior focus on the concept of alcoholism had distracted attention from the full range of alcohol problems that occur. This is not to imply that patients suffering from severe alcohol dependence should be ignored, only that the scope of treatment and preventive efforts should be broadened in an attempt to reach all those at risk and to reduce the aggregate of alcohol-related harm in society. Brief interventions in medical practice have a crucial role to play in this strategy.

Definitions

Hazardous and harmful drinking

In the International Statistical Classification of Diseases and Health-related Problems, 10th revision (ICD-10), harmful use of a psychoactive substance is defined as: 'A pattern of use which is already causing damage to health. The damage may be physical or mental.' ICD-10 guidelines go on to state that harmful use should be excluded in the presence of a dependence syndrome. Although not a diagnostic term in ICD-10, hazardous use is defined in the World Health Organization's lexicon of alcohol and drug terms as: 'A pattern of substance use that increases the risk of harmful consequences for the user.' Hazardous and harmful drinking are referred to together in this chapter as 'excessive drinking'.

Excessive drinking can be defined more precisely by drinking limits recommended by medical authorities in various countries, beginning with the level of consumption identified by epidemiological evidence as the point where the risk of harm begins to increase. In the United Kingdom, for example, a joint working group of the Royal Colleges of Physicians, Psychiatrists, and General Practitioners in 1995 defined low risk (or 'sensible') consumption as up to 21 units/week for men and 14 units/week for women, increasing risk (here hazardous) as 22 to 50 units/week for men and 15 to 35 units/week for women, and high risk (here harmful) consumption as above 50 units/week for men and above 35 units/week for women (one unit = 8 g ethyl alcohol). At about the same time, a United Kingdom government report on sensible drinking advised that, for men, consistently drinking 4 or more units a day and, for women, 3 or more units a day carries a progressive health risk. Hazardous and harmful drinking can also be defined by scores on the alcohol use disorders identification test (AUDIT) (see below).

Binge drinking

'Binge drinking' is a term that has entered into common parlance, although its precise meaning is often unclear. It was defined in the 1995 United Kingdom government report as drinking twice the daily limit (i.e. 8+ units for men/6+ for women) in one day.

Prevalence

In an alcohol needs assessment research project published in 2005, it was estimated that—in the general population of England—32% of men and 15% of women (23% overall) were hazardous or harmful drinkers. The level of excessive drinking in England and other countries of the United Kingdom is higher than in most other countries of the world. In the United Kingdom, binge drinking as defined above accounts for 40% of drinking occasions among men and 22% among women, again far higher than in many other countries. Although binge drinking is commonly associated with young people, it often persists into middle age.

Patients with alcohol problems consult their general practitioners nearly twice as often as the average, their most common problems being gastrointestinal, hypertensive, psychiatric, and accidents. Some 40 harmful drinkers and a further 100 hazardous drinkers would be expected in every 2000 patients in primary care, but it is likely that the primary care physician will be unaware of the problem in more than half of these. In surgical and general medical wards, estimates of excessive drinkers range up to 30% of all male admissions and 15% of female admissions. Again, few of these patients will be identified as hazardous or harmful drinkers. It is also well established that excessive drinkers are over-represented among patients of accident and emergency services, with an estimate in the United Kingdom of 40% of all admissions, rising to 70% at peak times.

Brief interventions

As delivered by nonalcohol specialists, brief interventions refer to a collection of methods incorporated into routine practice aimed at helping patients who drink excessively to reduce their consumption to low-risk levels. These interventions are often called 'opportunistic' because they take advantage of opportunities that arise when people present to a medical facility for reasons unconnected with a possible alcohol problem. Brief interventions are normally restricted to hazardous and harmful drinkers with no or only mild alcohol dependence or alcohol-related problems, those more seriously impaired usually being referred to specialist services. Although normally directed at a reduced drinking goal, there is no reason why brief interventions should not be targeted at total abstinence in appropriate circumstances or if the patient prefers it. However, for patients with relatively low levels of dependence and problems, insistence on abstinence is almost always a major disincentive to a change in behaviour.

Aims and targets of brief interventions

Opportunistic identification and brief intervention for excessive drinking are justified primarily as a means of early intercession and secondary prevention of alcohol problems. The attempt is made to help the patient reduce consumption or abstain before seriously adverse consequences arise, and before alcohol dependence and problems have reached levels that make intensive treatment difficult. However, as noted above, brief interventions can also be seen as making an important contribution to the public health approach to reducing alcohol-related harm at the population level. As public health measures, there is no incompatibility between the widespread implementation of brief interventions in medical practice and the adoption of fiscal, legislative, and other alcohol control policies. These two strategies can be seen as mutually reinforcing and as acting in combination to reduce and prevent alcohol-related harm.

Effectiveness of brief interventions

There is now abundant international evidence that brief interventions delivered in medical settings are efficacious in leading to reduced alcohol consumption. The most comprehensive systematic review of this evidence published so far, by Moyer and colleagues in the United States of America, considered 34 randomized controlled trials carried out in generalist settings among individuals not seeking treatment for alcohol problems. Small to medium aggregate effects were seen consistently across different follow-up points. At follow-ups of between 3 and 6 months inclusive, the effect for brief interventions compared to control conditions was significantly larger when patients showing more severe alcohol problems were excluded from the analysis.

A recent Cochrane Collaboration review by Kaner and colleagues showed that studies conducted in the 'real world' conditions of general practice do not show significantly less benefit than those carried out under optimal research conditions; hence brief interventions are effective in routine practice contexts. Equally impressive are the findings of randomized clinical trials (RCTs) carried out in emergency departments, with several large studies in the United States of America and United Kingdom showing the positive effects of brief intervention. Research in general hospital wards has been less extensive and evidence for the effectiveness of brief interventions is inconclusive at present, although there seems no good reason in principle why they should not also be effective there.

In general practice the 'number needed to treat' (NNT: the number of hazardous or harmful drinkers that need to receive a brief intervention for one to reduce drinking to low-risk levels) is about eight. This compares favourably with the NNT for physicians' advice to quit smoking. It may be that some doctors will find this success rate unacceptably low, recalling patients who have been advised to cut down but have ignored this advice. However, given that up to 80% of the population consult a health care professional at least once a year, brief interventions—if widely implemented—would undoubtedly represent a powerful means of reducing excessive drinking in the population at large. From the clinical perspective, patients who do not respond at first may do so on subsequent occasions, and even if advice seems to be ignored, it may well influence an evolving process of behaviour change.

Practical approach to brief interventions

Identifying hazardous and harmful drinkers

Screening is the process of identifying patients whose alcohol consumption places them at increased risk of physical, psychological, or social complications, and who might benefit from early detection and brief intervention. There are a number of laboratory indicators of excessive alcohol consumption, such as mean corpuscular volume (MCV), γ-glutamyl transferase (GGT), and carbohydrate-deficient transferrin (CDT). However, standardized questionnaires have been found to have a greater sensitivity and specificity than laboratory indicators in medical practice, and they are also far less intrusive and more acceptable to patients.

The alcohol use disorders identification test (AUDIT) was the first standardized instrument designed specifically to detect hazardous and harmful drinking in both primary and secondary health care settings. AUDIT is a 10-item questionnaire that includes items on drinking frequency and intensity (binge drinking), together with experience of alcohol-related problems and dependence (Fig. 26.7.2.1). At a score of 8+ out of a possible 40, the ability of AUDIT to detect genuine excessive drinkers (sensitivity) and to exclude false cases (specificity) is 92% and 93%, respectively.

While only 10 items, the full AUDIT might be considered too lengthy for use in routine practice, especially if screening is carried out during the consultation itself. For this reason, several shorter versions of the AUDIT have been developed, including the following:

- AUDIT-C—the first three (consumption) items of the AUDIT. A score of 5+ indicates hazardous or harmful drinking.

- Fast alcohol screening test (FAST)—a two-stage screening procedure based on four of the AUDIT items. Item 3 is asked first and classifies over half of respondents as either nonhazardous (Never) of hazardous (Less than monthly/monthly). Only those not classified at the first stage go on to the second stage which consists of AUDIT items 5, 8, and 10 (see Fig. 26.7.2.1). A response other than 'never' to any of these three items classifies the respondent as a hazardous drinker.

- Single alcohol screening questionnaire (SASQ)—'When was the last time you had more than 'x' drinks in one day?' (where x = eight for men and six for women)—Never/Over 12 months/3–12 months/ Within 3 months. The last response suggests hazardous or harmful drinking.

These short instruments are clearly less psychometrically efficient in varying degrees than the full AUDIT. They are therefore recommended as a prescreening procedure, followed by the full AUDIT in positive cases.

A current debate concerns the relative merits of two different approaches to screening—universal screening, aimed at all patients attending a medical facility, and targeted screening, aimed at predefined groups of patients such as those attending new patient registrations in general practice, special types of clinic or ward where hazardous and harmful drinkers are more likely to be found, and emergency department services where patients present with specific indications for hazardous or harmful drinking. Some research has shown that targeted screening is preferred by both practitioners and patients, but universal screening—if practicable—has the obvious advantage that excessive drinkers are less likely to be missed. The relative effectiveness, cost-effectiveness and acceptability of universal versus targeted screening in routine practice are the focus of ongoing research.

Types of brief intervention

While brief interventions studied in research have varied in length, contents, and theoretical orientation, research and practical considerations have identified two basic forms of intervention—simple brief intervention (simple, structured advice) and extended brief intervention (brief behavioural counselling). These two forms of brief intervention were identified in a review of the effectiveness of treatment for alcohol problems published in 2006 and are included in the Models of care for alcohol misusers issued by the United Kingdom's Department of Health.

Simple brief intervention

This consists of simple advice to cut down or abstain, personalized by taking into account the particular circumstances of the individual patient, their level of consumption in relation to population norms for their sex, and an appeal to any specific alcohol-related difficulties they may recognize as applying to them, including social and psychological as well as medical problems. The delivery of simple brief interventions should, as far as possible, follow the principles described by the acronym FRAMES:

- structured and personalized feedback on risk and harm

- emphasis on the patient's personal responsibility for change

- clear advice to the patient to make a change in drinking

- a menu of alternative strategies for making a change in behaviour

- delivered in an empathic and nonjudgemental fashion

- an attempt to increase the patient's confidence in being able to change behaviour ('self-efficacy')

Advice can be supported by the offer of self-help material, and a follow-up appointment to check on progress in cutting down will also be helpful. Successive feedback of GGT readings or other laboratory markers of alcohol consumption can be a powerful motivator. All this can be accomplished in a 3 to 5 min consultation, and specially developed brief intervention packages are available to assist this task. One such package is the 'How much is too much?' package, which was adapted from a WHO collaborative project on brief interventions in primary health care. It is available free of charge by email from the Institute of Health and Society at Newcastle University (http://www.ncl.ac.uk/ihs/enterprise). Competence in delivering a simple brief intervention does not need extensive training and one or two sessions of didactic and experiential training should suffice. A training programme developed in conjunction with the 'How much is too much?' package is available from the above website.

Simple brief intervention should be offered to patients who score between 8 and 15 on the full AUDIT, those whose drinking is within the hazardous range described above, and those whom the practitioner suspects on other grounds of drinking in a hazardous fashion. It should also be offered as a minimum to patients who

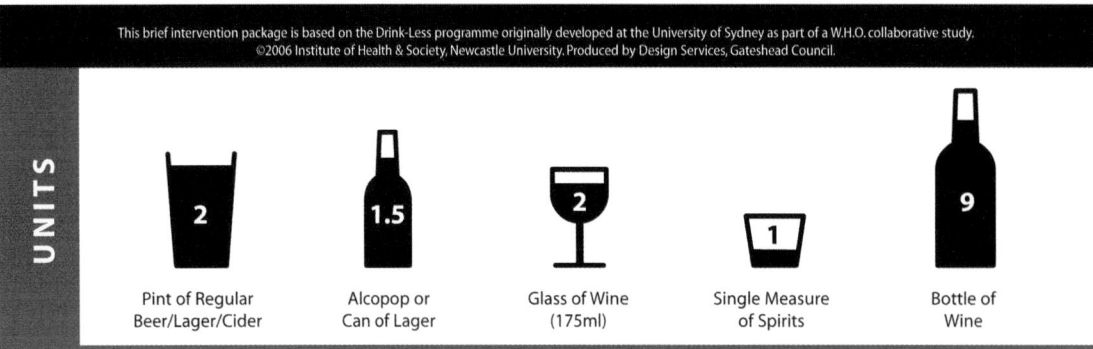

Alcohol Users Disorders Identification Test (AUDIT)

Questions	Scoring System					Your Score
	0	1	2	3	4	
How often do you have a drink that contains alcohol?	Never	Monthly or less	2 - 4 times per month	2 - 3 times per week	4+ times per week	
How many standard alcoholic drinks do you have on a typical day when you are drinking?	1 - 2	3 - 4	5 - 6	7 - 8	10+	
How often do you have 6 or more standard drinks on one occasion?	Never	Less than monthly	Monthly	Weekly	Daily or almost daily	
How often in the last year have you found you were not able to stop drinking once you had started?	Never	Less than monthly	Monthly	Weekly	Daily or almost daily	
How often in the last year have you failed to do what was expected of you because of drinking?	Never	Less than monthly	Monthly	Weekly	Daily or almost daily	
How often in the last year have you needed an alcoholic drink in the morning to get you going?	Never	Less than monthly	Monthly	Weekly	Daily or almost daily	
How often in the last year have you had a feeling of guilt or regret after drinking?	Never	Less than monthly	Monthly	Weekly	Daily or almost daily	
How often in the last year have you not been able to remember what happened when drinking the night before?	Never	Less than monthly	Monthly	Weekly	Daily or almost daily	
Have you or someone else been injured as a result of your drinking?	No		Yes, but not in the last year		Yes, during the last year	
Has a relative/friend/doctor/health worker been concerned about your drinking or advised you to cut down?	No		Yes, but not in the last year		Yes, during the last year	

Scoring: 0-7 = sensible drinking, 8-15 = hazardous drinking, 16-19 = harmful drinking and 20+ = possible dependence

How much is too much?   Screening Tools

Fig. 26.7.2.1 The AUDIT screening tool.
Saunders JB, Aasland OG, Babor TF, de la Fuente JR, Grant M. Development of the Alcohol Use Disorders Identification Test (AUDIT): WHO Collaborative Project on Early Detection of Persons with Harmful Alcohol Consumption-II. Addiction 1993; 88:791-804.

are thought to need more intensive intervention but who decline to accept it.

Extended brief intervention

An extended brief intervention typically takes 20 to 30 min to deliver and can involve a small number of repeat sessions. It is essentially a condensed form of 'motivational interviewing' in which an attempt is made to elicit, rather than impose, an increase in motivation to change behaviour. More specifically, extended brief intervention is based on generic principles of health behaviour change described by Rollnick and colleagues.

The level of training required to carry out this form of brief intervention effectively is substantially greater than that for simple advice and should involve an emphasis on experiential learning. Again, training materials are available from the website above. In addition, clinical guidelines on brief interventions and training materials are available from the Primary Healthcare European Project on Alcohol (http://www.phepa.net).

Extended brief intervention should be offered to harmful drinkers (AUDIT 16–19) whose level of alcohol-related harm indicates a need for it and who are willing to accept it. It may also be suitable for hazardous drinkers who are ambivalent about their drinking and wish to discuss it with a health care professional, or for those who do not respond to simple advice and wish further assistance in reducing drinking to safer levels. More generally, extended brief intervention is suitable for use by those practitioners (medical, nursing, or other health care professionals) who take a special interest in alcohol-related problems and have the time and commitment to learn and deliver it.

Implementing brief interventions

In a survey of general practitioners carried out in the English Midlands during 1995 to 1996, the main barriers to implementing brief interventions were stated as insufficient time and training, lack of appropriate reimbursement, and lack of help from government policy; the main incentives related to the availability of appropriate support services and the proven effectiveness of brief interventions. These barriers and incentives remain relevant today. As this chapter has shown, there is very good evidence for the effectiveness of brief interventions and it is clearly necessary to disseminate this information more widely. With regard to other barriers and incentives, strenuous efforts are now being made to persuade policy makers and decision makers at national, regional, and district levels to create the conditions needed to support the widespread implementation in routine medical practice of brief interventions against excessive alcohol consumption.

Possible dependence

Patients who score 20 or above on the full AUDIT should be assessed for the presence of an alcohol dependence syndrome and, if appropriate, referred on for specialist treatment of alcohol dependence. See Chapter 26.7.1 for further discussion.

Further reading

Bush K, et al. (1998). The AUDIT alcohol consumption questions (AUDIT-C): an effective brief screening test for problem drinking. Ambulatory Care Quality Improvement Project (ACQUIP). Alcohol Use Disorders Identification Test. Arch Intern Med, 158, 1789–95.

Department of Health (1995). Sensible drinking. The report of an interdepartmental working group. http://www.dh.gov.uk/prod_consum_dh/groups/dh_digitalassets/@dh/@en/documents/digitalasset/dh_4084702.pdf

Department of Health (2005). Alcohol needs assessment research project (ANARP). The 2004 national alcohol needs assessment for England. http://www.dh.gov.uk/prod_consum_dh/groups/dh_digitalassets/@dh/@en/documents/digitalasset/dh_4122239.pdf

Department of Health (2006). Models of care for alcohol misusers (MoCAM). http://www.dh.gov.uk/prod_consum_dh/groups/dh_digitalassets/@dh/@en/documents/digitalasset/dh_4136809.pdf

Heather N (2003). Brief interventions. In: Heather N, Stockwell T (eds) Essential handbook of treatment and prevention of alcohol problems, pp.117–138. Wiley Blackwell, Chichester.

Heather N, Robertson I (1997). Problem drinking, 3rd edition. Oxford University Press, Oxford.

Hodgson R, et al. (2002). The FAST Alcohol Screening Test. Alcohol Alcohol, 37, 61–6.

Kaner EF, et al. (1999). Intervention for excessive alcohol consumption in primary health care: attitudes and practices of English general practitioners. Alcohol Alcohol, 34, 559–66.

Kaner EF, et al. (2007). Brief interventions for excessive drinkers in primary health care settings. Cochrane Database of Systematic Reviews, Issue 2. Art No.: CD004148 DOI: 10.1002/14651858.CD004148.pub3.

Moyer A, et al. (2002). Brief interventions for alcohol problems: a meta-analytic review of controlled investigations in treatment-seeking and non-treatment seeking populations. Addiction, 97, 279–292.

Prime Minister's Strategy Unit (2003). Interim Analytical Report, Strategy Unit, Alcohol Harm Reduction Project. Cabinet Office, London. http://www.number10.gov.uk/files/pdf/SU%20interim_report2.pdf

Raistrick D, Heather N, Godfrey C (2006). Review of the effectiveness of treatment for alcohol problems. National Treatment Agency for Substance Misuse, London. http://www.nta.nhs.uk/publications/documents/nta_review_of_the_effectiveness_of_treatment_for_alcohol_problems_fullreport_2006_alcohol2.pdf

Rollnick S, Miller W, Butler C (2008). Motivational interviewing in health care: helping patients change. Guilford Press, New York.

Royal Colleges of Physicians, Psychiatrists, and General Practitioners (1995). Alcohol and the heart in perspective: sensible limits reaffirmed. Report of a joint working party. Royal College of Physicians, London.

Williams R, Vinson DC (2001). Validation of a single screening question for problem drinking. J Fam Pract, 50, 307–12.

SECTION 27

Forensic medicine

Forensic medicine and the practising doctor

Anthony Busuttil

Essentials

Doctors have to keep in mind their legal responsibilities and duties from the very first day of their practice. The services of a medical practitioner are often called upon when injuries and other forms of abuse have taken place, and also when death has occurred, particularly if death was sudden and unexpected. As a direct consequence, the doctor may acquire information that suggests a suspicious and potentially criminal event. In such instances, the doctor's duty of care and bond of confidentiality to the patient must be carefully balanced against their duties as a citizen of a country in which homicide cannot go undetected and crime cannot be condoned.

Duties at a death

When a doctor is called to a person thought to have died, six principal responsibilities have to be considered: (1) to confirm the fact of death and document the event at the time; (2) to exclude on medical grounds, where possible, any suspicions of foul play or negligence in relation to the death; (3) to identify whether there is a requirement to report the death to the appropriate authorities who have a duty to investigate deaths; (4) to issue a medical certificate of the causes of death when in a position to do so; (5) if unable to issue a death certificate, to refer the death to the legal authorities; and (6) if appropriate, and if the medical practitioner is suitably qualified, to issue other certification, which may be required in relation to the death and the disposal of the decedent.

In the recently deceased, formal clinical examination is required to ensure that the pumping action of the heart and breathing have both ceased by (1) auscultation over the chest for a timed period of about 2 min; (2) feeling the tension in the eyes, which decreases quite promptly after death; and (3) looking at the eyes—the pupils assume a mid position and the corneal and light reflexes disappear.

Other matters

This chapter includes sections on (1) particular causes of death—deaths resulting from and in the course of medical care, sudden infant deaths, sudden unexpected nocturnal deaths in adults, sudden death syndrome, cocaine abuse; (2) survivors of violence—including sexual assaults and the medical notes, with particular reference to wounding; (3) intoxication; (4) access to information; and (5) the forensic use of molecular biological techniques.

Introduction

The interface and borders between the law and the medical profession are becoming increasingly wider and their implications more far-reaching, and doctors have to keep in mind their legal responsibilities and duties from the very first day of their practice. Sound ethical principles should form the backbone of professional clinical practice, ensuring competence and integrity of the medical practitioner. The doctor–patient relationship is a partnership based on mutual trust, respect, and confidence, with the fundamental rights of every patient being adhered to always and respected fully. These patient rights are succinctly enshrined in the Declaration of Lisbon agreed to in September 1981 by the 34th Assembly of the World Medical Association (Box 27.1.1).

In addition to dealing with natural illnesses, the services of the medical practitioner, whether in primary care or in hospital practice, are often called upon when injuries and other forms of abuse have taken place, and also when death has occurred, particularly if death was sudden and unexpected. As a direct consequence, the doctor may acquire information that suggests a suspicious and potentially criminal event. In such instances the doctor's duty of care and bond of confidentiality to the patient must be carefully balanced against their duties as a citizen of a country in which homicide cannot go undetected and crime cannot be condoned. In the United Kingdom the General Medical Council (GMC) now formally places a duty on all registered doctors to assist the coroner or procurator fiscal by responding to their enquiries and by offering them relevant information about the deceased patient: you are only entitled to remain silent when your evidence may incriminate you or lead to court proceedings against you.

The courts

It is to be recalled at all times that the system in the courts in the United Kingdom, in contrast to other parts of Europe, is very firmly based on the so-called 'adversarial' system, with the sole

Box 27.1.1 Declaration of Lisbon

Recognizing that there may be practical, ethical, and legal difficulties, a physician should always act according to his or her conscience and always in the best interest of the patient. The following declaration represents some of the principal rights that the medical profession seeks to provide to patients. Whenever legislation or governmental action denies these rights of the patient, physicians should seek by appropriate means to assure and restore them.

♦ The patient has the right to choose his physician freely.

♦ The patient has the right to be cared for by a physician who is free to make clinical and ethical judgements without outside interference.

♦ The patient has the right to accept or refuse treatment after receiving adequate information.

♦ The patient has the right to expect that his physician will respect the confidential nature of his medical and personal details.

♦ The patient has the right to die with dignity.

♦ The patient has the right to receive or decline spiritual and moral comfort, including the help of a minister of an appropriate religion.

exception of the coroners' courts where an inquisitorial system is in place. In the adversarial system within the criminal courts, the object of the forensic exercise is for those acting for the prosecution on behalf of the State (Her Majesty in England, Wales, and Northern Ireland and the Lord Advocate—or procurator fiscal—in Scotland) to prove that the charges laid against the person in the dock (the 'plaintiff' in England and the 'accused' in Scotland) can be proved 'beyond reasonable doubt'. The charges are drafted in terms of alleged contraventions of the statutes of criminal law or of 'common law'. The common law is a universal system of unwritten law, applied commonly and universally throughout the land, which employs a set of principles, tenets, and maxims that can provide answers to legal problems and can be applied by the judiciary in deciding on cases. Over the years common law has been interpreted and remoulded by the decisions of one generation of judges after another; these decisions are recorded and can be alluded to and quoted in decisions and judgments made by other judges. As a hierarchy of courts developed, thereby enabling an appeal against a decision reached in a lower court to a more senior court, decisions taken by higher courts became binding on lower courts—the concept of 'precedent'. The courts do this by adducing evidence taken under oath or affirmation from witnesses in open court. This enables in minor (summary) cases, the judge, or in serious cases (indictable or solemn cases), the members of the jury (15 in Scotland in criminal cases, 12 in the rest of the United Kingdom) to come to decision. If the verdict is one of 'guilty', the judge will sentence the accused according to tariffs—fines, custodial sentences, community work, etc.—laid down in the statute. The object of the defence is to attempt to cast doubt and demolish the evidence that is being given: they do so through their own witnesses, of which the accused may be one, and by cross-examination of the

prosecution witnesses. They are entitled to instruct experts of their own in criminal cases, paid for, if needs be, by the public purse.

The expert witness

The medical practitioner in active employment is usually exempt from jury service but may have to give evidence to fact either as an 'ordinary' witness, like any other citizen, or as a 'professional' witness, by divulging to the court information which they have gathered in their professional capacity, e.g. about injuries, physical or mental illness of the persons in the dock, or other witnesses who have suffered injury. In matters of a scientific and medical nature, when the courts wish to be informed and have explained to them matters which do not fall within the ambit of common knowledge and common sense, persons of a sufficient experience and expertise in the particular subject who can suitably assist may be called as witnesses. By giving information about these matters to the court in this capacity the witness is referred to as an 'expert' (from the Latin *ex*, from; *peritia*, specialized skill). They are not there to come to a decision on behalf of the court, but solely to assist to the best of their capacity with information, and if required, also to give opinions based on their professional experience and expertise. Details of their qualifications and specialization would be brought to the attention of the courts at the commencement of the expert evidence. They are there as 'advocates for their opinion' and not 'to win cases for the side that has called them'.

The role of the medical expert witness has come under close scrutiny in Britain following the successful second appeal of Sally Clark against a conviction for homicide in which expert evidence was disputed. The GMC disciplined the expert witness and an appeal was heard in the Supreme Court of Judicature—Court of Appeal [Civil Division] on appeal from the High Court of Justice—*[2006] EWCA Civ 1390*. The court reiterated the standards expected of expert witnesses as classically defined in the judgement of Cresswell J in *National Justice CIA Naviera SA v Prudential Assurance Co. Ltd.(The Ikarian Reefer) [1993] 2 Lloyd's Reports 68, 81–82.* (Box 27.1.2).

In the coroners' courts, whose sole limit is the investigation of death, the questions are asked of all the witnesses by the coroner, who has to come to a decision at the end of the public 'inquest' as to the identity of the person who has died, when and where they died, and how they came about their death. There is no such office in Scotland, where death investigations are carried out in private by the procurator fiscal. There are no public inquests except for deaths in custody and in the course of work as a consequence of the employment; in all other cases the Lord Advocate decides whether 'in the public interest' a fatal accident inquiry is required.

In civil cases one party—persons, or company, or corporate body—sues another party, and the arbiter in almost all such cases is a judge or judges. Both sides can call witnesses, including expert witnesses, to give evidence, and all witnesses can be cross-examined. The only remedy in the civil courts is a pecuniary one, namely the award of monetary damages. The case requires to be proven 'on the balance of probabilities'.

Duties at a death

Death can be said to have occurred in the body of a person when there is either irreversible cessation of all function of the brain, or irreversible cessation of the circulation of blood.

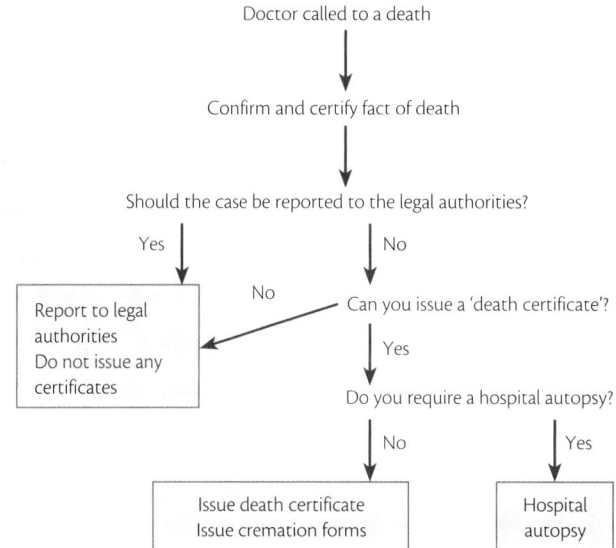

Fig. 27.1.1 The duties of a doctor called to a death.

6 If appropriate, and if the medical practitioner is suitably qualified, to issue other certification which may be required in relation to the death and the disposal of the decedent

Confirming and documenting death

In the recently deceased it is essential that a formal clinical examination is carried out to ensure that the pumping action of the heart and breathing have both ceased. This should be done by auscultation over the chest for a timed period of about 2 min. It is also useful to feel the tension in the eyes, which decreases quite promptly after death (due to a lack of blood pressure), and to look at the eyes—the pupils assume a mid position and the corneal and light reflexes disappear. If the cornea is still transparent and moist (usually until about 10 min after death if the eyelids were closed), and if in any doubt, it may be useful to examine the eye with an ophthalmoscope: the blood in the retinal veins breaks up into segments within 10 s of clinical death in most instances, a phenomenon variously referred to a 'railroading' or 'cattle-trucking'. In all deaths, there is also blanching of all retinal vessels if the eyeball is pressed with a finger.

In the presence of severe mutilation and burning, or if the body is showing obvious features of decomposition, these tests are obviously superfluous and to carry them out would not be sensible.

Great care must be taken in situations in which vital functions and general metabolism may have been decreased to such an extreme as to simulate death. For a doctor to be caught out in such situations is not only a major embarrassment but may lead to civil action for damages and disciplinary procedures for erroneous certification. Such 'apparent death' or 'suspended animation' can take place in instances where there has been an overdose of central nervous system depressant drugs, hypothermia from exposure or medical complaints, electrocution, drowning, or psychiatric catatonic states. When in any doubt, particularly when such conditions are present in combination, and particularly in the young, it is always wise to attempt full resuscitation (or 'reanimation' as it is referred to in continental Europe) (see Chapter 17.1).

In all situations when death has been medically confirmed, this must be fully documented in the case notes, with the entry timed,

In this country there is no statutory definition of death as exists elsewhere, e.g. in the United States of America or in New South Wales, Australia. There is also no statutory requirement that the diagnosis of the fact of death is invariably made by a doctor; it is, however, customary that all diagnoses of death are confirmed by a medical practitioner. This is no longer essential, and nurses and paramedics who have been specifically trained can verify that death has occurred.

When a doctor is called to a person thought to be have died, six principal responsibilities have to be considered (Fig. 27.1.1):

1 To confirm the fact of death and document this at the time

2 To exclude on medical grounds, where possible, any suspicions of foul play or negligence in relation to the death

3 To identify whether there is a requirement to report the death to the appropriate authorities who have a statutory (Her Majesty's coroners in England, Wales, and Northern Ireland) and/or 'common law' (procurators fiscal in Scotland) duty to investigate deaths

4 To issue a medical certificate of the causes of death (commonly referred to as the death certificate) when in a position to do so

5 If unable to issue a death certificate, to refer the death to the legal authorities

dated, and signed. This should be done at the time or as soon afterwards as is reasonable, and the entry should list the clinical tests carried out.

Brain death

The diagnosis of brain death (or 'brainstem death') in patients in an apnoeic coma should be done accurately and positively, even in the presence of a beating heart and machine-maintained respiration, by an appropriately qualified and suitably experienced medical practitioner (at least 5 years registration). Tests have to be carried by two doctors and on two occasions several hours apart. Details are discussed in Chapter 17.9, but in brief:

◆ Any potentially reversible condition that has led to cerebral depression must be positively excluded. The coma must not be due to central nervous system depressant drugs, neuromuscular blocking agents (muscle relaxants), hypothermia, or metabolic abnormalities, particularly hypoglycaemia, renal or hepatic failure.

Once all these conditions have been excluded, the simple tests used to confirm that brain death has occurred are that:

◆ Both pupils should be fixed, though not necessarily equal and rounded, and do not react to light.

◆ No response occurs to corneal stimulation with cotton wool.

◆ No response is found to the presence of the endotracheal tube, or any cough response to suction applied to the tracheal lumen.

◆ No eye movements occur when 20 ml of ice-cold water are injected into the external auditory meati, having previously established clear access to the eardrums.

◆ No motor cranial nerve responses are elicited to painful stimuli, e.g. earlobe pinching, supraorbital pressure.

◆ There is no spontaneous breathing with the onset of hypercapnia by disconnecting the respiratory support for a sufficiently lengthy period to allow the $Paco_2$ to build up.

If brain death is thus diagnosed, the time when this has first been definitively established can be taken as the 'time of death', and not the time that the respiratory support is withdrawn. Any subsequent harvesting of organs will therefore be carried out on a cadaver in whom artificial respiratory and other support has been retained.

The time of death

The actual time of death will always precede the time that 'life is pronounced extinct', and the duration of this period—often referred to as the 'post-mortem interval'—is frequently unknown and unknowable. Forensic pathologists are often involved in making estimates of this period by utilizing such phenomena as cooling of the body after death, the onset and distribution of rigor mortis, etc. This is an area fraught with problems and inaccuracies, and one that the non-forensically-qualified medical practitioner should best refrain from venturing into and giving any professional opinions on. In those instances where the estimation of the post-mortem interval is of specific importance, this matter should be referred to those who are forensically qualified.

Excluding foul play

Doctors, like other professional persons, have an overriding duty to the 'society' in which they practise, which allows breaches of medical confidentiality when it comes to ensuring that crime is prevented, fully investigated, and detected. Thus, if a medical practitioner suspects or has good reason to believe that a particular death was due to a criminal or negligent act, it is their unalienable public duty to ensure that this incident is reported to the police, and that no certification is completed, no matter how obvious the cause of death may be. If the doctor has acted in 'good faith' in such instances, even if their suspicions are eventually found to be unfounded on due investigation, they do not lay themselves open to civil litigation by informing about the death.

No matter the age of the decedent, but particularly so in elderly people and in children, other considerations should not obscure or sidetrack the doctor from accepting the possibility that death was due to a criminal or negligent act. In this respect it may be of some importance, as part of the diagnosis of the fact of death, to look carefully for petechial facial haemorrhages in all decedents, particularly around the eyes, behind the ears, on the labial mucosa, and specifically in the conjunctivae. In the absence of known coagulation problems their presence on the face should always be taken seriously, especially in babies, and if found should always raise the possibility of death being due to a mechanical form of asphyxia, suggesting the possibility of another party's involvement in the death.

Reporting deaths to the legal authorities

Certain categories of deaths are always reportable to the legal authorities. These include all violent deaths, deaths from all types of accidents, including medical mishaps, no matter how long before the death this accident took place; deaths from suicide and suspected suicide; deaths in legal custody and in secure mental institutions; deaths in fires and explosions, from suspected poisoning, from industrial diseases, and from other diseases which by law are notifiable—these include tuberculosis and hepatitis (but not HIV-related deaths). Deaths in which a medical, surgical, or therapeutic mishap may have contributed to or caused the death of the patient always have to be reported.

If the cause of death is not known and yet there is no other reason why the death should be reported, that death is an uncertified death and thus has to be reported. In such instances this notification should precede any attempts to secure an autopsy.

Death certification

The certification of death is a privilege accorded to doctors as a consequence of fulfilling the criteria for their registration with the GMC, and thus any misuse or abuse of this principle would render the doctor liable to a disciplinary procedure. The death certificate is an important statutory document and also a very important public health record: it should be filled in carefully and with all due consideration.

The certifier of the causes of death does so to 'the best of my knowledge and belief' and records both the immediate causes of death (Part I), these to be placed in a sequence with the initial line (a) being the condition which chronologically resulted from the condition in the second line (b) and so on. Other conditions that have contributed to the death or accelerated it should be listed in Part II of the certificate.

Terms describing the mode of dying, e.g. cardiac arrest, cardiac failure, coma, are inappropriate to use in this context, except if they are qualified by the underlying causative pathological condition, such as ischaemic heart disease. Terms such as 'senility' and 'old age' should strictly refer to decedents above the age of 80 years, and then only when there was no further recent superimposed pathology and if the patient had deteriorated gradually over a period of weeks prior to death. 'Natural causes' is not acceptable. However, it is accepted that in certain instances the determination of the cause of death would have to await laboratory studies, e.g. overdose deaths, and in such instances a death certificate indicating this may be acceptable.

Reporting to the legal authorities

People who have been recently bereaved are understandably often in a very distressed state, and great care and sensitivity should be exercised in ensuring that their grief is not made more acute. Any delays in certification would compound such grief, yet the doctor should not feel pressurized, and every effort should be made to follow the rules and regulations strictly. Religious observances and rites, and other social considerations and conventions, may also be brought to bear on the doctor. Although the family of the deceased should be heard out with deference and respect, the certifying doctor should not compromise his or her position in any way. If the doctor cannot certify the death or is bound to report it for any other reason, then the case should be referred further.

Consent to a hospital autopsy and to the retention of organs or tissues therefrom can only be sought if the cause of death is known and all other legal requirements have been abided by. This consent should be given in writing by the next of kin on the forms designated for this purpose. New parliamentary acts are now in force which covers these matters (Human Tissue Act 2004; Human Tissue (Scotland) Act 2006).

Other certification

In the United Kingdom the disposal of the deceased's body by cremation is covered by statute and statutory regulations. For human remains to be disposed of by cremation, a series of forms have to be endorsed by medical practitioners. Form B can be signed by any registered doctor and gives details of the death and its causes; Form C, a confirmatory certificate, can only be signed by a doctor who has been fully registered for 5 years. Both doctors need to have inspected the body after death and have conferred, and the second doctor needs to have spoken to some other person who had treated, nursed, or been otherwise directly involved in the patient's last illness. The duty of the 'Medical Referee to the Crematorium' is to scrutinize these certificates and the application for cremation (Form A), and if fully satisfied authorize the cremation to proceed. In cases reported to the legal authorities the coroner or procurator fiscal signs the forms that should otherwise have been signed by the two medical practitioners. In all instances, permanent pacemakers and radioactive implants have to be removed before cremation.

If the body has to be transported abroad or to other parts of the United Kingdom, there may be a requirement for further certificates to enable this to take place. These include certificates from the legal authorities enabling the movement of the body outwith their jurisdiction and confirming they require no further access to it, a 'freedom from infection' certificate, and often an 'embalming certificate'.

Particular causes of death

Deaths resulting from and in the course of medical care

No matter how vigilant and caring medical and surgical treatment may be, occasional deaths will occur in the course of treatment as a direct consequence of the treatment. This may due to an allergic or idiosyncratic response to medication, and much more rarely through error, such as giving an excessive dose of a drug, or from accidents (e.g. intra-arterial vs intravenous injection) or mishaps (e.g. internal bleeding after a liver biopsy). For this reason, deaths that occur during operation or in the early postoperative period, during investigative procedures, in the course of the administration of a general or local anaesthetic, or in the progress of clinical trials, invariably become the subject of a legal investigation.

Such deaths in the course of medical care raise the spectre of litigation and claims of medical negligence. There should be absolute transparency in divulging all the facts about such deaths, which should always be investigated by a pathologist who is completely independent of the hospital or other establishment in which the death has occurred, and who has some previous experience in such investigations. The investigating pathologist requires access to all the medical notes of the deceased patient, full statements from the doctors and nursing staff involved, detailing their involvement (disconcertingly, often acquired by the police), a thorough examination of any equipment used, access to batches of drugs used and blood samples collected before death. Such investigations will invariably require the assistance and participation of a number of 'experts' in other fields.

Sudden infant deaths

The careful investigation of death in infancy and childhood has led to major successful preventive campaigns; perhaps if unexpected adult deaths were to be looked at as carefully, similar measures could be implemented. These deaths have also led to the production of universally acceptable protocols for post-mortem examination that involve photography, radiology, microbiology, virology, immunology, genetics, etc. If this approach were to be emulated in other death investigations, the end-product therefrom would be much enhanced. A multi-agency working group convened by the Royal College of Pathologists and the Royal College of Paediatrics and Child Health under the chairmanship of Baroness Helena Kennedy QC reported in 2004 and called for changes:

> The investigation is to be carried out by specially trained individuals, with an emphasis on multi-agency working, involving close collaboration and the sharing of information between hospital- and community-based clinical staff, the pathologist, the police, social services and the coroner's service. The investigation will concentrate not just on the child, but will consider family history, past events and the circumstances in which the child lived.

As infectious diseases no longer take a major toll in infancy in most developed countries, and as serious congenital conditions are no longer so prevalent, the most important cause of the sudden death of infants after the first month of life and within the first year is the 'sudden infant death syndrome' (SIDS, sometimes referred to as 'cot death' or 'crib death'). The original definition, still applicable, is of 'sudden death of any young child—usually under 1 year of age—that is unexpected by the history, and in which a thorough post-mortem examination fails to demonstrate an adequate cause of death'. Most pathologists would also wish to have a thorough inspection of the scene of the death to exclude potentially noxious environmental agents, e.g. carbon monoxide exposure.

The diagnosis of SIDS is therefore only made by carefully and meticulously excluding any other causes, and is a morbid anatomical diagnosis rather than a clinical one; an autopsy is therefore a *sine qua non* to reach this diagnosis. It is especially important to exclude congenital metabolic abnormalities such as medium-chain acyl coenzyme A dehydrogenase (MCAD) deficiencies by appropriate testing (plasma/blood spot acylcarnitine profiles in MCAD deficiencies) and thus alert the family to possible further recurrences. Trauma and poisoning by alcohol, or with other sedative or anxiolytic preparations, also have to be excluded specifically on appropriate autopsy samples; fabricated or induced illness formerly known as 'Münchhausen syndrome by proxy', first described by Meadow in 1977, is another condition to be aware of.

The incidence of SIDS has decreased dramatically in many industrialized countries as a result of major public health educational campaigns advising parents about the risk factors and means of prevention. Overheating of the child is one such risk factor. Parents are instructed to prevent this by removing the child's headgear when indoors, and by ensuring that the sleeping child does not wear excessive clothing or have too many bedclothes, by preventing the ambient bedroom temperature from being too high, and by seeking medical advice when the child appears feverish. The dangers of cigarette smoking close to the baby have also been emphasized as an important risk factor for this and other childhood complaints. Cosleeping and the possibility of overlaying are also to be considered in the younger age groups, and if medication or other substances are taken which may increase depth of (the adult's) sleep. The 'back-to-sleep' campaign, i.e. ensuring that the child is placed in the prone sleeping position, is based on another epidemiologically established important risk factor. Paradoxically, immunization of the child for common childhood illnesses, once thought related to SIDS, has been shown to be protective and is thus further encouraged in this connection.

The actual pathogenetic cause of SIDS is still uncertain in most instances: hypoxia, cardiac arrhythmias, hypoglycaemia, loss of vascular tone, reflex apnoea, prolonged QT, cerebral problems, and heat shock have all been proposed, as well as the 'superantigen' effects of bacterial toxins. Other important aspects of the epidemiology of this condition is the seasonal incidence, the familial recurrence, the increased incidence in boys, and the increased association with certain ethnic groups, such as Native Americans and Australian Aborigines, and its absence in others, e.g. immigrant families from the Indian subcontinent. The pathognomonic feature of SIDS, which is yet to be explained, is the finding of diffuse, internal petechial haemorrhages overlying the thymus and beneath the pleura and the pericardium.

Sudden unexpected nocturnal deaths in adults

The syndrome of sudden unexpected nocturnal deaths (SUND) occurs in young adults and adolescents, mainly in immigrant workers from South-East Asia employed in Singapore and Saudi Arabia, and in refugees from eastern Asia. These decedents are usually employed in manual jobs in the building or the gardening trades, and have been residing in their adoptive country for several months. They are almost exclusively men who smoke or who are passively exposed to smoke in their environment, and who have a

recent history of a mild upper respiratory tract infection; petechiae may also be found internally. These deaths mostly occur during sleep and at night.

Various theories have been put forward, including vitamin B and other nutritional deficiencies, familial cardiac arrhythmias, brainstem epilepsy, *Pfeifferinella mallei* infection, stress and homesickness, and bacterial toxin production from nasopharyngeal colonization by *Staphylococcus aureus*, but no specific and recurring cause has been identified.

It is also the case that a full autopsy, with comprehensive toxicological and histological investigations, in the occasional sporadic death of an adolescent native of this country fails to yield a cause of death. Such deaths have been labelled as 'deaths from SUND' in the United Kingdom. However, it must be kept strictly in mind that this diagnosis is also one of exclusion, and should be used sparingly and appositely.

Sudden death syndrome

Sudden death syndrome is an umbrella term used for the many different causes of cardiac arrest in young people and is defined as a nontraumatic, nonviolent, unexpected occurrence resulting from cardiac arrest within as little as 6 h of previously witnessed normal health. The possible causes are listed with references in Box 27.1.3.

Cocaine abuse

Background

Cocaine is far from being a 'safe' recreational drug and is a powerfully addictive stimulant. Its illicit use has increased throughout the United Kingdom in recent years: its price on the street is lower and thus it is more easily affordable; it is no longer the drug of the rich. Cocaine (benzoylmethylecgonine, $C_{17}H_{21}NO_4$) is an alkaloid prepared from the leaves of the *Erythroxylon coca* plant by dissolving it in hydrochloric acid, thus forming a water-soluble salt, cocaine hydrochloride. It is sold illicitly as a fine white powder, or as crystals or granules. This has usually been mixed with inert substances such as cornstarch, talcum powder, sugars (e.g. lactose and mannitol), chemically related local anaesthetics (e.g. procaine and lignocaine), or other stimulants such as amphetamines. Cocaine can be 'freebased', before smoking, by dissolving it in ether or ammonia and then evaporating the volatile solvent; this form of cocaine was popular in the late 1970s. A further refinement, introduced in the United States of America during the 1980s, is the production of 'crack' cocaine by mixing cocaine hydrochloride with sodium bicarbonate (baking soda) and water, and then heating. On cooling, 'rocks' are precipitated, and these are smoked in crack pipes, or are heated on foil with the hot vapour inhaled.

Cocaine is abused in several ways: by snorting (inhalation through the nose with absorption into the bloodstream through the vascular submucosal nasal tissue); by smoking (which involves inhaling cocaine vapour or smoke into the lungs where absorption into the bloodstream is as rapid as by injection), when it is sometimes mixed with cannabis and also with heroin ('speedball' or 'snowball'); by application to the genitalia. With crack cocaine vapour is inhaled from a heated foil or pipe, and this may also be laced with marijuana. Each of these methods of administration poses great risks to the user. In the United Kingdom, cocaine is classified as a Class A controlled drug, by virtue of Schedule 2 of the Misuse of Drugs Act 1971 (as amended by the Misuse of Drugs Regulations 1985). It is a criminal offence to "unlawfully possess" (with or without intent to

Box 27.1.3 Possible causes of sudden death syndrome

◆ Hypertrophic cardiomyopathy
  • Nugent AW, *et al.* (2005). *Circulation*, **112**, 1332–8.
  • Bonne G, *et al.* (1998). *Circulation Res*, **83**, 580–93.
◆ Arrhythmogenic right ventricular cardiomyopathy
  • MacRae CA, *et al.* (2006). *J Clin Invest*, **116**, 1825–8.
◆ Dilated cardiomyopathy
  • Cohen N, *et al.* (2004). *Heart*, **90**, 835–41.
◆ Myocarditis
  • Feldman AM, *et al.*(2000). *N Engl J Med*, **343**, 1388–98.
◆ Coronary artery disease
  • Dolder MA, *et al.* (1975). *Br Heart J*, **37**, 493–504.
◆ Ion channelopathies:
  • *Brugada syndrome*
  • Butler JM, (2000). *J Accid Emerg Med*, **17**, 426–8.
  • *Long QT*
  • Schwartz PJ, *et al.* (1993), *Circulation*, 1993; **88**, 782–4.
  • Priori SG, *et al.* (2003). *N Engl J Med*, **348**,1866–1874.
  • *Progressive cardiac conduction defect (Lev–Lenegre syndrome)*
  • Vatta M, *et al.* (2002). *Hum Mol Genet*, **11**, 337–345.
  • *Idiopathic ventricular fibrillation (without Brugada ECG changes)*
  • Champagne J, *et al.* (2005). *BMC Med*, **3**, 1
  • *Catecholaminergic polymorphic VT*
  • Liu N, *et al.* (2006). *Circulation Res*, **99**, 292–8.
◆ Wolff–Parkinson–White syndrome
  • Gaita F, *et al.* (1992). *Drugs*, **43**, 185–200.
◆ Coronary artery anomalies
  • Manghat NE, *et al.* (2005). *Heart*, **91**, 1515–22.
◆ Marfan syndrome
  • Pyeritz RE (2000). *Annu Rev Med*, **51**, 481–510.
◆ Restrictive cardiomyopathy
  • Kushwaha SS, *et al.* (1997). *N Engl J Med*, **336**, 267–76.
◆ Endocardial fibroelastosis
  • Angelov A, *et al.* (1984). *Pathol Res Pract*, **178**, 384–8.
◆ Churgh–Strauss syndrome
  • Guillevin L, *et al.* (1999). *Medicine (Baltimore)*, **78**, 26–37.
◆ Right bundle branch block
  • Schaal SF, *et al.* (1973). *Ann Intern Med*, **79**, 63.

supply), to import or export the drug, or produce it, and the police have extensive 'stop and search' powers to enforce these offences. Cocaine is the most potent stimulant of natural origin.

Short-term effects of cocaine include constricted peripheral blood vessels, dilated pupils, increased temperature, heart rate, blood pressure, insomnia, loss of appetite, feelings of restlessness, irritability, and anxiety. The duration of cocaine's immediate euphoric effects, which include energy, reduced fatigue, and mental clarity, depends on how it is used. The faster the absorption, the more intense the high, but the shorter the 'high' lasts. The high from snorting cocaine may last 15 to 30 min, and that from smoking may last 5 to 10 min, but the effects are short lived and once the drug leaves the brain the user experiences a 'coke crash' that includes depression, irritability, and fatigue. High doses of cocaine and/or prolonged use can trigger paranoia, and smoking crack cocaine can produce a particularly aggressive paranoid behaviour in users. When addicted individuals stop using cocaine, they often become depressed. Prolonged cocaine snorting can result in ulceration of the mucous membrane of the nose.

Clinical and pathological aspects

The identification of cocaine or its metabolites in clinical specimens assists patient management. Toxicological analysis of urine is convenient and produces a longer-term chronological picture of drug use than does the analysis of blood or saliva. The half-life of cocaine is short, but cocaine and its metabolites remain in the urine for up to 14 days in a chronic user. False negatives may result from bleach and salt added to specimens, and those individuals with cholinesterase deficiencies continue to have detectable levels for a long time. The analysis of hair for toxicological purposes has now become quite well established, and initial concerns regarding external contamination of hair shafts by extraneous smoke and sweat containing cocaine have been allayed. Specimens need to be collected and preserved in sodium fluoride (or another pseudo-cholinesterase inhibitor), and refrigerated. Storage in a buffer at pH 5 can also prevent cocaine metabolism prior to analysis. Cocaine levels need to be interpreted with extreme care because it is rapidly metabolized in blood and continues to be broken down in post-mortem blood if incorrectly stored for analysis. Commercially available test kits are available for screening urine for cocaine metabolites, and positive samples are confirmed using gas chromatography–mass spectrometry, which has a lower limit of detection for cocaine in the blood of less than 0.5 µg/litre (or 0.5 ng/ml). Blood levels do not correlate well with psychological and physiological effects, unlike blood alcohol levels, as the measurement could represent a rising level associated with euphoria, or a falling level associated with dysphoria. A chronic user will also have built up tolerance to the effects of cocaine, and so a high blood concentration should not be interpreted as always having any specific effect on the user's mental state at the time the sample was taken. Benzoylecgonine, a metabolite of cocaine, is not freely permeable across the blood–brain barrier.

Sudden collapse and death in young people should begin with a consideration of the possible role of cocaine; considerable difficulties will be encountered in interpreting blood cocaine levels and cocaine metabolite levels and toxicological advice should be sought. In the United States of America, cocaine-related deaths were at one time considered to be 'accidental', with insurers thereby being rendered liable to pay out despite the policies excluding payment where death is due to the self-administration of drugs. Those with plasma pseudocholinesterase deficiency are at risk of sudden death when abusing cocaine because of their inability to effectively metabolize the drug.

Cocaine is directly toxic to cardiac myocytes; these effects are not dose-related, do not necessarily require large doses, and are not related to its route of administration. The changes may arise *de novo* or may be superimposed on pre-existing cardiovascular pathological changes. A genetic factor leading to an increased susceptibility to the cardiotoxic effect of cocaine has been proposed. Increased levels of circulating catecholamines, which are associated with the excitement brought about by cocaine use, also appear to damage the heart and great vessels. A cocaine-induced cardiomyopathy (resembling viral myocarditis) has been described, manifest as an enlarged heart, sometimes with patchy fibrosis.

Acute myocardial infarction may arise in cocaine use and often is of multifactorial pathogenesis, including focal vasoconstriction or spasm of coronary arteries due to direct and indirect effects on vascular smooth muscle via α-adrenergic stimulation (noradrenaline) and an independent, dose-related effect. Coronary artery spasm may not be severe enough to induce ischaemia in fit individuals, but in the presence of pre-existing coronary artery disease further reductions in flow can be catastrophic. Thrombotic occlusion of coronary arteries may also arise other than in association with atherosclerotic plaque rupture or haemorrhage: cocaine depletes protein C and antithrombin III, giving rise to a procoagulant effect, and increasing the risk of thrombus formation in vasoconstricted coronary arteries. All these problems can be worsened by coronary artery sclerosis due to cocaine-induced intimal hyperplasia, possible aetiologies of which include prolonged vasoconstriction, stimulation of smooth muscle growth factor, endothelial disruption or injury, and the action of noradrenaline or platelet-derived growth factor.

Large doses of cocaine are arrhythmogenic, possibly due to its effects on catecholamines rather than any direct effect of blocking sodium channels. Secondary arrhythmias can follow cardiac ischaemia due to prolonged coronary artery vasoconstriction, and another possible source of re-entry arrhythmias is the patchy fibrosis caused by chronic cocaine abuse. Cocaine abuse has been linked to sinus tachycardia, ventricular arrhythmias (extrasystoles, tachycardia, and fibrillation), asystole, postinfarction arrhythmias, and arrhythmias due to hyperpyrexia.

A massive increase in systolic blood pressure following an overdose of the drug may led to rupture of vascular malformations and aneurysms, particularly in the brain (berry aneurysms, arteriovenous malformations) and the aorta. Cerebrovascular accidents are other complications probably related to adrenergic stimulation, cerebral vasoconstriction and a sudden surge in blood pressure, but also possibly due to emboli secondary to cardiac arrhythmias or reperfusion injury following myocardial ischaemia or vasculitis. These may be haemorrhagic or ischaemic and can occur in the brain, spinal cord, or retina.

Respiratory findings include pulmonary oedema and congestion, possibly due to excess catecholamine release, also granulomas in the lungs (due to impurities in the drug or polydrug abuse), spontaneous pneumothorax, and spontaneous pneumopericardium. Crack cocaine abuse has been associated with haemoptysis, pulmonary hypertension (hypertrophy and hyperplasia of medium-sized pulmonary arteries), diffuse alveolar haemorrhage, intra-alveolar inflammatory infiltrates, prominent eosinophilia, and bronchiolitis obliterans. Thermal injury to the airway also occurs in crack smokers.

The pathological findings in the gastrointestinal tract are associated with high levels of catecholamines, including ulceration and perforation of the upper gastrointestinal tract (due to a disruption of the internal elastic lamina of the small vessels supplying the ulcerated areas), ischaemic colitis (often segmental), severe bowel ischaemia, and gangrene (due to vasoconstriction of mesenteric vasculature).

Renal infarction, haemolytic uraemic syndrome, and rhabdomyolysis with myoglobinuric renal failure (particularly in warm climates) are all potential renal complications of cocaine use. Mechanisms of rhabdomyolysis include pressure-related injury, vasospasm and myocyte necrosis, hypovolaemia, renal artery vasoconstriction, and myoglobinuria. A histological picture similar to acute tubular necrosis has also been reported (vacuolation, fragmentation, and desquamation of proximal tubular epithelial cells, with pigmented casts in some distal tubules), and cocaine use may be a risk factor for the development of glomerulosclerosis.

Cocaine's ability to produce hyperpyrexia, combined with its effects on neurotransmitters, means that the drug may contribute to seizures which occur in about 3% of cocaine users. These may be 'primary', due to cocaine lowering the seizure threshold, or 'secondary' to cardiac effects such as ventricular tachycardia and fibrillation. The convulsions can be generalized or partial, simple or complex, but most are single, generalized, induced by intravenous or crack cocaine, and not associated with any lasting neurological deficits. However, all routes of administration are associated with seizures, and seizures can be induced in some people by small quantities of cocaine.

Neuropsychiatric complications occur in about 40% of cocaine users. Psychiatric disturbances include depression, suicidal ideation, paranoia, kleptomania, violent antisocial behaviour, catatonia, and auditory or visual hallucinations. Hallucinations occurring with cocaine intoxication can be simple or complex, affecting various sensory categories (e.g. visual, auditory, cutaneous, visceral), and may be associated with delusions of persecution. Some addicts develop panic attacks.

Excited delirium leading to the deaths of an individual at the time of being taken into police custody or shortly after are well known in cocaine users, especially with concomitant alcohol and other stimulant abuse. A neurochemical explanation for excited delirium has been put forward by several researchers and involves differences in the distribution of dopamine D_1 and D_2 receptors, which are known to regulate temperature control. Loss of control of emotional interaction is a classic feature of excited delirium; these individuals have unexpected strength and endurance, apparently without fatigue, and they show an abnormal tolerance of pain, feel hot to touch, are agitated, sweat profusely, are very hostile and aggressive, and exhibit bizarre behaviour and speech.

In pregnant women placental vasoconstriction following cocaine administration leads to decreased blood flow to the fetus, and sometimes the onset of peripartum fetal distress and/or abruption of the placenta. Teratogenic effects and psychiatric abnormalities in babies born of cocaine-using mothers have also been described.

Survivors of violence

Sexual assaults

Over the last few decades the police in the United Kingdom have appropriately received positive and favourable publicity regarding the manner in which they now deal with the survivors of alleged sexual abuse, and investigate their formal complaints. This has enabled more of those who have been abused in this manner to come forward and report the abuse suffered. In spite of this, however, it is not infrequent that the first disclosure of such abuse, particularly abuse that occurred some time previously—on occasions, several years earlier—is initially made to a doctor in the course of a confidential consultation, perhaps on a totally unrelated matter. The medical practitioner is thus placed in a situation in which they are party to highly confidential and sensitive information relating to a potentially very serious crime, with a requirement for careful and specialized investigation. This requires the careful interviewing of the survivor of this crime, the description of general and genital injuries, the meticulous collection of trace evidence, and of course the presentation of all this expertly in the criminal courts.

In this situation—as in many other similarly problematic circumstances—doctors have to determine for themselves whether or not, in the eyes of the law, the person disclosing abuse has full competence to take decisions. In Scotland and the rest of the United Kingdom, the legal age above which legally valid consent to medical treatment can be given is 16 years. If the patient is competent in terms of age and of mental and physical faculties, then in all such instances the doctor must firmly put to them the option of immediately involving the police. The police are much more knowledgeable about the process of investigation of allegations of sexual abuse and better equipped for the purpose than any medical practitioner is likely to be. If after due consideration the patient does not wish to inform the police, for any reason or none, then patient confidentiality must be maintained, although this may be overruled in open court by a judge.

All efforts should be made to ensure that any problems related to possible sexual abuse are adequately dealt with, including any worries that the patient may have about the possibilities of an unwanted pregnancy, sexually transmitted diseases including HIV infection, and the physical and mental trauma sustained. If the police are brought into the picture, the patient may still require some further support. Very helpful guidelines on the medicolegal care to be given to victims of sexual violence have been published by the World Health Organization.

In Scotland, below the age of 16 years, the consent by a minor is only competent if in the view of the particular medical practitioner that patient fully understands the implications of the treatment being offered, and this consent can be extended to consent to medical procedures. Elsewhere, medical decisions of all types are also governed by the child's understanding of the proposed line of action or procedure—referred to as 'Gillick competence' in the United Kingdom. If the consent to involve the police is not forthcoming from a minor, then the doctor has to decide whether in the interest of the particular young patient, this decision should be overruled, and perhaps whether those with parental responsibility for the child are to become involved at this stage. This decision-taking tightrope has to be negotiated very carefully, with the best interests of the patient always paramount and with the medical practitioner acting 'in good faith'. Advice from more senior colleagues, from forensic medical practitioners, and from the medical defence unions is often invaluable in such instances.

In the case of young children who are 'not legally competent', appropriate multidisciplinary guidelines have been put together by every health authority and health board. In these a close cooperation between the health services, the police, the education department, and the local social work department forms the basis of investigation and further management. These guidelines should be adhered to strictly. All doctors now have an obligation imposed on them by the GMC to pass on to the relevant authorities or the social work department any disclosures may to them by children in this respect.

If the police are not involved it may be very difficult to collect evidence that would stand up in a court of law. If the doctor is inexperienced in such examinations then their competence and expertise will be called into serious question by the courts in any eventual adversarial criminal court case; a gynaecological or surgical colleague may have to be involved. For instance, the taking of swabs for seminal fluid analysis may fall short in terms of the unbroken continuity of the chain of evidence and the exclusion of cross-contamination that the courts would always require. These difficulties should be brought specifically to the attention of any patient who is reluctant to involve the police.

Another way to ensure that any physical evidence of injury to the genital area is recorded permanently at the time of the medical examination is to utilize videocolposcopy, as is now almost invariably performed in examinations of this type in prepubertal children to avoid problems with second examinations and nuances of varying interpretations.

It is a fact of life that a very significant number of prosecutions initiated in sexual assaults fail to produce a conviction. By the very nature of this crime, these incidents are usually perpetrated in private with no eye-witnesses to the event. It often boils down to the oral evidence given in court by the two parties, and which of the two—tested by cross-examination—the members of the jury are prepared to accept.

The medical notes

On the principle that contemporaneous recording will always provide good evidence in court, and in many cases that will be the best evidence, it is essential that all members of staff keep regularly annotated and thorough medical notes that are adequate, comprehensive, and comprehensible. Conciseness is not an issue at all in these instances: the notes made may be telegrammatic, provided that they convey all that has transpired on that occasion in terms of how the patient was dealt with and managed. An entry should accompany every single consultation with the patient by whichever grade of medical staff. It is important to record dates and timings, and to ensure that each page bears the name of the patient (or a sticker bearing their details).

In those patients who allege assault, or have been otherwise injured, the manner and method of presentation, as well as the triage procedures, all have to be documented in full. It may be said that some of these issues are normally attended to by other clerical staff; however, it does no harm when urgency and the vagaries of practice has put the system out of kilter, and indeed sometimes saves the day, for the doctor to record such important details, or at least ensure that they have been properly recorded.

The narrative given of the presenting complaint should be carefully recorded at the time, and—even more important—it is essential to document who gave the initial information that found its way on to the notes. If it is the ambulance crew or the accompanying relative or police officer from whom you obtained this information, indicate so, as this renders it second-hand or 'hearsay' information in a forensic context. If the patient has given you specific details about how their injuries were acquired, transcribe these into text. In cases that may end up in court it is important not to attempt to précis, filter, or alter the information as originally given, perhaps in an attempt to make it sound more plausible and coherent: it should be documented as it was imparted to the doctor at the time.

Always indicate the findings on clinical examination. State what you did and when, and the investigations that were carried out by you (e.g. blood pressure, peritoneal lavage), or asked for, either in the Emergency Department itself (such as breath testing for alcohol, urinalysis for blood), and/or elsewhere (such as blood gases, serum electrolytes). It is also important to ensure that when the reports of such tests are available they are quoted in the notes, even if this information has been given to you over the telephone.

If radiographs have been ordered, make sure that, in addition to your own viewing thereof and recording of the diagnosis made by you on your personal reading of them at the time, that the films are also subsequently reported on by the radiology department. These reports will serve as confirmation of your diagnosis and should always find their way into the patient's notes. For instance, it is of little assistance if you believe that there was a fracture of the maxilla or of the nasal bones, both clinically and on radiography, but this has not been confirmed anywhere in the notes in an 'official' radiological report.

If there has been a referral to other units (e.g. neurosurgery, maxillofacial surgery, or burns units), this must also be recorded, preferably with a copy of the letter of referral. Consultations with other colleagues, e.g. the physician on call or the otorhinolaryngological specialist registrar, should be fully documented for any future reference.

Describing wounds

It is absolutely essential that wounds in injured persons are carefully described in the medical notes. This holds true whether the presentation is in hospital or in primary care. Domestic violence is on the increase, and the setting up of units in the community run by primary care staff is becoming more frequent. It is not a valid excuse to claim that because the doctor to whom the patient presented initially was not an emergency physician, there was no obligation on them to record appropriate details (see Box 27.1.4).

A wound in the medicolegal sense is any traumatically induced abnormality, ranging from erythema to abrasion to cuts through the skin or mucous membranes to any internal injury. For each external 'wound', describe its shape (vertical, transverse, lozenge-shaped), and its exact location—the latter by reference to standard fixed anatomical sites (e.g. suprasternal notch, the prominence of the seventh cervical vertebra), and not variable ones such as the nipple or the umbilicus. The wound should be measured with some degree of accuracy, and if it happens to be oriented in any particular manner, this should also be recorded; similarly, document any collar of abrasion and bruising around it, and any pattern in the wound itself.

In forensic practice, trivial wounds that may not require any active treatment may be as important as those that are more serious. Abrasions in the form of fingernail scratches may be as important as any full-thickness lacerations that may be coexistent on the same patient, hence try to refer to all wounds in your description. Be careful to define each wound appropriately. By definition, a laceration indicates a wound with very irregular (and perhaps bruised)

> **Box 27.1.4** Wounds
>
> In a systematic way, for each wound:
>
> 1 Define the wound
> 2 Locate the wound in relation to fixed anatomical points
> 3 Measure the wound (with its edges in apposition)
> 4 Describe its edges, its immediate surroundings, and its floor
> 5 Describe the wound in terms of its orientation or pattern
> 6 State whether recent or old
> 7 Discuss its severity, either individually or collectively
> 8 Record the baseline general physiological parameters of the patient, e.g. pulse rate, blood pressure, respiratory rate, Glasgow Coma Scale
> 9 Consider sketching the wound freehand or on a line diagram
> 10 Consider photographing the wound

---

edges, and the presence of bridging of incompletely damaged tissue in its base. Furthermore, a laceration, again by definition, is also a wound caused by a blunt-force injury—i.e. a force that has stretched the skin excessively, and more usually over a bony point or surface, causing the elasticity of the epidermis and dermis, or of a mucosal surface (such as the lip, the vagina, or anus), to be so exceeded that as a consequence there is splitting and tearing apart of the skin or mucosa at the site of application of the force.

A sharp and pointed object will produce an incision or an incised wound with clean-cut, straight, undamaged edges. However, it is often impossible to indicate what specific weapon caused an injury: a sharp shard of glass, a kitchen knife, and the sharp edge of a tin can all produce incised wounds which look identical, even to someone with plenty of experience in wound interpretation. In the case of lacerations and bruises the difficulty may be even more pronounced. All that one can say with any degree of accuracy is that among other objects that could have produced the wound, its appearances are consistent with having been produced by the particular weapon that is being suggested.

If there is a penetrating stab wound, it is essential to record the length of the wound track after it has been probed or explored, also to what depth the wound has extended, and—if this has been identified—in which direction the track leads away from the skin. If the wound has penetrated beyond the skin, it is important to denote which layers have been breached.

Although it may prove impossible to record individually all the wounds sustained, the use of simple line drawings with the inclusion thereon of brief comments may be very effective. Remember that fractures, dislocations, and internal injuries come into the category of wounds in this context, also that any foreign bodies which have been retrieved from wounds, no matter how banal they may look (e.g. grit, glass), may have very important evidential value and should never be discarded.

Wounding in the legal context

Legal practitioners often have different priorities and different questions from medics in their mind when looking through descriptions of wounds. Occasionally, these may not be immediately apparent or deemed relevant by the medic, but these queries may be expressed in writing or in court. Samples of such questions include: 'How much force was required to produce the wound under review?'; 'Could the particular wound have been inflicted accidentally, or as part of a self-defence type of response by the patient to an assault on him?'; 'Was the wound inflicted by a right-handed or left-handed assailant?'; 'Were all the wounds inflicted in the course of one assault?' It is the counsel of perfection only to answer such questions if one feels experienced and fully competent to so do. An off-the-cuff remark on such matters that cannot be substantiated on robust cross-examination may cost dearly in lost face, and perhaps even in reputation, in the witness box.

It is important to be very circumspect about the ageing of wounds; interindividual variation is such that one can only provide general answers to questions on this matter. If a wound is showing healing, as demonstrated by scabbing, then it will be about 2 days old, and one which is scarred almost a week old, but statements must be as general as that. Ageing of bruises is particularly fraught, in that the colour change that can be seen as the haemoglobin that has extravasated into tissues is changed to bilirubin and biliverdin depends on a number of variable local and systemic factors.

Of specific importance to the criminal justice system are also such matters as the severity of the wound in question, and whether a particular wound could be considered as being life threatening. On the basis of the 'soil and seed' concept, severity should be assessed by the damage produced by the trauma, the amount of blood lost, the degree of surgical shock present; also on the amount of days lost from work, the age of the patient, associated medical conditions that decrease the rate of healing, the ease with which it could be dealt with medically, etc. Indeed, any answers to questions about severity should always be predicated by a series of reasons indicating why the opinion given is being proffered. In doing so it may be useful to distinguish between whether or not the particular wound is 'serious' and 'life-threatening', or whether wounds in that specific anatomical location (e.g. neck, anterior chest wall) in general terms are serious and life-threatening. For example, a penetrating stab wound of the chest may not have actually produced a pneumothorax, but had it been slightly deeper or its track slightly more medial or more lateral it could have: thus within these caveats, the wound can be considered as serious and potentially life-threatening. The fact that a particular injury can be salvaged with relative ease in a hospital does not necessarily detract from its degree of severity. Any inevitable or avoidable delay in seeking or obtaining medical help, any intervening wound infection, etc., should also be listed to enable a more balanced assessment of wound severity.

The aftereffects of the wounding are also of importance. Any scarring left behind by the wounding, which may be considered as cosmetically disfiguring, even if surgical in origin, can increase the 'legal' severity of the wound, and similarly any residual pain and stiffness of an injured joint.

Photographs of injury

Photographs of wounds may be extremely useful if in due course the case comes to a court hearing: pictures taken before stapling or suturing may clearly convey to a jury more poignantly the degree and variety of injury sustained. This may require close cooperation with the police, and above all the 'informed consent' of the patient, if at the time they are in a state in which they are legally capable to give this. If the patient is unconscious and the case is very likely to have been the result of criminal violence, there should be close cooperation with the police. If the management of the patient will not suffer adversely, any reasonable requests for photography made by the police should be considered—even if only a Polaroid—and if at all possible acquiesced to. In all such instances there must always be a careful and considered balance between one's professional obligation as a medical practitioner to provide optimal care and confidentiality for the patient, and one's duty as a citizen of a country in which violence cannot be condoned and for which its perpetrators are brought to justice in the course of a fair trial.

Photographs of wounds after they have been debrided and sutured may not be as useful as photographic documentation prior to such treatment, but they are better than nothing. Patterned injuries which may have to be matched to other weapons (e.g. footwear imprints, imprints from blows) may need to be photographed in black and white, in colour, and under different light sources (such as ultraviolet light). If photography cannot be used for any reason, then consider sketching the wound freehand or use anatomical outline drawings to indicate the location and appearances: this will also economize on text.

Human bites

Human bites may be the presenting injuries. In these instances photography may be essential, and valuable information can be gained from appropriately thorough and specialized examination. There may be enough material on the skin to secure a DNA profile of the perpetrator, and an odontological opinion may be able to produce a dental chart of the offending jaws for matching purposes. This cannot be done without the involvement of the police at an early stage, and—as always—the patient's own informed consent is required.

Intoxication

Alcohol tends to feature prominently in individuals who have been assaulted or accidentally injured, and it may be useful for the purposes of the courts to document the degree of intoxication observed in the victims or in the perpetrators. Although 'alcohol' can often be smelled on the breath, it must be remembered that it is not ethanol itself that is being picked up, but congeners such as esters and other organic compounds that have been consumed together with the alcohol. As with alcohol, these are excreted for a lengthy period after drinking has stopped.

Alcohol is absorbed from the upper gastrointestinal tract, mostly the duodenum, and disseminated uniformly and in an unimpeded fashion throughout all body compartments that contain water. Hence, the amount of water in the body, which relates to body weight and to gender, will influence the eventual concentration and therefore the effects of the alcohol consumed. Typically, the consumption of 1 pint (568 ml) of ordinary beer or a double public-house measure (c.55 ml) of spirits (40% (v/v) alcohol concentration) will result in a blood alcohol (ethanol) concentration of 30 mg of alcohol per 100 ml of blood, or 13 μg of alcohol per 100 ml of breath. The corresponding legally prescribed limits for driving in the United Kingdom are 80 mg/100 ml for blood and 35 μg/100 ml for breath.

One should only carry out a formal blood alcohol estimation if this has potential therapeutic indication, and then only with the knowledge and consent of the patient. Alcohol is a central nervous system depressant and the effects of alcohol intoxication can be elicited by tests of neuromuscular coordination and of higher central functions, including the Glasgow Coma Scale. The eyes will also show evidence of sustained lateral nystagmus and the pupils will be dilated.

In those who may be under the influence of 'controlled substances', with or without additional alcohol intoxication, a full neurological examination should be carried out and recorded. However, it is often unhelpful and profligate to carry out urinary or blood tests for the presence of drugs.

Access to information

The same rules of medical confidentiality apply wherever the patient is seen. Relay of information to others has to be carefully controlled. The police frequently seek information, either acutely and/or after the patient has been discharged. It is therefore important that some basic rules are laid down, enabling the police to know what information will and what will not be divulged to them, without the patient first having been approached and their formal consent obtained.

In terms of statute in the United Kingdom, the police have every right to ask for full details of those persons whom they believe have been driving a 'mechanically propelled vehicle' which has been involved in a collision, and who have been admitted to hospital. Similarly, in relation to acts of terrorism, the police have a right to obtain information. In other instances it is a question of whether, in terms of their inquiries, information should be divulged to police officers who are seeking it. The admission of a person who is likely to die (or as they would put it, 'a condition that is likely to prove fatal'), whether this is the result of an accident or a criminal assault, is cause enough to bring information to the attention of the police.

If the patient or their legal representative requests a copy of the medical notes, this legitimate request cannot be refused unless it can be shown—if need be to the scrutiny of a Crown Court judge (or a sheriff, in Scotland)—that disclosure of the notes may disclose the identify of a third party or be detrimental to the physical and/or mental heath of that particular patient. Barring this, such records should be handed over: staff in local hospital medical records' departments are trained to deal with such requests appropriately.

Forensic use of molecular biological techniques—DNA profiling evidence

DNA-based evidence has revolutionized forensic practice over the last few years. Based on the principles that all cells of an organism are derived from one fertilized ovum, and that mitotic division of cells is uniform and precise, all cells within an organism that contain a nucleus retain an identical DNA content. Thus, DNA from hair, buccal cells, semen, and white blood cells derived from the same individual is identical, and it is possible to determine the exact origin of a particular cell or group of cells if their DNA can be matched to that of some other cells of the same origin. Furthermore, as one-half of a cell's DNA has originated from each of the parents, it is also possible to derive the genetic origin of a particular cell by comparison of its DNA content with that of its parents.

Variable number of tandem-repeat loci

Groups of DNA loci that are used extensively in forensic analysis are those counting variable numbers of tandem repeats (VNTR).

These are not genes, since they do produce any known product, and those used in forensic analysis have no known biological role. They are thus less likely to be influenced by natural selection, which can lead to different frequencies in different populations. A typical VNTR region contains 500 to 10 000 base pairs, comprising many tandemly repeated units, each 15 to 35 bp in length. The exact number of repeats, and hence the length of the VNTR, varies from one allele to another, and different alleles may be identified by their relative lengths. VNTRs have a very high mutation rate, leading to changes in their length, with an individual mutation usually resulting in a change in length by only one or a few repeating units. This leads to a very large number of alleles, often 100 or more, no one of which is common, although only 15 to 25 can be distinguished practically. This means that the number of possible pairs of alleles forming the genotype at a locus is considerable, and given that testing of several different such loci can be combined, the total number of genotypes becomes enormous. For example, for n alleles there are n homozygous genotypes and $n(n - 1)/2$ heterozygous ones: in other words, if $n = 20$, there are a total of 210 genotypes, and if four loci are examined with 20 alleles each, then 210^4 or about 2 billion genotypes are possible (assuming that all four alleles are inherited independently).

The main uses of the DNA profiling method in forensic cases are:

- The identification of crime suspects from trace evidence left behind at the scene, e.g. a specimen of blood from the deceased is found to match stains on the clothing, etc. of the accused person.

- The elimination of crime suspects in crimes where there has been deposition of body fluids, e.g. the DNA profile of the seminal sample taken from the vagina of the victim does not match that obtained from the white cells of the peripheral blood of the alleged perpetrator of the rape.

- Paternity testing, when it is necessary to establish which one of two or more males is the actual biological father of a particular child, e.g. in incest or rape cases. Fetal tissue is also suitable for such testing (and is often used).

- Identification of an unknown person or of unknown mutilated human remains, by comparing material taken at post-mortem examination with material, such as hair or blood, which is authenticated as belonging to a particular person during life. This has been extended to buried remains, e.g. the Romanovs, Mengele.

- Mass disasters—this technique assists with the identification of individuals provided a pre-mortem sample is available for comparison, and has the ability to match together different and separated parts of the same body.

- Mass screening ('a genetic manhunt') of a well-circumscribed population from which the murderer or rapist is known to have originated: this was the first use of DNA profiling in a criminal context in the United Kingdom.

- DNA databases—allowing crimes committed by the same perpetrator in which body fluids have been deposited at the site of the crime to be associated, i.e. serial crimes and previous offenders to be linked with a specific 'new' crime, or resolution of historical unsolved cases.

- Disputed maternity, e.g. in cases of infanticide and child destruction, when it requires to be proven that a particular child is indeed the offspring of a particular woman.

◆ Settlement of immigration problems in relation to the admission into a country of blood relatives rather than 'friends'.

In the civil courts, DNA profiling has also been proving useful in such cases as:

◆ divorce (associated with alleged adultery)

◆ disputed paternity (and more rarely maternity) in settling estates after death

◆ immigration disputes (when a country only allows entry of certain closely related relatives, born outside that country, of newly established residents)

◆ disputed pedigrees of animals and origins of biological material.

Polymerase chain reaction techniques

The polymerase chain reaction (PCR) technique enables the rapid and specific *in vitro* enzymatic amplification of DNA fragments. It is so sensitive that even a very small amount of tissue, such as a single hair root, a single buccal cell, or a single spermatozoon, may be sufficient to produce a DNA profile that is adequate for matching purposes. It can also amplify denatured DNA, and even material from paraffin-embedded histology blocks and formalin-fixed tissue is suitable for replication. Very strict control of laboratory technique is required in conducting PCR procedures as any minute amount of DNA present in the sample will be replicated. Controls are of the essence in demonstrating the absence of contamination. Protective clothing is necessary when evidence is being collected at scenes of crime, as is careful attention to detail in terms of the collection of material for DNA analytical procedures.

HLA DQα

A further development is related to one of the genes that controls transplant rejection, *DQA*, coding for a protein HLA DQα that shows substantial variation in its base sequence from one individual to another. The most variable fragment of this gene may be readily amplified by PCR to distinguish eight different alleles, of which six are used in forensic practice, and thus 21 different combinations of 2 alleles—6 homozygous and 15 heterozygous. In practice, a reverse blot is used, with the nylon membrane containing pre-attached probes specific for the individual alleles, making a quick, reliable, and very useful preliminary test if one is required. On average the DQα profile of a person is identical with that of about 7% of the population.

Mitochondrial DNA

Mitochondrial DNA contains a segment called the control region, which is highly variable and has the following additional properties:

◆ It can survive in extensively decomposed tissues.

◆ It can be successfully amplified, even from the most unpromising tissues such as bones.

◆ It is strictly maternally inherited.

Analysis of mitochondrial DNA has been used most frequently in looking at historical cases, and in instances where nuclear DNA is in short supply or where it has been denatured e.g. by contact with soil and the bacteria therein.

Other advances

Microsatellites or short tandem-repeat loci

Microsatellites are much shorter than the minisatellites (VNTRs) and comprise 2- to 4-bp repeats only. They are very common, are distributed widely throughout the genome, and can be amplified singly or together by PCR. Individual specificity can be achieved by typing several loci sequentially. The method can be used with severely decomposed and burnt bodies, using the DNA from a portion of spared voluntary muscle or red bone marrow.

Amplitype polymarker DNA

This method analyses several loci simultaneously: LDLR (low-density lipoprotein receptor), GYPA (glycophorin A, the MN blood groups), HBGG (haemoglobin gammaglobulin), D7S8 (an anonymous genetic marker on chromosome 7), and GC (group-specific component). Each has two to three alleles per locus.

Minisatellite repeat mapping or digital typing

This analyses for length variation and detects sequence differences within the base sequences repeated in VNRTs.

DNA identikit

In the future it may be possible to describe physical (e.g. blue eyes, red hair) or other characteristics of a subject from their DNA sequence, thereby obtaining hints as to their actual identity.

Estimation of the population frequency of a DNA pattern

DNA 'exclusions' are easy to interpret: if technical artefacts can be excluded, a nonmatch is definitive proof that two samples have come from two different sources. However, 'DNA inclusions' cannot be interpreted without knowledge of how often a match might be expected to occur in the general population at random. In simple terms, if two DNA profiles match then there are two logical possibilities: first, that the DNA profile at the scene, on clothing, etc. is actually that of the suspect; and second, that it comes from someone else who has the same profile as the suspect. The commoner the particular DNA profile, the greater is the likelihood that it could come from someone other than the suspect; by contrast, if the suspect's profile happens to be a rare one, then the chances of this are much less likely. Thus the frequency of a particular profile in a particular population must be known to enable this comparison.

The statistical analysis of profiling data has caused problems to the courts—judiciary, jurors, and lawyers alike. Population frequencies of various profiles have been established, a standard method being to count occurrences in a random sample of the appropriate population and then to use classical statistical formulas to place upper and lower confidence limits on the estimate. Because estimates used in forensic science should avoid placing undue weight on incriminating evidence, an upper confidence limit of the frequency should be used in court, which is appropriate in the forensic context because any loss of power can be offset by studying additional loci.

The product rule should be used to estimate the frequency of a particular DNA profile frequency. If the ethnic origin of the particular individual is known, the database for that particular ethnicity should be used; if not, calculations for all prevalent racial groups should be used. The probability that two randomly chosen individuals have a particular phenotype is the square of its frequency in the population. The probability that two randomly chosen persons have the same unspecified genotype is the sum of the squares of the frequencies of all the genotypes. If there are n loci, and the sum of the squares of the genotype frequencies at locus 1 is p_1, then the exclusion power is $(1 - (p_1, p_2, ..., p_n))$.

Population frequencies that are quoted for DNA purposes are not based on actual counting but on theoretical models based on principles of population genetics. Each matching allele is assumed to provide statistically independent evidence, and the frequencies of the individual alleles are multiplied together to calculate a frequency of the complete DNA pattern. Although a databank might contain only 500 persons or less, multiplying the frequencies of enough separate events might result in an estimation frequency of their all occurring in the same person of 1 in 10^9. However, the scientific validity of this multiplication rule depends on whether the events are actually statistically independent. In organizing databanks it is essential that ethnic groups are considered separately, and in the United Kingdom databanks for whites, Afro-Caribbeans, Indians, Pakistanis, Chinese, etc. have yet to be established.

Further reading

Aitken CGG (1995). *Statistics and the evaluation of evidence for forensic scientists*. Wiley, Chichester.

Balarajan R, Reileigh VS, Botting B (1989). Sudden infant death syndrome and post neonatal mortality in immigrants in England and Wales. *BMJ*, **298**, 716–20.

Balding DJ, Donnelly P (1994). How convincing is DNA evidence? *Nature*, **368**, 285–6.

Beckwith JB (1970). Discussion of terminology and definition of the Sudden Infant Death Syndrome. In: Bergman AB, Beckwith JB, Ray GC (eds) *Proceedings of the Second International Conference on the Causes of Sudden Death in Infancy*, pp. 14–22. University of Washington Press, Seattle, WA.

Berenson AB, *et al.* (2000). A case control study of anatomic changes resulting from sexual abuse. *Am J Obstet and Gynecol*, **182**, 820–34.

Blackwell CC (1999). Sudden infant death syndrome. *FEMS Immunol Med Microbiol*, **25**(1–2), special issue.

Blackwell CC, *et al.* (1994). SUND among Thai immigrants in Singapore: the possible role of toxigenic bacteria. *Int J Legal Med*, **106**, 205–8.

Budowle B, *et al.* (1995). Validation and population studies of the loci LDRL, GYPA, HBGG, D7S8 and Gc (PM loci), and the HLD-DQα using a multiplex amplification and typing procedure. *J Forensic Sci*, **40**, 45–54.

Burst JCM (1993). Clinical, radiological, and pathological aspects of cerebrovascular diseases associated with drug abuse. *Stroke*, **24**, I-129–33.

Busuttil A (1993). Domestic violence. In: Mason JK (ed.) *The pathology of trauma*, 2nd edition, Chapter 10, pp. 121–37. Hodder & Stoughton, London.

Comey CT, *et al.* (1993). PCR amplification and typing of HLA-DQ α gene in forensic samples. *J Forensic Sci*, **38**, 239–49.

Eckart RE, *et al.* (2004). Sudden death in young adults: a 25-year review of autopsies in military recruits. *Ann Intern Med*, **141**, 829–34.

Editorial (2001). Fabricated or induced illness in children. *BMJ*, **323**, 296–7.

Evett IW, *et al.* (1996). Establishing the robustness of short-tandem-repeat statistics for forensic applications. *Am J Hum Genet*, **58**, 398–407.

Fleming PJ, Blair PS, Sidebotham PD, Hayler T (2004). Investigating sudden unexpected deaths in infancy and childhood and caring for bereaved families: an integrated multi-agency approach. *BMJ*, **328**, 331–4.

GMC (2006). *Good medical practice*. General Medical Council, London.

Hazelwood RR, Burgess AW (eds) (1995). *Practical aspects of rape investigation*. CRC Press, Boca Raton, FL.

Jeffreys AJ, *et al.* (1991). Minisatellite repeat coding as a digital approach to DNA typing. *Nature*, **354**, 204–9.

Kaku DA, Lowenstein DH (1990). Emergence of recreational drug abuse as a major risk factor for stroke in young adults. *Ann Intern Med*, **113**, 821–7.

Karlsson T, Ormastad K, Rajs J (1988). Patterns in sharp force fatalities—a comprehensive forensic medical study. *J Forensic Sci*, **33**, 448–61.

Kevorkian J (1961). The *fundus oculi* as a '*post mortem* clock'. *J Forensic Sci*, **6**, 261–8.

Killam AL (1993). Cardiovascular and thrombosis pathology associated with cocaine use. *Hematol Oncol Clin N Am*, **7**, 1143–51.

Knight B (ed.) (1995). *The estimation of the time since death in the early post-mortem period*. Edward Arnold, London.

Lander S, Budowle B (1994). DNA fingerprinting laid to rest. *Nature*, **371**, 735–8.

Langlois NEI, Gresham GA (1991). The ageing of bruises: a review and study of colour changes with time. *Forensic Sci Int*, **50**, 227–38.

Liberthson RR (1996). Sudden death from cardiac causes in children and young adults. *N Engl J Med*, **334**, 1039–44.

Marzuk PM, *et al.* (1995). Fatal injuries after cocaine use as a leading cause of death among young adults in New York City. *N Engl J Med*, **332**, 1753–7.

Millroy CM, Rutty GN (1997). If a wound is 'neatly incised' it is not a laceration? *BMJ*, **315**, 1312.

Morris JA, Haran D, Smith A (1987). Hypotheses: common bacterial toxins as a possible cause of the sudden infant death syndrome. *Med Hypotheses*, **22**, 211–22.

Ormstad K, *et al.* (1986). Patterns in sharp force fatalities—a comprehensive medical study. *J Forensic Sci*, **31**, 529–42.

Pallis C (1983). The ABC of brain stem death. *BMJ*, *London*.

Parrish R, *et al.* (1987). Sudden unexplained death syndrome in Southeast Asian refugees: a review of CDC surveillance. *MMWR*, **36**, 43–53.

Paterson DS, *et al.* (2006). Multiple serotonergic brainstem abnormalities in sudden infant death syndrome. *JAMA*, **296**, 2124–32.

Rao VG, Wetli CV (1988). The pathological significance of conjunctival petechiae. *Am J Forensic Med Pathol*, **9**, 32–4.

Raza NW, *et al.* (1999). Exposure to cigarette smoke, a major risk factor for SIDS: effects of cigarette smoke on inflammatory responses to viral infection and bacterial toxins. *FEMS Immunol Med Microbiol*, **25**, 145–54.

Royal College of Physicians and the Royal College of Pathologists (1982). Medical aspects of death certification. A Joint Report of the Royal College of Physicians and the Royal College of Pathologists. *J Royal Coll Phys, London*, **16**, 205–18.

Schwartz PJ, *et al.* (2000). A molecular link between the sudden infant death syndrome and the long-QT syndrome. *N Engl J Med*, **343**, 262–7.

Tomlin PJ (1967). 'Railroading' in retinal vessels. *Br Med J*, **3**(5567), 722–3.

Valdes-Dapena M (1992). A pathologist's perspective on the sudden infant death syndrome. *Pathol Annu*, **27**, 133–64.

Webb E, *et al.* (1999). A comparison of fatal with non-fatal injuries in Edinburgh. *Forensic Sci Int*, **99**, 179–87.

Wedikin H, *et al.* (2006). Sudden infant death syndrome and long QT syndrome: an epidemiological and genetic study. *Int J Legal Med*, **120**, 129–37.

Weir BS (1993). DNA fingerprinting report. *Science*, **260**, 473.

Weir BS, Hill WG (1993). Population genetics of DNA profiles. *J Forensic Sci*, **33**, 219–26.

Wilson MR, *et al.* (1993). Guidelines for the use of mitochondrial DNA sequencing in forensic science. *Crime Lab Digest*, **20**, 69–77.

Winton R (1982). The Declaration of Lisbon. *Med J Aust*, **1**, 101–4.

World Health Organization (2003) *Guidelines for medicolegal care for victims of sexual violence*. World Health Organization, Geneva.

Wroblewski B, Ellis M (1970). Eye changes after death. *Br J Surg*, **56**, 69–72.

Zhou W, *et al.* (2004). Acute arterial thrombosis associated with cocaine abuse. *J Vasc Surg*, **40**, 291–5.

SECTION 28

Sports medicine

Sports and exercise medicine

Roger L. Wolman

Essentials

Physicians are increasingly confronted with medical problems related to sport.

Female athlete triad—consists of disordered eating, amenorrhoea, and osteoporosis, which are most commonly seen in those pursuing endurance sports or gymnastics. Clinical assessment includes a nutritional screen to assess calorie and calcium intake, measurement of serum tri-iodothyronine level (typically low) and of bone density, along with exclusion of other causes of amenorrhoea. The most effective treatment is to re-establish natural menstruation with a combination of reducing training intensity and increasing calorie intake, both of which the athlete may find hard to accept.

Overtraining syndrome—is characterized by performance deterioration refractory to normal regeneration strategies and often associated with loss of appetite, depression and anxiety, sleep disturbance, fatigue, upper respiratory tract infections, and a raised resting heart rate. Treatment requires rest to allow regeneration and recovery, but most athletes will only accept absolute rest for a few days, hence it is important to follow this up with a period of relative rest that allows very low intensity training after which exercise can be slowly increased, but it may take up to 12 weeks to achieve full recovery.

Medical complications in sport—these include (1) delayed-onset muscle soreness, rhabdomyolysis, and heat stroke; (2) exercise-induced gastrointestinal symptoms including reflux/heartburn, intestinal cramps, the urge to defecate, and diarrhoea (sometimes bloody); (3) exercise-related anaemia, which can be due to faecal blood loss, also intravascular haemolysis caused by high impact forces on the feet; (4) hyponatraemia—a well-recognized problem in the marathon and other endurance events; can be severe, leading to encephalopathy, pulmonary oedema, and death; primarily caused by excessive fluid intake during the event; it is vital to measure the serum sodium concentration of any collapsed or confused competitor at the end of a race.

Overuse injuries—these are the most common type of injury seen in sports medicine clinics. Diagnosis is usually relatively straightforward by history and examination, but it is important to determine the aetiological factors responsible for the injury (training methods, equipment, and biomechanical factors) to prevent recurrence.

Drugs and nutritional supplements—these are widely used in competitive sports. Anabolic agents include anabolic–androgenic steroids, human growth hormone, β_2-agonists, and creatine. Stimulants include amphetamines, ephedrine, cocaine and caffeine. Other agents include β-blockers, diuretics, erythropoietin and blood doping, bicarbonate and β-hydoxy-β-methylbutyrate. Use of many of these agents is banned or restricted by sports governing bodies.

Introduction

Traditionally, sports medicine has concentrated on injuries that occur during exercise, and therefore has come under the umbrella of orthopaedics. However, with the pursuit of sporting excellence a range of different exercise-related medical disorders are now recognized. These are associated with intense levels of training and may have a detrimental effect on long-term health, as may drugs (and nutrients) that are frequently taken to enhance training and performance. Physicians are therefore increasingly being confronted with medical problems related to sport. This section will cover some of the medical disorders that occur with sport and physical training. It will also address the use of drugs and some of the common overuse injuries that occur with sport.

Developments in exercise physiology over the last 30 years have led to improved training regimes for athletes. A spin-off from this has been the recognition of the benefits of exercise in health promotion and disease management. Exercise prescription now forms an important part of some treatment programmes, with evidence for its use in the management of a range of disorders, including heart disease, diabetes, obesity, hypertension, osteoporosis, arthritis, back pain, chronic fatigue syndrome, and depression (for details see the relevant specific sections of this book).

Female athlete triad

History

Amenorrhoea in athletes was first recognized in the late 1970s. Before that it was unusual for women to train sufficiently hard to develop this syndrome. Since 1980, there has been a growth in the popularity of aerobic sports and in the number of endurance competitions for women, whose first Olympic marathon was in 1984 and first 10 000 m in 1988. The other important factor has been the fashion for thinness, which really began in the 1970s. These two changes in female behaviour are the main factors responsible for the development of this syndrome.

In the early 1980s it was thought that training intensity was the main underlying aetiological factor, but studies in the late 1980s indicate that many of these athletes also have disordered eating habits. It was also thought that the bone density of amenorrhoeic athletes would be normal, as the high levels of exercise would compensate for the low levels of oestrogen. However, studies from 1984 onwards have shown that amenorrhoeic athletes have low bone density. This female athlete triad therefore consists of disordered eating, amenorrhoea, and osteoporosis.

Incidence and aetiology

The female athlete triad occurs in endurance sports. The incidence of amenorrhoea varies in different sports and is a reflection of the requirements for that particular activity, in terms of training intensity, calorie restriction, and age group (Fig. 28.1.1).

Training intensity can be difficult to quantify in certain sports, but in runners it is relatively easy as the number of miles run per week provides an accurate estimate. Some work has shown that the incidence of amenorrhoea increases as weekly training mileage increases, with an incidence of about 50% in those running more than 80 miles (c.130 km) per week.

Disordered eating is commonly seen in female athletes and may occur in over 60% of competitors in sports such as gymnastics. In many cases, this is the result of constant pressure from coaches, and sometimes parents, to maintain a prescribed body weight and appearance. In some of these cases, the eventual outcome may

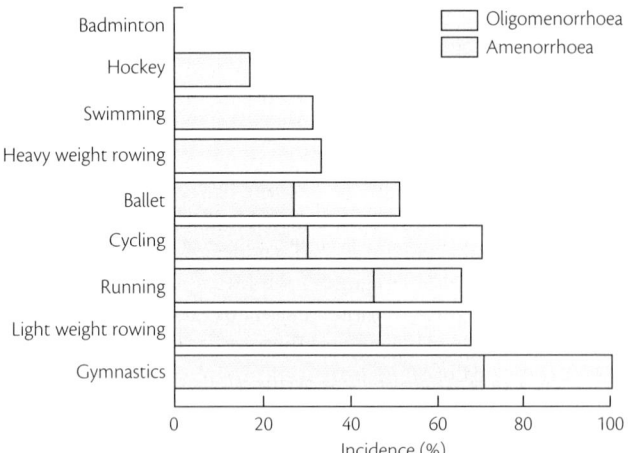

Fig. 28.1.1 The incidence of amenorrhoea among elite athletes in different sports.
Wolman RL, Harries MG (1989) Clinical Sports Medicine I, 95–000.

be an overt eating disorder and anorexia nervosa. The two most relevant nutritional deficiencies are of calories and calcium.

The importance of calorie restriction is seen in rowers, where the incidence of amenorrhoea is significantly higher amongst lightweights (who have to be below 59 kg in order to compete) than their heavyweight counterparts. Both groups have similar training regimes, but the lightweights frequently consume restricted diets in order to 'make the weight' for competition. Furthermore, nutritional studies on runners show that those with amenorrhoea have a lower daily calorie intake than their eumenorrhoeic counterparts.

Age is also important, with athletes in their late teens being more vulnerable to menstrual irregularity than those in their twenties. In activities such as gymnastics and ballet, where there are many teenage performers, there is a high incidence of amenorrhoea, both primary and secondary.

Pathophysiology

Endurance training is associated with menstrual dysfunction. At relatively low levels of training, a shortened luteal phase may occur, which can be associated with reduced progesterone levels and anovulatory cycles. These abnormalities become more frequent as training intensity increases and eventually cycles may become irregular (oligomenorrhoea) or absent (amenorrhoea). In those sports where training starts before puberty, there is often a delay in the menarche. Typically, this is seen in gymnasts and ballerinas where, on average, the menarche is delayed by 1 year. However, primary amenorrhoea may result, and in some cases the athlete may be in her twenties before menstruation begins.

There are many similarities between the female athlete triad and anorexia nervosa, and many believe that these are part of the same spectrum of ill health. In both disorders, the patient's psychological profile is very similar. Furthermore, in both there is disordered eating, energy imbalance, and low body weight. The aetiology of the amenorrhoea is also similar, with slowing of the gonadotropin-releasing hormone (GnRH) pulse generator in terms of both amplitude and frequency, leading to a reversible hypogonadotropic hypogonadism with severe impairment of oestrogen production, which seems to be a reversion to the prepubertal pattern of gonadotropin release.

Over the last 15 years or so, attention has been directed towards exploring the factors responsible for the suppression of the GnRH pulse generator. There are several hypotheses, including endorphin release, central 'stress', and energy deprivation, in each of which hormones are released that may influence hypothalamic function, including cortisol, insulin-like growth-factor binding protein-1 (IGFBP-1) and leptin (aside from endorphin). The inhibitory action of opioids on the GnRH pulse generator is now well established. However, although endorphin levels increase with acute aerobic training (which may account for the so-called 'runner's high'), there is much less evidence that they remain elevated with regular exercise, hence endorphin release alone is unlikely to account for the gonadal suppression seen in athletes.

Serum cortisol levels are elevated in amenorrhoeic athletes compared to their eumenorrhoeic counterparts. This represents central 'stress' and occurs as a result of the central activation of corticotropin-releasing hormone (CRH). CRH increases GnRH sensitivity to opioid inhibition, and therefore, in combination with endorphin release, provides a possible mechanism for amenorrhoea. The raised cortisol level may also adversely affect bone density (see following paragraphs).

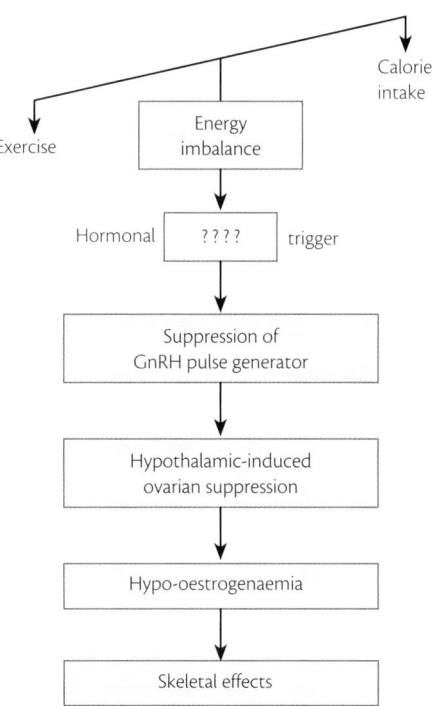

Fig. 28.1.2 The energy deprivation hypothesis for the female athlete triad.

An alternative hypothesis is that amenorrhoea occurs as a result of energy deprivation (Fig. 28.1.2). Energy balance occurs in young adults at an energy availability of about 45 kcal/kg (188 kJ/kg) of fat-free mass per day, and GnRH pulsatility is disrupted when this is reduced to 30 or below. Some amenorrhoeic athletes have an energy availability of as little as 16. This is similar to patients with anorexia nervosa and results in weight loss, a low body mass index (usually below 18), and low body fat (usually below 17%). Furthermore, they have reduced serum levels of glucose, insulin, insulin-like growth factor-1 (IGF-1), and tri-iodothyronine (changes that occur in situations of energy deprivation). It is uncertain whether any of these changes act as a metabolic signal influencing the release of GnRH.

Two other possible candidates are IGFBP-1 and leptin. The level of IGFBP-1 is directly suppressed by insulin, and in the amenorrhoeic athlete the level is elevated. Serum leptin levels are related to body fat and are reduced in anorexia nervosa and probably in the female athlete triad. Further work is needed to determine whether either of these hormones have a direct effect on the GnRH pulse generator.

Skeletal effects

Bone density
The bone density of amenorrhoeic athletes is reduced, most obviously in the spine where there is a high proportion of trabecular bone, but other sites such as the proximal femur and wrist may also be affected. The fall in bone density is predominantly due to low oestrogen levels, but other factors may be important since bone density does not always improve when oestrogen replacement is given (see below). In the female athlete triad levels of IGF-1, which has important anabolic effects on the skeleton, are reduced, while those of cortisol, which has a catabolic action, are elevated: either of these hormonal changes could enhance the fall in bone density.

The type of exercise undertaken modifies the fall in bone density. For example, amenorrhoeic rowers have a higher spinal bone density than amenorrhoeic runners, presumably due to intense exercise involving the trunk. Amenorrhoeic gymnasts have higher spinal and femoral neck bone density than amenorrhoeic runners, probably due to the weight training and jumping activity involved in gymnastic training.

With short episodes of amenorrhoea (6 to 12 months) the fall in bone density is reversible once normal menstruation is restored, but with longer episodes the changes may become irreversible and bone density remains persistently low. Occasionally the bone loss is severe, leading to bone densities similar to those seen in postmenopausal women, and in this subgroup, there is a significant risk of osteoporotic fracture. More commonly, bone density reduction is less extreme and the risk is of premature osteoporosis (10 to 15 years early).

Other skeletal effects
Stress fractures occur more frequently in amenorrhoeic athletes, which may be related to low bone density. Stress injuries to bone commonly occur in athletes: these are usually repaired, preventing the development of a full stress fracture. The repair mechanism may be less effective in those with amenorrhoea who have low levels of oestrogen and IGF-1, both of which are important in maintaining skeletal integrity.

Athletes with delayed menarche and primary amenorrhoea may have delayed skeletal maturation, including delayed epiphyseal closure that may increase the risk of epiphyseal injury.

Investigation and management
It is important to exclude other causes of amenorrhoea. This will include taking an accurate history to establish a relationship between training and menstrual abnormalities. Investigations should aim to exclude other causes of amenorrhoea (see Chapter 13.8.1) and the serum tri-iodothyronine level should be measured, which is likely to be low in the female athlete triad. A nutritional screen is helpful to assess calorie and calcium intake, and bone density should be measured (Box 28.1.1).

Once the diagnosis is established, the most effective treatment is to re-establish natural menstruation (Box 28.1.2). This can be achieved with a combination of reducing training intensity (with the help of the coach) and increasing calorie intake (with the aid of a dietitian). It is very important to educate the athlete about both the short- and long-term risks of remaining amenorrhoeic, otherwise many athletes will not accept this type of intervention. Psychological intervention may be necessary in those athletes where an eating disorder is apparent (see Chapter 26.5.6).

In those athletes who remain amenorrhoeic despite attempts at adjusting their training and diet, oestrogen replacement (either the oral contraceptive or hormone-replacement therapy) should

---

Box 28.1.1 Investigation of the female athlete triad

◆ Exclude other causes of amenorrhoea

◆ Serum tri-iodothyronine measurement

◆ Nutritional assessment for energy and calcium

◆ Bone mineral density

> **Box 28.1.2** Treatment of the female athlete triad
>
> ◆ Decrease amount of exercise, with the help of the coach
> ◆ Increase energy intake, with the help of a dietitian
> ◆ Consider psychological intervention
> ◆ Oestrogen replacement: HRT or oral contraceptive
> ◆ Calcium and vitamin D
> ◆ ?Bisphosphonates
> ◆ ?Raloxifene

be given. Unfortunately some athletes may have difficulty tolerating this, and anecdotal experience suggests that it is not always effective, probably for the reasons given earlier. Calcium supplements should be considered, especially in those with low intakes, and vitamin D supplements may also be helpful. Experience with bisphosphonates and other bone protective agents in this age group is too limited to offer clear advice.

Progress should be monitored with bone densitometry. In those who remain amenorrhoeic, either the progressive fall in bone density or recurrent injuries will eventually force them to make lifestyle adjustments in terms of training and nutrition. By then it may be too late, hence emphasis needs to be placed on education and counselling at an early stage.

Overtraining syndrome

This condition and its associated symptoms are well recognized in the athletic population, but the pathophysiology is poorly understood. It tends to occur in athletes doing high-intensity endurance training and is rarely seen in those who partake in strength and power sports. It is also known as the 'unexplained underperformance syndrome' and can be defined as a persistent decrement in athletic performance capacity despite 2 weeks of relative rest.

Aetiology

Athletes must train hard to improve their performance. This can lead to transient fatigue and underperformance, hence periods of intensive training should be followed by periods of relative rest to allow regeneration and recovery. This cyclical method of training is called 'periodization' and produces adaptation, allowing progressive increases in training intensity and performance. During the period of intense training, known as 'over-reaching', it is common for the athlete to complain of muscle soreness, fatigue, and stress-related symptoms. As part of the stress response serum cortisol may rise, testosterone may decrease, and creatine phosphokinase may be elevated as a reflection of transient muscle damage. These clinical and biochemical features should recover during the rest period. Over-reaching is a necessary part of training if the athlete's performance is going to improve.

In some situations, the athlete may not allow sufficient time for rest in between periods of heavy training. This leads to under-recovery and prevents full adaptation to increased training loads. This may occur when there is a rapid increase in training intensity, with very prolonged training, and at times of stressful competition. It may also occur when the athlete is exposed to other stresses, including intercurrent infection, travel across several time zones, or other unrelated psychoemotional stresses. In an adolescent athlete, it may be seen during a rapid growth spurt. This combination of stresses may lead to underperformance, which will usually respond to a rest period of 2 weeks, but if the athlete fails to recognize the early signs, the symptoms become more severe and may require a more prolonged rest period to achieve full recovery.

Pathophysiology

Over the last 25 years or so, there have been many studies investigating the pathophysiology of the overtraining syndrome, and these have generated several hypotheses. Unfortunately, studies are not always directly comparable because they use different definitions for the syndrome and may perform their evaluations at different stages in its evolution.

Neuroendocrinological features

Dysfunction of the hypothalamic–pituitary–adrenal (HPA) axis may occur, possibly as a result of a cytokine-induced inflammatory response due to localized muscle damage caused by intensive exercise. In some over-trained athletes, there is a rise in salivary cortisol levels, leading to a low testosterone:cortisol ratio, which correlates with the depressed mood state seen in some. There is a decreased pituitary ACTH response to insulin-induced hypoglycaemia, and reduced adrenal responsiveness to ACTH. The latter effect leads to a compensatory elevation of ACTH in the early stages of the overtraining syndrome, but at an advanced stage both ACTH release and the cortisol response may be blunted. There is also evidence of sympathetic involvement, with increased resting noradrenaline levels associated with decreased nocturnal excretion.

Central fatigue and the branched chain amino acids

Prolonged endurance exercise leads to a depletion of glycogen stores in muscles and liver, at which point muscle requires alternative sources of energy. Mobilization of fatty acids provides this, producing increased levels in plasma, where they are bound to albumin. The branched chain amino acids (valine, leucine, and isoleucine) are another alternative fuel for muscle, with an increased rate of oxidation during exercise. In plasma, fatty acids compete with tryptophan for binding to albumin; hence an increase of bound fatty acids leads to an increase in plasma levels of free tryptophan. Tryptophan and the branched chain amino acids cross the blood–brain barrier in competition for the same amino acid carrier, hence an increase in free plasma tryptophan and a decrease in branched chain amino acids favours the entry of free tryptophan into the brain, where it is converted to the neurotransmitter 5-hydroxytryptamine (5-HT, serotonin) which plays a role in the induction of sleep and fatigue and has an inhibitory effect on the hypothalamus. This hypothesis might therefore explain some of the effects that are seen in the overtraining syndrome, but human overtraining studies, including interventions with glycogen and with branched chain amino acids, have so far been inconclusive.

Glutamine and the immune system

The relationship between exercise and the immune system remains controversial. The leucocytosis of exercise is well recognized, and there is also evidence of impaired neutrophil function following intensive exercise, which may explain why upper respiratory tract infections are probably more common following a marathon. They also seem to be more frequent in the overtraining syndrome, although it is uncertain whether this is cause or effect.

Box 28.1.3 Symptoms of overtraining

- Underperformance
- Loss of appetite
- Depression and anxiety
- Sleep disturbance
- Fatigue
- Upper respiratory tract infections
- Raised resting heart rate

Glutamine metabolism provides one possible explanation for the relationship between immune function and exercise. Glutamine is a free amino acid that is utilized at high rates by rapidly dividing cells such as leucocytes, and therefore considered important for normal immune function. Plasma levels fall with intensive exercise, possibly due to the increased glutamine requirement for gluconeogenesis and increased uptake by the liver, gut, and kidney. There is evidence that glutamine supplements may reduce the risk of infection in endurance athletes and also that plasma glutamine levels can act as a marker of the overtraining syndrome, but more research is needed in this area.

Clinical features

The overtraining syndrome is characterized by performance deterioration refractory to normal regeneration strategies. Variable combinations of symptoms are seen in association with this (Box 28.1.3). The athlete will commonly complain of fatigue and heaviness in the muscles, which they tend to ignore in the early stages. Sleep disturbance is common, with difficulty getting off to sleep, early waking, and feeling unrefreshed on waking. They may complain of depression, anxiety, and irritability, with loss of appetite and of libido. There may also be a history of upper respiratory tract infections.

The resting heart rate may be elevated, but this gradually returns to normal (usually very low in an elite endurance athlete) as recovery occurs. Physiological testing may show an increased heart rate response to exercise, reduced maximum oxygen consumption (Vo_{2max}), and an impaired heart rate recovery following exercise. Maximum power output may also be reduced.

Blood tests show nonspecific changes consistent with heavy training such as dilutional anaemia and raised muscle enzymes (in some cases, the creatine phosphokinase level may be increased tenfold). There may be evidence of a recent viral illness, e.g. Epstein–Barr virus infection. It may also be possible to detect this syndrome by measuring pituitary hormonal responses to maximal exercise. A recent study showed that ACTH, growth hormone, and prolactin levels after each of two maximal exercise tests 4 h apart was different in overtrained athletes compared to controls.

It is also important to recognize that underperformance may be secondary to an underlying medical disorder such as anaemia, diabetes, or thyroid disease: these secondary causes are rare, but should always be considered.

Prevention

As our understanding of this syndrome improves, it may be possible to prevent it from occurring. This is not possible at present, because although it is related to prolonged intensive exercise, the ability to withstand the stress of training varies significantly between different athletes. Furthermore, there is currently no screening test that can reliably predict the onset of the syndrome. Resting heart rate can provide a guide: this is consistently low (within a couple of beats) in the healthy endurance athlete, but with over-reaching and overtraining this may increase significantly (by 5–10 beats/min) and only return to the previous low level when recovery occurs. Psychological assessment can also provide a guide, with the Profile of Mood State (POMS) questionnaire proving to be useful in this respect.

It is important to incorporate rest days into any training regime. Racehorses can develop a syndrome similar in many respects to the human overtraining syndrome, and in one study, where they were given an alternate-day regime of hard training day/easy training day the frequency of the equine equivalent of the overtraining syndrome decreased and performance improved. There have now been several human studies where rest days have been incorporated into the training regime (e.g. four heavy training days, two light training days, and one rest day per week): these seem to be associated with a reduction in the frequency of the syndrome.

It is also important to ensure that dietary intake is sufficient at times of intensive training, especially in terms of carbohydrate and hydration. It is surprising how many athletes are unaware of the nutritional components of diet and have an intake that is inadequate for the intensity of their training.

Treatment of the established syndrome

As many of the symptoms of this syndrome are nonspecific, it is important to exclude other causes of underperformance and fatigue (as described earlier), but in most cases tests for these disorders will be negative.

The treatment of the established syndrome requires rest to allow regeneration and recovery. Most athletes will only accept absolute rest for a few days; hence it is important to follow this up with a period of relative rest that allows very low intensity training. The exercise can then be slowly increased, but it may take up to 12 weeks to achieve full recovery. Many athletes are pleasantly surprised about how well they have maintained their performance despite 12 weeks of light training.

In addition to relative rest, it is important to adopt a holistic approach to treatment. This includes assessing other coexistent stresses and making use of relaxation techniques. Nutrition is important, and further advice on this should be offered as appropriate. Athletes should monitor their progress by measuring their resting heart rate, which will decrease as recovery occurs.

Medical complications in sport

Although injuries are the dominant feature of sports medicine, there are several well-recognized medical disorders that occur as a result of sport and physical activity. Some are associated with acute bouts of exercise and others with more prolonged periods of training. The female athlete triad is discussed earlier, and sudden cardiac death and exercise-induced asthma are dealt with elsewhere in this textbook.

Delayed-onset muscle soreness, rhabdomyolysis, and heat stroke

Strenuous exercise can produce transient damage to muscle. Delayed-onset muscle soreness can occur several hours after a bout of unaccustomed, intensive eccentric exercise, reaching a peak at between 1 and 3 days. It is associated with objective muscle weakness, which can last for up to 10 days. There are increased serum levels of creatine kinase and myoglobin, with muscle oedema and structural change revealed on magnetic resonance imaging (*T*2-weighted sequences) and muscle biopsy, respectively. These findings are most obvious after 2 to 3 days. The structural damage fully repairs and the symptoms and laboratory abnormalities resolve by 10 days. This phenomenon is commonly seen following marathon running, when creatine kinase levels may rise to more than 2000 IU/l (Fig. 28.1.3).

There is less muscle damage when a bout of similar intensive eccentric exercise is repeated. This is known as the 'repeated bout effect' and is probably due to a series of adaptations taking place at neural, connective tissue, and cellular levels. These changes make the muscle more resistant to damage with further bouts of intensive exercise.

It is rare for large amounts of myoglobin to be released from muscle during exercise ('exertional rhabdomyolysis'), but when it does occur, it can be life-threatening by causing acute renal failure, often with severe hyperkalaemia (see Chapters 21.2.2 and Chapter 21.5). This is associated with intensive eccentric exercise, dehydration, and hyperthermia and forms part of the syndrome of heat stroke.

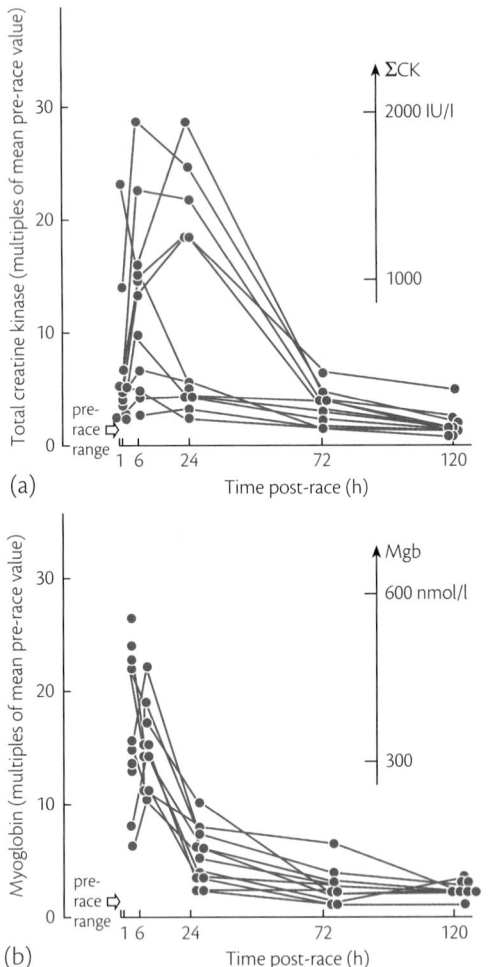

(a)

(b)

Fig. 28.1.3 Changes in: (a) serum total creatine kinase (CK) and (b) plasma myoglobin in young men who had completed a marathon (running times: mean, 194 min; range, 163–280 min).
From Young et al (1987). *European Journal of Clinical Investigation* Vol 17, Issue 4 pp 317–324, with permission from John Wiley and Sons.

There is high heat production with exercise: 75% of the energy expended during running is converted to heat. Heat dissipation therefore becomes extremely important, with evaporation through sweating being the most important mechanism, and anything that impairs sweat evaporation will put the athlete at risk of hyperthermia and heat stroke. This can occur in extreme environmental conditions such as high temperature and high humidity, and is more likely when the athlete is dehydrated. A poorly prepared athlete lacking fitness, who is inadequately acclimatized to the heat, has had a recent illness (e.g. a cold or gastroenteritis), or wears excessive clothing is more at risk. Nowadays heat stroke is more commonly seen in 'fun runs', when there are often a large number of poorly prepared participants, than in marathons. Furthermore, it can occur when the environmental conditions are not particularly extreme, suggesting that heat production during exercise is the most important factor.

The pathophysiology, clinical features, and management of heat stroke is dealt with elsewhere (Chapter 9.5.1). As patients with heat stroke require immediate treatment, on-site resuscitation facilities should be available at competitions and fun runs. Management includes the use of intravenous therapy and increasing heat loss through evaporation (the patient should be put in the shade and then wetted with lukewarm water and fanned). It is possible to minimize the risk of developing exertional heat stroke by paying attention to certain recommendations (Box 28.1.4).

Exercise-induced gastrointestinal symptoms

Up to 50% of long-distance runners will complain of gastrointestinal symptoms. These include reflux/heartburn, intestinal cramps, the urge to defecate, and diarrhoea, which may be bloody. The lower gastrointestinal symptoms are probably due to reduced blood flow (splanchnic blood flow decreases by up to 80% with intensive endurance activity) and possibly mechanical (jarring) stress on the gut (as symptoms are more common in runners than cyclists). The relative gut ischaemia may lead to the release of several gastrointestinal hormones including secretin, glucagon, and vasoactive intestinal polypeptide: the latter can remain elevated for up to 2 h after the termination of exercise. These hormones will increase secretion into the gut while also reducing absorption, effects that are enhanced by dehydration.

Box 28.1.4 Recommendations to minimize the risk of developing exertional heat stroke

◆ Organized competitions and events should avoid the hottest time of the year and the hottest part of the day.

◆ Training and fitness will improve thermoregulation during exercise, and hence participants should be given advice about how to prepare for an event.

◆ A minimum of 7–10 days acclimatization to heat should take place prior to the event.

◆ The athlete should be adequately hydrated prior to the event, and there should be opportunities to rehydrate during the event.

◆ Participants should avoid competitions and events when they are unwell, e.g. with an upper respiratory tract infection or gastroenteritis.

Exercise-induced gastrointestinal symptoms can usually be controlled with appropriate advice, and tend to decrease with adequate training. Adaptive changes occur with gradual increases in training volume and intensity, such that there may be an improvement in blood flow through the splanchnic circulation. It is also important for athletes to be adequately hydrated both before and during exercise: they should therefore take account of the ambient temperature and humidity and adapt their fluid intake accordingly. Hypertonic drinks should be avoided as they will tend to increase the risk of dehydration.

Exercise-related anaemia

Haemoglobin concentrations in highly trained endurance athletes are often at the lower end of the normal range or even just below it. In most cases this reflects a dilutional state where, although red cell mass increases with exercise, there is a proportionally greater increase in plasma volume. A true runners' anaemia may be caused by faecal blood loss (see earlier), also from intravascular haemolysis caused by high foot-impact forces ('march haemoglobinuria'). A similar traumatic haemoglobinuria also occurs in conga-drum players due to high impact on the hands.

Hyponatraemia

Hyponatraemia is a well-recognized problem in the marathon and other endurance events. In a study of the Boston marathon in 2002, 13% of 488 runners tested were hyponatraemic at the end of the race. In some cases this can be severe, leading to encephalopathy, pulmonary oedema, and death. Excessive fluid intake during the event is thought to be the primary risk factor, with the incidence being strongly correlated with weight gain (a measure of excessive fluid intake). It is also correlated with prolonged race times (a longer period of time for the athlete to ingest the fluid). As renal blood flow and glomerular filtration are both reduced during exercise the homeostatic mechanisms that prevent water intoxication may be impaired. Other factors may also be important (Box 28.1.5).

Traditional guidelines have recommended high fluid intake during endurance events in the belief that this would reduce the risk of dehydration and heatstroke, but this seems to have been a very important factor in provoking the problem of hyponatraemia. The International Marathon Medical Directors Association has recently recommended that fluid intake should be between 400 and 800 ml/h, with higher rates for faster runners in warmer conditions and lower rates for slow runners in cool conditions. It is difficult to give exact advice on the level of fluid intake as this will depend on the ambient conditions and the rate of losses from sweat, which will vary between runners. However, with a general reduction in

availability of fluid stations along marathon courses, there is some evidence of a reduction in the incidence of hyponatraemia without an increased risk of other complications.

In the emergency situation, e.g. with a collapsed or confused runner at the end of a race, it is vital to know the serum sodium concentration. Hypotonic intravenous fluids should be avoided. Isotonic saline should be given while awaiting the result of the sodium concentration. Hypertonic saline may then be appropriate in the hyponatraemic patient. See Chapter 21.2.1 for further discussion.

Fitness to exercise

Sudden death in sport

Although it often attracts headlines in the press, sudden death in sport is very rare, with frequency varying from about 0.5 to 6/100 000 per year, depending on the age group being assessed, the level of underlying fitness, and the intensity of activity. Fatal arrhythmia seems to be the most common mechanism of death (Box 28.1.6). Atherosclerotic coronary artery disease is the most common cause in those over 40 years of age: in younger athletes, underlying causes include hypertrophic cardiomyopathy, valvular heart disease, Marfan's syndrome and conduction defects, such as the long QT syndrome.

Myocarditis (see Chapter 16.7.1) is another possible cause of sudden death in sport. This is usually viral in origin, in particular cocksackie B virus, but a series of sudden death cases amongst Swedish orienteers was found to be associated with *Chlamydia pneumoniae* myocarditis.

Cardiac concussion is a rare cause of sudden death, thought to be due to arrhythmia resulting from a nonpenetrating precordial blow from a projectile, such as a cricket ball or an ice hockey puck.

Screening

Cardiac screening of athletes is of limited value because of the rarity of the cardiovascular abnormalities described earlier, the rarity of sudden death, and the cost of screening. It is estimated that 200 000 athletes would have to be screened to find one at-risk case. There is also limited predictive accuracy of some of the cardiac investigations. This is the case with electrocardiography, where it may be difficult to distinguish the physiological changes of the athlete's heart from the pathological changes seen with hypertrophic cardiomyopathy. Further cardiac investigation should probably be restricted to those with a history of cardiac and/or exercise-related symptoms, a relevant family history, or abnormalities found on cardiac auscultation.

Box 28.1.5 Factors associated with increased risk of running-related hyponatraemia

- Weight gain during the event
- Prolonged race time
- Female
- Low body mass index
- High body mass index
- Use of NSAIDs

Box 28.1.6 Cardiac causes of sudden death

- Coronary artery disease
- Hypertrophic cardiomyopathy
- Myocarditis
- Coronary artery anomalies
- Aortic rupture (Marfan's syndrome)
- Aortic valve stenosis
- Right ventricular cardiomyopathy
- Conduction defects

Prevention of sudden death in sport

Athletes with confirmed myocarditis should be withdrawn from competitive sports for at least 6 months, while those with more general viral illness should abstain from sport until they have recovered.

Patients with certain cardiovascular disorders (such as those described in Box 28.1.6) should avoid competitive sports and high-intensity activity (e.g. rock climbing and cross-country skiing). They should also avoid exercise in extremely adverse environmental conditions. Patients with Marfan's syndrome (due to weakening of the aortic media) and hypertrophic cardiomyopathy (due to left ventricular outflow obstruction) should avoid intense isometric exertion such as occurs in weight training.

Sudden death is most likely to occur in high-intensity competitive sports (e.g. squash), and in this situation, the athlete should be offered a basic medical assessment (personal and family history and physical examination) before competition. The need for a medical assessment is less important in those participating in recreational sports. Although acute bouts of exercise increase the risk of cardiac death, this transient increase in risk is outweighed by the cardiac benefits of habitual exercise. The importance of graded increases in exercise intensity, allowing cardiac and musculoskeletal adaptations to occur, should be stressed.

Overuse injuries

Overuse injuries are the most common type of injury seen in a sports medicine clinic. It is usually relatively straightforward to make the diagnosis from the history and examination. However, it is equally important to determine the aetiological factors responsible for the injury to prevent a recurrence. These can be divided into training methods, equipment, and biomechanical factors (see Table 28.1.1).

Table 28.1.1 Common overuse injuries seen in sport

Injury	Site	Sport	Aetiology	Treatment
Plantar fasciitis	Undersurface of the foot	Running	Overpronation	NSAID Physiotherapy Orthotic splint
Achilles tendinopathy	Posterior ankle	Running	Overpronation High arches Footwear	Physiotherapy NSAID Orthotics
Severs	Posterior ankle	Running	Early adolescence	Relative rest
Os trigonum	Posterior ankle	Dance Football	Repetitive plantar flexion	Excision
Flexor hallucis longus tendonitis	Medial ankle	Dance	Poor turnout Overpronation	Rest Physiotherapy
Compartment syndrome	Shin, calf	Running Walking Dance	Increased training intensity	Rest Physiotherapy Surgery
Patellofemoral joint syndrome	Anterior knee	Running Dance Cycling Swimming (breaststroke)	Overpronation Wide q angle Femoral neck Anteversion	Physiotherapy Orthotic Biomechanical correction
Osgood–Schlatter syndrome	Anterior knee—tibial tubercle	Running Jumping	Adolescence	Rest Physiotherapy
Patellar tendinopathy	Anterior knee	Jumping sports	Increased training intensity	Physiotherapy
ITB friction syndrome	Lateral knee	Running	Tight ITB Overpronation	Physiotherapy ITB stretches
Trochanteric bursitis	Lateral hip	Running Dance	Tight ITB Wide pelvis	Physiotherapy ITB stretches Steroid injection
Iliopsoas bursitis	Anterior hip	Dance	Poor trunk stability	Physiotherapy Steroid injection
Spondylolysis	Low back	Dance Tennis Gymnastics Cricket (bowling)	Increased lumbar lordosis Spinal hyperextension	Rest Physiotherapy ?Surgery
Subacromial impingement	Shoulder	Throwing sports Tennis Swimming	Hooked acromium Instability Poor scapula control	Physiotherapy Steroid injection Surgery

ITB, iliotibial band.

Injuries can occur when the training is increased too quickly, when there is an inadequate warm-up or cool-down period, and when there is inadequate flexibility training to complement the overall programme. Injuries can also occur when the athlete suddenly changes from one surface or gradient to another. Equipment factors are also important; this is especially the case for footwear in weight-bearing sport, where it is vital that the shoes provide adequate support for the sport being undertaken and are not overly worn out. In racket sports, the size, weight, and string tension of the racket are important factors that may influence the risk of injury.

It is important to consider biomechanical factors in athletes as the repetitive nature of their activities (e.g. running action, tennis serve, or cricket bowling) may magnify any minor misalignment. It is therefore necessary to assess for various factors, including leg-length difference, wide pelvis, pelvic tilt, femoral neck anteversion, and tibia varum. The shape of the foot on standing should also be considered, as either overpronated or rigid, high-arched feet can cause problems. Variations in anatomy of the bones may also increase the risk of injury, such as the hooked acromium and rotator cuff impingement in throwers and the os trigonum and posterior ankle impingement in dancers and footballers.

The type of injury will depend on the age of the athlete, as this determines the weakest point in the musculoskeletal chain. In the growing adolescent the point of attachment of the tendon to bone is vulnerable, and injuries such as Osgood–Schlatter disease at the tibial tubercle and Severs' disease at the calcaneus are commonly seen. In the young adult, tendinopathy and injuries at the musculotendinous junction are particularly common, while in elderly athletes degenerative injuries of the tendon and joint are seen.

Stress (or fatigue) fractures occur as a result of bone overload. They occur when training is increased too quickly, as in rapid preparation for a marathon, or when there are biomechanical factors that increase the stress load on bone, e.g. rigid, high-arched feet. They also occur more commonly in amenorrhoeic athletes than in their eumenorrhoeic counterparts. Clinically the athlete usually has point tenderness. A bone scan or MRI will allow an accurate diagnosis to be made, although the plain radiograph may be negative.

Drugs and ergogenic aids in sport

The use of drugs and nutritional supplements in competitive sports is widespread. The main reason for this is to enhance performance, but supplements are also taken to improve general health and to increase resistance to infection, which in theory would reduce the risk of developing coincidental medical problems and hence minimize interruptions to training. The scientific evidence for many of these substances is flimsy, but athletes are often prepared to try them on the basis of the anecdotal experience of fellow athletes or advice from their coach or even from suppliers at the local gym. Furthermore, surveys suggest that athletes are willing to take substances for short-term performance enhancement, even if it puts their long-term health at risk. The banning of some substances has had an effect on some athletes, but others continue to take them and are prepared go to extremes to avoid detection.

With most performance-enhancing drugs there is a large variation in interindividual response, but the cause for which is not fully understood. Studies on most drugs and nutritional supplements have therefore been unable to demonstrate consistent efficacy.

There is a large potential placebo effect, which may obscure any pharmacological action. Large randomized controlled trials would be helpful, but these are virtually impossible to do because most athletes would be unwilling to accept a placebo. Furthermore, if there is any possibility of the drug enhancing performance, it is likely already to have been banned by the sport's governing body. Studies on the nonathletic population, who exercise at much lower levels, may not be representative of the effects seen in athletes. Moreover, athletes often take a variety of substances in extremely large doses, making it difficult to compare the results with the lower doses given in the general population in terms of efficacy and (especially) safety.

Anabolic agents

Anabolic–androgenic steroids

Testosterone, first synthesized in the 1930s, has both anabolic and androgenic effects. Since then, several synthetic derivatives have been produced in an attempt to provide a steroid with predominant anabolic actions. The first recorded use of anabolic–androgenic steroids (AAS) was during the Second World War when they were given to German troops to increase their aggressiveness. In 1952, the Russian weightlifting team was suspected of taking them when they won three gold medals at the Helsinki Olympic Games. This increased the interest in these drugs, and by 1958, a United States pharmaceutical company had developed AAS. The dangers gradually became apparent, but it was not until 1975 that the International Olympic Committee banned their use.

AAS enhance muscle strength and power but have no effect on aerobic performance. They increase lean body mass and lead to a reduction of body fat. They are also thought to have psychological effects and can promote aggressiveness, which in its most extreme form may lead to 'roid rage'. Athletes may also experience euphoria and reduced fatigue while taking AAS, a combination of effects that may allow them to train harder and for longer.

Although AAS will increase muscle strength in nonexercising people, the greatest increases in strength occur when AAS are taken in conjunction with resistance exercise (Fig. 28.1.4). The reason for this may be that physiological stress occurs with intense resistance exercise and leads to increased levels of glucocorticoids, thereby producing a catabolic state with a negative nitrogen balance that anabolic steroids can reverse.

There is strong evidence of risk associated with their use, including cardiovascular disease, testicular atrophy, hepatocellular damage, and psychological disturbance.

The androgen precursors androstenedione and dehydroepiandrosterone are marketed as being able to increase the production of testosterone and lead to anabolic effects. However, studies have shown that this does not occur and there is no improvement in performance with either of these products.

Human growth hormone

The physiological effects of human growth hormone (HGH) include nitrogen retention, increased protein synthesis and tissue growth, and an increase in fat-free mass. Recombinant HGH was first produced in 1984, and although it is expensive its use by athletes has since increased.

The anabolic effects of HGH make it potentially valuable as an ergogenic aid for athletes participating in power sports. Furthermore, as it is not detected by most drug test screenings performed by sports governing bodies, it is a more attractive option

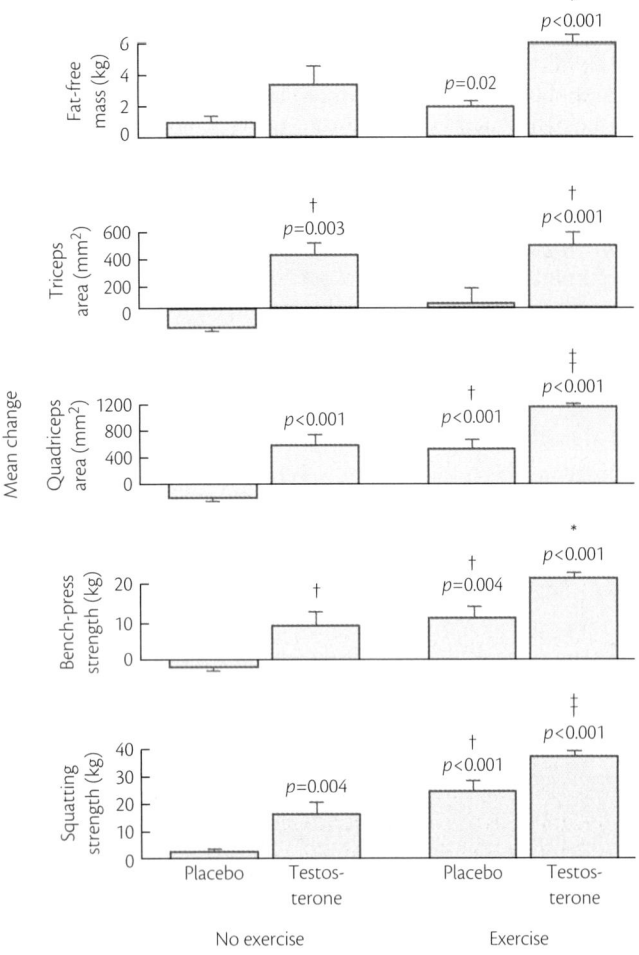

Fig. 28.1.4 A randomized trial of exercise and supraphysiological doses of testosterone in men over a 10-week period. Changes from baseline in mean (± SE) fat-free mass, triceps, and quadriceps cross-sectional areas, and muscle strength in the bench-press and squatting exercises. Note that the greatest effect is obtained with a combination of exercise and testosterone.

than anabolic steroids. However, so far there has been only limited research to determine its effectiveness, and although it leads to muscle hypertrophy, the evidence is lacking with regard to increasing muscle strength and power.

β$_2$-Agonists

This group of drugs was initially banned by the sporting bodies because of their stimulant action, but they have attracted interest as muscle strengthening agents when taken orally. During the 1992 Barcelona Olympics, two American power athletes were found to have taken clenbuterol, which can produce muscle hypertrophy in animal studies.

Studies of β$_2$-agonists in healthy men, in patients following lower limb surgery and those with spinal cord injury, all showed gains in muscle strength following an exercise programme when compared to a placebo group. However, there is very little data on their effect in highly trained athletes. Although they act as bronchodilators, there is no evidence that they can improve aerobic fitness in nonasthmatics.

Creatine

Creatine was first recognized as an ergogenic aid in the early 1990s and was used by athletes in the 1992 Barcelona Olympics. It is an amino acid present in meat, normal daily intake being less than 1 g. The highest concentration of creatine is in skeletal muscle, in particular in type-II muscle fibres, where most is in the form of creatine phosphate, providing a source of energy and assisting in the restoration of ATP following exercise. Creatine phosphate may also assist in buffering when the pH falls due to lactic acid accumulation during exercise.

Supplements are usually taken in high dosage for a limited period (e.g. 25 g for 6 days), following which muscle concentrations of free creatine and creatine phosphate remain elevated for several weeks. It is generally pointless to take high-dose supplementation beyond this period as most muscle creatine uptake occurs during the first few days, but some athletes take a maintenance dose of 2 g/day.

Following this regime many athletes report that they are able to increase their training loads, and studies suggest that supplementation does improve high-intensity performance, especially when repeated exercise bouts are carried out (e.g. repetitive sprinting and cycling). The ergogenic effects also extend to strength and power events such as weightlifting. No effect is seen in predominantly aerobic events.

Overall, there is only limited information on the effects of creatine supplementation, but these are consistent with the role of creatine phosphate in enhancing the restoration of ATP. The increase in muscle strength possibly occurs by allowing greater training intensity, leading to an enhanced training response. Within a few days of taking creatine, there is a weight gain of between 2 and 5 kg, a large proportion of which can be accounted for by an increase in intracellular fluid volume (it is well known that urine volume decreases during the period of supplementation), but there may also be an increase in fat-free mass.

There are theoretical concerns regarding the side effects of using large doses of creatine for prolonged periods. These include adverse effects on the kidney, although thus far there have been no confirmed reports of this. There are also anecdotal reports of increases in muscle cramps and concerns regarding the impact of weight gain, especially in athletes competing in weight-category sports (e.g. boxing and wrestling). In these sports, the athlete often has to lose weight rapidly to 'make the weight' for competition, and if they have gained extra weight with the use of creatine, they may have to severely dehydrate to achieve such weight reduction.

As supplementation with creatine seems capable of enhancing performance, there are ethical issues regarding its use. Some feel it should be banned, others argue against this on the basis that it is a component of a normal meat diet and is therefore no different to taking carbohydrate supplements.

Stimulants

Amphetamines, ephedrine, and cocaine

These stimulate the central and sympathetic nervous systems. As sympathomimetic agents they increase heart rate, blood pressure, metabolic rate, and plasma levels of free fatty acids. These actions could theoretically enhance aerobic performance, but not without risk. There were at least two amphetamine-related deaths in cyclists in the early years of their use (one in the Rome Olympic Games in 1960 and the other in the 1968 Tour de France) and there have also been several deaths in athletes associated with the use of both ephedrine and cocaine, whose side-effect profile includes ventricular arrhythmias, hypertension, and hallucinations. Despite this, they are commonly used in major league baseball.

Research on the use of amphetamines suggests that they have little direct physiological effect during exercise, but that they can mask pain and fatigue during activity. This may allow athletes to exercise closer to their limit, which may produce a positive effect, especially on endurance performance, but it could also have a detrimental effect on health by inhibiting the athlete's awareness of early warning signs (e.g. injury or dehydration). The same may apply to ephedrine and cocaine. Ephedrine is also used by athletes to reduce fat and increase fat-free mass, but there is little evidence for this effect. Cocaine can produce euphoria and also lead to addiction, which has caused great concern regarding its use amongst athletes.

Caffeine

Caffeine, which is chemically related to the theophyllines, is metabolized in the liver to produce dimethylxanthine. When used prior to prolonged exercise (in a dose of 3–6 mg/kg body weight, 1 h before exercise) it can delay fatigue and enhance endurance performance, although there is significant individual variation. Although caffeine is known to have effects on the central nervous system, adipose tissue, and skeletal muscle, the mechanism by which it reduces fatiguability is unclear. It has several unwanted effects, including insomnia, headache, and gastrointestinal irritation. Its diuretic effect, although of theoretical concern in endurance sports, appears to be attenuated by exercise.

The International Olympic Committee considers caffeine to be a performance-enhancing drug. However, it would be impossible to have an outright ban on a substance that is present in so many foods and drinks, hence only athletes found to have a urine concentration of more than 12 mg/litre are deemed to be guilty of a doping offence. This has its limitations. as some athletes can obtain a performance-enhancing effect at urine concentrations well below this level.

Other agents

β-Blockers

By reducing heart rate, this group of drugs reduces aerobic capacity and therefore decreases endurance. However, they are effective in skill sports, with studies confirming that shooters improve their performance when taking β-blockers. They probably exert their effect by reducing hand tremor and heart rate: top-class shooters tend to shoot between one heartbeat and the next, and therefore a reduction in heart rate is helpful. They have also been shown to be effective in treating stage fright in musicians.

Diuretics

Athletes use diuretics when they need to lose weight rapidly. This occurs in sports such as boxing, judo, and lightweight rowing, when the individual needs to make a particular weight classification for competition. They are very effective in producing short-term weight loss, of the order of 4% over 24 h, but such dehydration and electrolyte disturbance can affect performance. Frequently, the athlete will have up to 20 h between the weigh-in and competition: this gives sufficient time to replace the fluid loss, but is insufficient to re-establish normal electrolyte balance, which can lead to medical complications during competition, including renal failure, severe hyperkalaemia, and rhabdomyolysis.

Erythropoietin and blood doping

An increase in red cell mass of up to 5% occurs with adaptation to endurance training. This can take several months. However, some athletes artificially increase their red cell mass either by infusing previously stored red cells or by the use of erythropoietin. Infusing red cells has probably been used since the early 1970s in sports such as distance running, cycling, and cross-country skiing. In 1984, the United States men's cycling team confessed to using it during the Olympics, and won gold medals. Erythropoietin has probably been used by athletes since the late 1980s and may well have been responsible for a number of deaths of cyclists in the last 12 years.

Although homologous transfusions are used by athletes, autologous transfusion is probably more common. During this process, several units of blood are removed from the athlete and then stored for several weeks, while the blood count is naturally restored to normal. The red cells are then reinfused, thereby increasing the red cell count, which will be sustained for a few weeks. The alternative method of increasing red cell mass is to administer erythropoietin, when the red cell count rises gradually over several weeks and remains elevated as long as the treatment continues.

Physiological studies confirm improved exercise performance with the use of these techniques to increase the blood count. Maximal aerobic power, submaximal endurance, and race performance have all been shown to improve. Blood doping may also provide a thermoregulatory advantage for those exercising in the heat, and some benefit for those exercising at altitude.

Medical risks include those associated with transfusions. Even autologous infusions can cause problems through clerical errors and mishandling of the stored blood product. Risks also occur in association with the high haematocrit, with blood viscosity rising exponentially as the haematocrit increases above 30%, thus leading to an increased risk of thromboembolic events, and there have now been numerous deaths related to the use of blood doping by athletes.

Although blood doping is banned by all the main sports governing bodies, there is no reliable test for detecting either autologous red cell infusion or erythropoietin administration. It is therefore difficult to prove that an athlete has used this technique and to provide a consistent deterrent. One sport (cross-country skiing) has had some success by using an upper limit of haemoglobin as a rule for competition.

Bicarbonate

A metabolic acidosis occurs with anaerobic exercise and is thought to be responsible for the progressive fatigue that occurs. By inducing a metabolic alkalosis before exercise, it may be possible to delay the onset of fatigue and improve exercise performance. Several studies have been undertaken to assess the effect of pre-exercise bicarbonate ingestion on performance, with some showing benefit, others not. The reason for these differences is probably due to variations in the duration and intensity of exercise, the dosage of bicarbonate, and the length of time between taking bicarbonate and the onset of exercise. Bicarbonate is most likely to have an effect with exercise of only a few minutes' duration, when given 2 to 3 h before exercise, and at a dose of about 0.3 g of sodium bicarbonate per kg body weight. Side effects of this ingestion include vomiting and diarrhoea, which may limit the potential benefits. Bicarbonate is not banned by sports governing bodies.

β-Hydroxy-β-methylbutyrate

This is a metabolite of the essential amino acid leucine and is promoted for its possible anticatabolic actions. It is said to suppress protein breakdown in the recovery phase of a workout, thus leading to an increase in lean body mass. Several studies have shown reduced levels of muscle breakdown products (creatine phosphokinase and lactate dehydrogenase) following prolonged endurance exercise in athletes taking the supplements compared to controls. The mechanism of action is unclear, although there is some evidence that it may delay the onset of blood lactate accumulation during exercise, but it is not known whether this translates into improved performance.

Further reading

Almond CSD, *et al.* (2005). Hyponatremia among runners in the Boston marathon. *N Engl J Med*, **352**, 1550–6.

Bhasin S, *et al.* (1996). The effects of supraphysiologic doses of testosterone on muscle size and strength in normal men. *N Engl J Med*, **335**, 1–7.

Brouns F, Beckers E (1993). Is the gut an athletic organ? Digestion, absorption and exercise. *Sports Med*, **15**, 242–57.

Budgett R (1998). Fatigue and underperformance in athletes: the overtraining syndrome. *Br J Sports Med*, **32**, 107–10.

Budgett R, *et al.* (2000). Redefining the overtraining syndrome as the unexplained underperformance syndrome. *Br J Sports Med*, **34**, 67–8.

Clarkson PM, Thompson HS (1997). Drugs and sport. Research findings and limitations. *Sports Med*, **24**, 366–84.

Foster C, Lehmann M (1997). Training/overtraining: the first Ulm symposium. *Med Sci Sports Exerc*, **30**, 1137–78.

Futterman LG, Myerburg R (1998). Sudden death in athletes. *Sports Med*, **26**, 335–50.

Huston TP, *et al.* (1985). The athlete heart syndrome. *N Engl J Med*, **313**, 24–30.

Jenkins PJ, Grossman A (1993). The control of the gonadotrophin-releasing hormone pulse generator in relation to opioid and nutritional cues. *Hum Reprod*, **8**, 154–61.

Loucks AB. (2005). Essay: the female athlete triad. *Lancet*, **366**, S49– S50.

Maron BJ (1986). Structural features of the athletes' heart as defined by echocardiography. *J Am Coll Cardiol*, **7**, 190–203.

Maron BJ, *et al.* (2004). AHA Scientific Statement: Recommendations for physical activity and recreational sports participation for young patients with genetic cardiovascular diseases. *Circulation*, **109**, 2807–16.

Maughan RJ (1999). Nutritional ergogenic aids and exercise performance. *Nutr Res Rev*, **12**, 255–80.

McHugh MP, *et al.* (1999). Exercise-induced muscle damage and potential mechanisms for the repeated bout effect. *Sports Med*, **27**, 157–70.

Meeusen R, *et al.* (2004). Hormonal responses in athletes: the use of a two bout exercise protocol to detect differences in (over)training status. *Eur J Appl Physiol*, **91**, 140–6.

Mittleman MA, *et al.* (1993). Triggering myocardial infarction by heavy physical exertion. *N Engl J Med*, **329**, 1677–83.

Neely FG (1998). Biomechanical risk factors for exercise-related lower limb injuries. *Sports Med*, **26**, 395–413.

Noakes TD, Speedy DB (2006). Case proven: exercise associated hyponatraemia is due to overdrinking. So why did it take 20 years before the original evidence was accepted? *Br J Sports Med*, **40**, 567–72.

Otis CL, *et al.* (1997). American College of Sports Medicine position stand. The female athlete triad. *Med Sci Sport Exerc*, **29**, i–ix.

Redman LM, Loucks AB (2005). Menstrual disorders in athletes. *Sports Med*, **35**, 747–55.

Renstrom PAFH (1999). An introduction to chronic overuse injuries. In: Harries MG, *et al.* (eds) *Oxford textbook of sports medicine*, pp. 633–48. Oxford University Press, Oxford.

Robinson TL, *et al.* (1995). Gymnasts exhibit higher bone mass than runners despite similar prevalence of amenorrhoea and oligomenorrhoea. *J Bone Miner Res*, **10**, 26–35.

Sawka MN, *et al.* (1996). American College of Sports Medicine position stand. The use of blood doping as an ergogenic aid. *Med Sci Sport Exerc*, **28**, i–viii.

Tokish JM, *et al.* (2004). Ergogenic aids: a review of basic science, performance, side effects and status in sports. *Am J Sports Med*, **32**, 1543–53.

Walsh NP, *et al.* (1998). Glutamine, exercise and immune function. *Sports Med*, **26**, 177–91.

Wolman RL, *et al.* (1990). Menstrual status and exercise are important determinants of spinal trabecular bone density in female athletes. *BMJ*, **301**, 516–18.

Zanker CL, Swaine IL (1998). The relationship between serum oestradiol concentration and energy balance in young women distance runners. *Int J Sports Med*, **19**, 104–8.

SECTION 29

Geratology

Medicine in old age

Gordon Wilcock and Kenneth Rockwood

Essentials

Frailty

Frailty occurs in a mainly older or geriatric population, is linked to the accumulation of a number of different health-related problems, and may influence disease presentation. A frequently used clinical definition recognizes presentations comprising weight loss, exhaustion, slow movement, a low level of physical activity, and weakness. It can also be graded by degree of disability: (1) very mild frailty describes someone who has given up complex hobbies; (2) mild frailty implies some dependence on 'instrumental activities of daily living'; (3) moderate frailty involves intermediate self-care activities; and (4) severe frailty requires personal-care dependence. The complexity of frailty underlies the difficulties that often arise when managing the care of an older person. Understanding the concept and consequences of frailty is essential to the problems of and successful management of many older people.

Falls

Falls occur frequently in older people, especially women. Prevention, unfortunately often secondary prevention, is as important as managing the consequences of the fall that has brought someone to medical notice. A careful history should be taken from everyone who has fallen, and they should be carefully examined, including detailed examination of the central nervous system (CNS), rather than the frequently entered single comments 'CNS normal' or 'CNS NAD (no abnormality detected)'. Falls clinics make an important contribution both to the long-term well-being of patients and also to reducing hospital referral and the consequent costs. Helping patients overcome the fear of falling is often an important contribution to their well-being, as is teaching them how to get up after a fall. Careful assessment with appropriate management will often reduce the frequency of the falls, and also their consequences. Prognosis for many people who have been falling is good.

Pressure sores

A patient in hospital should never be allowed to develop a pressure sore. Those at risk should be carefully monitored and predisposing factors carefully managed. Most are multifactorial in aetiology, with important factors being pressure shearing forces, friction, and maceration from prolonged contact with moisture. Careful nursing,

the use of risk-factor scoring systems, and—where appropriate—pressure-relieving devices, will minimize their development. Once established, treatment should be directed not only at the pressure sore itself, but also to nutrition, fluid intake and predisposing factors such as incontinence and comorbidity that may impair healing. Infected and difficult pressure sores will often require expert advice from a microbiologist and/or plastic surgeon.

Delirium

Delirium is defined as a disturbance of consciousness and a change in cognition that develops acutely. It is common among older people, in whom it is a sensitive but nonspecific sign of illness, especially in older people who are frail. The American Psychiatric Association has developed widely used diagnostic criteria, emphasizing that delirium should be classified by its presumed cause.

Urinary incontinence

This is a frequent problem that is often under-reported. It can usually be classified into one of a number of causes, including (1) overflow incontinence, (2) stress incontinence, (3) urge incontinence and—probably most commonly—(4) mixed incontinence. Treatment depends upon the underlying cause or causes, and the ability to influence these. In many cases it will be possible to improve or resolve the incontinence, so improving the patient's quality of life. Long-term indwelling catheters always lead to infection and should be used only as a last resort.

Faecal incontinence

Faecal incontinence is much commoner than appreciated because people are reluctant to discuss an embarrassing condition. It can have a major effect on the quality of life of both patients and their relatives, and many can be helped by simple interventions, hence it is a symptom that should be sought directly during history taking in those particularly at risk, including (1) frail women who have had obstetric damage; (2) people with loose stools or diarrhoea (whatever the aetiology); (3) people with dementia or some neurological conditions; and (4) people with chronic constipation or faecal impaction. Management includes identifying and treating the underlying cause, but at the same time preserving the patient's dignity and offering appropriate psychological support.

Prescribing for older people

Dosing schedules of many drugs frequently prescribed for frail older patients are based on data obtained mainly from trials in younger patients. However, aside from issues of the effect of possibly impaired hepatic and renal function, older people often have comorbidities that are also treated with drugs, which may affect results of subsequent prescribing, and the tendency to do so without regular review is probably a significant cause of both morbidity and mortality. When a new drug is being prescribed, all existing treatments should be reviewed, and in most situations it is advisable to start with a low dose that is increased cautiously, monitoring the emergence of unwanted effects very carefully. Compliance is often a problem, for many reasons, and also needs careful monitoring.

Surgery and the older patient

Chronological age alone should never be considered a contraindication to surgical procedures. Careful preoperative assessment and evaluation of the relative fitness and frailty of patients will direct surgery towards improving the quality of life of many older people. Assessment requires a careful history and examination, also appropriate investigations, to identify the presence and extent of comorbidities (particularly cardiopulmonary) that may complicate the surgery and postsurgical recovery, with particular note taken of the patient's nutritional state. It is vitally important to have a careful understanding of the patient's prior state of function, and to assess both the patient's (and family's) and the surgeon's understanding of how the current level of function is likely to improve (or is threatened) by a given procedure. Making explicit the supposed goals of surgery also allows the patient and their family to have a role in making any decision about the appropriateness of surgical intervention.

Older people and driving

Driving skills decline in many older people, and in many countries this is taken into account when motor vehicle insurance and/or driving licences are renewed. However, the notion that older people are at greater risk on the road is not generally true, with the higher numbers of crashes per mile driven by older people being related more to their lower mileage than to age itself.

In many countries the driving licence authority must be notified, usually by self report, of the development of any condition that may affect driving skills, for some of which very definite guidelines have been formulated, e.g. cerebrovascular disease, seizures. Most people with early dementia can probably drive safely for the first 3 years after their diagnosis, but there is considerable variation between people and so assessment should be individualized. In the United Kingdom, the Driver and Vehicle Licensing Agency must be notified of all new diagnoses of dementia, usually by self report, but if necessary by the clinician involved. Cognitive testing in itself is not a good basis for judging driving skills, but identifies those who require formal on-the-road assessment. If the latter is not immediately available, a decision has to be made about whether the patient should continue to drive while awaiting their assessment.

Introduction

In the Western world, most people who are ill enough to be admitted to hospital are old, so it is natural to ask what makes a patient (or a clinical service) 'geriatric'. Just as there is much local variation in how specialized geriatric medicine services are labelled (e.g. 'clinical gerontology', 'elderly medicine', 'geriatric medicine'), the question of who or what is 'geriatric' is answered differently in different places.

Depending on local history and circumstances, some places run 'age-defined' specialized geriatric services, where chronological age, typically 70 or 75 years, makes someone 'geriatric'. Other specialized geriatric medicine services target certain conditions, such as delirium, falls, or functional decline. Elsewhere, the geriatric medicine service focuses more on rehabilitation, although this in turn prompts questions about what makes a patient suitable for 'geriatric rehabilitation' and not for the 'rehabilitation medicine' service. Others offer very little acute care, finding that the mandate of geriatric medicine in their area is best employed by focusing on patients who receive institutional long-term care. Wherever geriatric medicine is employed, however, patients tend to have in common their multiple, interacting medical and social problems that adversely affect their prognosis: worse health, impaired functional ability, and death.

The case for geriatric medicine can be restated as the care of elderly people who are frail. Above all, it is their complexity that justifies a separate speciality to care for frail elderly people. For many elderly people, the management of their medical conditions should be subject to the same principles as those applied in younger people, as described elsewhere in this textbook, but modified by the age-related principles discussed in the following paragraphs. Older people are prone to many diseases, few of which are specific to ageing although some occur more commonly in later life. It is the interaction of a number of factors, including multiple pathology, age-related changes in physiology, greater sensitivity to the effects of many drugs, often combined with an elderly person's social situation, that determines the presentation of illness. This chapter emphasizes the concept of frailty in older people, and some of the major problems that often lead to older people being admitted to hospital rather than specific medical conditions.

Frailty

Frailty and complexity

People who are frail are vulnerable because of the multiple deficits that they have accumulated. Conceptually, it is easy to understand how frail patients accumulate their deficits. In 1825, Gompertz observed the exponential increase in mortality rate with age. However, to understand the relationship between the Gompertz curve and frailty, it must be emphasized that the mortality rate is not expressed as an increase in the risk of sudden death. Elderly people commonly die having accumulated many health problems that themselves increase exponentially with age. This exponential accumulation of health problems defines frailty, just as frailty reflects vulnerability, including an increased risk of death.

In considering frailty in relation to the accumulation of health problems, many groups have defined health problems broadly, as deficits that can be symptoms, signs, illnesses, or disabilities. Deficits are combined into a single measure, the frailty index. Fig. 29.1.1 shows that, on average, the frailty index increases reproducibly by about 0.03 (3%) per year on a log-linear scale.

Several features make the reproducibility of this estimate noteworthy. First, estimates of the rate of deficit accumulation were gathered in different time periods (1970 to the late 1990s) in different developed countries: Australia, Canada, Sweden, and the United States of America. Such reproducibility across places and times supports both the internal validity and the generalizability of the approach. Secondly, and more challenging for traditionally trained physicians, the estimates of age-related increases in the rate of deficit accumulation are similar even though they were derived using different measurement instruments and approaches. Some of the surveys considered a frailty index comprising about 40 items, whereas in others it was based on 70 to 100 items. Thirdly, some of the surveys used only self-reported ('subjective') data, whereas others used clinical data, including from 'objective' tests such as blood pressure and pulse measures, electrocardiograms, and urinalysis. Even so, the rate of deficit accumulation was uniform.

The reproducibility in the rate of deficit accumulation captured by the varying frailty index variables is challenging because it seems to oppose the common sense notions that some deficits should be more important and therefore have a greater impact on health than others, and that more precise measurement of individual factors (e.g. the ECG more than clinically measured pulse rate more than self-report of a heart rhythm problem) should yield more useful information. Figure 29.1.2 confirms the validity of the frailty index. Among the four quartiles of the index, people have predictably different survival rates. The highest survival is seen consistently among those with fewest deficits and vice versa. What is especially noteworthy here is how the frailty index measures were defined: the different iterations of the frailty index displayed here show variables that have been selected at random. In consequence, the number of things wrong with a person seems to be at least as important as the nature of what is wrong.

How can we understand these apparent challenges to clinical common sense? Among people with one thing wrong in whom a single intervention is planned, it is obviously important to have as much precision as possible. It is less clear, however, that individual item precision is important when classifying individuals or considering groups. That is because of the redundancy of information in complex systems. For example, while it might seem obvious that in any frailty index a self report of 'cancer' should carry more weight than a self-report of 'skin disease', that is not necessarily so. Some cancers are benign and some fatal, but so too are some skin diseases. In older people, those with worse illnesses will tend to have more things wrong—e.g. they will rate their health poorly, report feeling sad or anxious, will have disabilities, mobility problems, will have had a recent fall, or will have lost weight.

Recognizing the redundancy of a biological system implies that interconnectedness will determine how that system begins to express failure. Interconnectedness has other clinical implications, including the difficulty of making a single intervention in the expectation of a single outcome. Multiple outcomes should be expected and sought, especially if some are likely to be adverse. Some specialists may regard a group of patients more prone to side effects as being a nuisance, but geriatricians consider them as people with complex needs whose care offers rewarding personal and professional challenges.

The frailty index approach reveals other patterns with potentially interesting clinical consequences. Although women survive longer than men, it is not because they have fewer deficits. At all ages, men and women accumulate problems at the same rate but women have more deficits. Women tolerate their deficits better, such that, at any given age, women with a given number of deficits are less likely to die than men with exactly the same level of accumulated deficits.

Another striking feature of considering the accumulation of deficits with age is that there appears to be a limit to deficit accumulation. In a frailty index that considered 40 items, less than 1% of people reported more than 26 items. This 99% limit of about 0.67 has held up in several additional studies and suggests that there is a limit beyond which further accumulation of deficits is impossible, the addition of more deficits usually resulting in death. If verified prospectively in clinical settings, this limit would help clinical decision making about the risks of interventions. Operative risks, for example, are currently expressed chiefly in relation to the risk of fatal and nonfatal cardiovascular or respiratory complications, or technical failures. However, the risk of delirium, functional decline, or hospitalization often plays only a minor role in evidence-based clinical decision making, even though it is of great importance to patients and families.

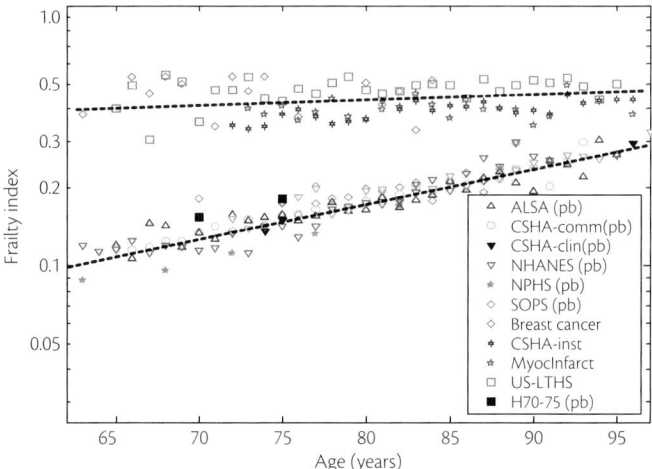

Fig. 29.1.1 Mean increase in the frailty index (y-axis) in relation to age (x-axis) for several community-dwelling samples (gradually increasing, lower line) and institutional or clinical samples (straight, upper line). On average, community-dwelling elderly people. The insert panel refers to the various samples form which the mean data points are drawn.
From Mitnitski A et al. (2005). *Relative fitness and frailty of elderly men and women in developed countries and their relationship with mortality.* J Am Geriatr Soc, **53**, 2184–9, with permission from John Wiley and Sons.

Defining frailty in clinical terms

It is generally agreed that the concept of frailty expresses both the features of multiple problems and the state of risk arising from those problems, but there is less consensus about clinical

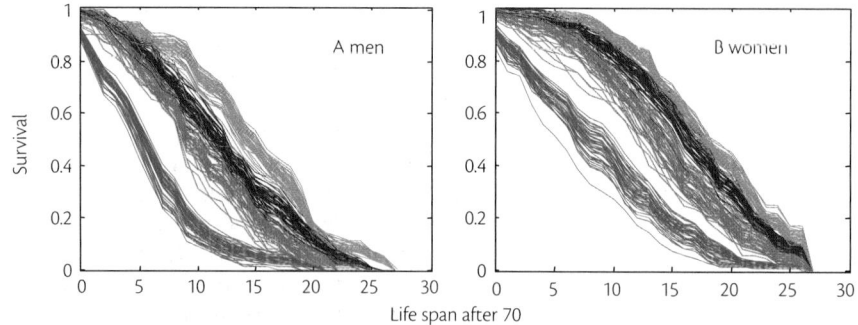

Fig. 29.1.2 Longer-term survival in relation to the frailty index. Gothenburg H-70 cohort, of people aged 70 at baseline, followed for 26 years. Panel A men, *n* = 448; Panel B, women, *n* = 518. Survival depends on the number of deficits accumulated, here presented as quartiles of the frailty index. Each line represents one Kaplan–Meyer survival curve, constructed from 70 deficits sampled at random.
(From Rockwood K *et al.* (2006). *Long-term risks of death and institutionalization of elderly people in relation to deficit accumulation at age 70*. J Am Geriatr Soc, **54**, 975–9. with permission from John Wiley and Sons.)

definitions of frailty. A popular view is that frailty describes a phenotype consisting of five features: weight loss, exhaustion, slow movement, low physical activity, and weakness. According to this view, only these features should define frailty, so that, e.g. the disability that often accompanies these features or the comorbidity that can give rise to them should be viewed separately. Although much work has been done to show that people who have three or more of the phenotypic characteristics have impaired stress responses, immune function and other physiological decrements, few empirical studies have explored the specificity of these attributes or whether they are detectable using other measures of frailty.

At least three other measures of frailty have been proposed. One is rules-based, prescribing certain characteristics that are present or absent. These include attributes that have been specifically excluded in the phenotype, such as disability, or those reflecting a mood disorder or impaired cognition. The phenotypic definition mainly describes physical frailty. A second definition of frailty is based on a single attribute, typically slow gait speed. A third approach defines frailty by the number of problems facing an elderly person, expressed either as an absolute number, or as a proportion in which the numerator is all the things that the person has wrong and the denominator is all the things that they might have wrong with them. 'All the things someone might have wrong with them' can be enumerated pragmatically, usually as 'All the things that were considered in producing the list of what was wrong'.

Frailty and disease presentation

Since the inception of their discipline, geriatricians have recognized that standard textbook descriptions of disease presentations often do not apply to frail elderly patients who become acutely ill. Core teaching in modern geriatrics surrounds the principal types of clinical presentation in elderly people, the so-called 'geriatric giants'. For many years, disease presentation in elderly people was epitomized as 'silent', as in the cases of patients whose ECGs or head CTs showed evidence of infarction despite the absence of any corresponding clinical history. However, it is now appreciated that while silent presentations are not rare, they are much less common than presentations such as delirium, falling, taking to bed, or functional decline that are not readily related to a single system. For example, a myocardial infarction is in the differential diagnosis of each of those presentations, whether or not chest pain, dyspnoea, or other 'properly cardiac' symptoms are present. Such disease presentations came to be described as 'atypical' even though they

can be the typical mode of presentation in frail elderly people. Commonly, the explanation for the 'geriatric giant' status of delirium, falls, immobility, and functional decline is that these syndromes are sensitive but nonspecific signs of illness. The disparity between sensitivity and specificity is partly explained by complexity. All human organisms are complex systems, and people who are frail are on the verge of failure. In many complex systems, the highest-order functions tend to fail first. At least from an evolutionary perspective, our highest-order functions are divided attention (arguably the basis of all high-order cognitive processes), upright bipedal ambulation, and opposable thumbs. Delirium, falls, and functional decline can therefore be seen as high-order presentations of systems failure, or signs that the patient has significant illness.

Frailty and patient management

The complexity of frailty is the rationale for geriatric medicine and also one of its major challenges. In managing complexity, a multidimensional approach known as 'comprehensive geriatric assessment' (CGA) has been employed. The CGA has been described as the prime technology of specialized geriatric interventions. A typical CGA form (Fig. 29.1.3) includes the evaluation of many aspects of a patient's function, from a cognitive assessment to an evaluation of bowel function, as well as some insight into daily function and social support.

Typically, the CGA contains enough information for a problem list to be developed, usually at a multidisciplinary team conference. There is an art to composing the problem list. Accounts that are too long and detailed can produce team paralysis, or commonly some arbitrariness in which problems should be given priority for intervention. Problem lists with insufficient detail do not provide the level of understanding necessary to set goals for intervention. Among other things, this makes it difficult to determine when a patient will be ready to be discharged. Obviously, the problem list becomes most useful when it is coupled with treatment and discharge plans. This clarification prevents situations in which teams react with hostility to a family whose relative's medical treatment course is over, but who 'won't take their mother home', only to find that the patient can't walk, or that the home has been sold.

Another important challenge is that our patients are often not seen as complex people with complex needs that require specialized approaches to their care. The idea that geriatrics is about 'second-rate patients cared for by second-rate doctors in second-rate facilities' is still sometimes endorsed, however quietly, by health care professionals

Comprehensive Geriatric Assessment
Division of Geriatric Medicine, Dalhousie University

Mental Status   ☐ WNL   ☐ Dementia   MMSE: _____
☐ CIND/MCI   ☐ Delirium   FAST: _____
Chief lifelong occupation: _____   Education (years): _____

Emotional   ☐ WNL   ☐ ↓ Mood   ☐ Depression   ☐ Anxiety   ☐ Other

Motivation   ☐ High ☐ Usual ☐ Low   **Health Attitude**   ☐ Excellent ☐ Good ☐ Fair ☐ Poor ☐ Couldn't say

Communication   **Speech** ☐ WNL ☐ Impaired   **Hearing** ☐ WNL ☐ Impaired   **Vision** ☐ WNL ☐ Impaired

		Baseline (two weeks ago)			Current (today)			Notes
Mobility	Transfer	I	A	D	I	A	D	
	Walking	I	A	D	I	A	D	
	AID	_____			_____			
Balance	Balance	WNL	IMPAIRED		WNL	IMPAIRED		
	Falls	N Y	#____		N Y	#____		
Elimination	Bowel	CONT	CONSTIP	INCONT	CONSTIP	CONT	INCONT	
	Bladder	CONT	CATHETER	INCONT	CATHETER	CONT	INCONT	
Nutrition	Weight	GOOD	UNDER OVER	OBESE	STABLE	LOSS	GAIN	
	Appetite	WNL	FAIR	POOR	WNL	FAIR	POOR	
ADLs	Feeding	I	A	D	I	A	D	
	Bathing	I	A	D	I	A	D	
	Dressing	I	A	D	I	A	D	
	Toileting	I	A	D	I	A	D	
IADLs	Cooking	I	A	D	I	A	D	
	Cleaning	I	A	D	I	A	D	
	Shopping	I	A	D	I	A	D	
	Medications	I	A	D	I	A	D	
	Driving	I	A	D	I	A	D	
	Banking	I	A	D	I	A	D	

Sleep   ☐ Normal   ☐ Disrupted   ☐ Daytime drowsiness

Social

Married/...	Lives	Supports	Home	Caregiver Relationship	Caregiver stress
☐ Married	Lives	☐ Informal	☐ Level house (#)	☐ Spouse	☐ None
☐ Divorced	☐ Alone	☐ HCNS	☐ Steps (#)	☐ Sibling	☐ Low
☐ Widowed	☐ Spouse	☐ Other	☐ Apartment	☐ Offspring	☐ Moderate
☐ Single	☐ Other	☐ Req. more support	☐ Assisted living	☐ Other	☐ High
		☐ None	☐ Nursing home		
			☐ Other		

Patient contact: (Pt.)
☐ Inpatient
☐ Clinic
☐ GDH
☐ NH
☐ Outreach
☐ Home
☐ Assisted living
☐ ER
☐ Other

How many months since well?

Current Frailty Score:

Scale	Pt.	CG
1. Very fit		
2. Well		
3. Well c̄ Rx'd co-morbid disease		
4. Apparently vulnerable		
5. Mildly frail		
6. Moderately frail		
7. Severely frail		
8. Terminally ill		

Caregiver occupation: (CG)

Problems:
1 RFR _____
2 _____
3 _____
4 _____
5 _____
6 _____
7 _____
8 _____
9 _____
10 _____
11 _____

Associated Medications: (*mark meds started in hospital with an asterisk)
_____
_____
_____
_____
_____
_____
_____
_____
_____
_____
_____

Assessor/Physician: _____   Date: _____
YYYY/MM/DD

Fig. 29.1.3 Comprehensive geriatric assessment (CGA) form. Commonly, this multidimensional assessment is supported by a multidisciplinary team, whose own detailed assessments can be summarized in the CGA. For example, physiotherapy assessments usually include precise descriptions of joint movement (e.g. '15° of abduction at the right hip'), whereas all that might be recorded in the CGA is 'narrow-based gait, stable with a cane'.

including physician colleagues and administrators. This deplorable attitude may reflect ambient ageism, ignorance, and a health care system with a single-system disease focus. The ageism long inherent in a youth-obsessed society will probably be attenuated somewhat as the 'baby boom' generation gets older. The lack of understanding by some health care professionals is not uncommonly reversed when they are directly exposed to specialized geriatric care following the failure of usual medical care of their parents.

A more fruitful approach to improved understanding of the complexities of the management of frail patients is reform of the system. The role of geriatricians as advocates for reform of the health care system is one of the oldest traditions of the discipline. For example, CGA can lead to a pragmatic treatment and discharge plan, which can be explained to patients and families in plain language. However, the efficacy of this form of effective care might not be readily measurable. As the measurement of health care effectiveness moves from measuring inputs (e.g. budget line items, length of stay) to measuring outcomes (proportion of people with hypertension in whom blood pressure control is achieved) it becomes essential to find outcome measures that themselves embrace the complexity of care. It is not unknown for an outcomes-orientated health systems manager to worry that the geriatric medicine service has a higher than average mortality rate without knowing whether a palliative care team is available. The apparently poor performance of the service may then be treated by budget cutbacks because of failure to recognize an above-average effort to provide humane care to people who are dying and who need more resources.

Even something as seemingly unassailable as 'proportion of people with hypertension in whom blood pressure control is achieved' might be an unrealistic target. Consider that many elderly people with dementia have a dysautonomia that renders them susceptible to orthostatic hypotension, even in the face of systolic hypertension while sitting. Outcome measures that exclude clinical judgement of individual patient's needs force physicians either to work against the interests of the patient by ignoring the arguably more lethal orthostatic hypotension in favour of the administratively correct 'blood pressure control' or against the interests of their service, by rationally not treating in the face of disabling orthostatic hypotension.

In some areas, a judgement-based outcome measure such as Goal Attainment Scaling has been used to provide the benefit of a measurable, quantifiable outcome with outcomes that are clinically meaningful and relevant to individual patients. With Goal Attainment Scaling, individually relevant target goals are negotiated between the multidisciplinary team and the patient. For example, in a patient with disabling orthostatic hypotension, the goal might be to relieve symptoms and lessen disability. Such a measure is readily open to audit (although it requires that the person doing such audits has the relevant experience necessary to assess the validity of clinical judgements). It can also be quantified, by a standardized means of quantifying the achievement of goals, or the occurrence of plausible adverse effects. In the case of the patient with orthostatic hypotension, the goal might be relief of symptoms 90% of the time, allowing general recovery of function; a compromise between the goal and the current state might be relief of symptoms 50% of the time, with improved function but some residual disability. Similarly, the worst outcome might be serious injury from a fall. In between that and the current state would be further restriction of activities. This approach arises logically from the problem list; integrates impairment, disability, and handicap; and is transparent to the patient, family team, and auditors, clarifying for team members in pursuit of their interventions, and time-saving in team conferences. It demonstrates to colleagues the complexity of patients' needs and of clinical decision making.

Falls

Falls are common in people over the age of 65 years. It has been estimated that as many as a half of those aged 80 years and over will have fallen at least once during the course of the preceding year. Recurrent falling is a significant indicator of frailty. Women are more at risk for a number of reasons including reduced muscular strength compared to men, and greater difficulty when employing corrective manoeuvres if balance is disturbed. The fall itself can lead to trauma, but many of the consequences of falls result from the person's inability to get up again. Prolonged periods of lying on the ground predispose to pressure sores, hypothermia, and rhabdomyolysis. Falls need to be taken into consideration when prescribing medication such as anticoagulants. Repeated falls force many older people to leave their home for institutional care.

Aetiology

The decrease in lean body mass with age is detectable in late middle life. It reduces muscle strength and power, particularly in women who, in most cases, have less muscle mass than men. Once off balance, the ability to regain equilibrium requires adequate muscle strength and the integrity of a number of other body systems. These include visual ability, intact cognition, proprioception, and joints that are stable, especially the knee joint. As people become frail, their ability to integrate these complex pathways becomes impaired. This probably reflects both the accumulation of age-related deficits, in addition to well-known contributory medical factors, some of which have been mentioned earlier, e.g. impairment of vision and proprioception. Others include disturbance of balance resulting from vestibular dysfunction, and postural hypotension with its myriad causes, including intrinsic disease and the prescription of a wide variety of drugs. Intrinsic medical problems include vertebrobasilar insufficiency, other forms of cerebrovascular disease including transient ischaemic attacks, neurological disorders such as Parkinson's disease, and peripheral neuropathy such as that associated with diabetes.

Environmental factors, such as poor lighting, loose mats, and inappropriate stairs, often contribute to falls.

Prevention

First, careful attention must be given to the environment in which an older person lives, as this will reduce the extrinsic factors contributing to falls. These include avoiding accident hazards such as loose mats and trailing flexes, ensuring adequate lighting, placing electrical sockets at a level that avoids the need to bend over, and installing chair lifts inside a dwelling or a lift within a block of flats where this is possible.

The patient's medical background is important, e.g. if they are taking medication that will cause postural hypotension or are suffering from neurological conditions such as Parkinson's disease or unstable joints requiring appropriate walking aids. This background knowledge will help prevent falls in the first place, and help with secondary prevention.

Assessment of a patient who has fallen

Careful assessment is necessary. This requires a careful history, particularly about the nature of the individual fall or the pattern of falling, if this is occurring frequently. Coexisting medical morbidity is important, as are the medications that the patient is taking, including their alcohol consumption. Physical examination may reveal postural hypotension, cardiac arrhythmias, valve lesions, or carotid bruits. Examination of the nervous system may also yield relevant information such as poor peripheral sensation, extrapyramidal disease, visual impairment, evidence of previous or perhaps recent cerebrovascular events, and cerebellar signs.

Careful musculoskeletal examination is essential, particularly muscle strength and mass and joint function and stability. Deconditioning is reflected by hip flexors that are weaker than knee extensors. A simple assessment of gait and the ability to transfer from bed to chair, and from chair to the upright position, is essential. In most cases, assessment by a physiotherapist and/or an occupational therapist is very valuable.

Investigations

To some extent, the investigations are determined by the precipitating factors discovered when taking a history and the findings on examination, but most people who have fallen will have a routine screen including full blood count, urea, creatinine, and electrolytes, random glucose, bone and thyroid biochemistry, and a vitamin B_{12} and folate estimation. A standard 12-lead ECG is often required, and where circumstances suggest it is appropriate, 24-h ECG monitoring and tilt-table testing may be necessary.

Management

This is multifactorial, depending to some extent on the circumstances of the fall and the patient's medical and social background. There are often treatable underlying medical causes. In most people treatment will involve both pharmacological and nonpharmacological strategies.

Reducing the risks in the patient's environment, provision of appropriate walking aids where required, improving strength where feasible, and balance training are important. What is needed is the multidisciplinary team assessment that is at the heart of much geriatric medicine. Polypharmacy should be addressed, and drugs that may contribute to falls should be stopped or changed to a less hazardous alternative wherever feasible. Lifestyle factors are also relevant, including whether the person who has fallen is prepared to accept more assistance where this is available, whether they should continue to live in their existing environment, and whether the intervention of a physiotherapist and occupational therapist might be helpful. Although moving into a different environment may reduce the frequency of falls, through improved lighting or fewer stairs, important medical components to falling must be addressed as well.

Fear of falling affects many older people and will often lead them to make a decision to move to where they feel more secure. In many cases, little can be done to overcome obvious distress, but sometimes careful attention to accident hazards, input from the physiotherapist and occupational therapist, and treatment of underlying contributory factors may help.

Restraints, whether these are employed when a person is sitting in a chair, or the more traditional cot sides and bed rails, should not be part of modern medical management of older people. They cause an increased risk of injury and are rarely helpful. Hip protectors have enjoyed a vogue, but it is becoming increasingly clear that they are not nearly as effective at reducing fracture rates as was initially hoped. One difficulty is putting them on in a reliable fashion.

Patients need to learn how to manage the situation after they have fallen, e.g. the best way of getting up from the floor. This is usually best undertaken by a physiotherapist. Similarly, the use of alarms, either within a room or of the pendant or wristwatch type, will reduce the length of time an elderly person stays on the floor. Monitoring by a warden, family members, or neighbours will also improve confidence. Appropriate management of osteoporosis is especially important and may reduce subsequent fractures.

The falls clinic

The important contributions that falls in older people make to morbidity and mortality, and consequently to quality of life, and the resulting cost to the community, have resulted in a move to establish falls clinics. This allows a multidisciplinary team to assess and advise those who have fallen. Different clinics have different styles of assessment, some concentrating more on 'funny turns', i.e. a syncope-based approach, while others are more general in their philosophy. However, it is important that all geriatric services are able adequately to assess and advise on the management of people who are falling. In the United Kingdom, the National Service Framework for Older People encourages falls clinics, but this should not used as an excuse for others to abdicate to such clinics their responsibility for investigating and managing falls, as the clinics cannot manage everyone who has fallen.

Prognosis

The prognosis for many people who are falling is good. It is often possible to reduce the rate of falling, either through treatment of underlying medical factors or by environmental adjustment, or both. Careful attention to reducing the consequence of falling is effective, e.g. a pendant alarm system minimizing the time the person spends on the floor with the consequent comorbidity that this introduces. However, falls are so often multifactorial in aetiology that for many the risk will be minimized not removed. It is important to remember that some aspects of management are intrusive to a person's lifestyle, and the patient must always be consulted about the level of risk they are prepared to accept.

Pressure sores

Pressure sores should almost never occur while a patient is in hospital, but some estimates put their prevalence as high as 5 to 10% among hospitalized patients. A high degree of awareness must be maintained and all older patients should have an assessment of their risk of developing pressure sores, particularly those who are relatively immobile. Pressure sores are particularly likely to occur where bony prominences lie close to the skin, e.g. sacrum, heels, and shoulders. Once established, they have important consequences for resources, notably increased length of hospital stay. The greatest cost is borne by the patient, but there is also a considerable financial burden in health care costs.

Prevention

This requires awareness of risk factors, notably increasing age and immobility. Other potential exacerbating factors include malnutrition, dehydration, lack of subcutaneous tissue, obesity, and vascular insufficiency. Patients who are continually wet because of incontinence are also more at risk, as are those who have impaired consciousness or a peripheral neuropathy. A number of protocols rate risk factors and produce scores for each patient. These are used routinely on many wards caring for elderly people. In the United Kingdom the National Institute for Health and Clinical Excellence (NICE) has produced guidelines recommending that those who are potentially at risk of developing a pressure sore should be assessed within 6 h of admission to hospital.

Types of pressure sore

Pressure sores are often classified into one of four types depending on their cause, but many are multifactorial. Some are caused predominantly by saturation of the skin, usually with urine but occasionally with perspiration. Faeces can be a problem, with increased risk of infection. The skin becomes macerated and breaks down. Other factors are friction and the shearing force that occurs when the skin is pulled or pushed away from its point of fixation to underlying bony prominences. A patient sitting up in bed may slip down, causing sacral and/or heel skin to be dragged away from its bony attachments. This damages the underlying supporting tissues, including small blood vessels. Excess pressure itself is a major factor, i.e. pressure sufficient to overcome the normal capillary pressure within the subcutaneous tissues. When external pressure exceeds 35 mmHg, the vascular system is compromised and ischaemia will result if this situation is allowed to continue.

Clinical features

Patients at risk should be regularly inspected for signs of hyperaemia—reddening of the skin around pressure points—which is often the earliest warning sign, especially if it does not blanch when gently pressured. This can be quickly followed by evidence of skin damage, a broken epidermis and dermis, progressing to ulceration through subcutaneous tissue and eventually down to other underlying structures such as bones and tendons.

Pressure sores often develop some considerable time after the damage that has caused them. Progression from the hyperaemic stage to significant ulceration may take days, and in some cases weeks. Precipitating factors need to be present for only a relatively short time, e.g. 2 to 3 h.

Treatment

Prevention is of paramount importance. In addition to the points already discussed, regular turning of the those at risk, e.g. every 2 h or so, has become part of the standard management. Although not evidence-based, it makes sense and seems to be helpful. However, turning itself can put a patient at risk. It is crucial to do this using appropriate procedures that do not themselves compromise the integrity of the skin, e.g. through friction and more especially shear forces.

A whole range of pressure-relieving devices are available in modern hospitals, many of which can also be found in the community. These include special mattresses with air pockets that are inflated intermittently so that no area of skin is under pressure for more than a relatively short period of time, mattresses filled with water, and foam mattresses that have been carefully designed to reduce the likelihood of pressure sores by spreading the distribution of weight.

Once a pressure sore is established, careful attention to nutrition and fluid intake is essential, as is management of underlying risk factors such as incontinence, and also other morbidity that may impair healing such as anaemia. Deep ulcers should be debrided of dead tissue. This is initiated with topical applications containing enzymes that break down dead tissue and slough. Surgical debridement is frequently required for extensive sores, and maggots, originally used in military medicine, are sometimes used.

A wide range of dressings can be used to help promote healing, some targeted at superficial pressure sores and others designed to promote healing where there are cavities. Advice from a nurse specialist is very valuable in this complex area.

Many pressure sores look as if they are infected, and smell unpleasant. In many cases, particularly those that have progressed to ulceration, bacterial colonization can be demonstrated, especially by staphylococci and mixed Gram-negative organisms such as bacteroides. Other common organisms include Gram-positive cocci and yeasts. There is an increasing risk of methicillin-resistant *Staphylococcus aureus* (MRSA). It is important to distinguish between colonization and an actively infected wound which should be considered when there is extensive cellulitis, and/or frank pus in a patient who is unwell. If this is suspected, the white count should be checked and blood cultures taken. Antibiotic treatment, when necessary, should cover a wide spectrum. It is also important to remember that infection from some ulcers spreads to underlying bone, causing osteomyelitis. If this situation arises, expert advice should be sought from a microbiologist.

Surgery and the older patient

Formerly, advanced age was regarded as a contraindication to many surgical procedures but advances in surgical techniques and intensive care procedures have changed this attitude. Biological, rather than chronological, age is the important factor, and many elderly people now undergo major surgical procedures and recover successfully. At least 25 to 30% of all surgery is undertaken in those aged 65 years and over. Increasingly, it is being recognized that it is not age itself, but rather the severity of the illness and the presence of comorbidity, that predicts complications and fatality.

Preoperative assessment and evaluation

The patient should be assessed for evidence of comorbidity and other risk factors that might influence surgical outcome. This is not necessarily to decide whether or not surgery is appropriate, but rather to plan the aftercare in a way that minimizes the impact of these risk factors. It is up to the patient and their family, together with the surgeon, to make the decision once they are in a position to make an informed decision.

Preoperative evaluation is best undertaken by considering the patient's history, conducting a physical examination, and assessing the relative laboratory investigations. In most cases, careful assessment of cardiopulmonary status is of major importance. Other important factors include the medications, both prescribed and over the counter, evidence of nutritional status, cognition, and evidence of psychiatric comorbidity such as depression, and also the patient's functional level and quality of life.

Investigations should include the usual laboratory screen covering basic haematological and biochemical indices and an ECG. Many would argue for a chest radiograph in appropriate circumstances, especially if there is clinical evidence of cardiac or pulmonary disease.

Peri- or intraoperative cardiovascular complications are usually the major concern. As already indicated, this is probably not a function of age itself, but rather that the latter may be a marker for presurgical cardiovascular pathology. The risk has to be put in the context of the nature of the surgery. It is also necessary to remember that there are physiological changes in the cardiovascular system as a person ages that may lead to an older person being less able to tolerate fluid overload, and hypotension. Another important point is that myocardial infarction in an older person may well be silent, and this should be considered a possibility in any person who shows signs of cardiac decompensation.

Major clinical predictors of increased risk from cardiovascular complications include recent myocardial infarction, significant or unstable angina, severe valvular disease, and significant arrhythmias. Their significance depends on the nature of the surgery that is contemplated. Where uncertainty exists, a full cardiovascular assessment by a cardiologist may be necessary, including exercise testing if this is practicable.

Pulmonary complications are the other major factor determining morbidity and mortality in a patient undergoing surgery. Again, it is not age itself, but the combination of the physiological changes associated with ageing and the presence of preexisting pulmonary comorbidity that are important, the consideration of biological as opposed simply to chronological age. A 70-year-old may have been smoking for 50 or 60 years while a 50-year-old smoker would have acquired 20 years less smoking-induced morbidity. Where there is evidence of respiratory disease, preoperative pulmonary function testing is essential if major surgery is under consideration. Where pulmonary disease constitutes a significant surgical risk, delaying surgery while optimizing treatment for the patient's pulmonary disorder will usually be worthwhile, especially if this can be accompanied by stopping smoking. As in the case of cardiovascular disease, early mobilization is valuable and will reduce the chance of postoperative lower respiratory tract infection and atelectasis.

Renal and hepatic function can contribute to perioperative risk. Careful attention must be given to fluid balance and electrolyte levels. It is unsatisfactory to rely upon a simple creatinine measurement as an indicator of presurgical renal function. Hepatic function, unless significantly impaired, is usually not a major consideration but one must bear in mind that many anaesthetic drugs are subject to hepatic metabolization and excreted via the biliary system.

The nutritional state of the patient is important, as a malnourished elderly patient has a significantly increased risk of infection, delayed wound healing, and death.

The expected level of function will depend on how the patient has functioned in the recent past, noting any functional decline and what improvement the surgery may achieve. The geriatrician may be the first to inquiry systematically into the patient's prior state of function. This can lead to a mediating role, between the perspectives of the patient, family, and the surgeon on how the current level of function might be improved, or even threatened, by a given procedure. An elective right total hip replacement might relieve pain, but is highly unlikely to improve walking if a left-hip flexion contracture has developed.

Antibiotic prophylaxis

This has proved effective in decreasing postoperative infection rates in a number of different surgical operations and may be particularly important in older people because of their age-related impairment of immunological function. Antibiotic prophylaxis is employed across a range of surgical procedures where the risk of infection, even if low, would create serious problems, e.g. where a foreign body such as a joint prosthesis is being implanted, and similarly for prosthetic valves. The antibiotic chosen is targeted against the most likely organisms to be involved. The dose is determined by the need to produce a high concentration around the time of surgery.

Prevention of endocarditis in those with damaged or prosthetic valves is an important consideration in older people, so many of whom have clinical evidence of possible valvular pathology. If necessary, further investigation such as echocardiography, may be required to discover whether a clinical finding, such as a bruit, is indicative of a damaged valve.

In general, the protocol for using antimicrobial prophylaxis for surgical procedures will be a standard part of the surgical protocol in each unit, often in conjunction with a microbiologist, and will probably not be determined by a physician's or a geriatrician's assessment.

Choice of anaesthetic procedure

This should usually be left to the anaesthetist. Sometimes, however, it requires a 'team' decision involving the geriatrician as well as the surgical and anaesthetic services, e.g. when deciding on general vs a more peripheral anaesthetic technique. Many older people will benefit from the latter, especially where there is cardiac or pulmonary comorbidity, even though this approach does not eliminate all the complications that are usually associated with general anaesthesia.

Postoperative management

A protocol for the postoperative management of elderly patients should rightly be a standard part of the surgical approach, and much will rely upon the nursing as well as the medical staff involved. The geriatrician's main contribution to postoperative management should begin at the preoperative stage, when a patient's particular postoperative risks are detailed and a strategy recommended to minimize them. These include delirium and its management, adequate pain control to facilitate respiratory function, and early mobilization to avoid venous thrombosis and pressure sores. Intraoperative use of indwelling catheters may lead to urinary tract infections, and postoperative urinary retention may be a problem in elderly men with prostatic hypertrophy.

Conclusions

Although a geriatrician is often asked to assess a patient preoperatively, particularly for surgical risks and their reduction, it is important to consider strategies to reduce postoperative complications and those occurring in the operating theatre. Surgery, even major surgery, should never be denied a person solely based on their chronological age. A balanced decision, involving the patient and their family as well as their medical attendants, should be made in each case depending upon biological age and comorbidities, severity of risks, quality of life, and the prognosis of the underlying condition requiring surgery. Many elderly people tolerate major surgery and if carefully managed return to a good quality of life.

Urinary incontinence

Urinary incontinence is embarrassing both for the person concerned and their families and carers. It occurs more frequently than is often appreciated, afflicting about 1 in 50 men and 1 in 10 women in middle age. The prevalence rises as the years increase and nearly 1 in 10 men and 1 in 6 women over the age of 75 years suffer with it. It may occur in as many as 50% of people living in care homes.

It is defined as the involuntary release of urine. During voluntary voiding, the sphincter of the bladder neck relaxes allowing the urine to escape. Bladder-emptying is under the control of the parasympathetic autonomic nervous system, and can usually be overridden by bringing higher mental function into play. This balance can be upset by a number of factors affecting the nervous system.

It is contributed to by a number of changes that increase as a person grows older including prostatic hypertrophy in men, pelvic floor weakness and vaginal atrophy in women, diminishing bladder

Box 29.1.1 Medical factors contributing to urinary incontinence

- Infection
- Drugs
- Cognitive impairment
- Constipation and faecal impaction
- Increased production of urine, including hyperglycaemia and hypercalcaemia
- Local bladder pathology such as tumours
- Urethral change associated with atrophic vaginitis
- Benign or malignant prostatic enlargement
- Detrusor overactivity
- Stress incontinence
- Some combinations: in many people there is more than one contributing factor

capacity, and contractility associated with an increased residual urinary volume. Ageing is accompanied by increasing frequency of bladder contractions. Incontinence can be exacerbated by a person's limited mobility, their inability to recognize a full bladder, dementia, severe constipation or faecal impaction, certain drugs, and the inability to manipulate appropriate clothing.

Assessment

This aims to identify critical factors contributing to incontinence (Box 29.1.1).

A careful history will often provide useful diagnostic information, including the mode of onset, whether any activity precipitates the incontinence, or whether there are associated symptoms such as dysuria or faecal incontinence. Past medical history is also important, e.g. damage occurring during childbirth, the presence of diabetes, or symptoms of prostatic enlargement. Medication, including diuretics, calcium channel blockers and anticholinergic drugs, can also play a part.

Physical examination should include neurological assessment, abdominal examination for bladder distension or other masses, and a careful pelvic examination in women. This is especially important as stress testing may reveal urinary leakage with a full bladder, e.g. after coughing.

Functional classification

Urinary incontinence is often classified into four major subtypes and, although this is an oversimplification, it can be helpful when assessing a patient or deciding about the management of their incontinence.

Overflow incontinence

This frequently results from bladder outlet obstruction, e.g. because of an enlarged prostate gland or impaired detrusor contractility. It is also a feature of some neurological conditions, e.g. spinal cord damage or the neuropathy that can occur in a number of conditions such as diabetes mellitus. It is usually marked by the continuous loss of small quantities of urine.

Stress incontinence

This occurs mainly in women and is most frequently associated with lack of support to the urethra because of weakness of the pelvic floor musculature. It may also occur, albeit less frequently, where there is an intrinsic weakness of the sphincter following pelvic surgery. In both situations, the sphincter is unable to hold back the urine flow when the abdominal pressure increases beyond a critical threshold, and urine may be lost when laughing, coughing, climbing stairs or other activities that increase intra-abdominal pressure.

Urge incontinence

This results from instability of the detrusor muscle resulting in hyperactivity and uninhibited bladder contractions. This phenomenon probably explains the incontinence that accompanies urinary tract infections. It can also result from damage to the higher inhibitory pathways of the central nervous system, e.g. following a cerebrovascular accident. Local bladder lesions such as stones or tumours can provoke detrusor hyperactivity. The patient usually experiences urgency and frequency leading to a sudden desire to void urine that is difficult to control, resulting in incontinence. In some older people this phenomenon may arise with little if any sensation of urge, but detrusor hyperactivity can still be present.

Mixed incontinence

This is most probably the commonest form of incontinence in women and results from coexistence of both urge and stress incontinence with symptoms that reflect this.

Other causes

These occur less frequently, particularly so in elderly people. They include results of trauma, especially pelvic fracture, surgical complications, and fistulas.

Investigation

Urine should always be screened for infection even in a person with long-standing incontinence, and in the absence of typical symptoms, since many elderly people escape these. It should also be checked for the presence of blood. General biochemical screening tests may reveal high plasma glucose levels, hypercalcaemia, or evidence of renal failure.

Ultrasonography may help detect and estimate the amount of residual postvoid urine, and the presence of stones or other abnormalities. In a normal older person, the maximum residual volume after urination should be no more than 100 ml. Residual volume is best investigated ultrasonographically, if possible, rather than by diagnostic catheterization. More sophisticated urodynamic studies may be required in some people if the cause of incontinence cannot be identified, or surgical intervention is being considered.

Treatment

A pragmatic approach is sometimes adopted to help elderly people with detrusor overactivity and an overactive bladder. Bladder retraining, by gradually increasing the time between the occasions when urine is passed, is sometimes helpful but needs a careful management plan and someone to monitor it. However, many people will need to be helped with medication, e.g. anticholinergic drugs such as tolterodine. The dose has to be titrated slowly and it may take 6 to 8 weeks before the maximum effect has been achieved.

Unfortunately, these drugs may precipitate urinary retention and other anticholinergic side effects such as a dry mouth, constipation, postural hypotension, and confusion. Other drugs in this category include trospium chloride and oxybutynin.

Stress incontinence should be treated first with pelvic floor exercises, although it can be difficult to persuade elderly people to adopt an effective programme. Even when they do, the benefits wear off after the exercises cease. To be successful, it must be a continuing programme. If pelvic floor exercises are unsuccessful, and the severity of the incontinence warrants it, surgery may have to be considered.

For men with overflow incontinence secondary to urinary tract obstruction, a transurethral prostatectomy maybe appropriate. However, in some patients, especially those who are frail and in whom there is significant prostatic enlargement, an antiandrogen may be worth trying first. Finasteride inhibits the conversion of testosterone to dihydrotestosterone, which is more potent than testosterone itself. This often results in a reduction in prostate size but improvement in urinary flow may take a period of several months so progress is slow. Antiandrogenic drugs may cause impotence and decrease libido.

α-Blockers such as doxazosin may relax smooth muscles sufficiently to increase urine flow rates and reduce obstructive symptoms in some men with benign prostatic hypertrophy. They may cause hypotension predisposing to postural instability and falls.

Patients who are particularly troubled by nocturnal incontinence or frequency may be helped by oral or intranasal synthetic vasopressin or other vasopressin-like analogues given at bed time. These will often produce an antidiuretic effect during the night, but can result in fluid retention and hyponatraemia, for which the patient must be carefully monitored. Other practical approaches to try and reduce the impact of nocturia include the judicious use of an alarm clock or other means of waking the patient up periodically through the night. This can enable some people to empty their bladder in a controlled rather than an involuntary fashion.

Some physicians recommend the use of a small dose of a rapidly acting diuretic between midday and evening, followed by fluid restriction after the evening meal until bedtime in an attempt to reduce urine production during the night. Occasionally, fluid restriction during the evening without the use of a diuretic earlier in the day will also help. Other simple practical measures include restriction of caffeine-containing drinks and alcohol, both of which can contribute to daytime and night-time incontinence.

Prognosis

Careful attention to the underlying nature of the incontinence and its likely aetiology will allow successful management in most cases, even if it cannot be completely resolved. The earlier it is assessed the more likely it is that a solution will be found.

Urinary catheters

Although they have an important part to play in the management of incontinence in some people, these are best avoided if possible and should never be used as the first line of response when managing incontinence. Every patient with incontinence should be properly assessed and a diagnosis of the underlying type and its aetiology made before considering treatment.

Pressure from staff in care homes for long-term catheterization of a resident simply on the grounds of nursing convenience should be resisted, not just because of the risk of chronic infection and stone formation, but also because of personal dignity, unless the patient makes a conscious decision that they would prefer catheterization. Other approaches include appropriate clothing and pads, programmed urination, improved access to the toilet such as a commode by the bed, or the use of a drainage sheath for men. The latter is especially useful for nocturnal incontinence where the patient is continent by day. In some circumstances, intermittent self-catheterization for the management of outflow obstruction may be considered, but this requires manual dexterity and normal cognitive ability.

When there is no alternative to catheterization, e.g. where there is a significant risk of pressure sores, or where a patient has chosen this route, it is important to change the catheter every 3 months, and in some cases even more frequently. Some patients prefer a valve on the end of the catheter rather than a permanent drainage bag. Where used, the latter should be of the leg bag type rather than one which is attached to a stand, informing everyone who passes about the patient's problems.

All catheters become colonized by bacteria but this does not mean that treatment with antibiotics is required. Only clinically significant infections should prompt antibiotic prescription. Inappropriate treatment will lead to the emergence of resistant organisms. Infection is not always indicated by dark and/or cloudy urine. The latter can result from concentrated urine secondary to dehydration.

If a significant infection arises, i.e. one with an accompanying fever, delirium, discomfort, and disturbed haematological or biochemical indicators, the catheter should be removed for 48 to 72 h, and the patient should be given an adequate fluid intake and an appropriate antibiotic. Reinsertion of the catheter may require a single dose of gentamicin. In those patients with indwelling catheters who develop repeated infections and morbidity, the incontinence should be managed without the use of a catheter if at all possible.

Faecal incontinence

Faecal incontinence is the involuntary passage of faecal material in inappropriate circumstances. It can be disastrous both for the person concerned and for those who look after them, and in some cases, may lead to admission to an institution for the provision of nursing home care. The aetiology of faecal incontinence is often multifactorial, e.g. a physical bowel problem that may be exacerbated by urgency in getting to the lavatory, a bowel infection, drugs, dietary factors, or lack of control or awareness of the need to empty the bowel in a person with dementia. Differentiating between incontinence associated with urgency and passive incontinence will often help to decide aetiology and hence management.

Faecal incontinence is much less frequent than urinary incontinence, which often accompanies it. Prevalence rates quoted in the literature vary widely, e.g. between 10% and 95% for elderly residents in institutional care. It has been estimated that up to 10% of those living in the community may have at least some minor degree of incontinence, but this is probably greatly under-reported because those affected are too embarrassed to seek help.

Continence is normally preserved by a variety of mechanisms including the anal and rectosigmoid sphincters, which have to relax to enable the passage of faecal material to the exterior. This relaxation can be over-ridden voluntarily, especially by contraction of the external anal sphincter, which consists of striated, i.e. voluntary, muscle. The activity of the sphincter mechanism is complemented by the puborectalis sling which ensures that there is an acute angle between the rectum and the anal canal, retarding passage of stool into the latter. Anal and rectal sensation are also important in helping to maintain continence, usually being adequate to distinguish flatus from faeces, although this may not be so easy in the presence of diarrhoea.

Aetiology

The commonest cause of faecal incontinence in older people is probably loading of the rectum and sigmoid colon from constipation. This can produce faecal impaction. Constipation in turn can be the consequence of conditions such as hypothyroidism or drugs, including many analgesics, and tricyclic antidepressants, which are associated with anticholinergic activity. Any cause of acute or chronic diarrhoea may result in incontinence as long as the diarrhoea persists, so that diverticulitis and late-onset inflammatory bowel diseases can present in this way. Physical conditions affecting the anal sphincter and lower rectum may cause or contribute to faecal incontinence as well as a number of neurological disorders affecting control of the sphincter mechanisms. These include a wide number of conditions, as can be seen from Box 29.1.2. Many causes of faecal incontinence should be curable through relatively simple measures such as relief of faecal impaction, attention to drug regimes, and treatment for underlying physical conditions.

Evaluation of the patient

The history should include details of pre-existing bowel conditions, medications, whether there is an associated passage of mucus and/or blood, and whether or not the patient is aware of the soiling. Regular bowel action does not necessarily exclude faecal impaction, which is often present in those with both faecal and urinary incontinence.

Examination starts by inspecting the anus for local pathology, followed by rectal examination. This allows assessment of anal tone, detection of a rectum full of faeces, or the presence of a tumour. Proctoscopy may be necessary. A routine abdominal examination is essential, particularly to assess the descending colon. Finally, examination of relevant parts of the nervous system is appropriate in those in whom there is a potential predisposing cause for neuropathy such as diabetes, or other relevant clinical predisposition.

Box 29.1.2 Physical conditions affecting faecal continence

- Anorectal abnormalities including prolapse, tumours, and constipation
- Neurological disorders
- Dementia
- Factors associated with urgency including diarrhoea, e.g. bowel disease and some drugs, reduced mobility
- Constipation or faecal impaction

Some patients will require a plain abdominal radiograph which may help to identify the extent of faecal loading. It can also act as a baseline for assessing subsequent treatment. It may indicate the possibility of 'high' impaction occurring at the rectosigmoid junction or above, which sometimes indicates neoplastic change or a stricture caused by other bowel conditions.

Treatment

In many cases this will involve treating underlying constipation, and its remediable underlying causes, e.g. alteration to the patient's drug regime, treatment of hypothyroidism, and attention to diet. Management of incontinence in those with neurological problems or dementia is more difficult. However, the situation can nearly always be significantly improved. Patients with dementia are very likely to have other contributory factors.

Where there is mild impaction, e.g. soft rather than hard stools are encountered in the rectum, laxatives may be adequate. In the presence of semi-solid stool, a stool softener may be required in addition. This approach, rather than the use of enemas, is preferable in very frail patients. If such a patient has hard stool, a stool-softening agent should be used first.

After clearing the bowel, a pattern of regular defecation may help, and can sometimes be facilitated by the use of a suppository. Paradoxically, this sometimes needs to be complemented by a small dose of a constipating agent such as loperamide to manage incontinence between bowel evacuations. The optimum dose will be found by titration, and if this is less than 2 mg, the syrup form may be preferable.

When there is refractory constipation or impaction, a phosphate enema may be needed daily or on alternate days, instead of a suppository. This is an unpleasant procedure both for the patient and for those caring for them. It should be avoided unless essential. This should be continued until rectal examination confirms that the rectum is clear, and palpation of the descending colon during abdominal examination shows no evidence of faecal loading. This may well take 7 to 10 days. If this fails, a more active approach using a bowel preparation such as sodium picosulphate may be required in order to avoid manual evacuation of faeces, an unpleasant and potentially dangerous procedure.

Sodium picosulphate is an osmotic laxative that draws fluid into the lower bowel. It is important that patient is well hydrated, and that the period of bowel evacuation should not be longer than 24 h to avoid water and electrolyte disturbance. It should not be used if there is any suggestion of intestinal obstruction, significant renal impairment, coexisting bowel pathology such as ulcerative colitis or Crohn's disease, or in the presence of hypocalcaemia.

A more sophisticated management approach, sacral nerve stimulation, is becoming better known. It involves low-level electrical stimulation of the nerve supply to the sphincters and also the smooth muscle of the lower bowel, which the patient can interrupt using an external magnet, allowing passage of the stool. It is appropriate for patients with a weak but structurally intact sphincter where all other measures have been unsuccessful.

Many patients will still require appropriate protective clothing even if the frequency and magnitude of the soiling is reduced. Finally, there are a small number of patients in whom only containment with appropriate padding and clothing will be possible.

Careful thought should be given to preventing recurrence of faecal loading by the judicious use of diet, laxatives, or in some people, even regular enemas. Patients must be managed individually.

Where possible, the patient should be carefully consulted about, and informed of, the management plan. Great care should be taken to preserve their dignity. Referral to a support group may be of value. Whenever necessary, a specialist adviser in faecal and urinary incontinence should be asked for their advice.

Prescribing medicine for older people

Two-thirds of people over the age of 65 take medication regularly. Although they account for about 15% of the population they are responsible for about 40% of the costs of drug prescribing. One-third of people aged 75 and over take at least three medications, and for those living in institutional care this number is on average doubled. There is a tendency to prescribe drugs for older people and then fail to review them. It is therefore not surprising that estimates suggest that about 1 in 10 hospital admissions of older people are caused by, or contributed to by, unwanted effects of drugs. The overall incidents and adverse reactions to drugs must be higher than this as in many incidences the problem will be dealt with in a primary care setting.

Preventing unwanted drug effects

The two most important questions to bear in mind when initiating a prescription are first: 'Is this treatment really necessary?', and secondly: 'If so, for how long should it be prescribed before review?' It can be surprisingly difficult to know what is necessary, as the evidence on which requirements are based must often be generalized from younger patients, or patients who are typically not as frail as those seen by geriatricians. For instance, while starting a patient on aspirin, a β-blocker, an angiotensin converting enzyme inhibitor, and a statin after a myocardial infarction may be good cardiology, it is often poor geriatrics. At present, there is no evidence to support the necessity for immediate polypharmacy. It is good practice to consider all the existing prescribed medication at the time of initiating a new treatment. It may well be possible to stop some of the existing medication, even if only on a trial basis. This will ensure that the prescriber does not forget to check for the presence of possible drug interactions.

Wherever possible, prescribe drugs that are part of the hospital's approved formulary, but be prepared to prescribe other medications if there is a genuine reason that can be objectively justified.

The well-known adage 'start low and go slow' is very important. The dose of each drug should be increased cautiously, depending upon the balance of benefit on the one hand, and unwanted effects on the other. Remember too the need to 'go slow, but go', i.e. to titrate upwards until the desired effect is achieved, lest the result is to expose the patient to the side effects of a drug without maximizing the potential for benefit.

Factors affecting drug efficacy

If the patient's condition does not respond to treatment as anticipated, there may be a number of reasons. First, ensure that the patient is actually taking the medication as prescribed. Poor vision, cognitive impairment, and sometimes difficulty in hearing are reasons why treatment is not taken properly. Some people will also be reluctant to take medication that tastes unpleasant, or if the individual capsules or tablets are large and difficult to swallow. It is also important to think about the total number of medications a person is taking, as polypharmacy easily contributes to confusion about the drug regime, e.g. where some medication is taken once a day, others more frequently, and if the individual dose consists of more than one tablet and/or capsule.

Absorption of drugs is largely unchanged with ageing, and this is less likely to contribute to lack of efficacy. This is certainly true for those drugs that diffuse passively across the intestinal mucosa, but even though there maybe some reduction in the transport mechanisms for those medications that are actively transported from the bowel lumen, this is usually not sufficient to make a major impact.

Other factors that affect the way drugs are metabolized include the ratio of lean body mass to fat, which has implications for the distribution of some drugs, especially those that are water soluble, and the binding of drugs to plasma proteins, which is often reduced in older people.

Hepatic metabolism and renal excretion of drugs are important considerations. Those that are absorbed from the gastrointestinal tract pass through the liver, whose mass and blood supply decrease with increasing age. Thus, there may be increased levels of some drugs in the systemic circulation because of reduced first-pass metabolism. This can be important, e.g. with some opiates. However, the individual metabolic pathways within hepatocytes for most drugs are probably affected little, if at all, by the ageing process.

Changes in renal function with age have a greater impact on prescribing than hepatic changes. Most older people experience a decline in glomerular filtration rate, which can be exacerbated by medication and illness. Hence, it is necessary to be aware of the patient's renal function and which drugs this may affect. Good examples are digoxin, gentamicin, and furosemide, which are cleared mainly through the kidneys. As already mentioned, comorbidity can affect renal function. This includes common conditions such as dehydration and renal infection.

Other factors that are important in the way drugs behave in older people include changes in sensitivity at a tissue and cellular level. This can be either a decrease in sensitivity, e.g. of the β-adrenoceptor, which has implications for the bradycardia produced by β-blockers or increased sensitivity such as often seen in the central nervous system to many centrally acting drugs including antidepressants, antiparkinsonian drugs, hypnotics, analgesics, and antipsychotics.

Compliance

In general terms, the simpler the regime the better the compliance. This obviously relates to the number of drugs and the frequency of their administration. As already mentioned, cognitive ability, sight, and vision are also important.

Sometimes, patients do not take their medication because they or their families do not really understand its importance. A careful explanation, ensuring that they understand the reasons for taking their medicine and also how it works, will often help. Sometimes, a written summary is also of value.

Where compliance appears to be erratic, family and friends can sometimes help, especially if a monitored dosing system is used, e.g. Nomad, or a dosette box i.e. a pill container with individual segments for different days and different times of day.

Finally, pragmatic issues are sometimes of importance, e.g. the patient may omit to take a powerful diuretic before going out to a social occasion where they are aware they may be not be able to find a lavatory in time. This situation can easily be avoided with a little common sense.

Where it proves necessary to investigate compliance, it is possible to check the number of tablets left in the bottle or a dosette box or similar. Blood or urinary levels of some medications are also relatively easily assayed, and in some situations measures of clinical efficacy may help, e.g. if bradycardia is induced by a β-blocker.

Older people and driving

As people age, the ability to drive safely declines in many. This is recognized in most countries; e.g. motor car insurance companies require a medical assessment on an elderly person, and/or enquiries are made by the driving licence issuing authority when an application is made to renew a licence, especially at the age of 70 years or over. In the United Kingdom, the maximum licence period after the age of 70 is 3 years. Many factors can contribute to deterioration in driving ability, including visual impairment, slowing down of reactions, and the development of cognitive impairment. The older driver is also subject to the same regulations that govern driving with other medical conditions such as seizures. These are covered in Chapters 13.11.1, 16.13.8, 24.5.1, and 24.13.1.

Driving and dementia

Whenever a person is diagnosed with dementia, it is essential to enquire about their driving status. The clinician must make a decision about whether the patient should be allowed to continue driving while awaiting a formal assessment by the licensing authority.

The diagnosis of dementia usually has negative connotations in the mind of most clinicians, but the risk of a crash is acceptably low during the first 3 years after diagnosis. After this, the risk rises significantly, but any patient who has evidence of cognitive impairment in modalities particularly relevant to safe driving, e.g. disorientation, impaired judgement, and visuospatial problems, should not be allowed to drive without a formal road test. Cognitive assessment tests are an inadequate basis for this decision and can only indicate the need for more formal assessment.

Elderly drivers who are developing cognitive impairment often present a particularly difficult problem, especially as they so often deny any memory impairment. In general terms, it is best to try and persuade them, possibly with help from their family, to inform the relevant authority, which then seeks additional information from the primary care physician or the hospital specialist. In the United Kingdom, for instance, it is mandatory that drivers report to the driving licence authority (DVLA) any condition that they have developed that may, currently or in the future, impair their driving skills. If people with dementia refuse to take any action, their doctor may have to inform the authority themselves. The authority should be able to provide advice about how best this can be done without offending confidentiality. It is ultimately the licensing authority's responsibility to decide whether or not a person should continue driving. However, if there is any doubt, it is best for the doctor to advise the patient not to drive until the authority has made that decision.

Ascertaining risk

Ascertainment of risk can be difficult and relies heavily upon a third-party history and also the impression gained during the consultation, e.g. the presence of obvious intellectual impairment that will impair judgement, or lead to situations where it is difficult to make appropriate decisions e.g. at a road junction.

Some spouses are reluctant to provide reliable information because they themselves depend upon their dementing partner for transport, or because they are afraid of the consequences when it becomes apparent that they have imparted this information.

Useful pointers from the history include recent accidents or near accidents, the person's behaviour while they are driving, whether family members generally feel happy to travel with the demented person, and, in particular, whether they would entrust the driver to take young children out in the car with them.

The type of journey is also important. Short journeys in the daylight within the home neighbourhood, e.g. to church or a shopping centre, are less likely to cause problems than negotiating busy roads in the dark. Other important factors may be found upon neuropsychological and physical examination. As well as impairment of important cognitive measures, other comorbidities are relevant, including vision, hearing, or a tendency to suffer syncopal episodes.

Where there is doubt in the face of denial by the driver, or where the driver wishes to dispute the decision of a licensing authority, a formal assessment of driving ability by a professional driving assessor may help resolve the issue. In some countries, there are special locations where the testing is undertaken, rather than on the open road.

Usually the person concerned will agree, albeit often very reluctantly, to inform the licensing authority or allow their family to do this on their behalf. However, it can cause great anger, often directed against the doctor imparting the advice. A rational explanation of the issues does not always help, nor does the explanation to someone with early dementia that the authority may well allow them to continue driving, but will require monitoring of the situation, and will probably request annual feedback. In many cases, families are relieved when the decision is made, especially if it is clear that this is the result of the medical assessment and not their responsibility.

Other conditions

Elderly people are subject to the same regulations as everyone else for driving with other medical conditions, including cerebrovascular disease and seizures. These may differ in different countries. In the United Kingdom, there are very clear guidelines, e.g. about driving after a cerebrovascular event. After a transient ischaemic attack or a stroke from which the person has fully recovered, driving must stop for 1 month; for recurrent ischaemic attacks, the period is extended to 3 months after the most recent event. Where there is continuing neurological impairment after a month following a stroke, the DVLA must be informed and they will decide on the basis of the individual details.

In the case of people who have had a seizure following a cerebrovascular event, the ban may be less than the 12 months usually required following spontaneous seizures.

As with cognitive impairment and dementia, every patient who suffers a seizure has to inform the driving licence authority, and in the United Kingdom, this will result in a 1 year ban. If the seizure results from comorbidity such as neurosurgery or a cerebrovascular event, the licensing authority may reduce the length of the ban. When someone stops taking medication for seizures, they will probably have to stop driving for 6 months.

Delirium

The criteria for delirium, as stated in the American Psychological Association's *Diagnostic and Statistical Manual*, are listed in Table 29.1.1.

Table 29.1.1 DSM-IV-TR criteria for delirium

A	Disturbance of consciousness (i.e. reduced clarity of awareness of the environment) with reduced ability to focus, sustain, or shift attention
B	A change in cognition (such as memory deficit, disorientation, language disturbance) or the development of a perceptual disturbance that is not better accounted for by a pre-existing, established, or evolving dementia
C	The disturbance develops over a short period of time (usually hours to days) and tends to fluctuate during the course of the day
D	DSM-IV-TR distinguishes between delirium due to general medical condition, substances (intoxication or withdrawal), multiple aetiologies and others. Thus D criterion varies with aetiology

DSM-IV-TR criteria for Delirium. American Psychiatric Association. Diagnostic and Statistical Manual of Mental Disorders (DSM-IV-TR). 4th ed. Washington, DC: American Psychiatric Association; 2000.

Definition

Clinically, the confusion assessment method (CAM) provides a means of standardizing the screening for delirium. The CAM establishes how the four features of acute onset and fluctuating course, inattention, disorganized thinking, and altered level of consciousness can be operationalized and recorded. It has become the standard for most academic studies of delirium. Even so, under-recognition of delirium has been a persistent problem. Most reports suggest that fewer than one in three people with delirium are recognized as having acutely disturbed consciousness and cognition.

Causes of delirium

Delirium can occur in anyone if the insult is specific enough (e.g. a head injury that affects the brainstem reticular activating system) or if the problem is severe enough (e.g. massive sepsis). However, in very young children or in elderly people who are frail, the precipitating insult can seem trivial and only quite uncommonly is localized to a focal brain lesion. So why is delirium so common in frail elderly patients who are acutely ill? In general, elderly people are predisposed to develop delirium for two reasons. Many have specific predisposing illnesses, i.e. they have brain disorders (especially dementia, but also parkinsonism or stroke or other structural lesions) that make the development of delirium more likely. Even frail older people with apparently intact brains can develop delirium with apparently trivial insults. In these people, the predisposition to delirium appears to be nonspecific. In such circumstances, delirium appears to reflect the failure of a high-order function of a complex system. Such failure of a high-order function reflects redundancy exhaustion. It is a sign of whole system failure and carries a poor prognosis. A vast number of causes can precipitate delirium. Different authors handle this nonspecificity of the causes of delirium in various ways. Many produce interminable lists of all reported causes, which have little practical merit. In contrast, simply recalling, and specifically searching for, the common causes of illness in older adults yields a precipitating cause within the first patient encounter in about two-thirds of cases. This proportion rises gradually over the next 48 h. In about 10 to 15% of cases, it is not possible to understand why a patient became delirious. Usually, this is not a good prognostic sign. Causes of illness in older patients without surgical problems include medications, heart problems, infection, metabolic abnormalities, and quite commonly, some combinations of these.

Medications that cause delirium come in many guises, not just prescription medications. Alcohol and over-the-counter medications can cause delirium and merit specific inquiry. While the dose of a given medication may be stable, the patient may not be. Drugs that are mainly excreted by the kidney can cause toxicity even when the dose has been stable. Errors in administering medications can cause toxicity in patients who report no changes in medications. Many medications have only small anticholinergic effects, but these effects can be cumulative.

Management of delirium

There is no specific treatment for delirium and despite its presumed cause or exacerbation by anticholinergic medications, cholinesterase inhibition has generally been a disappointing strategy. Instead, management focuses on prevention and on timely recognition, so that the precipitating cause can be identified and mitigated. An excellent set of guidelines for delirium management, which includes a considerable degree of documentation of the relevant evidence, is available online through the Canadian Coalition for Seniors Mental health (http://www.ccsmh.ca/en/natlGuidelines/delirium.cfm). Similarly, the British Geriatrics Society delirium guidelines can be accessed at http://www.bgs.org.uk/publications/clinicalguidelines.

The prevention of delirium requires a multifactorial approach. Judicious use of medications; clear, courteous and compassionate communication; attention to the environment in which patients find themselves (so that sleep deprivation and noise are minimized, for example); use of familiar objects; provision of hearing aids and glasses as needed; orientation by staff and visitors; and, especially when a patient is agitated, the presence of familiar reassuring people all have roles to play. In some jurisdictions agitated patients, or those at risk of running away, are assigned 'sitters', i.e. people who can provide individual supervision. Where this results in a caring interaction and the avoidance of sedating medications, it is especially welcome. Where, by dint of hospital regulations or contracts, the sitters are obliged simply to sit and watch the patient, alerting the nurses when the patient misbehaves, but not interacting with the patient in any meaningful way, the result appears to worsen delirium and specifically paranoia. Such expensive practices, which find no basis in evidence, should be avoided, whether 'nonpharmacological' or not.

Different authorities give different advice on which medications to use to manage a person who has delirium with psychomotor agitation. This is because, despite the problem being common and having a poor outlook (the risk of death, institutionalization, prolonged hospital stay, and disability are each increased in patients with delirium), delirium generally has been understudied. Despite the variability in specifics, all groups recommend the use of low doses of medications, combined with a supportive environment. Generally, some combination of a short-acting anxiolytic medication (usually lorazepam or a similar benzodiazepine) with or without a neuroleptic (usually haloperidol, if one is to be used at all) is proposed.

Common clinical challenges in patients with delirium

Even experienced clinicians can sometimes find the management of a patient with delirium to be challenging. Three particular hurdles are commonly encountered in diagnosis and another in management; these are outlined in the following paragraphs. The first is that the fluctuating nature of delirium can mean that it is missed on a single patient encounter if the patient is seen during a lucid period. The remedy for this is twofold. First, one should have a high index of suspicion; e.g. recalling that frailty, dementia, parkinsonism, and stroke are predisposing factors, and that their presence should alert an examining clinician to the possibility of delirium. Having a high index of suspicion also means being alert to when you, as the examiner, begin to fill in both sides of the conversation. It is better to press and to make any vagueness of meaning explicit than to assume that you know what the patient means. This is an acquired clinical skill; in our hurry, or even in our instinct to be polite, we often assume meaning rather than confront the patient about a statement that is vague or that does not entirely make sense. Having raised the suspicion of delirium, the next step is to test cognition, especially attention and concentration.

Axis I of Reisberg's Brief Cognitive Rating Scale provides an excellent attention and concentration battery. By this schema, a hierarchy can be established, with normal attention and concentration being the ability to subtract serial 7s from 100. At the next level of impairment comes serial 4s from 40, then 2s from 20, and then 10 to 1. At the lowest level of function, patients have difficulty even in counting from 1 to 10. Clinically, it is common to see patients deteriorate in performance on these tests as their delirium worsens, and improve as it resolves. The various subtests operate as a Guttman scale, so that people who can do serial 7s from 100 can do each of the items that is less difficult, and someone who, for example, can only correctly perform serial 2s from 20 will not be able to do the more difficult tasks. In consequence, with experience, it is possible to quickly narrow down which subtest a patient is likely to have difficulty with, and then to check that by testing the next lowest item. In this way, testing can be done quite rapidly—commonly in 60 to 90 s.

A second challenge in diagnosis is to distinguish patients with delirium from those with dementia. While for most patients this is not complicated, some dementias can affect consciousness. In practice, patients who have dementia with Lewy bodies and some with nondominant parietal lobe infarction can have presentations that look very much like delirium. This is particularly the case if there is no knowledgeable informant who can describe the premorbid cognitive and functional status. In such patients, time is often the best test.

Another pragmatic challenge to diagnosis occurs in the patient who is dying. Many patients experience a preterminal cognitive decline, or even restlessness prior to death. Knowing when there is a reversible cause can be tricky. In general, it is best to evaluate as noninvasively as possible and to be guided by the specificity of symptoms. Even so, this can be a difficult clinical challenge.

Sometimes, and especially in nursing homes, a patient can become delirious, the only apparent signs pointing to a urinary tract infection. The urine is often described as dark and foul-smelling, and although bacteriuria is present, there is no other sign of infection, either on the urine dipstick or clinically. (Note that while dipstick leucocytes do not necessarily indicate infection, their absence rules it out.) In such circumstances, it can be difficult to know whether the bacteriuria is implicated and the absence of other signs is to be considered as an 'atypical disease presentation'. However, a randomized controlled trial has established that, in long-term care institutions, antimicrobial prescriptions for suspected urinary tract infection can be reduced without adversely affecting hospital referral or mortality, by requiring some localizing features of infection before prescribing for the presumed cause of delirium.

There appears to be considerable variation in how delirium is investigated. In particular, some consider routine neuroimaging to be essential, while others favour its use only for specific indications (e.g. in the presence of focal or lateralizing signs, or in patients on anticoagulants, or who have fallen). Although there is some potential for specialized neuroimaging to elucidate the pathophysiology of delirium, its routine use cannot be recommended at present.

Conclusions

The care of elderly people, especially those who are frail, offers rewarding personal and professional opportunities for physicians who like complexity, who can handle uncertainty, who are interested in an approach to the whole patient, and who enjoy (or are at least skilled at) dealing with families. Good geriatric medicine is practised by balancing an understanding of the individual ailments faced by an older person with a sense of their overall needs. Geriatricians embrace the complexity of their patients through an approach rooted in comprehensive geriatric assessment, and by the evaluation of high-order, integrative activities such as cognition, function, mobility and balance, and drug handling. Societies' compelling need for geriatric medicine, and the considerable opportunities to make care better through a better understanding of what elderly people need, and what works best for them, will make this an exciting area of human endeavour for the foreseeable future.

Further reading

Bhat R, Rockwood K (2007). Delirium as a disorder of consciousness. *J Neurol Neurosurg Psychiatry*, **78**, 1167–70.

Breen DA, et al. (2007). Driving and dementia. *BMJ*, **334**, 1365–9.

Harari D, et al. (2007). Proactive Care of Older People Undergoing Surgery ('POPS'): Designing, embedding, evaluating and funding a comprehensive geriatric assessment service for older elective surgical patients. Reports on a proactive evidence based comprehensive geriatric assessment service for at-risk older elective surgical patients based upon the MRC framework for complex interventions. *Age Ageing*, **36**, 190–6.

Loeb M, et al. (2005). Effect of a multifaceted intervention on number of antimicrobial prescriptions for suspected urinary tract infections in residents of nursing homes: cluster randomised controlled trial. *BMJ*, **331**, 669.

Macmillan AK, et al. (2004). The prevalence of fecal incontinence in community-dwelling adults: a systematic review of the literature. *Dis Colon Rectum*, **47**, 1341–9.

Parker MJ, Gillespie WJ, Gillespie LD (2005). Hip protectors for preventing hip fractures in older people. *Cochrane Database Syst Rev*, **3**, CD001255.

Reisberg B, Ferris SH (1988). Brief Cognitive Rating Scale (BCRS). *Psychopharmacol Bull*, **24**, 629–36.

Rockwood K, Mitnitski A (2007). Frailty in relation to the accumulation of deficits. *J Gerontol A Biol Sci Med Sci*, **62**, 722–7.

Spinewine A, et al. (2007). Appropriate prescribing in elderly people: how well can it be measured and optimised? *Lancet*, **370**, 173–184.

Young J, Inouye SK (2007). Delirium in older people. *BMJ*, **334**, 842–6.

Websites

British Geriatrics Society (2006). *Guidelines for the prevention, diagnosis and management of delirium in older people in hospital.* http://www.bgs.org.uk/publications/clinicalguidelines

British Geriatrics Society (2007). *Behind closed doors: delivering dignity in toilet access and use*. http://www.bgs.org.uk/campaigns/dignitypress.htm

Canadian Coalition for Seniors Mental Health. *Assessment and treatment of delirium*. http://www.ccsmh.ca/en/natlGuidelines/delirium.cfm

Department of Health (UK) (2001a). *National Service Framework for older people*. http://www.dh.gov.uk/en/Publicationsandstatistics/Publications/PublicationsPolicyAndGuidance/DH_4003066 [A 10-year programme setting new national standards and service models of care across health and social services for all older people. It comprises eight standards including specific standards for general hospital care, stroke, and falls among others.]

Department of Health (UK) (2001b). *Medicines and older people*. http://www.dh.gov.uk/en/publicationsandstatistics/publications/publicationspolicyandguidance/DH_4008020 [Describes how the use of medicines for and by older people might be improved, and in particular relates to the National Service Framework for older people.]

Driver and Vehicle Licensing Agency (UK). *Rules on licensing and updating licences*. http://www.direct.gov.uk/en/motoring/index.htm

National Institute for Health and Clinical Excellence (2003). *The use of pressure-relieving devices (beds, mattresses and overlays) for the prevention of pressure ulcers in primary and secondary care*. NICE, London. [An extensive document which provides an evidence-based guideline for the use of pressure-relieving devices, particularly targeted at the NHS in England and Wales.] http://guidance.nice.org.uk/CG7/guidance/pdf/english

National Institute for Health and Clinical Excellence (2004). *Clinical Practice Guideline for the Assessment and Prevention of Falls in Older People*. NICE, London http://guidance.nice.org.uk/CG21/guidance/pdf/english [Presents a distillation of best guidance in relation to treatment and management of falls.]

National Institute for Health and Clinical Excellence (2006). *Urinary incontinence: the management of urinary incontinence in women*. NICE, London http://guidance.nice.org.uk/CG40/guidance/pdf/english [A comprehensive guide to the management of urinary incontinence in women, as its name suggests. Some of the principles inherent in the guideline are also applicable to incontinence in men. It also lists future research areas.]

National Institute for Health and Clinical Excellence (2007). *Faecal incontinence: the management of faecal incontinence in adults*. NICE, London. http://www.nice.org.uk/49

Mental disorders of old age

Robin Jacoby

Essentials

Mental disorders of old age are important because: (1) demographic trends in all countries show a marked increase in the number of older people, especially the very old; (2) this age group is particularly prone to debilitating mental illness—about 20% of people over 80 have dementia, and over 10% of people over 65 have pervasive depressive symptoms; (3) presentations of mental illness in older people may differ from those at younger ages and go unrecognized—assessment requires a reliable informant, examination of the mental state, and physical examination; (4) the pattern of morbidity differs, with older people suffering more from organic disorder—delirium and dementia; (5) mental and physical illness often occur together, the one sometimes masking the other.

Introduction

Elderly patients hospitalized in nonpsychiatric beds show high rates of mental disorder of various sorts. Community rates are also high. For instance, the prevalence of dementia is about 7% in people over 65 but approaches 20% in those over 80. For major depressive illness defined by the tenth edition of the World Health Organization's *International Classification of Diseases* (ICD-10) or the fourth edition of the American Psychiatric Association's *Diagnostic and Statistical Manual of Mental Disorders* (DSM-IV), the prevalence is not more than 3%, but for pervasive depressive symptoms, which most psychiatrists would consider in need of treatment, it is around 12%. There are no valid data for the prevalence of very late onset schizophrenia-like psychosis. The closure of large mental institutions in most developed countries has resulted in a greatly increased number of elderly patients in the community suffering from chronic schizophrenia that began much earlier in their lives.

Assessment

Factors to be considered are (1) where the patient is examined and (2) the patient's ability to provide information. The three pillars of assessment are (1) a reliable informant, (2) the mental state, and (3) the physical examination.

Assessing the patient at home gives invaluable clues about premorbid adjustment, activities of daily living, and even causes of an abnormal mental state, e.g. empty whisky bottles or multiple medication containers. Patients in general hospital wards should be assessed in a side room if possible. Many are unable to give a history. It is therefore essential to find reliable informants, even if this means disturbing neighbours or making long-distance telephone calls.

Examination of the mental state of an elderly person is essentially the same as for any adult, but with differences of emphasis. More attention is paid to the level of consciousness, particularly subtle fluctuations throughout 24 h. Brief cognitive assessment should be conducted in all cases, but for patients with suspected dementia a full cognitive examination is undertaken, frequently in several brief sessions because patients become easily fatigued and unable to cooperate. Tired, inattentive, or depressed patients may fail a test that they might otherwise have been able to perform satisfactorily. Systematic evaluation of all higher cerebral functions, such as memory, praxis and language, is essential because they are valuable indicators of organic cerebral impairment. On general hospital wards or home visits, the routine administration of standardized questionnaires is of value as an alerting mechanism but not a substitute for full evaluation. The Mini-Mental State Examination (MMSE) is widely used because it assesses a range of higher cerebral functions, not just memory and orientation. The respective short versions of the Geriatric Depression Scale (GDS) and the Informant Questionnaire on Cognitive Decline in the Elderly (IQCODE) also increase diagnostic capture.

Because the capacity to live independently may be a crucial determinant of social outcome, the patient's ability to perform activities of daily living (ADL)—dressing, feeding, elimination, etc.—must be assessed. The Bristol Activities of Daily Living Scale (BADLS) and the Barthel Scale are useful standardized instruments.

Delirium

The clinical features of delirium are described in Chapters 24.4.2 and 29.1. Older people are particularly susceptible to it because they more commonly suffer from the physical disorders that cause delirium: hypoxia, infections, toxicity (especially from drugs), and metabolic and central nervous system disorders. In addition, many have a decreased cerebral reserve because of incipient or overt dementia.

An underlying physical cause for delirium must be sought assiduously, as it is generally more important to treat this than the mental symptoms. Physical illnesses causing delirium can be relatively minor, e.g. a urinary tract infection, especially in patients with dementia. Because elderly people generally suffer high physical morbidity, they tend to receive more prescribed medication. Single or multiple drugs, as well as drug-withdrawal effects, are potent causes of delirium. Management is essentially that of the underlying cause and psychotropic drugs should be avoided whenever possible. However, short-term treatment of mental symptoms and behavioural disturbance with a small dose of a neuroleptic drug is sometimes unavoidable to allow medical treatment to proceed unhindered.

Dementia

The importance of dementia lies not only in the suffering it causes to patients but also in the demands it makes upon family caregivers and the medical and social services. The clinical features of the dementia syndrome are described in Chapter 24.4.2 and Chapter 29.1. Global impairment is required for diagnosis: memory loss alone, of which elderly people invariably complain, is not a sufficient criterion. Accurate diagnosis is required because:

♦ treatable or arrestable causes may be discovered

♦ management can be planned and implemented

♦ caregivers are helped by a clearer understanding of the process affecting the patient and its likely course

♦ knowledge of the underlying conditions is accrued and advanced

In some countries, patients are initially referred to memory clinics to decide whether central cholinesterase inhibitors (donepezil, rivastigmine, or galantamine) should be prescribed. Rational management requires an appreciation of the practical implications of cognitive impairment, e.g. ensuring nutrition in patients with dyspraxic inability to feed themselves. However, the noncognitive, behavioural, and psychiatric disturbances in dementia are the manifestations that cause most problems to caregivers and often require management by specialist services. Patients should be maintained at home for as long as possible, both for humane reasons and because they will have lost the capacity to adapt easily to a new environment. Intercurrent illness should be treated along with other medical problems, such as incontinence, which is often due to urinary tract infections and faecal impaction, rather than the underlying disease processes of dementia. Attention must be given to principal caregivers, most frequently spouses or adult daughters but sometimes unrelated neighbours, who show high levels of psychiatric morbidity themselves due to their burden of care.

Affective illness

Depression

Depressive illness in elderly people differs only in emphasis from that in earlier life, varying from mild dysthymia to major psychosis with high risk of suicide, especially in the oldest men. Psychosocial factors are as important but genetic loading is usually lower in patients with late-onset depression. Cerebral organic change is more common in late-onset cases.

Psychomotor retardation is frequent, as in younger patients, but anxiety and agitation are also characteristic. Delusions of guilt and unworthiness are typical, but hypochondriacal or nihilistic beliefs also often occur. Histrionic or other bizarre behaviour, which is out of premorbid character, is also seen. Some patients with severe depression perform badly on cognitive tests, so called 'depressive pseudodementia', which may lead to a wrong diagnosis of organic dementia. Hypochondriacal delusions together with anorexic weight loss can be mistaken for physical illness, such as cancer. Some patients may even deny low mood (masked depression), but the presence of other typical affective manifestations and a favourable response to antidepressant treatment reveal the correct diagnosis. The clinician should not avoid treating depression in patients, such as those with severe physical illnesses, simply because they appear to have a valid reason to be unhappy.

Elderly people are vulnerable to the unwanted effects of psychotropic drugs but respond well to standard antidepressants, although those with cerebral organic change are more resistant to treatment. Selective serotonin reuptake inhibitors (SSRIs) are usually preferred as first choice drugs because of safety and fewer side effects. Venlafaxine is effective but used more in secondary care because of potential toxicity. Mirtazepine is useful for agitation, being more sedative and promoting weight gain. Elderly patients also respond well to electroconvulsive therapy (ECT), regarded by many as the treatment of choice for deluded and/or suicidal patients. Extreme age, dementia, and physical infirmity are not contraindications to ECT. After recovery from an episode of major depression antidepressant treatment should be continued for at least 2 years, and probably indefinitely.

Bipolar disorder

Manic illness is usually less florid than in younger patients. Mixed manic and depressive pictures are seen. Cerebral organic disease is found in a high proportion of cases. Diagnosis is sometimes difficult to make because the presentation may be a rather nonspecific psychosis. The clinician should therefore enquire about a previous history of affective illness. Mania precipitated by physical illness or drug treatment in patients with no previous history of affective disorder may be mistaken for delirium or even bad behaviour. Patients respond well to treatment with neuroleptics and lithium carbonate in the acute phase. Lithium is also widely used to prevent relapse. Here, regular monitoring of renal and thyroid function is essential, and the serum lithium level should generally be maintained at relatively low levels, that is, between 0.2 and 0.6 mmol/litre. Other mood stabilizers, such as carbamazepine, valproate, and lamotrigine are also used.

Paranoid disorders

Ideas of persecution are common in dementia and affective disorder. In dementia, they tend to be transient, variable, and unsystematized. In affective disorder, they are usually mood-congruent, e.g. persecution deserved because of guilt. Persecutory ideas are also seen in paranoid personalities and acute paranoid reactions, but very-late-onset schizophrenia-like psychosis (the term used when onset is after age 60) is the main paranoid syndrome of old age. The following aetiological factors have been consistently reported:

- a high female-to-male ratio (up to 7:1)
- a family history of schizophrenia intermediate between the general population and younger schizophrenic patients
- social isolation and poor premorbid interpersonal relationships
- low marriage and fecundity rates compared with age-matched peers
- long-standing deafness

The patient usually presents with a few simple delusions and associated auditory hallucinations, e.g. hearing the neighbours through the wall plotting against her, or impugning her sexual virtue. Medication with atypical antipsychotic drugs, such as risperidone, olanzapine or quetiapine, to minimize the risk of extrapyramidal side effects, is the treatment of choice. However, neuroleptics rarely extinguish delusional beliefs: they become 'encapsulated', meaning set aside or compartmentalized and not intruding into so many aspects of mental and daily life as happens during the acute phase of illness. Adherence to treatment is often poor but can be improved with the help of a community psychiatric nurse, especially if the patient can be persuaded to accept a depot neuroleptic.

Neurotic, personality, and other disorders

It is essential to differentiate lifelong neurosis from neurotic symptoms of first onset in old age because the latter, predominantly anxiety and phobia, are most likely to indicate an underlying depressive illness. Those with lifelong neurosis have frequently adapted to their disability in spite of continued suffering. Mild and moderate personality deviations are common but severe disorders are occasionally encountered, such as the senile squalor (Diogenes) syndrome, which can require compulsory removal from home under mental or public health legislation. Illicit drug-taking is rare among the present generation of older people but abuse of prescribed drugs, notably benzodiazepines, is common. Alcohol abuse is increasingly recognized as a cause of mental and social disability in elderly people.

Abuse of older people

It is sad and shocking that older people are often subject to verbal, physical, financial, or even sexual abuse. Those suffering from dementia or extreme physical frailty are particularly vulnerable because they cannot defend themselves. Physicians and nurses need to have a high index of suspicion where bruising is not readily explained. The signing of wills or codicils by patients with terminal illness should also be treated with caution, since relatives might be coercing those who lack the mental capacity. If asked to do so, doctors should not witness wills unless they themselves know the legal tests for assessing capacity and are competent to do so.

Further reading

Burns A, Lawlor B, Craig S (eds.) (1999). *Assessment scales in old age psychiatry*. Martin Dunitz, London.
Jacoby R, Oppenheimer C, Dening T, Thomas A (eds.) (2008). *The Oxford textbook of old age psychiatry* (*Psychiatry in the elderly*, 4th edition). Oxford University Press, Oxford.

SECTION 30

Pain

Dealing with pain

Henry McQuay

Essentials

Pain is complex—it is too simple to view pain transmission as a hard-wired, line-labelled system, because that cannot explain complexities such as phantom limb pain. The crucial mechanistic distinction for clinical practice is between normal (nociceptive) and nerve damage (neuropathic) pain.

Types of analgesics—conventional analgesics, from paracetamol through to morphine, work well in nociceptive pain and less well in neuropathic pain. Unconventional analgesics, antidepressants, and antiepileptic drugs work well in neuropathic and less well in nociceptive pain.

Treating pain—most pains are dynamic rather than static, hence patients need to be able to deal with mild through to severe pain. In both nociceptive and neuropathic pain a three-stage algorithm provides a framework for both patient and prescriber. For nociceptive

pain: (1) mild pain—paracetamol (acetaminophen); (2) moderate pain—add (not substitute) weak opioid or non-steroidal anti-inflammatory drug; (3) severe pain—add (not substitute) strong opioid. For neuropathic pain: (1) mild pain—antidepressant; (2) moderate pain—add (not substitute) antiepileptic, e.g. gabapentin, pregabalin; (3) severe pain—add (not substitute) opioid.

Difficult pain—patients with complex pains, or with pain and complex needs, may need multidisciplinary approaches to untangle their pain, disability, and distress: tackling the elements singly is unlikely to succeed. There is no convincing evidence of the analgesic effectiveness of complementary approaches, but it is important to acknowledge that these interventions may make people feel better, although they rarely obviate the need for effective analgesia.

Pain sensation and transmission

The easiest way to think of pain in the nervous system is the idea of pain receptors and nerve cables dedicated to the transmission of pain signals; a hard-wired, line-labelled system. For most acute pain and chronic nociceptive pain, this simple idea works well. 'Nociceptive' here means pain caused by trauma as opposed to neuropathic pain that arises from nerve damage. The concept of specific cables whose transmission can be blocked is reinforced by everyday observations, e.g. the ability to perform surgery painlessly by using a local anaesthetic block. But the inadequacy of this simple explanation is exposed in chronic pain, particularly associated with nervous system damage. The return of pain after an initially successful cordotomy and the phenomenon of phantom limb pain are two examples. In a hard-wired, line-labelled system, the pain should not recur after the cordotomy and amputees should not feel pain in the absent foot or hand because the receptors and the cables are no longer there. The ability of the nervous system to rewire, known as plasticity, is recognized in the return of pain after destructive procedures, and the concept of 'pain memory' in the spinal cord and brain has to be invoked to explain phantom pain. Such phenomena mean that the simple view of a hard-wired, line-labelled system does not explain all kinds of pain.

Many treatments or interventions are used to treat both acute and chronic pain. Chronic pain, not surprisingly, is more convoluted, because its origins may be more complicated and because the nervous system can behave strangely if damaged or bombarded continuously by pain messages. The concept of plasticity has led to the adoption of some interventions and the rejection of others. Long-term destructive measures, such as cutting the nerves thought to carry a particular pain message, are going out of fashion. The reasoning is that the nervous system will 'rewire', the pain will re-emerge, and may well be more difficult to manage than it was in the first place. Better drug control of difficult pains has also reduced the necessity for destructive procedures.

Pain signals can be amplified or dampened by endogenous influences such as mood or endorphins, or exogenous factors such as drugs given or the circumstances of the injury. The classic damping-down scenario is the injured soldier who continues to get himself out of battle, despite a shattered leg. Conversely, a stubbed toe when you are tired and miserable is immeasurably more painful than the same injury on a cheerful morning. In chronic pain, it is sometimes very hard to disentangle depression from pain. Pain makes depression worse and depression makes pain worse. This pattern is all too familiar to those who manage pain. The thinking clinician needs to deal with both the pain and the depression. In chronic pain, distress and disability may also amplify the pain, and good pain relief will not improve disability. Expectations need to be realistic.

Pain is necessarily subjective. It is what one human being reports to another. There may be few objective signs to judge the severity of reported pain, and many patients have no visibly obvious handicap. The most important principle is that the patient and the doctor are best served if the doctor believes the patient's report. Their problems may be ill understood, even disbelieved, at work and at home. Chronic pain changes people, affecting their personal and working lives, and ultimately their personalities. Often, such changes are reversible with successful treatment. Much time and energy is wasted on procedures designed to 'catch the patient out'. Labelling patients as malingerers or the pain as psychogenic may be easier than admitting that there is no successful treatment.

Pain mechanisms and pain syndromes

Sacrificing precision for the sake of clarity, we can distinguish by mechanism two broad types of pain (Table 30.1.1). The distinction here is between normal or nociceptive pain and nerve damage or neuropathic pain. The importance of the distinction is that successful drug treatment of these two types requires different classes of drugs.

Conventional analgesics, from aspirin through to morphine, work well in nociceptive pain but not so well in neuropathic pain. Unconventional analgesics, antidepressants, or antiepileptics work well in neuropathic pain and not so well in nociceptive pain.

The incidences of each of the classic neuropathic pain conditions, postherpetic neuralgia, painful diabetic neuropathy, and trigeminal neuralgia (Table 30.1.1) is about 30 per 100 000 person-years observation. Neuropathic pain resulting from surgery and neuropathic pain as a consequence of back problems are very much commoner.

Further mechanistic subdivisions are possible, e.g. 'inflammatory pain' or 'visceral pain' are categories often used by scientists working on pain mechanisms, but pragmatically the same remedies work in these groupings as work in nociceptive pain generally, and the neuropathic remedies do not. Most difficult are the pain syndromes which are not clearly either nociceptive or neuropathic, but which undoubtedly impair function. Examples in this dysfunctional grouping include migraine, fibromyalgia, and irritable bowel syndrome. Migraine can be helped by the conventional analgesics used in nociceptive pain and it may respond to the triptans, which do not work in nociceptive pain, and can be prevented by antiepileptic drug prophylaxis. This crossover is apparent too in the effective treatment of fibromyalgia and irritable bowel syndrome with the unconventional analgesic classes of drugs.

Implicit in this scheme is the important distinction between acute, chronic, and 'acute on chronic' timing. Most pains wax and wane, and treatment needs to be sufficiently flexible to deal with both moderate and severe fluctuations. Most patients need a regime to deal with their baseline pain and a regime to deal with a flare of pain.

Pain histories

Asking whether sensation is normal in the painful area and whether the pain is shooting or stabbing in character may help to identify the pains variously known as dysaesthetic, deafferentational, or neuropathic. The distinction is important, because response to conventional analgesics is unlikely. These pains often have little pattern, but are less troublesome when the patient is distracted. Pain may be spontaneous or evoked in response to a normally nonpainful stimulus (allodynia) or it may be exaggerated in response to a marginally painful stimulus.

It is important to enquire specifically about the efficacy of each particular class of drug. This information prevents the inept prescription of drugs which have failed previously, and may give important clues to the kind of pain and its sensitivity to different classes of drugs.

It is also important to know the dose size, frequency, duration of prescription, and the side-effect problems for each drug that has

Table 30.1.1 Pain syndromes and mechanisms

| | 1. Nociceptive | 2. Neuropathic | | 3. Visceral | Combined |
		a. Peripheral	b. Central		
Acute	Postoperative Burns 'Sprains and strains'			'Stone' pain ulcer	
Intermittent/ Incidental	Headache Migraine Osteoarthritis	Trigeminal		Dysmenorrhea Endometriosis Pelvic IBS Dyspepsia	Cancer (1, 2, 3)
Chronic	Rheumatoid arthritis	PHN	Spinal cord injury	Pelvic	Cancer (1, 2, 3)
	Osteoarthritis	Diabetic mono/poly neuropathy	Central post stroke		LBP with radiculopathy (1, 2a)
	FM Myofascial (e.g. neck–shoulder) Low back pain	Nerve trauma	Multiple sclerosis Parkinson's disease		Whiplash (1, 2a)

FM, Fibromyalgia; IBS, irritable bowel syndrome; LBP, low back pain; PHN, postherpetic neuralgia.

been prescribed. Dose–response relationships apply with analgesics, and therapeutic failure should not be presumed if the dosage was inadequate. A good example is the use of carbamazepine in trigeminal neuralgia. The question we ask ourselves is, 'Has this patient had an adequate trial of this drug?', meaning has the dose been increased to the point of unmanageable or intolerable adverse effects without or precluding benefit. Is the patient taking drugs other than analgesics? Anticoagulation, for instance, is not only a virtually absolute contraindication to pain management by injection procedures, but also contraindicates most anti-inflammatory drugs.

It is important to be sure whether nerve blocks used previously were technically effective (e.g. did the patient have any numbness after an epidural which included local anaesthetic?), before dismissing them as being useless for this patient. Other measures, such as transcutaneous nerve stimulation (TENS), may not have been used correctly, and may succeed if the patient receives proper instruction in their use.

Recording pain

In cases of chronic pain, when patients record pain over long periods, we tend to use diaries with word categories, and ask about both pain intensity (none, mild, moderate, or severe) and pain relief (none, slight, moderate, good, or complete). Another useful scale is the patient's 'global report'. Using the same categories as the pain relief scale, this is a composite view encompassing both pain itself and any adverse effects of treatment. The clinician's 'global view' is notoriously unreliable and should not be used.

Most important and simplest is the idea of including a binary scale because of its clinical relevance. The question is phrased in various forms, around the idea: 'Is your pain at least 50% relieved?', to which the patient answers yes or no.

The argument for using pain charts as part of normal practice is to improve the quality of care. It is the fact of a chart rather than its form that is the more important. These should be completed, together with vital signs, and can then be used for both clinical care and for audit.

Some index of function is necessary as a baseline so that improvement or deterioration may be monitored. Useful clinical outcome measures are notoriously difficult, but simple pain charts and indices of activity can work well, using the patient's definition of impaired activity such as walking or gardening.

Treating pain

Drugs are the mainstay of treating both normal (nociceptive) and neuropathic pain. The menu of remedies also includes stimulation devices, from trans-cutaneous through to implanted stimulators, cognitive–behavioural therapy (pain programmes), complementary techniques, and invasive methods from injection through to surgery designed to block transmission of the pain message (Fig. 30.1.1).

Treating normal (nociceptive) pain

The basic algorithm for treating nociceptive pain, acute, chronic, or acute on chronic, is shown in Fig. 30.1.2, derived from the pain 'ladder' which is widely used in palliative care (see Section 31). This ladder was formulated originally in the 1980s under the aegis of the World Health Organization (WHO). In its raw form, it captured the treatment care pathway for pain by representing increasing strengths of analgesia as further steps or rungs up the ladder. At the

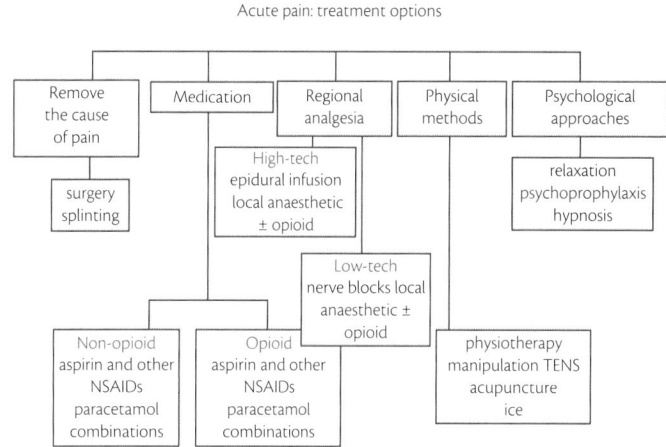

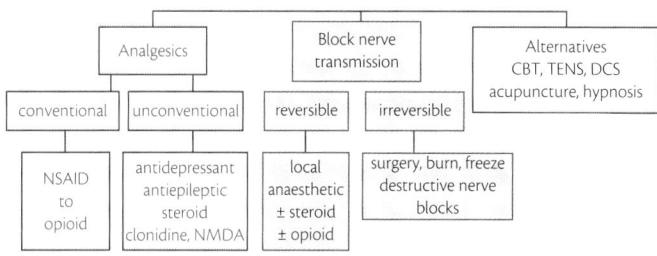

Fig. 30.1.1 Treatment options for acute and chronic pain.

bottom rung, or step 1, is a nonopioid analgesic, usually paracetamol (acetaminophen); at step 2, a nonsteroidal anti-inflammatory drug (NSAID) or a combination of minor opioid with paracetamol; and, at step 3, addition of a strong opioid, morphine by mouth or injection. This simple pathway has had enormous global impact in palliative care, even though the drugs that are available vary in different countries.

This algorithm is equally applicable and useful outside palliative care, e.g. in primary care and in postoperative pain. In acute pain, perioperative or traumatic, one is working right to left (in terms of Fig. 30.1.2) as pain decreases. In chronic pain, the patient

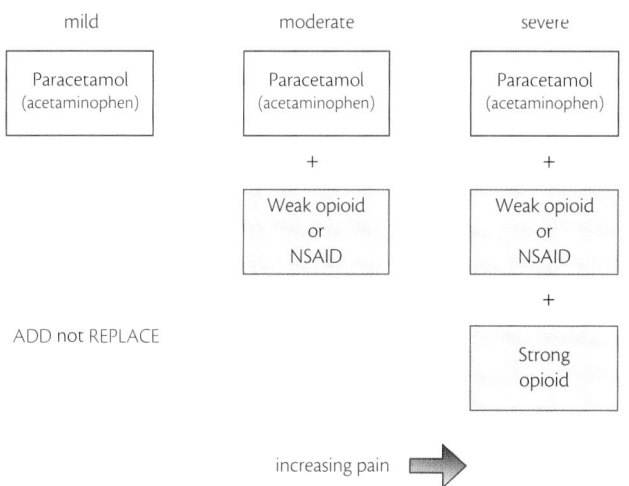

Fig. 30.1.2 Algorithm for analgesics in nociceptive pain.

needs to use the three strengths of analgesic as the pain increases or decreases, the 'three pot' system. The basic algorithm is thus the same across the different pain intensities, making teaching and implementation more effective, but the choice of particular drugs will vary locally with availability.

The visual presentation of the ladder differs from the original WHO palliative care ladder in two main ways. The first is that the analogy is with building blocks rather than with rungs on a ladder. What we wanted to convey visually was the principle of 'add rather than replace', by which we meant that if the pain becomes more severe you add a stronger analgesic to your other analgesics, adding rather than replacing. We believe that 'add rather than replace' is easier to understand using the building block analogy compared to rungs on a ladder, because one rarely stands simultaneously on multiple rungs on a ladder.

The second main difference is the inversion of the diagram. The basic building block (step 1) is at the top of the picture. This is different from the original WHO palliative care ladder, where the step 1 drug was at the bottom, to emphasize the 'add not replace' concept, because putting the step 1 drugs at the bottom of the algorithm makes it more likely that they will be overlooked and omitted in the management of moderate or severe pain.

Fleshing out the detail of the drugs and the route of administration for each of the drug choices for each section of the algorithm in each of the pain intensities, keeping as much in common as possible, will vary with available drug choice and clinical situation. Both choice of particular drug and dose might differ; e.g. lower starting doses might be used in older people. Some of the detail will rightly be determined by local custom and practice, and where the detail on the pathway is at variance with local belief, even if in just one tiny detail, then the whole pathway loses credibility. A simple example for trauma pain is the issue of NSAIDs and bone healing. When staff have been taught or instructed not to use NSAIDs because they are said to impair bone healing, including NSAIDs on the pathway will not work. Although many may doubt that NSAIDs have significant clinical impact on bone healing, the detailed algorithm will need to be subject to this local variation to give it the local ownership that it needs if it is to be part of everyday clinical practice.

The step 2 drugs in the algorithm are the NSAIDs and the minor opioids, such as codeine. NSAIDs are powerful analgesics. Standard oral NSAID doses provide analgesia equivalent to that from intramuscular morphine 10 mg. However, the adverse effects of NSAIDs at therapeutic doses limit their utility, particularly for extended use in chronic pain. In those for whom NSAIDs are contraindicated and paracetamol (acetaminophen) is not sufficient, a minor opioid should be added to the paracetamol to improve analgesia.

The choice of strong opioid will vary according to local availability, custom, and practice. Morphine is the gold standard, orally in chronic pain or by injection in acute pain, but other formulations or alternative opioids are used. When swallowing or gastrointestinal function is impaired, for instance, routes other than oral, such as injected, sublingual, topical, nasal or inhaled may be necessary. In perioperative care, patients self-administer strong opioid via patient-controlled analgesia systems. Pressing the button delivers an injected dose.

In chronic pain, modified-release oral formulations are convenient for patients, allowing the greater part of the daily opioid requirement to be taken just twice a day, using a normal-release formulation to deal with flares of pain. Faster-acting nasal and inhaled formulations to give improved control of these flares, 'breakthrough' pain, are emerging.

These drug regimes may fail to control pain. It is estimated that in cancer pain 5 to 10% of patients need a different approach. Perhaps the most important change in the last 30 years is the realization that destructive invasive techniques rarely produce long-term benefit because the system eventually rewires, and the pain may be more difficult to manage than before. Reversible invasive techniques such as long-term epidural infusions using local anaesthetic, opioids, and other drugs such as clonidine can provide the necessary control, and can be withdrawn if the pain improves, without making the situation worse.

Treating nerve damage (neuropathic) pain

Peripheral neuropathic pain can rarely be managed adequately over the long term with the conventional analgesics described earlier. The dose–response for opioids is shifted to the right in neuropathic pain compared to nociceptive pain, and response is often minimal. Precisely why is still a mystery. In central neuropathic pain, e.g. with multiple sclerosis, opioids may be more effective.

The unconventional analgesics listed in the lower panel of Fig. 30.1.1 are antidepressants and antiepileptics. Both classes of drugs have proved effective in a wide variety of neuropathic pain syndromes, and also in fibromyalgia and irritable bowel, which fall outside the usual lists of causes of neuropathic pain. An algorithm for drug management of neuropathic pain, using an analogous format to that for nociceptive pain, is shown in Fig. 30.1.3.

The evidence suggests that antidepressants have better (lower) numbers needed to treat (NNT) than antiepileptic drugs in the classic test beds of postherpetic neuralgia and painful diabetic neuropathy. This conclusion may be biased by the older, successful and small crossover trials of tricyclic antidepressants, producing NNTs of 3 or less for at least 50% pain relief over 6 to 8 weeks. The more recent and larger parallel group trials of antiepileptic and newer antidepressant drugs yielded NNTs of between 4 and 5.

Placing antidepressants at step 1 in the algorithm reflects these lower NNTs. Tricyclics are usually given as a single night-time dose, 1 h before lights out. The differences between tricyclics used to treat pain rather than depression are that onset of effect is in

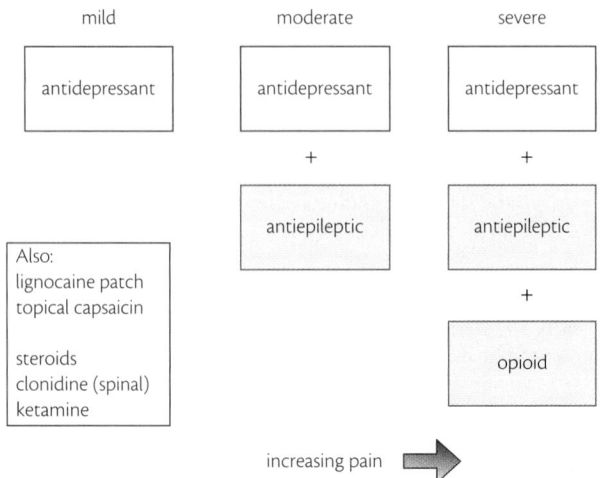

Fig. 30.1.3 Algorithm for analgesics in neuropathic pain.

days rather than weeks, the average effective dose is lower, and the analgesic effect is distinguishable from any mood effect. Titration to optimal dose, optimal balance between effect and adverse effect, can be managed by increasing the dose at weekly intervals, e.g. with 25-mg increments of amitriptyline. Continuing controversy exists over whether or not switching between different tricyclics to achieve a better balance is worthwhile, e.g. from amitriptyline to desipramine or nortriptyline; whether selective serotonin reuptake inhibitors are effective in these pain syndromes; and whether serotonin and noradrenaline (norepinephrine) reuptake inhibitors offer a better balance.

Gabapentin and pregabalin have become the first choice antiepileptic drugs, apart from carbamazepine in trigeminal neuralgia. Dosing is the same as in epilepsy. As with antidepressants, there is insufficient evidence about these drugs to allow certainty. Anecdote suggests that nonresponders may respond to antiepileptic drugs with a different mode of action, so that switching may be worthwhile.

There is evidence to support the use of both lidocaine (lignocaine) patches (in postherpetic neuralgia) and capsaicin. They may supplement antidepressant and antiepileptic analgesia. Oral steroids may be very effective, particularly in palliation of neuropathic pain from head and neck cancer. N-methyl-D-aspartate blockade with ketamine can also be useful to control severe neuropathic pain that is responding poorly to the algorithm. Regional blocks such as epidurals and spinals may be necessary to control really severe neuropathic pain. Clonidine given epidurally or intrathecally, usually with local anaesthetic and opioid, may usefully boost the analgesic effect.

Pain that is both nociceptive and neuropathic

The evidence for efficacy of complementary techniques is very poor. Perhaps the most important distinction is between remedies that make patients feel better, even if only for hours or days, and those that are effective in reducing pain. Studies of complementary techniques using pain outcomes show little sustained benefit, but may make people feel better. Similarly, the evidence for long-term efficacy of stimulation techniques is weak.

Cognitive behavioural therapy has proven benefit in helping patients to cope better with their pain.

Pains that resist treatment

Nothing so far in this chapter has acknowledged the awkward fact that there are many patients who complain of pain for which the diagnosis may never be made, or who fail to respond to any of the treatments described, or whose pain is part of a complicated mental health problem. More difficult still may be managing patients whose drug consumption seems extraordinarily high for the complaint, or indeed whose complaint is extraordinarily loud for the presenting problem. Another on the incomplete list is functional deficit that is greater than expected for the presenting problem.

Some humility is necessary, because each of us has been caught by the diagnosis missed, by the failure of our pattern recognition. That said, there are some constructive solutions. For these difficult pain problems, some form of multidisciplinary management can make a real difference.

The aim is for the patient to move from a distressed state, seeking a cure and bouncing round the health care system, to an acceptance that the best that can be done has been done. Unless a dramatic change occurs, a point will have been reached where all the possible tests have been done, and further treatments are likely to be fruitless. For this 'acceptance' conclusion to be reached there has to be a modicum of trust and reassurance. That point is much easier to achieve if and when the patient feels that they have been listened to and that all appropriate efforts have been made.

The ideal settings in which to reach this difficult goal are multidisciplinary assessment and multidisciplinary clinics. Assessment by an expert team may involve psychology, experienced nurses, physiotherapy, and occupational therapy, as well as the medical input. Such assessment may involve interacting with the patient over days and not just at a clinic appointment. The multidisciplinary clinic allows the patient to see the pain team with the specialist relevant to the complaint, so that a joint approach to further diagnostic efforts and to therapy, including a halt to both, can be achieved. Not all clinics need to be so grandiose; rather, the argument is for a 'hub and spoke' organization so that the patients with problematic pain unresolved at the spoke can be referred for the additional skill and experience at the hub.

In the end, not giving up on people and being accessible are important. Although an economic case can be made for the savings possible when patients do not have to rotate around the system to multiple clinics and multiple tests, the real yardstick is the quality of care.

Further reading

McMahon S, Koltzenburg M (eds.) (2006). *Wall and Melzack's textbook of pain*, 5th edition. Elsevier, Philadelphia, PA.

Moore A, *et al.* (2003). *Bandolier's little book of pain*. Oxford University Press, Oxford.

Twycross R, Wilcock A. (2007). *Palliative care formulary,* 3rd edition. http://palliativebooks.com.

Urch CE, Dickenson AH (2008). Neuropathic pain in cancer. *Eur J Cancer*, **44**, 1091–6.

Wall P (1999). *Pain: the science of suffering*. Weidenfeld & Nicolson, London.

SECTION 31

Palliative medicine

Palliative care

Bee Wee

Essentials

Palliative care addresses the physical, psychological, social, and spiritual needs of someone with advanced, progressive, and fatal disease. Good symptom control requires meticulous assessment, effective two-way communication, and the wise use of drugs, supported by other therapeutic interventions.

Common symptoms are (1) pain—one of the most feared symptoms in patients with advanced malignant disease; managed with disease modifying treatments, nondrug measures (e.g. heat pads), and/or analgesics (see also Chapter 30.1); (2) nausea and/or vomiting—after exclusion/treatment of reversible causes, management is with antiemetics chosen to target the receptors likely to be involved in the particular case and delivered by an appropriate route (oral or nonoral); (3) breathlessness—a disabling symptom in many patients with chronic and progressive illnesses; management requires dealing with reversible causes (e.g. anaemia, chest infection), nondrug

measures (e.g. relaxation techniques, fans), and/or drugs (e.g. strong opioids); (4) constipation—an under-recognized problem which must be handled proactively with rectal measures and/or oral laxatives; (5) depression—which is common but often not perceived; diagnosis and early treatment with antidepressants and psychological support are usually effective; (6) anorexia and fatigue—these are the 'Cinderellas' of symptom control, less amenable to drug therapy but requiring the management of the distress and frustration of the patient and family.

Medical emergencies are relatively uncommon in palliative care, but prompt diagnosis and (when appropriate) intervention are essential. However, it is vital to diagnose dying to avoid unrealistic attempts to cure or prolong life in hopeless situations. Once death is seen to be inevitable and imminent, the focus of care should change from sustaining life at all costs to supporting the natural process of dying.

Introduction and historical perspective

Palliative care is an approach that improves the quality of life of patients and their families facing the problem associated with life-threatening illness, through the prevention and relief of suffering by means of early identification and impeccable assessment and treatment of pain and other problems, physical, psychological, and spiritual.

(World Health Organization, http://www.who.int)

Palliative care is relevant to almost every aspect of clinical practice. Patients with advanced cancer as well as other progressive and ultimately fatal diseases face similar challenges. Their disease is incurable, progressive, and, put simply, physically and emotionally life-shattering. Those around them are also deeply affected. Even in developed countries, where patients may be buffered by relative affluence and privately or publicly funded comprehensive health care systems, they are not immune to suffering. Elsewhere, effective palliative care may be compromised by lack of access to simple effective drugs, inadequate training for professionals and systems which do not, or cannot, prioritize palliative care.

The modern hospice movement was established by Dame Cecily Saunders in the mid 20th century. However, the art of caring for the dying had been established in Our Lady's Hospice, Dublin and St Joseph's Hospice in the east end of London even before the First

World War. Terms used to describe this care started as 'terminal' or 'hospice' care but more recently, the term 'palliative' care has been used to emphasize its relevance throughout severe illness—not just at the dying stage (see Fig. 31.1.1).

So who provides palliative care? Although families, friends, and neighbours are almost always involved, this chapter focuses more on the medical management of these patients. Clearly, specialists in the underlying disease, e.g. oncologists, neurologists, physicians, or surgeons, are essential. In resource-rich countries, accredited palliative medicine physicians usually work alongside clinical nurse specialists, physiotherapists, occupational therapists, social workers, chaplains, and psychologists. In resource-poor countries, however, palliative care may be carried out by a single doctor and a single nurse or volunteer, often working in very difficult circumstances. Whatever the size of the team, palliative care must be delivered where the patient is—in hospital or at home.

This chapter is intended to guide the general physician in three aspects of palliative care:

- symptom management

- identification of emergencies

- end-of-life (terminal) care

Old model of 'terminal care'

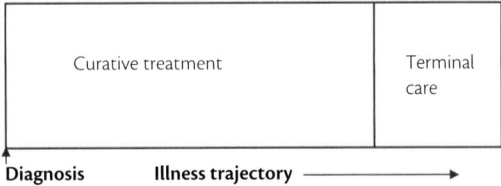

Contemporary model of 'palliative care'

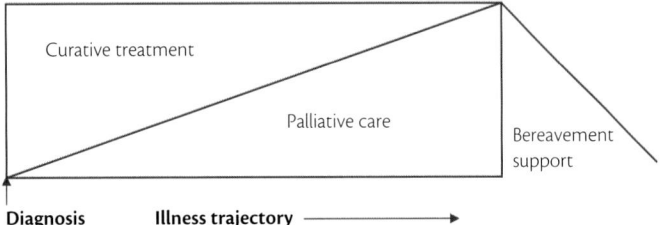

Fig. 31.1.1 Old and contemporary models of terminal and palliative care.

Approach to symptom management

Some tips are listed in Box 31.1.1.

Effective symptom management requires attention to the emotional and social impact of the symptoms as well as the physical issues. The prevalence of symptoms in patients suffering from cancer, as well as those who have progressive nonmalignant disease, is set out in Table 31.1.1.

Common symptoms discussed here include pain, nausea and vomiting, and breathlessness.

Pain

Clinical features

Pain is one of the most feared symptoms in patients diagnosed with advanced malignant disease. Careful history-taking and focused physical examination are fundamental to effective pain management.

Pain may be either (1) nociceptive—caused by physical and/or chemical stimulation of free nerve endings in soft tissue, viscera, bone, etc., or (2) neuropathic—caused by compression, infiltration, or injury to the peripheral nerve or central nervous system, commonly referred to as 'nerve pain'. The ways in which different pains are commonly described are set out in Table 31.1.2.

Each pain should be evaluated and documented separately, because different underlying mechanisms require different therapies. Questions to ask include:

- Pain: site, onset, severity, radiation, exacerbating and relieving factors, temporal factors, and impact on patient's daily living, sleep, and mood

- Analgesic history: effectiveness and side effects of previous and current analgesic drugs, including precisely how much and how frequently they are being taken—often different from what is prescribed

Pain in advanced disease may be continuous or acute-on-chronic. The management of continuous pain is described in the following paragraphs. The management of acute-on-chronic

---

Box 31.1.1 Tips on symptom management

Assessment

- Keep an open mind; symptoms may be caused by the disease, treatment, debility, or concurrent minor or major illness.

- Targeted examinations and investigations, particularly in weak and debilitated patients, are good and effective practice.

- Interventions are more likely to work if the choice of treatment is based on careful analysis of the mechanism of the symptoms.

- Consider whether there are reversible aspects of the problem.

Communication

- First, listen carefully; the best cues and clues come from the patient.

- Patients vary in the level and pace at which they desire information.

- Breaking bad news:

  Most doctors worry about doing badly and respond either by blurting out the whole truth in one shot or procrastinating and going round in circles; neither extreme works.

  The doctor who listens carefully to the patient, offers a warning shot, openly tackles questions, and remains sensitive to any hint that the patient has had enough is more likely to be successful.

  Go on a communication skills course if you feel you need to build your skills in this area.

Decision-making and management

- Listen carefully to the patient, relevant family members and other team members.

- Decision-making involves:

  Judgements based on the patient's best interest

  Balancing potential benefit with possible harm and burden of carrying out or withholding intervention

  Negotiation and clear explanations

- Management plans include:

  Correcting what is realistically reversible

  Targeting the symptom with drug and non-drug approaches

- Drug prescribing:

  Start with safe but sensible doses.

  Oral drugs are easier to manage in all settings, but nonoral routes may be required when the patient is unable to swallow or has nausea, vomiting, or severe diarrhoea.

  Some drugs, e.g. analgesia, require upward titration to achieve maximal symptom control with minimal side effects—warn the patient that it may take several steps to achieve this, otherwise they may get discouraged.

- Professional judgement needs to go beyond protocols and guidelines; decisions need to be about what is best for this patient in this situation at this time.

pain, though based on the same principles, require a particularly careful history to determine whether the pain is:

◆ due to an insufficient dose of the current analgesia, i.e. pain coming on shortly before the next dose is due (end-of-dose failure)

◆ triggered by particular movement or activity (movement-related pain)

◆ a spontaneous exacerbation against a background of chronic pain, occurring without apparent trigger (incident pain)

The first may be resolved by increasing the dose of current analgesia. The mechanism underpinning the other two is less well understood and current management involves a combination of analgesics and modification of lifestyle.

Management

The management of continuous pain consists of three approaches: disease-modifying treatment, nondrug measures, and analgesic drugs.

Disease-modifying treatment

This includes surgery, chemotherapy, radiotherapy, and hormonal therapy. These options should be regularly reconsidered and the balance of potential benefit weighed against any burden of treatment.

Non-drug measures

These involve simple noninvasive measures such as heat pads and physical interventions such as physiotherapy, acupuncture, or

Table 31.1.1 Prevalence of symptoms

Symptom	Percentage with symptom in last year of life	
	Cancer patients	Patients with progressive nonmalignant disease
Pain	87	67
Trouble with breathing	47	49
Vomiting or nausea	51	27
Sleeplessness	51	36
Mental confusion	33	38
Depression	38	36
Loss of appetite	71	38
Constipation	47	32
Bedsores	28	14
Loss of bladder control	37	33
Loss of bowel control	25	22
Unpleasant smell	19	13

Table 31.1.2 Pain: types and descriptors

Type of pain	Common descriptions
Visceral	Deep ache, poorly localized; may get referred pain
Soft tissue	More localized ache, throbbing
Bone	Well-localized pain, local tenderness; increased pain on weight-bearing if those bones are involved
Intestinal obstruction	Colicky, spasmodic abdominal pain, with or without background constant pain
Neuropathic	Classically pain in an area of numbness; burning; pins and needles; spontaneous stabbing pain

transcutaneous electrical nerve stimulation (TENS). Some patients find these helpful, usually in combination with analgesic drugs. Others benefit from specific interventions to interrupt the pain pathway, e.g. nerve blocks or neurolysis. Early involvement of the chronic pain anaesthetist is helpful in these situations.

Analgesic drugs

The rest of this section focuses on the mainstay of pain management, namely analgesic drugs. The World Health Organization (WHO) analgesic ladder (see Fig. 31.1.2) provides the fundamental basis for chronic pain management. It was devised for cancer pain but is relevant to pain from other progressive and incurable diseases. The groups of drugs used on the ladder and some common examples are:

◆ nonopioids: paracetamol or nonsteroidal anti-inflammatory drugs (NSAIDs)

◆ weak opioids: codeine, dextroprophyphene, dihydrocodeine, or tramadol

◆ strong opioids: morphine, methadone, fentanyl, hydromorphone, or oxycodone

◆ adjuvant analgesics: NSAIDs, steroids, tricyclic antidepressants, anticonvulsants, muscle relaxants, etc.

In theory, pain management should always begin at step 1 on the ladder. If this is unsuccessful, treatment should move sequentially to step 2, and then to step 3 as necessary. However, common sense has to prevail. A patient who is in severe pain from an advanced tumour will not obtain relief from paracetamol and will require

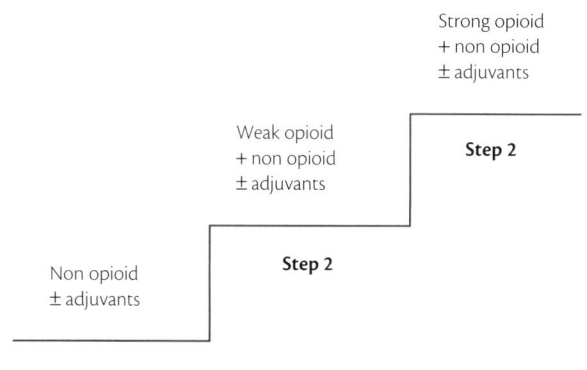

Fig. 31.1.2 World Health Organization analgesic ladder.
Adapted with permission from the World Health Organisation (WHO) http://www.who.int/cancer/palliative/painladder/en/

Table 31.1.3 Use of adjuvant analgesics

Type of pain	Adjuvant analgesics/therapy	Examples
Visceral or soft-tissue pain	Steroids if surrounding oedema is likely	Dexamethasone 4–8 mg daily orally
Bone pain	NSAIDs	Ibuprofen 400–800 mg three times daily orally; Diclofenac 50 mg three times daily orally
	Bisphosphonates (see 'Areas of uncertainty and controversy')	Zoledronic acid 4 mg by intravenous infusion every 3–4 weeks
	Radiotherapy and/or radioactive strontium (for prostate cancer)	Consult radiotherapist
Intestinal obstruction	Antispasmodic for colic	Hyoscine butylbromide 20–120 mg over 24 h by subcutaneous infusion
Neuropathic pain	Antidepressants	Amitriptyline 25–100 mg at night time
	Anticonvulsants	Sodium valproate 200–600 mg at night time; Gabapentin 100 mg three times daily, titrating up to 900 mg three times daily over 4 days (lower dose with renal impairment)
	Steroids	Dexamethasone 4–8 mg daily orally

a direct jump to step 2 or, often, step 3. In some countries, strong opioids are not readily available and clinicians have to work more creatively with nonopioids, weak opioids, and adjuvant drugs. In terms of clinical efficacy, there is little to choose between the various weak opioids. The use of adjuvant drugs is described in Table 31.1.3 and more comprehensive discussion about strong opioids follows.

Strong opioids Morphine remains the gold standard because there is a wealth of clinical experience with it, and it is also inexpensive. Alternative strong opioids are mentioned briefly at the end of this section.

An example of how to start a patient on morphine and titrate the dose upwards is set out in Box 31.1.2. Further tips on prescribing morphine are given in Box 31.1.3.

When patients cannot take drugs by mouth, other routes must be considered. Most commonly, these are:

- Subcutaneous: parenteral morphine may be given either as one-off injections or as subcutaneous infusions. The conversion ratio of oral to subcutaneous morphine is 2:1 (i.e. 10 mg orally = 5 mg by subcutaneous injection). Given adequate professional support, infusions may be carried out in hospital, at home, or in other institutions. In the United Kingdom, parenteral diamorphine is often used instead of morphine because it is more soluble, enabling lower volumes when high doses are required. The conversion ratio of oral morphine to subcutaneous diamorphine is 3:1 (i.e. 15 mg morphine orally = 5 mg diamorphine subcutaneously).

- Rectal: this is useful in resource-poor countries or where there is little or no access to professional support at home to offer subcutaneous injections or infusions. The conversion ratio of oral:rectal morphine is 1:1.

- Transdermal: fentanyl and buprenorphine are available by this route.

Intravenous, epidural, and intrathecal routes may occasionally be used but these are more difficult to achieve outside hospitals. Sublingual drugs is an alternative but absorption may be unreliable and proprietary preparations are expensive.

Although morphine is generally regarded as the gold standard for strong opioids, a number of other drugs are now available. None has demonstrated superior efficacy to morphine and most are more expensive. They should be considered in patients whose pain remains opioid-responsive but in whom upward dose titration is limited by unacceptable side effects which cannot be alleviated in other ways. On current evidence, these other drugs should remain second-line options.

- Transdermal fentanyl: less constipating than morphine; nonoral option; 72-h slow-release preparation; convenient but slow titration makes it less effective for rapid relief of severe pain.

Box 31.1.2 Starting and titrating morphine: an example

Matt is a 48-year-old man with lung cancer. He has a deep right chest pain which has not been adequately relieved with paracetamol and codeine (step 2 of the WHO analgesic ladder). Prescribe:

- immediate-release oral morphine 10 mg 4-hourly, and

- immediate-release oral morphine 10 mg as required for breakthrough pain; this is calculated as one-sixth of the total oral daily dose of regular morphine prescribed (60 mg/6 = 10 mg)

On review after 24 h, Matt has taken three additional 10-mg doses of breakthrough morphine. You calculate that the oral morphine requirements over the last 24 h has been 60 mg (from the regular doses) plus 30 mg (additional breakthrough doses) = 90 mg over 24 h. Redistributing this over a 24-h period, you now prescribe:

- immediate-release oral morphine 15 mg 4-hourly, and

- immediate-release oral morphine 15 mg as required for breakthrough pain

Continue titrating the dose upward, taking into account the amount of breakthrough analgesia required. One week later, Matt's pain is under control on immediate-release oral morphine 30 mg 4-hourly and he has not required additional breakthrough analgesia. For convenience, this may be converted to modified-release morphine. Now prescribe:

- modified-release oral morphine 90 mg 12-hourly, and

- immediate-release oral morphine 30 mg as required for breakthrough pain

---

Box 31.1.3 Tips for prescribing morphine

◆ Immediate-release morphine is quick acting and more suitable for rapid control of pain than modified-release preparations of morphine or other strong opioids.

◆ In theory, 4- hourly prescribing of immediate-release morphine requires round-the-clock prescribing. Taking a double dose at bedtime may obviate the need for a dose in the middle of the night, but most patients find that this is unnecessary once pain is under control.

◆ Constipation is a predictable side effect of morphine in almost all patients. Coprescribing of laxatives (softener and stimulant, see Table 31.1.8) is good practice.

◆ Nausea or vomiting persists in about one-third of patients taking morphine. Coprescribing of an antiemetic (e.g. haloperidol 1.5 mg at night or metoclopramide 10 mg three times daily, see Table 31.1.5) should be considered.

◆ Sleepiness tends to be a transient side effect, though it may recur briefly each time the dose is increased.

◆ Driving should be avoided until 2 weeks after the opioid dose has been stabilized or if the patient remains drowsy.

◆ Older, frail patients are more susceptible to side effects, especially when starting therapy. Starting with a lower dose (e.g. immediate-release oral morphine 2.5–5 mg 4-hourly) and titrating up gradually will usually circumvent this problem.

◆ Patients with mild to moderate renal failure should be prescribed morphine at lower doses and/or at longer dose intervals (e.g. immediate release oral morphine 5 mg 6-hourly) because the active metabolite of morphine accumulates. Those with more severe renal failure should be prescribed strong opioids which do not have active metabolites, e.g. methadone or alfentanil.

◆ Transdermal buprenorphine: relatively new on the market; also useful nonoral alternative; similar constraints as transdermal fentanyl.

◆ Methadone: difficult to use because of long and variable half-life. Titration and toxicity may be problematic; cheap and widely used in countries where morphine formulations are expensive or unavailable.

◆ Oxycodone: similar efficacy and side-effect profile to morphine; popular in North America.

◆ Hydromorphone: similar efficacy and side effect profile to morphine; popular in Ireland.

These drugs, with the exception of methadone, are more expensive than morphine. Given that they have not yet been shown to be more efficacious, cost remains an important issue.

Adjuvant analgesics These drugs may be useful and sometimes play an opioid-sparing role. Their mode of action in pain control is complex. The published literature is rapidly expanding, so that contemporary understanding is constantly being revised. Common adjuvant analgesics work in the following ways.

◆ NSAIDs and steroids suppress or modify inflammatory processes, e.g. in bone or inflammatory pain.

◆ Antidepressants and anticonvulsants dampen the hyperexcitability of damaged peripheral nerves; inhibit the glutamate excitatory system in the dorsal horn; and enhance the γ-aminobutyric acid (GABA) inhibitory system in the dorsal horn.

The clinical application of common adjuvant analgesics is shown in Table 31.1.3. Virtually all of these will have required the use of the WHO analgesic ladder up to step 3. In each case, the dose of the strong opioid, usually morphine, should be titrated up to maximum efficacy with tolerable side effects. One simple technique to achieve this is to identify the extent to which breakthrough doses of analgesic drugs alleviate pain. If breakthrough doses do not contribute to further pain relief but only cause additional side effects, the opioid responsiveness has probably reached saturation and focus should shift to adjuvant analgesics. When increasing the dose of opioids and introducing adjuvant analgesics, only one drug dose should be changed at a time to ascertain which one has been most effective.

Areas of uncertainty or controversy

Research into pain management continues to occupy the time and attention of many who specialize in palliative care and acute and chronic pain. Although there has been much progress over the past 20 years, much remains uncertain. Only areas that are particularly relevant to clinical practice are mentioned here.

Table 31.1.4 Common antiemetics and their receptor activity

Drug	D_2	H_1	Ach(m)	5-HT$_2$	5-HT$_3$	5-HT$_4$	GABA
Cyclizine		++	++				
Diazepam							++
Domperidone	++						
Haloperidol	+++						
Hyoscine			+++				
Levomepromazine	++	++	++	+++			
Metoclopromide	++				(+)	++	
Ondansetron					+++		
Prochlorperazine	++	+					

5-HT$_2$, 5-HT$_3$, 5-HT$_4$, serotonin types 2, type 3, and type 4 receptors; Ach(m), muscarinic anticholinergic receptors; D$_2$ = dopamine type 2 receptors; GABA, γ-amino-butyric acid receptors, H$_1$, histamine type 1 receptors.
+ slight affinity; ++ moderate affinity; +++ strong affinity.

The WHO analgesic ladder was originally devised as an educational tool. In developed countries, some advocate the abandonment of step 2, on the basis that it unnecessarily delays optimum pain management. Given that most patients eventually require strong opioids, this is reasonable for clinicians working in those countries. However, step 2 remains essential for those in countries where step 3 is irrelevant because strong opioids are either unavailable or unaffordable.

The use of bisphosphonates has risen exponentially in recent years. They have been shown to delay the onset of the first skeletal complication from bone metastases in multiple myeloma and breast and prostate cancer, e.g. pathological fracture and spinal cord compression. They also improve bone pain from these tumours. However, prolonged treatment is required for this benefit to accrue. The evidence that bisphosphonates benefit other tumours is currently weak. These are potent drugs and their potential benefit needs to be weighed against the burden of treatment (intravenous infusions every 3–4 weeks) and serious side effects, e.g. osteonecrosis of the jaw.

Opioid switching is a technique that has varied in popularity. The theoretical rationale rests on interindividual variation and cross-receptor activity. By switching between different opioids, responsiveness may be enhanced or maintained for longer periods. There is early evidence that this may have clinically meaningful outcomes for some patients, but this is insufficiently strong to support its widespread use by most clinicians. However, some patients do seem to tolerate one opioid better than another. In them, switching may be appropriate. There is emerging evidence that the genetic profile of individuals may influence this variability in response.

Nausea and vomiting

Clinical features

Nausea is persistent, often more distressing than vomiting itself. It is debilitating, distracting, and leaves the patient feeling continuously washed-out and fearful of doing anything that might make it worse, e.g. moving or eating. As with pain, successful management of nausea and vomiting requires close attention to detail. The history, analysis of the probable cause, the choice of antiemetic and route of administration, evaluation of effect and use of nondrug measures are all important. Even when the cause appears obvious, e.g. chemotherapy, effective management is rarely straightforward as there is often more than one cause in the same patient. Understanding the mechanism of emesis is helpful for a rational approach to management. A simple representation of this is set out in Fig. 31.1.3.

Management

First, reversible causes of nausea and vomiting should be corrected, e.g. urinary tract infection or hypercalcaemia. Secondly, managing the symptom should include the following steps:

1 Based on careful assessment, a hypothesis for the causes of nausea and vomiting is generated and reversible causes dealt with.

2 One antiemetic is chosen to target the receptors likely to be involved (see Tables 31.1.4 and 31.1.5).

3 Consider whether a nonoral route is required. Patients with established nausea and vomiting do not tolerate oral antiemetics. Parenteral or rectal antiemetics may be more appropriate, particularly when initiating therapy. Patients who suffer from nausea may not be absorbing their antiemetics normally; patients who vomit their oral medications certainly are not. A short course of antiemetics by subcutaneous infusion often breaks the cycle of nausea and vomiting.

4 Use one antiemetic to its full dosage before adding or substituting another.

5 Keep reviewing whether the hypothesis in step 1 was correct and whether a new trigger may have emerged in addition to, or instead of, the original cause.

Two situations which commonly face acute physicians and general practitioners merit particular mention. First is hypercalcaemia,

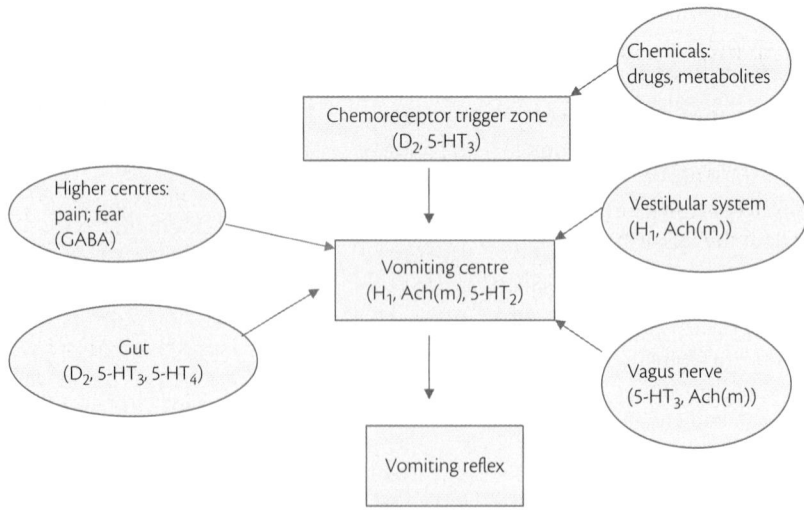

Key: D_2 – dopamine type 2 receptors
$5\text{-}HT_2$, $5\text{-}HT_3$, $5\text{-}HT_4$ – serotonin types 2, 3 and 4 receptors
H_1 – histamine type 1 receptors
Ach(m) – muscarinic anticholinergic receptors
GABA – gamma-amino-butyric receptors

Fig. 31.1.3 Mechanism of emesis.

Table 31.1.5 Nausea and vomiting: clinical pattern, likely causes and useful antiemetics

Characteristic description	Likely cause	Antiemetic management
Constant nausea but vomiting pattern variable	Chemically induced: drugs, metabolic (e.g. uraemia, hypercalcaemia)	Haloperidol 1.5–3 mg daily orally Haloperidol 2.5 mg immediate subcutaneous injection or 2.5–10 mg over 24 h by subcutaneous infusion Metoclopromide 10–20 mg 3–4 times daily orally Metoclopromide 10 mg immediate subcutaneous injection or 60 mg over 24 h by subcutaneous infusion
Nausea in the morning; projectile vomiting; worse on head movement	Raised intracranial pressure, e.g. brain metastases or haemorrhage	Dexamethasone 16 mg daily orally or subcutaneous injection (no good evidence that higher doses are more effective)
Nausea and vomiting worse when anxious	Anxiety	Diazepam 2–10 mg at night orally
Epigastric fullness, especially postprandial; symptoms eased by vomiting; nausea variable	Upper gastrointestinal stasis or outflow obstruction	Metoclopromide 10–20 mg three times daily orally Metoclopromide 10 mg immediate subcutaneous injection or 30–60 mg over 24 h by subcutaneous infusion Domperidone 10–20 mg 3–4 times daily orally Domperidone 30 mg 3–4 times daily per rectum
Periodic vomiting; minimal nausea; usually associated with abdominal colic, distension and constipation	Intestinal obstruction	If no colic present: Metoclopromide 30–60 mg over 24 h by subcutaneous infusion If colic present: Hyoscine butylbromide 60–120 mg over 24 h by subcutaneous infusion
Faeculent vomiting; nausea	Constipation	Deal with the constipation: rectal measures usually required

often presenting with nausea, vomiting, drowsiness, confusion, and thirst. Treatment involves intravenous hydration and intravenous bisphosphonates (see Table 31.1.9). The symptoms resolve rapidly once serum calcium levels begin to fall.

The second situation is intestinal obstruction caused by advanced malignant disease in the abdomen. This can be subacute or acute. Single-site obstruction in relatively fit patients may be amenable to surgery. If surgery is not an option, the old maxim of 'drip and suck' is inappropriate. Further management is symptomatic:

◆ nausea and vomiting: antiemetics (see Table 31.1.5)
◆ constipation: softener laxatives and rectal measures (see Table 31.1.8)
◆ pain: strong opioids for background pain and hyoscine butyl-bromide for colic
◆ thirst: ice chips and sips of fluid as required
◆ hunger: small amounts of food at short intervals is acceptable

Subacute intestinal obstruction often settles down with such conservative management. Full-blown obstruction is more intractable. Patients may have to settle for minimal nausea and possibly one or two vomits a day. If this is explained, most tolerate it well.

Finally, nondrug measures which patients have found helpful include:

◆ food being presented in small amounts, appetizingly and when the patient asks for it
◆ small amounts of cold or hot fluids, which seem better tolerated than lukewarm liquids
◆ ensuring that constipation is actively managed
◆ avoiding smells and situations that trigger nausea
◆ imbibing ginger
◆ aromatherapy and other forms of complementary therapy

Much of this is about personal preferences and individual patients will usually make their own choices.

Areas of uncertainty or controversy

5-HT₃ antagonists, e.g. ondansetron, are rightly used for the acute vomiting of chemotherapy. However, there is little evidence of their efficacy for chronic nausea and vomiting. Early evidence of the antiemetic action of agents such as propofol and neurokinin antagonists looks promising, but robust clinical data is awaited.

Breathlessness
Clinical features

Breathlessness is a disabling symptom in many patients with chronic and progressive illnesses. The pattern is commonly one of acute episodes of severe breathlessness against a background of chronic shortness of breath. Unlike pain, the breathless patient is unable to draw attention at the peak of distress through shouting or calling for help. Acute attacks of breathlessness can therefore be exceptionally frightening and isolating, often engendering panic.

Again, careful and patient history-taking will determine the severity and pattern of breathlessness, limitation of function and associated symptoms such as cough, wheeze, fatigue, weakness, and panic. Where every breath requires effort and energy, efficient and targeted physical examination and investigations must prevail. A key question in assessing breathless patients is to determine the extent to which the symptom is caused by the underlying disease, concurrent pathology, or as a consequence of treatment or frailty.

Management
To manage breathlessness, consider:

◆ reversible causes—e.g. anaemia, respiratory tract infection
◆ problems amenable to specific interventions (see Table 31.1.6)
◆ symptom management with drug and nondrug measures (see Table 31.1.7)

Table 31.1.6 Breathlessness: causes and specific interventions

Cause	Possible interventions
Pleural effusion	Pleural drainage and pleurodesis
Bronchial obstruction	Radiotherapy, stenting, surgery
Concurrent lung disease, e.g. asthma, COPD	Maximize standard therapy, seeking advice if necessary
Pulmonary embolus	Anticoagulation
Lymphangitis carcinomatosis	High dose steroids, e.g. dexamethasone 16 mg daily

Areas of uncertainty or controversy

Oxygen is routinely given to patients who complain of breathlessness, but evidence for its effectiveness in patients who are not hypoxic remains sparse. Studies have shown that some of these patients do benefit from oxygen therapy, but most also benefit from room air administered through nasal prongs. In clinical practice, oxygen should be offered to patients who are hypoxic and who report benefit. A trial of oxygen therapy may be offered to breathless patients who are not hypoxic, but only after room air has been tried and only if the oxygen is symptomatically beneficial. The disadvantages of oxygen are that it can be excessively drying for the airways, limits patient movement, and activity, is expensive and cumbersome, and induces dependence.

The use of nebulized opioids for dyspnoea, common in the 1990s, has now been abandoned as ineffective. Benzodiazepines are useful in breathlessness but it is uncertain whether they simply alleviate the anxiety provoked by shortness of breath or whether they have a specific role in diminishing the sensation of breathlessness. There is growing evidence that acupuncture and other complementary

Table 31.1.7 Breathlessness: symptom management

Drug measures	
Strong opioids to reduce the sensation of breathlessness	Immediate-release morphine 2.5 mg 4-hourly and as required orally, if opioid-naive Sustained release morphine 10 mg 12-hourly orally, if opioid-naive If already on opioids, e.g. for pain, increase that dose by 30–50%
Benzodiazepine	Lorazepam 0.5–1 mg as required orally or sublingually Diazepam 2–5 mg at night orally
Steroids	Dexamethasone 4–8 mg daily orally Can be helpful in improving breathlessness—mechanism unclear but remember to reduce dose and wean off or maintain as low as possible to minimize side effects
Oxygen	Consider whether this is necessary (see 'Areas of uncertainty or controversy')
Nondrug measures	
Explanation and reassurance	
Position patient in most comfortable position for breathing—often leaning forward	
Relaxation techniques and breathing exercises	
Involve physiotherapy and occupational therapy	
Keep window open or fan nearby	

therapies are helpful for some breathless patients. Convincing trials are awaited. Breathlessness clinics appear to be beneficial but, like complementary therapies, it is uncertain which is of primary benefit: the intervention itself or the undivided attention by the therapist.

Other common problems

Constipation

Most patients who are dying become constipated. This may be due to drugs, reduced mobility, and diminished intake of food and fluids. In addition, patients in hospitals may find that shared toilet facilities or the lack of privacy inhibits and disrupts their bowel habits. Physical causes of constipation include intestinal obstruction, hypercalcaemia, infection, and tumour invasion of the gut wall. Some of these may have reversible elements, e.g. correcting hypercalcaemia will usually improve the related constipation. Others may be harder to reverse. Careful history-taking needs to include questions about the stool consistency and colour and whether the patient is too weak to expel the stools. Examination of the abdomen should be carried out, including rectal examination to ascertain whether the rectum is empty, full, or impacted with faeces. The choice of oral laxatives (softeners, stimulants, or combinations) and rectal measures are guided by these findings. Commonly used oral laxatives and rectal measures are listed in Table 31.1.8.

Depression

Depression is underdiagnosed and undertreated in patients with advanced progressive disease. Although patients have understandable reasons for feeling sad, they may also be suffering from concurrent depression, which is amenable to therapy. The key symptoms of early morning waking, feeling depressed at specific times of day, and lack of normal enthusiasm and interest, e.g. in seeing grandchildren, are pointers to the diagnosis; weight loss, lack of energy, and reduced appetite are less so, as these are common symptoms of advanced cancer. The question, 'Are you depressed?' may be sufficient. A high index of suspicion and the

Table 31.1.8 Constipation: drug management

Main action	Examples
Oral laxatives	
Softeners (lubricant)[a]	Magnesium hydroxide 10–20 ml twice daily
Softeners (osmotic)[a]	Lactulose 10–20 ml twice daily Movicol 2–4 sachets daily
Stimulants[a]	Senna 2–4 tablets at night-time Bisacodyl 5–10 mg at night-time Docusate 100–200 mg once or twice daily
Combined softener and stimulant	Codanthrusate 50/60 1–3 capsules at night Codanthramer 25/200 or 37.5/500 1–2 capsules at night
Rectal measures	
Softeners	Glycerine suppositories
Stimulants	Bisacodyl suppositories
When rectum empty	Phosphate enemas
When rectum impacted	Manual evacuation under mild sedation

[a] Drug doses should be increased commensurate with need.

courage to ask direct questions about the patient's mood, depression, and suicidal thoughts are crucial.

Antidepressants require at least 2 weeks to achieve therapeutic effect, so prompt diagnosis and intervention is essential. Some patients may be already taking tricyclic antidepressants for neuropathic pain but the dose required for adjuvant analgesia (e.g. amitryptiline 25–100 mg daily) is not sufficient for treating depression (amitryptiline 150–200 mg daily). Rarely, the patient may be able to tolerate a sufficient increase in the dose of the tricyclic antidepressant. Selective serotonin reuptake inhibitors (SSRIs) are often better tolerated, e.g. citalopram 10–20 mg daily. A suitable alternative is mirtazapine 15 mg at night, a presynaptic α_2-antagonist.

Anorexia

Anorexia is common in advanced cancer and worries both patients and families. This is because eating represents far more than simply calorie intake. It is about survival and has cultural and social implications. For example, the loss of appetite and unwillingness to join in family meals means that patients can become isolated from the day-to-day family routine, which has been the glue of relationships. Managing anorexia is therefore important and requires:

- understanding and insight into the wider implications of food and feeding

- encouraging the patient to eat 'a little of what you fancy, but only when you fancy', and for the family to tolerate this

- treatment of reversible causes, e.g. mouth ulcers or oral thrush and provision of suitable dentures, spectacles, and appropriate utensils

- consideration of appetite stimulants such as steroids (prednisolone 15–20 mg daily or dexamethasone 2–4 mg daily). These are effective for only a few weeks at most.

Open acknowledgement of the upset induced by anorexia and the frustration it brings both to patients and families enables them to talk openly about it. This will relieve some of their accompanying, often silent, distress.

Fatigue

Debilitating fatigue is common: effective therapies are not. There is evidence that exercise and activity improve fatigue in the earlier stages of disease. However, this is difficult to achieve in patients who are more ill. In these patients, it is particularly important not to mislead them and their families into believing that fatigue can be improved by other factors, such as weight gain. Sensitive understanding, empathy, common sense, and encouraging patients to pace their activities and preserve energy for what is important to them are the key to managing fatigue in our present state of knowledge.

Palliative medicine emergencies

All palliative care problems require timely management: emergencies are urgent. Prompt recognition and treatment of these will often prevent serious consequences. Four situations that require urgent attention are summarized in Table 31.1.9.

Like any other situations in palliative care, the decision to intervene or not must again be guided by balancing potential benefit against the burden of treatment. For example, for a patient with advanced cancer and likely to die from this disease within the next week or so, palliative radiotherapy for spinal cord compression will be burdensome and of little benefit. On the other hand, for a patient who can still move about in bed and has a painful pathological fracture, fixing the fracture is obligatory to achieve effective pain control.

End-of-life (terminal) care

It is important to recognize when a patient is beginning to die. It enables appropriate decisions to be made about clinical management and engenders sensible, supportive, and realistic communication with the patient and their family. However, it is not always easy to recognize or acknowledge the point when the focus of care shifts from curative care to terminal or end-of-life care. Although this point may occur days or hours before death, it sometimes comes with little warning. However, families really value being prepared, because this allows them the opportunity to say their goodbyes, which can be an important part of their adjustment to death and loss. For some, this is crucial in working through bereavement.

Clinical features

The principles of end-of-life care are similar whatever the underlying disease. Although illness trajectories vary between patient and patient, distinct patterns are seen with different conditions (see Fig. 31.1.4).

The ability to recognize when a patient is deteriorating improves with clinical experience. Indicators listed in Box 31.1.4 may help

Table 31.1.9 Emergencies in palliative care

Situation	Key symptoms and signs	Consequences if not managed	Management
Spinal cord compression	Unremitting back pain; lower limb weakness; sensory deficit; urinary and/or faecal incontinence.	Paraplegia; double incontinence; consequences of paraplegia	Dexamethasone 16 mg daily; refer immediately for radiological confirmation, radiotherapy, or neurosurgery
Hypercalcaemia	Sudden confusion, drowsiness, nausea, vomiting, and thirst	Increasing confusion; dehydration; coma; death	Intravenous hydration, then intravenous bisphosphonates, e.g. pamidronate 30–90 mg or zoledronic acid 4 mg by intravenous infusion
Massive haemorrhage	Torrential bleed; may be heralded by minor bleeds	Death is inevitable but prompt management and control of the situation reduces distress	Subcutaneous or intravenous opioids and benzodiazepines, e.g. 5–10 mg morphine and 5–10 mg midazolam immediately
Pathological fracture	Sudden and severe pain; inability to move the affected limb (but in ill patients, may be less obvious)	Continuing pain; inability to mobilize	Fixation: internal or external

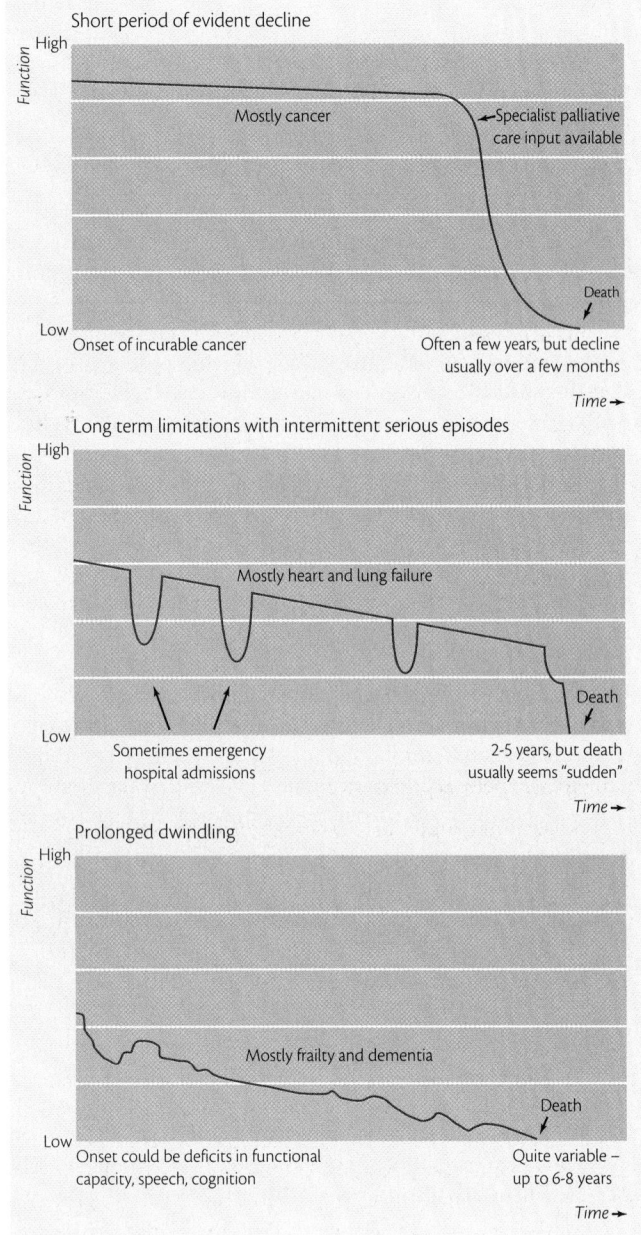

Fig. 31.1.4 Illness trajectories.
Reproduced from BMJ, Murray SA *et al*. Illness trajectories and palliative care, 330:1007–1111 (2005), as adapted from Lynn J, Adamson DM. (2003) Living well at the end of life, with permission from BMJ Publishing Group Ltd and the RAND Corporation.

those who are less experienced. Many Western families have never encountered dying people, and may need health professionals to guide them both practically and emotionally.

Management

Protocols and guidelines exist for terminal care but the real challenge is to recognize when the patient is dying and to individualize management for that patient. Key issues to consider include the following.

◆ Current drugs: which drugs are unnecessary at this stage? Is the burden of taking these greater than the benefit they confer? If some drugs remain necessary, can the patient swallow these or

◆ Spends more time in bed

◆ Less interested or able to engage with surroundings, including visitors

◆ Disorientation

◆ Less mobile in bed

◆ Profoundly weak and exhausted

◆ More difficulty in swallowing: choking, spluttering

◆ Drowsy and difficult to rouse

◆ Breathing pattern changes, in volume, rhythm, and quality of sound

◆ Skin changes, especially peripheries: becomes less perfused, cooler to touch

do they need to be administered by some other route, e.g. should oral analgesics now be administered subcutaneously or rectally?

◆ New drugs: additional analgesics and sedatives may be required to ensure the patient's comfort. Whether in hospital or at home, these need to be readily available (see Box 31.1.5), i.e. anticipatory prescribing.

◆ Monitoring and observations: if patients are in hospital, they may still be having their pulse rate, blood pressure, and temperature monitored. These are unnecessary and can be discontinued, as should other investigations.

◆ Physical care: is this at an appropriate level? If the patient is incontinent of urine, would an indwelling catheter be more comfortable than moving them to change the bedclothes? Is it necessary to turn the patient so frequently?

◆ Communication: are the family aware that the patient is dying? Have they had the opportunity to have their questions and concerns addressed? These are not one-off conversations but part of an ongoing process.

Intravenous hydration is a frequent concern, particularly from families. Their worries now often revolve around thirst and the likelihood of expediting death by dehydration. Professionals worry about these issues too. But, once again, the balance between the potential benefit and burden or harm to the patient needs to be weighed. Because of the old maxim 'thirst starts and stops at the mouth', comfort can be maintained by keeping the mouth moist with ice chips, sponge sticks, lip salve to minimize drying, and good caring nursing.

Patients who are artificially hydrated in the last 3 weeks of life do not have significantly different sodium, potassium, urea, and creatinine levels from those not given intravenous fluids. On the other hand, administration of intravenous fluid can be uncomfortable and restrictive and may disturb fluid balance. Current thinking suggests that artificial hydration in most dying patients causes more harm than benefit. Similar judgements need to be made about other issues which may arise, e.g. chest or urinary infection, pulmonary embolus, etc. The key consideration is how likely any intervention is to produce a net benefit for the patient at this stage

---

Box 31.1.5 Terminal care: problems that require attention

Pain management

Background analgesia

Patients who had been swallowing oral analgesia up to this point will need to continue this through an alternative route; e.g. a patient who has been on modified release morphine 30 mg 12-hourly orally may be converted to:

- subcutaneous morphine: conversion ratio 2:1, i.e. morphine 30 mg by subcutaneous infusion over 24 h

- rectal morphine: conversion ratio 1:1, i.e. morphine 10 mg 4-hourly suppositories or morphine 30 mg 12 hourly modified-release suppositories

Analgesia for breakthrough pain

This should be prescribed for all patients. In those who are opioid naive or who have not required any background analgesia so far, morphine 2.5 mg by subcutaneous injection suffices. For those who already require a background level of strong opioids, one-sixth of the total oral daily dose of morphine required should be calculated, divided by 2, and prescribed as morphine subcutaneous injection.

Death rattle

This is noisy, rattling breathing which may occur within hours or days of death.

- Chest infections and heart failure may make breathing noisier. Consider whether the patient's comfort would be improved by treating these.

- Observe whether the patient appears comfortable despite the sound; if so, drugs are unnecessary.

- Explain to relatives that the sound may be caused by air whistling past some secretions in the airways and/or the sound of

the patient's weakened muscles as s/he breathes; emphasize that the patient is not drowning in these secretions and will not choke to death.

- If the patient and/or family are disturbed by the sound, try repositioning and gentle upper airway suction. If necessary, drugs may be given by subcutaneous infusion:

    hysocine butylbromide 20–40 mg over 24 h

    glycopyrronium 400–800 μg over 24 h

    hyoscine hydrochloride 800–1200 μg over 24 h

Remember that these drugs have adverse effects, which the patient will not be able to report. They all cause excessive mouth dryness. Hyoscine hydrochloride crosses the blood–brain barrier and may cause excessive drowsiness and/or paradoxical agitation.

Terminal restlessness and agitation

- Rule out any reversible causes, e.g. urinary retention or constipation.

- Reassure patient.

- Control environment as far as possible: quiet, good lighting, etc.

- If drugs are necessary, consider:

    benzodiazepines orally or subcutaneously for sedation, e.g. diazepam 5–10 mg orally or midazolam 2.5–5 mg one-off subcutaneous injection or 5–10 mg over 24 h by subcutaneous infusion; haloperidol 2.5–5 mg orally or subcutaneously as one-off injections or by subcutaneous infusion over 24 h, if psychosis (e.g. hallucination or paranoia) is present

---

of their dying. Whatever decision is made, consultation and close communication with the family and other team members minimizes distress at this fraught and difficult time.

Likely future developments

The natural history of life-threatening illness, especially cancer, is changing radically. As a result of advances in antineoplastic therapy, more people are living longer with their tumours. In those who are not cured, metastases appear in uncommon sites, so the pattern of disability is changing. The range of diseases requiring input from palliative care clinicians has broadened to include a wide spectrum of nonmalignant disease. This involvement will grow over the next 10 years.

Research and clinical management have so far tended to focus on single symptoms. There is a growing recognition that some symptoms tend to cluster together, e.g. anorexia, cachexia, and fatigue. Over the next decade, more attention will focus on developing interventions to manage these symptom clusters.

The search for effective new drugs with minimal side effects continues, as with any other specialty. Advances in basic science research, especially in the area of genetics and pain pathways, and translational research will begin to allow more individualized, targeted therapies to be prescribed.

Research is difficult to carry out in this group of patients because of logistical and ethical problems. Up to recently, much of the evidence for management has been extrapolated from studies carried out on healthy volunteers, patients with nonmalignant disease, or those earlier in the illness trajectory. However, there is growing acceptance that to shy away from building the evidence base for clinical practice in terminal care is unethical. To deny patients the right to decide whether or not to participate in research, just because they are terminally ill, also undermines their dignity and integrity.

Finally, education and training in palliative care is forging ahead. Palliative care was first established and practised in the West. Experts from these countries then went out to teach others, often linking up with lone pioneers in developing countries. The balance has started to shift and will do so more radically over the next decade. Learning will become much more a two-way process, with practitioners in developed and developing countries learning from each other about innovative ways of delivering palliative care from which all patients with all diseases will ultimately benefit.

Further reading

Addington-Hall JM, Higginson I (2001). *Palliative care for non-cancer patients*. Oxford University Press, Oxford. [Useful summary and references for palliative care in specific nonmalignant conditions.]

American Thoracic Society (1999). Dyspnoea, mechanisms, assessment and management: a consensus statement. *Am J Resp Crit Care Med*, **159**, 321–40. [Older paper but offers a comprehensive consensus position.]

Eisenberg E, McNichol E, Carr DB (2006). Opioids for neuropathic pain. *Cochrane Database Syst Rev* CD001133. [Review of the evidence for use of opioids in neuropathic pain.]

Glare P, *et al.* (2004). Systematic review of the efficacy of antiemetics in the treatment of nausea in patients with far-advanced cancer. *Support Care Cancer*, **12**, 432–40. [Useful review of the evidence for antiemetics in advanced cancer.]

Hanks G, *et al.* (eds) (2009). *Oxford Textbook of Palliative Medicine*. Oxford University Press, Oxford. [Major reference work for palliative medicine.]

Jennings AL, *et al.* (2001). Opioids for the palliation of breathlessness in terminal illness. *Cochrane Database Syst Rev*, Issue 3, Art. No. CD002066. [Systematic review of the evidence for prescribing opioids for breathlessness.]

McQuay HJ, *et al.* (1999). Radiotherapy for the palliation of painful bone metastases. *Cochrane Database Syst Rev*, Issue 3, Art. No. CD001793. [Useful review of the evidence for efficacy of radiotherapy in management of bone pain, including comparison of different fractionation schedules.]

Moore A, *et al.* (2003). *Bandolier's little book of pain*. Oxford University Press, Oxford. [Concise summary of evidence for specific aspects of pain management, acute and chronic.]

Murray SA, *et al.* (2005). Illness trajectories and palliative care. *BMJ*, **330**, 1002–11. [Thought-provoking paper comparing illness trajectories in those suffering from cancer, heart failure, chronic obstructive pulmonary disease, and prolonged dwindling.]

Patchell R, *et al.* (2005). Direct decompressive surgical resection in the treatment of spinal cord compression caused by metastatic disease: a randomised trial. *Lancet*, **366**, 643–8. [Interesting study which has changed attitudes and clinical practice.]

Quigley C (2004). Opioid switching to improve pain relief and drug tolerability. *Cochrane Database Syst Rev*, Issue 3. Art. No. CD004847. [Reviews the evidence for the practice of opioid switching.]

Ross JR, *et al.* (2003). Systematic review of role of bisphosphonates on skeletal morbidity in metastatic cancer. *BMJ*, **327**, 469–74. [Useful review of the evidence for use of bisphosphonates.]

Twycross R, *et al.* (2007). *Palliative care formulary*. Radcliffe Publishing, Oxford. [Useful formulary for drugs commonly used in palliative care.]

Whiffen PJ, *et al.* (2007). Oral morphine for cancer pain. *Cochrane Database Syst Rev*, **4**, CD003868. [Systematic review of the effectiveness of morphine in managing cancer pain.]

Wong R, Whiffen PJ (2002). Bisphosphonates for the relief of pain secondary to bone metastases. *Cochrane Database Syst Rev*, **2**, CD002068. [Systematic review of the role of bisphosphonates in managing bone pain.]

SECTION 32

Biochemistry in medicine

Biochemistry in medicine—reference intervals: the use of biochemical analysis for diagnosis and management

P. Holloway and Heather Stoddart

Essentials

Biochemistry, biochemical testing, and specialist biochemical practitioners have an important role in clinical practice in both diagnosis and management, as emphasized by the fact that some discussion of biochemical testing appears in almost every chapter of this book. Included in this chapter are (1) a listing of the reference intervals (formerly termed reference ranges) for the most widely used biochemical tests, with conversion factors included (where appropriate) to convert intervals from SI to conventional units, and their grouping into organ system profiles in common usage; (2) description of the pitfalls and limitations of interpretation of reference intervals; and (3) some commonly used protocols for dynamic function tests.

Introduction

Biochemistry in medicine (variously known as chemical pathology, clinical biochemistry, or biochemical medicine) emerged from core clinical medicine in the middle of the 20th century and has developed into a major clinical pathology discipline. Huge advances in molecular and systems biology, analytical chemistry, and applied technology have placed this discipline in an indispensable position in medical practice. Along with these developments has been an increasing necessity for education and professional leadership in the use and interpretation of biochemistry in medicine. This chapter has been designed to assist in meeting this need.

Biochemistry in diagnosis and clinical management

Often quoted is an estimate that from 70 to 80% of clinical decisions affecting diagnosis or management are based on the results from a pathology investigation. Whatever the realistic figure for this influential role of the pathology services, the evolution of medical practice away from the reliance on 'clinical skills' and the fashion or fiscal drive to devolve clinical decision making to personnel with a lower level of training in clinical diagnostics necessitates a greater requirement for assistance from the diagnostics services. On a purely quantitative basis, the chemical pathology service predominates in this process and on the basis of the technology in use, this is increasing and spreading to embrace other pathology disciplines including immunology and microbiology.

Limitations

The results of biochemical analyses are used in screening for disease, as well as in diagnosis and for monitoring the response to therapy in established disease. Much diagnostic weight often rests on single determinations and patterns of biochemical tests. To this end it is important to consider biological variations between healthy individuals, inherent variations in laboratory methods, and the errors of sampling and hospital practice, which can influence every determination. The first (and the last) are the provinces of the physician ordering the test. The second is the concern of the laboratory, which provides quality assurance and the reference intervals for the test.

Point-of-care testing (POCT) is an important growth area in diagnostic pathology, particularly in the critical care environment. Technology has advanced to enable rapid analytical turnaround times in POCT, usually far less than 10 min from sample withdrawal to result, with consequent speeding up of clinical decision making. The laboratory's responsibility and functions for interpretation and overseeing test results are therefore partially devolved to the nurse or doctor at the bedside. As a result, there is greater need for an understanding of the appropriate reference intervals as well as of any limitations on the analytical precision when compared to central laboratory methods.

'Normal range' and 'abnormal' results

Clinical diagnostic decisions may depend equally upon finding a 'normal' result for any test requested. The physician should be clear as to the meaning of these terms. An important task of the clinical biochemist is therefore to provide relevant sets of reliable reference data. For any individual, the ideal reference value for an analyte should be that obtained when that individual is healthy, but in practice laboratory test results are interpreted by comparison to traditional but often inadequately defined reference intervals (formerly termed 'normal' ranges). The wide belief that biological data assume a Gaussian distribution is inappropriate. Most biological data are not symmetrically distributed and require statistical tools that assume other kinds of distribution or are independent of the form of the distribution. Ideally, each laboratory should establish sets of reference intervals derived from the local reference population, but this is seldom a practical option, particularly with restrictions on the use of surplus samples without patient consent, and reliance on intervals provided by diagnostic reagent companies has tended to become the norm.

Reference intervals

Reference intervals should not be used as a simple discriminator of 'normal' and 'abnormal' results; rather, results of biochemical investigations should always be interpreted in the context of the specific patient and the specific questions being posed. The significance of an 'abnormal' result may be evaluated by consideration of the evidence base for the diagnostic or discriminatory power of the test. This requires the application of likelihood ratios, a measure of the discriminatory power of the test. If the pretest odds of disease is known (usually equivalent to the prevalence of disease in a population appropriate to the patient), this can be multiplied by the likelihood ratio of the test to give the post-test odds of disease (either positive or negative). A test with a likelihood ratio of 1 is useless. The further the likelihood ratio from 1, the higher the discriminatory power of the test. Although this is rarely possible at the bedside, and there is little evidence of this kind for the usefulness of many older tests in wide use, the physician should be aware of this method of assessing the usefulness of a test and the importance of a positive or negative result.

Historically, many textbooks quoted a 'reference range' defined as the mean ± 2 standard deviations from the mean of results obtained from the reference population. This is, however, not now the commonest method applied to clinical biochemistry tests. Many of the 'intervals' quoted in clinical practice are in fact derived from a skew distribution calculated from the geometric mean to include

95% of values obtained from what is considered to be a 'healthy' population (95% confidence intervals). The merits of a diagnostic test are determined by the relationship between the data for healthy and unhealthy populations. By whatever criteria it is obtained, the reference interval is compounded of both physiological variation and the irreducible error. However, if this criterion of health (i.e. biochemical results within 95% limits for the given value) is applied to multiple tests in any individual, then with a battery of say 12 tests, only 50% of 'normal' individuals will be found to be 'healthy'. An important example of the limitations of strict referral to the 'reference interval' is highlighted by plasma total cholesterol measurements within certain populations, where established reference intervals may be considered to contain a considerable proportion of individuals with 'undesirable' or 'unhealthy' values. In such situations, it may be appropriate to define an 'ideal' or 'optimum' range for that variable. During pregnancy, intervals for variables such as creatinine, urea, uric acid, calcium, and albumin may decrease by more than 30%, and reproductive hormones change throughout pregnancy and during the menstrual cycle. Other difficulties arise from situations where the reference interval has not been constructed from a population of matched ethnic composition.

In conclusion, the use of the following tables of reference intervals for biochemical tests must include an appreciation of the limitations in reference intervals that derive from analytical variation (differences between methods of analysis), biological variables such as gender, age, posture and diet, as well as sampling, that contributes to such an operation. The diagnostics services are often criticized for failing to unify reference intervals for easy comparison of results from different laboratories, but the above-mentioned limitations illustrate the difficulties in achieving such a solution with adequate safety. In the UK a task force called Harmony has been established to achieve consensus for this. The physician should constantly bear in mind the need to see individual results of laboratory tests in their clinical context and not to hesitate to question an unexpected or unlikely result.

The reference intervals given here are established for laboratory investigations available at NHS hospitals in the United Kingdom, most of them from St Mary's Hospital (Imperial College Healthcare NHS Trust) in West London. Throughout the tables, intervals are given in Système International d'Unités (SI) and 'conventional' units together, wherever possible, with the factor for conversion from SI to conventional. The International medical community failed shamefully in the 1970's to agree on universal units of measurement for clinical practice and with globalization this now carries considerable clinical risk and needs urgent attention.

Table 32.1.1 Everyday tests (adult)

Determination	Sample	SI units		Conversion factor (SI to conventional)	Conventional units	
Alcohol						
Legal limit (UK)	P	<17.4	mmol/L	× 4.6	<80	mg/dL
Albumin	P	35–51	g/L	× 0.1	3.5–5.1	g/dL
Ammonia	p	10–50	µmol/L	× 1.4	14–70	µg/dL
Bilirubin	P	<17	µmol/L	× 0.058	<1.0	mg/dL
Bicarbonate[a]	P	22–27	mmol/L	× 1	22–27	mEq/L
Calcium						
Ionized	P	1.0–1.25	mmol/L	× 4.0	4.0–5.0	mg/dL
Total[b]	P	2.15–2.55	mmol/L	× 4.0	8.6–10.2	mg/dL
Chloride	P	95–105	mmol/L	× 1	95–105	mEq/L
Cholesterol[c]	P	See Table 32.1.10	mmol/L	× 38.6	See Table 32.1.10	mg/dL
Creatinine	P	60–125	µmol/L	× 0.011	0.66–1.375	mg/dL
eGFR [d]						
Normal GFR	P	>90	mL/min/1.73m^2			
Stage 1 CKD	P	>90	mL/min/1.73m^2	(with other evidence of chronic kidney damage)		
Stage 2 CKD	P	60–89	mL/min/1.73m^2	(with other evidence of chronic kidney damage)		
Stage 3 CKD	P	30–59	mL/min/1.73m^2			
Stage 4 CKD	P	15–29	mL/min/1.73m^2			
Stage 5 CKD	P	<15	mL/min/1.73m^2			
Ferritin	S	45–674	pmol/L	× 0.445	20–300	µg/L
Glucose (fasting)[e]	P	3.0–5.5	mmol/L	× 18	54–99	mg/dL
Glycated haemoglobin (HbA1C) (DCCT)[i]	B	<6.0%	%	× 1	<6.0%	%
HbA1c (IFCC)	B	<42	mmol/mol Hb	× 1	<42	mmol/mol Hb
Iron	S	9–29	µmol/L	× 5.59	50–162	µg/dL
Transferrin saturation	S	16–55%	%		16–55%	%
Lactate (venous)[b]	P	0.9–1.8	mmol/L	× 9.0	8.1–16.2	mg/dL
Magnesium	P	0.65–1.0	mmol/L	× 2.0	1.3–2.0	mEq/L
Osmolality	P	283–295	mosm/kg	× 1	283–295	mosm/kg
Phosphate (inorganic)[f]	P	0.8–1.4	mmol/L	× 3.1	2.48–4.30	mg/dL
Potassium[f]	P	3.5–5.0	mmol/L	× 1	3.5–5.0	mEq/L
Protein (total)	P	60–80	g/L	× 0.1	6.0–8.0	g/dL
Sodium	P	135–145	mmol/L	× 1	135–145	mEq/L
Troponin I[g]	P	<0.04	ng/mL	× 1	<0.04	ng/mL
Troponin T[h]	P	<0.01	ng/mL	× 1	<0.01	ng/mL
Urea	P	2.5–6.6	mmol/L	× 2.8	7.0–18.5	mg/dL
Uric acid	P	150–450	µmol/L	× 0.0169	2.5–7.6	mg/dL

B, whole blood; F, female M, male; P, plasma; S, serum; U, urine.

[a] See Table 32.1.4.

[b] Avoid use of tourniquet.

[c] Targets now quoted from JBS2—*Heart* (2005) **91**, Suppl V.

[d] eGFR (estimated glomerular filtration rate) calculated according to 4-variable MDRD equation; chronic kidney disease (CKD) as defined by UK guidelines for the management of CKD. For restrictions see Table 32.1.15.

[e] Collection tube must contain inhibitor of glycolysis (e.g. fluoride and oxalate).

[f] Avoid delayed separation and conditions inducing haemolysis (e.g. heat extremes, agitation).

[g] To exclude myocardial infarction 12–24 h from onset of chest pain.

[h] Same use as Troponin I. (Roche method.)

[i] Recommended target in diabetic patients is 7.5% or 58 mmol/mol Hb (Hb, Haemoglobin).

Table 32.1.2 Diagnostic enzymes

Enzyme		Sample	Reference intervals[b]	
Alkaline phosphatase[a]		P	30–130	U/L
Alanine-transaminase (ALT (SGPT))		P	<40	U/L
Amylase		P	<70	U/L
Angiotensin-converting enzyme (ACE)		S	20–90	U/L
Aspartate-transaminase (AST (SGOT))		P	<40	U/L
Creatine kinase (CK)		P	24–190	U/L
γ-Glutamyl transferase (GGT)[a]	M	P	11–50	U/L
	F	P	11–42	U/L
Lactate dehydrogenase (LDH) (total)		P	50–450	U/L
Pseudocholinesterase		P	2.25–6.9	kU/L

SGOT, serum glutamate oxaloacetate transaminase; SGPT, serum glutamate pyruvate
transaminase; other abbreviations as Table 32.1.1.
[a] Adult values. See Table 32.1.5 for intervals in paediatrics.
[b] Enzyme reference intervals are assay-dependent. Check with local laboratory.

Table 32.1.3 Organ system profiles: commonly used profiles and
supplementary components

Organ/system	Plasma/serum unless indicated	Function or process dysfunction demonstrated by test
Liver	Albumin	Estimate of protein synthesis
	Alkaline phosphatase (ALP)	Bile duct membrane transport and enzyme synthesis
	Alanine-transaminase (ALT(SGPT))	Hepatocellular damage
	Bilirubin	Ion transport, haemoglobin metabolism and bile duct integrity
	γ-Glutamyl transferase (γGT)	Bile duct membrane transport and enzyme synthesis
	Total protein	Estimate of protein and globulin synthesis
Other liver 'function' tests	Aspartate-transaminase (AST(SGOT))	Hepatocellular damage (less specificity than ALT)
	Bile acids	Hepatic blood flow and bile acid clearance
	Prothromin time	Clotting factor synthesis
Bone	Alkaline phosphatase	Osteoblast activity (total activity and thus relatively poor organ specificity)
	Calcium	Calcium homeostasis
	Phosphate	Phosphate homeostasis
	Albumin	For adjustment of total calcium to estimate ionized calcium
Other bone 'markers'	Bone-specific alkaline phosphatase (BALP)	Osteoblast activity (tissue specific, bone formation)
	Calcium (urine)	Calcium homeostasis

Table 32.1.3 (*Cont'd*) Organ system profiles: commonly used profiles
and supplementary components

Organ/system	Plasma/serum unless indicated	Function or process dysfunction demonstrated by test
	N-Telopeptide (urine) (NTX)	Bone resorption
	C-Telopeptide (CTX)	Bone resorption
	Procollagen 1N peptide (P1NP)	Bone formation
	Parathyroid hormone (PTH)	Key endocrine control of calcium homeostasis
	Vitamin D	Key endocrine control of calcium homeostasis
Kidney	Creatinine	Glomerular filtration rate (see eGFR in Table 32.1.1 and creatinine clearance calculation in Table 32.1.15)
	Potassium	Renal tubular function
	Sodium	Renal tubular function
	Urea	Glomerular filtration rate
Other kidney 'function' tests	Acidity (urine) (pH)	Renal tubular function/hydrogen handling
	Albumin and albumin/ creatinine (urine)	Glomerular membrane integrity, renal tubular function and endothelial damage
	Amino acids (urine)	Proximal renal tubular function
	Anion Gap (serum and urine)	Renal tubular function/acidosis
	Bicarbonate	Renal tubular function
	Chloride (serum and urine)	Renal tubular function
	Glucose (urine)	Renal tubular function
	Electrolytes (urine)	Renal electrolyte reabsorption/ function
	Osmolality (serum and urine)	Water reabsorption/concentrating ability
	Phosphate (serum and urine)	Proximal renal tubular function
	Protein and protein/ creatinine (urine)	Glomerular integrity
	Retinol binding protein (urine) (RBP)	Renal tubular function
Cardiac	Brain natriuretic peptide (BNP)	Heart failure
	Creatine kinase (MB isoenzyme) (CKMB)	Ischaemia: relatively poor cardiac specificity
	Myoglobin	Ischaemia: early but relatively poor cardiac specificity
	Troponin (I or T)	Ischaemia/injury: good cardiac specificity
Skeletal muscle	Aspartate transaminase (AST (SGOT))	Muscle damage/inflammation/ ischaemia: poor specificity

Table 32.1.3 *(Cont'd)* Organ system profiles: commonly used profiles and supplementary components

Organ/system	Plasma/serum unless indicated	Function or process dysfunction demonstrated by test
	Creatine kinase (CK)	Muscle damage/inflammation/ischaemia
Basic immune 'function' tests	Immunoglobulins (IgG, IgA and IgM)	B-cell activity and immunoglobulin synthesis
	Complement (C3 and C4)	Complement activation and synthesis
	C 1 inhibitor (antigenic)	C1 inhibitor (production and complement synthesis)
	C1 inhibitor (functional)	C1 inhibitor function
Specific immune 'function' tests	Specific antibodies: e.g. tetanus, *Haemophilus influenzae* type b, pneumococcal	Pinpoint pathogen specific antibody defects
	Lymphocyte subsets (T, B, and NK)	Cellular immunity
	Lymphocyte function tests	Cellular immune function
	Nitroblue tetrazolium test (NBT test)	Neutrophil oxidative burst function (innate immunity)
	CH100 and AP100	Classical and alternative complement pathway defects
	Mannose binding lectin (MBL)	Bacterial infection susceptibility (especially in children)
	Interferon-γ release assays	*Mycobacterium tuberculosis* exposure

Table 32.1.4 Blood gases

	SI units		Conversion factor (SI to conventional)	Conventional units	
Anion gap	12–16	mmol/L	× 1	12–16	mEq/L
$(Na^+ + K^+)—(HCO_3^- + Cl^-)$					
Arterial CO_2 ($PaCO_2$)	4.7–6.0	kPa	× 7.52	35–45	mmHg
Mixed venous CO_2 ($PvCO_2$)	5.5–6.8	kPa	× 7.52	41–51	mmHg
Arterial oxygen (PaO_2)	12.0–14.5	kPa	× 7.52	90–109	mmHg
Mixed venous oxygen (PvO_2)	4.0–6.0	kPa	× 7.52	30–45	mmHg
Newborn arterial oxygen	5.3–8.0	kPa	× 7.52	40–60	mmHg
H^+ ion activity	36–44	nmol/L	× 1	36–44	nmol/L
Arterial pH	7.35–7.45	pH units	× 1	7.35–7.45	pH units
Bicarbonate					
arterial—whole blood	19–24	mmol/L	× 1	19–24	mEq/L
venous—plasma	22–28	mmol/L	× 1	22–28	mEq/L
cord blood	14–22	mmol/L	× 1	14–22	mEq/L
Base excess	±2	mmol/L	× 1	±2	mEq/L
Strong ion difference (apparent) (SIDa)	38–42	mmol/L	× 1	38–42	mEq/L
$(Na^+ + K^+ + Ca(i)^{2+} + Mg(i)^{2+})—(lactate^- + Cl^-)$					

(i), ionized.

Table 32.1.5 Paediatric reference intervals (for immunoglobulins see Table 32.1.6)

	Sample	SI units		Conversion factor (SI to conventional)	Conventional units	
Alkaline phosphatase						
(p-nitrophenylphosphate method at 37°C)						
<1 year	P	71–247	IU/L	× 1	71–247	IU/L
1–5 years		105–275	IU/L	× 1	105–275	IU/L
5–10 years		90–290	IU/L	× 1	90–290	IU/L
10–16 years		30–317	IU/L	× 1	30–317	IU/L
Ammonia[a]						
0–4 weeks		10–100	µmol/L	× 1.4	14–140	µg/dL
>1 month		10–50	µmol/L	× 1.4	14–70	µg/dL
Aspartate transaminase (AST)						
<1 year	P	<50	IU/L	× 1	<50	IU/L
1–5 years		<45	IU/L	× 1	<45	IU/L
>5 years		<40	IU/L	× 1	<40	IU/L
Bicarbonate						
Infants	P	18–22	mmol/L	× 1	18–22	mEq/L
Older children		22–27	mmol/L	× 1	22–27	mEq/L
Bilirubin[b]						
First week of life	P	100–200	µmol/L (total)	× 0.058	6–11.6	mg/dL
After first week of life		<17	µmol/L (total)	× 0.058	<0.99	mg/dL
Throughout childhood		<5	µmol/L (direct)	× 0.058	<0.29	mg/dL
Calcium						
<1 year	P	2.13–2.62	mmol/L	× 4.0	8.52–10.48	mg/dL
1–5 years		2.20–2.53	mmol/L	× 4.0	8.80–10.12	mg/dL
5–10 years		2.17–2.58	mmol/L	× 4.0	8.68–10.32	mg/dL
10–16 years		2.21–2.57	mmol/L	× 4.0	8.84–10.27	mg/dL
β-Carotene[b]						
<1 year (upper limit falls with age up to 3.5 years)	S	1.3–6.3	µmol/L	× 53	69–334	µg/dL
3.5 years onwards		1.9–2.8	µmol/L	× 53	101–148	µg/dL
Creatinine[c]						
Cord blood	P	57–100	µmol/L	× 0.011	0.6–1.10	mg/dL
<1 year		19–66	µmol/L	× 0.011	0.21–0.73	mg/dL
1–5 years		22–72	µmol/L	× 0.011	0.24–0.79	mg/dL
5–10 years		34–88	µmol/L	× 0.011	0.37–0.97	mg/dL
10–16 years		44–108	µmol/L	× 0.011	0.48–1.19	mg/dL
Creatinine clearance						
3–13 years	U and P	94–142	mL/min per 1.73 m^2			
Creatine kinase (CK) (method: CK Boehringer at 37°C)						
Neonates	P	75–400	U/L	× 1	75–400	U/L
Infants 3–12 months		10–145	U/L	× 1	10–145	U/L
Children 1–15 years		15–130	U/L	× 1	15–130	U/L

Table 32.1.5 *(Cont'd)* Paediatric reference intervals (for immunoglobulins see Table 32.1.6)

	Sample	SI units		Conversion factor (SI to conventional)	Conventional units	
γ-Glutamyl transferase (GGT)						
0–1 month	P	12–271	U/L	× 1	12–271	U/L
1–2 months		9–159	U/L	× 1	9–159	U/L
2–4 months		7–98	U/L	× 1	7–98	U/L
4–7 months		5–45	U/L	× 1	5–45	U/L
7–12 months		4–27	U/L	× 1	4–27	U/L
1–15 years		3–30	U/L	× 1	3–30	U/L
Glucose (fasting)[d,e]						
Cord	P	2.5–5.3	mmol/L	× 18.0	45–95	mg/dL
Premature/low birth weight		1.1–3.3	mmol/L	× 18.0	20–60	mg/dL
Neonate		1.67–3.3	mmol/L	× 18.0	30–60	mg/dL
1 day		2.2–3.3	mmol/L	× 18.0	40–60	mg/dL
1–7 days		2.8–4.6	mmol/L	× 18.0	50–83	mg/dL
>7 days		3.3–5.5	mmol/L	× 18.0	60–100	mg/dL
Homovanillic acid (HVA): urine[f]						
Upper limits of normal in children:						
0–1 years	U	25	mmol/mol creat	× 1.6	40	μg/mg creat
1–3 years		17	mmol/mol creat	× 1.6	27	μg/mg creat
3–5 years		16	mmol/mol creat	× 1.6	26	μg/mg creat
5–8 years		14	mmol/mol creat	× 1.6	23	μg/mg creat
8–11 years		11.1	mmol/mol creat	× 1.6	18	μg/mg creat
>11 years		7		× 1.6	11	μg/mg creat
Lactate[e]	P—venous	0.5–2.2	mmol/L	× 9	4.5–19.8	mg/dL
	P—arterial	0.5–1.6	mmol/L	× 9	4.5–14.4	mg/dL
	B	0.5–1.7	mmol/L	× 9	4.5–15.3	mg/dL
	CSF	<2.8	mmol/L	× 9	<25.2	mg/dL
Phosphate (inorganic)[g,h]						
<1 year	P	1.60–2.90	mmol/L	× 3.1	5.0–9.0	mg/dL
1–5 years		1.25–1.90	mmol/L	× 3.1	3.9–5.9	mg/dL
5–10 years		1.25–1.70	mmol/L	× 3.1	3.9–5.3	mg/dL
10–16 years		0.8–1.70	mmol/L	× 3.1	2.5–5.3	mg/dL
Potassium[h]						
Newborn	P	up to 6.6	mmol/L	× 1	Up to 6.6	mmol/L
>1 month–6 years		4.1–5.6	mmol/L	× 1	4.1–5.6	mmol/L
Boys 7–16 years		3.3–4.7	mmol/L	× 1	3.3–4.7	mmol/L
Girls 7–16 years		3.4–4.5	mmol/L	× 1	3.4–4.5	mmol/L
Sweat sodium[i]		<70	mmol/L	× 1	<70	mEq/L
Sweat chloride[i]		<40	mmol/L	× 1	<40	mEq/L
Total protein						
1st month	P	51	g/L (mean)			
1st year		61	g/L (mean)			
1–6 years		61–78	g/L			
7–16 years		66–82	g/L			

(Continued)

Table 32.1.5 *(Cont'd)* Paediatric reference intervals (for immunoglobulins see Table 32.1.6)

	Sample	SI units		Conversion factor (SI to conventional)	Conventional units	
Thyroid-stimulating hormone (TSH)						
(outside neonatal period)[j]	S	0.5–5.0	mU/L	×1	0.5–5.0	µU/mL
Uric acid						
<1 year	P	0.06–0.24	mmol/L	× 16.8	1.0–4.0	mg/dL
1–5 years		0.18–0.29	mmol/L	× 16.8	3.0–4.9	mg/dL
5–10 years		0.12–0.36	mmol/L	× 16.8	2.0–6.0	mg/dL
10–16 years		0.16–0.39	mmol/L	× 16.8	2.7–6.6	mg/dL
Vanillylmandelic acid (VMA): urine[c]						
Upper limits of normal in children:						
0–1 years	U	13.9	mmol/mol creat	× 1.76	24.5	µg/mg creat
1–3 years		11	mmol/mol creat	× 1.76	19.4	µg/mg creat
3–5 years		10.5	mmol/mol creat	× 1.76	18.5	µg/mg creat
5–8 years		10	mmol/mol creat	× 1.76	17.6	µg/mg creat
8–11 years		7.5	mmol/mol creat	× 1.76	13.2	µg/mg creat
>11 years		7	mmol/mol creat	× 1.76	12.3	µg/mg creat

Creat, creatinine; other abbreviations as Table 32.1.1.

[a] Requires extra care in cleaning collection site and particularly avoidance of contamination with urine.

[b] Avoid exposure to light.

[c] Values depend also on gestational age.

[d] Typical definition of hypoglycaemia: low birth wt, <1.5 mmol/L × 18.0 <27 mg/dL; normal wt, 0–3 days, <1.7 mmol/L × 18.0 <31 mg/dL; >3 days, <2.2 mmol/L× 18.0 <40 mg/dL (SI units, conversion factor, conventional units, respectively).

[e] Collection tube must contain inhibitor of glycolysis (e.g. fluoride and oxalate).

[f] Collection must be into bottles containing acid.

[g] Affected by diet—particularly milk feed.

[h] Avoid delayed separation and conditions inducing haemolysis (e.g. heat extremes, agitation).

[i] Requires extra care in cleaning collection site with deionized water.

[j] TSH is elevated in the first few days of life reaching normal levels by day 5.

Table 32.1.6 Serum immunoglobulins

	Age	IgG (g/L)	IgA (g/L)	IgM (g/L)
Cord		5.2–18.0	< 0.02	0.02–0.20
Weeks	0–2	5.0–17.0	0.01–0.08	0.05–0.2
	2–6	3.9–13.0	0.02–0.15	0.08–0.4
	6–12	2.1–7.7	0.05–0.4	0.15–0.7
Months	3–6	2.4–8.8	0.10–0.5	0.2–1.0
	6–9	3.0–9.0	0.15–0.7	0.4–1.6
	9–12	3.0–10.9	0.2–0.7	0.6–2.1
Years	1–2	3.1–13.8	0.3–1.2	0.5–2.2
	2–3	3.7–15.8	0.3–1.3	0.5–2.2
	3–6	4.9–16.1	0.4–2.0	0.5–2.0
	6–9	5.4–16.1	0.5–2.4	0.5–1.8
	9–12	5.4–16.1	0.7–2.5	0.5–1.8
	12–15	5.4–16.1	0.8–2.8	0.5–1.9
Adult	15–45	6.0–16.0	0.8–2.8	0.5–1.9
	> 45	6.0–16.0	0.8–4.0	0.5–2.0

Values from *Handbook of clinical immunochemistry*, 9th edition 2007. PRU publications, Sheffield.

Table 32.1.7 Hormones

	Sample	SI units		Conversion factor (SI to conventional)	Conventional units	
ACTH[d]	P	3.3–15.4	pmol/L	× 4.55	15–70	ng/L
Adrenaline (epinephrine)[a,b]	P	0.03–1.31	nmol/L	× 183	5.5–240	pg/mL
Adrenaline (epinephrine)[c]	U	<100	nmol/24 h	× 0.183	<18.3	µg/24 h
Aldosterone						
Recumbent	P	100–450	pmol/L	× 0.03	3–14	ng/dL
Midday		100–800	pmol/L	× 0.03	3–24	ng/dL
Aldosterone	U	10–50	nmol/24 h	× 0.36	4–18	mg/24 h
Aldosterone/renin	P	<800	ratio		<24	ratio
Antidiuretic hormone (ADH)	P	0.2–2.0	pmol/L	× 1	0.2–2.0	ng/L
Brain natriuretic peptide (BNP)[d,e]	P	<29	pmol/L	× 3.45	100	ng/L
Catecholamines[c]	U	<2.6	µmol/24 h	× 169	<440	µg/24 h
Cortisol[a]						
00.00 h (midnight)	S	80–280	nmol/L	× 0.036	3–10	µg/dL
09.00 h		280–700	nmol/L	× 0.036	10–25	µg/dL
Free	U	<280	mmol/24 h	× 0.036	<10	µg/dL
Follicle-stimulating hormone (FSH)						
F—follicular phase	P/S	0.5–5.0	U/L	× 1	0.5–5.0	mIU/mL
F—ovulatory peak		8–15	U/L	× 1	8–15	mIU/mL
F—luteal phase		2–8	U/L	× 1	2–8	mIU/mL
F—post-menopausal		>30	U/L	× 1	>30	mIU/mL
M		0.5–5.0	U/L	× 1	0.5–5.0	mIU/mL
Growth hormone[a] (HGH)	S	<20	mU/L	× 1	<20	µU/mL
Homovanillinic acid (HVA)[c]	U	<43	µmol/24 h	× 0.18	<8	µg/24 h
Human chorionic gonadotrophin (HCG)	S	<5	U/L	× 1	<5	mIU/mL
Insulin (fasting)	P	<100	pmol/L	× 0.15	<15	µU/mL
Insulin C-peptide	P	<0.4	nmol/L	× 3.0	<1.2	ng/mL
(fasting) [b]		(undetectable in hypoglycaemia)				
Insulin-like growth factor-1 (IGF-1)	P	9–40	nmol/L	× 0.131	1.18–5.2	ng/dL
Luteinizing hormone						
F—pre-menopausal	P/S	6–13	U/L	× 1	6–13	mIU/mL
F—follicular phase		3–12	U/L	× 1	3–12	mIU/mL
F—ovulatory peak		20–80	U/L	× 1	20–80	mIU/mL
F—luteal phase		3–16	U/L	× 1	3–16	mIU/mL
F—post-menopausal		>30	U/L	× 1	>30	mIU/mL
M		3–8	U/L	× 1	3–8	mIU/mL
Metanephrine (metadrenaline) [c]	U	<2	µmol/24 h	× 0.195	<0.39	mg/24 h
(adults)	U (24h)	0.03–0.69	mmol/mol creat	× 1.74	0.05–1.20	µg/mg creat
3-Methoxytyramine (adults) [c]	U	<2	µmol/24 h	× 0.165	<0.33	mg/24 h
Noradrenaline[a,b]	P	0.47–4.14	mmol/L	× 169	79–700	ng/mL
Normetanephrine (normetadrenaline) [c]	U	<3	µmol/24 h	× 0.183	<0.55	ng/24 h
17-β-Oestradiol	S					
F—follicular phase		75–260	pmol/L	× 0.27	20–70	pg/mL
F—mid-cycle		370–1470	pmol/L	× 0.27	100–400	pg/mL
F—luteal phase		180–1100	pmol/L	× 0.27	50–300	pg/mL
M		<220	pmol/L	× 0.27	<60	pg/mL

(Continued)

Table 32.1.7 *(Cont'd)* Hormones

	Sample	SI units		Conversion factor (SI to conventional)	Conventional units	
Parathyroid hormone (PTH) (intact)	P (EDTA)	0.9–5.4	pmol/L	× 4.0	3.6–22	mg/dL
Procollagen 1 peptide (P1NP)						
F—pre-menopausal	P	15–60	µg/L	× 1	15–60	µg/L
F—post-menopausal		20–80	µg/L	× 1	20–80	µg/L
Procollagen type 3 (PIIINP)	P	1.7–4.2	µg/L	× 1	1.7–4.2	µg/L
Progesterone						
M	S	<5	nmol/L	× 0.314	<1.6	ng/mL
F—postovulation		15–77	nmol/L	× 0.314	4.7–24	ng/mL
F—follicular phase		<3	nmol/L	× 0.314	<1	ng/mL
17-Hydroxyprogesterone (newborn)	S	7–16	nmol/L	× 33.0	230–530	ng/dL
Prolactin [a]						
M	S	<450	U/L	× 1	<450	mIU/mL
F		<600	U/L	× 1	<600	mIU/mL
Renin activity						
Recumbent	P	0.5–2.2	pmol/mL per h	× 1.3	0.7–2.9	ng/mL per h
Erect after 30 min		3.0–4.3	pmol/mL per h	× 1.3	3.9–5.6	ng/mL per h
Random during day (depends on diuretics, salt intake, etc.)		0.5–3.5	pmol/mL per h	× 1.3	0.7–4.6	ng/mL per h
Sex-hormone binding protein (SHBG)						
M	S	17–52	nmol/L	× 0.027	0.5–1.4	µg/dL
F		35–104	nmol/L	× 0.027	1–3	µg/dL
Testosterone						
M	P/S	9–42	nmol/L	× 0.29	2.6–12.1	ng/mL
F		1–2.5	nmol/L	× 0.29	0.3–0.7	ng/mL
Thyroid-stimulating hormone	S	0.5–5.5	mU/L	× 1	0.5–5.5	mIU/mL
Thyroid-binding globulin	S	13–28	mg/L	× 1	13–28	mg/L
Free T_3 (FT$_3$)	S	3.3–8.2	pmol/L	× 65.0	214–533	pg/dL
Free T_4 (FT$_4$)	S	9–25	pmol/L	× 0.068	0.6–1.7	ng/dL
Vanillylmandelic acid (VMA) [c]	U	<35	µmol/24 h	× 0.20	<7	µg/24 h

Creat, creatinine; y, years of age; other abbreviations as Table 32.1.1.

[a] Should be collected under maximal resting conditions.

[b] Requires rapid separation and freezing.

[c] Collection must be into bottles containing acid.

[d] Method dependent and rises significantly with age.

[e] Guidelines for the diagnosis and treatment of acute and chronic heart failure, European Society of Cardiology *Eur Heart J*. 2008 Oct:29(19), 2388–442.

Table 32.1.8 Tumour markers

	Sample	Reference intervals	
α-Fetoprotein (AFP)	S	<6	kU/L
CA 125	S	<34	U/mL
CA 15–3	S	<13	kU/L
CA 19–9	S	<31	U/mL
Calcitonin	S	<2	mU/L
Carcinoembryonic antigen (CEA)	S	<5	µg/L
Chromogranin A [b]	S	<60	pmol/L
Chromogranin B [b]	S	<150	pmol/L
Gastrin [b]	S	<40	pmol/L
Glucagon [b]	S	<40	pmol/L

Table 32.1.8 *(Cont'd)* Tumour markers

	Sample	Reference intervals	
Human chorionic gonadotrophin (HCG)	S	<4	IU/L
Neurone-specific enolase (NSE)	S	<12.5	µg/L
Neurotensin [b]	S	<100	pmol/L
Pancreatic polypeptide (PP) [b]	S	<300	pmol/L
Prostatic-specific antigen (PSA)	S	<4 [a]	ng/mL
complexed PSA (cPSA)	S	<1.92 [a]	ng/mL
free PSA (fPSA)	S	<10%: high-risk	
		>20%: low-risk	
S100	S	<0.2	µg/L
Somatostatin [b]	S	<150	pmol/L
Squamous cell carcinoma antigen (SCC)	S	<1.8	µg/L
Tartrate-resistant acid phosphatase	S	<5	ng/mL
Thyroglobulin	S	<60	µg/L
Vasoactive intestinal polypeptide (VIP)[b]	S	<30	pmol/L

[a] Age-related reference ranges apply.
[b] Serum must be precipitated with aprotinin (Trasylol) or equivalent protease inhibitor immediately after venesection.

Table 32.1.9 Vitamins and related tests

Vitamin	Sample	SI units		Conversion factor (SI to conventional)	Conventional units	
Vitamin A (retinol)						
M	S	0.92–2.76	µmol/L	× 28.6	26–79	µg/dL
F		0.88–2.64	µmol/L	× 28.6	25–76	µg/dL
β-Carotene[a]						
M	S	0.01–6.52	µmol/L	× 53.7	0.5–350	µg/dL
F		0.019–2.93	µmol/L	× 53.7	12–158	µg/dL
Vitamin B						
Thiamine (B1)	P	66–200	nmol/L	× 0.034	2.22–6.74	µg/dL
as rbc thiamine diphosphate	B				275–675	ng/g Hb
Riboflavin (B$_2$)	S	100–630	nmol/L	× 0.038	4–24	µg/dL
as rbc glutathione reductase	B	6.6–17.9	U/L			
Pyridoxine (B$_6$)	P (EDTA)	20–120	nmol/L	× 0.247	5–30	ng/mL
as rbc aspartate transaminase	B	<150	% activation			
Vitamin B$_{12}$	S	92–441	nmol/L	× 1.36	125–600	ng/L
Folate	S	12–33	nmol/L	× 0.442	5.3–14.6	µg/L
	B (rbc)	362–1538	nmol/L	× 0.442	160–680	µg/L
Vitamin D metabolites	S					
25-(OH)D	deficient	<25	nmol/L	× 0.40	10	µg/L
	insufficient	25–50	nmol/L	× 0.40	10–20	µg/L
	sufficient	>50	nmol/L	× 0.40	20	µg/L
1,25-(OH)$_2$D$_3$		50–120	pmol/L	× 0.38	20–48	pg/mL
Vitamin E (α-tocopherol)						
M	S	13.0–36.2	µmol/L	× 0.043	0.56–1.56	mg/dL
F		11.6–36.7	µmol/L	× 0.043	0.50–1.58	mg/dL

rbc, red blood cells; EDTA, ethylene diamine tetra-acetic acid; other abbreviations as Table 32.1.1.
[a] For paediatric values, see Table 32.1.5.
Check with local laboratory for ideal collection conditions.

Table 32.1.10 Lipids and lipoproteins

	Sample	SI units Targets[a]			Conversion factor (SI to conventional)	Conventional units Targets		
		Minimum goal	High CVD risk goal			Minimum goal	High CVD risk goal	
Fasting								
Cholesterol[b]	P/S	<5.0	< 4.0	mmol/L	× 38.7	<194	<155	mg/dL
Triglyceride	P/S	<1.7	<1.7	mmol/L	× 88.4	<150	<150	mg/dL
Lipoproteins (as cholesterol)								
LDL	P/S	<3.0	<2.0	mmol/L	× 38.7	<116	<77	mg/dL
HDL								
M	P/S	>1	>1	mmol/L	× 38.7	>35	>35	mg/dL
F		>1.2	>1.2	mmol/L	× 38.7	>46	>46	mg/dL
Non-HDL	P/S	<4.0	<3.0	mmol/L	× 38.7	<155	<116	mg/dL
Total cholesterol/HDL								
Ideal	P/S	<5	<5	ratio		<5	<5	Ratio

HDL, high-density lipoproteins; LDL, low-density lipoproteins; other abbreviations as Table 32.1.1.
[a] Recommendations from JBS Guideline treatment targets: *Heart* (2005) **91**, Suppl V.
[b] Values increase with age.

Table 32.1.11 Specific proteins and immunoproteins

	Sample	Reference intervals	
Albumin	S/P	35–51	g/L
α_1-Antitrypsin	S	1.1–2.1	g/L
Complement			
C3	S/P	0.70–1.70	g/L
C4	S/P	0.15–0.50	g/L
Caeruloplasmin	S	0.24–0.71	g/L
C1 esterase inhibitor (antigenic)	S	150–350	mg/L
C1 esterase inhibitor (functional)	S	75–125	% normal reference sample
C-reactive protein (CRP)	S	<5	mg/L
Ferritin	S	20–300	µg/L
Fibrinogen	P	1.4–4.0	g/L
D-Dimer	S	<200	ng/mL
Haptoglobins	S	0.5–2.4	g/L
Immunoglobulins[a]			
IgG	S	5.8–16.3	g/L
IgA	S	0.7–3.5	g/L
IgM	S	0.5–2.4	g/L
IgE[b]		<120	kU/L
Mast-cell tryptase[c]	S/P[d]	2–14	µg/L
β_2-Microglobulin	S	1.2–2.4	mg/L
	U	<370	µg/L
Thyroid peroxisomal antibodies	S	<50	U/L
Transferrin	S	1.7–3.4	g/L

Abbreviations as Table 32.1.1.
[a] See Table 32.1.6.
[b] IgE specific to different antigens can be measured by immunoassay
[c] For anaphylaxis sample within 1 h and 3 h and 24 h after reaction. Systemic anaphylaxis >50 µg/L.
[d] EDTA plasma.

Table 32.1.12 Trace elements and metals

	Sample	SI units		Conversion factor (SI to conventional)	Conventional units	
Aluminium[a]	S	<0.3	μmol/L	× 27	<8	μg/L
Toxic		>7.4	μmol/L	× 27	>200	μg/L
	Dialysis fluid	<1.1	μmol/L	× 27	<30	μg/L
Arsenic	B (EDTA)	0.03–0.83	μmol/L	× 7.5	0.2–6.2	μg/dL
Bromide						
Unexposed	S	≤0.15	mmol/L	× 75	<11	mg/L
Toxic		>20	mmol/L	× 75	>1500	mg/L
Cadmium						
Non-smokers	B	2.7–10.7	nmol/L	× 0.11	0.3–1.2	μg/L
Smokers		5.6–34.7	nmol/L	× 0.11	0.6–3.9	μg/L
	U	<0.9	μmol/L	× 111.1	<100	μg/L
Chromium	S	<10	nmol/L	× 0.025	<0.25	μg/L
	U	<5	nmol/24 h	× 0.05	<0.25	μg/24 h
Cobalt	S	1.7–6.8	nmol/L	× 0.06	0.1–0.4	μg/L
	U[b]	<17.0	nmol/L	× 0.06	<1	μg/L
Copper						
0–6 months	P	3.0–11	μmol/L	× 6.54	20–72	μg/dL
6 months–6 years		14–30	μmol/L	× 6.54	92–196	μg/dL
6–12 years		12.6–25	μmol/L	× 6.54	82–164	μg/dL
Adult		11–22	μmol/L	× 6.54	72–144	μg/dL
Pregnancy		27–40	μmol/L	× 6.54	176–262	μg/dL
	U[b]	0.47–0.55	μmol/L	× 6.54	3.1–3.6	μg/L
Gold (therapeutic)	S	2.5–10.2	μmol/L	× 0.2	0.5–2.0	mg/L
Iron	S	9–29	μmol/L	× 5.5	50–160	μg/dL
Lead						
Environmental exposure						
Children	B	<1.2	μmol/L	× 20.5	<24	μg/dL
Adults	B	<1.4	μmol/L	× 20.5	<29	μg/dL
Significant exposure						
Women of reproductive age	B	≥0.1	μmol/L	× 20.5	≥20	μg/dL
Other	B	≥1.7	μmol/L	× 20.5	≥35	μg/L
Manganese[a]	B	80–200	nmol/L	× 0.057	4.6–11.4	μg/L
	S	9–24	nmol/L	× 0.057	0.5–1.3	μg/L
	U	2–27	nmol/L	× 0.057	0.1–1.5	μg/L
Mercury	B	<20	nmol/L	× 0.2	<4	μg/L
	U[b]	<50	nmol/24 h	× 0.2	<10	μg/24 h
	EMU	<5.5	nmol/mmol creat	× 2.0	<11	μg/g creat
Selenium	U	<3.8	μmol/24 h	× 7.9	<30	mg/g creat
Children [a]	P	0.44–1.43	μmol/L	× 79	35–113	μg/L
Adults [a]	P	0.89–1.65	μmol/L	× 79	70–130	μg/L
Silver	B	<2.8	nmol/L	× 0.107	<0.3	μg/L
Thallium	B	<5	nmol/L	× 0.2	<1	μg/L
	U	<5	nmol/L	× 0.2	<1	μg/L
Zinc	S	11–24	μmol/L	× 0.065	0.7–1.6	mg/L
	U	4.5–9	μmol/24 h	× 0.065	0.3–0.6	mg/24 h

EMU, early-morning urine sample; creat, creatinine; other abbreviations as Table 32.1.1.

[a] Usually requires special trace element free collection tube provided by laboratory.

[b] 24-h collection into bottle previously washed with nitric acid. Check with local laboratory for ideal collection conditions.

Table 32.1.13 Urinary and faecal reference intervals

	SI units		Conversion factor (SI to conventional)	Conventional units	
Aldosterone	10–50	nmol/24 h	× 0.36	4–18	µg/24 h
Albumin	<80	mg/24 h	× 1	<80	mg/24 h
M	<2.5	mg/mmol creat	× 12	<30	mg/g creat
F	<3.5	mg/mmol creat	× 12	<42	mg/g creat
Amylase					
secretion rate	<14	IU/h	× 1	<14	IU/h
Arginine	2–10	µmol/mol creat	× 1.49	3.0–14.9	mg/g creat
Ascorbic acid	110–170	µmol/L	× 0.179	19.7–30.4	mg/L
Calcium [d]	2.5–10.0	mmol/24 h	× 40	100–400	mg/24 h
	<0.75	mmol/mmol creat	× 40	<30	
Chloride	110–250	mmol/24 h	× 1	110–250	mEq/24 h
Copper[b]	0.047–0.55	µmol/24 h	× 6.54	3–35	µg/24 h
Cortisol	20–300	nmol/24 h	× 0.036	0.72–10.8	µg/24 h
Creatinine[e]	7–18	mmol/24 h	× 0.11	1–1.9	g/24 h
Cystine	5–25	µmol/mmol creat	× 2.0	10–50	mg/g creat
Faecal elastase	>200	µg/g dry weight	× 1	>200	µg/g dry weight
Glucose	0.06–0.84	mmol/L	× 18.0	1.1–15.1	mg/dL
Homovanillic acid (HVA) [d]	8–42	µmol/24 h	× 0.18	1.4–7.6	µg/24 h
Hydroxyindole acetic acid (5-HIAA) [d]	<40	µmol/24 h	× 0.19	<7.6	mg/24 h
Iron	<1.8	µmol/24 h	× 0.56	<1	mg/24 h
Lead	<0.4	µmol/L	× 200	<80	µg/L
Lysine	5–30	µmol/mmol creat	× 1.28	6.4–38.4	mg/g creat
Methylhistamine	10–25	ng/µmol creat			
β_2-Microglobulin[a]	<370	µg/L	× 1	<370	µg/L
Magnesium	0.6–4.8	mmol/24 h	× 24.5	15–118	mg/24 h
Ornithine	2–10	µmol/mmol creat	× 1.1	2.2–11	mg/g creat
Osmolality[f]	100–1000	mosm/kg	× 1	100–1000	mosm/kg
Oxalate [d]	0.1–0.46	mmol/24 h	× 9.0	0.9–4.14	mg/24 h
Phosphate (inorganic)	15–50	mmol/24 h	× 0.03	0.5–1.5	g/24 h
Porphyrins—urine[c]					
Coproporphyrin	50–350	nmol/24 h	× 0.67	34–234	µg/24 h
Porphobilinogen	<10	umol/24 h	× 0.23	<2.3	mg/24 h
Uroporphyrin	<49	nmol/24 h	× 0.83	<41	µg/24 h
Porphyrins—faeces[c]					
Uroporphyrin	<1200	nmol/24 h	× 0.83	<1000	µg/24 h
Coproporphyrin	<306	nmol/24 h	× 0.65	<199	µg/24 h
Protoporphyrin	<2.67	µmol/24 h	× 561	<1500	µg/24 h
Total porphyrin	10–200	nmol/g dry weight			
Potassium—urine [g]	20–60	mmol/L	× 1	20–60	mEq/L
	40–120	mmol/24 h	× 1	40–120	mEq/24 h
Potassium—faecal	~5	mmol/24 h	× 1	~5	mEq/24 h
Protein	<100	mg/24 h	× 1	<100	mg/24 h

Table 32.1.13 *(Cont'd)* Urinary and faecal reference intervals

	SI units		Conversion factor (SI to conventional)	Conventional units	
Sodium—urine [g]	50–125	mmol/L	× 1	50–125	mEq/L
	100–250	mmol/24 h	× 1	100–250	mEq/24 h
Sodium—faecal	<10	mmol/24 h	× 1	<10	mEq/24 h
Urea	250–500	mmol/24 h	× 0.06	15–30	g/24 h
Uric acid[e]	<5.0	mmol/24 h	× 0.167	<0.84	g/24 h
Vanillylmandelic acid (VMA) [d]	<35	μmol/24 h	× 0.20	<7	μg/24 h
Zinc	2.1–11	μmol/24 h	× 65.5	137–720	μg/24 h

mmol creat, mmol of creatinine. Other abbreviations as Table 32.1.1.

[a] Must be kept alkaline.
[b] 24-h collection into bottle previously washed with nitric acid.
[c] Avoid exposure to light.
[d] Collection must be into bottles containing acid.
[e] Partially influenced by diet.
[f] Range of young adults, declines with age.
[g] Urine electrolyte results must be interpreted in the light of concomitant serum electrolyte results.
Check with local laboratory for ideal collection conditions.

Table 32.1.14 Cerebrospinal fluid

	SI units		Conversion factor (SI to conventional)	Conventional units	
Glucose[a]	3.3–4.4	mmol/L	× 18.0	59–79	mg/dL
Protein	0.4–1.2	g/L	× 1	0.4–1.2	g/L
Lactate[a]	0.8–1.9	mmol/L	× 9.0	7.2–17.1	mg/dL
Tau protein	3–5	mg/L	× 1	3–5	mg/L
Xanthochromia[b,c]	Net bilirubin absorbance (NBA) ≤0.007 AU				

[a] Collection tube must contain inhibitor of glycolysis (e.g. fluoride and oxalate).
[b] Avoid exposure to light
[c] To exclude subarachnoid haemorrhage, specimen taken at least 12 h after onset of symptoms. NBA calculated according to the Chalmers modification of the Chalmers and Kiley method. See Cruikshank A *et al.* (2008). Revised national guidelines for analysis of cerebrospinal fluid for bilirubin in suspected subarachnoid haemorrhage, *Ann Clin Biochem*, **45**, 238–44.

Table 32.1.15 Dynamic function tests

Creatinine clearance	Normal: 90–120 mL/min Calculation:	[urine creatinine (mmol/L) × vol. (mL/min)]/ [plasma creatinine (mmol/L)]	
Renal functional capacity (GFR)	Male	age 20	105–270 mL/min per 1.73 m^2
		age 50	95–138 mL/min per 1.73 m^2
		age 70	70–110 mL/min per 1.73 m^2
	Female	age 20	104–158 mL/min per 1.73 m^2
		age 50	90–130 mL/min per 1.73 m^2
		age 70	74–114 mL/min per 1.73 m^2
Estimated GFR (eGFR) (see Table 32.1.1)			
Cautions for use for eGFR: Not suitable for: age <18 years, critically ill, pregnancy, malnourished, or patients with muscle loss.			
For age <18 years may use Schwartz equation requiring patient's age, sex, serum creatinine, and height. Same clinical restrictions for use apply.			
Maximum concentrating ability 800/1200 mosm/kg			
Minimum urinary pH 5.3 (after acid load)			

Table 32.1.15 *(Cont'd)* Dynamic function tests

Tubular phosphate reabsorption	Urine collection 08.00–12.00 h + plasma (fasting)			
(TRP)	Calculation:	TRP = 1—(phosphate clearance/ creatinine clearance) =		
		1– [(urine phosphate × plasma creatinine)/ (urine creatinine × plasma phosphate)] × 100		
		Adults† >80%		
Maximum tubular phosphate reabsorption (TM phosphate/GFR)	Calculated from nomogram[a] using TRP (decimal) and plasma phosphate			
		TM phos/GFR: adults,[b] 0.8–1.35 mmol/L (2.5–4.2mg/dL)		
Ischaemic lactate test	Fasting lactate:	0.5–1.5 mmol/L (4.5–13.5mg/dL)		
	Immediate post-exercise:	approximately 5 mmol/L (45mg/dL)		
	25 min post-exercise:	return to normal		
	Type V glycogen storage disease:	no response to exercise		
Dexamethasone suppression of adrenal cortex	(1) Overnight dexamethasone suppression—dose 2 mg at 24.00 h			
	Plasma cortisol at 09.00 h <200 nmol/L			
	(2) High dose: 2 mg dexamethasone every 6 h			
	NB Pituitary-dependent Cushing's disease: plasma and urine often gives values below 50% of basal level. Other aetiologies result in values above 50%			
Short Synacthen (tetracosactride)	Dose—0.25 mg IM:	plasma cortisol >580 nmol/L (>21 μg/dL) or increase of		
		>250 nmol/L (>9 μg/dL) at 30 and/or 60 minutes		
Depot Synacthen (tetracosactride + zinc)	Dose—1 mg IM:	Normal cortisol >900 nmol/L (>32.4 μg/dL) at 4–6 h:		
		ACTH-deficient patients may only reach this value at 24 h or after further injections.		
		Addison's disease results in <10% increment over basal at any of these times, even after further injections		
Response to insulin hypoglycaemia (plasma glucose <2.2 mmol/L (40 mg/dL)) plasma cortisol >600 nmol/L (>22 μg/dL) or 2× basal				
Growth hormone	(1) Fasting:	<20 mU/L		
	(2) Glucose suppression (75 g):	60 min, 90 min, 120 min: <5 mU/L		
	(3) Insulin hypoglycaemia:	peak >20 mU/L		
Glucose and insulin	Overnight fasting:	glucose 3.0–5.0mmol/L (54–90 mg/dL)		
	Overnight fasting:	plasma insulin 2–13 mU/mL (mean 5 mU/mL)		
Diabetes/impaired glucose tolerance(initial screen)	**Diabetes likely:**	**Diabetes uncertain**		**Diabetes unlikely**
Fasting venous plasma glucose	≥7.0 mmol/L (126 mg/dL)	≥5.5 mmol/L (100 mg/dL) and <7.0 mmol/L (126 mg/dL)		<5.5mmol/L (100mg/dL)
Random venous plasma glucose (follow-up—asymptomatic)	≥11 mmol/L (198 mg/dL)	≥5.5 mmol/L (100 mg/dL) and < 11.1 mmol/L (200 mg mg/dL)	<5.5mmol/L (100mg/dL)	
	Retest with fasting glucose (FG)	Oral Glucose Tolerance Test (OGTT)		Repeat FG if borderline

Table 32.1.15 *(Cont'd)* Dynamic function tests

Oral glucose tolerance test (OGTT)—Fasting plasma glucose (t=0), 75 g glucose orally followed by plasma glucose at 2 h (t=2 h) (60-min sample optional)[c]

Fasting glucose	2-h Glucose		Interpretation
≥7.0 mmol/L (126mg/dL)	and/ or	≥11.1 mmol/L (200mg/dL)	Diabetes Mellitus
≥6.1 mmol/L (110 mg/dL) and <7.0 mmol/L (126mg/dL)	and/ or	≥7.8 mmol/L (140 mg/dL) and <11.1 mmol/L (200 mg/dL)	Impaired glucose tolerance (IGT)
≥6.1 mmol/L (110 mg/dL) and <7.0 mmol/L (126mg/dL)	and	<7.8 mmol/L (140 mg/dL)	Impaired fasting glycaemia (IFG)

GFR, glomerular filtration rate; GTT, glucose tolerance text; IM, intramuscular; PCre, plasma creatinine; PPhos, plasma phosphate; UC, urine creatinine; UP, urine phosphate.
[a] From Walton and Bijvoet (1975). *Lancet*, **ii**, 309–10.
[b] Paediatric intervals are given in Kruse, Kracht, and Göpfert (1982). *Arch Dis Child*, **57**, 217–23.
[c] WHO (2006). *WHO definition, diagnosis and classification of diabetes mellitus and its complications.* WHO, Geneva.

Table 32.1.16 Therapeutic drugs

	Sample	SI units		Conversion factor (SI to conventional)	Conventional units	
Amikacin						
Trough	S	≤17	µmol/L	× 0.59	≤10	µg/mL
Peak		34–51	µmol/L	× 0.59	20–30	µg/mL
Amitryptiline	S	289–903	nmol/L	× 0.28	80–250	µg/L
Carbamazepine	P	17–43	µmol/L	× 0.235	4–10	µg/mL
Clonazepam[a]	fluoride/ oxalate	79–248	nmol/L	× 0.317	25–85	µg/L
Digoxin[b]	S	1–2.5	nmol/L	× 0.78	0.8–2.0	ng/mL
Ethosuximide	P	280–570	µmol/L	× 0.14	40–80	µg/mL
Gentamicin						
trough: adult	S	≤2	µmol/L	× 0.48	≤1	µg/mL
trough: neonate		≤4	µmol/L	× 0.48	≤2	µg/mL
peak		10–31	µmol/L	× 0.48	5–12	µg/mL
Lamotrigine	S	3.9–58.6	µmol/L	× 0.256	1–15.0	µg/mL
Lithium[c]						
Therapeutic	S	0.5–1	mmol/L	× 1	0.5–1	mEq/L
Toxic	S	>2.0	mmol/L	× 1	>2.0	mEq/L
Primidone	P	<59	µmol/L	× 0.22	<13	µg/mL
Phenobarbital	P	43–130	µmol/L	× 0.23	10–30	µg/mL
Phenytoin	P	40–80	µmol/L	× 0.24	10–20	µg/mL
Sodium valproate	P	0.35–0.70	µmol/L	× 144	50–100	µg/mL
Theophylline	P	55–110	µmol/L	× 0.18	10–20	µg/mL
Vancomycin						
trough	S	7–10	µmol/L	× 1.44	10–15	µg/mL
peak		29–58	µmol/L	× 1.44	20–40	µg/mL

Abbreviations as Table 32.1.1.
[a] NB: based on predose sample.
[b] NB: therapeutic range—sample taken at least 6h after dose
[c] NB: therapeutic range—sample taken at least 12h after dose.
Check with local laboratory for ideal collection conditions.
Samples should be taken predose, usually at least 6h after dose.

Table 32.1.17 Common drug toxicology

	Sample	SI units		Conversion factor (SI to conventional)	Conventional units	
Amphetamine	P	>1500	nmol/L	× 0.135	>200	μg/L
Cocaine	P	>3300	nmol/L	× 0.303	>1000	μg/L
Methadone	P	>6.5	μmol/L	× 310	>2000	μg/L
Paracetamol[a] (acetaminophen) (risk of liver damage)	P	>1.3	mmol/L	× 151	>200	mg/L
Salicylate (therapeutic limit)	P	<1.8	mmol/L	× 138	<250	mg/L

Abbreviations as Table 32.1.1.

[a] Sample taken 4-h post overdose.

SECTION 33

Acute medicine

33.1

Acute medical presentations

John D. Firth, David A. Warrell, and Timothy M. Cox

1 Heart and circulation

1.1 Cardiac arrest

See Chapter 17.1 in main text.

Clinical features	History
	(1) Sudden collapse
	Examination
	(1) Patient unresponsive
	(2) Airway, breathing—no respiration or agonal breathing
	(3) Circulation—pulse not palpable
Immediate management	See Figs. 33.1.1 and 33.1.2

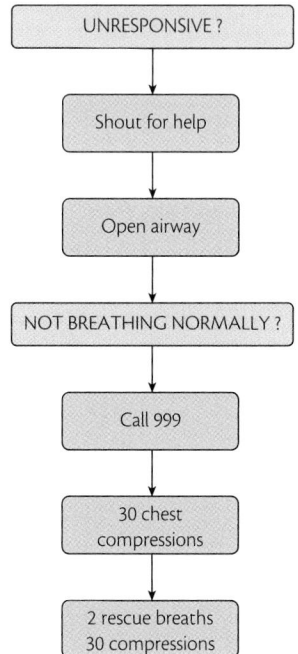

Fig. 33.1.1 The adult basic life support algorithm for use of a single rescuer out of hospital. (Note—'999' is the telephone number for emergency services in the United Kingdom.)
Reproduced with permission from the Resuscitation Council UK.

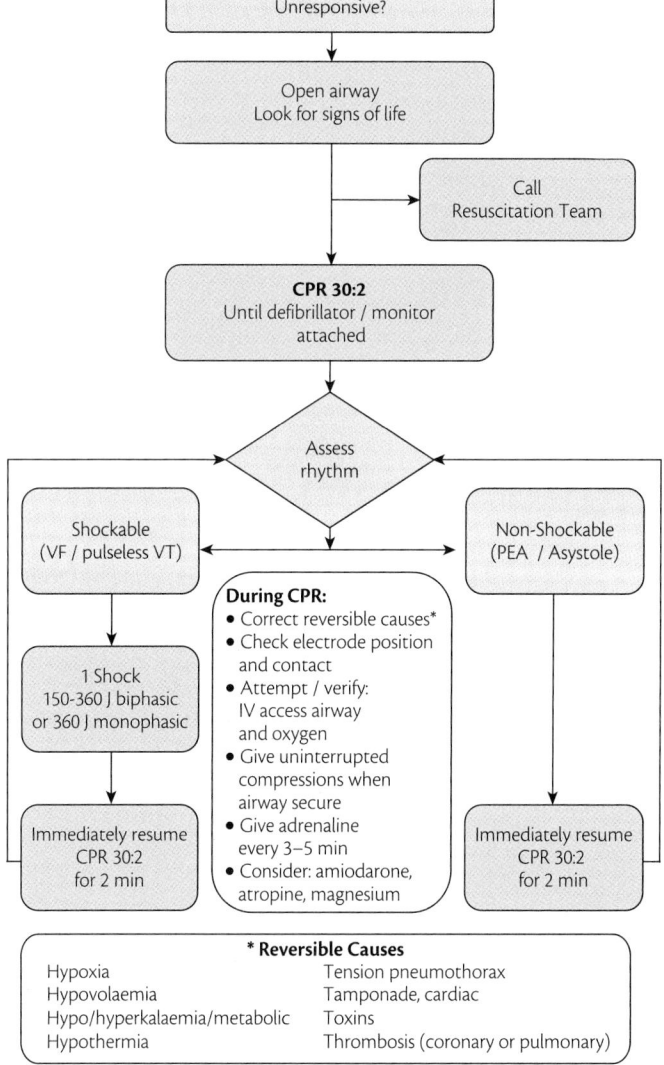

Fig. 33.1.2 The advanced life support algorithm.
Reproduced with permission from the Resuscitation Council UK.

1.2 Cardiorespiratory collapse: the patient *in extremis*

See Chapter 17.3 in main text.

Clinical features	**History** A patient who is *in extremis* is unlikely to be able to give a lucid history and may die during (unwise) interrogation, but the following clues may be elicited and be very useful diagnostically: (1) Chest pain—suggests myocardial infarction or other cardiorespiratory catastrophe (2) Chest and back pain—dissection of thoracic aorta must be seriously considered (3) Abdominal pain—suggests ruptured abdominal aortic aneurysm or other intra-abdominal emergency (4) Recent surgery—pulmonary embolism likely (5) High fever/rigors—suggests infective cause (6) Recent travel to relevant area—malaria until proven otherwise
	Examination Airway and breathing: (1) Is the airway patent? (2) Is the patient making a respiratory effort, and is the chest expanding with it? (3) Is the chest expanding symmetrically? Could there be a tension pneumothorax? (trachea deviated, mediastinum shifted, absent breath sounds on hyperinflated side of the chest; see 2.3 below) (4) Widespread crackles in the chest—suggests pulmonary oedema in this context (see 1.8 below). (5) Does the patient look as though they could keep this breathing up for the next 10 min?—If not, the patient is very likely to need respiratory support. Call for assistance from the ICU immediately

	Circulation
	(1) Do the peripheries feel cold or warm?—if warm, sepsis is likely
	(2) Pulse rate and rhythm—if rate <60/min or >120/min, consider whether arrhythmia is primary cause of hypotension
	(3) Blood pressure (BP)
	   ◆ Is there severe postural dizziness, a postural rise in pulse rate (>30 beats/min) or postural drop in BP (>20 mmHg) if the patient is moved from lying to being propped up? These indicate significant intravascular volume depletion in this context.
	   ◆ Does BP fall substantially on inspiration? If so, indicates large intrathoracic pressure swings with breathing (likely in upper airway obstruction or asthma) or cardiac tamponade
	(4) What is the jugular venous pressure (JVP)?
	   ◆ If low, indicates intravascular volume depletion or dilated circulation
	   ◆ If high, suggests primary cardiorespiratory problem

	General: (1) Rash—purpura suggests meningococcal or other septicaemia (2) Temperature—high fever suggests infection (3) Loss of left radial pulse, or BP lower in left arm than right arm, indicates aortic dissection (4) Abdominal tenderness/peritonism—suggests ruptured abdominal aortic aneurysm or other intra-abdominal emergency
	See Table 33.1.1 for further information
Immediate management	Airway and breathing: (1) Ensure airway is clear: consider oropharyngeal airway (2) Oxygen—high flow, with reservoir bag if needed, to achieve PaO_2 >92% (3) If tension pneumothorax, decompress immediately (see Chapter 33.1.2, 'Chest decompression') (4) Give intravenous (IV) naloxone (0.8–2.0 mg repeated at intervals of 2–3 min to a maximum of 10 mg) if there is any suspicion that patient has received opioids (5) Consider elective intubation and ventilation
	Circulation: Obtain IV access using a safe technique (see Chapter 33.1.2) Also: begin resuscitation according to volume status as indicated in Table 33.1.2 (1) Insert urinary catheter and monitor fluid input/output hourly in any patient with cardiorespiratory collapse. (2) Give broad spectrum antimicrobial cover to any patient with unexplained cardiorespiratory collapse, e.g. coamoxiclav 1.2g IV 6–8 hrly, as dictated by clinical suspicion of likely pathogen (see 7.7 below)
Key investigations	See Table 33.1.1
Further management	Determined by underlying condition

Table 33.1.1 Examination and investigation of the patient with cardiorespiratory collapse

Diagnosis		Key finding on examination	Key initial investigation	Definitive investigations
Cardiovascular	Myocardial infarction	No specific findings likely	ECG	ECG, cardiac enzymes
	Arrhythmia	Pulse rate and rhythm	ECG	ECG
	Aortic dissection	Absence or reduction in one or more peripheral pulse, especially left radial. Blood pressure lower in left arm than right	CXR showing widened mediastinum	Imaging of aorta, usually by CT or trans-oesophageal echocardiography
	Cardiac tamponade	Raised JVP. Pulsus paradoxus (pulse becomes impalpable on inspiration in extreme cases)	CXR may show globular heart. ECG may show low voltage complexes or electrical alternans	Echocardiography
Cardiorespiratory	Pulmonary embolus	Raised JVP. Right ventricular heave. Loud P2. Right ventricular gallop rhythm. Signs of DVT in leg	ECG may show features of acute right heart strain	Imaging of pulmonary vessels by CT (or ventilation / perfusion scanning, or [rarely] pulmonary angiography).
	Pulmonary oedema	Gallop rhythm, crackles	CXR	Usually cardiac—ECG, echocardiography
Respiratory	Tension pneumothorax	Tracheal deviation. Hyperexpansion of one side of chest. Mediastinal shift. Absent breath sounds on one side of chest	CXR—but should be treated on basis of clinical diagnosis (see text)	CXR—but should be treated on basis of clinical diagnosis (see text)
	Pneumonia	May have high fever. Signs of consolidation or pleurisy	CXR	CXR, blood culture, serological tests
	Asthma	Wheezes, but beware of silent chest	Response to treatment (β-agonist), but CXR excludes pneumothorax and other respiratory diagnoses	Peak flow measurements before and after β-agonist
	Exacerbation of COPD	Features of COPD	A clinical diagnosis, but CXR excludes other respiratory diagnoses	See Chapter 18.8
Abdominal	Gastrointestinal haemorrhage	Usually obvious, but don't forget rectal examination for blood/melaena in the patient with unexplained hypotension	A clinical diagnosis	Endoscopy
	Perforated viscus	Peritonism	Erect chest radiograph to look for free air under diaphragm	CT scan or laparotomy, depending on clinical situation
	Pancreatitis	Peritonism. Bruising in flanks	Serum amylase	Imaging of pancreas, usually by CT scan
	Ruptured abdominal aortic aneurysm	Peritonism. Palpable aneurysm. Bruising in flanks	A clinical diagnosis.	CT scan or laparotomy, depending on clinical situation
Sepsis		May have high fever. May have warm peripheries and bounding pulse, but could be cold and shut down. No specific findings likely, but look for rash or localized infection, e.g. abscess. Malaria if relevant travel history	A clinical diagnosis	Blood culture
Metabolic	Many possible causes, e.g. renal failure, hepatic failure, profound acidosis, but collectively these are rare causes of presentation with cardiorespiratory collapse	May have evidence of organ failure, or of drug overdose. May have no specific findings	Electrolytes, renal and liver function tests. Blood gases	As indicated following initial tests
Anaphylaxis		Facial, tongue and throat swelling. Stridor. Wheeze. Urticarial rash. Skin erythema or extreme pallor	A clinical diagnosis	Serum mast cell tryptase. Specific IgE for suspect allergens. See Chapter 17.2 for further discussion

COPD, chronic obstructive pulmonary disease; CXR, chest radiograph; GCS, Glasgow Coma Scale; JVP, jugular venous pressure.

Notes:

(1) Primarily neurological disorders may compromise the airway or ventilation, but rarely cause cardiovascular collapse. If a patient with cardiovascular collapse has a severely depressed conscious level (GCS <8) or focal neurological signs, then the assumption—until proven otherwise—should be that the neurological impairment is secondary to the cardiovascular collapse and not the cause of it.

(2) See other sections in Chapter 33 for further details of conditions listed in this table.

Table 33.1.2 Immediate clinical response to determination volume status in the patient with cardiorespiratory collapse

Main problem	Key clinical signs	Immediate management
Hypotension	Peripheries cool and shut down Postural rise in pulse rate ostural hypotension Low jugular venous pressure Lungs clear	Intravenous fluid (balanced salt solution, 0.9% saline or plasma expander) given rapidly (0.5 litre boluses) until there is clear evidence that physical signs are being restored to normal, then slow rate infusion
Breathing difficulty	High jugular venous pressure Gallop rhythm Basal crepitations	Do not give fluid Sit up Consider intravenous loop diuretic and/or venodilator Consider need for ventilation
Hypotension and breathing difficulty	Peripheries cool and shut down High jugular venous pressure May be gallop rhythm Basal crepitations	Will almost certainly need urgent ventilation Call for help from ICU/anaesthetist before the patient suffers cardiorespiratory arrest Trial of fluid infusion may be appropriate: give 250 ml of 0.9% balanced salt solution, saline or plasma expander, keeping patient under continuous observation and terminating infusion immediately in the event of clinical deterioration

ICU, intensive care unit.

Notes:

(1) All patients should be given high flow oxygen.

(2) Vigorous attempts should be made to diagnose and treat the underlying condition concurrent with efforts to resuscitate.

(3) Is resuscitation being effective in restoring organ perfusion? Do not forget the value of the urinary catheter: if the patient is passing urine, then their kidneys are being perfused effectively.

(4) If the patient remains hypotensive despite 'optimization' of intravascular volume then consideration can be given to the use of inotropes and vasoactive agents: see Chapter 17.4 for further discussion.

1.3 ST-segment elevation acute myocardial infarction (STEMI)

See Chapters 16.13.5 and 16.13.6 in main text.

Clinical features	**History** (1) Ischaemic chest pain (2) Cardiorespiratory collapse (3) May be nonspecific or silent, especially in elderly people or in diabetics
	Examination May be normal, but look for: (1) 'Pump failure'—cool peripheries, hypotension (2) Pulmonary oedema—see section 1.8 below (3) Cardiac—gallop rhythm, murmurs
Immediate management	If cardiorespiratory collapse, as described in 1.2 above Otherwise: (1) Oxygen—high flow, with reservoir bag if needed, to achieve PaO$_2$ >92% (2) Give aspirin 300 mg orally, chewed or dispersed in water (if not given before admission to hospital) (3) Give clopidogrel 300 mg orally (4) Analgesia—give adequate pain relief, e.g. (a) diamorphine by slow IV injection at 1 mg/min, usual maximum initial dose is 5 mg, but may be repeated if necessary, or (b) morphine by slow IV injection at 2 mg/min, usual maximum initial dose is 10 mg, but may be repeated if necessary. Both to be accompanied by appropriate antiemetic, e.g. metoclopramide 10 mg IV over 1–2 min, or cyclizine 50 mg IV over 1–2 min (caution in severe heart failure) (5) Reperfusion therapy—immediate triage to (a) primary percutaneous coronary intervention (PCI), if available in a timely manner (within 90 min of patient call) (Table 33.1.3), or (b) thrombolysis, if primary PCI not available (Table 33.1.4)
Key investigations	To establish the diagnosis: (1) ECG—looking for ST segment elevation and/or (presumed or proven) new bundle branch block (2) Cardiac biochemical markers (troponins, CK-MB) Other important tests: (1) As indicated by clinical examination, e.g. chest radiograph to look for pulmonary oedema; echocardiography to assess LV function or cause of pansystolic murmur (?mitral valve dysfunction, ?ventricular septal defect) (2) Assess modifiable risk factors for ischaemic heart disease, e.g. cholesterol

Further management	Consider:

Consider:
(1) Antiplatelet agents and anticoagulants
- Aspirin (75–325 mg daily)—continue long term (if not contraindicated)
- Clopidogrel (75 mg daily)—continue for at least 1 month after thrombolysis, or as determined by the type of stent implanted (if not contraindicated)
- Glycoprotein IIb/IIIa inhibitors—e.g abciximab, eptifibatide, tirofiban—are indicated in patients managed with primary PCI, but not after fibrinolysis
- Anticoagulants—patients treated with fibrinolytic therapy should receive low molecular weight heparin or fondaparinux (a factor Xa inhibitor)

(2) β-Blockade
- Early—if no contraindication (e.g. hypotension, heart failure, heart block) give, e.g. atenolol 5 mg IV over 5 min, repeated after 10–15 min
- Long term—if no contraindication continue oral β-blockade for at least 2–3 years

(3) Angiotensin converting enzyme (ACE) inhibition (or angiotensin receptor blockade)
- Early—start within 24 h in patients who are normotensive and continue for at least 5–6 weeks
- Long term—recommended for any patient with left ventricular dysfunction

(4) Lipid lowering—long-term treatment with statin will benefit most patients with coronary heart disease.
(5) Control of diabetes—evidence supports use of insulin in hospital and in the early post-hospital phase to maintain good control

Notes
(1) Treat complications, e.g. venodilator or diuretic for pulmonary oedema. Severe heart failure/shock may require ventilation, inotropes ± intra-aortic balloon pump
(2) Patients with diabetes will benefit from intensive insulin therapy during admission with acute myocardial infarction and afterwards
(3) For all patients: give advice regarding lifestyle issues before and after discharge from hospital—smoking, diet, exercise, management of obesity —also regarding resumption of normal activities. Consider referral to cardiac rehabilitation services
(4) Consider need for specialist cardiological opinion and/or investigation by cardiac stress test (e.g. treadmill exercise tolerance test) and/or coronary angiography

Table 33.1.3 Indications for primary percutaneous coronary intervention (PCI)

Primary PCI is the best management for STEMI when it can be performed:[a]
(1) within 60–90 min of admission
(2) by individuals skilled in the procedure (>75 cases/year)
(3) in a high-volume centre (>200 cases/year)

Primary PCI is specifically indicated when there is:
(1) Contraindication to thrombolysis
(2) Haemodynamic compromise

Primary PCI should be considered as:
(3) Salvage procedure after failed thrombolytic therapy

[a] American College Cardiology/American Heart Association guidelines.

Table 33.1.4 Thrombolysis in acute myocardial infarction (AMI)

Indications

Must satisfy three criteria:
(1) Typical chest pain at rest for >20 min
(2) ST elevation in two contiguous leads (≥1 mm inferiorly, ≥2 mm anteriorly), or (presumed or proven) new bundle branch block
(3) Within 12 h of onset, but consider at 12–24 h if continuing pain

Contraindications

Absolute contraindications
(1) Bleeding—active internal bleeding; proven active peptic ulcer
(2) Brain—cerebrovascular accident within the past 6 months (or at any time if haemorrhagic stroke); known intracranial neoplasm or aneurysm
(3) Suspected aortic dissection
(4) Uncontrolled hypertension—SBP >180 mmHg or DBP >110 mmHg after pain relief and nitrates
(5) Pregnancy

Relative contraindications
(1) Recent (<6 weeks) major trauma/surgery/injury or traumatic resuscitation (>10 min or sufficient to fracture rib)
(2) Symptoms suggesting active peptic ulceration
(3) Defective haemostasis
(4) Lactation/peripartum

Table 33.1.4 (Cont'd) Thrombolysis in acute myocardial infarction (AMI)

(5) Severe liver disease/oesophageal varices
(6) Severe renal disease
(7) Bacterial endocarditis
(8) Acute pancreatitis
(9) On warfarin with INR outside therapeutic range

Note that the following are not contraindications:
(1) Proliferative diabetic retinopathy
(2) Previous cardiopulmonary resuscitation, unless this is prolonged (>10 min) or associated with obvious trauma
(3) Therapeutic anticoagulation

Examples of agents

(1) Recombinant tissue-type plasminogen activator, **e.g.**

Alteplase	Accelerated regimen (within 6 h of AMI): 15 mg by IV injection, followed by IV infusion of 50 mg over 30 min, then 35 mg over 60 min (lower doses in patients <65 kg). This is the reference standard for comparison of other fibrinolytic agents/regimen Standard regimen (6–12 h from AMI): 10 mg by IV injection, followed by IV infusion of 50 mg over 60 min, then 40 mg over 120 min (lower doses in patients <65 kg)
Tenecteplase	30–50 mg (6000–10 000 units, depending on body weight) by intravenous injection over 10 s. This does not require infusion pump or refrigeration and is particularly suited for pre-hospital administration
Reteplase	10 units intravenously over not more than 2 min, followed 30 min later by another 10 units intravenously over not more than 2 min
(2) Streptokinase	1 500 000 units by IV infusion over 60 min. This remains the most widely used fibrinolytic agent internationally because it is relatively cheap

DBP, diastolic blood pressure; SBP, systolic blood pressure.
Notes:
(1) Use of rt-PA is preferred if anterior AMI presenting within 6 h of onset; cardiogenic shock (SBP <80 mmHg); streptokinase given more than 5 days previously; streptokinase allergy. In some health care systems use of rt-PA is restricted to younger patients because of cost considerations
(2) Most treatment regimen use 24 h of intravenous heparin as adjunctive therapy when recombinant tissue-type plasminogen activator is used (consult product literature)
(3) Problems during streptokinase infusion: see Table 33.1.5.

Table 33.1.5 Problems during streptokinase infusion

Problem	Immediate action	Further action
Common		
Hypotension (SBP<90 mmHg)	Stop infusion until blood pressure recovers	Recommence infusion more slowly (to complete over 2 h) OR switch to rt-PA regimen (see Table 33.1.4)
Rigors	Stop infusion until rigor settles	Recommence infusion more slowly (to complete over 2 h) OR switch to rt-PA regimen (see Table 33.1.4)
Ventricular fibrillation	Cardiovert	Continue infusion at usual rate
Uncommon		
Allergic reaction	Stop infusion	Recommence infusion more slowly if possible (to complete over 2 h) OR switch to rt-PA regimen (see Table 33.1.4)
	Give hydrocortisone 100 mg IV and chlorpheniramine 10 mg IV	
Haemorrhage (major)	Stop infusion	Consider fresh frozen plasma/cryoprecipitate
Stroke	Stop infusion	Urgent CT head

1.4 Acute coronary syndrome without ST segment elevation (unstable angina/non-STEMI)

See Chapters 16.13.5 and 16.13.6 in main text.

Clinical features	**History** (1) Ischaemic chest pain at rest or on minimal exertion (2) Chest tightness/breathlessness
	Examination Usually no specific signs, but may be: (1) 'Pump failure'—cool peripheries, hypotension (2) Pulmonary oedema—breathing difficulty, pulmonary crackles (see 1.8 below) (3) Cardiac—gallop rhythm, murmurs
Immediate management	**Triage into high, intermediate, and low risk categories** ♦ High risk—(1) typical clinical features of ischaemia and ST segment depression or transient ST segment elevation; (2) troponin elevation and a high risk score (risk calculator downloadable from http://www.outcomes.org/grace or http://www.timi.org/files/riskscore/ua_calculator.htm); (3) arrhythmias or haemodynamic compromise provoked by ischaemia ♦ Intermediate or low risk—clinical features of acute coronary syndrome and nonspecific ECG changes (T wave inversion, T wave flattening, minor conduction abnormalities) ♦ Low risk or an alternative diagnosis—normal electrocardiogram, normal biomarkers, normal cardiac examination and normal echo.
	High risk category (1) Oxygen—high flow, with reservoir bag if needed, to achieve PaO_2 >92% (2) Give aspirin 300 mg orally immediately, chewed or dispersed in water (if not given before admission to hospital) (3) Give clopidogrel 300 mg orally

(4) Give glycoprotein IIb/IIIa inhibitor—e.g abciximab, eptifibatide, tirofiban—probably benefits all high risk patients; definitely indicated in those undergoing revascularization.

(5) Give anticoagulation—low molecular weight heparin—e.g. enoxaparin 1 mg/kg (100 units/kg) every 12 h, or dalteparin 120 units/kg every 12 h (maximum 10 000 units twice daily)—or bivalirudin (a direct thrombin inhibitor). Continue for 48–72 h or after coronary angiography and revascularization.

(6) Give IV or oral β-blocker (see 1.3 above) unless contraindicated. Consider heart-rate-lowering calcium antagonist (e.g. diltiazem or verapamil) if β-blocker is contraindicated or not tolerated in patient without left ventricular dysfunction

(7) Nitrate—give if ongoing pain, e.g. (a) sublingual glyceryl trinitrate (GTN), 0.3–1 mg repeated as required; (b) buccal GTN, up to 5 mg, with tablet placed between upper lip and gum and left to dissolve; (c) IV infusion of isosorbide dinitrate at initial dose of 2 mg/h (increasing as necessary to maximum of 20 mg/h to relieve pain and as limited by hypotension)

(8) Analgesia—give adequate pain relief if ongoing pain not relieved by nitrate, e.g. (a) diamorphine by slow IV injection at 1 mg/min (usual maximum initial dose is 5 mg, but may be repeated if necessary), or (b) morphine by slow IV injection at 2 mg/min (usual maximum initial dose is 10 mg, but may be repeated if necessary). Both to be accompanied by appropriate antiemetic, e.g. metoclopramide 10 mg IV over 1–2 min, or cyclizine 50 mg IV over 1–2 min (caution in severe heart failure)

(9) Continuing ischaemia or haemodynamic instability—urgent PCI

	Intermediate risk category (1) As above for high risk, except do not give glycoprotein IIb/IIIa inhibitor. Patients who develop high risk features after initial presentation should be considered for urgent angiography and revascularization (within 24–72 h). Such patients also fulfill guideline criteria for GPIIb/IIIa inhibitors (initiated prior to angiography)
	Low risk category Clinically stable patients with minor or nonspecific ECG abnormalities and a low risk score (including negative repeat troponin) are at very low risk for in-hospital major cardiac events. Such patients may nevertheless have significant underlying coronary artery disease. They require stress testing or perfusion scanning, ideally prior to discharge
Key investigations	**To establish the diagnosis** (1) ECG—looking for transient ST segment shift with pain; T wave changes are less specific and ECG may be normal (2) Cardiac biochemical markers (troponins, CK-MB)
	Other important tests As for STEMI (see 1.3 above)
Further management	(1) Aspirin (75–325 mg daily)—continue long term (if not contraindicated) (2) ACE inhibition (or angiotensin receptor blockade)—recommended for any patient with left ventricular dysfunction

(3) Lipid lowering—long-term treatment with statin will benefit most patients with coronary heart disease

Consider:

(4) Clopidogrel (75 mg/day)—consider continuing for 1 year

Notes

(1) For all patients: give advice regarding lifestyle issues before and after discharge from hospital—smoking, diet, exercise, management of obesity—also regarding resumption of normal activities. Consider referral to cardiac rehabilitation services

(2) Consider need for specialist cardiological opinion and/or investigation by cardiac stress test (e.g. treadmill exercise tolerance test) and/or coronary angiography

1.5 Dissection of the thoracic aorta

See Chapter 16.14.1 in main text.

Clinical features	**History**
	(1) Chest pain, particularly if of sudden onset, tearing in quality, and radiating to the back
	(2) Collapse
	Examination
	(1) Patient will usually look very unwell and cool peripherally. BP may be low, normal, or raised. Pulse may be slow
	(2) Look for loss/reduction of one or more peripheral pulses: most likely is compromise of the left subclavian artery. Check left radial pulse in comparison with right; measure BP in both arms; any deficit on the left strongly supports the diagnosis of aortic dissection. Examine also for reduction of carotid or femoral pulse(s)
	(3) Look for signs of new aortic regurgitation—note that the diastolic murmur may be very short
	(4) Evidence of focal ischaemia, eg. focal neurological deficit ('stroke')
	(5) Could the patient have Marfan's syndrome? (risk factor)
Immediate management	If cardiorespiratory collapse, as described in 1.2 above
	(1) The key to correct management is a high index of clinical suspicion that aortic dissection might be the diagnosis. Most patients with chest pain and circulatory collapse have acute myocardial infarction, the management for which (thrombolysis) could clearly be fatal in the patient with aortic dissection
	(2) Oxygen—high flow, with reservoir bag if needed, to achieve PaO_2 >92%
	(3) Analgesia—give adequate pain relief, e.g. (a) diamorphine by slow IV injection at 1 mg/min (usual maximum initial dose is 5 mg, but may be repeated if necessary) or (b) morphine by slow IV injection at 2 mg/min (usual maximum initial dose is 10 mg, but may be repeated if necessary). Both to be accompanied by appropriate antiemetic, e.g. metoclopramide 10 mg IV over 1–2 min, or cyclizine 50 mg IV over 1–2 min (caution in severe heart failure)

Key investigations	**To establish the diagnosis:**
	(1) CT angiography of chest
	(2) Transoesophageal echocardiography
	(3) MRI of chest
	Other important tests:
	(1) Chest radiograph—look for widened mediastinum
	(2) ECG—may have features of acute myocardial infarction (usually inferior) if dissection has compromised a coronary artery (usually right coronary artery)
	(3) Cardiac biochemical markers—to exclude acute myocardial infarction, but note that elevation of troponin can occur
	(4) Full blood count, clotting screen, electrolytes, renal and liver function tests—may give a lead to an underlying medical condition and will establish baseline
	(5) Group and save/cross-match blood
Further management	(1) Reduce BP using agents that will not cause tachycardia or increase the rate of cardiac ejection, e.g. titrate IV labetolol (initial dose 50 mg bolus, followed by 1–2 mg/min) or esmolol (50–200 µg/kg per min) to achieve systolic BP <120 mmHg. If BP remains too high, add IV infusion of sodium nitroprusside (0.5–8 µg/kg per min) after β-blockade established (pulse <60/min)
	(2) Obtain opinion from cardiothoracic surgeon: immediate surgical repair will usually be the best management for patients with dissection of the ascending aorta (Stanford type A) who are in reasonable condition, but medical treatment is generally recommended (as long as the dissection does not progress) when the ascending aorta is spared (type B)

1.6 Bradycardia

See Chapters 16.2.2 and 16.4 in main text.

Clinical features	**History**
	(1) Syncope or presyncope
	(2) Fatigue/breathing difficulty
	(3) Drugs (especially β-blockers)
	Examination
	The most important immediate issue is to decide whether or not the circulation is compromised: is the patient cool peripherally? What are the rate, rhythm, and BP? Is there pulmonary oedema (see 1.8 below)?
	If seen in the presence of bradycardia, note rate and
	(1) Abnormal rhythm, e.g. dropped beats in second-degree AV block
	(2) Other cardiovascular abnormality, e.g. cannon waves in JVP in third-degree (complete) AV block
	(3) Temperature (hypothermia—see 9.4 below)
Immediate management	Obtain ECG
	If the patient is haemodynamically compromised:
	(1) Give atropine, 0.3–1.0 mg IV, repeated as necessary
	(2) Consider isoprenaline, 0.5–10 µg/min by IV infusion
	(3) Consider temporary pacing (see Chapter 33.2, 'Cardiac pacing (temporary)')
	(4) Consider glucagon 50–150 µg/kg IV in 5% glucose in cases of β-blocker overdose, with precautions to protect the airway in case of vomiting (NB unlicensed indication and dose)

Key investigations	**To establish the diagnosis:** 12-lead ECG
	Other important tests: (1) Electrolytes (particularly potassium) (2) Cardiac biochemical markers (depending on context) (3) Chest radiograph—look at heart size and for evidence of pulmonary oedema (4) 24h ECG monitor (if symptoms intermittent and 12-lead ECG not diagnostic) (5) Echocardiography (if clinical suspicion that heart is structurally abnormal)
Further management	Dependent on diagnosis. If not reversible, likely to require permanent pacing

1.7 Tachycardia

See Chapters 16.2.2 and 16.4 in main text.

Clinical features	**History** (1) Syncope or presyncope (2) Palpitations (3) Fatigue/breathing difficulty (4) Chest pain
	Examination The most important immediate issue is to decide whether or not the circulation is compromised: is the patient cool peripherally? What are the rate, rhythm, and BP? Is there pulmonary oedema (see 1.8 below)? Physical examination is unlikely to aid diagnosis of the particular type of tachycardia, excepting for the presence of an irregularly irregular rhythm in atrial fibrillation (AF), but note the following: (1) Jugular venous pulse—absence of 'a' waves in AF; rapid flutter waves in atrial flutter; cannon waves in ventricular tachycardia (2) First heart sound—variable intensity in AF (3) A dilated heart increases the chance that tachycardia is ventricular in origin
Immediate management	(1) Obtain ECG (2) If cardiorespiratory collapse, as described in 1.2 above (3) For any tachycardia that is poorly tolerated, synchronized DC shock (under deep sedation or general anaesthesia) is the treatment of choice and usually provides rapid relief (4) Management otherwise depends upon clinical context and type of tachycardia General rule—do not give more than one antiarrhythmic drug to a patient without seeking specialist advice; if a first line antiarrhythmic drug fails, the appropriate treatment will often be to proceed to DC cardioversion
Key investigations	**To establish the diagnosis:** (1) 12-lead ECG (see Table 33.1.6) (2) Uncertain of the diagnosis of a broad complex tachycardia? See Table 33.1.7 (3) IV adenosine (administered as described below)—transient AV block may (a) reveal (but rarely terminate) atrial tachycardia/fibrillation/flutter; (b) terminate atrioventricular nodal re-entry (AVNRT) and atrioventricular re-entry tachycardias (AVRT); (c) usually have no effect on ventricular tachycardia

	Other important tests: (1) Electrolytes (particularly potassium) (2) Cardiac biochemical markers (depending on context) (3) Chest radiograph—look at heart size and for evidence of pulmonary oedema (4) 24h ECG monitor (if symptoms intermittent and 12-lead ECG not diagnostic) (5) Echocardiography (if clinical suspicion that heart is structurally abnormal) (6) Thyroid function tests (in atrial fibrillation)
Further management if severe haemodynamic compromise	**Atrial fibrillation/flutter** ◆ DC cardioversion, or ◆ Amiodarone, 5 mg/kg over 20–120 min followed by 1200 mg/24h until sinus rhythm restored (into central venous catheter), or ◆ Sotalol, 1.5 mg/kg IV over 30 min **Atrioventricular nodal re-entry (AVNRT) and atrioventricular re-entry tachycardias (AVRT) (supra-ventricular tachycardias, SVTs)** ◆ Adenosine, 3 mg by fast IV injection, if necessary followed by 6 mg (also by fast IV injection) after 1–2 min, and then by 12 mg (also by fast IV injection) after a further 1–2 min (NB contraindicated in those with asthma, and patients taking dipyridamole are very sensitive, requiring reduced initial dose of 0.5–1 mg) ◆ Verapamil, 5–10 mg by slow IV injection over 2–3 min is an alternative in patients with asthma, but NOT in those who might have ventricular tachycardia, or in those who are receiving β-blockers **Ventricular tachycardia** ◆ DC cardioversion (see 1.1 above)
Further management if no severe haemodynamic compromise	**Atrial fibrillation/flutter** Duration <48 h or transoesophageal echocardiography shows no intracardiac thrombus: ◆ Consider prompt chemical or synchronized DC cardioversion ◆ Flecainide (class 1 C) 2 mg/kg IV over 30 min if there is no evidence of ischaemic heart disease or left ventricular dysfunction ◆ Amiodarone or sotalol (class III) can be used to restore sinus rhythm and maintain it ◆ Digoxin is useful for rate control only but will not restore sinus rhythm. If digoxin is ineffective in controlling ventricular rate, and cardioversion is unsuccessful or inappropriate, consider adding verapamil or β-blocker Duration >48 h or thrombus on transoesophageal echocardiography: ◆ Anticoagulate for 4–6 weeks before synchronized DC cardioversion **Note** Atrial fibrillation arising in the context of intercurrent illness is usually best managed by treatment of the underlying medical condition and with digoxin to control ventricular rate. The patient is likely to return to sinus rhythm when the underlying condition has resolved. **Atrioventricular nodal re-entry (AVNRT) and atrioventricular re-entry (AVRT) tachycardias (supraventricular tachycardias, SVTs)** ◆ Vagal stimulation by respiratory manoeuvres (Valsalva), prompt squatting, or pressure over one carotid sinus (but not the latter in those with recent ischaemia, digoxin toxicity, or in elderly patients) ◆ Adenosine if vagal stimulation fails ◆ Other options include verapamil, β-blocker, flecainide, sotalol, or amiodarone

Ventricular tachycardia

◆ Consider synchronized DC cardioversion.
◆ Lignocaine (lidocaine) 50–100 mg as IV bolus over a few min followed immediately by infusion of 4 mg/min for 30 min, 2 mg/min for 2 h, and then 1 mg/min up to 24 h.
◆ Other antiarrhythmics that can be used include amiodarone, sotalol, procainamide and disopyramide—but seek expert help

Torsade de pointes

This form of ventricular tachycardia requires particular treatment:

◆ Discontinue predisposing drugs and avoid empirical antiarrhythmic drug treatment
◆ Give magnesium sulphate, 8 mmol of magnesium over 10–15 min, repeated once if necessary
◆ If torsade is associated with bradycardia and pauses, consider isoprenaline infusion or overdrive atrial/ventricular pacing to increase heart rate

Table 33.1.6 ECG criteria to distinguish VT from SVT with aberrant conduction

Feature favouring diagnosis of VT	Notes	
AV dissociation-Capture/fusion beats	The most reliable criterion for VT Both occur rarely, but their presence usually secures the diagnosis of VT	
Wide QRS complex	QRS width (s)	Predictive value for VT (%)
	<0.12	14
	0.12–0.14	43
	>0.14	100
Concordance across chest leads	QRS complexes all positive or all negative is reliable pointer to VT	
Extreme left axis deviation and/or a definite axis shift compared with previous ECGs	Strong indicator of VT	

AV, atrioventricular; SVT, supraventricular tachycardia, VT, ventricular tachycardia.

Table 33.1.7 A practical clinical approach to broad-complex tachycardia

Clinical	Note	Working diagnosis
History	Myocardial infarction, ischaemic heart disease, or congestive heart failure present	VT
ECG	Features in Table 33.1.6 present	VT
Effect of adenosine	Inconclusive	VT
(given as described in section 1.7)	Reversion of tachycardia	AVNRT or AVRT (SVTs). May also reveal (but unlikely to revert) atrial flutter or fibrillation

AVNRT, atrioventricular nodal re-entry tachycardia; AVRT, atrioventricular re-entry tachycardia; SVT, supraventricular tachycardia.

Notes:

(1) Wrongly diagnosing an SVT is potentially disastrous, whereas manoeuvres to treat VT are unlikely to compromise the patient with SVT.
(2) History—patients with VT can have paroxysmal self-terminating episodes that are indistinguishable from those reported by patients with SVT.
(3) Examination—the haemodynamic state of the patient cannot be used to differentiate between VT and SVT: patients with VT can be haemodynamically stable, and those with haemodynamic compromise can have SVT.

1.8 Pulmonary oedema

See Chapter 16.15.3 in main text.

Clinical features	**History** (1) Breathing difficulty (2) Orthopnoea, paroxysmal nocturnal dyspnoea Other cardiac symptoms: (3) Palpitations (4) Chest pain (5) Ankle oedema (6) Any previous cardiac history **Examination** (1) How unwell is the patient? If very ill, see 1.2 above (2) Respiratory rate, cyanosis, peripheral circulation (cold, clammy), pulse rate and rhythm (?arrhythmia, see 1.6 and 1.7 above), BP (often elevated, but may be normal or low), JVP (likely to be elevated), apex beat (displaced in congestive cardiac failure), heart sounds (gallop rhythm, murmurs), crackles and/or wheezes in chest, peripheral oedema (suggests biventricular failure in this context) (3) Pulse oximetry
Immediate management	If cardiorespiratory collapse, as described in 1.2 above: (1) Position the patient 'trunk up, legs down' (2) Oxygen—high flow, with reservoir bag if needed, to achieve Pa_{O_2} >92% (3) Give furosemide 40–80 mg IV If not improving rapidly: (4) Give either: ◆ Diamorphine by slow IV injection at 1 mg/min (usual maximum initial dose is 5 mg, but may be repeated if necessary), or ◆ Morphine by slow IV injection at 2 mg/min (usual maximum initial dose is 10 mg, but may be repeated if necessary) ◆ Both to be accompanied by appropriate antiemetic, e.g. metoclopramide 10 mg IV over 1–2 min (not cyclizine in severe heart failure) (5) Unload with IV nitrate, e.g. isosorbide dinitrate 2–20 mg/h (6) Consider continuous positive airway pressure (CPAP) mask, noninvasive ventilation, or tracheal intubation and intermittent positive pressure ventilation (IPPV)
Key investigations	**To establish the diagnosis:** Chest radiograph **Other important tests:** (1) ECG—look for arrhythmia or acute myocardial infarction (2) Cardiac biochemical markers (3) Echocardiography—visualization of left ventricular size and function, also of other structural abnormalities, e.g. valve dysfunction (4) Invasive monitoring, e.g. pulmonary artery flow-directed (Swan Ganz) catheterization—to be considered only if the patient is failing to respond or when there is genuine doubt about cardiac filling pressures or diagnosis. A pulmonary capillary wedge pressure >18 mmHg supports the diagnosis of cardiogenic pulmonary oedema
Further management	Depending on clinical context: (1) Acute myocardial infarction—see 1.3 above (2) Arrhythmia—see 1.6 and 1.7 above (3) Acute mechanical cause—e.g. aortic incompetence, mitral regurgitation, ventricular septal defect—may require surgical intervention

1.9 Deep venous thrombosis and pulmonary embolus

See Chapters 16.16.1 and 16.16.2 in main text.

Clinical features	**History** Deep venous thrombosis (DVT): (1) Calf/leg pain (2) Calf/leg swelling (3) Features to suggest PE Pulmonary embolus (PE): (1) Shortness of breath, developing over hours, days, or (sometimes) weeks (2) Pleuritic chest pain, haemoptysis (lung infarction, peripheral emboli) (3) Circulatory collapse (massive PE) (4) Features to suggest DVT Deep venous thrombosis and pulmonary embolus: (1) Previous episodes of DVT and/or PE (2) Risk factors—immobilization, recent surgery, previous episodes, malignancy, travel, family history, etc. **Examination** Deep venous thrombosis: (1) Calf/leg swelling—measure circumference 10 cm below tibial tuberosity: difference between sides of >1.5 cm likely to be significant (2) Calf tenderness; palpable cord; positive Homan's sign (3) Dilated superficial veins; leg feels warmer than the other (4) Check for signs of PE (5) Consider alternative diagnoses—especially Baker's cyst, cellulitis, haematoma in muscle Pulmonary embolus: (1) May be no abnormal signs (2) Tachypnoea (50–70% of cases), crackles (18–50%), tachycardia (24–30%), pleural rub (<10%) (3) Circulatory collapse with cool peripheries, hypotension, and cyanosis. Look particularly for signs of right heart strain: elevated JVP, parasternal heave, S3 over right ventricle, loud P2 (4) Check for signs of DVT (5) Consider alternative diagnoses—especially pneumonia, musculoskeletal pain, pneumothorax **Notes** (1) Low-grade fever is common in both DVT and PE (2) In cases of DVT or PE—perform rectal/pelvic examination (before discharge from hospital)
Immediate management	(1) If cardiorespiratory collapse, as described in 1.2 above. Note that patients with massive PE require volume expansion even though their JVP is elevated (2) If index of clinical suspicion for PE is high, give treatment dose of low molecular weight heparin pending the results of investigation
Key investigations	**To establish the diagnosis:** Tests commonly used to demonstrate the presence of thrombus/embolus are as follows: ◆ DVT—venous ultrasonography, (contrast venography) ◆ PE— contrast enhanced spiral CT scan, (lung ventilation/perfusion [VQ] scan, pulmonary angiogram) **Other important tests:** Pulmonary embolus: (1) ECG—commonest abnormality is sinus tachycardia and/or nonspecific ST segment or T wave abnormalities. Look for signs of right heart strain, e.g. T wave inversion in V1/V2, S1Q3T3, axis shift (2) Chest radiograph—look for atelectasis or pulmonary parenchymal abnormality, also pleural effusion. May be normal (3) Arterial blood gases—look for hypoxia; but normoxia does not exclude PE Deep venous thrombosis and pulmonary embolus: (1) Full blood count, electrolytes, renal and liver function tests—may give a lead to an underlying medical condition and will establish baseline (2) At a later stage a thrombophilia screen may be appropriate, also investigations dictated by clinical findings or investigations detailed above
Clinical decision-making	Many patients referred for medical opinion have a low probability of having DVT or PE and not all require imaging to exclude DVT or PE. Follow management algorithms as follows: ◆ DVT—see Table 33.1.8 ◆ PE—see Table 33.1.9

Further management	(1) Anticoagulation with low molecular weight heparin (typical dose 200 IU/kg subcutaneous o.d., but see manufacturer's instructions) or standard (unfractionated) heparin (Table 33.1.10) until oral anticoagulation (usually with warfarin, Table 33.1.11) is established
	(2) In cases with circulatory collapse consider thrombolysis, e.g.:
	  ◆ Streptokinase by IV infusion of 250 000 units over 30 min, then 100 000 units/h for 24 h, or
	  ◆ Tissue plasminogen activator, 10 mg by IV infusion over 1–2 min, followed by 90 mg over 2 h (maximum 1.5 mg/kg in patients of <65 kg)
	(3) In cases with circulatory collapse and contraindication to thrombolysis, consider catheter extraction or fragmentation of embolus, or surgical embolectomy

	Notes (1) No monitoring of low molecular weight heparin treatment is required, excepting if used in patients with chronic kidney disease when monitoring of anti-Xa levels is required. (2) Methods of reversing anticoagulation are shown in Table 33.1.12

Table 33.1.8 Pretest clinical probability scoring system and care pathway for the patient with suspected DVT

(a) Pretest probability score

Criteria	Score
Active cancer	+1
Paralysis, plaster cast	+1
Bed rest >3 days, surgery within 4 weeks	+1
Tenderness along veins	+1
Entire leg swollen	+1
Calf swollen >3 cm	+1
Pitting oedema	+1
Collateral veins	+1
Alternative diagnosis likely	−2

Pre-test probability	
Low	0
Moderate	1–2
High	≥3

(b) Management algorithm

Pretest probability score	Action	Result	Further action
0 or 1	Perform D-dimer	Negative	No further investigation
		Positive	Perform ultrasonography
2 or more	Do not perform D-dimer		
	Perform ultrasonography	Negative	Withhold treatment and repeat ultrasonography in 10–14 days. If serial ultrasonography is negative, PE rarely occurs
		Positive	Diagnosis of DVT established

DVT, deep venous thrombosis; PE, pulmonary embolism.

Notes

(1) Reprinted from *The Lancet*, Vol. 350, Wells et al, *Value of assessment of pretest probability of deep-vein thrombosis in clinical management*, pp1795–8. Copyright (1997), with permission from Elsevier.

(2) If the physician's judgement is that DVT is very likely in a particular case, then they should proceed to investigations directed at detecting thrombus in leg veins whatever the scoring algorithm would suggest. If the result of ultrasonography is negative, and repeat ultrasonography in 10 to 14 days is also negative, pulmonary embolism rarely occurs.

(3) All patients who are discharged with 'DVT excluded' should be given written information describing how they can be reassessed if symptoms worsen or fail to settle over the next few days.

Table 33.1.9 Pretest clinical probability scoring system and care pathway for the patient with suspected PE

(a) Pretest probability score

Criteria	Score
Clinical signs and symptoms of deep venous thrombosis (objectively measured leg swelling and pain with palpation of deep vein region)	+3
PE as likely or more likely than alternative diagnosis	+3
Heart rate >100/min	+1.5
Immobilization >3 consecutive days (bedrest except access to bathroom) or surgery within 4 weeks	+1.5
Previous DVT or PE	+1.5

Table 33.1.9 *(Cont'd)* Pretest clinical probability scoring system and care pathway for the patient with suspected PE

(a) Pretest probability score

Criteria	Score
Haemoptysis	+1
Malignancy (cancer patients receiving treatment within 6 months or receiving palliative treatment)	+1

Pre-test probability	
Low (c.2–4% chance of PE)	0 or 1
Moderate (c.20% chance of PE)	2–6
High (c.60% chance of PE)	>6

(b) Management algorithm

Pretest probability score	Action	Result	Further action
0 or 1	Perform D-dimer	Negative	No further investigation
		Positive	Perform contrast enhanced spiral CT (see notes)
2 or more	Do not perform D-dimer		
	Perform contrast enhanced spiral CT scan (see notes)	Negative	PE is excluded
		Positive	Diagnosis of PE established

DVT, deep venous thrombosis; PE, pulmonary embolism.

Notes

(1) Pre-test probability score from Wells *et al.* (2001). Ann Intern Med 135, 98–107. http://www.annals.org/content/135/2/98.full.pdf+html

(2) If contrast enhanced spiral CT scan is not available or is contraindicated, then an alternative strategy is to image with ventilation-perfusion lung scanning: (a) normal scan—PE is excluded; (b) low / intermediate probability scan—scan is not diagnostic and further action determined by the pretest probability as follows: (i) if pretest probability is low (score 0 or 1), then perform bilateral venous ultrasonography—if this is negative, PE can be considered excluded without further testing; (ii) if pretest probability is high (score 2 or more), and the patient has adequate cardiopulmonary reserve, then serial ultrasonography of the leg veins over 10–14 days may be performed—if this is negative, PE rarely occurs. If cardiopulmonary reserve is inadequate, proceed to a definitive diagnostic test for PE (spiral CT or pulmonary angiography) (c) High probability scan—diagnosis of PE established

(3) If the physician's judgement is that PE is very likely in a particular case, then they should proceed to investigations directed at detecting PE, whatever the scoring algorithm would suggest

(4) All patients who are discharged with 'PE excluded' should be given written information describing how they can be reassessed if symptoms worsen or fail to settle over the next few days.

Table 33.1.10 A schedule for intravenous infusion of standard (unfractionated) heparin to obtain APTT ratio 1.5–2.5

(1) Measure APTT at start of therapy

(2) Give IV loading dose of 80 IU/kg by bolus injection, followed by

(3) IV infusion of heparin at 18 IU/kg/h—dilute 25 000 units heparin to 50 ml total volume with 0.9% saline (making solution of 500 IU/ml) and give at the following rate:

Body weight (kg)	Initial rate (ml/h)
50	1.8
60	2.2
70	2.5

(Continued)

Table 33.1.10 *(Cont'd)* A schedule for intravenous infusion of standard (unfractionated) heparin to obtain APTT ratio 1.5–2.5

Body weight (kg)	Initial rate (ml/h)
80	2.9
90	3.2
100	3.6
120	4.4

(4) Check APTT 6 h after start of treatment and then at least once daily, adjusting the infusion rate according to the APTT as follows:

APTT ratio	Continue infusion at
>7.0	Stop for 30 min and then reduce by 1.0 ml/h (check APTT 4 h later)
5.1–7.0	Reduce by 1.0 ml/h (check APTT 4 h later)
4.1–5.0	Reduce by 0.6 ml/h (check APTT 4 h later)
3.1–4.0	Reduce by 0.2 ml/h
2.6–3.0	Reduce by 0.1 ml/h
1.5–2.5	No change
1.2–1.4	Increase by 0.4 ml/h
<1.2	Increase by 0.8 ml/h (check APTT 4 h later)

Note:
(1) An alternative (but less well tried) regimen is to give unfractionated heparin (250 IU/kg) subcutaneously every 12 h, adjusting the dose according to the APTT measured 6 h after dosing.

Table 33.1.11 A warfarin induction regimen

Days 1 and 2	Day 3		Day 4	
	INR	Dose	INR	Dose
Give 5 mg each evening if baseline INR <1.4	<1.5	10 mg	<1.6	10 mg
	1.5–2.0	5 mg	1.6–1.7	7 mg
	2.1–2.5	3 mg	1.8–1.9	6 mg
	2.6–3.0	1 mg	2.0–2.3	5 mg
	>3.0	0 mg	2.4–2.7	4 mg
			2.8–3.0	3 mg
			3.1–3.5	2 mg
			3.6–4.0	1 mg
			>4.0	0 mg
	and seek advice on further management		and seek advice on further management	

Table 33.1.12 Reversal of anticoagulation

Anticoagulant	Method	Notes
Standard (unfractionated) heparin	(1) Stop heparin (2) Give protamine by slow IV injection: 1 mg neutralizes 100 units of heparin if given within 15 min of heparin. Give less if a longer time has elapsed because heparin is rapidly excreted. Maximum dose of protamine is 50 mg	(1) There is no point in giving FFP or other clotting concentrates: they do not contain heparin-neutralizing activity (2) Excess protamine is anticoagulant
LMWH	(1) Stop heparin (2) Administer protamine by slow IV injection, maximum 50 mg. This is less effective at neutralizing the effect of LMW heparin than it is for standard heparin. There is no good evidence on which to base dosage	(1) There is no point in giving FFP or other clotting concentrates: they do not contain heparin-neutralizing activity (2) Excess protamine is anticoagulant
Warfarin		
Immediate reversal (e.g. patient has major bleeding with high INR)		
	(1) Stop warfarin (2) Vitamin K 5 mg (IV) (3) FFP 15 ml/kg (IV), or PCC 50 IU/kg (IV). (4) Recheck INR	(1) Large volumes of FFP (up to 2 litres) can be required to effect complete reversal of warfarin (2) PCC should be used for life-threatening bleeding (3) Continue warfarin in lower dose if risk/benefit considerations indicate that continued anticoagulation is justified when INR back in therapeutic range
Controlled reversal (e.g. high INR but patient is not bleeding or has minor bleeding only)		
	(1) INR <8. Stop warfarin. Re-check INR in 3 days (2) INR 8–12. Stop warfarin. Give vitamin K 2.5 mg p.o or 0.5 mg IV. INR rechecked in 24 h should show a fall (3) INR >12. Stop warfarin. Give vitamin K 5 mg p.o. or 1 mg IV. INR rechecked in 24 h should show a fall	

FFP, fresh frozen plasma; LMWH, low molecular weight heparin; PCC, prothrombin complex concentrates; p.o, by mouth.

1.10 Cardiac tamponade

See Chapter 16.8 in main text.

Clinical features	**History**
	(1) Shortness of breath or circulatory collapse, but there are no specific symptoms
	(2) Can follow acute myocardial infarction, aortic dissection, cardiac trauma (including iatrogenic with cardiac catheterization)
	(3) There may be evidence of a condition that can cause pericardial effusion, e.g. tuberculosis, cancer, advanced renal failure
	Examination
	The key to making this rare but very important (because treatable) diagnosis is to consider it in any patient with unexplained cardiorespiratory collapse. Signs of tamponade are:
	(1) Grossly elevated JVP—which may rise further on inspiration (Kussmaul's sign)
	(2) Pulsus paradoxus—an exaggerated fall in systolic BP on inspiration (normal <10 mmHg), but a rapid screening test for severe cases is to ask 'Does the radial pulse disappear on inspiration'?
	Evidence of a (large) pericardial effusion, although these will not be present unless there is a pre-existing effusion
	(3) Increased area of cardiac dullness
	(4) Quiet heart sounds
Immediate management	If the patient is *in extremis* proceed as in 1.2 above
	(1) Give colloid, e.g. gelofusin 500 ml by rapid IV infusion, to support BP
	(2) Perform or arrange for immediate/urgent pericardial aspiration (see Chapter 33.2, 'Pericardiocentesis')
Key investigations	**To establish the diagnosis:**
	(1) Echocardiography
	◆ The most sensitive test for the presence of pericardial fluid
	◆ Diastolic collapse of right ventricle or right atrium indicate severe circulatory embarrassment
	(2) Cytology and culture of pericardial fluid
	Other important tests:
	(1) Chest radiograph—look for globular heart (almost invariably with clear lung fields)
	(2) ECG—look for low voltage QRS complexes and electrical alternans (in large pericardial effusion) and for evidence of acute myocardial infarction
Further management	As determined by underlying condition

1.11 Accelerated ('malignant') hypertension

See Chapter 16.17.5 in main text.

Clinical features	**History**
	(1) Headache
	(2) Blurring of vision
	(3) Drowsiness
	(4) Epileptic fits
	Examination
	(1) BP—will usually be grossly elevated with diastolic pressure >130 mmHg, but note that accelerated hypertension can occur at lower pressures than this and the diagnosis is established not by a particular elevation of BP but by signs of fibrinoid necrosis
	(2) Ocular fundi
	◆ Grade III retinopathy: flame-shaped superficial haemorrhages, 'dot and blot' haemorrhages, cotton wool spots (retinal microinfarcts), hard exudates
	◆ Grade IV retinopathy: as grade III + papilloedema
	◆ Note that there is no difference in management or prognosis of patients with grade III or grade IV disease
	(3) Urine—stix testing shows proteinuria and haematuria, microscopy may show red blood cell casts
	Also look for signs of:
	(4) Pulmonary oedema—see 1.8 above
	(5) Aortic dissection—see 1.5 above
	(6) Scleroderma—scleroderma renal crisis
Immediate management	In an uncomplicated case:
	(1) Admit to hospital
	(2) Bed rest
	(3) No smoking (causes an acute rise in BP)
	(4) Aim to lower diastolic pressure into range 100–105 mmHg over 2–3 days using:
	◆ Atenolol 25–50 mg orally, or
	◆ Nifedipine 10–20 mg of modified release preparation orally (tablets, not sublingual)
	◆ Further dosing determined by response
	◆ Maximum initial fall in BP should not exceed 25% of presenting value
	In a complicated case (aortic dissection, epileptic fitting, acute pulmonary oedema, oral medication not possible):
	(1), (2), and (3)—as above
	(4) Aim to lower diastolic pressure to less than 100–110 mmHg over several hours (depending on clinical context) using:
	◆ Labetolol, initial bolus of 20 mg IV, then at 20 mg/h, increased as necessary every 30 min to maximum of 120 mg/h, or
	◆ Sodium nitroprusside (IV) at initial dose of 0.25–0.5 µg/kg per min, increasing up to 8 µg/kg per min. This must only be given to patients with aortic dissection after β-blockade has been established with, e.g. esmolol (50–200 µg/kg per min)
Key investigations	**To establish the diagnosis:**
	Accelerated hypertension is a clinical diagnosis
	Other important tests:
	(1) ECG—looking for evidence of left ventricular hypertrophy and acute myocardial ischaemia
	(2) Chest radiograph—looking for heart size, pulmonary oedema, and (if chest/back pain) for aortic dissection
	(3) Electrolytes and renal function—if serum creatinine >250 µmol/litre renal function is likely to deteriorate further (at least in the short term)
	(4) 'Autoimmune/vasculitic' serology—ANCA, ANA, etc.—for evidence of multisystem disorder that can present with accelerated phase hypertension and which (if present) will require specific treatment
	(5) CT angiography of chest if aortic dissection suspected (or other imaging, see 1.5 above)
Further management	When acute emergency is controlled, all patients who have suffered from accelerated phase hypertension require thorough investigation for secondary causes of hypertension

1.12 Anaphylactic shock

See Chapter 17.2 in main text.

Clinical features	**History** (1) Premonitory aura—apprehension, light-headedness, dizziness, tingling or itching of skin (2) Facial, tongue or throat swelling (3) Stridor or wheeze (4) Syncope or collapse (5) Exposure to precipitant—foodstuffs (e.g. peanuts), hymenopteran stings, drugs (e.g. parenteral penicillins) **Examination** (1) Cyanosis (2) Hypotension (3) Facial, tongue, or throat swelling (4) Stridor or wheeze (5) Urticaria, angio-oedema, skin erythema, or extreme pallor

Immediate management	(1) Stop any potential causative agent immediately
	(2) Oxygen—high flow, with reservoir bag if needed, to achieve PaO_2 >92%
	(3) Adrenaline (epinephrine)
	   ◆ Give 0.3–0.5 ml of 1:1000 adrenaline (0.3–0.5 mg) intramuscularly into lateral thigh, repeated every 5–10 min as needed
	If this is ineffective, or if the patient is about to die:
	   ◆ Give 5 mg adrenaline (5 ml of undiluted 1:1000 adrenaline) nebulized with oxygen, and
	   ◆ Make up 1:100 000 preparation of adrenaline by diluting 0.5 mg adrenaline (0.5 ml of 1:1000 adrenaline) to total of 50 ml with 0.9% saline and give at 0.5–1.5 ml/min, titrated according to clinical response
	(4) Fluid—give balanced salt solution or 0.9% saline, 10–20 ml/kg, as rapid IV infusion if patient is hypotensive
	Second line therapy—can be considered after cardiorespiratory stability has been achieved (but no strong evidence that they are required):
	(5) H_1-blocker, eg. chlorpheniramine 10–20 mg IV, repeated up to 40 mg in 24 h (change to oral when patient tolerates)
	(6) H_2-blocker, e.g. ranitidine 50 mg IV three times daily (change to oral when patient tolerates)
	(7) Steroid, e.g. hydrocortisone 1.5–3 mg/kg IV, then repeated four times daily (change to oral prednisolone 40 mg daily when patient tolerates)
	(8) β_2-Agonist, e.g. salbutamol 5 mg (repeated as necessary) via oxygen-driven nebulizer if bronchospasm is a persistent problem

Key investigations	**To establish the diagnosis:** (1) Anaphylaxis is a clinical diagnosis (2) Mast cell tryptase—immediately after resuscitation, after 1–2 h, and after 24 h (or convalescent) **Other important tests:** ECG, chest radiograph, electrolytes, renal function, arterial blood gases (depending on context)
Further management	(1) Patients must be observed for 4–6 h after full recovery before discharge from immediate medical care (2) Determination of allergen (if any)—refer to allergy services; advice regarding avoidance; MedicAlert bracelet (3) Instruction regarding self-injection of adrenaline and supply of appropriate medication, e.g. EpiPen

2 Respiratory

2.1 Acute on chronic respiratory failure

See Chapters 17.5, 18.8, and 18.15 in main text.

Clinical features	**History**
	(1) Chronic respiratory condition—usually chronic obstructive pulmonary disease
	(2) Recent increase in breathlessness
	(3) Evidence of infection—fever, sweats, increased sputum production, increased sputum purulence
	(4) 'Cor pulmonale'—worsening ankle oedema
	Examination
	(1) Cyanosis
	(2) Respiratory rate
	(3) Temperature
	(4) Evidence of CO_2 retention—drowsiness, asterixis, metabolic flap
	(5) Chest signs—of chronic respiratory condition, of infection, and exclude pneumothorax
	(6) Signs of cor pulmonale—elevated JVP, right ventricular heave, right ventricular gallop, loud P2, congested liver, ascites, peripheral oedema
	(7) Check PEFR if patient is able to use PEF recorder
	(8) Check pulse oximetry. Is the patient getting exhausted? Remember that a 'normal' respiratory rate in the patient who looks very tired may mean that they are close to death
Immediate management	**The patient who is extremely ill**
	If the patient is *in extremis*, proceed as in 1.2 above, with the exception that a high concentration of inspired oxygen should NOT be given to patients who are KNOWN to have acute on chronic respiratory failure. If the patient is known to have chronic respiratory failure:
	(1) Give controlled oxygen (24–28% or 1–2 litre/min by nasal prongs), aiming to achieve PaO_2 >8 kPa (60 mmHg) or Sao_2 >90% without CO_2 retention or acidosis
	(2) Initiate other aspects of management listed below
	(3) Check arterial blood gases, adjusting inspired oxygen concentration if allowed by clinical response, PaO_2, $PaCO_2$, and pH (pH, not hypoxia, is the most important factor related to survival in patients with acute on chronic respiratory failure)
	Consider need for ventilatory support:
	◆ Noninvasive positive pressure ventilation (NIV)—particularly in patients with exacerbation of COPD who have persistent respiratory acidosis (pH<7.35) despite controlled oxygen therapy and maximal medical therapy—proceeding if required and if appropriate to
	◆ Endotracheal intubation and intermittent positive pressure ventilation
	Note—if it is uncertain whether or not a patient has acute on chronic respiratory failure, then high concentration oxygen should be given to all patients who are extremely ill. All such patients require continued close monitoring of their clinical state and arterial blood gases, allowing (amongst other things) detection of the few who will have acute on chronic respiratory failure and lose their respiratory drive in response to high concentration oxygen

The patient who is moderately unwell

(1) Give controlled oxygen (24–28% or 1–2 litre/min by nasal prongs), aiming to achieve PaO_2 > 8 kPa (60 mmHg) or Sao2 >90% without CO_2 retention or acidosis. Check arterial blood gases after 30–60 min

(2) Give nebulized β_2-agonist, e.g. salbutamol 2.5–5 mg, terbutaline 5–10 mg, using air as the driving gas, repeated as required, whilst continuing to deliver oxygen by nasal prongs at 1–2 litre/min

(3) Give nebulized anticholinergic, e.g. ipratropium bromide 500 µg (can be combined with β_2-agonist), repeated as required

(4) Give corticosteroid, e.g. hydrocortisone 100 mg IV twice daily or prednisolone 30 mg orally once daily (continued for 7–14 days)

(5) Give antibiotic that will cover likely respiratory pathogens if two of the following symptoms are present—increased breathlessness, increased sputum volume, or increased sputum purulence, e.g. amoxicillin 250 mg orally three times daily or (if allergic to penicillin) clarithromycin 250–500 mg orally twice daily (IV if oral administration not possible)

(6) Give diuretic, e.g. furosemide 40–80 mg IV, if evidence of fluid overload

(7) Consider aminophylline, loading dose (in patient not previously treated with theophylline) of 5 mg/kg given IV over 20 min, then an infusion of 0.5 mg/kg per h aiming for serum concentration in the range 10–20 mg/litre

(8) Consider need for ventilatory support, usually by NIV, if patient does not improve

Note—use IV fluids to correct and prevent dehydration

Key investigations	**To establish the diagnosis:**
	(1) Chest radiograph—looking for focal consolidation and to exclude pneumothorax
	(2) Sputum culture
	To determine severity and monitor response to treatment:
	(3) Arterial blood gases
	(4) Serial measurements of peak flow
	Other important tests:
	(1) Full blood count
	(2) Electrolytes, renal and liver function
	(3) ECG
Further management	(1) Optimization of treatment for chronic pulmonary condition, usually chronic obstructive pulmonary disease
	(2) Emphasize need to stop smoking

2.2 Tension pneumothorax

See Chapters 17.3 and 18.17 in main text.

Clinical features	**History**
	(1) Collapse with extreme difficulty in breathing
	Examination
	(1) Patient looks as though they are about to die
	(2) Gasping respiratory effort
	(3) Cyanosis
	(4) Chest looks asymmetrical, being prominent on side of tension
	(5) Tracheal deviation, away from side of tension
	(6) Mediastinal shift, away from side of tension, most reliably detected by percussion of cardiac dullness
	(7) Chest is silent on side of tension, the only breath sounds being heard in the opposite axilla
Immediate management	Insert needle to decompress chest; see Chapter 33.2, 'Chest decompression'

Key investigations	**To establish the diagnosis**
	(1) Tension pneumothorax is a clinical diagnosis to be treated immediately without delay for investigation
	Note:
	◆ The signs of tension pneumothorax are not subtle, but you will not make the diagnosis unless you consider it and seek the presence of the signs listed above
	◆ If a patient appears to be dying and you think that they might have a tension pneumothorax, then—after calling for help and initiating resuscitation (see 1.1 above)—there is nothing to be lost (and potentially much to be gained) from an attempt at chest decompression
	Other important tests:
	Chest radiograph will confirm diagnosis of pneumothorax after decompression
Further management	Insertion of chest drain (see Chapter 33.2, 'Chest drain') after tension has been relieved

2.3 Upper airway obstruction

See Chapter 18.5.1 in main text.

Clinical features	**History**
	(1) Extreme difficulty in breathing
	(2) Coughing/choking
	(3) Noisy breathing
	(4) Difficult/unable to speak
	(5) 'Something stuck'
	Examination
	(1) Extreme but ineffective respiratory effort
	(2) Cyanosis
	(3) Drooling (cannot swallow saliva)
	(4) Stridor
Immediate management	(1) Heimlich manoeuvre if the patient has inhaled a foreign body:
	◆ Patient sitting or standing—rescuer stands or kneels behind patient, encircling the patient's waist with their arms, placing one fist just above the navel (well below xiphoid process) and using their other hand to press the fist into the patient's abdomen with a quick upward thrust. Repeat as necessary
	◆ Patient lying—place patient on their back. Rescuer kneels astride patient and puts the palm of one hand between the navel and xiphisternum, places their other hand on top of this, and pushes upwards and inwards
	(2) If Heimlich manoeuvre is inappropriate or has failed:
	◆ If there is time and you have the expertise—spray the pharynx with local anaesthetic (e.g. 5% cocaine and adrenaline) and examine the pharynx and upper airway by indirect laryngoscopy to establish the cause of obstruction and allow (if possible) its removal (with finger sweep under direct vision or long-handled forceps) or passage of an endotracheal tube
	◆ If there is time and you are not experienced in upper airway management—call immediately for help from anaesthetic or ENT colleagues
	◆ If there is no time—call cardiac arrest team
Key investigations	**To establish the diagnosis**
	Upper airway obstruction is a clinical diagnosis
	Other important tests
	As dictated by cause of obstruction
Further management	As dictated by cause of obstruction; see Chapter 33.2, 'Cricothyroidotomy'

2.4 Asthma

See Chapter 18.7 in main text.

Clinical features	**History**
	(1) Worsening asthma
	(2) Increasing difficulty breathing
	(3) Decrease in exercise tolerance
	(4) Increasing wheeze
	(5) Chest tightness
	(6) Cough
	(7) Difficulty in speaking
	(8) Fall in self-monitored peak flow
	(9) Failure to obtain improvement with use of regular β_2-agonist
	(10) Precipitating factor—exposure to known precipitant, e.g. exercise, cold air, dusty environment, upper respiratory tract infection
	Examination
	Moderate uncontrolled acute asthma:
	(1) Breathlessness
	(2) Wheeze
	(3) Chest tightness
	(4) Peak flow 50–70% of predicted or personal best
	Acute severe attack:
	(1) Cannot complete sentences in one breath
	(2) Increased respiratory rate (>25 breaths/min)
	(3) Use of accessory muscles of respiration
	(4) Tachycardia (>110/min)
	(5) Peak flow <50% of predicted or personal best
	Life-threatening asthma:
	(1) Exhaustion, confusion, or coma
	(2) Inability to speak
	(3) Cyanosis
	(4) Bradycardia or hypotension
	(5) Silent chest
	(6) Peak flow <33% of predicted or personal best (or unrecordable)
	Notes
	(1) A 'normal' respiratory rate is consistent with the patient being near to death if they are exhausted
	(2) Always check carefully for signs of pneumothorax
	(3) Always check pulse oximetry
	(4) Asking the patient to count out loud as far as they can on a single breath provides a rapid, quantitative, and repeatable measure of respiratory function
Immediate management	If cardiorespiratory collapse, as described in 1.2 above
	Moderate uncontrolled acute asthma:
	(1) β_2-Agonist via spacer and mask or nebulizer (see below)
	(2) Oral prednisolone 30 mg once daily
	(3) Inhaled steroids—commence or increase dose
	Acute severe attack:
	(1) Oxygen—high flow, with reservoir bag if needed, to achieve PaO_2 >92%
	(2) Salbutamol 2.5–5 mg or terbutaline 5–10 mg via oxygen-driven nebulizer, repeated up to every 15–30 min as needed, and then 4 hourly
	(3) Steroids—hydrocortisone 200 mg IV four times daily or prednisolone 30–60 mg orally once daily
	Life-threatening attack or patient failing to improve:
	(1), (2), and (3) As for acute severe attack
	(4) Add ipatropium 0.5 mg to nebulized β_2-agonist
	(5) Consider magnesium sulphate 1.2–2 g IV over 20 min

(6) Consider aminophylline, loading dose (in patient not previously treated with theophylline) of 5 mg/kg given IV over 20 min, then an infusion of 0.5 mg/kg per h aiming for serum concentration in the range 10–20 mg/litre. Omit loading dose if patient already taking oral theophylline

(7) Consider IV salbutamol (3–20 μg/min) or terbutaline (1.5–5 μg/min) infusion

Notes

(1) Mechanical ventilation—if the patient is deteriorating, call for help from the ICU sooner rather than later. Elective endotracheal intubation and positive pressure ventilation is better than that done after cardiorespiratory arrest—indications are hypoxia (PaO_2 <8 kPa) despite FiO_2 60%, hypercapnoea ($PaCO_2$ >6 kPa), exhaustion with feeble respiratory effort, confusion/drowsiness, unconsiousness, respiratory arrest (to be avoided if possible)

(2) Fluids—give IV fluids to correct and prevent intravascular volume depletion/dehydration

Key investigations	**To establish the diagnosis:**
	Acute asthma is a clinical diagnosis
	Other important tests:
	(1) Chest radiograph—exclude pneumothorax
	(2) Arterial blood gases—markers for life-threatening asthma being normal or high $PaCO_2$ (>5 kPa), low pH or high H^+, severe hypoxia (PaO_2 <8 kPa) in spite of high flow oxygen treatment
	(3) Electrolytes, renal and liver function, full blood count
Further management	(1) Optimization of long-term asthma management
	(2) Education regarding how to recognize severe attacks and how to respond when they develop

2.5 Pneumonia

See Chapter 18.4.2 in main text.

Clinical features	**History**
	(1) Breathing difficulty
	(2) Flu-like prodrome
	(3) High fever, sweats, rigors
	(4) Pleuritic chest pain
	(5) Sputum production (but note that this is not expected in atypical pneumonia)
	(6) Travel
	(7) Pet birds
	Examination
	(1) Severity of illness—exhaustion, use of accessory muscles and inability to talk in sentences all indicate severe illness and probable need for management on HDU/ICU
	(2) Vital signs—temperature, pulse, BP—also peripheral perfusion (hot or cold)
	(3) Respiratory —cyanosis, respiratory rate, focal lung signs (consolidation, pleural rub, pleural effusion)
	(4) Sputum—inspect if any produced
	(5) Pulse oximetry
	Determination of severity
	(1) Can be estimated using the six-point CURB-65 score, with one point scored for each of (a) **C**onfusion; (b) **U**rea >7 mmol/litre; (c) **R**espiratory rate >30/min; (d) **S**ystolic **b**lood pressure <90 mmHg; (e) Diastolic **B**lood pressure <60 mmHg; (f) age >**65 years**.

(2) Depending on CURB-65 score, the risk of mortality or need for ICU admission is as follows: score 0, 0.7%; score 1, 3.2%; score 2, 13%; score 3, 17%; score 4, 41.5%; score 5, 57%

Immediate management	If cardiorespiratory collapse, as described in 1.2 above
	(1) Oxygen—high flow, with reservoir bag if needed, to achieve PaO_2 >92%
	(2) Appropriate antimicrobial agent

British Thoracic Society guidelines for treatment of community-acquired pneumonia:

♦ Mild/moderate pneumonia (CURB-65 score of 0–2)—oral therapy with extended spectrum penicillin (e.g. amoxicillin 250–500 mg three times daily) alone or with a macrolide (e.g. clarithromycin 250–500 mg twice daily). Omit the penicillin in patients with penicillin allergy

♦ Severe pneumonia (CURB-65 score of 3 or more)—IV therapy with a second- or third-generation cephalosporin (e.g. cefotaxime 1 g twice daily) plus a macrolide (e.g. erythromycin 500 mg four times daily)

♦ Suspected legionnaire's disease—high-dose IV erythromycin (1 g four times daily) plus consider adding oral rifampicin (0.6–1.2 g daily in two to four divided doses)

In areas/countries where there is serious concern that *Strep. pneumoniae* may be resistant to penicillin and other agents:

♦ Mild/moderate pneumonia (CURB-65 score of 0–2)—second- or third-generation cephalosporin (e.g. cefotaxime 1 g IV twice daily) plus macrolide (e.g. erythromycin 500 mg orally or IV four times daily), or fluoroquinolone (e.g. levofloxacin 500 mg orally or IV once or twice daily) alone

♦ Severe pneumonia (CURB-65 score of 3 or more)—second/third-generation cephalosporin (e.g. cefotaxime 1 g IV twice daily) plus macrolide (e.g. erythromycin 500 mg IV four times daily), or second-/third-generation cephalosporin (e.g. cefotaxime 1 g IV twice daily) plus fluoroquinolone (e.g. levofloxacin 500 mg IV twice daily)

Notes

(1) If staphylococcal pneumonia is suspected, add flucloxacillin 1 g IV four times daily (or vancomycin if methicillin-resistant *Staph. aureus* is proven or suspected)

(2) See Chapters 18.4.3 and 18.4.4 for discussion of antimicrobial treatment of patients with hospital-acquired pneumonia or pneumonia in immunocompromised patients

(3) Give IV fluids to maintain adequate intravascular volume/hydration

Key investigations	**To establish the diagnosis:**
	(1) Chest radiograph—looking for focal consolidation (lobar pneumonia) or more widespread interstitial shadowing
	(2) Blood culture
	(3) Sputum culture
	(4) Urinary pneumococcal antigen and legionella antigen tests
	To establish severity:
	Arterial blood gases—if patient is very ill or pulse oximetry shows PaO_2 <92%
	Other important tests:
	Full blood count, electrolytes, renal and liver function
Further management	Follow-up chest radiograph to ensure complete resolution

3 Gastrointestinal and hepatological

3.1 Upper gastrointestinal haemorrhage

See Chapter 15.4.2 in main text.

Clinical features	**History**
	(1) Haematemesis or 'coffee-ground' vomiting
	(2) Melaena
	(3) Presyncope
	(4) Indigestion or reflux or medication for these symptoms
	(5) Retching before haematemesis (consider Mallory–Weiss tear)
	(6) Previous upper gastrointestinal investigation or surgery
	(7) To suggest recent development of anaemia
	(8) Drugs that predispose to upper gastrointestinal haemorrhage—aspirin, nonsteroidal anti-inflammatory agents (NSAIDs), anticoagulants
	(9) Risk factors for, or presence of, chronic liver disease (consider varices)
	(10) Anorexia and weight loss (consider malignancy)
	Examination
	(1) State of circulation—temperature of peripheries, pulse rate, BP, JVP
	(2) Mucous membranes—chronic anaemia
	(3) Evidence of chronic liver disease—jaundice and other manifestations (consider varices)
	(4) Evidence of portal hypertension—especially splenomegally (consider varices)
	(5) Lymphadenopathy—especially in left supraclavicular fossa (consider malignancy)
	(6) Abdomen—for epigastic mass (consider malignancy)
	(7) Rectal examination—for blood/melaena
	Notes
	(1) The most reliable signs of intravascular volume depletion are severe postural (sitting vs lying, if standing not possible) dizziness, a postural rise in pulse rate of >30 beats/min, postural hypotension (>20 mmHg fall in systolic BP) and a low JVP
	(2) Clinical assessment of severity, see Table 33.1.13
	(3) Most likely diagnoses are peptic ulcer (35–50%), erosive disease (10–15%), oesophagitis (10%), Mallory–Weiss tear (5–10%) and oesophageal varices (5–10%). No cause can be established in 5–15% of cases
Immediate management	If cardiorespiratory collapse, as described in 1.2 above
	(1) Establish IV access with one or more large-bore peripheral venous cannulae (look in the antecubital fossae in the patient who is shut down). If you cannot do this, then insert a femoral venous catheter (see Chapter 33.2, 'Femoral vein cannulation'). DO NOT ATTEMPT TO INSERT AN INTERNAL JUGULAR OR SUBCLAVIAN VENOUS CATHETER INTO A PATIENT WHO OBVIOUSLY HAS SEVERE INTRAVASCULAR VOLUME DEPLETION (see Chapter 16.1 for discussion)
	(2) If clinical evidence of intravascular volume depletion, give 1000 ml of IV fluid (colloid, e.g Gelofusin, or 0.9% saline) as fast as possible. Repeat clinical examination. If the patient still has intravascular volume depletion, give further 500 ml of fluid as fast as possible. Repeat cycle until arterial pressure and JVP restored towards normal, then slow down rate of infusion. Use blood instead of colloid/saline as soon as it is available
	(3) Cross-match blood for transfusion

(4) Consider need for urgent upper gastrointestinal endoscopy

(5) If oesophageal varices—see Table 33.1.14

Also:

(1) Oxygen—high flow, with reservoir bag if needed, to achieve $PaO_2 > 92\%$

(2) Insert urinary catheter and monitor fluid input/output hourly in any patient with substantial gastrointestinal haemorrhage—a satisfactory urine output is the best gauge of adequate resuscitation

(3) Correct any coagulopathy—see 1.9 above, Table 33.1.3 (iatrogenic overanticoagulation) and 9.1 below (disseminated coagulation)

(4) Nurse to avoid aspiration, and do not insert nasogastric tube, which makes this more likely

Key investigations	**To establish the diagnosis (and also potentially therapeutic):** Upper gastrointestinal endoscopy:
	◆ Within 24 h of admission in anyone with a substantial gastrointestinal bleed
	◆ Urgently if oesophageal varices are suspected or the patient is actively bleeding
	◆ See Table 13.1.13 for assessment of risk of rebleeding and mortality after endoscopy
	Other important tests:
	(1) Full blood count—but remember that the initial haemoglobin concentration is a poor estimate of the volume of acute blood loss
	(2) Electrolytes, renal and liver function tests
	(3) Coagulation screen
	(4) To pursue possibility and causes of chronic liver disease (if clinically indicated)
Further management	(1) Immediately inform surgical colleagues of all cases of substantial gastrointestinal haemorrhage
	(2) Dependent on cause of haemorrhage, e.g.:
	◆ Acid suppression for ulcer healing—high-dose IV proton pump inhibitor, e.g. omeprazole 80 mg bolus followed by 8 mg/h for 72 h
	◆ Eradication of *H. pylori*

Table 33.1.13 Risk of rebleeding and mortality following upper gastrointestinal haemorrhage (Rockall score)

(a) Clinical and endoscopic parameters

Score	0	1	2	3
Clinical parameters				
Age (years)	<60	60–79	80+	
Shock	SBP >100 mmHg	SBP >100 mmHg	SBP <100 mmHg	
	Pulse <100/min	Pulse >100/min		
Comorbidity	None	Other	Cardiac failure	Renal failure
			Ischaemic heart disease	Liver failure
				Disseminated malignancy
Total clinical score	0	2	4	6
Mortality (%)	0.2	5	24	49

Table 33.1.13 (Cont'd) Risk of rebleeding and mortality following upper gastrointestinal haemorrhage (Rockall score)

Endoscopic parameters

Score	0	1	2
Diagnosis	No lesion seen and no stigmata of recent haemorrhage	Other diagnosis	Malignancy of upper gastrointestinal tract
	Mallory–Weiss tear		
Major stigmata of recent haemorrhage	None or dark spot only		Blood in upper gastrointestinal tract
			Adherent clot
			Visible or spurting vessel

(b) Total clinical and endoscopic score

	0	2	4	6	8+
Mortality (%)	0	0.2	5	17	41
Rebleeding (%)	5	5	14	32	41

SBP, systolic blood pressure.

Table 33.1.14 Management of bleeding from oesophageal varices

Resuscitation	As described in 3.1 above
Coagulopathy	Correct if present: Give vitamin K, 1 mg IV Maintain platelet count >25 × 10^9/l Give 2 units of FFP for every 4 units of blood or packed cells
Pharmacological measures to reduce haemorrhage	Consider: ◆ Vasopressin, 20 units IV over 15 min, followed by 20 U/h IV ◆ Terlipressin, 2–4 mg IV bolus, followed by 1–2 mg IV every 4–6 h as needed for up to 72 h ◆ Octreotide 50 µg IV bolus, followed by 50 µg/h IV for 5 days
	Note: Nitrates are often given (sublingually, as transdermal patch, or intravenously) concurrently with vasopressin to reduce side-effects
Urgent endoscopy	Banding or sclerotherapy can stop bleeding, hence immediate liaison with specialist gastroenterological/hepatological services is essential in cases of suspected variceal haemorrhage
Sengstaken–Blakemore tube	Consider if Haemorrhage is torrential Other factors prevent safe emergency endoscopy

FFP, fresh frozen plasma.

3.2 Lower gastrointestinal haemorrhage

See Chapter 15.4.2 in main text.

Clinical features	**History** (1) Haemorrhoids (2) Abdominal pain—if long-standing and intermittent may suggest diverticular disease, if severe may indicate mesenteric ischaemia (3) Previous lower gastrointestinal investigation or surgery (4) To suggest recent development of anaemia (5) Anorexia, weight loss, recent alteration in bowel habit (consider malignancy) (6) Drugs that predispose to gastrointestinal haemorrhage—aspirin, NSAIDs, anticoagulants (7) Risk factors for, or presence of, chronic liver disease (consider rectal varices) (8) Family history—colonic polyps/neoplasia, hereditary haemorrhagic telangiectasia **Examination** (1) State of circulation—temperature of peripheries, pulse rate, BP, JVP (2) Mucous membranes—chronic anaemia (3) Jaundice—suggests malignancy or chronic liver disease (4) Lymphadenopathy—suggests malignancy (5) Abdomen—for localized tenderness, peritonism, or palpable mass (6) Rectal examination—for piles and blood (7) Peripheral vasculature—generalized disease increases likelihood of mesenteric ischaemia (8) Telangiectasiae on skin or mucosae **Notes** (1) The most reliable signs of intravascular volume depletion are severe postural (sitting vs lying, if standing not possible) dizziness, a postural rise in pulse rate of >30 beats/min, postural hypotension (>20 mmHg fall in systolic BP) and a low JVP (2) Most likely diagnoses are diverticulosis (35%), colonic polyp or cancer (15%), inflammatory bowel disease (15%), benign anorectal conditions (10%), and angiodysplasia (10%).
Immediate management	If cardiorespiratory collapse, as described in 1.2 above (1) Establish IV access—as in 3.1 above (2) If clinical evidence of intravascular volume depletion, resuscitate as described in 3.1 above (3) Cross-match blood for transfusion Also: (4) Oxygen—high flow, with reservoir bag if needed, to achieve PaO$_2$ >92% (5) Insert urinary catheter and monitor fluid input/output hourly in any patient with substantial gastrointestinal haemorrhage—a satisfactory urine output is the best gauge of adequate resuscitation (6) Correct any coagulopathy—see 1.9 above, Table 33.1.3 (iatrogenic overanticoagulation) and 9.1 below (disseminated intravascular coagulation)
Key investigations	**To establish the diagnosis:** In all patients: (1) Proctoscopy and rigid sigmoidoscopy As required: (2) Colonoscopy (3) Mesenteric angiography **Other important tests** (1) Full blood count (2) Electrolytes, renal and liver function tests, coagulation screen, inflammatory markers (3) To pursue possibility and causes of chronic liver disease (if clinically indicated)
Further management	(1) Inform surgical colleagues of all cases of substantial gastrointestinal haemorrhage immediately (2) Dependent on cause of haemorrhage

3.3 Acute colitis

See Chapters 15.12 and 15.18 in main text.

Clinical features	**History**
	(1) Bowel motions—frequency and type (blood, mucus, pus)
	(2) Abdominal pain
	(3) Rapidity of onset
	(4) Systemic features—fever, malaise, anorexia
	(5) Previous episodes/known colitic disease
	(6) Recent diet (contaminated or infected food)
	(7) Have close contacts also been ill?
	(8) Recent antibiotic treatment (consider *C. difficile*)
	(9) Use of NSAIDs
	(10) Associated vomiting
	(11) Travel
	(12) Risk factors for HIV (in some cases)
	Examination
	(1) State of circulation—temperature of peripheries, pulse rate, BP, JVP
	(2) Signs of toxicity—fever
	(3) Mucous membranes—chronic anaemia, ulceration, candida
	(4) Abdomen—for distension, localized tenderness, peritonism or palpable mass, or altered bowel sounds (absent, reduced)
	(5) Rectal and perineal examination—for fistulas and nature of stool (blood, pus)
	(6) Peripheral vasculature—generalized disease increases likelihood of ischaemic colitis
	(7) Peripheral oedema—suggests hypoproteinaemia and chronic disease in this context
	Notes
	The most reliable signs of intravascular volume depletion are severe postural (sitting versus lying, if standing not possible) dizziness, a postural rise in pulse rate of >30 beats/min, postural hypotension (>20 mmHg fall in systolic BP) and a low JVP
Immediate management	If cardiorespiratory collapse, as described in 1.2 above
	(1) Fluid and potassium resuscitation as necessary—see 3.1 above and 5.5 below
	(2) Most cases of acute colitis do not require antimicrobial therapy and settle with rehydration and time, the results of stool culture and rectal biopsy (which should be available in 24–48 h) being used to guide further treatment decisions. However, patients who are very ill with marked systemic symptoms and bloody diarrhoea (indicating probable colitis) should be given antimicrobial therapy pending culture results. Treat empirically with, e.g. ciprofloxacin (500–750 mg orally twice daily, or 200–400 mg IV twice daily) and metronidazole (400 mg orally three times daily or 500 mg IV three times daily), or—in parts of the world where gastrointestinal pathogens are likely to be resistant to fluoroquinolones—with azithromycin 250–500 mg four times daily
	(3) Also, in cases of known colitis (and to be considered in those with new and undiagnosed presentations of colitis), give steroids to those who are very ill, e.g. hydrocortisone 100 mg IV every 6 h and 100 mg as rectal drip twice daily
	Note the features of a severe acute attack of ulcerative colitis (Table 33.1.15)
Key investigations	**To establish the diagnosis:**
	In all patients:
	(1) Abdominal radiograph—to assess extent of inflammation and to exclude toxic megacolon (required before proctoscopy/sigmoidoscopy), and erect chest radiograph—looking for air under diaphragm (perforation)
	(2) Flexible or rigid sigmoidoscopy and rectal biopsy
	(3) Stool—microscopy, culture, and testing for *C. difficile* toxin
	(4) Blood cultures
	Other important tests
	(1) Full blood count
	(2) Group and save or cross-match blood
	(3) Electrolytes, renal and liver function tests, inflammatory markers, coagulation screen
Further management	(1) Inform surgical colleagues of all cases of acute colitis, urgently if radiography shows perforation or toxic dilatation
	(2) Nurse with appropriate barrier precautions (if possible) until infective cause excluded
	(3) Further management dependent on cause of colitis
	(4) Note that suspected or proven food poisoning and typhoid are notifiable diseases in the UK

Table 33.1.15 Features that indicate a severe acute attack of ulcerative colitis

Bowels	Open >6 times per day, with blood in the motions
Pulse	>100/min
Fever	>38°C
Albumin	<30 g/l
CRP	>45 mg/dl
Abdominal Radiograph	Toxic megacolon
	Mucosal islands
	Dilated small bowel

3.4 Acute hepatic failure

See Chapter 15.22.4 in main text.

Clinical features	**Definitions**
	(1) Acute hepatic failure is hepatocellular jaundice, hypertransaminasaemia, and prolongation of the prothrombin time associated with an acute liver disease
	(2) Fulminant hepatic failure is acute liver failure with hepatic encephalopathy, most definitions specifying that this must occur within a particular time (variable) from the onset of clinical evidence of liver disease (usually jaundice)
	History
	(1) Jaundice—not always present in fulminant hepatic failure
	(2) Confusion/drowsiness—note timing of onset of mental changes in relation to jaundice
	(3) Relevant to cause of acute liver failure, e.g. paracetamol overdose, full drug history (prescribed and nonprescribed), risk factors for viral hepatitis
	(4) Is there a background of chronic liver disease?—alcohol, risk factors for viral hepatitis
	(5) Autoimmune conditions (associated with autoimmune chronic active hepatitis)
	(6) Family history (Wilson's disease is a rare cause of fulminant hepatic failure)
	Examination
	(1) State of circulation—vital signs are normal in the early stages. Tachycardia and hypotension occur later. Hypertension and bradycardia are very late and sinister signs of cerebral oedema
	(2) Jaundice
	(3) Liver—usually tender, but normal size or only slightly enlarged in acute hepatic failure. If hepatomegaly consider hepatic venous obstruction (Budd–Chiari), malignant infiltration, chronic liver disease

(4) Ascites—if substantial consider Budd–Chiari syndrome
(5) Encephalopathy
  ◆ Grade 1—mild confusion, irritability, decreased attention
  ◆ Grade 2—drowsiness, lethargy, inappropriate behaviour
  ◆ Grade 3—somnolent but rousable, disorientated
  ◆ Grade 4—coma
(6) Signs of chronic liver disease

Notes
Focal neurological signs are not expected in acute hepatic failure. If present they suggest a focal cerebral lesion, most likely haemorrhage in this context

Immediate management	If cardiorespiratory collapse, as described in 1.2 above Acute hepatic failure:

(1) Oxygen—high flow, with reservoir bag if needed, to achieve $PaO_2 > 92\%$
(2) Treat/prevent hypovolaemia—give 4.5% serum albumin IV to keep CVP at +10 cmH$_2$O. Give systemic vasopressor support (e.g. epinephrine, norepinephrine, dopamine) if fluid replacement fails to maintain mean arterial pressure of 50–60 mmHg.
(3) Treat/prevent hypoglycaemia—give 50% glucose IV (central line) at 5–10 ml/h (monitor BM stix regularly)
(4) Give prophylactic broad-spectrum antibiotic, e.g. cefotaxime 1 g IV twice daily
(5) Give prophylaxis against gastrointestinal stress ulceration, e.g. ranitidine (150 mg orally twice daily, 50 mg IV three times daily)
(6) Give N-acetylcysteine by IV infusion:
  ◆ Paracetamol overdose: 150 mg/kg in 200 ml 5% dextrose over 15 min, then 50 mg/kg in 500 ml 5% dextrose over 4 h, then 100 mg/kg in 1000 ml 5% dextrose over 16 h
  ◆ Other diagnosis: 150 mg/kg in 1000 ml 5% dextrose over 24 h
(7) Give corticosteroids, e.g. prednisolone 40–60 mg/day, if acute liver failure is due to autoimmune hepatitis.
Hepatic encephalopathy:
To prevent or treat:
(1) Removal or correction of precipitating factors
  ◆ Drugs—stop all if possible, particularly sedatives/hypnotics and diuretics
  ◆ Fluid and electrolyte balance—maintain carefully. Avoid/treat dehydration, hypoglycaemia, hypokalaemia, hypophosphataemia
(2) Minimize absorption of nitrogenous substances. The following treatments may be given:
  ◆ Enemas (MgSO$_4$ or phosphate) to encourage bowel emptying
  ◆ Disaccharide laxative, e.g. lactulose 30–50 ml three times daily, dosage then adjusted to produce 2–3 soft stools daily
  ◆ Broad-spectrum poorly-absorbed antibiotic, e.g. neomycin 1 g four times daily by mouth
(3) If grade 3 or 4 encephalopathy, also
  ◆ Intubate and ventilate
  ◆ Give parenteral feeding

Notes
(1) Hyponatraemia is common and due to water excess rather than sodium deficiency. It should be treated with fluid restriction and not by infusion of saline
(2) If there is a history of chronic high alcohol intake or malnourishment, give thiamine IV BEFORE giving glucose to avoid risk of precipitating Wernicke's encephalopathy, e.g. Pabrinex IV high-potency injection, 10 ml (2 ampoules) over 10 min (repeated three times daily)

(3) Insert urinary catheter and monitor fluid input/output hourly in any patient with acute hepatic failure
(4) Cerebral oedema:
  ◆ Avoidance—avoid overfilling with IV fluids
  ◆ Treatment—nurse in quiet room with trunk and head elevated at 40°; consider transfer to facility where intracranial pressure can be monitored; consider mannitol 1 g/kg as IV bolus of 20% solution (if plasma osmolality <315 mosmol/kg and the patient is not oliguric), repeated 4 hourly (0.5 g/kg) if previous infusion induced a diuresis

Key investigations	**To establish the presence of acute liver failure:**

(1) Liver blood tests—bilirubin, transaminases (ALT, AST, gGT)
(2) Prothrombin time/coagulation screen

To establish the cause of liver disease:
If no history of paracetamol overdose
(1) Hepatitis B core IgM, hepatitis A IgM, liver autoantibodies, immunoglobulins
(2) Abdominal ultrasound and Doppler of hepatic veins—looking for size/echogenicity of liver, splenomegaly, signs of Budd–Chiari
(3) If <40 years: serum copper and caeruloplasmin; ophthalmic examination for Kayser–Fleischer rings (Wilson's disease)

Notes
(1) Tap ascites if present—microscopy, culture, and sensitivity. Culture/swab blood, urine, nasal, high vagina
(2) Do not correct coagulopathy unless the patient is bleeding: the prothrombin time is an important prognostic indicator. If bleeding, or to cover invasive procedures, give vitamin K 10 mg IV, fresh frozen plasma and platelets, and maintain haematocrit 30–35% by blood transfusion.
(3) Where the prothrombin time (in s) is greater than the time after a paracetamol overdose (in h), there is a substantial risk of developing acute liver failure

Other important tests:
(1) Full blood count
(2) Glucose, renal function tests, amylase
(3) Arterial blood gases

Further management	(1) Discuss all cases of acute hepatic failure with a specialist (transplant) centre (see Table 33.1.16): urgent orthotopic liver transplantation may be required and appropriate (2) Dependent on cause of hepatic failure

Table 33.1.16 Guidelines for referral to a specialist (transplant) centre in case of paracetamol overdose

Parameter	Day 2 (24–48 h)	Day 3 (48–72 h)	Day 4 (72–96 h)
Arterial pH	<7.3	<7.3	–
INR	>3	>4.5	Any rise
Encephalopathy	Present	Present	Present
Creatinine	>200 µmol/litre	>200 µmol/litre	>250 µmol/litre
Hypoglycaemia	Present	Present	Present

3.5 The acute abdomen

See Chapter 15.4.1 in main text.

Clinical features	**History**
	(1) Abdominal pain—duration, constant or colicky, where is it worst (point with one finger), radiation
	(2) Gastrointestinal symptoms—anorexia, nausea, vomiting, diarrhoea, constipation (precisely when were the bowels last open), blood in vomit or stool
	(3) Urinary symptoms—frequency, pain on micturition, haematuria
	(4) Gynaecological symptoms—last menstrual period, vaginal discharge
	(5) To suggest sepsis—sweats, fevers, rigors
	(6) History of gastrointestinal problems—indigestion, peptic ulceration, gallstones, pancreatitis
	(7) History of atheromatous vascular disease—ischaemic heart disease, cerebrovascular disease, peripheral vascular disease (increase the likelihood of bowel ischaemia or of abdominal aortic aneurysm, also relevant to surgical risk)
	Examination
	(1) State of circulation—temperature of peripheries, pulse rate, BP, JVP
	(2) Signs of toxicity—fever
	(3) Foetor
	(4) Abdomen:
	♦ Inspection—distension, movement on respiration
	♦ Palpation—tenderness, guarding, rigidity, rebound tenderness, palpable mass
	♦ Auscultation—bowel sounds
	♦ Check all hernial orifices and abdominal aorta
	(5) Rectal examination—for tenderness and nature of stool, blood in stool
	(6) Vaginal examination—tenderness, pelvic mass
	(7) Test urine for blood
	Note
	The likely cause of abdominal pain depends on the context. Cases presenting in the community that require assessment in hospital will generally be referred directly to surgical services, and many will have 'obvious' diagnoses such as appendicitis. Patients presenting to medical services or who develop abdominal pain when already on a medical ward will generally be older and with multiple comorbidities, and are much more likely to have intestinal vascular events or obstruction due to malignancy
Immediate management	If cardiorespiratory collapse, as described in 1.2 above
	(1) Establish IV access—as in 3.1 above
	(2) If clinical evidence of intravascular volume depletion, resuscitate as described in 3.1 above
	(3) Urgent liaison with surgical colleagues
	(4) Analgesia—give adequate pain relief, e.g.:
	♦ NSAID: e.g. diclofenac 75 mg intramuscularly, repeated after 30 min if necessary
	♦ Opioid: e.g. morphine 5 mg subcutaneously plus 5 mg intramuscularly, repeated if necessary and accompanied by appropriate antiemetic, e.g. metoclopramide 10 mg IV over 1–2 min, or cyclizine 50 mg IV over 1–2 min
	(5) Nasogastric tube—when there is continued vomiting and/or suspected intestinal obstruction
	(6) Urinary catheter
Key investigations	**To establish the diagnosis:**
	(1) Supine abdominal radiograph—is there intestinal obstruction (seldom indicates cause)? Is there a urinary stone (CT preferred imaging technique)?
	(2) Erect chest radiograph—is there gas under the diaphragm indicating intestinal perforation?
	(3) Serum amylase—a substantial increase suggests pancreatitis
	(4) Abdominal CT scan—increasingly used in the management of patients with acute abdominal pain
	(5) Abdominal ultrasound—when acute gallbladder disease is suspected
	Note
	Patients with generalized peritonitis require an urgent laparotomy provided that pancreatitis has been excluded. Do not delay: if the patient requires resuscitation, then make arrangements for theatre whilst initiating resuscitation and continue to resuscitate in the anaesthetic room. Do not wait 'until the patient is a bit better' before involving anaesthetic and surgical colleagues
	Other important tests:
	(1) Full blood count
	(2) Group and save or cross-match blood
	(3) Electrolytes, renal and liver function tests
	(4) Coagulation screen
Further management	Dependent on the cause of the acute abdomen
	Notes
	(1) Adhesive small-bowel obstruction may resolve with conservative management
	(2) Remember rare 'medical' causes of abdominal pain, e.g. pneumonia, shingles, drugs (digoxin), diabetes, sickle cell crisis, porphyria, familial mediterranean fever—remember also that these are rare: if in doubt, diagnose a common condition

4 Renal

4.1 Acute kidney injury

See Chapter 21.5 in main text.

Clinical features	**History**
	(1) There are no specific features to suggest acute kidney injury: presentation is dominated by the precipitating condition
	(2) Previous renal or urinary tract disease
	(3) Drugs, prescribed and nonprescribed
	(4) Evidence of multisystem disease
	(5) Always seek the results of previous tests of renal function
	Examination
	(1) State of circulation—temperature of peripheries, pulse rate (+ postural change), BP (+ postural change), JVP
	(2) Evidence of infection—fever, localizing signs
	(3) Breathing—evidence of pulmonary oedema or acidosis (Kussmaul)
	(4) Abdominal—is the bladder palpable? (obstruction)
	(5) Rectal—is there pelvic malignancy? (obstruction)
	(6) General—signs indicating multisystem disorder: rash, joints, eyes, nose. Are muscles swollen/tender? (rhabdomyolysis)
	Note
	The most reliable signs of intravascular volume depletion are severe postural (sitting vs lying, if standing not possible) dizziness, a postural rise in pulse rate of >30 beats/min, postural hypotension (>20 mmHg fall in systolic BP) and a low JVP
Immediate management	If cardiorespiratory collapse, as described in 1.2 above
	Treatment of life-threatening complications:
	(1) Hyperkalaemia—see 5.4 below
	(2) Pulmonary oedema—see 1.8 above, but note that diuretics are not likely to induce diuresis in the context of acute kidney injury
	(3) Severe acidosis, causing circulatory compromise
	(4) 'Gross uraemia', causing encephalopathy or bleeding
	Note
	Aside from immediate life-saving medical treatments, patients with these features will need urgent renal replacement therapy (preferably by haemodialysis or haemofiltration, as dictated by clinical context) unless their renal function can be restored rapidly
	Resuscitation:
	(1) Optimization of intravascular volume—many patients presenting with acute kidney injury will be volume deplete
	Establish IV access—as in 3.1 above
	If clinical evidence of intravascular volume depletion, resuscitate as described in 3.1 above
	(2) Oxygen—high flow, with reservoir bag if needed, to achieve Pao_2 >92%
	Make diagnosis of cause of renal failure:
	(1) Is it acute or chronic?—previous biochemical measurements; renal size on ultrasonography (small kidneys indicate chronic disease)
	(2) Is it due to urinary obstruction?—history of lower urinary tract symptoms, heamaturia, urinary stones etc.; dilated pelvicalyceal system on ultrasonography (but beware of obstruction without dilatation)
	(3) Is it due to renal inflammation?—dipstick proteinuria and haematuria; urinary red cell casts
	(4) Is it due to prerenal failure/acute tubular necrosis?—clinical context; evidence of circulatory compromise/intrvascular volume depletion

	Notes
	(1) Stop all drugs that can be haemodynamically deleterious to renal function unless there is a very pressing indication for them, e.g. nonsteroidal anti-inflammatory agents, angiotensin converting enzyme inhibitors, angiotensin II receptor blockers; also stop all nephrotoxic agents (e.g. aminoglycosides) and substitute nontoxic alternative
	(2) Insert urinary catheter and monitor fluid input/output hourly in any patient with acute kidney injury—remove after 24 h if the patient is anuric/oliguric
Key investigations	To establish the diagnosis:
	Renal function tests—acute kidney injury is usually diagnosed clinically on the basis of rapid rise in serum creatinine
	Other important tests:
	(1) ECG—looking for manifestations of hyperkalaemia
	(2) Electrolytes—especially potassium
	(3) Full blood count, coagulation screen, liver function tests
	(4) Creatine kinase (rhabdomyolysis)
	(5) Blood and other cultures—if clinically indicated
	(6) Autoimmune/vasculitic screen (anti-GBM, ANCA, ANA, immunoglobulins, cryoglobulins)—if clinically indicated
	(7) Ultrasonography of urinary tract—to determine renal size and look for evidence of obstruction
	(8) Chest radiograph—looking for pulmonary oedema or (less likely) evidence of lung haemorrhage in pulmonary-renal syndrome
	(9) Arterial blood gases—quantitate acidosis
Further management	Dependent on the cause of acute kidney injury
	Notes
	(1) When intravascular volume has been restored to normal (JVP clearly visible/CVP in normal range; no postural rise in pulse rate or drop in BP), fluid input should then be given in equal volume to measured output of urine and other fluids, plus an allowance (500–1000 ml/day) for insensible losses. The prescription of fluid should be refined on the basis of (at least) twice daily clinical examination and daily measurement of the patient's weight
	(2) The patient is likely to have acute kidney injury due to renal inflammation if there is significant (2+) proteinuria and haematuria—urgent referral to a renal specialist is required. Precise diagnosis of glomerulonephritis, tubulointerstitial nephritis or vasculitis will probably require renal biopsy, with irreversible renal failure occurring in some patients in whom diagnosis is delayed
	(3) If imaging suggests urinary obstruction, then this requires urgent relief, e.g. by urethral catheterization, suprapubic catheterization or percutaneous antegrade nephrostomy as appropriate

4.2 Rhabdomyolysis

See Chapter 21.5 in main text.

Clinical features	Rhabdomyolysis is the breakdown of muscle fibres, when leakage of potentially toxic cellular contents into the circulation can lead to hypovolaemia, acidosis, hyperkalaemia, acute kidney injury, and disseminated intravascular coagulation.
	History
	Muscular symptoms:
	(1) Pain, tenderness—focal or generalized
	(2) May be none

Related to cause:

(1) Focal muscle damage:

- Obvious—e.g. crush injury, high-voltage electrical injury
- Not so obvious—e.g. ischaemic injury following arterial embolus to limb; pressure damage following prolonged immobilization (commonly coma)

(2) Generalized muscle damage:

- Excessive muscular activity—severe exercise—e.g. marathon running; prolonged epileptic fitting (see 6.5 below)
- Infections—septicaemia—see 7.7 below; viral myositis—e.g. influenza
- Toxins—prescribed drugs—e.g. HMG CoA reductase inhibitors; substance abuse—e.g. alcohol, barbiturates, opioids, methanol, ethylene glycol (antifreeze), cocaine, amphetamine, ecstacy (MDMA), lysergic acid diethylamide (LSD); other—e.g. snake bite, spider (black widow) bite, bee sting (multiple), carbon monoxide, toluene, hemlock (quail that have eaten hemlock)
- Heatstroke (see 9.3 below); malignant hyperpyrexia (see 9.3 below); neuroleptic malignant syndrome (see 9.3 below)
- Myopathies—consider particularly if rhabdomyolysis occurs without clear precipitant; metabolic—ask for history of intermittent muscular fatigue/pain, e.g. McCardle's syndrome; inflammatory—e.g. polymyositis
- Metabolic /endocrine—hypothyroidism; electrolyte disturbance—e.g. hypokalaemia; diabetic ketoacidosis

Examination

General:

(1) Vital signs—temperature, pulse rate, BP, respiratory rate
(2) Full physical examination
(3) Inspection of urine—looks dark brown ('Coca Cola')

For cause of rhabdomyolysis:

(1) Muscles—are any swollen or tender? Is there a compartment syndrome?
(2) Ischaemia—are legs and arms well perfused? Can you feel all peripheral pulses?
(3) Pressure damage—look especially at the back of the head, spine, pelvis, and heels—pressure sores indicate likelihood of pressure damage to muscles
(4) Systemic condition—rash—septicaemia (common), dermatomyositis (very rare); slow relaxing tendon jerks (hypothyroidism)

Immediate management

As for acute kidney injury: see 4.1 above
To prevent rhabdomyolysis from leading to renal failure:

(1) Restore intravascular volume rapidly: see 3.1 above
(2) Monitor—urine output—urethral catheter; urinary pH—dipstick
(3) Fluid—encourage brisk diuresis (urine output c.200 ml/h) by giving 0.9% saline or other balanced salt solution at initial rate of 1–2 litre/h, reducing to restrict urine output to 200–300 ml/h or at first sign of pulmonary oedema
(4) Consider alkali—e.g. 1.25% sodium bicarbonate (=150 mmol/litre each of sodium and bicarbonate) at 25 ml/h—adjust rate to achieve urinary pH >7.
(5) Consider mannitol—1 g/kg as 20% solution IV over 30–60 min
(6) Consider diuretic—if urine output remains low, e.g. furosemide 40 mg (push)–500 mg (over 2 h) IV

Notes

(1) If urine output remains low, then infusion of fluid as described here will inevitably lead to overload—fluid infusion must be stopped before pulmonary oedema develops. Then proceed as for acute kidney injury (see 4.1 above)

(2) Myoglobin is more soluble at elevated pH, but there is no substantial clinical evidence that mannitol/alkaline diuresis provides better outcome than saline diuresis.
(3) Close monitoring of serum electrolytes, particularly potassium and calcium, is required. Do not correct hypocalcaemia with calcium (risk of inducing/worsening metastatic calcification)

Key investigations

To establish the diagnosis:

(1) Urine—dipstick test positive for blood, but microscopy shows no red blood cells
(2) Blood—creatine kinase—grossly elevated (>10 000 IU/litre, with lesser elevation not diagnostic in the absence of other supporting evidence)

Other important tests:

(1) ECG—look for features of hyperkalaemia (see 5.4 below)
(2) Electrolytes—potassium (hyperkalaemia is potentially life-threatening and may develop rapidly; see 5.4 below), calcium (hypocalcaemia), phosphate (hyperphosphataemia)
(3) Biochemical screen—renal function; liver blood tests (elevated transaminases from muscle); LDH (elevated)
(4) Full blood count; coagulation screen (risk of disseminated intravascular coagulation)
(5) As dictated by clinical suspicion—e.g. blood cultures, thyroid function tests, muscle biopsy

Further management

(1) Dependent on the cause of rhabdomyolysis
(2) Compartment syndrome—measure compartment pressure; fasciotomy if elevated

5 Metabolic and endocrine

5.1 Hypoglycaemia

See Section 13.11.2 in main text.

Clinical features	**History**
	(1) Coma
	(2) Epileptic fitting
	(3) Confusion and/or delirium
	(4) Focal neurological signs (including hemiplegia, uncommon)
	The patient may not be able to give any useful history: obtain as much information as possible from others in attendance (relatives, friends, ambulance crew, bystanders, etc.). Ask in particular regarding:
	(1) Diabetes mellitus
	(2) Patient self-medication, and access to insulin/oral hypoglycaemic agents
	(3) Previous episodes
	(4) Alcohol and food consumption
	(5) Other medical conditions
	Examination
	Immediate priorities:
	(1) Airway, breathing, circulation
	(2) Glasgow Coma Score
	(3) Bedside stick test for blood glucose
	Other features:
	(4) Typically very pale and shut down peripherally with a cold sweat
	(5) Evidence that the patient is diabetic: search for MedicAlert bracelet/necklace, medication (insulin, oral hypoglycaemic agents), documentation (glucose monitoring, outpatient clinics), sites of insulin injection
	(6) Evidence of chronic liver disease or endocrine disorder
Immediate management	If cardiorespiratory collapse, as described in 1.2 above
	(1) Give glucose to symptomatic patient after establishing hypoglycaemia (<2.5 mmol/l) by bedside stick test, as follows:
	◆ Patient alert and cooperative: give glucose 10–20 g by mouth (2 teaspoons sugar, or 3 sugar lumps, or one 23 g oral ampoule of Hypostop gel)
	◆ If impaired consciousness and not protecting airway: give glucose 50% solution, 50 ml IV (note that the solution is viscous and irritant if extravasated, hence give through large-bore needle/cannula into large vein)
	◆ If impaired consciousness, not protecting airway and IV access not possible: give glucagon 1 unit (= 1 mg) intramuscularly
	(2) Repeat blood glucose measurement after 10 min and repeat glucose administration if still hypoglycaemic
	Notes
	(1) Hypoglycaemic symptoms are unusual if the plasma glucose is >2.5 mmol/litre, but the threshold varies from person to person, hence it is appropriate to administer one dose of glucose IV (50% solution, 50 ml) to any patient with impaired consciousness whose plasma glucose is <3.0 mmol/litre
	(2) Give hydrocortisone 100 mg IV if recovery delayed beyond 20 min

(3) Consider complication of cerebral oedema if patient does not recover as expected—refer to (neurological) intensive care; management requires infusion of glucose to keep within range 5–10 mmol/litre, IV mannitol, IV dexamethasone

Key investigations	**To establish the diagnosis:**
	Blood glucose—take sample through cannula before giving IV glucose: hypoglycaemia defined by glucose concentration <3 mmol/litre, acute symptoms possible at <2.5 mmol/litre
	Other important tests:
	(1) Serum sample for insulin and C-peptide levels— hypoglycaemia in a known diabetic is unlikely to require further investigation, but if the situation is not clear cut, then a serum sample should be taken before IV glucose (or intramuscular glucagon) is administered to determine whether hypoglycaemia is due to endogenous or exogenous insulin
	(2) Full blood count, clotting screen, electrolytes, creatinine, liver/bone blood tests—routine screen
	(3) Blood and other cultures—if clinical suspicion of sepsis
	(4) Tests for endocrine disease—adrenocortical insufficiency, hypothyroidism, hypopituitarism—if clinically appropriate
	(5) Salicylate level—if possibility of overdose
	(6) Chest radiograph—?aspiration in any patient who has been unconscious
Further management	Dependent on the cause of hypoglycaemia
	Notes
	(1) Hypoglycaemia may recur—patients who have been given IV glucose and recovered from hypoglycaemia should be observed for at least 12 h, longer if they have taken long acting insulin/oral hypoglycaemic agents
	(2) Education—most cases of hypoglycaemia occur in known diabetics and can be avoided by the patient checking their blood glucose and responding appropriately in the event of warning signals

5.2 Diabetic ketoacidosis

See Section 13.11.1 in main text.

Clinical features	**History**
	(1) Polyuria and polydipsia
	(2) Drowsiness
	(3) To suggest precipitating condition—often infection, but can be any acute illness
	(4) Monitoring and treatment of diabetes (in known diabetics)—in particular recent details of blood glucose measurements and medication with insulin or oral hypoglycaemic agents
	Examination
	(1) State of circulation/dehydration—temperature of peripheries, skin turgor, pulse rate, BP, tongue and mucous membranes, eyes, JVP
	(2) Breathing—in particular for indication of acidosis (Kussmaul) and for smell of ketones
	(3) Glasgow Coma Score
	(4) Evidence of infection—fever, localizing signs, including careful examination of feet and skin for ulceration/sepsis

Notes

(1) The most reliable signs of intravascular volume depletion are severe postural (sitting vs lying, if standing not possible) dizziness, a postural rise in pulse rate of >30 beats/min, postural hypotension (>20 mmHg fall in systolic BP) and a low JVP

(2) Examine carefully for evidence of long term complications of diabetes, but not in the immediate emergency setting

Immediate management	If cardiorespiratory collapse, as described in 1.2 above Restoration of intravascular volume/hydration (patients will typically have a total body fluid deficit of 3–6 litres):

- Establish IV access—as in 3.1 above
- Give 0.9% saline, 1–2 litre in 2 h, then
- Give 0.9% saline 1 litre in 4 h (with potassium, see below), then 4 litres in 24 h (each with potassium, see below)

Notes

(1) If hypotensive and shut down peripherally:
- Give 1 litre of 0.9% saline or colloid as fast as possible before starting fluid regimen detailed above
- When blood glucose 10–14 mmol/l, switch from 0.9% saline to 5% dextrose infusion until eating normally (Do NOT simply allow the glucose concentration to keep falling into the normal range, reducing the insulin infusion rate to low levels according to the sliding scale. The patient continues to require insulin in dosage sufficient to allow them to metabolize ketones effectively)
- If serum sodium >150 mmol/litre, consider replacing 0.9% saline with 0.45% saline

(2) Correction of electrolyte imbalance—all patients will have a very substantial deficit in body potassium, even though serum potassium concentration will usually be elevated at presentation. Replace potassium as follows, monitoring the serum concentration every few hours:

Serum potassium (mmol/litre)	Potassium (mmol) added to each litre of fluid replacement
<3.5	40
3.5–5.5	20
>5.5	None

(3) Correction of hyperglycaemia—give insulin (actrapid 50 units mixed in 50 ml of 0.9% saline) IV according to a sliding scale as follows:

Blood glucose, measured hourly (mmol/litre; fingerprick stick)	Insulin rate (units/h)
<4	0.5
4–7	1
7.1–11	2
11.1–15	4
15.1–20	6
>20	6—review if glucose failing to fall by 3–4 mmol/litre per h

Note—if not possible to give controlled infusion of IV insulin, then give 20 U soluble insulin IM, followed by 5–10 U IM each hour, titrated according to response

(4) Correction of acidosis—acidosis will correct with restoration of circulating volume and administration of insulin. Most cases do not require administration of bicarbonate, but consider giving sodium bicarbonate (1.26% solution, 500 ml by IV infusion over 1 h) if there is profound acidosis (e.g. arterial pH <7.0) that is thought to be causing circulatory compromise

Also:

(1) Empty the stomach with nasogastric tube if patient has nausea or vomiting—gastroparesis/acute gastric dilatation is a particular risk in diabetic ketoacidosis, with a high risk of vomiting and aspiration, which can be fatal

(2) Give prophylaxis against venous thromboembolism (high risk) with low molecular weight heparin, e.g. enoxaparin 40 mg by subcutaneous injection once daily

And:

Treat any precipitating condition vigorously. Note that surgical attention may be required, in particular when there is foot sepsis

Note

Hyperosmolar nonketotic diabetic coma (HONK):

- Typically occurs in elderly patients with type 2 diabetes
- Glucose usually >50 mmol/litre
- Not ketoacidotic (by definition)
- Look for plasma osmolality >350 mosmol/kg, calculated as $2 \times (Na+K) + urea + glucose$ (all measured in mmol/litre)
- Give colloid and 0.9% saline as for diabetic ketoacidosis, but switch to 0.45% saline when intravascular volume deficit is replaced (no postural rise in pulse rate or fall in BP, JVP clearly visible) if serum sodium remains >150 mmol/litre
- Insulin requirements are typically low: hence use a reduced dose of insulin on the sliding scale to avoid hypoglycaemia

Key investigations	**To establish the diagnosis:** (1) Blood glucose (2) Stick test of urine for ketones

Other important tests:
(1) Serum electrolytes
(2) Arterial blood gases
(3) Full blood count, renal and liver function tests
(4) 'Infection screen'—chest radiograph, urine and blood culture, swab any potentially infected site
(5) ECG (may have silent infarct)

Further management	Education—most cases of diabetic ketoacidosis occur in known diabetics and can be avoided. The key issue to emphasize is that illness increases insulin requirements, hence diabetics who are ill:

(1) Still need to take insulin, even if they are not eating
(2) Should check their blood glucose regularly (up to every 2 h or so)
(3) Should give themselves frequent appropriate doses of short-acting insulin if their blood glucose starts to rise
(4) Should have access to a phone number that they can call for advice if they run into problems

5.3 Metabolic acidosis

See Section 12.11 in main text.

Clinical features	**History** In the acute medicine context presents nonspecifically with: (1) Altered conscious level (2) Circulatory collapse (3) Hyperventilation Key points to establish: (1) In what circumstances was the patient found? (2) History of diabetes mellitus, particularly if treated with metformin (3) History of chronic renal failure (4) Overdose—most commonly salicylates (5) Consumption of poison—e.g. ethylene glycol, methanol, antifreeze **Notes** Medical conditions that can cause profound metabolic acidosis (with normal anion gap, see below) include: (1) Severe diarrhoeal illness (2) Renal tubular acidosis **Examination** (1) State of circulation—temperature of peripheries, pulse rate, BP, JVP (2) Breathing—in particular for indication of acidosis (Kussmaul) and for smell of ketones (3) Glasgow Coma Score
Immediate management	If cardiorespiratory collapse, as described in 1.2 above (1) Oxygen—high flow, with reservoir bag if needed, to achieve $PaO_2 > 92\%$ (2) Restoration of intravascular volume: ◆ Establish IV access—as in 3.1 above ◆ If clinical evidence of intravascular volume depletion, resuscitate as described in 3.1 above (3) Consider bicarbonate infusion—this is a contentious issue: if acidosis is severe (pH <7.0) and there is circulatory compromise, give IV sodium bicarbonate—e.g. 1.26% solution, 500 ml by IV infusion over 1 h (75 mmol of bicarbonate), or an equivalent amount of bicarbonate as a more concentrated solution if the patient is fluid overloaded); then assess clinical response and repeat estimation of arterial blood gases **Note** Correction of metabolic acidosis requires careful attention to serum potassium concentration: profound hypokalaemia can occur if this is neglected
Key investigations	To establish the diagnosis: (1) Arterial blood gases—show metabolic acidosis (by definition) (2) Plasma glucose and stick test for urinary ketones—to exclude diabetic ketoacidosis (see 5.2 above) (3) Plasma salicylate concentration—to exclude overdose (4) Serum creatinine and urea—to exclude renal failure and uraemic acidosis (5) Serum electrolytes—acidosis may be associated with hypokalaemia or hyperkalaemia, but with profound deficit in total body potassium in both situations. Close monitoring required (6) Blood lactate concentration—many types of severe illness are associated with lactic acidosis, especially overwhelming sepsis (7) Serum bicarbonate concentration

(8) Calculate the anion gap: are there unusual anions in the blood? The blood 'anion gap', calculated as $(Na^+ + K^+) - (Cl^- + HCO_3^-)$, usually equals 10–18 mmol/litre. If there is acidosis with a high anion gap, then there must be an unmeasured substance in the blood, in which case discuss measurement of specific toxins with a clinical biochemist if there is diagnostic doubt

Other important tests:
(1) Full blood count, clotting screen, electrolytes, liver and bone blood tests—routine screen
(2) Blood paracetamol level (rarely causes profound acidosis, but combined overdoses are common)—depending on clinical suspicion
(3) Serum sample—for toxicological analysis; depending on clinical suspicion
(4) Chest radiograph—consider aspiration in any patient with a depressed conscious level
(5) Abdominal radiograph—in cases of unexplained normal anion gap acidosis; renal tubular acidosis may be associated with nephrocalcinosis

Further management	Dependent on the cause of metabolic acidosis

5.4 Hyperkalaemia

See Chapters 21.2.2 and 21.5 in main text.

Clinical features	**History** (1) Hyperkalaemia does not produce specific symptoms. Patients may sometimes develop 'odd feelings' in their muscles, but these are rarely dramatic (2) Cardiac arrest (3) Context—almost always occurs in the context of acute or chronic renal failure **Examination** (1) Hyperkalaemia does not produce specific signs (2) Cardiac arrhythmia
Immediate management	If there are ECG changes that are more severe than tenting of the T waves: ◆ Give 10 ml of 10% calcium gluconate by slow IV injection, repeated as necessary until ECG shows clear evidence of returning towards normal If ECG changes are not severe, or after giving calcium gluconate: (1) Give 10–20 units of soluble insulin in 50 ml of 50% dextrose IV over 20 min, or (2) Give nebulized β_2-agonist, e.g salbutamol 10 mg These treatments will lower serum potassium concentration by 1–2 mmol/l over 20–30 min and buy a few hours of time, but hyperkalaemia will recur unless the cause can be treated rapidly, hence consider: (3) Urgent referral to nephrological services for renal replacement therapy **Notes** IV infusion of sodium bicarbonate 50–100 mmol (*c.*300–600 ml of 1.26% solution or *c.*50–100 ml of 8.4% solution) can usefully be employed to treat hyperkalaemia in the setting of severe acidosis. In other cases it has no advantage over insulin/dextrose or β_2-agonist and has the disadvantages of not only requiring a substantial sodium/fluid load (a problem in those who are already overloaded), but also that concentrated solutions are chemically irritant and hence must be administered through central venous lines

Key investigations	**To establish the diagnosis:**
	(1) ECG—the following changes occur progressively as the plasma potassium concentration rises:
	◆ Tenting of T waves
	◆ PR interval lengthens, P wave diminishes before disappearing, and QRS complex widens
	◆ 'Sine wave' pattern
	(2) Serum potassium—hyperkalaemia defined by concentration >5.5 mmol/l, but <7 mmol/l rarely life threatening
	Note
	The morphology of the ECG determines the risk of hyperkalaemia to the individual patient better than the absolute level of serum potassium
	Other important tests
	(1) Renal function tests
	(2) To determine cause of acute kidney injury—if clinical context is appropriate (see 4.1 above)
Further management	(1) Ion exchange resins, e.g. calcium resonium 15 g in water three or four times daily by mouth (with concurrent prescription of a laxative), or 30 g in methylcellulose solution given as an enema, retained for 9 h and then removed by irrigation—these can be helpful in patients with persistent (but not life-threatening) hyperkalaemia who would not otherwise require renal replacement therapy. Note, however, that ion exchange resins take at least 4 h to have any effect and are not a useful emergency treatment for hyperkalaemia
	(2) Stop all drugs that might exacerbate hyperkalaemia unless there is a very pressing need for them and no alternative is available, e.g. potassium supplements, potassium-sparing diuretics, ACE inhibitors, angiotensin II receptor antagonists, trimethoprim, heparin
	(3) Dependent on the cause of hyperkalaemia

5.5 Hypokalaemia

See Chapter 21.2.2 in main text.

Clinical features	**History**
	(1) In almost all cases of hypokalaemia there are no symptoms (or only nonspecific symptoms) attributable to the low plasma potassium concentration
	(2) Cardiac arrhythmia (rare)
	(3) Muscular paralysis (very rare)
	(4) Relevant to cause of hypokalaemia
	Examination
	(1) Hypokalaemia does not produce specific signs
	(2) Cardiac arrhythmia
	(3) Muscular paralysis (very rare)

Immediate management	Emergency treatment is rarely required
	If life-threatening cardiac arrhythmia or muscular paralysis:
	◆ Give 40 mmol of potassium IV via volumetric pump over 1 h, then repeat measurement of serum potassium concentration and adjust rate of potassium infusion as appropriate
	If thyrotoxic periodic paralysis:
	◆ Give propanolol 3 mg/kg orally
Key investigations	**To establish the diagnosis:**
	(1) Serum potassium—hypokalaemia defined by concentration <3.5 mmol/litre, severe <3.0 mmol/litre
	Other important tests:
	(1) ECG—looking for flattening of the T wave, depression of the ST segment, and the development of a prominent U wave, also for arrhythmia
	(2) To determine cause of hypokalaemia—see Chapter 21.2.2
Further management	Dependent on the cause of hypokalaemia

5.6 Hyponatraemia

See Chapter 21.2.1 in main text.

Clinical features	**History**
	(1) Does not produce specific symptoms
	(2) Altered consciousness, epileptic fitting
	(3) Relevant to cause of hyponatraemia
	Examination
	(1) Glasgow Coma Score
	(2) Fluid status:
	◆ Intravascular volume depletion—low JVP, postural hypotension/rise in pulse rate
	◆ Clinically normal volume status
	◆ Volume expansion—peripheral oedema
Immediate management of chronic asymptomatic hyponatraemia	Do not aim to correct rapidly
	(1) If intravascular volume depletion—give 0.9% saline IV until intravascular volume restored, then restrict water intake
	(2) If euvolaemic or hypervolaemic—restrict fluid intake to 1000 ml/day. Provide swabs to moisten the mouth and give the fluid allowance as ice cubes in aliquots throughout the day
Immediate management of acute symptomatic hyponatraemia	Severe cerebral oedema with active seizures or respiratory failure—give 3% saline, 100 ml IV over 10 mins; repeat until serum sodium increased by 2–4 mmol/litre or clinical improvement, then proceed as for:
	◆ Hyponatraemic encephalopathy with seizures (inactive), decreased GCS, headache, nausea, or vomiting—give 3% saline at 1 ml/kg/per h (or 1.8% saline at 1.7 ml/kg per h) by volumetric infusion pump
	◆ Check serum sodium every 2 h during infusion of hypertonic saline
	◆ Stop hypertonic saline when patient is symptom free or serum sodium has increased by 15–20 mmol/litre in the initial 48 h of therapy
	Notes
	(1) Do not attempt rapid correction of serum sodium concentration into the normal range (probably increases risk of central pontine myelinolysis)

	(2) No algorithm can accurately predict how much hypertonic saline a patient requires to correct hyponatraemia, or what the response of a particular patient will be to a given volume of hypertonic saline—hence the requirement for very close monitoring of serum sodium
	(3) Steroids—if glucocorticoid deficiency is possible, then give steroid replacement immediately, e.g. hydrocortisone 100 mg IV 6 hourly, until the diagnosis is excluded
Key investigations	**To establish the diagnosis:** Serum sodium—hyponatraemia defined by concentration <130 mmol/llitre; severe symptoms unlikely at >120 mmol/litre
	Other important tests: (1) Plasma and urinary osmolality (2) Urinary sodium concentration
Further management	(1) Stop diuretic (if relevant) (2) Dependent on the cause of hyponatraemia

5.7 Hypercalcaemia

See Chapter 13.6 in main text.

Clinical features	**History** (1) Does not produce specific symptoms (2) Acute hypercalcaemia—general malaise, anorexia, thirst, polyuria, constipation. In severe cases vomiting, confusion, coma (3) Chronic hypercalcaemia—urinary stones, abdominal pain, mental disturbance (4) Relevant to cause of hypercalcaemia
	Examination (1) Acute hypercalcaemia does not produce specific signs (2) Fluid status: ◆ Intravascular volume depletion—postural hypotension/ rise in pulse rate, low JVP ◆ Dehydration—reduced skin turgor, dry mucous membranes (3) Evidence of malignancy
Immediate management	If cardiorespiratory collapse, as described in 1.2 above (1) Restoration of intravascular volume (if necessary)—as described in 3.1 above (2) Saline diuresis—give 0.9% saline IV at a rate of 1 litre/6 h until calcium restored towards normal, assuming adequate urinary output (monitor carefully, and examine the patient regularly for signs of fluid overload). Give loop diuretic, e.g. furosemide 40–80 mg orally or IV twice daily, if urine output slow to increase. Watch carefully for signs of pulmonary oedema, particularly in elderly patients and those with heart disease, and stop saline if this develops
	When diuresis initiated: (2) Bisphosphonate, e.g. disodium pamidronate (60–90 mg by IV infusion at a rate of 1 mg/min) or zolendronic acid (4 mg IV)
	Also: Glucocorticoids, e.g. hydrocortisone 100 mg IV three times daily or prednisolone 40–60 mg orally daily, if hypercalcaemia is due to sarcoidosis, vitamin D toxicity, or haematological malignancy

	Notes (1) Consider glucocorticoid deficiency—if this is possible, then give steroid replacement immediately, e.g. hydrocortisone 100 mg IV 6 hourly, until the diagnosis is excluded (2) Consider dialysis with low-calcium (or zero-calcium, if available) dialysate if hypercalcaemia fails to respond to saline, furosemide and bisphosphonate (also in patients with renal failure)
Key investigations	**To establish the diagnosis:** (1) Serum calcium—hypercalcaemia defined by concentration >2.6 mmol/litre, acute symptomatic cases usually >3.0 mmol/litre.
	Other important tests: (1) Full blood count, electrolytes, renal and liver function tests (2) Serum PTH, immunoglobulins; protein electrophoresis of serum and urine (3) Chest radiograph (4) Directed by clinical suspicion of malignancy
Further management	Dependent on the cause of hypercalcaemia

5.8 Addisonian crisis

See Chapter 13.7.1 in main text.

Clinical features	**History** (1) Cardiovascular collapse (2) Context of nonspecific symptoms compatible with glucocorticoid deficiency: tiredness, weakness, dizziness, anorexia, weight loss, nausea, vomiting, diarrhoea, abdominal pain. May have salt craving (3) Related to cause—personal or family history of autoimmune/endocrine disease, steroid usage (and cessation), tuberculosis, recent flank pain (?adrenal haemorrhage/infarction) (4) Context of symptoms related to hypopituitarism (may be present in secondary but not primary adrenal insufficiency)—infertility, oligo-/amenorrhoea, poor libido (LH/FSH deficiency); weight gain, cold intolerance (TSH deficiency); hypoglycaemia (GH deficiency) (5) May occur in context of septicaemia
	Examination (1) State of circulation—temperature of peripheries, pulse rate, BP, JVP (2) Hyperpigmentation—palmar creases, scars, and buccal mucosae (present in primary but not secondary adrenal insufficiency) (3) Loss of axillary and pubic hair in women (4) Vitiligo
Immediate management	If cardiorespiratory collapse, as described in 1.2 above (1) Restoration of intravascular volume—give 0.9% saline IV as described in 3.1 above (2) Steroid, e.g. hydrocortisone 100 mg IV (give immediately, then every 6 h; give IM if IV not possible)
Key investigations	**To establish the diagnosis:** (1) Serum cortisol and ACTH—taken at the time of venous cannulation for resuscitation (2) Short synacthen test—performed later

Other important tests:

(1) Electrolytes (hyponatraemia, hyperkalaemia), glucose (hypoglycaemia), renal function tests (elevated urea), calcium, full blood count
(2) Autoantibodies (adrenal, thyroid, intrinsic factor)
(3) Thyroid function tests
(4) Plasma renin activity—to assess mineralocorticoid status (high renin in primary adrenal insufficiency; not high in secondary adrenal insufficiency, where mineralocorticoid reserve is normal)
(5) Chest radiograph—small heart, ?evidence of TB
(6) Adrenal CT scanning (where not available, abdominal radiograph—when adrenal calcification suggests TB)

Further management	(1) Long-term steroid replacement therapy: usually hydrocortisone (30 mg/day in divided doses), also fludrocortisone (50–150 μg/day) if mineralocorticoid deficient (2) Education—patients need to know that they will require increased steroid dosage at times of intercurrent illness. All patients must carry a steroid card. MedicAlert bracelet

5.9 Thyrotoxic crisis

See Chapter 13.4 in main text.

Clinical features	**History** (1) May have partially treated thyrotoxicosis (but many cases previously undiagnosed) (2) Compatible with thyrotoxicosis: weight loss, palpitations, heat intolerance, sweating, diarrhoea, tremor, agitation/anxiety/irritability (3) Precipitant of thyrotoxic crisis—acute illness or trauma, particularly if directed toward thyroid gland, e.g. radio-iodine treatment, iodinated contrast dyes, thyroid surgery (4) Personal or family history of autoimmune/endocrine disease
	Examination (1) Hyperpyrexia (>38.5°C) and profuse sweating (2) Jaundice (3) Extreme restlessness, confusion, psychosis, eventually progressing to coma (4) Cardiac arrhythmia—particularly fast atrial fibrillation. Eventually cardiorespiratory collapse (5) Signs of thyroid disorder—goitre, eye signs of Graves' disease

Immediate management	Thyrotoxic crisis is a potentially fatal disorder that requires immediate treatment on the basis of clinical suspicion
	♦ If cardiorespiratory collapse—as described in 1.2 above
	♦ Restoration of intravascular volume—as described in 3.1 above
	♦ Oxygen—high flow, with reservoir bag if needed, to achieve PaO_2 >92%
	Give:
	(1) Antithyroid drug: propylthiouracil is better than carbimazole in thyrotoxic crisis (but do not wait for hours to obtain propylthiouracil if carbimazole is available)
	  ♦ Propylthiouracil 600 mg orally or via NG tube given immediately, then 250 mg every 6 h (may also be given rectally if severe vomiting prevents oral/NG route), or
	  ♦ Carbimazole 20 mg orally or via NG tube given immediately, then 20 mg every 6 h

(2) Iodide, starting 1 h after the antithyroid drug
  ♦ Aqueous iodine oral solution, e.g. Lugol's (iodine 5%, potassium iodide 10% in purified water) 5 drops orally or via NG tube every 6 h
  ♦ Ipodate (oral cholecystographic agent) 500 mg every 12 h
(3) Propanolol, 2 mg IV or 40 mg orally every 4 h; careful monitoring required
(4) Steroid—dexamethasone 2 mg every 6 h
(5) Active cooling—cooling blankets, antipyretics (use paracetamol, not aspirin, which displaces thyroid hormone from thyroid-binding globulin)

Consider:
(6) Digoxin for atrial fibrillation—may need larger dose than usual
(7) Diuretics for pulmonary oedema

Also:
(1) Specific treatment of precipitating event (if possible), e.g. antibiotics for infection

Key investigations	**To establish the diagnosis:** Thyroid function tests—these confirm the diagnosis of hyperthyroidism, but note that the diagnosis of thyrotoxic crisis is made on clinical grounds. The severity of disturbance of the thyroid function tests does not correlate with the clinical picture
	Other important tests: (1) Full blood count, electrolytes, renal and liver function tests, calcium (2) Autoantibodies (adrenal, thyroid, intrinsic factor) (3) ECG—arrhythmia, especially atrial fibrillation (4) Chest radiograph—pulmonary oedema, infection
Further management	Dependent on the cause of thyrotoxicosis

5.10 Pituitary apoplexy

See Chapter 13.2 in main text.

Clinical features	**History**
	Most commonly: (1) Sudden onset retro-orbital headache (2) Visual disturbance—field defect and/or diplopia
	Sometimes: (3) Nausea and vomiting (4) Meningism (5) Altered conscious level
	Also: (6) Compatible with hypopituitarism or hyperprolactinaemia: lethargy, reduced libido, oligomenorrhoea/amenorrhoea, impotence, galactorrhoea
	Examination (1) Glasgow Coma Score (2) Vision—acuity and fields (3) Eye movements—looking for ophthalmoplegia (4) Signs of underlying pituitary disease, e.g. acromegaly, are rarely present
Immediate management	(1) If cardiorespiratory collapse, as described in 1.2 above (2) Oxygen—high flow, with reservoir bag if needed, to achieve PaO_2 >92%

On clinical suspicion of diagnosis:
(1) Serum cortisol—to establish baseline retrospectively
(2) Serum prolactin
(3) Assume anterior pituitary dysfunction and give corticosteroid, e.g. hydrocortisone 100 mg IV (immediately, then every 6 h)

Key investigations	**To establish the diagnosis:** MRI scan of pituitary fossa—looking for haemorrhage into pituitary adenoma or other tumour
	Other important tests: (1) Electrolytes (hyponatraemia common), glucose, renal function, calcium, full blood count, coagulation screen (2) Anterior pituitary function—baseline tests: cortisol, thyroid function tests, prolactin, LH, FSH, oestrogen/testosterone
Further management	All cases require: (1) Full endocrine evaluation (2) Management dependent on hormonal deficiencies and the cause of pituitary apoplexy: Prolactin <1500 mU/litre—if vision is severly affected—urgent surgical decompression; if vision is not severely affected—consider surgical decompression within 1 week (improves visual and endocrine outcomes) Prolactin >1500 mU/litre (suggests prolactinoma)—a conservative (nonsurgical) approach may be adopted if there is no progressive visual or neurological deficit and prolactin levels are very high; start immediate treatment with dopamine agonist such as bromocriptine or cabergoline

5.11 Acute porphyria

See Chapter 12.5 in main text.

Clinical features	**History** Intermittent episodes of: (1) Acute abdominal pain, vomiting and constipation; diarrhoea also occurs; most attacks in women—these usually occur in luteal phase premenstrually (2) Severe proximal limb and/or back pain (4) Altered urine colour in relation to attacks: occasionally red or even purple like permanganate solution—turns brown-red on standing, especially on exposure to light. (5) Seizures, coma (6) Psychiatric disturbance: anxiety, depression, hallucinations
	Notes (1) Family history—nearly all the acute porphyrias are dominantly inherited, but many carriers are latent (history of family illness as above) (2) Photosensitive skin eruption (exposed areas)—in variegate and hereditary coproporphyria (which can cause acute neurovisceral attacks) but not in acute intermittent porphyria (3) Precipitant—alcohol, sex steroids, other drugs (see Table 33.1.17), anaesthetic agents, starvation, recent infection or surgery

Examination
(1) Cardiovascular—seeking sinus tachycardia, hypertension
(2) Abdominal—may have signs indistinguishable from those of the acute 'surgical' abdomen, but tenderness is usually lacking; gratuitous gynaecological procedures are common
(3) Neurological—Glasgow Coma Score (if appropriate) motor neuropathy, respiratory muscle weakness with respiratory failure

Immediate management	◆ If cardiorespiratory collapse—as described in 1.2 above ◆ If coma—as described in 6.1 below ◆ Monitor ventilatory capacity (FEV1, as for demyelinating polyneuropathy, Guillain–Barré type) ◆ Oxygen—high flow, with reservoir bag if needed, to achieve Pao_2 >92% ◆ Check serum sodium twice daily in first instance (fulminant hyponatraemia)
	(1) Drugs—stop all known precipitant drugs, especially any that have recently been prescribed. Consult Table 33.1.17 before prescribing anything (2) Diet—give high-carbohydrate diet (suppresses haem biosynthesis). If patient unable to eat, seriously unwell or with sustained attack, then give haem arginate (3) Haem arginate—3 mg/kg once daily for 4 days (maximum 250 mg daily) by IV infusion in 0.9% saline over at least 30 min using inline filter. Protect from light and do not administer this agent other than freshly diluted immediately before use

Notes
(1) Supplies of haem arginate can be obtained from Orphan Europe Ltd (http://www.orphan-europe.com, +44 1491 414 333, info.ukorphan-europe.com). Also from the on-call pharmacist at the University College of Wales, Cardiff (029 2074 7747); St James' University Hospital, Leeds (0113 243 3144 or 0113 283 7010); St Thomas' Hospital, London (020 7928 9292)
(2) Seizures—pose difficulties since many anticonvulsants precipitate or worsen porphyric attacks: temazepam, lorazepam, and midazolam are probably safe
(3) Analgesia—morphine and pethidine can be used
(4) Distress/agitation—chlorpromazine can be used
(5) Hypertension/extreme tachycardia—propanolol, labetalolol can be used
(6) Dextrose—some authorities have advised administration of IV dextrose, 5% or 20%, to suppress haem biosynthesis, but this carries the risk of exacerbating/precipitating hyponatraemia (see below). Do not use if patient is hyponatraemic. Monitor serum sodium closely if used

Key investigations	**To establish the diagnosis:** Detection of porphyrin precursors (5-aminolaevulinate (ALA) and porphobilinogen (PBG)) in fresh urine (which may rarely become red/purple/brown on standing)
	Other important tests: (1) Electrolytes—there may be profound hyponatraemia. Monitor serum sodium daily in the acute phase and correct appropriately (2) Full blood count, renal and liver function tests, calcium (3) ECG

Further investigation to exclude serious abdominal or neurological disease will be determined by clinical presentation, especially if excretion of haem precursors is normal, e.g.

(4) Amylase/chest and abdominal radiograph/CT abdomen/ senior surgical opinion
(5) CT brain/lumbar puncture

Note
In a patient with known porphyria, the absence of excess PBG or ALA in the urine renders acute porphyria an unlikely cause of the current illness

Further management
(1) Seek expert advice to establish diagnosis and investigate family
(2) MedicAlert bracelet important as warning to health care personnel in the future
(3) Advise patient to stop smoking since it appears that this is associated with increased frequency of recurrent acute porphyric attacks

Table 33.1.17 Drugs unsafe for use in acute porphyrias

Drug/drug group	Comments
Unsafe drug groups (check this first)	
Amphetamines	
Anabolic steroids	
Antidepressants	Includes tricyclic (and related) antidepressants and MAOIs; fluoxetine and mianserin thought to be safe
Antihistamines	Alimemazine (trimeprazine), chlorphenamine, desloratadine, fexofenadine, ketotifen, loratadine, and promethazine thought to be safe
Barbiturates	Includes primidone and thiopental
Calcium channel blockers	Diltiazem may be used with caution if safer alternative not available
Contraceptives, hormonal	Progestogens are more porphyrinogenic than oestrogens; oestrogens may be safe at least in replacement doses.
	Progestogens should be avoided whenever possible by all women susceptible to acute porphyria; however, when nonhormonal contraception is inappropriate, progestogens may be used with extreme caution if the potential benefit outweighs risk. The risk of an acute attack is greatest in women who have had a previous attack or are aged <30 years. Long-acting progestogen preparations should never be used in those at risk of acute porphyria
Ergot derivatives	Includes ergometrine (oxytocin probably safe) and pergolide
Gold salts	
Hormone replacement therapy	See comments on contraceptives
Imidazole antifungals	Applies to oral and intravenous use; topical antifungals are thought to be safe due to low systemic exposure
Nonnucleoside reverse transcriptase inhibitors	Contact http://www.wmic.wales.nhs.uk/porphyria_info.php for further advice

Table 33.1.17 (*Cont'd*) Drugs unsafe for use in acute porphyrias

Drug/drug group	Comments
Progestogens	
Protease inhibitors	Contact http://www.wmic.wales.nhs.uk/porphyria_info.php for further advice
Statins	Rosuvastatin is thought to be safe
Sulphonamides	Includes co-trimoxazole and sulfasalazine
Sulphonylureas	Glipizide is thought to be safe
Tetracyclines	
Triazole antifungals	See comments on imidazole antifungals
Unsafe drugs (check groups above first)	
Aceclofenac	
Alcohol	
Amiodarone	
Azapropazone	
Bosentan	
Bromocriptine	
Buspirone	
Busulfan	
Cabergoline	
Carbamazepine	
Carisoprodol	
Chloral hydrate	Although evidence of hazard is uncertain, manufacturer advises avoid
Chlorambucil	May be used with caution if safer alternative not available
Chloramphenicol	
Chloroform	Small amounts in medicines probably safe
Clindamycin	
Clonidine	
Cocaine	
Colistin	
Cyclophosphamide	May be used with caution if safer alternative not available
Cycloserine	
Danazol	
Dapsone	
Dexfenfluramine	
Diazepam	Status epilepticus has been treated successfully with intravenous diazepam
Diclofenac	
Erythromycin	
Etamsylate	
Ethosuximide	

Table 33.1.17 *(Cont'd)* Drugs unsafe for use in acute porphyrias

Drug/drug group	Comments
Etomidate	
Fenfluramine	
Flupentixol	
Griseofulvin	
Halothane	
Hydralazine	
Indapamide	
Isometheptene mucate	
Isoniazid	
Ketamine	
Ketorolac	
Lidocaine (lignocaine)	When used for local anaesthesia, bupivacaine, lidocaine (lignocaine), procaine, prilocaine, and tetracaine are thought to be safe
Lisinopril	
Mebeverine	
Mefenamic acid	May be used with caution if safer alternative not available
Meprobamate	
Methyldopa	
Metoclopramide	May be used with caution if safer alternative not available
Metolazone	
Metronidazole	May be used with caution if safer alternative not available
Metyrapone	
Mifepristone	
Minoxidil	May be used with caution if safer alternative not available
Nalidixic acid	
Nitrofurantoin	
Orphenadrine	
Oxcarbazepine	
Oxybutynin	
Oxycodone	Buprenorphine, codeine, diamorphine, dihydrocodeine, fentanyl, methadone, morphine, and pethidine are thought to be safe
Pentazocine	Buprenorphine, codeine, diamorphine, dihydrocodeine, fentanyl, methadone, morphine, and pethidine are thought to be safe
Pentoxifylline (oxpentifylline)	
Phenoxybenzamine	
Phenytoin	
Pivmecillinam	

Table 33.1.17 *(Cont'd)* Drugs unsafe for use in acute porphyrias

Drug/drug group	Comments
Porfimer	
Probenecid	
Pyrazinamide	
Rifabutin	Rifamycins have been used in a few patients without evidence of harm—use with caution if safer alternative not available
Rifampicin[7]	Rifamycins have been used in a few patients without evidence of harm—use with caution if safer alternative not available
Spironolactone	
Sulfinpyrazone	
Sulpiride	
Tamoxifen	
Temoporfin	
Theophylline	Includes aminophylline
Tiagabine	
Tinidazole	
Topiramate	
Tramadol	Buprenorphine, codeine, diamorphine, dihydrocodeine, fentanyl, methadone, morphine, and pethidine are thought to be safe
Triclofos	Although evidence of hazard is uncertain, manufacturer advises avoid
Trimethoprim	
Valproate	Status epilepticus has been treated successfully with intravenous diazepam
Xipamide	
Zidovudine	Contact http://www.wmic.wales.nhs.uk/porphyria_info.php for further advice.
Zuclopenthixol	

Reproduced from British National Formulary (March 2009), 57, with addition of lisinopril to the list of unsafe drugs. The online website www.porphyria-europe.com is a source of useful consensus prescribing and practical information (and much more) for patients, their families and doctors.

6 Neurological

6.1 Coma

See Chapter 24.5.5 in main text

Clinical features	**History**
	Coma is defined as a Glasgow Coma Score (GCS) <8, hence the patient will not be able to give any useful history. Obtain as much information as possible from others in attendance (relatives, friends, ambulance crew, bystanders, etc.) or from notes (referring physician, paramedics). Ask in particular regarding:
	(1) The circumstances in which the patient was found
	(2) Alcohol consumption
	(3) Diabetes mellitus
	(4) Epilepsy
	(5) Drugs of abuse, in particular opioids
	(6) Head injury
	(7) Regular medications
	(8) Past medical history
	Examination
	Initial survey:
	(1) Airway, breathing, circulation
	(2) Finger prick stick test for blood glucose (?hypoglycaemia)
	(3) Check for small pupils and slow respiratory rate (?opioid overdose)
	(4) Check temperature (?hypothermia)
	(5) Head to toe screen
	(6) Look for MedicAlert bracelet or necklace
	(7) Glasgow Coma Score (Table 33.1.18)
	Further examination:
	(1) State of circulation—temperature of peripheries, pulse rate, BP, JVP
	(2) Respiratory—look for evidence of aspiration
	(3) Neurological:
	◆ Focal/lateralizing signs—a structural lesion is likely if these are present
	◆ Meningism
	◆ Movements (can be subtle)—status epilepticus
	(4) Tongue biting or incontinence of urine—suggest (but do not prove) epilepsy
	(5) Back of head and neck—for bruising or bleeding to suggest head injury
	(6) Ears and nose—for bleeding or cerebrospinal fluid leak to suggest basal skull fracture
	(7) Search pockets etc. for clues—e.g. anticonvulsant tablets
Immediate management	(1) If cardiorespiratory collapse—as described in 1.2 above
	(2) Nurse in recovery position (when injury to neck excluded)
	(3) Oxygen—high flow, with reservoir bag if needed, to achieve PaO_2 >92%
	(4) Airway—patients with a GCS <8 are likely to need endotracheal intubation to protect and maintain their airway if they do not respond to glucose or naloxone. This is obligatory if they need to be moved from an area where they can be given intensive nursing care to one where they cannot, e.g. CT scanner. Consider oropharyngeal airway, but do not attempt to force one in to a patient who resists (which means that they are protecting their airway)
	(5) Intravenous access—insert cannula
	(6) Consider and treat specific diagnoses
	◆ Hypoglycaemia—give 50 ml of 50% glucose (dextrose monohydrate) IV if blood glucose <2.5 mmol/litre
	◆ Opioid overdose—give naloxone 0.4–2 mg IV if this is a possible diagnosis
	◆ Hypothermia—start rewarming if temperature <35°C
Key investigations	**To establish the diagnosis:**
	(1) Blood glucose
	(2) CT brain—if diagnosis not clinically apparent and patient not improving rapidly. Look for:
	◆ Extradural, subdural, subarachnoid, or intracerebral haemorrhage
	◆ Signs of raised intracranial pressure
	◆ Focal ischaemia (may not be visible on early scan)
	(3) Blood film for malaria—if relevant travel history
	Other important tests:
	(1) Electrolytes (hyponatraemia), renal and liver function tests, calcium (hypo- or hypercalcaemia), full blood count
	(2) ECG—note that 'ischaemic' changes can occur in subarachnoid haemorrhage
	(3) Chest radiograph—?aspiration pneumonia
	(4) Arterial blood gases—if diagnosis not clear, or if PaO_2 <92% on air
	(5) Sepsis screen—selected cases
	(6) Lumbar puncture—selected cases, after CT has excluded raised intracranial pressure
	(7) EEG—selected cases; consider nonconvulsive status
Further management	Dependent on the cause of coma

6.2 Acute confusional state

See Chapter 24.8 and Section 29 in main text.

Clinical features	**History**
	Is the patient confused?:
	(1) Establish that the patient is not dysphasic rather than confused
	(2) Abbreviated Mental Test (AMT) score—a score of 6 or less is likely to indicate impaired cognition
	◆ Age
	◆ Time (to nearest hour)
	◆ What year is it?
	◆ Name of institution
	◆ Recognition of two persons (can the patient identify your job and that of a nurse?)
	◆ Date of birth (day and month)
	◆ Year of First World War
	◆ Name of present monarch
	◆ Count backwards from 20 to 1
	(3) Assessment of attention and concentration, which are typically impaired in acute confusional states:
	◆ Count backwards from 100 in 7's (93, 86, etc.)
	◆ Count backwards from 40 in 4's (36, 32, etc.)
	◆ Count backwards from 20 in 2's (18, 16, etc.)
	◆ Count backwards from 20 (19, 18, etc.)

Obtaining a history:

The patient who is confused cannot (by definition) give an accurate and reliable account of themselves, hence get as much information as possible from others in attendance (relatives, friends, ambulance crew, bystanders, etc.) or from notes (referring physician, paramedics). Ask in particular regarding:

(1) The situation in which the patient was found
(2) Any recent change in health, in particular:
   ◆ Symptoms to suggest infection
   ◆ Medications—especially any recent change
(3) Previous cognitive function
(4) Alcohol consumption—consider intoxication, withdrawal, Wernicke's encephalopathy
(5) Drugs of abuse (if relevant)
(6) Regular medications
(7) Past medical history
(8) Social circumstances

Examination

(1) General appearance—well-presented clothing and cleanliness indicates an acute problem or an assiduous carer
(2) Nutritional state—reflects previous weeks/months
(3) Hydration state—reflects previous 48 h
(4) Full physical examination—look in particular for:
   ◆ Temperature—pyrexia or hypothermia
   ◆ Pulse rate, BP, JVP—hypotension from any cause can lead to confusion
   ◆ Evidence of sepsis—in particular chest, urine, cellulitis
   ◆ Neurological—focal signs (indicating a focal neurological lesion, most commonly stroke), head injury, Wernicke's encephalopathy
   ◆ Evidence of organ failure—cardiac, respiratory, hepatic, renal
   ◆ Urinary retention or faecal impaction
   ◆ Hip or pelvic fracture

Immediate management

If cardiorespiratory collapse, as described in 1.2 above

Oxygen—high flow, with reservoir bag if needed, to achieve PaO_2 >92%

Hypoglycaemia—give 50 ml of 50% glucose (dextrose monohydrate) IV if blood glucose <2.5 mmol/litre

(1) Fluids—encourage oral intake, but if IV fluids are required, then insert venous cannula into flat site and bandage carefully
(2) Treat any obvious precipitating condition—if none apparent then consider initiating antibiotic treatment for, e.g. urinary infection, on a 'best guess' basis (e.g. coamoxiclav 250/125 mg orally twice daily, but note local hospital antibiotic policy)
(3) Anticipate and avoid problems:
   ◆ Do not exacerbate confusion—nurse in lit room (darkness makes confusion worse), expose to limited number of staff (many people 'popping in' increase confusion), enlist assistance from relatives/carers/friends (a sensible person that the patient knows can be enormously helpful)
   ◆ Pressure areas—appropriate mattress
   ◆ Urine—try to avoid catheterization if possible (will make any infection harder to clear), but need to strike a difficult balance with concern for skin/pressure areas
   ◆ Bowels—suppositories, laxatives, enemas as required
   ◆ Venous thromboembolism—low molecular weight heparin, e.g. enoxaparin 20 mg subcutaneously once daily

(4) Sedation—try to avoid if possible, but if necessary use risperidone 0.5 mg orally twice daily (increased in steps of 0.5 mg twice daily to 1–2 mg twice daily) or haloperidol 0.5–2 mg orally/intramuscularly two to three times daily. (Dosage of both drugs appropriate for elderly patients—higher doses likely to be required for younger patients)

Key investigations

To establish the diagnosis:
These will be guided by any clinical leads, but as nonspecific presentation is common, the following are advisable in almost all patients:
(1) Fingerprick stick test for blood glucose
(2) Oxygen saturation—check arterial blood gas if PaO_2 <92% on air
(3) Blood screen—full blood count, electrolytes, renal and liver function tests, calcium, phosphate, cardiac enzymes, glucose, thyroid function, inflammatory marker (CRP or ESR)
(4) Sepsis screen—urine dipstick test, urine and blood culture
(5) Chest radiograph
(6) ECG

Other important tests:
Guided by clinical findings or results of screening investigations, e.g. new focal neurological signs—imaging of brain by CT scan or MRI

Further management

Dependent on the cause of confusion

6.3 Acute stroke

See Chapter 24.10.1 in main text.

Clinical features

History
May be difficult to obtain, particularly if the patient has dysphasia. If this is the case, get as much information as possible from others in attendance (relatives, friends, ambulance crew, bystanders, etc.)
(1) Focal neurological deficit—usually of sudden onset
(2) Previous episodes—stroke, transient ischaemic attack, amaurosis fugax
(3) Risk factors
(4) Other medical conditions
(5) Medications
(6) Normal level of functioning—do they need help with activities of daily living?
(7) Social circumstances

Examination
(1) Airway, breathing, circulation
(2) Neurological
   ◆ Glasgow Coma Score (Table 33.1.18)
   ◆ Nature of focal deficit (Table 33.1.19)
(3) Cardiovascular—pulse rate and rhythm (?atrial fibrillation), BP, carotid bruits, cardiac murmurs, absent peripheral pulses

Immediate management

If cardiorespiratory collapse—as described in 1.2 above
(1) Nurse in recovery position if impairment of consciousness
(2) Oxygen—high flow, with reservoir bag if needed, to achieve PaO_2 >92%. Consider oropharyngeal airway
(3) Establish IV access
(4) Exclude hypoglycaemia—check fingerprick stick test for blood glucose and if <3 mmol/l give 50 ml of 50% glucose (dextrose monohydrate) IV.

(5) Consider thrombolysis—if time of onset can be clearly determined, and if the patient presents to centre with appropriate facilities within 3 h of onset (Table 33.1.20, 33.1.21)

(6) Reverse anticoagulation—if haemorraghic stroke and patient receiving anticoagulation (Table 33.1.12)

Notes

(1) Urgent neurosurgical assessment is required for patients with large cerebellar infarcts or haemorrhages, those with hydrocephalus, and for some cases with intracerebral haemorrhage

(2) There is no proven benefit for drugs in the limitation of neural damage, including corticosteroids, nimodipine, plasma volume expanders, barbiturates, or glutamate receptor antagonists: these (and similar agents) should only be given in the context of ethically approved clinical trials

Key investigations	**To establish the diagnosis:** CT or MRI brain—also to distinguish between infarction and haemorrhage **Other important tests:** (1) Full blood count, electrolytes, renal and liver function tests, calcium, inflammatory markers (CRP or ESR), coagulation screen (2) ECG—look for arrhythmia or signs of recent myocardial infarction (3) Chest radiograph—?aspiration pneumonia (4) Echocardiography; ultrasound/Doppler examination of carotid arteries—in selected cases

Further management	Short term:
	(1) Nursing and physiotherapy—protect pressure areas, attention to bladder and bowels, prevent contractures, aid recovery of function, psychological support
	(2) Hydration/nutrition—if swallowing impaired, stop oral feeding and start IV fluids
	(3) Blood pressure—this is commonly elevated immediately after a stroke, but cerebral autoregulation is impaired and aggressive attempts to reduce it are likely to cause more harm than good. There is much debate regarding best treatment:
	   ◆ Ischaemic stroke—if BP >220/130 mmHg then most physicians would treat—e.g. using modified release nifedipine 10 mg orally or IV labetolol (see 1.11 above)—but some would only do so if there was evidence that the hypertension were causing acute organ damage
	   ◆ Haemorrhagic stroke—if BP >180/110 mmHg then most physicians would treat—e.g. using modified release nifedipine 10 mg orally or IV labetolol (see 1.11 above)
	(4) Venous thromboembolism—high risk: use compression stockings
	(5) Antiplatelet therapy—usually aspirin 300 mg once daily—should be started to prevent recurrence as soon as haemorrhage has been excluded
	(6) Blood glucose—use IV sliding scale of insulin (see 5.2 above) to obtain good control in diabetics
	
	Medium/long term:
	(1) Rehabilitation and social support as required
	(2) Control of vascular risk factors—hypertension, hyperlipidaemia, cessation of cigarette smoking
	(3) Consider imaging of the carotid arteries in all patients who have made a reasonable recovery from a carotid territory stroke: endarterectomy may be indicated

Table 33.1.18 Glasgow Coma Scale

Eye opening	Score	Verbal	Score	Motor (best response in any limb)	Score
Spontaneously	4	Orientated	5	Obeys commands	6
To speech	3	Confused speech	4	Localizes to pain	5
To pain	2	Words	3	Withdraws to pain	4
None	1	Sounds	2	Flexor (decorticate) response to pain	3
		None	1	Extensor (decerebrate) response to pain	2
				None	1

Notes:
(1) The Glasgow Coma Score is obtained by adding the best eye, verbal and motor responses together: minimum = 3, maximum = 15, coma = 8 or less, significant deterioration = fall by 2 points or more.
(2) Painful stimulation: rub knuckles on sternum, squeeze pencil or biro against nail bed. Do not use methods that might lead to bleeding or bruising, which includes supraorbital pressure.
Reprinted from *The Lancet*, Vol. 304, Teasdale G, Jennett B, *Assessment of Coma and Impaired Consciousness: A Practical Scale*, pp 81–84. Copyright (1974), with permission from Elsevier.

Table 33.1.19 A practical classification of stroke (the Oxfordshire Community Stroke Subclassification System)

Total anterior syndrome circulation (TACS)	
Large cortical stroke in middle cerebral artery, or middle and anterior cerebral artery territories	New higher cerebral dysfunction (e.g. dysphasia, dyscalculia, visuospatial disorder)
	+
	Homonymous visual field defect
	+
	Ipsilateral motor and/orensory deficit involving two out of three of face, arm, or legs

Partial anterior circulation syndrome (PACS)	
Cortical stroke in middle or anterior cerebral artery territories	Two out of three components of TACS
	or
	New higher cerebral dysfunction alone
	or
	Motor/sensory deficit more restricted than those classified as LACS (e.g. monoparesis)

Lacunar syndrome (LACS)	
Subcortical stroke due to small-vessel disease	Pure motor stroke
	or
	Pure sensory stroke
	or
	Sensorimotor stroke
	or
	Ataxic hemiparesis
	or
	Dysarthria and clumsy hand
	Note that evidence of higher cortical involvement or disturbance of consciousness excludes a lacunar syndrome

Table 33.1.19 (Cont'd) A practical classification of stroke (the Oxfordshire Community Stroke Subclassification System)

Posterior circulation syndrome (PCS)

	Ipsilateral cranial nerve palsy with contralateral motor/sensory deficit
	or
	Bilateral motor and/or sensory deficit
	or
	Disorder of conjugate eye movement
	or
	Cerebellar dysfunction without ipsilateral pyramidal involvement (which would be an ataxic hemiparesis and classified as LACS)
	or
	Isolated homonymous visual field defect

Table 33.1.20 Thrombolysis for stroke

Parameter		Comment
Preconditions	Do not thrombolyse unless	The physician and other carers are trained and experienced in the administration of thrombolysis to stroke patients and are working in a centre with appropriate facilities The time of onset of stroke is known—if it was noticed when the patient woke from sleep, then the time of going to sleep is regarded as the time of onset Haemorrhagic stroke has been excluded by brain CT scan Thrombolysis can be started within 3 h of stroke onset
Stroke deficit	Exclude mild strokes	Dysphasia alone Hemianopia alone Inattention alone Ataxia alone
	Exclude very severe strokes	Clinical—no response to painful stimulation; NIH stroke score >25 (Table 33.1.21) Imaging shows large volume of ischaemia
Other considerations	Do not thrombolyse if	Patient heavily dependent on others for personal care before stroke Rapidly resolving neurological deficit Generalized seizure since onset of stroke History of stroke in last 3 months History of intracerebral bleed at any time Major surgery or haemorrhage in last 3 weeks BP >180/105 mmHg on repeated readings.
	Consent	From patient or next of kin—advise 10–20% chance of benefit vs 3% risk of significant bleed
Thrombolysis	Drug	Recombinant tissue plasminogen activator (rt-PA, Alteplase) 0.9 mg/kg IV, with 10% of dose given as initial bolus, the remainder infused over 60 min
Other care		Manage patient in acute stroke unit bed (or coronary care unit/high dependency unit) Check GCS, pulse and BP, every 15 min Do not give aspirin or other antiplatelet agents/anticoagulants for 24 h.

BP, blood pressure; GCS, Glasgow Coma Score.

Table 33.1.21 National Institutes of Health (NIH) stroke scale

Domain	Response	Scale	Maximum score
Level of consciousness	Keenly responsive	0	3
	Arousable by minor stimulation	1	
	Requires repeated stimulation to attend and/or strong/painful stimulation to make nonstereotyped movements	2	
	Unresponsive or reflex responses only	3	
Verbal response to questions What month is it? How old are you?	Answers both questions correctly	0	2
	Answers one question correctly	1	
	Answers neither question correctly	2	
Motor response to command (pantomime) Open and close your eyes Open and close your (nonparetic) hand	Performs both tasks correctly	0	2
	Performs one task correctly	1	
	Performs neither task correctly	2	
Gaze Only horizontal movements tested Voluntary or oculocephalic (reflex)	Normal	0	2
	Partial gaze palsy—gaze is abnormal in one or both eyes, but forced deviation or total gaze paresis is not present	1	
	Forced deviation or total gaze palsy not overcome by oculocephalic manoeuvre	2	
Visual fields Tested by confrontation	No visual loss	0	3
	Partial hemianopia	1	
	Complete hemianopia	2	
	Bilateral hemianopia (blind)	3	
Facial palsy Ask (pantomime) patient to show teeth, raise eyebrows and close eyes	Normal	0	3
	Minor paralysis—flattened nasolabial fold; asymmetry on smiling	1	
	Partial paralysis—total or near total paralysis of lower face	2	
	Total paralysis—absence of movement of upper and lower face (one or both sides)	3	
Motor arm Extend arms (palms down) at 90° (if sitting) or 45° (if supine)	No drift	0	4 for right arm + 4 for left arm
	Drift—within 10 s, but arm does not hit bed or other support	1	
	Some effort against gravity	2	
	No effort against gravity—arm falls	3	
	No movement	4	
Motor leg Hold leg at 30° (always tested with patient supine)	No drift	0	4 for right leg + 4 for left leg
	Drift—within 5 s, but leg does not hit bed	1	
	Some effort against gravity	2	
	No effort against gravity—leg falls	3	
	No movement	4	
Limb ataxia Finger-nose test Heel-shin test	Absent	0	2
	Present in one limb	1	
	Present in two limbs	2	

(Continued)

Table 33.1.21 *(Cont'd)* National Institutes of Health (NIH) stroke scale

Domain	Response	Scale	Maximum score
Sensory Pinprick Other noxious stimuli	Normal	0	2
	Mild / moderate sensory loss—pinprick is less sharp or dull on the affected side	1	
	Severe / total sensory loss—patient is not aware of being touched on the face, arm and leg	2	
Language Describe what is happening in the picture (provided) Name items on naming sheet (provided) Read list of sentences (provided)	Normal	0	3
	Mild-to-moderate dysphasia—obvious loss of fluency or comprehension	1	
	Severe dysphasia—all communication fragmentary	2	
	Mute, global aphasia	3	
Dysarthria Read or repeat words from list (provided) Spontaneous speech	None	0	2
	Mild-to-moderate—can be understood with some difficulty	1	
	Severe—unintelligible speech	2	

National Institutes of Health (NIH) stroke scale

Details available from http://www.ninds.nih.gov/doctors/NIH_Stroke_Scale.pdf (text version) or http://www.ninds.nih.gov/doctors/NIH_Stroke_Scale_Booklet.pdf (graphical version) - accessed 24/01/09.

6.4 Subarachnoid haemorrhage

See Chapter 24.10.1 in main text.

Clinical features	**History** (1) Presentation is very variable: typically severe headache ('worst ever') of sudden onset, but can vary from minor symptoms to collapse/coma or sudden death (2) Previous episodes; recent unusual headache (3) Risk factors—hypertension, cigarette smoking, alcohol (binge drinking), adult polycystic kidney disease, connective tissue disorders (some)

	Examination
	(1) Airway, breathing, circulation
	(2) Glasgow Coma Score
	(3) Focal neurological signs—in particular:
	   ♦ Third nerve palsy—posterior communicating artery aneurysm
	   ♦ Sixth nerve palsy—posterior fossa aneurysm, but usually a false localizing sign
	   ♦ Bilateral leg weakness—anterior communicating artery aneurysm
	   ♦ Dysphasia/hemiparesis—middle cerebral artery aneurysm
	(4) Neck rigidity
	(5) Retinal haemorrhages
	(6) Cardiovascular—arrhythmia, hypertension

Immediate management	If cardiorespiratory collapse—as described in 1.2 above (1) Nurse in recovery position if impairment of consciousness (2) Oxygen—high flow, with reservoir bag if needed, to achieve *Pao*₂ >92%. Consider oropharyngeal airway (3) Establish IV access and resuscitate if volume depleted or dehydrated: maintain total fluid input of 3 litres/day. (4) Bed rest for all patients

(5) Nimodipine 60 mg orally every 4 h, started within 4 days of subarachnoid haemorrhage and continued for 21 days, should be given to all patients with subarachnoid haemorrhage who are not hypotensive (systolic BP <110 mmHg). This is to prevent ischaemic neurological deficit

(6) Blood pressure—as with acute stroke there is much debate regarding best treatment. Most specialists advocate intervention at >180/110 mmHg (as for haemorrhagic stroke, see 6.3 above), with IV labetalol commonly employed (see 1.11 above)

(7) Analgesia—paracetamol, codeine if required

(8) Anxiety—short acting benzodiazepine if required

Key investigations	**To establish the diagnosis:** (1) CT brain, without contrast, taking thin cuts through the base (2) Lumbar puncture—perform not earlier than 12 h after the ictus if CT normal: look for xanthochromia after centrifugation of cerebrospinal fluid
	Other important tests: (1) Electrolytes, renal and liver function tests, full blood count, coagulation screen (2) ECG—note that 'ischaemic' changes can occur in subarachnoid haemorrhage (3) Chest radiograph—?aspiration pneumonia
Further management	(1) Neurosurgical referral—if GCS = 12 or more, or GCS <12 with space-occupying intracranial haemorrhage or hydrocephalus, then surgery should be considered in patients with proven intracranial aneurysms, hence discuss with neurosurgical colleagues with a view to arranging four-vessel angiography (CT angiograms may be done first, and sometimes instead) (2) Bowels—keep stools soft with adequate oral fluid intake and laxative if required (particularly if codeine given)

6.5 Status epilepticus

See Chapter 24.5.1 in main text.

Clinical features	**Definition** Continuous seizure for more than 30 min or serial (two or more) discrete seizures between which there is incomplete recovery of consciousness
	History The patient will not be able to give any useful history. Obtain as much information as possible from others in attendance (relatives, friends, ambulance crew, bystanders etc.). Ask in particular regarding: (1) Loss of consciousness, usually with obvious fitting (2) The circumstances in which the patient was found (3) Past history of epilepsy (4) Alcohol consumption (5) Any possible drug abuse (6) Diabetes mellitus (7) Regular medications (8) Any other medical history
	Examination Initial survey: (1) Airway, breathing, circulation (2) Signs of injury—especially of tongue, which can compromise breathing (3) Respiratory—?aspiration (4) Glasgow Coma Score (5) MedicAlert bracelet/necklace

Further examination:

(1) Vital signs—temperature, pulse rate, BP

(2) Neurological:
   ◆ Pupil size and reactions
   ◆ Other brainstem signs
   ◆ Symmetry of tone and reflexes in the limbs
   ◆ Neck stiffness
   ◆ Note that focal signs may indicate focal pathology, but can be seen as a postictal phenomenon (i.e. Todd's paresis)

(3) Search pockets, etc. for clues—e.g. anticonvulsant tablets

Immediate management

If cardiorespiratory collapse—as described in 1.2 above

(1) Place in recovery position (if possible)

(2) Oxygen—high flow, with reservoir bag if needed, to achieve PaO_2 >92%. Consider oropharyngeal airway, but do not try to insert one against resistance, i.e. when the patient is actually fitting

(3) Establish IV access.

(4) Fingerprick stick test for blood glucose — give 50 ml of 50% glucose (dextrose monohydrate) IV if glucose <3 mmol/litre

(5) Anticonvulsant—first line treatments:
   ◆ Lorazepam 0.1 mg/kg IV at 2 mg/min—this is the first line treatment of choice
   ◆ Diazepam 10–20 mg IV at a rate of 5 mg/min. This may be repeated after 30–60 min if necessary, and can be followed by infusion (add 10–40 mg of diazepam to 100 ml of 5% dextrose to make a solution containing 0.1–0.4 mg/ml) at a rate of e.g. 5 mg/h, adjusted according to clinical response, but with maximum dose of 3 mg/kg body weight over 24 h

(6) Anticonvulsant—second line treatments. If seizure activity still continues, consider:
   ◆ Fosphenytoin, 15 mg phenytoin-equivalent (PE)/kg body weight (fosphenytoin 1.5 mg = phenytoin 1 mg) by IV infusion at a rate of 100–150 mg PE/min, followed by 4–5 mg PE/kg daily in 1–2 divided doses. Dose adjusted according to clinical response and trough plasma phenytoin levels. This is the second line treatment of choice
   ◆ Phenytoin, 15 mg/kg body weight by IV infusion at a rate not exceeding 50 mg/min, followed by 100 mg every 6–8 h. Dose adjusted according to clinical response and trough plasma-phenytoin levels

(7) Anticonvulsant—third line treatments. If seizure activity still continues, consider:
   ◆ Phenobarbital (phenobarbitone), 20 mg/kg by IV infusion at a rate of not more than 50–75 mg/min, maximum dose 1000 mg. Note that this treatment may lead to respiratory depression. This is the third line treatment of choice
   ◆ Valproate, 25 mg/kg by IV infusion at a rate of 3–6 mg/kg per min
   ◆ Paraldehyde, 5–10 ml by deep intramuscular injection (not more than 5 ml at any one site), or 10–20 ml administered by enema as a 10% solution in physiological saline or mixed with an equal volume of olive oil. Note that this treatment is only to be used if other treatments detailed above are not available

(8) Anaesthesia—if seizure activity still continues after first, second, and third line treatments (or earlier if required to achieve adequate airway protection/ventilation):
   ◆ Call anaesthetist and arrange ICU admission for anaesthesia with thiopentone, propofol, or midazolam. Ventilate with EEG monitoring until clinical and EEG epileptic activity ceases

Note: Thiamine—give Pabrinex IV high potency over 10 min if suspicion of alcohol withdrawal

Key investigations

To establish the diagnosis:

Status epilepticus is a clinical diagnosis, although EEG is used to diagnose the very rare condition of nonconvulsive status in a patient with unexplained coma

Other important tests:

(1) Fingerprick stick test for blood glucose—should be performed in all patients

The requirement for further investigation depends on the context: the patient who is known to have epilepsy with frequent prolonged seizures does not require extensive investigation after each and every one. In other cases:

(2) Glucose, electrolytes, renal and liver function tests, calcium, creatine kinase, anticonvulsant level (if appropriate)

And consider:

(3) Arterial blood gases.

(4) Chest radiograph—?aspiration

(5) ECG

(6) Sepsis screen

(7) Toxicology screen

(8) CT or MRI brain

(9) Lumbar puncture—only after imaging to exclude raised intracranial pressure or intracerebral mass

Further management

Dependent on the cause of status epilepticus

6.6 Acute spinal cord dysfunction

See Chapters 24.13 and 24.13.1 in main text.

Clinical features

History

The immediate clinical priority is to exclude spinal cord compression:

(1) Motor symptoms—weakness; all limbs (quadriparesis) or legs only (paraparesis)

(2) Sensory symptoms — numbness, loss of sensation, tingling, incoordination (sensory ataxia)

(3) Autonomic—sphincter (particularly bladder) disturbance

Causes of cord compression:

(1) Nature of onset (sudden/gradual) and subsequent progression give important clues to likely cause, e.g. acute onset suggests trauma/mechanical or vascular pathology

(2) Back pain

(3) Intervertebral discs—any previous problem?

(4) Malignancy—any known previous, or any features to suggest this diagnosis, e.g. anorexia, malaise, weight loss

(5) Infection—sweats, fevers, rigors. Tuberculosis. Risk factors for osteomyelitis or abscess, e.g. previous septicaemia (particularly staphylococcal), IV drug abuse, haemodialysis

Other causes of spinal cord dysfunction:

◆ History to support the diagnosis of a demyelinating condition

Examination

(1) Motor—look for increased tone, weakness, and hyperreflexia below the site of the lesion. Do the plantars go up or down? Note that in acute lesions there may be flaccidity ('spinal shock'), later replaced by spasticity.

(2) Sensory—is there a sensory level, which can be suspended? In particular, check for sensory loss in the saddle area, which would suggest a cauda equina lesion

(3) Bladder—is this palpable?

Causes of cord compression:
(1) General examination for signs of malignancy—e.g. cachexia, clubbing, lymphadenopathy, pallor, jaundice, chest/abdominal examination, pelvic mass
(2) Suggestion of infective cause—temperature

Other causes of spinal cord dysfunction:
◆ Features to suggest a demyelinating condition, e.g. optic atrophy, internuclear ophthalmoplegia

Immediate management	(1) Nurse on pressure-relieving mattress
	(2) Relieve urinary retention with urethral catheter (if appropriate)
	(3) Emergency imaging and consultation with neurosurgical colleagues
	(4) If spinal cord compression, specific treatment depends on precise diagnosis:
	  ◆ Disc protrusion—surgical decompression
	  ◆ Metastasis—high dose steroids (e.g. methylprednisolone) and radiotherapy
	  ◆ Abscess—surgical decompression/drainage; antimicrobials. For an immunocompetent patient with a pyogenic abscess give IV antimicrobials as follows: third-generation cephalosporin, e.g. cefotaxime 1–2 g 12 hourly plus flucloxacillin 1–2 g 6 hourly plus metronidazole 500 mg 8 hourly. Modify regimen when microbiological results are available
	  ◆ Spinal cord tumours (rare)—neurosurgical intervention may be appropriate
	
	Note
	Acute spinal cord injury—consider methylprednisolone 30 mg/kg as IV bolus over 1 h, followed by 4.0 mg/kg per h for 23 h (but this treatment is contentious)

Key investigations	**To establish the diagnosis:** MRI spine, performed as an emergency (if this is not available, discuss best available imaging modality with radiological colleagues, e.g. CT scan, myelography) **Other important tests:** (1) Full blood count, electrolytes, renal/liver/bone function tests, inflammatory markers, coagulation screen (2) Chest radiograph—is there malignancy? Other tests as dictated by clinical suspicion, e.g. blood cultures, myeloma screen, autoimmune/vasculitic serology, MRI brain, visual/sensory/auditory evoked potentials, cerebrospinal fluid examination
Further management	Dependent on the cause of spinal cord dysfunction

6.7 Acute inflammatory polyneuritis (Guillain–Barré)

See Chapter 24.16 in main text.

Clinical features	**History** (1) Sensory symptoms— paraesthesiae and numbness, begin distally and ascend symmetrically (2) Motor symptoms —weakness, usually ascending (but can sometimes be proximal), symmetrical. Muscle pain is common (particularly lower back or interscapular) (3) Site of symptoms—legs usually worst affected, but sometimes arms; facial, bulbar, and ocular muscles may be involved

(4) Progression—usually occurs over days (no longer than 4 weeks, by definition), but can sometimes be more rapid
(5) Preceding illness—patients often have upper respiratory tract or diarrhoeal illness (especially *Campylobacter jejuni*) in the few weeks prior to onset

Examination
(1) Motor—reduced tone; lower motor neuron weakness, distal > proximal; areflexia. May have facial involvement and ophthalmoplegia (Miller–Fisher syndrome)
(2) Sensory—glove and stocking sensory disturbance, often mild
(3) Respiratory—respiratory failure due to muscle weakness is an avoidable cause of death: check forced vital capacity and monitor frequently
(4) Autonomic—look for variable pulse rate, variable arterial pressure, intestinal ileus, urinary retention
(5) Papilloedema—a rare feature

Immediate management	(1) Respiratory:
	  ◆ Consider elective assisted ventilation sooner rather than later if the patient is tiring
	  ◆ Note that tracheal suction can trigger hypotension or bradycardia in the presence of autonomic dysfunction
	(2) Cardiac:
	  ◆ Monitor ECG
	  ◆ Arrhythmias can be fatal—treat as appropriate
	  ◆ Use antihypertensive drugs with extreme caution (if at all) in the face of autonomic dysfunction
	(3) Fluids:
	  ◆ If gag reflex impaired—stop oral feeding and start IV fluids
	  ◆ Will need to consider PEG feeding as an early option
	(4) Nursing and physiotherapy:
	  ◆ Keep chest clear
	  ◆ Protect pressure areas
	  ◆ Attention to bladder and bowels
	  ◆ Prevent contractures: move all joints through their full range of movement daily
	  ◆ Aid recovery of function
	  ◆ Psychological support: emphasize that most cases recover well
	(5) Pain—give NSAIDs as required. Consider amitriptyline, carbamazepine, gabapentin
	(6) Compression stockings and low molecular weight heparin (e.g. enoxaparin 40 mg subcutaneously once daily)—to reduce the risk of venous thromboembolism
	(7) Intravenous immunoglobulin, 0.4 g/kg body weight/day, for 5 days—give to all patients, excepting those with very mild disease
	(8) Plasma exchange—consider in severe/refractory cases

Key investigations	**To establish the diagnosis:** Acute inflammatory polyneuritis (Guillain–Barré syndrome) is primarily a clinical diagnosis: investigation may confirm it, but initial management is dictated by clinical suspicion (1) Nerve conduction studies—the earliest abnormality is impersistence or absence of F waves. Peripheral demyelination starts proximally in the nerve roots, hence distal conduction velocities and motor latencies are often normal early in the illness, even when there is profound weakness (2) Lumbar puncture—look for elevated protein (but cells <50/μl)) (3) Anti GQ1b antibodies—present in all cases that are associated with ophthalmoplegia

Other important tests:

Relevant to cause:

(1) Stool culture and serology for *Campylobacter jejuni*
(2) Serology for atypical pneumonias
(3) cerebrospinal fluid analysis for viral infection

Need to exclude:

◆ Acute intermittent porphyria—see 5.11 above

General

(1) Full blood count, electrolytes, renal and liver function tests, plasma calcium, magnesium and phosphate concentrations
(2) ECG
(3) Chest radiograph

| **Further management** | Dependent on the nature of any residual disability. Significant weakness remains in about 10% of cases, especially those with the axonal form of disease |

6.8 Myasthenia gravis

See Chapter 24.23 in main text.

| **Clinical features** | **History**
Myasthenic crisis:
(1) Breathing difficulty due to muscular weakness in a patient with myasthenia.
Presentation of myasthenia:
(2) Muscular weakness—droopy eyelid(s)/double vision; difficulty chewing, swallowing, talking (nasal speech), holding the head up; limb weakness

(3) Diurnal variation—symptoms less severe in the morning, getting worse as the day goes on
(4) Exacerbating factors—intercurrent illness, pregnancy, menses, (some) drugs

Examination
Myasthenic crisis:
(1) Exhaustion
(2) Ineffective respiratory effort
(3) Inability to clear airway secretions
(4) Cyanosis
(5) Low vital capacity

Also:
(1) Check for focal lung signs

Myasthenia:
◆ Muscular weakness that becomes worse with repetitive effort (fatiguability) |
| **Immediate management** | Respiratory failure caused by muscular weakness in a patient with myasthenia can be due to a myasthenic crisis (attributable to the disease itself) or rarely to an overdose of anticholinesterases (cholinergic crisis). These cannot reliably be distinguished on clinical grounds, hence safe management consists of:
(1) Airway, breathing, circulation
(2) Intubate and ventilate
(3) Stop all anticholinesterases

If there is specialist expertise, and in conjunction with someone skilled in intubation, then edrophonium chloride, 2 mg by IV injection, can be used to discriminate between underdosage and overdosage of cholinergic drugs |

| **Key investigations** | **To establish the diagnosis:**
Myasthenic crisis is a clinical diagnosis

To establish the diagnosis of myasthenia gravis:
(1) Edrophonium chloride (Tensilon) test—after pretreatment with atropine (0.6 mg IV), give edrophonium 2 mg IV and look for transient improvement in e.g. ptosis, diplopia, dysarthria; if no improvement after 1–2 min give edrophonium 8 mg IV and watch for effect (limited sensitivity and specificity)
(2) Serum acetylcholine receptor antibodies—highly specific (present in 85% of patients with generalized myasthenia)
(3) Electromyography—look for increased jitter, also decremental response to repetitive nerve stimulation (good sensitivity and specificity)

Other important tests:
In myasthenic crisis:
(1) Arterial blood gases
(2) Chest radiograph
(3) Electrolytes, renal and liver function tests, calcium, phosphate, full blood count
(4) Sepsis screen (if appropriate) |
| **Further management** | Myasthenic crisis—consider the following:
(1) Plasma exchange—e.g. 50 ml/kg body weight per day for 4 or 5 days
(2) Intravenous immunoglobulin—e.g. 0.4 g/kg body weight per day, for 5 days

Myasthenia—consider the following for long-term treatment:
(1) Immunosuppression—usually prednisolone (starting at a low dose of e.g. 10 mg on alternate days) and azathioprine (2.5 mg/kg body weight per day)
(2) Anticholinesterase, e.g. pyridostigmine bromide 30–120 mg at suitable intervals throughout the day (total daily dose 0.3–1.2 g), together with antimuscarinic agent if needed
(3) Thymectomy |

6.9 Acute Wernicke's encephalopathy

See Chapter 24.19 in main text.

| **Clinical features** | **History**
(1) Alcoholism—usually, but also other states of nutritional deficiency and protracted vomiting (e.g. hyperemesis gravidarum)
(2) Motor—difficulty standing/walking
(3) Diplopia
(4) Higher cerebral function—lethargy, inattentiveness, confusion; the patient will almost certainly not be able to give a reliable history (corroborate as much information as possible from other sources, e.g. relatives, friends, general practitioner, etc.)

Examination
Related to Wernicke's encephalopathy, the classic triad of:
(1) Ophthalmoplegia:
◆ Horizontal and vertical nystagmus
◆ Weakness/paralysis of lateral rectus muscles
◆ Weakness/paralysis of conjugate gaze |

	(2) Ataxia—predominantly affecting stance and gait, often without clear-cut intention tremor (3) Confusion, confabulation
	Related to clinical context: (1) Cardiovascular—look for evidence of intravascular volume depletion and/or dehydration (2) Consider other complications of alcoholism—peripheral neuropathy; acute alcohol withdrawal; acute liver failure; chronic liver disease and its complications (3) Consider other causes of an acute confusional state—see 6.2 above (4) Nutritional status
Immediate management	Thiamine—give parenteral thiamine immediately, usually in combination with other vitamins B and C, e.g. Pabrinex I/V high potency, 2–3 pairs of ampoules IV over 10 min every 8 h (each pair of ampoules contains ascorbic acid 500 mg, anhydrous glucose 1 g, nicotinamide 160 mg, pyridoxine hydrochloride 50 mg, riboflavin 4 mg, and thiamine hydrochloride 250 mg in a total of 10 ml)
	Notes (1) Anaphylaxis—facilities for treating anaphylaxis should be available when giving Pabrinex (2) Glucose—alcoholics with stupor or coma must be given high-dose thiamine before receiving IV glucose; without thiamine they cannot handle a glucose load, with risk of death
Key investigations	**To establish the diagnosis:** (1) Wernicke's encephalopathy is a clinical diagnosis (2) Red cell transketolase—a reduced level confirms thiamine deficiency
	To exclude other conditions: CT scan brain—should be done in all cases because of the high incidence of structural lesions, e.g. subdural haematoma, in this group of patients
	Other important tests: Depending of clinical context, consider as for acute confusional state—see 6.2 above
Further management	(1) After 3–5 days, switch from IV to oral vitamin replacement, e.g. thiamine 50 mg once daily + vitamin B tablets, Compound, Strong, 1–2 tablets three times daily + vitamin C 100 mg once daily (2) If alcohol withdrawal—see 8.2 below (3) Other aspects: as for acute confusional state—see 6.2 above—except avoid antipsychotics which lower seizure threshold (4) Long term—measures to help alcoholism

7 Infectious disease

7.1 Malaria

See Chapter 7.8.2 in main text.

Clinical features	Falciparum malaria is the life-threatening form and the immediate concern in patients presenting to medical services in malarious areas, or who have travelled to such areas
	Transmitted to man by the bite of an infected anopheles mosquito. The interval between bite and first symptom is usually 7–14 days. Most patients with imported falciparum malaria present within 3 months of return from the malarious area, but a few present up to 1 year or more later
	History (1) Risk of exposure to malaria—anyone who has travelled to a malarious area and presents to medical attention with a febrile illness has malaria until proved otherwise Symptoms of malaria: (2) Early—malaise, headache, backache, myalgia, anorexia, fever (3) Later—dizziness, nausea, vomiting, abdominal discomfort, diarrhoea, rigors and drenching sweats (note that 'classical' tertian (48 h) or subtertian (36 h) periodicity of fever spikes are rarely seen in falciparum malaria) Symptoms of cerebral malaria: (4) Cerebral dysfunction—gradual decline in conscious level over several hours; generalized epileptic convulsion without postictal recovery of consciousness (present in 50% of adult cases)

	Examination
	(1) Vital signs—temperature, pulse rate, BP, respiratory rate. A high fever (rising to >39°C) is typical, which can be of any or no periodicity
	(2) General—anaemia, jaundice
	(3) Abdominal—look for moderate tender enlargement of liver and/or spleen
	(4) Neurological—look for signs of cerebral malaria
	  ◆ Glasgow Coma Score—reduced (by definition in cerebral malaria)
	  ◆ Focal signs—note presence of dysconjugate gaze, brisk tendon reflexes, ankle clonus, extensor plantar responses and absent abdominal reflexes; and of decorticate or decerebrate posturing in severe cases
	  ◆ Fundi—retinal haemorrhages are common (exudates and papilloedema also occur)

	Notes
	(1) The following are not found in malaria:
	  ◆ Lymphadenopathy
	  ◆ Rash—excepting herpes simplex 'cold sores' in some cases
	  ◆ Focal signs
	(2) Signs of hypoglycaemia may be misinterpreted as being manifestations of cerebral malaria

Immediate management	If cardiorespiratory collapse—as described in 1.2 above
	Oxygen—high flow, with reservoir bag if needed, to achieve PaO_2 >92%
	If clinical evidence of intravascular volume depletion—establish IV access and resuscitate as described in 3.1 above
	Correct hypoglycaemia—if fingerprick blood glucose <3 mmol/l, give 50 ml of 50% glucose (dextrose monohydrate) IV, followed by infusion of 10% glucose at sufficient rate to maintain blood glucose concentration >3 mmol/litre.

Antimalarial drugs for falciparum malaria (adult dosages)
◆ Assume chloroquine resistance

Patients who can swallow and retain tablets
Give one of the following regimen by mouth:
(1) Artemether with lumefantrine ('Riamet')—4 tablets (each containing 20 mg artemether and 120 mg lumefantrine) twice daily for 3 days
(2) Proguanil with atovaquone ('Malarone')—4 tablets (each containing 100 mg proguanil and 250 mg atovaquone) once daily for 3 days
(3) Quinine—the treatment of choice in many countries—600 mg of quinine salt every 8 h for 7 days, followed by tetracycline 250 mg four times daily for 7 days or doxycyline 100 mg daily for 7 days

Patients with severe malaria or who cannot swallow and retain tablets
Give one of the following regimens:
(1) Artesunate—by IV 'push': loading dose of 2.4 mg/kg followed by 1.2 mg/kg at 12 and 24 h, then 1.2 mg/kg daily for minimum of 3 days until patient can take oral therapy or another effective antimalarial
(2) Artemether—by intramuscular injection: loading dose of 3.2 mg/kg on the first day (in one or two doses), followed by 1.6 mg/kg/day for minimum of 3 days until patient can take oral therapy or another effective antimalarial
(3) Quinine—by IV infusion: (a) loading dose of 20 mg/kg dihydrochloride salt (maximum 1400 mg) diluted in 10 ml/kg isotonic fluid and given over 4 h, or (b) (in the intensive care unit) loading dose of 7 mg/kg dihydrochloride salt by infusion pump over 30 min, followed immediately by 10 mg/kg (maintenance dose) over 4 h; followed by (c) after 8 h give maintenance dose of 10 mg/kg (maximum 700 mg) over 4 h, repeated following further 8 h gaps until patient can swallow tablets to complete 7 day course; followed by (d) tetracycline 250 mg four times daily for 7 days or doxycycline 100 mg daily for 7 days

Other measures
(1) High fever—control by fanning, tepid sponging, cooling blankets, antipyretics (e.g. paracetamol 15 mg/kg in tablets, or powder washed down an NG tube, or as suppositories or ibuprofen 400 mg by IV injection 6 hourly)
(2) Anaemia—transfuse with whole blood or packed cells if haematocrit falls to <20% or if there is severe bleeding
(3) Urine output—insert urinary catheter to monitor closely
(4) Cerebral malaria—appropriate nursing care for the unconscious patient. Control convulsions (see 6.5 above). Consider elective intubation and ventilation if airway in danger of compromise
(5) Hyperparasitaemia—consider exchange transfusion or haemopheresis in nonimmune patients who are severely ill, who have deteriorated on conventional treatment, and who have parasitaemia >10%

| Key investigations | **To establish the diagnosis:**
Depends on the detection of parasitaemia (stop antimalarial chemoprophylaxis):
(1) Repeated examination of thick and thin blood films (8–12 hourly for 72 h) by an experienced microscopist
(2) Antibody detection technique, e.g. dipstick antigen-capture assay |

Note

If patient remains unwell and no other diagnosis can be made, consider therapeutic trial even if early smears are negative

Other important tests:

(1) Fingerprick stick test for blood glucose—?hypoglycaemia
(2) Full blood count—anaemia with evidence of haemolysis is usual. Neutrophilia is common, but white cell count can be normal or low
(3) Electrolytes, renal and liver function, glucose, coagulation screen—mild hyponatraemia is common
(4) Arterial blood gases
(5) Blood culture—to exclude secondary bacterial septicaemia in those with an obvious focus of such infection and in patients who are very unwell or have a raised blood white cell count
(6) Depending on clinical context (mainly to exclude differential diagnoses)—CT brain, lumbar puncture, chest radiograph

Further management	Emphasize need for avoidance and prophylaxis with any future travel to malarious areas

7.2 Meningitis

See Chapters 7.6.3, 7.6.5, 7.6.12, and 24.11.1 in main text.

Clinical features	Acute bacterial meningitis has a mortality of 70–100% if untreated and is the immediate concern in patients presenting to medical services

History

General symptoms:
(1) Early—malaise, headache, fever, vomiting, diarrhoea
(2) Later—increasingly severe headache, photophobia, drowsiness
(3) Very late—coma, convulsions

Localizing (if meningitis secondary to infection elsewhere):
(4) Respiratory—pneumococcal disease (pneumonia)
(5) Ear—*H. influenzae* (otitis media)

Also:
(6) Contact with a case of meningitis
(7) Previous history of meningitis
(8) History of immunodeficiency
(9) Pregnancy—increased risk of listeria
(10) Travel history—particularly meningococcal disease

Examination

(1) Vital signs—temperature, pulse rate, BP, respiratory rate
(2) General:
  ◆ Skin: petechiae/purpura—characteristic of meningococcal disease, but not specific
  ◆ Conjunctivae/palate: petechiae—characteristic of meningococcal disease, but not specific
  ◆ Posture—patients with severe meningism often lie with the back and neck in hyperextension

(3) Neurological
  ◆ Meningism—neck stiffness; Kernig's sign (with the leg flexed at the hip, an attempt by the clinician to passively extend the knee is resisted by hamstring spasm)
  ◆ Ocular fundi—papilloedema indicates raised intracranial pressure, but absence of papilloedema does not exclude this
  ◆ Cranial nerve lesions—most commonly sixth (false localizing sign)

(4) Other—in secondary meningitis there may be signs of primary focus, e.g. pneumonia, otitis media, cerebrospinal fluid shunts/reservoirs

Immediate management	(1) If cardiorespiratory collapse—as described in 1.2 above (2) Oxygen—high flow, with reservoir bag if needed, to achieve PaO_2 >92% (3) If clinical evidence of intravascular volume depletion, establish IV access and resuscitate as described in 3.1 above

Antimicrobial chemotherapy (empirical treatment, adult dosages)

(1) Spontaneous (community acquired) or post-traumatic meningitis

Drug	Dose	Route	Frequency	Duration
Cefotaxime	2 g	IV	4 hourly	2 weeks
or				
Ceftriaxone	2 g	IV	12 hourly	2 weeks

If high prevalence of penicillin-resistent pneumococci, then *add*

Ceftriaxone	2 g	IV	12 hourly	2 weeks
Vancomycin	1 g	IV	12 hourly	2 weeks

If underlying immunosuppression, pregnancy or age >50 years, then *add*

Ampicillin	2 g	IV	4–6 hourly	3 weeks

(2) Nosocomial meningitis

If probability of pseudomonas is high, give vancomycin plus

Ceftazidime	2 g	IV	8 hourly	3 weeks
or				
Meropenem	2 g	IV	8 hourly	3 weeks

If probability of pseudomonas is low, give vancomycin plus

Cefotaxime	2 g	IV	4 hourly	3 weeks
or				
Ceftriaxone	2 g	IV	12 hourly	3 weeks

(3) Shunt-associated meningitis

Treat as for nosocomial meningitis

Notes

(1) Antimicrobial therapy can be refined as soon as an organism is isolated, otherwise patients with suspected bacterial meningitis should receive treatment with the regimen indicated.
(2) Doses of antimicrobials need to be adjusted in patients with chronic kidney disease or acute renal impairment (especially vancomycin)

Corticosteroids	Currently available evidence does not support the use of adjunctive dexamethasone in adults with baterial meningitis (see Chapter 24.11.1)
Key investigations	**To establish the diagnosis:** (1) Epidemiological data (any current epidemics) (2) Lumbar puncture to obtain specimen of cerebrospinal fluid—looking in bacterial meningitis for: ◆ General appearance—cloudy or purulent, but can be clear ◆ Microscopy—(a) white cell count—usually raised (although can rarely be normal, i.e. <6 lymphocytes/μl) with neutrophils accounting for >80% of cells, but can have a lymphocytic pleocytosis in early bacterial meningitis or with *Listeria monocytogenes*; (b) Gram stain—shows organisms in 50–80% of cases ◆ Biochemical analysis—(a) glucose—usually reduced (<40% that of a parallel serum sample); (b) protein—usually elevated (>0.45 g/litre)

◆ Microbiological culture
◆ Other specific tests—antigen detection for common pathogens; PCR for meningococcal disease

Notes

(1) In cases of suspected meningococcal meningitis/septicaemia—give antibiotics immediately—before referral to hospital, and if in hospital before lumbar puncture

(2) Lumbar puncture should not be performed if there are any of the following:
◆ Symptoms or signs to suggest raised intracranial pressure, e.g. drowsiness/coma; focal neurological signs; loss of retinal vein pulsation/papilloedema; bradycardia/hypertension
◆ Local skin sepsis at the sight of puncture
◆ Clinical suspicion of spinal cord compression
◆ Bleeding diathesis

(3) If symptoms or signs suggest raised intracranial pressure—arrange for CT brain to exclude space occupying lesion or cerebral oedema

Other important tests:
For specific diagnosis
(1) Blood culture
(2) Throat swab—for viral and bacteriological culture
(3) Skin lesion—disrupt with needle and make contact slide for Gram stain.
(4) Blood sample—in EDTA (as full blood count) for bacterial PCR

Other:
(1) Full blood count
(2) Electrolytes, renal and liver function, glucose, clotting screen
(3) Arterial blood gases (severe cases)
(4) Chest radiography—?pneumonia (pneumococcal disease), ?aspiration (if impaired conscious level)
(5) CT/MRI brain—may demonstrate skull fractures or parameningeal septic foci

Further management	(1) Meningitis is a notifiable disease
	(2) If meningococcal meningitis
	◆ Household and other intimate contacts—give prophylaxis (e.g. rifampicin 600 mg orally twice daily for 2 days, or ciprofloxacin 750 mg orally as single dose) and immunize if serogroup A,C,Y or W135
	◆ Staff—prophylaxis is not required unless mouth to mouth resuscitation given

7.3 Encephalitis

See Chapters 7.5.2, 7.5.13, and 24.11.2 in main text.

| **Clinical features** | Encephalitis is an acute inflammation of the brain and/or spinal cord (encephalomyelitis) presenting as alteration of consciousness, convulsions and/or focal neurological signs. It is usually caused by an acute viral infection of the central nervous system (typically herpes simplex, Japanese encephalitis, or an arthropod-borne virus), or it complicates a systemic viral infection such as measles (postinfectious encephalomyelitis) or vaccination (postvaccinal encephalomyelitis). Case fatality is extremely variable but may exceed 40% when there is no antiviral therapy (e.g. Japanese encephalitis), and there is a high incidence of permanent neurological sequelae |

History

General symptoms (after incubation period of a few days to 2 weeks)
(1) Early—fever, headache, neck stiffness, vomiting
(2) Later—psychiatric symptoms, altered consciousness, convulsions

Localizing symptoms:
(3) Altered behaviour, hallucinations, temporal lobe seizures—herpes simplex encephalitis
(4) Rashes—preceding illness (e.g. measles, varicella, post-infectious encephalomyelitis); concurrent (e.g. West Nile virus encephalitis)

Also:
(5) Recent vaccination (vaccinia, nervous tissue rabies vaccine)
(6) Current seasonal epidemic (arthropod-borne encephalitides)
(7) Travel history—to endemic area (e.g. central Europe/Scandinavia—tick-borne encephalitis)

Examination

(1) Vital signs—temperature, pulse rate, BP, respiratory rate, Glasgow Coma Scale
(2) General
◆ Skin: rashes—West Nile virus, enteroviruses, etc.
◆ Mucous membranes: cold sores (herpes simplex encephalitis)
(3) Neurological:
◆ Meningism
◆ Ocular fundi—papilloedema indicates raised intracranial pressure, but absence of papilloedema does not exclude this
◆ Cranial nerve lesions—most commonly VI (false localizing sign)
(4) Other—in postinfectious encephalomyelitis there may be signs of the preceding illness, e.g measles, varicella, mumps, etc.

Immediate management	If cardiorespiratory collapse—as described in 1.2 above
	If convulsing—as described in 6.5 above
	Oxygen—high flow, with reservoir bag if needed, to achieve Pa_{O_2} >92%
	(1) Antiviral treatment:
	◆ Aciclovir—where it is affordable, treatment with aciclovir should be started immediately in all undiagnosed cases in which viral encephalitis is included in the differential diagnosis. Specifically, aciclovir is recommended for herpes simplex, herpes simiae (B), herpes zoster, and Epstein–Barr virus encephalitides: dose 10 mg/kg every 8 h by IV infusion (reduced in renal impairment)
	◆ Ribavirin (tribavirin)—for the rare encephalitides associated with RNA virus infections (e.g, Lassa fever, Argentine haemorrhagic fever, Hanta virus, Crimean–Congo haemorrhagic fever and Rift Valley fever) ribavirin (tribavirin) has been recommended: 2 g loading dose by IV infusion, then 1 g every 6 h for 4 days, then 0.5 g 8 hourly for 6 days
	(2) Other measures:
	◆ Corticosteroids—sometimes used for postvaccinal encephalomyelitis (controversial)
	◆ Reduction of severe intracranial hypertension—IV mannitol or mechanical hyperventilation

Key investigations	**To establish the diagnosis:**
	(1) Epidemiological data (any current epidemics)
	(2) Lumbar puncture to obtain specimen of cerebrospinal fluid—looking in viral encephalitis for:
	◆ Microscopy—(a) white cell count—usually raised (but normal in 10–15% of patients with herpes simplex encephalitis at first examination), with lymphocytes and other mononuclear cells predominant except in early infections; (b) Gram stain—to exclude bacterial meningoencephalitis
	◆ Biochemical analysis—(a) glucose—usually normal or increased, but low levels have been reported; (b) protein—usually elevated into range 0.5–1.5 g/l
	◆ Virological testing—(a) PCR; (b) specific viral IgM (microcapture technique); (c) viral isolation—e.g. mumps, enteroviruses, lymphocytic choriomeningitis virus
	(3) Other samples—(a) skin lesions—immunofluorescence (herpes zoster) and electron microscopy (herpesviruses); (b) nasopharyngeal aspirate—measles; (c) stool—enteroviruses; (d) serology (acute/ convalescent titres)—mumps, Coxsackie viruses, arthropod-borne viruses
	Other important tests:
	(1) Full blood count
	(2) Arterial blood gases (severe cases)
	(3) CT/MRI—may demonstrate focal lesions (e.g. herpes simplex encephalitis) or cerebral oedema
	Notes
	(1) The diagnosis of viral encephalitis should not be made too hastily as the differential diagnosis is broad and other treatable causes (e.g. cerebral malaria, bacterial or fungal meningoencephalitides) may be ignored
	(2) Lumbar puncture should not be performed if there are contraindications—see 7.3 above

7.4 Tetanus

See Chapter 7.6.22 in main text.

Clinical features	Tetanus, caused by toxins of *Clostridium tetani* in contaminated wounds, remains common in some developing countries but is preventable by vaccination. It is now rare in developed countries but, because it is decreasingly familiar, is less likely to be diagnosed. The case fatality ranges from 20 to 60%, although in expert hands this may be reduced to 6%, even in severe cases
	History
	(1) Recent wound, especially penetrating, contaminated, or with necrosis, is identified in 75–85% of cases
	(2) Problems in head, neck, mouth—trismus due to a painful local condition is an important differential diagnosis
	(3) Drugs—a dystonic drug reaction is an important differential diagnosis
	Symptoms of tetanus:
	After an incubation period of usually 6–10 days (<15 days in 90% of cases):
	◆ Nonspecific—malaise, fever, sweating, and headache
	◆ Suggestive—muscle stiffness (especially of the jaws), spasms, and dysphagia

Examination

Features of tetanus:

(1) Muscles—trismus, risus sardonicus, neck retraction; rigidity of erector spinae and abdominal muscles (board-like rigidity); opisthotonos; tonic contractions/spasms of the stiff muscles; spasms of respiratory muscles and larynx threaten to cause asphyxia; local tetanus may involve only muscles in the region of the wound, e.g. cephalic tetanus

(2) Autonomic nervous system—fluctuating heart rate, BP, and temperature, with sweating and hypersalivation

(3) Clinical grading—of prognostic significance:
   ◆ I (mild)—trismus and generalized stiffness without respiratory embarrassment or spasms
   ◆ II (moderate)—marked rigidity, brief spasms, mild respiratory embarrassment, and dysphagia
   ◆ III and IV—frequent prolonged spasms, respiratory embarrassment with apnoeic spells, severe dysphagia. and cardiovascular abnormalities

Also:
◆ Look for features of alternative diagnosis, e.g. local cause of trismus

Notes

(1) Incubation period less than 4 days and period of onset (trismus to first spasm) less than 48 h are associated with high mortality

(2) In developed countries, patients are often elderly (missed childhood vaccination)

Immediate management	◆ If cardiorespiratory collapse—as described in 1.2 above
	◆ If convulsing—as described in 6.5 above
	◆ Oxygen—high flow, with reservoir bag if needed, to achieve Pao_2 >92%

(1) Airway/ventilation—if apnoeic/asphyxiating/ hypoxaemic—may require emergency tracheostomy, assisted ventilation with oxygen, neuromuscular blockade (pancuronium/vecuronium). See Chapter 33.1.2 'Management of the airway'.

(2) Tetanus immune globulin—give in all cases before manipulating the wound, either (a) (preferably, if available) human tetanus immune globulin 100–300 U/kg intramuscularly, or (b) equine tetanus immune globulin 500–1000 U/kg intramuscularly (beware of anaphylaxis, see 1.12 above)

(3) Wound—give antibiotics to sterilize: metronidazole 500 mg, orally (if possible) or IV, three times a day for 10 days

(4) Wound—surgical debridement after tetanus immune globulin has been given

(5) Sedatives/muscle relaxants—give diazepam by continuous IV infusion (high doses may be required, up to 100 mg/h)

Notes

(1) Autonomic nervous system disturbances—(a) hypertension may require cautious use of low dose short-acting β-blockers; (b) brady/ tachyarrhythmias—treat only if causing significant haemodynamic disturbance: see 1.7 above; (c) IV magnesium sulphate (titrated to produce serum concentrations between 2 and 4 mmol/litre) improves cardiovascular stability

(2) Deep vein thrombosis prophylaxis—give low molecular weight heparin

Key investigations	Tetanus is a clinical diagnosis (1) Wound swab—but failure to culture *Clostridium tetani* from the wound does not exclude the diagnosis of tetanus (2) Lumbar puncture—the cerebrospinal fluid is normal
	Note The differential diagnosis includes the many local causes of trismus, dystonic reactions to drugs, tetany, strychnine poisoning, meningitis, and rabies (cephalic tetanus)
Further management	Infection does not confer immunity: give full course of active immunization (tetanus toxoid) after recovery

7.5 Rabies

See Chapter 7.5.10 in main text.

Clinical features	Rabies is a zoonotic viral infection of the central nervous system, endemic in domestic dogs and cats, wild carnivores, bats, etc., in most parts of the world. It is transmitted to humans by bites of rabid mammals, usually dogs. The case fatality of rabies encephalomyelitis is virtually 100%, but the disease is preventable by modern postexposure treatment started soon after the bite
	History (1) History of dog (or other mammal) bite (but may be distant or forgotten, especially with insectivorous bat bites in USA) or a lick by a mammal on broken skin (2) Travel history to rabies endemic area (3) Postexposure treatment—see 7.6 below

	Symptoms of rabies
	After an incubation period of usually 20–90 days (extreme range 4 days to 19 years):
	(1) Prodromal symptoms:
	    ♦ Nonspecific—fever, chills, malaise, weakness, tiredness, headache
	    ♦ Suggestive—itching, pain, or paraesthesiae at the site of the healed bite wound
	(2) A few days later:
	    ♦ Furious rabies—difficulty swallowing (especially water), causing spasms of breathing and great anxiety (with or without pain in the throat)
	    ♦ Extreme susceptibility to draughts, causing similar spasms
	    ♦ Bizarre behaviour
	    ♦ Periods of extreme excitement, hallucinations, terror, aggression with lucid intervals
	(3) After several more days:
	    ♦ Lapse into coma and convulsions
	    ♦ Sudden death during a hydrophobic spasm
	    ♦ Paralytic rabies—ascending weakness with sensory symptoms often starting in the bitten limb; sphincter problems; dysphagia, drooling, and respiratory weakness

	Examination
	(1) Wound:
	    ♦ Evidence of healed bite
	(2) Neurological:
	    ♦ Clinical examination may be normal
	    ♦ Excitable behaviour interspersed with lucid intervals
	    ♦ Furious rabies—violent, jerky spasms of inspiratory muscles associated with evident terror provoked by attempts to drink or exposure to a draught of air
	    ♦ Paralytic rabies—ascending flaccid paralysis with fasciculations, sensory loss, sphincter dysfunction
	    ♦ Weakness of muscles of deglutition and respiration
	    ♦ Excitable behaviour interspersed with lucid intervals

	(3) Autonomic nervous system: ♦ Signs of overactivity—hypersalivation, sweating, labile pulse rate and BP
Immediate management	(1) Although life can be prolonged by invasive, intensive care (tracheostomy, paralysis, mechanical ventilation, cardiac monitoring, etc.), the chances of a successful outcome are so low that there is a strong case for palliative care to relieve pain and anxiety (2) There is currently no evidence to support use of the 'Milwaukee Regimen' (sedation, antiviral drugs, etc.) that was administered to an American girl who recovered from rabies
Key investigations	**To establish the diagnosis during life:** (1) Skin punch biopsy (hairy area, e.g. nape of neck)—detection of virus by direct fluorescent antibody in nerves surrounding hair follicles (2) Saliva—virus may be isolated (3) Blood—rabies-neutralizing antibody titre—elevated in unvaccinated patient (but may be negative for 7 days after clinical illness has begun) (4) Cerebrospinal fluid analysis—(a) may be normal, but protein usually elevated, and may have elevated white blood cell count; (b) rapid PCR (experimental); (c) virus may be isolated; (d) rabies-neutralizing antibody titre—elevated in unvaccinated patient (but may be negative for 7 days after clinical illness has begun) (5) Exclusion of other diagnoses—given the appalling outcome of rabies it is important to pursue the possible differential diagnosis of a rapidly progressing encephalitis (see 7.3 above) if there is any doubt about the diagnosis
Further management	Attempt to identify/capture/examine (by veterinarian)/test the animal responsible for the bite—if the biting animal is available (usually dog), it should be euthanized and its brain immediately examined to detect rabies virus by direct fluorescent antibody labelling of brain smear, or by viral isolation. When possible, this is preferred to previous practice of observing the animal for onset of rabid symptoms over a 10-day period

7.6 Animal bites/stings

See Chapter 9.2 in main text.

Clinical features	A very wide range of animals may inflict bites and stings. Serious consequences may result from trauma, envenoming, allergy or infection
	History (1) Timing—the event is usually painful and memorable and so precisely timed by the victim

	Immediate symptoms:
	(2) Distress—associated with a terrifying event:
	(3) Trauma—pain, bleeding, dysfunction (depending on site and severity of injury)
	(4) Envenoming
	    ♦ Snake bite:
	      • Local—pain, swelling, persistent bleeding, bruising, blistering, painful enlargement of draining lymph nodes
	      • Systemic—syncope/collapse (may be early and transient), spontaneous systemic bleeding (gums, nose etc.), vomiting, progressive weakness starting with ptosis, blurred vision, inability to open mouth, swallow, speak etc., generalized muscle aches and tenderness, passage of black urine (rhabdomyolysis)

- Scorpion sting:
  - Local—very severe pain, mild swelling
  - Systemic—vomiting, sweating, faintness, difficulty with breathing, muscle spasms
- Spider bites:
  - Local—pain, sweating and gooseflesh (neurotoxic) or progressive skin changes (red, white, and blue sign; necrotic)
  - Systemic—vomiting, faintness, colic, and muscle spasms
- Jellyfish stings:
  - Local—severe pain, blistering, contact rash
  - Systemic—collapse, vomiting
- Fish stings:
  - Local—very severe pain
  - Systemic—rarely collapse

(5) Allergy:
- Hymenoptera stings (bees, wasps, hornets, yellowjackets, ants)
- Local—pain, swelling (may be negligible)
- Systemic—early syncope and collapse, raised, itchy rash, swelling of mouth, lips, tongue, and gums, chest tightness, wheezing, asthma attack, abdominal colic, vomiting, diarrhoea (all of these may develop within a few minutes of the sting)

(6) Infection:
- Symptoms attributable to infection are delayed, with earliest onset at about 12 h (*Pasteurella multocida*)
- Local—pain, swelling, redness, heat, purulent discharge
- Systemic—sometimes severe generalized symptoms (sepsis)

Examination

(1) Vital signs—temperature, pulse rate, BP, respiratory rate, Glasgow Coma Scale
(2) Trauma—injuries to soft tissues, joints, tendons, bones (crush fractures), body cavities (e.g. haemothorax), evisceration, dead tissue, foreign material in the wound (broken teeth, claws, earth, etc.). May be severe/life-threatening. May be associated with envenoming and/or allergy and/or infection (e.g. marine coral cuts, sting ray, and sea urchin injuries)
(3) Envenoming—see History
(4) Allergy—features of anaphylaxis (see 1.12 above)
(5) Infection—(a) local—pain, swelling, redness, heat, purulent discharge; (b) systemic—sepsis syndrome (see 7.7 above)

Notes

(1) Human bites:
- May be of medicolegal significance: document carefully, also any other evidence of injury (sketch and photograph)
- High risk of infection with group A β-haemolytic streptococci, *Staph. aureus* (40% of wounds), haemophilus, klebsiella, *Eikenella corrodens*, and anaerobes
- May be self-inflicted—typically lips, buccal cavity, fingers, clenched-fist injuries of knuckles

(2) Dog, cat/other mammal bites
- Associated with high risk of infection with a wide range of pathogens, notably *Pasteurella multocida*, *Capnocytophaga canimorsus*, *Staph. aureus*, *Clostridium tetani*, and other anaerobic bacteria, rabies virus, etc.

Immediate management

First aid

(1) Trauma:
- Control pain and bleeding, contain wound with bandaging, give plasma expander if available, transport to medical care

(2) Envenoming:
- Snake bite
  - Immobilize the patient, especially the bitten limb
  - Avoid harmful remedies—tourniquets, incisions, suction, electric shock, cryotherapy, snake stones, etc. should never be used
  - Transport the patient to medical care
  - Neurotoxic bites only—pressure immobilization and splinting with a long elasticated bandage
  - Venom ophthalmia (spitting cobras and rinkhals)—irrigate affected eye with liberal quantities of bland fluid (e.g. water, milk) and apply 1% adrenaline (epinephrine) or local anaesthetic drops for pain (if available)
- Other bites and stings:
  - Fish stings—immerse stung part in uncomfortably hot but not scalding water (maximum 45°C)
  - Scorpion stings and other painful bites and stings—local 1% lignocaine (lidocaine) with digital block or strong systemic analgesia (if available)
  - Jellyfish stings—(a) box jellyfish (North Australia, Indo-Pacific)—wash area with dilute acetic acid/vinegar; (b) Atlantic jellyfish—apply a slurry of baking powder (c) hot water immersion for pain (see fish stings above)
  - Bee stings—remove the sting as quickly as possible
  - Tick bites—apply surgical spirit to the animal and prise out the mouth parts with forceps

Hospital management

- If anaphylaxis—as described in 1.12 above
- If cardiorespiratory collapse—as described in 1.2 above
- Oxygen—high flow, with reservoir bag if needed, to achieve PaO_2 >92%
- If clinical evidence of intravascular volume depletion—establish IV access and resuscitate as described in 3.1 above

(1) Trauma:
- Explore wound under anaesthesia, debriding and removing foreign material.
- Treat specific injuries to vital structures
- Delayed primary suture

(2) Envenoming:
- Antivenom treatment—in cases of envenoming by snakes, fish, scorpions, spiders, box jellyfish, and ticks, administer antivenom IV (provided that an appropriate specific antivenom is available) if any of the following are present: paralysis (ptosis, etc.); spontaneous systemic bleeding (gums, GI tract etc); incoagulable blood; shock; ECG abnormalities; black urine (myoglobinuria, haemoglobinuria); severe/rapidly progressive local envenoming
- Antivenom reactions (anaphylactic or serum)—beware of these and treat/prevent as follows—(a) Treatment: give adrenaline (1/1000, 0.3–0.5 ml intramuscularly = 0.3–0.5 mg dose, repeated as necessary) plus anti-H_1 (e.g. chlorpheniramine 10–20 mg IV) plus corticosteroid (e.g. hydrocortisone 5 mg/kg IV) at the first sign of a reaction; (b) Prevention: do not give routine prophylaxis except in atopic subjects with severe asthma and those who have suffered previous reactions to antivenom. See 1.12 above

Key investigations	(1) Trauma:
	◆ Appropriate radiological imaging to define extent of the injury
	(2) Snake bites:
	◆ Simple 20 min whole blood clotting test or rapid coagulation screen
	◆ Stick test urine for blood—positive may indicate lysed red blood cells (?disseminated intravascular coagulation) or myoglobin (rhabdomyolysis)
	◆ Australia only—rapid EIA venom detection kit, using swab from the bite wound
	◆ Tensely-swollen limbs—measure intracompartmental pressure as guide to avoiding unnecessary fasciotomy

Other important tests:
◆ Depending on clinical context/severity—ECG, full blood count, electrolytes, renal and liver function tests, muscle enzymes (creatine kinase), arterial blood gases, chest radiograph

Further management	**Trauma (bites by large animals)**
	(1) Definitive wound closure with skin grafts, etc.
	(2) Infection risk:
	◆ Bacterial—prophylactic antibiotics for severe/multiple wounds or wounds of the fingers or in response to cultures: (a) amoxicillin/clavulanic acid—(expressed as) amoxicillin 250 mg three times daily by mouth (prophylaxis, mild case) to 1 g three times daily IV (treatment, severe case), or (b) second/third-generation cephalosporin, e.g. cefotaxime 1–2 g 6 hourly IV
	◆ Tetanus—give tetanus toxoid or, if unimmunized, consider tetanus immunoglobulin
	◆ Rabies—consider possibility of rabies exposure and (if appropriate) give rabies postexposure treatment: (a) thorough wound cleaning—scrub under running tap with soap and water; irrigate with plain water; (b) apply viricidal agent such as 40–50% alcohol or 1% iodine; (c) avoid suturing; (d) vaccination—start active vaccination using tissue culture vaccine (dividing one dose of 0.5–1 ml between 8 sites intradermally produces the most rapid antibody response) plus start passive immunization with equine rabies immunoglobulin (40 units/kg body weight) or (preferably if available) human rabies immunoglobulin (20 units/kg body weight) infiltrated around the wound, with the residue given intramuscularly distant from the site of rabies vaccination
	(3) Envenoming
	◆ Nursing—avoid elevation of the bitten limb
	◆ Surgery—debridement of necrotic tissue with immediate split skin grafting; avoid hasty and unjustified fasciotomy (especially if the blood is still incoagulable)
	◆ Myoglobinuric renal failure—try to prevent by correcting hypovolaemia and acidosis and encouraging diuresis (see 4.2 above)

7.7 Septic shock

See Chapters 7.2.1, 17.3, and 17.4 in main text.

Clinical features	Septic shock is a condition associated with severe infection in which there is hypotension (systolic BP <90 mmHg) unresponsive to fluids or requiring vasoactive drugs for its correction. The causative septicaemia may be with Gram-positive or Gram-negative bacteria, yeasts, viruses, or protozoa. Failure of one or more organ systems is common

History
(1) Systemic features—may develop rapidly (minutes–hours), e.g. meningococcaemia, or gradually
   ◆ Early—malaise, lethargy, nausea, vomiting, fever, sweating, shivering/rigors
   ◆ Later—restless, anxious, confused, agitated
(2) Localized features—related to causative infection—e.g pneumonia, urinary tract infection, infected intravascular catheter, meningitis, after large-bowel surgery, etc.
(3) Risk factors—complication of surgery, instrumentation, burns, or other trauma; complication of preceding illness, e.g flu predisposing to staphylococcal pneumonia; travel history—could the patient have malaria? (see 7.1 above)

Examination
(1) Vital signs—temperature (fever or hypothermia), tachycardia, tachypnoea, hypotension, peripheral perfusion—warm (vasodilated) or cold/cyanosis (vasoconstricted), Glasgow Coma Score
(2) Evidence of the causative infection—complete physical examination to look for focus of infection. Do not forget to examine the back and perineum/rectum (localized abscess)
(3) Evidence of organ failure:
   ◆ Respiratory—central cyanosis (check pulse oximetry), crackles. Risk of adult respiratory distress syndrome (ARDS)
   ◆ Renal—low urine output. Risk of prerenal renal failure or acute tubular necrosis
   ◆ Liver—jaundice
   ◆ Neurological—confusion
   ◆ Haematological—abnormal bleeding/gangrene of extremities

Notes
(1) Look for evidence of predisposition to infection—elderly, immunosuppressed, asplenic, malignant disease, artificial heart valve, prosthetic material, etc.
(2) Streptococcal toxic shock syndrome—erythematous rash, local severe pain and swelling (necrotizing fasciitis/myositis)
(3) Staphylococcal toxic shock syndrome—diarrhoea, myalgia, rash (desquamating), often associated with menstruation/tampon use

Immediate management	◆ If cardiorespiratory collapse—as described in 1.2 above
	◆ Oxygen—high flow, with reservoir bag if needed, to achieve Pa_{O_2} >92%
	◆ If clinical evidence of intravascular volume depletion, establish IV access and resuscitate as described in 3.1 above

(1) Fluid/circulatory:
- Targets for resuscitation are an Svo_2 >70% with a MAP >60 mmHg. Other reasonable goals include central venous pressure 8–12 mmHg and urine output >0.5 ml/kg per h
- Fluid—give repeated IV fluid boluses (e.g. 250 ml 0.9% saline or physiological salt solution) until BP and tissue perfusion are acceptable, or there is pulmonary oedema, or there is no further response
- Packed red blood cells—to restore haematocrit to 30%
- Vasopressor agents (e.g. dobutamine, norepinephrine, epinephrine, dopamine)—after giving fluid as above, restore arterial and venous vasomotor tone using α-adrenergic sympathomimetic agents
- Vasodilator agents (e.g. nitrates)—if there is impaired contractility then reduce afterload with vasodilators as tolerated, up to a decrease in MAP to about 70 mmHg, targeting pulmonary artery occlusion ('wedge') pressure <18 mmHg and Svo_2 >70%. In sepsis, Svo_2 is usually elevated following fluid resuscitation, hence resuscitation targets usually focus on reaching elevated levels of oxygen delivery (e.g. >450 ml/min per m²)
- Inotropes (e.g. dobutamine)—a trial of inotropic therapy is warranted if Svo2 remains <70% despite the interventions above

(2) Respiratory:
- Consider early intubation and mechanical ventilation

(3) Antibiotics—give broad-spectrum, empirical treatment

Community-acquired septicaemia:
- Aminoglycoside (e.g. gentamicin 5 mg/kg IV once daily, assuming normal renal function) + broad-spectrum penicillin (e.g. coamoxiclav 1.2g 6-8 hourly IV), or
- Broad-spectrum cephalosporin (e.g. cefotaxime, 1 g 12 hourly to 2 g 6 hourly, IV)

Hospital-acquired septicaemia:
- Aminoglycoside (e.g. gentamicin 5 mg/kg IV once daily, assuming normal renal function) + broad-spectrum anti-pseudomonal penicillin (e.g. Tazosin 2.25–4.5 g [= piperacillin 2–4 g + tazobactam 250–500 mg] 6 hourly IV), or
- Ceftazidime, 1g 12 hourly to 2 g 8 hourly, IV, or
- Meropenem 500 mg–1 g 12 hourly IV, or
- Imipenem with cilastatin, 500 mg–1 g (of imipenem) 6 hourly IV

Pseudomonas infection suspected:
- Aminoglycoside (e.g. gentamicin 5 mg/kg IV once daily, assuming normal renal function) + broad-spectrum anti-Pseudomonal penicillin (e.g. Tazosin 2.25–4.5 g [= Piperacillin 2–4 g + tazobactam 250–500 mg] 6 hourly IV)

Gram-positive infection suspected:
- Add flucloxacillin 1–2 g 12 hourly IV, or
- Vancomycin 1 g 12 hourly IV (assuming normal renal function)

Methicillin-resistant *Staph. aureus* (MRSA) suspected:
- Vancomycin 1 g 12 hourly IV (assuming normal renal function)

Anaerobic infection suspected:
- Add metronidazole 500 mg 8 hourly IV

Meningococcaemia:
- Benzylpenicillin 2.4 g 4 hourly IV, or
- Cefotaxime 2 g 6 hourly IV

Streptococcal toxic shock syndrome:
- Benzylpenicillin 1.2–2.4 g 6 hourly IV, or cefotaxime 2 g 6 hourly IV, both plus clindamycin 600–1200 mg 6 hourly IV

Notes

(1) Aminoglycosides, vancomycin—dosage dependent on renal function; always monitor levels
(2) Antibiotics—always refer to hospital protocols for antibiotic prescribing—these will take account of local epidemiology of infection and antimicrobial resistance patterns of pathogens
(3) Other aspects:
- Supportive treatment may be required for specific organ failure—mechanical ventilation, renal replacement therapy (haemofiltration, haemodialysis)
- Surgical—e.g. urgent fasciotomy and débridement for streptococcal necrotizing fasciitis/myositis
- Keep blood glucose in range 5.5–10 mmol/l (100–180 mg/dl) using IV infusion of actrapid insulin on sliding scale
- Consider recombinant human activated protein C in adult patients with high risk of death (APACHE score >25, multiple organ dysfunction, acute respiratory distress syndrome) (risk of bleeding)

Key investigations	**To establish the source of infection:** (1) Blood culture (2) Other cultures as determined by clinical signs or imaging, e.g. needle aspiration of fluid collections **Other:** (3) Full blood count—leucocytosis or leucopenia (4) Electrolytes, renal and liver function tests, glucose, clotting screen, muscle enzymes (creatine kinase, ? rhabdomyolysis) (5) Arterial blood gases—pH, pO_2, pCO_2, base excess

8 Psychiatry

8.1 Acute alcohol withdrawal

See Chapters 26.4 and 26.7.1 in main text.

Clinical features	**History**
	Related to alcohol withdrawal:
	(1) Agitation and anxiety
	(2) Tremor
	(3) Sweating
	(4) Insomnia
	(5) Nausea and vomiting
	(6) Hallucinations—tactile, visual, auditory
	(7) Grand mal seizures
	
	Also:
	(8) Drinking history—how much alcohol does the patient usually drink? Have they recently been drinking particularly heavily, or have they stopped?
	
	Examination
	Related to alcohol withdrawal:
	(1) Agitation and anxiety
	(2) Confusion
	(3) Tremor
	(4) Sweating
	(5) Tachycardia and hypertension
	
	Related to clinical context:
	(6) Cardiovascular—look for evidence of intravascular volume depletion and/or dehydration
	(7) Consider other complications of alcoholism:
	  ◆ Wernicke's encephalopathy—see 6.9 above
	  ◆ Acute liver failure
	  ◆ Chronic liver disease and its complications
	(8) Consider other causes of an acute confusional state—see 6.2 above
	(9) Nutritional status

Immediate management	(1) Sedation
	  ◆ Patient can take oral medication:
	    • Reducing schedule of chlordiazepoxide, e.g. 30 mg four times daily (day 1); 20 mg three times daily and 30 mg at night (day 2); 10 mg three times daily and 20 mg at night (day 3); 5 mg three times daily and 10 mg at night (day 4); 5 mg in the morning and 10 mg at night (day 5); 5 mg at night (day 6), then stop
	  ◆ Patient cannot take oral medication:
	    • Clomethiazole (chlormethiazole), 0.8% solution, initially 2.5–7.5 ml/min (20–60 mg/min) until light sleep is induced from which the patient can easily be roused, with the rate of infusion then reduced to the lowest possible to maintain this state. Note—careful monitoring for respiratory depression is required: resuscitation facilities must be available. Switch to oral sedation when possible
	(2) Thiamine
	  ◆ Give parenteral thiamine immediately, usually in combination with other vitamins B and C as Pabrinex I/V high potency, 2–3 pairs of ampoules IV over 10 min every 8 h (each pair of ampoules contains ascorbic acid 500 mg, anhydrous glucose 1 g, nicotinamide 160 mg, pyridoxine hydrochloride 50 mg, riboflavin 4 mg and thiamine hydrochloride 250 mg in a total of 10 ml). Note—facilities for treating anaphylaxis should be available

◆ Then
(3) Glucose—treat/prevent hypoglycaemia
  ◆ Do not give glucose before thiamine—danger of precipitating Wernicke's encephalopathy
  ◆ If blood glucose <3 mmol/litre, give 50 ml of 50% glucose (dextrose monohydrate) IV
  ◆ If not hypoglycaemic—start 5% dextrose infusion at 50 ml/h to prevent hypoglycaemia (if hyponatraemic used reduced volume of more concentrated dextrose solution)

Key investigations	**To establish the diagnosis:** Acute alcohol withdrawal is a clinical diagnosis **Other important tests:** Depending of clinical context, consider as for acute confusional state—see 6.2 above
Further management	(1) After 2 days, switch from IV to oral vitamin replacement, e.g. thiamine 50 mg once daily + vitamin B tablets, Compound, Strong, 1–2 tablets three times daily + Vitamin C 100 mg once daily (2) Other aspects: as for acute confusional state—see 6.2 above—except avoid antipsychotics which lower seizure threshold (3) Long term—measures to help alcoholism

8.2 Drug overdosage

See Chapter 9.1 in main text.

Clinical features	**History** The overdose: (1) Nature, time, and quantity of drug ingested (2) Circumstantial evidence (3) Concurrent alcohol consumption Also: (4) Assessment of intent (5) Past medical history, medications, and allergies (6) Past psychiatric history **Notes** (1) Be cautious in accepting the patient's account at face value (2) Assume that overdoses of multiple drugs are likely **Examination** Initial survey: (1) Airway, breathing, circulation (2) Fingerprick stick test for blood glucose (?hypoglycaemia) (3) Check for small pupils and slow respiratory rate (?opioid overdose) (4) Check temperature (?hypothermia) (5) Check Glasgow Coma Score (see Table 33.1.18) Further examination: (6) Look for features indicated in Table 33.1.22
Immediate management	If cardiorespiratory collapse, as described in 1.2 above ◆ Nurse in recovery position if Glasgow Coma Score impaired ◆ Oxygen—high flow, with reservoir bag if needed, to achieve PaO_2 >92%. ◆ Airway—consider oropharyngeal airway or cuffed endotracheal tube depending on level of consciousness

(1) Cardiac rhythm—place patient on ECG monitor, but do not treat arrhythmias unless these are associated with profound hypotension

(2) Establish IV access:
- If finger prick blood glucose <3 mmol/litre, give 50 ml of 50% glucose (dextrose monohydrate) IV
- If possibility of opioid overdose—give naloxone 0.4–2 mg IV, repeated at intervals of 2–3 min to a maximum of 10 mg. Treat if in doubt

(3) Consider hypothermia—start rewarming

(4) Prevention of drug absorption—see Table 33.1.23

(5) Specific antidote (if available)—see Table 33.1.24

If in doubt—discuss management with a Poisons Centre: the following single number for the UK National Poisons Information Service directs the caller to the relevant local centre: 0870 600 6266

Key investigations	**To establish the diagnosis:** (1) Serum drug levels, e.g. paracetamol, salicylates, iron, theophylline, lithium (2) Save serum sample for measurement of other toxins after discussion with clinical chemist, e.g. paraquat **Note** Record time of blood sampling accurately on specimen tube and in notes **Other important tests:** (1) Electrolytes; glucose; renal, liver, and bone function tests; full blood count; clotting screen (2) ECG Consider: (3) Arterial blood gases (4) Carboxyhaemoglobin level (5) Chest radiograph—look for evidence of aspiration or pulmonary oedema (6) Abdominal radiograph See Table 33.1.25
Further management	(1) Dependent on the nature of overdose taken (2) As dictated by psychiatric condition (if any)

Table 33.1.22 Clinical features of drug overdose

Clinical feature	Drug to consider
Vital signs	
Hypothermia	Alcohol
	Phenothiazines
Hyperthermia	Amphetamines
	Sympathomimetics, including cocaine
	Monoamine oxidase inhibitors
	Salicylates
	Ecstasy
General appearance	
Sweating	Salicylates
Venepuncture marks	Drug abuse

Table 33.1.22 (Cont'd) Clinical features of drug overdose

Clinical feature	Drug to consider
Cardiovascular	
Cardiac arrhythmia	Tricyclics
	Amphetamines
	Potassium
	Theophylline
	Digoxin
	β-Blockers
Hypertension and tachycardia	Amphetamines
	Sympathomimetics
Hypotension	Sedatives
	Narcotics
	Hypnotics
	Iron
	Tricyclics
	Alcohol
Respiratory	
Hyperventilation	Salicylates
Hypoventilation	Opioids
	Sedatives
	Hypnotics
Gastrointestinal	
Oral ulceration	Strong acids or alkalis
Haematemesis	Iron
	Salicylates
Eyes	
Pinpoint pupils	Opioids
Dilated pupils	Anticholinergics
	Tricyclics
	Cocaine
Neurological	
Drowsiness (depressed GCS)	Alcohol
	Sedatives
	Opioids
	Hypnotics
	Salicylates
	Tricyclics
Confusion	Alcohol
Ataxia	Tricyclics
Excitability	Antihistamines
	Salbutamol
	Solvents
Dystonia	Metoclopramide
	Haloperidol
	Phenothiazines

Table 33.1.23 Prevention of absorption of drugs taken in overdose

Indications	Contraindications	Notes
Gastric lavage		
Within 2 h of ingestion of life- threatening amount of toxic substance May be extended up to 6 h after drugs that delay gastric emptying (e.g. salicylates, opioid analgesics, anticholinergic drugs)	Inability to maintain the airway (unless intubated with cuffed endotracheal tube) Ingestion of corrosives or organic solvents	Save lavage sample for analysis
Ipecacuanha		
No indication (for use in adults)		No evidence of reduced drug absorption in poisoned patients
Activated charcoal		
Within 2 h of ingestion of life-threatening amount of toxic substance Consider repeat doses for some toxins, e.g. slow-release preparations, carbamazepine, dapsone, digoxin, paraquat, phenobarbitone, quinine, amanita phalloides (death cap mushroom)	Drugs that are not bound to charcoal, e.g. iron salts, lithium, ethanol, methanol, ethylene glycol, cyanide salts, acids/alkalis, organic solvents, mercury, lead, fluorides, potassium salts	Standard adult dose is 50 g Can be given after gastric lavage

Table 33.1.24 Antidotes used in drug overdose

Overdose	Antidote
β-Adrenoceptor blockers (if severe hypotension)	Atropine 0.6–3.0 mg IV If no response to atropine then give glucagon 50–150 μg/kg IV in 1 min, then 1–5 mg/h by IV infusion
Digoxin	Digoxin-specific Fab antibodies, IV over 30 min Dose determined in relation to patient's body weight and serum digoxin concentration (or 380–760 mg if potentially life-threatening toxicity and serum digoxin concentration not known)
Iron salts	Desferrioxamine mesilate 15 mg/kg/h IV (max 80 mg/kg over 24 h)
Opioids	Naloxone 0.8–2.0 mg IV/IM, repeated at intervals of 2–3 min to maximum 10 mg. If drowsiness recurs after arousal, consider IV infusion (2 mg in 500 ml 0.9% saline, rate adjusted according to response)
Paracetamol	Methionine 2.5 g orally, followed by 2.5 g 4 hourly (×3 further doses), or N-acetylcysteine 150 mg/kg IV in 15 min, then 50 mg/kg over 4 h, then 100 mg/kg over 16 h (in 5% dextrose)
Phenothiazines (dystonia)	Benzatropine mesilate 1–2 mg IV/IM or procyclidine 5–10 mg IV/IM
Warfarin	Vitamin K_1 (phytomenadione) 5 mg slow IV
Benzodiazepines	Flumazenil is a benzodiazepine antagonist but should not be given to patients when the identity of ingested drugs is not known: it can provoke withdrawal seizures in patients with benzodiazepine dependence and arrhythmias in patients who have also taken tricyclic antidepressants. If used then dosage is 0.2 mg IV over 15 s, then 0.1 mg at 60-s intervals (maximum total dose 1–2 mg), and if drowsiness recurs after arousal, consider IV infusion at 0.1–0.4 mg/h

Note:
(1) All dosages are for adults.

Table 33.1.25 Laboratory data in drug overdose

Abnormality	Drug to consider
Hypokalaemia	Sympathomimetic drugs
	Diuretics
Hyperkalaemia	Cardiac glycosides (e.g. digoxin)
	β-Blockers
	Potassium salts
Hypoglycaemia	Insulin
	Oral hypoglycaemic agents
	Ethanol
	Salicylates
Metabolic acidosis	Methanol
	Ethylene glycol
	Salicylates
	Tricyclics
	Carbon monoxide
	Cyanide
Carboxyhaemoglobin	Carbon monoxide
	Smoke
Chest radiograph—pulmonary oedema	Opioids
	Salicylates
	Inhalation of toxins (ammonia, chlorine, oxides of nitrogen)
Abdominal radiograph—radio-opacities	Button batteries
	Iron
	Sustained-release potassium tablets

9 Other conditions

9.1 Disseminated intravascular coagulation

See Chapters 22.6.2 and 22.6.5 in main text.

| Clinical features | Disseminated intravascular coagulation (DIC) is a systemic disorder in which haemorrhage (main problem in 90% of cases) and thrombosis can occur at the same time. It involves the generation of intravascular fibrin and the consumption of procoagulants and platelets. May be acute or chronic (only acute discussed here)

History
Presence of DIC:
(1) Bleeding
 ◆ Skin—extensive superficial bruising; oozing from venepuncture/intramuscular injection sites, around indwelling catheters/tubes
 ◆ Mucosa—mouth, nose, gastrointestinal tract, (lungs), (renal tract)
 ◆ Internal—brain, other organs
(2) Thrombosis:
 ◆ Microthrombotic lesions
 ◆ Skin—often on fingers/toes
 ◆ Internal organs—dysfunction of kidneys, liver, lungs, brain

Related to cause of DIC:
(1) Sepsis—bacterial, viral, fungal, parasitic (malaria)
(2) Major trauma—including burns, surgery
(3) Toxins—e.g. venoms (see 7.6 above)
(4) Obstetric—placental abruption, eclampsia, amniotic fluid embolism
(5) Cancer—metastatic carcinoma of stomach, colon, pancreas, breast, lung; mucin-secreting adenocarcinomas; leukaemia (especially acute promyelocytic leukaemia)
(6) Blood transfusion—incompatible, massive
(7) Liver disease—acute hepatic failure
(8) Others—heatstroke (see 9.3 below), prosthetic devices (e.g. shunts, ventricular assist devices)
(9) Idiopathic—purpura fulminans

Examination
(1) Vital signs
(2) Evidence of bleeding or thrombosis
(3) Related to possible cause (see above) |
| Immediate management | If cardiorespiratory collapse—as described in 1.2 above
(1) Underlying cause—DIC will not improve unless the underlying cause is treated effectively. Give broad-spectrum antimicrobials to cover sepsis if diagnosis not clear (see 7.7 above)
(2) DIC—treatment is justified in patients with serious bleeding, high risk of bleeding (e.g. postoperative), or who require invasive procedures
 ◆ Fresh frozen plasma—to keep prothrombin time and activated partial thromboplastin time below a value 1.5 times the upper limit of control values
 ◆ Cryoprecipitate/fibrinogen concentrates—to keep fibrinogen levels >1 g/litre
 ◆ Platelets—to keep platelets >50×10⁹/litre
 ◆ Blood (packed red blood cells)—to keep haematocrit >0.30 |

| Notes | (1) Heparin—if the main clinical problem is thrombotic, e.g. migratory thrombophlebitis or acral ischaemia, then consider giving heparin. On theoretical ground this would only be expected to be effective if patient's antithrombin III level is near normal, hence:
 ◆ If low antithrombin III—give antithrombin III in dose calculated according to manufacturer's instructions, aiming to maintain levels >80% of normal (unlicensed indication)
 ◆ Heparin, 500 units/h by continuous IV infusion, titrated to achieve activated partial thromboplastin time (aPTT) of about 45 seconds
(2) Protein C concentrate—consider in protein C deficiency (congenital or acquired, e.g. meningococcal septicaemia) associated with purpura fulminans
(3) Adrenal infarction (Waterhouse–Friederichson)— give steroid (e.g. hydrocortisone 50–100 mg 6 hourly IV) if circulatory compromise |
| Key investigations | **To establish the diagnosis:**
There is no single diagnostic test for DIC: the condition should be suspected in any patient with:
(1) Appropriate clinical context
(2) Platelet count—decreased
(3) Blood film—microangiopathic changes

The diagnosis is confirmed by laboratory demonstration of increased thrombin generation and increased fibrinolysis:
(1) Thrombin generation increased—fibrinogen decreased
(2) Fibrinolysis increased—elevated fibrinogen/fibrin degradation products; elevated D-dimer
(3) Prothrombin time— increased
(4) aPTT—increased
(5) Other haematological features that may be present include—reduced antithrombin III level; increased thrombin time; increased soluble fibrin monomers

Other important tests:
Dependent on clinical context |
| Further management | Dependent on clinical context |

9.2 Sickle cell crises

See Chapter 22.5.7 in main text.

| Clinical features | **History**
There are several clinical conditions:
(1) Pain crisis—severe pain in limbs, hips, back, chest, or abdomen; the pain is genuine, excruciating, and varies in character and location
(2) Chest/lung syndrome—breathlessness, pleuritic chest pain
(3) Brain/neurological syndrome—epileptic fits, transient ischaemic attacks, strokes

And less commonly in adults:
(4) Aplastic crisis—presents with breathlessness and fatigue. Usually seen in children. Associated with parvovirus infection
(5) Sequestration crisis—presents with profound anaemia. Usually seen in babies and young children when the spleen and/or liver enlarge rapidly due to trapping of red blood cells. Hepatic sequestration can occur in adults
(6) Priapism |

Also:

(7) Previous sickle cell crises

(8) Precipitating factors—extremes of heat and cold, infections/fever (often upper respiratory tract, flu), heavy exercise, emotional stress, any situation producing hypoxia

(9) Family history—patterns of crises may follow through generations

Note

Patients or their relatives/friends generally know that they have sickle cell disease and are often knowledgeable about the condition

Examination	(1) Airway, breathing, circulation (2) Glasgow Coma Scale (3) Vital signs—pulse rate, BP, respiratory rate, temperature Note particularly: (4) General examination—pallor (5) Chest—local tenderness and signs of infection. (6) Bones—tenderness (7) Liver or spleen—look for enlargement due to hepatosplenic sequestration (particularly in children, uncommon in adults) (8) Priapism (9) Infection—fever may be the only sign; there may be no localizing signs

Immediate management	If cardiorespiratory collapse, as described in 1.2 above
	(1) Oxygen—high flow, with reservoir bag if needed, to achieve PaO_2 >92%. Monitor with pulse oximeter.
	(2) Fluid—establish IV access (may be difficult, asking patient's advice on best site is often helpful) and give 1 litre of 0.9% saline rapidly, then repeat 4–6 hourly for duration of crisis (assuming satisfactory urine output)
	(3) Analgesia—give adequate pain relief
	   ◆ Intravenous e.g. (1) diamorphine by slow IV injection at 1 mg/min, usual maximum initial dose is 5 mg, but may be repeated if necessary, or (2) morphine by slow IV injection at 2 mg/min, usual maximum initial dose is 10 mg, but may be repeated if necessary. Both to be accompanied by appropriate antiemetic, e.g. metoclopramide 10 mg IV over 1–2 min, or cyclizine 50 mg IV over 1–2 min
	   ◆ Intramuscular/subcutaneous—if it is not possible to establish IV access, then give diamorphine (0.05 mg/kg) or morphine (0.1 mg/kg) subcutaneously, repeated after 1 h if necessary
	(4) Warmth—wrap in warm blankets if the patient feels cold
	(5) Antibiotics—as dictated by clinical context, e.g. appropriate cover for community acquired pneumonia, including atypical organisms
	(6) Prophylaxis against venous thromboembolism—give low molecular weight heparin, e.g. enoxaparin 20 mg subcutaneously once daily

Key investigations	**To establish the diagnosis** Sickle cell crisis is a clinical diagnosis Acute chest syndrome—tachypnoea/wheezing/cough; chest pain; fever >38.5°C; new pulmonary infiltrate involving at least one complete lung segment

Other important tests:

(1) Full blood count, reticulocytes, group and save

(2) Electrolytes, renal and liver function, glucose

(3) Cultures—blood, sputum, urine, throat swab

(4) Arterial blood gases

(5) Chest radiograph—may show widespread patchy infiltrate that is difficult to distinguish from infection

(6) HbS level (percentage of total Hb)—if exchange transfusion considered

(7) Abdominal radiograph, serum amylase (abdominal syndrome)

(8) Serology to detect acute parvovirus B19 infection (aplastic crisis)

Notes

(1) Other investigations as dictated by clinical context, e.g. CT scan brain if focal neurological signs

(2) Imaging—do not order plain radiographs of all sites of pain

Further management	(1) Seek expert advice if you are not familiar with managing patients with sickle cell crises (2) Exchange transfusion—chest syndrome with hypoxia, neurological symptoms or priapism (see Chapter 13.8.5) are indications for exchange transfusion to increase haematocrit to >30% and reduce HbS to <30% of total Hb (3) Education—patients should be taught to intiate treatment at the first hint of painful crisis with heating pads, increased oral fluids, analgesia (paracetamol, ibuprofen, mild opioid) (4) Hydroxyurea—reduces the frequency of painful crises

9.3 Heat stroke

See Chapters 9.5.1 and 26.6.1 in main text.

Clinical features	Hyperthermia is a failure of thermal homeostasis that allows the core temperature to rise above 40°C. It can result from exposure to environmental heat with/without prolonged physical exercise (especially if heat dissipating mechanisms are impaired) and/or from increased metabolic heat production. Heat stroke is hyperthermia with severe central nervous system abnormalities such as delirium, convulsions or coma, with case fatality ranging from 17 to 70%

History

Predisposing factors:

(1) Exposure to high ambient temperature ± high humidity (e.g. in a heatwave)

(2) Prolonged strenuous physical exercise at any ambient temperature, especially if insulation from clothing is excessive and the patient is unacclimatized

(3) Drugs:

   ◆ Neuroleptic malignant syndrome— caused by psychiatriac/recreational dopaminergic drugs, e.g. phenothiazines, thioxanthene, butyrophenones, amphetamines; usually develops over 1–3 days; often presents with delirium/confusion (evolving to coma)

   ◆ Malignant hyperpyrexia—occurs in people with a rare genetic predisposition (50% autosomal dominant due to mutation in skeletal muscle ryanodine receptor, RyR1) when exposed to various anaesthetic agents. Onset usually within 1 h of exposure.

(4) Previous history of heat intolerance

Symptoms

Heat exhaustion:

(1) General—irritability, weakness, lethargy, fatigue, dizziness, headache, muscle cramps/myalgias

(2) Gastrointestinal—nausea, vomiting, diarrhoea

(3) Respiratory—hyperventilation/tachypnoea

Heatstroke:

Any or all of the symptoms of heat exhaustion, plus

(4) Neurological dysfunction—impaired judgement, abnormal behaviour, disorientation, hallucinations, confusion, convulsions, loss of consciousness

Examination

(1) Vital signs—core (rectal) temperature >40°C (by definition), hypotension, tachycardia, tachypnoea

(2) Temperature control mechanisms—sweating can be present (>50% cases) or absent (<50%); piloerection; hot dry skin is a late finding

(3) General—weakness, dehydration, bleeding (DIC)

(4) Neurological—impaired consciousness (Glasgow Coma Scale), seizures, opisthotonus, decerebrate rigidity, cerebellar dysfunction, oculogyric crises, fixed dilated pupils

(5) Signs of predisposing condition—e.g. obesity, skin disease, thyrotoxicosis

Note

Muscular rigidity is a feature of neuroleptic malignant syndrome and malignant hyperpyrexia but not of heat stroke

Immediate management

♦ If cardiorespiratory collapse—as described in 1.2 above
♦ Oxygen—high flow, with reservoir bag if needed, to achieve PaO$_2$ >92%
♦ If clinical evidence of intravascular volume depletion, establish IV access and resuscitate using 0.9% saline as described in 3.1 above

(1) Cooling:
   ♦ Should be done rapidly
   ♦ Remove to shade or cooler place
   ♦ Remove clothes
   ♦ External methods—(as available) tepid sponging and fanning; ice packs to neck, axillae, groins; cover with wet sheet; hypothermia bed/blanket; immersion in cold water with vigorous massage (effective at lowering body temperature but associated with more complications than evaporative cooling and not generally recommended)
   ♦ Internal methods—(as available) ice water gastric lavage; ice water rectal lavage; ice water intraperitoneal lavage; mechanical ventilation with cooled gases; cardiac bypass (anecdotal success reported for these treatments)

(2) Fluids and electrolytes—correct volume depletion and electrolyte abnormalities (see below)

(3) Urine output—consider urethral catheter for monitoring

(4) Malignant hyperpyrexia and neuroleptic malignant syndrome:
   ♦ Stop drug/anaesthetic
   ♦ Treat muscle spasms/rigidity—give dantrolene sodium by rapid IV injection, 1–2 mg/kg repeated every 5 min as required to a cumulative maximum of 10 mg/kg (followed by 4–8 mg/kg per day orally in four divided doses)

Notes

(1) In the field—stop exertion at the first sign of heat exhaustion, remove excess clothing, move into shade, encourage oral fluids

(2) Do not give salicylates—which do not reduce body temperature and may exacerbate coagulopathy

(3) Do not give paracetamol (acetaminophen)—which does not reduce body temperature and may worsen hepatic damage

Key investigations

Heat stroke is a clinical diagnosis

Important tests:

(1) Electrolytes and renal function—risk of hypokalaemia, hyponatraemia, hypocalcaemia, hypomagnesaemia, hypophosphataemia, impaired renal function (hyperkalaemia if renal failure and rhabdomyolysis)

(2) Glucose—may have hyperglycaemia; also risk of hypoglycaemia

(3) Full blood count—high haematocrit indicates haemoconcentration

(4) Liver blood tests—transaminases are usually elevated in heatstroke and indicate hepatotoxicity and/or muscle damage

(5) Muscle enzymes—elevated creatine kinase indicates muscle damage (rhabdomyolysis)

(6) Albumin/serum proteins—elevated values indicate haemoconcentration

(7) Coagulation tests—evidence of DIC (see 9.1 above)

(8) Amylase—?pancreatitis

(9) ECG, troponin—evidence of myocardial damage

(10) Arterial blood gases—?lactic acidosis

Consider:

(11) Chest radiograph—?aspiration

(12) CT scan head—?alternative cause of CNS dysfunction

Further management

(1) Complications of active cooling—beware of seizures (see 6.5 above); beware of cardiac arrhythmias—only treat if causing significant haemodynamic compromise (see 1.7 above)

(2) Supportive care as appropriate—respiratory failure; circulatory failure (correct volume depletion, consider vasopressors); renal failure/rhabdomyolysis (see 4.1 and 4.2 above)

(3) Prevention—after recovery, give advice to prevent recurrence

(4) Genetic counselling—a diagnosis of malignant hyperpyrexia may have implications for family members

9.4 Hypothermia

See Chapter 9.5.2 in main text.

Clinical features

History

Two distinct contexts:

(1) Cold exposure—in patient of any age

(2) Multifactorial cause—often in elderly patients: immobility/falls; cognitive impairment; alcohol; vasodilating drugs; autonomic dysfunction, eg. diabetes mellitus; poor socio-economic conditions. Elderly patients with hypothermia have often been found on the floor at home following a fall

Examination

Initial survey:

(1) Airway, breathing, circulation

(2) Fingerprick stick test for blood glucose (?hypoglycaemia)

(3) Check for small pupils and slow respiratory rate (?opioid overdose)

(4) Temperature—using a low-range rectal thermometer: <35°C (by definition).

(5) Check Glasgow Coma Score (see Table 33.1.18)

Futher examination

(1) General appearance—cold, pale mottled skin (whereabouts on the body, if anywhere, does the skin feel warm?). At 32–35°C, shivering; at <32°C, muscular rigidity

(2) Cardiovascular—bradycardia and hypotension

(3) Respiratory—look for evidence of aspiration, pneumonia or pulmonary oedema

(4) Neurological—variable features ranging from mild incoordination to confusion, lethargy and coma. Pupils may be dilated and nonreactive. Focal/lateralizing signs may indicate stroke that has precipitated hypothermia.

(5) Endocrine—could the patient be hypothyroid?

Immediate management

Depends on the clinical context:

◆ If cardiorespiratory collapse—as described in 1.2 above

◆ Oxygen—high flow, with reservoir bag if needed, to achieve $PaO_2 > 92\%$

◆ Treat for hypoglycaemia and/or opioid overdose if appropriate

(1) Fluids— patients who are hypotensive should be given warmed IV fluids (see below, and as described in 3.1 above), but note risk of pulmonary oedema and check frequently for lung crackles and/or worsening gas exchange as resuscitation progresses. Adjust rate of infusion as determined by clinical response

(2) ECG monitoring—risk of ventricular tachycardia/fibrillation

(3) Antibiotics—as appropriate for pulmonary infection, which is common in this context, e.g. cefotaxime 1 g 12 hourly IV

(4) Rewarming—management depends on circumstances of hypothermia:

◆ Hypothermia of gradual onset (usually elderly, usually multifactorial cause)—rewarm slowly

◆ Nurse in warm room covered with a blanket or 'Bair Hugger' (do not use foil blankets, which retard rewarming)

◆ Cold exposure, severe hypothermia (<30°C), or hypothermia of any cause complicated by life-threatening arrhythmia—rewarm rapidly using both:

• Active external rewarming—apply heat to body surface, e.g. hot-water bottles/warmed IV bags (not too hot, must be comfortably bearable against your own skin) in groins and axillae, warmed blankets, radiant heaters

• Active core rewarming—give warmed (42–46°C) humidified oxygen and warmed (43°C) IV fluids; consider gastric, colonic, bladder, and peritoneal lavage with warmed (43°C) 0.9% saline solutions

• Extracorporeal blood re-warming—for potentially recoverable patients in cardiac arrest or others in extremis, use of venvenous rewarming, haemodialysis, continuous arteriovenous rewarming and cardiopulmonary bypass have been described

Notes

(1) Aim to rewarm at a rate of 0.5–2°C/h

(2) Patients with hypothermia are best managed in an ICU setting: they may require treatment of arrhythmia and/or ventilatory support

(3) Arrhythmias:

◆ Avoid use of catecholamines (arrhythmogenic)

◆ Only treat if life-threatening (ventricular fibrillation (VF) or asystole)—for VF, attempt defibrillation up to three times, but not more until core temperature >30°C. The drug of choice is probably bretylium 5–10 mg/kg IV over 15–30 min, repeated after 1–2 h to total dose of 30 mg/kg. Magnesium sulphate (8 mmol of magnesium) given IV over 10–15 min (repeated once if necessary) has also been reported to be effective. Lignocaine (lidocaine) is not effective in hypothermic VF, and the International Liaison Committee on Resuscitation guidelines suggest avoiding this drug, also adrenaline (epinephrine) and procainamide, because of the risk of accumulation to toxic levels

(4) Paradoxical fall in temperature—return of cold blood from the extremeties to the core circulation can lead to an initial paradoxical fall in temperature, hence apply active external rewarming to the trunk before the extremeties

(5) Diagnosis of death—this can be difficult. Patients with severe hypothermia can appear clinically dead. Resuscitative efforts must continue until the core temperature is 30–33°C, i.e. the patient is not dead until they are warm and dead

Key investigations

To establish the diagnosis:

Hypothermia is defined as a core temperature <35°C

Other important tests:

(1) Full blood count, electrolytes, glucose, renal and liver function tests—note that severe hyperkalaemia is common in profound hypothermia. Serum potassium must be monitored closely during rewarming, even if initially normal

(2) Calcium (low), amylase (high)—in pancreatitis, an important complication of hypothermia

(3) Thyroid function tests—?hypothyroid

(4) Arterial blood gases—to look for hypoxia and/or acidosis

(5) ECG—look for sinus bradycardia, J wave ('junctional' wave—a broad, slurred deflection that is superimposed on the distal limb of the QRS complex), prolonged QT interval. Note that the muscular tremor of shivering can lead to artefact on the ECG, which should not be confused with VF

(6) Chest radiograph—look for aspiration, pneumonia, pulmonary oedema

Further management

Dependent on the cause of hypothermia. Prevention of recurrence is likely to require socioeconomic intervention in elderly people, e.g. provision of heating, increased supervision

Practical procedures

John D. Firth, David A. Warrell, and Timothy M. Cox

Central vein cannulation, arterial cannulation, and invasive monitoring

The insertion of catheters into central veins is increasingly performed with ultrasonographic guidance. However, in some emergencies it may not be possible to use this even in the best-equipped hospital, and in many hospitals such imaging is simply not available. In these circumstances the central veins can be safely cannulated by landmark techniques, which are described in this section.

Femoral vein cannulation

The optimum position is with the patient supine, but their head and torso can be propped up to an angle of 15 to 30° if this is more comfortable. The key landmark is the femoral pulse, which should be palpated one finger-breadth below the crease of the groin. The femoral vein lies one finger-breadth medial to the femoral artery (the mnemonic NAVY, Nerve–Artery–Vein–Y-fronts, can be useful in remembering the anatomy). The needle should therefore enter the skin one finger-breadth medial to the femoral artery and one finger-breadth below the groin crease (Fig. 33.2.1). It should be advanced in the line of the leg, angled rostrally at about 60° to the skin, and with its bevel pointing forwards. When the vein is punctured the guidewire should pass directly up the femoral vein and into the inferior vena cava.

Internal jugular vein cannulation

Low lateral approach

The patient is supine with the head turned away from the side of the puncture. A towel may be placed under both shoulders to extend the neck. After preparation of the skin and drapes, and insertion of local anaesthetic, the bed is tilted to a 25° head-down position. The needle is inserted just lateral to the posterior border of the clavicular head of the sternocleidomastoid muscle, about one finger-breadth above the clavicle, with its bevel pointing caudally. It is then advanced parallel to the line of the clavicle and just behind the sternocleidomastoid muscle. The internal jugular vein, which lies superficially at this point, is cannulated close to its junction with the subclavian vein (Fig. 33.2.2a). As soon as the vein is entered the needle is angulated caudally to ease cannulation, the guide wire passing directly into the innominate vein. The risk of complications was lower with this technique than for any other

method of central venous cannulation used in one series of over 5400 cases (see Chapter 17.3).

Axial approach

The patient is positioned as described for the low lateral approach to the internal jugular vein (Fig. 33.2.2b). The needle is inserted in the centre of the triangle defined by the sternal and clavicular heads of the sternocleidomastoid muscle and the clavicle itself. It should be angulated caudally, at about 60° to the skin, and in a line pointing towards the ipsilateral anterior superior iliac spine.

Subclavian vein cannulation

Infraclavicular approach (Fig. 33.2.3a)

The patient is positioned as described for the low lateral approach to the internal jugular vein, excepting that instead of a towel being placed under both shoulders it should be positioned under the spine, allowing the shoulders to retract to reduce the risk of pneumothorax. The needle enters the skin below the midpoint of the lower border of the clavicle and is advanced under the clavicle towards the upper edge of the junction of the clavicle with the manubrium.

Supraclavicular approach (Fig. 33.2.3b)

The patient is positioned as described for the infraclavicular approach to the subclavian vein. The needle is inserted into the angle between the superior border of the clavicle and the posterior border of the clavicular head of sternocleidomastoid and advanced caudally, medially and ventrally.

Pulmonary artery flotation catheter

Central venous cannulation should be performed as described above and a pulmonary artery (PA) catheter introducer inserted. Ensure that the balloon at the end of the PA catheter inflates completely and uniformly, and then slowly advance the catheter whilst watching the pressure trace on the monitor. The balloon should be inflated when the catheter is advanced and deflated whenever the catheter is withdrawn. Pressure traces corresponding to the right atrium, the right ventricle, and the pulmonary artery should be seen (Fig. 33.2.4). As a rough guide, the waveform should change for every 10 cm that the catheter is advanced. Inflation of the balloon when the catheter is in a medium sized pulmonary artery allows it to 'wedge' and occlude distal flow. To obtain valid readings, the

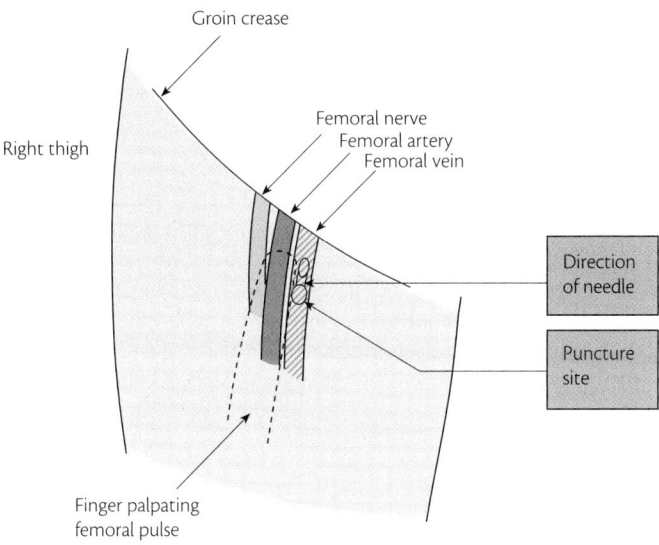

Fig. 33.2.1 The approach to the femoral vein.

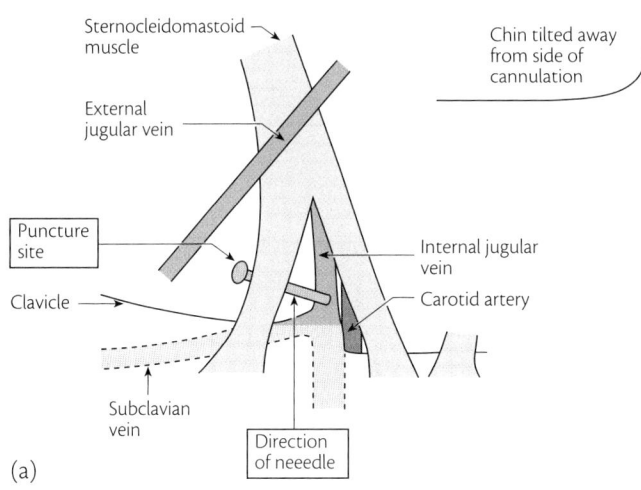

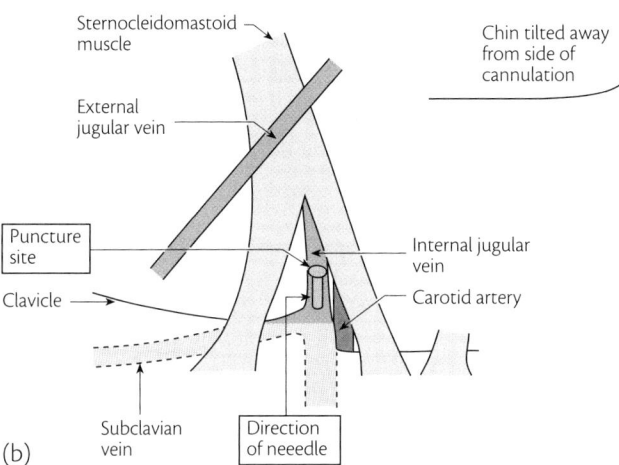

Fig. 33.2.2 (a) The low lateral approach to the internal jugular vein. (b) The axial approach to the internal jugular vein.

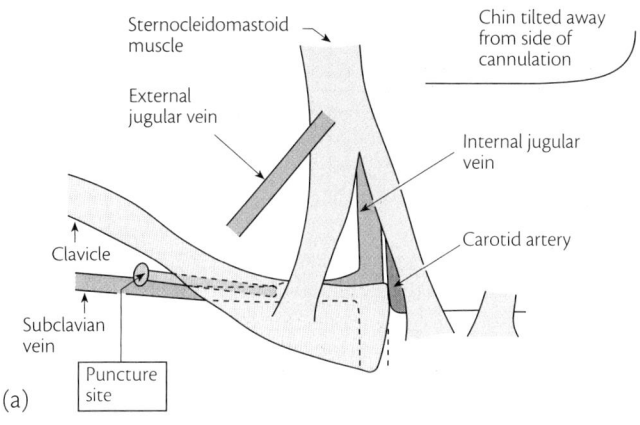

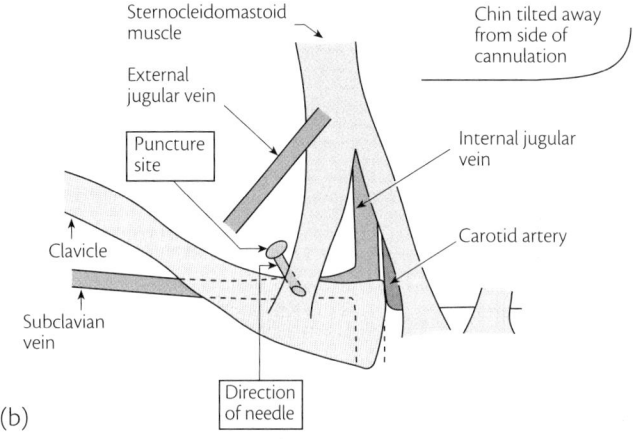

Fig. 33.2.3 (a) The infraclavicular approach to the subclavian vein. (b) The supraclavicular approach to the subclavian vein.

catheter tip should reside in a region of the lung where pulmonary venous pressure exceeds alveolar pressure. The pressure recorded at the tip of the catheter (pulmonary capillary wedge pressure, PCWP) provides indirect measurement of the left atrial pressure, which reflects left ventricular end-diastolic pressure if the chamber is not diseased. Values for cardiac output and mixed-venous blood chemistries may also be directly measured. A number of variables such as systemic vascular resistance and left ventricular stroke work may be derived from values measured with a PA catheter.

Arterial puncture/cannulation

Before attempting to puncture or cannulate the radial artery, check the patency of the ulnar artery by applying pressure to the radial

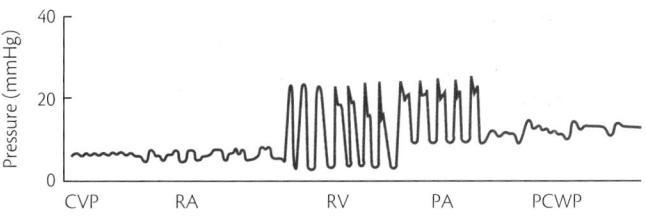

Fig. 33.2.4 Pressure tracings obtained on insertion of a pulmonary artery flotation catheter. CVP, central venous pressure; PA, pulmonary artery; PCWP, pulmonary capillary wedge pressure; RA, right atrium; RV, right ventricle.

artery and asking the patient to clench their fist firmly. On relaxing the fist, the hand should pink up within 10 s (Allen test).

A 25 G needle (orange) is perfectly adequate to obtain an arterial blood gas (ABG) sample from a radial artery; 18 G (green) or 23 G (blue) is needed for a femoral sample. Use either a preheparinized ABG syringe or draw up 1 ml of 1000 U/ml heparin into a syringe and then completely expel the heparin.

Lay the index and middle fingers of your nondominant hand along the line of the artery as a guide (Fig. 33.2.5). For radial and brachial samples, hold the syringe at 45 to 60° to the skin and slowly advance in the line of the artery. For femoral samples, hold the syringe at 90° to the skin. A flash of blood into the syringe indicates successful puncture. Some syringes will fill to a predetermined volume, others require aspiration of 1 to 2 ml.

After successful arterial puncture, press on the site for 3 min (5 min if anticoagulated) to prevent haematoma formation.

Arterial cannulation may be performed either with a cannula over a needle (similar to a venflon) or with a Seldinger technique. After preparation of the skin and insertion of local anaesthetic, the method of arterial puncture should be as described above, with the exception that for all arterial cannulations the needle should be inserted at 45° to the artery. Once arterial puncture has been confirmed, the cannula should be advanced over the needle, or the guide wire passed directly into the artery and the cannula then advanced over the guide wire.

Cardiac procedures

DC cardioversion

Synchronized cardioversion is the treatment of choice for symptomatic tachyarrhythmias. Conscious patients must be anaesthetized or sedated. Suitable monitoring and facilities for dealing with cardiac arrest should be available. Modern defibrillators incorporate a switch that allows the shock to be synchronized with the R wave of the ECG to reduce the risk of inducing ventricular fibrillation. Gel pads should be applied to the chest wall and cardioversion carried out in the same manner as for defibrillation. The energy required depends on the underlying rhythm. Synchronization means that there may be a delay between pressing the defibrillator buttons and the discharge of the shock when the next R wave occurs.

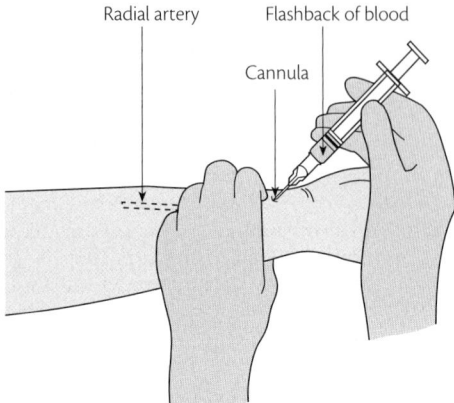

Fig. 33.2.5 Puncture of the radial artery.

Cardiac pacing (temporary)

Indications for emergency/acute temporary cardiac pacing are shown in Table 33.2.1.

External (transcutaneous) pacing
Percussion pacing
Percussion pacing can be used as a temporizing measure in some patients with profound bradycardia causing clinical cardiac arrest. It is particularly useful for ventricular standstill where P waves are visible on the ECG. A series of gentle blows should be applied to the lower left sternal edge using the closed fist. Using trial and error, a site can sometimes be found which results in stimulation of the ventricular myocardium. If percussion does not produce a cardiac output, orthodox pacing or CPR should be instituted immediately.

Transcutaneous pacing
Most modern transcutaneous pacing systems are integrated with an ECG monitor/defibrillator. Pacemaker electrodes should be placed in either an anterior–posterior position or in the conventional

Table 33.2.1 Indications for temporary transvenous cardiac pacing

Acute myocardial infarction
ACC/AHA Class I — pacing supported by evidence and/or general agreement
Asystole
Symptomatic bradycardia (includes sinus bradycardia with hypotension and type I second-degree AV block not responsive to atropine)
Bilateral BBB (alternating BBB or RBBB with alternating LAHB / LPHB)
Bifascicular block (RBBB with LAHB or LPHB, or LBBB) with first-degree AV block
Mobitz type II second-degree AV block
ACC/AHA Class IIa — weight of evidence and/or opinion favours pacing
RBBB with LAHB or LPHB
RBBB with first degree AV block
LBBB
Incessant VT, for overdrive pacing
Recurrent sinus pauses (>3 s) not responsive to atropine
ACC/AHA Class IIb— usefulness of pacing less well established
Bifascicular block of indeterminate age
Isolated RBB
ACC/AHA Class III—pacing not useful and may be harmful
First-degree AV block
Mobitz type I second-degree AV block with normal haemodynamics
Accelerated idioventricular rhythm
BBB or fascicular block known to be present before myocardial infarction
Bradycardia not associated with myocardial infarction
Asystole
Second- or third-degree AV block with haemodynamic disturbance or syncope at rest
Ventricular tachyarrhythmia secondary to bradycardia

ACC/AHA, American College of Cardiology/American Heart Association;
AV, atrioventricular block; BBB, bundle branch block; LAHB, left anterior hemiblock; LBBB, left bundle branch block; LPHB, left posterior hemiblock; RBBB, right bundle branch block; VT, ventricular tachycardia.
ACC/AHA, American College of Cardiology/American Heart Association

anterior–lateral configuration. The pacemaker should be set to demand pacing to prevent a stimulus from falling on the T wave following a spontaneous heartbeat, with the rate set at 60 to 90/min for adults. The pacemaker current should be set at the lowest setting and gradually increased to obtain capture of the myocardium and a palpable pulse. The current required to obtain capture is generally in the range 50 to 100 mA and will produce painful contraction of the patient's skeletal muscle. Conscious patients will require analgesia and/or sedation. If capture of the myocardium does not occur, alternative electrode placement should be tried.

Transcutaneous pacing is only a temporizing measure and arrangements should be made for urgent transvenous pacing.

Transvenous pacing (ventricular)

Temporary transvenous pacing can be achieved after cannulation of any central vein, but is most easily performed via the right internal jugular, right subclavian, or right femoral vein, which can be cannulated as described above.

The conventional Seldinger technique of guide wire and dilators is used to allow placement of a sheath (preferably haemostatic) of sufficient size to accept passage of the pacing wire in the vein that has been cannulated. The pacing wire is passed down the sheath and advanced towards the heart, the aim being to maneouvre it under fluoroscopic guidance into a position where its tip is at the apex of the right ventricule, angulated slightly downwards. Key aspects of the technique are shown in Fig. 33.2.6. Common problems and their solutions are described in Table 33.2.2.

After positioning the pacing wire, set the pacemaker to a rate of 70/min, or 10/min above the patient's ventricular rate, and to deliver a pulse of 3 V (or as directed by the manufacturer). A correctly positioned electrode should 'capture', such that each pacing spike is followed by a ventricular complex on the ECG. Establish the voltage threshold by gradually turning down the amplitude of the voltage delivered until capture is lost, which will usually be in the range 0.7 to 1.0 V. To allow a safety margin, it is then appropriate in most circumstances to set the pacemaker to deliver a voltage of at least twice the threshold. Sensing can be checked only if there is spontaneous ventricular activity: this is best done by setting the pacemaker rate to between 10 and 20/min below the spontaneous ventricular rate and looking on the ECG monitor and the pulse generator for evidence of pacing inhibition. Sensitivity is usually set to to its maximum. Common problems and their solutions are described in Table 33.2.3.

When the pacing wire is positioned appropriately and pacing is established, carefully remove the introducer sheath (in most cases), secure the wire with a strong suture (usually 2/0 silk), loop it once or twice on the skin, and then dress with a clear adhesive dressing.

Pericardiocentesis

Cardiac tamponade is the indication for pericardiocentesis as an emergency. Unless the patient is *in extremis* the procedure should, whenever possible, be performed with echocardiographic guidance by an operator experienced in the technique, as follows:

Two-dimensional echocardiography is used to assess the size, distribution, and haemodynamic effect of the effusion.

The ideal entry site for pericardiocentesis is the point on the skin where the effusion is closest to the transducer and the fluid accumulation is maximal. The distance from the skin to the pericardial space is estimated, with the needle trajectory defined by the angulation of the hand-held transducer. A straight path that best avoids

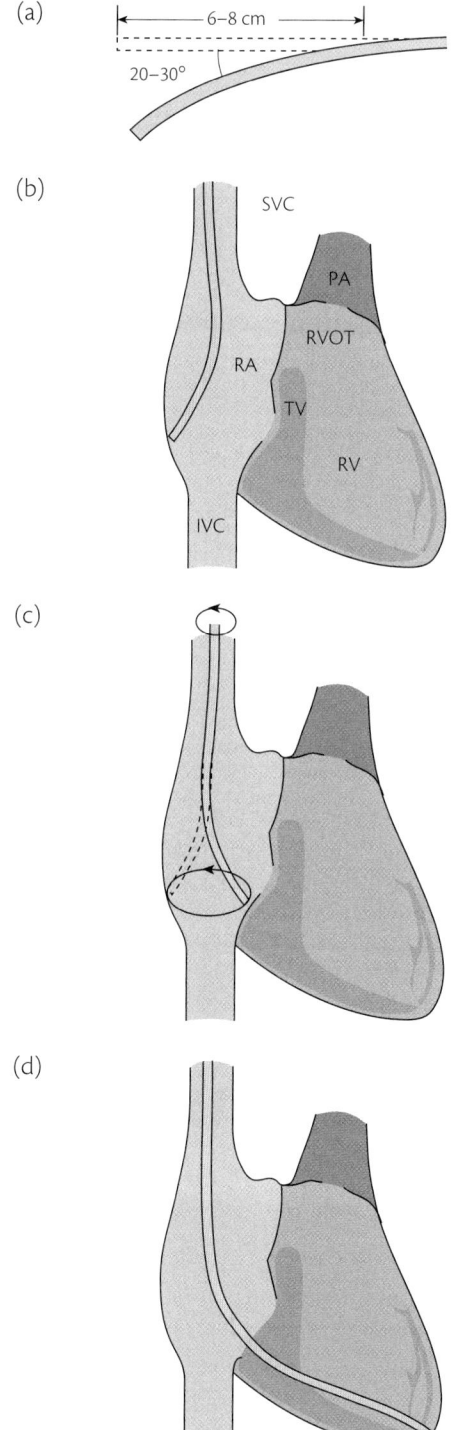

Fig. 33.2.6 Correct positioning of the electrode is helped if there is a 20 to 30° curve at the tip of the pacing wire. Mould the electrode to this shape using your fingers: it may need to be bent or straightened depending on its packaging. (a) Advance the wire until it lies vertically in the right atrium. It will usually assume a position where its tip points towards the free wall on the right side (b). Rotate the wire between your index finger and thumb until it points towards the patient's left (c). When it has done so, advance the wire steadily: it should pass through the tricuspid valve and along the floor of the right ventricle to the apex (d). IVC, inferior vena cava; RA, right atrium; RV, right ventricle; RVOT, right ventricular outflow tract; SVC, superior vena cava; TV, tricuspid valve.

Table 33.2.2 Common problems in temporary transvenous ventricular pacing

Problem	Possible solution
Wire will not cross the tricuspid valve	Feed the wire into the right atrium until it 'catches' and forms a large loop. It may pass into the IVC (if approaching from above) or SVC (if approaching from below), in which case it will need to be pulled back and then pushed forward until it does catch. When a large loop has been formed, rotate the wire until its tip flips through into the ventricle
Intubation of the coronary sinus	The wire appears to be in the right ventricle, but (sometimes) will not capture the ventricle at an acceptable voltage output. On fluoroscopy the electrode tip is directed upwards and towards the left shoulder (and on a lateral chest radiograph is directed posteriorly rather than anteriorly). If satisfactory pacing cannot be obtained, then the pacing wire must be withdrawn into the right atrium and further attempts made to advance it across the tricuspid valve
Wire is in the right ventricle, but it is difficult to get it positioned at the apex	Pass the tip of the wire into the right ventricular outflow tract, then gently withdraw it while rotating it between index finger and thumb. When the tip is angulated downwards, advance towards the apex of the ventricle. Note that it can be difficult to get a good position at the apex if the pacing wire is too bent to start off with, hence the injunction to mould the tip with the fingers to obtain an angulation of 20–30° at the beginning of the procedure

IVC, inferior vena cava; SVC, superior vena cava.

vital structures (also the internal mammary artery, which lies 3 to 5 cm lateral to the sternal margin) is chosen.

After preparation of the skin and insertion of local anaesthetic, a 16 to 18 gauge Polytef-sheathed (or similar) needle attached to a saline-filled syringe is advanced in the predetermined trajectory, with continued gentle aspiration as it moves forward. On entering the pericardial fluid, the needle is advanced approximately 2 mm further, when the sheath is advanced over the needle and the steel core withdrawn.

The position of the sheath in the pericardial space can be confirmed by injecting 5 ml of agitated saline through it, whilst

Table 33.2.3 Failure to pace

Problem	Causes	Solution
No spikes seen and no output	Battery/generator failure	Replace battery/generator
	Loose connections	Check and tighten
	Oversensing	Reduce sensitivity or go to fixed-rate pacing
Spikes seen, but no capture	Loose connections	Check and tighten
	Exit block (high threshold)	Increase output
		Check position of pacing wire (by fluoroscopy or plain radiograph)
		Consider repositioning of electrode

observing the pericardial space with two-dimensional echocardiography (optional).

Intrapericardial pressure can be directly measured with a manometer (optional); pericardial fluid can be sent for diagnostic tests (optional).

A guide wire is advanced through the Polytef sheath, which is removed over the guide wire. A small stab incision of the skin is made at the entry site, following which dilators are used to allow the insertion of a larger sheath (6–8 F) through which a pigtail angiocatheter can be introduced. After the pigtail catheter has been inserted the introducer sheath is removed, leaving only the smooth-walled pigtail catheter in the pericardial space. (Note that this technique is preferred to that of introducing the pigtail catheter directly over the guide wire because the catheter tip can occasionally pull the guide wire out of the pericardial sac, particularly if this is sclerotic.)

Pericardial fluid is drained completely by syringe suction and the pericardial catheter is secured to the chest wall by suture and appropriate dressing.

If left on continuous drainage, pericardial catheters become plugged. It is therefore better to perform intermittent aspiration, every 4 to 6 h or as clinically indicated, leaving the catheter flushed with saline in between times. It can be removed when drainage has been reduced to less than 25 to 30 ml/day and follow-up echocardiography shows no significant residual effusion (sooner if the catheter is causing problems).

If the patient is *in extremis* and/or echocardiography (with appropriate expertise) is not available, then a 'blind' subxiphoid approach is most often used:

- Sit the patient up at an angle of 45°.

- Insert the needle 3 cm below the xiphisternum at an angle of 30 to 45° to the skin and advance, applying gentle suction all the time (as above), in a line towards the patient's left shoulder.

- If the needle touches the heart, it will usually provoke ectopic beats. Some authorities recommend that the aspiration needle is attached to the 'V' lead terminal of an ECG cable (using insulated wire with a clip on each end, or simply with sticky tape) to allow continuous monitoring. If the needle touches the heart, then the character of the ECG changes, most particularly with the appearance of gross ST segment elevation if the needle touches the right or left ventricle.

- When fluid is obtained, proceed as described above.

Arterial blood gases

Parameters that may be measured or derived by blood gas machines are listed and commented on in Table 33.2.4.

Airway and respiratory procedures
Mechanical support of ventilation
Continuous positive airways pressure
Continual positive airway pressure (CPAP) exerts a dilating force on the upper airway (hence its use in obstructive sleep apnoea), and also recruits collapsed alveoli and increases functional residual capacity. This improves lung compliance, reducing the work of breathing, which is a benefit in a range of clinical circumstances.

Table 33.2.4 Blood gases—parameters

Normal range	Notes
pO₂ >10.6 kPa (80 mmHg),when breathing air	(1) Can only be interpreted if the inspired oxygen concentration is known (2) Hypoxia defined as pO_2 <8 kPa when patient breathing air. (3) If patient is breathing with supplemental oxygen, a 'hypoxaemia score' can be calculated as: Hypoxaemia score = pO_2 (mmHg)/FiO_2 If a patient was breathing air and had a pO_2 at the lower limit of the normal range, then their hypoxaemia score would equal $10.6 \times 7.6/0.21$, or c.380. If they had a pO_2 of 8 kPa, then their hypoxaemia score would be $8 \times 7.6/0.21$, or c.290. In assessing a patient breathing supplemental oxygen a value of <300 is usually taken as indicating significant compromise
pCO₂ 4.7–6.0 kPa (35–45 mmHg)	(1) pO_2 < 8 kPa with pCO_2 < 6.5 kPa = type 1 respiratory failure (2) pO_2 < 8 kPa with pCO_2 > 6.5 kPa = type 2 respiratory failure (3) Low pCO_2 indicates hyperventilation, which may be primary or secondary, the latter being indicated by a base excess more negative than −2 (see below) (4) High pCO_2 indicates hypoventilation, which may be primary or secondary, the latter being indicated by a base excess more positive than +2 (see below)
pH 7.37–7.43	(1) pH < 7.35 defines acidosis (2) pH > 7.45 defines alkalosis
H⁺ 37–43 nmol/l	(1) H^+ >45 nmol/litre defines acidosis (2) H^+ <35 nmol/litre defines alkalosis
HCO₃⁻ 19–24 mmol/l	(1) Measurement of arterial or venous (normal range 22–28 mmol/litre in plasma) bicarbonate concentration is often helpful in analysis of patients with acid–base disturbance (2) Changes in bicarbonate concentration occur slowly (over many hours or days), hence evidence of compensatory change, e.g. high bicarbonate concentration in the patient with elevated pCO_2, indicates that the respiratory abnormality is chronic
Base excess +2 to −2 mmol/litre	Are measured abnormalities of pH or pCO_2 due to metabolic or respiratory processes? Many blood gas machines display a value for the base excess (or deficit), which is a value derived from primary (directly measured) data using an algorithm, the principles of which are as follows: (1) Predict the pH that would arise in normal blood in the presence of the pCO_2 actually measured: if the pCO_2 is high, then the predicted pH is low, and vice versa (2) Calculate the amount of acid or base that would have to be added to the blood to change the predicted pH to the pH measured. This is the base deficit/excess and an estimate of the degree of 'metabolic' as opposed to 'respiratory' disturbance. A base excess more negative than −2 indicates metabolic acidosis; a value more positive than +2 indicates metabolic alkalosis

Note
1 kPa = 7.6 mmHg.

CPAP can be used for patients with acute or acute on chronic hypoxaemia who are not exhausted or in ventilatory failure (meaning elevated Pco_2), e.g. acute pulmonary oedema, postoperative atelectasis, pneumonia. It is not appropriate and is contraindicated for patients who are too obtunded to cooperate, who are unable to protect their airway, who have haemodynamic instability or life-threatening arrhythmias, life-threatening hypoxaemia, or exhaustion.

CPAP is applied via a tight-fitting face or nose mask, the usual range for pressure being 2.5 to 10 cmH₂O. Once the mask is applied, patient comfort, respiratory rate and arterial blood gases should be monitored. Some patients are unable to tolerate the face mask: gastric distension, vomiting, aspiration, eye irritation, conjunctivitis, and necrosis of the facial skin are other complications.

Noninvasive positive pressure ventilation

Masks that are used for CPAP can also be used to provide noninvasive positive pressure ventilation (NIPPV, often more simply referred to as NIV). The difference between the two treatments is that in CPAP a constant pressure is applied to the airway, but no airflow occurs in the absence of respiratory muscle activity. By contrast, in NIV a pulse of positive pressure is applied to assist respiration, the usual arrangement being that this is triggered by a sensor that detects a fall in pressure in the facial mask when the patient initiates a breath. If a positive pressure is also applied in the expiratory phase (EPAP) in addition to the pulse delivered to support inspiration, then then this is known as bilevel pressure support (BIPAP).

Contraindications for and complications of NIV are the same as those for CPAP.

Invasive ventilation

Invasive ventilation may be applied via a tracheal tube or tracheostomy. Ventilation can be adjusted by altering the minute volume (respiratory rate × tidal volume). Oxygenation is adjusted by altering inspired oxygen concentration and positive end-expiratory pressure (PEEP, which acts in a similar manner to CPAP by recruiting collapsed alveoli and reducing the work of breathing). Most ventilators for adults are volume generators that deliver a fixed tidal volume regardless of changes in lung mechanics. If the lungs become stiffer, then inflation pressure will increase to deliver the same tidal volume.

The change from inspiration to expiration is usually time cycled; that from expiration to inspiration is usually either time cycled or triggered by the patient if they are breathing spontaneously. The following values can be used as a guide when initially setting up a ventilator for an adult:

◆ Tidal volume should be 10–15 ml/kg

◆ Respiratory rate 10–12/min

◆ Ratio of inspiratory to expiratory time (I/E ratio) set at 1:2, but for patients with chronic obstructive pulmonary disease or asthma, a smaller I/E ratio is often used (e.g. 1:3) to prevent gas trapping and hyperinflation.

◆ Concentration of inspired oxygen depends on the clinical context: the patient with normal lungs who requires respiratory support because of respiratory muscle weakness does not need a high Fio_2 (start with say 28%), whereas the patient with severe problems with gas exchange, eg. bilateral pneumonia or acute respiratory distress syndrome, will require a high Fio_2 (start with say 60–80%).

Once ventilation is established, the various parameters should be adjusted (and others added, e.g. CPAP) according to the patient's clinical condition and the results of repeated measurement of arterial blood gases.

Management of the airway

Endotracheal intubation

Endotracheal intubation remains the gold standard for airway management as it provides a method of oxygenating and ventilating the patient, while securing the airway from vomitus and secretions.

Intubation should be preceded by ventilation with high-concentration oxygen. The neck should be slightly flexed and the head extended (an assistant holding the neck in a neutral position if trauma to the cervical spine is suspected). The mouth should be inspected for loose teeth or dentures, which should be removed, as should any secretions or vomitus (by suction). A trained assistant should apply cricoid pressure to prevent passive regurgitation.

The laryngoscope should be introduced over the right side of the tongue, moving the tongue to the left. The tip of the blade should be positioned in the valecula (between the epiglottis and the base of the tongue) and lifted upwards and away from the operator to expose the vocal cords (Fig. 33.2.7a). The endotracheal tube should be introduced so that the cuff is positioned just beyond the cords (Fig. 33.2.7b).

After successful intubation, the patient should be ventilated with high-concentration oxygen, the endotracheal tube secured, and the tube cuff inflated. Positioning of the endotracheal tube should be confirmed by listening over the apices and the bases of the lungs, and over the stomach. If available, an end-tidal CO_2 monitor should be attached to the endotracheal tube.

Laryngeal mask airway

The laryngeal mask airway (LMA) is used widely in routine anaesthetic practice and is increasingly used for immediate airway management in cardiac arrest. Pulmonary aspiration associated with the use of a LMA is uncommon provided high inflation pressures are avoided.

The patient should be supine with the neck slightly flexed and the head extended (an assistant holding the neck in a neutral position if trauma to the cervical spine is suspected). The LMA should be held like a pen, and introduced into the mouth with the distal aperture facing towards the patient's feet. The tip should be applied to the palate and advanced until it reaches the posterior pharynx. The LMA is then pressed backwards and downwards until the resistance of the hypopharynx is felt (Fig. 33.2.8), when the cuff of the LMA should be inflated. If insertion is satisfactory, the end of the LMA will rise slightly. Positioning of the LMA should be confirmed by listening over the apices and the bases of the lungs, and over the stomach. If available, an end-tidal CO_2 monitor should be attached.

Cricothyroidotomy
Needle cricothyroidotomy

Insertion of a needle or a cannula (typically a large-bore intravenous cannula) through the cricothyroid membrane is a useful emergency technique that allows short-term provision of oxygen until

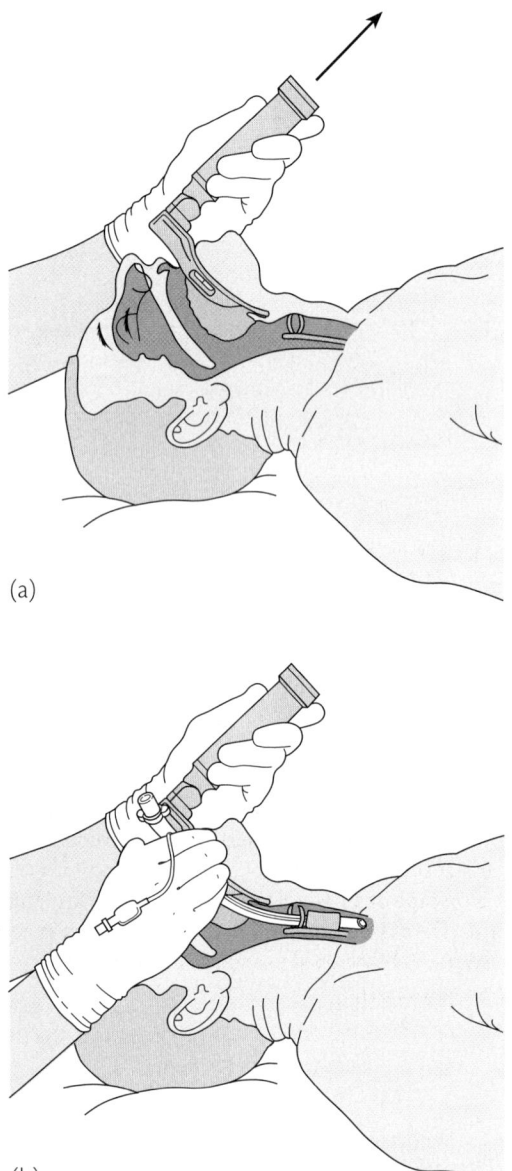

(a)

(b)

Fig. 33.2.7 (a) Position of the laryngoscope before insertion of the endotracheal tube. (b) Placement of the endotracheal tube.

a definitive airway can be placed. The cannula should be connected to high flow oxygen with either a Y connector or a side hole cut into the tubing between the cannula and the oxygen supply (Fig. 33.2.9). Intermittent insufflation can be achieved by closing the Y connector or side hole with a thumb for 1s and then releasing it for 3s. Inadequate exhalation leads to accumulation of CO_2, hence this technique of ventilation can only be used for 30 to 45 min.

Surgical cricothyroidotomy

The skin over the cricothyroid membrane should be cleaned and local anaesthetic inserted (in patients who are conscious). A horizontal skin incision is made and extended through the cricothyroid membrane (Fig. 33.2.10). A curved haemostat (forceps) is then used to dilate the opening and a small, cuffed endotracheal tube or tracheostomy tube inserted. The position of the tube should be confirmed by auscultation of the lungs and over the stomach, and the tube then secured.

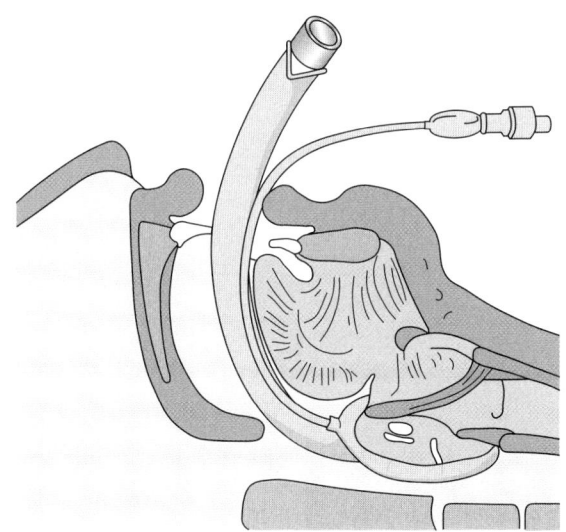

Fig. 33.2.8 Laryngeal mask airway inserted into the hypopharynx. The inflated cuff surrounds and isolates the entrance to the larynx.

Percutaneous procedures on the chest

Chest decompression

The rapidly deteriorating patient with clinical signs of a tension pneumothorax requires immediate needle decompression of the chest. The second intercostal space on the side of the tension pneumothorax should be identified, and an over-the-needle cannula or any hollow needle should be inserted in the midclavicular line, directing it just superior to the rib into the intercostal space. Listen for a sudden escape of air when the needle enters the pleural cavity. The cannula should be secured and arrangements made for an intercostal drain to be inserted as soon as the tension pneumothorax has been decompressed.

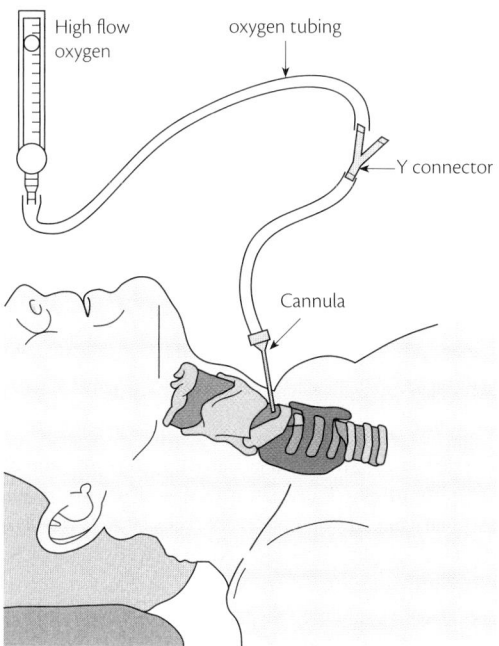

Fig. 33.2.9 Oxygenation via a cannula through the cricothyroid membrane.

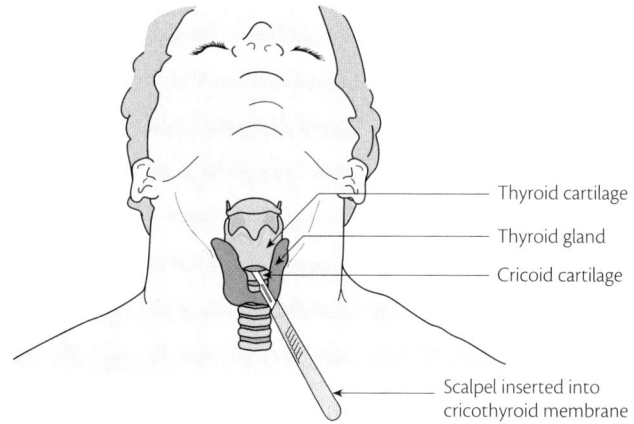

Fig. 33.2.10 Technique of surgical cricothyroidotomy.

Chest aspiration

Chest aspiration is recommended as first line treatment for all primary pneumothoraces that require intervention. The advantages over intercostal tube drainage are that, if successful, needle aspiration means a shorter hospital stay, less pain, and less scarring. Simple aspiration is less likely to succeed in those with secondary pneumothoraces and is only recommended in patients with underlying lung disease who are minimally breathless, les than 50 years of age, and with a small (<2 cm) pneumothorax.

An anterior approach using the second intercostal space in the midclavicular line can be used, or a posterior approach, with the patient in a sitting position with the arms gripping the knees, and using the second, third, or fourth intercostal space medial to the scapula.

The skin should be prepared and local anesthetic infiltrated down to the pleura. The cannula (either by a Seldinger over a guide wire technique, or using a cannula over-the-needle device) is inserted perpendicular to the skin and just over the superior border of the rib. It is then connected to a three-way tap, the second port of which is connected to a 50 ml syringe, and the third to a length of tubing that runs to open under the surface a container of sterile water (Fig. 33.2.11). Aspiration should be continued until resistance is felt, the patient coughs excessively, or a total of 4 litres of air has been aspirated.

The success (or otherwise) of aspiration can be determined by repeat chest radiography. The procedure may be repeated if not successful or if the pneumothorax recurs. Success is less likely for older patients and in those with chronic lung disease or recurrent pneumothorax, also after aspiration of more than 2.5 litres.

Chest drain

Always confirm the correct side for chest tube insertion. The usual site is the fourth to sixth intercostal space, just anterior to the midaxillary line. Position the patient supine with the head of the bed slightly elevated and the patient's arm behind their head. Clean and drape the area for tube insertion. Infiltrate local anaesthetic down to the parietal pleura (10–20 ml of 1% lignocaine (lidocaine)).

The technique for tube insertion depends on its type: those using a Seldinger over-a-wire mechanism should be placed according to the manufacturer's instructions; for trocar containing tubes, proceed as described below.

◆ Make a 2 to 3 cm transverse incision at the site and blunt dissect through the subcutaneous tissues, just over the superior surface

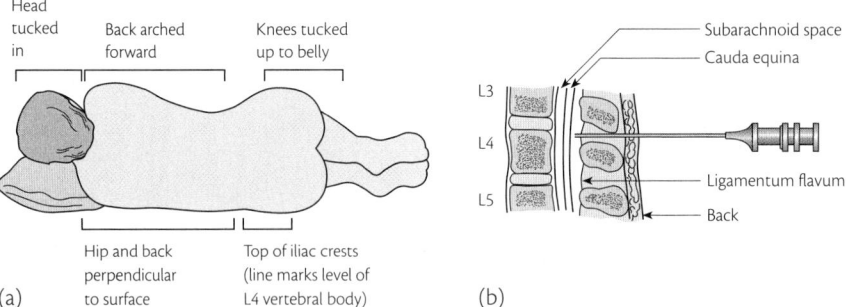

Fig. 33.2.12 (a) The patient should lie curled up to increase the space between the vertebrae. (b) The needle should be slowly advanced until it penetrates the ligamentum flavum.

of the rib. Puncture the parietal pleura with the end of the dissection forceps and insert a gloved finger into the incision to ensure that the pleural space has been entered.

- Remove the trocar from the intercostal drain and slide the drain over your finger into the pleural cavity, when 'fogging' of the tube should be seen. For pneumothorax the drain is angulated towards the apex of the lung; for pleural effusion/haemothorax it is angulated towards the base. Connect the end of the intercostal tube to an underwater-seal apparatus and confirm correct placement by ensuring that the fluid level is swinging with respiration.

- Insert two 3/0 monfilament sutures at 90° to the line of the skin incision, one on either side of the chest drain, but do not tie them. They will be used to close the skin when the chest drain is removed (and are much better for this purpose than a purse string suture, which produces an unsightly scar). Suture the tube in place with a separate 1/0 or 2/0 silk suture, tied around it as many times as its length allows. If the skin incision is gaping on either side of the drain, close this with one or more 3/0 sutures. Place a gauze dressing around the site and secure with strong tape, wrapping some of this around the tube to secure it firmly.

- Obtain a chest radiograph to confirm satisfactory placement and effect of the chest drain.

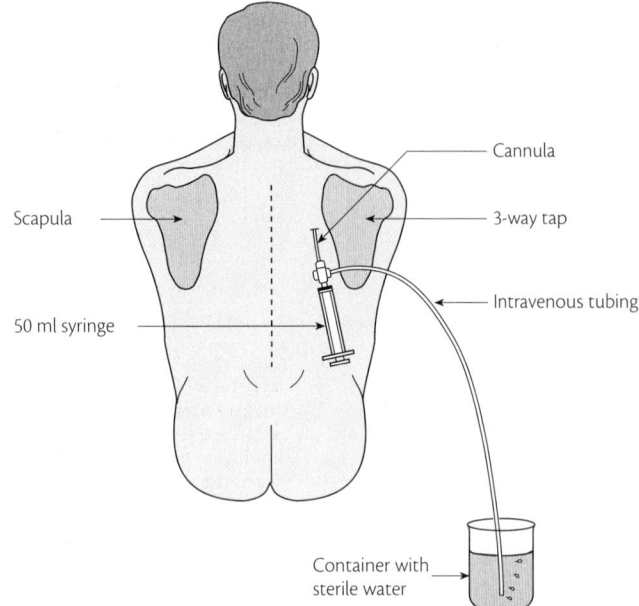

Fig. 33.2.11 Chest aspiration (posterior approach).

Note that inserting a chest drain is a risky procedure. Between January 2005 and March 2008 the (UK) National Patient Safety Agency received 12 reports of death and 15 of serious harm relating to chest drain insertion. All who insert chest drains must have been trained in the technique and familiar with the equipment that they are using. Ultrasound localization (when available) is recommended to guide the insertion of drains for pleural fluid.

Lumbar puncture

Ensure that there are no contraindications to lumbar puncture (LP), namely raised intracranial pressure, bleeding tendency, local sepsis, posterior fossa, or spinal cord mass lesion.

The patient should be positioned on the bed (Fig. 33.2.12a) in the lateral decubitus position with their knees drawn up towards the chest to open the space between the spinous processes and with their spine parallel to the bed. Prepare and drape the skin and locate the puncture site (L3/L4 or L4/L5).

Anaesthetize the skin and subcutaneous tissues using 5 to 10 ml of 1% lignocaine (lidocaine). Insert the LP needle at 90° to the skin. Advance slowly, aiming between two spinous processes (Fig. 33.2.12b). As the needle enters the dural space, there is a slight loss of resistance. Remove the stylet and ensure that cerebrospinal fluid drips freely from the needle. If it does not, insert the stylet and advance the needle a few millimetres then check again.

Check the opening cerebrospinal fluid pressure using a manometer (normally 6–15 cm H_2O) then collect cerebrospinal fluid samples. The red cell count in consecutive samples can sometimes help to distinguish subarachnoid haemorrhage from a bloody tap, but this is not always reliable and the sample should also be examined for xanthochromia (oxyhaemoglobin and bilirubin) when subarachnoid haemorrhage is possible. Always send blood samples for glucose and protein estimation at the same time, the cerebrospinal fluid glucose concentration normally being 60 to 80% of the blood level.

The patient should be asked to remain lying flat for 2 to 4 h to reduce the severity of post-LP headache.

Further reading

Temporary cardiac pacing

Fitzpatrick A, Sutton R (1992). A guide to temporary pacing. *BMJ*, **304**, 365–9.
Gammage MD (2000). Electrophysiology: temporary cardiac pacing. *Heart*, **83**, 715–20.

Pericardiocentesis

Tsang TS, Freeman WK, Sinak LJ, Seward JB (1998). Echocardiographically guided pericardiocentesis: evolution and state-of-the-art technique. *Mayo Clin Proc*, **73**, 647–52.

Index

Note: Numbers in italic refer to tables and/or illustrations separate from the text.

Species names for animals, plants, fungi and insects are listed by their Latin names, followed by their common name where appropriate.

cardiac 1772, 2785
cerebral 1770, *1770*
    Alzheimer's disease 1770
    hereditary cerebral amyloid
        angiopathy 1770
    prion disease 1771
    senile 1770
clinical 1767, *1767–8*
diagnosis and monitoring 1776
    histochemistry 1776
    nonhistological
        investigations 1777
dialysis patients 3942
endocrine 1772
haemodialysis-associated 1772,
    3942
hepatic involvement 2545
hereditary systemic 1771
    familial amyloid
        polyneuropathy 1771
    nonneuropathic 1771
immunoglobulin light-chain 4056
late gadolinium enhancement 2676
leprosy 4089
localized syndromes 1772
malabsorption 2221, *2221*
management 1778
monoclonal immunoglobulin
    light chain 1768
neuropathy 5086
primary 4353
    aetiology and epidemiology 4353
    clinical features 4353, *4354*
    diagnosis 4354, *4354*
    laboratory findings 4354
    prognosis 4354
    treatment 4354
pulmonary 3451
reactive systemic 1767
    associated conditions 1767,
        1768
    clinical features 1767
renal involvement 4075
and rheumatoid arthritis 3589
senile 1769
    focal 1769
    systemic (cardiac) 1769
amyotrophic lateral sclerosis 5070,
    5124, *384*, 5172
clinical features 5070
clinical variants 5071
differential diagnosis and
    investigation 5071
giving diagnosis 5072
pathology 5070
prognosis 5071
treatment 5072
anabolic steroids 5383, *5384*
    adverse effects,
        hepatotoxicity *2533*
    contraindication in porphyria 1641
anaemia 4374
    acquired pernicious 4408
    adaptation to 4375, *4375*
        cardiovascular changes 4377
        erythropoietin 4376
        pulmonary function 4377
        red cells 4376, *4376*
        tissue perfusion 4377
    aplastic *see* aplastic anaemia
    autoimmune haemolytic *276, 385*
    bartonellosis *937*
    cancer-associated *383*, 4548, 4549
    causes 4377, *4378*

blood loss 4379
cobalamin deficiency 4382
defective proliferation of red-
    cell precursors 4378, *4378*
defective red-cell matura-
    tion 4378
folate deficiency 4383
haemolytic 4379, *4379*
infection 4383
malabsorption 4384
of chronic disorders 4400
CKD 3923
    epidemiology and clinical
        significance 3924
    management 3924
    pathogenesis 3923, *3924*
clinical assessment 4380
clinical effects 4377
congenital dyserythropoietic 4449
consequences 4382
defective maturation of red
    cells 4445
definition 4375, *4382, 4382*
developing countries 4382, 4383
dialysis patients 3941
exercise-induced 5381
haematological
    investigation 4380, *4380*
haemolytic *see* haemolytic anaemia
and heart failure 2726
inherited 4384, *4384*
iron deficiency 4382
    pregnancy 2174
malaria 1063, *1065, 1067*
    treatment 1079
management 4381
megaloblastic *see* megaloblastic
    anaemia
microangiopathic
    haemolytic *385*, 4459, *4459*
normochromic,
    normocytic 4400, *4400*
    management 4401
pernicious *see* pernicious anaemia
pregnancy 2173
    aplastic 2177
    haemolytic 2177
    iron deficiency 2174
    vitamin B12 and folate
        deficiency 2174
prevalence 4375, 4382, *4382*
prevention 4385
refractory 4259
    with excess blasts 4260
    with ringed sideroblasts 4259
sideroblastic 4446
SLE 3659
vitamin deficiency 4418
and world health 4381
anaerobic bacteria 748
    antibiotic resistance *753*
    clinical spectrum 751
    definition 749
    diagnosis 752
    epidemiology 749
    history 748
    human commensal flora 749, *750*
    pathogenesis 750
    taxonomy 749, *749*
    treatment 752
Anaerobiospirillum spp. *962*
Anaerococcus spp. *962*
Anaeroglobus spp. *962*
Anaerorhabdus spp. *962*

anaesthesia
    and anaphylaxis 3108
    renal failure 4184
anaesthetics, topical 4736
anakinra 157
    rheumatoid arthritis 3598, *3599,
        3600*
anal sphincter, anatomy 2202
analgesia
    critical illness 3153
    hazards of 3154, *3155*
analgesic ladder 5413, *5421*
analgesic nephropathy 4008, *4008,
    4010*
analgesics
    antagonists 3156
    critical illness 3155, *3155*
    neuropathic pain 5414, *5414*
    nociceptive pain 5413, *5413*
    in renal failure 4182, *4182*
analphalipoproteinaemia 1657, 1671
anaphylactic shock
    malignant 5465
    see also anaphylaxis
anaphylactoid reactions 1466
anaphylatoxins 286
anaphylaxis 3106, 262, *262, 3107*
    aetiology 3107, *3108*
    allergist/immunologist
        referral 3113
    anaesthesia-related 3108
    clinical features 3109, *3110*
        cardiovascular
            manifestations 3110
        cutaneous and general
            reactions 3110, *3110*
        gastrointestinal
            manifestations 3110
        neurological
            manifestations 3110
        respiratory manifestations 3110
    continuing treatment 3113
    definition 3107, *3107*
    differential diagnosis 3110
    drug-induced 3108
    epidemiology 3109
    exercise-induced 3109
    fatal 3109
    food-induced 3108
    future developments 3114
    grading *3108*
    hospital admissions *260*, 3109
    hymenoptera stings 1350, 3108
    idiopathic 3109
    immediate treatment 3111, *3111*
        adrenaline 3111
        fluid replacement 3112
        oxygen and airway patency 3111
    investigations 3111
        IgE skin testing, *in vitro*
            testing and challenge
            testing 3111
        mast cell tryptase and
            histamine 3111
    latex-induced 3108
    observation 3112
    pathophysiology 3109
        mast cell/basophil inflammatory
            mediators 3109
        mediator actions 3109
    prevention 3113
        drug and allergen
            avoidance 3114
        education 3113

long-term desensitization
    (immunotherapy) 3113
pretreatment 3113
skin testing and short-term
    desensitization 3113
second-line treatments 3112
summation 3109
treatment 258
see also allergy
Anaplasma phagocytophilum 914,
    863, 903, 916
anaplasmosis 903, 914
    bacteriology, taxonomy and
        genomics 914, *915*
    human granulocytic 916, *917–18*
anaplastic large T/null-cell
    lymphoma 4328, 4332
anastrozole, breast cancer *1937*
Anatrichosoma spp. *1176*
ANCA-associated vasculitis 3855,
    4032, 4036–7, 4631
    aetiology and genetics 4034
    areas of uncertainty 4043
    clinical features 4036, *4037*
    differential diagnosis *4039, 4033,
        4039, 4042*
    epidemiology 4036, *4036*
    historical perspective 4034
    investigation 4038, *4039*
    pathogenesis and pathology 4034,
        4035
    prognosis 4042, *4042*
    quality of life 4042
    treatment 4040
        adverse events 4041
        induction therapy 4040
        maintenance therapy 4040
        refractory disease 4041
        renal transplantation 4041
    see also individual syndromes
ancrod 4540
Ancylostoma braziliense 1166
Ancylostoma caninum 1163, *1176*
    gastroenteritis 1166
Ancylostoma duodenale 1163, 1165
Ancylostoma malayanum 1176
Andersen syndrome 166, *1598*, 1602
Anderson-Fabry disease *see* Fabry's
    disease
Andes virus *581*
andioendothelioma, vasculitis 5162
androgen insensitivity
    syndrome *1917, 1966, 1971*
androgen receptor defects *1917*
androgen replacement 1921
    testosterone preparations 1921
androgens
    actions of *1915, 1966*
    biosynthesis *1965*
        defects in 1970
    deficiency *1915*
    maternal excess 1969
    resistance to 1971
Andrographis paniculata 68
andromedotoxins 1364
Anemonia sulcata 1347
anencephaly 5136
    antenatal screening *102*
aneuploidy 341
aneurysm
    abdominal aortic 2963
    Behçet's disease *3685*
    endovascular repair 2965
    syphilitic 2827

bromocriptine
  adverse effects,
      hepatotoxicity *2529, 2532*
  in breast milk *1469*
  prolactinoma 1811
  in pregnancy 2140
bronchi 3175, *3176*
  radiographic view 3207
bronchial adenoma 3532
bronchial carcinoid 3532
bronchial thermoplasty *3223, 3224*
bronchiectasis 3345
  aetiology and pathogenesis 3346,
      3346–7
    developmental defects 3346
    excessive immune
        response 3347
    immune deficiency 3347
    mechanical obstruction 3348
    mucociliary clearance
        disorders 3347
    postinfective 3348
    toxic insult 3348
  associated conditions 3348
  autoimmune rheumatic
      disorders *3390, 3391*
  complications 3351
  definition 3345
  epidemiology 3345
  examination 3348
  future developments 3352
  history 3348
  idiopathic 3348
  imaging *3215, 3215*
  investigation and diagnosis 3348
    cause of disease 3349, *3350*
    disease state 3349, *3349*
    radiological imaging 3348, *3349*
  management 3350, *3350–1*
    anti-inflammatory therapy 3351
    antibiotics 3350
    bronchodilators 3351
    monitoring response 3351
    surgery 3351
  pathology 3346
    microscopic features 3346
  prognosis 3352
  systemic sclerosis *3672*
bronchioles 3175, *3176*
  terminal 3178, *3179*
bronchiolitis obliterans
    syndrome *3483*
bronchiolitis obliterans *1599*, 3379,
    3383
  autoimmune rheumatic
      disorders *3390, 3391*
  clinical features 3383
  differential diagnosis 3384
  histopathology 3383, *3383*
  investigations 3383
    imaging 3383, *3384*
    lung function tests 3384
  and rheumatoid arthritis 3588
  treatment 3384
bronchiolitis 3321, *3321, 3368*
  follicular 3386
  obstructive 3312
  viral aetiology *474*
bronchitis
  chronic 3312, *3318, 3320*
    morbidity *3316*
bronchoalveolar lavage 3220, *3221*
  diffuse parenchymal lung
      disease 3373

organizing pneumonia 3385
  pulmonary fibrosis 3378
bronchoconstriction 3170
bronchodilatation 3170
bronchodilators
  acute asthma 3308
  in breast milk *2189*
  bronchiectasis 3351
  COPD 3334, *3335–6, 3342*
  cystic fibrosis 3360
  inhaled 3308
  intravenous 3308
  in renal failure 4181
bronchogenic cysts *3542, 3543*
bronchography, complications 3466
bronchoscopy 3216–17
  contraindications 3217
  diagnostic role 3222
    diffuse lung disease 3222
    lung cancer 3222
    respiratory infection 3223
  disinfection 3218
  equipment 3218
  indications 3217, *3217*
  lung cancer 3524
  patient preparation 3218, *3218*
  procedure 3219, *3219*
  techniques and sampling 3220
    bronchial biopsies 3220
    bronchial brushings 3220
    bronchial washings 3220
    bronchoalveolar lavage 3220,
        3221
    endobronchial
        ultrasound 3221, *3221*
    fine needle aspiration 3220
    fluorescence
        bronchoscopy 3222
    lung biopsy 3220
    magnetic navigation 3221, *3222*
  therapeutic role 3223
    asthma *3223, 3224*
    emphysema 3223, *3223*
    lung cancer 3223
bronchovascular bundle 2974
broom
  drug interactions *69*
  toxicity 68
Brown-Séquard syndrome 4743
Brown-Violetto-van Laere
    syndrome 5073
Brucella abortus 789
  renal toxicity 4086
Brucella canis 789
Brucella melitensis 789
Brucella spp. *962*
  infective endocarditis *2812*
  osteomyelitis 791, *793, 3789*
Brucella suis 789
brucellosis 789
  aetiological agent 789
  clinical features 790, *790*
  diagnosis 793
  epidemiology 789
  localizations 790, *791–3*
  mode of transmission 789
  pathogenesis 789
  prevention 794
  treatment 794
Brugada syndrome 2612, 2715
  sudden unexplained death during
    sleep 3840
Brugia malayi 1153–5
  renal toxicity 4088

Brugia spp. *1176*
Brugia timori 1153–5
Brugmansia suaveolens (angel's
    trumpet) *1362*
Bruton's agammaglobulinaemia
    tyrosine kinase (BTK) 244
bryostatin 1 *1939*
bubonic plague *see Yersinia pestis*
buccal drug administration 1452
Buchner, Eduard 11
Budd-Chiari syndrome 2483
  liver transplantation 2508
  pregnancy 2130
budesonide
  asthma 3300
  COPD 3334
  primary biliary cirrhosis *2467*
Buerger's disease 2960, 4687
Bukalasa bat virus *566*
bulimia nervosa 5319
  management 5323
bullae *4591*
Bulleidia spp. *962*
bullosis diabeticorum 2048
bullous emphysema 3343
bullous pemphigoid *4603*, 4606, *4606*
bumetanide, heart failure *2722*
bundle branch block 2650
  left 2650, *2651*, 2657
  right 2651, *2652*
bundle of His *see* His bundle
Bungarus caeruleus (common
    krait) 1328
  antivenom *1340*
Bunina bodies 5070
Bunostomum trigonocephalum 1176
Bunyamwera virus 580, *581*
Bunyaviridae 579
  Hantavirus 582
  Nairovirus 581, 585
  Orthobunyavirus 580
  Phlebovirus 581, 586
  viral taxonomy and vectors 580,
      581–2
  see also individual viruses
buprenorphine 1290
  palliative care 5423
buprioprion, adverse effects *5313*
Burkholderia cepacia, cystic
    fibrosis 3356
Burkholderia mallei 771
Burkholderia pseudomallei 768
  osteomyelitis 3789
  renal toxicity 4086
Burkitt's lymphoma 300
  endemic ('African') 502, 505, 1082
  sporadic 505
  translocations *341*
Burkitt's lymphoma/leukaemia 4227
burns
  electrical 1425
  lightning injuries 1424
  nutrition support 1542, *1543*
  radiation 1431
burr cells *4195*
bursitis
  anserine *3248, 3557*
  olecranon *3248*, 3588
  prepatellar *3248*
  septic 698, *700*
  trochanteric *3248*
Buruli ulcer 833, 848
  aetiology 848
  clinical features 849

disseminated disease 849
  localized disease 849, *849*
  differential diagnosis 849
  epidemiology and
      transmission 848
  laboratory diagnosis 850
  pathogenesis 849
  pathology 849
  prevention and control 850
  socioeconomic impact 850
  treatment 850
buspirone 5338
Bussuquara virus *566*
busulfan 398
  adverse effects,
      hepatotoxicity *2533, 2536*
  busulphan, carcinogenesis *307*
butcher's warts *4675*
butoconazole, candidiasis 1258
butterbur, migraine
    prevention 4916
butterfly stings 1351
Buttiauxella spp. *962*
Butvrivibrio spp. *962*
butyrophenones, poisoning 1283
Bwamba virus 581, 587
bystander apoptosis 596

C1 esterase inhibitor, reference
    values 5444
C1 inhibitor *216, 1753*
  antibodies 221
  deficiency 218, *254*
C1q, deficiency *254*
C1r, deficiency *254*
C1s *1753*
  deficiency *254*
C2, *1753*
  deficiency *254*
C3 224, *1753*
  deficiency *254*
  unregulated activation 219, *220*
C3 nephritic factor 221
C3a *286*
C3b *286*
C4 224, *1753*
  deficiency *254*
C4b *286*
C4-binding protein *216*
C5, deficiency *254*
C 56, *1753*
C5a *286*
C6, deficiency *254*
C7, deficiency *254*
C8, deficiency *254*
C9, deficiency *254*
CA125, reference values *5442*
CA19–9, reference values *5442*
Cabassou virus *558*
cabergoline
  prolactinoma 1811
  in pregnancy 2140
Cabot's rings *4195*
Cacipacore virus *566*
caclizumab 292
CADASIL 5110
cadmium
  carcinogenesis *308, 338*
  poisoning 1297, *3739, 4018*
  skeletal effects 3769
  reference values *5445*
  reproductive effects *1917*
caeruloplasmin *1753*
  reference values *5444*

Felty's syndrome 4307
  hepatic involvement 2544
  and rheumatoid arthritis 3589
female athlete triad 5376, *5376–7*
  history 5376
  incidence and aetiology 5376, *5376*
  investigation and
      management 5377, *5377–8*
  pathophysiology 5376, *5377*
  skeletal effects 5377
femfibrozil 1670
femoral nerve neuropathy 5084
femoral vein cannulation 5510, *5511*
fenbrufen, adverse effects,
      hepatotoxicity *2532*
fenofibrate 1670
  adverse effects,
      hepatotoxicity *2529*
fenoprofen
  and asthma *3289*
  rheumatoid arthritis *3594*
fenoterol
  asthma 3302
  COPD *3335*
fentanyl 3155, *3155*
  palliative care 5422
feprazon, adverse effects,
      hepatotoxicity *2532*
ferpexide, adverse effects,
      hepatotoxicity *2529*
ferritin 4389
  reference values *5435, 5444*
fertility *see* infertility
fetal alcohol syndrome *1468*, 2090,
      5146
fetal programming 2083
fetal switch 4201
α-fetoprotein, reference values *5442*
fetus
  adverse drug reactions 1468, 2187
  effects of maternal diabetes 2138
  growth and adult disease 2899
  thyroid function 2142
fever of unknown origin 423
  causes 423, *424–5*
      common diseases 426
      diagnostic spectrum 423
      subpopulations 423
  characteristics of 426
  definition 423, *424*
  drug-induced 426
  factious 426
  habitual hyperthermia 426
  imaging techniques 426
  immunocompromised host 435,
      435
  prognosis 427
  selective testing 427
  therapeutic trials 427
  watchful waiting 427
fever
  acute pancreatitis 2564
  cancer 382
  dialysis patients 3941
feverfew, migraine prevention *4916*
fexofenadine 3282
fibrates 1670
fibreoptic bronchoscopy 3135
fibrillary glomerulonephro-
      pathies 4060
fibrillin 1 mutations, Marfan's
      syndrome 2838, *3779, 3781*
fibrinectin *1753*
fibrinogen titre *4196*

fibrinogen *1753, 4490, 4494*, 4494,
      4503
  deficiency 4528
  laboratory tests *4522, 4504*
  plasma *4196*
  pregnancy *2126*
  reference values *5444*
fibrinolysis 416, 2601
  meningitis 721
  myocardial infarction *38*, 40, *42*
  venous thromboembolism 3020
fibrinolytic system 4496, *4496–7*
Fibrinolytic Therapy Trialists'
      Collaborative Group 38
fibroadenoma of breast 1940, *1940*
fibroblast growth factor 2601
fibrodysplasia ossificans
      progressiva 3713, *3721, 3765*
  clinical features *3731, 3765,
      3765–6*
  differential diagnosis 3765
  management 3766
  pathophysiology 3765
fibrogenesis imperfecta ossium 3769
  clinical features *3731*
fibroma, cardiac 2832
fibromatosis of breast 1941
fibropolycystic disease 2580
  choledochal cyst 2582, *2582*
  congenital hepatic fibrosis 2581
  microhamartomas 2582
  polycystic liver disease 2581, *2581*
fibrosing alveolitis
  cryptogenic 3375
  and rheumatoid arthritis 3588
  systemic sclerosis 3673, *3673*
fibrous dysplasia 3720, *3721, 3761,
      3762*
  clinical features *3731*
  monostotic 3762
  polyostotic 3762
fibrous erionite pneumoconiosis 3423
Fick principle 2681, *2682*
fifth disease 608
filarial nephropathy 4088
  clinical features 4088
  management 4089
  pathogenesis 4088
  pathology 4088
filariasis 3085
  cutaneous 1145
  lymphatic 1153, *1154*
      aetiology 1154
      clinical features 1155, *1156–7*
      diagnosis 1157
      epidemiology and
          transmission 1155
      Global Programme to
          Eliminate Lymphatic
          Filariasis 1158
      mosquito vectors *1154*, 1155
      pathogenesis 1155
      treatment 1159
  renal involvement 4075
  see also individual conditions
Filifactor spp. *962*
Filler formula 3871
Filodes fulvidorsalis 1236
filoviruses 595, 1442
  aetiology and genetics 596
  areas of uncertainty 599
  clinical features 598, *598–9*
  diagnosis/differential
      diagnosis 599, *599*

epidemiology 597
future developments 600
pathogenesis/pathology 596
prevention 597
prognosis 599
treatment 599
finasteride
  NNT *52*
  skin disorders 4739
fine needle aspiration
  bronchial 3220
  thyroid cancer 1847
Finegoldia spp. *962*
fingers
  boutonnière deformity 3587
  clubbing *see* digital clubbing
  dactylitis *3606*
  swan-neck deformity 3587
fire smoke 3457
first-pass metabolism 1456
Fischoederius elongatus 1223
fish allergy 263
fish odour syndrome 4677
fish oils
  in pregnancy 2090
  Raynaud's phenomenon *3671*
fish poisoning 1346
  carp gallbladder 1347
  diagnosis and treatment 1347
  gastrointestinal and neurotoxic
      syndromes 1346
  prevention 1346
fish stings 1325, *1344, 1344–5*
  clinical features 1345
  epidemiology 1344, *1345*
  incidence 1344
  prevention 1345
  treatment 1345
  venom composition 1345
Fisher's syndrome 5034, 5037, 5090
fitness factors 411
FitzHugh-Curtis syndrome 944,
      945, 1260
flail chest 3510
flatbush diabetes 2008
flavin adenine dinucleotide 1487–8
flaviviruses 564
  mosquito-borne 564–5
  taxonomy 566
  tick-transmitted 565
  see also individual viruses
Flavobacterium spp. *962*
flavoproteins 1490
flea-borne spotted fever 907
fleas 1225, *1232*, 1232
flecainide *2701*
  adverse effects,
      hepatotoxicity *2532*
  in renal failure *4179*
fleroxacin, typhoid fever *742*
Flexispira spp. *962*
Flexner, Abraham 11
flexor hallucis longus
      tendonitis *5382*
flies
  blood-sucking 1226, *1226*
  and hygiene 1236
FLIP protein 184
floods 121, 1440
flow-volume curves 3192, *3193*
  expiration 3193, *3193*
  inspiration 3193, *3193*
Flt-3, 4201
flucloxacillin *706*

adverse effects,
      hepatotoxicity *2533*
bacteraemia 703, *705*
endocarditis 704–5
epidural abscess *702*
infective endocarditis *2817, 2818*
osteomyelitis *701*
pharmacokinetics 449
pneumonia *702*, 3238
Raynaud's phenomenon *3671*
in renal failure *4185*
septic bursitis/arthritis *700*
spectrum of activity *446*
toxic shock syndrome 697
urinary tract infection *702*
fluconazole
  adverse effects,
      hepatotoxicity *2529*
  in breast milk *1469*
  candidiasis 1258
  coccidioidomycosis 1022
  cryptococcosis 1020
  dermatophytoses 1002
  disseminated candidosis 1013
  drug interactions *1471*
  oral candidiasis 2269
  prophylactic *440*
  in renal failure *4185*
flucytosine
  fungal infections 1016–17
  in renal failure *4185*
fludarabine 398
  lymphoma *4320*
fludrocortisone suppression
      test 3064
fludrocortisone
  congenital adrenal
      hyperplasia 1893
  orthostatic hypotension *5063*
fluid balance
  high altitude 1403
  malaria 1079
  pregnancy 2076
fluid replacement
  acute renal trauma 3892
  anaphylaxis 3112
  critical illness 3118
  diabetic ketoacidosis 2025
fluid restriction, heart failure 2720
fluid, requirements 1538, *1538*
flukes 1212
  intestinal 1219
  liver 1212
  lung 1216
  schistosomiasis 1202
flumazenil *1274*, 3156, 5265
  hepatic encephalopathy 2502
flunarizine, migraine
      prevention 4916
fluorescein angiography 5235
fluorescence bronchoscopy 3222
Fluorobacter spp. *962*
fluoroquinolone, pneumonia *3238*
fluorosis 3767
5-fluorouracil 398, 4736
  adverse effects *400*
      breast cancer *1937*
      resistance 399
fluoxetine
  adverse effects 5313
      hyperprolactinaemia 2068
  cataplexy *4833*
  poisoning 1281
  Raynaud's phenomenon *3671*

gyrate atrophy of choroid and
retina *1566*
gyromitrin *1367*, 1370

HAART therapy 3252
IRIS syndrome 640
see also antiretroviral therapy
Habershon's jaundice 2541
HACEK organisms, infective
endocarditis *2812*, 2816
haem arginate 1648
haem, biosynthesis 1637, *1639*
Haemagogus spp. *1226*
haemangioma
cardiac 2832
infantile 4693
intestinal 2585
liver 2520, *2520*
synovial 3713
Haemaphysalis concinna 1228
Haemaphysalis spinigera 1228
Haemaphysalis turturis 1228
haematemesis 2238, 2309
haematite lung 3424
haematocrit, infants and
children *4197*
haematological disease *see* blood
disorders
haematological values
adults *4196*
infants and children *4197*
haematopoietic growth factor
transfusion 4570
haematopoietic stem cell
transplantation
autologous, indications for 4578
conditioning 4575, *4575*
donors 4575
graft-vs-host disease 4576, *4576–7*
immune reconstitution and
infections 4577, *4577*
indications *4573*, 4578
lysosomal storage diseases 1697
multiple myeloma 4348
relapse 4578
Haematopota spp. *1226*
haematuria 3865
asymptomatic microscopic 3849
causes 3849, *3850*
management 3850
benign familial 4099
loin pain-haematuria
syndrome 3853
macroscopic 3852
causes *3851*
with proteinuria 3849
sickle cell disease 4070
haemochezia 2238
haemochromatosis 1673
adult 1673–4, *1674*
clinical features 1681,
1681–2
cardiac involvement 2787, *2840*
clinical features 1681
diagnosis 1682
family members 1682
laboratory investigations 1682,
1682
environmental cofactors 1683
epidemiology 1675
future directions 1685
genetics and molecular
biology 1679, *1680*
iron absorption 1678

iron storage 1677, *1677–8*
pathological 1674
iron toxicity 1677
juvenile 1675
neonatal *1674*, 1675
pathophysiology/
pathogenesis 1677
phenotypic expression 1676
prevalence 1675
prevention and control 1685
prognosis 1684
reproductive effects *1917*
secondary 4395, *4395*
treatment 1683
iron chelation therapy 1684,
4396
venesection 1683
haemodiafiltration 3935, *3935–6*
haemodialysis 3930
acute renal trauma 3893
adequacy of 3936
duration and frequency 3937,
3937
incremental dialysis 3937
quotidian dialysis 3937
target *Kt*/V 3937
urea kinetic modelling 3936,
3937
urea reduction ratio 3936,
3936
complications 3940
amyloidosis 1772, 3942
anaemia 3941
bone disease 3942
cardiovascular disease 3941
coagulation problems 3941
dialyser reactions 3941
disequilibration 3940
fevers 3941
hypotension 3941
development of 3931
adequacy 3931
changing demographics 3932
expanding services 3931, *3931–2*
impact of conservative
management 3932
impact of transplantation 3932
pioneers 3931
drug elimination 4175
future of 3942
hyperkalaemia *3891*
outcomes 3942
patient management 3938
diet and nutrition 3940
dry weight 3938
hyperlipidaemia 3940
hypertension 3939
infection control 3940
initiation of dialysis 3938
monitoring dialysis
delivery 3938
predialysis care 3938, *3938*
prescribing dialysis 3938
technical aspects 3932
anticoagulation 3935
control of ultrafiltration 3934,
3935
dialysis 3932
dialysis machine 3934
dialysis water and fluids 3933,
3933–4
extracorporeal circuit 3934, *3934*
membranes and dialysers 3932,
3933

techniques 3935
conventional
haemodialysis 3935
haemodiafiltration 3935,
3935–6
haemofiltration 3935
high-flux haemodialysis 3935
vascular access 3939
permanent 3939
recirculation 3940
temporary 3939
vs. peritoneal dialysis 3944
haemodilution 4515, 4535
haemodynamic homeostasis 3126,
3127
haemofiltration 3935
acute renal trauma 3893
drug elimination 4175
haemoglobin A2, *4196*
haemoglobin Alc 4445
haemoglobin Bart's hydrops
syndrome 4433, *4433*
haemoglobin H disease 4434
haemoglobin H 2176
haemoglobin Pb 4445
haemoglobin S *see* sickling
haemoglobinopathies
haemoglobin SC disease 4441
haemoglobin variants 4437, *4437*
abnormal oxygen binding 4442
haemolysis due to 4441
nomenclature 4437
sickling disorders 4437, *4437*
haemoglobin 4195, *4196*
fetal, in adult life 4445
function 4422
genetic control 4423, *4423–4*
glycated 2020
glycosylated 4445
high-affinity 4267
infants and children *4197*
nephrotoxicity 3899
plasma *4196*
structure 4422, *4445*
synthesis 4424, *4424*
variants, in pregnancy 2176
haemoglobin F *4196*
haemoglobinopathies 4420
classification 4424, *4424*
pregnancy 2173–4
screening *2175*
thalassaemias 2176
variant haemoglobins and sickle
cell syndromes 2176
skeletal involvement 3767
thalassaemias 4424
unstable haemoglobin disorders 4442, *4442*
see also haemoglobin variants
haemoglobin-oxygen dissociation
curve 3195, *3196, 3468*
haemoglobinuria 3853
malaria *1068*
march 4460
paroxysmal cold 4456
paroxysmal nocturnal 4298, 221,
4212
haemolysis
chemicals causing *4459*
hepatic involvement 2541
intravascular, malaria *1068*
thermal 4460
venom-induced 4460
haemolytic anaemia 4450, *4451*

acquired 4454
immune haemolytic
anaemias 4454, *4455*
nonimmune haemolytic
anaemias 4458, *4458–9*
alloimmune 4456
complement system in 222
congenital 4446
red cell enzyme disorders 4452,
4453–4
red cell membrane disor-
ders 4451
drug-induced 4456
pregnancy 2177
haemolytic disease of newborn 4457
antenatal screening *102*
haemolytic uraemic syndrome 4065,
3862, 4459, 4513
diagnosis 4066
diarrhoeal 4066
histopathology 4066
nondiarrhoeal 4067
drug-related 4068
familial 4067
HIV related 4068
idiopathic 4067
malignancy related 4068
post-renal
transplantation 4067
pregnancy related 4068
treatment 4068
pathogenesis 4066, *4066*
Haemonchus contortus 1176
haemoperfusion, poisoned
patients 1279
haemopexin *1753*
haemophagocytic lymphohistiocytosis 4362, *4362–3*, 4364
management 4365
haemophagocytic syndrome 4514,
4550
haemophilia A, pregnancy 2179
haemophilia B, pregnancy 2179
haemophilia 4518
antenatal screening *102*
arthralgia 3708
gene transfer 4524
treatment 4522
complications of 4523
Haemophilus aphrophilus 762, 859
Haemophilus ducreyi 764
Haemophilus influenzae 759
antibiotic resistance 761
antibiotic sensitivity *446*
clinical features 761
noncapsulate 761
type b 761, *761*
community-acquired
pneumonia *453*
cystic fibrosis 3356
description 759
epidemiology 760
nonapsulate/
nonwerotypeable 760
type b 760
HIV-associated infection *3247*
immunization *90–1*
laboratory diagnosis 762
pathogenicity 410, 760
pneumonia 760, 3231, *3232*, 3234
prevention and control 762
treatment 762, *3238*
Haemophilus parainfluenzae 762
Haemophilus paraphrophilus 762

Haemophilus segnis 762
Haemophilus spp. *962*
  osteomyelitis *3789*
haemopoiesis 4199
  fetal liver 4369
  phylogeny and ontogeny 4200
  spleen 4335
haemopoietic growth factors 4207
haemopoietic stem cell
    disorders 4199
  multilineage involvement 4209,
    4210
haemopoietic stem cell transplanta-
    tion 4571, *197, 4573*
  histocompatibility 4573
haemopoietic stem cells 4573
  plasticity 4575
  sources of 4574
    bone marrow 4574
    peripheral blood 4574
    umbilical cord blood 4574
haemoptysis 2848, *3184*
  cystic fibrosis 3361
  lung cancer 3518
haemorrhage
  leptospirosis 875
  peptic ulcer disease 2309
haemorrhagic diathesis 2496
  diagnosis 2500
  management 2504
haemosiderin 1677
haemosiderosis 1686
  idiopathic pulmonary 4558
haemostasis 4480
  assessment of 4502
  coagulation pathways 4494, *4494*
  coagulation proteins 4489, *4490–1*
  fibrinolytic system 4496, *4496–7*
  newborns 4541
  platelets in 4508
  screening assays *4533, 4535*
haemostatic defects
  pregnancy 2173, *2177*
    acquired factor VIII
        inhibitors 2179
    factor XI deficiency 2179
    haemophilias 2179
    thrombocytopenia 2177, *2177*
    von Willebrand's disease 2179
  snake bite 1332, *1331, 1333*
haemothorax 3486, 3497
  iatrogenic 3498, *3498*
  nontraumatic 3498
  traumatic 3497
Hafnia spp. *962*
Hailey-Hailey disease 4596
hair
  disorders of 4701
    alopecia areata 4702, *4703*
    eczema 4702
    fungal scalp disease 4702
    liver disease 4720
    scalp psoriasis 4701, *4702*
    scarring alopecia 4703
    systemic disease 4703
  greying 4662
  in pregnancy 2078, 2149
hairy cell leukaemia 4227
hairy leukoplakia 507
  oral *2266*
halitosis 2285
Hallervorden-Spatz disease 1686
hallucinations
  around sleep 4831

visual 4857
hallucinogens
  fungal 1368, *1368*
  plant-derived 1362, *1362*
haloperidol decanoate,
    schizophrenia 5325
haloperidol 3156, *5265, 5423*
  adverse effects,
      hepatotoxicity *2532, 2533*
  schizophrenia 5325
halothane
  adverse effects,
      hepatotoxicity *2529*
  hepatotoxicity *1385*
Haltia-Santavuori disease 1698
hamartin 367
hamartoma
  of breast 1941
  cardiac 2832
Hamman-Rich
    syndrome 3369, 3375
hand, foot and mouth disease 531,
    531, 2264
hand-arm vibration syndrome 1387
handedness 4787
hands
  diabetic hand syndrome 2047
  mechanic's *3694, 3694*
  osteoarthritis *3632, 3633*
  pain *3248*
  rheumatoid arthritis 3587, *3588*
Hand-Schüller-Christian
    disease 3446
Hansen's disease *see* leprosy
Hantaan virus *581*
hantavirus *581*, 582
  clinical features
    acute interstitial
        nephritis 3859, 3901
    pneumonia *3238*
    renal toxicity *4086*
  haemorrhagic fever with renal
      syndrome 582, *583*
  pulmonary syndrome 584, *584*
  renal involvement 4073
Haplorchis microchis 1222
Haplorchis pleurophocerca 1222
Haplorchis pumilio 1222
Haplorchis taichui 1222
Haplorchis vanissimus 1222
Haplorchis yokogawai 1222
HapMap project 149, 362
haptoglobin, serum *4196*
haptoglobins *1753*
  reference values *5444*
harlequin fetus 1698, 4598
Harmonia axyridis 1236
Hartnup's disease 1490, *4147, 4148*
harvest mites 1229
Harvey, William 10, 12
Hashimoto's thyroiditis 1834–5, 1847
Haverhill fever 858
  aetiology 858
  clinical features 859
hawthorn 68
  drug interactions *69*
hay fever *see* allergic rhinitis
Hazara virus *581*
hazard ratio 52
head and neck, infections,
    anaerobic 751
head injuries 4963
  cognitive impairment 5277, *5277*
  complications 4966

chronic subdural
    haematoma 4967
  cognitive symptoms 4966
  epilepsy 4967
  hydrocephalus 4967
  infection 4966
  intracranial haematoma 4966,
    4966
deteriorating conscious
    level 4964, *4965*
early management 4964
epidemiology 4963
follow-up 4966, *4967*
golden hour 4964, *4964*
primary and secondary 4963
severity 4964
head lice 1231, *1231*
headache 4911
  causes *4912*
  chronic daily 4923, *4923*
    new onset 4924, *4924*
  cluster 4918, *4918–20*
  CSF volume
    low 4925, *4925*
    raised 4926
  differential diagnosis *4920*
  hypertension 3040
  medication overuse 4924
  migraine *see* migraine
  pregnancy 2089, 2146
  primary syndromes 4912, *4912–14*
    cough headache 4921
    exertional headache 4921
    hypnic headache 4922
    sex headache 4921
    stabbing headache 4921
    thunderclap headache 4922
  secondary *4912, 4913, 4915*
    cervicogenic 4926
    food intolerance 2254
    giant cell arteritis 4926
    post-traumatic 4926
  SUNCT/SUNA 4921
  tension-type 4917
health advertising 109
  to patients 109
    food industry 110
    health care providers 110
    medical devices 110
    pharmaceutical companies 109
  to physicians 109
  USA 110
  rest of world 110
Health and Safety at Work etc. Act
    (1974), 1377, 1389
health anxiety 5301
health care costs 82
  components of *114*, 112–13
  consequences 115
  cost-control policies 114, *114*
  as policy issue 112
  reasons for interest 112
health care spending
  explanations of 113
  as share of GDP *113*
health education 110
health information 109
health, economic benefits 74
health-adjusted life years
    (HALYs) 55
healthcare provision 54
  health maximization vs health
    equity 58
  innovation 60

reasonableness in 57
  accountability 57
  societal investment 61
  spending 61–2
  see also medicines
hearing disorders 4865
  clinical examination 4867, *4867*
  investigations 4867, *4867–8*
  management 4868
  pathophysiology 4866, *4866–7*
  tinnitus 4869
heart disease
  amyloid 2785
  autoimmune rheumatic
      disorders 2783, *2783–4*
    antiphospholipid syn-
        drome 2783
    polymyositis and
        dermatomyositis 2784
    rheumatoid arthritis 2784
    seronegative
        arthropathies 2784
    systemic lupus
        erythematosus 2783
    systemic sclerosis 2783
  clinical investigation 2643
    catheterization and
        angiography 2678
    ECG 2643
    echocardiography 2662
    imaging techniques 2671
  clinical presentation 2628
    chest pain, breathlessness and
        fatigue 2628
    syncope and palpitations 2636
  clinical trials 43, *43*
  congenital *see* congenital heart
      disease
  endocrine disorders 2786
    diabetes 2786
    hyperthyroidism 2786
    hypothyroidism 2787
  haematological changes 4560
  HIV/AIDS 2822, *2822*
    assessment 2825
    cardiac tumours 2823
    coronary artery disease 2824
    endocardial disease 2823
    heart muscle 2823
    pericardium 2822
    pulmonary hypertension 2823,
        2824
    right ventricular
        dysfunction 2823, *2824*
    sudden death 2824
  inherited metabolic
      disorders 2787
    haemochromatosis 2787
    lysosomal diseases 2787
  leptospirosis 876
  malaria 1063
  myocarditis *276*, 2758
  myopathies *see* cardiomyopathy
  neuromuscular disorders 2787,
    2788
  pregnancy 2108
    antenatal care 2110
    aortopathy 2112, *2112*
    arrhythmias 2115
    cardiac surgery 2110
    cardiomyopathy 2110, *2111*
    congenital 2113, *2871, 2871*
    contraception 2115
    investigations 2109